OPERATIVE
TECHNIQUES IN
ORTHOPAEDIC
SURGERY

KW-018-817

ALSO AVAILABLE IN THIS SERIES

OPERATIVE TECHNIQUES IN
FOOT AND ANKLE SURGERY

Editor: Mark E. Easley
Editor-in-Chief: Sam W. Wiesel

ORTHOPAEDIC TECHNIQUES IN
PEDIATRIC ORTHOPAEDICS

Editor: John M. Flynn
Editor-in-Chief: Sam W. Wiesel

OPERATIVE TECHNIQUES IN
ORTHOPAEDIC TRAUMA

Editors: Paul Tornetta III
Gerald R. Williams & Matthew L. Ramsey
Thomas R. Hunt III
Editor-in-Chief: Sam W. Wiesel

OPERATIVE TECHNIQUES IN
SHOULDER AND ELBOW SURGERY

Editors: Gerald R. Williams & Matthew L. Ramsey
Editor-in-Chief: Sam W. Wiesel

OPERATIVE TECHNIQUES IN
SPORTS MEDICINE SURGERY

Editor: Mark D. Miller
Editor-in-Chief: Sam W. Wiesel

OPERATIVE TECHNIQUES IN
ADULT RECONSTRUCTION SURGERY

Editors: Javad Parvizi & Richard H. Rothman
Editor-in-Chief: Sam W. Wiesel

OPERATIVE TECHNIQUES IN
HAND, WRIST, AND FOREARM SURGERY

Editor: Thomas R. Hunt III
Associate Editor: Scott H. Kozin
Editor-in-Chief: Sam W. Wiesel

OPERATIVE TECHNIQUES IN ORTHOPAEDIC SURGERY

Sam W. Wiesel, MD

EDITOR-IN-CHIEF

Professor and Chair
Department of Orthopaedic Surgery
Georgetown University Medical School
Washington, DC

VOLUME THREE

Wolters Kluwer | Lippincott Williams & Wilkins
Health

Philadelphia • Baltimore • New York • London
Buenos Aires • Hong Kong • Sydney • Tokyo

Acquisitions Editor: Robert A. Hurley
Developmental Editor: Grace Caputo, Dovetail Content Solutions
Product Manager: Dave Murphy
Manufacturing Manager: Ben Rivera
Design Manager: Doug Smock
Compositor: Maryland Composition/ASI
Copyright 2011

© 2011 by **LIPPINCOTT WILLIAMS & WILKINS, a WOLTERS KLUWER business**
Two Commerce Square
2001 Market Street
Philadelphia, PA 19103

All rights reserved. This book is protected by copyright. No part of this book may be reproduced in any form by any means, including photocopying, or utilized by any information storage and retrieval system without written permission from the copyright owner, except for brief quotations embodied in critical articles and reviews. Materials appearing in this book prepared by individuals as part of their official duties as U.S. government employees are not covered by the above-mentioned copyright.

Printed in China

Operative techniques in orthopaedic surgery / editor-in-chief, Sam Wiesel.
    p. ; cm.
Includes bibliographical references and index.
ISBN 978-0-7817-6370-7
1. Orthopedic surgery. I. Wiesel, Sam W.
[DNLM: 1. Orthopedic Procedures. WE 190 O61 2010]
RD731.O845 2010
617.4'7—dc22

2010009690

Care has been taken to confirm the accuracy of the information presented and to describe generally accepted practices. However, the authors, editors, and publisher are not responsible for errors or omissions or for any consequences from application of the information in this book and make no warranty, expressed or implied, with respect to the currency, completeness, or accuracy of the contents of the publication. Application of the information in a particular situation remains the professional responsibility of the practitioner.

The authors, editors, and publisher have exerted every effort to ensure that drug selection and dosage set forth in this text are in accordance with current recommendations and practice at the time of publication. However, in view of ongoing research, changes in government regulations, and the constant flow of information relating to drug therapy and drug reactions, the reader is urged to check the package insert for each drug for any change in indications and dosage and for added warnings and precautions. This is particularly important when the recommended agent is a new or infrequently employed drug.

Some drugs and medical devices presented in the publication have Food and Drug Administration (FDA) clearance for limited use in restricted research settings. It is the responsibility of the health care provider to ascertain the FDA status of each drug or device planned for use in their clinical practice.

To purchase additional copies of this book, call our customer service department at (800) 638-3030 or fax orders to (301) 223-2320. International customers should call (301) 223-2300.

Visit Lippincott Williams & Wilkins on the Internet at LWW.com. Lippincott Williams & Wilkins customer service representatives are available from 8:30 am to 6 pm, EST.

10 9 8 7 6 5 4 3 2 1

CCS0610

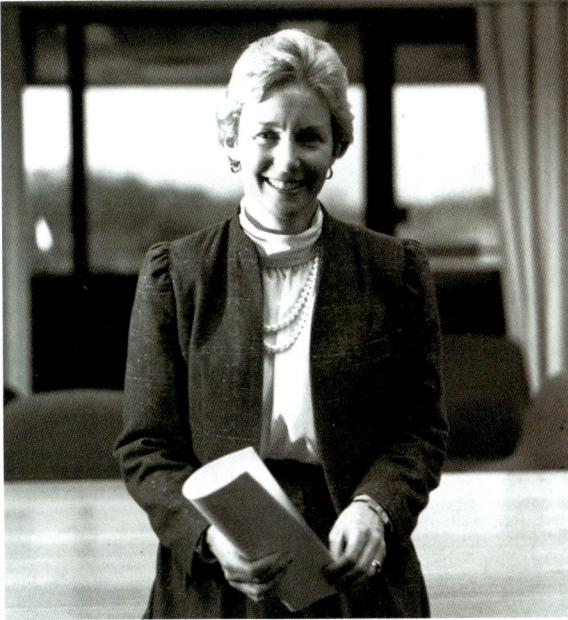

For Barbara Wiesel—confidante, advisor, best friend, and wife—thank you for a wonderful 39 years. With much love.

SWW

Dedication

To my beloved and inspiring family: Shelly, Yarden, Tom, Nimrod, and Dan —JB

To my family for the unending support of my academic endeavors. —SDB

To my orthopaedic mentors, especially Ed Hanley, John Hall, Jim Kasser, and Peter Waters, who have inspired me to write and teach and give back to orthopaedics, the way they have. —JMF

To Drs. Kenneth C. Francis, Ralph Marcove, and William F. Enneking, three great innovators, pioneers, developers, and critical thinkers in the field of orthopaedic oncology. I had the privilege to work with all three great pioneers and dedicate my work on this project to these world-class surgeons. —MMM

To my last child to leave the nest, Missy. I hope that all of our time together can be "quality time." — Your loving father, MDM

To my beautiful wife, Fariba, for her fortitude, devotion, and love. —JP

To my dear wife, Marcia, for always believing in and supporting me; to my children, Julia and James, for being my inspirations; to my parents, for always providing for me; and to God, for making it all possible. —JMR

To my mother, Phyllis, who found the best in people, had compassion for all, and whose insight, guidance, and love have always made me believe that anything is possible. —PT

To our wives, Robin and Nancy, and our children, Mark and Alexis and Chelsea, Alex, and Julia. —GRW and MLR

To my wife, Mary Lynne, and my children, Ford, Benson, and Charlotte, for patiently tolerating the time I spent away from them while I pursued this academic endeavor, and to my parents, Barbara and Dennis Easley, whose guidance and support prepared me for a career in academic medicine. —MEE

To my cherished wife Teri and our four extraordinary children, Thomas, William, Caitlin, and Christopher, for their love and understanding, and especially for their endless supply of smiles, laughter, and fun!—TRH

EDITORIAL BOARD

EDITOR-IN-CHIEF

Sam W. Wiesel, MD
Professor and Chair
Department of Orthopaedic Surgery
Georgetown University Medical School
Washington, District of Colombia

EDITORS

ADULT RECONSTRUCTION
Javad Parvizi, MD
The Rothman Institute
Professor, Department of Orthopaedic
    Surgery
Vice Chairman and Director of Research
Jefferson Medical College, Thomas
    Jefferson University
Philadelphia, Pennsylvania

Richard H. Rothman, MD
Founder, The Rothman Institute
The James Edwards Professor of the
    Department of Orthopaedic Surgery
Jefferson Medical College, Thomas
    Jefferson University
Philadelphia, Pennsylvania

FOOT AND ANKLE
Mark E. Easley, MD
Associate Professor of Orthopaedic Surgery
Co-Director, Foot and Ankle Fellowship
Duke University Medical Center
Durham, North Carolina

HAND, WRIST, AND FOREARM
Thomas R. Hunt III, MD
Professor of Surgery
John D. Sherrill Endowed Chair
    of Orthopaedic Surgery
Director, UAB Hand and Upper Extremity
Fellowship Director, Division of Orthopaedic
    Surgery
Surgeon-in-Chief, UAB Highlands Hospital
University of Alabama School of Medicine
Birmingham, Alabama

Associate Editor
Scott H. Kozin, MD
Professor of Orthopaedic Surgery
Temple University
Hand Surgeon, Shriners Hospital for Children
Philadelphia, Pennsylvania

ONCOLOGY
Martin M. Malawer, MD, FACS
Professor (Clinical Scholar) of Orthopaedics
Professor of Pediatrics (Hematology and
    Oncology)
Georgetown University School of Medicine
Professor of Orthopaedic Surgery
George Washington University
Director of Research and Development
Orthopaedic Oncology
Washington Cancer Institute
Orthopaedic Oncology
Children's National Medical Center
Washington, District of Columbia
Consultant (Pediatric and Surgery Branch)
National Cancer Institute, National
    Institutes of Health
Bethesda, Maryland

Jacob Bickels, MD
Professor, Orthopedic Surgery
National Unit of Orthopedic Oncology
Tel-Aviv Soursaky Medical Center
Tel Aviv, Israel

PEDIATRICS
John M. Flynn, MD
Associate Chief of Orthopaedic Surgery
The Children's Hospital of Philadelphia
Associate Professor of Orthopaedic Surgery
University of Pennsylvania School of
    Medicine
Philadelphia, Pennsylvania

**PELVIS AND LOWER EXTREMITY
TRAUMA**
Paul Tornetta III, MD
Professor and Vice Chairman
Department of Orthopaedic Surgery
Director of Orthopaedic Trauma
Boston University Medical Center
Boston, Massachusetts

SHOULDER AND ELBOW
Gerald R. Williams, MD
Professor of Orthopaedic Surgery
Chief, Shoulder and Elbow Service
The Rothman Institute
Jefferson Medical College, Thomas Jefferson
    University
Philadelphia, Pennsylvania

Matthew L. Ramsey, MD
Shoulder and Elbow Service
The Rothman Institute
Associate Professor of Orthopaedic Surgery
Jefferson Medical College, Thomas
    Jefferson University
Philadelphia, Pennsylvania

SPINE
John M. Rhee, MD
The Emory Clinic
Assistant Professor of Orthopaedic Surgery
Emory University
Atlanta, Georgia

Scott D. Boden, MD
The Emory Clinic
Professor of Orthopaedic Surgery
Director, Emory Orthopaedics & Spine
    Center
Staff Physician
Atlanta VA Medical Center
Atlanta, Georgia

SPORTS MEDICINE
Mark D. Miller, MD
S. Ward Casscells Professor of Orthopaedic
    Surgery
University of Virginia
Charlottesville, Virginia
Team Physician
James Madison University
Harrisonburg, Virginia

CONTENTS

Volume Two

PART 4 PEDIATRICS

SECTION I TRAUMA

SECTION II ARTHROSCOPIC AND SPORTS MEDICINE

SECTION III RECONSTRUCTION

Volume Three

PART 6 HAND, WRIST, AND FOREARM

Volume Four

PART 8 FOOT AND ANKLE

SECTION I FOREFOOT

SECTION II MIDFOOT

SECTION III HINDFOOT

SECTION IV ANKLE

PART 9 SPINE

SECTION I APPROACH TO THE SPINE

SECTION II CERVICAL SPINE SURGERY

SECTION III THORACOLUMBAR SPINE SURGERY

INDEX I-1

CONTRIBUTORS

PART 1 SPORTS MEDICINE

Christopher R. Adams, MD
Orthopaedic Surgeon
Advanced Shoulder Orthopaedics
Jupiter, Florida

Julie E. Adams, MD
Assistant Professor of Orthopaedic Surgery
University of Minnesota
Minneapolis, Minnesota

Christina R. Allen, MD
Associate Clinical Professor of
Orthopaedic Surgery
University of California
San Francisco, California

Michael J. Angel, MD
Orthopaedic Sports Medicine Fellow
Kerlan Jobe Orthopaedic Clinic
Los Angeles, California

Robert A. Arciero, MD
Professor of Orthopaedics
University of Connecticut Health Center
John Dempsey Hospital
Farmington, Connecticut

Steven A. Aviles, MD
Department of Orthopaedic Surgery
Iowa Orthopaedic Center
Mercy Hospital
Des Moines, Iowa

Frederick M. Azar, MD
Professor of Orthopaedic Surgery
University of Tennessee
Residency Program Director
Sports Medicine Fellowship Director
Campbell Clinic
Memphis, Tennessee

F. Alan Barber, MD
Fellowship Director
Plano Orthopedic Sports Medicine and
Spine Center
Plano, Texas

Mark J. Billante, MD
Physician
Greater Austin Orthopaedics
Austin, Texas

Matthew T. Boes, MD
Raleigh Orthopaedic Clinic
Raleigh, North Carolina

Kevin F. Bonner, MD
Assistant Professor
Eastern Virginia Medical School
Jordan-Young Institute
Sentara Leigh Hospital
Virginia Beach, Virginia

Jesse C. Botker, MD
Orthopaedic Surgery Chief Resident
University of Minnesota
Minneapolis, Minnesota

Craig R. Bottoni, MD
Chief of Surgery
Assistant Chief Medical Officer
Aspetar Orthopaedic & Sports Medicine
Hospital
Doha, Qatar

James P. Bradley, MD
Clinical Professor of Orthopaedic Surgery
University of Pittsburgh Medical Center
Pittsburgh, Pennsylvania

Anthony M. Buoncristiani, MD
Orthopaedic Surgeon
St. Luke's Wood River Medical Center
Ketchum, Idaho

Stephen S. Burkhart, MD
Director of Orthopaedic Education
The San Antonio Orthopaedic Group
The Orthopaedic Institute
San Antonio, Texas

Charles Bush-Joseph, MD, BA
Professor of Orthopaedic Surgery
Rush University Medical Center
Chicago, Illinois

J. W. Thomas Byrd, MD
Nashville Sports Medicine Foundation
Nashville, Tennessee

Eric W. Carson, MD
Associate Professor
Division of Sports Medicine
Department of Orthopaedic Surgery
University of Virginia
Charlottesville, Virginia

Mark S. Cohen, MD
Professor
Director, Hand and Elbow Section
Director, Orthopaedic Education
Department of Orthopaedic Surgery
Rush University Medical Center
Chicago, Illinois

Steven B. Cohen, MD
Assistant Professor of Orthopedic Surgery
Thomas Jefferson University
Rothman Institute Orthopaedics
Philadelphia, Pennsylvania

Brian Cole, MD, MBA
Professor
Section of Sports Medicine
Departments of Orthopaedic Surgery and
Anatomy & Cell Biology
Section Head, Cartilage Restoration Center
at Rush
Rush University Medical Center
Chicago, Illinois

Anne E. Colton, MD
Premier Orthopaedics
Broomall, Pennsylvania

John E. Conway, MD
Private Practice
Texas Health Harris Methodist Fort Worth
Hospital
Fort Worth, Texas

David A. Coons, DO
Multicare Orthopedics and Sports
Medicine
Tacoma, Washington

Andrew J. Cosgarea, MD
Professor, Orthopaedic Surgery
Director, Sports Medicine and Shoulder
Surgery
Department of Orthopaedic Surgery
Johns Hopkins University
Lutherville, Maryland

Thomas M. DeBerardino, MD
Associate Professor of Orthopaedic Surgery
University of Connecticut Health Center
Farmington, Connecticut

David R. Diduch, MS, MD
Professor of Orthopaedic Surgery
Head Orthopaedic Team Physician
University of Virginia
Charlottesville, Virginia

Ivica Ducic, MD, PhD
Associate Professor
Chief, Peripheral Nerve Surgery
Department of Plastic Surgery
Georgetown University Hospital
Washington, District of Columbia

Jeffrey S. Earhart, MD
Resident
Department of Orthopaedic Surgery
Feinberg School of Medicine
Northwestern University
Chicago, Illinois

Gregory C. Fanelli, MD
Orthopaedic Surgery
Geisinger Sports Medicine
Danville, Pennsylvania

David L. Feingold, MD
Chief, Department of Orthopaedics
Olive View Medical Center
West Hills, California

Larry D. Field, MD
Clinical Instructor
Department of Orthopaedic Surgery
University of Mississippi School of
Medicine
Director, Upper Extremity Service
Mississippi Sports Medicine and
Orthopaedic Center
Jackson, Mississippi

Donald C. Fithian, MD
Director, San Diego Knee and Sports
Medicine Fellowship
Kaiser Permanente, San Diego
El Cajon, California

Brett A. Freedman, MD
Orthopaedic Surgery
Walter Reed Army Medical Center
Washington, District of Columbia

Freddie H. Fu, MD, DSc, DPs (Hon)
Department of Orthopaedic Surgery
University of Pittsburgh Medical Center
Pittsburgh, Pennsylvania

John P. Fulkerson, MD
Clinical Professor of Orthopedic Surgery
University of Connecticut
Farmington, Connecticut

William E. Garrett, MD, PhD
Department of Orthopaedic Surgery
Duke University Medical Center
Durham, North Carolina

Jeffrey R. Giuliani, MD
Orthopaedic Surgery
Walter Reed Army Medical Center
Washington, District of Columbia

R. Timothy Greene, MD
Department of Orthopaedics
Orthopaedic and Neurosurgery Specialists
Greenwich, Connecticut

Christopher D. Harner, MD
Blue Cross of Western Pennsylvania
Professor
Department of Orthopaedic Surgery
UPMC Center for Sports Medicine
Pittsburgh, Pennsylvania

Justin D. Harris, MD
Nebraska Orthopaedic and Sports
Medicine
Lincoln, Nebraska

Laurence D. Higgins, MD
Department of Orthopaedic Surgery
Brigham and Women's Hospital
Boston, Massachusetts

MaCalus V. Hogan, MD
Resident Physician of Orthopaedic Surgery
Academic Orthopaedic Training Program
University of Virginia
Charlottesville, Virginia

Michael J. Huang, MD
Rocky Mountain Orthopaedic Associates,
PC
Grand Junction, Colorado

Jeffrey M. Jacobson, MD
Resident
Department of Plastic Surgery
Georgetown University Hospital
Washington, District of Columbia

David R. Joestling, MD, FACS
Surgical Consults, PA
Edina, Minnesota

Darren L. Johnson, MD
Professor and Chairman of Orthopaedic
Surgery
University of Kentucky
Lexington, Kentucky

Sean M. Jones-Quaidoo, MD
Resident
Department of Orthopaedic Surgery
University of Virginia
Charlottesville, Virginia

Spero G. Karas, MD
Associate Professor of Orthopaedic Surgery
Emory University
Atlanta, Georgia

Jay D. Keener, MD
Assistant Professor
Department of Orthopaedic Surgery
Washington University
St. Louis, Missouri

Roland S. Kent, MD
Corresponding Member of USUHS
Department of Surgery
Department of Orthopaedic Surgery
Navy Medical Center, Portsmouth
Uniformed Services University of Health
Sciences
Portsmouth, Virginia

Sami O. Khan, MD
Resurgens
Snellville, Georgia

Christopher A. Kurtz, MD
Assistant Professor of Surgery
Uniformed Services University of the
Health Sciences
Bethesda, Maryland
Chairman, Bone and Joint/Sports Medicine
Institute
Naval Medical Center Portsmouth
Portsmouth, Virginia

Robert F. LaPrade, MD, PhD
Professor of Orthopaedic Surgery
University of Minnesota
Minneapolis, Minnesota

Christopher M. Larson, MD
Director of Education
Minnesota Sports Medicine Orthopaedic
Sports Medicine Fellowship Program
Twin Cities Orthopaedics
Eden Prairie, Minnesota

Christian Lattermann, MD
Assistant Professor of Orthopaedic Surgery
and Sports Medicine
Director of Center for Cartilage Repair
and Restoration
University of Kentucky
Lexington, Kentucky

L. Scott Levin, MD, FACS
Chair of Orthopaedic Surgery
University of Pennsylvania School of
Medicine
Philadelphia, Pennsylvania

Krishna Mallik, MD
Orthopaedic Surgery Sports Medicine and
Arthroscopic Reconstruction
American Total Orthopedics
Scottsdale, Arizona

Elizabeth Matzkin, MD
Department of Orthopaedics
Tufts Medical Center
Boston, Massachusetts

Craig S. Mauro, MD
Chief Resident
Department of Orthopaedic Surgery
University of Pittsburgh Medical Center
Pittsburgh, Pennsylvania

Augustus D. Mazzocca, MD
Associate Professor
Department of Orthopaedics
University of Connecticut Health Center
John Dempsey Hospital
Farmington, Connecticut

David R. McAllister, MD
Professor of Orthopaedic Surgery and
Chief of Sports
David Geffen School of Medicine at UCLA
University of California, Los Angeles
Los Angeles, California

Eric C. McCarty, MD
Chief of Sports Medicine & Shoulder
Surgery
Associate Professor
Department of Orthopaedic Surgery
University of Colorado School of Medicine
Boulder, Colorado

Mark D. Miller, MD
S. Ward Casscells Professor
Department of Orthopaedic Surgery
University of Virginia
Charlottesville, Virginia
Team Physician
James Madison University
Harrisonburg, Virginia

Peter J. Millett, MD, MSc
Shoulder and Sports Medicine Specialist
Steadman-Hawkins Clinic
Vail, Colorado

Claude T. Moorman III, MD
Associate Professor of Surgery
Duke University
Durham, North Carolina

Craig D. Morgan, MD
Clinical Professor
Department of Orthopaedic Surgery
University of Pennsylvania School
of Medicine
Morgan-Kalman Clinic
Wilmington, Delaware

Amir Mostofi, MD
Department of Orthopaedic Surgery
University of Connecticut Health Center
Farmington, Connecticut

Kevin P. Murphy, MD
Heekin Orthopaedic Specialists
Jacksonville, Florida

Brett D. Owens, MD
Assistant Professor of Orthopaedic Surgery
Keller Army Hospital
West Point, New York

Samuel S. Park, MD
Orthopaedic Surgery
Good Samaritan Hospital
Downers Grove, Illinois

Ralph W. Passarelli, MD
Clinical Instructor
Department of Orthopaedic Surgery
University of Pittsburgh Medical Center
Pittsburgh, Pennsylvania

Matthew T. Provencher, MD
Associate Professor of Surgery
Director, Orthopaedic Shoulder and Sports
  Surgery
Department of Orthopaedic Surgery
Naval Medical Center San Diego
San Diego, California

R. David Rabalais, MD
Clinical Assistant Professor of Medicine
Department of Orthopaedic Surgery
Louisiana State University Health Science
  Center
New Orleans, Louisiana

William G. Rodkey, DVM, Diplomate
  ACVS
Chief Scientific Officer
Steadman Hawkins Research Foundation
Vail, Colorado

Anthony A. Romeo, MD
Department of Orthopaedic Surgery
Rush University Medical Center
Chicago, Illinois

J. R. Rudzki, MD
Clinical Assistant Professor
Department of Orthopaedic Surgery
George Washington University School of
  Medicine
Washington, District of Columbia

John-Paul Rue, MD, CDR, MC, USN
Assistant Professor
Department of Surgery
Uniformed Services University of Health
  Sciences
Director of Sports Medicine
Department of Orthopaedic Surgery
National Naval Medical Center
Bethesda, Maryland

Marc Safran, MD
Professor of Orthopaedic Surgery
Stanford University
Stanford, California

Felix H. Savoie, III, MD
Lee C. Schlesinger Professor of Clinical
  Orthopaedics
Tulane University School of Medicine
New Orleans, Louisiana

John A. Scanelli III, MD
Resident
Department of Orthopaedic Surgery
University of Virginia
Charlottesville, Virginia

Robert C. Schenck, MD
Professor and Chairman
Department of Orthopaedics and
  Rehabilitation
University of New Mexico
Albuquerque, New Mexico

Jon K. Sekiya, MD
Associate Professor
MedSport—Department of Orthopaedic
  Surgery
University of Michigan
Ann Arbor, Michigan

Nicholas A. Sgaglione, MD
Associate Clinical Professor of
  Orthopaedic Surgery
North Shore Long Island Jewish Health
  System
Great Neck, New York

Benjamin S. Shaffer, MD
Washington Orthopaedics & Sports
  Medicine
Chevy Chase, Maryland

Ryan W. Simovitch, MD
Palm Beach Orthopaedic Institute
Palm Beach Gardens, Florida

Jeffrey T. Spang, MD
Assistant Professor of Orthopaedics
University of North Carolina
Chapel Hill, North Carolina

Matthew A. Stanich, MD
Resident
University of California, San Francisco
San Francisco, California

Erick S. Stark, MD
Tri-City Orthopedics
Oceanside, California

J. Richard Steadman, MD
Orthopaedic Surgeon and Principal
Steadman Hawkins Clinic
Vail, Colorado

Scott P. Steinmann, MD
Professor of Orthopedic Surgery
Mayo Clinic College of Medicine
Rochester, Minnesota

Rebecca M. Stone, MS, ATC
Minnesota Sports Medicine
Twin Cities Orthopedics
Eden Prairie, Minnesota

Robert T. Sullivan, BS, MD
Orthopedic Surgeon/Sports Medicine
United States Air Force Academy
USAF Academy, Colorado

Kenneth G. Swan, Jr., MD
Department of Orthopaedic Surgery
Robert Wood Johnson University Hospital
New Brunswick, New Jersey

Robert Z. Tashjian, MD
Department of Orthopaedics
University of Utah Orthopaedic Center
Salt Lake City, Utah

Richard J. Thomas, MD
OrthoGeorgia Orthopaedic Specialists
Macon, Georgia

Fotios P. Tjoumakaris, MD
Assistant Professor of Orthopaedic Surgery
University of Pennsylvania School of
  Medicine/Penn Sports Medicine
Philadelphia, Pennsylvania

Michael S. Todd, MC
Orthopaedic Surgery Service
William Beaumont Army Medical Center
El Paso, Texas

Daniel J. Tomaszewski, MD
Department of Orthopaedic Surgery
Geisinger Clinic
Danville, Pennsylvania

Bradley B. Veazey, MD
Assistant Professor
Department of Orthopaedic Surgery and
  Rehabilitation
Texas Tech University
Lubbock, Texas

Christian J. H. Veillette, MD, MSc,
  FRCSC
Assistant Professor
Division of Orthopaedic Surgery
University of Toronto
Toronto Western Hospital
University Health Network
Toronto, Ontario, Canada

Andrew J. Veitch, MD
Assistant Professor
Department of Orthopaedics and
  Rehabilitation
University of New Mexico
Albuquerque, New Mexico

Winston J. Warme, MD
Associate Professor of Orthopaedics and
  Sports Medicine
Chief of Shoulder and Elbow Surgery
University of Washington
Seattle, Washington

Jon J. P. Warner, MD
Professor of Orthopaedic Surgery
Chief of Harvard Shoulder Service
Partner's Health Care System
Massachusetts General Hospital
Brigham and Women's Hospital
Boston, Massachusetts

Daniel C. Wascher, MD
Professor
Department of Orthopaedics and
  Rehabilitation
University of New Mexico
Albuquerque, New Mexico

Carl H. Wierks, MD
Orthopaedic Chief Resident
Johns Hopkins Hospital
Baltimore, Maryland

Jocelyn R. Wittstein, MD
Resident
Department of Orthopaedic Surgery
Duke University Medical Center
Durham, North Carolina

Ken Yamaguchi, MD
Professor of Orthopaedic Surgery
Sam and Marilyn Fox Distinguished
  Professor of Orthopaedic Surgery
Chief of Shoulder and Elbow Service
Washington University School of Medicine
St. Louis, Missouri

PART 2 PELVIS AND LOWER EXTREMITY TRAUMA

Animesh Agarwal, MD
Associate Professor of Orthopaedics
Chief, Division of Orthopaedic Trauma
University of Texas Health Science Center
  at San Antonio
San Antonio, Texas

Jeff Anglen, MD, FACS
Professor and Chairman of Orthopaedics
Indiana University School of Medicine
Indianapolis, Indiana

Michael R. Baumgaertner, MD
Professor
Chief, Orthopaedic Trauma Service
Department of Orthopaedics
Yale University School of Medicine
New Haven, Connecticut

James B. Carr, MD
Associate Clinical Professor
Department of Orthopedic Surgery
University of South Carolina
Columbia, South Carolina

Michael P. Clare, MD
Director of Fellowship Education
Foot and Ankle Fellowship
Florida Orthopaedic Institute
Tampa, Florida

Cory A. Collinge, MD
Director of Orthopedic Trauma
Harris Methodist Fort Worth Hospital
Staff Physician
John Petter Smith Orthopedic Residency
   Program
Fort Worth, Texas

William R. Creevy, MD
Vice Chairman and Associate Professor of
   Orthopaedic Surgery
Boston University School of Medicine
Boston Medical Center
Boston, Massachusetts

Brett D. Crist, MD
Assistant Professor
Department of Orthopaedic Surgery
University of Missouri
Columbia, Missouri

Nicholas Divaris, MD
Assistant Professor
Department of Orthopaedics
State University of New York at Stony
   Brook
Stony Brook, New York

Kenneth A. Egol, MD
Associate Professor
Vice Chairman
Department of Orthopaedic Surgery
NYU Hospital for Joint Diseases
New York, New York

Thomas Ellis, MD
Associate Professor of Orthopaedics
The Ohio State University College of
   Medicine
Columbus, Ohio

John C. P. Floyd, MD
Department of Orthopaedic Trauma
The Medical Center of Central Georgia
Macon, Georgia

Darin Friess, MD
Assistant Professor of Orthopaedics &
   Rehabilitation
Oregon Health & Science University
Portland, Oregon

Andrew Furey, MSc, MD, FRCSC
Assistant Professor
Department of Surgery
Memorial University of Newfoundland
St. John's, Newfoundland, Canada

Michael S. H. Kain, MD
Chief Resident, Orthopaedic Surgery
Boston University Medical Center
Boston, Massachusetts

David E. Karges, DO
Associate Professor
Department of Orthopaedic Surgery
St. Louis University
St. Louis, Missouri

Philipp Kobbe, MD
Department of Orthopaedic Surgery
University of Pittsburgh Medical Center
Pittsburgh, Pennsylvania

Stephen Kottmeier, MD
Associate Professor of Orthopaedics
University Hospital and Medical Center at
   Stony Brook
Stony Brook, New York

Ronald Lakatos, MD
Assistant Professor of Orthopaedics
The Ohio State University Medical Center
Columbus, Ohio

Mark A. Lee, MD
Associate Professor of Orthopaedic
   Surgery–Trauma
University of California, San Francisco
   School of Medicine
San Francisco, California

Seth P. Levitz, MD
Department of Orthopaedic Surgery
NorthShore University Health System
Evanston, Illinois

Brian Mullis, MD
Chief and Assistant Professor, Orthopaedic
   Trauma Service
Indiana University School of Medicine
Indianapolis, Indiana

Robert O'Toole, MD
Assistant Professor
Department of Orthopaedic Surgery
University of Maryland School of Medicine
Baltimore, Maryland

Matthew E. Oetgen, MD
Clinical Instructor
Department of Orthopaedic Surgery and
   Sports Medicine
Children's National Medical Center
Washington, District of Columbia

Hans Christoph Pape, MD
F. Pauwels Professor and Chairman
Department of Orthopaedic Surgery
University of Aachen Medical Center
Aachen, Germany

George Partal, MD
Department of Orthopaedics
Eastern Maine Medical Center
Bangor, Maine

Laura S. Phieffer, MD
Assistant Professor of Orthopaedics
The Ohio State University Medical Center
Columbus, Ohio

Michael Prayson, MD
Associate Professor of Orthopaedic Surgery
Wright State University Boonshoft School
   of Medicine
Miami Valley Hospital
Dayton, Ohio

William M. Ricci, MD
Associate Professor
Department of Orthopaedic Surgery
Washington University School of Medicine
St. Louis, Missouri

Toby M. Risko, MD
Assistant Professor of Orthopaedics
Texas Tech University
Lubbock, Texas

Thomas A. Russell, BS, MD
Professor of Orthopaedic Surgery
Campbell Clinic/University of Tennessee
   Department of Orthopaedics
Elvis Presley Trauma Center
University of Tennessee
Eads, Tennessee

Henry Claude Sagi, MD
Assistant Clinical Professor
Department of Orthopaedic Surgery and
   Orthopaedic Trauma Service
University of South Florida
Tampa General Hospital
Tampa, Florida

Roy W. Sanders, MD
Director, Orthopaedic Trauma Service
Tampa General Hospital
Florida Orthopaedic Institute
Tampa, Florida

Jodi Siegel, MD
Assistant Professor of Orthopaedics
Department of Orthopaedics and Physical
   Rehabilitation
University of Massachusetts Medical
   School
University of Massachusetts Memorial
   Medical Center
Worcester, Massachusetts

J. Benjamin Smucker, MD
Orthopaedic Resident
Metrohealth Hospital
Cleveland, Ohio

John K. Sontich, MD
Associate Professor of Surgery,
   Orthopaedics
Metrohealth Medical Center
Cleveland, Ohio

Natalie L. Talboo, MPAS, PA-C
Department of Orthopaedic Trauma
St. Elizabeth Health Center
Youngstown, Ohio

David C. Templeman, MD
Associate Professor of Orthopaedic Surgery
University of Minnesota
Hennepin County Medical Center
Minneapolis, Minnesota

Paul Tornetta III, MD
Professor and Vice Chairman
Department of Orthopaedic Surgery
Director of Orthopaedic Trauma
Boston University Medical Center
Boston, Massachusetts

J. Tracy Watson, MD
Professor of Orthopaedic Surgery
Chief, Division of Orthopaedic
   Traumatology
St. Louis University School of Medicine
St. Louis, Missouri

Bruce H. Ziran, MD
Associate Professor
Department of Orthopaedics
Northeastern Ohio Universities College of
    Medicine
Director of Orthopaedic Trauma
St. Elizabeth Health Center
Youngstown, Ohio

Navid M. Ziran, MD
Chief Resident of Orthopaedics
Strong Memorial Hospital of Rochester
Rochester, New York

PART 3 ADULT
RECONSTRUCTION

Anish K. Amin, MBChB, MRCSEd
Specialist Registrar
Department of Orthopaedic and Trauma
    Surgery
New Royal Infirmary of Edinburgh
Edinburgh, Scotland

Robert A. Arciero, MD
Professor and Chief of Sports Medicine
Department of Orthopaedic Surgery
University of Connecticut Health Center
Farmington, Connecticut

Matthew S. Austin, MD
Assistant Professor of Orthopaedic Surgery
Thomas Jefferson University Hospital
Rothman Institute
Philadelphia, Pennsylvania

B. Sonny Bal, MD, MBA
Associate Professor
Department of Orthopaedic Surgery
University of Missouri
Columbia, Missouri

Martin Beck, MD, PD, Dr.med.
Department of Orthopaedic Surgery
Canton Hospital Lucerne
Lucerne, Switzerland

Christopher P. Beauchamp, MD
Associate Professor of Orthopaedics
Mayo College of Medicine
Phoenix, Arizona

Benjamin Bender, MD
Joint Replacement Specialist
Assuta Hospital
Tel-Aviv, Israel

Keith R. Berend, MD
Clinical Assistant Professor
Department of Orthopaedics
The Ohio State University
New Albany, Ohio

Michael E. Berend, MD
Orthopaedic Surgeon
Center for Hip & Knee Surgery
St. Francis Hospital
Mooresville, Indiana

Hari P. Bezwada, MD
Assistant Clinical Professor
Department of Orthopaedic Surgery
University of Pennsylvania School of
    Medicine
Philadelphia, Pennsylvania

James Bicos, MD
Department of Orthopedics and Sports
    Medicine
St. Vincent Medical Center
Carmel, Indiana

Thomas E. Brown, MD
Associate Professor of Orthopaedic Surgery
University of Virginia School of Medicine
Charlottesville, Virginia

Shawn M. Brubaker, DO
Staff, Shasta Orthopaedics and Sports
    Center
Redding, California

Robert H. Cho, MD
Orthopaedic Resident
Department of Orthopaedic Surgery
Drexel University College of Medicine
Philadelphia, Pennsylvania

Christian P. Christensen, MD
Head, Adult Reconstruction
Lexington Clinic
Assistant Clinical Professor
University of Kentucky
Lexington, Kentucky

John C. Clohisy, MD
Professor of Orthopaedic Surgery
Washington University Medical School
St. Louis, Missouri

Janet D. Conway, MD
Head of Bone and Joint Infection
Rubin Institute for Advanced Orthopaedics
Sinai Hospital
Baltimore, Maryland

Marcus Crestani, MD
Department of Orthopaedics
Hospital Moinhos de Vento
Santa Casa, Brazil

Craig J. Della Valle, MD
Associate Professor of Orthopaedic Surgery
Rush University Medical Center
Westchester, Illinois

Jonathan Garino, MD
Associate Professor
Department of Orthopaedic Surgery
University of Pennsylvania School
    of Medicine
Philadelphia, Pennsylvania

Nelson V. Greidanus, MD, MPH, FRCSC
Assistant Professor
Department of Orthopaedics
University of British Columbia
Vancouver, British Columbia, Canada

David Gusmao, MD
Department of Orthopaedics
Hospital Moinhos de Vento
Santa Casa, Brazil

Mark A. Hartzband, MD
Senior Attending Director, Total Joint
    Replacement Service
Department of Orthopaedic Surgery
Hackensack University Medical Center
Hackensack, New Jersey

Philipp Henle, MD
Resident
Department of Orthopaedic Surgery
Inselspital, Bern University Hospital
Bern, Switzerland

Matthew S. Hepinstall, MD
Fellow, Adult Reconstruction & Joint
    Replacement
Department of Orthopedic Surgery
Hospital for Special Surgery
New York, New York

William J. Hozack, MD
Professor of Orthopedics
Department of Orthopedic Surgery
The Rothman Institute
Thomas Jefferson University Hospital
Philadelphia, Pennsylvania

Cale A. Jacobs, PhD
Director of Development
End Range of Motion Improvement, Inc.
Assistant Professor, Adjunct Title Series
College of Health Sciences
University of Kentucky
Suwanee, Georgia

S. Mehdi Jafari, MD
Assistant Professor
Department of Orthopaedic Surgery
Tehran University of Medical Sciences
Shariati Hospital
Tehran, Iran

Kang-Il Kim, MD, PhD
Associate Professor and Chief
Center for Joint Diseases
Department of Orthopaedic Surgery
Kyung Hee University School of Medicine
East-West Neo Medical Center
Seoul, Korea

Winston Y. Kim, MBChB, MSc, FRCS
Lecturer and Consultant Orthopaedic
    Surgeon
The Alexandra Hospital
University of Manchester
Cheadle, Cheshire, United Kingdom

Brian A. Klatt, MD
Assistant Professor
Department of Orthopaedic Surgery
University of Pittsburgh Medical Center
Pittsburgh, Pennsylvania

Gregg R. Klein, MD
Attending Physician
Department of Orthopaedic Surgery
Hackensack University Medical Center
Hackensack, New Jersey

Gwo-Chin Lee, MD
Assistant Professor
Department of Orthopaedic Surgery
University of Pennsylvania School of
    Medicine
Philadelphia, Pennsylvania

Michael Leunig, MD, PD, Dr.med.
Department of Orthopaedics
Schulthess Clinic
Zurich, Switzerland

Harlan B. Levine, MD
Attending Physician
Department of Orthopaedic Surgery
Hackensack University Medical Center
Hackensack, New Jersey

Adolph V. Lombardi, Jr., MD, FACS
Clinical Assistant Professor
Department of Orthopaedics
Department of Biomedical Engineering
The Ohio State University
New Albany, Ohio

Bassam A. Masri, MD, FRCSC
Professor and Head
Department of Orthopaedics
University of British Columbia
Vancouver, British Columbia, Canada

William M. Mihalko, MD, PhD
Department of Orthopaedics
Campbell Clinic
Germantown, Tennessee

S. M. Javad Mortazavi, MD
Associate Professor
Department of Orthopedic Surgery
Tehran University of Medical Sciences
Imam University Hospital
Tehran, Iran

David G. Nazarian, MD
Assistant Clinical Professor
Department of Orthopaedic Surgery
University of Pennsylvania School of
    Medicine
Philadelphia, Pennsylvania

Ali Oliashirazi, MD
Professor and Chairman
Department of Orthopaedic Surgery
Joan C. Edwards School of Medicine
Marshall University
Huntington, West Virginia

Alvin Ong, MD
Orthopaedic Surgeon
Specialist in Pelvis, Hip & Knee
    Reconstruction, Orthopaedic
    Traumatology
Director, Division of Orthopaedic Surgery
Jefferson University Hospital
Philadelphia, Pennsylvania
Atlanticare Regional Medical Center
Egg Harbor Township, New Jersey

Fabio Orozco, MD
Hip and Knee Surgeon
The Rothman Institute
Philadelphia, Pennsylvania

Javad Parvizi, MD, FRCS
Professor
Department of Orthopaedic Surgery
Rothman Institute at Thomas Jefferson
    University Hospital
Philadelphia, Pennsylvania

**James T. Patton, MBChB, FRCSEd
    (Tr&Orth)**
Consultant Orthopaedic Surgeon
Department of Orthopaedic and Trauma
    Surgery
New Royal Infirmary of Edinburgh
Edinburgh, Scotland

Trevor R. Pickering, MD
Center for Hip and Knee Surgery
St. Francis Hospital
Moorseville, Indiana

Ameet Pispati, MD
Visiting Surgeon
Center for Joint Diseases
Department of Orthopaedic Surgery
Kyung Hee University School of Medicine
East-West Neo Medical Center
Seoul, Korea

James J. Purtill, MD
Assistant Professor
Department of Orthopaedic Surgery
Thomas Jefferson University
Rothman Institute
Philadelphia, Pennsylvania

R. Lor Randall, MD
The L.B. & Olive S. Young Endowed
    Chair for Cancer Research
Professor
Department of Orthopaedic Surgery
Huntsman Cancer Institute
University of Utah
Salt Lake City, Utah

Camilo Restrepo, MD
Department of Orthopedic Surgery
Rothman Institute
Thomas Jefferson University
Philadelphia, Pennsylvania

José A. Rodriguez, MD
Chief of Adult Reconstruction
Department of Orthopaedic Surgery
Lenox Hill Hospital
New York, New York

Khaled J. Saleh, MD
Professor of Surgery
Chief of Orthopaedics and Rehabilitation
Southern Illinois University School of
    Medicine
Springfield, Illinois

Jeffrey W. Salin, DO
Kansas City Bone & Joint Clinic, Inc.
Overland Park, Kansas

Klaus A. Siebenrock, MD
Professor of Orthopaedic Surgery
Inselspital, Bern University Hospital
Bern, Switzerland

Franklin H. Sim, MD
Professor of Orthopedic Surgery
Mayo Clinic
Rochester, Minnesota

Mark J. Spangehl, MD
Assistant Professor of Orthopaedics
Mayo Clinic Arizona
Phoenix, Arizona

Moritz Tannast, MD
Resident
Department of Orthopaedic Surgery
Inselspital, Bern University Hospital
Bern, Switzerland

Marco Teloken, MD
Residency Instructor
Department of Orthopaedics
Hospital Moinhos de Vento
Santa Casa, Brazil

Brian Vannozzi, MD
Instructor
Department of Orthopaedic Surgery
University of Pennsylvania School
    of Medicine
Philadelphia, Pennsylvania

PART 4 PEDIATRICS

Behrooz Akbarnia, MD
Clinical Professor
University of California, San Diego
La Jolla, California

Jay C. Albright, MD
Director, Sports Medicine
Pediatric Orthopedic Specialty Practices
Arnold Palmer Hospital for Children
Orlando, Florida

Alexandre Arkader, MD
Assistant Professor of Clinical Orthopaedic
    Surgery
Children's Hospital Los Angeles
Keck School of Medicine
University of Southern California
Los Angeles, California

Donald S. Bae, MD
Assistant Professor
Department of Orthopaedic Surgery
Harvard Medical School
Children's Hospital Boston
Boston, Massachusetts

Robert M. Bernstein, MD
Associate Professor
Department of Surgery
Cedar-Sinai Medical Center
Los Angeles, California

Carla Baldrighi, MD
Department of Reconstructive
    Microsurgery
Ospedale CTO
Azienda Ospedaliero-Universitaria Careggi
Florence, Italy

R. Dale Blasier, MD, FRCS(C), MBA
Professor of Orthopaedic Surgery
Arkansas Children's Hospital
University of Arkansas for Medical
    Sciences
Little Rock, Arkansas

Arkady Blyakher, MD
Specialist Assistant
Department of Orthopedic Surgery
Hospital for Special Surgery
New York, New York

J. Richard Bowen, MD
Alfred I. duPont Hospital for Children
Department of Orthopaedics
Wilmington, Delaware

Richard E. Bowen, MD
Assistant Professor of Orthopaedic Surgery
Santa Monica/UCLA and Orthopaedic
    Hospital
Los Angeles, California

Michelle S. Caird, MD
Assistant Professor of Orthopaedic Surgery
University of Michigan Health System
Ann Arbor, Michigan

Gilbert Chan, MD
Clinical Fellow
Division of Orthopaedics
The Children's Hospital of Philadelphia
Philadelphia, Pennsylvania

Paul D. Choi, MD
Assistant Professor of Clinical
    Orthopaedics
Children's Hospital Los Angeles
University of Southern California Keck
    School of Medicine
Los Angeles, California

Roger Cornwall, MD
Assistant Professor of Orthopaedic Surgery
University of Cincinnati College of
    Medicine
Cincinnati, Ohio

Anna V. Cuomo, MD
Pediatric Orthopaedic Fellow
Division of Orthopaedic Surgery
Hospital for Sick Children
Toronto, Ontario, Canada

Kirk W. Dabney, MD
Associate Director of the Cerebral Palsy
    Program
Alfred I. duPont Hospital for Children
Wilmington, Delaware

Jon R. Davids, MD
Chief of Staff
Director, Motion Analysis Laboratory
Shriners Hospital for Children
Greenville, South Carolina

Richard S. Davidson, MD
Associate Professor
Division of Pediatric Orthopaedics
Department of Surgery
Children's Hospital of Philadelphia
University of Pennsylvania School of
    Medicine
Philadelphia, Pennsylvania

Matthew B. Dobbs, MD
Associate Professor of Orthopaedic Surgery
Washington University School of Medicine
Saint Louis, Missouri

John P. Dormans, MD
Chief of Orthopaedic Surgery
The Children's Hospital of Philadelphia
Philadelphia, Pennsylvania

Denis S. Drummond, MD
Professor of Orthopaedic Surgery
University of Pennsylvania School of
    Medicine
Attending Surgeon
Emeritus Chief of Orthopaedic Surgery
The Children's Hospital of Philadelphia
Philadelphia, Pennsylvania

Craig P. Eberson, MD
Assistant Professor and Division Chief
Division of Pediatric Orthopaedics
Department of Orthopaedics
Alpert Medical School of Brown University
Hasbro Children's Hospital
Providence, Rhode Island

John B. Emans, MD
Professor of Orthopedic Surgery
Children's Hospital Boston
Harvard Medical School
Boston, Massachusetts

Paul W. Esposito, MD
Professor of Orthopaedic Surgery and
    Pediatrics
University of Nebraska Medical Center
Children's Hospital and Medical Center
Omaha, Nebraska

Marybeth Ezaki, MD
Professor of Orthopaedic Surgery
Department of Hand Service
Texas Scottish Rite Hospital for Children
Dallas, Texas

Reginald S. Fayssoux, MD
Department of Orthopaedic Surgery
The Emory Spine Center
Emory University School of Medicine
Atlanta, Georgia

Fabio Ferri-De-Barros, MD, FSBOT
Clinical Fellow, PhD Student
Department of Orthopaedics
Hospital for Sick Children
Toronto, Ontario, Canada

John M. Flynn, MD
Associate Chief of Orthopaedic Surgery
The Children's Hospital of Philadelphia
Associate Professor of Orthopaedic Surgery
University of Pennsylvania School of
    Medicine
Philadelphia, Pennsylvania

Jenny M. Frances, MD, MPH
Assistant Professor of Orthopaedic Surgery
New York University Hospital for Joint
    Diseases
New York, New York

John Frino, MD
Assistant Professor of Orthopaedic Surgery
Wake Forest University School of Medicine
Winston-Salem, North Carolina

Theodore J. Ganley, MD
Associate Professor of Orthopaedic Surgery
University of Pennsylvania School of
    Medicine
Attending Surgeon
Director of Sports Medicine
The Children's Hospital of Philadelphia
Philadelphia, Pennsylvania

Matthew R. Garner, BS
The Children's Hospital of Philadelphia
Philadelphia, Pennsylvania

Purushottam A. Gholve, MD, MBMS,
    MRCS
Assistant Professor of Orthopaedics
Floating Hospital for Children at Tufts
    Medical Center
Tufts University School of Medicine
Boston, Massachusetts

J. Anthony Gonzales, Jr., BS, MD
Department of Pediatric Orthopedics
Children's Hospital of New Orleans
New Orleans, Louisiana

J. Eric Gordon, MD
Associate Professor of Medicine
Department of Orthopedics
Washington University School of
    Medicine/St. Louis Children's Hospital
St. Louis, Missouri

James T. Guille, MD
Division of Spinal Disorders
Brandywine Institute of Orthopaedics
Pottstown, Pennsylvania

Aaron B. Heath, MD
Division of Orthopaedic Surgery
The Children's Hospital of Philadelphia
Philadelphia, Pennsylvania

Daniel J. Hedequist, MD
Associate Professor of Orthopedic Surgery
Department of Orthopedics
Children's Hospital Boston/Harvard
    Medical School
Boston, Massachusetts

B. David Horn, MD
Assistant Professor
Department of Orthopaedic Surgery
University of Pennsylvania School of
    Medicine
Philadelphia, Pennsylvania

Victor Hsu, BA, MD
Attending Spine Surgeon
Department of Orthopaedic Surgery
Orthopaedic Specialty Center
Willow Grove, Pennsylvania

Lori A. Karol, MD
Professor of Orthopaedic Surgery
Texas Scottish Rite Hospital for Children
Dallas, Texas

Kathryn A. Keeler, MD
Assistant Professor
Department of Orthopedic Surgery
Washington University School of Medicine
St. Louis, Missouri

Young-Jo Kim, MD, PhD
Assistant Professor of Orthopaedic Surgery
Harvard Medical School
Children's Hospital Boston
Boston, Massachusetts

Mininder S. Kocher, MD, MPH
Associate Director
Division of Sports Medicine
Department of Orthopaedic Surgery
Children's Hospital Boston
Associate Professor of Orthopaedic Surgery
Harvard Medical School
Harvard School of Public Health
Boston, Massachusetts

J. Todd R. Lawrence, MD, PhD
Fellow, Pediatric Orthopaedic Surgery
The Children's Hospital of Philadelphia
Philadelphia, Pennsylvania

Bryan T. Leek, MD
Fellow
Department of Orthopedic Surgery
University of California, San Diego
San Diego, California

Noppachart Limpaphayom, MD
Instructor
Department of Orthopedics
Chulalongkorn University
Bangkok, Thailand

Jeffrey E. Martus, MD
Assistant Professor
Department of Orthopedics and
    Rehabilitation
Vanderbilt Children's Hospital
Nashville, Tennessee

Travis H. Matheney, MD
Instructor in Orthopaedic Surgery
Harvard Medical School
Children's Hospital Boston
Boston, Massachusetts

James J. McCarthy, MD
Faculty
University of Wisconsin School of
    Medicine
    and Public Health
University of Wisconsin Hospital and
    Clinics
American Family Children's Hospital
Rosemont, Illinois

Richard E. McCarthy, MD
Professor
Chief of Spinal Deformities
Department of Orthopaedics
Arkansas Children's Hospital
Little Rock, Arkansas

Charles T. Mehlman, DO, MPH
Professor
Department of Pediatric Orthopaedic
  Surgery
Cincinnati Children's Hospital Medical
  Center
Cincinnati, Ohio

Gokce Mik, MD
Department of Orthopaedic Surgery
The Children's Hospital of Philadelphia
Philadelphia, Pennsylvania

Freeman Miller, MD
Al duPont Hospital for Children
Wilmington, Delaware

Michael B. Millis, MD
Associate Professor of Orthopaedic Surgery
Harvard Medical School
Children's Hospital Boston
Boston, Massachusetts

Vincent S. Mosca, MD
Associate Professor of Orthopedics
University of Washington School of
  Medicine
Seattle Children's Hospital
Seattle, Washington

Scott J. Mubarak, MD
Clinical Professor
Department of Orthopedics
University of California
San Diego Medical Center
San Diego, California

Stuart M. Myers, MD
Department of Orthopedic Surgery
The Johns Hopkins University School of
  Medicine
Baltimore, Maryland

Karen S. Myung, MD, PhD
Assistant Professor
Children's Orthopedic Center
Children's Hospital of Los Angeles
Los Angeles, California

**Unni G. Narayanan, MBBS, MSc,
  FRCS(C)**
Assistant Professor of Surgery
Division of Orthopaedic Surgery
University of Toronto
The Hospital for Sick Children
Toronto, Ontario, Canada

Blaise Nemeth, MA, MS
Assistant Professor (CHS)
Department of Orthopedics
University of Wisconsin School of
  Medicine and
  Public Health
Madison, Wisconsin

Kenneth Noonan, MD
Associate Professor
Department of Orthopaedics
University of Wisconsin School of
  Medicine and
  Public Health
Madison, Wisconsin

Tom F. Novacheck, MD
Associate Professor
Director, Center for Gait and Motion
  Analysis
Department of Orthopaedic Surgery
University of Minnesota
Gillette Children's Specialty Healthcare
St. Paul, Minnesota

Scott N. Oishi, MD
Assistant Professor of Plastic Sugery
Department of Hand Service
Texas Scottish Rite Hospital for Children
Dallas, Texas

Brad Olney, MD
Professor and Chief
Department of Orthopaedics
Children's Mercy Hospital
Kansas City, Missouri

Norman Y. Otsuka, MD
Clinical Professor
Department of Orthopedic Surgery
University of California, Los Angeles
Shriners Hospitals for Children
Los Angeles, California

Dror Paley, MD, FRCSC
Director
Paley Advanced Limb Lengthening
  Institute
St. Mary's Hospital
West Palm Beach, Florida

Kristan A. Pierz, MD
Assistant Professor of Orthopaedics
Connecticut Children's Medical Center
University of Connecticut School of Medicine
Hartford, Connecticut

Maya E. Pring, MD
Clinical Instructor of Orthopedic Surgery
University of California San Diego
Rady Children's Hospital San Diego
San Diego, California

Ellen M. Raney, MD
Clinical Professor of Surgery
Department of Surgery
Clinical Professor of Pediatrics
Department of Pediatrics
University of Hawaii John A. Burns School
  of Medicine
Shriners Hospital for Children
Honolulu, Hawaii

Margaret M. Rich, MD, PhD
Shriners Hospitals for Children—St. Louis
St. Louis, Missouri

James R. Romanowski, MD
Fellow, Orthopaedic Sports Medicine
Department of Orthopaedic Surgery
University of Pittsburgh Medical Center
Pittsburgh, Pennsylvania

Anthony A. Scaduto, MD
Pediatric Orthopaedics
Los Angeles Orthopaedic Hospital
Los Angeles, California

David Scher, MD
Associate Professor of Clinical Orthopaedics
Division of Pediatric Orthopaedic Surgery
Department of Orthopaedic Surgery
Weill Cornell School of Medicine
Hospital for Special Surgery
New York, New York

Perry L. Schoenecker, MD
Professor and Chief of Pediatric
  Orthopaedics
Washington University School of Medicine
Shriners Hospital for Children
St. Louis, Missouri

Tim Schrader, MD
Medical Director, Hip Program
Children's Healthcare of Atlanta
Atlanta, Georgia

Richard M. Schwend, MD
Professor
Department of Orthopaedics
Children's Mercy Hospital
Kansas City, Missouri

Eric D. Shirley, MD
Attending Pediatric Orthopaedic Surgery
Bone and Joint Institute
Naval Medical Center Portsmouth
Virginia Beach, Virginia

Om Prasad Shrestha, MBBS
Clinical Fellow
Division of Orthopaedics
The Children's Hospital of Philadelphia
Philadelphia, Pennsylvania

Ernest L. Sink, MD
Associate Professor
Department of Orthopaedics
The Children's Hospital
University of Colorado
Aurora, Colorado

David L. Skaggs, MD
Professor of Orthopaedic Surgery
University of Southern California
Chief of Orthopaedic Surgery
Children's Hospital Los Angeles
Los Angeles, California

Brian G. Smith, MD
Associate Professor of Orthopaedics and
  Rehabilitation
Director, Yale Pediatric Orthopaedics and
  Rehabilitation
Yale School of Medicine
New Haven, Connecticut

Brian Snyder, MD, PhD
Associate Professor
Department of Orthopaedic Surgery
Harvard Medical School
Children's Hospital Boston
Boston, Massachusetts

David A. Spiegel, MD
Assistant Professor of Orthopaedic Surgery
Children's Hospital of Philadelphia
University of Philadelphia School of
  Medicine
Philadelphia, Pennsylvania

Shawn C. Standard, MD
Head of Pediatric Orthopedics
International Center for Limb Lengthening
Rubin Institute for Advanced Orthopedics
Sinai Hospital of Baltimore
Baltimore, Maryland

Anthony A. Stans, MD
Assistant Professor of Medicine
Chair, Division of Pediatric Orthopedics
Mayo Clinic
Rochester, Minnesota

Peter M. Stevens, MD
Professor of Orthopaedics
University of Utah
Salt Lake City, Utah

Joshua A. Strassberg, MD
Associate Attending
Department of Orthopedic Surgery
Morristown Memorial Hospital
Cedar Knolls, New Jersey

Daniel J. Sucato, MD, MS
Associate Professor
University of Texas at Southwestern
    Medical Center
Staff Orthopaedic Surgeon
Texas Scottish Rite Hospital
Dallas, Texas

Ann E. Van Heest, MD
Professor of Orthopaedic Surgery
University of Minnesota
Minneapolis, Minnesota

Thanapong Waitayawinyu, MD
Assistant Professor of Orthopaedics
Thammasat University
Klongluang, Pathumthani, Thailand

Eric J. Wall, MD
Director of Orthopaedic Surgery
Cincinnati Children's Hospital Medical
    Center
Cincinnati, Ohio

Lawrence Wells, MD
Assistant Professor of Orthopaedic Surgery
University of Pennsylvania School of
    Medicine
Children's Hospital of Philadelphia
Philadelphia, Pennsylvania

Dennis R. Wenger, MD
Clinical Professor of Orthopedic Surgery
University of California San Diego
Rady Children's Hospital San Diego
San Diego, California

Roger F. Widmann, MD
Associate Professor of Clinical
    Orthopaedic Surgery
Division of Pediatric Orthopaedic Surgery
Weill Cornell Medical College
Hospital for Special Surgery
New York, New York

Jennifer J. Winell, MD
Assistant Professor of Orthopaedic Surgery
Children's Hospital of Philadelphia
Philadelphia, Pennsylvania

Yi-Meng Yen, MD, PhD
Instructor in Orthopedic Surgery
Harvard Medical School
Orthopedic Surgery/Sports Medicine
Children's Hospital Boston
Boston, Massachusetts

PART 5 ONCOLOGY

Adesegun Abudu, FRCS
Royal Orthopaedic Hospital Oncology
    Service
Northfield, Birmingham, United Kingdom

Aharon Amir, MD
Attending Surgeon
Department of Plastic Surgery
Tel-Aviv Sourasky Medical Center
Tel-Aviv, Israel

Jacob Bickels, MD
Head, Service for the Management of
    Metastatic Bone Disease
Attending Surgeon, National Unit of
    Orthopedic Oncology
Tel-Aviv Sourasky Medical Center
Professor of Orthopedic Surgery
Sackler School of Medicine, Tel-Aviv
    University
Tel-Aviv, Israel

Loretta B. Chou, MD
Professor of Orthopaedic Surgery
Stanford University
Chief, Foot and Ankle Service
Lucile Packard Children's Hospital at
    Stanford
Palo Alto, California

Ernest U. Conrad III, MD
Professor of Orthopaedics
University of Washington
Director, Bone Tumor Clinic
Children's Hospital and Regional Medical
    Center
Seattle, Washington

Jeffrey J. Eckardt, MD
Director, Orthopaedic Oncology
UCLA Santa Monica Orthopaedic Center
Santa Monica, California

Steven Gitelis, MD
Professor and Vice Chairman of
    Orthopaedic Surgery
Director, Section of Orthopaedic Oncology
Rush University Medical Center
Chicago, Illinois

Robert Grimer, FRCS
Consultant Orthopaedic Surgeon
Royal Orthopaedic Hospital
Northfield, Birmingham, United Kingdom

Eyal Gur, MD
Director, Unit of Microsurgery
Department of Plastic Surgery
Tel-Aviv Sourasky Medical Center
Senior Lecturer
Sackler School of Medicine
Tel-Aviv University
Tel-Aviv, Israel

Lee Jeys, MB, ChB, MSc, FRCS
Consultant Orthopaedic Surgeon
Specialist in Hip, Knee, and Oncology
    Surgery
Midland Hip & Knee Clinic
Royal Orthopaedic Hospital
Northfield, Birmingham, United Kingdom

Robert M. Henshaw, MD
Associate Clinical Professor of
    Orthopaedic Surgery
Georgetown University Medical Center
Director, Orthopaedic Oncology
Director, Fellowship Program in
    Orthopaedic Oncology
Washington Cancer Institute
Washington, District of Columbia

Yvette Ho
Research Assistant
Washington Musculoskeletal Tumor Center
Washington Cancer Institute
Washington, District of Columbia

Norio Kawahara, MD, PhD
Clinical Professor
Department of Orthopaedic Surgery
Kanazawa University School of Medicine
Ishikawa, Japan

Kristen Kellar-Graney, MS
Tumor Biologist and Clinical Research
    Coordinator
Washington Cancer Institute
Washington, District of Columbia

Piya Kiatsevi, MD
Orthopaedic Oncology Unit
Institute of Orthopaedics
Lerdsin Hospital
Bangkok, Thailand

Yehuda Kollender, MD
Attending Surgeon, National Unit of
    Orthopedic Oncology
Tel-Aviv Sourasky Medical Center
Senior Lecturer
Sackler School of Medicine, Tel-Aviv
    University
Tel-Aviv, Israel

Jennifer Lisle, MD
Assistant Professor of Orthopedics,
    Rehabilitation, and Pediatrics
University of Vermont College of Medicine
Vermont Children's Hospital at Fletcher
    Allen Health Care
Burlington, Vermont

Martin M. Malawer, MD, FACS
Professor (Clinical Scholar) of
    Orthopaedics
Professor of Pediatrics (Hematology and
    Oncology)
Georgetown University Medical Center
Professor of Orthopaedic Surgery
George Washington University
Director of Research and Development
Orthopaedic Oncology
Washington Cancer Institute
Orthopaedic Oncology
Children's National Medical Center
Washington, District of Columbia
Consultant (Pediatric and Surgery Branch)
National Cancer Institute, National
    Institutes of Health
Bethesda, Maryland

Isaac Meller, MD
Director, National Unit of Orthopedic
    Oncology
Tel-Aviv Sourasky Medical Center
Professor of Orthopedic Surgery
Sackler School of Medicine, Tel-Aviv
    University
Tel-Aviv, Israel

Benjamin J. Miller, MD
Rush Orthopaedic Oncology
Rush University Medical Center
Chicago, Illinois

Hideki Murakami, MD
Lecturer of Orthopaedic Surgery
Department of Orthopaedic Surgery
Kanazawa University School of Medicine
Ishikawa, Japan

Gregory P. Nicholson, MD
Associate Professor of Orthopaedic Surgery
Rush University Medical Center
Chicago, Illinois

Tamir Pritsch, MD
Department of Orthopaedic Surgery
Tel Aviv Sourasky Medical Center
Tel Aviv, Israel

Amir Sternheim, MD
Orthopedic Oncology
Washington Cancer Institute
Washington, District of Columbia

H. Thomas Temple, MD
Professor of Orthopaedics and Pathology
Vice Chair and Chief, Oncology Division
Director, University of Miami Tissue Bank
University of Miami Leonard M. Miller
  School of Medicine
Miami, Florida

Daria Brooks Terrell, MD
Attending Physician
Department of Orthopaedic Oncology
Washington Hospital Center
Washington, District of Columbia
Consultant (Pediatric and Surgery Branch)
National Cancer Institute, National
  Institutes of Health
Bethesda, Maryland

Katsuro Tomita, MD
Professor of Orthopaedic Surgery
Department of Orthopaedic Surgery
Kanazawa University School of Medicine
Ishikawa, Japan

Jason Weisstein, MD, MPH, FACS
Assistant Professor of Orthopaedics and
  Sports Medicine
Co-Director, Northwest Tissue Center
University of Washington
Seattle, Washington

James C. Wittig, MD
Associate Professor of Orthopedic Surgery
Chief of Orthopedic Oncology and
  Sarcoma Program
Mount Sinai Medical Center
New York, New York

Yehuda Wolf, MD
Director, Department of Vascular Surgery
Tel-Aviv Sourasky Medical Center
Professor of Surgery
Sackler School of Medicine, Tel-Aviv
  University
Tel-Aviv, Israel

Walter W. Virkus, MD
Associate Professor of Orthopaedic Surgery
Associate Attending Surgeon (Orthopedic
  Surgery)
Rush University Medical Center
Chicago, Illinois

Arik Zaretski, MD
Attending Surgeon
Department of Plastic Surgery
Tel-Aviv Sourasky Medical Center
Tel-Aviv, Israel

PART 6 HAND, WRIST, AND FOREARM

Brian D. Adams, MD
Professor of Orthopedic Surgery and
  Bioengineering
University of Iowa
Iowa City, Iowa

Christopher H. Allan, MD
Associate Professor of Orthopaedics and
  Sports Medicine
University of Washington
Seattle, Washington

Edward A. Athanasian, MD
Associate Professor of Clinical
  Orthopaedic Surgery
Weill Cornell Medical College
Associate Attending Orthopaedic Surgeon
Hospital for Special Surgery
New York, New York

Mark N. Awantang, MD
Orthopedic Associates
Washington, District of Columbia

Alejandro Badia, MD, FACS
Badia Hand to Shoulder Center
Chief of Hand Surgery
Baptist Hospital
Miami, Florida

Mark E. Baratz, MD
Professor and Executive Vice Chairman
Chief, Upper Extremity Service
Director of Orthopaedic Residency and
  Upper Extremity Fellowship
Department of Orthopaedic Surgery
Drexel University College of Medicine
Allegheny General Hospital
Pittsburgh, Pennsylvania

Asheesh Bedi, MD
Assistant Professor of Orthopaedic Surgery
University of Michigan Health System
Ann Arbor, Michigan

Michael S. Bednar, MD
Professor of Orthopaedic Surgery
  and Rehabilitation
Stritch School of Medicine
Loyola University–Chicago
Maywood, Illinois

Kerry Bemers, CHT
University Orthopedics
Providence, Rhode Island

Leon S. Benson, MD
Professor of Clinical Orthopaedic Surgery
University of Chicago Pritzker School of
  Medicine
Illinois Bone and Joint Institute
Glenview, Illinois

Pedro K. Beredjiklian, MD
Associate Professor of Orthopaedic Surgery
Thomas Jefferson School of Medicine
Chief, Hand Surgery Division
The Rothman Institute
Thomas Jefferson School of Medicine
Philadelphia, Pennsylvania

Randy R. Bindra, MD
Professor of Orthopaedic Surgery
Loyola University Medical Center
Maywood, Illinois

Philip E. Blazar, MD
Assistant Professor of Orthopedic Surgery
Brigham and Women's Hospital
Boston, Massachusetts

Michael R. Boland, MBChB, FRCS,
  FRACS
Assistant Professor of Orthopaedic Surgery
University of Kentucky College of
  Medicine
Lexington, Kentucky

Benjamin J. Boudreaux, MD
Assistant Clinical Professor of Plastic
  Surgery
Louisiana State University
Baton Rouge, Louisiana

Martin I. Boyer, MD
Carole B. and Jerome T. Loeb Professor of
  Orthopaedic Surgery
Department of Orthopaedic Surgery
Washington University School of Medicine
St. Louis, Missouri

David J. Bozentka, MD
Associate Professor of Orthopaedic Surgery
University of Pennsylvania
Chief, Orthopaedic Surgery
Penn Presbyterian Medical Center
Philadelphia, Pennsylvania

Jay T. Bridgeman, MD
Assistant Professor of Orthopaedics
Penn State Hershey Bone and Joint
  Institute
Hershey, Pennsylvania

John S. Bucchieri, MD
Private Practice, Lake Health
Willoughby, Ohio

Jeffrey E. Budoff, MD
Director, Orthopaedic Hand and Upper
  Extremity Service
Houston VA Medical Center
Southwest Orthopaedic Group
Houston, Texas

Reuben A. Bueno, Jr., MD
Assistant Professor of Plastic Surgery
Southern Illinois University School of
  Medicine
Springfield, Illinois

John T. Capo, MD
Associate Professor of Orthopaedics
Chief, Division of Hand and Microvascular
  Surgery
UMDNJ-New Jersey Medical School
Newark, New Jersey

Charles Cassidy, MD
Henry H. Banks Associate Professor and
  Chairman
Tufts University School of Medicine
Orthopaedist in Chief at Tufts Medical
  Center
Boston, Massachusetts

Louis W. Catalano III, MD
Assistant Clinical Professor
Columbia University
C. V. Staff
Hand Surgery Center
Roosevelt Hospital
New York, New York

Edwin Y. Chang, MD
Spokane Plastic Surgeons
Spokane, Washington

Nilesh M. Chaudhari, MD
Assistant Professor of Surgery
Department of Orthopaedic Surgery
University of Alabama, Birmingham
Birmingham, Alabama

Neal C. Chen, MD
Clinical Instructor
Department of Orthopaedic Surgery
University of Michigan
Ann Arbor, Michigan

Andrew Chin, MD FRCS
Consultant Hand Surgeon
Hand Surgery Unit
Singapore General Hospital
Singapore

Kevin C. Chung, MD, MS
Professor of Surgery
Section of Plastic Surgery
University of Michigan
Ann Arbor, Michigan

Evan D. Collins, MD
Assistant Professor of Orthopaedics
Weill Cornell Medical College
New York, New York
Staff Physician
Department of Orthopaedics
The Methodist Hospital
Houston, Texas

Cari Cordell, MD
Fellow
Department of Orthopaedics
Loyola University Medical Center
Maywood, Illinois

Andrew W. Cross, DVM, MD
Hand Surgery Specialists, Inc.
Cincinnati, Ohio

Randall W. Culp, MD
Professor of Orthopaedic Hand and
    Microsurgery
Department of Orthopaedics
Thomas Jefferson University Hospital
Philadelphia, Pennsylvania

Catherine M. Curtin, MD
Assistant Professor of Plastic Surgery
Stanford University
Pal Alto, California

Leonard L. D'Addesi, MD
Orthopaedic Associates of Reading
Reading Hospital and Medical Center
West Reading, Pennsylvania

Jorge de la Torre, MD
Professor of Surgery
Chief, Plastic Surgery
Division of Plastic Surgery
Department of Surgery
University of Alabama at Birmingham
Birmingham VA Medical Center
Birmingham, Alabama

Anthony M. DeLuise, Jr., MD
Fellow
Department of Orthopaedic Surgery
Thomas Jefferson University Hospital
Philadelphia, Pennsylvania

Edward Diao, MD
Professor Emeritus of Orthopaedic Surgery
    and Neurosurgery
University of California, San Francisco
San Francisco, California

John A. Dilger, MD
Department of Anesthesiology
Mayo Clinic
Rochester, Minnesota

Christopher Doumas, MD
Clinical Assistant Professor of Orthopaedic
    Surgery
Robert Wood Johnson Medical School
University of Medicine and Dentistry of
    New Jersey
New Brunswick, New Jersey

Christopher J. Dy, MD, MSPH
Resident Physician
Department of Orthopaedic Surgery
Hospital for Special Surgery
New York, New York

John C. Elfar, MD
Assistant Professor
Department of Orthopaedics
University of Rochester
Rochester, New York

Peter J. Evans, MD, PhD, FRCSC
Director, Hand and Upper Extremity
Department of Orthopaedics
Cleveland Clinic
Cleveland, Ohio

Paul Feldon, MD
Clinical Associate Professor of
    Orthopaedics
Tufts University School of Medicine
New England Baptist Hospital
Boston, Massachusetts

Diego Fernandez, MD
Lindenhof Hospital
Bern, Switzerland

John J. Fernandez, MD
Assistant Professor of Orthopaedic Surgery
Division of Hand, Wrist, and Elbow
Rush University Medical Center
Chicago, Illinois

Angel Ferreres, MD, PhD
Consultant Hand Surgeon
Hand Surgery Unit
Institut Kaplan
Barcelona, Spain

Rimma Finkel, MD
Chandler, Arizona

Christian Ford, MD
Chief Resident
Department of Plastic Surgery
Stanford Hospitals and Clinics
Palo Alto, California

Christopher L. Forthman, MD
Consultant, Curtis National Hand Center
Department of Orthopaedic Surgery
Union Memorial Hospital
Baltimore, Maryland

Jeffrey B. Friedrich, MD
Assistant Professor of Surgery and
    Orthopedics (Adjunct)
University of Washington
Seattle, Washington

Marc García-Elías, MD, PhD
Consultant Hand Surgeon
Hand Surgery Unit
Institut Kaplan
Barcelona, Spain

William B. Geissler, MD
Professor and Chief
Division of Hand and Upper Extremity
    Surgery
Chief
Arthroscopic Surgery and Sports Medicine
Department of Orthopaedic Surgery and
    Rehabilitation
University of Mississippi Medical Center
Jackson, Mississippi

Harris Gellman, MD
Voluntary Professor
Department of Orthopedic and Plastic
    Surgery
University of Miami
Miami, Florida

**Grey Giddins, MBBCh, FRCS(Orth),
    EDHS**
Consultant Orthopaedic and Hand
    Surgeon
Department of Orthopaedics
Royal United Hospital
Bath, England

Steven Z. Glickel, MD
Clinical Professor of Orthopaedic Surgery
C. V. Staff
Hand Surgery Center
Roosevelt Hospital
New York, New York

Charles A. Goldfarb, MD
Associate Professor
Department of Orthopaedic Surgery
Washington University School of Medicine
St. Louis, Missouri

Mark Goleski, MD
Resident of Internal Medicine
UT Southwestern Medical Center
Dallas, Texas

Christopher R. Goll, MD
Heekin Orthopaedics
Jacksonville, Florida

Thomas J. Graham, MD
Associate Professor
Department of Orthopaedic Surgery
Department of Plastic Surgery
Johns Hopkins School of Medicine
Chief, The Curtis National Hand Center
Vice-Chair, Department of Orthopaedic
    Surgery
Director, MedStar SportsHealth
Founder and Surgeon-in-Chief, Arnold
    Palmer SportsHealth Center
Union Memorial Hospital
Baltimore, Maryland

Jennifer Green, MD
Hand and Upper Extremity Surgeon
Newton Wellesley Orthopaedic Association
Newton, Massachusetts

Jeffrey A. Greenberg, MD, MS
Clinical Assistant Professor
Department of Orthopedics
Indiana University
Indiana Hand Center
Indianapolis, Indiana

Warren C. Hammert, MD
Associate Professor of Orthopaedic Surgery
  and Plastic Surgery
Department of Orthopaedic Surgery and
  Rehabilitation
University of Rochester Medical Center
Rochester, New York

Douglas P. Hanel, MD
Professor of Orthopaedics and Sports
  Medicine
University of Washington
Head, Pediatric Hand Surgery Program
Children's Hospital Medical Center
Seattle, Washington

Scott L. Hansen, MD
Assistant Professor of Surgery
Division of Plastic and Reconstructive
  Surgery
University of California, San Francisco
San Francisco, California

Timothy W. Harman, BA, DO
Associate Clinical Professor
Assistant Program Director
Department of Orthopedics
Ohio University
Dayton, Ohio

Colin Harris, MD
Department of Orthopaedics
UMDNJ-New Jersey Medical School
Newark, New Jersey

Mark F. Hendrickson, MD
Section Head, Hand Surgery
Cleveland Clinic
Cleveland, Ohio

**Carlos Heras-Palou, MD,
  FRCS(Trau&Orth)**
Pulvertaft Hand Centre
Royal Derby Hospital
Derby, England

Eric P. Hofmeister, MD
Assistant Professor of Surgery
Uniformed Services University of the
  Health Sciences
Vice Chairman and Director, Hand and
  Microvascular Service
Department of Orthopaedic Surgery
Naval Medical Center, San Diego
San Diego, California

Samuel C. Hoxie, MD
Department of Orthopaedic Surgery
Mayo Clinic
Rochester, Minnesota

Harry A. Hoyen, MD
Assistant Professor of Orthopaedic Surgery
Case Western Reserve University
MetroHealth Medical Center
Cleveland, Ohio

Thomas Hughes, MD
Assistant Professor
Department of Orthopaedic Surgery
Drexel University College of Medicine
Philadelphia, Pennsylvania
Allegheny General Hospital
Pittsburgh, Pennsylvania

Thomas R. Hunt III, MD
Professor of Surgery
John D. Sherrill Endowed Chair of
  Orthopaedic Surgery
Director, UAB Hand and Upper Extremity
Fellowship Director, Division of
  Orthopaedic Surgery
Surgeon-in-Chief, UAB Highlands Hospital
University of Alabama School of Medicine
Birmingham, Alabama

Asif M. Ilyas, MD
Director, Temple Hand Center
Assistant Professor
Department of Orthopaedic Surgery
Temple University Hospital
Philadelphia, Pennsylvania

Joseph E. Imbriglia, MD
Clinical Professor
Department of Orthopaedic Surgery
University of Pittsburgh Medical Center
Pittsburgh, Pennsylvania

Robert E. Ivy, MD
Knoxville, Tennessee

Peter J. L. Jebson, MD
Associate Professor
Chief, Division of Elbow and Hand Surgery
Department of Orthopaedic Surgery
University of Michigan Health System
Ann Arbor, Michigan

Nelson L. Jenkins, MD
Hand Surgery Fellow
Department of Orthopedics
University of Massachusetts
Worcester, Massachusetts

Jeff W. Johnson, MD
Adjunct Assistant Clinical Professor
Department of Orthopaedic Surgery
University of Arkansas for Medical Sciences
Ozark Orthopaedic Associates
Fayetteville, Arkansas

Marci D. Jones, MD
Associate Professor
Department of Orthopedic Surgery and
  Rehabilitation
Department of Cell Biology
University of Massachusetts
Worcester, Massachusetts

Neil F. Jones, MD
Professor of Orthopaedic Surgery
Chief of Hand Surgery
University of California
Irvine Medical Center
Orange, California

Jesse B. Jupiter, MD
Hanstorg Wyss/AO Professor of
  Orthopaedic Surgery
Harvard Medical School
Chief, Hand and Upper Limb Service
Massachusetts General Hospital
Boston, Massachusetts

Emese Kalnoki-Kis, MD
Resident, Plastic Surgery
Phoenix Integrated Surgical Residency
Phoenix, Arizona

Morton Kasdan, BA, MD
Clinical Professor
Division of Plastic Surgery
University of Louisville
Louisville, Kentucky

Mohamed Khalid, MD
Fellow, UAB Hand and Upper Extemity
  Fellowship
Department of Orthopaedic Surgery
University of Alabama, Birmingham
Birmingham, Alabama

Prakash Khanchandani, MD
Hand Fellow
Miami Hand Center
Miami, Florida

Thomas R. Kiefhaber, MD
Hand Surgery Specialists
Cincinnati, Ohio

Richard Y. Kim, MD
Director of Hand Surgery
Departments of Plastic & Reconstructive
  Surgery and Orthopaedic Surgery
Hackensack University Medical Center
Hackensack, New Jersey

Hervey L. Kimball III, MD
Clinical Instructor of Orthopaedics
Tufts University School of Medicine
New England Baptist Hospital
Boston, Massachusetts

Joel C. Klena, MD
Director of Hand Division
Department of Orthopaedic Surgery
Geisinger Medical Center
Danville, Pennsylvania

Scott H. Kozin, MD
Professor of Orthopaedic Surgery
Temple University School of Medicine
Hand Surgeon
Shriners Hospital for Children
Philadelphia, Pennsylvania

Mark A. Krahe, DO
Professor of Orthopaedic Surgery
Hamot Hospital
Erie, Pennsylvania

Leo T. Kroonen, MD
Staff Surgeon
Division of Hand and Microvascular
  Surgery
Department of Orthopaedic Surgery
Naval Medical Center, San Diego
San Diego, California

Amy L. Ladd, MD
Professor of Orthopaedic Surgery
Chief, Chase Hand & Upper Limb Center
Stanford University School of Medicine
Chief of the Children's Hand Clinic
Lucile Packard Children's Hospital
Palo Alto, California

Jeffrey Lawton, MD
Hand and Upper Extremity Surgeon
Department of Orthopaedic Surgery
Cleveland Clinic Foundation
Cleveland, Ohio

Charles K. Lee, MD
Assistant Clinical Professor of Surgery
Department of Plastic and Reconstructive
   Surgery
University of California, San Francisco
San Francisco, California

Daniel J. Lee, MD
Department of Orthopaedic Surgery
Pomona Valley Hospital Medical Center
Southern California Orthopaedic Center
Pomona, California

Albert Leung, MD
Brigham and Women's Hospital
Boston, Massachusetts

Fraser J. Leversedge, MD
Assistant Professor
Division of Orthopaedic Surgery
Duke University
Durham, North Carolina

L. Scott Levin, MD, FACS
Chair of Orthopaedic Surgery
University of Pennsylvania School of
   Medicine
Philadelphia, Pennsylvania

R. Gordon Lewis, Jr., MD
Private Practice
Department of Plastic Surgery
CJW Hospital
Richmond, Virginia

Soma I. Lilly, MD
Orthopaedic and Neurosurgical Center of
   the Cascades
Bend, Oregon

Tommy Lindau, MD, PhD
Assistant Professor in Hand Surgery
The Pulvertaft Hand Unit
Royal Derby Hospital
Derby, United Kingdom

Andrew J. Logan, MB, BCh
Department of Orthopaedics
University Hospital of Wales
Cardiff, Wales

James N. Long, MD
Assistant Professor
Department of Plastic and Reconstructive
   Surgery
University of Alabama at Birmingham
Birmingham, Alabama

John D. Lubahn, MD
Hand Microsurgery and
   Reconstructive Orthopaedics
Erie, Pennsylvania

Shai Luria, MD
Assistant Professor
Department of Orthopaedic Surgery
Hadassah-Hebrew University Medical
   Center
Hand and Microvascular Surgeon
Department of Orthopaedic Surgery
Hadassah Medical Organization
Jerusalem, Israel

David H. MacDonald, DO
Hand and Upper Extremity Specialist
Department of Orthopaedic Surgery
Naval Hospital Jacksonville
Jacksonville, Florida

Anna-Lena Makowski,
   Histotechnologist, HTL
Miami International Hand Surgical
   Services
North Miami Beach, Florida

Kevin J. Malone, MD
Assistant Professor
Department of Orthopaedic Surgery
MetroHealth Medical Center
CWRU School of Medicine
Cleveland, Ohio

Alexander M. Marcus, MD
Orthopedic Associates of Central Jersey, PA
Edison, New Jersey

Andrew D. Markiewitz, MD, MBA
Assistant Professor
Department of Surgery
Uniformed Services University of the
   Health Sciences
Clinical Assistant Professor
University of Cincinnati
Cincinnati, Ohio

Paul A. Martineau, MD, FRCSC
Assistant Professor
Section of Sport Medicine
Section of Upper Extremity Surgery
Department of Orthopaedic Surgery
McGill University Health Center
Montreal, Quebec, Canada

Kristofer S. Matullo, MD
Department of Orthopaedic Surgery
St. Luke's Hospital
Bethlehem, Pennsylvania

Kenneth R. Means, Jr., MD
Attending Surgeon
Curtis National Hand Center
Union Memorial Hospital
Baltimore, Maryland

Robert J. Medoff, MD
Windward Orthopedic Group
Kailua, Hawaii

Greg Merrell, MD
Indiana Hand to Shoulder Center
Indianapolis, Indiana

Alex M. Meyers, MD
Reconstructive Hand Surgeons of Indiana
Carmel, Indiana

Alexander D. Mih, MD
Associate Professor of Orthopaedic Surgery
Indiana University School of Medicine
Indianapolis, Indiana

Bruce A. Monaghan, MD
Advanced Orthopedic Centers
Woodbury, New Jersey

Chaitanya S. Mudgal, MD, MS(Orth.),
   MCh(Orth.)
Instructor, Orthopaedic Surgery
Department of Orthopaedics
Harvard Medical School
Massachusetts General Hospital
Boston, Massachusetts

Peter M. Murray, MD
Professor of Orthopaedic Surgery
Mayo Clinic
Jacksonville, Florida

Daniel J. Nagle, MD
Professor of Clinical Orthopedics
Northwestern University Feinberg School
   of Medicine
Northwestern Memorial Hospital
Chicago, Illinois

Mitchell E. Nahra, MD
Lake Orthopaedic Associates, Inc.
Mentor, Ohio

Sanjiv Naidu, MD, PhD
Pinnacle Hand Center
Mechanicsburg, Pennsylvania

Brian Najarian, MD
Associate Clinical Professor
Department of Orthopaedic Surgery
St. John Providence Hospital & Medical
   Center
Southfield, Michigan

A. Lee Osterman, MD
Professor
Hand and Orthopedic Surgeon
Thomas Jefferson University
The Philadelphia Hand Center
King of Prussia, Pennsylvania

E. Anne Ouellette, MD, MBA
Miami International Hand Surgical
   Services
North Miami Beach, Florida

Patrick Owens, MD
Assistant Professor of Clinical
   Orthopaedics
Hand and Upper Extremity Surgery
University of Miami Leonard M. School of
   Medicine
Miami, Florida

Andrew K. Palmer, MD
Department of Orthopaedic Surgery
College of Medicine
State University of New York
Syracuse, New York

Alexander H. Payatakes, MD
Assistant Professor of Orthopaedics
Penn State College of Medicine
Penn State Milton S. Hershey Medical
   Center
Hershey, Pennsylvania

Craig S. Phillips, MD
Illinois Bone & Joint Institute
Glenview, Illinois

Vimala Ramachandran, MD
Northern Arizona Orthopaedics
Flagstaff, Arizona

Ghazi Rayan, MD
Clinical Professor of Orthopedic Surgery
Adjunct Professor
Department of Anatomy/Cell Biology
Oklahoma University
Director, Oklahoma Hand Fellowship
   Program
Chair, Division of Hand Surgery
INTEGRIS Baptist Medical Center
Oklahoma City, Oklahoma

Marc Richard, MD
Assistant Professor
Department of Orthopaedic Surgery
Duke University Medical Center
Durham, North Carolina

Ross J. Richer, MD
Orthopaedic Specialty Group, PC
Fairfield, Connecticut

David Ring, MD, PhD
Associate Professor of Orthopaedic Surgery
Harvard Medical School
Orthopaedic Hand and Upper Extremity
    Unit
Massachusetts General Hospital
Boston, Massachusetts

Kyle P. Ritter, MD
Hendricks Orthopaedics and Sports
    Medicine
Danville, Indiana

Joseph E. Robison, MD
Fayetteville Orthopaedics and Sports
    Medicine
Fayetteville, North Carolina

Matthew J. Robon, MD
Proliance Orthopaedics & Sports Medicine
Bellevue, Washington

Melvin P. Rosenwasser, MD
Robert E. Carroll Professor of Orthopedic
    Surgery
Chief
Orthopedic Hand and Trauma Surgery
Department of Orthopedic Surgery
Columbia University College of Physicians
    and Surgeons
New York, New York

Justin M. Sacks, MD
Assistant Professor
Department of Plastic Surgery
The University of Texas/MD Anderson
    Cancer Center
Houston, Texas

Rodrigo Santamarina, MD
Plastic Surgeon
Fellowship-trained Hand Surgeon
Assistant Professor of Surgery
University of Massachusetts
Berkshire Medical Center
Pittsfield, Massachusetts

Keith A. Segalman, MD
Assistant Professor of Orthopaedic Surgery
Johns Hopkins School of Medicine
Baltimore, Maryland
Greater Chesapeake Hand Specialists
Lutherville, Maryland

David B. Shapiro, MD
Section of Hand and Upper Extremity
    Surgery
Department of Orthopaedic Surgery
The Cleveland Clinic
Cleveland, Ohio

Joseph M. Sherrill, MD
Chairman of Surgery
Healthsouth Medical Center
Alabama Orthopaedic Institute
Birmingham, Alabama

Alexander Y. Shin, MD
Professor of Orthopedic Surgery
Mayo Clinic
Rochester, Minnesota

Joseph F. Slade III, MD
Professor of Orthopaedics and Plastic
    Surgery
Department of Orthopaedics and
    Rehabilitation
Yale University School of Medicine
Guilford, Connecticut

Robert R. Slater, Jr., MD
Associate Clinical Professor
Department of Orthopaedic Surgery
University of California, Davis
Folsom, California

David J. Slutsky, MD, FRCS(C)
Assistant Clinical Professor
David Geffen UCLA School of Medicine
Chief of Reconstructive Hand Surgery
Department of Orthopaedics
Harbor-UCLA Medical Center
The Hand and Wrist Institute
Torrance, California

Hugh M. Smith, MD
Assistant Professor of Anesthesiology
Mayo Clinic
Rochester, Minnesota

Dean G. Sotereanos, MD
Professor of Orthopaedic Surgery
Drexel University College of Medicine
Allegheny General Hospital
Pittsburgh, Pennsylvania

Edwin E. Spencer, Jr., MD
Attending Surgeon
Shoulder and Elbow Center
Knoxville Orthopaedic Clinic
Knoxville, Tennessee

Rena L. Stewart, MD
Assistant Professor
Department of Surgery/Orthopaedics
University Hospital (University of Alabama)
Birmingham, Alabama

Robert J. Strauch, MD
Professor of Clinical Orthopaedic Surgery
Columbia University Medical Center
New York, New York

James W. Strickland, MD
Clinical Professor of Orthopaedic Surgery
Indiana University School of Medicine
Reconstructive Hand Surgeons of Indiana
Carmel, Indiana

Eric Stuffmann, MD
Chief Resident of Orthopaedic Surgery
Stanford University Medical Center
Redwood City, California

Robert M. Szabo, MD, MPH
Professor of Orthopaedic Surgery and
    Plastic Surgery
Chief, Hand, Upper Extremity, &
    Microvascular Surgery
Department of Orthopaedic Surgery
University of California, Davis School of
    Medicine
Sacramento, California

Jane S. Tan, MD
Department of Orthopaedic Surgery
Kaiser Permanente
Denver, Colorado

John S. Taras, MD
Associate Professor
Department of Orthopaedic Surgery
Thomas Jefferson University
Chief, Division of Hand and Surgery
Associate Professor
Department of Orthopaedic Surgery
Drexel University
Philadelphia, Pennsylvania

Andrew L. Terrono, MD
Clinical Professor of Orthopaedics
Tufts University School of Medicine
New England Baptist Hospital
Boston, Massachusetts

Joseph J. Thoder, MD
Professor
Department of Orthopaedic Surgery
Temple University Hospital
Philadelphia, Pennsylvania

Christopher J. Thomson, MD
Birmingham, Alabama

E. Bruce Toby, MD
Department of Orthopaedic Surgery
The University of Kansas Hospital
Kansas City, Kansas

Matthew M. Tomaino, MD
Tomaino Orthopaedic Care for Shoulder,
    Hand, & Elbow
Rochester General Health System
Rochester, New York

Thomas Trumble, BA, MD
Professor and Chief, Hand and Upper
    Extremity Surgery
Department of Orthopaedics/Sports
    Medicine
University of Washington School of
    Medicine
Seattle, Washington

Richard L. Uhl, MD
Professor of Surgery
Division of Orthopaedic Surgery
Albany Medical College
Albany, New York

Thomas F. Varecka, MD
Assistant Professor of Orthopaedic Surgery
University of Minnesota
Director, Hand and Microsurgery
Hennepin County Medical Center
Minneapolis, Minnesota

Luis O. Vasconez, MD
Professor of Surgery
Division of Plastic Surgery
University of Alabama at Birmingham
Birmingham, Alabama

John J. Walsh IV, MD
Associate Professor
Department of Orthopaedics
University of South Carolina School of
    Medicine
Columbia, South Carolina

Christina M. Ward, MD
Department of Orthopaedic Surgery
University of Minnesota
Minneapolis, Minnesota

Lance G. Warhold, MD
Division Director, Upper Extremity
Department of Orthopaedic Surgery
Dartmouth-Hitchcock Medical Center
Lebanon, New Hampshire

Arnold-Peter Weiss, MD
R. Scot Sellers Scholar of Hand Surgery
Professor of Orthopaedics
Associate Dean of Medicine
Brown University Medical School
Providence, Rhode Island

Mark Wilczynski, MD
Department of Orthopaedic Surgery
Washington University School of Medicine
St. Louis, Missouri

D. Patrick Williams, DO
Hand Microsurgery & Reconstructive
    Orthopaedics
Erie, Pennsylvania

Rafael M. M. Williams, MD
Wilson, Wyoming

Andrew Wong, MD
Private Practice
Arrowhead Orthopaedics
Redlands, California
Assistant Professor—Clinical
Department of Orthopaedic Surgery
Loma Linda University
Loma Linda, California

Jeffrey Yao, MD
Assistant Professor
Department of Orthopaedic Surgery
Stanford University Medical Center
Redwood City, California

Elvin G. Zook, MD
Professor Emeritus
Division of Plastic Surgery
Department of Surgery
Southern Illinois University School of
    Medicine
Springfield, Illinois

PART 7 SHOULDER AND ELBOW

Joseph A. Abboud, MD
Clinical Assistant Professor of Orthopaedic
    Surgery
University of Pennsylvania Health System
Philadelphia, Pennsylvania

Aymeric André, MD
Resident
Department of Plastic Surgery
University Hospital Rangueil
Paul-Sabatier University
Toulouse, France

Carl Basamania, MD, FACS
The Polyclinic First Hill
Seattle, Washington

Robert H. Bell, MD
Associate Professor of Orthopaedics
Crystal Clinic
Orthopaedic Surgeons, Inc.
Akron, Ohio

Ryan T. Bicknell, MD, MSc, FRCS(C)
Assistant Professor of Orthopaedic Surgery
Queen's University
Kingston General Hospital
Kingston, Ontario, Canada

Louis U. Bigliani, MD
Frank E. Stinchfield Professor and
    Chairman of Orthopedic Surgery
Columbia University
Director of the Orthopedic Surgery Service
New York-Presbyterian Hospital/Columbia
    University Medical Center
New York, New York

Theodore A. Blaine, MD
Associate Professor of Orthopaedic Surgery
Brown Alpert Medical School
Attending Orthopaedic Surgeon
Rhode Island Hospital
Providence, Rhode Island

Kamal I. Bohsali, MD
Attending Orthopaedic Surgeon, Shoulder
    and Elbow Reconstruction
Department of Orthopaedics
Memorial Hospital
St. Luke's Hospital
St. Vincent's Hospital
Jacksonville, Florida

Nicolas Bonnevialle, MD
Clinical Assistant in Orthopedic Surgery
Department of Orthopedics and
    Traumatology
University Hospital Purpan
Paul-Sabatier University
Toulouse, France

Christopher T. Born, MD
Professor of Orthopaedic Surgery
The Warren Alpert Medical School of
    Brown University
Rhode Island Hospital
Providence, Rhode Island

Joanna G. Branstetter, MD
Orthopaedic Surgeon
Madigan Army Medical Center
San Antonio, Texas

Juan Castellanos-Rosas, MD
Orthopaedic Surgeon
Department of Trauma Surgery
Hospital General Regional
Col Girasoles, Coyoacán, Mexico

Michael J. Codsi, MD
Department of Orthopaedic Surgery
The Everett Clinic
Everett, Washington

Mark S. Cohen, MD
Professor and Director
Section of Hand and Elbow Surgery
Rush University Medical Center
Chicago, Illinois

J. Dean Cole, MD
Medical Director
Florida Hospital Orthopaedic Institute
    Fracture Care Center
Orlando, Florida

Patrick M. Connor, MD
Clinical Faculty
Shoulder and Elbow Surgery, Sports
    Medicine, and Trauma
Department of Orthopaedic Surgery
Carolinas Medical Center
Charlotte, North Carolina

Allen Deutsch, MD
Clinical Assistant Professor
Department of Orthopaedic Surgery
Baylor College of Medicine
Kelsey-Seybold Clinic
Houston, Texas

Mark T. Dillon, MD
Fellow, Shoulder and Elbow Surgery
Department of Orthopaedic Surgery
University of Pennsylvania Presbyterian
    Medical Center
Philadelphia, Pennsylvania

Bassem Elhassan, MD
Assistant Professor of Orthopedics
Mayo Clinic
Rochester, Minnesota

Evan L. Flatow, MD
Professor of Orthopaedic Surgery
Mount Sinai Medical Center
New York, New York

Leesa M. Galatz, MD
Associate Professor
Department of Orthopaedic Surgery
Washington University School of Medicine
St. Louis, Missouri

Matthew J. Garberina, MD
Department of Orthopaedic Surgery
Summit Medical Group
Berkeley Heights, New Jersey

Charles L. Getz, MD
Assistant Professor of Orthopaedic Surgery
Thomas Jefferson University Hospital
Rothman Institute
Philadelphia, Pennsylvania

Filippos S. Giannoulis, MD
Department of Upper Extremity and
    Microsurgery
KAT Hospital
Athens, Greece

David L. Glaser, MD
Assistant Professor of Orthopaedic Surgery
University of Pennsylvania
Chief, Shoulder and Elbow Service
Penn Presbyterian Medical Center
Philadelphia, Pennsylvania

Andreas H. Gomoll, MD
Assistant Professor of Orthopaedic Surgery
Brigham and Women's Hospital
Harvard Medical School
Boston, Massachusetts

Thomas P. Goss, MD
Professor of Orthopaedic Surgery
Department of Orthopaedics and Physical
    Rehabilitation
University of Massachusetts Medical
    School
Worcester, Massachusetts

Andrew Green, MD
Associate Professor of Orthopaedic Surgery
Brown Alpert Medical School
Chief, Shoulder and Elbow Surgery
Rhode Island Hospital
Providence, Rhode Island

George Frederick Hatch III, MD
USC Orthopaedic Surgery Associates
Los Angeles, California

Laurence D. Higgins, MD
Associate Professor
Chief, Sports Medicine and Shoulder
 Service
Department of Orthopedic Surgery
Brigham & Women's Hospital
Boston, Massachusetts

Joseph P. Iannotti, MD, PhD
Maynard Madden Professor of
 Orthopaedic Surgery
Chairman, Orthopaedic and
 Rheumatologic Institute
The Cleveland Clinic
Cleveland, Ohio

Asif M. Ilyas, MD
Director, Temple Hand Center
Assistant Professor, Orthopaedic Surgery
Temple University Hospital
Philadelphia, Pennsylvania

John M. Itamura, MD
Associate Professor
Department of Orthopaedic Surgery
University of Southern California
Keck School of Medicine
Los Angeles, California

Jesse B. Jupiter, MD
Hanstorg Wyss/AO Professor of
 Orthopaedic Surgery
Harvard Medical School
Chief, Hand and Upper Limb Service
Massachusetts General Hospital
Boston, Massachusetts

Steven P. Kalandiak, MD
Assistant Professor of Clinical
 Orthopaedics
University of Miami
Miami, Florida

**Srinath Kamineni, MBBCh, BSc(Hons),
 FRCS-Orth**
Associate Professor of Elbow and Shoulder
 Surgery
Professor of Bioengineering
Department of Sports, Orthopaedics, and
 Trauma
Kentucky Clinic
University of Kentucky
Lexington, Kentucky

Leonid I. Katolik, MD
Philadelphia Hand Center
Philadelphia, Pennsylvania

Graham J. W. King, MD, MSc, FRCSC
Professor of Surgery
Division of Orthopaedic Surgery
University of Western Ontario
Hand and Upper Limb Centre
St. Joseph's Health Centre
London, Ontario, Canada

Raymond A. Klug, MD
Active Staff
Department of Orthopaedic Surgery
Los Alamitos Medical Center
Los Alamitos, Califonia

Thomas J. Kovack, DO
Department of Orthopaedic Surgery
Doctors Hospital
Hillard, Ohio

Sumant G. Krishnan, MD
Fellowship Director
Department of Shoulder Service
The Carrell Clinic
Dallas, Texas

John E. Kuhn, MD
Associate Professor
Chief of Shoulder Surgery
Department of Orthopaedics and
 Rehabilitation
Vanderbilt University Medical Center
Nashville, Tennessee

Phillip Langer, MD, MS
Assistant Team Physician and Orthopedic
 Surgeon
NFL Atlanta Falcons
NHL Atlanta Thrashers
Atlanta Sports Medicine & Orthopedic
 Center
Atlanta, Georgia

Jonathan H. Lee, MD
Fellow in Adult Reconstruction
Department of Orthopaedic Surgery
Hospital for Special Surgery
New York, New York

William N. Levine, MD
Vice Chairman and Professor
Residency Director and Director of Sports
 Medicine
Department of Orthopaedic Surgery
Columbia University Medical Center
New York, New York

Steven B. Lippitt, MD
Professor of Orthopaedic Surgery
Northeastern Ohio Universities College of
 Medicine
Akron General Medical Center
Akron, Ohio

Bryan J. Loeffler, MD
Department of Orthopaedic Surgery
Carolinas Medical Center
Charlotte, North Carolina

John Lunn, FRCSI
Department of Orthopaedics
Hermitage Medical Clinic
Dublin, Ireland

Pierre Mansat, MD, PhD
Professor of Orthopedic Surgery
Department of Orthopedics and
 Traumatology
University Hospital Purpan
Paul-Sabatier University
Toulouse, France

Frederick A. Matsen III, MD
Professor and Chair
Department of Orthopaedics and Sports
 Medicine
University of Washington
Seattle, Washington

Jesse A. McCarron, MD
Associate Professor
Department of Orthopaedic Surgery
The Cleveland Clinic
Cleveland, Ohio

Michael D. McKee, MD, FRCS(c)
Professor
Division of Orthopaedics
Department of Surgery
University of Toronto
Toronto, Ontario, Canada

Mark A. Mighell, MD
Associate Director of Shoulder and Elbow
 Fellowship
Florida Orthopaedic Institute
Associate Professor
Department of Upper Extremity Surgery
University of South Florida
Tampa, Florida

Steven Milos, MD
Department of Orthopaedics
Swedish American Hospital
Rockford, Illinois

Anthony Miniaci, MD, FRCSC
Professor of Surgery
Cleveland Clinic Lerner College of
 Medicine
Director, Case Western Reserve University
 Center
Head, Sports Medicine
Cleveland Clinic Sports Health Center
Orthopaedic and Rheumatologic Institute
Garfield Heights, Ohio

Anand M. Murthi, MD
Assistant Professor of Orthopaedics
Chief of Shoulder and Elbow Service
Department of Orthopaedics
University of Maryland School of Medicine
Baltimore, Maryland

Andrew S. Neviaser, MD
Resident
Department of Orthopaedic Surgery
Hospital for Special Surgery
New York, New York

Robert J. Neviaser, MD
Professor and Chairman
Department of Orthopaedic Surgery
George Washington University
Washington, District of Columbia

Daniel D. Noble, BA
Research Assistant
Crystal Clinic
Orthopaedic Surgeons, Inc.
Akron, Ohio

Jeffrey S. Noble, MD
Associate Professor of Orthopaedics
Crystal Clinic
Orthopaedic Surgeons, Inc.
Akron, Ohio

Brett D. Owens, MD
Assistant Professor
Department of Orthopaedic Surgery
    Service
Keller Army Hospital
West Point, New York

Bradford O. Parsons, MD
Assistant Professor of Orthopaedic Surgery
Mount Sinai Medical Center
New York, New York

Jubin B. Payandeh, MD, FRCS(c)
Staff Surgeon
Department of Surgery
Big Thunder Orthopaedics
Thunder Bay, Ontario, Canada

Alexander H. Payatakes, MD
Assistant Professor
Hand and Wrist Service
Department of Orthopaedics
Penn State College of Medicine
Penn State Milton S. Hershey Medical
    Center
Hershey, Pennsylvania

Matthew D. Pepe, MD
Sports Medicine Surgeon
The Rothman Institute
Voorhees, New Jersey

Matthew L. Ramsey, MD
Associate Professor of Orthopaedic Surgery
Rothman Institute Shoulder and Elbow
    Surgery
Thomas Jefferson University
Philadelphia, Pennsylvania

Michael A. Rauh, MD
Clinical Assistant Professor of Orthopaedic
    Surgery
State University of New York at Buffalo
Buffalo, New York

David Ring, MD, PhD
Associate Professor of Orthopaedic Surgery
Harvard Medical School
Department of Orthopaedic Surgery
Massachusetts General Hospital
Boston, Massachusetts

Robin R. Richards, MD, FRCSC
Professor
Department of Surgery
University of Toronto
Sunnybrook Health Sciences Center
Toronto, Ontario, Canada

Charles A. Rockwood, MD
Professor and Chairman Emeritus of
    Orthopaedics
The University of Texas Health Science
    Center at San Antonio
San Antonio, Texas

Anthony A. Romeo, MD
Associate Professor of Orthopaedic Surgery
Director, Section of Shoulder & Elbow
Rush University Medical Center
Chicago, Illinois

Yishai Rosenblatt, MD
Orthopaedic Surgeon
Hand and Upper Limb Surgeon
The Unit of Hand Surgery and
    Orthopaedic Surgery
Tel-Aviv Sourasky Medical Center
The Sackler Faculty of Medicine
Tel-Aviv University
Tel-Aviv, Israel

Joaquin Sanchez-Sotelo, MD, PhD
Associate Professor
Department of Orthopedic Surgery
Mayo Clinic
Rochester, Minnesota

Shadley C. Schiffern, MD
Attending Orthopaedic Surgeon
NorthEast Orthopedics, PA
Concord, North Carolina

Ryan W. Simovitch, MD
Shoulder and Elbow Service
Palm Beach Orthopaedic Institute
Palm Beach Gardens, Florida

Anshu Singh, MD
Shoulder and Elbow Surgeon
Kaiser Permanente
San Diego, California

Dean G. Sotereanos, MD
Professor of Orthopaedic Surgery
Drexel University College of Medicine
Allegheny General Hospital
Pittsburgh, Pennsylvania

Edwin E. Spencer, Jr., MD
Knoxville Orthopaedic Clinic
Knoxville, Tennessee

Jason A. Stein, MD
Assistant Professor
Department of Orthopaedics
University of Maryland
Baltimore, Maryland

Scott P. Steinmann, MD
Professor of Orthopaedics
Mayo Clinic
Rochester, Minnesota

Bradford S. Tucker, MD
Clinical Instructor
Department of Orthopaedic Surgery
Thomas Jefferson University Hospital
Egg Harbor Township, New Jersey

Gilles Walch, MD
Department of Shoulder Surgery
Centre Orthopédique Santy
Hopital Privé J Mermoz
Lyon, France

Jon J. P. Warner, MD
Chief, The Harvard Shoulder Service
Professor of Orthopaedics
Massachusetts General Hospital
Boston, Massachusetts

Brent B. Wiesel, MD
Chief, Shoulder Service
Department of Orthopaedic Surgery
Georgetown University Hospital
Washington, District of Columbia

Gerald R. Williams, MD
Professor of Orthopaedic Surgery
Chief, Shoulder and Elbow Service
The Rothman Institute
Jefferson Medical College
Philadelphia, Pennsylvania

Michael A. Wirth, MD
Professor of Orthopaedics
The Charles A. Rockwood, Jr., MD Chair
University of Texas Health Science Center
San Antonio, Texas

PART 8 FOOT AND ANKLE

Jorge I. Acevedo, MD
Associate Clinical Faculty
Department of Orthopedic Surgery
University of Miami
Wellington Regional Medical Center
Royal Palm Beach, Florida

Samuel B. Adams, Jr., MD
Resident
Department of Orthopaedic Surgery
Duke University Medical Center
Durham, North Carolina

Robert S. Adelaar, MD
Medical College of Virginia
Richmond, Virginia

Oladapo Alade, MD
Private Practice
Houston, Texas

Richard Alvarez, MD
Southern Orthopedic Foot Center
Chattanooga, Tennessee

Annunziato Amendola, MD
Professor and Callaghan Chair
Department of Orthopaedic Surgery
University of Iowa
Iowa City, Iowa

John G. Anderson, MD
Associate Professor
Michigan State University College of
    Human Medicine
Co-Director
Grand Rapids Orthopaedic Foot and Ankle
    Fellowship
Assistant Program Director
Grand Rapids Orthopaedic Residency
    Program
Orthopaedic Associates of Michigan
Grand Rapids, Michigan

Robert B. Anderson, MD
Chief, Foot and Ankle Service
Department of Orthopaedic Surgery
Carolinas Medical Center, OrthoCarolina
Charlotte, North Carolina

Michael S. Aronow, MD
Associate Professor
Department of Orthopaedic Surgery
University of Connecticut Health Center
Farmington, Connecticut

Mathieu Assal, MD
Orthopaedic Surgery Service
Geneva University Hospital
Geneva, Switzerland

Vikrant Azad, MD
Research Fellow
Department of Orthopaedics
University of Medicine and Dentistry of
   New Jersey
NJ Medical School
Newark, New Jersey

Alexej Barg, MD
Orthopaedic Clinic
Kantonsspital
Lirstal, Switzerland

Michael Barnett, MD
Assistant Professor of Orthopaedic Surgery
Director of Undergraduate Orthopaedic
   Education
Wright State University Boonshoft School
   of Medicine
Dayton, Ohio

Heather Barske, MD
Department of Orthopaedic Surgery
University of Manitoba
Winnipeg, Manitoba, Canada

Douglas N. Beaman, MD
Clinical Assistant Professor
Department of Orthopaedic Surgery
Oregon Health Sciences University
Summit Orthopaedics
Portland, Oregon

Christoph Becher, MD
Department of Orthopaedic Surgery
Hannover Medical School
Hannover, Germany

Karl Bergmann, MD
Department of Orthopaedics
University of Medicine and Dentistry of
   New Jersey
NJ Medical School
Newark, New Jersey

Gregory C. Berlet, MD, FRCS(C)
Chief, Foot and Ankle
Department of Orthopedics
Orthopedic Foot and Ankle Center
Ohio State University
Westerville, Ohio

James L. Beskin, MD
Clinical Assistant Professor
Department of Orthopedics
Tulane University
Director, Foot & Ankle Section
Orthopedic Residency Program
Atlanta Medical Center
Atlanta, Georgia

Eric M. Bluman, MD, PhD
Assistant Professor
Department of Orthopaedic Surgery
Harvard University
Brigham and Women's Hospital
Boston, Massachusetts

Donald R. Bohay, MD
Associate Professor
Department of Orthopaedic Surgery
Michigan State University
Orthopaedic Associates of Michigan
Grand Rapids, Michigan

Michel Bonnin, MD
Department of Orthopaedic Surgery
Centre Orthopédique Santy
Lyon, France

Michael E. Brage, MD
Assistant Professor of Clinical Orthopedics
Director, Foot and Ankle Services
Department of Orthopaedic Surgery
University of California, San Diego
South County Orthopaedic Specialists
Laguna Woods, California

Lloyd C. Briggs, Jr., MD
Associate Clinical Professor
Department of Orthopaedic Surgery
Orthopaedic Institute of Ohio
Lima, Ohio

Matteo Cadossi, MD
PhD Student
Department of Human Anatomy and
   Pathophysiology of Musculoskeletal
   System
2nd Orthopaedic Department
Istituto Orthopedico Rizzoli
University of Bologna
Bologna, Italy

John T. Campbell, MD
Institute for Foot and Ankle
   Reconstruction at Mercy
Mercy Medical Center
Baltimore, Maryland

Fabio Catani, MD
Professor of Orthopaedics
Department of Orthopaedic Surgery
Istituto Orthopedico Rizzoli
University of Bologna
Bologna, Italy

Wen Chao, MD
Department of Orthopaedic Surgery
PennCare—Pennsylvania Orthopaedic Foot
   and Ankle Surgeons
Philadelphia, Pennsylvania

Timothy Charlton, MD
Assistant Professor of Clinical
   Orthopaedics
Keck School of Medicine
University of Southern California
USC Orthopaedic Surgery Associates
Los Angeles, California

Christopher P. Chiodo, MD
Brigham Foot and Ankle Center at Faulkner
   Hospital
Boston, Massachusetts

Thomas O. Clanton, MD
Professor of Orthopaedic Surgery
The University of Texas Medical School at
   Houston
Director, Foot and Ankle Sports Medicine
The Steadman Clinic
Vail, Colorado

Michael P. Clare, MD
Director of Fellowship Education, Foot &
   Ankle Fellowship
Florida Orthopaedic Institute
Tampa, Florida

J. Chris Coetzee, MD, FRSCS
Minnesota Orthopedic Sports Medicine
   Institute
Eden Prairie, Minnesota

Bruce Cohen, MD
Department of Orthopedic Surgery
Carolina Medical Center
Charlotte, North Carolina

Jean-Alain Colombier, MD
Department of Orthopaedic Surgery
Clinique de L'Union
Saint Jean, France

Michael J. Coughlin, MD
Chief of Orthopaedics
St. Alphonsus Regional Medical Center
Clinical Professor of Surgery
Department of Orthopaedics
Oregon Health Sciences University
Boise, Idaho

Justin S. Cummins, MD, MS
Department of Orthopedic Surgery
SMDC Health System
Duluth, Minnesota

Richard J. deAsla, MD
Co-Director, Foot and Ankle Unit
Instructor
Department of Orthopaedic Surgery
Harvard Medical School
Boston, Massachusetts

Bryan D. Den Hartog, MD
Assistant Clinical Professor
Department of Orthopaedics
Sanford School of Medicine
Rapid City, South Dakota

Jonathan T. Deland, MD
Chief, Foot and Ankle Service
Associate Attending Orthopaedic Surgeon
Hospital for Special Surgery
Associate Professor
Department of Orthopaedic Surgery
Weill Cornell Medical College
New York, New York

James K. DeOrio, MD
Associate Professor
Division of Orthopedic Surgery
Department of Surgery
Duke University
Durham, North Carolina

Matthew J. DeOrio, MD
The Orthopedic Center
Huntsville, Alabama

Benedict F. DiGiovanni, MD
Associate Professor of Orthopaedics
University of Rochester Medical Center
Rochester, New York

Christopher W. DiGiovanni, MD
Director and Professor
Brown University Orthopaedic Residency
    Program
Chief, Foot and Ankle Service
Department of Orthopaedic Surgery
The Warren Alpert School of Medicine
Brown University
Rhode Island Hospital
Providence, Rhode Island

Brian Donley, MD
Director, Center for Foot and Ankle
Department of Orthopaedic Surgery
Cleveland Clinic
Cleveland, Ohio

Thomas Dreher, MD
Orthopaedic Department
University of Heidelberg
Heidelberg, Germany

Brad Dresher, MD
Department of Orthopaedics
Penrose St. Francis Medical Center
Colorado Springs, Colorado

Mark E. Easley, MD
Associate Professor of Orthopaedic Surgery
Co-Director, Foot and Ankle Fellowship
Duke University Medical Center
Durham, North Carolina

Patrick Ebeling, MD
Associate Clinical Instructor
Department of Orthopaedic Surgery
University of Minnesota
Burnsville, Minnesota

Andrew J. Elliott, MD
Assistant Professor
Department of Orthopaedic Surgery
Hospital for Special Surgery
New York, New York

Cesare Faldini, MD
Professor of Orthopaedics
Department of Human Anatomy and
    Pathophysiology of Musculoskeletal
    System
2nd Orthopaedic Department
Istituto Orthopedico Rizzoli
University of Bologna
Bologna, Italy

Nicholas A. Ferran, MBBS, MRCSEd
Specialist Registrar
Department of Trauma and Orthopaedics
Lincoln County Hospital
Lincolnshire, United Kingdom

Lamar L. Fleming, MD
Professor and Chairman
Department of Orthopaedics
Emory University School of Medicine
Atlanta, Georgia

Adolph S. Flemister, Jr., MD
Associate Professor
Department of Orthopaedics
University of Rochester
Rochester, New York

Austin T. Fragomen, MD
Limb Lengthening Specialist
Fellowship Director, Director of
    Education, and Director of Limb
    Lengthening and Deformity Service
Hospital for Special Surgery
New York, New York

Carol Frey, MD
Assistant Clinical Professor of Orthopedic
    Surgery (Volunteer)
University of California, Los Angeles
Manhattan Beach, California

Delan Gaines, MD
Department of Sports Medicine
Southeastern Orthopedic Center
Savannah, Georgia

Richard E. Gellman, MD
Clinical Assistant Professor
Department of Orthopaedic Surgery
Oregon Health Sciences University
Summit Orthopaedics
Portland, Oregon

Sandro Giannini, MD
Professor of Orthopaedics
Department of Human Anatomy and
    Pathophysiology of Musculoskeletal
    System
2nd Orthopaedic Department
Istituto Orthopedico Rizzoli
University of Bologna
Bologna, Italy

Brian D. Giordano, MD
Department of Orthopaedics
University of Rochester
Rochester, New York

Jason P. Glover, DPM
Department of Foot and Ankle Surgery
Rutherford Hospital
Rutherfordton, North Carolina

John S. Gould, MD
Professor of Surgery/Orthopaedics
University of Alabama at Birmingham
Birmingham, Alabama

Gregory P. Guyton, MD
Department of Orthopedic Surgery
Union Memorial Hospital
Baltimore, Maryland

Steven L. Haddad, MD
Associate Professor of Clinical
    Orthopaedic Surgery
University of Chicago Pritzker School of
    Medicine
Section Head, Foot and Ankle Surgery
NorthShore University HealthCare Systems
Illinois Bone and Joint Institute, LLC
Glenview, Illinois

Sigvard T. Hansen, Jr., MD
Professor
Director, Sigvard T. Hansen, Jr., MD Foot
    and Ankle Institute
Department of Orthopaedics and Sports
    Medicine
University of Washington
Seattle, Washington

Paul Hamilton, BMedSci, FRCS(Tr&Orth)
Senior Clinical Fellow
Department of Orthopaedics
Guy's and St. Thomas' NHS Foundation
    Trust
London, England

William G. Hamilton, MD
Clinical Professor
Department of Orthopedic Surgery
Columbia University College of Physicians
    and Surgeons
New York, New York

Thomas G. Harris, MD
Assistant Professor
Department of Orthopaedics
UCLA-Harbor Medical Center
Torrance, California

Paul J. Hecht, MD
Associate Professor
Department of Orthopaedic Surgery
Dartmouth Hitchcock Medical Center
Lebanon, New Hampshire

W. Bryce Henderson, BSc, MD, FRCSC
Chief of Orthopedics
Department of Orthopedic Surgery
Red Deer Hospital, Central Alberta
Alberta, Canada

John E. Herzenberg, MD, FRCSC
Director, International Center for Limb
    Lengthening
Rubin Institute for Advanced Orthopedics
Sinai Hospital of Baltimore
Baltimore, Maryland

Beat Hintermann, MD
Associate Professor of Medicine
Orthopaedic Clinic
University of Basel
Liestal, Switzerland

Stefan G. Hofstaetter, MD
Orthopaedic Senior Resident
Department of Orthopaedics
Klinikum Wels-Grieskirchen
Wels, Austria

George B. Holmes, Jr., MD
Assistant Professor
Director, Section of Foot and Ankle
Rush University Medical Center
Westchester, Illinois

Jason M. Hurst, MD
Associate Partner
Joint Implant Surgeons
New Albany, Ohio

James J. Hutson, Jr., MD
Associate Clinical Professor
Department of Orthopedic Surgery
Miller School of Medicine
University of Miami
Miami, Florida

Christopher F. Hyer, DPM, FACFAS
Co-Director, Foot and Ankle Fellowship
Orthopedic Foot & Ankle Center
Westerville, Ohio

Clifford L. Jeng, MD
Institute for Foot and Ankle
 Reconstruction
Mercy Medical Center
Baltimore, Maryland

Shine John, DPM, AACFAS
Private Practitioner
Foot Specialists
Georgetown, Texas

Catherine E. Johnson, MD
Department of Orthopaedic Surgery
Massachusetts General Hospital
Watertown, Massachusetts

Jeffrey E. Johnson, MD
Associate Professor
Chief, Foot and Ankle Service
Department of Orthopaedic Surgery
Barnes-Jewish Hospital at Washington
 University Medical Center
St. Louis, Missouri

Thierry Judet, MD
Chief
Department of Orthopedics
Hopital Raymond Poincare
Garches, France

Kevin L. Kirk, DO
Chief
Orthopedic Surgery Service
San Antonio Military Medical Center
Houston, Texas

Alex J. Kline, MD
Department of Orthopaedic Surgery
University of Pittsburgh Medical Center
Pittsburgh, Pennsylvania

Markus Knupp, MD
Department of Orthopaedics
Kantonsspital Liestal
Liestal, Switzerland

Sameh A. Labib, MD
Assistant Professor of Orthopedic Surgery
Director of Foot and Ankle Service
Emory University
Atlanta, Georgia

Bradley M. Lamm, DPM, FACFAS
Head, Foot and Ankle Surgery
International Center for Limb Lengthening
Rubin Institute for Advanced Orthopedics
Sinai Hospital of Baltimore
Baltimore, Maryland

Geoffrey S. Landis, DO
Tucson Orthopaedic Institute Oro Valley
Oro Valley, Arizona

Johnny T. C. Lau, MD, MSc, FRCSC
Assistant Professor of Surgery
University Health Network – Toronto
 Western Division
Toronto, Ontario, Canada

Ian L. D. Le, MD
Department of Orthopaedic Surgery
Duke University Medical Center
Durham, North Carolina

Alberto Leardini, DPhil
Movement Analysis Laboratory
Istituto Orthopedico Rizzoli
Bologna, Italy

Simon Lee, MD
Assistant Professor
Department of Orthopaedic Surgery
Rush University Medical Center
Westchester, Illinois

Johnny Lin, MD
Assistant Professor
Department of Orthopaedic Surgery
Rush University Medical Center
Westchester, Illinois

Sheldon Lin, MD
Associate Professor
Department of Orthopaedics
University of Medicine and Dentistry of
 New Jersey
NJ Medical School
Newark, New Jersey

Umile Giuseppe Longo, MD
Consultant
Department of Orthopaedic and Trauma
 Surgery
Campus Biomedico University
Rome, Italy

Deianira Luciani, MD
PhD Student
Department of Human Anatomy and
 Pathophysiology of Musculoskeletal
 System
2nd Orthopaedic Department
Istituto Orthopedico Rizzoli
University of Bologna
Bologna, Italy

**Nicola Maffulli, MD, MS, PhD,
 FRCS(Orth.)**
Professor of Orthopaedic and Trauma
 Surgery
Centre for Sports and Exercise Medicine
Barts and The London School of Medicine
 and Dentistry
London, England

Ansar Mahmood, MD
Department of Trauma and Orthopaedic
 Surgery
Keele University School of Medicine
Stoke on Trent, Staffordshire, United
 Kingdom

Peter Mangone, MD
Department of Orthopaedic Surgery
Mission Hospitals Health System
Asheville, North Carolina
Margaret R. Pardee Hospital
Hendersonville, North Carolina

Jeffrey A. Mann, MD
Private Practice
Oakland, California

Roger A. Mann, MD
Department of Orthopaedic Surgery
Oakland Bone and Joint Specialists
Oakland, California

Arthur Manoli, MD
Department of Orthopedic Surgery
Michigan International Foot & Ankle
 Center
Pontiac, Michigan

Javier Maquirriain, MD, PhD
Director, Orthopaedic Department
Director, Sports Medicine Research
 Department
Centro Nacional de Alto Rendimiento
 Deportivo
Buenos Aires, Argentina

Richard M. Marks, MD, FACS
Assistant Professor
Department of Orthopaedic Surgery
Medical College of Wisconsin
Milwaukee, Wisconsin

William C. McGarvey, MD
Associate Professor
Residency Program Director
Department of Orthopaedic Surgery
University of Texas Medical School at
 Houston
Houston, Texas

Angus M. McBryde, MD
Director
Ankle and Foot Fellowship
American Sports Medicine Institute
St. Vincent's – Birmingham
Birmingham, Alabama

**Ronan McKeown, MB, BCh, BAO, MD,
 FRCSI(T&O)**
Craigavon Area Hospital
Portadown
Co. Armagh, Ireland

Siddhant Mehta
Research Fellow
Department of Orthopaedics
University of Medicine and Dentistry of
 New Jersey
NJ Medical School
Newark, New Jersey

Marc Merian-Genast, MD
Clinical Assistant Professor
Department of Orthopedics
University of Saskatoon
Regina, Saskatchewan, Canada

Stuart D. Miller, MD
Attending
Department of Orthopaedic Surgery
Union Memorial Hospital
Baltimore, Maryland

Andrew P. Molloy, FRCS(Tr & Orth), MR
Department of Trauma and Orthopaedics
University Hospital Aintree
Liverpool, England

Mark S. Myerson, MD
Institute for Foot and Ankle
 Reconstruction at Mercy
Mercy Medical Centre
Baltimore, Maryland

Caio Nery, MD
Professor of Medicine
Department of Orthopaedics and
 Traumatology
Federal University of São Paulo, Brazil
São Paulo, Brazil

Christopher W. Nicholson, MD
Department of Orthopedics
The Doctors Hospital of Tatnall
Savannah, Georgia

Florian Nickisch, MD
Assistant Professor of Orthopaedic Surgery
Department of Orthopaedics
University of Utah
Salt Lake City, Utah

James A. Nunley II, MD
Chairman and Professor
Department of Orthopaedic Surgery
Duke University
Durham, North Carolina

Tahir Öğüt, MD
Associate Professor of Medicine
Department of Orthopaedics and
    Traumatology
Istanbul University Cerrahpasa Medical
    Faculty
Istanbul, Turkey

Blake L. Ohlson, MD
Fellow
Department of Orthopaedics
Union Memorial Hospital
Baltimore, Maryland

Martin J. O'Malley, MD
Associate Professor of Orthopaedics
Hospital for Special Surgery
New York, New York

Enyi Okereke, MD†
Associate Professor of Orthopedic Surgery
University of Pennsylvania School of
    Medicine
Chief, Division of Foot and Ankle Surgery
University of Pennsylvania Health Systems
Philadelphia, Pennsylvania

Justin Orr, MD
Division of Orthopaedic Surgery
Department of Surgery
William Beaumont Army Medical Center
El Paso, Texas

Fred W. Ortmann, MD
Greensboro Orthopaedics
Greensboro, North Carolina

Thomas G. Padanilam, MD
Clinical Assistant Professor
Department of Orthopaedic Surgery
University of Toledo
Toledo, Ohio

Geert I. Pagenstert, MD
Assistant Professor
Department of Orthopaedic Surgery
University Hospital Basel
Basel, Switzerland

Dror Paley, MD, FRCSC
Director, Paley Advanced Limb
    Lengthening Institute
St. Mary's Hospital
West Palm Beach, Florida

Selene G. Parekh, MD, MBA
Associate Professor
Division of Orthopaedics
Department of Surgery
Duke University
Durham, North Carolina

Terrence M. Philbin, DO
Clinical Assistant Professor
Department of Orthopaedic Surgery
The Ohio State University College of
    Medicine and Public Health
Orthopedic Foot and Ankle Center
Weiterville, Ohio

Phinit Phisitkul, MD
Clinical Assistant Professor
Department of Orthopaedics
University of Iowa
Iowa City, Iowa

Michael S. Pinzur, MD
Professor
Department of Orthopaedic Surgery and
    Rehabilitation
Loyola University Medical Center
Maywood, Illinois

Gregory C. Pomeroy, MD
New England Foot and Ankle Specialists
Portland, Maine

George E. Quill, Jr., MD
Clinical Instructor of Orthopaedics
University of Louisville School of Medicine
Director of Foot and Ankle Services
Louisville Orthopaedic Clinic
Louisville, Kentucky

Steven M. Raikin, MD
Associate Professor
Director, Foot and Ankle Service
Department of Orthopaedic Surgery
Rothman Institute at Thomas Jefferson
    University Hospital
Philadelphia, Pennsylvania

Keri A. Reese, MD
South Bay Orthopaedic Specialists
Clinical Instructor, Volunteer
Department of Orthopaedic Surgery
University of California, Irvine, School of
    Medicine
Torrance, California

David R. Richardson, MD
Assistant Professor
Resident Program Director
Department of Orthopaedic Surgery
University of Tennessee—Campbell Clinic
Memphis, Tennessee

Mark A. Reiley, MD
Department of Orthopaedic Surgery
Berkeley Orthopaedic Medical Group, Inc.
Berkeley, California

Pascal Rippstein, MD
Department for Foot and Ankle Surgery
Schulthess Clinic
Zurich, Switzerland

Mark Ritter, MD
Department of Orthopedic Surgery
Methodist Sports Medicine Center
Indianapolis, Indiana

Venus R. Rivera, MD
Foot and Ankle Fellow
Department of Orthopaedic Surgery
Union Memorial Hospital
Baltimore, Maryland

Robert Rochman, MD
Private Practice
Royal Palm Beach, Florida

Matteo Romagnoli, MD
2nd Clinic of Orthopaedic Surgery
Istituto Orthopedico Rizzoli
Bologna, Italy

Michael M. Romash, MD
Orthopedic Surgeon
Orthopedic Foot and Ankle Center of
    Hampton Roads
Sports Medicine and Orthopedic Center
Chesapeake, Virginia

S. Robert Rozbruch, MD
Institute for Limb Lengthening and
    Complex Reconstruction
Hospital for Special Surgery
Weill Cornell Medical College
New York, New York

S. Robert Rozbruch, MD
Institute for Limb Lengthening
    and Complex Reconstruction
Hospital for Special Surgery
Weill Cornell Medical College
New York, New York

G. James Sammarco, MD, FACS
Professor
Department of Orthopaedic Surgery
Tulane University School of Medicine
Clinical Professor
Department of Orthopaedic Surgery
University of Cincinnati Medical Center
Cincinnati, Ohio

Vincent James Sammarco, MD
Department of Orthopedic Surgery
Cincinnati Sports Medicine and
    Orthopaedic Center
Cincinnati, Ohio

Thomas P. San Giovanni, MD
Department of Orthopedic Surgery
UHZ Sports Medicine Institute
Coral Gables, Florida

Amy Sanders, RN, BSN/PAC
Physician's Assistant
Columbia Orthopaedic Group
Columbia, Missouri

Roy W. Sanders, MD
Clinical Professor of Orthopaedics
University of South Florida
Chief, Department of Orthopaedics
Tampa General Hospital
Director, Orthopaedic Trauma Services
Florida Orthopaedic Institute
Tampa, Florida

Bruce J. Sangeorzan, MD
Professor of Orthopedics and Sports
    Medicine
University of Washington/Harborview
    Medical Center
Seattle, Washington

James Santangelo, MD
Staff Orthopaedic Surgeon
Womack Army Medical Center
Fort Bragg, North Carolina

† deceased

Michael Scherb, MD
Fellow
Department of Orthopaedics
Union Memorial Hospital
Baltimore, Maryland

Aaron T. Scott, MD
Assistant Professor
Department of Orthopaedic Surgery
Wake Forest University Baptist Medical
 Center
Winston-Salem, North Carolina

Steven L. Shapiro, MD
Savannah, Georgia

Scott B. Shawen, MD
Assistant Professor
Department of Surgery
Uniformed Services University of Health
 Sciences
Bethesda, Maryland

Paul S. Shurnas, MD
Director, Foot and Ankle
Columbia Orthopaedic Group
Columbia, Missouri

Sam Singh, MD
Director, CathLab and Continuing Medical
 Education
San Joaquin Community Hospital
Bakersfield, California

Bertil W. Smith, MD
Department of Orthopaedic Surgery
University of California at San Diego
San Diego, California

Ronald W. Smith, MD
Associate Clinical Professor
Department of Orthopaedic Surgery
University of California at Los Angeles
Balance Orthopaedic Foot and Ankle
 Center
Long Beach, California

**Emmanouil D. Stamatis, Lt Colonel MD,
 FHCOS, FACS, PhD**
Orthopaedic Department
General Army Hospital
Athens, Greece

**Michael M. Stephens, MSc(Bioeng.),
 FRCSI**
Associate Professor
Department of Orthopaedic Surgery
Cappagh National Orthopaedic Hospital
Dublin, Ireland

Karen M. Sutton, MD
Assistant Professor
Department of Orthopaedic Surgery
Yale University
New Haven, Connecticut

Yoshinori Takakura, MD
Department of Orthopaedic Surgery
Nara Medical University
Nara, Japan

Virak Tan, MD
Associate Professor
Department of Orthopaedics
University of Medicine and Dentistry of
 New Jersey
NJ Medical School
Newark, New Jersey

Yasuhito Tanaka, MD
Department of Orthopaedic Surgery
Nara Medical University
Nara, Japan

James P. Tasto, MD
Clinical Professor
Department of Orthopaedic Surgery
University of California at San Diego
Founder, San Diego Sports Medicine &
 Orthopaedic Center
San Diego, California

Dean C. Taylor, MD
Professor of Orthopaedic Surgery
Co-Director, Sports Medicine Fellowship
Duke University Medical Center
Durham, North Carolina

Ahmed M. Thabet, MD, PhD
Lecturer of Orthopaedic Surgery
Benha University
Benha, Egypt

Hajo Thermann, MD, PhD
Professor
Center for Knee and Foot Surgery/Sports
 Trauma
ATOS Clinic Center
Heidelberg, Germany

Sandra L. Tomak, MD
Department of Orthopedic Surgery
Center for Orthopaedics
New Haven, Connecticut

Brian C. Toolan, MD
Associate Professor of Surgery, Foot and
 Ankle
Director, Residency Program of
 Orthopaedic Surgery
The University of Chicago Hospitals
Chicago, Illinois

Hans-Joerg Trnka, Univ. Doz. Dr.
Foot and Ankle Center
Vienna, Austria

H. Robert Tuten, MD
Associate Clinical Professor
Department of Orthopedic Surgery
Medical College of Virginia
Richmond, Virginia

Victor Valderrabano, MD, PhD
Professor and Chairman
Orthopaedic Department
University Hospital Basel
Basel, Switzerland

C. Niek van Dijk, MD, PhD
Professor of Medicine
Department of Orthopaedic Surgery
Academic Medical Center
University of Amsterdam
Amsterdam, The Netherlands

Francesca Vannini, MD, PhD
2nd Orthopaedic Department
Istituto Orthopedico Rizzoli
Bologna, Italy

Emilio Wagner, MD
Associate Professor
Department of Orthopedic and Trauma
 Surgery
Universidad del Desarrollo/Clinica Allemana
Santiago, Chile

Markus Walther, MD, PhD
Professor of Orthopaedic Surgery
Orthopaedic Hospital Munich-Harlaching
Munich, Germany

Keith L. Wapner, MD
Clinical Professor
Department of Orthopedic Surgery
Pennsylvania Hospital
University of Pennsylvania
Philadelphia, Pennsylvania

Anthony Watson, MD
Assistant Professor
Department of Orthopaedic Surgery
Drexel University College of Medicine
Philadelphia, Pennsylvania

Troy Watson, MD
Director, Foot and Ankle Institute
Department of Orthopaedic Surgery
Institute of Orthopaedic Surgery
Las Vegas, Nevada

Wolfram Wenz, MD
Head of Unit for Pediatric Orthopaedics
 and Foot Surgery
Department of Orthopaedics
University of Heidelberg
Heidelberg, Germany

Michael G. Wilson, MD
Assistant Professor
Department of Orthopaedic Surgery
Harvard Medical School
Brigham and Women's Hospital
Boston, Massachusetts

Dane K. Wukich, MD
Assistant Professor
Department of Orthopaedic Surgery
UPMC Cancer Center Physicians
Pittsburgh, Pennsylvania

Gilbert Yee, MD, Med, MBA, FRCSC
Department of Surgery
The Scarborough Hospital
Toronto, Ontario, Canada

**Alastair Younger, MD, ChB, MSc, ChM,
FRCS(C)**
Ambulatory Care Physician Leader
Providence Health Care
Director, BC Foot and Ankle Clinic
Vancouver, British Columbia, Canada

PART 9 SPINE

Todd J. Albert, MD
Richard H. Rothman Professor and
 Chairman
Department of Orthopaedic Surgery
Professor of Neurosurgery
Thomas Jefferson University Hospital
Rothman Institute
Philadelphia, Pennsylvania

Maneesh Bawa, MD
Department of Orthopaedics
Emory University School of Medicine
Atlanta, Georgia

Jacob M. Buchowski, MD, MS
Assistant Professor of Orthopaedic and
 Neurological Surgery
Washington University in St. Louis
St. Louis, Missouri

Patrick Cahill, MD
Staff Surgeon
Shriners Hospital for Children
Philadelphia, Pennsylvania

Saad B. Chaudhary, MD, MBA
Center for Spine Health
The Cleveland Clinic
Cleveland, Ohio

Morgan N. Chen, MD
Orthopedic Associates of Long Island, LLP
East Setauket, New York

Mark Dumonski, MD
Resident
Department of Orthopaedic Surgery
Rush University Medical Center
Chicago, Illinois

Ira L. Fedder, DPharm, MD
Scoliosis and Spine Center of Maryland
Towson Orthopaedic Associates
Towson, Maryland

James S. Harrop, MD
Associate Professor of Neurological and
    Orthopedic Surgery
Thomas Jefferson University
Philadelphia, Pennsylvania

Andrew C. Hecht, MD
Co-Chief, Spine Surgery
Assistant Professor of Orthopaedic and
    Neurosurgery
Mt. Sinai Medical Center and School of
    Medicine
New York, New York

John Heflin, MD
Resident
Department of Orthopaedic Surgery
Emory University School of Medicine
Atlanta, Georgia

John G. Heller, MD
Professor of Orthopaedic Surgery
Spine Fellowship Director
The Emory Spine Center
Emory University School of Medicine
Emory University Orthopaedics & Spine
    Hospital
Atlanta, Georgia

Claude Jarrett, MD
Resident
Department of Orthopaedic Surgery
Emory University School of Medicine
Atlanta, Georgia

James S. Kercher, MD
Resident
Department of Orthopaedic Surgery
Emory University
Atlanta, Georgia

Youjeong Kim, MD
Orthopaedic Consultants of North Texas
Baylor University Medical Center
Dallas, Texas

Michael J. Lee, MD
Assistant Professor
Department of Sports Medicine and
    Orthopaedic Surgery
University of Washington Medical Center
Seattle, Washington

Ronald A. Lehman, Jr., MD
Director
Pediatric and Adult Spine
Assistant Professor of Surgery, USUHS
Department of Orthopaedics and
    Rehabilitation
Walter Reed Army Medical Center
Potomac, Maryland

Satyajit V. Marawar, MD
Fellow in Spine Surgery
Department of Orthopaedic Surgery
Medical College of Wisconsin
Milwaukee, Wisconsin

Paul C. McAfee, MD
Chief of Spine Surgery
St. Joseph's Hospital
Towson, Maryland

Daniel Park, MD
Resident
Department of Orthopaedic Surgery
Rush University Medical Center
Chicago, Illinois

Sheeraz A. Qureshi, MD
Assistant Professor of Orthopaedic Surgery
Mount Sinai Hospital
Chief, Spinal Trauma
Elmhurst Hospital Center
New York, New York

Raj Rao, MD
Professor of Orthopaedic Surgery
Medical College of Wisconsin
Milwaukee, Wisconsin

Mitchell F. Reiter, MD
Assistant Professor of Orthopedic Surgery
The New Jersey Medical School/UMDNJ
Summit, New Jersey

John M. Rhee, MD
Assistant Professor
Department of Orthopaedic Surgery
Emory University School of Medicine
Atlanta, Georgia

K. Daniel Riew, MD
Mildred B. Simon Distinguished Professor
    of Orthopaedic Surgery
Professor of Neurological Surgery
Chief, Cervical Spine Surgery
Washington University Orthopedics
Director, Orthopedic-Rehab Institute for
    Cervical Spine Surgery
St. Louis, Missouri

Samer Saiedy, MD
Department of Surgery
Towson, Maryland

**Matthew N. Scott-Young, MBBS, FRACS,
    FAOrthA**
Associate Professor
Faculty of Health Science and Medicine
Bond University
Gold Coast, Australia

Kern Singh, MD
Assistant Professor
Department of Orthopaedic Surgery
Rush University Medical Center
Chicago, Illinois

Thomas Stanley, MD
Resident
Department of Orthopaedic Surgery
Rush University Medical Center
Chicago, Illinois

P. Justin Tortolani, BA, MD
Towson Orthopaedic Associates
Towson, Maryland

Bradley K. Weiner, MD
Associate Professor
Chief of Spinal Surgery
Department of Orthopaedic Surgery
The Methodist Hospital
Houston, Texas

Andrew P. White, MD
Instructor
Harvard Medical School
Department of Orthopaedic Surgery
Beth Israel Deaconess Medical Center
Boston, Massachusetts

Sam W. Wiesel, MD
Professor and Chair
Department of Orthopaedic Surgery
Georgetown University Medical School
Washington, District of Columbia

Bart Wojewnik, MD
Resident
Department of Orthopaedic Surgery
Loyola University Health System
Maywood, Illinois

S. Tim Yoon, MD, PhD
Assistant Professor
Department of Orthopaedic Surgery
Emory University
Atlanta, Georgia

Aristidis Zibis, MD
Fellow in Spinal Surgery
Department of Orthopaedic Surgery
Penn State Hershey Medical School
Hershey, Pennsylvania

PREFACE

When a surgeon contemplates performing a procedure, there are three major questions to consider: Why is the surgery being done? When in the course of a disease process should it be performed? And, finally, what are the technical steps involved? The purpose of this text is to describe in a detailed, step-by-step manner the "how to do it" of the vast majority of orthopaedic procedures. The "why" and "when" are covered in outline form at the beginning of each procedure. However, it is assumed that the surgeon understands the basics of "why" and "when," and has made the definitive decision to undertake a specific case. This text is designed to review and make clear the detailed steps of the anticipated operation.

Operative Techniques in Orthopaedic Surgery differs from other books because it is mainly visual. Each procedure is described in a systematic way that makes liberal use of focused, original artwork. It is hoped that the surgeon will be able to visualize each significant step of a procedure as it unfolds during a case.

The text is divided into nine major topics: Adult Reconstruction; Foot and Ankle; Hand, Wrist, and Forearm; Oncology; Pediatrics; Shoulder and Elbow; Sports Medicine; Spine; and Pelvis and Lower Extremity Trauma. Each chapter has been edited by a specialist who has specific expertise and experience in the discipline. It has taken a tremendous amount of work for each editor to enlist talented authors for each procedure and then review the final work. It has been very stimulating to work with all of these wonderful and talented people, and I am honored to have taken part in this rewarding experience.

Finally, I would like to thank everyone who has contributed to the development of this book. Specifically, Grace Caputo at Dovetail Content Solutions, and Dave Murphy and Eileen Wolfberg at Lippincott Williams & Wilkins, who have been very helpful and generous with their input. Special thanks, as well, goes to Bob Hurley at LWW, who has adeptly guided this textbook from original concept to publication.

SWW
January 1, 2010

ACKNOWLEDGMENTS

I would like to acknowledge my wife, Mary, and my children Erin, Colleen, John, and Kelly, who tolerate all the orthopaedic "homework" required to write and teach orthopaedics.

—JMF

I greatly acknowledge the never-ending hard work, dedication, and enthusiasm of Ms. Kristen Kellar-Graney, who has been my right-hand woman for over 12 years.

—MMM

All book projects are a challenge and I certainly could not get as involved with them as I am without a lot of help. To my partners (especially David), my PAs (Jen and Jerry), the residents and fellows, and everyone I have had the pleasure to teach and learn alongside. Thank you!

—MDM

With appreciation to my great mentor, Richard Rothman, MD, PhD, the most amazing human and scholar I have known.

—JP

I acknowledge my mentors and colleagues, Mark Myerson, Lew Schon, Robert Anderson, Hodges Davis, Jim Nunley, and Jim DeOrio, whose tireless commitment to academic orthopaedic surgery continues to inspire me, and the tremendous contributions of the authors who shared their expertise to make this textbook possible.

—MEE

RESIDENCY ADVISORY BOARD

The editors and the publisher would like to thank the resident reviewers who participated in the reviews of the manuscript and page proofs. Their detailed review and analysis was invaluable in helping to make certain this text meets the needs of residents today and in the future.

Daniel Galat, MD
Dr. Galat is a graduate of Ohio State University College of Medicine and the Mayo Clinic Department of Orthopedic Surgery residency program.
He is currently serving at Tenwek Hospital in Kenya as an orthopedic surgeon.

Lawrence V. Gulotta, MD
Fellow in Sports Medicine/Shoulder Surgery
Hospital for Special Surgery
New York, New York

Dara Chafik, MD, PhD
Southwest Shoulder, Elbow and Hand Center PC
Tuscon, Arizona

Gautam Yagnik, MD
Attending Physician
Orthopaedic Surgery
DRMC Sports Medicine
Dubois, Pennsylvania

Gregg T. Nicandri, M.D.
Assistant Professor
Department of Orthopaedics (SMD)
University of Rochester
School of Medicine and Dentistry
Rochester, New York

Catherine M. Robertson, MD
Assistant Clinical Professor
UCSD Orthopaedic Surgery—Sports Medicine
San Diego, California

Jonathan Schoenecker, MD
Assistant Professor
Departments of Orthopaedics, Pharmacology and Pediatrics
Vanderbilt University
Nashville, Tennessee

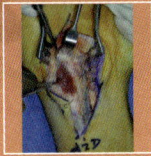

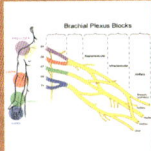

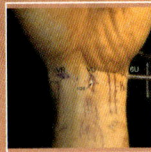

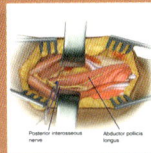

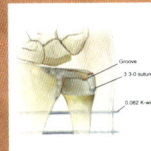

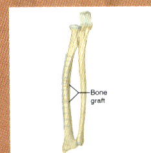

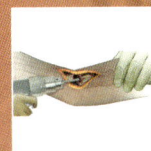

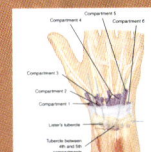

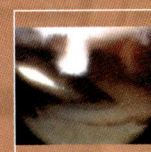

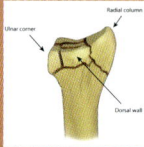

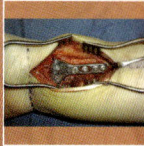

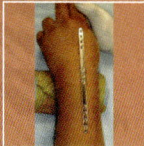

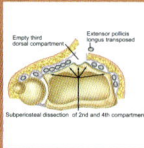

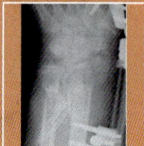

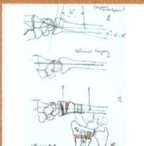

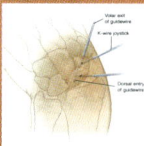

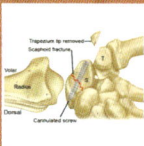

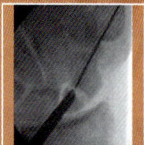

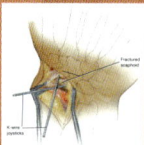

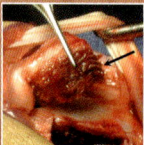

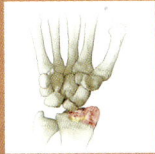

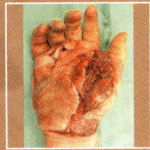

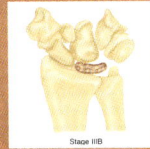

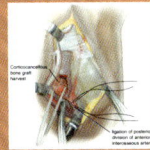

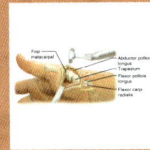

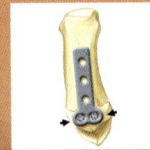

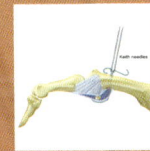

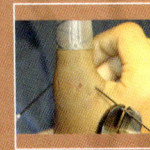

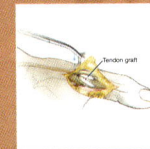

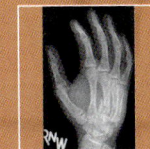

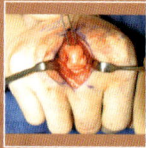

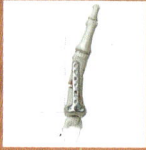

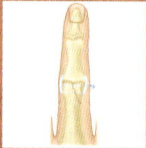

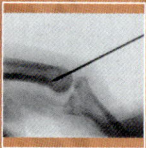

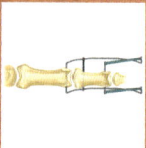

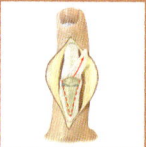

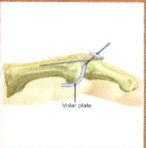

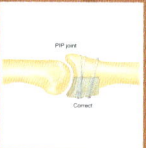

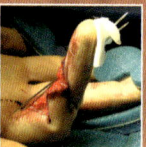

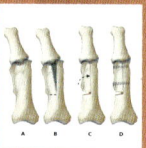

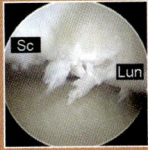

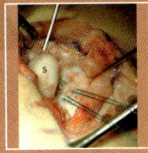

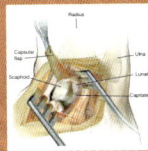

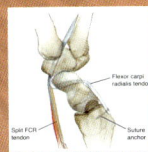

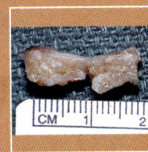

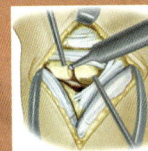

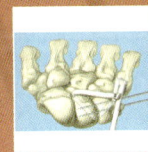

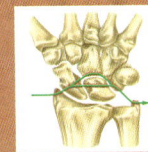

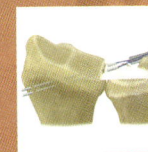

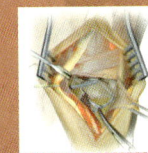

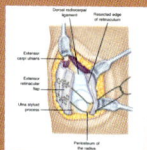

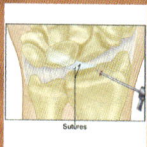

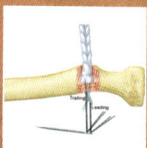

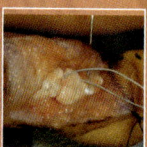

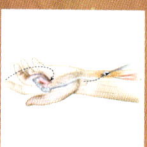

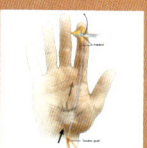

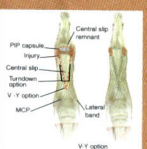

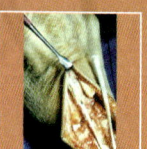

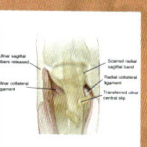

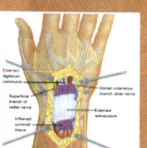

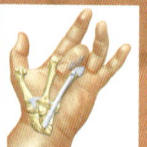

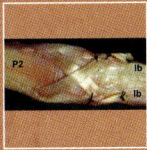

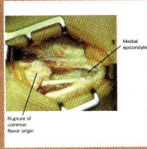

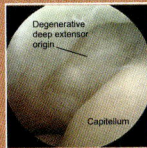

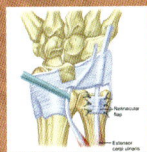

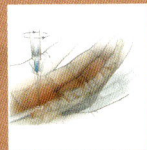

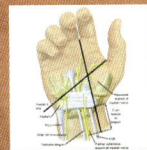

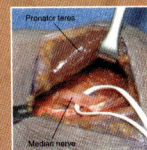

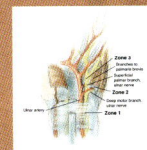

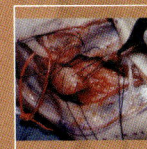

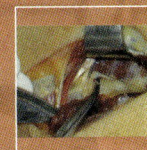

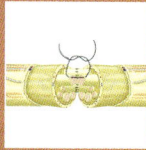

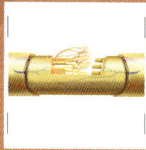

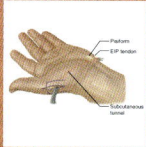

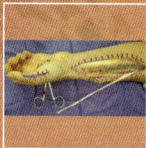

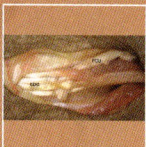

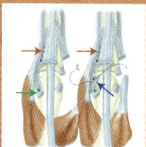

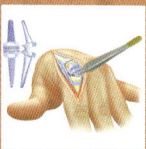

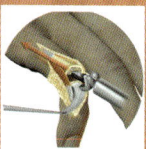

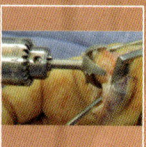

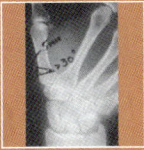

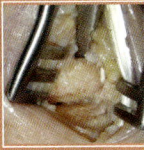

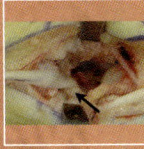

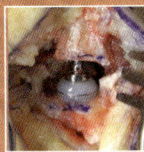

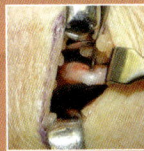

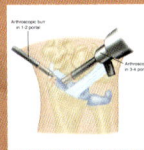

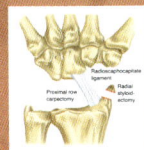

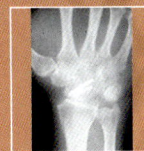

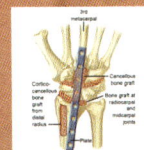

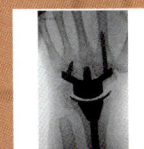

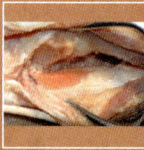

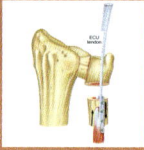

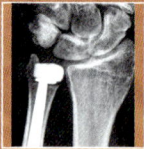

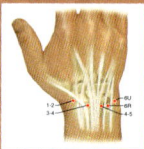

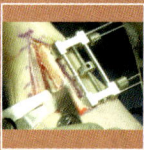

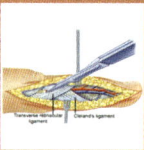

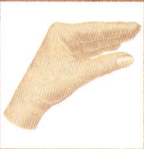

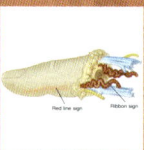

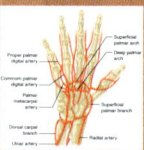

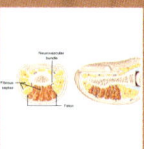

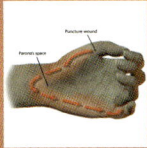

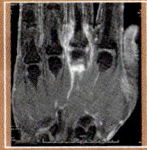

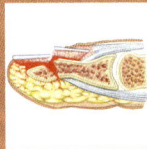

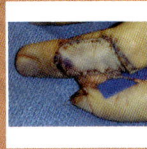

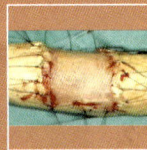

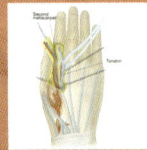

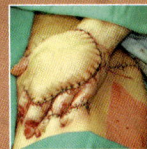

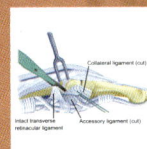

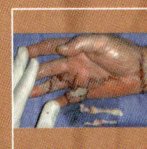

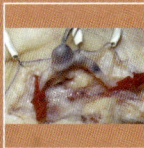

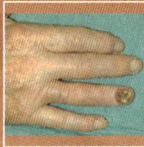

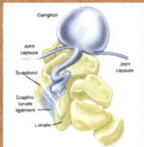

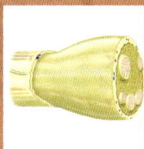

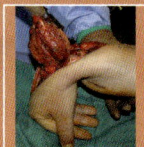

Anatomy and Surgical Approaches of the Forearm, Wrist, and Hand

Asif M. Ilyas, Neal C. Chen, and Chaitanya S. Mudgal

DEFINITION

- Safe surgical dissection and exposure require an in-depth knowledge of anatomy. In no place is this more relevant than in the surgical approaches to the hand, wrist, and forearm.
- The critical aspect of successful surgical approaches is the use of internervous planes.
  - These planes lie between muscles that are innervated by different nerves.
  - This allows extensive mobilization and exposure without risk of muscle denervation.

- Unique to the hand, wrist, and forearm is the complex relationship of not only the muscles overlying bone but also the close proximity and delicate balance of accessory anatomic structures, including tendons, vessels, and nerves.

ANATOMY

- The anatomy of the hand, wrist, and forearm is intricate and can be discussed in many ways and in extensive detail. For the discussion in this chapter, anatomy will focus on the compartments of the hand and forearm, and their relevance to surgical approaches (Table 1).

Table 1	Compartments of the Hand and Forearm		
Compartments	**Origin**	**Insertion**	**Innervation**
Thenar			
Abductor pollicis brevis	Trapezium/scaphoid	Radial base of thumb P1	Median (recurrent motor branch)
Flexor pollicis brevis	Trapezium	Base of thumb P1	Median (recurrent motor branch)
Opponens pollicis	Trapezium	Radial base of thumb P1	Median (recurrent motor branch)
Adductor			
Adductor pollicis	Capitate/third metacarpal	Ulnar base of thumb P1	Ulnar
Hypothenar			
Abductor digiti minimi	Pisiform	Ulnar base of small P1	Ulnar
Flexor digiti minimi brevis	Hook of hamate	Base of small P1	Ulnar
Opponens digiti minimi	Hook of hamate	Ulnar base of small P1	Ulnar
Interosseous			
Dorsal interossei (4)	#2, 3, 4, 5 metacarpals	Radial or ulnar base of P1	Ulnar
Volar interossei (3)	#2, 4, 5 metacarpals	Radial or ulnar base of P1	Ulnar
Carpal Tunnel			
Lumbricals/Flexor tendons/median nerve	Flexor digitorum profundus tendons	Lateral bands	Median and ulnar
Superficial Volar Forearm			
Pronator teres	Medial epicondyle	Mid third of radius	Median
Flexor carpi radialis	Medial epicondyle	Base of #2 metacarpal	Median
Palmaris longus	Medial epicondyle	Palmar fascia of hand	Median
Flexor carpi ulnaris	Medial epicondyle	Pisiform/base of #5	Median
Flexor digitorum superficialis	Medial epicondyle	Base of #2, 3, 4, 5 P2	Median
Deep Volar Forearm			
Flexor digitorum profundus	Ulna/Interosseus membrane	Base of #2, 3, 4, 5 P3	Median (ant. interosseous branch)
Flexor pollicis longus	Distal third of radius	Base of thumb P2	Median (ant. interosseous branch)
Pronator quadratus	Distal third of ulna	Distal third of radius	Median (ant. interosseous branch)
Dorsal Forearm			
Abductor pollicis longus	Mid-third dorsal radius	Radial base of thumb MC	Radial (post. interosseous branch)
Extensor pollicis brevis	Mid-third dorsal radius	Dorsal base of thumb P1	Radial (post. interosseous branch)
Extensor pollicis longus	Dorsal ulna	Dorsal base of thumb P2	Radial (post. interosseous branch)
Extensor digitorum communis	Lateral epicondyle	Dorsal base of #2, 3, 4, 5 P3	Radial (post. interosseous branch)
Extensor indicis proprius	Dorsal ulna	Dorsal base of #2 P3	Radial (post. interosseous branch)
Extensor digiti quinti	Lateral epicondyle	Dorsal base of #5 P3	Radial (post. interosseous branch)
Extensor carpi ulnaris	Lateral epicondyle	Dorsal base of #5 MC	Radial (post. interosseous branch)
Supinator	Lateral epicondyle	Proximal third of radius	Radial (post. interosseous branch)
Mobile Wad			
Brachioradialis	Lat. condyle humerus	Distal radius styloid	Radial
Extensor carpi radialis longus	Lat. condyle humerus	Dorsal base of #2 MC	Radial
Extensor carpi radialis brevis	Lat. condyle humerus	Dorsal base of #3 MC	Radial (post. interosseous branch

SURGICAL MANAGEMENT

- All surgical approaches to the hand, wrist, and forearm warrant sound understanding of surface and deep anatomy, internervous planes, and surgical technique.
- Planning the surgical approach begins by identifying reliable surface anatomy.

Preoperative Planning

- Arrangements for instruments, sutures, microscope, imaging support, implants, and assistants should be made before the day of surgery.
- Anatomy, radiographic templating, surgical approach, procedure, and alternatives should be reviewed.

Positioning

- Most approaches to the hand, wrist, and forearm can be performed with the patient supine and the operative extremity extended on a hand table and the surgeon and assistants seated.

- The hand table should be stable and well secured and should allow adequate space for both the operative limb and the surgeon's elbow and forearm to minimize fatigue and enhance stability.
- The stool should be stable and comfortable, with the height set such that the knees are level with the hips and the feet are resting flat on the ground.
- The lights should be angled directly over the hand table, and not from behind the surgeon or assistant's shoulder, to prevent shadows on the operative field.
- The use of a pneumatic tourniquet is advised to maintain a bloodless field and clear visualization of all anatomic structures.

Approach

- Multiple approaches to the hand, wrist, and forearm exist and are best divided into the anatomic site and direction of exposure.
- The approach should be chosen based on the indication for surgery.

TECHNIQUES

SKIN INCISIONS OF THE HAND

- Incisions in the hand can be placed almost anywhere as long as certain principles are respected.
- Incisions should be outlined by sterile surgical markers before making the actual incision to confirm appropriate position, to confirm the adequacy of skin bridges should multiple incisions be used, and to help guide closure.
- Incisions can be made in skin creases on the volar aspect of the hand but incisions in deep creases should be avoided due to the thin subcutaneous tissue, tendency

for maceration due to moisture, and tendency toward poor apposition of skin edges on closure.
- Incisions perpendicular to a volar flexion crease should be avoided to prevent scar formation and secondary skin contractures that can lead to loss of motion and functional impairment (**TECH FIG 1A,B**).
- Incisions on the dorsal surface of the hand can be smaller due to the more mobile and loose nature of the dorsal skin (**TECH FIG 1C**).

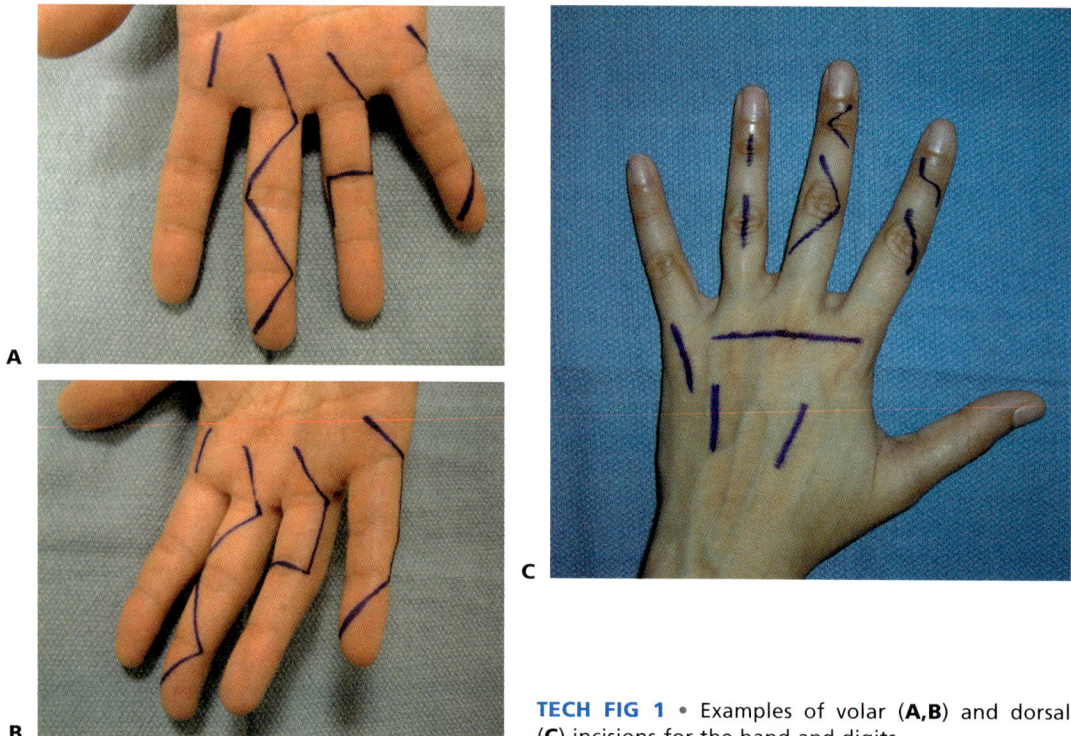

TECH FIG 1 • Examples of volar (**A,B**) and dorsal (**C**) incisions for the hand and digits.

- Vertical, horizontal, and curved incisions can all be used with good facility as long as adequate skin bridges are maintained.
- Fingers can be exposed dorsally, volarly, or midaxially.
  - Dorsal incisions can be longitudinal or curvilinear.
  - Volar incisions are best facilitated by a zigzag pattern that crosses creases laterally and at angles.

- Midaxial incisions are best placed at the junction of glabrous and nonglabrous skin, with attention being paid to the neurovascular bundle that sits in the plane of the flexor sheath. The neurovascular bundle can be taken volarly with the volar flap or can be left in place by carrying the dissection superficial to it.

APPROACH TO THE INTERPHALANGEAL JOINTS

- Straight dorsal longitudinal incisions can be made or a variety of curved incisions can be used, including an S-type and a chevron style (**TECH FIG 2A**).
- In the distal interphalangeal joint, caution must be paid to the germinal matrix, which is about 1 mm distal to the attachment of the extensor tendon.
- At the proximal interphalangeal joint, there is no internervous plane and the extensor mechanism should be immediately evident (**TECH FIG 2B**).
- The integrity of the central slip inserting in the middle phalanx guides exposure of the proximal interphalangeal joint.

- Three techniques can be employed to approach the joint:
  - The lateral bands can be freed and gently retracted dorsally, allowing a lateral approach into the joint.
  - When more exposure is required, the lateral bands can be incised in line with the extensor mechanism and repaired later.
  - Lastly, to maximize exposure of the joint, the extensor mechanism is cut dorsally in a long distally based V-shaped flap, raised, and later repaired.
- It is critical not to detach the central slip distally and to maintain continuity of the extensor mechanism through the lateral bands on each side (**TECH FIG 2C**).

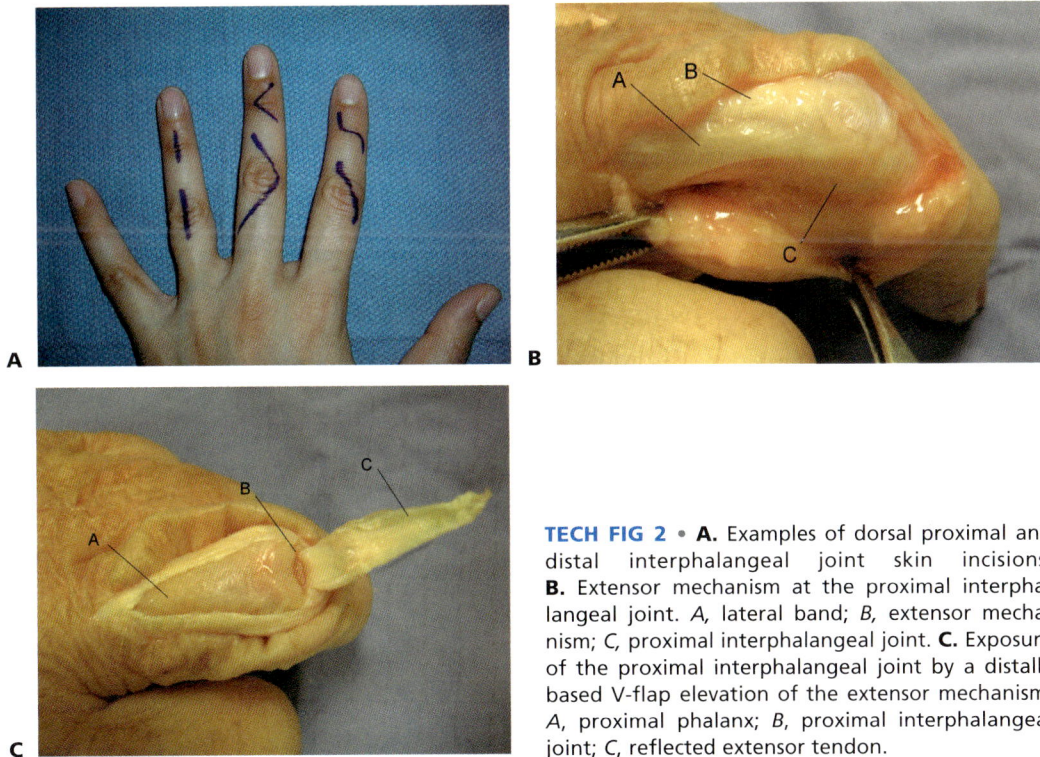

TECH FIG 2 • **A.** Examples of dorsal proximal and distal interphalangeal joint skin incisions. **B.** Extensor mechanism at the proximal interphalangeal joint. *A,* lateral band; *B,* extensor mechanism; *C,* proximal interphalangeal joint. **C.** Exposure of the proximal interphalangeal joint by a distally based V-flap elevation of the extensor mechanism. *A,* proximal phalanx; *B,* proximal interphalangeal joint; *C,* reflected extensor tendon.

APPROACH TO THE METACARPOPHALANGEAL JOINT

- With the metacarpophalangeal joint flexed, identify the apex of the joint, which is the metacarpal head, and the extensor tendon.
- Make a straight dorsal longitudinal incision centered over the metacarpophalangeal joint.

- If multiple joints are being approached, a transverse incision centered dorsally connecting each of the joints may be used (**TECH FIG 3A**).
- There is no internervous plane. The extensor mechanism should be immediately evident. Sensory branches of

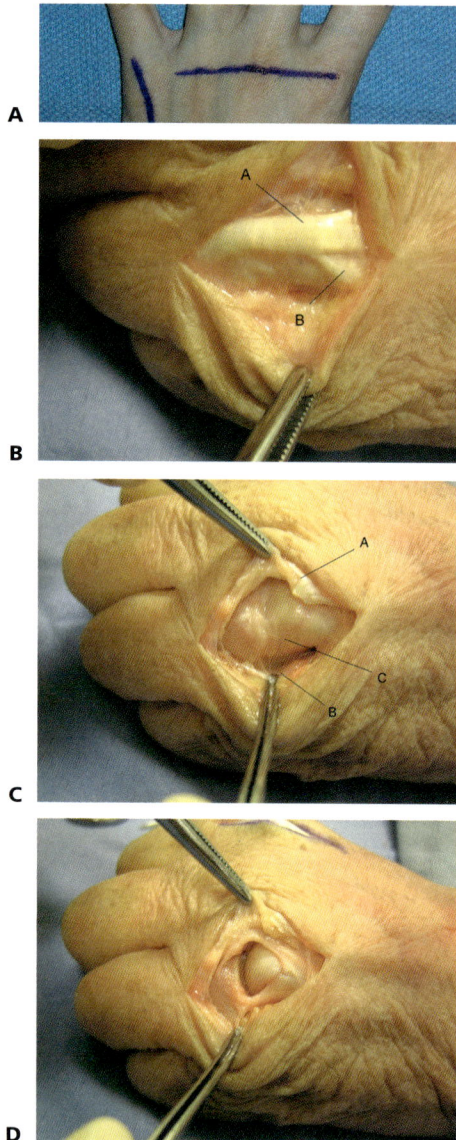

either the radial or ulnar nerve, depending on which joint is being approached, should be identified and protected (**TECH FIG 3B**).

- Three techniques can be employed to approach the metacarpophalangeal joint:
  - The sagittal band that runs like a sling around the joint can be freed and retracted distally, exposing the dorsal capsule of the metacarpophalangeal joint.
    - This technique is best used for a dorsal capsulotomy or capsulectomy.
  - When further exposure is required, the extensor mechanism is incised centrally and longitudinally through the substance of the tendon. Extensile exposure of the joint will be obtained immediately deep to the tendon.
    - This technique maintains balance of the extensor mechanism and avoids postoperative subluxation and deviation.
    - The tendon split should stop before the level of the proximal interphalangeal joint to avoid compromise of the central slip.
  - The extensor mechanism can be incised along the ulnar sagittal band in line with the tendon.
    - Release of the radial sagittal band should be avoided to prevent postoperative ulnar subluxation of the tendon.
    - This technique also provides extensile exposure of the metacarpophalangeal joint as well as the collateral ligaments but risks postoperative tendon subluxation or finger deviation (**TECH FIG 3C,D**).

TECH FIG 3 • **A.** Examples of metacarpophalangeal skin incisions. A straight longitudinal incision can be placed over each joint. If multiple joints are being approached, a single straight transverse incision can be used. **B.** Extensor mechanism overlying the metacarpophalangeal joint. *A*, extensor tendon; *B*, ulnar sagittal band. **C.** The ulnar sagittal band is incised in line with the extensor mechanism revealing the metacarpophalangeal joint. *A*, extensor tendon; *B*, reflected ulnar sagittal band; *C*, metacarpophalangeal joint. **D.** The metacarpophalangeal joint is arthrotomized dorsal to the collaterals.

APPROACH TO THE METACARPALS

- Palpate the metacarpal subcutaneously. Identify overlying extensor tendons.
- Make a straight dorsal longitudinal incision over the metacarpal. If more than one metacarpal is being approached, then place the incision between adjacent metacarpals (**TECH FIG 4**).
- There is no true internervous plane. Overlying extensor tendons must be identified and protected.
- Juncturae tendinae may cross over the field while connecting two tendons. They should be maintained if possible; if not, they should be released and tagged for repair before closure.
- Dorsal interossei are attached to either side of the metacarpal.
- Incise the periosteum of the metacarpal longitudinally along its exposed dorsal ridge and raise the interossei medially and laterally in a subperiosteal fashion.

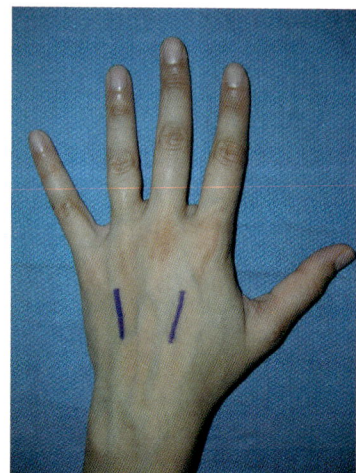

TECH FIG 4 • Incision for approaching multiple metacarpals.

APPROACH TO THE CARPAL TUNNEL

- The carpal tunnel is an enclosed fibro-osseous tunnel that contains nine flexor tendons and the median nerve. Its borders include the transverse carpal ligament (the roof), the carpal bones (the floor), the hook of hamate (ulnar wall), and the scaphoid (radial wall).
    - The proximal extent of the tunnel lies at the level of the distal wrist crease.
- Identify the interthenar depression, which lies between the thenar eminence radially and the hypothenar eminence ulnarly (**TECH FIG 5A**).
- Palpate the hook of hamate and pisiform bone along the ulnar base of the hand.
- Determine the cardinal line of Kaplan, the estimated distal extent of the transverse carpal ligament.[4] The cardinal line of Kaplan runs from the base of the first web space (with the thumb abducted in the plane of the palm) parallel to the proximal palmar crease toward the hook of hamate.
- Multiple incisions can be used depending on the surgeon's preference, ranging from a limited approach (**TECH FIG 5B**) to an extensile one.
- The incision should be centered within the interthenar depression and in line with the third web space to avoid injury to the palmar cutaneous branches of the median and ulnar nerves.[8]
- The internervous plane occurs between the palmar cutaneous branches of the ulnar and median nerves.

- Incise the subcutaneous fat in line with the skin incision. Deep to the fat lies the longitudinally oriented superficial palmar fascia (**TECH FIG 5C**).
    - Incise this fascia in line with the incision.
    - Avoid raising flaps radially or ulnarly to prevent skin devitalization and injury to branches of the palmar cutaneous branch of the median and ulnar nerves.
- Deep to the superficial palmar fascia lies the thick transverse carpal ligament.
    - Release this ligament in line with the skin incision, paying attention to the median nerve lying deep to it as well as being cautious of the recurrent motor branch of the median nerve, which could cross through or across the transverse carpal ligament (**TECH FIG 5D**).
- Distal to the transverse carpal ligament, confirm release of the ligament both proximally and distally.
    - Distal release is confirmed on visualization of the "sentinel" pad of fat, which has a distinct yellow color different from that of the subcutaneous fat.
    - Proximal release is confirmed both visually and by feel and usually corresponds to the confluence of the transverse carpal ligament with the deep forearm fascia, generally located at the level of the distal wrist crease.

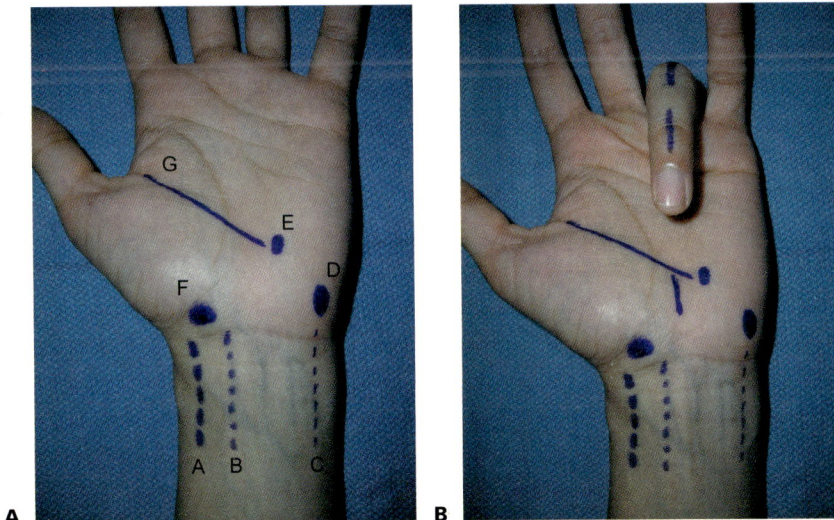

A

B

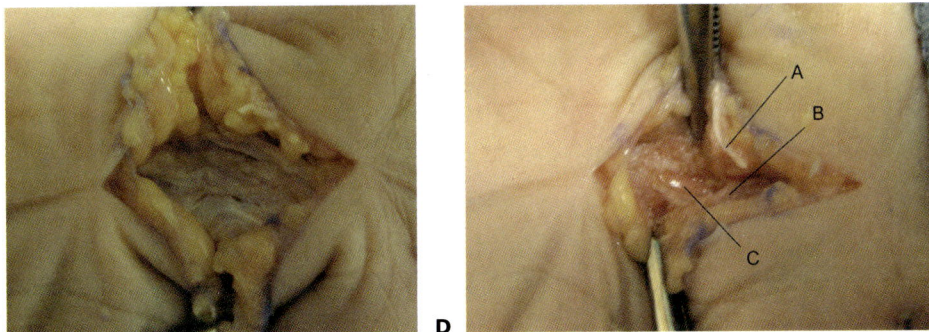

C

D

TECH FIG 5 • A. Surface anatomy of the volar hand. *A*, radial artery; *B*, flexor carpi radialis tendon; *C*, flexor carpi ulnaris tendon; *D*, pisiform; *E*, hook of hamate; *F*, distal pole of scaphoid; *G*, cardinal line of Kaplan. **B.** Incision for the limited incision carpal tunnel approach. **C.** Superficial palmar fascia of the hand. **D.** Partial release of the transverse carpal ligament with the median nerve lying deep to it. *A*, retracted superficial palmar fascia; *B*, partially released transverse carpal ligament; *C*, median nerve.

APPROACH TO CANAL OF GUYON

- The canal of Guyon is an enclosed fibro-osseous space at the ulnar base of the hand through which the ulnar neurovascular structures travel before innervating and perfusing the intrinsic structures of the hand.
  - Its borders include the volar carpal ligament (the roof), the transverse carpal ligament (the floor), the pisiform (ulnar wall), and the hook of hamate (radial wall).
- Palpate the pisiform bone, which lies subcutaneously at the ulnar base of the hand immediately distal to the wrist flexion crease in line with the flexor carpi ulnaris (see **TECH FIG 5A**).
- Palpate the hook of hamate, which lies about 2 cm distal and 2 cm radial to the pisiform bone.
  - This may be difficult to palpate in patients with large hands or those with well-developed hypothenar musculature.
- Palpate the flexor carpi ulnaris tendon, which runs along the ulnar aspect of the forearm and inserts into the pisiform upon crossing the wrist flexion crease.
- Make a zigzag or curved incision between the pisiform and hook of hamate and extend it proximally (**TECH FIG 6A**).

- Avoid crossing the wrist flexion crease perpendicularly. Extend it proximally along the radial border of the flexor carpi ulnaris tendon (**TECH FIG 6B**).
- Identify the flexor carpi ulnaris proximal to the wrist flexion crease and mobilize it ulnarly by releasing the fascia along its radial border. The ulnar artery and nerve will lie just deep and radial to the tendon, with the nerve more superficial and ulnar to the artery.
- Follow the ulnar artery and nerve distally into the hand.
  - In the hand, the flexor carpi ulnaris tendon will insert into the pisiform and the ulnar artery and nerve will dive deep to the volar carpal ligament.
- Releasing the volar carpal ligament radial to the pisiform opens the roof of the canal of Guyon and decompresses the ulnar artery and nerve. In the canal of Guyon, the nerve splits into its motor and sensory branches. The motor branch of the ulnar nerve dives below a fibrous arch formed by the hypothenar musculature originating from the hook of hamate (**TECH FIG 6C**).
- There is a high frequency of anatomic variations of the ulnar neurovascular structures within the canal of Guyon, and a release of the canal must include not only the roof but also the distal extent of it as it enters below the fibrous arch below the hypothenar muscles.[5]

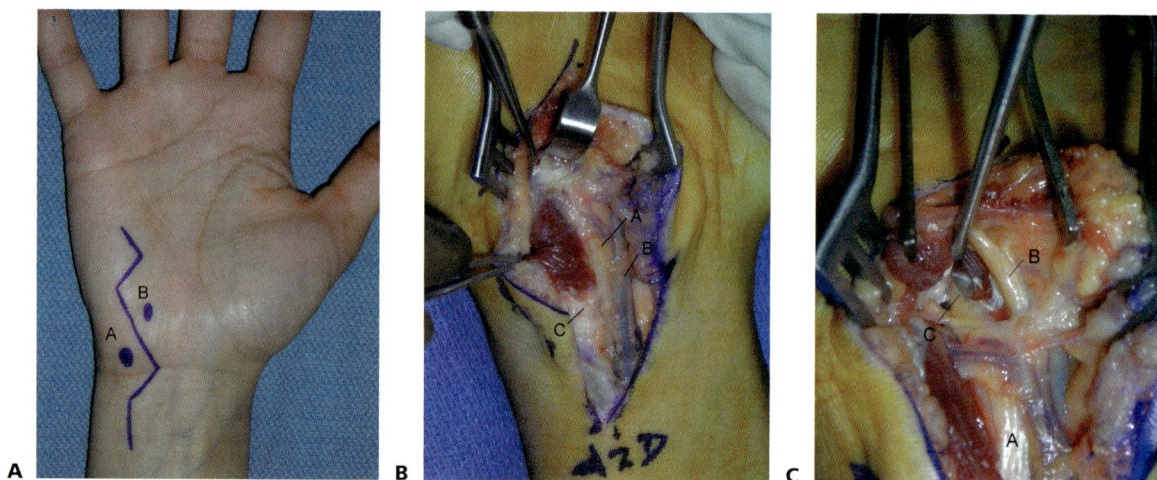

TECH FIG 6 • A. Surface anatomy and incision for the approach to the canal of Guyon. *A,* pisiform; *B,* hook of hamate. **B.** The ulnar neurovascular structures in the base of the hand after release of the volar carpal ligament. *A,* ulnar nerve; *B,* ulnar artery and vein; *C,* pisiform with origin of the hypothenar muscles. **C.** Fibrous arch formed by the hypothenar muscles over the motor branch of the ulnar nerve. *A,* ulnar nerve; *B,* sensory branch of ulnar nerve; *C,* motor branch of ulnar nerve.

VOLAR APPROACH TO THE RADIUS

- Identify the flexor carpi radialis at the wrist flexion crease distally and follow it subcutaneously proximally (**TECH FIG 7A**).
  - Its tendinous nature will give way to muscle at roughly the middle of the forearm.
- Identify the brachioradialis, which originates along the lateral epicondylar ridge of the distal humerus and is the

most superficial muscle mass along the lateral forearm. Distally and laterally it has a broad insertion along the flare of the radial border of the radius.
- Identify the biceps tendon, which is the broad and taut extension of the biceps tendon that crosses anterior to the elbow joint and dives toward its insertion into the radius medial to the brachioradialis.

- Identify the radial artery at the wrist. It is found between the flexor carpi radialis and brachioradialis tendons.
- With the forearm supinated, begin the incision proximal to the wrist flexion crease and immediately radial to the flexor carpi radialis tendon and extend the incision proximally parallel to the tendon.
  - The incision can end lateral to the biceps tendon and distal to the elbow flexion crease.
  - The incision can be extended as shown by the dotted extensions in Techniques Figure 7A.
  - The length of the incision depends on the extent of bone that needs to be exposed.
- As described by Henry,[3] the internervous plane distally occurs between the flexor carpi radialis (median nerve) and the brachioradialis (radial nerve). Proximally it occurs between the pronator teres (median nerve) and the brachioradialis (radial nerve).
  - Distally the interval between the flexor carpi radialis and the brachioradialis is developed (**TECH FIG 7B**).
  - The radial artery lies just ulnar to the brachioradialis tendon and lies underneath the brachioradialis in the middle of the forearm. Dissection should not drift ulnar to the flexor carpi radialis, for the median nerve lies just deep and ulnar to this tendon.
  - The superficial radial sensory nerve exits from under the brachioradialis at the middle of the forearm, about 8 to 10 cm proximal to the radial styloid, and travels adjacent to the tendon distally.[1] The nerve arborizes proximal to the wrist joint.
  - Proximally the interval between the pronator teres and brachioradialis is developed.
- An alternative to the volar approach of Henry is the trans–flexor carpi radialis approach.
  - In this approach, the incision is placed directly over the flexor carpi radialis tendon.
  - The flexor carpi radialis sheath is opened sharply in line with the tendon.
  - The tendon is retracted ulnarly and the floor of the tendon sheath is opened sharply, leading directly into the deep layer between the finger flexors and the pronator quadratus, also known as the space of Parona.[6]
- Several muscles lie over the radius in the deep layer. Distally, the pronator quadratus and flexor pollicis longus cover the radius (**TECH FIG 7C**). On the middle third of the radius lie the flexor carpi radialis and pronator teres.
- To expose the radius, these muscles are released along the volar radial aspect of the radius and are raised in a subperiosteal fashion ulnarly.
- Proximally, the supinator muscle covers the radius. Through its substance travels the posterior interosseous

nerve as it travels to the dorsal compartment of the forearm.
- To expose the radius proximally, the forearm must be fully supinated and the supinator is released along the ulnar border of the radius and raised radially. The forearm must be kept fully supinated to protect the posterior interosseous nerve.

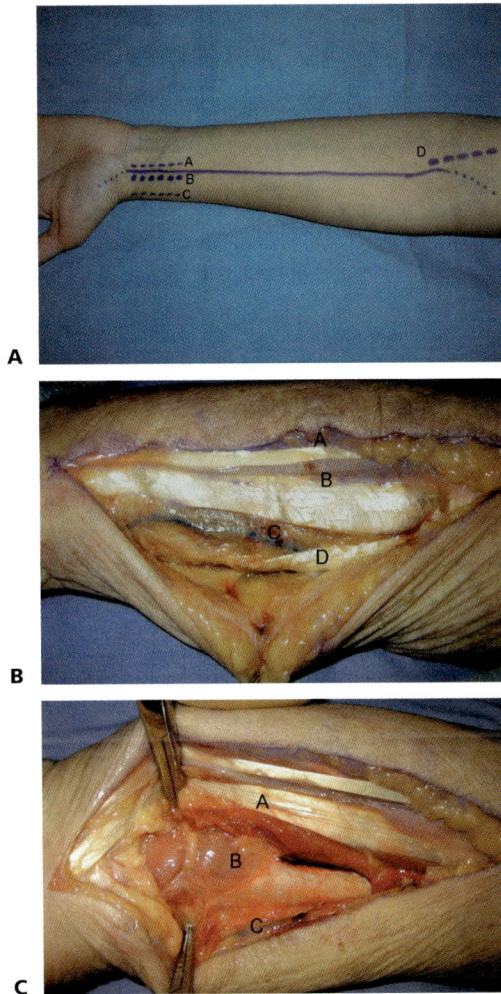

TECH FIG 7 • A. Surface anatomy and incision of the volar forearm. *A*, flexor carpi radialis; *B*, radial artery; *C*, brachioradialis; *D*, biceps tendon. **B.** Superficial exposure of the volar radius showing the palmaris longus (*A*) and the internervous plane between the flexor carpi radialis (*B*) and the brachioradialis (*D*). *C*, radial artery. **C.** Deep exposure of the volar distal radius showing the pronator quadratus (*B*) covering the distal radius. *A*, flexor carpi radialis; *C*, radial artery.

DORSAL APPROACH TO THE RADIUS

- Identify the tubercle of Lister at the distal and radial aspect of the radius. It is the most prominent bony protuberance on the dorsal distal radius, and the extensor pollicis longus tendon curves around it (**TECH FIG 8A**).
- Identify the "mobile wad of three," which is the common muscle mass composed of the brachioradialis and the extensor carpi radialis longus and brevis.[3]

- Identify the lateral epicondyle of the distal humerus, which is the bony prominence most easily palpable proximal to the radial head along the lateral aspect of the elbow.
- With the forearm pronated, make the incision from the tubercle of Lister and extend it proximally along the medial border of the "mobile wad" toward the lateral epicondyle.

TECHNIQUES

- The length of the incision depends on the extent of bone that needs to be exposed (**TECH FIG 8A**).
- As described by Thompson, the internervous plane distally occurs between the extensor carpi radialis brevis (radial nerve, posterior interosseous nerve, or both) and the extensor pollicis longus (posterior interosseous nerve).[7]
  - Proximally it occurs between the extensor carpi radialis brevis (radial nerve; inconsistent innervation) and the extensor digitorum communis (posterior interosseous nerve).
- Distally, develop the interval between the extensor carpi radialis brevis and the extensor pollicis longus with the tubercle of Lister positioned between them (**TECH FIG 8B**).
- Exposing proximally, the interval between the extensor carpi radialis brevis and the extensor digitorum communis is identified by the emergence of the outcropping abductor pollicis longus and the extensor pollicis brevis (**TECH FIG 8C**).
- Distally the radius sits immediately below the superficial extensor tendons.
  - To expose the distal radius, the extensor retinaculum and the sheath of the extensor pollicis longus tendon is opened and the tendon is retracted radially.
  - The floor of the tendon sheath is incised longitudinally and the extensor tendons are raised subperiosteally, with the extensor carpi radialis longus and brevis taken radially and the finger extensors taken ulnarly.
- Proximally, the abductor pollicis longus and extensor pollicis brevis cover the middle third of the radius.
  - To expose the radius, these muscles are released along their radial border, to avoid denervation, and raised ulnarly.
  - The proximal third of the radius is covered by the supinator. Within its substance and between its two heads runs the posterior interosseous nerve.
- Exposure of the dorsal radius proximally requires exposure and protection of this nerve before elevating the supinator off the radius.
  - First, identify the nerve as it exits between the two heads of the supinator.
  - Follow the nerve proximally through the substance of the supinator's superficial head while taking care to preserve all its branches.
  - Once the nerve is identified along its entire course, the supinator can be released along its radial border and raised ulnarly.

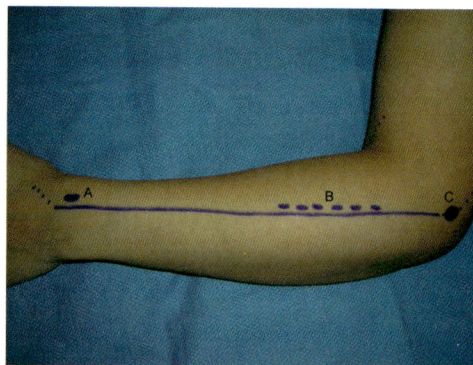

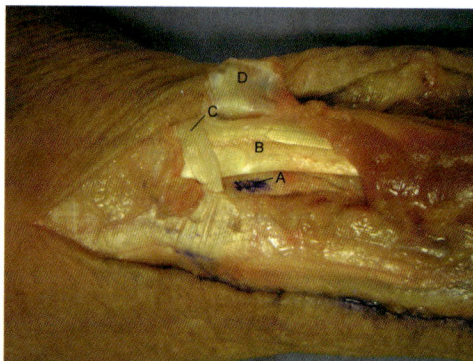

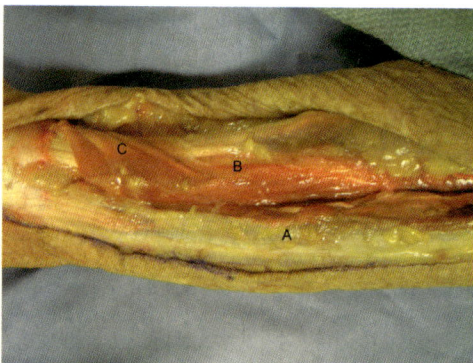

TECH FIG 8 • **A.** Surface anatomy and incision of the dorsal forearm. *A,* tubercle of Lister; *B,* ulnar border of the "mobile wad of three"; C, lateral epicondyle. **B.** Superficial exposure of the dorsal distal radius. *A,* tubercle of Lister; *B,* extensor carpi radialis longus and brevis; *C,* extensor pollicis longus; *D,* reflected extensor retinaculum. **C.** Musculature of the dorsal forearm. *A,* extensor digitorum communis; *B,* extensor carpi radialis brevis; *C,* abductor pollicis longus and extensor pollicis brevis.

APPROACH TO THE ULNA

- Identify the ulnar head and styloid distally with the forearm in neutral rotation (**TECH FIG 9**).
- Identify the subcutaneous border of the ulna.
- Identify the tip of the olecranon proximally.
- With the forearm in neutral rotation, begin the incision at the level of the head of the ulna but proximal to the styloid. Extend the incision across the subcutaneous border of the ulna proximally toward the olecranon. The length of incision depends on the extent of the bone that needs to be exposed.

- Distally, the internervous plane occurs between the flexor carpi ulnaris (ulnar nerve) and the extensor carpi ulnaris (posterior interosseous nerve).
  - Proximally, at the level of the olecranon, the internervous plan occurs for a short length between the flexor carpi ulnaris (ulnar nerve) and the anconeus (radial nerve).
- Distally, the interval between the flexor carpi ulnaris and the extensor carpi ulnaris occurs along the subcutaneous border of the ulna.

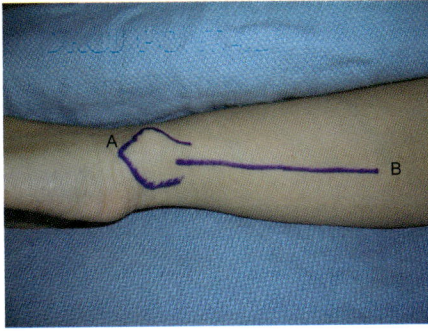

TECH FIG 9 • Surface anatomy and incision for the ulnar shaft. *A,* ulnar head and styloid; *B,* subcutaneous border of ulna.

- Both muscles can be raised volarly and dorsally off the ulna, respectively, in a subperiosteal fashion.
- The ulnar artery and nerve travel deep and radial to the flexor carpi ulnaris. The nerve is protected by careful subperiosteal elevation of the flexor carpi ulnaris.

- The dorsal branch of the ulnar nerve branches about 8 cm proximal to the pisiform and crosses the subcutaneous border of the ulna as it travels dorsally about 5 cm proximal to the pisiform.[2]
- Proximally the interval remains along the subcutaneous border of the ulna.
- The proximal aspect of the ulna receives the insertion of the triceps tendon.
- When exposing the ulna proximally during deep dissection, the integrity of the triceps tendon is maintained by incising the tendon in line with its fibers across the border of the ulna and raising it medially and laterally in a subperiosteal fashion.
- The ulnar nerve travels around the medial epicondyle and dives between the two heads of the flexor carpi ulnaris.
- Before exposing the ulna's most proximal and medial portion, the ulnar nerve should be identified and protected, followed by subperiosteal elevation of the flexor carpi ulnaris.

PEARLS AND PITFALLS

Approach to the interphalangeal joints (proximal and distal)	■ Protect the germinal matrix and terminal tendon at the base of the distal phalanx. ■ Protect the central slip at the base of the middle phalanx.
Approach to the metacarpophalangeal joints	■ If necessary, release the ulnar sagittal band at the joint. Avoid releasing the radial sagittal band.
Approach to the carpal tunnel	■ Protect branches of the palmar cutaneous branch of the median and ulnar nerves in the subcutaneous tissue by centering the incision in the interthenar eminence. ■ Remain vigilant for a transligamentous recurrent motor branch of the median nerve.
Volar approach to the radius	■ Dissection should not drift ulnar to the flexor carpi radialis tendon to protect the median nerve and its cutaneous branches.
Dorsal approach to the radius	■ The posterior interosseous nerve ends at the level of the wrist dorsally in line with the fourth metacarpal and is easily approached for denervation for postoperative pain relief.

REFERENCES

1. Abrams RA, Brown RA, Botte MJ. The superficial branch of the radial nerve: an anatomic study with surgical implications. J Hand Surg 1992;17:1037–1041.
2. Botte MJ, Cohen MS, Lavernia CJ, et al. The dorsal branch of the ulnar nerve: an anatomic study. J Hand Surg 1990;15:603–607.
3. Henry AK. Extensile exposure, 2nd ed. Edinburgh: E&S Livingstone, 1966.
4. Kaplan EB. Functional and surgical anatomy of the hand, 2nd ed. Philadelphia: JB Lippincott, 1965.
5. Konig PS, Hage JJ, Bloem JJ, et al. Variations of the ulnar nerve and ulnar artery in Guyon's canal: a cadaveric study. J Hand Surg 1994;19:617–622.
6. Parona F. Dell'oncotomia negli accessi profundi diffuse dell'avambrachio. Annali Universali di Medicina e Chirurgia Milano, 1876.
7. Thompson JE. Anatomical methods of approach in operations on the long bones of the extremities. Ann Surg 1918;68:309–329.
8. Watchmaker GP, Weber D, Mackinnon SE. Avoidance of transection of the palmar cutaneous branch of the median nerve in carpal tunnel release. J Hand Surg 1996;21:644–650.

TECHNIQUES

Chapter 2

Anesthetic Considerations for Surgery of the Upper Extremity

John A. Dilger and Hugh M. Smith

BACKGROUND

- Orthopaedic surgery makes up a considerable portion of the 70% of procedures done on an ambulatory basis in the United States.[9]
- Several factors have fueled this growth in outpatient orthopaedic surgery, including less invasive surgical approaches, changes in practice patterns, and the introduction of anesthetic agents associated with fewer postoperative side effects.
- Postoperative pain management represents a particular challenge with ambulatory surgery, as 40% of patients experience severe pain despite treatment.[5]
- Regional anesthesia techniques have been used to solve this problem.
  - Anesthetic techniques incorporating peripheral nerve blocks are associated with superior analgesia and a lower incidence of postoperative nausea and vomiting.[12,15]
  - Regional anesthetic techniques result in increased patient satisfaction and fewer unanticipated hospital admissions.[23]
- Peripheral nerve blocks administered with a single dose of long-acting local anesthetic (bupivacaine or ropivacaine) have frequently been used to provide postoperative pain control. However, patients and surgeons alike become frustrated when these blocks dissipate in the middle of the night, resulting in the return of severe pain. In these situations, the pain state is longer than the duration of the block.
- Despite the selection of long-acting local anesthetics (14 to 24 hours of analgesia), about 20% of patients after orthopaedic surgery have significant pain requiring opioids after 7 days.[14]
  - Continuous regional analgesia, using an indwelling nerve catheter and local anesthetic pump, can maintain analgesia until the pain state dissipates.
- The frustration with the limited analgesia provided by a single dose of local anesthetic causes some physicians to avoid nerve blocks altogether. They choose instead to use an opioid strategy begun preoperatively with sustained-release analgesics (oxycodone SR).
  - This approach is associated with increased side effects such as urinary retention, pruritus, ileus, nausea, and vomiting.
- If continuous regional analgesia is selected, it may be used for anesthesia and postoperative analgesia.
- The continuous peripheral nerve catheter offers prolonged analgesia and minimal side effects and eliminates the problem of block resolution and the return of severe pain. The nerve block is maintained with a continuous infusion of local anesthetic agents.
  - Pumps have been developed allowing outpatient infusions, and these elastometric pumps are ideal because they are compact, simple to operate, and designed to provide safe infusion rates of local anesthetic in the uncontrolled home environment.

PREOPERATIVE EVALUATION

Rheumatoid Arthritis

- In advanced rheumatoid arthritis, atlantoaxial subluxation may develop from erosion of ligaments at the odontoid process of C2 as it is attached to C1. This C1 and C2 instability may produce subluxation, resulting in cord compression and paralysis.
  - Anatomic changes involving the cervical spine, temporomandibular joint, or arytenoids may necessitate awake airway management with a fiberoptic bronchoscope (Table 1).
    - Preoperative flexion and extension films are indicated with advanced rheumatoid arthritis, and cervical fusion of C1 to the occiput may be required before the procedure.
  - Regional anesthesia may avoid the airway challenges of general anesthesia, but it may be difficult in these patients if the loss of range of motion in the joints prevents proper needle placement.
- Rheumatoid arthritis is associated with cardiovascular disease, and atherosclerosis occurs at an accelerated rate in rheumatoid arthritis, resulting in a greater risk of myocardial infarction and cerebrovascular accident.[7]
  - The rate of cardiovascular morbidity and mortality in rheumatoid arthritis is higher than the general population.[19]
- Rheumatoid arthritis also causes deteriorations in respiratory performance as the lungs become affected, resulting in restrictive pulmonary disease.[17]
- Preoperative evaluations including an echocardiogram and cardiac stress and pulmonary function testing should be considered in patients with severe rheumatoid arthritis.

Trauma

- Surgical emergencies may require general anesthesia before completing radiologic evaluations.
  - An uncleared cervical spine requires in-line manual stabilization during the endotracheal intubation, regardless of

Table 1	Factors Associated with Difficult Endotracheal Intubation
	Anatomic abnormalities: micrognathia, limited jaw or neck mobility
	Cervical spine fusion
	Trauma
	Ankylosing spondylitis
	Juvenile rheumatoid arthritis
	Adult rheumatoid arthritis
	Achondroplasia
	Acromegaly
	Pierre Robin syndrome
	Treacher Collins syndrome
	Goldenhar syndrome

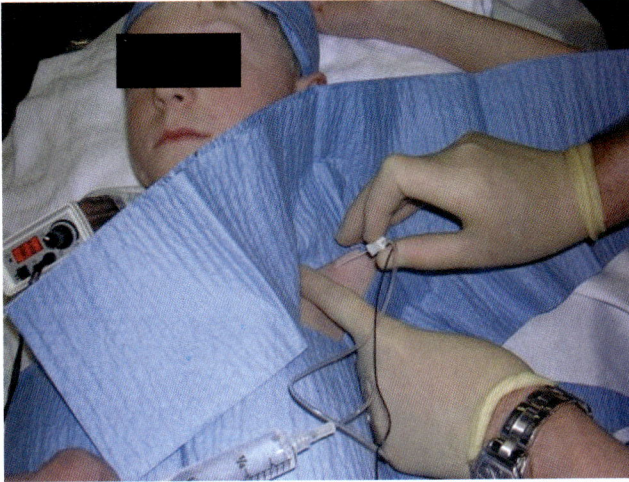

FIG 1 • Pediatric axillary brachial plexus block.

Table 2	Fasting Guidelines for Pediatric Patients	
	Fasting Time (hr)	
Age	**Milk and Solids**	**Clear Liquids**
<6 mo	4	2
6–36 mo	6	3
>36 mo	8	3

whether the intubation is performed with the patient awake or asleep.

▪ General anesthesia is frequently used for orthopaedic trauma. Factors that influence this decision include surgery on more than one extremity, unknown duration of procedure, the need to assess postoperative neurologic function, and surgeon or patient preference.

▪ Nerve blocks with concentrated local anesthesia (bupivacaine or ropivacaine 0.5% or higher) can mask symptoms of compartment syndrome and should be avoided in patients at risk.

▪ Advantages of regional anesthesia for upper extremity trauma surgery include:

  ▪ Increased blood flow in anesthetized area
  ▪ Lower incidence of deep venous thrombosis with neuraxial blocks
  ▪ Decreased blood loss
  ▪ Decreased postoperative nausea and vomiting
  ▪ Avoidance of difficult endotracheal intubation
  ▪ Decreased phantom limb pain following amputation by preventing pain centralization

Pediatrics

▪ General anesthesia is often used in pediatric surgery because children lack the emotional and intellectual maturity to be conscious during the procedure (**FIG 1**).

▪ Regional anesthesia may be performed in a child during general anesthesia, but the loss of patient feedback regarding pain and paresthesia increases the risk of neural injury.

▪ Regional anesthesia decreases anesthetic and opioid requirements, resulting in shorter wakeup times with general anesthesia.

▪ Caudal and spinal blocks have been the most commonly used regional techniques due to the anesthesiologist familiarity and their relative safety when performed in the anesthetized patient.

▪ Nerve blocks may provide preemptive analgesia by blocking painful stimuli and lead to lower stress hormone levels and less overall pain.[18]

  ▪ Nerve blocks done while the patient is under anesthesia have caused severe injury in adults, but these injuries are much less common in children.[16]

  ▪ Ultrasound-guided nerve blocks during general anesthesia may reduce the risk of nerve injury, allowing direct visualization of neural targets.

▪ Pediatric regional techniques require smaller needles, which have only recently become available, but continuous blocks are done with adult equipment, a less-than-optimal situation.

▪ Pediatric patients require cautious local anesthetic selection and administration to avoid toxicity.

  ▪ Epinephrine is typically added to enable the diagnosis of an intravascular injection of local anesthetic and to decrease its systemic absorption.

▪ Fasting guidelines for children up to 3 years old are given in Table 2.

▪ Pediatric doses of local anesthetics are summarized in Table 3.

▪ Continuous peripheral nerve catheters offer the same advantages in pediatric patients as in adults.

  ▪ Recommended infusion rates begin at 0.15 mL/kg per hour of bupivacaine 0.25%.[22]

  ▪ Continuous peripheral nerve catheters may be dosed with dilute local anesthetics (bupivacaine or ropivacaine 0.1%) because of incomplete myelinization of neural fibers, permitting greater local anesthetic penetration. This will decrease the risks of local anesthetic toxicity.

Table 3	Pediatric Doses of Clinical Characteristics of Commonly Used Local Anesthetics*					
Local Anesthetic	**Usual Concentration (%)**	**Usual Doses (mg/kg)**	**Maximum Dose, Plain[†] (mg/kg)**	**Maximum Dose with Epinephrine[†] (mg/kg)**	**Latency (min)**	**Duration of Effects (hr)**
Lidocaine	0.5–2.0	5	7.5	10	5–15	0.75–2.0
Prilocaine	0.5–1.5	5	7.0	10	15–25	0.75–2.0
Mepivacaine	0.5–1.5	5–7	8.0	10	5–15	1–1.25
Bupivacaine	0.25–0.5	2	2.5	3	15–30	2.5–6.0
Ropivacaine	0.2–10.0	3	3.5	NA	7–20	2.5–5.0

*Data are not applicable to spinal anesthesia or intravenous regional anesthesia.
[†]Maximum doses vary; free and unbound local causes toxicity, not total dose. Do not apply if previously injected or local anesthetic infusion maintained.

ANESTHESIA SELECTION FOR UPPER EXTREMITY PROCEDURES

- Anesthesia for arm and hand surgery may be general, regional, or a combination of techniques.
- The potential benefits of an upper extremity nerve block are less nausea, a shorter recovery, and faster discharge from the hospital, in part due to improved postoperative analgesia, requiring fewer narcotics for pain.[8]
- The anesthetic plan may also be based on factors unrelated to evidence-based medicine, such as anxiety, extended case duration, or the need for immediate neurologic examination after surgery.

General Anesthesia

- Easier to apply and no anesthetic failures
- Provides unconsciousness for the long procedure or uncomfortable position
- Pediatric and mentally retarded patients are easier to manage.
- Cadaveric conditions when the surgery requires no movement
- Procedure and graft harvest can be in different anatomic locations.
- Nerve function can be immediately assessed.
- Efficient anesthesia recovery with anesthetics such as propofol, sevoflurane, or desflurane

Regional Anesthesia

- Increases operating room efficiency: nerve blocks are done before entering the operating room, eliminating the time needed for induction and emergence from anesthesia
- Simplified perioperative management with conditions such as malignant hyperthermia, cardiomyopathy, and obstructive or restrictive lung conditions
- Continuous nerve blocks may provide anesthesia and be used for postoperative pain control.
- Propofol may be administered with regional blocks for light or heavy sedation.
- Less postoperative nausea and vomiting
- Faster recovery from anesthesia and earlier discharge
- Less postoperative cognitive dysfunction than from general anesthesia due to superior pain control, fewer sleep disturbances, and fewer unplanned admissions to the hospital
  - By avoiding unplanned admissions to the hospital, the incidence of postoperative cognitive dysfunction is lowered from 9.8% to 3.5%.[3]
- American Society of Regional Anesthesia and Pain Medicine guidelines on anticoagulation are given in Table 4.

Table 5	**Nerve Blocks for Surgery**
Procedure	**Block**
Shoulder surgery	Interscalene
Elbow surgery	Interscalene, supraclavicular, or infraclavicular
Forearm and hand surgery	Intraclavicular, axillary or IV regional (short procedures <1 hour)

- No contraindication
  - Carpel tunnel syndrome
  - Multiple sclerosis (spinal anesthesia contraindicated)
  - Stroke
  - Diabetes mellitus

Contraindications

- Absolute
  - Acute or resolving nerve injury in the regional block distribution
  - Progressive peripheral neuropathy
  - Infection at the puncture site for the block
  - Patient refusal
  - Bleeding disorder: full anticoagulation, thrombolytic therapy, and hemophilia
- Relative
  - Stable nerve impairment
  - Interscalene blocks with severe chronic obstructive pulmonary disease
  - Fever, bacteremia

REGIONAL ANESTHESIA FOR UPPER EXTREMITY SURGERY

- Nerve blocks for upper extremity surgery are summarized in Table 5.

Shoulder Surgery

- Because of the intense perioperative pain, particularly with arthroplasty or open rotator cuff operations, general anesthesia is rarely the sole technique for shoulder surgery.
- Performing regional anesthesia for shoulder surgery requires knowledge of the anatomy and the surgical approach.
  - The shoulder is innervated primarily by the brachial plexus, with minor contributions of sensory innervation from the superficial cervical plexus (**FIG 2**).

Table 4	**American Society of Regional Anesthesia Guidelines for Anticoagulation**
Medication	**Discontinuation Recommendation**
Herbal medications: ginkgo, ginseng, and garlic (greatest effect)	No discontinuation
Nonsteroidal anti-inflammatories and acetaminophen	No discontinuation
Ticlopidine and clopidogrel	14 days
Heparin	
SQ	No discontinuation
IV	Stop and 1 hour after block
Low-molecular-weight heparin	12 hours after last dose
Coumadin	Discontinue 4 days
Thrombolytics	Avoid regional

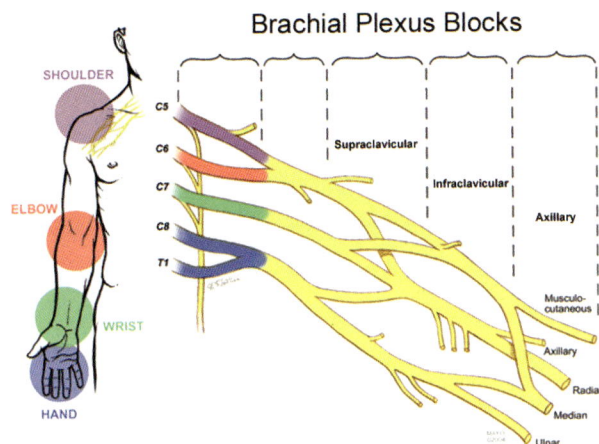

FIG 2 • Brachial plexus blocks. (By permission of Mayo Foundation for Medical Education and Research. All rights reserved.)

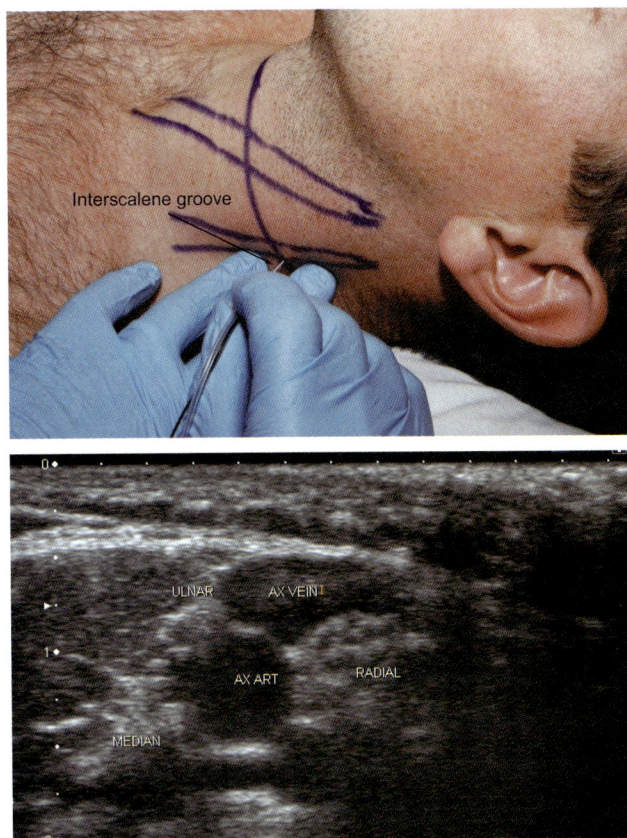

FIG 3 • **A.** Interscalene block superficial landmarks. **B.** Axillary artery and surrounding nerves of brachial plexus.

■ The interscalene block is done at the level of the trunks and blocks the superior and middle trunks along with the superficial cervical plexus.

■ Identification of superficial landmarks and the needle puncture site is done by palpating the space created by the trunks between the anterior and middle scalene muscles at the level of the cricoid cartilage (**FIG 3A**).

■ The nerves can be localized using paresthesia, nerve stimulator, or ultrasound (**FIG 3B**).

■ Once the needle is in approximation to the brachial plexus trunks, local anesthetic is incrementally injected, resulting in anesthesia of the shoulder and proximal arm.

■ Interscalene blocks with bupivacaine or ropivacaine provide perioperative analgesia.

■ Interscalene blocks cause a sympathectomy and resultant redistribution of blood away from the surgical site, decreasing intraoperative blood loss.

■ Incisions and port holes are occasionally outside the block's anesthetic distribution, requiring local anesthetic to be injected by the surgical team into the affected area.

■ Intra-articular local anesthetic and narcotic infusions may be helpful but must be combined with interscalene blocks for maximum postoperative analgesia

■ The semisitting position is often selected for the surgery, and the table must be equipped with a head piece securing the patient's head with a padded strap at the forehead.

■ The semisitting and lateral decubitus positions place the operative site above the heart, rarely resulting in air embolism.

■ Head and neck positioning is crucial to avoid spinal cord compression and neurologic deficits. However, the anesthesiologist may be hampered by this position because the proximity of the surgical incision allows little access to the head.

■ It may be very difficult to convert to general anesthesia without disrupting the sterile surgical field when a patient with a regional anesthetic must be put to sleep in the middle of the procedure. General anesthesia can be administered without endotracheal intubation either by holding a mask on the face or by inserting a laryngeal mask airway while the patient remains in the semisitting position.

■ Although this does not provide protection from stomach content aspiration, it offers some control of the airway without putting the patient supine and taking down the drapes for endotracheal intubation.

■ Because of this potential problem, many anesthesiologists and surgeons alike prefer to use general anesthesia with an endotracheal tube in combination with an interscalene block.

■ This combined anesthetic would also be chosen with complicated reoperations or where induced hypotension is needed.

■ Continuous interscalene blocks may be done to provide analgesia for a prolonged period.

■ Typically 48 hours of postoperative pain is adequate, and catheters are then removed.

■ Prolonged interscalene analgesia may be required in acute surgical shoulder pain in the chronic pain patient or in a patient with a frozen shoulder requiring mobilization therapy.

■ Continuous interscalene blocks have been associated with enhanced physical rehabilitation after shoulder surgery due to superior pain control.[6]

■ Interscalene block side effects include phrenic nerve, recurrent laryngeal nerve, and stellate ganglion blockade.

■ These may result in transient loss of ipsilateral diaphragm function, weak voice, miosis, ptosis, and anhydrosis (Horner syndrome).

Elbow Surgery

■ Surgical procedures at the elbow, whether for arthroplasty or the reattachment of a biceps brachii tendon, frequently require general anesthesia despite the advantages of regional anesthesia.

- The proximity of nerves to the surgical incision is concerning to surgeons who may wish to examine neurologic function in the immediate postoperative period, which is not possible with a nerve block.
  - Regional techniques are often performed in the recovery area after nerve function is assessed.
- Functional outcomes after elbow surgery often depend on early rehabilitation using continuous passive motion devices.
  - This therapy can be facilitated with continuous brachial plexus analgesia. The infraclavicular and the axillary approaches to the brachial plexus are options for catheter placement.
- The infraclavicular block is performed by placing the needle 1 inch distal to the midclavicle, with the needle advanced toward the axillary pulsation until twitch or paresthesia is obtained (**FIG 4**).
  - Continuous infraclavicular blocks are ideal as they cover the brachial plexus, including the musculocutaneous nerves, providing anesthesia of the entire arm.
  - Continuous axillary nerve blocks cover the brachial plexus, with the exception of the musculocutaneous nerve. This may result in pain during continuous passive motion and it may need to be separately blocked.
- Surgery with brachial plexus blocks may require supplementation at the musculocutaneous and intercostobrachial nerves.

Hand Surgery

- Hand procedures are frequently done with nerve blocks because of the ideal operating conditions and early discharge times postoperatively.
  - General anesthesia is reserved for extremely long cases and is combined with brachial plexus analgesia.
- Carpel tunnel release surgery is one of the most common hand procedures and may be done with an intravenous regional block (Bier block).
  - Bier blocks are impractical for the efficient outpatient practice. Local infiltration by the surgeon combined with intravenous sedation is a more common and efficient anesthetic approach.
- The axillary approach to the brachial plexus is ideal for more extensive hand procedures (**FIG 5A**).
  - The block may be placed easily, sets up quickly, covers all of the nerves of the hand, and is associated with low complication rates.
  - The nerves in the axilla have a predictable anatomic relationship to the axillary artery.
  - The block may be done with paresthesia, nerve stimulation, or transarterial approaches.
- Ultrasound guidance more recently has been used to provide real-time visualization of both the needle and the neural targets (**FIG 5B,C**).
  - The success of the block can be predicted by confirming circumferential spread of local anesthetic around the nerves.
- Continuous peripheral nerve catheters may be placed if the procedure is prolonged, a sympathectomy is needed, or significant pain is expected.
- Brachial plexus anesthesia with an intercostobrachial nerve block will prevent tourniquet pain, unlike general anesthesia.

Supplementing Nerve Blocks

- It is preferable to place blocks outside the operating room so that block efficacy can be evaluated.

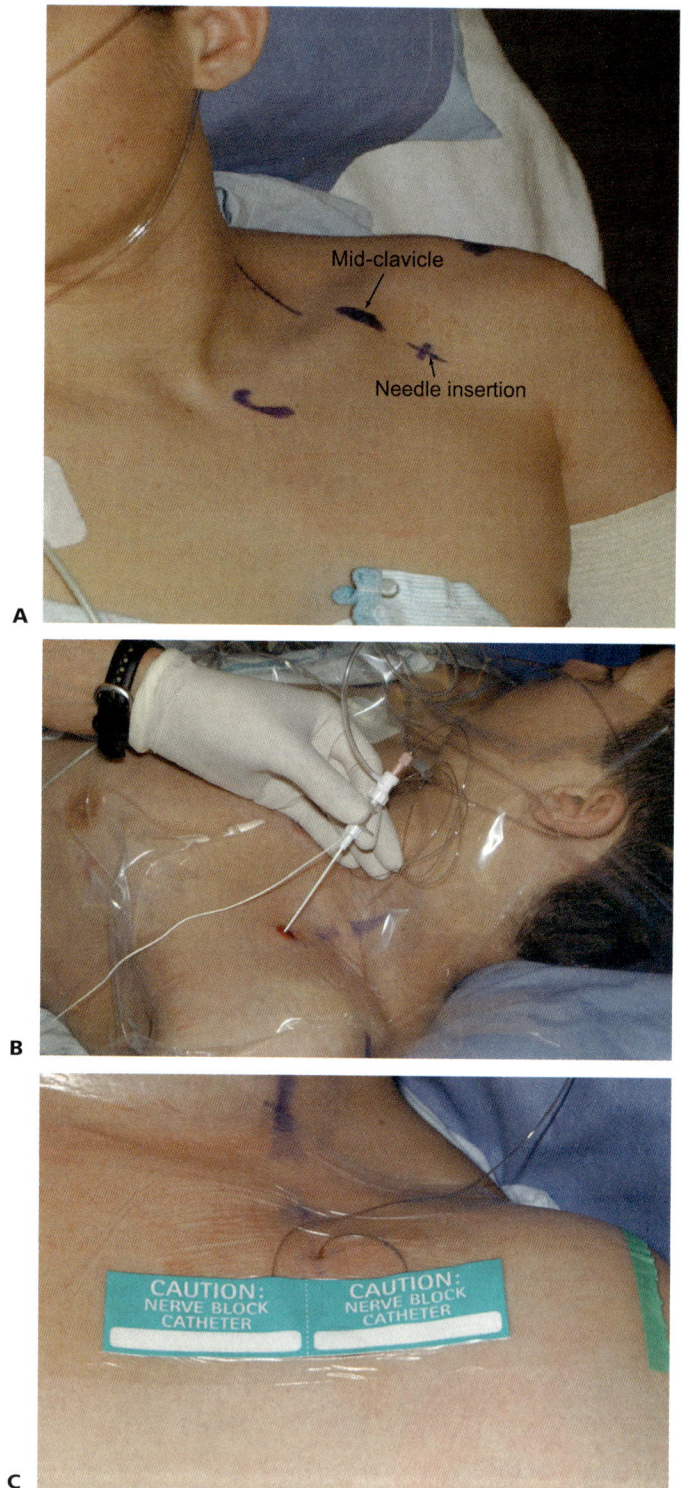

A

B

C

FIG 4 • **A.** Infraclavicular block superficial landmarks. **B.** Continuous infraclavicular block catheter needle insertion. **C.** Infraclavicular continuous catheter secured and labeled.

- Often a "failed" block is simply the result of inadequate time for local anesthetic distribution to nerve targets.
- Insufficient blocks can be supplemented, and again ultrasound offers a safe option for this.
- Propofol infusions will allow control of anxiety and can turn an incomplete block into an intraoperative success.

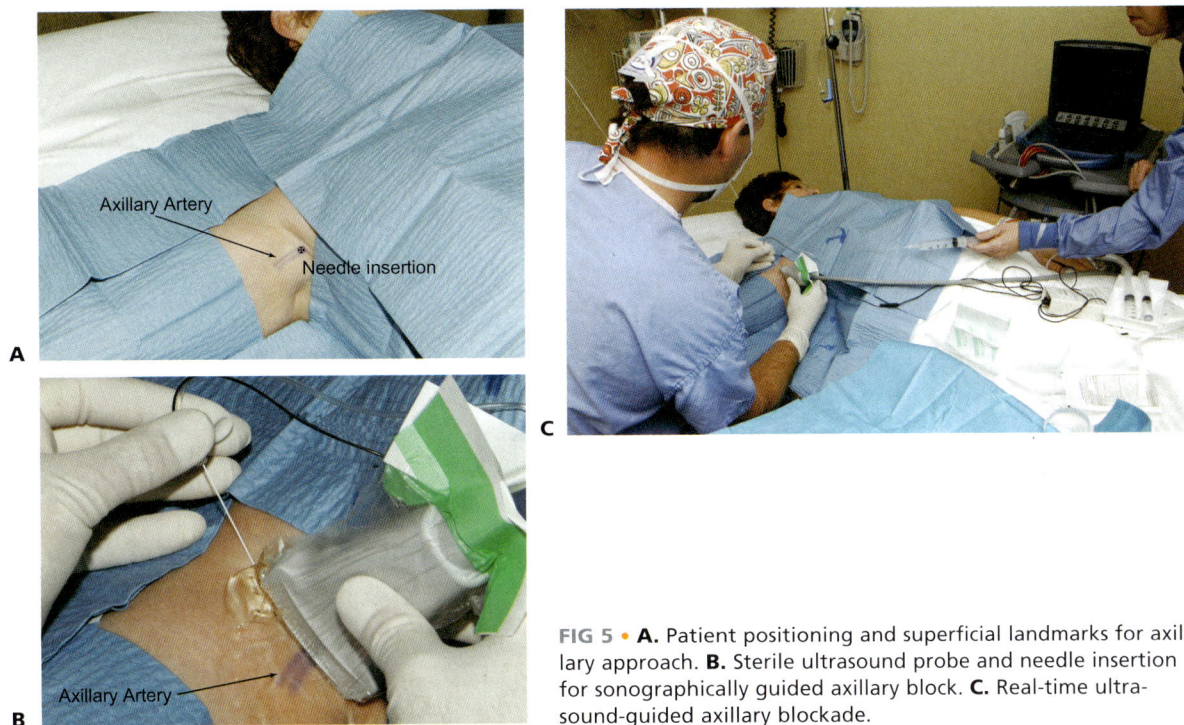

FIG 5 • A. Patient positioning and superficial landmarks for axillary approach. **B.** Sterile ultrasound probe and needle insertion for sonographically guided axillary block. **C.** Real-time ultrasound-guided axillary blockade.

Continuous Nerve Blocks

- Postoperative pain control after a single injection of local anesthesia is limited to 16 hours, and this limits its usefulness for postoperative pain management.
  - In a procedure associated with moderate to severe postoperative pain, patients experience significant pain when the block resolves.
  - Undertreated pain may result in more refractory pain states, such as chronic pain or complex regional pain syndromes.
- Because of the anatomic relationships of the upper extremity, a single catheter may provide continuous analgesia in the distribution of surgical pain.
  - The catheter is placed and local anesthetic administered preoperatively and combined with other analgesic interventions.
  - The surgical pain is not amplified at the tissue level or centrally in the spinal cord, so the pain is less intense and of shorter duration.[20]
- Continuous blocks may be maintained in the hospital as well as at home using disposable infusion pumps. To ensure success with home-going regional anesthesia, instructions and teaching must begin in the preoperative period.
  - Patients must be counseled about the danger of injury in the absence of normal pain responses. They are instructed to avoid working with extreme heat or cold and to avoid driving.
  - Patients are educated about symptoms of local anesthetic toxicity, and phone numbers are provided with instructions to call in the event of problems.
  - When continuous peripheral nerve catheters are part of a multimodal pain therapy consisting of nonsteroidal anti-inflammatory medications, acetaminophen, cryotherapy, and weak opioids, greater analgesia and patient satisfaction may be achieved.

- The efficacy of continuous interscalene blocks was demonstrated in patients treated with ropivacaine 0.2% after open rotator cuff surgery; they achieved pain scores averaging 1 out of 10 compared to placebo.[13]
  - Similar results were achieved with outpatient shoulder patients sent home with continuous interscalene blocks.[11]
- The efficacy of continuous infraclavicular blocks was demonstrated when ropivacaine 0.2% was administered to outpatients with moderately painful orthopaedic procedures; they achieved pain scores of 2 versus 6 in the placebo control group. The blocks were associated with less pain, resulting in fewer sleep disturbances, less opioid consumption, and fewer side effects.[10]
- Infusion pumps maintain the block by infusing dilute local anesthetic (bupivacaine 0.1% and ropivacaine 0.2%) at 10 cc/hr.
- Local anesthetic toxicity resulting from the continuous infusion is very rare. Local anesthetic toxicity is most likely during the initial injection (bolus with 30 to 40 cc of bupivacaine or ropivacaine 0.5%).

Local Anesthetics and Additives

- Local anesthetics produce anesthesia by inhibiting excitation of nerve endings and blocking conduction in peripheral nerves due to the binding and inactivation of both sodium and potassium channels. This prevents the sodium influx through these channels that is necessary for the depolarization of nerve cell membranes and propagation of impulses along the course of the nerve.
- There are two classes of local anesthetics, named for their linkage between the carbon chain and aromatic chain.
  - The amino amides have an amide link between the chain and the aromatic end, and amino esters have an ester link between the chain and the aromatic end.
  - The amino esters are metabolized in the plasma via pseudocholinesterases, and amino amides are metabolized in the liver.

Table 6	Local Anesthetic Dosages					
Local Anesthetic	Usual Concentration (%)	Usual Doses (mg/kg)	Maximum Dose, Plain[†] (mg/kg)	Maximum Dose with Epinephrine[†] (mg/kg)	Latency (min)	Duration of Effects (hr)
Lidocaine	0.5–2.0	5	7.5	10	5–15	0.75–2
Mepivacaine	0.5–1.5	5–7	7.5	10	5–15	1–1.25
Bupivacaine	0.25–0.5	2	2.5	3	15–30	2.5–6.0 (peripheral nerve block 15)
Ropivacaine	0.2–10.0	3	3.5	NA	10–20	2.5–5.0 (peripheral nerve block 14)

[†]Epinephrine is 1:200,000 concentration.

- Amino esters are eliminated rapidly compared with amides, decreasing the possibility of toxicity.
  - Amino esters are much more likely than amino amides to cause true allergic reactions due to metabolites like para-aminobenzoic acid.
- Varying the concentration of local anesthetics will produce a differential block. Higher concentrations produce an intense motor and sensory block. More dilute locals result in a sensory block with little motor blockade.
- Toxicity from local anesthesia occurs when a peak plasma level is reached, typically from inadvertent intravascular administration of anesthetic.
  - Toxicity from rapid absorption is also possible, especially in vascular areas (intercostal, epidural, or interscalene), and epinephrine is added to the local anesthetic to signal intravascular injection and decrease the vascular absorption of the local anesthetic.
  - The inadvertent intravascular injection of bupivacaine or ropivacaine may result in cardiovascular collapse (ventricular tachycardia or fibrillation).
    - Because of their potent binding to the heart, these arrests can be difficult to treat.
    - Cardiotoxicity from bupivacaine has been successfully treated with 2 mL/kg of 20% lipid emulsion in a case report.[21] The mechanism of the lipid emulsion is the binding of bupivacaine in the plasma and tissues. In other cases patients have required cardiopulmonary bypass until the conduction blockade resolved.
- Recommended doses of local anesthetics are given in Table 6.
- The use of additives with local anesthetics has increased as regional analgesia has become a standard method for managing postoperative pain.
  - Some additives prolong the duration of the block and therefore the postoperative pain control (Table 7).

EQUIPMENT

Airway Management

- For 30 minutes after a nerve block, patients must be closely monitored for signs of systemic toxicity.
- Medications to treat seizures and to establish general anesthesia must be immediately available.
- Induction drugs such as propofol and succinylcholine and airway equipment, including oxygen, an Ambu-bag with mask for positive-pressure ventilation, and a laryngoscope with assorted endotracheal tubes, should be nearby.

Monitoring

- The rare occurrence of local anesthetic toxicity mandates full monitoring in the operating room and in areas where blocks may be done before surgery.
- Pulse oximetry measures blood oxygen saturation in response to sedatives and analgesics, and the electrocardiogram is required to diagnose rhythm changes in the unlikely event of cardiac toxicity.
- Observation of the patient for early signs of central nervous system excitation is perhaps the best monitoring practice.

Regional Equipment

- The practice of regional anesthesia requires special equipment designed for peripheral nerve blockade.
- The nerve stimulator allows confirmation of the needle position adjacent to the nerve when a motor response is seen with low current output (0.5 mA; **FIG 6**).
  - In today's clinical practice, continuous nerve blocks for pain control are commonly placed using nerve stimulation.
- A newer technique uses ultrasound to visualize the nerve to be blocked.
  - With ultrasound, it is possible to visualize, in real time, images of the nerve, the needle approaching the nerve, and

Table 7	Additives to Local Anesthetics	
Additive	**Dosage**	**Effect on Intermediate Local Anesthetic**
Epinephrine	2.5 μg/mL	Prolonged
Clonidine	1.0 μg/kg	Prolonged
Opioids (alfentanil, sufentanil, morphine)		None
Buprenorphine	0.3 mg	None
Neostigmine		None
Ketamine		None
Sodium bicarbonate	1.0 mEq/10.0 mL	Faster onset

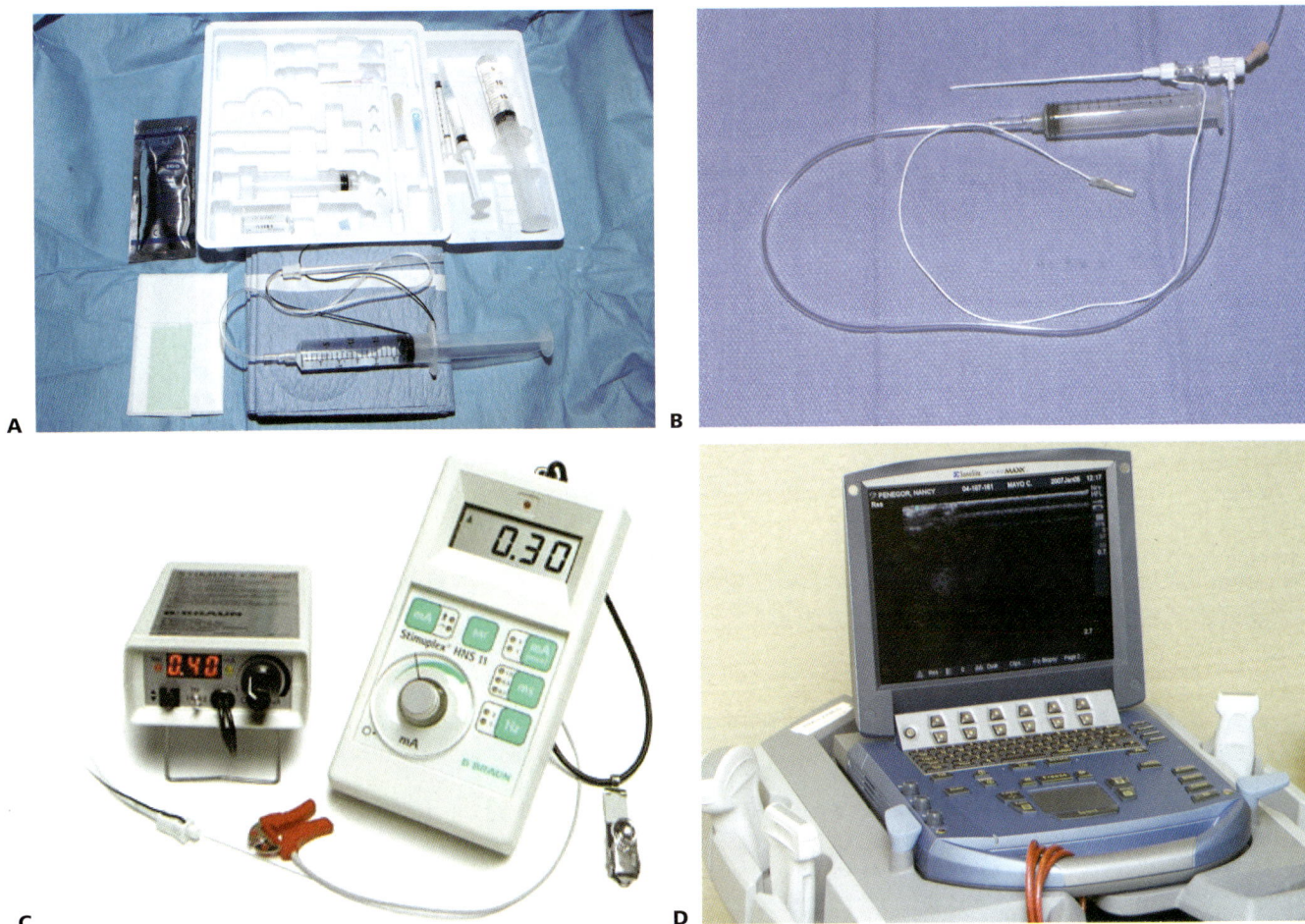

FIG 6 • **A.** Regional anesthesia sterile tray and stimulating needle. **B.** Regional anesthesia stimulating needle and catheter. **C.** Nerve stimulator. **D.** Portable ultrasound machine and transducers.

the local anesthesia or catheter being placed in the space around the nerve.

PAIN MANAGEMENT

Preemptive Analgesia

▪ Preemptive analgesia is implemented before a painful stimulus, which limits the sensitization of the nervous system to the pain. This should result in less intense pain of shorter duration.

▪ A dense, sustained nerve block inhibits the transmission of noxious afferent stimuli from the operative site to the spinal cord and brain.

▪ Multimodal pain control uses multiple analgesics affecting multiple pathways to maximize analgesia (Table 8).

   ▪ These interventions complement each other and often allow smaller individual drug doses to be used, thereby minimizing side effects.

Table 8	Nonopioid Analgesics				
Analgesic	**Dosage**	**Interval**	**Route**	**Maximum Dose**	**Comments**
Oral					
Aspirin	300–600	q4–6h	PO	3600 mg	
Acetaminophen	500–1000 mg	q4–6h	PO	4000 mg/d	Avoid in liver disease and glucose-6-phosphate deficiency.
Ibuprofen	200–400	q4–6h	PO	3200 mg	Avoid in renal insufficiency.
Naproxen	250–500 mg	q12	PO	1000 mg	
Celecoxib	400 mg initial; 200 mg	q12h	PO	800 mg	Avoid in renal insufficiency.
Tramadol	50–100 mg	q6h	PO	400 mg	Lower dosing in renal and hepatic disease
Gabapentin	600 mg initial; 300 mg	q8h	PO	2400 mg	
Parenteral					
Ketorolac	15 mg	q4–6h	IM/IV	<65 yr, 90 mg; >65 yr, 60 mg	Avoid in renal insufficiency.

Table 9	Narcotic Dosage Comparison	
	Dose (mg)	
Drug	**Oral**	**Parenteral**
Fentanyl	—	0.1
Meperidine	300	100
Morphine	30	10
Hydromorphone	7.5	1.5
Methadone	20	10
Tramadol	100	—
Codeine	200	130
Oxycodone	25	15

- The primary goal is to avoid hyperalgesia, allodynia, and increased pain.
- Acetaminophen is a weak analgesic, but it should be given preoperatively and postoperatively (1 g every 8 hours) unless contraindicated.
  - The drug acts on prostaglandin synthesis centrally, so there are no concerns with hyper- or hypo-coagulation side effects perioperatively.
- Celecoxib is currently the only available cyclooxygenase inhibitor available for clinical use.
  - It is an ideal nonsteroidal anti-inflammatory as it has no platelet and few gastrointestinal effects.
  - Caution should be exercised with chronic administration: strokes and myocardial infarctions have been reported after 18 months of regular use.
- Gabapentin has been shown to reduce pain and analgesic requirements when given preoperatively.
  - The drug is an N-methyl-D-aspartic acid antagonist, and it reduces hyperexcitability of dorsal horn neurons induced by tissue trauma.
  - Gabapentin is active only where there is tissue trauma and sensitization of nociceptive pathways, which distinguishes it from other analgesics.
  - Mild side effects include slight dizziness and somnolence.

Multimodal Analgesia Perioperative Pain Control

- Table 9 covers equianalgesic dosages of opioids.
- Table 10 summarizes multimodal postoperative pain control methods.

Chronic Pain

- Patients with chronic pain can be expected to have higher analgesic requirements after surgery.
- These patients are tolerant to the effects of opioids and tend to have very low thresholds for pain.
- Plans for pain management, in consultation between the surgeon, anesthesiologist, and patient, should be made preoperatively to optimally manage this acute-on-chronic pain state.
- The patient's chronic narcotic therapy should be continued and increased 30% to 40%, depending on the expected severity of the postoperative pain.
- Multimodal analgesia should be implemented before the procedure.
- Continuous peripheral nerve blocks are critical in the treatment of this population of patients.
- Reasonable expectations for analgesia should be discussed by the care team with the patient, and the goal for pain control should be to reach his or her average pain score.
  - The concept of pain as the "fifth vital sign" (postoperative pain score of 3 or less out of 10) will not apply to these patients.

INFORMED CONSENT

- The anesthesiologist must separately articulate both the risks and benefits of regional and general anesthetic options.
  - Patients are most often accepting of a regional technique once it has been explained properly and they understand the benefits of superior pain management and the avoidance of postoperative nausea and vomiting.
- The patient may make the final decision, but it is important for the surgical and anesthesia staff to recommend techniques associated with positive outcomes.
- The clinical impression is that regional anesthesia is safer than general anesthesia.
  - Numerous studies have examined the complication rate for general and regional anesthesia.
  - These studies have compared long-term outcomes between both techniques and have found no difference between regional and general anesthesia in terms of nonfatal myocardial infarction, unstable angina, or 6-month mortality.
  - This is reassuring, but there are other outcomes important when choosing an anesthetic plan.

Table 10	Multimodal Postoperative Pain Management		
Drug	**Mild Postoperative Pain**	**Moderate Postoperative Pain**	**Severe Postoperative Pain**
Acetaminophen	Preop: 1000 mg Postop: 1000 mg q8h	Preop: 1000 mg Postop: 1000 mg q8h	Preop: 1000 mg Postop: 1000 mg q8h
Celecoxib	Preop: 400 mg Postop: 200 mg q12h	Preop: 400 mg Postop: 200 mg q12h	Preop: 400 mg Postop: 200 mg q12h
Gabapentin		600 mg	600 mg/300 mg q8h
Oxycodone SR			
Pt <65 yr		Preop: 10 mg Postop: 10 mg q12h	Preop: 20 mg Postop: 20 mg q12h
Pt >65 yr			Preop: 10 mg Postop: 10 mg q12h
Oxycodone IR		Assess pain score (0–10) 4 or 5: 5 mg q4h 6–10: 10 mg q4h	Assess pain score (0–10) 4 or 5: 5 mg q2h 6–10: 10 mg q2h

COMPLICATIONS

General Anesthesia

- The perceived efficiencies of general anesthesia may not be evident in the postoperative period where more complications must be managed, and the level of postoperative care with general anesthesia will be dictated by these complications.

Postoperative Nausea and Vomiting

- Avoiding postoperative nausea and vomiting (PONV) is a high priority because of the expense resulting from treatments and subsequent delays.
  - PONV may not respond to treatment, leading to an unplanned hospital admission.
  - Patient satisfaction surveys have determined that patients often find PONV more unpleasant than postoperative pain.
- Postoperative nausea and vomiting risk is related to age.
  - There is a low risk in children less than 2 years old, but the risk increases until puberty and then drops as aging occurs.
- Patients with prior PONV or who have motion sickness have a higher risk of PONV with general anesthesia.
  - Women have a higher incidence of PONV.
  - Nonsmokers have a higher risk of PONV.
- The risk of PONV varies with the type of surgery.
  - Ear, nose, and throat and dental procedures have a high incidence of PONV, followed by orthopaedic and plastic surgery.
  - Procedures such as strabismus, peritoneal, testicular, and middle ear surgeries are associated with PONV.
- The risk of PONV is higher with general anesthesia than regional anesthesia.
  - General anesthetics such as the inhalational gasses (nitrous oxide, sevoflurane, and desflurane) increase the incidence of PONV compared to propofol.
- Droperidol (0.625 mg) has been a PONV treatment mainstay because of its efficacy and low cost.
  - However, as a result of isolated cardiac events with large doses of droperidol (1.25 to 2.5 mg) in the presence of prolonged Q-T syndrome, the U.S. Food and Drug Administration has issued a black box warning for its clinical use.
- Table 11 summarizes factors related to patient and surgery and lists treatment guidelines.

Urine Retention

- Voiding difficulty is common after spinal anesthesia and in patients with prostatic hypertrophy as well as in urology, inguinal hernia, and genital procedures.
- The use of parenteral opioids to control significant pain will increase the incidence of urine retention.
- For procedures associated with a low risk of urine retention, patients may be discharged without demonstration of voiding.
- Patients must be instructed to return for evaluation if they have not voided in a specified time frame.

Postanesthetic Injuries

- Corneal abrasion
  - Corneal abrasion may occur due to drying of the cornea or incidental trauma during mask ventilation or intubation or as a result of the patient rubbing the eyes after the procedure.

Table 11	Postoperative Nausea and Vomiting Prophylaxis and Treatment

Factors

Patient
  Premenopausal female
  History of motion sickness
  History of PONV
  Nonsmoker
Surgical
  Laparoscopic/laparotomy
  Plastic surgery
  Otolaryngology
  Strabismus surgery

Treatment

Monitored anesthesia care or regional anesthesia
  No treatment required
Two factors
  Dexamethasone 8 mg at induction of anesthesia
  Odansetron (Zofran) 4 mg at end of surgery
Three or four factors
  Dexamethasone 8 mg at induction of anesthesia
  Droperidol 0.625 mg at induction of anesthesia (Q-T interval less than 440 msec)
Five factors
  Dexamethasone 8 mg at induction of anesthesia
  Droperidol 0.625 mg at induction of anesthesia (Q-T interval less than 440 msec)
  Odansetron (Zofran) 4 mg at end of surgery
  Total intravenous anesthesia with propofol

- The symptoms of corneal abrasion include redness, tearing, photophobia, decreased visual acuity, and pain.
- They are usually self-limited, resolving in 24 to 48 hours, and artificial tears and an eye patch are standard treatments.
- Severe abrasions may warrant ophthalmologic consultation as they may lead to cataract formation.
- Pharyngeal injuries
  - Endotracheal intubation may cause a sore throat in 20% to 50% of patients, depending on the amount of trauma during laryngoscopy or oropharyngeal suctioning.
  - Local anesthetic ointments during anesthesia, once thought to prevent sore throats, may also result in airway irritation. This may present as pain or as unquenchable thirst.
  - Mucosal trauma may also be the result of the laryngeal mask airway, despite the impression that they are less invasive and traumatic than endotracheal tubes.
  - Dental damage may occur during the induction or emergence from anesthesia.
    - Any dental damage should be carefully documented, and dental consultation may be needed depending on the extent of the injury.
    - Lip, gum, or tongue damage may be treated with ice to manage the pain and inflammation.
- Nerve injuries
  - Nerve injuries may occur during general anesthesia from improper positioning and padding during the procedure.
  - Injury may occur from compression or stretch of the neural tissue.

- Nerve injury is usually thought to be associated with regional anesthesia, but the incidence of nerve injury is higher with general anesthesia (ulnar nerve).

Regional Anesthesia

Nerve Injury

- The incidence of nerve injury was evaluated in a large retrospective European study involving over 150,000 regional anesthetics.[1]
  - The anesthetics were administered over a 10-month period; over 50,000 were peripheral nerve blocks. The incidence of peripheral nerve injury was 0.04% (4/10,000). Peripheral nerve injury occurred in 12 patients, and the symptoms were present after 6 months in 7 patients.
  - Much has been written about the risks of nerve injury after peripheral nerve blocks, but it is only recently that the positive merits of these techniques have been discussed.
- Peripheral nerve injury with regional anesthesia may be the result of direct needle or catheter trauma, local anesthetic toxicity, or vasoconstrictors added to the local solution.
- Severe injuries occurred, in adult patients under general anesthesia, when local anesthetic was inadvertently injected into the spinal cord. This resulted in irreversible paralysis.[2]
- Short-beveled needles do not result in fewer cases of nerve injury compared with long-beveled needles, as had previously been believed.
  - The neural repair appears more rapid after injury from a long-beveled needle according to animal data, although there are no clinical data to support this.
- Patient factors increasing the risk of nerve injury include diabetes mellitus, pre-existing nerve injury, male sex, and older age.
- Surgical factors associated with a higher rate of nerve injury include trauma, stretch, positioning, tourniquet ischemia, and cast compression.
- Neurologic changes should be evaluated urgently so that treatable causes such as hematoma, constrictive dressings, and abscess formation may be diagnosed and treated, limiting the extent of injury.
- If significant nerve injury is suspected, documentation of neurologic status and neurology consultation with early and late electromyography are advisable.

Infectious Complications

- Infection may result after a nerve block from the contamination of the needle or local anesthetics as well as from bacteremia.
  - This would be less likely with a single injection block because the local anesthetics used in regional anesthesia are bactericidal (bupivacaine at a concentration of at least 0.25%).
  - Infection is more likely with a continuous block as the catheter is a track for bacteria and dilute local anesthetics are less bactericidal.
  - Local infection at the site of the block is a clear contraindication to a regional anesthetic, especially catheter placement.
- Bacterial colonization of continuous nerve blocks was examined by Capdevila et al.[4]
  - In the 969 catheters that were cultured, bacterial colonization was found to be present in 28.7% (278), but only 3% of the patients had signs of local inflammation at the site.
  - The bacteria most often identified were coagulase-negative staphylococci (*Staphylococcus epidermidis*; 61%),

gram-negative bacillus (21.6%), and *Staphylococcus aureus* (17.6%).
- Localized inflammation or infection at the site is associated with factors such as catheter duration greater than 48 hours, male sex, absence of antibiotic prophylaxis, and postoperative monitoring in the intensive care unit.[4]
  - It is our practice to limit the peripheral nerve catheter and infusion to 48 hours.
  - Catheters are tunneled under the skin for prolonged analgesia, preventing bacteria from migrating to deeper tissue planes.

Hemorrhagic Complications

- The risk of bleeding during regional anesthesia, although rare, is always present because of the anatomic relationships of nerves and vascular structures.
- Hematoma formation has been reported with almost every nerve block approach, and superficial bruising is very common.
- A high index of suspicion will allow early diagnosis and treatment, avoiding permanent injury.
- Patients at particularly high risk for hemorrhagic complications are those receiving low-molecular-weight heparins, antiplatelet drugs such as clopidogrel (Plavix), therapeutic Coumadin levels, and antithrombolytic drugs.
- Hematomas should be considered in the setting of an evolving neural deficit and obviously if vascular injury occurred during the technique.
- Acute hematoma formation may be handled conservatively by holding pressure for at least 5 minutes and continued observation.
- A large hematoma that continues to expand or is causing acute neural deficits will require surgical drainage to preserve nerve function.
  - Imaging such as ultrasound or CT scanning may confirm the diagnosis before surgery if there is doubt.

Local Anesthetic Toxicity

- Local anesthetics in the proper concentration and dosage are safe. When local anesthesia is inadvertently injected intravascularly, seizures may occur.
- Seizures result due to high concentration of local anesthesia in the plasma despite binding by albumin and alpha-1 acid glycoprotein.
- The seizures tend to be short with the prompt administration of benzodiazepines and positive-pressure ventilation.
- When a significant portion of a bupivacaine dose becomes intravascular, death has occurred as a result of the cardiac conduction being blocked, which resulted in cardiovascular collapse.
- Factors affecting toxicity of local anesthetics
  - Location of block (intercostal, epidural, or interscalene)
  - Patient characteristics (extremes of age, parturients, hypoalbuminemia)
  - Pharmacologic factors
- Toxicity: bupivacaine> ropivacaine >> mepivacaine>> lidocaine

Perioperative Considerations

- The proper selection of anesthetic techniques for orthopaedic surgery begins with the consideration of surgical and patient factors. Additionally, factors such as safety, cost-effectiveness, and efficiency are considered.

- A well-organized surgical and anesthetic practice allows patients to receive nerve blocks before going to the operating room.
  - Peripheral nerve blocks need not delay surgery or fail if proper utilization of the induction room occurs.
  - Operating room efficiency and turnover are increased in this manner. The patient will be sedated and have monitors, intravenous access, and a functional regional block in place when he or she enters the operating room.
- The regional patient will also bypass the postanesthesia care unit and may move to the outpatient or regular nursing area without delay.
  - The upper extremity is uniquely suited for regional anesthesia because the brachial plexus may be anesthetized with one injection, and continuous blocks may be maintained postoperatively, providing extended analgesia.
- Whether general, regional, or a combination is selected for anesthesia, patients' perioperative experiences are improving.
  - In the past, regional anesthesia was selected for safety reasons, and now regional anesthesia is being administered for its superior pain control.
  - In the future, anesthetics may be selected based on the patient's genotype, and the patient may have surgery and postoperative pain control without needles, catheters, or even a general anesthesia. Until then, regional techniques, in conjunction with multimodal analgesic protocols, will continue to be the care standard after orthopaedic surgery.

REFERENCES

1. Auroy Y, Benhamou D, Barques L, et al. Major complications of regional anesthesia in France. Anesthesiology 2002;97:1274–1280.
2. Benumof JL. Permanent loss of cervical spinal cord function associated with interscalene block performed under general anesthesia. Anesthesiology 2000;93:1541–1544.
3. Canet J, Raeder J, Rasmussen LS, et al. Cognitive dysfunction after minor surgery in the elderly. Acta Anaesth Scand 2003;47:1204–1210.
4. Capdevila X, Pirat P, Bringuier S, et al. Continuous peripheral nerve blocks in hospital wards after orthopedic surgery: a multicenter prospective analysis of the quality of postoperative analgesia and complications in 1,416 patients. Anesthesiology 2005;103:1035–1045.
5. Chung F, Ritchie E, Su J. Postoperative pain in ambulatory surgery. Anesth Analg 1997;85:808–816.
6. Cohen NP, Levine WN, Marra G, et al. Indwelling interscalene catheter anesthesia in the surgical management of stiff shoulder: a report of 100 consecutive cases. J Shoulder Elbow Surg 2000;9: 268–274.
7. Del Rincon ID, Williams K, Stern MP, et al. High incidence of cardiovascular events in a rheumatoid arthritis cohort not explained by traditional cardiac risk factors. Arthritis Rheum 2001;44:2737–2745.
8. Hadzic A, Arliss J, Kerimoglu B, et al. A comparison of infraclavicular nerve block versus general anesthesia for hand and wrist day-case surgeries. Anesthesiology 2004;101:127–132.
9. Hall MJ, Lawrence L. Ambulatory surgery in the United States, 1996. Adv Data 1998;300:1–16.
10. Ilfeld BM, Morey TE, Enneking FK. Continuous infraclavicular brachial plexus block for postoperative pain control at home: a randomized, double-blinded, placebo-controlled study. Anesthesiology 2002;96:1297–1304.
11. Ilfeld BM, Morey TE, Wright TW, et al. Continuous interscalene brachial plexus block for postoperative pain control at home: a randomized, double-blinded, placebo-controlled study. Anesth Analg 2003;96:1089–1095.
12. Klein SM, Bergh A, Steele S. Thoracic paravertebral block for breast surgery. Anesth Analg 2000;90:1402–1405.
13. Klein SM, Grant SA, Greengrass RA, et al. Interscalene brachial plexus block with a continuous catheter insertion system and a disposable infusion pump. Anesth Analg 2000;91:1473–1478.
14. Klein SM, Nielson KC, Greengrass R. Ambulatory discharge after long-acting peripheral nerve blockade. Anesth Analg 2002;94:65–70.
15. Larson S, Lundberg D. A prospective survey of nausea and vomiting. Act Anesth Scand 1995;39:539–545.
16. Lee LA, Domino KB, Caplan RA. Complications associated with peripheral nerve blocks: lessons From the ASA Closed Claims Project. Anesthesiology 2004;101:143–152.
17. Maione S, Valentini G, Giunta A, et al. Cardiac involvement in rheumatoid arthritis: an echocardiographic study. Cardiology 1993; 83:234–239.
18. McNeely JK, Farber NE, Rusy LM, et al. Epidural analgesia improves outcome following pediatric fundoplication. Reg Anesth 1997;22: 16–23.
19. Navarro-Cano G, Del Rincon I, Pogosian S, et al. Association of mortality with disease severity in rheumatoid arthritis, independent of comorbidity. Arthritis Rheum 2003;48:2425–2433.
20. Ong CK, Lirk P, Seymour RA, et al. The efficacy of preemptive analgesia for acute postoperative pain management: a meta-analysis. Anesthesia Analgesia 2005;100:757–773.
21. Rosenblatt MA, Abel M, Fischer GW, et al. Successful use of a 20% lipid emulsion to resuscitate a patient after a presumed bupivacaine-related cardiac arrest. Anesthesiology 2006;105:217–218.
22. Tobias JD. Continuous femoral nerve block to provide analgesia following femur fracture in a pediatric ICU population. Anaesth Intensive Care 1994;22:616–618.
23. Weltz CR, Greengrass R, Lyerly H. Ambulatory surgery management of breast carcinoma using paravertebral block. Ann Surg 1995;222:19–26.

Chapter 3

Arthroscopy of the Hand and Wrist

David J. Slutsky

BACKGROUND

- Since its inception, wrist arthroscopy has continued to evolve. The initial emphasis on viewing the wrist from the dorsal aspect arose from the relative lack of neurovascular structures as well as the familiarity of most surgeons with dorsal approaches to the radiocarpal joint.
- Anatomic studies provided a better understanding of both the interosseous ligaments as well as carpal kinematics, which led to the development of midcarpal arthroscopy.
- Innovative surgeons continue to push the envelope through the development of techniques for treating intracarpal pathology, which in turn has culminated in a plethora of new accessory portals.

ANATOMY

- The standard portals for wrist arthroscopy are dorsal (**FIG 1A–C**). This is in part due to the relative lack of neurovascular structures on the dorsum of the wrist as well as the initial emphasis on assessing the volar wrist ligaments. The dorsal portals that allow access to the radiocarpal joint are so named in relation to the tendons of the dorsal extensor compartments.
  - The 1–2 portal lies between the first extensor compartment tendons, which include the extensor pollicis brevis and the abductor pollicis longus, and the second extensor compartment, which contains the extensor carpi radialis brevis and longus (**FIG 1D**).

- The 3–4 portal is named for the interval between the third dorsal extensor compartment, which contains the extensor pollicis longus tendon, and the fourth extensor compartment, which contains the extensor digitorum communis (EDC) tendons.
- The 4–5 portal is located between the EDC and the extensor digiti minimi (EDM).
- The 6R portal is located on the radial side of the extensor carpi ulnaris (ECU) tendon; the 6U portal is located on the ulnar side.
- The midcarpal joint is assessed through two portals, which allows triangulation of the arthroscope and the instrumentation.
  - The midcarpal radial portal is located 1 cm distal to the 3–4 portal and is bounded radially by the extensor carpi radialis brevis and ulnarly by the EDC.
  - The midcarpal ulnar portal is similarly located 1 to 2 cm distal to the 4–5 portal and is bounded by the EDC and the EDM.
- The triquetrohamate portal enters the midcarpal joint at the level of the triquetrohamate joint ulnar to the ECU tendon. The entry site is both ulnar and distal to the midcarpal ulnar portal. Branches of the dorsal cutaneous branch of the ulnar nerve are most at risk (**FIG 2A**).
- The dorsal radioulnar joint portal lies between the ECU and the EDM tendons. Transverse branches of the dorsal cutaneous branch of the ulnar nerve are the only sensory

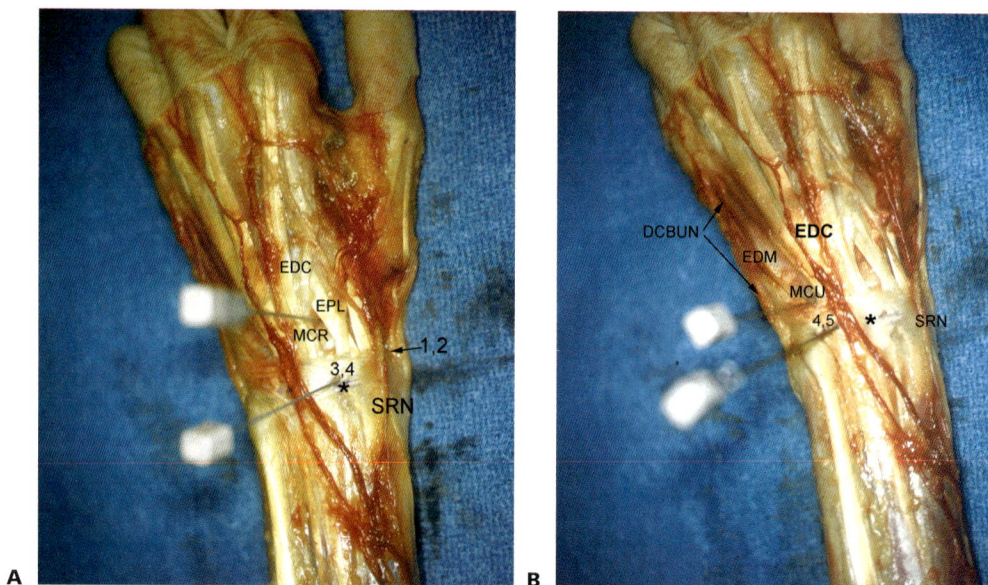

A

B

FIG 1 • Dorsal portal anatomy. **A.** Cadaver dissection of the dorsal aspect of a left wrist demonstrating the relative positions of the dorsoradial portals. *EDC*, extensor digitorum communis; *EPL*, extensor pollicis longus; *SRN*, superficial radial nerve; *, tubercle of Lister. **B.** Relative positions of the dorsoulnar portals. *EDM*, extensor digiti minimi; *DCBUN*, dorsal cutaneous branch of the ulnar nerve. *(continued)*

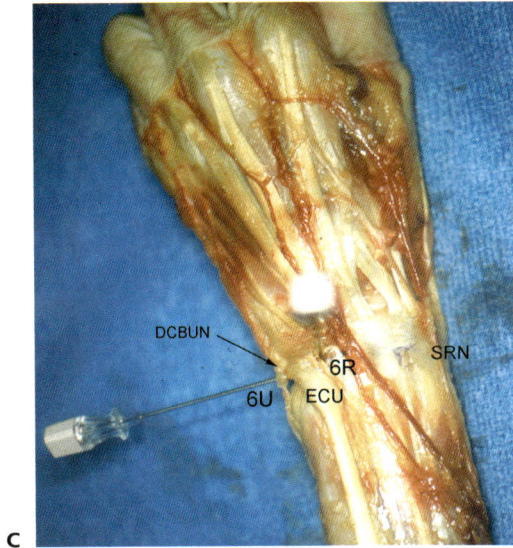

C

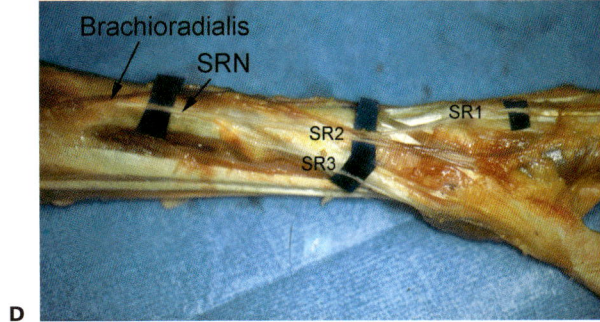

D

FIG 1 • *(continued)* C. Positions of the 6R and 6U portals. **D.** Branches of the superficial radial nerve (SRN). *SR1*, minor dorsal branch; *SR2*, major dorsal branch; *SR3*, major palmar branch. (From Slutsky DJ. Wrist arthroscopy portals. In Slutsky DJ, Nagle DJ, eds. Techniques in Hand and Wrist Arthroscopy. Philadelphia: Elsevier, 2007.)

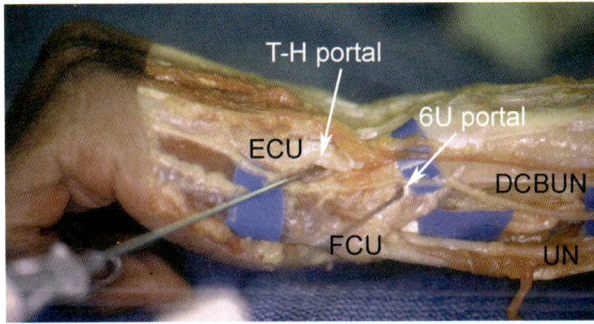

A

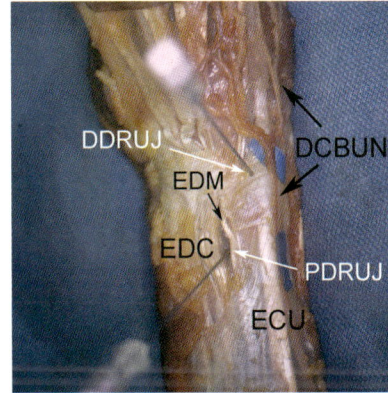

B

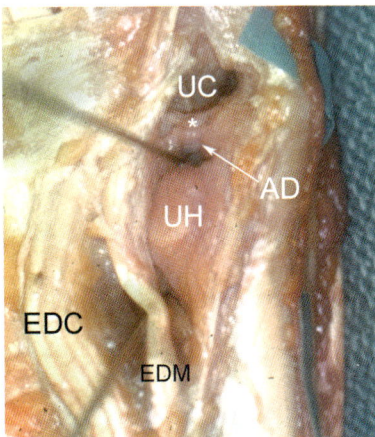

C

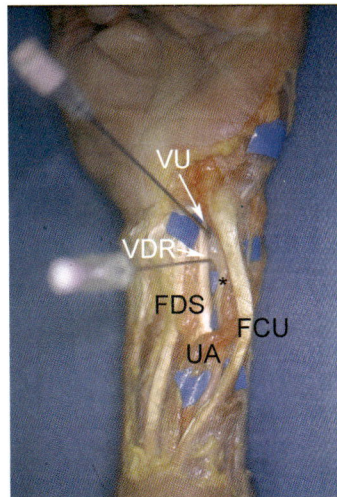

D

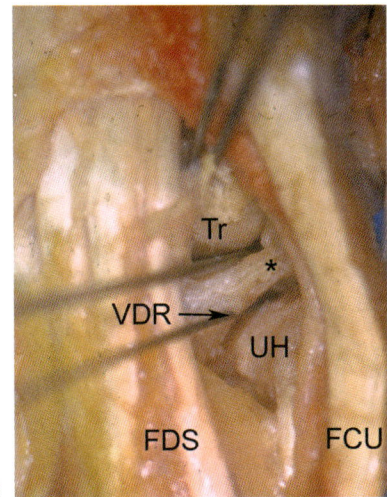

E

FIG 2 • A. Ulnar aspect of a left wrist demonstrating the relative positions of the triquetrohamate (T-H) portal and the 6U portal. *DCBUN*, dorsal cutaneous branch of the ulnar nerve; *UN*, ulnar nerve. **B,C.** Dorsal distal radioulnar joint (DRUJ) portal anatomy. **B.** Relative position of the proximal (PDRUJ) and distal (DDRUJ) portals. **C.** Close-up with the dorsal capsule removed demonstrating the position of the needles in relation to the dorsal radioulnar ligament (*). *AD*, articular disc; *UC*, ulnocarpal joint; *UH*, ulnar head. **D,E.** Volar DRUJ portals. **D.** Volar aspect of a left wrist demonstrating the relative positions of the volar ulnar (VU) and volar DRUJ (VDR) portals in relation to the ulnar nerve (*) and ulnar artery (UA). *FDS*, flexor digitorum sublimis; *FCU*, flexor carpi ulnaris. **E.** Close-up view after the volar capsule is removed showing position of needles in relation to the volar radioulnar ligament (*). *Tr*, triquetrum; *UH*, ulnar head. (From Slutsky DJ. Wrist arthroscopy portals. In Slutsky DJ, Nagle DJ, eds. Techniques in Hand and Wrist Arthroscopy. Philadelphia: Elsevier, 2007.)

nerves in proximity to the dorsal radioulnar portal, at a mean of 17.5 mm distally (range 10–20 mm) (**FIG 2B,C**).

- There are two volar portals that can be used to access the radiocarpal joint.

  - The volar radial portal is accessed through the floor of the flexor carpi radialis tendon sheath at the level of the proximal wrist crease.[5,7,9]

    - Anatomic studies revealed that there is a safe zone free of any neurovascular structures, equal to the width of the flexor carpi radialis tendon plus at least 3 mm in all directions.

    - The volar aspect of the midcarpal joint can be accessed through the volar radial midcarpal portal. The same skin incision is used but the capsular entry point is about 1 cm distal.

  - The volar ulnar portal is located underneath the ulnar border of the flexor tendons at the level of the proximal wrist crease.[6]

- The volar aspect of the distal radioulnar joint (DRUJ) can be accessed through the volar distal radioulnar portal using the same skin incision, but the capsular entry point for the volar distal radioulnar portal lies 5 mm to 1 cm proximal to the ulnocarpal entry point (**FIG 2D,E**).

AUTHOR'S EXPERIENCE

- The volar radial portal has been used in 111 patients since 1998.[4]

  - Additional pathology was evident in 61 of the patients that was not visible from any standard dorsal portals. This included 1 case of hypertrophic synovitis of the dorsal capsule (**FIG 3A**), 1 patient with an avulsion of the radioscapholunate ligament that exposed the volar scapholunate cleft (**FIG 3B**), 2 patients with tears restricted to the palmar region of the scapholunate interosseous ligament (SLIL), and 57 patients with tears of the dorsal radiocarpal ligament (DRCL). In 16 patients an isolated DRCL tear alone was responsible for chronic dorsal wrist pain (**FIG 3C,D**).

- The midcarpal joint was accessed from the volar radial portal in three cases. In one patient with Preiser disease, the use of the volar radial midcarpal portal allowed a more complete assessment of the distal articular surface of the

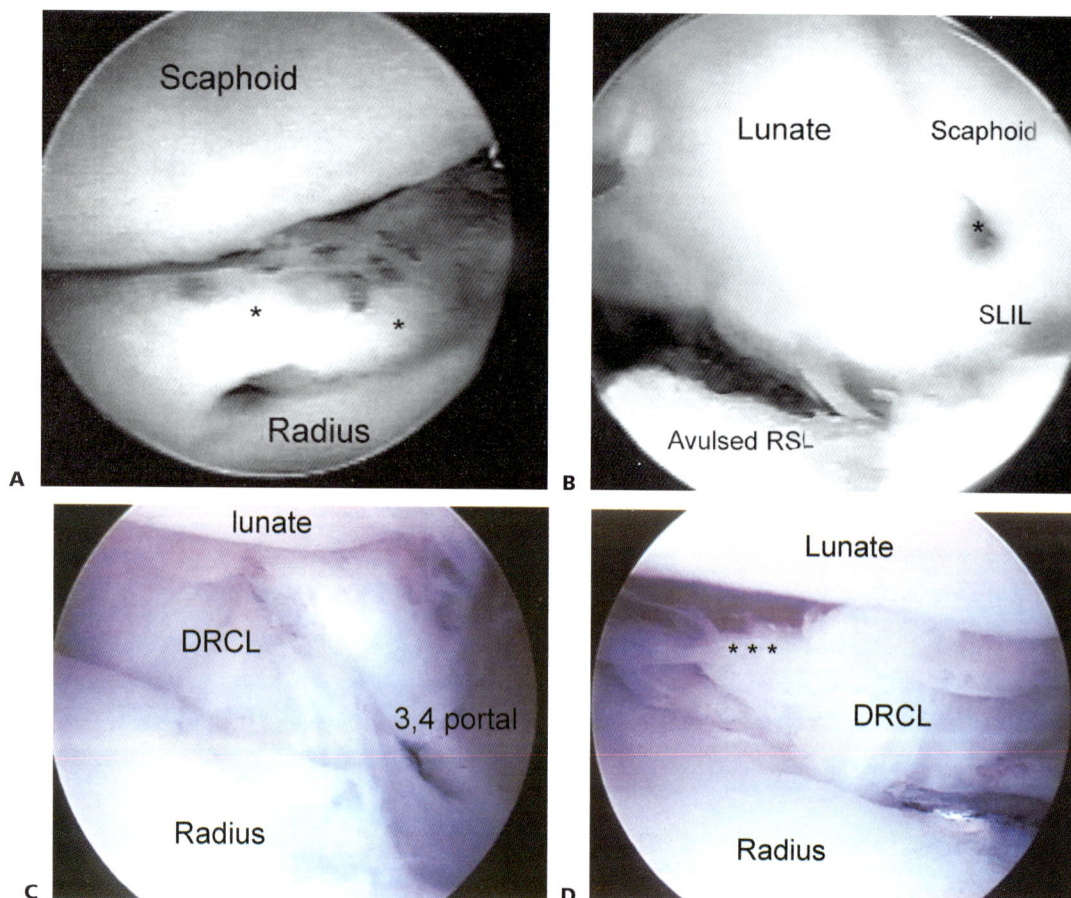

FIG 3 • A. Hypertrophic synovitis (*) of the dorsal capsule in a case of Presier disease as seen through the volar radial portal. **B.** Radioscapholunate ligament avulsion. Note unmasking of the palmar cleft (*) between the scaphoid and lunate. *SLIL,* scapholunate interosseous ligament; *RSL,* radioscapholunate ligament. **C,D.** Volar radial portal view. **C.** Normal dorsal radiocarpal ligament. Hook probe is inserted through the 3–4 portal. *SLIL,* scapholunate interosseous ligament; *DRCL,* dorsal radiocarpal ligament. **D.** DRCL tear (*). Hook probe inserted through the 3–4 portal. *(continued)*

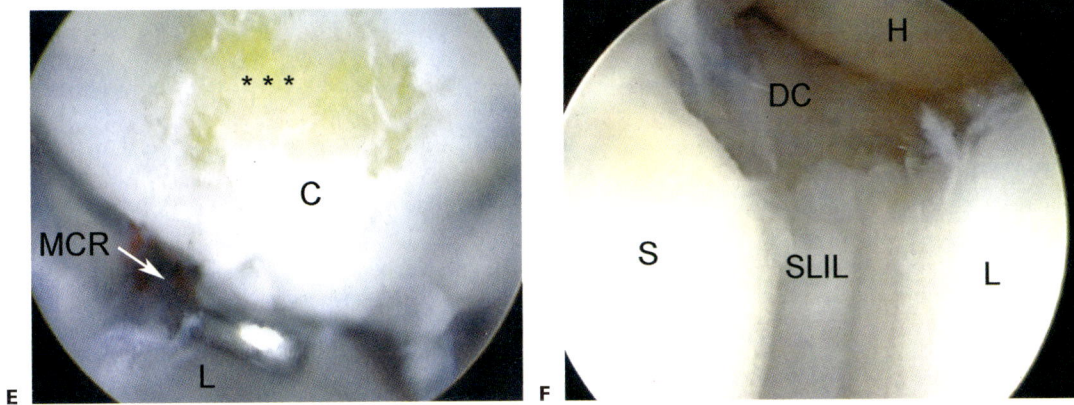

FIG 3 • *(continued)* Volar midcarpal portal. **E.** Chondromalacia of the palmar capitate (C). Probe is in the midcarpal radial portal (MCR). *L,* lunate. **F.** Tear of the palmar region of the scapholunate interosseous ligament (SLIL), as viewed from the volar radial midcarpal portal. Note the intact dorsal fibers of the SLIL. *S,* scaphoid; *L,* lunate; *H,* hamate; *DC,* dorsal capsule. (**A,B**: From Slutsky DJ. Wrist arthroscopy through a volar radial portal. Arthroscopy 2002;18:624–630, with permission.)

scaphoid. Another patient had unrecognized chondromalacia of the palmar capitate following a perilunate dislocation (**FIG 3E**). The volar radial midcarpal portal admirably demonstrated the intact dorsal portion of the SLIL in the patient with the palmar tear (**FIG 3F**).

■ The volar ulnar portal has been used in 61 patients since 1998.[8]

▪ The ulnar-sided pathology included 21 tears of the lunotriquetral interosseous ligament (LTIL) (**FIG 4A**), 19 triangular fibrocartilage complex (TFCC) tears, and 2 ulnolunate ligament tears. In one patient a TFCC tear was found to extend into the dorsoulnar ligament (**FIG 4B,C**). The volar ulnar portal facilitated débridement of the palmar region of the LTIL ligament through the 6R or 6U portals. In three of these

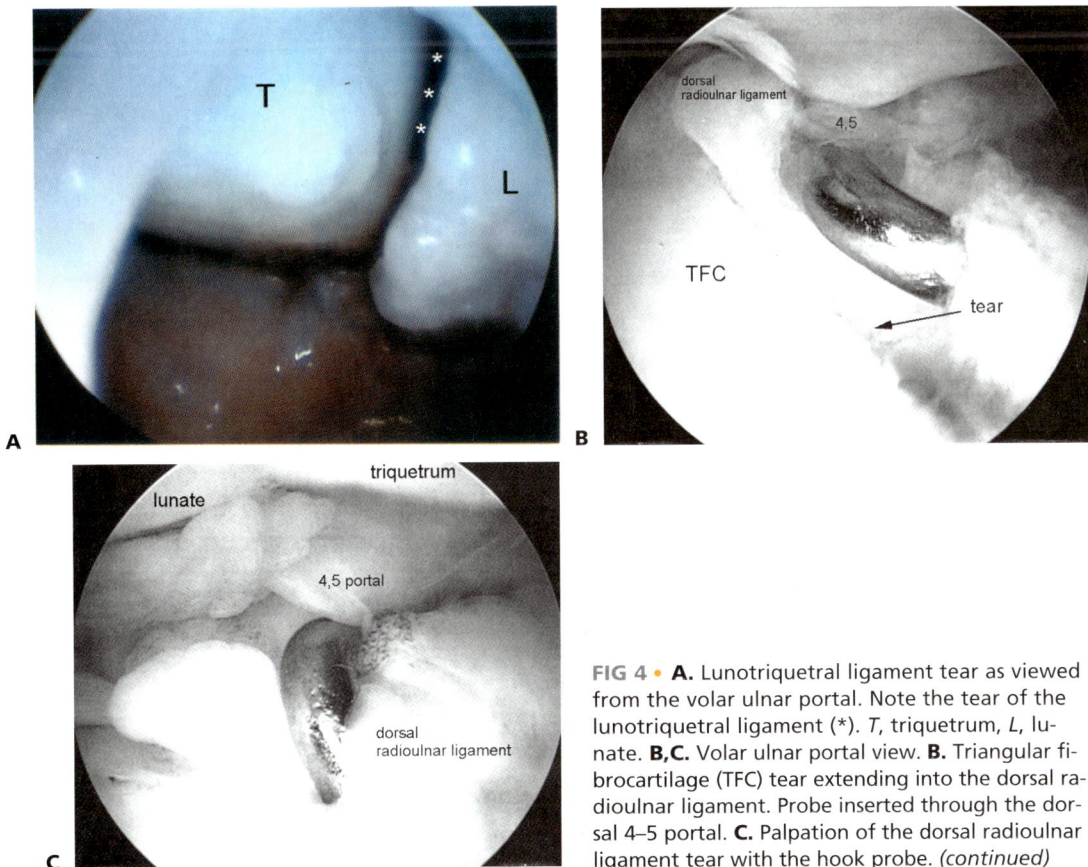

FIG 4 • A. Lunotriquetral ligament tear as viewed from the volar ulnar portal. Note the tear of the lunotriquetral ligament (*). *T,* triquetrum, *L,* lunate. **B,C.** Volar ulnar portal view. **B.** Triangular fibrocartilage (TFC) tear extending into the dorsal radioulnar ligament. Probe inserted through the dorsal 4–5 portal. **C.** Palpation of the dorsal radioulnar ligament tear with the hook probe. *(continued)*

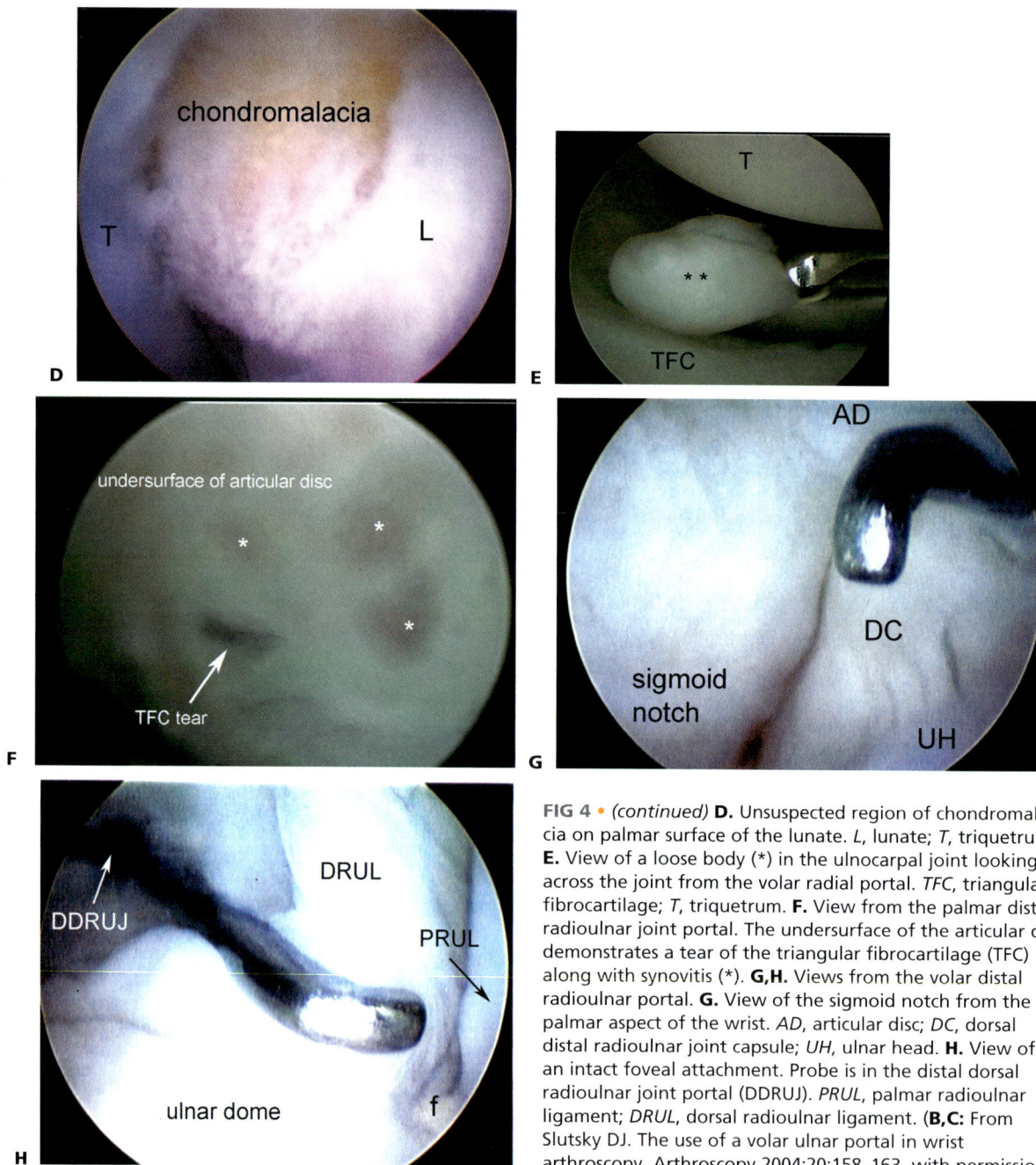

FIG 4 • *(continued)* **D.** Unsuspected region of chondromalacia on palmar surface of the lunate. *L*, lunate; *T*, triquetrum. **E.** View of a loose body (*) in the ulnocarpal joint looking across the joint from the volar radial portal. *TFC*, triangular fibrocartilage; *T*, triquetrum. **F.** View from the palmar distal radioulnar joint portal. The undersurface of the articular disc demonstrates a tear of the triangular fibrocartilage (TFC) along with synovitis (*). **G,H.** Views from the volar distal radioulnar portal. **G.** View of the sigmoid notch from the palmar aspect of the wrist. *AD*, articular disc; *DC*, dorsal distal radioulnar joint capsule; *UH*, ulnar head. **H.** View of an intact foveal attachment. Probe is in the distal dorsal radioulnar joint portal (DDRUJ). *PRUL*, palmar radioulnar ligament; *DRUL*, dorsal radioulnar ligament. (**B,C:** From Slutsky DJ. The use of a volar ulnar portal in wrist arthroscopy. Arthroscopy 2004;20:158–163, with permission.)

patients unrecognized chondromalacia of the palmar aspect of the lunate was identified (**FIG 4D**), and one patient had chondromalacia of the palmar triquetrum. One patient was found to have a loose body in the ulnocarpal joint (**FIG 4E**).

■ The volar aspect of the DRUJ was accessed in eight of these patients to rule out a peripheral TFCC tear. The DRUJ was well visualized, demonstrating an intact articular disc in four and a full-thickness tear with undersurface fibrillation in one (**FIG 4F**). The foveal attachment of the TFCC was seen to be intact in each case (**FIG 4G,H**).

NONOPERATIVE MANAGEMENT

■ In general, wrist arthroscopy is indicated as a diagnostic technique in any patient with persistent wrist pain that has not responded to an appropriate trial of conservative measures:

   ■ Nonsteroidal anti-inflammatories and activity modification
   ■ Cortisone injection

■ Wrist arthroscopy is used as an adjuvant procedure for the treatment of acute fractures of the distal radius or scaphoid, or for staging degenerative disorders involving the carpus.

Indications

■ The indications for the use of the standard dorsal portals are intertwined with the indications for wrist arthroscopy and depend largely on the condition that is being treated.

   ■ A typical arthroscopic examination of the wrist will include variable combinations of the 3–4 portal, the 4–5 portal, and the 6R and 6U portals.

- The 3–4 and 4–5 portals are the main viewing portals for the radial aspect of the radiocarpal joint and for instrumentation.
  - The 4–5 and 6R portals are used to access the ulnocarpal joint.
  - The 6U portal is typically used for outflow.
- The volar radial portal is indicated for the evaluation of the DRCL and the palmar portion of the SLIL. The volar radial portal also facilitates arthroscopic reduction of intra-articular fractures of the distal radius fractures by providing a clear view of the dorsal rim fragments.
- The volar ulnar portal is indicated for visualizing and débriding palmar tears of the lunotriquetral ligament. It also aids in the repair or débridement of dorsally located TFCC tears since the proximity of the 4–5 and 6R portals makes triangulation of the instruments difficult.
- Midcarpal arthroscopy through the dorsal midcarpal portals is essential in making the diagnoses of scapholunate and lunotriquetral instability.
  - The grading scale reported by Geissler and colleagues[2] provides a means for staging the degree of instability and provides an algorithm for treatment.
  - Midcarpal arthroscopy is likewise employed for the assessment and treatment of chondral lesions of the proximal hamate.
  - The triquetrohamate joint can also be accessed through another special-use midcarpal portal.[1]
- The volar radial midcarpal portal is occasionally used as an accessory portal for visualizing the palmar aspects of the capitate and hamate in cases of avascular necrosis or osteochondral injury.
  - This portal facilitates visualization of the palmar aspect of the capitohamate interosseous ligament, which is important in minimizing translational motion and has an essential role in providing stability to the transverse carpal arch.
- The volar distal radioulnar portal is useful for assessing the deep foveal attachment of the TFCC, which would normally require an open capsulotomy.
  - It may be employed if the suspicion of a peripheral TFCC detachment remains despite the absence of any visible TFCC tears through the standard ulnocarpal portals.

- The dorsal DRUJ portals may be used in concert with the volar distal radioulnar portal to more completely assess the status of the articular cartilage of the ulnar head and sigmoid notch as well as for instrumentation.
- The number of conditions amenable to arthroscopic treatment continues to grow. Many arthroscopic procedures are now common, while others await clinical validation. Table 1 provides a list of the more standard procedures.

Contraindications

- Contraindications to the use of dorsal or volar portals would include marked swelling, which distorts the topographic anatomy; large capsular tears, which might lead to extravasation of irrigation fluid; neurovascular compromise; bleeding disorders; or infection.
- Unfamiliarity with the regional anatomy is a relative contraindication.

SURGICAL MANAGEMENT

- It is useful to have a systematic approach to viewing the wrist.
- The structures that should be visualized as a part of a standard examination include the radius articular surface; the proximal scaphoid, lunate, and triquetrum; the SLIL and LTIL, both palmar and dorsal; the radioscaphocapitate ligament; the long radiolunate ligament; the radioscapholunate ligament; the ulnolunate ligament; the ulnotriquetral ligament; the articular disc; and the radial and peripheral TFCC attachments.
- It is my practice to establish the dorsal portals first but then to start the arthroscopic examination with the volar radial portal to visualize the palmar SLIL and the DRCL ligament to minimize any error from iatrogenic trauma to the dorsal capsular structures.
- In patients with ulnar-sided wrist pain, the volar ulnar portal is used to assess the palmar LTIL and dorsal radioulnar ligament, the region of the extensor carpi ulnaris subsheath, and the radial TFCC attachment.
  - The scope is then inserted in the 3–4 portal followed by various combinations of the 4–5 portal and 6R portal. The 6U portal is mostly used for outflow, but it may be used for instrumentation when débriding palmar LTIL tears.
- Midcarpal arthroscopy is then performed to probe the SLIL and LTIL joint spaces for instability, the capitohamate interosseous ligament, and to look for chondral lesions on the proximal capitate and hamate and loose bodies (**FIG 5**).
  - The special-use portals such as the dorsal and volar DRUJ portals and the 1–2 portal are used as needed.

Preoperative Planning

- A 2.7-mm, 30-degree-angled scope along with a camera attachment is used.
  - Table 2 describes the typical field of view as seen through a 2.7-mm arthroscope under ideal conditions.[1,4]
  - A 1.9-mm scope is sometimes beneficial, especially for evaluation of the DRUJ.
- A fiberoptic light source, video monitor, and printer have become the standard of care.
- Digital systems allow direct writing to a CD and superior video quality as compared to analog cameras.
- A 3-mm hook probe is needed for palpation of intracarpal structures.

Table 1	Arthroscopic Wrist Procedures

Ganglion resection: volar and dorsal
Release of wrist contracture
Arthroscopic synovectomy
Staging of degenerative arthritis (scapholunate advanced collapse or scaphoid nonunion advanced collapse, Kienbock disease)
Radial styloidectomy
Proximal pole of hamate resection
Dorsal radiocarpal ligament repair
Evaluation and treatment of carpal instability: scapholunate, lunotriquetral, midcarpal
Triangular fibrocartilage tears: repair vs. débridement
Arthroscopic wafer resection
Arthroscopic reduction and internal fixation of distal radius fractures
Arthroscopic-guided fixation of scaphoid fractures

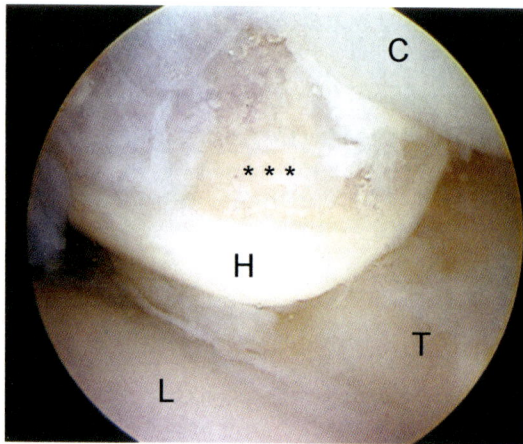

FIG 5 • Chondromalacia (*) on the proximal pole of the hamate (H). C, capitate; L, lunate; T, triquetrum.

- A motorized shaver or diathermy unit such as the Oratec probe (Smith & Nephew, NY) is useful for débridement.
- Ancillary equipment is largely procedure-dependent.
  - A motorized 2.9-mm burr is needed for bony resection.
  - There are a variety of commercially available suture repair kits, including the TFCC repair kit by Linvatec

(Conmed–Linvatec Corporation, Largo, FL). Ligament repairs can also be facilitated by use of a Tuohy needle, which is generally found in any anesthesia cart.

Positioning

- The patient is positioned supine on the operating table with the involved arm abducted on an arm table.
- A tourniquet is placed as far proximal on the arm as feasible.
- Traction is useful:
  - A shoulder holder along with 5- to 10-lb sand bags attached to an arm sling
  - A commercially available traction tower such as the Linvatec tower (Conmed–Linvatec Corporation, Utica, NY) or the ARC traction tower (Arc Surgical LLC, Hillsboro, OR)
- For the dorsal portals the surgeon faces the dorsum of the wrist and is seated by the patient's head. For the volar portals the surgeon faces the palm and is seated in the patient's axillary region.

Approach

- Portals are established by palpating and identifying anatomic landmarks and then inserting a 22-gauge needle into the joint space. The joint is then injected with 5 cc of saline. The ability to draw the saline back into the syringe serves as evidence that the needle is in the joint.

Table 2 | **Field of View**

Portal	Radial	Central	Volar	Dorsal /Distal	Ulnar
1–2	Scaphoid and lunate fossa, dorsal rim of radius	Proximal and radial scaphoid, proximal lunate	Oblique views of RSC, LRL, SRL	Oblique views of DRCL	TFCC poorly visualized
3–4	Scaphoid and lunate fossa, volar rim of radius	Proximal scaphoid and lunate, dorsal and membranous SLIL	RSC, RSL, LRL, ULL	Oblique views of the DRCL insertion onto the dorsal SLIL	TFCC radial insertion, central disc, ulnar attachment, PRUL, DRUL, PSO, PTR
4–5	Lunate fossa, volar rim of radius	Proximal lunate, triquetrum, dorsal and membranous LTIL	RSL, LRL, ULL	Poorly seen	TFCC radial insertion, central disc, ulnar attachment, PRUL, DRUL, PSO, PTR
6R	Poorly seen	Proximal lunate, triquetrum, dorsal and membranous LTIL	ULL, ULT	Poorly seen	TFCC radial insertion, central disc, ulnar attachment, PRUL, DRUL, PSO, PTR
6U	Sigmoid notch	Proximal triquetrum, membranous LTIL	Oblique views of ULL, ULT	Oblique views of DRCL	TFCC oblique views of the radial insertion, central disc, ulnar attachment, PRUL, DRUL
Volar radial	Scaphoid and lunate fossa, dorsal rim of radius	Scaphoid and lunate fossa, dorsal rim of radius	Palmar scaphoid and lunate, palmar SLIL	Oblique views of RSL, LRL, ULL	Oblique views of the radial insertion, central disc, ulnar attachment, PRUL, DRUL
Midcarpal radial	Scaphotrapezotrape-zoidal joint, distal scaphoid pole	SLIL joint, distal scaphoid, distal lunate	Radial limb of arcuate ligament (ie, continuation of the RSC ligament)	Proximal capitate, CHIL, oblique views of proximal hamate	LTIL joint, partial triquetrum
Midcarpal ulnar	Distal articular surface of the lunate and triquetrum and partial scaphoid	SLIL joint	Volar limb of arcuate ligament (ie, continuation of the triquetro-capito-lunate)	Oblique views of proximal capitate, CHIL, proximal hamate	LTIL joint, triquetrum
Dorsal distal radioulnar joint	Sigmoid notch, radial attachment of TFCC	Ulnar head	Palmar radioulnar ligament	Proximal surface of articular disc	Limited view of deep DRUL
Volar distal radioulnar joint	Sigmoid notch, radial attachment of TFCC	Ulnar head	Dorsal radioulnar ligament	Proximal surface of articular disc	Foveal attachment of deep fibers of TFCC (ie, DRUL,PRUL)

CHIL, capitohamate ligament; DRCL, dorsal radiocarpal ligament; DRUL, dorsal radioulnar ligament; LRL, long radiolunate ligament; LTIL, lunotriquetral interosseous ligament; PRUL, palmar radioulnar ligament; PSR, prestyloid recess; PTO, piso-triquetral orifice; RSC, radioscaphocapitate ligament; RSL, radioscapholunate ligament; SLIL, scapholunate interosseous ligament; SRL, short radiolunate ligament; TFCC, triangular fibrocartilage complex; ULL, ulnolunate ligament; ULT, ulnotriquetral ligament.
Adapted from Slutsky DJ. Wrist arthroscopy portals. In Slutsky DJ, Nagle DJ, eds. Techniques in Hand and Wrist Arthroscopy. Philadelphia: Elsevier, 2007.

- Shallow incisions avoid injury to sensory nerve branches and tendons. Soft tissues are dissected using a blunt mosquito clamp or a pair of small curved scissors. The dorsal capsule is pierced with these same instruments, providing access to the joint.
- A blunt trocar is used to introduce the scope cannula, which will house the scope and the inflow.

- Routinely, an 18-gauge needle is placed in the 6U portal for outflow.
- Synovitis, fractures, ligament tears, and a tight wrist joint may limit the field of view and necessitate the use of more portals to adequately assess the entire wrist.

3–4 PORTAL

- The concavity overlying the lunate between the extensor pollicis longus and the EDC is located just distal to the tubercle of Lister, in line with the second web space.
- The radiocarpal joint is identified with a 22-gauge needle that is inserted 10 degrees palmar to account for the volar inclination of the radius.
- The vascular tuft of the radioscapholunate ligament is directly in line with this portal. Superior to the radioscapholunate ligament is the membranous portion of the SLIL.

- By rotating the scope dorsally while looking in an ulnar direction, the insertion of the dorsal capsule onto the dorsal aspect of the SLIL can often be visualized. This is a common origin for the stalk of a dorsal ganglion.
- The radioscapholunate ligament and the long radiolunate ligament are radial to the portal and can be probed with a hook in the 4–5 portal.
- The LTIL, TFCC, and ulnolunate ligament are ulnar to the portal.

4–5 PORTAL

- The interval for the 4–5 portal is identified with the 22-gauge needle between the EDC and EDM, in line with the ring metacarpal.
- Because of the normal radial inclination of the distal radius, this portal lies slightly proximal and about 1 cm ulnar to the 3–4 portal.
- Care must be taken when inserting the scope since the LTIL lies directly ahead of this portal.
- One encounters the ulnar half of the lunate when moving the scope radially, and the oblique surface of the triquetrum in a superior and ulnar direction.
- The LTIL is seen obliquely from this portal and is often difficult to differentiate from the carpal bones without probing, unless a tear is present.

- The ulnolunate ligament and the ulnotriquetral ligament can be seen on the far end of the joint.
- Proximally, the radial insertion of the TFCC blends imperceptibly with the sigmoid notch of the radius, but it can be palpated with a hook probe in either the 3–4 or 6R portal.
- The peripheral insertion of the TFCC slopes upward into the ulnar capsule. Peripheral TFCC tears are often located ulnarly and dorsally.
- The palmar radioulnar ligament can be probed and visualized (especially if torn), but the dorsal radioulnar ligament is poorly seen.
- The pisotriquetral recess can sometimes be identified by a small tuft of protruding synovium and when probed may yield views of the articular facet of the pisiform.

6R AND 6U PORTALS

- The 6R portal is identified on the radial side of the ECU tendon, just distal to the ulnar head.
  - The scope should be angled 10 degrees proximally to avoid hitting the triquetrum. The TFCC is immediately below the entry site.
  - The LTIL is located radially and superiorly, whereas the ulnar capsule is immediately adjacent to the scope.

- The 6U portal is found on the ulnar side of the ECU tendon. Angling the needle distally and ulnar deviation of the wrist helps avoid running into the triquetrum.
  - This portal can be used to view the dorsal rim of the TFCC or for instrumentation when débriding the palmar LTIL.

TECHNIQUES

TECHNIQUES

1–2 PORTAL

- The relevant landmarks in the snuff box are palpated and outlined, including the distal edge of the radial styloid, the abductor pollicis longus, extensor pollicis brevis, and extensor pollicis longus tendons, and the radial artery in the snuff box.
- To minimize the risk of injury to branches of the superficial radial nerve and the radial artery, the 1–2 portal should be no more than 4.5 mm dorsal to the first extensor compartment and within 4.5 mm of the radial styloid (**TECH FIG 1**).[10]
- A blunt trocar and cannula are inserted with the wrist in ulnar deviation to minimize damage to the proximal scaphoid.

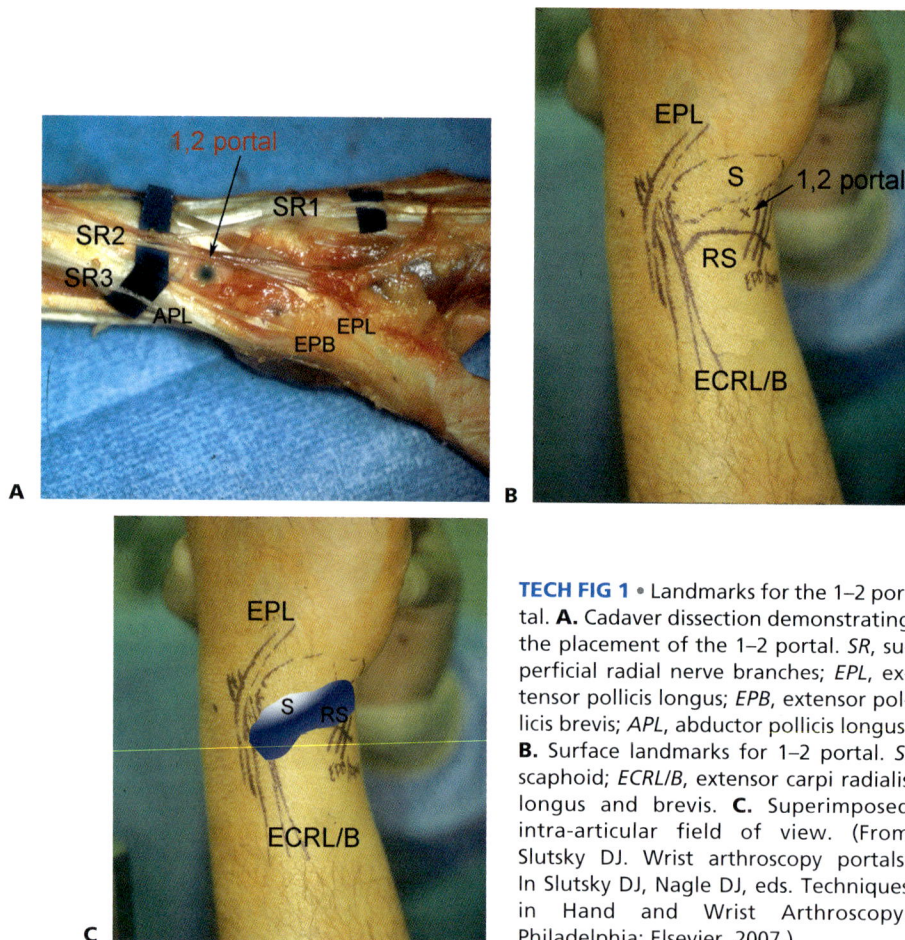

TECH FIG 1 • Landmarks for the 1–2 portal. **A.** Cadaver dissection demonstrating the placement of the 1–2 portal. *SR*, superficial radial nerve branches; *EPL*, extensor pollicis longus; *EPB*, extensor pollicis brevis; *APL*, abductor pollicis longus. **B.** Surface landmarks for 1–2 portal. *S*, scaphoid; *ECRL/B*, extensor carpi radialis longus and brevis. **C.** Superimposed intra-articular field of view. (From Slutsky DJ. Wrist arthroscopy portals. In Slutsky DJ, Nagle DJ, eds. Techniques in Hand and Wrist Arthroscopy. Philadelphia: Elsevier, 2007.)

MIDCARPAL RADIAL PORTAL

- The midcarpal radial portal is found 1 cm distal to the 3–4 portal.
- Flexing the wrist and firm thumb pressure helps identify the soft spot between the distal pole of the scaphoid and the proximal capitate.
- The scaphotrapezial trapezoidal joint lies radially and can be seen by rotating the scope dorsally.
- The scapholunate articulation can be seen proximally and ulnarly; it can be probed for instability or step-off.
- Further ulnarly, the lunotriquetral articulation is visualized.
- Moving the scope superiorly yields oblique views of the proximal surface capitate and hamate as well as the capitohamate interosseous ligament.
- The continuation of the radioscaphocapitate ligament, which forms the radial arm of the arcuate ligament (ie, the scaphocapitate ligament) can occasionally be seen across the midcarpal space.

TECHNIQUES

MIDCARPAL ULNAR PORTAL

- The midcarpal ulnar port is found 1 cm distal to the 4–5 portal and 1.5 cm ulnar and slightly proximal to the midcarpal radial portal, in line with the ring metacarpal axis.
- This entry site is at the intersection of the lunate, triquetrum, hamate, and capitate with a type I lunate facet and directly over the lunotriquetral joint with a type II lunate facet.[11]
  - This portal provides preferential views of the lunotriquetral articulation.
- Directly anteriorly, the ulnar limb of the arcuate ligament (ie, the triquetro-hamate-capitate ligament) can be seen as it crosses obliquely from the triquetrum, across the proximal corner of the hamate to the palmar neck of the capitate.
  - This is especially important in midcarpal instability.
  - Normally there is very little step-off between the distal articular surfaces of the scaphoid and lunate.
  - Direct pressure from the scope combined with traction may force the carpal joints out of alignment.
- The traction should be released and the scapholunate joint should be viewed with the scope in the midcarpal ulnar portal, whereas the lunotriquetral joint should be viewed with the scope in the midcarpal radial portal.

VOLAR RADIAL PORTAL

- A 2-cm transverse or longitudinal incision is made in the proximal wrist crease overlying the flexor carpi radialis tendon. The portal is established in the usual manner (**TECH FIG 2**).
- It is not necessary to specifically identify the adjacent neurovascular structures, provided that the anatomic landmarks are adhered to.
- A hook probe is inserted through the 3–4 portal and used to assess the palmar aspect of the SLIL and the DRCL.
- A useful landmark when viewing from the volar radial portal is the intersulcal ridge between the scaphoid and lunate fossae.
  - The radial origin of the DRCL is seen immediately ulnar to this, just proximal to the lunate.

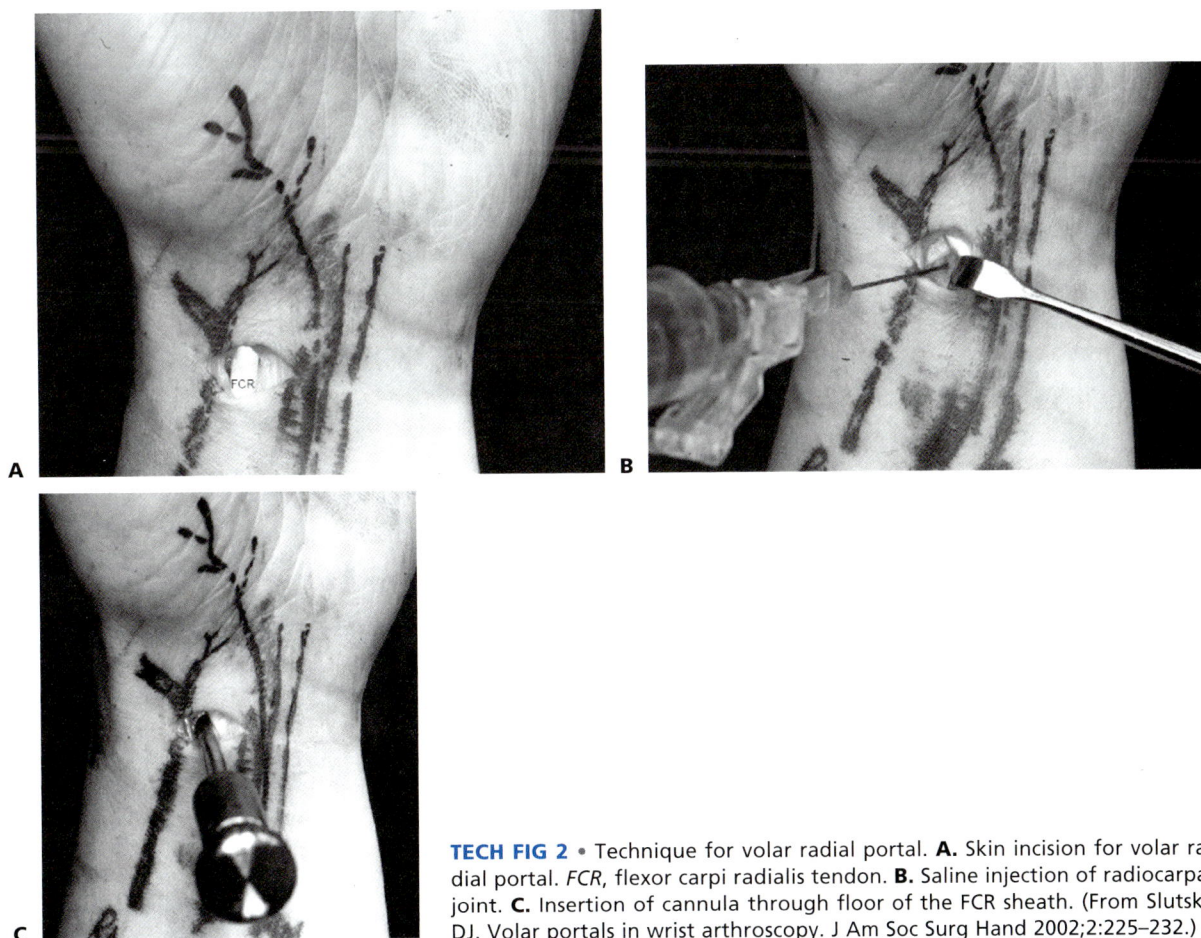

TECH FIG 2 • Technique for volar radial portal. **A.** Skin incision for volar radial portal. *FCR*, flexor carpi radialis tendon. **B.** Saline injection of radiocarpal joint. **C.** Insertion of cannula through floor of the FCR sheath. (From Slutsky DJ. Volar portals in wrist arthroscopy. J Am Soc Surg Hand 2002;2:225–232.)

TECHNIQUES

VOLAR RADIAL MIDCARPAL PORTAL

- The volar aspect of the midcarpal joint can be accessed through the same skin incision as the volar radial portal.
- The capsular entry site through the volar radial midcarpal portal is entered by angling the trocar 1 cm distally and about 5 degrees ulnarward to the radiocarpal site.

- A hook probe can be inserted dorsally in the midcarpal radial portal for palpation.
- With tears of the palmar SLIL one can see the intact dorsal fibers and the volar surface of the capitate.

VOLAR ULNAR PORTAL

- The volar ulnar portal is established via a 2-cm longitudinal incision centered over the proximal wrist crease along the ulnar edge of the finger flexor tendons (**TECH FIG 3**).
- The tendons are retracted to the radial side and the radiocarpal joint space is identified with a 22-gauge needle.
- Care is taken to situate the portal underneath the ulnar edge of the flexor tendons and to apply retraction in a radial direction alone to avoid injury to the ulnar nerve and artery.
- The median nerve is protected by the interposed flexor tendons.
- The palmar region of the LTIL can usually be seen slightly distal and radial to the portal.
- A hook probe is inserted through the 6R or 6U portal.

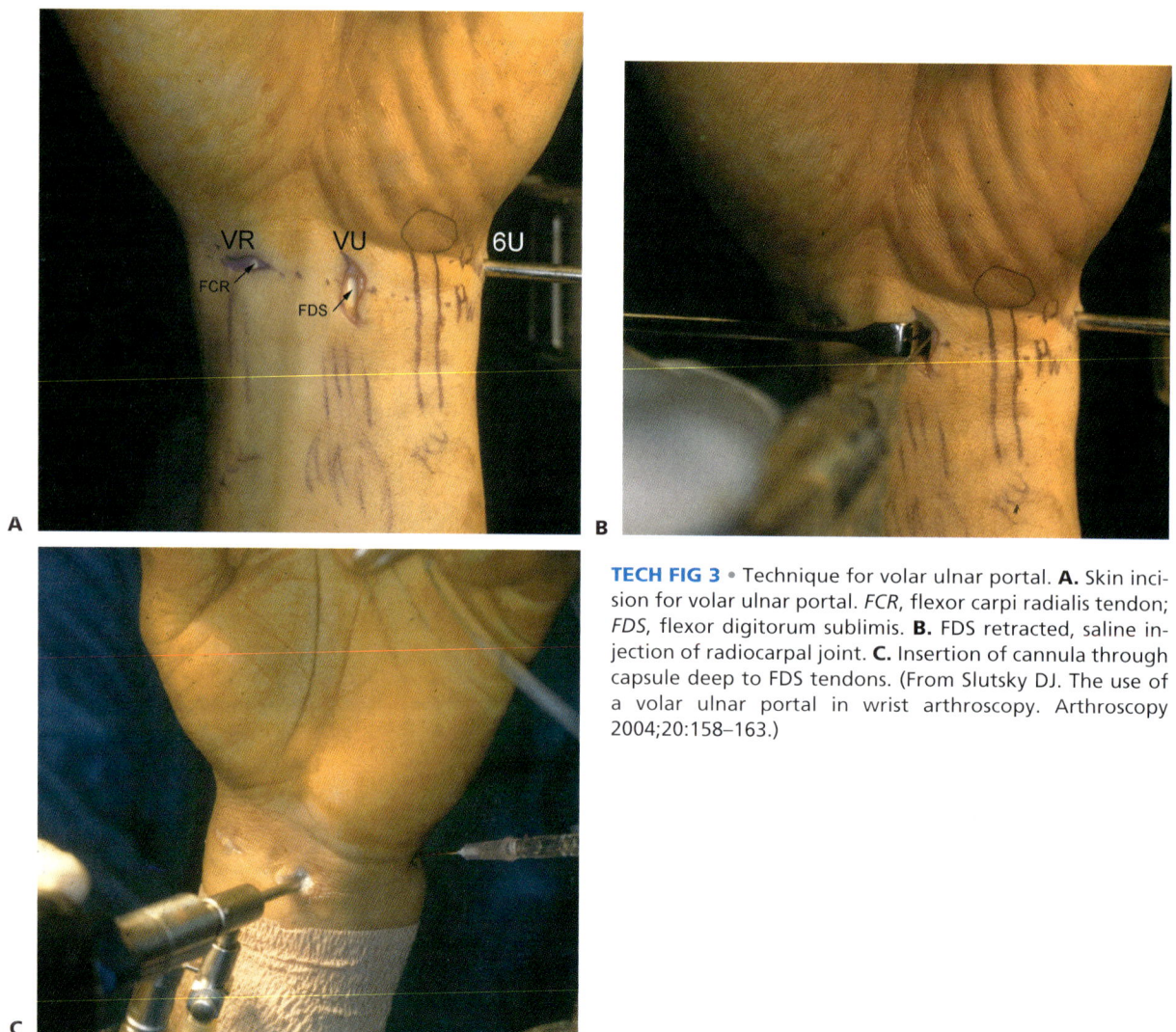

TECH FIG 3 • Technique for volar ulnar portal. **A.** Skin incision for volar ulnar portal. *FCR*, flexor carpi radialis tendon; *FDS*, flexor digitorum sublimis. **B.** FDS retracted, saline injection of radiocarpal joint. **C.** Insertion of cannula through capsule deep to FDS tendons. (From Slutsky DJ. The use of a volar ulnar portal in wrist arthroscopy. Arthroscopy 2004;20:158–163.)

VOLAR DRUJ PORTAL

- The volar DRUJ portal is accessed through the volar ulnar skin incision.
  - The joint is entered by angling the 22-gauge needle 45 degrees proximally.
    - It is useful to leave a needle or cannula in the ulnocarpal joint for reference.
  - Alternatively, a probe can be placed in the distal DRUJ portal and advanced through the palmar incision to act as a switching stick over which the cannula can be threaded.[3]
- Initially, the space appears quite limited, but over the course of 3 to 5 minutes the fluid irrigation expands the joint space, which improves visibility.
- A 3-mm hook probe is inserted through the dorsal distal DRUJ portal for palpation.
  - A burr or thermal probe can be substituted as necessary.

- Direct visualization of the foveal attachment prevents accidental injury to this structure.
- The articular disc is seen superiorly.
- Proximal surface tears of the TFCC, which are usually caused by severe axial load, may be detected through this portal.
- The dome of the ulnar head lies inferiorly.
- The TFCC attachment to the sigmoid notch can be palpated with a hook probe in the distal dorsal DRUJ portal as it penetrates the dorsal DRUJ capsule.
- The deep attachments of the dorsal radioulnar ligament can be seen as it inserts into the fovea.
- In ideal cases, the conjoined tendon of the dorsal radioulnar ligament, ulnar collateral ligament, and palmar radioulnar ligament can be visualized.

DORSAL DRUJ PORTALS

- The dorsal aspect of the DRUJ can be accessed through proximal and distal portals.
- The proximal DRUJ portal is located in the axilla of the joint, just proximal to the sigmoid notch and the flare of the ulnar metaphysis.
  - This portal is easier to penetrate and should be used initially to prevent chondral injury from insertion of the trocar.
  - The forearm is held in supination to relax the dorsal capsule, to move the ulnar head volarly, and to lift the central disc distally from the head of the ulna.
  - Reducing the traction to 1 to 2 pounds permits better views between the ulna and the sigmoid notch by reducing the compressive force caused by axial traction.
  - The joint space is entered by inserting a 22-gauge needle horizontally at the neck of the distal ulna.
    - Fluoroscopy facilitates needle placement.

- The distal dorsal DRUJ portal is identified 6 to 8 mm distally with the 22-gauge needle, and just proximal to the 6R portal.
  - This portal can be used for outflow drainage or for instrumentation.
  - It lies on top of the ulnar head but underneath the TFCC and so is difficult to use in the presence of positive ulnar variance.
  - The TFCC has the least tension in neutral rotation of the forearm, which is the optimal position for visualizing the articular dome of the ulnar head, the undersurface of the TFCC, and the proximal radioulnar ligament from its attachment to the sigmoid notch to its insertion into the fovea of the ulna.
  - Because of the dorsal entry of the arthroscope, the course of the dorsal radioulnar ligament is not visible until its attachment into the fovea is encountered.
  - Entry into this portal provides views of the proximal sigmoid notch cartilage and the articular surface of the neck of the ulna.

PEARLS AND PITFALLS

- Use shallow skin incisions.
- Use the wound spread technique to protect surrounding sensory nerves.
- If the trocar does not insert easily, reposition to avoid chondral injury.
- Wrist traction often diminishes during the procedure and should be readjusted as needed to avoid scraping the articular surface.
- Use of a standard methodologic approach ensures a complete and thorough examination.

POSTOPERATIVE CARE

- The postoperative rehabilitation depends on the specific procedure that is performed.
- After diagnostic arthroscopy, with or without débridement, the patient is splinted for comfort for a brief period of 4 to 7 days.

- Active wrist motion is encouraged after this period and patients are allowed activities of daily living, followed by gradual strengthening.
- If a ligament repair or TFCC repair has been performed or if there is interosseous pinning, the protocol is adjusted as necessary and typically involves an initial period of immobilization before instituting wrist motion.

COMPLICATIONS

- Most of the complications related to use of the dorsal portals are related to injury to the sensory branches of the superficial radial nerve and the dorsal cutaneous branch of the ulnar nerve.
    - The palmar cutaneous branch of the ulnar nerve is at risk with the volar radial portal, although the interposed flexor carpi radialis tendon mitigates this risk.
    - There is no true internervous plane when using the volar ulnar portal; hence, sensory branches of the palmar cutaneous branches of the ulnar nerve or nerve of Henle are always at risk. Thus, proper wound spread technique is paramount.
    - The ulnar neurovascular bundle is also potentially at risk with overzealous retraction or poor portal placement.
- Venous bleeding, loss of wrist motion (especially forearm supination), complications related to fluid extravasation, and infection are general risks attendant to any arthroscopic procedure.
    - These can be minimized by fastidious surgical technique, aggressive rehabilitation as necessary, and diligent follow-up in the early postoperative period.

REFERENCES

1. Berger RA. Arthroscopic anatomy of the wrist and distal radioulnar joint. Hand Clin 1999;15:393–413.
2. Geissler WB, Freeland AE, Savoie FH, et al. Intracarpal soft-tissue lesions associated with an intra-articular fracture of the distal end of the radius. J Bone Joint Surg Am 1996;78A:357–365.
3. Slutsky DJ. Distal radioulnar joint arthroscopy and the volar ulnar portal. Tech Hand Up Extrem Surg 2007;11:38–44.
4. Slutsky DJ. Arthroscopy portals: volar and dorsal. In Budoff J, Slade JF, Trumble TE, eds. Master's Techniques in Wrist and Elbow Arthroscopy. Chicago: American Society for Surgery of the Hand, 2006.
5. Slutsky DJ. Clinical applications of volar portals in wrist arthroscopy. Tech Hand Up Extrem Surg 2004;8:229–238.
6. Slutsky DJ. Management of dorsoradiocarpal ligament repairs. J Am Soc Surg Hand 2005;5:167–174.
7. Slutsky DJ. Volar portals in wrist arthroscopy. J Am Soc Surg Hand 2002;2:225–232.
8. Slutsky DJ. Wrist arthroscopy portals. In Slutsky DJ, Nagel DJ, eds. Techniques in Hand and Wrist Arthroscopy. Philadelphia: Elsevier, 2007.
9. Slutsky DJ. Wrist arthroscopy through a volar radial portal. Arthroscopy 2002;18:624–630.
10. Steinberg BD, Plancher KD, Idler RS. Percutaneous Kirschner wire fixation through the snuff box: an anatomic study. J Hand Surg Am 1995;20A:57–62.
11. Viegas SF. Midcarpal arthroscopy: anatomy and portals. Hand Clin 1994;10:577–587.

Chapter 4

Open Reduction and Internal Fixation of Diaphyseal Forearm Fractures

Michael R. Boland

DEFINITION

- Motion in the human forearm is a complex interaction between the radius and ulna produced by the combination of multiple muscles working coherently and hinged at the proximal and distal radioulnar joints.
- Surgical reconstruction of diaphyseal forearm fractures requires precise realignment of both radius and ulna to minimize complications and maximize function.
- Ingenious surgical approaches have been described that allow the surgeon to follow defined internervous planes to the bones for internal fixation. The design of the forearm allows near 180-degree rotation combining with considerable elbow flexion–extension and wrist circumduction. To achieve this, the ulna is enlarged proximally, making it a principal bone of the elbow, and is smaller distally, while the reverse is true for the radius, with the enlarged radius being the primary articulation with the carpus. The result for the diaphysis of each bone is that the proximal ulna is metaphyseal for about 25% to 30% of its length but distally less than 10%, with the reverse holding true for the radius. Implant design has taken these differences into account, with many whole systems available for metaphyseal distal radius and proximal ulna fractures.
- The importance of maintaining the radial and ulnar heads has only recently been understood. New developments are taking place, therefore, for the management of distal ulna and proximal radius fractures.
- This chapter discusses ulna fractures distal to the junction of the proximal and middle thirds to the distal margin of the pronator quadratus (PQ) and radius fractures distal to the biceps tuberosity down to the distal flare of the radius.
  - Pediatric fractures, distal radius and ulna fractures, olecranon and radial head fractures are not covered.
- Diaphyseal forearm fractures usually are classified according to the AO classification.

ANATOMY

- The surgical approaches to the forearm bones for fracture osteosynthesis involve five steps:
  - Finding an interval between longitudinally oriented superficial muscles
  - Finding and preserving vessels and nerves
  - Understanding the anatomy of deeper muscles that cross the forearm obliquely or transversely
  - Knowing where to lift these muscles to expose the bone
  - Understanding the shape of the bones themselves and their relation to one another

Radius and Ulna

- Motion of the forearm involves a complex interaction between the radius and ulna.
  - The radius rotates around a longitudinal axis that passes through the center of the radial head at the proximal radioulnar joint and through the center of the ulnar head distally.

- With rotation, the radius rotates around the ulna, and the ulna moves in a varus–valgus direction about 9 degrees at the elbow. This allows the ulnar head to move out of the way of the rotating radius distally.
- At the distal radioulnar joint (DRUJ), motion between 50 degrees pronation and 50 degrees supination is almost pure rotation, but at the extremes the radius translates in a dorsal direction during pronation and a palmar direction during supination.
- Movement at the proximal radioulnar joint (PRUJ) is primarily rotation.
- The radius and ulna have two bows that assist in getting out of the other's way. Schemitsch and Richards[22] quantified the importance of the distal of the two bows in the radius. Restoration of this bow is the single most important step in reconstruction of the forearm after diaphyseal fracture.
  - To determine whether the bow has been restored after osteosynthesis, draw a line from the biceps tuberosity to the sigmoid notch. A perpendicular line from the apex can then be measured (**FIG 1**). The normal range of bow is 15.3 ± 0.3 mm at a point at 60% of the radius measured between the bicipital tuberosity and the distal radius at the sigmoid notch.
  - At the apex of this bow on the convex side is the insertion of the pronator teres. This provides a biomechanical advantage for pronation.
  - The biceps insertion is at the apex of a smaller proximal bow. As a result, the biceps needs to be much larger to overcome the disadvantage of insertion into a small bow for balanced supination.
  - The arrangement in the ulna is the converse of the radius: a longer shallower proximal bow (the anconeus inserts into the apex for valgus of the elbow), and a small distal bow for the insertion of the PQ.
- The radius and ulna are bound together essentially throughout their length, with the annular ligament at the PRUJ, the interosseous ligament through the middle 75%, and the ligaments of the triangular fibrocartilage complex

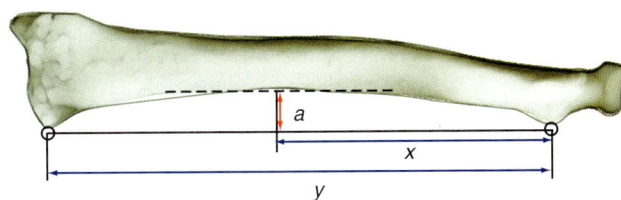

Maximum radial bow a (mm)
Location of maximum radial bow (%) $\frac{x}{y}$ x 100

FIG 1 • The method of Schemitsch and Richards for quantifying the maximum radial bow and its location relative to the length of the entire radius.[1]

(TFCC) distally. The TFCC ligaments are the palmar and dorsal radioulnar ligaments, which attach to the distal rim of the sigmoid notch and the fovea of the ulna. Disruption of these ligaments often is associated with fractures of the radius and ulna and may lead to DRUJ incongruity (ie, Galeazzi fractures) or radial head dislocation (ie, Monteggia fractures).

Muscles and Ligaments

- The forearm is criss-crossed with longitudinal, oblique, and transversely directed musculotendinous units. These muscles are in layers, with longitudinal muscles more superficial and crossing muscles deeper.
- Most activities performed by the forearm, wrist, and hand occur from the midpronation position, with the wrist moving into extension and radial deviation (ERD), then in an arc accelerating past neutral again, to flexion and ulnar deviation (FUD, end of deceleration) before returning to wrist neutral. The forearm is designed to maximize the ability to perform this motion. This wrist motion is commonly known as the "dart thrower's motion" or primary wrist motion.
- The extensor carpi radialis longus (ECRL), the cocking or lifting muscle of primary wrist motion, originates proximal to the lateral epicondyle on the supracondylar ridge, is positioned "above" the forearm, and inserts into the radial and dorsal aspect of the index metacarpal.
- On either side of the ECRL is the brachioradialis (BR), which originates high on the lateral supracondylar ridge, inserting on the radial styloid deep to the first dorsal compartment, and the extensor carpi radialis brevis (ECRB), which originates more distally just above the lateral epicondyle and inserts into the long finger metacarpal. ECRL and ECRB share the second dorsal compartment at the wrist.
- Together the BR, ECRL, and ECRB form a mobile wad above the forearm (in the functional position). They are innervated directly by the radial nerve and are best palpated just distal to the elbow.
  - In a posterior approach to the radius, which is performed in pronation, after incising the deep fascia, the dissection interval is between the ECRB and the extensor digitorum communis (EDC) muscle. The EDC originates from the lateral epicondyle (where it shares a common origin with the extensor digiti minimi) and passes essentially in a straight line down the forearm, then through the fourth dorsal compartment at the wrist, just ulnar to Lister's tubercle.
  - In an anterior approach, which is performed in supination, the deep fascia is incised along the medial border of the BR. The BR is then mobilized radially and the interval between it and flexor carpi radialis is developed. The FCR, like the EDC, has a straight course in the forearm from the medial epicondyle to the scaphoid tubercle (where it passes en route to the index metacarpal).
- The muscle of utmost importance in approaches to the ulna is the flexor carpi ulnaris (FCU). It is the primary accelerator of the wrist, and thus has a large tendon (equal to the mechanical strength of the ECRL and ECRB combined), which originates from two heads, one from the medial epicondyle and one from the ulna. It proceeds straight down the forearm along the ulna border and inserts into the pisiform. From the distal tip of the lateral epicondyle originates the extensor carpi ulnaris, which runs down the forearm on the extensor

side of the subcutaneous border of the ulna, sharing a septum with the FCU.
  - The ulna is approached along this septum. The anterior surface and posterior aspects of the ulna can be approached this way. The true anterior approach to the ulna is along the radial edge of the FCU, mobilizing the ulna neurovascular bundle and going between the FCU and the flexor digitorum profundus (FDP). The FDP occupies the floor of most of the flexor compartment of the forearm.
- Crossing the forearm in its deepest parts are a series of obliquely oriented muscles. The supinator plays a role in both the anterior and posterior approaches to the radius. It has two heads of origin and probably can be thought of as two muscles, because the fibers of each head traverse in different directions.
  - The ulnar head attaches to the supinator crest on the radial side of the ulna. Its fibers are transverse (like those of the PQ distally) and attach to the most proximal part of the radius, deep to the posterior interosseous nerve (PIN).
  - The humeral head attaches to the lateral epicondyle, deep to the ECU and anconeus. Its fibers slope down the forearm more longitudinally, and wrap over the deep or ulnar head to attach to the radius distal to the ulnar head of the supinator and proximal to the insertion of the pronator teres.
  - In an anterior approach to the radius, the forearm is supinated, protecting the PIN, and the humeral head of the supinator is lifted from its most ulnar attachment.
- The pronator teres originates mainly from the medial supracondylar ridge, arches obliquely across the ulnar artery and median nerve, and inserts into the apex of the larger bow of the radius. Proximally, it is superficial, but distally, where it must be lifted from the radius, it is deep to the BR muscle (**FIG 2**). It must be lifted from the most radial aspect of the radius in the anterior approach.
- Distally in the floor of the anterior compartment the PQ muscle comes into play in anterior approaches to the radius and ulna. It must be lifted from the radial border in an approach to the radius and the ulna border in an approach to the ulna.
- In a posterior approach to the radius, the abductor pollicis longus muscle drapes across the radius just distal to its midpoint. It can be lifted to allow plate fixation to this part of the radius. Its ulnar origin is always left intact.

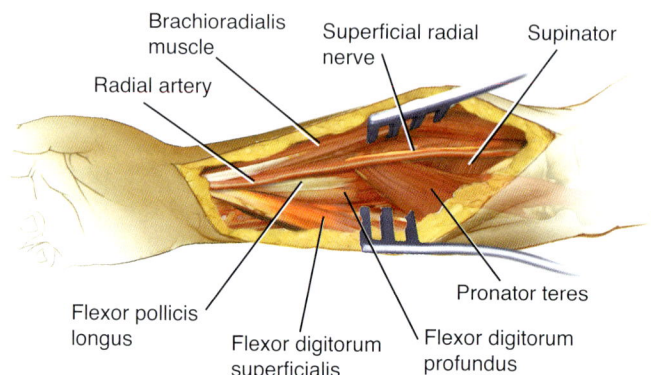

FIG 2 • Anterior approach. The interval between the brachioradialis and flexor carpi radialis is entered, and the radial artery is retracted laterally. The supinator, pronator teres, flexor pollicis longus, and flexor digitorum superficialis can be seen.

Nerves

- The forearm is traversed longitudinally with three major nerves plus an additional three sensory nerves, only one of which is of surgical importance. Once the interval between muscles is breached, care is taken to find these nerves. Each nerve enters the forearm from the arm in a predictable place, and each gives off key branches that must be protected.
- Although the radial nerve supplies all the extensor muscles of the arm and forearm, it is an anterior structure after it pierces the lateral intermuscular septum 10 cm above the elbow.
  - At the elbow the radial nerve lies between the BR and the brachialis and gives off the PIN.
  - The radial sensory nerve continues deep to the BR muscle, on its undersurface. Here, the nerve generally lies close to the radial artery. The anterior approach to the radius is through the interval between the nerve and artery.
  - The posterior interosseous branch leaves the main nerve just distal to the elbow and passes through the supinator muscle, between its two heads, to enter the dorsal or extensor compartment of the forearm.
    - As it leaves the supinator, it fans into multiple variable branches to supply the EDC, EDM, and ECU, with the majority of the nerve continuing distally deep to the interval between EDC and ECRB.
- The course of the ulnar nerve is represented by a line drawn from the medial epicondyle to the pisiform. Throughout the forearm the nerve is deep to the FCU muscle and lies deep and slightly radial to the tendon of this muscle at the wrist. Throughout most of the forearm the nerve is between the FCU and the FDP.
- The median nerve enters the forearm between the brachial artery and the tendon of the biceps brachii. It lies deep to the pronator teres, then passes deep to the fibrous arch of the FDS. The nerve is closely associated with the undersurface of the FDS as it travels distally.

Blood Supply

- The vascular anatomy is of critical importance in the flexor compartment.
  - The brachial artery enters the forearm deep to the lacertus fibrosus, next to the median nerve. It almost immediately branches into radial and ulnar arteries.
  - The ulnar artery passes deep to the arch of origin of the FDS to lie next to the ulnar nerve throughout the distal two thirds of the forearm.
  - The radial artery is pushed more superficial by the bulk of the FDS and the pronator teres lying just deep to the fascia along the medial border of the BR muscle.

PATHOGENESIS

- The degree of injury and specifics of the fracture are directly related to the magnitude, direction, and duration of energy.
  - Both-bone forearm fractures are common in motor vehicle trauma.
  - Industrial trauma often is associated with a high level of soft tissue injury.
  - Forearm fractures occur relatively commonly in some sports, eg, rugby in all its forms and wrestling.
- The most common mechanism of injury is a direct blow to the mid-forearm. If this blow is directed primarily at the ulna, an isolated ulna shaft fracture results ("nightstick" fracture).

- An isolated radius fracture often is associated with a fall onto an outstretched hand.

NATURAL HISTORY

- Normal function of the human forearm requires the radius to rotate around the ulna.
- Matthews[15] showed in a cadaveric study that 10 degrees of angulation of one or both bones of the forearm results in a loss of 20 degrees of pronation and supination. Thus, the natural history is highly dependent on the position of healing of the two forearm bones.
- It is reasonable to consider nonoperative treatment of an isolated ulna fracture with less than 10 degrees angulation,[21] but nonoperative treatment of both-bone forearm fractures has a poor outcome.[8,13]

PATIENT HISTORY AND PHYSICAL FINDINGS

- In most cases, the initial presentation of a radius or ulna diaphyseal fracture makes the diagnosis obvious. Most fractures are displaced due to the high-energy nature of the traumatic event and, therefore, deformity is common. Patients with nondisplaced fractures usually have considerable pain and swelling in the forearm.
  - Despite the ease of initial diagnosis, the treating physician must be on guard for significant associated injuries and complications, not only of the bone and joint but also of soft tissue.
- A systems approach to these associated injuries is as follows:
  - *Skin:* Look at the skin for any evidence of laceration or abrasion. A laceration may communicate with the fracture site; therefore, a contaminated abrasion at the site of surgical incision should be allowed to heal before surgery.
  - *Fascia:* Tense tissues to palpation over the flexor or extensor compartments and pain with passive finger extension are evidence of compartment syndrome, and compartment release must be considered.
  - *Vascular:* Radial and ulnar pulses distal to the site of injury must be palpated and compared to the uninjured side. These pulses can be difficult to palpate due to the proximity of the fractures, so checking capillary refill in the digits is the next step. In the multiply injured patient, the peripheries are shut down, making capillary refill and pulses difficult to perform. In such a situation, a needle stick to the digit should reveal bright red blood.
  - *Nerve:* Assessment of nerve injury is summarized later in this chapter.
  - *Bone:* The joints above and below the fracture must be palpated for associated joint disruption.
- For any upper extremity injury, a history of the causative event is essential to understand the degree of energy that the limb has had to absorb. Given the common association with high energy, the patient must be assessed according to an appropriate trauma checklist protocol.
- The patient must be questioned specifically regarding elbow or wrist pain, and neurologic symptoms of numbness, tingling, or unusual sensation in the hand. Severe pain should suggest the possibility of compartment syndrome or vascular injury.
- Palpation of the mid-forearm should be gentle, step by step feeling along the radius and ulna. A tense forearm may indicate a compartment syndrome.

■ Palpation should then proceed over the DRUJ and ulnar head plus PRUJ and radial head. Palpation should be performed of the medial and lateral epicondyles, of the scaphoid in the snuff box, and over carpal bones and the carpometacarpal joints.

■ A systematic examination of the median, ulnar, and radial nerves involves examination of sensory and motor aspects (Table 1).

■ The sensory examination involves static two-point discrimination of the digital nerves and light touch over the autogenous zones of each nerve.

■ Motor examination is graded by Medical Research Council (MRC) grading and is done by stressing the appropriate joint and palpating the affected muscle.

IMAGING AND OTHER DIAGNOSTIC STUDIES

■ High-quality plain radiographs of the forearm, wrist, and elbow are the mainstay of diagnosis of diaphyseal radius and ulna fractures.

■ Mino[16] described a technique to interpret the lateral wrist radiograph whereby the radial styloid is aligned with the center of the lunate, and an assessment of the overlap of the radius and ulna is made. The head of the ulna should be completely obscured by the radius. If only part of the ulnar head is obscured by the radius, then there is subluxation of the head; if the ulnar head is clearly seen, there is dislocation. Any shift in the ulnar head is a subluxation and, when combined with a radius fracture, represents a Galeazzi fracture-dislocation.[9]

■ A CT scan in neutral, pronation, and supination is useful in interpreting the degree of DRUJ congruity. This is rarely used in the acute setting.

■ On a lateral radiograph of the elbow, the radial head should align directly with the capitellum of the distal humerus. Monteggia[17] in 1814 described a fracture of the proximal third of the ulna with an anterior radial head dislocation, and Bado[2] later subclassified these according to direction (**FIG 3**).

DIFFERENTIAL DIAGNOSIS

■ Pathologic fracture may result from a number of causes.

■ *Metabolic causes:* osteoporosis, estrogen deficiency, renal transplantation, vitamin D deficiency, parathyroid disease, Cushing disease, hyperthyroidism, hypogonadism, hypophosphatasia

■ *Primary tumors:* osteosarcoma, Ewing sarcoma and primitive neuroectodermal tumors, chondrosarcoma, myeloma, fibrous histiocytoma, desmoplastic fibroma, hemangioma, intraosseous lipoma, acute myeloid leukemia, Langerhans' cell histiocytosis, fibrous dysplasia, chondroblastoma

■ *Metastatic tumors:* breast, thyroid, lung, prostate, melanoma

■ *Infection:* osteomyelitis, tuberculosis

■ *Congenital disorders:* Turner syndrome, neurofibromatosis pseudoarthrosis, osteogenesis imperfecta

■ *Iatrogenic fracture:* post–plate/screw removal; post–osteocutaneous radial forearm flap; post–elbow, forearm, and wrist manipulation

■ Stress fracture

NONOPERATIVE MANAGEMENT

■ Slight deviations in the spatial orientation of the radius and ulna will significantly decrease the forearm's ability to rotate, impairing hand function.

Table 1	Methods for Neurologic Examination After Radius and Ulna Fracture

Examination	Technique	Grading	Significance
Median nerve autogenous zone	Light palpation over the palmar aspect of the index MP joint crease	Compare sides: can be considered normal, absent, or altered.	If altered or absent, consider median nerve palsy. Examine median distribution two-point discrimination.
Ulnar nerve autogenous zone	Light palpation over the palmar aspect of the small finger MP joint crease	Compare sides: can be considered normal, absent, or altered.	If altered or absent, consider ulnar nerve palsy. Examine ulnar distribution two-point discrimination.
Radial nerve autogenous zone	Light palpation over dorsal first interosseous space	Compare sides: can be considered normal, absent, or altered.	If absent, consider radial nerve palsy.
First dorsal interosseous muscle test	Abduction of first dorsal interosseous against resistance	MRC muscle grading	If weak, consider ulnar nerve lesion.
Abductor pollicis brevis muscle test	Abduction of thumb against resistance with palpation of thenar space	MRC grading	If weak, consider median nerve lesion.
Extensor pollicis longus muscle test	Extend the interphalangeal joint of the thumb against resistance and hyperadduct thumb while palpating the extensor pollicis longus tendon.	MRC grading	If weak, consider radial nerve palsy.
Flexor pollicis longus muscle test	Flex interphalangeal joint of thumb against resistance.	MRC grading	If weak, consider palsy to anterior interosseous branch of median nerve.
Passive stretch test	Passively extend all fingers.	Severe pain may indicate compartment syndrome.	Consider intracompartmental pressure monitoring.

MRC, Medical Research Council system.

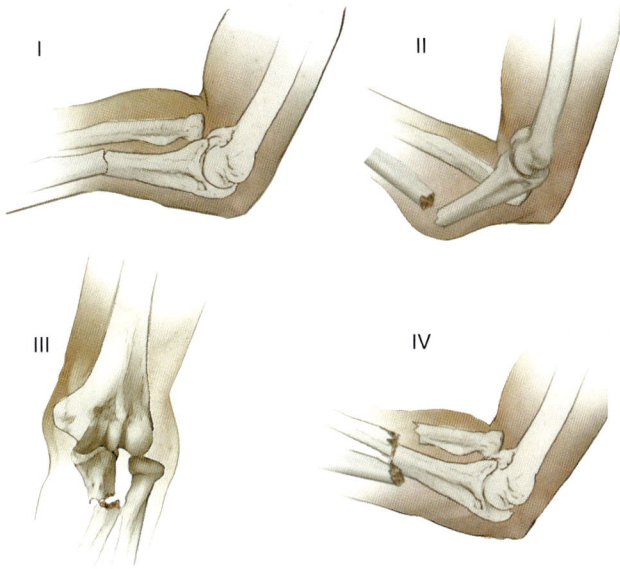

FIG 3 • The Bado classification of Monteggia lesions lists four types, depending on the direction of the radial head. In type I lesions the head is anterior to the distal humerus. In type II lesions it is posterior, and in type III lesions it is lateral. Type IV fracture-dislocations involve a dislocation of the radial head associated with a fracture of both the radius and the ulna.

- Fractures of the radius and ulna can be regarded as articular fractures in the sense that functional restoration requires anatomic reduction.
- The only indication for nonoperative treatment is a nondisplaced fracture of the ulna,[14,21] or if the patient's general condition makes operative treatment ill advised.
  - In the case of a displaced fracture, closed reduction and cast immobilization sometimes is possible but is unreliable. Loss of initial satisfactory reduction is common.[3,8,12,13]
- The treatment of choice for adult diaphyseal forearm fractures is open reduction and internal fixation.[1,7,20]

SURGICAL MANAGEMENT

- The most common scenario is fractures of the radius and ulna in the middle third of both bones. The most common questions confronting the surgeon are considered here.
  - Which approach should be used?
    - The anterior surface of the radius and ulna is the best location for a plate. This surface is broad and flat on both bones, and a plate on this surface is covered with muscle, resulting in less plate irritation for the patient.
    - Consequently, I prefer the anterior approach to both the radius and the ulna. In addition, the patient is positioned supine for these approaches, reducing the need to reposition the patient during the procedure.
  - Should one or two incisions be used?
    - Use of two incisions markedly decreases the risk of synostosis, decreases the length of the incision, and reduces tension on the skin and soft tissue by retractors.
  - Which bone should be stabilized first?
    - The fracture with the least comminution should be approached first and stabilized. This allows for length to be restored in the forearm, allowing easier judgment of length in the more comminuted bone.

- Where there is equal comminution or no comminution, the radius is generally approached first.
- Should fixation be completed on one bone before approaching the other?
  - I recommend not completing fixation but stabilizing one bone before proceeding to the next. This allows reduction of the second bone.
  - In a stable, non-comminuted fracture, "temporary stability" may mean a plate and one screw through two cortices on each side of the fracture. In a comminuted fracture, it may mean four cortices and two screws on each side.
  - Completion of fixation should occur after the second bone is reduced and stabilized.
- What implant and what length of implant should be used?
  - The plate must span the fracture complex and provide six cortices of fixation in stable bone, both proximally and distally.
  - Non-comminuted transverse fractures require at least a six-hole small fragment limited contact–dynamic compression (LC-DC) or locking plate.
  - Oblique fractures and comminuted fractures require a longer plate. Oblique fractures are treated with an interfragmentary screw or screws at right angles to the fracture line and a seven-hole plate.
  - A unicortical locked screw can be considered "bicortical," but practically speaking, this rule is used only for the screw hole furthest from the fracture. In almost all situations there must be three screw holes in the plate over stable bone away from the fracture complex.
  - In distal metaphyseal, diaphyseal fractures of the ulna, it often is impossible to get six cortices of fixation. In this situation, two mini fragment plates (with 2.7-mm screws) applied at a 90-degree angle to each other provides excellent fixation.
- Anterior and posterior approaches can be used to treat fractures along the entire length of each bone. The anterior approach to the radius is preferred when possible.
  - This location allows for excellent soft tissue coverage, reducing the need for plate removal.
- Most diaphyseal forearm fractures are best stabilized by plates and screws, but other implants sometimes are indicated.
- External fixation may be used in the following settings:
  - Open fractures with severe soft tissue damage, as a temporizing measure until reconstruction can safely be undertaken
  - Maintenance of length in fractures with severe bone loss (this usually occurs in open fractures)
  - Patients with multiple injuries ("damage control" surgery)
  - The Ilizarov technique is useful in segmental fractures, especially when the fractures are very close to the wrist and elbow joints.
- Intermedullary nailing is used in the following settings:
  - Young women who desire a better cosmetic result
  - Segmental fractures
  - Re-fracture at the bone plate interface in a contact athlete or following plate removal

Preoperative Planning

- The surgeon must develop a strategy to achieve satisfactory alignment of the radius and ulna with congruency of the PRUJ and DRUJ.

- Factors that must be considered include the following:
  - Operating room time and availability (ideally within 7 days of the injury)
  - Implant and equipment availability (eg, a distraction device)
  - Patient factors and patient support factors (in outpatient surgery a supportive family or friend is needed in the early postoperative period)
  - Regional versus general anesthesia
- Standard AO planning[18] consists of drawing the fragments on transparent paper; superimposing the transparent sheets to align the bones; adding a chosen implant template; and drawing the final outcome corresponding to the expected postoperative radiograph. With experience in fracture management, these steps are intuitive.
- AO principles of internal fixation using plates and screws should be reviewed by the surgeon before attempting internal fixation.

Positioning

- Generally, the patient is positioned supine and the hand table is attached to the main table so the midpoint of the hand table is directly opposite the patient's shoulder. The shoulder is directly over the adjoining point of the hand and main tables. The arm is abducted to 90 degrees at the shoulder, so the entire arm lies across the midpoint of the hand table.
- In the case of a posterior approach to the proximal ulna, the patient is positioned supine and a pillow is placed across his or her chest and secured with broad paper tape to the operating table. A hand table is used to rest the instruments rather than support the upper extremity. If other forearm fractures are present, however, the arm table may then be available.
- A non-sterile tourniquet is applied to the upper arm before prepping and draping the patient.
- The surgeon usually is seated on the side of the hand table closest to the bone being reduced and stabilized.
- For the anterior approach to the radius, the surgeon is on the side of the table closest to the patient's head. The forearm is supinated and the elbow extended. For a posterior approach to the radius, the forearm is pronated and the elbow extended.
- For a posterior or subcutaneous approach to the ulna, the elbow is flexed, and the forearm is in a neutral position.

Approach

- The anterior approach to the radius is the standard approach for a radius fracture, but the posterior approach is useful when soft tissue lesions are posterior or the anterior approach is compromised in some way.
- The posterior or subcutaneous approach to the ulna is the common approach. I prefer an anterior approach, however, because the anterior border of the ulna is flat, and, therefore, the plate fits better and is buried deep to the FCU and FDP muscles, reducing plate irritation.
- In general, the incision is 2 cm longer than the implant to be utilized.

TECHNIQUES

ANTERIOR APPROACH TO THE RADIUS

- The anterior approach to the radius, first described by Henry,[17] is one of the classic approaches in orthopaedic surgery.
- A straight metallic instrument is placed on the forearm skin, and a C-arm image is taken to judge the position of the fracture. The skin is marked (**TECH FIG 1A**).
- The biceps tendon and radial styloid are found and marked. The diathermy cord is extended between these points (**TECH FIG 1B**), and the skin incision is marked centered on the fracture site (**TECH FIG 1C**).

A

TECH FIG 1 • Anterior approach to the radius. **A.** The patient is positioned supine, with the forearm supinated. In this image the elbow is to the left and the wrist to the right. A straight metal instrument is placed across the forearm, and a C-arm fluoroscopic image is taken to confirm the level of the fracture. *(continued)*

- The skin is incised, and the superficial tissues are carefully dissected, looking for the lateral antebrachial cutaneous nerve (lateral cutaneous nerve of the forearm) (**TECH FIG 1D**).
- At the level of the deep fascia, a Raytech (Raytech Industries, Middletown, CT) is used to sweep the soft tissues so that the ulnar edge of the BR can be seen (**TECH FIG 1E**).
- The deep fascia is incised along the ulnar edge of the BR, and the BR is mobilized and lifted (**TECH FIG 1F**). The radial nerve and radial artery are found deep to the BR.
- The interval between the radial artery and nerve is opened (**TECH FIG 1G,H**), exposing the radius.
- The radial aspect of the pronator teres insertion is dissected off the radial shaft, in this case exposing the distal fragment (**TECH FIG 1I**).
  - For more proximal exposure, follow the radial sensory nerve proximally to the place where it and the posterior interosseous nerve bifurcate (**TECH FIG 1J**).
  - The supinator is dissected off the ulnar aspect of the radius to protect the PIN, thus exposing the proximal fragment (**TECH FIG 1K**).
- The fracture is then reduced and held following AO principles. I prefer six cortices of screw fixation on either side of the fracture and currently use the Synthes Small Fragment Locking Compression Plates as fixation.

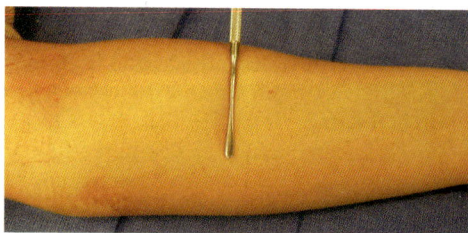

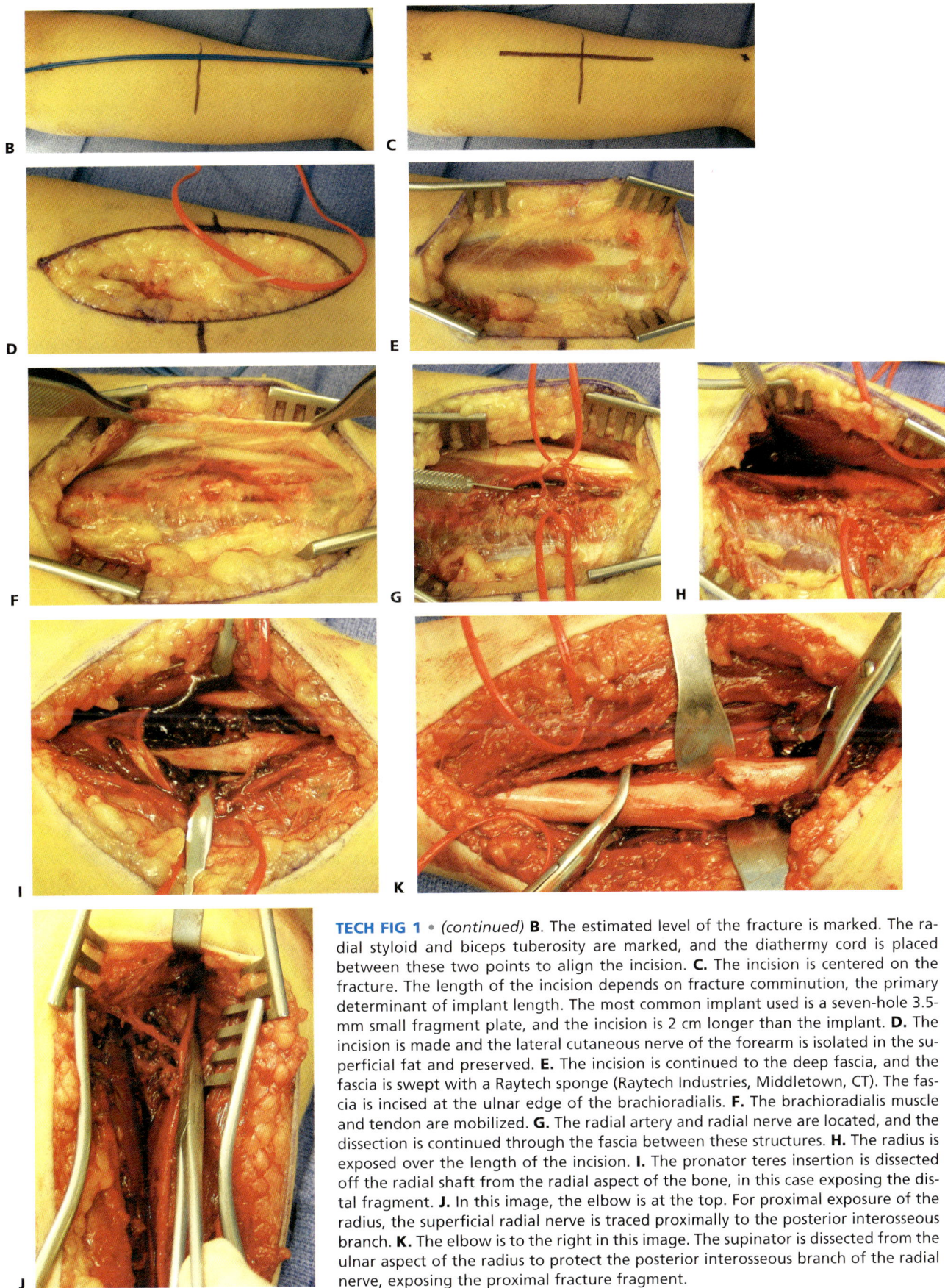

TECH FIG 1 • *(continued)* **B.** The estimated level of the fracture is marked. The radial styloid and biceps tuberosity are marked, and the diathermy cord is placed between these two points to align the incision. **C.** The incision is centered on the fracture. The length of the incision depends on fracture comminution, the primary determinant of implant length. The most common implant used is a seven-hole 3.5-mm small fragment plate, and the incision is 2 cm longer than the implant. **D.** The incision is made and the lateral cutaneous nerve of the forearm is isolated in the superficial fat and preserved. **E.** The incision is continued to the deep fascia, and the fascia is swept with a Raytech sponge (Raytech Industries, Middletown, CT). The fascia is incised at the ulnar edge of the brachioradialis. **F.** The brachioradialis muscle and tendon are mobilized. **G.** The radial artery and radial nerve are located, and the dissection is continued through the fascia between these structures. **H.** The radius is exposed over the length of the incision. **I.** The pronator teres insertion is dissected off the radial shaft from the radial aspect of the bone, in this case exposing the distal fragment. **J.** In this image, the elbow is at the top. For proximal exposure of the radius, the superficial radial nerve is traced proximally to the posterior interosseous branch. **K.** The elbow is to the right in this image. The supinator is dissected from the ulnar aspect of the radius to protect the posterior interosseous branch of the radial nerve, exposing the proximal fracture fragment.

POSTERIOR APPROACH TO THE RADIUS

- The posterior approach to the radius also is known as the dorsolateral approach or Thompson's approach.[24]
- Lister's tubercle is palpated at the dorsal aspect of the distal radius and marked. The lateral epicondyle of the humerus is palpated and marked.
  - The diathermy cord is extended between these bony prominences, and the skin incision is centered on the fracture site.
  - A straight metal instrument is placed transverse to the forearm, and fluoroscopy is used to find the level of the fracture site, which is marked with a transverse line.
- The approach uses the theoretical internervous plane between the ECRB (radial nerve) and the extensor digitorum (PIN; **TECH FIG 2A**).

- The ECRB is part of the mobile wad of Henry,[10] which also includes the BR and the ECRL. This usually can be palpated and can help guide placement of the skin incision.
- After the skin incision and superficial dissection are performed, the interval between the ECRB and EDC is opened distally where the abductor pollicis longus transversely spans the forearm (**TECH FIG 2B**).
- Extending the interval proximally reveals the PIN as it leaves the supinator. Here, it is always accompanied by a leash of vessels, the posterior interosseous artery, and its venae communicantes.
  - The surgeon must be cautious at this stage, because as it leaves the supinator, the PIN quickly gives off small branches to the EDC and ECU. The main nerve at

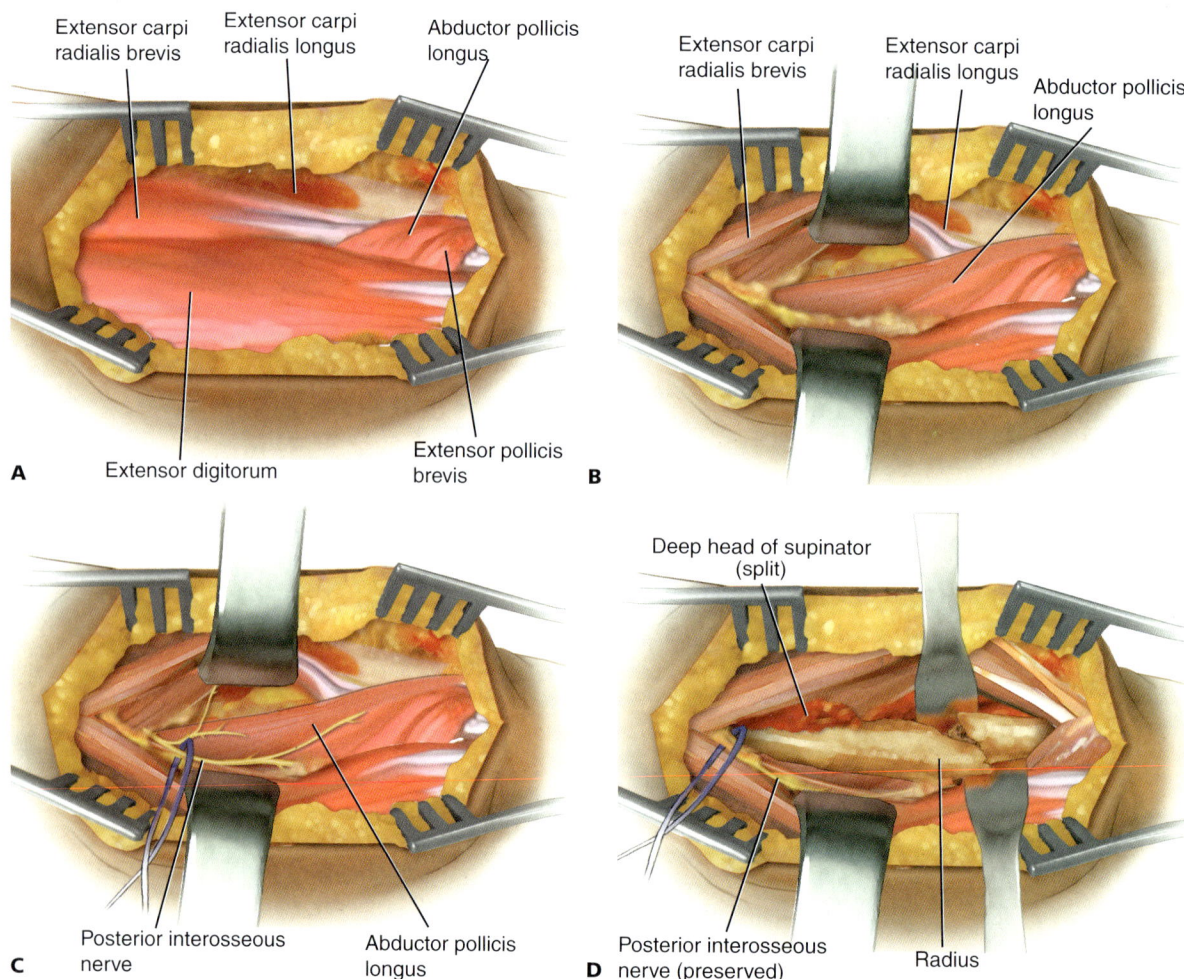

TECH FIG 2 • Posterior approach to the radius. **A.** After incising the deep fascia, the interval between the extensor carpi radialis brevis and the extensor digitorum communis muscles is identified. **B.** The interval between the extensor carpi radialis brevis and extensor digitorum is developed. **C.** Further dissection of the interval proximally with splitting of the aponeurotic origin of the extensors reveals the supinator and the posterior interosseous nerve as it leaves the arcade of Frohse. **D.** Development of the interval between extensor carpi radialis brevis and extensor pollicis longus reveals the radius distal to the extensor pollicis brevis. Proximally, the nerve can be mobilized where it exits the supinator if required. The posterior interosseous nerve should be identified and protected throughout the whole procedure.

this stage can become relatively small, taking on the appearance of a branch.

- Branches to the long muscles to the thumb also can come off relatively high, giving a fan-like appearance to the nerves and branches (**TECH FIG 2C**).
- The PIN must be mobilized from the deep head of supinator. The deep head is then split to reach the radius proximally. Fibers of the pronator teres encroach

into the field over the middle radius, and distally the abductor pollicis longus must be carefully lifted from the radius to provide room for the plate (**TECH FIG 2D**).

- The fracture is then reduced and held with a plate and screws. I prefer a locked small fragment plate (Synthes) with six cortices on either side of the fracture.
- The deep fascia is closed, followed by the skin.

ANTERIOR APPROACH TO THE ULNA

- The anterior approach is my preferred approach for fixation of the distal two thirds of the ulna, because the plate is buried deep to the FCU and FDP muscles and the anterior surface of the ulna is flat, much like the anterior surface of the radius. This allows for minimal contouring of the plate and minimal overhang of the plate over the borders of the bone.
- The bony landmarks for the incision are the medial epicondyle of the humerus and the ulnar aspect of the pisiform at the wrist.
    - As with the radius approach, the diathermy cord can be extended between these two points, a straight

metal instrument can be placed on the patient transverse to the long axis of the forearm, and a C-arm image taken to confirm that the incision is centered on the fracture site (**TECH FIG 3A**).

- The skin incision should be through skin and dermis only.
- If the fracture is relatively distal, care should be taken to avoid injuring the dorsal branch of the ulnar nerve, which exits between the FCU and the ulna about 4 cm proximal to the ulnar head.
- The dissection continues directly deep down to the fascia overlying the FCU muscle. The epimysium and fascia are incised in the line of the incision (**TECH FIG 3B**), and the

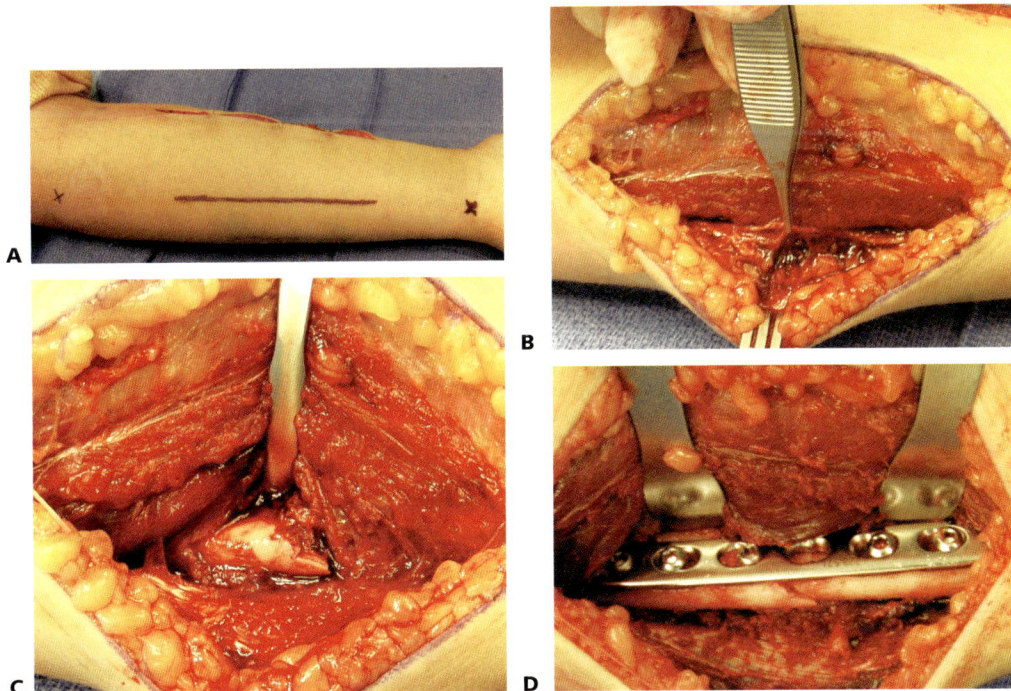

TECH FIG 3 • Anterior approach to the ulna. **A.** The radial incision has been temporarily closed with staples. The medial epicondyle and ulnar aspect of the pisiform are marked. Using a similar technique to that described in Tech Fig 1A, with C-arm fluoroscopy and diathermy lead, the incision is centered on the fracture. **B.** The deep fascia and epimysium of the flexor carpi ulnaris are opened. The fascia is mobilized off the FCU and followed around the ulnar border of the muscle. **C.** The interval between the flexor carpi ulnaris and extensor carpi ulnaris is incised, and the ulna exposed subperiosteally at the level of the fracture site. A Hohmann retractor lifts the FCU. **D.** The flexor digitorum profundus and distally the pronator quadratus are lifted, the fracture is reduced, and a locked small fragment plate applied. (The elbow is to the left and the wrist to the right.)

- dissection continues superficial to the FCU muscle ulnarly around onto the ulna (**TECH FIG 3C**).
- Dissection is continued proximally and distally in the interval between the FCU and ECU, and the fracture is reduced and held with a locked small fragment plate (Synthes; **TECH FIG 3D**).

- I prefer to use six cortices of fixation on either side of the fracture, but this is not possible within 3 cm of the ulnar head. In this situation, two 2.7-mm mini-fragment plates are placed at right angles to each other.
- The fascia and epimysium are closed together, and skin closure follows.

POSTERIOR APPROACH TO THE ULNA

- The posterior approach is preferred for fractures of the proximal third of the ulna diaphysis but can be used to expose the entire ulna.
  - Distally, the dorsal branch of the ulna nerve is at risk where it exits between the FCU and the ulna, but it usually passes distal to the head of the ulna where it crosses the ECU tendon sheath and the extensor retinaculum.
- The interval for the approach is between the ECU and FCU, which share a short fascial septum along most of the length of the ulna.
- The olecranon and ulnar head can be palpated on all patients, and marked. In slim individuals, the fracture and the

entire subcutaneous border of the ulna can be palpated. The incision is centered on the fracture, over the subcutaneous border or in line with the olecranon and ulnar head.

- The incision is deepened down to the fascia, and in most cases the epimysium over the ECU is opened. The ulna is exposed in the interval between the ECU and FCU distally and between the FCU and anconeus proximally.
- The fracture is reduced and held following AO principles with a locked small fragment plate. The plate usually is placed on the lateral surface of the ulna.

FRACTURE REDUCTION AND FIXATION

- Once the bone is reached by an anterior or posterior approach, reduction and fixation are performed.
- Bone-holding clamps allow delivery of the fracture ends into the wound (**TECH FIG 4A**).
  - For an oblique fracture, a lobster claw bone reduction clamp is placed on either side of the fracture site and angled about 30 degrees to the longitudinal axis of the bone. This allows control of both fracture fragments.
- The fracture fragments are completely cleaned of all soft tissue debris (**TECH FIG 4B**).
- The fracture fragments are reduced using longitudinal traction and rotation (**TECH FIG 4C**).
- Once this is accomplished provisional stability is obtained using a bone clamp across the fracture site (**TECH FIG 4D**).

- The clamp is then lifted and the plate slid beneath and the clamp replaced (**TECH FIG 4E**).
  - In its mid-portion the radius is bowed, but the plate is straight. The plate will always appear to sit obliquely even when properly applied.
- The two screw holes closest to the fracture are filled first, followed by placement of an interfragmentary screw (**TECH FIG 4F**).
- In both-bone fractures, the second bone is now approached and stabilized in a similar manner before final fixation of the first fracture.
- Locking (**TECH FIG 4G**) or non-locking screws are placed in the remaining open screw holes, and fixation is complete (**TECH FIG 4H**).

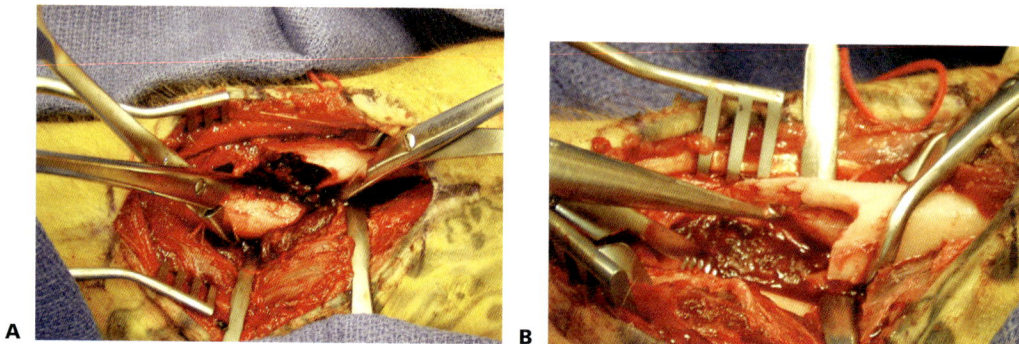

A **B**

TECH FIG 4 • Reduction of an oblique fracture. **A.** A lobster-claw bone reduction clamp is placed on either side of the fracture site and angled about 30 degrees to the longitudinal axis of the bone. Each end of the fracture is delivered into the wound. **B.** The fracture fragments are completely cleaned of all soft tissue debris. *(continued)*

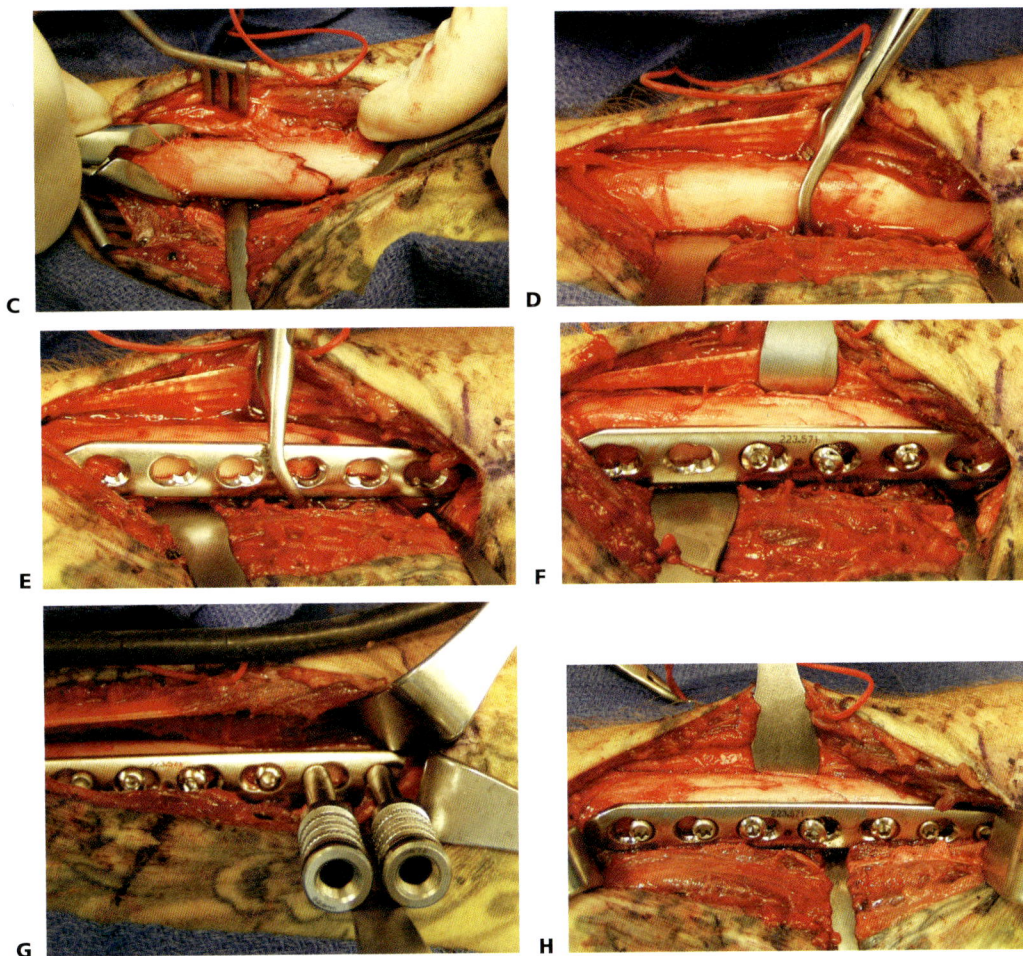

TECH FIG 4 • *(continued)* **C.** Fracture reduction is obtained using longitudinal traction, and rotation applied through the lobster clamps. **D.** The lobster-claw bone clamp temporarily secures the fracture site. **E.** The clamp is lifted and the plate slid beneath. **F.** One screw on each side of the fracture and closest to the fracture is placed first, followed by an interfragmentary screw. **G.** Locking guides attached to the proximal two holes allow placement of the locking screws in this Synthes plate. **H.** Fixation is complete.

PEARLS AND PITFALLS

Plate irritation on the subcutaneous border of the ulna	■ Use an anterior approach on the distal half to two thirds of the diaphysis and place the plate on the anterior (volar) surface. Be very diligent about screw length, because long screws can be felt dorsally. Place the plate more proximally on the lateral surface.
Proximal exposure of the radius and the posterior interosseous nerve	■ When in doubt, find the nerve. This is mandatory in a posterior approach, but in an anterior approach follow the superficial radial nerve to its bifurcation proximally.
The wound is tight and difficult to close.	■ Leave the wound open, admit the patient to the hospital for strict elevation, and revisit the operating room in 48 to 72 hours. The wound usually will have closed at that time. This scenario is far more predictable and easier to deal with than a compartment problem and a wound slough.
Should the fascia be closed?	■ In most patients, the fascia can be safely closed, but when it is tense, leave open and consider the above.
Distal radioulnar joint and forearm rotation	■ Always examine the DRUJ for stability at the end of the case, and put the forearm through a range of motion. Then obtain radiographs of the wrist. ■ DRUJ instability can be subtle and may not be picked up until late. ■ DRUJ problems can occur in the presence of an ulna fracture. ■ If the forearm is not able to complete a full ROM (compare opposite forearm), that usually means the radial bow has not been preserved.
Proximal radioulnar joint	■ As with the DRUJ an elbow AP and lateral should be performed at the end of the case.

POSTOPERATIVE CARE

- The key points in immediate postoperative care are splinting, pain relief, elevation of the extremity, and watching for signs of complications.
  - The patient usually receives axillary block anesthesia, which allows him or her to return home pain-free.
  - A sugartong splint is placed at the time of surgery and is worn for 2 weeks, at which time the patient returns to the office for a removal of splint and sutures.
  - Narcotic pain relief usually is ceased at 2 weeks.
  - Radiographs of the wrist, elbow, and forearm are ordered at the 2-week visit.
- At the 2-week visit the patient is referred for physical therapy and rehabilitation to work on ROM of the elbow, forearm, and wrist using active and gentle active assisted exercises.
- From 2 to 6 weeks, the patient is given a 5-pound weight lifting restriction and is placed on restricted work duty, including no repetitive forearm twisting, until union occurs.
- At 6 weeks, simple two-part fractures usually are united and all lifting and twisting restrictions are removed. If there is no evidence of union, the patient is placed on a 20-pound weight restriction until union has occurred.

OUTCOMES

- In two-part fracture of the radius and ulna, patients can expect over 95% problem-free consolidation before 6 months. In a study by Hertel,[11] out of 132 patients there were two delayed unions and two non-unions that required reoperation. Plates were removed from 70 patients (53%) at a mean of 33.1 months (range 8–122 months) after the first operation. In this group, there were three refractures (4.3%) occurring at a mean of 8.7 months (range 0–14) after plate removal. In another study by Chapman,[7] 98% of the fractures united, and 92% of the patients achieved an excellent or satisfactory functional result.
- Nonunion rates are much higher in comminuted fractures, approximately 12%, but it has been shown that bone grafting primarily does not lead to improved outcomes.[19]

COMPLICATIONS

- Complications of forearm fractures include compartment syndrome,[6] malunion,[25] nonunion,[5] and radioulnar synostosis.[4] The rate of infection is about 2%.[7]
- In a study by Stern[23] of 64 adult patients with 87 diaphyseal forearm fractures treated by plating, 18 patients (28%) had a major complication. There was a nonunion rate four times higher for bones plated with four screws than six screws, and screws loosened in three fractures, all involving the ulna. Radioulnar synostosis occurred in seven forearms, and in five of these the forearm injuries were associated with multiple-system trauma involving head injury. Two patients had osteomyelitis.
- The surgeon must be aware of the DRUJ and PRUJ dislocation associated with either an isolated or both-bone forearm fracture.

- With attention to detail, using the appropriate anatomic approach, accurate reduction, and the use of hardware that provides adequate bone stability, outcomes from diaphyseal fractures of the forearm are as good as any in orthopaedic surgery.

REFERENCES

1. Anderson LD, Sisk D, Tooms RE, et al. Compression-plate fixation in acute diaphyseal fractures of the radius and ulna. J Bone Joint Surg Am 1975;57:287.
2. Bado JL. The Monteggia lesion. Clin Orthop Relat Res 1967; 50:71–86.
3. Bolton H, Quinlan AG. The conservative treatment of fractures of the shaft of the radius and the ulna in adults. Lancet 1952;1:700.
4. Botting TD. Posttraumatic radio-ulna cross union. J Trauma 1970; 10:16–24.
5. Brakenbury H, Corea JR, Blakemore ME. Nonunion of the isolated fracture of the ulnar shafts in adults. Injury 1985;12:371.
6. Brostrom LA, Stark A, Svartengren G. Acute compartment syndrome in forearm fractures. Acta Orthop Scand 1990;61:50–53.
7. Chapman MW, Gordon JE, Zissimos AG. Compression-plate fixation of acute fractures of the diaphyses of the radius and ulna. J Bone Joint Surg Am 1989;71A:159–169.
8. Evans EM. Rotational deformities in the treatment of fractures of both bones of the forearm. J Bone Joint Surg Am 1945;27A:373–379.
9. Galeazzi R. Uber ein Besonderes Syndrom bei Verltzunger im Bereich der Unteraumknochen. Arch OrthoUnfallchir 1934;35:557–562.
10. Henry AK. Extensile Exposure, 2nd ed. Baltimore: Williams & Wilkins, 1970.
11. Hertel R, Pisan M, Lambert S, et al. Plate osteosynthesis of diaphyseal fractures of the radius and ulna. Injury 1996;27:545–548.
12. Hughston JC. Fracture of the distal radial shaft: Mistakes in management. J Bone Joint Surg Am 1957;39:249–264.
13. Knight RA, Purvis GD. Fractures of both bones of the forearm in adults. J Bone Joint Surg Am 1949;31A:755–764.
14. Mackay D, Wood L, Rangan A. The treatment of isolated ulnar fractures in adults: a systematic review. Injury 2000;31:565–570.
15. Matthews LS, Kaufer H, Garver DF, et al. The effect on supination-pronation of angular malalignment of fractures of both bones of the forearm. J Bone Joint Surg Am 1982;64A:14–17.
16. Mino DE, Palmar AK, Levinsohn EM. The role of radiography and computerized tomography in the diagnosis of subluxation and dislocation of the distal radioulnar joint. J Hand Surg Am 1983;8:23–31.
17. Monteggia GB. Instituzioni Chirurgiche Vol. 5. Milano: Maspero, 1814.
18. Muller ME, Allgower M, Schneider R, et al. Manual of Internal Fixation: Techniques Recommended by the AO-ASIF Group. New York: Springer-Verlag, 1991.
19. Ring D, Rhim R, Carpenter C, et al. Comminuted diaphyseal fractures of the radius and ulna: Does bone grafting affect nonunion rate? J Trauma 2005;59:438–441.
20. Rosacker JA, Kopta JA. Both bone fractures of the forearm: A review of surgical variables associated with union. Orthopaedics 1981; 4:1353–1356.
21. Sarmiento A, Latta LL, Zych G, et al. Isolated ulnar shaft fractures treated with functional braces. J Orthop Trauma 1998;12:420–423.
22. Schemitsch EH, Richards RR. The effect of malunion on functional outcome after plate fixation of fractures of both bones of the forearm in adults. J Bone Joint Surg Am 1992;74:1068–1078.
23. Stern PJ, Drury WJ. Complications of plate fixation of forearm fractures. Clin Orthop Relat Res 1983;175:25–29.
24. Thompson JE. Anatomical methods of approach in operations on the long bones of the extremities. Ann Surg 1918;68:309.
25. Trousdale RT, Linscheid RL. Operative treatment of malunited fractures of the forearm. J Bone Joint Surg Am 1995;77A:894–902.

Chapter 5

Reduction and Stabilization of the Distal Radioulnar Joint Following Galeazzi Fractures

Michael R. Boland

DEFINITION

- In 1934 Galeazzi[7] described a fracture of the junction of the middle and distal thirds of the radius and called attention to the associated dislocation or subluxation of the distal radioulnar joint (DRUJ).
- Garcia-Elias and Dobyns[8] divided DRUJ dislocations into three types:
  - Type I: Pure soft tissue dislocations
  - Type II: Intra-articular fracture dislocations where there is a fracture involving the joint surface of the sigmoid notch of the radius
  - Type III: Extra-articular DRUJ fracture dislocations for subdivided
  - Type III fracture-dislocations can be subdivided as follows:
    - IIIa: abnormal joint surface orientation; usually involve fractures of the distal two thirds of the radius without complete longitudinal disruption of the forearm
    - IIIb: radioulnar length discrepancy; fractures of the distal two thirds of the radius with complete longitudinal disruption of the forearm; also known as Essex-Lopresti injuries
- In this chapter, the term *Galeazzi fracture-dislocation* refers to a type IIIa (extra-articular) fracture of the distal two thirds of the radius with any disruption at all of the congruency of the DRUJ due to soft tissue injury.
- Management of the fractured radius is discussed elsewhere (see Chaps. HA-8 to HA-13). A fracture of the ulna styloid commonly is associated with a distal radius fracture. Reduction and fixation of this fracture is covered in Chapter HA-14.

ANATOMY

- During forearm rotation a complex interaction occurs between the radius and the ulna.
  - From about 50 degrees pronation to 50 degrees supination there is a nearly pure rotation of the radius around the ulna, with the center of rotation through the middle of the ulna head. The ulna moves out of the way of the radius by virtue of a 9-degree varus–valgus motion that occurs at the elbow.
  - At 50 degrees supination or pronation, a translational slide of the radius occurs on the ulna at the DRUJ.
  - In full pronation the radius slides volar, making the ulna head prominent dorsally. The opposite takes place in full supination.
- The head of the ulna is the keystone of the DRUJ. It is flattened distally adjacent to the triangular fibrocartilage disc and rounded radially articulating with the sigmoid notch of the radius. The sigmoid notch of the radius is only mildly concave but is functionally deepened by a horseshoe-shaped labrum. A flimsy, somewhat loose capsule attached to this labrum allows the nearly 180 degrees of rotation required of the forearm.

- The capsule is relevant only when it is thickened, causing a contracture and limitation in forearm motion.[12]
- Considerable incongruity exists between the curvature of the ulna head and sigmoid notch, which, along with the weak capsule, results in an inherently lax joint.
- The triangular fibrocartilage is a specialized structure, part meniscus (to allow compression accommodating the relative shortening of the radius in pronation) and part ligament. It has palmar and dorsal fibrous thickenings known as the palmar and dorsal radioulnar ligaments. These attach to the distal palmar and dorsal rims of the sigmoid notch as separate bundles, and have superficial fibers that attach to the ulna styloid and deep fibers that criss-cross to form a weave as they attach to the foveal fossa of the distal ulna adjacent to the head. These ligaments, along with the distal aspect of the interosseous membrane, are the most important primary stabilizers of the DRUJ.
  - During rotation, the deep interdigitating fibers create a screw home mechanism, similar to the cruciate ligaments of the knee.
  - In pronation the deep fibers of the dorsal radioulnar ligament are taut and the superficial fibers are lax, whereas the superficial fibers of the palmar radioulnar ligament are taut and the deep fibers are lax.[10]
  - The opposite is true in supination. Avulsion of the foveal attachment is common in Galeazzi injuries.

PATHOGENESIS

- The most common mechanism of injury is an axial load in pronation, associated with wrist hyperextension.
- Acute dislocations of the DRUJ also can occur in supination. This usually happens after a fall with a rotating body on an outstretched hand, but also can occur in the workplace when the forearm is twisted by rotating machinery.[8]
- The direction of force is radial to ulnar and proximal to distal, through the radius fracture down the interosseous membrane, and through the DRUJ.
  - The DRUJ zone of injury includes the capsule, avulsion of the foveal attachment of the palmar and dorsal radioulnar ligament, and tear of the extensor carpi ulnaris (ECU) subsheath.

NATURAL HISTORY

- Hughston,[9] in 1957, brought attention to the poor outcome of these fracture-dislocations without surgical intervention. The criteria used for a perfect result were very strict, leading to a judgment of poor results in 92% of cases. This injury complex has been termed "the fracture of necessity," meaning open reduction and internal fixation of the radius is necessary for a good result.[22]
- Mikic[15] drew attention to the significance of the DRUJ injury. He advocated reduction and percutaneous K-wire fixation, noting poor results otherwise.

- Experiments have shown that with an artificial osteotomy of the radius, up to 5 mm of radial shortening occurs.[18] Shortening of more than 10 mm does not occur unless both the interosseous ligament and the triangular ligament are sectioned.
- Alexander and Lichtman[2] added another subcategory of Galeazzi injury, those in which closed reduction cannot be achieved. The natural history of injuries in this subcategory depends on the recognition and appropriate management of neurologic and vascular complications, in addition to the adequacy of reduction and the degree of DRUJ instability.
- The DRUJ component of Galeazzi fracture dislocations, after anatomic reduction and fixation of the radius, can be considered simple (ie, able to be reduced closed) or complex (ie, requiring open reduction).[19] Once reduced, the DRUJ is re-examined and judged stable or unstable.

PATIENT HISTORY AND PHYSICAL FINDINGS

- Lister[13] stated "nothing influences the eventual recovery of hand function more than the mechanism and the force of the injury." This is certainly true for forearm injuries.
  - Accurate anatomic bone anatomy is required for perfect functioning of the forearm during rotation.
- Patients with a Galeazzi fracture-dislocation usually present acutely to an emergency department due to the severity of the pain.
- Three common mechanisms lead to Galeazzi injuries: falls, industrial accidents, and motor vehicle trauma.

- It is important to elicit information regarding the degree of energy associated with the injury. A fall off a ladder from a height or from a roof is associated with much greater energy than a ground-level fall.
- In industrial accidents, the worker will tend to use technical jargon in referring to machinery, but the examiner must obtain a layman's description of the machinery and get an accurate idea of the force the machinery will generate.
  - Any motor vehicle accident is associated with high energy.
  - Any crushing component to the injury must be elicited.
- Initially, the fracture pain may overwhelm both the patient and the examiner. Reassessment of the patient following a radiograph showing a radius fracture in the presence of an intact ulna should direct the examiner to the DRUJ as a site of pathology.
- The patient must be asked about neurologic symptoms in the hand, in particular numbness and tingling in the median nerve distribution.
  - Acute carpal tunnel syndrome and forearm and hand compartment syndromes must be ruled out in the Emergency Department.
- Forearm swelling and tenderness with dorsal prominence of the distal ulna (ie, caput ulna deformity) will be observed.
- The entire carpus and the elbow should be palpated to rule out any longitudinal forearm injury (ie, Essex Lopresti injury).
- Forearm, wrist, and digital motion often are extremely limited due to pain.

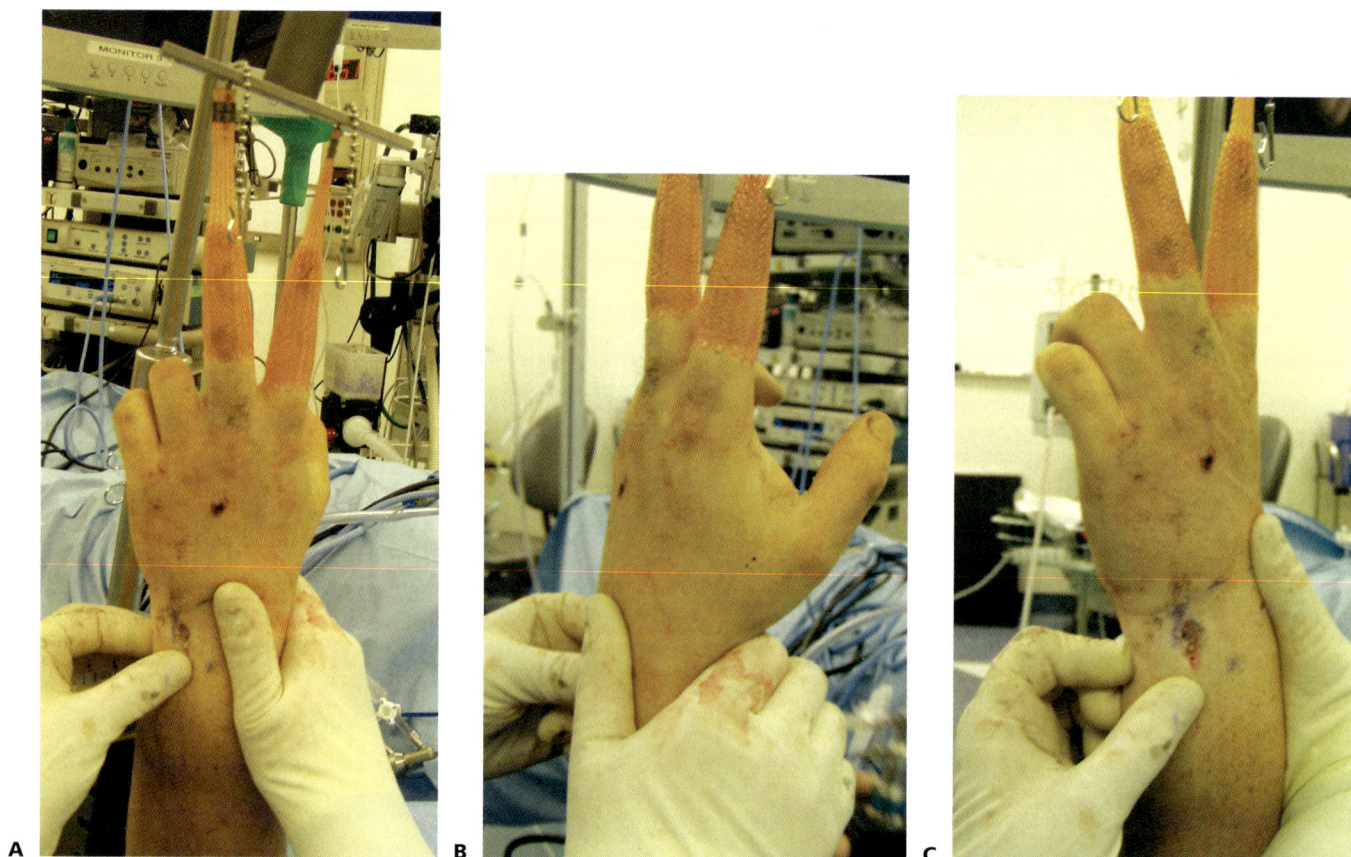

FIG 1 • Intraoperative distal radioulnar joint (DRUJ) shuck test. The head of the ulna is held with a chuck pinch grip, and the wrist and distal radius are held with a span grasp with the thumb extended across the wrist joint. The radius is held firmly and the ulna is moved back and forth in a palmar-dorsal direction. The test is done first in neutral (**A**), then in supination (**B**) and in pronation (**C**).

Table 1	Shuck Test		
Grade	**Description**	**Pathogenesis/Diagnosis**	**Management**
I	<0.5 cm motion at extremes; firm endpoint	Probable intrasubstance tearing of either the PRUL or DRUL	Cast in neutral rotation
II	>0.5 cm motion at extremes; soft endpoint but no dislocation	Usually associated with foveal avulsion of the TFCC; can be confirmed by arthroscopy of the DRUJ and repaired. No rupture of the distal interosseous membrane.	Cast in midpronation
III	Reduced joint seen before stress, with dislocation of the DRUJ at extremes	Rupture of distal aspect of interosseous membrane	Repair foveal avulsion as for grade II; pin DRUJ in midsupination.
IV	Dislocated joint	"Mushy" feeling on stressing joint	Reducible with rotation, consider malposition of radius fragments if easily dislocatable. If truly mushy throughout forearm rotation, there is interposition of soft tissue, and open treatment is required.

DRUJ, distal radioulnar joint; *DRUL,* distal radioulnar ligament; *PRUL,* proximal radioulnar ligament.

- A sensory examination using static two-point testing is the most reliable Emergency Department examination for sensation. Vascularity is best assessed by examination of radial and ulnar pulses together with capillary refill in the fingers.
  - Often the fingers are pale in this situation. A needle stick to the digital pulp should cause bright red bleeding.
- The fingers must be passively extended to rule out a forearm compartment syndrome. Inability to extend the fingers combined with tense forearm swelling are the best indicators of a compartment syndrome, which if present, necessitates urgent surgery.
- Patients presenting late, in the office, usually complain of ulnar-sided wrist pain, pain with activities requiring pronosupination, and DRUJ instability. In these situations the radius often is malunited or there is unrecognized bowing of the ulna.
- The DRUJ is examined initially by direct observation, looking for a caput ulna deformity. Palpation begins at the radial head, along the interosseous membrane to the ulnar head. Tenderness at the DRUJ proper is elicited by palpating the head of the ulna with the examiner's thumb and sliding the thumb off the head in a radial direction. Tenderness just distal to the head dorsally is associated with a dorsal tear of the triangular fibrocartilage complex (TFCC). A volar tear of the TFCC is tender on palpation of the ulnar head between the FCU and ECU and when the examiner slides his or her thumb distally over the head.
- DRUJ laxity is assessed with the elbow flexed 90 degrees. A shuck test is done on the DRUJ at neutral, full pronation, and full supination (**FIG 1**), and then compared with the uninjured wrist.
  - At full rotation, there should be no motion of the radius relative to the ulna. At neutral, the DRUJ ligaments are loose and there is about 1 cm of shuck (Table 1).

IMAGING AND OTHER DIAGNOSTIC STUDIES

- Imaging of the patient with a suspected Galeazzi injury consists of plain radiographs of the elbow, forearm, and wrist.
  - The forearm views help in preoperative planning for fixation of the radius fracture.
  - The wrist views help to determine the degree of disruption to the DRUJ. On a posteroanterior (PA) view of the wrist, the degree of ulna shortening has been shown to differ depending on which structures are torn at the DRUJ.[18] Less than 5 mm of positive variance of the ulna indicates that TFCC disruption is unlikely; more than 1 cm indicates interosseous membrane disruption.
- Mino et al[16] described a technique for interpreting the lateral wrist radiograph whereby the radial styloid is aligned with the center of the lunate and an assessment of the overlap of the radius and ulna is made. The head of the ulna should be completely obscured by the radius. If only part of the ulna head is obscured by the radius, then there is subluxation of the head, and if the ulnar head is clearly seen, then the joint is dislocated. In the operating room a C-arm image in neutral forearm rotation is obtained with the radial styloid in the mid-lunate position to interpret DRUJ subluxation.
- A CT scan is very useful in measuring the degree of subluxation or dislocation of the DRUJ. A CT scan in the acute situation can be useful in interpreting the degree of DRUJ congruity, but the test is more often performed in the setting of a chronic injury.
  - This is most reliably interpreted by the radioulnar ratio (**FIG 2**), calculated as follows:
    - The center of the ulnar head is found using concentric circles.
    - A line similar to that used in the epicenter method is drawn from the dorsal and volar margins of the sigmoid notch (line A-B).
    - A line perpendicular to this line is drawn to the center of the ulnar head (line C).
    - The AD:AB ratio is the radioulnar ratio. The normal ratios are 0.5 to 0.71 for pronation, 0.42 to 0.58 for neutral, and 0.19 to 0.55 for supination.

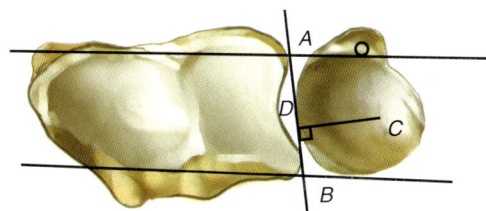

FIG 2 • Radioulnar ratio method to measure DRUJ subluxation on a CT scan. See text for details. (Adapted from Lo IK, MacDermid JC, Bennett JD, et al. The radioulnar ratio: A new method of quantifying distal radioulnar joint subluxation. J Hand Surg Am 2001;26:236–243.)

- MRI shows foveal avulsion injuries well and is useful for the assessment of the TFCC.

DIFFERENTIAL DIAGNOSIS

- The differential diagnosis of ulnar wrist pain in the presence of a radius fracture includes:
  - Fracture of the ulna: shaft, metaphysis, head, styloid
  - Triangular fibrocartilage complex injury. Any of the following structures may be injured: fibrocartilage disc, palmar and dorsal radioulnar ligaments, ulnotriquetral ligament, ulnolunate ligament, ECU subsheath.
  - Lunotriquetral ligament: isolated and as part of either a perilunate dislocation or a longitudinal wrist
  - Carpal fractures: triquetrum, hamate, lunate
- Essex-Lopresti injury
- Monteggia fracture-dislocation
- Elbow fracture-dislocation
- Stress and pathologic fractures of the radius

NONOPERATIVE MANAGEMENT

- The only time the radius is not internally fixed is when other patient factors make such surgery unsafe.
- In the Emergency Department, the longitudinal injury to the forearm should be reduced and held in a splint.
  - The reduction maneuver is performed under conscious sedation with the thumb and index fingers placed in finger traps and 10 pounds of traction applied.
  - A sugartong or long-arm splint with an interosseous mold is applied.
  - Radiographs must be obtained to confirm reduction.
- If the DRUJ is reduced, then surgery can be delayed for up to 2 weeks. If the DRUJ remains dislocated, surgery should be performed within 72 hours.
  - This interval allows an MRI or CT scan to be ordered and interpreted to plan for the operative procedure.
- Options for nonoperative management of the DRUJ after fixation of the radius are discussed later in this chapter.

SURGICAL MANAGEMENT

- The key to the management of a Galeazzi fracture is determination of the degree of injury to the DRUJ. It can be classified as stable, unstable but reducible, or unstable and irreducible.
- The following information is considered in deciding whether the DRUJ is unstable:
  - If, on the initial pre-reduction PA radiograph, the ulna variance is more than 5 mm positive
  - If frank dislocation remains after evaluation of the postreduction lateral radiograph using the Mino technique (discussed under Imaging And Other Diagnostic Studies)

- A foveal avulsion of the TFCC is noted on the preoperative MRI scan.
- Intraoperative fluoroscopic examination of the DRUJ after fracture fixation
  - Intra-operative C-arm assessment includes PA and lateral views in neutral rotation. In most cases the DRUJ should be reduced following fixation.
  - If increased ulna variance, joint diastasis, or subluxation of the ulna head is seen, the first possibility to consider is a malreduction of the radius fracture.
- Most importantly, instability is determined by intraoperative physical examination after fracture fixation.
  - Grade I: less than 0.5 cm motion at extremes, with a firm endpoint. Probable intrasubstance tearing of either the proximal radioulnar ligament or the DRUL. Management is in a cast in neutral rotation.
  - Grade II: more than 0.5 cm motion at extremes, with a soft endpoint but no dislocation. This injury usually is associated with foveal avulsion of the TFCC, which can be confirmed by arthroscopy of the DRUJ and repaired. The distal interosseous membrane is not ruptured. Cast in midsupination.[3]
  - Grade III: reduced joint prior to stress with dislocation of the DRUJ at extremes. Requires rupture of the distal aspect of the interosseous membrane. Repair the foveal avulsion as in grade II and pin the DRUJ in mid-supination.
  - Grade IV: dislocated joint. "Mushy" feeling with stressing joint. This joint may be reducible with rotation; consider malposition of radius fragments if easily dislocatable. If truly mushy throughout forearm rotation, then there is interposition of soft tissue, and open treatment is required.

Positioning

- The patient is positioned supine on the operating table with a hand table, and the affected extremity is abducted at the shoulder and extended across the table.
  - The hand table is positioned so that it adjoins the main table at the level of the shoulder. When the extremity is abducted 90 degrees, it lies in the mid portion of the table.
- A tourniquet is applied at the mid-humerus level, and a layer of towels is placed between the humerus and the arm. A layer of padding is placed on the upper arm just proximal to the elbow, and the arm is taped firmly to the hand table. This allows traction to be applied along the axis of the forearm for arthroscopy.
- Following fixation of the radius, finger traps are applied to the long and index fingers, and 10 to 12 lb of traction is applied.

Approach

- The DRUJ can be approached using arthroscopy,[28] a miniopen technique,[6] or an open dorsal approach.[22]

TECHNIQUES

ARTHROSCOPICALLY ASSISTED REPAIR OF FOVEAL TFCC AVULSIONS

Arthroscopy of the Distal Radioulnar Joint

- A 1.9-mm scope and 2.0-mm shaver are the working instruments for DRUJ arthroscopy.
- Two principal portals are used.
  - The dorsal-proximal DRUJ (PDRUJ) portal is located in the axilla of the joint, just proximal to the sigmoid

notch of the radius and the flare of the metaphysis of the ulna. It is easily palpated with the wrist supinated, which relaxes the dorsal capsule and facilitates introduction of the trocar and scope sheath.

- The joint is insufflated with about 3 mL of saline (which helps as a direction guide), the skin is incised with a no. 15 blade, and a hemostat pierces the deep fascia and capsule, followed by scope sheath insertion.

- After initial joint penetration, the scope is withdrawn slightly until the sigmoid notch and neck of the ulna are brought into view.
- Systematically, the steps of a diagnostic arthroscopy are as follows
  - Evaluate the sigmoid notch while in supination.
  - Look down into the axilla of the joint (loose bodies sometimes hide here).
- The scope is then swept distally over the head of the ulna and pushed anteriorly between the disc of the TFCC and the seat of the head while relaxing the rotation of the forearm to neutral.
- Rotate into pronation and visualize the anterior compartment of the DRUJ.
- Then slightly withdraw the scope and visualize the foveal region.
- The distal DRUJ (DDRUJ) portal is located just distal to the seat of the ulna between the fifth and sixth dorsal compartments. It is about 5 mm proximal to the 6R portal.
  - The DDRUJ portal allows entry of the scope between the disc of the TFCC and the head of the ulna.
  - A 21-gauge hypodermic needle is inserted as a direction finder with the scope in the PDRUJ portal.
- A probe can be inserted to stress the undersurface of the TFCC disc and ligament insertion into the fovea.
- A shaver and other instruments also can be introduced through the DDRUJ portal.

Repair of Foveal TFCC Avulsion

- Diagnostic arthroscopy of the radiocarpal joint may reveal a peripheral tear in the TFCC.
- Mid-carpal arthroscopy is performed primarily to evaluate the integrity of the lunotriquetral ligament.
- DRUJ arthroscopy shows the status of the proximal surface of the TFCC and confirms a foveal tear of the TFCC (**TECH FIG 1A**).
- A shaver is introduced through the DDRUJ portal to débride this area (**TECH FIG 1B**), and the mini C-arm is brought in to confirm position over the fovea.
- A curette is used to freshen the ulna at the foveal insertion.
- Using a C-arm and arthroscopic guidance, a 1.8-mm drill hole is made (**TECH FIG 1C–E**).
- The DDRUJ portal is then enlarged to about 1 cm in size with the drill bit in place (**TECH FIG 1F**).
- The deep fascia and capsule are opened in line with the incision. A Mitek Mini QuickAnchor (Mitek Products, Norwood, MA) is inserted into the drill hole (**TECH FIG 1G**).
- Each suture end is placed through the TFCC, and the needle is brought out the 6R window made in the radiocarpal capsule.
- The suture is then tied, pulling the TFCC back to its anatomic position.
- A DRUJ shuck test is performed to ensure restoration of stability, the wounds are closed, and a long-arm splint is added in mid-supination.

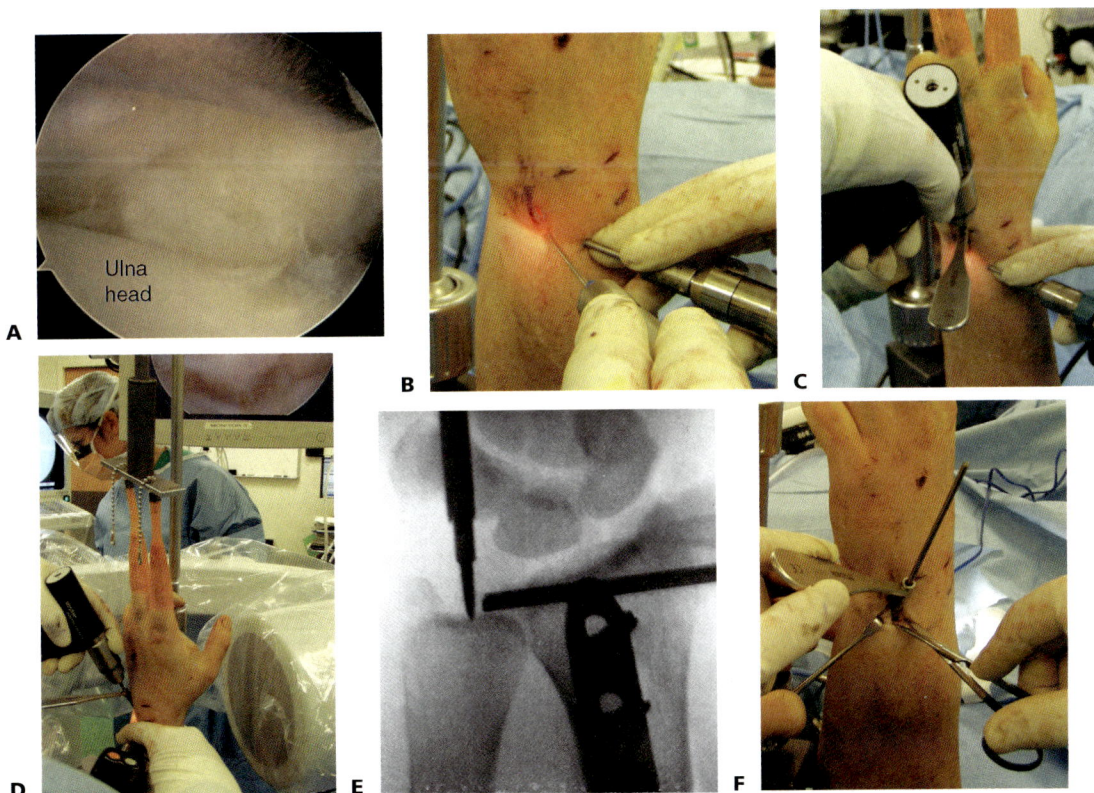

TECH FIG 1 • Diagnostic arthroscopy and distal radioulnar joint (DRUJ) arthroscope-assisted repair of the triangular fibrocartilage complex (TFCC). **A.** Foveal avulsion tear. **B.** Hand placement and portal position using 1.9-mm scope and 2.0-mm shaver. **C.** Hand placement for drilling before Mitek anchor insertion. **D.** Position of the mini–C-arm, which is brought in to confirm placement of the drill bit in the fovea for insertion of the Mitek anchor. **E.** C-arm image confirming placement of the drill bit at the foveal insertion of the TFCC. **F.** The distal DRUJ portal is opened to about 1 cm, and dissection is carried down through the deep fascia in line with the incision. Care is taken to avoid the dorsal branch of the ulnar nerve. *(continued)*

TECHNIQUES

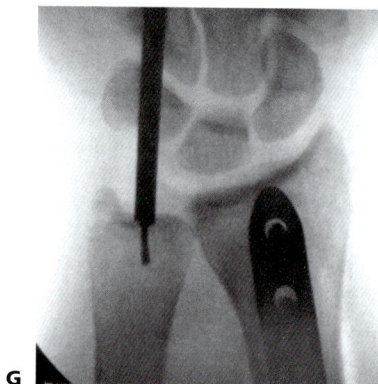

TECH FIG 1 • *(continued)* **G.** C-arm image confirming placement of the Mitek anchor.

ARTHROSCOPICALLY ASSISTED REPAIR OF FOVEAL TFCC AVULSION WITH RADIOCARPAL ARTHROSCOPY AND OPEN TECHNIQUES

Mini-Open Approach

- In the mini-open approach, a diagnostic arthroscopy of the radiocarpal joint is carried out.
- The 6R portal should be made in a longitudinal orientation. This is a guide for creation of a longitudinal 2- to 3-cm incision incorporating the 6R portal.
  - The incision usually is about 5 mm distal to the 6R portal and 2 cm proximal.
  - The dorsal branch of the ulnar nerve is found in the soft tissues at the distal end of the incision and is preserved.
- The deep fascia is incised in line with the incision.
- A 21-gauge needle is inserted through the capsule of the DRUJ into the interval between the head and the proximal edge of the TFCC.
- The joint capsule is incised from just proximal to the TFCC disc to the metaphysis of the ulna.
- A 21-gauge needle is then inserted just distal to the TFCC disc into the radiocarpal joint.
- The radiocarpal joint capsule is incised transversely about 6 or 7 mm (not quite to the lunate).

- The 6R portal also can be enlarged to see the distal aspect of the TFCC disc. This gives the surgeon good visualization of both surfaces of the TFCC disc and associated ligaments.

Repair of Foveal TFCC Avulsion

- The avulsed TFCC is identified and débrided.
- The ulnar fovea is roughened with a curette and drilled with a 1.8-mm bit, after which a single Mitek Mini QuickAnchor (Mitek Products, Norwood, MA) is inserted into the drill hole.
- The torn ulnar border of the TFCC is then advanced and sutured down to the ulnar fovea (**TECH FIG 2**). The suture on the Mitek Quick Anchor is double ended. Each needle is passed from a proximal to distal direction about 5 mm apart, and then the needles are cut off and the sutures tied within the radiocarpal joint. I use a one-handed suture-tying technique. No additional suturing is necessary.
- The capsule, retinaculum, and skin are closed, and a sterile dressing and long-arm splint are applied.

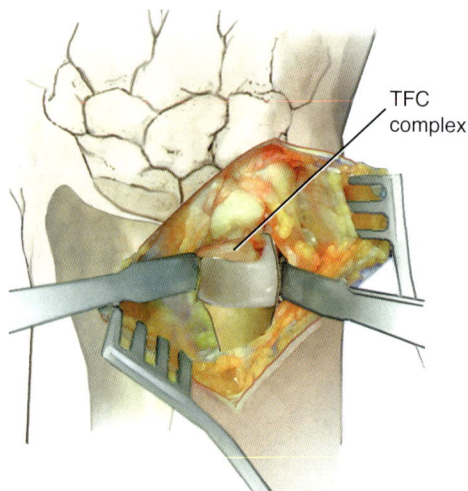

TFC complex

TECH FIG 2 • Sotereanos triangular fibrocartilage complex repair. The technique involves a 3-cm incision centered on the distal aspect of the head of the ulna. Small windows are created in the capsule of the DRUJ and the radiocarpal joint, and the foveal tear of the TFCC is identified. *(continued)*

C

Drill guide

Drill

D

E

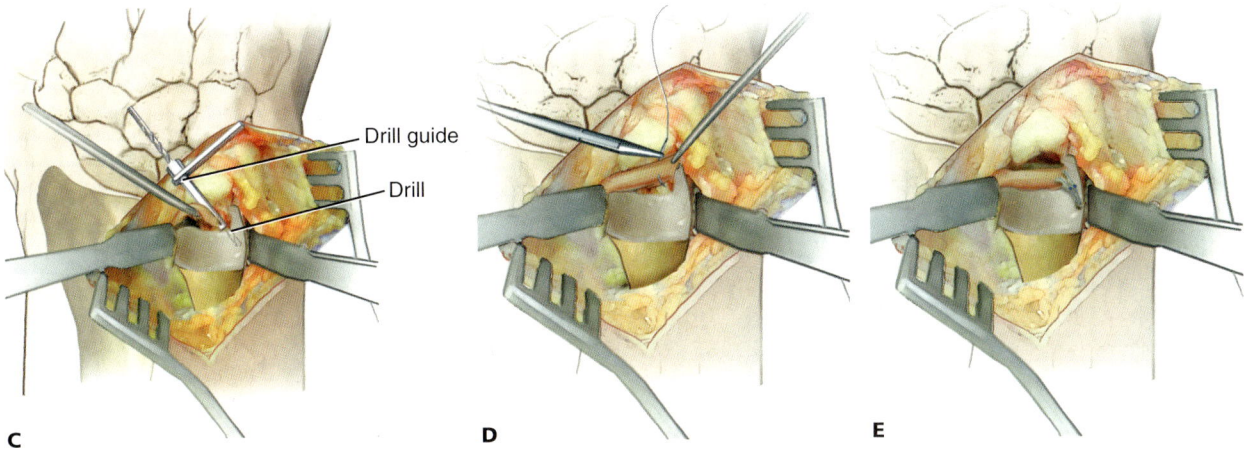

TECH FIG 2 • *(continued)* **C.** The TFCC is lifted and the fovea cleared of soft tissue debris. A bone anchor (usually a 2-0 suture mini-Mitek) is placed in the head of the ulna at the fovea. **D.** The sutures are passed through the TFCC. **E.** The sutures are tied, repairing the TFCC back to its foveal insertion.

OPEN DRUJ ARTHROTOMY AND TFCC REPAIR[11]

Two-Window Exposure of the DRUJ

- The forearm is pronated and extended at the elbow.
- A dorsal incision is made beginning 3 cm distal to the ulnar styloid.
    - The incision is carried proximally at 45 degrees to the long axis of the forearm in a radial direction until it reaches the dorsal aspect of the radius at the sigmoid notch.
    - At this point it is continued proximally, longitudinally down the forearm for about 7 cm (**TECH FIG 3A**).
- The soft tissues are spread, taking care to preserve the dorsal sensory branch of the ulnar nerve, which passes onto the dorsum of the hand about 1 to 2 cm distal to the ulna styloid.

- At the level of the deep fascia the soft tissues are swept off the fascia in the region of the ulna head (**TECH FIG 3B**).
- The distal aspect of the antebrachial fascia and the proximal 50% of the extensor retinaculum are incised longitudinally between the EDM and ECU tendons, and an ulnarly based flap is created (**TECH FIG 3C**).
    - A 21-gauge needle can be inserted to assess the proximal and distal margins of the TFCC disc.

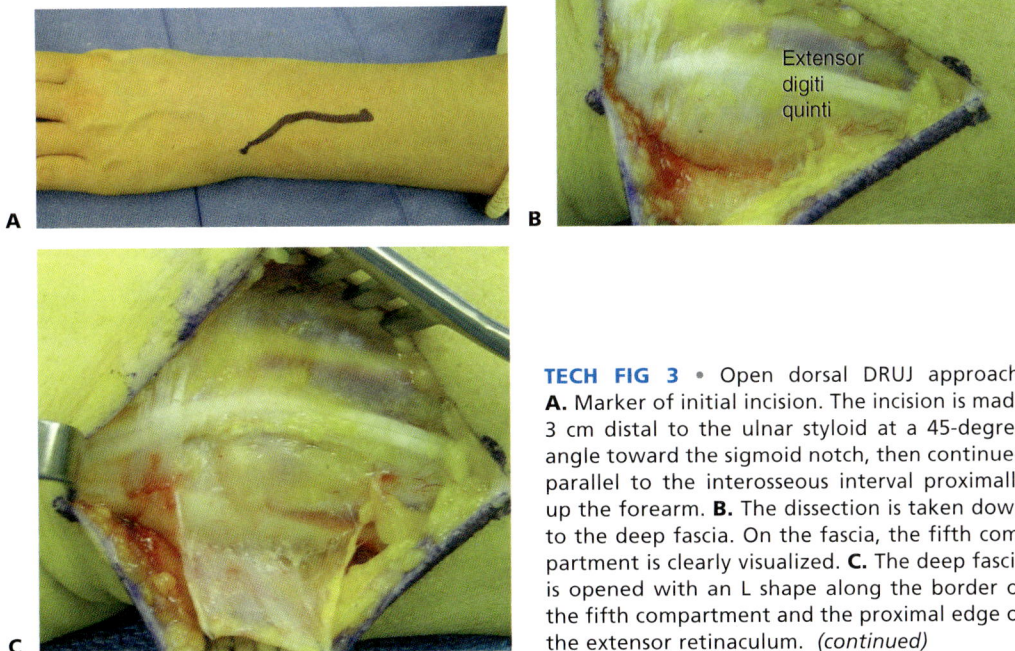

A

Extensor
digiti
quinti

B

C

TECH FIG 3 • Open dorsal DRUJ approach. **A.** Marker of initial incision. The incision is made 3 cm distal to the ulnar styloid at a 45-degree angle toward the sigmoid notch, then continued parallel to the interosseous interval proximally up the forearm. **B.** The dissection is taken down to the deep fascia. On the fascia, the fifth compartment is clearly visualized. **C.** The deep fascia is opened with an L shape along the border of the fifth compartment and the proximal edge of the extensor retinaculum. *(continued)*

TECHNIQUES

TECHNIQUES

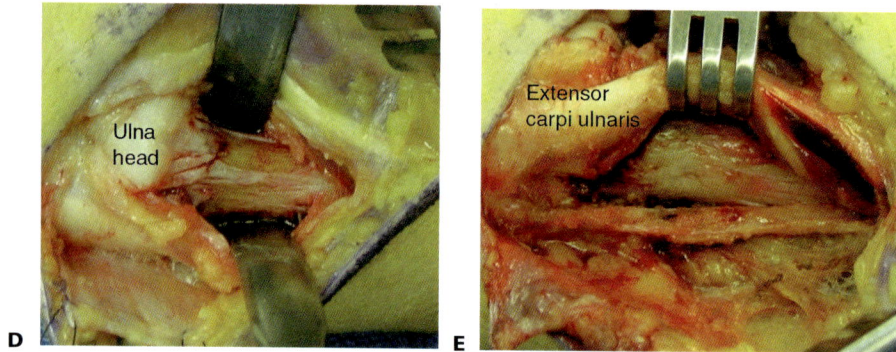

TECH FIG 3 • *(continued)* **D.** The dorsal capsule of the DRUJ and periosteum of the distal ulna are opened longitudinally from the proximal edge of the TFCC. **E.** A second window is created ulnar to the ECU tendon from the styloid. The length of this window usually is 2 to 3 cm.

- The capsule of the DRUJ is incised proximal to the TFCC disc to the point where it blends with the periosteum over the metaphysis of the ulna (**TECH FIG 3D**).
- The ulnocarpal joint capsule is opened to the lunotriquetrum.
  - Both capsular incisions are in line with retinaculum–fascial incision.
- The TFCC disc and associated ligaments, the DRUJ, and ulnar aspect of the radiocarpal joint can be inspected.
- A second, more ulnar window to the distal ulna can be made by sharp dissection to the ulna styloid and carried proximally parallel with the ECU sheath (**TECH FIG 3E**).
  - Care is taken to avoid opening the EDM and ECU sheaths.

TFCC Repair

- The peripheral foveal avulsion is débrided, and the fovea freshened with a curette.

- Two drill holes are made with 0.045-inch K-wires at a 45-degree angle about 1 cm from the articular surface of the head of the ulna, directed from the medial cortex of the ulna and exiting at the ulnar fovea.
  - The holes are parallel, beginning 1 cm apart, and converge toward the fovea.
- A transverse arthrotomy is made in the radiocarpal capsule at the distal edge of the TFCC disc.
- Three separate loops of a 3-0 braided nylon suture are passed through one hole, through the peripheral TFCC, and back out the other hole, and tied individually over the medial ulna.
- The capsulotomy incisions are closed first, then the retinaculum is closed, and finally the skin is closed.
- Two 0.062-inch K-wires are placed through the ulna and into the radius in a neutral position (**TECH FIG 4**).
- The capsule, retinaculum–fascia, and skin are closed in layers.

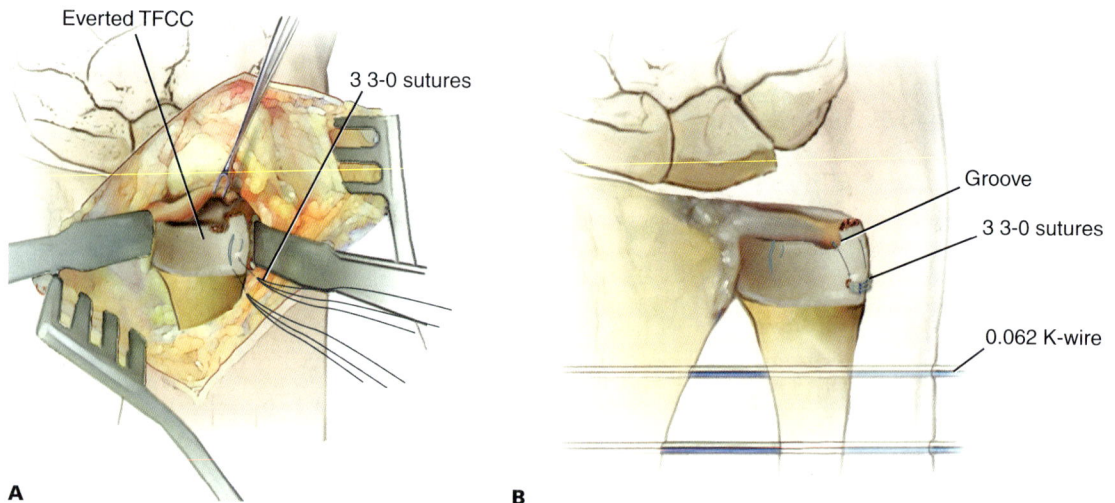

TECH FIG 4 • Repair of the TFCC. **A.** Three 3-0 nonabsorbable sutures are placed through the retracted medial TFCC and passed through holes at the medial base of the ulna styloid. **B.** Before tightly suturing the TFC to the prepared trough, the distal radioulnar relationship is secured by two percutaneous 0.062-inch K-wires placed through the ulna into the radius in neutral position. Care must be exercised to avoid injury to the DRUJ.

OPEN DRUJ ARTHROTOMY AND TFCC RECONSTRUCTION USING A PALMARIS GRAFT[1]

- Rarely, the TFCC can be completely shredded in a high-energy injury. In this instance the TFCC is excised and reconstructed using a palmaris graft.

PEARLS AND PITFALLS

Assessment of DRUJ instability	■ The initial PA view of the wrist will show more than 5 mm of ulna shortening. The initial lateral radiograph will show dorsal subluxation of the ulna. A preoperative MRI scan will show increased signal (white) in the TFCC and an avulsion of the TFCC at the fovea. A positive shuck test will be present intraoperatively (this is the most important test). A subluxed ulna will be seen in the lateral intraoperative C-arm view.
Irreducible DRUJ after radial fixation	■ Consider lack of anatomic reduction of the radius. Radial bow will not have been fully restored. This is especially prevalent in the segmental or comminuted radius. If convinced the radius is anatomic, then explore the DRUJ with open technique. The ECU and the extensor digitis minimi of the ulnar styloid are commonly in the joint.
Difficulty interpreting DRUJ shuck test	■ Ensure forearm is in full supination or pronation. There should be no motion at the DRUJ between the radius and the ulna. If there is any motion then there is likely to be instability, and at the very least, a long-arm cast in mid-supination should be applied.
Difficulty in getting into the joint for DRUJ arthroscopy	■ Reduce traction to about 5 lb. Use a 1.9-mm scope, and use a 21-gauge needle and saline to insufflate the joint. Place the forearm in supination. Push the trocar into the neck of the ulna (ie, between the radius and ulna).

POSTOPERATIVE CARE

■ All of the following protocols assume that rigid and stable fixation of the radius fracture has been obtained.
■ Stable DRUJ
 ■ The patient is placed in a sugar-tong splint for 2 weeks, and is given a Carter block arm pillow for strict elevation and encouragement of finger and thumb motion.
 ■ At 2 weeks, the patient returns to the office for suture and splint removal.
 ■ The patient is referred to a hand therapist for active, passive, and gentle resisted motion up to 10 lbs resistance.
 ■ Motion of all joints from the elbow distally is encouraged.
 ■ Further resistance and weight bearing depend on union of the radius.
 ■ Usually, union occurs by 6 weeks and restrictions are lifted.
 ■ Return to work status depends on the level of repetition and lifting required by the patient's job.
■ Rehabilitation following bone anchor fixation of a foveal avulsion of the TFCC and full palmaris graft reconstruction
 ■ Long-arm splint, elbow at 90 degrees, forearm in mid-supination, wrist neutral; fingers not included
 ■ At 2 weeks the patient returns to the office for suture removal and the arm is placed in a cast in the same position.
 ■ Four weeks later (ie, 6 weeks postoperatively), the cast is removed and active gentle passive motion is begun to all joints from the elbow distally.
 ■ At 12 weeks postoperatively, graduated lifting activity is begun, and continues for 6 more weeks.
 ■ At week 18 all restrictions are removed.
■ Open foveal repair and K-wire
 ■ At 6 weeks, K-wires are removed.
 ■ Begin protocol as for bone anchor fixation.

OUTCOMES

■ The key to a successful outcome of acute Galeazzi fracture-dislocations is accurate reduction and rigid fixation of the radius along with recognition and appropriate repair or reconstruction of the disrupted DRUJ.[15] Conservative management seems to be successful only in children.
 ■ In a classic article by Mikic,[15] conservative management in adults resulted in failure in 80% of cases. The results of operative treatment were much better, and the conclusion

was that rigid internal fixation is necessary for the dislocation as well as the fracture.
■ So-called "isolated" fractures of the radial diaphysis, where there is less than 5 mm of positive ulna variance, are more common than true Galeazzi fractures. Fractures without identifiable radioulnar disruption can be treated without specific treatment of the DRUJ and with immediate mobilization.[23] In this situation, patients with anatomic fracture reduction have minimal sequelae and better or equal functional results than patients with imperfect reduction.[20]
 ■ In a series of 50 Galeazzi fracture dislocations treated by early open reduction and internal fixation, Mohan et al[17] found, at 1 year, 40 good, 8 fair, and 2 poor results. Their conclusion was that early open reduction and rigid internal fixation re-establishes the normal relation of the fractured fragments and the DRUJ without repair of the ligaments. Thus, in many situations, ligament repair is unnecessary. (However, in Mohan et al's series, 1 in 5 had a less than good result.)
■ Rettig and Raskin,[21] in a more recent series, found that the more distal the fracture the greater the likelihood of DRUJ disruption. In this series, 12 out of 22 fractures within 7.5 cm of the midarticular surface of the distal radius had intraoperative DRUJ instability, whereas only one of 18 more proximally were unstable. Their conclusion was that a high index of suspicion, early recognition, and acute treatment of DRUJ instability will avoid chronic problems in this complex injury.
■ This high index of suspicion will lead to the recognition that dislocations of the DRUJ associated with fractures of the forearm often are irreducible.[5] These have been termed "complex" DRUJ dislocations: dislocations characterized by obvious irreducibility, recurrent subluxation, or "mushy" reduction caused by soft tissue or bone interposition.
■ With the advent of internal fixation of the radius, most Galeazzi fractures are predictably reduced. It is mandatory that the DRUJ be evaluated and managed according to the degree of instability to the joint. A high index of suspicion means the outcome is associated more with the degree of energy involved in the injury than with any inability on the part of the surgeon to care for the DRUJ appropriately.

COMPLICATIONS

■ The most common complication of a Galeazzi fracture is malunion of the radius and residual DRUJ instability,[9] due to malrotation and residual angulation of the radial shaft.[8] In most cases a DRUJ-stabilizing tenodesis cannot restore the joint, and a corrective osteotomy is required.[4]

- A preoperative three-dimensional CT reconstruction of the bones of the entire forearm is very helpful in this situation.
- Management of a missed dislocation[5] depends on the timing of presentation.
  - If less than 10 weeks after the injury, open reduction and repair usually is possible.
  - After 10 weeks, reconstruction with ligament grafting is required.
- The incidence of radius nonunion is directly related to the number of screws used: the rate is four times higher for bones plated with four screws compared to those plated with five or more screws.[26]
- Radioulnar synostosis may be seen, particularly in patients with multiple system trauma involving head injury.
- Osteomyelitis may develop in open and crush injuries.
- Nerve palsies, including the anterior interosseous and ulna nerves, have been associated with Galeazzi fractures,[24,25] and acute carpal tunnel syndrome is a common complication, particularly in crush and high-energy injuries.
- Compartment syndrome of the forearm also is a known complication.
- Osteoarthritis of the DRUJ is a long-term complication and can be managed by arthroscopy, interposition arthroplasty, ulna shortening, ulna head replacement, or total joint arthroplasty, depending on severity of the injury and age of the patient.
- Complications in Galeazzi fracture-dislocations can be minimized with attention to detail, in particular accurate anatomic reduction of the radius fracture, thorough assessment and repair of instability of the DRUJ, and appropriate postoperative rehabilitation.

REFERENCES

1. Adams BD, Berger R. An anatomic reconstruction of the distal radioulnar ligaments for posttraumatic distal radioulnar joint instability. J Hand Surg 2002;27:243–251.
2. Alexander AH, Lichtman DM. Irreducible distal radioulnar joint occurring in a Galeazzi fracture—case report. J Hand Surg Am 1981;6:258–261.
3. Boland MR, Bader J, Pienkowski D. Joint reaction forces at the distal radioulnar joint: A biomechanical model presentation at the ASSH Annual Meeting 2006, Washington, DC.
4. Bowers WH. Instability of the distal radioulnar articulation. Hand Clin 1991;7:311–327.
5. Bruckner JD, Lichtman DM, Alexander AH. Complex dislocations of the distal radioulnar joint. Recognition and management. Clin Orthop Relat Res 1992;275:90–103.
6. Chow KH, Sarris IK, Sotereanos DG. Suture anchor repair of ulnar-sided triangular fibrocartilage complex tears. J Hand Surg Br 2003;28:546–550.
7. Galeazzi R. Uber ein Besonderes Syndrom bei Verltzunger im Bereich der Unteraumknochen. Arch OrthoUnfallchir 1934;35:557–562.
8. Garcia-Elias M, Dobyns J. Dorsal and palmar dislocations of the distal radioulnar joint. In Cooney WP, Linscheid RL, Dobyns JH, eds. The Wrist: Diagnosis and Operative Treatment. St. Louis: Mosby, 1998.
9. Hughston JC. Fracture of the distal radial shaft: Mistakes in management. J Bone Joint Surg Am 1957;39A:249–264.
10. Ishii S, Palmer AK, Werner FW, et al. An anatomic study of the ligamentous structure of the triangular fibrocartilage complex. J Hand Surg Am 1998;23:977–985.
11. Kleinman WB. Repair of chronic peripheral tears/avulsions of the triangular fibrocartilage. In Blair W, ed. Techniques in Hand Surgery. Baltimore: Williams & Wilkins, 1996.
12. Kleinman WB, Graham TJ. The distal radioulnar joint capsule: Clinical anatomy and role in posttraumatic limitation of forearm motion. J Hand Surg Am 1998;23:588–599.
13. Lister G. The Hand: Diagnosis and Indications. Edinburgh: Churchill Livingstone, 993:2.
14. Lo IK, MacDermid JC, Bennett JD, et al. The radioulnar ratio: A new method of quantifying distal radioulnar joint subluxation. J Hand Surg 2001;26:236–243.
15. Mikic ZD. Galeazzi Fracture-Dislocations. J Bone Joint Surg Am 1975;57A:1071–1080.
16. Mino DE, Palmar AK, Levinsohn EM. The role of radiography and computerized tomography in the diagnosis of subluxation and dislocation of the distal radioulnar joint. J Hand Surg Am 1983;8:23–31.
17. Mohan K, Gupta AK, Sharma J, et al. Internal fixation in 50 cases of Galeazzi fracture. Acta Orthop Scand 1988;59:318–320.
18. Moore TM, Lester DK, Sarmiento A. The stabilizing effect of soft-tissue constraints in artificial Galeazzi fractures. Clin Orthop Relat Res 1985;194:189–194.
19. Nicolaidis SC, Hildreth DH, Lichtman DM. Acute injuries of the distal radioulnar joint. Hand Clin 2000;16:449–459.
20. Reckling FW. Unstable fracture-dislocations of the forearm (Monteggia and Galeazzi lesions). J Bone Joint Surg Am 1982;64A:857–863.
21. Rettig ME, Raskin KB. Galeazzi fracture-dislocation: A new treatment-oriented classification. J Hand Surg Am 2001;26:228–235.
22. Richards RR, Corley FG. Fractures of the shafts of the radius and ulna. In Rockwood CA, Green DP, Buckholz RW, et al, eds. Rockwood and Green's Fractures in Adults, ed 4. Philadelphia: Lippincott-Raven, 1996.
23. Ring D, Rhim R, Carpenter C, et al. Isolated radial shaft fractures are more common than Galeazzi fractures. J Hand Surg Am 2006;31:17–21.
24. Saitoh S, Seki H, Murakami N, et al. Tardy ulnar tunnel syndrome caused by Galeazzi fracture-dislocation: neuropathy with a new pathomechanism. J Orthop Trauma 2000;14:66–70.
25. Stahl S, Freiman S, Volpin G. Anterior interosseous nerve palsy associated with Galeazzi fracture. J Pediatr Orthop B 2000;9:45–46.
26. Stern PJ, Drury WJ. Complications of plate fixation of forearm fractures. Clin Orthop Relat Res 1983;175:25–29.
27. Strehle J, Gerber C. Distal radioulnar joint function after Galeazzi fracture-dislocations treated by open reduction and internal plate fixation. Clin Orthop Relat Res 1993;293:240–245.
28. Whipple TL. Arthroscopy of the distal radioulnar joint. Hand Clinics 1994;10:589–592.

Chapter 6

Corrective Osteotomy for Radius and Ulna Diaphyseal Malunions

Vimala Ramachandran and Thomas F. Varecka

DEFINITION

- Malunion of the radial or ulnar shaft can lead to pain, loss of motion, loss of strength, and instability at the level of the wrist or elbow.
- Malrotation, angulation (with narrowing of the interosseous space between the radius and ulna), shortening, and loss of the radial bow have been shown in various studies to lead to decreased functional outcomes.[4,5,9,10,12]
- Arthritis has been reported at the level of the proximal radioulnar joint (PRUJ) with longstanding malunions, although the distal radioulnar joint (DRUJ) is most commonly affected by forearm malunions.[11]

ANATOMY

- The forearm can be thought of as a ring, connected at the PRUJ, the interosseous membrane, and the DRUJ (**FIG 1**).
- Force transmission occurs through the interosseous membrane from the radius distally to the ulna proximally.
- Radius
  - The radius lies parallel to the ulna in supination. With pronation, it rotates around the ulna while the ulna maintains its position throughout forearm rotation.
  - The radius shaft is triangular in cross section, with the apex toward the attachment of the interosseous membrane.
  - It contains three surfaces: anterior, lateral, and posterior.

- The shaft possesses a gentle bow, with the volar surface concave and the dorsal and lateral surfaces convex.[1]
- Schemitsch and Richards[9] devised a formula that locates the apex and defines the magnitude of the radial bow for each individual (**FIG 2**).
- Ulna[1]
  - The ulna is a long bone that has a triangular cross section in the proximal two thirds and a circular cross section distally.
  - It possesses three surfaces: anterior, posterior, and medial.
  - The proximal half of the shaft is slightly concave volarly. The distal half is relatively straight.
- The PRUJ consists of the radial head, the radial notch, the annular ligament, and the quadrate ligament.
- The DRUJ consists of the sigmoid notch, the ulnar head, the dorsal and volar radioulnar ligaments, the extensor carpi ulnaris (ECU) subsheath, and the triangular fibrocartilage complex (TFCC).

PATHOGENESIS

- Both-bone forearm fractures occur through a variety of mechanisms, including indirect trauma (such as falls on an outstretched arm or motor vehicle accidents) and direct trauma (such as blows to the forearm).

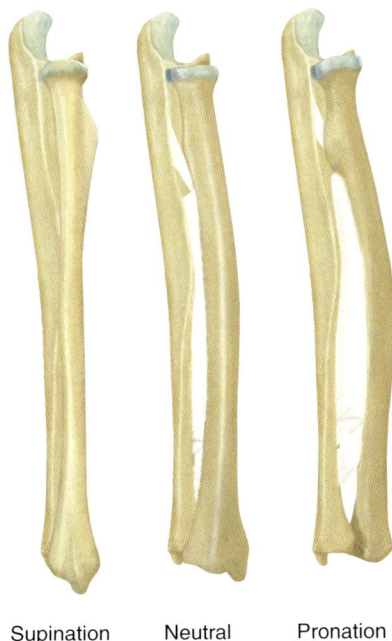

FIG 1 • Lateral projection of the radius and ulna. Relationship of the interosseous membrane to the radius and ulna during forearm rotation. The fibers of the interosseous membrane are longest with the forearm in neutral position and shorten in both pronation and supination.

Supination   Neutral   Pronation

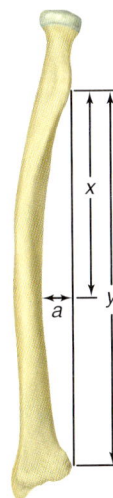

FIG 2 • Measurement of the location and magnitude of the radial bow. The distance *y* represents the length of the radius as measured from the bicipital tuberosity to the ulnar aspect of the radius. Line *a*, drawn perpendicular to *y* from the point of greatest curvature of the radius, represents the magnitude of the radial bow (expressed in millimeters). The distance *x* represents the length of the radius from the bicipital tuberosity to the point where *a* intersects *y*. The location of the radial bow is calculated by $x/y \times 100$. (Adapted from Schemitsch EH, Richards RR. The effect of malunion on functional outcome after plate fixation of fractures of both bones of the forearm in adults. J Bone Joint Surg Am 1992;74A:1068–1078.)

■ Acute fractures treated closed or with intramedullary nailing techniques are more likely to heal malunited.[7,8]

■ Radius malunions have a greater effect on forearm rotation than ulna malunions.[10,12]

■ A torsional deformity of greater than 30 degrees in the radius leads to significant loss of forearm motion.[4]

■ Changes in the length–tension curve of the interosseous membrane may also account for loss of rotation.[12]

NATURAL HISTORY

■ Fifty degrees of supination and 50 degrees of pronation are needed for activities of daily living.[6]

■ Patients with untreated forearm malunions may experience loss of forearm rotation, PRUJ or DRUJ instability, wrist pain, loss of strength, and arthritis at the PRUJ.[11] The severity of the symptoms depends on the degree of malunion and the corresponding alteration in degree and location of the bow of the radius.

■ Malunions of 10 degrees or less lead to less than a 20-degree loss of forearm rotation and hence are clinically insignificant.[7]

■ Angular malalignment of more than 20 degrees in the radius or ulna results in clinically significant loss of motion. Greater than 15 degrees of malalignment leads to inability to perform activities of daily living.[5,7,10]

■ Patients with greater than 15 degrees of malalignment or loss of the radial bow will have clinically significant loss of motion and strength if left untreated.

PATIENT HISTORY AND PHYSICAL FINDINGS

■ The preoperative evaluation for patients with forearm malunions includes a detailed assessment of the patient's functional limitations as well as documentation of elbow and wrist range of motion, the supination–pronation arc of the forearm, and the stability of the PRUJ and DRUJ.

■ Physical examination

■ The skin is inspected for scarring or previous incision sites.

■ Muscle bulk and tone are examined.

■ The wrist, elbow, and malunion site are palpated for tenderness.

■ Range of motion

■ The flexion–extension arc of the elbow is measured with the shoulder at 30 degrees of forward flexion.

■ Rotation of the forearm is ascertained with the humerus stabilized against the chest wall and the elbow at 90 degrees of flexion.

■ Wrist flexion and extension are determined with the forearm in neutral rotation.

■ Joint loss of motion may indicate location of pathology.

■ A high degree of motion loss will lead to functional deficits.

■ PRUJ and DRUJ

■ Stability of the PRUJ is assessed by palpation during passive pronation and supination.

■ The DRUJ is evaluated by stressing the ulna volarly and dorsally while stabilizing the radius.

■ Subluxation of the ulnar head or the ECU is evaluated during passive range of motion (ECU subluxation test).

■ The piano key test can also be used to assess for an unstable DRUJ. Patients with a positive piano key sign will have an ulnar head that shifts volarly with a minimal volarly directed force and then rebounds dorsally once that force is removed, much like a key in a piano.

■ Pain with compression of the radius and ulna at the level of the DRUJ may also be indicative of DRUJ instability or arthritis (DRUJ compression test).

■ Neurovascular examination

■ The examiner should check for anterior interosseous nerve (OK sign), posterior interosseous nerve (thumb extension), and ulnar nerve (abduction–adduction of fingers) function.

■ Inability to perform tasks identifies nerve injury.

IMAGING AND OTHER DIAGNOSTIC STUDIES

■ AP and lateral radiographs of both forearms should be obtained (**FIG 3A,B**).

■ Both the bicipital tuberosity and the radial styloid should be visualized for the film to be adequate.

■ The degree of angulation and comminution can be calculated from these films.

■ Contralateral forearm films provide a comparison for the amount of shortening as well as for the location and angle of the radial bow.[9]

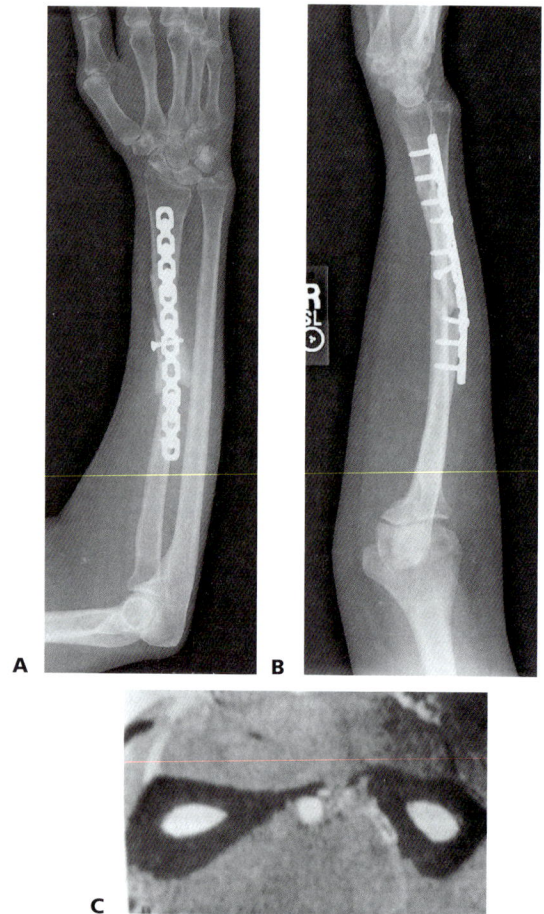

A B

C

FIG 3 • **A,B.** AP and lateral radiographs demonstrate a segmental radius shaft fracture resulting in a malunion both proximally and distally despite open reduction and internal fixation. Note the loss of radial bow in both direction and magnitude, narrowing of the interosseous space between the radius and ulna, dorsal positioning of the distal ulna, and nonunion of the basilar ulnar styloid fracture. The patient was unable to supinate to neutral and demonstrated instability at the distal radioulnar joint. **C.** CT scan demonstrates narrowing of the interosseous space with heterotopic bone formation.

■ A CT (**FIG 3C**) scan or MRI can also be obtained to assess for malrotation.[2]

DIFFERENTIAL DIAGNOSIS

■ DRUJ injury or instability
■ PRUJ injury or instability
■ Injury to the interosseous membrane
■ Synostosis
■ Nonunion

NONOPERATIVE MANAGEMENT

■ Nonoperative treatment of malunions depends on the patient's symptoms and includes occupational therapy for strengthening and range of motion, removable off-the-shelf braces, non-narcotic medications, and custom molded DRUJ orthoses.

SURGICAL MANAGEMENT

■ Operative intervention for forearm malunions depends on the functional limitations of the patient, not the degree of deformity apparent on radiographs.
■ Indications for surgery include loss of forearm rotation that leads to a functional deficit (rotational arc less than 100 degrees), DRUJ instability, unacceptable cosmesis, and painful nonunion.
■ Risks to the patient include vascular injury, nerve injury or paresthesias (specifically the superficial radial nerve), infection, nonunion, delayed union, need for iliac crest bone graft, synostosis, loss of motion, and DRUJ instability.
■ Patients treated within 1 year of the initial injury may be more likely to improve functionally and have a lower surgical complication rate.[11]
■ Malunions of the radius and ulna are generally treated with an open approach, corrective osteotomy of one or both bones, compression plating, and bone grafting as necessary.
  ■ Generally, the more deformed bone is corrected first. If after correction of the first bone forearm rotation is still lacking, an osteotomy is performed on the second bone.
  ■ If both bones are equally deformed, the ulna is osteotomized and provisionally plated first to provide a working length for the radius.
■ Restoration of the radial bow in large part determines functional outcome.
  ■ Patients whose radial bow is restored within 1.5 mm of magnitude and located within 4.3% of the contralateral forearm regain 80% of normal motion.
  ■ Eighty percent of grip strength is regained if the radial bow is located within 5% of the contralateral side.[9]
■ Anatomic realignment of the radius and ulna will not improve functional deficits if a synostosis or significant scarring and contracture involving the soft tissues has occurred.
  ■ Occult injury to or contracture of the DRUJ and PRUJ must be identified and treated at the time of surgery.

Preoperative Planning

■ Radiographs of the affected and contralateral extremity should be reviewed.
  ■ A CT scan is helpful to assess for rotational deformity.
■ A corrective three-dimensional osteotomy is planned using standard AO technique (**FIG 4**).
■ The need for corticocancellous iliac crest bone graft should be determined by the degree of shortening.
■ The surgeon should be familiar with techniques for reconstruction or stabilization of the DRUJ should it remain unstable after correction of the malunion.

Positioning

■ The patient is positioned supine on the operating table. A radiolucent hand board is attached to the table, centered on the patient's axilla. The affected extremity is then extended and can be positioned for either a volar or dorsal approach to the radius by rotating through the shoulder.
■ The subcutaneous border of the ulna can be visualized by flexing the arm at the elbow or by placing the arm across the chest.
■ A nonsterile tourniquet may be used on the arm.

Approach

■ Radius shaft malunions may be approached either volarly or dorsally.
■ The volar (Henry) approach is best suited for midshaft and distal radius shaft malunions.
  ■ The proximal radius shaft can be approached volarly in this manner; however, injury to the posterior interosseous nerve (PIN) can occur when dissecting the supinator muscle off the radius.
  ■ The approach is extensile and can be used to expose not only the entire length of the radius but also the wrist joint.[3]
■ The dorsal (Thompson) approach to the radius is used most commonly for proximal malunions.
  ■ It provides access to the PIN, allowing the surgeon to isolate the nerve and retract it out of harm's way for the remainder of the procedure.
  ■ This approach may be of value for midshaft exposure of the radius, especially in the case of a midshaft segmental malunion (see Fig 3A,B).
  ■ The entire dorsal surface of the radius can be exposed through this approach.[3]
■ The ulna is approached along its subcutaneous border.
  ■ The entire length of the ulna can easily be exposed through this approach.

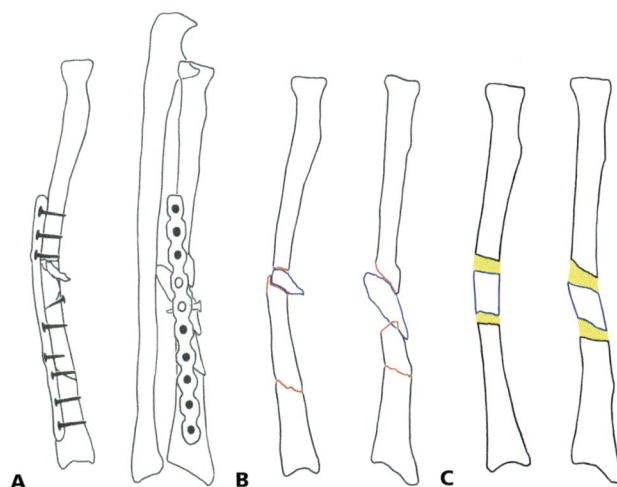

FIG 4 • Preoperative planning using AO technique for correction of the malunion of the case in Figure 3. **A.** The malunion is first sketched out from the preoperative radiographs. **B.** Each fragment is then drawn out separately. **C.** The osteotomy sites are noted on both the AP and lateral views. The radius is then realigned through the planned osteotomy sites and bone graft (*yellow*) is inserted to restore the normal magnitude and location of the radial bow.

TECHNIQUES

VOLAR APPROACH TO THE RADIUS

- Landmarks: biceps tendon, brachioradialis (BR), radial styloid
- Center the skin incision over the malunion site and follow a line that begins lateral to the biceps tendon, continues over the medial edge of the BR, and ends distally at the level of the radial styloid.
  - The length of the incision depends on the amount of exposure needed to take down the malunion and plate the osteotomy.
- To expose the midshaft, dissect between the BR and the pronator teres (PT) proximally (**TECH FIG 1**).
  - The superficial radial nerve lies on the undersurface of the BR and must be protected.

- Ligate the recurrent radial artery to retract the BR laterally.
- Pronate the forearm and release the PT insertion.
- Dissect the PT muscle subperiosteally from a lateral to medial direction to expose the volar surface of the radius.
- To expose the distal radius, the surgical interval lies between the flexor carpi radialis (FCR) and the radial artery.
- Retract the FCR medially and the radial artery laterally to expose the flexor pollicis longus (FPL) and the pronator quadratus (PQ).
- Retract the FPL medially.
- Release the PQ from its radial insertion and dissect the muscle belly from the volar distal radius.

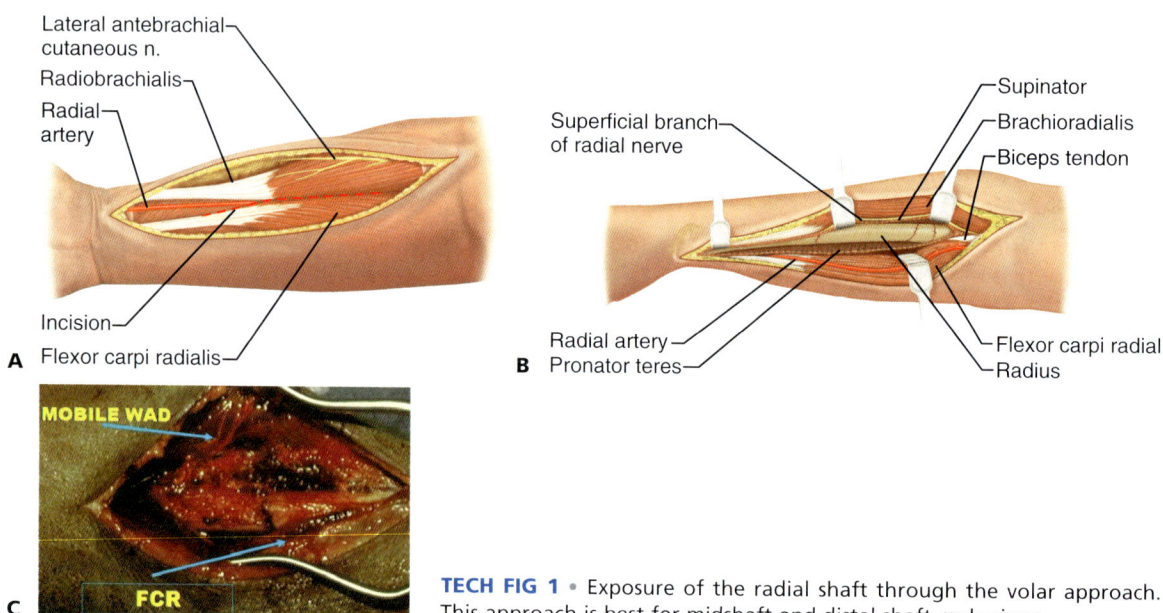

TECH FIG 1 • Exposure of the radial shaft through the volar approach. This approach is best for midshaft and distal shaft malunions.

DORSAL APPROACH TO THE RADIUS

- Landmarks: lateral epicondyle, tubercle of Lister
- The skin incision is centered over the malunion and follows a gently curved line starting just anterior to the lateral epicondyle and ending just distal and ulnar to the tubercle of Lister at the wrist (**TECH FIG 2A**).
- Incise the fascia in line with the skin incision.
- Dissect between the extensor digitorum communis (EDC) and the extensor carpi radialis brevis (ECRB) proximally.
- Pronate the forearm.
- Identify the PIN as it emerges from the supinator 1 cm proximal to the distal edge of the muscle (**TECH FIG 2B**).
  - Follow the nerve in a distal to proximal direction through the supinator, carefully preserving its motor branches.

- Once the nerve is fully mobilized and protected, supinate the arm and release the supinator from the anterior surface of the radius in a medial to lateral direction.
- To expose the midshaft of the radius dorsally, the abductor pollicis longus (APL) and the extensor pollicis brevis (EPB) must be mobilized as they cross radially over the dorsal shaft of the radius.
- Incise the fascia along the inferior and superior borders of the two muscles and lift them off the radius.
  - Retract them distally or proximally as needed for exposure of the malunion.

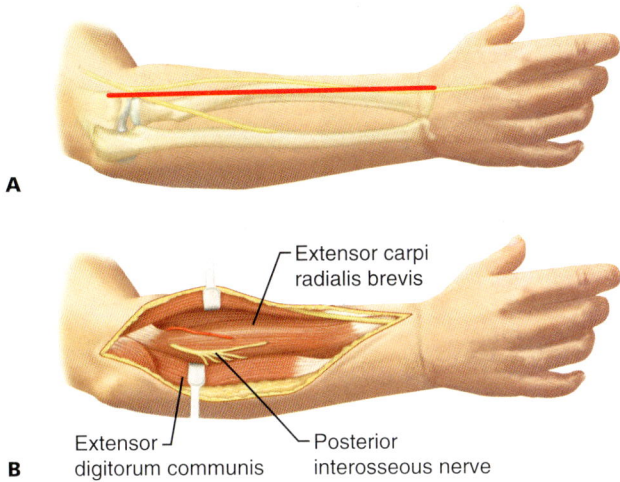

A

B

- Extensor carpi radialis brevis
- Extensor digitorum communis
- Posterior interosseous nerve

TECH FIG 2 • Exposure of the radius through the dorsal approach. This approach is best for proximal shaft malunions. **A.** Skin incision on dorsal surface, running from tip of lateral epicondyle toward radial styloid. **B.** The posterior interosseous nerve is followed through the supinator, with its branches preserved.

APPROACH TO THE ULNA

- Landmark: subcutaneous border of the ulna
- Make a longitudinal incision along the subcutaneous border of the ulna (**TECH FIG 3A**).
- Incise the fascia in line with the skin incision.
- Dissect between the extensor carpi ulnaris (ECU) dorsally and the flexor carpi radialis (FCU) volarly (**TECH FIG 3B**).
  - Take care to avoid disrupting the ECU subsheath distally over the ulna head.

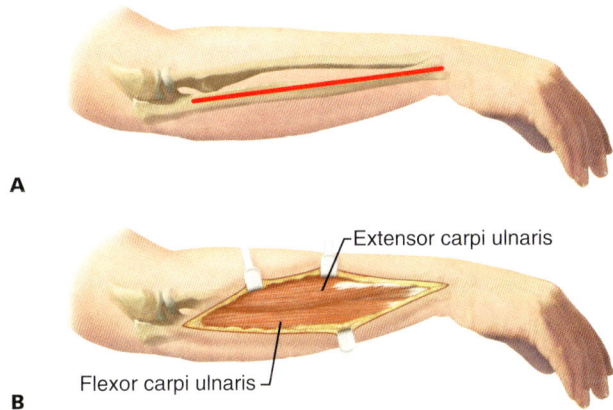

A

B

- Extensor carpi ulnaris
- Flexor carpi ulnaris

TECH FIG 3 • Exposure of the ulna. **A.** Skin incision along subcutaneous border of ulna. **B.** Dissection is performed between the extensor carpi ulnaris dorsally and the flexor carpi radialis volarly.

REDUCTION, PLATING, AND BONE GRAFTING

- Based on the preoperative scheme, perform the planned osteotomy at the site of malunion using a combination of a water-cooled saw and osteotomies.
- Bring the radius out to length and insert bone graft as necessary (**TECH FIG 4A**).
- Make a template for plate contouring so as to match the radial bow (**TECH FIG 4B,C**).

- Plate the malunion using a 3.5-mm compression plate and AO compression plating techniques (**TECH FIG 4D–G**).
  - Obtain a minimum of six cortices of fixation proximal and distal to the malunion.
  - In smaller patients, a 2.7 DC plate may be used instead.

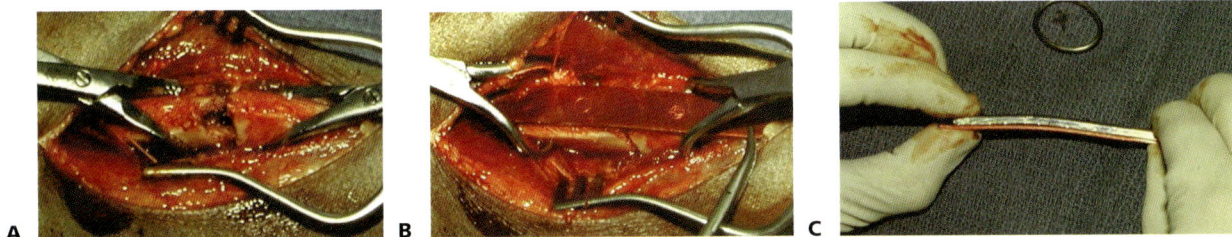

A

B

C

TECH FIG 4 • **A.** Reduction after osteotomy of the midshaft segmental radius malunion through a volar exposure in the patient in Figures 3 and 4. Because of the segmental nature of this malunion, fixation was accomplished by plating both volarly and dorsally. **B.** A metal template is placed on the volar surface of the corrected radius. **C.** The template is used to precisely contour the plate so that when applied, the normal curvature of the radius is restored. *(continued)*

TECHNIQUES

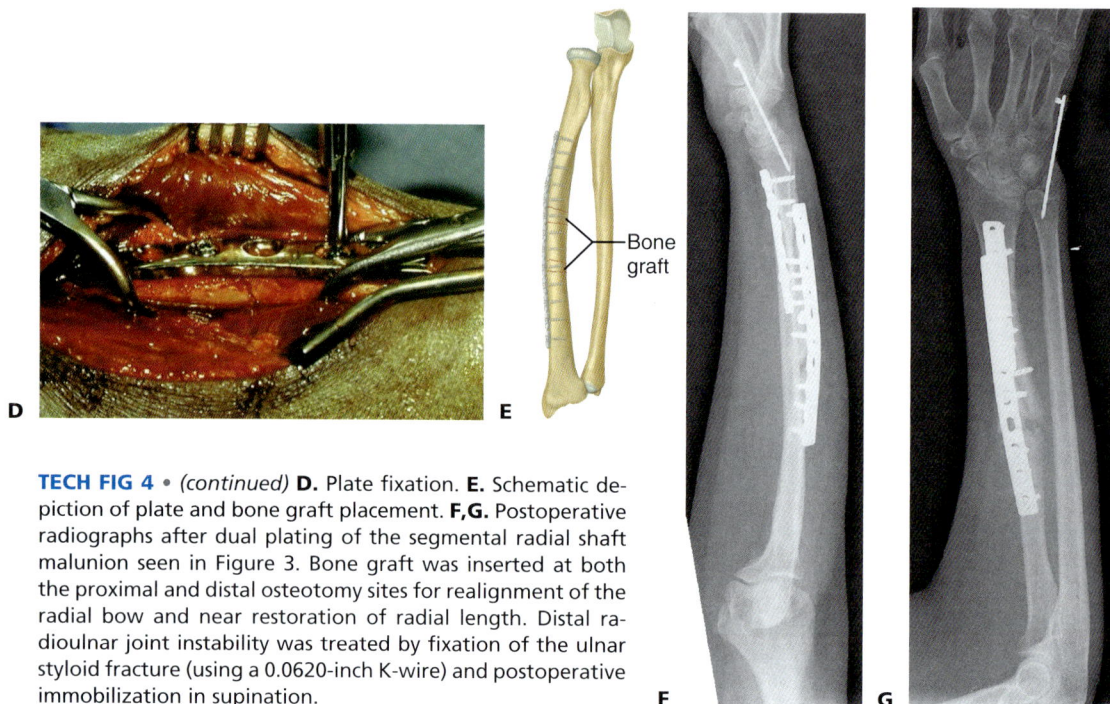

Bone graft

TECH FIG 4 • *(continued)* **D.** Plate fixation. **E.** Schematic depiction of plate and bone graft placement. **F,G.** Postoperative radiographs after dual plating of the segmental radial shaft malunion seen in Figure 3. Bone graft was inserted at both the proximal and distal osteotomy sites for realignment of the radial bow and near restoration of radial length. Distal radioulnar joint instability was treated by fixation of the ulnar styloid fracture (using a 0.0620-inch K-wire) and postoperative immobilization in supination.

- After fixation, take the forearm through a full supination–pronation arc.
  - Blocks to motion result from an uncorrected ulnar malunion, DRUJ incongruency or instability, failure to restore the radial bow, synostosis, and soft tissue or interosseous membrane scarring and contracture.
- If an ulna osteotomy is required, the plate can be placed on the volar surface of the ulna or on its subcutaneous border in the manner detailed above.
- If the DRUJ is unstable, consider palmar capsular reefing, reconstruction with tendon graft, fixation of an ulnar styloid base nonunion, or pinning of the joint in full supination.

- If the joint is incongruent or arthritic, consider ulna shortening, matched resection arthroplasty, Darrach resection, or the Sauve-Kapandji procedure.
- Reapproximate tendon insertions. For example, in the case of a volar exposure to the distal radius, repair the PQ to its radial insertion using absorbable suture.
- Close the subcutaneous tissues and skin.
  - To minimize the risk of compartment syndrome, do not close the fascia.
- Apply a volar splint.
  - In patients with concomitant DRUJ instability, a sugar-tong splint with the forearm in full supination is placed.

PEARLS AND PITFALLS

Indications	▪ Assess DRUJ stability. ▪ Determine that lack of motion is not due to soft tissue contracture, synostosis, or interosseous membrane scarring, for which realignment of the malunion would not improve motion.
Osteotomy	▪ Obtain contralateral forearm films to determine location and magnitude of radial bow. ▪ Obtain CT or MRI if concerned for rotational malunion. ▪ Perform detailed preoperative drawings to determine the ideal location for the osteotomy, the degree and direction of correction required, and the need for bone graft. ▪ Obtain consent for bone graft.
Approach	▪ If a volar approach to the proximal radius is chosen, avoid injury to the PIN by careful subperiosteal stripping of the supinator from the radius and gentle retraction of the supinator laterally to prevent a traction neurapraxia. Avoid placing a retractor around radial neck as this can compress the PIN (or cause a traction injury of the nerve). Gently retract the superficial radial nerve and radial artery. ▪ Protect the PIN during dissection when approaching the proximal radius dorsally. The nerve lies directly on bone dorsally, opposite of the bicipital tuberosity in 25% of patients. Avoid trapping the nerve between the plate and bone when placing a plate proximally.
DRUJ	▪ Determine the cause of instability of the DRUJ once malalignment is restored. ▪ Perform a procedure that addresses the precise cause of the DRUJ instability.

POSTOPERATIVE CARE

- In a compliant patient with secure fixation, the splint may be removed 5 to 7 days after surgery and range-of-motion exercises initiated.
  - A removable orthosis is worn for the next 4 to 5 weeks.
- Strengthening exercises are begun 6 weeks after surgery.
  - Resistive strength training is delayed until radiographic evidence of healing is present (usually 8 to 12 weeks postoperatively).
- Normal activities are resumed when a solid union is present.
- Plates are generally not removed in adults.
- If concomitant DRUJ instability is present:
  - A Munster cast is applied at the first postoperative visit. The forearm is held in full supination for 6 weeks.
  - Finger range-of-motion and elbow flexion–extension exercises are begun at the first postoperative visit.
  - At 6 weeks, any pins in the DRUJ are removed, and supination–pronation exercises are initiated.

OUTCOMES

- Trousdale and Linscheid retrospectively reviewed 27 patients with corrective osteotomies for forearm malunions. Indications for surgery included loss of rotation (20 patients), unstable DRUJ (6 patients), and cosmesis (1 patient).[11]
  - Of the six patients with DRUJ instability, five had stable wrist joints at follow-up. Three patients were stabilized with correction of the deformity alone, and three required reefing of the palmar capsule and temporary pinning of the DRUJ with Kirschner wires (K-wires).
  - The patient who underwent the procedure for cosmesis lost 10 degrees of rotation but was happy with the overall appearance and function.
  - The age of the patient at the time of injury, location of the malunion, and involvement of one or both bones were not associated with the final outcome.
  - Shorter time from injury to corrective surgery (less than 12 months) was associated with improved forearm rotation and a lower complication rate.

COMPLICATIONS

- A 48% complication rate was noted in Trousdale and Linscheid's study.[11]
- Infection
- Wrist pain
- Loss of motion
- Heterotopic ossification
- DRUJ instability
- Delayed union or nonunion
- Superficial radial nerve paresthesias

REFERENCES

1. Botte M. Skeletal anatomy. In: Doyle J, Botte M, eds. Surgical Anatomy of the Hand and Upper Extremity. Philadelphia: Lippincott Williams & Wilkins, 2003:3–91.
2. Dumont CE, Pfirrmann CW, Ziegler D, et al. Assessment of radial and ulnar torsion profiles with cross-sectional magnetic resonance imaging. J Bone Joint Surg Am 2006;88A:1582–1588.
3. The forearm. In: Hoppenfeld S, DeBoer P, eds. Surgical Exposures in Orthopaedics, 2nd ed. Philadelphia: Lippincott Williams & Wilkins, 1994:117–146.
4. Kasten P, Krefft M, Hesselbach J, et al. How does torsional deformity of the radial shaft influence the rotation of the forearm? A biomechanical study. J Orthop Trauma 2003;17:57–60.
5. Matthews LS, Kaufer H, Garver DF, et al. The effect on supination-pronation of angular malalignment of fractures of both bones of the forearm. J Bone Joint Surg Am 1982;64A:14–17.
6. Morrey BF, Askew LJ, An KN, et al. A biomechanical study of normal functional elbow motion. J Bone Joint Surg Am 1981;63A:872–877.
7. Sarmiento A, Ebramzadeh E, Brys D, et al. Angular deformities and forearm function. J Orthop Res 1992;10:121–133.
8. Schemitsch EH, Jones D, Henley MB. A comparison of malreduction after plate and intramedullary nail fixation of forearm fractures. J Orthop Trauma 1995;9:8–16.
9. Schemitsch EH, Richards RR. The effect of malunion on functional outcome after plate fixation of fractures of both bones of the forearm in adults. J Bone Joint Surg Am 1992;74A:1068–1078.
10. Tarr RR, Garfinkel AI, Sarmiento A. The effects of angular and rotational deformities of both bones of the forearm. J Bone Joint Surg Am 1984;66A:65–70.
11. Trousdale RT, Linscheid RL. Operative treatment of malunited fractures of the forearm. J Bone Joint Surg Am 1995;77A:894–902.
12. Tynan MC, Fornalski S, McMahon PJ, et al. The effects of ulnar axial malalignment on supination and pronation. J Bone Joint Surg Am 2000;82A:1726–1731.

Chapter 7

Operative Treatment of Radius and Ulna Diaphyseal Nonunions

Rena L. Stewart

DEFINITION

- A diaphyseal forearm fracture is generally considered to be a nonunion if healing has not taken place within 6 months.
- Nonunions are generally classified as hypertrophic or atrophic, an important distinction in treatment selection.
  - Hypertrophic nonunions have abundant callus and a rich blood supply and result from inadequate stability of fracture fixation. This type of nonunion is rare in the forearm and constitutes less than 10% of nonunion cases.[9]
  - Atrophic nonunions are characterized by poor blood supply and little or no callus formation.
- Nonunion of the forearm diaphysis is rare because of the success of current techniques of plate and screw fixation. Nonunion rates of only 2% in the radius and 4% in the ulna are reported.[2]

ANATOMY

- The forearm consists of the radius and ulna, joined at either end by the proximal and distal radioulnar joints (PRUJ and DRUJ, respectively) (**FIG 1**).
- The ulna is straight, while the radius has both an apex radial and apex dorsal curvature.
- It can help to think of the forearm as a joint rather than a pair of long bones.
  - Pronation and supination are achieved by rotation of the curved radius about the straight ulna.

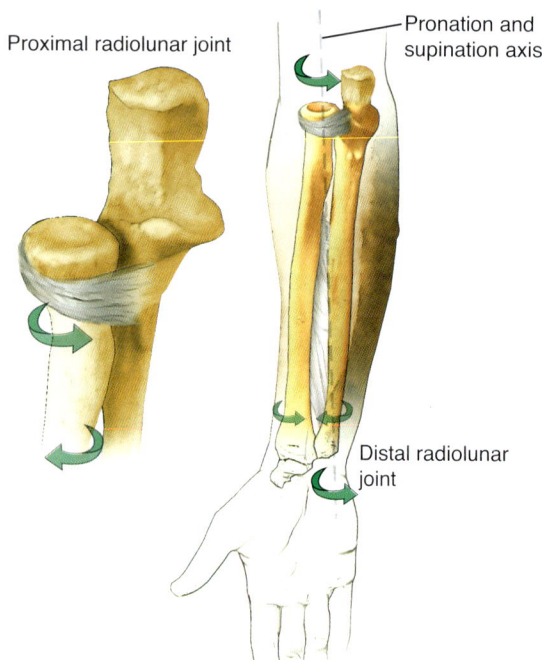

Proximal radiolunar joint

Pronation and supination axis

Distal radiolunar joint

FIG 1 • The two bones of the forearm form a functional unit, with the axis of rotation extending from the radiocapitellar joint to the distal radioulnar joint.

- Both the curvature of the radius and the integrity of the interosseous space and interosseous membrane (IOM) must be maintained for the forearm "joint" to function optimally.
- The diaphyseal portions of the radius and ulna are surrounded by complex anatomy, including neural and vascular structures, that must be considered during any surgical approach. Both radius and ulna are covered by muscle proximally, while the ulna emerges distally to be subcutaneous.

PATHOGENESIS

- Nonunions of the diaphysis of the forearm are rare and result most commonly from incorrect or inadequate treatment.
  - Inadequate fixation, generally less than six cortices of screw fixation proximal and distal to the fracture, will increase the rate of nonunion.
  - Lack of attention to critical surgical principles such as creating compression across the fracture site (either with the use of an interfragmentary screw or a compression plate) also leads to nonunion.
  - Nonoperative treatment results in markedly increased rates of nonunion and other complications.[2] With the exception of isolated, minimally displaced ulnar shaft fractures, all adult diaphyseal forearm fractures require operative management.
- Comminution increases the risk of nonunion, with 12% of comminuted, diaphyseal fractures going on to develop nonunion after treatment with dynamic compression plates.[11]
- Fracture characteristics that increase the risk of nonunion include extensive devascularization and periosteal stripping, bone loss, and infection.
  - Open, comminuted fractures with bone loss have the highest rate of nonunion.[7]
- Patient comorbidities known to increase rates of nonunion include diabetes mellitus, steroid use, malnutrition, and renal dysfunction.

NATURAL HISTORY

- Once a nonunion of the forearm is established, it will not go on to heal spontaneously.
- If significant shortening of either the radius or ulna occurs, the intricate anatomy of the entire forearm "joint" can be disrupted. Malalignment of the DRUJ secondary to such shortening can cause pain and lead to loss of motion at the wrist.
- Loss of motion secondary to pain, particularly pronation and supination, can lead to shortening and fibrosis of the IOM. This can lead to permanent loss of rotational motion in the forearm.

PATIENT HISTORY AND PHYSICAL FINDINGS

- Patients with nonunion of the diaphysis of the radius or ulna most commonly present with pain.
  - This pain frequently worsens with attempts to use the extremity for lifting or pushing, but may also occur at rest.

- Resisted rotational movements are frequently painful, such as turning a key in a lock.
- It is important to explore whether infection could be the cause of the nonunion. Important history includes whether or not the original fracture was open, whether postoperative complications or drainage developed, and whether the patient has received antibiotics.
- During the physical examination, the examiner should do the following:
  - Palpate the nonunion site for pain.
  - Grasp the bone on either side of the nonunion and attempt to flex and extend the nonunion to assess fracture stability and healing. Palpable motion and increased pain indicate lack of union.
  - Loss of flexion–extension in the elbow may result from pain. Loss of pronation and supination indicates deranged forearm anatomy or pain.
  - Loss of flexion or extension at the wrist may indicate pain or scarring of muscle and tendons or IOM around the nonunion. Loss of radioulnar deviation may indicate DRUJ abnormality secondary to shortening at the nonunion site.

IMAGING AND OTHER DIAGNOSTIC STUDIES

- Plain radiographs are essential for diagnosis. This should include AP and lateral views of the forearm, elbow, and wrist.
  - Comparative views of the contralateral forearm, elbow, and wrist are also essential for preoperative planning.
  - Plain radiographs will allow the surgeon to determine if the nonunion is hypertrophic (**FIG 2A**) or atrophic (**FIG 2B**).
- CT is helpful in identifying synostosis, assessing rotational deformity, and evaluating the size of the gap between bone ends at the nonunion site. CT also allows assessment of the DRUJ and PRUJ.
  - The metal suppression CT technique minimizes the bright scatter created by retained hardware.

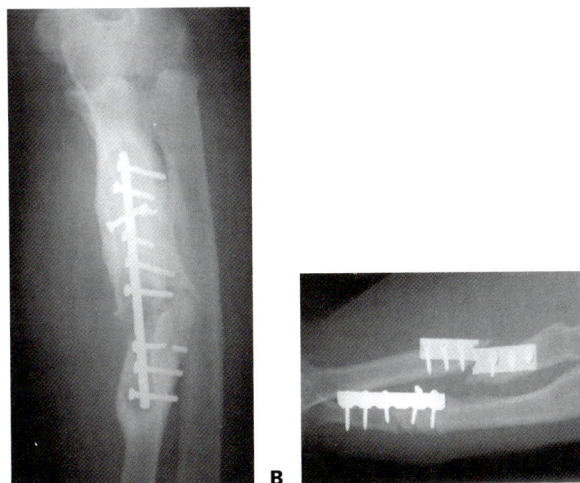

FIG 2 • **A.** Radiograph showing an infected, hypertrophic nonunion. The abundant callus formation indicates a biologically active nonunion. **B.** Radiograph showing an atrophic nonunion. There is complete absence of callus at the fracture site. The problem in an atrophic nonunion is lack of biologic activity. (Courtesy of Thomas R. Hunt III, MD.)

- MRI is rarely used but can allow further evaluation of the IOM.
- A technetium-99m bone scan followed by an indium-111–labeled leukocyte scan may be indicated when suspicion of an infected nonunion exists.
  - False-positive and false-negative results occur.

DIFFERENTIAL DIAGNOSIS

- Malunion
- Infection
- IOM injury
- Painful hardware

NONOPERATIVE MANAGEMENT

- The goal of treatment is to alleviate pain and restore function to the forearm. This can rarely be accomplished without surgical intervention.
- In rare circumstances (if the patient is a high risk for surgery due to comorbidities, for example), an external bone stimulator can be used.
- A minority of patients develop a stable, fibrous nonunion that is painless and allows good function. Nonoperative management can be considered in such patients.

SURGICAL MANAGEMENT

- In all nonunions of the forearm, the first considerations are the patient's level of pain and function.
  - The surgeon should not elect to operate based on radiographic findings alone.
- All patients with nonunions should undergo a workup to determine if the cause of the nonunion is infection, particularly after open fractures.
  - The workup should include careful history of open fracture, drainage, or postoperative complications after initial surgery.
  - Blood should be obtained for a complete blood count, erythrocyte sedimentation rate, and C-reactive protein.
  - Nuclear medicine imaging should be performed if the suspicion of infection is high.

Preoperative Planning

- All imaging studies should be reviewed and pathoanatomy recognized.
- Plain radiographs should be reviewed for presence or absence of callus in order to categorize the nonunion as hypertrophic or atrophic.
  - If a nonunion of the forearm is hypertrophic (which is rare), it may be treated by simple revision of hardware, creating compression across the fracture site with either a compression screw or a compression plate. This is the same technique that should be used for initial management of radius or ulna fractures (see Chap. HA-4).
- If any possibility of infection at the nonunion site exists, plans must be made to search for infection when the nonunion site is opened, and to have an alternative treatment plan if infection is encountered.
  - Preoperative antibiotics may be held until cultures are obtained from the nonunion site (ensure the tourniquet is not inflated if antibiotics are administered later in the case).

- Intraoperative culture swabs and tissue for aerobic, anaerobic, and fungal cultures should be obtained from sites within the nonunion.
- Patients should be made aware that if severe infection is encountered, the planned procedure may need to be altered. For example, if frank purulence is encountered, the nonunion repair may be abandoned in favor of débridement and irrigation with possible antibiotic bead placement and even external fixation if stability is compromised.
- Template the radiographs to ensure selection of proper plate size and length.
  - DCP, LCDCP, and combination locking plates are all appropriate.
  - A minimum of six cortices of screw purchase proximal and distal to the nonunion is critical. This may require plates longer than those available in a standard plating set.
  - In osteoporotic bone, the use of locking plates should be considered.
- If bone graft will be required, the type of graft should be determined preoperatively. While autograft is still considered the gold standard, a vast array of bone graft substitutes are now available. The surgeon's preference and familiarity with various bone graft substitutes may guide this choice. It is important to determine if a structural graft will be required, as this may necessitate the use of autograft.
- Patients should be counseled regarding the possible need for (and risks associated with) various types of autograft, including the possible need for a tricortical iliac crest or fibula graft if significant bone loss is encountered.
  - A vascularized fibula graft may be used to fill large defects, especially those associated with infection.[1,4,6,12]
- A complete examination of range of motion of the elbow and wrist, including pronation and supination, should be performed under anesthesia.

Positioning

- The patient should be positioned supine with the operative arm extended on a radiolucent arm table.
- A nonsterile or sterile tourniquet may be applied, but full access to the elbow is necessary.
- Because restoration of the radial bow is a critical component in restoring forearm motion, intraoperative radiographs showing the entire radius are essential. For this reason, use of the mini C-arm should be avoided in favor of regular fluoroscopy, with its much larger field of view.
- The selected site for harvest of autograft should also be prepared and draped.

Approach

- The approach to either the radius or ulna should generally be through the original surgical incisions.
- Approach to the radius is most commonly volar through the standard Henry approach. Proximal nonunions of the radius may be more easily accessed via a dorsal Thompson approach, particularly in muscular individuals.
  - Care should be taken to identify and protect the posterior interosseous nerve during this approach.
- The ulna is accessed along the subcutaneous border in the interval between the flexor carpi ulnaris and the extensor carpi ulnaris.
  - Care should be taken to identify and protect the dorsal cutaneous branch of the ulnar nerve distally.
- In all cases, preservation of blood supply is key to healing of a nonunion. Therefore, periosteal stripping should be kept to a minimum and the use of cautery should be restricted to vessel coagulation.

TECHNIQUES

PLATE FIXATION FOR TREATMENT OF FOREARM NONUNIONS

Preparation of the Nonunion

- Determine the correct length of the radius or ulna by measuring the corresponding contralateral bone.
- Expose the nonunion site and search for evidence of infection. If found, send specimens for Gram stain and culture and abort the planned procedure. Perform a two-stage reconstruction.
  - Thoroughly débride all necrotic and infected bone and soft tissue. Remove all hardware.
  - Place antibiotic-loaded PMMA beads in the gap.
  - Begin a multiweek course of antibiotics before proceeding with definitive nonunion repair.
- If infection is considered unlikely, after removal of all hardware, thoroughly débride the nonunion site of all necrotic and inflammatory tissue, synovial membranes, and sclerotic or avascular bone (**TECH FIG 1A**).
  - Tools such as curved curettes, small rongeurs, and a small high-speed burr (with copious irrigation to prevent thermal injury to the bone) are helpful.
  - Flatten the bone ends to allow for excellent fragment-to-fragment contact with compression.
- Open the sclerotic bone ends using sequentially larger diameter drills.
  - Pass these drills proximally and distally as far as possible to open the medullary canals (**TECH FIG 1B**).
- Restrict elevation of muscle and periosteum to only what is needed to thoroughly débride the nonunion and to realign the bone.
- Realign the bone and restore length by manipulating fragments with bone-holding forceps.
  - Use of a small skeletal distractor, small external fixator, or lamina spreader aids in restoration of length.[10]
- Measure the length of the residual bone defect directly and, taking into consideration the preoperative plan, determine the appropriate bone graft to use.

Compression Plating Without Bone Graft

- In rare cases with minimal or no bone loss at the nonunion site, the bone may be plated in situ without causing shortening. Because the bone remains at normal

TECHNIQUES

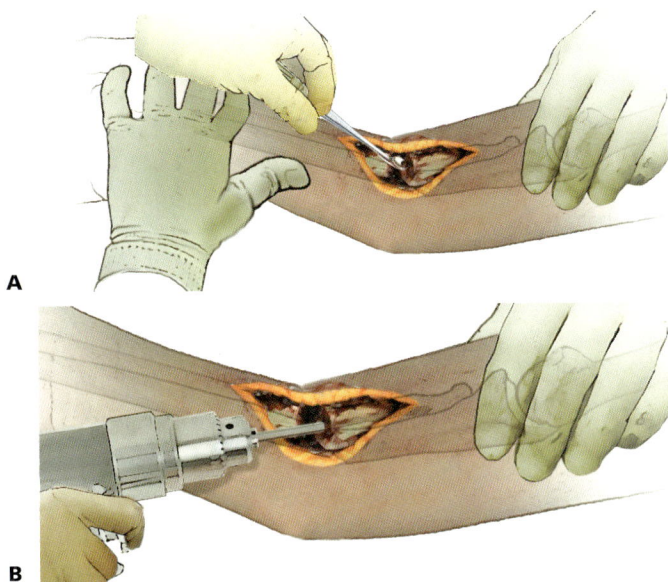

TECH FIG 1 • **A.** Complete débridement of the nonunion site is the essential first step. Any fibrous or necrotic material must be removed and the bone ends delivered. **B.** Medullary canals are opened using increasing-diameter drill bits to allow vascular ingrowth.

length, the relationship of the radius and ulna at both the DRUJ and the PRUJ is not disrupted and rotation will be preserved.

- This technique may also be used if there is nonunion of both the radius and the ulna. Both bones may then be shortened a symmetrical distance.

- After bone preparation as detailed above, anatomically align the bone ends and precisely apply a compression plate using the same technique employed for acute forearm fractures.

  - Ensure that compression of the bone ends is achieved.

- If a small bone gap exists after compression, the other forearm bone may then be shortened to restore the length relationship.

  - Because this approach involves surgery on a normal bone, this strategy should be used with caution.

Cancellous Bone Grafting

- Cancellous bone grafting is generally used for small defects up to 3 cm that can be effectively stabilized with a plate.

  - Gaps of up to 6 cm have been successfully treated using cancellous bone for grafting.[9]

- Firmly pack the cancellous autograft into the residual nonunion defect after the plate is applied.

- Ensure the graft does not escape from the nonunion site and come to lie on the IOM (**TECH FIG 2**).

Structural Corticocancellous Autograft Bone Grafting

- Structural autograft harvested from the anterior or posterior iliac crest is used for larger defects.

- Expose the superior crest and define the inner and outer tables.

- Utilize a water-cooled sagittal saw and osteotomes to harvest a tricortical block of bone from the iliac crest. Additionally, harvest cancellous bone to fill defects that may present.

- The graft should be slightly larger than that required based on preoperative planning.

- Precisely contour the graft to fit snugly into the defect. Square the ends of the graft to match the ends of the bone fragments.[5]

  - Alternatively, cut both the bone ends of the radius or ulna and of the bone block chamfered, or on the bias, to increase the area of bony contact.[3] This also allows the graft to be wedged securely in place.

- Insert the graft before plate fixation and fill any residual gaps with cancellous bone after plate application.

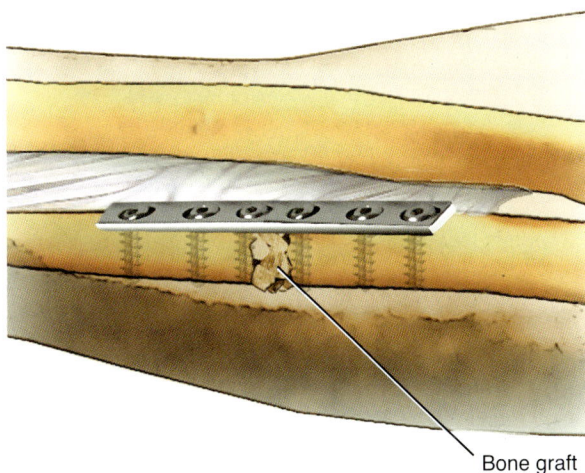

Bone graft

TECH FIG 2 • The nonunion gap is distracted if necessary to recreate the normal anatomic bone length. A 3.5-mm plate with a minimum of three screws proximal and distal should be used. Cancellous bone graft is inserted and packed in the nonunion gap.

TECHNIQUES

Nonvascularized Structural Fibula Autograft With Cortical Allograft Bone Grafting

- An appropriate-length segmental graft is harvested from the fibula and placed into the defect.
- The fibula is approached laterally, via the intramuscular plane between the peroneal muscles and the soleus.
- A cuff of muscle 2 to 3 mm in thickness should be left to protect the periosteum.
- The IOM is incised longitudinally, taking care to avoid the posterior neurovascular bundle.
- The fibula is osteotomized proximally and distally to create an appropriate-length graft.
  - Complications of fibular harvest are rare but include transient motor weakness, peroneal nerve palsy, and flexor hallucis longus (FHL) contracture.
  - A minimum of 6 cm of the distal fibula must be retained to avoid adversely affecting the distal tibiofibular syndesmosis and ankle joint function.
- Insert the fibula graft into the defect and then apply the plate as described below, first placing the two screws just proximal and just distal to the nonunion to gain initial compression.
- Select a cortical allograft several centimeters longer than the defect.

TECH FIG 3 • Combined intercalary autograft and allograft strut technique described by Moroni et al.[8] After débridement of the nonunion site, an intercalary graft of appropriate length is harvested from the patient's fibula and placed in the gap. A cortical allograft is placed opposite to the plate, and screws are placed passing though the plate, the patient's radius or ulna, and finally the allograft strut.

- Tibial allograft is recommended due to its suitable thickness and mechanical characteristics, which provide excellent screw purchase.[8]
- Place the cortical allograft along the outer cortex of the bone, opposite the plate, spanning beyond the length of the fibula allograft.
- Insert the remainder of the screws so that they pass through the plate and then the patient's bone and finally into the cortical allograft on the opposite side (**TECH FIG 3**).

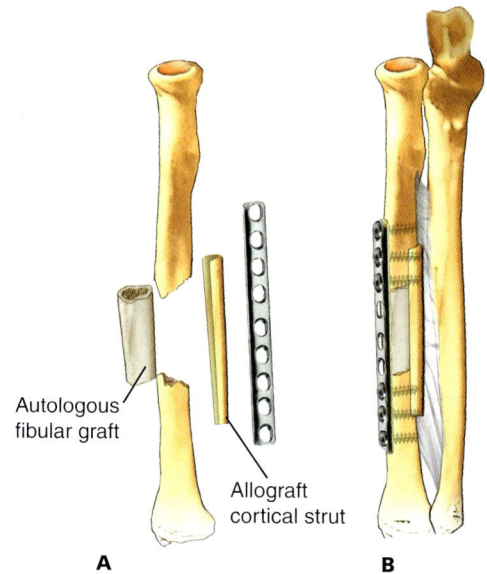

Autologous fibular graft

Allograft cortical strut

A   **B**

COMPRESSION PLATE FIXATION

- Select a 3.5-mm (small fragment) compression plate of adequate length to ensure a minimum of three or four screws (six to eight cortices) on either side of the nonunion.
  - Always err on the side of a longer plate.
  - Thinner locking plates may be considered when structural fibular autografts are combined with cortical allograft struts.
- Fix the plate to the bone in compression (ensuring that proper length is maintained) with one screw proximal and one screw distal to the nonunion, then use full-length fluoroscopic views or radiographs of the forearm to ensure restoration of length, bow, and joint alignment.
  - Compare with the contralateral forearm.
- Insert the remaining screws.
  - Ideally, screws are not placed into the graft itself and the graft is stabilized by the compression created by the plate (**TECH FIG 4**).
- Close the wound routinely and apply an above-elbow or sugartong splint.

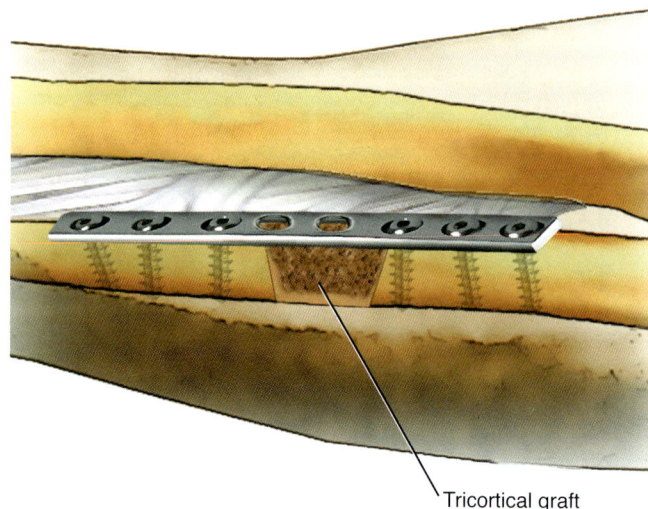

Tricortical graft

TECH FIG 4 • Modified Nicoll technique with tricortical iliac crest graft. The graft is chamfered, allowing the graft to be compressed as the plate is applied.

PEARLS AND PITFALLS

Indications	■ Careful evaluation of the patient's pain and functional limitations must be done before surgical management is planned.
Radiographs	■ Differentiation should be made between hypertrophic and atrophic nonunions, as treatment differs. ■ Contralateral radiographs must be used to determine the appropriate length of the forearm bones and degree of radial bow. ■ Anatomic restoration of length and bow is necessary to allow full rotational motion of the forearm.
Diagnosis of infection	■ A complete preoperative infection workup should be done for all patients with a nonunion. ■ A negative preoperative workup does not rule out infection. ■ An intraoperative infection workup, including Gram stain and culture, should be performed and an alternative plan should be available if infection is encountered.
Nonunion site preparation	■ Débridement of all necrotic, sclerotic, and avascular tissue from the nonunion site is essential. ■ Opening the sclerotic bone ends and gentle reaming of the medullary canals promotes ingrowth of medullary blood vessels. ■ Periosteal stripping and cautery must be minimized to preserve periosteal blood supply.
Graft selection	■ Defects up to 3 cm are successfully managed with cancellous autograft and appropriate fixation. ■ Bone graft substitutes may offer alternatives to autograft, but no comparative studies exist at this time.
Compression of structural grafts	■ Compression must be created across all structural grafts.

POSTOPERATIVE CARE

■ The longer motion is delayed after surgery, the greater the chance the patient will develop stiffness. Therefore, early active range of motion (ROM) should be initiated at the first postoperative visit, except in cases with more tenuous fixation.

■ Use of the arm for activities of daily living is encouraged.

■ If the patient has difficulty in achieving satisfactory ROM with active, active-assisted, and gentle passive ROM, static progressive splints may be used.

■ Having the patient sleep in a static extension splint may significantly improve elbow extension.

■ Heavy lifting, pushing, and weight bearing are delayed until radiographic evidence of healing is present, often 3 to 6 months after the index procedure.

OUTCOMES

■ When precise surgical techniques are used, such as creating stable compression across structural grafts, high rates of union are expected.

■ Rates of healing from 95% to 100% are reported for all of the methods described in this chapter.[3,8,9]

■ Failure of union is related to recurrence of previous infection in nearly all cases. The prognosis for infected nonunions should be guarded.

■ Patient satisfaction does not correlate directly with bony healing. In multiple studies only two thirds of patients achieved good or excellent results.[3,5,8,9]

■ Unsatisfactory results are associated with poor postoperative motion in the majority of cases.

■ Other injuries to the upper extremity (common in high-energy trauma associated with nonunions) contributed to unsatisfactory overall function in a minority of patients.[9,10]

■ Because nonunion of the forearm diaphysis is a rare condition, no comparative studies of treatment methods exist, including the use of bone graft substitutes.

COMPLICATIONS

■ Infection
■ Graft displacement
■ Recurrent nonunion and hardware failure
■ Loss of motion
■ Synostosis
■ Pain or other complications at the autograft harvest site

REFERENCES

1. Adani R, Delcroix L, Innocenti M, et al. Reconstruction of large post-traumatic skeletal defects of the forearm by vascularized free fibular graft. Microsurgery 2004;24:423–429.
2. Chapman MW, Gordon JE, Zissimos AG. Compression-plate fixation of acute fractures of the diaphyses of the radius and ulna. J Bone Joint Surg Am 1989;71A:159–169.
3. Davey PA, Simonis RB. Modification of the Nicoll bone-grafting technique for nonunion of the radius and/or ulna. J Bone Joint Surg Br 2002;84B:30–33.
4. Dell PC, Sheppard JE. Vascularized bone grafts in the treatment of infected forearm nonunion. J Hand Surg Am 1984;9A:653–658.
5. Grace TG, Eversman WW. The management of segmental bone loss associated with forearm fractures. J Bone Joint Surg Am 1980;62A:1150–1155.
6. Jupiter JB, Gerhard HJ, Guerrero J, et al. Treatment of segmental defects of the radius with use of the vascularized osteoseptocutaneous fibular autogenous graft. J Bone Joint Surg Am 1997;79A:542–550.
7. Moed BR, Kellam JF, Foster JR, et al. Immediate internal fixation of open fractures of the diaphysis of the forearm. J Bone Joint Surg Am 1986;68A:1008–1017.
8. Moroni AG, Rollo G, Guzzardella M, et al. Surgical treatment of isolated forearm non-union with segmental bone loss. Injury 1997;28:497–504.
9. Ring D, Allende C, Jafarnia K, et al. Ununited diaphyseal forearm fractures with segmental defects: plate fixation and autogenous cancellous bone-grafting. J Bone Joint Surg Am 2004;86A:2440–2445.
10. Ring D, Jupiter JB, Gulotta L. Atrophic nonunions of the proximal ulna. Clin Orthop Relat Res 2003;409:268–274.
11. Ring D, Rhim R, Carpenter C, et al. Comminuted diaphyseal fractures of the radius and ulna: does bone grafting affect nonunion rate? J Trauma 2005;59:436–440.
12. Safoury Y. Free vascularized fibula for the treatment of traumatic bone defects and nonunions of the forearm bones. J Hand Surg Br 2005;30B:67–72.

Chapter 8

K-Wire Fixation of Distal Radius Fractures With and Without External Fixation

Christopher Doumas and David J. Bozentka

DEFINITION

- Distal radius fractures occur at the distal end of the bone, originating in the metaphyseal region and often extending to the radiocarpal and distal radioulnar joints.
- Distal radius fractures can be classified as stable or unstable and extra- or intra-articular to assist in treatment decisions.
- Fractures may angulate dorsal or volar and may have significant comminution, depending on the energy of the injury and the quality of the bone.
- Percutaneous pins or K-wires, typically 0.062- or 0.045-inch, can be used for unstable intra-articular or extra-articular fractures with mild comminution and no osteoporosis.
- Percutaneous pins can aid reduction and stabilize the fragments in a minimally invasive manner.
- Percutaneous pins can support the subchondral area of the distal radius and maintain the articular reduction in highly comminuted fractures, which is useful in combined fixation methods.
- Smooth percutaneous pins may also be placed across the physis to maintain a reduction in children without causing a growth arrest.
- Highly comminuted fractures are more difficult to fix rigidly and often require internal and external fixation to maintain alignment during healing.
- External fixators can be hinged or static, and may or may not bridge the wrist joint.

ANATOMY

- The distal radius consists of three articular surfaces: the scaphoid fossa, the lunate fossa, and the sigmoid notch.
- Ligamentotaxis aids in the reduction of intra-articular and comminuted fractures.
  - Volar ligamentous attachments include the radioscaphocapitate, long radiolunate, and short radiolunate ligaments.
  - Dorsal ligamentous attachments include the dorsal intercarpal and radiocarpal ligaments.
- Dorsal and radial to the second metacarpal lie the first dorsal interosseous muscle and the terminal branches of the radial sensory nerve.

- The distal radial sensory nerve branches lie superficial to the distal radius and should be protected during dissection and pin placement.
- The radial sensory nerve emerges between the brachioradialis and the extensor carpi radialis longus (ECRL) muscle bellies (**FIG 1**).
- The terminal branches of the lateral antebrachial cutaneous nerve lie superficial to the forearm fascia at the radial wrist.
- There is a bare spot of bone between the first and second dorsal compartments in the region of the radial styloid.
- The brachioradialis tendon inserts onto the radial styloid adjacent to the first dorsal compartment.
- The extensor carpi radialis longus and the extensor carpi radialis brevis lie dorsal to the brachioradialis in the second dorsal compartment.
- Lister's tubercle is dorsal, with the extensor pollicis longus (EPL) tendon on its ulnar side, in the third dorsal compartment.
- The extensor digitorum communis tendons lie over the dorsal ulnar half of the distal radius in the fourth dorsal compartment.
- The extensor digiti minimi lies over the distal radioulnar joint (DRUJ) in the fifth dorsal compartment.

PATHOGENESIS

- Distal radius fractures are the most common fractures of the upper extremity in adults, representing about 20% of all fractures seen in the emergency room.[17]
- Mechanism of injury typically is a fall on an outstretched hand with axial loading, but other common histories include motor vehicle accidents or pathologic fractures.
- Higher-energy injuries cause increased comminution, angulation, and displacement.
- Osteoporosis, tumors, and metabolic bone diseases are risk factors for sustaining pathologic distal radius fractures.
- In children, fractures typically occur along the physis due to its relative weakness compared to the surrounding ligaments.

NATURAL HISTORY

- Distal radius fractures needing no reduction and those that are stable after reduction typically recover functional range of motion with minimal long-term sequelae.

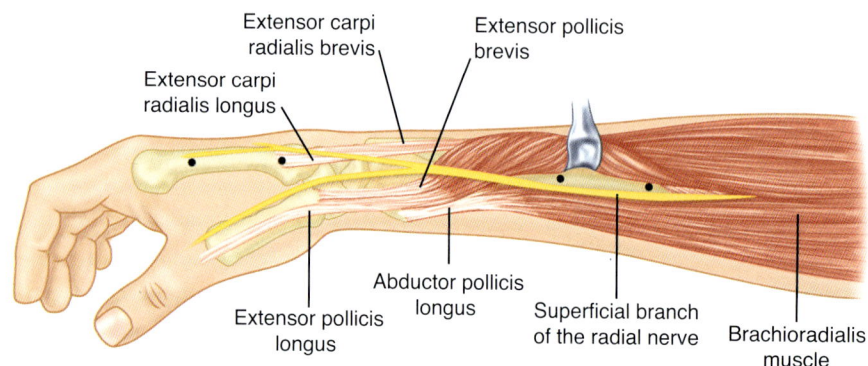

FIG 1 • Anatomy surrounding the radial sensory nerve branch in the forearm.

- Three parameters that affect outcome include articular congruity, angulation, and shortening.[16,20]
    - 1 to 2 mm of articular surface incongruity of the distal radius can lead to degenerative changes, pain, and stiffness.
    - Dorsal angulation can lead to decreased range of motion and increased load transfer to the ulna.
    - Radial shortening can lead to decreased range of motion, pain, and ulnar impaction of the carpus.

PATIENT HISTORY AND PHYSICAL FINDINGS

- The history of a fall on an outstretched hand is the most common presentation for a patient with a distal radius fracture.
- Motor vehicle or motorcycle accidents and osteoporosis account for most comminuted fractures.
- It may be clinically indicated to implement a workup for osteoporosis.
- Pain, tenderness, swelling, crepitus, deformity, ecchymosis, and decreased range of motion at the wrist are typical symptoms and warrant radiographic evaluation.
- Physical examination should include the following:
    - Inspection: Evaluate the integrity of the skin, cascade of the digits, direction of displacement, and presence of any swelling.
    - Identify points of maximal tenderness to differentiate between distal radius injuries and carpal or ligamentous injuries.
        - Touch or press specific areas of the wrist and hand to differentiate distal intra-articular, DRUJ, and carpal injuries.
    - Two-point discrimination: Higher than normal (5 mm) results in the form of progressive neurologic deficit may signify an acute carpal tunnel syndrome or ulnar neuropathy.
    - Passive finger stretch test to assist with diagnosis of compartment syndrome.
    - EPL tendon function should be evaluated.
    - EPL assessment: Assess the resting position of the thumb interphalangeal joint and the patient's ability to lift the thumb off of a flat surface to determine the continuity of the EPL tendon.
    - Palpation of forearm and elbow to assess for concomitant injury proximally.
    - The DRUJ must be assessed for displacement.
    - The bony anatomy must be carefully evaluated to avoid missing minimally displaced fractures, which may displace without treatment.
        - Skin should be assessed to avoid missing an open fracture.
        - Swelling should be monitored to allow for early diagnosis of compartment syndrome.
        - Sensory examination should be monitored for progressive changes, which may represent acute carpal tunnel syndrome.

IMAGING AND OTHER DIAGNOSTIC STUDIES

- Radiographic evaluation should include posteroanterior (PA), lateral, and oblique views to assess displacement, angulation, comminution, and intra-articular involvement, and allow for radiologic measurements.[14,17]
    - Lateral articular (volar) tilt is the angle between the radial shaft and a tangential line parallel to the articular margin as seen on the lateral view (**FIG 2A**). The normal angle is 11 degrees.
    - Radial inclination, measured on the PA view (**FIG 2B**), is the angle between a line perpendicular to the shaft of the radius at the ulnar articular margin and the tangential line

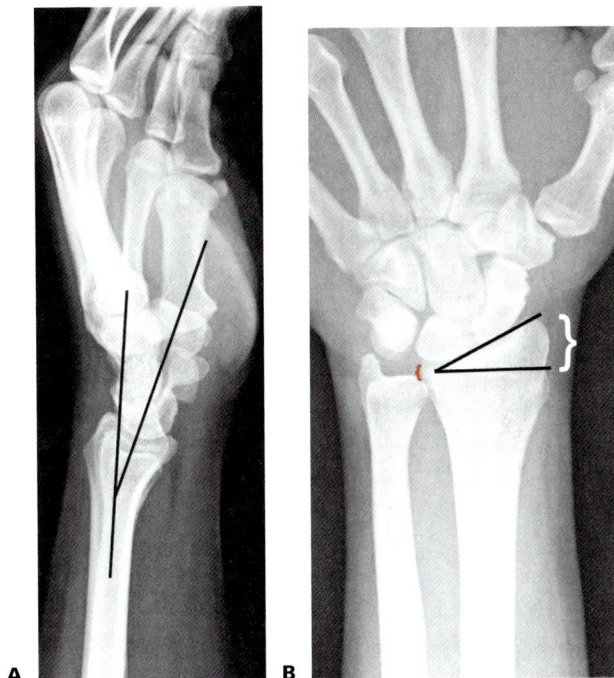

FIG 2 • **A.** Lateral radiograph of the wrist demonstrating volar tilt (*black lines*). **B.** PA radiograph demonstrating radial inclination (*black lines*), ulnar variance (*red bracket*), and radial height (*white bracket*).

along the radial styloid to the ulnar articular margin. The normal angle is 22 degrees.
    - Ulnar variance, also measured on the PA view (see Fig 2B), is the distance between the radial and ulnar articular surfaces. Ulnar variance is compared to the contralateral side.
- Traction radiographs help assess intra-articular involvement, intercarpal ligamentous injury, and potential fracture reduction through ligamentotaxis.
- CT scans are useful in fully elucidating the anatomy of the fracture, including impaction, comminution, and size of the fragments.
    - CT scans often significantly alter the original treatment plan.[11]
- MRI is rarely performed acutely but can diagnose concomitant ligamentous injuries, triangular fibrocartilage complex injuries, and occult carpal fractures.

DIFFERENTIAL DIAGNOSIS

- Bony contusion
- Radiocarpal dislocation
- Scaphoid or other carpal fracture
- Perilunate or lunate fracture dislocation
- Distal ulna fracture
- Wrist ligament or triangular fibrocartilage complex injury
- DRUJ injury

NONOPERATIVE MANAGEMENT

- Conservative treatment consists of splinting or casting for stable fracture patterns using a three-point mold.
- Fractures amenable to nonoperative treatment include fractures that are stable after reduction with minimal metaphyseal comminution, shortening, angulation, and displacement.

- Evaluation for secondary displacement weekly for 2 to 3 weeks is critical as the swelling subsides.
- Unstable patterns will displace if not surgically stabilized.
  - There is little role for nonoperative treatment in highly comminuted fractures.
- The physiologic age, medical comorbidities, and functional level of the patient should be considered in determining the need for surgical treatment.
- Early range of motion of the nonimmobilized joints is essential in the nonoperative treatment of all fractures near the wrist to prevent contracture.
  - The cast or splint must not extend past the metacarpophalangeal joints so as to allow digital motion.

SURGICAL MANAGEMENT

- Surgical treatments are indicated to prevent malunion and improve pain control, function, and range of motion.
- Surgery is reserved for unstable fractures, including displaced, intra-articular, comminuted, or severely angulated injuries and fractures that displace following attempted closed management.
- Percutaneous pinning can assist in obtaining and maintaining reduction of displaced fractures with limited comminution in a minimally invasive manner.
- External fixators maintain radius length but cannot always control angulation and displacement; therefore, supplementation with percutaneous pins is typically performed.[2]
- Conversely, external fixators may augment percutaneous pins and plate fixation when extensive comminution is present.
  - Supplemental external fixation should be considered for fractures with comminution of over 50% of the diameter of the radius on a lateral view.
- External fixation may be used as a neutralization device, because the distraction forces decrease soon after fracture reduction.
- External fixators also are useful for "damage control orthopaedics" to temporarily stabilize wrist fractures, especially for complex, combined, open injuries.
- For nonbridging external fixation, there must be at least 1 cm of volar cortex intact and adequate fragment sizes to allow proper pin placement.
- A relative contraindication to pin fixation with or without external fixation is a volar shear injury, which should be reduced and stabilized using a volar plate and screws.

Preoperative Planning

- All radiographs should be reviewed before surgery and brought into the operating room.
- Analysis of the pattern and presumed stability of the fracture fragments determines whether percutaneous fixation, with or without external fixation, is suitable.
- For intra-articular fractures, the specific fragments to be reduced and fixed must be identified preoperatively to avoid incomplete reduction of the joint surface.
- The surgeon must be prepared to change his or her management decision intraoperatively if the fracture behavior is different than anticipated. A variety of fixation devices should be available in the operating room.

Positioning

- The patient is positioned supine on the operating table with a radiolucent arm board.

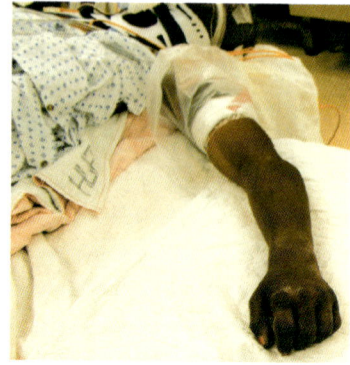

FIG 3 • Positioning of patient supine on the hand table with tourniquet in place.

- A tourniquet is applied near the axilla with the splint still in place (**FIG 3**).
- Fluoroscopy should be used for reduction confirmation and fixation throughout the procedure.
- There must be enough range of motion of the shoulder and elbow to allow standard AP, lateral, and oblique images.

Approach

- Various approaches can be used in the application of external fixators and the insertion of percutaneous pins.
- Distal external fixator half-pins may be placed directly into the second metacarpal or into other carpal bones (for injuries including the second metacarpal). Wires and half-pins, which are non-bridging fixators, may be placed in the distal radius itself.
- Percutaneous pins can be inserted through the radial styloid between the first and second dorsal compartments, through Lister's tubercle, through the interval between the fourth and fifth dorsal compartments, and across the DRUJ (**FIG 4**).
  - Caution is taken to avoid skewering tendons and nerves and to avoid penetrating the articular surface.

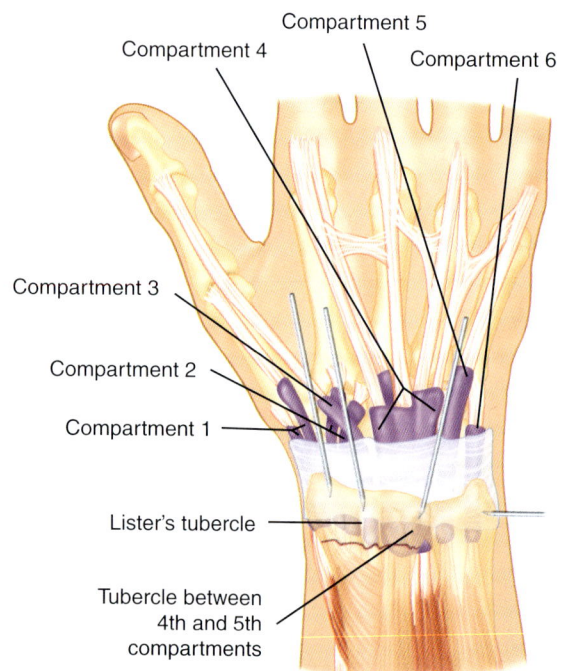

FIG 4 • Areas for K-wire insertion at the distal radius.

CLOSED REDUCTION OF A DISTAL RADIUS FRACTURE

- Closed reduction should be performed before fixation using distraction and palmar translation of the distal radius fragment and carpus.[1]
- Use of a padded bump or towel roll will aid in the reduction (**TECH FIG 1**).
- Overdistraction will cause increased dorsal angulation due to the intact short, stout volar ligaments.[1]
- Excessive palmar flexion of the wrist can restore volar tilt but leads to an increased incidence of stiffness and carpal tunnel syndrome.[7]
- Overdistraction can be assessed by measuring the carpal height index, measuring the radioscaphoid and midcarpal joint spaces, checking full finger flexion into the palm, or evaluating index finger extrinsic extensor tightness.[8]

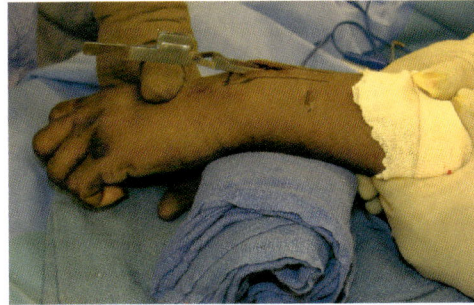

TECH FIG 1 • Closed reduction over a towel bump using traction and palmar translation.

KAPANDJI TECHNIQUE FOR PERCUTANEOUS PINNING

- Closed reduction is obtained using a bump, and the reduction is confirmed using fluoroscopy.
- This technique should be employed in patients younger than 55 years of age with minimal comminution. It should not be used in osteoporotic, elderly patients or those with comminution secondary to a higher loss of reduction. External fixation should be used to supplement pinning in these populations.[21]

- A stab incision is made radially, and a 0.062-inch pin is manually inserted into the fracture site, taking care to protect the sensory nerve branches and the first dorsal compartment tendons (**TECH FIG 2A**).
  - The pin is angled distal, levering the bone back into its normal position and restoring the radial inclination (**TECH FIG 2B**). The pin is advanced through the far cortex using power, acting as a buttress to prevent loss of radial inclination (**TECH FIG 2C**).

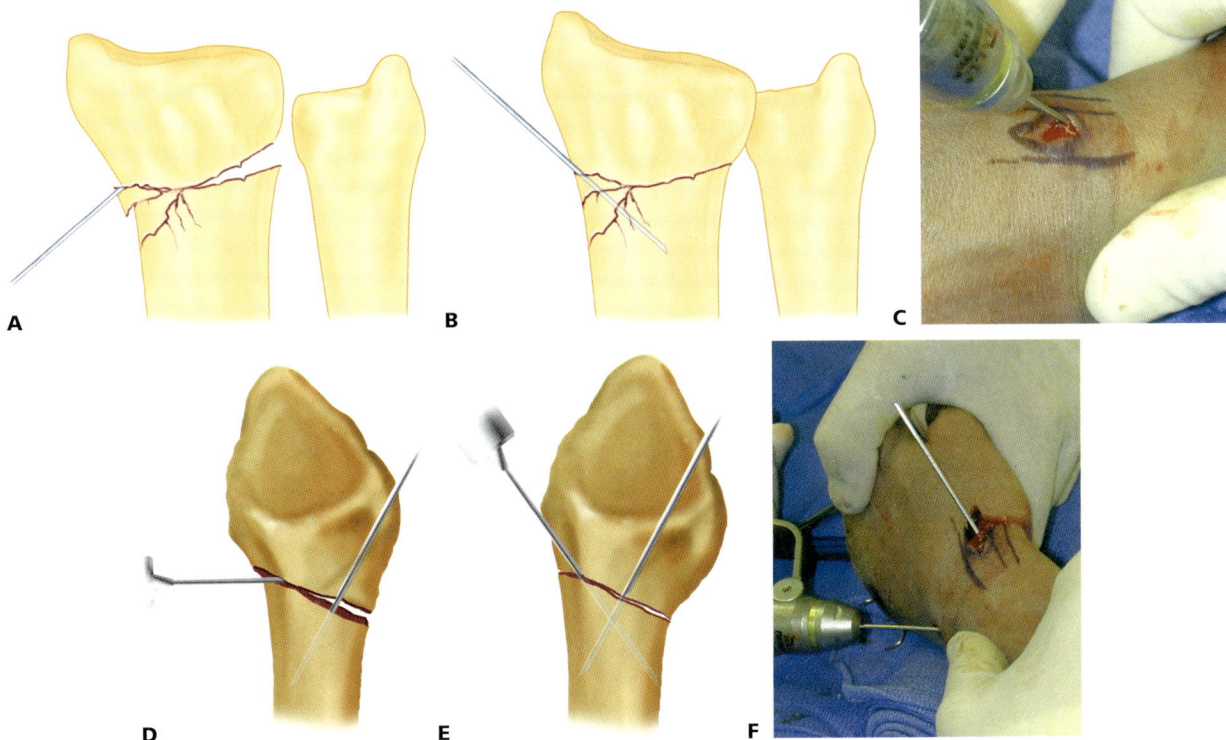

TECH FIG 2 • **A.** An incision is made over the radial styloid and a K-wire is manually inserted into the fracture site. **B.** The wire is levered distally to correct the radial inclination. **C.** The wire is advanced proximally, using power, into cortical bone. **D.** An incision is made over Lister's tubercle, and a wire is inserted into the fracture site. **E,F.** The wire is levered distally to correct the dorsal angulation and advanced proximally using power into cortical bone.

- A second stab incision is placed dorsally, and a second pin is manually inserted into the fracture (**TECH FIG 2D**).
  - The pin is angled distal, levering the bone back into its normal position and restoring the volar tilt (**TECH FIG 2E**). The pin is advanced through the volar cortex using power, acting as a buttress to prevent loss of volar tilt (**TECH FIG 2F**).
- Using the modified technique, a third pin is placed retrograde using power, starting at the radial styloid and pro-

ceeding into the ulnar cortex of the radius proximal to the fracture line.

- The pins are buried and cut just below the skin, and the skin is sutured.
  - Alternatively, the pins may be bent using two needle drivers and left outside the skin.
- The pins are then cut and covered with pin caps or antibiotic gauze.
- A sterile dressing is applied, followed by a splint.

AUTHOR'S PREFERRED TECHNIQUE FOR PERCUTANEOUS PINNING

- Closed reduction is obtained using a bump, and the reduction is confirmed using fluoroscopy (**TECH FIG 3A,B**).
- A small incision is placed over the bare spot on the radial styloid between the first and second dorsal compartments (**TECH FIG 3C**).
- Two 0.062-inch smooth K-wires are placed retrograde from the radial styloid across the reduced fracture, engaging the opposite cortex in a divergent fashion (**TECH FIG 3D,E**).
- A small incision is placed over the interval between the fourth and fifth dorsal compartments.

- One or two K-wires are placed retrograde from the dorsal ulnar corner of the distal radius across the reduced fracture, engaging the opposite cortex in a divergent fashion (**TECH FIG 3F–H**).
- The pins are cut just beneath the skin, which is closed with a 5-0 nylon suture.
- Alternatively, the pins are bent and cut and left outside the skin (**TECH FIG 3I**).
- A dressing and splint are then applied.

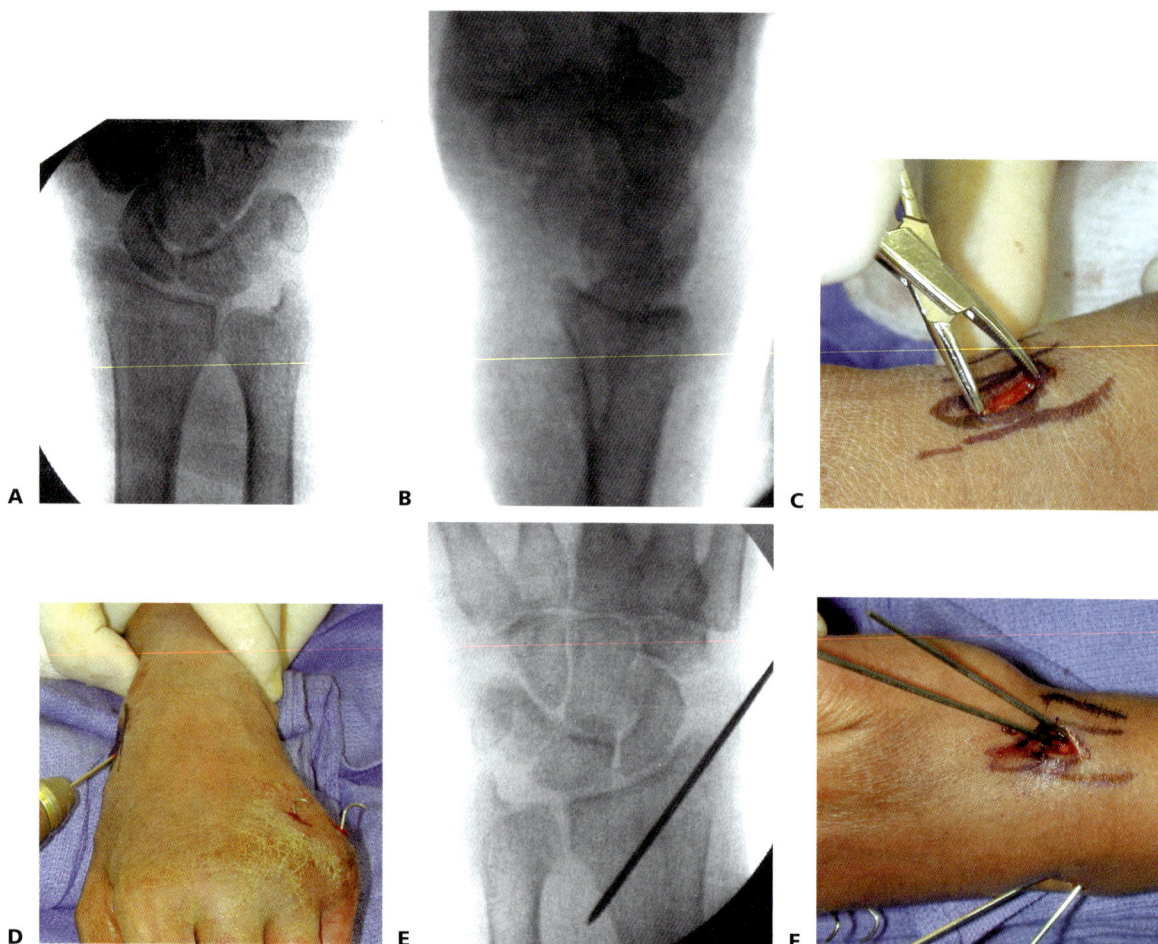

TECH FIG 3 • **A,B.** PA and lateral views demonstrating reduction of distal radius fracture. **C.** The incision is made over the radial styloid. **D.** A pin is inserted retrograde into the radial styloid. **E.** PA radiograph demonstrating the course of the radial styloid wire. **F.** Two radial styloid wires and two dorsoulnar wires are in place. *(continued)*

G H I

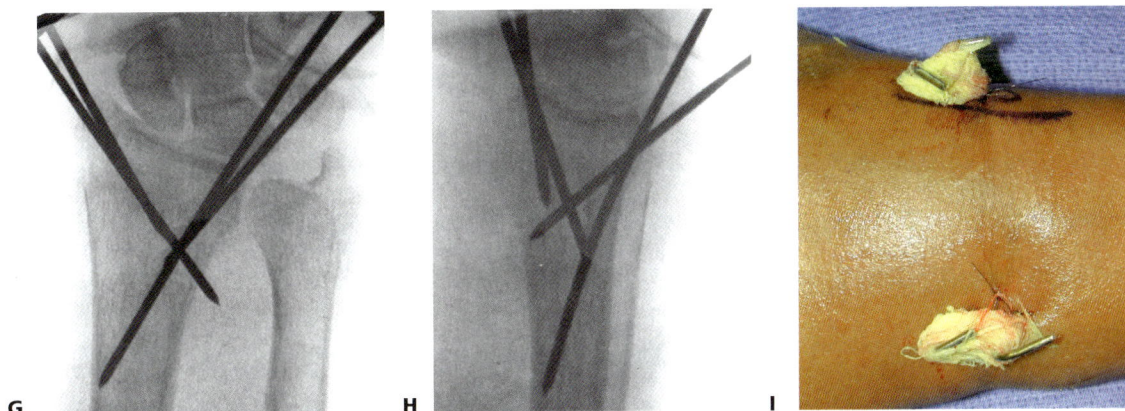

TECH FIG 3 • *(continued)* **G.** PA view showing fixation and the path of the wires. **H.** Lateral view showing fixation and path of wires. **I.** Pins are bent, cut, and covered above the skin.

BRIDGING EXTERNAL FIXATOR APPLICATION

Distal Pin Placement

- A 3-cm incision is made over the dorsal index metacarpal, exposing the proximal two thirds.
- The distal sensory nerve branches are retracted, and the first dorsal interosseous muscle is elevated from the metacarpal to identify the insertion of the ECRL (**TECH FIG 4A**).

- The index metacarpophalangeal joint is flexed to protect the sagittal band and first dorsal interosseous aponeurosis.
- The metacarpal drill guide is placed on the radial base of the index metacarpal at the flare of the metaphysis. Partially threaded 3- to 4-mm pins are used, with or without predrilling.

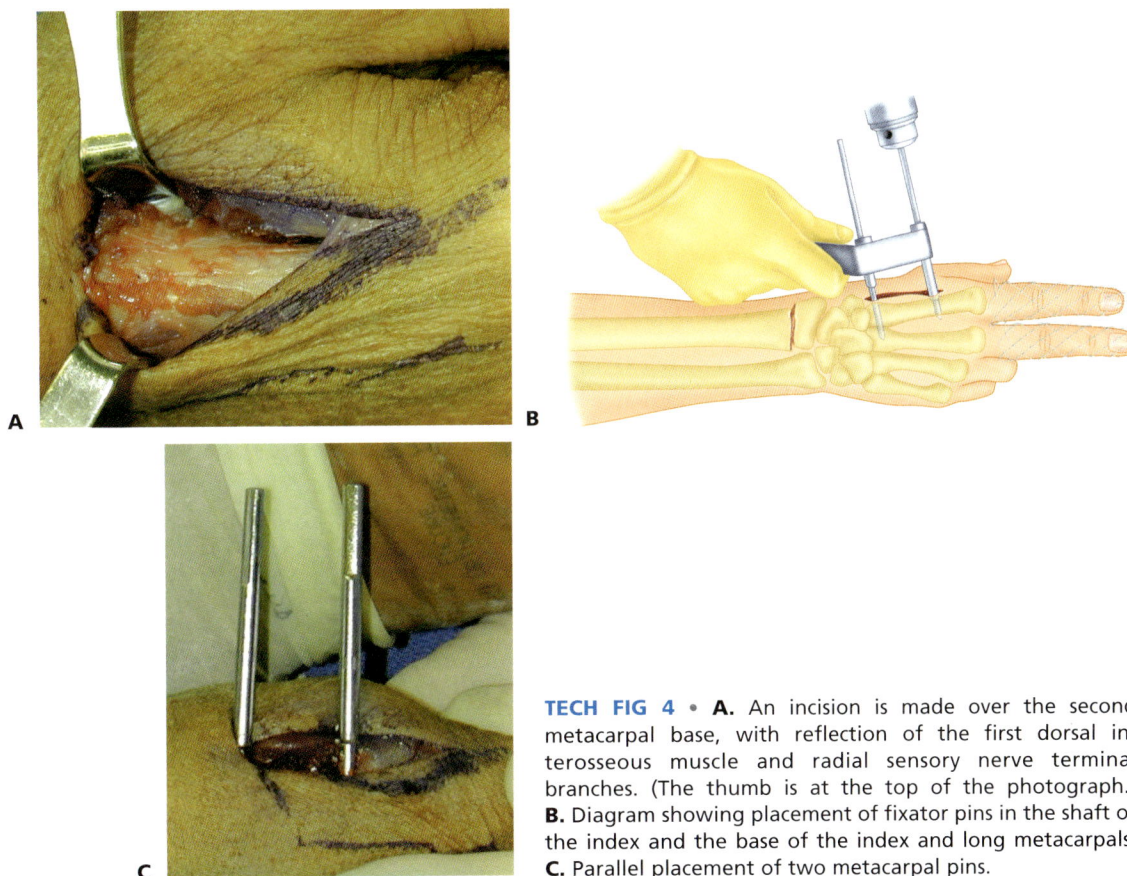

A B

C

TECH FIG 4 • **A.** An incision is made over the second metacarpal base, with reflection of the first dorsal interosseous muscle and radial sensory nerve terminal branches. (The thumb is at the top of the photograph.) **B.** Diagram showing placement of fixator pins in the shaft of the index and the base of the index and long metacarpals. **C.** Parallel placement of two metacarpal pins.

- A long threaded pin is placed through the index and long metacarpal bases, obtaining three cortices of fixation.
  - Care is taken not to enter the carpometacarpal joint.
- The double drill guide is then placed over the first pin, and the distal short threaded pin is placed through both cortices of the index metacarpal shaft (**TECH FIG 4B,C**).
- Fluoroscopy confirms placement and length of the pins.

Proximal Pin Placement and Frame Construction

- A 4- to 5-cm incision is made over the radial forearm, proximal to the first dorsal compartment musculature, through skin and subcutaneous tissue, avoiding the lateral antebrachial cutaneous nerve branches.
- The fascia overlying the interval between the brachioradialis and the ECRL is divided, and the radial sensory nerve is identified and retracted (**TECH FIG 5A**).
  - The interval between the ECRL and ECRB also may be used to avoid the radial sensory branch.

- The double drill guide is placed onto the diaphysis of the radius between the brachioradialis and the radial wrist extensors or between the ECRL and ECRB (**TECH FIG 5B**).
- Threaded 3- to 4-mm pins are placed, with or without predrilling.
  - The fracture should be reduced, and the pins placed parallel to the metacarpal pins to facilitate alignment of the fracture.
  - The proximal pin should be placed bicortically, just distal to the tendon of the pronator teres.
  - The distal pin is then drilled bicortically through the double drill guide.
- Pin placement is confirmed using fluoroscopy.
- The incisions are closed using nylon suture, ensuring no tension is on the skin at the pin sites.
- Clamps and rods or adjustable fixators may then be applied to the pins to achieve and maintain final reduction (**TECH FIG 5C**).
- Supplementary K-wire fixation is added before or after external fixation (**TECH FIG 5D**).

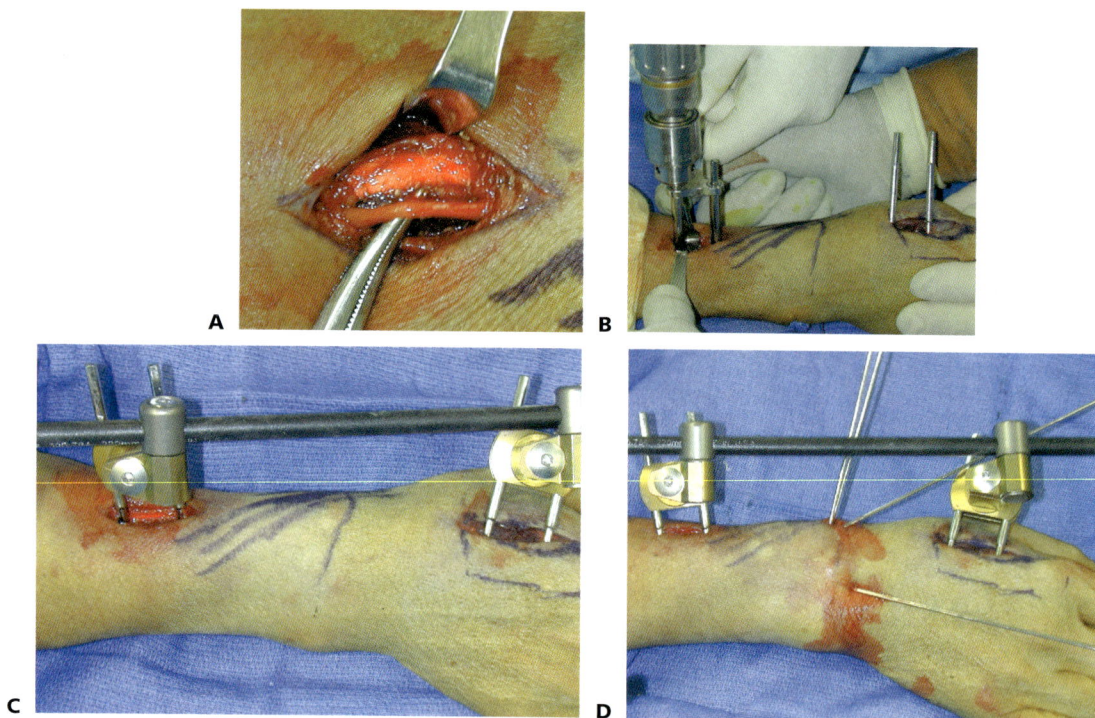

TECH FIG 5 • **A.** Incision over the radial forearm demonstrating the radial sensory nerve branch deep to the fascia. (The hand is to the right.) **B.** The double drill guide is placed onto the radius. **C.** Final reduction is maintained by the addition of clamps and rods. **D.** K-wires are used for supplemental fixation when necessary.

NONBRIDGING EXTERNAL FIXATOR APPLICATION

- Fracture reduction can be performed after insertion of the distal pins, allowing direct control of the distal fragment.
- The wrist is placed for a lateral fluoroscopic view, and a marker is used to determine the level of incision halfway between the radiocarpal joint and the fracture. A short transverse skin incision is made just proximal to the radiocarpal joint.

- A longitudinal incision is then made through the retinaculum on either side of Lister's tubercle, and the EPL is protected.
- The first distal pin is drilled using power, parallel to the radiocarpal joint on the lateral view, halfway between the fracture and the joint surface (**TECH FIG 6A**).

TECHNIQUES

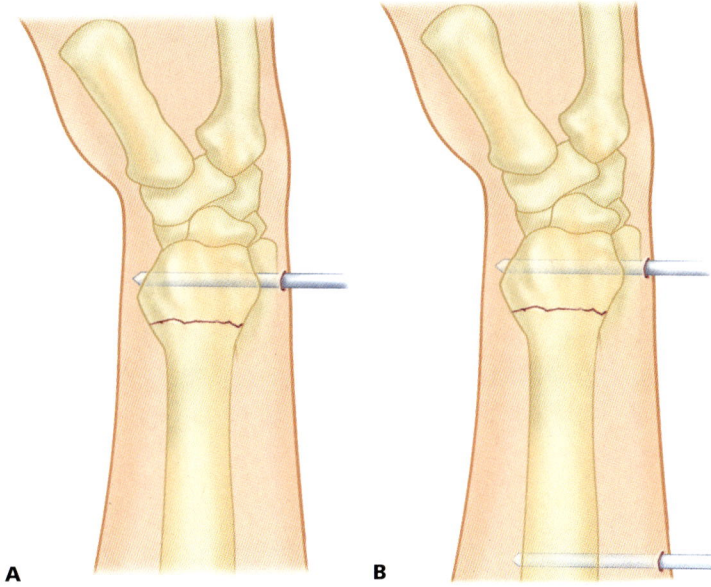

TECH FIG 6 • **A.** Distal pin placement. **B.** Final reduction with nonbridged external fixator in place.

- The second distal pin is placed between the second and third dorsal compartments, between the radial wrist extensors and the EPL tendon.
- This pin should be placed parallel to the first pin in both planes, with the starting point halfway between the radiocarpal joint and the fracture.
- The two proximal radius pins are placed using the technique described for placement of a bridging external fixator.

- The incisions are closed, after which the clamps are applied but not tightened.
- Reduction is achieved by manipulation of the distal pins and clamps.
  - Pushing the pins in the dorsal/volar plane corrects dorsal tilt.
  - Adjusting the pin clamp can correct radial inclination.
- Reduction is confirmed using fluoroscopy, and the clamps are tightened (**TECH FIG 6B**).

PEARLS AND PITFALLS

Indications	▪ Determine stability. ▪ Determine comminution and supplement fixation with external or internal fixation as necessary.
Surgical approach	▪ Make skin incisions for pin placement to avoid sensory nerves, tendons, and crossing veins. ▪ Obtain adequate exposure of the radial sensory branch at forearm and hand to avoid injury.
Hardware placement	▪ Choose pins of appropriate diameter. ▪ Supplement fixation with pins, using external or internal fixation as necessary. ▪ Do not leave pins more than 1 to 2 mm out of the cortex, and keep all pins extra-articular. ▪ If placing the proximal metacarpal pin in metaphyseal bone, ensure that three cortices are penetrated. ▪ Do not back out conical pins, because fixation will be lost. ▪ Evaluate the DRUJ after fixation to determine stability. ▪ Subcutaneous pins are more costly to remove, because that requires a second procedure, but they have a lower infection rate. Therefore, if fixation is needed for an extended period, bury the pins. ▪ Overdistraction of the carpus must be avoided, because it is associated with chronic pain–mediated syndromes and nonunion.
Postoperative management	▪ Allow for adequate immobilization. ▪ Encourage early range of motion of the fingers, elbow, and shoulder whenever possible. ▪ Educate the patient regarding appropriate pin care. ▪ Begin strengthening only after healing is complete and range of motion is maximized.

POSTOPERATIVE CARE

- After fixation with percutaneous pins, alone the wrist is immobilized in a short-arm splint to allow for swelling but provide stability. A cast is applied after the swelling goes down.
- Isolated radial styloid fractures fixed with pins can be placed in a volar wrist splint.

- External fixation devices typically require no additional immobilization, although a volar forearm–based Orthoplast (Johnson & Johnson, Langhorne, PA) splint may be used for support and patient comfort.
- The splint or cast is continued for 4 to 8 weeks, until healing occurs and the pins are removed.

- K-wires and half pins should be inspected and cleaned regularly using either soap and water or half-strength hydrogen peroxide and water.
- Finger, elbow, and shoulder range of motion are begun immediately, and wrist range of motion is begun as the fracture heals.

OUTCOMES

- A prospective randomized trial comparing percutaneous pinning and casting versus external fixation with augmentation (eg, pins, screws, bone graft) found no difference in clinical outcomes for fractures with minimal articular displacement.[9]
- In patients over 60 years of age, percutaneous pinning has been shown to provide only marginal radiographic improvement over cast immobilization alone, with no correlation with clinical outcome.[4]
- Ebraheim et al[5] reported excellent outcomes for restoration of radiographic parameters and functional outcomes with intrafocal pinning and trans-styloid augmentation.
- An evaluation of percutaneous pinning outcomes found the best results for metaphyseal fractures. Good results were found for intra-articular fractures. The worst results were seen in fractures with associated ulnar styloid fractures and fractures in elderly persons.[15]
- A retrospective review of radiographic and clinical outcomes of open reduction internal fixation (volar and dorsal) versus external fixation revealed no significant differences, except that palmar tilt was more effectively restored with dorsal plating.[22]
- A meta-analysis found no evidence for the use of internal fixation over external fixation for unstable distal radius fractures.[12]
- Women over 55 years of age with unstable intra-articular distal radius fractures treated with external fixation have a high rate of secondary displacement but can have acceptable functional outcomes.[10]
- Patients over the age of 55 years have better results with external fixation and pinning than with pinning alone. Younger patients with two or more sides having comminution also have better results with supplemental external fixation.[21]
- Nonbridging external fixation has been shown to maintain volar tilt and carpal alignment better than bridging external fixation while having significantly better function during the first year.[13]
- Nonbridging external fixation was shown to have no clinical advantage in patients over 60 years of age with moderately or severely displaced distal radius fractures.[3]
- A prospective, randomized comparison of bridging versus nonbridging external fixation revealed more complications in the nonbridging fixators and better outcomes in the bridged fixator group.[18]
- A prospective study compared unrepaired ulnar styloid fractures to those without ulnar styloid fractures and found no significant differences in clinical outcome. However, DRUJ instability was not evaluated.[19]

COMPLICATIONS

- Infection (pin tract or deep). Pin tract infections occur in 10% to 30% of patients.[8,9]
- Injury to tendons, vessels, and nerves due to percutaneous technique. Stiffness may result if tendons are inadvertently skewered, and the radial sensory branch can be injured.

- Loss of range of motion
- Posttraumatic arthritis
- Weakness in grip or pinch
- Tenosynovitis and tendon rupture
- Malunion or nonunion
- Compartment syndrome
- Carpal tunnel syndrome
- Hardware failure
- Nonunion (associated with overdistraction with an external fixator)
- Complex regional pain syndrome type I (associated with overdistraction with an external fixator)

REFERENCES

1. Agee JM. Distal radius fractures. Multiplanar ligamentotaxis. Hand Clin 1993;9:577–585.
2. Anderson JT, Lucas GL, Buhr BR. Complications of treating distal radius fractures with external fixation: a community experience. Iowa Orthop J 2004;24:53–59.
3. Atroshi I, Brogren E, Larsson GU, et al. Wrist-bridging versus non-bridging external fixation for displaced distal radius fractures: a randomized assessor-blind clinical trial of 38 patients followed for 1 year. Acta Orthop 2006;77:445–453.
4. Azzopardi T, Ehrendorfer S, Coulton T, et al. Unstable extra-articular fractures of the distal radius: a prospective, randomised study of immobilisation in a cast versus supplementary percutaneous pinning. J Bone Joint Surg Br 2005;87B:837–840.
5. Ebraheim NA, Ali SS, Gove NK. Fixation of unstable distal radius fractures with intrafocal pins and trans-styloid augmentation: a retrospective review and radiographic analysis. Am J Orthop 2006; 35:362–368.
6. Gupta A. The treatment of Colles' fracture. Immobilisation with the wrist dorsiflexed. J Bone Joint Surg Br 1991;73B:312–315.
7. Gupta R, Bozentka DJ, Bora FW. The evaluation of tension in an experimental model of external fixation of distal radius fractures. J Hand Surg Am 1999;24:108–112.
8. Hargreaves DG, Drew SJ, Eckersley R. Kirschner wire pin tract infection rates: A randomized controlled trial between percutaneous and buried wires. J Hand Surg Br 2004;29:374–376.
9. Harley BJ, Scharfenberger A, Beaupre LA, et al. Augmented external fixation versus percutaneous pinning and casting for unstable fractures of the distal radius—a prospective randomized trial. J Hand Surg Am 2004;29:815–824.
10. Hegeman JH, Oskam J, Vierhout PA, et al. External fixation for unstable intra-articular distal radial fractures in women older than 55 years. Acceptable functional end results in the majority of the patients despite significant secondary displacement. Injury 2005;36:339–344.
11. Katz MA, Beredjiklian PK, Bozentka DJ, et al. Computed tomography scanning of intra-articular distal radius fractures: does it influence treatment? J Hand Surg Am 2001;26:412–421.
12. Margaliot Z, Haase SC, Kotsis SV, et al. Meta-analysis of outcomes of external fixation versus plate osteosynthesis for unstable distal radius fractures. J Hand Surg Am 2005;30:1185–1199.
13. McQueen MM. Redisplaced unstable fractures of the distal radius. A randomised, prospective study of bridging versus nonbridging external fixation. J Bone Joint Surg Br 1998;80B:665–669.
14. Nana AD, Joshi A, Lichtman DM. Plating of the distal radius. J Am Acad Orthop Surg 2005;13:159–171.
15. Rosati M, Bertagnini S, Digrandi G, et al. Percutaneous pinning for fractures of the distal radius. Acta Orthop Belg 2006;72:138–146.
16. Short WH, Palmer AK, Werner FW, et al. A biomechanical study of distal radial fractures. J Hand Surg Am 1987;12:529–534.
17. Simic PM, Weiland AJ. Fractures of the distal aspect of the radius: changes in treatment over the past two decades. J Bone Joint Surg Am 2003;85A:552–564.
18. Sommerkamp TG, Seeman M, Silliman J, et al. Dynamic external fixation of unstable fractures of the distal part of the radius. A prospective, randomized comparison with static external fixation. J Bone Joint Surg Am 1994;76A:1149–1161.

19. Souer S, Ring D, Matschke S, et al. Effect of an unrepaired fracture of the ulnar styloid base on outcome after plate and screw fixation of a distal radius fracture. J Bone Joint Surg Am 2009;91:830–838.

20. Trumble TE, Schmitt SR, Vedder NB. Factors affecting functional outcome of displaced intra-articular distal radius fractures. J Hand Surg Am 1994;19:325–340.

21. Trumble TE, Wagner W, Hanel DP, et al. Intrafocal (Kapandji) pinning of distal radius fractures with and without external fixation. J Hand Surg Am 1998;23:381–394.

22. Westphal T, Piatek S, Schubert S, et al. Outcome after surgery of distal radius fractures: no differences between external fixation and ORIF. Arch Orthop Trauma Surg 2005;125:507–514.

Chapter 9

Arthroscopic Reduction and Fixation of Distal Radius and Ulnar Styloid Fractures

William B. Geissler

DEFINITION

- A bimodal age distribution exists for patients with distal radius fractures (ie, young adults vs elderly persons), and they frequently have a different mechanism of injury.
- Patients 65 years of age or older have an annual incidence of 8 to 10 fractures of the distal radius per 1000 person-years.
  - The incidence is seven times higher in women than in men.
  - Sixteen percent of white women and 23% of white men will sustain a fracture of the distal radius after the age of 50 years.
- Fractures of the distal radius are one of the most common skeletal injuries treated by orthopaedic surgeons.
- These injuries account for one-sixth of all fractures that are evaluated in the Emergency Department.
- Displaced intra-articular fractures of the distal radius are a unique subset of radius fractures.[18]
  - These fractures are a high-energy injury.
  - This high-energy injury results in comminuted fracture patterns.
  - These fractures are less amenable to traditional closed manipulation and casting.
- The prognosis for these fractures depends on the amount of residual radius shortening, both radiocarpal and radioulnar articular congruity, and associated soft tissue injuries.[22,24]

ANATOMY

- The distal radius serves as a plateau to support the carpus.
- The distal radius has three concave articular surfaces: the scaphoid fossa, the lunate fossa, and the sigmoid notch.
- The distal articular surface of the radius has a radial inclination averaging 22 degrees and palmar tilt averaging 11 degrees.
- Radial-based volar and dorsal ligaments arise from the distal radius to support the wrist.
- The sigmoid notch of the distal radius articulates with the ulnar head about which it rotates.
  - The distal radioulnar joint (DRUJ) is primarily stabilized by the triangular fibrocartilage complex (TFCC).
- The sigmoid notch angles distally and medially at an average of 22 degrees.

PATHOGENESIS

- The biomechanical characteristics of each fracture type depend on the mechanism of injury.
- Fernandez and Geissler[4] developed a classification based on the mechanism of injury. They noted that the associated ligamentous lesions, subluxations, and associated carpal fractures are related directly to the degree of energy absorbed by the distal radius.

- Type I fractures are bending fractures of the metaphysis in which one cortex fails to tensile stress and the opposite one undergoes a certain degree of comminution (eg, extra-articular Smith or Colles' fractures).
- Type II fractures are shearing fractures of the joint surface (eg, radial styloid fractures, Barton's fracture).
- Type III fractures are compression fractures of the joint surface with impaction of the subcondral and metaphyseal cancellous bone (ie, intra-articular comminuted fractures).
- Type IV fractures are avulsion fractures of ligamentous attachments, including radial styloid and ulnar styloid fractures, and are associated with radiocarpal fracture-dislocations.
- Type V fractures are high-energy injuries that involve a combination of bending, compression, shearing, and avulsion mechanisms or bone loss.
- Several studies have shown that a high incidence of associated soft tissue injuries is seen with displaced intra-articular distal radius fractures.[9,11–13,17,19,20]
  - Arthroscopic studies demonstrate a high incidence of injury to the triangular fibrocartilage complex, followed by the scapholunate interosseous ligament, and then the lunotriquetral interosseous ligament (which is the least injured).
  - A spectrum of injury occurs to the interosseous ligament in which it attenuates and eventually tears and the degree of rotation between the carpal bones increases.
  - Geissler et al defined an arthroscopic classification of interosseous ligament tears that helps define the degree of ligament injury and secondary instability as well as proposes treatment (Table 1; see also Chap. HA-41).

NATURAL HISTORY

- Intra-articular fractures of the distal radius have two pathologies: the associated global injury to the soft tissues and the injury to the bone itself.
- The natural history for an intra-articular fracture of the distal radius depends on restoration of anatomy as well as detection and management of any associated soft tissue injuries.[1,4]
- Knirk and Jupiter[13] documented the importance of articular restoration over extra-articular orientation in predicting outcomes for fractures of the distal radius.
  - They showed solid evidence that the largest tolerable articular step-off is 2 mm.
  - They demonstrate that the better the restoration of the articular surface, the better the outcome.
- A loss in radius length of 2.5 mm will shift the normal load transmitted across the ulna from 20% to 42%, which may lead to various stages of ulnar impaction syndrome.

Table 1	Geissler Arthroscopic Classification of Carpal Instability		
Grade	**Definition**	**Arthroscopic Findings**	**Management**
I	Attenuation/hemorrhage of interosseous ligament as seen from the radiocarpal joint. No incongruency of carpal alignment in the midcarpal space.	There is a loss of the normal concave appearance between the carpal bones, and the interosseous ligament attenuates and becomes convex as seen from the radiocarpal space. In midcarpal space, the interval between the carpal bones will still be tight and congruent, with no step-off.	Immobilization
II	Attenuation/hemorrhage of the interosseous ligament as seen from the radiocarpal joint. Incongruency/step-off as seen from the midcarpal space. A slight gap between the carpal bones may be present.	A slight gap (less than the width of a probe) between the carpal bones may be present. The interosseous ligament continues to become attenuated and is convex as seen from the radial carpal space. In the midcarpal space, the interval between the involved carpal bones is no longer congruent, and a step-off is present. In scapholunate instability, palmar flexion of the dorsal lip of the scaphoid will be seen as compared to the lunate. In lunotriquetral instability, increased translation between the triquetrum and lunate will be seen when palpated with a probe.	Arthroscopic reduction and pinning
III	Incongruency/step-off of carpal alignment is seen in both the radiocarpal and midcarpal spaces.	The interosseous ligament has started to tear, usually from volar to dorsal, and a gap is seen between the carpal bones in the radiocarpal space. A probe often is helpful to separate the involved carpal bones in the radiocarpal space. In the midcarpal space, a 2-mm probe may be placed between the carpal bones and twisted.	Arthroscopic/open reduction and pinning
IV	Incongruency/step-off of carpal alignment is seen in both the radiocarpal and midcarpal spaces. Gross instability with manipulation is noted.	A 2.7-mm arthroscope may be passed through the gap between the carpal bones. The interosseous ligament is completely detached between the involved carpal bones. This is the "drive-through" sign, when the arthroscope may be freely passed from the radiocarpal space through the tear to the midcarpal space.	Open reduction and repair

- Untreated complete tears of the scapholunate interosseous ligament, which are highly associated with radial styloid fractures, may progress to a wrist with scapholunate advanced collapse.

PATIENT HISTORY AND PHYSICAL FINDINGS

- A thorough history should be obtained, including the circumstances surrounding the injury as well as any additional injuries.
    - Neurologic basis
    - Cardiac basis
    - Patients' level of independence, dominant hand, status with assisted devices, work, activity level, and support structure should be determined.
- Physical examination, while concentrating on the wrist, should also include the hand, elbow, and shoulder to check for concomitant injuries.
    - The hand, wrist, arm, and shoulder must be carefully inspected for open injury so that tetanus and antibiotic prophylaxis may be initiated if necessary.
    - Thorough distal sensory and motor function examination should be carried out in an organized manner.
    - Vascular examination should include palpation of both the radial and ulnar pulses and determination of capillary refill time.
    - Precise palpation is used to define areas of potential trauma.

- Diminished sensibility, pallor, altered capillary refill, increased tenseness of the soft tissues, and pain out of proportion should raise suspicion for significant soft tissue injury, including compartment syndrome.

IMAGING AND OTHER DIAGNOSTIC STUDIES

- Posteroanterior (PA), oblique, and lateral radiographs are the primary radiographic workup for distal radius fractures.
    - Contralateral radiographs of the uninvolved extremity are useful to compare radial inclination, ulnar variance, and sigmoid notch anatomy.
    - PA projections are useful to evaluate the radial inclination, radius height, presence of ulnar styloid fractures, widening of the DRUJ, widening of intracarpal spaces, and intra-articular involvement (**FIG 1A**).
        - Standard radiographic parameters of the distal radius include radial inclination of 23 degrees (range 13–30), radius length of 12 mm (range 8–18 mm), and volar tilt of 12 degrees (range 1–21 degrees).
        - Ulnar variance should be measured with the shoulder in 90 degrees of abduction, the elbow at 90 degrees of flexion, and the wrist in neutral pronation-supination.
    - A lateral projection is used to assess volar and dorsal tilt of the distal fragment, dislocation or subluxation of the DRUJ or carpus, lunate angulation, and dorsal comminution (**FIG 1B**).

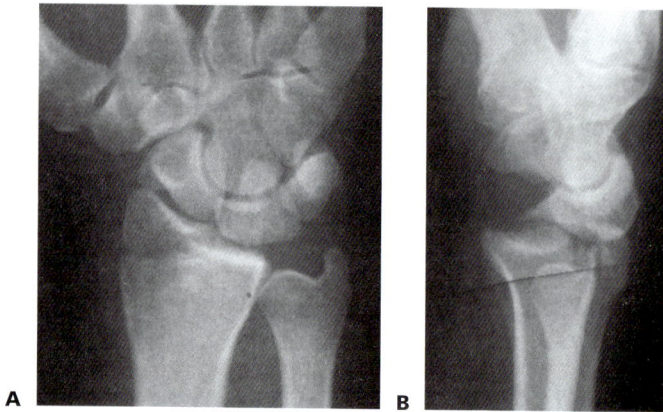

FIG 1 • **A.** PA radiographic view showing a minimally displaced radial styloid fracture fragment. **B.** The lateral view shows a complete fracture-dislocation of the wrist.

■ A modified lateral radiograph with the beam angulating 10 to 30 degrees proximally improves visualization of the articular surface and evaluation of the volar rim of the lunate facet represented by the anterior teardrop.

■ An additional 30-degree anteroposterior (AP) cephalic projection is useful to evaluate the dorsal ulnar margin of the distal radius.

■ Oblique radiographs are very helpful, because major fracture fragments may be rotated out of their anatomic planes.

■ CT evaluation, particularly three-dimensional CT, can further delineate fragment location, joint compression, and rotation.

■ MRI evaluation is useful in assessing for associated soft tissue injuries such as TFCC tears, interosseous ligament injuries, and carpal fractures.

■ Radiographic signs that demonstrate that the distal radius fracture is likely unstable and closed reduction would be insufficient include[15]:

■ Lateral tilt greater than 20 degrees dorsal
■ Dorsal comminution greater than 50% of the width
■ Initial fragment displacement greater than 1 cm
■ Volar translation greater than 2 mm
■ Initial radius shortening more than 5 mm
■ Intra-articular step-off greater than 2 mm
■ Associated ulna fracture
■ Severe osteoporosis.
■ Age greater than 60 years

DIFFERENTIAL DIAGNOSIS

■ Carpal bone fracture
■ Metacarpal or phalangeal fracture
■ DRUJ disruption
■ Essex-Lopresti lesion
■ Interosseous ligament tear
■ Carpal dislocation (perilunate)

NONOPERATIVE MANAGEMENT

■ Displaced fractures of the distal radius are reduced using an adequate anesthetic agent.

■ Knowledge of the mechanisms of injury helps facilitate manual reduction. Force is applied opposite the force that caused the fracture.
■ Gentle traction is necessary to disimpact the fracture fragments, followed by palmar translation of the hand and carpus in respect to the radius.
■ The radius articular surface will rotate around the intact volar cortical lip to restore volar inclination with palmar translation.
■ Care must be taken to avoid trauma to the skin during the reduction maneuver, particularly in elderly patients where the skin may be fragile.
■ A splint is supplied following the reduction. No consensus has been established regarding wrist or forearm position, long-arm versus short-arm immobilization, or splint versus cast.
■ Extreme positions of wrist flexion and ulnar deviation should be avoided.
■ Postreduction radiographs are taken in plaster.
■ Depending on stability of the fracture, most patients treated nonoperatively require weekly visits for the first 3 weeks to monitor fracture reduction.
■ In patients older than 65 years, one third of initially undisplaced fractures subsequently collapsed to some degree.
■ One study of elderly patients with moderately displaced fractures of the distal radius found that two thirds of the correction obtained by closed manipulation was lost at 5 weeks.
■ Patients with minimally displaced or nondisplaced fractures of the distal radius treated nonoperatively must be made aware of possible complications, including rupture of the extensor pollicis longus tendon, carpal tunnel syndrome, and compartment syndrome.

SURGICAL MANAGEMENT

■ Distal radius fractures without extensive metaphyseal comminution are ideal candidates for arthroscopic-assisted fixation with K-wires or cannulated screws.[7,8]
■ Radial styloid fractures
■ Impacted fractures
■ Die punch fractures
■ Three-part T-type fractures and four-part fractures with metaphyseal comminution are best treated with a combination of volar plate stabilization. Wrist arthroscopy is used as an adjunct to fine-tune the articular reduction and evaluate for associated soft tissue lesions.
■ Distal radius fractures that may be minimally displaced, and fractures with strongly suspected associated soft tissue injury, also are candidates for arthroscopic-assisted fixation to stabilize the fracture but, more importantly, to evaluate and treat the acute associated soft tissue injury.
■ Stabilization of associated ulnar styloid fragments is controversial.[13] Wrist arthroscopy provides a rationale as to when to stabilize an ulnar styloid fragment.

Preoperative Planning

■ All radiographic studies are reviewed.
■ Equipment needed for arthroscopic treatment and for open stabilization is made available.
■ Small joint instrumentation is essential for arthroscopic-assisted fixation of distal radius fractures. The small joint arthroscope is approximately 2.7 mm in diameter, and even

smaller scopes may be used if desired. In addition, a small joint shaver (3.5 mm or less) is useful to clear fracture debris and hematoma.

- The ideal timing for arthroscopic-assisted fixation of distal radius fractures is 3 to 10 days following injury.[6]
  - Earlier attempts at fixation may be complicated by soft tissue swelling and troublesome bleeding, obscuring visualization.
  - After 10 days, the fracture fragments start to become sticky and more difficult to percutaneously elevate and reduce.

Positioning

- Arthroscopic-assisted fixation of distal radius fractures may be performed with the arm suspended vertically in a traction tower, horizontally in a traction tower, or with finger traps applied attached to weights hanging over the edge of the hand table.
  - Wrist arthroscopy in the horizontal position may make it easier to simultaneously monitor the reduction fluoroscopically and place hardware. However, it does not allow for simultaneous volar access to the wrist.
  - Suspending the wrist in a vertical position with a traction tower allows simultaneous access to both the volar and dorsal aspects of the wrist. This is particularly useful when wrist arthroscopy is used as an adjunct to volar plate fixation of the distal radius fracture.
- A new traction tower has been designed to allow simultaneous evaluatation of the intra-articular reduction of the distal radius arthroscopically and fluoroscopically (**FIG 2A**).
  - The surgeon may stabilize a comminuted fracture of the distal radius with a plate and simultaneously evaluate the articular reduction arthroscopically.
  - The traction tower allows for traction of the wrist in either the vertical or horizontal planes, depending on the surgeon's preference (**FIG 2B**).

Approach

- The wrist is suspended in a traction tower, and the standard dorsal 3/4 viewing portal, 4/5 or 6R working portal, and 6U inflow portal are made.

- It is difficult to palpate the normal extensor tendon landmarks for traditional wrist arthroscopy in patients who sustain a fracture of the distal radius because of swelling.[10] However, the bony landmarks usually can still be palpated. These bony landmarks include the bases of the metacarpals, the dorsal lip of the radius, and the ulnar head.
- The 3/4 portal is made in line with the radial border of the long finger. It is very useful to place a no. 18 needle into the proposed location of the 3/4 portal before making a skin incision.
  - If the portal is placed too proximal, the arthroscope may be placed within the fracture pattern itself. If it is placed too distal, it can injure the articular surface of the carpus.
- Once the precise ideal location of the portal is located, the portal is made by pulling the skin with the sugeon's thumb against the tip of a no. 11 blade. Blunt dissection is carried down with a hemostat, and the arthroscope, with a blunt trocar, is introduced into the dorsal 3/4 portal.
  - This technique decreases potential injury to cutaneous nerves.
- Thorough irrigation of the joint is necessary to wash out fracture hematoma and debris and improve visualization. Inflow may be provided through the arthroscope cannula or separately through a no. 14 needle into the 6U portal.
  - Use of a separate 6U inflow portal is recommended. The small-joint arthroscopy cannula does not allow as much space between the cannula and the arthroscope, limiting the amount of flow through the cannula.
  - Outflow to the wrist is provided through intervenous extension tubing connected to the arthroscope cannula.
- The 4/5 working portal is made in line with the mid-axis of the ring metacarpal. Alternatively, the 6R working portal is made just radial to the palpable extensor carpi ulnaris tendon.
  - A no. 18 needle is placed into the joint and should lie just distal to the articular disc.
  - A 4/5 or 6R portal usually is located just proximal to the 3/4 portal because of the natural radial slope of the distal radius.

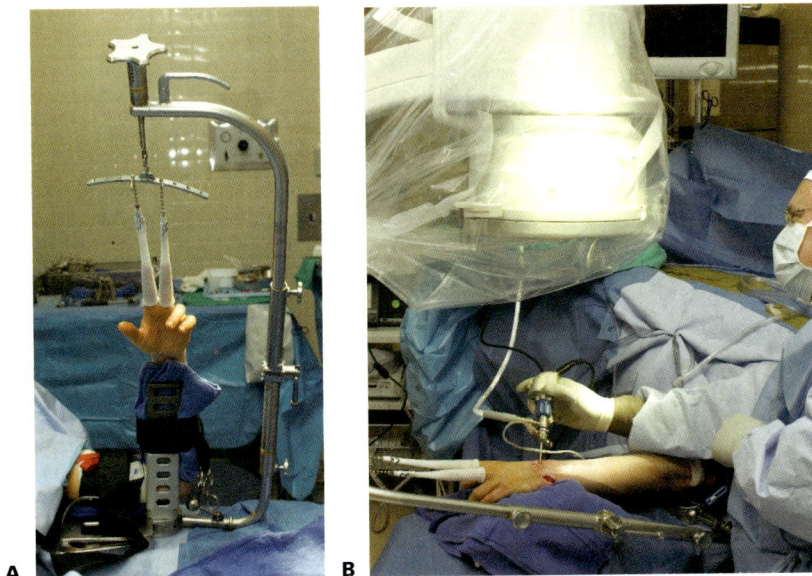

FIG 2 • **A.** This traction tower (Acumed, Hillsboro, OR) uses a suspension bar at the side rather than at the center of the wrist. This allows easy fluoroscopic evaluation of the fracture reduction, with simultaneous full access to the volar and dorsal aspects of the wrist. **B.** The tower can be flexed into a horizontal position for surgeons who prefer to treat distal radius fractures in that position.

RADIAL STYLOID FRACTURES

- An isolated fracture of the radial styloid is an ideal fracture pattern to manage arthroscopically, especially for the surgeon beginning to gain experience in arthroscope-assisted fixation of distal radius fractures.

- In addition, radial styloid fractures have a high incidence of associated injury to the scapholunate interosseous ligament, which is best assessed arthroscopically.

- Insert one or two guidewires from a cannulated screw system percutaneously into the radial styloid—not across the fracture site—using a wire driver in oscillation mode.

  - Evaluate the position of the wires under fluoroscopy to ensure they are centered in the radial styloid fragment.

- Suspend the wrist in a traction tower and establish the standard arthroscopic portals.

- Insert the scope in the dorsal 3/4 portal and clear the joint of debris and hematoma.

- Transfer the arthroscope to the 6R or 4/5 portal to look across the wrist and effectively judge rotation and reduction of the radial styloid fragment.

- Using the previously placed guidewires as joysticks, manipulate and anatomically reduce the fracture fragment under direct arthroscopic observation.

  - A trocar can be inserted through the 3/4 portal to help further guide the reduction of the radial styloid fragment (**TECH FIG 1A,B**).

- Once the fracture is judged to be absolutely anatomic, the guidewires are advanced across the fracture site into the radius shaft and evaluated under fluoroscopy (**TECH FIG 1C**).

  - In many cases, the fracture reduction may look anatomic under fluoroscopy, but when viewed arthroscopically, the radial styloid fragment is seen to be slightly rotated.[3]

- Guidewires alone can be used to stabilize the fracture, but cannulated screws (with or without heads) are recommended (**TECH FIG 1D,E**).

  - Cannulated screws decrease soft tissue irritation and potential pin track infection as compared with K-wires.

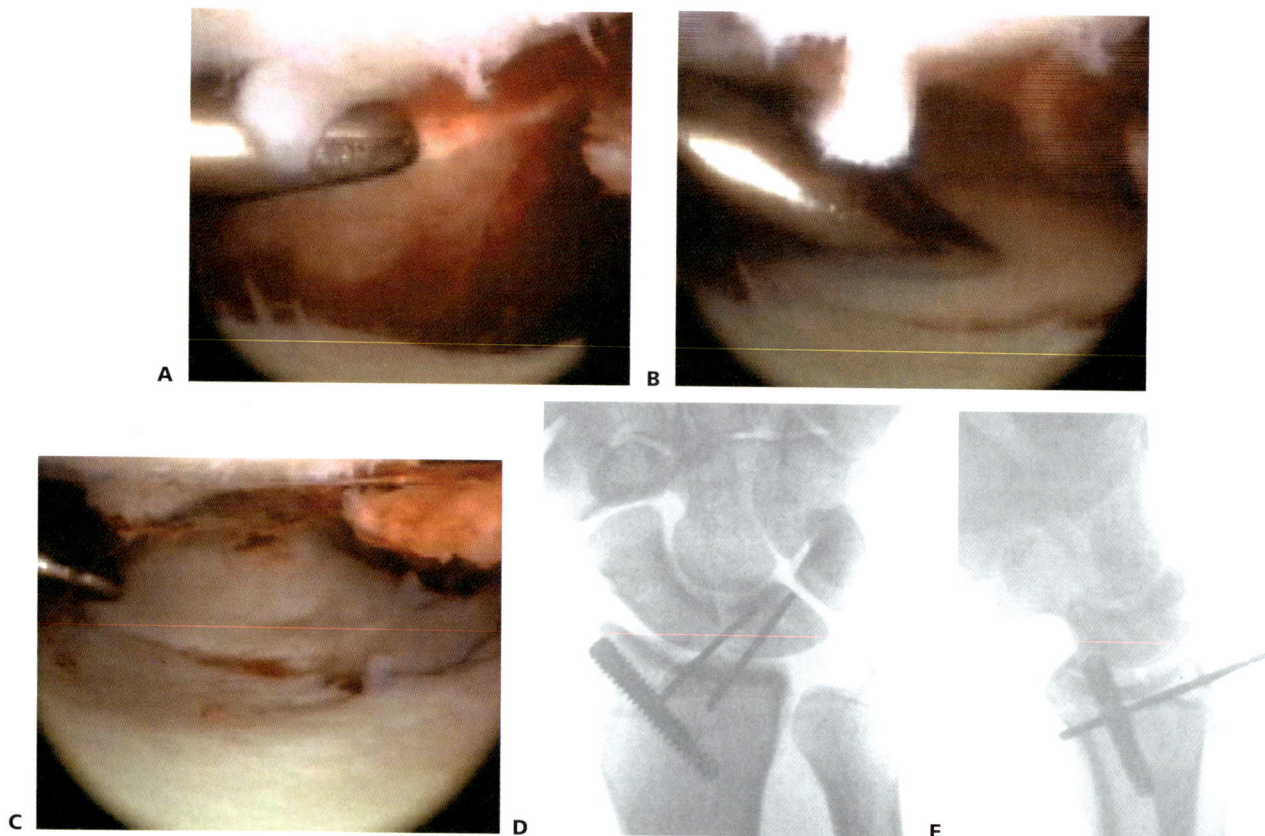

TECH FIG 1 • A. Arthroscopic view of the patient whose radiographs are seen in Figure 1. The arthroscope is in the 6R portal looking across the wrist, and a blunt trochar is in the 3/4 portal. The displaced radial styloid fragment is well visualized. **B.** A combination of joysticks inserted into the radial styloid fragment and a trochar inserted into the 3/4 portal allows anatomic reduction of the displaced radial styloid fragment and radiocarpal joint. **C.** The radial styloid fragment is anatomically reduced (with no residual rotation) and stabilized. **D.** PA view demonstrating anatomic reduction to the radial styloid fragment. Headless cannulated screws are used, if possible, to avoid soft tissue irritation. **E.** Lateral view showing anatomic restoration to the radial styloid fragment and restoration of the carpus in line with the radius.

THREE-PART FRACTURES

- Three-part fractures that involve a displaced fracture of the radial styloid and a lunate facet fragment without metaphyseal communtion are ideal for arthroscopic-assisted reduction (**TECH FIG 2A,B**).
- Reduce and provisionally stabilize the radial styloid fragment with guidewires under fluoroscopic guidance.
  - The radial styloid serves as a landmark to which the depressed lunate facet fragment is reduced.
- Suspend the wrist in the traction tower, establish portals, and evacuate the fracture debris and hematoma.
  - The depressed lunate facet fragment is best seen with the arthroscope in the 3/4 portal (**TECH FIG 2C,D**).
- Percutaneously place a no. 18 needle directly over the depressed fragment as viewed arthroscopically.
- Insert a large K-wire about 2 cm proximal to the previously placed no. 18 needle to percutaneously elevate the depressed lunate facet fragment.

- Use a bone tenaculum to further diminish the gap between the radial styloid and lunate facet fragments.
- Place guidewires transversely under the subchondral surface of the radius from the radial styloid into the anatomically reduced lunate facet fragment.
  - It is important to pronate and supinate the wrist following placement of the transverse pins to ensure the guidewires have not violated the DRUJ. The concave nature of the DRUJ makes radiographic assessment difficult.
- Consider insertion of bone graft to support the reduced lunate fragment and avoid late settling.
  - Make a small incision between the fourth and fifth dorsal compartments.
  - Use cancellous allograft bone chips or bone substitutes.
- If feasible, place headless cannulated screws to stabilize both the radial styloid and the impacted lunate facet fragments (**TECH FIG 2E–H**).

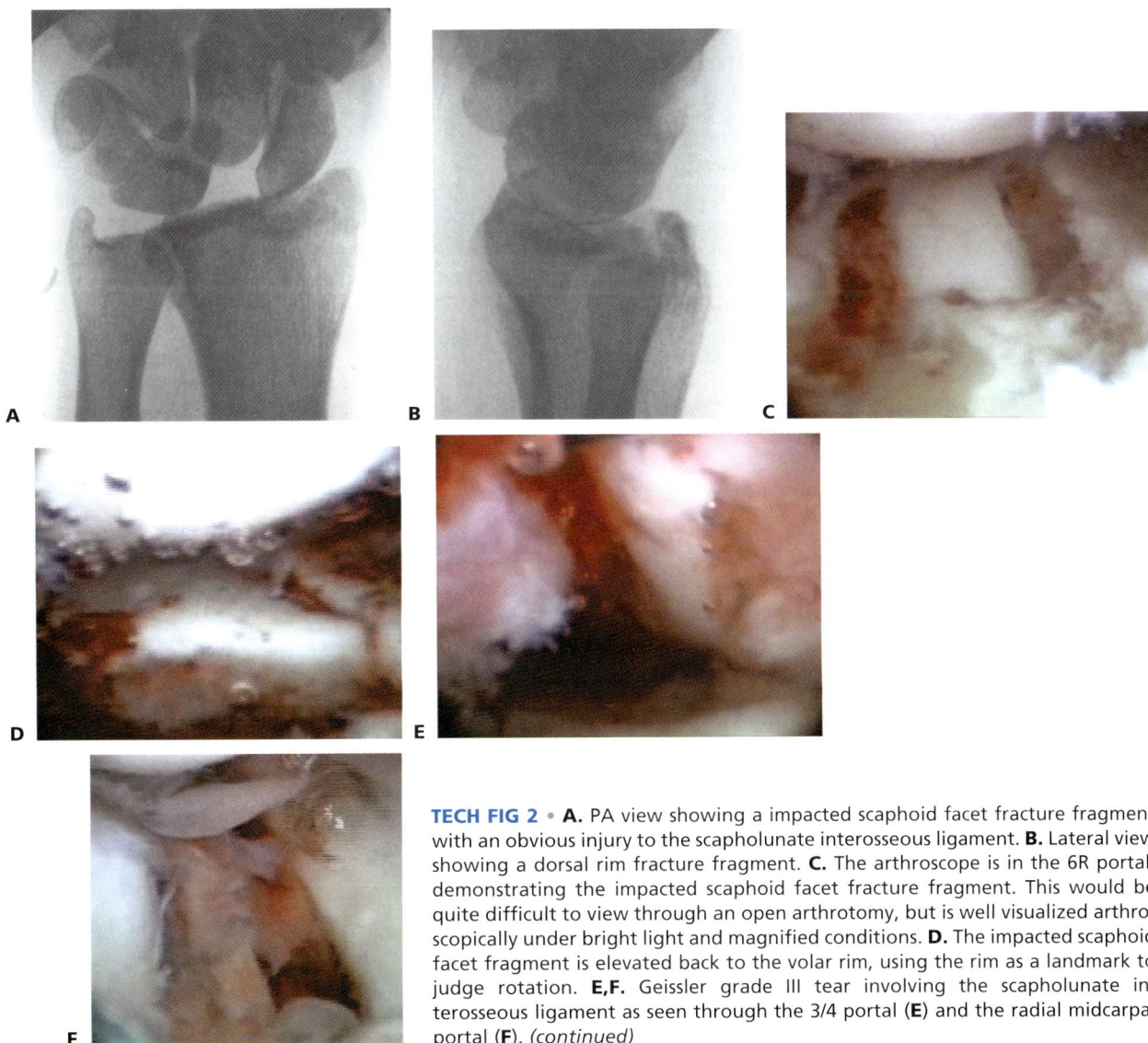

TECH FIG 2 • A. PA view showing a impacted scaphoid facet fracture fragment with an obvious injury to the scapholunate interosseous ligament. **B.** Lateral view showing a dorsal rim fracture fragment. **C.** The arthroscope is in the 6R portal, demonstrating the impacted scaphoid facet fracture fragment. This would be quite difficult to view through an open arthrotomy, but is well visualized arthroscopically under bright light and magnified conditions. **D.** The impacted scaphoid facet fragment is elevated back to the volar rim, using the rim as a landmark to judge rotation. **E,F.** Geissler grade III tear involving the scapholunate interosseous ligament as seen through the 3/4 portal (**E**) and the radial midcarpal portal (**F**). *(continued)*

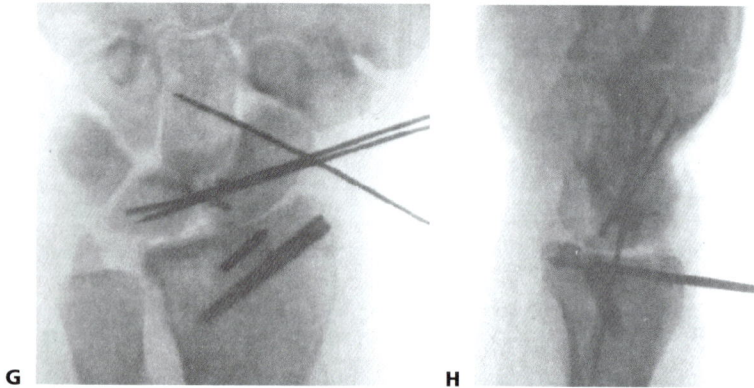

G   **H**

TECH FIG 2 • *(continued)* **G,H.** PA and lateral radiographs showing anatomic reduction to the impacted scaphoid facet fracture. (The tear of the scapholunate interosseous ligament also was acutely repaired.)

THREE- AND FOUR-PART FRACTURES WITH METAPHYSEAL COMMINUTION

- A combination of open surgery, using a volar plate for stability, and arthroscopy, as an adjunct to assist the articular reduction, is used if metaphyseal comminution is present (**TECH FIG 3**).
- Volar plate stabilization is very stable and allows for early range of motion and rehabilitation as compared to K-wires or headless screws alone.

Open Reduction and Stabilization

- Perform a standard volar approach and do not open the radiocarpal joint capsule (**TECH FIG 4A**).
- The radial styloid fragment and the volar ulnar fragment are reduced to the shaft under direct visualization. The radial styloid fragment is provisionally pinned.
- Apply a volar distal radius locking plate to stabilize the volar bone fragments (**TECH FIG 4B**).
  - Place a screw in the proximal portion of the plate first, to reduce the plate to the shaft.

- Provisionally pin the distal fragments through the plate.
- Manipulate the articular fragments under fluoroscopy to obtain as anatomic a reduction as possible (**TECH FIG 4C,D**).
- Suspend the wrist in the traction tower and reduce the articular fragments arthroscopically (**TECH FIG 4E,F**).
  - If articular reduction is not anatomic, remove the pins and fine-tune the reduction.
- Once the fracture reduction is thought to be anatomic, place the distal screws through the plate (**TECH FIG 4G–I**).
  - It is important that the fracture be reduced to the plate, with no gap between the plate and the bone. This can be achieved by flexion of the wrist in the tower and by insertion of a non-locking screw first, before the insertion of standard locking screws.
- Place the remaining proximal and distal screws if the reduction is anatomic under both fluoroscopy and arthroscopy.

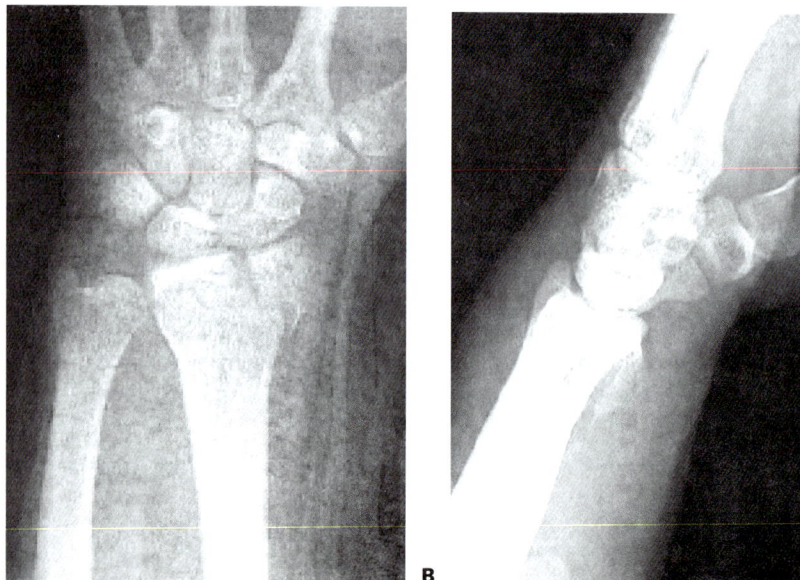

A   **B**

TECH FIG 3 • **A.** The PA radiograph shows a displaced fracture of the radial styloid. **B.** This lateral radiograph shows metaphyseal comminution associated with the displaced radial styloid fragment. Because of the metaphyseal comminution, it was decided to stabilize the fracture using a volar plate.

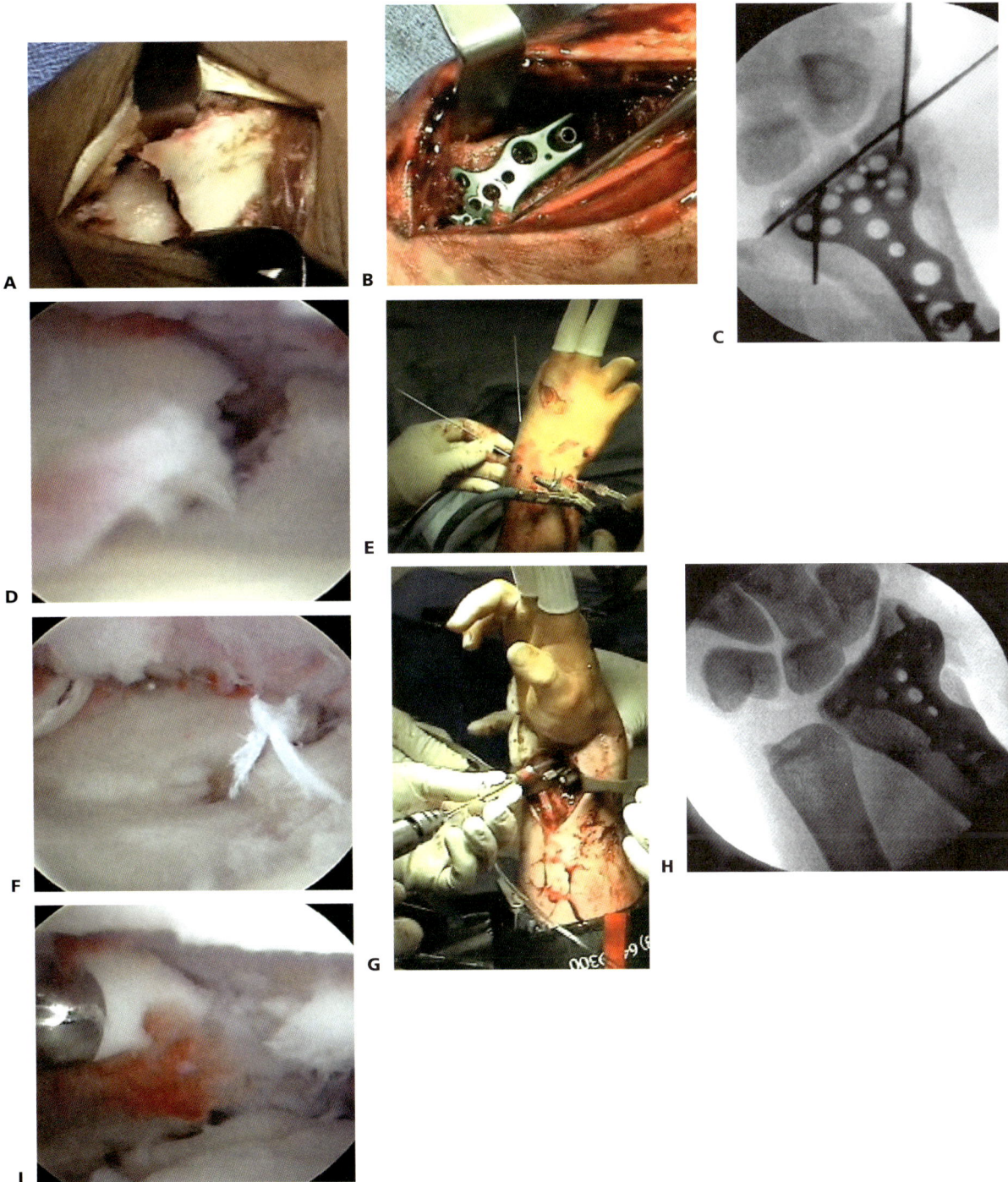

TECH FIG 4 • A. A standard volar approach is made, centered over the flexor carpi radialis tendon, and the fracture site is exposed. **B.** A volar distal radius locking plate (Acumed, Hillsboro, OR) is applied. The initial screw is placed through the proximal plate to secure the plate to the shaft. **C.** The intra-articular reduction is viewed under fluoroscopy and provisionally pinned. A displaced intra-articular fracture fragment can still be identified. **D.** The arthroscope is in the 3/4 portal, showing the volar capsule blocking reduction of the radial styloid fragment. **E.** Joysticks previously inserted into the radial styloid fragment are then used to control and anatomically reduce the radial styloid fragment. **F.** The arthroscope is in the 6R portal looking across the wrist. Anatomic reduction of the radial styloid fragment is documented. **G.** Once the anatomic restoration of the articular surface is evaluated both arthroscopically and fluoroscopically, the distal screws are placed in the plate. **H.** Fluoroscopic view showing anatomic restoration to the articular surface of the distal radius. **I.** The patient had an associated osteochondral fracture of the lunate, not visible on plain radiographs. The displaced fragment is arthroscopically removed.

TECHNIQUES

Reduction and Stabilization of a Dorsal Die Punch Fragment

- It is not possible to see the reduction of a dorsal die punch fragment through the volar approach when stabilized with a plate. Arthroscopy can be helpful in this scenario.
- Insert the volar plate as previously described and provisionally fix the device to the radius.
  - Frequently, the dorsal fragment may still be slightly proximal in relation to the radial shaft.

- The dorsal die punch fragment is best seen with the arthroscope in the 6R portal.
- Establish the volar radial portal between the radioscaphocapitate ligament and the long radiolunate ligment, as viewed directly through the previous performed volar approach.[16]
- Percutaneously elevate and anatomically reduce the dorsal die punch fragment as viewed arthroscopically.
- Once this has been achieved, place the screws into the plate and observe their path arthroscopically to ensure adequate stabilization of the dorsal die punch fragment.

ULNAR STYLOID FRACTURES

- Following anatomic reduction of the distal radius fracture, insert the arthroscope in the dorsal 3/4 portal and the probe in the 6R portal. Palpate the tension of the articular disc.
  - Good tension indicates that the majority of the peripheral TFCC fibers are intact or still attached to the proximal ulna.
  - A peripheral tear of the articular disc is repaired arthroscopically when detected.[21]
- Stabilization of a large ulnar styloid fragment is considered when the articular disc is lax by palpation and no peripheral TFCC is identified (**TECH FIG 5**).
  - In this instance, the majority of the fibers of the TFCC are attached to the displaced ulnar styloid fragment.
- Make a small incision between the extensor carpi ulnaris and the flexor carpi ulnaris tendons and identify the fracture site.
- Retrieve the distal fragment, which often displaces in a distal and radial direction.
- Mobilize the styloid fragment using a no. 15 blade, taking care to protect the TFCC insertion.
- Reduce the fragment anatomically, under direct visualization, and insert a guidewire in a retrograde manner for provisional stability.
- Stabilize the ulnar styloid fragment using either a tension band technique (with wire and two K-wires) or, preferably, using a micro headless cannulated screw.

- Place the cannulated headless screw over the guidewire and verify fracture reduction with fluoroscopy.
- Insert the arthroscope into the 3/4 portal and the probe into the 6R portal to document restoration of TFCC tension.

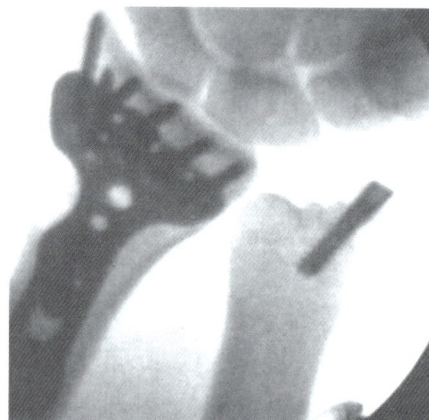

TECH FIG 5 • In this case, following reduction to the distal radius fracture, the articular disc was palpated and found to be lax but with no peripheral tear. The large ulnar styloid fragment was reduced with a micro Acutrak screw (Acumed, Hillsboro, OR).

PEARLS AND PITFALLS

Timing of reduction	■ Arthroscopically assisted reduction of distal radius fractures is most ideal between 3 and 10 days following injury. Assisted fixation before 3 days usually is complicated by bleeding that can obscure visualization. Percutaneous fracture reduction more than 10 days after the injury is exceedingly difficult and often unsuccessful.
Arthroscopic visualization	■ It is important to take the time to thoroughly irrigate and débride the joint of hematoma and debris. This especially helps visualization of fragment rotation. Irrigation through a separte 6U inflow portal is helpful. A Coban wrap (3M, St. Paul, MN) may be wrapped around the forearm to limit fluid extravasation into the soft tissues.
Instrumentation	■ Large-joint instrumentation will damage the articular cartilage and is not appropriate. A mobile traction tower is extremely helpful in arthroscopic-assisted management of distal radius fractures.
Fixation	■ Do not substitute poor fixation for an arthroscopically assisted procedure. Fixation should be chosen to fit the personality of the fracture. For example, K-wires should not be used to stabilize a volar Barton's fracture when volar plate stabilization is the obvious choice. While K-wires are easy to insert, they hinder rehabilitation and have the potential for pin track infections.

	■ Cannulated screws are recommended when arthroscopically stabilizing a fracture of the distal radius without metaphyseal comminution. ■ Volar plate fixation is recommended when metaphyseal comminution is present. ■ Arthroscopic evaluation of the wrist while the distal screws are being placed offers the advantage of seeing the screws penetrate into the fracture fragments, thereby ensuring stability. Arthroscopic evaluation is helpful in variable-angle volar locking plates to ensure the screws do not violate the joint.
Observation	■ It is imperative following arthroscopically assisted reduction of the distal radius in the radiocarpal space to evaluate the midcarpal space. The midcarpal space is the most sensitive and ideal location to evaluate intercarpal stability. In addition, loose bodies from the capitate or hamate occasionally are seen, particularly in association with lunate die punch fractures. Arthroscopic evaluation also aids in determining when to fix the ulnar styloid.

POSTOPERATIVE CARE

■ The degree of postoperative immobilization depends on numerous factors, including the mode of fracture stabilization, the quality of the bone for internal fixation, the stability of the fixation, and the management of any associated soft tissue injuries that were addressed during the arthroscopic evaluation.
■ Immediate range of motion of the digits and wrist is initiated in patients with volar plate fixation with good bone stock and solid fixation.
■ In patients with soft osteopenic bone with volar plate fixation, digital range of motion exercises are initiated immediately, but wrist range of motion is delayed approximately 3 to 4 weeks to permit some fracture healing.
  ■ Soft bone may collapse around the rigid plate.
■ In patients without metaphyseal comminution treated by arthroscopically assisted stabilization with cannulated screws, range of motion is initiated as the patient tolerates.
■ In patients treated with percutaneous K-wires, the wrist is immobilized until the wires are removed, usually 4 to 6 weeks after surgery.
■ A patient with an unstable DRUJ treated by TFCC repair or ulnar styloid reduction and fixation is restricted from pronation and supination for 2 to 4 weeks.

OUTCOMES

■ The literature is relatively sparse regarding the results of arthroscopically assisted fixation of displaced intra-articular distal radius fractures.
■ A comparison study of 12 open and 12 arthroscopic reductions of comminuted AO type VII and VIII fractures of the distal radius found that the arthroscopic group had increased range of motion as compared to the open stabilization group.[23]
■ A second comparison study of 38 patients who underwent arthroscopically assisted fixation compared to open reduction found the arthroscopically assisted group had better results and improved range of motion.[2]
■ One study compared 15 patients with arthroscopically assisted fixation to 15 patients who underwent closed reduction and external fixation.[21] In this study, there were 10 tears of the triangular fibrocartilage complex in the group that underwent arthroscopic reduction, of which seven were peripheral and repaired. There were no signs of distal radioulnar joint instability at final follow-up visit. In the 15 patients who underwent stabilization by external fixation alone, four patients had continued complaints of instability of the distal radial joint, very possibly the result of undiagnosed and untreated TFCC tears.

COMPLICATIONS

■ Failure of fixation
■ Late settling of the fracture despite fixation
■ Flexor and extensor tendon irritation
■ Painful metal requiring removal
■ Neuromas of the dorsal sensory branch of the radial and ulnar nerves
■ Carpal tunnel syndrome
■ Reflex sympathetic dystrophy
■ Wrist and hand stiffness

REFERENCES

 1. Bradway JK, Amadio PC, Cooney WP. Open reduction and internal fixation of displaced comminuted intraarticular fractures of the distal end of the radius. J Bone Joint Surg Am 1989;71A:839–847.
 2. Doi K, Hatturi T, Otsuka K, et al. Intraarticular fractures of the distal aspect of the radius arthroscopically assisted reduction compared with open reduction and internal fixation. J Bone Joint Surg Am 1999;81A:1093–1110.
 3. Edwards CC III, Harasztic J, McGillivary GR, et al. Intraarticular distal radius fractures: arthroscopic assessment of radiographically assisted reduction. J Hand Surg Am 2001;26A:1036–1041.
 4. Fernandez DL, Geissler WB. Treatment of displaced articular fractures of the radius. J Hand Surg Am 1991;16:375–384.
 5. Geissler WB. Arthroscopically assisted reduction of intra-articular fractures of the distal radius. Hand Clin 1995;11:19–29.
 6. Geissler WB. Intra-articular distal radius fractures: the role of arthroscopy? Hand Clin 2005;21:407–416.
 7. Geissler WB, Freeland AE. Arthroscopically assisted reduction of intra-articular distal radial fractures. Clin Orthop Relat Res 1996;327:125–134.
 8. Geissler WB, Freeland AE, Savoie FH, et al. Intracarpal soft-tissue lesions associated with an intra-articular fracture of the distal end of the radius. J Bone Joint Surg Am 1996;78A:357–365.
 9. Geissler WB, Savoie FH. Arthroscopic techniques of the wrist. Mediguide to Orthopedics 1992;11:1–8.
10. Hanker GJ. Wrist arthroscopy in distal radius fractures. Proceedings of the Arthroscopy Association North America Annual Meeting, Albuquerque, NM, October 7–9, 1993.
11. Hixon ML, Fitzrandolph R, McAndrew M, et al. Acute ligamentous tears of the wrist associated with Colles fractures. Proceedings of the Annual Meeting of the American Society for Surgery of the Hand, Baltimore, 1989.
12. Hollingworth R, Morris J. The importance of the ulnar side of the wrist in fractures of the distal end of the radius. Injury 1976;7:263.
13. Knirk JL, Jupiter JB. Intra-articular fractures of the distal end of the radius in young adults. J Bone Joint Surg Am 1986;68A:647–658.
14. Lafontaine M, Hardy D, Delince P. Stability assessment of distal radius fractures. Injury 1989;20:208–210.
15. Levy HJ, Glickel SZ. Arthroscopic assisted internal fixation of intra-articular wrist fractures. Arthroscopy 1993;9:122–123.
16. Lindau T. Treatment of injuries to the ulnar side of the wrist occurring with distal radial fractures. Hand Clin 2005;21:417–425.

17. Melone CP. Articular fractures of the distal radius. Orthop Clin North Am 1984;15:217–235.
18. Mohanti RC, Kar N. Study of triangular fibrocartilage of the wrist joint in Colles fracture. Injury 1979;11:311–324.
19. Mudgal CS, Jones WA. Scapholunate diastasis: a component of fractures of the distal radius. J Hand Surg Br 1990;15:503–505.
20. Ruch DS, Vallee J, Poehling GG, et al. Arthroscopic reduction versus fluoroscopic reduction in the management of intra-articular distal radius fractures. Arthroscopy 2004;20:225–230.
21. Short WH, Palmer AK, Werner FW, et al. A biomechanical study of distal radial fractures. J Hand Surg Am 1987;12:529–534.
22. Stewart NJ, Berger RA. Comparison study of arthroscopic as open reduction of comminuted distal radius fractures. Abstract. Presented at the 53rd Annual Meeting of the American Society for Surgery of the Hand. January 11, 1998, Scottsdale, AZ.
23. Trumble TE, Schmitt SR, Vedder NB. Factors affecting functional outcome of displaced intra-articular distal radius fractures. J Hand Surg Am 1994;19:325–340.

Chapter 10

Fragment-Specific Fixation of Distal Radius Fractures

Robert J. Medoff

DEFINITION

- Fragment-specific fixation is a treatment approach in which each major fracture component is identified and fixed independently using low-profile implants with a certain degree of "spring-like" elasticity.
- Each fracture component has a unique implant specifically designed for that particular fracture element (**FIG 1**).
- Surgical planning is extremely important to determine whether a single approach or a combination of surgical approaches is needed to visualize and fix each of the main fracture components present in a particular injury.
- At the start of surgery, a complete set of implants should be available to address fractures of the radial column, ulnar corner, volar rim, dorsal wall, and free impacted articular fragments. In addition, identification and treatment of distal radioulnar joint (DRUJ) disruptions or unstable fractures of the ulnar column may be required.
- As a rule, this technique avoids creating large holes in small distal fragments, with fixation based and often triangulated to the stable ipsilateral cortex of the proximal fragment.

- The goal of fragment-specific fixation is to create a multiplanar, load-sharing construct that anatomically restores the articular surface and has enough stability to allow immediate motion after surgery.

ANATOMY

- The radial column fragment is formed from the pillar of bone along the radial border (**FIG 2**). This fracture component is important to maintain radial length to support the carpus in its normal spatial position. The brachioradialis inserts on the base of the radial column and may result in shortening of the radial column fragment, leading to impaction of the carpus into remaining fragments. Metaphyseal comminution may also contribute to radial column instability.
- The volar rim of the lunate facet is a primary load-bearing structure of the articular surface. Instability of the volar rim occurs in two patterns:
  - In the volar instability pattern, shortening and volar translation of the volar rim result in secondary volar subluxation of the carpus.

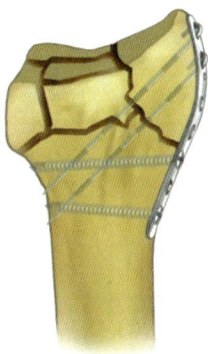

Radial pin plate

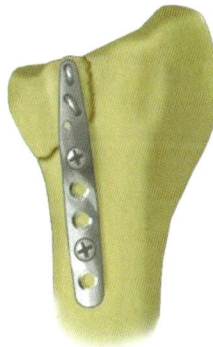

Ulnar pin plate

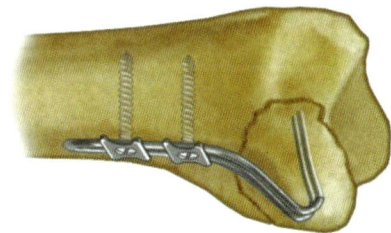

Volar buttress pin

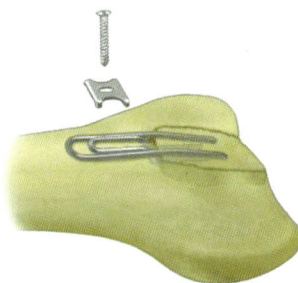

Small fragment clamp

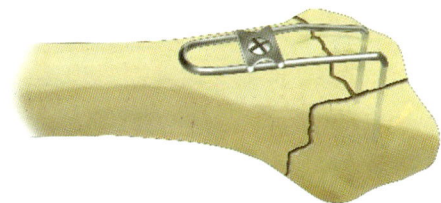

Dorsal buttress pin

FIG 1 • Fragment-specific implants.

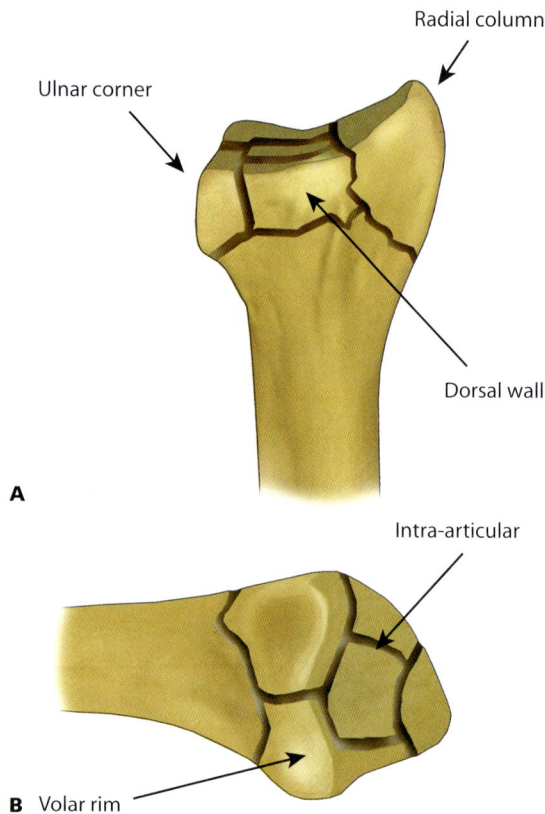

FIG 2 • Articular fracture components.

- In the axial instability pattern of the volar rim, axial impaction of the carpus drives the volar rim into dorsiflexion, resulting in secondary axial and dorsal subluxation of the carpus.
- The ulnar corner fragment involves the dorsal half of the sigmoid notch. Typically a result of impaction of the lunate into the articular surface, this fragment migrates dorsally and shortens proximally. Residual displacement of the ulnar corner can result in instability of the DRUJ as well as restriction of forearm rotation.
- Dorsal wall fragmentation typically occurs with either dorsal bending injuries or axial loading injuries and may contribute to fracture instability.
- Free articular fragments may be impacted within the metaphyseal cavity and result in incongruity of the articular surface.

PATHOGENESIS

- Dorsal bending injuries result in extra-articular fractures with dorsal displacement (**FIG 3A**). Comminution of the metaphyseal cavity or dorsal wall usually suggests a dorsally unstable fracture pattern.
- Volar bending injuries result in extra-articular fractures with volar displacement (**FIG 3B**). Fractures with significant volar displacement are nearly always unstable and require some type of intervention to obtain and hold a reduction until union.
- Dorsal shearing injuries present as fractures of the dorsal rim and are often associated with dorsal instability of the carpus (**FIG 3C**).
- Volar shearing injuries present as displaced fractures of the volar rim and result in volar instability of the carpus (**FIG 3D**). Often, this pattern is comminuted and highly unstable and not suited to closed methods of treatment.
- Simple three-part fractures are usually the result of low-energy injuries that combine an axial loading and dorsal bending mechanism (**FIG 3E**). This pattern is characterized by the presence of an ulnar corner fragment that involves the dorsal portion of the sigmoid notch, a main articular fragment, and a proximal shaft fragment.
- Unstable fractures with complex involvement of the articular surface to simplify complex articular fractures. In addition to articular comminution, this pattern may often generate a significant defect in the metaphyseal cavity or complete disruption of the DRUJ (**FIG 3F**).

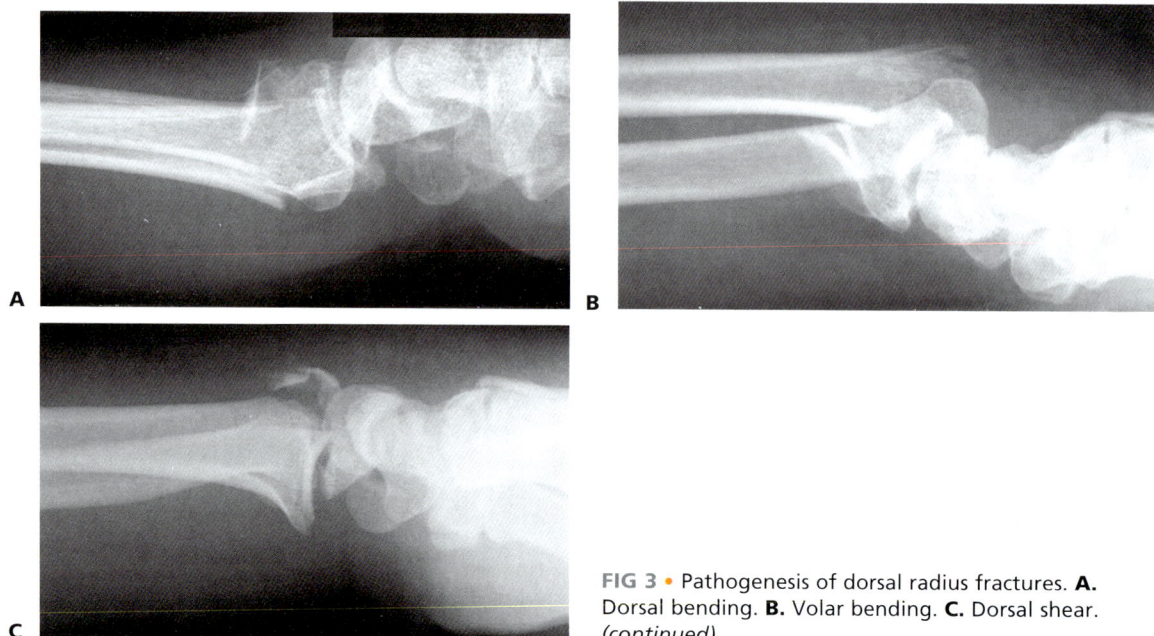

FIG 3 • Pathogenesis of dorsal radius fractures. **A.** Dorsal bending. **B.** Volar bending. **C.** Dorsal shear. *(continued)*

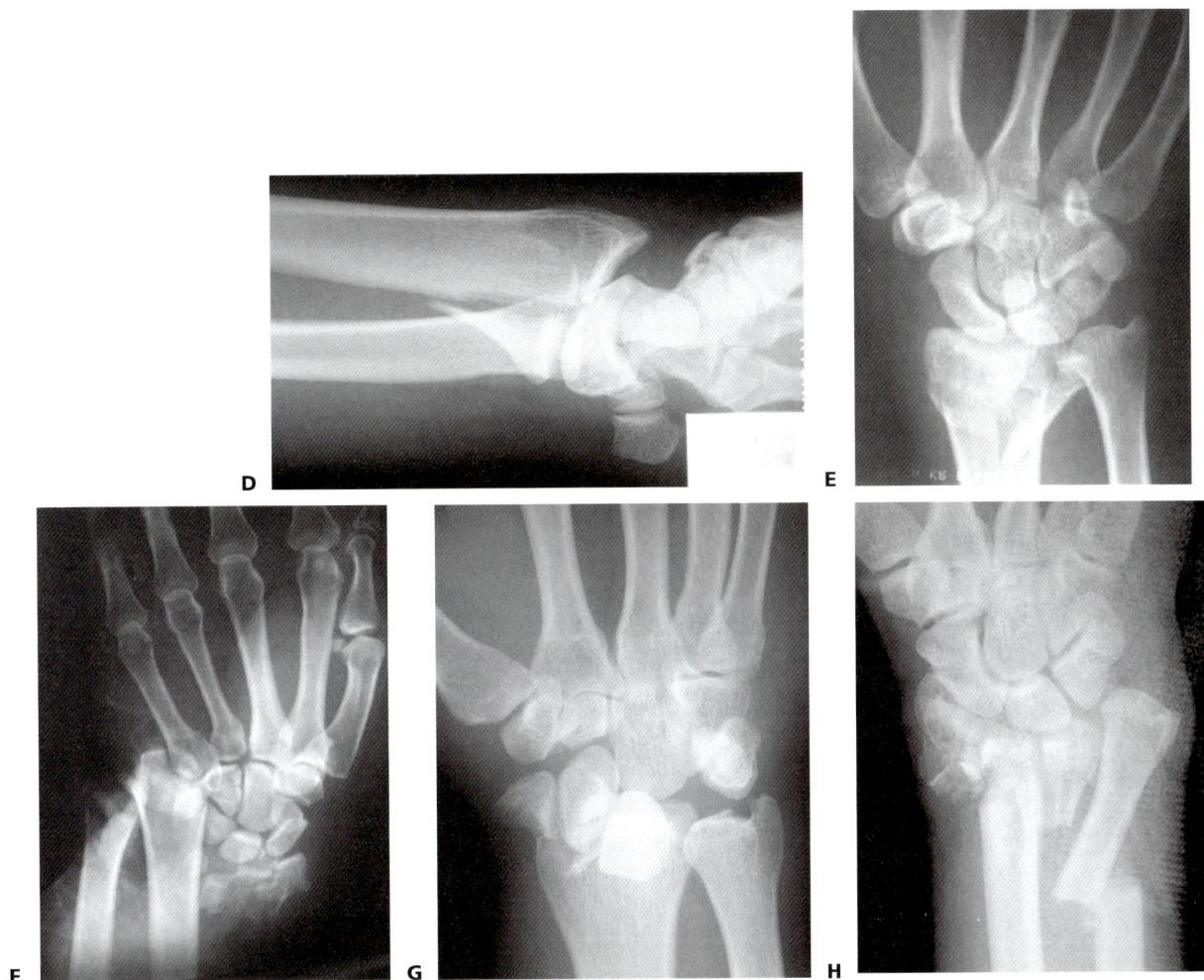

FIG 3 • *(continued)* **D.** Volar shear. **E.** Three-part articular. **F.** Comminuted articular. **G.** Carpal avulsion. **H.** High energy.

- The avulsion and carpal instability pattern is primarily a ligamentous injury of the carpus that has associated osseous avulsions of the distal radius (**FIG 3G**).
- Extremely high-energy injuries present as complex fractures involving comminution of the articular surface as well as extension into the radial or ulnar shaft (**FIG 3H**).

IMAGING AND OTHER DIAGNOSTIC STUDIES

- Posteroanterior (PA), standard lateral (**FIG 4A,B**), and 10-degree lateral views are routine views for radiographic evaluation of the distal radius. The 10-degree lateral view (**FIG 4C,D**) clearly visualizes the ulnar two thirds of the articular surface from the base of the scaphoid facet through the entire lunate facet. Oblique views may also be helpful for evaluating the injury.
- The radiographic features of distal radius fractures include the following:
  - Carpal facet horizon (**FIG 5A,B**). This is the radiodense horizontal landmark that is used to identify the volar and dorsal rim on the PA view. If the articular surface is in palmar tilt, the x-ray beam is parallel to the subchondral bone of the volar half of the lunate facet and the carpal facet horizon identifies the volar rim. However, if the articular surface is in dorsal tilt, the x-ray beam is parallel to the subchondral bone of the dorsal half of the lunate facet and the carpal facet horizon identifies the dorsal rim (not shown). The carpal facet horizon is the portion of the articular surface that is visualized on the 10-degree lateral x-ray projection.
  - Teardrop angle (normal 70 ± 5 degrees; **FIG 5C,D**). The teardrop angle is used to identify dorsiflexion of the volar rim of the lunate facet. Depression of the teardrop angle to a value less than 45 degrees indicates that the volar rim of the lunate facet has rotated dorsally and impacted into the metaphyseal cavity (axial instability pattern of the volar rim). This may be associated with axial and dorsal subluxation of the carpus. Restoration of the teardrop angle is necessary to correct this type of malreduction.
  - Articular concentricity (**FIG 5E,F**). The subchondral outline of the articular surface of the distal radius is normally congruent and concentric with the subchondral outline of the base of the lunate; a uniform joint interval should be present between the radius and lunate along the entire articular surface. When these articular surfaces are

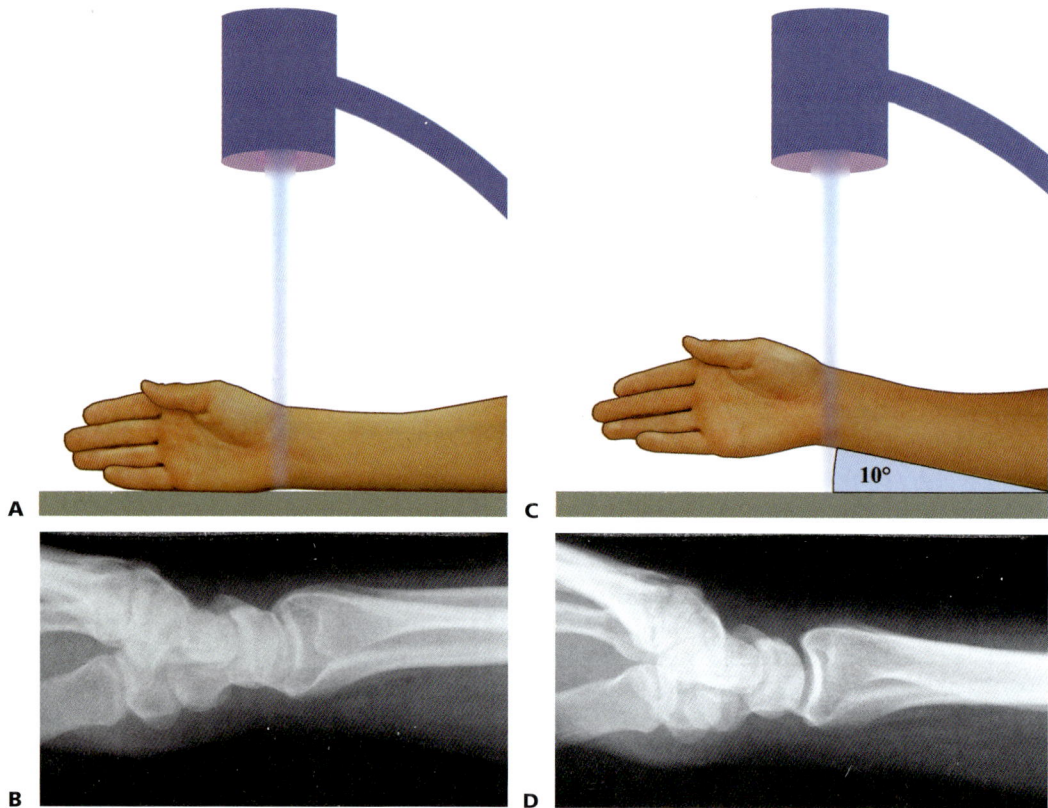

FIG 4 • **A.** Positioning for standard lateral radiography. **B.** Standard lateral radiograph. **C.** Positioning for 10-degree lateral radiography. **D.** Ten-degree lateral radiograph. Note the improved visualization of the articular surface of the base of the scaphoid facet and the entire lunate facet.

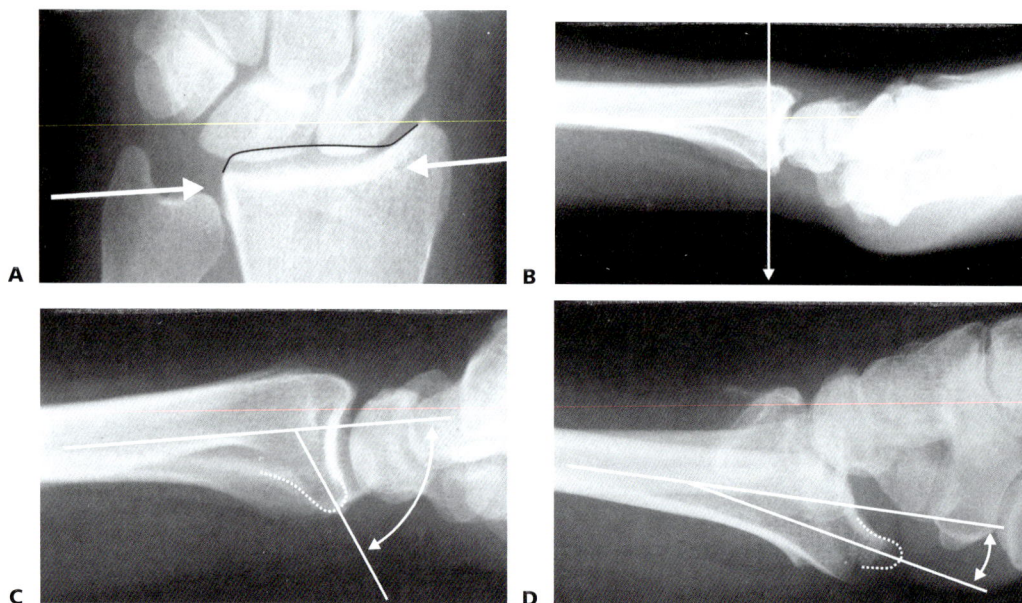

FIG 5 • **A.** Carpal facet horizon (*arrows*). Used to differentiate between the volar and dorsal rim on the PA projection. **B.** Origin of carpal facet horizon. The carpal facet horizon is formed by that part of the articular surface that is parallel to the x-ray beam and depends on whether the articular surface is in volar or dorsal tilt. **C.** Normal teardrop angle. **D.** Depressed teardrop angle, in this case caused by axial instability of the volar rim. *(continued)*

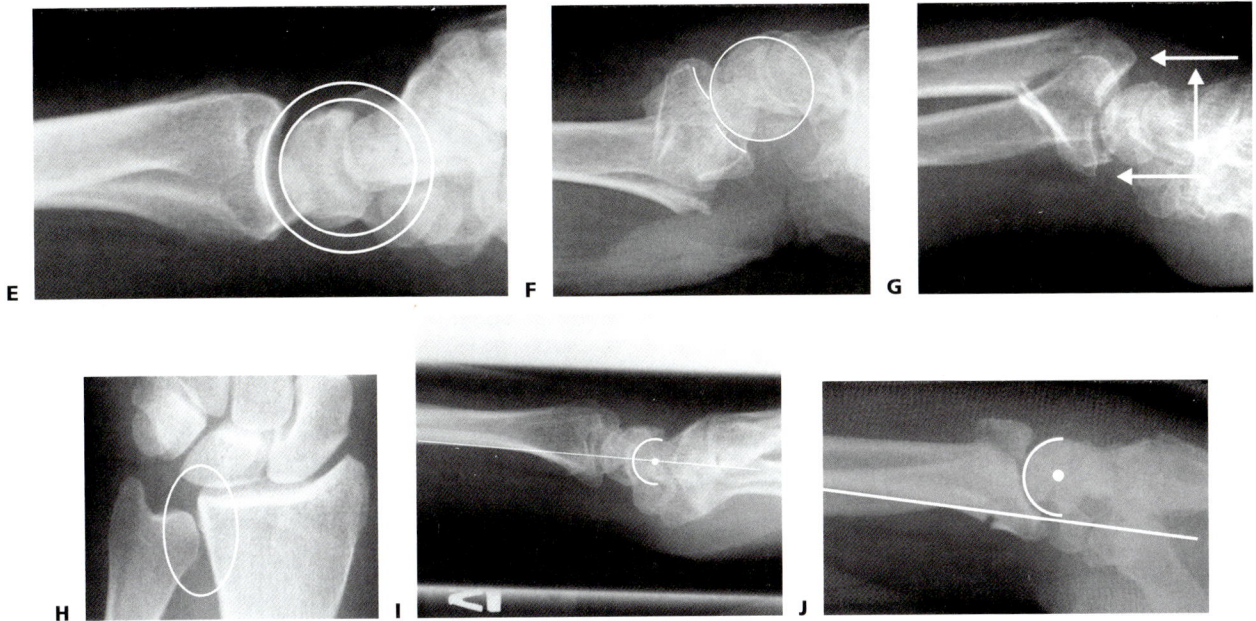

FIG 5 • *(continued)* **E.** Normal articular concentricity. **F.** Abnormal articular concentricity, indicating disruption across the volar and dorsal surfaces of the lunate facet. **G.** AP interval is the point-to-point distance between the corners of the dorsal and volar rim. **H.** Distal radioulnar joint interval. **I.** Normal lateral carpal alignment. **J.** Dorsal subluxation of the carpus.

not concentric, discontinuity and disruption of the lunate facet has occurred.

- AP distance (normal: females 18 ± 1 mm, males 20 ± 1 mm; **FIG 5G**). The AP distance is the point-to-point distance from the dorsal corner of the lunate facet to the palmar corner of the lunate facet. It is best evaluated on the 10-degree lateral view. Elevation of the AP distance indicates disruption of the volar and dorsal portion of the lunate facet.
- DRUJ interval (**FIG 5H**). The DRUJ interval measures the apposition between the head of the ulna and the sigmoid notch. Significant widening of the DRUJ interval implies disruption of the DRUJ capsule and triangular fibrocartilage complex (TFCC).
- Lateral carpal alignment (**FIG 5I,J**). The center of rotation of the capitate normally lines up with a line extended from the volar surface of the radial shaft with the wrist in neutral position. Dorsal rotation of the volar rim results in dorsal subluxation of the carpus from this normal position, placing the flexor tendons at a mechanical disadvantage, which may affect grip strength.
- In addition to the injury films, it is important to reassess postreduction views to determine the personality and specific components of the fracture.
- CT scans allow higher resolution and definition of fracture characteristics, particularly for highly comminuted fractures. Preferably, an attempt at closed reduction is done before a CT scan is obtained to limit distortion of the image. CT scans are particularly helpful for visualizing intra-articular fragments as well as DRUJ disruption.
- Clinical and radiographic evaluations of the carpus, interosseous membrane, and elbow are used to identify the

presence of other associated injuries that may affect the decision for a particular treatment.

SURGICAL MANAGEMENT

Operative Indications

- General parameters:
  - Shortening of more than 5 mm
  - Radial inclination of less than 15 degrees
  - Dorsal angulation of more than 10 degrees
  - Articular stepoff of more than 1 to 2 mm
  - Depression of teardrop angle of less than 45 degrees
- Volar instability
- DRUJ instability
- Displaced articular fractures
- Young, active patients are generally less tolerant of residual deformity and malposition.

Preoperative Planning

- Extra-articular fractures: multiple options:
  - Volar plating through a volar approach
  - Dorsal plating through a dorsal approach
  - Fragment-specific fixation
    - Radial pin plate (TriMed, Inc., Valencia, CA) and volar buttress pin (TriMed, Inc.) fixation through a limited incision volar or standard volar approach
    - Radial pin plate and either an ulnar pin plate dorsally or a dorsal buttress pin through a dorsal or combined approach
- Intra-articular fractures: surgical approach is based on the fragmentation pattern
  - Unstable volar rim fragments require a standard volar or ulnar-volar approach for adequate visualization.

▪ Fixation of the radial column can be done through either a limited-incision volar-radial approach, a volar approach with a radial extension combined with pronation of the forearm, or a dorsal approach with radial extension combined with supination of the forearm.

▪ Fixation of dorsal, ulnar corner, and free intra-articular fragments can be done through a dorsal approach.

Positioning

▪ The patient is supine.
▪ The affected arm is on an armboard out to the side.
▪ C-arm
  ▪ If the armboard is radiolucent, the C-arm can be brought in from the end of the armboard and images taken directly with the wrist on the armboard.
  ▪ If the armboard is not radiolucent, the C-arm is brought in along the side of the table from the foot, and the arm is brought off the armboard for each image.

Operative Sequence

▪ Radial column length is restored first with traction; a transstyloid pin is inserted to hold the reduction if needed.
▪ The volar rim is reduced and fixed.
▪ The dorsal ulnar corner is reduced and fixed.
▪ Free intra-articular fragments and the dorsal wall if needed are reduced and stabilized.
▪ Bone graft is applied if the metaphyseal defect is large.
▪ Fixation is completed with a radial column plate.

Approach

▪ The repair is undertaken by means of one of the following approaches:
  ▪ Limited-incision volar approach
  ▪ Dorsal approach
  ▪ Extensile volar approach
  ▪ Volar-ulnar approach

TECHNIQUES

LIMITED-INCISION VOLAR APPROACH

▪ Make a longitudinal incision along the radial side of the radial artery.
▪ Proximally, insert the tip of a tenotomy scissors over the surface of the first dorsal compartment sheath and sweep distally to elevate a radial skin flap.
▪ Pronate the forearm and sharply expose the bone over the radial styloid in the interval between the first and second dorsal compartments (**TECH FIG 1A**).
▪ Leaving the distal 1 cm of sheath intact, open the first dorsal compartment proximally and mobilize the tendons.

▪ Reflect the insertion of brachioradialis to expose the radial column (**TECH FIG 1B**).
▪ If needed, the dissection can be continued through the floor of the incision to expose the volar surface. Detach the insertion of the pronator quadratus radially and distally and reflect it to the ulnar side. Alternatively, create an ulnar skin flap superficial to the artery and continue the exposure through a standard volar approach.
▪ This approach cannot be used to access the ulnar side of the volar rim.

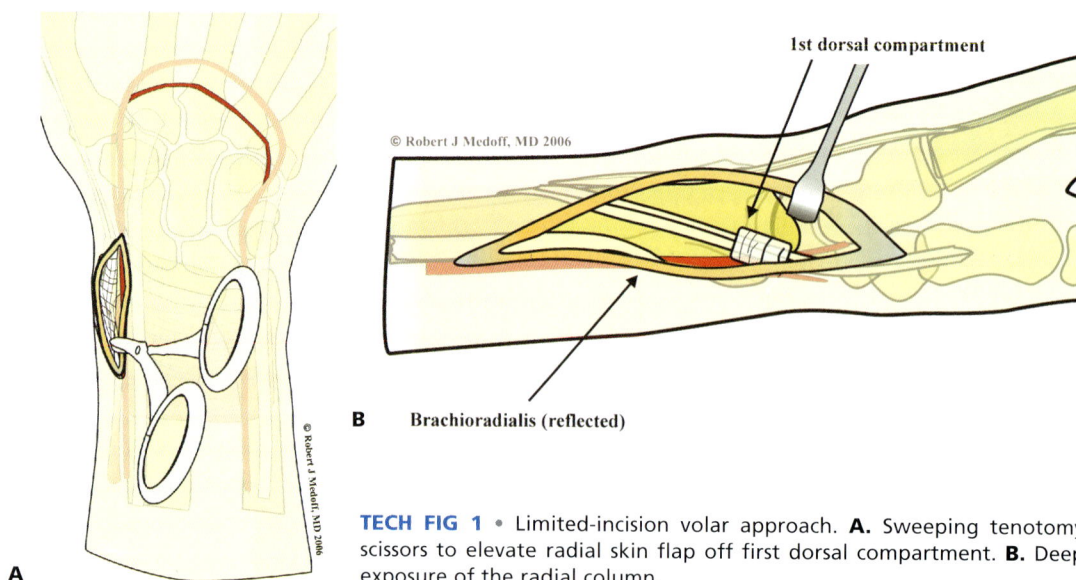

TECH FIG 1 • Limited-incision volar approach. **A.** Sweeping tenotomy scissors to elevate radial skin flap off first dorsal compartment. **B.** Deep exposure of the radial column.

TECHNIQUES

DORSAL APPROACH

- Make a longitudinal skin incision dorsally along the ulnar side of the tubercle of Lister (**TECH FIG 2A**).
- Identify the extensor digitorum communis (EDC) tendons visible proximally through the translucent extensor sheath. Incise the dorsal retinacular sheath.
- Develop the interval between the third and fourth compartment tendons for access to dorsal wall and free, impacted articular fragments. Resect a segment of the terminal branch of the posterior interosseous nerve (**TECH FIG 2B**).
- Transpose the extensor pollicis longus (EPL) from the tubercle of Lister if required for additional exposure.

- Develop the interval between the fourth and fifth extensor compartments to gain access to the ulnar corner fragment.
- A dorsal capsulotomy can be done to visualize the articular surface and carpus if necessary.
- To gain access to the radial column through a dorsal exposure, extend the incision as needed and elevate a radial subcutaneous flap and supinate the wrist.
- To gain access to the distal ulna, extend the incision as needed and elevate an ulnar subcutaneous flap.

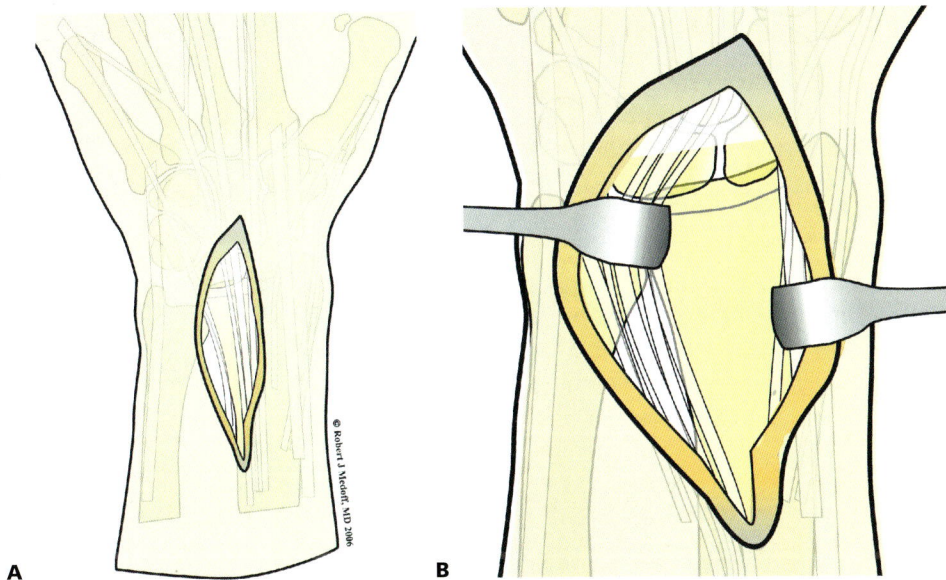

TECH FIG 2 • Dorsal approach. **A.** Initial incision. **B.** Deep exposure.

EXTENSILE VOLAR APPROACH

- Start the skin incision at the distal pole of the scaphoid and angle it toward the radial border of the flexor wrist crease, then extend it proximally along the flexor carpi radialis (FCR) tendon (**TECH FIG 3A**).
- Open the FCR tendon sheath both proximally and distally and continue in the plane between the FCR tendon and the radial artery (**TECH FIG 3B**).
- Use blunt dissection with a finger or sponge to separate the interval between the contents of the carpal tunnel and the surface of the pronator quadratus. Retract the FCR, median nerve, and flexor tendons to the ulnar side.
- Divide the radial and distal attachment of the pronator quadratus and reflect it to the ulnar side. Limit the distal dissection to no more than 1 or 2 mm beyond the distal radial ridge to avoid detachment of the volar wrist capsular ligaments (**TECH FIG 3C**).
- Reflect the brachioradialis from its insertion on the distal fragment if needed. Bone graft can be applied through the radial fracture defect.

- If access to the radial column is needed, elevate a radial subcutaneous flap superficial to the radial artery and first dorsal compartment tendon sheath. Pronate the wrist and retract the radial skin flap to expose the radial column.

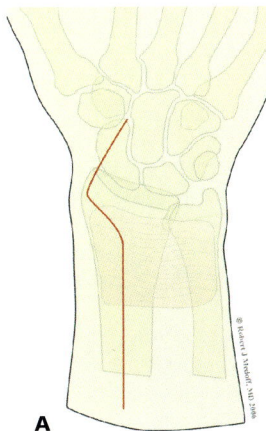

TECH FIG 3 • Extensile volar approach. **A.** Initial incision. *(continued)*

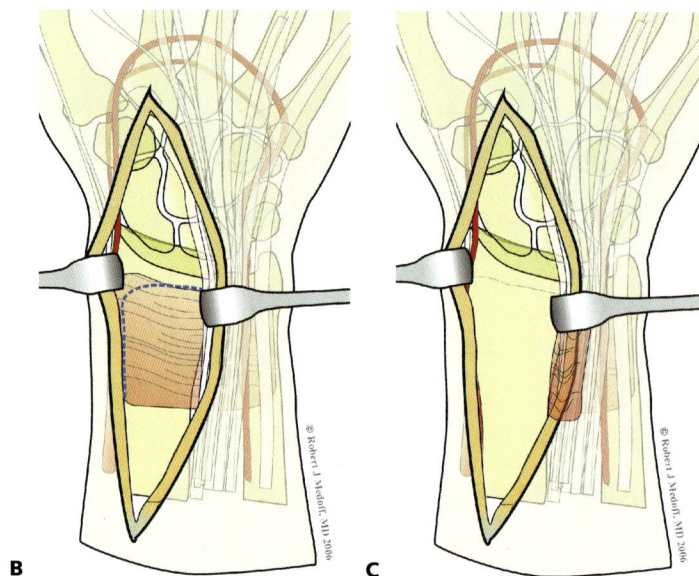

TECH FIG 3 • *(continued)* **B.** Line of incision in pronator quadratus. **C.** Deep exposure.

VOLAR-ULNAR APPROACH

- Make a longitudinal skin incision along the ulnar border of the flexor carpi ulnaris (FCU) tendon (**TECH FIG 4A**).
- Reflect the FCU tendon and the ulnar artery and nerve to the ulnar side (**TECH FIG 4B**).
- With blunt finger or sponge dissection, develop the plane on the superficial surface of the pronator quadratus.
- Retract the contents of the carpal tunnel to the radial side (**TECH FIG 4C**).
- Reflect the pronator quadratus from its ulnar and distal attachment. Do not dissect more than 1 to 2 mm beyond the distal radial ridge to avoid detaching the volar wrist capsule.

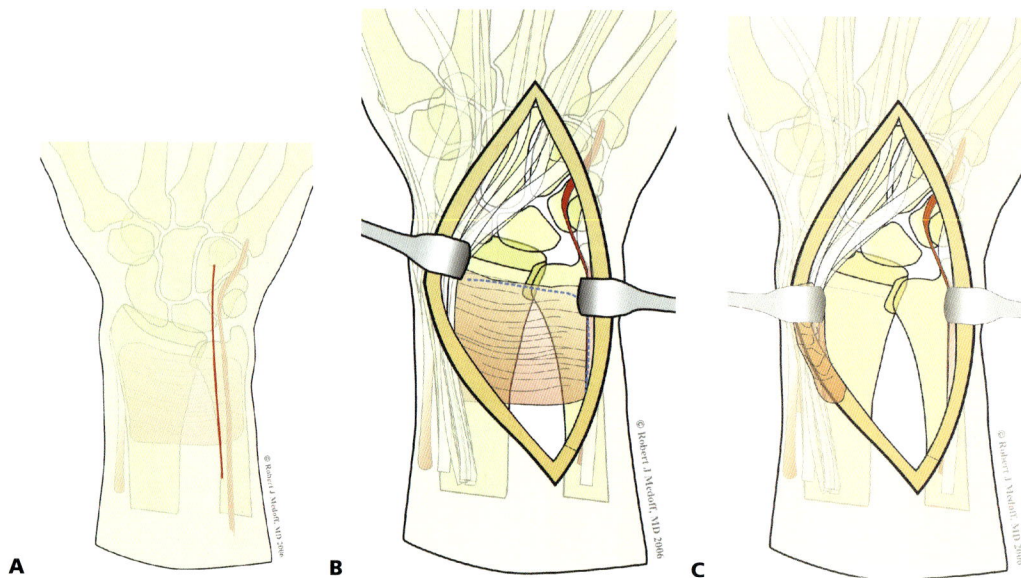

TECH FIG 4 • Volar-ulnar approach. **A.** Incision. **B.** Initial exposure. **C.** Completed exposure.

RADIAL COLUMN FIXATION WITH RADIAL PIN PLATE

- Expose the radial column with any of the approaches previously described. Sharply expose the interval between the first and second dorsal compartments over the tip of the radial styloid. Release the tendon sheath of the first dorsal compartment proximally, leaving the last 1 cm of tendon sheath intact.
- Retract the tendons of the first dorsal compartment dorsally or volarly as needed. Release the terminal insertion

of the brachioradialis to complete exposure of the radial column.

- After the initial fracture exposure, restore radial length with traction and ulnar deviation of the wrist. If needed, structural bone graft can be inserted through the radial fracture defect.
- Insert a 0.045-inch transstyloid Kirschner wire angled to engage the far cortex of the proximal fragment (**TECH FIG 5A**). When the advancing tip of the Kirschner wire hits the far cortex, place a drill sleeve over the Kirschner wire to use as a drill stop to limit penetration of the far cortex to 1 to 2 mm.
- Once the radial column is temporarily fixed with a transstyloid Kirschner wire, reduce and stabilize other volar, dorsal, and articular fracture elements before completing fixation of the radial column.
- Select a distal pin hole and slide a radial pin plate over the transstyloid Kirschner wire. Proximally, guide the plate under the tendons of the first dorsal compartment and secure it initially with a single 2.3-mm bone screw.
- Insert a second transstyloid Kirschner wire through a non-adjacent distal pin hole. Use the previous technique to limit penetration of the Kirschner wire through the far cortex to 1 to 2 mm.

- Mark a reference point where the Kirschner wire crosses the surface of the plate. Withdraw the Kirschner wire 1 cm and cut it 1 cm or more above the reference mark (**TECH FIG 5B**).
- Position the reference mark between the lower two posts of a wire bender and create a hook (**TECH FIG 5C**). The bend should start at the reference mark to make a Kirschner wire of proper length when completed.
- Complete the bend with a pin clamp, overbending slightly to allow the hook to snap into an adjacent pin hole or over the edge of the plate. With a free 0.045-inch Kirschner wire, predrill a hole to accept the end of the hook (**TECH FIG 5D**).
- Impact the Kirschner wire with a pin impactor and fully seat the hook (**TECH FIG 5E**). Repeat the procedure with the second Kirschner wire.
- Complete proximal fixation with 2.3-mm cortical bone screws (**TECH FIG 5F,G**).

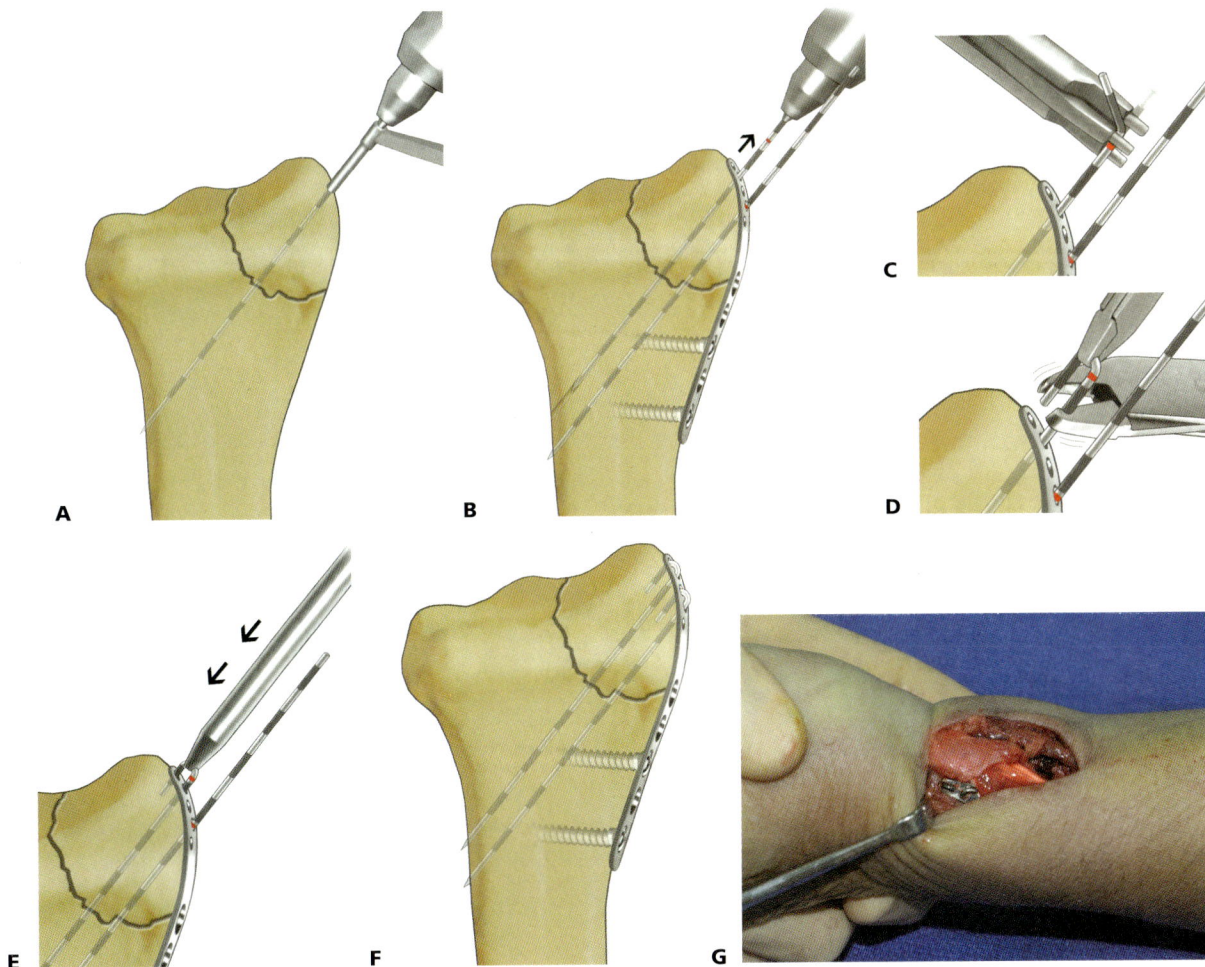

TECH FIG 5 • Radial column fixation. **A.** Insertion of transstyloid Kirschner wire. **B,C.** Creation of pin hook. **D,E.** Completion and impaction of pin hook. **F,G.** Completed radial column fixation.

ULNAR CORNER AND DORSAL WALL FIXATION

Ulnar Pin Plate

- Through a dorsal approach, expose and reduce the dorsal ulnar corner fragment, dorsal wall fragment, or both.
- Insert a 0.045-inch Kirschner wire through the fragment (**TECH FIG 6A**), angled proximally and slightly radially to purchase the far cortex of the proximal fragment.
- Insert structural bone graft into the metaphyseal defect if present to support the subarticular surface.
- If the plate is aligned over the ulnar half of the shaft, add a 15-degree torsional bend to the plate (twist the proximal end of the plate into slight supination). Often, a little extra extension can be contoured at the distal end of the plate (**TECH FIG 6B**).

- Slide the plate over the Kirschner wire and fix it proximally with a 2.3-mm bone screw (**TECH FIG 6C**).
- Insert a second Kirschner wire if the fragment is large enough. Create and impact hooks as described for the radial pin plate (**TECH FIG 6D–E**).
- If the Kirschner wire tips protrude beyond the volar cortex, they can be cut flush to the bone surface through a volar incision.

Dorsal Buttress Pin

- Through a dorsal approach, expose and reduce the dorsal ulnar corner fragment, dorsal wall fragment, or both.

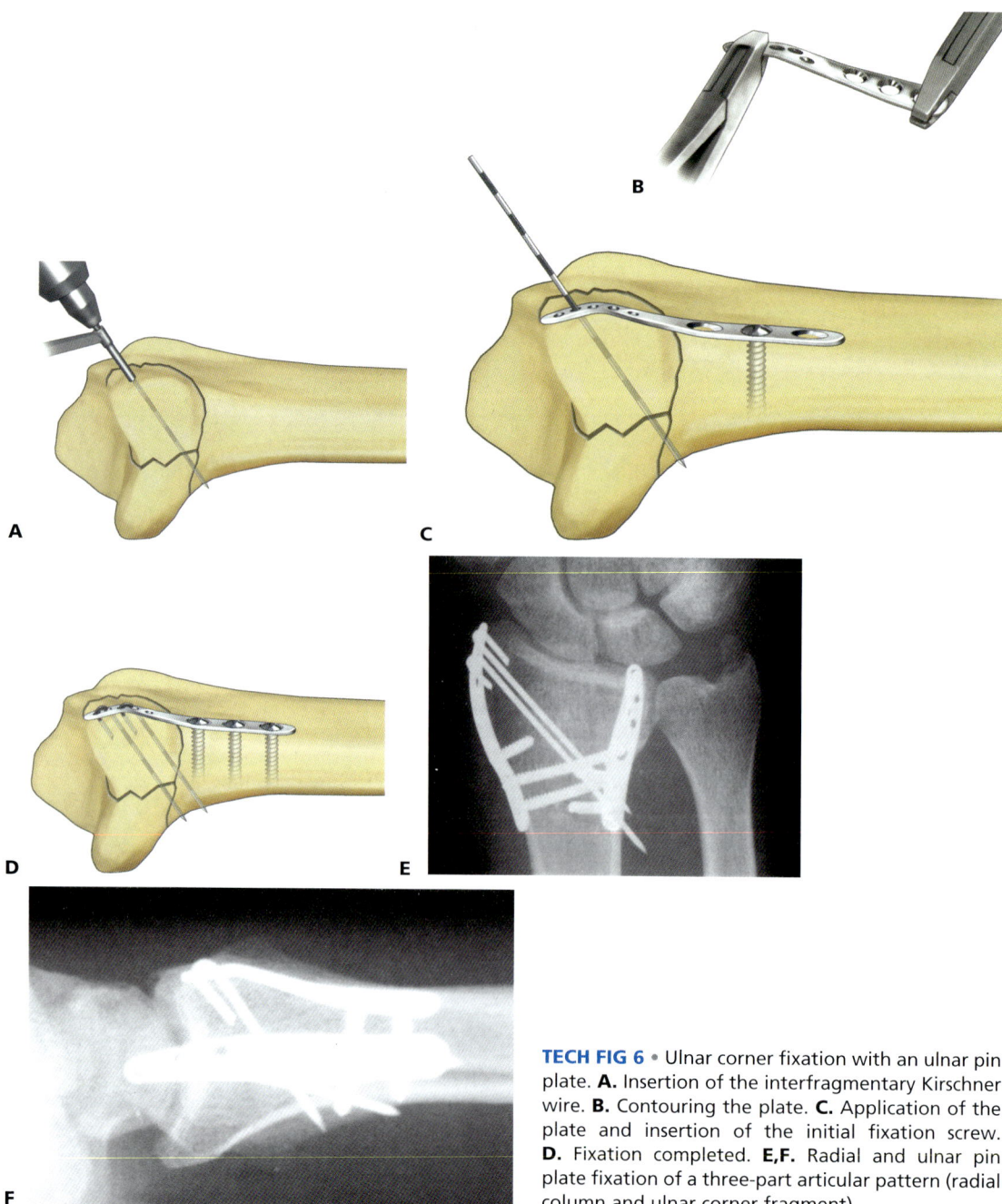

TECH FIG 6 • Ulnar corner fixation with an ulnar pin plate. **A.** Insertion of the interfragmentary Kirschner wire. **B.** Contouring the plate. **C.** Application of the plate and insertion of the initial fixation screw. **D.** Fixation completed. **E,F.** Radial and ulnar pin plate fixation of a three-part articular pattern (radial column and ulnar corner fragment).

TECHNIQUES

- Insert structural bone graft into the metaphyseal defect if present to support the subarticular surface.
- Insert two 0.045-inch Kirschner wires through the dorsal cortex and behind the subchondral bone; check the position with the C-arm (**TECH FIG 7A**). The Kirschner wires should be separated by about 1 cm and should be transverse to the longitudinal axis of the shaft. Initially placing a dorsal buttress pin upside-down on the bone is helpful to use as a template to visualize the proper position and insertion angle of the Kirschner wires (**TECH FIG 7B**).
- Ensure that the leading tips of the legs of the dorsal buttress pin are straight and cut to the required length (**TECH FIG 7C**). Leave the ulnar leg 2 to 3 mm longer than the radial leg so one leg can be engaged at a time.
- Place the ulnar leg of the buttress pin adjacent to the insertion site of the ulnar Kirschner wire, and then withdraw the Kirschner wire and immediately engage the leg in the hole. Repeat with the radial Kirschner wire to engage the radial leg of the buttress pin. Impact and seat the buttress pin (**TECH FIG 7D**).
- Fine-tune the reduction and complete the fixation proximally with one or two 2.3-mm cortical bone screws and washers (**TECH FIG 7E,F**). If needed, a blocking screw can be placed just proximal to the end of the buttress pin to prevent shortening of the fragment.

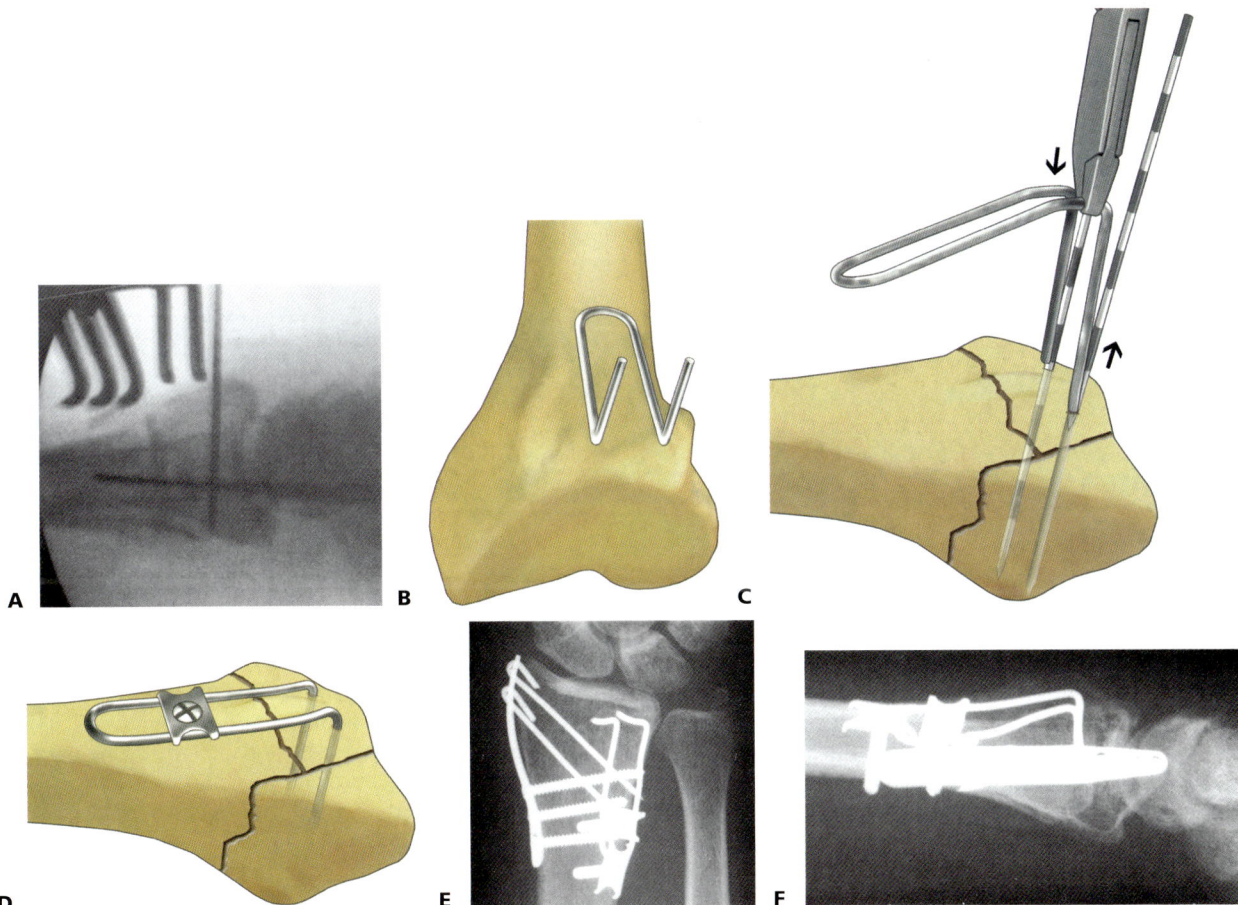

TECH FIG 7 • Dorsal buttress pin fixation. **A.** The position of the Kirschner wires is checked with a C-arm before inserting the implant. **B.** Placing an implant upside-down on bone to template the trajectory of the Kirschner wires. **C.** Inserting the dorsal buttress pin. **D.** Buttress pin fixation completed. **E,F.** Fixation of a three-part articular fracture with radial column and ulnar corner fragment with radial column plate and dorsal buttress pin.

VOLAR RIM FRAGMENT

Small-Fragment Plate Fixation

- Small-fragment volar plate fixation may be indicated for treatment of a volar instability pattern of the volar rim. The fragment must be of adequate size to allow buttressing on the volar surface by the plate (**TECH FIG 8A,B**).
- If volar rim fragmentation is associated with an axial instability pattern, the fragment must be of adequate size

and strength to allow distal locked screw purchase to obtain angular correction of the dorsiflexion deformity.
- An appropriate volar approach is used to expose the volar rim fragment. If a shortened radial column fragment is present, first restore radial length and provisionally hold it with a transstyloid Kirschner wire to unload the lunate facet.

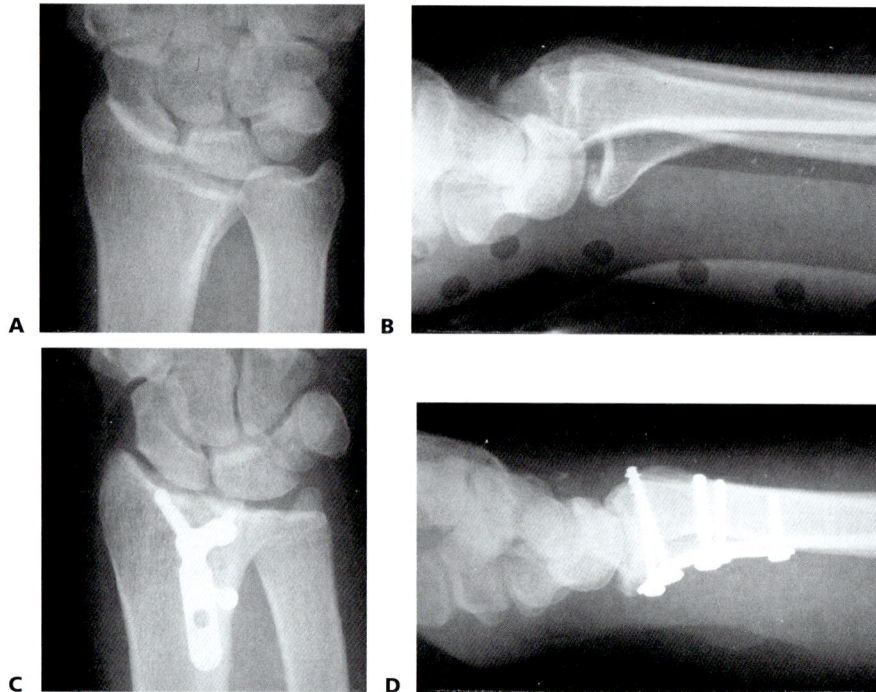

TECH FIG 8 • Volar rim fixation with small-fragment plate. **A,B.** Shear fracture of volar rim with volar instability pattern. **C,D.** Fixation with small-fragment plate.

- Reduce the volar rim fragment; this should restore normal carpal alignment.
- Apply a small-fragment volar plate and fix it proximally with cortical bone screws. If needed, secure the distal fragment with standard or locking bone screws (**TECH FIG 8C,D**).

Volar Buttress Pin Fixation

- Volar buttress pin fixation is indicated for unstable volar rim fragments and can be a particularly effective technique when faced with small distal fragments or axial instability patterns of the volar rim (depressed teardrop angle; **TECH FIG 9A,B**).
- Use an appropriate volar approach to expose the volar rim fragment. If necessary, restore radial length and provisionally hold it with a transstyloid Kirschner wire to unload the lunate facet (**TECH FIG 9C**).
- Continue exposure for up to 1 to 2 mm beyond the distal radial ridge. Reduce the volar rim fragment as much

as possible and note the orientation of the teardrop on the 10-degree lateral view.

- Insert two 0.045-inch Kirschner wires transverse to one another starting at an entry site 1 to 2 mm beyond the distal radial ridge. They should be placed within the center of the teardrop on the lateral view. Confirm the position of the Kirschner wires with C-arm.
- If necessary, the volar buttress pin may be contoured with a wire bender to match the flare of the volar surface of the distal radius. Adjust the trajectory of the legs of the implant to make a 70-degree angle with the base of the wire form. Cut the legs to appropriate length, leaving the ulnar leg 2 to 3 mm longer than the radial leg (**TECH FIG 9D,E**).
- Noting the entry site of the Kirschner wire, carefully remove the ulnar Kirschner wire and engage the ulnar leg of the volar buttress pin. Repeat the procedure with the radial leg. Impact and seat the implant into the volar rim fragment (**TECH FIG 9F**).
- Fine-tune the reduction and fix it proximally with a minimum of two screws and washers (**TECH FIG 9G,H**).

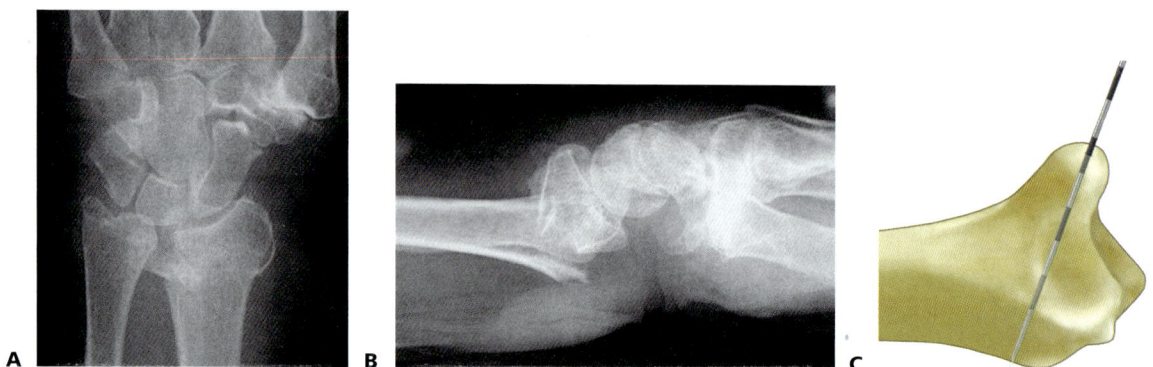

TECH FIG 9 • Volar rim fixation with a volar buttress pin. **A,B.** Articular fracture with axial instability pattern of volar rim. **C.** Insertion of Kirschner wires. *(continued)*

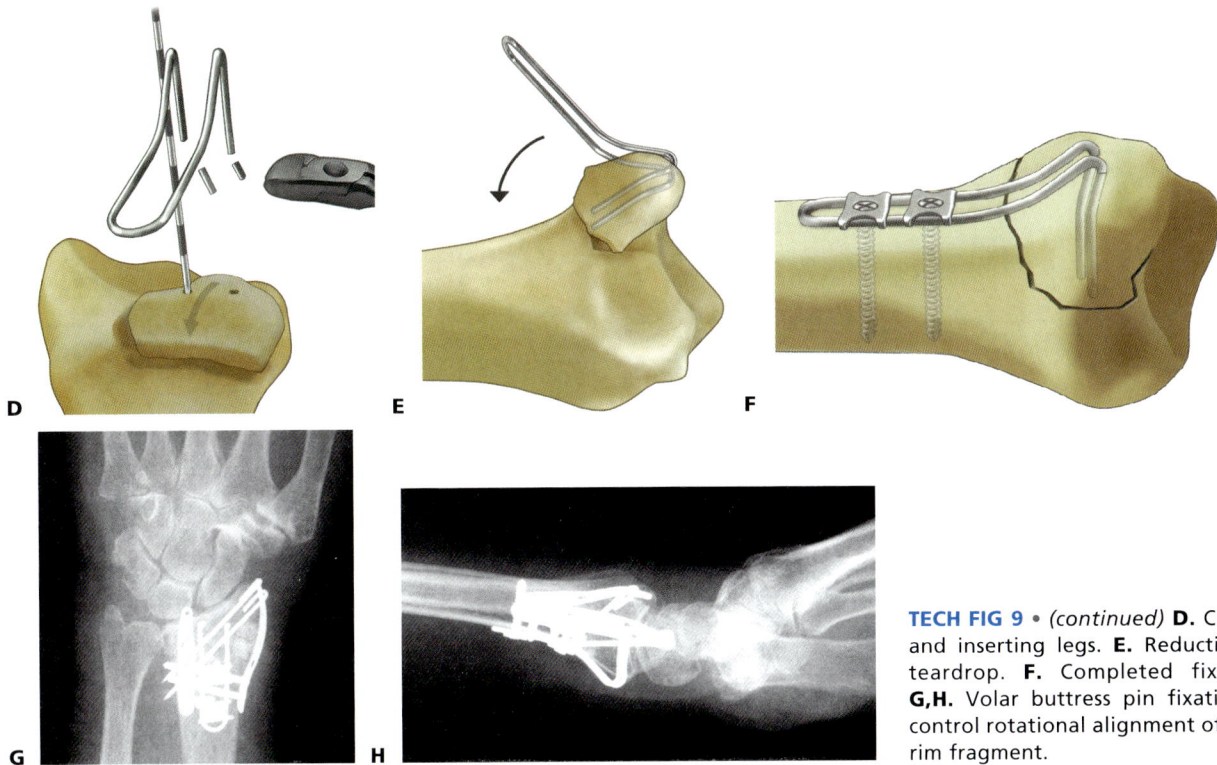

TECH FIG 9 • *(continued)* **D.** Cutting and inserting legs. **E.** Reduction of teardrop. **F.** Completed fixation. **G,H.** Volar buttress pin fixation to control rotational alignment of volar rim fragment.

FREE ARTICULAR FRAGMENT SUPPORT WITH A BUTTRESS PIN

- Free articular fragments impacted into the metaphyseal cavity require both a buttress to support the subchondral surface and circumferential peripheral cortical stability to prevent displacement (**TECH FIG 10A**).

- In some cases, impacted free articular fragments may be adequately supported by a properly applied locking plate that provides subchondral support.

- An alternative method is to use structural bone graft to support the free articular fragment in combination with fragment-specific fixation of the surrounding cortical shell, resulting in containment of the graft within the metaphysis.

- The dorsal buttress pin can also be used for direct subchondral support of impacted articular fragments. The legs of the implant are cut to length and inserted through the dorsal defect, slid distally directly behind the articular fragment, and then fixed proximally with a screw and washer (**TECH FIG 10B**). The articular fragment is sandwiched between the base of the lunate and the legs of the implant (**TECH FIG 10C**).

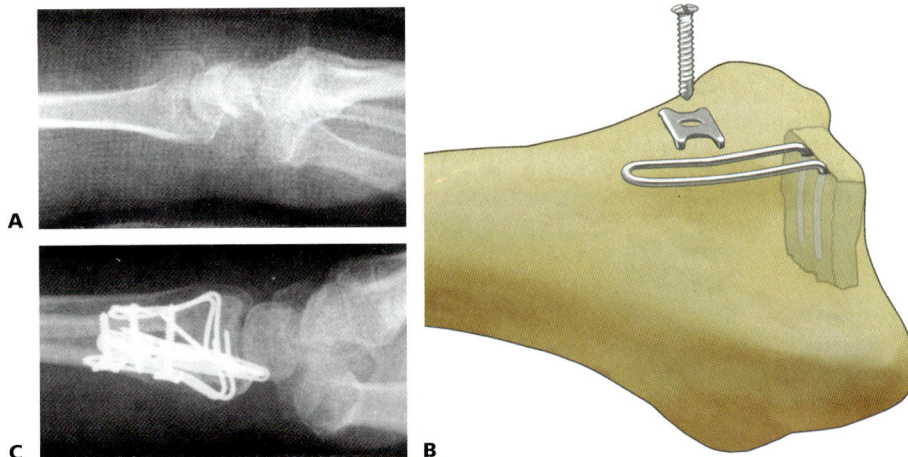

TECH FIG 10 • **A.** Depressed articular fragment. **B.** Support of free articular fragment with a buttress pin. **C.** Dorsal buttress pin to support fragment from endosteal surface.

PEARLS AND PITFALLS

Determining whether a fragment is volar or dorsal on the PA view	▪ Correlate the carpal facet horizon with the lateral view to determine whether a fragment is dorsal or volar.
	  ▪ If the articular surface is tilted dorsally, the carpal facet horizon identifies the dorsal rim.
	  ▪ If the articular surface is tilted volarly, the carpal facet horizon identifies the volar rim.

Reduction of unstable fracture pattern	▪ Identify and start reduction with the fragment that stabilizes the carpus to its normal spatial relationship. Often, initial reduction of the radial column with a provisional transstyloid Kirschner wire will restore carpal length. Alternatively, when this fragment is comminuted, fixation of the volar rim is often successful for reduction of the carpus. ▪ Adding structural bone graft, either through the fracture line at the base of the radial column or through a dorsal defect, can help stabilize the reduction during operative fixation.
Widening of the DRUJ or carpal translation	▪ Make sure the distal articular fragments are translated toward the ulna before completing volar fixation. ▪ An elastic, slightly overcontoured radial column plate can help close sagittal fracture gaps and seat the sigmoid notch against the ulnar head. ▪ Assess the clinical stability of the DRUJ and consider TFCC repair or suture or fixation of the ulnar styloid if needed.
Small or dorsally rotated volar rim fragment; loss of fixation of small volar-ulnar fragment	▪ Ensure adequate fixation of volar-ulnar corner fragment. ▪ Consider volar buttress pin fixation for an extremely distal or dorsally rotated volar rim fragment. ▪ Avoid release of the volar wrist capsule. When necessary, the legs of the implant can be inserted through the capsule. ▪ If needed, the volar buttress pin can be contoured as needed to match the arc of curve of the flare of the volar shaft.
Unrecognized carpal ligament injury	▪ Maintain a high index of suspicion for ligamentous injuries of the carpus. Consider arthroscopic evaluation, particularly in the context of radial or dorsal shear fractures, carpal avulsion and instability patterns, or articular fractures associated with a significant longitudinal stepoff between the scaphoid and lunate facets.
Complications	
Missed fragment: fracture displacement after surgery	▪ Careful analysis of radiographic features both before and during reduction; CT scan when needed ▪ Preoperative planning to select approaches that allow complete visualization of all major fragments ▪ Complete set of implants and instruments available before surgery
Loss of radial length: proximal migration of articular surface	▪ Graft the metaphyseal defect when needed with structural bone graft. ▪ Use implants that buttress the subchondral bone.
DRUJ dysfunction: pain, instability, or limitation of forearm rotation	▪ Assess clinical stability of DRUJ at end of procedure. ▪ Use radial column plate to push distal fragment against ulna to seat sigmoid notch against ulnar head. ▪ Evaluate and repair TFCC and capsular tears when necessary. ▪ Reduce and fix ulnar corner and volar rim fragments to restore congruity of sigmoid notch. ▪ Ensure that radial length is restored.
Stiffness: slow, restricted return of movement of wrist, forearm, and fingers, often associated with pain	▪ Early range of motion and mobilization of soft tissues ▪ Avoidance of constricting bandages and postoperative swelling
Tendinitis or rupture: pain with resisted motion, loss of tendon function, clicking and pain	▪ Use implants that have a low distal profile. ▪ Avoid placing sharp, bulky edges of hardware in proximity to tendons. ▪ Cover plates distally with retinacular flap when needed. ▪ Consider use of buttress pins (which have a very low profile) when possible. ▪ Remove any pins or hardware that back out or become prominent postoperatively. ▪ Ensure that volar plates do not extend up beyond distal volar ridge into soft tissues. ▪ Avoid long screws or pins, particularly when placed from volar to dorsal. Distal screws should normally be 2 to 4 mm shy of the dorsal cortical margin.

POSTOPERATIVE CARE

▪ At the end of the surgical procedure, confirm the stability of fixation as well as the stability of the DRUJ.

▪ If stable, apply a removable wrist brace and instruct the patient to initiate gentle range-of-motion exercises of the fingers, wrist, and forearm twice or more daily as tolerated. For non-compliant patients or injuries with tenuous fixation, use a cast for 2 to 3 weeks postoperatively.

▪ Avoid resistive loading across the wrist until signs of radiographic healing are present; typically this occurs by 4 weeks postoperatively. Specifically instruct older patients not to push up out of a chair or lift heavy objects after surgery.

- If there is persistent stiffness after 4 weeks, initiate physical and occupational therapy.

OUTCOMES

- Konrath and Bahler[4] reported 27 patients with at least 2 years of follow-up:
  - One fracture lost reduction.
  - Patient satisfaction was high (average DASH scores 17 and PRWE scores 19 at follow-up).
  - In only three cases was hardware removed; no tendon ruptures occurred.
- Schnall et al[7] reported on two groups of patients: group I had sustained high-energy trauma and group II had lower-energy injuries.
  - Group I patients averaged return to work in 6 weeks, with all fractures uniting without loss of position or deformity.
  - Two patients in group I required removal of painful hardware.
  - Group II patients averaged 2 degrees of loss of volar tilt, a 0.3-mm change in ulnar variance, and no loss of joint congruity at follow-up.
  - Grip strength in group II patients was 67% of the contralateral side.
- Benson et al[2] reported on 85 intra-articular fractures in 81 patients with a mean follow-up of 32 months.
  - There were 64 excellent and 24 good results, with an average DASH score of 9 at final follow-up.
  - Flexion and extension motion was 85% and 91% of the opposite side at final follow-up.
  - Grip strength was 92% of the opposite side at final follow-up.
  - Sixty-two percent of patients had a 100-degree arc of flexion–extension and normal forearm rotation by 6 weeks postoperatively.
  - Postoperative radiographic alignment was maintained at follow-up.
  - There were no cases of symptomatic arthritis.

COMPLICATIONS

- Stiffness: common early, uncommon at follow-up
  - Recovery can be accelerated by anatomic fixation that is stable enough to start motion immediately after surgery. The relative degree of trauma to the bone and soft tissues, combined with underlying physiologic factors, is also a critical factor that can lead to slow recovery of motion or residual stiffness.
- Malunion or nonunion: rare
  - Loss of reduction may occur, particularly if a major fracture component is missed and left untreated. In addition,

osteoporosis, failure to graft the metaphyseal defect, and associated DRUJ injuries may contribute to loss of reduction or malunion.
  - Pin plates are able to resist translational displacements but are less effective for preventing loss of length; they require osseous contact between the proximal and distal fragments or additional support by a secondary implant that will buttress the subchondral surface.
  - Nonunions are extremely rare.
- Tendinitis or tendon rupture: uncommon
  - If pins are noted postoperatively to back out, they should be removed. Leaving the distal 1 cm of tendon sheath of the first dorsal compartment intact helps avoid tendon contact with hardware.
  - Using low-profile implants dorsally, covering the distal ends with a strip of retinacular sheath, or both is also helpful.
  - The surgeon should avoid leaving screws or pins protruding from the dorsal or volar surfaces of the bone.
- Painful hardware: rare
  - Painful hardware can be related to migration of a pin or settling of the fracture proximally. Overbending pin hooks and using bone graft or buttressing implants can help avoid this problem.
  - Remove hardware when painful.
- Late arthritis is uncommon and probably related to the quality of the articular restoration.
- Infections, bleeding, carpal tunnel syndrome, and other nerve injuries are uncommon and often related to the primary injury.
- Complex regional pain syndrome is rare and may be related to initiation of early motion after surgery.

REFERENCES

1. Barrie K, Wolfe S. Internal fixation for intraarticular distal radius fractures. Tech Hand Up Extrem Surg 2002;6:10–20.
2. Benson LS, Minihane KP, Stern LA, et al. The outcome of intra-articular distal radius fractures treated with fragment-specific fixation. J Hand Surg Am 2006;31A:1333–1339.
3. Fernandez DL, Jupiter JB. Fractures of the Distal Radius, 2nd ed. Springer, 2001:42–50.
4. Konrath G, Bahler S. Open reduction and internal fixation of unstable distal radius fractures: results using the TriMed system. J Orthop Trauma 2002;16:578–585.
5. Leslie BM, Medoff RJ. Fracture-specific fixation of distal radius fractures. Tech Orthop 2000;15:336–352.
6. Medoff R. Essential radiographic evaluation for distal radius fractures. Hand Clin 2005;21:279–288.
7. Schnall S, Kim B, Abramo A, et al. Fixation of distal radius fractures using a fragment specific system. Clin Orthop Relat Res 2006;445:51–57.
8. Swigart C, Wolfe S. Limited incision open techniques for distal radius fracture management. Orthop Clin North Am 2001;30:317–327.

Chapter 11

Intramedullary and Dorsal Plate Fixation of Distal Radius Fractures

Pedro K. Beredjiklian and Christopher Doumas

DEFINITION

- Distal radius fractures typically originate in the radial metaphysis and occasionally enter the radiocarpal joint and distal radioulnar joint.
- These fractures may be stable or unstable, intra-articular or extra-articular, and can be associated with various other bony and soft tissue injuries about the wrist.
- Distal radius fractures are most commonly dorsally displaced or angulated (apex volar).
- Treatment is based on fracture stability, comminution, articular segment displacement, articular surface displacement, and the functional demand of the patient.
- Stability is related to initial dorsal angulation, residual dorsal angulation after closed reduction, dorsal comminution, age of the patient, and associated distal ulna fracture and intra-articular fracture extension.[7,8]

ANATOMY

- The distal radius has articulations at the scaphoid fossa, lunate fossa, and sigmoid notch.
- The normal bony anatomy includes volar tilt of 10 degrees, radial height of 11 mm, and radial inclination of 22 degrees.
- Ulnar variance (the length of the radius relative to the ulnar head at the sigmoid notch) is variable and patient dependent.
- Dorsal ligamentous structures include the dorsal intercarpal ligament and the dorsal radiocarpal ligament.
- The dorsal radiocarpal ligament originates from the dorsal lip of the radius and attaches on the ulnar carpus.
- The dorsal intercarpal ligament represents a capsular thickening on the dorsum of the carpus, with fiber alignment perpendicular to the long axis of the radius.
- Volar ligamentous origins include the radioscaphocapitate ligament, the long radiolunate ligament, and the short radiolunate ligament, among others.
- The triangular fibrocartilage complex (TFCC) consists of the triangular fibrocartilage and volar radioulnar and dorsal radioulnar ligaments.
- The volar radioulnar and dorsal radioulnar ligaments originate form the volar and dorsal edges of the sigmoid notch respectively, and become confluent and insert at the base of the ulnar styloid.
- The extensor retinaculum lies superficial to the extensor tendons and deep to the subcutaneous tissues. It has septations creating six dorsal compartments (**FIG 1**).
  - The first compartment lies over the radial styloid and contains the abductor pollicis longus and the extensor pollicis brevis tendons (each may have multiple slips).
  - The second compartment, containing the extensor carpi radialis longus and extensor carpi radialis brevis, lies radial to the tubercle of Lister.
  - The third compartment, containing the extensor pollicis longus, lies ulnar to the tubercle of Lister.
  - The fourth compartment, containing the extensor indicis proprius and extensor digitorum communis, lies over the dorsal-ulnar distal radius.
  - The fifth compartment, containing the extensor digiti minimi, lies over the distal radioulnar joint.
  - The sixth compartment, containing the extensor carpi ulnaris, lies over the distal ulna.

PATHOGENESIS

- Distal radius fractures typically occur due to a fall on an outstretched hand.
- Fractures occur when the force of axial loading exceeds the failure strength of cortical and trabecular bone.[9]
- The fracture pattern is determined by the magnitude and direction of the force applied and the position of the hand during impact.[3]
- Dorsally displaced or angulated fractures occur when the wrist is neutral or extended and an axial or dorsally directed force is applied to the carpus.
- Osteoporosis, metabolic bone diseases, and bony tumors are risk factors for fracture.

NATURAL HISTORY

- Distal radius fractures are either stable or unstable.
- Stable fractures, treated nonoperatively, historically have excellent outcomes in terms of range of motion, pain, strength, and function.[1]
  - Nonoperative management consists of immobilization with either a cast or a splint, molded to prevent dorsal displacement.
- Displaced, unstable, and comminuted fractures often require operative treatment.
- The goals of surgical treatment are to provide stability and improve bony alignment in order to achieve pain control, improve range of motion, and increase function.[1,6]

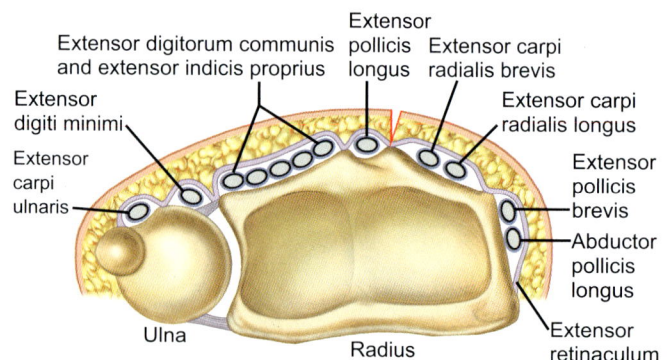

FIG 1 • Anatomy of the distal radius. The six dorsal extensor compartments at the level of the extensor retinaculum.

- One to 2 mm or more of displacement of the articular surface of the distal radius leads to degenerative changes in young adults.[6]
- Dorsal angulation of more than 20 degrees from normal (10 degrees dorsal tilt) can lead to pain, decreased range of motion, and decreased grip strength.[10]
- Radial shortening can decrease range of motion and cause pain with ulnar impaction of the carpus.[10]

PATIENT HISTORY AND PHYSICAL FINDINGS

- A history of trauma is the most common patient presentation.
- Pathologic fractures may occur with minimal stress or trauma.
- Patients complain of localized pain and present with swelling, decreased range of motion, and ecchymosis about the fracture.
- A history of previous fractures in an older patient should alert the physician to the possibility of underlying osteoporosis.
- The skin should be carefully examined to rule out the presence of an open fracture and to assess swelling before surgery or casting. If the wrist is markedly swollen or if swelling is anticipated, casting should be delayed and a splint should be placed.
- Neurologic symptoms in the form of numbness, tingling, and radiating pain into the digits should alert the physician to the possibility of acute carpal tunnel syndrome. Careful neurologic assessments should be performed to rule out the presence of a progressive neurologic deficit.
- Acute carpal tunnel syndrome represents a surgical emergency.
- Examination:
  - Remove splints and dressings to visualize all areas of skin.
  - Palpate for areas of tenderness or deformity. Palpate anatomic snuffbox.
  - Visualize and palpate the elbow for swelling, ecchymosis, tenderness, crepitus, and deformity.
  - Visualize and palpate the hand and fingers for swelling, ecchymosis, tenderness, crepitus, and deformity.
  - Use two-point tool or paper clip bent to 5 mm and touch radial and ulnar aspects of all fingers with one or two points. Greater than normal (5 mm) two-point testing in the form of progressive neurologic deficit may signify an acute or chronic carpal tunnel syndrome.

IMAGING AND OTHER DIAGNOSTIC STUDIES

- Posteroanterior (PA), lateral, and oblique radiographic views are critical in evaluating all suspected distal radius fractures.
  - Consider imaging the uninjured wrist for comparison and to serve as a template for surgical reconstruction.
  - Radiographs of the elbow should be obtained in almost all cases, especially if any tenderness, swelling, or deformity is detected clinically.
- Radiographic measurements taken from the PA view (**FIG 2A**) include[9,13]:
  - Radial inclination, which is the angle between a line perpendicular to the shaft of the radius at the articular margin and a line along the radial articular margin
    - Normal angle = 21 degrees
  - Radial length, which is the distance from a line tangential to the ulnar articular margin to a line drawn perpendicular to the long axis of the radius at the radial styloid tip
    - Normal length = 11 mm
  - Ulnar variance, which is the distance from a line perpendicular to the long axis of the radius at the sigmoid notch and a line tangential to the ulnar articular surface
    - Ulnar variance is variable, so to establish a normal value, radiographs of the normal contralateral side should be obtained.
- Lateral articular (volar) tilt is the angle between a line for the articular surface of the radius and a perpendicular line to the long axis of the radius.
  - Normal angle = 11 degrees volar tilt (**FIG 2B**)[9,13]
- CT scans can fully elucidate the anatomy of the fracture, particularly articular disruption or incongruity, and also help to determine the necessary surgical approach based on the location and extent of comminution.
  - CT scans increase the interobserver reliability of treatment plans and may actually alter the initial treatment plan based on plain radiographs.[5]
- MRI can be useful in evaluating for concomitant ligamentous injuries, TFCC injuries, stress fractures, and occult carpal fractures.

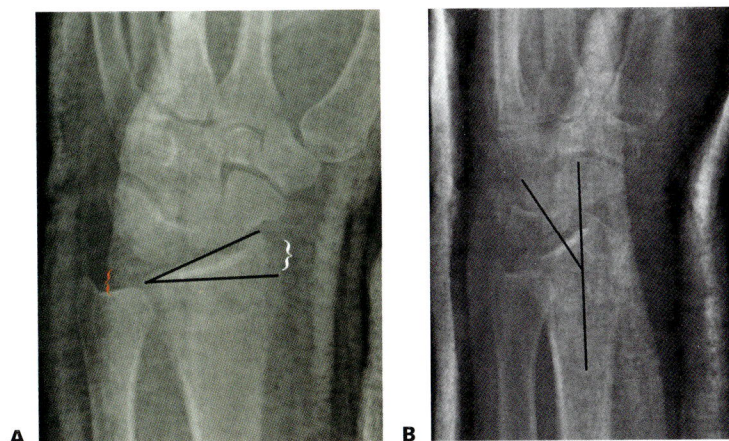

FIG 2 • A. PA radiograph demonstrating radial inclination, *(black lines)*, ulnar variance *(red)*, and radial height *(white bracket)*. **B.** Lateral radiograph of the wrist demonstrating volar tilt *(black lines)*.

DIFFERENTIAL DIAGNOSIS

- Bony contusion
- Wrist dislocation
- Scaphoid or other carpal fracture
- Carpal instability or dislocation
- Distal ulna fracture
- Wrist ligament or TFCC sprain or tear

NONOPERATIVE MANAGEMENT

- Closed reduction should be performed in the emergency department with longitudinal axial traction followed by volar displacement of the carpus. A bivalved, short-arm, well-molded cast or sugar-tong splint should be applied.
- Casting is the most commonly used method to definitively treat distal radius fractures and is preferred for nondisplaced or minimally displaced fractures and those that are stable after a reduction maneuver (ie, restored volar tilt with minimal dorsal comminution). A precise three-point mold is required to maintain fracture reduction.
- Removable splinting can be considered when treating completely nondisplaced stable fractures in young adults.
- If nonoperative treatment is chosen, repeat radiographs should be taken on a weekly basis for the first 3 weeks to ensure that the reduction is maintained. The physician should have a low threshold for changing the cast.
- Any sign of dorsal migration indicates instability, and operative stabilization should be considered.
- Finger range of motion is begun immediately and wrist range of motion can be started as the fracture heals and is managed in a removable splint.

SURGICAL MANAGEMENT

- Open reduction and internal fixation with a dorsal plate can be used successfully in the treatment of displaced, unstable, comminuted fractures of the distal radius that fail to respond to closed treatment.
  - Dorsal plating buttresses the fracture to correct deformity and maintain fracture reduction.
  - New intramedullary implants have been designed to alleviate some of the complications associated with traditional dorsal plates and allow a less invasive option for fixation of dorsally displaced fractures (**FIG 3A,B**).
- Indications for dorsal plating include:
  - Severe initial dorsal displacement (>20 degrees from normal, 10 degrees dorsal tilt)
  - Marked dorsal comminution (greater than or equal to 50% of the diameter of the radius shaft on the lateral radiograph)
  - Residual (after reduction) dorsal tilt greater than 10 degrees past neutral
  - 10 mm of radius shortening
  - Dorsal intra-articular fragments displaced more than 1 mm[1,6]
- Stabilization using an intramedullary device is indicated for distal radius fractures without extensive articular involvement in which a limited incision and shorter procedure are desired (see Tech Fig 4E).
  - Comminution of the volar metaphysis is a relative contraindication for the use of a dorsal intramedullary implant.
- The surgeon should be prepared to change management intraoperatively and must have additional stabilization options available, if necessary, such as percutaneous pins or an external fixator.

Preoperative Planning

- All radiographic imaging must be reviewed before surgery.
  - It is helpful to compare radiographs of the injured wrist to the uninjured wrist.
  - Displaced intra-articular fragments must be identified.
  - Dorsal comminution must be evaluated to determine fracture stability and the need for bone grafting.
  - The distal extent of the fracture must be determined to enable the buttress plate to function properly.
- Bone should be evaluated for osteopenia, osteoporosis, and tumors.

Positioning

- The patient is placed supine on a regular operating table.
- A tourniquet is placed near the axilla with the splint in place.

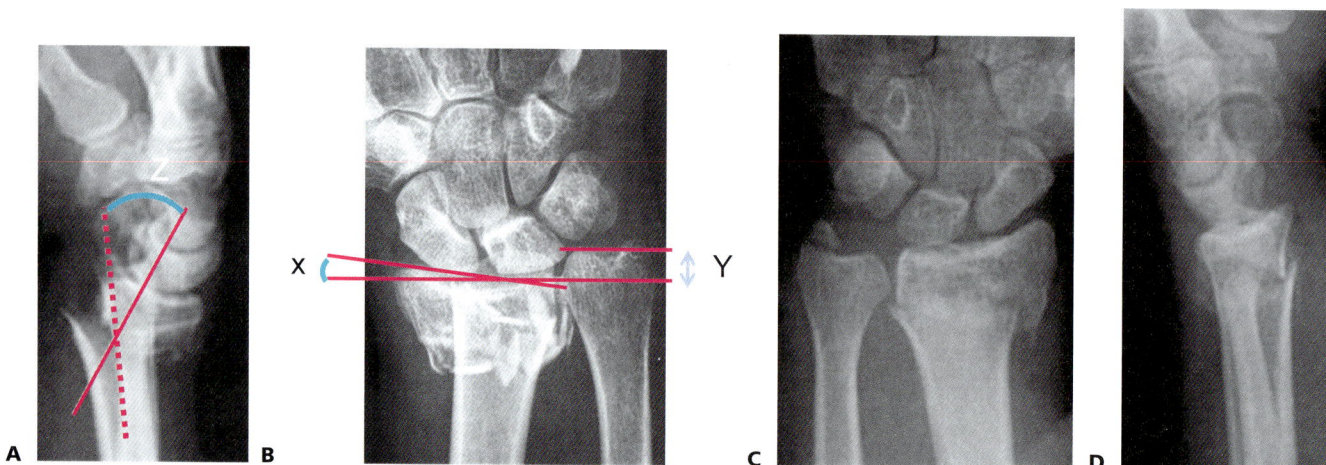

FIG 3 • PA radiograph (**A**) and lateral radiograph (**B**) of a healed distal radius fracture fixed with an intramedullary plate. **C,D.** PA and lateral radiographs showing an unstable metaphyseal distal radius fracture. (**C,D**: copyright Thomas R. Hunt III, MD.)

- After anesthesia has been administered, the arm is placed on a radiolucent hand table (**FIG 4**).
- Motion of the shoulder and elbow should be adequate to allow adequate reduction and positioning.
- Image intensification using fluoroscopy should be performed throughout the procedure to assess fracture reduction and the position of the hardware.

Approach

- The dorsal approach to the distal radius through the third dorsal compartment with subperiosteal elevation of the compartments provides the exposure needed to place a dorsal plate while protecting the extensor tendons from the plate and screws.
  - This approach helps to minimize adhesions and the risk of tenosynovitis and tendon rupture.
- The approach used to place an intramedullary device depends on the nature of the implant and the location and extent of the fracture.
  - Dorsal intramedullary implants are placed through a limited dorsal approach through the third extensor compartment.
  - Radial intramedullary implants are placed through a small radial incision with careful protection of the radial sensory nerve.

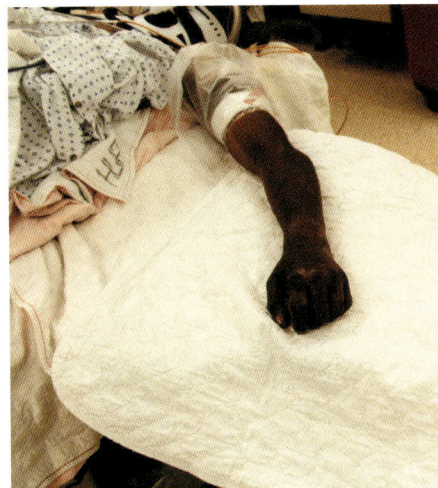

FIG 4 • Patient is positioned supine with arm on a hand table and tourniquet applied on proximal arm.

DORSAL PLATE FIXATION OF DISTAL RADIUS FRACTURES

Incision and Dissection

- The skin incision is centered over the tubercle of Lister (**TECH FIG 1A**).
- The subcutaneous tissues are dissected down to extensor retinaculum, with care to preserve any sensory nerve branches while obtaining hemostasis with bipolar electrocautery (**TECH FIG 1B**).
- The extensor retinaculum is incised just ulnar to the tubercle of Lister, exposing the extensor pollicis longus (EPL) tendon (**TECH FIG 1C**).
- The hematoma is evacuated and the EPL tendon is freed proximally and distally by incising the septa of the third compartment (**TECH FIG 1D**).

- The EPL tendon can then be removed from the third compartment and protected for the rest of the surgical procedure.
- The extensor compartments are subperiosteally elevated using a scalpel in radial and ulnar directions to expose the dorsal cortex of the distal radius (**TECH FIG 1E,F**).
  - If properly maintained, the periosteum of the extensor compartments can be repaired after placement of the fixation device and will serve as a barrier between the dorsal plate and the extensor tendons.
- The tubercle of Lister is almost invariably involved in the fracture and should be completely removed using a rongeur (**TECH FIG 1G**).

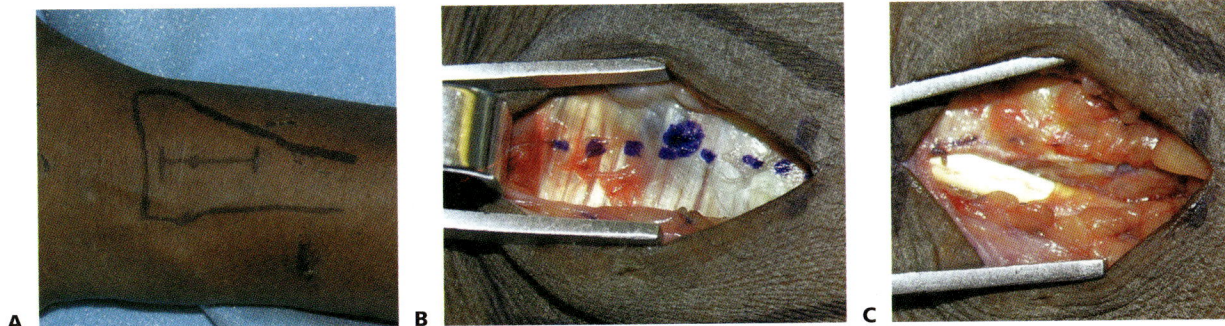

TECH FIG 1 • **A.** Skin incision is drawn in relation to the tubercle of Lister. **B.** Skin incision is carried down to extensor retinaculum. Tubercle of Lister and retinacular incision are drawn. **C.** The retinaculum is incised and the EPL tendon is exposed. Hematoma has already been evacuated. *(continued)*

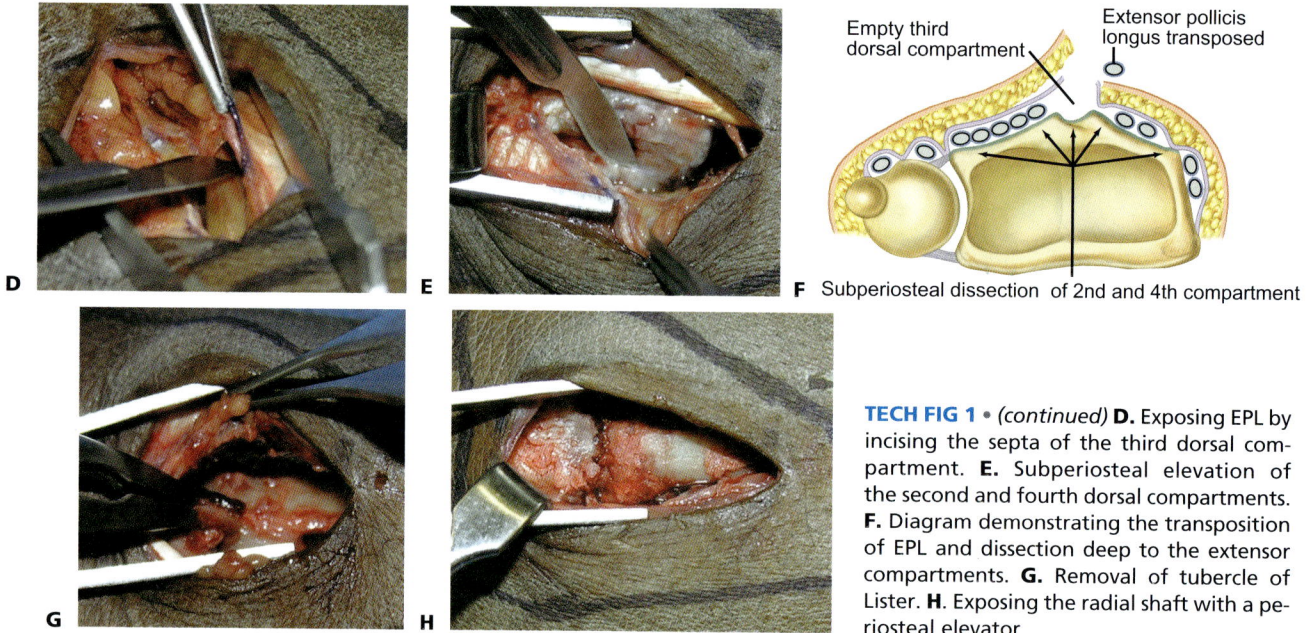

D

E

F Subperiosteal dissection of 2nd and 4th compartment

Empty third dorsal compartment

Extensor pollicis longus transposed

G

H

TECH FIG 1 • *(continued)* **D.** Exposing EPL by incising the septa of the third dorsal compartment. **E.** Subperiosteal elevation of the second and fourth dorsal compartments. **F.** Diagram demonstrating the transposition of EPL and dissection deep to the extensor compartments. **G.** Removal of tubercle of Lister. **H.** Exposing the radial shaft with a periosteal elevator.

- The radius shaft is exposed with a periosteal elevator (**TECH FIG 1H**).

Reduction and Plate Fixation

- Reduction is obtained and confirmed using axial traction and palmar translation of the hand (**TECH FIG 2A**).
- If reduction of articular fragments is needed, the radial portion of the origin of the dorsal radiocarpal ligament can be elevated sharply off the radius to evaluate the articular surfaces.

- Kirschner wires can be used for temporary fixation.
- Bone graft is inserted to support reduced articular fragments.
- The dorsal plate is applied directly on the radius (**TECH FIG 2B**).
- The plate is secured beginning with a bicortical screw in the oval sliding hole.
- Fracture reduction and placement of the plate are confirmed using fluoroscopy.
- The plate is secured to the distal fragment with one or two cancellous screws. The surgeon should avoid placing

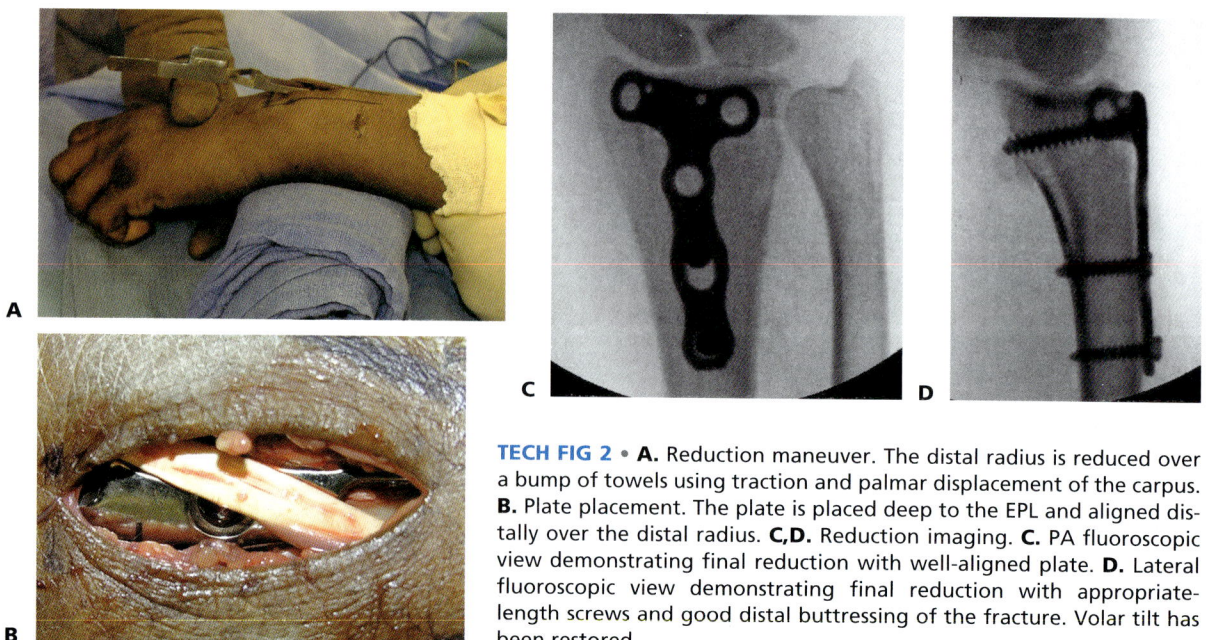

A

B

C

D

TECH FIG 2 • **A.** Reduction maneuver. The distal radius is reduced over a bump of towels using traction and palmar displacement of the carpus. **B.** Plate placement. The plate is placed deep to the EPL and aligned distally over the distal radius. **C,D.** Reduction imaging. **C.** PA fluoroscopic view demonstrating final reduction with well-aligned plate. **D.** Lateral fluoroscopic view demonstrating final reduction with appropriate-length screws and good distal buttressing of the fracture. Volar tilt has been restored.

the distal, ulnar screw if possible as this may irritate the overlying digital extensor tendons in the fourth dorsal compartment.
- Additional cortical screws are added in the radius shaft.
- Reduction and stability are confirmed (**TECH FIG 2C,D**).

Wound Closure

- The wound is copiously irrigated.
- The retinaculum is closed deep to the transposed EPL tendon, incorporating the periosteal layer that forms the floor of the extensor compartments (**TECH FIG 3A**).
- The skin is closed with nylon suture (**TECH FIG 3B**).
- A volar splint is applied.

TECH FIG 3 • A. Retinacular closure. The extensor retinaculum is closed deep to the EPL with a nonabsorbable suture. **B.** Skin closure. The skin is closed with a horizontal mattress stitch to evert the skin edges.

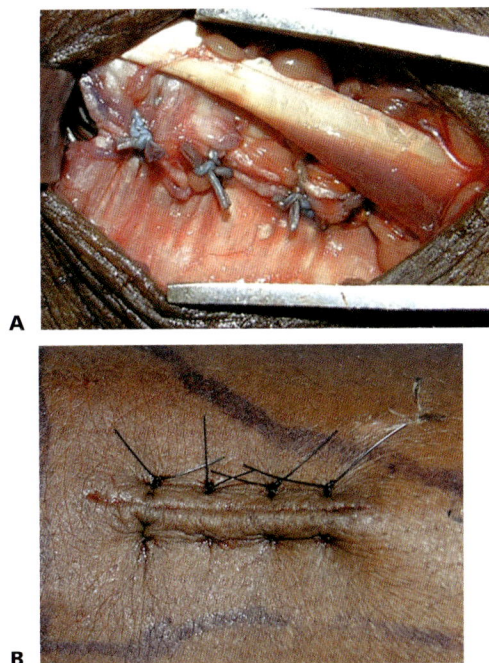

FIXATION OF DISTAL RADIUS FRACTURES USING A DORSAL INTRAMEDULLARY DEVICE (TORNIER)

- The fracture is exposed using a limited version of the incision detailed for placement of a dorsal plate (**TECH FIG 4A**).
  - The extensor retinaculum is incised just ulnar to the tubercle of Lister, exposing the EPL tendon.
  - The EPL tendon is freed proximally and distally by incising the septa of the third compartment.
  - The EPL tendon can then be transposed for the rest of the surgical procedure.
- A scalpel is used to subperiosteally elevate the fourth and portions of the second extensor compartment in radial and ulnar directions.
  - The dorsal cortex of the distal radius is exposed and room is created for seating of the extramedullary portion of the device.
- The tubercle of Lister is removed and an awl is used to create an entry point in the dorsal cortex (**TECH FIG 4B**).
  - This usually involves a portion of the fracture line.
- The canal is rasped until the rasp may be fully seated (**TECH FIG 4C**).
- The implant is placed using the insertion device to control rotation (**TECH FIG 4D**).
  - Fracture reduction is typically achieved as the device is inserted and seated due to its buttress effect and three-point fixation in the canal.
- Lag screws are inserted as required, followed by a cover lock to create fixed angle stability.
- Reduction and stabilization are confirmed radiographically (**TECH FIG 4E,F**).
- Wound closure and splinting are as described above.

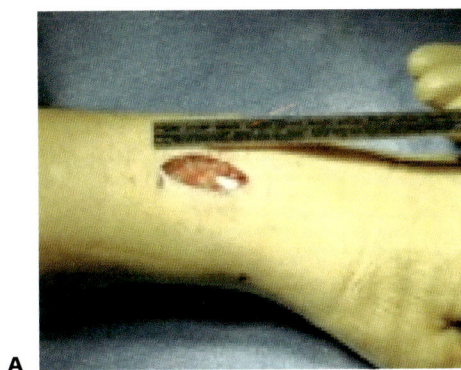

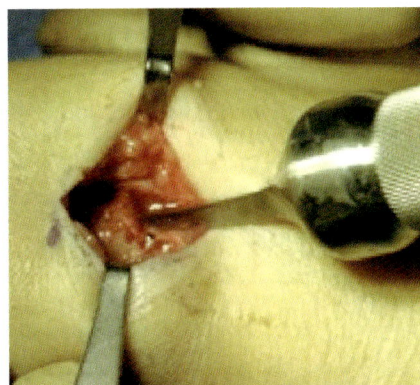

TECH FIG 4 • A. A 2.5-cm dorsal incision is used for exposure. **B.** The awl is inserted through the fracture site after removal of the tubercle of Lister. *(continued)*

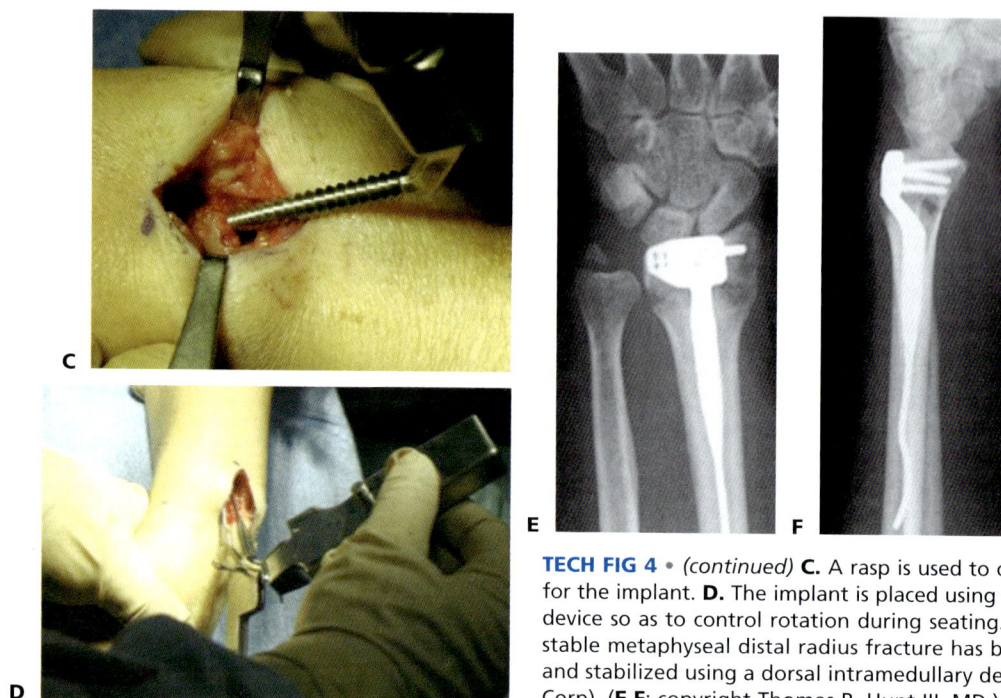

TECH FIG 4 • *(continued)* **C.** A rasp is used to create a path for the implant. **D.** The implant is placed using the insertion device so as to control rotation during seating. **E,F.** An unstable metaphyseal distal radius fracture has been reduced and stabilized using a dorsal intramedullary device (Tornier Corp). (**E,F**: copyright Thomas R. Hunt III, MD.)

FIXATION OF DISTAL RADIUS FRACTURES USING A RADIAL INTRAMEDULLARY DEVICE (WRIGHT MEDICAL)

- A 2- to 3-cm incision is made over the radial styloid, between the first and second extensor compartments.
- Care is taken to protect branches of the radial sensory nerve.
- A cannulated drill is used to penetrate the cortex 2 to 3 mm proximal to the radiocarpal joint line to create the entry point.
- After insertion of a starter awl, the canal is broached sequentially under fluoroscopic guidance to fit the medullary canal.
- The implant is then inserted with the insertion jig, making sure the implant is countersunk into the radial styloid.

- The proximal interlocking screws are then placed using the insertion jig, using small incisions of the dorsal aspect of the forearm.
- The distal interlocking screws are placed last using the insertion jig.
  - Small adjustments to radial height and tilt can be made at this time.
- Reduction and stabilization are confirmed radiographically.
- Wound closure and splinting are as described above.

PEARLS AND PITFALLS

Indications	▪ Determine the direction of fracture stability. ▪ Determine the area and extent of comminution. ▪ Ensure that an acute carpal tunnel syndrome does not exist.
Surgical approach	▪ Incise the extensor retinaculum sharply to allow easier repair. ▪ Expose only the third dorsal compartment. ▪ Remove the tubercle of Lister to allow better plate contouring.
Hardware choice and placement	▪ Choose a low-profile implant system that offers the flexibility needed to stabilize the fracture. ▪ Place the plate distally to ensure buttress effect. ▪ Place the oval plate hole screw initially. ▪ Do not place the plate distal to the dorsal lip of the distal radius. ▪ Avoid placing the distal, ulnar screw. ▪ Although titanium implants and their particulate debris have been implicated in the development of tenosynovitis and other tendon pathology, there is no clear scientific evidence to substantiate these claims.
Postoperative management	▪ Avoid casting for long periods. ▪ Encourage early active range of motion of the wrist and fingers. ▪ Avoid using a sling to prevent unnecessary shoulder and elbow stiffness. ▪ Do not begin strengthening until range of motion is restored.

POSTOPERATIVE CARE

- Postoperatively the patient is placed in a bulky dressing that allows motion of the digits, elbow, and shoulder. A volar resting splint may be used to support the wrist if there is any concern about fixation strength.
- The patient is encouraged to begin finger range-of-motion exercises immediately after surgery.
- Seven to 10 days after surgery the sutures are removed, Steri-Strips are applied, and the incision is allowed to get wet.
- The patient is evaluated by an occupational therapist, who provides a thermoplastic splint, and can start active and active-assisted range-of-motion exercises depending on fracture stability.
- When the fracture heals at about 6 weeks, gentle passive range of motion and strengthening may be started.

OUTCOMES

- Dorsal plating has recently been shown biomechanically to be stronger and stiffer than volar plating for dorsally unstable fractures.[12]
- Dorsal plating has been associated with a higher complication rate than other means of stabilization.[2,9,10]
  - Extensor tenosynovitis and tendon rupture have been prevalent in the past, mainly due to bulky implants.
- There has been renewed interest in dorsal plating of the distal radius as it has been shown to have a low rate of tendon-related complications with the use of low-profile, anatomic implants.[4,10,11]
- Clinical reports have suggested that low-profile systems are more important in satisfactory outcomes for dorsal plating, with a much lower rate of complications.[10]
- Fixation with low-profile dorsal plates can result in at least 80% of contralateral wrist range of motion, about 80% to 90% of grip strength, and over 90% pinch strength, with minimal risk of tendon rupture.[4,11]

COMPLICATIONS

- Infection (pin tract or deep)
- Injury to tendons, vessels, and nerves
- Stiffness
- Posttraumatic arthritis
- Weakness in grip or pinch
- Tenosynovitis and tendon ruptures
- Malunion or nonunion
- Compartment syndrome
- Carpal tunnel syndrome
- Late tendon rupture, potentially related to implant design and material
- Hardware failure
- Complex regional pain syndrome type I

DISCLOSURE

Dr. Beredjiklian is a stockholder with and consultant for Tornier, Inc.

REFERENCES

1. Glowacki KA, Weiss AP, Akelman E. Distal radius fractures: concepts and complications. Orthopedics 1996;19:601–608.
2. Grewal R, Perey B, Wilmink M, Stothers K. A randomized prospective study on the treatment of intra-articular distal radius fractures: open reduction and internal fixation with dorsal plating versus mini open reduction, percutaneous fixation, and external fixation. J Hand Surg Am 2005;30A:764–772.
3. Jupiter JB, Fernandez DL. Comparative classification for fractures of the distal end of the radius. J. Hand Surg Am 1997;22A:563–571.
4. Kamath AF, Zurakowski D, Day CS. Low-profile dorsal plating for dorsally angulated distal radius fractures: an outcomes study. J Hand Surg Am 2006;31A:1061–1067.
5. Katz MA, Beredjiklian PK, Bozentka DJ, et al. Computed tomography scanning of intra-articular distal radius fractures: does it influence treatment? J Hand Surg Am 2001;26A:412–421.
6. Knirk JL, Jupiter JB. Intra-articular fractures of the distal end of the radius in young adults. J Bone Joint Surg am 1986;68A:647–659.
7. Lafontaine M, Hardy D, Delince P. Stability assessment of distal radial fractures. Injury 1989;20:208–210.
8. Mackenney PJ, McQueen MM, Elton R. Prediction of instability in distal radial fractures. J Bone Joint Surg Am 2006;88A:1944–1951.
9. Nana AD, Joshi A, Lichtman DM. Plating of the distal radius. J Am Acad Orthop Surg 2005;13:159–171.
10. Rozental TD, Beredjiklian PK, Bozentka DJ. Functional outcome and complications following two types of dorsal plating for unstable fractures of the distal part of the radius. J Bone Joint Surg Am 2003;85A:1956–1960.
11. Simic PM, Robison J, Gardner MJ, et al. Treatment of distal radius fractures with a low-profile dorsal plating system: an outcomes assessment. Hand Surg Am 2006;31A:382–386.
12. Trease C, McIff T, Toby EB. Locking versus nonlocking T-plates for dorsal and volar fixation of dorsally comminuted distal radius fractures: a biomechanical study. Hand Surg Am 2005;30A:756–763.
13. Trumble TE, Culp R, Hanel DP, et al. Intra-articular fractures of the distal aspect of the radius. J Bone Joint Surg Am 1998;80A:582–600.

Chapter 12

Volar Plating of Distal Radius Fractures

John J. Fernandez

DEFINITION

- Distal radius fractures are defined by their involvement of the metaphysis of the distal radius.
- They are assessed on the basis of fracture pattern, alignment, and stability:
  - Articular versus nonarticular
  - Reducible versus irreducible
  - Stable versus unstable
- Irreducible or unstable fractures require surgical reduction and stable fixation.
- Volar plating historically has been the method of choice for volar shear-type fractures.
  - Recently developed fixed-angle plates have now made it a preferred method of fixation for most types of distal radius fractures.

ANATOMY

- The distal radius serves as a buttress for the proximal carpus, transmitting 75% to 80% of its forces into the forearm.
  - The remaining 20% to 25% of force is transmitted through the distal ulna and the triangular fibrocartilage complex (TFCC).
- Dorsally
  - The distal radius is the origin for the dorsal radiocarpal ligament.
  - It is the floor of the fibro-osseous extensor tendon compartments and includes Lister's tubercle, assisting in extensor pollicis longus function (**FIG 1A**).
  - The extensor tendons are in immediate contact with the dorsal surface of the distal radius.
- Volarly
  - The distal radius is the origin for the extrinsic ligaments of the carpus, including the radioscaphocapitate ligament.
  - It also is the origin of the pronator quadratus.
  - The flexor tendons are separated from the distal radius by the pronator quadratus.
- Ulnarly
  - The distal radius is the origin for the radial triangular fibrocartilage (**FIG 1A**).
  - It also contains the sigmoid notch, which articulates with the head of the distal ulna, contributing to forearm rotation.
- Distally
  - The surface is divided into a triangular, radioscaphoid fossa and a square, radiolunate fossa articulating with the respective carpal bones (**FIG 1B**).
- The distal articular surface is inclined approximately 22 degrees ulnarly in the coronal plane and 11 degrees volarly in the sagittal plane (**FIG 1C,D**).
- The metaphysis is defined by the distal radius within a length of the articular surface that is equivalent to the widest portion of the entire wrist.

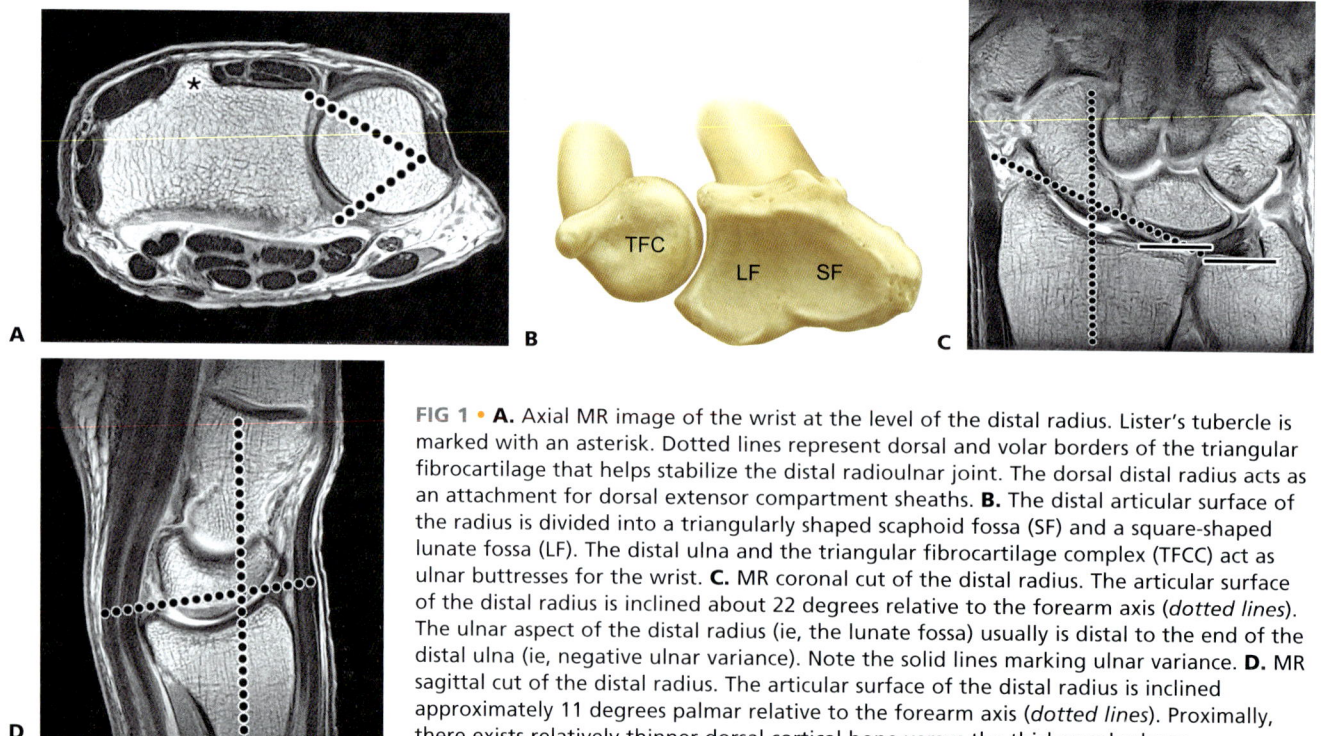

FIG 1 • **A.** Axial MR image of the wrist at the level of the distal radius. Lister's tubercle is marked with an asterisk. Dotted lines represent dorsal and volar borders of the triangular fibrocartilage that helps stabilize the distal radioulnar joint. The dorsal distal radius acts as an attachment for dorsal extensor compartment sheaths. **B.** The distal articular surface of the radius is divided into a triangularly shaped scaphoid fossa (SF) and a square-shaped lunate fossa (LF). The distal ulna and the triangular fibrocartilage complex (TFCC) act as ulnar buttresses for the wrist. **C.** MR coronal cut of the distal radius. The articular surface of the distal radius is inclined about 22 degrees relative to the forearm axis (*dotted lines*). The ulnar aspect of the distal radius (ie, the lunate fossa) usually is distal to the end of the distal ulna (ie, negative ulnar variance). Note the solid lines marking ulnar variance. **D.** MR sagittal cut of the distal radius. The articular surface of the distal radius is inclined approximately 11 degrees palmar relative to the forearm axis (*dotted lines*). Proximally, there exists relatively thinner dorsal cortical bone versus the thicker volar bone.

- The dorsal cortical bone is less substantial than the volar cortical bone, contributing to the characteristic dorsal-bending fracture pattern of distal radius fractures.

PATHOGENESIS

- The mechanism of injury in a distal radius fracture is an axial force across the wrist, with the pattern of injury determined by bone density, the position of the wrist, and the magnitude and direction of force.
- Most distal radius fractures result from falls with the wrist extended and pronated, which places a dorsal bending moment across the distal radius.
  - Relatively weaker, thinner dorsal bone collapses under compression, whereas stronger volar bone fails under tension, resulting in a characteristic "triangle" of bone comminution with the apex volar and greater comminution dorsal.
- Other possible mechanisms form a basis for some fracture classifications such as the one proposed by Jupiter and Fernandez.[5]
  - Bending
  - Compression
  - Shear
  - Avulsion
  - Combinations
- Articular involvement and its severity are the basis of some fracture classifications, such as the AO[9] and Melone[8] classifications.
- Articular involvement splits the distal radius into distinct fragments separate from the radius shaft (**FIG 2**):
  - Scaphoid fossa fragment
  - Lunate fossa fragment. Further comminution can split the lunate fossa fragment into dorsal and volar segments, creating the so-called four-part fracture.

NATURAL HISTORY

- Clinical outcome usually, but not always, correlates with deformity.
  - Variable residual deformity can be tolerated best by individuals with fewer functional demands.

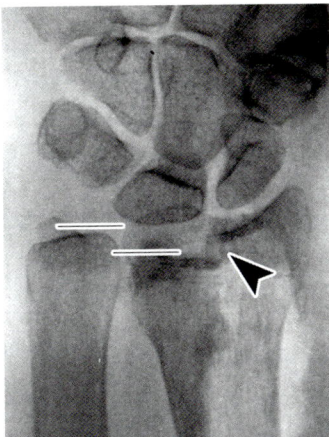

FIG 2 • The arrowhead points to the articular split. Articular displacement of the scaphoid fossa fragment radially and the lunate fossa fragment ulnarly is apparent, as is significant shortening (ulnar positive variance) as outlined by the lines.

- As wrist deformity increases, physiologic function is progressively altered.
  - Intra-articular displacement of 1 to 2 mm results in an increased risk of osteoarthritis.[3,6]
  - Radial shortening of 3 to 5 mm or more results in increased loading of the ulnar complex.[1,12]
  - Dorsal angulation greater than 10 degrees shifts contact forces to the dorsal scaphoid fossa and the ulnar complex, causing increased disability.[13,16]
- The incidence of associated intracarpal injuries increases with fracture severity. Such injuries can account for poor outcomes. These injuries often are not recognized at first, with the result that treatment is delayed.[4,14]
  - Triangular fibrocartilage (TFC) tears
  - Scapholunate and lunotriquetral ligament tears
  - Chondral injuries involving the carpal surfaces
  - Distal radioulnar joint injury
  - Distal ulna fractures
- By predicting the stability of a distal radius fracture, deformity and its complications can be minimized. Several risk factors have been suggested by LaFontaine et al[7] and others. The presence of three or more indicates instability:
  - Dorsal angulation greater than 20 degrees
  - Dorsal comminution
  - Intra-articular extension
  - Associated ulna fracture
  - Patient age over 60 years

PATIENT HISTORY AND PHYSICAL FINDINGS

- The mechanism of injury should be sought, to assist in assessing the energy and level of destruction.
- Associated injuries are not uncommon and should be carefully ruled out.
  - Injuries to the hand, carpus, and proximal arm, including other fractures or dislocations
  - Injuries to other extremities or the head, neck, and torso
- Establish the patient's functional and occupational demands.
- Document co-existing medical conditions that may affect healing, such as osteoporosis or diabetes.
- Determine possible risk factors for anesthesia and surgery, such as cardiac disease.
- The physical examination should document the following:
  - Condition of surrounding soft tissues (ie, skin and subcutaneous tissues)
  - Quality of vascular perfusion and pulses
  - Integrity of nerve function
  - Sensory two-point discrimination or threshold sensory testing
  - Motor function of intrinsic, thenar, and hypothenar muscles of the hand
- Examination of the distal ulna, TFCC, and distal radioulnar joint should rule out disruption and instability.
- Reliable physical examination of the carpus often is difficult, making radiographic review even more critical and follow-up examinations important.

IMAGING AND OTHER DIAGNOSTIC STUDIES

- Imaging establishes fracture severity, helps determine stability, and guides the operative approach and choice of fixation.

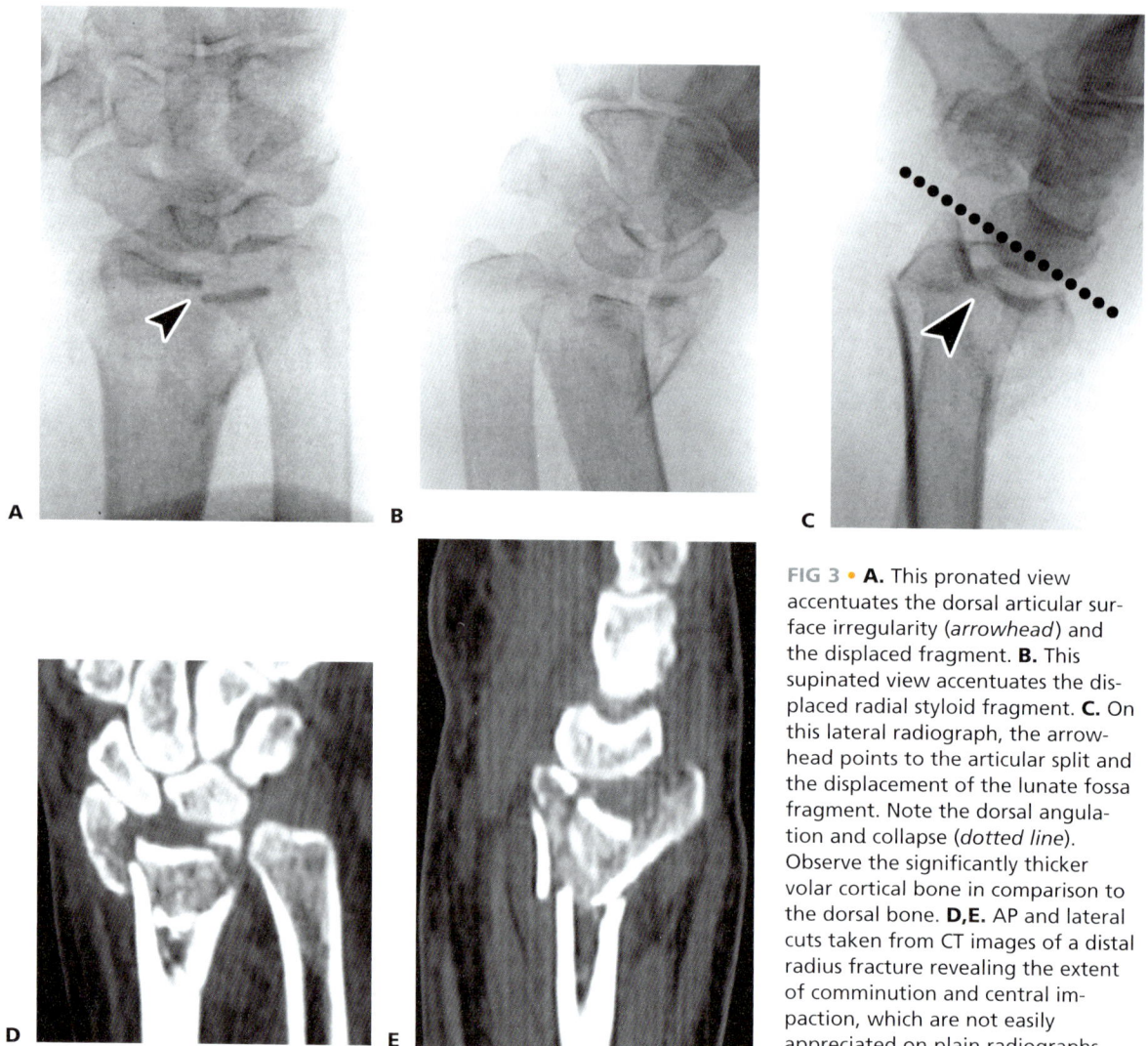

FIG 3 • **A.** This pronated view accentuates the dorsal articular surface irregularity (*arrowhead*) and the displaced fragment. **B.** This supinated view accentuates the displaced radial styloid fragment. **C.** On this lateral radiograph, the arrowhead points to the articular split and the displacement of the lunate fossa fragment. Note the dorsal angulation and collapse (*dotted line*). Observe the significantly thicker volar cortical bone in comparison to the dorsal bone. **D,E.** AP and lateral cuts taken from CT images of a distal radius fracture revealing the extent of comminution and central impaction, which are not easily appreciated on plain radiographs.

- Plain radiographs should be obtained before and after reduction: PA, lateral, and two separate oblique views.
  - Oblique views, in particular, help evaluate articular involvement, particularly the lunate fossa fragment (**FIG 3A,B**).
  - The lateral view should be modified with the forearm inclined 15 to 20 degrees to best visualize the articular surface (**FIG 3C**; see Tech Fig 5BC).
- Fluoroscopic evaluation can be useful, because it gives a complete circumferential view of the wrist and, with traction applied, can help evaluate injuries of the carpus.
- CT helps define intra-articular involvement and helps detect small or impacted fragments, which may not be apparent on plain radiographs, particularly those involving the central portion of the distal radius (**FIG 3D,E**).

DIFFERENTIAL DIAGNOSIS

- Diagnosis is directly confirmed by radiographs.
- Associated and contributory injuries should always be considered.
  - Pathologic fracture (eg, related to tumor, infection)
  - Associated injuries to the carpus (eg, scaphoid fracture, scapholunate ligament injury)

NONOPERATIVE MANAGEMENT

- Nonoperative treatment is reserved for distal radius fractures that are reducible and stable based on the criteria previously discussed.
- The goal of nonoperative treatment is to immobilize the wrist using a method that will maintain acceptable alignment until the fracture is healed.
  - Radial inclination greater than 10 degrees
  - Ulnar variance less than 4 mm positive
  - Palmar tilt less than 15 degrees dorsal or 20 degrees volar
  - Articular congruity less than 2-mm gap or step-off

SURGICAL MANAGEMENT

- The goal of operative treatment is to achieve acceptable alignment and stable fixation.
- Various methods of fixation are available: pins, external fixators, dorsal plates, intramedullary devices, and volar plates.

Preoperative Planning

- The standard preoperative medical and anesthesia evaluation for concurrent medical problems is done.

■ Discontinue blood thinning medications (anticoagulants and nonsteroidal anti-inflammatory drugs).

■ Request necessary equipment, including fluoroscopic and power equipment.

■ Confirm the plate fixation system to be used and check the equipment before beginning surgery for completeness (ie, all appropriate drills, plates, and screws).

■ Have a contingency plan or additional fixation (external fixator, bone graft, or bone graft substitute).

■ Review previous radiographic studies.

■ Consider use of a regional anesthetic for postoperative pain control.

Positioning

■ Place the patient in the supine position with the affected extremity on an arm table.

■ Apply an upper arm tourniquet, preferably within the sterile field.

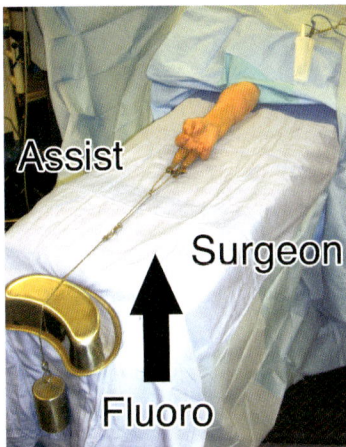

FIG 4 • Traction is applied over the arm table with finger traps and hanging weights. The surgeon sits on the volar side, and the assistant on the dorsal side. Fluoroscopy can be brought in from any direction, but preferably from the side adjacent or the opposite surgeon.

■ Incorporate weights or a traction system to apply distraction across the fracture (**FIG 4**).

■ The surgeon is seated on the side, toward the patient's head, particularly if he or she is right-hand dominant.

■ The assistant is seated opposite the surgeon.

■ The fluoroscopy unit is brought in from the end or corner of the table.

Approach

■ Dorsal exposure allows for direct visualization of the articular surface when necessary.

■ Fracture comminution is more severe dorsally, making overall alignment more difficult to judge.

■ The thicker volar cortex is less comminuted, allowing for more precise reduction and buttressing of bone fragments.

■ Sometimes both dorsal and volar exposures may be necessary to achieve articular congruency and volar reduction and fixation, respectively.

■ An extended volar–ulnar exposure may be necessary to perform a carpal tunnel release if indicated.

■ The techniques described in this chapter use the volar approach to distal radius, as described by Henry (**FIG 5**).

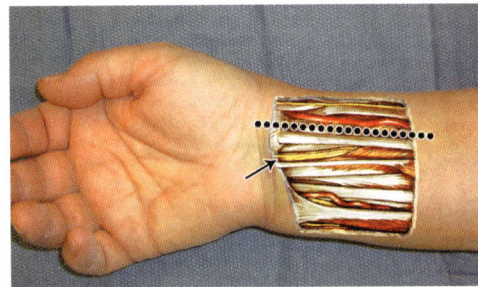

FIG 5 • The volar incision is represented by the dotted line just proximal to the wrist flexion creases and radial to the flexor carpi radialis longus. Care is exercised to avoid dissection ulnar to the flexor carpi radialis, because the palmar cutaneous nerve branch of the median nerve (*arrow*) is at risk.

VOLAR FIXED-ANGLE PLATE FIXATION OF THE DISTAL RADIUS

Incision and Dissection

■ Palpate the flexor carpi radialis tendon and make a 4- to 8-cm longitudinal incision from the proximal wrist flexion crease, extending proximally along the radial border of the flexor carpi radialis tendon.

   ■ If the incision must cross the wrist flexion creases, use a zigzag incision in that area.

■ Carefully avoid the palmar cutaneous branch of the median nerve along the ulnar side of the flexor carpi radialis within 10 cm of the wrist flexion crease.

   ■ Branches of the dorsal radial sensory nerve and lateral antebrachial cutaneous nerve sometimes appear along the path of the incision and also need to be protected.

■ At the distal end of the incision, protect the palmar branch of the radial artery to the deep arch.

   ■ It usually is not necessary to dissect out the radial artery (**TECH FIG 1A**).

■ Incise the anterior sheath of the flexor carpi radialis tendon and retract the tendon ulnarly to help protect the median nerve (**TECH FIG 1B**).

■ Incise the posterior sheath of the flexor carpi radialis tendon.

   ■ The deep tissues likely will bulge out from the pressure of swelling and fracture hematoma.

   ■ The median nerve lies within the subcutaneous tissues along the ulnar portion of the wound (**TECH FIG 1C,D**).

   ■ The flexor pollicis longus tendon sits along the radial margin of the wound.

■ Using blunt dissection with a gauze-covered finger, sweep the tendons and the nerve ulnarly.

   ■ A self-retaining retractor is carefully placed between the radial artery radially and the tendons and median nerve ulnarly.

TECHNIQUES

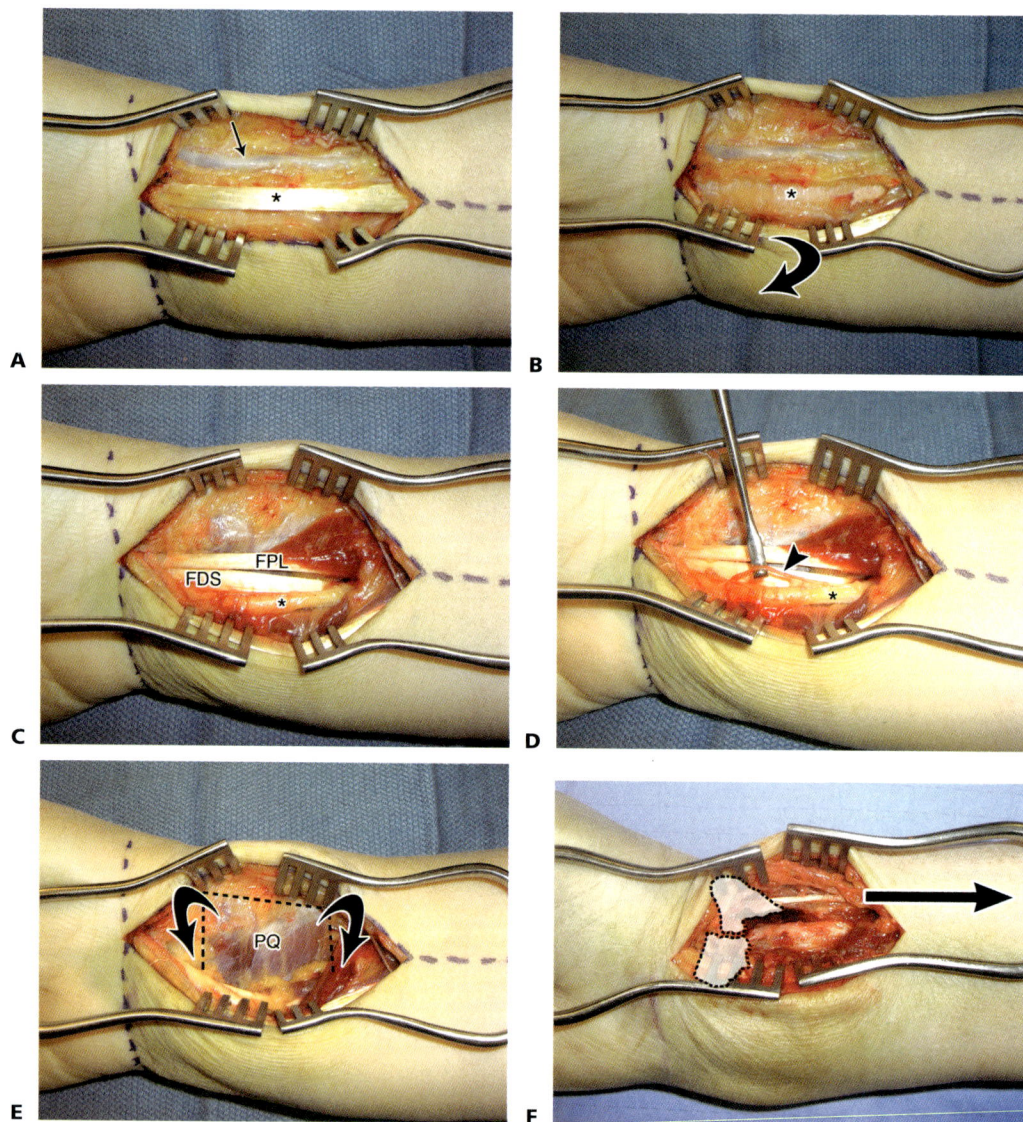

TECH FIG 1 • **A.** The interval between the radial artery (*arrow*) and the flexor carpi radialis tendon (*) is seen. **B.** The posterior sheath (*) of the flexor carpi radialis is visible after retracting the flexor carpi radialis ulnarly (*arrow*). Be careful during deeper dissection, because swelling and hematoma may distort the position of the median nerve beneath the sheath. **C.** Following incision in the flexor carpi radialis posterior sheath, the deep tendons are visible, including the flexor pollicis longus (FPL) and the flexor digitorum superficialis of the index finger (FDS). The median nerve also is visible (*). **D.** The palmar cutaneous nerve branches of the median nerve (*arrow*) and median nerve (*asterisk*) are both at risk for injury during this approach. Be careful regarding placement of retractors and during dissection and plate placement. **E.** The pronator quadratus (PQ) is incised distally, radially, and proximally and then reflected ulnarly after dissection off the volar distal radius. **F.** The brachio-radialis (*arrow*) can be a deforming force, especially in comminuted fractures and in those for which treatment has been delayed. This tendon can be released if necessary.

- The pronator quadratus is now visualized at the floor of the wound.
- Incise the pronator quadratus at its radial insertion, leaving fascial tissue on either side to aid in closure. Also, determine the proximal and distal extent of the muscle, and make horizontal incisions at both of those points (**TECH FIG 1E**).
  - The distal margin of the pronator quadratus attaches along the distal volar lip of the distal radius, along the "teardrop."

- The radial margin is in proximity to the tendons of the first dorsal compartment and the brachio-radialis.
- Subperiosteally dissect the pronator quadratus off the volar surface of the distal radius as an ulnarly based flap with a knife or elevator.
- Retract the pronator ulnarly with the flexor tendons and median nerve.
- Particularly if significant shortening of radial-sided fracture fragments has occurred, incise the broad insertion

of the brachioradialis to eliminate the deforming force (**TECH FIG 1F**).

- Release the first dorsal compartment and retract the tendons before releasing the brachioradialis.
- Alternatively, Z-lengthen the brachioradialis tendon to allow for repair at the completion of the case.

Fracture Reduction and Provisional Fixation

- Apply a lobster-claw clamp around the radius shaft at a perpendicular angle to the volar surface at the most proximal portion of the wound (**TECH FIG 2A**).
  - This allows for excellent control of the proximal shaft for rotation and translation.
  - It also provides an excellent counterforce when correcting the dorsal angulation collapse.
- With the fracture now exposed, apply traction distally to distract and disimpact the fragments.

- Carefully clean the fracture of any interposed muscle, fascia, hematoma, or callus while maintaining the bony contours.
- In the case of significant volar comminution, reduce and provisionally stabilize the fragments with K-wires.
  - Take plate positioning into account when placing these K-wires.
- The articular surface is first reduced, if necessary.
- Under fluoroscopic guidance, manipulate the articular fragments through the fracture with a periosteal elevator, osteotome, or K-wires (**TECH FIG 2B,C**).
  - Longitudinal traction is important during this reduction phase. It can be performed by an assistant or using cross-table weights and finger-traps.
  - A dorsal exposure is performed at this stage if there is significant impaction, particularly centrally, that cannot be corrected using the extra-articular technique described here.

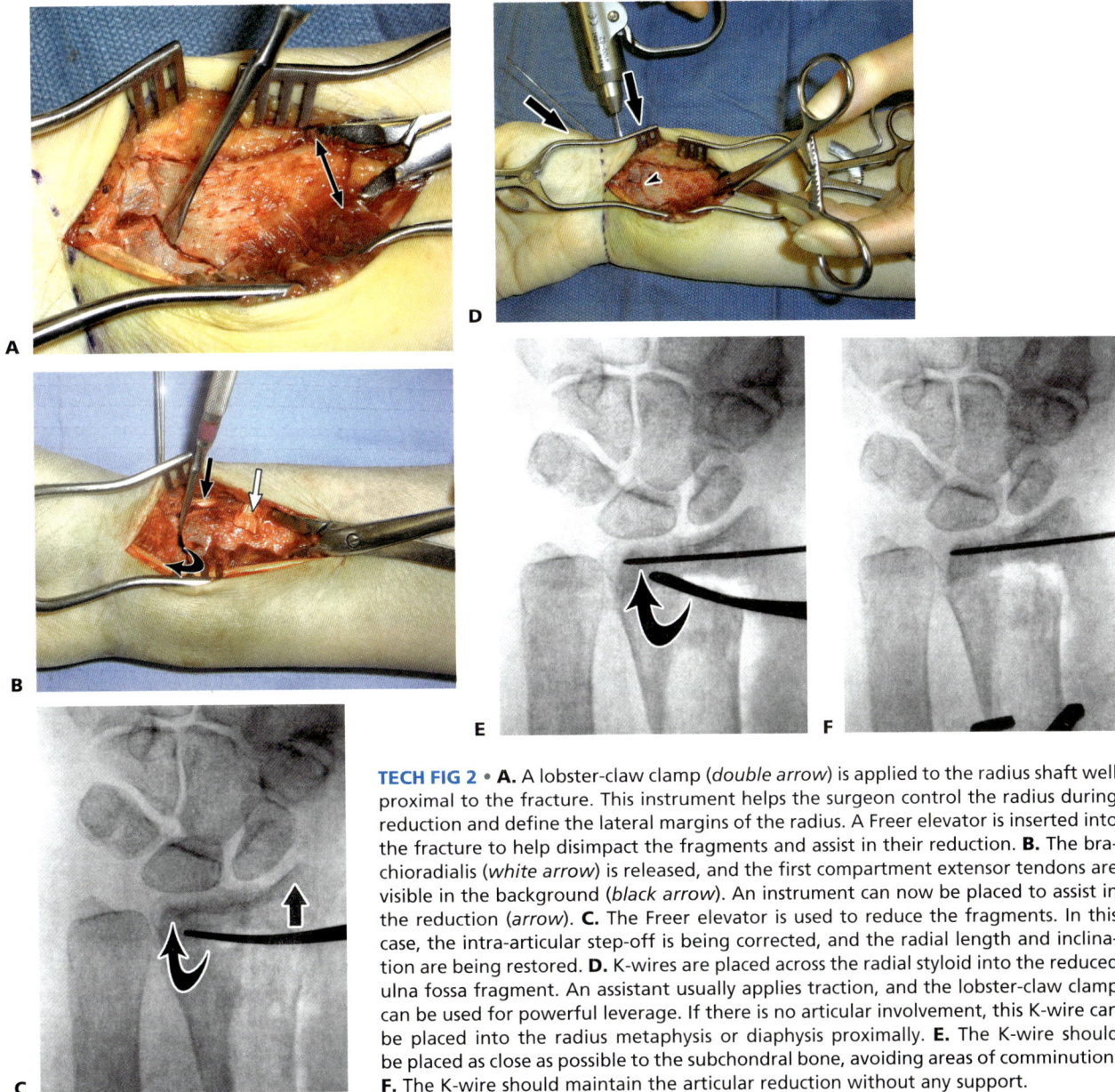

TECH FIG 2 • A. A lobster-claw clamp (*double arrow*) is applied to the radius shaft well proximal to the fracture. This instrument helps the surgeon control the radius during reduction and define the lateral margins of the radius. A Freer elevator is inserted into the fracture to help disimpact the fragments and assist in their reduction. **B.** The brachioradialis (*white arrow*) is released, and the first compartment extensor tendons are visible in the background (*black arrow*). An instrument can now be placed to assist in the reduction (*arrow*). **C.** The Freer elevator is used to reduce the fragments. In this case, the intra-articular step-off is being corrected, and the radial length and inclination are being restored. **D.** K-wires are placed across the radial styloid into the reduced ulna fossa fragment. An assistant usually applies traction, and the lobster-claw clamp can be used for powerful leverage. If there is no articular involvement, this K-wire can be placed into the radius metaphysis or diaphysis proximally. **E.** The K-wire should be placed as close as possible to the subchondral bone, avoiding areas of comminution. **F.** The K-wire should maintain the articular reduction without any support.

TECHNIQUES

- Place K-wires from the radial styloid fragment into the lunate fossa fragment to maintain the articular reduction (**TECH FIG 2D**).
  - The K-wires should be placed as close as possible to the subchondral plate (**TECH FIG 2E,F**).
- Once the distal articular reduction is complete, reduce the distal radius as a single unit to the radius shaft.
- Insert K-wires as required to maintain the provisional reduction between the distal fragments and the proximal shaft fragment.
  - If radial collapse and translation are prominent, a large K-wire can be introduced into the radial portion of the fracture and advanced proximally and ulnarly to behave like an intrafocal pin and provide a radial buttress by pushing the distal fragment ulnarly.
  - A similar technique can be applied through the dorsal fracture to assist in maintaining the palmar tilt correction.

Plate Application

- Apply a fixed-angle volar plate to the volar surface of the distal radius and shaft. Position the plate to accommodate for the unique design characteristics of the plating system as well as the location of the fracture fragments.
  - Each plating system has unique characteristics that determine its optimal placement.
  - Ideally, the plate should be placed as close to the articular margin as possible without the distal locking pegs or screws penetrating the joint.
  - If the fracture has not yet been fully reduced, this must be taken into account when placing the device.
- Clamp the previously applied lobster claw to the proximal portion of the plate to keep the plate centralized on the radius shaft.
- Place provisional K-wires through the plate to maintain position (**TECH FIG 3**). Then fluoroscopically confirm proper plate position in both the distal–proximal and radioulnar directions.
  - Proper alignment of the plate can be determined only using a true anteroposterior (AP) image in which the distal radioulnar joint is well visualized.

- The K-wires allow for fine adjustment in plate position before committing to insertion of a screw.
- Drill and insert a provisional screw in the oblong hole in the plate.
  - If the bone is osteopenic, a screw longer than the initial measurement should be placed to ensure that both cortices are engaged. Otherwise, the plate may not be held securely, and the reduction will be compromised. After the remaining screws have been secured, this screw can be replaced with one of the appropriate length.
- Insert at least one additional proximal screw and remove the provisional K-wires holding the plate in place.

Distal Fragment Reduction

- Once the proximal plate has been secured, execute any additional reduction needed.
  - A well-designed plate serves as an excellent buttress for correction of the palmar tilt (**TECH FIG 4A**).
- Apply counterforce through the lobster-claw clamp in a dorsal direction while the distal hand and wrist are translated palmarly and flexed (**TECH FIG 4B**).
  - This maneuver reduces the distal radius to the plate, effectively restoring volar tilt by pushing the lunate against the volar lip of the distal radius (**TECH FIG 4C,D**).
- Additional distraction and ulnar deviation correct radial collapse and loss of radial inclination.

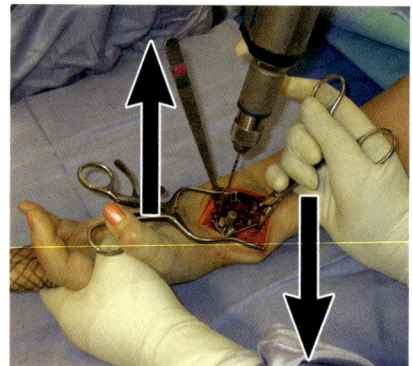

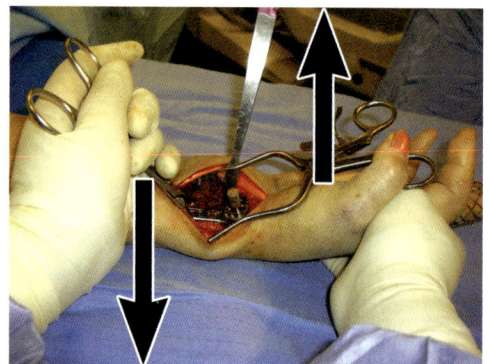

TECH FIG 4 • A. The final reduction is performed with traction on the hand and with the radius held proximally with a clamp. Once the reduction is confirmed radiographically, the assistant places the distal screws or K-wires. **B.** The hand is translated (not appreciably flexed) palmarly while the radius shaft is held with the clamp. *(continued)*

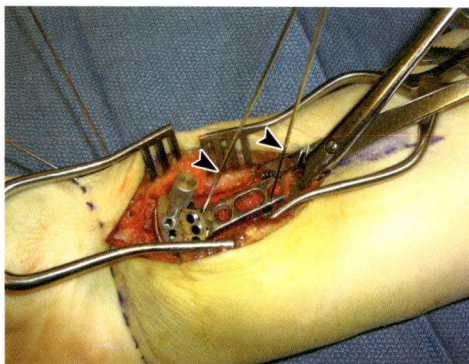

TECH FIG 3 • Keep the plate centered on the radius and as distal as possible. The lobster-claw clamp helps keep the plate centered. K-wires (*arrows*) are helpful as provision fixation until alignment can be confirmed radiographically and screws placed.

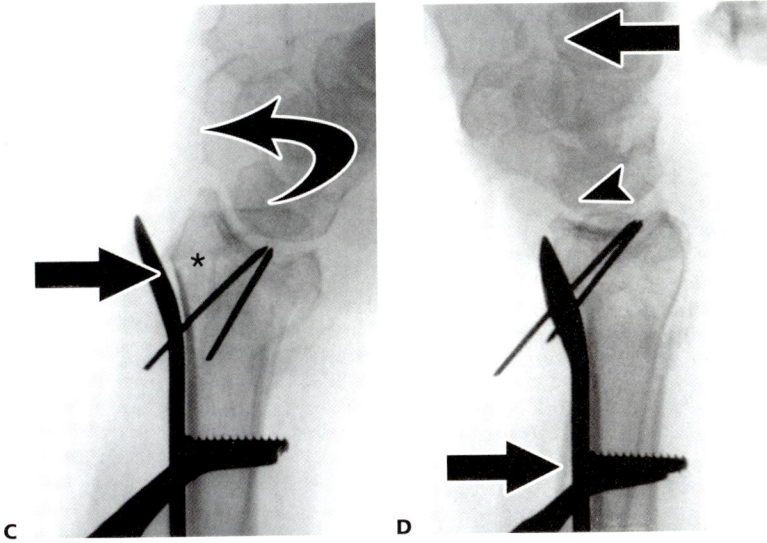

C **D**

TECH FIG 4 • *(continued)* Prereduction (**C**) and postreduction (**D**) radiographs demonstrating the palmar translation reduction maneuver. The volar plate acts as a strong buttress (*arrow*), allowing the translated lunate to push on the volar radius (*) and correct the dorsal angulation deformity.

Plate Fixation

- While the reduction is held, drill the holes in the distal plate (**TECH FIG 5A**).
  - Some plate systems allow for provisional fixation using K-wires placed through the distal plate.
  - Do not penetrate the dorsal distal radius with the drill, to protect the dorsal extensor tendons.
- Drill and place the distal ulnar screws first and then proceed radially and proximally.
- Judge the placement of all distal screws or pegs precisely using fluoroscopic imaging in multiple planes.
  - Perform a "true" lateral view of the wrist with the x-ray beam at a 20-degree angle to the radius shaft

(**TECH FIG 5B,C**). This is facilitated by lifting the wrist off the table with the elbow maintained on the table and the forearm at a 20-degree angle to the table (**TECH FIG 5D,E**).
  - Lister's tubercle can be mistaken for the dorsal cortex, resulting in screws that are too long.
  - The extensor pollicis longus is at greatest risk of injury from a protruding screw.
- Sequentially insert the remaining distal screws or pegs, followed by the remaining proximal plate screws (**TECH FIG 5F**).
- If necessary, add bone graft or bone graft substitute around the plate into the fracture site or through a small dorsal incision.

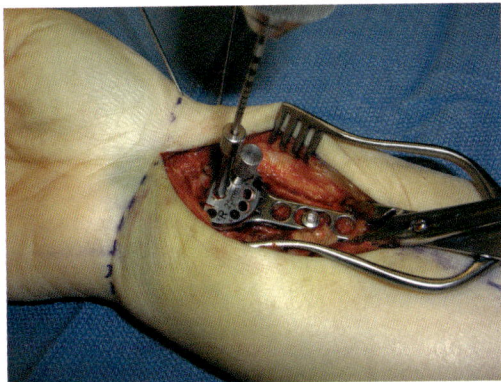

A

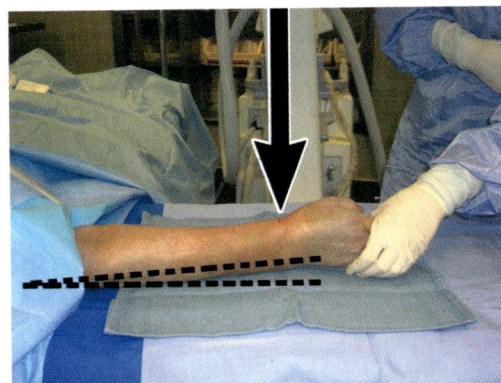

D

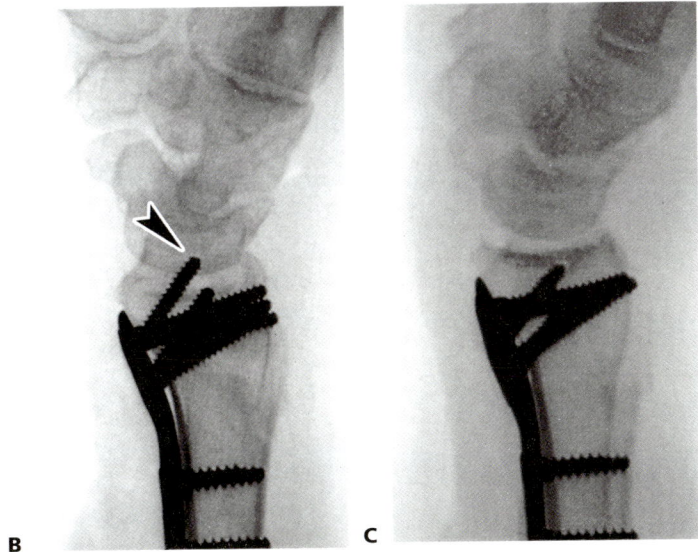

B **C**

TECH FIG 5 • **A.** The remaining holes can now be drilled and screws placed where needed. **B.** This screw (*arrow*) looks as though it has penetrated the joint when in reality it is simply the angle of the radiographic beam that throws its projection into the joint. **C.** A true lateral view of the distal radius is necessary to judge placement of the radial screws. **D.** A radiograph is being taken with the wrist perpendicular to the x-ray beam (*arrow*). This is not a true lateral image, because the distal surface of the radius is inclined 20 degrees radially. *(continued)*

TECHNIQUES

E

F

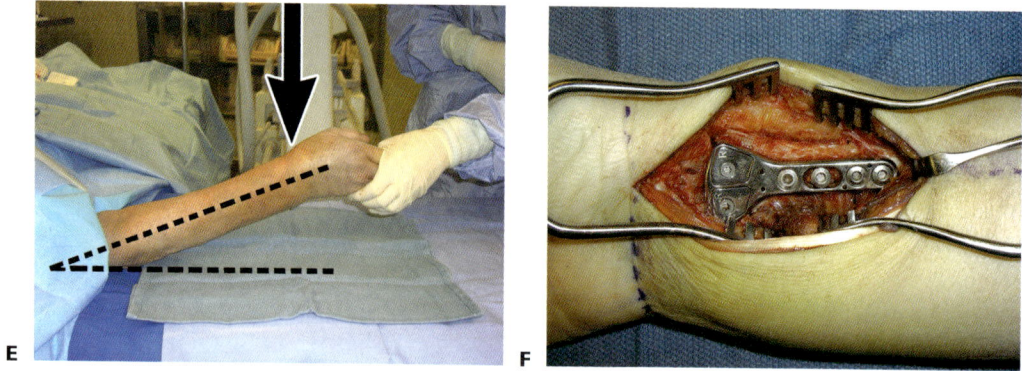

TECH FIG 5 • *(continued)* **E.** By lifting the hand and wrist 20 degrees off the table, a "true" lateral image can be achieved. The x-ray beam is now perpendicular to the joint *(arrow)*. **F.** The remaining screws have been placed.

- Precisely assess the stability of the construct after the plate has been applied. If appropriate, remove the provisional K-wires.
    - If the K-wires are deemed critical for fracture stability, they can be left in place and removed 4 to 8 weeks later
    - If residual instability exists, add additional fixation with K-wires, an external fixator, a dorsal plate, or a combination.

Closure

- Repair the pronator quadratus to its insertion site with a series of 3-0 absorbable horizontal mattress sutures (**TECH FIG 6A**).
    - In many cases it is impossible to repair the pronator quadratus because the muscle and fascia are extremely thin or the muscle is damaged. In this situation, the muscle can be debrided or simply left in place.

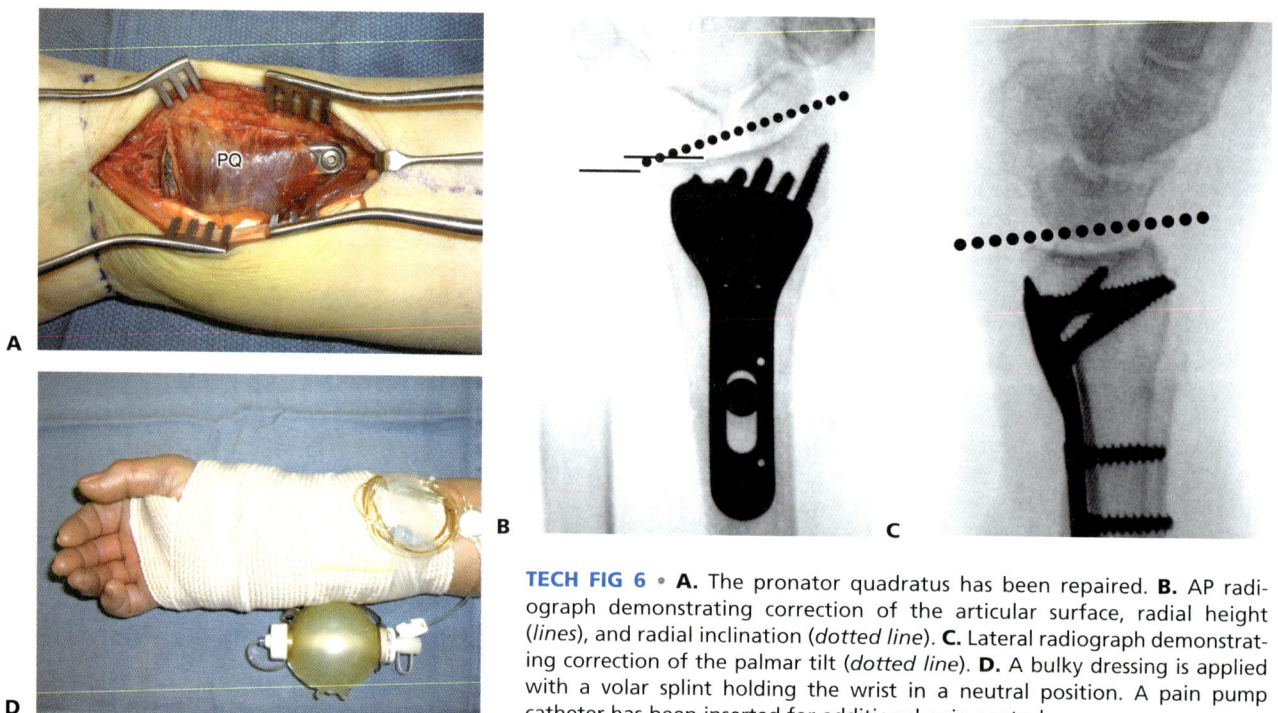

- Before skin closure, obtain final radiographs (**TECH FIG 6B,C**), and assess stability of the distal radioulnar joint.
- Place a drain only if excessive bleeding is anticipated.
- Consider methods to minimize postoperative pain:
    - Percutaneous placement of a pain pump catheter
    - Injection of a long-acting local anesthetic
- Close the subcutaneous tissues with 4-0 absorbable suture and reapproximate the skin with interrupted 4-0 or 5-0 nylon sutures or a running subcuticular stitch.
- Place two layers of gauze and a nonadherent gauze over the wound, wrap the wrist and forearm with thick Webril (Kendall, Mansfield, MA), and apply a below-elbow splint in a neutral wrist position (**TECH FIG 6D**).
    - If there is injury to the ulnar wrist (eg, ulna styloid fracture, distal radioulnar joint injury), immobilize the forearm with an above-elbow or Munster splint.

A

B

C

D

TECH FIG 6 • **A.** The pronator quadratus has been repaired. **B.** AP radiograph demonstrating correction of the articular surface, radial height *(lines)*, and radial inclination *(dotted line)*. **C.** Lateral radiograph demonstrating correction of the palmar tilt *(dotted line)*. **D.** A bulky dressing is applied with a volar splint holding the wrist in a neutral position. A pain pump catheter has been inserted for additional pain control.

VOLAR FIXED-ANGLE PLATE USING THE PLATE AS REDUCTION TOOL

- We do not recommend use of the volar fixed-angle plate as a reduction tool in the acute setting. It is best employed (if at all) for a malunion, or perhaps for a fracture with minimal articular comminution.
  - This technique is difficult, because it has to account for the longitudinal and translational alignment of the plate before the reduction has been achieved.
- Perform the surgical approach previously described.
- Address first any distal articular involvement with reduction and K-wire fixation.

- Affix the plate to the distal fragment, accounting for where the plate will sit on the radius shaft once the reduction is completed.
- Place the screws so that they are parallel to the articular surface on the lateral x-ray view (**TECH FIG7A,B**).
- On the AP radiograph, align the plate with the perpendicular of the radial inclination of the distal radius (20 degrees; **TECH FIG 7C,D**).
- Once distal fixation is complete, secure the proximal plate to the radius shaft, thereby completing the reduction.
- Close and splint as described previously.

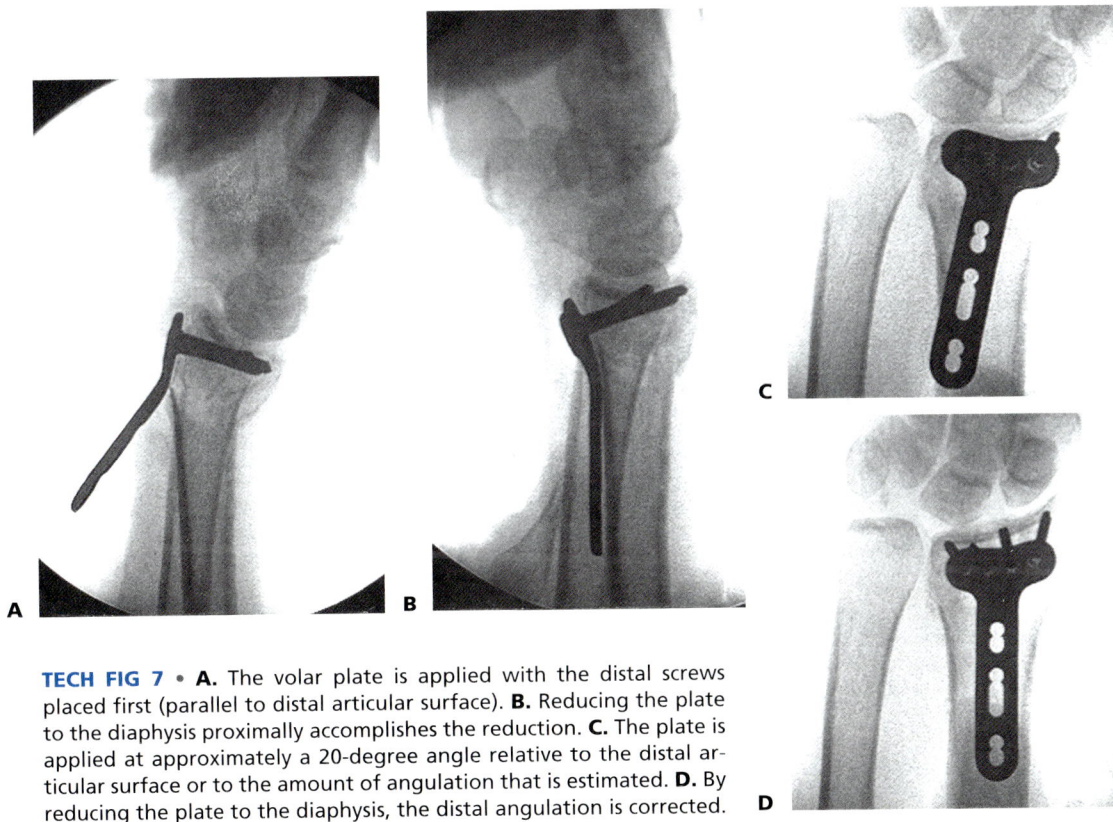

TECH FIG 7 • **A.** The volar plate is applied with the distal screws placed first (parallel to distal articular surface). **B.** Reducing the plate to the diaphysis proximally accomplishes the reduction. **C.** The plate is applied at approximately a 20-degree angle relative to the distal articular surface or to the amount of angulation that is estimated. **D.** By reducing the plate to the diaphysis, the distal angulation is corrected.

PEARLS AND PITFALLS

Preoperative planning	■ Obtain multiple radiographs in different positions (eg, several oblique views), especially in the setting of comminution or articular involvement. ■ Obtain a CT scan if assessing the pattern of fracture when radiographs alone are difficult or uncertain.
Surgical approach	■ Avoid crossing the distal flexion creases of the wrist. ■ Avoid exposure ulnar to the midline of the flexor carpi radialis. ■ Use extra care with deep dissection in the presence of hematoma or significant swelling.
Fracture reduction	■ Employ traction across the wrist with a device or weights. ■ Use a lobster-claw clamp on the proximal radius shaft for control of the forearm and as a reference for the lateral margins. ■ Use instruments to disimpact and reduce articular fragments through the fracture itself, either volarly, dorsally, or both. ■ Employ a temporary K-wire to stabilize the reduction before placement of the plate.
Plate alignment	■ Confirm appropriate radial–ulnar positioning of the proximal plate using a true AP radiograph (ie, forearm in supination with open view of the distal radioulnar joint).

	▪ Confirm proper distal plate position on a true lateral view (ie, forearm 20 degrees off the table). ▪ Place the plate as distal as possible, up to the volar tear drop of the distal radius, if possible. ▪ Evaluate the screws for possible joint penetration using 360-degree fluoroscopic images.
Plate fixation	▪ Use K-wires to fix the plate provisionally to the proximal radius. ▪ The initial "oblong hole" screw should be slightly longer than the measured length to ensure better initial fixation.
Postoperative	▪ Closure of the pronator quadratus is not critical and should be reserved for more substantial muscles with limited trauma. ▪ Begin immediate range of motion (ROM) to digits with edema.

POSTOPERATIVE CARE

▪ The wrist is splinted in a neutral position, leaving the digits free.

  ▪ If the fracture is particularly tenuous or there is injury to the ulnar wrist, a long-arm or Munster splint is applied.

▪ The patient is instructed to perform active ROM exercises for the digits every hour and to engage in strict elevation for at least 3 days.

  ▪ It is critical to emphasize edema prevention and immediate ROM of the digits.

▪ At 1 week postoperatively, the splint is removed and the wound is examined.

▪ If swelling permits, the therapist fabricates a molded Orthoplast splint (Johnson & Johnson Orthopedics, New Brunswick, NJ) to be worn at all times.

▪ Active ROM exercises of the wrist are implemented 1 week postoperatively.

▪ At 4 to 6 weeks, putty and grip exercises are added.

▪ At 6 to 8 weeks, the splint is discontinued, and progressive strengthening exercises are advanced.

▪ If necessary, progressive passive ROM can begin, including use of dynamic splints.

▪ At 10 to 12 weeks, the patient usually can be discharged to all activities as tolerated.

OUTCOMES

▪ Overall good to excellent results can be expected in over 80% of patients with ROM, strength, and outcomes scoring.[10,11,15,17]

▪ Studies comparing volar fixation to other forms of fixation (eg, external fixators, pins, and dorsal plating) have revealed similar if not superior results.

  ▪ Results appear to be superior in the early recovery period, with the final outcome yielding equivalent results among all fixation groups.

  ▪ Some studies suggest better maintenance in overall reduction compared to other forms of fixation.

COMPLICATIONS

▪ Complication rates as high as 27% have been reported.

▪ Complications can be categorized into those involving hardware, fracture, soft tissues, nerves, and tendons.[2]

▪ Failures of hardware, such as plate or screw breakage, can occur but are rare. Usually such failures are an indication of other problems, such as nonunion.

▪ The hardware becomes unacceptably prominent in a minority of patients.

  ▪ This complication may become evident only after some time has elapsed, as swelling of fibrous tissue subsides and bone remodels.

  ▪ The most common sites include the dorsal wrist, when screws have been inserted, and the radial wrist, when a plate has been used.

  ▪ It can be avoided with careful screw and plate placement and radiographic verification of their position.

▪ Nonunion and delayed union are unusual. Consider a diagnosis of osteomyelitis or other risk factors such as smoking.

▪ Loss of fracture reduction and fixation can occur, and is most common in patients with osteopenic bone or comminuted and articular fractures.

  ▪ This can be avoided with frequent and early follow-up with repeat radiographs.

  ▪ If instability is suspected, the fracture can be casted.

  ▪ In the operating room, if instability is suspected, additional fixation should be considered (eg, external fixator, pins, bone graft).

▪ Soft tissue complications are proportional to the energy of the initial injury.

▪ Open wounds usually can be addressed with local measures.

▪ Significant swelling must be addressed with early and aggressive modalities. Swelling can lead to other complications, such as joint stiffness and tendon adhesions.

▪ Nerve injuries can be the result of initial trauma or subsequent surgical trauma.

  ▪ Assess and document neurologic status before surgery.

  ▪ Avoid further injury to nerves with careful placement of retractors.

  ▪ The palmar cutaneous branch of the median nerve can be injured during incision and exposure.

  ▪ Postoperative neuromas can cause pain and sensitivity along scar.

  ▪ Avoid the nerve with a well-placed incision radial to the flexor carpi radialis and careful deep dissection.

▪ Postoperative swelling also can lead to median neuropathy. Carpal tunnel release should be performed if there is any suspected compression neuropathy or if this is to be anticipated as a result of postoperative swelling.

▪ Tendon complications include adhesions and ruptures.

▪ Most tendon adhesions involve the dorsal extensor tendons resulting in extrinsic extensor tightness.

▪ Flexor tendon adhesions are uncommon and involve primarily the flexor pollicis longus.

▪ Tendon ruptures have been described, especially involving the flexor pollicis longus and the extensor pollicis longus, as a result of plate and screw prominence, respectively.

  ▪ The distal screws must not be left prominent, and caution must be applied when drilling.

  ▪ The sagittal and coronal profiles of the plate being used must be taken into consideration—some plates are very prominent and extend far radially.

REFERENCES

1. Aro HT, Koivunen T. Minor axial shortening of the radius affects outcome of Colles' fracture treatment. J Hand Surg Am 1991;16:392–398.

2. Arora R, Lutz M, Hennerbichler A, et al. Complications following internal fixation of unstable distal radius fracture with a palmar locking plate. J Orthop Trauma 2007;21:316–322.

3. Fernandez JJ, Gruen GS, Herndon JH. Outcome of distal radius fractures using the Short Form 36 health survey. Clin Orthop Relat Res 1997;341:36–41.

4. Geissler WB, Freeland AE, Savoie FH, et al. Intracarpal soft-tissue lesions associated with an intra-articular fracture of the distal end of the radius. J Bone Joint Surg Am 1996;78:357–365.

5. Jupiter JB, Fernandez DL. Comparative classification for fractures of the distal end of the radius. J Hand Surg Am 1997;22:563–571.

6. Knirk JL, Jupiter JB. Intra-articular fractures of the distal end of the radius in young adults. J Bone Joint Surg Am 1986;68:647–659.

7. LaFontaine M, Hardy D, Delince PH. Stability assessment of distal radius fractures. Injury 1989;20:208–210.

8. Melone CP Jr. Articular fractures of the distal radius. Orthop Clin North Am 1984;15:217–236.

9. Muller ME, Nazarian S, Koch P, et al. The Comprehensive Classification of Fractures of Long Bones. New York: Springer-Verlag, 1990.

10. Musgrave DS, Idler RS. Volar fixation of dorsally displaced distal radius fractures using the 2.4-mm locking compression plates. J Hand Surg Am 2005;30:743–749.

11. Orbay JL, Fernandez DL. Volar fixed-angle plate fixation for unstable distal radius fractures in the elderly patient. J Hand Surg Am 2004;29:96–102.

12. Pogue DL, Viegas SF, Patterson RM, et al. Effects of distal radius fracture malunion on wrist joint mechanics. J Hand Surg Am 1990;15:721–727.

13. Porter M, Stockley I. Fractures of the distal radius. Intermediate and end result in relation to radiologic parameters. Clin Orthop Relat Res 1987;220:241–252.

14. Richards RS, Bennett JD, Roth JH, et al. Arthroscopic diagnosis of intra-articular soft tissue injuries associated with distal radius fractures. J Hand Surg Am 1997;22:772–776.

15. Rozental TD, Blazar PE. Functional outcome and complications after volar plating for dorsally displaced, unstable fractures of the distal radius. J Hand Surg Am 2006;31:359–365.

16. Short WH, Palmer AK, Werner FW, et al. A biomechanical study of distal radius fractures. J Hand Surg Am 1987;12:529–534.

17. Wright TW, Horodyski M, Smith DW. Functional outcome of unstable distal radius fractures: ORIF with a volar fixed-angle tine plate versus external fixation. J Hand Surg Am 2005;30:629.

Chapter 13

Bridge Plating of Distal Radius Fractures

Paul A. Martineau, Kevin J. Malone, and Douglas P. Hanel

DEFINITION

- High-energy fractures of the distal aspect of the radius with extensive comminution of the articular surface and extension into the diaphysis represent a major treatment challenge. Standard plates and techniques may be inadequate for the management of such fractures.
- Before the introduction of the bridge plating technique, treatment of these injuries was limited to cast immobilization or external fixation with or without Kirschner wire augmentation. Both of these methods are associated with unacceptably high complication rates.

ANATOMY

- The articular surface of the distal radius is tilted 21 degrees in the anteroposterior plane and 5 to 11 degrees in the lateral plane.
- The dorsal cortex surface of the radius thickens to form the tubercle of Lister.
- A central ridge divides the articular surface of the radius into a scaphoid facet and a lunate facet.
- Because of the different areas of bone thickness and density, fractures tend to occur in the relatively weaker metaphyseal bone and propagate intra-articularly between the scaphoid and lunate facets.
- The degree, direction, and magnitude of applied load may cause coronal or sagittal splits within the lunate or scaphoid facets.

PATHOGENESIS

- Two subsets of patients with distal radius fractures continue to represent unique treatment challenges:
  - Patients with high-energy wrist injuries with fracture extension into the radial diaphysis
  - Patients with multiple injuries who require load bearing through the injured wrist to assist with mobilization and nursing care

NATURAL HISTORY

- Lafontaine et al[13] showed that the end results of comminuted distal radius fractures treated by closed methods resembled the prereduction radiographs more than any other radiographs during treatment, even when the reduction successfully restored wrist anatomy.
- A number of studies clearly show that restoration of normal anatomy after distal radius fracture provides better function.[4,6–8,10–12,14]
- Functional outcome scores in patients without anatomic reduction are poor.[4,15]
- Malunion of the distal radius has been associated with pain, stiffness, weak grip strength, and carpal instability in a substantial percentage of patients.[8] Long-term consequences include degenerative arthritis in up to 50% of patients with even minimal displacement in the young adult population.[16]
- As surgical treatment (plating in particular) ensures more consistent correction of displacement and maintenance of reduction, there has been a trend toward operative treatment in both the elderly and the young population.

PATIENT HISTORY AND PHYSICAL FINDINGS

- In the management of high-energy distal radius fractures, a complete history should include the mechanism of injury. These fractures are commonly the result of axial loading as opposed to the bending forces, which are all low-velocity fractures.
- Examination of the soft tissue envelope of the wrist should be performed to rule out open fractures.
- Because of the high-energy nature of these fractures, patients are at increased risk of neurovascular compromise. Careful examination for signs of impending compartment syndrome as well as median nerve dysfunction from an acute carpal tunnel syndrome should be clearly documented.
- Associated injuries should be ruled out, and appropriate patient clearance according to advanced trauma life support guidelines should be obtained.

IMAGING AND OTHER DIAGNOSTIC STUDIES

- Good-quality pre- and post-reduction wrist radiographs should be obtained preoperatively to assess the fracture pattern and rule out associated injuries to the carpus or distal radioulnar joint (DRUJ).
- CT scans may be helpful to assess complex intra-articular distal radius fractures.

NONOPERATIVE MANAGEMENT

- There is no acceptable nonoperative management for high-energy comminuted distal radius fractures.

SURGICAL MANAGEMENT

- The use of internal distraction plating or bridge plating for distal radius fractures was introduced by Burke and Singer.[3] The technique was expanded by Ruch et al,[17] who described the use of a 12- to 16-hole 3.5-mm plate dynamic compression plate (DCP) (Synthes, Paoli, PA) placed in the floor of the fourth dorsal extensor compartment to span from the intact radius diaphysis to the third metacarpal.[5,17]
- The bridge plating technique provides strong fixation and allows for distraction across impacted articular segments.
- The technique can be combined with a limited articular fixation approach for fracture patterns with intra-articular extension.

Table 1	Indications for Bridge Plating of Distal Radius Fractures
Indication	**Explanation**
Metadiaphyseal comminution of the radius	Extensive comminution in metadiaphyseal region is difficult to treat with standard implants used for distal radius fractures.
Need for weight bearing through the upper extremity	Patients with associated lower limb injuries may require the need for early weight bearing through the upper extremities.
Polytrauma	Nursing care of the multiply injured patient may be easier with spanning internal fixation than with external fixation.
Augmented fixation	In osteoporotic bone, bridge plating can be used to augment tenuous fixation.
Carpal instability	Carpal instability, particularly radiocarpal, isolated or in combination with a distal radius fracture, may be held in a reduced position with the help of spanning internal fixation.

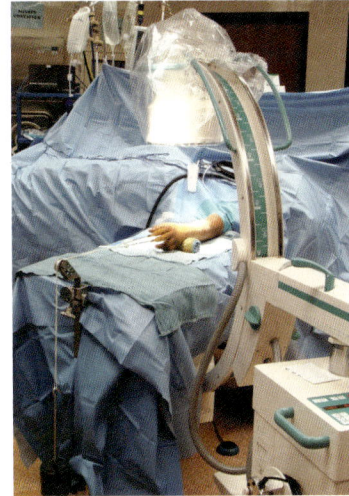

FIG 1 • Setup for this procedure, with longitudinal traction applied through finger traps and the C-arm coming in from above or below the hand table.

■ Bridge plating of the distal radius was further refined by Hanel et al.[9] The authors described a variant of the bridge plating technique using 2.4-mm AO plates passed extra-articularly through the second dorsal compartment and secured onto the dorsal-radial aspect of the radius diaphysis and the second metacarpal (Table 1).

Preoperative Planning

■ A 22-hole 2.4-mm titanium mandibular reconstruction plate (Synthes, Paoli, PA) or a 2.4-mm stainless steel plate specifically designed for use as a distal radius bridge plate (DRB plate, Synthes, Paoli, PA) is used for distal radius bridge plating.
■ The mandibular reconstruction plate is made of titanium and has square ends and scalloped edges and threaded holes to accept locking screws. The DRB plate that the authors currently use is made of stainless steel and has tapered ends to facilitate sliding the plate within the extensor compartment; it also has locking screws.

Positioning

■ With the patient anesthetized and supine on the operating table, the involved extremity is draped free and centered on a radiolucent hand table.
■ Finger traps are applied to the index and middle fingers and 4.5 kg of longitudinal traction is applied through a rope and pulley system.
■ A C-arm comes in from above or below the hand table (**FIG 1**).

Approach

■ Under image intensification, the closed reduction maneuver described by Agee[1] is performed.
■ Plates are passed extra-articularly through the second dorsal compartment and secured onto the dorsal-radial aspect of the radius diaphysis and the second metacarpal.
■ The interval between the extensor carpi radialis longus (ECRL) and brevis (ECRB) is developed and the diaphysis of the radius exposed.
■ The DRB plate is introduced beneath the muscle bellies of the outcroppers extraperiosteally and advanced distally between the ECRL and ECRB tendons.

CLOSED REDUCTION MANEUVER OF AGEE

■ Longitudinal traction is first used to restore length and to assess the benefit of ligamentotaxis for the restoration of articular stepoff (**TECH FIG 1A,B**).
■ Next, the hand is translated palmarly relative to the forearm to restore sagittal tilt and to assess the integrity of the volar lip of the radius (**TECH FIG 1C–F**).
■ Finally, pronation of the hand relative to the forearm is performed to correct the supination deformity.
■ Once the initial reduction maneuver is completed, the bridge plate is then applied.

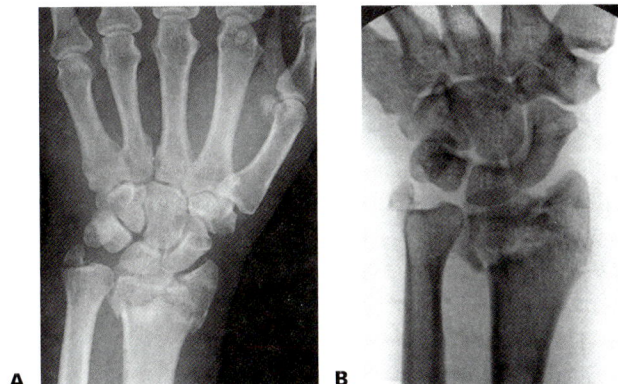

TECH FIG 1 • Radiographs show an AP projection of the wrist injury before (**A**) and after (**B**) distraction is applied. *(continued)*

A   B

TECHNIQUES

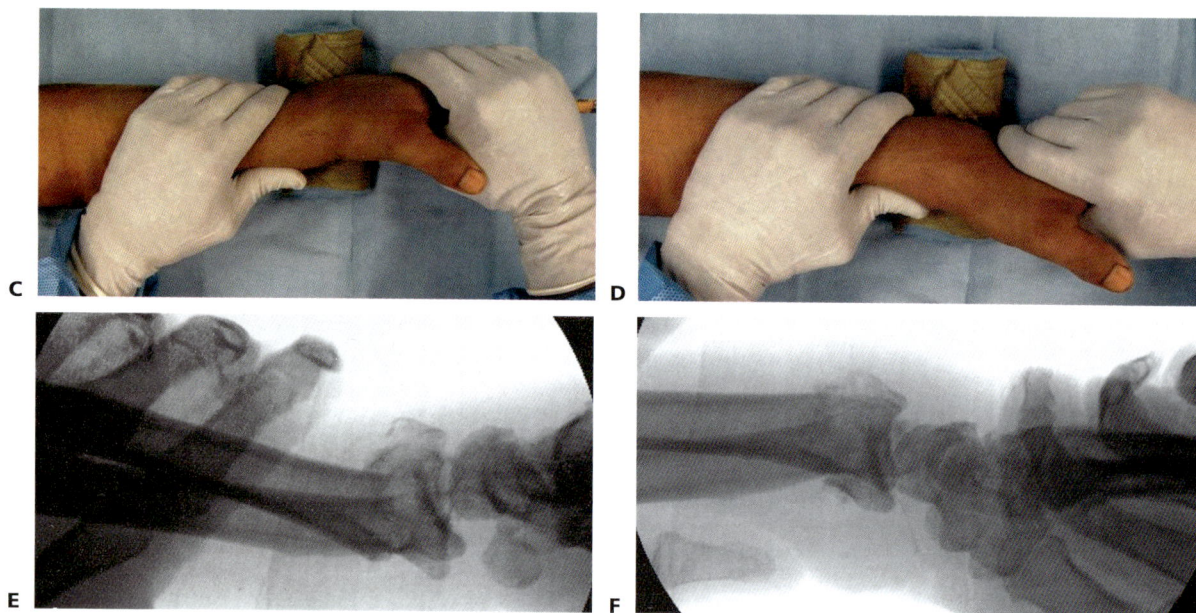

TECH FIG 1 • *(continued)* Clinical pictures show the wrist deformity before (**C**) and after (**D**) application of the Agee reduction maneuver, which is a combination of longitudinal traction and volar translation of the carpus. Radiographs show the wrist deformity before (**E**) and after (**F**) application of the Agee reduction maneuver.

APPROACH AND PLATE INSERTION

- The DRB plate is superimposed on the skin from the radial diaphysis to the distal metadiaphysis of the second metacarpal. The position of the plate is verified with image intensification and markings are placed on the skin at the level of the proximal and distal four screw holes of the plate (**TECH FIG 2A–C**).

- The subcutaneous tissues are infiltrated with 0.25% bupivacaine with epinephrine to promote hemostasis.

- A 5-cm incision is made at the base of the second metacarpal and continued along the second metacarpal shaft. In the depths of this incision, the insertions of the ECRL and ECRB are identified as they pass beneath the distal edge of the second dorsal wrist compartment to insert on the second and third metacarpal bases respectively.

- A second incision is made just proximal to the outcropper muscle bellies (abductor pollicis longus and extensor pollicis brevis), in line with ECRL and ECRB tendons. The interval between the ECRL and ECRB is developed and the diaphysis of the radius exposed (**TECH FIG 2D,E**).

- The DRB plate is introduced beneath the muscle bellies of the outcroppers extraperiosteally and advanced distally between the ECRL and ECRB tendons (**TECH FIG 2F**).

- Some resistance may be encountered as the plate emerges distally but can usually be easily overcome with gentle manipulation of the plate (**TECH FIG 2G**).

  - Occasionally, the plate will not pass through the compartment. In these cases, a guidewire or stout suture

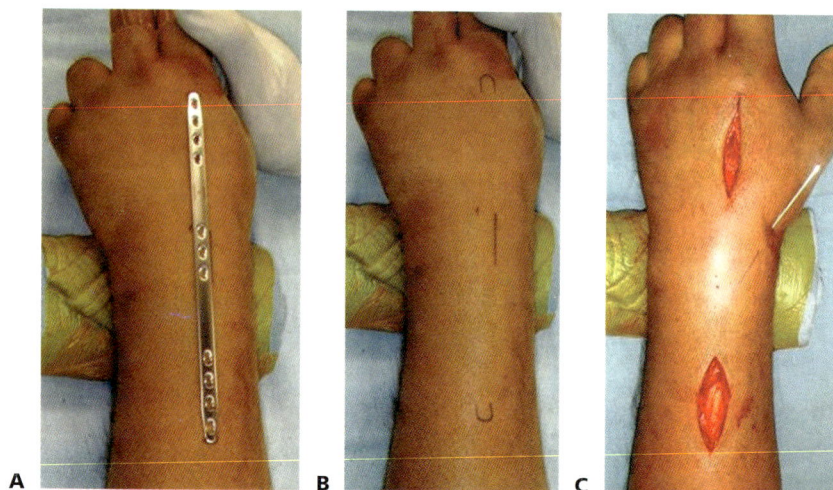

TECH FIG 2 • **A.** The plate is placed over the forearm and hand. Radiographs can be taken to confirm the position of the plate. The plate should be centered over the second metacarpal distally and the radius proximally. This will be along the course of the extensor carpi radialis longus (ECRL). **B.** Outline of the plate. **C.** Incisions are made over the second metacarpal and the radius. *(continued)*

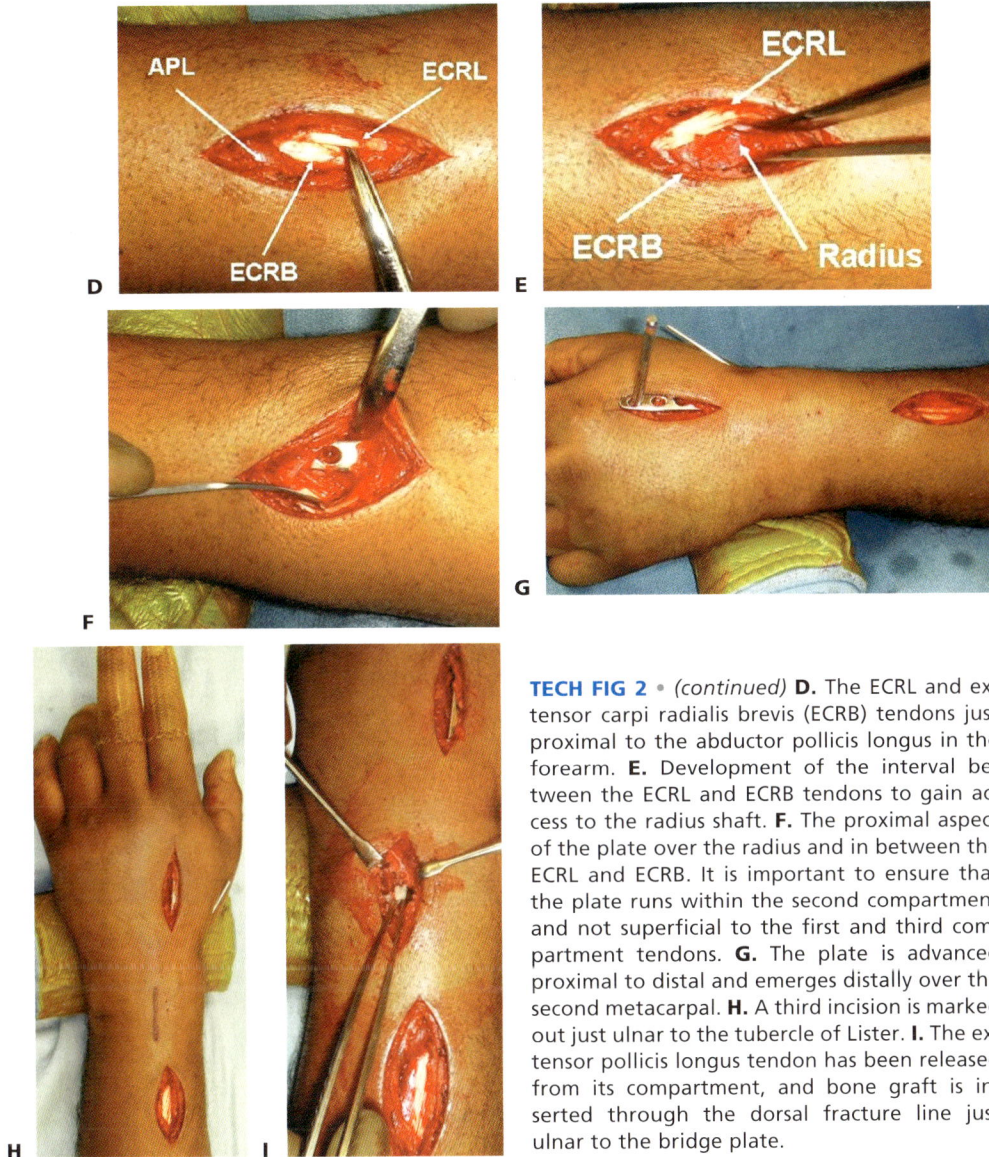

TECH FIG 2 • *(continued)* **D.** The ECRL and extensor carpi radialis brevis (ECRB) tendons just proximal to the abductor pollicis longus in the forearm. **E.** Development of the interval between the ECRL and ECRB tendons to gain access to the radius shaft. **F.** The proximal aspect of the plate over the radius and in between the ECRL and ECRB. It is important to ensure that the plate runs within the second compartment and not superficial to the first and third compartment tendons. **G.** The plate is advanced proximal to distal and emerges distally over the second metacarpal. **H.** A third incision is marked out just ulnar to the tubercle of Lister. **I.** The extensor pollicis longus tendon has been released from its compartment, and bone graft is inserted through the dorsal fracture line just ulnar to the bridge plate.

retriever is passed along the compartment from distal to proximal. The plate is secured to the distal end of the wire and delivered into the hand.

■ In the rare instance that these measures fail, a third incision is made directly over the metaphysis of the ra-

dius, the proximal half of the second compartment is incised, and the plate is passed under direct vision.

■ The third, or periarticular, incision may also be used to assess the articular surface, reduce die-punch fragments, and introduce bone graft (**TECH FIG 2H,I**).

PLATE FIXATION AND ARTICULAR FIXATION

■ After the bridge plate is passed, it is then secured to the second metacarpal by placing a nonlocking fully threaded 2.4-mm cortical screw through the most distal plate hole. The proximal end of the plate is then identified in the forearm.

■ If the radial length has not been restored, then the plate, secured to the second metacarpal, is pushed distally until the length is reestablished and a fully threaded 2.4-mm nonlocking screw is placed in the most proximal plate hole. By using nonlocking screws the plate is effectively lagged onto the intact bone.

■ Plate alignment along the longitudinal axis of the radius is guaranteed by securing the most distal and most proximal screw holes first.

■ The remaining holes are secured with fully threaded locking screws inserted with bicortical purchase.

■ It has been our experience that as the plate is passed along the radial diaphysis, through the second compartment and along the second metacarpal, extra-articular alignment, radial inclination, volar tilt, and radial length are restored.

■ Intra-articular reduction may be further adjusted by using limited periarticular incisions to allow for direct manipulation of articular fragments, placement of sub-chondral bone grafts, repair of intercarpal ligament injuries, and augmentation of fracture fixation with Kirschner wires and periarticular plates.

■ Displaced volar medial fracture fragments that are not reduced with this technique require a separate volar incision and appropriate buttress support.

■ The biomechanical stability of spanning plates is strong and predictable. Behrens et al,[2] studying the rigidity of external fixator configurations, demonstrated that

rigidity is directly proportional to how close the longitudinal fixator bar is to the bone and the fracture. A bridge plate, resting directly against the radius proximally and metacarpals distally, therefore optimizes the conditions to obtain the strongest possible fixator construct.

■ A DRB plate fixed with a minimum of three screws at either end of the plate confers significantly more stability than would an external fixator used to stabilize a comparable fracture (**TECH FIG 3**).[18]

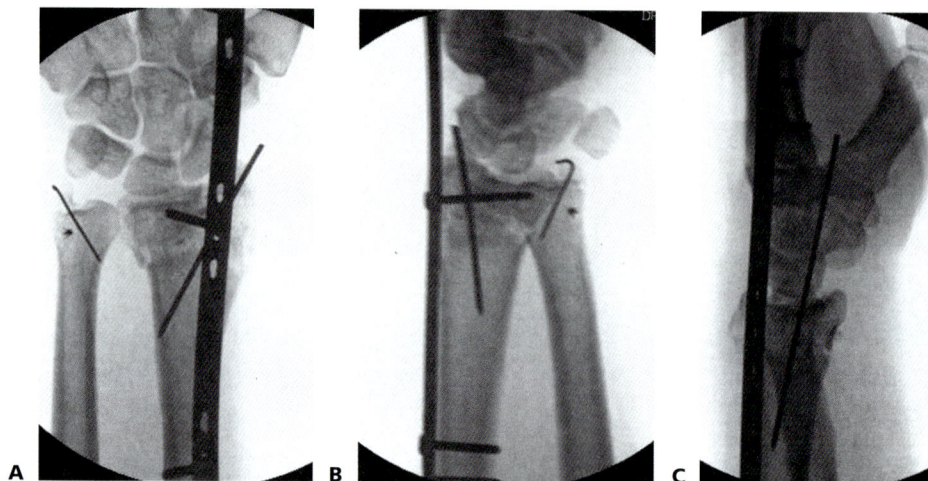

TECH FIG 3 • Final AP (**A**), oblique (**B**), and lateral (**C**) radiographic images.

DISTAL RADIOULNAR JOINT MANAGEMENT

■ DRUJ stability is assessed after radius reconstruction. If the DRUJ is stable, the limb is immobilized in a long-arm splint with the forearm in supination for the first 10 to 14 days postoperatively.

■ If the DRUJ is unstable, and there are no contraindications to prolonging the operation, repair or reconstruction of DRUJ and triangular fibrocartilage complex is undertaken.

■ If however, the patient's condition does not allow the operation to be prolonged, the ulnar head is reduced manually into the sigmoid notch and the ulna is transfixed to the radius with a minimum of two 1.6-mm Kirschner wires passed proximal to the DRUJ.

PEARLS AND PITFALLS

Hardware removal	■ At the time of hardware extraction, if a mandibular reconstruction plate was used, the screws are removed and the plate is twisted axially 720 degrees to break up the soft tissue adhesions and callus that tend to grow around and onto the scalloped edges of the titanium plate. This maneuver is not usually required when the smooth-edged stainless steel DRB is used. ■ A removable short-arm splint is worn for 2 to 3 weeks after plate removal. Hand therapy at this point is directed at regaining motion and strength.

POSTOPERATIVE CARE

■ Digit range-of-motion exercises start within 24 hours of surgery. Load bearing through the forearm and elbow is allowed immediately, as well as the use of a platform crutch when the patient is physiologically stable. One month postop-

eratively the platform is removed and weight bearing is allowed through the hand grip of regular crutches. Lifting and carrying are restricted to about 4.5 kg until fracture healing.

■ DRUJ stability and forearm motion are assessed 2 weeks after reduction. If the patient can supinate the forearm with little effort and the DRUJ is stable, then splinting is discontinued and axial loading through the extremity is allowed at this point.

- If the patient has difficulty maintaining supination, or if the DRUJ was reconstructed acutely, a removable long-arm splint is fabricated.
- If the DRUJ was transfixed with Kirschner wires, then the wires are removed on the third postoperative week and DRUJ stability is reassessed.
- Supplemental Kirschner wires for articular fixation are removed 6 weeks postoperatively.
- The DRB plate and screws are removed usually no earlier than 12 weeks after injury.

OUTCOMES

- The bridge plating technique for distal radius fractures was reviewed in a retrospective study consisting of 62 consecutive patients treated in this fashion.[9] The series represents the senior author's 10-year experience with the technique at a Level 1 trauma center. Patients managed with bridge plating either for distal radius fractures with extensive metadiaphyseal comminution or for distal radius fractures associated with other injuries requiring weight bearing through the affected extremity represented 13% of distal radius fractures treated with operative fixation during this period. Fracture healing occurred in all 62 patients.
  - In each case radial length was within 5 mm of neutral ulnar variance, radial inclination was greater than 5 degrees, and palmar tilt was at least neutral.
  - There were also no articular gaps or stepoffs greater than 2 mm and the DRUJ was stable in all cases.
  - The plates were removed on average 112 days after placement.
  - Forty-one of the 62 patients have returned to their previous levels of employment. Of the remaining 21 patients, 8 were unemployed at the time of injury and remain so.
  - Thirteen patients sustained multiple injuries requiring considerable changes in occupation and lifestyle. Only 1 of these 13 patients considers the wrist fracture to be the limiting factor in failing to return to work.
  - Overall these results compare favorably with the findings of Burke and Singer[3] and Ruch et al.[17]
- Similarly, Ruch et al[17] showed that 64% of patients obtained excellent radiographic and functional results and another 27% of patients obtained good results in their prospective cohort of patients with comparable pathology.
- The authors of each of these studies propose that distraction plating allows fracture reduction and fixation over a broad metadiaphyseal area while effectively diverting compression forces away from the fracture site.
- The use of bridge plating in the treatment of distal radius fractures avoids the complications of external fixation. A bridge plate can remain implanted for extended periods without deleterious effects on functional outcome. All patients in our series went on to heal with acceptable metadiaphyseal and intra-articular alignment. In patients with multiple traumatic injuries, bridge plating allowed earlier postoperative load bearing across the affected wrist. This enabled independent transfers and the use of ambulatory aids. Application of bridge plates is simple and surgical time is comparable with the application of an external fixator.

COMPLICATIONS

- There was one documented hardware failure in the series in a patient who initially refused to have the implant taken out and continued to work in heavy manual labor for 19 months before the bridge plate failed.
- In addition, there were no cases of excessive postoperative finger stiffness or reflex sympathetic dystrophy.
- This reflects the overall infrequent complications reported in the literature for bridge plating of the distal radius. In fact, Burke and Singer[3] reported no complications, and Ruch et al[17] reported no hardware failures and only three patients who developed long finger extensor lag of 10 to 15 degrees.

REFERENCES

1. Agee JM. Distal radius fractures: multiplanar ligamentotaxis. Hand Clin 1993;9:577–585.
2. Behrens F, Johnson W. Unilateral external fixation: methods to increase and reduce frame stiffness. Clin Orthop Relat Res 1989;241:48–56.
3. Burke EF, Singer RM. Treatment of comminuted distal radius with the use of an internal distraction plate. Tech Hand Up Extrem Surg 1998;2:248–252.
4. Drobetz H, Bryant AL, Pokorny T, et al. Volar fixed-angle plating of distal radius extension fractures: influence of plate position on secondary loss of reduction: a biomechanic study in a cadaveric model. J Hand Surg Am 2006;31A:615–622.
5. Ginn TA, Ruch DS, Yang CC, et al. Use of a distraction plate for distal radial fractures with metaphyseal and diaphyseal comminution: surgical technique. J Bone Joint Surg Am 2006;88A(Suppl 1 Pt 1):29–36.
6. Gradl G, Jupiter JB, Gierer P, et al. Fractures of the distal radius treated with a nonbridging external fixation technique using multiplanar K-wires. J Hand Surg Am 2005;30A:960–968.
7. Graff S, Jupiter J. Fracture of the distal radius: classification of treatment and indications for external fixation. Injury 1994;25(Suppl 4):11 25.
8. Handoll HH, Madhok R. Surgical interventions for treating distal radial fractures in adults. Cochrane Database Syst Rev 2003(3):CD003209.
9. Hanel DP, Lu TS, Weil WM. Bridge plating of distal radius fractures: the Harborview method. Clin Orthop Relat Res 2006;445:91–99.
10. Hastings H II, Leibovic SJ. Indications and techniques of open reduction: internal fixation of distal radius fractures. Orthop Clin North Am 1993;24:309–326.
11. Kamath AF, Zurakowski D, Day CS. Low-profile dorsal plating for dorsally angulated distal radius fractures: an outcomes study. J Hand Surg Am 2006;31:1061–1067.
12. Konrath GA, Bahler S. Open reduction and internal fixation of unstable distal radius fractures: results using the Trimed fixation system. J Orthop Trauma 2002;16:578–585.
13. Lafontaine M, Hardy D, Delince P. Stability assessment of distal radius fractures. Injury 1989;20:208–210.
14. McQueen MM. Non-spanning external fixation of the distal radius. Hand Clin 2005;21:375–380.
15. McQueen MM, Simpson D, Court-Brown CM. Use of the Hoffman 2 compact external fixator in the treatment of redisplaced unstable distal radial fractures. J Orthop Trauma 1999;13:501–505.
16. Orbay JL, Touhami A. Current concepts in volar fixed-angle fixation of unstable distal radius fractures. Clin Orthop Relat Res 2006;445:58–67.
17. Ruch DS, Ginn TA, Yang CC, et al. Use of a distraction plate for distal radial fractures with metaphyseal and diaphyseal comminution. J Bone Joint Surg Am 2005;87A:945–954.
18. Wolf JC, Weil WM, Hanel DP, et al. A biomechanic comparison of an internal radiocarpal-spanning 2.4-mm locking plate and external fixation in a model of distal radius fractures. J Hand Surg Am 2006;31:1578–1586.

Open Reduction and Internal Fixation of Ulnar Styloid, Head, and Metadiaphyseal Fractures

Tommy Lindau and Andrew J. Logan

DEFINITION

- The distal ulna is the fixed point[3] around which the radius and the hand function (**FIG 1A**).
- Fractures of the distal ulna are often inadequately treated in comparison to its larger counterpart, the radius (**FIG 1B,C**).
- The current literature gives little guidance as to the management of these fractures and associated injuries.

ANATOMY

- The ulnar head forms the fixed point on which the hand and radius rest[3] (**FIG 2A**).
- The radius rotates around the ulnar head through the distal radioulnar joint (DRUJ) during forearm pronation and supination.[3,4]
- This joint is connected to the carpus by a complicated ligament apparatus, the triangular fibrocartilage complex (TFCC).
- The stability of the DRUJ is achieved through bony congruity between the sigmoid notch of the radius and the ulnar head supported by the ulnoradial ligaments[1,4] (**FIG 2B**).
  - The spheres of the two articular surfaces differ (**FIG 2C**).
  - Sixty percent of the joint surfaces are in contact in neutral forearm position.[1]
  - In full pronation and supination there is only 10% bony contact.[1]
  - The ligaments run from the fovea of the ulnar head and the base of the ulnar styloid to the dorsal and palmar edges of the sigmoid notch on the distal radius[1,9] (Fig 2B).

PATHOGENESIS

- Isolated ulnar fractures most commonly occur when the forearm is struck by an object, explaining the eponym "nightstick fracture."
- Distal ulnar fractures are most often due to a fall on an outstretched hand.
- It is a common understanding that ulnar-sided injuries are more often caused by falls backward in which the forearm is in supination, loading the ulnar side of the distal forearm and wrist and causing distal ulnar fractures, triquetral chip fractures, TFCC injuries, and so forth.
  - In contrast, radial-sided injuries are more often caused by falls forward, loading the radial side of the forearm and wrist and causing scaphoid fractures, distal radius fractures, and so forth.

NATURAL HISTORY

- Many distal ulnar fractures leave only marginal long-term problems.
- Some distal ulnar malunions cause DRUJ incongruency with subsequent instability or blocked forearm rotation (**FIG 3**). This is why management of these deceptive fractures is important.

IMAGING AND OTHER DIAGNOSTIC STUDIES

- Posteroanterior, lateral, and oblique radiographs typically reveal the pathology.

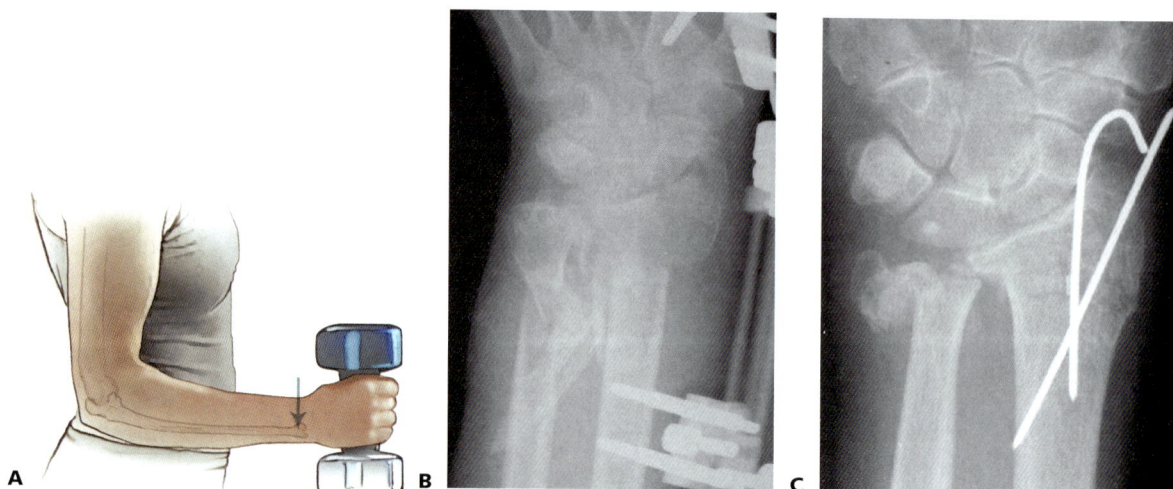

FIG 1 • **A.** The distal ulna is the fixed point upon which performance of most daily hand activities depends. **B,C.** Fractures of the distal ulna are often neglected in comparison to those of its larger counterpart, the radius, which always attracts attention and treatment efforts. The outcome after distal forearm fractures could be improved if the fixed point—the distal ulna—is addressed surgically at the same time as the radius is operated on.

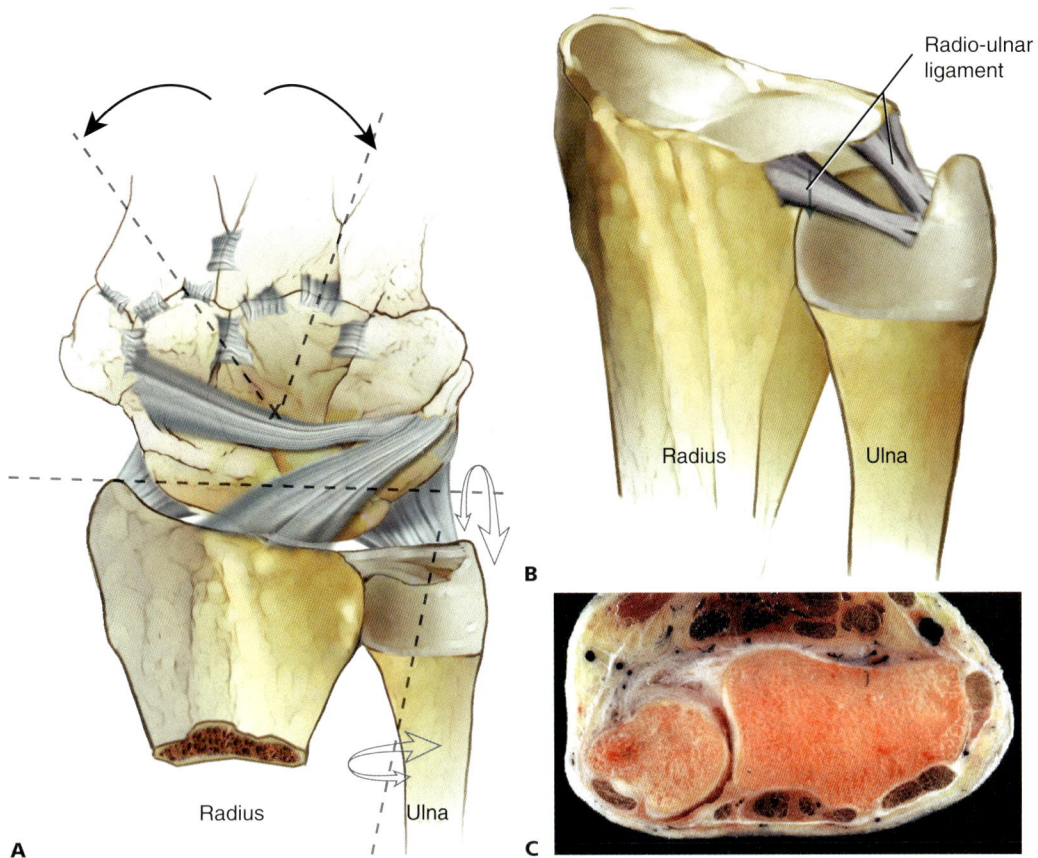

FIG 2 • A. The distal ulna is the fixed point around which the radius rotates in pronation and supination. Through the ulnocarpal ligament the distal ulna relates to the hand, allowing daily hand activities. **B.** The distal radioulnar joint is stable because of bony congruity between the ulnar head and the sigmoid notch on the radius. The ulnoradial ligament inserts in the fovea and the base of the ulnar styloid and has a dorsal and palmar ligament attached to the dorsal and palmar part of the sigmoid notch respectively. They act as reins in the pronation and supination motion. **C.** The spheres of the two articular surfaces differ: the curvature of the ulnar head has a shorter radius, whereas the curvature of the sigmoid notch has a greater radius.

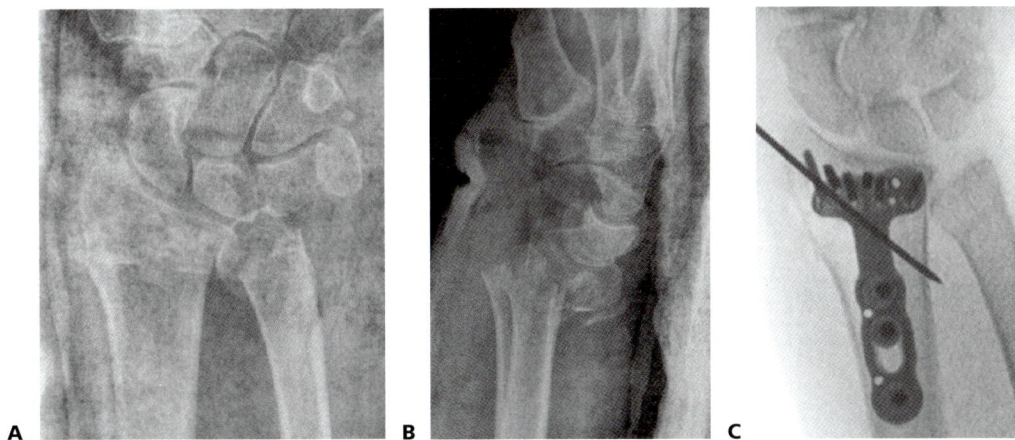

FIG 3 • A,B. Radiographs showing a distal radius fracture together with an ulnar head and styloid fracture. The complexity of the ulnar-sided injury was underappreciated. **C.** Intraoperative fluoroscopic image after fixation of the distal radius fracture, revealing displaced and unstable ulnar fractures. *(continued)*

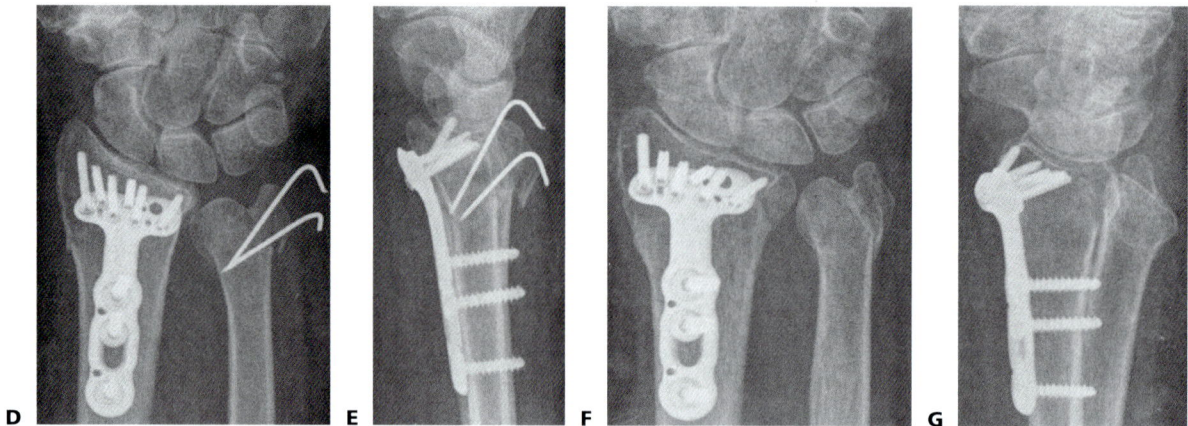

FIG 3 • *(continued)* **D,E.** The distal radius fracture was stabilized using a volar locking plate. The ulnar head and styloid fractures were partially reduced and fixed with two Kirschner wires. The surgeon adequately secured the ulnar styloid fracture but not the ulnar head fracture and postoperatively did not restrict forearm rotation. **F,G.** These radiographs reveal the eventual ulnar head malunion that resulted in distal radioulnar joint instability and diminished forearm rotation. The situation was salvaged using an ulnar head replacement prosthesis.

- CT is useful in examining articular fractures of the ulnar head.
- MRI is sometimes needed to evaluate the integrity of the TFCC.
- Arthroscopy should be considered if a radiograph leads the physician to suspect DRUJ dissociation without radiographic explanations, such as a displaced ulnar styloid base fracture.

SURGICAL MANAGEMENT

Findings and Indications

DRUJ Dissociation

- Radiographs occasionally reveal DRUJ dissociation in the absence of an ulnar-sided fracture (**FIG 4**). This results from detachment of the ulnoradial ligament[8] (**FIG 5A**).
  - Such ulnoradial ligament injuries have been found to cause DRUJ laxity and a worse outcome after distal radius fractures in patients without osteoporosis[7] (**FIG 5B**).
  - Arthroscopically assisted repair or open repair and reattachment of the ulnoradial ligament to the fovea of the ulnar head are required to restore stability in the DRUJ (**FIG 5C**) (see Chap. HA-49).

Ulnar Styloid Fractures

- The importance of ulnar styloid fractures and the need for operative intervention depends on the involvement of the ulnoradial ligament insertion site around the fovea of the ulnar head at the base of the styloid (**FIG 6A**).
  - Generally, ulnar styloid fractures should be operated on if the fracture is at the base of the ulnar styloid and is displaced more than 2 mm[11] (**FIG 6B,C**).
  - Radial translation of the fractured ulnar styloid is caused by the detachment of the ulnoradial ligament. This increases the indication (**FIG 6D**) more than axial, distal fracture displacement (detaching the ulnotriquetral collateral ligament).
  - Ulnar styloid fractures at the tip are likely to be stable and do not require fixation, as the ulnoradial ligament remains attached to the ulnar head at the base of the styloid (**FIG 6E,F**).
- Ulnar-sided injuries associated with distal radius fractures should be carefully assessed radiographically and clinically after open reduction and internal fixation (ORIF) of the radius fracture.
  - Ulnar fracture reduction and DRUJ joint stability are often improved after treatment of the radius fracture.
  - Stable DRUJ means that the ulnoradial ligament is not attached to the fractured ulnar styloid and therefore can be treated nonoperatively.
  - Unstable DRUJ indicates that the ulnoradial ligament is detached *with* the styloid fracture. The styloid should be reduced and stabilized or the ligament reattached.

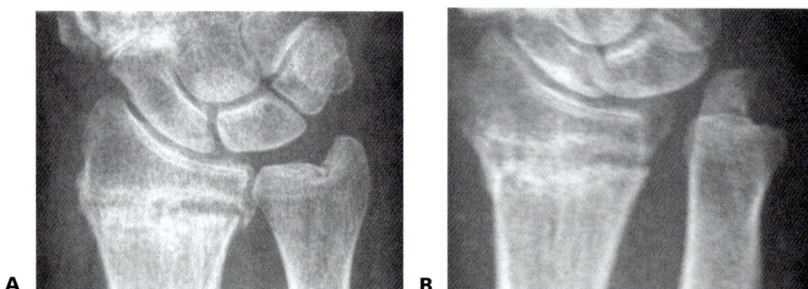

FIG 4 • **A.** An undisplaced distal radius fracture with no obvious distal ulna pathology. **B.** The same fracture with a stress test to the distal radioulnar joint (DRUJ), and an obvious DRUJ dissociation is seen as a sign of a complete ulnoradial ligament detachment in the absence of an ulnar styloid fracture.

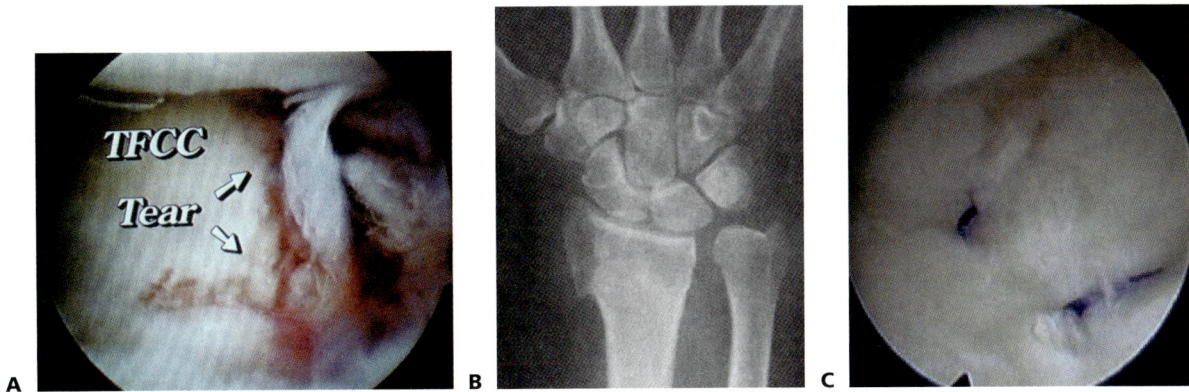

FIG 5 • A. Arthroscopic view of an ulnoradial (peripheral triangular fibrocartilage complex) detachment. The lunate is seen at the top, the radius below, and the detached surface with bleeding at the right side. **B.** Distal radioulnar joint dissociation after a distal radius fracture with a complete detachment of the ulnoradial ligament in the absence of any ulnar-sided fracture. **C.** Arthroscopic view of an arthroscopically assisted repair and reattachment of an avulsed ulnoradial ligament. The lunotriquetral interval is seen on top, the radius joint surface is seen in the lower left corner, and the blue sutures are bringing down the ligament toward the fovea of the ulnar head, which is not seen arthroscopically.

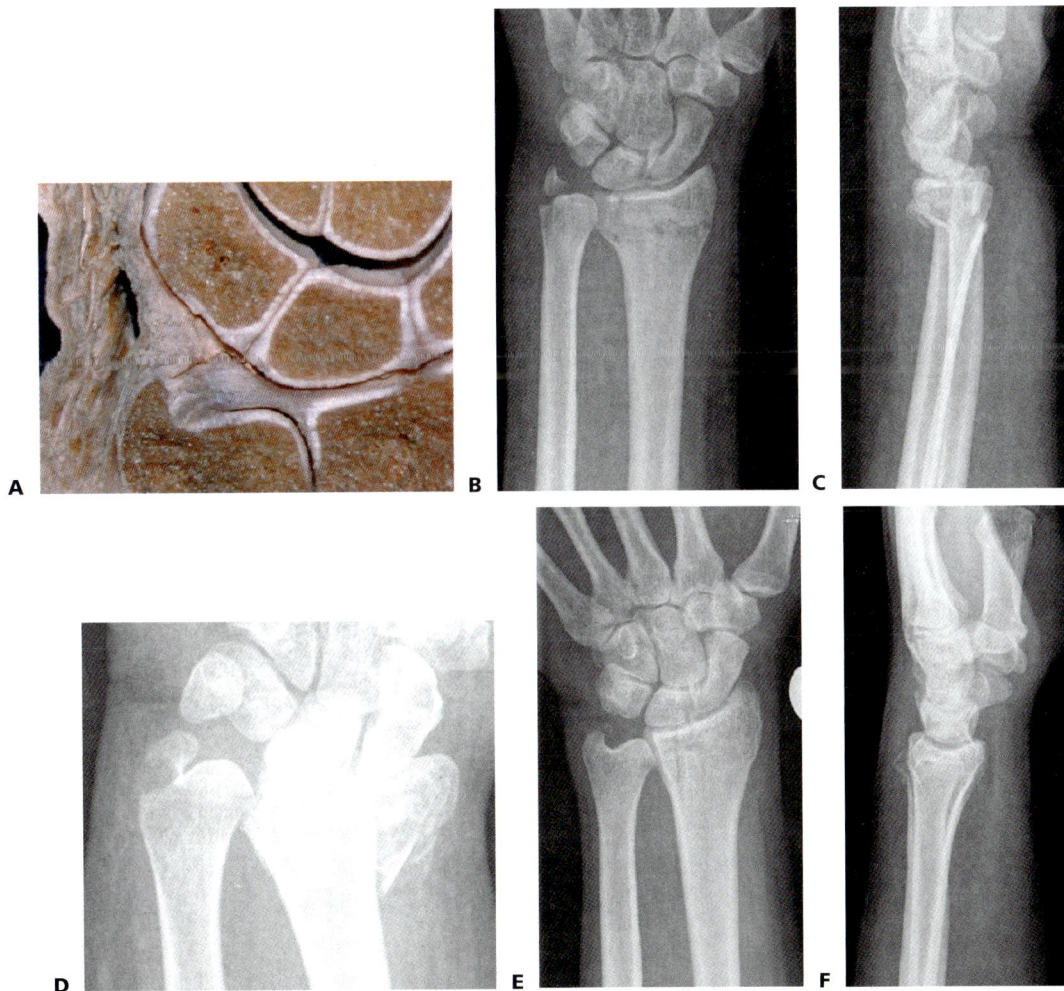

FIG 6 • A. The ulnoradial ligament has superficial and deeper components, which insert at the fovea of the ulnar head and partly attach to the base of the ulnar styloid. Consequently, a fracture at the base of the ulnar styloid may or may not detach the main distal radioulnar joint-stabilizing ligament. **B,C.** Ulnar styloid fractures at the base may detach the ulnoradial ligament and should be operated on if they are displaced more than 2 mm.[11] **D.** Radial displacement (detaching the ulnoradial ligament) increases the indication for surgical treatment. **E,F.** Ulnar styloid tip fractures represent avulsion fractures from the ulnotriquetral collateral ligament. They demand no further treatment.

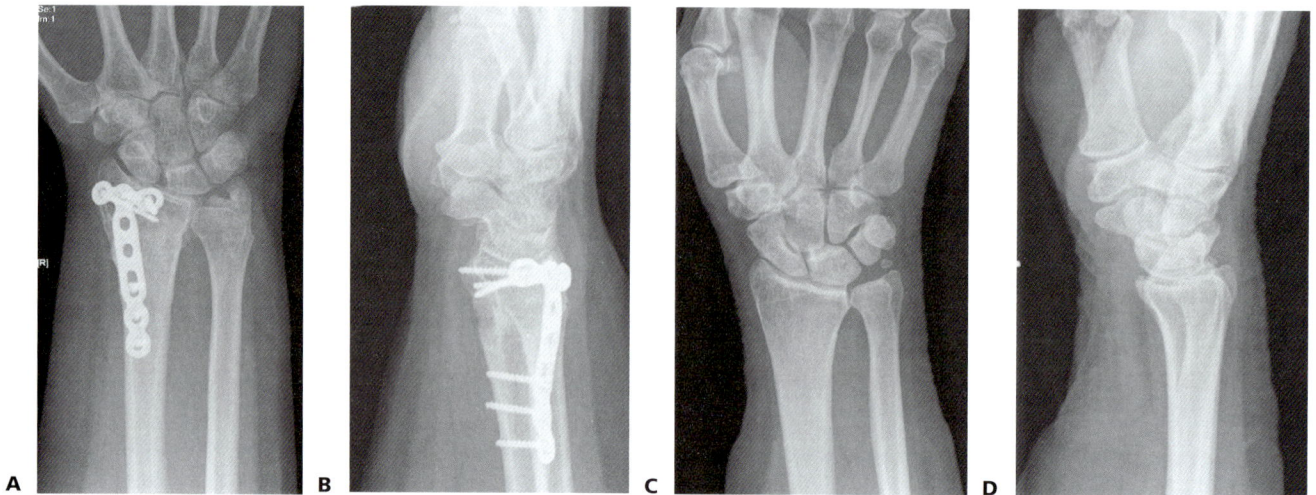

FIG 7 • **A,B.** Abutment of the ulnar styloid into the triquetrum on the ulnar side of the carpus. **C,D.** An ulnar styloid nonunion causing problems as a loose body.

Ulnar Styloid Nonunion

■ The main physical findings of ulnar styloid nonunion are ulnar-sided wrist pain worse with loading in rotation and tenderness over the ulnar styloid.[5] Symptoms from an ulnar styloid nonunion are related to the following:

■ DRUJ instability from a malfunctioning ulnoradial ligament (peripheral TFCC detachment)[5] (Fig 5B)
■ Impingement of the overlying extensor carpi ulnaris (ECU) tendon
■ Abutment on the carpus[5] (**FIG 7A,B**)
■ Soft tissue irritation from the loose body (**FIG 7C,D**)

Ulnar Head Fractures

■ Ulnar head fractures are most often associated with distal radius fractures, and the pattern of the distal radius fracture will have a strong influence on the overall functional outcome.
■ Ulnar head fractures are seen either alone or with involvement of extra-articular portions of the distal ulna, proximally toward the diaphysis or distally including the styloid (Fig 3A,B).

Distal Ulnar Neck and Shaft Fractures

■ A distal ulnar neck or distal shaft fracture is a fracture that occurs within 4 cm of the distal dome of the ulnar head (**FIG 8A–D**).

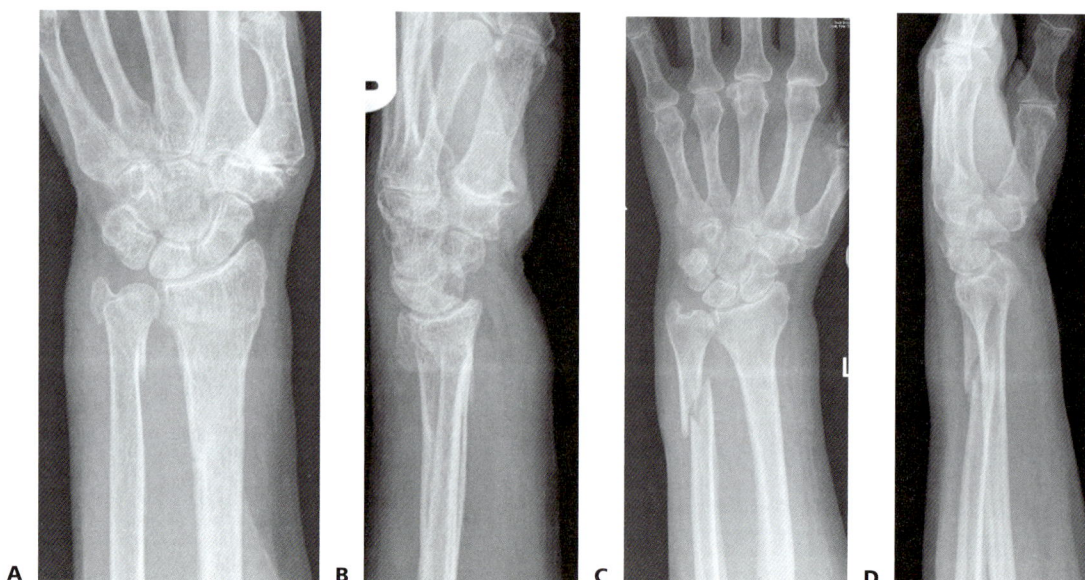

FIG 8 • **A,B.** This ulnar shaft fracture is by definition within 4 cm of the distal dome of the ulnar head. **C,D.** This ulnar shaft fracture is more proximal and should be considered an isolated ulnar fracture. However, there may still be involvement in the distal radioulnar joint (DRUJ), which needs to be taken into account. The DRUJ should be examined for stability after open reduction and internal fixation. *(continued)*

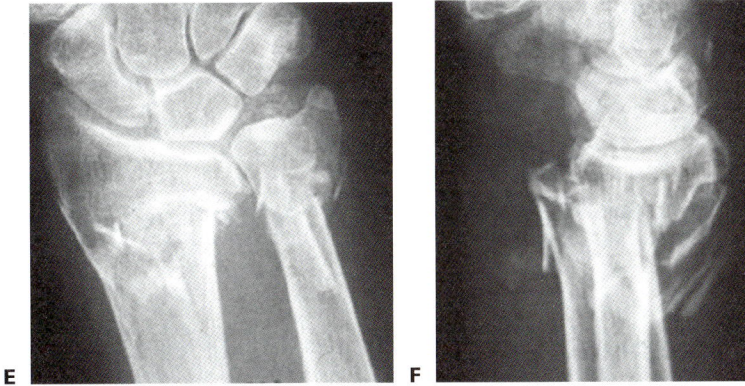

FIG 8 • *(continued)* **E,F.** Unstable distal radius and ulnar fractures are difficult to immobilize with casts alone. AP and lateral views show comminution and dorsal displacement in both fractures. This fracture cannot be treated conservatively.

- Some distal ulnar fractures in association with distal radius fractures realign after manipulation and are considered to be stable once the radius is reduced.[10]
- It is difficult to immobilize unstable fractures with a cast alone. Three-point fixation, even in an above-elbow cast, is not effective (**FIG 8E,F**).

Comminuted Intra-Articular Distal Ulnar Fractures

- Comminuted distal ulnar fractures that are irreducible and cannot be reconstructed have been mentioned in the literature in only one case report.[2]

- It is generally recommended that the initial approach be geared toward restoring the anatomy and maintaining the overall alignment of the ulna and DRUJ.

Approach

- The described approach is used for all distal ulnar fractures, including the ones extending into the neck of the ulna and into the distal shaft.
- This approach can, for instance, access an ulnar styloid fracture or nonunion and at the same time visualize, assess, and allow treatment of any associated TFCC pathology.

INCISION AND EXPOSURE

- Approach the distal ulna through a dorsal zigzag incision centered over the DRUJ (**TECH FIG 1AB**).
    - This approach allows reattachment of all crucial stabilizing structures at the time of wound closure.
    - Carefully protect the dorsal sensory branches of the ulnar nerve (**TECH FIG 1C**).
- Incise the retinaculum overlying the fifth extensor compartment (**TECH FIG 1D**).

- Elevate the ulnar retinacular flap in the interval between the extensor retinaculum and the separate dorsal sheet for the ECU tendon.
    - Preserve the integrity of the separate ECU compartment (**TECH FIG 1E**).
- Open the dorsal capsule of the DRUJ using an ulnarly based flap raised from the 4–5 septum (**TECH FIG 1F**).
- Identify the 4–5 intercompartmental artery.

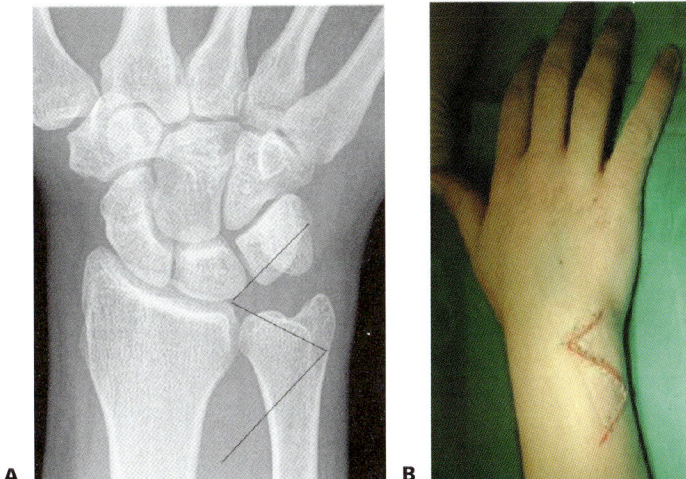

TECH FIG 1 • Surgical approach to all distal ulnar fractures. **A,B.** A dorsal zigzag incision is made with the center directed toward the distal radioulnar joint. *(continued)*

TECHNIQUES

C

D

F

Radius

Ulna

Retinacular
flap

Compartment VI

Compartment V
opened

E

G

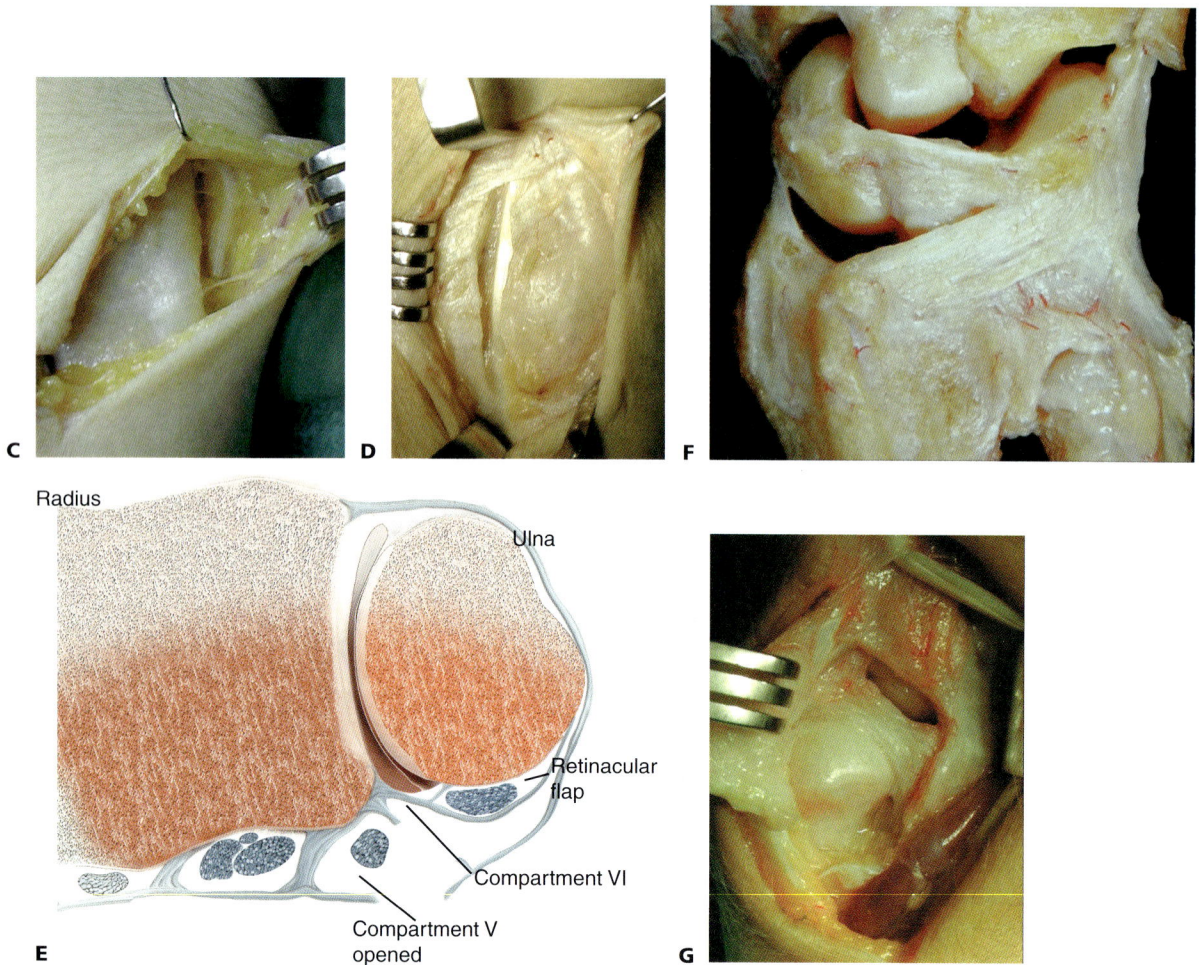

TECH FIG 1 • *(continued)* **C.** Subcutaneous dissection should be performed so that the dorsal cutaneous branch from the ulnar nerve is protected. **D.** The retinaculum is identified and an approach through the fifth extensor compartment is done. **E.** The retinaculum is elevated as an ulnarly based flap between the true retinaculum and the separate dorsal sheet for the extensor carpi ulnaris (ECU) tendon (which should be preserved). The ECU is thereby kept in its tendon sheath. **F.** An ulnarly based capsular flap is raised from the 4–5 septum to gain access to the distal ulna. **G.** As shown in this dissected specimen, the ulnocarpal joint is often hidden behind the synovium over the meniscus homolog. (**C,D:** Courtesy of M. Garcia-Elias, Spain.)

- Begin the capsular incision at the neck of the ulna and extend it to the 4–5 intercompartmental artery, which is diathermied.
- The incision continues along this line to the level of the radiocarpal joint, where it then extends distally and ulnarly along the dorsal radiotriquetral ligament to the triquetrum.
  - By staying in a flat layer along the dorsal cortex of the radius, the dorsal ulnoradial ligament attachment is not violated.
- The DRUJ and the spanning TFCC are then readily visualized. The ulnocarpal joint is often hidden behind the synovium over the meniscus homolog (**TECH FIG 1G**).
  - If required, remove the synovium dorsal to the ulnoradial ligament to gain access to the ulnar styloid and the ulnocarpal joint.
- In cases of a distal neck fracture without any intra-articular involvement or soft tissue components, the approach stays proximal to the capsular flap. However, the retinacular flap needs to be raised to address the distal metaphyseal fractures.

ULNAR STYLOID FRACTURES

- Options for fixation of ulnar styloid base fractures include the following:
  - Single or double Kirschner wires (**TECH FIG 2A,B**)
- Tension band wiring (**TECH FIG 2C**)
- Wire loop or suture
- Screw fixation (**TECH FIG 2D**)

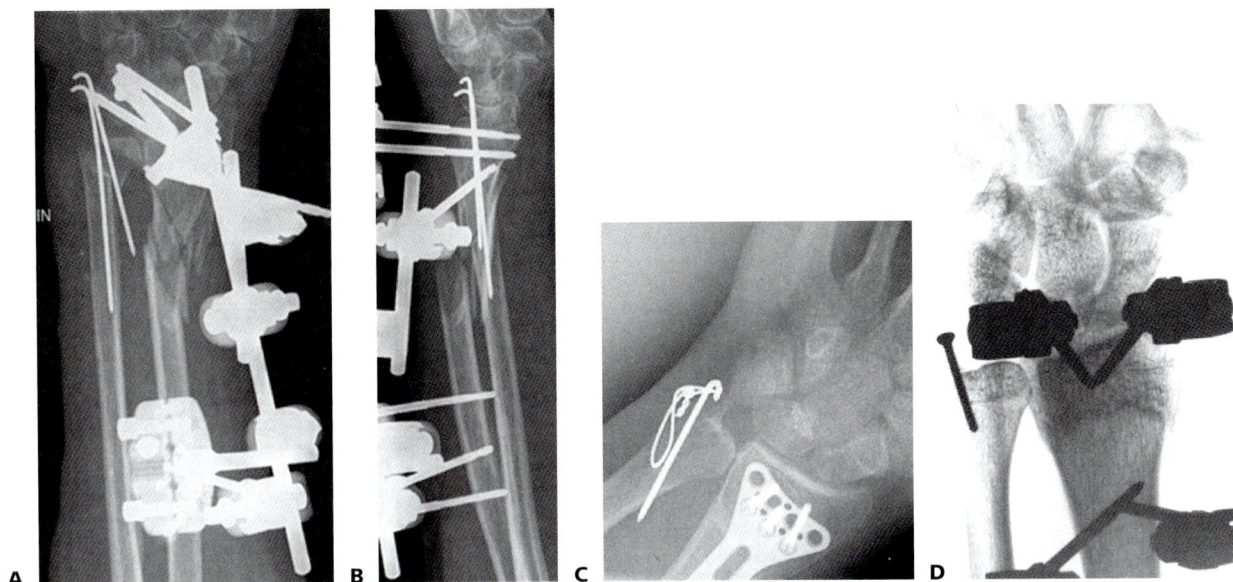

TECH FIG 2 • The ulnar styloid can be fixed in various ways to secure reattachment of the ulnoradial ligament and thereby stabilize the distal radioulnar joint. **A,B.** Single (not rotationally stable) or double Kirschner wires. **C.** Tension band wiring. **D.** Screw fixation (not rotationally stable).

ULNAR STYLOID NONUNIONS

- Reattachment of the nonunited fragment to the ulnar head is indicated if the fragment is large.[5]
- If the fragment is small, it should be excised and the ulnoradial ligament reattached directly to the fovea of the ulnar head.[5]

- If the fragment is small and located distally and there is no DRUJ instability, the ulnar styloid can be excised without any associated ligament procedure.[5]

ULNAR HEAD FRACTURES

- Ulnar head fractures without a proximal extra-articular component
  - Fractures that are displaced (with an intra-articular stepoff) or unstable are treated with ORIF using buried headless compression screws[6] or Kirschner wires.
  - Immobilization after fixation depends on the stability of the fracture and its fixation.
- Ulnar head fractures with a proximal extra-articular component

- The intra-articular component is reduced and stabilized.
- If the extra-articular component extends proximally toward the neck of the distal ulna a condylar blade plate is recommended (**TECH FIG 3**), whereas tension band wiring is recommended if the extra-articular component involves the ulnar styloid (Tech Fig 2C).
- Immobilization after fixation depends on the stability of the fracture and its fixation.

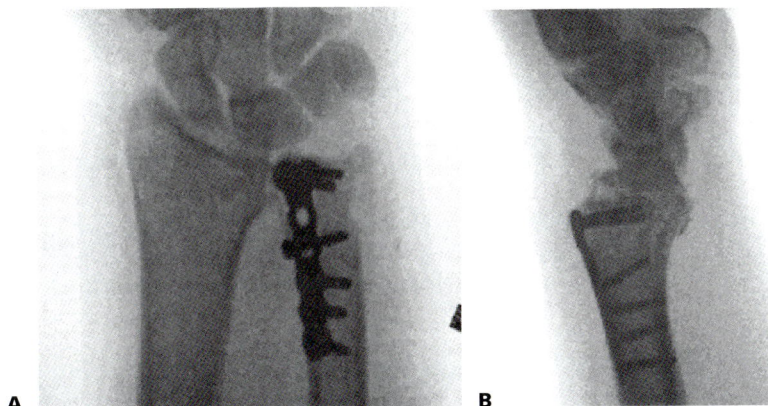

TECH FIG 3 • Irreducible or unstable distal forearm fractures require open reduction and internal fixation.[10] AP and lateral radiographs show a dorsally displaced distal forearm fracture fixed with a blade plate.

TECHNIQUES

DISTAL ULNAR NECK AND SHAFT FRACTURES

- Irreducible or unstable fractures require ORIF.[10]
- This can be achieved using either a condylar blade plate[10] (Tech Fig 3) or tension band wiring supplemented by intrafragmentary screws (**TECH FIG 4**).

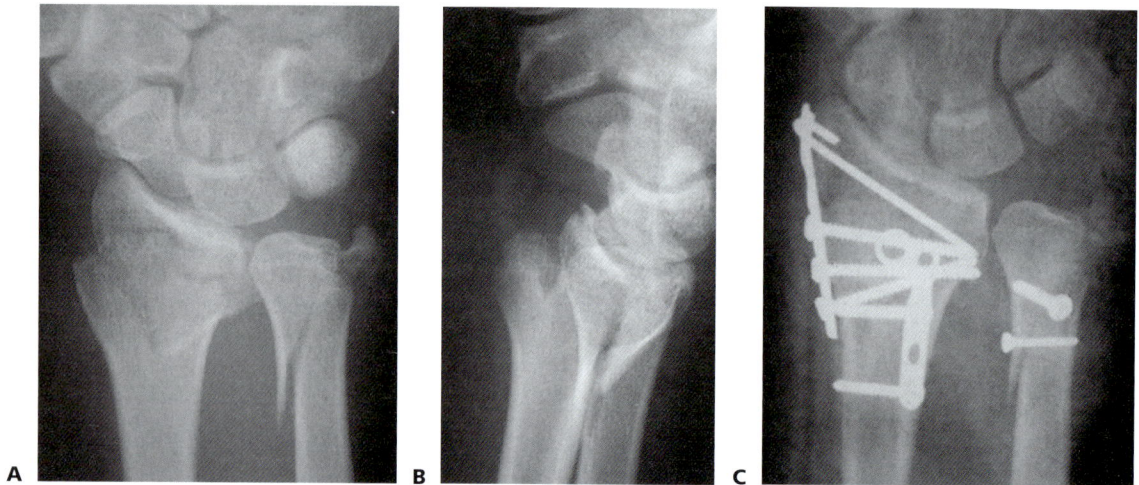

TECH FIG 4 • **A,B.** AP and lateral radiographs show a dorsally displaced distal forearm fracture. Open reduction and internal fixation was performed using both a dorsoradial and a dorsoulnar approach to stabilize the fractures. **C.** Because of the comminution around the ulnar styloid base, fixation was achieved with a suture loop.

COMMINUTED INTRA-ARTICULAR DISTAL ULNAR FRACTURES

- Three treatment options exist for comminuted intra-articular distal ulnar fractures:
  - Restoration of the anatomy and overall alignment of the ulna and DRUJ as mentioned above
    - This can be accomplished with manipulation and above-elbow cast immobilization alone or alternatively by surgical means with temporary wiring or external fixation.
    - The potential problems with this management technique are wrist stiffness and reduced forearm rotation that may not be corrected with a late salvage procedure.
  - Primary distal ulnar head replacement[2]
    - The theoretical advantage is reduced stiffness (from having early movement) and less DRUJ pain.
  - Total or partial excision of the ulnar head as well as DRUJ arthrodesis with distal ulnar neck resection (Sauve-Kapandji procedure)

POSTOPERATIVE CARE

- Stable fixation of the distal ulnar complex still requires protection postoperatively with a below-elbow splint.
- Intermediate stable fixation requires 4 weeks of protection using a sugartong-type splint to allow flexion and extension of the elbow but protect against uncontrolled pronation and supination.
- Unstable fixation after internal, external, or nonoperative treatment requires above-elbow protection in neutral forearm rotation to limit movement for the first 6 weeks. There is otherwise a risk that rotational forces will cause a nonunion or malunion.

OUTCOMES

- Outcome is influenced by the fact that most distal ulnar fractures are neglected in comparison to the more common and more extensively treated distal radius fractures.

- The outcome can surely be improved if distal ulnar fractures are treated more directly and aggressively.
- The outcome will also improve if the relationship between the ulnar styloid and the ulnoradial ligament is fully understood and addressed.

COMPLICATIONS

- Stiffness of the DRUJ with limited pronation and supination
- Infection
- Nonunion
- Malunion

REFERENCES

1. af Ekenstam F, Hagert CG. Anatomical studies on the geometry and stability of the distal radio ulnar joint. Scand J Plast Reconstr Surg 1985;19:17–25.

2. Grechenig W, Peicha G, Fellinger M. Primary ulnar head prosthesis for the treatment of an irreparable ulnar head fracture dislocation. J Hand Surg Br 2001;26B:269–271.

3. Hagert CG. The distal radioulnar joint in relation to the whole forearm. Clin Orthop Relat Res 1992;275:56–64.

4. Hagert CG. Current concepts of the functional anatomy of the distal radioulnar joint, including the ulnocarpal junction. In: Büchler U, ed. Wrist Instability. Berlin: Martin Dunitz, 1996:15–21.

5. Hauck RM, Skahen III J, Palmer AK. Classification and treatment of ulnar styloid nonunion. J Hand Surg Am 1996;21A:418–422.

6. Jakab E, Ganos DL, Gagnon S. Isolated intra-articular fractures of the ulnar head. J Orthop Trauma 1993;7:290–292.

7. Lindau T, Adlercreutz C, Aspenberg P. Peripheral tears of the triangular fibrocartilage complex cause distal radioulnar instability after distal radius fractures. J Hand Surg Am 2000;25A:464–468.

8. Lindau T, Arner M, Hagberg L. Intraarticular lesions in distal fractures of the radius in young adults: a descriptive arthroscopic study in 50 patients. J Hand Surg Br 1997;22B:638–643.

9. Palmer AK, Werner FW. The triangular fibrocartilage complex of the wrist: anatomy and function. J Hand Surg Am 1981;6A:153–162.

10. Ring D, McCarty PL, Campbell D, et al. Condylar blade plate fixation of unstable fractures of the distal ulna associated with fractures of the distal radius. J Hand Surg Am 2004;29A:103–109.

11. May MM, Lawton JN, Blazar PE. Ulnar styloid fractures associated with distal radius fractures: incidence and implications for distal radioulnar joint instability. J Hand Surg Am 2002;27A:965–971.

David Ring, Diego Fernandez, and Jesse B. Jupiter

DEFINITION

- Distal radius malunion is best defined as malalignment associated with dysfunction.
  - Malalignment does not always result in dysfunction. In particular, the vast majority of older, low-demand patients function very well with deformity.
- Dysfunction can include loss of motion, loss of strength, or pain.[1,2,5]
- Pain can be the most difficult to associate with deformity. Osteotomy for pain—as with any surgery for pain—is relatively unpredictable and should be undertaken with caution. Carpal malalignment, ulnocarpal impaction, and distal radioulnar joint malalignment are all potentially painful and can be variably addressed.
- The relationship between distal radius malunion and carpal tunnel syndrome is disputed. Some surgeons claim a direct causal relationship as well as the ability to improve carpal tunnel syndrome with osteotomy alone.

ANATOMY

- Loss of alignment can be measured on radiographs.
- Angulation of the articular surface on the lateral view is measured as the angle between a line connecting the dorsal and palmar lips of the distal radius articular surface on the lateral view and a line perpendicular to the radius shaft.
- Ulnarward inclination (often called radial inclination, a misnomer since the articular surface tilts toward the ulna) is measured as the angle between a line connecting the ulnar limit and the radial limit of the distal radius articular surface on the posteroanterior (PA) view and a line perpendicular to the radial shaft.
- Ulnar variance is a better measure of shortening of the radius than radial length. It is measured as the distance between two lines drawn perpendicular to the radial shaft on the PA view, one at the level of the most ulnar corner of the lunate facet and the other at the distal limit of the ulnar head.
  - Positive ulnar variance means that the ulna is longer than the radius. Negative means the ulna is shorter.
- Loss of articular surface alignment can be measured on radiographs as gap, step, or subluxation.
  - This is most accurately measured using CT images (**FIG 1**).
- Sources of variability in radiographic measurements include variation in the radiographs, imprecision in the measurement techniques, and imprecision in the selection of the points of reference.

PATHOGENESIS

- Fractures of the distal radius heal rapidly. A malaligned healing fracture can be considered a malunion within 4 to 6 weeks of injury.
- Risk factors for fracture instability, loss of reduction, and malunion include age over 60 years, more than 20 degrees of dorsal angulation, dorsal metaphyseal comminution, comminution extending to the volar metaphyseal cortex, associated fracture of the ulna, and displaced articular fracture.

- Risk factors for fracture instability include age, metaphyseal comminution, dorsal tilt, ulnar variance, and lack of functional independence.
- Manipulation of previously reduced fractures that redisplace in a cast or splint signifies instability and is not worthwhile.
- Limitations of various treatment techniques may contribute to creation of a malunion.
  - Percutaneous pins alone may not be sufficient to maintain alignment when there is substantial metaphyseal comminution.
  - External fixation alone without ancillary percutaneous pin fixation of the fracture
  - Early removal of pins or an external fixator. Settling of the fracture can also be observed after implant removal more than 6 weeks after injury, particularly when there is substantial metaphyseal comminution.
  - Nonlocked plates may loosen in the osteopenic metaphyseal bone.
- Complacence must be avoided. Many older patients desire optimal wrist alignment and function, and treatment decisions should not be made on chronological age alone.

NATURAL HISTORY

- Ulnar-sided wrist pain can improve for a year or more after fracture of the distal radius, so patience is warranted.
- Lack of forearm rotation may be related to capsular contracture or bony malalignment. For slight malunions, patience with exercises and rehabilitation is advisable.

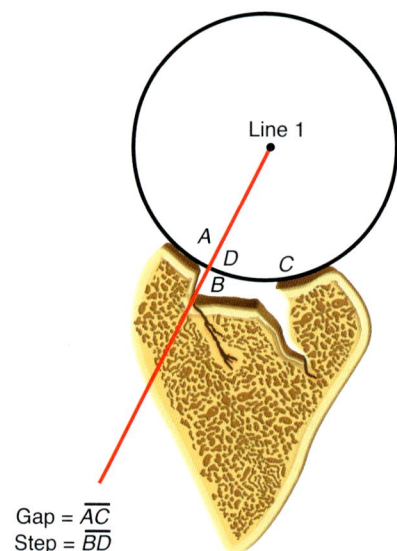

FIG 1 • The arc method for measuring articular malalignment of the distal radius. The distance between *B* and *D* is the articular step, and the distance between *A* and *C* is the maximum articular gap. (After Catalano LW III, Cole RJ, Gelberman RH, et al. Displaced intra-articular fractures of the distal aspect of the radius: long-term results in young adults after open reduction and internal fixation. J Bone Joint Surg Am 1997;79A:1290–1302.)

- While it is often stated that an extra-articular distal radius malunion leads to future arthrosis, there are no data to support this contention.
  - After a recovery period of 1 to 2 years from fracture, the functional deficits seem fairly stable.
- Articular incongruity or subluxation in relatively nonarticular areas can be reasonably well tolerated, but in most cases intra-articular incongruity will lead to arthrosis, pain, and dysfunction. There is no clear time frame for these changes—indeed, symptoms do not correlate well with radiographic anatomy and the predictors of arthrosis are not well established.

PATIENT HISTORY AND PHYSICAL FINDINGS

- Pain should be very discrete and specific. It is important that there be a direct correlation of the pain with a clear operative target. Vague, diffuse, or disproportionate pain should not be treated with osteotomy. Pain alone is not a good indication for osteotomy, so the interview should elicit specific aspects of the pain for which there is a good operative target and the risks of surgery are justified.
- Lack of motion should be clearly due to malalignment and not due to pain or squeamishness—likewise for instability of the distal radioulnar joint (DRUJ).
- Range of motion: A goniometer is used to measure wrist flexion, extension, radial and ulnar deviation, supination, and pronation.
- Ulnocarpal compression: The carpus is forcefully ulnarly deviated toward the ulna.
  - Consistent reproduction of usual pain with ulnar deviation tasks is consistent with ulnocarpal impaction.
- The examiner can test for DRUJ instability by stabilizing the radius and trying to subluxate the distal ulna dorsal and volar from the sigmoid notch of the radius.
  - Substantially less stability than the opposite side may correlate with symptomatic DRUJ instability, but this is a very difficult and subjective test.
- Scaphoid shift test: Instability would indicate a possible scapholunate interosseous ligament tear, indicating a potential dissociative rather than the typical nondissociative carpal malalignment usually associated with distal radius malunion.
- Grip strength is one measure of wrist dysfunction, but it is largely determined by pain and effort—both strongly influenced by psychosocial factors.

IMAGING AND OTHER DIAGNOSTIC STUDIES

- Posteroanterior and lateral radiographs of the wrist (**FIG 2A–D**) can be supplemented by specific radiographs for evaluation of the joint surface, particularly for potential articular malunions.
  - Comparison with the opposite, uninjured wrist is useful and serves as a template for surgical correction.
- CT, particularly three-dimensional CT, is useful to precisely evaluate the joint surfaces (**FIG 2E**).
- Neurophysiologic tests (nerve conduction velocity and electromyography) are ordered to evaluate any symptoms or signs of carpal tunnel syndrome that may need to be addressed.

DIFFERENTIAL DIAGNOSIS

- Stiffness: capsular stiffness and tendon adhesions
- Numbness: idiopathic carpal tunnel syndrome
- Pain: another discrete source of pain or even idiopathic pain

NONOPERATIVE MANAGEMENT

- Nonoperative management is appropriate for low-demand and infirm individuals. Splints are weaned after 6 weeks of cast immobilization. Patients who struggle to regain motion may benefit from working with an occupational therapist or a certified hand therapist. Normal activities are resumed in 3 or 4 months. The patient may return every 2 or 4 months or so until satisfied with the result.
- Patience is warranted in many situations, particularly for patients with ulnar-sided wrist pain thought due to an extra-articular malunion.
  - This discomfort is the last pain to go away after a distal radius fracture and routinely lasts up to a year.

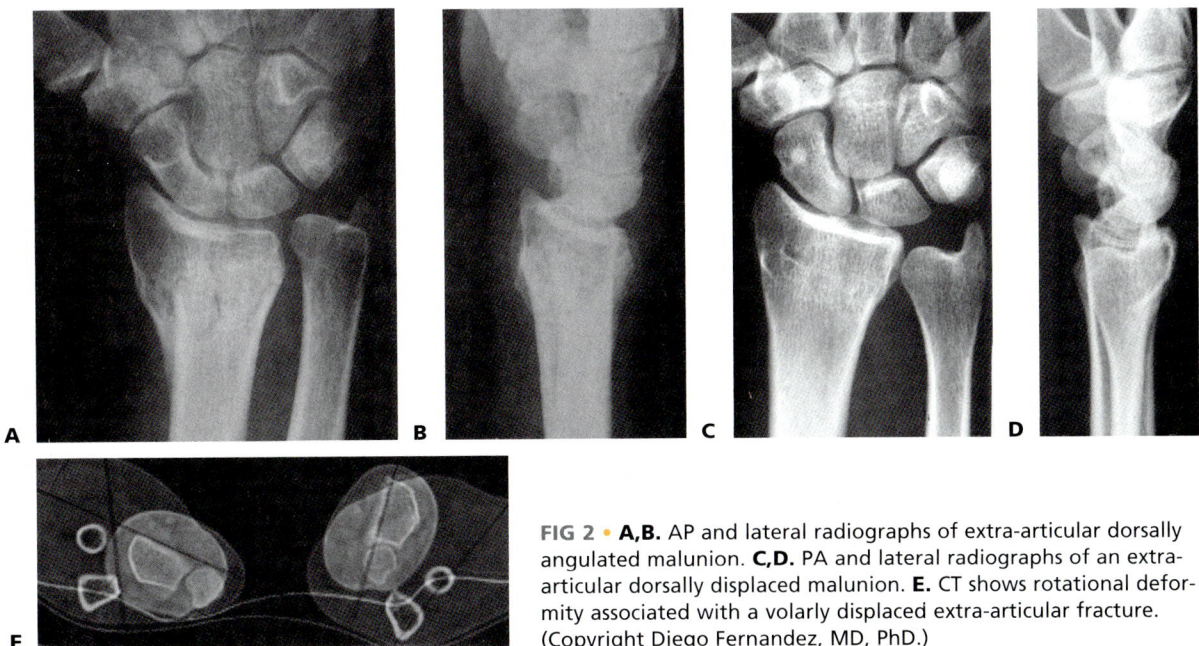

FIG 2 • A,B. AP and lateral radiographs of extra-articular dorsally angulated malunion. **C,D.** PA and lateral radiographs of an extra-articular dorsally displaced malunion. **E.** CT shows rotational deformity associated with a volarly displaced extra-articular fracture. (Copyright Diego Fernandez, MD, PhD.)

SURGICAL MANAGEMENT

- Surgery is appropriate when a radiographic deformity correlates with a specific anatomically correctable problem and the deformity is associated with a substantial risk of dysfunction and arthrosis.
  - The patient must understand the risks and benefits of intervening.
  - The surgeon should be wary of pain as the primary complaint, because pain is strongly influenced by psychosocial factors, and pain relief is an achievable goal only when consistent with an objective, correctable anatomic deformity such as discomfort clearly associated with a substantial ulnocarpal impingement.
  - When the issue is restriction of motion and there is less than 20 degrees of dorsal tilt or less than 5 mm of ulnar positive variance, a nonoperative approach may be warranted.
- There are no fixed rules or thresholds for acceptable alignment. The correlation with symptoms and dysfunction is more important.
- Intra-articular osteotomies should be considered only when the malalignment is simple and the planned correction is straightforward.
  - For instance, malalignment of volar shearing fracture would be considered when the fragment is large, there is little or no articular comminution or impaction, and the dorsal fragments are not healed in a malaligned position.

- Distal radius osteotomy need not be performed urgently. The patient should have demonstrated excellent exercise skills and full finger motion, and there should be no significant nerve or tendon dysfunction or edema.
  - In the case of an intra-articular malunion, intervening early (optimally within 6 months, definitely within 1 year of the fracture) when the fracture is not completely healed may take precedence over these concerns.

Preoperative Planning

- The desired angular, rotational, and length corrections are planned based on preoperative radiologic studies, including a radiograph of the opposite wrist if uninjured (**FIG 3A,B**).
- It can be useful to draw and write out a reconstruction plan, particularly for complex malunions (**FIG 3C–E**). In that way every contingency is anticipated and the surgery is likely to go more smoothly.

Positioning

- The patient is positioned supine with the arm supported on a hand table.
- A nonsterile pneumatic tourniquet is used and inflated after exsanguination and before the skin incision.

Approach

- The operative approach is either dorsal or volar, depending on the deformity and the chosen surgical technique.

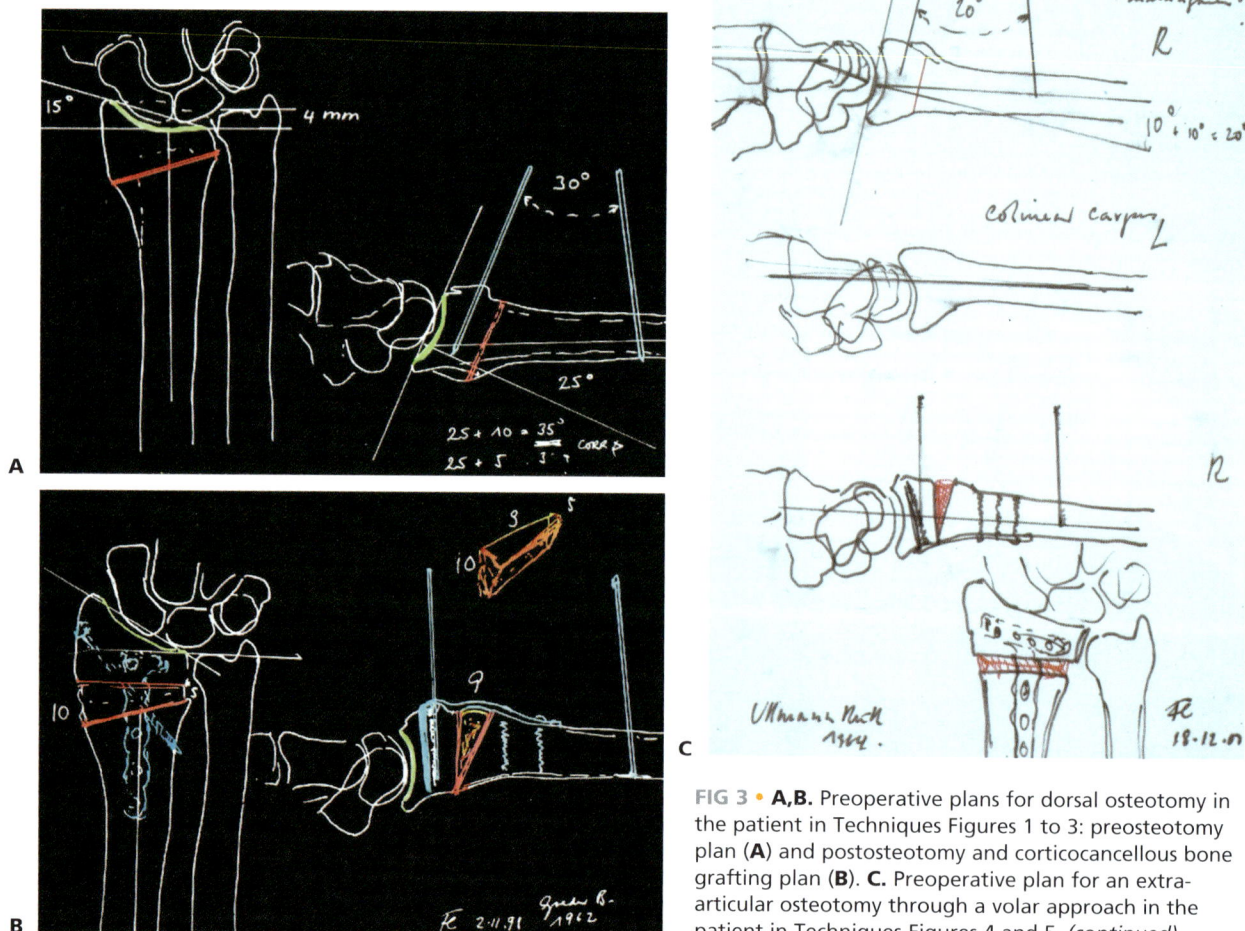

FIG 3 • **A,B.** Preoperative plans for dorsal osteotomy in the patient in Techniques Figures 1 to 3: preosteotomy plan (**A**) and postosteotomy and corticocancellous bone grafting plan (**B**). **C.** Preoperative plan for an extra-articular osteotomy through a volar approach in the patient in Techniques Figures 4 and 5. *(continued)*

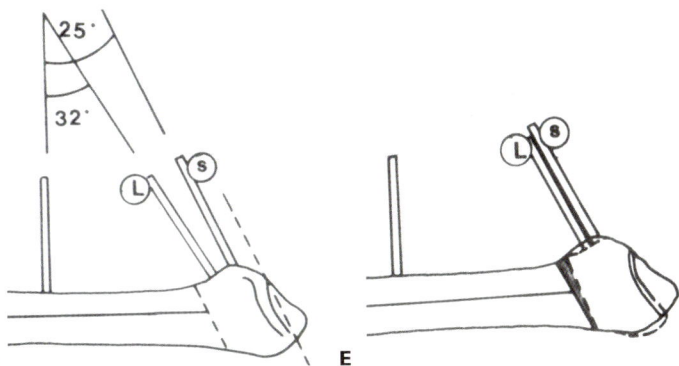

FIG 3 • *(continued)* **D,E.** Preoperative plans for an intra-articular dorsally angulated malunion in the patient in Techniques Figure 6. (Copyright Diego Fernandez, MD, PhD.)

TECHNIQUES

DORSAL EXTRA-ARTICULAR DISTAL RADIUS OSTEOTOMY: CORTICOCANCELLOUS GRAFT

Exposure

- Make a longitudinal incision centered over the tubercle of Lister, in line with the third metacarpal (**TECH FIG 1A**).
- Elevate skin flaps, taking care to protect the branches of the superficial radial nerve in the radial skin flap.
- Incise the retinaculum over the third extensor compartment. Remove the tendon of the extensor pollicis longus (EPL) and transpose it radialward (**TECH FIG 1B**).
  - The EPL tendon will be left in the subcutaneous tissues at the completion of the procedure.

- Elevate the fourth dorsal compartment and its tendons subperiosteally.
  - Preserve the integrity of this compartment.
- It is usually not possible to elevate the second dorsal compartment subperiosteally, so simply retract the extensor carpi radialis brevis and longus tendons radialward after opening the compartment.

Osteotomy and Realignment

- Kirschner wires drilled parallel to the articular surface can facilitate monitoring of realignment (**TECH FIG 2A**).
- A distractor or small external fixator may facilitate realignment and provisionally stabilize the fracture.
  - The proximal threaded pin is drilled into the radial diaphysis perpendicularly in a position that will not interfere with implant application.
  - The distal threaded pin is drilled at an angle equal to the desired correction of the lateral tilt of the distal radius articular surface so that distraction of the two pins will bring this pin parallel to the proximal pin (perpendicular to the radius), thereby restoring alignment.
  - The pins should be drilled so that they also help restore the appropriate ulnarward inclination of the distal radius articular surface when distracted.
  - Planned angular corrections can be monitored with sterile geometric templates.
- The osteotomy is made parallel with the distal Kirschner wire and as close to the original fracture site as possible using an oscillating saw (**TECH FIG 2B**).
- If the fracture is not yet completely healed (nascent malunion—usually within 4 months of injury), recreate the original fracture line by carefully removing fracture callus at the fracture site.
  - This callus can be saved and used as bone graft.
- If the fracture is solidly healed, attempt to identify the prior fracture site. If this is uncertain, choose a site that creates a distal fragment large enough to facilitate manipulation and internal fixation while trying to stay distal enough to take advantage of the healing capacity of metaphyseal bone.

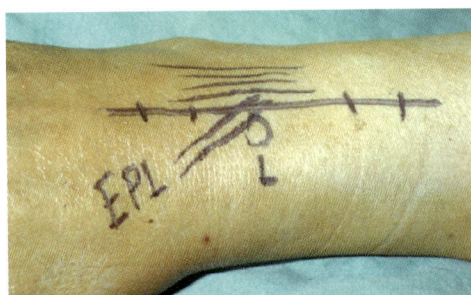

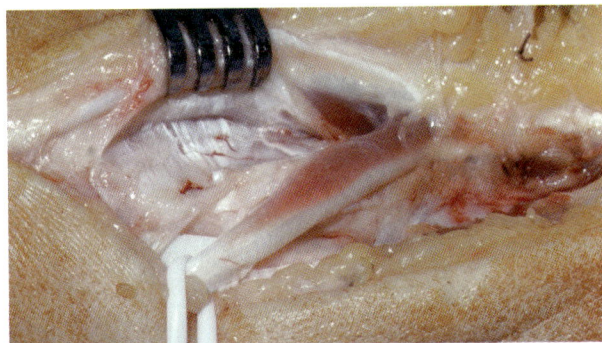

TECH FIG 1 • Correction of extra-articular dorsally angulated malunion in the patient in Figure 2A,B. **A.** Straight longitudinal skin incision. **B.** The extensor pollicis longus is mobilized and transposed dorsoradially into the subcutaneous tissues. (Copyright Diego Fernandez, MD, PhD.)

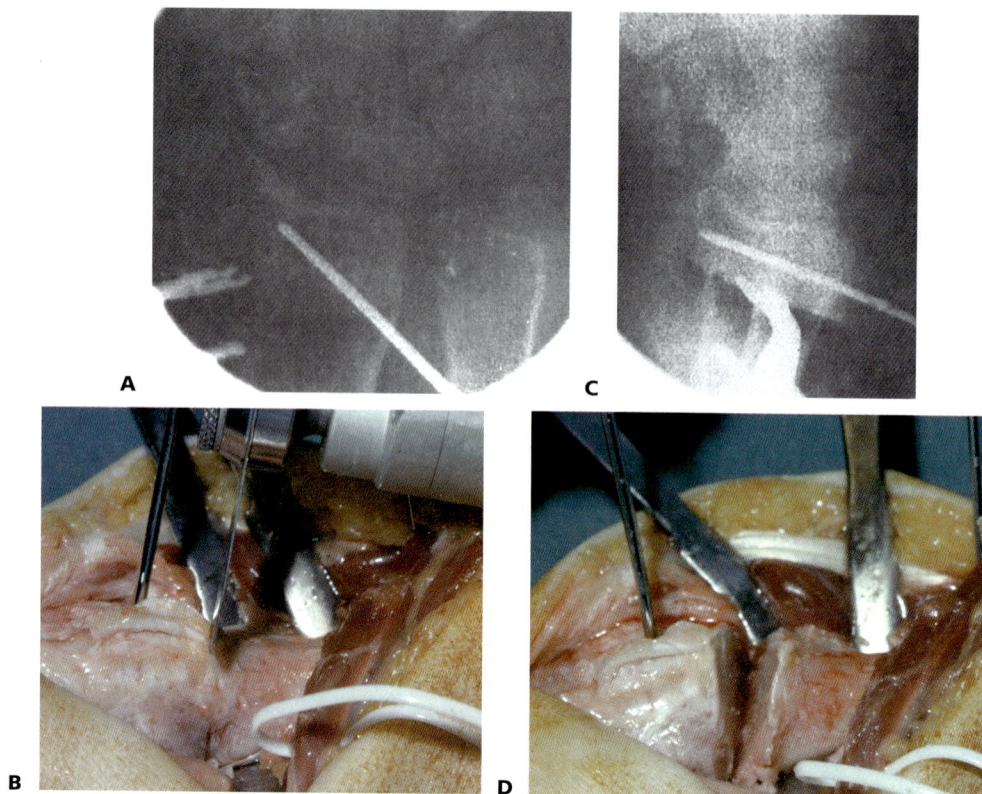

TECH FIG 2 • **A.** Kirschner wires are placed parallel to the articular surface. Fluoroscopic image showing pin placement. **B.** The osteotomy is made with a saw as close as possible to the original fracture site. **C.** Lateral fluoroscopic image showing use of a lamina spreader to realign the distal fragment. **D.** The osteotomy has been opened and is ready for graft placement. (Copyright Diego Fernandez, MD, PhD.)

- A lamina spreader can be used to help realign the distal fragment as well (**TECH FIG 2C,D**).
  - Care must be taken when operating on osteoporotic bone.
- Additional provisional stability can be provided by placing 1.6-mm smooth Kirschner wires.
- If the ulnar variance can be restored with angular realignment alone, the volar cortex can be cracked and hinged open in an attempt to maintain some stability of the osteotomy. If lengthening of the volar cortex is required to restore ulnar variance, a second distractor in another plane (eg, direct radial) may prove useful for obtaining and maintaining alignment.

Graft Insertion and Fixation

- Once the osteotomy is created and the radius realigned, bone graft is inserted.
- Harvest bone graft (**TECH FIG 3A**). Either a corticocancellous (structural) bone graft or cancellous bone graft can be used.
  - Potential advantages of a structural graft include immediate structural support (**TECH FIG 3B**) and the possibility of using a smaller implant and thereby avoiding tendon irritation.
  - A cancellous (nonstructural) bone graft can be harvested using trephines (**TECH FIG 3C**). This avoids tedious, difficult, and unpredictable harvest and contouring of corticocancellous grafts, as well as the

morbidity associated with harvest of a standard iliac crest bone graft.

- Apply a single T- or Pi-shaped plate or two 2.0- or 2.4-mm plates (one applied dorsally, ulnar to the tubercle of Lister, and the other applied radially between the first and second dorsal compartments).
  - When a structural, corticocancellous bone graft is used, a single plate or a plate and separate screw may be adequate (**TECH FIG 3D–H**).
  - Plates with angular stable screws or blades in the distal fragment may be more reliable than standard screws, particularly if the bone is of poor quality and if nonstructural graft is chosen.
- Once implants are placed and stability is ensured, remove all provisional fixation devices.
- This entire process is monitored using image intensification to confirm appropriate osteotomy site, correction of alignment, and implant placement.
- Repair the extensor retinaculum with absorbable suture.
  - In some cases, a flap of retinaculum is brought deep to the tendons to add a layer of protection between the implants and extensor tendons.
  - We usually do not close the retinaculum, and we no longer make retinacular flaps.
- The tourniquet is deflated and hemostasis ensured.
- The skin is closed.
- A bulky dressing incorporating a volar plaster wrist splint is applied.

TECHNIQUES

TECHNIQUES

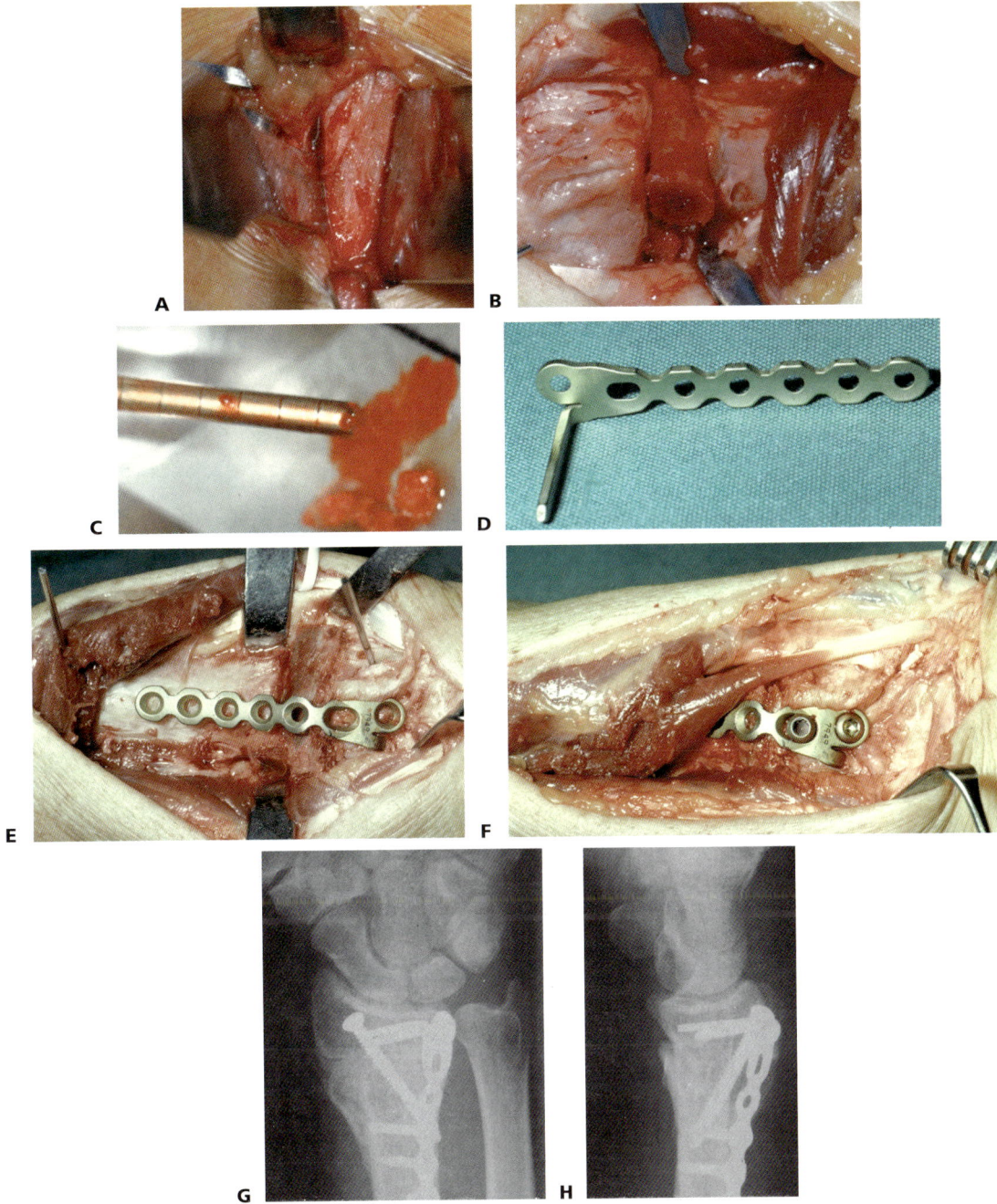

TECH FIG 3 • **A.** Corticocancellous bone graft is harvested from the iliac crest. **B.** After final sculpting it is applied to the osteotomy site. **C.** Autogenous cancellous bone graft is harvested from the iliac crest using a trephine. **D.** A 2.0-mm condylar blade plate can provide fixed-angle internal fixation. **E,F.** Intraoperative photographs of the fixation. **G,H.** Final AP and lateral radiographs. (Copyright Diego Fernandez, MD, PhD.)

VOLAR EXTRA-ARTICULAR DISTAL RADIUS OSTEOTOMY

Exposure

- Use a volar-radial Henry (flexor carpi radialis [FCR]) approach for both dorsally and volarly angulated malunions (see Fig 2C,D).
- Make a 5- to 7-cm longitudinal incision over the FCR tendon ending at the wrist flexion crease.
- If more exposure is required, the incision is angled or zigzagged at least 45 degrees toward the scaphoid distal pole.
- Incise the FCR sheath, retract the tendon ulnarly, and incise the floor.
    - Leave the radial artery undissected and protected in the radial soft tissues.

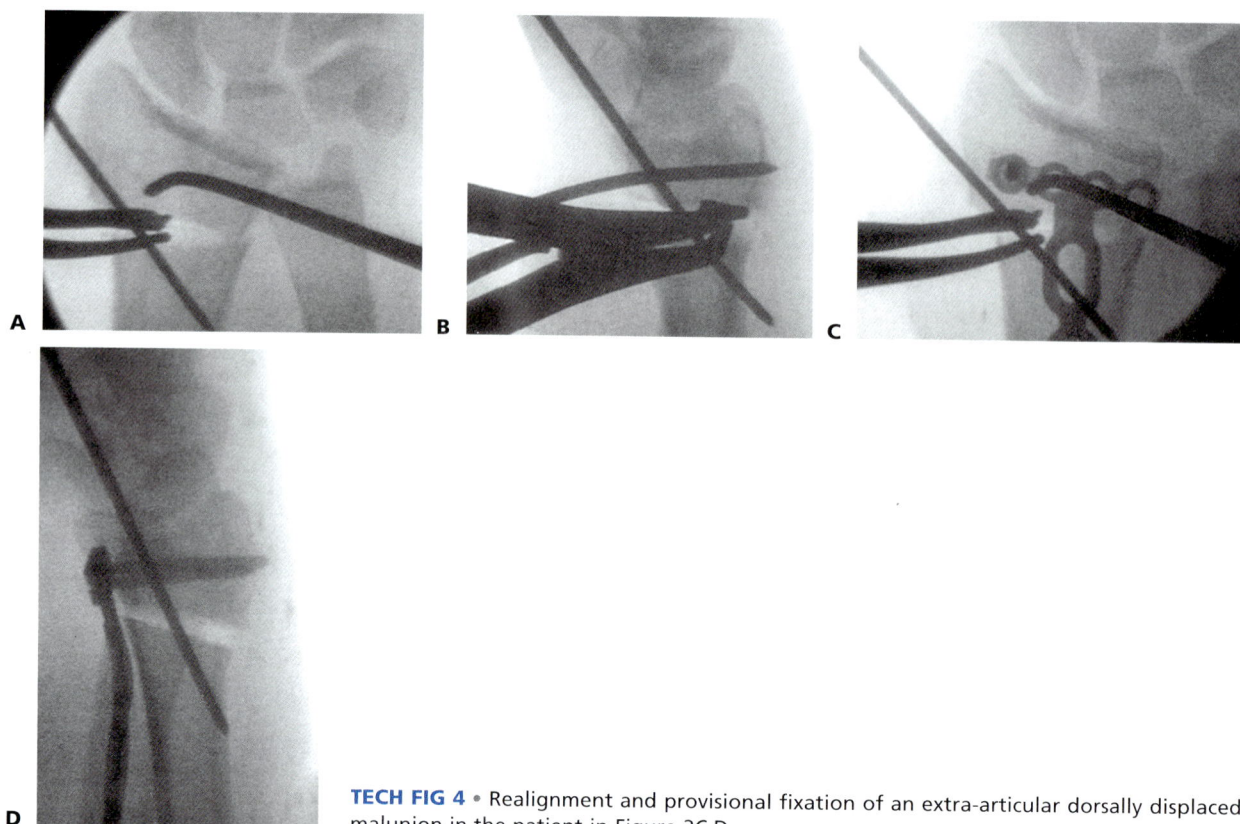

TECH FIG 4 • Realignment and provisional fixation of an extra-articular dorsally displaced malunion in the patient in Figure 2C,D.

- Sweep the fat overlying the pronator quadratus together with the digital flexors and median nerve ulnarward with a sponge or blunt elevator.
- Proximally in the incision, elevate the most distal aspect of the origin of the flexor pollicis longus from the volar distal radius (taking care to cauterize a consistent artery in this region) and retract it ulnarly with a small Hohmann retractor placed around the ulnar border of the radius.
- Expose the radial border of the radius using a blunt elevator and Hohmann retractors.
- Incise the pronator quadratus over its most radial and distal limits (L-shaped incision) and elevate it subperiosteally.
  - Leaving the periosteum with the muscle can facilitate later repair.
- For dorsally angulated malunions, release of the radial and dorsal soft tissues facilitates realignment.
  - The brachioradialis is Z-lengthened and the periosteum is elevated from the radius shaft proximally.
- After osteotomy in the manner detailed above (for the dorsal approach to malunions), pronate the proximal radius shaft out of the wound, providing access to the dorsal periosteum, which can be isolated and divided.
  - With the release of the brachioradialis and the dorsal periosteum, realignment of the radius is usually comparable to an acute fracture.
- Volarly angulated malunions do not need an extensive soft tissue release in most cases. The plate can facilitate

realignment by pushing the distal fragments into position as the proximal screws are tightened.

Realignment and Provisional Fixation

- The fragments are realigned using the techniques described above (**TECH FIG 4**).
  - The techniques are similar to those for acute fractures once an adequate soft tissue release has been performed.
- Apply a fixed-angle volar implant.
- Insert provisional Kirschner wires either through or adjacent to the plate (see Tech Fig 4).

Plate Fixation

- Placement of the plate will frequently help reduce the proximal and distal fragments (**TECH FIG 5A,B**).
- After final plate fixation and removal of provisional fixation, apply cancellous graft to the osteotomy site (**TECH FIG 5C–F**).
  - Excellent access is available radially for placement of the bone graft.
- The tourniquet is deflated and hemostasis ensured.
- Repair the pronator quadratus if possible.
  - It can be sutured to the brachioradialis tendon.
- The skin is closed.
- A bulky dressing incorporating a volar plaster wrist splint is applied.

TECHNIQUES

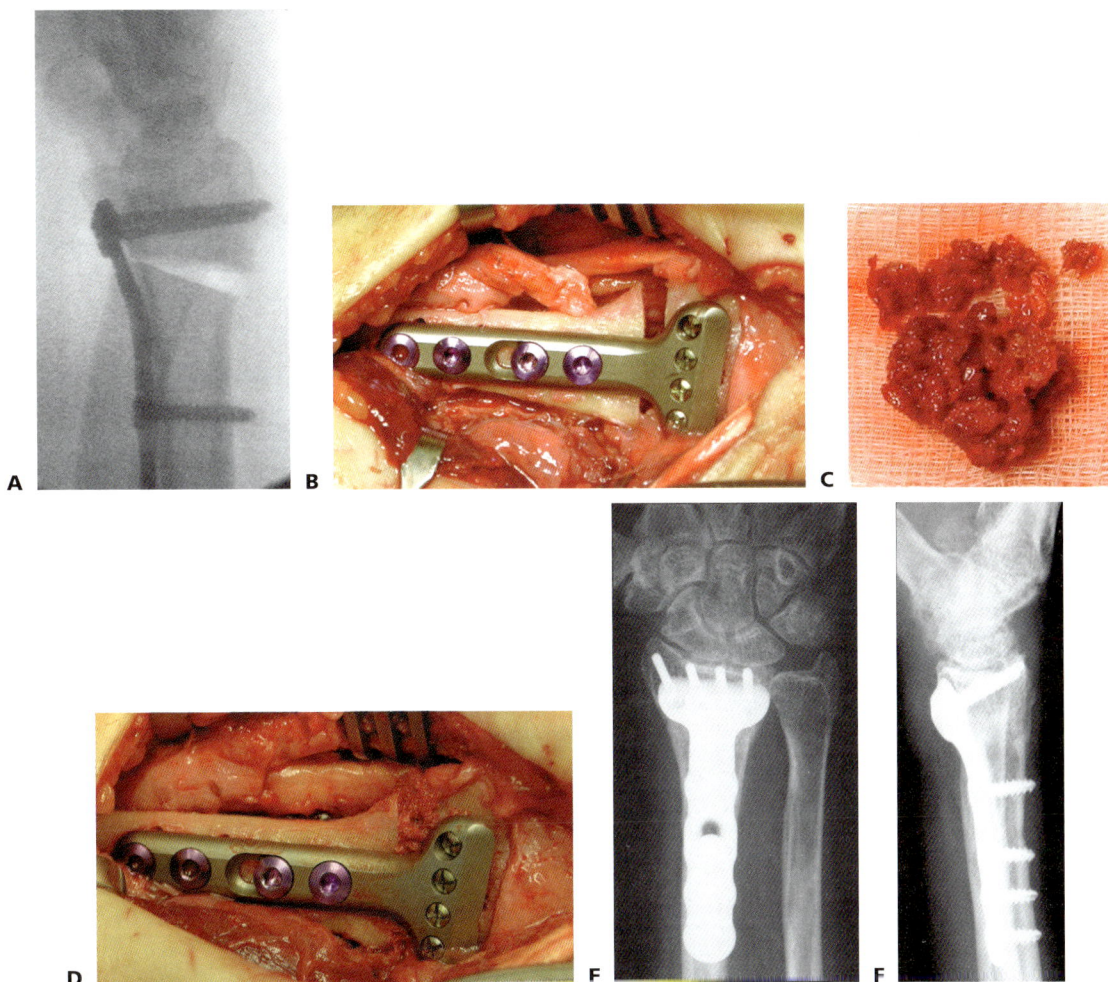

TECH FIG 5 • **A.** Fluoroscopic image of plate fixation and realignment. **B.** Defect after correction. Autogenous cancellous graft. (**C**) and graft placement (**D**), showing final clinical appearance. **E,F.** Final PA and lateral radiographs. (Copyright Diego Fernandez, MD, PhD.)

INTRA-ARTICULAR DISTAL RADIUS OSTEOTOMY

- Intra-articular osteotomy should be attempted only when there is a simple fracture line that can be clearly identified by direct visualization as well as under image intensification (**TECH FIG 6A–C**).
  - Incompletely healed fractures (fewer than 3 to 4 months since injury) are ideal.
- Depending on the locations of the malunited articular fragments, perform either a dorsal or a volar exposure in the manner detailed above.
  - When a dorsal exposure is used, a transverse capsulotomy allows access to the joint and monitoring of the articular osteotomy and realignment.
  - In the case of a volar exposure, the capsule is not incised, but articular exposure may be possible through the osteotomy site.
- The osteotomy should recreate the original fracture line. This is monitored directly and under image intensification.
- Reduction is accomplished by soft tissue release and direct fragment manipulation. For many malunions it is

necessary to remove bone or callus from the fracture site to realign the fracture fragment. Callus or bone is removed until the fracture fragment fits properly (**TECH FIG 6D**).
- Provisional Kirschner wires are used to hold the reduction (**TECH FIG 6E,F**).
- The implants are then applied.
  - Dorsally a single T- or Pi-shaped plate or two 2.0- or 2.4-mm plates (one applied dorsally, ulnar to the tubercle of Lister, and the other applied radially between the first and second dorsal compartments) can be used (**TECH FIG 6G,H**).
  - Volarly, a T-shaped plate is usually used.
  - After final plate fixation, provisional fixation is removed.
- This entire process is monitored using image intensification to confirm appropriate osteotomy site, correction of alignment, and implant placement.
- Deflate the tourniquet, close the wound, and apply the splint in the manner detailed above.

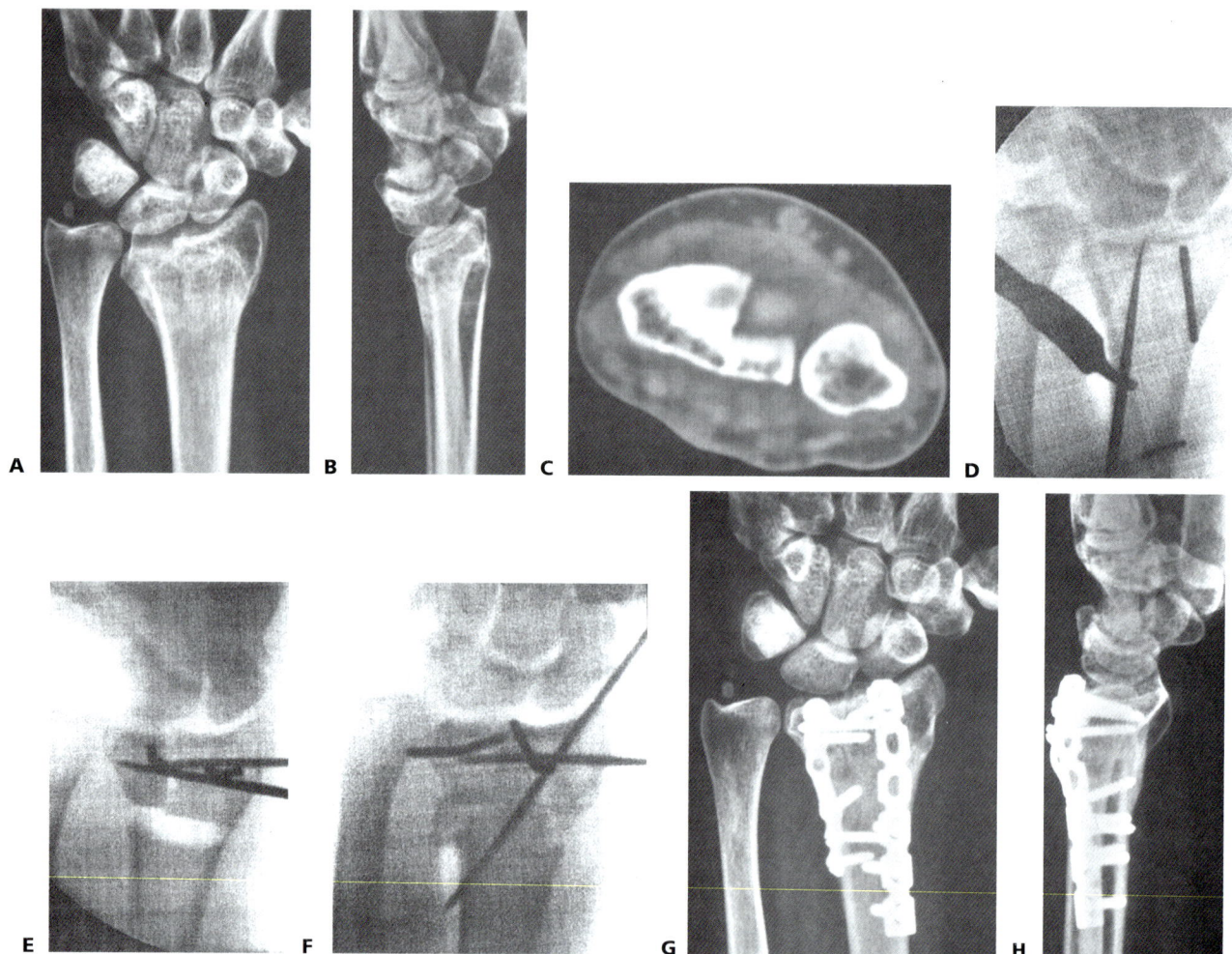

TECH FIG 6 • **A–C.** PA and lateral radiographs and CT of an intra-articular dorsally angulated malunion. **D.** A Freer elevator is used under fluoroscopy to reposition the articular fragment. **E,F.** Intraoperative fluoroscopic views showing provisional correction and fixation. **G,H.** Final plate and screw fixation. (Copyright Diego Fernandez, MD, PhD.)

PEARLS AND PITFALLS

Preoperative plan	▪ A poor or incomplete preoperative plan will increase the amount of uncertainty and hesitation during surgery. This will increase the operative time and the frustration level and will decrease the satisfaction with the surgery. ▪ Making a detailed preoperative plan will improve the efficiency and efficacy of the procedure.
Extra-articular malunions	▪ Manipulating the distal fragment can be much more difficult with poor-quality bone. ▪ The use of a distractor or small external fixator greatly facilitates realignment and provisional stabilization of the fragments. ▪ Consider using two distractors in perpendicular planes (eg, one dorsal and one direct radial) to help obtain and maintain alignment. ▪ Restoration of length in addition to that gained with angular realignment (ie, lengthening of both the dorsal and volar cortices) is much more difficult. ▪ The most difficult part of performing an osteotomy for a dorsal angulated malunion from a volar approach is realignment of the bone. ▪ An extended FCR exposure allows release of the dorsal periosteum and Z-lengthening of the brachioradialis, both of which facilitate realignment of the radius.
Intra-articular malunions	▪ Handling small articular fracture fragments can be difficult. ▪ Each fragment can be realigned using a Kirschner wire as a joystick. ▪ The articular osteotomy is easiest when the original fracture lines can be identified. ▪ Try to intervene within 3 months of injury when articular malunion is identified.

POSTOPERATIVE CARE

- Active and active-assisted exercise of the fingers and forearm, finger exercises to reduce swelling, and active functional use of the limb for light tasks are encouraged immediately.
- The initial plaster splint is exchanged for a custom Orthoplast removable splint 2 weeks after the surgery.
- The patient gradually weans out of the splint between 4 and 6 weeks after surgery and initiates active and active-assisted wrist exercises.
- Strengthening and forceful use of the arm are restricted until early radiographic union is apparent.
- Unrestricted use of the limb is allowed when solid union is present clinically and radiographically.

OUTCOMES

- Fernandez' articles describing dorsal osteotomy with cortico-cancellous bone graft with[1] and without[2] Bower arthroplasty of the DRUJ established the value of the technique for improving function in patients with symptomatic distal radius malunions.
  - He documented good or excellent results in 75% and 80% of patients respectively, noting that satisfactory results depend upon the absence of degenerative changes in the radiocarpal and intercarpal joints, and the presence of adequate preoperative range of motion of the wrist.
  - Corrective osteotomy with carefully preoperatively planned structural corticocancellous bone graft does not reliably achieve the planned correction.[12]
  - Nonunions, loss of alignment, and major complications were not reported in these series.
- Jupiter and Ring[5] demonstrated that early correction of distal radius deformity shortened the period of disability without increasing complications, and that the combination of cancellous autograft and locking plates was as reliable as corticocancellous bone grafting.[9]
  - Nonunions, loss of alignment, and major complications were not reported in these series.
- Several small articles have established the safety and efficacy of volar osteotomy for a dorsally displaced fracture.[4,6]
- Shea et al[10] established the safety and efficacy of osteotomy for volar extra-articular malunions in a case series.
- Fernandez et al[3] established the safety and efficacy of osteotomy for a radially deviated extra-articular malunion in a case series.
- Several case series have documented the safety and efficacy of intra-articular osteotomy.[7,8,11]

COMPLICATIONS

- Nonunion
- Loss of alignment
- Loss of fixation
- Infection
- Wound problems
- Nerve injury

REFERENCES

1. Fernandez DL. Correction of posttraumatic wrist deformity in adults by osteotomy, bone grafting and internal fixation. J Bone Joint Surg Am 1982;64A:1164–1178.
2. Fernandez DL. Radial osteotomy and Bowers arthroplasty for malunited fractures of the distal end of the radius. J Bone Joint Surg 1988;70A:1538–1551.
3. Fernandez DL, Capo JT, Gonzalez E. Corrective osteotomy for symptomatic increased ulnar tilt of the distal end of the radius. J Hand Surg Am 2001;26A:722–732.
4. Henry M. Immediate mobilisation following corrective osteotomy of distal radius malunions with cancellous graft and volar fixed angle plates. J Hand Surg Eur Vol 2007;32:88–92.
5. Jupiter JB, Ring D. A comparison of early and late reconstruction of the distal end of the radius. J Bone Joint Surg 1996;78A:739–748.
6. Malone KJ, Magnell TD, Freeman DC, et al. Surgical correction of dorsally angulated distal radius malunions with fixed angle volar plating: a case series. J Hand Surg Am 2006;31A:366–372.
7. Marx RG, Axelrod TS. Intraarticular osteotomy of distal radial malunions. Clin Orthop Relat Res 1996;327:152–157.
8. Ring D, Prommersberger KJ, Gonzalez del Pino J, et al. Corrective osteotomy for intra-articular malunion of the distal part of the radius. J Bone Joint Surg Am 2005;87A:1503–1509.
9. Ring D, Roberge C, Morgan T, et al. Comparison of structural and non-structural bone graft for corrective osteotomy of distal radius malunion. J Hand Surg Am 2002;27A:216–222.
10. Shea K, Fernandez DL, Jupiter JB, et al. Corrective osteotomy for malunited, volarly displaced fractures of the distal end of the radius. J Bone Joint Surg Am 1997;79A:1816–1826.
11. Thivaios GC, McKee MD. Sliding osteotomy for deformity correction following malunion of volarly displaced distal radial fractures. J Orthop Trauma 2003;17:326–333.
12. von Campe A, Nagy L, Arbab D, et al. Corrective osteotomies in malunions of the distal radius: do we get what we planned? Clin Orthop Relat Res 2006;450:179–185.

Percutaneous Fixation of Acute Scaphoid Fractures

Peter J.L. Jebson, Jane S. Tan, and Andrew Wong

DEFINITION

- Located in the proximal carpal row, the scaphoid serves as an important link between the proximal and distal carpal rows. It is the most commonly fractured carpal bone, accounting for about 1 in every 100,000 emergency room visits.[12]
- There are about 345,000 scaphoid fractures annually in the United States.
- A scaphoid fracture classically occurs in a young, active adult due to a fall onto an outstretched hand.
- The Herbert classification categorizes scaphoid fractures into acute stable, acute unstable, delayed union, and established nonunion patterns.

ANATOMY

- The scaphoid has a complex three-dimensional geometry that has been described as a "twisted peanut."[8] Anatomically the scaphoid is organized into proximal pole, waist, and distal pole regions.
- The scaphoid articulates with the radius, lunate, capitate, trapezium, and trapezoid; thus, its surface is almost completely covered with hyaline cartilage. This feature has several important implications, including articular disruption during wire or screw insertion, paucity of vascular supply, and the absence of periosteum.
  - Lacking periosteum, the scaphoid heals almost completely by primary bone healing, resulting in minimal callus and a biomechanically weak early union.[17]
  - Blood supply comes from branches of the radial artery that enter the scaphoid via two main routes[7]:
    - A dorsal branch, which enters the scaphoid via the dorsal ridge, provides the primary supply and 70% to 80% of the overall vascularity, including the entire proximal pole (via retrograde endosteal branches).
    - A volar branch, which enters through the tubercle, supplies 20% to 30% of the internal vascularity, all in the distal pole.
- The precarious blood supply contributes to the high incidence of nonunion after a fracture at the scaphoid waist or proximal pole. It also places the proximal pole at risk for the development of avascular necrosis.

PATHOGENESIS

- The typical mechanism of injury involves a fall onto the wrist. Studies have demonstrated that wrist extension of more than 95 degrees combined with more than 10 degrees of radial deviation is required for a scaphoid fracture to occur. In this position, the scaphoid abuts the distal radius, resulting in fracture.
- Seventy to 80% of scaphoid fractures occur at the waist region, while 10% to 20% involve the proximal pole and 5% occur at the distal pole and tuberosity.
- In children, the most common location for a scaphoid fracture is the distal pole.[2]

NATURAL HISTORY

- The true natural history of an untreated scaphoid fracture is unknown due to limitations in the existing literature, particularly with respect to study design.[11] However, several retrospective studies have suggested that if a nonunion occurs, a predictable pattern of wrist arthritis develops usually within 10 years of the injury.[14,16]
- Unrecognized, untreated, or inadequately treated scaphoid fractures have an increased likelihood of nonunion and secondary carpal instability. A fracture through the proximal pole has the highest likelihood of nonunion, followed by a fracture of the scaphoid waist.
- If the scaphoid fracture is unstable, extension forces at the proximal fragment (via the lunate and scapholunate ligament) and flexion forces at the distal fragment result in a flexion ("humpback") deformity of the scaphoid.
  - This loss of scaphoid support results in carpal instability, most frequently a dorsal intercalated segment instability (DISI) pattern, which eventually leads to arthritis as previously described.
- The overall incidence of nonunion after fracture of the scaphoid waist region is about 5% to 10%.[13]

PATIENT HISTORY AND PHYSICAL FINDINGS

- A patient with an acute or subacute scaphoid fracture presents with radial-sided wrist pain, swelling, and loss of motion, particularly with dorsiflexion.
- Classic physical examination findings include:
  - Edema over the dorsoradial aspect of the wrist
  - Tenderness to palpation between the first and third dorsal compartments (the "anatomic snuffbox")
  - Tenderness with palpation volarly over the distal tubercle
  - Pain with axial compression of the wrist (scaphoid compression test)
  - Acutely, swelling and ecchymoses over the volar radial wrist

IMAGING AND OTHER DIAGNOSTIC STUDIES

- Initial imaging studies for a suspected scaphoid fracture should include a posteroanterior (PA) view with the wrist in ulnar deviation, semipronated and semisupinated 45-degree oblique views, and a lateral view.
  - The PA ulnar deviation view produces scaphoid extension, permitting visualization of the entire scaphoid.
  - The semipronated view permits visualization of the waist and distal-third regions.
  - The semisupinated view provides visualization of the dorsal ridge.
  - The lateral view can demonstrate a waist fracture, fracture displacement and angulation, and overall carpal alignment.

- Displaced and unstable fractures are defined by the following criteria:
  - At least 1 mm of displacement
  - More than 10 degrees of angular displacement
  - Fracture comminution
  - Radiolunate angle of more than 15 degrees
  - Scapholunate angle of more than 60 degrees
  - Intrascaphoid angle of more than 35 degrees
- CT scan is helpful in identifying and characterizing an acute fracture and evaluating for a nonunion. Thin 1-mm cuts are obtained in the sagittal and coronal planes.
- MRI is useful for diagnosing an occult fracture and, when combined with gadolinium administration, can be used to assess the vascularity of the proximal pole and the presence of avascular necrosis.
- Technetium bone scan has been shown to be up to 100% sensitive in identifying occult fractures but lacks specificity. It is optimally used 48 hours after injury.

DIFFERENTIAL DIAGNOSIS

- Scapholunate injury
- Wrist sprain
- Wrist contusion
- Fracture of other carpal bones
- Distal radius fracture

NONOPERATIVE MANAGEMENT

- Nonoperative management, specifically cast immobilization, is indicated for a nondisplaced, acute (less than 4 weeks from injury) fracture of the distal pole. For a nondisplaced, acute waist fracture, there is debate regarding the preferred treatment approach—cast immobilization or surgical stabilization.
- With cast immobilization, there is no consensus regarding the preferred position of the wrist, the need to immobilize other joints besides the wrist, and the duration of immobilization.[4]
  - Clinical studies have demonstrated no benefit with thumb immobilization, nor any influence of wrist position on the rate of union.
  - Studies have also demonstrated no difference in union rates with use of a long-arm versus short-arm cast; however, a small randomized prospective study by Gellman et al[9] demonstrated a shorter time to union and fewer nonunions and delayed unions with the initial use of a long-arm cast.

- In general, cast immobilization is required for 6 weeks after a distal pole fracture and 10 to 12 weeks following a nondisplaced waist fracture.
  - Confirmation of fracture union requires serial plain radiographs demonstrating progressive obliteration of the fracture line and clear trabeculation across the fracture site.[6]
- If there is any question regarding fracture union, a CT scan should be obtained.

SURGICAL MANAGEMENT

- Operative treatment is advocated for fractures that are unstable or displaced (see above criteria) and following a significant treatment delay.
- Percutaneous fixation is indicated for:
  - Nondisplaced fractures of the scaphoid waist
  - Displaced fractures of the scaphoid waist
  - Proximal pole fractures
- Percutaneous stabilization of scaphoid fractures may be performed using either the dorsal arthroscopically assisted reduction and fixation (AARF) approach[17–19] or the volar approach.[3,10]
  - Regardless of the technique used, the screw must be inserted in the middle third or central axis of the scaphoid, as this provides the greatest stability and stiffness, improves fracture alignment, and decreases time to union.[1,20,21]

Preoperative Planning

- All imaging studies should be reviewed to identify the location of the fracture and the size of the scaphoid, both of which influence implant selection.
- Plain radiographs should be templated to determine the approximate screw length.
- Required equipment:
  - Portable mini-fluoroscopy unit
  - Kirschner wires
  - Cannulated headless compression screw system
  - Wrist arthroscopy equipment for AARF

Positioning

- The patient is positioned supine on the operating table, with the shoulder abducted 90 degrees and the arm on a radiolucent hand table.
- A pneumatic tourniquet is applied to the upper arm.
- The portable fluoroscopy unit is positioned at the end of the hand table.

DORSAL ARTHROSCOPY-ASSISTED REDUCTION AND FIXATION

Nondisplaced Fracture of the Scaphoid Waist or Proximal Pole

- Position the wrist to obtain a PA view of the wrist.
- Under fluoroscopic guidance, gently pronate the wrist until the scaphoid appears as an oblong cylinder, indicating that the proximal and distal poles are aligned.
- Flex the wrist about 45 degrees until the cylinder rotates into the plane of imaging, forming a "ring" sign. The center of the ring indicates the central axis of the scaphoid (**TECH FIG 1**).

- Using a 14-gauge angiocatheter as a guide for wire insertion, place the tip of a 0.045-inch guidewire through the catheter and onto the proximal pole of the scaphoid, at the center of the scaphoid ring. Confirm correct positioning with fluoroscopy.
- Insert the guidewire down the central axis of the scaphoid using a wire-driver. Keep the wrist flexed to avoid bending the wire.
- Insert the guidewire through the trapezium and advance it until the proximal tip of the guidewire clears the radiocarpal joint such that the wrist can be extended for arthroscopic examination.

TECHNIQUES

TECHNIQUES

A

B

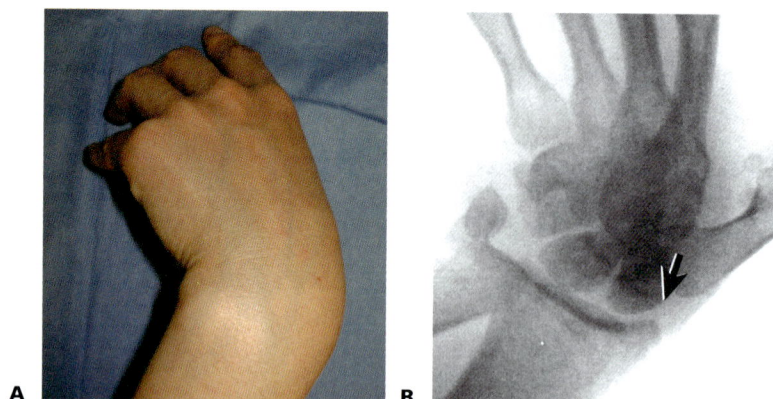

TECH FIG 1 • The scaphoid ring sign indicates the central axis of the scaphoid, which is critical for accurate insertion of the cannulated compression screw. The wrist is positioned in flexion and pronation until the scaphoid appears as a "ring" (*arrow*) on fluoroscopic imaging. A 0.045-inch guidewire is inserted through the center of the ring.

- Confirm correct wire position with fluoroscopy.
- The radial midcarpal portal is used to evaluate the accuracy of fracture reduction.
- The 3-4 and 4-5 portals are used to assess the integrity of the radiocarpal and intercarpal ligaments.
- Suspend the hand vertically in finger traps and apply 10 lb of traction to the upper arm to distract the radiocarpal and midcarpal articulations.
- Create a small longitudinal incision over each portal site, and bluntly dissect down to the capsule with a hemostat. Enter the capsule with a blunt trocar.
- Perform a diagnostic arthroscopy to assess for any associated injuries and to evaluate the fracture reduction.
- Remove the hand from traction for screw insertion.
- Position the wrist again to obtain the "ring" sign, and maintain the wrist in flexion.
- Drive the guidewire from dorsal to volar, perpendicular to the fracture line, until the distal tip lies just within the distal pole of the scaphoid (**TECH FIG 2A–C**).
- Place a second guidewire of equal length against the tip of the proximal pole, parallel and next to the first guidewire. The difference between lengths of the protruding wires represents the length of the scaphoid.

- Subtract at least 4 mm from the length of the scaphoid to obtain the desired screw length.
- Make a small longitudinal incision around the guidewire, and bluntly dissect down to the joint capsule. Carefully retract the extensor pollicis longus and extensor digitorum communis tendons away from the surgical site.
- Use the cannulated reamer to ream to 2 mm short of the distal articular. It is critical not to ream closer than 2 mm, as this may cause loss of fracture compression during screw insertion.
- Insert an Acutrak or mini-Acutrak screw (Acumed, Beaverton, OR) of appropriate length (at least 4 mm shorter than the measured scaphoid length) to within 1 to 2 mm of the distal surface.
  - The tip of the screw should not penetrate the distal surface, and the proximal end of the screw should rest 2 mm deep to the proximal articular cartilage (**TECH FIG 2D,E**).
- Confirm satisfactory screw position and fracture reduction with fluoroscopy. The screw should be inserted down the central axis of the scaphoid. If any doubt exists, use the arthroscopic portals to confirm that the screw is buried in the scaphoid.

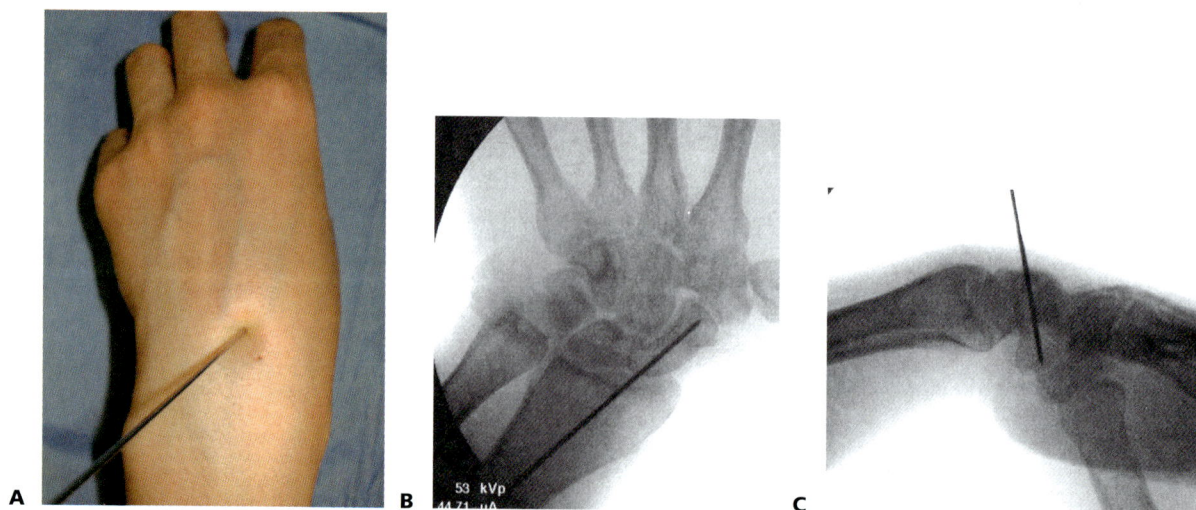

A

B

C

TECH FIG 2 • **A–C.** Before screw insertion, the position of the Kirschner wire must be changed from its position used for arthroscopy. The Kirschner wire should be driven from volar to dorsal until the distal end lies just beneath the articular surface of the scaphoid. *(continued)*

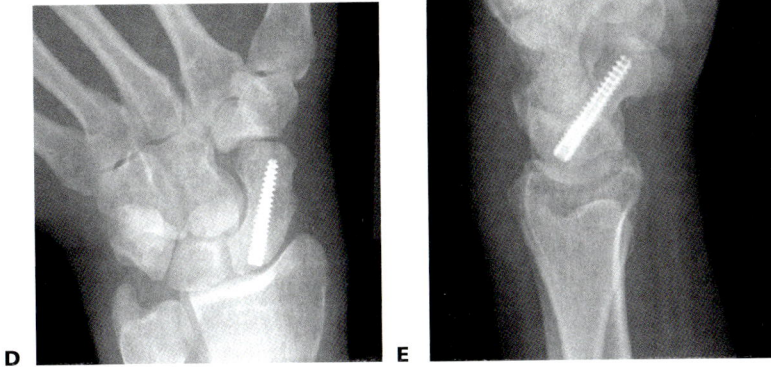

D **E**

TECH FIG 2 • (continued) D,E. Screw fixation of minimally displaced scaphoid fracture via the dorsal percutaneous technique. The screw tip should rest within 1 to 2 mm of the distal cortex. Excellent compression should be obtained with this technique.

- The 3-4 portal and the radial midcarpal portals provide the best view to ensure that the fracture is adequately reduced and that there is no violation of the midcarpal joint.

Displaced Scaphoid Waist Fracture

- Insert two percutaneous 0.062-inch smooth Kirschner wires dorsally into each fragment perpendicular to the long axis of the scaphoid to be used as joysticks to reduce the fracture (**TECH FIG 3A,B**).
- Position the wrist as previously described.

- The guidewire from the Acutrak system is inserted from proximal to distal, starting dorsally and aiming for the central axis of the distal fragment.
  - The guidewire is driven through the distal fragment and out through the volar skin of the hand. The protruding tip is then pulled volarly until the wire is only in the distal fragment (**TECH FIG 3C**).
- The proximal fragment, which is now freely mobile, is reduced manually using the Kirschner wire joysticks.
  - Once the fracture is reduced, the central guidewire is driven from volar to dorsal into the proximal fragment, securing it in place (**TECH FIG 3D**).

TECH FIG 3 • A. Reduction of a displaced scaphoid waist fracture using Kirschner wire joysticks. **B.** The Kirschner wire joystick technique for fracture reduction. **C.** The guidewire is pulled volarly until it remains only in the distal fragment. **(continued)**

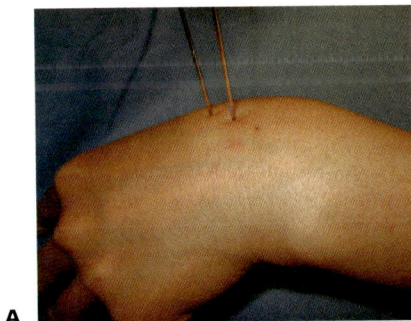

A

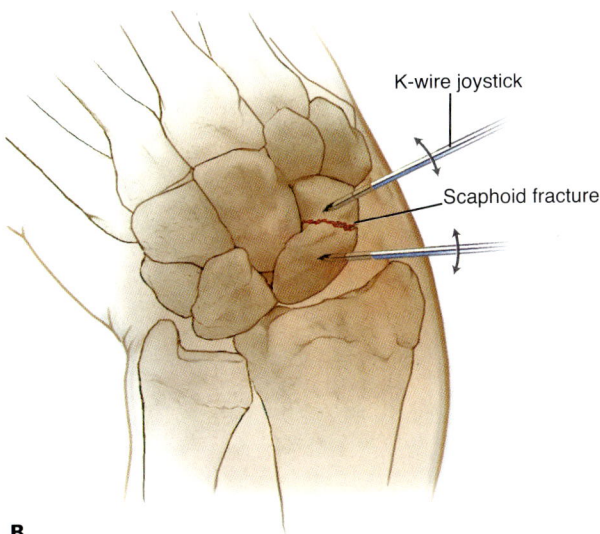

B

K-wire joystick

Scaphoid fracture

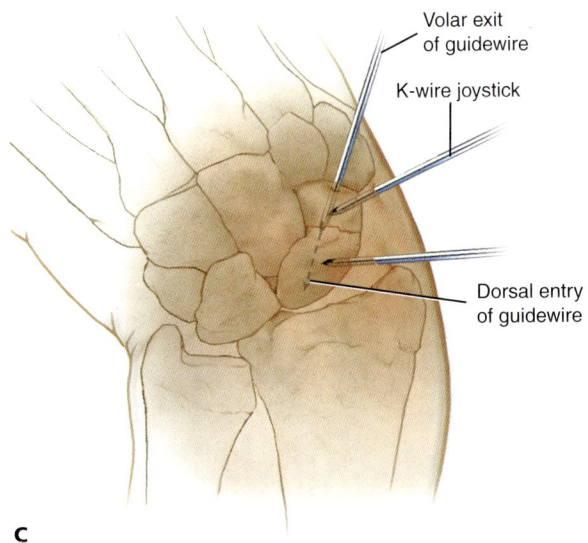

C

Volar exit of guidewire

K-wire joystick

Dorsal entry of guidewire

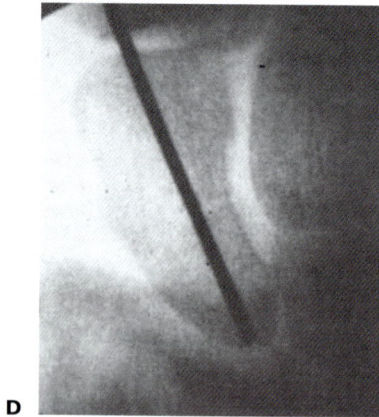

- The guidewire is further advanced from volar to dorsal until its distal tip is just within the subchondral bone of the distal articular surface. This allows for measurement of the screw length as previously described.
- An additional 0.045-inch Kirschner wire is inserted parallel to the guidewire to prevent rotation of the scaphoid fragments during reaming and screw implantation.
  - Maintenance of reduction during and after screw insertion is confirmed with fluoroscopy, and all wires are subsequently removed.

TECH FIG 3 • (continued) **D.** The guidewire is driven from volar to dorsal, transfixing the proximal fragment.

VOLAR PERCUTANEOUS APPROACH

- Position the patient in a supine position with the shoulder abducted and the forearm in supination. The wrist is placed into an extended and ulnarly deviated position over a rolled towel to gain access to the distal pole of the scaphoid.
- Position the portable fluoroscopy unit such that PA and lateral views of the wrist can be obtained. Image intensification is used to locate the distal scaphoid tuberosity.
- A small longitudinal stab incision is made at this point, and the soft tissues are bluntly dissected down to the scaphotrapezial articulation.
- Introduce the guidewire on the distal scaphoid tuberosity. Under image guidance, the wire is advanced toward the center of the proximal pole, aiming for the tubercle of Lister (**TECH FIG 4**).
  - The volar prominence of the trapezium may be partially excised to facilitate the correct starting point and trajectory for the guidewire.

- Alternatively, the guidewire may be placed directly through the trapezium into the scaphoid distal pole. We do not prefer this approach due to concerns about the development of scaphotrapezial arthritis.
- Advance the guidewire to the subchondral bone of the proximal pole.
- Place a second guidewire of equal length against the surface of the distal scaphoid, adjacent and parallel to the first guidewire. The difference between the lengths of the wires represents the length of the scaphoid.
- Subtract 4 mm from the length of the scaphoid to obtain the desired screw length.
- Use the cannulated reamer to ream to within 2 mm of the proximal cortex. It is critical not to ream closer than 2 mm from the proximal cortex, as this may result in a lack of compression during screw insertion.
- Insert an Acutrak or mini-Acutrak screw of appropriate length, remove the guidewire, and confirm satisfactory screw position and fracture reduction with fluoroscopy.

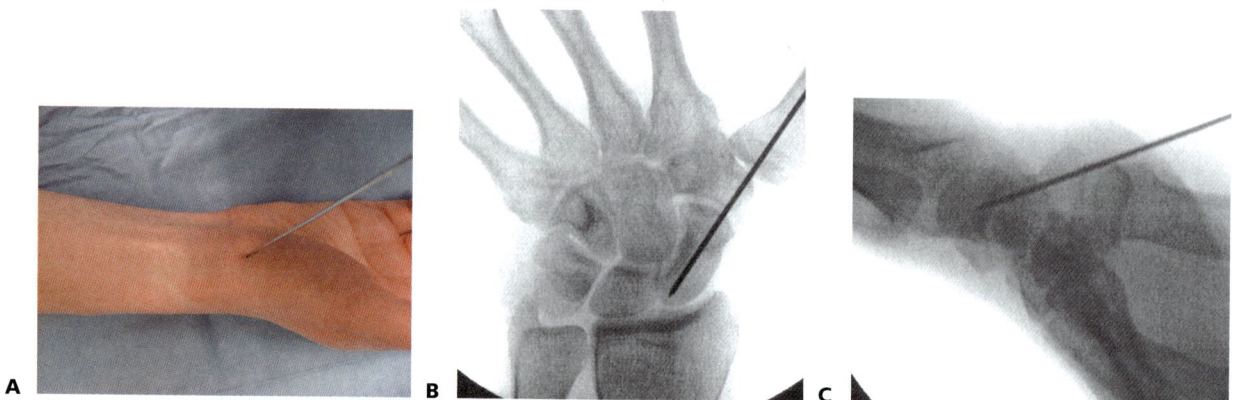

TECH FIG 4 • In the percutaneous volar approach, the guidewire is inserted into the scaphoid at the scaphotrapezial joint, and into the center of the proximal pole. The wire should be inserted aiming for the tubercle of Lister.

PEARLS AND PITFALLS

Dorsal technique	
Injury to dorsal structures	▪ Blunt dissection through the capsule minimizes the risk of injury.
Malpositioning of guidewire	▪ Pronate and flex the wrist until the "ring" sign is noted; the center of the ring is the insertion point for the guidewire.
Screw penetration	▪ Select a screw that is at least 4 mm shorter than the measured length of the scaphoid. ▪ A common mistake is to place a screw that ends up too long once the screw compresses the fragments. ▪ Ream to 2 mm short of the distal cortex. ▪ Confirm central position of guidewire via fluoroscopy.
Reduction of unstable fracture	▪ Kirschner wires may be used as joysticks for reduction. ▪ A derotational Kirschner wire should be placed before reaming and screw insertion if the fragments are unstable.
Extremely small proximal pole fractures	▪ Use a mini-Acutrak screw to prevent comminution of the proximal fracture fragment.
Volar technique	
Injury to volar structures	▪ Blunt dissection to the scaphoid minimizes the risk of injury.
Malpositioning of guidewire	▪ A central starting point on the distal scaphoid tuberosity can be hindered by the trapezium. ▪ Part of the volar trapezium can be resected to achieve a correct starting point for trajectory of the guidewire, or the wire may be inserted through the trapezium.
Screw penetration	▪ Select a screw that is at least 4 mm shorter than the measured length of the scaphoid. ▪ Ream to 2 mm short of the proximal articular surface. ▪ Confirm central position of guidewire via fluoroscopy.

POSTOPERATIVE CARE

▪ Dressings are applied and the limb is immobilized in a forearm-based splint, immobilizing only the wrist. The thumb and fingers remain free for range-of-motion exercises.

▪ The patient is instructed in the importance of limb elevation and finger range-of-motion exercises.

▪ At 2 weeks postoperatively, the sutures are removed, a removable wrist splint is applied, and a wrist range-of-motion exercise program is initiated.

▪ If the patient is noncompliant, the fracture is deemed unstable, or the fixation is less than ideal, then a short-arm cast is applied for at least 6 weeks.

▪ Plain radiographs are obtained at 2, 6, 12, and 24 weeks postoperatively.

▪ The splint (or cast) is discontinued when union is confirmed on serial plain radiographs. If there is any question regarding fracture union, a CT scan is obtained.

▪ Unprotected strenuous activity or contact sports are not permitted until 3 months postoperatively.

OUTCOMES

▪ Results of contemporary techniques of percutaneous fixation are excellent; it has been shown to allow for earlier mobilization and return to activity and high satisfaction rates compared to nonoperative measures.[5,17,22]

▪ Earlier mobilization avoids complications such as muscle atrophy and joint stiffness.

▪ Percutaneous techniques result in decreased soft tissue damage compared to conventional open techniques.[22]

▪ In a recent series of 27 consecutive patients, the union rate (confirmed by CT) was 100%. The average time to union was 12 weeks, with a prolonged time to union noted in patients with a proximal pole fracture.[18]

COMPLICATIONS

▪ Complications are rare with percutaneous fixation techniques. The risks associated with open reduction and internal fixation, such as damage to the ligamentous support of the carpus and disruption of the dorsal blood supply, are minimized.

▪ Possible complications include[15,19]:
  ▪ Nonunion
  ▪ Malunion
  ▪ Injury to the dorsal sensory branch of the radial nerve
  ▪ Extensor tendon injury
  ▪ Infection
  ▪ Technical problems: screw protrusion, screw malposition, bending or breakage of guidewire
  ▪ Erosion of the trapezium and discomfort from the head of the screw has been reported with the use of a percutaneous cannulated screw inserted via the volar approach.[22]

REFERENCES

1. Adams BD, Blair WF, Reagan DS, et al. Technical factors related to Herbert screw fixation. J Hand Surg Am 1988;13A:893–899.
2. Amadio PC, Moran SL. Fractures of the carpal bones. In Green D, Hotchkiss R, Pederson WC, eds. Green's Operative Hand Surgery, 5th ed. Philadelphia: Churchill Livingstone, 2005:711–740.
3. Bond CD, Shin CA. Percutaneous cannulated screw fixation of acute scaphoid fractures. Tech Hand Up Extrem Surg 2000;4:81–87.
4. Burge P. Closed cast treatment of scaphoid fractures. Hand Clin 2001;17:541–552.
5. Chen AC, Chao EK, Hung SS, et al. Percutaneous screw fixation for unstable scaphoid fractures. J Trauma 2005;59:184–187.
6. Dias JJ, Taylor M, Thompson J, et al. Radiographic signs of union of scaphoid fractures: an analysis of inter-observer agreement and reproducibility. J Bone Joint Surg Br 1988;70:299–301.
7. Gelberman RH, Menon J. The vascularity of the scaphoid bone. J Hand Surg Am 1980;5:508–513.

8. Gelberman RH, Wolock BS, Siegel DB. Fractures and non-unions of the carpal scaphoid. J Bone Joint Surg Am 1989;71A:1560–1565.

9. Gellman H, Caputo RJ, Carter V, et al. Comparison of short and long thumb-spica casts for non-displaced fractures of the carpal scaphoid. J Bone Joint Surg Am 1989;71A:354–357.

10. Haddad FS, Goddard NJ. Acute percutaneous scaphoid fixation: a pilot study. J Bone Joint Surg Br 1998;80B:95–99.

11. Kerluke L, McCabe SJ. Nonunion of the scaphoid: a critical analysis of recent natural history studies. J Hand Surg Am 1993;18A:1–3.

12. Kozin SH. Incidence, mechanism, and natural history of scaphoid fractures. Hand Clin 2001;17:515–523.

13. Leslie IJ, Dickson RA. The fractured carpal scaphoid: natural history and factors influencing outcome. J Bone Joint Surg Br 1981;63B: 225–230.

14. Mack GR, Bosse MJ, Gelberman RH, et al. The natural history of scaphoid nonunion. J Bone Joint Surg Am 1984;66A:504–509.

15. Martus J, Bedi A, Jebson PJL. Cannulated variable pitch compression screw fixation of scaphoid fractures using a limited dorsal approach. Tech Hand Upper Ext Surg 2005;9:202–206.

16. Ruby LK, Stinson J, Belsky MR. The natural history of scaphoid nonunion: a review of fifty-five cases. J Bone Joint Surg Am 1985;67A: 428–432.

17. Slade JF III, Dodds SD. Minimally invasive management of scaphoid nonunions. Clin Orthop 2006;445:108–119.

18. Slade JF III, Gutow AP, Geissler WB. Percutaneous internal fixation of scaphoid fractures via an arthroscopically assisted dorsal approach. J Bone Joint Surg Am 2002;84:21–36.

19. Slade JF III, Jaskwhich D. Percutaneous fixation of scaphoid fractures. Hand Clin 2001;17:553–574.

20. Trumble TE, Clarke T, Kreder HJ. Non-union of the scaphoid: treatment with cannulated screws compared with treatment with Herbert screws. J Bone Joint Surg Am 1996;78A:1829–1837.

21. Trumble TE, Gilbert M, Murray LW, et al. Displaced scaphoid fractures treated with open reduction and internal fixation with a cannulated screw. J Bone Joint Surg Am 2000;82A:633–641.

22. Yip HSF, Wu WC, Chang RYP, et al. Percutaneous cannulated screw fixation of acute scaphoid waist fracture. J Hand Surg Br 2002;27B: 42–46.

Chapter 17

Open Reduction and Internal Fixation of Scaphoid Fractures

Asheesh Bedi and Peter J.L. Jebson

DEFINITION

- The scaphoid is the most commonly fractured carpal bone, accounting for 1 in every 100,000 emergency department visits.[12]
- Scaphoid fractures typically result from a fall on an outstretched hand.
- Scaphoid nonunion or proximal pole avascular necrosis (AVN) after a fracture has been associated with considerable morbidity and a predictable pattern of wrist arthritis.[15,17,18]
- The complex anatomy and tenuous blood supply to the scaphoid make operative management of these fractures technically challenging.[18]
- The Herbert classification system organizes scaphoid fractures into four groups: acute stable, acute unstable, delayed union, and established nonunion.

ANATOMY

- The scaphoid has a complex three-dimensional geometry that has been likened to a "twisted peanut." It can be divided into three regions: proximal pole, waist, and distal pole.
- The scaphoid functions as the primary link between the forearm and the distal carpal row and therefore plays a critical role in maintaining normal carpal kinematics.
- Articulating with the scaphoid fossa of the radius, the lunate, capitate, trapezium, and trapezoid, more than 70% of the scaphoid is covered with articular cartilage.
- Gelberman and Menon[8] have described the vascular supply of the scaphoid. The main arterial supply is from the radial artery; it enters the scaphoid via two main branches:
  - A dorsal branch, entering through the dorsal ridge, is the primary supply and provides 70% to 80% of the vascularity, including the entire proximal pole via retrograde endosteal branches.
  - A volar branch, entering through the tubercle, supplies the remaining 20% to 30%, predominantly the distal pole and tuberosity.
- The proximal pole is at increased risk for avascular necrosis (AVN) secondary to disruption of its tenuous retrograde blood supply after a fracture of the scaphoid waist or proximal pole.
- Due to its tenuous vascular supply, the scaphoid heals almost entirely by primary bone healing, resulting in minimal callus formation.
- The size and shape of the scaphoid, in combination with its precarious blood supply, demands attention to detail and accurate implantation of fixation devices during fracture fixation.

PATHOGENESIS

- Scaphoid fractures are most commonly seen in young, active males who fall on an outstretched upper extremity.[12]
- With the wrist dorsiflexed greater than 95 degrees, in combination with 10 degrees or more of radial deviation, the distal radius abuts the scaphoid and precipitates a fracture.[12]

- Most of these fractures occur at the waist region, although 10% to 20% occur in the proximal pole.
  - Proximal pole fractures are associated with an increased risk of nonunion, delayed union, and AVN.
- In children, scaphoid fractures are less common and are most frequently seen in the distal pole.

NATURAL HISTORY

- An untreated or inadequately treated scaphoid fracture has a higher likelihood of nonunion. The overall incidence of nonunion is estimated at 5% to 10%, but the risk is significantly increased with nonoperative treatment of a displaced waist or proximal pole fracture.
- The natural history of scaphoid nonunions is controversial, but they are believed to result in a predictable pattern of progressive radiocarpal and midcarpal arthritis.[8,9,11,14,15,17,18]
- In an established scaphoid nonunion, the distal portion of the scaphoid may flex, producing a "humpback" deformity of the scaphoid. The loss of scaphoid integrity can result in carpal instability and abnormal carpal kinematics, most frequently manifesting as a dorsal intercalated segment instability (DISI) pattern.
  - The pattern of carpal instability and secondary arthrosis due to an unstable scaphoid nonunion has been termed a SNAC wrist (scaphoid nonunion advanced collapse pattern of wrist arthritis).[11,17]
  - In the SNAC wrist, there is a loss of carpal height with proximal capitate migration, flexion and pronation of the scaphoid, and secondary midcarpal arthritis.[17]
- Factors associated with the development of a scaphoid fracture nonunion include[14]:
  - Delayed diagnosis or treatment
  - Inadequate immobilization
  - Proximal fracture
  - Initial and progressive fracture displacement
  - Fracture comminution
  - Presence of associated carpal injuries (ie, perilunate injury)

PATIENT HISTORY AND PHYSICAL FINDINGS

- Scaphoid fractures classically occur in the active, young adult population after a fall onto an outstretched hand. Patients present with radial-sided wrist pain.
- Classic physical examination findings include:
  - Swelling over the dorsoradial aspect of the wrist
  - Erythema over the volar radial aspect of the wrist
  - Tenderness to palpation in the "anatomic snuffbox"
  - Tenderness with palpation volarly over the distal tubercle
  - Pain with axial compression of the wrist (scaphoid compression test)
- Scaphoid fractures can be part of a greater arc injury.
  - The physician should examine the entire wrist carefully for areas of tenderness and swelling.

2251

- Plain radiographs are scrutinized for an associated ligamentous injury or disruption of the midcarpal joint as seen in the transscaphoid perilunate fracture-dislocation.

IMAGING AND OTHER DIAGNOSTIC STUDIES

- The following plain radiographs should routinely be ordered in the patient with a suspected scaphoid fracture: posteroanterior (PA), oblique, lateral, and dedicated scaphoid views.
  - The PA view allows visualization of the proximal pole of the scaphoid.
  - The semipronated oblique view provides the best visualization of the waist and distal pole regions.
  - The semisupinated oblique view provides the best visualization of the dorsal ridge.
  - The lateral view permits an assessment of fracture angulation, carpal alignment, and carpal instability.
  - The dedicated scaphoid view is a PA view with the wrist in ulnar deviation. This results in scaphoid extension, allowing visualization of the scaphoid in profile (**FIG 1A**).
- The following criteria define a displaced or unstable fracture as noted on plain radiographs[2,9,14]:
  - At least 1 mm of displacement
  - More than 10 degrees of angular displacement
  - Fracture comminution
  - Radiolunate angle of more than 15 degrees
  - Scapholunate angle of more than 60 degrees
  - Intrascaphoid angle of more than 35 degrees
- CT with reconstruction images in multiple planes is used to identify an acute fracture not detected on plain radiographs (**FIG 1B,C**).
  - CT is most useful in evaluating an established scaphoid nonunion or malunion.[6]

- Since plain radiographs are often unreliable, CT is preferred for confirming union after a scaphoid fracture.
- MRI may be indicated in the evaluation of a suspected scaphoid fracture not detected on plain radiographs (**FIG 1D,E**). MRI is highly sensitive, with a specificity approaching 100% when performed within 48 hours of injury.[13]
  - MRI with gadolinium contrast is helpful in assessing the vascularity of the proximal pole, particularly in the patient with an established nonunion.
- A technetium bone scan has been shown to be up to 100% sensitive in identifying an occult fracture.[20] Unfortunately, it is also associated with a low specificity and often will not be positive immediately after the fracture.

DIFFERENTIAL DIAGNOSIS

- Scapholunate injury
- Wrist sprain
- Wrist contusion
- Fracture of other carpal bone
- Greater arc injury
- Distal radius fracture

NONOPERATIVE MANAGEMENT

- Nonoperative management is indicated for a nondisplaced, stable scaphoid waist or distal pole fracture. Unstable fractures and nondisplaced fractures of the proximal pole are indications for internal fixation based on studies that have demonstrated a poor outcome with nonoperative treatment.[2,4,14]
- The appropriate type and duration of cast immobilization remain controversial. We recommend a long-arm thumb spica cast for the first 6 weeks, followed by a short-arm thumb spica

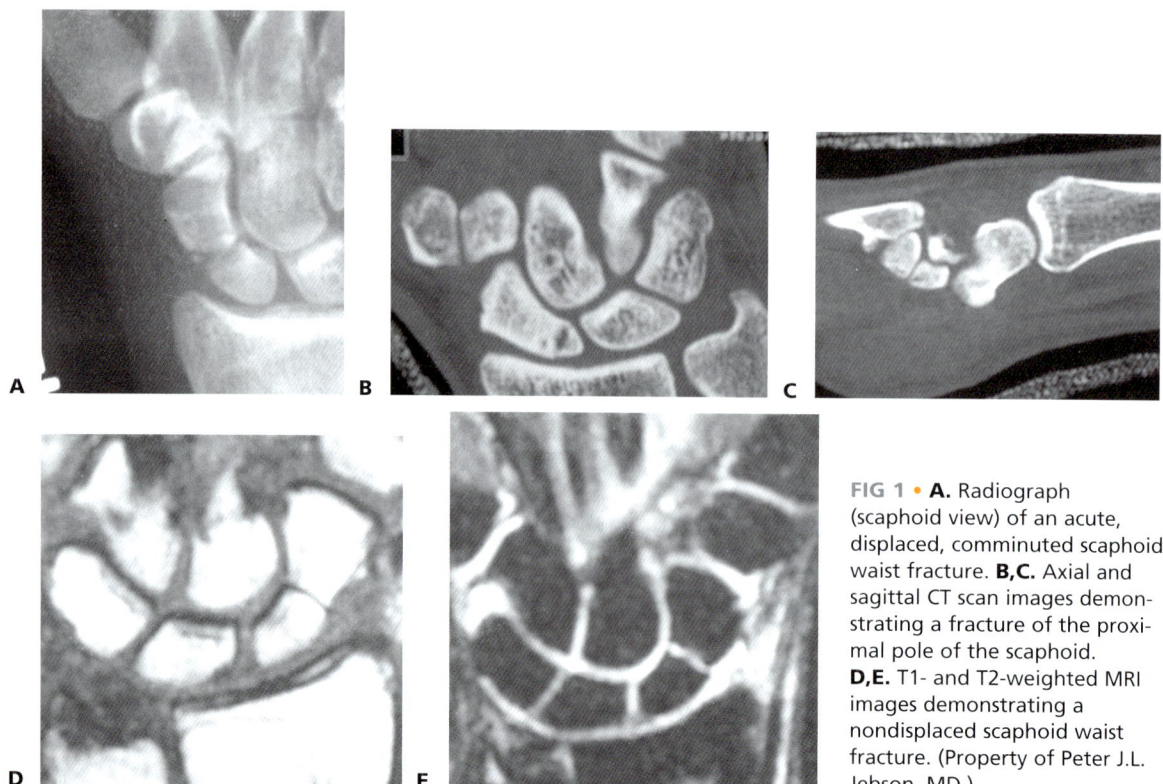

FIG 1 • **A.** Radiograph (scaphoid view) of an acute, displaced, comminuted scaphoid waist fracture. **B,C.** Axial and sagittal CT scan images demonstrating a fracture of the proximal pole of the scaphoid. **D,E.** T1- and T2-weighted MRI images demonstrating a nondisplaced scaphoid waist fracture. (Property of Peter J.L. Jebson, MD.)

cast until the clinical examination and radiologic studies (usually a CT scan) confirm fracture union.

- Clinical studies have failed to demonstrate any benefit from including the thumb or fingers in the cast.[2,4]
- Similarly, wrist position has not been proven to improve scaphoid fracture healing.
- Numerous studies have revealed no difference in union rates for a long-arm versus short-arm cast; however, a randomized prospective study by Gellman et al[10] documented a shorter time to union and fewer nonunions and delayed unions with initial use of a long-arm cast.
- The morbidity of a nonoperative approach, specifically cast immobilization, has become of increasing concern. A prolonged duration of immobilization is often required for waist fractures, and this can be accompanied by muscle atrophy, stiffness, reduced grip strength, and residual pain. In addition, cast immobilization can cause significant inconvenience for the patient and interference with activities of daily living. The prolonged duration of immobilization is of particular concern in the young laborer, athlete, or military personnel, who typically desire expedient functional recovery.[5,16,21]
- If the clinical history and physical examination are suggestive of a scaphoid fracture but initial radiographs are negative, the wrist should be immobilized for 2 weeks. Repeat radiographs are then obtained. If a fracture is present, resorption at the fracture may be noted. If wrist pain and "snuffbox" tenderness persist but radiographs are negative, a bone scan may be obtained. A negative scan excludes the presence of a scaphoid fracture. A positive scan may indicate an occult fracture or ligamentous injury. CT or MRI is usually indicated for further evaluation.[13,20]
- Alternatively, if there is a high index of suspicion at initial presentation and there is a need to know the status of the scaphoid, MRI or CT of the wrist is obtained.

SURGICAL MANAGEMENT

- Indications for open reduction and internal fixation (ORIF) of scaphoid fractures include[2,14]:
  - Any proximal pole fracture
  - A displaced, unstable fracture of the scaphoid waist
  - Associated carpal instability or perilunar instability
  - Associated distal radius fracture
  - Delayed presentation (more than 3 to 4 weeks) with no prior treatment
  - A nondisplaced, stable scaphoid waist fracture (Herbert A2 type) in a patient who wishes to avoid the morbidity of cast immobilization. In this clinical scenario, operative treatment should occur only after an explanation of the rationale for, and the risks and benefits of, operative treatment versus cast immobilization.

Preoperative Planning

- All imaging studies should be reviewed to accurately define the fracture pattern.
- Required equipment:
  - Portable mini-fluoroscopy unit
  - Kirschner wires
  - Cannulated headless compression screw system. We prefer to use the Acutrak or mini-Acutrak screw system (Accumed, Beaverton, OR), but any cannulated screw system that permits screw insertion beneath the articular surface may be used.

Positioning

- General or regional anesthesia may be used.
- The patient is positioned supine on the operating table with a radiolucent hand table at the shoulder level.
- The fluoroscopy unit is draped and positioned at the end of the hand table.
- A pneumatic tourniquet is carefully applied to the proximal arm.
- An intravenous antibiotic is provided before inflation of the tourniquet as prophylaxis for infection.
- The limb is prepared and draped, followed by exsanguination of the limb with an Esmarch bandage and tourniquet inflation, usually to a pressure of 250 mm Hg.

Approach

- ORIF of scaphoid fractures can be performed through either a dorsal or volar approach.
- The specific approaches that will be described include:
  - Open dorsal approach[16]
  - Open volar approach

OPEN DORSAL APPROACH (AUTHORS' PREFERRED APPROACH)

Exposure

- If the fragments are displaced, requiring reduction, pronate the forearm and make a longitudinal skin incision, about 3 to 4 cm long, beginning at the proximal aspect of the tubercle of Lister and extending distally along the axis of the third metacarpal (**TECH FIG 1A**).
  - If the fracture is nondisplaced, a smaller skin incision and capsulotomy may be used.
- Raise skin flaps at the level of the extensor retinaculum.
- Incise the extensor retinaculum overlying the third compartment immediately distal to the tubercle of Lister and carefully release the fascia overlying the extensor pollicis longus (EPL) tendon, permitting gentle retraction of the

EPL radially. Similarly incise the dorsal hand fascia longitudinally.

- Gently retract the extensor digitorum communis (EDC) tendons ulnarly while retracting the extensor carpi radialis brevis (ECRB) and longus (ECRL) tendons radially with the EPL, thus exposing the underlying radiocarpal joint capsule (**TECH FIG 1B**).
- Make a limited inverted T-shaped capsulotomy with the transverse limb placed just distal to the dorsal rim of the radius and the longitudinal limb directly over the scapholunate articulation (**TECH FIG 1C**).
  - The tubercle of Lister is helpful in locating the articulation.

TECHNIQUES

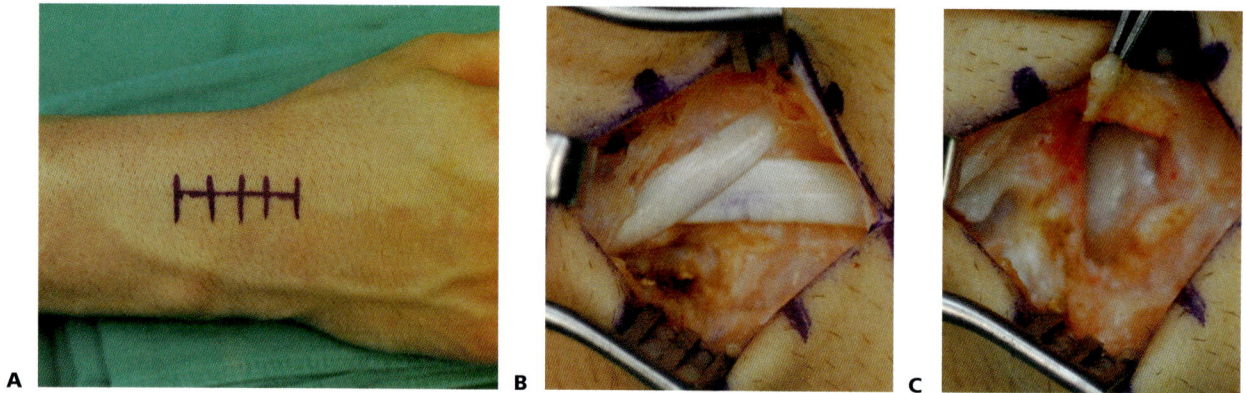

TECH FIG 1 • **A.** Skin incision used for ORIF of scaphoid fractures via the dorsal approach. **B.** Retracting the thumb and wrist extensor tendons radially and the finger extensor tendons ulnarly facilitates exposure of the underlying capsule. **C.** A limited capsulotomy should be performed to expose the proximal scaphoid and scapholunate ligament. (Property of Peter J.L. Jebson, MD.)

- Carefully elevate the capsular flaps from the dorsal lunate, the dorsal component of the scapholunate ligament, and the proximal pole of the scaphoid.
    - Evacuate fracture hematoma.
    - It is often helpful to extend the longitudinal limb of the capsulotomy to expose the scaphocapitate articulation and the radial aspect of the midcarpal joint.
    - Especially when elevating the radial flap, take care to avoid stripping the dorsal ridge vessels entering at the scaphoid waist region.

Fracture Reduction and Provisional Fixation

- Distract the carpus manually via longitudinal traction on the index and long fingers.
- If the fracture is displaced, insert 0.045-inch Kirschner wire joysticks perpendicularly into the proximal and distal scaphoid fragments to assist in the reduction (**TECH FIG 2A**).
    - The accuracy of the reduction can be determined by assessing congruency of the radioscaphoid and scaphocapitate articulations.

- When a satisfactory reduction has been achieved, obtain provisional fixation with derotational 0.045-inch Kirschner wires.
    - The first wire is inserted dorsal and ulnar to the central axis of the scaphoid, into the trapezium for enhanced stability.
    - The second derotational wire may be inserted volar and radial to the anticipated central axis insertion site if more fixation is needed.
    - The derotational wires must be placed such that they will not interfere with central axis guidewire placement, reaming, and screw insertion (**TECH FIG 2B**).

Guidewire Placement

- The starting position for guidewire is at the membranous portion of the scapholunate ligament origin (**TECH FIG 3A,B**).
    - In very proximal fractures, the starting point for the guidewire is as far proximally in the scaphoid as possible, at the mid-aspect of the membranous portion of the scapholunate ligament complex. This point is critical to avoid propagation of the fracture into the proximal scaphoid during insertion of the screw.

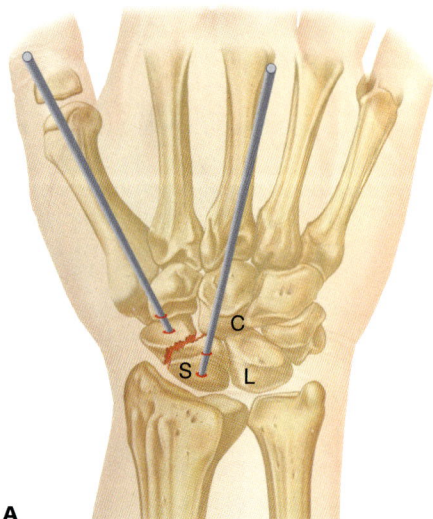

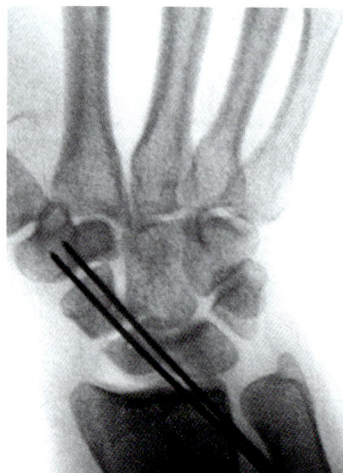

TECH FIG 2 • **A.** Percutaneous insertion of Kirschner wires into the proximal and distal scaphoid (*S*) fragments is helpful to facilitate manual reduction of a displaced fracture. *C*, capitate; *L*, lunate. **B.** A displaced scaphoid waist fracture has been stabilized with a derotational Kirschner wire placed dorsal and ulnar to the guidewire. The derotational Kirschner wire does not interfere with insertion of the screw in the central axis. (Radiograph is the property of Peter J.L. Jebson, MD.)

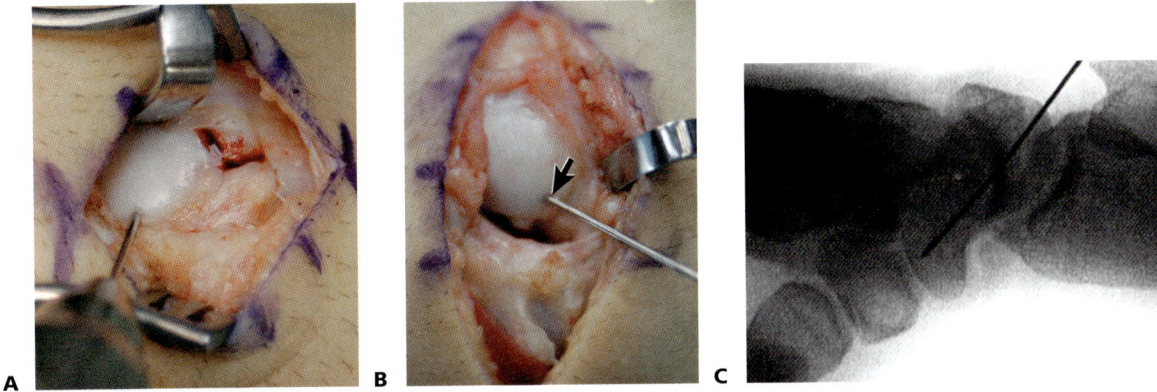

TECH FIG 3 • **A,B.** Note the starting point at the membranous portion of the scapholunate ligament (*arrow*). **C.** The 30-degree pronated oblique view demonstrating guidewire placement down the central axis of the scaphoid. (Property of Peter J.L. Jebson, MD.)

- With the wrist flexed over a bolster, insert the guidewire down the central axis of the scaphoid in line with the thumb metacarpal.
  - Be very patient with this important step; proceed with reaming and screw insertion only after central placement has been confirmed on the PA, lateral, and 30-degree pronated lateral views (**TECH FIG 3C**).
  - It is critical to insert the wire in the optimal position in all three views to avoid violating the midcarpal joint or the volar surface of the scaphoid.
  - Take care to avoid bending the guidewire.
- Advance the wire up to but not into the scaphotrapezial joint.

Screw Insertion

- Determine screw length by measuring the guidewire (**TECH FIG 4A**).
  - In the case of minimal fragment separation, subtract 4 mm from the measured length of the wire to allow recession of the proximal screw beneath the articular surface.
  - If fragments are more displaced, consider compression and choose an even shorter screw.
- Advance the wire into the trapezium to avoid loss of position during drilling.

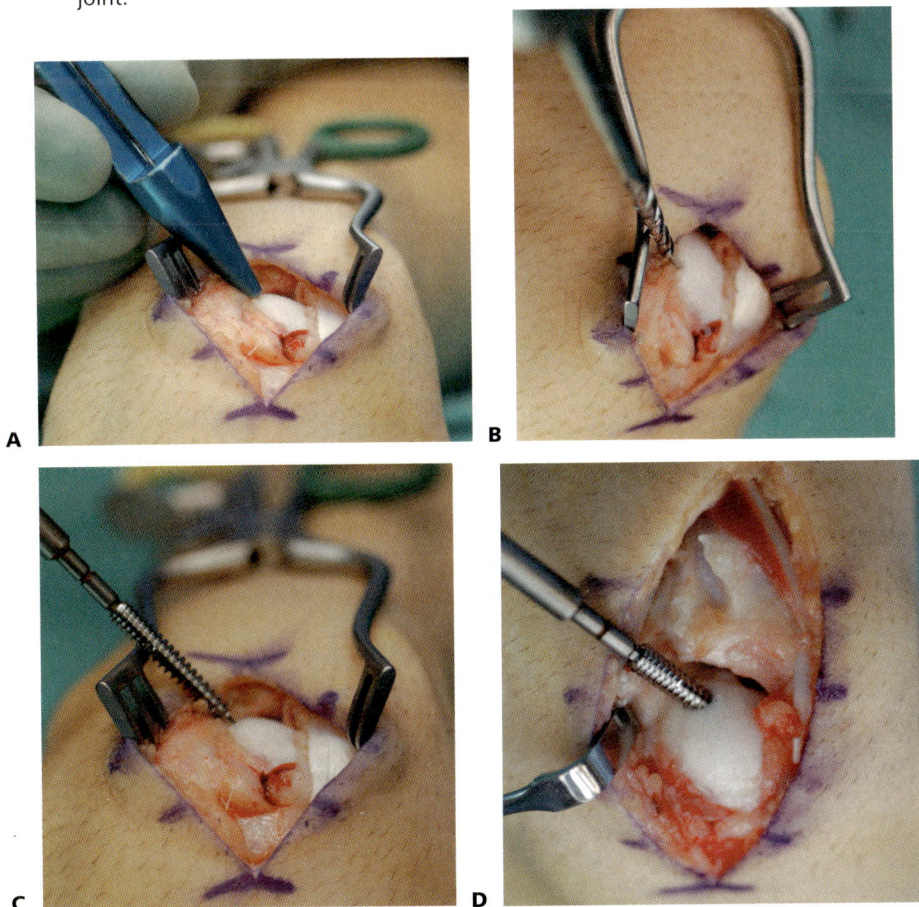

TECH FIG 4 • **A.** Determining the appropriate screw length. **B.** Reaming with the cannulated reamer. **C,D.** Insertion of the screw. (Property of Peter J.L. Jebson, MD.)

- Use the cannulated drill (**TECH FIG 4B**), tap the bone if necessary, and manually insert the screw (**TECH FIG 4C,D**).
  - We use the larger Acutrak screw when feasible, but the mini-Acutrak system may be necessary in patients with a small scaphoid or if the fracture is located proximally such that insertion of an Acutrak screw may result in inadvertent propagation of the fracture to the insertion site with fragmentation of the proximal scaphoid.
  - Remove the guidewire and assess screw position via fluoroscopy using the same views.

OPEN VOLAR APPROACH

Exposure

- Radially deviate the wrist and palpate the scaphoid tubercle.
- Make a 3- to 4-cm incision centered over the scaphoid tubercle, directed distally toward the base of the thumb and proximally over the flexor carpi radialis (FCR) tendon sheath. If the superficial volar branch of the radial artery is encountered, cauterize it at the level of the wrist flexion crease.
- Open the FCR sheath and retract the tendon ulnarly. Open the floor of the sheath distally to expose the underlying volar wrist capsule.
- Distally, develop the interval by splitting the origin of the thenar muscles in line with their fibers over the distal scaphoid and trapezium.
- Incise the capsule longitudinally, taking care to avoid damage to the underlying articular cartilage.
  - Proximally, divide the thickened radiolunate and radioscaphocapitate ligaments to allow exposure of the proximal scaphoid pole.
- Identify the scaphotrapezial joint with a Freer elevator and bluntly expose it.
  - Dissection over the radial aspect of the scaphoid is limited to avoid injury to the dorsal ridge vessel.
- Define and clear the fracture site by irrigation, sharp excision of periosteal flaps, and curetting of debris and hematoma.
  - Assess the instability of the fracture by wrist manipulation.
  - It is critical to identify any bone loss, as compression during screw placement can result in an iatrogenic malunion.

Fracture Reduction and Fixation

- Obtain correct fracture alignment through longitudinal traction followed by wrist manipulation.
  - An anatomic reduction may also be achieved by direct manipulation of the fragments with a dental pick, pointed reduction forceps, or joystick Kirschner wires.

- Place a provisional 0.045-inch Kirschner wire to secure the reduction. Insert the wire in a retrograde manner from volar distal to dorsal proximal, gaining fixation in the proximal pole.
  - It is critical to place this wire such that it does not interfere with central axis screw placement.
- The central axis guidewire is placed, taking into consideration all the factors detailed above.
- To gain the needed dorsal starting position in the distal scaphoid pole, displace the trapezium dorsally with an elevator or resect a small portion of the proximal volar trapezium with a rongeur (**TECH FIG 5**).
- The cannulated compression screw may be inserted using a freehand technique or a commercial device, which may facilitate simultaneous fracture reduction and guidewire positioning.
  - Fluoroscopy is invaluable during wire and screw insertion and to confirm accurate placement and fracture reduction as described above.
- Precisely repair the volar wrist capsule and radiolunate and radioscaphocapitate ligaments with permanent suture.

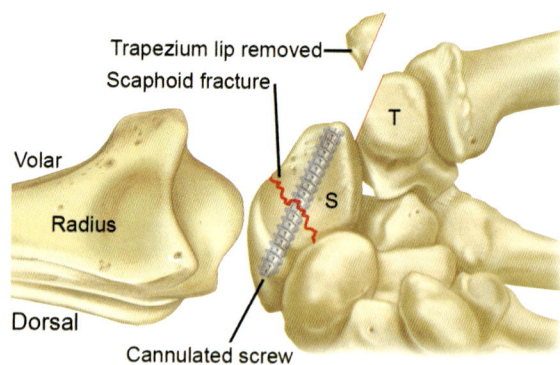

TECH FIG 5 • Accurate insertion of a screw via the volar approach usually requires partial resection or dorsal displacement of the volar trapezium to expose the distal scaphoid.

PEARLS AND PITFALLS

Injury to the scaphoid blood supply	■ Meticulous limited dissection of the capsule. Avoid any dissection on the dorsal ridge of the scaphoid.
Malpositioning of guidewire	■ Pronate and flex wrist during the dorsal approach to allow appropriate trajectory. Confirm position on multiple views to ensure insertion in the central axis of the scaphoid.
Screw position	■ Select a screw that is 4 mm shorter than measured length unless fracture fragments are separated; in that case choose a shorter screw. Drill 2 mm short of the distal pole.

Reduction of an unstable fracture	▪ Perpendicular Kirschner wire joysticks inserted into the proximal and distal scaphoid fragments are useful to obtain a reduction. ▪ Provisional derotational Kirschner wires placed before screw insertion can be used to stabilize fragments during screw insertion. ▪ Recognize comminution and bone loss to avoid inadvertent shortening or malreduction with screw compression.
Small proximal pole fracture	▪ Use of a small screw (ie, mini-Acutrak) may be necessary to prevent comminution of the proximal fragment. ▪ Confirm central axis screw position, especially in the proximal pole.

POSTOPERATIVE CARE

▪ The patient is immobilized in a below-elbow volar thumb spica splint and discharged to home with instructions on strict limb elevation and frequent digital range-of-motion exercises.
▪ At 2 weeks, the patient returns for suture removal. Range-of-motion exercises are begun and a removable forearm-based thumb spica splint is worn. The splint is discontinued at 4 to 6 weeks postoperatively.
   ▪ If the fracture involves the proximal pole or if significant comminution was noted at surgery and there is concern regarding stability of the fixation, immobilization in a short-arm cast for 6 to 10 weeks is indicated. Typically, such fractures take longer to achieve union.
▪ After cast removal, a formal supervised therapy program is initiated to achieve satisfactory range of motion, strength, and function.
▪ Fracture healing is assessed at 2, 6, and 12 weeks postoperatively with plain radiography. Fracture union is defined as progressive obliteration of the fracture and clear trabeculation across the fracture site (**FIG 2**).
▪ If there is any question regarding fracture union, a CT scan is obtained at 3 months postoperatively or before the patient is allowed to return to unrestricted sporting activities.

OUTCOMES

▪ Surgical fixation of unstable, displaced scaphoid fractures has been increasingly advocated, given the unsatisfactory outcomes that have been reported with nonoperative management.[2,4,14]

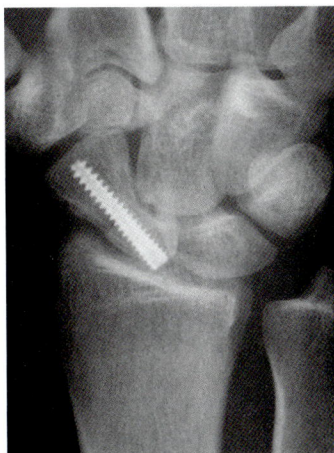

FIG 2 • A healed scaphoid waist fracture after ORIF via the dorsal approach. Although the screw may appear slightly long, both the proximal scaphoid and distal scaphoid are covered with hyaline cartilage not detected on diagnostic imaging. (Property of Peter J.L. Jebson, MD.)

Rigid internal fixation allows for early physiotherapy throughout the healing phase, a more rapid time to union, improved range of motion, and rapid functional recovery.[5,10,16,21] Several studies have reported a high rate of union and excellent clinical outcome with minimal morbidity using both limited open and percutaneous techniques.[1,3,5,10,19,19,21]
▪ Clinical and biomechanical studies have also recently documented the importance of screw position after fixation of scaphoid fractures.[7,18] Central placement of the screw is biomechanically advantageous, with greater stiffness and load to failure.[7] Trumble et al[18] demonstrated more rapid progression to union with central screw position in cases of scaphoid nonunion.
▪ A volar approach has traditionally been used for screw insertion. However, recent studies have raised potential concerns regarding eccentric screw placement and damage to the scaphotrapezial articulation with this approach.[21]
▪ Our preferred technique for fixation of a scaphoid proximal pole or waist region fracture involves a limited dorsal approach with compression screw fixation.[16] The technique is simple and permits visualization of a reliable starting point for screw placement within the central axis of the scaphoid, offering a significant potential advantage over the volar approach. We recently reported our clinical experience in a consecutive series of nondisplaced scaphoid waist fractures.[3]

COMPLICATIONS

▪ Postoperative wound infections are rare and can be prevented with routine preoperative antibiotic prophylaxis, thorough wound irrigation, and appropriate soft tissue management.
▪ Intraoperative technical problems
   ▪ Inadvertent bending or breakage of the guidewire can occur if the wrist is dorsiflexed with the wire in position or during drilling before screw insertion.
   ▪ Care should be taken to confirm that the screw is fully seated beneath the articular cartilage to avoid prominence and erosion of the distal radius articular surface. Similarly, failure to carefully judge accurate screw length intraoperatively can result in prominence and erosion of the scaphotrapezial articulation.
▪ Nonunion with or without AVN can occur despite compression screw fixation, particularly with a proximal pole or displaced waist fracture. Stripping of the dorsal ridge vasculature should be avoided. Supplemental cancellous bone graft from the distal radius may be used at the time of fixation if desired.
▪ Other potential but rare complications
   ▪ Hypertrophic scar
   ▪ Injury to the dorsal branches of the superficial radial nerve
   ▪ Damage to the scaphotrapezial articulation
   ▪ Proximal pole fragment comminution

REFERENCES

1. Adams BD, Blair WF, Reagan DS, et al. Technical factors related to Herbert screw fixation. J Hand Surg Am 1988;13A:893–899.
2. Amadio PC, Moran SL. Fractures of the carpal bones. In Green D, Hotchkiss R, Pederson WC, eds. Green's Operative Hand Surgery, 5th ed. Philadelphia: Churchill Livingstone, 2005:711–740.
3. Bedi A, Jebson PJL, Hayden RJ, et al. Internal fixation of acute, nondisplaced scaphoid waist fractures via a limited dorsal approach: an assessment of radiographic and functional outcomes. J Hand Surg Am 2007;32A:326–333.
4. Burge P. Closed cast treatment of scaphoid fractures. Hand Clin 2001;17:541–552.
5. Chen AC, Chao EK, Hung SS, et al. Percutaneous screw fixation for unstable scaphoid fractures. J Trauma 2005;59:184–187.
6. Dias JJ, Taylor M, Thompson J, et al. Radiographic signs of union of scaphoid fractures: an analysis of inter-observer agreement and re-producibility. J Bone Joint Surg Br 1988;70B:299–301.
7. Dodds SD, Panjabi MM, Slade JF 3rd. Screw fixation of scaphoid fractures: a biomechanical assessment of screw length and screw aug-mentation. J Hand Surg Am 2006;31A:405–413.
8. Gelberman RH, Menon J. The vascularity of the scaphoid bone. J Hand Surg Am 1980;5A:508–513.
9. Gelberman RH, Wolock BS, Siegel DB. Fractures and non-unions of the carpal scaphoid. J Bone Joint Surg Am 1989;71A:1560–1565.
10. Gellman H, Caputo RJ, Carter V, et al. Comparison of short and long thumb-spica casts for non-displaced fractures of the carpal scaphoid. J Bone Joint Surg Am 1989;71A:354–357.
11. Kerluke L, McCabe SJ. Nonunion of the scaphoid: a critical analysis of recent natural history studies. J Hand Surg Am 1993;18A:1–3.
12. Kozin SH. Incidence, mechanism, and natural history of scaphoid fractures. Hand Clin 2001;17:515–523.
13. Kukla C, Gaebler C, Breitenseher MJ, et al. Occult fractures of the scaphoid: the diagnostic usefulness and indirect economic repercus-sions of radiography versus magnetic resonance scanning. J Hand Surg Br 1997;22B:810–813.
14. Leslie IJ, Dickson RA. The fractured carpal scaphoid: natural history and factors influencing outcome. J Bone Joint Surg Br 1981;63B:225–230.
15. Mack GR, Bosse MJ, Gelberman RH, et al. The natural history of scaphoid nonunion. J Bone Joint Surg Am 1984;66A:504–509.
16. Martus J, Bedi A, Jebson PJL. Cannulated variable pitch compression screw fixation of scaphoid fractures using a limited dorsal approach. Tech Hand Upper Ext Surg 2005;9:202–206.
17. Ruby LK, Stinson J, Belsky MR. The natural history of scaphoid non-union: a review of fifty-five cases. J Bone Joint Surg Am 1985;67A:428–432.
18. Trumble TE, Clarke T, Kreder HJ. Non-union of the scaphoid: treat-ment with cannulated screws compared with treatment with Herbert screws. J Bone Joint Surg Am 1996;78A:1829–1837.
19. Trumble TE, Gilbert M, Murray LW, et al. Displaced scaphoid frac-tures treated with open reduction and internal fixation with a cannu-lated screw. J Bone Joint Surg Am 2000;82A:633–641.
20. Waizenegger M, Wastie ML, Barton NJ, et al. Scintigraphy in the evaluation of the "clinical" scaphoid fracture. J Hand Surg Br 1994;19B:750–753.
21. Yip HSF, Wu WC, Chang RYP, et al. Percutaneous cannulated screw fixation of acute scaphoid waist fracture. J Hand Surg Br 2002;27B:42–46.

Chapter 18

Percutaneous Treatment of Grade I to III Scaphoid Nonunions

Joseph F. Slade III, and Greg Merrell

DEFINITION

- Scaphoid nonunion describes a wide spectrum of conditions.
- The classification system shown in Table 1 describes them in the context of treatment options.

ANATOMY

- The scaphoid is almost entirely covered with cartilage and provides the mechanical link between proximal and distal carpal rows.
- Blood supply is from volar and dorsal, entering distally. The volar artery supplies only the distal tubercle region. The proximal pole is primarily dependent on intraosseous blood supply, similar to the head of the proximal femur.

PATHOGENESIS

- Mechanical instability and decreased perfusion are the most common causes of scaphoid nonunion.
- These factors work to exacerbate each other. Micromotion disrupts vascular perforators (often the only blood supply), leading to bone resorption and further decrease in mechanical stability.
- Proximal pole fractures are particularly at risk for nonunion for both mechanical (long distal lever arm and a small proximal contact area) and vascular reasons.
- Infection is rarely a cause of scaphoid nonunion but should not be forgotten in the workup and treatment.

NATURAL HISTORY

- Although progression is variable, patients often develop a dorsal intercalated segment instability (DISI) deformity (as described for scapholunate ligament injuries) and advance through stages of degeneration (scaphoid nonunion advanced collapse [SNAC] wrist arthritis) over decades.
    - SNAC wrist stage I: affects only radial styloid; stage II: arthritis at radioscaphoid joint; stage III: involvement of the scaphocapitate and capitolunate joints; stage IV: pancarpal arthritis with preservation of the radiolunate joint

PATIENT HISTORY AND PHYSICAL FINDINGS

- In established nonunions, patients present with wrist pain and in many cases are unaware of their original injury many years before.
- Findings on examination typically include radial-sided wrist tenderness on palpation and decreased range of motion, particularly extension (secondary to the DISI deformity of the carpus).
- Other than information regarding previous operative and nonoperative treatments, the additional information for evaluation and treatment decisions comes more from imaging.

IMAGING AND OTHER DIAGNOSTIC STUDIES

- CT scan with 1-mm slices in the plane of the scaphoid can help delineate bony anatomy in established nonunions and can determine if there is any evidence of healing in early nonunions.
- MR with intravenous contrast will help determine proximal pole vascularity.
    - The time and equipment required for vascularized bone grafting are more substantial than those needed for simple open reduction and internal fixation (ORIF) of the scaphoid with nonvascularized bone graft.

DIFFERENTIAL DIAGNOSIS

- Bone cyst
- Infection
- Acute fracture
- Pressier disease (scaphoid avascular necrosis [AVN])

NONOPERATIVE MANAGEMENT

- If a nonunion has not previously been given a trial of conservative care and if there is no significant resorption, casting and a bone stimulator could be attempted prior to surgical fixation.

SURGICAL MANAGEMENT

- Surgical treatment must solve three obstacles:
    - Re-establishment of local perfusion
    - Replacement of necrotic tissue with an osteoconductive and osteoinductive matrix
    - Stable fixation
- Not all proximal pole nonunions with AVN require a vascularized graft.
    - If the distal scaphoid is well perfused and good fixation can be achieved, healing can proceed via creeping substitution.
    - Guidewire placement and reaming for screw fixation helps re-establish vascular channels.
- Palmar flexion of the distal fragment and DISI position of the carpus must be corrected at the time of surgery.
- The surgical technique described in this chapter is appropriate to repair grade I to III scaphoid nonunions.
    - If a grade IV nonunion lacks significant flexion deformity and has an intact fibrous shell to contain bone graft, one may consider treatment of these fractures using the minimally invasive method reviewed in this chapter.
    - Grade V and VI nonunions are characterized by substantial bone loss, synovial nonunion, and significant flexion deformity. They are therefore not suitable for percutaneous treatment.

Preoperative Planning

- Advanced degenerative changes secondary to scaphoid nonunion are a relative contraindication to repair of a nonunion.

Table 1	Classification of Scaphoid Nonunion			
Classification Grade	**Illustration**	**Category**	**Characteristics**	**Treatment**
I		Delayed presentation	Fractures presenting 4–12 weeks after injury	Screw fixation alone usually sufficient
II		Fibrous	Intact cartilaginous envelope and no sclerosis or resorption	Percutaneous débridement, bone graft, and fixation
III		Minimal sclerosis	Resorption <1 mm with minimal sclerosis	Percutaneous débridement, bone graft, and fixation
IV		Moderate resorption and sclerosis	Resorption <5 mm, maintained alignment	Either percutaneous or open depending on intact envelope around fracture site
V		Extensive resorption and sclerosis	Resorption 5–10 mm but maintained alignment	Typically requires open bone grafting and fixation
VI		Pseudarthrosis	Profound resorption, deformity, independent fragment motion	Open fixation and strut grafting
Subtype				
a		Proximal pole	Greater risk of nonunion and AVN	Dorsal approach, may require supplemental fixation to decrease micromotion
b		AVN	Confirmed on gadolinium-enhanced MR or lack of punctate bleeding. Decreased mechanical strength and difficulty healing.	Early AVN may be suitable to rigid fixation and grafting; more advanced AVN may require vascularized graft or salvage operation

Table 1	(continued)			
Classification Grade	**Illustration**	**Category**	**Characteristics**	**Treatment**
c		Ligamentous injury	Suggested by static and dynamic imaging or direct arthroscopic observation	Débridement, pinning, or direct repair depending on grade
d		Deformity	Humpback flexion deformity must be corrected.	This typically requires cortical strut graft and rigid fixation.

■ Advanced imaging, as discussed earlier, is crucial for appropriate preoperative planning.

Positioning

■ The patient is placed supine.
■ Traction for arthroscopy can be performed with either a traction tower or a simple horizontal pulley traction system.

Approach

■ A dorsal approach is used for proximal pole fractures to provide the most secure fixation (as a basic principle, think of securing the island to the mainland).
■ Waist fractures can be treated either dorsally or volarly.
  ■ The dorsal approach is preferred.
■ Nonunion of a distal pole scaphoid fracture, although rare, is best approached volarly.

PLACEMENT OF THE TARGETING GUIDEWIRES

■ A fluoroscopic survey is undertaken to evaluate the fracture, scaphoid alignment, and fragment mobility.
  ■ Other occult carpal fractures are sought.
■ The wrist is ulnarly deviated to extend the distal fragment. A smooth 0.062-inch dorsal-to-volar targeting Kirschner

wire is placed in the distal fragment in the center position.
■ A smooth 0.062-inch lateral targeting wire is placed in the center of the distal fragment from radial to ulnar.
■ These Kirschner wires form a "crosshair" target to guide placement of the central axis guidewire (**TECH FIG 1**).

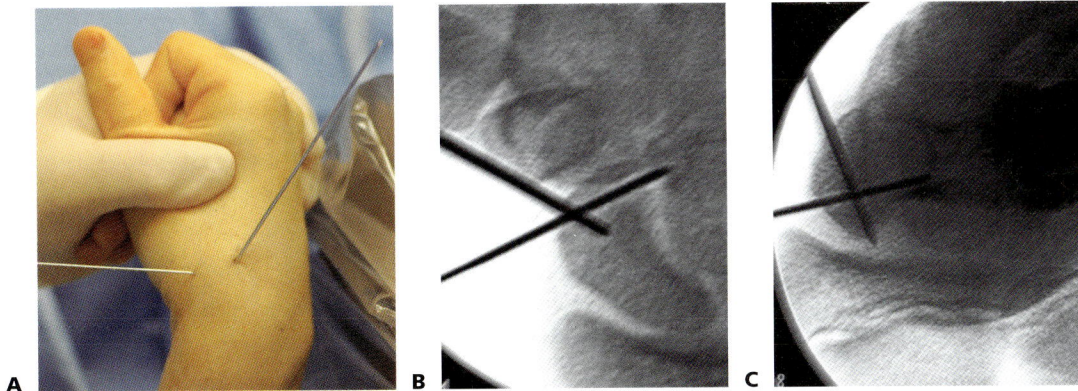

TECH FIG 1 • Crosshair targeting guide. **A.** External view. **B.** AP view. **C.** Central axis view.

PLACEMENT OF THE DISTAL CENTRAL AXIS DEROTATION WIRE

■ Placement of the first central axis wire in the distal fragment is undertaken.
■ Place a 19-gauge needle into the fracture site and confirm position fluoroscopically.
■ Use the position of the needle to introduce a double-cut 0.045-inch Kirschner wire into the fracture site and down the medullary canal of the distal fragment, using the distal crossed targeting Kirschner wires as guides.

■ Exit at the base of the thumb in an area devoid of neurovascular structures and withdraw it until the proximal tip is at the fracture site.
■ This first Kirschner wire will be used only to maintain a reduction and serve as a derotation wire, so perfect central axis placement is not necessary.

TECHNIQUES

TECHNIQUES

FRACTURE REDUCTION

- From dorsal to volar drive a 0.062-inch Kirschner wire into the proximal fragment to serve as the proximal joystick.
- Flex the distal dorsal-to-volar targeting Kirschner wire toward the proximal fragment joystick wire to correct the flexion deformity of the distal fragment (**TECH FIG 2A,B**).
  - Sometimes a percutaneous snap may need to be introduced for additional leverage or to correct translational deformities.
- Confirm fragment position fluoroscopically while holding the reduction.
- Drive the distal fragment wire that is at the base of the thumb retrograde into the proximal fragment to secure the reduction (**TECH FIG 2C**).
  - Again, perfect placement in the proximal pole is not necessary, as this wire is used only temporarily.

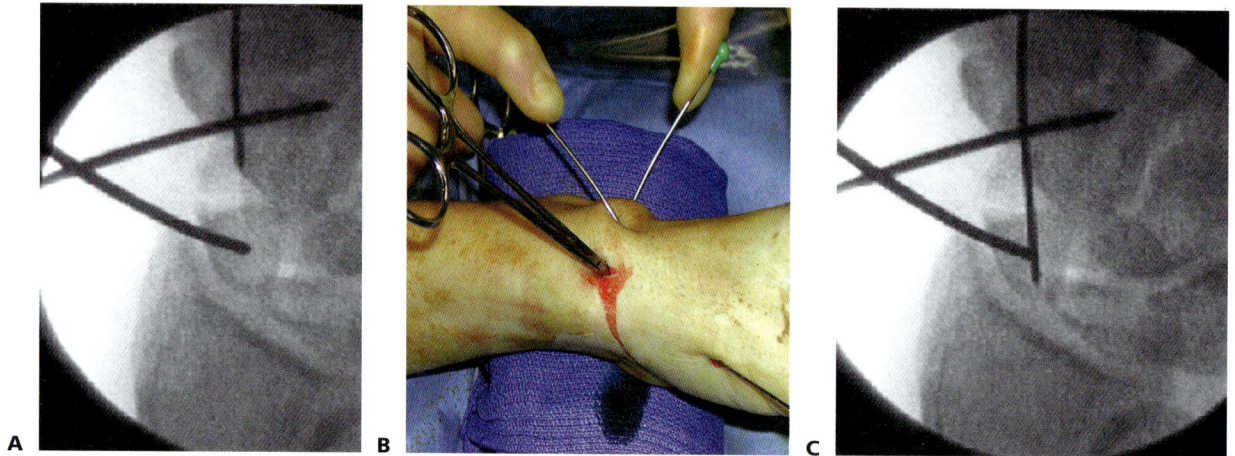

TECH FIG 2 • A. Fracture during reduction showing Kirschner wire positioned distally to capture reduction. **B.** Fracture reduction with joysticks. **C.** Radiograph of reduced fracture secured with a Kirschner wire.

PLACEMENT OF THE PROXIMAL CENTRAL AXIS GUIDEWIRE

- With the wrist partially flexed and under fluoroscopy, impale a 19-gauge needle into the proximal ulnar corner of the proximal pole (**TECH FIG 3A,B**).
- Drive a 0.045-inch Kirschner wire toward the thumb base, correcting its direction based on the external crossed-wire targeting guide.
- A successfully placed central axis scaphoid wire will hit the crossing wires in the distal scaphoid.
- The guidewire is driven volarly past this intersection, through the trapezium, and exits at the thumb base in a zone devoid of neurovascular structures.

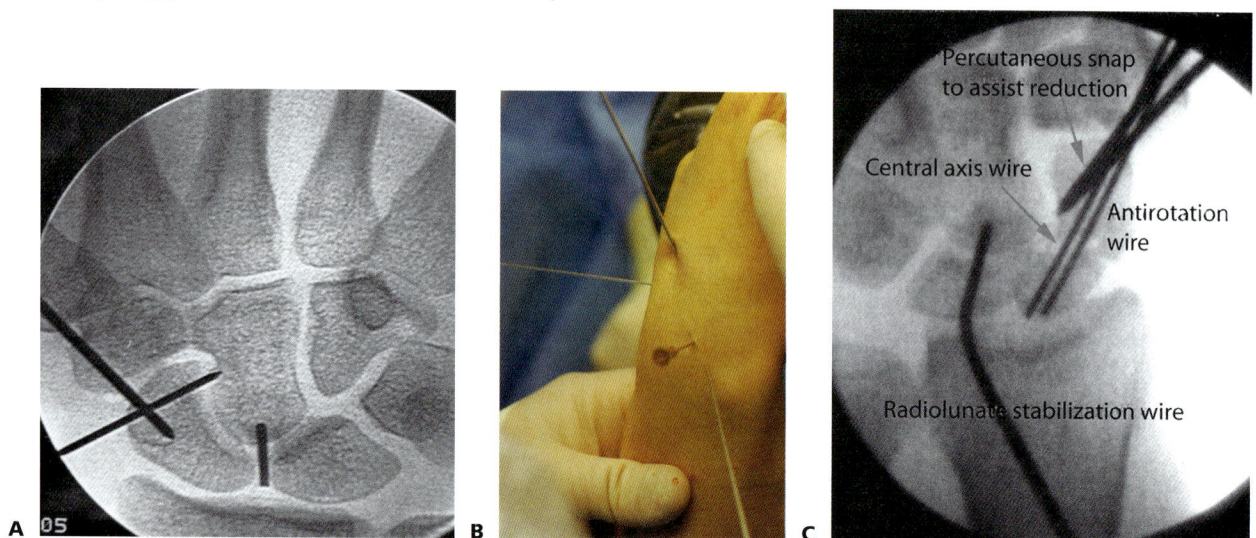

TECH FIG 3 • A. Radiograph of a needle used to identify starting position for central axis wire. **B.** External view of starting position for central axis wire. **C.** Reduced fracture with antirotation wire.

- The guidewire is withdrawn until the trailing edge crosses the radiocarpal joint and the wrist can be safely extended without bending the wire.
- There are now two intramedullary Kirschner wires down the length of the scaphoid, one used to capture the initial

reduction and the other placed down the long axis to be used as a guide for eventual screw insertion (**TECH FIG 3C**).
- The use of two Kirschner wires limits bending forces and acts as an antirotation construct during scaphoid reaming and screw placement.

ARTHROSCOPIC EVALUATION AND REAMING

- The arm is exsanguinated and the extremity is placed in a traction tower with 12 pounds distributed between four finger traps.
- Fluoroscopy can be used with 19-gauge needles to identify the radiocarpal and midcarpal portals.
  - This maneuver limits iatrogenic injury to the joint, which can result from multiple attempts to introduce a blunt trocar blindly.
- A small hemostat is used to separate the soft tissue and enter the wrist joint. A blunt trocar is placed at the radial midcarpal portal and a small joint angled arthroscope is introduced.
- Additional 19-gauge needles are inserted to establish outflow.
- A probe is introduced at the ulnar midcarpal portal, and the competency of the carpal ligaments is evaluated by directly stressing their attachments to detect partial and complete tears.
- Any scapholunate interosseous ligament (SLIL) injury detected is graded using the Geissler grading system.[2]
  - Grade I and II ligament injuries are treated with débridement and shrinkage alone.
  - Grade III injuries are treated with débridement and, after fracture repair, carpal pinning for 6 weeks.
  - Grade IV instability requires open repair of the dorsal SLIL ligament with or without capsulodesis.

- Tears of the triangular fibrocartilage complex are classified using the Palmer classification and are treated based on established guidelines.
- Fracture reduction is thoroughly evaluated arthroscopically.
- It is important to determine the presence of a fibrous capsule around the nonunion site. If there is no fibrous capsule, percutaneous bone graft is contraindicated as it will dissipate into the surrounding synovial fluid.
- If vascularity of the proximal fragment is in question, flex the wrist in the traction tower.
- Drive the central axis guidewire retrograde through the proximal fragment, ream over the wire to the level of the nonunion site.
- Withdraw the central axis wire to the fracture site (while keeping the derotation Kirschner wire in place to maintain reduction) and introduce the scope into the proximal fragment through the previously reamed tract.
- Stop the inflow and let down the tourniquet. Inspect the cancellous bone of the proximal pole with the scope for the appearance of punctate bleeding (**TECH FIG 4**).
- Keep the wrist in a flexed position and retrograde the central axis wire so it is equally exposed dorsally and volarly.
- Hand ream, under fluoroscopy, to within 2 mm of the distal cortex. Then withdraw the central axis wire volarly back to the level of the fracture site.

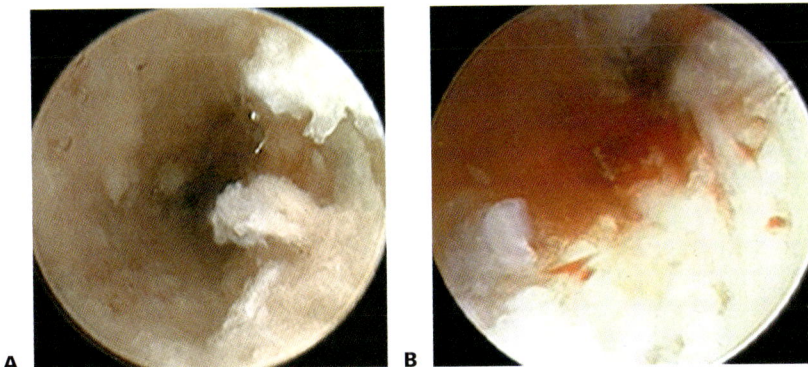

A   B

TECH FIG 4 • Inspect the cancellous bone of the proximal pole with the scope for the appearance of punctate bleeding. **A.** Devascularized proximal pole with no punctate bleeding. **B.** Vascularized proximal pole.

DÉBRIDEMENT OF THE NONUNION SITE AND BONE GRAFTING

- A grade I scaphoid nonunion (delayed presentation) typically does not require débridement or bone grafting.
- For grade II or III nonunions, insert a small curved curette through the path that was just reamed and débride the nonunion site (**TECH FIG 5A**).
  - Avoid disrupting the peripheral fibrous shell so there is a contained cavity within which to pack bone graft.

- Using an 8-gauge bone biopsy needle, harvest cores of cancellous bone from either the distal radius or iliac crest. Introduce the bone biopsy cannula into the reamed proximal pole tract.
- Pack plugs of bone graft through the cannula into the nonunion site until the radiolucent image of the nonunion site becomes radiopaque (**TECH FIG 5B**).

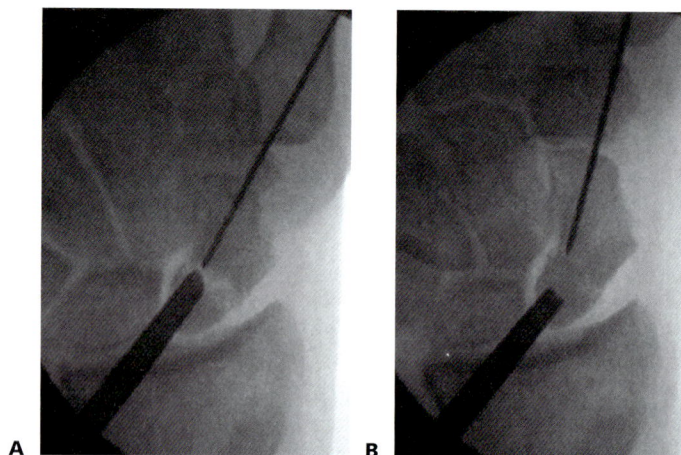

TECH FIG 5 • **A.** Percutaneous curette of nonunion. **B.** Nonunion site filled with percutaneous bone graft.

FIXATION

- The wrist is flexed and the central axis scaphoid guidewire at the base of the thumb is driven dorsally.
  - The wire is adjusted until the trailing end is in the subchondral bone of the distal scaphoid pole.
- A second wire of equal length is placed percutaneously against the proximal scaphoid pole, next to and parallel with the guidewire.
- The difference in length between the trailing end of each wire represents the scaphoid length. The screw length selected should be 4 mm less than the scaphoid length.
  - This permits 2 mm of clearance of the screw at each end of the scaphoid, thus ensuring complete implantation without screw prominence.
  - The most common reported complication of percutaneous screw stabilization for scaphoid fractures is implantation of a screw that is too long.[1]
- Advance the central axis wire so it is exposed equally volar and dorsal.
- Re-ream the entire path of the screw to within 2 mm of the opposite cortex. This creates a path through the bone graft for the screw and prevents exploding the graft through the cortical shell with a blunt screw.
  - The scaphoid should never be reamed to the opposite bone cortex (overdrilling). This reduces fracture compression and increases the risk of motion at the fracture site.
- Place the headless cannulated screw. If the screw is advanced to the distal cortex, attempts to advance the screw further will force the fracture fragments to gap and separate.
  - A standard-size Acutrak screw will best resist flexion moments.[4]
  - In unstable nonunions, as the screw is advanced it is advisable to use the joysticks to maintain a counterforce compression at the fracture site.
- If screw fixation provides only modest stability, additional fixation is advantageous.
  - In proximal pole nonunions the bending forces of the long lever arm of the distal scaphoid can be neutralized with a Kirschner wire or screw from the distal scaphoid into the capitate (**TECH FIG 6A**).
  - Micromotion can be decreased with a Kirschner wire down the second or third web space locking the capitolunate articulation.
  - With the wrist partially flexed the radiolunate joint can be secured with a Kirschner wire, preventing the tendency of DISI position (**TECH FIG 6B**).

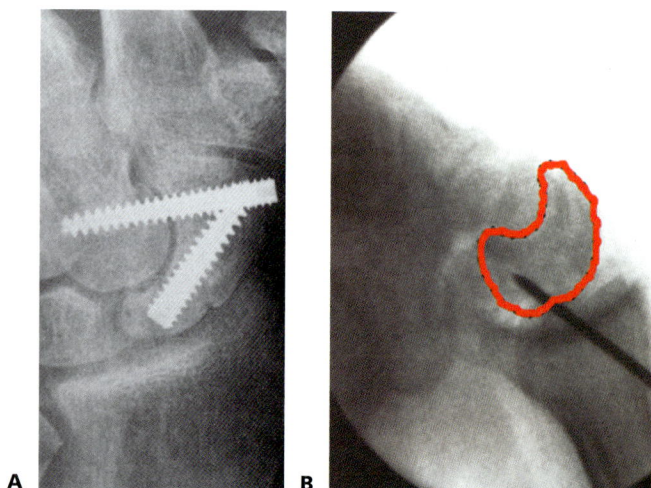

TECH FIG 6 • **A.** Decreasing lever arm with scaphocapitate screw. **B.** Helping dorsal intercalated segment instability (DISI) reduction by pinning lunate with wrist flexed.

PEARLS AND PITFALLS

Central wire placement	▪ Use the crossed Kirschner wire targeting guide in the distal fragment.
Achieving and maintaining reduction	▪ Ignore the proximal fragment first and place a wire down the distal fragment. ▪ Use joysticks and percutaneous hemostats for the reduction, then drive the wire retrograde to capture the reduced proximal fragment. ▪ A DISI deformity can be corrected and a deforming force minimized on the nonunion by flexing the wrist, thereby reducing the lunate and then capturing it by a Kirschner wire from the radius into the lunate.
Avoid over-reaming	▪ This reduces compression at the fracture site. Ream under fluoroscopy and stay 2 mm short of the opposite cortex.
Place the correct screw length	▪ A screw needs to be long enough to maximize mechanical fixation while being short enough to avoid pushing against the opposite cortex and distracting the fracture, and to avoid intra-articular prominence. Measure 4 mm less than the scaphoid along the central axis guidewire.
Decrease "windshield wipering"	▪ Use a headless screw with a large shank diameter (eg, regular Acutrak).
Decrease micromotion	▪ Add supplemental fixation as needed between the scaphocapitate, capitolunate, or radiolunate articulations.

POSTOPERATIVE CARE

▪ A short-arm volar splint and bulky dressing are applied in the operating room and the patient returns in 1 week for suture removal.

▪ If fixation is secure (as in a waist nonunion), then additional immobilization is not necessary.

▪ Proximal pole nonunions, especially those with AVN, or other unstable patterns are protected with a short-arm cast until bridging bone is visible on CT scan.

▪ Early finger motion and gentle hand strengthening are encouraged to reduce swelling and promote axial loading, encouraging fracture healing.

▪ Serial CT scans can be performed every 6 weeks to assess healing.

▪ Plain radiographs are not reliable for assessing healing.

▪ Clinical symptoms are also not a reliable indicator of healing. Rigid fixation alone may provide a painless wrist after surgery before actual bridging bone has occurred.

▪ Contact sports and heavy labor are restricted until healing is confirmed on CT.

OUTCOMES

▪ The only published series of nonunions treated percutaneously is a select series of 15 patients with minimal resorption treated with screw fixation alone. All healed, as demonstrated by bridging bone on CT scans.[3]

▪ Many grade I to IV nonunions have been successfully treated with this technique (data not yet published).

▪ As more case series are reported, we will be better able to define the functional outcomes, indications, contraindications, and rate of union of percutaneous treatment of these injuries.

COMPLICATIONS

▪ Complications are often related to screw placement.

▪ Screws placed outside the central axis have less stable fixation and therefore an increased risk of nonunion.

▪ A screw that is too long risks wear of the radioscaphoid joint.

▪ Infection and scar tenderness are reported complications but are uncommon.

REFERENCES

1. Bond CD, Shin AY, McBride MT, et al. Percutaneous screw fixation or cast immobilization for nondisplaced scaphoid fractures. J Bone Joint Surg Am 2001;83:483–488.
2. Geissler WB, Freeland AE, Savoie FH, et al. Intracarpal soft-tissue lesions associated with an intra-articular fracture of the distal end of the radius. J Bone Joint Surg Am 1996;78A:357–365.
3. Slade JF III, Geissler WB, Gutow AP, et al. Percutaneous internal fixation of selected scaphoid nonunions with an arthroscopically assisted dorsal approach. J Bone Joint Surg Am 2003;85A(Suppl 4):20–32.
4. Toby EB, Butler TE, McCormack TJ, et al. A comparison of fixation screws for the scaphoid during application of cyclic bending loads. J Bone Joint Surg Am 1997;79A:1190–1197.

Chapter 19

Volar Wedge Bone Grafting and Internal Fixation of Scaphoid Nonunions

Evan D. Collins

DEFINITION

- The scaphoid is the most commonly fractured carpal bone in the wrist. Scaphoid fractures that fail to heal after 6 months of treatment are categorized as nonunions and represent about 5% to 10% of all scaphoid fractures.
- Untreated nonunions have been reported to lead to progressive arthrosis and wrist pain.[6]
- Volar wedge bone grafting is an effective surgical technique in the treatment of certain scaphoid nonunions based on:
  - Location of the fracture
  - Degree of the deformity
  - Vascularity of the scaphoid
- This general technique can also be adapted to increase its versatility.

ANATOMY

- Nearly 80% of the scaphoid's surface is covered by articular cartilage.[6]
- Through ligamentous connections, the scaphoid serves as the bridge or link between the proximal and distal rows. Due to these strong tethers proximally and distally, it is highly susceptible to an acute fracture after a fall on an outstretched hand (**FIG 1**).[18]
- Other key factors that influence scaphoid fracture healing are its tenuous vascular supply and its unique bony architecture.
  - The vulnerable vascularity of the scaphoid, especially the proximal pole, is well described in the literature.[8,14,15,16,20] This is due to the fact that the scaphoid has a retrograde blood supply, with 70% of the vascular supply through the dorsal ridge vessel and 30% provided through branches to the scaphoid tubercle (at the level of the radiocarpal joint via superficial palmar branch perforators off the radial artery).
  - The complex geometry of the bone makes it difficult to anatomically reduce the bone fragments.

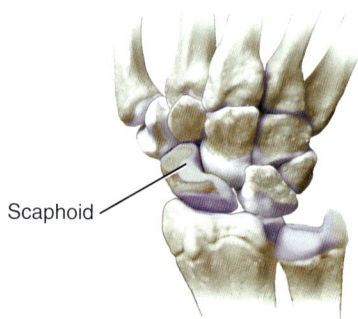

FIG 1 • Anatomy of the wrist joint. The scaphoid bridges the proximal and distal carpal rows and is largely covered by articular cartilage.

PATHOGENESIS

- Although there may be a variety of reasons for the development of a scaphoid nonunion, a fractured scaphoid usually fails to heal for three primary reasons:
  - The fracture is either undetected or untreated within the first 4 weeks after the injury.
  - The location of the fracture is proximal, resulting in poor vascularity of the most proximal fragment.
  - The fracture is displaced more than 1 mm.

NATURAL HISTORY

- Scaphoid nonunion advanced collapse (SNAC), described in the literature, is a predictable sequence of changes that occurs as a result of scaphoid nonunion leading to wrist arthrosis, often associated with pain and limitation of motion.[4,5]
- In studying patients with painful wrists over a 15-year period to determine who will develop symptoms, it is evident that the incidence of symptomatic wrist pathology requiring reconstruction is significantly higher for scaphoid nonunions that have gone untreated.[1]
- Techniques used to detect an acute scaphoid fracture and its susceptibility to nonunion, wrist pain, and corresponding arthrosis have been discussed in great detail in the literature.[14,15,20]

PATIENT HISTORY AND PHYSICAL FINDINGS

- The patient who presents with a scaphoid nonunion is usually a man between the ages of 18 and 25.
  - Unrecognized injuries in adolescence may present with pain related to early SNAC wrist arthrosis in the middle-aged adult.
- Patients generally complain of wrist pain that limits range of motion or hinders activities such as pushups, weightlifting, and opening a door. Moderate to heavy pinch and grip pain have also been described.
- A specific event resulting in the original scaphoid fracture years before is rarely cited by the patient on presentation.
- Consistent physical examination findings include subtle tenderness in the region of the scaphoid tubercle or the anatomic snuffbox, limited wrist extension compared to the contralateral side, and localized pain on the radial side along the radiostyloid or scaphoid with loaded wrist extension.

IMAGING AND OTHER DIAGNOSTIC STUDIES

- Standard radiographs include posteroanterior (PA), lateral, and scaphoid oblique 45- and 60-degree pronated views (**FIG 2**). Such views:
  - Confirm the diagnosis
  - Provide information regarding displacement, angulation, shortening, and the presence of a "humpback deformity"

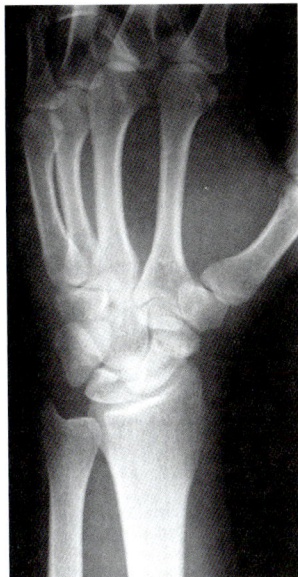

FIG 2 • An oblique view of a scaphoid that has not healed.

- Reveal compensatory carpal instability, dorsal intercalated segment instability (DISI)
- As part of a treatment algorithm, dividing scaphoid fractures into either proximal, middle, or distal is very helpful.
- Other factors considered in diagnostic assessment include previous wrist fracture or sprain later becoming symptomatic; tenderness on the scaphoid tubercle or in the anatomic snuffbox; localized pain to the radial side of the wrist along the radiostyloid or scaphoid itself, with a loaded dorsiflexed wrist; and pinching and heavy grip pain.
- Once the scaphoid nonunion is diagnosed, often a CT scan performed in the plane of the scaphoid helps define bony architecture. Sagittal and coronal images are particularly helpful in characterizing the nonunion site and its orientation, displacement, and degree of bone loss.
  - Scaphoid collapse (or "humpback deformity") is most clearly determined by measuring the lateral intrascaphoid angle on the sagittal CT views.
- MR imaging, especially when combined with intravenous gadolinium, is helpful in defining the presence or absence of osteonecrosis and any associated ligamentous or cartilaginous injuries. If osteonecrosis of the proximal fragment is seen, the surgeon should consider a vascularized bone graft[10] (see Chap. HA-20) rather than the nonvascularized grafting procedure described in this chapter.

DIFFERENTIAL DIAGNOSIS

- De Quervain's tendinitis
- Scaphotrapeziotrapezoidal arthritis
- Scaphoid lunate instability, static and dynamic
- Radial styloid fracture
- Trapezial ridge fracture

NONOPERATIVE MANAGEMENT

- Surgery is generally indicated for established scaphoid nonunions that are displaced and symptomatic because of the strong likelihood that radiocarpal arthrosis may develop with this type of persistent nonunion.[18,20]

- Nonoperative management may be appropriate for minimally symptomatic scaphoid nonunions. All factors should be taken into consideration when determining the most appropriate treatment: scaphoid nonunion alone is not an absolute reason for surgery.[12]

SURGICAL MANAGEMENT

- Volar wedge bone grafting is the preferred surgical technique for treatment of a scaphoid nonunion without osteonecrosis but with shortening, an increased intrascaphoid angle causing a "humpback deformity," and concomitant carpal collapse. Although many scaphoid nonunions without deformity can be effectively treated with the described procedure, other approaches and grafting techniques that are less invasive may be an option, especially for proximal pole nonunions.[2]
- Determining which bone graft is necessary depends on how much shortening is anticipated.[3]
  - The benefits of distal radius bone grafting include its location within the same surgical site and the fact that it is not limited in size and can be harvested as a vascularized or nonvascularized graft. One important disadvantage is the creation of a relatively large defect and stress riser within the distal radius. Also, the surgical incision is more extensile and it is not possible to get a bicortical or tricortical piece of bone for a more structural bone graft.
  - Iliac crest bone graft may be harvested in large quantities and as a bicortical or tricortical piece of bone. It is relatively simple to procure and has a long history of success in such cases, a standard by which all others are currently measured. The disadvantages of this type of bone graft include a separate incision with associated morbidity, as well as a reported risk of cutaneous nerve injuries. Also, it cannot be converted to a vascularized pedicle bone graft.
- When an MRI reveals the presence of osteonecrosis, a vascularized procedure should be considered (see Chap. HA-20).[14,15,20]

Preoperative Planning

- After assessing all diagnostic studies, including plain films, MRI and CT scans, the type of bone graft is determined.
- Two types of fixation screws can be used.
  - One type of screw has a smooth shank and two threaded heads. This screw is strong and creates high compression but may not be appropriate for all nonunions. The scaphoid nonunion fragments must be large enough to ensure that no threads of the screw cross into the bone graft site.
  - The other type of compression screw uses a deferential pitch between the proximal and distal portion of the screw. This screw may be more versatile, although it lacks compression strength compared to the above-mentioned screw.
- If compression screws are not deemed appropriate for the type of nonunion that exists, multiple Kirschner wires can be used.
- A regional anesthetic block is used for most patients and is helpful for alleviating postoperative pain. When iliac crest grafting is chosen, additional general anesthesia is needed.
- All radiographic studies are reviewed and brought to the operating room for re-evaluation during the case.

Positioning

- The patient is placed in the supine position with the upper extremity positioned on a hand table.
- If an ipsilateral iliac crest bone graft is used, the hip on the same side as the affected hand is prepared and draped. A small bump is placed under the hip for patients with significant adipose tissue.
- A tourniquet is applied to the proximal arm.

Approach

- The location of the scaphoid nonunion helps determine the surgical approach. Wedge bone grafting of a waist nonunion is performed using a standard volar approach.
- For proximal pole fractures with evidence of osteonecrosis, a dorsal approach with possibly a vascularized bone graft would be a more amenable surgical approach.[13,19]

VOLAR WEDGE BONE GRAFTING USING DISTAL RADIUS BONE GRAFT AND INTRAOSSEOUS COMPRESSION SCREW FIXATION

Incision and Initial Dissection

- An incision is drawn over the flexor carpi radialis (FCR) tendon and extended distally between the glabrous skin of the thenar eminence, angled across the wrist flexion crease (**TECH FIG 1A**).
- After exsanguination the skin is incised and the FCR tendon is identified. Distally in the wound a volar branch of the radial artery is often sacrificed to gain exposure (**TECH FIG 1B**).
- The floor of the FCR tendon is sharply incised over the entire course of the incision and the digital flexors and median nerve are swept ulnarly. They are carefully protected throughout the case. A blunt Wheatlander is used to maintain visualization of this interval between the radial artery and the FCR tendon.
  - The volar extrinsic ligaments, the radioscaphocapitate (RSC) and long radiolunate (LRL), are identified and precisely incised. Much of the LRL and a portion of the RSC are left intact, helping to stabilize the proximal pole (**TECH FIG 1C**).
  - This stability facilitates the reduction of the distal fragment to the proximal fragment.

- Preserving this ligamentous support also helps maintain fracture reduction during the placement of an intraosseous compression screw by counteracting the torque created during screw insertion.
- Deep dissection proceeds to the scaphotrapezial joint. This interval is exposed using a transverse capsular incision for later insertion of the intraosseous screw.
- The articulation between the scaphoid and capitate is carefully exposed. This visualization will be important during reduction of the scaphoid fragments.
- During exposure it is critical to avoid dissection over the distal dorsoradial scaphoid to avoid interrupting the contribution by the dorsal ridge vessel.

Nonunion Exposure and Preparation

- A no. 64 Beaver blade and Freer elevator are used to define the location of the nonunion and the borders of the scaphoid itself. Time spent here makes reduction and bone graft placement simpler later (**TECH FIG 2A,B**).
- Two joystick K-wires are placed, one angled proximally in the proximal fragment and one angled distally in the distal fragment (**TECH FIG 2C**).

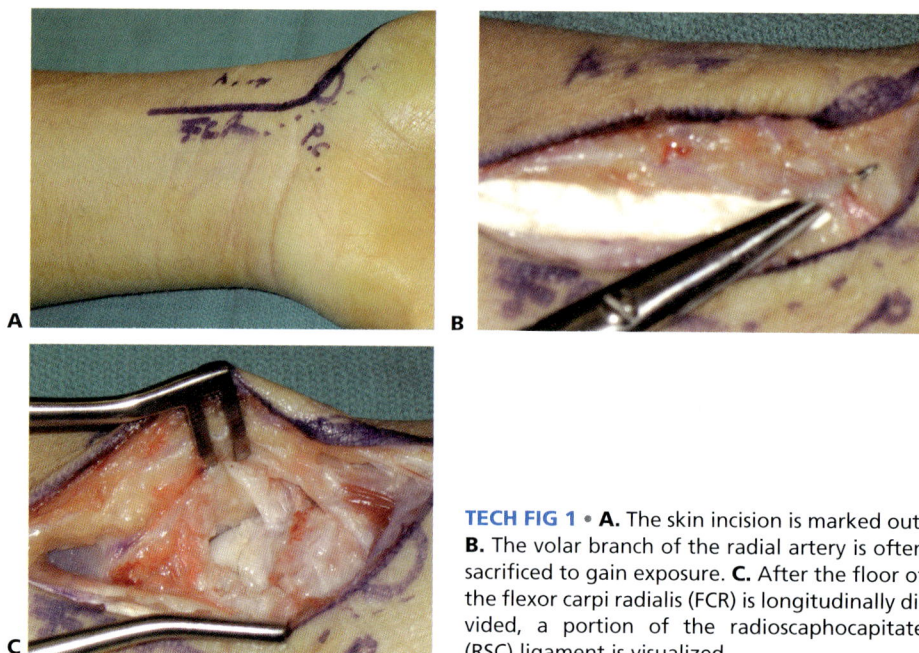

TECH FIG 1 • **A.** The skin incision is marked out. **B.** The volar branch of the radial artery is often sacrificed to gain exposure. **C.** After the floor of the flexor carpi radialis (FCR) is longitudinally divided, a portion of the radioscaphocapitate (RSC) ligament is visualized.

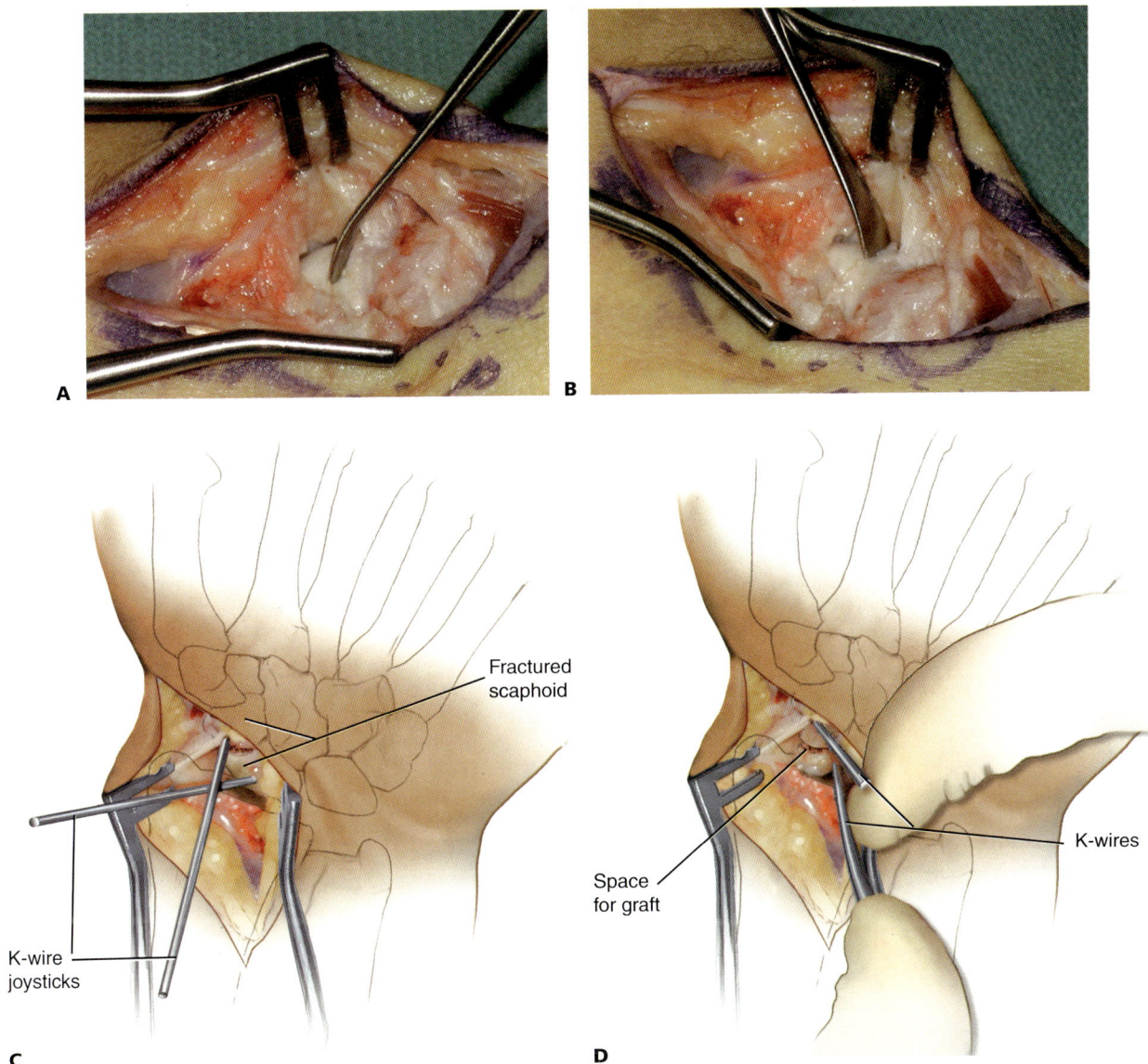

TECH FIG 2 • A,B. A Freer elevator identifies the nonunion site. **C.** K-wires are used as joysticks to control the scaphoid proximal and distal fragments. **D.** Manipulation of the K-wires allows for access to the nonunion site for débridement and then graft placement.

- These K-wires facilitate manipulation of the fragments and therefore access to the nonunion site for débridement (**TECH FIG 2D**).
- The proximal and distal poles are examined carefully for osteolysis and sclerosis. A small curette or rongeur is used for débridement and removal of intervening fibrous tissue. Débridement is complete once good punctate bleeding is noted. In some situations deflating the tourniquet temporarily can be of value in assessing viability of the fragments.

Fracture Reduction and Preliminary Stabilization

- By bringing the joystick/crossed K-wires into a more parallel position (relative to one another) and rotating the distal K-wire into slight supination, initial fracture reduction is often accomplished by removing the humpback (**TECH FIG 3**).

- A retrograde K-wire may be inserted along the longitudinal axis of the scaphoid to temporarily hold the reduction.
  - If placed in an appropriately eccentric position this K-wire may serve effectively as the derotation K-wire (used later to avoid fragment rotation during screw insertion) and yet remain out of the path of the screw.
- Restoration of scaphoid length and anatomic reduction of the fragments are best assessed by direct visualization and fluoroscopy.
  - Lateral images will reveal correction of the DISI deformity.
  - PA images document proper length of the scaphoid and determine if the Gilula lines are re-established.[9]
- The size of the volar wedge graft needed to maintain the reduction is now determined based on the volar defect noted after the reduction is accomplished.

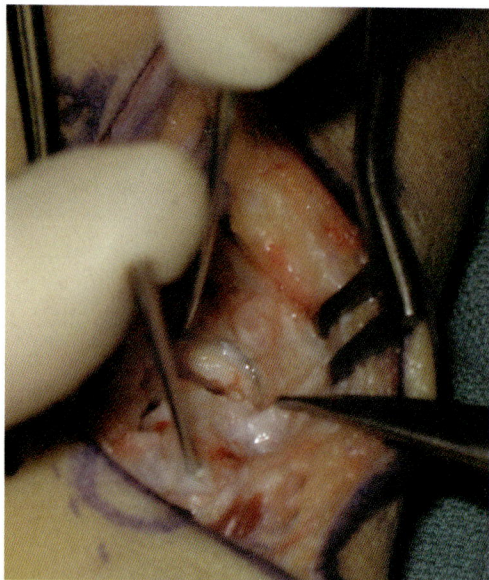

TECH FIG 3 • The scaphoid joysticks are used to reduce the fracture, and the length is estimated to determine the size of the volar wedge graft.

Distal Radius Graft Harvest

- A two-fingerbreadths incision is made more proximally than initially described. This provides the necessary access to the distal radius.
- The pronator quadratus is elevated using cautery, and the distal radius is perforated using K-wires to outline the size of the graft needed to fill the volar defect.
  - Great care is taken to avoid destabilizing the radial cortex of the radius.
- A curved osteotome introduced on three sides allows harvest of the corticocancellous wedge.
- A curette is then used to harvest as much cancellous bone as necessary.

Graft Contouring and Insertion

- The volar cortical defect in the reduced scaphoid is "regularized" using a small water-cooled sagittal saw or a fine rongeur.
  - Very little bone is removed from the fracture fragments to create a standard-shaped trough.
  - Creating such a "regular" defect makes insertion of the wedge graft easier and more secure.
- The same saw or rongeur is used to shape the corticocancellous graft to match the "regularized" defect.
- The prepared proximal and distal fragments are packed with cancellous bone and the corticocancellous graft is tapped into place (**TECH FIG 4A**).
  - Before graft insertion, the longitudinal K-wire, whether it is the K-wire placed to maintain reduction or the K-wire over which the cannulated compression screw is to be placed, is withdrawn into the distal pole and then reinserted after placement of the graft into the trough.

Cannulated Intraosseous Compression Screw Fixation

- At the level of the scaphotrapezial joint a small rongeur is used to remove a portion of the trapezial lip.[20]
  - This facilitates the placement of the K-wire and screw down the longitudinal access of the scaphoid, helping secure center placement of the screw within the bone. A center screw position has been demonstrated to lead to increased healing rates.
- A K-wire from the compression screw system is then inserted in a retrograde direction (distal to proximal) into the center of the scaphoid, perpendicular to the fracture line.
  - If the K-wire is not perpendicular to the fracture, compression generated from the screw may malreduce the fragments.
- Once the K-wire is in perfect position, as judged fluoroscopically, and is fixed in the far (proximal) cortex of the scaphoid, the length is measured.
  - Factors such as cartilage thickness and distance between the fracture fragments is taken into account. It is critical that the screw not be too long and enter the radiocarpal joint.
- While some surgeons advocate advancing the K-wire into the distal radius after the measurement is taken so that the wire remains in position during drilling, that practice is dangerous. It is preferable to leave the K-wire in the scaphoid.
  - Advancing the K-wire can result in cutting the guidewire during drilling or screw placement (particularly with a second-generation compression screw that has cutting flutes at the distal end).
- If not already present, an eccentric K-wire is placed to maintain the reduction during screw insertion.
- Under fluoroscopic guidance, a cannulated drill is used followed, in some cases, by a cannulated bone tap. The screw is then placed over the K-wire and the guidewire is removed.
  - Especially during drilling, the surgeon must be careful to remain parallel with the wire.
  - The corticocancellous bone graft must be visualized at all times during these procedures to make certain position is maintained. Maintaining finger pressure over the graft during screw insertion is helpful.
- Imaging confirms proper screw location, fracture reduction, and construct stability. The K-wire is removed from the cannulated screw and the eccentric K-wire is removed (**TECH FIG 4B,C**).
- The wound is then irrigated and the volar extrinsic ligaments are repaired precisely with permanent suture. The remainder of the joint capsule may be closed with an absorbable suture.
- Bone filler, preferably cadaver dried cancellous bone chips, can be inserted into the distal radius harvest site with a small tamp to compress and fill the defect. This potentially decreases the risk of hematoma formation. The periosteal sleeve is then closed over the distal radius with absorbable suture.
- Skin is closed using nylon suture, and the tourniquet is then deflated after placement of a thumb spica splint.

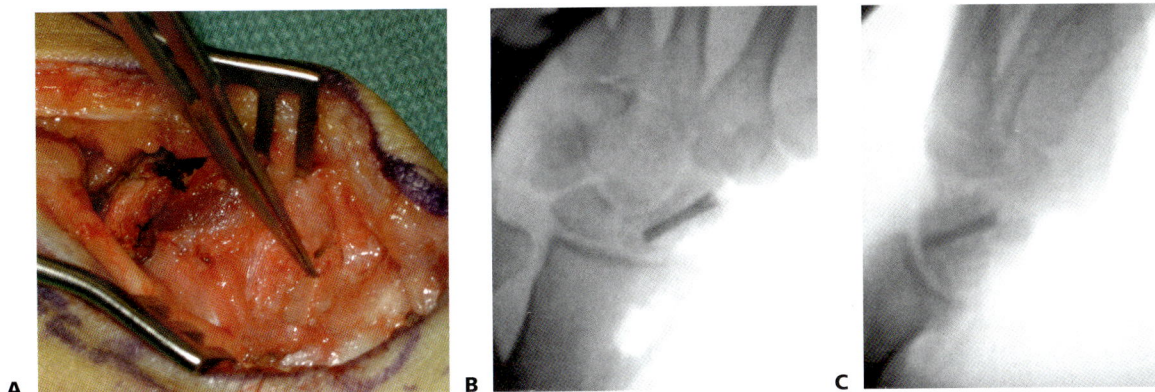

TECH FIG 4 • **A.** The wedge placement is complete. **B,C.** Posteroanterior and lateral views of the compression bone screw after harvesting the bone graft from the distal radius.

K-WIRE FIXATION

- If compression screw fixation is not feasible, then retrograde, nonthreaded K-wires are recommended and placed in the same manner as described above for the bone screw.
  - The wires should be left under the skin and removed once the bone has healed.
- K-wires provide adequate stability and may be a better fixation choice with large bone grafts.

Iliac Crest Graft Harvest

- Rather than obtaining bone graft from the distal radius, a standard technique of harvesting bone from the iliac crest may be used.[16,20]
- A 2- to 3-cm incision is made just inferior to the superior border of the iliac crest just posterior to the anterior superior iliac spine (ASIS).
  - The incision is kept below the belt line to minimize postoperative incisional tenderness.
  - The incision is posterior to the ASIS to avoid iatrogenic nerve injury and subsequent numbness and pain over the proximal lateral thigh.
- Dissection is accomplished using cautery through the deep fascia down to the crest. The superior crest is exposed and muscles are released from a portion of the outer table using cautery and an elevator.
- A water-cooled sagittal saw and a curved osteotome are used to harvest a bicortical segment of corticocancellous graft.
  - The graft is slightly larger than the measured defect in the scaphoid.
  - The inner table is left intact.
  - The harvested outer table will be volar when the graft is placed in the scaphoid and the superior crest will be radial.
- A curette is used to harvest cancellous bone graft.
- The wound is copiously irrigated and temporarily packed with thrombin-soaked Gelfoam while attention is redirected to the scaphoid.
- After the scaphoid is reconstructed, the Gelfoam is removed and the wound again irrigated.
- If indicated, a small suction drain is placed below the fascia.
- The wound is closed in layers with a running locking stitch used for the fascia.
- A local anesthetic with epinephrine may be injected before harvest of the graft or after closure.

PEARLS AND PITFALLS

When MRI reveals osteonecrosis in a scaphoid nonunion	■ Volar wedge bone grafting and internal fixation is the treatment option that is most effective when applied to scaphoid waist fractures, distal-third fractures of the scaphoid without osteonecrosis, or scaphoid waist fractures with concomitant carpal collapse and a nondissociated DISI pattern. When osteonecrosis is present, a vascularized procedure is preferable.
Surgeon prefers an adaptable graft should physical findings during the procedure reveal osteonecrosis not revealed on MRI	■ The advantage of harvesting from the distal radius rather than the iliac crest exists when the MRI is inconsistent with physical examination findings during the procedure. Harvesting from the distal radius allows the surgeon to use a modified pedicle technique using the pronator quadratus and the periosteum of the distal radius and place it into the volar defect as a vascularized bone graft if necessary.[20]
Fixation for greatest chance of bone healing	■ While either compression bone screws or K-wires can be used as effective fixation in this procedure, compression screws are believed to improve chances of overall bone healing.[7,11,18]

POSTOPERATIVE CARE

▪ When a screw is placed for internal fixation, a thumb spica splint is applied after the procedure.

▪ The patient returns for a follow-up visit 10 days after surgery. During this visit, the hand is examined for swelling and sutures may be removed.

▪ A thumb spica, short-arm cast is applied, leaving the interphalangeal joint free. The patient is followed radiographically at intervals of 3 to 4 weeks.

▪ CT scans are the most predictable way to determine if the scaphoid has healed. This evaluation is recommended before allowing the patient to resume vigorous activities.

OUTCOMES

▪ Symptomatic scaphoid nonunions with shortening respond well to volar wedge bone grafting with internal fixation, particularly when scaphoid length is restored and when any bony union is achieved.

▪ A higher rate of bone healing is achieved when a compression bone screw is used as the internal fixation. Reported results show that internal fixation leads to better functional results than standard techniques of bone grafting.[7,11,16–18]

▪ Bones failing to heal after the procedure have been shown to respond well to vascularized grafts. Other options for failure to heal include partial scaphoid excision, complete scaphoid excision with four-corner fusion, proximal row carpectomy, radial styloidectomy, and complete wrist fusion.

COMPLICATIONS

▪ Radiographic findings may not match the findings at surgery. This affects the outcome to varying degrees, depending on the type of graft harvested.

▪ Persistent nonunion and osteonecrosis resulting in wrist arthrosis

▪ Scarring associated with repair of the capsule, causing some postoperative stiffness

REFERENCES

1. Allende BT. Osteoarthritis of the wrist secondary to non-union of the scaphoid. Int Orthop 1988;12:201–211.
2. Amandio PC, Berquist TH, Smith DK, et al. Scaphoid malunion. J Hand Surg Am 1989;14A:679–687.
3. Barton N. Experience with scaphoid grafting. J Hand Surg Br 1997;22B:153–160.
4. Cooney WP III, Dobyns JH, Linscheid RL. Nonunion of the scaphoid: analysis of the results from bone grafting. J Hand Surg Am 1980;5:343–354.
5. Cooney WP, Linscheid RL, Dobyns JH. Scaphoid fractures: problems associated with nonunion and avascular necrosis. Orthop Clin North Am 1984;15:381–391.
6. Duppe H, Johnell O, Lundborg G, et al. Long-term results of fracture of the scaphoid: a follow-up study of more than thirty years. J Bone Joint Surg Am 1994;76A:249–252.
7. Filan SL, Herbert TJ. Herbert screw fixation of scaphoid fractures. J Bone Joint Surg Br 1996;78B:519–529.
8. Gelberman RH, Menon J. The vascularity of the scaphoid bone. J Hand Surg Am 1980;5:508–513.
9. Gilula LA, Destouet JM, Weeks PM, et al. Roentgenographic diagnosis of the painful wrist. Clin Orthop Relat Res 1984;187:52–64.
10. Hunter JC, Escobedo EM, Wilson AJ, et al. MR imaging of clinically suspected scaphoid fractures. AJR Am J Roentgenol 1997;168:1287–1293.
11. Inoue G, Shionoya K, Kuwahata Y. Herbert screw fixation for scaphoid nonunions. Clin Orthop Relat Res 1997;343:99–106.
12. Kerluke L, McCabe SJ. Nonunion of the scaphoid: a critical analysis of recent natural history studies. J Hand Surg Am 1993;18:1–3.
13. Kuhlmann JN, Mimoun M, Boabighl A, et al. Vascularized bone graft pedicled on the volar carpal artery for non-union of the scaphoid. J Hand Surg Br 1987;12:203–210.
14. Lindstrom G, Nystrom A. Natural history of scaphoid non-union with special reference to "asymptomatic" cases. J Hand Surg Br 1992;17:697–700.
15. Moreno R, Gupta A. Scaphoid fractures. First Hand News, a publication of the Christine M. Kleinert Institute for Hand and Microsurgery, Inc., Summer 2004.
16. Mulier T, Adrianssens N, Nijs S, et al. Scaphoid delayed unions and nonunions: a prospective study comparing different treatment methods. Folia Traumatologica Lovaniensia 2003;84–93.
17. Rajagopalan BM, Squire DS, Samuels LO. Results of Herbert-screw fixation with bone-grafting for the treatment of nonunion of the scaphoid. J Bone Joint Surg Am 1999;81:48–52.
18. Ring D, Jupiter JB, Herndon JH. Acute fractures of the scaphoid. J Am Acad Orthop Surg 2000;8:225–231.
19. Sawaizumi T, Nanno M, Nanbu A, et al. Vascularised bone graft from the base of the second metacarpal for refractory nonunion of the scaphoid. J Bone Joint Surg Br 2004;66B:1007–1012.
20. Trumble TE, Salas P, Barthel T, Robert KQ III. Management of scaphoid nonunions. J Am Acad Orthop Surg 2003;11:380–391.

Chapter 20

Vascularized Bone Grafting of Avascular Scaphoid Nonunions

Alexander D. Mih

DEFINITION

- Scaphoid fractures account for 60% of carpal bone fractures.
- Nonunions occur in up to 15% of scaphoid fractures and often result from delayed treatment, inadequate immobilization, displacement of the fracture, or proximal pole involvement or in the setting of avascular necrosis (AVN).

ANATOMY

- The blood supply to the scaphoid travels in a distal to proximal direction and emanates from the radial artery. Intraosseous vessels traverse the scaphoid to supply the proximal pole.
  - In about 30% of scaphoids, there is either a single or no vascular channel found reaching the proximal pole.
- Studies of vascularity of the distal radius have identified several sources of vascularized bone graft available for nonunion treatment.
- Animal studies of vascularized bone grafts have documented a significant increase in blood flow present when compared to nonvascularized grafts.

PATHOGENESIS

- Without adequate blood flow, the normal bone healing response cannot be completed. The scaphoid fracture site fills with fibrous connective tissue and motion persists at the site of the fracture.
- In some cases, the bone undergoes changes of AVN with cellular death, edema, and the eventual loss of trabecular architecture.
  - Studies have shown that in cases in which the trabecular bone pattern has been lost, union may be difficult if not impossible to achieve.

NATURAL HISTORY

- Nonunion of the scaphoid severely alters the normal carpal biomechanics and subjects the cartilage to shear forces detrimental to its survival.

PATIENT HISTORY AND PHYSICAL FINDINGS

- Often patients recall injuring their wrists several years before developing pain severe enough to seek medical attention.
- Patients usually complain of limited range of wrist motion and pain, often with grip or weight bearing. The patients have often significantly reduced their activity level due to persistent pain.
- In most cases the patient will experience tenderness to palpation at the anatomic snuffbox (**FIG 1A**), the radial styloid–scaphoid joint (**FIG 1B**), or the distal pole of the scaphoid (**FIG 1C**), which is palpable on the palmar side of the wrist.
- Wrists with established scaphoid nonunions have an arc of motion that is significantly reduced from the uninvolved side, primarily in extension.

IMAGING AND OTHER DIAGNOSTIC STUDIES

- Standard radiographic studies include posteroanterior (PA), lateral, and scaphoid (ulnar deviation) views (**FIG 2**).
  - Classic radiographic findings begin at the radial styloid–distal pole of scaphoid interface and proceed to involve the entire scaphoid fossa, the midcarpal joint, and eventually the entire radiocarpal articulation.
- CT is essential for determining union as well as for identifying patients in whom the normal trabecular bone pattern has been lost.
- MRI is useful in evaluating the scaphoid for vascularity, although definitive determination of avascularity may be difficult.

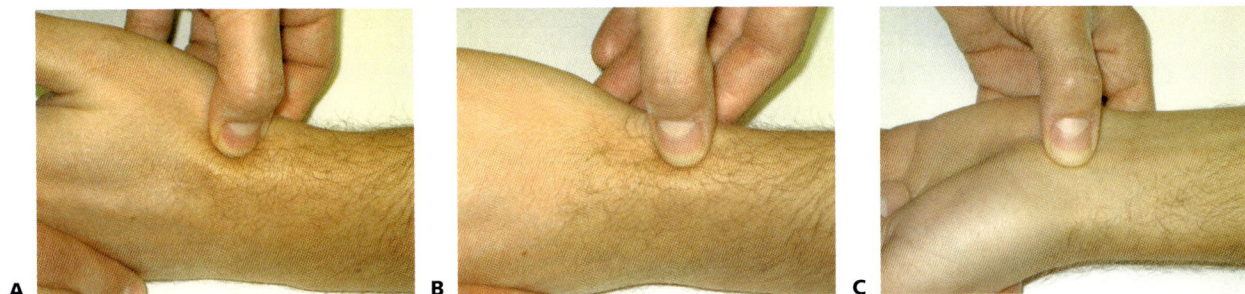

FIG 1 • **A.** Tenderness at the anatomic snuffbox is a classic finding of scaphoid nonunion. **B.** The radial styloid–scaphoid interface is the earliest site of degenerative change in scaphoid nonunions, and patients will often display tenderness at that location. **C.** The distal pole of the scaphoid is palpable at the base of the thumb on the palmar aspect of the wrist. Tenderness at this region is usually found in cases of scaphoid nonunion.

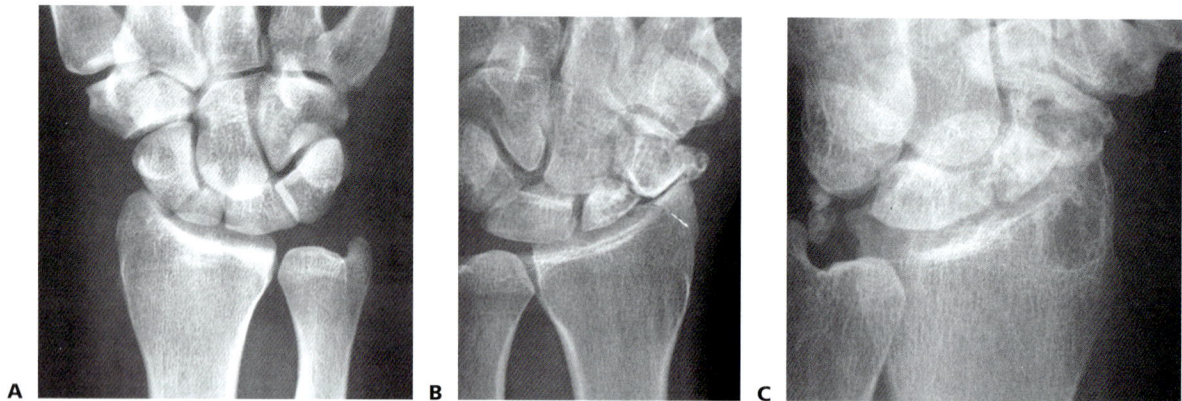

FIG 2 • **A.** Early radiographic appearance of scaphoid nonunion before degenerative change. **B.** Development of degenerative changes at the radial styloid–scaphoid interface. **C.** Advanced changes involving the entire scaphoid fossa.

Conflicting reports regarding the usefulness of gadolinium enhancement have been published over the past several years.

DIFFERENTIAL DIAGNOSIS

- Ligamentous injury to the wrist
- Wrist synovitis
- Intraosseous ganglia
- Primary AVN of the scaphoid

NONOPERATIVE MANAGEMENT

- Nonoperative treatment is limited for established nonunions.
- Investigators have attempted the use of bone stimulators, which use either electrical stimulation or ultrasound.
    - There is little evidence in the literature supporting the use of these units for treatment of established scaphoid nonunions.

SURGICAL MANAGEMENT

- A vascularized distal radial bone graft is indicated for scaphoid nonunions with and without evidence of avascularity.
- Correction of a "humpback deformity" requires extensive mobilization of the pedicle when attempting the use of a dorsally sourced graft, and a palmar vascularized graft may be more appropriate.

- For significant collapse, a nonvascular iliac crest graft may be required to create a compression-resistant construct.
- When early degenerative changes are present, a radial styloidectomy should accompany the use of a vascularized distal radial graft.
- The presence of more advanced degenerative joint disease or carpal malalignment is a contraindication to performing surgery to obtain bony union.

Preoperative Planning

- Radiographs must be evaluated to rule out degenerative joint changes or carpal instability patterns, which are often found in established nonunions.

Positioning

- The patient is placed supine on the operating table with the arm placed on an armboard.
- Surgery is performed under tourniquet control.

Approach

- Vascularized grafting is carried out through a dorsal approach. Anatomic studies have shown that the dorsal irrigating vessels are of greater diameter and are further from the articular surface than irrigating vessels on the palmar surface of the radius.

TECHNIQUES

VASCULARIZED DISTAL RADIUS BONE GRAFTING USING THE 1,2-INTER-COMPARTMENTAL SUPRARETINACULAR ARTERY[7]

Exposure

- A curvilinear incision is made over the dorsoradial aspect of the wrist, centered between the first and second extensor compartments (**TECH FIG 1A**).
- The 1,2-intercompartmental supraretinacular artery (1,2 IC SRA) lies on the surface of the retinaculum between the first and second compartments (**TECH FIG 1B**).
    - The irrigating branch enters the distal radius and supplies bone distal and dorsal to the brachioradialis insertion.
    - Avoidance of exsanguination before tourniquet inflation facilitates its identification.

- The first and second compartments are unroofed on their radial and ulnar aspects, respectively, to avoid damage to this irrigating vessel.

Graft Harvest

- The periosteum is scored with a scalpel to outline the graft shape, which measures 1.5 cm in the longitudinal dimension and 0.5 to 0.75 cm in the transverse dimensions (**TECH FIG 2A**). The distal graft margin extends to a point 0.5 to 1 cm from the articular surface.
- Osteotomes are used to elevate the cortical cancellous graft.

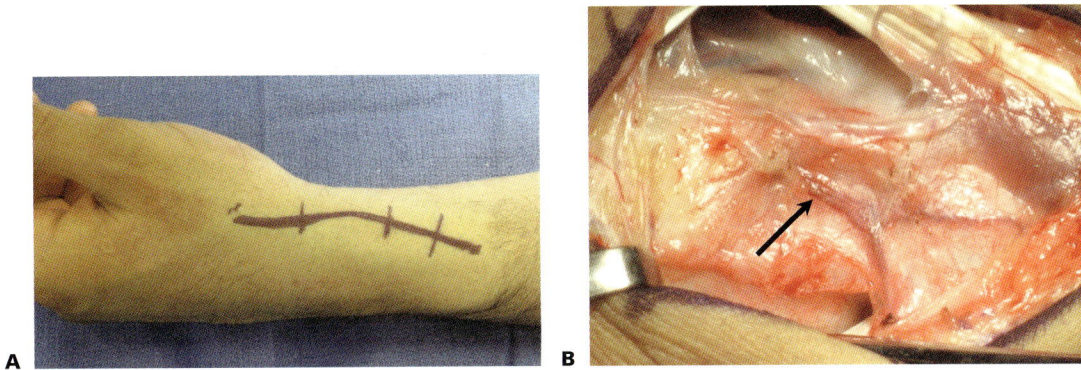

TECH FIG 1 • A. The incision is made over the dorsoradial aspect of the distal radius. **B.** 1,2-intercompartmental supraretinacular artery is visible between the first and second compartments (*arrow*).

- The soft tissue envelope containing the vessel is elevated from the radial periosteum distal to the site of graft harvest (**TECH FIG 2B**). This can usually be accomplished with a scalpel or Freer elevator.
  - The 1,2 IC SRA is not dissected free; rather, it is left as part of the retinacular septum.
- The tourniquet is deflated and perfusion of the vascularized bone graft is ensured (**TECH FIG 2C**).

Graft Placement

- The joint capsule is incised in the distal portion of the incision and the scaphoid nonunion is identified.
  - A radial styloidectomy greatly increases the exposure of the scaphoid and eliminates the possibility of bone graft impingement.
- Intervening fibrous tissue and sclerotic bone are removed

from the nonunion site using rongeurs and curettes to prepare the scaphoid for graft placement.

- Cancellous bone graft from the distal radius is packed proximally and distally to fill voids created by débriding sclerotic bone.
- The carefully contoured vascularized graft is then rotated into the nonunion site and pressfit into position, taking care to avoid torsion of the vascular pedicle (**TECH FIG 3A**).
- Kirschner wires are advanced from the distal pole of the scaphoid to the proximal pole to secure the graft in place (**TECH FIG 3B**).
- The radial capsule is closed loosely with absorbable suture and the skin is closed in a routine fashion.
  - The pedicle must not be compressed.
- The patient is placed in a short-arm thumb spica splint.

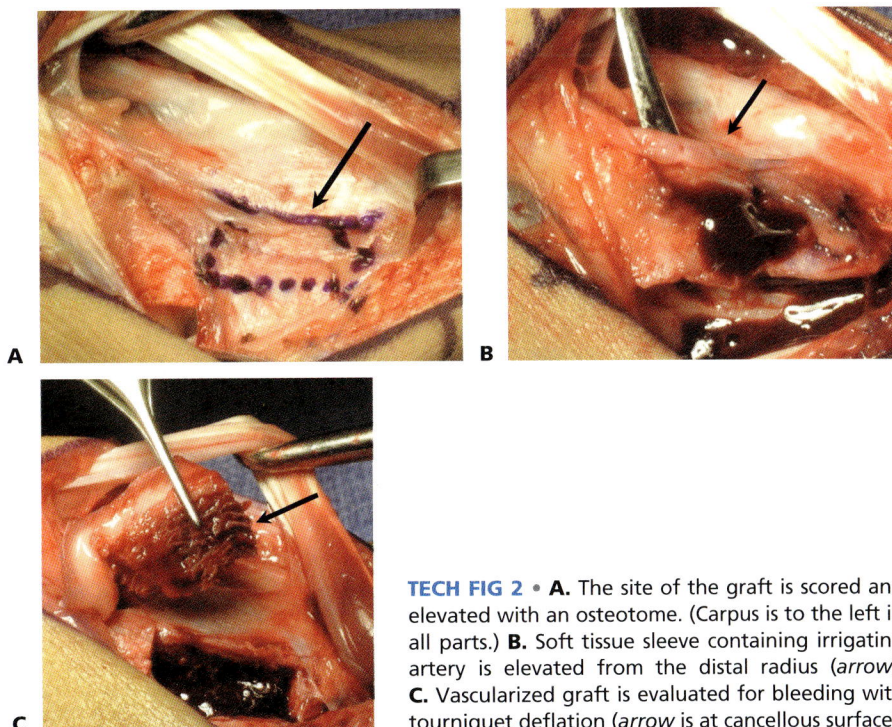

TECH FIG 2 • A. The site of the graft is scored and elevated with an osteotome. (Carpus is to the left in all parts.) **B.** Soft tissue sleeve containing irrigating artery is elevated from the distal radius (*arrow*). **C.** Vascularized graft is evaluated for bleeding with tourniquet deflation (*arrow* is at cancellous surface).

TECHNIQUES

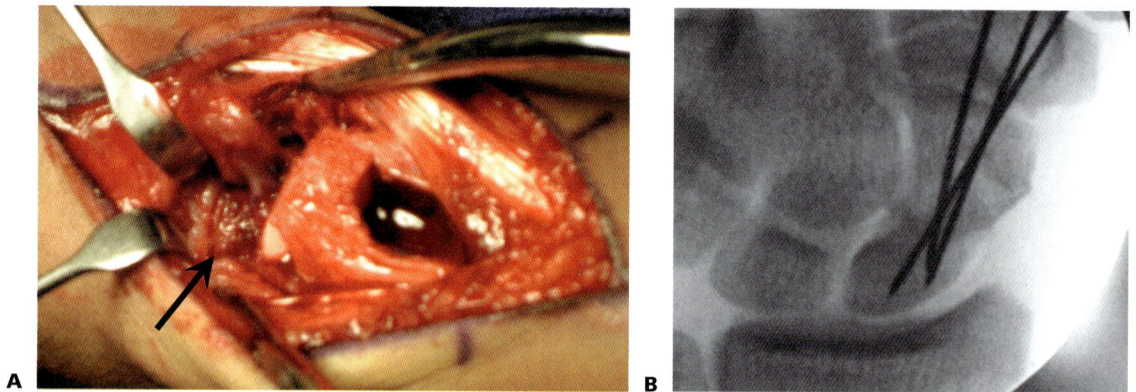

TECH FIG 3 • A. The vascularized graft is rotated into the nonunion site (*arrow*) and pressfit into position. **B.** Kirschner wire placement is percutaneous, from distal to proximal.

PEARLS AND PITFALLS

Avoid compression screw fixation.	■ Graft fracture often will occur. ■ Kirschner wire removal facilitates imaging studies.
Perform a radial styloidectomy.	■ Improves exposure and reduces the chance of graft impingement
Do not exsanguinate before tourniquet inflation.	■ Visibility of the irrigating artery is enhanced with blood present in the vessels.
The retinaculum is opened over the radial side of the first compartment and the ulnar side of the second compartment.	■ This diminishes chances of damaging the irrigating artery. ■ Graft is harvested from the radius distal and dorsal to the brachioradialis insertion.

POSTOPERATIVE CARE

■ Kirschner wires are removed when healing is observed, usually 4 to 6 weeks after surgery.
■ CT scanning may be required to document complete healing before the patient resumes risky activities.
■ MRI may be useful in evaluating the scaphoid for vascularity and may be done after Kirschner wire removal.

OUTCOMES

■ A recent meta-analysis[2] found a scaphoid union rate of 88% with the use of a vascularized bone graft. Individual series report union rates ranging from 60% to 100%.
■ Previous reports have shown that patients with MRI evidence of AVN or loss of trabecular bone pattern noted on CT have a decreased level of success with reconstructive surgery. Treatment is rarely successful when both findings are present.
■ A recent study[1] has identified risk factures for failure: proximal pole AVN, radiographic degenerative changes, loss of carpal alignment, inadequate fracture fixation, tobacco use, advanced age, and female gender.

COMPLICATIONS

■ Failure to gain union
■ Progressive degenerative changes

■ Impingement of bone on radial styloid
■ Infection

REFERENCES

1. Chang MA, Bishop AT, Moran SL, et al. The outcomes and complications of 1,2-intercompartmental supraretinacular artery pedicled vascularized bone grafting of scaphoid nonunions. J Hand Surg Am 2006;31A:387–396.
2. Merrell GA, Wolfe SW, Slade JF III. Treatment of scaphoid nonunions: quantitative meta-analysis of the literature. J Hand Surg Am 2002;27A:685–691.
3. Sheetz KK, Bishop AT, Berger RA. The arterial blood supply of the distal radius and ulna and its potential use in vascularized pedicled bone grafts. J Hand Surg Am 1995;20A:902–914.
4. Shin AY, Bishop AT. Pedicled vascularized bone grafts for disorders of the carpus: scaphoid nonunion and Kienbock's disease. J Am Acad Orthop Surg 2002;10:210–216.
5. Steinmann SP, Bishop AT, Berger RA. Use of the 1,2 intercompartmental supraretinacular artery as a vascularized pedicle bone graft for difficult scaphoid nonunion. J Hand Surg Am 2002;27:391–401.
6. Waters PM, Stewart SL. Surgical treatment of nonunion and avascular necrosis of the proximal part of the scaphoid in adolescents. J Bone Joint Surg Am 2002;84A:915–920.
7. Zaidemberg C, Siebert JW, Angrigiani C. A new vascularized bone graft for scaphoid nonunion. J Hand Surg Am 1991;16A:474–478.

Chapter 21

Partial Scaphoid Excision of Scaphoid Nonunions

Joseph E. Imbriglia and Justin M. Sacks

DEFINITION

- The scaphoid is the most frequently fractured bone in the carpus. In acute fractures, appropriate treatment yields union rates greater than 90%.[1] However, without proper diagnosis and treatment scaphoid fractures frequently result in nonunion.
- Initial treatment for a scaphoid nonunion is typically open reduction and internal fixation (ORIF) with bone graft, vascularized or unvascularized.
  - Despite appropriate internal fixation and bone grafting, failure rates of 15% have been documented.[4]
- If internal fixation and bone grafting fails, the surgeon is then left with difficult choices:

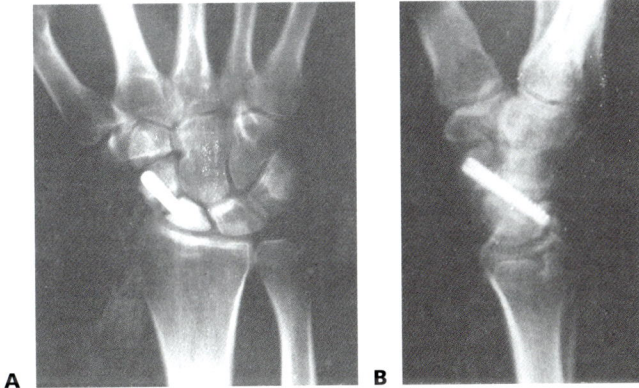

FIG 1 • Failed open reduction and internal fixation of a scaphoid nonunion (PA and lateral views).

- Revision ORIF with bone grafting (failure rate of 50%)[2]
- A salvage procedure with lower morbidity and a higher rate of satisfactory results
- Currently, there are no acceptable prostheses available to replace the scaphoid.
- When the index treatment or procedure has failed and the patient has persistent pain caused by a chronic scaphoid nonunion (**FIG 1**) with posttraumatic arthritis limited to the distal pole of the scaphoid and radius, partial scaphoid excision (distal fragment) provides a reasonable, low-morbidity alternative treatment option.[3–5]

ANATOMY

- The carpus is divided into proximal (scaphoid, lunate, triquetrum, pisiform) and distal (trapezium, trapezoid, capitate, hamate) rows.
- The scaphoid bone represents the bridge between these two rows. Largely covered by articular cartilage, it has important intrinsic and extrinsic ligamentous attachments (radioscaphocapitate, long radiolunate, scapholunate, and scaphotrapezialtrapezoid). In its precarious position as an intercalated rod between the proximal and distal carpal row, the scaphoid is at mechanical risk for fracture when an abnormal stress is applied (eg, forced dorsiflexion).
- After a fracture of the scaphoid, the vascular anatomy specific to this bone contributes to problems in bone healing.[7] Taleisnik and Kelly describe three groups of vessels responsible for scaphoid blood supply: laterovolar, dorsal, and distal vessels (**FIG 2**). The laterovolar vessels are the main contributors to the intraosseous blood supply.

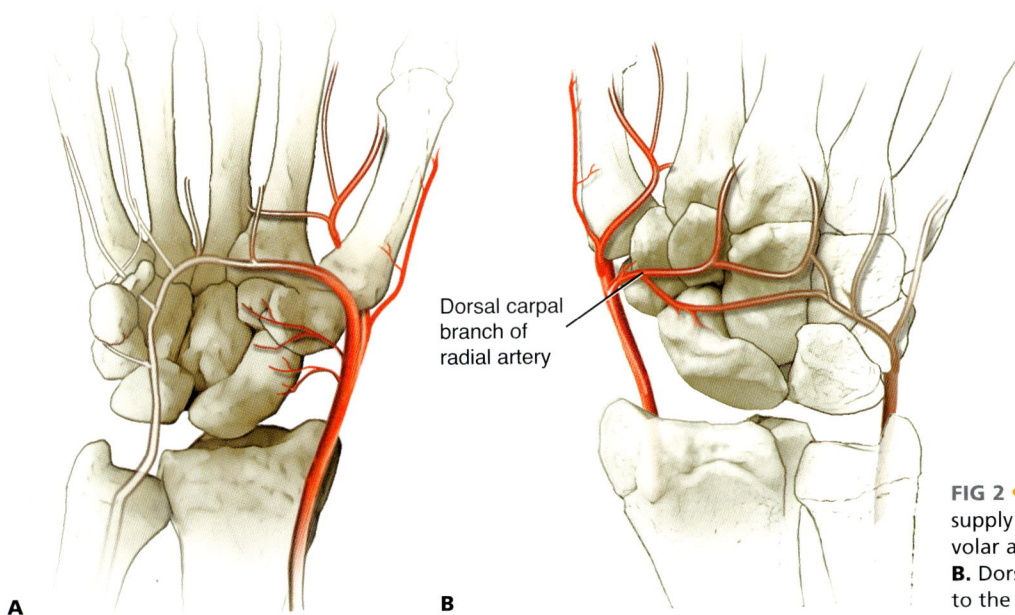

Dorsal carpal branch of radial artery

FIG 2 • **A.** Volar intraosseous blood supply to the scaphoid with laterovolar and distal vessels visualized. **B.** Dorsal intraosseous blood supply to the scaphoid.

- Variations exist in the exact number and locations of the volar vessels entering the scaphoid, but in all studies the most significant vessels enter the scaphoid distal to its waist.
- The proximal pole is at risk secondary to its tenuous blood supply.[7]

PATHOGENESIS

- Based on its retrograde pattern of blood supply, a more proximal fracture of the scaphoid will have an increased potential to form a nonunion.
- Patients with scaphoid fractures who present with delays in both diagnosis and treatment can develop a nonunion. In addition, patients with comminution, displacement, or improper immobilization of the scaphoid fracture can develop nonunions.

NATURAL HISTORY

- A scaphoid nonunion leads to the development of posttraumatic arthritis in the region of the radioscaphoid joint. How quickly this arthritis develops and progresses varies, but most patients will show radiographic evidence of degenerative changes within 5 to 10 years of their nonunion.
- Arthritis first develops between the distal pole of the scaphoid and the radial styloid (scaphoid nonunion advanced collapse [SNAC] wrist stage I; **FIG 3A**).
  - The degenerative changes occur at this location due to the abnormal motion between the ununited distal scaphoid fragment and the radial styloid.
- Left untreated, stage I SNAC will progress to involve the entire radioscaphoid articulation (SNAC stage II) and eventually diffuse arthritis of the wrist (SNAC stages III and IV) (**FIG 3B–D**).

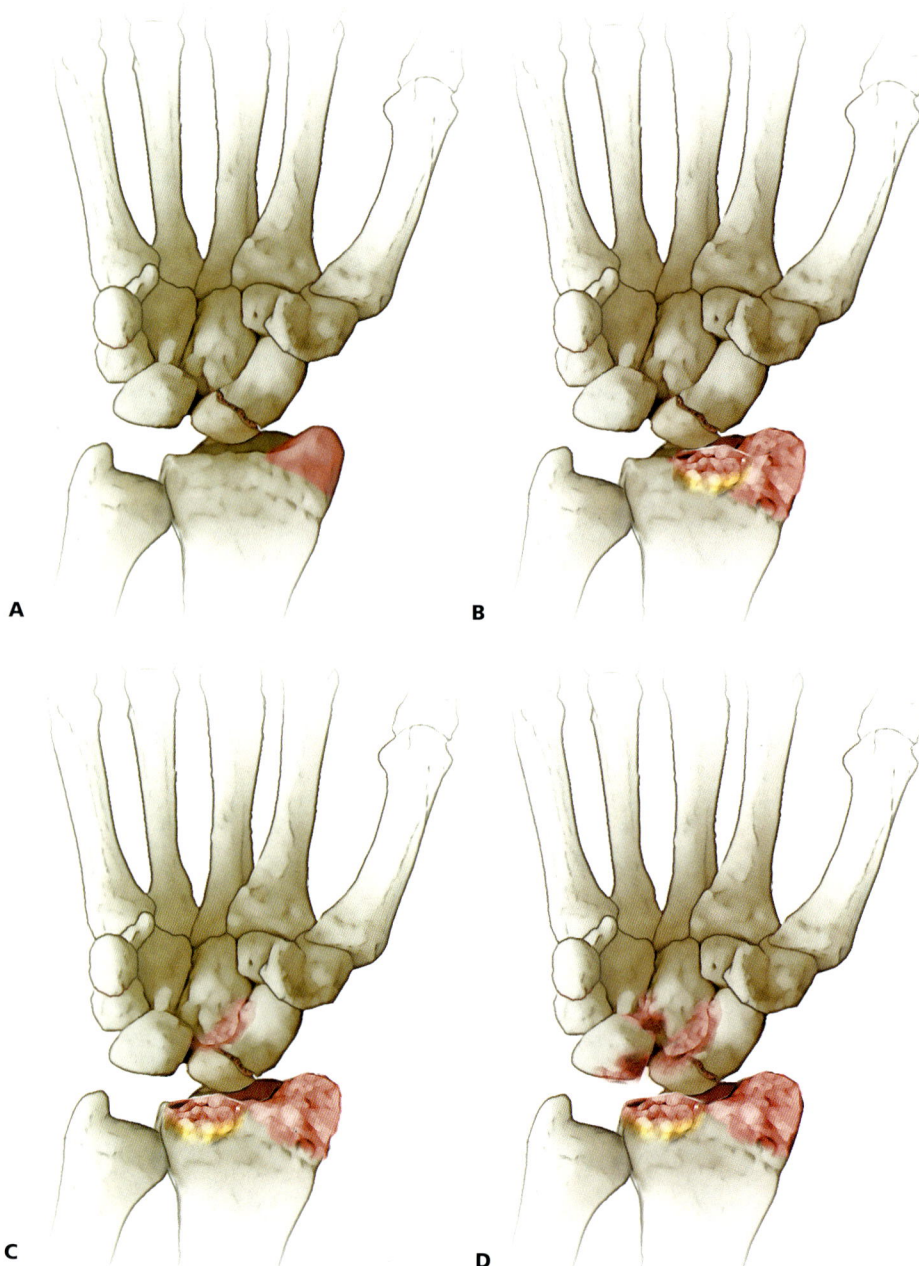

A

B

C

D

FIG 3 • **A.** Arthritis observed between the distal pole of the scaphoid and the radial styloid (scaphoid nonunion advanced collapse [SNAC] grade I). **B–D.** Stage I SNAC can progress to involve the entire radioscaphoid articulation (SNAC grade II) with eventual diffuse arthritis of the wrist (SNAC grade III and IV).

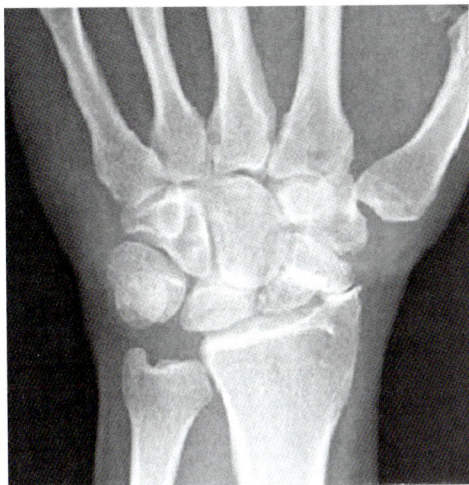

FIG 4 • Chronic nonunion of the scaphoid with scaphoid non-union advanced collapse (SNAC) in a patient with no previous treatment.

■ Patients sometimes do not seek medical care until pain and decreased range of motion in the wrist become increasingly severe. In these cases, initial radiographic studies reveal a scaphoid nonunion and associated arthritis.

PATIENT HISTORY AND PHYSICAL FINDINGS

■ Most patients are young to middle-aged men who sustained a dorsiflexion injury to their involved wrist. Some patients will present with no previous treatment and a chronic nonunion (**FIG 4**), and some will have failed to respond to either operative or nonoperative therapy.
  ■ Pain aggravated by motion and use, loss of motion, and loss of grip strength, all slowly worsening over the preceding years, are consistent presenting complaints.

■ It is critical to know the patient's smoking history, occupation, and previous operations, as these will dictate future interventions.
■ The examiner should palpate the anatomic snuffbox, which lies on the dorsum of the wrist between the extensor pollicis longus and extensor pollicis brevis tendons. Pain in this region is indicative of a fracture.
■ Measurements of grip strength and range of motion (ROM) need to be ascertained.
  ■ Strength is often decreased by as much as 30% to 40% if the patient is experiencing pain.
  ■ There will often be a decrease in extension and radial deviation of the wrist relative to the contralateral unaffected side.
  ■ Limited active ROM of the wrist can indicate carpal pathology.
  ■ Decreased grip strength in association with physical findings can indicate carpal pathology.
■ During palmar flexion the examiner may notice both a fullness and a hard bone excrescence on the dorsal radial aspect of the wrist. This fullness is secondary to synovitis and the hard excrescence is the result of the hypertrophic distal pole of the scaphoid.

IMAGING AND OTHER DIAGNOSTIC STUDIES

■ We routinely order true posteroanterior (PA), lateral, and ulnar and radial deviation views of the wrist. These views assist in determining whether a partial scaphoid excision is indicated.
  ■ The lateral plain radiograph allows one to determine the degree of dorsal intercalated segment instability (DISI) (**FIG 5A**).
  ■ If the radiographs reveal intercarpal arthritis (**FIG 5B**) or a small avascular proximal pole, partial scaphoid excision may be contraindicated.
  ■ If no radioscaphoid arthritis is observed, another procedure (eg, vascularized bone graft) to salvage the scaphoid might be considered.
■ MRI is helpful in evaluating the joint surfaces and the blood supply of the proximal scaphoid fragment.

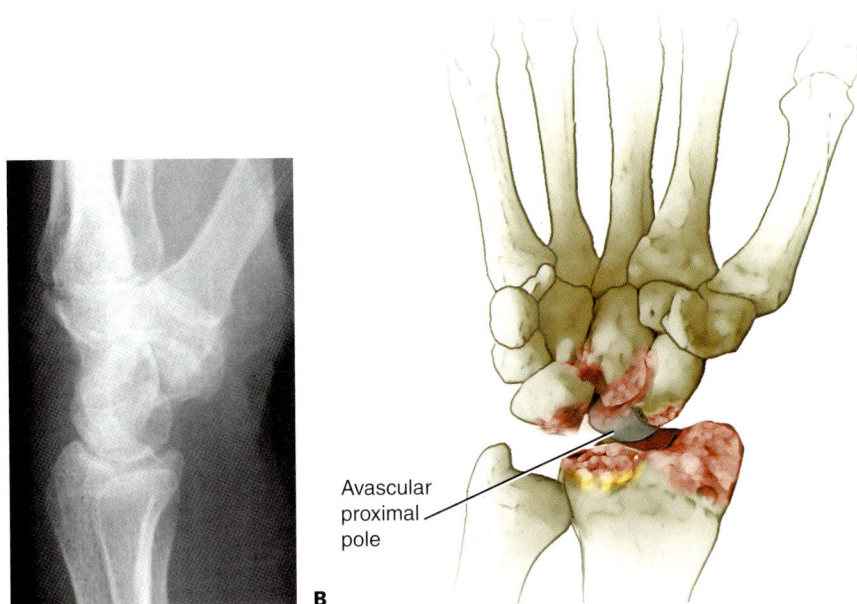

Avascular proximal pole

A   **B**

FIG 5 • **A.** Lateral plain radiograph displaying a dorsal intercalated segment instability (DISI) deformity. **B.** When intercarpal arthritis (SNAC grade III or IV) or an avascular proximal pole are found, partial scaphoid excision may be contraindicated.

■ However, MRIs rarely change the decision to perform a distal pole excision, as plain radiographs most often give adequate and accurate information.

■ From a radiographic perspective, the ideal candidate for distal pole excision of the scaphoid has a nonunion of the scaphoid fracture in the midwaist or distal pole with concomitant degenerative joint disease between the distal radius and distal pole only.

DIFFERENTIAL DIAGNOSIS

■ Scaphoid fracture
■ Scaphoid nonunion
■ Radioscaphoid arthritis
■ Midcarpal arthritis
■ Carpometacarpal arthritis

NONOPERATIVE MANAGEMENT

■ Nonoperative management of chronic wrist pain should be considered before any surgical intervention. Chronic wrist pain is never an emergency and simple noninvasive techniques can be used to control pain.

■ The treatment of any painful joint begins with intermittent immobilization (wrist splinting), activity modification, and nonsteroidal anti-inflammatory medications (NSAIDs).

■ If immobilization and NSAIDs are ineffective, temporary pain relief can almost always be gained with a steroid injection. These temporizing treatments also put the pain in perspective for the patient. The patient may conclude that medication and splinting is all that is necessary.

■ During the nonoperative management period, the surgeon gains a perspective on the degree of patient discomfort and simultaneously gauges the patient's expectations.

   ■ The operation will work better and the patient will be more satisfied if the patient's expectations and surgeon's expectations are similar.

SURGICAL MANAGEMENT

■ Surgical options to treat persistent pain resulting in compromised function in a patient with a scaphoid nonunion and arthritis limited to the area between the distal fragment of the scaphoid and the radial styloid (stage I SNAC wrist arthritis) include:

   ■ Open reduction and internal fixation (ORIF) combined with radial styloidectomy
   ■ Resection of the distal scaphoid fragment

■ A patient with an untreated scaphoid nonunion and no arthritis most often has ORIF of the scaphoid with bone grafting as the initial procedure. In a patient with SNAC wrist grade II, it is too late for distal pole excision; this patient may require a proximal row carpectomy or scaphoid excision with intercarpal fusion.

■ Most patients requiring excision of the distal pole have undergone prior treatment that has failed and both the surgeon and the patient are searching for a reliable procedure with low morbidity to help alleviate the patient's pain and augment function.

■ Distal scaphoid excision requires that the robust and taut radioscaphoid and long radiolunate ligaments exist to support the remaining proximal carpus and prevent collapse (dorsal intercalated segment instability [DISI]) of the wrist.

■ Contraindications to distal pole excision include:
   ■ Pre-existing significant DISI deformity. The DISI deformity may indeed get worse with distal pole excision in an individual with poor ligamentous support.
   ■ Proximal pole that is less than half the entire size of the scaphoid. If the distal fragment is greater than 50% of the size of the scaphoid, resultant collapse of the carpus may occur with severe morbidity.

Preoperative Planning

■ Before deciding if distal pole excision of the scaphoid is a reasonable choice, radiographs or other images (eg, CT or MRI) must be carefully reviewed.

■ If the distal pole is to be excised, there must be enough proximal pole left to support the capitate and the remainder of the carpus. At least one third of the scaphoid must remain. If only a very small (and possibly an avascular) proximal pole remains, the carpus is likely to collapse, resulting in failure of the procedure.

Positioning

■ The patient is placed in the supine position with application of a pneumatic tourniquet.

Approach

■ The distal pole of the scaphoid can be excised through either a dorsal or palmar approach. The approach may be dictated by existing scars.

   ■ The palmar approach is the preferred method due to the relatively accessible palmar position of the distal fragment.
   ■ An advantage of the dorsal approach is the ease of excision of the posterior interosseous nerve for wrist denervation.
   ■ A radial styloidectomy can be performed through either approach.

VOLAR APPROACH TO DISTAL POLE OF SCAPHOID EXCISION

Incision and Scaphoid Excision

■ An incision is made directly over the flexor carpi radialis (FCR) tendon, incorporating any previous incisions (**TECH FIG 1A,B**).

■ The tendon is retracted ulnarly and the subsheath of the tendon incised longitudinally (**TECH FIG 1C**).

■ The radiocarpal joint capsule is opened longitudinally and the distal pole of the scaphoid is excised with osteotomies and rongeurs (**TECH FIG 1D–G**).

Radial Styloidectomy

■ If indicated, a radial styloidectomy can be performed at this point using an osteotome.

■ In this situation, the distal pole may be too large to excise and a radial styloidectomy can accomplish the same purpose.

■ The styloidectomy should be large enough so that the arthritic distal pole no longer touches the radius in radial deviation.

Wound Closure

■ The capsule and volar extrinsic ligaments are closed with interrupted absorbable 4-0 sutures.

■ The skin is closed with interrupted nonabsorbable 4-0 sutures.

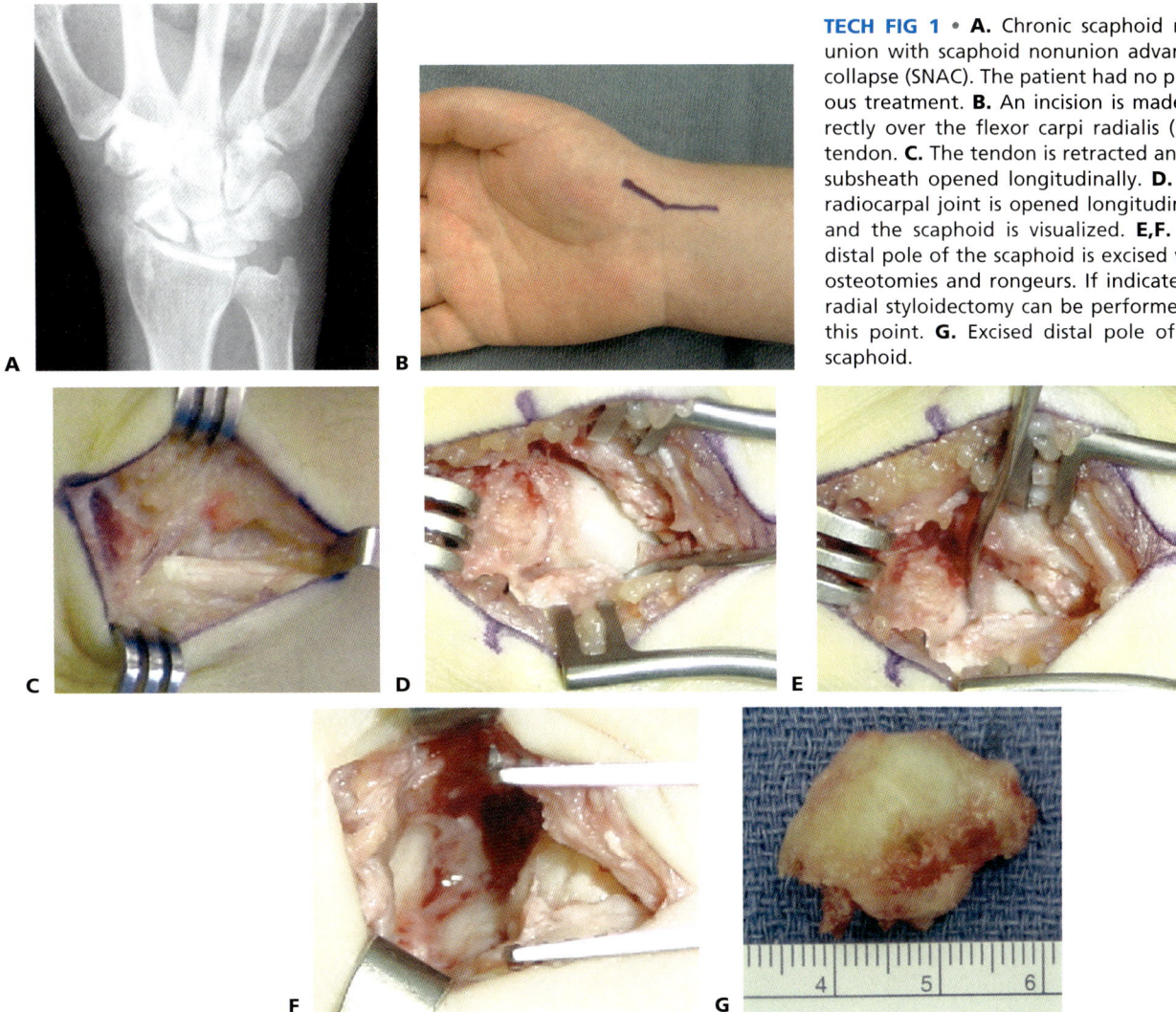

TECH FIG 1 • **A.** Chronic scaphoid nonunion with scaphoid nonunion advanced collapse (SNAC). The patient had no previous treatment. **B.** An incision is made directly over the flexor carpi radialis (FCR) tendon. **C.** The tendon is retracted and its subsheath opened longitudinally. **D.** The radiocarpal joint is opened longitudinally and the scaphoid is visualized. **E,F.** The distal pole of the scaphoid is excised with osteotomies and rongeurs. If indicated, a radial styloidectomy can be performed at this point. **G.** Excised distal pole of the scaphoid.

DORSAL APPROACH TO DISTAL POLE OF SCAPHOID EXCISION

- An incision is made over the radial aspect of the carpus, incorporating any old incisions (**TECH FIG 2**).
- The radial sensory nerve is identified and retracted.

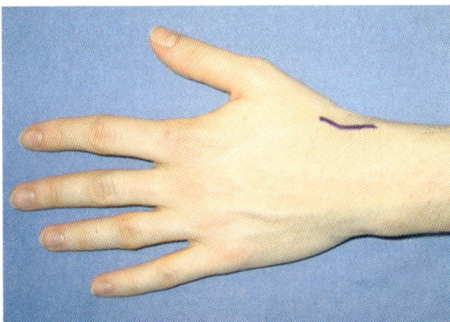

TECH FIG 2 • An incision over the dorsoradial aspect of the wrist may be used when prior surgery has been performed.

- The interval between the extensor pollicis longus and the radial wrist extensors is entered.
- The radial artery and its branches are retracted and protected, and then the joint capsule is incised.
- The distal scaphoid fragment will be deep and is best removed using rongeurs after defining its borders with a no. 15 blade.
- A radial styloidectomy can be performed if necessary as mentioned above.
- The capsule is closed with absorbable 4-0 suture.
- The skin is closed with interrupted nonabsorbable 4-0 sutures.
- The patient is placed in a well-padded forearm-based splint, leaving the finger metacarpophalangeal joints and thumb interphalangeal joint free. This volar splint is placed after either the volar or dorsal approach.

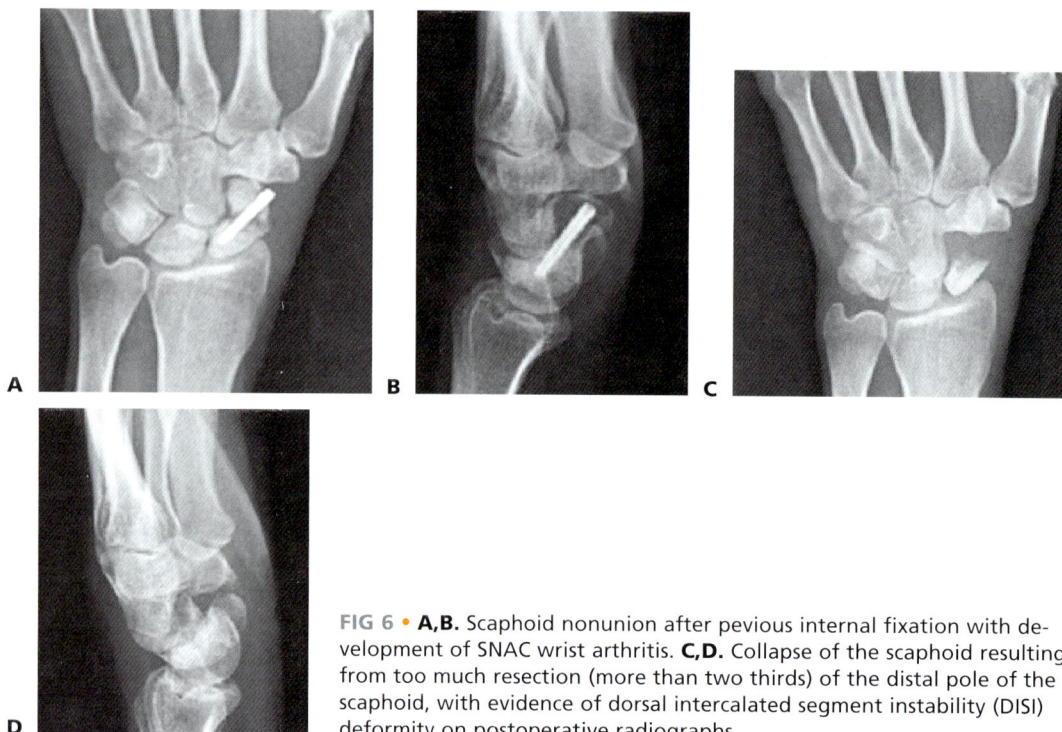

FIG 6 • A,B. Scaphoid nonunion after pevious internal fixation with development of SNAC wrist arthritis. **C,D.** Collapse of the scaphoid resulting from too much resection (more than two thirds) of the distal pole of the scaphoid, with evidence of dorsal intercalated segment instability (DISI) deformity on postoperative radiographs.

PEARLS AND PITFALLS

Indications	▪ It is critical to observe that arthritis does not involve the midcarpal joint.
	▪ There must be enough proximal scaphoid remaining to support the carpus. A third to a half of the remaining proximal pole of the scaphoid should be sufficient to support the capitate and the remaining carpus (**FIG 6**).
Technique	▪ The procedure is simpler to perform through a palmar approach.
	▪ Avoid injury to either the radial sensory nerve or radial artery.
	▪ Interpositional material in the space left by the resected distal pole of the scaphoid is not necessary.

POSTOPERATIVE CARE

▪ Patients are immobilized for 2 weeks in a well-padded volar splint.

▪ The splint and sutures are removed 2 weeks after the procedure.

▪ A removable orthosis is applied and the patient is instructed on active and passive ROM exercises.

▪ Once active and passive ROM has been achieved, strength exercises are started (usually at 4 weeks postoperatively).

▪ Regaining full ROM and strength typically takes about 3 months.

▪ Pain relief is noticeable within 2 to 4 weeks of surgery.

OUTCOMES

▪ Review of outcomes in the literature suggest that both ROM and grip strength improve postoperatively.[3–5]

▪ Pain relief can be expected if the proper indications for surgery are followed.

▪ All patients have some degree of DISI preoperatively, and this pattern of deformity may worsen after excision of the distal pole of the scaphoid. DISI deformities that are severe can result in both loss of motion and pain. This problem is not well documented in the literature but certainly exists.[5]

▪ In the patient undergoing multiple procedures, outcomes of distal pole excision are better than attempting another bone graft and internal fixation, where the failure rate can approach 50%.[1]

COMPLICATIONS

▪ The presence of midcarpal arthritis undiagnosed before distal pole excision can lead to persistent pain.

▪ Resection of too large a distal pole (more than two thirds) can result in collapse of the scaphoid.

▪ If the procedure is performed in a very loose-jointed individual, the DISI pattern may significantly worsen, leading to persistent pain.

REFERENCES

1. Bishop AT. Vascularized bone grafts. In Green DG, Hotchkiss R, Pederson W, eds. Green's Operative Hand Surgery. New York: Churchill Livingstone, 1999.
2. Chang MA, Bishop AT, Moran SL, et al. The outcomes and complications of 1,2 intercompartmental supraretinacular artery pedicled vascularized bone grafting of scaphoid nonunions. J Hand Surg Am 2006;31A:387–396.

3. Drac P, Manak P, Pieranova L. Distal scaphoid resection arthroplasty for scaphoid nonunion with radioscaphoid arthritis. Biomed Pap Med Fac Univ Palacky Olomouc Czech Repub 2006;150: 143–145.

4. Malerich MM, Clifford J, Eaton B, et al. Distal scaphoid resection arthroplasty for the treatment of degenerative arthritis secondary to scaphoid nonunion. J Hand Surg Am 1999;24A: 1196–1205.

5. Ruch DS, Papadonikolakis A. Resection of the scaphoid distal pole for symptomatic scaphoid nonunion after failed previous surgical treatment. J Hand Surg Am 2006;31A:588–593.

6. Smith BS, Cooney WP. Revision of failed bone grafting for nonunion of the scaphoid: treatment options and results. Clin Orthop Relat Res 1996;327:98–109.

7. Taleisnik J, Kelly PJ. The extraosseous and intraosseous blood supply of the scaphoid bone. J Bone Joint Surg Am 1966;48A:1125.

Chapter 22

Surgical Treatment of Carpal Bone Fractures, Excluding the Scaphoid

Kenneth R. Means, Jr. and Thomas J. Graham

DEFINITION

- These injuries include fractures of the lunate, triquetrum, pisiform, hamate body or hook, capitate, trapezoid, and trapezial body or ridge.
- Any fracture involving the carpal bones should raise suspicion of associated carpal instability.

ANATOMY

- Certain anatomic features of the carpal bones make them more susceptible to injury. These include the unique osteologic regions of some of the carpal bones, such as the hook of the hamate, the ridge or tubercle of the trapezium, and the neck of the capitate.
- The slender shape and projection of the hamate hook make it an obvious injury target for direct trauma to the palmar-ulnar surface of the wrist (**FIG 1A**). The hook can be identified before incision by placing the interphalangeal joint of the surgeon's thumb on the pisiform and flexing the thumb toward the first web space. The surgeon's thumb tip will land directly on top of the hook.
- The trapezial ridge may be considered a radial-sided analogue to the hamate hook in that it is a relatively prominent volar projection, further accentuated by the deep groove for the flexor carpi radialis tendon that runs along its ulnar side (**FIG 1B**).
- The strong, inelastic transverse carpal ligament attaches to the hamate hook ulnarly and the trapezial tubercle radially.
- These facts make the ridge of the trapezium more susceptible to fracture after direct trauma to the thenar region of the hand.
- The constricted neck portion of the capitate lies between the dense head proximally and the body distally. The body, which accounts for the distal half of the capitate, is rigidly constrained

by its associations with the index, middle, and ring finger metacarpal bases, the trapezoid, and the hamate. As a result the capitate neck is a biomechanically vulnerable area.

- Transverse plane fractures through the capitate neck are reported as being the most common.
- Fractures across the neck place the head at risk for avascular necrosis because the blood supply to the capitate flows retrograde toward the head proximally.

PATHOGENESIS

- Traumatic fractures of the carpal bones may occur via direct or indirect mechanisms.
- Direct mechanisms include crush injuries, which should alert the physician to the possible development of compartment syndrome of the hand. Compressive trauma to the hand in the anteroposterior plane will flatten the palmarly directed concave longitudinal and horizontal arches of the carpus and should raise suspicion for potential carpal body fractures and axial disruptions.
  - The presence of a seemingly unusual carpal bone fracture may be a herald of a globally destructive injury to the hand and other associated injuries, such as carpometacarpal (CMC) fracture-dislocations, longitudinal fractures of the metacarpals, severe thumb damage, and significant soft tissue injuries. This constellation of pathologies has been referred to as the "exploded hand" (**FIG 2**).
- More focused direct trauma to individual carpal bones may also cause a fracture. Examples of this include direct blows to the dorsum of the hand, causing capitate fractures, or direct injury from a racquet or club, causing a hamate hook fracture.

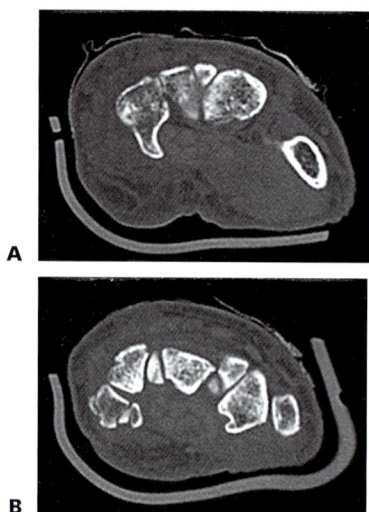

FIG 1 • A. CT scan showing hamate hook. **B.** CT scan showing trapezial ridge.

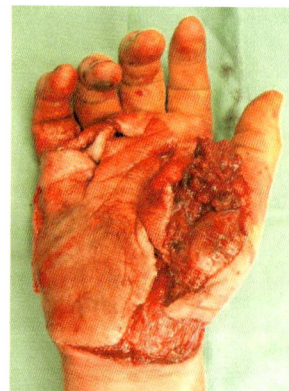

FIG 2 • "Exploded hand" is a constellation of injuries that can include carpometacarpal fracture-dislocations, longitudinal fractures of the metacarpals, severe thumb damage, and significant soft tissue damage. (Reprinted from Graham TJ. The exploded hand syndrome: logical evaluation and comprehensive treatment of the severely crushed hand. J Hand Surg Am 2006;31A: 1012–1023; copyright 2006, with permission from Elsevier.)

- Indirect trauma includes the progressive perilunate instability patterns that are well described and may lead to fractures of the lunate, capitate, triquetrum, or other carpal bones.
  - Scaphocapitate syndrome involves a dorsiflexion and radial deviation mechanism by which the scaphoid bone fractures and is followed by a fracture of the capitate through the neck in the coronal plane. The capitate head may rotate up to 180 degrees from its anatomic position.
  - A progressive perilunate instability pattern can produce a similar coronal fracture through the capitate neck but normally without such a severe degree of capitate head rotation.
- More minor indirect trauma mechanisms can cause isolated carpal bone fractures.
  - The commonly seen avulsion fractures from the dorsum of the triquetrum may occur when a fall onto the palmar-flexed wrist causes the dorsal radiotriquetral (also known as dorsal radiocarpal) ligament to avulse a portion of the dorsal cortex.
  - An impaction type of fracture of the triquetrum may be seen more often in patients with an elongated ulnar styloid.

NATURAL HISTORY

- The natural history of carpal bone fractures depends both on the specific bone in question as well as associated impairment of other structures.
- All of the carpal bones have at least three articular surfaces, except the pisiform, which articulates only with the triquetrum. Anatomic reduction of articular facets is a primary surgical goal in an effort to decrease the incidence and severity of post-traumatic arthritis.
- Avascular necrosis can have a profoundly negative impact on final outcome after carpal bone fracture.
  - Concerns of vascular disruption arise when lunate and capitate fractures occur, although generally fractures of the lunate are not associated with avascularity.
- The potential for nonunion is most often seen with hamate hook fractures, capitate neck fractures, and trapezial ridge fractures, especially Palmer type II fractures that involve the tip and not the base of the ridge.
- Barring nonunion, the related instabilities and involvement of other hand components are the most troublesome and will most significantly affect patient outcome.

PATIENT HISTORY AND PHYSICAL FINDINGS

- Ascertaining the mechanism of injury is the most important component of the patient history.
- Neurovascular symptoms should be explored, especially when a severe crush or high-energy mechanism is involved, or in cases of hamate hook or pisiform fractures, with special attention to the ulnar neurovascular structures within the canal of Guyon.
  - A complete evaluation of the median, radial, ulnar, and digital nerves is warranted. Assessment of capillary refill, color, temperature, and Doppler signal determines the vascular status.
- The examiner should observe the patient's hand and wrist for swelling, deformity, and skin and soft tissue injuries, including possible open fractures or fracture-dislocations.
  - Swelling and soft tissue damage give an indication as to the severity of the injury. The presence of deformity alerts the examiner to possible carpal dislocations that require emergent reduction. Open fractures and fracture-dislocations will guide surgical management.

- The examiner should ask the patient where the pain is most significant. The examination should start away from and progress toward this point. The hand, forearm, and elbow should also be palpated to assess for possible associated injuries.
  - The most obvious area of pain and tenderness is usually the most structurally significant. However, it may mask other more subtle injuries that should be detected by a more thorough global examination.

IMAGING AND OTHER DIAGNOSTIC STUDIES

- Routine AP, lateral, and oblique views of the wrist and hand are obtained (**FIG 3A**).
  - Radiographs of the elbow and forearm are ordered if indicated.
- Fluoroscopic images, including dynamic stress and distraction views, help to rule out carpal instability.
- Special views, often best performed with fluoroscopy, help to profile difficult-to-see structures.
  - The hook of the hamate is evaluated with the carpal tunnel view and supinated and oblique lateral view with the wrist in radial deviation and the thumb abducted, as if the patient was holding a cup (referred to as the papillon view) (**FIG 3B**).
  - The trapezial ridge is visualized on the carpal tunnel view (**FIG 3C**).
  - The pisotriquetral joint is best seen on a 45-degree supinated lateral view of the wrist.
- CT scans effectively assess osseous detail and will often detect more subtle associated carpal fractures that may be missed on routine radiographs.
  - CT is considered the imaging modality of choice for confirming a hamate hook fracture if plain films are non-diagnostic.

NONOPERATIVE MANAGEMENT

- Isolated carpal bone fractures without associated carpal instability, significant displacement, or intra-articular stepoff may be managed nonoperatively.
  - This usually includes use of a cast or brace for several weeks (usually 4 to 6 weeks) until symptoms have improved, tenderness is resolving, and radiographs are stable.
  - Short-arm thumb spica casts or splints have been recommended for isolated trapezium and capitate fractures. The digits should be left free.
- A specific fracture of note is the hamate hook.
  - These fractures can be treated with cast immobilization if nondisplaced and acute (less than 1 month).
  - There is a relatively high rate of symptomatic nonunion, and surgical intervention may eventually be necessary.
- Similar to the treatment of the hamate hook, trapezial ridge fractures may be initially immobilized and later excised if symptomatic nonunion develops.

SURGICAL MANAGEMENT

Indications

- Indications for surgical management of these fractures include those that significantly involve an articular surface or are structurally destabilizing to the remainder of the carpus, such as a displaced or unstable capitate body fracture.
  - Other operative indications include those that are true for most fractures, such as open injuries and those requiring nerve, vessel, tendon, ligament, or soft tissue repair.

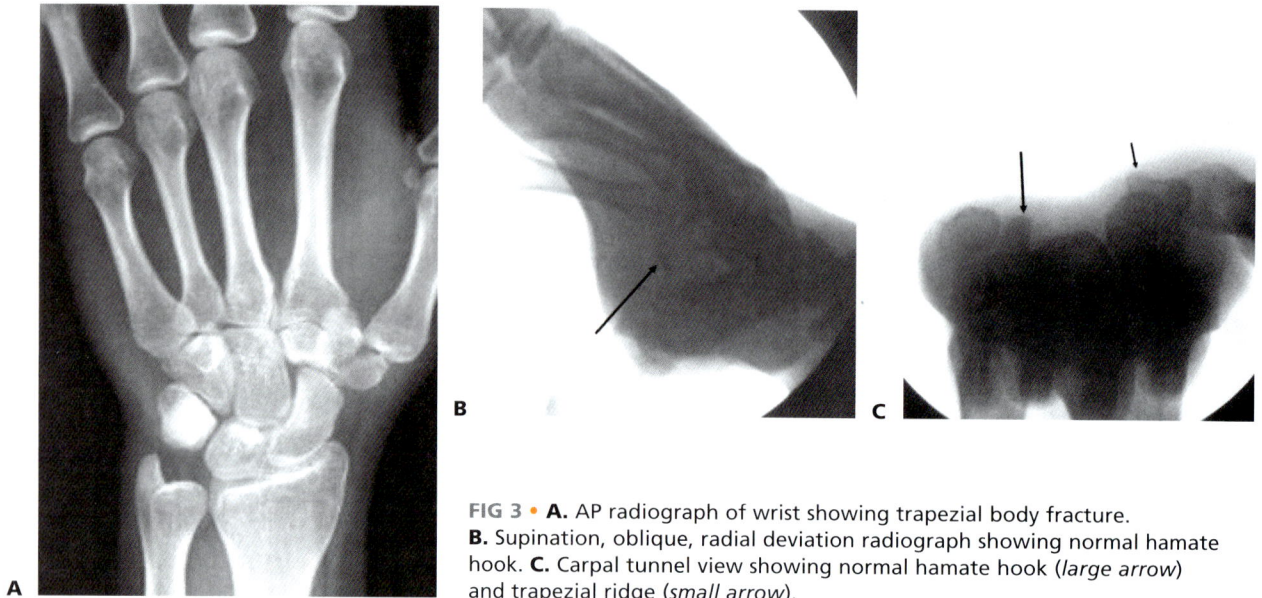

FIG 3 • **A.** AP radiograph of wrist showing trapezial body fracture. **B.** Supination, oblique, radial deviation radiograph showing normal hamate hook. **C.** Carpal tunnel view showing normal hamate hook (*large arrow*) and trapezial ridge (*small arrow*).

▪ If stable and near-anatomic reduction of carpal fractures is not possible, primary limited arthrodesis or carpectomy may be indicated.

▪ Because of the unique nature of each carpal bone, more specific indications will be considered for each fracture.

▪ Late reconstructive options include partial or total wrist arthrodesis or proximal row carpectomy for symptomatic arthritic changes.

　▪ Trapezial excision with thumb metacarpal suspension-plasty may be used for posttraumatic arthritis after trapezial body fractures.

　▪ Total or hemi-wrist arthroplasty for select cases may become a more popular option as techniques improve.

Lunate Fractures

▪ In general, fractures that are of sufficient size and displacement should be reduced and internally fixed.

▪ Fractures that involve the palmar surface of the lunate where stout volar extrinsic wrist ligaments (long and short radiolunate) and vascular conduits (radioscapholunate ligament of Testut) attach should be stabilized.

▪ If the capitate is subluxated volarly relative to the lunate and radius, such as when there is a lunate palmar lip fracture, this must be corrected with reduction and fixation of the lunate palmar fragment.

　▪ These fractures are routinely approached palmarly as described in Techniques.

　▪ Alternatively, a standard 3–4 interval dorsal exposure (described under capitate fractures) can be used if the fracture pattern dictates a dorsal approach and fixation.

Triquetral Fractures

▪ In general, displaced fractures of the triquetral body that are of sufficient size are best treated by open reduction and internal fixation (ORIF).

　▪ This can be accomplished through use of pins or screws into the triquetrum alone or in combination with pinning to the lunate or to the hamate as dictated by the fracture.

▪ The triquetrum may be removed in its entirety if it is not amenable to repair.

▪ An apparently isolated fracture of the triquetrum may in fact be part of a reverse perilunate instability pattern (in which the portal of energy entry is at the ulnar wrist) and may be associated with other fractures and ligament disruptions.

Pisiform Fractures

▪ The pisiform, similar to another sesamoid bone, the patella, most often fractures in a transverse pattern via an indirect avulsion mechanism through the flexor carpi ulnaris (FCU) or in a pattern of comminution from a direct blow.

▪ Virtually all pisiform fractures are treated nonoperatively initially and then excised late if immobilization of the fracture fails to relieve symptoms after 2 or 3 months.

　▪ Fractures that are of sufficient size and displacement can be reduced and internally fixed, although this is rarely indicated.

　▪ The approach described in Techniques can be used for fixation or excision of the pisiform.

▪ The pisiform is the last carpal bone to ossify, usually by age 12, and may have a nonpathologic fragmented appearance before complete ossification.

Hook of Hamate Fractures

▪ Like pisiform fractures, most acute hamate fractures are treated nonoperatively initially. If the fracture remains persistently symptomatic or nonunited, excision is indicated, even for base fractures (**FIG 4A**).

▪ ORIF is associated with relatively high complication rates and provides little or no advantage over simple fragment excision.

　▪ If ORIF is desired, the hamulus is exposed as described in Techniques and standard internal screw fixation principles are used.

Hamate Body Fractures

▪ Fractures of the hamate body are often associated with fourth or fifth CMC dislocations (**FIG 4B,C**). ORIF is recommended to reduce the articular surfaces and stabilize the CMC joints.

▪ These injuries most often result from a dorsal shear mechanism with fracture of the hamate body in the frontal plane. The metacarpals displace dorsally and proximally with the dorsal hamate fracture fragment.

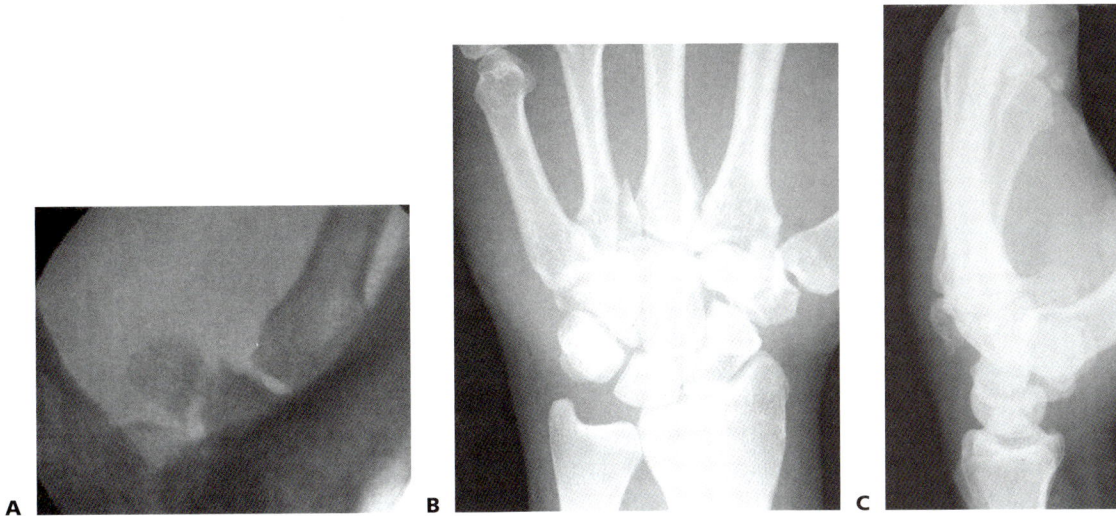

FIG 4 • Hamate fractures. **A.** Supination, oblique, radial deviation radiograph showing hamate hook fracture. **B,C.** AP and lateral radiographs of a hamate body dorsal shear fracture associated with the small finger and ring finger carpometacarpal articulation as well as a fracture of the base of the ring finger metacarpal.

Capitate Fractures

- Capitate fractures are by and large associated with significant trauma to the wrist.
  - In addition to fractures associated with progressive perilunate instability patterns and the scaphocapitate syndrome, capitate fractures may also occur due to axial loading along the middle finger ray or via direct trauma.
  - If caused by axially directed forces, the fracture line is often in the frontal plane, similar to the hamate dorsal shear fractures described earlier. The capitate may be essentially divided in half in this frontal plane.
  - In these cases, ORIF is performed through a dorsal approach.
- Truly isolated capitate fractures with minimal displacement heal by immobilization, but this often takes time.

Trapezoid Fractures

- The trapezoid is believed to be the least frequently fractured carpal bone.
- As with the other bones of the distal carpal row, assessment of the associated index CMC joint is necessary to rule out a fracture-dislocation.
  - Frontal plane dorsal shear fractures of the trapezoid can destabilize the index CMC.
- These fractures and fracture-dislocations can often be treated by closed reduction and pinning.
- If an open approach is required to reduce the articular surface and CMC joint, a standard 3–4 dorsal approach may be used. Fixation can be accomplished with pins or screws.
  - A limited exposure (as described below) is an alternative.

Trapezium Fractures

- Fractures of the body of the trapezium nearly always involve one of its four articular facets and frequently lead to subluxation of the thumb CMC joint (**FIG 5**).
- If internal fixation is not possible, trapezial excision and palmar oblique ligament reconstruction, or an alternative procedure used for routine thumb CMC osteoarthritis, is performed.

Preoperative Planning

- Examination under anesthesia, possibly with concomitant fluoroscopic imaging, helps confirm whether carpal instability coexists.
- The surgeon should ensure that all needed fixation implants and systems are available before bringing the patient to the operating room.
- A hand table, a well-padded upper arm tourniquet, and a mobile mini-fluoroscopy unit are used.
- Anesthesia and analgesia may be obtained through regional or general methods.

Approach

- Carpal fractures may be approached dorsally, palmarly, radially, or ulnarly depending on the reduction needs, implants used, and fracture location and characteristics.
- Some surgeons use wrist or small joint arthroscopy as an aid to fracture reduction and management.

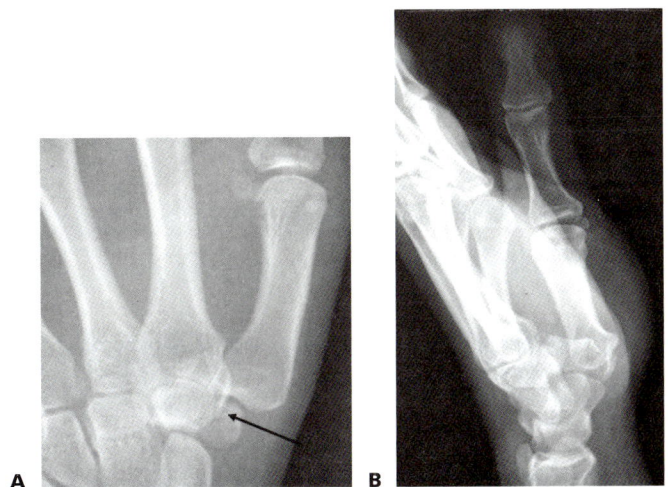

FIG 5 • Trapezial body fractures.

ORIF OF LUNATE FRACTURES

Incision and Dissection

- An extended carpal tunnel approach is used for palmar exposure.
- The incision begins in the palm, just ulnar to the thenar crease and in line with the radial border of the ring finger. If the surgeon is comfortable with the deep anatomy, especially the possible anatomic variations involving the thenar motor branch, the incision in the palm may also be along the thenar crease itself.
- It is extended proximally until the distal volar wrist crease is reached.
- A curved or zigzag continuation of the incision is made at the crease so as to avoid crossing perpendicular to the wrist crease, which might cause excessive scarring and a flexion contracture.
- The incision may be continued into the distal forearm, staying ulnar to the palmaris longus so as to avoid damage to the palmar cutaneous branch of the median nerve (**TECH FIG 1A**).
- It is deepened distally until the palmar fascia is encountered (**TECH FIG 1B**). This fascia is incised in line with the skin incision.

- The transverse carpal ligament is opened longitudinally, just radial to the hamate hook.
- The incision is continued proximally, releasing the distal volar forearm fascia, again staying ulnar to the palmaris longus.
  - The contents of the carpal canal are now visualized (**TECH FIG 1C**).
- The digital flexors and median nerve are gently and bluntly retracted radially, revealing the floor of the canal that overlies the volar carpus (**TECH FIG 1D**).
- The volar capsule of the wrist joint is incised longitudinally, providing exposure of the volar carpus and radiocarpal joint.

Reduction and Fixation

- The palmar lip fracture of the lunate is identified, cleaned, and anatomically reduced.
- The fracture may be fixed with small interfragment screws or buried Kirschner wires (**TECH FIG 2**).
  - Screws are favored if at all possible to minimize chances of hardware migration into the carpal tunnel.

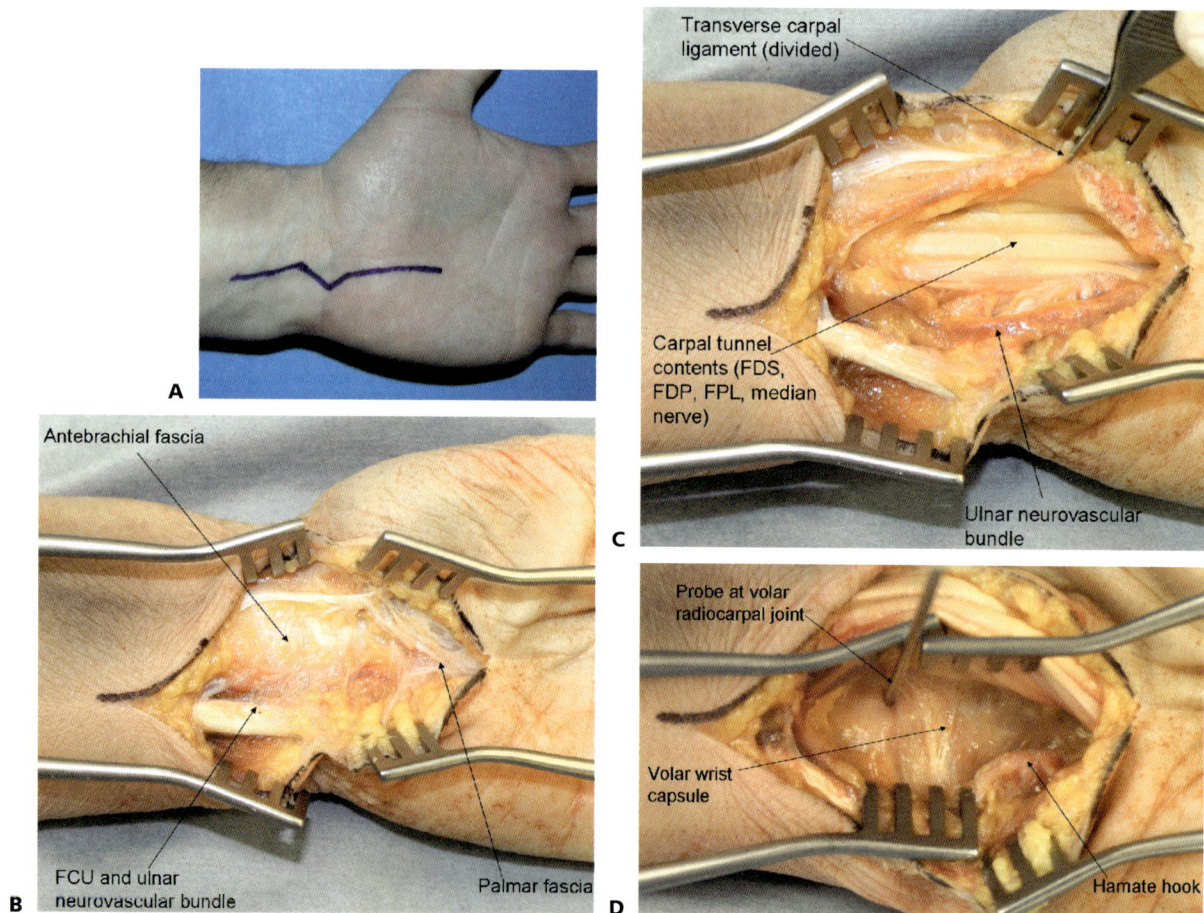

TECH FIG 1 • Fixation of lunate palmar lip fractures. **A.** Carpal tunnel approach. The incision can be continued into the distal forearm, staying ulnar to the palmaris longus to avoid damage to the palmar cutaneous branch of the median nerve. **B.** Palmar fascia and antebrachial fascia exposed. **C.** Transverse carpal ligament released from hamate hook. **D.** Volar wrist capsule exposed.

TECHNIQUES

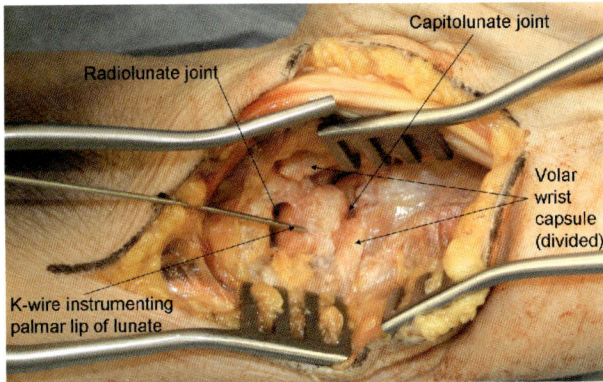

TECH FIG 2 • Palmar lunate lip exposed and instrumented.

- Fluoroscopic images are necessary to confirm that the volar carpal subluxation has been corrected with fixation of the lunate fracture.
- The volar wrist capsule is repaired with permanent suture and the median nerve and digital flexors are allowed to return to their normal resting position.
- The transverse carpal ligament may be repaired in a lengthened fashion or left divided (our preference).
- Subcutaneous tissue and skin closure is performed according to the surgeon's routine.

ORIF OF TRIQUETRAL FRACTURES

- Access to the triquetrum is usually achieved through the standard dorsal approach to the wrist that is described for capitate fractures.
- If there is truly isolated triquetral pathology, a more limited dorsal approach between the fifth and sixth extensor compartments is used.
  - This incision is centered distal to that which would be used for distal radioulnar joint (DRUJ) exposure.
- The fifth compartment (extensor digiti minimi [EDM]) is retracted radially while the sixth compartment (extensor carpi ulnaris [ECU]) is retracted ulnarly.

- The carpal capsule is incised longitudinally or obliquely depending on the fracture and the integrity of the dorsal radiotriquetral ligament.
- The triquetral fracture may now be cleaned, reduced, and fixed with mini-screws or Kirschner wires as the fracture pattern prescribes.
- Supplemental pinning to the lunate or hamate is performed as needed.
- The capsule is closed with nonabsorbable suture, followed by routine subcutaneous tissue and skin closure.

EXCISION OR ORIF OF PISIFORM FRACTURES

- A curvilinear incision is made with special care not to cross the distal volar wrist crease perpendicularly. The incision is made centered on or just radial to the pisiform.
- The ulnar neurovascular bundle is identified proximally and traced distally just past the pisiform body.
- The pisohamate ligament is divided.
- The flexor carpi ulnaris (FCU) tendon insertion, if intact, is divided longitudinally and subperiosteally elevated from the radial and ulnar margins of the pisiform.

- At this point the pisiform can be excised or internally fixed with mini-fragment screws or Kirschner wires.
  - The risk for hardware migration, penetration into the pisotriquetral joint, and other complications in the region of the ulnar neurovascular bundle must be weighed against the good results expected with simple excision.
- The split FCU is closed with a nonabsorbable suture and the subcutaneous tissue and skin are sutured in routine fashion.

HOOK OF HAMATE EXCISION

- The hook can be identified before incision by placing the interphalangeal joint of the surgeon's thumb on the pisiform and flexing the thumb toward the first web space. The surgeon's thumb tip will land directly on top of the hook.
- The hamate hook can be approached through a volar incision (preferred) or directly ulnar, proceeding palmar to the small finger metacarpal and dorsal to the abductor digiti minimi.
- A longitudinal or curvilinear skin incision is made, centered over the hook (**TECH FIG 3A**).
- The ulnar nerve and artery are identified proximally first and then traced distally, ulnar and superficial to the hamate hook (**TECH FIG 3B–D**).

- Once the level of the hook is reached distally, the ulnar neurovascular bundle is gently retracted ulnarly.
- Soft tissue attachments to the tip of the hook are incised longitudinally, including the transverse carpal ligament radially and the pisohamate ligament ulnarly and proximally.
- The deep motor branch of the ulnar nerve should be identified as it passes distally around the base of the hamate hook in an ulnar-to-radial direction and must be protected during excision (**TECH FIG 3E**).
- The digital flexors within the carpal canal are identified. The ring and small finger flexors, especially the profundus tendons, are inspected to ensure integrity and should be débrided or repaired as needed (**TECH FIG 3F**).
  - The tendons are then gently retracted radially.

TECHNIQUES

Transverse carpal ligament
Hook of hamate
Pisohamate ligament (cut)
Pisiform
Palmar carpal ligament (cut)

Ulnar nerve
Ulnar artery

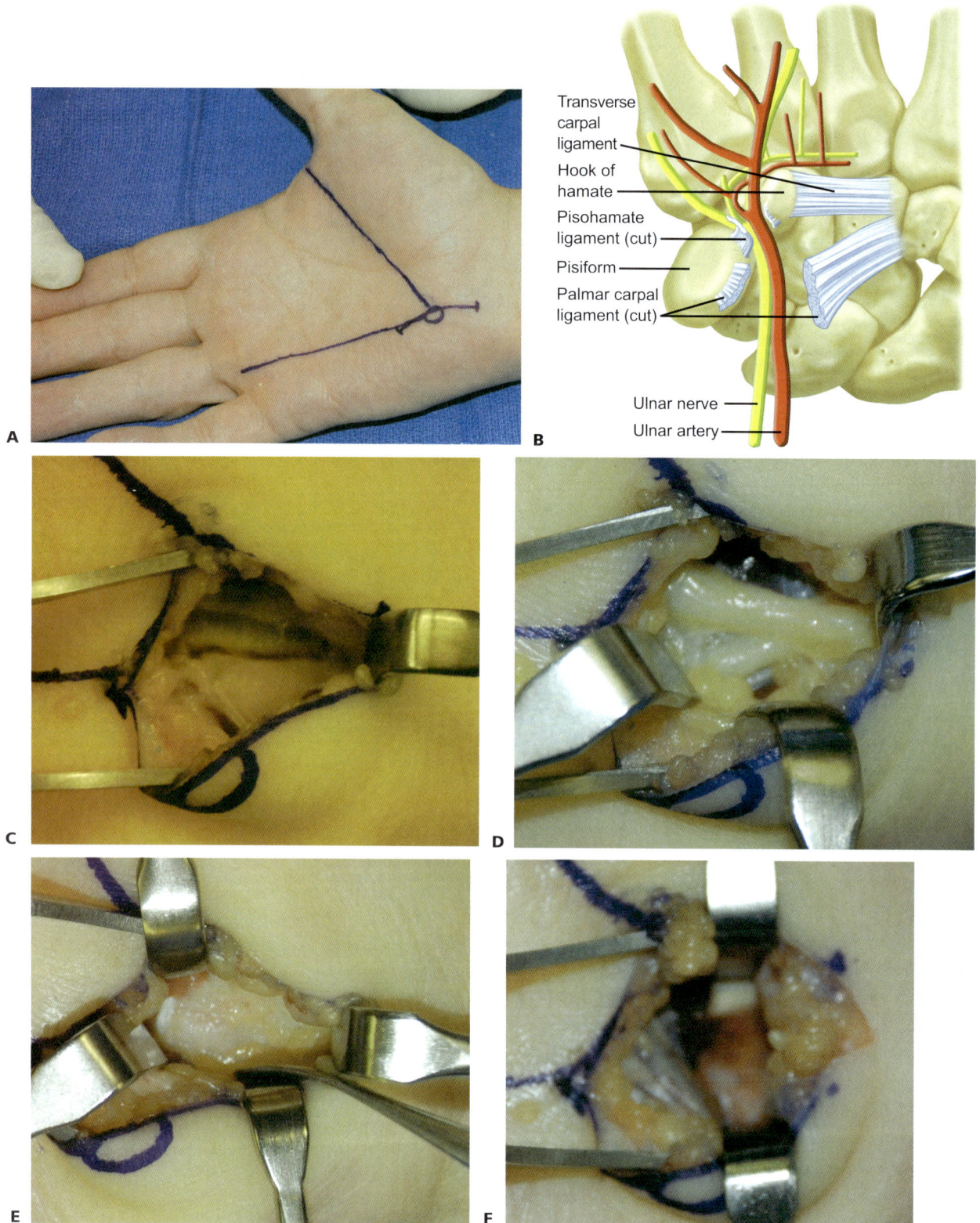

TECH FIG 3 • Excision of hamate hook fractures. **A.** The cardinal line of Kaplan, drawn from the apex of the first web space to the ulnar border of the hand, intersects a second line drawn along the ulnar margin of the ring digit at the hamate hook (*circle*). A 3-cm incision is centered over the hamate hook, gently curving with the radial border of the hypothenar eminence. **B.** The ulnar nerve and artery can be found proximally first and then traced distally, ulnar and superficial to the hamate hook. **C.** The ulnar artery is encountered first, volar and radial to the ulnar nerve. **D.** With the artery retracted ulnarly, the common digital nerve to the fourth web space and the small digit ulnar sensory nerve are visualized. The deep motor branch and the hypothenar motor branch have already been given off. **E.** The hamate hook is subperiosteally exposed and its margins are palpated with an elevator. The deep motor branch curves radially, closely associated with the distal surface of the hook. **F.** Care is also taken to protect the flexor tendons during exposure and resection, seen here on the radial margin of the hook.

- The hook is cleared of all soft tissue attachments down to the level of the fracture site.
  - A no. 69 Beaver blade helps make this exposure precise.
- Using a rongeur or similar tool, the fractured hook is removed piecemeal, again with care to protect the deep ulnar motor branch and other structures.

- Once the fragment is removed, the remaining base is inspected and smoothed with a rongeur, curette, or similar tool until there are no sharp bony prominences.
- The surrounding periosteum is closed if possible.
- Subcutaneous tissue and skin closure is performed in a routine manner.

HAMATE BODY FRACTURES

- A dorsal longitudinal or curvilinear incision is made centered over the ring or small finger CMC joints (**TECH FIG 4A**).
- The ring and small finger extensor tendons are retracted radially or ulnarly together or individually as needed.
  - There can be significant variation in the anatomic appearance and interconnections of the extensor digitorum communis tendons to the ring and small fingers as well as the EDM (**TECH FIG 4B**). These variations usually dictate which direction to retract the tendons and whether to retract them together or individually to give the best access to the CMC joints.
- The CMC joint capsule and dorsal CMC ligaments are incised longitudinally. The CMC joint is cleared of any hematoma and bone fragments (**TECH FIG 4C**).
- The fracture site is cleared of hematoma and reduced while directly visualizing the distal articular surface.
  - A dental pick is useful to reduce small fragments.
- The fracture is temporarily stabilized with Kirschner wires and fluoroscopic images are taken to confirm reduction (**TECH FIG 4D,E**).

- If there is a large dorsal fragment, two or more dorsal-to-volar lag screws (usually 2.0-mm screws or smaller) are placed perpendicular to the fracture line into the hamate body (**TECH FIG 4F,G**).
- If there are several small fragments, individual screws may be used for each piece, or a dorsal plate may be more effective (**TECH FIG 4H**).
- Fluoroscopic images are necessary to confirm that the screws do not protrude outside of the hamate hook, potentially damaging ulnar neurovascular structures or flexor tendons.
- The dorsal capsuloligamentous sleeve is closed if possible, thus providing a smooth gliding surface between the extensor tendons and the CMC joint and hardware.
- The CMC joints may be pinned temporarily if still unstable.
  - In the acute setting, if the dorsal hamate fracture is of sufficient size and securely stabilized and the joint capsule is closed, this is usually not necessary.
- Soft tissues and skin are closed in a routine manner.

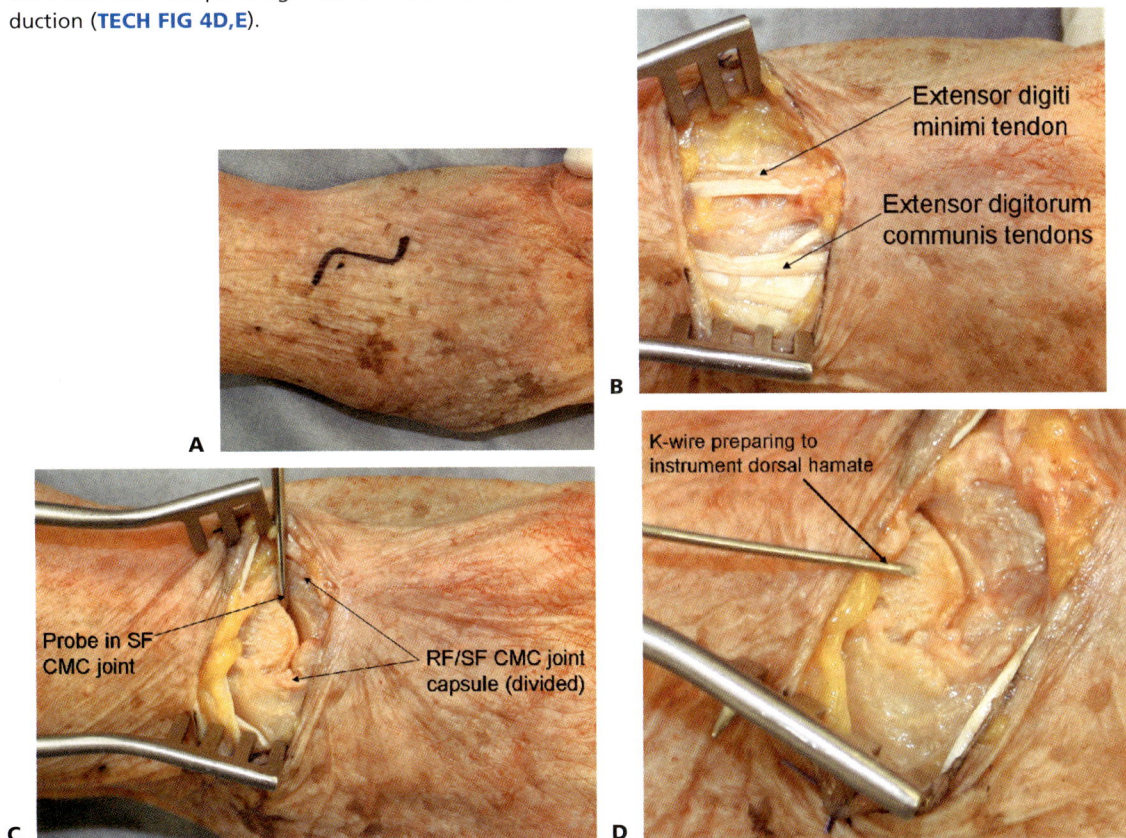

Extensor digiti minimi tendon

Extensor digitorum communis tendons

Probe in SF CMC joint

RF/SF CMC joint capsule (divided)

K-wire preparing to instrument dorsal hamate

TECH FIG 4 • Fixation of hamate dorsal shear fractures. **A.** Dorsal curvilinear incision centered on ring finger–small finger carpometacarpal joint. **B.** Extensor tendons exposed. **C.** Ring finger–small finger carpometacarpal joint exposed. **D.** Dorsal hamate reduced and instrumented. *(continued)*

TECHNIQUES

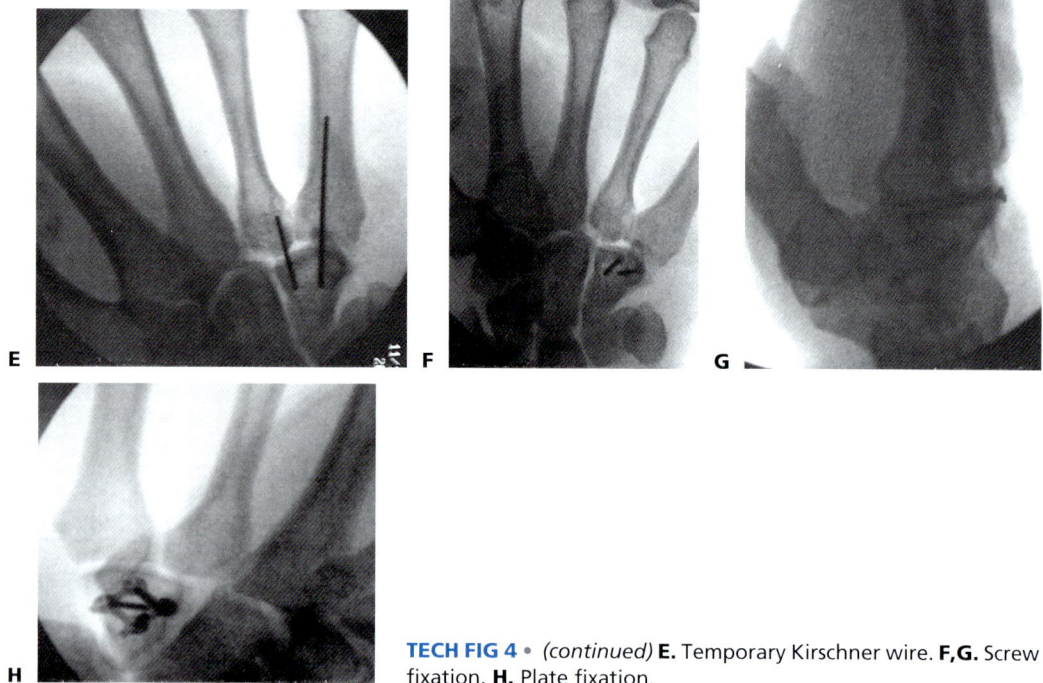

TECH FIG 4 • *(continued)* **E.** Temporary Kirschner wire. **F,G.** Screw fixation. **H.** Plate fixation.

CAPITATE FRACTURES

- Often a standard approach to the dorsal carpus is required and is carried out through the routine 3–4 extensor compartment interval.
- A dorsal midline longitudinal or curvilinear skin incision is made, in line with the middle finger ray and centered on the capitate.
- Full-thickness skin flaps are elevated radially and ulnarly.
- The extensor pollicis longus (EPL) is identified, released from its third extensor compartment, and transposed radially.
- The plane between the extensor tendons and the wrist capsule is developed by elevating the second and fourth compartments radially and ulnarly, respectively.
- The joint capsule and dorsal intercarpal ligament are usually divided longitudinally for access to the capitate body.
  - Alternatively, the capsule can be opened longitudinally distal to the dorsal intercarpal ligament (**TECH FIG 5**).
  - The capsule can be incised transversely distal to the ligament and in line with its fibers, provided that exposure of the capitate is adequate for reduction and fixation of the fracture.
- The fracture site is explored, cleaned as necessary, and stabilized with mini-screws, plates, or pins as indicated.
- The capsule and dorsal intercarpal ligament, if divided, are repaired.

- The EPL tendon is left transposed, superficial to the extensor retinaculum.
- The retinaculum is closed over the second and fourth compartments, followed by routine closure of subcutaneous tissue and skin.

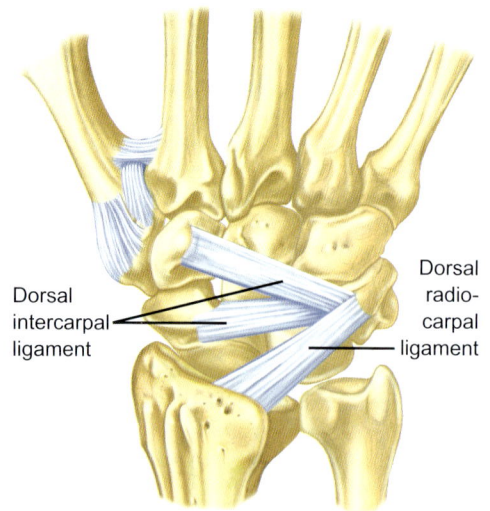

TECH FIG 5 • Dorsal intercarpal ligament anatomy.

TRAPEZOID FRACTURES

- The trapezoid is approached through a limited dorsal longitudinal or curvilinear incision centered over the index CMC.
  - Care must be exercised to identify and protect dorsal radial sensory nerve branches.
- The EPL tendon is identified, released, and transposed radially if needed.
  - In the case of limited exposure of the trapezoid, simple retraction of the EPL distal to the extensor retinaculum is effective.

- A longitudinal interval is developed between the extensor carpi radialis longus (ECRL) and brevis (ECRB) tendons with radial and ulnar retraction, respectively.
  - It is important to stay ulnar to the ECRL to avoid inadvertent damage to the dorsal branch of the radial artery.
- The capsule is divided longitudinally, exposing the trapezoid and the index CMC joint.
- Fracture fixation is carried out with mini-screws or pins, the capsule is closed, and routine subcutaneous tissue and skin closure is performed.

TRAPEZIUM FRACTURES

- Fractures of sufficient size and significant displacement are internally fixed (**TECH FIG 6**).
  - Excision rather than internal fixation may be warranted based on preoperative and intraoperative considerations.
- Unless the fracture planes dictate a specific approach for fixation, the surgeon has the option of using whichever approach he or she is most comfortable with for routine surgical treatment of thumb CMC arthritis (see Chap. HA-102).
  - The Wagner approach (described below) is one such approach frequently used for surgical reconstruction of thumb CMC arthritis and is an effective exposure for internal fixation of body fractures.
  - Isolated trapezial ridge fractures and nonunions are best approached using the flexor carpi radialis (FCR)

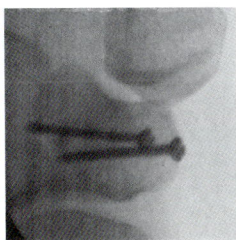

TECH FIG 6 • Open reduction and internal fixation of a trapezial body fracture.

approach centered on the scaphotrapezial joint, with retraction of the FCR ulnarly or radially out of its trapezial groove to gain access to the ridge. The Wagner approach is also effective.
- For the Wagner approach, an incision is made along the radial border of the thumb metacarpal at the glabrous skin border.
- At the distal volar wrist crease, the incision is continued ulnarly to the level of the FCR tendon.
  - Superficial radial sensory nerve and lateral antebrachial cutaneous nerve branches may be encountered and should be carefully preserved.
- The thenar musculature is elevated in a radial-to-ulnar direction off the thumb metacarpal base.
- Once the FCR tendon sheath is reached, it is incised longitudinally and the tendon is retracted ulnarly if necessary.
- The capsule overlying the trapeziometacarpal and scaphotrapezial joints is opened and the joints are visualized.
- The entire length of the trapezium may be exposed if needed, but it is critical to avoid subperiosteal dissection where not necessary for accurate fracture reduction.
  - Extensive exposure may result in delayed union or nonunion.
- At this point, internal fixation is performed if technically feasible, usually using lag screw fixation.
- The capsule is carefully reapproximated and the subcutaneous tissues and skin are closed.

PEARLS AND PITFALLS

Carpal instability	▪ Be aware of the carpal instability patterns that can accompany these fractures and treat accordingly. ▪ Failure to recognize an associated carpal instability pattern can lead to progressive carpal collapse and degeneration.
Fracture identification	▪ Preoperative imaging is critical so that all fractures that require stabilization are identified; consider CT scanning if plain radiographs are insufficient. ▪ Failing to identify all unstable fractures before or during surgery can necessitate a return to the operating room.

Screw size	▪ Use small interfragmentary screws or even small plates for fracture fixation whenever possible to decrease chances for hardware migration and to increase stability and possibly allow earlier range of motion.
Excision versus fixation	▪ We recommend hamate hook excision as opposed to fixation due to the minimal, if any, added benefit with fixation and the concern for significant nerve and tendon injuries with internal fixation.
Future surgery	▪ Be sure the patient is aware of the possible need for further surgery in the future, such as for hamate hook excision, addressing capitate avascular necrosis, excisional arthroplasty or arthrodesis for post-traumatic articular degeneration of any joints involved with the initial trauma, and so forth.

POSTOPERATIVE CARE

▪ Patients are placed in a well-padded volar plaster wrist splint postoperatively.

▪ The digits, including the metacarpophalangeal (MCP) joints, are left free unless there is some contraindication, like a dorsal hamate fracture with CMC dislocation, which may require inclusion of MCP joints.

▪ This allows early digital range of motion and elevation.

▪ Following ORIF of a trapezial fracture, a short-arm thumb spica splint is applied.

▪ Two weeks postoperatively the patient is placed in a custom fabricated splint (assuming there is no associated carpal instability).

▪ If pins were used and are left outside of the skin, pin care is initiated at this time. Pins are usually removed 4 to 8 weeks postoperatively.

▪ In the case of a CMC joint fracture in which relatively large fracture fragments are anatomically stabilized with rigid internal fixation, near-immediate postoperative range of motion is initiated.

▪ For most other fractures, a total of about 6 weeks of wrist immobilization is followed by progressive range of motion.

OUTCOMES

▪ Most isolated carpal bone body fractures unite, and it is generally thought that these patients do quite well with regard to symptomatic and functional recovery.

▪ The potentially symptomatic exceptions involving the hamate hook and trapezial ridge are easily treated by excision. Posttraumatic symptoms from other fractures, such as of the pisiform, trapezium, or triquetrum, may usually be addressed with isolated carpal bone excision with or without reconstruction, depending on the bone in question and other soft tissue and ligamentous considerations. For those carpal bones that cannot typically be simply excised, such as the hamate body and capitate, symptomatic posttraumatic changes may require partial or total wrist arthrodesis or other reconstructive options.

▪ Associated injuries are often the most problematic, and patients must understand the guarded prognosis for severe destabilizing carpal injuries.

COMPLICATIONS

▪ Those complications common to all surgical procedures may occur, including but not limited to bleeding, infection, damage to structures, failure of surgery, potential need for more surgery, and untoward effects of anesthesia.

▪ Patients must also understand the relative severity of their injuries and risk for pain, stiffness, and loss of function.

▪ Capitate neck fractures are sometimes associated with nonunion or delayed union (up to 50% or more of isolated fractures) and may be analogous to scaphoid proximal pole fractures.

▪ Treatment of such nonunions is similar for both entities.

▪ Although rare, avascular necrosis of the capitate head may follow a capitate neck fracture that disrupts the vascular supply.

▪ The capitate head may be excised with or without interpositional arthroplasty if attaining union is not likely because of avascularity or other issues.

▪ Intra-articular fractures of the carpal bones are often complicated by posttraumatic arthritis. When symptomatic, treatment with traditional arthritis remedies, such as activity modification, anti-inflammatory medications, immobilization, or steroid injection, can be tried. If these fail to relieve the patient's symptoms to his or her satisfaction, the patient may elect to proceed with partial or total wrist arthrodesis, partial carpectomy, whether of the proximal row or otherwise, or selective arthroplasties as indicated.

REFERENCES

1. Adler JB, Shaftan GW. Fractures of the capitate. J Bone Joint Surg Am 1962;44A:1537–1547.
2. Amadio PC, Moran SL. Fractures of the carpal bones. In Green DP, ed. Operative Hand Surgery, 5th ed. Philadelphia: Elsevier, 2005.
3. Cohen MS. Fractures of the carpal bones. Hand Clin 1997;13:587–599.
4. Gelberman RH, Gross MS. The vascularity of the wrist: identification of arterial patterns at risk. Clin Orthop Relat Res 1986;202:40–49.
5. Hoppenfeld S, deBoer P. Surgical Exposures in Orthopaedics: The Anatomic Approach, 2nd ed. Philadelphia: Lippincott, 1994.
6. Vigler M, Aviles A, Lee SK. Carpal fractures excluding the scaphoid. Hand Clin 2006;22:501–516.
7. Yu HL, Chase RA, Strauch B. Atlas of Hand Anatomy and Clinical Implications. St. Louis, MO: Mosby, 2004.

Chapter 23

Osteotomy of the Radius for Treatment of Kienböck Disease

Jeffrey E. Budoff

DEFINITION

- Kienböck disease is a disorder of undetermined etiology that results in avascular necrosis (AVN) of the lunate.[5]

ANATOMY

Lunate Vascularity

- The extraosseous blood supply of the lunate is extensive: branches of the radial and anterior interosseous arteries form a dorsal lunate plexus and branches of the radial, ulnar, and anterior interosseous arteries as well as the recurrent deep palmar arch form a volar plexus.
- The intraosseous blood supply is variable. Because the lunate is covered by cartilage proximally and distally, vessels can enter the bone only at its dorsal and volar poles.[1,13]
  - Three studies have identified "lunates at risk" from a vascular standpoint. The vulnerable lunate is one that has large areas of bone dependent on a single intraosseous vessel, which occurs in 7% to 20%. In addition, 31% of lunates have no internal arterial branching.[6,7,16] These internal vascular arrangements may render the lunate more vulnerable to AVN, as injury to the single vessel could not be compensated for by collateral flow.

Ulnar Variance

- The standard posteroanterior (PA) wrist radiograph is taken with the shoulder and elbow at 90 degrees and the forearm in neutral rotation.
- In this view, the length of the distal ulna with respect to the distal radius is called ulnar variance (**FIG 1**).
  - When the ulna is the same length as the radius, it is said to have neutral ulnar variance. When the ulna is shorter than the radius, it is referred to as negative ulnar variance, and when the ulna is longer than the radius it is referred to as positive ulnar variance.
- Theoretically, a negative ulna variance increases shear forces on the lunate.
  - The triangular fibrocartilage complex (TFCC) is thicker in these patients and the difference in compliance between it and the ulnar edge of the radius is accentuated, leading to greater shear force.
  - In addition, loads across the radiocarpal joint are borne disproportionately by the radius.[5]
- In the North American population, Kienböck disease is associated with an ulnar negative variance.
  - This relationship does not hold true in the Japanese literature.[1]
- Other authors have noted a tendency toward smaller lunates in patients with Kienböck disease.[3]

PATHOGENESIS

- The cause of Kienböck disease is incompletely understood. Current thinking is that acute or repetitive trauma causes excessive shear forces on a lunate at risk, interrupting its intraosseous vascularity and leading to AVN.[1,2]
- While a history of injury is elicited in over 50% of cases, the absence of a single traumatic event is still very common.
  - Fracture of the lunate has been reported in up to 82% of lunates with Kienböck disease.[1] However, it remains unclear whether these fractures are the cause or the result of AVN.
  - Kienböck disease is not seen after lunate or perilunate dislocations.[5,13]
    - Although transient ischemia may be seen after carpal fracture-dislocations, this spontaneously resolves after 5 to 32 months and should be treated expectantly.[1,2]
    - The key feature of transient ischemia is that no progressive radiographic collapse occurs, as opposed to Kienböck disease, where radiographic changes and collapse are predictable.
- It has been suggested that Kienböck disease may be due to venous outflow obstruction with intraosseous vascular congestion, rather than arterial insufficiency. Increased intraosseous pressure has been shown in lunates with Kienböck disease, as well as in femoral heads with AVN.

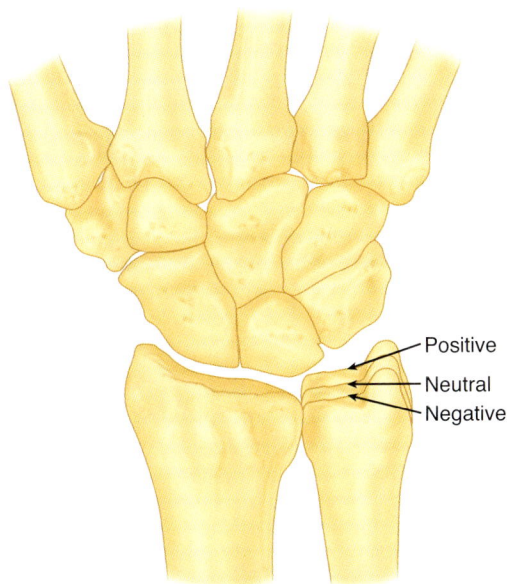

FIG 1 • Measurement of ulnar variance. Ulnar variance is determined by extending a line from the radius's articular surface ulnarward and measuring the distance between this line and the distal surface of the ulnar head. Neutral ulnar variance occurs when the carpal surface of the radius and ulna are equal in height. If the ulna is shorter than the radius, negative ulnar variance exists; if the ulna is longer than the radius, positive ulnar variance exists.

- This is more consistent with venous stasis than arterial compromise.
  - This increased pressure could also be due to bony collapse.[3,5]
- Once the lunate becomes avascular, stress fractures occur first in the proximal lunate adjacent to the radial articular surface, where the blood supply is poorest.[1,6,13] Consequently, the proximal lunate is usually more involved and more flattened than the distal lunate. In addition, the radial lunate that articulates with the distal radius is usually more involved than the ulnar lunate that overlies the triangular fibrocartilage, probably because of the difference in compliance between the two supporting surfaces. This difference is accentuated in patients with ulnar-negative variants.[13]
- Lunate collapse leads to loss of carpal height. If a coronal plane fracture is present, the compressive forces of the capitate displace these two fragments volarly and dorsally.[13]

NATURAL HISTORY

- The natural history of Kienböck disease is one of progressive fragmentation and collapse of the lunate, loss of carpal height with scaphoid flexion, and proximal capitate migration leading to perilunate arthritis. However, these changes do not universally lead to a poor clinical outcome.[5]
- A follow-up study of 49 patients compared 23 wrists treated with mean 8 weeks of immobilization and 26 without treatment.[5,11]
  - In both groups, the majority reported a gradual decrease in symptoms over time.
  - At mean 20.5 years of follow-up, 83% of the wrists in the immobilized group were pain-free or were painful only with heavy work.
  - In the nontreated group, this was true for 77%.
  - In all wrists, the lunate was deformed and 67% developed radiocarpal arthritis on radiographs.
  - The authors concluded that Kienböck disease has a naturally benign course.
  - There was no correlation between residual symptoms and the radiographic appearance, including the appearance of arthritis.
  - In this study, immobilization did not lead to any long-term benefit.

PATIENT HISTORY AND PHYSICAL FINDINGS

- Most patients with Kienböck disease are young, active patients between 20 to 40 years of age.
  - This has led to significant concerns about the long-term effects of this disorder.
- The male–female ratio is approximately 3:1 to 7:1. It is rarely bilateral.[3,21]
  - Regardless of gender, more than 95% of patients are engaged in heavy manual labor.[21]
- The most common complaints are dorsal central wrist pain, stiffness, and significant weakness of grip, which is often reduced to 50% of the opposite hand.[1,5,13]
  - There may be a long history of symptoms before presentation.
  - The pain may vary in intensity from mild discomfort to constant, debilitating pain. It is often activity-related and improves with rest and immobilization.
  - A history of trauma is variable.[1,5]

- The wrist is typically mildly swollen dorsally, consistent with synovitis, and is tender over the lunate.
- Flexion and extension are predictably diminished.
  - Wrist flexion is more likely to be limited than extension because the volar pole of the lunate often extrudes so that it impinges against the volar rim of the distal radius.
    - Forearm rotation is not affected.[13]
- While Kienböck disease has been reported in association with steroid use, septic emboli, sickle cell disease, gout, carpal coalition, and cerebral palsy, there is no well-defined correlation with any systemic or neuromuscular process that warrants screening when considering the diagnosis.[3]

IMAGING AND OTHER DIAGNOSTIC STUDIES

Radiographic Classification

- Kienböck disease is diagnosed radiographically,[12] and staging is based on plain radiographs.
- In 1977, Lichtman and Degnan[12] modified Stahle's original radiographic classification in an attempt to help guide treatment decisions (**FIG 2**).
- Stage I
  - Radiographs are normal, although a linear fracture without sclerosis or lunate collapse is occasionally present.
  - MRI shows the characteristic changes of AVN (**FIG 3A**).[5,21]
- Stage II
  - The lunate becomes sclerotic and radiodense, similar to the radiologic appearance of other bones with AVN (**FIG 3B**). A coronal fracture splitting the lunate into dorsal and volar fragments may be noted.
  - Late in stage II, some loss of lunate height on the radial side may be evident.
  - The lunate retains its overall shape, and its anatomic relationship to the other carpal bones is not significantly altered.[12,21]
- Stage III
  - The lunate collapses in the coronal plane and elongates in the sagittal plane. The carpal architecture is altered and the capitate begins to migrate proximally.
  - Stage IIIA
    - Lunate collapse has occurred, but carpal height is relatively unchanged and carpal collapse has not yet led to proximal migration of the capitate or scaphoid flexion. Therefore, the carpal kinematics have not yet been significantly altered.
  - Stage IIIB
    - The carpal collapse with proximal capitate migration has led to fixed scaphoid flexion, which may be noted on the AP radiograph as the "cortical ring sign."[3,12,21]
- Stage IV
  - Arthritis of the radiocarpal or midcarpal joint has resulted from the collapse, fractures, and altered carpal kinematics, leading to joint space narrowing, osteophyte formation, subchondral sclerosis, and degenerative cysts.[3,21]

MRI and CT

- MRI is extremely sensitive in detecting changes in marrow fat that are consistent with, but not diagnostic of, AVN.
- Decreased signal on T1 sequences represents replacement of the normal fatty marrow by dead bone or fibrous tissue.[21]

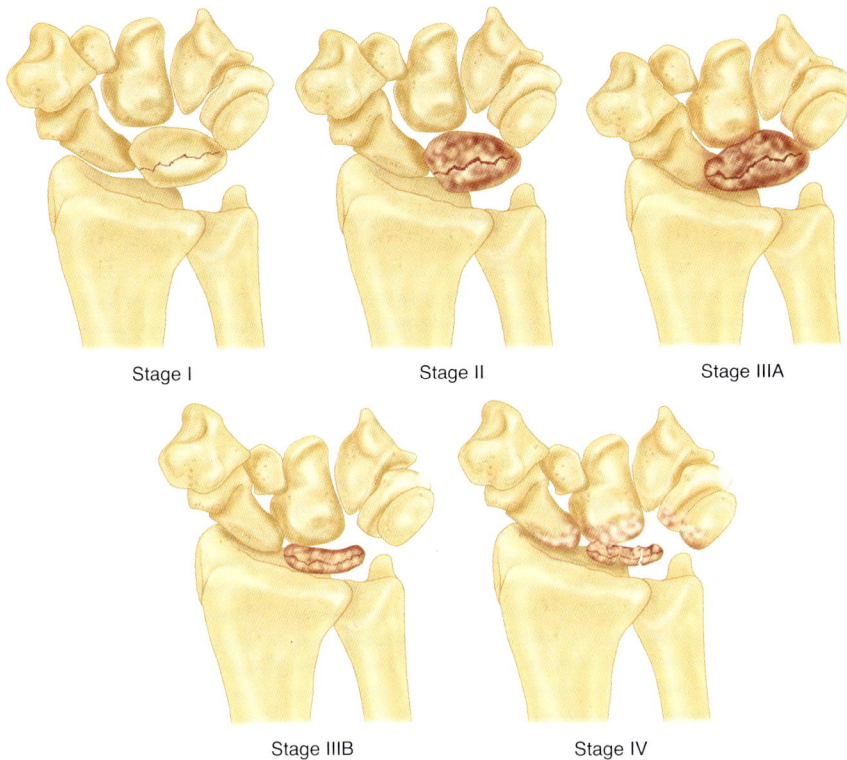

FIG 2 • Kienböck disease stage classification based on radiographic appearance.

■ Because MRI detects only the loss of marrow fat and not AVN specifically, to consider an MRI diagnostic for Kienböck disease over 50% of the lunate should be hypointense on T1 because the changes of Kienböck disease are diffuse, as opposed to other conditions such as ulnocarpal impaction, fractures, and intraosseous tumors, which cause more focal MRI changes.[4,20,22]

■ It is possible that a large enchondroma, interosseous ganglion, or other marrow-replacing lesion could lead to MRI changes in over 50% of the lunate. Thus, there is currently no truly pathognomonic imaging sign for Kienböck disease.[4]

■ T2 images typically show low signal intensity, which represents replacement of the normal fatty marrow by fibrosis.[21]

■ An increased T2 signal may occur if intramedullary edema is present or if revascularization is occurring.[3,4,20]

Thus, when the T2 images show normal or increased signal intensity, an earlier stage of disease with a better prognosis can be inferred.[20,21]

■ Although it cannot diagnose AVN directly, MRI is still the optimal imaging modality and gold standard for diagnosing Kienböck disease, especially before trabecular bone has been destroyed.

■ Gadolinium-enhanced MRI may provide a more sensitive means of evaluating lunate vascularity.

■ CT may upstage the disease compared with radiographs in 89% of those originally considered to have stage I, 71% with apparent stage II, and 9% with apparent stage III disease on radiographs.[3]

■ Once lunate collapse has occurred, CT best reveals the extent of necrosis and trabecular destruction.[3]

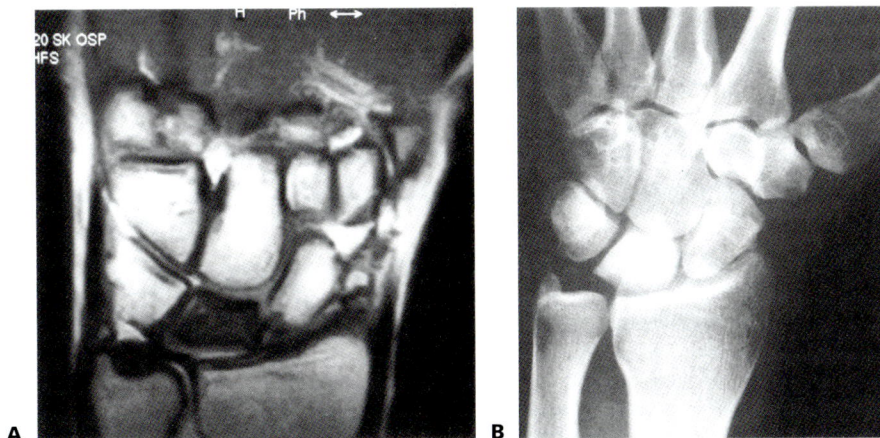

FIG 3 • **A.** Magnetic resonance image of wrist with Kienböck disease demonstrates diminished signal intensity of the lunate. **B.** Radiograph showing density changes in the lunate in Kienböck disease. (From Bishop AT, Pelzer M. Avascular necrosis. In: Berger RA, Weiss A-PC, eds. Hand surgery. Vol 1. Philadelphia: Lippincott Williams & Wilkins, 2004:554.)

DIFFERENTIAL DIAGNOSIS

- Ulnocarpal impaction
- Rheumatoid arthritis
- Radial-sided triangular fibrocartilage tears
- Posttraumatic arthritis
- Acute fracture
- Carpal instability
- Lunate fracture
- Enchondroma
- Osteoid osteoma
- Bone island
- Occult or intraosseous ganglion
- Intraosseous cyst
- Transient ischemia
- "Bone bruise"
- Paget disease
- Gaucher disease[4]

NONOPERATIVE MANAGEMENT

- A trial of 2 weeks to 3 months of immobilization may be attempted for patients with stage I Kienböck disease, especially young patients with hyperintense lunates on T2 MR images.
  - The theory behind the use of immobilization is that by decreasing the forces across the carpus, the lunate may be able to revascularize.[12]
  - Most series report poor results with immobilization, and progressive collapse is common.
  - There is no study of immobilization consisting of patients with only stage I Kienböck disease. Consequently, the efficacy of immobilization in patients with stage I disease is anecdotal.
- Immobilization does not decrease compressive forces across the lunate, which are imparted by the capitate. The capitate may still force any fracture fragments apart, leading to collapse and displacement.
  - Immobilization leads to stiffness.
  - The earlier the lunate is unloaded, the less collapse is anticipated. For this reason, early surgical decompression may be considered rather than immobilization, and many clinicians treat stage I disease surgically.[13]
- In Trumble and Irving's series of 22 patients with various stages of Kienböck disease treated with immobilization, 17 showed disease progression with continued collapse of the lunate and 5 showed no improvement.[22]
  - In Lichtman et al's series, 19 of 22 had unsatisfactory results.[2,3]
- When immobilization fails to reverse the avascular changes, the process will almost always advance to stage II, where surgical management is strongly recommended.[2,3]
  - In a series of patients with stage II or more advanced disease treated with immobilization, 76% (19/25) had either undergone total wrist arthrodesis or experienced daily problems with their wrists at mean 8 (1–11) year follow-up.[15]
- A study of 18 patients with stage II or III disease treated nonoperatively were compared with those treated by radius shortening.
  - Patients treated surgically had less pain and better grip strength.
  - In some patients with stage III disease treated nonoperatively there was rapid deterioration to carpal collapse.
  - Although radius shortening did not reverse or prevent carpal collapse, it slowed the process.[18]

SURGICAL MANAGEMENT

- There is no agreement on the optimal way to treat Kienböck disease.[5] Multiple options for surgical management exist and the results do not vary significantly between the different procedures.
  - The mainstays of treatment are radius-shortening osteotomy and proximal row carpectomy.[5]
  - Two major radiographic features influence treatment choice: the stage of the disease and ulnar variance.[12]
- Radius-shortening osteotomy is currently the benchmark against which other treatments are judged.[13]
  - For stages I to IIIB, radius-shortening osteotomy is a very popular option in patients who are ulnar negative. While the use of radius shortening in stage IIIB is controversial, because lunate height and normal carpal kinematics will not be re-established, potentially leading to progressive degenerative changes, very good results have been demonstrated in these patients with this procedure.[2,24,25] Radius shortening is contraindicated for stage IV disease unless symptoms are severe and salvage procedures are not desired.[24]
  - Radius shortening decreases joint compression forces at the radiolunate joint by redistributing them to the radioscaphoid and ulnolunate joints. In addition, it relatively lengthens the tendons crossing the wrist, diminishing overall joint compressive forces.[17]
    - As opposed to ulnar lengthening, no intercalary bone graft is required and only one interface needs to heal, instead of two.
    - In addition, radial shortening leads to a relative lengthening of the musculotendinous units crossing the wrist, resulting in less force transmission across the carpus. Ulnar lengthening does not provide this particular advantage.[24]
    - After radial shortening, the ulnar head and TFCC support more of the wrist's compressive load through the triquetrum and the ulnar aspect of the lunate. The TFC is thicker in patients with ulna-minus variance, which provides a compliant pad to support the ulnar carpus.
  - Because radial-shortening osteotomy is an extra-articular procedure, it does not alter normal carpal joints or interfere with intracarpal relationships. It "burns no bridges," and intracarpal procedures can always be undertaken at a later date if the radial shortening is ineffective and disease progression occurs.[24]
- In patients who are ulnar-neutral or ulnar-positive, a radial closing wedge osteotomy (**FIG 4**) or capitate shortening with or without capitohamate fusion can be performed.
  - While radius shortening in patients with neutral or positive ulnar variance is not advised, good results have been reported even in these patients.[1,24]
- For stages I to IIIA, revascularization using a vascularized pedicle or bone graft may be performed and may be combined with radius shortening or another unloading procedure (see Chap. HA-24).
- In patients with stage IIIB disease, proximal row carpectomy, scaphotrapeziotrapezoid fusion, or scaphocapitate fusion may be performed with or without lunate excision and soft tissue interposition.
- For stage IV disease, proximal row carpectomy or total wrist fusion may be indicated. A study of arthroscopic débridement for stage III or IV disease showed some pain relief at 19 months of follow-up.[14]

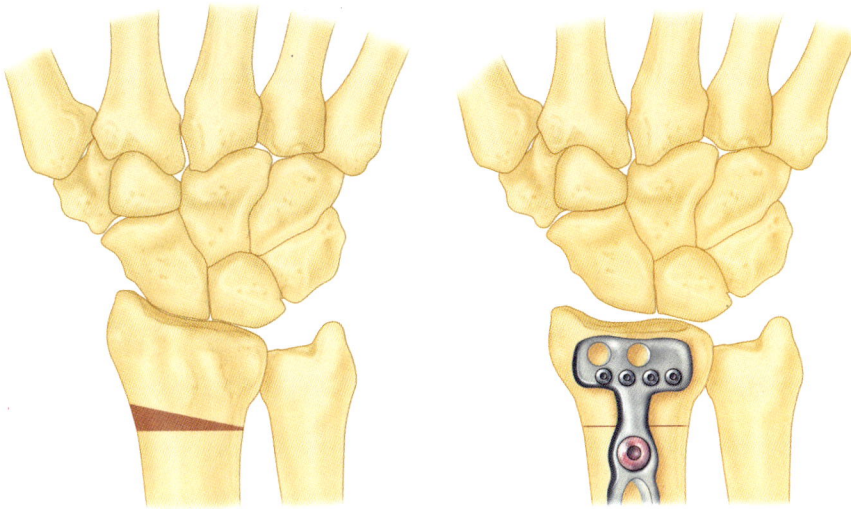

FIG 4 • Lateral closing wedge osteotomy. (Adapted from Soejima O, Iida H, Komine S, et al. Lateral closing wedge osteotomy of the distal radius for advanced stages of Kienbock's disease. J Hand Surg Am 2002;27A:31–36.)

- Based on the hypothesis that Kienböck disease is due to venous obstruction, "metaphyseal core decompression" of the distal radius has also been reported with good results.[8]
- Wrist denervation may also be considered and can be used as an adjunct at any stage.[3]
- Lateral closing wedge osteotomies increase lunate coverage (joint contact area) in proportion to the decrease in radial inclination.
  - This transfers the compressive forces of the capitate from the lunate to the scaphoid, decreasing pressure at the radiolunate joint.[17,23]
  - To keep the wrist straight in relation to the forearm, the patient is forced to ulnarly deviate the wrist, extending the scaphoid, which may further transfer forces from the capitate to the scaphoid and decrease forces on the lunate.[19]

Preoperative Planning

- Good-quality, standard preoperative PA radiographs should be taken with the shoulder and elbow flexed 90 degrees and the forearm in neutral rotation.
- While many authors have recommended removing sufficient bone during radial shortening to result in an ulnar-neutral to 1-mm-positive variance,[3] 90% of the strain reduction occurs within the first 2 mm of shortening.[1,5]

- Good results with excellent relief of symptoms have been reported removing only 2 mm of bone, regardless of variance. This has the advantages of technical ease and decreases the risk of distal radioulnar joint (DRUJ) incongruity and ulnocarpal impaction, which may occur with excessive shortening.
- In patients with significant obliquity of the sigmoid notch, radial shortening should be limited to 2 mm to avoid overcompressing the DRUJ.
- Postoperative ulnocarpal impaction and DRUJ incongruity are especially likely with shortenings of 4 mm or more, leading to pain with forearm rotation or limitation of forearm rotation.[24] Therefore, shortening of the radius by over 4 mm is not recommended.
  - Patients with more than 4 mm of shortening and age greater than 30 years were found to be more likely to have poor results.[1]

Positioning

- The patient is positioned supine with the arm on a radiolucent armboard.

Approach

- A volar approach to the radius is performed.

VOLAR APPROACH

- A longitudinal incision is made over the flexor carpi radialis (FCR) tendon, ending distally at the distal volar wrist crease (**TECH FIG 1A**).
- The approach is continued through the FCR sheath (**TECH FIG 1B**), with the FCR tendon retracted ulnarly to protect the palmar cutaneous branch of the median nerve (**TECH FIG 1C**).
- The plane between the FCR and deep muscles of the radius (pronator quadratus and FCR) is bluntly dissected (**TECH FIG 1D**).

- The distal border of the pronator quadratus and the radial insertions of the pronator quadratus and flexor pollicis longus muscles are incised with Bovie electrocautery, with care taken to retract and protect the radial artery, which does not need to be formally identified.
- The volar surface of the radius is then subperiosteally exposed in a radial to ulnar direction (**TECH FIG 1E**).
- Circumferential subperiosteal dissection should be avoided to preserve maximal blood supply to the osteotomy.

TECHNIQUES

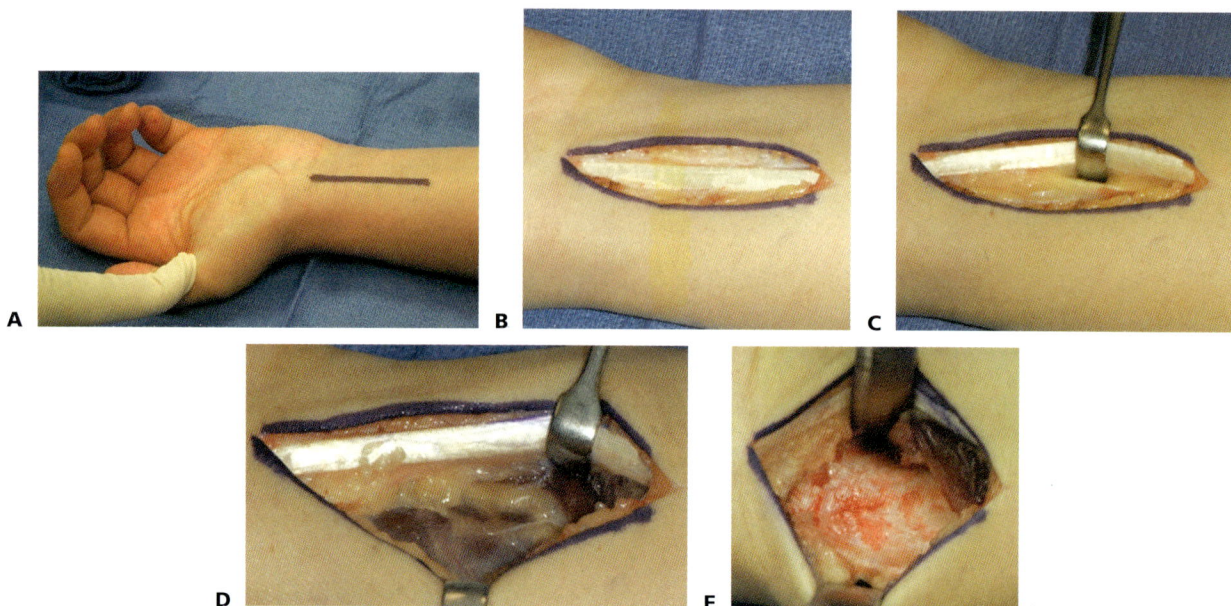

TECH FIG 1 • **A.** Incision. **B.** Dissection proceeds through the flexor carpi radialis (FCR) sheath. **C.** The FCR is retracted ulnarly to protect the palmar cutaneous branch of the median nerve. **D.** The pronator quadratus is exposed. **E.** The volar distal radius is subperiosteally exposed.

RADIUS-SHORTENING OSTEOTOMY

Initial Plate Application

- Traditionally, a seven-hole 3.5-mm dynamic compression plate is placed as far distally as possible without riding up the volar lip of the distal radius.[24]
  - However, the newer fixed-angle volar plates used for fixation of distal radius fractures work very well and allow the osteotomy to be placed in metaphyseal bone.
- To decrease the risk of nonunion, the osteotomy should be performed as distal as possible to be through metaphyseal cancellous bone, staying proximal to the DRUJ.
- The plate is placed over the distal radius so that its distal fixation will be within 2 to 3 mm of the subchondral bone, without intra-articular penetration. The plate is provisionally fixed with Kirschner wires (**TECH FIG 2**).

- Following fluoroscopic confirmation of appropriate placement, four fixed-angle screws are placed distally.

Radius Osteotomy

- The osteotomy is marked proximal to the distal fixation and proximal to the DRUJ (**TECH FIG 3A**).
- The plate is removed and the osteotomy is made at a 45-degree angle, from distal volar to proximal dorsal (**TECH FIG 3B**).
  - An oblique osteotomy has less potential for nonunion than a transverse osteotomy[1] and allows placement of an interfragmentary compression screw for additional fixation.

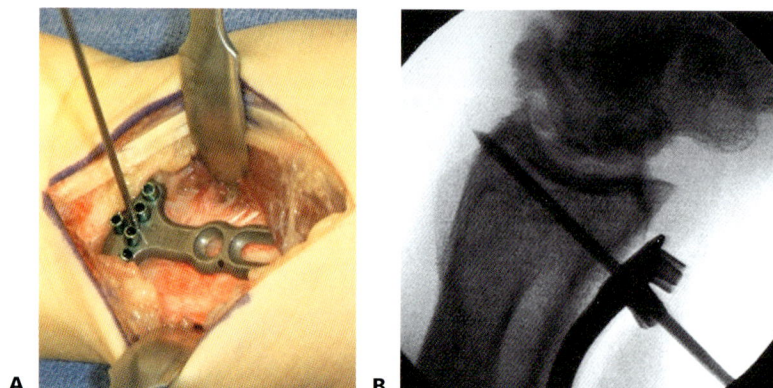

TECH FIG 2 • **A,B.** The volar locking plate is placed so that its distal fixation (represented radiographically by a Kirschner wire) travels just proximal to the subchondral surface. Distal locking screw fixation is placed but not fully tightened.

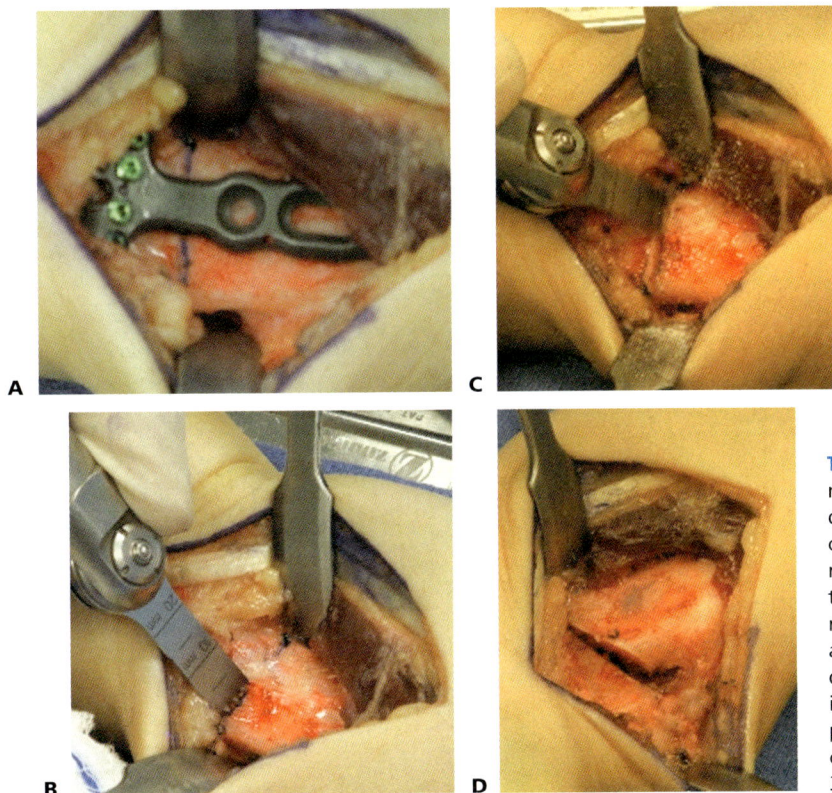

TECH FIG 3 • **A.** The osteotomy site is marked between the plate's proximal and distal fixation. When using a plate specifically designed for the fixation of distal radius fractures, this automatically places the osteotomy proximal to the distal radioulnar joint. **B.** The osteotomy is created with a saw at a 45-degree angle from distal volar to proximal dorsal. **C.** The saw is used to remove 2 to 3 mm of bone, proceeding from volar to dorsal. **D.** The oblique osteotomy is finished and 2 to 3 mm of dorsal cortex is removed.

- A longitudinal line may be marked across the osteotomy site to allow rotational assessment. However, the flat surface of the volar cortex allows for easy assessment of rotation.
- An elevator can be placed on the dorsal surface of the osteotomy to protect the extensor tendons from the saw.
- Two to 3 mm of shortening may be appropriate regardless of the amount of negative ulnar variance present.
  - For the reasons noted above, I prefer to shorten the radius by only 2 to 3 mm.
  - Excellent results have been reported with osteotomies that do not fully correct the radius length to neutral variance.[24,25]

- The 2 to 3 mm to be taken is measured out and marked and the full amount of bone to be taken is removed from volar to dorsal so that the dorsal cortex remains intact to stabilize the bone during bone removal (**TECH FIG 3C**).
- The dorsal cortex is then removed last (**TECH FIG 3D**).
  - During the osteotomy, constant cool irrigant is used to avoid thermal osteonecrosis.
- While a slight (1 mm) concave bend in the plate over the osteotomy site may occasionally be needed to achieve compression of the dorsal osteotomy surface, this is not usually necessary.

Final Plate Application and Osteotomy Fixation

- The plate and its distal fixation are then replaced.
- Approximation of the two bone ends may also be facilitated by radial deviation of the wrist[24] and use of a Verbrugge clamp.
  - A bicortical screw is placed 1 cm proximal to (not through) the plate (**TECH FIG 4A**).

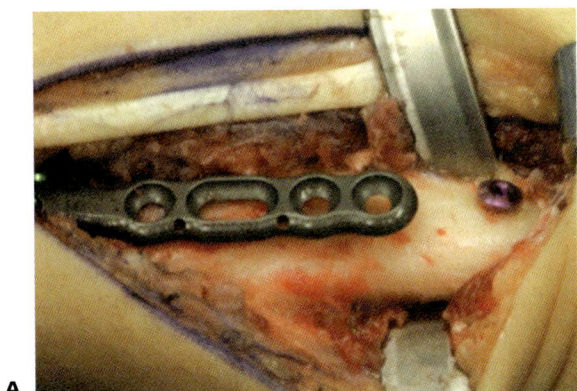

TECH FIG 4 • **A.** The plate and its distal fixation are replaced. A bicortical screw a few millimeters longer than the bone width is placed 2 to 3 cm proximal to the plate and left proud. A retractor may provide the necessary proximal exposure without lengthening the incision. *(continued)*

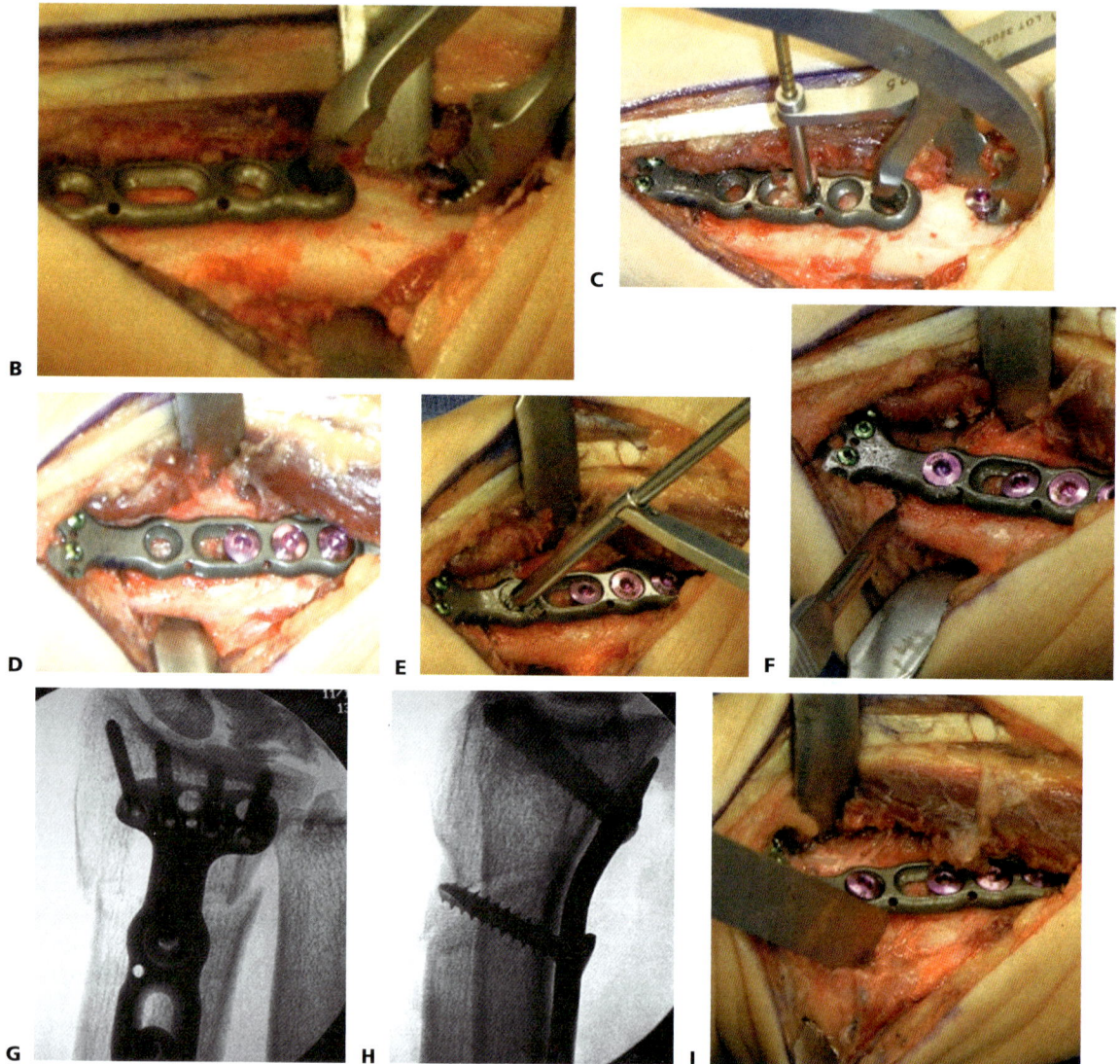

TECH FIG 4 • *(continued)* **B.** A Verbrugge clamp is placed in the most proximal plate hole and around the proximal screw. Squeezing the clamp provides a tremendous mechanical advantage to facilitate osteotomy closure. **C.** With the clamp compressing the osteotomy, the first proximal screw is drilled eccentrically through the most proximal aspect of a plate hole to provide additional compression. **D.** Three proximal bicortical screws are placed. **E.** The most distal of the proximal screws may be placed in lag fashion, overdrilling the near cortex. **F.** A stably fixed and well-compressed osteotomy. The tip of a scalpel blade could not be forced into the osteotomy. **G,H.** Intraoperative PA and lateral radiographs. The significant obliquity of the distal radioulnar joint (DRUJ) led to some radial displacement of the distal fragment. This should be allowed, as it "decompresses" the DRUJ. In patients with significant DRUJ obliquity, only 2 mm of shortening should be performed. **I.** Osteoperiosteal shingling of the volar cortex, which may facilitate osteotomy healing. Synthetic bone substitute was then placed over the shingled volar cortex.

- The hooked end of the Verbrugge is placed in the plate's most proximal screw hole and the bifid end is placed around the screw proximal to the plate (**TECH FIG 4B**).
- The Verbrugge clamp is closed manually, imparting tremendous mechanical advantage to compress the osteotomy.
- The first screw is placed in a compression mode eccentrically in the plate hole just proximal to the osteotomy (**TECH FIG 4C**).

- Reduction of the osteotomy and fixation are evaluated fluoroscopically.
- Adjustments are made as necessary and the remaining screws are placed (**TECH FIG 4D**).
- A lag screw is placed obliquely across the osteotomy through the most distal of the proximal plate holes for additional fixation (**TECH FIG 4E–H**).
- After irrigation, osteoperiosteal shingling may be performed with allograft or bone substitute placed over the shingled cortex to facilitate healing (**TECH FIG 4I**).

- Forearm rotation should be checked to ensure that it is full.
  - If forearm rotation is limited after osteotomy, the radius should be translated radially or a lateral closing wedge component added.[17]
- Radiographs often show some mild residual gap at the osteotomy site even with full compression under direct vision.[24]
- Intraoperative radiographs may not demonstrate the eventual ulnar variance (amount of radial shortening) because of soft tissue restraints at the DRUJ. In these cases, postoperative radiographs will demonstrate the anticipated correction.[17]

RADIUS CLOSING WEDGE OSTEOTOMY

- A radial closing wedge osteotomy may be performed through the same approach with the same fixation.
- A 15-degree radial closing wedge osteotomy is performed 4 to 5 cm proximal to the tip of the radial styloid and proximal to the DRUJ.[23]

PEARLS AND PITFALLS

Radial shortening	- Two to 3 mm of shortening is all that is needed in the vast majority of cases. Shortening the radius by only 2 to 3 mm makes compression of the osteotomy easier. - In cases of significant DRUJ obliquity, shortening the radius greater than 2 mm may lead to DRUJ problems.
Fragment handling	- If rotation is not full or the DRUJ is compromised after osteotomy, radial translation of the distal fragment should be considered.
Verbrugge clamp	- Use of a Verbrugge clamp compressing against a screw proximal to the plate gives the surgeon a tremendous mechanical advantage in shortening the osteotomy.

POSTOPERATIVE CARE

- The extra-articular nature of this procedure combined with stable internal fixation allows for quick postoperative rehabilitation.
- The wrist is splinted for 2 weeks, after which a removable splint may be used and gentle motion started.
- The osteotomy usually heals in 2 to 3 months, although 4 or 5 months is occasionally required.

OUTCOMES

- A review of the reported series by Weiss[24] in 1993 included 121 patients treated with radius shortening, with about 85% good or excellent results at just over 4 years of follow-up.
- One study reviewed 30 wrists after radial shortening osteotomy for stages I to IIIB Kienböck disease at mean 3.8 years of follow-up.[25]
  - Pain decreased in 87% and grip strength improved in 49%. However, the radiographic appearance of the lunate changed little if at all.
  - The authors noted that good results could be obtained by shortening less than that required to attain neutral ulnar variance.
  - The exact amount of radius shortening may not be as important as the relative unloading of the lunate resulting from the shortening of the radius. The amount of shortening needed to be effective may be only about 2 mm. Radial shortening may therefore be used in ulnar-neutral wrists.
  - In addition, excellent results were realized in patients with stage IIIA and IIIB disease. There was one nonunion. Only 10 of 30 wrists had evidence of possible lunate

revascularization, as indicated by decreased sclerosis and a more normal trabecular pattern.
- Clinical improvement after radius shortening or radial wedge osteotomy does not necessarily correlate with the radiographic results.[1,5,19] It appears that the lunate "stands still in time" after radius shortening, with no significant further deterioration or improvement in the lunate architecture or height.[24]
- Another study reviewed 68 radius-shortening osteotomies at a mean of 52 months of follow-up.[17]
  - Pain was diminished in 93%, grip strength was improved in 74%, and motion was improved in 52% and worsened in 19%.
  - Twenty-five patients had undergone one or more additional procedures concurrently, which did not lead to a significant difference in clinical outcomes.
  - Complications were uncommon; there were no nonunions, but ulnocarpal impaction developed in two patients.
  - Lunate density was improved in 40%, unchanged in 46%, and increased (worsened) in 14%.
  - Fifty-five percent of wrists that underwent concurrent vascularized bone grafting of the lunate had an improved radiographic appearance, compared to only 20% that underwent isolated radius shortening.
- It has been suggested that prognosis is improved in younger patients due to increased remodeling potential.[12]
  - Teenage patients (aged 11 to 19 years) were treated by radius shortening or lateral closing wedge osteotomy.[9] Two had neutral or positive ulnar variance. At a mean 50 months of follow-up, 10 of 11 were pain-free. Five of six with stage IIIB disease had excellent outcomes.

- The other patient had moderate wrist pain during strenuous activity, leading to only a fair result after lateral closing wedge osteotomy for stage IIIB disease.
- Radiographic improvement, indicating possible lunate revascularization, was seen in 8 of 11 patients.
- There were no complications of radial overgrowth or growth abnormalities in these patients.
- Twenty-five patients were followed for a minimum of 10 years (mean 14.5 years) after radial osteotomy.[10]
  - Ninety-six percent had good or excellent results.
  - Pain, motion, and grip strength were all significantly improved after surgery and the results were maintained.
  - Although radiologic improvement was not drastic and carpal height did not significantly improve, sclerosis and bone cysts improved and there was evidence of improved lunate revascularization over time.
  - Osteoarthritic changes were observed in 54% at 5 years and in 73% at the time of final follow-up, but the arthrosis was generally mild and did not affect the clinical results.
  - Severe osteoarthritis and proximal migration of the capitate were avoided.
  - Radius shortening was used for patients with ulnar-negative variants and closing wedge osteotomy for those with ulnar-positive variants. These procedures gave identical outcomes.
- Iwasaki et al[9] also noted that both radius shortening and lateral closing wedge osteotomies gave equally acceptable results in adult patients.
- Good long-term results were reported in 100% of 13 patients at a mean of 14 years after radial closing wedge osteotomy.[23]
  - Pain relief was good, and improvements in grip strength and range of motion were seen.
  - Radiographic changes improved in one, did not change in four, and advanced in eight.

COMPLICATIONS

- Nonunion has been reported in up to 6% of cases.[5]
  - If the fixation remains stable, treatment should consist of autogenous cancellous bone grafting if healing has not occurred by 5 or 6 months.
- A second operation may occasionally be necessary for plate removal, but this is uncommon.
- Care must be taken not to overshorten the radius, or DRUJ incongruity or ulnocarpal impaction may occur.[24]

REFERENCES

1. Alexander CE, Alexander AH, Lichtman DM. Kienbock's disease and idiopathic necrosis of carpal bones. In: Lichtman DM, ed. The Wrist and Its Disorders, 2nd ed. Philadelphia: WB Saunders, 1997: 329–346.
2. Alexander AH, Lichtman DM. Kienbock's disease. Orthop Clin North Am 1986;17:461–472.
3. Allan CH, Joshi A, Lichtman DM. Kienbock's disease: diagnosis and treatment. J Am Acad Orthop Surg 2001;9:128–136.
4. Budoff JE, Lichtman DM. Spontaneous wrist fusion: an unusual complication of Kienbock's disease. J Hand Surg Am 2005;30A:59–64.
5. Divelbiss B, Baratz ME. Kienbock's disease. J Am Soc Surg Hand 2000;1:1–12.
6. Gelberman RH, Bauman TD, Menon J, et al. The vascularity of the lunate bone and Kienbock's disease. J Hand Surg 1980;5A:272–278.
7. Gelberman RH, Szabo RM. Kienbock's disease. Orthop Clin North Am 1984;15:355–367.
8. Illarramendi AA, Schulz C, De Carli P. The surgical treatment of Kienbock's disease by radius and ulna metaphyseal core decompression. J Hand Surg Am 2001;26A:252–260.
9. Iwasaki N, Minami A, Ishikawa J, et al. Radial osteotomies for teenage patients with Kienbock disease. Clin Orthop Relat Res 2005; 439:116–122.
10. Koh S, Nakamura R, Horii E, Nakao E, et al. Surgical outcome of radial osteotomy for Kienbock's disease: minimum 10 years of follow-up. J Hand Surg Am 2003;28A:910–916.
11. Kristensen SS, Thomassen E, Christensen F. Kienbock's disease: late results by non-surgical treatment: a follow-up study. J Hand Surg Br 1986;11B:422–425.
12. Lichtman DM, Degnan GG. Staging and its use in the determination of treatment modalities for Kienbock's disease. Hand Clin 1993;9: 409–416.
13. Linscheid RL. Kienbock's disease. AAOS Instr Course Lect 1992; 41:45–53.
14. Menth-Chiari WA, Poehling GG, Wiesler ER, et al. Arthroscopic debridement for the treatment of Kienbock's disease. Arthroscopy 1999;15:12–19.
15. Mikkelsen SS, Gelineck J. Poor function after nonoperative treatment of Kienbock's disease. Acta Orthop Scand 1987;58:241–243.
16. Panagis JS, Gelberman RH, Taleisnik J, et al. The arterial anatomy of the human carpus. Part II: The intraosseous vascularity. J Hand Surg Am 1983;8A:375–382.
17. Quenzer DE, Dobyns JH, Linscheid RL, et al. Radial recession osteotomy for Kienbock's disease. J Hand Surg Am 1997;22A: 386–395.
18. Salmon J, Stanley JK, Trail IA. Kienbock's disease: conservative management versus radial shortening. J Bone Joint Surg Br 2000;82B: 820–823.
19. Soejima O, Iida H, Komine S, et al. Lateral closing wedge osteotomy of the distal radius for advanced stages of Kienbock's disease. J Hand Surg Am 2002;27A:31–36.
20. Sowa DT, Holder LE, Patt PG, et al. Application of magnetic resonance imaging to ischemic necrosis of the lunate. J Hand Surg 1989; 14A:1008–1016.
21. Szabo RM, Greenspan A. Diagnosis and clinical findings of Kienbock's disease. Hand Clin 1993;9:399–408.
22. Trumble TE, Irving J. Histologic and magnetic resonance imaging correlations in Kienbock's disease. J Hand Surg Am 1990;15A: 879–884.
23. Wada A, Miura H, Kubota H, et al. Radial closing wedge osteotomy for Kienbock's disease: an over-10-year clinical and radiographic follow-up. J Hand Surg Br 2002;27B:175–179.
24. Weiss AP. Radial shortening. Hand Clin 1993;9:475–482.
25. Weiss AP, Weiland AJ, Moore JR, et al. Radial shortening for Kienbock disease. J Bone Joint Surg Am 1991;73A:384–391.

Chapter 24

Vascularized Bone Grafting and Capitate Shortening Osteotomy for Treatment of Kienböck Disease

Nilesh M. Chaudhari, Mohamed Khalid, and Thomas R. Hunt III

DEFINITION

- Lunate revascularization for Kienböck disease involves transfer of either a vessel or a pedicled bone graft to the lunate in an attempt to reverse avascular necrosis.
- Vascularized bone grafts from the pisiform, volar and dorsal radius metaphysis, second metacarpal head,[6] and iliac crest (via free microvascular graft)[2] have all been reported.
- Unloading procedures, like a capitate shortening osteotomy, are often combined with a revascularization procedure to protect the graft and to alter forces through the lunate.

ANATOMY

Vascular Anatomy of the Dorsal Distal Radius

- The dorsal distal radius is primarily supplied by the branches of the radial artery and the posterior division of the anterior interosseous artery (pAIA) (**FIG 1**).
- The 2, 3 intercompartmental, supraretinacular artery (2, 3 ICSRA) is superficial to the extensor retinaculum and passes between the second and third extensor compartments (Fig 1).
- The fourth extensor compartment artery (ECA) is located deep to the extensor retinaculum in the fourth extensor compartment (Fig 1).
  - It lies directly adjacent to the posterior interosseous nerve on the radial floor of that compartment.
  - It originates from the pAIA or the fifth ECA.
  - It anastomoses with the dorsal intercarpal arch and the dorsal radiocarpal arch.
  - The fourth ECA is a source of numerous small nutrient arteries to the dorsal radius at the level of the fourth extensor compartment that penetrate deeply into cancellous bone.
- The fifth ECA is located deep to the extensor retinaculum in the fifth extensor compartment or within the septum between the fourth and fifth extensor compartments (Fig 1).
  - It is the largest of the four dorsal vessels.
  - It originates from the pAIA and anastomoses distally with the fourth ECA, the dorsal intercarpal arch, the radiocarpal arch, the 2, 3 ICSRA, and/or the oblique dorsal artery of the distal ulna.
- The fourth and fifth ECA pedicle is ideal for use in grafting the lunate because of the large diameter of the fifth ECA, the length of combined pedicle, the ulnar location of the fifth ECA (away from necessary incisions), and the multiple anastomoses, which provide retrograde flow.
  - The fifth ECA by itself seldom provides direct nutrient branches to the radius.
  - A 2, 3 ICSRA graft based on antegrade flow through the fifth ECA can be used if the fourth ECA is damaged or not present.

Vascular Anatomy of the Dorsal Hand

- The blood supply to the hand consists of a series of anastomotic arches over the carpus that form the dorsal carpal arch, usually with contributions from both the radial and ulnar arteries (Fig 1).[3,8]
- The dorsal carpal arch lies distal and deep to the extensor retinaculum.
- The dorsal metacarpal arteries lie just deep to the fascia overlying the interossei muscles.
- The second, third, and fourth dorsal metacarpal arteries arise from the dorsal carpal arch. They terminate by dividing into digital arteries.

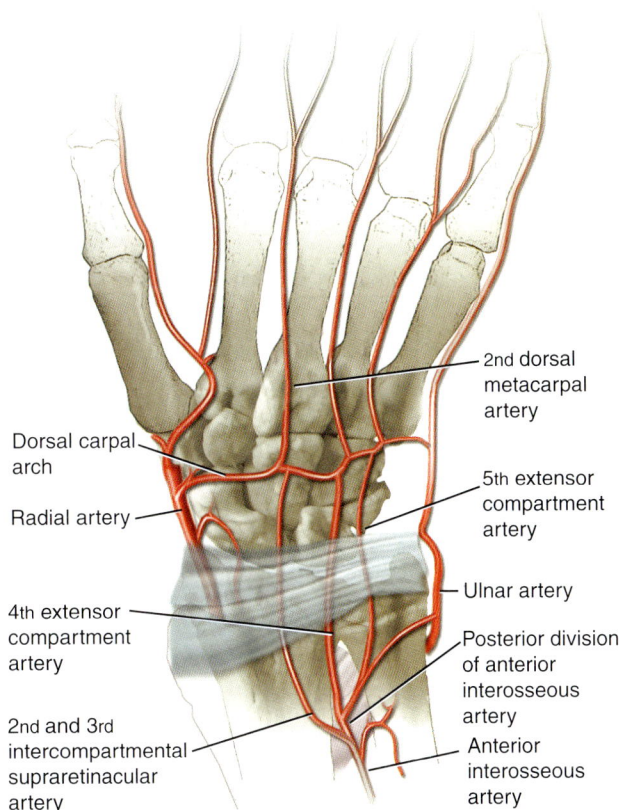

FIG 1 • Arterial anatomy of the dorsal distal radius and wrist. RA, radial artery; UA, ulnar artery; AIA, anterior interosseous artery; pAIA, posterior division of anterior interosseous artery; 4th ECA, fourth extensor compartment artery; 5th ECA, fifth extensor compartment artery; 2, 3 ICSRA, 2, 3 intercompartmental supraretinacular artery.

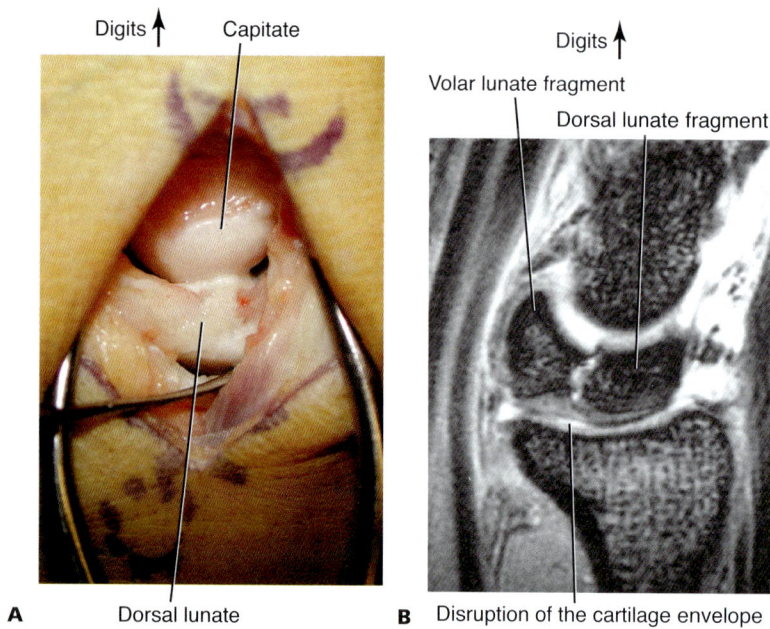

FIG 2 • **A.** At the time of surgery the articular surfaces are carefully evaluated. **B.** T2-weighted MRI sagittal image of the lunate revealing a coronal plane fracture line, separation of volar and dorsal fragments, and interruption in the cartilaginous envelope. (Copyright Thomas R. Hunt, III, MD.)

- The digital arteries are also supplied by perforating branches from the deep palmar arch.
- The first and fifth dorsal metacarpal arteries are direct branches from the radial and ulnar arteries respectively.
- The second dorsal metacarpal artery is the preferred vascular source for vessel implantation due to its size and predictable presence.
  - If this vessel is damaged or cannot be found, the third dorsal metacarpal artery may be used.

SURGICAL MANAGEMENT

- Treatment of Kienböck disease is based on the following factors:
  - Lichtman stage
  - Ulna variance
  - Presence of arthritic changes
  - Integrity of the lunate's cartilaginous shell (**FIG 2**)
  - Patient symptoms and other patient-specific factors

- Nonsmokers with Stage I to IIIA Kienböck disease, an intact lunate cartilaginous shell (as determined using sagittal images and at surgery), and limited arthritic changes are suitable candidates for treatment using a vascularized grafting procedure (**FIG 3**).
- Relative contraindications to vascularized grafting include:
  - Previous surgery with exposure of the dorsal aspect of the hand and wrist
  - Age more than 60 years
  - History of peripheral vascular diseases or poorly controlled diabetes
- Vascular grafting is accompanied by a lunate unloading procedure.
  - Unloading has been shown to improve symptoms related to Kienböck disease (see Chap. HA-23).
  - Altering force distribution through the lunate serves to protect the vascular grafts and to encourage revascularization.

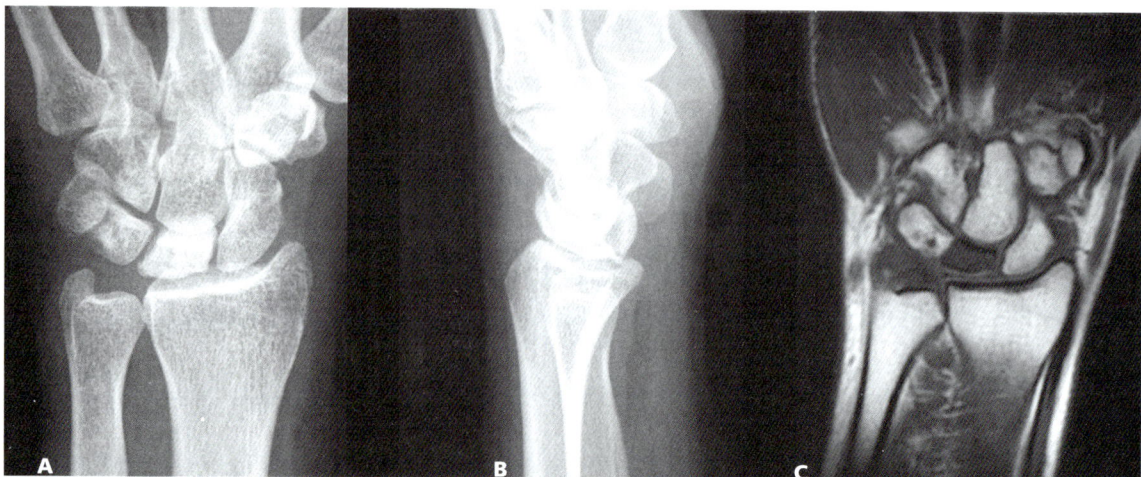

FIG 3 • **A, B.** AP and lateral radiographs showing stage II–III Kienböck disease with sclerosis and subtle, early collapse. There is no evidence of a coronal plane fracture line. **C.** T1-weighted MRI coronal image showing loss of marrow signal of the lunate. (Copyright Thomas R. Hunt, III, MD.)

■ Unloading procedures commonly used in conjunction with a vascular procedure include:

   ■ Capitate shortening osteotomy is our preferred choice in patients with positive or neutral ulna variance. This procedure is completed before inserting the vascular graft or vessel.

   ■ Scaphocapitate pinning or external fixation (4 to 6 weeks) is used when ulna variance is positive and a contraindication to capitate shortening osteotomy exists.

   ■ Radius shortening and angular osteotomy is used when ulna variance is negative (see Chap. HA-23).

   ■ Intercarpal arthrodesis (see Chap. HA-88).

Preoperative Planning

■ The surgeon should review all imaging studies to determine the stage of the disease, ulna variance, and the status of the lunate's articular shell.

Positioning

■ The patient is positioned supine with the arm on a radiolucent armboard.

■ A proximal arm tourniquet is applied. Gravity exsanguination of the limb before tourniquet inflation allows visualization of the vessels.

Approach

■ The surgeon should consider arthroscopic assessment before the open approach if the status of the lunate articular shell is in question.

   ■ The 4-5 portal and ulnar midcarpal portal should be avoided as they may damage 4+5 ECA.

■ Dorsal approaches to the hand and the wrist are used.

■ Specific incision placement varies based on the graft choice and associated lunate unloading procedure.

VASCULARIZED BONE GRAFTING

Exposure and Identification of the Fourth and Fifth Extensor Compartment Arteries

■ Make a 5- to 6-cm longitudinal skin incision between fourth and fifth extensor compartments, ending distally between the third and fourth metacarpal bases.

■ Incise the fifth extensor compartment.

■ Identify the fifth ECA and its venae comitantes on the radial aspect of the compartment lying adjacent to or partially within the septum and separating the fourth and fifth extensor compartments (**TECH FIG 1**).

■ Trace the fifth ECA proximally to its origin from the posterior division of the anterior interosseous artery as it emerges from the interosseous membrane.

■ Identify the fourth ECA arising from the same feeding vessel.

■ Trace the fourth ECA distally and identify the area of greatest vascular penetration into bone, typically 1 cm proximal to the radiocarpal joint.

Lunate Preparation

■ Elevate the extensor retinaculum as a radial-based flap from the fifth through the second extensor compartments to allow joint capsulotomy.

   ■ Carefully protect the dorsal carpal arch.

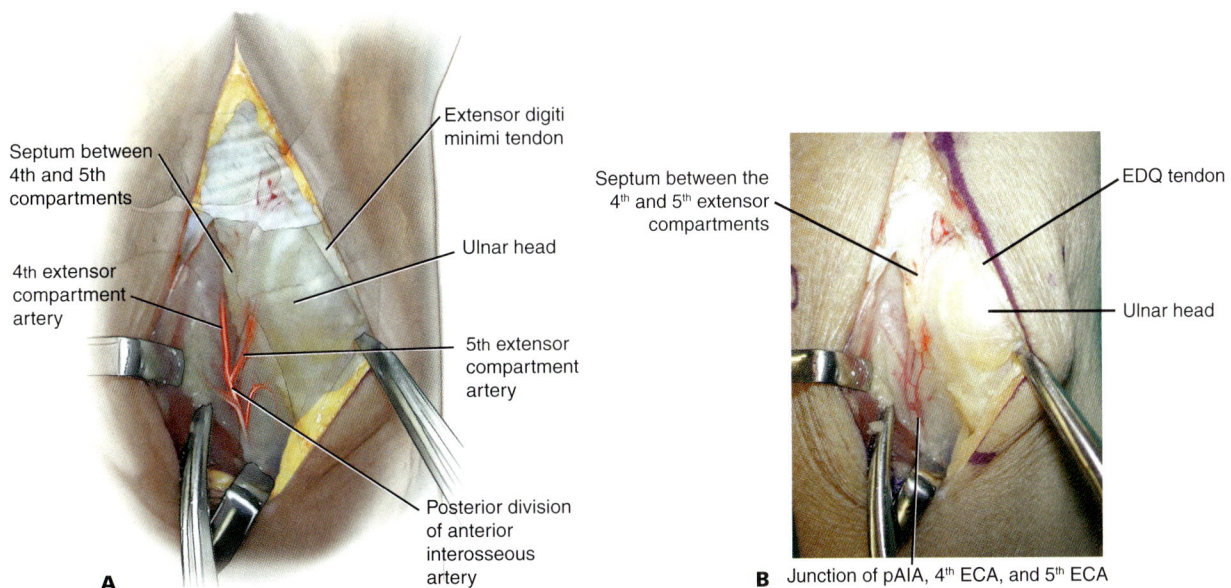

TECH FIG 1 • A. The fifth extensor compartment artery is identified and carefully traced proximally to its origin from the posterior division of the anterior interosseous artery. **B.** Matching clinical photograph showing fourth and fifth extensor compartment arteries. (**B:** Copyright Thomas R. Hunt, III, MD.)

- Perform a ligament-splitting capsulotomy and protect the scapholunate and lunotriquetral ligaments.
- Inspect the lunate, its cartilage shell, and surrounding articular surfaces.
  - Consider vascularized bone grafting only if the shell is not compromised, the bone is not fragmented, and the joint is not arthritic.
- Enter the noncartilaginous portion of the dorsal lunate cortex using a small curette or a 2- to 3-mm round burr.
- Through this dorsal cortical window and under direct visualization and fluoroscopic guidance, carefully remove necrotic bone from the lunate by hand with curved and straight curettes.
  - Leave a shell of intact subchondral bone.
- If the lunate is collapsed, expand it gently using a small blunt-ended lamina spreader.
  - The amount of expansion obtained is highly variable.
  - Use of a lamina spreader in this manner is not suggested in cases with bone fragmentation.
- Determine the graft size required by measuring the dorsal excavated area of the lunate.

Elevation of the Vascularized Bone Graft

- Using a smooth 0.045-inch Kirschner wire, outline the area of the distal radius most infiltrated by nutrient vessels from the fourth ECA.
  - The size of the graft is influenced by the nutrient vessels and the earlier measurement.
- Ligate the posterior division of the anterior interosseous artery proximal to the fourth and fifth ECA branches (**TECH FIG 2**).

- Sharply elevate the vascular pedicle from the bone while protecting the nutrient vessels at the graft site.
- Complete elevation of the corticocancellous graft using sharp osteotomes, with judicious handling of the vascularized pedicle (Tech Fig 2).
- Deflate the tourniquet to verify blood flow to the graft.
- Protect the pedicle graft in a moist sponge.

Placement of the Vascularized Bone Graft into the Lunate

- Obtain cancellous bone graft from the donor site in the distal radius and pack this graft into the lunate cavity using fluoroscopic images for guidance.
- Using small, precise rongeurs, contour the corticocancellous pedicle graft to the size needed.
- Insert the vascularized bone graft with the cortical surface arranged in a proximal–distal orientation and without tension on the vascular leash (**TECH FIG 3**).
  - This allows the graft to serve as a strut to help maintain lunate height during revascularization.
  - No internal fixation is necessary to secure the graft in the lunate.

Closure

- Repair the capsule using absorbable suture, taking great care to avoid pressure on the vascular pedicle.
- Close the extensor retinaculum with absorbable suture and the skin with Prolene.
- Apply a nonocclusive dressing and a volar, below-elbow splint.

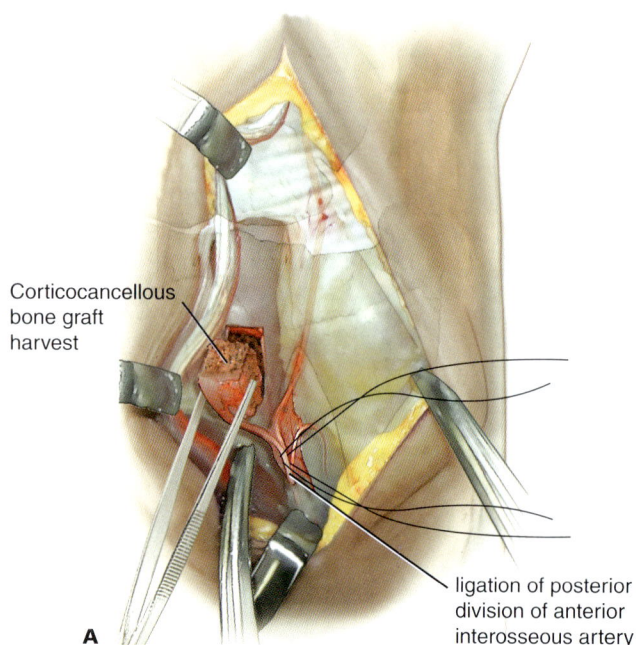

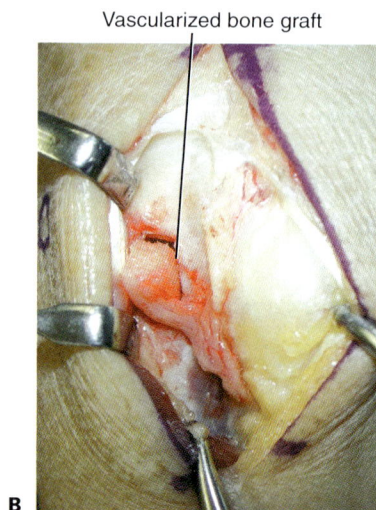

TECH FIG 2 • A, B. Drawing and clinical picture after ligation of the posterior division of anterior interosseous artery (pAIA) and harvest of the corticocancellous bone graft. (**B:** Copyright Thomas R. Hunt, III, MD.)

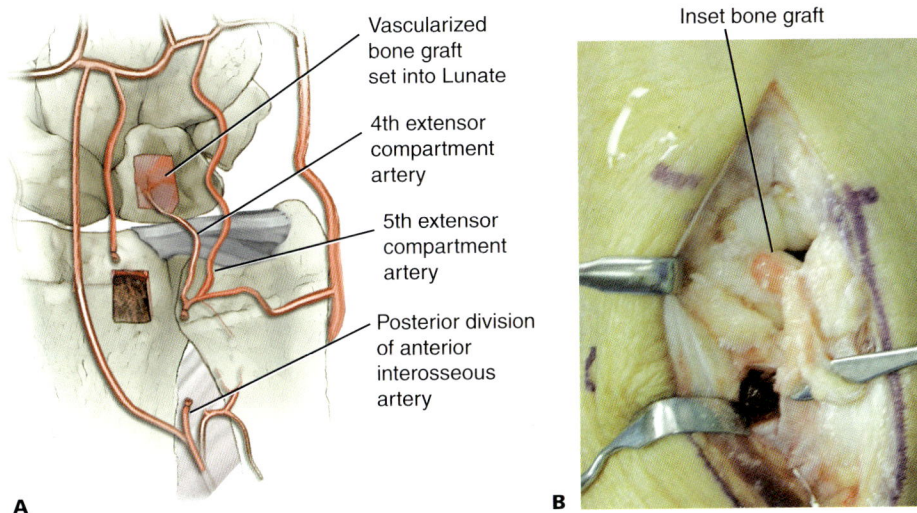

TECH FIG 3 • A, B. Drawing and corresponding clinical picture showing inset of the vascularized bone graft into the prepared lunate. Note the proximal–distal orientation of the cortex. (**B:** Copyright Thomas R. Hunt, III, MD.)

VASCULAR BUNDLE IMPLANTATION

Incision and Approach

- Make an extensive dorsoradial incision extending from the second metacarpophalangeal joint to a point about 4 cm proximal to the wrist, which gently slopes ulnarly around the tubercle of Lister.
  - Visualize and protect the dorsal sensory branch of the radial nerve.
- Incise the extensor retinaculum over the third compartment and transpose the extensor pollicis longus into a subcutaneous position.
- Retract the contents of the fourth extensor compartment ulnarly and the second extensor compartment radially.
- Use fluoroscopy to confirm the lunate's location.
- Perform a standard ligament-splitting capsulotomy.
  - Take care to avoid injury to the transverse basal dorsal metacarpal arch from which the vascular pedicle arises.
- Inspect the lunate and surrounding joints. Perform a synovectomy as required.

Elevation of the Second Dorsal Metacarpal Vascular Pedicle

- In the interval between the second and third metacarpals, incise the interosseous muscle fascia from proximal to distal.
  - The vessels lie underneath the aponeurosis that covers the interosseous muscles.
- Elevate the artery and venae comitantes along with a thin layer of surrounding perivascular areolar tissue from

the second dorsal web space to the dorsal carpal arch (**TECH FIG 4A**).
- Identify and coagulate all branches off this main metacarpal artery.
- Ligate the vessel at its most distal location.
  - This should provide a 5- to 6-cm vessel of adequate length to reach the dorsal lunate.

Lunate Preparation and Implantation of the Vascular Bundle

- Curette and expand the lunate as discussed earlier.
- Pack autogenous cancellous bone graft into the lunate.
- Use a 2.7-mm bit and drill from dorsal to volar through the body of the lunate.
- Sew a 5-0 monofilament suture to the end of the mobilized vessel, then place the suture ends through the eye of a straight needle.
- Feed the vessel into the avascular portion of the lunate by passing the needle from dorsal to volar through the previously drilled hole, exiting the palmar skin just ulnar to the flexor carpi radialis tendon (**TECH FIG 4B**).
- Make a small skin incision over the needle and tie the suture over the palmar antebrachial fascia.
- Release the tourniquet to assess vessel patency.
- Achieve hemostasis and close the capsule, retinaculum, and skin in the manner described earlier.
- Apply a nonocclusive dressing and a volar, below-elbow splint.

TECHNIQUES

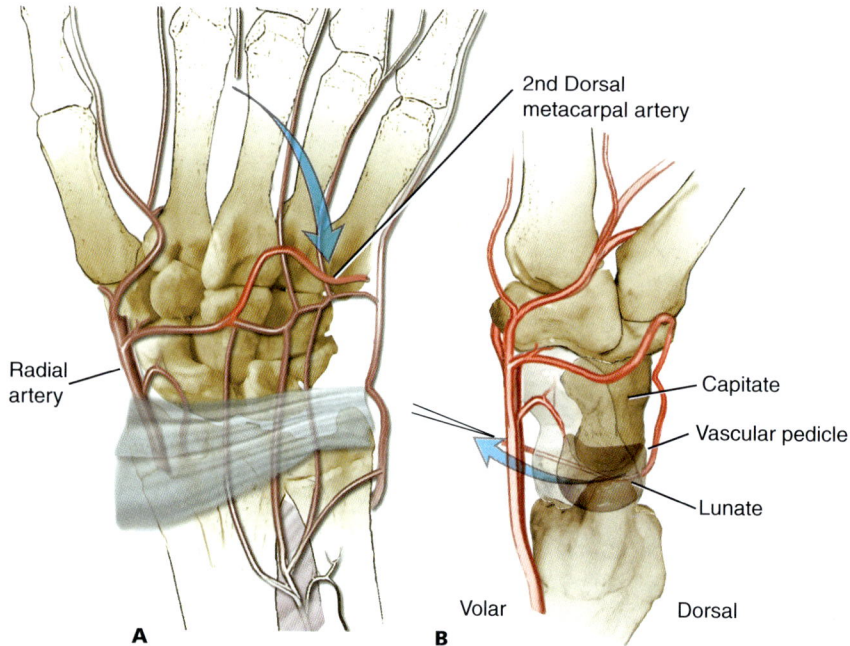

2nd Dorsal metacarpal artery

Radial artery

Capitate

Vascular pedicle

Lunate

Volar   Dorsal

A   B

TECH FIG 4 • A. The artery has been ligated distally and mobilized proximally along with its perivascular tissue. **B.** Fine suture is sewn to the edge of the vessel lumen and placed into a straight Keith needle for insertion into the lunate from a dorsal to volar direction.

CAPITATE SHORTENING OSTEOTOMY

Capitate Osteotomy

- After the capsular-sparing incision is performed for the vascular procedure but before the graft or vessel is inset into the lunate, identify the waist of the capitate and confirm the osteotomy site with fluoroscopic imaging.
  - The osteotomy should correspond to the level of the scaphotrapeziotrapezoidal joints (**TECH FIG 5A**).
- Use a sharp osteotome, a fine water-cooled saw, or both to resect a 2.0-mm wafer bone from the capitate (**TECH FIG 5B**).
  - Complete the proximal cut before the distal cut.
- Perform a trial reduction using a Freer elevator in the midcarpal joint to control and compress the proximal capitate fragment.

- If this trial reduction reveals that the proximal hamate is prominent in the midcarpal joint or the hamate–lunate articulation is incongruous, perform a hamate osteotomy in the same manner and at the same level as the capitate osteotomy.

Osteotomy Fixation

- Compress the two cut surfaces of the capitate manually as discussed earlier in preparation for placement of a cannulated, headless compression screw.
- Place the guidewire across the osteotomy site of the capitate from proximal to distal.
  - Wrist flexion helps present the capitate head into the field. Be careful to avoid distraction of the osteotomy with this maneuver.

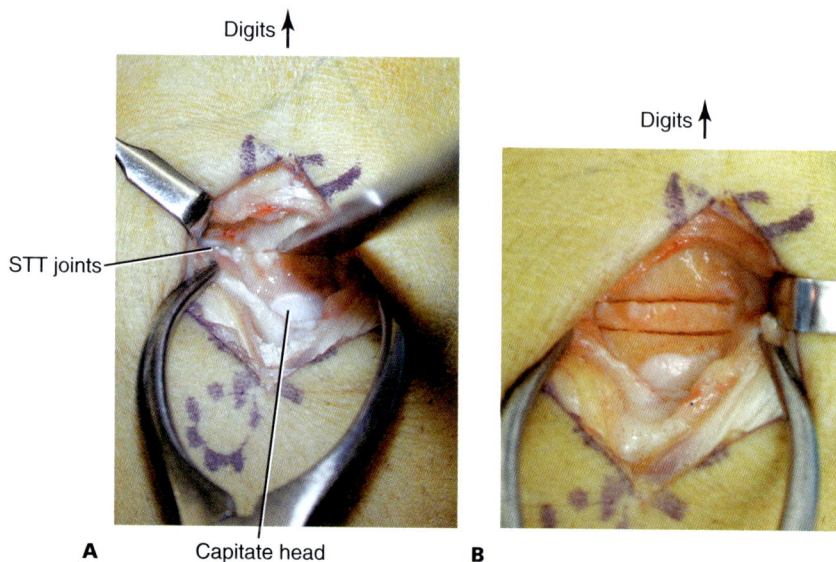

Digits ↑

Digits ↑

STT joints

A   Capitate head   B

TECH FIG 5 • A. The capitate osteotomy is performed at the waist, which corresponds to the level of the scaphotrapeziotrapezoidal joints. **B.** A 2-mm wafer of bone is removed from the capitate. The proximal cut is completed first. The cuts must be parallel to ensure precise reduction. (Copyright Thomas R. Hunt, III, MD.)

- Confirm the placement of the guidewire with fluoroscopy.
- Insert the headless compression screw over the guidewire and achieve compression across the osteotomy site (**TECH FIG 6A**).

- Complete the vascular procedure as indicated and close the wrist capsule, the extensor retinaculum, and the skin (**TECH FIG 6B**).
- Apply a bulky hand dressing with a volar splint.

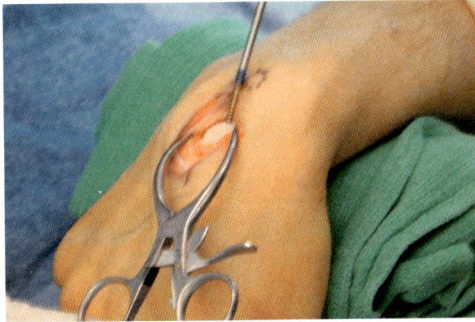

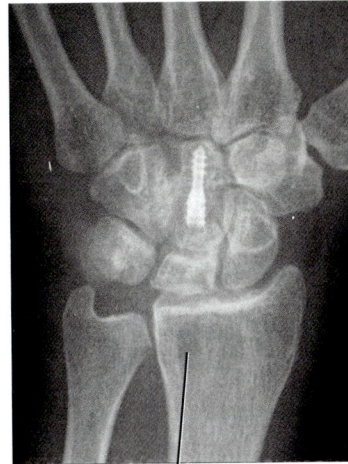

Site of bone graft harvest

TECH FIG 6 • **A.** A headless compression screw is inserted antegrade. Wrist flexion provides access to the capitate head. **B.** Posteroanterior radiograph after vascularized bone grafting and capitate shortening osteotomy. (Copyright Thomas R. Hunt, III, MD.)

PEARLS AND PITFALLS

Tourniquet	▪ Gravity exsanguination allows visualization of the vessels, simplifying exposure and harvest.
Lunate preparation	▪ Examine the cartilage shell of the lunate before harvesting the vascularized graft. Separation of dorsal and volar fragments can take place during débridement and bone expansion if performed in patients with a fracture line noted on the sagittal MRI views.
Elevation of vascularized bone graft	▪ Elevate the vascular pedicle with its perivascular tissue sufficiently to allow tension-free placement of the graft.
Capitate osteotomy	▪ Evaluate the prominence of the hamate at the midcarpal joint. If present, consider performing a hamate shortening osteotomy as well.

POSTOPERATIVE CARE

- Remove the dressing 10 to 14 days postoperatively and apply a below-elbow cast for 3 weeks.
- Remove the cast 4 to 5 weeks after surgery and initiate supervised therapy emphasizing active wrist motion. Over the next 4 weeks the patient can progress to active assisted and then passive range-of-motion exercises.
  - A removable splint is used for 3 to 4 weeks.
- Evaluate the progress of healing using serial radiographs.
- Strengthening is initiated at 3 months after surgery and slowly progressed.
- Patients undergoing revascularization of the lunate are followed for 1 to 3 years.

OUTCOMES

- Lunate revascularization techniques have demonstrated promising clinical results for Kienböck disease.[1,7]
- Mazur et al[4] described the results of nine reverse-flow pedicle grafts obtained from the radius metaphysis in patients with stage IIIA Kienböck disease.

- Grip strength was improved by 25%, ultimately measuring 60% to 100% of the opposite side.
- Range of motion of the wrist joint was not significantly different from the preoperative status.
- Radiographic measurements demonstrated no change in the modified carpal height ratio, lunate index, or scapholunate angle.
- MRI data demonstrated progressive signs of revascularization over time. Normalization of T2 values was seen initially by 18 months, followed by normalization of T1 values by 36 months.
- Moran et al[5] retrospectively reviewed the results of 24 patients treated with vascularized bone graft using 4+5 extensor compartment artery (4+5 ECA).
  - Grip strength improved from 50% to 89% of the unaffected side.
  - Ninety-two percent of the patients had significant improvement in their pain.
  - Seventy-seven percent of patients showed no further collapse on postsurgical radiographs.

- Seventy-one percent of the patients showed evidence of revascularization with improvement in the T2 signal, T1 signal, or both.
- Waitayawinyu et al[9] described the results of 14 patients who had capitate shortening osteotomy with vascularized bone grafting for Kienböck disease; all had positive ulna variance.
  - Grip strength was improved from 58% to 78% of the normal side.
  - Average time to osteotomy healing was 48 days.

COMPLICATIONS

- Failure of revascularization of the lunate or progression of disease may necessitate a second procedure such as intercarpal arthrodesis, proximal row carpectomy, total wrist arthrodesis, or wrist denervation.
- Continued inflammation or disease progression may cause persistent pain, which may require brief periods of splinting during symptomatic flares.

REFERENCES

1. Bouchud RC, Buchler U. Kienböck's disease, early stage 3-height reconstruction and core revascularization of the lunate. J Hand Surg Br 1994;19B:466–478.
2. Galb M, Reinhart C, Lutz M, et al. Vascularized bone graft from the iliac crest for the treatment of nonunion of the proximal part of the scaphoid with an avascular fragment. J Bone Joint Surg Am 1999; 81A:1414–1428.
3. Hori Y, Tamai S, Okuda H, et al. Blood vessel transplantation to bone. J Hand Surg Am 1979;4A:23–33.
4. Mazur KU, Bishop AT, Berger RA. Vascularized bone grafting for Kienböck's disease: method and results of retrograde-flow metaphyseal grafts. American Society for Surgery of the Hand 51st Annual Meeting, Nashville, TN, 1996.
5. Moran SL, Cooney WP, Berger RA, et al. The use of the 4+5 extensor compartmental vascularized bone graft for the treatment of Kienböck's disease. J Hand Surg Am 2005;30A:50–58.
6. Sheetz KK, Bishop AT, Berger RA. The arterial blood supply of the distal radius and ulna and its potential use in vascularized pedicle bone grafts. J Hand Surg Am 1995;20A:902–914.
7. Shin AY, Bishop AT. Vascularized bone grafts for scaphoid nonunions and Kienböck's disease. Orthop Clin North Am 2001;32: 263–277.
8. Tamai H, Yajima H, Mizumoto S, et al. Treament of Kienböck's disease with vascular bundle implantation. Transaction of the American Society of Surgery of the Hand 1980;3:69.
9. Waitayawinyu T, Chin SH, Luria S, et al. Capitate shortening osteotomy with vascularized bone grafting for the treatment of Kienböck's disease in the ulnar positive wrist. J Hand Surg Am 2008;33A:1267–1273.

Chapter 25

Ligament Stabilization of the Unstable Thumb Carpometacarpal Joint

Richard Y. Kim and Robert J. Strauch

DEFINITION

- Thumb carpometacarpal (CMC) joint instability can occur as a result of ligament laxity or trauma.
- Regardless of the cause, injury to the stabilizing ligaments surrounding the CMC joint leads to instability and dorsoradial subluxation or dislocation of the thumb metacarpal.

ANATOMY

- The thumb CMC joint is a biconcave-convex joint similar to a horseback rider's saddle.[4]
- The base of the thumb metacarpal has a prominent volar styloid process (beak) that articulates with a recess in the volar trapezium when in flexion.
- There are 16 ligaments that provide stability to the thumb CMC joint.[1] Of these ligaments, the two that provide the most restraint against dorsoradial subluxation of the thumb metacarpal are the dorsoradial and volar beak ligaments (**FIG 1**).[1,4,12,15]
  - The volar beak ligament (deep anterior oblique ligament, palmar ligament, ulnar ligament) originates from the volar central apex of the trapezium and inserts onto the volar beak of the thumb metacarpal.[1] It lies immediately under a more widely based superficial anterior oblique ligament, which is located immediately deep to the thenar musculature and has a broad insertion across the base of the thumb metacarpal.
  - The dorsoradial ligament originates from the dorsoradial tubercle of the trapezium and inserts onto the dorsal base of

the thumb metacarpal. It is the thickest, widest, shortest, and strongest of the CMC ligaments.[4]

PATHOGENESIS

- The biconcave-convex nature of the thumb CMC joint allows for a wide range of thumb motion but is inherently unstable.[7] Laxity or incompetence of the supporting ligaments, especially the volar beak or dorsoradial ligaments, will cause instability of the thumb CMC joint.[10,12] Especially in middle-aged women, the cause of the laxity is often idiopathic.
- In addition, there is a population of patients who have inherent ligament laxity, such as those with collagen disorders like Ehlers-Danlos syndrome.
- In the setting of trauma, acute thumb CMC joint dislocation occurs with axial loading and flexion of the thumb metacarpal. In all reported cases, the dislocation occurs in a dorsoradial direction.[11,12]

NATURAL HISTORY

- Ligamentous laxity at the thumb CMC joint may cause degenerative changes to the joint cartilage and lead to arthritis, corresponding to higher stages in the Eaton–Littler staging system.[2]
  - If the ligamentous laxity is symptomatic and causing pain, ligament reconstruction can be successful in reducing pain in over 90% of patients. Ligament reconstruction has also been shown to potentially halt the progression of arthritis.[5]

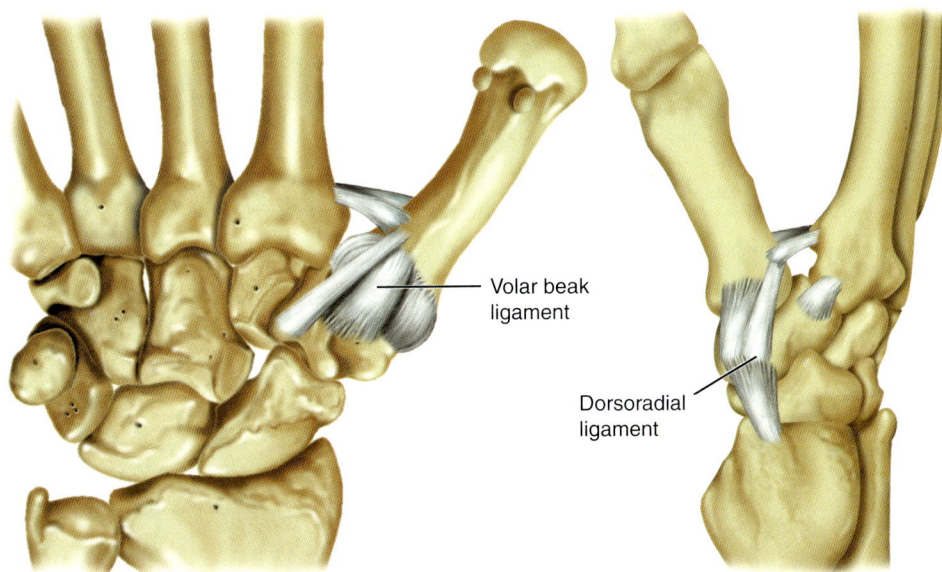

Volar beak ligament

Dorsoradial ligament

FIG 1 • The stabilizing ligaments of the thumb carpometacarpal joint. Of these, the dorsoradial and volar beak ligaments are the most important in preventing dorsoradial subluxation of the thumb metacarpal.

■ For traumatic dislocations, a stable reduction is important for thumb function. If the thumb CMC joint remains unstable, functions such as key pinch and grasp may be compromised.

   ■ Open ligament reconstruction of these unstable thumb CMC joint dislocations may decrease the incidence of recurrent instability and joint degeneration compared to closed reduction and pinning.[11]

PATIENT HISTORY AND PHYSICAL FINDINGS

Nontraumatic Ligamentous Laxity

■ The history should include questions about ligament laxity involving other joints. Metabolic diseases such as Ehlers-Danlos syndrome are notable.

■ Radiographic findings often do not correlate with symptomatology. Therefore, it is important to elicit from the patient the exact symptoms and their severity.

■ Any history of previous nonoperative treatments should be noted. If splinting and steroid injections have not been attempted, it may be beneficial to attempt these treatment modalities before discussing surgery.

■ The physical examination should determine the degree of subluxation and reducibility of the thumb CMC joint.

■ The thumb metacarpophalangeal (MCP) joint should also be examined for possible hyperextension laxity.

■ Pinch strength and opposition should be tested and compared to the contralateral side.

■ The hand should also be evaluated for concomitant carpal tunnel syndrome, flexor carpi radialis tunnel syndrome, and DeQuervain tenosynovitis, as these may also need to be addressed.

Traumatic Injuries

■ In addition to the evaluation cited for nontraumatic laxity, the history and physical examination should include the following:

   ■ Time and nature of the injury

   ■ Status of the thumb before injury

   ■ Stability of joint reduction: This is of major concern in the physical examination because assessment of stability will determine the treatment path.

   ■ Associated MCP joint collateral ligament injury and stability

■ Other associated hand injuries are important to note as well.

■ Tests to perform include the ballottement test and the grind test.

   ■ Tenderness associated with dorsal pressure indicates symptomatic subluxation.

   ■ Crepitance and pain are positive indicators of CMC pathology.

IMAGING AND OTHER DIAGNOSTIC STUDIES

■ AP, lateral, and oblique views of both thumbs should be obtained.

   ■ A true AP (Robert) view is taken with the forearm in maximal pronation and the dorsum of the thumb resting on the imaging table. The beam is then angled 15 degrees from distal to proximal.[4]

   ■ A true lateral film of the thumb is one in which the sesamoids volar to the thumb MCP joint overlap each other.

   ■ A 30-degree oblique stress view of the thumb CMC joint is performed by pressing the radial side of the thumb tips together. This maneuver will subluxate the thumb metacarpal base radially, thereby demonstrating the degree of laxity in the radial direction.[14]

DIFFERENTIAL DIAGNOSIS

■ De Quervain tenosynovitis
■ Flexor carpi radialis tunnel syndrome
■ C6 radiculopathy
■ Trigger thumb

NONOPERATIVE MANAGEMENT

■ For symptomatic ligament laxity and stage I or II basal joint disease, conservative management should first be attempted. This includes thumb spica splint immobilization and anti-inflammatory medications.[6,13]

■ If the symptoms do not improve, a steroid injection into the CMC joint can be attempted. The number of injections should be limited to a maximum of three; theoretically more than three injections increases joint morbidity.

■ In the scenario of acute trauma, reduction of the CMC joint should be performed by applying axial traction and palmar-directed pressure to the base of the thumb metacarpal, along with pronation of the thumb metacarpal. After reduction, if the joint remains reduced, the injury can be treated with cast immobilization.

   ■ If the joint is unstable at all after an attempt at closed reduction, surgical management is indicated.[11]

SURGICAL MANAGEMENT

■ Freedman et al[5] have demonstrated that ligament reconstruction for symptomatic thumb CMC joint laxity can halt or slow the progression to degenerative arthritis. By providing joint stability, shear forces on the CMC joint and translation of the metacarpal on the trapezium can be minimized.

■ In the presence of articular pathology, arthroplasty may be the treatment of choice, depending on the degree of chondromalacia.

■ If greater than 20 degrees of MCP hyperextension is present with lateral pinch, MCP capsulodesis or arthrodesis may also need to be considered.[14]

■ If carpal tunnel syndrome or De Quervain tenosynovitis is present, carpal tunnel release or first dorsal compartment release may be need to be addressed at the time of surgery.

■ For traumatic thumb CMC joint dislocations, Simonian and Trumble have shown that ligament reconstruction was superior to percutaneous pinning of unstable joints.[11]

■ When the injury pattern results in fracture-dislocations such as unstable Bennett and Rolando fractures, percutaneous pinning or open reduction and internal fixation may be the treatment of choice.

Preoperative Planning

■ Plain films should be reviewed.

■ In the case of acute trauma, associated fractures and hand injuries should be addressed.

- A preoperative Allen test should be performed since all procedures involving the thumb CMC joint are in close vicinity to the radial artery, and iatrogenic injury may occur.

Positioning

- The procedure is performed with the patient supine and the arm on a standard hand table.
- The operating table should be turned away from the anesthesia machines to allow the surgeon and assistant to sit across from each other at the hand table.

Approach

- A number of techniques have been described for ligament reconstruction of the thumb CMC joint using a variety of different tendons, including the flexor carpi radialis, palmaris longus, extensor carpi radialis longus, extensor pollicis brevis, and abductor pollicis longus (APL).
- The technique presented here is the classic volar ligament reconstruction described by Eaton and Littler.[3] This method effectively reconstructs both the volar and dorsal ligaments using the flexor carpi radialis.

MODIFIED WAGNER APPROACH TO THE THUMB CMC JOINT

- The incision is started longitudinally along the radial side of the thenar mass, at the junction between the glabrous and nonglabrous skin. The distal extent of the incision is near the midportion of the thumb metacarpal (**TECH FIG 1A**).
- Proximally at the wrist crease, the incision is brought transversely across the wrist to the ulnar side of the flexor carpi radialis tendon.
- Once through the skin, care should be taken to avoid transection of superficial radial sensory nerve branches that may be crossing the operative field.

- The soft tissue is bluntly dissected until the thenar musculature is identified (**TECH FIG 1B**). The radial border of the thenar muscle mass is incised and the muscles are elevated extraperiosteally to expose the CMC joint capsule. The capsule is incised and the thumb metacarpal base, the CMC joint, and the trapezium exposed (**TECH FIG 1C**).
- Blunt dissection is continued dorsally toward the extensor pollicis longus and brevis tendons. The dorsal metacarpal cortex is exposed between these tendons.

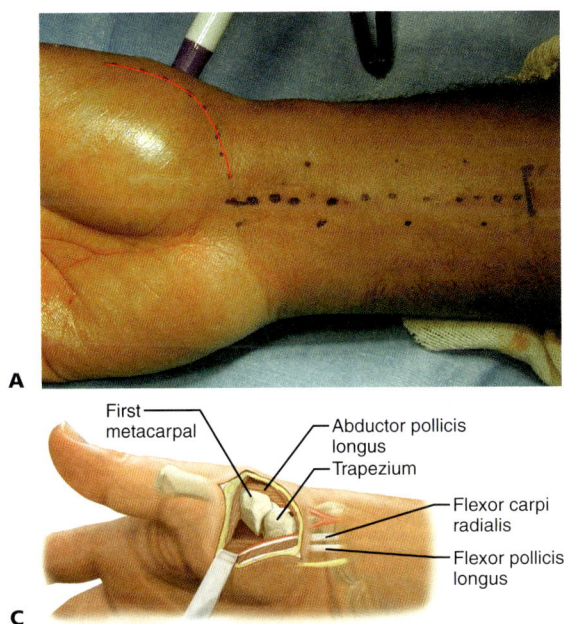

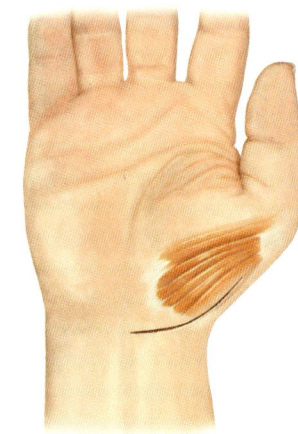

A

B

C

First metacarpal
Abductor pollicis longus
Trapezium
Flexor carpi radialis
Flexor pollicis longus

TECH FIG 1 • A. Modified Wagner incision. **B.** Thenar musculature. **C.** The radial border of the thenar muscles is incised and elevated, exposing the thumb carpometacarpal joint.

FLEXOR CARPI RADIALIS GRAFT HARVEST

- The flexor carpi radialis tendon is identified just radial to the palmaris longus tendon at the wrist crease. The tendon sheath is then opened.
- A transverse incision is made proximally in the forearm overlying the flexor carpi radialis musculotendinous junction, about 8 to 10 cm proximal to the wrist crease (**TECH FIG 2A,B**).

- The soft tissue is bluntly dissected until the tendon sheath is identified and opened. The flexor carpi radialis tendon is then exposed.
- A longitudinal split is made in the midline of the tendon just proximal to its insertion onto the trapezium. A 0 Prolene suture is then passed through the longitudinal split (**TECH FIG 2C**).

- A pediatric feeding tube is now passed from the proximal wound into the distal wound, just underneath the flexor carpi radialis tendon sheath but superficial to the flexor carpi radialis tendon fibers. The tip of the feeding tube is cut off, and the two ends of the Prolene suture are passed through the end of the feeding tube from distal to proximal. Once the suture is seen in the proximal wound, the feeding tube can be removed, leaving the ends of the Prolene suture in the proximal wound site (**TECH FIG 2D–F**).

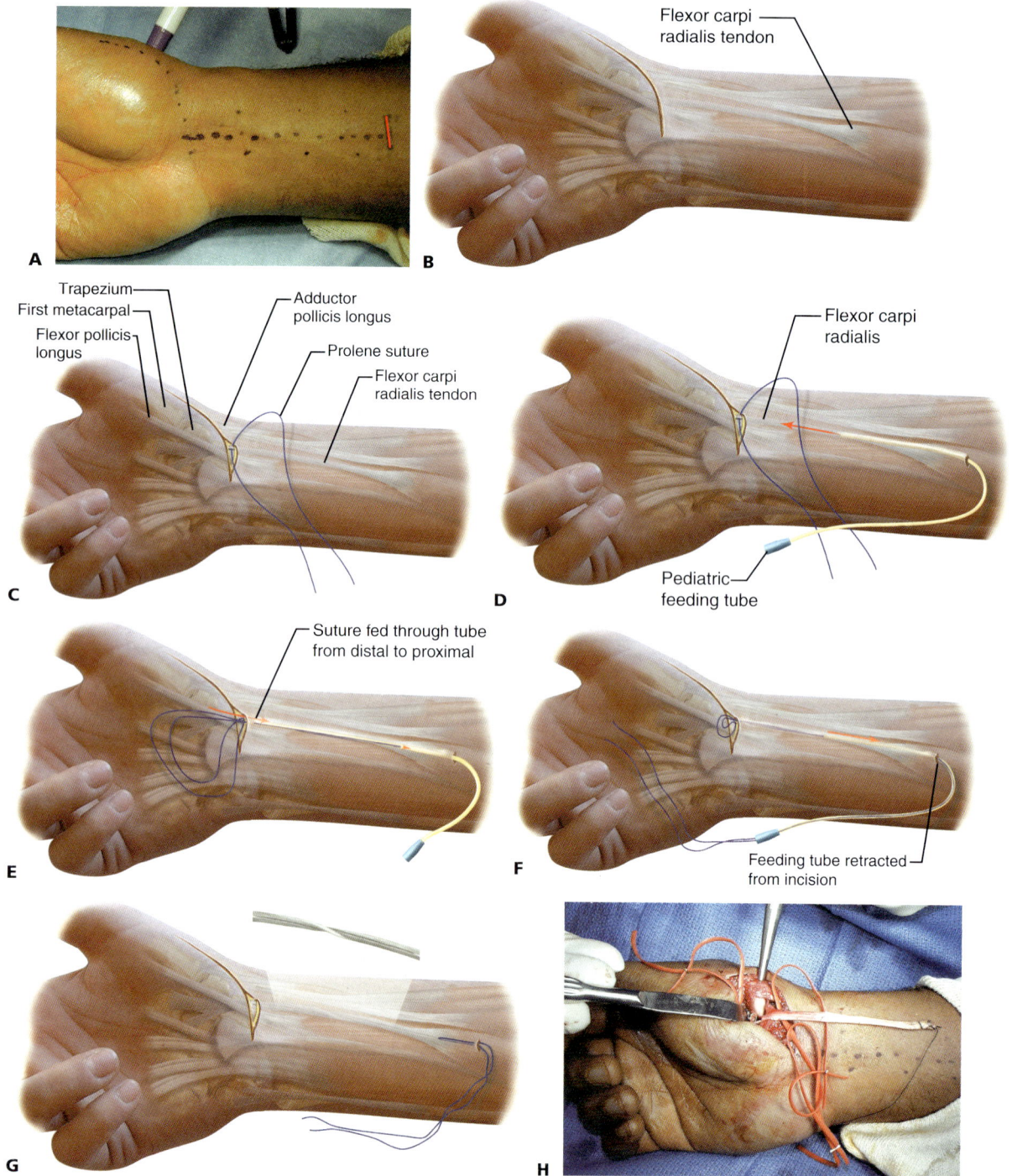

TECH FIG 2 • **A.** Flexor carpi radialis harvest incision is made 8 to 10 cm proximal to the wrist crease. **B.** Flexor carpi radialis musculotendinous junction. **C.** A longitudinal split is made through the flexor carpi radialis distally and a 0 Prolene suture is passed through it. **D.** A pediatric feeding tube is passed from the proximal to the distal wound. **E.** The Prolene suture is then passed through the feeding tube from distal to proximal. **F.** The feeding tube is removed, leaving the Prolene suture ends in the proximal wound. **G.** The two suture ends are pulled, thereby dividing the flexor carpi radialis tendon in half until the proximal wound is reached. The flexor carpi radialis tendon spirals, so the distal radial half corresponds to the proximal ulnar half of the tendon. **H.** The split flexor carpi radialis tendon is delivered into the distal wound.

- The two suture ends in the proximal wound are now pulled so that the rest of the suture is delivered from the distal to the proximal wound. In so doing, the suture will divide the flexor carpi radialis tendon in half along its course into the proximal wound (**TECH FIG 2G**).
- At this time, the ulnar half of the tendon is transected proximally just after the musculotendinous junction. The fibers of the flexor carpi radialis tendon spiral, so the ulnar half of the tendon will continue to become the radial half of the tendon distally at the wrist. Before transection, traction should be applied to the proximal ulnar half of the tendon to ensure that it corresponds to the distal radial half of the tendon.
- The split flexor carpi radialis tendon is finally delivered into the distal wound (**TECH FIG 2H**).

METACARPAL TUNNEL PLACEMENT AND FLEXOR CARPI RADIALIS GRAFT PASSAGE AND FIXATION

- A tunnel is made from dorsal to volar in the thumb metacarpal, 1 cm distal to the articular base. The tunnel should start dorsal to the APL insertion and then course parallel to the articular surface, exiting volarly just distal to the insertion of the volar beak ligament onto the metacarpal base.
  - The tunnel is started by first drilling a 0.045 Kirschner wire from dorsal to volar in the manner described. The tunnel is enlarged by drilling a 0.062 Kirschner wire, followed by a 3.5-mm drill (**TECH FIG 3A,B**).
- Once completed, a nylon whipstitch is placed in the end of the flexor carpi radialis graft. The ends of the stitch are passed through the metacarpal tunnel from a volar to dorsal direction. The stitch is pulled dorsally, delivering the flexor carpi radialis graft through the metacarpal tunnel to the dorsum (**TECH FIG 3C**).
- As the graft exits the dorsal hole in the metacarpal, the thumb is extended and abducted. The graft is pulled tightly and then allowed to relax 2 to 3 mm to set the appropriate tension.

- Once the graft tension is set, the graft is sutured to the metacarpal periosteum where it exits the dorsal hole using nonabsorbable 3-0 suture material.
- The flexor carpi radialis graft is then passed under the APL tendon radially toward the volar side of the wrist. The graft is sutured to the APL with similar nonabsorbable 3-0 suture material as it is passed underneath it.
- The graft is then passed underneath and around the ulnar portion of the flexor carpi radialis tendon that has remained intact. The graft is also sutured to the flexor carpi radialis tendon as it is looped around it.
- If there is additional length to the graft, it is brought back dorsally and again passed underneath and sutured to the APL (**TECH FIG 3D**).
- A 0.045-inch Kirschner wire is drilled from the radial thumb metacarpal base into the trapezium to immobilize the CMC joint. The wire is removed after 5 weeks once adequate soft tissue healing has occurred (**TECH FIG 3E**).

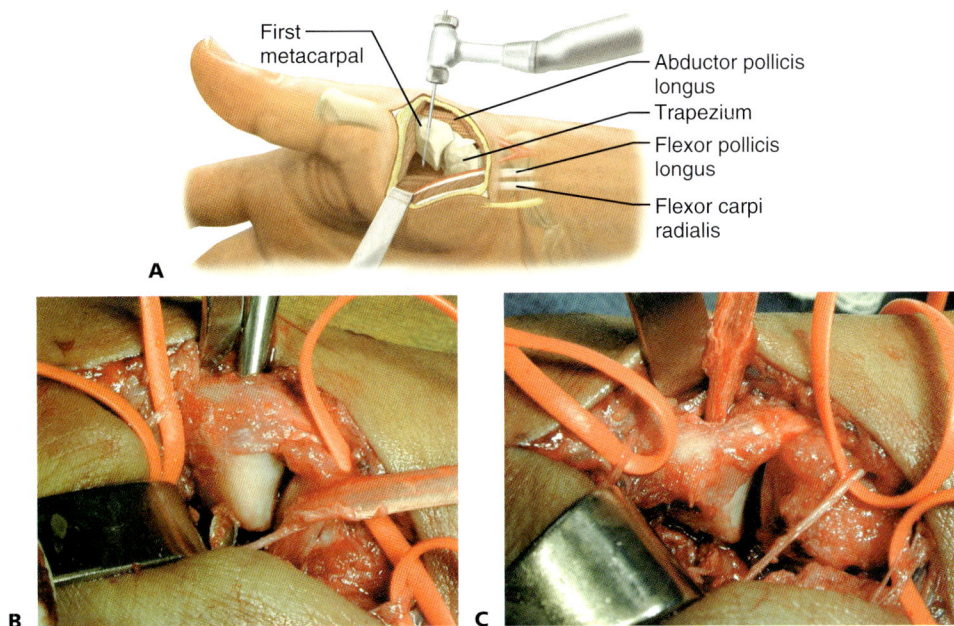

TECH FIG 3 • A. The tunnel is drilled from dorsal to volar, staying parallel and 1 cm distal to the metacarpal articular base. **B.** A curette is shown in the metacarpal tunnel to illustrate its size and direction. **C.** The flexor carpi radialis graft is passed through the tunnel from volar to dorsal. *(continued)*

TECHNIQUES

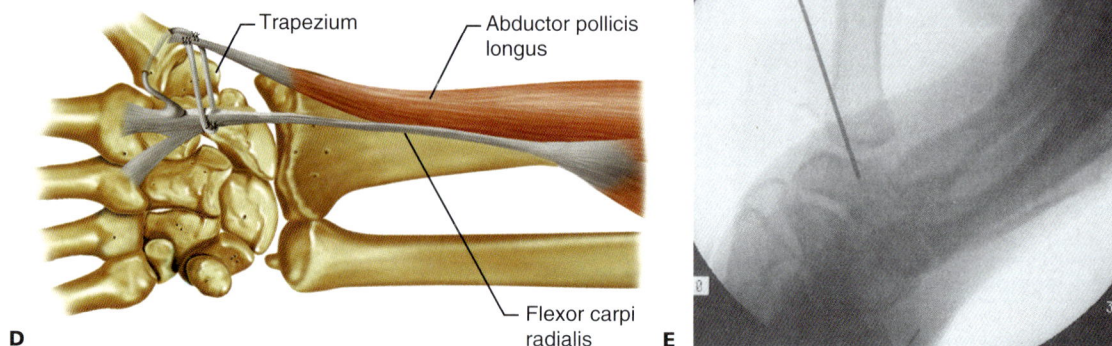

Trapezium

Abductor pollicis longus

Flexor carpi radialis

D

E

TECH FIG 3 • *(continued)* **D.** The flexor carpi radialis graft is passed underneath and sutured to the abductor pollicis longus, the remaining flexor carpi radialis, and back dorsally to the abductor pollicis longus if the graft length permits. **E.** A 0.045 Kirschner wire is drilled from the thumb metacarpal into the trapezium to protect the ligament repair.

WOUND CLOSURE

- The thenar muscle mass is reapproximated and sutured using synthetic absorbable 3-0 suture material.
- The proximal and distal skin incisions are closed with 5-0 nylon sutures (**TECH FIG 4**).
- The hand is then placed in a short-arm thumb spica splint.

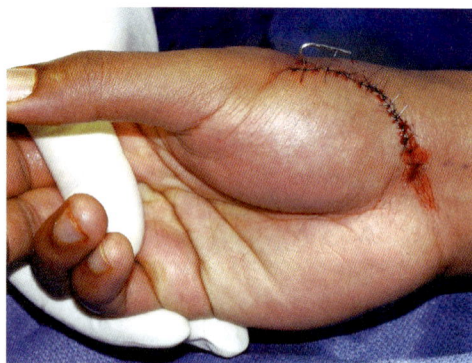

TECH FIG 4 • Final wound closure with nylon sutures.

PEARLS AND PITFALLS

Indications	■ In the setting of stage I or II basal joint disease and ligament laxity, the status of the articular cartilage must be carefully assessed intraoperatively. If significant cartilage damage is present, arthroplasty may be preferred.
Approach	■ Care must be taken to identify and preserve the superficial radial sensory nerve and lateral antebrachial cutaneous nerve branches to prevent neuroma formation.
Flexor carpi radialis graft harvest	■ The entire insertion of the flexor carpi radialis onto the second metacarpal base must be left intact. ■ Transect the proximal portion of the graft near the musculotendinous junction to ensure that adequate graft length will be obtained. ■ Once the graft harvest is completed, the graft should occasionally be moistened through the remainder of the procedure to prevent desiccation and tenocyte injury.
Metacarpal tunnel placement	■ Start with a small-diameter tunnel. Gradually increase the diameter of the tunnel until the graft fits snugly through it. ■ When creating the tunnel, be careful not to injure the insertion of the APL onto the radial base of the thumb metacarpal.
Flexor carpi radialis graft passage and fixation	■ It is important to set the appropriate graft tension. After placing a few periosteal sutures to hold the graft, make sure that the thumb can still be brought back into a neutral position. ■ Before weaving the graft under the APL and around the intact flexor carpi radialis tendons, check an image to ensure that the CMC is adequately reduced. ■ Braided synthetic suture such as Ethibond is soft and may be less palpable than stiffer suture such as Prolene.

POSTOPERATIVE CARE

- AP, lateral, and oblique films or fluoroscopic mini C-arm views are obtained intraoperatively to evaluate CMC joint congruency and Kirschner wire placement.
- The thumb spica splint is left in place for 2 weeks. At 2 weeks of follow-up, the dressings are taken down, sutures are removed, and a new thumb spica splint is applied.
- At 5 weeks of follow-up, the Kirschner wire is removed and a removable thumb splint is used for protection. The splint can be removed for therapy, which can be started at this time.
- Therapy should start with active range-of-motion exercises of the wrist, thumb CMC, MCP, and interphalangeal joints. Thumb abduction, flexion, and opposition are emphasized.
- Strengthening exercises can be started at 2 months after surgery, and full activity without restrictions can begin at 3 months.

OUTCOMES

- When performed for stage I basal joint disease, ligament reconstruction has been shown to improve pain and establish joint stability.
  - In a number of long-term follow-up studies of over 5 years, 87% to 100% of patients demonstrated joint stability against stress testing, 29% to 67% of patients reported no pain, and 83% to 100% reported marked improvement in pain. Interestingly, only 0% to 37% of patients progressed to a higher stage of arthritis.[5,8]
  - Freedman et al[5] reviewed their long-term results of 24 thumbs that underwent ligament reconstruction for stage I or II disease. After a minimum of 10 years of follow-up, 29% of patients reported no pain, 54% reported pain with strenuous activity only, and 17% of patients had pain during activities of daily living. When tested against stress, 87% demonstrated joint stability.
- Simonian and Trumble[11] found that 89% of patients who underwent ligament reconstruction after traumatic thumb CMC dislocation had no pain with work at 2 years of follow-up. Also, none of the patients in this treatment group had any evidence of joint instability, and no revision procedures were required. This is in contrast to 50% of patients who had residual joint instability and pain after closed reduction and percutaneous pinning. Of this treatment group, 38% required revision surgery and underwent ligament reconstruction. 12% of these patients required CMC arthrodesis.

COMPLICATIONS

- Residual joint instability
- Residual pain, likely due to untreated arthritis involving surrounding joint articulations, such as the scaphotrapezial joint
- Radial artery injury
- Superficial radial nerve or lateral antebrachial cutaneous nerve injury
- Pin tract infection

REFERENCES

1. Bettinger PC, Linscheid RL, Berger RA, et al. An anatomic study of the stabilizing ligaments of the trapezium and trapeziometacarpal joint. J Hand Surg Am 1999;24A:786–798.
2. Eaton RG, Glickel SZ, Littler JW. Tendon interposition arthroplasty for degenerative arthritis of the trapeziometacarpal joint of the thumb. J Hand Surg Am 1985;10A:645–654.
3. Eaton RG, Littler JW. Ligament reconstruction for the painful thumb carpometacarpal joint. J Bone Joint Surg Am 1973;55A:1655–1666.
4. Edmunds JO. Traumatic dislocations and instability of the trapeziometacarpal joint of the thumb. Hand Clin 2006;22:365–392.
5. Freedman DM, Eaton RG, Glickel SZ. Long-term results of volar ligament reconstruction for symptomatic basal joint laxity. J Hand Surg Am 2000;25:297–304.
6. Glickel SZ, Gupta S. Ligament reconstruction. Hand Clin 2006;22: 143–151.
7. Imaeda T, An KN, Cooney WP 3rd. Functional anatomy and biomechanics of the thumb. Hand Clin 1992;8:9–15.
8. Lane LB, Eaton RG. Ligament reconstruction for the painful "prearthritic" thumb carpometacarpal joint. Clin Orthop Relat Res 1987;220:52–57.
9. Pellegrini VD Jr. Osteoarthritis of the trapeziometacarpal joint: the pathophysiology of articular cartilage degeneration. I. Anatomy and pathology of the aging joint. J Hand Surg Am 1991;16:967–974.
10. Pellegrini VD Jr. Pathomechanics of the thumb trapeziometacarpal joint. Hand Clin 2001;17:175–184.
11. Simonian PT, Trumble TE. Traumatic dislocation of the thumb carpometacarpal joint: early ligamentous reconstruction versus closed reduction and pinning. J Hand Surg Am 1996;21:802–806.
12. Strauch RJ, Behrman MJ, Rosenwasser MP. Acute dislocation of the carpometacarpal joint of the thumb: an anatomic and cadaver study. J Hand Surg Am 1994;19:93–98.
13. Swigart CR, Eaton RG, Glickel SZ, et al. Splinting in the treatment of arthritis of the first carpometacarpal joint. J Hand Surg Am 1999;24:86–91.
14. Tomaino MM, King J, Leit M. Thumb basal joint arthritis. In Green DP, ed. Green's Operative Hand Surgery, 5th ed. Philadelphia: Elsevier/Churchill Livingstone, 2005.
15. Van Brenk B, Richards RR, Mackay MB, et al. A biomechanical assessment of ligaments preventing dorsoradial subluxation of the trapeziometacarpal joint. J Hand Surg Am 1998;23:607–611.

Chapter 26

Operative Treatment of Thumb Carpometacarpal Joint Fractures

John T. Capo and Colin Harris

DEFINITION

- The first carpometacarpal (CMC) joint comprises the thumb metacarpal base and the trapezium.
- The thumb CMC joint is vital to the function of the hand, and injuries can result in pain, weakness, and loss of grip or pinch strength.
- Two fracture-dislocation patterns commonly result from trauma to the thumb CMC joint: Bennett and Rolando fractures.
  - Bennett fractures are intra-articular fractures in which the metacarpal shaft is radially displaced by the pull of the abductor pollicis longus tendon, leaving an intact ulnar fragment at the base of the thumb metacarpal that is held reduced by the strong volar beak ligament (**FIG 1A**).
  - Rolando fractures are complex intra-articular fractures involving the base of the thumb metacarpal that often have a T- or Y-type pattern. These fractures are classically described as being three-part; however, the name also applies to more comminuted fracture variants (**FIG 1B**).[8]

ANATOMY

- Understanding the deforming forces in these fracture-dislocations is important when deciding on treatment options and determining prognosis.
- The thumb metacarpal serves as the site of attachment for several tendons, including the abductor pollicis longus (APL) at the proximal base, the adductor pollicis (AP) distally, and the thenar muscles volarly.[15]
- The articular surfaces of the thumb metacarpal base and trapezium resemble reciprocally interlocking saddles and allow motion in many planes.[10,15]
- Joint stability is maintained by five primary ligaments: the anterior-volar (beak), the posterior oblique, the dorsal radial, and the anterior and posterior intermetacarpal ligaments (**FIG 2**).[18]

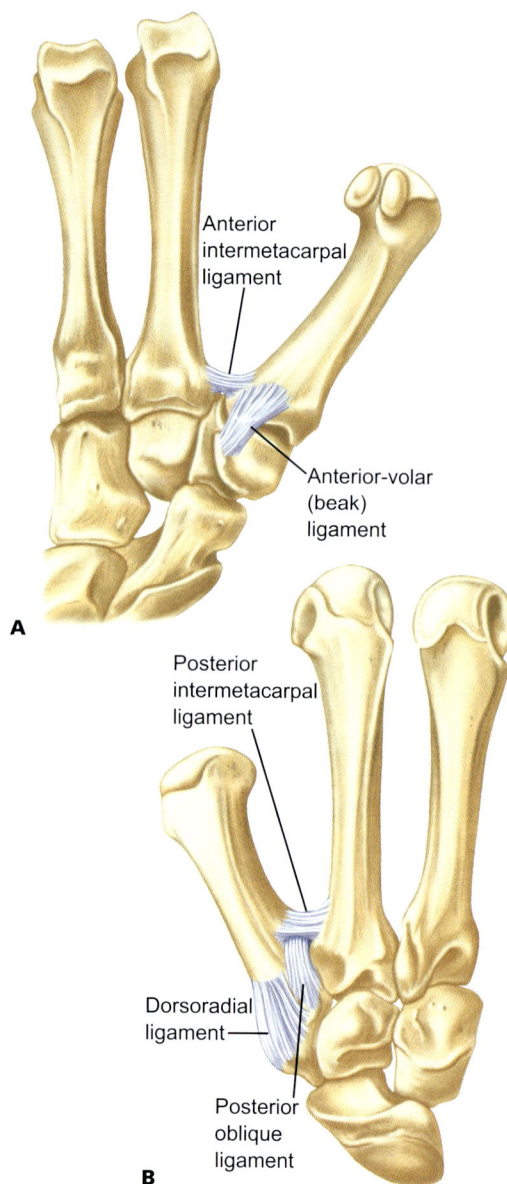

FIG 2 • **A,B.** Anterior and posterior views of the thumb basal joint stabilizing ligamentous structures. The crucial anterior, volar-oblique (beak) ligament is often attached to the displaced Bennett fragment.

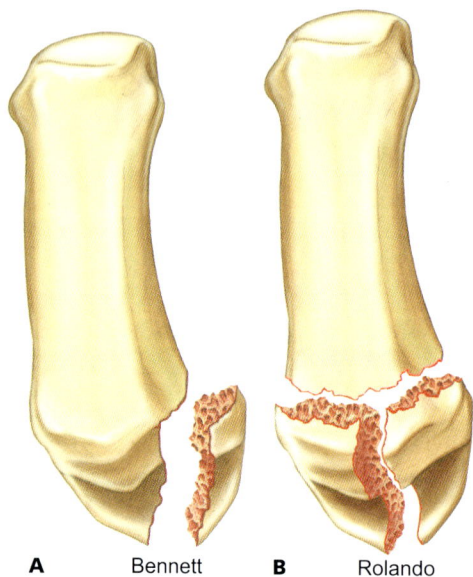

FIG 1 • **A.** A typical Bennett fracture is a unicondylar fracture of the base of the first metacarpal with the fracture fragment consisting of the volar-ulnar corner of the proximal metacarpal. **B.** A Rolando fracture is multifragmentary, with the entire articular base of the metacarpal being involved. By definition, no portion of the metacarpal shaft is in continuity with the carpometacarpal joint.

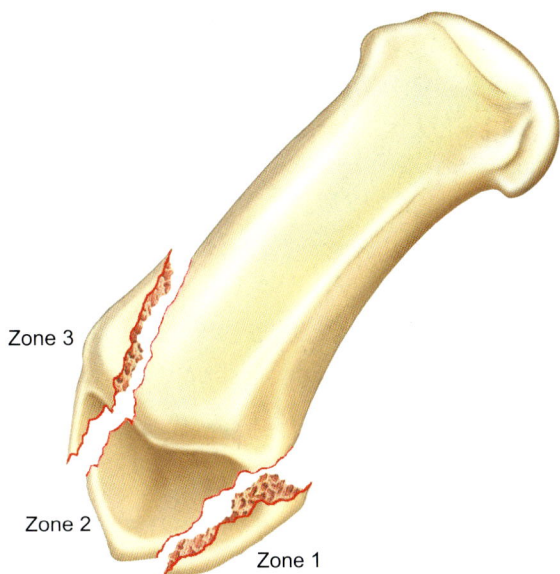

FIG 3 • The three zones found in fractures of the first metacarpal base. The central zone 2 is critical for joint stability and if involved usually requires open reduction and internal fixation.

- Buchler et al[2] described three zones at the base of the thumb metacarpal (**FIG 3**):
  - Zone 2 represents the central portion of the joint that is normally loaded.
  - Zone 1 includes the volar aspect of the joint.
  - Zone 3 involves the dorsal aspect of the joint.
- The trapezium has several important adjacent articulations. These include the first metacarpal base, the radial aspect of the second metacarpal base, the scaphoid, and the trapezoid (along with the trapezium, these last two make up the STT joint).

PATHOGENESIS

- Bennett fractures occur when the partially flexed thumb metacarpal is axially loaded, resulting in a Bennett articular fragment (the volar-ulnar portion of the metacarpal base) and the remainder of the metacarpal that displaces dorsally, proximally, and radially.
- Rolando fractures result from a similar injury mechanism and may have a variable degree of comminution at the base of the thumb metacarpal.
- In Bennett-type fractures, the thumb metacarpal shaft is displaced dorsally and proximally by the pull of the APL at the metacarpal base, and angulated ulnarly by the AP and the extensor pollicis longus (EPL) tendons, which insert more distally on the digit.[15]
- Rolando-type fractures are subject to the same deforming forces, except that the APL can sometimes displace both the shaft and the dorsal-radial basilar articular fragment.
- Due to the deforming forces that act on the fracture fragments, both injury patterns are usually unstable and difficult to reduce and stabilize by closed means.

NATURAL HISTORY

- Injuries to the thumb CMC joint are the most common of all thumb fractures.[4,8]

- Nonoperative treatment is generally reserved for nondisplaced fractures. There is a low likelihood of maintaining reduction using closed means in displaced fractures.
- Residual subluxation of the metacarpal shaft leads to basal joint incongruity and the potential for developing posttraumatic arthrosis.[5] In addition, residual intra-articular step-off greater than 1 mm may predispose to the development of arthrosis, although this has not been found to be true in all studies.[5,6,19]

PATIENT HISTORY AND PHYSICAL FINDINGS

- Most of these fractures occur with direct trauma to the thumb tip, often from a fall or sports-related injury.
- The injury is most common in young males, and two thirds occur in the dominant hand.[8,15]
- The history should reveal whether the patient had preexisting basal joint arthritis, which is common and will affect treatment options and expected results.
- Common physical examination findings include tenderness and ecchymosis surrounding the thumb CMC joint, crepitus with attempted motion, instability, and a "shelf" deformity resulting from displacement of the metacarpal shaft dorsally (**FIG 4**).[16]
  - Metacarpal subluxation or dislocation represents an unstable fracture.
- Range of motion is decreased and may be associated with crepitus. Adjacent joints may also have arthrosis and decreased range of motion.
- It is important to perform a complete neurovascular examination and to search for associated pathology such as wrist ligamentous injuries.
  - Neurovascular injuries are uncommon but compartment syndrome should be suspected in higher-energy injuries.
- Tendon function should be examined, specifically the EPL, flexor pollicis longus (FPL), and extensor pollicis brevis (EPB).

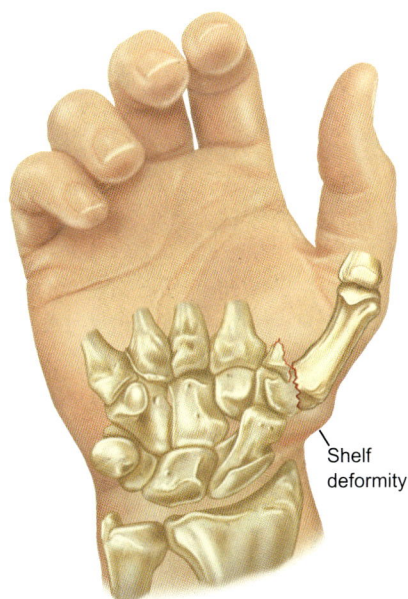

FIG 4 • A typical shelf deformity is depicted in a Bennett fracture. When viewing the thumb from the lateral perspective, the thumb metacarpal shaft can be seen riding dorsally as it displaces from the unstable carpometacarpal joint.

IMAGING AND OTHER DIAGNOSTIC STUDIES

- AP, lateral, and oblique images of the hand should be obtained, although the oblique plane of the thumb in relation to the hand may make these images difficult to interpret.
  - A true AP view of the thumb CMC joint can be obtained with the forearm maximally pronated with the dorsum of the thumb placed on the cassette (**FIG 5A**).[17]
  - A true lateral view, advocated by Billing and Gedda,[1] is obtained with the hand pronated 20 degrees and the thumb positioned flat on the cassette. The x-ray beam is tilted 10 degrees from vertical in a distal-to-proximal direction (**FIG 5B**).
  - Radiographs of the contralateral, uninjured basal joint are helpful in certain cases as a template for reconstruction.
- Computed tomography may be indicated if a significant amount of articular comminution is present or when plain films inadequately demonstrate the pathology.
- A traction view may be helpful in Rolando-type fractures in which nonoperative treatment is being considered and tomography is not available (**FIG 5C**).
- Fluoroscopy alone should be used with caution in ensuring anatomic reduction as this has recently been shown to be less accurate than plain x-rays or direct visualization.[3]

DIFFERENTIAL DIAGNOSIS

- Bennett-type fracture
- Rolando-type fracture
- Basal joint degenerative joint disease
- STT joint arthrosis
- Thumb CMC joint ligamentous injury
- Trapezial body fracture
- De Quervain tenosynovitis

NONOPERATIVE MANAGEMENT

- Nondisplaced, minimally comminuted fractures may be treated with closed reduction and thumb spica casting, but precise molding of the cast and close observation for fracture displacement are necessary.
- In a Bennett fracture, closed treatment may be indicated if there is minimal displacement between the volar ulnar fragment and the metacarpal shaft. Most importantly, a concentric reduction of the metacarpal base in Bennett fractures must be maintained.[6]
- Several factors make closed treatment of these intra-articular fractures problematic and worsen results:
  - Difficulty in providing accurate three-point molding of the thumb metacarpal
  - Treatment of patients 4 or more days after the initial injury
  - Difficulty assessing the adequacy of reduction with radiographs taken through the cast[4,9]
- Some studies looking at closed treatment have demonstrated decreased motion, grip strength, and radiographic evidence of degenerative joint disease at long-term follow-up.[14]
- Development of degenerative changes may occur if there is any residual subluxation of the thumb metacarpal shaft.[5,8]

SURGICAL MANAGEMENT

- The majority of displaced Bennett fractures and almost all Rolando fractures require percutaneous Kirschner wire fixation or open reduction and internal fixation.
- The goals of surgery are to restore the articular congruity of the thumb CMC joint and to align the first metacarpal base articular surface with the trapezium.
- In thumb CMC joint fractures associated with trapezial body fractures, the trapezial articular surface should first be reduced anatomically before proceeding to the thumb metacarpal fracture.[16]

Bennett Fractures

- Closed reduction and percutaneous pinning is the preferred treatment for most Bennett fractures with displaced fracture fragments representing less than 25% to 30% of the articular surface.[16,18]

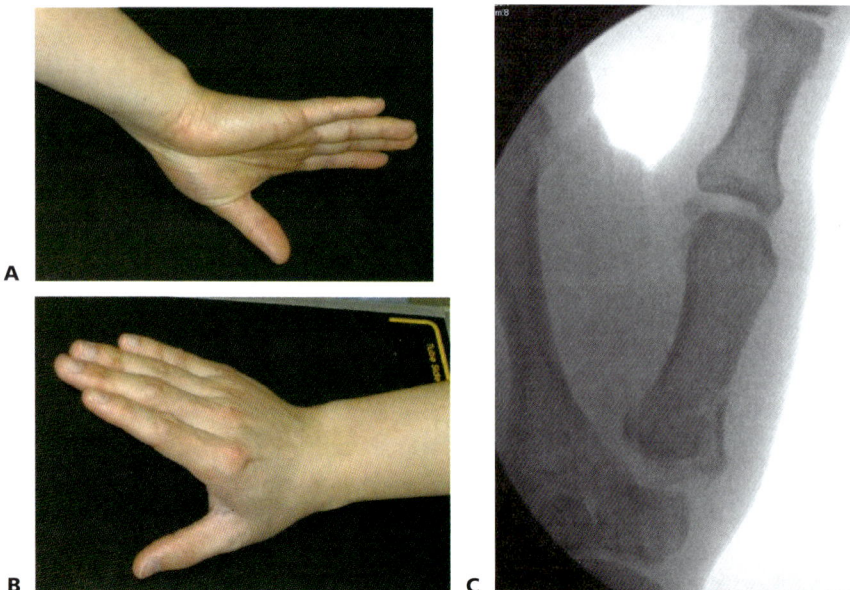

FIG 5 • **A.** An ideal AP view of the thumb and carpometacarpal joint is taken with the forearm hyperpronated and the dorsum of the thumb on the cassette. **B.** A true lateral view of the carpometacarpal joint is obtained with the radial aspect of the thumb on the cassette and the other fingers clear of the x-ray beam. **C.** A fluoroscopic view of a Rolando fracture with traction applied. Distraction at the carpometacarpal joint helps to delineate the fragments at the base of the metacarpal. (Copyright John Capo, MD.)

- The metacarpal base often needs to be pinned to the unfractured second metacarpal, trapezoid, or trapezium to lessen the deforming forces on the fracture.
- Residual displacement of the joint surface greater than 2 mm after attempted closed reduction and percutaneous pinning or impaction in the force-bearing aspect of the joint surface (Buchler zone 2) necessitates open reduction.[15]

Rolando Fractures

- Closed reduction with longitudinal traction and percutaneous pinning is indicated if successful reduction can be achieved under fluoroscopic guidance; however, this is usually successful only when large T- or Y-type fragments are present.
- If the joint cannot be reduced by closed methods, open reduction and internal fixation with a combination of smooth wires, screws, and 1.5- to 2.7-mm L, T, or blade plates is indicated.
- Significant comminution may require either external fixation or a combination of external fixation, limited internal fixation with Kirschner wires and small (1.3 or 1.5 mm) screws, and cancellous bone grafting as advocated by Buchler et al.[2]
- An additional option is tension-band wiring with or without external fixation, as described by Howard.[11] The external fixator maintains length and alignment, while the tension-band construct provides stability to the fracture fragments.

Preoperative Planning

- A thorough history and physical examination are mandatory to choose the appropriate treatment and rule out associated injuries.
- True AP, lateral, and oblique radiographs of the thumb should be obtained in all cases. Traction radiographs help assess the effects of ligamentotaxis on fracture reduction.
- Surgery may be performed acutely, but if significant soft tissue swelling is present, elevation in a well-padded thumb spica splint for 2 to 5 days may be necessary before undergoing operative fixation.[16]

Positioning

- The patient is placed supine on the operating room table.
- A radiolucent hand table is used to allow for intraoperative fluoroscopy.
- The patient is moved toward the operative side to center the hand on the table.
- A non-sterile tourniquet is placed on the upper arm.
- General, regional (axillary or infraclavicular), or local (wrist block with local infiltration) anesthesia can be used, although muscle relaxation is often necessary to obtain proper reduction.[16,18]

Approach

- The Wagner approach can be used for both Bennett and Rolando fractures in which open reduction is necessary.

CLOSED REDUCTION AND PERCUTANEOUS PINNING OF BENNETT AND ROLANDO FRACTURES

- Longitudinal traction, abduction, and pronation of the thumb is performed while applying direct manual pressure over the metacarpal base.[16]

- Traction is maintained and the reduction is held while fluoroscopy is used to verify acceptable fracture reduction and alignment of the articular surface (**TECH FIG 1A,B**).

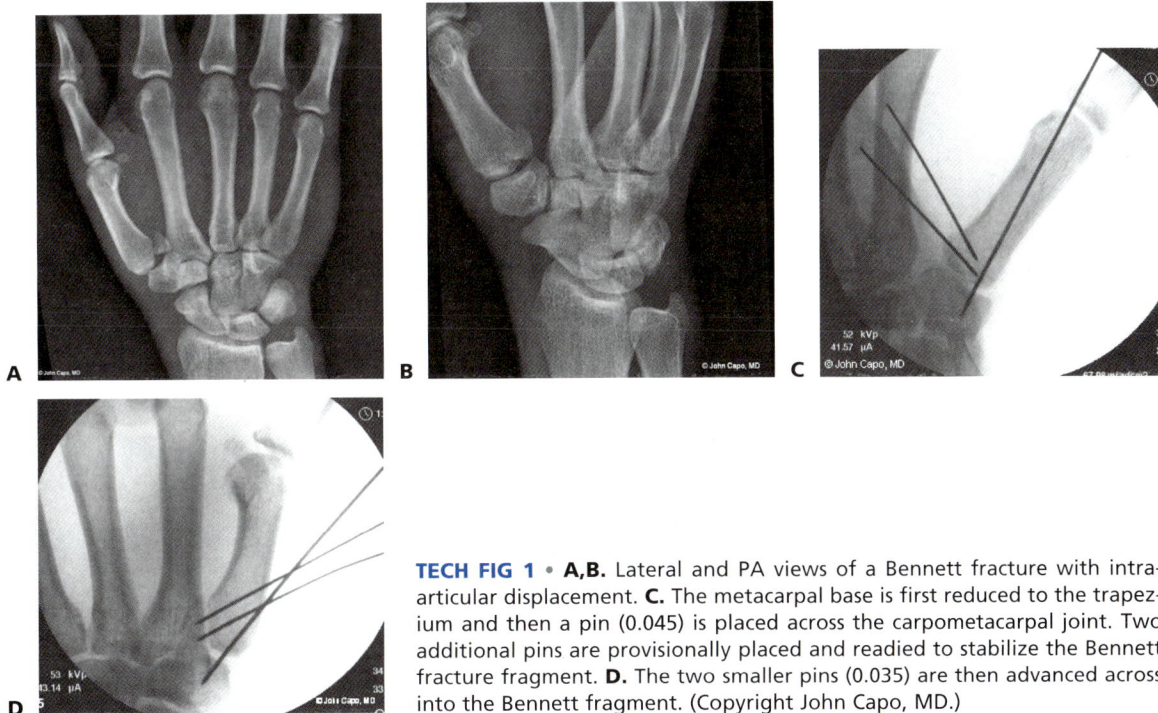

TECH FIG 1 • **A,B.** Lateral and PA views of a Bennett fracture with intra-articular displacement. **C.** The metacarpal base is first reduced to the trapezium and then a pin (0.045) is placed across the carpometacarpal joint. Two additional pins are provisionally placed and readied to stabilize the Bennett fracture fragment. **D.** The two smaller pins (0.035) are then advanced across into the Bennett fragment. (Copyright John Capo, MD.)

TECHNIQUES

TECHNIQUES

- Smooth 0.045-inch Kirschner wires are inserted from the proximal thumb metacarpal shaft into the uninjured index metacarpal base or trapezium. These wires stabilize the concentrically reduced metacarpal shaft and CMC joint (**TECH FIG 1C**).
- The size of the articular Bennett fracture determines whether fixation to this fragment is needed (**TECH FIG 1D**).
- Large fragments may be manipulated percutaneously with Kirschner wire "joysticks" and then stabilized.

- The wires are bent and cut outside of the skin, followed by application of a well-padded thumb spica splint with the thumb in abduction and wrist in extension.
- If less than 2 mm of step-off cannot be obtained by closed reduction, the surgeon should consider abandoning this technique for an open reduction and internal fixation.[16,18]
- In rare instances, a similar technique can be used for Rolando fractures, with large T- or Y-type fracture patterns with minimal comminution.

OPEN REDUCTION AND INTERNAL FIXATION OF BENNETT FRACTURES

Incision and Dissection

- A Wagner approach is used for open reduction of a Bennett fracture (**TECH FIG 2A**).
- An incision is made on the dorsal-radial aspect of the thumb CMC joint, at the junction of the glabrous and nonglabrous skin, and curved in a volar direction toward the distal wrist crease to the flexor carpi radialis (FCR) tendon sheath (**TECH FIG 2B**).
  - The palmar cutaneous branch of the median nerve, the superficial radial nerve, and distal branches of the lateral antebrachial cutaneous nerve are at risk in this approach and should be carefully protected (**TECH FIG 2C**).
- The thenar muscles are elevated extraperiosteally from the CMC joint and a longitudinal capsulotomy is made to expose the joint and the fracture fragments.
- An effort should be made to preserve all soft tissue attachments to the fracture fragments (**TECH FIG 2D**).
- The fracture line is exposed and cleaned of all hematoma and early callus.
  - This often requires abduction, supination, and dorsal displacement of the metacarpal shaft to expose the volar-ulnar Bennett fragment.

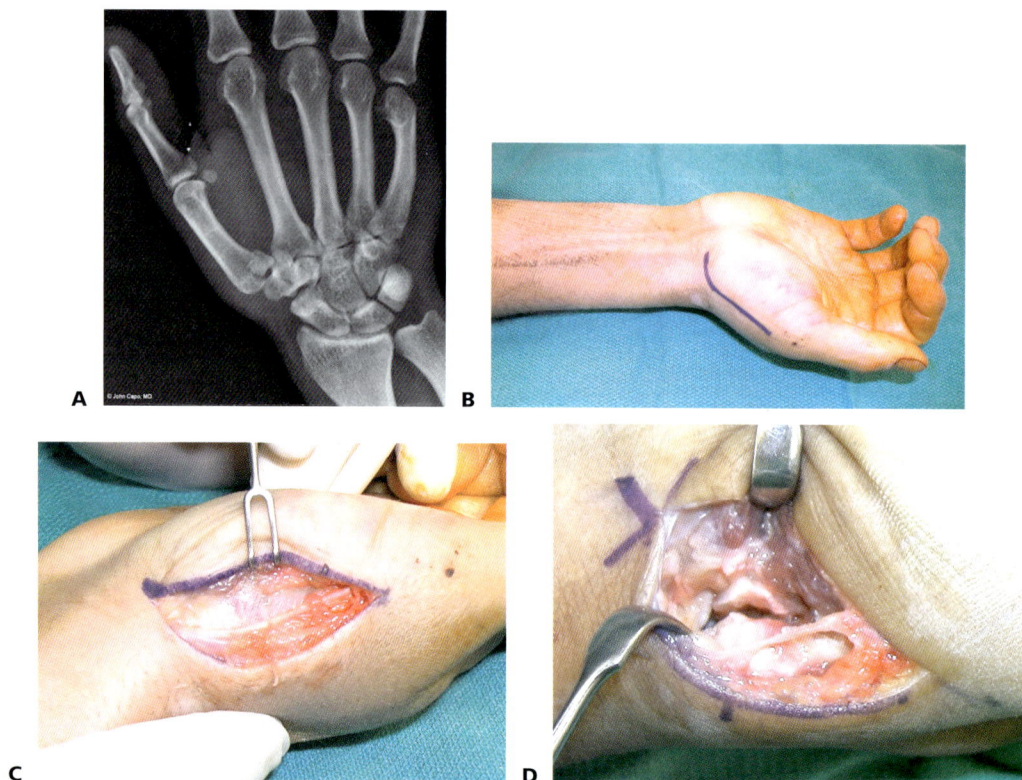

TECH FIG 2 • A. A preoperative radiograph demonstrating a large (~40%) Bennett fracture with intra-articular displacement. **B.** The typical incision for open reduction and internal fixation of a Bennett or Rolando fracture. The proximal aspect starts at the flexor carpi radialis tendon sheath. In the case of a Rolando fracture, especially one treated by plate fixation, the distal portion of the incision should extend along the thumb metacarpal. **C.** Distal nerve branches are seen during the exposure of these fractures. The nerves can usually be retracted dorsally to allow exposure of the carpometacarpal joint. **D.** The thenar muscles are reflected volarly and the carpometacarpal joint is entered. The volar, oblique fracture is now clearly visualized. Care is taken to maintain soft tissue attachments. (Copyright John Capo, MD.)

TECHNIQUES

Reduction and Fixation

- The displaced thumb metacarpal shaft should be reduced to the volar-ulnar fragment under direct visualization and secured with fine reduction clamps or Kirschner wires (**TECH FIG 3A**).
- One or two 0.045-inch smooth Kirschner wires are used to provisionally hold the reduction, or in certain fracture patterns they can serve as the definitive means of fixation.
- Alternatively, 1.3- to 2.0-mm screws can be placed in an interfragmentary compression fashion for added stability (**TECH FIG 3B**).[7]
  - One Kirschner wire is removed at a time and replaced with a screw.
  - Generally, the path of the removed Kirschner wire effectively guides the drill in the appropriate direction. Use of a mini-fluoroscopy unit is helpful.

- Care should be exercised to avoid overcompression, which may cause an alteration in the arc of curvature of the articular surface.
- If fixation is tenuous, the metacarpal base can be pinned to the second metacarpal or to the carpus for added stability.
- Anatomic reduction of the articular surface is verified under direct visualization.
- The wound is closed in layers with absorbable suture in the capsule, followed by nylon sutures in the skin. A thumb spica splint is applied.
- The screws should be precisely evaluated fluoroscopically to be certain they are not in the CMC joint or adjacent second metacarpal base (**TECH FIG 3C,D**).

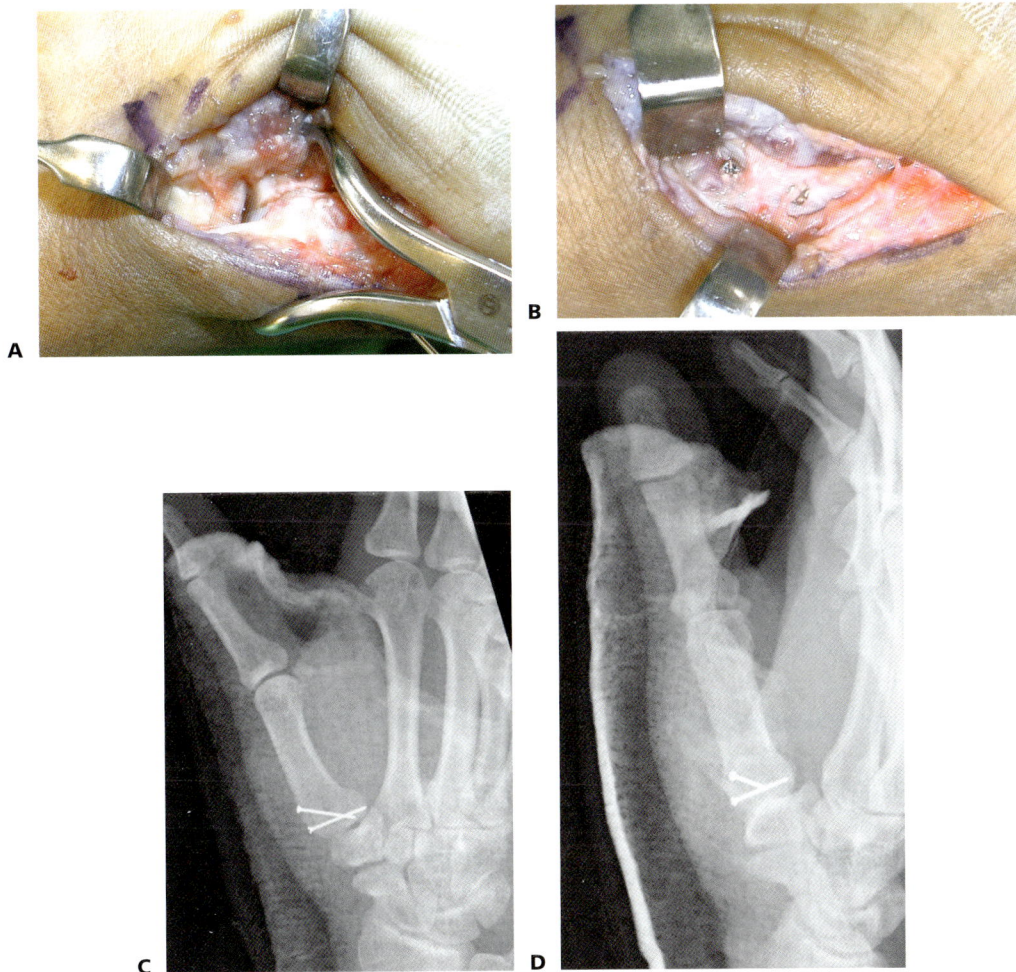

TECH FIG 3 • A. The fracture is cleared of hematoma and then reduced with a pointed reduction forceps. A provisional Kirschner wire is placed percutaneously from the dorsal metacarpal shaft into the fragment. **B.** Two screws of 1.3 mm diameter are placed in a lag fashion from the metacarpal shaft into the fracture fragment. **C,D.** Lateral and AP postoperative views showing reduction of the fracture and articular surface with two screws inserted in different planes. (Copyright John Capo, MD.)

TECHNIQUES

OPEN REDUCTION AND INTERNAL FIXATION OF ROLANDO FRACTURES

Incision and Dissection

- The previously described Wagner approach is used to expose the thumb CMC joint (**TECH FIG 4A,B**).
- The radial portion of the incision is extended distally to expose the diaphysis of the thumb metacarpal. Branches of the radial sensory nerve must be protected at this stage (**TECH FIG 4C**).

Reduction and Fixation

- The basilar-articular fragments are then reduced under direct visualization and provisional fixation is performed with Kirschner wires or bone reduction clamps (**TECH FIG 5A**).
- A lag screw can be placed in a transverse direction by overdrilling the proximal cortex to compress the basilar fragments together, followed by application of a minifragment neutralization plate or by additional Kirschner wires to stabilize the shaft (**TECH FIG 5B,C**).[6,16]
- If greater fracture stability is desired, a small (1.5 to 2.7 mm) T, L, or blade plate can be used alone.
  - The palmar radial incision is extended further distally to expose the thumb metacarpal shaft to accommodate the plate.
  - Reduction is obtained using the above techniques, with axial traction to maintain appropriate length

and bone reduction forceps or smooth Kirschner wires to provisionally hold the articular reduction.
- Once the fracture fragments are aligned, the plate is secured to the thumb metacarpal, with the transverse portion of the plate placed over the basilar fracture fragments.[16]
- The most palmar and dorsal proximal holes of the T portion of the plate can be drilled eccentrically to allow for compression at the fracture site between the basilar fragments,[7,13] followed by fixation of the plate to the metacarpal shaft with cortical screws (**TECH FIG 5D,E**).
- Additionally, a lag screw can be placed between the shaft and the basilar fragment either within or outside of the plate. An appropriate bit is used for overdrilling of the shaft fragment, followed by core drilling of the distal basilar fragment. This interfragmentary screw increases the stability of the construct and may allow for earlier functional range of motion (**TECH FIG 5F–I**).
- The joint surface reduction is visualized directly with distal traction of the thumb and ensured to be anatomic.
- The wound is then irrigated and closed in layers, followed by immobilization in a well-padded thumb spica splint.

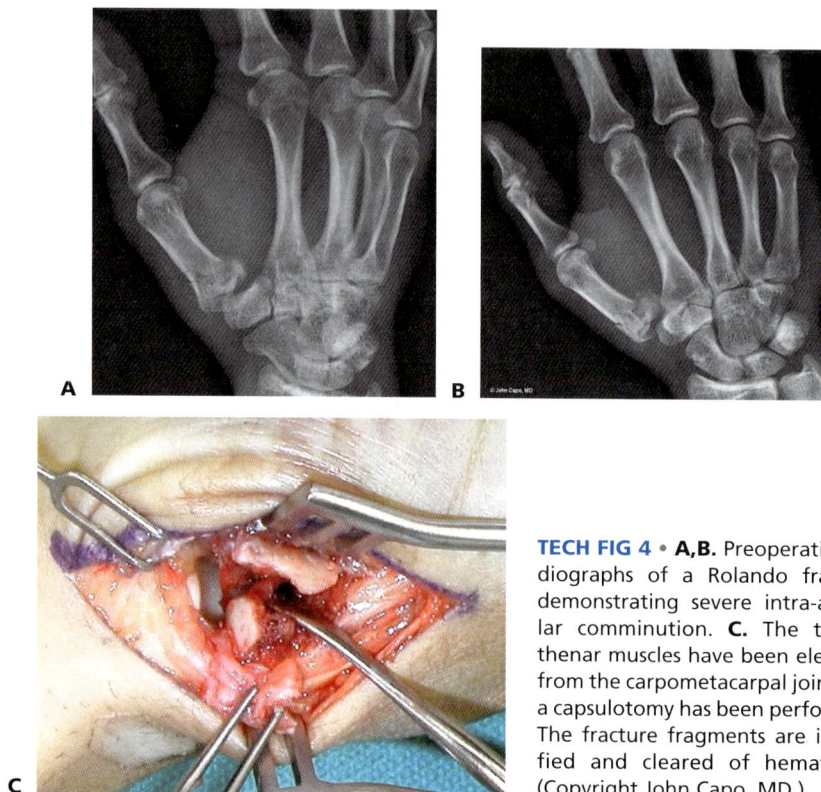

TECH FIG 4 • **A,B.** Preoperative radiographs of a Rolando fracture demonstrating severe intra-articular comminution. **C.** The thumb thenar muscles have been elevated from the carpometacarpal joint and a capsulotomy has been performed. The fracture fragments are identified and cleared of hematoma. (Copyright John Capo, MD.)

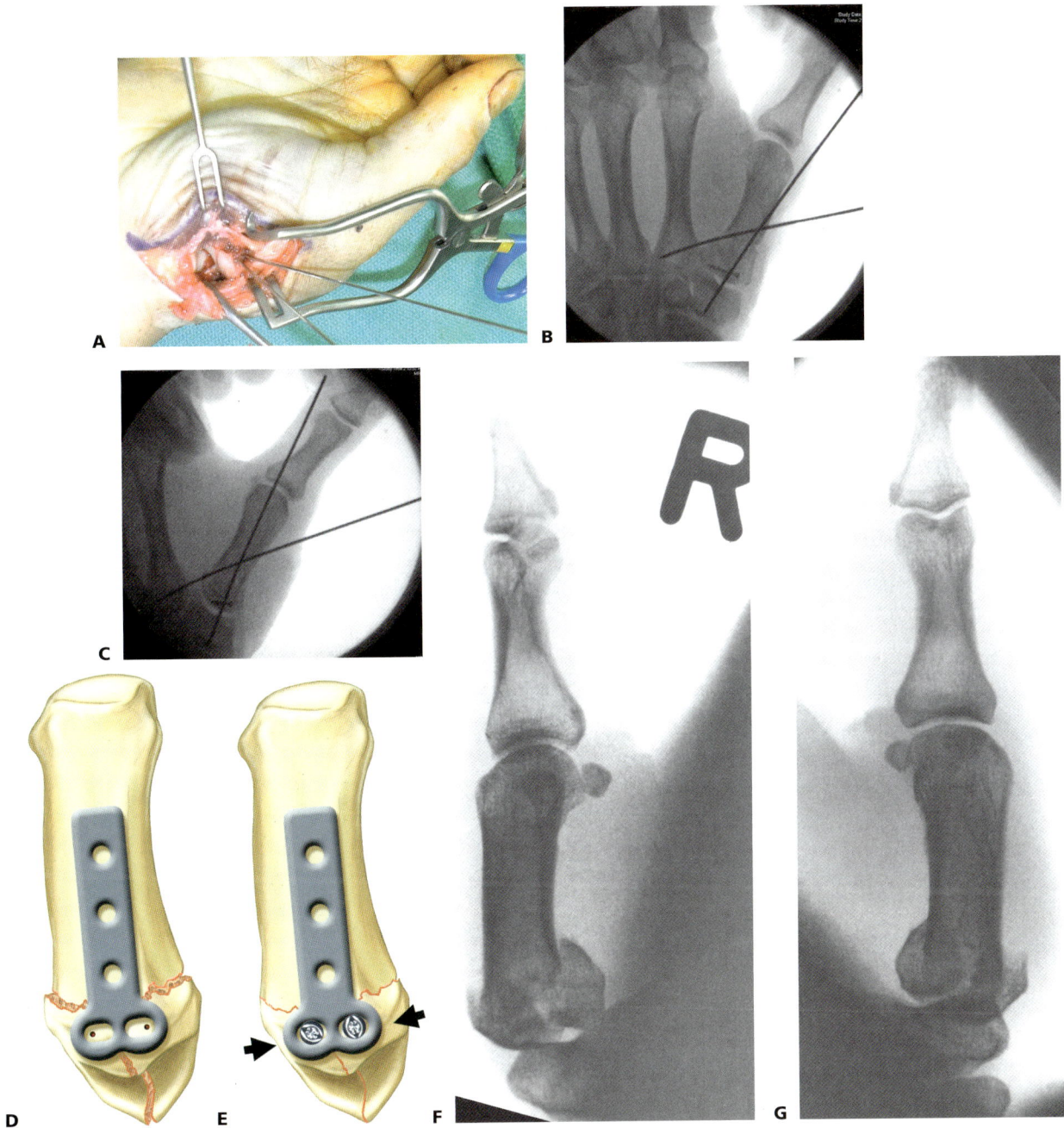

TECH FIG 5 • **A.** The articular surface is first reduced and provisionally stabilized with multiple small Kirschner wires. **B,C.** Intraoperative fluoroscopic lateral and AP views demonstrate excellent restoration of the joint surface. Kirschner wires have been placed from the thumb metacarpal into the trapezium and second metacarpal to stabilize the construct. **D.** The two proximal holes of the T plate are drilled offset for articular fragment reduction. **E.** The two proximal screws are tightened to compress the proximal fragments. **F,G.** AP and lateral views of a comminuted, displaced Rolando fracture. *(continued)*

TECHNIQUES

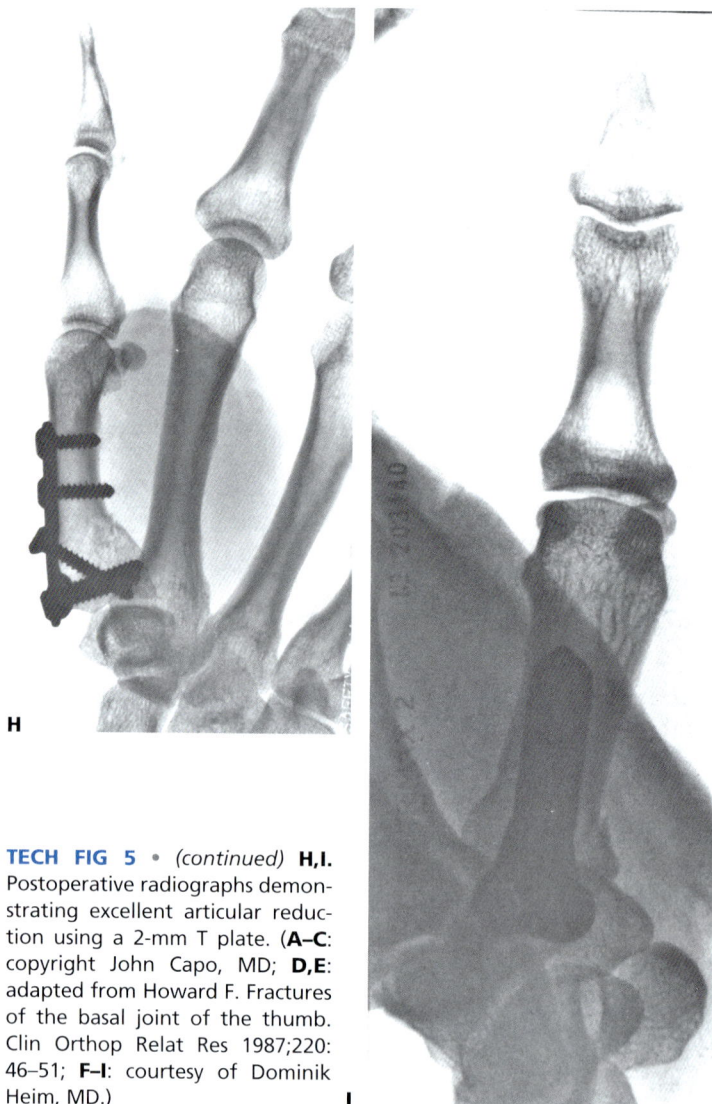

H

TECH FIG 5 • (continued) **H,I.** Postoperative radiographs demonstrating excellent articular reduction using a 2-mm T plate. (**A–C**: copyright John Capo, MD; **D,E**: adapted from Howard F. Fractures of the basal joint of the thumb. Clin Orthop Relat Res 1987;220: 46–51; **F–I**: courtesy of Dominik Heim, MD.)

I

APPLICATION OF AN EXTERNAL FIXATOR FOR COMMINUTED ROLANDO FRACTURES

- Before this procedure, a radiograph of the contralateral thumb CMC joint is advised for templating and to judge postreduction length.
- A mini-external fixator (2.0- to 2.5-mm pins) is applied to the thumb and index metacarpals using standard technique with a quadrilateral frame configuration.[2,12]
- Exposure and open reduction are then performed as discussed previously.
- Distraction is maintained using the external fixator, and the depressed joint fragments are elevated and aligned using the preoperative radiograph of the opposite side as a guide.
    - A sharp dental pick is an excellent tool to manipulate small fragments.

- 0.045-inch smooth Kirschner wires or interfragmentary screws can then be used to secure the fracture fragments.
- The external fixator is loosened to decrease the flexion deformity of the thumb metacarpal shaft, and to ensure the base of the thumb is maintained in the proper position. It should be co-linear with the base of the second metacarpal base.
- At the end of the procedure the thumb should be in 45 degrees of palmar and radial abduction and about 120 degrees of pronation in relation to the plane of the hand (**TECH FIG 6**).
- The incision is irrigated and closed in layers.

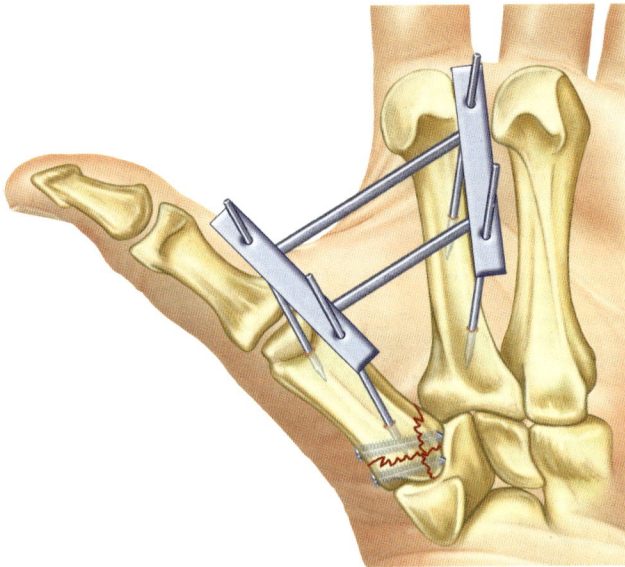

TECH FIG 6 • A schematic of an external fixator frame used for stabilization of a comminuted Rolando-type fracture. Care should be taken to place the thumb in a functional position with wide palmar and radial abduction.

PEARLS AND PITFALLS

Indications	▪ Operative treatment should be considered if greater than 2 mm of step-off persists after closed reduction. Displaced Bennett fractures greater than 20% to 25% of joint surface usually require open reduction and internal fixation for optimal reduction.
Preoperative evaluation	▪ Proper radiographs, including a true lateral view and an AP hyperpronated view, must be obtained before operative treatment. CT scanning is usually indicated only if significant comminution is present or if plain radiographs are difficult to interpret.
Thumb position	▪ The thumb should be placed in a position of function with pinning and postoperative splinting. This position is palmar and radial abduction of 45 degrees and pronation of 120 degrees.
Joint reduction	▪ Joint reduction must be obtained because residual displacement leads to poor outcomes. If adequate joint reduction cannot be verified by fluoroscopy, then open treatment and direct visualization is mandatory. Percutaneous methods may be inadequate for fractures involving more than 25% to 30% of the joint surface.[15]
Postoperative management	▪ Thumb spica casting for 4 to 6 weeks is necessary if percutaneous Kirschner wire fixation is used. Excessively early motion may break Kirschner wires that span the adjacent joints. Range-of-motion exercises can be begun 1 to 2 weeks postoperatively if stable plate fixation is used.

POSTOPERATIVE CARE

Bennett Fractures

▪ A thumb spica splint is applied in the operating room. Pin sites are inspected at 1 week and a thumb spica cast is applied for 4 to 6 weeks, until fracture union.

▪ Hand therapy is begun early for thumb IP and MP joint motion and index through small finger range of motion.

▪ Pins are removed at 4 to 6 weeks and therapy is advanced to the CMC joint along with intermittent immobilization using a removable thumb spica splint.[16]

▪ In patients treated with interfragmentary compression screws and therefore more stable fixation, active range-of-motion exercises can by started at 1 to 2 weeks postoperatively with a removable splint for protection.

Rolando Fractures

▪ Patients treated with closed reduction and percutaneous pinning are placed in a thumb spica splint, which is removed at 1 week for pin inspection. A thumb spica cast is applied for an additional 4 to 5 weeks.

▪ The pins are removed in the outpatient office at 6 weeks after surgery. A removable splint may be continued for 2 to 4 additional weeks while active range-of-motion exercises are advanced.[16]

▪ In patients treated with stable plate fixation, active range-of-motion exercises may be instituted at 1 to 2 weeks after surgery. Patients typically wear a removable splint for 2 to 4 weeks.

▪ If a severe injury dictated the use of external fixation, the pins and frame should remain in place for about 6 weeks, or until fracture stability is adequate based on interval radiographs. A removable thumb spica splint can then be worn for an additional 4 to 6 weeks.

OUTCOMES

▪ The majority of patients can expect a successful recovery after operative treatment of Bennett or Rolando fractures (**FIG 6**).

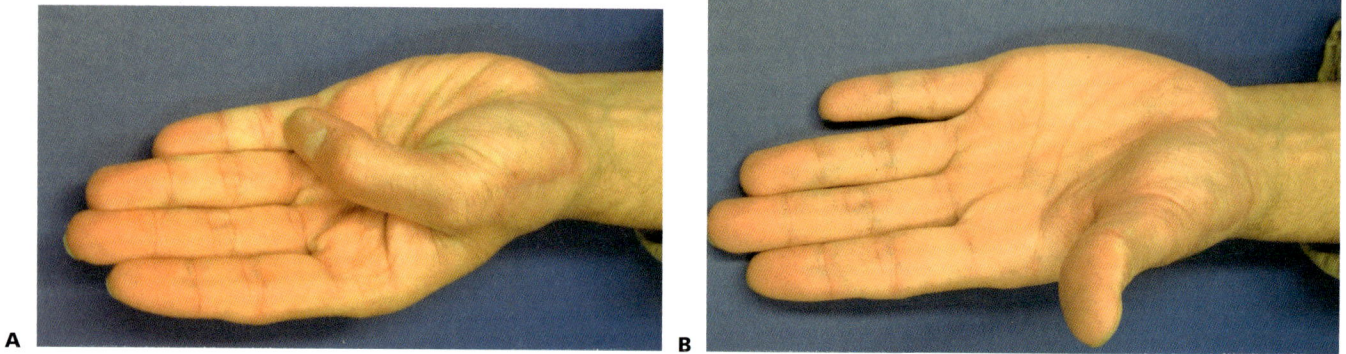

FIG 6 • Clinical photographs of a patient with a Rolando fracture who had undergone open reduction and internal fixation 8 months previously, demonstrating a functional range of flexion (**A**) and extension (**B**). (Copyright John Capo, MD.)

▪ Superior results are seen in operatively treated fractures in which there is no residual subluxation of the thumb metacarpal shaft and less than 2 mm of intra-articular displacement.[5,15]

▪ It is generally agreed that if pain and articular incongruity persist after 6 months of observation after closed or open treatment, arthrodesis of the thumb metacarpal to the trapezium or basal joint arthroplasty may be indicated.

  ▪ CMC joint fusion is durable, but patients have difficulty with placing their hand on a flat surface and getting the hand into a pants pocket.

  ▪ Basal joint arthroplasty for acute fractures should be reserved for older, lower-demand patients.

COMPLICATIONS

▪ Malunion and subsequent arthrosis resulting from inadequate articular reduction

▪ Pin tract infection

▪ Injury to the superficial cutaneous nerves during open dissection and percutaneous fixation

▪ Contracture of the first web space from immobilization or pinning of the thumb in an adducted position

REFERENCES

1. Billing L, Gedda K. Roentgen examination of Bennett's fracture. Acta Radiol 1952;38:471–476.
2. Buchler U, McCollam S, Oppikofer C. Comminuted fractures of the basilar joint of the thumb: combined treatment by external fixation, limited internal fixation, and bone grafting. J Hand Surg Am 1991; 16A:556–560.
3. Capo JT, Kinchelow T, Orillaza NS, Rossy W. Accuracy of fluoroscopy in closed reduction and percutaneous fixation of simulated Bennett's fracture. J Hand Surg (Am), 2009;34(4):637-41.
4. Charnley J. The Closed Treatment of Common Fractures, 3rd ed. Edinburgh: Churchill Livingstone, 1974:150.
5. Cannon S, Dowd G, Williams D, Scott J. A long-term study following Bennett's fracture. J Hand Surg Br 1986;11:426–431.
6. Cullen J, Parentis M, Chinchilli V, et al. Simulated Bennett fracture treated with closed reduction and percutaneous pinning: a biomechanical analysis of residual incongruity of the joint. J Bone Joint Surg Am 1997;79:413–420.
7. Foster R, Hastings H. Treatment of Bennett, Rolando, and vertical intra-articular trapezial fractures. Clin Orthop Relat Res 1987;214: 121–129.
8. Gedda K. Studies on Bennett fractures: anatomy, roentgenology, and therapy. Acta Chir Scand Suppl 1954;193:5.
9. Griffiths J. Fractures of the base of the first metacarpal bone. J Bone Joint Surg Br 1964;46B:712–719.
10. Haines R. The mechanism of rotation at the first carpometacarpal joint. J Anat 1944;78:4.
11. Howard F. Fractures of the basal joint of the thumb. Clin Orthop Relat Res 1987;220:46–51.
12. Jobe M, Calandruccio J. The hand: fractures, dislocations, and ligamentous injuries. In Canale T, ed. Campbell's Operative Orthopedics, 10th ed. Philadelphia: Elsevier, 2003:3489.
13. Jupiter J, Axelrod T, Belsky M. Fractures and dislocations of the hand. In Browner B, Jupiter J, Levine A, Trafton P, eds. Skeletal Trauma: Basic Science, Management, and Reconstruction, 3rd ed. Philadelphia: Elsevier, 2003:1196.
14. Livesley J. The conservative management of Bennett's fracture-dislocation: a 26-year follow-up. J Bone Joint Surg Br 1990;15B: 291–294.
15. Pellegrini V. Fractures at the base of the thumb. Hand Clin 1988;4: 87–102.
16. Raskin K, Shin S. Surgical treatment of fractures of the thumb metacarpal base: Bennett's and Rolando's fractures. In Strickland J, Graham T, eds. The Hand (Master's Techniques in Orthopaedic Surgery). Philadelphia: Lippincott Williams & Wilkins, 2005:125–135.
17. Roberts P. Bulletins et memoires de la Societe de Radiologie Medicale de France, 1936;24:687.
18. Stern P. Fractures of the metacarpals and phalanges. In Green D, Hotchkiss R, Pederson W, et al, eds. Green's Operative Hand Surgery, 5th ed. Philadelphia: Elsevier, 2005:332–338.
19. Thurston A, Dempsey S. Bennett's fracture: a medium to long-term review. Aust NZ J Surg 1993;63:120–123.

Dislocations and Chronic Volar Instability of the Thumb Metacarpophalangeal Joint

Robert R. Slater, Jr.

DEFINITION

- Disruption of the restraining structures on the volar surface of the joint between the metacarpal and proximal phalanx of the thumb may result in excessive joint motion and abnormal hyperextension.
- Often painful, this instability frequently causes significant functional deficits because so much of what humans do with their hands depends on having a stable, pain-free thumb to oppose the other digits.
- Acute injuries, including joint dislocations, must be treated correctly and promptly to afford the best chance for successful outcomes.
- Chronic volar instability is seen less often than is collateral ligament incompetence, but it should not be overlooked. It can be treated effectively with a variety of techniques, which will be discussed in this chapter.

ANATOMY

- The thumb metacarpophalangeal (MP) joint has features of both a ginglymus (hinge) joint and a condyloid joint. The joint moves mostly in a flexion–extension mode (ginglymus-style), but there are also elements of rotation and abduction–-adduction in the normal joint (condyloid).
- Thumb MP joint motion varies widely from individual to individual because of the spectrum of metacarpal head geometry seen in "normal" hands.
  - Some metacarpal heads are more rounded and allow greater flexion, extension, and rotation, while others are flatter and allow relatively less range of motion (ROM).
- The joint derives its stability mostly from soft tissue constraints, not bony architecture (**FIG 1**).
- The proper collateral ligaments originate from the region of the lateral condyles of the MC and pass palmarly and obliquely to insert on the palmar portion of the proximal phalanx.
- The accessory collateral ligaments originate from the same region but slightly more proximal and traverse distally and palmarly in an oblique fashion to insert on the volar plate and sesamoids.
- The volar plate serves as the floor of the MP joint. The adductor pollicis inserting into the ulnar styloid sesamoid at the distal edge of the volar plate and the insertions of the flexor pollicis brevis and abductor pollicis brevis into the radial sesamoid at the radial-distal edge of the volar plate provide additional volar support.
  - Those muscles also contribute fibers to the extensor mechanism by way of the adductor and abductor aponeuroses and thus provide a modicum of lateral joint stability.

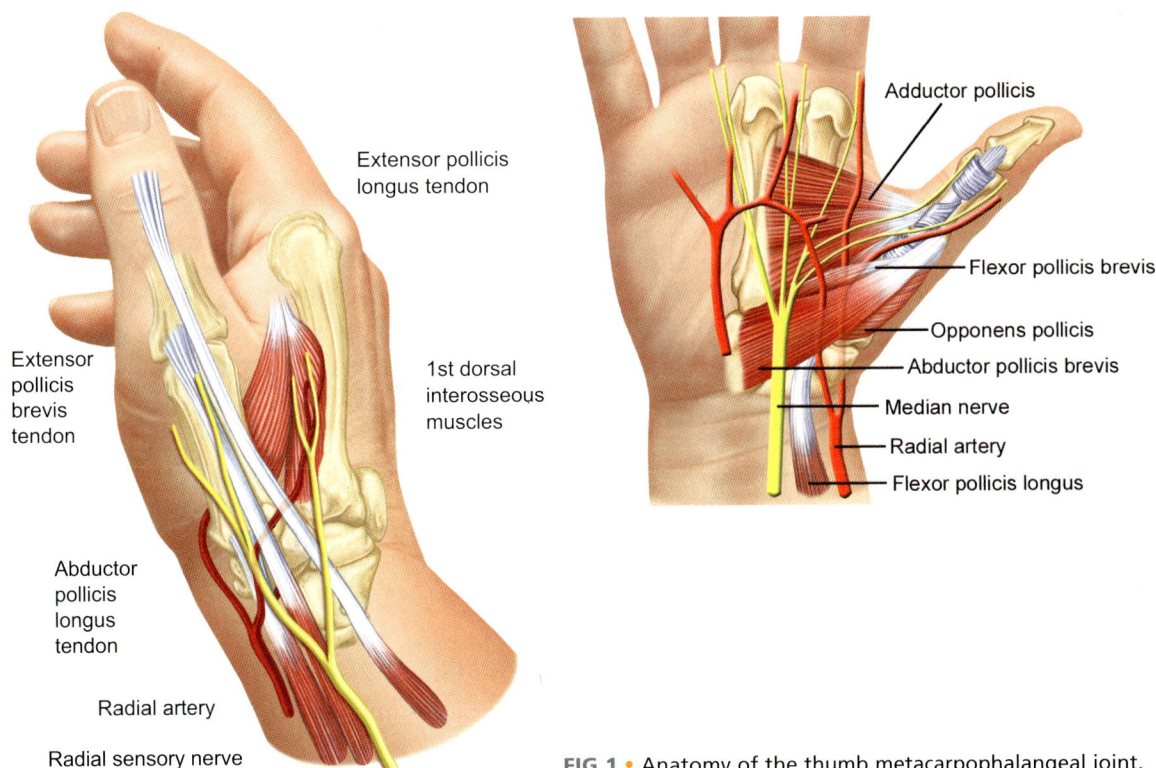

Extensor pollicis longus tendon

Extensor pollicis brevis tendon

1st dorsal interosseous muscles

Abductor pollicis longus tendon

Radial artery

Radial sensory nerve

Adductor pollicis

Flexor pollicis brevis

Opponens pollicis

Abductor pollicis brevis

Median nerve

Radial artery

Flexor pollicis longus

FIG 1 • Anatomy of the thumb metacarpophalangeal joint.

- Dorsally, the extensor pollicis brevis inserts onto the base of the thumb proximal phalanx and the extensor pollicis longus inserts at the base of the thumb distal phalanx; both traverse the MP joint and add to the stabilizing forces surrounding the joint.
- The MP joint capsule itself surrounds the joint and contributes slightly to stability.

PATHOGENESIS

- Dorsal dislocations of the thumb MP joint are much more common than are volar dislocations.[4,5]
- The typical mechanism is a hyperextension force strong enough to rupture the volar plate and joint capsule.
  - For example, when a ball strikes a player's thumb or when there is a direct blow or fall that drives the phalanx into sudden hyperextension
- Occasionally the radial or ulnar collateral ligaments (or both) of the MP joint are ruptured along with the volar plate. Their treatment is addressed in other chapters.
- Sometimes the instability occurs in the setting of a patient with generalized ligamentous laxity such as Ehlers-Danlos syndrome (or other collagen disorders), but in those situations symptoms are less common and patients typically learn to compensate for the joint laxity.

NATURAL HISTORY

- Posttraumatic instability left untreated may result in weakness of pinch and grip and progress to painful arthrosis due to the abnormal biomechanics of the damaged joint.

HISTORY AND PHYSICAL EXAMINATION

- In traumatic cases it is important to inquire about the mechanism of injury.

- If patients recall which way the thumb was "pointing" at the time of injury, it helps the examiner determine which structures were likely injured.
- Was the joint dislocated and did it reduce spontaneously or with assistance from a coach, trainer, or the patient?
- How difficult was the reduction?
- Physical examination should include an assessment of ROM and grip and pinch strength, particularly in comparison with the contralateral thumb. Focal areas of tenderness should be ascertained. Residual tenderness along the volar plate may persist long after the injury.
  - The examiner should observe the resting joint posture; dislocated joints exhibit obvious deformity.
  - The examiner should check for open wounds and assess vascular status. Open wounds or vascular compromise mandate emergent treatment.
  - Limited or absent interphalangeal joint ROM suggests flexor pollicis longus tendon entrapment.
  - Dislocated or painful MP joints will have limited ROM.
  - Volar plate stability is assessed, since instability must be recognized and treated appropriately to maximize outcomes.
  - Severe collateral ligament injury is uncommon in conjunction with volar plate instability but must be recognized and treated where indicated.
  - An acute dislocation is rarely subtle, but when patients present with chronic instability symptoms, there may be guarding against full joint extension and soft tissue thickening in areas of chronic pathology.

IMAGING AND DIAGNOSTIC STUDIES

- Plain radiographs of the thumb in three views (AP, lateral, and oblique) are requisite.
  - Injury films will reveal the direction of joint dislocation and any associated fractures (**FIG 2A–C**).

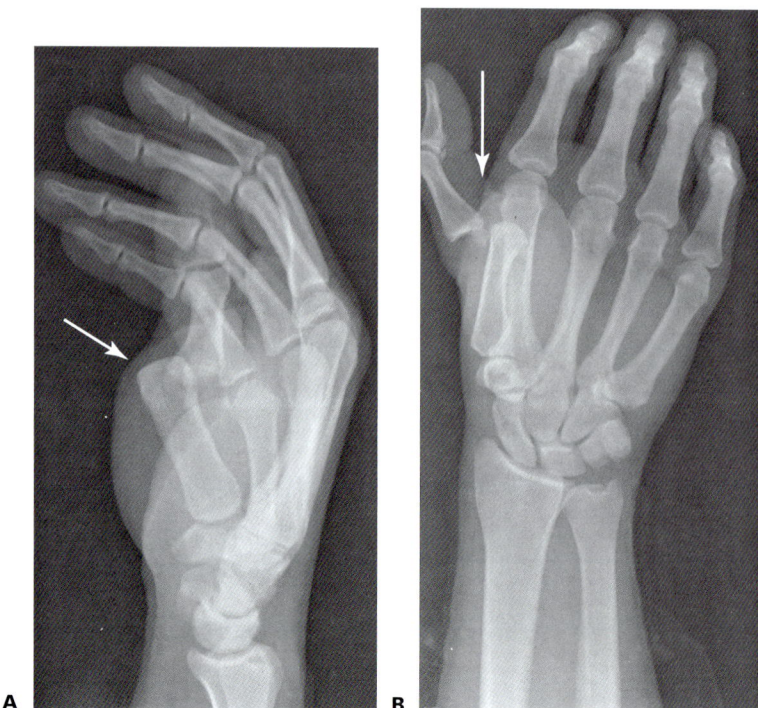

A

B

FIG 2 • (**A**) AP and (**B**) lateral injury films. *(continued)*

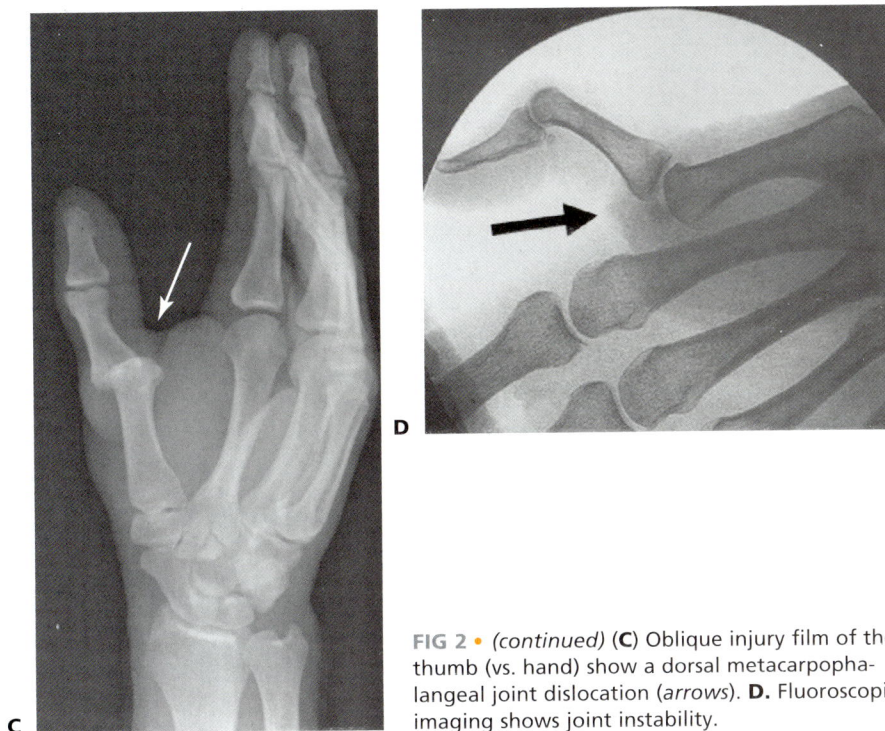

FIG 2 • *(continued)* (**C**) Oblique injury film of the thumb (vs. hand) show a dorsal metacarpophalangeal joint dislocation (*arrows*). **D.** Fluoroscopic imaging shows joint instability.

- In the chronic setting, films may show evidence of prior fractures or bony injuries as well as the positions of the sesamoid bones relative to the joint space. In cases of chronic volar plate instability, the proximal phalanx may show subtle dorsal subluxation on the metacarpal head (that is more commonly noted when there has been injury to the dorsal capsule in association with collateral ligament damage).
- Arthritic changes at the MP joint seen on the plain films will alter the treatment options. If the chronically unstable joint is already arthritic at the time of presentation, then an arthrodesis will be a better option than a soft tissue reconstruction.
- Fluoroscopic real-time imaging and stress testing may confirm the suspected joint instability (**FIG 2D**).
  - A digital block may be placed to facilitate an adequate examination.
- Ultrasound, MR imaging, and arthrography[6–8] are advocated by some, but these studies are rarely of additional value in the assessment of thumb MP joint stability.

DIFFERENTIAL DIAGNOSIS

- Fracture
- Collateral ligament injury
- Ligament laxity, generalized (eg, Ehlers-Danlos syndrome)
- Arthritis
- Locked trigger thumb (stenosing tenosynovitis)

NONOPERATIVE MANAGEMENT

- Most acute thumb MP dislocations can be reduced closed.
- The reduction maneuver for a dorsal dislocation involves very slight hyperextension of the MP joint followed by direct volarly directed pressure on the base of the proximal phalanx to gently slide the phalanx over the metacarpal head and back into proper alignment.

- Subtle, slight rotation (pronation and supination) at the same time may help ease any interposed soft tissue out of the way as the phalanx reduces.
- Longitudinal traction and excessive hyperextension should be avoided because the soft tissue tension generated may cause one or more structures surrounding the joint to slip between the metacarpal head and the proximal phalanx, blocking reduction.
  - The volar plate, the flexor pollicis longus, and one or both sesamoid bones have all been described as culprits that have become incarcerated in the joint space, preventing reduction.[2,3,5,9]
- Once the joint is reduced, the patient should be able to flex and extend the thumb joints and the radiographs should show concentrically reduced and congruent joint surfaces (**FIG 3**).
  - If either of those conditions is not met, it suggests there may be residual soft tissue interposed in the joint, an indication for open reduction.
- After successful closed reduction, the thumb should be splinted in flexion to relax the injured volar structures.
- After a few days, when the acute swelling has dissipated, the splint may be changed to a thumb spica cast, again with the MP joint flexed, for an additional 2 to 3 weeks. Rehabilitation can commence thereafter, emphasizing ROM exercises within a safe zone of motion from full flexion to just short of neutral extension and then increasing gradually to unrestricted ROM and hand use by 6 weeks after injury.
  - For patients engaged in activities that risk forced hyperextension of the thumb, taping or splinting may be required during these endeavors for an additional period.
- Failure to recognize or treat the acute instability or overly aggressive progression to full, unlimited hand use may result in chronic volar instability.

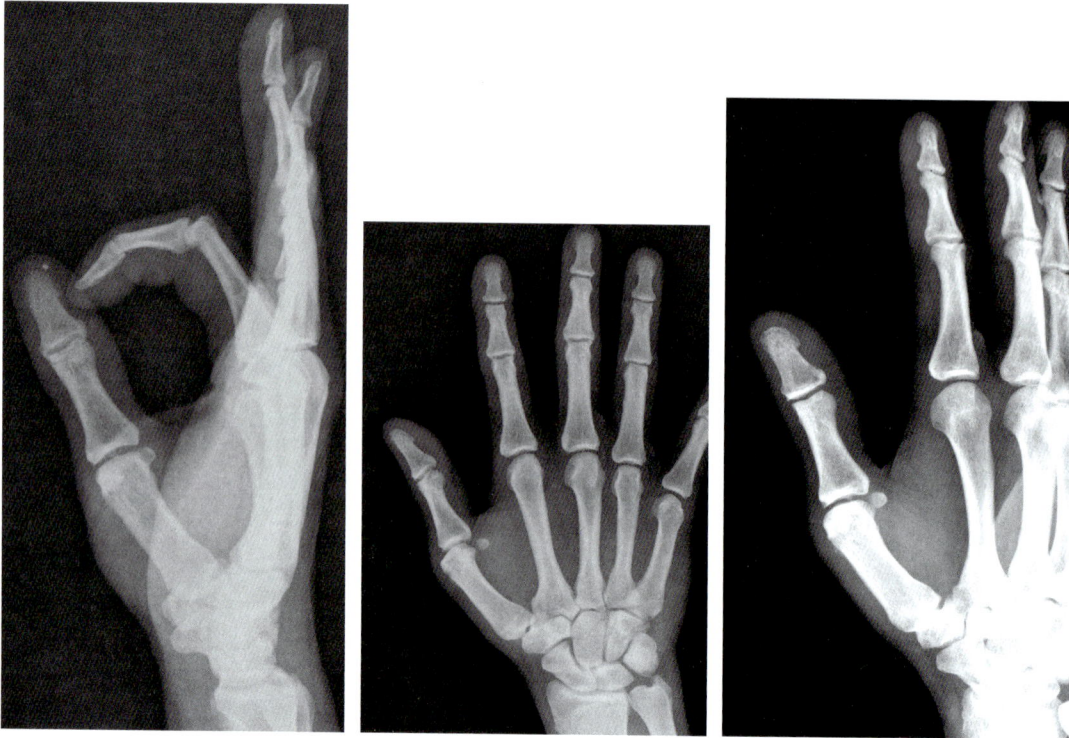

FIG 3 • Postreduction views of the patient in Figure 2 confirm congruent joint surfaces and satisfactory alignment, including the sesamoid bone positions.

■ Nonoperative management then is limited to providing the patient with a custom-molded splint to prevent hyperextension of the MP joint.

■ A properly trained hand therapist is invaluable in assisting patients who prefer to manage the problem nonoperatively and use a protective splint rather than proceeding with surgical treatment for their chronic instability.

■ Volar dislocation is very rare. There are only a few cases reported in the literature, and all required open reduction.[4,5]

SURGICAL MANAGEMENT

■ Open reduction is required when attempts at closed manipulation and reduction of acute dislocations fail.

■ Failure is typically the result of soft tissue interposition in the joint that blocks reduction. Tissue interposition may have happened at the time of the original injury or as a result of a well-meaning coach, friend, or medical colleague trying to reduce the dislocation by applying vigorous traction, which can cause the soft tissues to become incarcerated.

■ Chronic instability, which is persistently symptomatic despite nonoperative treatment, is best treated with a soft tissue stabilization technique unless moderate to severe arthrosis is present or the instability is global and exceedingly severe. In those cases, arthrodesis is the treatment of choice.

Preoperative Planning

■ The physician should review all imaging studies. In most cases, those will be limited to plain radiographs and perhaps spot films from fluoroscopic evaluations.

■ Films should be reviewed for any bony abnormalities, especially nondisplaced fractures. One should avoid fracture displacement during intraoperative manipulation of the thumb.

■ In fracture-dislocations of the MP joint, larger fragments are stabilized using Kirschner wires or screws and smaller avulsion-type fragments are excised and the ligament is secured to the bone.

■ For chronic cases, it is important to review the films and rule out osteoarthrosis, which would warrant different treatment strategies.

■ Examination under anesthesia with the assistance of fluoroscopy can be useful to confirm the degree and direction of joint instability.

■ Spot films obtained before and after surgical stabilization can be helpful visual aids for use in postoperative discussions with the patient and his or her family to explain again the nature of the problem and how it was treated.

Positioning

■ The patient should be supine on the operating table with a standard hand table attached and projecting out from the operating table to support the operative hand.

■ A tourniquet should be placed on the operative arm and checked for proper function and pressure before initiation of the surgery (typically 250 mm Hg or 100 mm Hg greater than systolic blood pressure).

Approach

■ Acute, irreducible MP joint dislocations are best approached from the volar side of the joint so that any soft tissues that may be trapped in the joint can be identified and carefully protected, *before* they are injured by approaching them "blindly" from the dorsal side!

■ That assumes there are no open wounds, which then would alter one's approach accordingly by incorporating the traumatic wound into the surgical incision.

- A lateral approach is also possible, but less often used.
- Chronic MP joint volar instability that is amenable to soft tissue stabilization should also be approached from the volar aspect of the joint so the pathology can be visualized and addressed directly.

- If chronic MP joint instability has resulted in arthritis, arthrodesis is a better solution. This may be accomplished in a variety of ways using a variety of hardware options, including screws, plates, and wires. All are best placed through a dorsal approach.

OPEN REDUCTION OF ACUTE MP JOINT DISLOCATIONS

- Make a zigzag (Bruner-type) incision, centered at the level of the MP joint.
- Gently elevate the skin flaps to expose the underlying soft tissues, which will by definition be displaced from their usual locations (**TECH FIG 1**).
- Identify the neurovascular bundles and mobilize them enough to ensure their protection.
    - Small rubber loops can be placed around them if desired both for protection and for easy identification.

- Retract the soft tissues enough to identify whatever structure is interposed into the MP joint and reflect it out of the joint.
    - Most often that is the flexor pollicis longus tendon or the volar plate. The volar plate may have the sesamoids still attached to its distal edge if it has failed proximally.
- Reduce the joint and check for smooth, congruent joint motion.
- Check the stability of the collateral ligaments. Providing the joint does not gap open more than 25 degrees due to

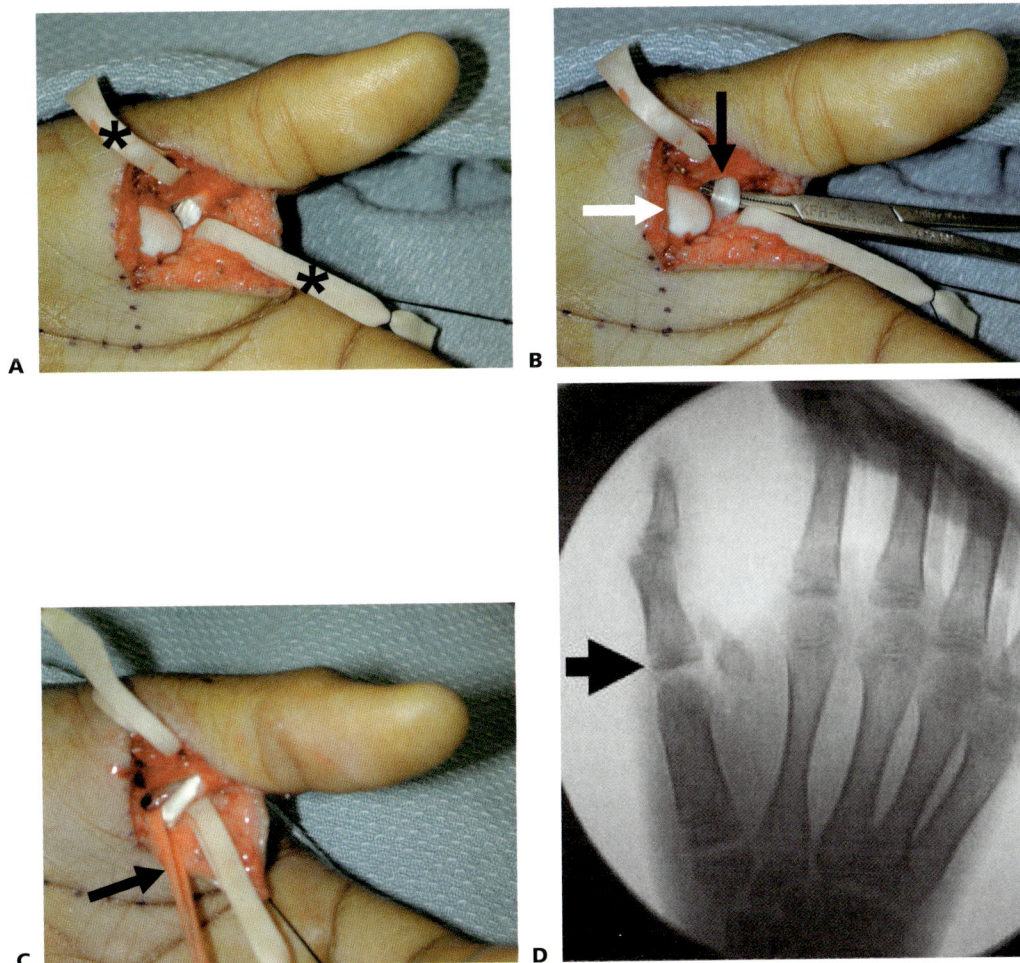

TECH FIG 1 • Open reduction of dorsal thumb metacarpophalangeal joint dislocation. **A.** Make a volar surgical approach and carefully identify the neurovascular bundles; tag and protect them with soft rubber loops (*). **B.** The flexor pollicis longus (*solid arrow*) is interposed and trapped behind the metacarpal head (*open arrow*). **C.** Umbilical tape (*arrow*) passed around the flexor pollicis longus delivers the tendon safely out of harm's way, allowing the joint to be reduced. **D.** Intraoperative fluoroscopy is helpful for verifying anatomic reduction (*arrow*) with congruent joint surfaces and smooth gliding through a safe range of motion.

collateral ligament damage (rare), no further treatment for that component of the joint injury is needed.

- In some cases it may be possible to place sutures through the volar plate at its torn proximal or distal edge and tack that back to its normal insertion point. Otherwise, simply replacing the plate in normal alignment will be adequate when combined with proper rehabilitation (discussed later in the chapter).

- Replace the neurovascular bundles and flexor pollicis longus into their proper locations and close the wound in routine fashion.

CHRONIC VOLAR INSTABILITY

Volar Plate Advancement and Sesamoid Arthrodesis

- The Tonkin procedure[11] was originally described to treat MP instability resulting secondarily from osteoarthrosis of the thumb carpometacarpal joint or in patients with cerebral palsy, but it is now considered a valuable technique or treating posttraumatic instability of the MP joint.
- Approach the MP joint through a volar or volar-radial incision (**TECH FIG 2A**).
- Divide the accessory radial collateral ligament at its insertion into the volar plate and mobilize the plate to advance it proximally (**TECH FIG 2B**).
- Denude the articular surface of the sesamoid bones. A Beaver blade works well.

- Decorticate a trough along the retrocondylar fossa of the metacarpal neck to accept the sesamoids.
- Drill Keith needles through that area of the retrocondylar fossa using a wire driver. The needles should exit the metacarpal dorsally (**TECH FIG 2C**).
- Advance the sesamoids and volar plate into the prepared trough and secure the sutures dorsally (**TECH FIG 2D**).
- Variations:
  - Schuurman and Bos[10]: Place sutures through the proximal edge of the volar plate and pass them through the metacarpal via the Keith needles. Reinforce the construct with nonabsorbable sutures to local tissue where possible.

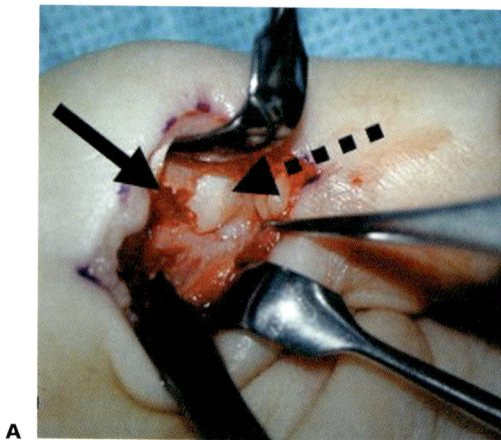

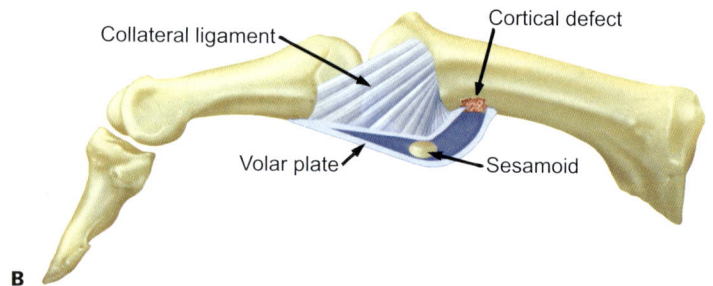

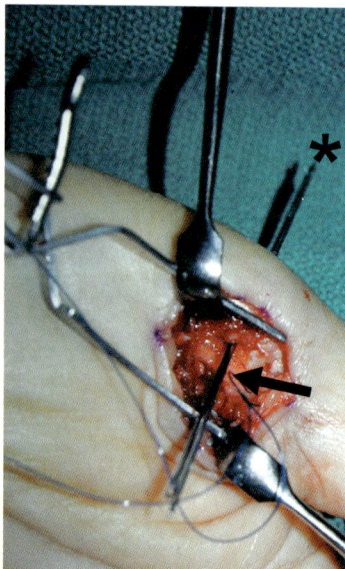

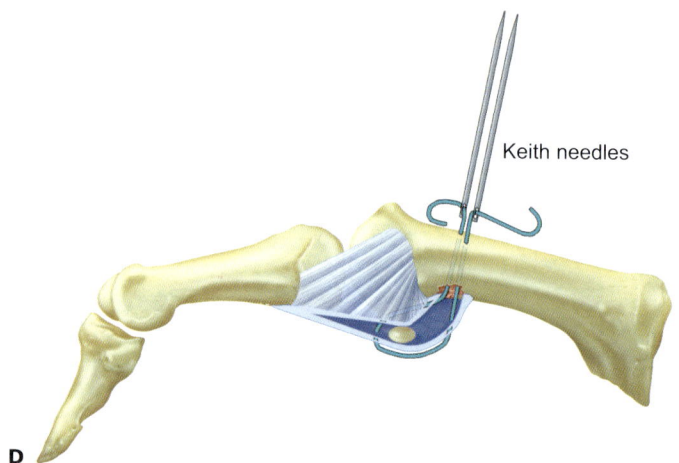

TECH FIG 2 • Sesamoid arthrodesis in the manner of Tonkin. **A,B.** Through a volar or radial lateral approach, create a cortical defect in the metacarpal retrocondylar fossa (*solid arrow*), which will accept the denuded sesamoids while preserving the articular surface of the metacarpal head (*dashed arrow*). **C.** Advance and secure the volar construct including the sesamoids into the prepared trough (*arrow*), using sutures in the volar plate that are brought through the metacarpal neck via Keith needles drilled through the bone. **D.** The sutures are tensioned and tied over the dorsal metacarpal (*). *(continued)*

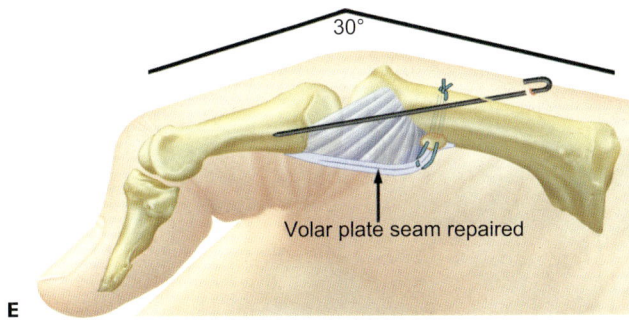

TECH FIG 2 • *(continued)* **E.** A Kirschner wire is drilled across the metacarpophalangeal joint to keep it flexed 30 degrees, protecting the repaired volar structures during initial healing.

- Eaton and Floyd[1]: Place sutures in the proximal corner of the volar plate and pass them subperiosteally from volar to dorsal around the metacarpal and secure them to advance the volar plate snugly into the prepared retrocondylar fossa.

- Pin the MP joint in about 30 degrees of flexion using a Kirschner wire (**TECH FIG 2E**).
- Close the wound in routine fashion and apply dressings and a thumb spica splint.
- Remove the sutures at 10 to 14 days as usual and apply a thumb spica cast.
- Remove the Kirschner wire and cast at 4 to 6 weeks and begin active flexion exercises.

Tendon Graft Tenodesis

- A procedure used by Littler and cited by Glickel et al[3] has been described whereby a free tendon graft (usually the palmaris longus) is woven through drill holes in the proximal phalanx and metacarpal and secured in place to provide a passive restraint against MP joint hyperextension.
  - However, the bulk of soft tissue that results from this procedure and the amount of dissection needed to perform it have caused this operation to fall out of favor.
  - Local tissue mobilization in conjunction with suture anchors provides a better solution.

ARTHRODESIS

Cannulated Headless Compression Screw Fixation

- Make a dorsal longitudinal approach (**TECH FIG 3A–D**).
  - Split the interval between extensor pollicis longus and brevis.
  - Split the joint capsule longitudinally.

- Mobilize the joint adequately. That requires releasing the remaining collateral ligaments and recessing the volar plate enough to deliver the metacarpal head fully into view.
- Use a water-cooled oscillating saw to remove the metacarpal head. Angle the cut from dorsal-distal to

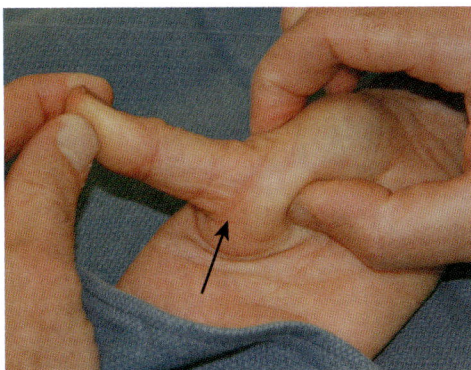

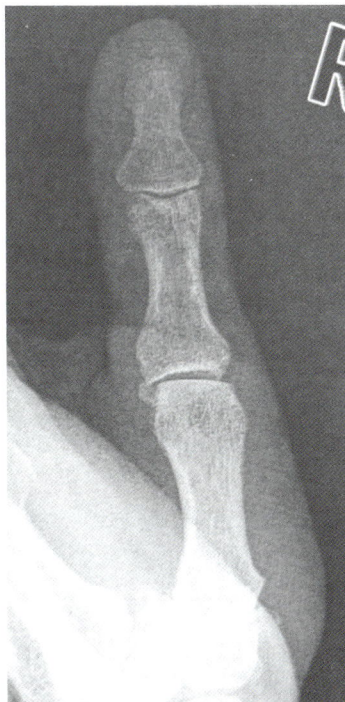

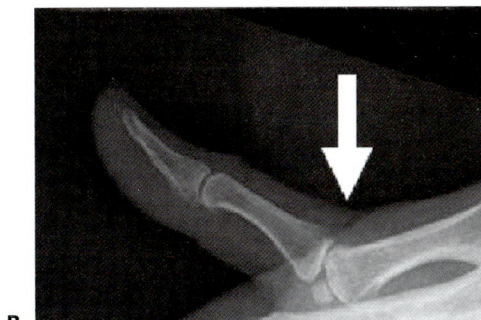

TECH FIG 3 • Clinical examination (**A**) shows metacarpophalangeal joint hyperextension (*arrow*), but in this case it is chronic and associated with joint space narrowing and asymmetry indicative of osteoarthrosis, as seen on radiographs (**B,C**), as well as hyperextension (*arrow* in **B**). *(continued)*

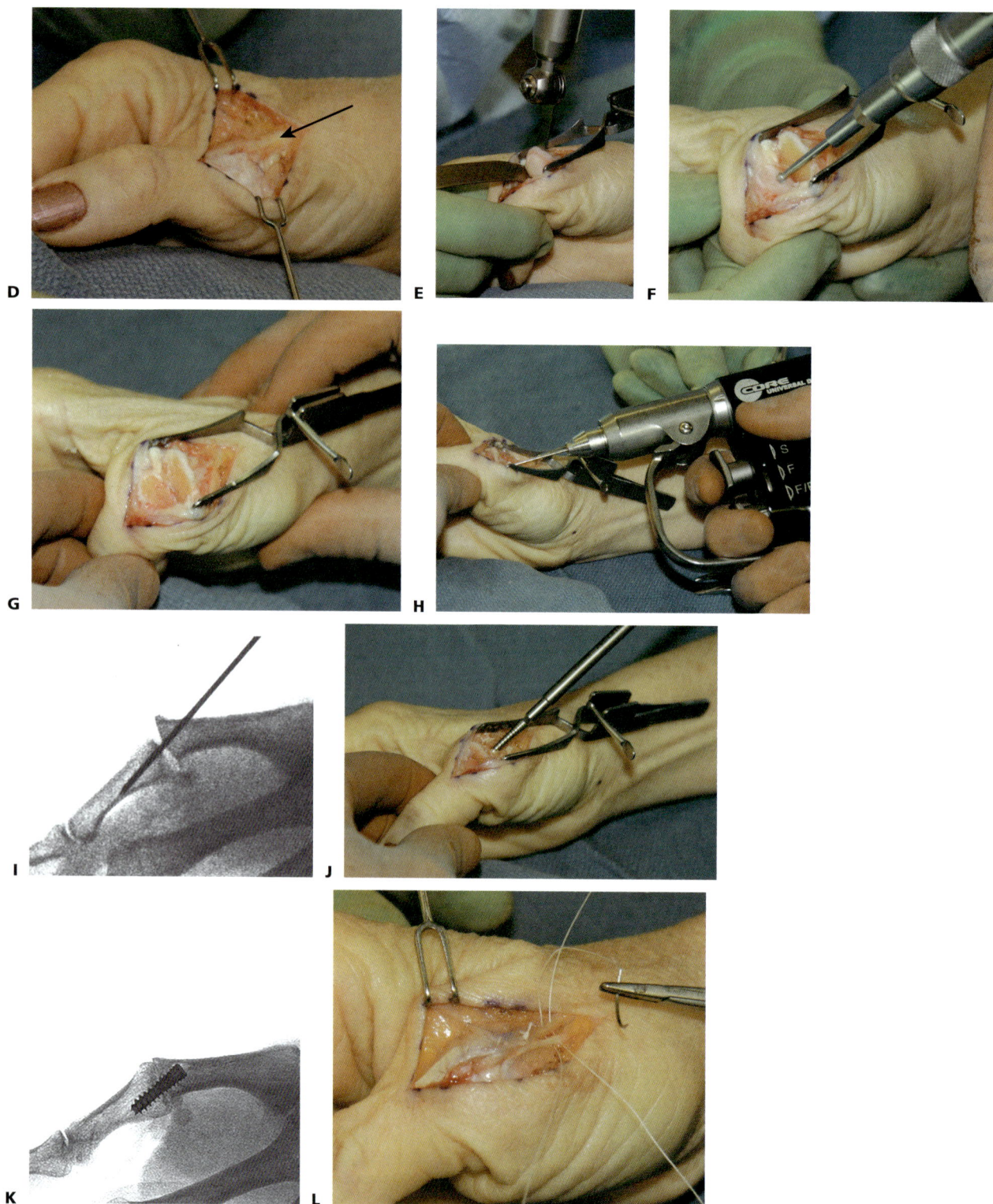

TECH FIG 3 • *(continued)* **D.** Through a dorsal approach, the interval between the extensor pollicis brevis and longus *(arrow)* is developed and the joint is entered. **E.** Remove the metacarpal head with an oscillating saw. **F.** Prepare the base of the proximal phalanx with a burr. **G.** The opposing bone surfaces should be flush-cut and angled slightly so the final arthrodesis position is 15 to 20 degrees of flexion. **H.** The guidewire for the chosen cannulated screw is drilled across from metacarpal into the medullary canal of the proximal phalanx. **I.** Its position is checked with fluoroscopy. **J.** After the proper implant length is measured and the leading cortex overdrilled, the screw is inserted over the guidewire. **K.** Confirm correct final positioning with fluoroscopy. **L.** The joint capsule is closed and the extensor mechanism reapproximated.

palmar-proximal so that the final positioning will leave the MP joint surface flexed about 15 degrees (**TECH FIG 3E**).

- All the flexion for the arthrodesis will be accomplished by this cut. Preparation of the proximal phalanx base will be perpendicular to the longitudinal axis of that bone and will not add flexion.

- Use a burr to prepare the base of the proximal phalanx, removing any remaining articular cartilage and eburnated subchondral bone (**TECH FIG 3F**). Osteophytes and ridges should be trimmed away also to make a flush surface that will oppose the MC surface (**TECH FIG 3G**).
  - Alternatively, carefully protect the underlying flexor pollicis longus and use a water-cooled oscillating saw to remove the needed bone.

- Avoid excessive bone resection that will shorten the thumb. Cup and cone reamers are an alternative to straight bone cuts and may minimize shortening and maximize flexibility in positioning the arthrodesis.

- Reduce the fusion surfaces and drive a guidewire for the selected cannulated screw set from the metacarpal into the medullary cavity of the proximal phalanx (**TECH FIG 3H**).
  - Be certain that the starting point for the guidewire is sufficiently proximal on the dorsal surface of the metacarpal that the screw does not fracture the cortical bridge when inserted.
  - Alternatively, the guidewire may be drilled in a retrograde fashion starting at the cut end of the metacarpal head. The fusion surfaces are then reduced and the guidewire is advanced into the phalanx in an antegrade manner.
  - Consider placing a second temporary Kirschner wire to increase stability and minimize rotation during screw insertion.

- Confirm that the overall alignment is satisfactory radiographically and clinically (**TECH FIG 3I**).
  - The metacarpal and phalanx should be co-linear in the AP plane and flexed about 15 to 20 degrees in the lateral plane. Rotation should be neutral or slight pronation for pinch.
  - Intraoperative fluoroscopy is helpful to confirm correct alignment.

- Adjust the position of the guidewire for the cannulated screw such that its distal tip is just past the narrowest portion of the proximal phalanx. A screw ending at this level will experience excellent purchase and gain maximum stability. Measure the Kirschner wire length, choose the screw (keeping in mind the likelihood of compression at the arthrodesis site), and then advance the guidewire distally into the cortex.

- Drill, tap, and place the selected screw, avoiding any prominence over the dorsal metacarpal. Tighten securely while the reduction is compressed manually (**TECH FIG 3J**).

- Reconfirm correct alignment in all planes, paying particular attention to rotation. Confirm satisfactory hardware positioning (**TECH FIG 3K**).

- Morselized bone graft can be harvested from the resected metacarpal head and packed in and around the arthrodesis site if needed.

- Close the joint capsule with absorbable suture to minimize extensor tendon adhesions.

- Approximate the extensor tendon interval with interrupted, inverted permanent suture and close the wound in a routine fashion (**TECH FIG 3L**).

- Place a forearm-based thumb spica splint.

Plate and Screw Fixation

- It may be desirable to use plate and screw fixation rather than cannulated screws in such cases as nonunion after attempted arthrodesis, failure of implant arthroplasty, and traumatic injuries with severe deformity, bone loss, or segmental defects (**TECH FIG 4**).
  - The advantage of plates and screws is that more rigid, secure fixation can be achieved immediately, avoiding the concern for rotation or loosening around a single cannulated screw.
  - The disadvantage of that technique is that hardware prominence and tendon irritation and adhesions are more often a subsequent source of trouble.

- If plate and screw fixation is chosen as the desired technique, then the overall approach and bone preparation are similar to that described for the cannulated screw technique.

- With the arthrodesis site reduced and temporarily stabilized with a Kirschner wire, a 2.0-mm, five-hole compression plate is contoured to the dorsal surface of the bones.

- The plate is first secured distally and then applied proximally using compression technique principles.
  - It is critical to avoid long screws and irritation of the flexor pollicis longus.

- Closure and postoperative care are similar to that described earlier.

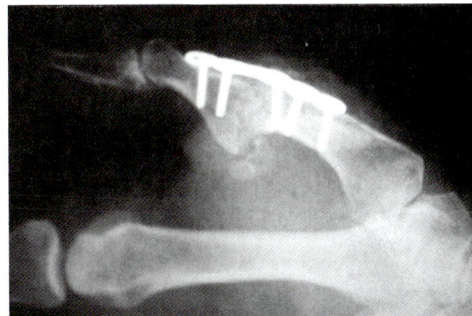

TECH FIG 4 • Arthrodesis with plate and screw fixation.

TECHNIQUES

PEARLS AND PITFALLS

Initial treatment	■ Acute MP joint dislocations should be reduced promptly, but straight traction should be avoided because it can result in soft tissue entrapment and turn a simple dislocation into a complex, irreducible injury requiring open reduction. ■ The joint should be immobilized and protected long enough and rehabilitated carefully enough to avoid chronic volar instability.
Treatment indications	■ Chronic volar instability without arthritic change can be treated with a variety of capsulodesis procedures. ■ When arthritic changes have developed as a result of chronic instability, MP joint arthrodesis should be done.
Hardware problems	■ Cannulated screws work well for MP arthrodesis and leave the hardware buried. ■ Plates and screws, Kirschner wire fixation, and transosseous wiring techniques can be effective ways of achieving arthrodesis but are more likely to cause hardware problems requiring subsequent treatment.

POSTOPERATIVE CARE

Acute Dislocation

■ The MP joint is generally stable once a dislocation is reduced acutely, whether by closed or open methods.

■ The MP joint should be held in about 30 degrees of flexion in a short-arm thumb spica splint or cast for 2 weeks.

■ ROM exercises can begin thereafter, using a removable thumb spica splint for an additional 4 weeks, gradually weaning out of the splint and advancing activities as symptoms allow.

■ Supervised hand therapy is often helpful for patients to guide their recovery of motion and strength and optimize their outcomes.

Chronic Instability

■ Volar plate advancement procedures and the Tonkin sesamoid arthrodesis procedure should be protected with the thumb MP joint flexed in a cast for 4 to 6 weeks, depending on the surgeon's assessment of tissue quality and patient compliance. Then supervised ROM can begin, but MP joint hyperextension forces should be avoided for 8 to 12 weeks.

■ MP joint arthrodesis procedures require longer protection so that the fusion site is not stressed or disrupted before final bony union.

■ Generally it is best to use a thumb spica splint (plaster) for the first 10 to 14 days after surgery until the swelling decreases and the sutures are removed.

■ Then a thumb spica cast can be used for an additional 3.5 to 4 weeks, at which time a custom-molded, removable splint can be used to protect the arthrodesis site but allow ROM of the uninvolved adjacent joints of the hand to prevent undue stiffness.

■ By 12 weeks most arthrodeses are healed solidly enough to allow unrestricted hand use.

OUTCOMES

■ Acute volar instability and dorsal dislocations of the MP joint that are treated appropriately can be expected to have a good prognosis.[2,3,9] Whether the dislocation is reduced closed or open reduction is required, once the joint is reduced it is usually stable.

■ Following rehabilitation as outlined above, there well may be some residual joint stiffness. While that may continue to improve for up to 1 year after injury, the lost range of motion is rarely a functional problem.

■ Tonkin et al[11] reported successful outcomes in 38 of 42 cases (90%) of sesamoid arthrodeses for chronic MP joint volar instability. Those results compare favorably with outcomes following other capsulodesis and volar plate reinforcing procedures. The advantage of all such procedures is that hyperextension is blocked, restoring stability to the joint, while still allowing the MP joint to flex. Mean loss of flexion compared with the preoperative condition was 8 degrees in the series reported by Tonkin et al.[11]

■ Outcomes after arthrodesis for chronic volar instability must be viewed with the proper surgical goal in mind. The goal is to relieve pain (from instability and arthritic change) and provide stability to the thumb ray. Success rates are high, barring any unfortunate complications as discussed next.

COMPLICATIONS

■ Complications following MP joint dislocations are uncommon and mostly limited to the sequelae of concomitant soft tissue injuries.

■ Damage to the adjacent neurovascular structures can result from the initial traumatic injury or careless surgical technique at the time of open reduction.

■ Damage to the flexor pollicis longus tendon may occur when it gets trapped in the joint or again when it is manipulated surgically during an open reduction.

■ A complication encountered more often is persistent, chronic instability of the MP joint that results from failure to recognize the nature of the original injury or rehabilitate it properly.

■ Complications after treatment for chronic MP joint volar instability are likewise uncommon and generally related to failure of the chosen procedure.

■ Volar plate advancement can fail due to stretching out over time or a second trauma that causes acute rupture of the repair or sutures.

■ Nonunion of attempted arthrodesis is always a risk, but fortunately in the small joints of the hand, including thumb MP joints, it is uncommon. Nonunion rates range from 0% to 12% in several reported series.[12]

■ Hardware causing soft tissue irritation is a potential complication. That can be from superficial pin tract infections in cases where Kirschner wires are used to maintain joint reduction to extensor tendon irritation when fusions are done using plates and screws.

REFERENCES

1. Eaton RG, Floyd WE. Thumb metacarpophalangeal capsulodesis: an adjunct procedure to basal joint arthroplasty for collapse deformity of the first ray. J Hand Surg Am 1988;13A:449–453.
2. Glickel SZ. Metacarpophalangeal and interphalangeal joint injuries and instabilities. In Peimer CA, ed. Surgery of the Hand and Upper Extremity. New York: McGraw-Hill, 1996:1043–1067.
3. Glickel SZ, Barron OA, Eaton RG. Dislocations and ligament injuries in the digits. In Green DP, Hotchkiss RN, Pederson WC, eds. Green's Operative Hand Surgery. Philadelphia: Churchill Livingstone, 1999: 772–808.
4. Gunther SF, Zielinski CJ. Irreducible palmar dislocation of the proximal phalanx of the thumb: case report. J Hand Surg Am 1982;7A: 515–517.
5. Hirata H, Takegami K, Nagakura T, et al. Irreducible volar subluxation of the metacarpophalangeal joint of the thumb. J Hand Surg Am 2004;29A:921–924.
6. Kahler DM, McCue FC. Metacarpophalangeal and proximal interphalangeal joint injuries of the hand, including the thumb. Clin Sports Med 1992;11:57–76.
7. Kijowski R, DeSmet AA. The role of ultrasound in the evaluation of sports medicine injuries of the upper extremity. Clin Sports Med 2006;25:569–590.
8. Masson JA, Golimbu CN, Grossman JA. MR imaging of the metacarpophalangeal joints. Magn Reson Imaging Clin North Am 1995;3: 313–325.
9. Posner MA, Retaillaud J-L. Metacarpophalangeal joint injuries of the thumb. Hand Clin 1992;8:713–732.
10. Schuurman AH, Bos KE. Treatment of volar instability of the metacarpophalangeal joint of the thumb by volar capsulodesis. J Hand Surg Br 1993;18B:346–349.
11. Tonkin MA, Beard AJ, Kemp SJ, et al. Sesamoid arthrodesis for hyperextension of the thumb metacarpophalangeal joint. J Hand Surg Am 1995;20A:334–338.
12. Weiland AJ. Small joint arthrodesis. In Green DP, Hotchkiss RN, Pederson WC, eds. Green's Operative Hand Surgery. Philadelphia: Churchill Livingstone, 1999:95–107.

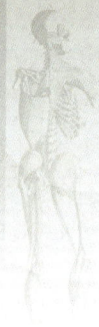

Chapter 28

Arthroscopic and Open Primary Repair of Acute Thumb Metacarpophalangeal Joint Radial and Ulnar Collateral Ligament Disruptions

Alejandro Badia and Prakash Khanchandani

DEFINITION

- Ulnar collateral ligament (UCL) and radial collateral ligament (RCL) tears of the thumb metacarpophalangeal joint (MCP) are common injuries resulting from disruption of the continuity of these ligaments.
- These disruptions are frequently the result of an athletic injury, a fall, or a motor vehicle accident.

ANATOMY

- The MCP joint of the thumb is transitional between a condyloid and ginglymus joint. The articulating surface of the base of the proximal phalanx is a shallow concavity that provides relatively little intrinsic stability. Hence, most of the joint's stability is afforded by its ligament and capsular supports.
- The RCL and UCL are both structurally similar, composed of both proper and accessory components, and are the main stabilizers of the thumb MCP joint.[27]
- The proper collateral ligaments, which originate from a fossa in the metacarpal neck dorsal to the axis of rotation, are the primary ligamentous supports. They fan out from their proximal origins to distal insertions on the lateral and volar aspect of the base of proximal phalanx.
- The accessory collateral ligaments act as supplementary supports originating from the palmar aspect of the metacarpal neck fossa and inserting into the volar plate and the sesamoid on respective sides of the joint.[27]
- The collateral ligaments provide not only medial and lateral stability but also stability in the dorsovolar plane by virtue of their dorsal origin and their volar insertion.[26]
- The volar plate is a central fibrocartilaginous structure extending from the neck of the metacarpal proximally to the base of the proximal phalanx distally.
- One difference between the ulnar and radial sides of the MCP joint is related to the aponeurosis. The broad abductor aponeurosis covers the entire radial side of the MCP joint, whereas the much narrower adductor aponeurotic sheath spans the ulnar side of the joint.

PATHOGENESIS

- Acute injury of the UCL usually results from sudden forceful abduction and extension at the thumb MCP joint.[21,25]
  - This can take place during a fall on an outstretched hand with the thumb abducted, as seen in skiers,[8] or in baseball players when the glove strikes the ground while fielding.
  - The extent of the injury and the grade of the injury depend on the loading force at the time of impact. The most common injury of the thumb MCP joint is a partial disruption or sprain of the UCL.
- Tears of the UCL can occur anywhere within the ligament's substance, although most take place at or near the site of insertion into the proximal phalanx, sometimes with an avulsion fracture (**FIG 1A**).[4,9,29]
- The narrower adductor sheath on the ulnar aspect of the joint allows superficial displacement and entrapment of the torn proximal end of UCL, termed a Stener lesion (**FIG 1B**).[29] Because of the broader abductor aponeurosis, however, such a lesion is not seen on the radial side.[11]
- RCL injuries are generally caused by sudden adduction and extension of the MCP joint, commonly occurring during athletic injuries.[5] They can also occur by direct blunt impact to the lateral side of the thumb.
  - The RCL is more often injured close to its origin on the dorsal radial metacarpal head. It may also be disrupted in its midsubstance.

NATURAL HISTORY

- Untreated UCL injuries are relatively common. Patients are often sent away being told they simply have a "sprain." If instability is present and not corrected, the patient may experience pinch weakness and eventually chronic pain.
- Untreated RCL tears are even more common and often result in late degenerative arthritis, commonly requiring MCP arthrodesis.
  - Less severe avulsions may lead to prominent osteophytes on the dorsoradial aspect of the metacarpal neck, suggesting the prior injury.
- Mondry[19] first described the unstable thumb MCP joint in 1940, while Watson-Jones[30] mentioned the importance of the UCL in relation to stability of the MCP joint of the thumb.
  - Campbell[6] described gamekeeper's thumb as a chronic instability of the UCL in Scottish gamekeepers.
  - Gerber et al[13] popularized the term *skier's thumb* to refer to acute UCL injuries.
  - Stener[29] outlined the ligamentous anatomy of the thumb MCP joint and subsequent pathoanatomy of the lesion now termed the Stener lesion. Stener also described avulsion of the UCL leading to articular fracture of the proximal phalanx, now popularly referred to as a "bony gamekeeper's thumb."[28]
  - Moberg and Stener[18] reported that UCL disruption is 10 times more common than RCL disruption. This frequency has been widely confirmed.[9,23,26]

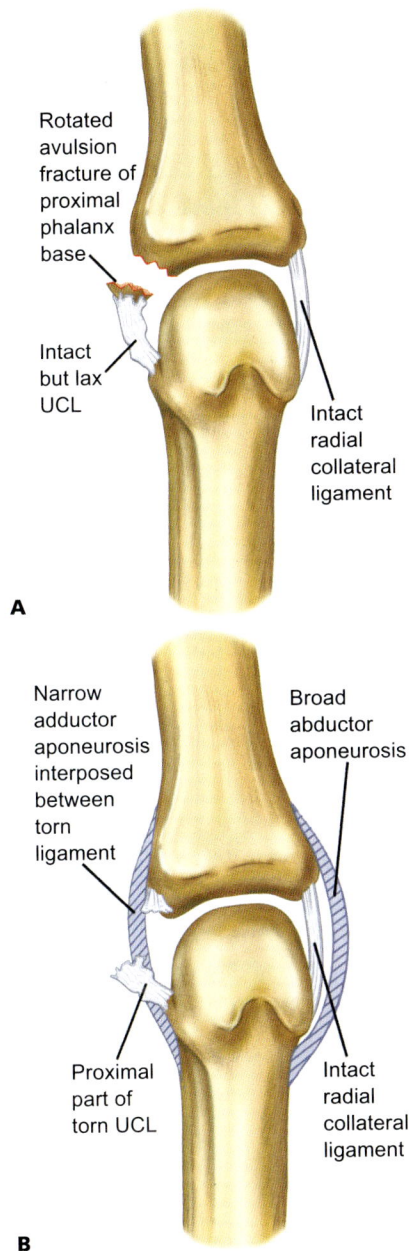

Rotated avulsion fracture of proximal phalanx base

Intact but lax UCL

Intact radial collateral ligament

A

Narrow adductor aponeurosis interposed between torn ligament

Broad abductor aponeurosis

Proximal part of torn UCL

Intact radial collateral ligament

B

FIG 1 • A. A bony gamekeeper's thumb. **B.** The narrow adductor aponeurosis is interposed between the avulsed ligament–bone and the site of attachment.

- Frank and Dobyns[12] reported that RCL injuries are somewhat more common than initially thought, with incidences ranging from 23% to 35% of collateral ligament injuries.
  - This has echoed our experiences with the more subtle RCL injuries often being neglected, causing late morbidity.

PATIENT HISTORY AND PHYSICAL FINDINGS

UCL Tears

- Patients with UCL tears present with pain, stiffness, tenderness, and swelling of the MCP joint. The defining symptom, however, may be marked pinch weakness.

- On examination there is discrete tenderness over the ulnar joint line, at the ulnar side of the metacarpal neck, and most classically at the volar ulnar base of the proximal phalanx.[2]
- Physical examination is critical in establishing the need for surgical treatment by distinguishing between a partial and a complete ligament tear.
- A valgus stress examination comparing the stability of the injured versus the uninjured UCL is the best method to detect a complete tear.
  - The stress test may be aided by live fluoroscopy and the use of a local anesthetic block.
  - The presence of an associated fracture should not deter the examiner from performing a stress test. Nondisplaced avulsion fractures at the insertion site of the proper collateral ligament may coexist with a complete ligament tear.
  - The results of the stress test are based on angular instability of the joint and the quality of the "end point."
  - Laxity of more than 30 degrees in extension and 15 degrees in flexion as compared to the contralateral side should be highly suggestive of a complete tear of the UCL.[15]
- The presence of fullness or a palpable mass on the ulnar aspect of the metacarpal head and neck, representing a Stener lesion,[1] is strongly suggestive of a completely disrupted and retracted UCL.
- Volar subluxation of the MCP joint signifies loss of the dorsal volar stabilizing effect of the collateral ligament and is also consistent with a complete tear.

RCL Tears

- RCL tears present as localized tenderness over the radial base of the proximal phalanx but more commonly over the metacarpal head.
- The dorsoradial aspect of the metacarpal head may be prominent due to soft tissue swelling.
- Acute RCL injuries are assessed in the same manner as discussed for UCL injuries.
  - For the stress test of the RCL in extension and 30 degrees of flexion, laxity of the joint greater than 30 degrees as compared to the uninjured side suggests a complete tear of the RCL.
- The emphasis on distinguishing partial tears from complete tears does not directly affect treatment and therefore is less important than for UCL injuries. Even complete RCL tears are not capable of retracting behind the aponeurosis and therefore may be treated nonoperatively.
- RCL injuries are more common than often thought. Significant radial-sided pain with laxity or subtle radiographic signs of dorsal capsule avulsion necessitate treatment (**FIG 2**).

IMAGING AND OTHER DIAGNOSTIC STUDIES

- Radiographs include posteroanterior, lateral, and oblique views of the thumb. Images of the contralateral thumb are used for comparison and may reveal subtle joint subluxation.
- Stress radiographs of the MCP joint in full extension and in 30 degrees of flexion are rarely required though occasionally

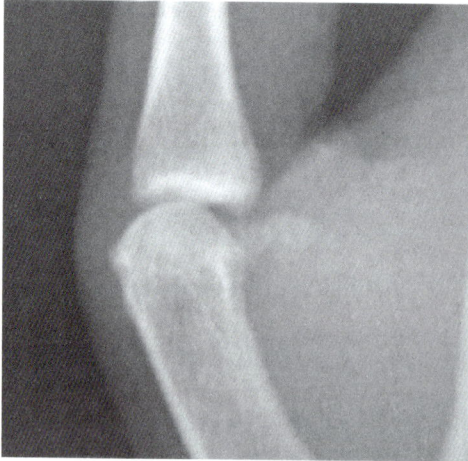

FIG 2 • Radiograph showing a chronic neglected radial collateral ligament tear. There is subtle volar subluxation of the proximal phalanx. Oblique views often demonstrate a small bony prominence on the metacarpal neck dorsum.

can help distinguish between a partial and complete ligament injury.[4,12]

- MCP joint arthrography, MRI, and ultrasound have all been used to determine the degree of ligament injury and displacement but are almost never required.
  - On MRI, a Stener lesion is characterized by a "yo-yo on a string" sign.

DIFFERENTIAL DIAGNOSIS

- Diffuse capsular injury without discrete ligament tear
- Fracture or articular cartilage injury
  - The articular surface is best assessed via arthroscopy or perhaps MRI.
- Arthritis
  - Diffuse soft tissue injury involving a previously asymptomatic but arthritic joint can result in persistent pain.

NONOPERATIVE MANAGEMENT

- Treatment depends on the severity of injury, the type of tear,[7,14,16,17,20,22] and the presence of an avulsion fracture involving a significant portion of the articular surface or an open physis.
- Partial UCL and partial and complete RCL tears without volar subluxation of the proximal phalanx can be effectively managed by immobilization, then protected mobilization using a removable splint for a total of 4 to 6 weeks.
  - Initial immobilization is traditionally accomplished using a thumb spica cast. Such a cast allowing wrist motion is preferable.
  - Alternatively, a customized thermoplastic splint that immobilizes only the thumb MCP joint and leaves the wrist and interphalangeal joint free can be used for reliable patients with less severe injuries.

SURGICAL MANAGEMENT

- Complete UCL disruption, especially if denoted by a Stener lesion or joint subluxation, should be treated surgically. Additionally, a displaced avulsion fracture involving a significant portion of the articular surface should be reduced and stabilized operatively.
- An avulsion fracture of the proximal phalanx can be effectively managed by arthroscopic techniques.[3,23,24] Occasionally, it is necessary for an arthroscopic procedure to be converted to an open procedure if reduction of a large or comminuted fracture fragment in the proximal phalanx is not feasible (**FIG 3**).
- Injuries associated with a Stener lesion warrant open repair.
- Partial tears of RCL are best managed by cast immobilization, whereas complete tears associated with palmer subluxation require open surgical repair of the ligament and dorsal capsule.[10]
- Arthroscopy can also be a useful adjunct to open procedures as it allows a more thorough débridement and evaluation of concomitant pathology.
- A regional anesthetic combined with light intravenous sedation is generally adequate for the procedures detailed below.

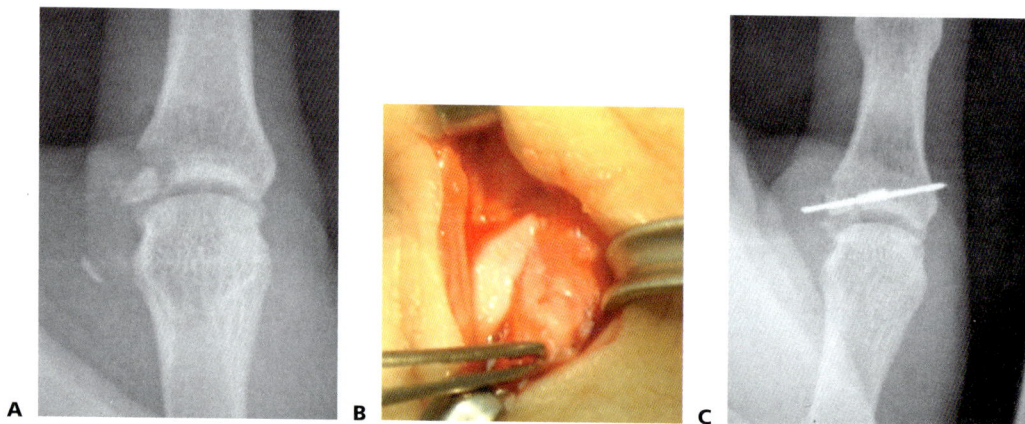

FIG 3 • **A.** Preoperative radiograph showing an avulsion fracture at the ulnar collateral ligament insertion site. **B.** Arthroscopic reduction failed and an open procedure was performed because of the interposition of the adductor aponeurosis at the fracture site and unrecognized fracture comminution. **C.** Postoperative radiograph showing fixation of the fragment and attachment of the ligament using a Kirschner wire and a bone anchor.

ACUTE UCL DISRUPTIONS

Arthroscopic Treatment of UCL Avulsion Fractures

- Traction is applied using a finger trap placed on the thumb with 5 pounds of counterforce.
  - A traction tower is not used in order to facilitate fluoroscopy.
- Palpate the joint and then inject 1 to 2 mL of lidocaine using an 18-gauge needle.
  - Take care to avoid injuring the articular cartilage.
- Insert a 1.9-mm 30-degree arthroscope via a longitudinal portal stab wound on the radial side of the extensor pollicis longus tendon.
  - This allows the best visualization of the ulnar-sided pathology.
- Insert a 2-mm full-radius shaver in the ulnar portal and evacuate the hematoma and any minute bone fragments that may prevent visualization.
- Perform a synovectomy, with emphasis on the ulnar side. This allows clear delineation of the avulsed fracture fragment (**TECH FIG 1A**).
- Insert a small probe through the ulnar portal and hook the fragment on its radial side, within the fracture site. Gentle proximal and radial traction on the ulnar fragment typically accomplishes the reduction.
  - Preoperative radiographs help to plan the specific maneuver necessary for fracture reduction, but the arthroscopic picture will ultimately determine the direction of fragment derotation required to achieve anatomic reduction of the joint.
- Reintroduce the shaver as needed for débridement and to assist fracture reduction.
- Insert a 0.035-inch Kirschner wire percutaneously into the joint just proximal and ulnar to the reduced bony fragment (**TECH FIG 1B**).
- Arthroscopic visualization aids in placement and orientation of the transfixing Kirschner wire using the wire driver (**TECH FIG 1C**).
- Using the wire driver, engage the radial cortex to stabilize the fracture fragment.
- Use both fluoroscopy and arthroscopy to determine the adequacy of fragment reduction as well as to confirm proper wire placement and fracture stability (**TECH FIG 1D,E**).
- Cut the wire just underneath the skin (**TECH FIG 1F**).
- Close the skin and apply a bulky thumb spica plaster splint while the thumb is still suspended.
- Final fluoroscopic pictures are taken and the tourniquet is released.

Open Repair of Complete UCL Disruptions

- Make a curvilinear or a longitudinal lazy-Z incision with the superior or dorsal portion proximal.
  - The UCL origin is more dorsal and fans out in volar fashion.

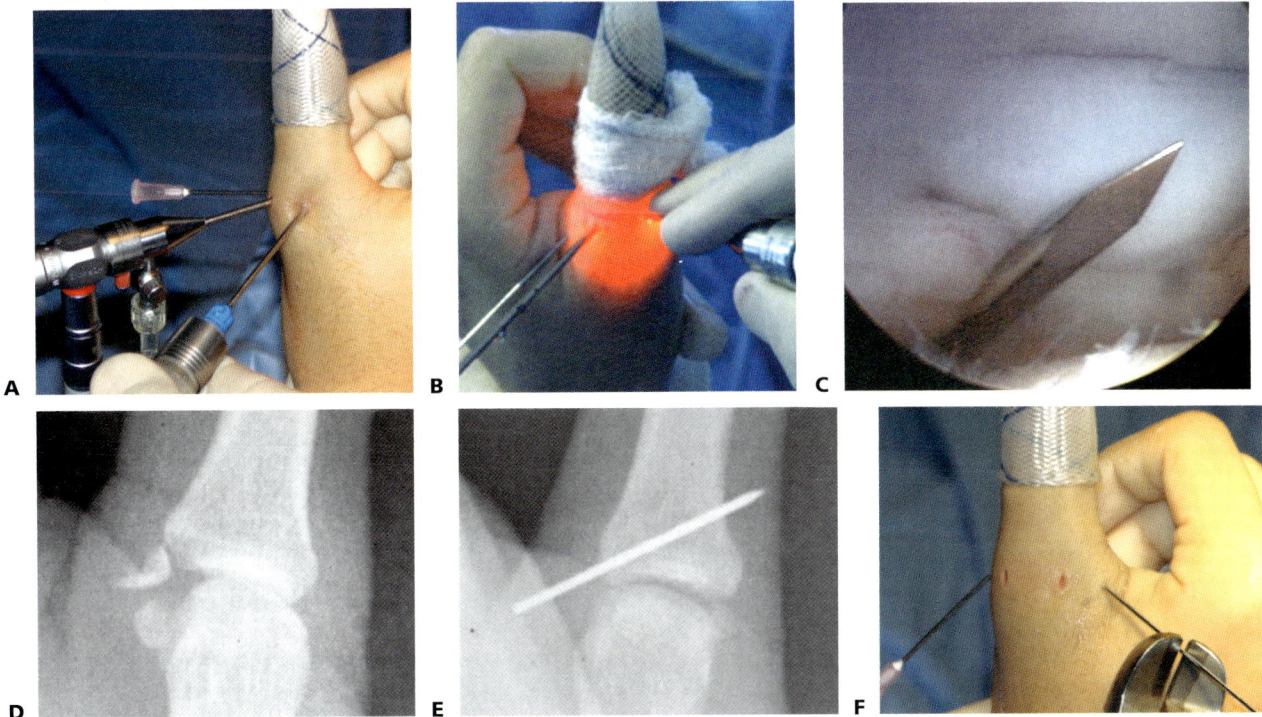

TECH FIG 1 • **A.** With the arthroscope in the dorsoradial portal and the shaver in the dorsoulnar portal, arthroscopic débridement is performed before reduction of the fragment. **B.** The fragment is reduced arthroscopically and stabilized with a Kirschner wire. **C.** Arthroscopic view showing the Kirschner wire and the fracture fragment before reduction. **D.** This displaced and rotated bony avulsion fracture at the attachment of the UCL is reduced arthroscopically and stabilized. **E.** Radiograph showing anatomic arthroscopic reduction and pinning. **F.** The Kirschner wire, fixing the avulsed fragment, is cut beneath the skin.

- Dissect the subcutaneous tissues with small tenotomy scissors, taking care to maintain hemostasis using a bipolar cautery.
  - Identify the dorsal radial sensory nerve branches and gently retract them dorsally.
- Take note of the oblique transverse fibers of the adductor aponeurosis. In more severe injuries the aponeurosis my be torn, revealing the underlying UCL.
- Divide the adductor aponeurosis longitudinally, allowing the muscular origin of the adductor pollicis to pull back the fascia and facilitate posterior retraction of the aponeurosis.
  - The torn UCL is seen directly under the incised adductor aponeurosis (**TECH FIG 2A**).
  - In the case of a Stener lesion, the retracted and displaced stump of the UCL is visualized just superficial to the proximal edge of the adductor aponeurosis before incision.
- Determine the direction of the UCL fibers and incise the joint capsule on the ligament's dorsal margin.
- Inspect the joint, and perform a limited débridement and synovectomy as indicated.
- Precisely determine the location and degree of UCL injury.
  - Less common intrasubstance tears are repaired primarily with 3-0 or 4-0 permanent suture in a mattress or figure of 8 configuration.
  - Avulsion of the ligament attachment from the base of the proximal phalanx is most frequently encountered and is treated by reattaching the ligament's insertion.

- Isolate the anatomic insertion site for the proper collateral ligament on the volar ulnar base of the proximal phalanx and prepare the site for ligament attachment by débriding the remaining soft tissue down to bleeding bone.
  - Creating a small bony trough at the insertion site helps stimulate bleeding and ligament attachment (**TECH FIG 2B**).
- Prepare the UCL stump by mobilizing it on its margins and freshening the distal end with a no. 15 blade.
- Insert a 2-mm or smaller suture anchor into the prepared bony site and verify its position with fluoroscopy.
- While the thumb is deviated in an ulnar direction, reattach the ligament stump to the proximal phalanx by placing a horizontal mattress stitch using the suture from the anchor.
- Repair the accessory portion of the UCL by placing 3-0 or 4-0 permanent suture from the ligament into the ulnar margin of the volar plate.
- Additional permanent sutures may be placed to secure the repaired UCL to surrounding soft tissues.
- Close the capsule to the dorsal margin of the ligament using 4-0 absorbable suture.
- Precisely reconstruct the adductor aponeurosis with 4-0 inverted interrupted permanent suture and close the skin.
- Ensure restoration of stability and maintenance of full MCP joint flexion.
- Place a forearm-based thumb spica splint.
- Very severe injuries with extensive disruption of soft tissue stabilizers may rarely require augmentation with a temporary Kirschner wire.

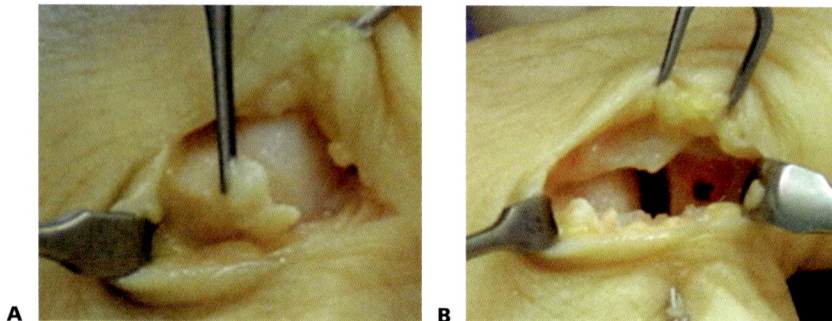

TECH FIG 2 • **A.** Avulsed ulnar collateral ligament (Stener lesion) is well visualized after division of the adductor aponeurosis. **B.** At the anatomic site of ulnar collateral ligament insertion, the bone is prepared and a bone anchor inserted.

ACUTE RCL DISRUPTIONS

- Make a dorsoradial curvilinear or a longitudinal lazy-Z incision similar to that used for the repair of UCL disruptions, and dissect the soft tissues as detailed earlier.
- Incise the abductor aponeurosis in line with the RCL.
- Radial-sided lesions are often coupled with concomitant avulsions of the dorsal capsule. If the capsule is intact, incise it along the dorsal margin of the RCL to inspect the joint.
- Isolate the ligament and its point of disruption, and then mobilize the structure to allow for anatomic repair.
  - Typically, disruptions take place at the proximal origin (**TECH FIG 3A**).

- Débride the bone and ligament stump in the manner detailed for open repair of UCL avulsions.
  - Remove reactive bone and early osteophytes at the site of ligament or capsule avulsion with a rongeur.
- Place a 2.0-mm or smaller suture anchor in the collateral recess, the dorsoradial distal metacarpal.
  - Ensure proper placement radiographically.
- Reattach the ligament to its anatomic point of origin using the suture from the anchor (**TECH FIG 3B**).
- Repair the capsule and further secure the RCL to surrounding soft tissue with 3-0 or 4-0 permanent suture (**TECH FIG 3C**).

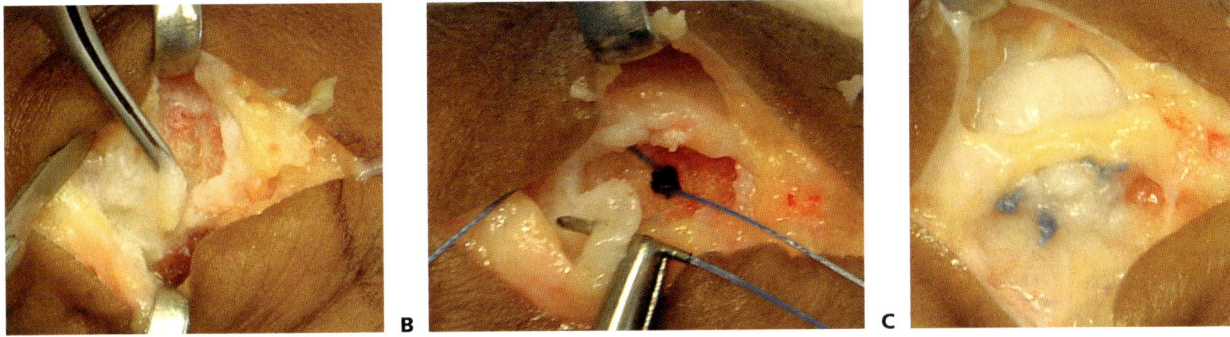

TECH FIG 3 • **A.** Dorsal capsule to be repaired to the metacarpal head with decortication in a chronic radial collateral ligament injury. **B.** Anchors placed in the bone with the ligament ready to be sutured. **C.** Completed reconstruction of the radial collateral ligament with repaired abductor aponeurosis and demonstrated course of the radial sensory nerve, which is protected throughout the procedure.

- Repair the abductor aponeurosis and skin as described earlier.
- Ensure restoration of stability and maintenance of full MCP joint flexion.

- Place a forearm-based thumb spica splint.
- Very severe injuries with extensive disruption of soft tissue stabilizers may rarely require augmentation with a temporary Kirschner wire.

PEARLS AND PITFALLS

- MCP ligamentous lesions require a high index of suspicion.
- The obvious lesions with instability will likely get appropriate repairs with subsequent rehabilitation programs.
- Missing a significant ligament tear may cause few physical problems short term but may become a chronic painful lesion long term.
  - This is where arthroscopy may also play a good role. The chronically painful lesions may not demonstrate laxity or even a gross physical problem. Nevertheless, the pain is present and repeat corticosteroid injections are certainly not a solution. Arthroscopic synovectomy or capsular or ligamentous débridement will alter the articular milieu enough to allow for resolution of chronic pain and swelling. All this is coupled with rapid resolution of symptoms and recovery of range of motion.

POSTOPERATIVE MANAGEMENT

- Bony gamekeeper's thumb
  - A fiberglass thumb spica cast is applied at 1 week postoperatively and the pin is removed under local anesthesia at about 5 weeks postoperatively.
  - A brief course of physical therapy is initiated. The patient is given a hand-based thumb–carpometacarpal type of removable splint to be used during strenuous activities.
  - Therapy is usually short term owing to less swelling and stiffness as compared with open approaches.
  - All unrestricted activities are permitted at 8 weeks.
- UCL and RCL injuries: True ligament-to-bone healing is necessary, so 6 weeks of postoperative thumb spica immobilization is critical to success.

OUTCOMES

- Clinical results after a combined arthroscopic and open procedure can be excellent.
- Functional outcome after repair of either UCL or RCL injuries tends to be excellent. Perhaps this is because thumb stability, not MCP motion, is critical to hand function.
  - While the MCP joint often remains fairly stiff long after immobilization is discontinued, the resultant disability is minimal, considering that people demonstrate a wide range of normal MCP arc of motion.

- Many contralateral thumbs display a flexion arc of less than 20%; therefore, the normal restoration of full motion is not the goal. Good stability without pain should be the aim.
- RCL injuries of the thumb tend to have a higher tendency to develop posttraumatic arthritis.
  - Our long-term experience has shown the need for late arthrodesis on only two occasions. These are cases in which significant volar subluxation is present, and the articular wear at time of surgery was likely predictive of this long-term outcome.
  - A chronically painful thumb, with any degenerative changes on radiographs, coupled with volar posturing of the phalanx, should likely be considered straightaway for fusion.
  - Thorough counseling of the patient indicating the minimal deficit produced by arthrodesis is helpful.

COMPLICATIONS

- Careful surgical dissection should avoid the most common complication, which would be iatrogenic trauma to the dorsal sensory nerve. Once done, there are minimal complications associated with this area of hand surgery.
- Other complications can include stiffness, as previously discussed, infection, persistent instability, or chronic pain syndromes.
- Recalcitrant pain or instability can simply be managed by arthrodesis, still portending a good functional outcome.

REFERENCES

1. Abrahamson S, Sollerman C, Lundborg G, et al. Diagnosis of displaced ulnar collateral ligament of the metacarpophalangeal joint of the thumb. J Hand Surg Am 1990;15A:457–460.
2. Arnold DM, Cooney WP, Wood ME. Surgical management of chronic ulnar collateral ligament injury of the thumb metacarpophalangeal joint. Orthop Rev 1992;21:583–588.
3. Badia A. Arthroscopic reduction and internal fixation of bony gamekeepers thumb. Orthopedics 2006;29:675–678.
4. Bowers WH, Hurst LC. Gamekeeper's thumb: evaluation by arthrography and stress roentgenography. J Bone Joint Surg Am 1977;59A:519–524.
5. Camp RA, Weatherwax RJ, Miller EB. Chronic post-traumatic radial instability of the thumb metacarpophalangeal joint. J Hand Surg Am 1980;5A:221–225.
6. Campbell CS. Gamekeeper's thumb. J Bone Joint Surg Br 1955;37B:148–149.
7. Campbell JD, Feagin JA, King P, et al. Ulnar collateral ligament injury of the thumb: treatment with glove spica cast. Am J Sports Med 1992;20:29–30.
8. Carr D, Johnson RJ, Pope MH. Upper extremity injuries in skiing. Am J Sports Med 1981;9:378–383.
9. Coonrad RW, Goldner JL. A study of the pathological findings and treatment in soft tissue injuries of the thumb metacarpophalangeal joint. J Bone Joint Surg Am 1968;50A:439–451.
10. Dray GJ, Eaton RG. Dislocations and ligament injuries in the digits. In Green DP, ed. Green's Operative Hand Surgery, 2nd ed. New York: Churchill Livingstone, 1988:777–811.
11. Durham JW, Khuri S, Kim MH. Acute and late radial collateral ligament injuries of the thumb metacarpophalangeal joint. J Hand Surg Am 1993;18A:232–237.
12. Frank WE, Dobyns J. Surgical pathology of collateral ligamentous injuries of thumb. Clin Orthop Relat Res 1972;83:102–114.
13. Gerber C, Senn E, Matter P. Skier's thumb: surgical treatment of the recent injuries to the ulnar collateral ligament of the thumbs metacarpophalangeal joint. Am J Sports Med 1981;993:171–177.
14. Glickel SZ, Malerich M, Pearce SM, et al. Ligament replacement for chronic instability of the ulnar collateral ligament of the metacarpophalangeal joint of the thumb. J Hand Surg Am 1993;18:930–941.
15. Heyman P, Gelberman RH, Duncan K, et al. Injuries of the ulnar collateral ligament of the thumb metacarpophalangeal joint: biomechanical and the prospective clinical studies on the usefulness of the valgus stress testing. Clin Orthop Relat Res 1993;292:165–171.
16. Kozin SH. Treatment of thumb ulnar collateral ligament ruptures with the Mitek bone anchor. Ann Plast Surg 1995;35:1–5.
17. Kozin SH, Bishop AT. Tension wire fixation of avulsion fractures at the thumb metacarpophalangeal joint. J Hand Surg Am 1994;19A:1027–1031.
18. Moberg E, Stener B. Injuries to the ligaments of the thumb and fingers: diagnosis, treatment and prognosis. Acta Chir Scand 1953;106:166–186.
19. Mondry F. Beitrag fur Operative Behandlung des Wackeldaumens. Zentralbl Chir 1940;67:1532.
20. Neviaser RJ, Wilson JN, Lievano A. Rupture of the ulnar collateral ligament of the thumb (gamekeeper's thumb): correction by dynamic repair. J Bone Joint Surg Am 1971;53A:1357–1364.
21. Parikh M, Nahigian S, Froimson A. Gamekeeper's thumb. Plast Reconstr Surg 1980;58:24–31.
22. Pichora DR, McMurtry RY, Bell MJ. Gamekeeper's thumb: a prospective study of functional bracing. J Hand Surg Am 1989;14A:567–573.
23. Rozmaryn LM, Wei N. Metacarpophalangeal arthroscopy. Arthroscopy 1999;15:333–337.
24. Ryu J, Fagan R. Arthroscopic treatment of acute complete thumb metacarpophalangeal ulnar collateral ligament tears. J Hand Surg Am 1995;20A:1037–1042.
25. Smith MA. The mechanism of acute ulnar stability of the metacarpophalangeal joint of the thumb. Hand 1980;12:225–230.
26. Smith RJ. Posttraumatic instability of the metacarpal joint of the thumb. J Bone Joint Surg Am 1977;59A:14–21.
27. Smith RJ, Desantolo A. Lateral instability at the metacarpophalangeal joint of the thumb. Handchirurgie 1972;4:95–98.
28. Stener B. Hyperextension injuries of the metacarpophalangeal joint of the thumb-rupture of flexor pollicis brevis: an anatomic and clinical study. Acta Chir Scand 1963;125:275–293.
29. Stener B. Displacement of the ruptured ulnar collateral ligament of the metacarpophalangeal joint of the thumb: a clinical and anatomical study. J Bone Joint Surg Br 1962;44B:869–879.
30. Watson-Jones R. Fractures and Joint Injuries, 4th ed. Baltimore: Williams & Wilkins, 1955.

Chapter 29

Reconstruction of Chronic Radial and Ulnar Instability of the Thumb Metacarpophalangeal Joint

Steven Z. Glickel and Louis W. Catalano III

DEFINITION

- Chronic instability of the ulnar collateral ligament (UCL) and the radial collateral ligament (RCL) of the metacarpophalangeal (MCP) joint of the thumb usually results from unrecognized or untreated acute tears of the ligament.
- Persistent laxity may cause pain and weakness and, eventually, osteoarthritis resulting from asymmetrical wear of the articular cartilage.

ANATOMY

- The MCP joint of the thumb has characteristics of both a condyloid and a ginglymus joint. The radial condyle is taller in the dorsovolar dimension than the ulnar condyle.
- The dorsoulnar and dorsoradial digital nerves are terminal branches of the superficial sensory branch of the radial nerve and invariably cross the operative field in the plane immediately superficial to the adductor and abductor aponeuroses, respectively.
  - They are at risk during reconstruction of the collateral ligaments. During the exposure of the joint, the nerve should be mobilized and gently retracted.
- The adductor aponeurosis is an extension of the tendon of the adductor pollicis muscle, which contributes obliquely oriented fibers to the extensor mechanism distal to the vertical fibers.
- The abductor aponeurosis is an extension of the tendon of the abductor pollicis brevis muscle, which contributes obliquely oriented fibers to the extensor mechanism distal to the vertical fibers.
- The proper ulnar and radial collateral ligaments originate from fossae of the condyle of the metacarpal head on the radial and ulnar sides and pass obliquely from dorsal proximal to volar distal to insert on the volar third of the base of the proximal phalanx. The ligament widens as it goes from its metacarpal origin to its proximal phalangeal insertion.
  - The proper collateral ligaments are tight in MCP joint flexion and lax in extension.
- The accessory collateral ligaments originate on the metacarpal head contiguous with but just volar to the proper collateral ligament and extend obliquely across the MCP joint, inserting on the sesamoid and volar plate.
  - The accessory collateral ligaments are tight in extension and lax in flexion.
- By definition, to have a complete ligament rupture, both the proper and the accessory collateral ligaments must be torn.
- The Stener lesion is a palpable soft tissue mass on the ulnar aspect of the MCP joint. It results from a tear of the UCL caused by forceful radial deviation of the proximal phalanx, angulating the MCP joint 70 degrees or more. The ligament tears distally at or near its insertion on the volar ulnar base of the proximal phalanx. As the proximal phalanx deviates radially, the ruptured UCL stump retracts proximal and superficial to the adductor aponeurosis. Hence, the avulsed ligament is separated from its deep insertion by the aponeurosis, preventing ligament healing.
- The abductor aponeurosis is wider than the adductor aponeurosis. When the RCL tears, the ends of the torn ligament remain deep to the abductor aponeurosis. Hence, a Stener type of lesion rarely occurs on the radial side.

PATHOGENESIS

- The UCL of the MCP joint of the thumb is usually torn by forceful abduction and extension of the thumb, as in a fall on the outstretched hand with the thumb abducted. The proximal phalanx deviates radially and, if there is sufficient force, the UCL either avulses from its insertion on the base of the proximal phalanx or, less commonly, tears in its midsubstance or from its origin on the metacarpal head.[19]
  - Two primary causes of chronic instability of the UCL exist.
    - Inadequate treatment of an acute, complete UCL disruption, with or without an associated Stener lesion
    - Progressive attenuation of the ligament due to repetitive trauma
- Tears of the RCL typically result from forceful ulnar deviation and extension of the MCP joint.
  - Proximal and distal avulsions of the ligament occur with roughly equal frequency.
  - Intrasubstance tears occur infrequently.
- Chronic instability of the radial RCL has three primary causes.
  - Most commonly, chronic laxity is due to lack of recognition of the pathology and therefore inadequate or late treatment.
  - Even when recognized, conservative management may fail.
  - Chronic attenuation due to repetitive trauma is less common.

NATURAL HISTORY

- Over time, chronic tears of the collateral ligaments of the thumb MCP joints cause weakness of pinch and grip due to lack of stability and pain.
  - Incompetence of the UCL diminishes the thumb's ability to act as a stable post against which to pinch with the index finger. Patients often have difficulty holding large objects that require counterpressure by a stable thumb.
  - Patients with chronic RCL instability often have pain with torsional motions like unscrewing jar tops.

2349

- Chronic laxity may cause incongruity and asymmetrical wear of the MCP joint, which may progress to posttraumatic osteoarthritis of the joint.
  - Arthritis of the joint causes pain, stiffness, and progressive weakness.

PATIENT HISTORY AND PHYSICAL FINDINGS

- Obtaining a relevant history from patients with chronic instability of the thumb MCP joint includes eliciting a history of trauma to the thumb in the recent or distant past.
- Patients are questioned about pain in the thumb, particularly if it is exacerbated by forceful pinch and grasp and torsional activities like turning keys in locks, turning doorknobs, or unscrewing jar tops.
  - The examine should establish the chronicity of the symptoms and whether they are increasing in severity.
- Assessment of instability of the thumb MCP collateral ligaments is primarily clinical.
- Clinical examination begins with observation.
  - The resting posture of the thumb at the MP joint is occasionally indicative of pathology. The joint may be angulated or rotated in its resting posture if the collateral ligament is grossly incompetent and the instability is chronic.
  - In thumbs with chronic RCL instability, there is often a dorsal prominence on the radial aspect of the metacarpal head. Such a prominence is generally not present in cases of chronic UCL instability.
- The involved side of the joint is usually tender to palpation.
- Palpation of a fullness or soft tissue mass on the ulnar side of the metacarpal head is strongly suggestive of a Stener lesion.
- Stability of the collateral ligament is tested in extension and 30 degrees of MCP joint flexion (under local anesthesia if needed). There is no consensus in the literature concerning the degree of instability that is diagnostic of a complete tear.
  - Valgus stress of the MCP joint in flexion is used to assess the stability of the proper UCL, whereas stress with the joint in extension is used to assess the accessory UCL as well.
  - The criteria for diagnosis of a complete ligament disruption that are most accurate were described by Heyman et al[12] and include 30 to 35 degrees of laxity of the ulnar side of the MCP joint when stressed in extension and 15 degrees more laxity than the contralateral thumb when stressed in 30 degrees of flexion.
  - Laxity in extension suggests that the accessory and proper collateral ligaments are both torn.
  - A more subtle, but often more helpful, finding is the presence or absence of a discrete endpoint to joint opening when stressed. Absence of a solid endpoint is strongly suggestive of a complete ligament tear.
- To test for joint degeneration, the MP joint is passively moved in extension and flexion combined with radial and ulnar deviation. The joint is axially loaded as it is deviated. Crepitus and pain strongly suggest the presence of osteoarthritis, a contraindication to reconstruction of an unstable MCP joint.

IMAGING AND OTHER DIAGNOSTIC STUDIES

- Radiographic evaluation includes PA, lateral, and oblique radiographs of both thumbs.
  - Fractures should be ruled out.

- The lateral view may show volar subluxation of the MCP joint, which is fairly common and may be the result of extension of the collateral ligament tear to involve the dorsal capsule. This may occur with UCL or RCL tears. An isolated tear of the dorsal joint capsule very rarely causes volar subluxation without an associated collateral ligament injury.
  - A comparison lateral radiograph of the contralateral thumb is extremely helpful if volar subluxation is suspected.
- Stress views of the MP joint have been recommended to radiographically demonstrate instability.
  - Most experienced clinicians rely almost exclusively on physical examination and static plain radiographs to make the diagnosis.
- MRI, ultrasound, and arthrography are rarely indicated to assess completeness of the UCL tear, particularly in the setting of a chronic injury.
- The use of arthroscopy as a diagnostic and treatment modality in the setting of chronic UCL instability remains investigational.

DIFFERENTIAL DIAGNOSIS

- Fracture of the metacarpal head or base of the proximal phalanx
- Synovitis of the MCP joint
- Chronic partial tear of the UCL or RCL
- MCP joint arthrosis

NONOPERATIVE MANAGEMENT

- Customized hand-based thermoplastic splints, nonsteroidal anti-inflammatory medication, and corticosteroid injections may improve the synovitis and pain resulting from chronic instability and early degenerative arthritis.

SURGICAL MANAGEMENT

- The indication for reconstruction of chronic UCL or RCL disruption is failure of conservative treatment, with persistent pain and instability of the MCP joint.
- Instability alone is a soft indication for surgery.
  - Theoretically, the asymmetric wear of the articular cartilage resulting from chronic laxity causes degeneration of the articular cartilage. This can be used as an argument for prophylactic reconstruction.
  - Most patients without pain are hesitant to consider surgery and the prolonged rehabilitation required after surgery.
- Contraindications to reconstruction of UCL or RCL tears include osteoarthritis, "multidirectional" instability, and fixed subluxation of the joint.
  - Mild chondromalacia is a relative contraindication to reconstruction and may be better treated by MCP arthrodesis.
    - If an arthritic joint is stabilized, pain is likely to persist and increase over time, necessitating conversion to an arthrodesis.
  - Fixed instability of the MCP joint is an uncommon contraindication to ligament reconstruction.
  - Reconstruction of the incompetent ligament in this scenario requires an extensive joint release, creating "multidirectional" instability.
  - Failure to release the joint adequately results in rapid recurrence of the preoperative deformity and instability.

- Reconstruction of chronic instability may involve mobilization of the disrupted ligament, mobilization of local tissues, or ligament replacement using a tendon graft.
  - The decision is made at the time of surgery.
  - The more chronic the injury and the more dramatic the laxity and deformity, the more likely the need for replacement of the ligament with a graft.

Preoperative Planning

- The patient is asked to actively bring all five digits together and simultaneously flex the wrist against resistance. The volar wrist is inspected for the presence of a palmaris longus tendon.

- Examination under anesthesia may show even greater joint laxity than expected.

Positioning

- The patient is supine on the operating room table with the arm on a hand table at an angle slightly less than perpendicular to the torso.

Approach

- Lazy-S incision centered over the MCP joint
- Midaxial incision
- Chevron-shaped incision centered over the midaxial point of the MCP joint

RECONSTRUCTION OF CHRONIC UCL DISRUPTIONS USING TENDON GRAFT

Exposure

- Incise the skin over the ulnar joint line (**TECH FIG 1A,B**).
- Elevate skin flaps and retract them with 4-0 silk sutures.
- Identify and protect the branch of the dorsoulnar digital nerve that invariably crosses the wound (**TECH FIG 1C**).
- Identify the frequently fibrotic adductor aponeurosis.
  - The proximal stump of the torn UCL may be visualized at the proximal margin of the adductor aponeurosis if a Stener lesion is present.
- Incise the adductor aponeurosis longitudinally, exposing the underlying torn UCL (**TECH FIG 1D**).

- If the ligament cannot be defined and mobilized sufficiently for direct repair or reinsertion the remnant of the ligament is excised, exposing the ulnar side of the distal metacarpal head, the base of the proximal phalanx, and the MCP joint (**TECH FIG 1E**).
- The MCP joint is "booked open" to visualize the articular cartilage.
  - Significant degenerative disease is a contraindication to reconstruction (**TECH FIG 1F**).

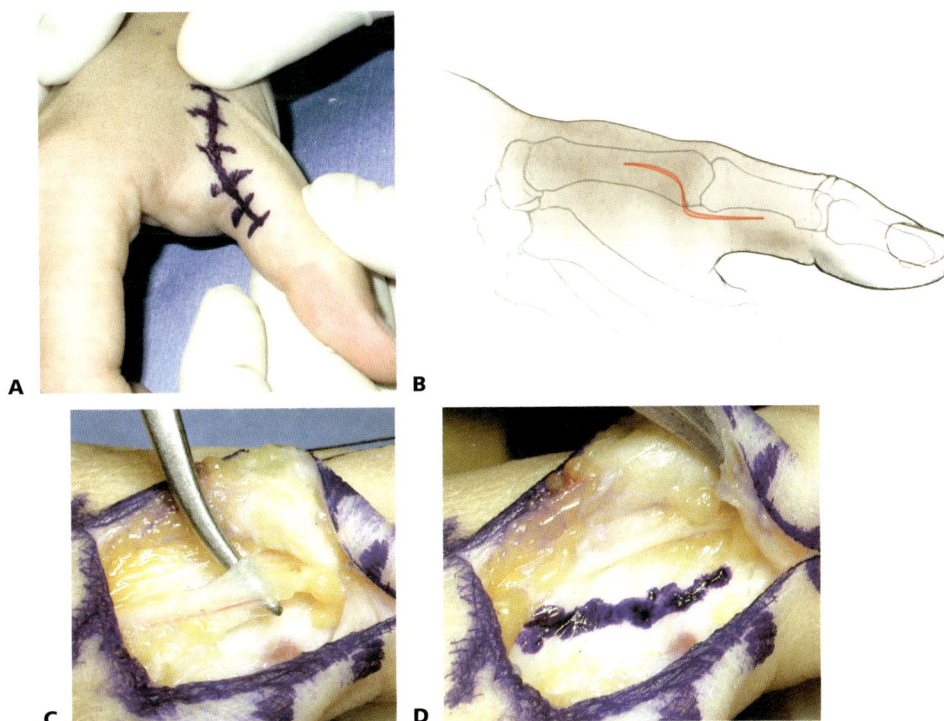

TECH FIG 1 • **A.** The lazy-S incision used for ulnar collateral ligament reconstruction. The proximal incision is dorsal and the distal incision is midaxial. **B.** A chevron-shaped incision is made centered over the ulnar side of the metacarpophalangeal joint. **C.** A dorsal ulnar sensory nerve branch is identified and protected throughout the surgery. **D.** The adductor aponeurosis is incised longitudinally about 2 mm from the extensor expansion, providing a cuff of tissue dorsally to facilitate an adequate repair at the end of the procedure. *(continued)*

TECHNIQUES

TECHNIQUES

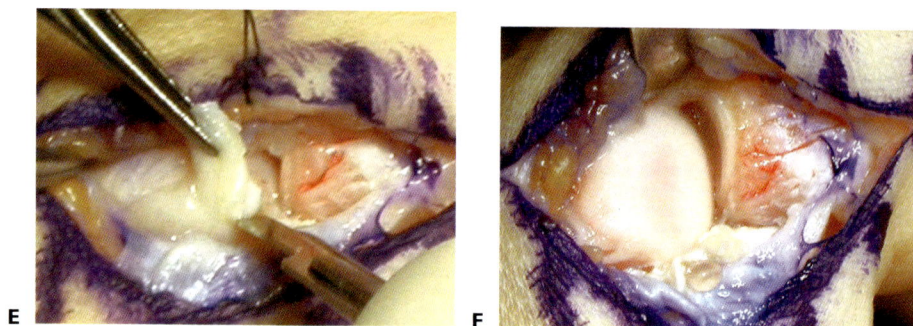

TECH FIG 1 • *(continued)* **E.** Excision of the ulnar collateral ligament remnants exposes the metacarpophalangeal joint, the metacarpal head, and the base of the proximal phalanx. **F.** The metacarpophalangeal joint is inspected for degenerative changes. Extensive degenerative disease is a contraindication to reconstruction. Arthrodesis is appropriate in the setting of an arthritic metacarpophalangeal joint. This joint shows no evidence of arthritis.

Bone Preparation

- Make two holes in the ulnar base of the proximal phalanx using hand-held gouges of increasing diameter (**TECH FIG 2A**).
  - The diameter of the hole required depends on the size of the tendon graft to be used for reconstruction.
  - The preferred donor is the palmaris longus, which is usually fairly thin and can fit in a relatively small hole.
- The gouge holes must be made far enough apart to preserve a substantial bony bridge between the holes.
  - A bridge that is too narrow can fracture during passage of the tendon graft.
- Place the holes at the 7 and 11 o'clock positions in the base of the proximal phalanx if looking at the right thumb end on. Make the holes at an angle of about 45 degrees to the bone surface and direct them toward each other in order to converge within the medullary canal and create a bone tunnel.

- Prebend a 28-gauge stainless steel wire into the approximate arc of curvature of the bone tunnel to facilitate its passage.
- Pass the wire through the bone tunnel and secure the ends with a hemostat.
- Create a second bone tunnel in the metacarpal neck. Use the gouges beginning at the fossa from which the UCL normally originates and extending slightly obliquely, from distal to proximal, across the metacarpal, exiting radially (**TECH FIG 2B,C**).
  - Most often the small, medium, and large gouges are used to create one large hole since both ends of the tendon graft are passed through this hole.

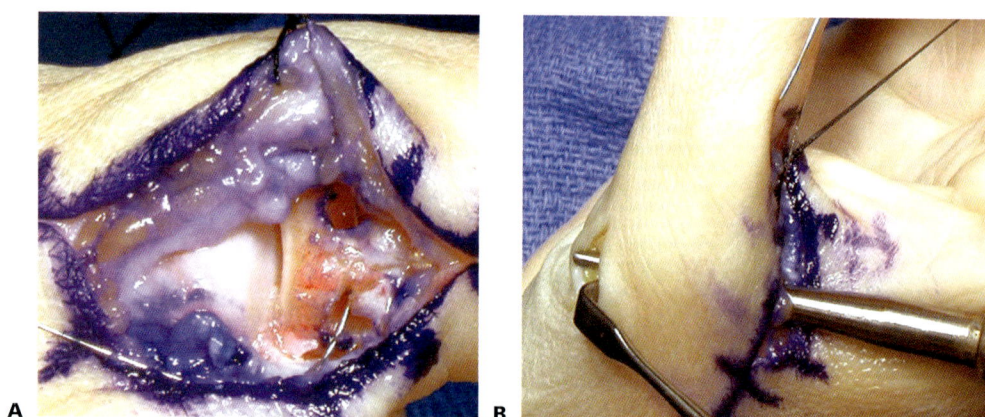

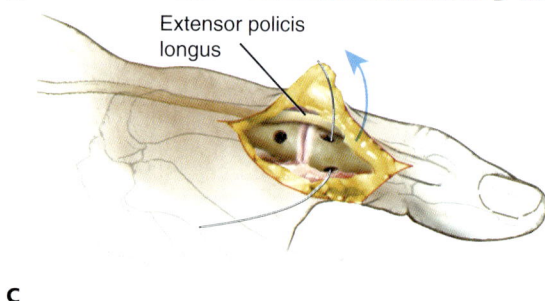

TECH FIG 2 • **A.** The proximal phalangeal holes are made at the 7 and 11 o'clock position; the surgeon must be careful to make a wide bone bridge to avoid fracture. A 28-gauge wire is placed into the bone tunnel to assist with passage of the tendon graft. **B.** A large gouge is used to create a single hole in the metacarpal head. An incision is made radially over the end of the gouge to allow for fixation of the graft. **C.** The adductor aponeurosis has been divided and the collateral ligament remnants have been excised. Gouge holes have been made in the base of the proximal metacarpal head.

- A second 28-gauge stainless steel wire is placed through this bone tunnel and the ends are secured with another hemostat.
- Preset a 0.045-inch Kirschner wire (sharp at both ends) in the metacarpal head for later advancement across the MCP joint.
  - Radially deviate the proximal phalanx to expose the metacarpal head.
  - Starting in the center of the metacarpal head and aiming at an angle of about 45 degrees, advance the wire retrograde through the radial cortex of the metacarpal shaft until it is just below the articular surface of the metacarpal head.

Tendon Graft Harvest and Passage

- Harvest the palmaris longus (PL) for use as a graft.
  - If the palmaris is absent, use half of the flexor carpi radialis (FCR) tendon or the plantaris tendon.
  - The obvious advantage of the FCR is its availability without requiring a second surgical site.
- Make a short transverse incision over the PL tendon at the distal wrist flexion crease (**TECH FIG 3A**) and mobilize the tendon distally.
- Make a second, proximal incision over the PL musculotendinous junction and mobilize the tendon at this level and under the skin bridge.
  - Use of a tendon stripper is an alternative method of harvest.
- After incising the PL as distal as possible, apply firm traction and withdraw the tendon through the proximal incision, and then divide the tendon at the musculotendinous junction.
- Secure the tendon graft to the limb of the stainless steel wire emerging from the more volar of the two proximal phalangeal gouge holes by tying a knot around one end of the tendon graft (**TECH FIG 3B**) or by using a grasping suture placed through the graft.
- Moisten the tendon graft with saline.
- Pull the wire to draw the tendon into and through the bone tunnel, emerging from the dorsal hole (**TECH FIG 3C**).

- The tendon is pulled using moderately firm traction and a circular motion of the wire.
- Avoid fracturing the bony bridge between the gouge holes by pulling too firmly on the wire with a vector of pull away from the bone.
- The wire is removed from the end of the tendon.
- Remove this wire and tie the ulnar end of the wire previously placed in the metacarpal bone tunnel around both ends of the tendon graft.
- Using the same technique combining lubrication, traction, and rotation of the wire, bring the two ends of the graft together and through the metacarpal gouge hole, exiting radially (**TECH FIG 3D,E**).
- Set the tension of the reconstruction by pulling on both limbs of the graft simultaneously and stressing the joint with radially directed force on the proximal phalanx.
  - Flexion and extension should not be limited and the joint should open minimally with stress.
- When the desired tension is achieved, tie the ends of the graft in a knot (**TECH FIG 3F**).
- Suture the knot to the adjacent periosteum with two mattress sutures stitches of 3-0 braided synthetic suture.
  - Alternatively, place a bone anchor adjacent to the metacarpal tunnel on the radial side and use the loaded sutures to secure the knot.
- Transfix the MCP joint by driving the previously placed Kirschner wire antegrade, across the joint into the proximal phalanx (**TECH FIG 3G,H**).
- Bend and cut the proximal end of the Kirschner wire superficial to the skin.
- Suture the tendon graft to the native collateral ligament remnants using 3-0 braided suture (**TECH FIG 3I**).
- Repair the adductor aponeurosis with 5-0 absorbable PDS suture (**TECH FIG 3J**).
- Reapproximate the skin with either subcuticular 4-0 Prolene or interrupted, absorbable 5-0 suture.
- A forearm-based thumb spica splint is applied, leaving the thumb interphalangeal joint free.

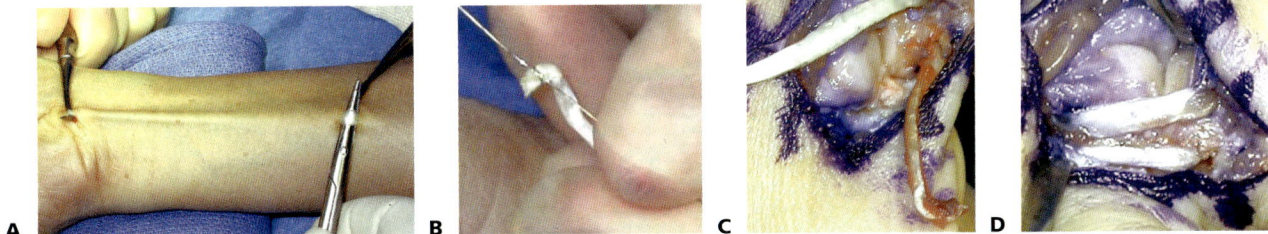

TECH FIG 3 • A. If it is present, the palmaris longus tendon is harvested with two small transverse incisions. Great care is taken to protect the median nerve during harvest. **B.** The wire is tied over the end of the tendon graft and is used to pull the graft through the bone tunnel in the proximal phalanx for reconstruction of the radial collateral ligament in this case. **C.** The palmaris longus tendon is placed through the proximal phalangeal holes using the previously placed wire. Care is taken not to pull against the bone bridge during graft placement. **D.** Both ends of the tendon graft are passed together through the hole in the metacarpal head. *(continued)*

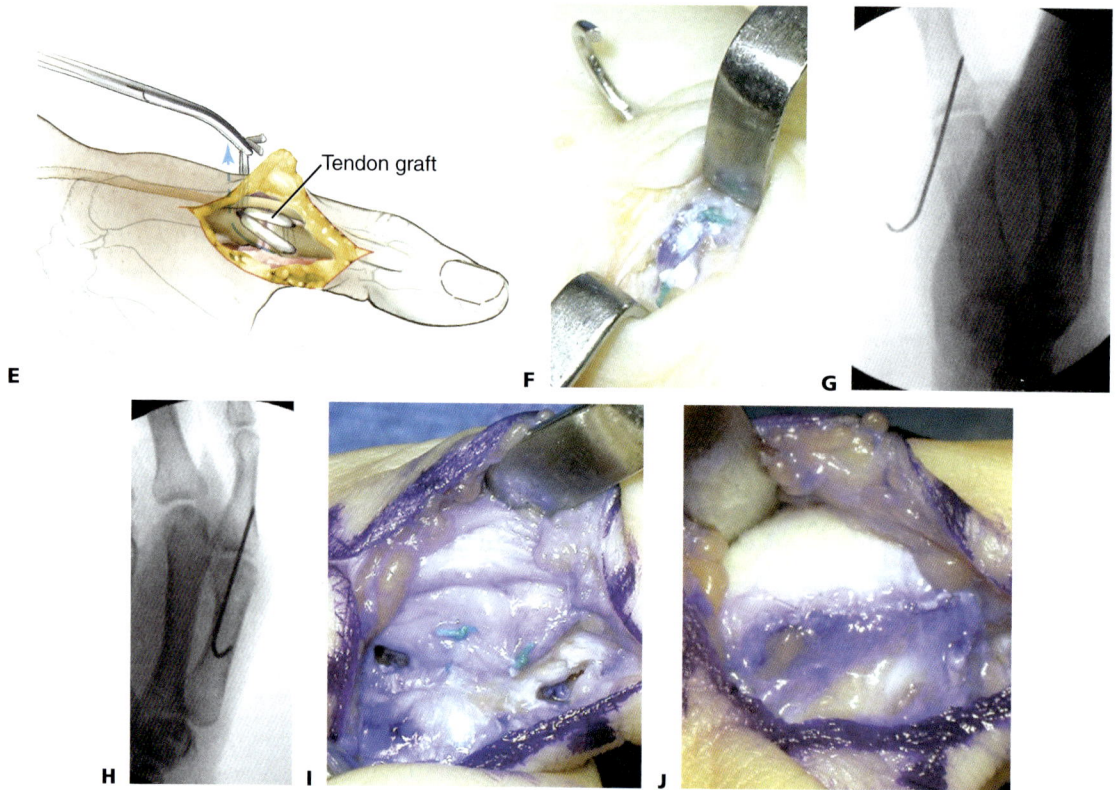

TECH FIG 3 • *(continued)* **E.** The graft has been passed through the gouge holes and is secured on the radial side of the thump metacarpophalangeal joint by tying the ends into a knot; it is further secured with sutures to local tissue. **F.** The graft ends are tied into a knot and secured to the local periosteum with 3-0 nonabsorbable suture. **G,H.** AP and lateral radiographs verify concentric joint reduction and proper placement of the transfixing 0.045-inch Kirschner wire. The Kirschner wire is left in place for 6 weeks. **I.** The tendon graft is sutured to the dorsal and volar remnants of the native collateral ligament for additional fixation. **J.** The adductor aponeurosis is repaired with 5-0 absorbable suture. This layer must be repaired separately from the collateral ligament as differential gliding between the two layers occurs with thumb motion.

RECONSTRUCTION OF CHRONIC RCL DISRUPTIONS USING TENDON GRAFT

- The steps used to stabilize the radial MCP joint using a tendon graft are much the same as those detailed for reconstruction of chronic UCL disruptions.

Exposure

- Center the skin incision over the radial MCP joint line (**TECH FIG 4A**).

- Identify and protect the branch of the dorsoradial digital nerve (**TECH FIG 4B**).
- Incise the abductor aponeurosis longitudinally, exposing the underlying torn RCL.
  - In thumbs with chronic instability the RCL may be densely fibrotic and adherent to the underlying ligament.

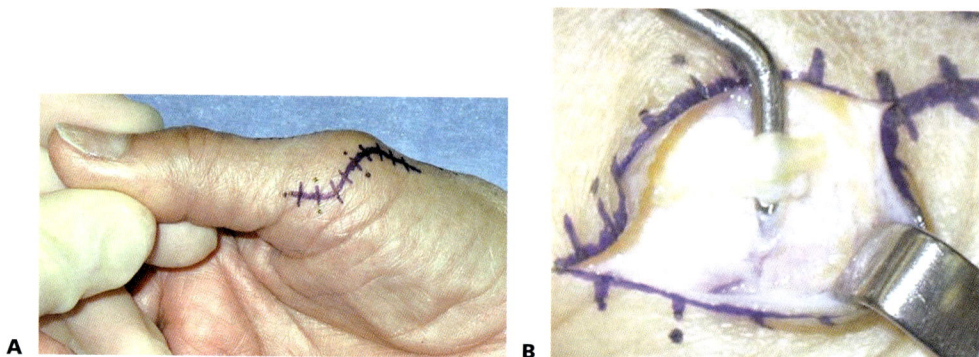

TECH FIG 4 • A. A lazy-S incision is used for radial collateral ligament reconstruction. **B.** A dorsal radial sensory nerve branch is identified and protected.

TECHNIQUES

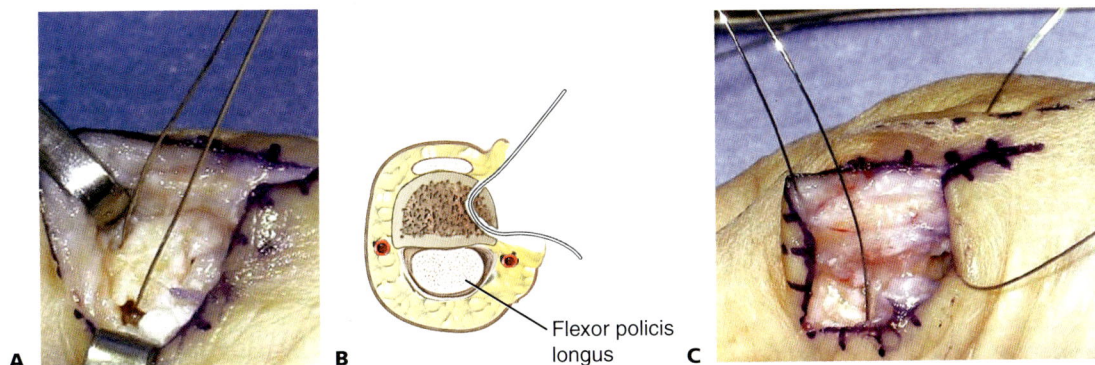

TECH FIG 5 • **A.** Two holes are made in the base of the proximal phalanx using a small, then a medium gouge. A 28-gauge wire is placed through the bone tunnel to be used later for passage of the graft. **B.** An axial view of the proximal phalanx of a right thumb demonstrating the 1 and 5 o'clock positions of the gouge holes when viewed from the side. **C.** A single large hole is made in the metacarpal neck and another 28-gauge wire is placed through this hole, exiting ulnarly.

- Excise the remnant of the RCL, exposing the radial side of the metacarpal head, base of the proximal phalanx, and MCP joint.
- Deviate the MCP joint to visualize the articular cartilage and ensure the absence of significant arthrosis.

Bone Preparation

- Using hand-held gouges of increasing diameter in the manner previously detailed, make two holes in the radial base of the proximal phalanx.
  - The holes are made at the 1 and 5 o'clock positions in the base of the proximal phalanx if looking at the right thumb end on (**TECH FIG 5A,B**).
  - The holes are made at an angle of about 45 degrees directed toward each other to create a continuous bone tunnel within the medullary canal.
  - The holes must be spaced far enough apart to maintain a substantial bony bridge.
  - A 28-gauge stainless steel wire is passed from one hole to the other through the medullary canal to be used for later passage of the tendon graft in the manner described above for UCL reconstruction.

- Create a bone tunnel in the metacarpal neck beginning at the fossa from which the RCL normally originates on the radial side of the metacarpal head and extending slightly obliquely, from distal to proximal, across the metacarpal, exiting ulnarly (**TECH FIG 5C**).
  - A second 28-gauge stainless steel wire is placed through this hole and the ends are secured with a second hemostat.
- Preset a 0.045-inch Kirschner wire in the metacarpal head to be used later for transfixing the MCP joint.

Tendon Graft Passage

- Introduce the tendon graft into the prepared bone tunnels using the techniques described for UCL reconstruction (**TECH FIG 6A,B**).
- The tension of the reconstruction is set and the graft secured in the manner reviewed.
- The MCP joint is transfixed and the wound closed (**TECH FIG 6C**).
- A forearm-based thumb spica splint is applied, leaving the thumb interphalangeal joint free.

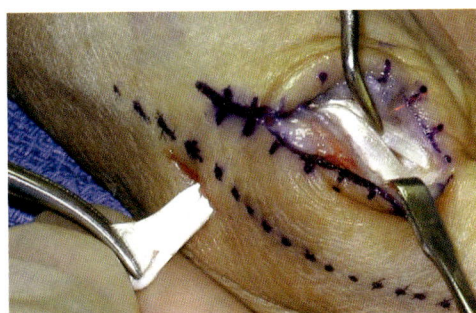

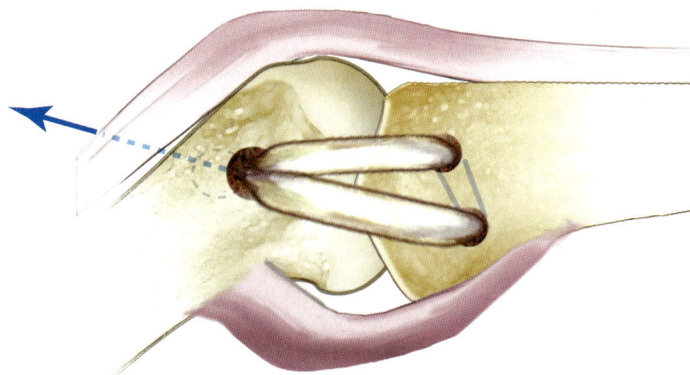

TECH FIG 6 • **A.** Both tendon ends are pulled together through the metacarpal head, exiting ulnarly. **B.** Converging gouge holes are made at the base of the proximal phalanx and an oblique hole is made in the metacarpal head. Subsequently, the graft is passed through these holes. *(continued)*

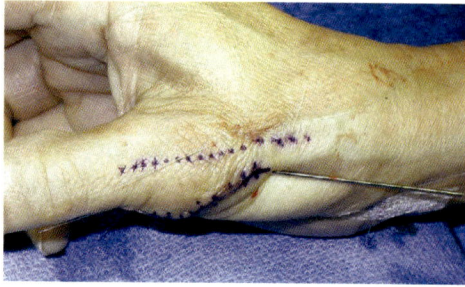

TECH FIG 6 • *(continued)* **C.** The final photograph after wound closure and pin placement.

PEARLS AND PITFALLS

Traction on the dorsoulnar digital nerve	▪ Excessive traction on the dorsoulnar digital nerve may cause numbness, paresthesias, and dysesthesia on the dorsoulnar aspect of the thumb distal to the incision.
Tools	▪ Using hand-held gouges gives the operator good control of the direction and progressive enlargement of the holes in the proximal phalanx and metacarpal. ▪ If power tools are used to make the holes, soft tissue adjacent to the holes can be inadvertently wrapped up in the spinning instrument. The heat generated by a burr may also burn the bone.
Making holes in the proximal phalanx	▪ The most important aspect of making the holes in the base of the proximal phalanx is to make them wide enough apart to maintain a substantial bone bridge. ▪ The greatest risk is making the holes too close together. The consequence is that the bridge fractures when the tendon graft is pulled through the holes.
Tying the wire	▪ The wire used for passage of the tendon graft should be tied with hemostats, not manually; it can cut the skin of the surgeon's fingers if done manually.
Graft tension	▪ The graft can be made too tight, limiting motion of the MP joint and possibly causing pain postoperatively. The knot in the graft should be sutured after the tension has been set and felt to be appropriate. Less likely is the possibility that the graft is too loose, allowing persistent laxity of the joint. ▪ After the tension is set, the joint should be flexed and extended to ascertain that the reconstruction is not too tight to allow motion or too loose to adequately correct the instability.

POSTOPERATIVE CARE

▪ The thumb is immobilized in a thumb spica cast for 6 weeks postoperatively.
▪ At 6 weeks after surgery, the cast and pin are removed.
  ▪ The thumb is immobilized after cast removal in a customized, thermoplastic short opponens splint fashioned by the hand therapist.
  ▪ The splint is worn most of the time except when the patient is exercising the thumb or is sedentary.
▪ Therapeutic exercise is done with the therapist and at home and includes active and active assisted range of motion in flexion and extension, avoiding force on the proximal phalanx, which would stress the reconstruction.
  ▪ Patients are instructed to do 12 repetitions four or more times per day.
▪ After 2 weeks, the thermoplastic splint is eliminated except for strenuous activity.
▪ Patients continue range-of-motion exercises and begin strengthening with soft putty and light gripping.
▪ At 12 weeks after surgery, pinch and grip strengthening and light free weights are initiated.
▪ Full, unrestricted activity is allowed 16 weeks postoperatively.

▪ Patients are expected to regain about 80% of the range of motion of the contralateral thumb MP joint and nearly full range of motion of the interphalangeal joint.
  ▪ Key pinch strength should be more than 90% of the contralateral, uninjured thumb at final follow-up.

OUTCOMES

▪ Reconstruction of the UCL using the technique described in this chapter produces results only slightly less favorable than UCL repair.
▪ Range of motion of the MCP joint averaged 80% of the uninjured side. Motion of the interphalangeal joint is often limited initially after reconstruction but at final follow-up was 94% of the unoperated thumb.[11]
▪ Key pinch strength averaged 95% and grip strength averaged 103% of the unoperated thumb not corrected for handedness.[11]
▪ Sixty-nine percent of patients had no pain postoperatively and the remainder had mild or intermittent pain. Eighty-eight percent of patients had no functional limitations, 8% had minimal limitations, and 2% had moderate functional limitation.[11]

- None of the reconstructions that had normal or minimally degenerated cartilage required revision due to development or progression of degenerative disease.[11]
- Results of RCL reconstruction in the hands of the same authors were similar to those of UCL reconstruction.[6]
- Range of motion of the MCP joint on the operated side was 59% of the unoperated side and interphalangeal range of motion was 94% of the unoperated thumb.[6]
- Both grip and key pinch strength were equal in the operated and unoperated thumbs.[6]
- The MCP joints were equally stable to stress in operated and unoperated thumbs.[6]
- Patients had minimal pain and no significant functional limitations. All returned to their preoperative occupations.[6]

COMPLICATIONS

- Some patients develop transient hypesthesia on the dorsal aspect of the thumb distal to the incision due to intraoperative traction on a branch of the radial sensory nerve.
  - This generally resolves over several weeks.
- Occasionally, patients develop stiffness of the MP joint that is persistent. This may be the result of the reconstruction being too tight.
- The MCP joint occasionally develops some laxity postoperatively, which may be a consequence of the reconstruction being too loose or the patient being too aggressive during rehabilitation.
- The bony bridge between the proximal phalangeal gouge holes can theoretically crack intraoperatively, but this has not happened to the authors or their colleagues.
  - If it did occur, an alternative form of fixation of the graft to the proximal phalanx would have to be used, like suturing the graft to the adjacent periosteum, pulling it out through a gouge hole on the opposite side of the phalanx, or employing a suture anchor.

REFERENCES

1. Alldred AJ. Rupture of the collateral ligament of the metacarpophalangeal joint of the thumb. J Bone Joint Surg Br 1955;37B:443–445.
2. Bean CHG, Tencer AF, Trumble TE. The effect of thumb metacarpophalangeal ulnar collateral ligament attachment site on joint range of motion: an in vitro study. J Hand Surg Am 1999;24A:283–287.
3. Breek JC, Tan AM, Van Thiel TPH, et al. Free tendon grafting to repair the metacarpophalangeal joint of the thumb. J Bone Joint Surg Br 1989;71B:383–387.
4. Camp RA, Weatherwax RJ, Miller EB. Chronic posttraumatic radial instability of the thumb metacarpophalangeal joint. J Hand Surg Am 1980;5A:221–225.
5. Campbell CS. Gamekeeper's thumb. J Bone Joint Surg Br 1955;37B:148–149.
6. Catalano LW III, Cardon L, Patenaude N, et al. Results of surgical treatment of acute and chronic grade III tears of the radial collateral ligament of the thumb metacarpophalangeal joint. J Hand Surg Am 2006;31A:68–75.
7. Coonrad RN, Goldner JL. A study of the pathological findings and treatment in soft-tissue injury of the thumb metacarpophalangeal joint. J Bone Joint Surg Am 1968;50A:439–454.
8. Coyle MP Jr. Grade III radial collateral ligament injuries of the thumb metacarpophalangeal joint: treatment by soft tissue advancement and bony reattachment. J Hand Surg Am 2003;28A:14–20.
9. Durham JW, Khuri S, Kim MH. Acute and late radial collateral ligament injuries of the thumb metacarpophalangeal joint. J Hand Surg Am 1993;18A:232–237.
10. Glickel SZ. Metacarpophalangeal and interphalangeal joint injuries and instabilities. In Peimer CA, ed. Surgery of the Hand and Upper Extremity. New York: McGraw-Hill, 1996:1043–1068.
11. Glickel SZ, Malerich M, Pearce SM, et al. Ligament replacement for chronic instability of the ulnar collateral ligament of the metacarpophalangeal joint of the thumb. J Hand Surg Am 1993;18A:930–941.
12. Heyman P, Gelberman RH, Duncan K, et al. Injuries of the ulnar collateral ligament of the thumb metacarpophalangeal joint—biomechanical and prospective clinical studies on the usefulness of valgus stress testing. Clin Orthop Relat Res 1993;292:165–171.
13. Kaplan EB, Riordan DC. The thumb. In Spinner M, ed. Kaplan's Functional and Surgical Anatomy of the Hand, 3rd ed. Philadelphia: JB Lippincott, 1984:116–117.
14. Lyons RP, Kozin SH, Failla JM. The anatomy of the radial side of the thumb static restraints in preventing subluxation and rotation after injury. Am J Orthop 1998;27:759–763.
15. Melone CP, Beldner S, Basuk RS. Thumb collateral ligament injuries: an anatomic basis for treatment. Hand Clin 2000;16:345–357.
16. Mitsionis GI, Varitimidis SE, Sotereanos GG. Treatment of chronic injuries of the ulnar collateral ligament of the thumb using a free tendon graft and bone suture anchors. J Hand Surg Br 2000;25B:208–211.
17. Osterman AL, Hayken GD, Bora FW. A quantitative evaluation of thumb function after ulnar collateral ligament repair and reconstruction. J Trauma 1981;21:854–861.
18. Smith RJ. Post-traumatic instability of the metacarpophalangeal joint of the thumb. J Bone Joint Surg Am 1977;59A:14–21.
19. Stener B. Displacement of the ruptured ulnar collateral ligament of the metacarpo-phalangeal joint of the thumb: a clinical and anatomical study. J Bone Joint Surg Br 1962;44B:869–879.

John J. Walsh IV

DEFINITION

- Fractures and dislocations of the carpometacarpal (CMC) joints of the index through small fingers involve intra-articular fractures at the base of the metacarpals or pure dislocations between the metacarpals and carpus. The fracture can involve the base of the metacarpal or the trapezoid, capitate, or hamate articular surface.
- These fractures and dislocations can result in instability and articular incongruity (**FIG 1**).

ANATOMY

- The CMC joints connect the metacarpals and the distal carpal row.
- The shape and degree of constraint present in the joints differ from finger to finger.
  - The index and middle fingers have highly constrained articulations due to the shape of the index CMC articulation and supporting soft tissues.[4] These include the flexor carpi radialis tendon, extensor carpi radialis longus and brevis tendons, and very strong capsular insertions. This provides for a strong radial column for the hand, and efficient force transfer to the radius (**FIG 2A**).
  - The ring and small fingers have a gliding articulation on the hamate, which allows for the closure of the hand around objects and is very important in power grip. This mobility makes them more susceptible to injury. The extensor carpi ulnaris tendon attaches to the base of the small finger metacarpal.[4]

- The deep motor branch of the ulnar nerve crosses around the base of the hamate hook and runs along the volar surface of the CMC joints (**FIG 2B**). It is vulnerable at the time of injury or during fixation.

PATHOGENESIS

- Injuries of the CMC joints may be divided into two broad categories.
  - The first, involving a load applied to a flexed metacarpal, is by far the most common mechanism. This injury usually involves the ring and small fingers displacing dorsally as a unit relative to the hamate. This may occur as a dislocation only or include a marginal fracture of the hamate.[8]
  - The second mechanism involves an axially directed force that creates a comminuted fracture of the articular surface (**FIG 3A**). Severe crushing injuries can cause multiple dislocations and fractures diffusely throughout the CMC region[1,7] (**FIG 3B,C**).

NATURAL HISTORY

- The natural result of an untreated fixation dislocation is progressive arthritis of the involved joints.

PATIENT HISTORY AND PHYSICAL FINDINGS

- The patient's history is important to assess the mechanism of injury, which provides further clues regarding concomitant injuries in the extremity.

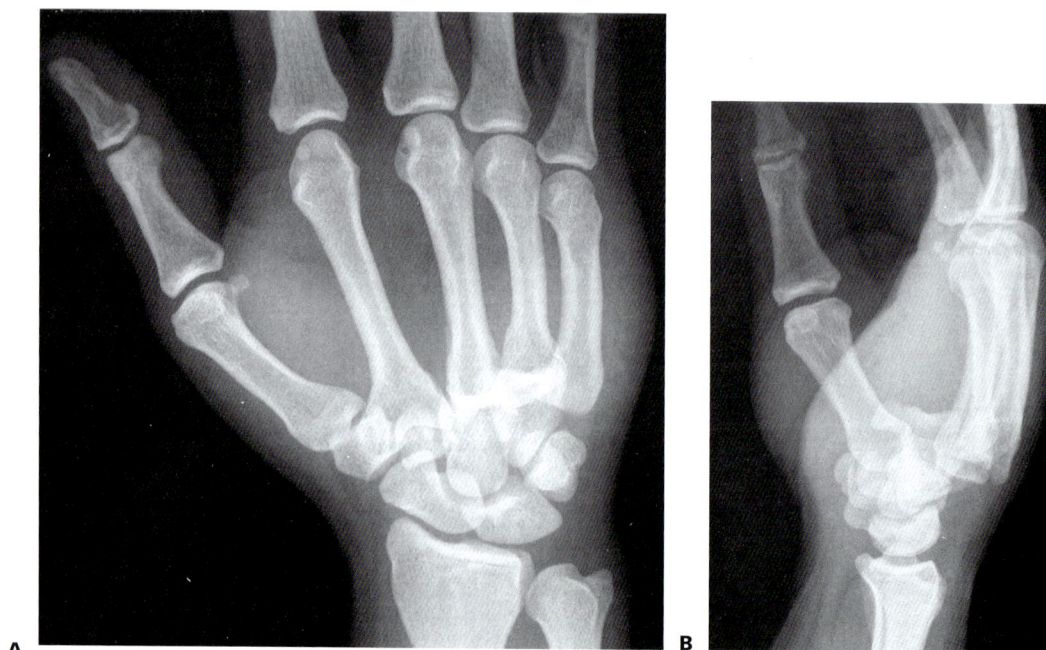

A   B

FIG 1 • Multiple dorsal carpometacarpal (CMC) dislocations involving the index through small fingers.

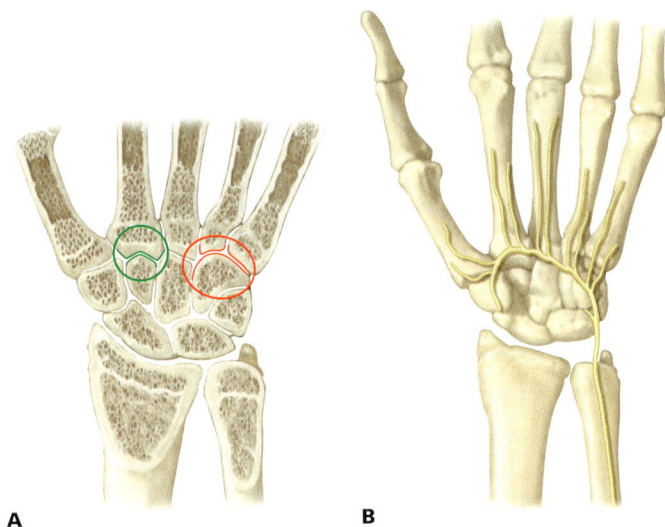

FIG 2 • A. Variable articular congruity of the various CMC joints. **B.** Deep motor branch of the ulnar nerve adjacent to the metacarpal bases.

- Examine the hand for tenderness and local swelling.
- Assess neurovascular integrity, especially function of the deep branch of the ulnar nerve (first dorsal interosseous contraction).
- Examine the limb for other injuries.
- Associated injuries should be detected by examination and verified by radiographs.
- Preoperative notation of nerve function is important when comparing function following reduction and fixation.

IMAGING AND OTHER DIAGNOSTIC STUDIES

- Radiographs of the CMC joints require careful positioning to assess each joint.

- The transverse metacarpal arch causes the CMC joints of the index and middle fingers to appear in an oblique projection when a standard PA radiograph is obtained of the ring and small finger CMC joints, and vice versa (**FIG 4A**).
- A true frontal radiograph is most easily obtained by positioning the hand in an AP projection with the dorsum of the hand placed flat on the cassette (or image intensifier, if using fluoroscopy). The base of the affected metacarpal should lie on the cassette (**FIG 4B**). This will result in a far more accurate portrayal of the joint, essential for assessing the fracture as well as checking hardware position after fixation.
- Visualization of the joint surfaces at the base of the ring and small fingers differs in a typical PA projection (**FIG 4C**) and a properly positioned film of the same patient (**FIG 4D**).

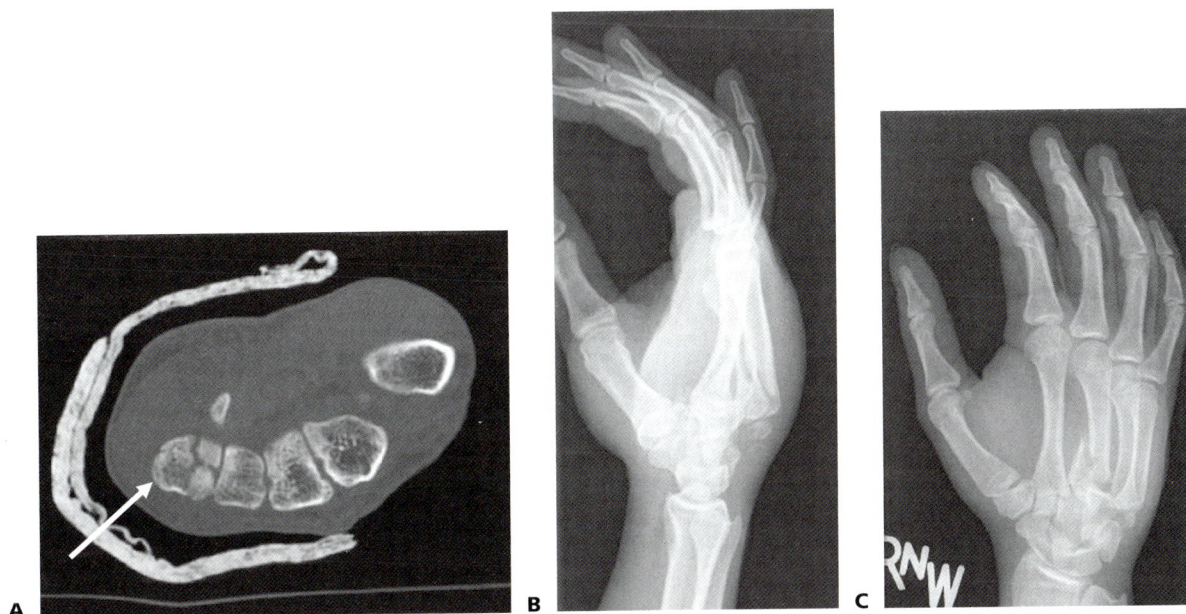

FIG 3 • A. Comminuted fracture of the fifth metacarpal base. **B,C.** Multiple fractures and dislocations involving the ulnar side of the hand.

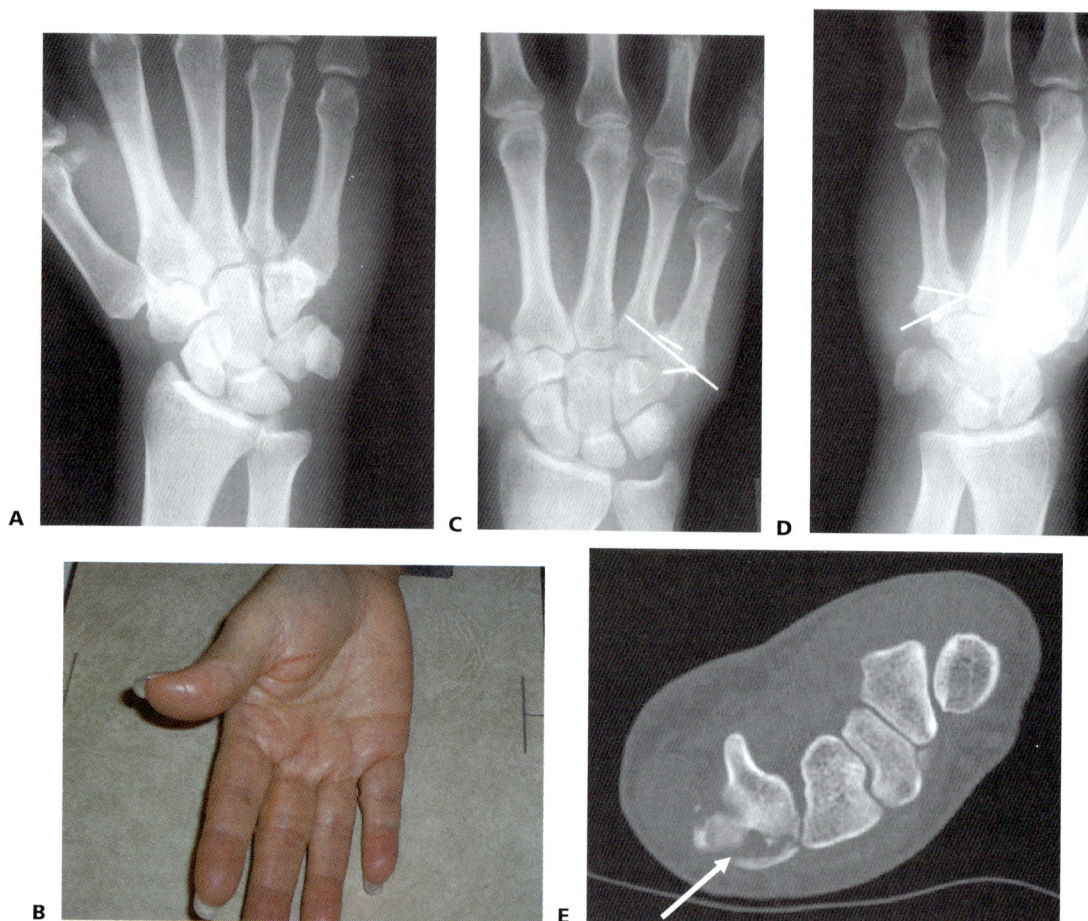

FIG 4 • A. A conventional PA view of the hand creates an oblique view of the ring and small finger bases. **B.** Hand properly positioned for AP view of the ring and small finger CMC joints. **C.** Postoperative PA film after open reduction with internal fixation of the ring and small finger CMC joints. **D.** AP projection clearly shows the joint reduction in the same patient shown in **C. E.** CT scan of the fracture of the dorsal lip of the hamate.

■ The same principle holds for obtaining lateral radiographs. A semisupinated lateral view will best visualize the base of the index and middle CMC joints,[5] and a semipronated lateral view will best show the bases of the ring and small finger CMC joints.[2]

■ A CT scan should be obtained in most cases to assess for articular injury. CT also is especially helpful for visualizing impacted articular surface fragments. The best visualization and determination of fracture patterns will be possible if the scan is obtained after preliminary reduction of any displaced fractures or dislocations associated with a fracture (**FIG 4E**).[10]

DIFFERENTIAL DIAGNOSIS

■ Metacarpal fracture
■ Carpal bone fracture
■ Carpometacarpal fracture/dislocation
■ Fracture associated with neurovascular injury

NONOPERATIVE MANAGEMENT

■ Nondisplaced fractures can be treated in a below-elbow cast that incorporates the affected digit or digits and one adjacent digit.[5,9] Special attention should be paid to positioning the hand in an intrinsic-plus position. Capsular contractures of the

metacarpophalangeal (MCP) joints can develop relatively rapidly in hands with the MCP joints immobilized in extension.

■ Radiographs following cast immobilization should be checked carefully to ensure that no dorsal subluxation is present and should be repeated at weekly intervals for the first 2 weeks to prevent healing in a displaced position.

■ These injuries, especially those involving a dislocation, have a known propensity for recurrent dorsal subluxation following reduction. Most will require operative fixation.[2,4,9] Some authors believe nonoperative management does have a role despite intra-articular displacement and shortening.[4,13]

SURGICAL MANAGEMENT

Preoperative Planning

■ Careful review of all imaging studies will facilitate planning of fracture fragment exposure and identify sites for internal fixation.

Positioning

■ The patient is positioned supine on the operating table with a standard arm table.

■ The surgeon often is more comfortable seated on the head side of the arm table. This avoids the neck strain that may

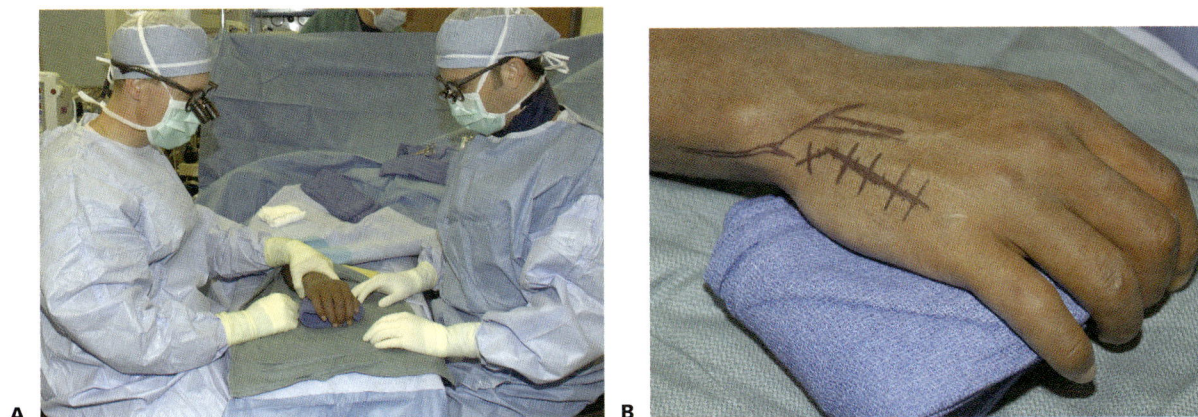

FIG 5 • **A.** Positioning of the surgeon (on left) and assistant (right). **B.** Skin incision marked with probable course of nerve.

result from looking "over the top" that happens when the arm externally rotates and the surgeon is seated on the axilla side of the table (**FIG 5A**).

Approach

■ A dorsal extensile approach provides satisfactory exposure of any of the CMC joints.

■ Incisions placed between metacarpals allow access to two adjacent joints.
■ Cross the wrist with oblique extensions if necessary.
■ Marking out the anticipated locations of nearby nerve branches can be helpful (**FIG 5B**).

DORSAL EXPOSURE

■ Following incision of the skin, careful spreading dissection should be used to locate and protect the dorsal cutaneous nerve branches in the operative field.
  ■ Ulnar sensory nerves are most commonly encountered during exposure of the CMC joints of the ring and small fingers (**TECH FIG 1**), and radial sensory nerves during exposure of the index and middle finger CMC joints.
■ Extensor tendons are mobilized and retracted.

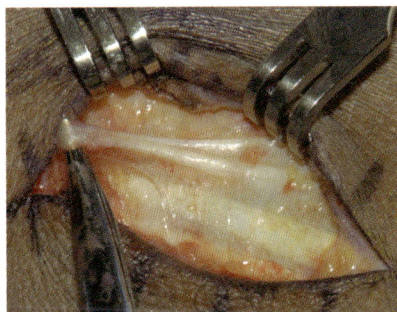

TECH FIG 1 • Dorsal cutaneous branch of the ulnar nerve crossing the incision.

FRACTURE EXPOSURE

■ Careful mobilization of the fracture fragments with minimal soft tissue stripping is important.
■ This can be facilitated by the use of a Beaver blade, a dental pick, and a fine synovial rongeur.

■ The rongeur is useful because it is helpful to débride fracture callus and hematoma.

FRACTURE REDUCTION

■ The fracture is then reduced and held provisionally using fine K-wires (**TECH FIG 2A**). The surgeon must be aware of the planned location for definitive hardware placement, given the limited room available.
  ■ Pins temporarily driven across the base of an articular fragment into the corresponding carpal bone can be

helpful in stabilizing any mobile pieces of bone (**TECH FIG 2B**).
■ The conventional technique of first reconstructing the articular surface, followed by securing the shaft to the reassembled joint surface, is useful.

TECHNIQUES

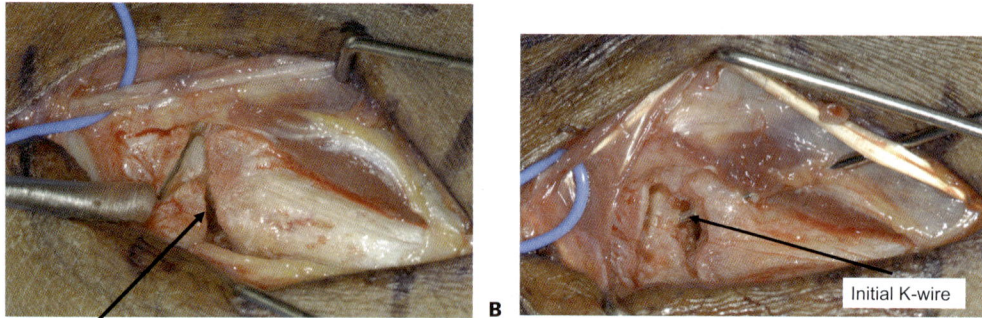

A Fracture line   **B** Initial K-wire

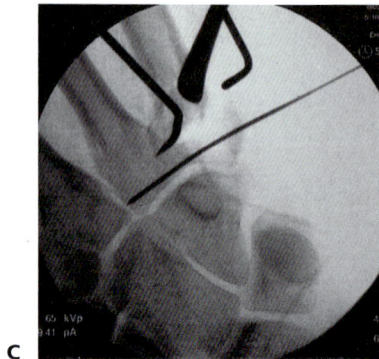

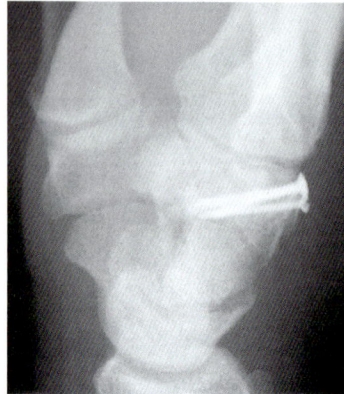

C   **D**

TECH FIG 2 • **A.** Provisional fracture reduction using the hamate surface as a mold for articular reduction of the metacarpal base. **B.** Initial reduction of the shaft and stabilization of the articular surface. **C.** Fluoroscopic view of articular reduction. **D.** Dorsal hamate lip fixation with three screws.

- Confirmation of the provisional reduction should be obtained with fluoroscopy before any definitive screw placement (**TECH FIG 2C**).
- The corresponding articular surface on the uninjured bone is used as a mold for the fragments, serving as a guide to reassembly of the injured bone.

- This technique works regardless of whether the injury is in the metacarpal base, as pictured in these figures, or in a distal articular injury of one of the carpal bones (**TECH FIG 2D**).

DEFINITIVE FIXATION

- Wires can be replaced by screws if fragment size permits (**TECH FIG 3A**).
  - Placing the fragments under compression manually and inserting screws sometimes is preferable to using the lag screw technique, which requires overdrilling the near side and may risk iatrogenic comminution.

- Simple K-wire fixation is satisfactory for isolated dislocations with fracture (**TECH FIG 3B**).
  - The insertion point for a percutaneous wire often is quite distant from the dislocation site in crushed and severely swollen hands.

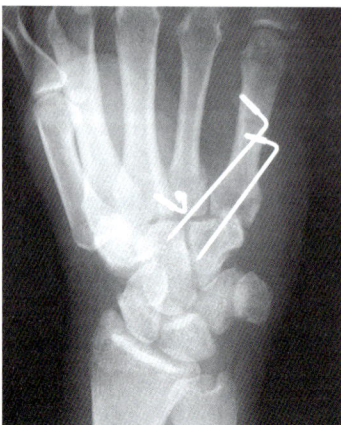

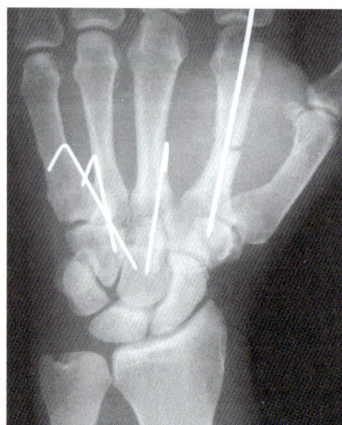

A   **B**

TECH FIG 3 • **A.** Fracture-dislocation of the ring and small finger metacarpal bases using pins and a screw. **B.** Percutaneous K-wire fixation of a metacarpal shaft fracture and CMC dislocation.

ADJUNCTIVE TECHNIQUES

- The construct can be protected by placing the affected metacarpal under slight distraction and pinning it to the adjacent metacarpal.
- Alternatively, the proximally directed deforming force of the extensor carpi ulnaris can be reduced by detaching it from the base of the small finger metacarpal at the beginning of the procedure, and securing it to the hamate at the close, thereby avoiding proximal pull on the base of the small finger metacarpal.
  - I have never found it necessary to use this alternative approach, but it may be helpful in a delayed presentation, where myostatic contractures due to shortening are present.

PEARLS AND PITFALLS

Imaging	■ Ensure that adequate radiographs are available for intraoperative review. ■ If necessary, obtain a CT scan.
Positioning	■ It is often easier for the surgeon to be seated on the outside of the hand table, instead of in the axilla between the table and patient, due to the limited internal rotation present in the shoulder, which can make visualization difficult from the usual seating position.
Exposure	■ The dorsal cutaneous branch of the ulnar nerve crosses the incision obliquely and lies immediately across the operative field for exposure of the fourth and fifth CMC joints. Cutting this nerve often is associated with very symptomatic neuromas, although the sensory deficit is well tolerated.
Fracture management	■ Fragments can be small, and periosteal stripping can result in devitalization. Use fracture lines for visualization of the articular surface as much as possible. A dental pick, fine K-wire joysticks, and provisional fixation before final screw insertion can be helpful. Provisional fixation should be done with careful attention to the anticipated location of definitive fixation. Avoid malrotation of the shaft during reduction by grasping it together with one or two adjacent metacarpals when aligning it relative to the joint. Small degrees of malrotation at the base of the metacarpal can result in substantial distal overlap of the digits.
Postoperative protection	■ Consider placing a temporary distraction K-wire between adjacent metacarpals to limit the load placed on the articular surface before it has healed.

POSTOPERATIVE CARE

- Aftercare following operative fixation falls into three general phases: acute swelling control and wound healing (10–14 days), fracture consolidation and maintenance of digit range of motion (4–6 weeks), and restoration of global hand function and strength (2–6 months).
- Immediate measures following surgery include strict elevation and range-of-motion exercises through a full arc of motion.[4] This limits swelling, reduces pain, and prevents accumulation of protein-rich edema fluid that will slow rehabilitation.
- The relative speed at which the hand can be mobilized during the weeks after surgery depends on a number of factors, including the magnitude of the original injury, stability of fixation, reliability of the patient, and specific occupational or athletic needs.
- The radiograph in Tech Fig 2D shows the hand of a physician with stable fixation of a dorsal hamate injury who was mobilized and given a 1-pound lifting restriction shortly after surgery to allow continuation of his residency training.
  - In contrast, unreliable patients require immobilization for 6 weeks in a cast (see Tech Fig 3B).
- Patients should be warned that full grip strength is the last thing that will recover and may take months.[2] It is not uncommon for patients to report pain with a handshake for an extended period of time.

OUTCOMES

- Opinions on outcomes vary with regard to overall success. A dichotomy exists between recommendation for operative and nonsurgical treatment. Kjaer-Petersen and colleagues[11] found that, regardless of treatment, long-term symptoms were present in 38% of patients at 4.3 years of follow-up.
- Petrie and Lamb,[13] who used immediate, unrestricted motion, reported on results at 4.5 years. Even with metacarpal shortening and irregularities in the articular surface, only one patient had work limitations.
- Another study found that pain was related to the degree of posttraumatic arthritis secondary to articular incongruity and advocated anatomic reductor and internal fixation.[12]
- Multiple CMC dislocations were reviewed by Lawliss and Gunther, and poor results were noted in dislocations of the second and third CMC joints (which require higher energy for dislocation) and in those patients with an ulnar nerve injury.[7]

COMPLICATIONS

- Complications include those common to any periarticular surgery:
  - Failure of wound healing
  - Hematoma formation
  - Neurovascular injury

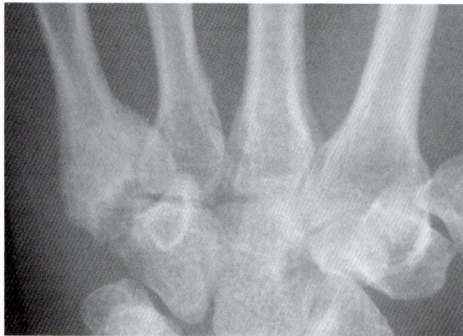

FIG 6 • Radiograph taken several months following K-wire fixation of a fracture-dislocation of the fifth CMC joint. Fragments were too small for screw fixation and were resorbed.

- Neuroma formation
- Tendon adhesions
- Posttraumatic arthritis
- Nonunion or malunion
- Joint stiffness
- Weakness

■ Occasionally small fragments may resorb, leading to collapse and articular incongruity (**FIG 6**).

■ Long-term arthritis can be treated with fusion of the affected joint.[4]

■ Alternatively, an interposition "anchovy" using the palmaris longus as a biologic spacer can be inserted after resection of the arthritic joint surfaces, analogous to that performed for thumb basal joint arthritis.[3]

REFERENCES

1. Bergfield TG, DuPuy TE, Aulicino PL. Fracture-dislocations of all five carpometacarpal joints: a case report. J Hand Surg Am 1985;10:76–78.
2. Bora FW Jr, Didizian NH. The treatment of injuries to the carpometacarpal joint of the little finger. J Bone Joint Surg Am 1974;56A:1459–1463.
3. Gainor BJ, Stark HH, Ashworth CR, et al. Tendon arthroplasty of the fifth carpometacarpal joint for treatment of posttraumatic arthritis. J Hand Surg Am 1991;16:520–524.
4. Glickel SZ, Barron OA, Catalano LW. Dislocations and ligament injuries in the digits. In Green DP, Hotchkiss RN, Pederson WC, et al, eds. Green's Operative Hand Surgery, ed 5. Philadelphia: Churchill Livingstone, 2005:364–366.
5. Hsu JD, Curtis RM. Carpometacarpal dislocations on the ulnar side of the hand. J Bone Joint Surg Am 1970;52:927–930.
6. Kjaer-Petersen K, Jurik AG, Petersen LK. Intra-articular fractures at the base of the fifth metacarpal: a clinical and radiographical study of 64 cases. J Hand Surg Br 1992;17:144–147.
7. Lawliss JF III, Gunther SF. Carpometacarpal dislocations. J Bone Joint Surg Am 1991;73A:52–58.
8. Lilling M, Weinberg H. The mechanism of dorsal fracture dislocation of the fifth carpometacarpal joint. J Hand Surg Am 1979;4:340–342.
9. Lundeen JM, Shin AY. Clinical results of intraarticular fractures of the base of the fifth metacarpal treated by closed reduction and cast immobilization. J Hand Surg Br 2000;25:258–261.
10. Marck KW, Klasen HJ. Fracture-dislocation of the hamatometacarpal joint: A case report. J Hand Surg Am 1986;11:128–130.
11. Niechajev I. Dislocated intra-articular fracture of the base of the fifth metacarpal: a clinical study of 23 patients. Plast Reconstr Surg 1985;75:406–410.
12. Papaloizos MY, Le Moine PH, Prues-Latour V, et al. Proximal fractures of the fifth metacarpal: a retrospective analysis of 25 operated cases. J Hand Surg Br 2000;25:253–257.
13. Petrie PWR, Lamb DW. Fracture-subluxation of the base of the fifth metacarpal. Hand 1974;6:82–86.

Chapter 31

Operative Treatment of Metacarpal Fractures

Christopher L. Forthman and Thomas J. Graham

DEFINITION

- Metacarpal fractures are most significant when they disrupt function of the associated digit.
- The treatment of metacarpal fractures affects finger function and must be weighed against the sequelae of the fracture itself.
- Intra-articular fractures may involve the carpometacarpal (CMC) joint or metacarpophalangeal (MCP) joint.
  - CMC joint injuries are discussed in other chapters.
- Intra-articular MCP joint fractures have an increased risk of stiffness and posttraumatic arthritis.

ANATOMY

- The metacarpals are long tubular bones with relatively flat surfaces dorsally. The medial and lateral cortices converge volarly, making the cross-section triangular. The bone may be quite narrow in the mid-diaphyseal region, with the fourth metacarpal being particularly gracile.
- Dorsal and volar interossei muscles envelop the medial and lateral surfaces. When undisturbed, the muscles provide abundant blood supply to the underlying bone (**FIG 1A**). When severely disrupted, the muscles have the potential for disabling scarring and "intrinsic contracture."
- Deep transverse intermetacarpal ligaments lie at the level of the metacarpal neck and limit deformity with typical low-energy injuries.
  - Intact ligaments limit shortening to about 5 mm.

- The extensor apparatus envelops the MCP joint (**FIG 1B**). Proper collateral ligaments originate from a tubercle on the metacarpal head and may contribute to posttraumatic MCP joint contracture (see Chapter HA-108). The adjacent lateral furrow or so-called collateral recess allows passage of the interosseous tendon and may serve as a portal of entry for Kirschner wire fixation into the intramedullary canal.

PATHOGENESIS

- Metacarpal fractures typically result from one of two mechanisms of injury:
  - Most commonly, an axial load is transmitted from the MCP joint down the shaft of the metacarpal. Such injuries include the spectrum of fractures from a low-energy fifth metacarpal neck "boxer's fracture" to a high-energy comminuted shaft fracture caused by a blow from the steering wheel in a motor vehicle collision.
  - The metacarpal less commonly is injured by a crush-type injury that flattens the metacarpal arch bridging the carpus to the phalanges. Crush injuries typically involve multiple metacarpals and are often associated with other fractures and significant soft tissue trauma.[4]
- Extra-articular fracture orientation may be characterized as transverse, oblique, or spiral, and with or without comminution. As with other long tubular bones, the exact pattern depends on the degree of shear and torsion associated with the applied load. The fracture typically has apex-dorsal malalignment secondary to the flexion force applied by the lumbrical and interossei muscles.

NATURAL HISTORY

- Most metacarpal fractures heal uneventfully without surgery.
- Low-energy transverse or oblique fractures of a single metacarpal usually maintain acceptable alignment and heal without any measurable functional deficit.
- Spiral fractures, comminuted fractures, and fractures of multiple metacarpals are more likely to shorten and rotate, resulting in tendon imbalance and overlapping of the fingers.
- Fractures of the metacarpal neck (usually the fourth or fifth) may have varying degrees of apex-dorsal malalignment.
  - Flexion of the fourth or fifth metacarpal heads beyond 30 and 45 degrees, respectively, results in a visible pseudo-extensor lag and sometimes pain in the palm during grasping.
  - Less angulation is tolerated in the index and middle metacarpals as there is less compensatory motion available at the radial-sided CMC joints.
- Cadaveric studies of fifth metacarpal neck "boxer's fractures" have demonstrated that every 2 mm of shortening causes an average of 7 degrees of extensor lag,[6] and 30 degrees of angulation results in 22% loss of finger range of motion.[1]
- Nevertheless, there is no well-defined relationship between angular fracture malalignment and symptoms. However,

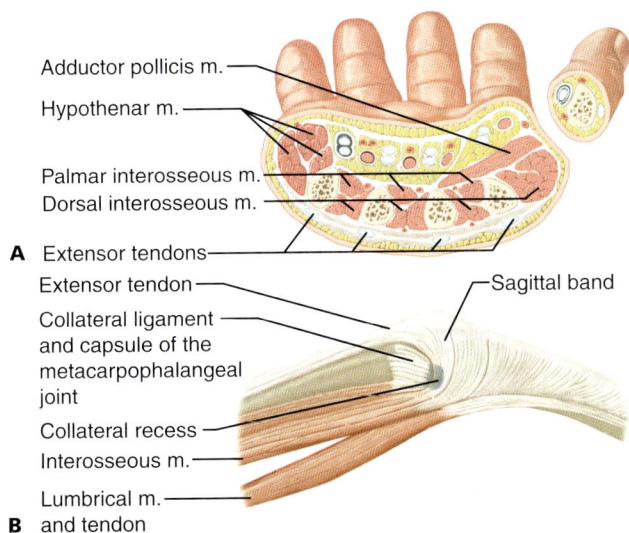

Adductor pollicis m.
Hypothenar m.
Palmar interosseous m.
Dorsal interosseous m.
A Extensor tendons

Extensor tendon
Collateral ligament and capsule of the metacarpophalangeal joint
Collateral recess
Interosseous m.
Lumbrical m.
B and tendon
Sagittal band

FIG 1 • A. Anatomy of the metacarpals. Each metacarpal cross-section is roughly triangular, with intrinsic musculature on both sides and the extensor tendon on the dorsal surface. **B.** The metacarpophalangeal joint movers. The metacarpophalangeal joint is enveloped by a complex system of motors, including the extension moment generated by the extensor apparatus and the flexion power provided by the intrinsic muscles of the hand.

rotational malalignment is poorly tolerated as it results in digital scissoring and difficulty with grasp.

PATIENT HISTORY AND PHYSICAL FINDINGS

- Physical examination methods include:
  - Inspection. The examiner should visualize the fingers as the patient carries them through an arc of motion. All nail beds should point toward the scaphoid tubercle with finger flexion.
  - Extensor lag. The examiner should assess the resting posture of the MCP joint and active MCP extension. Apex-dorsal malangulation results in some loss of active MCP joint extension.
  - Palpation. The examiner should determine the degree of dorsal fracture eminence or palmar metacarpal head prominence. Dorsal callus is usually only a cosmetic concern. The palmar head prominence may be painful with grasp.
- The examination is not complete without carefully assessing for associated injuries:
  - Open wound: The most common (and often missed) open wound results from a tooth puncture into the MCP, the so-called fight bite. These injuries should be treated urgently with surgical débridement *before* infection develops.
  - CMC dislocation: Metacarpal base fractures are often associated with CMC joint subluxation or dislocation. These injuries may go unrecognized until a true lateral radiograph of the hand is inspected.
  - Carpal tunnel and compartment syndromes: High-energy fractures may result in compartment syndrome, necessitating fasciotomy of the involved intrinsic muscles. Carpal tunnel syndrome may also result, particularly with an associated wrist injury such as a perilunate dislocation.

IMAGING AND OTHER DIAGNOSTIC STUDIES

- Plain radiographs including AP, lateral, and oblique views usually suffice. Radiographs of the contralateral hand may be valuable for comparison at the time of surgery.
  - AP view: Sagittal plane malalignment is underestimated. Any coronal plane angular malalignment is likely to be clinically relevant.
  - Lateral view: Metacarpal overlap makes the lateral view difficult to analyze. It may be omitted unless there is specific concern for subluxation at the MCP or CMC joints.
  - Oblique view: A partially pronated radiograph is the most telling perspective and may be used to measure flexion deformity at the fracture site.

- Traction views may be performed to assess the degree of comminution at the fracture site or to check the mobility of subacute fractures.
- Cross-sectional imaging (CT or MRI) may be considered to evaluate a potentially pathologic fracture or to further define articular fractures and subluxations.

DIFFERENTIAL DIAGNOSIS

- CMC fracture-dislocation
- MCP dislocation
- Fight bite
- Pathologic fracture (eg, enchondroma)

NONOPERATIVE MANAGEMENT

- Nondisplaced and minimally displaced metacarpal fractures should be protected in a thermoplast splint or cast for 3 to 4 weeks, followed by gradual mobilization. The MCP joints should be immobilized in flexion to (1) relax the intrinsic muscles and prevent further deformity at the fracture site and (2) place the MCP collateral ligaments on stretch.
- Apex-dorsal malalignment of the border metacarpals may be partially corrected with reduction and splinting.
- Rotational malalignment cannot be reliably corrected with nonoperative means.

Jahss Maneuver

- Reduction is accomplished under a hematoma block with this maneuver[5] (**FIG 2**).
- The metacarpal shaft is stabilized and the MCP joint flexed 90 degrees.
- While distracting at the fracture site, upward force is applied to the proximal phalanx and metacarpal head to realign the neck and shaft.
- A splint with three-point molding is applied with dorsal compression at the fracture site and volar support for the metacarpal head and base.
- A cast is applied 10 to 14 days later.
- Joint mobilization begins at 4 weeks.

SURGICAL MANAGEMENT

- Surgical reduction and stabilization is indicated for malrotated fractures, open fractures, unstable fractures (especially involving the border metacarpals), or fractures associated with joint disruption, tendon injury, or neurovascular injury.
  - Relative indications for surgery include fractures associated with significant extensor lag, palmar metacarpal head

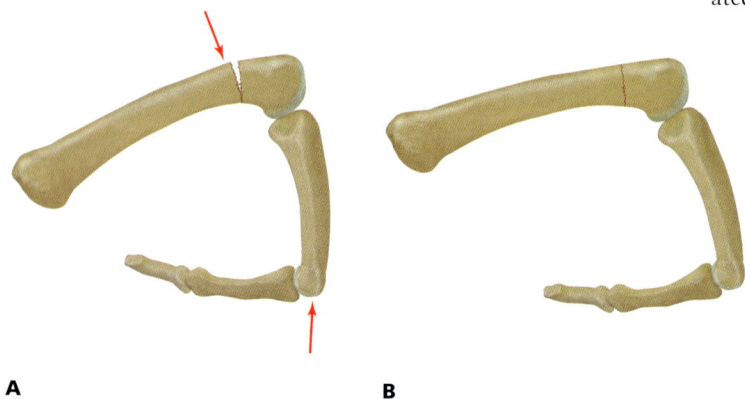

A   **B**

FIG 2 • Jahss maneuver: correction of apex dorsal malalignment as shown by Jahss in 1938.

prominence, more than 5 mm of shortening, and the presence of multiple displaced metacarpal fractures.

■ Percutaneous surgical techniques are often adequate for low-energy metacarpal shaft fractures and for most metacarpal neck fractures.

■ Open reduction and internal fixation should be considered for open fractures, shaft fractures with significant comminution, and fractures associated with joint disruption, tendon injury, or neurovascular injury.

  ▪ Dorsal plating is the most biomechanically stable fixation,[2] although it is potentially more disruptive to the soft tissues than other methods, such as crossed Kirschner wires or interosseous wires.

■ Crush-type injuries flatten the bony arch of the hand, often resulting in open metacarpal neck fractures with varying degrees of soft tissue injury. Carpal and CMC joint injuries also occur and are discussed in other chapters.

■ Crush fractures associated with mild to moderate soft tissue injury with or without disruption of the extensor mechanism may be stabilized by conventional pinning techniques or by a T-type plate applied distally up to the proximal margin of the joint capsule (**FIG 3A,B**).

  ▪ Occasionally, crush injuries result in long oblique neck fractures, which may be stabilized with lag screws alone (**FIG 3C**).

  ▪ More stable internal fixation is recommended over percutaneous pins when early motion is necessary (eg, associated extensor laceration).

■ Crush fractures associated with severe soft tissue injury or internal degloving are best pinned percutaneously (**FIG 3D–F**).

  ▪ The dorsal soft tissues are often tenuous and surgical incisions can result in necrosis and the need for otherwise unnecessary soft tissue coverage procedures.

■ Metacarpal fractures resulting from projectiles are graded as either low or high energy.

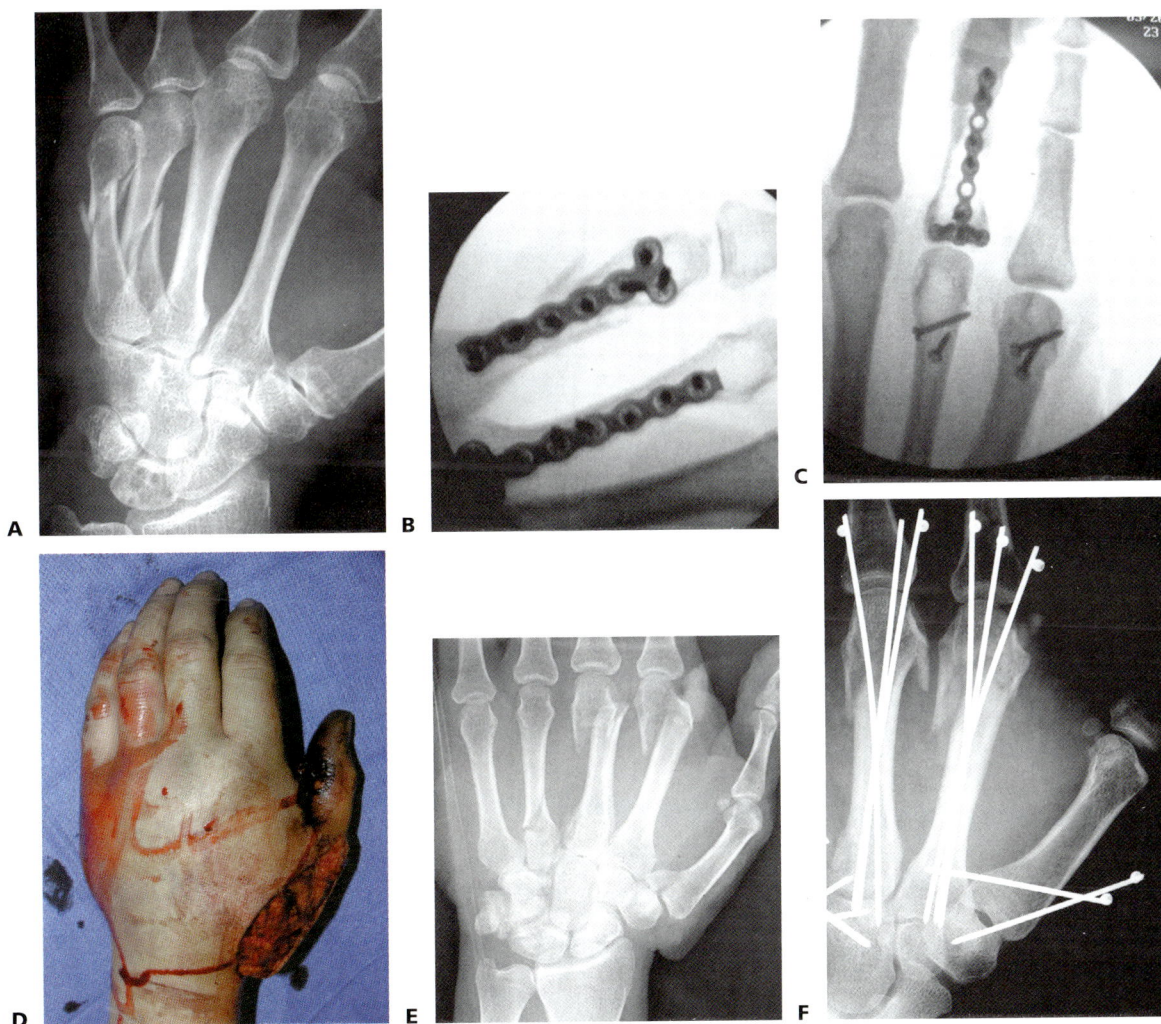

FIG 3 • **A.** Oblique view of the hand demonstrates fourth and fifth metacarpal shaft fractures. **B.** Repair may be achieved with conventional plates using a T-shape to gain additional fixation in the metaphyseal bone near the metacarpal head or base. **C.** Long oblique fractures of the fourth and fifth metacarpal heads have been stabilized with multiple lag screws. An adjacent transverse fracture of the ring finger proximal phalanx has been repaired with a plate. **D.** Clinical photograph of a crushed hand reveals global swelling and splitting of the skin indicative of severe internal degloving. **E.** Radiograph confirms fracture of all five metacarpals and the carpus. **F.** Fractures are stabilized with percutaneous pins to avoid additional trauma from surgical dissection.

▪ Simple comminuted fractures cased by low-energy projectiles with small entry or exit wounds are best treated with limited exposure and débridement, and fracture pinning (**FIG 4A**).
  ▪ Callus usually forms because the fracture fragments, although comminuted, remain vascularized.
  ▪ If there is a large area of bone loss, more rigid plate and screw fixation supplemented with bone graft may be safely performed.[3]
▪ Complex, comminuted fractures resulting from high-energy projectiles and associated with large open wounds and metal debris should be carefully cleansed, taking measures to minimize devascularization of the fracture fragments.
  ▪ Tendons, nerves, and vessels may need to be repaired.
  ▪ Provisional fixation with Kirschner wires may be considered if serial débridements are anticipated.
  ▪ If and when soft tissues allow, consideration should be given to rigid stabilization of the fractures with a bridge plate technique to facilitate mobilization (**FIG 4B**).
  ▪ Bone grafting may be necessary but can be delayed until there is minimal risk of wound infection (**FIG 4C**).
▪ Simple thumb metacarpal shaft fractures usually heal in acceptable alignment with nonoperative management. The massively comminuted thumb metacarpal may be difficult to control in a splint or cast alone. Spanning external fixators are effective for these injuries in order to maintain the first web space while fracture consolidation occurs (**FIG 4D,E**).

Preoperative Planning

▪ A surgical technique is selected based on the clinical examination, radiographs, and the surgeon's preference.
▪ The "best" technique is usually the method that is least disruptive to the soft tissues while allowing early digital mobilization.
▪ The "best" technique depends on patient factors. For example, a grossly contaminated and devitalized open metacarpal fracture may be treated with percutaneous Kirschner wires to minimize further soft tissue stripping. In contrast, a simple closed transverse metacarpal fracture in a dentist would be considered for dorsal plating to facilitate a prompt return to work.
▪ The "best" technique also depends on surgeon factors. A surgeon facile with the technique of collateral recess pinning may quickly stabilize multiple metacarpal fractures. A surgeon inexperienced in this technique may spend considerable time and frustration trying to pass wires. Poorly placed percutaneous wires in any technique may cause more soft tissue problems (eg, infection) than open reduction and fixation.

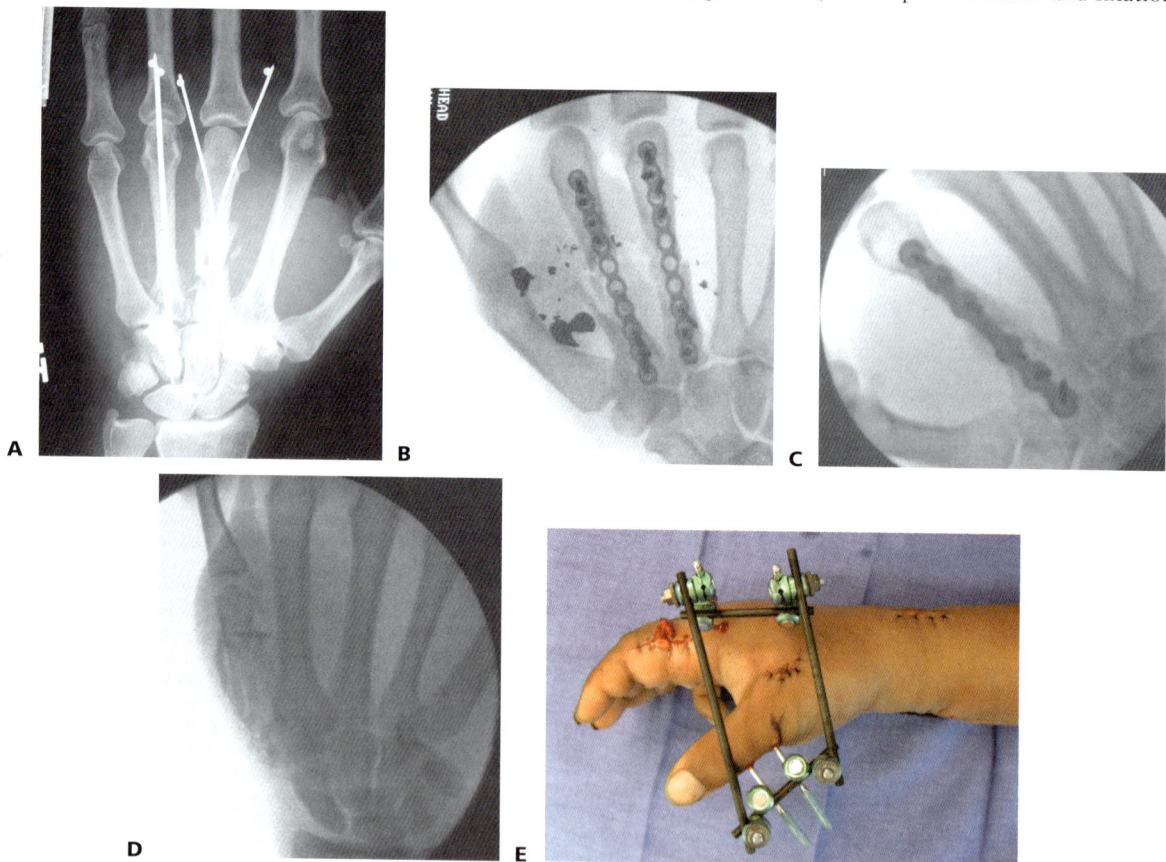

FIG 4 • **A.** A radiograph of the hand shows percutaneous fixation of displaced metacarpal fractures from a gunshot wound. **B.** Higher-energy projectiles may cause considerable displacement and comminution, as shown in this radiograph. Bridge plating is performed to improve alignment while minimizing soft tissue dissection. **C.** This index metacarpal developed a nonunion and segmental defect after nonoperative treatment of a gunshot-related fracture. A locking plate applied with cancellous bone graft to fill the void resulted in solid healing. **D.** Fractures of the first ray, as shown in this radiograph, often result in contraction of the thumb–index web space. **E.** A clinical photograph shows application of an external fixator to allow fracture consolidation in a functional position.

■ In the operating room, the contralateral hand is examined, note is made of the patient's native digital rotation, and contralateral radiographs are reviewed to assess appropriate metacarpal length.

Positioning

■ The patient is positioned supine with the affected extremity placed on a hand table. A brachial tourniquet is applied.

■ Surgery may be performed under regional or general anesthesia.

Approach

■ Percutaneous landmarks are described in the Techniques section.

■ A single extra-articular metacarpal fracture is approached with a dorsal longitudinal incision.

■ Crossing dorsal sensory nerves are sought and avoided, particularly as they pass over the bases of the border metacarpals.

■ The extensor mechanism is retracted to one side and the underlying metacarpal exposed in an extraperiosteal fashion.

■ At closure, hardware may often be covered by the fascia of the interosseous muscles.

■ Multiple metacarpal fractures are exposed by way of separate dorsal longitudinal incisions placed between affected metacarpals. If necessary, each incision may be extended as a Y distally to facilitate exposure of each metacarpal head and neck. Alternatively, the incision may be designed as a lazy S to facilitate exposure of both metacarpals (**FIG 5A,B**).

■ Intra-articular fractures are approached by longitudinally splitting the extensor tendon over the MCP (**FIG 5C**).

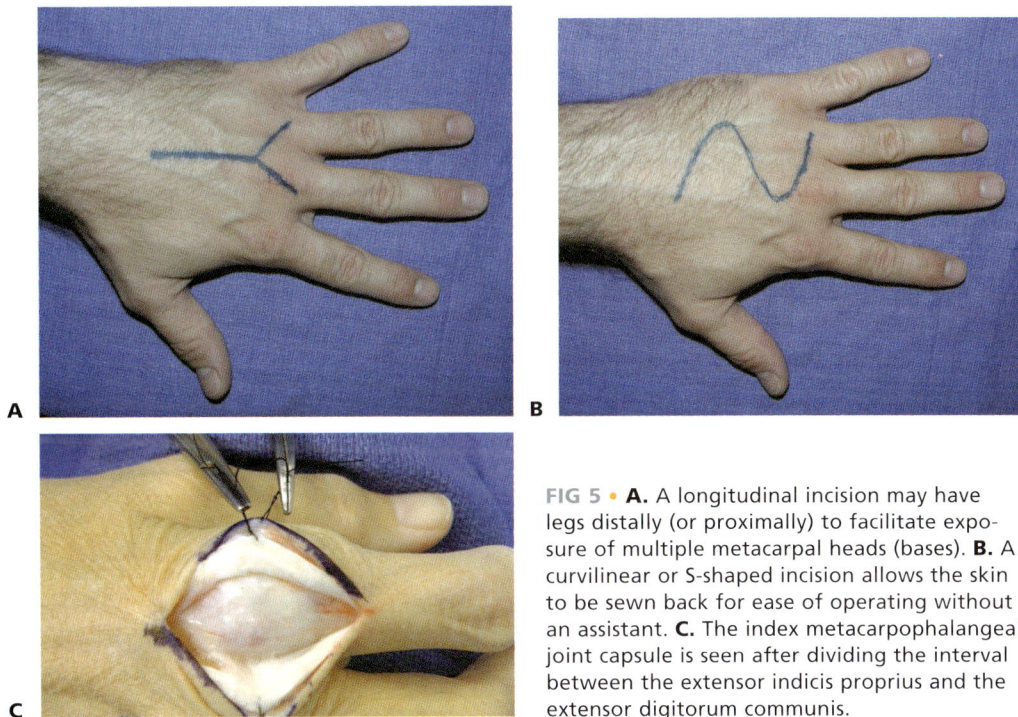

FIG 5 • **A.** A longitudinal incision may have legs distally (or proximally) to facilitate exposure of multiple metacarpal heads (bases). **B.** A curvilinear or S-shaped incision allows the skin to be sewn back for ease of operating without an assistant. **C.** The index metacarpophalangeal joint capsule is seen after dividing the interval between the extensor indicis proprius and the extensor digitorum communis.

CLOSED REDUCTION AND PINNING OF METACARPAL FRACTURES

■ A multitude of methods for pinning metacarpal fractures have been described.

   ■ We have found collateral recess pinning to be an expedient and elegant technique for managing the wide spectrum of closed and open, simple and comminuted, single and multiple metacarpal shaft fractures.

   ■ In contrast, a technique called bouquet pinning is uniquely suited for neck fractures of the border metacarpals.

   ■ These two techniques are illustrated in view of the technical challenge associated with these procedures.

Collateral Recess Pinning of Metacarpal Shaft or Neck Fractures

■ Obtain gross alignment in a closed fashion (**TECH FIG 1A**).

■ Flex the MCP joint to facilitate control of the distal fragment and subsequent pin placement (**TECH FIG 1B**).

■ Place a 0.045-inch smooth Kirschner wire by hand onto the radial (or ulnar) collateral recess and confirm appropriate placement at the deepest concavity of the collateral recess (**TECH FIG 1C**).

   ■ An oblique or near true lateral view confirms placement in the sagittal plane.

TECHNIQUES

TECHNIQUES

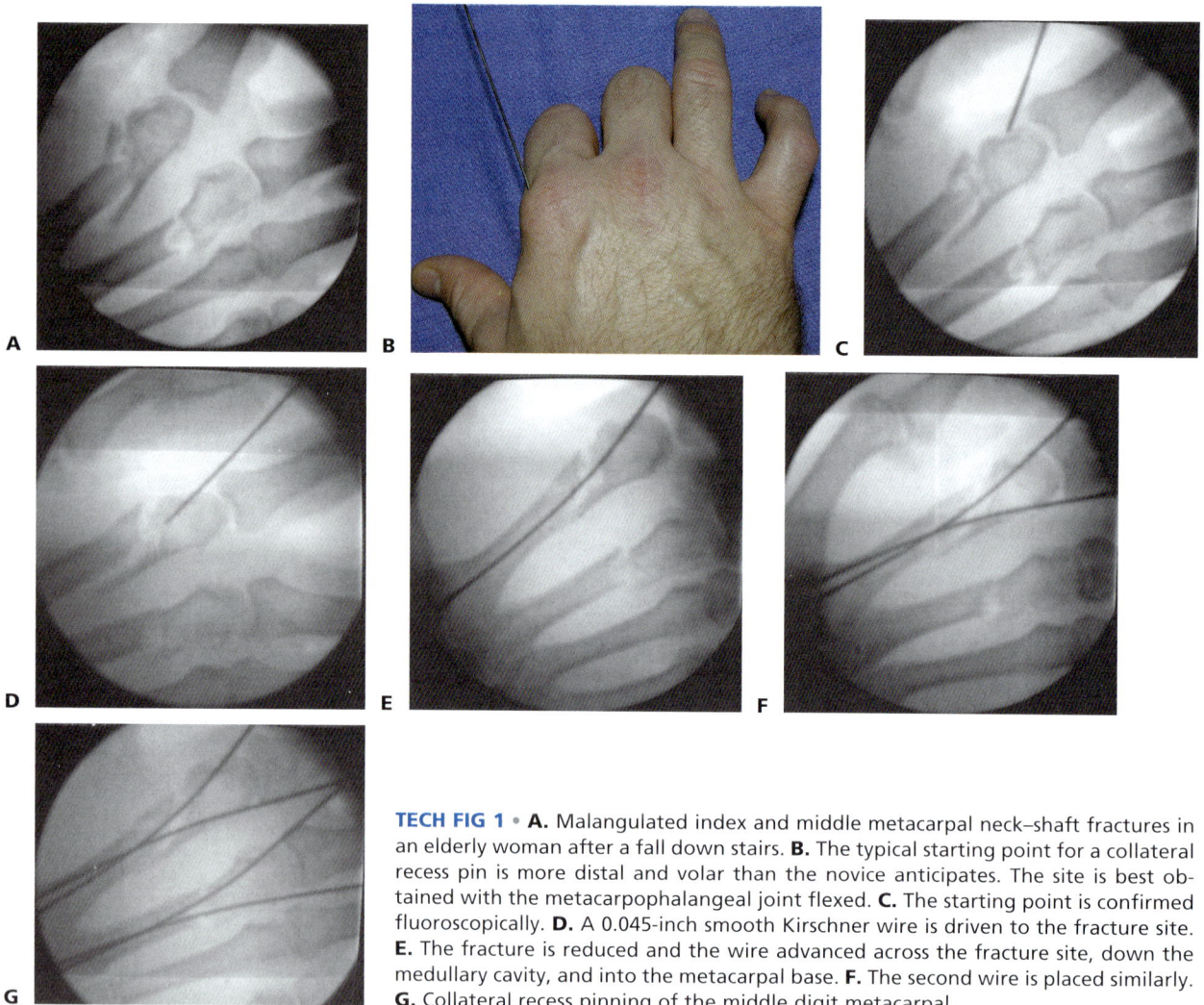

TECH FIG 1 • A. Malangulated index and middle metacarpal neck–shaft fractures in an elderly woman after a fall down stairs. **B.** The typical starting point for a collateral recess pin is more distal and volar than the novice anticipates. The site is best obtained with the metacarpophalangeal joint flexed. **C.** The starting point is confirmed fluoroscopically. **D.** A 0.045-inch smooth Kirschner wire is driven to the fracture site. **E.** The fracture is reduced and the wire advanced across the fracture site, down the medullary cavity, and into the metacarpal base. **F.** The second wire is placed similarly. **G.** Collateral recess pinning of the middle digit metacarpal.

- Advance the wire with power into the shoulder of the metacarpal and down the intramedullary canal to the fracture site (**TECH FIG 1D**).
- Reduce the fracture and advance the wire, keeping it intramedullary and seating it in the bone of the metacarpal base (**TECH FIG 1E**).
  - Consider advancing the wire using a mallet rather than power in order to "bounce" off the far cortex and remain intramedullary.
- Pass a second wire, completing fracture stabilization (**TECH FIG 1F,G**).
  - Reduction and fixation is optimized when the wires cross the fracture site.

Bouquet Pinning of Metacarpal Neck Fracture

- Make a longitudinal 2-cm incision over the radial aspect of the second metacarpal base and CMC joint (**TECH FIG 2A,B**) for the index or on the corresponding ulnar side of the small metacarpal base.
  - The wrist extensor is elevated partially but not completely detached.
- Prepare a 0.045-inch smooth Kirschner wire by cutting off the sharp tip, gently bending the pin along its length, and

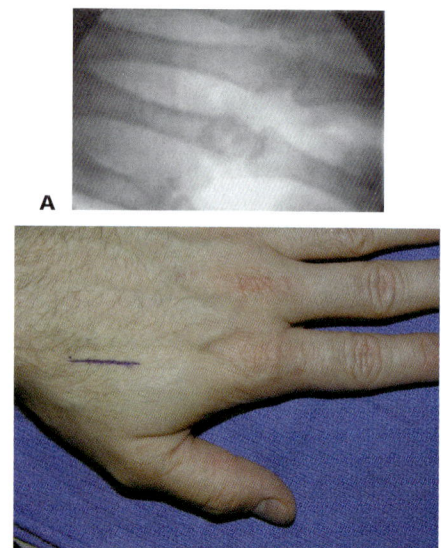

TECH FIG 2 • A. The contour of the index metacarpal head is distorted on this radiograph due to flexion of the distal fragment in this metacarpal neck fracture. **B.** A small incision site is marked at the palpable radial base of the index metacarpal. *(continued)*

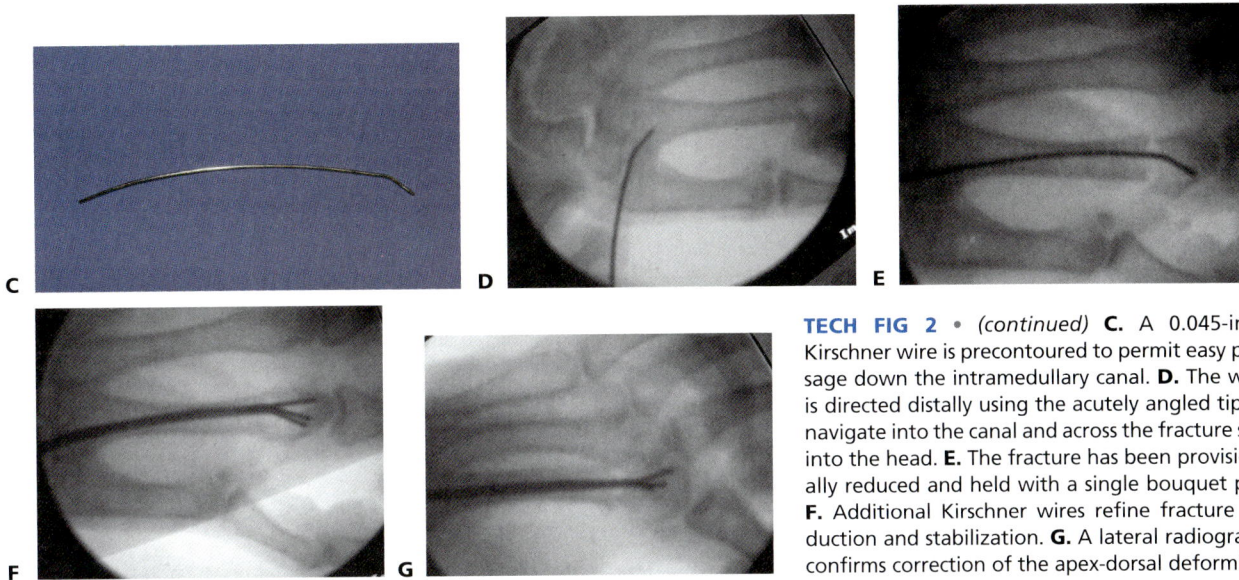

TECH FIG 2 • *(continued)* **C.** A 0.045-inch Kirschner wire is precontoured to permit easy passage down the intramedullary canal. **D.** The wire is directed distally using the acutely angled tip to navigate into the canal and across the fracture site into the head. **E.** The fracture has been provisionally reduced and held with a single bouquet pin. **F.** Additional Kirschner wires refine fracture reduction and stabilization. **G.** A lateral radiograph confirms correction of the apex-dorsal deformity.

creating a deflection of the pin in the plane of the original bend about 3 mm from its leading end (**TECH FIG 2C**).

- Locate an entry site into the medullary canal at the proximal aspect of the metaphysis using fluoroscopy.
- Enter the canal with a 2-mm drill and enlarge the introitus to about 5 mm.
- Introduce the precontoured 0.045-inch Kirschner wire and direct it distally, at the most acute angle possible (**TECH FIG 2D**).
- Advance and direct the wire down the canal and across the reduced fracture site using two large needle holders (**TECH FIG 2E**).
- Insert several additional 0.045- or 0.035-inch Kirschner wires to complete the bouquet and maintain the reduction.

- The goal is to tension the wires off the intact proximal cortex and enter the distal fragment in varied locations, creating a "bouquet" effect.
- Cut the pins flush with the canal and "nudge" them inside with a bone tamp (**TECH FIG 2F**).
- A lateral radiograph confirms correction of the preoperative apex-dorsal angulation (**TECH FIG 2G**).

Alternative Methods

- The combination of a longitudinal "collateral recess" pin and a transverse pin is a technically simple method of fixation for certain border metacarpal neck and base fractures (**TECH FIG 3**).

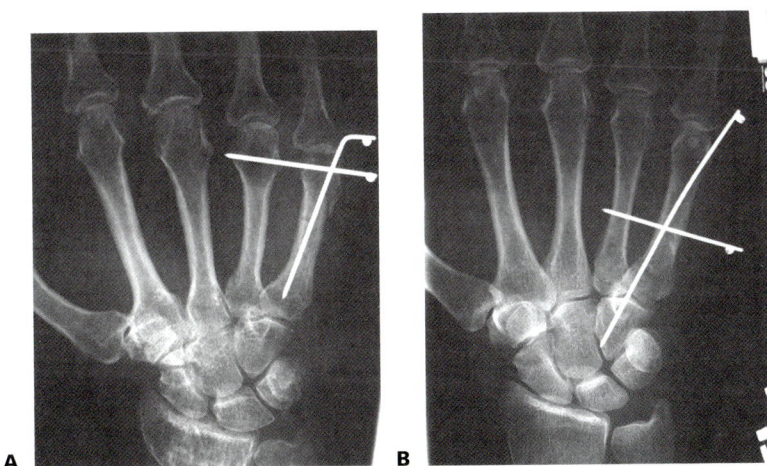

TECH FIG 3 • A transverse Kirschner wire may be used in lieu of a second collateral recess pin to stabilize metacarpal neck (**A**) or shaft fractures (**B**).

OPEN REDUCTION AND INTERNAL FIXATION OF METACARPAL FRACTURES

- Traditional AO techniques may be used to stabilize metacarpal fractures: long oblique or spiral fractures are secured with multiple screws, while short oblique and transverse fracture patterns require plate fixation.

Dynamic Compression Plating for Transverse Fractures

- Dynamic compression plating is performed using a dorsal longitudinal approach.

- Incorporate open wounds or previous incisions as needed (**TECH FIG 4A**).
- Identify and protect dorsal sensory nerve branches (**TECH FIG 4B**).
- Expose the fracture in an extraperiosteal fashion.
  - In addition to the dorsum, visualize both the radial and ulnar margins to help guide reduction.
- Apply the appropriately sized dynamic compression plate to the dorsum of the distal fracture fragment and clamp it proximally to obtain provisional fracture reduction (**TECH FIG 4C**).
  - Plate size and length depend on the patient and the fracture. The most commonly used are 2.0 to 2.5 mm.

- Add a subtle concave bend to the plate before application to the bone to help compress the volar cortices.
- Assess sagittal and coronal plane alignment by direct inspection of the fracture site; assess rotation clinically with the aid of tenodesis (**TECH FIG 4D**).
- Fill screw holes in compression mode, achieving at least four cortices of fixation in both the proximal and distal fragments (**TECH FIG 4E**).
- Fluoroscopy confirms anatomic fracture reduction and appropriate hardware placement (**TECH FIG 4F,G**).
- Close the periosteum and interosseous muscle fascia over the plate to provide a smooth gliding surface for the extensor mechanism (**TECH FIG 4H**).

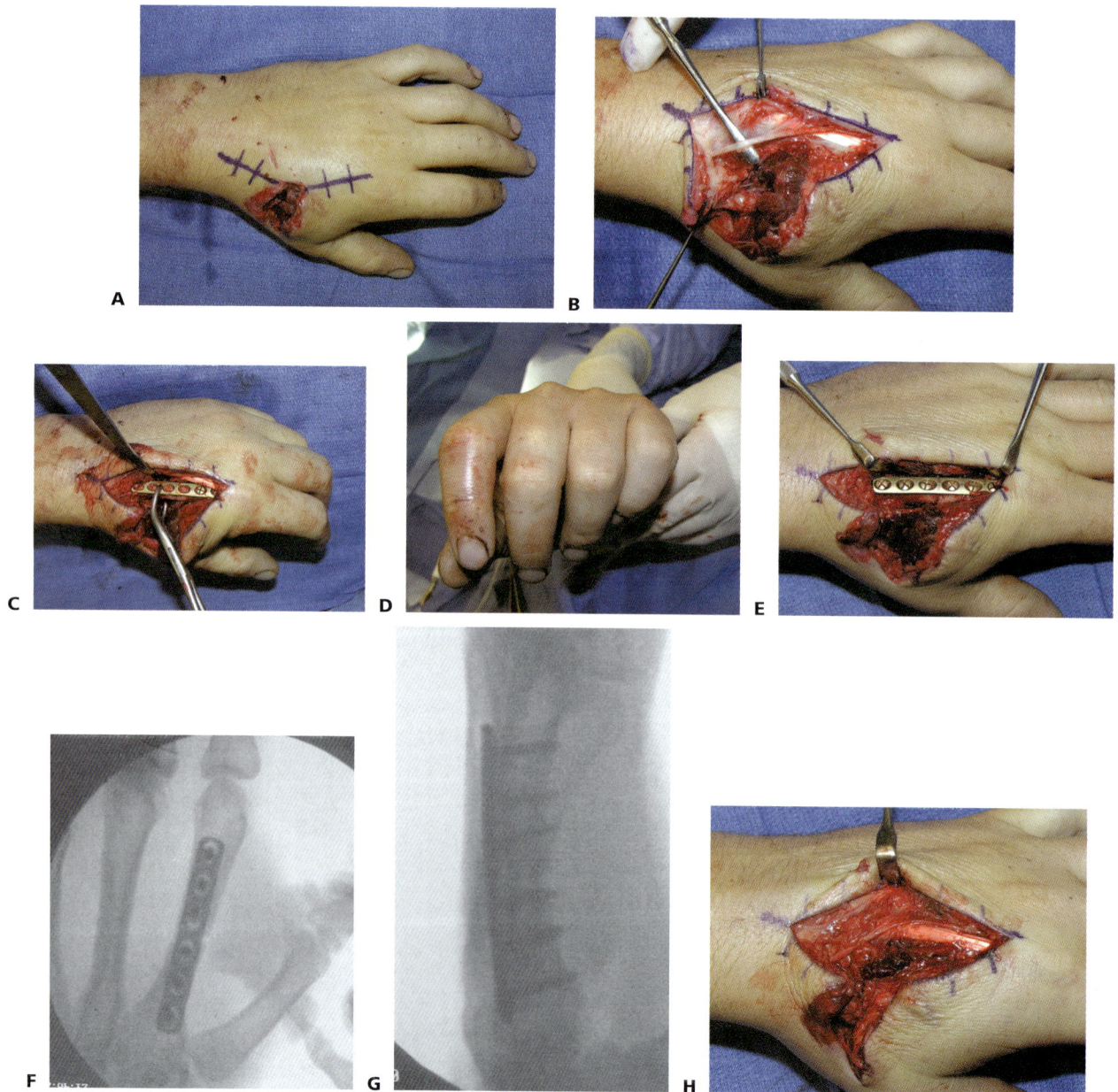

TECH FIG 4 • **A.** A malrotated open index metacarpal fracture from an industrial machine accident. **B.** A branch of the radial sensory nerve crosses the metacarpal. **C.** A 2.4-mm dynamic compression plate is secured distally with a screw and proximally with a clamp to obtain provisional reduction. **D.** Digital rotation is inspected. **E.** In the absence of comminution, the plate may be applied in compression mode. **F,G.** AP and lateral views demonstrate anatomic reduction and appropriate screw lengths. **H.** The plate is covered by fascia to minimize extensor tendon irritation.

TECHNIQUES

Neutralization Plating with Lag Screw Fixation for Short Oblique Fractures

- A short oblique fracture can be compressed with a lag screw and protected with a neutralization plate. In this case of pathologic fracture, a lag screw crosses an enchondroma cavity filled with bone graft. A T-type plate has been selected to optimize distal fixation without disrupting the MCP joint capsule (**TECH FIG 5A**).
- The exposure of short oblique metacarpal fractures is similar to transverse fractures. Adequate bone must be exposed proximal and distal to the fracture site to allow at least four cortices of screw fixation (**TECH FIG 5B,C**).

- Provisional fracture reduction can usually be achieved with a fracture reduction clamp. If fracture geometry allows, a plate (2.0 to 2.5 mm) can be contoured and held in place without disturbing the reduction (**TECH FIG 5D**).
- A lag screw may be placed alone or through the plate. Lag screw placement through the plate reduces soft tissue dissection and improves stability (**TECH FIG 5E,F**).
- Screw holes are filled in the remainder of the plate to protect the fracture site (**TECH FIG 5G,H**). Standard cortical screws may be used, although many modern plate systems also have the option for locking screws to improve fixation in metaphyseal bone.

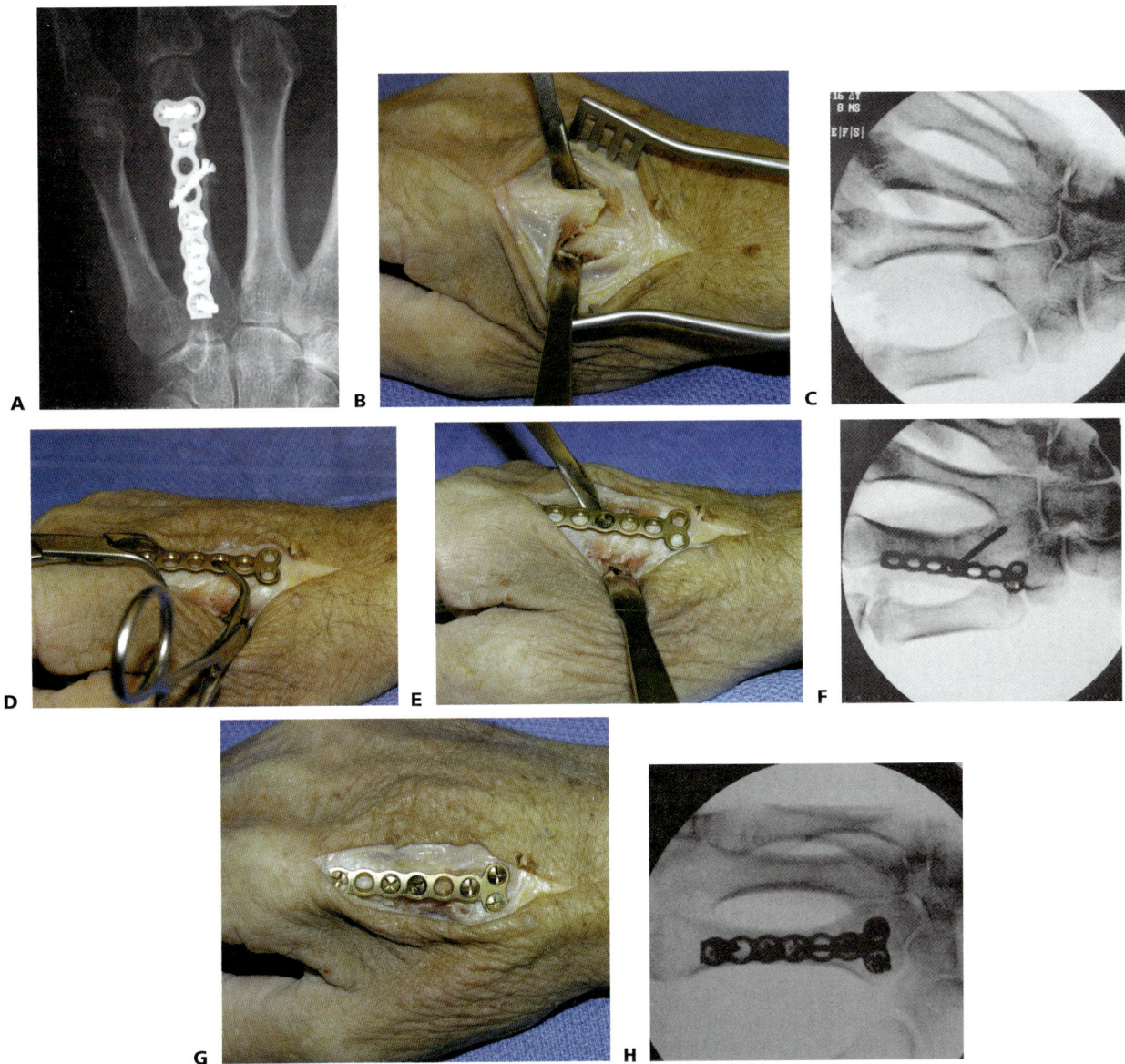

TECH FIG 5 • A. Short oblique fractures can be lagged together before placement of a dorsal plate. **B.** This cadaver specimen demonstrates a short oblique fracture at the proximal metadiaphyseal junction of the index metacarpal. **C.** Fluoroscopy reveals the proximity of the fracture to the carpometacarpal joint. **D.** The unstable distal fragment is controlled by a small pointed clamp to facilitate reduction. The reduction is maintained by a second clamp, which may also be used to hold a plate. **E.** A screw is inserted across the fracture site with lag technique to achieve optimal compression. **F.** Fluoroscopy confirms the reduction. **G.** Additional screws are placed, neutralizing forces at the fracture site. **H.** Final radiograph.

TECHNIQUES

Lag Screw Fixation for Long Oblique and Spiral Fractures

- Lag screws obviate the need for excessively long plates (**TECH FIG 6A**). Ideally, one screw is placed perpendicular to the fracture to maximize compression and another screw is placed perpendicular to the intramedullary axis of the metacarpal to resist axial loads.
- A long oblique ring metacarpal fracture is exposed enough to see the length of the fracture line; however, further proximal and distal dissection is unnecessary as a plate will not be used (**TECH FIG 6B**). The distal extent of the volar fracture fragment approaches the metacarpal head as clarified by careful fluoroscopic imaging (**TECH FIG 6C**).

- Long spiral and oblique fractures typically key into position easily with the aid of a pointed clamp (**TECH FIG 6D**).
- Fluoroscopy may be used to confirm reduction as the entire fracture length may be difficult to visualize (**TECH FIG 6E**). Rotational alignment should also be assessed clinically as described above.
- Lag screws are placed in different planes to achieve fracture compression and resist loads applied to the metacarpal (**TECH FIG 6F**).
- A final lag screw is placed proximally with strict adherence to good technique in order to avoid splintering of the metacarpal (**TECH FIG 6G–I**).
- Live fluoroscopy is best to confirm reduction and screw lengths when there are multiple screws in different planes (**TECH FIG 6J**).

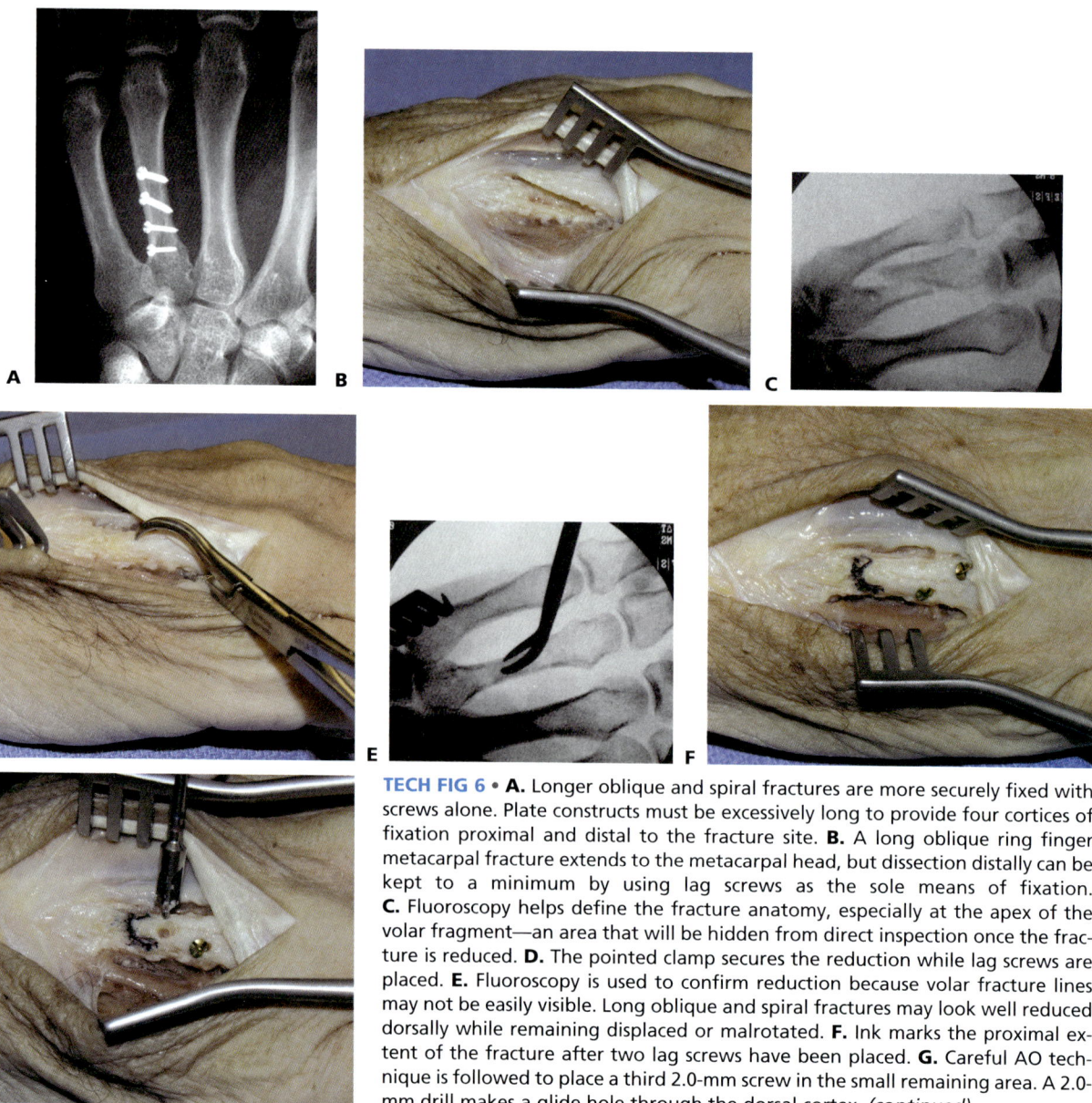

TECH FIG 6 • A. Longer oblique and spiral fractures are more securely fixed with screws alone. Plate constructs must be excessively long to provide four cortices of fixation proximal and distal to the fracture site. **B.** A long oblique ring finger metacarpal fracture extends to the metacarpal head, but dissection distally can be kept to a minimum by using lag screws as the sole means of fixation. **C.** Fluoroscopy helps define the fracture anatomy, especially at the apex of the volar fragment—an area that will be hidden from direct inspection once the fracture is reduced. **D.** The pointed clamp secures the reduction while lag screws are placed. **E.** Fluoroscopy is used to confirm reduction because volar fracture lines may not be easily visible. Long oblique and spiral fractures may look well reduced dorsally while remaining displaced or malrotated. **F.** Ink marks the proximal extent of the fracture after two lag screws have been placed. **G.** Careful AO technique is followed to place a third 2.0-mm screw in the small remaining area. A 2.0-mm drill makes a glide hole through the dorsal cortex. *(continued)*

H   **I**   **J**

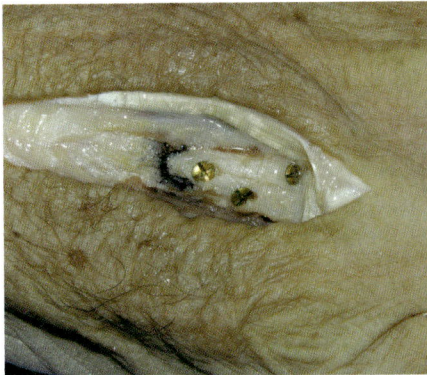

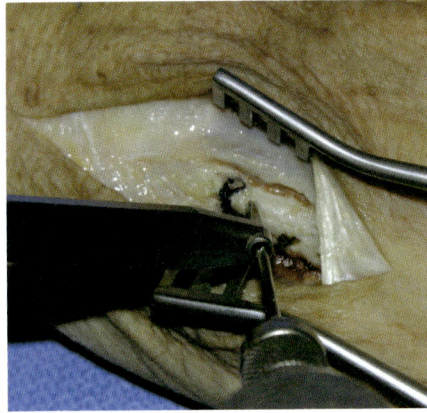

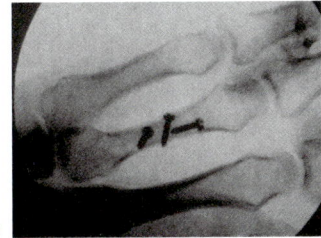

TECH FIG 6 • *(continued)* **H.** A 1.5-mm drill creates the threaded hole through the volar cortex. **I.** A countersink disperses forces about the screw head to prevent an iatrogenic fracture of the dorsal lip of bone. **J.** Radiograph confirms an anatomic reduction.

OPEN REDUCTION AND INTERNAL FIXATION OF METACARPAL HEAD FRACTURES

- Metacarpal head fractures often occur in the coronal plane (**TECH FIG 7A**) and may be associated with fractures of the neck or shaft.
- Make a longitudinal or curvilinear incision over the metacarpal head (**TECH FIG 7B**).
- Split the extensor mechanism and incise the capsule longitudinally (**TECH FIG 7C**).
- Flex the MCP joint to facilitate exposure of the fracture (**TECH FIG 7D**).
- Reduce the fracture with a dental pick or small pointed reduction forceps.

- Insert guidewires from a cannulated headless screw set to maintain the reduction (**TECH FIG 7E**).
- Insert headless screws over the guidewires (**TECH FIG 7F**).
- Close the extensor mechanism with 4-0 nonabsorbable suture (**TECH FIG 7G**).
- Confirm appropriate screw placement and fracture reduction radiographically (**TECH FIG 7H,I**).

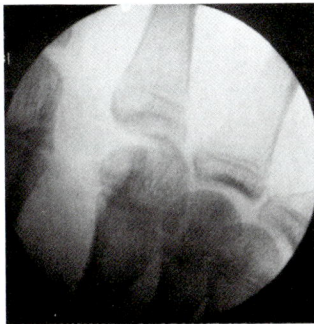

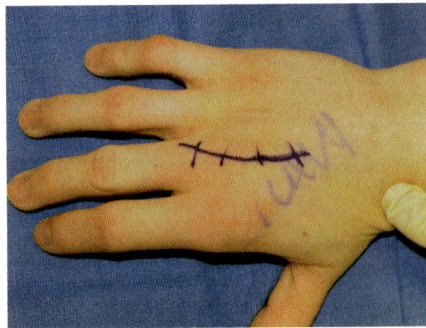

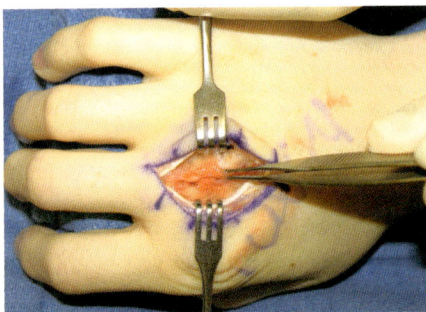

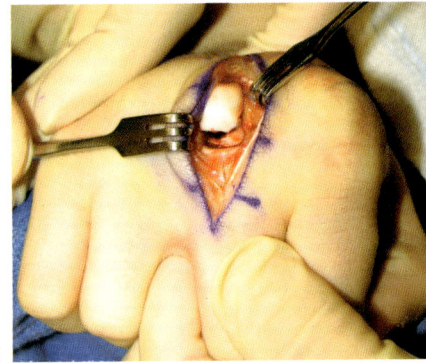

A   **B**

C   **D**

TECH FIG 7 • A. A volar coronal shear fracture in an adolescent boy has resulted in several millimeters of joint incongruity. **B.** A dorsal approach is chosen, although this fracture may also be seen well volarly. **C.** The extensor mechanism and capsule are incised. **D.** The fracture fragment is small but critical for flexion stability of the metacarpophalangeal joint. *(continued)*

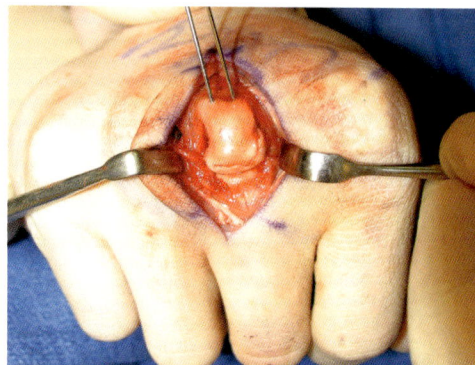

TECH FIG 7 • *(continued)* **E.** The fracture has been reduced with the proximal phalangeal base to restore metacarpal head congruity. Provisional fixation is achieved with two guidewires. **F.** Definitive fixation with cannulated headless screws facilitates early rehabilitation. **G.** The repaired extensor incision will tolerate active and active assisted motion immediately. **H, I.** AP and lateral views reveal a smooth articulation.

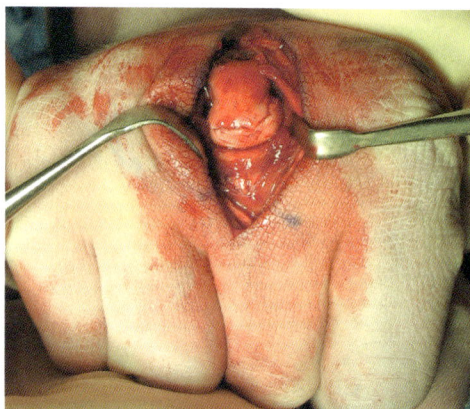

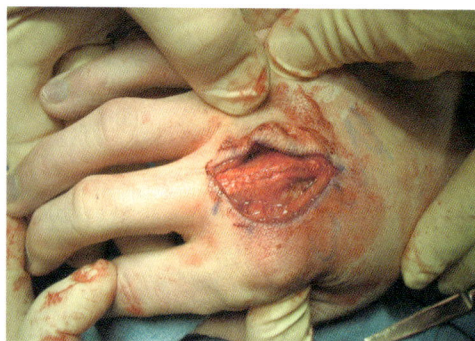

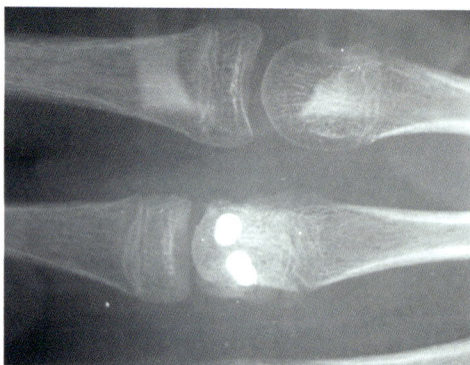

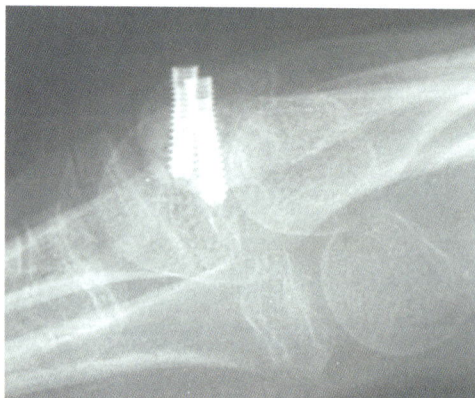

PEARLS AND PITFALLS

Indications	■ Most metacarpal fractures have good functional results with nonoperative treatment. ■ Surgery always causes some disturbance in the extensor mechanism, MCP joint capsule, or intrinsic muscles.
History	■ Antecedent pain or minimal precipitating trauma should raise the possibility of a pathologic fracture. ■ A fight-related injury may have an associated open wound. Some of these patients will have prior fracture deformities, which may be confused with an acute injury.

Examination	■ Rotational malalignment is poorly tolerated and must not be overlooked.
	■ Crush injuries of the metacarpals may be associated with:
	  ■ Fractures and dislocations of the carpus and CMC area
	  ■ Compartment syndrome and carpal tunnel syndrome

Exposure	■ Metacarpals heal quickly when exposure is limited and the bone remains within the well-vascularized bed of intrinsic musculature. ■ Massive crush and high-energy projectile injuries cause the MOST internal tissue disruption and are often best treated with the LEAST surgical tissue dissection.

TECHNIQUES

Fixation problems	■ Although popular, two parallel transverse Kirschner wires usually provide inadequate control of border metacarpal fractures. We recommend the bouquet technique or using an oblique or intramedullary "collateral recess" pin to improve stability. ■ Plate and screw fixation of long oblique or spiral metacarpal fractures may, to the surgeon's surprise, fail. It is easy to overlook the need for four cortices of fixation proximal and distal to the fracture line.
Soft tissue problems	■ Pin tract infections are particularly common around mobile skin (eg, the MCP joint). Pins should be kept clean (not dry and wrapped up) and local irritation and cellulitis treated with an oral antibiotic. ■ Fractures associated with contamination and full-thickness dorsal tissue loss may be provisionally stabilized with Kirschner wires until the wound has been serially débrided. When definitive coverage is performed, the pins may be exchanged for plates and screws to facilitate postoperative mobilization. In most hand wounds, there is no greater likelihood of infection with a fasciocutaneous flap (eg, pedicled radial forearm or free anterolateral thigh) compared with a more conventional muscle flap.

POSTOPERATIVE CARE

■ Protective splints or casts are typically worn for 4 to 6 weeks after surgery depending on the stability of fixation, the soft tissue envelope, and treatment of associated injuries.

■ The interphalangeal joints should undergo immediate active and active assisted motion to promote tendon gliding and prevent capsular contracture.

■ It is also important to mobilize the MCP joint as this allows the greatest extensor excursion over the fracture site. If necessary due to swelling, comminution of the metacarpal neck, or troubles with soft tissue healing, the MCP joint may be immobilized in the safe position (flexed 70 degrees) for about 3 weeks.

■ Kirschner wires are removed about 4 weeks after surgery. When callus is slow to form on radiographs and the fracture site remains tender, wires may be left in place for several more weeks if the pin sites remain free of infection.

■ Bone grafting should be considered if union is not achieved by 8 to 12 weeks.

■ Plates may be removed 4 to 6 months after surgery if they are causing pain or extensor tendon irritation.

OUTCOMES

■ The literature provides no conclusive evidence that either of the methods of fixation of metacarpal fractures is superior.

■ Surgical stabilization of a single closed extra-articular metacarpal fracture generally results in a good functional outcome. Nonoperative management of these injuries will also result in a good functional outcome, behooving the surgeon to identify an appropriate surgical indication—most commonly malrotation.

■ Outcome after surgical management of multiple or open metacarpal fractures is less predictable and mostly depends on the patient's long-term digital motion. Peritendinous adhesions and capsular contracture can be minimized by even small amounts of motion during the early postoperative period.

■ Nonunion is rare and usually is associated with infection, segmental bone loss, or a compromised soft tissue envelope. Occasionally, an innocuous-appearing transverse fracture may be slow to heal due to the combination of soft tissue stripping for plate fixation and the small surface area of the fracture.

COMPLICATIONS

■ Malunion (flexion or rotational deformity)
■ Delayed union or nonunion (more common with surgery)
■ Pin site or surgical wound infection
■ Extensor tendon adhesions or rupture
■ MCP or interphalangeal capsular contractures

REFERENCES

1. Ali A, Hamman J, Mass DP. The biomechanical effects of angulated boxer's fractures. J Hand Surg Am 1999;24A:835–844.
2. Black D, Mann RJ, Constein R, et al. Comparison of internal fixation techniques in metacarpal fractures. J Hand Surg Am 1985;10A: 466–472.
3. Gonzalez MH, McKay W, Hall RF Jr. Low-velocity gunshot wounds of the metacarpal: treatment by early stable fixation and bone grafting. J Hand Surg Am 1993;18A:267–270.
4. Graham TJ. The exploded hand syndrome: logical evaluation and comprehensive treatment of the severely crushed hand. J Hand Surg Am 2006;31A:1012–1023.
5. Jahss SA. Fractures of the metacarpals: a new method of reduction and immobilization. J Bone Joint Surg Am 1938;20A:178–186.
6. Strauch RJ, Rosenwasser MP, Lunt JG. Metacarpal shaft fractures: the effect of shortening on the extensor tendon mechanism. J Hand Surg Am 1998;23A:519–523.

Chapter 32

Operative Treatment of Extra-articular Phalangeal Fractures

Timothy W. Harman, Thomas J. Graham, and Richard L. Uhl

DEFINITION

- Extra-articular fractures of the phalanges include metaphyseal and diaphyseal fractures of the proximal, middle, and distal phalanges.
- Extra-articular fractures of the phalanx can range from an isolated injury, which is relatively simple to treat, to a complex trauma involving multiple structures; these latter injuries are often profoundly difficult to reconstruct and can severely affect the function of the hand.

ANATOMY

- The phalanges are the long, tubular bones of the hand that enable a functional arc of motion.
  - While each phalanx of each ray is similar, there are anatomic differences that account for the normal cascade and curvature of the digits, allowing for flexion and extension.
- The extensor mechanism of the finger glides directly on top of the phalanges, with only a thin layer of periosteum and peritenon between bone and tendon (**FIG 1**).
  - Fractures of the phalanges and the resultant bleeding, swelling, and scarring can greatly inhibit extensor function.
  - Early motion of the extensor mechanism can help minimize adhesions between bone and tendon. This is an essential principle that must be kept in mind when treating these injuries.
  - Hardware, particularly a plate, placed dorsally beneath the tendon may interfere with extensor tendon function and risk its integrity. This has led many to recommend alternate fixation methods as well as plate placement on the lateral aspect of the bone.

- A dorsal implant may abrade the tendon, especially if the end of the plate is at the level of the proximal interphalangeal joint.
- Even a low-profile dorsal plate can lead to extensor imbalance. A plate on the proximal phalanx effectively shortens and tightens the central slip tendon, leading to limited proximal interphalangeal flexion.
- There is even less room to place a dorsal plate under the triangular ligament and terminal tendon over the middle phalanx (**FIG 2**).

PATHOGENESIS

- Because the fingers project from the hand, they are subject to bending and twisting forces in a wide variety of situations.
- The fracture pattern depends on the position of the digit at the time of injury and the direction and degree of force applied.
  - As a rule, long spiral fractures tend to result from torsional forces and transverse fractures tend to occur after angular and three-point bending forces.
- Fingers are also subject to direct trauma, such as a blow from a hammer, crush injury from a window or door, or even a gunshot.
  - These injuries are often associated with skin, tendon, nerve, and artery injuries, all of which worsen the prognosis for recovery of function.
  - Most distal phalanx fractures are comminuted in nature and result from a crush mechanism. Significant displacement of the fragments is associated with a nail bed disruption.

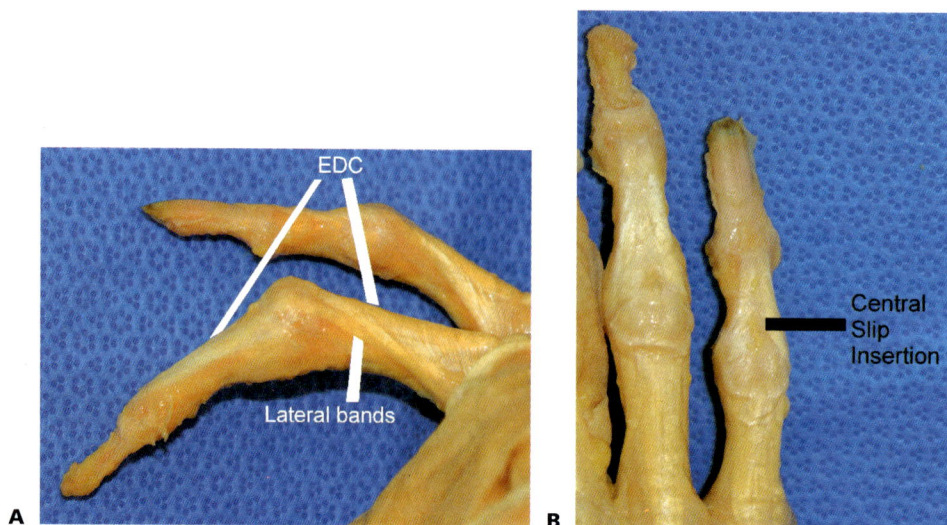

FIG 1 • **A.** Anatomic dissection of a digit showing the relationship and position of the lateral bands and extensor digitorum communis (EDC). **B.** Anatomic dissection showing the EDC with the important insertion of the central slip, which should not be detached if possible during the surgical approach.

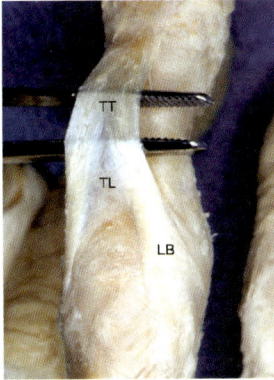

FIG 2 • The terminal tendon (*TT*) is formed by a confluence of the lateral bands (*LB*). The triangular ligament (*TL*) keeps the tendons on the dorsal aspect of the finger. The terminal tendon is intimately associated with the middle phalanx.

- Fractures of the proximal phalanx will generally assume a position of apex volar angulation.
  - The intrinsic muscle tendons, inserting on the proximal phalanx base, pull the proximal fragment into flexion and the central slip pulls the distal fragment into extension (**FIG 3**).
- Fractures of the middle phalanx deform less predictably but often assume an apex volar angulation due to the pull of the flexor digitorum sublimis tendon on the volar base of the middle phalanx proximal fragment and the force exerted by the terminal extensor tendon on the distal fragment.
- Both the extensor and flexor tendons insert on the distal phalanx at the base only. The flexor tendon insertion is more distal than the extensor tendon insertion. It is possible to have an extra-articular fracture between the two insertion sites, a so-called Seymour fracture, which angulates in a dorsal apex direction.

NATURAL HISTORY

- Extra-articular fractures of the phalanges usually heal without treatment, but often with deformity.

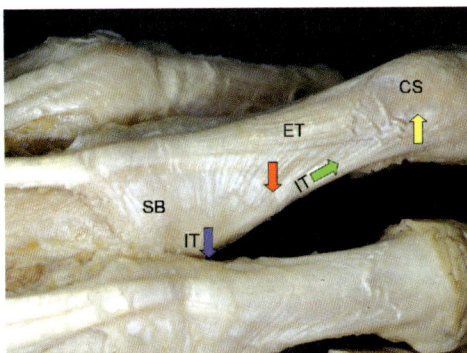

FIG 3 • Most proximal phalanx fractures assume an apex volar angulation (*red arrow*). This is due to a combination of tendon forces. The intrinsic tendon (*IT*) insertion at the base of the proximal phalanx pulls the proximal fragment into flexion (*blue arrow*). The central slip (*CS*) is formed from the extensor tendon (*ET*) and contribution from the intrinsic tendon (*IT*) as they cross dorsally (*green arrow*). The central slip pulls the distal fragment into extension (*yellow arrow*), resulting in an apex volar angulation (*red arrow*). *SB*, sagittal bond.

- It has been shown that there is a linear relationship between the degree of proximal phalanx angulation and the extensor lag.[13]
  - The correction of such deformity must be balanced with the potential for stiffness after surgical intervention as well as other potential surgical complications.

PATIENT HISTORY AND PHYSICAL FINDINGS:

- Knowledge of the mechanism of injury, time from injury to treatment, previous treatments rendered, and the injury's impact on the patient's career and hobby skill set is critical.
- It must be determined whether the patient has previously injured the digit and what, if any, preinjury functional limitations existed.
- The clinician should evaluate the cascade of the digits, looking for subtle changes in the attitude and position of the fingers. This may help to localize areas of injury.
- Pain with palpation helps localize the area of injury if there is no clear deformity of the digit and assesses fracture healing.
- Phalangeal fractures can be displaced in an AP or lateral plane, rotated, or shortened or can exhibit a combination of these deformities.
  - Resultant hand function will depend on the specific deformity and its location along the skeleton.
  - The more proximal the fracture, the greater the potential deformity at the fingertip.
  - Rotational deformity affects ultimate function the greatest, especially if it causes the fingers to scissor (**FIG 4A**).
    - Rotation can be evaluated by asking the patient to flex and extend the digits as a unit. The clinician should compare the relative position of the injured digit to adjacent digits on the injured and uninjured hand.
    - A digital anesthetic block can facilitate the examination.
    - The digits should generally point toward the distal pole of the scaphoid during flexion.

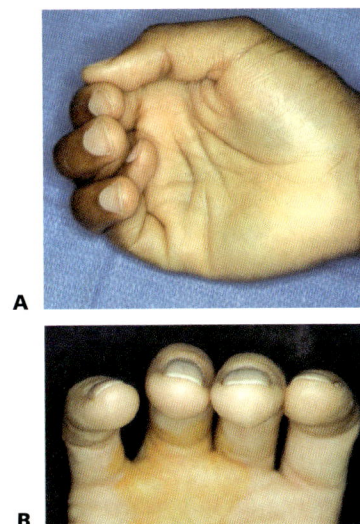

FIG 4 • **A.** Rotational deformity is the least tolerated deformity in the fingers. Assessment can be difficult, however, if the patient cannot make a fist. **B.** Rotation can be assessed by observing the planes of the fingernails to each other. The nail that is rotated out of the plane of the others (in this case the ring finger) indicates a rotational deformity of that digit.

■ It is often difficult for the patient to make a fist at the initial assessment due to pain and swelling. In these cases, comparing the plane of the nail bed of the injured finger to the adjacent nail beds and comparing with the other hand can provide a valuable clue to the presence of a rotational deformity (**FIG 4B**).

■ Neurocirculatory status
  ■ Altered skin color and diminished turgor and capillary refill of the digit are clear indicators of vascular compromise.
  ■ Two-point discrimination can be used to assess innervation density and is an excellent method for evaluating the integrity of digital nerves.

■ Condition of the soft tissue envelope
  ■ The skin may be visibly damaged with lacerations, degloving, or burns. Its condition will influence treatment.
  ■ A subungual hematoma is common with a distal phalanx fracture.

■ Unstable fracture patterns must be recognized (Table 1).

IMAGING AND OTHER DIAGNOSTIC STUDIES:

■ AP, oblique, and lateral radiographs will provide sufficient imaging for the majority of extra-articular phalangeal fractures.
  ■ Critical evaluation may show subtle rotational malalignment if a true lateral view of either the base or the condyles of a phalanx does not match up across its corresponding joint.
  ■ Slightly obliqued lateral views are useful for imaging fractures at the base of the proximal phalanx, where the overlap on a true lateral view makes evaluation difficult.

■ A mobile, small fluoroscopy unit allows magnification to help characterize subtle injuries and dynamic evaluation to gauge fragment stability.

■ More sophisticated imaging (MRI, CT, ultrasound) is rarely needed to make the diagnosis of a phalangeal fracture or to guide treatment.

DIFFERENTIAL DIAGNOSIS

■ While there are other causes of hand pain and deformity (eg, osteoarthritis, congenital deformity, tumor, infection), the patient history and plain radiographs should leave little doubt that the patient has a phalanx fracture.

■ If a fracture is not evident, all the following diagnoses should be considered:
  ■ Acute sprains
  ■ Metacarpophalangeal (MP) and interphalangeal dislocations
  ■ Mallet finger
  ■ Phalangeal contusions
  ■ Benign and malignant lesions of the digits
  ■ Soft tissue injuries
  ■ Collateral ligament injury
  ■ Boutonnière or swan-neck injuries
  ■ Sagittal band ruptures
  ■ Tendon ruptures
  ■ Pulley ruptures
  ■ Stenosing tenosynovitis or trigger finger
  ■ Acute infection

NONOPERATIVE MANAGEMENT

■ Many phalangeal fractures are stable and can be treated effectively by closed means. Each fracture must be addressed individually, taking into account the condition of the soft tissue envelope, the fracture characteristics, and the functional needs of the patient.
  ■ Mild (nonrotational) deformities do well with immobilization and protection while the fractures heal, but unstable or malrotated fractures benefit from surgical intervention.
  ■ Distal phalanx fractures are most commonly amenable to nonoperative treatment.

Table 1	Unstable Extra-articular Fracture Patterns of the Phalanx	
Fracture Pattern	**Cause (Forces)**	**Technique**
Spiral oblique fractures	Inherently unstable	Long oblique – Lag screws Short oblique – Lag screws - Kirschner wires - Plate and screws - +/− lag screw
P1 short transverse fractures	Intrinsic interossei tend to pull the proximal fragment into flexion. The distal segment is pulled into extension by the action of the central slip insertion into the base of the middle phalanx.	- Intrafocal pinning—intramedullary pinning across the metacarpophalangeal joint in flexion - Eaton-Belsky pinning - Oblique/crossed Kirschner wires - Plate and screws - Tension banding
P2 short transverse fractures	Fractures proximal to the flexor digitorum superficialis (FDS) insertion cause extension of the proximal fragment and flexion of the distal fragment. Fractures distal to the FDS insertion become flexed due to the strong pull of the FDS.	- Oblique/crossed Kirchner wires - Plate and screws - Retrograde intramedullary pinning across the distal interphalangeal joint - +/− oblique Kirschner wire - Tension banding
P3 transverse fractures proximal to the tuft	Instability possible with loss of support to the nail bed Action of the flexor digitorum profundus to the proximal fragment with a floating distal fragment	- Retrograde intramedullary pinning across the distal interphalangeal joint - Spanning with plate and screws - Blade plate and screws
Comminuted fractures	Inherently unstable	- External fixator

- Results are good or excellent in more than 70% of extra-articular phalangeal fractures treated nonoperatively.[1,5,7,10]
- Early motion is always desirable, but it is somewhat less important with closed treatment.
  - Immobilization beyond 3 weeks has been shown to increase stiffness[12] and lead to worse outcomes.
- Closed treatment
  - Less scarring to the extensor mechanism
  - Less ability to move early, unless the fracture is very stable
  - Minimal ability to hold a corrected deformity
- Internal fixation
  - Greater scarring of the extensors, especially with a dorsal approach and a dorsal implant
  - Early motion essential
  - Greatest ability to hold the fracture in a stable, corrected position
- If a fracture is incomplete, complete but nondisplaced, or impacted (such as the metaphysis at the base of the proximal phalanx), a short period (1 to 2 weeks) of splinting followed by buddy taping to the adjacent digit is appropriate (**FIG 5**).
- A fracture that can be adequately reduced but is relatively unstable can occasionally be held reduced with a splint.
  - This has the advantage of avoiding a trip to the operating room and the possible complications of surgical fixation but requires close follow-up and serial radiographs to ensure that reduction is maintained (**FIG 6**).

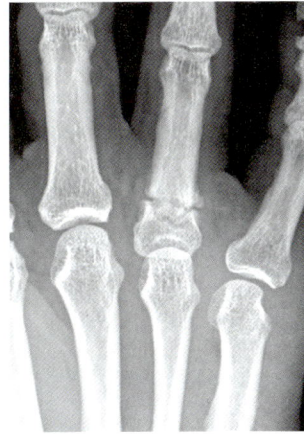

FIG 5 • This fracture is stable because it is well aligned (on the AP and lateral radiographs) and that alignment does not change with motion. This fracture was treated with splinting for 2 weeks and buddy taping for 2 more weeks.

SURGICAL MANAGEMENT

- When considering any surgery, it is necessary to balance the potential benefits of surgery with the risks of the procedure.
  - The goal of surgery is to restore alignment and to stabilize the fracture to a degree sufficient to begin early motion.

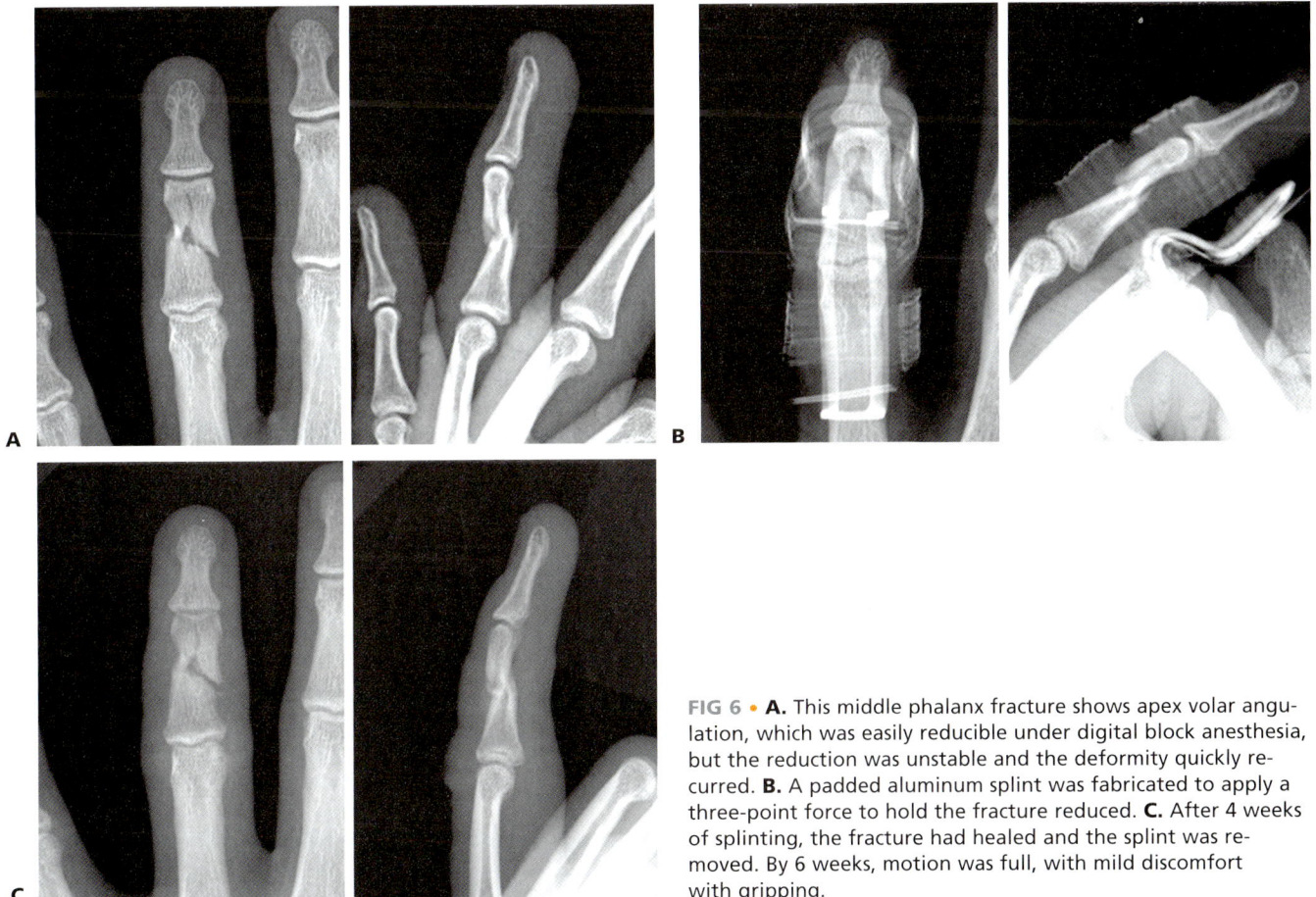

FIG 6 • **A.** This middle phalanx fracture shows apex volar angulation, which was easily reducible under digital block anesthesia, but the reduction was unstable and the deformity quickly recurred. **B.** A padded aluminum splint was fabricated to apply a three-point force to hold the fracture reduced. **C.** After 4 weeks of splinting, the fracture had healed and the splint was removed. By 6 weeks, motion was full, with mild discomfort with gripping.

- Any phalangeal fracture with a significant injury to the soft tissue envelope has a worse prognosis.
  - Stable fixation (to the degree that it does not further compromise the soft tissues) and early motion assume a greater importance in phalangeal fractures with associated soft tissue injuries.
  - Patients with open fractures are treated with the appropriate intravenous antibiotic therapy.[11]
- Once the decision is made to surgically intervene, the surgeon must decide which mode of fixation will best suit the fracture pattern (Table 1).
  - This decision is often made intraoperatively and is frequently based on the ability of the fracture to be adequately reduced closed.
- Fractures that are reduced closed are stabilized externally with a cast or fixator or are held with Kirschner wires placed percutaneously.
  - Kirschner wiring and external fixation are techniques that, when appropriately applied, will result in acceptable outcomes without potential soft tissue surgical interruption and scarring.[4]
- Open reduction and internal fixation with plates and screws will potentially provide stable fixation but without early mobilization could result in decreased range of motion.
  - Overly aggressive soft tissue stripping will cause extensor tendon adhesions, and bulky implants will affect extensor tendon balance and function.[9]
- An algorithm can be used to aid in the decision-making process (**FIG 7**).

Methods

Percutaneous Wire Fixation

- Closed reduction with percutaneous fixation can be used to treat the majority of unstable spiral fractures of the phalanges.
- The technique is also suitable for transverse metaphyseal fractures, but it may be less suited for transverse diaphyseal fractures.
- When the wires are inserted radial and ulnar to the extensor mechanism, percutaneous wire fixation offers the advantage of minimal disruption of the soft tissues in general, and the extensor mechanism in particular.
- This technique is best suited for fractures less than 10 days old. After that time, early healing makes accurate closed reduction more difficult.
- Kirschner wires provide less stable fixation than plates and screws and may restrict soft tissue gliding due to their prominence. This restriction of early motion may lead to increased stiffness.

Interosseous Wire Fixation

- Interosseous wire fixation is more rigid than Kirschner wire fixation but requires open reduction and additional dissection to expose the bone surfaces.
  - This method of fixation is less bulky than a plate and, as such, is particularly well suited for fractures of the middle phalanx when percutaneous pinning is not possible.
- Interosseous wiring works best with a transverse fracture. The wires provide compression to stabilize the fracture. Interosseous wiring will not work if the fracture is comminuted. Interosseous wiring is made more stable when it is combined with pin fixation and placed in a 90-degree configuration.

Lag Screw Fixation

- Lag screw fixation is best suited for oblique and simple spiral fractures.
  - Lag screws can be used alone if the length of the fracture is greater than twice the diameter of the bone at the level of the fracture.
  - If the obliquity is less, a neutralization plate should be added.
- Comminuted and transverse fractures are not amenable to lag screw fixation.
- Contemporary lag screws are extremely low profile, making them an excellent fixation option in the phalanx, especially the middle phalanx.
- Lag screw fixation is more rigid than Kirschner wire fixation, and unlike wires, the screws do not need to be removed.
- Lag screws can be inserted percutaneously, but the procedure can be technically challenging.
- Usually, an oblique fracture will be visualized best in the AP plane and the screws inserted from the lateral aspects.
  - Spiral fractures frequently require the screws to be placed in two planes.
  - Multiplanar screw fixation greatly increases the biomechanical stability (**FIG 8**).

Plate Fixation

- Plate fixation is best suited for transverse fractures, short oblique fractures, periarticular metaphyseal fractures, and comminuted fractures, in which the plate serves as a bridge to maintain phalangeal length.
  - Midshaft, transverse fractures are fixed with a straight plate. At least two screws should be placed in either side of the fracture site with fixation of four cortices (**FIG 9**).
  - If close to the metaphysis, a T plate, a Y plate, or a condylar blade plate will allow improved fixation compared with a straight plate.

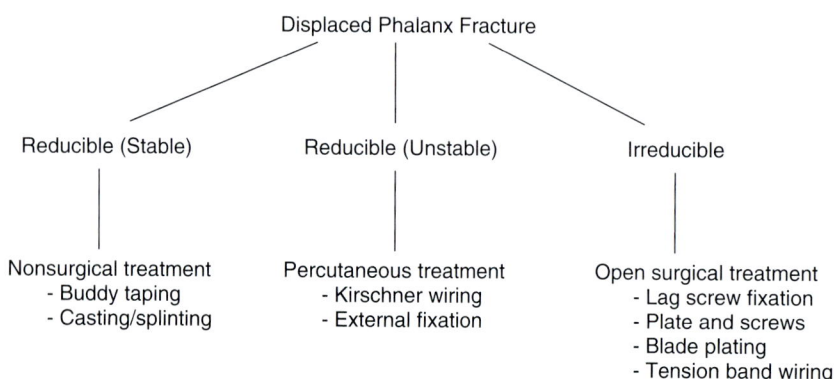

Displaced Phalanx Fracture

Reducible (Stable) — Reducible (Unstable) — Irreducible

Nonsurgical treatment
- Buddy taping
- Casting/splinting

Percutaneous treatment
- Kirschner wiring
- External fixation

Open surgical treatment
- Lag screw fixation
- Plate and screws
- Blade plating
- Tension band wiring

FIG 7 • Decision algorithm for the progression to open surgical treatment for phalangeal fractures and the subsequent treatment options for fixation.

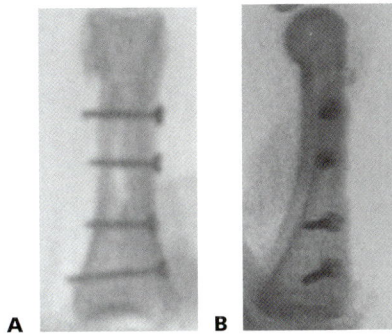

FIG 8 • Lag screw fixation of a proximal phalanx. The placement of the screws prevents prominence to the extensor mechanism (**A**), and the multiplanar placement of the screws adds to the biomechanical stability of the fracture fixation (**B**).

- Adding a lag screw across an oblique fracture, either through the plate or as an adjunct to plate fixation, will add to the rigidity of the construct.
  - Compression, obtained by eccentrically drilling one or more of the screws in the plate, will increase fracture stability.
- Plate fixation requires more extensive soft tissue dissection and increases the risk of postoperative extensor scarring.
  - Immediate motion of the digits is essential to minimize the scarring.
- Plates are more bulky and may lead to extensor mechanism imbalance, especially near the central slip insertion and on the middle phalanx.

Preoperative Planning

- Preoperative posteroanterior, lateral, and oblique radiographs are essential.
  - Evaluation of these studies helps determine the plane of the fracture and the size of the fracture fragments, allowing the surgeon to choose the best surgical approach and the ideal fixation technique.

- The surgeon must be certain that all potential implants are available. Surgical error can frequently be traced to implant availability problems.
  - Many sets include only one or two plates of a given size and shape. In the case of multiple digit involvement, extra plates and screws are helpful.
- Intraoperative imaging using a mini fluoroscopy unit is essential, and its availability should be ensured.
- The surgeon should plan for alternative approaches and means of fixation should comminution or soft tissue problems preclude the original plan.

Positioning

- The patient is placed supine on the operating table with a radiolucent hand table attached.
- A padded arm or forearm tourniquet is used for all cases.

Approach

- The phalanx is most commonly approached laterally or dorsally. The exact approach used for open reduction is often based on the location of the fracture as it relates to the extensor mechanism (**FIG 10**).
- The sagittal bands at the MP joint, the central slip insertion, and the triangular ligament should be preserved whenever possible (**FIG 11**).
  - Motion is necessarily delayed after surgery if these structures are incised and subsequently repaired.
  - A portion of the lateral band may be excised rather than repaired as part of the midaxial approach (**FIG 12**).
  - Longitudinal incisions in the midportion of the extensor tendon and especially in the midaxial interval between the extensor and the lateral band allow early motion.
- At the middle phalanx level, a midaxial approach on the edge of the terminal tendon is preferred so that the tendon can be pulled to the side, exposing the bone (**FIG 13**).
  - The midaxial approach is also useful when using lag screw fixation, as the screws are usually inserted on the lateral aspect of the bone.

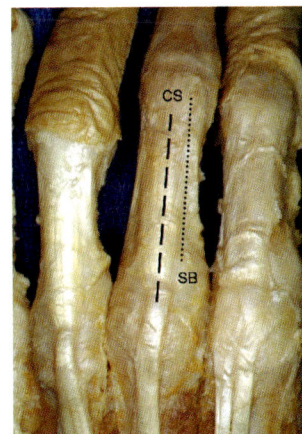

FIG 10 • The surgical approach to the proximal phalanx can be straight dorsal, through the extensor tendon (*dashed line*), or midaxial (*dotted line*), between the dorsal tendon and the intrinsic contribution. Care must be taken not to disrupt the central slip (*CS*) with the dorsal approach, and not to disrupt the sagittal bands (*SB*) with the midaxial approach. Thus, the dorsal approach is better suited for the more proximal fractures and the midaxial approach is better for the more distal fractures.

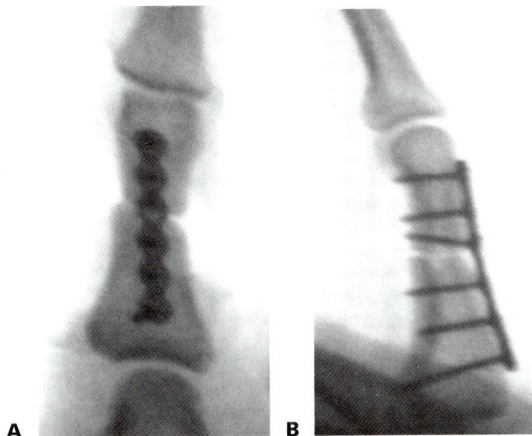

FIG 9 • Posteroanterior (**A**) and lateral (**B**) radiographs after plate and screw fixation of an unstable fracture pattern. The length of the screws is crucial to obtain bicortical fixation without prominence that will wear on the flexor tendon mechanism.

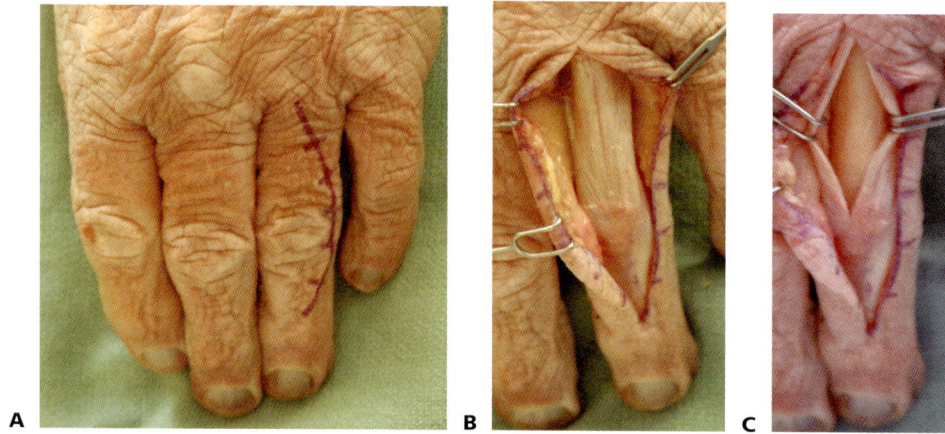

FIG 11 • **A.** Utilitarian dorsal curvilinear approach to the proximal phalanx. **B.** The extensor digitorum communis (EDC) tendon is fully visualized. **C.** A midline incision is made in the EDC, exposing the proximal phalanx, but protecting the sagittal band and the central slip insertion.

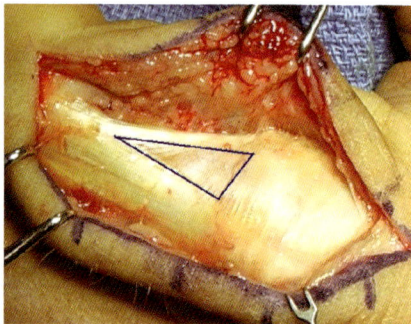

FIG 12 • A dorsolateral surgical approach to an index finger that demonstrates the sagittal fibers and extensor digitorum and lateral bands. The portion of the lateral bands outlined by the triangle may safely be excised.

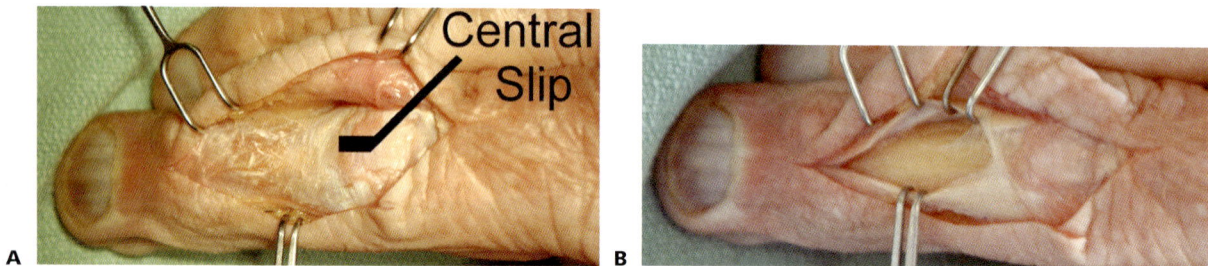

FIG 13 • **A.** Utilitarian dorsal curvilinear approach to the middle phalanx with exposure of the extensor digitorum communis (EDC). **B.** A midline incision is made in the EDC, exposing the middle phalanx, but leaving the central slip and terminal extensor tendon insertions intact.

TECHNIQUES

PERCUTANEOUS KIRSCHNER WIRE FIXATION

Fracture Reduction

- Before performing any reduction maneuver, obtain posteroanterior and lateral C-arm images for reference.
  - If the fracture is very close to the MP joint, a slightly oblique lateral view will show the fracture better by avoiding some of the overlap of the other MP joints.
- Unstable spiral fractures of the phalanges are usually shortened, rotated, and angulated (**TECH FIG 1A**).
- Begin the reduction by applying longitudinal traction.

- This can be accomplished with direct traction on the digit. Use a moist gauze, fingertraps, or a pointed towel clip applied distal to the fracture.
- While traction is applied, correct the rotational deformity (**TECH FIG 1B**). Any angular deformity is then corrected before placing a reduction clamp across the fracture.
  - Flexing the MP joint stabilizes the proximal P-1 fragment by tightening the collateral ligaments.
- Apply a reduction clamp (a towel clip-like device with sharp points) across the fracture percutaneously to hold the reduction.

A   **B**

TECH FIG 2 • Posteroanterior and lateral radiographs showing a spiral proximal phalanx fracture treated with percutaneous pinning using the method described.

- Usually 0.045-inch Kirschner wires are used in the proximal phalanx, although fixation in the small finger and in the more distal phalanges may require the smaller 0.035-inch Kirschner wire size (**TECH FIG 2**).
- Diamond-tipped smooth Kirschner wires are preferred.
- Crossed wires can be used to secure transverse fractures.
  - This method is useful for metaphyseal fractures (**TECH FIG 3**) and to stabilize middle phalanx fractures to avoid the need for plate fixation (**TECH FIG 4**).
  - Avoid distraction at the fracture site when using crossed wires.

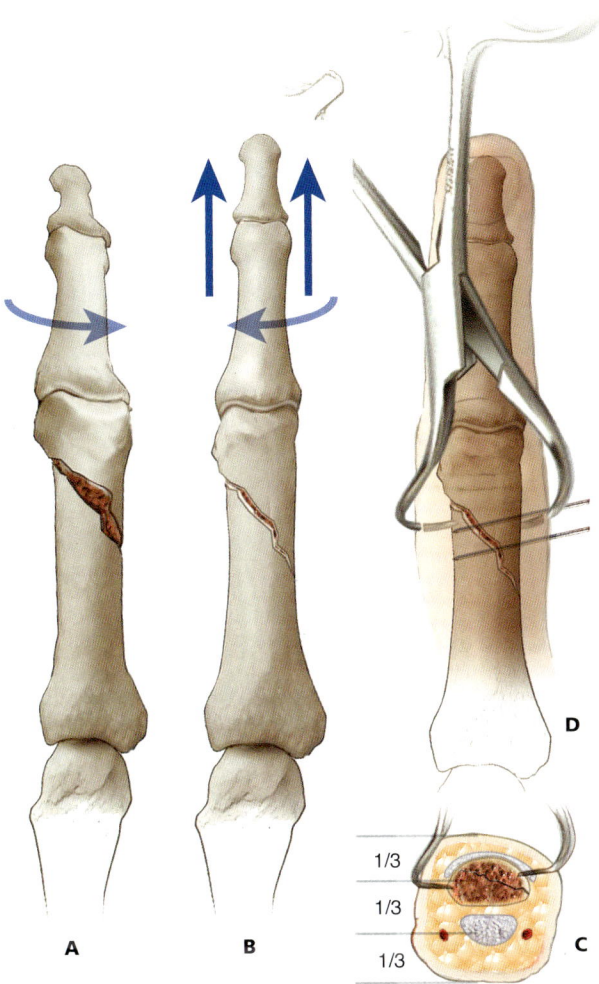

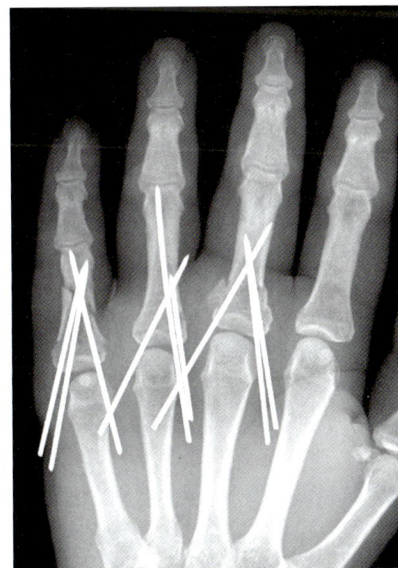

TECH FIG 1 • **A.** Unstable phalangeal fractures deform with shortening, rotation, and angulation. **B.** Longitudinal traction is applied first, and then the rotation and angulation are corrected. **C.** The bone is in the dorsal two thirds of the finger rather than in the middle. The neurovascular bundles are in the volar third and should, of course, be avoided when the reduction clamp is applied. **D.** When the fracture is reduced and compressed with the reduction clamp, the pins are drilled across the fracture site.

- When considering the cross-sectional anatomy of the finger, remember that the bone lies in the dorsal two thirds, not in the midline (**TECH FIG 1C**). Thus, the clamp tips should enter the skin dorsal to the midlateral line.
- Placing the clamp at a slight angle so that it is more perpendicular to the fracture will aid stability of the reduction through fracture compression.
- Reduction can further be fine-tuned by twisting the clamp slightly when tightening.

Fracture Stabilization

- After checking the reduction with the fluoroscope, drill the Kirschner wires across the fracture site until they gain purchase in the far cortex (**TECH FIG 1D**).

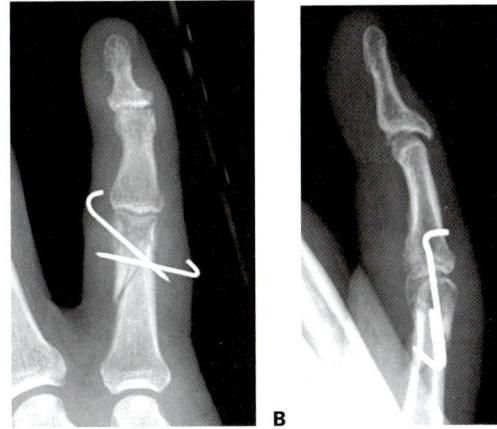

TECH FIG 3 • This patient sustained a crush injury to the hand resulting in fractures of the middle, ring, and small fingers. The fingers were reduced by pinning them in flexion and passing the pins between the metacarpal heads rather than spearing the extensor tendons. This held the metacarpophalangeal joints in a flexed position once pinned. Active motion of the proximal and distal interphalangeal joints was started in the immediate postoperative period.

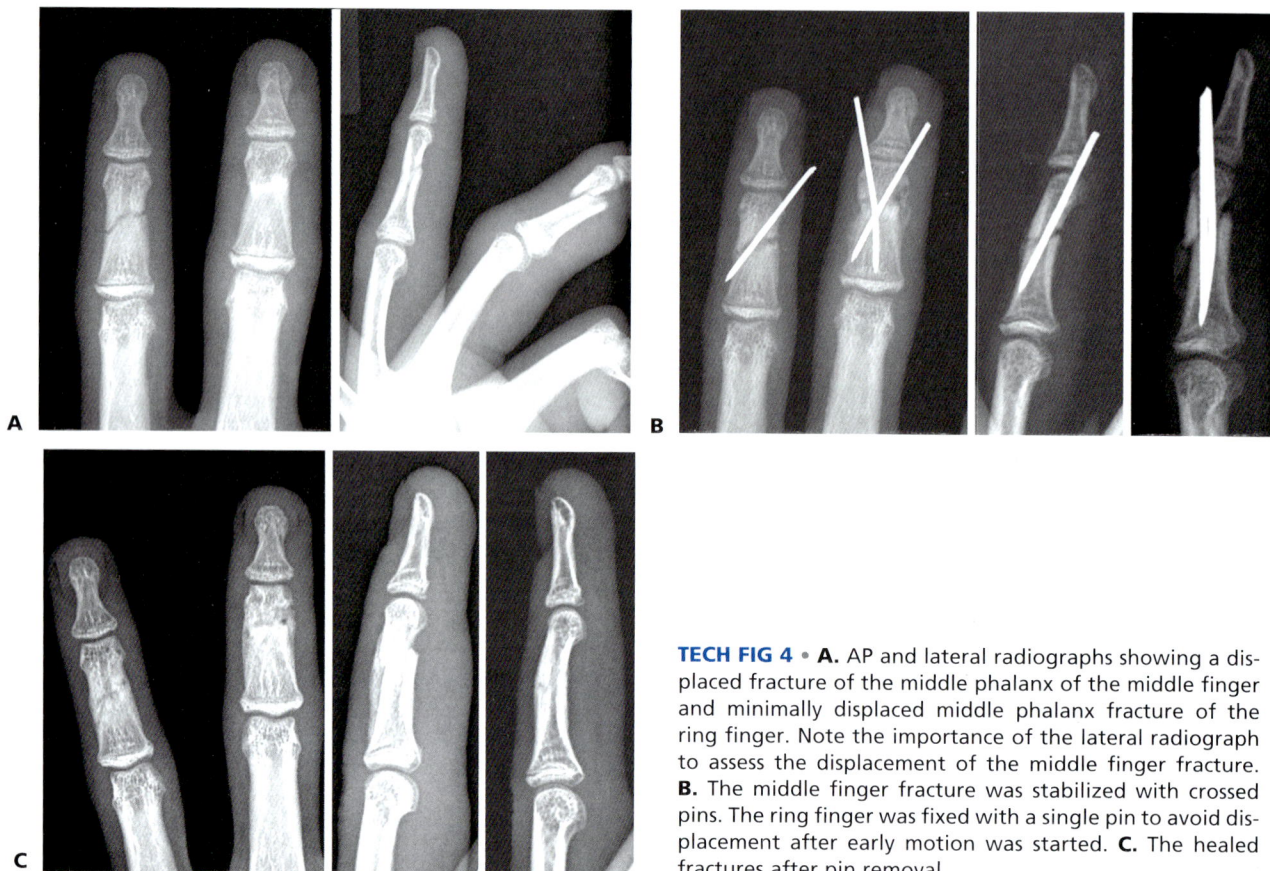

TECH FIG 4 • **A.** AP and lateral radiographs showing a displaced fracture of the middle phalanx of the middle finger and minimally displaced middle phalanx fracture of the ring finger. Note the importance of the lateral radiograph to assess the displacement of the middle finger fracture. **B.** The middle finger fracture was stabilized with crossed pins. The ring finger was fixed with a single pin to avoid displacement after early motion was started. **C.** The healed fractures after pin removal.

INTEROSSEOUS WIRE FIXATION

Exposure

- Open reduction and fairly extensive fracture exposure is required for placement of the intraosseous wires, especially when using a dorsovolar wire.
- Expose the fracture using either a dorsal or midaxial approach.
- Place the bone in the "shotgun" position (apex dorsal) and gently elevate the soft tissues from the proximal and distal fragments 3 to 5 mm at the fracture site.
- Drill transverse and anteroposterior holes 2 to 5 mm away from the fracture site using a 0.045 smooth Kirschner wire.

Fracture Reduction and Stabilization

- Reduce the fracture and verify reduction through direct observation and with a mini C-arm.
- Pass a 24-gauge steel wire through the transverse hole and a second wire though the anteroposterior holes.
- Tighten the wire loops sequentially by pulling the wire away from the fracture and twisting slowly to stabilize and compress the fracture (**TECH FIG 5**).
    - Do not fully tighten the first wire until the second wire has been at least partially tightened.

- Plan placement of the wire loops so as to lay them flat against bone and minimize soft tissue irritation.
- If greater stability is required, drill a 0.035 to 0.045 smooth Kirschner wire obliquely across the fracture.

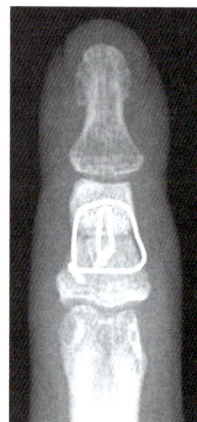

TECH FIG 5 • AP radiograph of a middle phalanx infected nonunion treated by débridement, squaring of the fracture ends, and 90-90 interosseous wiring.

LAG SCREW FIXATION

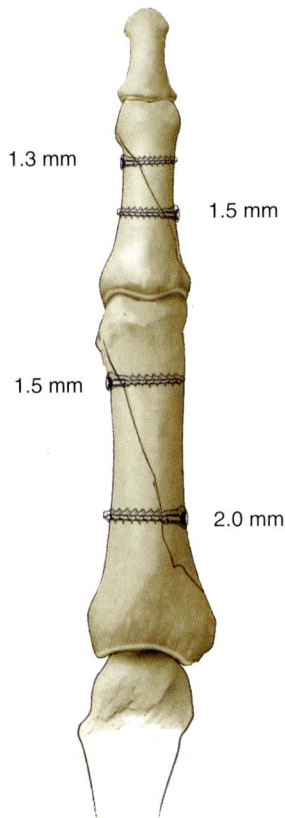

- 1.3 mm
- 1.5 mm
- 1.5 mm
- 2.0 mm

- Lag screws can be inserted percutaneously, but the procedure is technically challenging. Precise reduction of the fracture is the first priority and should not be sacrificed in an attempt to limit incision length.
- Most often, the midaxial approach will provide the best exposure with the least amount of soft tissue stripping.
- Screw size and number are determined based on fracture location, fracture characteristics, and the size of the bone fragments (**TECH FIG 6**).
  - When considering the use of multiple screws and screw location within the fragment, screws should be placed at least two diameters from the tip of the fracture and centered within the fragment.
  - The distance between screws should be at least two screw diameters.
  - The screws' orientation should be between perpendicular to the fracture line and perpendicular to the bone itself.
    - Screws placed perpendicular to the fracture provide maximal compression.
    - Screws placed more perpendicular to the bone provide axial stability.
  - Screws should always be drilled along a diameter (ie, crossing though the middle of the bone).
- Reduce and hold the fracture with a clamp while the drill is advanced across the fracture site into the opposite cortex (**TECH FIG 7A**).
- To gain a lag effect, create a gliding hole in the near cortex using a drill bit that is the same size as the screw's outer diameter (**TECH FIG 7B**).

TECH FIG 6 • Screw size is determined by the bone size. Usually 1.5-mm or 2.0-mm screws are used in the proximal phalanx and 1.3-mm or 1.5-mm screws in the middle phalanx.

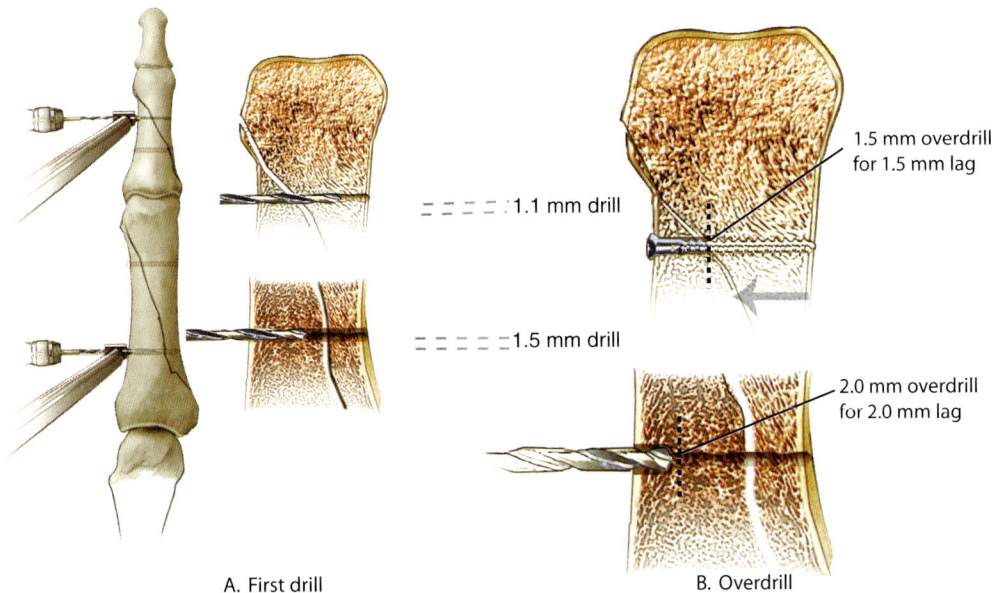

1.1 mm drill

1.5 mm drill

1.5 mm overdrill for 1.5 mm lag

2.0 mm overdrill for 2.0 mm lag

A. First drill

B. Overdrill

TECH FIG 7 • **A.** The tap drill for the chosen screw size is drilled from the near cortex, across the fracture and into the far cortex. The hole should be oriented so the drill crosses through the center of the bone and is centered in the far fragment as well. **B.** To gain a lag effect, the near cortex is opened to the outer diameter of the screw (overdrilled) so the screw threads will engage only in the far cortex, compressing the fractures as the screw is tightened.

TECHNIQUES

- Countersink the screw head to disperse forces as compression is applied and decrease screw head prominence.
  - Because the cortex is thin, countersinking is not recommended in the metaphysis.
- Insert a self-tapping screw through the gliding hole and into the far cortex.
- When the screw is tightened, the fracture is compressed.
  - Remain colinear with the screw to avoid deforming the soft titanium.

- During final tightening, exert steady forward pressure and turn the screw slowly to avoid stripping the far cortex.
- Repeat the procedure for additional screws (**TECH FIG 8**).
- Alternatively, reduce the fracture with a clamp, then stabilize it with a Kirschner wire smaller than the core diameter of the screw. Place the first lag screw as described, then remove the Kirschner wire and insert the second screw through the predrilled Kirschner wire hole.

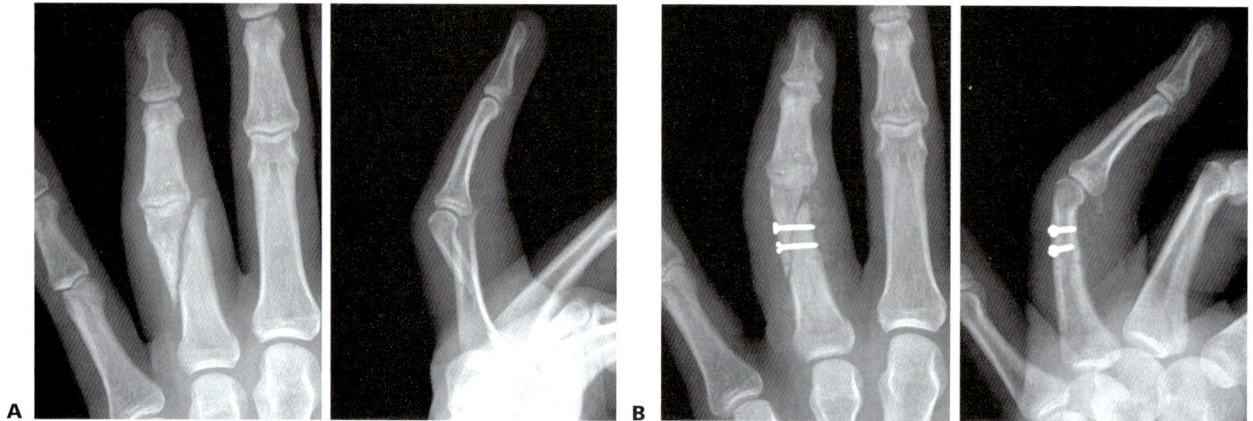

TECH FIG 8 • Preoperative (**A**) and postoperative (**B**) radiographs of a spiral fracture of the proximal phalanx fixed with two lag screws.

PLATE FIXATION

- Plates can be placed either dorsally or laterally on the bone.
- Lateral placement via the midaxial approach has the advantage of less extensor disruption and potentially fewer adhesions. Lateral plate placement effectively resists compressive forces.[6]
- If the plate is applied to the dorsal surface, avoid overdrilling and placement of a long screw that may damage the flexor tendons.
- Once exposed, clear the fracture site of soft tissue and reduce the fracture.

- Insert the remaining screws (**TECH FIG 9C**).
- In the case of comminution, the plate is used to bridge the fracture fragments (**TECH FIG 10**).

Fixation of Metaphyseal Fractures: T-Plate Technique

- Provisionally place the plate on the bone using a pointed reduction clamp, a specialized plate-holding clamp, or a screw at one end of the plate.
- Insert the screw in the middle of the T plate first, but before screw tightening align the plate perpendicular to the adjacent joint (**TECH FIG 9A**).
- Perform the final fracture reduction and insert a screw on the other side of the fracture (**TECH FIG 9B**).
- Assess the length, angulation, and most importantly the rotation clinically and radiographically.

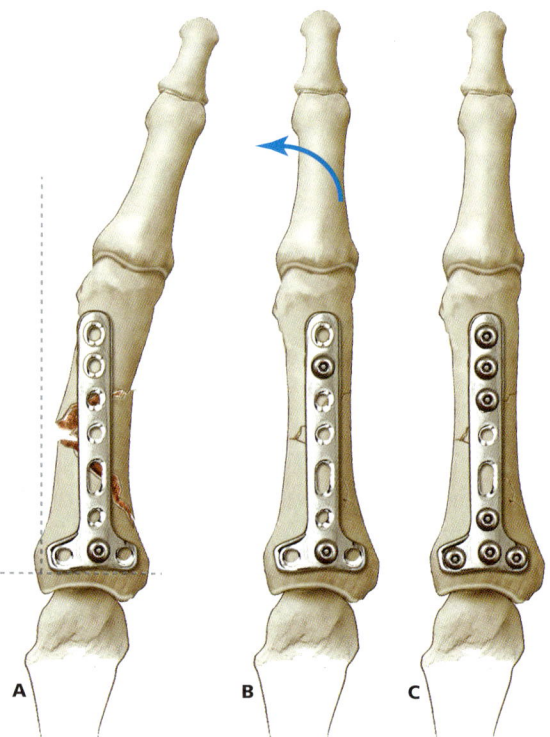

TECH FIG 9 • **A.** The T plate is aligned perpendicular to the joint line and secured with a single screw. **B.** The distal portion of the fracture is brought into alignment and secured with one additional screw. **C.** Length, angulation, and rotational correction are all confirmed before insertion of the remaining screws.

TECHNIQUES

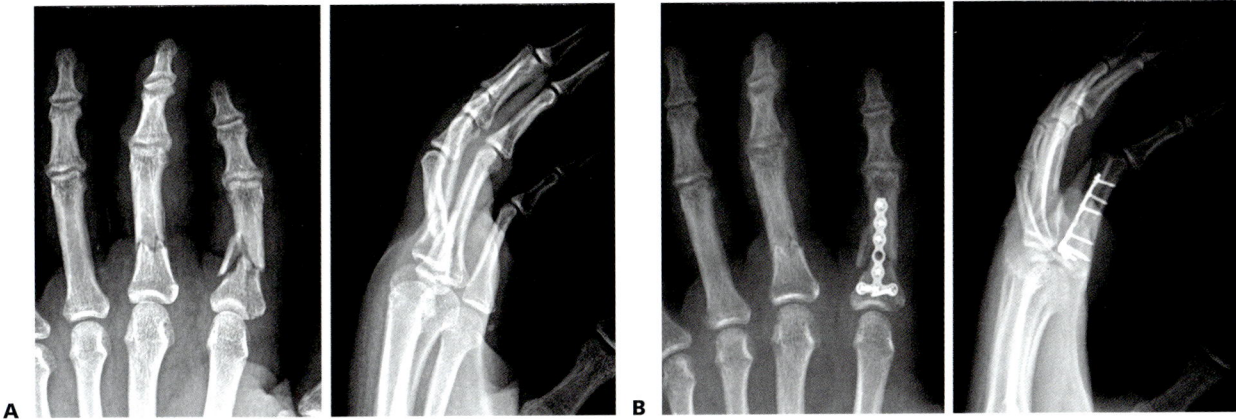

TECH FIG 10 • **A.** Preoperative posteroanterior and lateral radiographs showing a comminuted index finger proximal phalanx fracture with significant shortening, angulation, and rotation, and a middle finger proximal phalanx fracture with reasonable alignment. The middle finger had a significant crush injury and a large volar wound. **B.** The index finger proximal phalanx fracture is fixed with a T plate, which is used to restore alignment, length, and rotation while bridging the fracture. Rather than risking additional vascular compromise to the middle finger with pins or open reduction, the relatively stable fracture of the middle proximal phalanx was treated by closed means. Active motion of both fingers was started 1 week after open reduction and internal fixation.

OTHER METHODS

- Some authors have described using Kirschner wires as stacked intramedullary nails to secure phalangeal fractures. Intrafocal pinning is an excellent way to stabilize juxta-articular fractures of the proximal phalanx.[3]
  - By placing several wires along the canal, the fracture can be stabilized sufficiently to allow early motion.
  - Inserting the wires along the sides minimizes extensor tendon injury (**TECH FIG 12A**).
- Other methods of fixation not commonly used for extra-articular phalangeal fractures include external fixation and bridging Kirschner wire fixation (**TECH FIG 12B**).
  - These rarely used methods are most useful for temporary fixation while allowing the soft tissue injuries to heal.
  - External fixation is more advantageous for border digits. For treatment of extra-articular phalangeal fractures, these fixators should not be placed across a joint if at all possible.

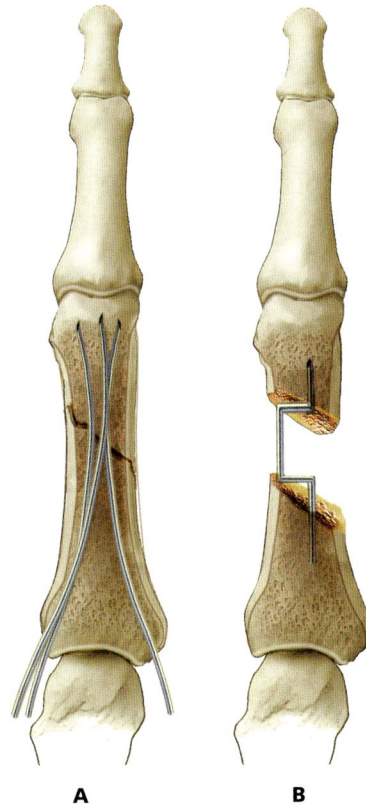

TECH FIG 11 • **A.** Intramedullary Kirschner wires can be stacked in the canal to provide intramedullary support to a phalangeal fracture. Wires are inserted from the sides to minimize extensor tendon damage. **B.** In the case of soft tissue damage with bone loss, a square U-shaped bend in a Kirschner wire can be used to temporarily maintain length while the soft tissue heals.

PEARLS AND PITFALLS

Indications	• Thorough history and physical must be obtained. • Recognizing malalignment and especially rotation is crucial.
Choice of technique	• Preoperative planning is critical. • Choose the least invasive method that will align and stabilize the fracture. • If open reduction is planned, and especially if plate fixation is chosen, stable fixation must be obtained to allow early motion.

Kirschner wiring	■ Avoid placing crossed pins with their intersection at the level of the fracture, as this may cause rigid distraction. ■ Smooth pin wiring is not without complications.[2]
Plate fixation	■ Placing the plate laterally or dorsolaterally may minimize the negative effects on the extensor mechanism. ■ Do not detach the insertion of the central slip at the dorsal base of the middle phalanx. ■ Augmenting fixation with a lag screw either through or adjacent to the plate markedly increases fracture stability. ■ If plating dorsally, avoid placing overly long screws, which may damage flexor tendons. ■ Always check plate placement and length fluoroscopically. ■ Thoughtful placement of temporary Kirschner wires will avoid frustration with simultaneous fracture reduction and plate placement. ■ Temporary Kirschner wire placement can maintain fracture reduction as well as take the place of predrilling for screws; replace the Kirschner wire with an appropriately sized screw. ■ After a midaxial approach and placement of a plate on the proximal phalanx, excise rather than repair the lateral band to minimize scarring and maximize motion.
External fixation	■ Useful in markedly comminuted fractures with bone loss ■ Avoid spanning joints if possible. ■ Most applicable for border digits
Distal phalanx fractures	■ Nonunions can be painful. ■ Support of the nail bed can help prevent later nail deformities. ■ Temporary pinning through the distal interphalangeal joint can provide stability and is an easier technique than cross-pinning in the distal phalanx.
Problems	■ Recognize and correct malalignment in the operating room. Clinical and radiographic assessment is required throughout the process of fracture reduction and stabilization. Always compare with the contralateral hand. ■ With postoperative swelling, it is our practice to always include more than one digit in the postoperative dressing to avoid potential vascular complications.
Postoperative care	■ Early evaluation and treatment by an experienced hand therapist will improve outcome. ■ Diligent pin care in Kirschner wire and external fixator constructs is necessary to avoid infection.

POSTOPERATIVE CARE

■ Postoperative care depends on the location of the injury and the bony fixation.

■ The best outcomes are achieved with restoration of anatomic alignment, respect for the soft tissue envelope, and early range of motion.

■ Treatment by an experienced hand therapist is a key component.

 ■ In the early phases, therapy consists of edema control and mobilization of adjacent digits and joints.

 ■ If adequate fracture stabilization is obtained, then mobilization of the involved digit is started almost immediately.

 ■ If fracture fixation is not ideal, active motion of the involved segment should be started no later than 3 to 4 weeks after surgery regardless of the radiographic appearance.

 ■ Protected mobilization should include removable splints that allow motion of adjacent digits and joints. As healing progresses, these splints are eliminated and buddy taping is employed.

■ Return to full activity is usually possible by 8 weeks.

OUTCOMES

■ Virtually all phalangeal fractures will heal in 4 to 6 weeks. Malalignment, especially rotation, and stiffness will diminish the outcome.

■ Most simple fractures treated with splinting, percutaneous pinning, or open reduction and internal fixation will regain near-full motion in 2 to 6 months, if the principles are followed and the proper intraoperative and postoperative techniques are employed.

■ In complex injuries where early motion is delayed because of concomitant soft tissue injury or prolonged splinting, the final outcome will be worse.

■ Sometimes hardware removal, tenolysis, and joint release are needed to improve motion.

 ■ Such procedures should be attempted only after tissue equilibrium has been reached (usually at least 4 months after the initial injury or surgery).

COMPLICATIONS

■ Loss of motion

 ■ Surgical: careful soft tissue handling with avoidance of prominent hardware

 ■ Postoperative: Elevation, ice, early motion of all non-injured joints, and controlled mobilization of injured segments as soon as possible are the best preventive measures.

 ■ If the problem persists and despite good therapy passive motion greatly exceeds active motion, tenolysis is a reliable method of treatment.

■ Malunion

 ■ Malreduction is common and, once secured with a plate and screws, difficult to correct. It is important to assess rotation on all phalangeal fractures before final fixation.

 ■ Accurate assessment is often difficult because the patient cannot make a full fist. Therefore, a reduction that was thought to be adequate in the face of restricted motion may prove inadequate once full motion is regained.

- If significant enough, osteotomy should be considered.
- Neurovascular injury while pinning a fracture
  - By observing the cross-sectional anatomy of the digit, damage to the neurovascular bundle can usually be avoided when inserting the wires.
  - Care must be taken when the wire passes through the second cortex, as it will usually be heading directly toward the neurovascular bundle.
  - Inserting the wires initially by hand until bone contact is made and using small open incisions may decrease the chance of injury when inserting the wire close to the neurovascular bundle.
- Complex regional pain syndrome
  - Early recognition and treatment are essential.
  - A high index of suspicion is needed to identify key symptoms:
    - Swelling despite elevation and other edema-control efforts
    - Stiffness, especially in adjacent digits, despite efforts toward early mobilization
    - Color changes in the hand
    - Mottling or shiny appearance of the skin
    - Abnormal hair growth
    - Burning pain in the hand
- Tendon rupture
- Nonunion
- Infection
- Pin loosening and migration
- Implant failure
- Pain and symptoms from retained hardware

REFERENCES

1. Barton NJ. Fractures of the shafts of the phalanxes of the hand. Hand 1979;11:119–133.
2. Botte MJ, Davis JL, Rose BA, et al. Complications of smooth pin fixation of fractures and dislocations in the hand and wrist. Clin Orthop 1992;276:194–201.
3. Crofoot CD, Saing M, Raphael J. Intrafocal pinning for juxtaarticular phalanx fractures. Tech Hand Up Extrem Surg 2005;9:164–168.
4. Eaton RG, Hastings HH. Point/counterpoint: closed reduction and internal fixation versus open reduction and internal fixation for displaced oblique proximal phalangeal fractures. Orthopedics 1989;12:911–916.
5. Ebinger T, Erhard N, Kinzl L, et al. Dynamic treatment of displaced proximal phalangeal fractures. J Hand Surg Am 1999;24:1254–1262.
6. Lins RE, Myers BS, Spinner RJ, et al. A comparative mechanical analysis of plate fixation in a proximal phalangeal fracture model. J Hand Surg Am 1996;21:1059–1064.
7. Maitra A, Burdett-Smith P. The conservative management of proximal phalanx fractures of the hand in an accident and emergency department. J Hand Surg Br 1992;17B:332–336.
8. Margic K. External fixation of closed metacarpal and phalangeal fractures of digits: a prospective study of one hundred consecutive patients. J Hand Surg Br 2006;31B:30–40.
9. Pa Pehlivan O, Kiral A, Solakoglu C, et al. Tension band wiring of unstable transverse fractures of the proximal and middle phalanges of the hand. J Hand Surg Br 2004;29:130–141.
10. Reyes FA, Latta LL. Conservative management of difficult phalangeal fractures. Clin Orthop Relat Res 1987;214:23–30.
11. Sloan JP, Dove AF, Maheson M, et al. Antibiotics in open fractures of the distal phalanx? J Hand Surg Br 1987;12B:123–124.
12. Strickland JW, Steichen JB, Kleinman WB, et al. Phalangeal fractures: factors influencing digital performance. Orthop Rev 1982;11:39–50.
13. Vahey JW, Wegner DA, Hastings H III. Effect of proximal phalangeal fracture deformity on extensor tendon function. J Hand Surg Am 1998;23A:673–681.

Chapter 33

Open Reduction and Internal Fixation of Phalangeal Condylar Fractures

Greg Merrell, Kerry Bemers, and Arnold-Peter Weiss

DEFINITION

- Phalangeal condylar fractures include unicondylar and bicondylar intra-articular fracture of the distal ends of the proximal and middle phalanx. Proximal phalangeal condylar fractures are more common.
- Table 1 demonstrates the variety of condylar fracture patterns typically observed.

ANATOMY

- Collateral ligaments, finger position, and direction of force play a role in both fracture pattern and the direction of displacement (**FIG 1**).

- Blood is supplied to the condyles by a branch of the digital artery and vein that travels with the collateral ligaments.
  - Care must be taken not to disrupt this blood supply or to strip small fragments of their soft tissue attachments.

PATHOGENESIS

- These fractures often are sports-related injuries.
- The mechanism is hypothesized to be tension or rotation force through the collateral ligaments for an oblique fracture and compression and subluxation in the case of a coronal fracture.[1,5]
- Fractures often are unstable because there is a minimal periosteal sleeve, and forces seen at the joint are substantial.

Table 1	Condylar Fracture Patterns			
Fracture Configuration	**Illustration**	**Characteristics**	**Fixation**	
			Nondisplaced Fracture	**Displaced Fracture**
Type I: unicondylar short oblique		Unstable Fracture exits just proximal to collateral ligaments Deformity is oblique to coronal and sagittal planes	Could consider nonoperative treatment, but must follow closely. Otherwise, two percutaneous K-wires	Joystick closed reduction and K-wires, or open reduction and screws, or K-wires
Type II: unicondylar long oblique		Unstable, but fixation a little easier than type I	Could consider nonoperative treatment, but must follow closely. Otherwise two or three percutaneous K-wires	Joystick closed reduction and K-wires, or open reduction and screws, or K-wires

(continued)

| Table 1 | Condylar Fracture Patterns *(continued)* | | | |

Fracture Configuration	Illustration	Characteristics	Fixation	
			Nondisplaced Fracture	**Displaced Fracture**
Type III: dorsal coronal		Often stable	<25% and stable joint: consider nonoperative treatment or excision. >25% and nondisplaced: could consider nonoperative treatment, but must follow closely. Otherwise, two percutaneous K-wires.	>25% and displaced or <25% with subluxed joint: joystick closed reduction and K-wires, or open reduction and K-wires (rarely screws)
Type III: dorsal coronal		Unstable	<25% and stable joint: consider nonoperative treatment or excision. >25% and nondisplaced: could consider nonoperative treatment, but must follow closely. Otherwise, two percutaneous K-wires.	>25% and displaced or <25% with subluxed joint: joystick closed reduction and K-wires or open reduction and K-wires (rarely screws)
Type V: bicondylar		Unstable	A nondisplaced fracture: could consider K-wires.	Usually requires open reduction and screws, plates, or K-wires
Type IV: triplane-type bicondylar		Unstable	Percutaneous K-wires	Usually requires open reduction with dorsal-to-volar screws

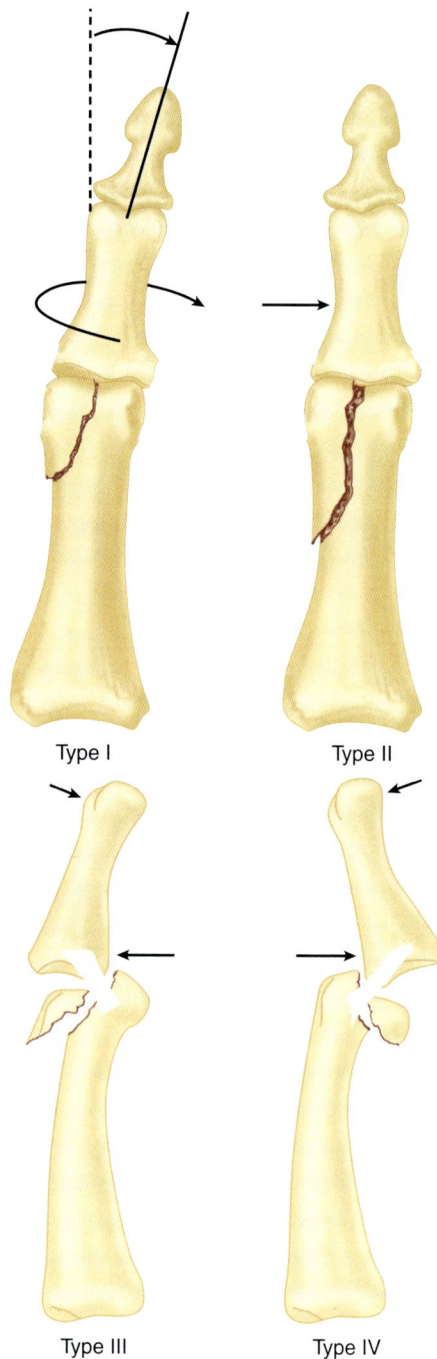

Type I   Type II

Type III   Type IV

FIG 1 • Direction of applied force determines the fracture type.

■ Most commonly, the condyle toward the midline of the hand (ie, the middle finger axis) is fractured: the ulnar condyle in the index finger and thumb and the radial condyle in the ring and small fingers.

NATURAL HISTORY

■ In developed countries, these fractures rarely go untreated, but they often are *under*treated given that their presentation may be interpreted as a "minimally displaced finger fracture."
■ Similar to any proximal interphalangeal (PIP) joint injury, lack of immobilization in full extension or prolonged immobilization will likely lead to a stiff finger.

■ If treated conservatively, displacement of the fracture, a common occurrence, will lead either to early painful arthritic changes, or rotational malalignment on full flexion, or both.

PATIENT HISTORY AND PHYSICAL FINDINGS

■ A typical patient is a 24-year-old male baseball player who has sustained an angular impact to the finger from the ball.
■ A high index of suspicion is required when evaluating these patients. The patient often is still able to bend the finger, and the fracture line can be subtle, but even nondisplaced fractures are prone to subsequent displacement.
■ Joint subluxation is an absolute indication for surgery and must be assessed carefully both radiographically and clinically.
■ With any fracture displacement, a rotational deformity of the finger usually occurs, best assessed either looking end on at the digit or evaluating position with PIP flexion (**FIG 2A**).
■ Subtle joint depression may lead to angular deformity; this is best assessed by examining fingers in full extension (**FIG 2B**).

IMAGING AND OTHER DIAGNOSTIC STUDIES

■ The fracture pattern dictates the type of fixation or treatment.
■ Multiple views should be obtained as needed to understand the geometry. Fluoroscopy often is helpful in obtaining precise views.
　■ Osteochondral fragments often are larger than they appear, because the cartilage is radiolucent.
　■ Hidden fracture lines are common and often are not visualized until surgery.
■ CT occasionally is helpful.

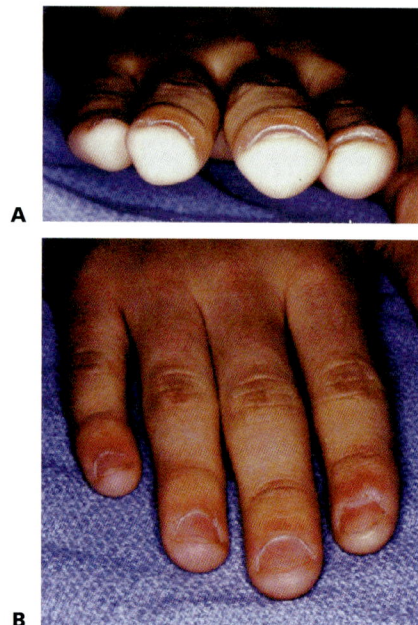

FIG 2 • **A.** End-on observation of the fingers can demonstrate subtle rotational deformities. **B.** Observation of the fingers in full extension can demonstrate subtle angular deformities caused by a displaced condyle.

DIFFERENTIAL DIAGNOSIS

- Collateral ligament or volar plate avulsion
- PIP dislocation
- Distal shaft fracture

NONOPERATIVE MANAGEMENT

- Reports regarding the results of nonoperative treatment present conflicting results.
  - Weiss et al[5] found five of seven nondisplaced fractures treated conservatively went on to displace and required surgery.
  - In an 11-year follow-up study, using a functional outcome score, O'Rourke et al.[4] demonstrated several interesting points:
    - 27% of patients experienced joint aching in cold weather.
    - Four patients at 1 year follow-up had moderate pain and considered arthrodesis. However, by the time they got off the waiting list their symptoms had subsided to the point that they declined surgery.
    - No patient had less movement in the joint at year 11 than at year 1.
    - 25% of patients had continued improvement in range of motion after 12 months follow-up.
    - Three patients with displaced bicondylar fractures treated conservatively had outcomes of good, fair, and poor, respectively.
    - Three patients with displaced unicondylar fractures treated conservatively had a good outcome; however, in O'Rourke et al's discussion, they conclude that these fractures should be treated with reduction and fixation.[4]
- Operating on nondisplaced or minimally displaced fractures can be viewed in two ways:
  - On the one hand, a percentage of patients would be subjected to a procedure that they did not need. Also, with close follow-up, if a fracture were to displace later, it could be addressed at that point, although it would require slightly more work to regain reduction and functional restoration.
  - On the other hand, there is minimal morbidity in percutaneous pinning, and that would minimize the likelihood of displacement in a fracture that often is unstable.
  - Given the propensity for displacement and the potential functional difficulties with malunion, we recommend, at a minimum, percutaneous stabilization of most condylar fractures.
- Several review texts suggest that coronal fractures of less than 25% of the joint surface with a stable congruent joint can be treated nonoperatively or with fragment excision. Although this may be true, there are few biomechanical or clinical outcomes data to support the statement.

SURGICAL MANAGEMENT

Preoperative Planning

- Preoperative planning should be mindful of the goals of treatment of any articular fracture established by the AO:
  - Anatomic reduction of the articular surface
  - Restoration of stability
  - Minimizing soft tissue injury
  - Early mobilization
- Access to a mini C-arm is highly advantageous.
  - Fluoroscopic examination under anesthesia provides a good sense of joint stability and fracture fragment orientation.
  - Fracture reduction, implant placement, and fracture stability are effectively evaluated fluoroscopically.

Positioning

- The patient is positioned supine with a hand table.
- If an assistant is unavailable, finger-trap traction also may be helpful.

Approach

- A unicondylar fracture typically is approached either between the central slip and lateral band (**FIG 3**) or via a midaxial approach.

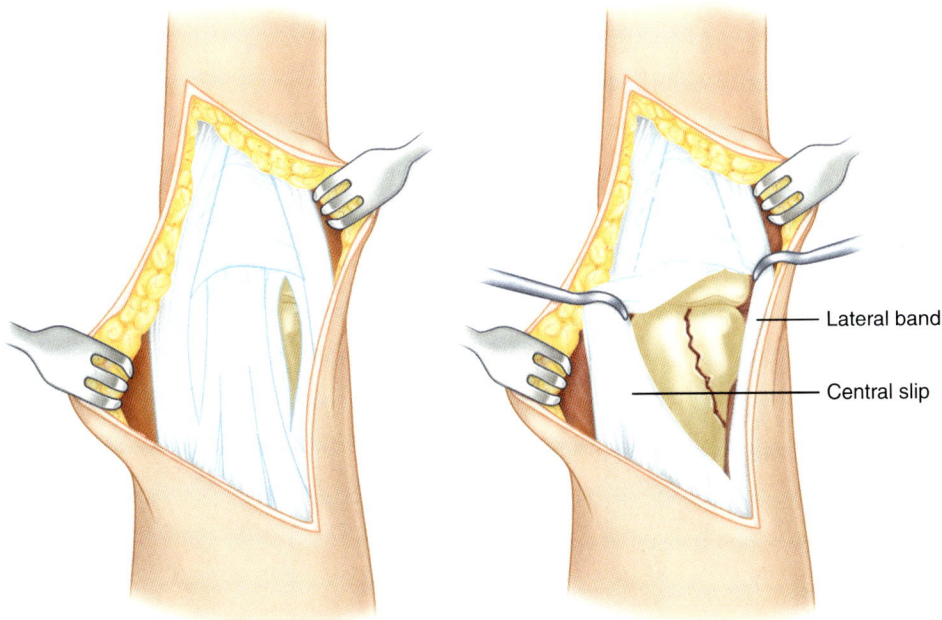

A   B

— Lateral band

— Central slip

FIG 3 • A dorsal-lateral incision (**A**) with dissection between the lateral band and extensor mechanism (**B**) provides excellent exposure.

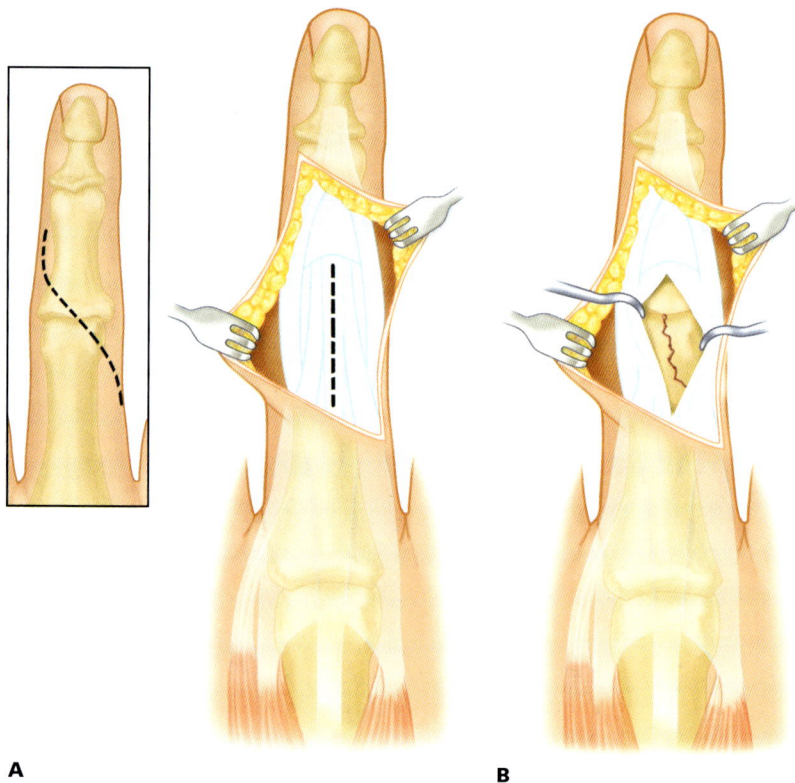

A   **B**

FIG 4 • A dorsal-lateral incision (**A**) with midline incision in the extensor mechanism (**B**) can provide additional exposure if needed.

■ The lateral (mid-axial) approach is suggested as a means to minimize extensor mechanism scarring, but only if significant joint incongruity or comminution is absent.
■ If more extensive joint visualization is needed, the extensor mechanism can be incised and repaired later (**FIG 4**).
■ A bicondylar or triplane fracture requires a more global joint and fragment exposure.
■ A dorsal, slightly curvilinear incision is made.
■ The extensor tendon may be split longitudinally, but preferably incisions are made on its borders, allowing mobilization and excellent joint exposure.
■ A palmar approach is rarely used except for volar coronal shear fractures.

■ If necessary, make a Brunner-style volar incision, and retract the flexor tendons to expose the volar plate.
■ If possible, reflect the volar plate on one side and a little up the lateral edge for exposure via a triangle-shaped flap.
■ If more complete exposure is needed, make a transverse incision along the proximal edge of the volar plate, leaving enough proximal cuff to reattach the volar plate.
■ Elevate the volar plate on a distal hinge, repair the fracture, and then reattach the volar plate.
■ The PIP joint is prone to stiffness from injury, so every effort should be made to minimize surgical injury to the soft tissues.
■ Avoid at all costs stripping soft tissue attachments from small fracture fragments.

SHORT AND LONG OBLIQUE FRACTURE WITH PERCUTANEOUS REDUCTION, K-WIRES, MINIFRAGMENT SCREWS, OR CANNULATED HEADLESS COMPRESSION SCREWS

Tips for Achieving Fixation

■ Visualize the fracture well using live fluoroscopy.
■ Fracture displacement typically is in an oblique plane, sometimes not well appreciated on the straight anteroposterior or lateral views.
■ Use of the view on live fluoroscopy that best shows the displacement will make it possible to determine when reduction has truly been achieved.
■ Apply traction and rotation to the distal aspect of the finger to assist reduction through ligamentotaxis (**TECH FIG 1A**).

■ Try percutaneous manipulation of the fragment with a dental pick.
■ If reduction is achieved, place either a pointed reduction clamp or the first K-wire to hold it.
■ If the dental pick does not work, place one prong of a pointed reduction clamp through the skin into the stable condyle, then place the other prong into the fragment and try to reduce the fragment with a slight rotation of the clamp (**TECH FIG 1B**).
■ Resist the urge to use clamp compression to force a reduction, because the small fragments shatter easily.

TECHNIQUES

TECHNIQUES

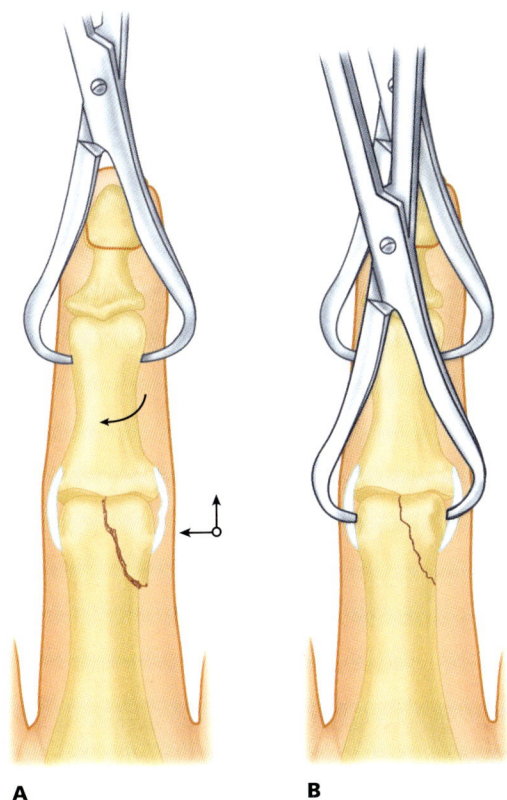

A   **B**

TECH FIG 1 • Percutaneous fracture reduction with traction and rotational correction (**A**), followed by percutaneous clamping (**B**).

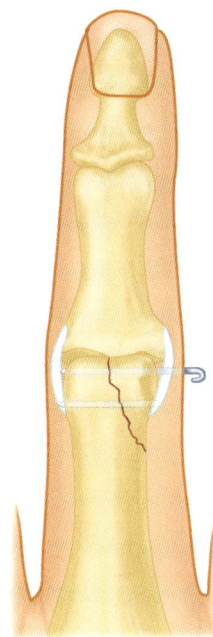

TECH FIG 2 • Pinning with K-wires.

- Avoid placing the clamp volar to the mid-axial line to avoid iatrogenic injury to the neurovascular bundle.
- If that does not succeed, try a 0.035 K-wire joystick or proceed with an open reduction.

Fixation Choices

- In our practice, if we can achieve a percutaneous reduction, we prefer the use of multiple 0.028-inch K-wires.
- If we have to open to achieve the reduction, we prefer the stability of screw fixation.
  - Occasionally, fragments are too small or comminuted for screw fixation, necessitating the use of K-wires.

K-Wire Fixation

- A single K-wire is not sufficient fixation.
- Drive two K-wires from the fragment into the shaft either transversely or obliquely depending on the fracture orientation (**TECH FIG 2**).
  - The first wire should be placed perpendicular to the fracture line to maximize fixation and minimize displacement while capturing the reduction.
  - Additional wires should be placed slightly oblique to the first wire so that the fracture fragment cannot displace along the axis of two parallel wires.
  - The best bone quality is found distal and volar; therefore, to avoid injury, insert wires from contralateral

dorsal side of the intact condyle and advance distally and volarly.
- Hold the PIP joint in extension while driving wires.
  - This position keeps the lateral bands dorsal, and the entry of the K-wire can be just volar to the lateral bands.
  - The condyle, as viewed on a lateral image, is the area with the least excursion of the collateral ligaments; therefore, K-wires in the volar position cause the least restriction of motion.
- The use of 0.028-inch K-wires avoids further fragmentation of fragments and usually provides sufficient fixation.

Screw Fixation

- Screw fixation should avoid the collateral ligaments by one of four methods (**TECH FIG 3**):
  - Flexing the joint and passing the screw distal and dorsal to the collateral ligaments
  - Keeping the joint in extension, with subperiosteal stripping of a limited portion of the collateral ligament origin from proximal to distal
  - Excising a small window in the collateral ligament for the screw head, which is gently countersunk
  - Placing the screw proximal to the collateral ligament if the fracture extends far enough proximally
- Screw fixation must not impinge on the collateral ligaments through any of the four methods listed, or the screw will cause permanent difficulties with joint motion.
- Screw fixation should be with 1.0- or 1.3-mm screws placed in lag fashion (**TECH FIG 4A–E**).
- For longer oblique fractures, make a stab incision, spread with a snap, and place three screws or three or more wires spaced along the fracture (**TECH FIG 4F**).

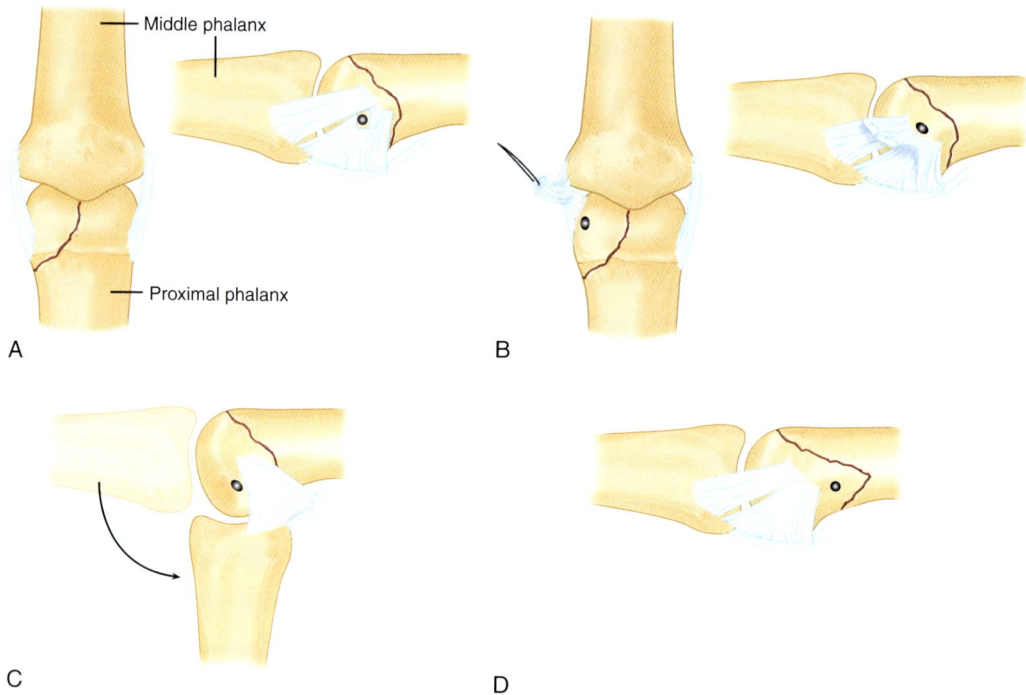

A — Middle phalanx

— Proximal phalanx

B

C

D

TECH FIG 3 • The four methods for screw placement to minimize impingement on collaterals. Methods **A** and **C** require seating the screw head almost flush with the bone. **A.** Creation of a small window in the collateral for screw placement. **B.** Reflection of the proximal part of the collateral ligament for screw placement. **C.** Flexion to allow exposure of the condyle for screw placement. **D.** In a longer fracture, placement of the screw proximal to collateral insertion.

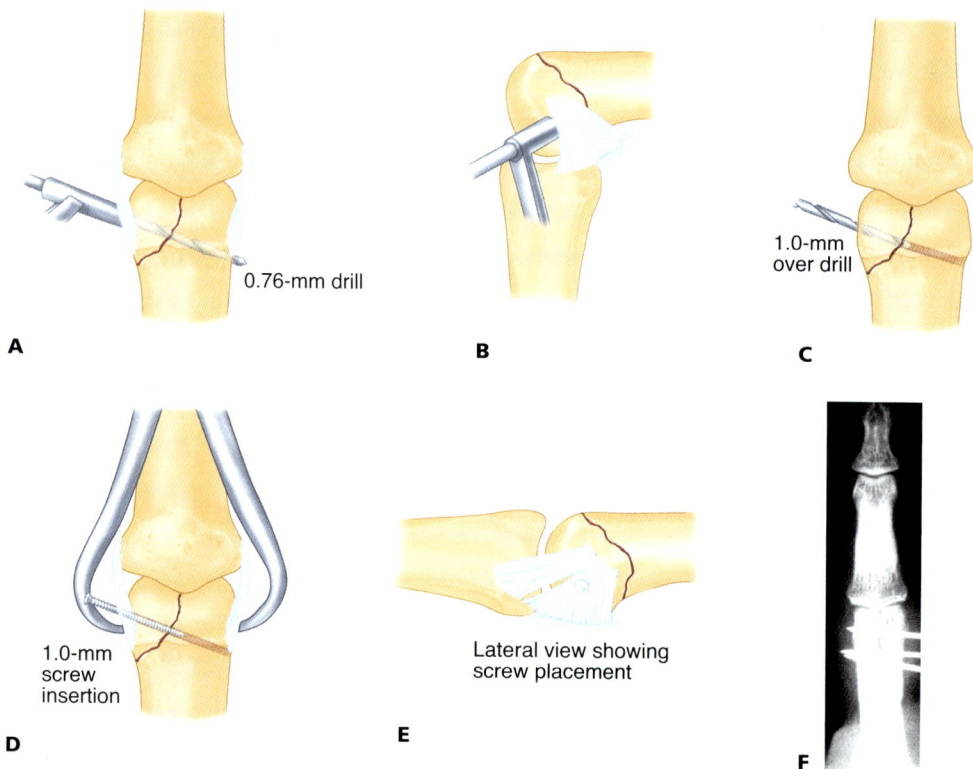

A — 0.76-mm drill

B

C — 1.0-mm over drill

D — 1.0-mm screw insertion

E — Lateral view showing screw placement

F

TECH FIG 4 • Placement of a lag screw. **A.** 0.076-inch drilling is done through both cortices. **B.** The joint is flexed to permit placement of the screw out of the way of the collateral ligaments. **C.** Overdrilling only the proximal cortex with a 1.0-mm drill. **D.** Compression of fragments by a reduction clamp while placing the lag screw. **E.** Position of the screw head after extension of the joint. **F.** Long oblique fracture maintained with three 0.028-inch K-wires.

- The first screw should be placed in lag mode, perpendicular to the fracture line, to prevent displacement of the fracture during compression.
- If there is good compression, the second and third screws can be in neutralization mode.
- If compression from the first screw was poor, additional screws can be placed in the lag mode.

- Consider placing one screw more perpendicular to the long axis of the phalanx to resist axial forces.
- While screws are being placed, the reduction can be held either by a reduction clamp or with a temporary K-wire. The hole made by the temporary K-wire, after removal, can be used for the last screw.

DORSAL AND VOLAR CORONAL SHEAR FRACTURE WITH SCREWS OR K-WIRES

- A dorsal approach typically is used for dorsal fractures and a volar approach for volar fractures.
- Dental picks are used for all fragment manipulation and reduction.
- Traction generally does not help reduction.
- Because fragments usually are very small, fixation with 0.028-inch K-wires may involve crossing the joint surface.
- Typically, a trade-off must be made in terms of implant position.
  - For example, in a dorsal shear fragment, it may be necessary for a K-wire to pass through the dorsal articular

surface of the fragment into the condyle below. Try to stay as dorsal as possible to minimize impingement in extension, while still securing the fragment adequately. It is possible to bury a screw beneath the articular surface, but if it is possible to use K-wires, they are preferred for their small and temporary footprint. A dorsal shear fracture with a nonarticular component would be a better choice for screw fixation than an all-articular fragment.
- We do not have experience with absorbable implants, but would be concerned about their use due to the small size of the fragments and resorption products.

BICONDYLAR FRACTURE WITH OPEN REDUCTION AND INTERNAL FIXATION

- Use a dental pick to align the condylar fragments and secure with a K-wire or screw.
  - Similar to previous discussion, if reduction is achieved percutaneously, one or two K-wires may be used to secure the condyles to each other.
  - Typically, open reduction is required, in which case screws are preferred whenever possible.
  - Occasionally, if it is difficult to the secure the two condylar fragments to each other, try reducing the

largest condylar piece to the shaft and hold it with a K-wire. Then reduce the smaller condylar piece or pieces to the main construct. Once the entire reduction is achieved and held with clamps or K-wires, a screw can be placed transversely across the condyles.
- If minimal metaphyseal comminution is present, the condylar fragments are secured to the shaft using K-wires (**TECH FIG 5**).

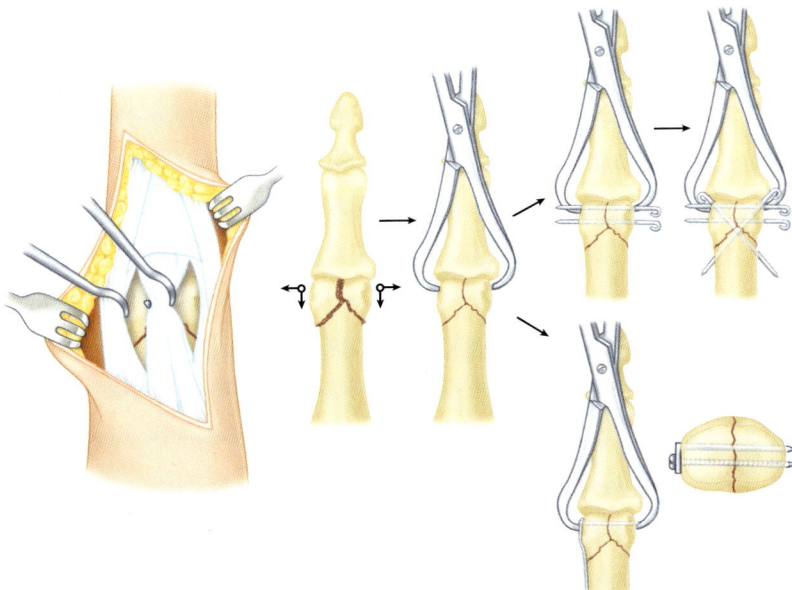

TECH FIG 5 • Reduction of bicondylar fractures begins with reduction of the condyles to each other. The condyles are then secured to the shaft.

TECHNIQUES

Condylar Plate

- If metaphyseal comminution is present, consider a condylar plate (**TECH FIG 6**).
- The reduction starts with the condylar fragments, ignoring any proximal comminution.

- These fragments are held temporarily while the condylar plate is drilled and placed into just the distal fragment.
- Care must be taken to align the plate on the condyles so that the plate aligns with the shaft, once the condylar/plate construct is reduced to the shaft, bypassing the comminution.

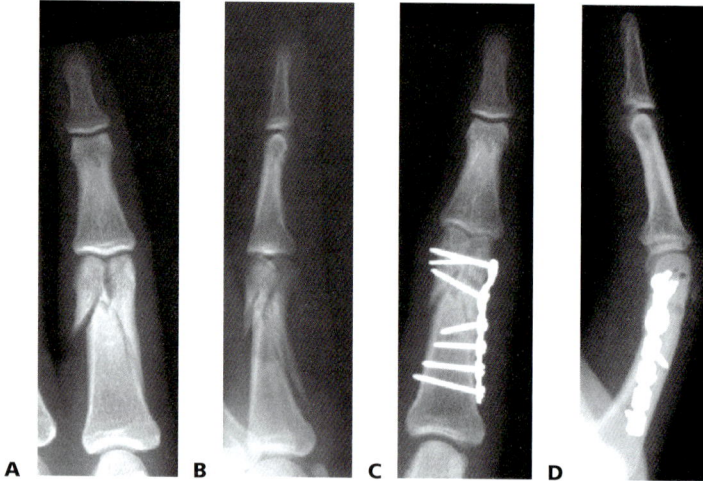

TECH FIG 6 • **A,B.** Radiographs of a bicondylar fracture. **C,D.** Postoperative radiographs after reduction and application of a condylar plate fixation. (Courtesy of Alan Freeland, MD.)

TRIPLANE FRACTURE WITH OPEN REDUCTION AND FIXATION USING LAG SCREWS AND K-WIRES

- An extensile dorsal approach is used.
- **TECH FIG 7** shows a triplane fracture in a 42-year-old carpenter with a table saw injury, who was treated as follows:
  - The collateral ligaments were attached to the two volar condylar pieces.

- Lag screws were placed into each condyle from dorsal to volar.
- A K-wire was used to secure the condyles to the shaft and keep the joint reduced.
- Metaphyseal comminution has been treated with bone grafting and, in some cases, distraction external fixation for 3 weeks, after which motion is commenced.[1]

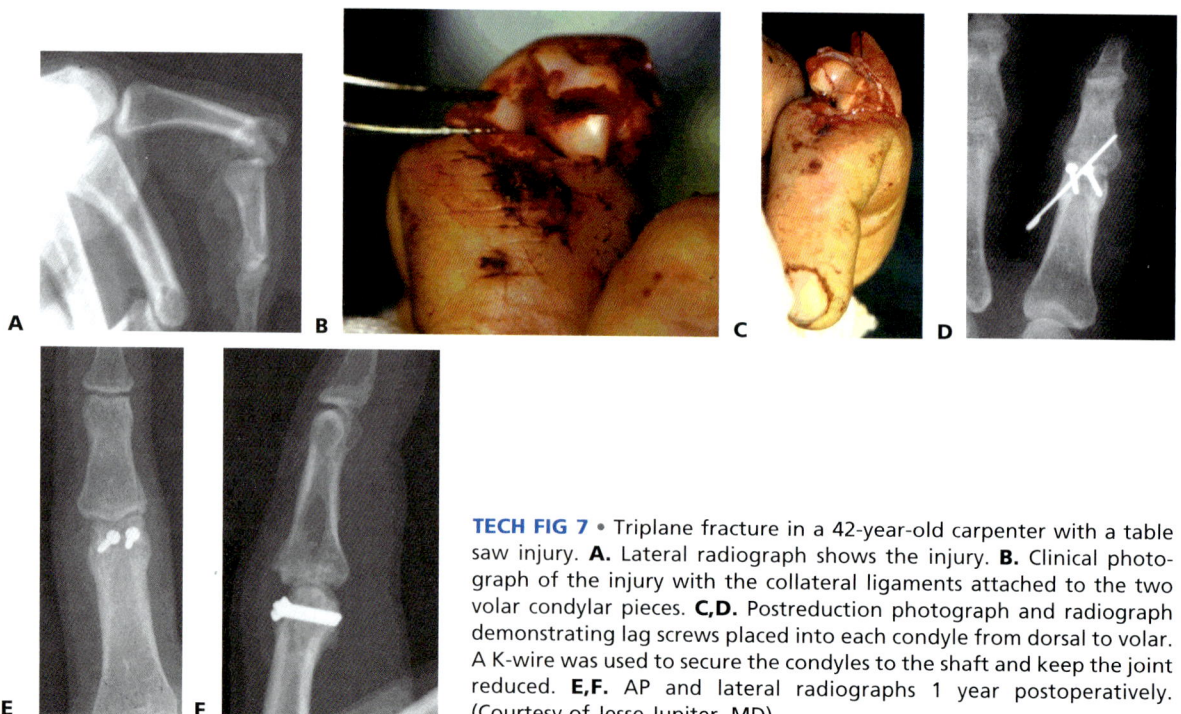

TECH FIG 7 • Triplane fracture in a 42-year-old carpenter with a table saw injury. **A.** Lateral radiograph shows the injury. **B.** Clinical photograph of the injury with the collateral ligaments attached to the two volar condylar pieces. **C,D.** Postreduction photograph and radiograph demonstrating lag screws placed into each condyle from dorsal to volar. A K-wire was used to secure the condyles to the shaft and keep the joint reduced. **E,F.** AP and lateral radiographs 1 year postoperatively. (Courtesy of Jesse Jupiter, MD)

PEARLS AND PITFALLS

Difficulties with closed reduction and pinning	▪ Try using traction with rotation, a dental pick, pointed reduction clamp, or a K-wire as a joystick into the displaced fragment.
Preventing fracture of a small fragment	▪ Make sure the screw diameter is no more than one third the size of the fragment and is placed one screw diameter from the edge of the fragment.
Maintaining reduction and pinning small fragments	▪ Use a cannulated reduction forceps.
Obtaining maximum mechanical stability	▪ Place the screw from the fragment into the phalanx, "from the island to the mainland."
Maximizing reduction with small intra-articular fragments	▪ Reduce the large fragments first. Often the smaller pieces then fall into place with soft tissue tensioning or can be excised: "Rule of Vassals, or Majority Rule."
Minimizing postoperative adhesions	▪ Avoid plating the phalanges whenever possible. Meticulous handling of soft tissue, and sharp dissection where possible rather than blunt spreading minimizes tissue trauma and permits early active range of motion (AROM).

POSTOPERATIVE CARE

▪ Fracture stability dictates the protocol, but most patients should be started on AROM within 1 week, with extension splinting of the PIP joint while at rest.
   ▪ It is important for the surgeon and therapist to communicate regarding the extent of injuries, type of fracture fixation used, and co-existing conditions, because these variables will affect the rate of healing and progression of therapy.
   ▪ Exercises should be performed at least six times per day.
   ▪ When immobilization is involved, it is extremely important for the patient to perform AROM to all noninvolved joints to prevent secondary weakness and stiff joints in the involved extremity, as well as to aid edema control.
▪ 1–7 days after surgery
   ▪ Control edema with Coban wraps (3M, St. Paul, MN), compressive digit sleeves, elevation and AROM, and contrast baths (if no pin or sutures are present).
   ▪ A hand-based safe-position splint including the involved digit and an adjacent digit is worn between exercises and at night. Use a forearm-based splint including all digits if multiple digits are involved.
   ▪ AROM exercises are used based on the stability of fracture:
      ▪ Composite flexion and extension of the digits
      ▪ Blocking of the PIP and DIP joints to provide differential gliding of the flexor digitorum superficialis and profundus tendons (especially important following a volar exposure)
      ▪ Reverse blocking (metaphalangeal [MP] joints passively flexed with active interphalangeal [IP] joint extension), flexor and extensor tendon glides
▪ 7–14 days post-surgery
   ▪ Gentle assisted AROM and passive ROM may begin as tolerated, again based on fracture stability. Passive ROM should not begin with K-wires in place.
   ▪ Avoid painful ROM and monitor splints closely for excessive forces on the PIP joint. This can result in a counterproductive inflammatory and fibroblastic response.
▪ Early scar management (approximately 10–14 days)
   ▪ When the incision or pin site has healed, begin scar massage with lotion.
   ▪ Superficial heat application applied before scar massage helps increase scar pliability.

▪ If scar sensitivity develops, introduce scar desensitization, to include stimulation of the sensitive scar with graded textures and tactile pressure and tapping of scar, progressing as the patient develops increased tolerance to each stimulus.
▪ If scar adherence persists, use iontophoresis with Iodex (Baar Products, Inc., Downingtown, PA) to soften the scar.
▪ For a raised scar, encourage scar remodeling by use of a nocturnal scar pad, such as elastomere or Otoform K (AliMed, Deham, MA).
▪ After initial fracture healing (about 4–6 weeks)
   ▪ Assisted and passive ROM should be started if they have not been initiated earlier.
   ▪ Continue the "safe position" splint between exercises and at night.
   ▪ As the patient's pain level decreases and functional use of the involved digit increases, reduce the splint to a gutter splint worn at night to prevent PIP flexion contracture.
   ▪ If a flexion contracture develops at the PIP joint, consider serial extension casting of the involved digit. The contracture should be no more than 45 degrees, because the patient will have difficulty donning the serial cast with any greater degree of joint contracture. Dynamic splinting or static progressive splinting by day may be used as needed.
   ▪ Progressively wean splints as passive ROM improves, and encourage active ROM.
▪ Strengthening (about 8 weeks)
   ▪ Progressive strengthening can be initiated with light putty and further progressed with activities appropriate for the patient's occupation.
▪ About 10 weeks
   ▪ Discharge all splinting.
   ▪ Encourage unrestricted use of the involved digit and hand.
▪ In closed fractures, with a good soft tissue envelope and blood supply, K-wires should be removed at about 3 weeks to facilitate rehabilitation.

Overcoming Issues Related to Rehabilitation

Decreased PIP Joint Flexion

▪ The reason for decreased flexion at the PIP joint must be determined. If the joint has full PIP joint flexion on passive ROM and decreased PIP joint flexion on active ROM, the problem most likely is caused by adhesions.

- Treatment should attempt to regain ROM through active exercise:
  - Before treatments, application of heat is useful to increase tissue extensibility for increased ROM gains and assist the patient with increased tolerance to exercise.
  - Superficial modalities such as moist hot pack, paraffin, and fluidotherapy may be used. Benefits of fluidotherapy include the ability to actively stretch with application of heat.
  - Ultrasound may be used to heat deeper tissues.
- Exercises
  - Tendon glides
  - Isolated blocking of the flexor digitorum superficialis and profundus tendons to maximize differential tendon gliding
  - Active flexion of the digit against resistance, such as hook fist exercises performed with therapeutic putty, or raking the digits through putty
  - Blocking splint for exercise: the MP joints are blocked in extension by a splint with the PIP joints free. The patient performs active PIP flexion and extension to increase differential glide of the tendons (**FIG 5A**).
  - Neuromuscular electrostimulation of the flexor digitorum superficialis and profundus may be used to assist active ROM and tendon glide.
- If the fracture is healed and passive ROM of the joint is limited in flexion, passive ROM exercises and splinting alternatives will assist to progressively stretch a tight joint capsule and elongate shortened ligaments. Splinting options include:
  - Static progressive splinting
  - Use of a dynamic flexion splint (**FIG 5B**)

- Passive ROM and joint mobilizations are appropriate if the fracture is healed.
  - Use of heat (as discussed earlier) to increase tissue extensibility will make the patient more comfortable and help increase ROM. To assist stretch into flexion with heat, try wrapping the digit(s) in flexion with Coban and dipping them in paraffin.

Decreased PIP Joint Extension

- The appropriate treatment approach depends on the structures involved. If the PIP joint can be passively placed into full extension but is unable to actively extend, the extensor apparatus may be scarred down.
- The following treatments are beneficial to increase active extension of the PIP joint.
  - Before beginning the exercises, use of superficial heat modalities and ultrasound will assist to increase tissue extensibility, ROM gains, and the patient's tolerance to exercises.
  - Active exercises include:
    - Active reverse blocking (passively flex the MP joints while actively extending the IP joints to transmit the extension force to the IP joints).
    - A reverse blocking splint is helpful to assist the patient with reverse blocking (**FIG 5C**).
    - Block the MP joint in flexion while actively extending the PIP joint into extension with simultaneous neuromuscular electrostimulation of the extensor digitorum communis muscle and the intrinsic muscles.
    - Active extension against resistance, such as theraputty

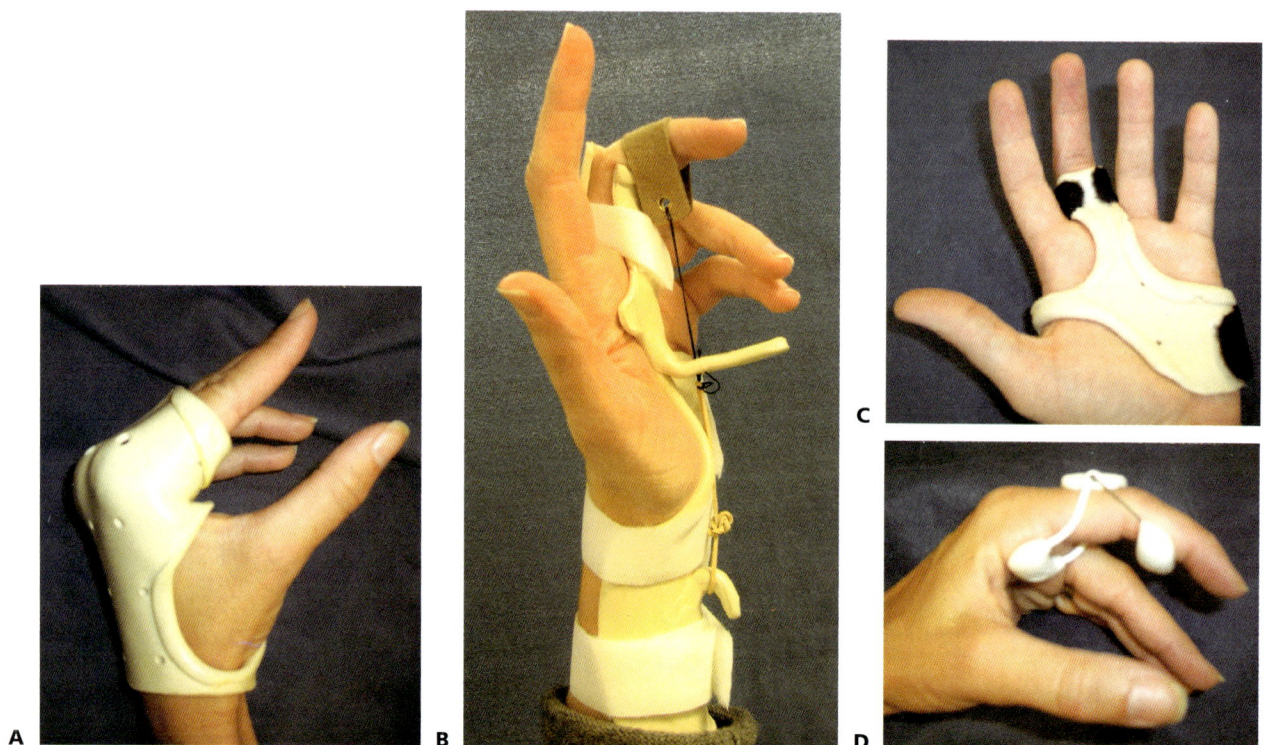

FIG 5 • A. MP blocking splint. **B.** Dynamic flexion splint. **C.** Reverse blocking splint. **D.** Finger-based dynamic PIP extension splint.

- If the fracture is healed and passive ROM of the PIP is limited with extension, exercises and splinting can assist with improving passive ROM.
  - Serial casting PIP into extension
  - Finger-based dynamic PIP extension splint (**FIG 5D**)
  - Dynamic extension splint with MP block in flexion
- Passive ROM and joint mobilizations with heat applied before these manual activities are appropriate if the fracture is healed.

Scar Adhesions Limiting Tendon Glide

- Active ROM, including extensor/flexor tendon glides, and scar massage and reverse scar massage (opposite the direction of the adhesion with active ROM) are key to decreasing adhesions of the tendon.
- These modalities work well in conjunction and may be used individually or in combination based on the patient's individual needs.
  - Superficial heat (eg, fluidotherapy, moist heat, paraffin)
  - Ultrasound
  - Scar pad (eg, elastomere, Otoform K)
  - Iontophoresis with Iodex to soften scar

OUTCOMES

- In one series of 36 patients, the arc of motion of the PIP joint averaged 72 degrees with a 13-degree extensor lag. Patients with volar coronal fractures fared worse, with an average arc of 57 degrees.[5]

- In the McCue series of 32 patients treated with open reduction and two K-wires, flexion averaged greater than 93 degrees and extensor lag averaged less than 5 degrees.[3]

COMPLICATIONS

- Loss of PIP joint motion is the most common complication.
  - Fixation must be secure enough to allow early motion.
  - Delay of motion of the hand by more than a few weeks significantly decreases final outcome.[2] Ideally, motion should be initiated in the immediate postoperative period.
  - Increases in motion may be obtained up to 1 year after the injury, although opportunity does decrease with time.[2]
  - Dorsal capsulotomies and extensor tenolysis are options for patients lacking flexion.
- Loss of reduction is common if fractures are not stabilized or are stabilized with only one point of fixation.[5]

REFERENCES

1. Chin KR, Jupiter JB. Treatment of triplane fractures of the head of the proximal phalanx. J Hand Surg Am 1999;24:1263–1268.
2. Freeland AE, Benois LA. Open reduction and internal fixation method for fractures at the proximal interphalangeal joint. Hand Clinics 1994;10:239–250.
3. McCue FC, Honner R, Johnson MC, et al. Athletic injuries of the proximal interphalangeal joint requiring surgical treatment. J Bone Joint Surg Am 1970;52A:937–956.
4. O'Rourke SK, Gaur S, Barton NJ. Long-term outcome of articular fractures of the phalanges: an eleven year follow-up. J Hand Surg Br 1989;14:183–193.
5. Weiss APC, Hastings HH. Distal unicondylar fractures of the proximal phalanx. J Hand Surg Am 1993;18:594–599.

Chapter 34

Dorsal Block Pinning of Proximal Interphalangeal Joint Fracture-Dislocations

Mark Goleski and Jeffrey Lawton

DEFINITION

- The laymen's term "jammed finger" often is used to indicate an injury sustained to the proximal interphalangeal (PIP) joint. If the force behind this injury is sufficient, the joint may suffer a fracture-dislocation, an injury that may be difficult to treat.
- PIP fracture-dislocations in the dorsal direction is caused by disruption of the volar fibrocartilaginous plate, fragmentation of the middle phalanx where it attaches to this plate, and damage to the collateral ligaments on each side of the joint. Instability with dorsal displacement of the middle phalanx may result, accentuated by the unbalanced pull of the central slip.
- Stiffness, pain, persistent subluxation, osteoarthritis, and permanent dysfunction are common sequelae, even with dedicated treatment in the best of circumstances.
- Dynamic external skeletal traction, extension block splinting or pinning, transarticular pinning, open reduction with internal fixation (ORIF), and volar plate arthroplasty are the techniques most often used to address this problem.
  - None of these techniques have proven to be satisfactory for all patients in all instances.
- Extension block pinning has been used with reasonable success to reduce and stabilize unstable PIP fracture-dislocations.
  - A K-wire is placed into the head of the proximal phalanx, mechanically blocking full extension and thereby preventing dorsal subluxation of the middle phalanx.
  - The advantages of this technique include its simplicity and the early mobility it affords an injured joint. It can be used alone or in combination with volar plate arthroplasty or ORIF.

ANATOMY

- The PIP joint acts mostly as a hinge joint in the sagittal plane, although it does possess a few additional degrees of motion in the coronal and axial planes.[17] It has an average range of flexion–extension of 105 degrees.[16]
- The joint has a great deal of stability throughout its range of motion.[16]
- When healthy, the joint is most stable in full extension.
  - A tongue-and-groove structure, formed by the bicondylar head of the proximal phalanx and the reciprocal concave surfaces of the middle phalanx, contours closely in this position.[16]
- As the joint flexes, the ligamentous elements take up responsibility for maintaining stability.[16]
  - The volar plate, a structure that is ligamentous at its origin on the proximal phalanx and cartilaginous at its insertion on the middle phalanx, and the two collateral ligaments, one on the radial and one on the ulnar side of the joint, are the most important (**FIG 1**).
  - Two out of three of these structures must be impaired for displacement of the middle phalanx to occur.

PATHOGENESIS

- Although the PIP joint may become dislocated in any direction, displacement of the middle phalanx dorsally is the most common.
- Simultaneous hyperextension and compression forces—such as those seen when a ball strikes the tip of the finger—stress the volar plate and the collateral ligaments.
- Type I injury
  - If the force of injury is mild, partial disruption of the collateral ligaments and the volar plate at its distal insertion on the middle phalanx are the only consequences.
  - The articular surfaces remain intact and the joint is stable.
  - If appropriate treatment is initiated promptly, an excellent long-term result is anticipated.[13]
- Type II injury
  - If the force of injury is more substantial, bilateral longitudinal splitting of the collateral ligaments may occur in addition to rupture of the volar plate. Complete dorsal displacement of the middle phalanx is then possible due to unopposed pull of the central slip.
  - The joint can be readily reduced and usually is stable following the reduction.
- Type III injury—stable
  - If an avulsion fracture of the middle phalanx occurs at the attachment of the volar plate, the joint may still remain stable. When less than 30% to 40% of the joint surface is involved, the joint is stable following reduction because collateral ligament integrity is maintained.[4,15]
- Type III injury—unstable
  - If the fracture at the base of the middle phalanx involves more than 40% to 50% of the articular surface, collateral ligament support is lost. The joint exhibits persistent dorsal subluxation of the middle phalanx due to unopposed pull of the extensor tendon and lack of volar restraints.

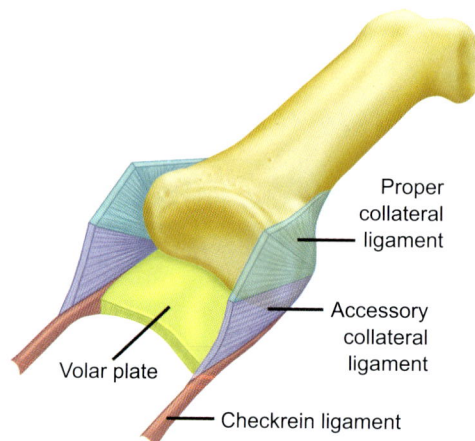

FIG 1 • Anatomy of the proximal interphalangeal joint.

- Closed reduction may not be possible, and treatment is more difficult, often leading to unsatisfactory overall results.[20]

NATURAL HISTORY

- The outcome following even a minor injury is often less satisfactory than the patient anticipates. Although it is possible for a PIP joint that has suffered a fracture-dislocation to regain fully normal function, this often is not the case. Persistence of a stiff joint with a cosmetically thickened outline is common.
    - Delay in treatment or lack of vigilant care negatively affects outcome.[10]
    - Prolonged immobilization of the joint following reduction leads to stiffness. Early mobilization can avoid stiffness and promote nutrition of the damaged articular cartilage.[19]
- Patients should be reassured, however, that carefully planned treatment and compliance with the postoperative therapy regimen leads to long-term satisfactory results in most cases.[10]

PATIENT HISTORY AND PHYSICAL FINDINGS

- The history should elicit the manner in which the digit was injured, the nature of any medical treatment or manipulation of the digit before the current visit, and how much time has elapsed since the injury.
    - The likelihood of a favorable result diminishes with increased time from injury, particularly beyond 6 weeks.[9]
- The digit will look surprisingly normal at presentation in many cases, particularly if it was previously reduced.
    - A transverse skin injury on the volar side of the PIP joint may indicate that the volar plate has been disrupted.[25]
- The integrity of the neurovascular status should be documented on examination before digital anesthetic block and reduction.[18]
- With the forearm supinated and the hand relaxed, observe the position of the patient's fingers. Note the axial and rotational alignment of the digit.
    - The uninjured, quiescent hand has increasing flexion tone in the digits from the radial side to the ulnar side,[2] a phenomenon known as the *flexion or resting cascade* (**FIG 2A**).
- Observe the patient's fingers directly and fluoroscopically as he or she attempts to move them through a normal range of motion. Dorsal subluxation often can be detected visually and through palpation.

- Digital or wrist block anesthesia can be used to relieve discomfort associated with motion (**FIG 2B**).
- If the joint can be moved through a full arc of motion without subluxation, adequate joint stability remains, and only brief immobilization will be required.
- If redisplacement occurs, significant instability results. The position of redisplacement is a clue both to the specific site of ligament injury and the optimal position for joint immobilization.[8] Loss of active extension implies central slip injury.
- For grossly stable digits, manipulate the joint passively through the normal range of motion. Gentle lateral and dorsovolar shearing stresses are applied at full extension and at 30 degrees of flexion. The findings are compared to those of the contralateral uninjured digit (**FIG 2C**).
    - The position of the PIP joint at the point of instability suggests which of the soft tissue supports has been injured. Instability at more than 70 degrees of flexion indicates damage to the collateral ligaments. Instability in extension indicates disruption of both the collateral ligaments and the volar plate. The degree of joint laxity suggests the extent of injury to the ligaments, from microscopic tearing to complete rupture.
- Palpate the PIP joint from all sides to determine point tenderness. Point tenderness often is valuable in localizing the injured structure.
    - Absence of point tenderness on the condyles may rule out significant injury to these structures. If the volar lip of the middle phalanx has been fractured, minor tenderness over the dorsum of the middle phalanx and greater tenderness volarly and laterally will be present.[5]

IMAGING AND OTHER DIAGNOSTIC STUDIES

- Obtain anteroposterior, lateral, and oblique radiographs of the injured digit. Assess the digit for joint dislocation, subluxation, and fracture.[18]
    - Evaluate the radiographs before performing the physical examination to detect potentially unstable fractures or dislocations before they are manipulated.[18]
    - Radiographs of the hand as a whole (eg, the "fanned four-finger lateral" view) are not adequate. Subtle fracture-dislocations may be missed due to poor depiction of the areas of suspected pathology.[23]
- Fluoroscopy is extremely valuable in defining the pathoanatomy and determining stability.

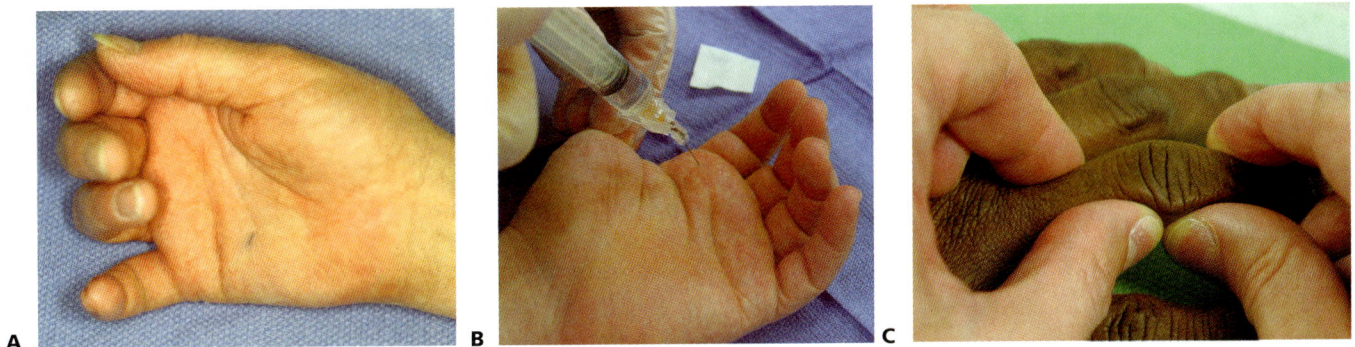

FIG 2 • **A.** Disruption of resting flexor cascade. **B.** Digital block technique. **C.** Passive stability evaluation.

■ CT scanning occasionally is indicated, particularly to assess suspected articular depression.[10]

DIFFERENTIAL DIAGNOSIS

■ Fracture
■ Fracture-dislocation
■ PIP dislocation
■ Collateral ligament and PIP joint sprain
■ PIP volar plate injury
■ PIP joint infection
■ Localized soft tissue infection
■ Flexor digitorum profundus tendon rupture
■ Extensor tendon central slip injury
■ Closed pulley rupture (flexor sheath)
■ Swan neck/boutonniere deformity

NONOPERATIVE MANAGEMENT

■ Most type I, type II, and type III stable injuries (and some type III unstable injuries) are amenable to nonoperative treatment.
■ The joint can be immobilized for a short time to afford the patient comfort and to allow soft tissue recovery.
  ■ A dorsal splint is applied to the digit at 20 to 30 degrees of flexion, avoiding immobilization beyond 30 degrees to lessen the risk of flexion contracture.
  ■ The duration of immobilization reflects the minimum amount of time needed to effect healing and obtain joint stability. Type I injuries are immobilized for several days; type III injuries may be immobilized for up to 3 weeks.
  ■ Avoidance of prolonged immobilization and patient education are the most important aspects of this treatment, because stiffness and contracture are very common.
■ Extension block splinting allows early motion of a joint while preventing extension past an angle where instability is possible.[7,12,13,21]
  ■ First, the position in which the joint re-displaces is determined.
  ■ A length of aluminum splint is then bent to an angle 10 or 15 degrees greater than this point of redisplacement and secured to the dorsum of the hand with adhesive tape or as part of a short-arm cast. The hand is positioned with 25 degrees of extension at the wrist and 45 to 60 degrees of flexion at the metacarpophalangeal joint[7] (**FIG 3A,B**).
    ■ If the angle of the splint is greater than 60 degrees, the arc of motion may be insufficient for the patient to achieve adequate flexibility, and it may be necessary to consider another treatment regimen.
  ■ An extension block splint made from two pieces of AlumaFoam (Hartmann International, Rock Hill, SC) and spanning only the finger itself is another option (**FIG 3C,D**).
    ■ The two Alumafoam pieces are held to each side of the PIP joint with adhesive tape and are bent such that they

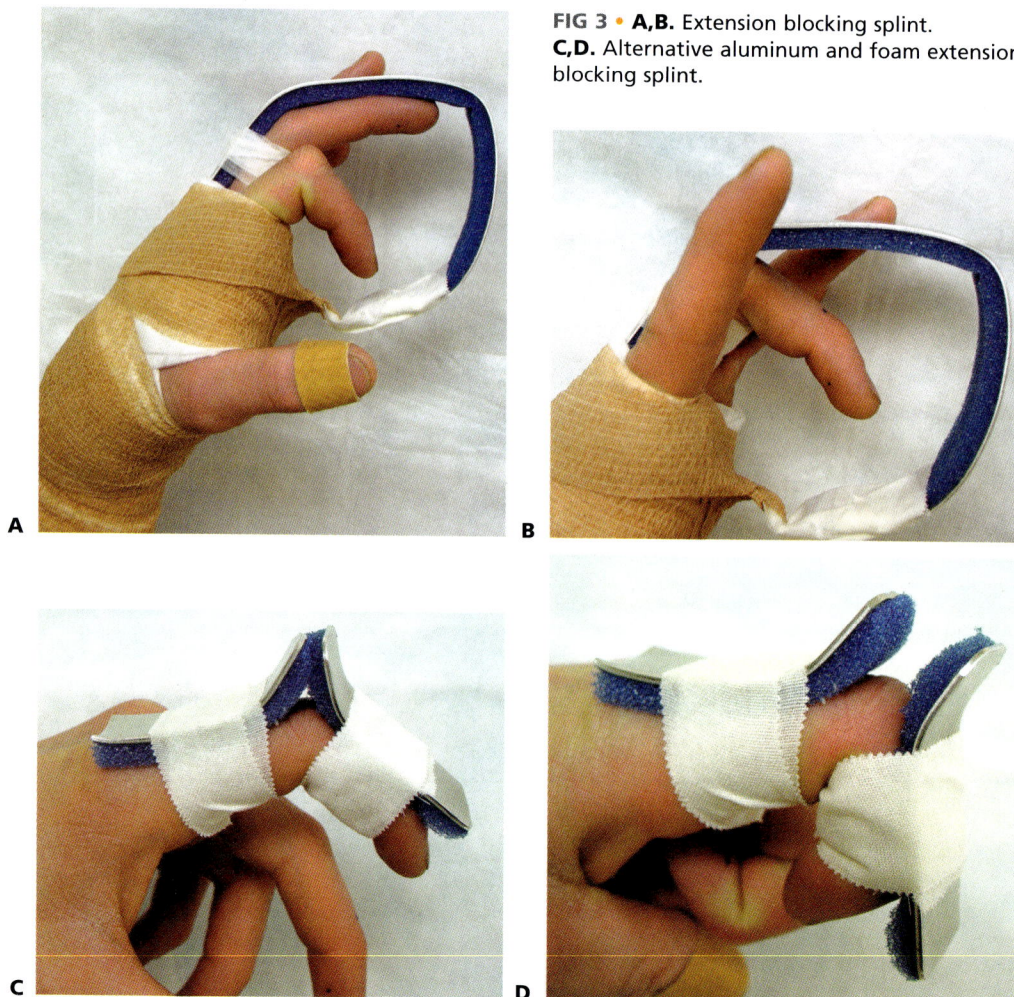

FIG 3 • **A,B.** Extension blocking splint. **C,D.** Alternative aluminum and foam extension blocking splint.

come into contact with each other at a particular degree of extension, thus preventing motion beyond that point.[21]

■ In general, extension block splinting is recommended for fractures involving less than 40% of the articular surface. Successful results have been noted, however, with fractures involving up to 75% of the joint.[12]

■ Following application of the splint, radiographs are taken to confirm satisfactory reduction, and the patient is encouraged to flex the finger as much as the swelling allows.

■ As the fracture-dislocation heals, the extension block splint is progressively adjusted toward full extension, usually during a period of 3 to 8 weeks.[7] Weekly radiographs and splint adjustments are required.

■ In certain instances, the digit may be too short, stocky, or swollen for such treatment, or patient compliance and sophistication for such a regimen may be in question. In such a case, extension block pinning may be the better option.

■ Because of the possibility of recurrent subluxation, the use of conservative treatment must be matched with frequent and careful assessment of the joint. Serial radiographs should be obtained weekly to document continued reduction of the joint and progressive healing of any fractures.[7]

SURGICAL MANAGEMENT

■ Operative treatment is indicated for those unstable fracture-dislocations in which closed treatment does not provide a congruent reduction of the joint. This includes most type III unstable injuries with fractures that involve more than 40% to 50% of the volar articular surface.

■ As noted earlier, many surgical options are available. The choice of procedure is based on the exact nature of the injury and the surgeon's comfort with each option.

■ Dynamic skeletal traction methods, which use the principle of ligamentotaxis to maintain concentric joint reduction, are especially useful when the fracture is significantly comminuted.[1]

■ These methods allow early active range of motion.

■ Drawbacks include the following:

■ Significant prowess on the part of the surgeon is required, as are close postoperative supervision and adjustment.

■ The external device may be cumbersome for the patient.

■ ORIF is especially useful when the avulsed volar fragment is large and minimally comminuted.[11] If the joint is stabilized with transarticular pinning as part of the ORIF procedure, however, stiffness usually results.

■ Volar plate arthroplasty, or the use of the distal aspect of the fibrocartilaginous volar plate to resurface the comminuted

volar articular surface of the middle phalanx, is another option that can be employed when comminution of the volar fragment makes other techniques infeasible.[3] Most authors have reported reasonably favorable results, but residual stiffness and contracture have been reported as well.[6]

■ Simple reduction with transarticular pinning (with no attempt at articular reconstruction) may be useful in injuries with less than 40% articular involvement. Extension block splinting may be just as effective in these milder instances, however, and it enjoys a lower risk of joint contracture.[10]

■ Extension block pinning is a viable alternative for mild to moderately unstable fracture-dislocations under the following circumstances:

■ The fracture-dislocation cannot be reduced and stabilized effectively with an extension block splint.[14,22,24]

■ Patient compliance is uncertain.

■ The finger is too short or swollen to fit appropriately into an extension block splint.

■ It may be used alone or in combination with an ORIF or a volar plate arthroplasty procedure.[3]

Preoperative Planning

■ Before the operation, the patient should be provided realistic expectations regarding outcome.

■ He or she should be aware of the possibility that immobilization, splinting, and long-term rehabilitation may be necessary.

■ The patient should be instructed to keep the injured hand clean before the procedure and to avoid additional skin injury to minimize the potential for infection. Fingernails should be trimmed and cleaned and the hands thoroughly scrubbed with antiseptic soap before the operation.

■ Intraoperative decision-making often is necessary. The surgeon should be comfortable in the performance of a number of alternative procedures and should have the necessary equipment available should findings require an alteration in the original surgical plan.

Positioning

■ The method of preparing, draping, and positioning the upper extremity is the same as for most hand surgeries.

■ A well-padded, proximal upper extremity tourniquet is applied.

Approach

■ Because extension block pinning is a percutaneous technique, no approach is required.

EXTENSION BLOCK PINNING[14,22,24]

■ The PIP joint is reduced by flexing the joint to 90 degrees and applying axial traction.

■ Concentric reduction of the joint is confirmed with fluoroscopy (**TECH FIG 1A**).

■ If an open wound is present or the joint cannot be manipulated into an acceptable reduction, such as may occur with soft tissue entrapment, open reduction becomes necessary.

■ Following reduction through either open or closed methods, and with the joint flexed 90 degrees or more, a smooth 0.035- to 0.045-inch K-wire is placed percutaneously into the distal, dorsal aspect of the proximal

phalanx across the dorsal lip of the base of the middle phalanx (**TECH FIG 1B**).

■ The wire is inserted in a retrograde direction, approximately 30 degrees off the long axis of the proximal phalanx.

■ When placing the K-wire centrally, hyperflexing the PIP joint prevents tethering of the extensor mechanism to the proximal phalanx, which would limit joint flexion. Alternatively, the K-wire can be placed to one side of the central tendon to avoid tethering the extensor mechanism.

TECHNIQUES

- The wire is guided with fluoroscopy through the shaft of the proximal phalanx and is left protruding from the head of the bone. Fluoroscopy is used to confirm a congruous joint reduction following the procedure.
- The joint is then passively extended to the limit of the K-wire, and the reduction of the joint is again critically evaluated fluoroscopically (**TECH FIG 1C**).
  - If the joint continues to subluxate dorsally at extension, a V-shaped gap between the articular surfaces of the head of the proximal phalanx and the dorsal lip of the middle phalanx will be seen on radiograph.[16]
- With the pin in this position (**TECH FIG 1D**), the patient will be able to move the finger actively but will not be able to extend the digit beyond the point where subluxation is possible due to mechanical blockage by the pin (**TECH FIG 1E,F**).
  - An arc of more than 60 degrees is ideal.

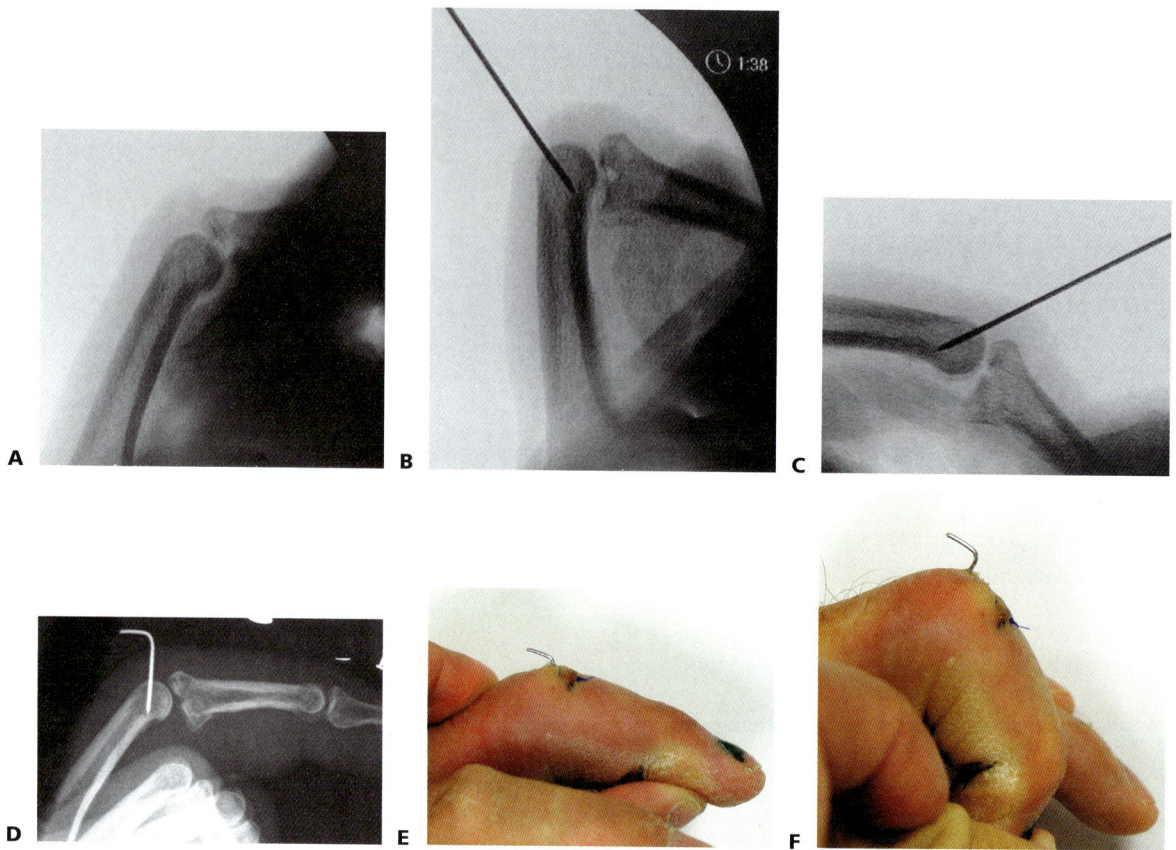

TECH FIG 1 • Dorsal block pinning. **A.** Fluoroscopic view confirms adequate joint reduction. Note that fracture reduction is not anatomic but is considered acceptable in this clinical scenario. **B.** Insertion of the retrograde K-wire with the joint hyperflexed to avoid tethering the extensor mechanism. **C.** Passive intraoperative extension of the joint to the level of the K-wire. The dorsal joint remains concentrically reduced. **D.** The K-wire is left protruding through the bone, and its placement is confirmed by fluoroscopy. **E,F.** The patient should be able to move the finger through an arc of about 60 degrees.

PEARLS AND PITFALLS

- The patient's ability to comply with fairly complex and intensive hand therapy should be confirmed before surgery.
- The insertion point for the K-wire can be located by a freehand technique and then confirmed with fluoroscopy.
- Easy passive flexion of the joint through an arc of 60 degrees or greater should be confirmed following pin insertion.
- The surgeon should remain hypervigilant for the presence of a V sign in full passive extension.
- The surgeon should ensure that the skin is not tented by the Kirschner wire.

POSTOPERATIVE CARE

- The patient should have a thermoplastic splint fabricated for protection and should begin a supervised program with a hand therapist 3 to 5 days after surgery.
  - Gentle active range-of-motion exercises are allowed immediately and should be encouraged in most cases.
    - If the injury is especially serious—eg, injuries that required volar plate arthroplasty or that contained significant comminution—immobilization for up to 2 weeks may be indicated.[14]
- Pin care must be explained carefully and performed regularly.
- The pin is removed 3 weeks after surgery, and vigorous active flexion and extension are encouraged. Reverse blocking is initiated.
  - Full extension should be limited for 1 additional week.[14]
- Active and passive joint exercises, including dynamic extension splinting, is initiated after 6 to 8 weeks of therapy, until full motion is achieved.
- Buddy taping or wrapping can be used, if added, longer-term protection is needed.

OUTCOMES

- The outcome for intervention into PIP fracture-dislocations depends mostly on the severity of the initial injury.
- Because few cases of extension block pinning used as the sole intervention are available in the literature, it is difficult to assess the long-term outcome of the procedure.
- Inoue and Tamara[14] reported the use of extension block pinning in 14 cases of fracture-dislocation of the PIP joint with an average fracture fragment size of 38% of the articular surface (range 25% to 60%). Ten patients regained full range of motion, and four patients regained a more limited range (89, 65, 64, and 40 degrees, respectively). The average ROM for all patients was 94.4 degrees.
  - The authors attributed the four cases with less satisfactory results to the use of a 60-degree extension block splint postoperatively in one patient and significant comminution in the other three patients.
- Viegas[24] reported the use of this technique in three cases of fracture-dislocation of the PIP joint. One case involved a 45% single fragment fracture seen 1 day postinjury and another a 35% comminuted fracture seen 17 days post-injury. Following pin removal and 1 month of passive and active exercises, both patients regained full range of motion. A third case involved a 75% comminuted fracture seen 2 days post-injury. The patient's ROM after pin removal was 30 to 65 degrees. Because the patient did not return for further care, no final outcome was available.
- Twyman and David[22] reported the use of this technique in two cases of fracture-dislocation of the PIP joint. The extent of injury in each patient was not specified, but quick recovery to satisfactory ROM in both patients was reported (20 to 100 degrees and 15 to 110 degrees, respectively).

COMPLICATIONS

- Persistent pain and swelling
- Stiffness
- Flexion contracture and extensor lag
- Redisplacement of the joint and persistent subluxation
- Angulation and rotation of the middle phalanx
- Weakness
- Boutonniere deformity
- Post-traumatic arthritis (not necessarily symptomatic)

REFERENCES

1. Agee JM. Unstable fracture dislocations of the proximal interphalangeal joint: treatment with the force couple splint. Clin Orthop Relat Res 1987;214:101–112.
2. American Society for Surgery of the Hand. General principles of management. In The Hand: Primary Care of Common Problems. New York: Churchill Livingstone, 1985:1–17.
3. Blazar PE, Robbe R, Lawton JN. Treatment of dorsal fracture/dislocations of the proximal interphalangeal joint by volar plate arthroplasty. Tech Hand Up Extrem Surg 2001;5:148–152.
4. Deitch MA, Kiefhaber TR, Comisar BR, et al. Dorsal fracture dislocations of the proximal interphalangeal joint: surgical complications and long-term results. J Hand Surg Am 1999;24A:914–923.
5. Dias JJ. Intraarticular injuries of the distal and proximal interphalangeal joints. In: Berger RA, Weiss AC, eds. Hand Surgery. Baltimore: Lippincott Williams & Wilkins, 2004:153–174.
6. Dionysian E, Eaton RG. The long-term outcome of volar plate arthroplasty of the proximal interphalangeal joint. J Hand Surg Am 2000;25:429–437.
7. Dobyns JH, McElfresh EC. Extension block splinting. Hand Clin 1994;10:229–237.
8. Eaton RG, Littler JW. Joint injuries and their sequelae. Clin Plast Surg 1976;3:85–98.
9. Eaton RG, Malerich MM. Volar plate arthroplasty for the proximal interphalangeal joint: a review of ten years' experience. J Hand Surg Am 1980;5:260–268.
10. Glickel SZ, Barron OA, Catalano LW III. Dislocations and ligament injuries in the digits. In Green DP, Hotchkiss RN, Pederson WC, et al, eds. Green's Operative Hand Surgery, ed 5. Philadelphia: Elsevier, 2005:343–388.
11. Green A, Smith J, Redding M, et al. Acute open reduction and rigid internal fixation of proximal interphalangeal joint fracture dislocation. J Hand Surg Am 1992;17:512–517.
12. Hamer DW, Quinton DN. Dorsal fracture subluxation of the proximal interphalangeal joints treated by extension block splintage. J Hand Surg Br 1992;17:586–590.
13. Incavo SJ, Mogan JV, Hilfrank BC. Extension splinting of palmar plate avulsion injuries of the proximal interphalangeal joint. J Hand Surg Am 1989;14:659–661.
14. Inoue G, Tamura Y. Treatment of fracture-dislocation of the proximal interphalangeal joint using extension-block Kirschner wire. Ann Chir Main Memb Super 1991;10:564–568.
15. Kiefhaber TR, Stern PJ. Fracture dislocations of the proximal interphalangeal joint. J Hand Surg Am 1998;23:368–380.
16. Kraemer BA, Gilula LA. Phalangeal fractures and dislocations. In Gilula LA, ed. The Traumatized Hand and Wrist: Radiographic and Anatomic Correlation. Philadelphia: WB Saunders, 1992:105–170.
17. Leibovic SJ, Bowers WH. Anatomy of the proximal interphalangeal joint. Hand Clin 1994;10:169–178.
18. Robinson ME Jammed finger. eMedicine web site. http://www.emedicine.com/sports/topic55.htm. Updated April 27, 2006. Accessed August 16, 2006.
19. Salter RB, Simmonds DF, Malcolm BW, et al. The biological effect of continuous passive motion on the healing of full-thickness defects in articular cartilage: an experimental investigation in the rabbit. J Bone Joint Surg Am 1980;62A:1232–1251.
20. Schenck RR. Classification of fractures and dislocations of the proximal interphalangeal joint. Hand Clin 1994;10:179–185.
21. Strong ML. A new method of extension-block splinting for the proximal interphalangeal joint. J Hand Surg Am 1980;5:606–607.
22. Twyman RS, David HG. The doorstop procedure: A technique for treating unstable fracture dislocations of the proximal interphalangeal joint. J Hand Surg Br 1993;18:714–715.
23. Vercillo AP, Squier RC, Ritland GD, et al. Finger dislocations in alcoholics. Conn Med 1987;51:293–295.
24. Viegas SF. Extension block pinning for proximal interphalangeal joint fracture dislocations: Preliminary report of a new technique. J Hand Surg Am 1992;17:896–901.
25. Zook EG, Van Beek AL, Wavak P. Transverse volar skin laceration of the finger: Sign of volar plate injury. Hand 1979;11:213–216.

Dynamic External Fixation of Proximal Interphalangeal Joint Fracture-Dislocations

Grey Giddins

DEFINITION

- Proximal interphalangeal (PIP) joint bone injuries may affect the convex side of the joint (end of the proximal phalanx) or the concave side of the joint (base of the middle phalanx).
- Convex-side injuries are typically simple (two-fragment) injuries best treated with open reduction and internal fixation if surgery is required.
- Concave-side injuries tend to be comminuted (multifragmented), presenting either as fracture-subluxations or dislocations or a pilon fracture.
- Fracture subluxations-dislocations typically involve dorsal displacement of the main (dorsal) fragment of the middle phalanx (**FIG 1A**), although volar and lateral subluxations and dislocations are less common (**FIG 1B,C**).
  - Dorsal fracture-dislocations typically occur after a hyperextension injury of the PIP joint.

- Pilon fractures are compression fractures of the base of the middle phalanx (rarely the distal phalanx) and are characterized by depression of the central articular component and splaying of the articular margins.
  - This may be associated with longitudinal fracture extension that may reach most of the length of the middle phalanx.
  - There is typically marked comminution of the base of the middle phalanx (**FIG 1D,E**).
  - The fracture typically occurs due to a longitudinal (end-on) force, crushing the base of the middle phalanx (rarely the distal phalanx or thumb proximal phalanx). This may occur due to a fall or miscatching a ball (eg, at cricket or baseball).

ANATOMY

- The distal end of the proximal phalanx is a convex surface made up of two condyles. The proximal end of the middle phalanx is a concave surface (**FIG 2A**).

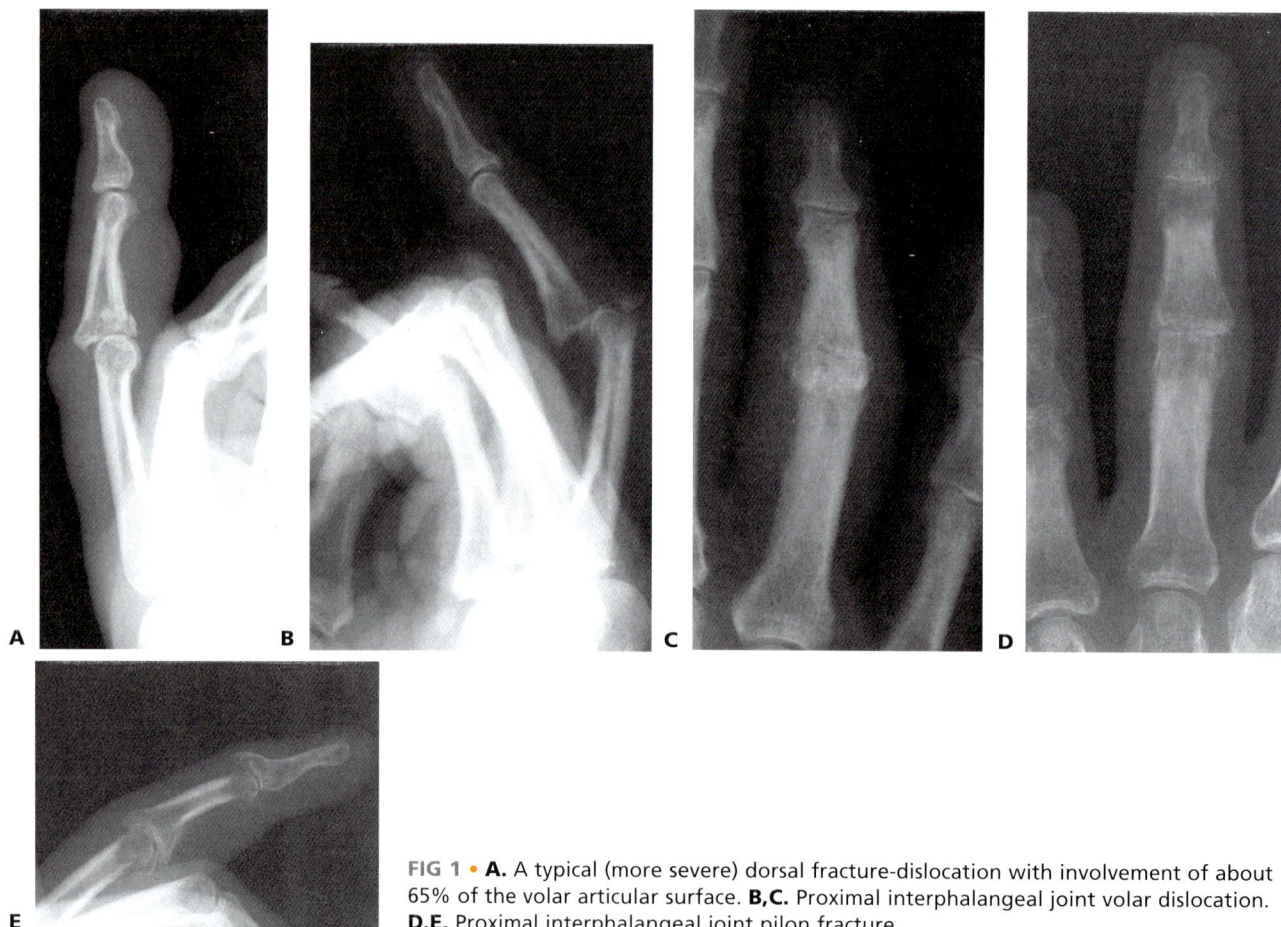

A **B** **C** **D** **E**

FIG 1 • A. A typical (more severe) dorsal fracture-dislocation with involvement of about 65% of the volar articular surface. **B,C.** Proximal interphalangeal joint volar dislocation. **D,E.** Proximal interphalangeal joint pilon fracture.

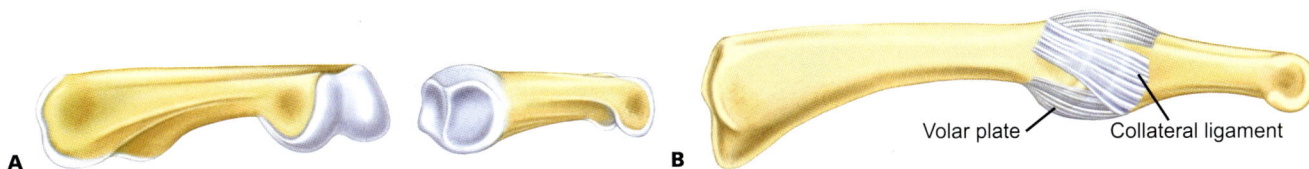

FIG 2 • **A.** The distal end of the proximal phalanx is a convex surface made up of two condyles. The proximal end of the middle phalanx is a concave surface. The two are linked by ligaments. **B.** The strongest is the volar plate and the volar part of the lateral collateral ligaments. These resist dorsal subluxation of the proximal interphalangeal joint when loaded.

- The two bones are linked and stabilized by ligaments (**FIG 2B**).
- These structures resist dorsal subluxation of the PIP joint when loaded:
  - Volar plate
  - Collateral ligaments (radial and ulnar)

PATHOGENESIS

- The tendon attachments are dorsal proximal and weak through the central slip and volar distal and strong through the flexor digitorum superficialis tendon slips. Thus, the flexor forces dominate the extensor forces.
- The shape of the joint and the soft tissue restraints allow a powerful lever arm to work for flexion. If, however, the volar restraint fails (particularly in a dorsal fracture-dislocation), the resultant forces lead to dorsal subluxation and proximal migration of the main dorsal fracture fragment of the middle phalanx (**FIG 3A**).
  - Research work and clinical experience have shown that the joint will be stable if up to 42% of the volar half of the middle phalanx articular surface is damaged as measured on a lateral radiograph (**FIG 3B**).
  - In practice, subluxation can occur with as little as 10% to 15% of joint surface loss, but that is uncommon.
- For pilon fractures, the condyles of the proximal phalanx are driven up into the base of the middle phalanx, displacing the central part of the articular surface distally and splaying the dorsal-volar and lateral margins of the middle phalanx joint surface. This injury is longitudinally unstable and results in proximal migration and diminution or obliteration of the joint space, usually with significant articular incongruity.

PATIENT HISTORY AND PHYSICAL FINDINGS

- Most patients present within a few days, although later presenters (up to 2 to 3 weeks) are common and some very late presenters (after 6 weeks) are also seen.
  - The delays are usually due to underestimation of the severity of the injury either by the patient (who thinks he or she has a sprain and it will resolve) or medical/paramedical staff (who fail to perform or interpret properly an adequate radiograph).
- The finger will be swollen and tender, centered around the PIP joint.
- An angular deformity may be evident.
- Subluxation of the joint may be clinically evident, visually or by palpation.
- There will be reduced range of movement throughout the finger and particularly in the PIP joint.

Fracture-Dislocation Involving the Proximal Interphalangeal Joint

- Most are mild injuries with limited volar plate avulsion that reduce either spontaneously or with assistance, usually under local anesthesia (**FIG 4A–D**). Radiographs may reveal a small volar bone avulsion from the base of the middle phalanx. These injuries are longitudinally stable.
  - The examiner must test for stability through a full arc of motion.
  - If there is a tendency for subluxation, the position of the joint that allows this instability is recorded.
- More severe injuries (ie, involving a greater part of the volar lip) may be longitudinally unstable, resulting in persistent subluxation of the PIP joint with attendant clinical findings as described above.

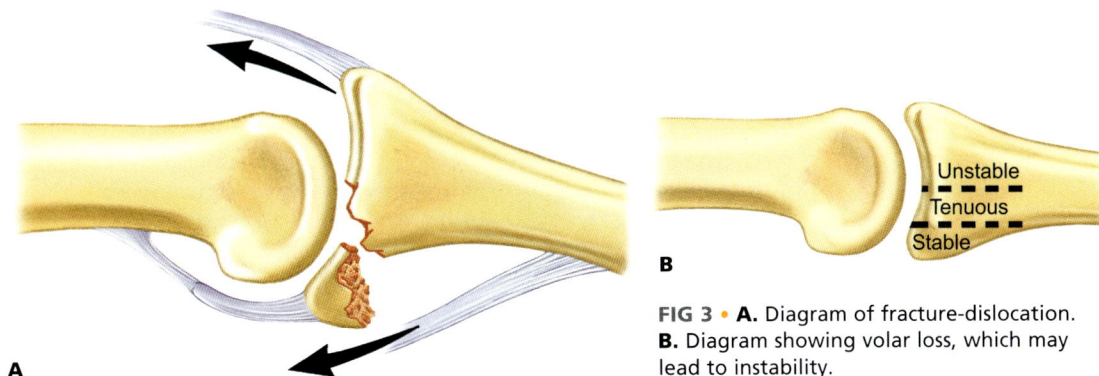

FIG 3 • **A.** Diagram of fracture-dislocation. **B.** Diagram showing volar loss, which may lead to instability.

Unstable
Tenuous
Stable

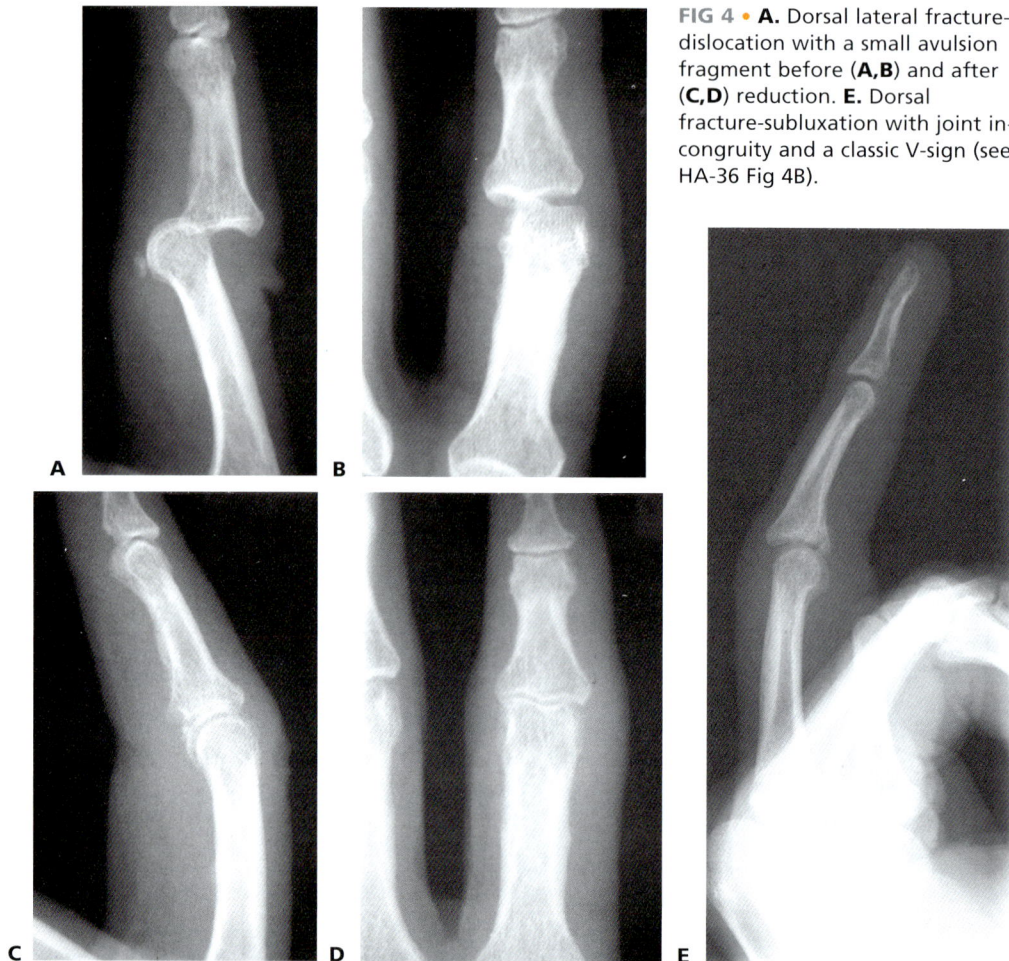

FIG 4 • A. Dorsal lateral fracture-dislocation with a small avulsion fragment before (**A,B**) and after (**C,D**) reduction. **E.** Dorsal fracture-subluxation with joint incongruity and a classic V-sign (see HA-36 Fig 4B).

- Subluxation and dislocation are best visualized on the lateral radiograph and may be quite subtle, appearing as joint incongruity at the dorsum of the joint (the triangle sign, due to dorsal overhang of the base of the middle phalanx) (**FIG 4E**).

IMAGING AND OTHER DIAGNOSTIC STUDIES

- The key investigation is plain radiology.
- Often only radiographs of the hand are taken in the emergency department. These are not adequate. Posteroanterior and lateral radiographs need to be taken, centered on the PIP joint of the injured finger (**FIG 5**).
- The key information obtained from the radiographs (supplemented by physical examination) can be used to differentiate stable from unstable injuries, either of fracture-subluxations or dislocations or pilon fractures.
- Fluoroscopy can be of great value in assessing the injury and joint stability.

DIFFERENTIAL DIAGNOSIS

- Soft tissue
  - Volar plate injury
  - Collateral ligament injury
  - Central slip injury

- Bone
  - Proximal phalanx condylar injury
  - Proximal phalanx distal diaphyseal injury
  - Middle phalanx proximal diaphyseal injury

NONOPERATIVE MANAGEMENT

- If the injury is stable, early protected mobilization can start within 1 week of injury.

Fracture-Dislocation

- A stable injury (the majority of cases) can be treated with early mobilization concentrating on regaining extension, which is commonly lost.
  - Only if there is significant pre-existing volar plate laxity (often occurs in young women) is there a need for an extension block splint for up to 6 weeks.
- Most patients regain full or nearly full movement but may be left with minor swelling and stiffness and mild cold discomfort.
  - Heavy activity may cause discomfort.
  - In approximately 5% of patients the joint remains significantly swollen and uncomfortable beyond 6 weeks. This is probably due to persistent joint synovitis, which usually resolves with a steroid injection.
- If the joint is unstable but there is limited volar joint damage (less than about 30 degrees), it may reduce when held in flexion with a dorsal block splint.

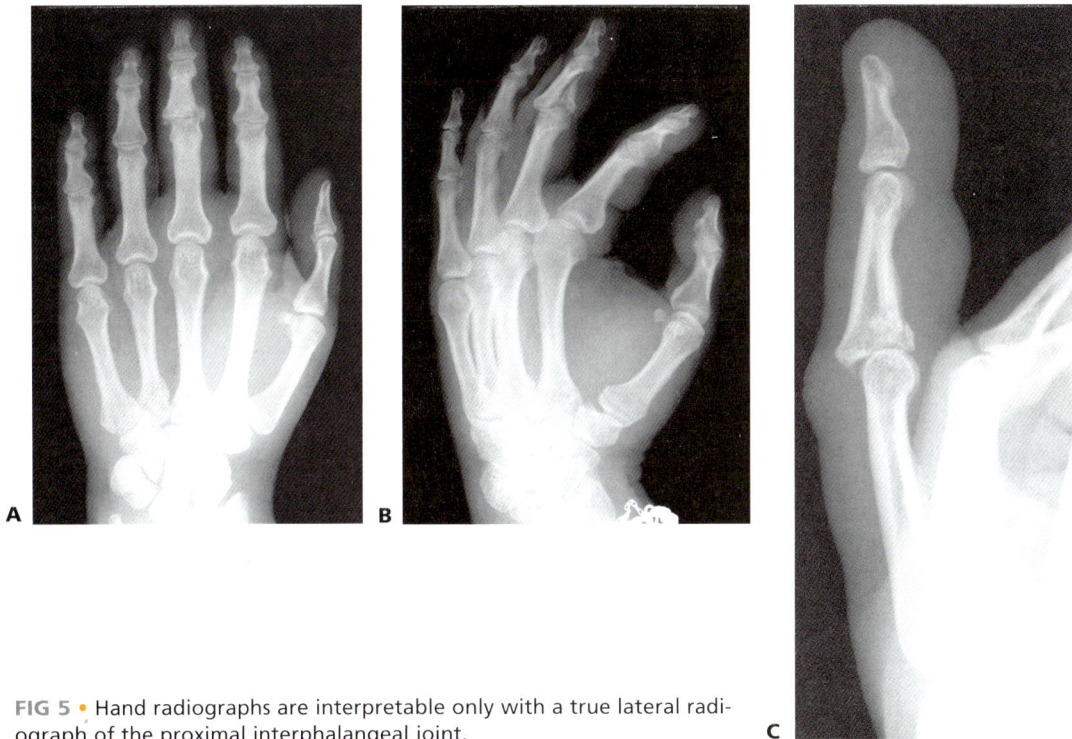

FIG 5 • Hand radiographs are interpretable only with a true lateral radiograph of the proximal interphalangeal joint.

■ Joint reduction and congruity must be documented radiologically and should not require more than about 50 degrees of joint flexion, or unacceptable PIP joint stiffness may result.

■ Patients should be encouraged to flex and extend to the splint. They should be seen weekly for 4 weeks. Flexion of the splint is reduced by about 10 degrees each week. At each increase in extension, the reduction needs to be precisely checked radiologically.

■ A reasonable range of movement with only a mild flexion contracture and loss of flexion is anticipated.

Pilon Fractures

■ The minority of pilon fractures have minimal displacement (less than 1 mm) and a reasonable joint space (**FIG 6**). These are usually stable injuries but must be carefully assessed clinically.

■ Most of these patients can achieve a range of movement from 10 to 20 degrees short of full extension to 70 to 80 degrees of flexion with only mild discomfort.

■ Patients can start early gentle mobilization with part-time protection in a splint at night and outdoors for 4 weeks.

■ Patients treated with early, protected mobilization need clinical and radiologic review weekly for at least 2 to 3 weeks.

■ Most patients will achieve a nearly full range of motion with minimal pain, stiffness, or swelling.

■ If there is greater displacement, then surgery is almost always needed to achieve longitudinal stability and early movement.

SURGICAL MANAGEMENT

Preoperative Planning

■ The proximal wire is always placed at or near the center of rotation of the injured joint.

■ Distal wire placement needs to be planned.

■ For fractures localized to the base of the middle phalanx, the distal wire can be anywhere from the midpart of the middle phalanx or more distal. In fact, the middle phalanx is narrowest at this point, so the wire is more easily placed distally.

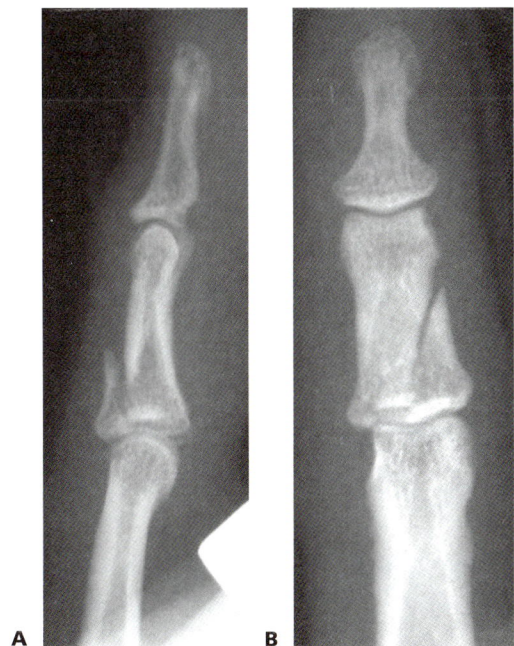

FIG 6 • Pilon fracture that was sufficiently congruent and comfortable to respond to early mobilization with a good long-term result. This could not have been predicted radiologically, and all cases require clinical assessment.

■ If the fracture extends distally, as can easily occur with pilon fractures, the distal wire should be distal to that extension to ensure adequate fixation and stability. The distal wire can be placed as far distal as the head of the middle phalanx.

■ I have never had a fracture so distal that the distal wire could not gain adequate fixation.

■ The procedure is best performed under local anesthesia. This allows the patient to participate during the operation. The patients also understands what has happened and is often clearer about the postoperative regimen.

■ At least 10 mL of plain 0.5% bupivacaine is injected at the midmetacarpal level. Bupivacaine works more slowly than lidocaine, but if given before skin preparation, it usually works completely by the time surgery starts. It then provides prolonged anesthesia for 12 to 36 hours. This helps reduce postoperative pain.

Positioning

■ Informed consent is needed, with a discussion of the risks and benefits of the various conservative (nonoperative) and surgical options.

■ Risks include infection, nerve injury, stiffness, scar tenderness, nonunion, malunion, the need for revision procedures, and the risk associated with any operation (ie, making the patient worse).

■ The digit needs to be marked very clearly, especially if the patient is receiving general anesthesia (the minority of patients).

■ Typically 1.5 g of cefuroxime is administered preoperatively. There is no need for postoperative antibiotics.

■ The patient lies supine with the affected hand out on an armboard at 90 degrees to the table (ie, standard position for hand surgery).

■ A proximal arm tourniquet is applied as a backup to the digital tourniquet.

■ The skin is prepared with chlorhexidine in an alcohol solution with a pink dye to ensure that all the fingers have been fully painted. If the finger has had adhesive dressings on it or has not been well cleaned, the anesthetized finger is scrubbed before skin preparation.

■ The operated arm is draped sterilely.

Approach

■ The operation is performed closed with insertion of percutaneous wires.

TECHNIQUES

INSERTING THE WIRES

■ I use 1.1-mm K-wires: 0.9-mm wires are too flexible and 1.6-mm wires are too rigid. I know that 1.2-mm wires have been used successfully. I suspect that wires from 1.0 to 1.3 mm are fine, but I recommend 1.1-mm wires.

■ Identify the level of the center of rotation of the PIP joint with the image intensifier and mark this level on the skin (**TECH FIG 1A,B**).

■ Insert the wire partially through the proximal phalanx and check carefully on the image intensifier with true posteroanterior and lateral projections (**TECH FIG 1C**).

■ Aim 1 to 2 mm proximal rather than distal to remain extracapsular (the capsule of the joint reflects proximally). A distal wire may risk a joint infection if pin track sepsis develops.

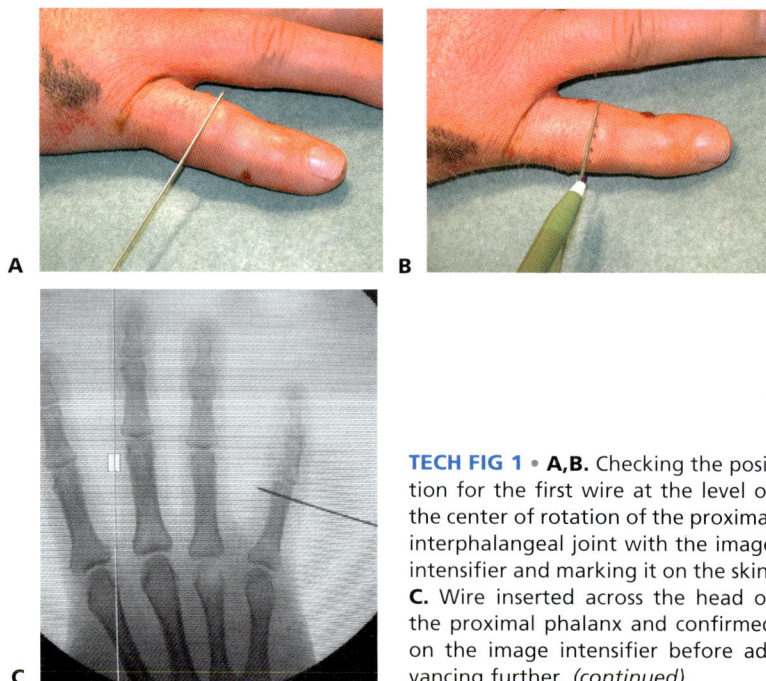

TECH FIG 1 • A,B. Checking the position for the first wire at the level of the center of rotation of the proximal interphalangeal joint with the image intensifier and marking it on the skin. **C.** Wire inserted across the head of the proximal phalanx and confirmed on the image intensifier before advancing further. *(continued)*

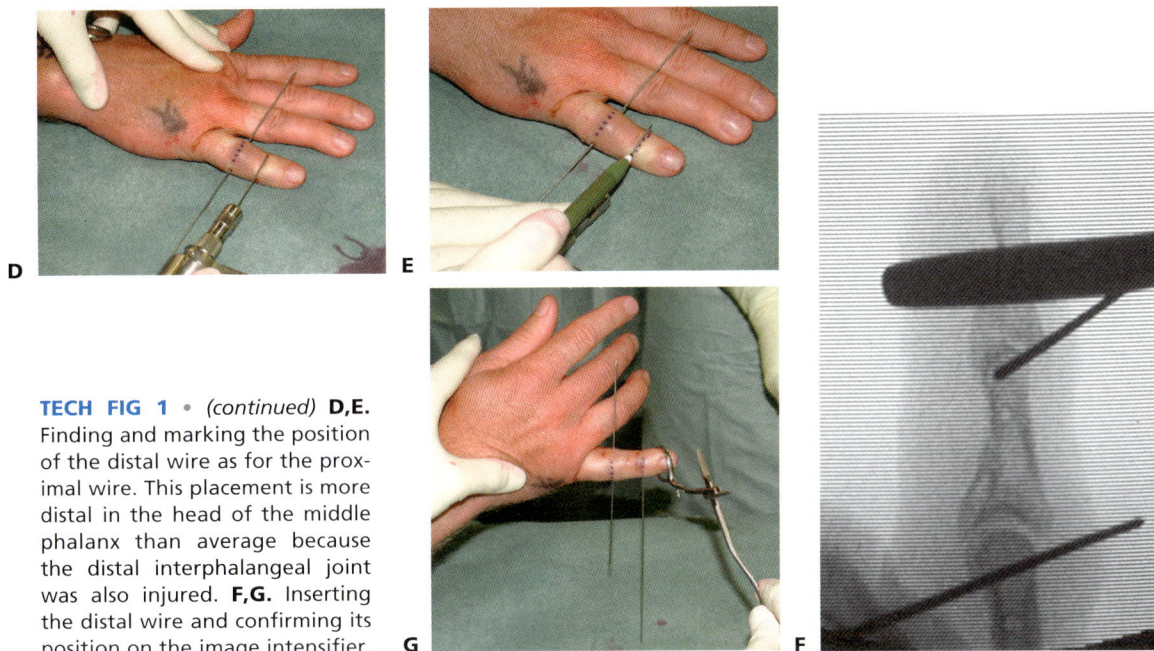

TECH FIG 1 • *(continued)* **D,E.** Finding and marking the position of the distal wire as for the proximal wire. This placement is more distal in the head of the middle phalanx than average because the distal interphalangeal joint was also injured. **F,G.** Inserting the distal wire and confirming its position on the image intensifier.

- Placing this wire too far proximal of the construct will restrict full joint movement. *This is the most important step in the whole procedure.*
- Identify an appropriate level in the distal half to two thirds of the middle phalanx, distal to any fracture extension in the shaft of the middle phalanx, with the image intensifier.
  - Mark this level on the skin.
  - This wire may be inserted near the center of rotation of the distal interphalangeal (DIP) joint, in the distal middle phalanx. This is acceptable because the bone is wider and provides more margin for error (**TECH FIG 1D,E**).

- Insert the wire partially through the middle phalanx and check carefully (posteroanterior and lateral) on the image intensifier (**TECH FIG 1F,G**).
  - Aim to be perpendicular to the long axis of the finger and parallel to both the plane of rotation and the first wire (which should also be in the plane of rotation).
  - Insert the wire so equal lengths are present on either side of the finger (by doing this for the proximal wire, where it is less important, you will have a guide for the distal wire). This helps in the wire bending. If one end is too short it can become difficult to bend, especially in patients with long fingers.

BENDING THE WIRE

- Wire bending is the more technically demanding part of the procedure. It is important to understand and follow the steps carefully.
  - One may create the construct in reverse of that described below, but this results in motion on the proximal wire rather than the distal wire, which in theory increases the risk of pin track and PIP joint sepsis.
- To ensure enough but not too much clearance from the finger, the wire is held with a medium needle holder against the skin, then manually bent past a right angle (because there is spring in the wire).
  - Bend the opposite half of the wire to the same degree and in the same direction.
- Bend the distal wire on each side through 90 degrees (**TECH FIG 2A,B**).
- Bend each half of the distal wires to make the linkage between the wires (**TECH FIG 2C,D**).
  - It is *critical* that this bend is sufficiently distal in the wire (proximal relative to the finger) to ensure that

the construct is long enough and provides adequate joint distraction.
  - If the bend is not distal enough, it is difficult to salvage, and you will probably need to remove the distal wire and insert a new wire.
- Grip the distal wires with the medium needle holder just after the second bend and bend the distal end back up about 135 degrees, creating a Z shape (**TECH FIG 2E**).
  - The proximal wire will sit in the distal narrow angle of the Z.
  - It important to put the Zs at the same level, although the construct can tolerate some mismatch.
  - If the Zs are at different levels, careful unbending or further bending of the wires should help.
- The proximal wire is flicked into place in the distal angle of the Z (**TECH FIG 2F**).
  - It should bow, showing that tension has been applied across the construct and thus traction across the joint.
  - Improved fracture and joint alignment can be visualized on the image intensifier.

TECHNIQUES

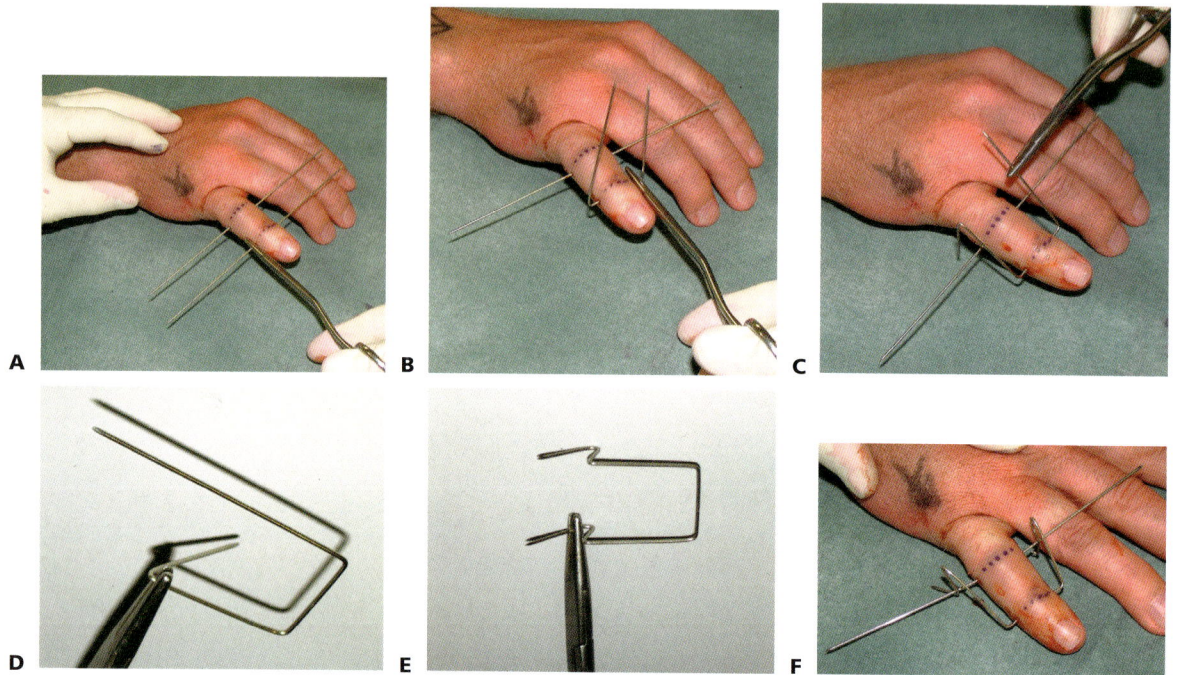

TECH FIG 2 • **A,B.** Grasping the distal wire with the needle holder and making the first bend. **C,D.** Start and completion of the second wire bend. **E.** Third wire bend shown on a freestanding wire. **F.** The properly bent distal wire is placed around the proximal wire distracting the joint.

TIDYING UP AND ENSURING THE CONSTRUCT DOES NOT DISENGAGE

Proximal Wire

- Bend the proximal wire down. Place the medium needle holder on the wire, pushing the Z construct of the distal wire against the skin (**TECH FIG 3A,B**).
  - This ensures that the construct is neither too bulky nor too close to the finger, allowing for some swelling.
  - A distance of about 3 to 4 mm is effective.
- Bend the proximal wire down about 135 degrees (**TECH FIG 3C**).
- Cut the proximal wire with wire cutters about 3 mm after the bend and crimp the cut ends (**TECH FIG 3D,E**).
  - If too short, it cannot be bent; if too long, it will abut the finger.

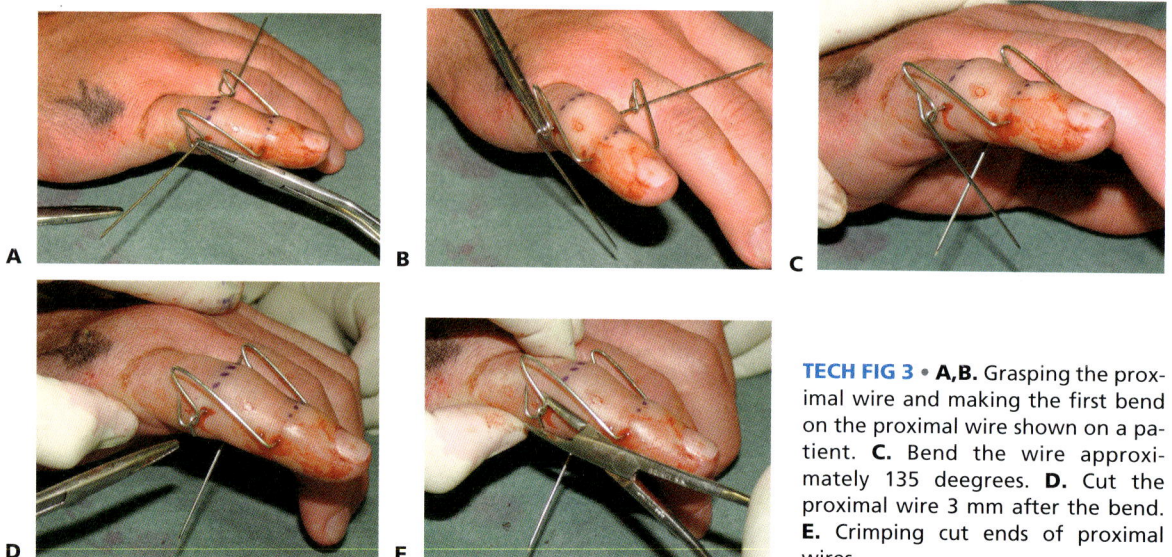

TECH FIG 3 • **A,B.** Grasping the proximal wire and making the first bend on the proximal wire shown on a patient. **C.** Bend the wire approximately 135 deegrees. **D.** Cut the proximal wire 3 mm after the bend. **E.** Crimping cut ends of proximal wires.

Distal Wire

- Crimp the distal point of the wire and the part of the proximal wire just outside the skin down together with the medium needle holders (**TECH FIG 4A**).
  - Do not crimp too far or the middle phalanx wire will be gripped and not allow full rotation.
  - The wire has to be bent enough to ensure that the construct cannot disengage.
- Bend the distal tail of each Z over to ensure that the proximal wire cannot disengage (**TECH FIG 4B**).
- This process leaves slightly irregular cut wire ends. These need to be kept close to the construct and typically do not cause problems, but if they do they can be covered postoperatively.
- Check the final fracture position on the image intensifier (**TECH FIG 4C,D**).

- At the end of the operation, if the patient is under local anesthesia, ask him or her to watch the injured digit while extending the PIP joint to neutral and flexing to at least 90 degrees.
  - This method of educating the patient is painless and gives him or her greater confidence in the postoperative period.

Force Couple

- Some surgeons advocate a force couple—that is, a third wire in the proximal end of the middle phalanx that hooks under the bent distal middle phalanx wire to force the middle phalanx volar and improve dorsal joint subluxation (**TECH FIG 5**).
- We have not needed a force couple, nor is there any evidence as yet to support its use.

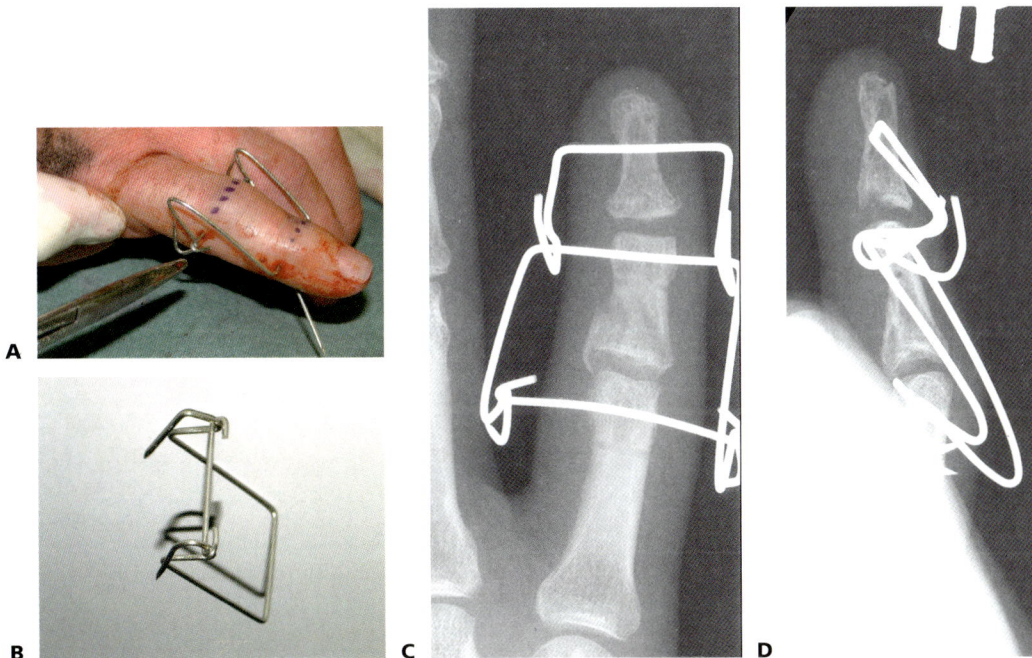

TECH FIG 4 • **A,B.** Distal wire bends completed. The fourth bend is just to prevent disengagement of the construct. **C,D.** The position of the final construct on a patient on whom, for the only time in my practice, I used a double fixator on one finger. The proximal interphalangeal joint had a pilon fracture, which is well but not perfectly reduced. The distal interphalangeal joint had a fracture-dislocation that is also well but not perfectly reduced.

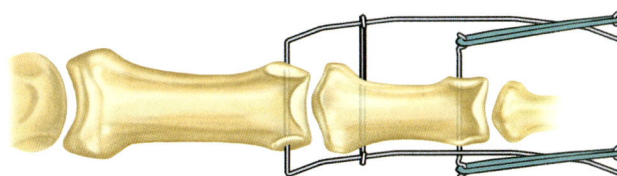

TECH FIG 5 • Drawing of a Suzuki frame showing a third (middle) wire in position, where it can act as a force couple.

PEARLS AND PITFALLS

- External fixation is typically very reliable and flexible in the treatment of PIP fractures and dislocations. The indications for open reduction and internal fixation are extremely limited due to the degree of fracture comminution and the morbidity associated with even limited open methods of treatment.
- At operation the key is to place the proximal wire at or just proximal to the center of rotation of the PIP joint in the head of the proximal phalanx.
- Bending of the wires requires practice but with experience becomes easy. It is important to avoid putting twist into the wires to optimize motion in the construct.
- Sufficient tension in the construct and across the joint is critical.
- If inadequate, the wire bends may be adjusted, but probably the distal wire will need to be replaced.

POSTOPERATIVE CARE

- The construct should not disimpact if made properly. If it does, it can usually be adjusted in clinic with further wire bending. Local anesthesia may be needed.
- The hand is elevated maximally for 3 to 5 days and movement is started once the patient is comfortable.
- The use of a long-acting local anesthetic means the patient can go home and start taking simple oral analgesics (eg, ibuprofen and diclofenac, paracetamol and codeine, or both).
  - Opiate analgesics are rarely required, and almost no patient complains of significant pain.
  - The analgesics should continue for at least 24 hours but not longer than 1 week.
- Long slow stretches both into extension and into flexion are emphasized. They should be performed hourly.
  - The stretches should be held for 5 minutes at a time. They should not be painful, although they need to be at least on the edge of discomfort or in the mildly uncomfortable range. Painful stretches will lead to more swelling, increase the risk of complex regional pain syndrome type I, and discourage the patient from performing exercises.
  - Formal therapy visits begin the second postoperative week. In addition to PIP motion, DIP motion is emphasized. The therapist works with these patients at least weekly.
- The patient is checked after 5 to 7 days.
  - The dressing is removed and radiographs are performed to ensure that the reduction has been maintained.
  - The dressings are left off and the patient is instructed in pin track care (see below), care of the sharp wire points (ie, covering them with tape if necessary), and stretching exercises, supported by a hand therapist.
- The pins are cleaned and dried as one would for their hand day to day.
  - Assuming the pin tracks stay dry, nothing more needs to be done.
  - If the pin tracks start oozing, clean with preboiled water four times a day.
  - If the pin sites do not improve within 24 hours, I advise the patient to seek medical help for antibiotics.
  - The redness and oozing should resolve within 2 to 3 days. If not, the patient may require intravenous antibiotics and early pin removal, but this is extremely rare.
- The patient is checked again about 2 weeks postoperatively.
  - At this stage the finger will still be mildly swollen.
  - There should be minimal or no pain except with stretches.
  - The pin tracks should be clean and dry.
  - The range of movement should be in the PIP joint a fixed flexion deformity of no more than 10 degrees and flexion to at least 50 degrees, and in the DIP joint full extension and flexion to at least 50 degrees.
- If this has been achieved, the patient returns to the office 4 to 5 weeks postoperatively for wire removal. There appears no good reason to leave the wires in longer, and the incidence of pin track sepsis increases after 4 weeks.
- Final review takes place 10 to 12 weeks after surgery.

OUTCOMES

- The finger will still be mildly swollen; this will never resolve fully.
- The final range of movement will have been achieved; it should be about 10 to 90 degrees in the PIP joint and full (0 to 70 degrees) in the DIP joint. There should be no rest pain but there will probably be some achiness with heavy use. The pin tracks should have healed with minimal if any tenderness or cosmetic abnormality.
- Pilon fractures typically reduce only in part, with at least one impacted fragment remaining impacted in the middle phalanx.
  - Because the concave side of the joint seems to tolerate some incongruity well, this fragment is not routinely disimpacted.
- Fracture-dislocations also tend to reduce incompletely, with some mild residual dorsal subluxation of the joint surface (ie, widening of the joint on the lateral view). If mild, this too is well tolerated.
- Traction devices generally give reliable results, with range of motion of about 89 degrees and only 2% poor results; open reduction and internal fixation gives range of motion of 79 degrees and 10% to 12% poor results.

COMPLICATIONS

- Complications are uncommon but recovery is never full, as indicated above.
- Pin track infection is the most common risk, but if the wires are removed between 4 and 5 weeks it is uncommon (less than 10% of cases). It typically resolves with cleaning, elevation, and 2 to 3 days of oral antibiotics (typically flucloxacillin 500 mg four times a day and amoxicillin 500 mg three times a day).
- Mild malunion is accepted and well tolerated.
- Nonunion has not occurred as a functional problem, although radiographs may show odd ununited peripheral fragments of bone.
- Nerve injury may occur.
- Significant poor results and persistent rest pain occur in only about 3% to 5% of patients.

REFERENCES

1. Agee JM. Unstable fracture dislocation of the proximal interphalangeal joint. Clin Orthop Relat Res 1987;214:101–112.
2. Aladin A, Davis TR. Dorsal fracture-dislocation of the proximal interphalangeal joint: a comparative study of percutaneous Kirschner wire fixation versus open reduction and internal fixation. J Hand Surg Br 2005;30B:120–128.
3. Allison DM. Fractures of the base of the middle phalanx treated by dynamic external fixation. J Hand Surg Br 1996;21B:305–310.
4. Badia A, Riano F, Ravikoff J, et al. Dynamic intradigital external fixation for proximal interphalangeal joint fracture dislocations. J Hand Surg Am 2005;30A:154–160.
5. Deitch M, Kiefhaber T, Rodney Comisar B, et al. Dorsal fracture dislocations of the proximal interphalangeal joint: surgical complications and long-term results. J Hand Surg Am 1999;24A:914–923.
6. Deshmukh SC, Kumar D, Mathur K, et al. Complex fracture-dislocation of the proximal interphalangeal joint of the hand: results of a modified pins and rubbers traction system. J Bone Joint Surg 2004;86B:406–412.
7. De Smet L, Boone P. Treatment of fracture-dislocation of the proximal interphalangeal joint using the Suzuki external fixator. J Orthop Trauma 2002;16(9):668–671.
8. de Soras X, de Mourgues P, Guinard D, et al. Pins and rubbers traction system. J Hand Surg Br 1997;22B:730–735.
9. Duteille F, Pasquier P, Lim A, et al. Treatment of complex interphalangeal joint fractures with dynamic external traction: a series of 20 cases. Plast Reconstr Surg 2003;15:1623–1629.
10. Fahmy NRM. The Stockport serpentine spring system for the treatment of displaced comminuted intra-articular phalangeal fractures. J Hand Surg Br 1990;15B:303–311.
11. Grant I, Berger AC, Tham SK. Internal fixation of unstable fracture dislocations of the proximal interphalangeal joint. J Hand Surg Br 2005;30B:492–498.
12. Hamilton SC, Stern PJ, Fassler PR, et al. Mini-screw fixation for the treatment of proximal interphalangeal joint dorsal fracture-dislocations. J Hand Surg Am 2006;31A:1349–1354.
13. Hastings H, Carroll C. Treatment of closed articular fractures of the metacarpophalangeal and proximal interphalangeal joints. Hand Clin 1988;4(3):503–527.
14. Inanami H, Ninomiya S, Okutsu I, et al. Dynamic external finger fixator for fracture dislocation of the proximal interphalangeal joint. J Hand Surg Am 1993;18A:160–164.
15. Kiefhaber T, Stern PJ. Fracture-dislocations of the proximal interphalangeal joint. J Hand Surg Am 1998;23A:368–380.
16. Krakauer JD, Stern PJ. Hinged device for fractures involving the proximal interphalangeal joint. Clin Orthop Relat Res 1996;327:29–37.
17. Schenk RR. The dynamic traction method: combined movement and traction for interarticular fractures of the phalanges. Hand Clin 1994;10:187–198.
18. Seno N, Hashizume H, Inoue H, et al. Fractures of the base of the middle phalanx of the finger: classification, management and long-term results. J Bone Joint Surg Br 1997;79B:758–763.
19. Weiss AP. Cerclage fixation for fracture dislocation of the proximal interphalangeal joint. Clin Orthop Relat Res 1996;327:21–28.

Chapter 36

Open Reduction and Internal Fixation of Proximal Interphalangeal Joint Fracture-Dislocations

Brian Najarian and Jeffrey Lawton

DEFINITION

- Proximal interphalangeal (PIP) joint fracture-dislocations are intra-articular injuries that include a concomitant soft tissue injury to the surrounding capsular and ligamentous structures.
- The injury can result from axial, bending, and torsional loads, or combinations thereof.
- These injuries of the finger are relatively common and potentially disabling, and may result in:
  - Joint stiffness
  - Persistent subluxation
  - Posttraumatic arthritis
  - Chronic pain
- Stability and alignment are more important goals than articular congruency in determining a successful outcome.[18]
- Evaluation and treatment may be delayed, with the injury dismissed as a "jammed finger."

ANATOMY

- The PIP joint is a hinge joint, consisting of radial and ulnar condyles on the proximal phalanx, with matching concavities on the middle phalangeal base. This construction allows for a wide range of motion (ROM) in flexion and extension, but relative rigidity in abduction and adduction.
  - The PIP joint has an arc of motion of 120 degrees and accounts for 85% of the motion required to grasp an object.[2]

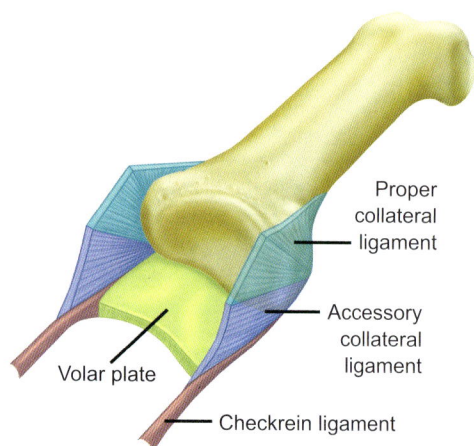

FIG 1 • Diagram of proximal interphalangeal (PIP) joint anatomy. The PIP joint is a hinge joint that derives its stability from bony articular congruence of the proximal and middle phalanx and soft tissue restraints: the volar plate and its checkrein ligament extensions, the proper and accessory collateral ligaments, and the extensor complex (not shown).

- The joint derives its stability from its bony articular congruence and its soft tissue restraints (**FIG 1**).
  - The volar plate resists dorsal stress, is taut in extension, and often fails distally from bone.
    - Checkrein ligaments are slender proximal extensions of the volar plate under which branches of the digital arteries pass, supplying the joint and vincula and nourishing the flexor tendons.
  - Collateral ligaments, the primary soft tissue restraints, have two components:
    - The proper collateral ligaments (radial and ulnar), which insert on the middle phalanx, provide the principal resistance to abduction/adduction stress. These ligaments are commonly injured in dorsal dislocations. Injury to the radial collateral ligament is more common than injury to the ulnar collateral ligament by nearly six-fold.
    - The accessory collateral ligaments arise from a conjoined origin just volar to the proper collateral ligament and insert on the volar plate.
  - The extensor complex limits volarly directed stress.
    - The central slip attaches to the dorsal tubercle on the base of the middle phalanx.
    - The conjoint lateral bands run obliquely on each side of the joint.
    - The transverse retinacular ligament connects the central slip and the conjoint lateral bands and extends laterally.
  - For a dislocation to occur, at least one, often two, and sometimes all three of these structures must be significantly disrupted.

PATHOGENESIS AND CLASSIFICATION

- The PIP joint is uniquely susceptible to injury.
- The pattern of joint injury depends on the direction, degree, and rate of force application.
- The three main groups of PIP fracture dislocations are defined by the mechanism of injury force and the direction of deformity (**FIG 2**).
  - *Dorsal* subluxation, or dislocation of the middle, the most common type, is caused by hyperextension and axial loading of the middle phalanx against the head of the proximal phalanx. The result is a fracture involving the base of the middle phalanx and dorsal positioning of the middle phalanx.

    This injury can be subclassified into three types based on the amount of volar middle phalanx articular surface involved, as determined on a lateral radiograph.[13] The degree of instability is directly proportional to volar lip fragment size due to the loss of collateral ligament support, and the articular buttress (see Fig 3B in Chap. HA-35).
    - *Stable:* less than 30% of the articular surface, reduced in extension

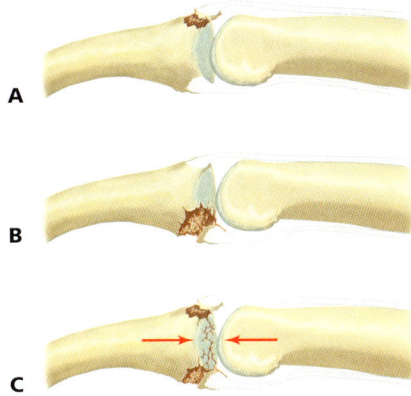

FIG 2 • PIP fracture-dislocation classifications. The three main groups of PIP fracture-dislocations are volar (**A**), dorsal (**B**), and pilon (**C**).

Tenuous: 30% to 50% of the articular surface, reduction maintained with less than 30 degrees of flexion

Unstable: either more than 50% of the articular surface *or* 30% to 50% of the articular surface, but requiring more than 30 degrees of flexion to maintain reduction

- *Volar* subluxation, or dislocation of the middle phalanx, is less common and is thought to be caused by forced flexion of an extended joint.

  Stable: joint reduction in extension

  Unstable: palmar subluxation of middle phalanx with the joint extended

- *Pilon injuries* are not associated with significant subluxation or dislocation. They are caused by an axial force on a partially flexed PIP joint, resulting in comminution of the articular surface of the middle phalanx (most commonly, volar and dorsal articular fragments surrounding a central depressed fragment)

- Unicondylar fractures of the head of the proximal phalanx, another variant of this injury type, are included in a classification system proposed by Weiss and Hastings[21] (see Chap. HA-33).

  These injuries also can be accompanied by dislocation of the PIP joint and nearly always are unstable and require operative fixation. They often are amenable to the same approaches and fixation methods presented here.

NATURAL HISTORY

- Following injury, the PIP joint quickly stiffens. Pain and instability limit motion initially; then the joint capsule and ligaments become fibrotic.
- Over time the unreduced PIP joint will become arthritic and painful.

HISTORY AND PHYSICAL FINDINGS

- Patients present following a traumatic event to the digit, frequently one that occurred some time ago.

  In the acute setting, the primary complaints are pain and swelling of the joint and digit.

  Patients with subacute and chronic injuries are focused primarily on stiffness, loss of function, and persistent swelling, and secondarily on pain.

  The history must include a detailed description of the mechanism of injury and any previous treatment.

- Inspection

  Evaluate the skin and soft tissues for swelling and for any open or healed wounds that could indicate an open fracture-dislocation.

  Deformity in extension or flexion indicates whether the dislocation is volar or dorsal, respectively.

  Axial or rotational malalignment may result from articular depression of a condyle. This can be recognized clinically as subtle angulation when full digital extension is attempted.

- Tenderness

  The acute location of greatest tenderness on palpation may indicate which soft tissue structures are injured.

- ROM

  Adequate evaluation may be difficult in the acute setting due to pain. After neurologic examination, a digital block may be necessary.

  Elson test (**FIG 3**)

  From a 90-degree flexed position over the edge of a table, ask the patient to actively extend the PIP joint of the involved finger against resistance. If the central slip is intact, the examiner will feel an extension force from the middle phalanx. In addition, the distal interphalangeal (DIP)

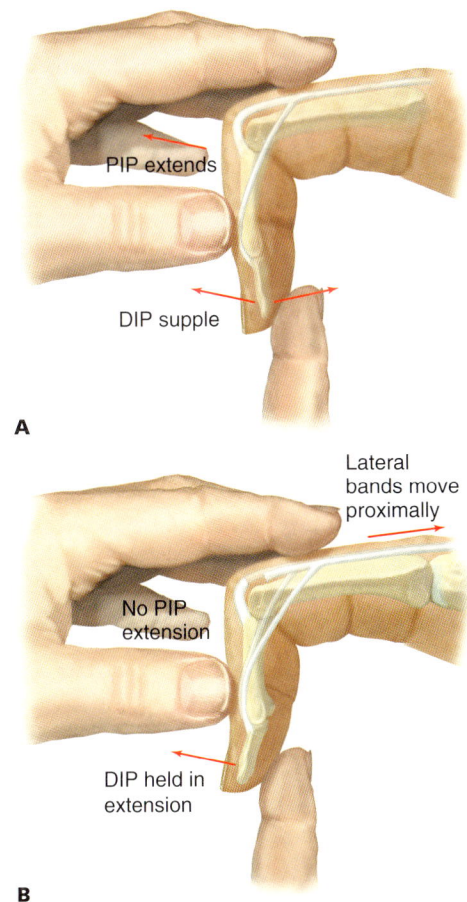

FIG 3 • Elson test. **A.** Intact central slip. From a 90-degree flexed position, the patient can actively extend the PIP joint of the involved finger against resistance. The distal interphalangeal (DIP) joint is supple. **B.** Ruptured central slip. The patient cannot actively extend the PIP joint against resistance and has fixed extension at the DIP joint, due to the extensor action of the lateral bands alone.

joint remains flail during this effort, because the competent central slip prevents the lateral bands from acting distally.

■ An *absence* of extension force at the PIP joint and fixed extension at the DIP joint (due to the extensor action of the lateral bands alone) is diagnostic of a complete rupture of the central slip. In the acute setting, the patient may be reluctant to perform this test due to pain, but this can be relieved by proximal infiltration with local anesthetic around the dorsal sensory nerves of the digit.[7]

■ Note the range of motion through which the joint remains reduced. In the case of a dorsal dislocation, the degree of extension that results in instability or redislocation determines the angle for the extension block splint.

■ An irreducible joint is consistent with entrapment of a soft tissue structure (eg, volar plate, collateral ligament, flexor or extensor tendon) in the joint, which usually necessitates urgent surgery.

■ The neurovascular examination usually is normal.

　■ Subjective complaints of paresthesias and objective measure of capillary refill should be noted, both pre- and post-reduction.

IMAGING AND OTHER DIAGNOSTIC STUDIES

■ Posteroanterior (PA), lateral, and partially supinated and pronated oblique radiographs of the involved digit(s) are required.

　■ Oblique views help to identify fracture planes and determine the extent of comminution, valuable for surgical planning.

　■ It is critical to determine amount of articular involvement on a true lateral film in full PIP joint extension to evaluate stability of the joint.

　■ Radiographs can be misleading, suggesting that a very simple fracture involving only a small fragment of the bone has occurred. This fragment is potentially the major attachment of a collateral ligament, the volar plate, or a tendon. The resultant incompetence of these structures can render the joint grossly or potentially unstable (**FIG 4A**).

■ V sign[13] (**FIG 4B**)

　■ On a postreduction true lateral radiograph of the digit, divergence of the dorsal articular surfaces from the central portion of the joint creates a V-shaped gap between the articular surfaces of the head of the proximal phalanx and the undamaged portion of the middle phalanx base.

　■ The presence of this sign indicates an incompletely reduced joint.

■ Dynamic fluoroscopy is extremely valuable in evaluating the reduction and its stability.

　■ Hinged flexion is a variant of the V sign in which congruent rotation of the joint is replaced by abnormal translation as the joint is actively flexed and extended across the flattened fracture segments.

　■ The joint position that results in instability or redislocation is best determined fluoroscopically.

DIFFERENTIAL DIAGNOSIS

■ Pure dislocation (simple or complex)
■ Extra-articular fractures
■ "Jammed finger"—collateral sprain[9,14,23]
■ Volar plate injury
■ Central slip injury

NONOPERATIVE MANAGEMENT

■ Prompt recognition of the complexity of injury and an understanding of the appropriate treatment options are essential for optimal management of these fractures.

■ Although fractures and dislocations of the PIP joint have the potential to be disabling, most can be treated with closed reduction, splinting, early motion, and close follow-up.

■ Closed reduction is almost always successful for acute dorsal PIP dislocations. Volar dislocations are more problematic, especially if the deformity has a rotary component.

　■ Reductions performed immediately after the injury often can be accomplished without anesthesia. If reduction is delayed, a digital block with 1% lidocaine (without epinephrine) is helpful.

　■ Always make sure to complete a careful neurologic examination of the digit before performing an anesthetic block. Confirm adequate anesthesia before manipulation.

　■ Be gentle, and limit the number of attempts. Irreducible dislocations usually are caused by soft tissue interposition.

■ Dorsal dislocations can be reduced with gentle traction on the finger with the wrist in the neutral position, followed by pressing the base of the middle phalanx in a volar direction while holding the proximal phalanx steady.

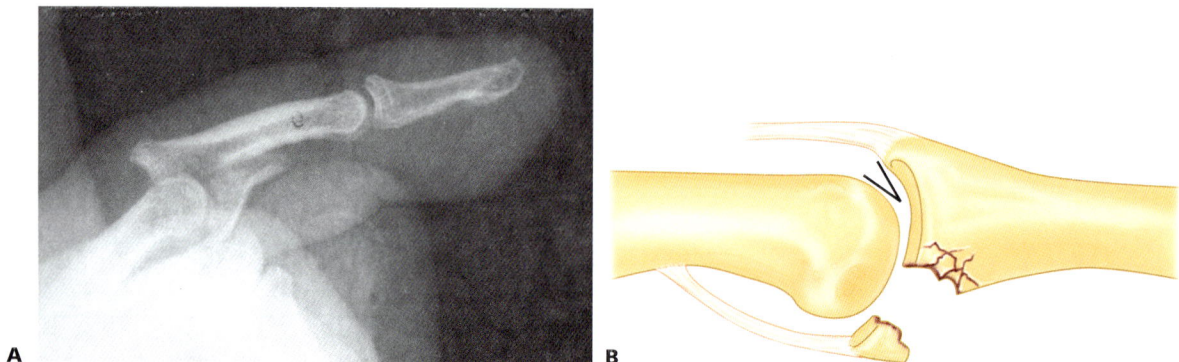

FIG 4 • **A.** Unstable dorsal PIP fracture-dislocation. This lateral radiograph of a typical PIP joint fracture, demonstrates dorsal dislocation of the middle phalanx on the proximal phalanx due to the large amount of volar articular surface involved (over 50%). **B.** The V-sign in an incompletely reduced dorsal fracture-dislocation. Divergence of the dorsal articular surfaces from the central portion of the joint creates a V-shaped gap, which can be demonstrated on a lateral radiograph.

■ Volar dislocations *without* a rotatory component usually are reducible with gentle traction.

■ Place the wrist in the neutral position and apply a dorsally directed force to the middle phalanx and a volarly directed force on the proximal phalanx.

■ These dislocations, which usually can be treated with closed reduction, commonly involve an avulsion of the central slip.

■ Volar dislocations *with* a rotatory component often are difficult to reduce by closed means. The head of the proximal phalanx becomes trapped between the central slip and one of the lateral bands of the extensor mechanism.

■ These injuries occasionally can be reduced closed by placing the metacarpophalangeal (MCP) and PIP joints in 90 degrees of flexion with the wrist extended, applying light traction, and rotating the middle phalanx in the direction opposite to the deformity.

SURGICAL MANAGEMENT

■ Surgical management is difficult for two reasons:

■ The fracture fragments can be small and comminuted, making anatomic reduction and stabilization with implants difficult.

■ The need for early mobilization of the joint to prevent stiffness requires rigid fixation of these fragments.

■ These fractures have a high risk of redisplacement, and patients must be warned of the possibility that repeat surgical treatment of the fracture may be necessary.

■ The specific injury and fracture pattern often dictate the most appropriate method of treatment. Some methods can be used in combination.

■ For stable, reducible fractures, typically involving less than 30% of the articular surface, treatment includes:

■ Extension block splinting and pinning

■ Traction, dynamic or static (see Chap. HA-35).

■ Unstable, irreducible fractures, typically involving more than 30% to 50% of the joint, require:

■ External fixation

■ Percutaneous fixation

■ Open reduction with internal fixation using K-wires, screws, cerclage wires

■ When dorsal fracture-dislocations are associated with bone loss or fracture comminution to such a degree that a stable reduction is unobtainable using the methods listed earlier, two salvage procedures are commonly employed.

■ *Volar plate arthroplasty.* The volar plate is advanced into the middle phalangeal defect, simultaneously restoring stability and resurfacing the damaged articular surface[6,15](see Chap. HA-37).

■ *Hemi-hamate autograft reconstruction.* The fractured middle phalangeal base is débrided, and the defect is replaced using a size-matched portion of the dorsal/distal hamate osteoarticular surface and secured with mini-fragment screws[22] (see Chap. HA-38).

■ Table 1 illustrates some of the indications, advantages, and disadvantages of open reduction and internal fixation and some of the salvage options discussed in this chapter.[8]

Indications

■ Unstable and tenuous fractures requiring more than 30 degrees of flexion to maintain reduction

■ Closed management of these fractures requires extreme flexion to prevent redislocation is likely to result in a flexion contracture.

■ Fractures with fragments that are irreducible by closed methods and amenable to internal fixation with available hardware

■ Significant articular depression, displacement, or incongruity

Goals

■ Stable, anatomic fixation of the fracture resulting in a concentric reduction of the PIP joint

■ Early range of motion designed to enhance cartilage and soft tissue healing, enhance joint remodeling, and minimize adhesions and contractures

■ Anatomic restoration of the congruous joint surface is a desirable but less important treatment goal and does not supersede a concentric PIP reduction and early motion.

Preoperative Planning

■ Radiographic evaluation, as discussed earlier

■ The surgeon must be adept at using the various techniques, and the patient should be counseled that intraoperative observations will dictate the definitive method of fixation.

Positioning

■ The patient is placed supine with a radiolucent hand table.

■ A brachial tourniquet is placed on the upper arm before draping and is inflated to 250 mm Hg just before the incision is made.

Table 1	Advantages and Disadvantages of Techniques for Repair of PIP Joint Fracture-Dislocation			
Technique	**Indications**	**Advantages**	**Disadvantages**	**Pearls**
ORIF	Minimal comminution	Anatomic reduction	Technically difficult if multiple fragments	Consider other options in older patients (>60 yo), eg, dorsal block pinning.
	Intact dorsal cortex	Can use bone graft Early ROM	Increased risk of infection	
Volar plate arthroplasty	<50% articular surface involved	Proven track record	Redislocation (especially if >50% P-2 base fractured	Careful patient selection
	Comminution base of P-2	Restores volar buttress	Stiffness Arthritis	
Osteochondral autograft (ie, hemihamate, radial styloid, toes)	Highly unstable dislocations: • >60% of articular surface involvement • Acute or chronic dislocation	Biologic replacement of articular surface	Donor morbidity Technically demanding	Consider osteochondral autograft if >50% involved. Short-term results promising

ORIF, open reduction with internal fixation; P-2, middle phalanx; ROM, range of motion.

■ Surgery can be performed under a wrist or digital block, but an axillary block is preferred to obtain adequate sensory anesthesia and motor relaxation of the flexors and extensors.

■ The operative hand is supinated, and a "lead hand" can be used to hold it in place.

Operative Equipment

■ A mini C-arm fluoroscopy unit is necessary to confirm fracture reduction, joint reduction, and correct placement of implants.

■ Mini-fragment plate and screw set

■ 24-gauge wire
■ K-wires

Approach

■ The volar (Bruner) approach, the dorsal (Chamay) approach, and the mid-axial approach are all useful.

■ The approach is chosen based on the fracture pattern and the direction of instability.

  ■ When most of the fracture comminution is dorsal, a Chamay or mid-axial approach is selected.

  ■ When most of the comminution is volar, as is more common with dorsal fracture-dislocations, a volar Bruner incision is employed.

TECHNIQUES

EXPOSURE

Volar Approach (Bruner)[3,10]

■ A palmar zigzag skin incision is made from the MCP joint crease across the PIP joint to the DIP flexion crease. In a larger or longer digit, two limbs of a Bruner incision may be necessary between the flexion creases (**TECH FIG 1A,B**).

■ An ulnarly based, thick subcutaneous flap is mobilized at the level of the flexor sheath.

■ The digital neurovascular structures are mobilized from the flexor sheath apparatus.

  ■ These procedures are necessary to avoid traction on the associated structures if the joint is dorsally displaced during exposure and fixation.

■ The flexor sheath over the PIP joint (including the A3 pulley) is incised on three sides, creating a rectangular flap between the A2 and A4 pulleys (**TECH FIG 1C**).

  ■ Alternatively, the flexor sheath may be split longitudinally to expose the underlying flexor tendons.

■ The flexor digitorum profundus and flexor digitorum superficialis tendons are retracted to the side to expose the volar plate (**TECH FIG 1D**).

  ■ A Penrose drain placed around the tendons permits atraumatic retraction.

■ The PIP joint and bare surface of the volar fragment are exposed by dividing the volar plate in the transverse plane just proximal to its distal insertion.

  ■ Make sure to leave a small amount of the distal portion attached to the bony fragment of the middle phalanx for later repair.

  ■ Retract the main portion of the volar plate proximally, creating a proximally based flap. The volar plate is *not* excised.

■ Sharp recession of the collateral ligaments at their proximal or distal volar attachments may be required to access fragments that are more dorsal than the volar third of the middle phalangeal base or to reduce chronic subluxations.

  ■ Most often, the collateral ligaments are elevated only from their middle phalangeal insertion.

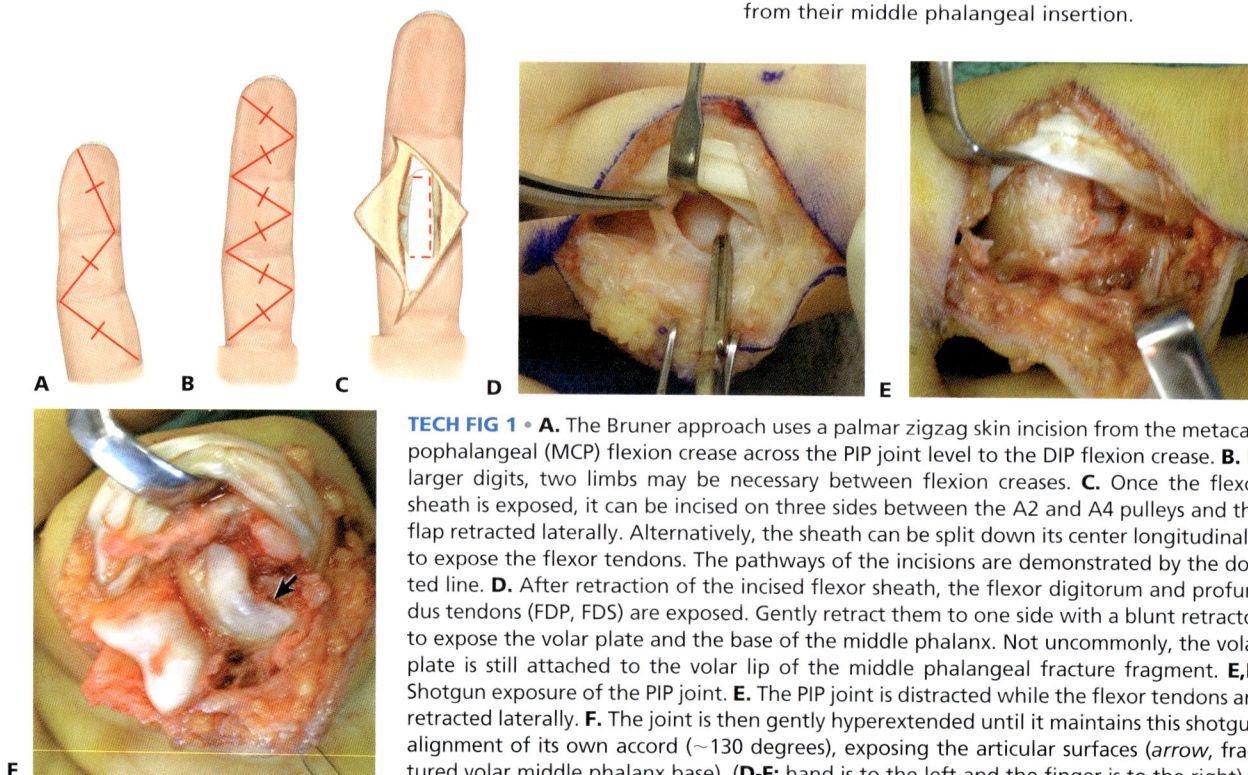

TECH FIG 1 • A. The Bruner approach uses a palmar zigzag skin incision from the metacarpophalangeal (MCP) flexion crease across the PIP joint level to the DIP flexion crease. **B.** In larger digits, two limbs may be necessary between flexion creases. **C.** Once the flexor sheath is exposed, it can be incised on three sides between the A2 and A4 pulleys and the flap retracted laterally. Alternatively, the sheath can be split down its center longitudinally to expose the flexor tendons. The pathways of the incisions are demonstrated by the dotted line. **D.** After retraction of the incised flexor sheath, the flexor digitorum and profundus tendons (FDP, FDS) are exposed. Gently retract them to one side with a blunt retractor to expose the volar plate and the base of the middle phalanx. Not uncommonly, the volar plate is still attached to the volar lip of the middle phalangeal fracture fragment. **E,F.** Shotgun exposure of the PIP joint. **E.** The PIP joint is distracted while the flexor tendons are retracted laterally. **F.** The joint is then gently hyperextended until it maintains this shotgun alignment of its own accord (~130 degrees), exposing the articular surfaces (*arrow,* fractured volar middle phalanx base). (**D-F:** hand is to the left and the finger is to the right).

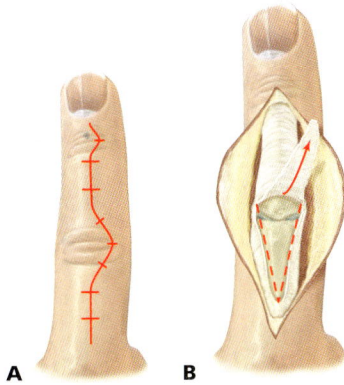

TECH FIG 2 • Dorsal (Chamay) approach. **A.** A longitudinal skin incision is made midline over the dorsal aspect of the proximal phalanx proximally and then is curved laterally and distally around the dorsal aspect of the PIP joint. **B.** After superficial dissection is carried down to expose the extensor mechanism, a distally based, V-shaped flap of central slip is created, with the apex of the flap extending to the proximal third of the proximal phalanx. This pedicle flap of central slip is then pulled distally with a hooked retractor to expose the PIP joint.

- If comprehensive exposure of the PIP joint is required, the collateral ligaments are released from their site of insertion, and the PIP joint is distracted and then gently hyperextended until it maintains this alignment of its own accord (about 130 degrees). This has been referred to as "shotgun" exposure of the joint[6] (**TECH FIG 1E,F**).
  - Watch the neurovascular bundles closely during this hyperextension maneuver to ensure they can easily subluxate dorsally.

Dorsal Approach (Chamay)[4]

- A longitudinal skin incision is made over the dorsal aspect of the PIP joint along the midline proximally and distally curving around the dorsal aspect of the PIP joint, exposing the extensor mechanism (**TECH FIG 2A**).
- A distally based, V-shaped flap of central slip with the pedicle extending as far as the proximal third of the proximal phalanx is made (**TECH FIG 2B**).
- The extensor flap is reflected distally, allowing the intact lateral bands to slip palmarly and laterally, providing a wide exposure of the PIP joint.
- On completion of the surgery, the central slip is securely sutured in place with 4-0 nonabsorbable suture.
- The repair is strong and will allow early active motion within the first 48 hours.

Mid-Axial Approach

- Identify the midaxial line by marking the axes of the IP joints and drawing a line through these points proximally and distally (**TECH FIG 3A**).

- Make the skin incision on this midaxial line. The digital nerve and artery lie about 2 mm volar to the margin of the incision (**TECH FIG 3B**).
- Avoid a radial-sided incision on the index finger and an ulnar-sided incision on the small finger. These surfaces are important for contact and should be protected from potential scar sensitivity.
- The first structure encountered in the subcutaneous fat is Cleland's ligament, which contains fibers that run volar to dorsal and consist of thin fascial layers surrounding the digital nerve and artery with skin. It can be isolated from adjacent fat at the level of the PIP joint.
- Once Cleland's ligament is divided, carry the dissection slightly volarward, deep to the neurovascular bundle, and expose the lateral aspect of the middle phalanx and lateral margin of the flexor sheath.
  - The neurovascular bundle remains in the volar flap.
- Enter the joint between the volar plate and the accessory collateral ligament and inspect the joint.
- Additional exposure is gained by elevating the collateral ligament at the origin or the insertion.

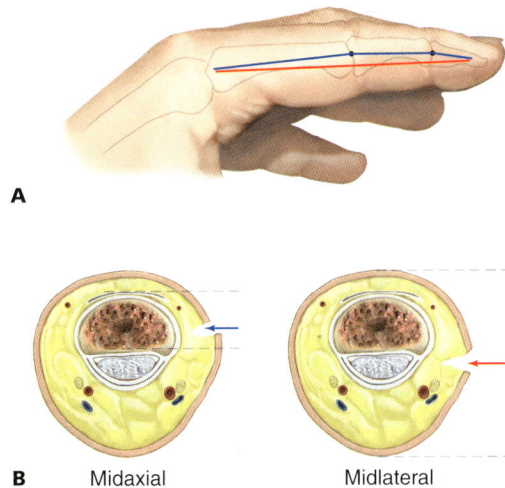

TECH FIG 3 • **A.** Diagrams demonstrating the midaxial (*blue line*) and midlateral (*red line*) approaches. The midlateral approach is shown for reference, but the midaxial approach is the one most often used clinically. Midaxial approach (*blue*): flex the finger and mark the motion axes of the IP joints by marking the points at the IP joints where the flexion creases end dorsally. Draw a line through these points proximally and distally (*blue line*). **B.** In a cross-section diagram of these approaches, the midaxial dissection will be dorsal to the neurovascular bundle and the midlateral dissection will be at the level of the neurovascular bundle.

FRACTURE AND JOINT REDUCTION

- The joint and fractures are exposed, cleansed of hematoma, and fully evaluated.
  - If soft tissues are interposed, a fine curved hemostat or dental pick may be introduced to clear the fracture site.

- A dental pick or Freer elevator may be used to carefully manipulate and elevate depressed articular fragments, restoring articular congruity.
  - Maintain cancellous and subchondral bone on the articular cartilage-bearing fragments.

- Cancellous bone grafting may be required to prevent articular surface collapse in highly comminuted fractures.
  - Allo- or autograft (often harvested from the dorsal distal radius) can be used. The graft material is packed into the metaphysis through either direct application or a cortical window.
- Small 0.045- or 0.030-inch K-wires may be used to provisionally stabilize the reduction.
- Preliminary joint reduction, fracture reduction, and articular restoration are confirmed under direct vision and with fluoroscopy.
- Fracture fixation may proceed through various methods, depending on fracture pattern and surgeon-preference.

- Following definitive fixation, the digit is put through full ROM under fluoroscopy to ensure a stable concentric reduction has been achieved without sign of abnormal joint motion.
  - Close evaluation of lateral fluoroscopic images is critical to ensure that the PIP joint does not remain dorsally subluxated.
  - If the joint is not concentrically reduced or the internal fixation of the fracture is tenuous, it may be augmented with dynamic external fixation,[13] extension block pinning, or a transarticular K-wire.[5]

MINI-FRAGMENT FIXATION

- Screw fixation, if attainable, provides excellent stability and may allow earlier ROM and improved functional restoration. This form of stabilization is indicated for larger and fewer fragments (**TECH FIG 4A–D**).
  - Be aware that these fragments are often more comminuted than believed, and screws may further comminute the bone, making ultimate fixation difficult.[8]
- After anatomic reduction of the fragments is achieved by careful manipulation and the fragments are stabilized with clamps or K-wires (as needed), appropriately sized screws, typically in the 1.0- to 1.7-mm range, are chosen.
- The screw hole is drilled as perpendicular to the fracture plane as possible.
- The depth is measured.

- If possible, an interfragmentary lag technique is preferred. This is done by overdrilling the near fragment cortex with a drill equal to the screw's outer diameter.
- A self-tapping, minifragment cortical screw is placed.
  - Countersinking of screws or use of headless screws may be helpful to avoid soft tissue tethering and tendon irritation (**TECH FIG 4E**).
- If the fragment is large enough, two screws, or a screw and a supplementary threaded K-wire (0.028 inch), can be used to prevent rotation of the fragment (**TECH FIG 4F,G**).
- After the procedure, PIP joint ROM usually is compromised, with a residual flexion contracture occurring in more than 80% of cases of volar fracture and dorsal instability.[11]

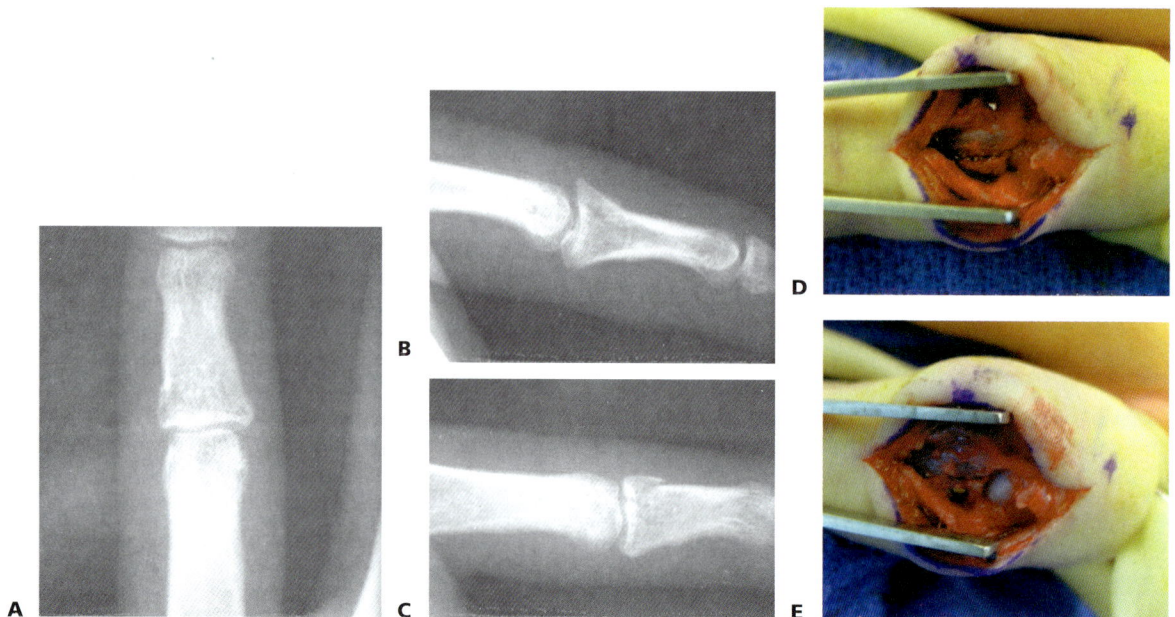

TECH FIG 4 • **A–C.** Preoperative AP, lateral, and oblique radiographs demonstrating a displaced small finger PIP intra-articular fracture with a large dorsal/ulnar fragment. **D,E.** Intraoperative photos show the dorsal approach to the PIP joint. **D.** The fragment was large enough to be amenable to microscrew fixation. **E.** Using standard AO technique, a 1.7-mm screw was placed to achieve stable fixation of the fragment. The head of the screw has been countersunk. (continued)

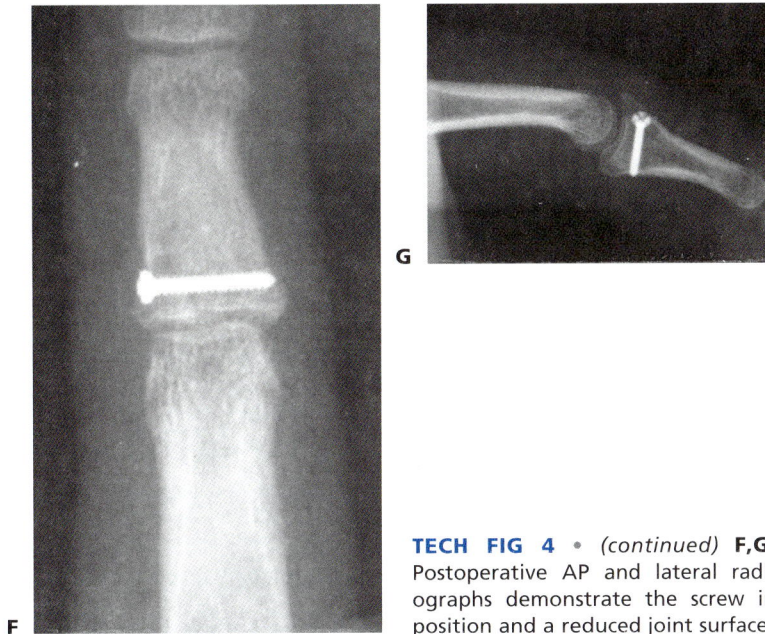

TECH FIG 4 • *(continued)* **F,G.** Postoperative AP and lateral radiographs demonstrate the screw in position and a reduced joint surface.

CERCLAGE WIRE TECHNIQUE

- The cerclage wire technique[20] allows reduction of multiple small articular fragments and provides adequate fixation to allow early ROM exercises (**TECH FIG 5A**).
  - A thorough joint release is required, which carries the risk of increased fibrosis and stiffness postoperatively.
- A volar incision with a "shotgun" exposure of the PIP joint is used (**TECH FIG 5B**).
- Judicious elevation of the central slip is performed.

- A thin ring of periosteum around the bony fragments of the middle phalanx is cleared by sharp dissection.
  - This allows the wire loop to seat directly against bone, providing firm fixation of the fracture fragments.
  - The normal shape of the base of the middle phalanx (reverse funnel contour) also aids in fixation of the wire and prevents postoperative slippage, even with early ROM.

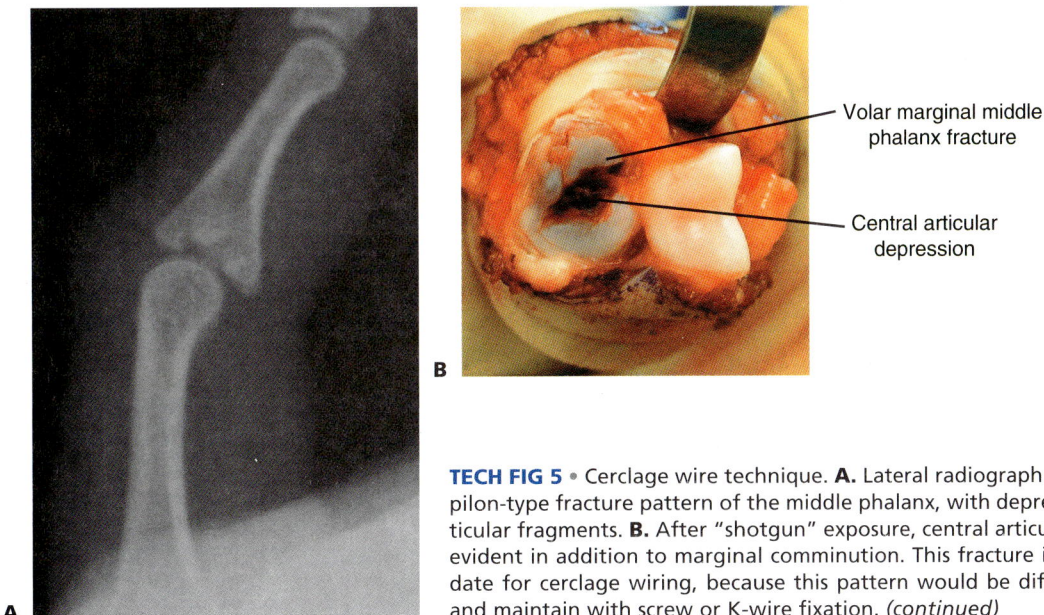

TECH FIG 5 • Cerclage wire technique. **A.** Lateral radiograph demonstrates a pilon-type fracture pattern of the middle phalanx, with depressed central articular fragments. **B.** After "shotgun" exposure, central articular impaction is evident in addition to marginal comminution. This fracture is a good candidate for cerclage wiring, because this pattern would be difficult to reduce and maintain with screw or K-wire fixation. *(continued)*

TECHNIQUES

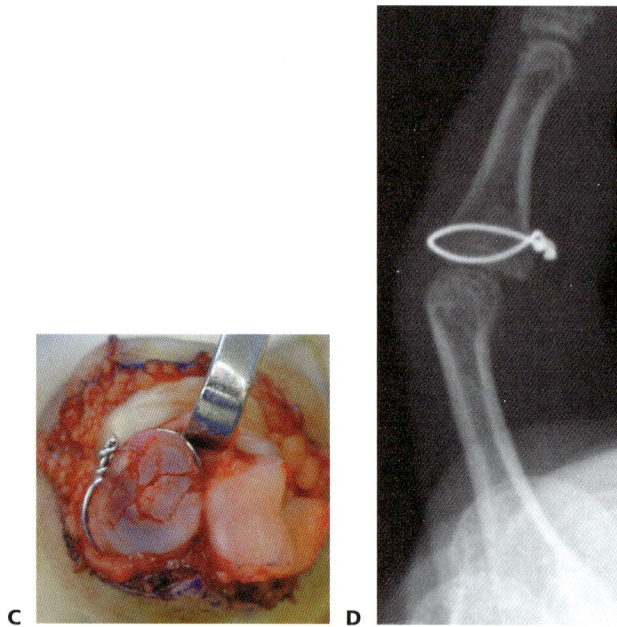

TECH FIG 5 • *(continued)* **C.** The central fragment has been reduced and a 24-gauge steel wire was formed into a loop and gently placed, allowing circumferential compression of the fracture fragments. **D.** A postoperative lateral radiograph confirms correction of the central articular depression.

- 24-gauge steel wire is formed into a loop and twisted on itself until the loop is partially closed, just larger than the base of the middle phalanx.
- After fracture reduction, the loop of wire is seated and gently tightened, allowing circumferential compression of the fracture fragments (**TECH FIG 5C**).
- Final confirmation of articular reduction is made, with careful attention to the correction of central depression and joint subluxation (**TECH FIG 5D**).
- The twisted portion of the loop is placed on the volar or volar lateral surface or the middle phalanx base, flush to the cortex, at the edge of the volar plate.
- The wire is covered by the repaired volar plate to prevent mechanical irritation of the flexor tendons.

Supplementary K-Wire Addition

- A supplementary K-wire may be necessary, depending on fracture configuration (**TECH FIG 6A,B**).
- The cerclage wire is loosely twisted around the base of the middle phalanx, maintaining the position of the articular fragments prior to the replacement of the central and volar depressed fragment (**TECH FIG 6C**).
- After replacement of the central fragment and further fixation with a K-wire, the cerclage wire is tightened (**TECH FIG 6D,E**) and the tail cut.

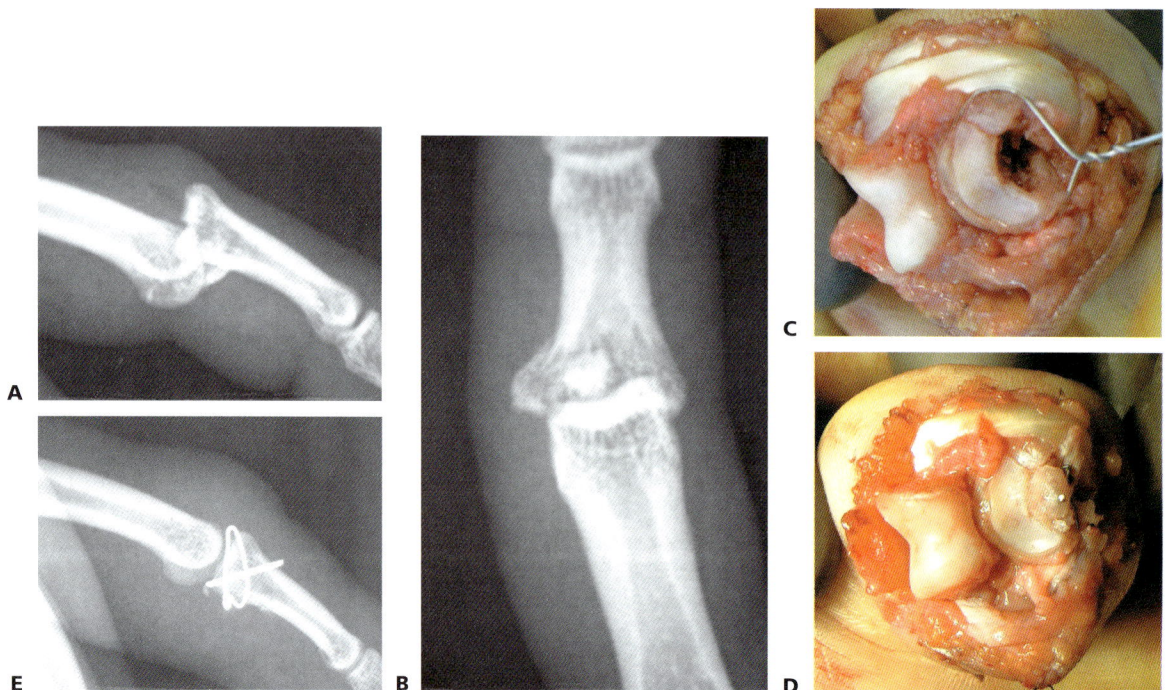

TECH FIG 6 • Cerclage wire technique with K-wire supplementation. **A,B.** Preoperative lateral and AP injury radiographs demonstrating a dorsal fracture-dislocation with central and volar articular depression and comminution. **C.** The cerclage wire is twisted loosely to around the base of the middle phalanx, maintaining the position of the articular fragments before reduction of the central and volar depressed fragment. **D.** After reduction of the central fragment and further fixation with a K-wire, the cerclage wire is tightened. The "tail" is then turned 90 degrees so that it is flush with the bone and cut. **E.** A postoperative lateral radiograph demonstrates restoration of the articular surface and reduction of the dislocation.

CLOSURE AND SPLINTING

- The volar plate and central slip flaps are closed with a 4-0 nonabsorbable suture.
- The flexor tendon sheath is closed using either absorbable or nonabsorbable 5-0 or 6-0 suture.
- The tourniquet is deflated, and hemostasis is achieved with bipolar cautery.
- The skin is closed with 5-0 nylon suture.
- The patient is placed into an intrinsic-plus volar splint. Usually, the MP joints are flexed 70 to 90 degrees and the IP joints are extended based on the stability of fixation and joint reduction.

PEARLS AND PITFALLS

- PIP fracture-dislocations often are missed by athletic trainers and patients, dismissed as a "jammed finger."[9,14,23]
- Avoid forceful passive testing for stability, which can convert a partial tear to a complete one. Instability of any of these structures to passive stress is unlikely to change the management of an injury that is stable with active range of motion. The one potential exception to this is complete rupture of the radial collateral ligament of the index finger PIP joint in a young active patient. This injury may be surgically repaired primarily because stability at this joint (required for a normal pinch grip) may be more important than full ROM.[10]
- Make sure to preserve the A2 and A4 pulleys. Failure to do so will result in bowstringing of the flexor tendons and a failed outcome.
- Screw fixation should not be attempted for fracture fragments that are too small or too comminuted (eg, more than three fragments).
- Make sure to angle the K-wire or screw toward the distal dorsal cortex to maximize screw length and purchase.
- Fracture fragments are delicate. Take your time and select the correct starting location and track of the screws and K-wires. Multiple passes will result in poor fixation and further fracture fragmentation.
- After screw or K-wire insertion, check a lateral radiograph to ensure that the implant does not violate the extensor mechanism.
- To avoid recurrent dislocation, any bony defect remaining behind the repaired volar plate complex should be filled with bone graft. Otherwise, the head of the proximal phalanx will fall into the defect, resulting in recurrent dorsal subluxation of the middle phalanx.

POSTOPERATIVE CARE

- Progressive active and active assisted range of motion does not begin until postoperative day 2 to 5, depending on initial patient comfort.
  - A thermoplastic splint provides protected mobilization.
  - Relatively more aggressive flexion than extension (less than 30 degrees) is pursued with the therapist.
- Close weekly follow-up for the first 3 weeks is necessary to monitor for any loss of reduction.
- All restrictions on motion are removed at 5 to 6 weeks, and radiographic signs of healing are followed.
- Therapy is continued for 1 to 2 months after removal of the splint, to recover motion and strengthen the hand.

OUTCOMES

- Green and Akelman reported on two patients with dorsal fracture-dislocations who underwent ORIF and reported an average active range of motion of 95 degrees at 1-year follow-up, with neither patient demonstrating any evidence of subluxation.[10,13]
- Hastings and Carroll[12] reported on 15 patients treated with ORIF using various combinations of K-wire fixation, tension band wire fixation, and screw fixation. Eventual average postoperative ROM was 17 to 90 degrees.
- Dietch et al[5] reported on 24 patients with unstable dorsal fracture dislocations of the PIP joint treated with two methods, volar plate arthroplasty and ORIF. At an average follow-up of 46 months, results indicated that if reduction of the joint is maintained, patients could expect few functional deficits despite radiographic degenerative changes and loss of mobility.
- Weiss[20] reported on 12 patients with dorsal fracture-dislocations treated with cerclage wire fixation and reported an average ROM of 89 degrees at 2 years follow-up, with no complications and only one patient with evidence of radiographic degenerative changes.
- Stern et al[19] reported on 20 patients with pilon fracture-dislocations of the PIP joint. They used three treatment methods: splinting, skeletal traction, and open reduction with K-wire fixation. After a clinical and radiographic follow-up of 25 months, skeletal traction led to fewer complications and clinically comparable outcomes to open reduction (achieving an average ROM of 80 degrees vs. 70 degrees, respectively).
- While clinical experience supports anatomic reduction of intra-articular fractures in weight-bearing joints such as the hip or knee, most laboratory and clinical reports support the theory that anatomic surface restoration is unnecessary if subluxation is corrected and motion is instituted shortly after injury.[1,11,17]

COMPLICATIONS

- Degenerative arthritis
- Loss of PIP joint motion, stiffness, flexion contracture, and extensor lag
- Loss of fixation or redisplacement
- Persistent subluxation or dislocation
- Infection
- Malunion
- Boutonnière deformity
- Pain

REFERENCES

1. Agee JM. Unstable fracture dislocations of the proximal interphalangeal joint. Treatment with the force couple splint. Clin Orthop Relat Res 1987;214:101–112.
2. Blazar PE, Steinberg DR. Fractures of the proximal interphalangeal joint. J Am Acad Orthop Surg 2000;8:383–390.
3. Bruner JM. Surgical exposure of the flexor tendons in the hand. Ann R Coll Surg Engl 1973;53:84–94.
4. Chamay A. A distally based dorsal and triangular tendinous flap for direct access to proximal interphalangeal joint. Ann Chir Main 1988;7:179–183.
5. Deitch MA, Kiefhaber TR, Stern PJ. Dorsal fracture dislocations of the proximal interphalangeal joint: surgical complications and long-term results. J Hand Surg Am 1999;24:914–923.
6. Eaton RG, Malerich MM. Volar plate arthroplasty for the proximal interphalangeal joint: A review of ten years' experience. J Hand Surg Am 1980;5:260–268.
7. Elson RA. Rupture of the central slip of the extensor hood of the finger. A test for early diagnosis. J Bone Joint Surg Br 1986;68B:229–231.
8. Freeland AE, Benoist LA. Open reduction and internal fixation method for fractures at the proximal interphalangeal joint. Hand Clin 1994;10:239–250.
9. Glickel SZ, Barron OA. Proximal interphalangeal joint fracture dislocations. Hand Clinics 2000;16:333–344.
10. Green A, Akelman E, et al. Acute open reduction and rigid internal fixation of proximal interphalangeal joint fracture dislocation. J Hand Surg Am 1992;17:512–517.
11. Hamilton SC, Stern PJ, Fassler PR, et al. Mini-screw fixation of proximal interphalangeal joint dorsal fracture-dislocations. J Hand Surg Am 2006;31:1349–1354.
12. Hastings H, Carroll C. Treatment of closed articular fractures of the metacarpophalangeal and proximal interphalangeal joints. Hand Clin 1999;6:429–453.
13. Kiefhaber TR, Stern PJ. Fracture dislocations of the proximal interphalangeal joint. J Hand Surg Am 1998;23:368–380.
14. Kiefhaber TR, Stern PJ, Grood ES. Lateral stability of the proximal interphalangeal joint. J Hand Surg Am 1986;11:661–669.
15. Malerich MM, Eaton RG. The volar plate reconstruction for fracture-dislocation of the proximal interphalangeal joint. Hand Clin 1994;10:251–260.
16. McCue FC, Honner R, Johnson MC, et al. Athletic injuries of the proximal interphalangeal joint requiring surgical treatment. J Bone Joint Surg Am 1970;52A:937–956.
17. Morgan JP, et. al. Dynamic digital traction for unstable comminuted intraarticular fracture-dislocations of the proximal interphalangeal joint. J Hand Surg Am 1995;20:565–573.
18. Schenck RR. Dynamic traction and early passive movement for fractures of the proximal interphalangeal joint. J Hand Surg Am 1986;11:850–858.
19. Stern PJ, Roman RJ, Kiefhaber TR, et al. Pilon fractures of the proximal interphalangeal joint. J Hand Surg Am 1991;16:844–850.
20. Weiss AP. Cerclage fixation for fracture dislocation of the proximal interphalangeal joint. Clin Orthop Relat Res 1996;327:21–28.
21. Weiss AP, Hastings H 2nd. Distal unicondylar fractures of the proximal phalanx. J Hand Surg Am 1993;18:594–599.
22. Williams RM, Kiefhaber TR, Sommerkamp TG, et al. Treatment of unstable dorsal proximal interphalangeal fracture/dislocations using hemi-hamate autograft. J Hand Surg Am 2003;28:856–865.
23. Wolfe SW, Katz LD. Intra-articular impaction fractures of the phalanges. J Hand Surg Am 1995;20:327–333.

Chapter 37

Volar Plate Arthroplasty

Albert Leung and Philip E. Blazar

DEFINITION

- Volar plate arthroplasty (VPA) provides a volar restraint to dorsal subluxation and dislocation of either the middle or distal phalanx base to maintain reduction of the proximal interphalangeal (PIP) or distal interphalangeal (DIP) joint. It resurfaces the volar portion of the injured joint using local tissue (volar plate).
- VPA is used much more commonly for PIP joint stability than DIP joint stability.

ANATOMY

- The volar plate, which is the primary restraint against hyperextension instability, lies palmar to both the PIP and DIP joints, separating the joint from the flexor tendon(s).
  - At its origin, the volar plate is "swallowtail" shaped and connected only by proximal checkrein ligaments to the phalanx and fiberosseous tendon sheath (**FIG 1A**).
  - Distally, the VP is primarily cartilaginous. It inserts centrally via the periosteum and laterally with a conjoined insertion through the collateral ligaments (**FIG 1B**).
  - The volar plate glides proximally and distally with joint motion.
- The collateral ligaments originate on the dorsal radial and dorsal ulnar surfaces proximal to the joint. The proper collateral ligaments insert on the volar radial and volar ulnar surface distal to the joint, and the accessory collateral ligaments insert into the lateral margin of the volar plate, creating a box-type configuration (see Fig 1B).
  - In subacute or chronic cases of dorsal joint subluxation or dislocation, these ligaments contract, thereby accentuating the deformity by virtue of their oblique orientation.
- The flexor digitorum superficialis (FDS) inserts just distal to the volar plate on the middle phalanx.
  - Due to the direction of pull, forces exerted by the FDS may accentuate dorsal subluxation of the middle phalanx base when the volar restraints are lost.

PATHOGENESIS

- Injuries to the PIP and DIP are caused by longitudinal compression or hyperextension forces (common in sports injuries) and typically occur in young, active individuals.
- Dorsal fracture dislocations of the PIP occur with damage to the volar articular surface of the middle phalanx when a force drives it dorsally against the condyles of the proximal phalanx.
- Chronic subluxation or dislocation (more than 6 weeks) often occurs, especially with the PIP joint when the injury is perceived as minor and is considered a "sprain."

NATURAL HISTORY

- Chronic subluxation of the PIP joint leads to poor function and degenerative arthritis.
  - Flexion of the joint is limited and painful.

- Despite optimal surgical treatment, PIP joint fracture-dislocations often result in some loss of PIP or DIP joint motion.
- PIP joint injuries, even those that do not require surgical treatment, commonly result in a protracted period of symptoms (eg, swelling, stiffness, pain) beyond what patients expect from a "minor" injury.

PATIENT HISTORY AND PHYSICAL FINDINGS

- When taking the patient's history, ask about the mechanism of injury, time since injury, any prior injuries, and the direction of deformity. Time since injury and mechanism of injury help determine the most appropriate treatment for any particular PIP joint injury.

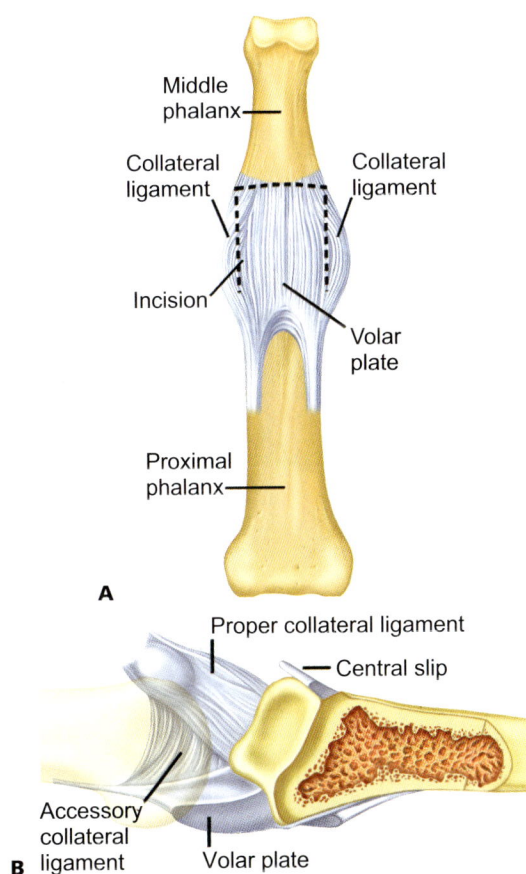

FIG 1 • **A.** Volar view of the PIP joint. The PIP joint is supported by ligamentous structures that include the collateral ligaments on each side, with the volar plate and flexor tendons underneath. **B.** Sagittal view of the PIP joint showing the relative positions of the central slip, volar plate, collateral ligaments, and accessory collateral ligaments.

2431

- Inspect the finger for any swelling or deformity. Clinical deformity may be subtle, even with significant subluxation.
- Examine range of motion, noting degrees of PIP motion. With joint subluxation, patients will have painful and limited flexion.
- Examine joint stability; joints that are dislocatable will need intervention for stability (eg, extension block splinting, VPA).

IMAGING AND OTHER DIAGNOSTIC STUDIES

- Every patient with a PIP injury must have anteroposterior, lateral, and oblique radiographs to evaluate for a PIP joint fracture or subluxation (**FIG 2A**).
  - The severity of the fracture and degree of involvement of the middle phalanx often are much greater than they appear on these radiographs.
- In evaluating for a subluxation by radiographs, a true lateral view of the PIP joint is mandatory. A dorsal V sign at the joint indicates that the articular surfaces are neither congruent nor parallel (**FIG 2B**).
- Fluoroscopy allows dynamic evaluation of the joint and its stability and often is also the best way to obtain magnified images and a perfect lateral view.
- CT scans rarely are needed but can effectively evaluate the articular surfaces and define the bone loss.

DIFFERENTIAL DIAGNOSIS

- Acute central slip injury (ie, boutonniere deformity)
- PIP joint fracture

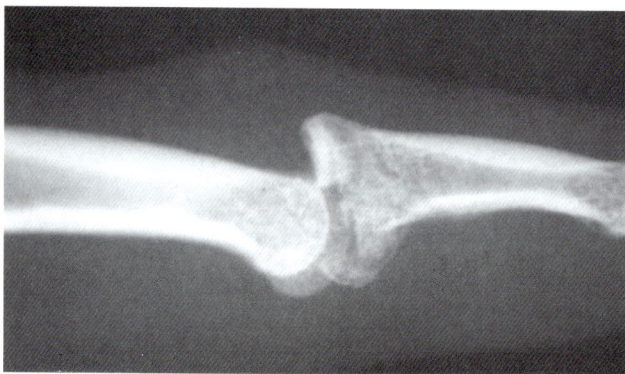

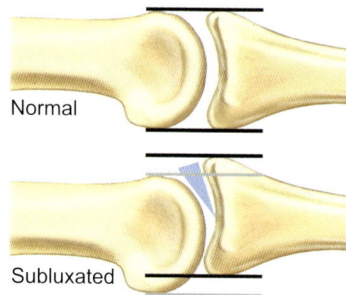

FIG 2 • A. Lateral radiograph of subluxation of the PIP joint. **B.** PIP joint subluxations typically display a signature dorsal V sign on the lateral radiograph, as described by Light.[6]

- PIP dislocation
- Volar plate or collateral ligament sprain without instability

NONOPERATIVE MANAGEMENT

- Closed reduction and extension block splinting are appropriate for PIP fracture subluxations when a stable concentric joint reduction is obtained and maintained in an acceptable position.
  - If more than 65 degrees of flexion is required to maintain reduction, surgical reconstruction should be strongly considered.
- Articular defects will often dramatically remodel in a concentrically reduced, mobilized joint.

SURGICAL MANAGEMENT

- For simplicity, the techniques here describe VPA for the PIP joint, but the same principles may apply to the DIP joint. The primary difference is that the FDP insertion on the volar base of the distal phalanx makes exposure of the volar plate more complicated.
- Indications
  - Acute fracture-dislocations that are unstable after closed reduction of the PIP joint in cases in which the volar base of the middle phalanx is not reconstructable, or if surgical reconstruction is less likely to achieve a functional result
  - Chronic subluxations or dislocations up to 2 years following trauma
  - A normal articular contour of the proximal phalanx is a prerequisite.
  - An intact dorsal cortex and dorsal articular surface are required.
  - Some authors (eg, Burton[4]) use VPA for chronic osteoarthritis in select situations.

Preoperative Planning

- Fractures typically involve over 30% of the surface of the middle phalanx base, and the joint is subluxated or dislocated. If the fracture involves under 30% of the joint surface, it typically can be managed either in a closed manner or with less invasive techniques for the acute scenario.
- The literature is unclear whether a specific degree of involvement of the articular surface precludes VPA (ie, is too large), but involvement of the dorsal cortex is a contraindication.
  - VPA is a less successful treatment for injuries involving over 50% to 60% of the middle phalanx articular surface. In these cases, recurrent subluxation is common.
- In chronic dislocations, soft tissue contracture and heterotopic bone may make dissection and relocation more complex.

Positioning

- The patient is positioned supine on the operating table with the affected arm on a hand table.
- Intraoperative fluoroscopy is critical to this procedure, and it is important to position the hand relative to the fluoroscopy unit so that a true lateral view of the injured PIP joint may easily be obtained.
- The surgery is performed under tourniquet control.

PRIMARY INCISIONS AND EXCISIONS ON THE VOLAR SIDE

- The joint is exposed using two limbs of a Bruner incision centered at the PIP flexion crease, elevating a radially based flap (**TECH FIG 1A**).
- The radial and ulnar neurovascular bundles are identified and mobilized throughout the field to prevent a traction injury when the PIP joint is hyperextended to achieve optimal visualization (**TECH FIG 1B**).

- The flexor sheath is incised as a rectangular flap between the A2 and A4 pulleys and protected for later repair.
- The flexor tendons are atraumatically retracted radially or ulnarly, as needed to visualize the volar plate (**TECH FIG 1C,D**).

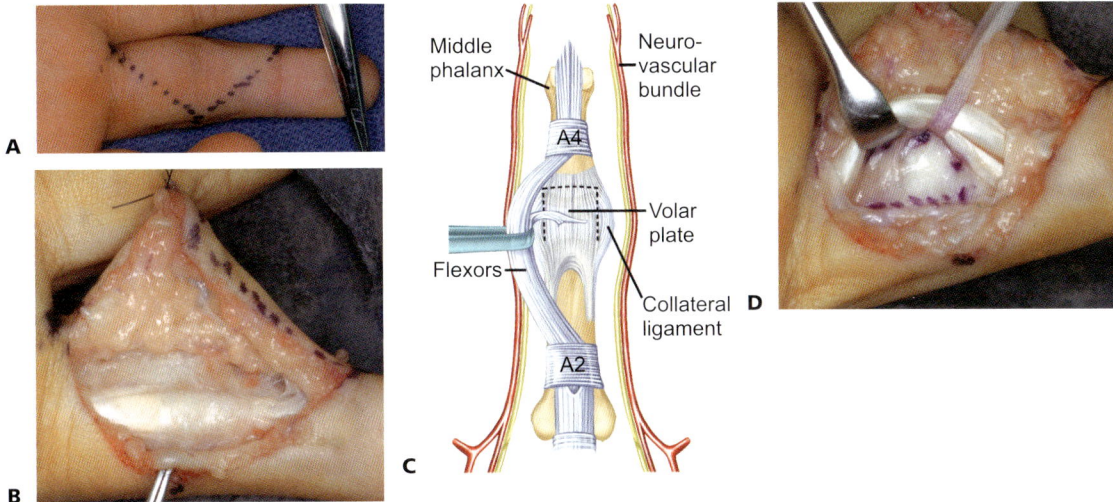

TECH FIG 1 • A. The Bruner incision is centered over the PIP flexion crease, with the vertex on the ulnar side. **B.** To prevent traction injuries, mobilization of the neurovascular bundles is necessary. **C.** Illustration of retraction of the flexor tendons and neurovascular bundles relative to the volar plate. **D.** The flexor tendons must be retracted radially and ulnarly to access the volar plate. The proposed incision to detach and mobilize the volar plate is outlined in pen.

DETACHMENT OF THE VOLAR PLATE

- The volar plate is detached from the middle phalanx or fracture fragments, including as much tissue as possible.
- The volar plate is incised from the proper and accessory collateral ligaments through an incision along its radial- and ulnar-most margins (Tech Fig 1D).
- The volar plate flap must be as long and broad as possible to maintain adequate stability of the arthroplasty. It should be symmetrical radially and ulnarly to avoid angular deformities.
- The collateral ligaments are excised.
- The joint is then hyperextended approximately 180 degrees ("shotgunning") to achieve maximum visualization of the base of the middle phalanx (**TECH FIG 2**).
- Small fragments of depressed articular cartilage or subchondral bone are débrided and saved for possible later use.
- Care is taken to avoid over-resection and loss of the dorsal articular support.

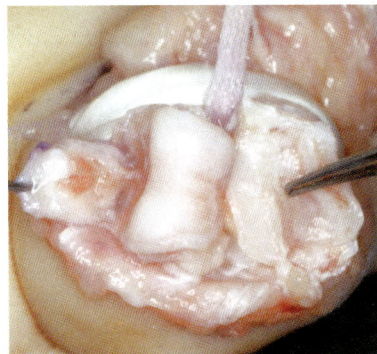

TECH FIG 2 • Shotgunning. Hyperextending the joint allows clear visualization of the volar plate to the left, the avulsed bone, and the articular surface of each phalanx. The trough is fashioned symmetrically in the coronal plane, at the dorsal-most aspect of the articular defect to the right.

TECHNIQUES

SHAPING THE ARTICULAR SURFACE OF THE MIDDLE PHALANX

- A transverse trough is fashioned with an osteotome or a rongeur across the middle phalanx and finished with a small curette, at the juncture between the intact articular surface and the fracture defect (Tech Fig 2).

- This trough must be symmetric in the coronal plane to avoid angular deformity. The depth of the trough at its dorsal side should be the thickness of the volar plate, thereby allowing a smooth transition from articular cartilage to transposed volar plate.

TRANSPOSING THE VOLAR PLATE

- A 3-0 nonabsorbable grasping suture (eg, Bunnell fashion) is placed in both the ulnar- and radial-most margins of the volar plate flap (**TECH FIG 3A**).
- Two straight Keith needles are passed through each side of the base of the middle phalanx using a wire driver. They are placed as far radially, ulnarly, and distally in the bone defect as possible, and directed centrally to penetrate the cortex distal to the central slip insertion (**TECH FIG 3B**).
  - The sutures are tensioned as the middle phalanx is flexed, bringing the volar plate into the defect at a level that produces a smooth transition from the intact dorsal base of the middle phalanx to the volar plate.

- The joint should remain flexed about 20 to 25 degrees so the volar plate can advance both distally and dorsally.
- Examine the reduction with a true lateral fluoroscopic view on a mini C-arm (**TECH FIG 3C**).
  - The base of the middle phalanx should glide over the head of the proximal phalanx and should not hinge open dorsally.
  - The fingertip should be able to touch the distal palmar crease (110 degrees of flexion).
- If the PIP joint lacks substantial extension or has inadequate flexion, it may be necessary to advance the volar plate distally by teasing the checkrein ligaments from their origin or by fractional lengthening through step-cutting (Tech Fig 3A).

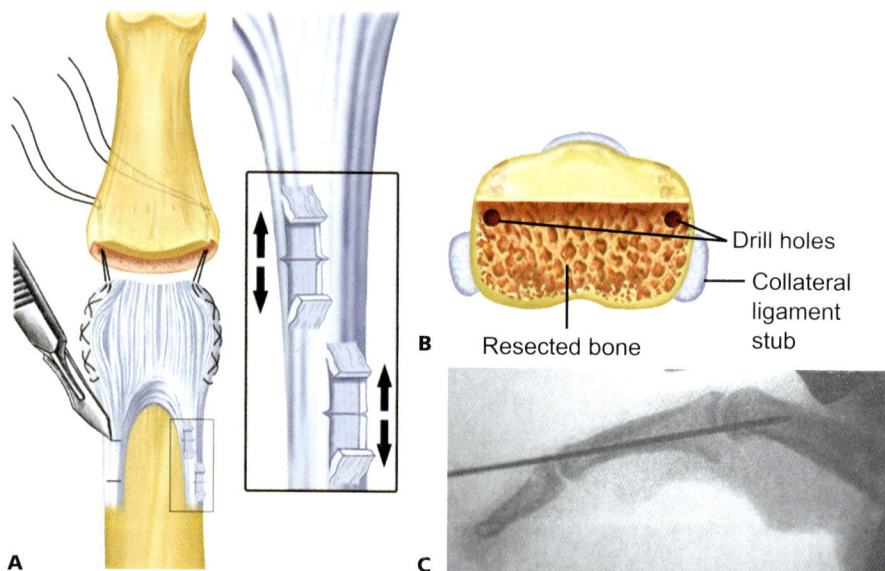

B Resected bone

Drill holes

Collateral ligament stub

A

C

TECH FIG 3 • A. Suturing the volar plate. Sutures are passed through the margins of the volar plate and through the base of the middle phalanx using straight Keith needles. The volar plate is advanced into the trough, resurfacing the PIP joint. It may be necessary to advance the volar plate by step-cut lengthening of the checkrein ligaments. **B.** Bone resection. This diagram shows the needle holes in relation to the resected bone, the collateral ligament stubs, and the extensor mechanism central tendon. The holes in the middle phalanx should be as far dorsal and lateral as possible for maximum stability. **C.** The PIP joint has now been reduced and stabilized as shown.

SECURING THE VOLAR PLATE

- The sutures may be tied over a button dorsally.
  - Alternatively, the sutures may be tied directly onto periosteum via a small incision distal to the central slip insertion. Care must be taken to ensure the sutures do not entrap the lateral bands or injure the central slip.

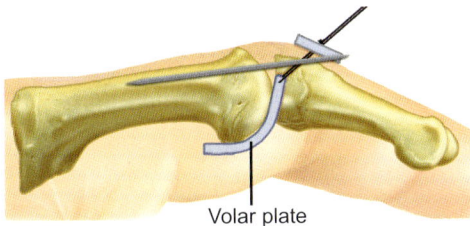

Volar plate

- In the acute setting, fractured bone fragments collected during the volar plate detachment may be placed in the defect of the middle phalanx, distal to the advanced volar plate. This provides support to the base of the phalanx.
- A K-wire is used with the joint in slight flexion to maintain reduction for 3 weeks (**TECH FIG 4**).
  - Alternatively, the joint reduction can be maintained with an articulated external fixator to allow for early motion.

TECH FIG 4 • Lateral diagram of VPA. The overall diagram of this procedure illustrates the joint with a double-ended K-wire for stability and the volar plate secured by sutures.

PEARLS AND PITFALLS

Angular deformity	■ The trough must be transverse, and tension of the volar plate flap must be symmetric on the two sides.
Recurrent subluxation	■ Fixation with a K-wire or articulated fixator for 2 to 3 weeks is recommended.
Loss of flexion	■ Aggressive range of motion to restore flexion at both the PIP and DIP joints is essential and safe, because these injuries typically are more stable in flexion.
Neurologic injury	■ Meticulous dissection of both neurovascular bundles is required before "shotgunning" the joint open.
Loss of extension	■ Some loss of extension is expected. Failure to lengthen the checkrein ligaments may lead to an unacceptable contracture.

POSTOPERATIVE CARE

- The K-wire PIP joint fixation is removed at 2 to 3 weeks, when active flexion and extension are begun.
- An extension block splint is used during weeks 3 to 6 after the operation.
- Motion of the DIP is encouraged before K-wire removal, because deficits in DIP motion have been reported after VPA.
- After 6 weeks, the pullout suture, if one was used, is removed.
- A dynamic extension splint may be used at 6 weeks if the achieved extension is not as expected based on intraoperative range of motion.

OUTCOMES

- More normal PIP motion is restored in acute injuries than in chronic injuries: 85 degrees of active PIP motion versus 60 degrees.
- Patients can expect to see continued improvement in range of motion up to 1 year after VPA.
- Mild contractures of the DIP joint (10 to 20 degrees) are common. Patients are encouraged in DIP motion during rehabilitation.

COMPLICATIONS

- Resubluxation or dislocation
- Flexion contracture of the PIP or DIP joint

- Angular deformities
- Pin and wire track infections
- Pain
- Stiffness
- Degenerative arthrosis

REFERENCES

1. Blazar PE, Robbe R, Lawton JN. Treatment of dorsal fracture/dislocations of the proximal interphalangeal joint by volar plate arthroplasty. Tech Hand Up Extrem Surg 2001;5:148–152.
2. Blazar PE, Steinberg DR. Fractures of the proximal interphalangeal joint. J Am Acad Orthop Surg 2000;8:383–390.
3. Bowers WH, Wolf JW, Nehil JL, et al. The proximal interphalangeal joint volar plate. I. An anatomical and biomechanical study. J Hand Surg Am 1980;5:79–88.
4. Burton RI, Campolattaro RM, Ronchetti PJ. Volar plate arthroplasty for osteoarthritis of the proximal interphalangeal joint: a preliminary report. J Hand Surg Am 2002;27:1065–1072.
5. Eaton RG, Malerich MM. Volar plate arthroplasty of the proximal interphalangeal joint: a review of ten years' experience. J Hand Surg Am 1980;5:260–268.
6. Light TR. Buttress pinning techniques. Orthop Rev 1981;10:49–55.
7. Malerich MM, Eaton RG. The volar plate reconstruction for fracture-dislocation of the proximal interphalangeal joint. Hand Clin 1994;10:251–260.
8. Rettig ME, Dassa G, Raskin KB. Volar plate arthroplasty of the distal interphalangeal joint. J Hand Surg Am 2001;26:940–944.

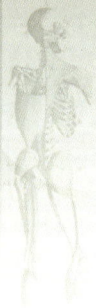

Chapter 38

Hemi-Hamate Autograft Reconstruction of Unstable Dorsal Proximal Interphalangeal Joint Fracture-Dislocations

Thomas R. Kiefhaber, Rafael M. M. Williams, and Soma I. Lilly

DEFINITION

- Proximal interphalangeal (PIP) joint fracture-dislocations occur with the following fracture patterns[9]:
  - Palmar lip fracture-dislocations: Fracture of the middle phalanx palmar lip with dorsal subluxation of the middle phalanx on the head of the proximal phalanx
  - Dorsal lip fracture-dislocations: Fracture of the dorsal lip of the middle phalanx with palmar subluxation of the middle phalanx
  - Pilon fractures: Pilon fractures include a loss of continuity of both the dorsal and palmar cortical margins of the middle phalangeal articular surface. The base of the middle phalanx usually is highly comminuted, and the articular fragments may be significantly impacted.
- PIP fractures are further classified as "stable" or "unstable."
  - Stable fractures maintain concentric joint reduction throughout the range of motion (ROM).
  - Unstable fractures sublux or dislocate during parts of the motion arc.
- Dorsal lip fracture treatment is complicated by the need to re-establish continuity of the extensor tendon insertion onto the middle phalanx.
- Pilon fractures are best treated with some form of traction and early motion.
- Unstable palmar lip fractures are amenable to treatment with hemi-hamate autograft and are the focus of this chapter.

ANATOMY

- The PIP joint is a complex hinge articulation that provides more than 95 degrees of flexion while maintaining stable, concentric reduction of the joint surfaces.
- Several forces encourage dorsal migration of the middle phalanx: the extensor tendon lifts the middle phalanx and the mid-middle phalanx superficialis insertion levers the middle phalanx dorsally[5] (**FIG 1A**).
- The only restraints on middle phalangeal dorsal translation are the palmar plate and the cup-shaped geometry of the middle phalanx articular surface. The middle phalangeal palmar lip wraps around the proximal phalanx head and acts as a hook, preventing dorsal translation.
- Palmar lip fractures disrupt both of the restraints to dorsal subluxation. The palmar plate is no longer attached, and the middle phalangeal palmar lip is disrupted. The slope of the remaining middle phalangeal articular surface encourages the middle phalanx to travel up and over the proximal phalangeal head.
- A direct relation exists between the amount of palmar articular surface disrupted and stability (**FIG 1B**).
  - Hastings[6] has shown that when 42% of the palmar articular surface is damaged, the joint always exhibits dorsal instability.
  - In the clinical setting, fractures with as little as 30% articular surface involvement can be unstable.

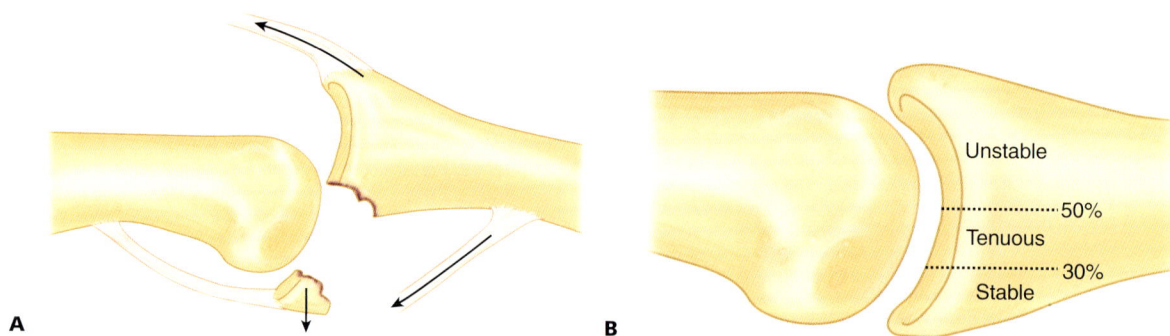

FIG 1 • A. Unstable PIP fracture-dislocation. The upward pull of the central tendon insertion and the distal superficialis insertion pull and push the middle phalanx up and over the proximal phalangeal head. The only forces preventing dorsal subluxation are the middle phalanx palmar lip and the palmar plate, both of which are lost in an unstable PIP palmar lip fracture. **B.** PIP instability after a fracture. A direct relation exists between the amount of middle phalanx palmar lip destroyed by the fracture and the resultant PIP joint stability. Articular damage in excess of 50% of the joint surface always renders the joint unstable, whereas fractures involving less than 30% usually are stable. Tenuous fractures (ie, those with articular damage of 30% to 50% of the joint surface), must be assessed with lateral radiographs. If the joint will not stay reduced with less than 30 degrees of flexion, it must be classified as "unstable."

■ Hemi-hamate arthroplasty restores stability by rebuilding the cup-shaped geometry of the middle phalangeal base and restoring the palmar plate attachment.

PATHOGENESIS

■ The middle phalangeal palmar lip fracture that is associated with unstable dorsal PIP fracture-dislocations is created by either avulsion of the fracture fragment or an impaction shear mechanism.

■ Avulsion fractures result from PIP joint hyperextension and traction through the palmar plate attachment (**FIG 2A**).

  ■ The fracture fragment is not comminuted and represents less than 30% of the articular surface.

  ■ These injuries usually are stable and rarely require surgical intervention. If the joint is unstable, osteosynthesis with lag screws often is possible because of the lack of comminution and the substantial size of the fragment.

■ Impaction shear PIP fracture-dislocations result from a longitudinally applied load to the tip of the finger with the PIP joint slightly flexed, such as in a mishandled ball catch. The force drives the middle phalanx into and over the proximal phalanx head, resulting in a middle phalangeal palmar lip fracture that is highly comminuted (**FIG 2B**).

  ■ Up to 80% of the joint surface can be involved, and the articular fragments are often deeply impacted into the soft metaphyseal bone.

■ Disruption of the terminal extensor tendon (mallet finger) often occurs in association with unstable dorsal PIP fracture-dislocations.

NATURAL HISTORY

■ The long-term prognosis for PIP fracture-dislocations is theoretically affected by the quality of the joint surface restoration and the maintenance of concentric reduction of the middle phalanx on the proximal phalangeal head.

  ■ The PIP joint seems to tolerate less than perfect restoration of a smooth joint surface. As long as motion is initiated quickly, small gaps and step-offs seem to be tolerated. Long-term, some remodeling occurs, and most patients do not need to be treated for symptomatic posttraumatic degenerative arthritis.

  ■ Joint reduction that is less than perfect is not well tolerated. When the middle phalanx rides dorsally on the proximal phalangeal head, PIP flexion occurs by "hinging" at the fracture margin.[9] The joint pivots on the palmar edge of the fracture, and the proximal phalanx falls into the fracture defect at the palmar base of the middle phalanx. The proximal phalangeal articular cartilage suffers accelerated wear, while the remaining undamaged middle phalangeal articular surface remains unused throughout the motion arc (**FIG 3**).

■ Treatment of unstable PIP palmar lip fractures is directed toward re-establishing joint stability so that flexion occurs by "gliding" of the remaining middle phalangeal articular cartilage on the head of the proximal phalanx.

PATIENT HISTORY AND PHYSICAL FINDINGS

■ Assess alignment in the coronal plane. Lateral deviation suggests asymmetric compression of articular fragments.

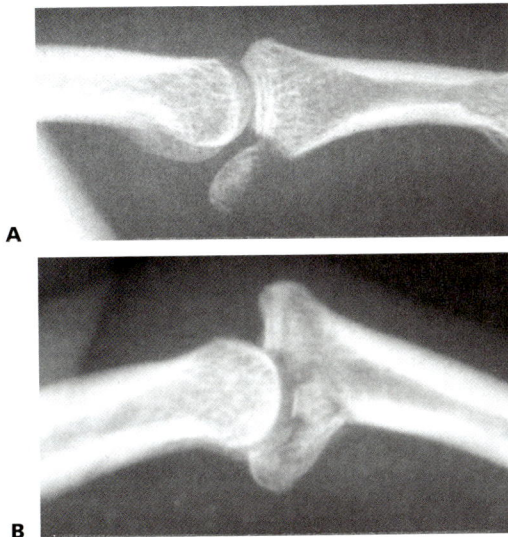

FIG 2 • Fracture types. **A.** Avulsion fracture. Avulsion fractures usually are caused by a forced PIP joint hyperextension. The fragment is not comminuted and involves less than 30% of the joint surface. The PIP joint is most often stable. **B.** Impaction shear fracture. This type of PIP fracture-dislocation is caused by a longitudinal load to the joint. The fracture fragments are comminuted and impacted into the middle phalanx. The joint reduction often is unstable.

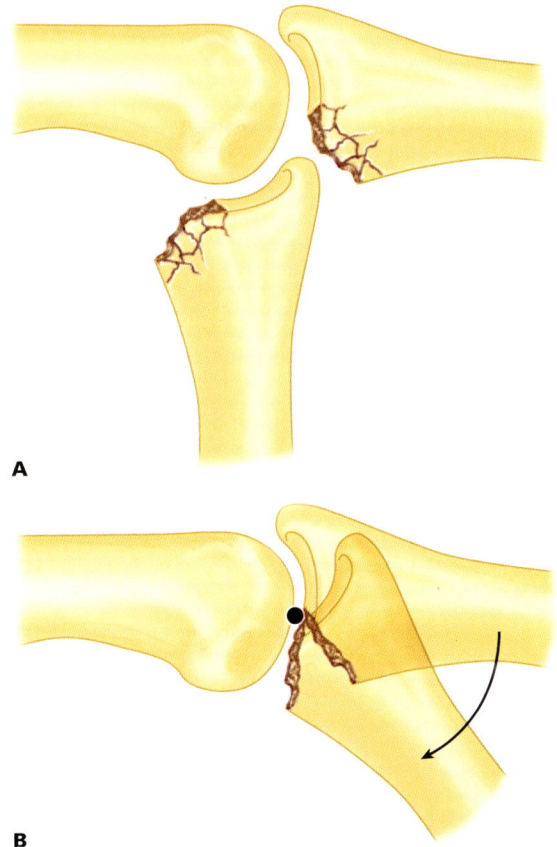

FIG 3 • Gliding or hinging. **A.** Normal PIP flexion occurs as the middle phalanx glides around the proximal phalanx head. **B.** When the middle phalanx palmar lip is lost, PIP flexion can occur by hinging at the fracture margin. Treatment of unstable PIP fracture-dislocations must rebuild the cup-shaped middle phalanx base and restore a normal gliding motion.

- Assess alignment in the sagittal plane. Lack of colinearity of the middle and proximal phalanx suggests persistent joint subluxation or dislocation.
- Associated mallet injuries must be treated concurrently with a DIP extension splint.

IMAGING AND OTHER DIAGNOSTIC STUDIES

- Plain radiographs in the posteroanterior (PA) and lateral planes provide the mainstay of radiographic evaluation of PIP fracture-dislocations.
- Inspect the lateral radiograph to determine the percentage of joint surface fractured and the quality of the reduction.
  - If the joint is not concentrically reduced with less than 30 degrees of flexion, the joint is classified as unstable and must be treated appropriately (see Fig 1B).
- On every lateral radiograph taken throughout the treatment course, carefully scrutinize the quality of the reduction. The remaining articular cartilage on the middle phalanx base must be in full contact with the proximal phalanx head. Any dorsal gap between the two surfaces—a "V" sign—indicates persistent instability and must be corrected (**FIG 4**).
- The percentage of the middle phalanx articular surface consumed by the fracture can be used to predict joint reduction stability[5,6,9] (see Fig 1B):
  - Less than 30%: The reduction usually is stable. The middle phalanx almost always remains concentrically reduced on the head of the proximal phalanx throughout a full ROM.
  - 30% to 50%: The reduction is tenuous. The middle phalanx may or may not subluxate dorsally when the PIP joint is extended. If any subluxation is noted on the lateral radiograph with the PIP joint fully extended, flex the joint to 30 degrees and repeat the lateral radiograph.
    - If concentric reduction is achieved and the palmar fragments are sitting where they will reconstitute a palmar lip, some form of extension block treatment may be employed.
    - If the joint will not stay reduced with less than 30 degrees of flexion, the joint is unstable and must be treated accordingly.
  - Over 50%: The PIP joint is unstable, and surgical intervention usually is required to rebuild the cup-shaped geometry of the middle phalanx base and to reattach the palmar plate.

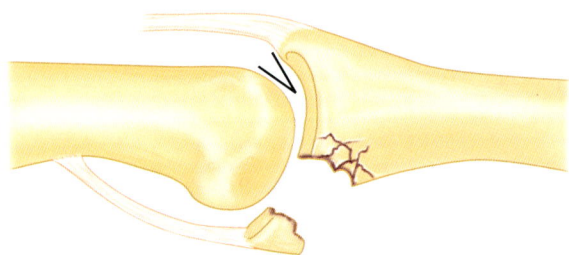

FIG 4 • Unstable PIP palmar lip fracture-dislocation. Extensive damage has occurred to the palmar lip of the middle phalanx, but the dorsal cortical margin and a small amount of dorsal articular cartilage remain intact. Even slight dorsal subluxation can be detected by looking for a V-shaped gap between the middle and proximal phalanges.

- Inspect the PA view to determine asymmetric compression of middle phalanx articular fragments leading to varus or valgus angulation.
- CT or MRI evaluation rarely is necessary.

DIFFERENTIAL DIAGNOSIS

- In patients with a history of recent trauma and radiographic confirmation of a large PIP palmar lip fracture associated with dorsal subluxation, the diagnosis of an unstable PIP dorsal fracture-dislocation is obvious.
- Dorsal dislocation and disruption of the middle phalanx palmar lip also may be seen in chronic PIP fracture-dislocations and occasionally in association with various forms of arthritis.

NONOPERATIVE MANAGEMENT

- Unstable PIP fracture-dislocations rarely can be managed nonoperatively. When over 50% of the middle phalanx articular surface is consumed by fracture, all restraints to dorsal subluxation are lost. The cup-shaped geometry of the middle phalanx base must be restored and the palmar plate reattached. Both goals can be accomplished with osteosynthesis of a single large fragment,[2,3,8] palmar plate arthroplasty,[1] or a hemi-hamate osteochondral autograft.[4,15,16]
- Stable PIP fracture-dislocations are treated nonoperatively. If the joint does not hyperextend and the lateral radiograph in full extension confirms concentric reduction, buddy tape the fingers and allow early ROM. If the joint hyperextends, some flexion must be maintained for 3 weeks while the fracture fragments consolidate enough to restore functional palmar plate continuity. Apply a dorsal blocking splint that prevents PIP hyperextension but allows full active flexion.
- Nonoperative treatment of tenuous PIP fracture-dislocations requires careful thought, patient cooperation, and meticulous follow-up.
  - The primary treatment goal is to maintain joint reduction while the middle phalanx palmar fragments consolidate and restore the cup-shaped geometry of the middle phalanx base. Joint reduction must be achievable with less than 30 degrees of flexion, and the palmar fragments must fall into a position that will restore the middle phalanx palmar lip.
  - A secondary goal is to provide immediate active ROM. Any treatment method that prevents extension past 30 degrees and allows full flexion can be employed. Options range from simple extension block splints[11] or pins[14] to external traction[12,13] or complex frame constructions.[7,10]

SURGICAL MANAGEMENT

- Hemi-hamate osteochondral autograft is indicated for the treatment of unstable PIP fracture-dislocations. The middle phalanx dorsal cortex must be intact.
- Hemi-hamate arthroplasty is a valuable salvage procedure for treatment that has failed with traction, external fixation devices, extension block splinting, or palmar plate arthroplasty.
- Chronic PIP dorsal dislocations also are amenable to treatment with hemi-hamate autograft if enough intact cartilage remains on both sides of the joint. Undamaged cartilage must be present on the palmar 50% of the proximal phalanx head and on at least a small rim of the middle phalanx dorsal articular surface.

Preoperative Planning

- Review the radiographs to determine the extent of articular surface damaged by the fracture, joint stability, and the quality of the remaining articular surface.
- Patients with extensive pre-existing degenerative arthritis may be better served with a PIP arthrodesis or total joint arthroplasty than with hemi-hamate arthroplasty.
- Assess the finger for radial or ulnar deviation. If coronal plane angulation is observed, it will be necessary to level the middle phalangeal joint surface during fracture site preparation and graft placement.
- Examine the patient for a mallet finger. If the terminal extensor tendon has been damaged, plan to include a mallet splint in the postoperative regimen.

Positioning

- Position the patient supine with the arm extended onto a radiolucent hand table.

- A mini C-arm is required for the procedure.
- Either regional or general anesthesia may be used, depending on the patient's or surgeon's preference.
- Perioperative antibiotics are provided.
- An upper arm tourniquet is applied. This is preferred over a forearm tourniquet, which puts pressure on the flexor muscles and causes excessive finger flexion.
- If necessary, the dorsum of the hand is shaved at the fourth and fifth carpometacarpal (CMC) joints to facilitate harvesting of the graft.

Approach

- We recommend performing the PIP portion of the procedure through a Brunner incision, because this incision provides excellent visualization of the fracture, the pulley system, and the neurovascular bundles.
- The hamate graft is harvested through a transverse incision at the level of the fourth and fifth CMC joints.

FRACTURE SITE PREPARATION

- Use a lead hand to position the hand palm up with the fingers extended. It will be necessary to remove the lead hand intermittently to facilitate use of fluoroscopy.
- Make a Brunner incision from the base of the finger to the DIP flexor crease (**TECH FIG 1A**)
- Coagulate intervening vessels with bipolar cautery as the full-thickness flaps are elevated.
- Identify the neurovascular bundles proximally and mobilize them away from the flexor sheath throughout the length of the dissection.
- Divide Cleland's ligaments dorsal to the neurovascular bundles. This allows full visualization of the collateral ligaments and facilitates retraction of the neurovascular bundles without excessive traction.
- Retract skin flaps with 5-0 nylon suture.
- Open the flexor tendon sheath from the distal end of the A2 pulley to the proximal edge of the A4 pulley. Start the dissection with a longitudinal incision along the edge of the flexor tendon sheath that is closest to the surgeon.
  - Create a flexor tendon sheath flap by making transverse incisions at the proximal end of A4 and the distal margin of A2. Elevate the flexor tendon sheath flap away from the surgeon (**TECH FIG 1B**).
  - Take care to prevent superficial damage to the flexor tendons while incising the flexor sheath.
- With the flexor tendons retracted away from the midline, make longitudinal incisions down the lateral margins of the palmar plate to separate the palmar plate from the accessory collateral ligaments. The distal attachment of the palmar plate will already be detached (ie, avulsed) as a result of the injury, but it still may need to be gently mobilized. Leave any remaining bone fragments attached to the distal edge of the palmar plate.
  - If the fragments are large enough to accept interfragmentary screws, consider open reduction and internal

fixation instead of proceeding with the hemi-hamate autograft.
- Release the collateral ligaments distally. Leave a small stump on the middle phalanx to facilitate repair at the end of the procedure.
- "Shotgun" the joint open (**TECH FIG 1C**).
  - Retract the flexor tendons away from the midline.
  - Hyperextend the PIP joint to expose the base of the middle phalanx and the head of the proximal phalanx.
  - If necessary, use a Freer elevator to prevent impingement of the intact dorsal base of the middle phalanx against the head of the proximal phalanx.
    - Caution: forceful hyperextension may lead to fracture of the dorsal articular fragment.
  - Only if absolutely necessary, release 1 to 2 mm of the A4 pulley to facilitate adequate mobilization of the flexor tendons. The A4 pulley is essential for finger function and must not be released completely.
- Assess the damage to the articular surfaces of the middle phalanx and the head of the proximal phalanx.
- Prepare the middle phalanx to receive the autograft (see Tech Fig 1C).
  - Elevate and excise impacted fragments of articular cartilage.
  - Use an oscillating saw to level the surface of the bony defect and to remove sufficient bone to allow graft placement. Make the cuts parallel to the dorsal margin of the articular surface and the long axis of the phalangeal shaft. Make the height of the intact articular surfaces equal at both the radial and ulnar margins. Limit thermal osteonecrosis with liberal use of irrigation.
  - The proximal to distal length of the cut usually is only about 5 to 7 mm. Take care to avoid notching the dorsal or distal portion of the cut, because this may weaken the shaft.
- Carefully measure the defect in the middle phalanx base to determine the appropriate graft size. Make notes of

TECHNIQUES

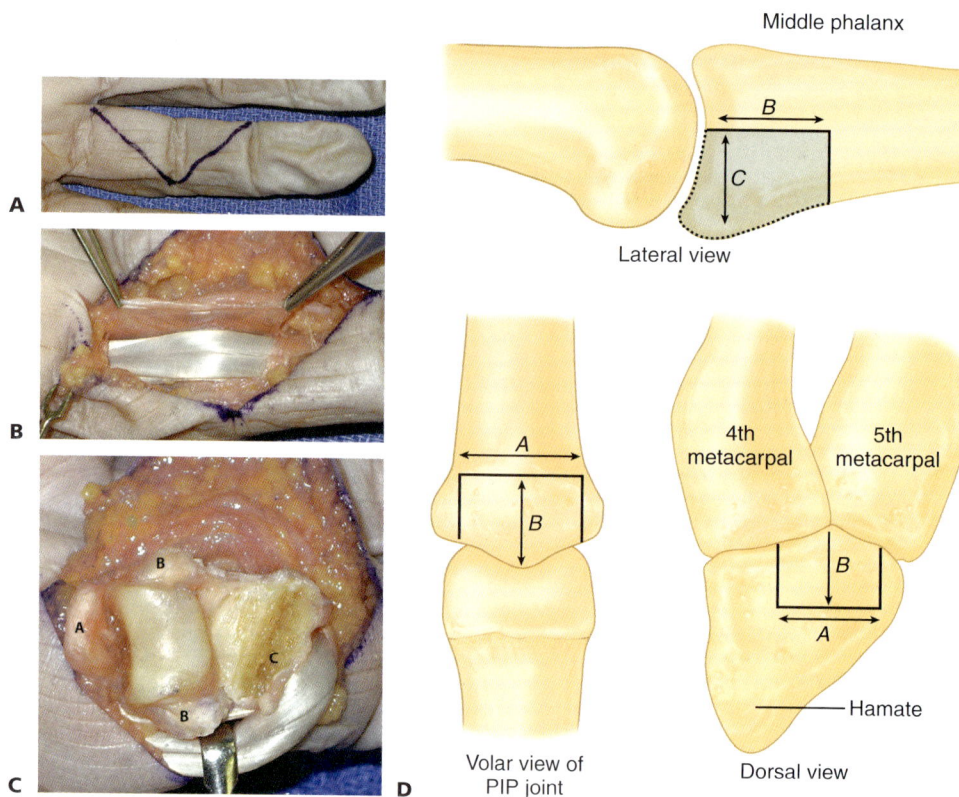

TECH FIG 1 • A. A Brunner incision, as depicted in this cadaver dissection, provides excellent visualization of the neurovascular structures, the flexor tendons, and the fracture site. **B.** Creating a flexor tendon sheath flap. Elevate a flap of the flexor tendon sheath from the distal end of the A2 pulley to the proximal edge of the A4 pulley. Preserve the flap so that it may be used to cover the palmar plate and the graft during closure. **C.** "Shotgun" the joint and prepare the fracture site. The PIP joint has been hyperextended 180 degrees to expose the fracture site. Note the palmar plate (*A*), the collateral ligaments (*B*) and the fracture defect (*C*). The fracture defect must be prepared so that it is of equal height and thickness on the radial and ulnar sides of the middle phalanx. **D.** Measuring graft dimensions. Measure the fracture defect to determine the medial-to-lateral width (*A*), proximal-to-distal depth (*B*). and anterior-to-posterior height (*C*) of the needed graft. Transfer these measurements to the dorsal surface of the hamate.

the dimensions on a drawing created on the back table (**TECH FIG 1D**).

- **A**: Width of the fracture defect. Measure the distance from the radial margin to the ulnar margin of the fracture defect. The graft must be centered on the central ridge of the proximal phalanx. Prepare the fracture site so that radial and ulnar extent of the fracture defect are equal.
- **B**: The proximal-to-distal size of the defect. To avoid creating an uneven joint surface that causes angulation in the coronal plane, the proximal-to-distal de-

fect size should be equal on the radial and ulnar margins or the middle phalanx.

- **C**: Height of articular surface at the central ridge. Measure the distance from the dorsal aspect of the fracture defect to what would be the most palmar extent of the middle phalanx palmar lip. It will be necessary to estimate this based on a lateral view of the proximal phalanx and from the preoperative radiographs (percentage of joint involvement).
- Return the joint to neutral and place a moist sponge on the finger incision while the graft is harvested.

HARVESTING THE HAMATE GRAFT

- Identify the distal articular margin of the hamate with fluoroscopy and mark the skin with a transverse line.
- Make a transverse 2-cm incision just proximal to the articular line.
- Bluntly dissect to mobilize the subcutaneous nerves, vessels, and extensor tendons.

- Longitudinally incise the hamate-CMC joint capsule, and then subperiosteally elevate the flaps to provide adequate visualization of the articular surfaces and the dorsum of the hamate (**TECH FIG 2A**)
- The apex of the distal articular surface between the fourth and fifth metacarpal articular surfaces will become the

new central ridge of the middle phalangeal base once the graft is transferred.

- A 12-mm segment is trimmed from the flexible plastic ruler that accompanies the marking pen. A fine-tipped marker is preferred, because it will not bleed as much on the bone. Less soft tissue on the dorsum of the hamate also helps prevent the ink from bleeding.

- Using a fine-tip marker and ruler, mark the dimensions of the graft on the hamate. To ensure stability of the CMC joints, leave at least 2 mm of the radial edge of the fourth metacarpal–hamate articulation and 2 mm of the ulnar edge of the fifth metacarpal–hamate surface.

- Harvest a graft that is of adequate height to fill the middle phalanx defect, but do not fracture the dorsal cortex of the hamate.

- Use an oscillating saw to make the cuts in the hamate very carefully. Alternatively, define the graft dimensions with a series of holes made with a K-wire, and then make the cuts with an osteotome (**TECH FIG 2B**).
  - To ensure that the graft is not too small, make the osteotomies on the outside of the measured lines.
  - Protect the articular surfaces at the base of the fourth and fifth metacarpals with a Freer elevator.

- Estimate the depth of the cuts by marking the saw blade or osteotome and measuring how deeply it penetrates the hamate.

- Create a notch in the hamate cortex proximal to the most proximal cut using a rongeur or by making an angled cut from proximal to distal with the saw. The notch is necessary to allow the final coronal cut to be made with a curved osteotome (**TECH FIG 2C**).

- Using extreme care, make the final cut in the hamate and complete the graft harvest.
  - Gently advance an angled osteotome from proximal to distal, aiming to complete the cut through the distal hamate articular surface at the predetermined depth.
  - Protect the metacarpal articular surfaces with an elevator.
  - Take slightly more bone than needed. It is easier to trim excess than to deal with a graft that is too small.

- Keep the graft protected in a moist saline sponge during wound closure.

- After the wound is irrigated, securely close the capsule over the fourth and fifth CMC joints with a 4-0 braided, nonabsorbable suture. Close the skin in layers.

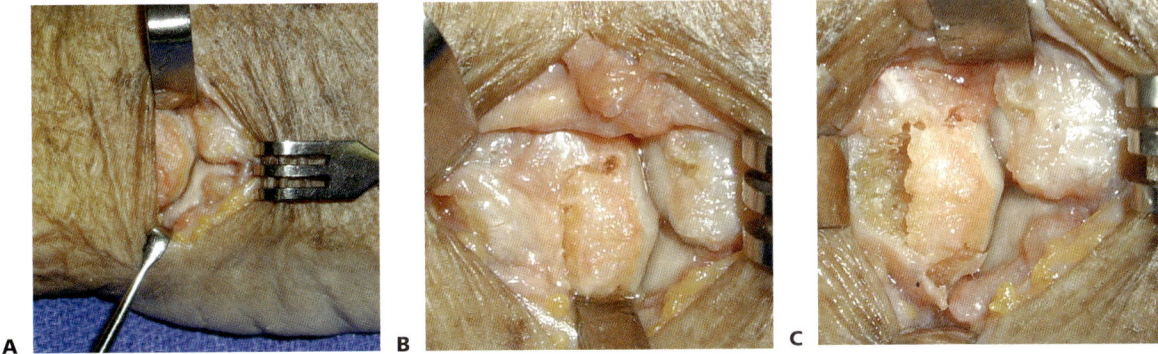

TECH FIG 2 • A. Exposure of the fourth and fifth metacarpal–hamate joints. Through a transverse skin incision and longitudinal capsular incision, as demonstrated in this cadaver dissection, expose the distal hamate articular surface and mark the graft dimensions. **B.** Use an oscillating saw or, as depicted in this cadaver dissection, K-wire holes and an osteotome, to make the cortical cuts in the dorsal surface of the hamate. **C.** Making the final hamate cut. A curved osteotome is used to make the final coronal cut that separates the graft from the hamate. It is necessary to make a back cut in the proximal hamate cortex to allow the osteotome to approach the cut at the proper angle. (**A–C:** wrist is to the left and fingers are to the right.)

GRAFT FIXATION

- "Shotgun" the PIP joint open to expose the fracture site.

- Carefully trim the graft with a rongeur or oscillating saw so that it fits precisely into the prepared defect at the middle phalanx base.

- It is very important to tailor the graft so that it restores the cup-shaped contour of the middle phalanx base. Joint stability will be restored only by restoring a concave middle phalanx articular surface that includes a stout palmar lip (**TECH FIG 3A–C**).

- A common error is to set the graft at an angle that creates a dorsal–proximal to palmar–distal slope. This carpentry error fails to restore joint stability and encourages the dorsal migration of the middle phalanx on the proximal phalangeal head (**TECH FIG 3D,E**).

- Temporarily fix the graft with a centrally placed 0.028-inch K-wire.

- Lag 1.0- or 1.3-mm screws on either side of the provisional K-wire.

- If the graft is large enough, augment the fixation with a third screw placed into the hole that remains once the K-wire is removed (**TECH FIG 3F**).

- Relocate the middle phalanx on the proximal phalanx, and assess the joint for stability and alignment.
  - The joint should remain in position throughout a full ROM. Dorsal subluxation suggests that the graft has been set too flat, failing to restore a concave articular surface.

TECHNIQUES

- The joint should exhibit neutral alignment. Varus or valgus angulation suggests that the graft has not been set perpendicular to the long axis of the middle phalanx.
- Assess screw length and graft placement with fluoroscopy. The hamate articular cartilage is thicker than the middle phalanx cartilage. This discrepancy creates the illusion that the hamate has not been set flush with the middle phalanx, but a lack of step-off already has been confirmed by direct inspection of the joint surface (**TECH FIG 3G**).
- Often, the distal edge of the graft protrudes beyond the volar cortex of the middle phalanx fracture defect. Shave the graft edge to smooth the transition from graft to middle phalanx.

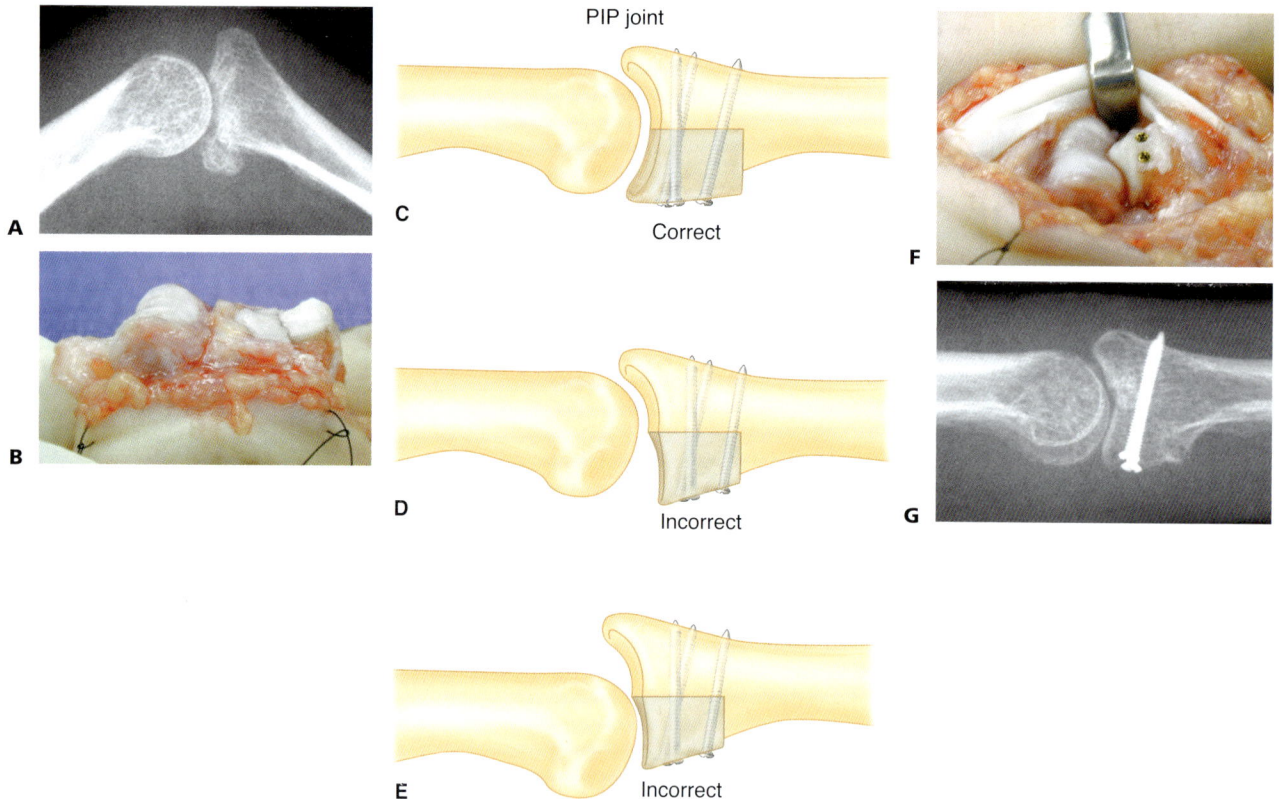

TECH FIG 3 • **A.** This lateral preoperative radiograph demonstrates a chronic, unstable PIP fracture-dislocation in a 19-year-old woman. Joint flexion occurs as the middle phalanx hinges at the palmar fracture margin and the proximal phalanx falls into the fracture defect. **B.** The graft has been inset to recreate a middle phalanx articular surface that is concave and matches the curvature of the proximal phalanx head. **C.** The graft must be contoured and set into the middle phalanx in a manner that restores the cup-shaped geometry of the middle phalanx base. Failure to restore a concave joint surface creates a flat surface (**D**) that encourages dorsal subluxation of the middle phalanx (**E**). **F.** Relocation of the joint. The joint has been relocated and stability confirmed by taking the joint through a full range of motion and ensuring that subluxation does not occur. Note how nicely the hamate graft recreates the palmar lip of the middle phalanx. **G.** Lateral radiograph of the graft. The lateral radiograph gives the false appearance that a step-off exists between the graft and the remaining middle phalangeal articular cartilage.

CLOSURE

- Repair the palmar plate and palmar margin of the middle phalanx. It may be necessary to secure the sutures through small drill holes.
- Repair the collateral ligaments to the stumps that were left on the middle phalanx during the approach.
- Interpose the flexor tendon sheath flap under the flexor tendons and over the PIP joint.
- Obtain hemostasis after the tourniquet is deflated.
- Close the skin.
- Apply a bulky dressing and splint holding the PIP joint in slight flexion.

PEARLS AND PITFALLS

Recurrent dorsal subluxation	▪ This is most commonly caused by failure to inset the graft in a position that restores the cup-shaped middle phalanx base. ▪ Failure to repair the palmar plate also may contribute to recurrent dorsal subluxation.
Angulation in the coronal plane	▪ The graft must be positioned perpendicular to the long axis of the middle phalanx. After provisional graft fixation, clinically assess the finger for varus or valgus angulation and adjust the graft to achieve neutral alignment.

POSTOPERATIVE CARE

▪ The goal of hemi-hamate arthroplasty is to operatively restore osseous PIP stability. Assuming that this goal has been attained and confirmed with lateral radiographs in extension that demonstrate concentric reduction, ROM is begun within the first week.
▪ Apply a postoperative dressing that controls edema and supports the PIP joint in a slightly flexed posture.
▪ Within the first week, begin active PIP flexion within an extension block splint that prevents extension past 20 degrees. The therapists may choose to fabricate a hand-based dorsal extension block splint if swelling is excessive, but a figure-eight splint is preferable.
▪ Encourage full active and passive motion at the MP and DIP. If a concomitant mallet injury is being treated, splint the DIP joint in full extension, but do not inhibit motion at the other joints.
▪ If the radiographs at 3 weeks show concentric joint reduction and solid graft fixation, begin gentle active assisted ROM.
▪ At 6 weeks postoperatively, again confirm solid graft fixation and concentric joint reduction radiographically, discontinue figure-eight splinting, and then begin passive ROM into flexion and correction of an excessive PIP flexion contracture with dynamic extension splinting.

OUTCOMES

▪ We have previously reported the outcome of 13 patients with unstable PIP dorsal fracture-dislocations treated with hemi-hamate autograft.[16] The original results were extremely encouraging, and our long-term results have not dampened our enthusiasm for the procedure.
▪ Eleven of the 13 patients returned for examination and final radiographs, one patient's results were assessed by chart review, and one patient was lost to follow-up.
▪ Pain
  ▪ Pain in the injured digit was minimal, and was rated at an average of 1.3. Two patients had regular pain, and six noted occasional aching discomfort.
  ▪ Graft donor site aching discomfort was noted only rarely in three patients. The remaining patients were asymptomatic.
▪ Motion
  ▪ ROM in the PIP averaged 85 degrees (range 65 degrees to 100 degrees).
  ▪ Most patients had a slight PIP flexion contracture that averaged 9 degrees (range 0 degrees to 25 degrees).
  ▪ The ROM of the MP joint averaged 90 degrees (range 75 degrees to 100 degrees), and the motion at the DIP joint averaged 60 degrees (range 35 degrees to 80 degrees).
▪ Stability
  ▪ Two of 12 patients demonstrated slight dorsal subluxation on the lateral radiograph, but neither patient had symptoms or functional problems.

  ▪ One of the two patients with dorsal subluxation also demonstrated 20 degrees of ulnar instability, but she was not symptomatic from this abnormality.
▪ Radiographs
  ▪ An apparent articular surface step-off between the graft and native middle phalanx cartilage commonly is observed. This phenomenon is caused by the greater thickness of the cartilage on the graft compared to the middle phalanx cartilage.
  ▪ All grafts united, as demonstrated by bridging trabeculae.
  ▪ None of the grafts demonstrated sclerosis that suggested osteonecrosis.
  ▪ Graft reabsorption was not observed.
▪ Long-term outcome
  ▪ Our experience with PIP hemi-hamate arthroplasty is too short to definitively determine the ultimate fate of the transferred articular cartilage.
  ▪ Early results do not suggest that autograft will lead to excessive rates of cartilage degeneration causing symptomatic posttraumatic changes.

COMPLICATIONS

▪ The complication rate in our original patient cohort was low.[16]
  ▪ No patients developed infection, and no patients required subsequent surgery.
  ▪ Dorsal subluxation was noted in 2 of 12 patients. One was believed to have been caused by an incompetent palmar plate. The other case of dorsal subluxation was attributed to a graft that was not appropriately contoured to restore the cup-shaped geometry of the middle phalanx base.
▪ Donor site morbidity has not occurred. To date, no patient has had instability or significant pain at the fourth or fifth CMC joints.
▪ We have maintained an acceptably low complication rate in our subsequent experience.

REFERENCES

1. Eaton RG, Malerich MM. Volar plate arthroplasty for the proximal interphalangeal joint: a ten year review. J Hand Surg Am 1980;5:260–268.
2. Freeland AE, Benoist LA. Open reduction and internal fixation method for fractures at the proximal interphalangeal joint. Hand Clin 1994;10:239–250.
3. Hamilton SC, Stern PJ, Fassler PR, et al. Mini-screw fixation for the treatment of proximal interphalangeal joint dorsal fracture-dislocations. J Hand Surg Am 2006;8:1349–1354.
4. Hastings H, Capo J, Steinberg B, et al. Hemicondylar hamate replacement arthroplasty for proximal interphalangeal joint fracture-dislocations. Abstract. Presented at the 54th annual meeting of The American Society for Surgery of the Hand, September 3–5, 1999, Boston, MA.
5. Hastings H II, Carroll C IV. Treatment of closed articular fractures of the metacarpophalangeal and proximal interphalangeal joints. Hand Clin 1988;4:503–527.

6. Hastings J II, Hamlet WP. Critical assessment of PIP joint stability after palmar lip fractures dislocations. Abstract. Presented at the 56th Annual Meeting of The American Society for Surgery of the Hand, October 3–6, 2001, Baltimore, MD.

7. Inanami H, Ninomiya S, Okutsu I, et al. Dynamic external finger fixator for fracture-dislocation of the proximal interphalangeal joint. J Hand Surg Am 1993;18:160–194.

8. Jupiter JB, Sheppard JE. Tendon wire fixation of avulsion fractures in the hand. Clin Orthop Relat Res 1987;214:113–120.

9. Kiefhaber TR, Stern PJ. Fracture-dislocations of the proximal interphalangeal joint. J Hand Surg Am 1998;23:368–380.

10. Krakauer JD, Stern PJ. Hinged device for fracture involving the proximal interphalangeal joint. Clin Orthop Relat Res 1996;327:29–37.

11. McElfresh EC, Dobyns JH, O'Brien ET. Management of fracture-dislocations of the proximal interphalangeal joints by extension-block splinting. J Bone Joint Surg Am 1972;54:1705–1711.

12. Morgan JP, Gordon DA, Klug MS, et al. Dynamic digital traction for unstable comminuted intra-articular fracture-dislocations of the proximal interphalangeal joint. J Hand Surg Am 1995; 20:565–573.

13. Schenck RR. Dynamic traction and early passive movement for fractures of the proximal interphalangeal joint. J Hand Surg Am 1986;11:850–858.

14. Viegas SF. Extension block pinning for proximal interphalangeal joint fracture-dislocations: preliminary report of a new technique. J Hand Surg Am 1992;17:896–901.

15. Williams RMM, Hastings H II, Kiefhaber TR. PIP fracture-dislocations treatment technique: use of a hemi-hamate resurfacing arthroplasty. Tech Hand Up Extrem Surg 2002;6:185–192.

16. Williams RMM, Kiefhaber TR, Sommerkamp TG, et al. Treatment of unstable dorsal proximal interphalangeal fracture/dislocations using a hemi-hamate autograft. J Hand Surg Am 2003;28:856–865.

Chapter 39

Operative Treatment of Distal Interphalangeal Joint Fracture-Dislocations

Leo T. Kroonen and Eric P. Hofmeister

DEFINITION

- Injuries about the distal interphalangeal joint (DIP) consist of avulsion injuries of the terminal extensor tendon or the flexor digitorum profundus (FDP) tendon, or isolated dislocations of the DIP joint.
- Isolated dislocations of the DIP joint are rare injuries in which the distal phalanx is dislocated either dorsal or volar relative to the middle phalanx.
- A "bony" mallet finger (ie, mallet fracture) is an intraarticular bony avulsion at the insertion site of the terminal extensor tendon on the dorsal base of the distal phalanx that results in inability to actively extend the DIP joint.
- A "non-bony" mallet finger is an injury to the extensor mechanism at or near the insertion onto the distal phalanx that typically results in inability to actively extend the DIP joint.
- "Jersey finger" is an avulsion of the FDP tendon, with or without its bony attachment, from the volar base of the distal phalanx. It typically results in inability to actively flex the DIP joint.

ANATOMY

- The DIP joint is stabilized by the radial and ulnar collateral ligaments, the volar plate, and the firm insertions of the FDP and terminal tendons of the extensor mechanism.
- The extensor mechanism terminates with the confluence of the lateral bands into a single terminal tendon, which inserts on the dorsal base of the distal phalanx. The terminal tendon is a strong, flat, thin segment that averages 10.1 mm in length and 5.6 mm in width.[8]
- The terminal tendon insertion, on average, is 1.4 mm proximal to the germinal matrix of the fingernail.[9]
- The volar surface of the terminal tendon usually is adherent to the dorsal capsule of the DIP joint.[9]
- The FDP tendon inserts on the volar surface of the base of the distal phalanx. It is surrounded by the flexor tendon sheath. The A4, A5, and C3 pulleys secure the FDP tendon around the level of the DIP joint.
- The vinculum longus profundus and vinculum brevis profundus are thin mesenteries providing vascular supply to the distal portion of the FDP tendon. They also provide a weak attachment of the FDP tendon to the flexor tendon sheath.[4]

PATHOGENESIS

- Mallet finger injuries are the result of a disruption to the extensor mechanism at or near the insertion to the base of the distal phalanx. Such disruptions can occur as a result of a laceration or a sudden flexion force to an extended DIP joint. The disruption of the extensor mechanism leaves the pull of the FDP unopposed, leaving the DIP joint in a flexed posture.

The views expressed in this chapter are those of the authors and do not reflect the official policy or position of the Department of the Navy, Department of Defense, or the United States Government.

- Dislocations of the DIP joint are rare due to the inherent stability provided by the collateral ligaments, the volar plate, and the flexor and extensor tendon insertions. However, when a dislocation does occur, the distal end of the middle phalanx usually "buttonholes" through these structures, making reduction more difficult.
- "Jersey finger" injuries occur as a result of disruption to the FDP, from either a laceration or a sudden extension force applied to a flexed DIP joint, causing an eccentric contraction. The disruption of the FDP tendon leaves the pull of the extensor mechanism unopposed, resulting in an extended posture of the DIP joint.

NATURAL HISTORY

- Mallet finger injuries can occur in any finger, but most commonly are seen in the three most ulnar digits.
  - Left untreated, a mallet finger injury can progress to a secondary "swan neck" deformity.
    - With the disruption of the extensor mechanism at the DIP joint, the pull of the lateral bands adds to the extension force of the central slip at the PIP joint, thereby creating an imbalance in forces at the PIP joint and a hyperextension deformity at that joint.[11]
  - Despite treatment, residual deformity, usually in the form of a dorsal prominence, can be seen in up to 80% of cases.[11]
- About 75% of cases of FDP avulsions involve the ring finger. Although some researchers hypothesize that this happens because the ring finger protrudes the farthest when the hand is held in a flexed position, this theory has never been proven.
  - Leddy and Packard[3] proposed the classification system that is still widely used today for FDP avulsion injuries, based on the level of retraction of the tendon. Other authors since have made modifications, including the addition of a fourth type of injury.[10]
    - Type I FDP avulsions retract into the palm, thereby disrupting the vincular system and leading to poor blood supply. Surgery should be performed within 7 to 10 days.
    - Type II injuries retract to the level of the PIP joint or distal A2 pulley. An associated small bony fleck often is seen on the lateral radiograph. Because the proximal blood supply is preserved through the long vincula, these injuries can be successfully treated as late as 6 weeks from the time of injury.
    - Type III injuries usually are associated with a bony avulsion, and as a result, do not retract proximal to the A4 pulley. These injuries are treated as bony injuries with open reduction and internal fixation and can be treated late if required.
    - Type IV injuries are bony avulsion injuries in which the tendon also has separated from the avulsed bony fragment. Time to treatment depends on the level of tendon retraction.

PATIENT HISTORY AND PHYSICAL FINDINGS

■ As with all hand injuries, patients should be questioned about their hand dominance and occupational requirements so the surgeon can better understand individual needs and goals.

■ The following examinations should be performed to determine possible injuries:

■ FDP function

■ Inability to flex at the DIP joint implies disruption of the FDP tendon.

■ Limited, weak, or painful flexion may indicate a partial injury or a complete disruption with intact vinculae or pseudotendon.

■ DIP joint extensor mechanism function

■ Inability to extend at the DIP joint implies disruption of the terminal extensor tendon. Weak extension implies a partial or less severe injury. Loss of passive extension indicates a possible fracture or dislocation.

■ Axial injuries to an extended DIP joint often are the culprit in mallet finger injuries.

■ The history often reveals an axial blow to the fingertip, such as when catching a ball.

■ The patient will be unable to actively extend at the DIP joint.

■ "Jersey finger" injuries often are the result of a sudden extension force on a flexed DIP joint, such as when grabbing for another player's shirt while playing football.

■ These patients will be unable to actively flex through the DIP joint.

■ Active PIP flexion will be present but may be moderately diminished due to pain or stiffness.

■ Most dislocations of the DIP joint are the result of sporting injuries.[7,8]

IMAGING AND OTHER DIAGNOSTIC STUDIES

■ Plain radiographs of the affected hand (PA, lateral, and oblique) and dedicated views of the affected finger (PA, lateral, and oblique) should be obtained, and usually are sufficient for making the diagnosis in association with a thorough clinical examination.

■ Mallet finger injuries can be associated with a bony avulsion. Any joint subluxation should be noted, and the size of the avulsed fragment should be estimated (**FIG 1**).

■ In FDP avulsion injuries, the location of the retracted flexor tendon often can be appreciated by finding a bony fragment on the lateral radiograph of the affected digit (**FIG 2A**).

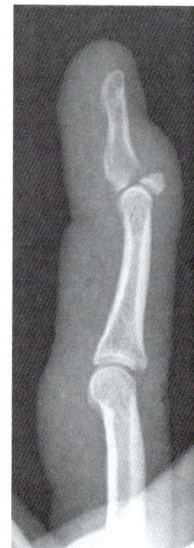

FIG 1 • Lateral radiographs usually are the most helpful in identifying a mallet fracture. Note that in this image, the avulsed fragment includes more than 50% of the articular surface. There is no significant volar subluxation in this case.

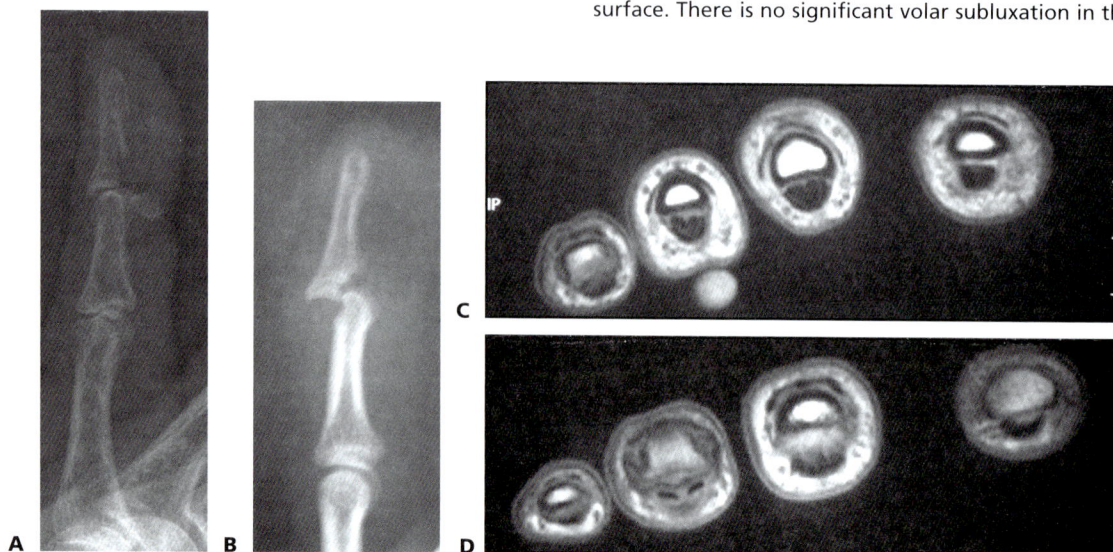

FIG 2 • **A.** Flexor digitorum profundus (FDP) avulsion in which a bony fragment has been caught up at the A4 pulley. **B.** Lateral radiograph of a finger demonstrates chronic dorsal dislocation of the DIP joint, with associated arthrosis. **C.** Axial cut MRI at the level of the proximal phalanx shows both FDP and flexor digitorum superficialis (FDS) tendons are present. **D.** At the level of the middle phalanx, only the FDS tendon can be seen. (**B-D:** Copyright Thomas R. Hunt III, MD.)

- Ultrasound sometimes can be helpful in determining continuity of the flexor tendon or identifying the location of the retracted proximal flexor tendon stump.
- MRI also is valuable in determining flexor tendon continuity and level of tendon retraction (**FIG 2C,D**).

DIFFERENTIAL DIAGNOSIS

- Osteoarthritis
- Inflammatory arthropathy
- FDP rupture
- FDP laceration
- Terminal extensor tendon rupture (mallet finger)
- Mallet fracture

NONOPERATIVE MANAGEMENT

- For tendinous mallet fingers and mallet fractures involving less than one third of the articular surface and without joint subluxation, a variety of splints are available.
  - We prefer immobilizing the DIP joint with a prefabricated polyethylene extension splint.
  - Casting of the DIP joint also has been described.
  - Full-time splinting in extension is recommended for 6 weeks, followed by 6 weeks of part-time splinting. During this second 6 weeks, we advise our patients to wear the splint for any heavy activity and at night, and we emphasize the inclusion of gentle DIP joint flexion, not exceeding 20 degrees in the first 2 weeks, and then gradually increasing to full flexion over the course of 6 weeks. If any loss of extension is experienced during this time, we advise the patient to return immediately to full-time splinting and to follow up in our clinic.
- Nonoperative treatment of acute FDP lacerations or ruptures at the DIP joint is not recommended unless the patient is unwilling to comply with postoperative splinting or rehabilitation.
- In subacute and chronic FDP lacerations or avulsions, the functional necessity of DIP joint motion should be carefully considered, and nonoperative treatment should be considered.
  - Literature directing treatment in cases of delayed diagnosis is scarce.
  - If the patient does not have any functional limitations as a result of the injury, we prefer to defer surgical management.
  - If the patient is troubled by a tender mass in the palm but the hand is functional, we recommend excision of the tendon alone.
  - Instability and weakness of pinch can become problematic. In such cases, we recommend tenodesis or arthrodesis.
  - Only if the function of the DIP is *crucial* to the performance of daily activities do we recommend a staged reconstruction of the flexor tendon.

- Closed reduction of isolated DIP joint dislocations can be attempted under a digital block.
  - For dorsal dislocations, the FDP tendon or the volar plate can be interposed, blocking the reduction as the head of the middle phalanx buttonholes through the interval between the FDP tendon and the collateral ligament.[8]
    - For dorsal dislocations, gentle traction and extension through the DIP joint can assist in reducing the interposed volar plate.
  - In volar dislocations, the head of the middle phalanx can buttonhole through the interval between the terminal extensor tendon and the collateral ligament.[7]
    - For volar dislocations, gentle traction can be used while guiding the condyle of the middle phalanx back through the interval between the terminal extensor tendon and the collateral ligament.
  - In either case, a gentle reduction maneuver should be attempted, keeping in mind the structures that are likely to be interposed in the joint. Care should be taken to avoid excessive traction, which may tighten the tendon and ligament, preventing reduction.

SURGICAL MANAGEMENT

- Surgical treatment of mallet fractures is reserved for those fractures associated with joint subluxation.
- Operative treatment is recommended for all acute flexor tendon avulsions at the DIP joint and selected subacute or chronic cases.
  - The level of retraction of the tendon on the flexor side determines the urgency with which the injury needs to be addressed (see Table 1). Although Type I and II injuries can be treated up to 6 weeks with good results, we recommend treating these injuries sooner when possible to optimize recovery and function.
- For isolated dislocations of the DIP joint, surgical management is indicated in those cases where closed reduction is unsuccessful. Generally, no surgical stabilization is required.

Preoperative Planning

- All images should be reviewed.
- For isolated dislocations, a review of the relevant anatomy, including the volar plate, flexor and extensor tendons, and collateral ligaments, is essential to understand which structures might be interposed in the DIP joint.

Positioning

- The patient is placed supine on the operating room table with the affected arm outstretched on an arm board. When

Table 1	Classification of Flexor Digitorum Profundus Avulsion Injuries		
Type	**Level of Tendon Retraction**	**Vascularity**	**Approximate Time to Surgery**
I	Palm	Vinculae are disrupted, leading to dysvascularity of tendon	7–10 days
II	Distal A-2 pulley or PIP joint	Vinculae remain intact, providing vascularity and preventing further retraction	Up to 6 weeks
III	A-4 pulley	Bony attachment prevents retraction beyond the A-4 pulley	6 weeks +
IV	The tendon is avulsed from a bony avulsion fracture, and can retract to any level	Determined by the level of tendon retraction	Determined by the level of tendon retraction

treating a flexor tendon injury, a flexible aluminum hand-holder can be useful for positioning the hand during the exploration.

- A well-padded tourniquet is placed high on the arm.

Approach

- Mallet fingers
  - We prefer to treat mallet fingers with percutaneous techniques.
    - Percutaneous treatment is more likely to succeed if the injury is treated within the first 3 to 5 days after the injury, although we have successfully treated cases at as late as 6 weeks.
  - If open treatment is to be attempted, a variety of incisions can be used, including straight longitudinal, lazy-S type, H-type, and Bruner incisions. Meticulous soft tissue handling

is vital to minimize trauma to the skin. Great care must be taken to avoid injury to the germinal matrix proximal to the nail fold.

- "Jersey fingers"
  - A volar Bruner incision is used and is extended proximal enough to identify or retrieve the proximal tendon stump.
  - In type I injuries, one oblique limb of the Bruner incision over the A1 pulley region often is used to retrieve the retracted tendon.
  - Care is taken to preserve the A2 and A4 pulleys.
- For open reduction of isolated DIP dislocations, the approach is dictated by the direction of the dislocation.
  - Dorsal dislocations are approached volarly, and volar dislocations are approached dorsally.

TECHNIQUES

TREATMENT OF MALLET FINGERS

Extension-Block Pinning of Mallet Fractures

- The DIP joint is flexed initially, pulling the avulsed fragment volarly.
- A dorsal block pin is inserted obliquely from distal to proximal under fluoroscopy. A 0.045-inch K-wire usually is ideal, although 0.035-inch K-wires are sometimes preferred if the finger is small.
  - The pin should enter at the dorsal edge of the articular surface of the middle phalanx, and bicortical purchase should be obtained (**TECH FIG 1A,B**). The dorsal blocking pin should not actually engage the fracture fragment, because this may result in comminution of the bone.

- Anteroposterior and lateral views on fluoroscopy should be obtained to ensure appropriate positioning (**TECH FIG 1C**).
- The distal phalanx is then extended, reducing and compressing the fracture.
- A second K-wire is inserted in a retrograde manner from the distal tip of the distal phalanx to the level of the DIP joint (**TECH FIG 1D**).
- While holding the digit extended with the fracture and DIP joint reduced, the second smooth K-wire is advanced retrograde across the DIP joint into the middle phalanx (**TECH FIG 1E,F**).
- The K-wires are cut, and protective plastic caps are placed over the exposed ends.
- The finger is then placed in a protective dressing.

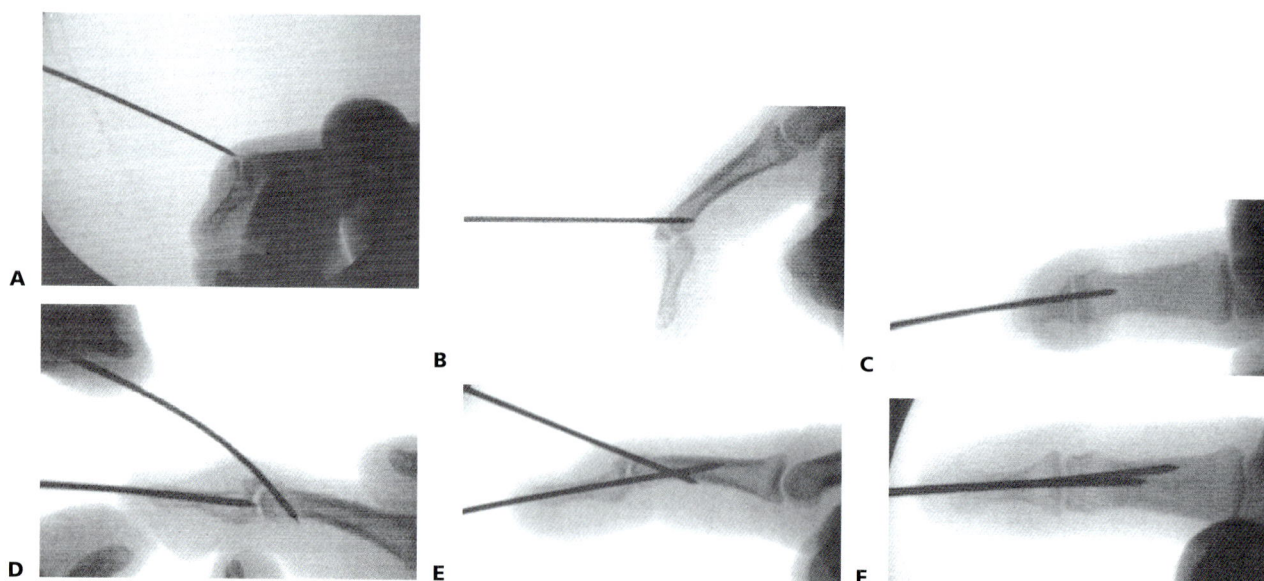

TECH FIG 1 • **A** With the DIP joint flexed, a K-wire is inserted at the dorsal edge of the articular surface of the middle phalanx. **B.** Bicortical purchase is obtained. **C.** PA fluoroscopic image confirms good bony purchase in both the dorsal and volar phalanx. **D.** With the DIP joint extended, a retrograde K-wire is introduced through the tip of the distal phalanx. **E.** Once reduction is confirmed, this retrograde pin is advanced into the middle phalanx. **F.** A final PA image confirms good placement of pins.

Pinning of Non-Bony Mallet Fingers

- For patients whose compliance is in doubt, or to assist with occupational requirements, a single 0.045- or 0.062-inch K-wire can be inserted in a retrograde manner through an extended DIP joint.
- The pin can be left either protruding through the skin and covered with a pin cap, or under the skin.

Pull-Through Button Technique for Flexor Digitorum Profundus Avulsions

- The fingers are held in an extended position using an aluminum hand.
- The volar surface of the injured finger is exposed through a Bruner incision, and the edges of the avulsed tendon are identified (**TECH FIG 2A**).
- The proximal segment of the tendon is retrieved, pulled out to length, and secured using a small-gauge needle directed transversely across the tendon (**TECH FIG 2B**).
- Using a 2-0 monofilament nonabsorbable suture (or other permanent suture appropriate for tendon repair), the proximal segment of the avulsed tendon is captured using a Krakow or Bunnell suture technique (**TECH FIG 2C**).
- The proximal segment of tendon is then threaded through the flexor pulley system.
- The volar base of the distal phalanx is prepared with a rongeur to expose bleeding bone.
- Two straight Keith needles are introduced into the volar wound and, using a wire driver, driven from the volar base of the distal phalanx, through the nailbed, and exiting through the center of the fingernail on the dorsal side (**TECH FIG 2D,E**).
- A small square of sterile felt and a plastic sterile button are placed over the exposed tips of the Keith needles (**TECH FIG 2F**).
- The two free ends of suture are threaded through the eyelets of the Keith needles, and the needles are advanced through the nailbed, felt, and button.
- The distal end of the avulsed tendon is pulled into its prepared footprint at the volar base of the distal phalanx, and the suture is then carefully tied over the button (**TECH FIG 2G,H**).
  - Additional fixation is obtained by securing the tendon to tendon remnants at the insertion site.
- As an alternative to tying over the nail and a button, the Keith needles may be advanced through the proximal portion of the distal phalanx, avoiding the germinal matrix. A 3-mm transverse incision is then made over the exiting Keith needles, and the suture is tied down on bone.
- The wound is closed in standard fashion, and the hand is secured in a dorsal extension blocking splint (**TECH FIG 2I**).

Suture Anchor Technique for Flexor Digitorum Profundus Avulsions

- The approach, identification, and suture of the avulsed profundus tendon are the same as in the pull-through button technique.
- Two small suture anchors are introduced into the volar base of the distal phalanx in a trajectory from proximal-volar to distal-dorsal, or, as recently described by McAllister et al,[6] may be placed in a distal-volar to proximal-dorsal

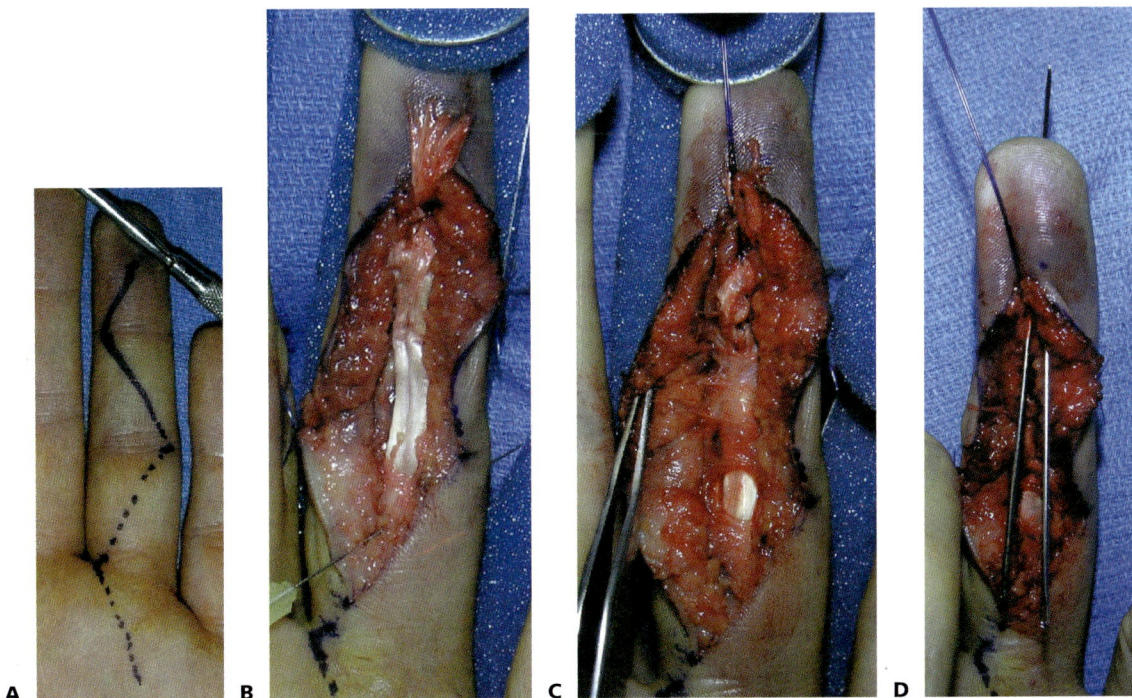

TECH FIG 2 • **A.** A volar Bruner incision is planned. **B.** The avulsed tendon is identified and held in the wound with a small-gauge needle. **C.** The avulsed tendon is captured with a Krakow technique. **D.** Keith needles are advanced through the volar wound to exit in the center of the fingernail. *(continued)*

TECHNIQUES

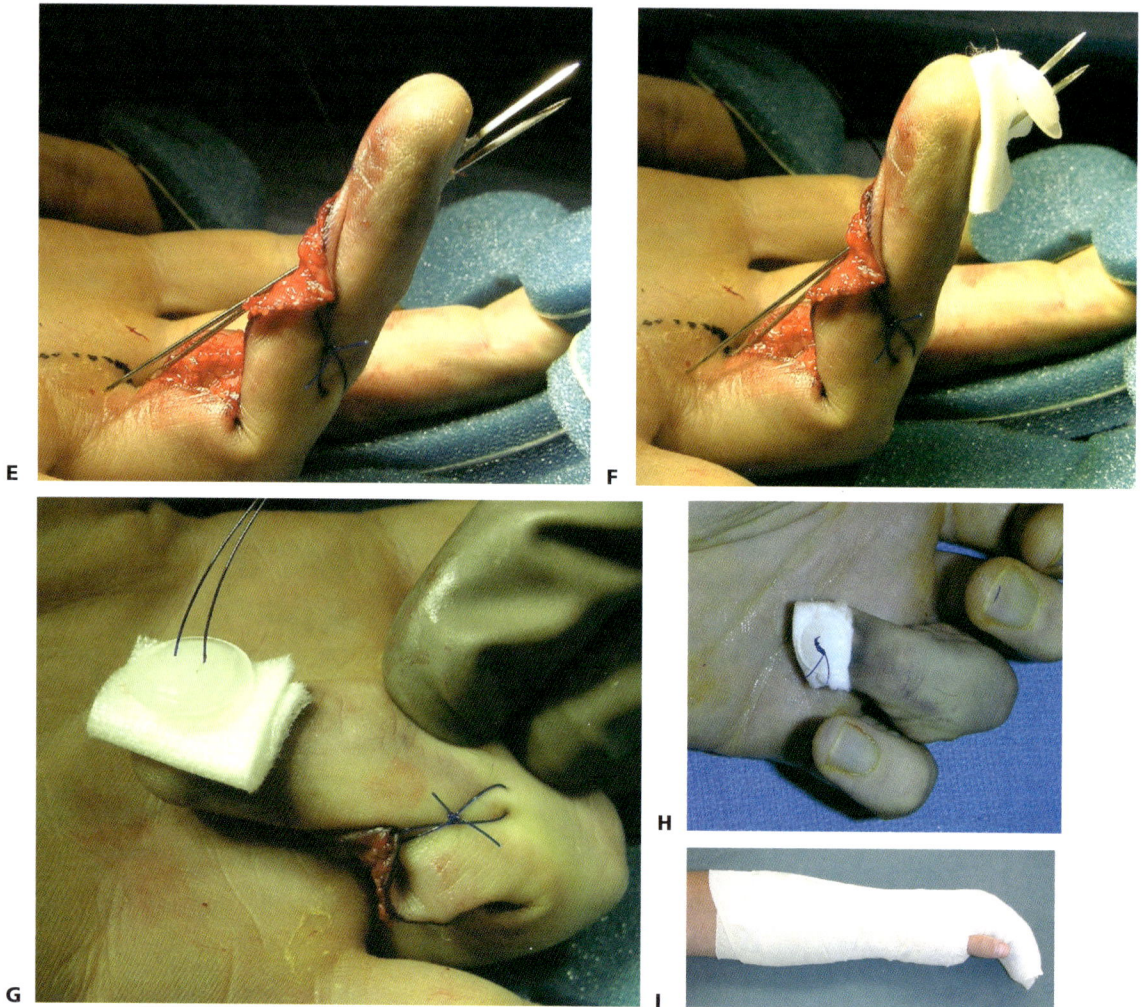

TECH FIG 2 • *(continued)* **E.** A side view shows the Keith needles exiting through the fingernail. **F.** Sterile felt and a plastic button are threaded over the needles. **G.** The finger is flexed down, and the sutures are pulled through. **H.** The suture is securely tied over the button. **I.** The patient is immobilized initially in an extension block splint.

direction, taking special care not to violate the dorsal cortex. This placement ensures maximum bony purchase in the thickest portion of the distal phalanx and ensures maximum pullout strength.

- Fluoroscopic imaging can be used to ensure proper anchor placement and document that the suture anchors have not violated the dorsal cortex or the joint.
- A modified Kessler pattern of suturing can then be used to secure the FDP tendon in place at the base of the distal phalanx.
- The wound is closed and the splint applied in the manner described.

Treatment Technique for Flexor Digitorum Profundus Disruption With Bony Avulsion

- If the avulsed fragment is large enough, some authors recommend open reduction and internal fixation using small screws or wires.
- It is recommended that the fragment have a diameter at least 2½ times the diameter of the screw to avoid comminution of the bony fragment.[5]
- Intraoperative radiographs are imperative to confirm reduction.

PEARLS AND PITFALLS

Prevent proximal pin migration in nonbony mallet fingers	▪ For cases in which we bury the pin, we prefer to make a small 90-degree bend in the distal end of the wire to prevent proximal migration of the pin into the phalanges.
Tendon retrieval in FDP avulsions	▪ It is helpful to use a "milking" technique from proximal to distal in the forearm and palm, with the wrist in a flexed position, to deliver the proximal end of the tendon. Doing so can often decrease the length of the incision that is required for the repair.
Skin irritation with use of button	▪ It is recommended to place a small piece of felt between the patient's nail and the button to decrease irritation (see Tech Fig 2F,G).
PIP flexion contracture	▪ Delayed treatment of a type I FDP avulsion can result in a PIP flexion contracture. If nearly full passive joint extension is not obtainable following tendon reinsertion, the repair should be abandoned.
Extension block pinning	▪ Full DIP extension is not required to achieve reduction of the fracture. ▪ Avoid multiple attempts at K-wire placement. ▪ Avoid forced extension of the DIP joint, which may result in fracture at the entrance site of the dorsal block K-wire. ▪ Early treatment is easier and more effective.

POSTOPERATIVE CARE

▪ Mallet fractures
  ▪ The patient is allowed nearly full activity immediately postoperatively, including PIP joint and MCP joint motion.
  ▪ An antibiotic ointment may be applied to the pin sites twice daily.
  ▪ The patient should be counseled thoroughly on keeping pin sites clean.
  ▪ The patient is seen for follow-up around postoperative day 10, and as needed for 4 weeks.
  ▪ Pins are removed in the office setting when there is no tenderness to palpation at the fracture site and there is evidence of bridging trabeculae at the fracture site (usually about 4 to 5 weeks).
▪ FDP avulsions/lacerations
  ▪ The patient is evaluated 3 to 5 days postoperatively, and if a strong repair has been accomplished and the patient is deemed compliant, a forearm-based dorsal extension block splint is fitted and the patient is enrolled into a directed hand therapy rehabilitation protocol with immediate edema control.
  ▪ In the compliant patient, place-and-hold exercises, initially in the splint and then with the wrist in slight extension, are started between postoperative days 5 and 7.
  ▪ Further progression is based on the protocol described by Cannon and Strickland,[1] and typically includes tendon glides and wrist tenodesis activities at 5 weeks, and progressive strengthening at 7 to 8 weeks.

OUTCOMES

▪ For extension block pinning of mallet fractures, one study by the primary author reported average time to bony union of 35 days.
  ▪ At an average follow-up time of 74 weeks, range of motion averaged 4 to 78 degrees.[2]
▪ For isolated dislocations of the DIP joint, case studies suggest that active range of motion at the DIP joint from 0 to 65 degrees is regained by 4 to 12 months postreduction.[7,8]
▪ Most patients with FDP avulsions treated acutely are able to work between 8 and 18 weeks after the surgery, with some

studies suggesting that an earlier return to work is seen with a suture anchor repair.
  ▪ An 8- to 10-degree flexion contracture and a similar lack of terminal flexion at the DIP joint often are encountered.[6]

COMPLICATIONS

▪ Pin tract infection
▪ Migration of pins
▪ Loss of reduction
▪ Nail deformity
▪ Dorsal skin necrosis from splinting
▪ Joint stiffness
▪ Loss of grip strength
▪ Tendon adherence
▪ Tendon rupture

REFERENCES

1. Cannon NM, Strickland JW. Therapy following flexor tendon surgery. Hand Clin 1985;1:147–165.
2. Hofmeister EP, Mazurek MT, Shin AY, et al. Extension block pinning for large mallet fractures. J Hand Surg Am 2003;28:453–459.
3. Leddy JP, Packer JW. Avulsion of the profundus tendon insertion in athletes. J Hand Surg Am 1977;2:66–69.
4. Leversedge FJ, Ditsios K, Goldfarb CA, et al. Vascular anatomy of the human flexor digitorum profundus tendon insertion. J Hand Surg Am 2002;27:806–812.
5. Lubahn JD, Hood JM. Fractures of the distal interphalangeal joint. Clin Orthop Relat Res 1996;327:12–20.
6. McCallister WV, Ambrose HC, Katolik LI, et al. Comparison of pullout button versus suture anchor for zone I flexor tendon repair. J Hand Surg Am 2006;31:246–251.
7. Morisawa Y, Ikegami H, Izumida R. Irreducible palmar dislocation of the distal interphalangeal joint. J Hand Surg Br 2006;31:296–297.
8. Pohl AL. Irreducible dislocation of a distal interphalangeal joint. Br J Plas Surg 1976;29:227–229.
9. Schweitzer TP, Rayan GM. The terminal tendon of the digital extensor mechanism: Part I, anatomic study. J Hand Surg Am 2004;29:898–902.
10. Smith JH. Avulsion of the profundus tendon with simultaneous intraarticular fracture of the distal phalanx—case report. J Hand Surg Am 1981;6:600–601.
11. Wehbe MA, Schneider LH. Mallet fractures. J Bone Joint Surg Am 1984;66A:658–669.

Chapter 40

Corrective Osteotomy for Metacarpal and Phalangeal Malunion

Mohamed Khalid, Nilesh M. Chaudhari, and Thomas R. Hunt III

DEFINITION

- *Malunion* results when a fracture fragment heals in incorrect anatomic alignment.

ANATOMY

- Metacarpals and phalanges are tubular structures with a smooth dorsal surface covered by the extensor tendon and its expansions.
- Metacarpals are triangular in cross section. The medial and lateral surfaces meet at the volar ridge, providing attachment to the interossei. These attachments together with the intermetacarpal ligaments proximally and distally help splint fractured bones, making functionally significant malunions of the ring and small metacarpals less common.
- Phalanges are bean-shaped in cross section. The volar aspects of the proximal and middle phalanges are in intimate relation to the flexor digitorum profundus (FDP) and superficialis (FDS) tendons, particularly in the region of the annular pulleys (**FIG 1**).
  - As a result, the tendons are vulnerable to damage from drills and screws used in a dorsovolar direction. This problem is especially significant in the region of the annular pulleys, where the tendons are strapped against the volar cortex, rendering them vulnerable to damage.

PATHOGENESIS

- Malunions most often occur secondary to lack of treatment or inadequate nonoperative care.
  - Malunion following internal fixation is uncommon, but when present usually results from inadequate stability or poor patient compliance.

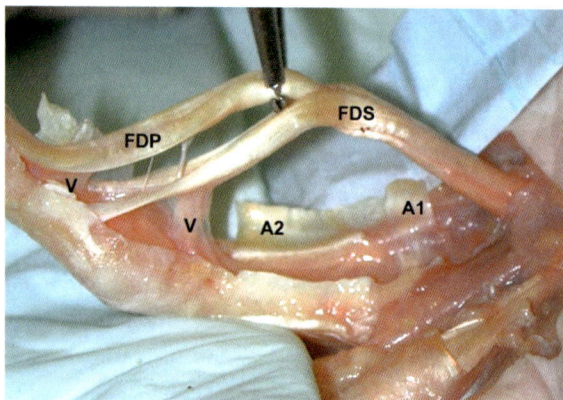

FIG 1 • Structures on the volar aspect of the metacarpals and phalanges. The flexor digitorum profundus (FDP) and flexor digitorum superficialis (FDS) tendons are intimately associated with the volar aspect of the phalanges and, to a lesser extent, the metacarpals. This dissected specimen also depicts the vinculae (V) and the A-1 and A-2 annular pulleys. (From http://www.turntillburn.ch.)

- Extra-articular malunions (EAM) often are multiplanar, but usually there is one major component to the deformity that causes the functional deficit.[5]
- The more proximal the malunion, the greater the deformity.
  - Just 1 degree of rotation at the fracture site may translate to 5 degrees at the finger tip.[4]
  - 5 degrees of fracture malrotation can cause 1.5 cm of digital overlap when the fingers are flexed.[2]
- Soft tissue pathology such as neurovascular deficits, trophic changes, joint contractures, and tendon adhesions can coexist.
  - Results of corrective osteotomy are significantly poorer in the presence of such complicating factors.[1]

NATURAL HISTORY

- Significant EAM can cause crossing or scissoring of fingers, pain due to distortion of joints, disturbance of muscle/tendon balance, and reduction of grip strength.[1]
- EAMs associated with shortening can lead to an extension lag proportional to the degree of shortening. The effect is more pronounced in proximal phalanges compared to metacarpals.[10]
- Intra-articular malunion (IAM) with a significant step (0.5 mm) or gap (1 mm) may cause joint surface incongruity, synovitis, capsular loosening or stiffness, and, ultimately, painful posttraumatic arthrosis.[1,3]

PATIENT HISTORY AND PHYSICAL FINDINGS

- The value of a good history and physical examination cannot be overemphasized. The decision as to whether surgical treatment is to be offered depends almost entirely on a history suggestive of a significant functional impairment or pain.
- Injury specifics
  - The original injury and method(s) of treatment
  - Location
    - Phalanx versus metacarpal
    - Extra-articular versus intra-articular versus combined deformities
  - History of complicating factors, eg, infection and chronic mediated pain syndrome
  - Duration of malunion, particularly relevant in deciding surgical strategy (reducing the fracture vs osteotomy)
  - Associated injuries such as soft tissue defects and neurovascular injuries
- Specific patient characteristics
  - Skeletal maturity
  - Hand dominance
  - Degree of deformity, swelling, stiffness, weakness of grip, and pain
  - Occupation and avocational pursuits as well as patient expectations and goals
  - Ability to cooperate with postoperative therapy regimen

IMAGING AND OTHER DIAGNOSTIC STUDIES

- Good-quality radiographs taken in three precise planes (anteroposterior, lateral, and oblique) are sufficient for simple EAMs.
  - Radiographs of the opposite hand are helpful in preoperative planning for complex EAMs.
- IAMs and combined malunions may require CT scans with three-dimensional reconstruction.

DIFFERENTIAL DIAGNOSIS

- Fibrous nonunion
- Nonunion with soft tissue contracture
- Sequelae of epiphyseal injury or growth arrest
- Erosive arthritis

NONOPERATIVE MANAGEMENT

- Hand therapy is directed toward maximizing the range of motion (ROM) of the digits, promoting optimal tendon excursion, and improving the grip strength.
- In less dramatic deformities, physical therapy is the first line treatment. Many patients will gain enough functional improvement that they decide to "live with" the deformity.
- Initiation of therapy allows the opportunity to assess the patient's personality with respect to compliance and realistic expectations.

SURGICAL MANAGEMENT

Timing of Correction

- Treatment of nascent malunions results in improved outcomes.
- IAMs must be corrected as soon as possible if there is a significant articular step and no overwhelming technical difficulties are anticipated.[1]
- In the case of an EAM, after 6 to 8 weeks from the injury, a "wait and watch" policy before osteotomy is advisable to see whether the malunion causes significant functional or cosmetic problems.

Location of Correction

- At or near the apex of the deformity for angular and complex EAMs
- In the proximal metaphysis of the malunited bone for rotational EAMs. With improved osteotomy techniques and fixation implants, a proximal metacarpal osteotomy is no longer recommended for treatment of a P-1 rotational malunion.[1]

Type of Osteotomy

- For angular EAMs, a closing wedge osteotomy is preferable, especially in the setting of intrinsic tightness. This approach is most commonly used for dorsal apex metacarpal malunions. An opening wedge osteotomy is best in the setting of an extension lag and pseudoclaw deformity, which are more commonly seen in apex volar phalangeal malunions. An incomplete osteotomy may be used for either of these cases.
- For rotational and combined rotational/angular EAM correction, a complete osteotomy is required.[4] Metacarpal neck EAM from a previous Boxer's fracture without significant shortening may be corrected with a pivot osteotomy.[9]

- Condylar advancement osteotomy[8] is suitable for IAM correction in many cases.

Severity of Deformity

- Malunion does not always mandate a corrective osteotomy. Patients possess a significant capacity to adapt to minor deformities. For instance, slight overlap of adjacent digits due to rotational malunion may be unsettling and unsightly, but it is consistent with good hand function.[5] Similarly, a proximal diaphyseal malunion of the small-finger metacarpal can contribute to tendon imbalance and flexion contracture of the proximal interphalangeal joint, but the hand may function effectively.[7]
- Multifragment IAMs and those with established posttraumatic arthrosis are best treated by arthrodesis or arthroplasty rather than repositioning osteotomy.

Preoperative Planning

- In addition to precise evaluation of the bony deformity, careful assessment of the soft tissue envelope, gliding capacity of the flexor and extensor tendons, joint mobility, and neurovascular status is critical.
  - Plan for adjunct procedures (eg, tenolysis, capsulotomy) that may be required.
  - Determine the optimal location for placement of internal fixation.
  - Decide on opening or closing wedge osteotomy. In the presence of an extension lag, an opening wedge is preferred, whereas, in the presence of intrinsic tightness, a closing wedge is preferred.
  - Provide for soft tissue coverage as needed.
- Preoperative templates are created for bony correction.
  - The proximal and distal fragments are each outlined then superimposed over an outline of the contralateral uninjured bone.
  - The type and location of the osteotomy, the size of the bone graft needed (in the case of an opening wedge osteotomy), as well as the method of fixation are determined.
  - In the rare cases requiring large corticocancellous interposition grafts, iliac crest bone graft harvest is planned.

Positioning

- The patient is positioned supine with the shoulder abducted to 90 degrees, elbow extended, and the extremity on an arm table.
- Place a proximal arm, non-sterile tourniquet.
- If required, prep for ipsilateral iliac crest graft harvest.
- Perform an examination under anesthesia to determine joint ROM and stability.

Approach

- A dorsal approach through a dorsal skin incision in the intermetacarpal space is used for the second through fourth metacarpals (**FIG 2A**).
- A midaxial approach through a midaxial skin incision at the junction of the wrinkled dorsal and smooth volar skin is used for the fifth metacarpal and the proximal and middle phalanges (**FIG 2B**).
  - Coronal plane correction is best accomplished with a lateral buttress plate placed over the bone graft (**FIG 2C,D**).
  - Dorsal plates should be avoided in the phalanges due to extensor tendon adhesions and resulting loss of motion.

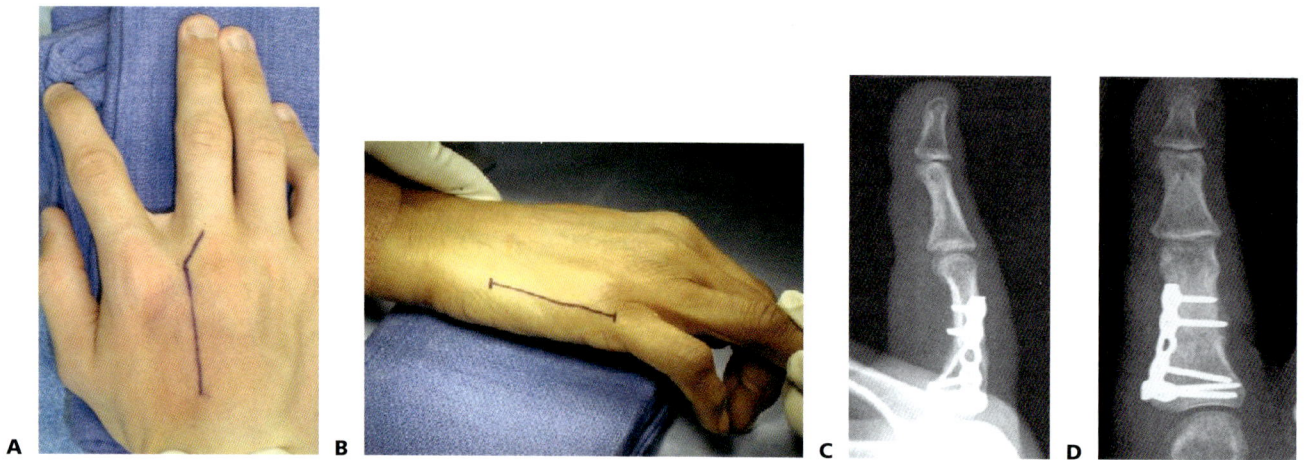

FIG 2 • A. Skin incision used for a dorsal approach to a third metacarpal malunion. The longitudinal limb of the skin incision runs between the metacarpals, and depending on whether the malunion is proximal or distal, the appropriate end is curved. **B.** Skin incision at the junction of the glabrous skin for an osteotomy of the fifth metacarpal. A similar mid-axial incision is employed for phalangeal malunion correction. **C,D.** Coronal plane correction of a proximal phalangeal malunion. The plate has been placed laterally to avoid interfering with the extensor mechanism, as well to avoid damage to the flexor tendons while drilling and inserting screws.

INCOMPLETE OSTEOTOMY FOR ANGULAR CORRECTION

Metacarpal Closing Wedge Osteotomy

- Make a dorsal incision in the interval between either the index–long or ring–small metacarpals. depending on the bone to be treated (see Fig 2A).
  - An incision at the junction of the glabrous skin often is appropriate for small metacarpal malunion correction (see Fig 2B).
- Retract the extensor tendon to expose the metacarpal (**TECH FIG 1A**).
- Make a dorsolateral incision through the metacarpal's periosteum, and carefully free this layer from the dorsum of the metacarpal with a no. 15 blade (**TECH FIG 1B**).
  - At completion of the operation, this periosteal and muscle layer will be closed, serving to protect the extensor tendons from the underlying internal fixation.
- Subperiosteally expose the circumference of the bone at the planned osteotomy site.
- Pass two small Hohmann retractors, one radially and one ulnarly, to protect the tendons and neurovascular structures.
  - Take care not to put undue tension on these structures.
- Precisely identify the apex of the deformity by determining the intersection between the true anatomic axis of both the proximal and distal fragments.
  - Place a 0.35-mm K-wire parallel to the proximal fragment and under radiographic guidance mark the anatomic axis using diathermy or a marking pen.
  - Mark the distal fragment in a similar manner.

- Design the osteotomy around the intersection of these two marks (**TECH FIG 1C**).
  - Plan the cuts perpendicular to the long axis of each fragment.
  - The size of the bone wedge to be removed is determined based on preoperative templates and intraoperative measurements.
- Center and apply a six- or seven-hole 2.0- to 2.7-mm compression plate to the dorsum of one fragment using two screws.
  - Moderately tighten the screws.
  - Plan for six cortices of fixation proximal and distal to the osteotomy if possible.
  - Juxta-articular osteotomies are best stabilized using condylar plates, T-plates, or Y-plates. Locking plates also may be of value in these cases.
- Remove one screw and rotate the plate away from the osteotomy site.
- Create an incomplete osteotomy, starting on the dorsal convex surface and using a water-cooled sagittal saw or sharp osteotome.
  - Complete the distal bone cut before making the proximal bone cut.
  - An elastic pillar of bone is left intact volarly on the concave side to act as a hinge.
  - In some cases, complete correction and osteotomy reduction can be obtained only if the volar cortex is cut and only the volar periosteum is left intact as the hinge.
- Correction is adequate when the true anatomic axes of the proximal and distal fragments are parallel (**TECH FIG 1D**).
  - The dorsal plate often will serve as a guide to reduction when it sits flat on the dorsum of both fragments.

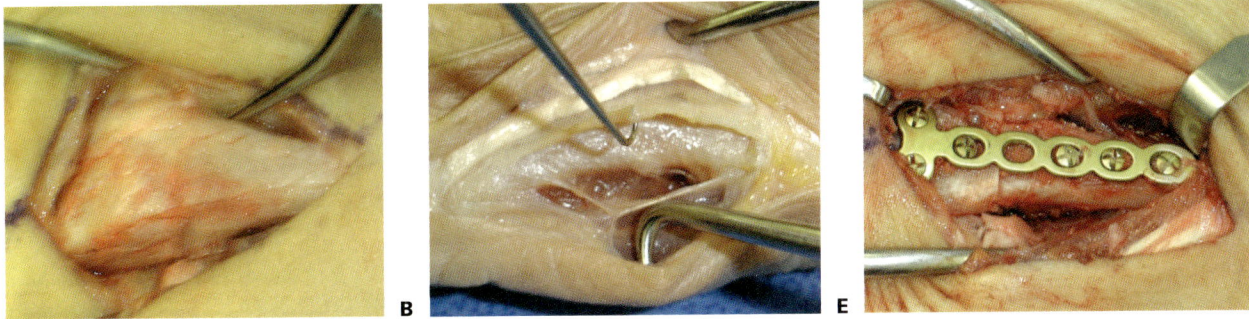

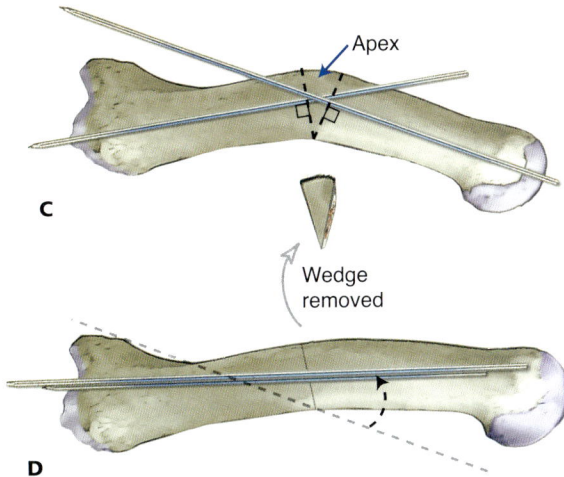

TECH FIG 1 • **A.** Extensor tendons have been retracted to expose the dorsal surface of the metacarpal sagittal plane malunion. **B.** The deep subtendinous layer of the metacarpal is demonstrated. Note that the periosteum is still intact. This layer is repaired covering the implant to prevent tendon adhesions. **C,D.** Method of using K-wires to determine the apex of the deformity. After removing a wedge, the size of which is determined by preoperative templating (**C**), deformity correction is confirmed when the K-wire markings are observed to be parallel (**D**). **E.** Dorsally applied T-plate with three screws distal and three screws proximal to the osteotomy.

- Re-apply the plate, tightening the two screws. Reduce the osteotomy, and secure the other fragment by applying the other side of the plate in compression (**TECH FIG 1E**).
- Insert the remaining screws and assess reduction clinically and radiographically.
- Close the periosteal and muscle layer between the plate and the extensor tendons with absorbable suture, and close the skin in the usual manner.
- Place a forearm-based splint with the wrist mildly extended and the metacarpophalangeal (MP) joints immobilized in 60 to 70 degrees of flexion. The proximal interphalangeal (PIP) joints are left free.

Phalangeal Opening Wedge Osteotomy

- Make a mid-axial skin incision (**TECH FIG 2A**).
- Protect against injury to the dorsal sensory nerve branch (**TECH FIG 2B**).

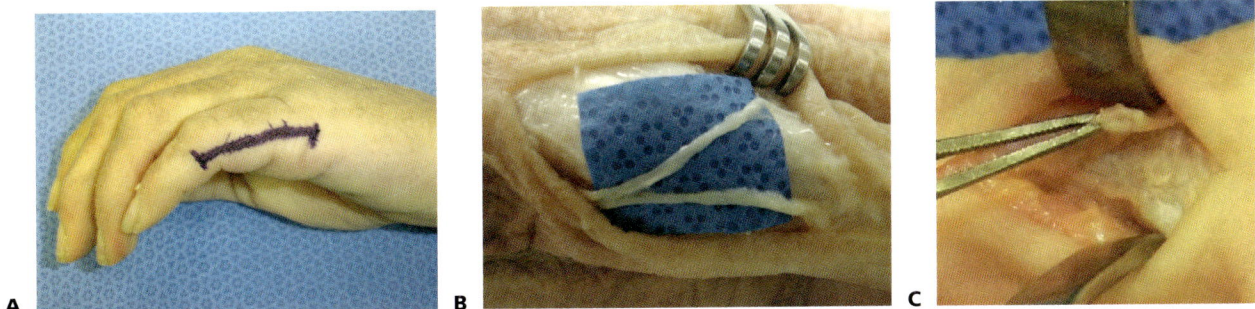

- Incise the lateral band as required (**TECH FIG 2C**), and expose the circumference of the bone subperiosteally at the site of the planned osteotomy.
- Use a "no touch" technique with the extensors and insert small Hohmann retractors to visualize the bone and the deformity.
- Apply K-wires to precisely locate the site of the deformity and serve as a guide for correction in the manner detailed earlier (**TECH FIG 2D,E**).
- Make an incomplete osteotomy on the concave side at the apex of the deformity perpendicular to the distal fragment.
  - Contouring of the bone graft is simplified if the osteotomy is made perpendicular to the distal fragment. This leaves only the proximal portion of the graft irregular.
- Provisionally stabilize the fragments with a longitudinal K-wire and assess clinically and radiographically.

TECH FIG 2 • **A.** Lateral incision for proximal phalangeal osteotomy. **B.** Dorsal cutaneous nerve. **C.** Lateral approach to the proximal phalanx. The sagittal band has been cut and elevated to expose the proximal phalanx. *(continued)*

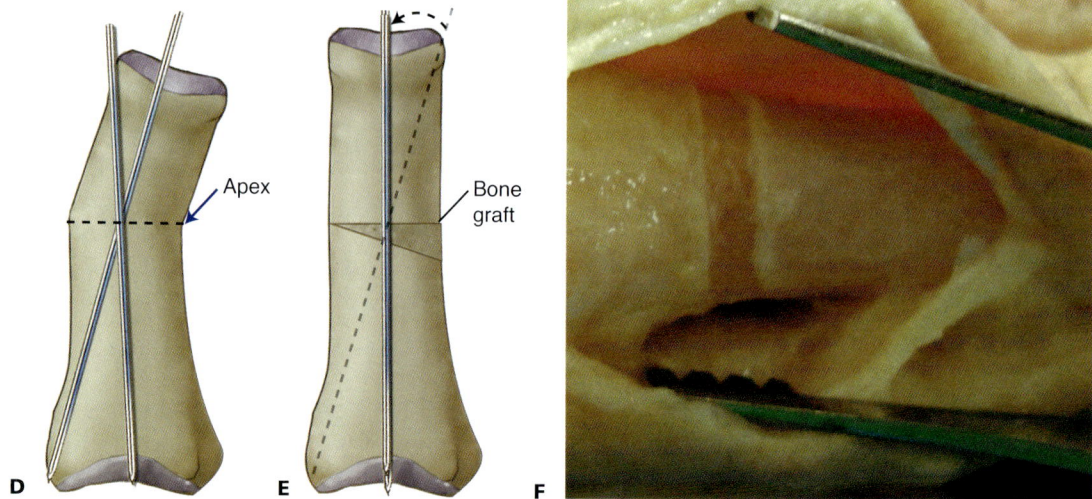

TECH FIG 2 • (continued) **D.** Method of determining the apex of the deformity for an opening wedge osteotomy. **E.** With the deformity adequately corrected, the wire markings are parallel or overlapping. **F.** The corticocancellous graft has been inserted into the defect correcting the deformity.

- Harvest either a corticocancellous wedge of bone or cancellous bone from the dorsal distal radius just proximal and ulnar to Lister's tubercle.
  - The size of the graft is determined by preoperative templating and intraoperative measurement.
- Contour the graft using a water-cooled sagittal saw.
- Insert the graft to correct the deformity and apply a lateral six-or seven-hole 1.5- to 2.0-mm compression plate (**TECH FIG 2F**).
  - Plan for six cortices of fixation proximal and distal to the osteotomy, if possible.

- Juxta-articular osteotomies are best stabilized using condylar plates, T-plates, or Y-plates. Locking plates also may be of value.
- If possible, close the thin periosteal layer between the plate and the extensor tendons with absorbable suture, and close the skin in the usual manner.
- Do not repair the lateral band. Check the correction clinically and compare with the preoperative pictures.
- Place a forearm-based splint with the wrist mildly extended and the MP joints immobilized in 60 to 70 degrees of flexion. The IP joints are immobilized in full extension.

COMPLETE OSTEOTOMY FOR ROTATIONAL AND COMBINED ROTATIONAL/ANGULAR MALUNIONS

- Perform a dorsal approach for malunions of the second through fourth metacarpals and a lateral approach for the fifth metacarpal and phalangeal malunions, as detailed earlier.
- Identify and mark the true anatomic axis of the proximal and distal fragments using 0.35-mm K-wires under radiographic guidance in the manner already reviewed. Define the apex of the angular deformity (see Tech Figs 1C and 2D,E).
- Insert one K-wire proximal and one distal to the malunion, perpendicular to the long axis and in a true dorsal-volar direction. This defines the rotational deformity.
- In the manner detailed previously, perform the osteotomy (opening vs closing) needed to correct the angular portion of the malunion using a water-cooled sagittal saw or a sharp osteotome.
  - Insert a longitudinal K-wire to temporarily stabilize the fragments.
  - Early correction of the angular malunion aids in plate contouring and placement.

- Select a suitable plate (1.5 to 2 mm for P-1 and 2.0 to 2.7 mm for metacarpals), contour it to the lateral bony surface of the proximal fragment, align it to the anatomic axis, and insert screws through the plate fixing it to that fragment.
- Harvest, contour, and insert bone graft if required.
- Remove the longitudinal K-wire and correct the rotational portion of the malunion by bringing the dorsal-volar K-wires into a parallel position while still maintaining angular correction (**TECH FIG 3A**).
- Secure the distal fragment to the plate in a compression mode.
- Fine-tune the rotational alignment while maintaining the angular correction by using a gliding hole rotation plate (**TECH FIG 3B,C**).
- Check the correction and range of motion clinically (**TECH FIG 3D**).
- Close the wound and splint as previously discussed.

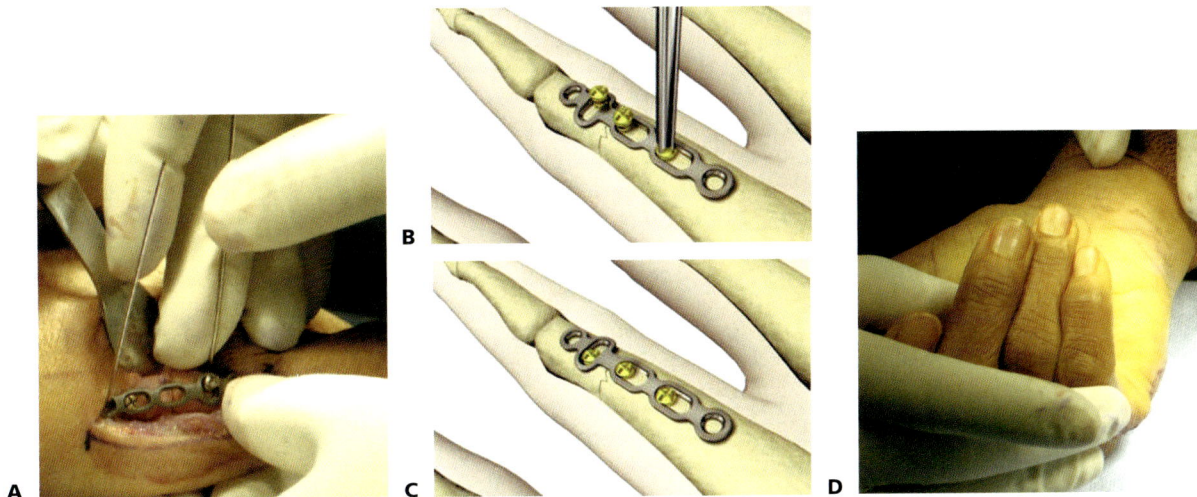

TECH FIG 3 • **A.** K-wires previously were inserted in the dorsovolar plane, perpendicular to the dorsal surface of the proximal and distal fragments. The position of these K-wires defines the degree of rotational malunion. After correction of the sagittal plane deformity, the K-wires are manipulated into a parallel position to achieve rotational correction. **B,C.** Use of the rotation plates (in this case, VariAx Hand Locking Plate Module [Stryker]). The screw in the perpendicular gliding hole is positioned (but not tightened) ulnar or radial, depending on the direction of the rotational correction desired. The osteotomy is compressed, and the screws in the parallel oblong holes are tightened first. The rotational correction is then obtained, and the gliding hole screw is tightened to obtain controlled correction. **D.** View after correction of a combined rotational and angular malunion of the fifth metacarpal. (**B,C:** Courtesy of Stryker Osteosynthesis.)

CONDYLAR ADVANCEMENT OSTEOTOMY

- Condylar advancement osteotomy avoids the problem of handling a small condylar malunion (**TECH FIG 4A**), which is difficult to fix securely and is susceptible to osteonecrosis.[9]
- Make a sweeping dorsal, curved skin incision over the involved MP or PIP joint.
  - MP: Incise the sagittal band and then the capsule.
  - PIP: Enter the interval between the lateral band and the central slip and incise the capsule.
  - Protect the origin of the collateral ligament and its accompanying vascularity.
- Carefully dissect the extensor tendon gently off the bone over the region of the proposed osteotomy.

- Evaluate the condition of the joint. If significant arthrosis is present, consider a salvage procedure rather than a repositioning osteotomy.
- Resect a wedge of bone between the condyles with a water-cooled sagittal saw (**TECH FIG 4B**).
- Make a counter-cut in the diaphysis and advance the mal-united condyle distally to restore articular congruity (**TECH FIG 4C**).
- Stabilize the mobilized fragment using interfragmentary screws (**TECH FIG 4D**).
  - Insert the first screw parallel with the joint to ensure precise joint reduction.

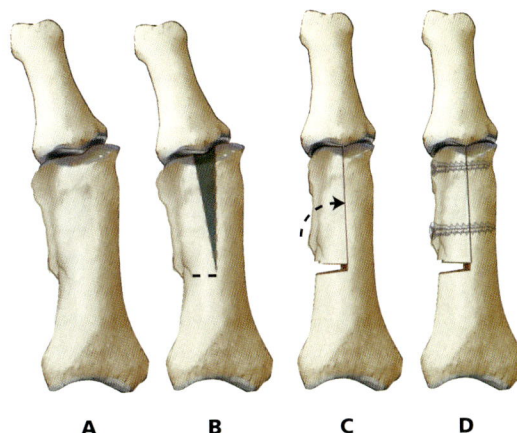

TECH FIG 4 • Condylar advancement osteotomy for unicondylar malunion.

PEARLS AND PITFALLS

Indications	▪ Define the goals of treatment with the patient, and ensure that they are realistic. ▪ In the case of an intra-articular malunion, consider a salvage procedure rather than a repositioning osteotomy in the face of arthrosis.
Preoperative assessment	▪ Understand the "personality" of the malunion as well as the patient. Bony as well as soft tissue aspects of the deformity must be understood.
Operative planning	▪ The plane of the deformity and the different components of the deformity, as well as the true extent of the deformity, must be factored in planning the location, orientation, and extent of the osteotomy.
Operative technique	▪ Atraumatic bone and soft tissue handling is critical, especially in regard to the extensor mechanism overlying P-1. An oscillating power saw with a thin blade and a field of excursion similar to the diameter of the bone is needed. Copious saline irrigation is used to prevent thermal necrosis. ▪ Accurate plate and screw placement is essential. A screw offset of 1 mm can cause as much as 10 degrees of rotation.[4]
Implants	▪ Stable fixation is needed to allow early range of motion. ▪ Consider using implants a size larger than used for acute fractures, particularly if extensive soft tissue release has been performed. ▪ Newer-generation locking plates and screws are valuable when fixation in the metaphysis is required.
Postoperative	▪ Institute early postoperative therapy.

POSTOPERATIVE CARE

▪ If adequate stability is obtained at the time of surgery, remove the postoperative splint 3 to 5 days after surgery and initiate protected motion.

   ▪ Initiate an early active and active assisted ROM program.

   ▪ When not performing ROM exercises, rest the hand in a volar splint in a functional position (MP joints flexed to 60–70 degrees and IP joints fully extended), apply a compression bandage, and elevate.

▪ Progress to passive ROM exercises, and use reverse blocking exercises to strengthen and rebalance the extensors.

▪ If needed, and if healing is progressing appropriately, use static or dynamic splints to address pending joint contractures.

▪ Encourage functional use of the hand long before the radiographs show complete bony consolidation.

OUTCOMES

▪ Encouraging results have been reported. In the largest reported series of 59 osteotomies Buchler et al[4] reported the following:

   ▪ A 100% union rate
   ▪ Satisfactory correction of the deformity in 76% of cases
   ▪ A net gain in active ROM in 89% of the patients
   ▪ Excellent and good functional results in 96% of patients requiring bony corrections only and 64% for those requiring bony and soft tissue correction

COMPLICATIONS

▪ Incomplete or inadequate correction (up to 24% of patients)
▪ Iatrogenic damage to soft tissues (up to 4% of patients)
▪ Residual stiffness

REFERENCES

1. Büchler U, Gupta A, Ruf S. Corrective osteotomy for posttraumatic malunion of the phalanges in the hand. J Hand Surg Br 1996;21:33–42.
2. Freeland AE, Jabaley ME, Hughes JL. Fracture repair: metacarpals and carpals. In Freeland A, Jabaley M, Hughes J, eds. Stable Fixation of the Hand and Wrist. New York: Springer-Verlage, 1986:35–71.
3. Light TR. Salvage of intra-articular malunions of the hand and wrist. The role of realignment osteotomy. Clin Orthop Relat Res 1987;214:130–135.
4. Opgrande JD, Westphal SA. Fractures of the hand. Orthop Clin North Am 1983;14:779–792.
5. Ring D. Malunion and nonunion of the metacarpals and phalanges. J Bone Joint Surg Am 2005;87A:1380–1388.
6. Rosenwasser MP, Quitkin HM. Malunion and other posttraumatic complications in the hand. In: Berger R, Weiss A, eds. Hand Surgery. Philadelphia: Lippincott Williams & Wilkins, 2003:207–230.
7. Strauch RJ, Rosenwasser MP, Lunt JG. Metacarpal shaft fractures: The effect of shortening on the extensor tendon mechanism. J Hand Surg Am 1998;23:519–523.
8. Teoh LC, Yong FC, Chong KC. Condylar advancement osteotomy for correcting condylar malunion of the finger. J Hand Surg Br 2002;27:31–35.
9. Thurston AJ. Pivot osteotomy for the correction of malunion of metacarpal neck fractures. J Hand Surg Br 1992;17:580–582.
10. Vahey JW, Wegner DA, Hastings H. Effect of proximal phalangeal fracture deformity on extensor tendon function. J Hand Surg Am 1998;23:673–681.

Arthroscopic Evaluation and Treatment of Scapholunate and Lunotriquetral Ligament Disruptions

Alexander H. Payatakes, Alex M. Meyers, and Dean G. Sotereanos

DEFINITION

- Scapholunate and lunotriquetral interosseous ligament tears are common wrist injuries occurring in isolation or as part of the perilunate injury pattern.
- Interosseous ligament injuries are being diagnosed with an increased frequency as a result of recent advances in imaging and arthroscopy.
- Management of these injuries has proven to be a difficult clinical problem. Surgical management has been more reliable in pain relief than in altering the natural history.

ANATOMY

- The scapholunate complex is subject to significant loads, since the scaphoid is the only carpal bone to span from the proximal to the distal carpal row.
- The proximal carpal row flexes with radial deviation and extends with ulnar deviation.
  - The scaphoid "wants" to flex and the triquetrum "wants" to extend.
  - The lunate (the intercalated segment) is tethered between the scaphoid and triquetrum. A large amount of potential energy exists in the proximal carpal row.
- Stability is provided to the scapholunate complex by the intrinsic scapholunate interosseous ligament (SLIL) as well as extrinsic capsular ligaments, especially the dorsal radiocarpal (DRC), dorsal intercarpal (DIC) ligament, and volar radioscaphocapitate (RSC) and scaphotrapezium-trapezoid (STT) ligaments.
- The SLIL is a C-shaped structure consisting of a stronger dorsal ligamentous portion (2 to 3 mm thick), a volar ligamentous portion (1 mm thick), and a proximal fibrocartilaginous (membranous) portion.[2]
- Isolated injuries to the SLIL appear to be associated with dynamic instability, whereas static instability usually indicates additional injury to the secondary ligamentous stabilizers, including the DIC ligament.[16]
- The lunotriquetral complex is also stabilized by an intrinsic lunotriquetral ligament (LTIL) and extrinsic (volar and dorsal) capsular ligaments.
- The LTIL is C-shaped, analogous to the SLIL, consisting of dorsal and volar ligamentous portions and a membranous proximal portion. In contrast to the SLIL, the volar ligamentous portion of the LTIL is stronger and more significant functionally.[12]
- As with the scapholunate complex, isolated injuries to the LTIL are usually insufficient for the development of static instability. Presence of a static deformity indicates additional injury to extrinsic ligamentous structures (volar ulnotriquetral, ulnolunate, and ulnocapitate ligaments or the dorsal radiocarpal and intercarpal ligaments).[7,20]

PATHOGENESIS

- Mayfield et al[9] postulated that scapholunate disruption is the initial component of the lesser arc perilunate injury pattern, which occurs when force is applied to the thenar area with the wrist in extension, supination, and ulnar deviation.
  - Depending on the amount of kinetic energy involved, the injury may or may not extend to the ulnar side of the wrist.
- SLIL injuries can be sprains, partial tears, or complete tears (with or without injury to the extrinsic ligament stabilizers).
  - With complete SLIL tears the scaphoid flexes and the lunate is pulled by the triquetrum into extension (dorsal intercalated segment instability [DISI] pattern).
  - With complete SLIL tears the ligament usually fails at the bone–ligament interface off the scaphoid.
- Arthroscopic evaluation has revealed associated SLIL injuries in up to 30% of intra-articular distal radius fractures.[5]
- LTIL disruption may be traumatic or atraumatic in origin.
  - Traumatic LTIL rupture may occur as the final component of a greater or lesser arc perilunate injury pattern.[9]
  - Isolated LTIL tears may result from a fall on an outstretched hand in extension, pronation, and radial deviation (reverse perilunate injury)[11] or from a dorsally applied force on a flexed wrist.[25]
  - Atraumatic ruptures of the LTIL may occur secondary to inflammatory arthritis or ulnar impaction syndrome.[18]

NATURAL HISTORY

- Tears of the SLIL or LTIL, with or without extrinsic ligamentous injury, may lead to various degrees of carpal instability (predynamic, dynamic, or static), alteration of normal carpal mechanics and kinematics, and early degenerative changes in the radiocarpal and midcarpal joints.
- A complete SLIL tear is associated with the development of a DISI deformity, which may be dynamic or static (indicates additional injury to the extrinsic ligaments).
  - As a DISI deformity forms, abnormal radiocarpal contact loading occurs as the proximal carpal bones shift in position and lose congruency.
  - Abnormal flexion and hypermobility of the scaphoid over time leads to degenerative changes of the radioscaphoid and capitolunate joints and ultimately collapse, termed scapholunate advanced collapse (SLAC) wrist degeneration.[22,23]
  - These degenerative changes have been documented to begin as early as 3 months after injury.

- A complete LTIL tear is associated with the development of a volar intercalated segment instability (VISI) deformity.
- The natural history of partial tears of the SLIL or LTIL is at present poorly defined.
    - Partial scapholunate and LT injuries may cause chronic, activity-related wrist pain in the absence of radiologic findings.[23]
- Predynamic or dynamic instability may cause attenuation of extrinsic ligaments with progressive development of further instability and static changes.[29,30]
    - There is evidence that this process typically requires many years.[10]

PATIENT HISTORY AND PHYSICAL FINDINGS

- Dorsoradial or ulnar-sided wrist pain with a history of a fall, sudden loading, or twisting of the wrist should raise suspicion for a SLIL or LTIL tear, respectively. However, it is not uncommon for the patient to deny any significant injury.
- Patients frequently complain of weakness, swelling, and loss of range of motion of the wrist.
- A sensation of instability or "giving way" is often reported, occasionally associated with a painful clunk.
- A detailed physical examination of the wrist may provide significant information for the diagnosis of ligamentous injuries and help to rule out other wrist pathology.
- Examination of the wrist begins with evaluation for any deformity or swelling and determination of wrist range of motion.
- Key tests and maneuvers specifically evaluating the scapholunate and lunotriquetral ligaments are as follows:
    - Grip strength and pain: Diminished grip strength correlates with wrist pathology.
    - The presence of pain at the central aspect of the wrist with attempted grip has also been associated with scapholunate ligament pathology.
    - Deep palpation of scapholunate interval: Point tenderness indicates SLIL injury, scaphoid injury, or ganglion cyst.
    - Watson's scaphoid shift test: Pain with or without a clunk or catch sensation is highly suggestive of scapholunate instability.
    - Scaphoid ballottement test: Pain and increased anteroposterior laxity are highly suggestive of scapholunate instability.
    - Deep palpation of lunotriquetral interval: Point tenderness indicates LTIL injury or triangular fibrocartilage complex (TFCC) pathology.
    - Ulnar wrist loading: A painful snap indicates lunotriquetral instability, midcarpal instability, or TFCC complex pathology. This maneuver will also be painful if ulnar impaction is present.
    - Triquetrum ballottement test: Pain and increased anteroposterior laxity are highly suggestive of lunotriquetral instability.
    - "Ulnar snuffbox" tenderness: Pain with or without crepitus indicates lunotriquetral instability, TFCC complex pathology, or triquetrohamate pathology.

IMAGING AND OTHER DIAGNOSTIC STUDIES

- Initial imaging of the wrist should always include AP and lateral radiographs, combined with special views depending on the suspected pathology. If scapholunate pathology is suspected, a bilateral pronated grip anteroposterior (Mayo Clinic) view should be obtained for comparison to the contralateral side.
- Abnormal findings in static scapholunate instability include:
    - AP view: increased scapholunate interval (3 mm or more; comparison to contralateral wrist), scaphoid cortical "ring sign," and triangular appearance of lunate
    - Lateral view: flexion of scaphoid and dorsiflexion of lunate, as determined by increased scapholunate angle (more than 60 degrees) and increased lunocapitate angle (over 10 degrees) with dorsal translation of capitate
- Radiographic findings in patients with lunotriquetral tears are often normal. Abnormal findings in static lunotriquetral instability include:
    - AP view: proximal translation of triquetrum or lunotriquetral overlap without gapping, and interruption of Gilula's arc
    - Lateral view: flexion of scaphoid and lunate, as determined by normal or decreased scapholunate angle (less than 45 degrees), increased lunocapitate angle (more than 10 degrees) with volar translation of capitate, and a negative lunotriquetral angle
- Provocative views (radial-ulnar deviation, flexion–extension views) or videofluoroscopy may demonstrate asynchronous scapholunate motion (dynamic scapholunate instability) in cases with suspected SLIL injury and normal standard views. Increased, synchronous mobility of the scapholunate complex with diminished motion of the triquetrum indicate an LTIL injury.
- Wrist arthrography has a sensitivity of only 60% compared to arthroscopy and cannot determine the extent of any tear present.[26]
- MRI (with or without arthrography) has limited value in evaluating interosseous ligament injuries. Reported sensitivity rates for SLIL injuries range from 40% to 65% compared to arthroscopy.[17] MRI is even less reliable in diagnosing LTIL injuries.
- Arthroscopy (radiocarpal, midcarpal with probing) remains the gold standard in evaluation of SLIL and LTIL injuries.

DIFFERENTIAL DIAGNOSIS

- Differential diagnosis of scapholunate injuries and radial-sided wrist pain[21]
    - Scaphoid fracture or nonunion
    - Scaphotrapezial arthritis
    - Radiocarpal arthritis
    - De Quervain's tenosynovitis
    - Dorsal ganglion cyst
    - Dorsal wrist impaction syndrome
    - Perilunate instability
    - Isolated DRC ligament tear
- Differential diagnosis of lunotriquetral injuries and ulnar-sided wrist pain[18]
    - TFCC injury
    - Distal radioulnar joint (DRUJ) instability or arthritis
    - Ulnar impaction syndrome or chondromalacia
    - Ulnar styloid impingement syndrome
    - Extensor carpi ulnaris (ECU) tendon subluxation
    - Pisotriquetral arthritis
    - Triquetrohamate instability

- Hamate fracture
- Ulnar neurovascular syndromes

NONOPERATIVE MANAGEMENT

- SLIL and lunotriquetral injuries associated with dynamic instability may respond to initial nonoperative treatment for 6 to 12 weeks.
- Conservative management typically includes a combination of the following:
  - Splinting
  - Nonsteroidal anti-inflammatories
  - Intra-articular (radiocarpal) corticosteroid injections
  - Occupational therapy and work restrictions
  - Re-education of wrist proprioception with flexor carpi radialis strengthening

SURGICAL MANAGEMENT

- The selection of surgical treatment for SLIL and LTIL injuries is based on the severity of symptoms, the degree of instability (dynamic or static), chronicity (acute, subacute, or chronic), arthroscopic findings (Geissler grade; see **TECH FIG 1**), and reparability of the ligament.
- Dynamic instability (based on positive physical findings with provocative maneuvers, abnormal stress radiographs, arthroscopic findings) that has failed to respond to nonoperative treatment may be treated arthroscopically.
  - Arthroscopic options include simple débridement, débridement with thermal shrinkage, and débridement (with or without shrinkage) with percutaneous pinning.
- Static instability and severe dynamic instability are indications for open surgery.
  - Surgical options include open repair or augmentation (especially of acute or subacute injuries), capsulodesis, and tenodesis.
- Patients developing carpal collapse with arthritic changes require salvage procedures such as radial styloidectomy, proximal row carpectomy, and limited wrist fusions (eg, STT, scaphocapitate, scaphoidectomy plus four-corner fusion, reduction-association scapholunate [RASL] procedure, lunotriquetral fusion).
- The focus of this chapter is on arthroscopic procedures described for management of dynamic scapholunate or lunotriquetral instability. Newer arthroscopic alternatives advocated for management of more advanced pathology are also described.

Arthroscopic Procedures

- Arthroscopic débridement of SLIL and LTIL injuries
  - Indications: Predynamic or dynamic instability; arthroscopic findings of a partial ligament tear with an unstable tissue flap (Geissler grade II); with or without synovitis[15,27]
  - The ideal patient for this technique is one with mechanical symptoms (pain with crepitance or clicking) attributable to impingement of unstable tissue flaps and resulting synovitis.
- Arthroscopic débridement and thermal shrinkage of SLIL and LTIL disruptions
  - Indications: Predynamic or dynamic instability; arthroscopic finding of a partial ligament tear (Geissler grade I or II).[5,7] The dorsal segment of the SLIL should be intact for this procedure.

- This technique provides an option for the management of lax, redundant ligaments with no frank tear (Geissler grade I) where simple débridement is not an option.
  - Thermal shrinkage is performed in an attempt to increase stability and improve long-term outcome compared to simple débridement.
  - Radiofrequency probes use a high-frequency alternating current to generate heat. This leads to denaturation (uncoiling) of the collagen triple helix with reduction in overall ligament length.
    - Use of this device is contraindicated in patients with pacemakers or other implantable electronic devices.
- Arthroscopic débridement and percutaneous pinning of SLIL and LTIL disruptions
  - Indications: Acute or subacute dynamic instability (Geissler grades II and III)[3,28]
  - This technique aims to induce the formation of fibrous union between the two involved carpal bones.
- Arthroscopic radial styloidectomy
  - Indications: Early (stage I) scapholunate advanced collapse (SLAC) wrist (ie, radial styloid–scaphoid impingement or arthritis) with focal and reproducible clinical findings of radial styloid pain exacerbated by wrist flexion and radial deviation
  - This procedure may provide significant pain relief until a salvage procedure (proximal row carpectomy, scaphoid excision, four-corner fusion) becomes necessary.
- Arthroscopic RASL procedure (see Chap. HA-46) and lunotriquetral fusion
  - Indications: Static instability (Geissler grade IV); lunotriquetral arthritis[13,14]
  - Early (stage I) SLAC wrist is not a contraindication.
  - The RASL procedure aims to achieve fibrous union while maintaining mild rotation at the scapholunate joint, thus approximating normal wrist kinematics. On the other hand, bony fusion is the goal in the lunotriquetral joint.

Preoperative Planning

- A careful review of the patient's history, physical findings, as well as static and stress radiographs may provide the surgeon with a reasonable impression of what will be required.
  - In most cases, however, a decision on the type of procedure to be performed is made intraoperatively based on the arthroscopic findings and associated pathology.
- Consideration must therefore be given to have the following available: radiofrequency probes, mini C-arm, drills, Kirschner wires of various widths, and headless compression screws.

Positioning

- The patient is placed in the supine position with the extremity on a hand table.
- Any possible donor site for ligament reconstruction or augmentation should also be prepared and draped in a sterile fashion.
- The extremity is placed in a tower distraction device with 10 to 12 lb (5 to 6 kg) of distraction and 12 to 15 degrees of wrist flexion (**FIG 1**).
- The arthroscope monitor is placed on the opposite side of the hand table from the surgeon.

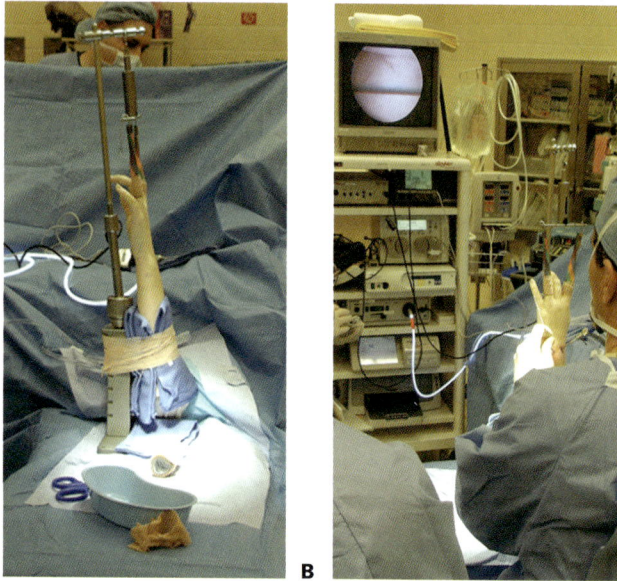

- If percutaneous pinning or use of other implants is anticipated, a small fluoroscopy unit is placed adjacent to the head of the operating table.

Approach

- Arthroscopic evaluation and management of scapholunate and lunotriquetral injuries can typically be performed through standard dorsal wrist portals (3–4, 4–5, 6R, midcarpal).
- The additional use of a radial volar portal through the flexor carpi radialis (FCR) sheath has been advocated for better visualization of the volar portions of the SLIL and LTIL, as well as the DRC and DIC ligaments.[1,19]

FIG 1 • A. Positioning for arthroscopy of the wrist. **B.** The monitor should be visible to the surgeon. If use of fluoroscopy is anticipated, the C-arm is placed adjacent to the head of the operating table.

ARTHROSCOPIC EVALUATION

- An 18-gauge needle is used to distend the radiocarpal joint with 7 to 10 mL of normal saline.
- A 2.7-mm, 30-degree arthroscope is preferred for wrist arthroscopy.
- Typical working portals include the 3–4, 4–5, 6R, and midcarpal portals. Outflow is established through the 6U or 6R portal.
- The entire radiocarpal joint is evaluated in a systematic manner, usually from radial to ulnar.

- The SLIL is best visualized through the 3–4 portal with probe insertion through the 4–5 or 6R portal. The 4–5 portal is used for instrumentation.
  - Occasionally the avulsed portion of the SLIL may make visualization through the 3–4 portal difficult. In this situation, the arthroscope is transferred to the 6R portal and directed radially.
- The proximal portion of the SLIL is easily visualized by following the radioscapholunate ligament (ligament of

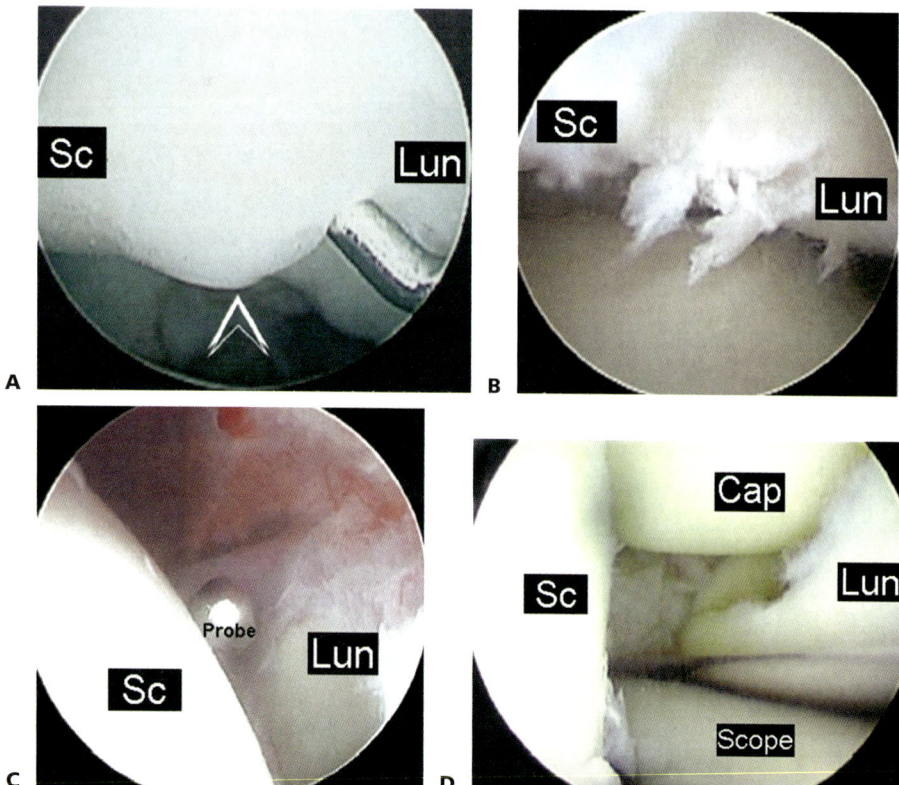

TECH FIG 1 • Geissler arthroscopic classification of interosseous ligament injuries of the wrist. The scapholunate joint is depicted here but the classification is also applicable to the lunotriquetral joint. **A.** Grade I: Attenuation of the scapholunate interosseous ligament as visualized in the radiocarpal joint. No incongruence is noted in the midcarpal joint. **B.** Grade II: Partial full-thickness tear with unstable flap but minimal joint incongruity. **C.** Grade III: Complete tear of the scapholunate interosseous ligament with moderate joint incongruity. A 1.5-mm probe can enter the joint (view from midcarpal portal). **D.** Grade IV: Complete tear with marked incongruity. The 2.7-mm arthroscope can "drive through" the joint.

TECHNIQUES

Testut) to its insertion. The volar radioscapholunate and long radiolunate ligaments (wider) are visualized radially, and the short radiolunate is located ulnar to the ligament of Testut.

- The LTIL is best visualized through the 4–5 or 6R portal, with use of the 3–4 and 6R for instrumentation.
- Both ligaments should be evaluated in their entirety (dorsal, proximal, and volar portions).
    - If visualization of the volar portions of the SLIL and LTIL is inadequate, an additional volar portal through the FCR sheath may be used,[1] but this has rarely been necessary in our experience.
- In patients with gross scapholunate instability, the arthroscope is finally turned toward the dorsum of the scaphoid and lunate to identify possible avulsion of the DIC or DRC ligament.[16]

- Evaluation of carpal congruence and stability is incomplete without performance of midcarpal arthroscopy.
- The midcarpal portals are placed 1 cm distal to the 3–4 and 4–5 portals.
- The 2.7-mm, 30-degree arthroscope is aimed proximal.
    - The scapholunate joint is visualized radially and the lunotriquetral joint ulnarly.
    - Both joints are evaluated for congruity.
    - Stability is evaluated with a 1-mm arthroscopic probe and the 2.7-mm arthroscope.
    - A Watson scaphoid shift test may be performed while visualizing the scapholunate joint.
- The Geissler arthroscopic classification of wrist interosseous ligament tears is shown in Techniques Figure 1.[5]

ARTHROSCOPIC DÉBRIDEMENT

- A thorough diagnostic arthroscopy (radiocarpal plus midcarpal) is performed to verify the diagnosis and rule out instability or other associated pathology.
- The inflamed synovium is excised with a 2.5- or 2.7-mm full-radius resector.
- Any unstable tissue flaps are resected with a suction punch or synovial resector.
- Redundant tissue is then resected to a stable rim with the synovial resector or bipolar radiofrequency probe.

- A probe is then inserted through the 4–5 or 6R portal to reassess stability from both the radiocarpal and midcarpal joint.
- Débridement should generally be limited to the proximal membranous portion of the SLIL or LTIL.
- Unwarranted débridement of the dorsal (SLIL) or volar (LTIL) portions of the ligamentous complex may lead to further instability.
- Carpal stability should be assessed both before and after débridement.

ARTHROSCOPIC DÉBRIDEMENT AND THERMAL SHRINKAGE

- Diagnostic arthroscopy is performed as previously described.
- Geissler grade II tears are débrided with a synovial resector to a stable rim (**TECH FIG 2A**). Thermal shrinkage of the intact portion of the ligament is then performed with a 2.3-mm bipolar radiofrequency probe.
    - Attenuated ligaments (Geissler grade I) are treated with thermal shrinkage alone.
- Thermal shrinkage is performed by applying the radiofrequency probe in a paintbrush fashion (2.3-mm radiofrequency probe [Mitek VAPR®, Westwood, MA]) (**TECH FIG 2B**). The goal is to evenly distribute the thermal

energy throughout the ligament.
    - The 4–5 portal is preferred for this procedure for optimal access to the SLIL.
    - Ligament shrinkage is visually confirmed by a change in its color and consistency (**TECH FIG 2C**).
- Intermittent application of the probe (a few seconds at a time) with adequate outflow prevents ablation of the ligament and overheating of the joint.
    - Radiofrequency probes specially designed for thermal shrinkage have recently become available. They offer additional safety by not reaching ablation temperature.

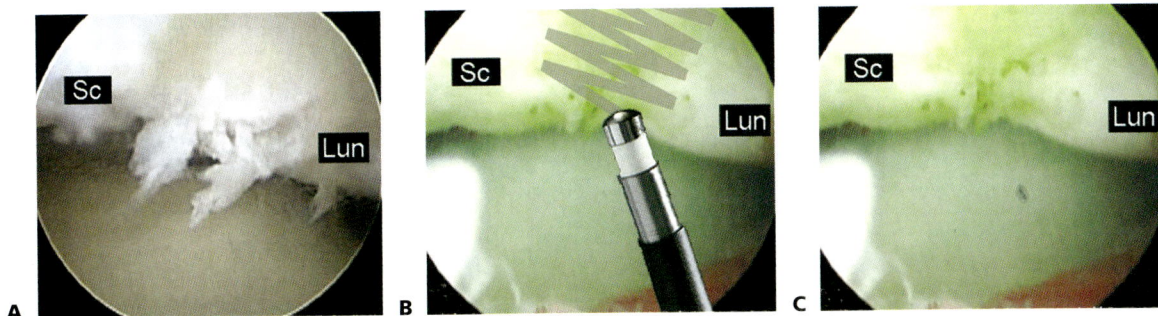

TECH FIG 2 • Débridement and thermal shrinkage. **A.** Geissler grade II scapholunate interosseous ligament tear as seen through 3–4 portal. **B.** "Paintbrush" technique for thermal shrinkage. The probe is applied intermittently to avoid overheating. **C.** The same ligament after débridement and thermal shrinkage. Note apparent change in color and consistency.

TECHNIQUES

ARTHROSCOPIC DÉBRIDEMENT AND PERCUTANEOUS PINNING

- Diagnostic arthroscopy is performed as previously described.
- All residual tissue of the torn ligament (SLIL or LTIL) is debrided with a 2.5- or 2.7-mm full-radius resector.
- The cartilage of the apposing surfaces of the involved carpal bones is then débrided to bleeding bone with a 2.5- or 2.7-mm aggressive full-radius resector and a 2.9-mm barrel abrader (**TECH FIG 3A**).
- The extremity is then removed from the distraction tower.
- If necessary, congruity of the joint is improved by external (pressure on the distal pole of scaphoid) or internal maneuvers (percutaneous Kirschner wires used as joysticks).

- The joint is stabilized by percutaneously inserting three or four 0.045-inch (1.1-mm) Kirschner wires under fluoroscopic control.
- The scapholunate joint is typically stabilized with two Kirschner wires across the scapholunate joint (radial to ulnar) followed by one or two Kirschner wires across the scaphocapitate joint (**TECH FIG 3B**).
- The lunotriquetral joint is similarly stabilized with two Kirschner wires across the lunotriquetral joint (ulnar to radial) followed by one or two Kirschner wires across the lunocapitate joint.
- The pins are then cut subcutaneously or bent outside the skin per surgeon preference.

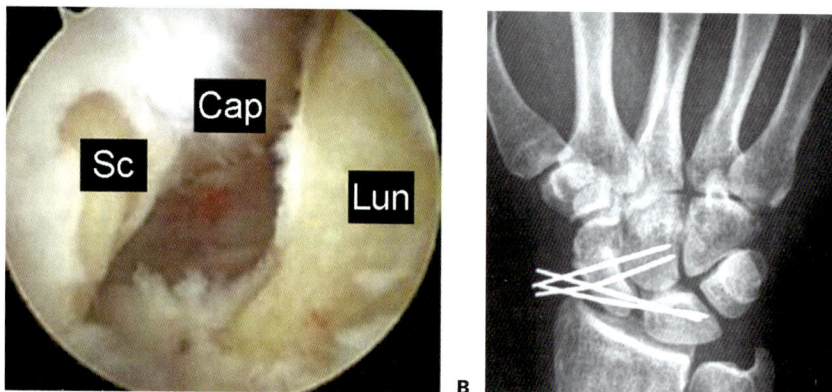

TECH FIG 3 • Débridement and percutaneous pinning. **A.** Remnants of ligament and articular cartilage of apposing surfaces are débrided to bleeding bone. **B.** The joint is stabilized with three or four Kirschner wires placed under fluoroscopic guidance.

ARTHROSCOPIC RADIAL STYLOIDECTOMY

- Diagnostic arthroscopy is initially performed to delineate the chondral lesions and accurately stage the SLAC wrist.[22]
- The arthroscope is placed in the 3–4 or 4–5 portal.
- Excision of the radial styloid is performed through the 1–2 (or 3–4) portal with a side-cutting 3.5-mm sheathed burr.

- Arthroscopic evaluation of articular cartilage and intraoperative radiographs should be used to determine the extent of resection.
  - The origin of the radioscaphocapitate ligament is visualized and preserved during bone resection.
- Although the tendency is to overestimate the amount of bone resected, excision of more than 4 mm may jeopardize the ligament and result in ulnar carpal dislocation.

ARTHROSCOPIC RASL PROCEDURE AND LUNOTRIQUETRAL FUSION

- Diagnostic arthroscopy with evaluation of chondral lesions is performed as described previously.
- The apposing surfaces of the joint to be fused are débrided to bleeding bone with a 2.5- or 2.7-mm aggressive full-radius resector and a 2.9-mm barrel abrader.
  - Complete decortication is verified from both the radiocarpal and midcarpal joints.
- In the case of the RASL procedure, a side-cutting 3.5-mm sheathed burr is then used to perform an arthroscopic radial styloidectomy through the 1–2 (or 3–4) portal as described previously.

- Kirschner wires (0.062 inch or 1.6 mm) are then inserted percutaneously from the dorsum into the involved carpal bones (distal scaphoid-lunate or lunate-triquetrum). Positioning of the wires should be slightly eccentric to allow for subsequent placement of the screw centrally. The Kirschner wires are used as joysticks to reduce the joint under fluoroscopic (with or without arthroscopic) control.
  - It is essential to verify adequate reduction of the capitolunate joint on the lateral view.
  - A Köcher clamp may be placed across the Kirschner wires to maintain reduction.

- An additional 0.045-inch (1.1-mm) Kirschner wire may be inserted through the dorsal rim of the distal radius into the lunate for provisional stabilization of the lunate.
- A 0.035-inch (0.9-mm) guidewire is then placed across the joint (scapholunate or lunotriquetral) under fluoroscopic control.
- In the case of the RASL procedure, the guidewire should be placed through the 1–2 portal, across the scaphoid waist toward the proximal-ulnar corner of the lunate, thus approximating the normal axis of rotation of the scapholunate joint (**TECH FIG 4**).
- A cannulated headless compression screw is then placed across the joint. Length measurement should be reduced by about 4 mm to accommodate for joint compression and to ensure that the screw is completely countersunk into bone.
- After satisfactory reduction and fixation are verified, the wrist capsule incision is repaired.
- In patients with lunotriquetral instability as a result of ulnar impaction syndrome, fusion of the lunotriquetral joint must be combined with an arthroscopic wafer procedure or an ulnar shortening.

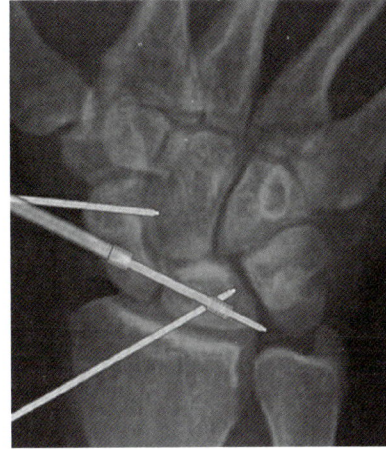

TECH FIG 4 • RASL technique. Scapholunate joint reduction is achieved using two Kirschner wires as joysticks. Optimal positioning of a compression screw is through the scaphoid waist toward the proximal-ulnar corner of the lunate, and fully countersunk.

PEARLS AND PITFALLS

Diagnosis	■ Meticulous examination and arthroscopy of the entire wrist are necessary to ensure diagnosis and treatment of concomitant pathology.
Indications	■ Arthroscopic débridement with or without thermal shrinkage is not adequate management for static scapholunate or lunotriquetral instability.
Contraindications	■ Use of radiofrequency probes for débridement or thermal shrinkage is contraindicated in patients with pacemakers or implantable electronic devices.
Surgical technique	■ Wrist arthroscopy for evaluation of SLIL or LTIL tears must include arthroscopy of the midcarpal joint. ■ Carpal stability should be assessed both before and after any débridement of the SLIL or LTIL. ■ Débridement of functionally significant portions of the SLIL (dorsal) or LTIL (volar) should be kept to a minimum to prevent further destabilization. ■ Thermal shrinkage should be performed with specially designed radiofrequency probes. Otherwise, the probe should be applied in a paintbrush fashion for only a few seconds at a time with adequate outflow to avoid reaching ablation temperatures.
Rehabilitation	■ If thermal shrinkage is performed, the wrist should be immobilized for at least 2 weeks postoperatively and protected for an additional 4 weeks to allow healing of treated tissue.

POSTOPERATIVE CARE

■ Patients treated with arthroscopic débridement alone are placed in a cock-up wrist splint postoperatively and instructed to initiate range-of-motion exercises at 48 hours.

■ Patients treated with arthroscopic débridement and thermal shrinkage are placed in a full-time short-arm splint postoperatively. Range-of-motion exercises are initiated at 2 to 4 weeks, with use of a removable cock-up splint between sessions. Strengthening exercises are initiated at 4 to 6 weeks.

■ Patients treated with arthroscopic débridement and percutaneous pinning are placed in a short-arm splint, changed to a short-arm cast after suture removal. The cast is maintained until pin removal, which is performed at 8 to 10 weeks for the scapholunate and at 4 to 6 weeks for the lunotriquetral joint. Range-of-motion exercises are then initiated, with progression to strengthening as tolerated.

■ Patients treated with an arthroscopic RASL procedure are placed in a short-arm splint for only 2 or 3 weeks. Range-of-motion exercises are then initiated, with progression to strengthening as tolerated. Conversely, patients treated with arthroscopic fusion of the lunotriquetral joint are immobilized until radiographic fusion is obtained.

OUTCOMES

■ Ruch and Poehling[15] reported excellent results with arthroscopic débridement alone in 14 patients with partial SLIL or lunotriquetral tears, or both, and predominantly mechanical symptoms. At a minimum follow-up of 2 years, all patients reported complete relief of their mechanical symptoms, while pain was significantly reduced and grip strength was restored.

■ Weiss et al[27] have treated both partial and complete SLIL and lunotriquetral tears with arthroscopic débridement alone in an attempt to elicit scar formation with some degree of stabilization. Excellent pain relief and increased strength were achieved in 17 of 19 patients with partial tears, but only in 17 of 24 patients with complete tears. No radiologic progression was noted at 27 months follow-up.

- Darlis et al[4] reported substantial pain relief in 14 of 16 patients with Geissler grade I or II SLIL tears treated with arthroscopic débridement and thermal shrinkage. Wrist motion was maintained and there was no radiologic evidence of instability at 19 months of follow-up.
- Hirsh et al[6] reported excellent results in 9 of 10 patients with Geissler grade II SLIL tears treated with arthroscopic débridement and thermal shrinkage at 28 months of follow-up.
- Whipple[28] reported his results with percutaneous pinning in patients with scapholunate instability. Symptom duration of more than 3 months and a side-to-side gap difference of more than 3 mm were associated with poor outcomes. Pain relief was satisfactory in only 53% of patients with both of these factors.
- Darlis et al[3] reported management of chronic (longer than 3 months) dynamic scapholunate instability (Geissler grades III, IV) with arthroscopic débridement and percutaneous pinning in patients who did not wish to undergo open surgery. Results were suboptimal, with significant pain relief and improved grip strength in 6 of 11 patients. At 33 months of follow-up there was no radiologic evidence of progression to static instability, but three patients required additional surgery to address persistent pain.
- Clinical experience with the arthroscopic RASL procedure and lunotriquetral fusion is limited. Rosenwasser et al[14] reported excellent results using the open RASL technique in 20 patients with static instability. At 54 months of follow-up, patients had achieved 91% of their normal wrist motion and 87% of contralateral grip strength. The authors noted that the procedure may be performed arthroscopically, but thought that experience with the open technique should first be obtained.

COMPLICATIONS

- Injury to branches of superficial radial sensory nerve (especially with use of 1–2 portal) or dorsal branch of ulnar nerve (6R, 6U portals)
- Injury to radial artery (radial volar portal). This portal should be established through the floor of the FCR sheath.
- Persistent pain or instability
- Need for additional surgery (ligament reconstruction, capsulodesis, tenodesis, proximal row carpectomy, partial or complete wrist fusion)

REFERENCES

1. Abe Y, Doi K, Hattori Y, et al. Arthroscopic assessment of the volar region of the scapholunate interosseous ligament through a volar portal. J Hand Surg Am 2003;28A:69–73.
2. Berger RA. The gross and histologic anatomy of the scapholunate interosseous ligament. J Hand Surg Am 1996;21A:170–178.
3. Darlis NA, Kaufmann RA, Giannoulis F, et al. Arthroscopic debridement and closed pinning for chronic dynamic scapholunate instability. J Hand Surg Am 2006;31A:418–424.
4. Darlis NA, Weiser RW, Sotereanos DG. Partial scapholunate ligament injuries treated with arthroscopic debridement and thermal shrinkage. J Hand Surg Am 2005;30A:908–914.
5. Geissler WB, Freeland AE. Arthroscopically assisted reduction of intraarticular distal radial fractures. Clin Orthop Relat Res 1996;327:125–134.
6. Hirsh L, Sodha S, Bozentka D, et al. Arthroscopic electrothermal collagen shrinkage for symptomatic laxity of the scapholunate interosseous ligament. J Hand Surg Br 2005;30B:643.
7. Horii E, Garcia-Elias M, An KN, et al. A kinematic study of lunotriquetral dissociations. J Hand Surg Am 1991;16A:355–362.
8. Mathiowetz V, Kashman N, Volland G, et al. Grip and pinch strength: normative data for adults. Arch Phys Med Rehabil 1985;66:69–74.
9. Mayfield JK, Johnson RP, Kilcoyne RK. Carpal dislocations: pathomechanics and progressive perilunar instability. J Hand Surg Am 1980;5A:226–241.
10. O'Meeghan CJ, Stuart W, Mamo V, et al. The natural history of an untreated isolated scapholunate interosseus ligament injury. J Hand Surg Br 2003;28B:307–310.
11. Reagan DS, Linscheid RL, Dobyns JH. Lunotriquetral sprains. J Hand Surg Am 1984;9A:502–514.
12. Ritt MJ, Bishop AT, Berger RA, et al. Lunotriquetral ligament properties: a comparison of three anatomic subregions. J Hand Surg Am 1998;23A:425–431.
13. Ritt MJ, Maas M, Bos KE. Minnaar type 1 symptomatic lunotriquetral coalition: a report of nine patients. J Hand Surg Am 2001;26A:261–270.
14. Rosenwasser MP, Miyasajsa KC, Strauch RJ. The RASL procedure: reduction and association of the scaphoid and lunate using the Herbert screw. Tech Hand Up Extrem Surg 1997;1:263–272.
15. Ruch DS, Poehling GG. Arthroscopic management of partial scapholunate and lunotriquetral injuries of the wrist. J Hand Surg Am 1996;21A:412–417.
16. Ruch DS, Smith BP. Arthroscopic and open management of dynamic scaphoid instability. Orthop Clin North Am 2001;32:233–240.
17. Schaedel-Hoepfner M, Iwinska-Zelder J, Braus T, et al. MRI versus arthroscopy in the diagnosis of scapholunate ligament injury. J Hand Surg Br 2001;26B:17–21.
18. Shin AY, Battaglia MJ, Bishop AT. Lunotriquetral instability: diagnosis and treatment. J Am Acad Orthop Surg 2000;8:170–179.
19. Slutsky DJ. Arthroscopic dorsal radiocarpal ligament repair. Arthroscopy 2005;21:1486.
20. Trumble TE, Bour CJ, Smith RJ, et al. Kinematics of the ulnar carpus related to the volar intercalated segment instability pattern. J Hand Surg Am 1990;15A:384–392.
21. Walsh JJ, Berger RA, Cooney WP. Current status of scapholunate interosseous ligament injuries. J Am Acad Orthop Surg 2002;10:32–42.
22. Watson HK, Ballet FL. The SLAC wrist: scapholunate advanced collapse pattern of degenerative arthritis. J Hand Surg Am 1984;9A:358–365.
23. Watson H, Ottoni L, Pitts EC, et al. Rotary subluxation of the scaphoid: a spectrum of instability. J Hand Surg Br 1993;18B:62–64.
24. Watson HK, Weinzweig J, Zeppieri J. The natural progression of scaphoid instability. Hand Clin 1997;13:39–49.
25. Weber ER. Wrist mechanics and its association with ligamentous instability. In: Lichtman DM, ed. The Wrist and its Disorders. Philadelphia: Saunders; 1988:41–52.
26. Weiss AP, Akelman E, Lambiase R. Comparison of the findings of triple-injection cinearthrography of the wrist with those of arthroscopy. J Bone Joint Surg Am 1996;78A:348–356.
27. Weiss AP, Sachar K, Glowacki KA. Arthroscopic debridement alone for intercarpal ligament tears. J Hand Surg Am 1997;22A:344–349.
28. Whipple TL. The role of arthroscopy in the treatment of scapholunate instability. Hand Clin 1995;11:37–40.
29. Wolfe SW, Katz LD, Crisco JJ. Radiographic progression to dorsal intercalated segment instability. Orthopedics 1996;19:691–695.
30. Zachee B, De Smet L, Fabry G. Frayed ulno-triquetral and ulno-lunate ligaments as an arthroscopic sign of longstanding triquetrolunate ligament rupture. J Hand Surg Br 1994;19B:570–571.

Chapter 42

Open Scapholunate Ligament Repair and Augmentation

Alex M. Meyers, Alexander H. Payatakes, and Dean G. Sotereanos

DEFINITION

- Scapholunate instability is the most common form of carpal instability.
- Scapholunate interosseous ligament (SLIL) injury can result in a predictable pattern of arthritis over time: scapholunate advanced collapse (SLAC).[12]
- Acute tears (<6 weeks from injury) versus chronic tears (>6 weeks from injury)
  - Acute tears tend to be amenable to primary ligament repair.
  - Chronic tears tend to require ligament reconstruction procedures.
- Static or dynamic instability
  - Static instability: any or all of the five characteristic changes on standard plain radiographs (see below)
  - Dynamic instability: normal plain radiographs; however, with loaded (grip view) plain radiographs, any or all of the five characteristic changes may become present.[10]
- Fixed versus reducible deformity
  - Fixed deformity: the static radiographic changes are not passively correctible
  - Reducible deformity: the static radiographic changes are passively correctible
    - This distinction can be determined preoperatively by noting improvement in the static changes on plain radiographs of the wrist in radial deviation compared with AP views of the wrist.

ANATOMY, PATHOGENESIS, AND NATURAL HISTORY

- See Chapter HA-41.

PATIENT HISTORY AND PHYSICAL FINDINGS

- Typical presentation follows a fall on an outstretched hand with acute onset of wrist pain and mild dorsal wrist swelling.
- Key physical examination findings are reviewed in Chapter HA-41.

IMAGING AND OTHER DIAGNOSTIC STUDIES

- Plain radiographs may reveal five characteristic findings suggestive of SLIL pathology (**FIG 1**).
  - Terry Thomas sign: gap between the scaphoid and lunate of more than 3 mm on posteroanterior (PA) radiograph
  - Cortical ring sign: Cortical hyperdensity is seen on PA radiograph as the scaphoid moves into increasing flexion.[1]
  - Angular changes in the carpal rows
    - Scapholunate angle: Normal is 30 to 60 degrees (mean 46 degrees); with SLIL injury, more than 60 degrees[6]
    - Capitolunate angle: Normal is −15 to 15 degrees (mean 0 degrees); with SLIL injury, more than 15 degrees

- Radiolunate angle: Normal is −10 to 10 degrees (mean 0 degrees); with SLIL injury, more than 10 degrees
  - Quadrangular lunate: As the lunate moves into extension it assumes a rectangular appearance on PA radiograph.
  - Disruption of Gilula's lines: Gentle concentric arcs follow the proximal and midcarpal rows. These lines are disrupted with SLIL tears as the relationship of the proximal row is lost.
- Arthrography: sensitivity 56%, specificity 83%, accuracy 60%[13]
  - False-positive results have been documented with communication of contrast shown in asymptomatic patients.[1]
- CT arthrography: sensitivity 86% to 100% (100% sensitive in the detection of dorsal ligament tears), specificity 50% to 79% (79% specific in the detection of dorsal ligament tears), accuracy 78% to 83%[7]
- MRI: sensitivity 25% to 60%, specificity 77% to 100%, accuracy 64% to 78%[8]
  - Specifically, palmar tears of the SLIL were identified with a sensitivity of 60% and specificity of 77% in a cadaveric study. However, the more important stabilizing dorsal portion tears were seen in 0 of 9 specimens.[7]
- Ultrasound: sensitivity 46%, specificity 100%, accuracy 89%[2]
- A negative result with various imaging studies does not prove an absence of ligamentous injury. Arthroscopy has become the gold standard for the diagnosis of SLIL tears.

DIFFERENTIAL DIAGNOSIS

- Dynamic SLIL instability or partial SLIL tear
- Radiocarpal arthritis
- Scaphoid fracture
- Keinböck or Preiser disease

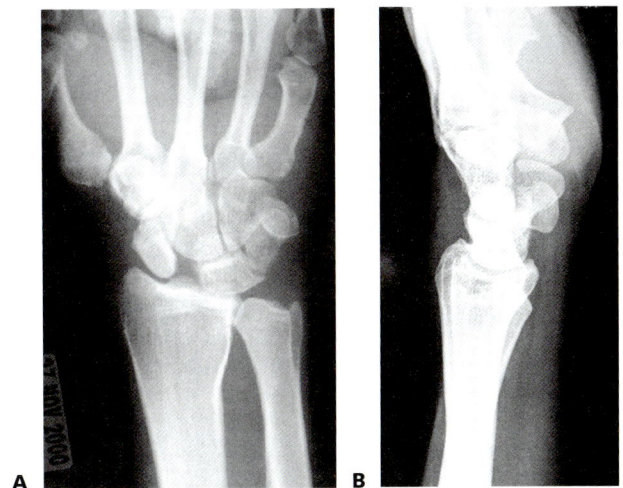

FIG 1 • AP and lateral plain radiographs of a patient with scapholunate ligament tear.

NONOPERATIVE MANAGEMENT

- Nonoperative methods are unsuccessful in treating dynamic or static acute scapholunate ligament injuries.
  - 0 of 19 patients with dynamic instability treated with immobilization, nonsteroidal anti-inflammatories, and activity modification had substantial reduction in symptoms even up to 12 weeks into treatment.[14]

SURGICAL MANAGEMENT

- Indications
  - Wrist pain with an acute tear (<6 weeks)
    - These patients may or may not have static radiographic changes.
    - Should static radiographic changes be present, plain radiographs in radial deviation can show if the radiographic changes are fixed (and therefore are not amenable to soft tissue repairs) or correct in radial deviation (and therefore are amenable to soft tissue repairs).
  - Wrist pain with dynamic instability
  - We advocate diagnostic arthroscopy before open treatment.

Preoperative Planning

- General or regional anesthesia
- Equipment
  - Mini suture anchors (1.8 mm)
  - Kirschner wire driver and smooth wires (0.045 and 0.062 inch)
  - Arthroscopic equipment (see Chap. HA-41)
  - Mini C-arm

Positioning

- The patient is positioned supine with a hand table.
- The bed is turned such that the hand table faces the corner opposite anesthesia.
- Fluoroscopy can then move in and out from the opposite corner perpendicular to the patient.
- An upper arm nonsterile tourniquet should be placed.
- The operative arm is prepared and draped. Slack is left in the armboard portion of the drape to allow the sterile wrist traction tower to slide under the arm above the elbow.
- The operative wrist is suspended in a wrist traction tower.

Approach

- A preoperative examination of both wrists is performed and documented, noting passive range of motion, swelling, and the Watson scaphoid shift test.
- Arthroscopy is recommended before open reconstruction because of the lack of diagnostic accuracy of available imaging modalities.
  - Wrist arthroscopy is considered the gold standard for diagnosis of SLIL pathology and can confirm the diagnosis and degree of instability before making a larger skin incision.
  - Geissler staging of SLIL tears[3] is covered in Chapter HA-41.

TECHNIQUES

DIAGNOSTIC WRIST ARTHROSCOPY

- See Chapter HA-41.
- The 3–4 portal is used for viewing.
- The 6U portal is used for outflow (typically an 18-gauge needle with sterile IV tubing).
- The 4–5 is used for placement of instruments.

- The SLIL is probed in the radiocarpal and midcarpal joints.
  - A 1-mm arthroscopic probe passable in the scapholunate interval and rotated 360 degrees is indicative of a grade III Geissler lesion.
  - A "drive-through" sign with a 2.7-mm arthroscope is indicative of a grade IV Geissler lesion.
  - Midcarpal arthroscopy most effectively reveals the degree of instability.

DIRECT SLIL REPAIR

- Specific indications for direct SLIL repair with or without dorsal capsulodesis
  - Geissler III or IV complete SLIL tear
  - Injury less than 6 weeks old
    - It is rare that a repairable ligament is available more than 3 months after injury.
  - Minimal degenerative changes in the radiocarpal and midcarpal joints
  - Static radiographic changes that are not fixed
  - Adequate SLIL tissue
- Make a standard longitudinal dorsal incision just ulnar to the tubercle of Lister and dissect to the extensor retinaculum.
- Raise flaps at the level of the extensor retinaculum, exposing the retinacular edges proximally and distally.
  - Superficial radial and ulnar dorsal cutaneous nerve branches will be within these flaps.
- Incise the extensor retinaculum over the third extensor compartment and transpose the extensor pollicis longus (EPL) tendon into the radial subcutaneous space.

- Expose the dorsal capsule and dorsal extrinsic radiocarpal ligaments (dorsal radiocarpal [DRC] and dorsal intercarpal [DIC] ligaments).
- Incise the dorsal capsule, leaving a 1- to 1.5-cm ulnar-based flap (**TECH FIG 1A**).
  - Leaving the capsule attached ulnarly provides a capsular flap available for capsulodesis or augmentation of a repair if desired.
  - This flap of tissue will parallel the DIC and include the capsule and portions of the DIC and DRC.
- With the scaphoid, SLIL, and lunate exposed, note any arthritic changes, the location of the SLIL disruption (typically it avulses off the scaphoid) (**TECH FIG 1B,C**), and any injury to the DIC ligament.
  - In cases of high energy the DIC may avulse off its scaphoid and lunate attachment.
- Place joystick Kirschner wires (0.062 inch) into the scaphoid and the lunate.

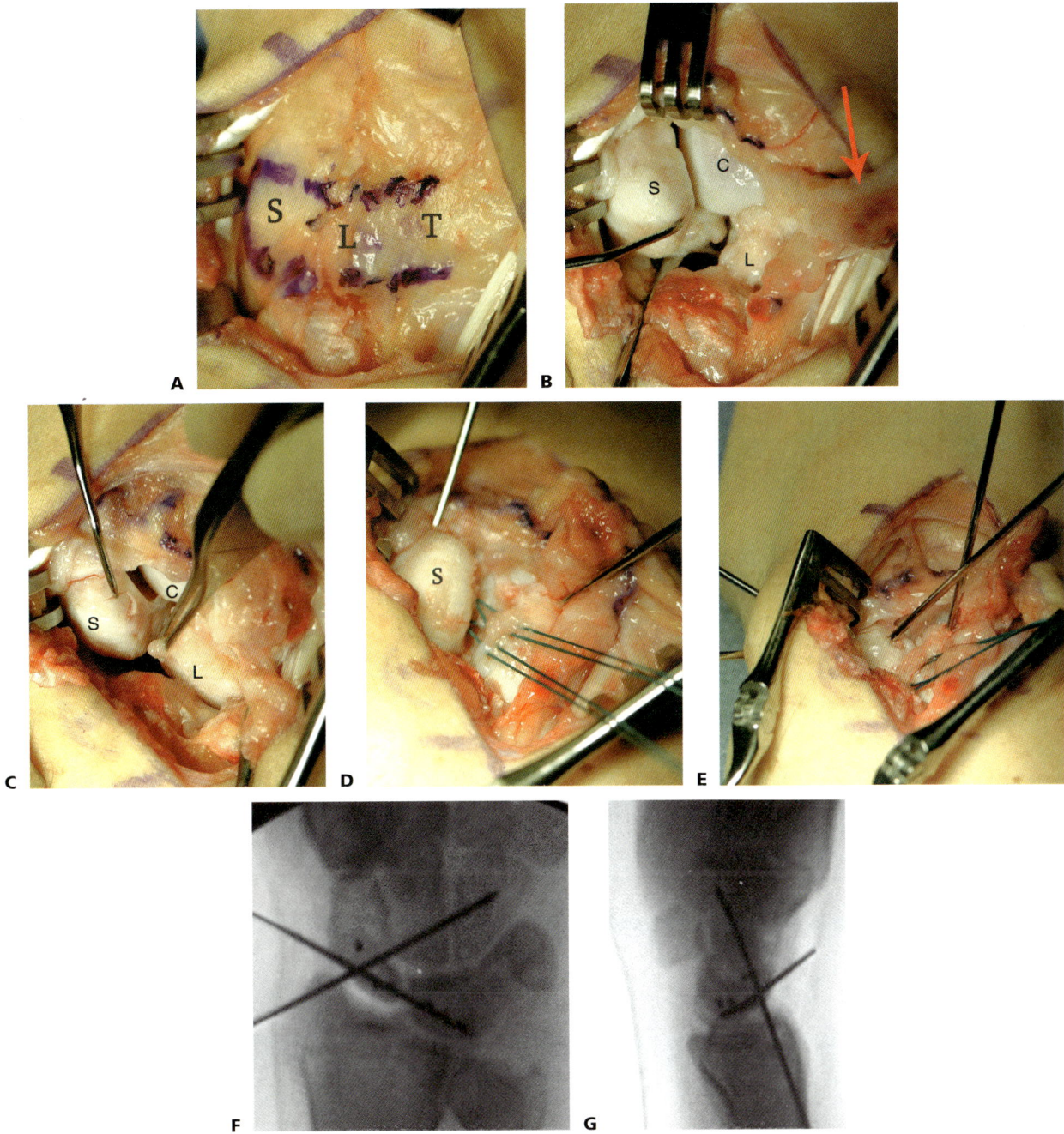

TECH FIG 1 • A. Intraoperative photo demonstrating the exposure and location of the dorsal capsular ulnar-based flap. The DIC parallels the more distal transverse limb of the flap. *S*, scaphoid; *L*, lunate; *T*, triquetrum. **B.** Intraoperative photo demonstrating the flexed scaphoid (*S*), the capitate (*C*), and the extended lunate (*L*). A complete disruption of the scapholunate interosseous ligament (SLIL) is noted. The *arrow* points at the ulnar-based capsular flap. **C.** Intraoperative photo showing the scaphoid on the left and the SLIL still attached to the lunate on the right (held by forceps). The capitate head is seen distal to the lunate at the top of the photo. **D.** Intraoperative photo after suture anchor placement into the scaphoid at the dorsal SLIL footprint on the left, then passed through the SLIL shown on the right. The joystick Kirschner wires are placed into the scaphoid and the lunate in such a manner that when they are brought together, the dorsal intercalated segment instability (DISI) deformity will be corrected and the joint reduced. **E.** Intraoperative photo after reduction of the joint and DISI deformity using the joystick Kirschner wires and suture repair of the avulsed SLIL. The Kirschner wires in the scaphoid and in the lunate have been brought together from their divergent positions and are now in the same plane, correcting the DISI deformity. The two Kirschner wires have been placed from radial to ulnar (seen on the left of the image), passing through the scapholunate interval and scaphocapitate interval. **F,G.** AP and lateral intraoperative fluoroscopic images demonstrating Kirschner wire placement across the scaphocapitate joint and the reduced scapholunate joint. Suture anchors can be seen in the scaphoid at the dorsal SLIL footprint. This example shows a third, more distal suture anchor at the scaphoid that was used for dorsal capsule augmentation.

- Place these wires parallel to the scapholunate joint about 5 mm from the articular surface.
- The scaphoid joystick should angle proximally and the lunate joystick should angle distally (**TECH FIG 1D**).
- The Kirschner wire joysticks are brought together, taking the scaphoid out of flexion and the lunate out of extension to correct any dorsal intercalated segmental instability deformity and reduce the joint.

- Preliminarily reduce the scapholunate joint and identify the anatomic insertion site for the SLIL.
- Roughen the SLIL footprint to bleeding bone on the dorsal ulnar portion of the scaphoid and insert one or more mini suture anchors (2.0 or 2.5 mm).
- Pass the sutures from the suture anchor through the SLIL stump but do not tie them (**TECH FIG 1D**).
- With the joint reduced via the joysticks, drive two 0.045-inch smooth Kirschner wires from the scaphoid into the lunate across the reduced scapholunate joint and drive one or two 0.045-inch Kirschner wires through the waist of the scaphoid into the capitate (**TECH FIG 1E–G**).

- Secure the SLIL to the prepared site by tying the suture anchor sutures.
- Remove the joystick Kirschner wires and cut the remainder of the Kirschner wires below the skin.
- Suture anchors are placed at the DIC footprint on the dorsal more distal scaphoid should it be avulsed and need repair or should capsular flap augmentation be desired (see Direct SLIL Repair with Dorsal Capsulodesis).
- Close the capsule with 3–0 absorbable suture.
- Transpose the EPL tendon subcutaneously and repair the extensor retinaculum with 3–0 absorbable suture.

DIRECT SLIL REPAIR WITH DORSAL CAPSULODESIS

- Indications
  - Tenuous SLIL repair
  - Chronic scapholunate dissociation (>6 weeks) without arthritis
    - The deformity must be reducible and not fixed.
- Should capsulodesis be required for augmentation, perform the SLIL repair as described above, making the same ulnar-based dorsal capsular incision.
- After the SLIL is repaired, swing the ulnarly based capsular flap over the scapholunate interval and plan the location for its attachment to the scaphoid waist.
  - Plan to secure the flap under tension to further stabilize the scapholunate joint.
- Place one or two mini suture anchors (1.8 or 2.0 mm) into the scaphoid at the determined location and another mini suture anchor dorsal-central into the lunate.
- With the capsular flap pulled taut, pass the scaphoid suture anchor sutures through the flap. Then pass the lunate sutures through the central aspect of the flap, estimating suture location to maximize stabilization of the scapholunate joint.
- Once all sutures from the scaphoid and the lunate are placed through the capsular flap, tie them down (**TECH FIG 2**).

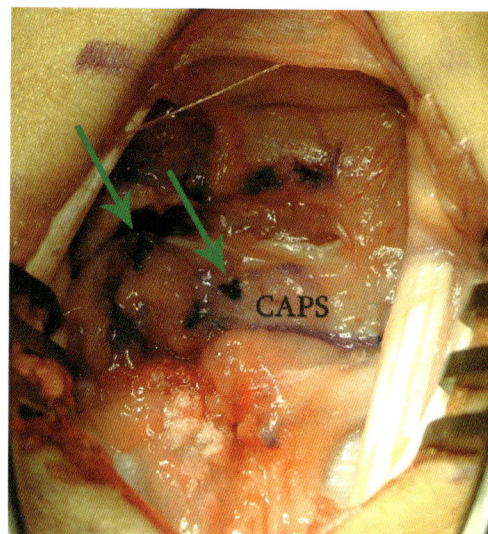

TECH FIG 2 • Repair augmentation with ulnar-based capsular (*CAPS*) flap. Note the suture anchor knots (*arrows*) and the location of the distal suture anchor at the scaphoid at the footprint of the dorsal intercarpal ligament.

PEARLS AND PITFALLS

Fluoroscopy	• By moving the fluoroscopy unit perpendicular to the patient with the C-arm parallel to the floor and locking all the joints but the most distal fulcrum, the amount of "fighting" with the fluoroscopy unit is minimized. • Drape the fluoroscope and keep the C-arm parallel and elevated above the floor (this allows you to keep the fluoroscope sterile and above the hand table).
Buried Kirschner wires	• Buried Kirschner wires require removal in the operating room but minimize the risk of pin tract infection.
Posterior interosseous nerve neurectomy	• Consider performing a posterior interosseous nerve neurectomy during the procedure. Identify the nerve on the floor of the fourth extensor compartment, cauterize it and its accompanying vessel, then resect a segment.
Joystick placement during reduction of the scapholunate joint	• Place the scaphoid Kirschner wire distal in the scaphoid, angling proximally. Remember the scaphoid is flexed and most of the cartilage you will see initially is the radiocarpal articular portion of the scaphoid. Similarly, place the lunate Kirschner wire proximally, angling in a distal direction to correct its extended position.

	■ Place the joystick Kirschner wires at positions where they will not impede the path of the transarticular scapholunate Kirschner wires.
Kirschner wire placement	■ Place the Kirschner wires distal and slightly volar to prevent them from affecting the placement of the suture anchors. A 1-cm longitudinal skin incision with blunt dissection and a guide should be considered to prevent injury to superficial radial nerve branches.
Capsular flap creation	■ When performing dorsal capsulodesis, keep the flap of capsular tissue at least 1 cm wide (this provides a broad enough tether for the scaphoid) and plan the flap length carefully to create a flap with enough length to cross the scapholunate joint and reach the scaphoid waist.

POSTOPERATIVE CARE

■ The wrist is immobilized in a short-arm thumb spica splint immediately after surgery.
■ Sutures are removed at 2 weeks and the wrist is placed into a short-arm thumb spica cast for 8 weeks.
   ■ Radiographs are obtained at 2 and 4 weeks to evaluate reduction and any pin migration.
■ Pins are removed at 8 weeks and the wrist is placed back into a short-arm thumb spica splint.
   ■ Gentle active range-of-motion exercises are allowed at 8 weeks, out of the splint for exercises only.
■ Immobilization is discontinued at 12 weeks.
■ Full activities are allowed at 4 to 6 months.
   ■ Forced hyperextension (push-ups) and axial loading are especially restricted during the 4- to 6-month postoperative period.

OUTCOMES

■ Results following direct SLIL repair with capsulodesis are highly variable.
■ By not crossing the radiocarpal joint with the capsulodesis, theoretically wrist motion will be maximized.
   ■ Szabo et al[9] showed mean loss of wrist flexion of 10 degrees, extension of 15 degrees, radial deviation of 20 degrees, and ulnar deviation of 11 degrees at 2 years of follow-up for chronic (>6 weeks) SLIL tears treated with DIC capsulodesis.
      ■ Grip strength was unchanged from the preoperative assessment (mean 41).
■ Results of the procedure typically do not hold over time radiographically.
   ■ Minimum 5-year follow-up for chronic SLIL tears treated with DIC capsulodesis showed[4]:
      ■ Immediate postoperative scapholunate angle of 56 degrees at 5 years increased to 62 degrees
      ■ Immediate postoperative scapholunate gap of 2.6 mm at 5 years increased to 3.5 mm
   ■ Also, 50% of wrists show arthritic changes at 5 years.
■ Radiographic changes have not correlated with clinical results over time.[4]
   ■ Wrist flexion decreased 19 degrees at 5-year follow-up compared with preoperative values.
   ■ Extension and radial and ulnar deviation remained unchanged at 5 years from the immediate postoperative values shown above.[9]
   ■ Grip strength remained unchanged at 5 years (mean 43).
   ■ Outcome instrument scores at 5 years (Mayo Wrist Score)
      ■ 38% excellent, 19% good, 31% fair, 12% poor outcomes
   ■ No correlation between subjective pain scores and radiographic changes has been shown at 5 years.

COMPLICATIONS

■ Pin tract infections (this risk is minimized with buried pins)
■ Superficial radial nerve injury
   ■ The surgeon should keep skin flaps thick when dissecting on top of the extensor retinaculum (this keeps the superficial radial nerve branches within the flaps).
   ■ The surgeon should make a small stab incision to bluntly dissect down to bone to minimize risk of nerve injury during pin placement.
■ Loss of scapholunate reduction
■ Arthritic changes in the radiocarpal and midcarpal joints

REFERENCES

1. Blatt G. Capsulodesis in reconstructive hand surgery: dorsal capsulodesis for the unstable scaphoid and volar capsulodesis following excision of the distal ulna. Hand Clin 1987;3:81–102.
2. Dao KD, Solomon DJ, Shin AY, et al. The efficacy of ultrasound in the evaluation of dynamic scapholunate ligamentous instability. J Bone Joint Surg Am 2004;86A:1473–1478.
3. Darlis NA, Weiser RW, Sotereanos DG. Partial scapholunate ligament injuries treated with arthroscopic debridement and thermal shrinkage. J Hand Surg Am 2005;30A:908–914.
4. Gajendran VK, Peterson B, Slater RR, et al. Long-term outcome of dorsal intercarpal ligament capsulodesis for chronic scapholunate dissociation. J Hand Surg Am 2007;32A:1323–1333.
5. Geissler WB, Freeland AE, Savoie FH, et al. Intracarpal soft tissue lesions associated with an intra-articular fracture of the distal end of the radius. J Bone Joint Surg Am 1996;78A:357–365.
6. Linscheid RL, Dobyns JH, Beabout JW, et al. Traumatic instability of the wrist: diagnosis, classification, and pathomechanics. J Bone Joint Surg Am 1972;54A:1612–1632.
7. Schmid MR, Schertler T, Pfirrmann CW, et al. Interosseous ligament tears of the wrist: comparison of multi-detector row CT arthrography and MR imaging. Radiology 2005;237:1008–1013.
8. Schweitzer ME, Brahme SK, Hodler J, et al. Chronic wrist pain: spin-echo and short tau inversion recovery MR imaging and conventional MR arthrography. Radiology 1992;182:205–211.
9. Szabo RM, Slater RJ, Palumbo CF, et al. Dorsal intercarpal ligament capsulodesis for chronic, static scapholunate dissociation: clinical results. J Hand Surg Am 2002;27A:978–984.
10. Taleisnik J. Post-traumatic carpal instability. Clin Orthop Relat Res 1980;149:73–82.
11. Viegas SF, Patterson RM, Hokanson JA, et al. Wrist anatomy: incidence, distribution, and correlation of anatomic variations, tears, and arthrosis. J Hand Surg Am 1993;18:463–475.
12. Watson K, Ballet FL. The SLAC wrist: scapholunate advanced collapse pattern of degenerative arthritis. J Hand Surg Am 1984; 9:358–365.
13. Weiss AP, Akelman E, Lambiase R. Comparison of the findings of triple-injection cinearthrography of the wrist with those of arthroscopy. J Bone Joint Surg Am 1996;78A:348–356.
14. Wintman BI, Gelberman RH, Katz JN. Dynamic scapholunate instability: results of operative treatment with dorsal capsulodesis. J Hand Surg Am 1995;20:971–979.

Chapter 43

Capsulodesis for Treatment of Scapholunate Instability

Angel Ferreres, Marc García-Elías, and Andrew Chin

DEFINITION

- Scapholunate dissociation (SLD) is the rupture of the anatomic linkage between the scaphoid and lunate and its subsequent progressive dysfunction, with or without carpal malalignment.
- Classical radiographic signs occur only when there is permanent carpal malalignment. This is preceded by complete scapholunate disruption together with failure of the secondary scaphoid stabilizers, namely the scaphotrapezial-trapezoid ligament (STT), the scaphocapitate (SC) ligament, and the radioscaphocapitate (RSC) ligament.
- However, in many cases, only partial tears or ligament sprains occur and do not produce positive radiologic signs. These injuries are often seen only arthroscopically.
- Dorsal capsulodesis of the radioscaphoid joint was first described by Blatt.[2] Now it is one of the most commonly used techniques in the treatment of carpal instability. This procedure involves the creation of a dorsal capsular flap.

ANATOMY

- Scapholunate ligaments are divided into three fibrous structures:
  - Dorsal ligament
  - Volar ligament
  - Thin proximal membrane
- Anatomically, the dorsal scapholunate ligament is the thickest and shortest of the fibrous structures, measuring 2 to 3 mm thick and 2 to 5 mm long. Biomechanically, it is the strongest and most resistant to failure under load (**FIG 1A**).[1] The radioscapholunate (Testut) ligament is only a path for vascularization and innervation of the scaphoid and lunate.
- Scaphoid position and relationship with lunate and distal carpal row is maintained by the scapholunate ligaments and by the secondary stabilizers (STT, SC, and RSC ligaments), which prevent excessive scaphoid flexion. These are called secondary stabilizers (**FIG 1B**).
- The flexor carpi radialis tendon is closely related to the scapholunate joint and acts as a crucial dynamic stabilizer of the scaphoid, preventing it from going into excessive flexion and pronation during a firm grip of an object (**FIG 1C**).

PATHOGENESIS

- Injury to the scapholunate ligaments occurs when the wrist is hyperextended, ulnarly deviated, and supinated during a fall on an outstretched hand. Because of the osseous configuration and disposition of the bones of the proximal carpal row, when the hand hits the floor, the tubercle of the scaphoid is pushed dorsally and extended. The lunate is held in position by the volar radiolunate (RL) ligaments and resists the tendency to extension transmitted by the scaphoid. The impact of the hand on the floor also pushes the pisiform against the triquetrum and because of the configuration of the joint between

the triquetrum and the hamate, the former turns into flexion. If forces exceed the ligaments' resistance, they will rupture.
- The sequence of failure of the ligaments is from palmar to dorsal. The first to tear is the volar scapholunate ligament, the weaker of the two scapholunate ligaments, followed by the dorsal scapholunate ligament.[4]
- The participation of the dorsal intercarpal ligament (DICL) in scapholunate instability has been recently supported by the studies of Mitsuyasu et al.[8]

NATURAL HISTORY

- Most SLDs present as the initial stage of a progressive carpal destabilization. The mechanism of injury produces a spectrum of injuries, ranging from mild scapholunate sprains to complete perilunar dislocations, all being different stages of the same progressive perilunar destabilization process as described by Mayfield et al.[9]
- If only the palmar scapholunate ligament and the proximal membrane are disrupted, minor kinematic alterations result in predynamic instability. There is no gross carpal malalignment but because there is an increased motion between the scaphoid and lunate causing shear stress, these injuries may be sufficient to promote painful synovial inflammation.
- Complete disruption of the scapholunate ligament complex leads to substantial alteration in kinematic and force transmission parameters (demonstrated in cadaver specimens), but not necessarily static carpal malalignment.[8,13] This results in a dynamic instability. The scaphoid is unconstrained at the proximal end, resulting in increased radiolunate motion and correspondingly decreased radioscaphoid motion. This is accentuated in a loaded wrist.
- When the secondary stabilizers start to attenuate after repeated use of the wrist, carpal malalignment develops, eventually resulting in static instability. Initially the scaphoid is still reducible, but over time it becomes permanently flexed and pronated (see "Imaging and Other Diagnostic Studies").
- If the alteration in the motion of the scaphoid persists, the cartilage degenerates and arthrosis develops. This pattern of degeneration is known as scapholunate advanced collapse (SLAC).
- Once arthrosis is present, surgical techniques directed at replacing or reconstructing the injured ligaments are no longer options.
- SLD is a progressive entity. Therefore, reconstruction is advocated as soon as it is diagnosed.

PATIENT HISTORY AND PHYSICAL FINDINGS

- Almost always, patients present after a fall on their outstretched hand. The patient complains of dorsal hand and wrist pain when loading the affected wrist, such as when standing up from a chair.

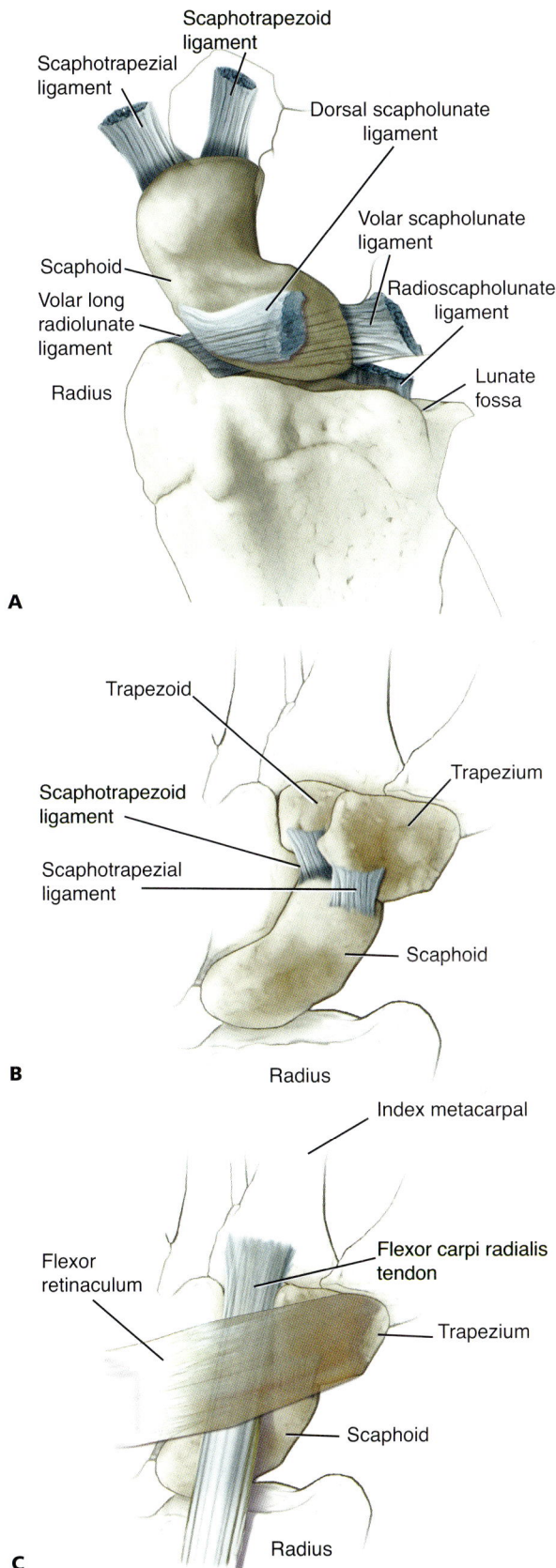

FIG 1 • **A.** The elements that maintain the scaphoid in its normal position. **B.** Volar view of secondary stabilizers. **C.** The dynamic stabilizer of the scaphoid.

■ Predynamic and dynamic stages of SLD are often missed or overlooked. The injury usually is the result of isolated trauma, which the patient does not clearly remember, or is masked by other more severe or obvious injuries (eg, fractured scaphoid and distal radius). A high index of suspicion is required.

■ Weakness of grip strength, occasional swelling over the dorsoradial wrist, point tenderness over the scapholunate interval (more pronounced with gripping), and radial-sided wrist pain after excessive or heavy use are common but subtle physical examination findings.

  ■ The examiner should palpate the scapholunate interval dorsally (1 cm distal to the tubercle of Lister) with the wrist in 30 to 50 degrees of flexion.

  ■ On palpation of the anatomic snuffbox and palmar scaphoid tubercle, tenderness may also be present, suggesting ligament involvement, synovitis, or an occult ganglion.

■ Provocative tests such as the Watson scaphoid shift test and resisted finger extension test reinforce the possibility of the diagnosis.

■ Watson scaphoid shift test: The scaphoid flexes as the wrist goes from ulnar to radial deviation. The examiner's thumb prevents the scaphoid from flexing and if the scapholunate ligament is torn or incompetent, the proximal pole subluxates dorsally out of the scaphoid fossa, causing pain. When the thumb pressure is released, there may be a snap, signifying spontaneous reduction of the scaphoid back into the scaphoid fossa. This test is not highly specific and may signify synovitis, an occult ganglia, or radioscaphoid impingement.

■ Sharp pain on the resisted finger extension test has low specificity but high sensitivity.

IMAGING AND OTHER DIAGNOSTIC STUDIES

■ Radiographs
  ■ Posteroanterior (PA) view
    ▪ Elbow flexed at 90 degrees, neutral prono-supination, and the middle finger aligned with the forearm axis. The palm of the hand is in full contact on the film case.
    ▪ Scapholunate gap greater than 3 mm or wider than the contralateral normal side and a cortical "ring" sign suggest static scapholunate dissociation.
    ▪ Decreased space between the radius and the scaphoid signifies cartilage loss and arthrosis.
  ■ Anteroposterior (AP) view
    ▪ Forearm is in maximal supination.
    ▪ This projection puts the scapholunate interval aligned with the beam of the ray.
  ■ Lateral view
    ▪ Elbow at 90 degrees of flexion, middle finger aligned with the forearm, and wrist at 0 degrees of extension or flexion
    ▪ This projection allows measurement of the scapholunate angle. An angle greater than 60 degrees indicates disruption of the scapholunate ligaments and often corresponds with widening on the PA and AP views.
  ■ Clenched-fist AP view demonstrates a widened scapholunate gap compared to the normal side (**FIG 2A**).
  ■ Cineradiography reveals abnormal movements between the scaphoid and lunate and an increase in the scapholunate gap as the wrist moves from radial to ulnar deviation.

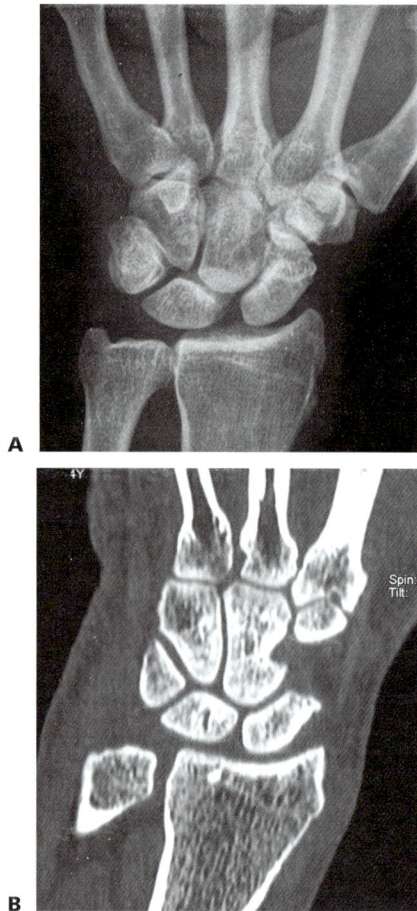

FIG 2 • **A.** Clenched-fist PA view with the wrist in supination that shows a significant increase of the scapholunate interval space. **B**. CT scan of a patient with pain over the dorsal aspect of his left radiocarpal joint, showing a nonwidened space between scaphoid and lunate.

- Arthrography is not specific and may be positive in conditions such as degenerative perforations of the scapholunate membrane and osteochondral defects.
- Magnetic resonance imaging does not provide much additional information. Minor, degenerative perforation of the scapholunate membrane may result in a positive test.
    - Scapholunate ligaments can be seen clearly only on transverse cuts that pass through the two horns of the lunate.
    - MRI plays an important role in excluding other differential diagnoses.
- Computed tomography scans do not give additional information except for providing a more accurate measurement of the parameters involved in the diagnosis of static SLD (eg, scapholunate distance and angle; **FIG 2B**).
    - It is useful in looking for other osseous anomalies of the wrist (eg, impacted fracture of the radius, scaphoid fracture).
- Arthroscopy is the gold standard for diagnosing and staging SLD. It allows grading of the instability (Geissler classification) and therefore determination of the degree of injury to the ligament complex.[4]
    - It is also useful in assessing the condition of the cartilage and in locating concomitant carpal injuries that might negatively affect the outcome of a capsulodesis (Table 1).

DIFFERENTIAL DIAGNOSIS

- Occult ganglia
- Synovitis
- Scaphoid fracture, nonunion, and avascular necrosis
- Radiocarpal arthrosis
- Radioscaphoid impingement

NONOPERATIVE MANAGEMENT

- Initial conservative management aims at resting the injured limb and decreasing edema. Adequate immobilization with casting or splinting is advocated.
    - This immobilization is frequently therapeutic for patients with predynamic SLD.
    - Elevation of the limb and active finger motion minimize edema.
    - Anti-inflammatory medications can be given for pain relief.
- Physiotherapy may have a role if a Geissler grade 1 is diagnosed by arthroscopy. As the ligaments have not lost their integrity, a period of short immobilization (2 weeks), followed by proprioception re-education of the flexor carpi radialis (FCR), as dynamic stabilizer of the scaphoid, is suggested.
- Nonoperative treatment is seldom indicated when a significant disruption is diagnosed.

SURGICAL MANAGEMENT

- Capsulodesis is part of the surgical armamentarium for the treatment of SLD. It is indicated for predynamic SLD, resulting from an isolated partial tear of the scapholunate ligament, and for dynamic SLD when the following criteria are fulfilled:
    - Complete disruption of all scapholunate components (palmar and dorsal)
    - Technically repairable dorsal ligament that has good healing potential
    - Intact secondary stabilizers
    - No cartilage degeneration
- Capsulodesis is not indicated when static SLD is present.

Table 1	Arthroscopic (Geissler) Grading of Interosseous Ligament Tears

Grade	Description
1	Attenuation or hemorrhage of interosseous ligament as seen from the radiocarpal joint. No incongruency of carpal alignment in midcarpal space.
2	Attenuation or hemorrhage of interosseous ligament as seen from the radiocarpal joint. Incongruency or stepoff as seen from midcarpal space. Slight gap (less than width of 1-mm probe) between the carpal bones.
3	Incongruency or stepoff as seen from both radiocarpal and midcarpal spaces. The 1-mm probe is able to pass through the gap between the carpal bones.
4	Incongruency or stepoff as seen from both radiocarpal and midcarpal spaces. Gross instability with manipulation noted. A 2.7-mm probe is able to pass through the gap between the carpal bones.

See also Chap. HA-41.

- Capsulodesis is used either as an isolated procedure together with Kirschner wire stabilization of the scapholunate joint in predynamic cases, or in combination to augment a direct repair of the dorsal scapholunate ligament in dynamic cases.
- Due to its structure and position within the wrist, the scaphoid has an inherent tendency to flex and pronate, especially when the wrist is in flexion and radial deviation. The capsular flap created during dorsal capsulodesis acts as a checkrein to tether the scaphoid, preventing it from going into excessive flexion and pronation.

Preoperative Planning

- All preoperative radiographs and diagnostic studies, especially arthroscopic findings, are reviewed.

Positioning

- The patient is under anesthesia and in the supine position with hips and knees flexed at 30 degrees for low back comfort. The arm is exsanguinated and the tourniquet inflated at 250 mm Hg.
- The arm is on the hand table in pronation, presenting the dorsal aspect of the wrist.

BLATT CAPSULODESIS

Exposure

- The tubercle of Lister and the radial styloid are identified by palpation.
- An oblique skin incision is made following a line from a point 1 cm distal and ulnar with respect to the tubercle of Lister, to a point 1 cm distal to the radial styloid (**TECH FIG 1**).
- Veins are coagulated or ligated.
- Care is taken to identify the branches of the superficial radial nerve and mobilize and retract them with the subcutaneous tissue. This is accomplished taking all the fat with the skin as a flap.
- Communicating vessels from the superficial layers to the deep arches are divided and coagulated.
- The extensor retinaculum overlying the fourth dorsal extensor compartment is incised. The extensor retinaculum is then raised as two flaps, radially and ulnarly based, to free the extensor tendons from the second to fourth compartments.
- A neurectomy of the posterior interosseous nerve can be performed at this point.
- The extensor digitorum communis (EDC) is retracted ulnarly and the extensor pollicis longus (EPL) and extensor carpi radialis brevis (ECRB) radially to expose the dorsal capsule.

Creation of the Capsular Flap

- A rectangular capsular flap, 25 mm long and 10 mm wide, is created by making a transverse capsular incision just proximal to the vascular dorsal carpal arch and elevating the tissue in a distal to proximal direction, leaving the proximal end still attached to the dorsal rim of the distal radius (**TECH FIG 2A**).
- As the flap is elevated, the scaphoid is exposed (**TECH FIG 2B**).
- At the dorsum of the scaphoid, a trough is created at a point distal to the axis of rotation of the scaphoid (scaphoid neck) (**TECH FIG 2C**).

Reducing the Instability

- If the instability is acute, a primary repair of the scapholunate ligament is performed.
- The space between scaphoid and lunate is reduced, using a 1.1-mm Kirschner wire inserted in the scaphoid as a joystick, and then another Kirschner wire is placed in the scaphoid and fixed to the lunate.
  - This step should be performed under radiologic guidance. The scapholunate angle in which these bones are fixed should be 45 ± 5 degrees.
- When fixing the scaphoid to the lunate, ensure that the lunate is in a neutral position.

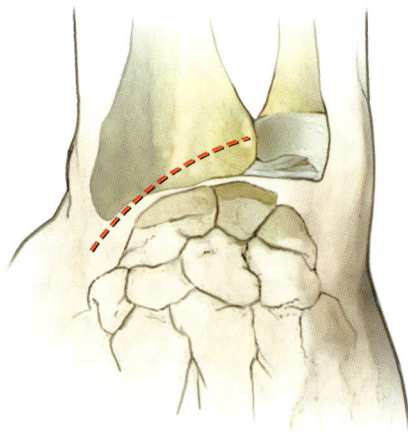

TECH FIG 1 • Incision site.

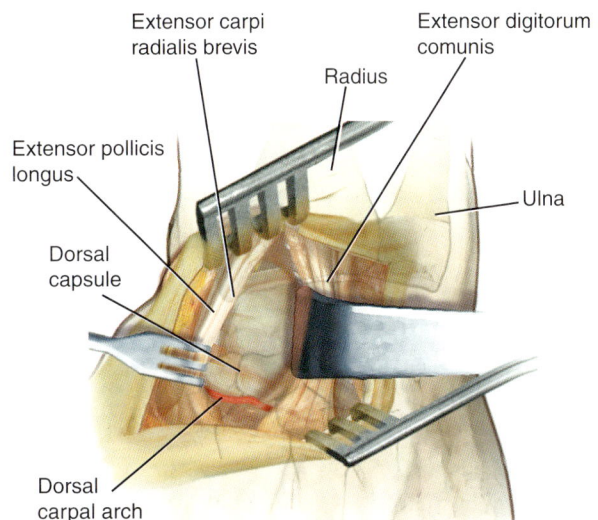

TECH FIG 2 • **A.** The vascular dorsal arch. *(continued)*

B

C

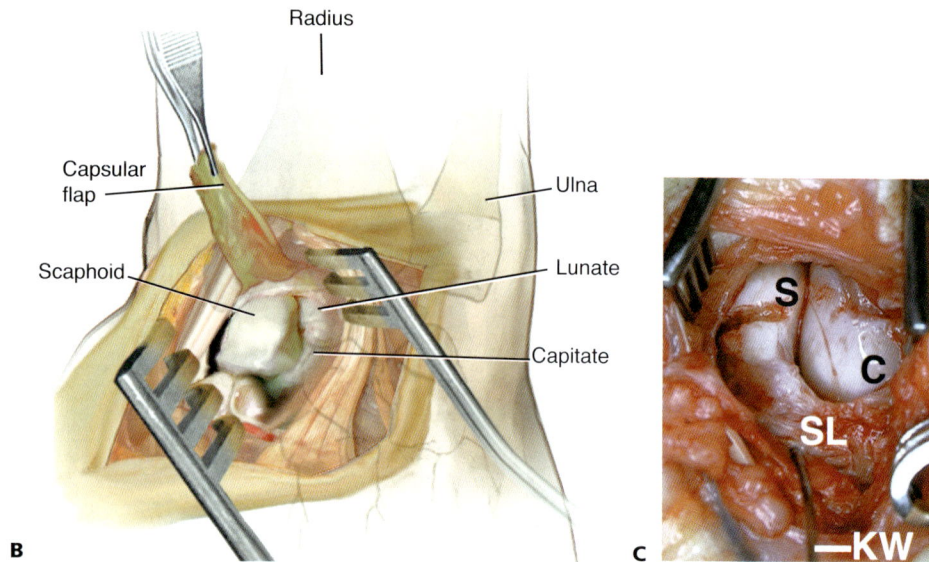

TECH FIG 2 • (continued) **B.** Capsular flap is elevated, allowing visualization of the scaphoid, lunate, and head of the capitate. **C.** Intraoperative photo showing the scaphoid (*S*), the capitate (*C*), and the dorsal scapholunate ligament (*SL*). A bone trough has been created in the distal scaphoid for insertion of the capsular flap. *KW*, Kirschner wire in the lunate. (**C**: Courtesy of A. Lluch, Institut Kaplan.)

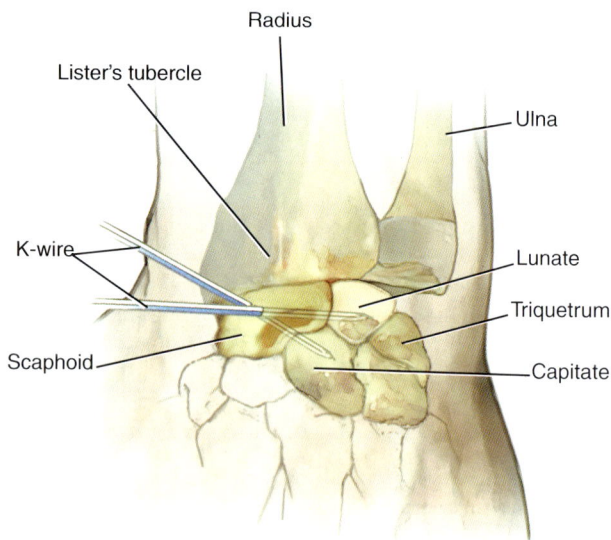

TECH FIG 3 • Orientation of the Kirschner wires recommended to stabilize the joints and protect the capsulodesis.

- If the capsulodesis is being performed for predynamic instability, the scaphoid is fixed to the lunate in its normal alignment. This is also accomplished by means of a Kirschner wire as described earlier.
- Another Kirschner wire is passed from the scaphoid into the capitate to avoid flexion and pronation (**TECH FIG 3**).

Securing the Capsular Flap and Wound Closure

- The flap is tightly inserted into the notch created on the dorsum of the scaphoid.
- There are two ways of securing the proximally based capsular flap to the scaphoid:
  - The flap is secured through holes created in the notch and transosseous sutures that are tied on the volar surface of the scaphoid tubercle.
  - The flap is secured to the sutures of a bone anchor (authors' preferred method) (**TECH FIG 4**).
- The dorsal capsule is left in situ. The extensor retinaculum is closed with resorbable sutures.
- Layered closure of the wound and skin is performed.

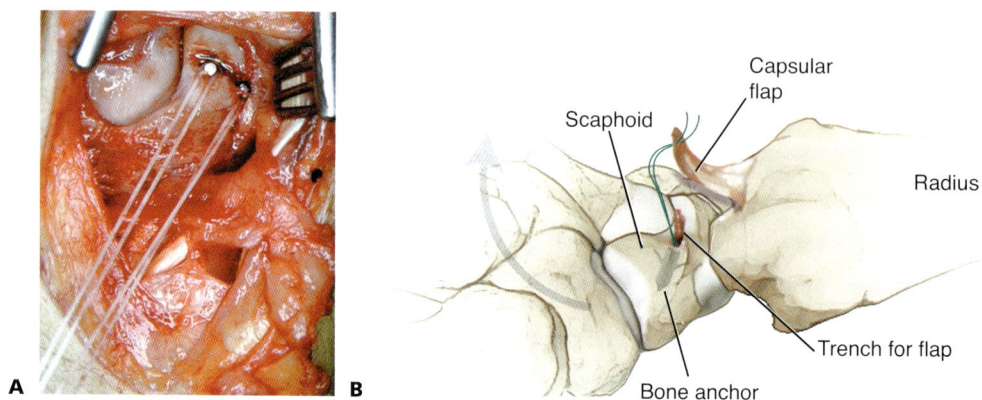

A

B

TECH FIG 4 • **A.** Placement of two bone anchors in the distal dorsal scaphoid. **B.** The proximally based capsular flap is prepared for insertion. (continued)

TECHNIQUES

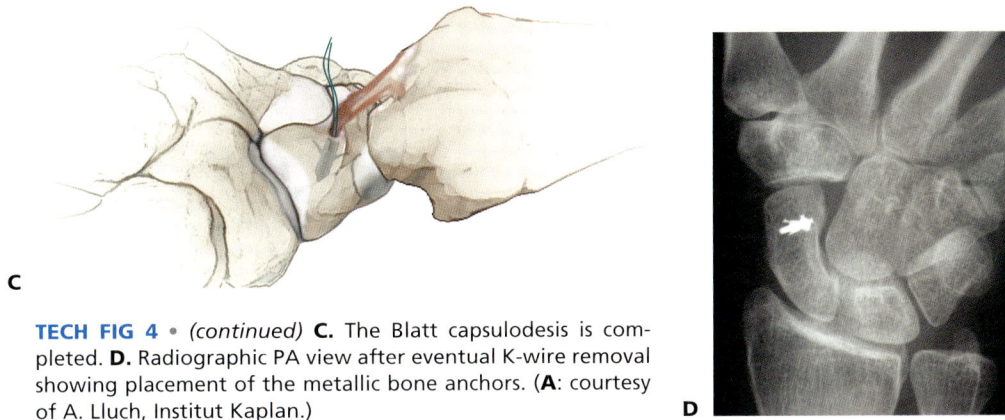

TECH FIG 4 • *(continued)* **C.** The Blatt capsulodesis is completed. **D.** Radiographic PA view after eventual K-wire removal showing placement of the metallic bone anchors. (**A:** courtesy of A. Lluch, Institut Kaplan.)

HERBERT TECHNIQUE

- This method is very similar to Blatt's technique, the difference being that the capsular flap is distally based.
  - There is no clear advantage to this technique over that described by Blatt.

- The same approach is used and the same capsular flap created except that the tissue is left attached to the distal third of the scaphoid.
- The flap is incised at the radiocarpal joint, tensioned proximally, and anchored to the dorsal radius using a suture anchor. This force extends the distal pole of the scaphoid, reducing the scapholunate joint (**TECH FIG 5**).[6]

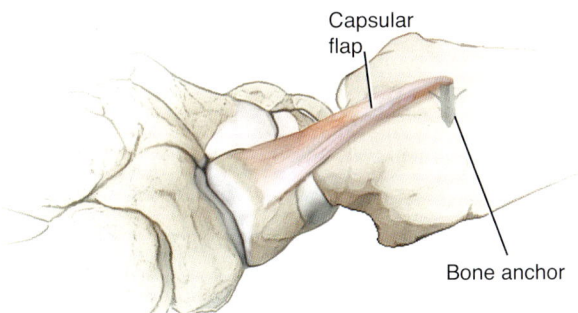

TECH FIG 5 • Drawing depicting the distally based capsulodesis described by Herbert.

BERGER CAPSULODESIS

- Use the same approach and exposure as described for the Blatt capsulodesis.
- Raise a rectangular, radially based, capsular flap to allow exposure of the carpus. Its ulnar margin is the radiotriquetral ligament, its proximal margin is the radius, and its distal margin is the midsubstance of the DICL.
- This elevated flap includes the proximal half of the DICL. Separate this portion of the DICL from the capsular tissue in an ulnar to radial direction, maintaining the radial insertion of the ligament.
- Transfer this strip of ligament to the dorsum of the lunate into a prepared cancellous trough (**TECH FIG 6**).
  - This will create a link between scaphoid and lunate, preventing scaphoid flexion and pronation.
- The ligament is secured by tying to the suture anchor(s) in the lunate.
- This technique represents a variation of a previous version described by Taleisnik and Linscheid[15,17] in which the flap was attached to the dorsum of the distal radius.

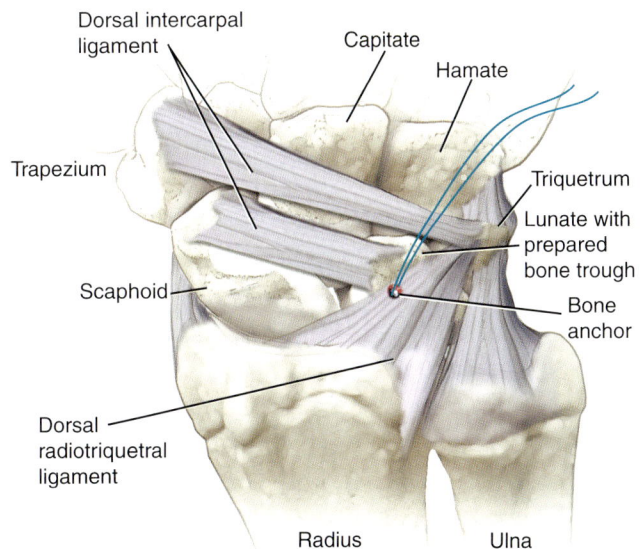

TECH FIG 6 • Berger's technique involves transfer of the proximal half of the dorsal intercarpal ligament to the dorsum of the lunate.

SZABO TECHNIQUE

- The DICL is used to stabilize the scapholunate interval as above except the ligamentous tissue is ulnarly based and is inserted into the scaphoid rather than the lunate (**TECH FIG 7**).
- Typically a longitudinal capsular incision is used to expose the carpus.
  - Care is taken to avoid incising the DICL.
- The DICL is defined and its proximal half separated.

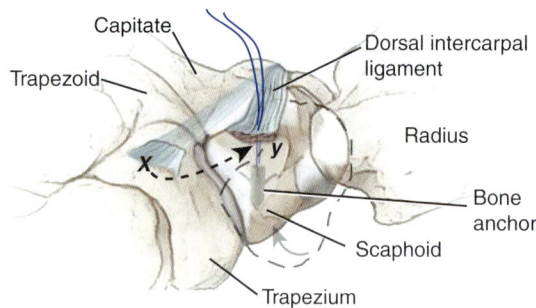

- The radial insertion is incised at the level of the trapezium, trapezoid, and distal third of the scaphoid and then transferred to the scaphoid at the level of the scapholunate ligament insertion.
  - The transferred ligament may also be integrated into the scapholunate ligament repair more proximally.
- The transferred ligament is secured using suture anchor(s) into a cancellous trough in the scaphoid.
- Like the Berger capsulodesis, this technique does not specifically limit wrist flexion as it does not cross the radiocarpal joint.[14]

TECH FIG 7 • Szabo's technique involves transfer of the distal half of the dorsal intercarpal ligament from its attachment to the trapezium and trapezoid (*x*) to the distal third of the dorsum of the scaphoid (*y*).

PEARLS AND PITFALLS

Indication	- This procedure should be used only in cases of predynamic and dynamic instability; it is not recommended for static instability.
Approach	- Dorsal and oblique from proximal to distal and ulnar to radial
Preparation of the flap	- Less than 10 mm wide is not adequate.
Preparation of the scaphoid	- Roughen the dorsal aspect of the distal third of the scaphoid. - Use bone anchors; it is the simplest and fastest. - If making holes for attaching the capsule, direct them distally, to the tubercle. Then tie the sutures directly on the bone and leave the stitch under the skin.
Reducing instability	- If the lunate is not reduced, flexion of the wrist may be limited postoperatively. When securing the scaphoid to the lunate, be sure not to place the scaphoid in more than 70 degrees of extension. This will also limit flexion postoperatively.
Fixing the flap	- Tension is adjusted with the wrist in a neutral position.

POSTOPERATIVE CARE

- Blatt recommended wearing a thumb spica cast for 2 months, after which active range-of-motion exercises were begun. The Kirschner wires were left in place for another month before removal, allowing intercarpal motion at 3 months postoperatively. Forceful stress was discouraged for up to 6 months postoperatively.
- We prefer 6 weeks of immobilization in a rigid splint, avoiding extreme motions for one additional month. Kirschner wires can be removed at 8 weeks from the time of surgery.

OUTCOMES

- A number of clinical series have reported good results with these procedures.[2–4,6,7,10–12,14,16,18,19] The agreement of these series is that tensioning or augmenting the dorsal radioscaphoid capsule offers less surgical morbidity than other alternatives.

- At an average of 2 years of follow-up, these studies noted an absence of symptoms in two thirds of patients, with 75% grip strength compared to the contralateral side.
- When examined with MRI, these patients demonstrate an increased capsular thickening that prevents rotary subluxation of the scaphoid but with the drawback of limiting wrist flexion by an average of 20 degrees.
- The long-term stabilizing efficacy of this capsule, however, has yet to be determined.
- Poor results have been reported in some series. This may be due to the use of the technique in cases of static instability or even in irreducible forms of SLD.[3,10,11,18,19] This procedure is not recommended if the SLD has progressed to the static form because the pathomechanics from the permanent malalignment will increase the risk of a failed procedure. Studies reporting more favorable outcomes are those in which capsulodesis is used mainly for dynamic SLD.[2,7,12,16]

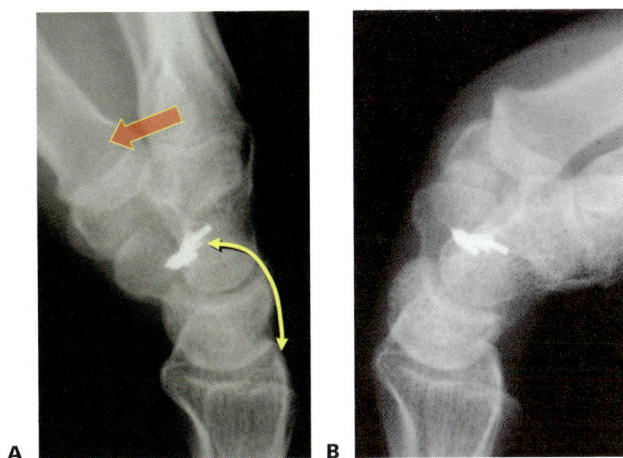

FIG 3 • **A.** The amount of flexion is reduced because of the dorsal restraint. The *yellow arrow* indicates the origin and insertion of the capsular flap. **B.** Extension is not restricted by the capsulodesis.

COMPLICATIONS

- Reduction of wrist flexion (**FIG 3**)
- Failure
- Progression of SLD

REFERENCES

1. Berger RA. Ligament anatomy. In Cooney WP, Linsheid RL, Dobyns JH, eds. The Wrist: Diagnosis and Operative Treatment. St. Louis: Mosby, 1998:73–105.
2. Blatt G. Capsulodesis in reconstructive hand surgery. Hand Clin 1987;3:81–102.
3. Deshmukh SC, Givissis P, Belloso D, et al. Blatt's capsulodesis for chronic scapholunate dissociation. J Hand Surg Br 1999;24B: 215–220.
4. Garcia-Elias M, Geissler WB. Carpal instability. In Green DP, Hotchkiss RN, Pederson WC, et al, eds. Green's Operative Hand Surgery, 5th ed. Philadelphia: Elsevier, 2005:535–604.
5. Garcia-Elias M, Lluch AL, Stanley JK. Three-ligament tenodesis for treatment of scapholunate dissociation: indications and surgical technique. J Hand Surg Am 2006;31A:125–134.
6. Herbert TJ, Hargreaves IC, Clarke AM. A new surgical technique for treating rotatory instability of the scaphoid. Hand Surg 1996;1: 75–77.
7. Lavernia CJ, Cohen MS, Taleisnik J. Treatment of scapholunate dissociation by ligamentous repair and capsulodesis. J Hand Surg Am 1992;17A:354–359.
8. Mitsuyasu H, Patterson RH, Shah MA, et al. The role of the dorsal intercarpal ligament in dynamic and static scapholunate instability. J Hand Surg Am 2004;29A:279–288.
9. Mayfield JK, Johnson RP, Kilcoyne RK. Carpal dislocations: pathomechanics and progressive perilunar instability. J Hand Surg Am 1980;5A:226–241.
10. Moran SL, Cooney WP, Berger RA, et al. Capsulodesis for the treatment of chronic scapholunate instability. J Hand Surg Am 2005; 30A:16–23.
11. Moran SL, Ford KS, Wulf CA, et al. Outcomes of dorsal capsulodesis and tenodesis for treatment of scapholunate instability. J Hand Surg Am 2006;31A:1438–1446.
12. Pomerance J. Outcome after repair of the scapholunate interosseous ligament and dorsal capsulodesis for dynamic scapholunate instability due to trauma. J Hand Surg Am 2006;31A:1380–1386.
13. Short WH, Werner FW, Green JK, et al. Biomechanical evaluation of ligamentous stabilizers of the scaphoid and lunate. J Hand Surg Am 2002;27A:991–1002.
14. Slater RR, Szabo RM. Scapholunate dissociation: treatment with the dorsal intercarpal ligament capsulodesis. Tech Hand Up Extrem Surg 1999;3:222–228.
15. Taleisnik J, Linscheid RL. Scapholunate instability. In Cooney WP, Linsheid RL, Dobyns JH, eds. The Wrist: Diagnosis and Operative Treatment. St. Louis: Mosby, 1998:501–526.
16. Wintman BI, Gelberman RH, Katz JN. Dynamic scapholunate instability: results of operative treatment with dorsal capsulodesis. J Hand Surg Am 1995;20A:971–979.
17. Walsh JJ, Berger RA, Cooney WP. Current status of scapholunate interosseous ligament injuries. J Am Acad Orthop Surg 2002;10:32–42.
18. Wyrick JD, Youse BD, Kiefhaber TR. Scapholunate ligament repair and capsulodesis for the treatment of static scapholunate dissociation. J Hand Surg Br 1998;23B:776–780.
19. Zarkadas PC, Gropper PT, White NJ, et al. A survey of the surgical management of acute and chronic scapholunate instability. J Hand Surg Am 2004;29A:848–857.

Chapter 44

Tenodesis for Treatment of Scapholunate Instability

Marc García-Elías and Angel Ferreres

DEFINITION

- Scapholunate dissociation (SLD) is a symptomatic wrist dysfunction that results from partial or total rupture of the scapholunate ligamentous complex, with or without carpal malalignment.
- It may appear either as an isolated injury, or associated with distal radius fractures or displaced scaphoid fractures. Usually the result of trauma (hyperextension and ulnar deviation injury to the wrist), SLD may also result from a chronic inflammatory arthropathy (rheumatoid arthritis, chondrocalcinosis).

ANATOMY

- Under load the scaphoid is inherently unstable owing to its oblique alignment relative to the direction of axial forces being transmitted across the wrist.[6] The amount of instability depends on the following factors:
  - The geometry of the radioscaphoid joint (the deeper the scaphoid fossa, the less unstable)
  - The stabilizing efficacy of the periscaphoid ligaments (proximal scapholunate interosseous ligament complex, dorsal scaphotriquetral [STq], palmar scaphocapitate [SC] and lateral scapho-trapezial-trapezoidal [STT] ligaments)[7]

- The indirect action of the flexor carpi radialis (FCR) muscle
- The scapholunate interosseous ligament complex consists of three structures: the two scapholunate ligaments (palmar and dorsal) and the proximal fibrocartilaginous membrane.
  - The proximal membrane connects the two adjacent convex borders of the two bones from dorsal to palmar, separating the radiocarpal and midcarpal joint spaces (**FIG 1**).
  - The dorsal scapholunate ligament is formed by dense, slightly oblique connective fibers that link the dorsal aspects of the scaphoid and lunate bones.
  - The palmar scapholunate ligament has longer, more obliquely oriented fibers, allowing substantial rotation of the scaphoid relative to the lunate.
  - The dorsal scapholunate ligament has the greatest yield strength (260 Newtons [N] on average), followed by the palmar scapholunate ligament (118 N) and the proximal membrane (63 N).[2]
  - The proximal portion of the membrane often appears perforated in middle-aged and older individuals, which does not cause instability.

PATHOGENESIS

- When axially loaded, the three proximal bones do not react equally in terms of direction of rotation. The scaphoid tends to rotate into flexion and pronation while the triquetrum is pulled into extension by the dorsally subluxing hamate bone (**FIG 2A**).
  - If both the palmar and dorsal scapholunate and lunotriquetral (LTq) ligaments are intact, such differences in reactive motion generate increasing torques at both scapholunate and LTq levels, resulting in an increasing coaptation of these joints. Such an increased coaptation further contributes to the proximal carpal row stability (**FIG 2B**).
- If the scapholunate ligaments are completely torn, the scaphoid no longer appears constrained by the rest of the proximal row, and tends to collapse into an abnormally flexed and pronated posture ("rotatory subluxation of the scaphoid").
  - By contrast, the lunate and triquetrum translate ulnarly while rotating abnormally into extension, a pattern of carpal malalignment known as a dorsal intercalated segment instability (DISI) (**FIG 2C**).

NATURAL HISTORY

- Partial scapholunate ligament injury may not be radiologically demonstrable and may not produce symptoms unless the wrist is overloaded (predynamic instability).
- If left untreated, a partial scapholunate tear may progress toward a more complete disruption of all three elements of the scapholunate joint, in which case a symptomatic dysfunction usually appears.
  - Radiographically, a gap between the scaphoid and lunate may be seen. This, however, is visible only under certain loading conditions (dynamic instability).

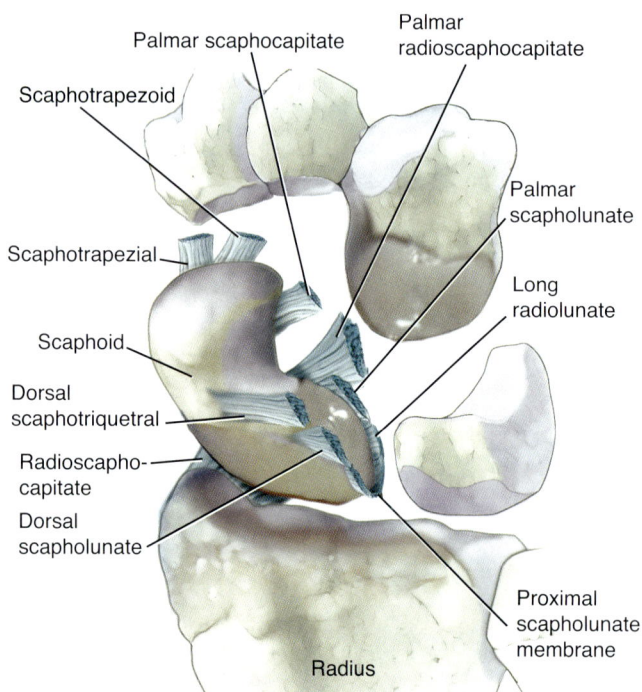

FIG 1 • Schematic representation of the periscaphoid ligaments seen from a dorsoulnar perspective. Both the lunate and the distal row have been drawn away from the scaphoid to better expose the ligaments.

Palmar scaphocapitate
Palmar radioscaphocapitate
Scaphotrapezoid
Palmar scapholunate
Scaphotrapezial
Long radiolunate
Scaphoid
Dorsal scaphotriquetral
Radioscapho-capitate
Dorsal scapholunate
Proximal scapholunate membrane
Radius

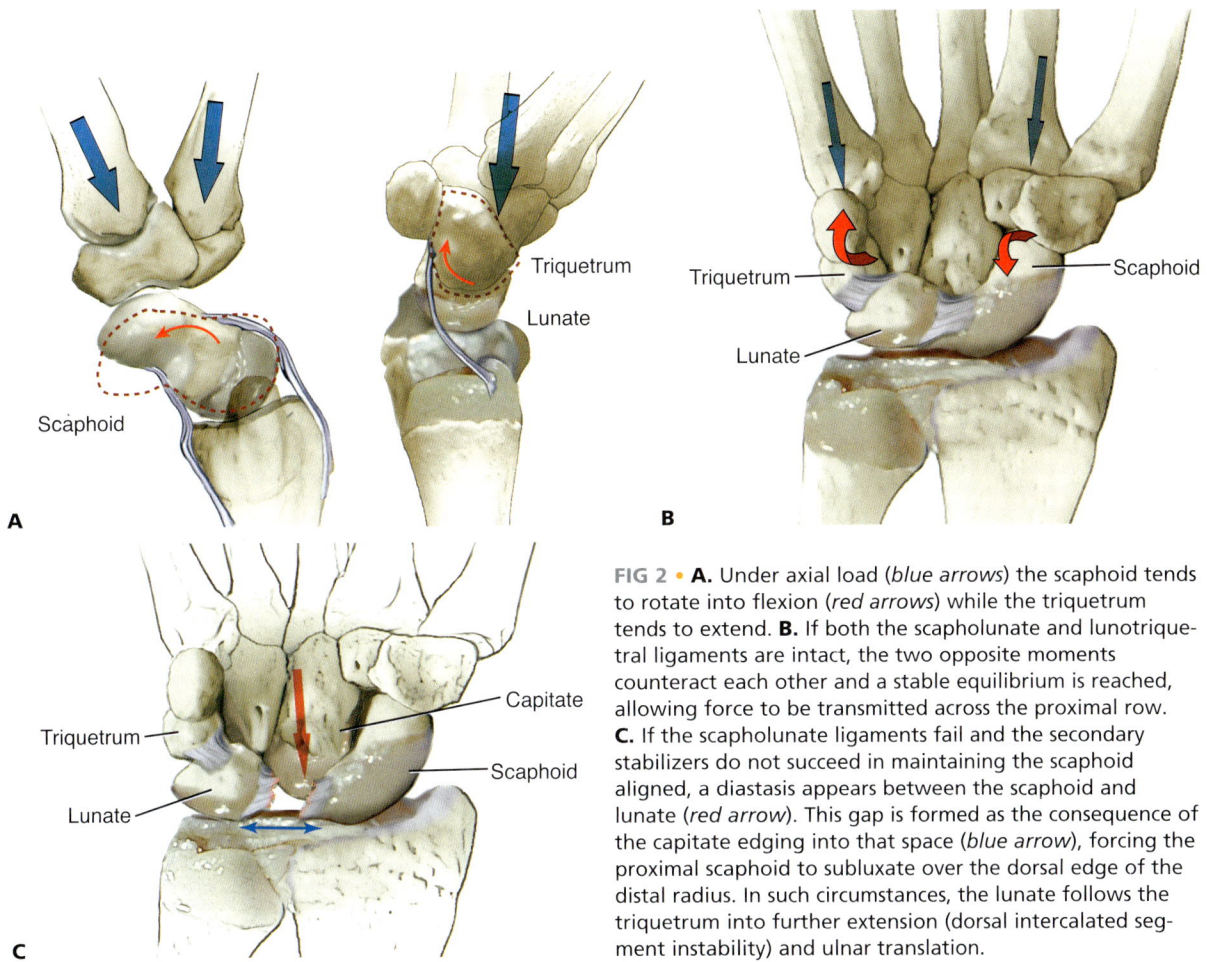

FIG 2 • **A.** Under axial load (*blue arrows*) the scaphoid tends to rotate into flexion (*red arrows*) while the triquetrum tends to extend. **B.** If both the scapholunate and lunotrique-tral ligaments are intact, the two opposite moments counteract each other and a stable equilibrium is reached, allowing force to be transmitted across the proximal row. **C.** If the scapholunate ligaments fail and the secondary stabilizers do not succeed in maintaining the scaphoid aligned, a diastasis appears between the scaphoid and lunate (*red arrow*). This gap is formed as the consequence of the capitate edging into that space (*blue arrow*), forcing the proximal scaphoid to subluxate over the dorsal edge of the distal radius. In such circumstances, the lunate follows the triquetrum into further extension (dorsal intercalated seg-ment instability) and ulnar translation.

■ With time, the secondary stabilizers (STT and SC ligaments) may stretch out and become inefficient. In such circumstances, the wrist may progress toward permanent malalignment (static instability) (**FIG 3A,B**).

　■ The wrist moves abnormally, with the lunate decreasing its range while progressively adopting an extended posi-tion (DISI).

　■ Conversely, the scaphoid adopts a flexed collapsed posi-tion, with its proximal pole subluxing dorsoradially over the edge of the radioscaphoid fossa (**FIG 3C**).

■ The abnormal joint contact between radius and scaphoid may cause cartilage deterioration of the proximal pole of the scaphoid and the reactive formation of an osteophyte at the tip of the radial styloid. This condition is known as scapholunate advanced collapse (SLAC), stage 1.

■ If untreated, SLAC stage 1 may progress toward a more ex-tended cartilage loss involving the entire scaphoid fossa (SLAC stage 2).

■ As the lunate becomes fixed in DISI, the dorsally subluxing capitate may present with cartilage deterioration progressing

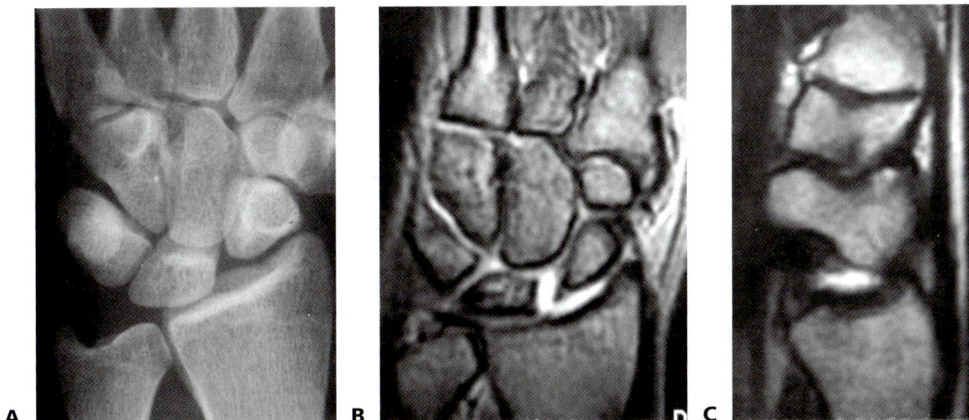

FIG 3 • **A.** PA radiographic view demonstrating a scapholunate gap and a foreshortened scaphoid with the classic ring sign indicating static scapholunate dissociation. **B.** Coronal MRI showing the remnants of the disrupted proximal membrane hanging into the scapholunate gap, which is filled with fluid. **C.** Sagittal MRI showing the ab-normal dorsal subluxation of the proximal scaphoid over the edge of the radius.

from radial to ulnar until it involves the entire capitolunate joint (SLAC stage 3).

PATIENT HISTORY AND PHYSICAL FINDINGS

- Two clinical situations lead to a diagnosis of SLD. One is the patient who presents following violent trauma, such as a fall from a height or a motorcycle accident, who is likely to have a major carpal derangement. Another is the patient who may not recall specific trauma and yet presents with symptoms.
  - In the first case, the diagnosis of a major SLD may be obvious.
  - In the second case, identification of the true nature of dysfunction may require a high index of suspicion, careful examination, and appropriate diagnostic tools.
  - Not uncommonly, arthroscopy is the only way to fully assess the extent of ligament derangement (see Chap. HA-41).
- In both dynamic and static SLD, swelling may be moderate. In acute cases, range of motion may be limited by pain, whereas it may be normal in chronic cases.
- Scapholunate point tenderness: If sharp pain is elicited by pressing this area, the probability of localized synovitis is high. Not all synovitis represents an injury to the scapholunate joint. Occult ganglia may present with a similar type of pain on palpation.
- The resisted finger extension test[9] has low specificity but excellent sensitivity. In the presence of scapholunate injury, sharp pain is elicited at the scapholunate area, representing dorsal subluxation of the scaphoid.
- Scaphoid shift test[9]: If the scapholunate ligaments are completely torn, the proximal pole may sublux dorsally out of the radius, inducing pain on the dorsoradial aspect of the wrist. This test has low specificity: occult ganglia, hyperlaxity, or radioscaphoid degenerative arthritis may produce similar symptoms.

IMAGING AND OTHER DIAGNOSTIC STUDIES

- Posteroanterior radiographic view of the neutral positioned wrist
  - Increased scapholunate joint space compared with the contralateral side (Terry Thomas sign) suggests static SLD.
  - A foreshortened appearance of the scaphoid with the scaphoid tuberosity projected in the form of a ring over the distal two thirds of the scaphoid (ring sign) indicates rotatory subluxation of the scaphoid. The ring sign is not specific for SLD; it may also be present in static LTq dissociations.
- Lateral radiographic view
  - Increased scapholunate angle compared with the contralateral side. For this to be significant, the wrist needs to be in strict neutral alignment and neutral prono-supination.
- Arthroscopy is the gold standard technique in the diagnosis of SLD. It is also useful in describing the degree of injury to the interosseous ligaments.[4]
- Magnetic resonance imaging may provide useful information regarding ligament integrity, bone vascularity, presence of local synovitis, and other soft tissue status.

Staging

- SLD stage 1: Partial scapholunate ligament injury. Normal wrist alignment. Usually diagnosed by arthroscopy. No abnormal scapholunate gap (Table 1).[4,5]

Table 1	Staging of Scapholunate Dissociation					
			Stage			
Criteria	1	2	3	4	5	6
Partial rupture with normal dorsal scapholunate ligament	Yes	No	No	No	No	No
If ruptured, dorsal scapholunate ligament is reparable	Yes	Yes	No	No	No	No
Scaphoid normally aligned (ie, 45 degrees or less)	Yes	Yes	Yes	No	No	No
Carpal malalignment easily reducible	Yes	Yes	Yes	Yes	No	No
Normal cartilage at both RC and MC joints	Yes	Yes	Yes	Yes	Yes	No

Modified from Garcia-Elias M, Lluch A, Stanley KJ. Three-ligament tenodesis for the treatment of scapholunate dissociation: Indications and surgical technique. J Hand Surg Am 2006;31A:125–134.

- SLD stage 2: Complete scapholunate ligament injury, reparable. Complete disruption of scapholunate ligaments, the dorsal one being still reparable, with good healing potential. Normal wrist alignment.
- SLD stage 3: Complete scapholunate ligament injury, nonreparable, normally aligned scaphoid. Dorsal scapholunate ligament with poor healing capability. Normal carpal alignment.
- SLD stage 4: Complete scapholunate ligament injury, nonreparable, reducible rotary subluxation of the scaphoid. Complete SLD plus detachment of the dorsal STq ligament off the distal margin of the lunate, plus insufficiency of the distal scaphoid stabilizers (STT and SC ligaments). Rotary subluxation of the scaphoid. Radioscaphoid angle greater than 45 degrees. The lunate may appear abnormally ulnarly translated and in DISI.
- SLD stage 5: Complete scapholunate ligament injury with irreducible malalignment, but normal cartilage. Fixed, irreducible long-lasting malalignment, without cartilage degeneration.
- SLD stage 6: Complete scapholunate ligament injury with irreducible malalignment and cartilage degeneration. Chronic dysfunctional wrists with cartilage degeneration (SLAC).

NONOPERATIVE MANAGEMENT

- Acute, minimally dysfunctional SLD, stage 1, may respond well to a period of 3 to 5 weeks of wrist immobilization, anti-inflammatory medication, and subsequent physical rehabilitation.
- Re-education of the dynamic scaphoid stabilizing capability of the FCR muscle may be helpful in minimal scapholunate dysfunctions. The FCR uses the scaphoid tuberosity as a hinge toward its distal insertion into the second metacarpal base. Its contraction generates a dorsally directed vector to the unstable scaphoid that prevents its collapse into flexion. Optimization of the time response of the FCR muscle to wrist loading may prevent progression of scapholunate ligament disruption (**FIG 4**).[4]

SURGICAL MANAGEMENT

- Partial ligament injuries may create discomfort from joint irritation by the ligament remnants. Arthroscopic débridement of these fragments may solve this problem.
- Electrothermal shrinkage of stretched scapholunate ligaments has been shown to be beneficial in selected cases of dynamic

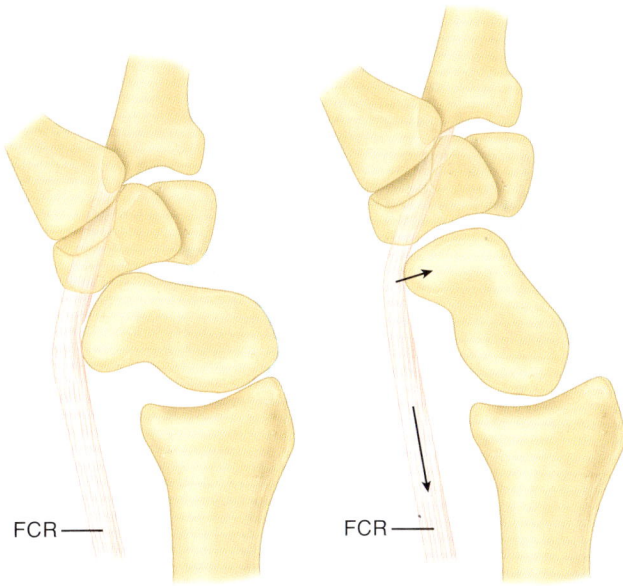

FIG 4 • The flexor carpi radialis (FCR) tendon is in close relationship to the scaphoid tuberosity. Based on this, the scaphoid flexion tendency that appears when the bone is unstable can be effectively compensated by the dynamic action of the FCR muscle. Indeed, proprioception re-education of this muscle may be useful in stage 1 scapholunate dissociation.

instability. Careful control of intra-articular fluid temperature is mandatory. Burns are not rare if lasers are carelessly applied.[4]
- Tendon reconstruction of the scapholunate linkage is recommended only in SLD stages 3 or 4—that is, when there is a nonreparable complete scapholunate ligament injury causing carpal malalignment. For this to be successful, however, it is very important that:
  - The malalignment is easily reducible, and
  - The periscaphoid cartilages are completely normal
- No soft tissue reconstruction can achieve effective carpal stability if the malalignment cannot be reduced with minimal force.
  - Intra-articular fibrosis is the most common cause of irreducibility.
- Heavy manual workers are not good candidates for this treatment modality; they may require a more solid form of stabilization, such as a partial fusion.
  - Tendon reconstruction cannot solve the loss of protective capsular proprioception, and therefore tenodeses are likely to deteriorate with time if chronically overstressed.

Preoperative Planning
- A complete set of plain radiographic views and stress views are mandatory.
- Arthroscans (tomograms taken after three-compartment injection of dye) are very useful to assess cartilage status.
- Best-quality magnetic resonance imaging may provide useful accessory information regarding bone vascularity, synovitis effects, and soft tissue status.
- Arthroscopy is by far the best tool for preoperative planning.

Positioning
- An axillary block is used. The patient is in the supine position. The arm is exsanguinated.

Approach
- An 8-cm dorsal zigzag, lazy S, or longitudinal incision of the skin and subcutaneous tissue is centered on the tubercle of Lister.
- The dorsal sensory branches of the radial and ulnar nerves are identified and protected.
- The extensor retinaculum is divided along the third compartment and the extensor pollicis longus tendon is retracted radially.
- The retinacular septa between compartments II and V are sectioned and the two retinacular flaps so created are retracted. Most septa contain intraseptal vertical vessels that need to be carefully coagulated (**FIG 5**).

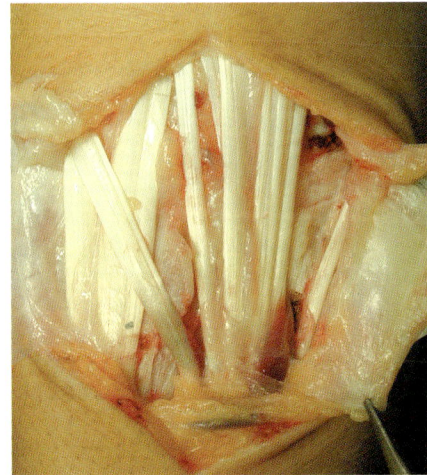

FIG 5 • Dorsal approach to the wrist through a longitudinal incision. The extensor retinaculum has been divided along the third compartment and retracted in the form of two flaps, radial and ulnar. Extensor tendons are uncovered.

DORSAL LIGAMENT-SPLITTING CAPSULOTOMY (BERGER ET AL[1])

- The first incision is made along the dorsal rim of the radius to the center of the lunate fossa.
- The second incision is made from the end of the first incision following the fibers of the dorsal radiotriquetral ligament to its distal insertion onto the dorsal ridge of the triquetrum (**TECH FIG 1A**).
- The third incision is made from the STT joint progressing medially along the dorsal intercarpal ligament to its insertion onto the dorsum of the triquetrum.

- By connecting the last two incisions, a radially based capsular flap is created. This flap is carefully elevated by sectioning its connections to the dorsal edge of the three bones of the proximal row (**TECH FIG 1B**).
- It is important to leave enough dorsal RTq ligament attached to the triquetrum in order to facilitate later tensioning of the tendon reconstruction.

TECHNIQUES

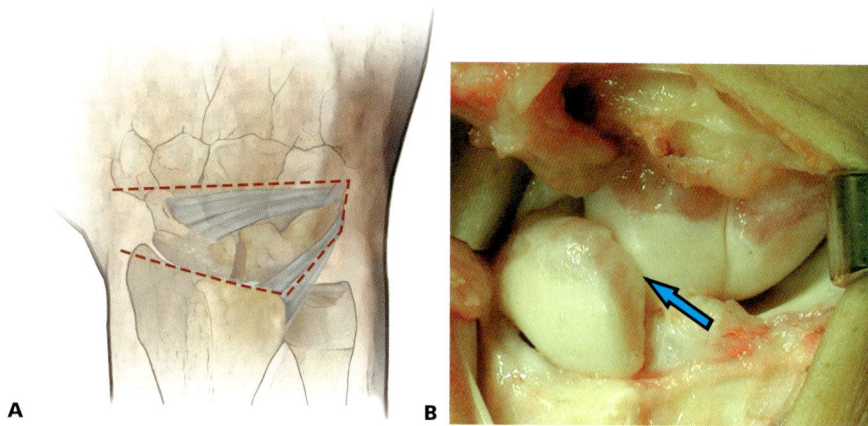

TECH FIG 1 • **A.** A radially based capsular flap is created by incising the dorsal capsule along the fibers of both the dorsal radiotriquetral ligament and the dorsal intercarpal ligament. **B.** Once the capsular flap is retracted radially, the scapholunate injury can be inspected (*arrow*) and a final therapeutic decision can be made.

PALMAR SCAPHOTRAPEZOID PLUS DORSAL RADIOSCAPHOID TENODESIS (BRUNELLI AND BRUNELLI[3])

- Beginning at the level of the distal pole of the scaphoid, using small transverse palmar incisions along the course of the FCR, a strip of the FCR tendon is obtained.
  - The strip is incised at the musculotendinous junction and left attached distally.
  - The size of graft harvested depends on the size of the scaphoid and bone tunnel created.
- A 2.7- to 3.2-mm drill hole is started volarly at the distal pole of the scaphoid, entering at the front of the scaphoid tuberosity to emerge dorsally at the level of the scaphoid neck.
- Using a tendon passer or a wire loop, the tendon strip is passed through the bone tunnel.
- While maintaining the proximal pole of the scaphoid reduced on its fossa, two Kirschner wires are passed across the scaphocapitate joint.
- Fluoroscopic assessment of reduction is important. Slight overreduction (radioscaphoid angle of about 60 degrees) is recommended.
  - Later stretch of the tenodesis is likely, in which case the scaphoid will recover its ideal alignment of 45 degrees.
- While the wrist is maintained in neutral position, the tendon is tightly anchored to the area of the tubercle of Lister using transosseous nonabsorbable sutures or metal suture anchors (**TECH FIG 2**).
- The capsular flap is passed underneath the tenodesis and reattached to its origins by absorbable sutures.

- The extensor retinaculum is repaired, leaving subretinacular drains. The extensor pollicis longus is usually left superficial to the extensor retinaculum.

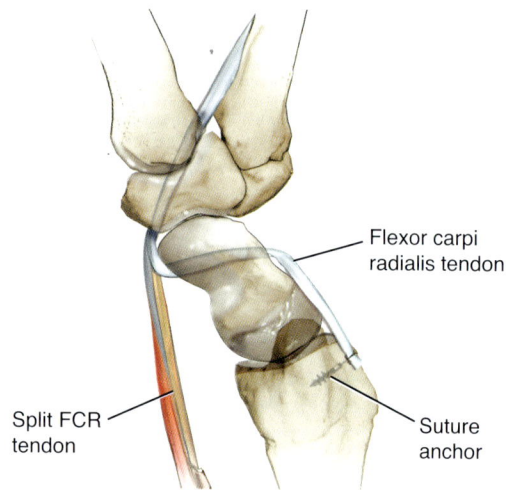

TECH FIG 2 • Schematic representation of the palmar scaphotrapezoid plus dorsal radioscaphoid tenodesis (Brunelli and Brunelli's technique) as seen from a lateral view. Note the location and direction of the bone tunnel as well as the placement of the suture anchor.

THREE-LIGAMENT TENODESIS (MODIFIED BRUNELLI'S TENODESIS[5,8])

- The transscaphoid tunnel is not transverse across the distal scaphoid (as detailed above), but oblique along the longitudinal axis of bone, from dorsal to palmar, entering at the level of the original insertion site of the dorsal scapholunate ligament, aiming at the palmar tuberosity (**TECH FIG 3A**).
  - So as not to damage the medial or lateral articular surfaces of the scaphoid, we recommend using a 2.7- to 3.2-mm cannulated drill over a Kirschner wire preset under fluoroscopy control.

- The FCR tendon strip is passed through the oblique scaphoid tunnel using a wire loop or a tendon passer (**TECH FIG 3B**).
- A transverse trough or channel is then made over the dorsum of the lunate with a rongeur. This trough needs to uncover cancellous bone, the only tissue able to generate proper healing of the tendon into bone (**TECH FIG 3C**).
- To obtain intimate contact between the tendon strip and the lunate cancellous bone, a small anchor suture is placed into the floor of the trough.

- The distal end of the dorsal radiotriquetral ligament is then localized. By its insertion on the bone, a slit is created through which the tendon strip is passed volar to dorsal (**TECH FIG 3D**).
  - The dorsal radiotriquetral ligament is used as a pulley to tension the ligament strip.
- The scaphoid, lunate, and capitate are reduced and stabilized with two 1.5-mm Kirschner wires prior to tensioning the tendon graft. One wire is placed across the scapholunate joint and one across the SC joint.
  - It is critical to ensure reduction of the scaphoid and the lunate, elimination of any DISI deformity, and proper placement of the wires using fluoroscopy.
- Radially directed tension is applied to the tendon graft already placed around and through the dorsal radiotriquetral ligament (**TECH FIG 3E**).

- The tendon graft is secured tightly into the cancellous bone channel created in the lunate using the suture anchor (**TECH FIG 3F**).
- The end of the tendon strip is sutured onto itself with nonabsorbable 3–0 sutures (**TECH FIG 3G,H**).
- The capsular flap is brought back, over the tendon reconstruction, to its original position by suturing side-by-side the split fibers of the two ligaments involved in the capsulotomy. Some sutures are also placed connecting the capsule and the tendon loop to re-establish the normal capsular attachment to the dorsum of the scapholunate joint.
- The extensor retinaculum is finally reconstructed, drains are placed, and the skin is closed.

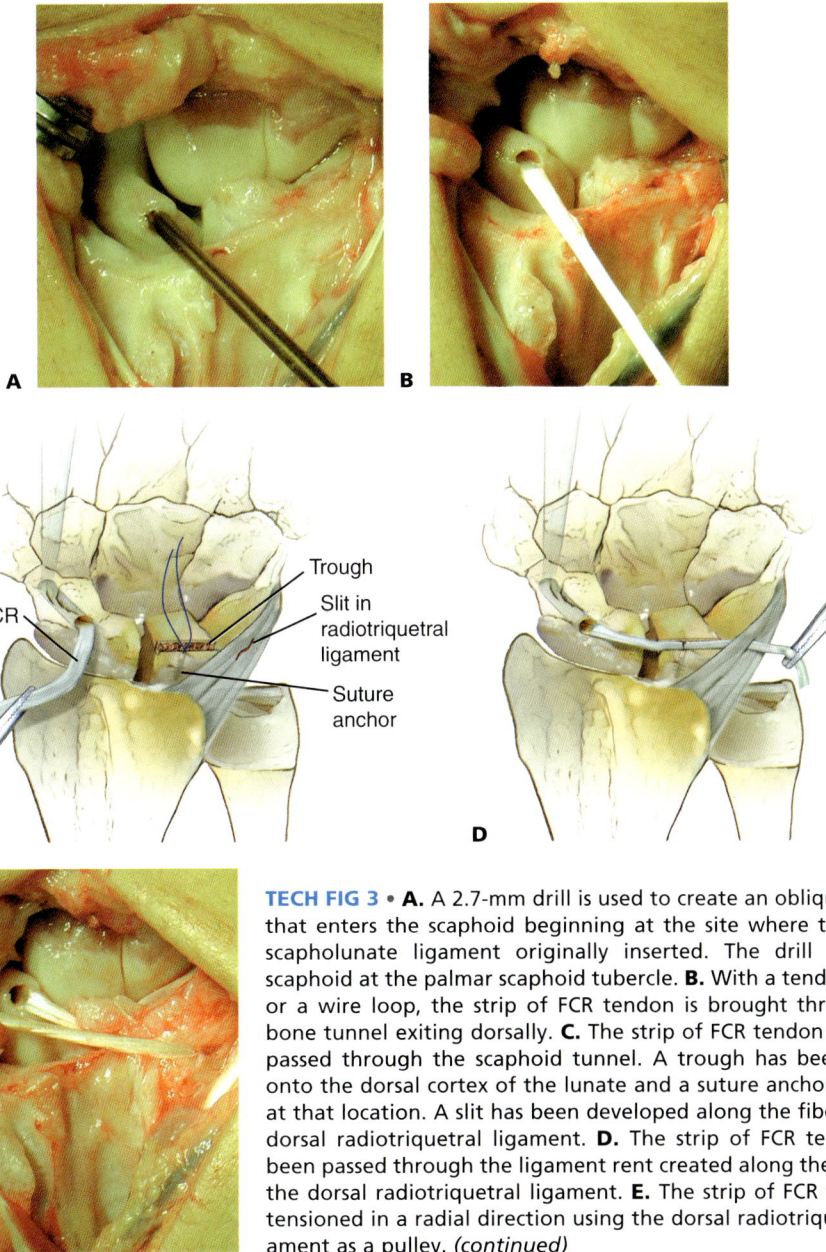

TECH FIG 3 • A. A 2.7-mm drill is used to create an oblique tunnel that enters the scaphoid beginning at the site where the dorsal scapholunate ligament originally inserted. The drill exits the scaphoid at the palmar scaphoid tubercle. **B.** With a tendon passer or a wire loop, the strip of FCR tendon is brought through the bone tunnel exiting dorsally. **C.** The strip of FCR tendon has been passed through the scaphoid tunnel. A trough has been carved onto the dorsal cortex of the lunate and a suture anchor inserted at that location. A slit has been developed along the fibers of the dorsal radiotriquetral ligament. **D.** The strip of FCR tendon has been passed through the ligament rent created along the fibers of the dorsal radiotriquetral ligament. **E.** The strip of FCR tendon is tensioned in a radial direction using the dorsal radiotriquetral ligament as a pulley. *(continued)*

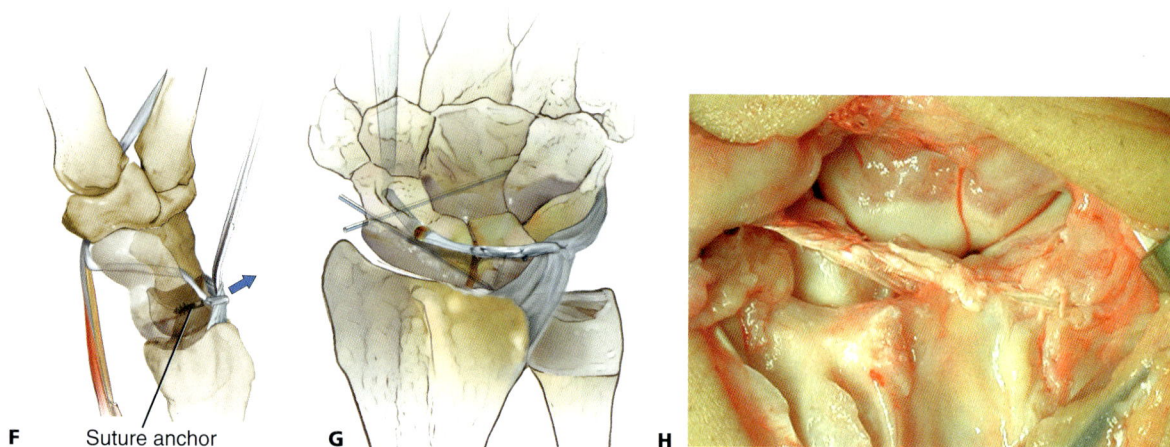

TECH FIG 3 • *(continued)* **F.** Lateral depiction of the tendon graft secured to the dorsal lunate utilizing the suture anchor. **G.** After stabilization of the scaphoid, lunate, and capitate with two Kirschner wires, tensioning of the graft, and suturing of the graft into the lunate trough, the strip of FCR tendon is sutured back to itself. **H.** Final clinical appearance of the tenodesis.

PEARLS AND PITFALLS

Indications	■ Never perform a tenodesis if the malalignment is not easily reducible, or if there is cartilage wear at the periscaphoid joints.
Scaphoid tunnel placement	■ Drill a Kirschner wire from dorsal to palmar and from proximal to distal, aiming at the tuberosity. After fluoroscopy control, use a cannulated 2.7- or 3.2-mm drill depending on the size of the tendon strip obtained. It is best to have a tighter fit rather than a looser fit in the tunnel so that there is less "slop" in the system and potentially less likelihood of loss of reduction. The bone tunnel size, therefore, depends on the tendon graft thickness and also on the size of the scaphoid.
Pin stabilization	■ One 1.5-mm Kirschner wire enters from the dorsoradial corner of the scaphoid across the scaphoid, aiming at the hook of the hamate. ■ A second Kirschner wire enters from the palmar-radial corner of the scaphoid tuberosity, aiming at the lunate. ■ Avoid Kirschner wires across the anatomic snuffbox (radial artery at risk).
Fixation of the split tendon to the lunate	■ The anchor suture in the lunate is not to be used as anchor point for tendon tensioning, but only as a means to maintain the split tendon in full contact to cancellous bone. Tension of the tenodesis relies on the dorsal radiotriquetral ligament.
Tensioning of the tenodesis	■ Avoid excessive reduction of the DISI by applying too much tension to the graft. A "volar intercalated segment instability" may be created, aside from affecting motion, or may even lead to necrosis.

POSTOPERATIVE CARE

■ The wrist is immobilized in a well-padded splint including the metacarpophalangeal joint of the thumb for 10 days.
■ After stitch removal, the wrist is maintained in a short-arm thumb spica cast for 5 more weeks.
■ A protective removable splint is then fabricated. This will allow resting the joint between sessions of supervised physiotherapy. The splint is used for an additional 4 weeks.
■ Before wire removal, at 8 weeks, therapy consists of only gentle radiocarpal mobilization. After pin removal, global active mobilization is emphasized. Aggressive passive mobilization is never recommended.

■ Muscle strengthening exercises are not initiated until 10 weeks after surgery.
■ Contact sports are to be avoided for 6 months after surgery.

OUTCOMES

■ A recently published review of 38 patients with a symptomatic SLD who had a three-ligament tenodesis procedure, with a mean follow-up of 46 months, showed an average range of motion of about 75% of the contralateral side.[5] Average grip strength was 65%. Pain relief at rest was obtained in 28 patients, with 8 complaining of mild discomfort during strenuous activity, and 2 having pain in most activities of daily life. Twenty-nine resumed their normal occupational-vocational activities. There were no signs of scaphoid necrosis. Recurrence of carpal collapse occurred in only two wrists. Nine patients showed mild signs of degenerative osteoarthritis at the tip of the radial styloid, but none had substantial symptoms.

COMPLICATIONS

- Recurrence of the malalignment and subsequent development of degenerative arthritis is common when the technique is used inappropriately, in cases with a poorly reducible SLD (stage 5), or when cartilage deterioration is already present (SLAC).
- When reducibility is in doubt, a more aggressive treatment (partial fusion or proximal row carpectomy) is recommended.

REFERENCES

1. Berger RA, Bishop AT, Bettinger PC. New dorsal capsulotomy for the surgical exposure of the wrist. Ann Plast Surg 1995;35:54–59.
2. Berger RA, Imaeda T, Berglund L, et al. Constraint and material properties of the subregions of the scapholunate interosseous ligament. J Hand Surg Am 1999;24A:953–962.
3. Brunelli GA, Brunelli GR. A new technique to correct carpal instability with scaphoid rotary subluxation: a preliminary report. J Hand Surg Am 1995;20A:S82–S85.
4. Garcia-Elias M, Geissler WB. Carpal instabilities. In: Green DP, Hotchkiss RN, Pederson WC, et al, eds. Green's Operative Hand Surgery, 5th ed. Philadelphia: Elsevier-Churchill Livingstone, 2005:535–604.
5. Garcia-Elias M, Lluch A, Stanley KJ. Three-ligament tenodesis for the treatment of scapholunate dissociation: indications and surgical technique. J Hand Surg Am 2006;31A:125–134.
6. Linscheid RL, Dobyns JH, Beabout JW, et al. Traumatic instability of the wrist: diagnosis, classification, and pathomechanics. J Bone Joint Surg Am 1972;54A:1612–1632.
7. Short WH, Werner FW, Green JK, et al. Biomechanical evaluation of ligamentous stabilizers of the scaphoid and lunate. J Hand Surg Am 2002;27A:991–1002.
8. Van Den Abbeele KLS, Loh YC, Stanley JK, et al. Early results of a modified Brunelli procedure for scapholunate instability. J Hand Surg Br 1998;23B:258–261.
9. Watson HK, Ashmead D IV, Makhlouf MV. Examination of the scaphoid. J Hand Surg Am 1988;13A:657–660.

Chapter 45

Bone–Ligament–Bone Reconstruction of the Scapholunate Ligament

Anthony M. DeLuise, Jr. and Randall W. Culp

DEFINITION

- Scapholunate ligament tears are the most common form of carpal instability.
- If left untreated, this injury will cause degenerative changes in the wrist.[3,6,8,13]
- Complete tears of the scapholunate ligament exist, yet partial tears, or dynamic instability, occur as well. This diagnosis requires a high index of suspicion and specific imaging. Dynamic instability is defined as a wrist that maintains normal alignment at rest but will collapse with applied load. Consequently, stress radiographs or diagnostic arthroscopy is needed to make the diagnosis.[3,13]
- Treatments of scapholunate ligament tears include primary repair, dorsal capsulodesis, tendon grafting, ligament reconstruction, proximal row carpectomy (PRC), and limited carpal arthrodesis.
  - Primary repair may not be possible if the remnant ligament is not amenable to repair.
  - Tendon weaves are technically challenging and do not recreate the unique motion between the scaphoid and lunate and thus may yield new problems. A PRC alters kinematics and may decrease grip strength.
  - Limited arthrodesis for the chronic scapholunate ligament tear with coincident radiocarpal arthrosis relieves pain but creates a decrease in range of motion and alters the mechanics of the wrist joint, potentially leading to degenerative changes in adjacent joints.[3,6,13]

ANATOMY

- The scapholunate ligament is one of the many intrinsic ligaments of the wrist. It is intra-articular and is composed of collagen fascicles. It consists of three main parts: dorsal, membranous (or proximal), and volar (**FIG 1**).[1,11]
- The dorsal portion is the strongest of the three. It is 2 to 3 mm thick and 3 to 5 mm long. Its collagen bundles are ori-

ented transversely. It is most important in limiting dorsal–palmar translation. The most dorsal area always merges with the wrist articular capsule. More than 300 Newtons (N) of tensile stress is required for failure.
- The proximal or membranous portion is weak and thin. It is composed of mostly fibrocartilage and there are no neurovascular bundles within it (avascular). Only 25 N of stress will cause this portion of the scapholunate ligament to fail.
- The volar portion of the scapholunate ligament is only 1 mm thick and 4 to 5 mm long. Its collagen bundles are oriented obliquely. The volar and proximal portions are most important in limiting dorsal–palmar rotation. The volar and membranous portions of the scapholunate ligament are intersected by the loose radioscapholunate ligament (ligament of Testut). The amount of stress to failure here is 150 N.
- The scaphocapitate, scaphotrapezium–trapezoid (intrinsic), radioscaphocapitate, long and short radiolunate (volar extrinsic), dorsal radiocarpal, and dorsal intercarpal (dorsal extrinsic) ligaments also provide support and stability in this area.

PATHOGENESIS

- The mechanism of injury is often a fall on an outstretched hand. Mayfield et al[9] described this injury occurring with an axial load in excessive dorsiflexion, ulnar deviation, and midcarpal supination. This position causes the capitate to separate the scaphoid (radial and dorsal) and lunate (ulnar and palmar).
- An ipsilateral distal radius fracture or scaphoid fracture can occur up to 30% of the time.[3,4]
- The lunate will naturally flex with the scaphoid and extend with the triquetrum. In a patient with a scapholunate ligament injury, the connection to the scaphoid is lacking, the scaphoid will flex and rotate away from the lunate because of its other attachments, and the lunate will fall into a dorsal intercalated segment instability (DISI) pattern. For this rotational instability to occur, the dorsal capsular ligaments must be injured as well.
  - An acute scapholunate injury may or may not coincide with an injury to the surrounding ligaments (ie, dorsal extrinsics). If it does, a DISI pattern may be noted soon after injury. If there is no injury to the surrounding structures, attenuation of these structures over time may occur and then subsequently cause a DISI pattern. When DISI does occur, this pattern of carpal instability must be corrected for any treatment of this injury to be successful.

NATURAL HISTORY

- The natural history of the wrist with a scapholunate ligament injury has been described by several authors. Pain and instability can result from a static injury. A DISI pattern deformity as described earlier will develop, and a very specific sequential pattern of wrist arthrosis will progress (scapholunate advanced collapse [SLAC]):
  - Stage IA: radial styloid with or without scaphoid arthrosis
  - Stage IB: radioscaphoid arthrosis

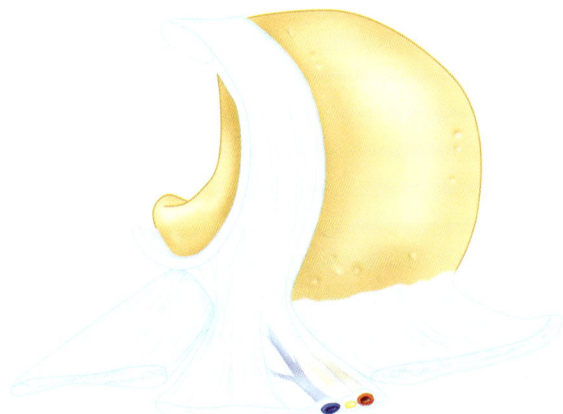

FIG 1 • The scapholunate ligament viewed from the proximal-radial side with the scaphoid removed.

- Stage II: capitolunate arthrosis
- Stage III: pan-arthritis
- The radiolunate joint is typically spared.[14,15]

PATIENT HISTORY AND PHYSICAL FINDINGS

- Commonly, the patient will describe radial-sided wrist pain, pain with loading activities, and weakness.
- Physical examination methods include the following:
  - Observation and palpation of gross edema
  - Wrist range of motion in extension, flexion, ulnar, and radial directions. Decreased range of motion or pain with extremes of motion will be evident.
  - Palpation just distal to the tubercle of Lister to assess for scapholunate interval tenderness
  - Ballottement test: Pain or instability here is concerning for a scapholunate ligament tear
  - Watson test: Pressure on the scaphoid tuberosity during ulnar-to-radial deviation of the wrist prevents the scaphoid from normally flexing. In a wrist with a scapholunate ligament tear, the proximal pole of the scaphoid will dorsally subluxate out of the scaphoid fossa with this maneuver, causing a clunk. A palpable clunk is indicative of instability.
  - Grip strength weakness is sensitive but not specific for scapholunate ligament disruption.
- A complete examination of the wrist should also include evaluation of associated injuries and ruling out differential diagnoses. This includes but is not limited to the following:
  - Lunatotriquetral tears: pain with "shuck" of the lunate and triquetrum
  - Masses: examine carefully for any cysts or masses that may be causing pain
  - Distal radius or scaphoid fracture: tenderness at the distal end of the radius or the snuffbox as well as a fracture noted on radiographs
  - Triangular fibrocartilage complex (TFCC) tears: pain with a TFCC stress test, which is an axially applied load via ulnar deviation while moving the wrist through a flexion–extension arc

IMAGING AND OTHER DIAGNOSTIC STUDIES

- Plain radiographs include posteroanterior (PA), lateral, and scaphoid views, although some authors will advocate the "complete" series to include a clenched-fist PA, a radial deviation PA, and flexion and extension lateral radiographs. It is helpful to compare the radiographs with the contralateral extremity.[3,13]
  - A static scapholunate ligament injury will reveal an increased space between the scaphoid and lunate on a PA radiograph. The normal scapholunate distance is less than 3 mm. If this interval is greater than 3 mm, the patient has what is known as the Terry Thomas sign. Additionally, as mentioned earlier, the scaphoid will collapse into flexion and the tuberosity will project in the coronal plane, revealing a scaphoid ring sign. The astute observer may also note the volar lip of the extended lunate overlapping with the capitate (**FIG 2A–C**).
  - The lateral radiograph may reveal an increased scapholunate angle. This angle is found by drawing lines through the longitudinal axes of the scaphoid and lunate and measuring the angle. Normally, it falls between 30 and 60 degrees. A radiolunate angle greater than 15 degrees indicates a DISI deformity (**FIG 2D**).
  - Flexion and extension lateral radiographs will show motion occurring at the lunocapitate joint and an uncoupling of the normally synchronous scapholunate motion.
  - Radial and ulnar deviation radiographs and a clenched-fist radiograph may portray a dynamic instability picture in that a static radiograph reveals no deformity (ie, normal scapholunate gap), but one of these views will reveal an abnormal scapholunate diastasis.
  - The chronic scapholunate injury may have evidence of arthritis on any of these views and the physician must recognize these findings, which indicate an old injury (**FIG 2E,F**).
- Magnetic resonance imaging has become valuable in assessing acute or chronic scapholunate ligament tears (**FIG 2G**).
- Arthroscopy is the imaging method of choice. It allows the experienced surgeon to diagnose most wrist pathology as well as affording the ability to possibly treat it (**FIG 2H**).
  - Geissler et al[4] published four stages of scapholunate ligament tears based on arthroscopic examination (see Chap. HA-41).

DIFFERENTIAL DIAGNOSIS

- Distal radius fracture
- Scaphoid fracture
- Radioscaphoid arthritis
- Scaphotrapezial arthritis

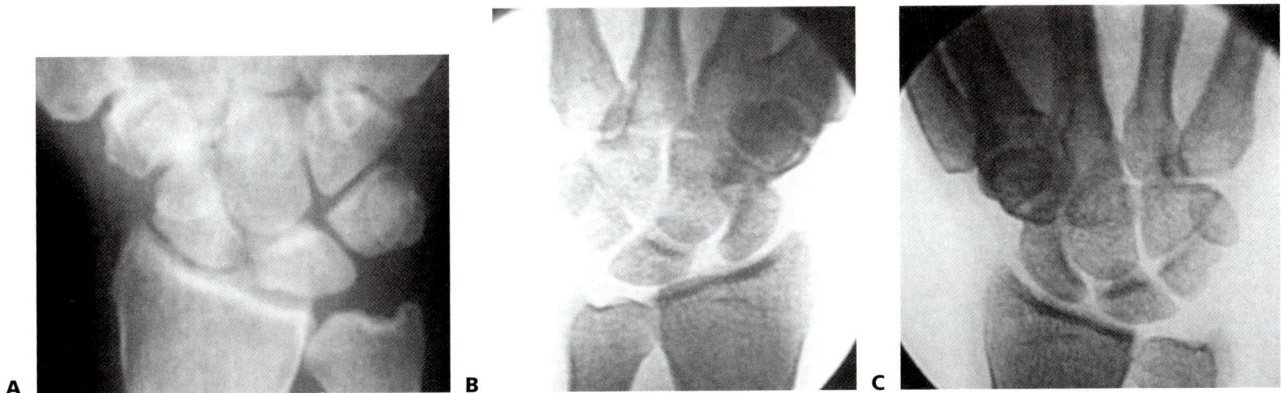

FIG 2 • A. PA radiograph demonstrating an increased scapholunate gap and a scaphoid ring sign. **B.** A fluoroscopic image of another example of an increased scapholunate gap. **C.** The contralateral wrist demonstrates a normal scapholunate interval. *(continued)*

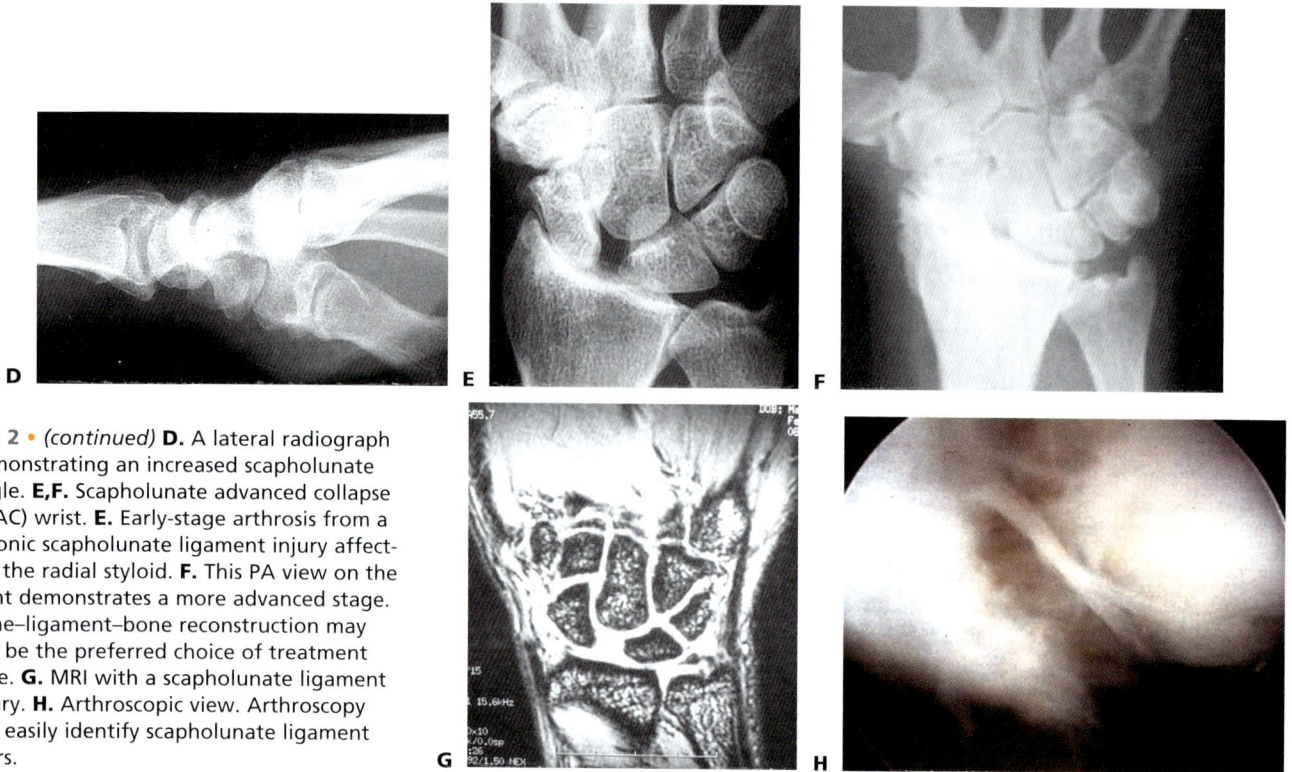

FIG 2 • *(continued)* **D.** A lateral radiograph demonstrating an increased scapholunate angle. **E,F.** Scapholunate advanced collapse (SLAC) wrist. **E.** Early-stage arthrosis from a chronic scapholunate ligament injury affecting the radial styloid. **F.** This PA view on the right demonstrates a more advanced stage. Bone–ligament–bone reconstruction may not be the preferred choice of treatment here. **G.** MRI with a scapholunate ligament injury. **H.** Arthroscopic view. Arthroscopy can easily identify scapholunate ligament tears.

- deQuervain tenosynovitis
- Dorsal wrist impaction syndrome
- Dorsal ganglion cyst
- Lunatotriquetral instability
- Midcarpal instability

NONOPERATIVE MANAGEMENT

■ Nonoperative management of a scapholunate injury is seldom indicated. Geissler grade 1 injuries are the only injuries treated with just immobilization. We prefer a removable volar splint worn full time for 4 weeks followed by 4 weeks of splinting and removal of the splint for active range-of-motion exercises of the wrist. At the conclusion of 8 weeks, passive range of motion is initiated if necessary, followed by strengthening.

SURGICAL MANAGEMENT

■ Less invasive surgical procedures are used for partial scapholunate ligament tears and the wrist with dynamic instability. This can consist of thermal shrinkage through the arthroscope, arthroscopic débridement, and percutaneous pinning of the scaphoid and lunate in a reduced position. A capsulodesis may be considered.

■ The surgical treatment of complete scapholunate ligament tears depends on the chronicity of the injury and the presence of joint arthrosis. Ligament injuries older than 3 weeks have a lower rate of healing because of the ligament's lack of vascularity. In these more subacute or chronic injuries, it may be difficult to obtain a good outcome when performing a primary direct repair of the ligament.[3]

■ In addition, repair or reconstruction of the scapholunate ligament is a futile exercise in those joints with SLAC arthrosis, demonstrated by imaging studies preoperatively or arthroscopic findings intraoperatively. These procedures will not address arthritic pain.

■ Our algorithm is given in Table 1.

■ The purpose of this chapter is to review the techniques for bone-ligament-bone reconstruction of the scapholunate ligament.

■ The advantages of this technique compared to other techniques are a more anatomic reconstruction, better approximating carpal kinematics; bone-to-bone healing as opposed to tendon-to-bone healing; and local availability.

Table 1	Algorithm for Treatment of Scapholunate Ligament Injuries
Injury Type	**Treatment**
Acute (<3–4 wk)	
Dynamic	Immobilization vs. arthroscopic shrinkage +/− percutaneous pinning +/− capsulodesis
Static	Open repair of scapholunate interosseous ligament (treatment of choice) if possible vs. bone–ligament–bone reconstruction vs. tendon weave +/− capsulodesis
Subacute (4–24 wk)	Reconstruction vs. tendon weave +/− capsulodesis (open repair can be done if enough remnant ligament is available)
Chronic (>24 wk)	
No arthrosis	Reconstruction vs. tendon weave +/− capsulodesis
With arthrosis	Salvage (ie, scapholunate advanced collapse procedure, proximal row carpectomy, intercarpal arthrodesis*)

* Intercarpal arthrodesis examples include scapho–trapezium–trapezoid, scaphocapitate, scapholunate, and scapholunate–capitate.

Preoperative Planning

- The surgeon should review radiographs for any evidence of arthrosis. MRI is reviewed for pathology.
- Associated fractures or other soft tissue pathology should be addressed.
- Any evidence of joint arthrosis should indicate to the surgeon that a salvage procedure should be performed rather than a ligament reconstruction.
- A Watson shift test is performed while the patient is under anesthesia. The examiner may better appreciate a clunk while the patient is under anesthesia in contrast to the awake patient where pain may be present, making it difficult for the examiner to perform this maneuver well.

Positioning

- Often, a diagnostic wrist arthroscopy is performed initially.
- The patient is positioned supine. A hand table is appropriately positioned. A nonsterile tourniquet (set to 250 mm Hg) is placed on the upper arm.
- After preparation and draping, the wrist is placed in the arthroscopic tower. About 10 to 15 pounds of traction is used to distract the joint for the arthroscopy.
- Arthroscopy aids in evaluating the extent of the injury to the scapholunate ligament, assessing the quality of tissue remaining, and diagnosing concomitant injuries (**FIG 3**).

FIG 3 • Arthroscopic setup. The arthroscopic tower uses plastic hook-and-eye straps and finger traps. About 10 to 15 lb of traction is used to distract the joint for the diagnostic arthroscopy.

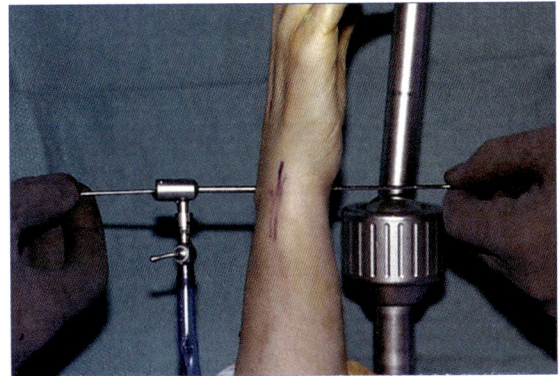

- Once the diagnostic arthroscopy is completed and the decision to perform a reconstruction is made, the wrist is taken out of the tower and placed pronated on the hand table.

Approach

- There are several dorsal approaches to the wrist. Some prefer a trans-fourth compartment approach. We prefer an approach between the second and fourth compartments while transposing the extensor pollicis longus.
- Another decision to be made is where to obtain the bone–ligament–bone graft. We prefer local tissue, such as the capitohamate ligament, while some would advocate autograft from the foot. Autograft from the foot creates two operative sites and thus a second potential site of morbidity. In addition, there have been no clinical studies at this point verifying its merit; however, biomechanical studies are encouraging.[2,12]

APPROACH TO THE DORSAL WRIST

- An incision of about 6 to 8 cm is made just ulnar to the tubercle of Lister, extending distally to include the third metacarpal (**TECH FIG 1A**).
- The extensor pollicis longus sheath is incised and the tendon is transposed in a radial direction (**TECH FIG 1B**).
- The interval continues between the second and fourth compartment.

- The posterior interosseous nerve is excised to decrease residual pain.
- A ligament-splitting dorsal wrist capsulotomy described is made through the dorsal intercarpal and dorsal radiocarpal ligaments (**TECH FIG 1C**).[1,3,13]
- Direct visual inspection and probing allows the surgeon to further assess the scapholunate ligament for direct primary repair versus reconstruction.

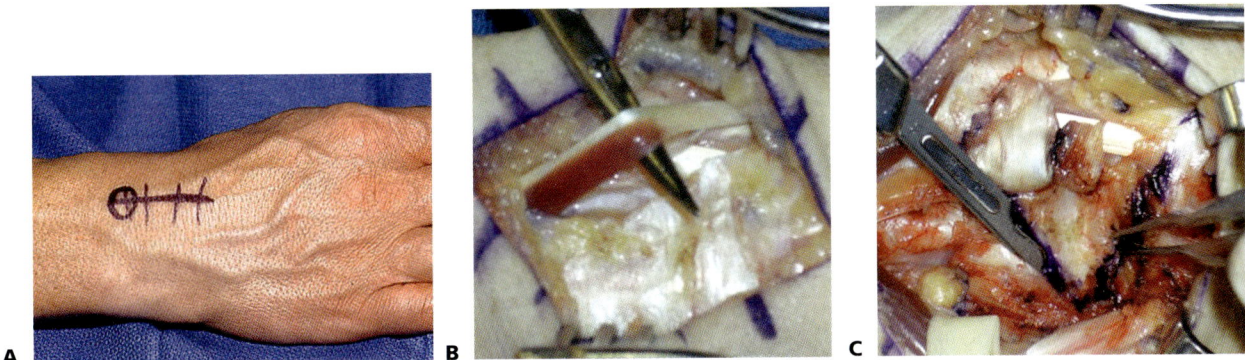

TECH FIG 1 • Approach. **A.** A 6- to 8-cm incision is made ulnar to the tubercle of Lister, extending distally. **B.** The third extensor compartment is incised and the tendon is radialized. **C.** A ligament-splitting incision is made in the capsule.

TECHNIQUES

TECHNIQUES

GRAFT HARVESTING

- Fluoroscopy and an 18-gauge needle can help identify the capitohamate ligament.
- Using a quarter-inch osteotome, a portion of the ligament with bone blocks (10 × 5 × 5 mm) is taken. This concept is quite similar to a bone–patellar tendon–bone autograft for anterior cruciate ligament reconstructions (**TECH FIG 2A,B**).
- Other ligaments from the upper extremity that can be used include the third metacarpal–capitate ligament, the capito–trapezoid ligament, the second metacarpal–trapezoid ligament, and the dorsal extensor retinaculum bone block.[10,16] This last choice was the weakest of all in a biomechanical study.[7]

- The dorsal tarsometatarsal ligaments between the lateral cuneiform and the third metatarsal or the ligament between the navicular and the first cuneiform of the foot have also been shown to be both geometrically and biomechanically similar to the scapholunate ligament, and they remain an option for grafting.[2,12]
- If the surgeon prefers this dorsal foot graft, a longitudinal incision is made over the base of the third metatarsal. Sharp dissection is used for exposure to the joint. An osteotome is used to harvest the ligament with large bone blocks as close to the size of the scapholunate recipient site as possible—typically no greater than a 5- to 8-mm-wide section. The remainder of the dorsal ligament as well as the plantar ligament remains in place, ensuring maintained stability for the foot (**TECH FIG 2C**).

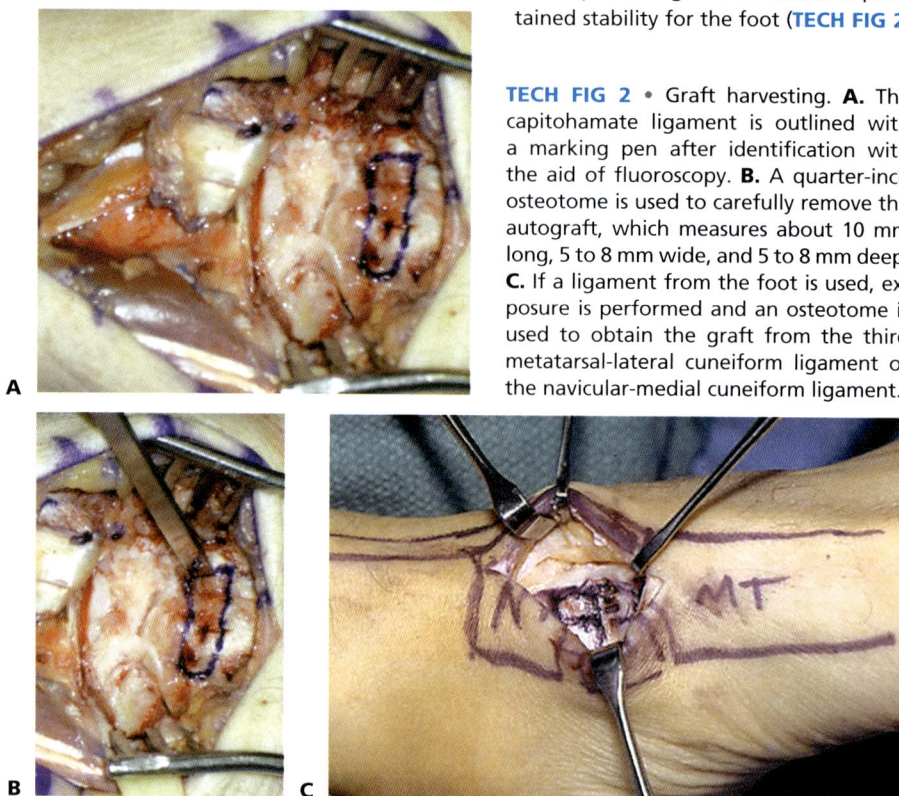

TECH FIG 2 • Graft harvesting. **A.** The capitohamate ligament is outlined with a marking pen after identification with the aid of fluoroscopy. **B.** A quarter-inch osteotome is used to carefully remove the autograft, which measures about 10 mm long, 5 to 8 mm wide, and 5 to 8 mm deep. **C.** If a ligament from the foot is used, exposure is performed and an osteotome is used to obtain the graft from the third metatarsal-lateral cuneiform ligament or the navicular-medial cuneiform ligament.

PREPARATION OF THE RECIPIENT SITE AND FIXATION

- Using fluoroscopic guidance, 0.062 Kirschner wires are used to reduce the DISI (ie, joysticks) and hold the scaphoid and lunate in position (**TECH FIG 3A**).
- Two Kirschner wires from scaphoid to lunate and, if required, one from scaphoid to capitate to stabilize the reduced scapholunate interval (**TECH FIG 3B**). More recently, we have been using a cannulated scapholunate screw for fixation.
- A trough is cut in the dorsal aspect of the scaphoid and lunate using an osteotome (**TECH FIG 3C**). The trough must be large enough to accept the bone blocks of the bone–ligament–bone autograft. We aim to make the trough as equal to the bone blocks as possible.

- The bone blocks are placed into the trough with digital pressure and they are held with a 1.5-mm screw in each bone. It is important to ensure that full flexion and extension of the wrist is still possible after fixation (**TECH FIG 3D–F**).
- Another option would be to acquire a "press fit" with the bone blocks, thereby bypassing the need for screws. This will decrease the possibility of fragmenting the bone block with the screws. However, we prefer obtaining a larger bone block autograft and using screws for added stability.
- A dorsal capsulodesis (see Chap. HA-43) can be performed for added stability. We prefer using a portion of the dorsal intercarpal ligament. This technique is described elsewhere in this part.

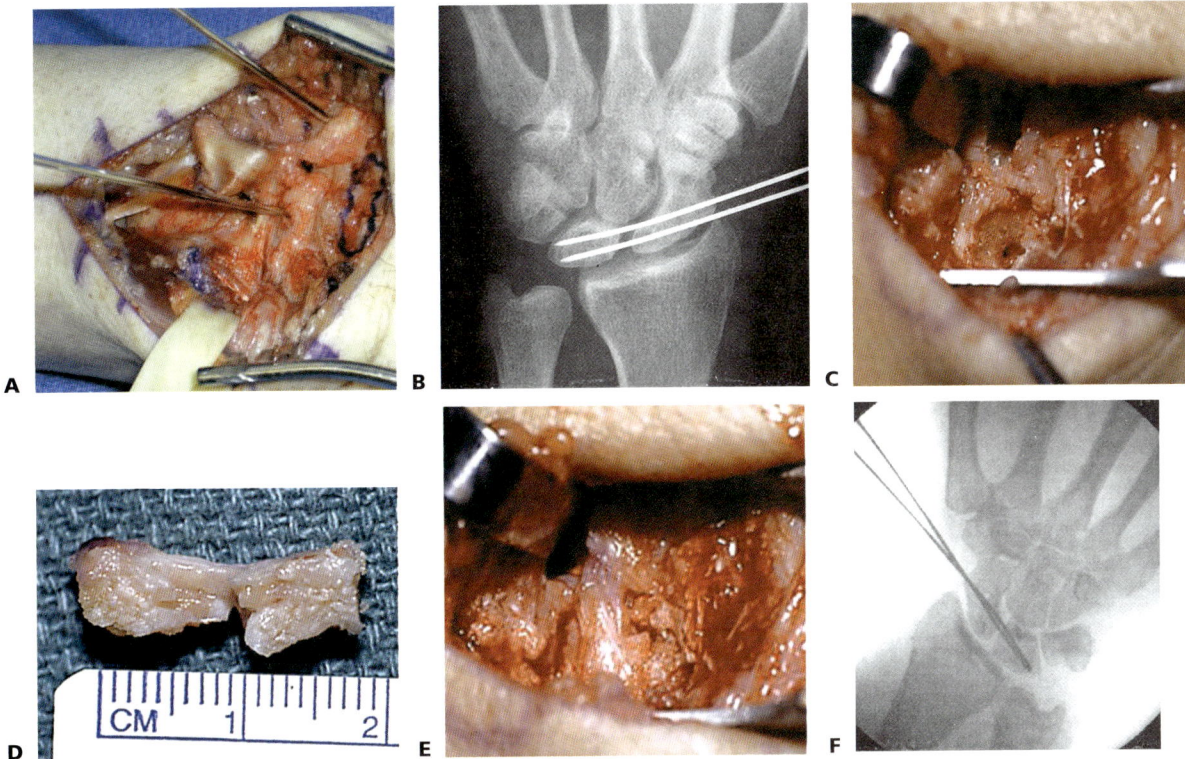

TECH FIG 3 • Preparation of the recipient site and fixation. **A.** Using fluoroscopic guidance, 0.062-inch Kirschner wires are placed into the scaphoid and lunate and used as joysticks to reduce and hold position. **B.** Two 0.045-inch Kirschner wires are placed from scaphoid to lunate and one is placed from scaphoid to capitate for additional fixation. The joysticks are removed. **C.** A trough is cut in the dorsal aspect of the scaphoid and lunate using a quarter-inch osteotome; the surgeon should try to make the trough as equal to the bone blocks as possible. **D.** Bone–ligament–bone autograft. **E.** The bone blocks are placed into the trough with digital pressure. **F.** A 1.5-mm screw is placed in each bone. It is important to still have the ability of full flexion and extension.

CLOSURE

- We prefer to deflate the tourniquet and obtain hemostasis before closure. Once hemostasis is achieved, the capsule and extensor retinaculum are closed.
- The extensor pollicis longus tendon is left out of its sheath so swelling will not cause any attenuation and possible attritional rupture in its watershed area.
- The skin is closed. Kirschner wires are cut under the skin to prevent pin tract infection.

- Final radiographs should demonstrate screws to be adequately placed and the scaphoid and lunate to be in good position by noting a decreased scapholunate interval, a reduced scapholunate angle, and no evidence of DISI.
- The wrist is splinted in neutral or 30 degrees of extension; theoretically, the dorsal rim of the radius buttresses the graft for additional support in this slightly extended position.

PEARLS AND PITFALLS

Indications	▪ Carefully review the history for assessment of chronicity of the injury to determine whether a repair versus a reconstruction is needed. ▪ Carefully review all imaging studies preoperatively to assess for any arthritic changes that may preclude bone–ligament–bone reconstruction.
Approach	▪ It is helpful to transpose the extensor pollicis longus.
Donor graft	▪ The bone blocks should be large enough to accommodate a 1.5-mm screw without the risk of fragment fracture.
Recipient site	▪ The trough should be large enough to accept the bone blocks without being so large that the scaphoid or lunate would lose their dimensions. ▪ The scaphoid and lunate must be reduced and pinned before stabilization of the graft; otherwise the graft will be tensioned incorrectly.
Postoperative care	▪ A good outcome will be predicated on supervised postoperative therapy after healing.

POSTOPERATIVE CARE

- The wrist is strictly immobilized for 8 weeks. Finger and elbow range of motion is encouraged.
- Pins are removed at 8 weeks and gentle active range-of-motion exercises are started. A removable splint is still worn when not exercising for an additional 4 weeks.
- Passive range of motion begins at 12 weeks, followed by strengthening.

OUTCOMES

- Patients with a partial tear or dynamic component and patients with a shorter time from injury to treatment have a better outcome.
- Weiss[16] reported excellent results at a minimum of 2 years of follow-up in 13 of 14 patients with scapholunate gaps of less than 8 mm using a bone–retinaculum–bone autograft, even though it has been shown to be biomechanically weaker than the native scapholunate ligament. This may be due to graft remodeling or hypertrophy in vivo.
- Lutz al[18] used a periosteal flap of iliac crest as the autograft. With an average follow-up of 29 months, they reported 6 of 11 patients to be clinically excellent or good and 5 as fair. Average radiographic parameters improved.
- Hanel[5] reported that all 39 of his patients treated with the bone-ligament-bone reconstruction outlined in this chapter returned to work, but some had difficulty with return to some sports. All patients would have the surgery again as it had helped their day-to-day activities.
- Although there are no long-term clinical outcome studies in the literature on bone–ligament–bone reconstruction, short-term results are promising. A larger number of patients with a longer follow-up is required to fully recommend this technique for most scapholunate injuries.

COMPLICATIONS

- Fragmentation of the bone block intraoperatively or postoperatively
- Failure of graft to incorporate if the trough made in the scaphoid or lunate is not deep enough to cause punctate bleeding for the incorporation of the graft
- Pin tract infections (which are treated with oral antibiotics)
- Failure to achieve normal carpal alignment

REFERENCES

1. Berger RA. The ligaments of the wrist: a current overview of anatomy with considerations of their potential functions. Hand Clin 1997; 13:63–82.
2. Davis CA, Culp RW, Hume EL, et al. Reconstruction of the scapholunate ligament in a cadaver model using a bone-ligament-bone autograft from the foot. J Hand Surg Am 1998;23A:884–892.
3. Garcia-Elias M, Geissler WB. Carpal instability. In: Green DP, Pederson WC, Hotchkiss RN, et al, eds. Green's Operative Hand Surgery, 5th ed. Philadelphia: Elsevier Churchill Livingstone, 2005:535–604.
4. Geissler WB, Freeland AE, Savoie FH, et al. Intracarpal soft tissue lesions associated with an intra-articular fracture of the distal end of the radius. J Bone Joint Surg Am 1996;78A:357–365.
5. Harvey EJ. Hand-based autograft replacement of the scapholunate ligament: early outcome (meeting transcript). American Society for Surgery of the Hand. Seattle, 2000.
6. Harvey EJ, Hanel DP. Bone-ligament-bone reconstruction for scapholunate disruption. Tech Hand Upper Extr Surg 2002;6:2–5.
7. Harvey EJ, Hanel DP. Autograft replacements for the scapholunate ligament: a biomechanical comparison of hand based autografts. J Hand Surg Am 1999;24A:963–967.
8. Mayfield JK. Wrist ligamentous anatomy and pathogenesis of carpal instability. Orthop Clin 1984;15:209–216.
9. Mayfield JK, Johnson RP, Kilcoyne RK. Carpal dislocations: pathomechanics and progressive perilunar instability. J Hand Surg Am 1980;5:226–241.
10. Shin SS, Moore DC, McGovern RD, et al. Scapholunate ligament reconstruction using a bone-retinaculum-bone autograft: a biomechanic and histologic study. J Hand Surg Am 1998;23:216–221.
11. Sokolow C, Saffar P. Anatomy and histology of the scapholunate ligament. Hand Clin 2001;17:77–81.
12. Svoboda SJ, Eglseder A, Belkoff SM. Autografts from the foot for reconstruction of the scapholunate interosseous ligament. J Hand Surg Am 1995;20A:980–985.
13. Walsh JJ, Berger RA, Cooney WP. Current status of scapholunate interosseous ligament injuries. J Am Acad Orthop Surg 2002;10:32–42.
14. Watson HK, Ballet FL. The SLAC wrist: scapholunate advanced collapse pattern of degenerative arthritis. J Hand Surg Am 1984;9A: 358–365.
15. Watson HK, Weinzweig J, Zeppieri J. The natural progression of scaphoid instability. Hand Clin 1997;13:39–49.
16. Weiss APC. Scapholunate ligament reconstruction using a bone-retinaculum-bone autograft. J Hand Surg Am 1998;23A:205–215.
17. Wolf JM, Weiss APC. Bone-retinaculum-bone reconstruction of scapholunate ligament injuries. Orthop Clin North Am 2001;32: 241–246.
18. Lutz M, Kralinger F, Goldhahn J, et al. Dorsal scapholunate ligament reconstruction using a periosteal flap of iliac crest. Arch Orthop Trauma Surg 2004;124:197–202.

Reduction and Association of the Scaphoid and the Lunate for Scapholunate Instability

Richard Y. Kim and Melvin P. Rosenwasser

DEFINITION

- Scapholunate instability occurs as a result of injury to the scapholunate interosseous ligament (SLIL).
- Instability can be categorized based on physical and radiographic findings.
  - Static instability: abnormal alignment of the scaphoid and lunate evident on routine radiographs
  - Dynamic instability: abnormal alignment of the scaphoid and lunate present only on stress radiographs
  - Predynamic instability: no radiographic abnormalities present, but history and physical findings consistent with a SLIL injury
- Reduction and association of the scaphoid and the lunate (the RASL procedure) is used to correct scapholunate instability.

ANATOMY

- The SLIL can be divided into three components: dorsal, palmar, and proximal. Of these, the dorsal component is the thickest and contributes the most to scapholunate stability.[1]
- Normally, the interval between the scaphoid and the lunate measures less than 3 mm, but this can vary between patients. The interval should be compared to the contralateral wrist (**FIG 1A**).

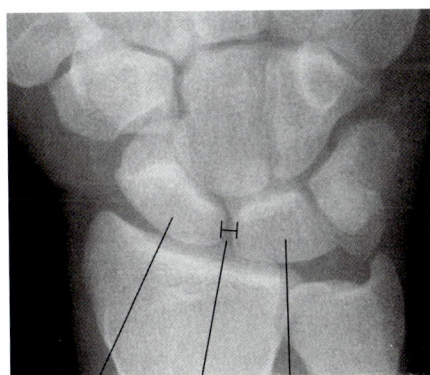

A Scaphoid   <3 mm   Lunate

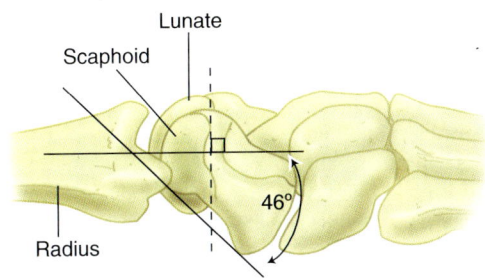

B

FIG 1 • A. The scapholunate interval normally measures less than 3 mm. **B.** The scapholunate angle normally measures 46 degrees with the wrist in neutral position.

- The normal angle between the scaphoid and the lunate measures 46 degrees with the wrist in neutral position (**FIG 1B**).[5]
- With wrist flexion and extension, there is 25 degrees of obligatory rotation motion between the scaphoid and the lunate. With radial and ulnar deviation, there is 10 degrees of normal motion.[7]

PATHOGENESIS

- SLIL injury typically occurs after a fall onto an extended wrist. The combination of axial load, wrist extension, intercarpal supination, and ulnar deviation leads to supraphysiologic loads across the SLIL.
- Injury can also occur in association with other injuries, such as the constellation seen in perilunate dislocations and distal radius fractures.

NATURAL HISTORY

- The motion of the scaphoid and that of the lunate are linked, such that both bones flex with wrist flexion and radial deviation and extend with wrist extension and ulnar deviation.[2] After SLIL injury, the synchronous movement between the scaphoid and lunate is lost and the scaphoid flexes while the lunate extends.
  - Increased scaphoid flexion leads to point stress at the radiostylo–scaphoid juncture. This is the path to scapholunate advanced collapse and osteoarthritis.
  - Dorsal intercalated segment instability (DISI) occurs because of unlinked lunate extension, which creates a scapholunate diastasis and allows for descent and altered kinematics (**FIG 2**). This results in pain, weakness, and progressive osteoarthritis.
- Over time, a progressive pattern of degenerative arthritis termed scapholunate advanced collapse (SLAC) occurs.[10]
  - Arthritic changes first arise between the radial styloid and the scaphoid (stage 1), followed by progression of arthritis into the proximal scaphoid fossa (stage 2). Next, the midcarpal joint becomes involved (stage 3), in particular the capitolunate joint, and eventually pancarpal arthritis is the final result (stage 4).

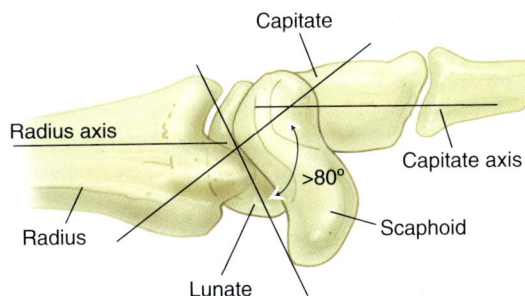

FIG 2 • Dorsal intercalated segment instability (DISI) occurs as a result of lunate extension. Consequently, the capitate and distal carpal row migrate proximally and translate dorsally.

PATIENT HISTORY AND PHYSICAL FINDINGS

- History should include details of prior wrist trauma, especially in regard to mechanism and timing.
  - Acute injuries are those that have occurred within 3 weeks, subacute between 3 weeks and 3 months, and chronic greater than 3 months before presentation.[3] Dates are unreliable, but radiographic changes suggest many are acute-on-chronic injuries.
  - After acute trauma, there is usually a repairable scapholunate ligament, whereas in the setting of subacute or chronic injury, the ligament is resorbed or mechanically unsound. The presence of adequate ligament tissue for repair outweighs the reported time since injury.
  - Instability may be the result of cumulative trauma, and the patient may present with a history of multiple wrist sprains that ultimately produce chronic wrist pain.
- Physical examination includes the following:
  - Direct palpation of the wrist: Tenderness in this region corresponds to scapholunate ligament injury. May also see fullness or thickness, corresponding to dorsal capsule synovitis.
  - Range of motion: Pain with range of motion may indicate instability, synovitis, and chondral wear.
  - Watson scaphoid shift test: Pain over the scaphoid tubercle with radial deviation indicates SLIL injury.
  - Assessment of both normal and aberrant motion
  - Provocative maneuvers
- Examination of the contralateral uninjured wrist is essential to assess radiographic findings of minimal diastasis or DISI, which may be part of a hyperlaxity syndrome.

IMAGING AND OTHER DIAGNOSTIC STUDIES

- Plain radiographs and stress views are critical in diagnosis and consist of:
  - Neutral posteroanterior (PA), lateral, and oblique views
  - PA views in ulnar and radial deviation
  - Clenched-fist PA view in pronation
- Contralateral wrist films should always be taken for comparison.
- Radiographic evidence of SLIL injury includes:
  - Scapholunate diastasis greater than 3 mm. Comparison should be made with the contralateral side, as ligamentous laxity can produce a normal scapholunate interval of greater than 3 mm (**FIG 3A**).[4]
  - Scaphoid cortical ring sign, which occurs when the scaphoid is in a flexed posture and the distal tubercle aligns with the proximal scaphoid (**FIG 3A**).
  - Scapholunate angle greater than 60 degrees (**FIG 3B**)[6]
  - DISI deformity pattern with capitate dorsal translation and decreased carpal height measurements
- The accuracy of MRI is affected by the strength of the magnet and the use of dedicated wrist coils.
  - Sensitivity ranges from 63% to 92%.
  - Specificity ranges from 86% to 100%, depending on the degree of injury and the type of MRI used.[6,8]

DIFFERENTIAL DIAGNOSIS

- Scaphoid fracture
- Capitolunate arthritis
- Scaphotrapeziotrapezoidal (STT) arthritis

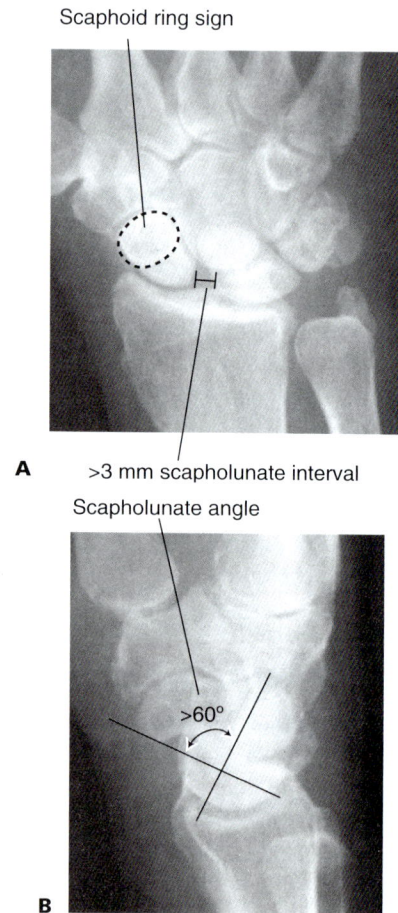

FIG 3 • A. A widened scapholunate interval (>3 mm) and a scaphoid cortical ring sign are seen on an AP view of the wrist. **B.** An obtuse scapholunate angle (>60 degrees) is appreciated on a lateral view of the wrist.

- Midcarpal instability
- Dorsal carpal ganglion
- Dorsal impaction syndrome

NONOPERATIVE MANAGEMENT

- Normal clinical alignment with persistent wrist pain with or without a Watson sign is managed with resting splints until symptoms resolve.
- Occasionally intra-articular steroid injections are performed.

SURGICAL MANAGEMENT

Contraindications to RASL

- A repairable SLIL
  - A primary ligament repair is preferable if a ligament of adequate tissue quality is present.
  - This is most likely seen in acute injuries (less than 3 weeks) but may be possible in chronic injuries. For this reason, arthroscopy is recommended before performing a RASL procedure to evaluate the quality of the SLIL.
- Presence of significant capitolunate or pancarpal arthritis
  - If significant midcarpal, radiolunate, or radioscaphoid arthritis is present, a salvage procedure, such as a proximal row carpectomy or a limited wrist fusion, may be a better treatment option.

■ Focal arthritis between the scaphoid and radial styloid is not a contraindication since a radial styloidectomy is routinely performed during the RASL procedure.

Positioning

■ The procedure is performed with the patient supine and the arm on a standard hand table.

■ The operating table should be rotated 90 degrees to facilitate the use of the image intensifier during the procedure.

Approach

■ The RASL procedure can be performed either arthroscopically or via an open dorsal approach.

■ The arthroscopic RASL should be attempted only after obtaining experience with the open technique, or if already a master arthroscopist.

■ The open technique is performed using a dorsal intercarpal ligament–sparing approach.

TECHNIQUES

DORSAL LIGAMENT–SPARING CAPSULOTOMY

■ Make a longitudinal incision on the dorsal wrist, staying just ulnar to the tubercle of Lister (**TECH FIG 1A**).

■ Bluntly dissect the soft tissue down to the level of the extensor retinaculum, taking care to preserve any dorsal veins and cutaneous nerve branches wherever possible.

■ Incise obliquely the extensor retinaculum parallel to the course of the extensor pollicis longus (EPL) tendon (**TECH FIG 1B**).

  ■ This will open the third and fourth extensor compartments.

  ■ The EPL is retracted radially and the fourth compartment tendons are retracted ulnarly.

■ Make an oblique incision through the dorsal wrist capsule parallel and proximal to the dorsal intercarpal ligament (DIC) (**TECH FIG 1C**).

  ■ The dorsal radiocarpal ligament (DRC) should be identified and preserved.

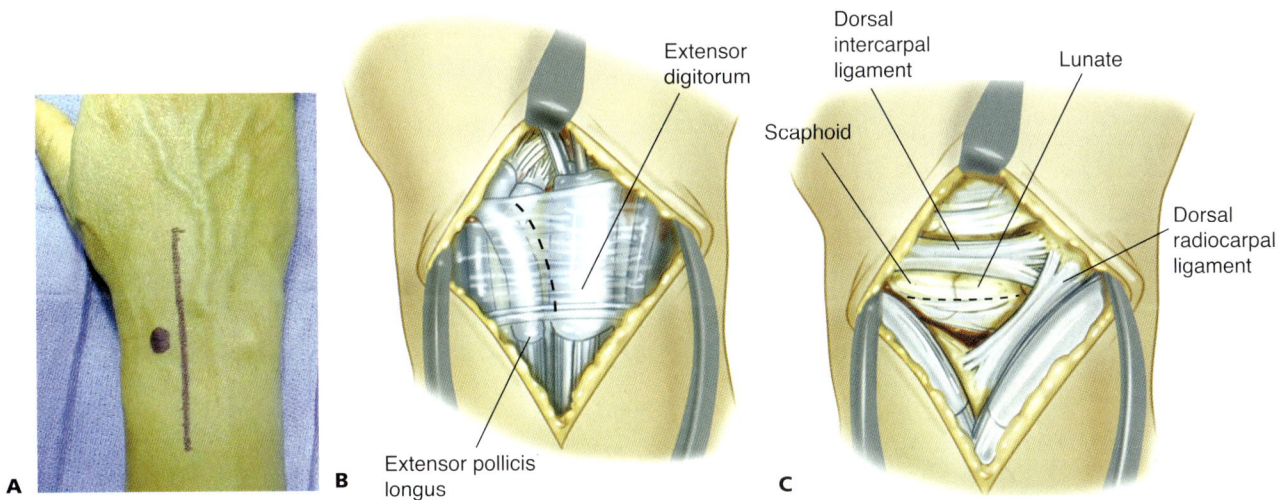

TECH FIG 1 • **A.** A dorsal midline incision is made just ulnar to the tubercle of Lister. **B.** An oblique incision is made through the extensor retinaculum parallel to the extensor pollicis longus (EPL) tendon. The EPL is retracted radially and the fourth compartment tendons are retracted ulnarly. **C.** An oblique incision is made through the dorsal wrist capsule parallel and proximal to the dorsal intercarpal ligament. The dorsal radiocarpal ligament should also be identified and preserved.

STYLOIDECTOMY

■ Once the capsulotomy is performed, identify the scapholunate interval and the SLIL and inspect the radiocarpal and intercarpal joints.

  ■ If significant arthrosis is present in areas other than the radiostyloscaphoid articulation, a salvage procedure is indicated.

■ Perform a second incision in the midaxial line over the first dorsal compartment (**TECH FIG 2A**).

  ■ The major branch of the superficial radial nerve should be seen and isolated with a vessel loupe.

■ Release the first compartment retinaculum and retract the tendons dorsally.

■ Incise the capsule longitudinally through the wrist capsule, thereby exposing the radial styloid (**TECH FIG 2B**).

■ Elevate the periosteum overlying the radial styloid and use an osteotome to perform a radial styloidectomy.

  ■ Remove enough of the radial styloid that radial deviation of the wrist does not cause impingement of the scaphoid and radius.

  ■ Too aggressive of a radial styloidectomy will compromise the volar radioscaphocapitate ligament, which originates from the base of the radial styloid.

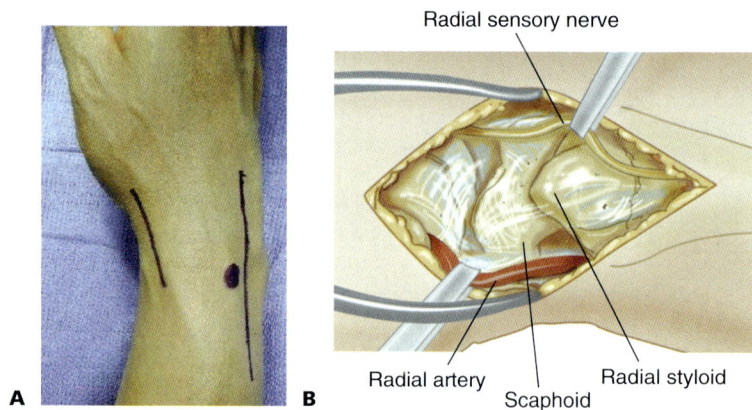

TECH FIG 2 • **A.** A longitudinal incision is made over the first dorsal extensor compartment. **B.** The first compartment is released and a longitudinal incision is made down to the radial styloid.

PREPARATION AND REDUCTION OF THE SCAPHOLUNATE JOINT

- Place a 0.062-inch Kirschner wire in the lunate and another in the scaphoid to serve as joysticks (**TECH FIG 3A**).
  - To bring the lunate out of extension, place the Kirschner wire in the most proximal portion of the exposed dorsal surface, angled from proximal to distal.
  - Similarly, to bring the scaphoid out of flexion, place the Kirschner wire in the most distal portion of the exposed dorsal surface, angled from distal to proximal.
  - Keep in mind the eventual path of the Herbert screw when placing the Kirschner wires and try to avoid this area in both bones.

- Remove the articular cartilage of the scapholunate joint using a side-cutting burr (**TECH FIG 3B**).
  - The joysticks can be used to separate the two bones to better visualize the articular surfaces.
  - Remove the cartilage until cancellous bone and punctate bleeding are visualized.
- Reduce the scaphoid and lunate by flexing the lunate and extending the scaphoid (**TECH FIG 3C**).
  - A Köcher clamp is used to hold the reduction (**TECH FIG 3D**).
- Verify the reduction with an image intensifier (**TECH FIG 3E**).

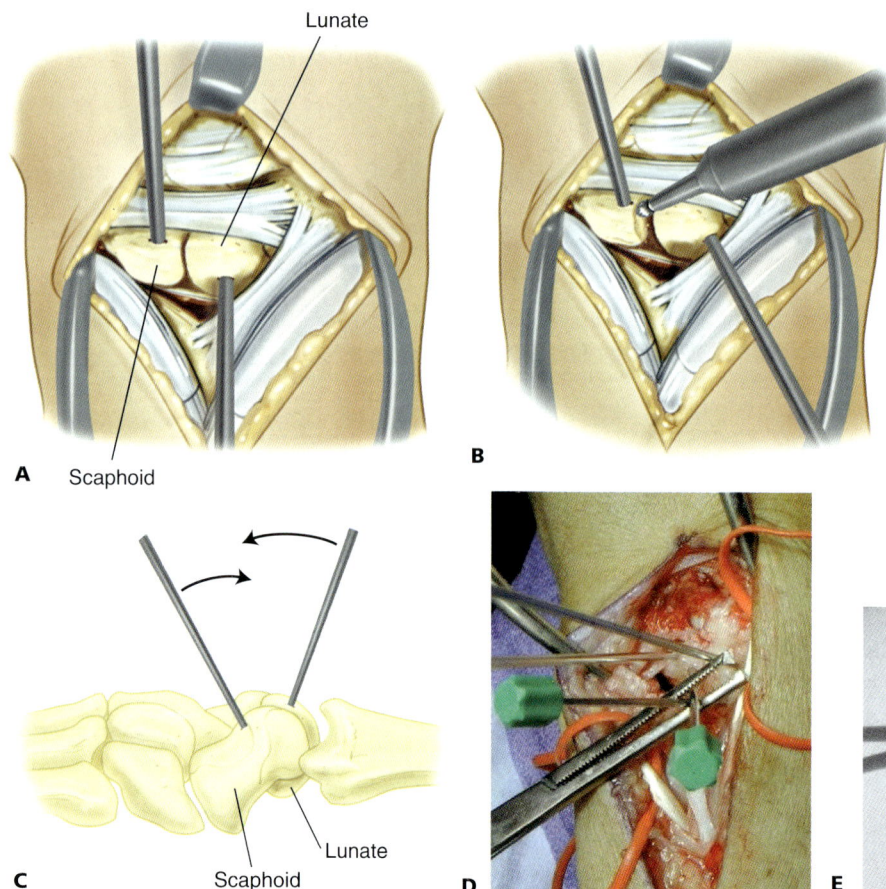

TECH FIG 3 • **A.** 0.062-inch Kirschner wires are placed in the lunate and scaphoid to serve as joysticks. **B.** A side-cutting burr is used to remove the cartilage within the scapholunate joint. **C.** The joysticks are used to extend the scaphoid and to flex the lunate. **D.** A Köcher clamp is used to hold the reduction. **E.** The reduction is verified with an image intensifier.

HERBERT SCREW PLACEMENT

- The path of the Herbert screw should be through the center of rotation of both the scaphoid and the lunate.
- Introduce the Herbert jig through the radial incision and place the insertion point of the jig on the scaphoid waist.
- Through the dorsal incision, introduce the end of the jig and rest it on the proximal ulnar corner of the lunate.
  - Do not violate the lunotriquetral interosseous ligament.
- The insertion angle of the screw should be roughly parallel to the radial inclination of the distal radius, 20 degrees (**TECH FIG 4A**).

- Once the jig is in proper position and both bones are properly measured, drilled, and tapped, insert the Herbert screw.
  - Countersink the screw into the scaphoid so that it is not palpable.
  - Correct screw placement should be confirmed by fluoroscopy (**TECH FIG 4B,C**).
- Remove the Köcher clamp and the joystick wires.
- Take the wrist through a full range of motion to assess for any restrictions in motion and to confirm that the scaphoid and lunate remain reduced.

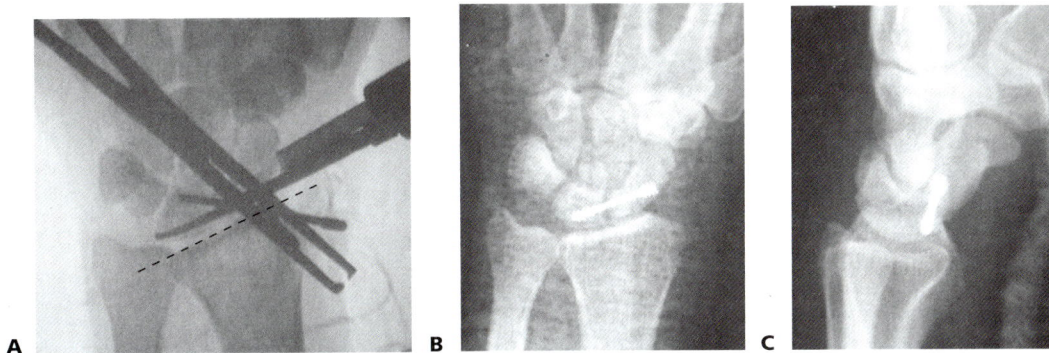

TECH FIG 4 • **A.** The insertion angle of the Herbert screw should be roughly parallel to the radial inclination of 20 degrees. **B,C.** The position of the screw is verified with an image intensifier.

WOUND CLOSURE

- Release the tourniquet and achieve hemostasis using Bovie or bipolar electrocautery.
- Close the dorsal and radial capsular incisions and extensor retinaculum (once the EPL and fourth compartment

tendons are placed back into their respective compartments) using 3-0 absorbable monofilament suture.
- Close the skin using 5-0 nylon suture and apply a sterile bulky dressing and volar thumb spica splint.

PEARLS AND PITFALLS

Indications	■ Carefully evaluate both radiographically and intraoperatively for the presence of significant arthrosis.
Dorsal and radial approaches	■ Identify and protect all neurovascular structures, especially superficial radial sensory nerve branches through the radial incision. ■ Identify the dorsal radial artery just distal to the screw insertion site before screw placement.
Radial styloidectomy	■ Avoid removing too much of the radial styloid since this may destabilize the radioscaphocapitate and long radiolunate volar ligaments. ■ Remove just enough to prevent radioscaphoid impingement.
Kirschner wire joystick placement	■ Do not place the Kirschner wires in the centers of the scaphoid and lunate. ■ Aim for the proximal ulnar corner of the lunate and the distal radial corner of the scaphoid to avoid interfering with the eventual path of the screw.
Bone preparation	■ When burring down the chondral surfaces of the scaphoid and lunate before screw placement, remove only the cartilage and dense subchondral bone. ■ Removing too much bone will decrease the amount of bony contact between the scaphoid and lunate after reduction.
Screw placement	■ After placing the jig, inspect its position both visually and by fluoroscopy. ■ The axis of the jig should cross the central portions of the scaphoid and lunate. ■ The screw should be directed toward the proximal ulnar corner of the lunate.

POSTOPERATIVE CARE

- The wrist is kept immobilized for 4 to 6 weeks.
- After 4 to 6 weeks, the thumb spica splint is removed, a removable splint is applied, and range-of-motion therapy is initiated.
- Over time, therapy is advanced to strengthening exercises around 3 months postoperatively.

OUTCOMES

- Rosenwasser et al[3] reported on a series of 21 patients with a mean of 32 months of follow-up.
  - In this group, 95% of patients returned to their previous occupations. One-year postoperative scapholunate angles and intervals were corrected to within normal limits, with the scapholunate angle being corrected from 69 degrees preoperatively to 40 degrees postoperatively, and the scapholunate interval being corrected from 4.1 mm preoperatively to 1.4 mm postoperatively.
  - One patient was converted to a partial wrist fusion secondary to screw migration and failure of reduction. Another patient required removal of the screw 4 years postoperatively secondary to radial impingement and still demonstrated scapholunate stability after screw removal.

COMPLICATIONS

- Residual instability
- Screw migration
- Superficial radial sensory nerve injury

REFERENCES

1. Berger RA, Imeada T, Berglund L, et al. Constraint and material properties of the subregions of the scapholunate interosseous ligament. J Hand Surg Am 1999;24A:953–962.
2. Garcia-Elias M, Geissler WB. In Green DP, ed. Green's Operative Hand Surgery, 5th ed. Philadelphia: Elsevier/Churchill Livingstone, 2005.
3. Lipton CB, Ugwonali OF, Sarwahi V, et al. Reduction and association of the scaphoid and lunate for scapholunate ligament injuries (RASL). Atlas Hand Clin 2003;8:249–260.
4. Linscheid RL. Scapholunate ligamentous instabilities (dissociations, subdislocations, dislocations). Ann Chir Main 1984;3:323–330.
5. Linscheid RL, Dobyns JH, Beabout JW, et al. Traumatic instability of the wrist: diagnosis, classification, and pathomechanics. J Bone Joint Surg Am 1972;54A:1612–1632.
6. Rosenwasser MP, Miyasajsa KC, Strauch RJ. The RASL procedure: reduction and association of the scaphoid and lunate using the Herbert screw. Tech Hand Up Extrem Surg 1997;1:263–272.
7. Ruby LK, Cooney WP III, An KN, et al. Relative motion of selected carpal bones: a kinematic analysis of the normal wrist. J Hand Surg Am 1988;13A:1–10.
8. Schädel-Höpfner M, Iwinska-Zelder J, Braus T, et al. MRI versus arthroscopy in the diagnosis of scapholunate ligament injury. J Hand Surg Br 2001;26:17–21.
9. Schmitt R, Christopoulos G, Meier R, et al. Direct MR arthrography of the wrist in comparison with arthroscopy: a prospective study on 125 patients [in German]. Rofo 2003;175:911–919.
10. Watson HK, Weinzweig J, Zeppieri J. The natural progression of scaphoid instability. Hand Clin 1997;13:39–49.

Chapter 47

Lunotriquetral Ligament Repair and Augmentation

Samuel C. Hoxie and Alexander Y. Shin

DEFINITION

- Isolated injury of the lunotriquetral interosseous ligament complex is less common and less well understood compared with the other proximal row ligament injury, scapholunate dissociation.
- Lunotriquetral ligament disruption can occur in isolation or in combination with other wrist pathology, such as a perilunate dislocation.
- It may result from acute trauma or chronic degenerative or inflammatory processes.
- Injuries to the lunotriquetral ligament occur in a spectrum of severity ranging from partial tears with dynamic dysfunction (most common) to complete dissociation with static collapse.
  - Lunotriquetral instability can occur when the ligament complex is intact but incompetent or attenuated. If the ligament is stretched and attenuated from chronic or inflammatory degradation, instability can occur in the absence of ligament dissociation (complete disruption).
- When the lunotriquetral ligament is completely ruptured (both dorsal and volar regions), it is called a lunotriquetral dissociation.
- When the dorsal radiotriquetral ligament (and other secondary restraints) is also compromised and the entire ligament complex is disrupted, carpal collapse results. This deformity is termed volar intercalated segment instability (VISI). VISI carpal collapse cannot be reproduced by simply sectioning the dorsal and palmar subregions of the lunotriquetral ligament. Loss of integrity of the radiotriquetral ligament restraint is required to create static carpal instability (**FIG 1**).

ANATOMY AND KINEMATICS

- Like the scapholunate ligament, the lunotriquetral interosseous ligament is C-shaped, spanning the dorsal, proximal, and palmar edges of the joint surface.
- The palmar portion of the lunotriquetral ligament is the thickest and most biomechanically important region of the

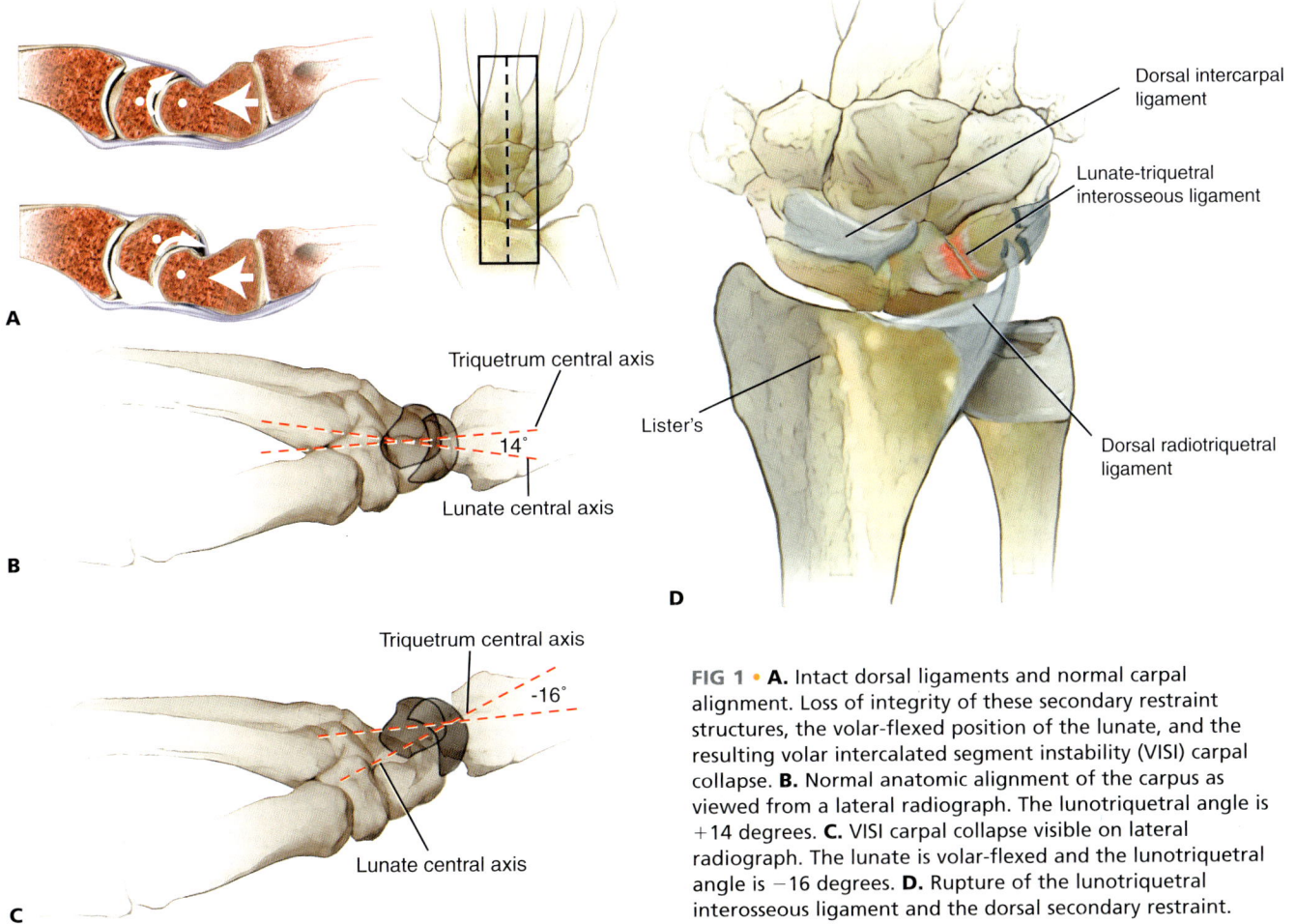

FIG 1 • **A.** Intact dorsal ligaments and normal carpal alignment. Loss of integrity of these secondary restraint structures, the volar-flexed position of the lunate, and the resulting volar intercalated segment instability (VISI) carpal collapse. **B.** Normal anatomic alignment of the carpus as viewed from a lateral radiograph. The lunotriquetral angle is +14 degrees. **C.** VISI carpal collapse visible on lateral radiograph. The lunate is volar-flexed and the lunotriquetral angle is −16 degrees. **D.** Rupture of the lunotriquetral interosseous ligament and the dorsal secondary restraint.

2501

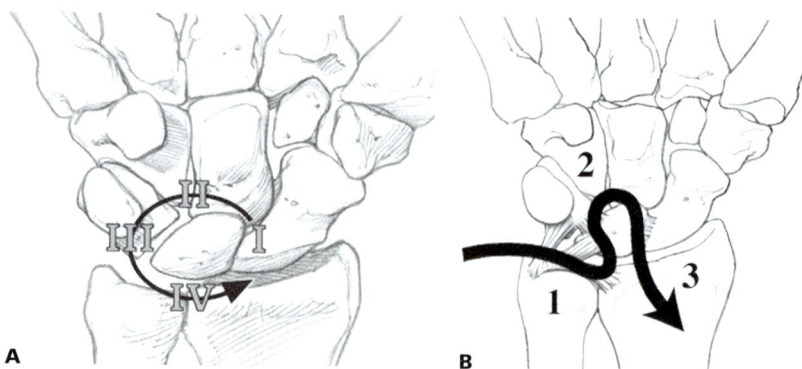

FIG 2 • **A.** Perilunate dislocation. **B.** Reverse perilunate injury (with permission, Mayo Foundation.)

entire complex.[12] In contrast, the dorsal component of the scapholunate ligament has been shown to be the strongest.[3]

- The dorsal lunotriquetral ligament is important as a rotational constraint, while the palmar portion is the strongest and transmits the extension moment of the triquetrum as it engages the hamate.
- The membranous region has little effect on rotation, translation, or distraction.
- These findings illustrate the "balanced lunate" concept, which describes the lunate as torque suspended between the scaphoid and triquetrum. The scaphoid has a tendency to palmar flex, while the triquetrum has a tendency to extend. Through the lunotriquetral and scapholunate ligaments the two forces are balanced and the entire proximal carpal row is balanced about the lunate.

PATHOGENESIS

- The exact mechanism of traumatic lunotriquetral ligament injuries is not fully understood. Many mechanisms may play a role.

- Lunotriquetral ligament injuries can occur in Mayfield III and IV perilunate injuries (**FIG 2A**).
- An isolated traumatic lunotriquetral ligament injury may occur in a reverse perilunate injury (**FIG 2B**).[11]
- In the absence of trauma, degenerative lunotriquetral instability can result from inflammatory arthritis.[16]
- Positive ulnar variance may lead to lunotriquetral ligament degeneration by wear mechanisms or altered intercarpal kinematics (ulnar impaction syndrome).[10]

NATURAL HISTORY

- The natural history of these injuries has not been fully elucidated but they may lead to degenerative joint changes.

PATIENT HISTORY AND PHYSICAL FINDINGS

- Lunotriquetral ligament injuries present as vague ulnar-sided wrist pain either acutely after trauma or as generalized ulnar-sided chronic wrist pain.[14]

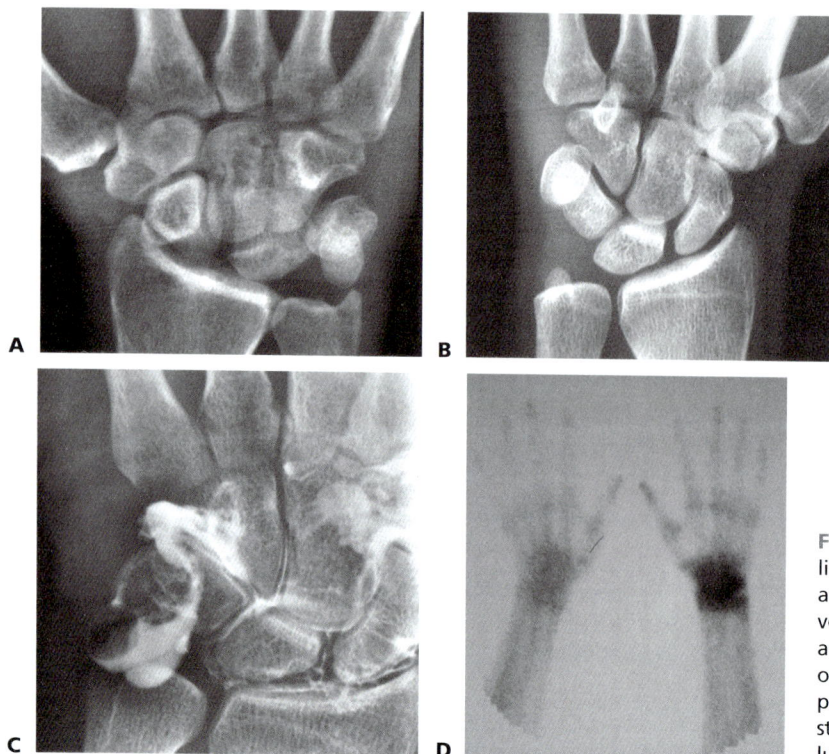

FIG 3 • AP projections of patients with lunotriquetral ligament dissociation. **A.** The proximal row appears abnormal because both the lunate and scaphoid are volar-flexed. **B.** Disruption of the arcs of Gilula. **C.** Wrist arthrography showing contrast dye pooling, indicative of a lunotriquetral ligament injury. **D.** Bone scan of a patient with lunotriquetral ligament injury demonstrates increased radiotracer uptake centered at the lunotriquetral joint.

Table 1	Perilunate and Reverse Perilunate Injury
Stage **Perilunate Injury**	**Ligament or Bony Injury**
1	Scapholunate ligament and long radiolunate disruption or scaphoid fracture
2	Volar capitolunate capsule tear in the space of Poirer
3	Lunotriquetral ligament dissociation
4	Dorsal radiolunate capsule tear and lunate subluxation
Reverse Perilunate Injury	
1	Ulnolunate and ulnotriquetral
2	Lunotriquetral
3	Midcarpal joint and scapholunate

- The examination should encompass the entire wrist, especially the ulnar side.
- Dorsal lunotriquetral joint tenderness should be elicited in lunotriquetral joint injuries.[8,11]
- Ulnar deviation with pronation and axial compression may elicit dynamic instability with a painful snap "catch-up" clunk.
- A palpable wrist click is occasionally significant, particularly if painful and occurring with radioulnar deviation.
- Provocative tests that demonstrate lunotriquetral laxity, crepitus, and pain are helpful to accurately localize the site of pathology. Three useful tests to perform include:
  - Ballottement[11]: The test is positive if increased anteroposterior laxity and pain occur.
  - Compression: Pain with this maneuver may indicate pathology of the lunotriquetral or triquetral hamate joints.[1]
  - Shear test[7]: Positive with pain, crepitance, and abnormal mobility of the lunotriquetral joint
- Other common findings on physical examination include limited range of motion and diminished grip strength.[8]
- Comparison of findings with the contralateral wrist is essential.

IMAGING AND OTHER DIAGNOSTIC STUDIES

- Plain radiographs are often normal in lunotriquetral ligament injuries because the most common presentation is dynamic dysfunction that manifests only with loading or certain positions of the hand and wrist.
  - Dissociation of the lunotriquetral ligament can lead to disruption of Gilula arcs I and II, demonstrating proximal translation of the triquetrum, with or without lunotriquetral overlap (**FIG 3A,B**).
  - Often, no lunotriquetral gap occurs, in contrast to scapholunate injuries.
  - A static VISI deformity indicates not only lunotriquetral interosseous ligament injury but also damage to the dorsal radiotriquetral ligament.
  - Radial and ulnar deviation together with clenched-fist anteroposterior views are often helpful. Lunotriquetral dissociation leads to lessened triquetral motion and increased movement of the lunate, scaphoid, and distal row.[2]

- Injection of local anesthetic into the midcarpal space can be useful to localize the cause of the patient's pain.
  - Addition of corticosteroid to the injection may provide temporary relief by decreasing local inflammation.
- Arthrographic dye pooling or leakage at the lunotriquetral interspace can indicate ligamentous injury (**FIG 3C**). However, age-dependent degenerative changes and asymptomatic lunotriquetral instability have been reported. Correlation with physical examination is required.
- Real-time videofluoroscopy can illustrate the site of a "clunk" that occurs with wrist deviation. This occurs in lunotriquetral injuries when the triquetrum "catches up" when the wrist is moved into maximal ulnar deviation.
- Technetium-99m diphosphate bone scan can aid in the localization of an acute injury but has been shown to be less specific than arthrography (**FIG 3D**).[6]
- Magnetic resonance imaging is improving but is not yet reliable for imaging of lunotriquetral ligament injuries.

DIFFERENTIAL DIAGNOSIS

- The differential diagnosis of ulnar-sided wrist pain can be divided into six categories: osseous, ligamentous, tendinous, vascular, neurologic, and miscellaneous.
- Osseous injuries include the sequelae of fractures (ie, nonunion or malunion) and degenerative processes. Fracture nonunions can affect the hamate, pisiform, triquetrum, base of the fifth metacarpal, ulnar styloid process, and distal part of the ulna or radius.
- Degenerative processes at the pisotriquetral joint, midcarpal (triquetrohamate) articulation, fifth carpometacarpal joint, or distal radioulnar joint can also result in substantial ulnar-sided wrist pain. Ulnar impaction or abutment into the radius or carpus has been reported as well.
- Ligamentous injuries can occur in any of the ulnar-sided intrinsic (lunotriquetral or capitohamate) or extrinsic (ulnolunate, triquetrocapitate, or triquetrohamate) ligaments as well as the triangular fibrocartilage complex.
- Tendinopathy of the extensor carpi ulnaris or flexor carpi ulnaris
- Vascular lesions such as ulnar artery thrombosis or hemangiomas
- Neurologic processes such as entrapment of the ulnar nerve in Guyon's canal, neuritis of the dorsal sensory branch of the ulnar nerve, and complex regional pain syndromes
- The miscellaneous group includes the very unusual etiologies such as tumors, including osteoid osteomas, chondroblastomas, and aneurysmal bone cysts.

NONOPERATIVE MANAGEMENT

- Initial care for most lunotriquetral ligament injuries is immobilization with a splint or cast with a pisiform lift. Initially the wrist is immobilized in a long-arm cast for 4 weeks and then a short-arm cast for an additional 4 weeks. Care should be taken to mold a pad underneath the pisiform (pisiform lift) to maintain optimal alignment as the ligament heals.
  - Acute injuries without radiographic changes may be successfully treated nonoperatively.
  - Symptoms of chronic injuries often improve with immobilization.
- Midcarpal injections with local anesthetic and corticosteroid often provide significant relief for a prolonged time.

■ If conservative management fails for either acute or chronic injuries, surgical treatment can be performed. A trial of non-operative treatment does not seem to jeopardize the outcome of subsequent surgical intervention.

SURGICAL MANAGEMENT

■ Operative management is indicated in acute or chronic injuries unresponsive to conservative treatment.
■ The goal of surgery is to return rotational stability of the proximal carpal row and restore the natural alignment of the lunocapitate axis.
■ Functional reconstruction of the lunotriquetral ligament can be accomplished with direct ligament repair, ligament reconstruction with a strip of extensor carpi ulnaris tendon graft, or arthrodesis.
■ The choice of intervention should be discussed with the patient. Our preference, based on outcomes studies performed at our institution, is tendon repair or reconstruction.[13]
   ■ Arthrodesis is avoided whenever possible secondary to higher complication rates and lower patient satisfaction.
■ If significant degenerative changes have occurred in the lunotriquetral, radiocarpal, or midcarpal joints, partial or total carpal arthrodesis or proximal row carpectomy may be indicated.
■ In the presence of significant VISI deformity that cannot be easily reduced (ie, static VISI), intercarpal arthrodesis is recommended.
■ In cases of significant ulna-positive or ulna-negative variance, ulna shortening or lengthening may be indicated as well.

Preoperative Planning

■ The senior author's preference is to perform diagnostic arthroscopy on patients with lunotriquetral ligament injuries to evaluate the articular surface and assess other intercarpal pathology.
   ■ Anterior interosseous and posterior interosseous nerve neurectomies can be performed at this time as well.
   ■ The findings of the arthroscopy are discussed with the patient at a second meeting and a reconstructive or salvage procedure can then be performed 6 weeks later.
   ■ Alternatively, a definitive surgical procedure can be performed at a single surgical setting following a thorough preoperative discussion with the patient.
■ When a lunotriquetral dorsal ligament repair is planned, preparations should also be made to proceed with ligament reconstruction if the quality of the lunotriquetral ligament is poor.

Positioning

■ The patient is positioned supine on a standard operating room table with the affected arm on a hand table.
■ A long-acting axillary regional anesthetic block placed preoperatively is helpful with postoperative pain control.
■ A nonsterile tourniquet is applied above the surgical drapes.
■ Preoperative intravenous antibiotics are routinely administered before beginning the procedure.
■ The hand and arm are prepared and draped in standard fashion.
■ An examination under anesthesia is always performed initially to evaluate for "catch-up" intercarpal clunks and well as radioulnar clunks.

TECHNIQUES

DIRECT LUNOTRIQUETRAL LIGAMENT REPAIR

Incision and Dissection

■ A longitudinal incision is made over the third extensor compartment (**TECH FIG 1**).
   ■ Alternatively, a curvilinear incision can be used.
■ The dorsal sensory branch of the ulnar nerve is identified and protected.

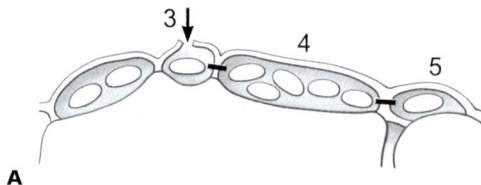

■ The extensor retinaculum is divided over the extensor pollicis longus, releasing it from the third compartment (**TECH FIG 2**).
■ Ulnar-based flaps of extensor retinaculum are developed by dividing the septa separating the third through the fifth extensor compartments (**TECH FIG 3**).

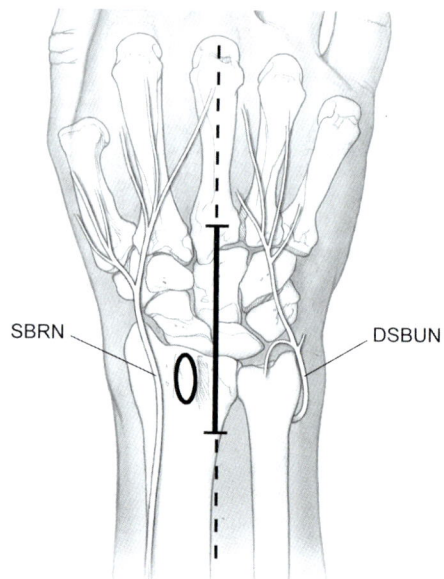

TECH FIG 1 • A. Axial image of dorsal wrist compartments with *arrow* indicating location for skin incision over third compartment. **B.** Skin incision centered over third dorsal compartment with superficial branch of the radial nerve (SBRN) and dorsal sensory branch of the ulnar nerve (DSBUN). *Oval* indicates tubercle of Lister. (Copyright © Mayo Clinic.)

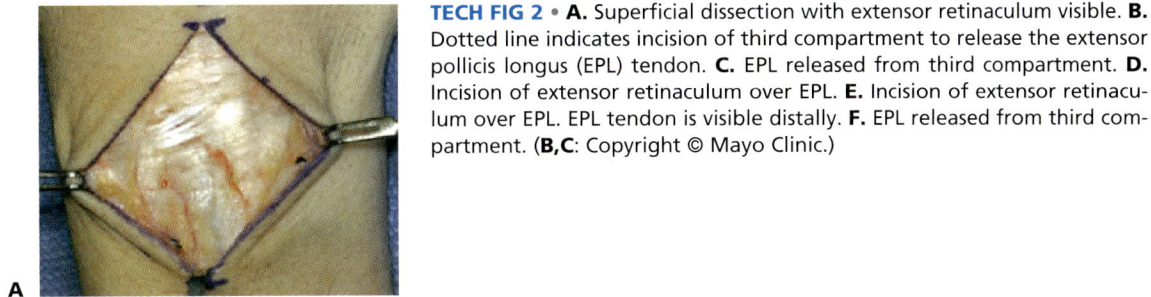

TECH FIG 2 • A. Superficial dissection with extensor retinaculum visible. **B.** Dotted line indicates incision of third compartment to release the extensor pollicis longus (EPL) tendon. **C.** EPL released from third compartment. **D.** Incision of extensor retinaculum over EPL. **E.** Incision of extensor retinaculum over EPL. EPL tendon is visible distally. **F.** EPL released from third compartment. (**B,C**: Copyright © Mayo Clinic.)

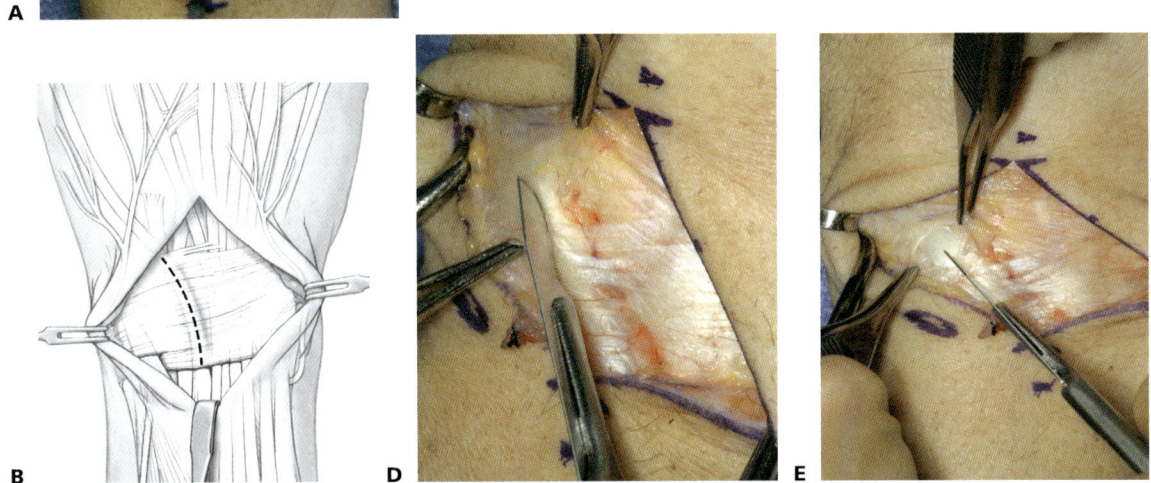

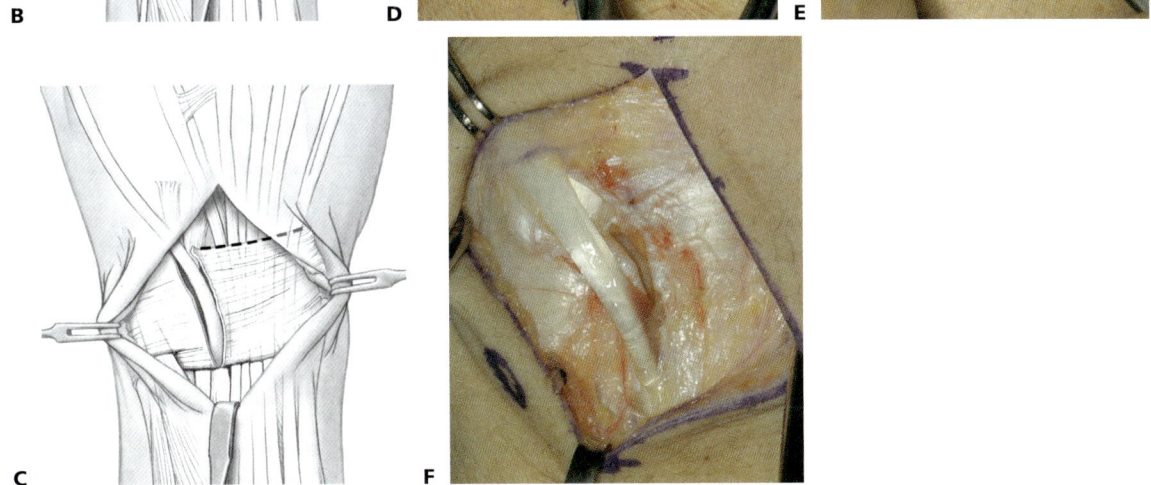

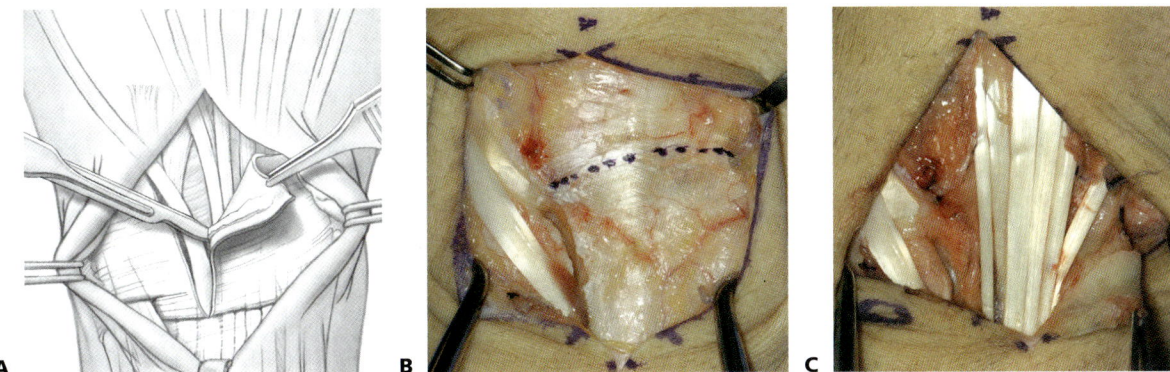

TECH FIG 3 • A. Dissection of septa to create ulnar-based flap of extensor retinaculum. **B.** Preparing to reflect extensor retinaculum. **C.** Retinaculum has been reflected ulnarly and extensor tendons are released. (**A**: Copyright © Mayo Clinic.)

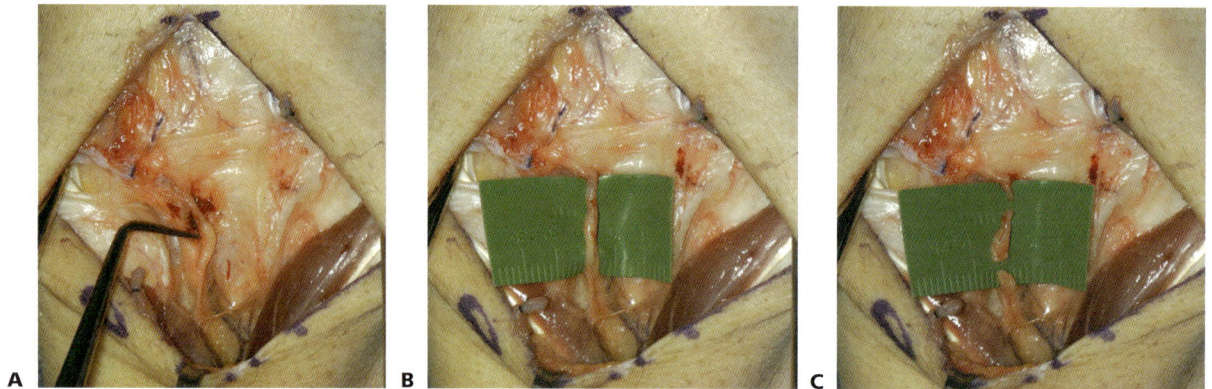

TECH FIG 4 • **A.** Posterior interosseous nerve (PIN) visible overlying wrist capsule. **B.** PIN identified and isolated. **C.** Segment resected from PIN.

- If not previously performed, a posterior interosseous neurectomy is performed to partially denervate the dorsal wrist capsule (**TECH FIG 4**).
- The dorsal radiocarpal and intercarpal ligaments are identified and a ligament-splitting capsulotomy made as described by Berger and Bishop[4] (**TECH FIG 5A–D**).
- When elevating the capsule it is important not to dissect too deep over the region of the lunotriquetral area. The lunotriquetral ligament is intimately related to the radiotriquetral ligament and can be injured if attention is not paid during the capsulotomy.
- The midcarpal and radiocarpal joint surfaces are exposed and examined for arthritic changes (**TECH FIG 5E**).
- The scapholunate and lunotriquetral ligament are thoroughly examined.
  - The dorsal aspect of the lunotriquetral ligament is inspected to determine if it is suitable for repair. The midcarpal joint is also inspected.

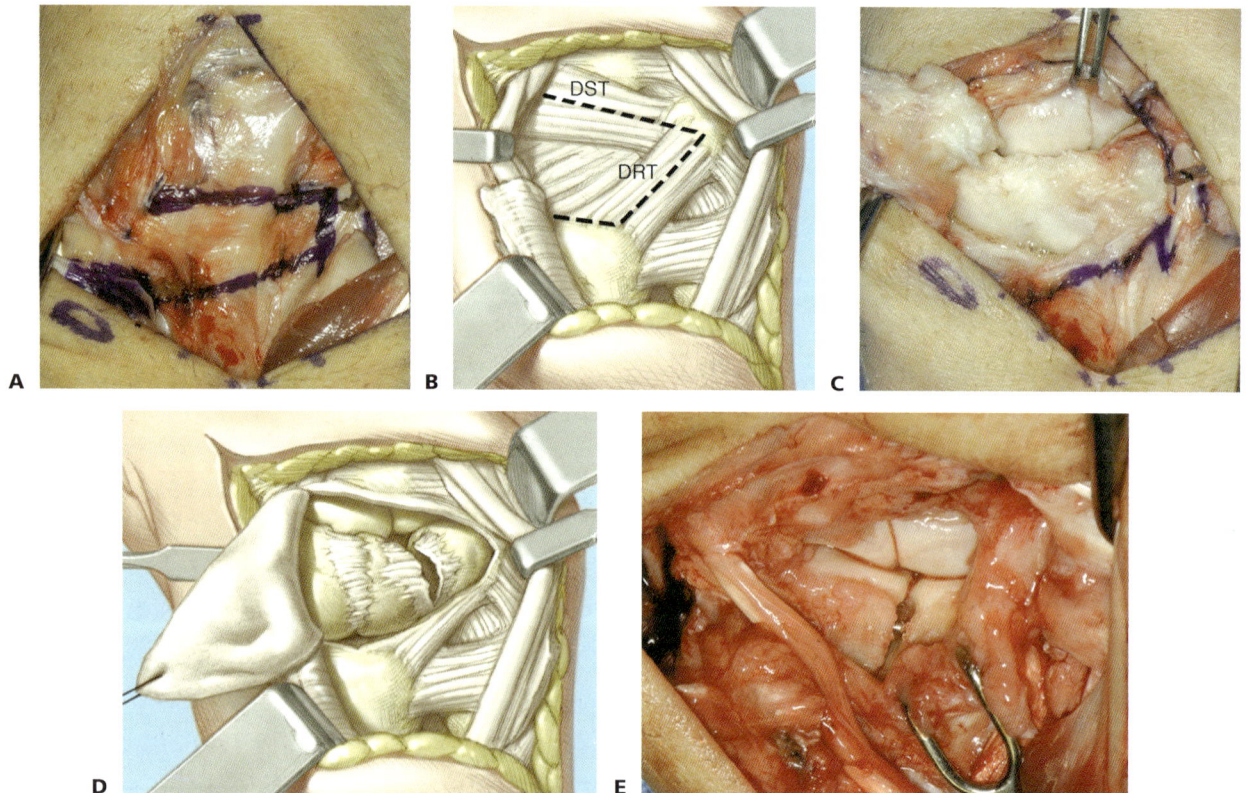

TECH FIG 5 • **A.** Dorsal ligament-splitting capsulotomy planned. **B.** Dorsal ligament-splitting capsulotomy showing location of the dorsal radiotriquetral and scaphotriquetral ligaments. **C.** Dorsal capsule reflected radially. **D.** Dorsal capsule reflected radially showing lunotriquetral ligament disruption. **E.** Dorsal capsulotomy performed. The dorsal lunotriquetral ligament is visibly torn. (**B,D**: Copyright © Mayo Clinic.)

- The volar portion of the lunotriquetral joint is examined, and the integrity of the volar lunotriquetral ligament is indirectly inspected. If it is completely incompetent, then a direct repair of the dorsal lunotriquetral ligament is contraindicated and one should proceed to a ligament reconstruction as described later in this chapter.
- Intra-articular step-off of the lunotriquetral articulation is also assessed, as well as the presence of a separate lunate facet (type II lunate).

Reattaching the Ligament

- The lunotriquetral ligament is reattached to the site of avulsion, usually the triquetrum.
- Two techniques for reattachment of the ligament exist: the use of drill holes or suture anchors. Multiple horizontal drill holes or suture anchors are placed in the dorsal, nonarticular, surface of the triquetrum (**TECH FIG 6A**).

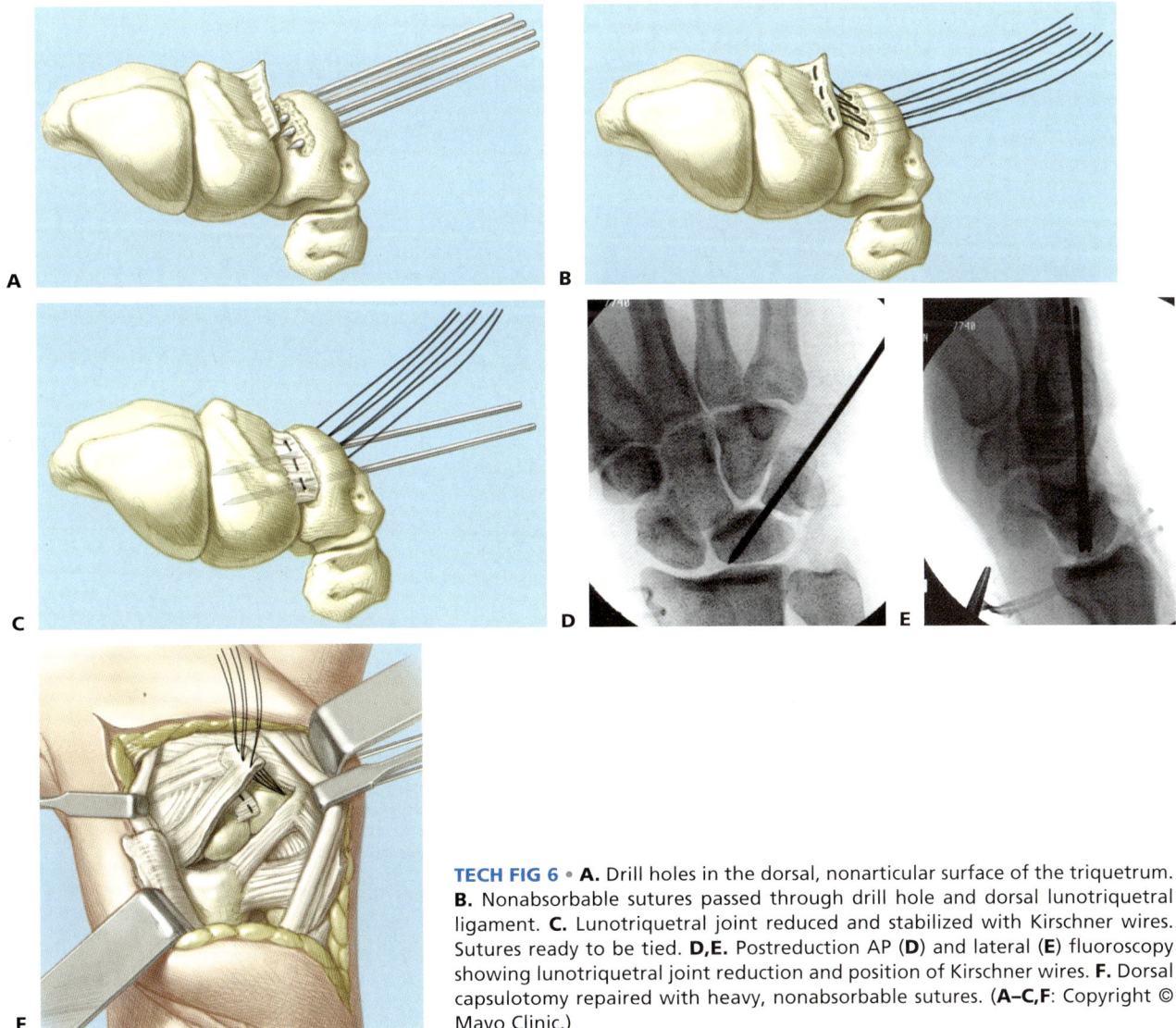

- Numerous strands of nonabsorbable suture (size 2-0) are used to repair the avulsed ligament (**TECH FIG 6B**).
- Before tensioning and tying the sutures, the diastasis of the lunotriquetral joint must be reduced and the articular congruity at the midcarpal joint reduced. The reduction is secured by two 0.045-inch smooth Kirschner wires (**TECH FIG 6C–E**).
- The sutures are then tensioned and tied, but not cut short.
- Dorsal capsulodesis is then performed to augment the lunotriquetral ligament. A portion of the radiotriquetral ligament can be used to augment the lunotriquetral ligament repair by placing additional suture anchors into the lunate and triquetrum and sewing the radiotriquetral ligament to the lunotriquetral ligament
- The ligament-splitting capsulotomy is repaired with nonabsorbable sutures (**TECH FIG 6F**).
- The extensor retinaculum is repaired with the extensor pollicis longus dorsally transposed.
- The skin is closed.
- A long-arm, bulky splint is applied.

TECH FIG 6 • **A.** Drill holes in the dorsal, nonarticular surface of the triquetrum. **B.** Nonabsorbable sutures passed through drill hole and dorsal lunotriquetral ligament. **C.** Lunotriquetral joint reduced and stabilized with Kirschner wires. Sutures ready to be tied. **D,E.** Postreduction AP (**D**) and lateral (**E**) fluoroscopy showing lunotriquetral joint reduction and position of Kirschner wires. **F.** Dorsal capsulotomy repaired with heavy, nonabsorbable sutures. (**A–C,F**: Copyright © Mayo Clinic.)

LUNOTRIQUETRAL LIGAMENT RECONSTRUCTION WITH DISTALLY BASED EXTENSOR CARPI ULNARIS STRIP

Harvesting the Graft

- To avoid disrupting the extensor carpi ulnaris (ECU) subsheath,[15] a 2-cm transverse incision is made through the skin and the ECU sheath 6 cm proximal to the ulnar styloid. The ECU tendon is identified (**TECH FIG 7A**).
- A small right-angle clamp or 90-degree retractor is used to isolate and elevate the ECU tendon (**TECH FIG 7B**).
- A 4-mm incision is made on the radial side of the ECU tendon to create a strip of tendon graft. A piece of 28-gauge wire is tied to the free end of the tendon graft (**TECH FIG 7C**).
- The ECU sheath is opened at the level of the carpometacarpal joint. The wire is looped and passed from proximal to distal through the sheath into the distal incision. The wire and tendon are gently pulled distally, creating a distally based tendon graft (**TECH FIG 7D**).
- The graft is passed deep to the extensor retinaculum.
- The 28-gauge wire is left tied to the end of the graft and a moist sponge is wrapped around the graft while the bone tunnels are prepared.

Bone Tunnel Creation and Graft Passage

- 0.045-inch Kirschner wires are advanced through the lunate and the triquetrum.
  - The correct starting points for these Kirschner wires are the dorsal ulnar aspect of the triquetrum and the dorsal radial edge of the lunate.
  - The holes should converge at the volar margin of the lunotriquetral joint and must *not* be intra-articular (**TECH FIG 8A**).
- If a reducible VISI deformity exists, it is important to place the Kirschner wires while the deformity is held reduced. Joysticks in the scaphoid and triquetrum are useful to maintain the reduction while the lunate and triquetral wires are placed (**TECH FIG 8B**).
- The position of the wires is checked with fluoroscopy to confirm the ability to safely enlarge the drill holes without fracture.
- The tunnels are created using a series of sharp awls or drill bits, gradually increasing the diameter until a 4- to 5-mm tunnel is created in both the lunate and triquetrum (**TECH FIG 8C**).
  - Alternatively, a cannulated drill system can be used.

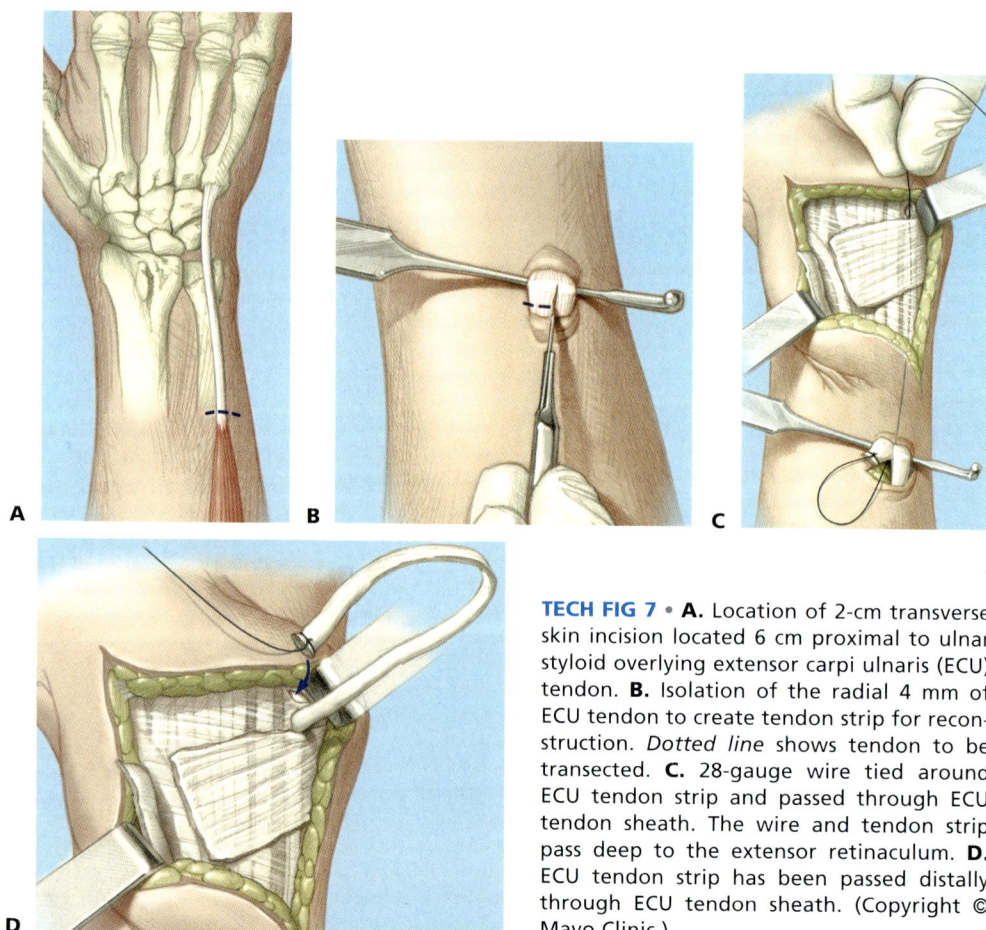

A   B   C

D

TECH FIG 7 • **A.** Location of 2-cm transverse skin incision located 6 cm proximal to ulnar styloid overlying extensor carpi ulnaris (ECU) tendon. **B.** Isolation of the radial 4 mm of ECU tendon to create tendon strip for reconstruction. *Dotted line* shows tendon to be transected. **C.** 28-gauge wire tied around ECU tendon strip and passed through ECU tendon sheath. The wire and tendon strip pass deep to the extensor retinaculum. **D.** ECU tendon strip has been passed distally through ECU tendon sheath. (Copyright © Mayo Clinic.)

A **B**

C

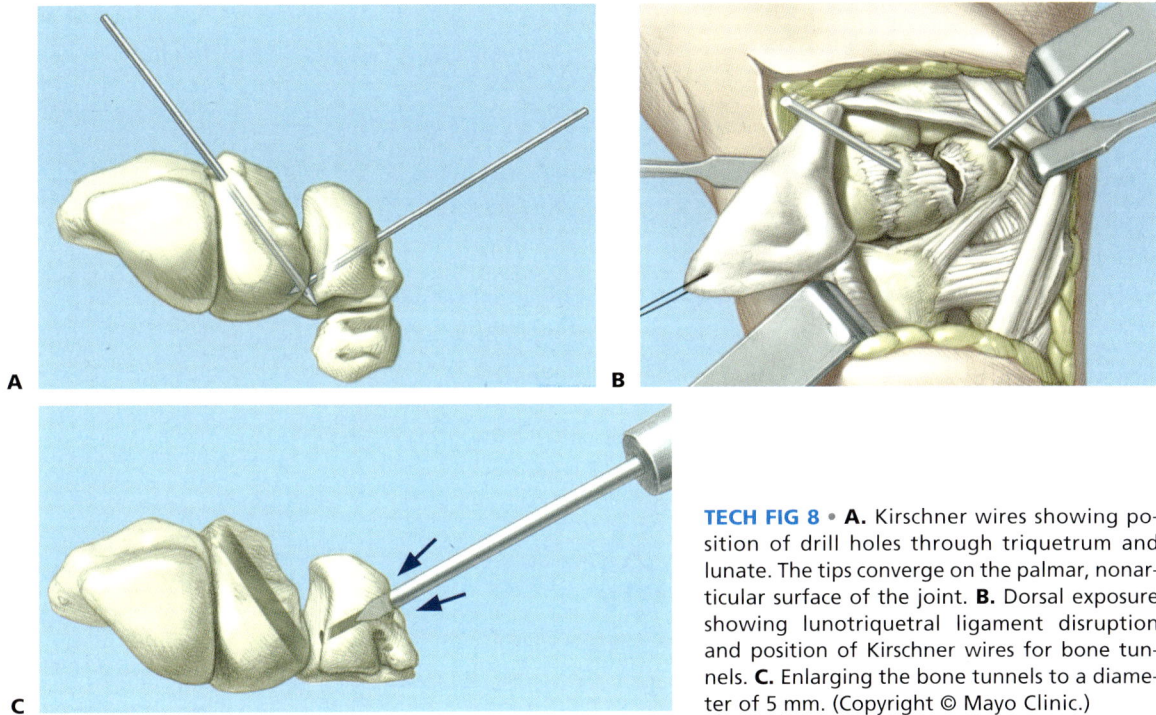

TECH FIG 8 • A. Kirschner wires showing position of drill holes through triquetrum and lunate. The tips converge on the palmar, nonarticular surface of the joint. **B.** Dorsal exposure showing lunotriquetral ligament disruption and position of Kirschner wires for bone tunnels. **C.** Enlarging the bone tunnels to a diameter of 5 mm. (Copyright © Mayo Clinic.)

- The wire previously secured to the end of the graft is looped and passed through the triquetral tunnel toward the lunate (**TECH FIG 9A–C**).
- An arthroscopic hook or probe is useful to hook the wire loop and pull it through the lunate bone tunnel (**TECH FIG 9D,E**).
- The wire is used to pass the tendon graft through the tunnels (**TECH FIG 10A**).
- While maintaining tension on the tendon graft, the articular surfaces of the lunate and triquetrum are reduced

and two 0.045-inch Kirschner wires are passed percutaneously across the lunotriquetral joint.
- Reduction, pin position, and length are checked with fluoroscopy.
- The tendon graft is then woven through itself on the dorsum of the lunate and triquetrum and firmly secured with nonabsorbable suture (**TECH FIG 10B,C**).
- Excess tendon is trimmed, and the wound is irrigated with normal saline solution.
- The wound is closed as previously described in the ligament repair section.

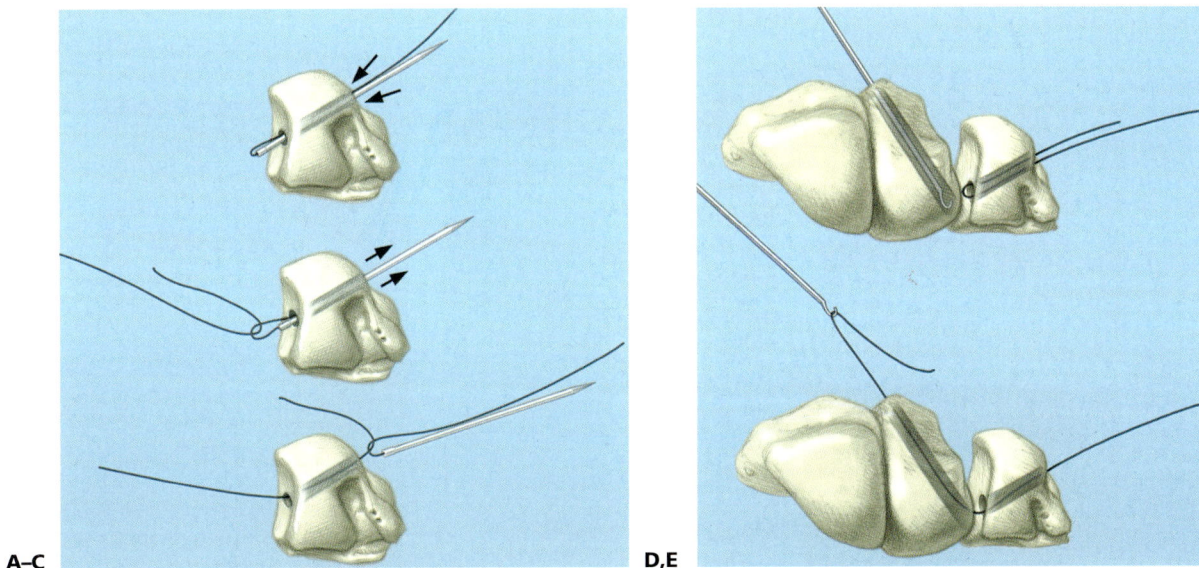

A–C **D,E**

TECH FIG 9 • A–C. Straight Keith needle used to shuttle wire or heavy suture to assist in passing the extensor carpi ulnaris (ECU) tendon strip through bone tunnels—first through the triquetrum and then through the lunate. **D,E.** Arthroscopic hook used to pass wire or heavy suture through bone tunnels. (Copyright © Mayo Clinic.)

TECHNIQUES

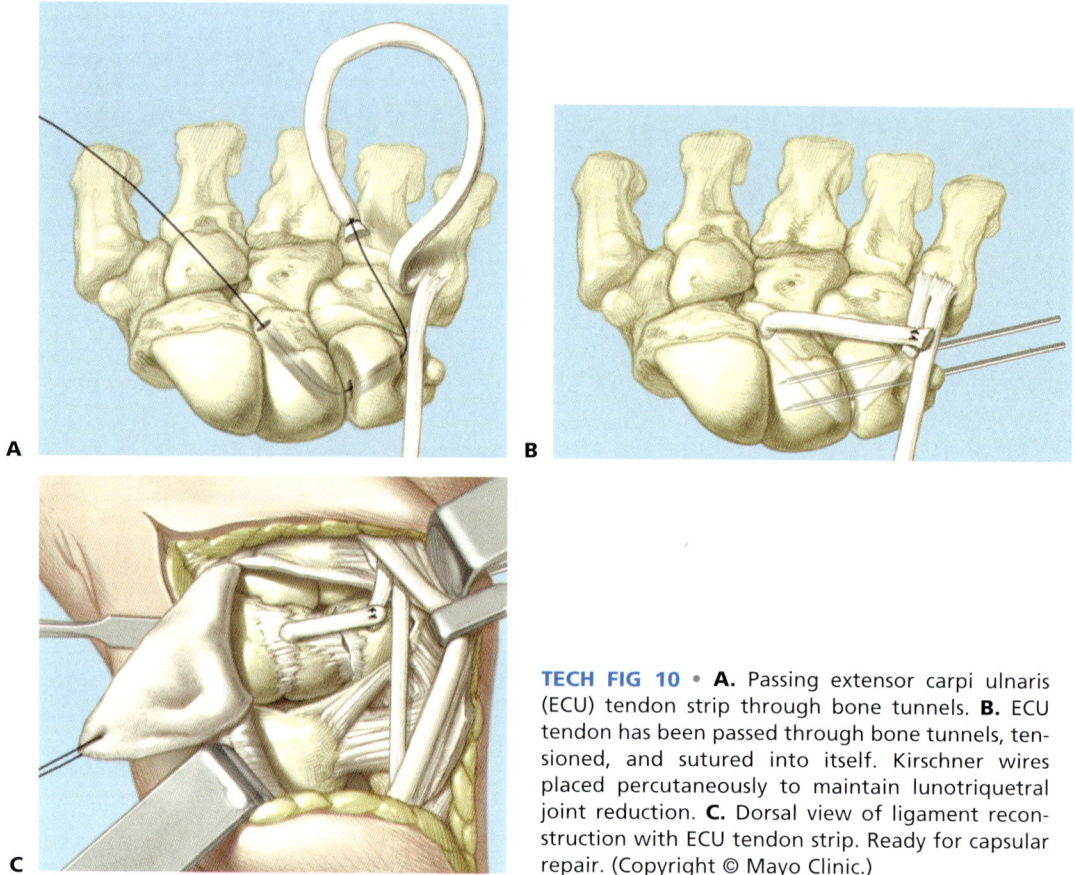

TECH FIG 10 • A. Passing extensor carpi ulnaris (ECU) tendon strip through bone tunnels. **B.** ECU tendon has been passed through bone tunnels, tensioned, and sutured into itself. Kirschner wires placed percutaneously to maintain lunotriquetral joint reduction. **C.** Dorsal view of ligament reconstruction with ECU tendon strip. Ready for capsular repair. (Copyright © Mayo Clinic.)

COMBINED REPAIR

- Ligament reconstruction with an ECU tendon strip can be combined with direct ligament repair to provide additional strength for the repair (**TECH FIG 11**).

- This is especially useful when the volar region of the lunotriquetral ligament is disrupted and the dorsal aspect of the ligament is attenuated.

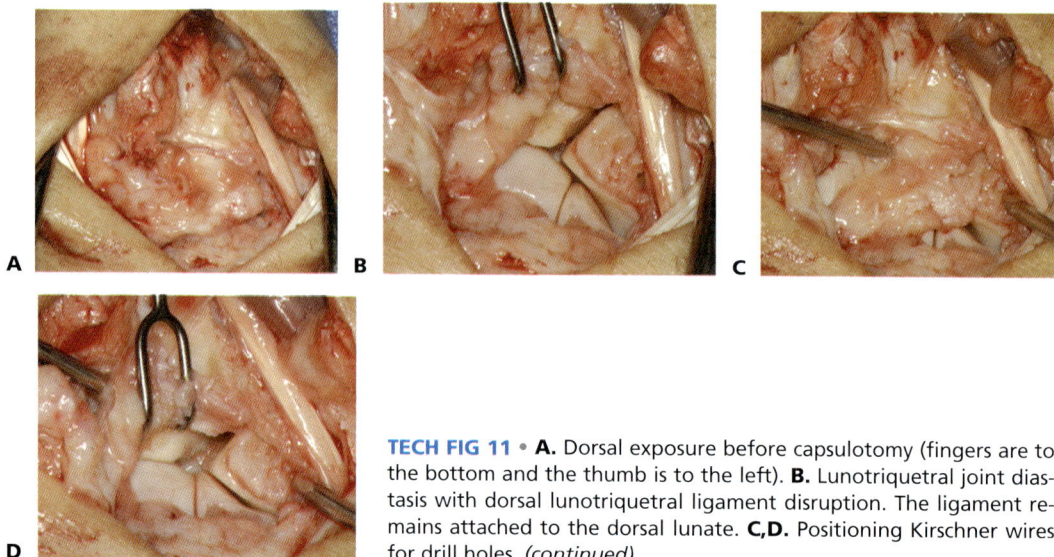

TECH FIG 11 • A. Dorsal exposure before capsulotomy (fingers are to the bottom and the thumb is to the left). **B.** Lunotriquetral joint diastasis with dorsal lunotriquetral ligament disruption. The ligament remains attached to the dorsal lunate. **C,D.** Positioning Kirschner wires for drill holes. *(continued)*

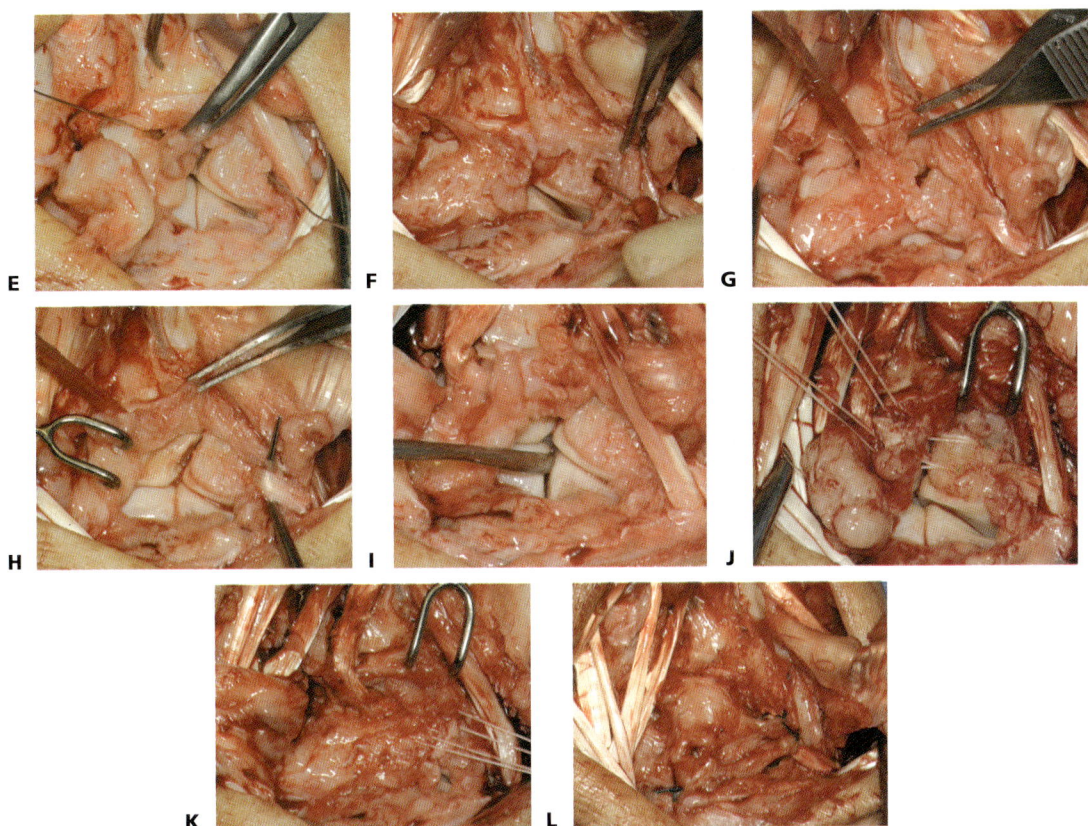

TECH FIG 11 • *(continued)* **E.** 28-gauge wire passes through bone tunnels. **F,G.** The tendon graft is first advanced through the triquetrum and then through the lunate. **H.** The tendon graft is tensioned. **I.** Reduction should be verified and maintained with lunotriquetral Kirschner wires before final ligament tensioning and suture placement. **J.** Direct repair of dorsal lunotriquetral ligament utilizing suture form anchors placed into the triquetrum. **K.** Tensioning direct lunotriquetral ligament repair. **L.** Final view of the reconstruction after capsulotomy repair. Heavy nonabsorbable sutures secure the capsular repair.

PEARLS AND PITFALLS

Direct repair	■ Position the drill holes in the triquetrum so that a strong bridge of bone remains to support the sutures and knots. Holes placed too close to the edge of the bone will allow the suture to pull through when tensioned. ■ Pass the sutures through sufficient substance of the lunotriquetral tendon so that the suture does not tear or pull out of the tendon. ■ The use of heavy, nonabsorbable suture is important for an adequate capsular repair. ■ It is important to visualize and ensure the adequacy of the reduction before placing the Kirschner wires across the lunotriquetral joint. ■ The senior author prefers to cut the Kirschner wire below the level of the skin. Other authors advocate percutaneous placement for easy removal.
Ligament reconstruction with distally based ECU strip	■ Positioning the ECU tendon strip through the drill holes can be difficult. Stainless-steel wire or heavy monofilament suture can be passed first and used to shuttle the strip of tendon in the correct position. ■ Tensioning the tendon and suturing it into itself can be challenging. A surgical clamp such as a Köcher or Allis can be attached to the proximal free edge of the tendon strip and used as a handle to apply traction to the tendon strip as it is being secured. ■ Tension the tendon strip while the lunotriquetral joint is reduced. ■ It is important to visualize and ensure the adequacy of the reduction before placing the Kirschner wires across the lunotriquetral joint. ■ Adequate duration of postoperative immobilization is important to ensure a successful outcome.

POSTOPERATIVE CARE

- Edema control and range-of-motion exercises of the digits are initiated immediately postoperatively.
- Seven to 10 days after the procedure, the surgical splint is removed, sutures are removed, and a long-arm cast is applied for 6 weeks. A short-arm cast is then applied for an additional 4 to 6 weeks for a total period of immobilization of 10 to 12 weeks.
- The Kirschner wires are removed at 10 to 12 weeks and wrist range-of-motion exercises are commenced.

OUTCOMES

- A high-quality tendon repair is vital for a successful outcome of the lunotriquetral tenodesis.
- Several studies have shown that direct lunotriquetral ligament repair results in a successful clinical result.[5,9,11,15]
- Reagan et al[11] reported that six of seven cases of direct lunotriquetral ligament repairs were successful.
- Favero et al[5] reported patient satisfaction of 90% with only one failure in 21 cases.
- In high-demand patients such as laborers and athletes, re-rupture or attenuation can occur and lead to late failure. Reconstruction with a strip of ECU tendon should be considered in this patient subgroup.
- A review of clinical outcomes comparing lunotriquetral ligament repair, ligament reconstruction, and lunotriquetral joint arthrodesis at our institution showed that patients treated with ligament reconstruction have the lowest reoperation rate.[13]
  - Rerupture after trauma and late attenuation appear to be common modes of long-term failure of direct repair.
- Review of the clinical outcomes at our institution showed that reconstruction with a strip of ECU tendon as described can be an effective treatment.[3]

REFERENCES

1. Beckenbaugh RD. Accurate evaluation and management of the painful wrist following injury. Orthop Clin 1984;15:289–306.
2. Beckenbaugh RD. Accurate evaluation and management of the painful wrist following injury: an approach to carpal instability. Orthop Clin North Am 1984;15:289–306.
3. Berger RA. The gross and histologic anatomy of the scapholunate interosseous ligament. J Hand Surg Am 1996;21A:170–178.
4. Berger RA, Bishop AT. A fiber-splitting capsulotomy technique for dorsal exposure of the wrist. Tech Hand Upper Extrem Surg 1997;1:2–10.
5. Favero KJ, Bishop AT, Linscheid RL. Lunotriquetral ligament disruption: a comparative study of treatment methods [abstract SS-80]. American Society for Surgery of the Hand, 46th Annual Meeting, 1991, Orlando.
6. Gilula LA, Weeks PM. Post-traumatic ligamentous instabilities of the wrist. Radiology 1978;129:641–651.
7. Kleinman WB. Diagnostic exams for ligamentous injuries. American Society for Surgery of the Hand, Correspondence Club Newsletter, 1985. No. 51.
8. Linscheid RL, Dobyns JH. Athletic injuries of the wrist. Clin Orthop Relat Res 1985;198:141–151.
9. Palmer AK, Dobyns JH, Linscheid RL. Management of post-traumatic instability of the wrist secondary to ligament rupture. J Hand Surg Am 1978;3A:507–532.
10. Palmer AK, Werner RW. Biomechanics of the distal radioulnar joint. Clin Orthop Relat Res 1984;187:26–35.
11. Reagan DS, Linscheid RL, Dobyns JH. Lunotriquetral sprains. J Hand Surg Am 1984;9A:502–514.
12. Ritt MJ, Bishop AT, Berger RA, et al. Lunotriquetral ligament properties: a comparison of three anatomic subregions. J Hand Surg Am 1998;23A:425–431.
13. Shin AY, Weinstein LP, Berger RA, et al. Treatment of isolated injuries of the lunotriquetral ligament: a comparison of arthrodesis, ligament reconstruction and ligament repair. J Bone Joint Surg Br 2001; 83B:1023–1028.
14. Shin AY, Deitch MA, Sachar K, et al. Ulnar-sided wrist pain: diagnosis and treatment. AAOS Instr Course Lect 2005;54:115–128.
15. Shin AY, Bishop AT. Treatment options for lunotriquetral dissociation. Tech Hand Upper Extrem Surg 1998;2:2–17.
16. Taleisnik J, Malerich M, Prietto M. Palmar carpal instability secondary to dislocation of scaphoid and lunate: report of case and review of the literature. J Hand Surg Am 1982;7A:606–612.

Chapter 48

Operative Treatment of Lesser and Greater Arc Injuries

Leonard L. D'Addesi, Joseph J. Thoder, and Kristofer S. Matullo

DEFINITION

▪ The carpus is a complex, intercalated system of dual rows that allow paired motion within the radial–ulnar and flexion–extension plane. A disruption of the intrinsic ligaments of the carpus or a combination of ligamentous and osseous structures leads to a spectrum of injuries ranging from "wrist sprains" to complex perilunate injuries including lesser and greater arc injuries.

▪ Lesser arc injuries are purely capsuloligamentous.

▪ Greater arc injuries include a range of associated carpal fractures.

▪ Disruptions of the normal kinematics and stability of the carpal row lead to acute failure with a predictable pattern of posttraumatic degenerative changes.

ANATOMY

▪ There are eight carpal bones without tendinous insertions, whose motion is passively transmitted and guided by precise ligamentous architecture and bony geometry.

▪ Volar extrinsic ligaments are the prime stabilizers of the carpus and are oriented in a double-V arrangement with a relative weakness between these V's called the space of Poirier.

  ▪ The volar extrinsic ligaments include the inner-V ligaments: long radiolunate (LRL), radioscapholunate (RSL), short radiolunate (SRL), and ulnolunate (UL). The outer V consists of the radioscaphocapitate (RSC) and the ulnotriquetrocapitate complex (UTCC) (**FIG 1A**).[7]

  ▪ The dorsal extrinsic ligaments provide less structural stability and include the radiotriquetral (RT) and dorsal intercarpal (DIC) ligaments (**FIG 1B**).

▪ The intrinsic ligaments are direct intercarpal connections that provide intra-row stability.

  ▪ These include the lunotriquetral and the scapholunate ligaments.

▪ Complex, three-dimensional motion occurs with wrist movement: radial deviation and wrist dorsiflexion are paired, as are ulnar deviation and wrist volarflexion.

PATHOGENESIS

▪ These may involve high-energy injuries in which an axial load is applied to a hyperextended and ulnarly deviated wrist, placing the volar structures under tension and the dorsal structures under compression and shear.

▪ The energy dissipates in a radial to ulnar direction.

▪ Lesser arc injuries are purely ligamentous and advance through four progressive stages as originally described by Mayfield et al[4] (**FIG 2A**):

  ▪ Stage I: the scapholunate ligament
  ▪ Stage II: the space of Poirier
  ▪ Stage III: the UTCC and UL ligament
  ▪ Stage IV: lunate dislocation

▪ Greater arc injuries proceed in the same direction but involve fractures through the radial styloid, scaphoid, lunate,

capitate, triquetrum, and ulna, either solely or in combination (**FIG 2B**).

▪ Perilunate dislocations most commonly occur as dorsal dislocations of the capitate and surrounding carpus with respect to the lunate, which remains in the lunate fossa of the distal radius.

▪ A lunate dislocation often involves volar displacement of the lunate into the carpal tunnel, with the capitate articulating in the lunate fossa of the radius. Median neuropathy is common. The lunate is ousted from the wrist joint through the space of Poirier, creating a rent in the volar capsule that extends medially and laterally along the interval between the V ligaments. The rent is semilunar or crescentic in appearance.

NATURAL HISTORY

▪ Nonoperative management yields predictably poor results, with loss of reduction and progression to wrist deformity and pain.[1,2]

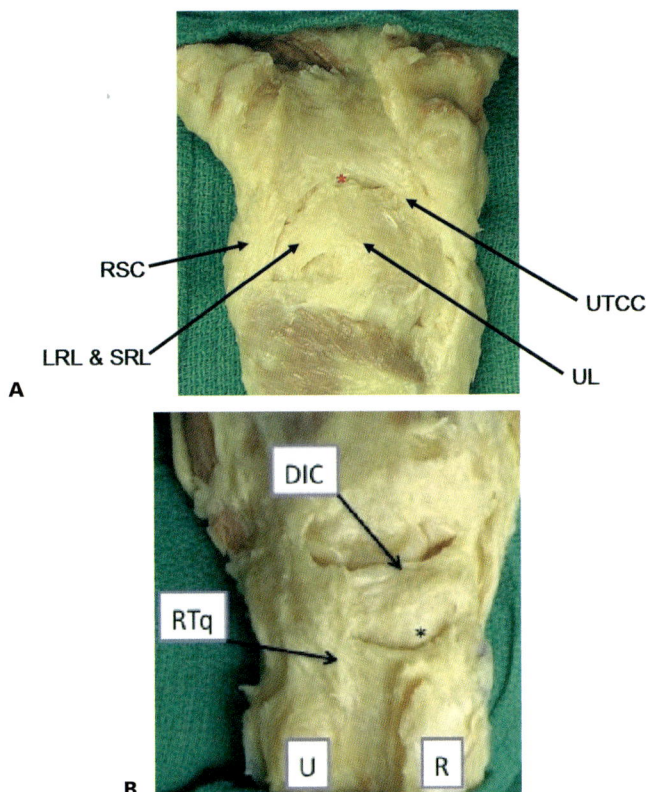

FIG 1 • A. Volar extrinsic carpal ligaments. *LRL,* long radiolunate ligament; *SRL,* short radiolunate; *RSC,* radioscaphocapitate ligament; *UL,* ulnolunate ligament; *UTCC,* ulnotriquetrocapitate complex; *,* space of Poirier. **B.** Dorsal extrinsic carpal ligaments. *RTq,* radiotriquetral ligament; *DIC,* dorsal intercarpal ligament; *,* scaphoid.

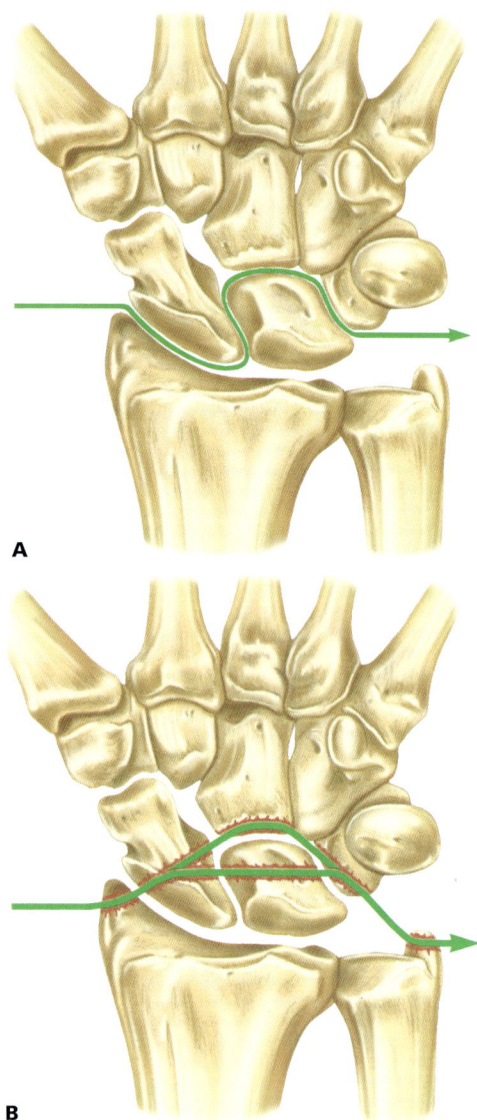

FIG 2 • A. Lesser arc injury. Progression of capsuloligamentous injury from radial to ulnar direction. **B.** Greater arc injury. Transscaphoid perilunate injury pattern.

- Typical instability patterns (depending on extent of injury) include scapholunate advanced collapse, scaphoid nonunion advanced collapse, and volar or dorsal intercalated segmental instability.
- Definitive treatment is operative intervention.

PATIENT HISTORY AND PHYSICAL FINDINGS

- A typical history may range from a fall and twist on an extended hand to a high-energy event with extreme forces transferred to the wrist. Patients complain of pain and stiffness.
- Physical examination findings depend on the level of injury and the elapsed time from injury to presentation.
  - Stiffness, tenderness, crepitus, swelling, and resistance to motion are common findings. Deformity is usually minimal.
  - Depending on the severity of injury, the findings can be subtle and easily missed. The examiner must maintain a high index of suspicion.

- A thorough neurologic examination is critical. Median neuropathy is relatively common and ranges from dysesthesia to overt motor dysfunction. This finding is more common in cases associated with lunate dislocation.
- Palpation of individual carpal bones in a greater arc injury may reveal tenderness over specific fractures.
- Specific testing of intrinsic and extrinsic ligaments (eg, the Watson test, the lunotriquetral shuck, and the ulnar catch-up) may prove difficult and of little value in an acute setting.

IMAGING AND OTHER DIAGNOSTIC STUDIES

- True posteroanterior (PA) and true lateral radiographs should be obtained. The diagnosis is made primarily with these views. These radiographs should be compared with identical radiographs of the uninjured wrist.
  - Other views such as radial–ulnar deviation, flexion–extension, supinated, and clenched-fist views are often difficult to obtain and are of little additional value.
- Perilunate dislocations involve disruption of the lines of Gilula, best seen on the PA radiograph. The lunate assumes a triangular shape, different from its standard trapezoidal shape. On the lateral radiograph, the concentricity of the C's, representing the distal radius, lunate, and capitate, is lost, indicating a dorsal dislocation of the capitate from the lunate fossa (**FIG 3A,B**).
- A lunate dislocation is represented by the "spilled tea cup" sign on the lateral radiograph. The lunate is volarly displaced and flexed. It often lies anterior to the volar cortex of the distal radius. The capitate articulates with the lunate fossa of the radius (**FIG 3C,D**).
- Greater arc injuries must be ruled out. Scaphoid fractures are most common. Capitate and triquetral fractures have been described.
- MRI, arthrography, arthroscopy, and bone scan are not indicated in the acute setting after major trauma to the wrist.

DIFFERENTIAL DIAGNOSIS

- Given the severity of this injury pattern and the frequency with which it is missed, greater and lesser arc injuries must be ruled out in any situation in which the wrist is traumatized.
- Wrist sprain
- Triangular fibrocartilage complex (TFCC) injury
- Extrinsic or intrinsic ligament disruptions
- Carpal fractures
- Distal radius or ulna fracture
- Median neuropathy
- Kienböck disease
- Ulnar impaction syndrome
- DeQuervain tenosynovitis
- Basal joint arthritis

NONOPERATIVE MANAGEMENT

- Closed reduction of perilunate dislocations may be achieved by in-line traction and gentle wrist manipulation as described by Tavernier.[6]
  - In-line traction is helpful for muscle relaxation before reduction and can be applied using finger traps and weights suspended from the arm with the elbow flexed 90 degrees for 10 minutes.
  - The surgeon extends the wrist and applies gentle manual traction. The surgeon's thumb stabilizes the lunate volarly

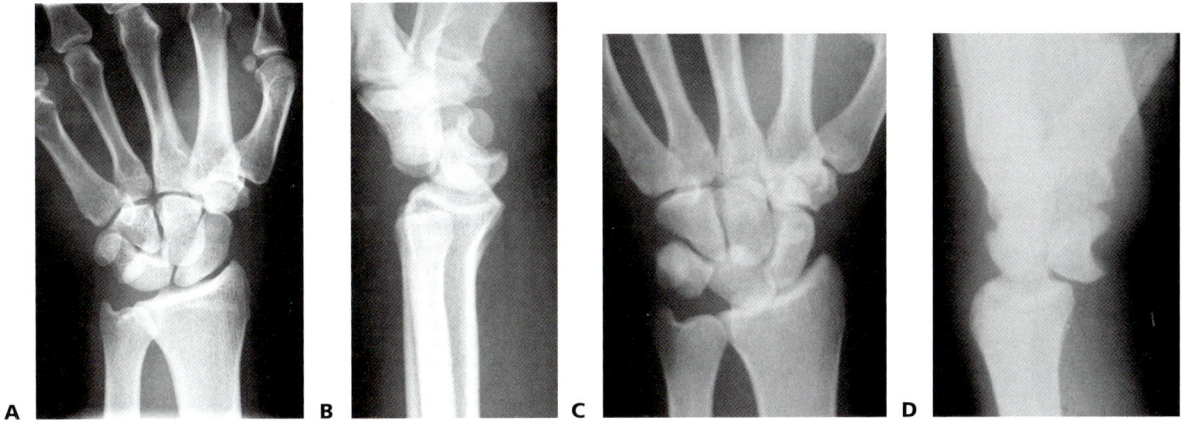

FIG 3 • A,B. Perilunate dislocation. **A.** AP projection demonstrates loss of lines of Gilula. **B.** Dorsal dislocation of the capitate out of the lunate fossa. **C,D.** Lunate dislocation. AP and lateral projections demonstrating loss of lines of Gilula and volar dislocation of the lunate into the carpal tunnel, with the capitate articulating in the radial fossa.

and rotates the lunate into extension. The capitate is then translated up and over the lunate while simultaneously flexing the wrist. A snapping sound may be heard when the capitate reduces over the lunate.

- Closed reductions of lunate dislocations are frequently unsuccessful. As traction is applied to the wrist, the volar rent narrows to prevent reduction of the lunate into the wrist joint.
  - Acute carpal tunnel syndrome in this scenario is a surgical emergency.
- Long-term outcomes of closed reduction have been shown to be suboptimal, and surgical treatment is warranted.

SURGICAL MANAGEMENT

Preoperative Planning

- All radiographs are reviewed.
- The surgeon should determine what ligaments are damaged and whether biosuture anchors are needed to augment repair.
- The surgeon should assess osseous structures and determine whether fractures need to be stabilized with hardware such as Kirschner wires or dual-pitch screws.
- If median neuropathy is present or impending, a carpal tunnel release should be performed.

Positioning

- Supine positioning with a well-padded pneumatic tourniquet on the upper arm
- The use of a radiolucent hand table with fluoroscopic imaging aids in repair and reduction.

Approach

- Surgical approaches to this injury include dorsal approach, volar approach, and combined dorsal and volar approach.
- The dorsal approach uses the universal dorsal wrist incision and the interval between the third and fourth compartments to expose the dorsal capsule and gain access to the joint.
  - The dorsal approach is helpful for open reduction of the dislocation and direct assessment of articular injuries. However, great difficulty may be encountered if attempting to reduce a lunate dislocation through only a dorsal approach.
  - Direct or augmented repair of the scapholunate ligament and open reduction and internal fixation of any concomitant carpal fractures are accomplished through this approach.
- The volar approach is performed through an extended carpal tunnel incision. Retraction of the carpal tunnel contents allows visualization of the volar capsuloligamentous structures and the semilunar rent. Decompression of the carpal tunnel, evacuation of any hematoma, and tenosynovectomy of the digital flexor tendons is accomplished.
  - Open reduction of a volar lunate dislocation is facilitated by this approach.
  - Repair of the volar capsuloligamentous injuries can also be performed to further stabilize the carpus.
  - An exclusive volar approach does not allow precise repair of the intercarpal ligaments, and bony fixation is difficult.
- The combined dorsal and volar approach is preferred: this is the only method that allows true assessment of the pathology and anatomic repair of all injured structures.

DORSAL APPROACH

Incision and Dissection

- A universal dorsal skin incision is made under tourniquet control. The extensor retinaculum is exposed, raising medial and lateral skin flaps. Access to the dorsal capsule is gained through the 3–4 extensor compartment interval (**TECH FIG 1A**).
- The extensor pollicis longus (EPL) tendon is dissected distal to the extensor retinaculum and the third compartment is incised. The EPL is transposed radially to prevent

injury to the tendon during manipulation and stabilization of the carpus (**TECH FIG 1B**).
- The fourth extensor compartment is incised longitudinally and the tendons are retracted. The dorsal capsule is now visible.
  - One centimeter of the posterior interosseous nerve is excised as part of the procedure (**TECH FIG 1C**).
- A transverse rent extending through the dorsal capsule and radiotriquetral ligament is often found. This rent

TECHNIQUES

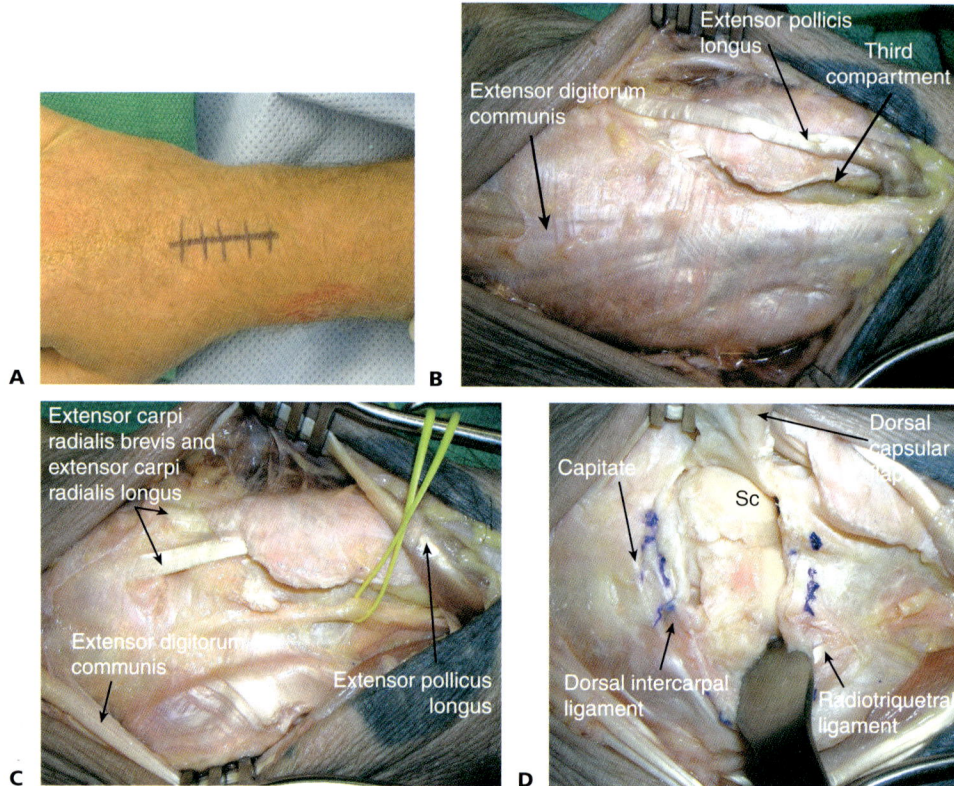

TECH FIG 1 • **A.** Universal dorsal skin incision for the dorsal approach. **B.** The third extensor compartment is incised and the extensor pollicis longus (EPL) is transposed radially. The extensor digitorum communis (EDC) tendons are visible. (Thumb is at top left and wrist is to the right.) **C.** The fourth extensor compartment is incised and the EDC tendons are retracted ulnarly. The sensory branch of the posterior interosseous nerve to the wrist (vessel loop) is sacrificed. **D.** A ligament-sparing capsular incision may be made to visualize the carpus. *Sc*, scaphoid.

should be extended in both the radial and ulnar directions to allow visualization of the capitolunate interval.

- A more extensile ligament-sparing incision can also be used to gain considerable access to the carpus.
  - Incise the capsule in a radial direction along the dorsal distal radial lip, leaving a small cuff of tissue attached to the radius for later repair.
  - Incise ulnarly, along the dorsal radiotriquetral ligament and dorsal intercarpal ligament. This generates a radially based capsular flap (**TECH FIG 1D**).
- If the dislocation was not reducible closed, the capitate is prominent and the absence of the lunate is evident.
- The articular injury can now be assessed.

Reduction and Fixation

- Before reduction of the dislocation–subluxation, 0.045- or 0.062-inch Kirschner wire transfixation pins are inserted into the triquetrum and scaphoid through the dorsal incision in an in-to-out fashion. These pins are later driven back into the lunate to stabilize the reduction.
  - The starting point for these pins is through the centroid of the aspect of the proximal pole of the scaphoid and triquetrum that articulates with the lunate (**TECH FIG 2**).
  - Transfixation pins are unnecessary in the scaphoid if it

is fractured since a screw in the scaphoid will stabilize the radial side of the carpus.
- In combination with manual traction and volar pressure on the lunate, insert a Freer elevator into the capitolunate

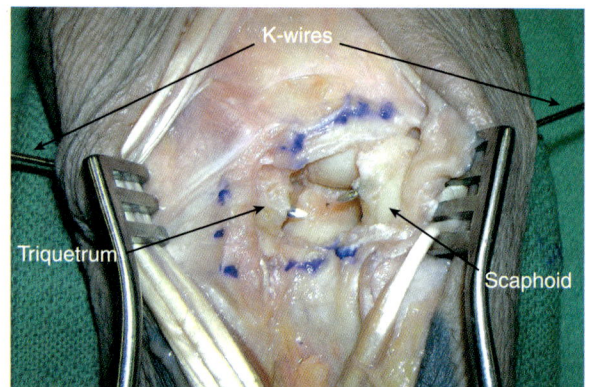

TECH FIG 2 • Transfixation pins are placed through the scaphoid and triquetrum before reduction of the lunate. This facilitates placement of these Kirschner wires and advancement into the lunate after reduction. The entry point is the centroid of the intercarpal joint on the scaphoid and triquetrum. The tips of the Kirschner wires are seen slightly protruding from the scaphoid and triquetrum. The lunate is displaced volarly and is not visible.

joint around the proximal pole of the capitate and shoehorn the lunate into place.
- Reduce and stabilize carpal fractures.
- Attention is first directed toward fixation of an associated scaphoid fracture using proximal to distal (antegrade) fixation.
  - The scaphoid is usually fractured at its waist or proximal pole.
  - In a noncomminuted fracture, stabilization is accomplished with a cannulated headless compression screw.
  - If comminution exists, autologous cancellous bone graft is applied before final tightening of the screw.

Ligament Repair
- Intercarpal ligament injuries may now be repaired.
- In a transscaphoid perilunate dislocation, the proximal pole of the scaphoid remains attached to the lunate with an intact scapholunate ligament. However, in lesser arc injuries, the scapholunate and the lunotriquetral ligament are disrupted.
- Before ligamentous repair, anatomic carpal realignment is ensured.
  - 0.045-mm Kirschner wires are introduced into the scaphoid, lunate, and triquetrum and used as joysticks to align these bones.
- The previously set Kirschner wires used as transfixation pins are then advanced from the scaphoid and triquetrum into the lunate.

- Transfixation pins are also percutaneously introduced to stabilize the scaphoid and triquetrum to the capitate (**TECH FIG 3A**).
- Intraoperative fluoroscopy aids alignment and placement of Kirschner wires.
  - The scapholunate angle (40 to 60 degrees), capitolunate angle (less than 15 degrees), and radiolunate angle (less than 15 degrees) should be reduced and verified.
  - The C shape of the distal radius, lunate, and capitate should be concentric (**TECH FIG 3B**).
- Small (about 2 mm) suture anchors with nonabsorbable suture (2-0 to 3-0) are inserted for reattachment of the scapholunate and lunotriquetral ligaments, avoiding the Kirschner wires.
  - Most often the ligaments avulse from the scaphoid and the triquetrum; therefore, the anchors are placed in those locations.
  - When the intercarpal ligaments are beyond repair, suture anchors are unnecessary, and stability is established via extrinsic capsuloligamentous healing.
- The dorsal capsular injury and extended capsulotomy is closed with nonabsorbable suture.
- The EPL tendon is left transposed in a subcutaneous location (**TECH FIG 3C**).
- The subcutaneous tissue and skin are closed in a standard fashion.

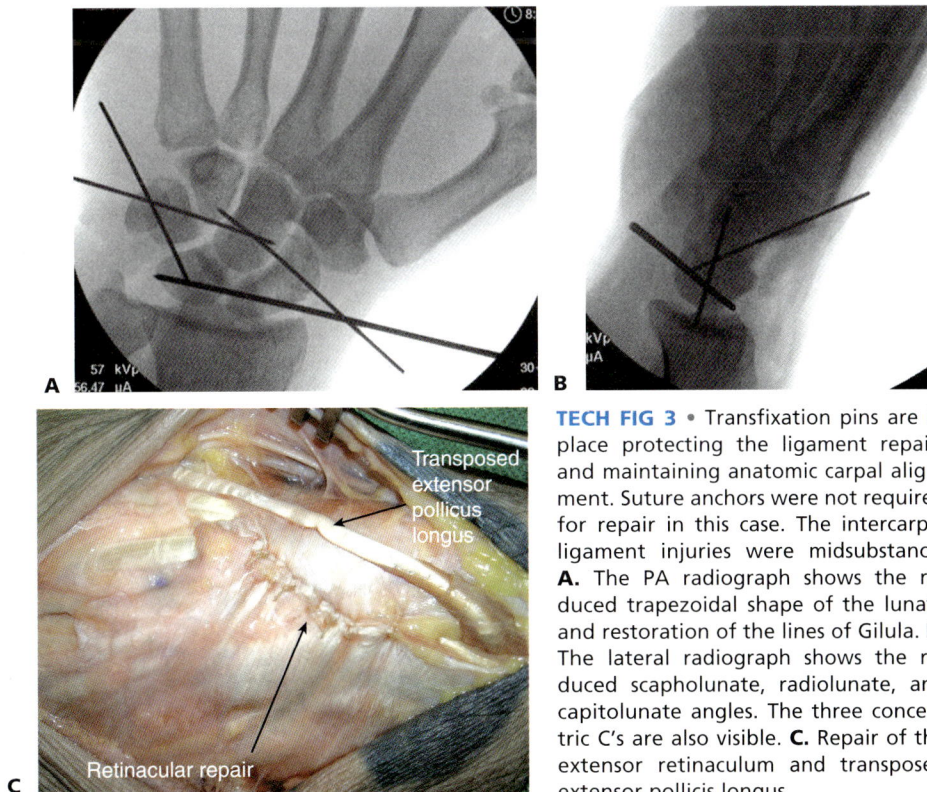

TECH FIG 3 • Transfixation pins are in place protecting the ligament repairs and maintaining anatomic carpal alignment. Suture anchors were not required for repair in this case. The intercarpal ligament injuries were midsubstance. **A.** The PA radiograph shows the reduced trapezoidal shape of the lunate and restoration of the lines of Gilula. **B.** The lateral radiograph shows the reduced scapholunate, radiolunate, and capitolunate angles. The three concentric C's are also visible. **C.** Repair of the extensor retinaculum and transposed extensor pollicis longus.

TECHNIQUES

COMBINED DORSAL AND VOLAR APPROACH (AUTHORS' PREFERRED APPROACH)

Incision and Dissection

- A standard extended carpal tunnel approach is performed under tourniquet control (**TECH FIG 4A**).
  - The median nerve is completely decompressed.
- The contents of the carpal canal are retracted and hematoma is evacuated.
- The volar capsuloligamentous injury, which is represented by an apex-distal, semilunar rent, is visualized (**TECH FIG 4B**).
  - This rent courses between the RSC and LRL radially, and between the UTCC and ulnolunate ligaments ulnarly.
  - In the case of a lunate dislocation, the lunate can be visualized within the carpal canal, having been extruded through the capsular tear.

- Next, the wrist is exposed dorsally as described above.
- The degree of injury is assessed.

Reduction, Fixation, and Repair

- Preset transfixation Kirschner wires as previously described.
- Reduce the carpus under direct visualization, with wrist extension and the aid of a Freer elevator to shoehorn the capitate into the lunate fossa.
  - The volar approach facilitates the reduction by allowing direct access to the lunate.
  - Surgical extension of the capsular tear between the RSC and LRL ligaments or between the UTCC and ulnolunate ligaments allows greater access to the wrist without further disruption of extrinsic ligaments.
- Through the dorsal incision, reduce, stabilize, and repair any associated carpal fractures and intercarpal ligament injuries in the manner described above.
- The volar capsuloligamentous rent is closed with nonabsorbable suture (**TECH FIG 5**).
- The flexor tendons may now be assessed. Often the tenosynovium surrounding the tendons within the carpal tunnel is thickened. A tenosynovectomy may be performed.
- The EPL should be left transposed dorsally.
- The subcutaneous tissue and skin are closed in a standard fashion.

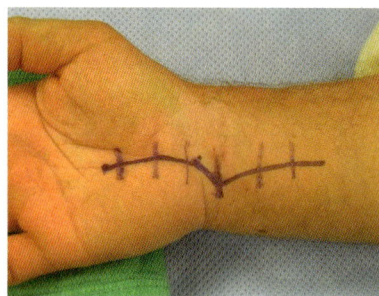

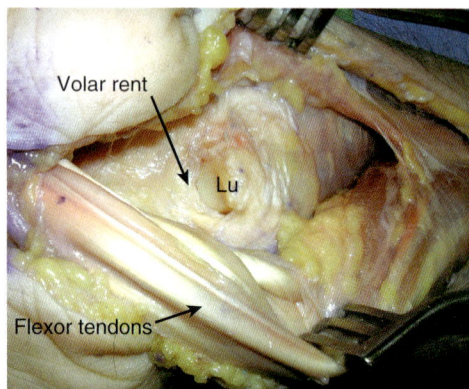

TECH FIG 4 • **A.** Extended carpal tunnel incision used for the volar approach. **B.** A volar, semilunar, apex-distal, capsuloligamentous rent is visible at the space of Poirier. The lunate (*Lu*) is seen protruding from the rent.

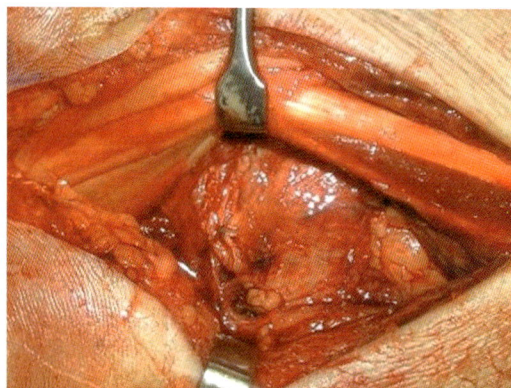

TECH FIG 5 • The volar capsule is closed with nonabsorbable suture.

PEARLS AND PITFALLS

Radiographs	▪ This injury is easily missed; therefore, true lateral and posteroanterior radiographs are necessary to avoid the "bag of bones" appearance on oblique views.
Timing	▪ Although not a surgical emergency, definitive stabilization should be carried out as soon as possible for technical ease and improved postoperative outcomes, especially in the presence of median nerve symptoms.
Intraoperative reduction	▪ The ever-elusive lunate may be stabilized during reduction by placing the thumb through the dorsal incision and the index finger through the volar incision (when a dual-incision approach is used). This facilitates stabilization by transfixion pins in an anatomic position.
Soft tissue repair	▪ The bony architecture should be reduced and stabilized in an anatomic position before capsuloligamentous repair. This will ensure proper tension of the soft tissue repair. Overtensioning of the soft tissues by repairing them first may prevent accurate reduction of the carpus.

POSTOPERATIVE CARE

▪ The immediate postoperative dressing includes a well-padded splint immobilizing the wrist and forearm in a neutral rotational position with about 20 degrees of wrist extension.

▪ Edema control and prevention of skin maceration can be accomplished with the addition of sterile gauze dressings between the digits and a bulky dressing within the palm.

▪ Active and passive digital range-of-motion exercises are encouraged immediately to prevent flexor tendon adhesions and digital stiffness.

▪ Sutures are removed at 10 to 14 days and full-time cast or splint immobilization is continued for a total of 8 weeks postoperatively.

▪ Pins may be removed at 8 weeks, and the patient may be converted to a removable splint to promote range of motion of the wrist.

▪ At 12 weeks, strengthening is permitted with progressive resistance as tolerated.

▪ Anticipated return to activities is 6 to 12 months.

OUTCOMES

▪ Outcomes will vary with regard to stiffness and grip strength.

▪ More accurate anatomic reduction will lead to improved results. Sotereanos et al[5] used a dorsal–volar approach in 11 patients with perilunate dislocations and fracture-dislocations. Good to excellent results were achieved in 9 of 11 patients.

▪ Up to 50% loss of flexion–extension motion arc can be anticipated.[3]

▪ Up to 60% diminished grip strength can be anticipated.[3]

COMPLICATIONS

▪ Missed diagnosis
▪ Postoperative pin-tract infections
▪ Median nerve injury
▪ Transient ischemia of lunate
▪ Chondral injury or chondrolysis
▪ Late carpal instability
▪ Nonunion or malunion of the scaphoid
▪ Posttraumatic arthritis

REFERENCES

1. Adkison JW, Chapman MW. Treatment of acute lunate and perilunate dislocations. Clin Orthop Relat Res 1982;164:199–207.
2. Apergis E, Maris J, Theodoratos G, et al. Perilunate dislocations and fracture dislocations: closed and early open reduction compared in 28 cases. Acta Orthop Scand Suppl 1997;275:55–59.
3. Cooney WP, Bussey R, Dobyns JH, et al. Difficult wrist fractures: perilunate fracture-dislocations of the wrist. Clin Orthop Relat Res 1987;214:136–147.
4. Mayfield JK, Johnson RP, Kilcoyne RK. Carpal dislocations: pathomechanics and progressive perilunar instability. J Hand Surg Am 1980;5:226–241.
5. Sotereanos DG, Mitsionis GJ, Giannakopoulos PN, et al. Perilunate dislocation and fracture dislocation: a critical analysis of the volar-dorsal approach. J Hand Surg Am 1997;22A:49–56.
6. Tavernier L. Les deplacements tramatiques du semilunaire. Theses, Lyons, 1906:138–139.
7. Walsh JJ, Berger RA, Cooney WP. Current status of scapholunate interosseous ligament injuries. JAAOS 2002;10:32–42.

Chapter 49

Arthroscopic and Open Triangular Fibrocartilage Complex Repair

A. Lee Osterman

DEFINITION

- The triangular fibrocartilage complex (TFCC) is a complex anatomic structure located at the ulnar side of the wrist. It has several important biomechanical functions:
  - Extends the gliding surface of the radiocarpal joint
  - Cushions and stabilizes the ulnar carpus
  - Stabilizes the distal radioulnar joint (DRUJ)
- Disorders of the TFCC are responsible for the ulnar-sided wrist symptoms of pain, weakness, and instability that affect the patient's function.
- The diagnosis and treatment of these injuries to the TFCC will restore stability, resulting in pain relief and a generally good prognosis for functional return.

ANATOMY

- The TFCC is a cartilaginous and ligamentous structure interposed between the ulnar carpus and the distal ulna (**FIG 1A**). It arises from the distal aspect of the sigmoid notch of the radius and inserts into the base of the ulnar styloid.[17]
- The TFCC attaches to the ulnar carpus via the ulnocarpal ligament complex (ulnolunate, ulnotriquetral, and ulnar collateral ligament) (**FIG 1B**).
- The radioulnar ligaments stabilize the DRUJ, limiting rotation as well as axial migration.[7]
  - The dorsal and volar radioulnar ligaments are fibrous thickenings within the substance of the TFCC.
  - As a result of this anatomic configuration, they function as a unit rather than as independent ligaments.
- The central, horizontal portion of the TFCC is the thinnest portion, composed of interwoven obliquely oriented sheets of collagen fibers for the resistance of multidirectional stress.
- The vascularity of the TFCC has been carefully studied.[3] The TFCC receives its blood supply from the ulnar artery through its radiocarpal branches and the dorsal and palmar branches of the anterior interosseous artery. These vessels supply the TFCC in a radial fashion (see Bednar et al[3] for a good image of TFCC vascularity).
  - Histologic sections demonstrate that these vessels penetrate only the peripheral 10% to 40% of the TFCC. The central section and radial attachment are avascular.
  - This vascular anatomy supports the concept that peripheral injuries can heal if injured and treated appropriately, whereas tears of the central portion do not heal if sutured and are usually débrided.

Biomechanics

- The TFCC has several important biomechanical functions: it transmits 20% of an axially applied load from the ulnar carpus to the distal ulna; it is the major stabilizer of the DRUJ; and it is a stabilizer of the ulna.[1,6,18,19]

- The amount of the load transferred to the distal ulna varies with ulnar variance. A greater amount is transferred in positive ulnar variance than negative.
  - This results in a corresponding decreased thickness of the central portion of the TFCC in ulnar-positive wrists.
- There is a variable load placed on the TFCC with forearm rotation. Supination causes a negative ulnar variance due to the proximal migration of the ulna. This is reversed with pronation as the ulna moves distally, causing it to become ulnar-positive.
- The ulnar head also moves within the sigmoid notch in a dorsal direction with pronation and a volar direction with supination.
  - The dorsal and volar radioulnar ligaments, which form the peripheral portion of the TFCC, serve as major stabilizers to translation at the DRUJ during forearm rotation.

PATHOGENESIS

- Traumatic injuries of the TFCC result from either the application of an extension, pronation force to the axially loaded wrist or a distraction force to the ulnar aspect of the wrist.

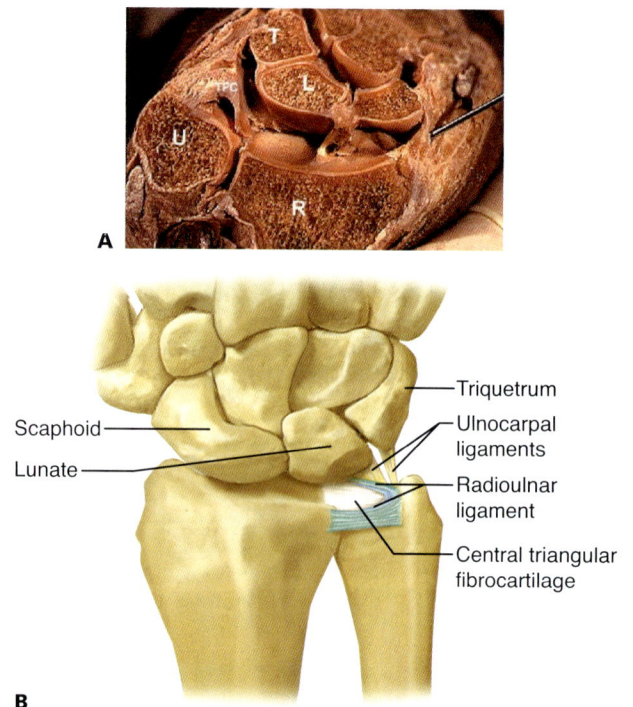

FIG 1 • **A.** Anatomic coronal section demonstrating the triangular fibrocartilage (*TFC*) and its relation to the lunate (*L*), triquetrum (*T*), distal ulna (*U*), and radius (*R*). **B.** Triangular fibrocartilage complex.

Labels on FIG 1B: Scaphoid, Lunate, Triquetrum, Ulnocarpal ligaments, Radioulnar ligament, Central triangular fibrocartilage

- This will most commonly occur with a fall on the outstretched hand or a resisted torque force.
- The lesions are more common with ulnar-positive and neutral patients and are frequently found in patients with fractures of the distal radius.
- Several authors have examined the incidence of intracarpal soft tissue injuries associated with distal radial fractures.
  - Geissler et al[8] studied 60 patients, finding a TFCC injury in 26 (43%).
  - In Lindau et al's series of 51 patients,[13] 43 had a TFCC injury (84%): 24 had a peripheral tear, 10 had a central perforation, and 9 had a combined central and peripheral tear.
- In a study of 180 wrist joints in 100 cadavers ranging in age from fetuses to 94 years, Mikic[14] found that degeneration of the TFCC begins in the third decade of life.
  - This degeneration increases in frequency and severity as people age.
  - After the fifth decade of life, 100% of TFCCs appear abnormal.
  - However, these age-related TFCC lesions are often asymptomatic.[6]

NATURAL HISTORY

- The classification system described by Palmer[16] is the most useful for describing TFCC injuries, dividing them into traumatic and degenerative.
- Traumatic lesions are classified according to the location of the tear within the TFCC. The traumatic class has been designated by Palmer as class 1, with subclasses of A, B, C, and D assigned to anatomic lesions within the TFCC (**FIG 2A**).
  - A class 1A lesion represents a tear in the horizontal or central portion of the TFCC. The tear is 2 to 3 mm medial to the radial attachment of the cartilage. It is usually oriented from dorsal to volar.
  - A class 1B lesion represents an avulsion of the peripheral aspect of the TFCC from its insertion onto the distal ulna. This can occur either with a fracture of the ulnar styloid or as a pure avulsion from its bony attachment. This type of injury disrupts the stabilizing effect of the TFCC on the DRUJ, resulting in clinical instability.
  - A class 1C lesion represents an avulsion of the TFCC attachment to the ulnar carpus by disruption of the ulnocarpal ligaments. These lesions result in ulnar carpal instability with volar translocation of the carpus.
  - A class 1D lesion represents an avulsion of the TFCC from its radial attachment. Isolated disc tears should be differentiated from disruption of the dorsal and volar radioulnar ligaments. Such global TFCC injury will result in DRUJ instability.
- Degenerative type 2 lesions are age-related, nontraumatic lesions to the TFCC, typically characterized by central perforations and positive ulnar variance.[6,23]
- The natural history of such degenerative lesions, when and if they become symptomatic, is a progressive cascade of degenerative changes, as reflected in Palmer's type 2 classification (**FIG 2B**).
  - The deterioration proceeds from TFC wear through central perforation (type 2C) to lunatotriquetral ligament tear and arthritic changes of the lunate, triquetrum, and distal ulna (type 2D or E).
  - Treatment is based on the stage of involvement.

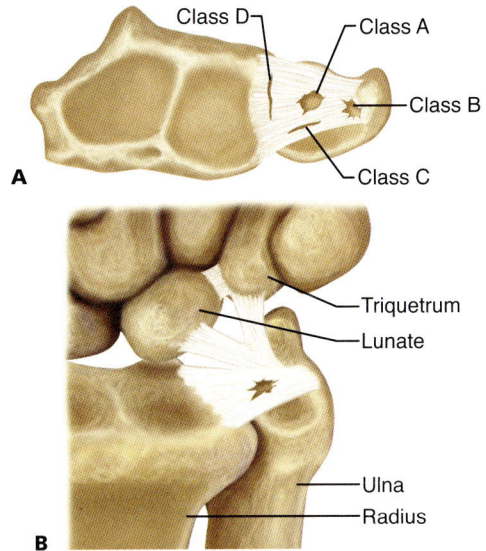

FIG 2 • A. Axial drawing looking at the radius platform and the TFCC. Dorsal is up and volar is down. Palmer classification for acute triangular fibrocartilage complex (TFCC) injuries. A class 1A lesion involves a tear in the central, horizontal portion of the TFCC. A class 1B lesion is a tear of the TFCC from the distal ulna with or without an ulnar styloid fracture. A class 1C lesion is a tear of the TFCC distal attachment to the lunate and triquetrum through the ulnolunate and ulnotriquetral ligaments. A class 1D lesion is a detachment of the TFCC from its insertion on to the radius at the distal sigmoid notch. **B.** Palmer classification for degenerative TFCC lesions, usually related to positive ulnar variance and ulnocarpal impaction syndrome. The degeneration occurs in a progressive cascade: types 2A and 2B, TFC wear; type 2C, fibrillated central TFC lesion; types 2D and 2E, arthritic chondral changes of the distal ulna and lunate and disruption of the lunatotriquetral ligament. (**A**: Modified From Palmer AK. Triangular fibrocartilage complex lesions: a classification. J Hand Surg Am 1989;14A:601.)

- Degenerative and traumatic lesions can coexist, and injury can render a degenerative lesion symptomatic.

PATIENT HISTORY AND PHYSICAL FINDINGS

- Symptoms consist of ulnar-sided wrist pain, frequently with clicking, that typically occurs after a fall.
- The initial physical examination reveals swelling over the ulnar aspect of the wrist with inflammation of the tendon of the extensor carpi ulnaris.
- Point tenderness is present over the TFCC and distal ulna. The more isolated the point of maximal tenderness, the more specific the diagnosis.
  - A fovea sign (point tenderness directly over the ulnar TFC origin) indicates a type 1A or IB TFC injury or an ulnar extrinsic injury type [1C]).
- Ulnar deviation and axial loading of the wrist (TFCC compression test) will elicit a painful response and a click with forearm rotation.
- The DRUJ must be assessed for instability. Instability is best assessed with the forearm in neutral rotation, but it is also checked in full supination and full pronation.
  - The examiner stabilizes the distal radius with one hand and applies a force to the distal ulna, moving it dorsal and

volar, looking for increased motion or subluxation of the distal ulna relative to the radius and comparing it with the opposite uninjured wrist.

- Significant instability can present as laxity of the distal ulna with a positive "piano key" sign and dorsal prominence of the distal ulna. This may be due to a significant tear or detachment of the dorsal or volar radioulnar ligaments.

- A click produced by ulnar deviation and supination over the extensor carpi ulnaris (ECU) sheath at the distal ulna indicates ECU instability with subluxation out of its sixth extensor compartment.

- A visual carpal supination deformity with ulnar prominence that can be passively corrected by a dorsally applied force to the pisiform indicates an ulnar extrinsic ligament tear.

- TFCC injuries do not occur in isolation; they are often a component of a spectrum of injury to the ulnar side of the wrist. The examiner must therefore evaluate all of the commonly injured structures on the ulnar side of the wrist.

  - The lunatotriquetral joint must be assessed for instability due to a lunatotriquetral ligament tear. This would cause tenderness over the lunatotriquetral interval with a positive shuck test (painful click as the lunate and triquetrum slide abnormally).

  - Point tenderness over the triquetrum may signify a triquetral avulsion fracture.

  - An audible clunk and visual subluxation of the carpus that occur with active ulnar deviation suggest that a midcarpal instability is present.

- Crepitus and pain over the pisotriquetral joint on the shear test may indicate pisotriquetral arthritis.

- The other soft tissue structures around the ulnar wrist should be examined, including the ulnar nerve, the dorsal ulnar sensory nerve branch, and the ulnar artery.

- Grip strength measurements using a Jamar dynamometer, while subjective, are helpful in quantitating patient effort and as a parameter to follow therapeutic progress.

IMAGING AND OTHER DIAGNOSTIC STUDIES

- The diagnostic workup should include plain radiographs and a neutral rotation posteroanterior and lateral view.

  - This will allow assessment for fracture, ligament instability resulting in carpal malalignment, and ulnar variance. It is important to determine ulnar variance because it will influence treatment options (**FIG 3A**).

  - The DRUJ must also be examined radiographically to determine if subluxation, arthritis, or ulnar styloid abnormalities such as an acute or chronic nonunited fracture fragment are present.

- MRI is useful in the diagnosis of TFCC tears, especially the class 1A and D lesions.[9,11] T2-weighted images in the coronal plane are of the greatest diagnostic value (**FIG 3B**).

  - The TFCC has a homogenous low signal intensity. The synovial fluid of the joint appears as a bright image on T2 and will outline tears in the TFCC.

  - A gadolinium arthrogram enhances the visualization of TFCC tears.

- The reported sensitivity and specificity of MRI in diagnosing injuries of the TFCC in the literature is variable.

  - Golimbu et al[9] reported a 95% accuracy of MRI in the detection of TFCC tears. MRI findings were verified arthroscopically.

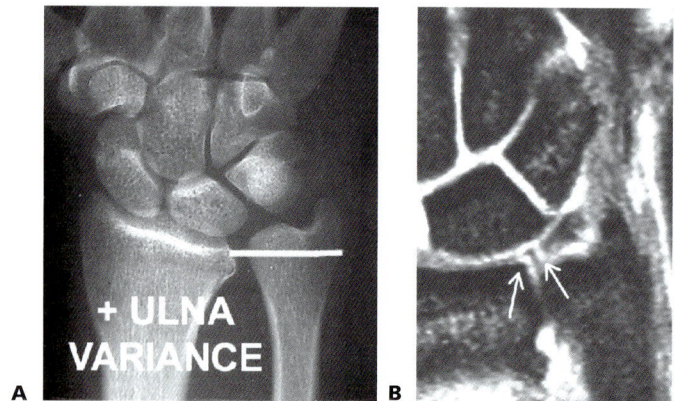

FIG 3 • **A.** Positive ulnar variance is often associated with degenerative triangular fibrocartilage (TFC) tears and ulnocarpal impaction syndrome. The radiograph should be taken in neutral rotation. **B.** Coronal T2 MRI wrist image. High signal of the joint fluid outlines the low-signal substance of the TFC complex. Tears will show as high signal within the central region (*arrow at right*) or TFCC periphery. There is a normal clear area (*arrow at left*) at the insertion of the radial TFC into the medial articular cartilage of the radius.

- Schweitzer et al[20] reported a sensitivity of 72%, a specificity of 95%, and an accuracy of 89%.

- Arthroscopic findings were correlated with the MRI and clinical examination in a series of patients with TFC injuries reported by Bednar et al.[2] The MRI sensitivity was 44% (the probability of a positive MRI when a TFCC lesion is present) and the specificity was 75% (the probability of a negative MRI when a TFCC lesion is absent). The clinical examination sensitivity was 95%. The MRI correlated with arthroscopic findings in 45% of the wrists studied.

- Joshy et al[11] reported on a series of patients with a clinical suspicion of a TFCC tear studied by MR arthrography and then wrist arthroscopy. The MR arthrography sensitivity was 74% and its specificity was 80%. They caution that negative results of MR arthrography in patients with clinical suspicion of TFCC tear should be interpreted with caution.

- Wrist arthroscopy has recently become the criterion standard for both diagnosing and treating lesions of the TFCC.[6]

  - When compared to MRI and arthrography, arthroscopy most accurately determines the location of lesions and the size of tears and allows determination of whether a flap is unstable.

  - Wrist arthroscopy can determine the coexistence of other lesions such as tears within the lunotriquetral interosseous ligament, ECU subsheath, or chondral lesions.

DIFFERENTIAL DIAGNOSIS

- ECU subluxation
- Ulnar extrinsic ligament tear
- DRUJ instability
- Triquetral avulsion fracture
- Lunatotriquetral ligament injury
- Pisotriquetral arthritis
- Ulnar artery thrombosis
- Ulnar neuropathy at the canal of Guyon
- Dorsal ulnar sensory neuritis

NONOPERATIVE MANAGEMENT

- The initial treatment of acute TFCC injuries includes immobilization of the wrist and DRUJ.
  - The patient must be examined carefully to look for DRUJ instability or ECU subluxation.
- If the radiographs are negative and instability is not present, then immobilization for 4 to 6 weeks is recommended to allow healing of the TFCC disruption.
- A peripheral tear is expected to heal if the torn edges are held in close contact, due to the good vascularity of the periphery of the TFCC. Many central tears also become asymptomatic with immobilization even though there is no significant vascularity to the central portion.
- After immobilization, a therapy program involving range-of-motion exercises and gradual strengthening is initiated. Forceful grasp or torque is restricted for 8 weeks.
- If there is ongoing synovitis, a well-placed cortisone shot can further help to quiet this inflammation.
- Tears involving the ligamentous portion of the TFCC or those that heal with a flap of cartilage that impinges on the carpus or distal ulna will fail to respond to conservative treatment and will require operative intervention.
  - It is reasonable to wait 3 to 4 months before proceeding to surgical treatment.
- Class 1B lesions without an ulnar styloid fracture and a stable DRUJ can be immobilized for 4 weeks in a cast. If an ulnar styloid fracture is present, closed reduction should be attempted. If adequate reduction is achieved, then cast immobilization is sufficient. If the styloid remains displaced, then open reduction and internal fixation is required.

SURGICAL MANAGEMENT

- Patients who remain symptomatic after adequate immobilization should undergo further workup, including MRI with or without gadolinium.
- The specific treatment for each traumatic class 1 lesion is determined by the type of tear found arthroscopically.
  - Arthroscopic treatment has become increasingly the method of choice for many traumatic lesions.
- The treatment of traumatic radial detachment of the TFCC from the sigmoid notch of the distal radius is controversial. There appears to be no vascularity to this portion of the TFCC, so theoretically a reattached cartilage would not heal at this repair site. However, clinical experience with open repair of these tears has been positive.[6,21] This may be attributed to vascular ingrowth from the bony radial insertion site that occurs with abrasion of the attachment site, stimulating the formation of new vessels.

  - If the radial tear includes disruption of one or both of the radioulnar ligaments, repair is required to prevent chronic DRUJ instability.
- The algorithm for the treatment of degenerative type 2 tears proceeds from arthroscopy to ulnar-shortening osteotomy (see Chaps. HA-94 and HA-95).
  - Plain films should identify the ulnar variance, DRUJ alignment, abnormalities of the ulnar styloid, or the presence of arthritic changes. Positive ulnar variance has a strong association with degenerative tears.

Preoperative Planning

- All physical examination findings and radiographic study results must be reviewed.
- Examination under anesthesia is performed, including the tests discussed earlier, before positioning in the arthroscopy tower.

Positioning

- Wrist arthroscopy requires distraction, and the wrist is positioned in the traction tower (**FIG 4**).

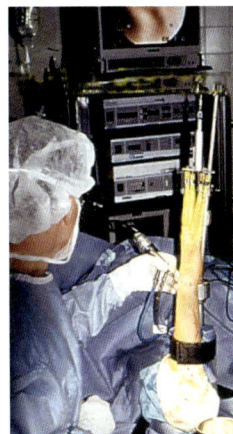

FIG 4 • Positioning for standard wrist arthroscopy. Distraction of the wrist using a wrist traction tower.

WRIST ARTHROSCOPY

- Diagnostic wrist arthroscopy of the radiocarpal and midcarpal joints is completed and all pathology is identified.
- Recognize the appearance of a normal TFC (**TECH FIG 1**).
- The type of TFC injury is identified.
  - A trampoline test is positive when the surgeon's probe sinks into the TFCC rather than bouncing off it like a drumstick on a snare drum. Such loss of disc compliance is often seen with a peripheral tear.[10] However, laxity of the TFCC does not necessarily translate into DRUJ instability.
- Loose bodies, if present, are removed.
- Inflamed synovium is removed with a shaver or radiofrequency probe.

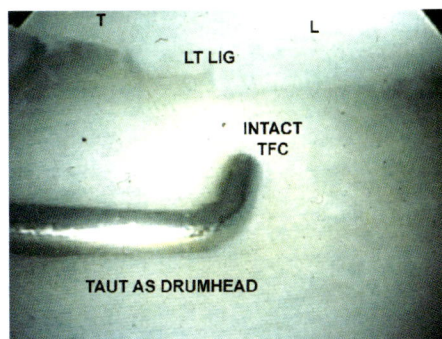

TECH FIG 1 • Normal arthroscopic view of the intact triangular fibrocartilage (*TFC*) with normal "trampoline" tension when probed.

TECHNIQUES

TECHNIQUES

ARTHROSCOPIC REPAIR OF PERIPHERAL TFC TEARS

- Peripheral TFC tears are well vascularized and amenable to repair using arthroscopic techniques. A two-needle method similar to that employed for the repair of a knee meniscus is described here (**TECH FIG 2A**).
- Visualize the tear through the 3–4 portal.
- Initial arthroscopic evaluation may not reveal a tear of the TFCC periphery, but often synovitis and a thin scar will be seen along the periphery of the TFCC at the location of the tear (**TECH FIG 2B**).
  - A probe placed through the 6R portal will demonstrate loss of the normal trampoline effect of the TFCC, indicating a peripheral tear and loss of mechanical function of the TFCC (**TECH FIG 2C**).
- Débride the edges of the tear and undersurface scarring with a shaver to create mobile edges with fresh areas for healing.
  - Adhesions may be present between the undersurface of the TFCC and the distal ulna. These must be released and the TFC mobilized sufficiently to allow advancement to reattach it and to restore proper tension.
- After débridement, a 1-cm longitudinal incision is made extending the 6R portal.

- Avoid injury to branches of the dorsal ulnar sensory nerve.
- Open the sixth extensor compartment radially for 1 cm and retract the extensor carpi ulnaris ulnarly, providing access to its subsheath.
  - The repair includes the subsheath of the ECU compartment as this is intimately associated with the peripheral TFC.
- Two needles are passed across the tear under arthroscopic vision (**TECH FIG 2D**).
- A wire loop is passed through one needle to retrieve a 2-0 PDS suture, which is passed through the other needle.
  - This allows the placement of a horizontal mattress suture across the tear (author's preference) (**TECH FIG 2E**).
  - Alternatively, multiple simple vertical sutures placed at the periphery of the TFCC may approximate the torn edges and restore tension to the TFCC. The suture is tied either under the skin over the dorsal wrist capsule (preferred) or out of the skin over a bolster. Usually two or three sutures are placed.
- Postoperatively, a short-arm splint is applied.
  - I have not found a significant difference between use of a short-arm splint and use of a long-arm or sugar-tong splint in regard to healing and outcome.

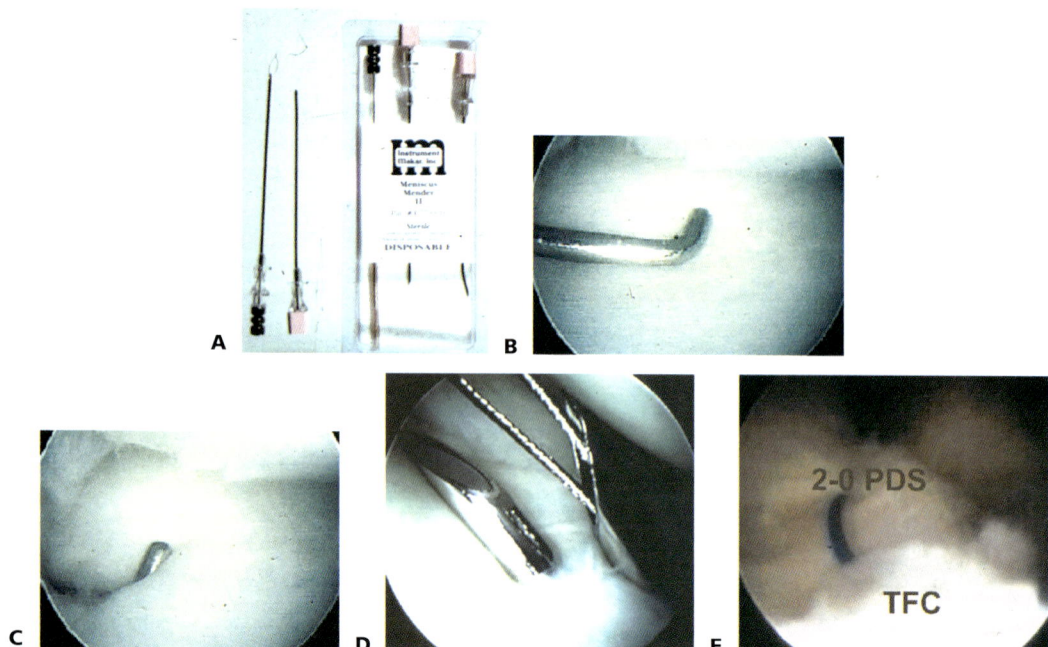

TECH FIG 2 • **A.** Meniscus repair needles with 2-0 PDS suture used for an out-to-in repair. **B,C.** Peripheral TFC tear with loss of compliance such that the probe sinks into the lax surface. Unlike a central tear, fibrous tissue and incomplete healing obscure the actual tear. **D.** Arthroscopic repair of a type 1B peripheral TFC complex tear. Two hollow needles are passed across the tear. A wire loop in one needle is used to pass 2-0 suture across the tear. The suture is tied over the capsule. **E.** The suture approximates the tear and restores tension to the TFCC.

OPEN REPAIR OF PERIPHERAL TFC TEARS WITHOUT ULNAR STYLOID FRACTURE

- If there is significant DRUJ instability and avulsion of the TFC from the ulna fovea, an open repair is preferred.
- Expose the fifth extensor compartment and retract the extensor digiti quinti minimi tendon.
- Create an L-shaped capsulotomy of the DRUJ and identify the foveal attachment site of the TFC (**TECH FIG 3A**).

- Reattach the TFC with a bone anchor or bone suture (**TECH FIG 3B–D**).
- Postoperative care mirrors that of arthroscopic TFC repair.[10]

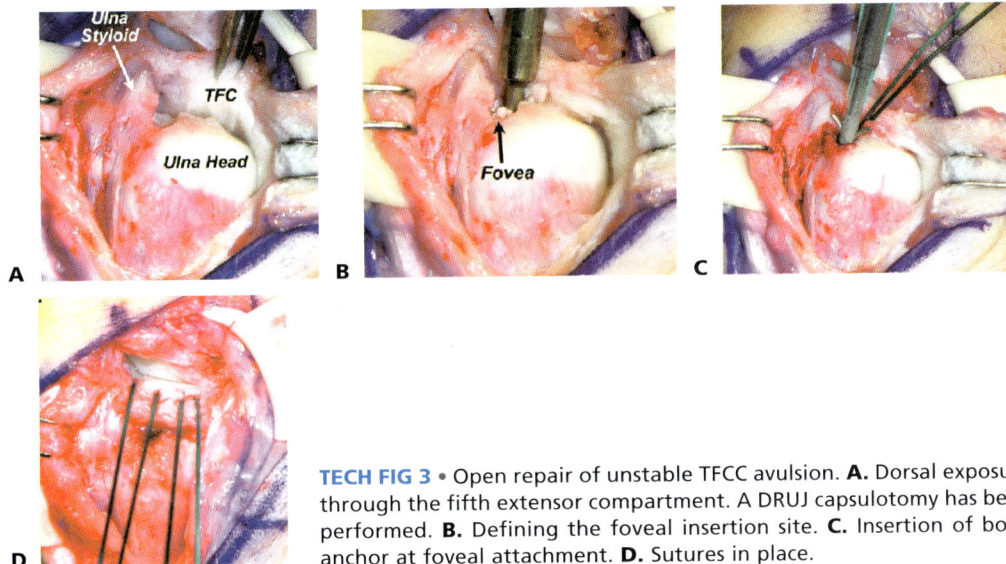

TECH FIG 3 • Open repair of unstable TFCC avulsion. **A.** Dorsal exposure through the fifth extensor compartment. A DRUJ capsulotomy has been performed. **B.** Defining the foveal insertion site. **C.** Insertion of bone anchor at foveal attachment. **D.** Sutures in place.

OPEN REPAIR OF PERIPHERAL TFC TEARS WITH ULNAR STYLOID FRACTURE

- Expose the ulnar styloid using an incision just volar and parallel to the ECU tendon.
  - Protect the dorsal ulnar sensory nerve and preserve the ECU sheath.
- Base the method of fixation (longitudinal Kirschner wire, screw, bone anchor, or tension band) on fragment size and surgeon comfort.
  - If the ulnar styloid is comminuted and will not allow stable fixation, it can be excised and the TFCC attached to the ulna by a suture placed through drill holes in the ulna proximal to the fracture or using the suture anchor technique described earlier.
- The patient is immobilized in a short-arm splint or cast for 4 weeks before starting rotational motion.

Surgery for Radial-Sided TFC Avulsion Tears

- Assess the tear arthroscopically (**TECH FIG 4A**) and repair it in the manner detailed below if instability is present.
- Place a burr through the 6R portal to roughen the radial attachment of the TFCC (**TECH FIG 4B**).
- Drill two holes using a 0.062-inch Kirschner wire in a retrograde manner, starting at the TFC insertion site. These holes will allow placement of the repair suture.

- The wires must exit the radius on its radial border, just volar to the first extensor compartment.
- An incision is made over the exiting Kirschner wire to retract and protect the radial sensory nerve and the tendons of the first extensor compartment.
- A cannula is placed in the 6R portal, through which a meniscal repair suture (2-0 PDS suture with a long straight needle at each end) is passed through the torn radial aspect of the TFCC in a horizontal mattress fashion, with each needle passing through the predrilled holes in the radius. (**TECH FIG 4C**).
  - The placement of the needles into the predrilled holes can be challenging since the holes are not visible by the scope in the 3-4 portal. Two 18-gauge spinal needles can be placed from the radial side of the radius through the bone until they can be seen in the joint at the attachment site for the TFCC. The needles provide a visible target for the meniscal repair suture needles.
- If the meniscal repair suture with long straight needles is not available, pass 18-gauge needles through the bone tunnels, then directly through the torn radial TFC. A 2-0 PDS suture is passed from one 18-gauge needle to the other using a wire retrieval loop.
- The suture is tied over the radius (**TECH FIG 4D**).
- A short-arm splint is applied.

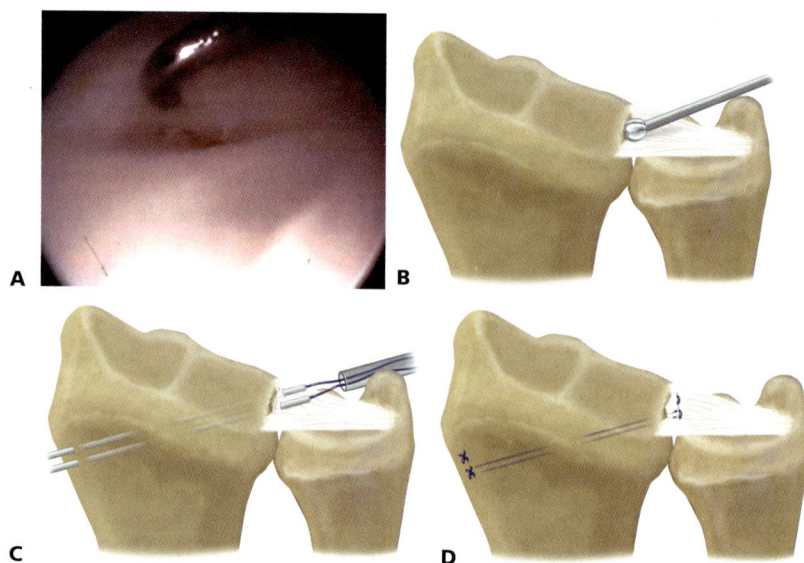

TECH FIG 4 • A. Traumatic radial TFC tear. Such an isolated tear can be débrided or repaired based on the degree of instability. **B.** Radial TFC tear repair. Burring of the attachment site along the sigmoid notch of the radius to bleeding bone is necessary to introduce additional vascularity and promote wound healing. **C,D.** Radial tears are repaired with suture on meniscal needles, tied over a bone bridge on the radial aspect of the distal radius.

PEARLS AND PITFALLS

Indications	▪ Traumatic and degenerative TFC lesions with sufficient symptoms ▪ If the DRUJ is stable, allow 3 to 4 months of nonoperative treatment.
Preoperative evaluation	▪ Assess ulna variance. ▪ Physical examination under anesthesia ▪ Complete diagnostic wrist arthroscopy of both radiocarpal and midcarpal joints ▪ A complete history and physical examination of ulnar wrist pain causes
Treatment options relate to type of TFC lesion	▪ 1A: arthroscopic débridement ▪ 1B without fracture: arthroscopic or open repair (DRUJ instability) ▪ 1B with ulna styloid fracture and instability: reattach ulna styloid ▪ 1C: Rare 1B repair plus ulnar extrinsic ligament repair ▪ 1D: If isolated, débride; if unstable, repair ▪ Degenerative lesions: arthroscopic wafer or ulna-shortening osteotomy
Pitfalls	▪ Excise only unstable central TFC portion. ▪ Protect dorsal sensory nerves and extensor tendons.

POSTOPERATIVE CARE

▪ After open or arthroscopic TFC repair, a short-arm splint or cast is applied for 4 to 6 weeks.

▪ Range-of-motion exercises are then progressed, using a removable splint for protection initially.

▪ Forceful wrist use is restricted for 3 months.

OUTCOMES

▪ Arthroscopic limited débridement of the central portion of the tear will provide excellent relief of symptoms, with 80% to 85% of patients having a good to excellent result.[15]

▪ The biomechanical effect of excision of the central portion of the TFCC has been examined.[1,6] The excision of the central two thirds of the TFCC with maintenance of the dorsal and volar radioulnar ligaments as well as the ulnocarpal ligaments had no statistical significant effect on forearm axial load transmission. The removal of greater than two thirds will unload the ulnar column, shifting load to the distal radius and destabilizing the DRUJ.

▪ Adams[1] further emphasized that the peripheral 2 mm of the TFCC must be maintained during central débridement in order not to have a biomechanical effect on load transfer.

▪ The results of arthroscopic repair of 1B TFCC lesions are equivalent to those reported for open repair. Gratifying outcomes are reached 85% to 90% of the time.[5,6,22]

▪ The treatment of radial detachment of the TFCC from the sigmoid notch of the distal radius remains controversial.

▪ Débridement of an isolated radial tear not associated with joint instability, similar to that for 1A lesions, yields excellent results.[15]

▪ Clinical experience with open repair of radial TFC avulsion tears has also been good.[6,21] Short[21] reported 79% excellent and good results in his series, with return of grip strength to 90%, after arthroscopic repair of radial TFCC tears.

COMPLICATIONS

▪ Failure to make a complete diagnosis (eg, associated ECU subluxation)

- Failure to appreciate DRUJ instability
- Loss of wrist motion
- Injury to dorsal sensory nerves
- Nonunion of the ulnar styloid or ulnar osteotomy

REFERENCES

1. Adams BD. Partial excision of the triangular fibrocartilage complex articular disk: a biomechanical study. J. Hand Surg Am 1993; 18A:334–340.
2. Bednar JM, Bos M, Giacobetti F. Comparison of the Accuracy of Clinical Exam and MRI in Diagnosing TFCC Lesions. Presented at the ASSH 52nd Annual Meeting, Sept. 11, 1997, Denver, Colorado.
3. Bednar MS, Arnoczky SP, Weiland AJ. The microvasculature of the triangular fibrocartilage complex: its clinical significance. J. Hand Surg Am 1991;16A:1101–1105.
4. Chun S, Palmer AK. The ulnar impaction syndrome: follow up of ulnar shortening osteotomy. J Hand Surg Am 1993;18A:46–53.
5. Corso SJ, Savoie FH, Geissler WB, et al. Arthroscopic repair of peripheral avulsions of the triangular fibrocartilage complex of the wrist: a multicenter study. Arthroscopy 1997;13:78–84.
6. Culp R, Osterman L, Kaufmann R. Wrist arthroscopy: operative procedures. In: Green D, Hotchkiss R, Pederson W, et al, eds. Green's Operative Hand Surgery, 5th ed, vol. 1. Philadelphia: Elsevier, 2005.
7. Ekenstein FW, Palmer AK, Glisson RR. The load on the radius and ulna in different positions of the wrist and forearm. Acta Orthop Scand 1984;55:363–365.
8. Geissler WB, Freeland AE, Savoie FH, et al. Intracarpal soft-tissue lesions associated with an intra-articular fracture of the distal end of the radius. J Bone Joint Surg Am 1996;78A:357–365.
9. Golimbu CN, Firoznia H, Melone CP Jr, et al. Tears of the triangular fibrocartilage of the wrist: MR imaging. Radiology 1989;173: 731–733.
10. Hermansdorfer JD, Kleinman WB. Management of chronic peripheral tears of the triangular fibrocartilage complex. J Hand Surg Am 1991;16A:340–346.
11. Joshy S, Ghosh S, Lee K, et al. Accuracy of direct magnetic resonance arthrography in the diagnosis of triangular fibrocartilage complex tears of the wrist. Int Orthop 2008;32:251–253 [e-pub Jan. 11, 2007].
12. Kostas JC, Tomaino MM, Herndon JH, et al. Comparison of ulnar shortening osteotomy and the wafer resection as a treatment for ulnar impaction syndrome. J Hand Surg Am 2000;25A:55–60.
13. Lindau T, Adlercreutz C, Aspenberg P. Peripheral tears of the triangular fibrocartilage complex cause distal radioulnar joint instability after distal radial fracture. J Hand Surg Am 2000;25A:464–468.
14. Mikic ZD. Age changes in the triangular fibrocartilage of the wrist joint. J Anat 1978;126:367–384.
15. Osterman AL. Arthroscopic debridement of triangular fibrocartilage complex tears. Arthroscopy 1990;6:120–124.
16. Palmer AK. Triangular fibrocartilage complex lesions: a classification. J Hand Surg Am 1989;14A:594–606.
17. Palmer AK, Werner FW. The triangular fibrocartilage complex of the wrist: anatomy and function. J. Hand Surg Am 1981;6A:153–162.
18. Palmer AK, Werner FW. Biomechanics of the distal radioulnar joint. Clin Orthop Relat Res 1984;187:26–34.
19. Schuind F, An KN, Berglund L, et al. The distal radioulnar ligaments: a biomechanical study. J Hand Surg Am 1991;16A:1106–1114.
20. Schweitzer ME, Brahme SK, Hodler J, et al. Chronic wrist pain: spin-echo and short tau inversion recovery MR imaging and conventional and MR arthrography. Radiology 1992;182:205–211.
21. Short WH. Arthroscopic repair of radial-sided triangular fibrocartilage complex tears. J Am Soc Surg Hand 2001;1:258–266.
22. Trumble TE, Gilbert M, Vedder N. Ulnar shortening combined with arthroscopic repairs in the delayed management of triangular fibrocartilage complex tears. J Hand Surg Am 1997;22A:807–813.
23. Viegas SF, Ballantyne G. Attritional lesions of the wrist joint. J Hand Surg Am 1987;12A:1025–1029.

Chapter 50

Intra-articular Radioulnar Ligament Reconstruction

Brian D. Adams and Christina M. Ward

DEFINITION

- Distal radioulnar joint (DRUJ) instability may be classified as acute or chronic, unidirectional (volar or dorsal) or bidirectional, and isolated or in association with other injuries.
- There is no consensus regarding the definition of clinically significant instability, though various radiographic criteria have been used. In general, the key physical finding is the presence of increased anteroposterior translation of the DRUJ with passive manipulation when compared with the normal side.
- Although the radius actually rotates around the stable ulna, by convention DRUJ dislocation or instability is described by the position of the ulnar head relative to the distal radius.

ANATOMY

- The DRUJ consists of the articulation between the ulnar head and the sigmoid notch of the distal radius and the associated supporting soft tissues.
- The DRUJ is not a congruent joint. The shallow sigmoid notch has a radius of curvature that is on average 50% greater than the ulnar head. Joint surface contact area is maximized at neutral rotation.[3] Though the sigmoid notch is relatively flat, the dorsal and volar rims, which are typically augmented by fibrocartilaginous extensions, do provide an important contribution to joint stability (**FIG 1A**).[13]
- The soft tissue structures that contribute to DRUJ stability are the pronator quadratus, extensor carpi ulnaris (ECU) and its sheath, interosseous membrane, DRUJ capsule, and several components of the triangular fibrocartilage complex (TFCC). Multiple structures must be injured to result in joint instability.[5]

- The palmar and dorsal radioulnar ligaments are the prime components of the TFCC that stabilize the DRUJ.[11] They are thickenings at the combined junctures of the triangular fibrocartilage articular disc, DRUJ capsule, and ulnocarpal capsule.
- As each radioulnar ligament passes ulnarly, it divides in the coronal plane into two limbs. The deep or proximal limbs of the radioulnar ligaments attach at the fovea and the superficial or distal limbs attach to the base and midportion of the ulnar styloid (**FIG 1B**).
- The total pronation–supination arc in a normal individual varies between 150 and 180 degrees. Normal pronation and supination involves a combination of rotation and dorsal-palmar translation of the distal radius on the stable ulna.

PATHOGENESIS

- The most common cause of DRUJ disruption is a fracture of the distal radius.
- Distal radius angulation greater than 20 or 30 degrees creates DRUJ incongruity, distorts the TFCC, and alters joint kinematics.[1,4] More than 5 to 7 mm of radial shortening results in rupture of at least one of the radioulnar ligaments.[1]
- Fractures of the tip of the ulnar styloid are not typically associated with DRUJ instability. Fractures of the base of the ulnar styloid can result in disruption of the radioulnar ligaments, causing DRUJ instability.[8]
- Most isolated DRUJ dislocations (not associated with a fracture) are dorsal and caused by forceful hyperpronation and wrist extension, such as with a fall on an outstretched hand or the sudden torque of a rotating power tool.

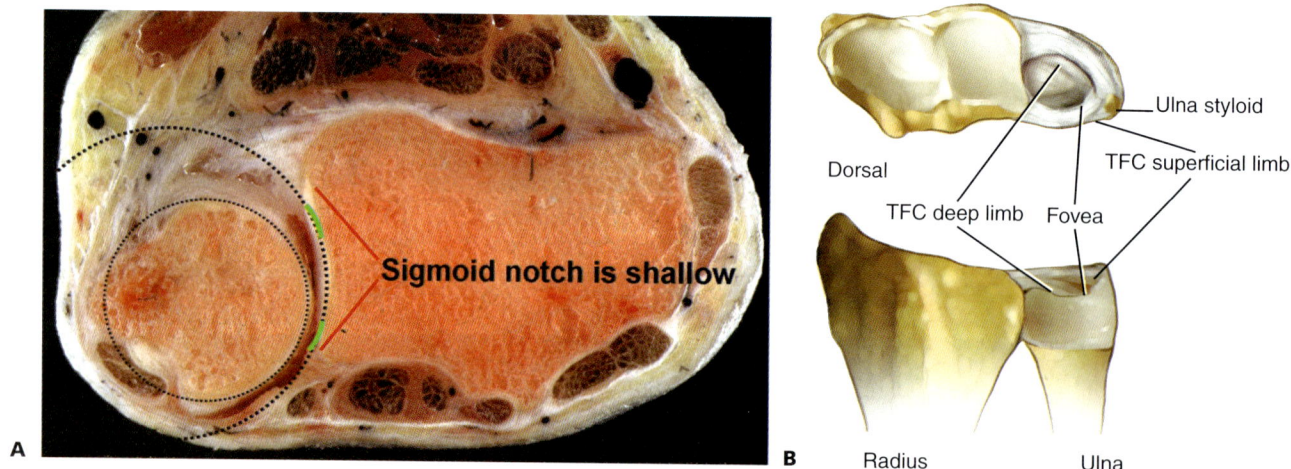

FIG 1 • **A.** Distal radioulnar joint (DRUJ) cross-section. The radius of curvature of the sigmoid notch is much greater than the radius of curvature of the ulnar head. **B.** DRUJ ligaments. (The disk component of the triangular fibrocartilage complex has been removed to show the deep limbs of the radioulnar ligaments.) The volar and dorsal radiopalmar ligaments, the major soft tissue stabilizers of the DRUJ, insert at the fovea and onto the base of the ulnar styloid.

- Isolated volar DRUJ dislocations occur with an injury to the supinated forearm or a direct blow to the ulnar aspect of the forearm.

NATURAL HISTORY

- Delayed diagnosis and treatment of DRUJ injuries associated with distal radius fractures results in worse outcomes.[7]
- Chronic instability rarely improves spontaneously.
- Although there is no proven association between DRUJ instability and the development of symptomatic arthritis, some degeneration should be expected in recurrent dislocators.

PATIENT HISTORY AND PHYSICAL FINDINGS

- Patients may report falling on an outstretched hand or a forced rotation of the hand followed by ulnar-sided wrist pain and swelling.
- Patients with chronic instability may report a clunk at the wrist with forearm rotation.
- Pain and weakness is exacerbated by activities requiring forceful rotation while gripping, such as turning a screwdriver.
- Increased passive volar-dorsal translation of the ulna relative to the radius is evidence of DRUJ instability.
- When treating an acute distal radius fracture with evidence of DRUJ disruption, the fracture should be reduced and stabilized first, followed by assessment of the DRUJ, as the fracture management alone usually provides adequate treatment for the DRUJ.
- In the absence of DRUJ arthritis, patients with DRUJ instability typically have full or nearly full wrist range of motion, including flexion, extension, pronation, and supination.
- A thorough patient examination should include the following tests:
    - Passive translation ("piano key" sign). Perform the test and compare results to the unaffected side. A positive test result indicates DRUJ instability, which is seen in 14 of 14 patients treated by ligament reconstruction.[2]
    - Modified press test. Increased depression of ulnar head on affected side ("dimple" sign) indicates instability.[2] Pain without increased depression may indicate a TFCC tear.[6]
    - Passive forearm rotation. A painful clunk indicates gross DRUJ instability. This should not be confused with more subtle ECU subluxation.

IMAGING AND OTHER DIAGNOSTIC STUDIES

- A zero-rotation posteroanterior view is obtained by abducting the humerus 90 degrees, flexing the elbow 90 degrees, and placing the forearm on a flat surface. Signs of DRUJ instability on this view include:
    - Displaced fracture at the base of the ulnar styloid
    - Fleck fracture from the fovea of the ulnar head
    - Widening of the DRUJ
    - Greater than 5 mm of acquired ulnar or positive variance compared to the opposite wrist
- A true lateral radiograph is performed with the arm at the patient's side and the elbow flexed 90 degrees. Obtaining a true lateral radiograph is important to avoid inaccurate assessment of DRUJ alignment. Mino et al[9] showed that only 10 degrees of rotation from neutral resulted in an inability to correctly diagnose DRUJ dislocation on the lateral radiograph.

- On a true lateral wrist radiograph, the lunate, proximal pole of the scaphoid, and triquetrum should overlap completely and there should be no space between the triquetrum and pisiform.
- CT must be performed on both wrists, with each image obtained with the forearm in identical rotation to allow comparison between the normal and symptomatic joints (**FIG 2**).
- The addition of applied stress to the joint during imaging may aid in detection of subtle instability.[10]
- MRI (with or without intra-articular dye) may be used to detect TFCC tears, although the reported sensitivity and specificity for such injuries is variable. MRI can also be used instead of CT to assess the shape of the sigmoid notch and joint stability.

DIFFERENTIAL DIAGNOSIS

- ECU tendinitis or subluxation
- Ulnar impaction syndrome
- DRUJ arthritis
- Pisotriquetral arthritis
- Lunotriquetral ligament injuries
- TFCC disc tears

NONOPERATIVE MANAGEMENT

- Patients with mild chronic instability may benefit from a course of nonsteroidal anti-inflammatories, a splint that limits forearm rotation, and a forearm strengthening program.
- Patients with generalized ligamentous laxity and bilateral DRUJ instability have less predictable results with operative reconstruction. In such patients, all attempts at conservative management should be exhausted before considering surgery.

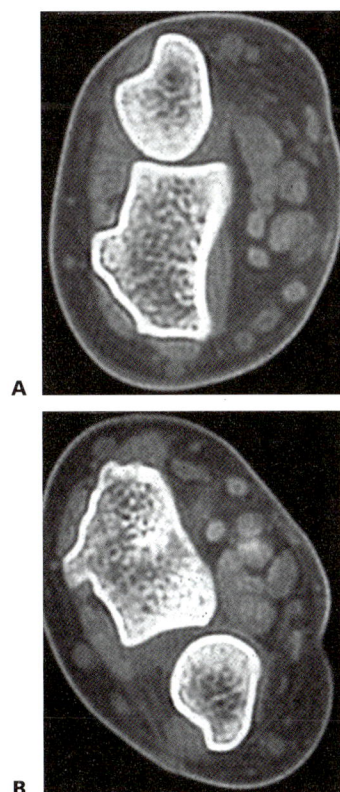

FIG 2 • CT of distal radioulnar joint (DRUJ). **A.** Well-reduced asymptomatic DRUJ. **B.** Subluxated DRUJ on the symptomatic side. (**A, B:** dorsal is left and volar is right.)

SURGICAL MANAGEMENT

▪ Distal radioulnar ligament reconstruction is indicated in cases of chronic DRUJ instability where tissues are inadequate for primary repair of the TFCC.

▪ The goal of ligament reconstruction is to restore DRUJ stability and provide a full, painless arc of forearm motion.

▪ The technique described creates stability by near-anatomic reconstruction of the dorsal and volar radioulnar ligaments.

▪ If present, osseous malalignment must be addressed at the time of ligament reconstruction to obtain a good result.

Preoperative Planning

▪ The surgeon should review imaging studies for evidence of osseous deformity or degeneration of the DRUJ articular surfaces. Soft tissue reconstruction in the presence of substantial residual bony deformity or arthritis will yield poor results.

▪ Intra-articular radioulnar ligament reconstruction requires a competent sigmoid notch for success. A notch that is developmentally flat or that has posttraumatic deficiency of either rim should be treated with a sigmoid notch osteoplasty at the time of ligament reconstruction.

▪ The surgeon should determine the presence of suitable tendon graft. The palmaris longus (PL) tendon is typically used. Alternative graft sources include plantaris, extensor digitorum longus, or most commonly a strip of the flexor carpi ulnaris tendon.

▪ The PL tendon can be identified by having the patient flex the wrist while holding the tips of the thumb and small finger together.

Positioning

▪ The patient is positioned supine with the affected limb resting on a hand table. Additional positioning may be necessary to allow access to graft harvest sites.

▪ A well-padded tourniquet is placed on the upper arm.

PALMARIS TENDON GRAFT HARVEST

▪ The PL tendon is identified by palpation. It is one of the most superficial structures at the distal wrist crease and lies just ulnar to the flexor carpi radialis tendon (**TECH FIG 1A**).

▪ A single 1-cm transverse incision is made at the proximal volar wrist crease overlying the PL tendon (**TECH FIG 1B**).

▪ A shepherd's hook is used to pull tension on the tendon and absolutely confirm its identity.

▪ The tendon is clamped with a hemostat and transected just distal to the hemostat.

▪ A small tendon stripper is passed distal to proximal along the PL tendon in the forearm to complete the harvest.

▪ Alternatively, a strip of the flexor carpi ulnaris tendon can be harvested using a tendon stripper through the same volar incision for graft passage.

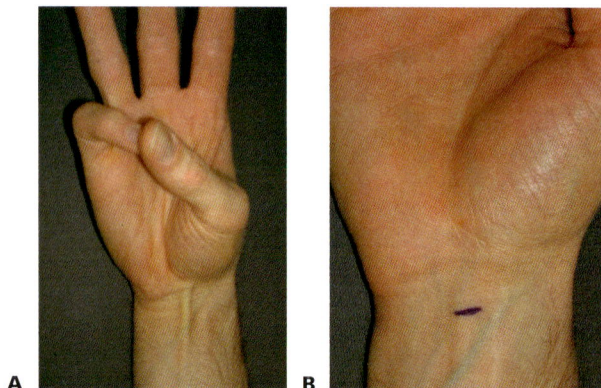

A   **B**

TECH FIG 1 • Graft harvest. **A.** The palmaris tendon can be brought into relief by having the patient touch the thumb and small fingers while flexing the wrist slightly. **B.** A small transverse incision is made at the proximal wrist crease.

DORSAL APPROACH

▪ A 5-cm skin incision is made between the fifth and sixth extensor compartments overlying the DRUJ (**TECH FIG 2A**).

▪ The fifth compartment is opened and the extensor digiti minimi is retracted.

▪ An L-shaped capsulotomy is made in the DRUJ capsule

with one limb in line with the sigmoid notch and the other just proximal and parallel to the TFCC (**TECH FIG 2B**). The ECU tendon sheath marks the ulnar limit of the capsulotomy.

▪ The ECU tendon sheath is not disrupted during this approach.

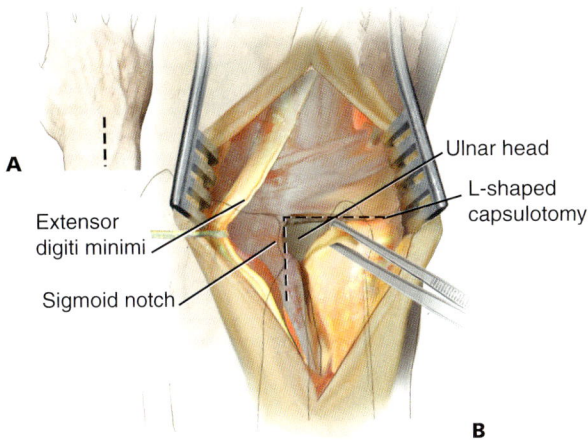

A

B

Ulnar head

L-shaped capsulotomy

Extensor digiti minimi

Sigmoid notch

TECH FIG 2 • Dorsal approach to distal radioulnar joint (DRUJ). **A.** Dorsal skin incision. **B.** Capsulotomy over the DRUJ.

BONE TUNNEL PLACEMENT

- Careful subperiosteal dissection is used to elevate the soft tissue from the dorsal edge of the sigmoid notch for several millimeters.
- A guidewire for a 3.5-mm cannulated drill bit is driven from dorsal to volar through the radius.
  - The tunnel should begin several millimeters proximal to the lunate fossa and about 5 mm radial to the articular surface of the sigmoid notch (**TECH FIG 3A**).
  - The tunnel should be parallel to the articular surfaces of both the sigmoid notch and lunate fossa.
- Fluoroscopy is used to confirm guidewire placement, and the tunnel is made with a 3.5-mm cannulated drill bit (**TECH FIG 3B**).
- If a corrective osteotomy of the radius is planned, it is easier to make the bone tunnels before performing an osteotomy, but the tendon graft should not be placed or tensioned until the osteotomy is completed.

- The ulnar flap of the DRUJ capsulotomy is elevated to expose the ulnar head and neck, being careful not to interrupt the ECU tendon sheath.
- The ulnar bone hole travels from the ulnar fovea to exit on the lateral ulnar neck just volar to the ECU tendon (see Tech Fig 3A). Flex the wrist pronate the forearm, and retract the TFCC remnant to reveal the ulnar fovea. Pass a guidewire retrograde from the ulnar fovea to exit on the lateral ulnar neck just volar to the ECU tendon. Confirm the guidewire position with fluoroscopy. If flexing the wrist does not provide adequate exposure, the tunnel may be created antegrade from ulnar neck to fovea, while carefully protecting any TFCC remnant and the ulnar carpus (**TECH FIG 3C**).
- Standard drill bits may be used to enlarge the bone tunnels to accommodate the previously harvested graft. The ulnar bone tunnel must accommodate both limbs of the tendon graft.

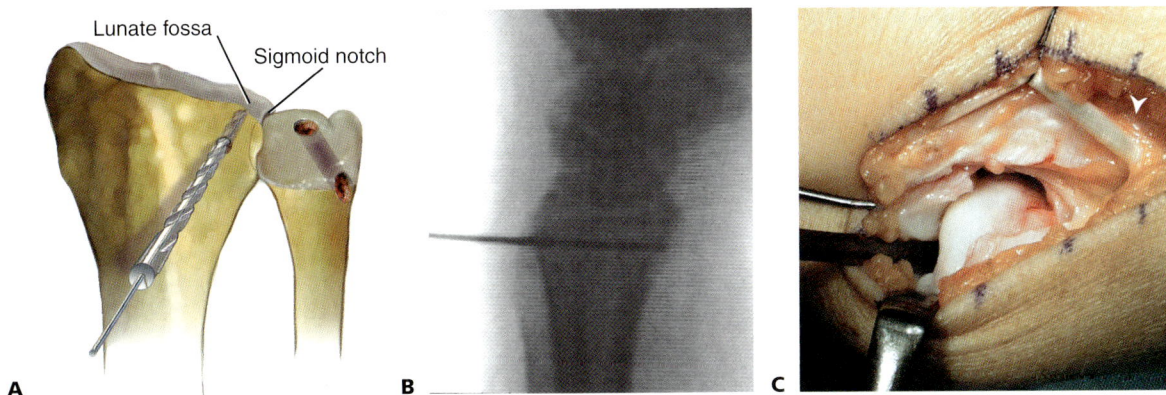

A

B

C

Lunate fossa

Sigmoid notch

TECH FIG 3 • Tunnel placement. **A.** Bone tunnels are placed to mimic the normal anatomic attachments of the dorsal and volar radioulnar ligaments. **B.** Fluoroscopy is used to confirm bone tunnel placement. **C.** The probe indicates the location of the fovea on the ulnar head where the drill should exit. The *arrowhead* indicates the extensor carpi ulnaris tendon being retracted.

GRAFT PASSAGE

- A second exposure is made to visualize the volar aspect of the radius bone tunnel.
- A 3-cm longitudinal incision is made extending proximally from the proximal wrist crease (TECH FIG 4A).
- Dissection is carried down between the ulnar neurovascular bundle and finger flexor tendons to reach the volar surface of the radius.
- A suture passer is passed through the radius bone tunnel from dorsal to volar and used to pull one end of the tendon graft back through the distal radius (TECH FIG 4B).
- A straight hemostat is passed over the ulnar head, dorsal to volar, to bluntly pierce the volar DRUJ capsule just

distal to the ulnar head. The other end of the graft is grasped and pulled back through the capsule.
- At this point, both tendon ends should be visible through the dorsal wound. The suture retriever is used to pass both tendon ends through the ulna bone tunnel from the fovea to exit at the ulnar neck (TECH FIG 4C).
- A curved hemostat is used to guide the tendon ends around a portion of the ulnar neck in opposite directions, with one limb of the graft passing deep to the ECU sheath and the other around the volar neck (TECH FIG 4D).
- Avoid entrapping any nearby neurovascular structures.

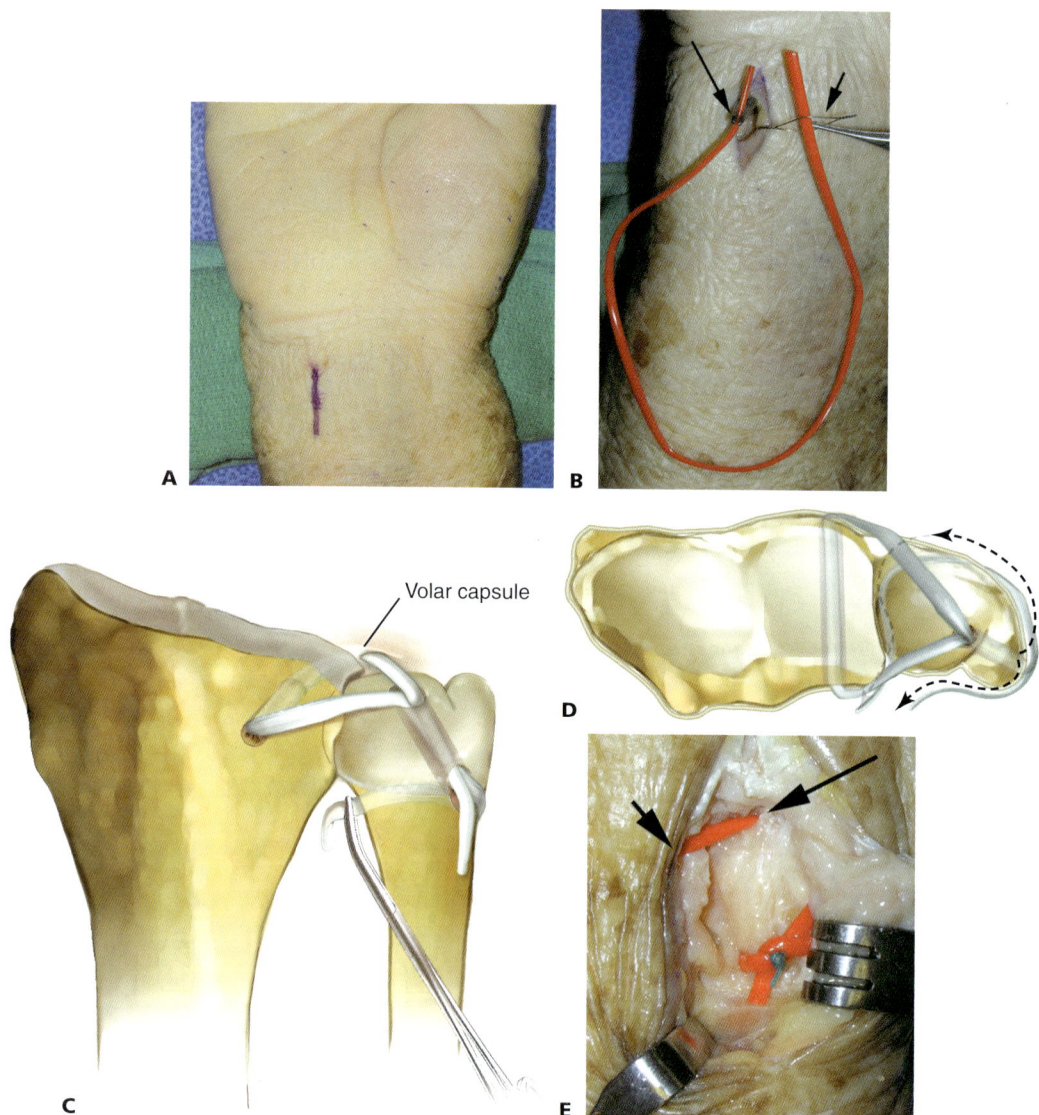

TECH FIG 4 • Graft passage. **A.** A small volar approach is necessary to allow graft passage. **B.** A suture passer travels through the radial bone tunnel (dorsal to volar) to retrieve one limb of the graft (indicated by a red vessel loop). **C.** In this dorsal view, the graft is brought through the volar capsule into the ulnocarpal joint then the two ends are fed into the ulna tunnel. **D.** In this axial drawing the course of the free graft is visualized. The graft provides a near-anatomic reconstruction of the volar and dorsal radioulnar ligaments. **E.** The graft (red vessel loop) exits the radial bone hole (*short arrow*) into the dorsal wound and then enters the ulnar bone hole through the fovea (*long arrow*). The ends of the graft are then wrapped around the ulna neck.

TECHNIQUES

GRAFT TENSIONING AND FIXATION

- The forearm is held in neutral rotation and the DRUJ is manually compressed.
- The two graft limbs are pulled taut and a half-hitch knot is made against the dorsal aspect of the ulnar neck.
- While maintaining firm tension in the graft, the half-hitch is secured with 3-0 nonabsorbable sutures (**TECH FIG 5**).

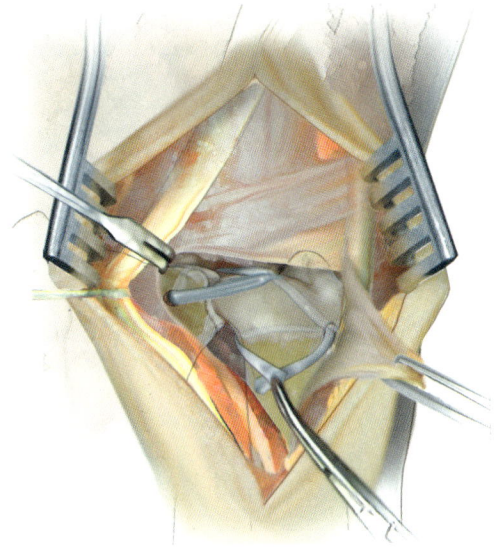

TECH FIG 5 • Graft tensioning. Tension is held on the graft while the knot is secured with a suture.

PEARLS AND PITFALLS

Indications	▪ Patients with chronic DRUJ instability in whom the TFCC cannot be repaired
	▪ Confirm the patient does not have DRUJ arthritis or a deficient sigmoid notch.
Graft management	▪ Harvest the graft early to determine bone tunnel size.
	▪ Use a suture passer to facilitate graft passage.
Tunnel placement	▪ Place the tunnel an adequate distance from the articular surfaces of the DRUJ and lunate fossa to prevent fracturing into the joint.
	▪ If concurrently performing a corrective osteotomy, make the bone tunnels before completing the osteotomy.

POSTOPERATIVE CARE

- The patient is placed in a long-arm splint with the forearm in neutral to slight pronation or supination, depending on the most stable DRUJ position. At the first postoperative visit, the patient is transitioned to a long-arm cast for 3 weeks.
- At 4 weeks postoperatively, the patient is placed in a well-molded short-arm cast for an additional 2 weeks.
- At 6 weeks after surgery, the cast is changed to a removable splint, which is worn for an additional 4 weeks.
- The patient should be able to return to most activities by 4 months after surgery, but heavy lifting and impact loading are avoided until 6 months postoperatively.

OUTCOMES

- Patients with a deficient sigmoid notch are more likely to experience recurrent instability if the deficits are not corrected.
- Most patients experience decreased pain and improved strength and stability while maintaining near normal range of motion. However, full recovery may require 6 to 9 months.
  - The described technique effectively restored stability in 12 of 14 patients while providing about 85% of the strength and range of motion of the contralateral unaffected side.[2] The two failures resulted from deficiencies of the sigmoid notch that were not recognized preoperatively.

- Teoh and Yam[12] reported similar results, with restoration of stability in seven of nine patients using a similar reconstructive method.

COMPLICATIONS

- Joint stiffness
- Recurrent instability
- Persistent pain
- Weakness of grasp
- Infection
- Complex regional pain syndrome

REFERENCES

1. Adams BD. Effects of radial deformity on distal radioulnar joint mechanics. J Hand Surg Am 1993;18A:492–498.
2. Adams BD, Berger RA. An anatomic reconstruction of the distal radioulnar ligaments for posttraumatic distal radioulnar joint instability. J Hand Surg Am 2002;27A:243–251.
3. Ekenstam F. Anatomy of the distal radioulnar joint. Clin Orthop Relat Res 1992;275:14–18.
4. Kihara H, Palmer AK, Werner FW, et al. The effect of dorsally angulated distal radius fractures on distal radioulnar joint congruency and forearm rotation. J Hand Surg Am 1996;21A:40–47.
5. Kihara H, Short WH, Werner FW, et al. The stabilizing mechanism of the distal radioulnar joint during pronation and supination. J Hand Surg Am 1995;20A:930–936.

6. Lester B, Halbrecht J, Levy IM, et al. "Press test" for office diagnosis of triangular fibrocartilage complex tears of the wrist. Ann Plast Surg 1995;35:41–45.

7. Lindau T, Hagberg L, Adlercreutz C, et al. Distal radioulnar instability is an independent worsening factor in distal radial fractures. Clin Orthop Relat Res 2000;376:229–235.

8. May MM, Lawton JN, Blazar PE. Ulnar styloid fractures associated with distal radius fractures: incidence and implications for distal radioulnar joint instability. J Hand Surg Am 2002;27A:965–971.

9. Mino DE, Palmer AK, Levinsohn EM. Radiography and computerized tomography in the diagnosis of incongruity of the distal radio-ulnar joint: a prospective study. J Bone Joint Surg Am 1985;67A:247–252.

10. Pirela-Cruz MA, Goll SR, Klug M, et al. Stress computed tomography analysis of the distal radioulnar joint: a diagnostic tool for determining translational motion. J Hand Surg Am 1991;16A:75–82.

11. Stuart PR, Berger RA, Linscheid RL, et al. The dorsopalmar stability of the distal radioulnar joint. J Hand Surg Am 2000;25A:689–699.

12. Teoh LC, Yam AKT. Anatomic reconstruction of the distal radioulnar ligaments: long-term results. J Hand Surg Br 2005;30B:185–193.

13. Tolat AR, Stanley JK, Trail IA. A cadaveric study of the anatomy and stability of the distal radioulnar joint in the coronal and transverse planes. J Hand Surg Br 1996;21B:587–594.

Chapter 51

Extra-articular Reconstructive Techniques for the Distal Radioulnar and Ulnocarpal Joints

Christopher J. Dy, E. Anne Ouellette, and Anna-Lena Makowski

DEFINITION

- The diagnostic and therapeutic challenge presented by instability of the ulnocarpal joint reflects the inherent biomechanical and anatomic incongruity of the articulation.
- The triangular fibrocartilage complex (TFCC) provides the majority of anatomic and functional stability of the distal radioulnar and ulnocarpal joints.[1,16]
- As expected, the consequences of TFCC lesions reflect a disruption of its normal function. The Hui-Linscheid procedure and the modified Herbert reconstruction are two approaches to achieve surgical stabilization of the distal radioulnar joint (DRUJ). The Hui-Linscheid reconstruction stabilizes the DRUJ by augmenting function of the ulnocarpal ligament,[6] while the modified Herbert reconstruction restores the radioulnar and ulnocarpal functions of the TFCC by ligamentotaxic constraint of the ulnar carpus.[3]

ANATOMY

- The ulnar carpus does not directly articulate with the distal ulna; instead, the ulnar carpus is suspended from the ulnar head by the TFCC.
- The TFCC is a collection of soft tissue structures that stabilizes the radial-ulnar-carpal unit (**FIG 1**). It consists of fibers originating from the subsheath of the extensor carpi ulnaris, the ulnocarpal ligaments, the dorsal and palmar radioulnar ligaments, and the triangular fibrocartilage proper.
- The TFCC provides a continuous gliding surface that spans the distal surfaces of the radius and ulna, allowing carpal movements and acting as a dynamic stabilizer of the forearm during pronation and supination.[12,18] In addition to its radioulnar function, the TFCC stabilizes the ulnar side of the carpus, aids in load transference from the ulnar carpus to the ulna, and cushions ulnocarpal forces.[16]
- The dorsal and volar distal radioulnar ligaments, which are often referred to as the marginal ligaments, help to stabilize the radioulnar joint through its extremes of motion.
  - While controversy exists concerning the exact role of each marginal ligament, several authors have agreed that the ligaments act in concert to stabilize the DRUJ during pronosupination.
- The extensor retinaculum is a thick fibrous band of tissue that holds the extensor tendons against the distal radius and ulna to prevent bowstringing and displacement of the tendons (**FIG 2**). It is continuous with the palmar carpal ligament and shares connecting fibers with the flexor retinaculum just proximal to the pisiform. The extensor retinaculum attaches to the pisiform and triquetrum medially and to the lateral margin of the radius laterally. It is positioned from a radial-proximal to ulnar-distal direction.[15,19]

PATHOGENESIS

- Injuries to the TFCC can occur secondary to trauma, such as a fall on the outstretched hand, or from degenerative changes caused by repetitive loading, especially in patients with rheumatoid arthritis. Palmer has classified TFCC abnormalities by differentiating between traumatic and degenerative pathologies, with further specification within each group.[11]
- Dorsal subluxation of the ulnar head, with or without supination deformity of the radiocarpal complex and ulnocarpal instability, can occur with attenuation or tears of the dorsal radioulnar ligaments.[16,18] The Hui-Linscheid reconstruction repairs these defects through augmentation of ulnocarpal ligament

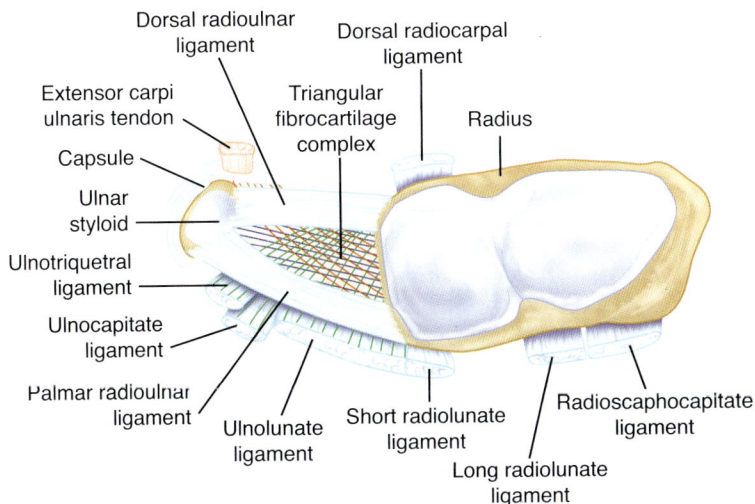

FIG 1 • The soft tissue structures encompassing the triangular fibrocartilage complex of the wrist stabilizing the radial-ulnar-carpal unit. The triangular fibrocartilage proper originates from the radius medially and attaches to the base of the ulnar styloid. Fibers originating from the subsheath of the extensor carpi ulnaris dorsally cross paths with fibers originating from the ulnocarpal ligaments volarly and blend with the triangular fibrocartilage proper.

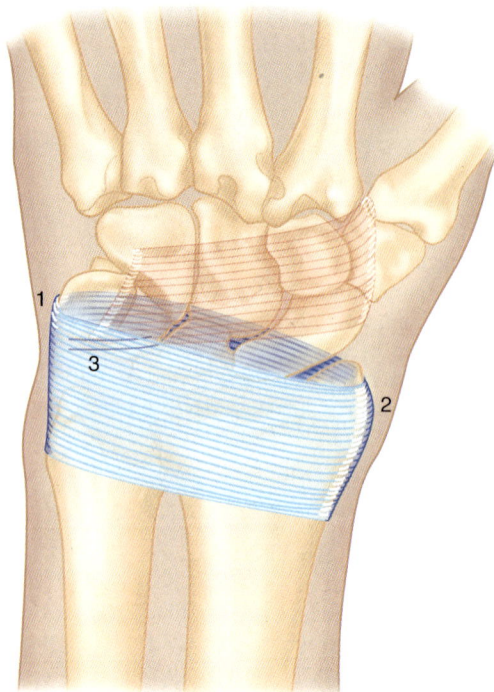

FIG 2 • Extensor retinaculum (*light blue*), flexor retinaculum (*shaded red*), and palmar carpal ligament (*dark blue*). The extensor retinaculum inserts in the pisiform and triquetrum bones (*1*) medially and connects with the lateral margin of the radius laterally (*2*), causing its orientation to be radial-proximal to ulnar-distal. The extensor and flexor retinaculum connects proximal to the pisiform (*3*). The extensor retinaculum is continuous with the palmar carpal ligament, which is superficial to and proximal to the flexor retinaculum.

function and an optional imbrication of the attenuated dorsal radioulnar ligament.[4,6]

■ Ulnocarpal instability may also result from incompetence of the ulnocarpal ligaments, either secondary to acute trauma or from accumulative attrition.[1,7] The modified Herbert reconstruction addresses ulnocarpal instability by using ligamentotaxis to stabilize both the ulnocarpal and radioulnar aspects of the DRUJ.[3,13]

NATURAL HISTORY

■ Ulnocarpal instability is a relatively common finding in the general population. Approximately two thirds of asymptomatic volunteers were found to have some form of ulnocarpal instability on physical examination.[10] Medical or surgical intervention is necessary if symptoms are present or are worsening.

■ The unstable ulnocarpal joint uses the radiocarpal joint as a pivot. The abnormal rotation in this pathologic state leads to increased pain, weakness, and loss of function during wrist supination. In addition, an ulnar-sided supination deformity may be present.

PATIENT HISTORY AND PHYSICAL FINDINGS

■ In both acute and chronic cases, the clinical presentation of the ulnocarpal instability consists of ulnar-sided wrist pain with or without clicking, especially with forearm pronation–supination activities, such as putting topspin on a tennis ball with a forehand shot.

■ There may be demonstrable laxity during supination and weakness in passive or active pronation–supination movements. These symptoms may hinder range of motion and function of the wrist.

■ On physical examination, patients often localize tenderness to the ulnar carpus on palpation.

  ▪ The examiner should palpate the ulnar styloid.

  ▪ The examiner should palpate between the ulnar styloid and triquetrum.

■ Visual inspection of the ulnocarpal area is important, looking for swelling and alignment of the carpal area in relation to the ulna. Swelling may be the result of acute injury. Position of tissues indicates stability or instability.

■ In the absence of concomitant pathology, provocative maneuvers such as Watson and shuck tests are negative.

  ▪ Watson test: Pain and movement of the scaphoid despite blocking its normal capacity to flex in radial deviation is an indication of scapholunate tear or laxity.

  ▪ The Shuck test is performed to evaluate lunotriquetral instabilities.

  ▪ A positive piano key test indicates a complete peripheral tear of the TFCC and/or dorsal radioulnar ligament tear.

  ▪ Midcarpal instability can be ruled out with a negative wrist pivot shift test, as first described by Lichtman et al.[9]

■ In patients with ulnocarpal instability, the wrist assumes an ulnar-sided supination deformity similar to that seen in rheumatoid arthritis.

■ A key to diagnosing ulnocarpal instability is the supination test, which is a diagnostic maneuver developed by the first author. This examination is performed by stabilizing the affected DRUJ with a firm grasp while stressing the wrist in supination and volar translation.

  ▪ When the wrist is loaded axially and returned through neutral in ulnar deviation, the patient's pain is reproduced. The wrist may also "clunk" back into reduction.

  ▪ The contralateral wrist is also tested for comparison.

IMAGING AND OTHER DIAGNOSTIC STUDIES

■ Standard posteroanterior and lateral radiographs have poor diagnostic value for ulnocarpal joint instabilities but can be used to rule out scapholunate interosseous ligament (SLIL) and lunatotriquetral interosseous ligament (LTIL) tears. On a pure lateral view, if there is DRUJ instability, the ulna will be dorsally positioned relative to the radius instead of being seen superimposed on the radius.

■ Computed tomography is useful for visualizing joint congruity and fractures as well as subluxation or dislocation of the DRUJ.

■ Live fluoroscopy during the supination test allows the examiner to evaluate and visualize the presence and amount of ulnocarpal joint instability (**FIG 3**).

  ▪ The changing appearance of the triquetrum, demonstrated by its decreased length while in a position of supination, indicates ulnocarpal instability.

  ▪ The pisiform's location in relation to the triquetrum may also indicate the type of ligamentous tear or laxity by either moving together with the triquetrum during the supination test or appearing to be stationary as the triquetrum is moving.[5]

■ Triple-injection arthrography of the midcarpal row, radiocarpal joint, and DRUJ can be useful in showing SLIL or

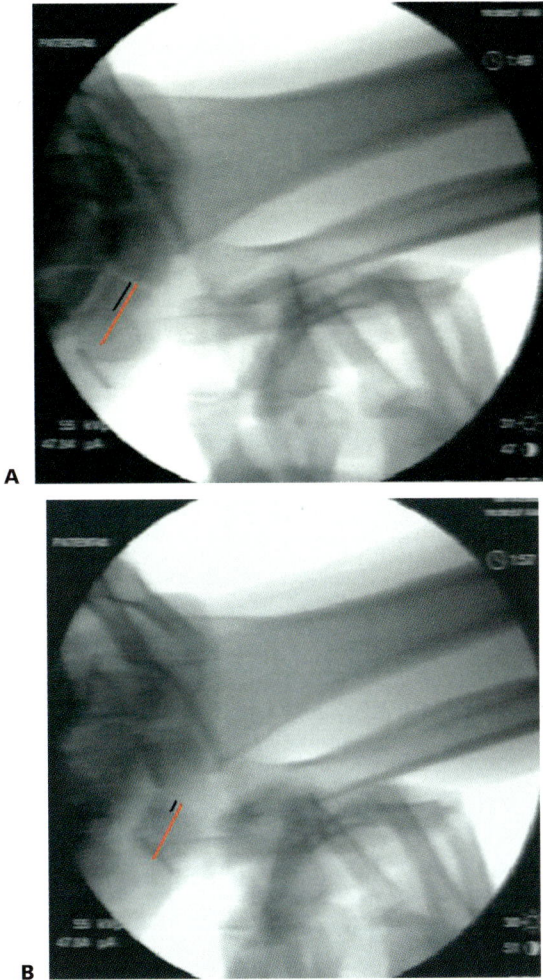

FIG 3 • The still photographs shown have been captured from a fluoroscopy video of a wrist with ulnocarpal instability during the supination test. **A.** Top of the examination cycle with the wrist in neutral position. **B.** Bottom of the examination cycle. In both images, the *black line* represents the distance between proximal edges of pisiform and triquetrum. The *red line* indicates the length of the triquetrum. The shorter length of the red and black lines in **B** compared with **A** demonstrates the ulnocarpal instability present during dynamic testing.

LTIL tears, TFCC tears, and ulnar-sided TFCC tears, respectively.

■ The findings must correlate with symptoms for accurate diagnosis.[8,17]

■ Standard magnetic resonance (MR) imaging effectively demonstrates the normal anatomy of the TFCC as well as the intrinsic and extrinsic ligaments of the wrist.

■ Abnormalities of these structures can be detected with experience, but the radiographic literature has reported shortcomings of standard MR in diagnosing peripheral TFCC tears.

■ MR arthrography, with injection of contrast into the DRUJ, has been shown as an adequate way of diagnosing peripheral TFCC tears, with a sensitivity of 85% and specificity of 76% when compared to wrist arthroscopy.[14]

■ Wrist arthroscopy is widely considered the gold standard of diagnostic studies of the wrist joint. Arthroscopic visualization

allows for the determination of the size, location, and extent of ligamentous injuries of the wrist.

■ Comparison of arthroscopy to arthrography by Cooney[2] revealed arthroscopy to be the superior method of diagnosing injuries of the TFCC and interosseous ligaments.

DIFFERENTIAL DIAGNOSIS

■ Fracture
■ DRUJ instability
■ Extensor carpi ulnaris subluxation
■ TFCC lesions
■ Ulnar impaction syndrome
■ Degenerative changes of DRUJ and ulnar carpus
■ Carpal instability, scapholunate tear (dorsal intercalated segment instability [DISI]), lunotriquetral tear (volar intercalated segment instability [VISI])
■ Tendinitis
■ Chondromalacia
■ Ligament injuries
■ Ulnocarpal instability

NONOPERATIVE MANAGEMENT

■ Conservative treatment includes the use of a removable soft leather splint that minimizes motion of the wrist, such as those originally designed for use by gymnasts.

■ If the patient wishes to return to athletic activities, he or she should proceed with cautious limitation while wearing a sports splint.

■ Although these splints allow for motion of the wrist and for the use of athletic tools, the patient must understand that he or she must reduce the intensity of activity to a level that the wrist will tolerate.

■ When activity levels are limited or more support is needed, such as while sleeping, a static splint is advised.

■ Physical or occupational therapy, including training to increase range of motion and to strengthen the muscles spanning the ulnocarpal and distal radioulnar joints, may be beneficial.

■ Nonsteroidal anti-inflammatories are also recommended before deciding on surgery, with an initial trial of 4 to 6 weeks.

SURGICAL MANAGEMENT

■ The main indication for surgery is a painful ulnocarpal joint with diminished grip or pronosupination strength (or both) that does not respond to conservative treatment.

■ Individuals with high demand for strong wrist function in weight-bearing supination (eg, golfers, tennis players, certain skilled labor professions) may be considered for surgery even without first receiving conservative treatment.

Preoperative Planning

■ The surgeon should review all imaging studies to identify any concomitant pathology of the wrist joint.

■ Arthroscopic examination of the wrist is generally undertaken immediately before ulnocarpal reconstruction to address any concomitant lesions or synovitis within the wrist.

■ Diagnostic physical examination maneuvers are repeated while the patient is under anesthesia. These maneuvers include the piano key test and ulnocarpal supination test, as described earlier.

Positioning

▪ Using an arm board, the patient is positioned with the forearm in pronation and the elbow flexed at 45 degrees. The dorsal aspect of the wrist joint is prepared in a sterile manner.

Approach

▪ Modified Herbert reconstruction
  ▪ Exposure of the dorsal surface of the wrist joint is the only surgical approach needed for the Herbert sling repair.
  ▪ The Herbert sling procedure consists of the development of an ulnar-based flap of the extensor retinaculum, advanced at a 30- to 40-degree angle from distal ulnar to proximal radial by securing into the distal radial retinacular attachments.
▪ This reduces the radioulnar joint and the carpus to the ulna with a single advancement of the extensor retinaculum (**FIG 4**).
▪ Hui-Linscheid reconstruction
  ▪ A standard incision on the dorsal surface of the wrist is used to access the ulnocarpal articulation, the ulnar head, and the flexor carpi ulnaris.
  ▪ A tendon graft is harvested from the flexor carpi ulnaris and passed through the tunnel in the ulnar head and looped back to its proximal insertion on the pisiform.

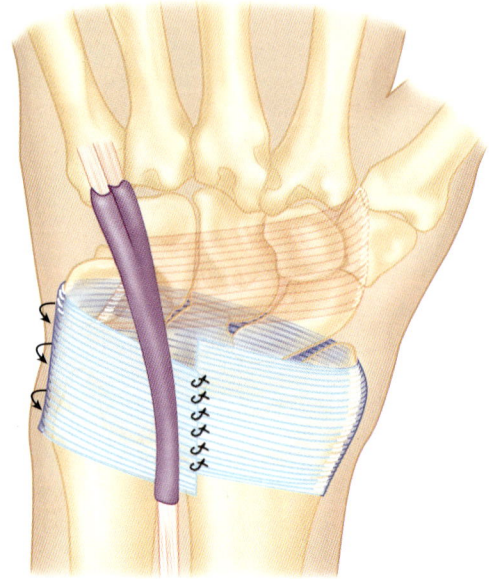

FIG 4 • The extensor digiti quinti is relocated dorsally of the extensor retinaculum. This procedure uses ligament materials to create an effective sling, providing support to the distal radioulnar and ulnocarpal joints. The ulnar-based extensor retinaculum flap is advanced in a distal-ulnar to radial-proximal direction. *Arrows* illustrate the direction of the ligamentotaxis.

TECHNIQUES

MODIFIED HERBERT RECONSTRUCTION

▪ Create a longitudinal incision over the fifth extensor compartment at the level of the wrist (**TECH FIG 1A**).
▪ Incise the extensor retinaculum between the fourth and fifth compartments, taking care not to enter the fourth compartment (**TECH FIG 1B**).
▪ Raise an ulnarly based flap of the distal two thirds of the retinaculum, and prepare the extensor digiti quinti (EDQ) for transposition dorsal to the retinaculum flap (**TECH FIG 1C**).

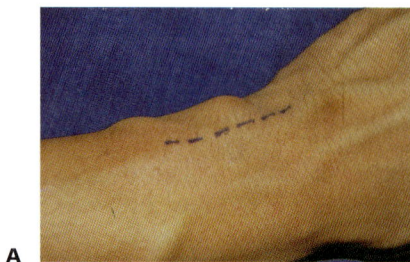

A

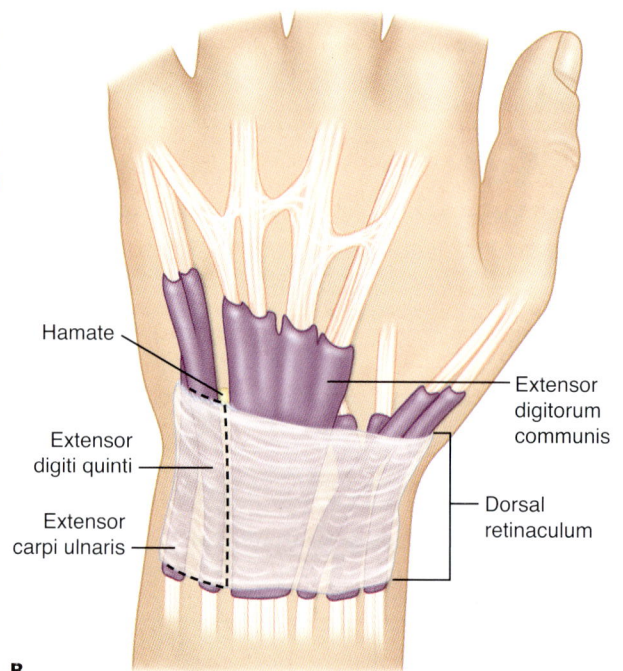

B

TECH FIG 1 • Modified Herbert reconstruction. **A.** A longitudinal incision over the fifth extensor compartment at the wrist is created. **B.** Plan the transection of the extensor retinaculum along the extensor digiti quinti. Incise the extensor retinaculum, taking care not to enter the fourth compartment. *(continued)*

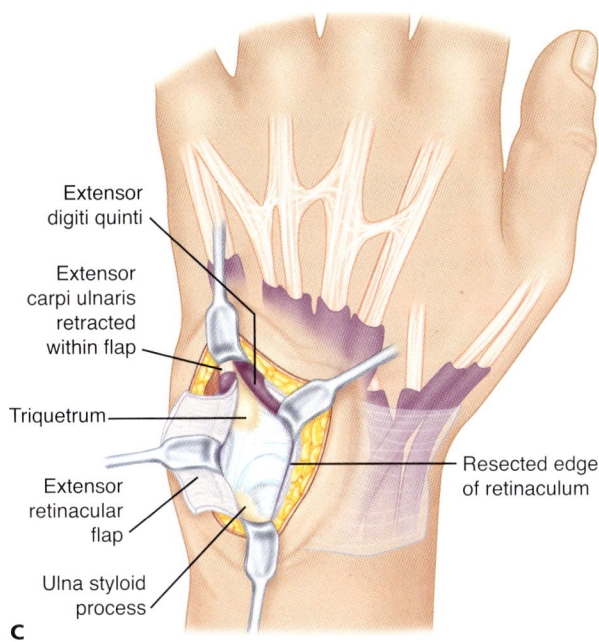

C

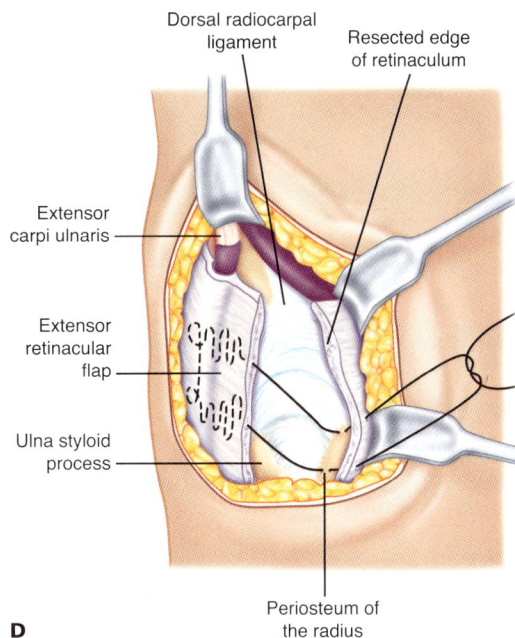

D

TECH FIG 1 • *(continued)* **C.** Raise an ulnar-based flap. Prepare the extensor digiti quinti to be transposed dorsal to the extensor retinaculum. **D.** The retinacular flap is sutured to the periosteum of the ulnar border on the distal radius. **E.** Imbricate the extensor retinaculum obliquely in a distal-ulnar to radial-proximal direction. The extensor digiti quinti should remain dorsally of the imbricated extensor retinaculum flap.

- Place the wrist in neutral and apply downward force on the distal ulna to reduce the DRUJ.
- Translate the retinacular flap proximally and suture it to the periosteum of the ulnar border of the distal radius using 2-0 PDS absorbable sutures (**TECH FIG 1D**).
  - Carefully imbricate the extensor retinaculum in an oblique fashion (30 to 40 degrees) from distal-ulnar to radial-proximal (**TECH FIG 1E**).
  - The EDQ is relocated dorsally of the imbricated extensor retinaculum flap.

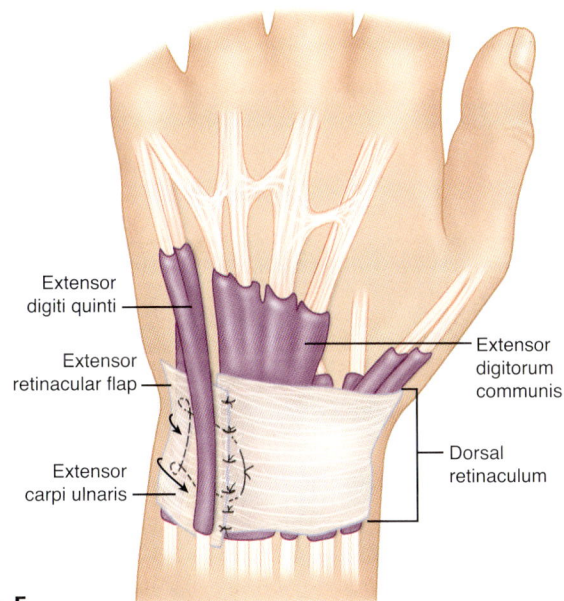

E

HUI-LINSCHEID RECONSTRUCTION
Incision and Dissection

- Start the incision at the level of the fifth carpometacarpal joint. Curve the incision over the ulnocarpal joint to reach the far ulnar border and continue to the middorsal forearm for exposure of the dorsal carpal ligament (**TECH FIG 2A**).
- Locate and protect the dorsal sensory branch of the ulnar nerve (**TECH FIG 2B,C**).
- Incise the extensor retinaculum over the sixth extensor compartment, taking care to protect the underlying extensor carpi ulnaris tendon and subsheath.
- Retract the extensor retinaculum medially to expose the capsule over the ulnocarpal joint and the subluxated ulnar head, creating an ulnarly based flap of retinaculum (**TECH FIG 2D**).

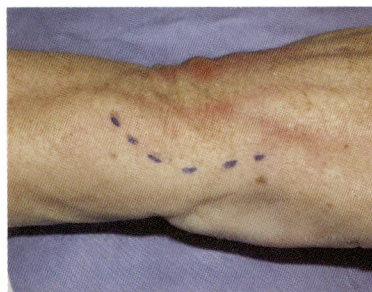

A

TECH FIG 2 • Hui-Linscheid reconstruction. **A.** Make a slightly curving incision over the ulnocarpal joint to reach the lateral ulnar border and continue it to the middorsal forearm for exposure of the dorsal carpal ligament. *(continued)*

B
Extensor retinaculum
Dorsal branch of ulnar sensory nerve
Incision

C

D

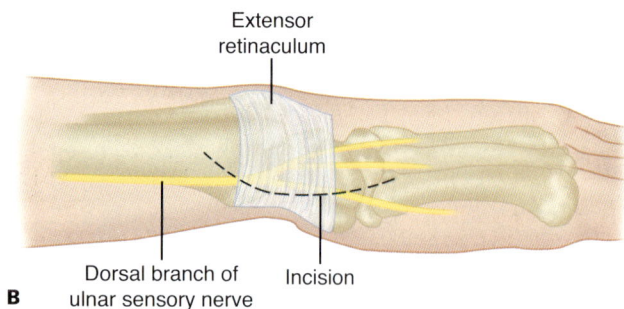

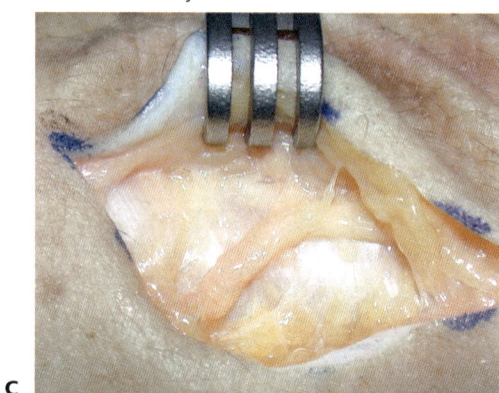

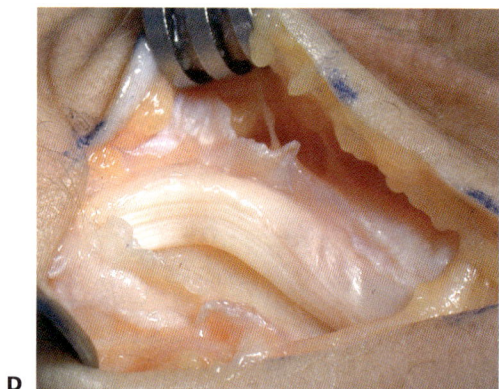

TECH FIG 2 • (*continued*) **B.** Take care not to injure the dorsal branch of the ulnar sensory branch during the incision and throughout the procedure. **C.** The ulnar nerve is located volar to the incision. The extensor retinaculum is incised at the fifth dorsal compartment. Protect the underlying extensor carpi ulnaris tendon and subsheath. **D.** Retract the extensor retinaculum medially to expose the capsule over the ulnocarpal joint and the subluxated ulnar head, creating an ulnar-based flap. **E.** Incise the capsule to expose the distal radioulnar joint while preserving the dorsal radioulnar ligament and taking care not to injure the extensor carpi ulnaris. **F.** Drill a 0.625-inch Kirscher wire through the ulnar head in a distal-to-proximal direction. The guidewire should be inserted obliquely starting from the base of ulnar styloid and aiming toward the synovial reflection proximally.

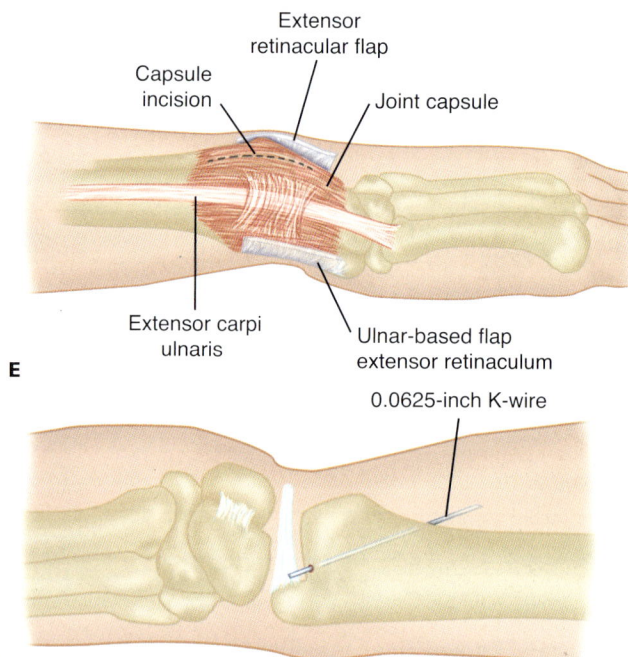

Capsule incision
Extensor retinacular flap
Joint capsule
Extensor carpi ulnaris
Ulnar-based flap extensor retinaculum
E

0.0625-inch K-wire
F

- Make a longitudinal incision in the capsule to expose the DRUJ while preserving the dorsal radioulnar ligament (**TECH FIG 2E**).
- Drill a 0.0625-inch Kirschner wire obliquely through the ulnar head beginning near the base of ulnar styloid to the ulnar fovea proximally (**TECH FIG 2F**).
- Placement of the Kirschner wire is confirmed visually and sequential hand awls are used to create a 4- to 5-mm bone tunnel.

Tendon Graft Harvest

- Locate the flexor carpi ulnaris (FCU) in the incision distally and trace it to the musculotendinous junction. This will allow about 10 cm of tendon graft for harvest (**TECH FIG 3A**).
  - If needed, a separate longitudinal incision on the palmar area of the wrist can be used.
  - Alternatively, a free tendon graft from the palmaris longus or other donor area may be used if the FCU tendon is inadequate.
- Split the FCU tendon longitudinally and cut the graft proximally at the musculotendinous junction. Leave the

distal portion still attached at its insertion onto the pisiform (**TECH FIG 3B**).
- Perforate the pisotriquetral capsule in a dorsal to volar direction (**TECH FIG 3C**).

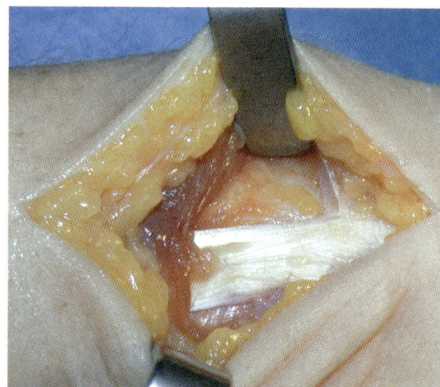

A

TECH FIG 3 • Hui-Linscheid tendon harvest. **A.** The flexor carpi ulnaris (FCU) is located distally and traced into the muscle belly to obtain about 10 cm of tendon graft. (*continued*)

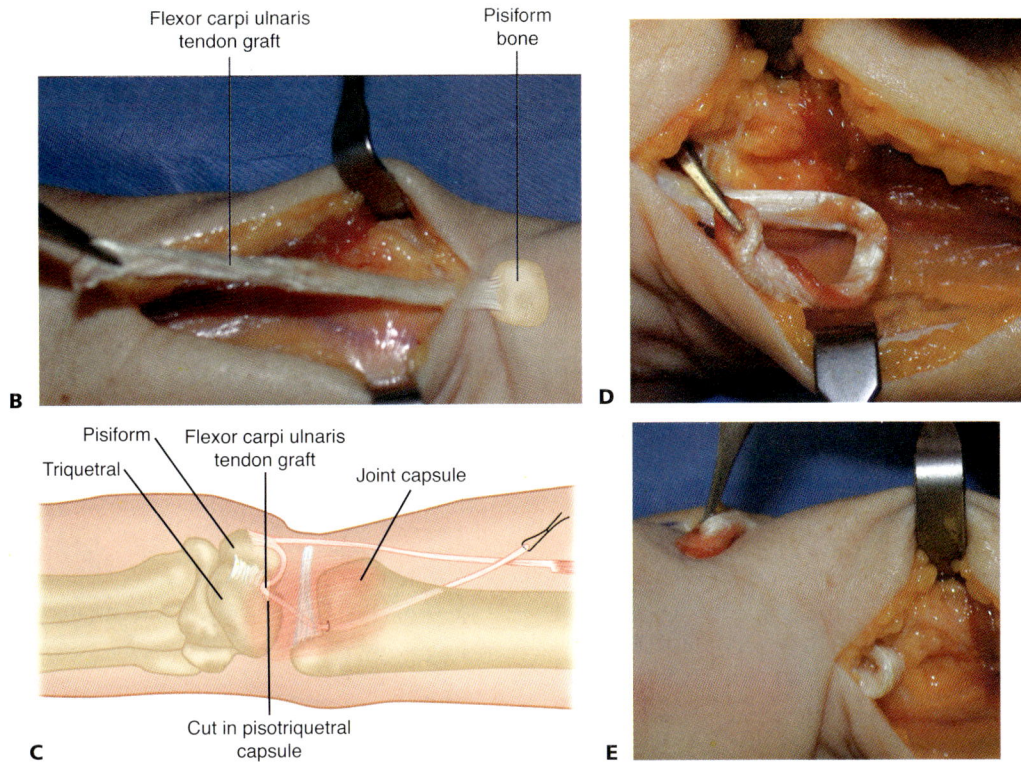

Flexor carpi ulnaris tendon graft

Pisiform bone

B

D

Pisiform

Triquetral

Flexor carpi ulnaris tendon graft

Joint capsule

Cut in pisotriquetral capsule

C

E

TECH FIG 3 • (*continued*) **B.** Cut the FCU graft proximally, leaving the distal portion attached distally in its insertion onto the pisiform. **C.** Pass the FCU tendon intracapsularly. **D, E.** Ensure that the graft is not placing any tension on the ulnar artery or nerve.

- The FCU tendon is passed intracapsularly using a tendon passer or by placing a Kessler suture into the tendon edge and using the suture to pull the tendon through the capsular perforation.
  - Ensure that the graft does not place any tension on the ulnar artery or nerve (**TECH FIG 3D,E**).
- The FCU tendon graft is passed through the TFCC if it is perforated or through an enlargement of the prestyloid recess of the TFCC and through the drill hole in the distal end of the ulna.

Completion of the Reconstruction

- The carpal supination and the ulnar head dorsal subluxation is reduced by pulling the FCU tendon graft taut from its pisiform insertion.
- Hold this reduction by placing the forearm in supination and transfix the distal ulna to the distal radius with two parallel 0.062-inch Kirschner wires.
- Close the DRUJ capsule incision using a 3-0 nonabsorbable suture.
- The FCU tendon graft is pulled taut through the drill hole and then secured to the periosteum adjacent to the ulna bone tunnel using a 2-0 nonabsorbable suture.
- The FCU graft is doubled back superficially to the radioulnar capsule (**TECH FIG 4A**) and sewn to its pisotriquetral insertion (**TECH FIG 4B**).
- If the dorsal radioulnar ligament is found to be attenuated, imbrication of the ligament is performed.
- The extensor retinaculum is imbricated using a nonabsorbable 3-0 suture.

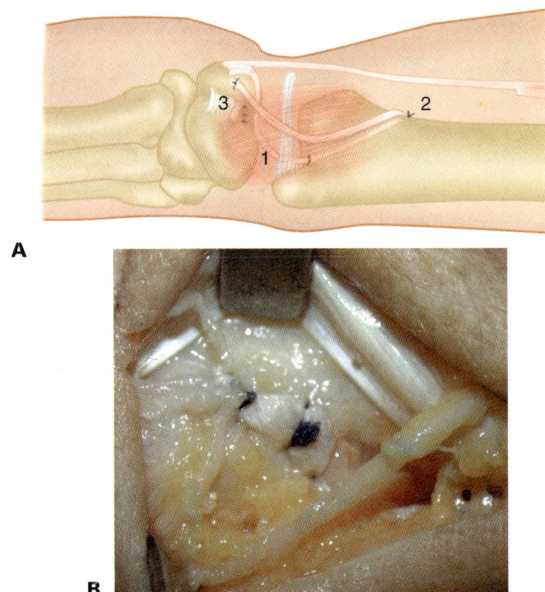

A

B

TECH FIG 4 • Hui-Linscheid completion. **A.** The flexor carpi ulnaris (FCU) tendon graft is passed through the triangular fibrocartilage complex (TFCC) if it is perforated or through an enlargement of the prestyloid recess of the TFCC (*1*) and through the drill hole in the distal end of the ulna (*2*). The FCU tendon graft is doubled backed superficially to the radioulnar capsule and approached to its proximal insertion in pisiform (*3*). **B.** The FCU graft is pulled through the tunnel in the ulna and is sewn to its pisotriquetral insertion.

PEARLS AND PITFALLS

Modified Herbert Reconstruction

Orientation of the capsulorrhaphy	■ Imbricate the extensor retinaculum in an oblique fashion (distal-ulnar to proximal-radial) to maximize the ulnocarpal ligamentotaxis effect of the repair. This will minimize the risk of postoperative supination deformity. If imbrication occurs at 90 degrees perpendicular to the DRUJ, only the DRUJ will be stabilized, not the ulnocarpal instability.
Placement of sutures in extensor retinaculum	■ Avoid injury to surrounding tissues or nerve structures (the dorsal branch of the ulnar nerve and the posterior interosseous nerve, terminal branch) when placing sutures in the extensor retinaculum (**FIG 5**). This will minimize the risk of postoperative wrist pain and dysesthesia.
EDQ tendinitis	■ The tendinitis usually resolves within 6 months.
Postoperative therapy	■ Advise the patient to avoid aggressive strengthening too soon after surgery, which may lead to loosening of the extensor retinaculum imbrication and failure of the Herbert sling repair.

Hui-Linscheid Reconstruction

Preservation of the nerve	■ The risk of damaging the dorsal branch of the ulnar nerve can be minimized by being aware of the dorsal ulnar nerve's location during surgical incision, manipulation, and drilling.
Postoperative ulnar fracture	■ In the postoperative period, the FCU tendon graft may migrate within the ulnar tunnel, which may predispose the distal ulna to fracture. This risk can be minimized by sewing the FCU tendon graft to the ulnar periosteum and local soft tissues around the drill hole, decreasing the chance of the tendon gliding within the tunnel.
Nerve adherence	■ The ulnar nerve may adhere to surrounding scar tissue at the closing site of soft tissue.

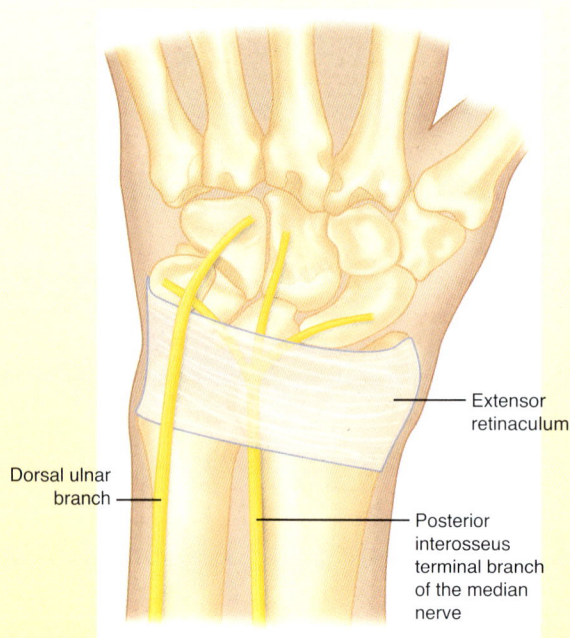

FIG 5 • Note the location of the dorsal branch of the ulnar nerve and the posterior interosseous nerve, terminal branch.

POSTOPERATIVE CARE

Modified Herbert Reconstruction

■ Six weeks in a thumb spica Muenster cast with the forearm and wrist both positioned in neutral, followed by 6 weeks in a removable thumb spica splint

Hui-Linscheid Reconstruction

■ Long-arm plaster cast for 6 weeks with the forearm and wrist both positioned in neutral. The cast and Kirschner wire are removed after 6 weeks.

■ After 6 weeks, an ulnar gutter splint with "boost" padding is applied to the ulnar head dorsally and pisiform palmarly to support the wrist between mobilization exercises (**FIG 6**).

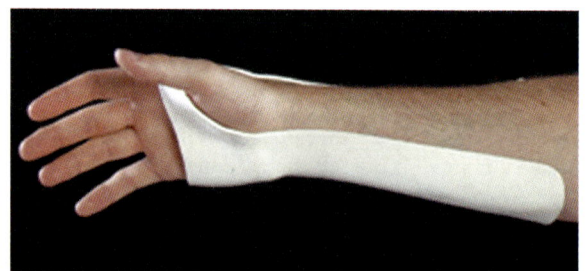

FIG 6 • An ulnar gutter splint with "boost" padding applied to the ulnar head dorsally and pisiform palmarly can be used in the postoperative period to support the wrist between mobilization exercises.

General Suggestions

- Gentle active rotatory motion during temporary splint removal is introduced at 6 weeks postoperatively at the patient's discretion. Passive motion with a physical or occupational therapist is not necessary at this point.
- No heavy lifting or aggressive motion is permitted until 3 months postoperatively.
- Vigorous strengthening exercises to regain pronation are begun 3 months after the operation with a physical or occupational therapist at a pace with which the patient is comfortable, with exercise intensity increased gradually.
- A warm, moist wrap can be used around the wrist to provide additional stretching of the wrist before activities. Ice and nonsteroidal anti-inflammatory agents can be used to provide relief after each session.
- Examples of exercises:
  - Pronation and supination: Stretching can be achieved by holding a hammer or frying pan as a weight during the motions.
  - Wrist flexion and extension: Stretching can be achieved using bucket exercises. The patient places his or her arm on a table with the wrist hanging off the edge while holding an empty bucket. The bucket is filled with water until the point of discomfort. The patient holds the bucket for 2 to 3 minutes and repeats the exercise twice daily in flexion and extension.
- If the patient's preoperative activities included sports such as golf and tennis, these activities should be gradually incorporated into the strengthening program.
- A Silastic sheet can be applied to aid scar remodeling. Scar massage may be started after the first 6 weeks.

OUTCOMES

- Modified Herbert reconstruction
  - A recent long-term follow-up study, ranging from 1 month to 13 years, of 39 wrists showed that 85% of the wrists remained stable at the ulnocarpal joint (in preparation for publication).
- Hui-Linscheid reconstruction
  - Successful short-term clinical outcomes have been reported in a small patient series by Hui and Linscheid, with patients reporting satisfactory and excellent outcomes.[6]
  - Mild limitations in pronation may be expected.

COMPLICATIONS

- The sling repair can loosen if aggressive strengthening occurs too quickly.
- If imbrication of the extensor retinaculum is not performed in an oblique direction, the ulnocarpal effect of the sling is lost, and a supination deformity of the wrist may occur or recur.
- Pain and dysesthesias at dorsal branch of ulnar nerve: Care must be taken when placing sutures for imbrication of the extensor retinaculum to avoid injury to surrounding tissues or nerve structures.
- EDQ tendinitis usually resolves 6 months after the operation.
- Damage to the ulnar nerve during the surgical procedure is concerning because of its anatomic location. The nerve is immediately exposed after the opening incision and is vulnerable during drilling of the ulnar tunnel. Dorsal ulnar nerve damage ranging from irritation to neuroma may occur.
  - Additionally, the nerve will be passing directly over an area of soft tissue closure and may be affected by the surrounding scar tissue.
  - A protective covering (such as those used for recurrent nerve entrapments) to protect the dorsal ulnar nerve may minimize damage to the nerve.
- Other potential complications may occur as a result of the Kirschner wire, such as migration, infection, and nerve injury.

REFERENCES

1. Adams BD. Partial excision of the triangular fibrocartilage complex articular disk: a biomechanical study. J Hand Surg Am 1993;18A:334–340.
2. Cooney WP. Evaluation of wrist pain by arthrogram, arthroscopy, and arthrotomy. J Hand Surg Am 1993;18A:815–822.
3. Dy CJ, Ouellette EA, Malik A, et al. Mechanical Testing of Distal Radioulnar Instability Repair: Ligament Reconstruction vs. Capsulorrhaphy. Proceedings of the Annual Meeting of the American Academy of Orthopaedic Surgeons, Feb. 16, 2007.
4. Glowacki KA, Shin AY. Stabilization of the unstable distal ulna: the Linscheid-Hui procedure. Tech Hand Upper Extr Surg 1993;4:229–236.
5. Harrison RJ, Ouellette EA, Latta LL, et al. The Biomechanics of Diagnosing and Treating Peripheral TFCC Instability. Proceedings of the Annual Meeting of the American Society for Surgery of the Hand, Sept. 9, 2004.
6. Hui FC, Linscheid RL. Ulnotriquetral augmentation tenodesis: a reconstructive procedure for dorsal subluxation of the distal radioulnar joint. J Hand Surg Am 1982;7A:230–236.
7. Kapindji AI, Martin-Bouyer Y, Verdeille S. Etude du carpe au scanner a trois dimensions sous contraintes de prono-supination (Three-dimensional CT study of the carpus under pronation-supination constraint). Ann Chir Main 1991;10:36–47.
8. Levinsohn EM, Rosen DI, Palmer AK. Wrist arthrography: value of the three-compartment injection method. Radiology 1991;179:231–239.
9. Lichtman DM, Bruckner JD, Culp RW, et al. Palmar midcarpal instability: results of surgical reconstruction. J Hand Surg Am 1993;18A:307–315.
10. Ouellette EA. Distal Radioulnar Joint and Ulnocarpal Instability. Proceedings of the International Wrist Investigators Workshop, American Society for Surgery of the Hand. Washington, DC, Sept. 6, 2006.
11. Palmer AK. Triangular fibrocartilage complex lesions: a classification. J Hand Surg Am 1989;14A:594–606.
12. Palmer AK, Werner FW. The triangular fibrocartilage complex of the wrist: anatomy and function. J Hand Surg Am 1981;6A:153–162.
13. Ritt MJ, Stuart PR, Berglund LJ, et al. Rotational stability of the carpus relative to the forearm. J Hand Surg Am 2000;20A:305–311.
14. Ruegger C, Schmidt MR, Pfirrmann CW, et al. Peripheral tear of the triangular fibrocartilage: depiction with MR arthrography of the distal radioulnar joint. AJR Am J Roentgenol 2007;188:187–192.
15. Schmidt HM, Lahl J. Studies on the tendinous compartments of the extensor muscles on the back of the human hand and their tendon sheaths. Gegenbaurs Morphol Jahrb 1988;134:155–173.
16. Schuind F, An KN, Berglund L, et al. The distal radioulnar ligaments: a biomechanical study. J Hand Surg Am 1991;16A:110.
17. Weiss AP, Akelman E, Lambiase R. Comparison of the findings of triple-injection cinearthrography of the wrist with those of arthroscopy. J Bone Joint Surg Am 1996;78A:348–356.
18. Wiesner L, Rumehart C, Pham E, et al. Experimentally induced ulnocarpal instability: a study on 13 cadaver wrists. J Hand Surg Br 1996;21B:24–29.
19. Zancolli EA, Elbio PC. Atlas of Surgical Anatomy of the Hand. Churchill Livingstone, 1991.

Chapter 52

Arthroscopic Dorsal Radiocarpal Ligament Repair

David J. Slutsky

DEFINITION

- Tears of the dorsal radiocarpal ligament (DRCL) are more common than previously suspected. They are best seen through a volar radial portal and are amenable to arthroscopic repair.
- Tears of the DRCL have been implicated in both volar and dorsal intercalated segmental instabilities, and they also have a role in midcarpal instability.[3,5]
- DRCL tears appear to be part of a spectrum of radial- and ulnar-sided carpal instability, as evidenced by the frequent association with scapholunate and lunotriquetral ligament injuries as well as triangular fibrocartilage (TFC) tears.
- Isolated DRCL tears can be solely responsible for wrist pain. The presence of an associated DRCL tear when seen in combination with a scapholunate, lunotriquetral, or TFC tear connotes a greater degree or duration of carpal instability and portends a poorer prognosis after treatment.[12]
- Good results are obtained after arthroscopic repair of isolated DRCL tears. Results of DRCL repairs are less predictable when seen in combination with other types of carpal pathology.[11]
- Recognition of this condition and further research into treatment methods is needed.

ANATOMY

- The DRCL is an extracapsular ligament on the dorsum of the wrist. It originates on the tubercle of Lister and moves obliquely in a distal and ulnar direction to attach to the tubercle of the triquetrum. Its radial fibers attach to the lunate and lunotriquetral interosseous ligament.[4]
- The dorsal intercarpal (DIC) ligament originates from the triquetrum and extends radially to attach onto the lunate, the dorsal groove of the scaphoid, and then the trapezium.
- The lateral V configuration of the DRCL and the DIC functions as a dorsal radioscaphoid ligament.
  - It can vary its length by changing the angle between the two arms while maintaining its stabilizing effect on the scapholunate joint during wrist flexion and extension.

- This would require changes in length far greater than any single fixed ligament could accomplish.[14]
- When viewed from a volar radial portal, the DRCL is seen immediately ulnar to the 3-4 portal, just underneath the lunate (**FIG 1A**).
- The actual fibers of the DRCL may not be seen unless there is a tear present, since it is normally covered by an epiligamentous sheath (**FIG 1B**).

PATHOGENESIS

- It is instructive to consider the wrist as having a number of primary and secondary stabilizers.
  - The scapholunate interosseous ligament (SLIL), the lunotriquetral interosseous ligament (LTIL), and the triangular fibrocartilaginous complex (TFCC) are the primary stabilizers.
- The capsular ligaments, including the radioscaphocapitate, radiolunotriquetral, ulnolunate, ulnotriquetral, dorsal radiocarpal, and dorsal intercarpal ligaments, can be thought of as secondary stabilizers.[6]
- A chronic tear of a primary stabilizer may culminate in the attenuation or tearing of the secondary stabilizer.
  - This is seen in patients with a triquetrolunate dissociation of more than 6 months' duration, in whom arthroscopy often reveals fraying of the ulnolunate ligaments and ulnotriquetral ligaments.[17]
- DRCL tears appear to be part of a spectrum of radial- and ulnar-sided carpal instability, as evidenced by the frequent association with SLIL, LTIL, or TFC tears. They have also been associated with midcarpal instability.[10]
- The DRCL tear may occur after or precede these injuries.
- In a recent study, 35 of 64 patients who underwent arthroscopy for the diagnosis and treatment of refractory wrist pain were noted to have associated DRCL tears, for an overall incidence of 55%.[9]
  - Five patients had an isolated DRCL tear.
  - 13 patients in this series had SLIL instability, tear, or both; 7 of 13 (54%) also had a DRCL tear. Of this subgroup four

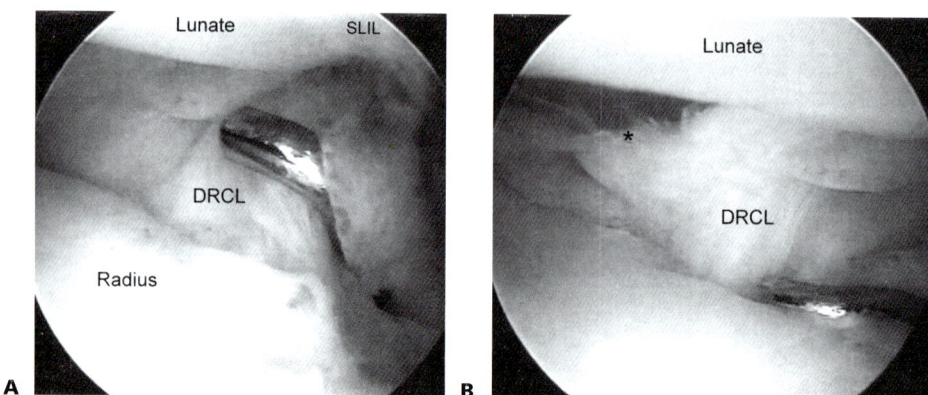

FIG 1 • **A.** View of an intact dorsoradiocarpal ligament (*DRCL*) from the VR portal. *SLIL*, scapholunate interosseous ligament. The hook-probe is in the 3-4 portal. **B.** DRCL tear (*). (From Slutsky DJ. Arthroscopic repair of dorsal radiocarpal ligament tears. Arthroscopy J Arthroscopic Relat Surg 2002;18:E49.)

patients had Geissler stage 1 or 2 instability and three had a Geissler stage 3 or 4 tear.

▪ Seven patients had LTIL instability, tear, or both; 2 of 7 (28%) also had a DRCL tear. Of this subgroup one patient had Geissler stage 2 instability and one had a Geissler stage 3 or 4 tear.

▪ Two patients had a capitohamate ligament tear; one of these patients also had a DRCL tear.

▪ Seven patients had a solitary TFCC tear; 6 of 7 (86%) were in association with a DRCL tear. One patient had a chronic ulnar styloid nonunion and a DRCL tear. There was TFCC fraying but no tear or detachment.

▪ Two or more lesions were present in 23 patients; DRCL tears were present in 12 patients (52%). Sixty-two percent of the combined lesions that were associated with a DRCL tear also included a TFCC tear.

NATURAL HISTORY

▪ The natural history of DRCL tears is not completely certain.[9]

▪ Unrecognized DRCL tears may be a cause for treatment failures in patients with persistent dorsal wrist pain.

▪ In nondissociative carpal instability, the pain is believed to be caused by dynamic joint incongruity.[1] Chronic detachment of the ulnar sling on the triquetrum has been implicated as a cause of wrist pain in these cases.[16] It is plausible that impingement of the torn edge of the DRCL against the lunate can have a similar effect.

▪ The DRCL, DIC, and dorsal SLIL are richly innervated, and 80% of nerve endings are in the epiligamentous sheath.[2]

▪ DRCL repair may allow a reinnervation of nerve endings and proprioceptive restoration (similar to anterior cruciate ligament repairs).

▪ The frequent observation of a DRCL tear in association with the altered kinematics caused by chronic radiocarpal or ulnocarpal instability might be attributed to plastic deformation of the DRCL with cyclical wrist motion that ultimately culminates in a tear.[6]

▪ When combined with other wrist pathology, the presence of a DRCL tear signifies a greater degree or longer duration of carpal instability and connotes a worse prognosis with regard to treatment.

▪ A classification of DRCL tears was devised based on the presence or absence of associated carpal pathology (Table 1).[7]

▪ Each successive stage denotes a longer standing or more severe condition, and this has a negative impact on the prognosis.

▪ An isolated DRCL tear does not necessarily lead to other intracarpal ligament or TFCC tears.[8]

PATIENT HISTORY AND PHYSICAL FINDINGS

▪ A typical patient with an isolated DRCL tear presents with complaints of intermittent dorsal midline wrist pain that may be sporadic but last 2 or 3 days; the pain is precipitated by repetitive loading or torquing movements of the wrist.

▪ When there is an underlying SLIL or LTIL tear or instability or TFCC tear, the pain may be more persistent and localized to the radial or ulnar side of the wrist.

▪ There are no physical findings that are pathognomonic of a DRCL tear. When there is no other associated wrist pathology, the diagnosis can be made only at the time of arthroscopy.

▪ Patients with isolated DRCL tears tend not to have localizing carpal tenderness and typically have a normal wrist examination, although some are mildly tender over the tubercle of Lister.[11,12]

▪ Positive physical findings are usually related to any associated wrist pathology. In patients who have scapholunate instability, scaphoid tenderness and a positive scaphoid shift test are usually present.

▪ When there is an associated TFC tear, the patient will often have tenderness over the ulnar capsule and may have crepitus and pain with ulnar loading of the pronated wrist.

▪ If midcarpal instability is present, the patient may have a positive midcarpal shift test.

IMAGING AND OTHER DIAGNOSTIC STUDIES

▪ Imaging studies are of mostly of value for ruling out associated carpal pathology since they are ineffective at making the diagnosis of an isolated DRCL tear.

▪ Plain radiographs and arthrograms are normal.

▪ The MRI is typically normal, although in one patient in the author's series an MRI was wrongly interpreted as showing a dorsal ganglion due to a high fluid signal intensity over the dorsal capsule (**FIG 2**).

Table 1	Classification of Dorsal Radiocarpal Ligament Tears
Stage*	**Description**
1	Isolated DRCL tear
2	DRCL tear with associated SLIL or LTIL (Geissler stage 1 or 2) or TFCC tear
3A	DRCL tear with associated SLIL and/or LTIL (Geissler stage 3) and/or TFCC tear
3B	DRCL tear with SLIL and/or LTIL (Geissler stage 4) and/or TFCC tear
4	Chondromalacia with widespread carpal pathology

*The ligament with the highest Geissler grade determines the stage.
DRCL, dorsal radiocarpal ligament; LTIL, lunotriquetral interosseous ligament; SLIL, scapholunate interosseous ligament; TFCC, triangular fibrocartilage complex.
(Adapted from Slutsky DJ. Wrist arthroscopy portals. In: Slutsky DJ, Nagle DJ, eds. Techniques in Hand and Wrist Arthroscopy. Philadelphia: Elsevier, 2007.)

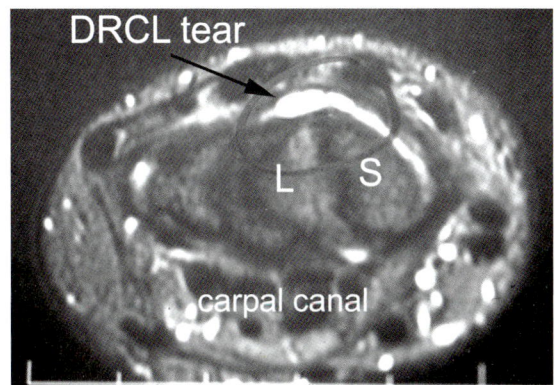

FIG 2 • MRI of an axial view of the carpus at the level of the carpal canal depicting a dorsoradiocarpal ligament tear. S, scaphoid; L, lunate.

DIFFERENTIAL DIAGNOSIS

- Dynamic scapholunate instability
- Scapholunate ligament tear
- Dorsal wrist syndrome[15]

NONOPERATIVE MANAGEMENT

- Patients should be treated with at least 1 month of wrist splinting, nonsteroidal anti-inflammatories, and activity modification with avoidance of repetitive gripping and lifting.
- Failure to respond is an indication for a radiocarpal cortisone injection followed by 1 additional month of splinting.
- Patients who continue to have wrist pain should then undergo imaging studies to rule out associated intracarpal pathology.

SURGICAL MANAGEMENT

- An arthroscopic repair is especially indicated for stage 1 (ie, isolated) DRCL tears, since the results are quite favorable.
- Repairs may also be considered in stage 2 and 3A DRCL tears, where the associated interosseous ligament tear or TFCC tear is treated arthroscopically.
- Stage 3B and stage 4 tears will likely be unresponsive to a DRCL repair since the outcomes are quite variable in the face of combined pathologies (Table 2).

Preoperative Planning

- Preoperative investigations should include plain radiographs to rule out a static carpal instability pattern.
- A double-row wrist arthrogram or an MR arthrogram is performed to assess the intracarpal ligaments and TFC.

Positioning

- The patient is positioned supine on the operating table with the arm abducted.
- Some method of overhead traction is useful. This may include traction from the overhead lights or a shoulder holder along with 5- to 10-lb sand bags attached to an arm sling. A traction tower such as the Linvatec tower (Conmed, Linvatec Corp, Largo, FL) or the ARC wrist traction tower designed by Dr. William Geissler (Arc Surgical LLC, Hillsboro, OR) greatly facilitates instrumentation.
- A 2.7-mm 30-degree angled arthroscope with a camera attachment is necessary.
  - A fiberoptic light source, video monitor, and printer are also standard equipment.

Table 2	Treatment of DRCL Tears

Stage	Description
1	Arthroscopic DRCL repair
2	Arthroscopic DRCL repair, SLIL or LTIL debridement ± shrinkage, TFCC repair or débridement
3A	Arthroscopic DRCL repair, SLIL or LTIL shrinkage + pinning, TFCC repair or débridement ± wafer (consider STT shrinkage)
3B	Open SLIL repair or reconstruction ± capsulodesis, LTIL repair or reconstruction, TFCC repair or débridement ± wafer or ulnar shortening
4	Partial carpal fusion versus proximal row carpectomy

DRCL, dorsal radiocarpal ligament; LTIL, lunotriquetral interosseous ligament; SLIL, scapholunate interosseous ligament; TFCC, triangular fibrocartilage complex; STT, scaphotrapeziotrapezoidal.
(Adapted from Slutsky DJ. Wrist arthroscopy portals. In: Slutsky DJ, Nagle DJ, eds. Techniques in Hand and Wrist Arthroscopy. Philadelphia: Elsevier, 2007.)

- Newer digital systems provide superior video quality compared with analog cameras and allow direct writing to a CD or DVD.
- A 3-mm hook-probe is needed for palpation of intracarpal structures.
- A motorized shaver and suction punch forceps are useful for débridement.
- Some type of diathermy unit such as the Oratec radiofrequency probe (Smith and Nephew, NY) is needed if augmentation of the repair with capsular shrinkage is desired.
- A variety of curved and straight 18-gauge spinal needles are used for passage of an absorbable 2-0 suture for the outside-in repair.
  - A suture lasso or grasper is needed to retrieve the suture ends.

Approach

- An inside-out arthroscopic repair technique of the DRCL ligament was initially performed.
  - An outside-in technique is technically easier and is now preferred.
- The standard dorsal portals are established, including the 3-4 and 4-5 portals, a midcarpal radial portal, and a midcarpal ulnar portal.
- A 6U portal is used for outflow.
- A standard arthroscopic survey is performed.

TECHNIQUES

VR PORTAL[16]

- A 2-cm longitudinal incision is made in the proximal wrist crease, exposing the flexor carpi radialis (FCR) tendon sheath (**TECH FIG 1A**).
- The sheath is divided and the FCR tendon retracted ulnarly.
- The radiocarpal joint space is identified with a 22-gauge needle and the joint inflated with saline (**TECH FIG 1B**).

- A blunt trocar and a cannula are introduced through the floor of the FCR sheath, which overlies the interligamentous sulcus between the radioscaphocapitate ligament and the long radiolunate ligament.
- A 2.7-mm 30-degree angled arthroscope is inserted through the cannula (**TECH FIG 1C**).

TECHNIQUES

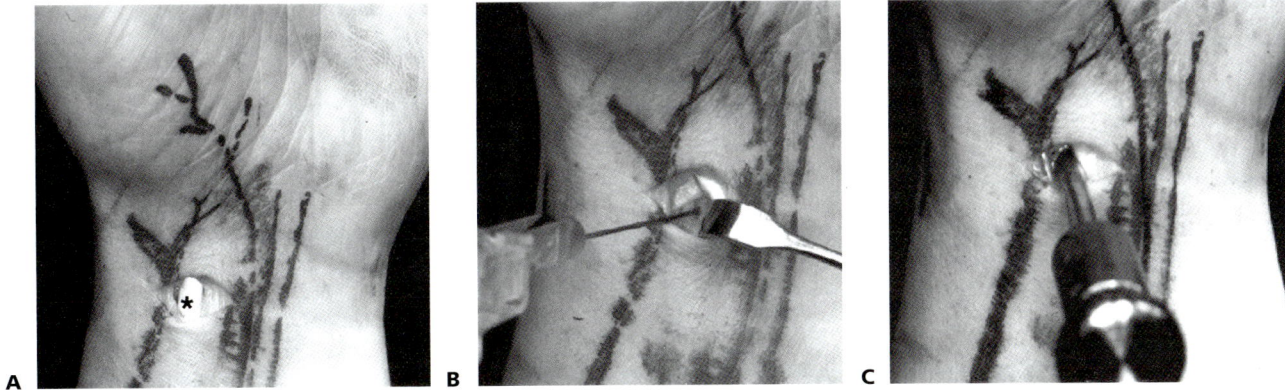

TECH FIG 1 • Establishing the volar radial portal. **A.** Skin incision for VR portal. *FCR*, flexor carpi radialis tendon. **B.** Saline injection of radiocarpal joint. **C.** Insertion of cannula through floor of the FCR sheath. (From Slutsky DJ. Volar portals in wrist arthroscopy. J Am Soc Surg Hand 2002;2:225–232.)

LIGAMENT REPAIR

- The repair is performed by inserting a curved 21-gauge spinal needle through the 4-5 portal while viewing through the arthroscope, which is inserted in the VR portal (**TECH FIG 2A–C**).
- A 2-0 absorbable suture is threaded through the spinal needle and retrieved with a grasper or suture snare inserted through the 3-4 portal (**TECH FIG 2D, E**).

- A curved hemostat is used to pull either end of the suture underneath the extensor tendons, and the knot is tied either at the 3-4 or 4-5 portal (**TECH FIG 2F**).
- With dorsal traction, the encircling suture pulls the torn DRCL up against the dorsal capsule, preventing it from impinging into the joint.
- The repair may be augmented with thermal shrinkage if the torn edge of the DRCL is voluminous (**TECH FIG 2G**).

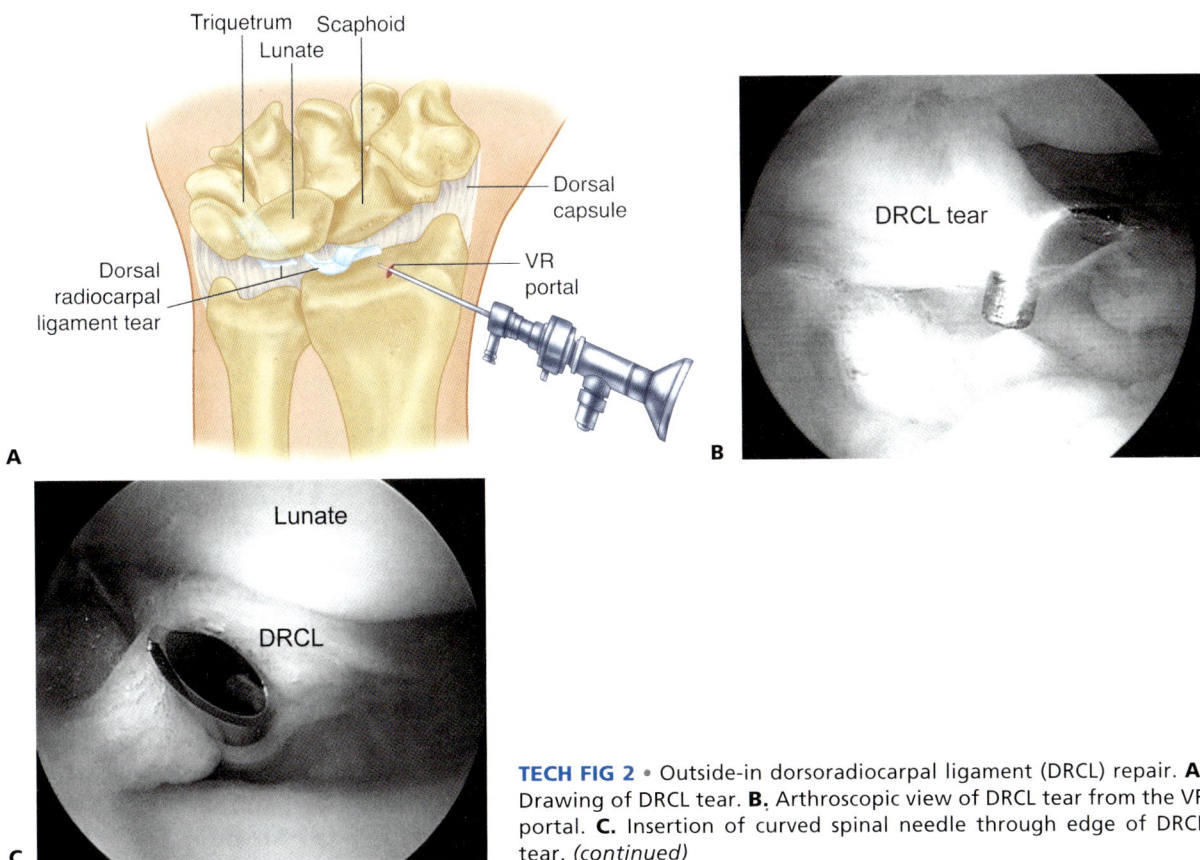

TECH FIG 2 • Outside-in dorsoradiocarpal ligament (DRCL) repair. **A.** Drawing of DRCL tear. **B.** Arthroscopic view of DRCL tear from the VR portal. **C.** Insertion of curved spinal needle through edge of DRCL tear. *(continued)*

TECHNIQUES

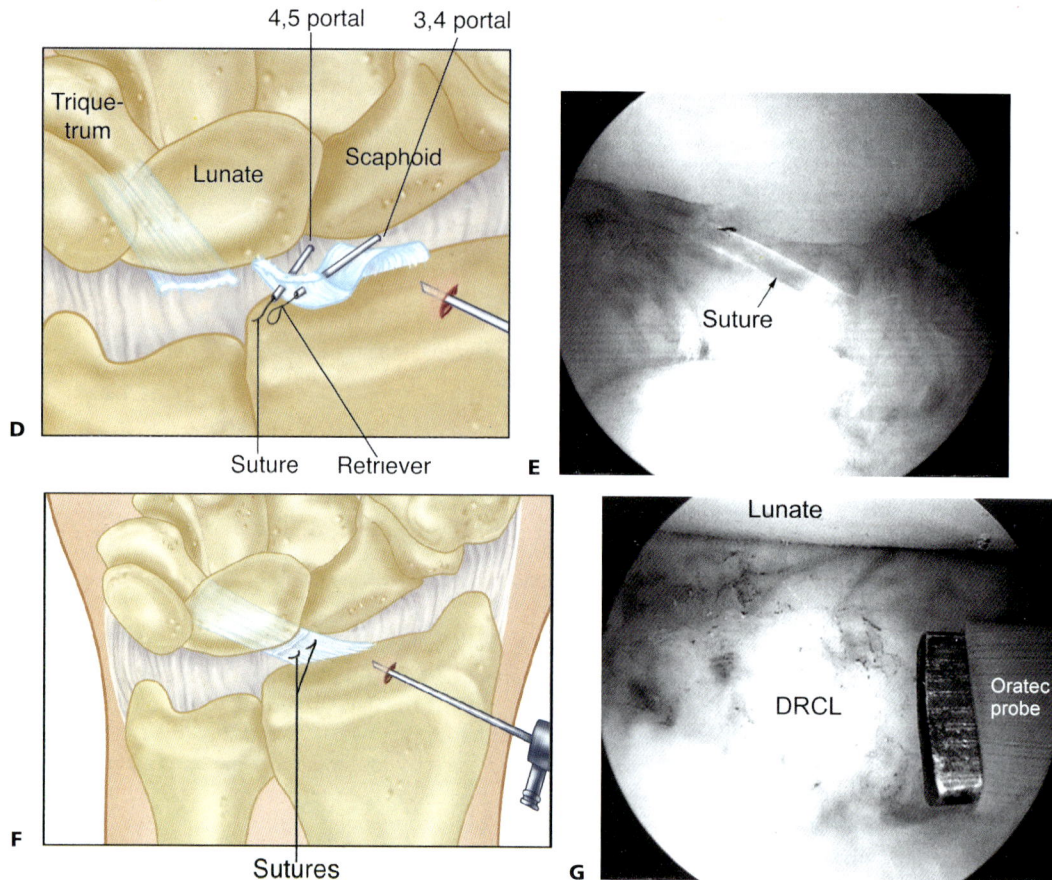

TECH FIG 2 • *(continued)* **D.** Outside-in technique using two spinal needles and a suture retriever. **E.** Arthroscopic view of suture loop before tying. **F.** Drawing of completed repair. **G.** Repair augmented with thermal shrinkage after suture has been tied. (**B,C,E,G:** Courtesy of Slutsky DJ. Clinical applications of volar portals in wrist arthroscopy. Tech Hand Up Extrem Surg 2004;18:229–238.)

PEARLS AND PITFALLS

Procedural tips
- Use the hook probe in the 3-4 portal to palpate the DRCL. Tears may not be evident until the free edge is pulled into the joint.
- Be sure to assess the scapholunate and lunotriquetral intervals from the midcarpal joint to assess any dynamic instability. Consideration may be given to thermal shrinkage of the palmar aspect of the scapholunate ligament when there is an associated dynamic scapholunate instability.
- To ensure that the extensor tendons are not entrapped, use a hemostat to thread either end of the suture underneath the extensor compartment. Tie the suture under the skin only after the wrist traction is backed off.
- When performing capsular shrinkage, use copious irrigation to prevent thermal chondral damage. Monitor the temperature of the outflow fluid.

POSTOPERATIVE CARE

- After an isolated DRCL repair the patient is placed in a below-elbow splint with the wrist in neutral rotation.
- Finger motion and edema control are instituted immediately. At the first postoperative visit the sutures are removed and the patient is placed in a below-elbow cast for a total immobilization time of 6 weeks.
- Wrist motion with use of a removable splint for comfort is instituted after cast removal.
- Gradual strengthening exercises are added after 8 weeks.
- Dynamic wrist splinting is instituted at 10 weeks if needed.

OUTCOMES

- The five patients who underwent an isolated DRCL repair graded their pain as none or mild.[9]
  - No patient required pain medication and all had returned to their previous occupation without restriction.
  - The pre- and postoperative wrist motion was unchanged in four of these patients, with less than 15% loss of motion in the fourth patient.
  - Grip strengths were 90% to 130% of the opposite side.
- A dorsal capsulodesis was performed in the seven patients with scapholunate instability.

- Three of these patients graded their pain level as none or mild, with both returning to full duty.
  - Four graded their pain as moderate or severe, with all four changing their occupation.
- Four patients underwent DRCL repair or shrinkage and LTIL pinning.
  - Two patients had no pain, and two had chronic, moderate pain.
- Seven patients underwent DRCL repair and TFCC repair or débridement, wafer resection, or both.
  - Two had no pain (with wafer resection), two had occasional mild pain, and three had chronic moderate pain.
- Of the patients with combined injuries who underwent a DRCL repair and treatment for associated tears of the SLIL, LTIL, or TFCC, seven of nine had chronic moderate pain.

COMPLICATIONS

- There were no complications related to the DRCL repair as described.
- Potential complications from use of a volar radial portal would include injury to the radial artery or the palmar cutaneous branch of the median nerve.
- Use of capsular shrinkage is still unproven and cannot as yet be considered a standard of care of the treatment of intercarpal ligament injuries.

REFERENCES

1. Bednar JM, Osterman AL. Carpal instability: evaluation and treatment. J Am Acad Orthop Surg 1993;1:10–17.
2. Hagert E, Garcia-Elia M, Forsgren S, et al. Immunohistochemical analysis of wrist ligament innervation in relation to their structural composition. J Hand Surg Am 2007;32A:30–36.
3. Horii E, Garcia-Elias M, An KN, et al. A kinematic study of lunotriquetral dissociations. J Hand Surg Am 1991;16A:355–362.
4. Mitsuyasu H, Patterson RM, Shah MA, et al. The role of the dorsal intercarpal ligament in dynamic and static scapholunate instability. J Hand Surg Am 2004;29A:279–288.
5. Moritomo H, Viegas SF, Elder KW, et al. Scaphoid nonunions: A 3-dimensional analysis of patterns of deformity. J Hand Surg Am 2000;25A:520–528.
6. Short WH, Werner FW, Green JK, et al. Biomechanical evaluation of the ligamentous stabilizers of the scaphoid and lunate, part III. J Hand Surg Am 2007;32A:297–309.
7. Slutsky DJ. Arthroscopic dorsal radiocarpal ligament repair. In: Slutsky DJ, Nagle DJ, eds. Techniques in Hand and Wrist Arthroscopy. Philadelphia: Elsevier, 2007.
8. Slutsky DJ. The incidence of dorsal radiocarpal ligament tears in patients having diagnostic wrist arthroscopy for wrist pain. J Hand Surg Am 2008;33A:332–334.
9. Slutsky DJ. The incidence of dorsal radiocarpal ligament tears in the presence of other intercarpal derangements. Arthroscopy 2008;24:526–533.
10. Slutsky D. Arthroscopic repair of dorsoradiocarpal ligament tears. J Arthroscopic Relat Surg 2005;21:86e1–86e8.
11. Slutsky DJ. Management of dorsoradiocarpal ligament repairs. J Am Soc Surg Hand 2005;5:167–174.
12. Slutsky DJ. Arthroscopic repair of dorsal radiocarpal ligament tears. Arthroscopy 2002;18:E49.
13. Slutsky DJ. Wrist arthroscopy through a volar radial portal. Arthroscopy 2002;18:624–630.
14. Viegas SF, Yamaguchi S, Boyd NL, et al. The dorsal ligaments of the wrist: anatomy, mechanical properties, and function. J Hand Surg Am 1999;24A:456–468.
15. Watson HK, Weinzweig J. Physical examination of the wrist. Hand Clin 1997;13:17–34.
16. Watson HK, Weinzweig J. Triquetral impingement ligament tear (tilt). J Hand Surg Br 1999;24B:321–324.
17. Zachee B, De Smet L, Fabry G. Frayed ulno-triquetral and ulno-lunate ligaments as an arthroscopic sign of longstanding triquetro-lunate ligament rupture. J Hand Surg Br 1994;19B:570–571.

Chapter 53

Distal Biceps Tendon Disruptions: Acute and Delayed Reconstruction

Robert E. Ivy and Edwin E. Spencer, Jr.

DEFINITION

- Disruption of distal biceps tendon at its insertion

ANATOMY

- Distal tendon inserts into the biceps tuberosity on the proximal radius.
- A relatively avascular zone exists just proximal to the tendon's insertion site.[15]

PATHOGENESIS

- Injury typically results from an eccentric muscle contraction. The forearm is forced into extension from a flexed position as the biceps muscle fires
- Avascular changes in the distal tendon and possible impingement in the interosseous space between the tuberosity and the proximal ulna may contribute to rupture.[15]

NATURAL HISTORY

- Complete ruptures
  - Distal biceps tendon ruptures usually occur in middle-aged men, similar to pectoralis major tendon ruptures and Achilles tendon ruptures.
  - The initial pain subsides quickly but there is usually a noticeable deformity in the anterior brachium as the biceps muscle contracts and retracts. The degree of the retraction can be mitigated by the lacertus fibrosus, which may remain intact.
  - The patient usually reports loss of flexion and supination strength. This is especially noted in patients who require repetitive supination, such as mechanics and plumbers. Pain is usually not a predominant complaint, although some patients will experience fatigue-type pain and cramping in the retracted muscle belly.
  - Studies have revealed a 25% reduction in flexion strength and a 40% loss of supination strength.[2,11]
- Partial ruptures
  - Partial distal biceps tendon injuries are usually more painful than complete tears. Patients usually present with pain in the antecubital fossa, especially with resisted flexion and supination. There is an absence of clinical deformity.
  - Partial tears can progress to complete tears.

PATIENT HISTORY AND PHYSICAL FINDINGS

- History of a rapid eccentric load on the involved extremity
- In acute cases of a complete distal biceps tendon rupture, there is usually a significant amount of ecchymosis in the antecubital fossa, distal arm, and proximal forearm.
- The distal biceps tendon is not palpable in the antecubital fossa. Comparison to the uninvolved side is helpful.
- Local edema can make the diagnosis a little more difficult, but the "hook test" has been found to be a very reliable diagnostic tool. To perform the test, the patient actively supinates the forearm while the examiner attempts to "hook" the distal biceps tendon from the lateral side.[12]
- The degree of proximal retraction of the tendon can be mitigated by the lacertus fibrosus.

IMAGING AND OTHER DIAGNOSTIC STUDIES

- MRI is usually not necessary to make the diagnosis. The only caveat is that if the examiner feels that the distal biceps tendon is intact, the injury might be more proximal at the myotendinous junction or only a partial tear at its insertion.
  - It is important to make the distinction between the common complete avulsion from the radial tuberosity and an injury at the myotendinous junction, as the more proximal injuries are best treated nonoperatively.[14]
- Partial tears occur at the radial tuberosity, are usually not associated with ecchymosis, and demonstrate no proximal retraction. They present late with pain with resisted flexion and supination. The distal biceps tendon is palpable and frequently tender.
  - MRI can aid in the diagnosis of partial tendon ruptures.

NONOPERATIVE MANAGEMENT

- Nonoperative management of complete distal biceps tendon ruptures entails the use of modalities to reduce pain and swelling and simply allowing the patient to use the extremity as tolerated. Strengthening should focus on elbow flexion and supination.
- The surgeon should discuss with the patient that complete distal biceps tendon ruptures are not usually associated with residual pain but rather loss of flexion (30%) and supination (40%) strength.[2,11] If that is compatible with the patient's job and lifestyle, nonoperative management is acceptable.
- Partial biceps tendon ruptures and ruptures at the myotendinous junction are treated in a similar manner. The patient should proceed to strengthening when full painless range of motion is obtained.
- Operative intervention is considered when nonoperative management fails for partial ruptures. Usually a minimum 3 to 4 months of observation is appropriate. Patients should be counseled that pain is more of a predominant complaint with these partial injuries.

SURGICAL MANAGEMENT

Complete and Partial Ruptures

- The EndoButton (Smith & Nephew, Andover, MA) method of fixation has been shown to have the highest ultimate tensile load.[10,16] Clinical studies with the EndoButton have also demonstrated good results with few complications.[1,4]
- Other methods are suture anchor and interference screw fixation.

Chronic Disruptions

- The definition of "chronic" is vague. Some authors have stated that greater than 8 weeks is chronic and that a graft is needed in these situations. However, we have been able to primarily repair distal biceps tendon ruptures out to 3 months. In these situations the elbow might not extend beyond 60 degrees on the table, but within 3 months after the repair the patient's range of motion is full. The biceps brachii, like the pectoralis major, has a significant ability to stretch back out over time.
- The surgeon should discuss with the patient that a more chronic rupture might require graft and should discuss the type of graft to be used. Semitendinosus (either autograft or allograft),[16] Achilles tendon allograft[13] (with the bone plug inserted into the radial tuberosity or just soft tissue repair), flexor carpi radialis autograft,[9] and fascia lata[6] have been described.

- Any of the techniques of radial tuberosity fixation described in the acute section can be used. We use the EndoButton for the chronic reconstructions.

Positioning

- The patient is placed in the supine position on an armboard with a sterile tourniquet on the upper arm.

Approach

- The approach depends on the surgeon's preferred method of fixation.
- Classic two-incision techniques had complications such as heterotopic ossification and posterior interosseous nerve palsy. Therefore, single-incision anterior approaches were developed with various methods of fixation, including suture anchors, interference screws, and the EndoButton.

ENDOBUTTON

- A longitudinal 4- to 5-cm anterior incision starting at the antecubital fossa and extending distally along the ulnar border of the brachioradialis is used. The lateral antebrachial cutaneous nerve and superficial radial nerve are identified and protected.
- The distal biceps tendon is retrieved into the wound. This can be accomplished by flexing the elbow and using a retractor to lift the skin of the distal arm for exposure.
  - The tendon can be adherent to the adjacent tissues or the lacertus fibrosus. This may require a limited tenolysis to mobilize the tendon stump. Protect and isolate the lateral antebrachial cutaneous nerve and the brachial artery.
- On occasion, the biceps tendon cannot be retrieved through the anterior incision. In that case, an incision can be made medially along the distal aspect of the arm. The tendon is isolated and prepared and then passed into the distal wound.
- Once the tendon is isolated, a no. 2 nonabsorbable suture is woven into the distal biceps tendon using a locking Krackow technique or other locking suture technique. The locking sutures should extend 4 to 5 cm above

the stump. The goal is to create a locking stitch proximally and allow about 1 cm of the distal biceps tendon to be unlocked.
- The two sutures extending from the tendon stump are then passed through the two central holes of the EndoButton.
- The sutures are tied, leaving no space between the end of the tendon and the EndoButton (**TECH FIG 1A**).
  - Alternatively, one suture from the tendon can be passed through one of the central holes of the EndoButton and then back through the other central hole and the knot is then tied, thus placing the knot between the EndoButton and the tendon stump.
  - Passing sutures (kite strings) are placed in the other two holes of the EndoButton.
- The radial tuberosity is exposed, and a burr is used to create an oval cortical window roughly the same dimension as the distal tendon stump. This is performed while an assistant holds the forearm in full supination. Two small Bennett retractors can be placed on either side of the radial tuberosity. Then, the EndoButton drill is used to create a hole in the far cortex to pass the button.

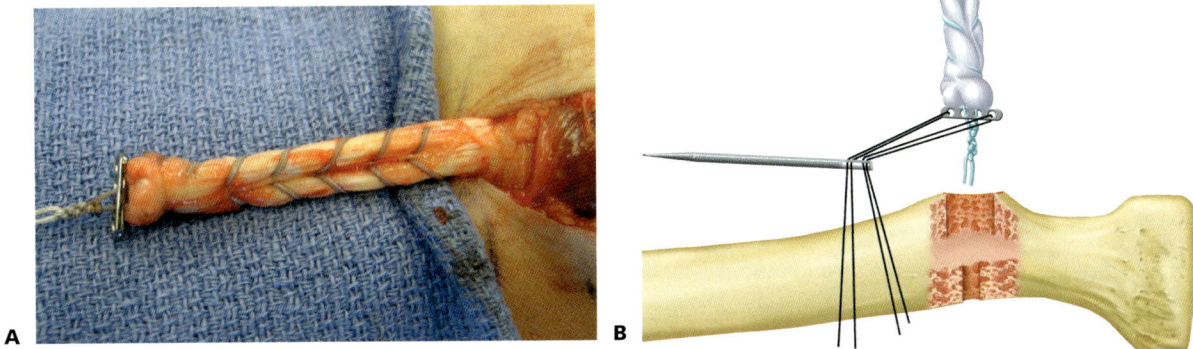

TECH FIG 1 • A. EndoButton attached to the distal end of the biceps tendon. **B.** A Keith needle is placed to pass the suture. (*continued*)

- Keith needles or a Beath needle are used to pass the passing sutures (kite strings) through the bicortical hole and are retrieved as they pass through the skin on the dorsal side of the forearm (**TECH FIG 1B**).
- One of the passing sutures is independently pulled, drawing the tendon into the radial tuberosity. Continued

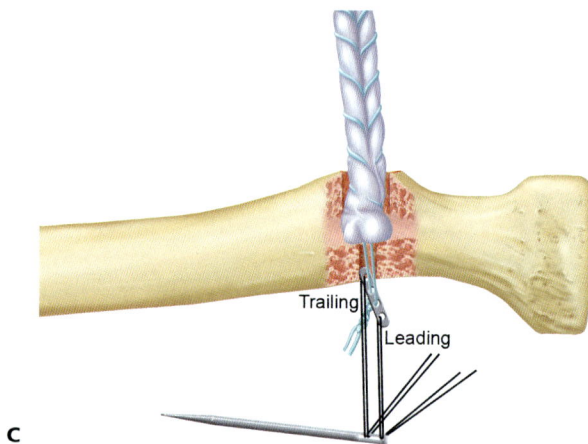

tension on this kite string draws the EndoButton in its vertical orientation through the hole in the far cortex of the radius (**TECH FIG 1C**).

- Once the EndoButton is on the far side of the radius, the other suture is pulled to flip it and lock it in its horizontal orientation on the far side of the radius (**TECH FIG 1D**).
- We use fluoroscopy to confirm placement of the button.
- The passing sutures are then pulled completely out after anatomic tendon placement is visually confirmed.

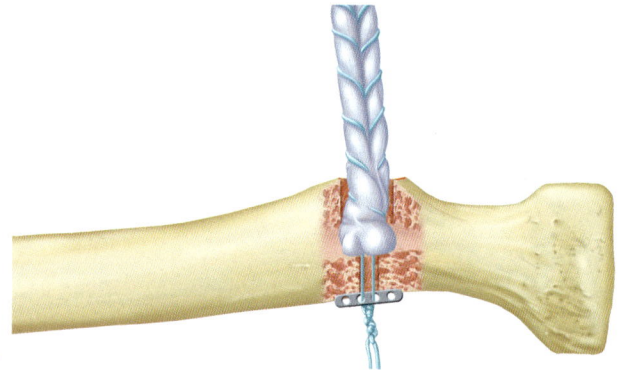

C   **D**

TECH FIG 1 • (continued) **C.** The tendon is pulled into the proximal radial hole as the EndoButton is advanced through the distal hole. **D.** The EndoButton is flipped to secure it on the other side of the radial cortex.

SUTURE ANCHOR OR INTERFERENCE SCREW FIXATION

- The same anterior approach is used, and the tendon is retrieved in a similar manner with both suture anchor and interference screw fixation. However, the radial tuberosity is prepared differently.
- In the case of interference screw fixation, a hole is drilled in the radial tuberosity. The diameter of the hole

depends on the system (and the size of the screw) being used.

- In the case of suture anchor fixation, the radial tuberosity is lightly decorticated and suture anchors of choice are placed. Some authors use two suture anchors, and most use some kind of a sliding knot to advance the tendon onto the bone.

TWO-INCISION TECHNIQUE

- The anterior incision is made transverse in the antecubital flexion crease and used to locate the distal tendon stump. A second longitudinal incision is made 1 cm radial to the subcutaneous border of the radius in the proximal forearm at the level of the biceps tuberosity.
- Dissection is initially made in the extensor carpi ulnaris muscle and then through the supinator muscle. Take great care to avoid subperiosteal dissection on the ulna to decrease the risk of synostosis.

- The forearm is placed in maximal pronation and an oval cavity is created in the biceps tuberosity with a burr. Drill holes are then placed into this cavity with the forearm in supination.
- A no. 2 Fiberwire suture is then placed in the distal tendon in a Krackow technique.
- The sutures are then passed from anterior to the posterior incision with a long hemostat and retrieved. It is critical to pass the sutures in the interosseous space.
- The sutures are then passed through the drill holes and tied over bone with the forearm in supination.

CHRONIC DISTAL BICEPS TENDON RECONSTRUCTIONS

- More exposure of the biceps tendon and the myotendinous junction is required for the chronic reconstructions. This can be accomplished by creating a second incision at the medial aspect of the distal arm.
  - One could connect the two anterior incisions, but this risks creating additional scarring.
- A more meticulous dissection is required to protect the lateral antebrachial cutaneous and musculocutaneous

nerves. Invariably there will be considerable scarring and adhesions, especially between the biceps tendon and lacertus fibrosus. Some of the lacertus can be used in the reconstruction.

- We have used semitendinosus autograft, which is harvested in a fashion similar to that used with anterior cruciate ligament reconstructions.

- The tendon is doubled up and the two free ends are woven into the remaining distal biceps tendon and the myotendinous junction (**TECH FIG 2A**).
- A Bunnell tendon passer is very effective at passing the tendon ends.
- The length of the graft is chosen so that the reconstruction is tight at 60 degrees of elbow flexion. This can be accomplished by fixing it distally first and then performing the weave, or vice versa.
- A nonabsorbable suture is passed through the graft–tendon construct, and this is secured to the radial tuberosity (**TECH FIG 2B**).

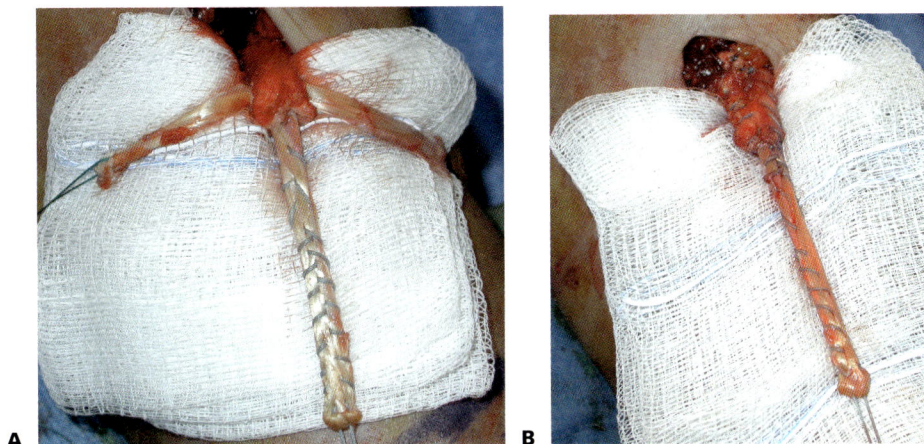

TECH FIG 2 • A. Hamstring tendon is doubled up and folded on itself and the free ends are passed into the distal end of the biceps tendon stump to add length. The free ends of the tendon graft exit laterally. **B.** The free ends of the hamstrings tendon graft are woven into the biceps tendon stump.

PEARLS AND PITFALLS

One-incision technique	• Avoid excessive retraction on the radial side to avoid injury to the lateral antebrachial cutaneous nerve. • Prepare the biceps tendon before the radial tuberosity. • Use fluoroscopic guidance to pass the EndoButton.
Two-incision technique	• Avoid subperiosteal dissection on the ulna.

POSTOPERATIVE CARE

- Radiographs are obtained at the time of surgery and at the first postoperative visit to ensure that the fixation (EndoButton or anchors) is in good position.
- For the EndoButton repair we remove the splint at 2 weeks and allow active and passive range of motion but no lifting greater than a cup of coffee for 6 weeks. Strengthening is then started, but rarely is formal physical therapy necessary.
- Other authors have reported good results with early range-of-motion therapy.[1]
- Others use a more conservative approach and limit full extension until 6 to 8 weeks after surgery.

OUTCOMES

- Patient-weighted outcome measures such as the DASH and the MEPS have been used in many studies and have demonstrated excellent results with primary repair.[1,5]
- Objective data including strength testing have also demonstrated good results with anatomic repair, especially with regard to restoring supination strength.[8]
- Chronic repairs or reconstructions have also performed well.[17]

COMPLICATIONS

- Reruptures are rare in most series irrespective of the method of fixation.

- Certain fixation methods have been associated with a higher occurrence of certain complications.
  - Classic two-incision technique: Heterotopic ossification, radioulnar synostosis, and posterior interosseous nerve palsies. Heterotopic ossification and radioulnar synostosis rates have been decreased by avoiding the ulnar periosteum.[3,7]
  - Single-incision technique: Lateral antebrachial cutaneous and superficial radial nerve palsies
- Loss of motion

REFERENCES

1. Bain GI, Prem H, Heptinstall RJ, et al. Repair of distal biceps tendon rupture: a new technique using the EndoButton. J Shoulder Elbow Surg 2000;9:120–126.
2. Baker BE, Bierwagen D. Rupture of the distal tendon of the biceps brachii: operative versus non-operative treatment. J Bone Joint Surg Am 1985;67A:414–417.
3. Failla JM, Amadio PC, Morrey BF, et al. Proximal radioulnar synostosis after repair of distal biceps brachii rupture by the two-incision technique: report of four cases. Clin Orthop Relat Res 1990;253:133–136.
4. Greenberg JA, Fernandez JJ, Wang T, et al. EndoButton-assisted repair of distal biceps tendon ruptures. J Shoulder Elbow Surg 2003;12:484–490.
5. John CK, Field LD, Weiss KS, et al. Single-incision repair of acute distal biceps ruptures by use of suture anchors. J Shoulder Elbow Surg 2007;16:78–83.

6. Kaplan FT, Rokito AS, Birdzell MG, et al. Reconstruction of chronic distal biceps tendon rupture with use of fascia lata combined with a ligament augmentation device: a report of 3 cases. J Shoulder Elbow Surg 2002;11:633–636.

7. Kelly EW, Morrey BF, O'Driscoll SW. Complications of repair of the distal biceps tendon with the modified two-incision technique. J Bone Joint Surg Am 2000;82A:1575–1581.

8. Klonz A, Loitz D, Wohler P, et al. Rupture of the distal biceps brachii tendon: isokinetic power analysis and complications after anatomic reinsertion compared with fixation to the brachialis muscle. J Shoulder Elbow Surg 2003;12:607–611.

9. Levy HJ, Mashoof AA, Morgan D. Repair of chronic ruptures of the distal biceps tendon using flexor carpi radialis tendon graft. Am J Sports Med 2000;28:538–540.

10. Mazzocca AD, Burton KJ, Romeo AA, et al. Biomechanical evaluation of 4 techniques of distal biceps brachii tendon repair. Am J Sports Med 2007;35:252–258.

11. Morrey BF, Askew LJ, An KN, et al. Rupture of the distal tendon of the biceps brachii: a biomechanical study. J Bone Joint Surg Am 1985;67A:418–421.

12. O'Driscoll SW, Goncalves LB, Dietz P. The hook test for distal biceps tendon avulsion. Am J Sports Med 2007;35:1865–1869.

13. Sanchez-Sotelo J, Morrey BF, Adams RA, et al. Reconstruction of chronic ruptures of the distal biceps tendon with use of an Achilles tendon allograft. J Bone Joint Surg Am 2002;84A:999–1005.

14. Schamblin ML, Safran MR. Injury of the distal biceps at the musculo-tendinous junction. J Shoulder Elbow Surg 2007;16:208–212 [e-pub Dec. 13, 2006].

15. Seiler JG 3rd, Parker LM, Chamberland PD, et al. The distal biceps tendon. Two potential mechanisms involved in its rupture: arterial supply and mechanical impingement. J Shoulder Elbow Surg 1995; 4:149–156.

16. Spang JT, Weinhold PS, Karas SG. A biomechanical comparison of EndoButton versus suture anchor repair of distal biceps tendon injuries. J Shoulder Elbow Surg 2006;15:509–514.

17. Wiley WB, Noble JS, Dulaney TD, et al. Late reconstruction of chronic distal biceps tendon ruptures with a semitendinosus autograft technique. J Shoulder Elbow Surg 2006;15:440–444.

Chapter 54

Repair of Acute Digital Flexor Tendon Disruptions

Christopher H. Allan

DEFINITION

▪ Flexor tendon injuries can occur in any of the five described zones within the finger, hand, wrist, or forearm. All such injuries require surgical repair to restore active finger flexion.

▪ The most challenging injuries to manage are those in zone II, where two flexor tendons occupy a narrow fibro-osseous sheath. Successful repair requires meticulous technique and a careful postoperative therapy regimen balancing the risks of adhesion formation versus rupture.

ANATOMY

▪ The flexor tendons form two layers in the forearm (zone V; **FIG 1A**), with the thumb's flexor pollicis longus (FPL) and the fingers' flexor digitorum profundus (FDP) muscles deep to the flexor digitorum superficialis (FDS) muscle. At the wrist the FPL and FDP tendons remain deep, with the index and small FDS tendons above, and the middle and ring FDS tendons most superficial.

▪ The median nerve runs down the forearm beneath the fascia of the FDS on its undersurface, becoming superficial within the carpal tunnel just proximal to the volar wrist crease (zone IV), with the flexor tendons closely packed together.

▪ Exiting the carpal tunnel, the flexor tendons cross the palm (zone III) toward the individual digits.

▪ The two tendons of each non-thumb digit (the thumb has just the FPL) enter the fibro-osseous sheath (zone II) at the level of the metacarpophalangeal (MP) joint. The FDS then divides into two slips to form the decussation termed the chiasm of Camper, through which the FDP passes from deep to superficial (**FIG 1B**).

▪ The two slips of the FDS insert along the proximal aspect of the volar surface of the middle phalanx, and the FDP proceeds distally to insert along the volar surface of the base of the distal phalanx.

▪ The flexor sheath extends from the level of the MP joint to the distal interphalangeal (DIP) joint. Multiple condensations of discrete fibers are found along its course and are named as either annular or cruciate pulleys, reflecting the orientation of the fibers forming the pulley (**FIG 1C**).

▪ The thicker, annular (A1 through A5, from proximal to distal) pulleys hold the tendons close to bone while the more slender cruciate (C1 through C3) pulleys collapse with digit flexion, allowing the sheath to shorten without buckling. Zone II is that part of the sheath where both FDS and FDP tendons are present, and zone I is distal to the FDS insertion.

▪ Tendon nutrition within the sheath is provided indirectly via synovial fluid and directly via vascular inflow through mesenteric folds called vinculae, with one vinculum longus and one vinculum brevis to each flexor tendon.

PATHOGENESIS

▪ Most acute flexor tendon injuries are the result of open trauma, with sharp transection of the tendon. In such cases, other structures are often injured as well. In particular, examination should include assessment of sensibility and capillary

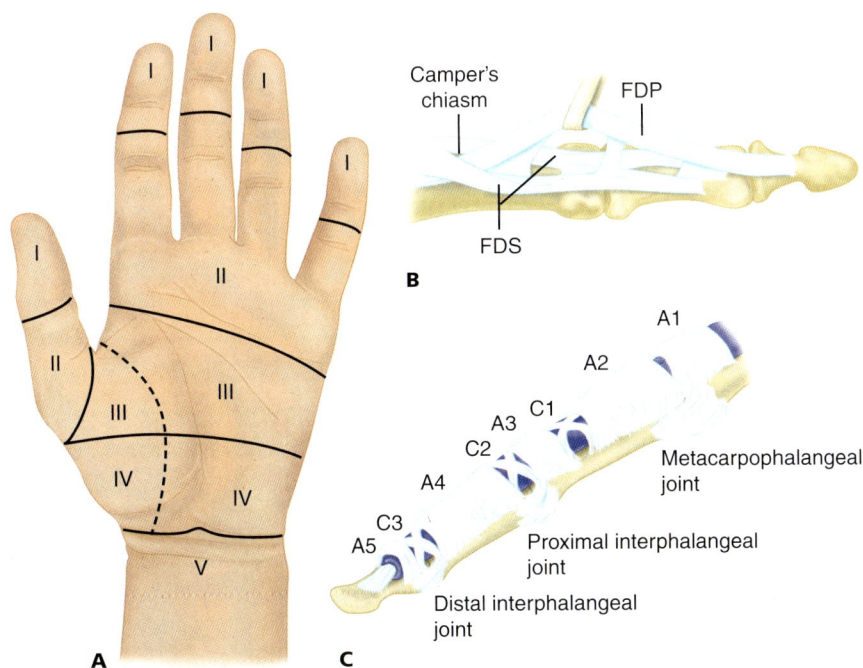

FIG 1 • **A.** Flexor tendon zones. **B.** Flexor tendon anatomy in zone II. **C.** Flexor sheath pulley anatomy and distribution in zones I and II.

refill to identify injury to the digital nerves and vessels that would affect preoperative planning.

▪ A less common injury mechanism is closed avulsion of the FDP from its distal attachment to bone. The term "jersey finger" is sometimes used for this injury, as it is often the result of an athlete's fingers forcibly flexing to grab an opponent's jersey, followed by sudden and forceful extension of the DIP joint against resistance as the opponent pulls away. This avulsion injury is addressed elsewhere.

NATURAL HISTORY

▪ Flexor tendon injuries require surgical repair to restore active digit flexion. Early repair is crucial, with several studies pointing to better results when repairs are performed within the first 7 days after injury.[3,7]

▪ Outcomes aside, as a practical matter it is easiest to repair the tendon before proximal tendon retraction occurs, requiring additional incisions. Late repair with tendon retraction and muscle shortening can also result in tension at the repair site, leading to gapping of the repair (which increases the failure rate) or influencing the surgeon to splint the wrist or digits in excessive flexion, leading to joint contractures.

PATIENT HISTORY AND PHYSICAL FINDINGS

▪ Methods for examining the hand or upper extremity with an acute flexor tendon injury
  ▪ Isolate FDP: While maintaining the injured digit's proximal interphalangeal joint extended, the examiner asks the patient to actively flex the DIP joint (**FIG 2A**).
  ▪ Isolate FDS: While maintaining all uninjured digits in full extension, the examiner asks the patient to actively flex the injured digit's proximal interphalangeal joint (**FIG 2B**).
▪ Uncooperative or unresponsive patient
  ▪ Tenodesis effect: The examiner extends the wrist; flexion is observed at the interphalangeal joints if the flexor tendons are intact.
  ▪ Forearm compression: Pressure applied to flexor tendon muscle bellies results in interphalangeal joint flexion if flexor tendons are intact.
  ▪ The examiner inspects for normal flexion arcade (**FIG 2C**).
▪ Examination of the digit to rule out associated digital nerve injury is required.

PHYSICAL FINDINGS

▪ Laceration
▪ Affected digit held in unopposed extension
▪ Inability to actively flex interphalangeal joints (if both tendons are cut), isolated DIP joint (if FDP only is cut) or isolated PIP joint (if FDS only is cut)

IMAGING AND OTHER DIAGNOSTIC STUDIES

▪ The sudden loss of active flexion after a laceration overlying the flexor sheath almost always represents a tendon injury. Radiographs should be obtained to rule out associated fractures that would require treatment at the time of tendon repair. Lacerations due to glass, metal fragments, and so forth should be imaged to localize any residual foreign bodies for removal.

▪ In the setting of a closed injury with the sudden loss of active flexion, one must consider the possibility of a tendon avulsion from its insertion. Radiographs may demonstrate an avulsed fleck of bone. In the more common cases of an FDP avulsion, this bone fragment may remain in the region of the distal phalanx or may be pulled proximally into the flexor sheath. If no bony fragment is seen on a plain radiograph and the diagnosis is still in doubt, ultrasound may help.

DIFFERENTIAL DIAGNOSIS

▪ Pain after injury may cause a patient (especially a child) to hold a digit or hand immobile, mimicking tendon injury.

▪ Testing for the tenodesis effect (digits passively flex with wrist extension) or compressing the flexor musculature in the forearm should help with diagnosis in these situations.

NONOPERATIVE MANAGEMENT

▪ There is no nonoperative means of restoring active flexion to a digit whose flexors have been cut, as the tendon ends retract and do not heal to one another.

▪ If a flexor tendon laceration is encountered within the first 4 weeks after injury, it is probably worthwhile attempting primary repair. After that time, discussion should be held with the patient regarding other options.

▪ For late presentation of an isolated FDP laceration in zone I, it may be practical to do nothing, as full proximal interphalangeal motion should still be present. If the DIP joint is or

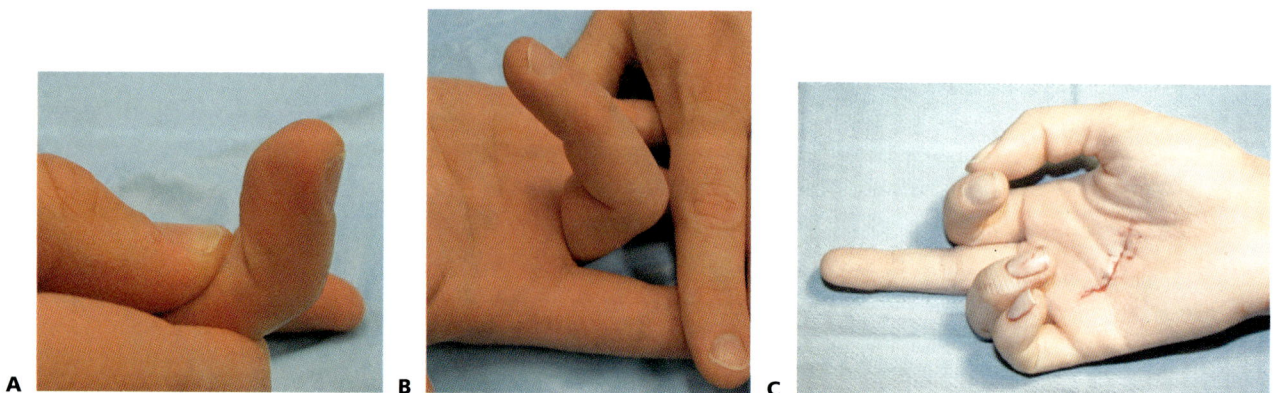

FIG 2 • **A.** Isolation of distal interphalangeal flexion to test flexor digitorum profundus integrity. **B.** Isolation of proximal interphalangeal flexion to test flexor digitorum superficialis integrity. **C.** Loss of normal flexion cascade after tendon laceration in palm.

becomes unstable, a DIP joint fusion or tenodesis of the distal FDP stump can be performed. One large series reported successful primary tendon grafting for isolated FDP lacerations even in zone II, but this is not widely performed.

- For late presentation of zone II injuries involving both tendons, staged tendon reconstruction (see Chap. HA-55) may be an option.

SURGICAL MANAGEMENT

- The goal of flexor tendon surgery is a repair that will allow early motion, will not fail due to gap formation or suture pullout, and will not develop adhesions limiting final range of motion.
- Several variables under control of the surgeon contribute to repair strength:
  - Number of strands (most important determinant; a four-strand repair with an epitenon suture added has been shown in laboratory studies to withstand limited early active motion)[6,11]
  - Suture size (3-0 or 4-0 is sufficient; larger suture increases resistance to gliding)
  - Configuration of repair (cruciate repair requires only one knot, buries the knot within the repair site, and allows for equal distribution of force across all four strands)[5]
  - Use of locking stitches (adds resistance to suture pullout)
  - Addition of an epitenon suture (increases repair strength and decreases gap formation and gliding resistance)[6]
  - Presence of a gap (greater than 3 mm at any point will likely result in rupture)
  - Bunching of repair (due to taking too large a "bite" of tendon end; increases gliding resistance and therefore risk of rupture)
  - Integrity of pulleys (at least half of both A2 and A4 should be preserved to maintain tendon excursion and allow tip-to-palm contact)
  - Repair of one versus both tendons (if repair of both FDS slips impedes gliding, one slip should be resected, or the FDS not repaired at all)
- It is well accepted that core suture strength is directly related to the number of suture strands crossing the repair site between proximal and distal tendon ends; all else being equal, using more strands means a stronger repair.[11]
  - This concept must be balanced against other factors: too many sutures crossing the repair site limits the available surface area for exposed tendon ends to heal; more sutures and knots increase the gliding resistance of the tendon; and the more sutures placed, the longer the surgical time, which is associated with risks such as infection and anesthesia-related issues.

- Strickland[6] showed that a four-strand zone II repair with an epitenon suture is strong enough to tolerate an immediate light active range-of-motion protocol, which allows for early gliding of the repair and decreases the risk of adhesion formation.
- Suture size contributes to repair strength, but one study showed 3-0 and 4-0 suture to resist repair rupture equally well and 2-0 suture to increase gliding resistance significantly.[1]
- Adding at least one locking stitch (making an additional pass to capture more tendon fibers) has been shown to increase repair strength and minimize gap formation.
- Multiple studies suggest that when both tendons are cut in zone II, repair of the FDP and only one slip of FDS rather than both slips results in decreased gliding resistance and improved range of motion.[9,10,13]
  - My present compromise is a four-strand cruciate repair using 3-0 nonabsorbable suture, with a 6-0 Prolene running epitenon suture, with repair of one slip of FDS and resection of the other slip when both tendons are lacerated in zone II.

Preoperative Planning

- As noted previously, it is usually preferable to perform tendon repair early (if other circumstances allow).[3,7] The upper limit of time past which proximal stump contracture is likely to cause technical difficulty is variable. Although 3 to 4 weeks is a commonly cited limit for primary tendon repair, in rare cases the vinculae may prevent retraction and allow repair even later.
- Patients presenting late should be fully counseled regarding other options, including the potential for intraoperative changes in plan.

Positioning

- Flexor tendon surgery, like most hand surgery, is generally performed with the affected extremity on a hand table, with the shoulder abducted 90 degrees and the elbow extended. The forearm is supinated, exposing the volar surface of the digits.
- A positioning device such as a lead hand can be helpful in stabilizing digits for surgery (once tendon ends have been delivered into the wound) and keeping other digits out of the way.

Approach

- Incisions should be planned so as to incorporate the laceration into the exposure.
  - Zigzag (Bruner) or midlateral approaches both work well; they can be combined if needed.
  - Midlateral incisions extending proximally on one side of the digit and distally on the other can give large flaps and excellent exposure.
- The chief concern is not to cross a flexion crease at a right angle since the resultant scar will tend to contract and limit extension.

PRIMARY REPAIR IN ZONE II

Retrieval of Tendon Ends

- A zigzag or Bruner incision is made, sometimes in combination with mid-lateral incisions (**TECH FIG 1A**).
- Often some manipulation is needed to bring the tendon ends into the wound; for the proximal tendon end, wrist flexion and "milking" of the forearm may succeed. The distal stump is best exposed by extending the incision so that the repair can be performed without holding the digit flexed.

- Initial exposure should include both digital neurovascular bundles, whether or not they were injured along with the tendon or tendons.
  - If digital nerve or artery repair is needed, this should be done after the tendon repair so that the more delicate microsuture used is not disrupted with manipulation of the digit. Exposure of these bundles even when uninjured allows much more freedom for manipulating the cut tendon ends.

TECHNIQUES

TECHNIQUES

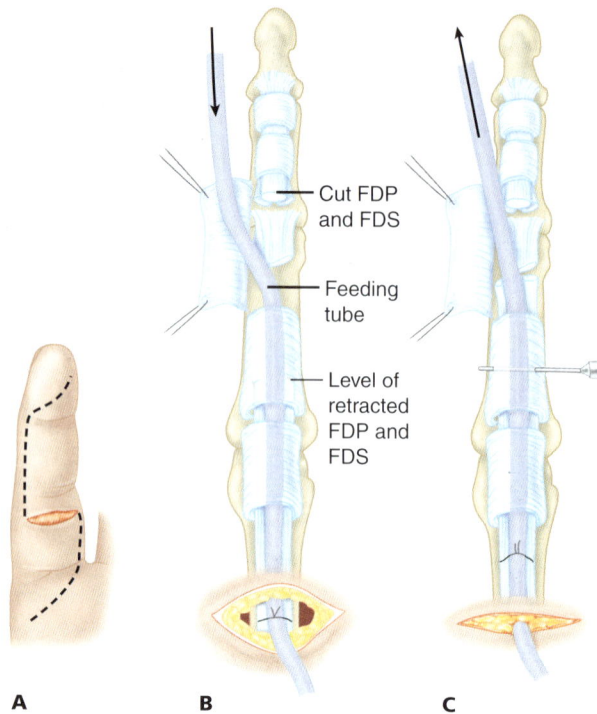

- Cut FDP and FDS
- Feeding tube
- Level of retracted FDP and FDS

A   **B**   **C**

TECH FIG 1 • Exposure (**A**), retrieval (**B**), and temporary transverse pinning through sheath of cut tendon ends (**C**) to allow tension-free repair.

- Once the neurovascular bundles are exposed and protected, the sheath should be cleared of overlying soft tissues and inspected. The sheath laceration can be extended with a sidecut to form an L-shaped flap, always preserving as much as possible of the A2 and A4 pulleys. Creating such flaps can facilitate retrieving the tendon ends.

- Because most flexor tendon injuries occur with the digit in flexion, the skin laceration is generally more proximal than the tendon laceration. This means that exposure of the distal stump often requires considerable distal extension of the incision, often to the level of the DIP joint and obliquely across the pulp of the distal phalanx.

- The proximal tendon end may be held in place near the laceration by its vinculae, but it will often have retracted well proximally.
  - It is reasonable to make several attempts to retrieve the proximal tendon end through the sheath with an appropriately small instrument (curved tendon passer, small hemostat, etc.), keeping in mind that the less damage to the tendon end, the easier the repair and the less scarring that will result. Flexing the wrist and "milking" the forearm will sometimes encourage a proximally migrated tendon to protrude into the wound.
  - If these measures fail, a short transverse incision along the distal palmar crease can be made, as if exposing the A1 pulley for a trigger finger release, and the tendon exposed at this level.
- A pediatric feeding tube can be threaded from one wound to the other and sutured to the tendon in the proximal wound (**TECH FIG 1B**).
- The tube and flexor tendon can then be retrieved into the distal wound and the tube and suture cut free.
- Once the proximal end is in the planned repair site, the tendon can be pinned with a 25-gauge needle to prevent retraction back into the sheath (**TECH FIG 1C**).
- Often the distal location of the distal stump requires that the proximal tendon end be threaded past the original laceration site to a more distal "window" made in the sheath for tendon repair. This, coupled with flexion of the DIP joint, should allow for apposition of the tendon ends and repair under minimal tension.

Tendon Repair

- Four-strand cruciate repair is effected using 3-0 nonabsorbable suture, with a 6-0 Prolene running locking epitendon suture, and repair of one slip of FDS (**TECH FIG 2**).

Epitenon-First Repair

- For very oblique lacerations it may be easier to perform an epitenon-first repair, coapting the cut tendon ends smoothly, and then performing the core stitch beginning through a slit on the outside of the tendon, burying the knot in this same slit (**TECH FIG 3**).
- The repair is otherwise the same as a four-strand cruciate repair.

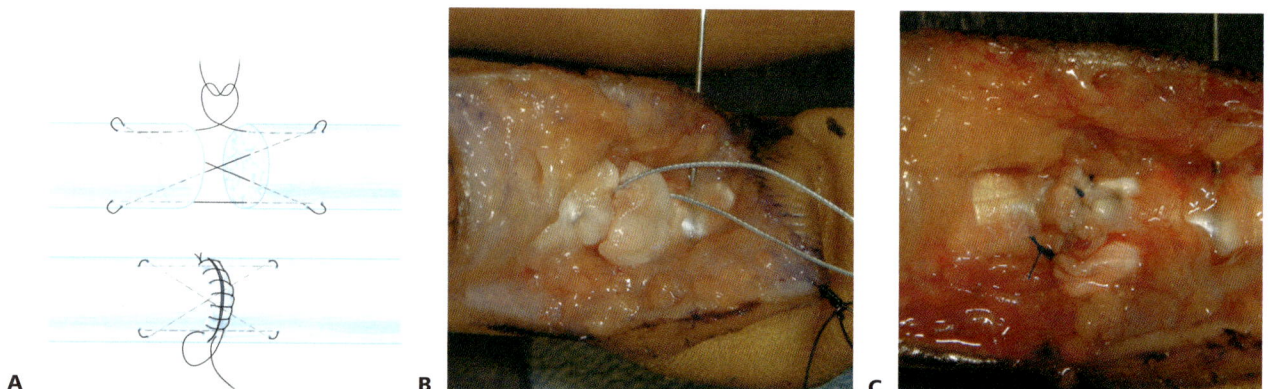

A   **B**   **C**

TECH FIG 2 • **A.** Four-strand cruciate repair with epitenon stitch. **B,C.** The hand is to the right and the fingertips to the left. **B.** Distal zone II flexor digitorum profundus laceration with tendon ends pinned in place and core stitch being placed. **C.** Completed repair with epitenon stitch.

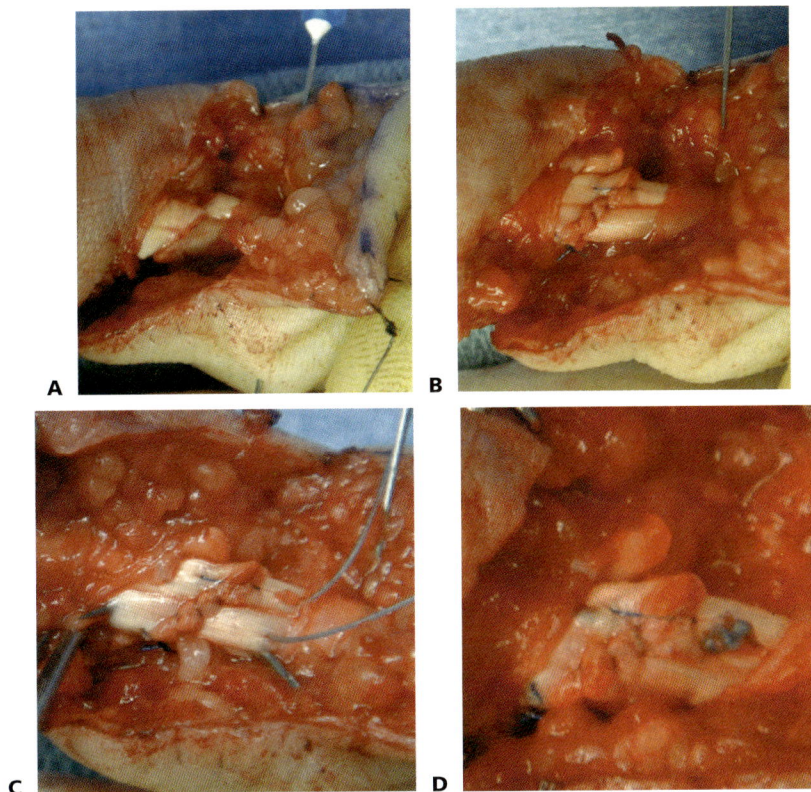

TECH FIG 3 • **A–D.** The hand is to the right and the fingertips to the left. **A.** Oblique laceration of flexor tendons in zone II; tendon ends retrieved and pinned in place for repair. **B.** Epitenon repair performed first. **C.** Core suture begun via small incision in tendon proximal to repair; otherwise similar to standard cruciate repair. **D.** Core stitch completed and knot buried in small incision used for starting point.

PEARLS AND PITFALLS

- Early repair is easiest and gives best results.
- Midlateral incisions give wide exposure.
- Hold tendon ends in place with 25-gauge needles to allow tension-free repair.
- A four-strand locking cruciate repair using 3-0 nonabsorbable suture combined with a 6-0 absorbable running epitenon stitch will allow protected early active motion and has been shown to maximize the outcome.
- Limiting repair of FDS to one slip minimizes overcrowding in zone II and allows better tendon gliding.
- For partial lacerations, no repair is necessary unless greater than 60% of the cross-sectional area of the tendon has been divided. Any flap of tendon should be trimmed to prevent later triggering.[2,4,12]

POSTOPERATIVE CARE

- If a primary repair has been performed as described above, an immediate light active "place and hold" therapy regimen can usually begin safely as long as the patient is reliable.

OUTCOMES

- A recent meta-analysis of multiple studies over the past 15 years found a rupture rate of 4% to 10% and good to excellent results in about three quarters of patients.[8] Present-day techniques should allow for continued improvement in these results.
- Injury mechanism is a predictor of outcome and is beyond the surgeon's control. An uncomplicated, isolated sharp flexor tendon laceration that is treated acutely represents the best possible scenario for a highly functional digit. Additional injury to bone, tendon, or nerve negatively affects outcome.

COMPLICATIONS

- Two extremes of bad outcomes are tendon rupture and tendon adhesions. Ruptures are rare, but adhesions, and resultant limited motion, are common.
- If ruptures are noticed immediately, a repeat repair should be performed, although the patient and surgeon should be prepared for the need to proceed intraoperatively with other reconstructive options.

■ The management of tendon adhesions is discussed in Chapter HA-55.

REFERENCES

1. Alavanja G, Dailey E, Mass DP. Repair of zone II flexor digitorum profundus lacerations using varying suture sizes: a comparative biomechanical study. J Hand Surg Am 2005;30A:448–454.
2. Erhard L, Zobitz ME, Zhao C, et al. Treatment of partial lacerations in flexor tendons by trimming: a biomechanical in vitro study. J Bone Joint Surg Am 2002;84A:1006–1012.
3. Gorriz GJ, Cooke J. Assessment of the influence of the timing of repair on flexor tendon injuries in chickens. Br J Plast Surg 1976;29:82–84.
4. Hariharan JS, Diao E, Soejima O, et al. Partial lacerations of human digital flexor tendons: a biomechanical analysis. J Hand Surg Am 1997;22A:1011–1015.
5. McLarney E, Hoffman H, Wolfe SW. Biomechanical analysis of the cruciate four-strand flexor tendon repair. J Hand Surg Am 1999;24A: 295–301.
6. Strickland JW. Flexor tendon injuries: I. Foundations of treatment. J Am Acad Orthop Surg 1995;3:44–54.
7. Tang J, Shi D, Gu Y. Flexor tendon repair: timing of surgery and sheath management. Zhonghua Wai Ke Za Zhi 1995;33:532–535.
8. Tang JB. Clinical outcomes associated with flexor tendon repair. Hand Clin 2005;21:199–210.
9. Tang JB. Flexor tendon repair in zone 2C. J Hand Surg Br 1994;19B:72–75.
10. Tang JB, Xie RG, Cao Y, et al. A2 pulley incision or one slip of the superficialis improves flexor tendon repairs. Clin Orthop Relat Res 2006;456:121–127.
11. Thurman RT, Trumble TE, Hanel DP, et al. Two-, four-, and six-strand zone II flexor tendon repairs: an in situ biomechanical comparison using a cadaver model. J Hand Surg Am 1998;23A:261–265.
12. Wray RC Jr, Weeks PM. Treatment of partial tendon lacerations. Hand 1980;12:163–166.
13. Zhao C, Amadio PC, Zobitz ME, et al. Resection of the flexor digitorum superficialis reduces gliding resistance after zone II flexor digitorum profundus repair in vitro. J Hand Surg Am 2002;27A:316–321.

Chapter 55

Tenolysis Following Injury and Repair of Digital Flexor Tendons

Shai Luria and Christopher H. Allan

DEFINITION

- Flexor tendon trauma and repair are commonly complicated by adhesions, limiting the gliding capacity of the tendons.
  - These injuries have long been highly challenging.
  - The infamous "no man's land" or zone II injuries were treated in the past only after the acute phase, when the delay in treatment was perceived to minimize the development of adhesions.
- Tendon adhesions result in limited excursion of the tendon in its sheath and occur when the tendon surface is violated either through the injury itself or secondary to surgical manipulation. When limited digital function is the consequence, and no further improvement with therapy is seen, surgical treatment should be considered.
- The spectrum of treatment of flexor tendon adhesions ranges from nonoperative treatment to different surgical modalities, from tenolysis to a two-stage tendon reconstruction.
  - The operative decision is based on different factors, such as the quality of the tendon involved and the integrity of the surrounding sheath. Some of these factors can be evaluated only during the operation.
  - All treatment options should be discussed preoperatively and the surgeon should be prepared to make the final decision based on operative findings.
- Tenolysis consists of surgical release of tendon adhesions to restore tendon gliding and digital motion. This can be a very satisfying procedure in selected cases, particularly when adhesions are localized to just a portion of the sheath.
- Proper patient selection is crucial and several questions must be asked: Will the patient cooperate with extensive hand therapy? Is the functional improvement after this complex and time-intensive process likely to be better and more rapid than with fusion of an interphalangeal (IP) joint or even with amputation of the digit?

ANATOMY

- Refer to Chapter HA-54.

PATHOGENESIS

- Injury (or repair) of the tendon and its synovial sheath is the basis for the development of adhesions.
- The initial mode of inflammatory reaction is similar to that after any tissue injury. Initiation of adhesion formation begins with deposition of a fibrin matrix that typically occurs during the coagulation process.
  - This matrix is gradually replaced by vascular granulation tissue containing macrophages, fibroblasts, and giant cells.
  - The clots are slow to achieve complete organization. In this process, they consist of erythrocytes separated by masses of fibrin that are covered with layers of flattened cells and contain a patchy infiltrate of mononuclear cells.
  - The adhesion matures into a fibrous band, often containing small nodules of calcification.

- Mature adhesions are often covered by mesothelium, are vascularized, and contain other connective tissue fibers, such as elastin.[12]
- The extracellular matrix, which is composed of collagen, proteoglycans, fibronectin, and elastin, plays a central role in the management of tendon healing as well as the development of adhesions. Degradation products in the matrix are chemotactic for fibroblasts, leukocytes, and endothelial cells.[12]
- During the first few days after trauma, T cells and macrophages accumulate in the location of injury and stimulate the synovial cells to produce fibronectin. Collagen types 1 and 3 accumulate between tenocytes and around the tendon by 1 week after trauma. Adhesions between the tendon and its sheath can be seen by this time as a thickening of the epitenon to five to seven cell layers. Fibronectin is present as well and serves as scaffolding for the developing scar.[12]
- The process described occurs to a lesser extent in the proximal zones of the flexor tendons. Zone II tendon injuries occur in the milieu of two tendons gliding in a constrictive fibroosseous tunnel. In other zones, this potential for development of adhesions exists to a much lesser extent.
- Three types of adhesions have been described:
  - Loose adhesions arising from subcutaneous tissue and allowing some glide of the tendons
  - Moderately dense adhesions from the synovial sheath or pulleys that are remarkably restrictive of tendon motion
  - Dense adhesions arising from the bony floor or volar plate, penetrating the dorsal aspect of the tendon
  - Both dense and moderately dense adhesions prevent tendon motion and jeopardize healing.[23]
- The role of different cytokines has been evaluated in the pathogenesis of adhesions in general and tendon adhesions in specific.[16,26]
  - Transforming growth factor-beta (TGF-β) has been shown to be a prominent regulator of tendon healing, although its precise role is still unclear and under extensive research.[27] In the laboratory, these factors have been shown to be regulated by physical factors such as shear stress[7] as well as by specific neutralizing antibodies[32] or chemical modulators such as 5-fluorouracil.[18]

NATURAL HISTORY

- Symptomatic adhesions result in substantial morbidity such as decreased range of motion, joint contracture, decreased strength, and substantial decrease in hand and upper extremity function. Adhesions occur with every tendon injury and depend on the extent of injury, the mobilization of digits after the injury, and the treatment applied. They are especially severe and symptomatic in injuries in zone II. Before the widespread use of early and intensive mobilization protocols after injury and repair, limited success was achieved and tenolysis was frequently required.
- Strickland and Glogovac[21] reported in 1980 on the advantage of early mobilization of zone II flexor tendon injuries.

In their report, by 160 days after repair, 10 of 25 patients achieved less than 70% of the expected range of motion of the proximal and distal IP joints. Although there are limited reports regarding the natural history of these injuries when untreated, this report gives us a sense of the typical outcome of flexor tendon repair in the era before early motion protocols.

- Tenolysis is by far the most common secondary procedure performed after digit replantation, according to a recent meta-analysis.[29] Although stiffness of a replanted finger is a result of multiple causes, the adhesion of tendons is a leading cause of this problem.
- Tang[3] estimates that 10% of repaired flexor tendons will need surgical treatment of adhesions. Moderately dense adhesions of the synovial sheath or pulley and dense adhesions of the bone to tendon are difficult to alter once they have formed. These adhesions should be treated surgically.
- Proximal to zone II, the limitation in range of motion and need for flexor tenolysis are less common, even in the setting of a severe injury.[30]

PATIENT HISTORY AND PHYSICAL FINDINGS

- Evaluate both passive and active range of motion.
- Note the skin integrity and the location and condition of scars and previous surgical incisions.
- Look for other deforming conditions, such as malaligned fractures.
- The examiner should search for other factors limiting range of motion, such as intra-articular pathology, scar contracture of the skin, extensor tendon contracture or adhesions, interosseous muscle contractures, or capsular and collateral ligament contractures.
- The neurovascular status of the digit is documented.
- The continuity of both flexor tendons in all digits is evaluated:
- Continuity of the flexor digitorum superficialis (FDS) tendon
- Active flexion of the proximal interphalangeal (PIP) joint is evaluated for each digit separately. The adjacent digits are held in full extension by the examiner at the metacarpophalangeal (MP), PIP, and distal interphalangeal (DIP) joints to assess for intact fibers of the FDS inserting into the middle phalanx. This does not exclude a partial tear of the tendon.
- Continuity of the flexor digitorum profundus (FDP) tendon
- Active flexion of the DIP while the examiner grasps the middle phalanx to assess for intact fibers of the FDP inserting into the distal phalanx. This does not exclude a partial tear of the tendon.
- Range of motion (ROM): If passive ROM exceeds active, the pathology is at least partly musculotendinous (tendon adherent, incompetent, or both).
- The "seesaw effect": The examiner should passively extend and flex the DIP, PIP, and MP joints. Extend one joint followed by the other to assess for the seesaw effect. Nonarticular contracture is revealed when one joint is flexed, the other can be extended, and vice versa.
- The Bunnell intrinsic tightness test is performed to evaluate flexion of the PIP joint with the MP joint extended and then flexed. With intrinsic tightness, there is less passive flexion of the PIP joint when the MP joint is held extended than when the MP joint is flexed (therefore, the surgeon may need to release the intrinsics as part of treatment).

- Evaluate for lumbrical contracture: An intrinsic tightness test is performed with the fingers radially or ulnarly deviated. With lumbrical contracture, there is less passive flexion of the PIP joint with the finger deviated or with the DIP joint flexed in comparison to intrinsic testing. If present, this suggests lumbrical muscle contracture as part of the pathology.
- Alternatively, the test is performed with the DIP joint flexed as well as the PIP joint.
- Evaluate for extensor contractures: The examiner flexes the wrist and MP joints and examines flexion of the PIP and DIP joints. With extensor contractures there will be limited flexion of the digit IP joints with flexed wrist and MP joints.
- Evaluate for flexor contractures: The examiner extends the wrist and MP joints and examines extension of the IP joints. With flexor contracture, there will be limited extension of the digit IP joints with extension of the wrist and MP joints.
- The Landsmeer test is performed for evaluation of contracture of the oblique retinacular ligament (extending from the volar aspect of the PIP joint to the dorsal aspect of the DIP joint). In a positive test, passive extension of the PIP joint will result in extension of the DIP joint as well. Continued shortening of the ligament will result in a boutonnière deformity.

IMAGING AND OTHER DIAGNOSTIC STUDIES

- Radiographs of the hand are taken to evaluate for bony and articular pathology as well as the presence and location of implants. Skeletal deformity secondary to avulsion injuries may be seen.
- CT scans may be helpful in selected cases for bony and articular pathology.
- Magnetic resonance imaging (MRI) or ultrasound may be useful in identifying tendon or capsular injury as well as aiding in the differential diagnosis of severe tendon adhesions versus rupture.

DIFFERENTIAL DIAGNOSIS

- Intrinsic muscle contracture
- Capsular or collateral ligament contractures
- Malalignment of fracture
- Extensor tendon adhesions
- Rheumatoid arthritis
- Dupuytren's disease
- Neurologic causes
- Burns
- Congenital anomalies
- Complex regional pain syndrome

NONOPERATIVE MANAGEMENT

- ROM exercises as well as pain management play a role in several clinical situations:
  - During the period after repair of the injury
  - When the functional results are satisfactory to the patient and meet his or her needs
  - Delayed healing of soft tissue or bony injury
  - Limited passive range of motion
  - When the patient is uncooperative with perioperative care and therapy
- The therapy should include full active as well as resistive exercises designed at maximizing the active ROM achieved, before surgical treatment.

SURGICAL MANAGEMENT

- Tenolysis of the flexor tendon requires intact tendons and pulleys in order to succeed. Patients for whom tenolysis is appropriate have reached a plateau in function despite appropriate therapy, and have significantly greater passive than active range of motion.
- Prerequisites for tenolysis also include healing of all fractures and wounds with soft, pliable skin and minimal inflammatory reaction around scars.
- The timing of tenolysis is the subject of debate. Recommendations range from 3 to 9 months after the tendon repair or grafting. Strickland[20] recommends waiting at least 3 months after repair, with 4 to 8 weeks without measurable improvement in active motion with intensive therapy.
- Concomitant procedures should be considered carefully and limited to those procedures that will not affect postoperative therapy.
    - Capsulotomies of the PIP or DIP are often necessary in these cases and may be performed,[20] although some authors warn of inferior results with this addition.[24]
    - Pulley reconstruction with tenolysis should be avoided if possible, although successful combined procedures have been described.[8]
    - Procedures requiring immobilization should not be performed concomitantly with the tenolysis. Examples include tendon lengthening or shortening, free skin grafts, or osteotomies.[8,28]
- Local anesthetic supplemented by intravenous analgesia and tranquilizing drugs was popularized by Schneider.[19] This allows the surgeon to evaluate the extent of adhesiolysis achieved by having the patient actively flexing the digit during surgery. The patient can also see the results, motivating him or her to achieve a similar range of motion postoperatively.
    - Anesthetic options include local infiltration into the palm and a wrist block.
    - The use of local anesthesia is limited by the use of a tourniquet, which causes paralysis of the muscles after 30 minutes and may be difficult for the patient to tolerate past that time. To deal with these problems, a sterile forearm tourniquet may be elevated 30 minutes into the procedure, releasing the arm tourniquet.
- Regional and general anesthesia are additional techniques suitable for a tenolysis procedure. General anesthesia is necessary in cases of questionable patient cooperation, tolerance to pain or other contraindication to local or regional anesthesia, or where time to completion of tenolysis (and any associated procedures) is expected to exceed the likely duration of a local or regional block.
- Foucher et al[8] report that they have abandoned local anesthesia or "selective sensory blocks" except in late tenolysis where they have doubts about the performance of the muscle. Instead, they use a separate incision in the palm or forearm to test flexion at the end of the procedure.

Preoperative Planning

- Surgical supplies including implants necessary to perform a staged tendon reconstruction should be available.

Positioning

- The patient is positioned supine with the upper extremity on a hand table. A lead hand splint is recommended.

Approach

- Wide exposure of the flexor tendon is necessary. This may be accomplished either by a zigzag (Brunner-type) incision or by a midlateral incision (**FIG 1**).[1]
- The Brunner zigzag incision provides the best exposure of the tendon and pulley system.
- A midlateral exposure will protect the neurovascular structures dorsally and will cause less scar directly over the tendon. It may also cause less wound tension during early therapy.

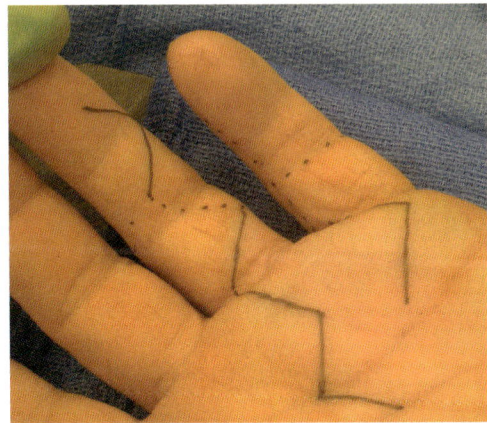

FIG 1 • Either a zigzag (Brunner-type) incision or a midlateral incision can be used to expose the tendons. The incisions are designed taking into account the previous scars. In this case, the ring finger palmar scars (marked with a *dotted line*) were extended (*solid line*) to a Brunner-type exposure. In the small finger, the scars (*dotted lines*) were midlateral and the exposure was planned in that fashion. (Courtesy of Dr. T.E. Trumble.)

FLEXOR TENOLYSIS

- Expose the flexor tendons starting from the unaffected region and proceeding to the involved areas (**TECH FIG 1A**).
- Define the borders of the tendons (**TECH FIG 1B**).
- Raise both flexor tendons as one, carefully lysing the adhesions around them.
    - This may be performed using a scalpel, tenotomy scissors, or a Freer elevator (**TECH FIG 1C**).
- Retraction and manipulation of the elevated tendons should be accomplished in as atraumatic a fashion as possible using a Penrose drain or blunt instrument.

- If possible, separate FDS from FDP tendons.
    - The FDS tendon may need to be sacrificed if the scarring is extremely severe[19] in order to achieve adhesiolysis under the pulleys and smooth gliding of the tendon.
    - Resection of a slip of FDS has been shown to improve FDP gliding after repair in zone II injuries.[33]
    - In some cases it may be preferable not to separate severely adhesed tendons, allowing them to act as one, where a single combined tendon is mobilized to its insertion.

TECHNIQUES

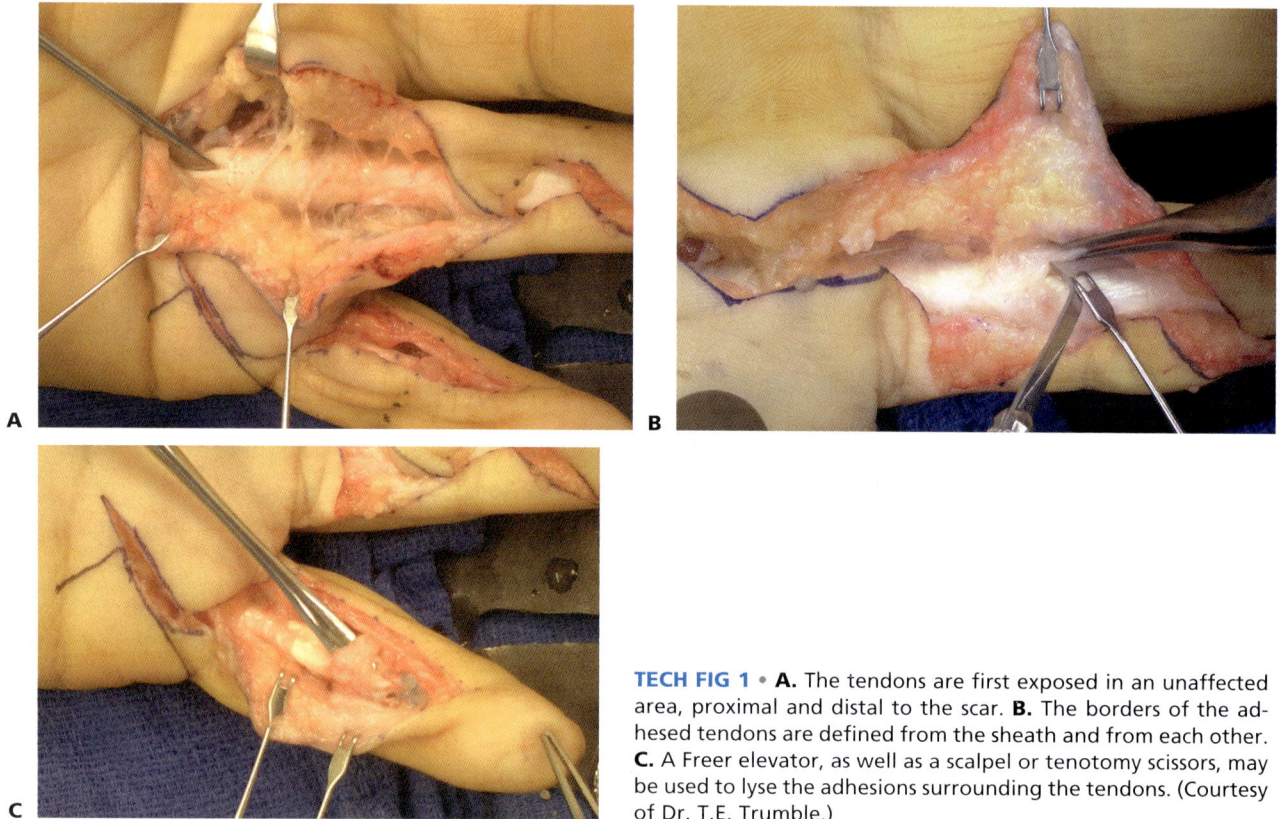

TECH FIG 1 • **A.** The tendons are first exposed in an unaffected area, proximal and distal to the scar. **B.** The borders of the adhesed tendons are defined from the sheath and from each other. **C.** A Freer elevator, as well as a scalpel or tenotomy scissors, may be used to lyse the adhesions surrounding the tendons. (Courtesy of Dr. T.E. Trumble.)

ADHESIOLYSIS

- Adhesiolysis may be facilitated using these instruments and techniques:
  - A modified 69 Beaver blade (McDonough and Stern 45-degree Beaver blade) with an angle of 45 degrees (**TECH FIG 2A**).
  - Schreiber knee arthroscopy blades.
  - Braided suture (0 Mersilene, 2-0 Prolene) or dental wire may be inserted between the tendon and phalanx[2] and used as a Gigli saw to separate the tendon from bone by pulling on the suture ends back and forth along the tendon (**TECH FIG 2B**).
    - This technique may be advantageous when separating adhesed FDP and FDS tendons or when performing tenolysis under a pulley or preserved sheath.
    - Alternatives to collect and pass the suture include use of a blunt elevator with a hole at its distal tip, which may be inserted under the pulley from a proximal to distal direction,[6] and a wire loop or a needle inserted backward in the gutter between the phalanx, the tendon, and the sheath.[2]
  - Meals developed a set of instruments specifically designed for tenolysis (George Tiemann & Co, Hauppauge, NY).
    - The necks of these tenolysis knives follow the natural curvature of the finger and have semisharp blades that conform to the circumference of the

tendon sheath with either a convex or a concave edge[1] (**TECH FIG 2C**).

- Débride the tendons free of previous suture material or frayed edges.

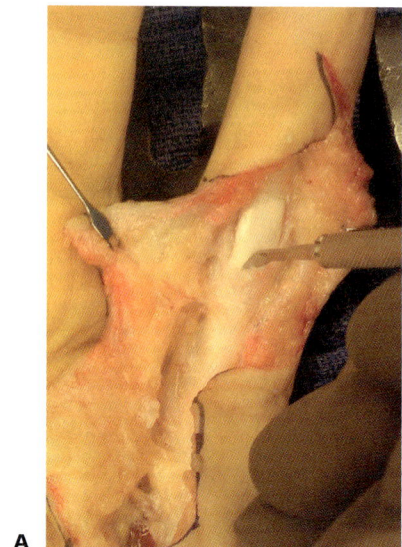

TECH FIG 2 • **A.** A modified 69 Beaver blade with an angle of 45 degrees is at a comfortable angle to perform the adhesiolysis of the tendons. *(continued)*

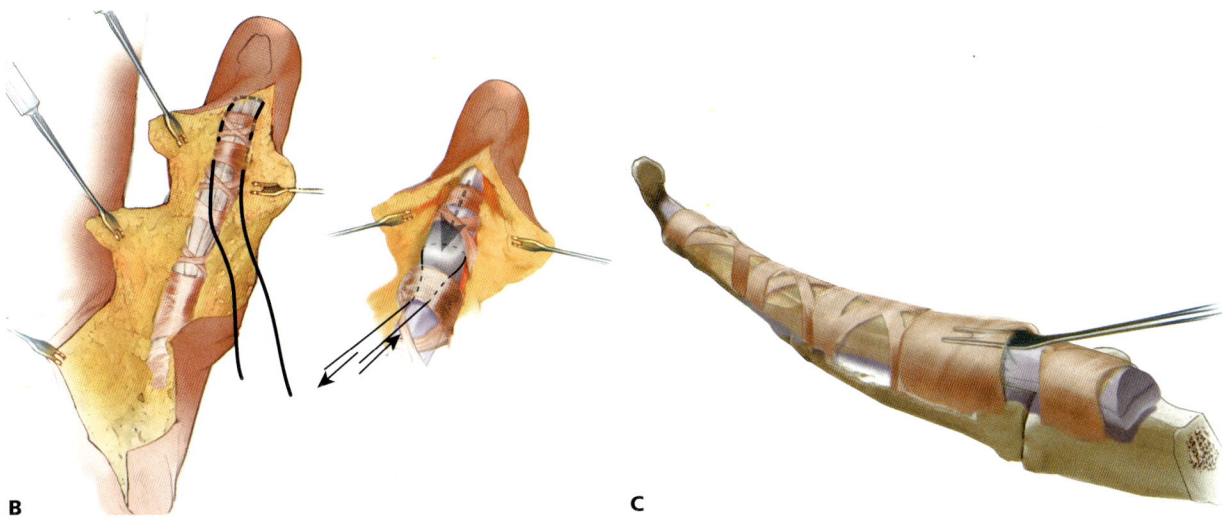

B

C

TECH FIG 2 • (*continued*) **B.** A suture or a dental wire may be inserted between the tendons or between the tendons and phalanx or sheath and pulled under the pulleys (as a Gigli saw) to lyse the adhesions while preserving the pulleys. **C.** Flexor tenolysis with a Meals tenolysis knife. (**A:** Courtesy of Dr. T.E. Trumble.)

ADDRESSING THE PULLEY SYSTEM

- Preserve as much of the pulley system as possible. It is crucial to preserve the A2 and A4 pulleys to prevent bowstringing and loss of tip-to-palm contact in full flexion. This may be performed by creating transverse windows along the course of the tendon. Some resection of the pulleys is possible (**TECH FIG 3**).

- In case sacrifice of part of these pulleys is crucial to achieve better tendon excursion or to facilitate the release of adhesions, about half of a pulley can be incised.[17]
- Widening of the pulleys may be performed with small pediatric urethral dilators or cardiac coronary artery dilators.

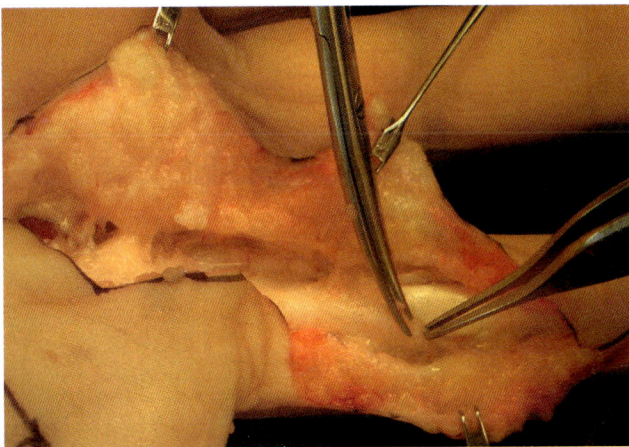

TECH FIG 3 • Exposing the tendons while preserving the pulleys is performed by creating transverse windows along the course of the tendon. (Courtesy of Dr. T.E. Trumble.)

EVALUTION OF ADEQUACY OF RELEASE

- Adequacy of release must be evaluated and may be assessed using several techniques.
- If the patient is awake, he or she can actively flex the digit. Otherwise a traction flexion check should be performed for each of the flexor tendons separately.
- Through the palmar extension of the exposure, pull on the tendon with a blunt tendon hook or retractor (**TECH FIG 4A**).

- If the expected excursion cannot be tested through the palmar incision, proximal exposure of the tendon may be necessary through a separate incision proximal to the wrist (**TECH FIG 4B**).
  - An Allis clamp may be placed around the tendon and pulled gently to examine the tendon's excursion.

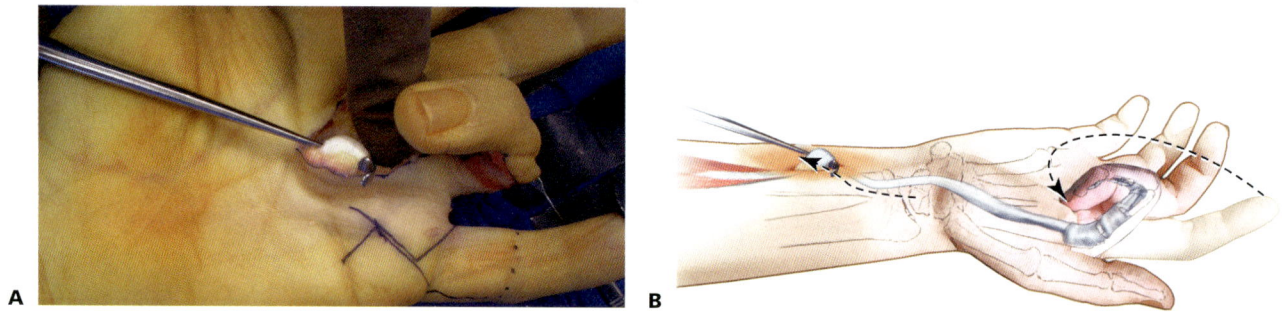

TECH FIG 4 • A. A traction flexion check may be performed through the palmar extension of the exposure, pulling on each tendon with a blunt hooked instrument. **B.** If the expected excursion cannot be tested through the palmar incision, proximal exposure of the tendon may be necessary, through a separate incision proximal to the wrist. (**A:** Courtesy of Dr. T.E. Trumble.)

CLOSURE

- The tourniquet is deflated before closure to ensure adequate hemostasis. If needed, a Penrose drain is placed and removed the next day.
  - Hematoma formation will lead to scarring and have a negative impact on the final result.

- The skin is closed using nonabsorbable suture and a soft, mildly compressive dressing is applied that allows for early range of motion.

PEARLS AND PITFALLS

Indications	■ Negative prognostic indicators are age older than 40 years, nerve suture, late tenolysis (more than 1 year postoperatively), and tenolysis requiring a prolonged operative time.[28]
Intraoperative evaluation	■ A tendon gap filled with scar, or a tendon with more than a third of its width missing, should probably be treated with staged reconstruction or immediate grafting. ■ Attenuated or destroyed critical pulleys should be reconstructed. This may be an additional reason to perform a staged reconstruction.
Separate tendon from scar	■ Start from unaffected and work toward affected areas.
Poor-quality tendon	■ It is possible to place a rod adjacent to the tendon. In the event of tendon rupture, only the second stage of the reconstruction will need to be performed.[20]
Operative evaluation of results	■ Marking the tendon with a marking pen and following the mark throughout digit motion may aid in the evaluation of the excursion and the quality of the adhesiolysis.

POSTOPERATIVE CARE

- Hand therapy is initiated the day of surgery in the postanesthesia care unit if an isolated tenolysis is performed without pulley reconstruction.
- A detailed referral note or discussion with the therapist is necessary to plan the rehabilitation program for each patient. Patient history, type of injury, surgical intervention and intraoperative findings, motivation, and pain tolerance should be discussed. The condition of the tendon and pulley system and the vascularity of the digit may alter the course of therapy and should be reported.
- It is crucial that the patient be motivated and understand the therapy protocol, the need for frequent meetings with the therapist, and the daily exercises to be performed independently.

- Adequate pain control is ensured.
- Local blocks may be used in selected cases to allow early mobilization.[15]
- Transcutaneous nerve stimulators are recommended by some for postoperative pain reduction in combination with oral medication.
- Wound care education should be part of the first therapy meetings.
- Edema control is frequently necessary. The patient should be instructed to elevate the hand during the first days after surgery as well as to perform hourly fist pumps with the hand elevated. Gentle compression with a glove, Coban wrap, or elastic bandages should be considered.
- Early mobilization of the tendon is crucial to the success of the procedure, although the quality of the tendon should be taken into account. A weak tendon should limit the therapy to

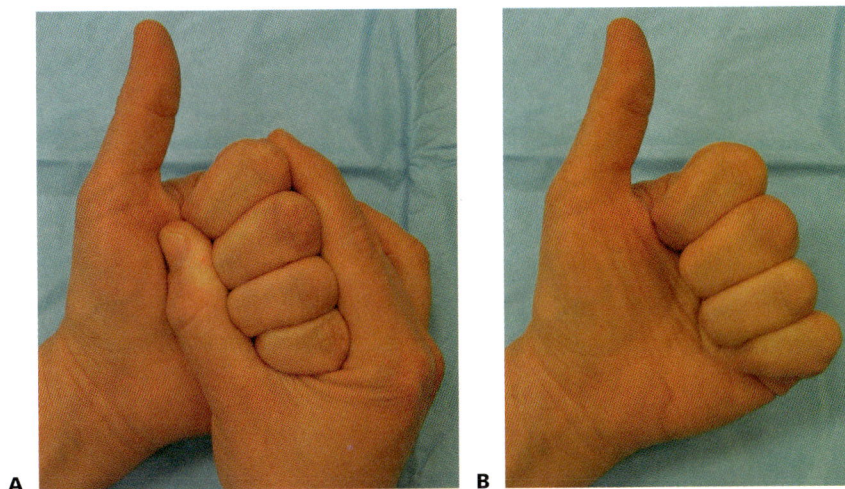

FIG 2 • In "place and hold" exercises, the digits are passively flexed (**A**) and then actively held in place by the patient (**B**).

a limited exercise protocol, although this may be an indication in itself for staged reconstruction or grafting rather than simple tenolysis.

- Various protocols have been described[8,10,25] that balance the maintenance of active flexion ROM achieved in the operating room, maintaining the mobility of the joints as well as the full ROM of active extension. The common protocols achieve a small differential gliding of the FDS versus the FDP tendon.[11]
- Blocking and strengthening exercises should be added at a later date. This may depend on the quality of the lysed tendon, although usually after 4 to 6 weeks these exercises are considered not to endanger the tendons' continuity.[8,20]
  - Trumble and Sailer[25] begin light resistive exercises at 6 weeks and add progressively more resistance after 8 weeks.
- Continuous passive motion (CPM) is under investigation. There have been reports of increased risk of tendon rupture and force required for passive ROM.[1] CPM should not be used in place of active ROM exercises. However, it may be of value if passive ROM is limited or the patient is apprehensive about moving actively. It may also minimize edema and scar formation.[25]
- A protective resting wrist-based splint may be necessary in cases with a thin or damaged tendon. A closely supervised therapy program is important in these cases. Static–progressive or dynamic splints may be needed to treat patients with joint stiffness or contractures.
- A fabricated pulley ring may be used during active motion exercises if the pulleys are tenuous.[25]
- In patients with a weak tendon, therapy should begin with "place and hold" exercises (**FIG 2**). In these exercises, the digit is passively flexed and then actively held in place by the patient.
  - This minimizes the tensile forces on the weak tendon while passing it through its maximal excursion. Further protection may be added when the exercises are performed with the wrist or MP joints flexed. This program should be carried out for 4 to 6 weeks. Active ROM exercises may be added later on.
- Hourly exercises by the patient should be part of any protocol.

OUTCOMES

- Good outcomes after flexor tenolysis have been reported, but outcome measures have varied across reports (Table 1).

Significant complications have been reported in all series, including a significant number of patients with either no improvement or with postoperative worsening. Less information is available but poorer results have been reported after tenolysis in children (under 11) and for the thumb.

- Strickland[20] reported that 64% of tenolysed digits after zone II injury had at least 50% improvement in active ROM. Twenty percent of the patients had no improvement and 8% had rupture of the tendon.
- Jupiter et al[13] used the Strickland formula (Table 1) for the evaluation of 37 replanted digits and 4 replanted thumbs treated with flexor tenolysis. They reported good to excellent results with 24 of the 37 digits. Only poor or fair results were found after thumb flexor tenolysis.
  - Several factors negatively influenced the final results: classification of injury, inferior results of tenolysis with avulsion or crush injuries, number of amputated digits, capsulotomy, level of injury (inferior results with zone II injuries), digit injured (inferior results with thumb procedures), and multiple tenolysed digits.
  - The authors recommend tenolysis of digit flexors when indicated, but not of the thumb flexor.
- Foucher et al[8] reported their results after the treatment of 78 digits, 9 of which were thumbs, and excluding replanted digits. They implemented both their technique of pulley reconstruction and of therapy. The therapy included the use of percutaneous catheters for additional pain control for 3 weeks and passive extension exercises beginning 2 days following the tenolysis surgery. A splint providing some flexion (of MP and IP joints) was removed hourly for exercise. The result after a mean period of 21.5 months was graded both by total active motion (TAM) measurement and the Swanson method for functional evaluation (Table 1). Of the 78 digits, 3% were unimproved and 13% were made worse by the tenolysis. For the remainder of the cases, the TAM improved from 135 degrees to 203 degrees. Using Swanson's assessment the functional deficit improved from 41% to 20%. The thumbs achieved less success, with two cases unimproved, while the rest resulted in an improvement of 65 degrees to 115 degrees, or a decrease in deficit from 12% to 2% according to Swanson. The authors did not separate the results according to the zone of injury and did not report the results for the entire group of patients.

Table 1   Formulas for Outcome Measurement of Flexor Tenolysis

Measurement	Formula	Notes
Total active motion (TAM)	TAM = (active flexion of MP + PIP + DIP) − (extension deficit of MP + PIP + DIP)	For thumb, include MP and IP joints. TAM will not take into account the limited passive ROM that may precede the procedure.
Potential active motion (PAM)	PAM = TAM / TPM	In this formula, the potential ROM after a tenolysis procedure takes into account possible limits in passive ROM.
Strickland et al[21] formula	$(100 - [TPM_{pre} - TAM_{post}]/[TPM_{pre} - TAM_{pre}]) \times 100$	May be performed with or without the MP joint for the calculation of the TAM or TPM. The comparison between the passive and active ROM achieved with the procedure is expressed as a percentage of the preoperative ROM. This may be expressed in a qualitative manner, from poor to excellent (excellent, 75% to 100%; good, 50% to 74%; fair, 25% to 49%; and poor, <24%).
Buck-Gramcko scoring system[5,6]		Qualitative system that grades in points the distance of digits from the palmar crease in flexion, the extension deficit, and the TAM.
Combined angular measurement of finger flexion (Swanson et al[8,22])	A% + B% (100 − A%)	This is based on the combined angular measurement principle.
		This system was designed to evaluate impairment in the hand and upper extremity due to different pathologies. This evaluation of limited ROM of the digits is based on Boyes' linear measurement of the distance between finger pulp and middle palmar crease relating to the percentage of combined impairment of finger flexion.
		Swanson et al[22] combined the impairment value for a finger and correlated it with Boyes' linear measurements to create charts that could be used for everyday clinical practice. This measurement is based on the principle that each impaired joint affects the other joints, and for that reason their ROM cannot be simply summed.
		The values are expressed in percentage of impairment and not classified (as poor, fair, etc.) as the previous measurement systems.

DIP, dorsal interphalangeal; IP, interphalangeal; MP, metacarpophalangeal; PIP, proximal interphalangeal; ROM, range of motion; TPM, total passive motion.

■ Eggli et al[6] evaluated the change in ROM of each joint of the digit in 8 digits treated with flexor tenolysis out of a group of 32 digits with varying zone II injuries requiring tenolysis. They found a decrease of 5 degrees of MP active ROM and an increase of 25 and 35 degrees of PIP and DIP active ROM, respectively. TAM improved by 55 degrees. They found an additional improvement in TAM when the tenolysis was combined with PIP capsulolysis. The authors compared the results of flexor tenolysis with patients treated with flexor and extensor tenolysis in the same digit and found better total active motion (63-degree improvement) and better extension with the second group. The five patients with palmar injury alone achieved 80% good to excellent results according to the Buck-Gramcko scoring system, while only 55% good to excellent results were seen in digits tenolysed after replantation.

■ Reports of tenolysis in children are rare. Birnie and Idler[4] compared treatment of children under and over the age of 11 after repair of zone II and III flexor tendon injuries. They concluded, by using Strickland's method (Table 1) that under age 11, tenolysis was of no significant benefit. Of the 21 digits of children between the ages of 11 and 16, 13 had good to excellent results, 5 were graded poor, and 2 suffered rupture of the tendon. Of the eight digits of children ages 10 and under, two had fair results and six had poor results. They explained that under the age of 11, the cooperation of the patient necessary for the success of the procedure cannot be expected. Early therapy was more difficult in this group, resulting in inferior results. Within a group of 12 children after flexor tendon repair, Kato et al[14] described one successful tenolysis after zone II injury in a child age 3 years 10 months.

They reported that the tenolysis was performed 9 months after the initial injury and repair and that the result of the tenolysis was excellent.

COMPLICATIONS

■ Rupture of the flexor tendon may be the result of poor-quality tendon or aggressive therapy as well as patient noncompliance. It may be prevented by limiting tenolysis only to tendons of good quality. Eggli et al[6] reported rupture in 3 of 16 flexor tendons tenolysed that were treated successfully with two-stage reconstruction. Jupiter et al[13] reported 2 ruptured tendons of 37 replanted digits, both in zone II injuries. Others have claimed this to be a rare yet disastrous complication.[1]

■ Rupture of a pulley, more significantly A2 or A4 pulleys, may result from narrowing or fraying of the pulleys as part of the trauma or further compromise with surgical intervention.

■ Multiple surgical treatments of the digits involved in various trauma mechanisms may result in significant scarring, decreased vascularity, delayed wound healing, and infection, further compromising the functional results. Adherence to careful surgical technique, including atraumatic handling of tissue, is crucial to minimize these complications.[1,19]

■ Foucher et al[8] reported eight complications in 72 patients (78 digits): two with delayed healing, two with flexor tendon exposure, two with rupture, and two diagnosed using bone scan to have a localized form of reflex sympathetic dystrophy.

Prevention of Recurrence

■ Bathing the tendon in a steroid solution to prevent recurrence of adhesions has been suggested but has only anecdotal evidence of efficacy. Others have reported that corticosteroids may be associated with smaller, weaker tendons, diminished wound healing, and decreased resistance to infection.[16]

■ Biologic and artificial membranes have been used to wrap the repair site and mechanically isolate the tendon. Cellophane, polyethylene film, silicone, paratenon, amniotic membrane, gelatin sponge, and hyaluronic acid derivatives have been studied with mixed results and limited clinical support. Promising results were achieved with ADCON-T/N (Gliatech, Cleveland, OH), a bioresorbable gel of gelatin and carbohydrate polymer that acts as a physical barrier.[9] A disappointing prospective double-blind, randomized, controlled clinical trial assessing flexor tendon repair in zone II found no statistically significant effect on TAM. The patients treated with ADCON-T/N did achieve their final range of motion significantly earlier than the control group. The authors also reported a higher rate (although not statistically significant) of tendon rupture with the ADCON-T/N.

REFERENCES

1. Azari KK, Meals RA. Flexor tenolysis. Hand Clin 2005;21:211–217.
2. Bain GI, Allen BD, Berger AC. Flexor tenolysis using a free suture. Tech Hand Up Extrem Surg 2003;7:61–62.
3. Bayat A, Shaaban H, Giakas G, et al. The pulley system of the thumb: anatomic and biomechanical study. J Hand Surg Am 2002;27:628–635.
4. Birnie RH, Idler RS. Flexor tenolysis in children. J Hand Surg Am 1995;20A:254–257.
5. Buck-Gramcko D, Dietrich FE, Gogge S. Evaluation criteria in follow-up studies of flexor tendon therapy [in German]. Handchirurgie 1976;8:65–69.
6. Eggli S, Dietsche A, Eggli S, et al. Tenolysis after combined digital injuries in zone II. Ann Plast Surg 2005;55:266–271.
7. Fong KD, Trindade MC, Wang Z, et al. Microarray analysis of mechanical shear effects on flexor tendon cells. Plast Reconstr Surg 2005;116:1393–1404.
8. Foucher G, Lenoble E, Ben Youssef K, et al. A post-operative regime after digital flexor tenolysis: a series of 72 patients. J Hand Surg Br 1993;18B:35–40.
9. Golash A, Kay A, Warner JG, et al. Efficacy of ADCON-T/N after primary flexor tendon repair in zone II: a controlled clinical trial. J Hand Surg Br 2003;28B:113–115.
10. Goloborod'ko SA. Postoperative management of flexor tenolysis. J Hand Ther 1999;12:330–332.
11. Horii E, Lin GT, Cooney WP, et al. Comparative flexor tendon excursion after passive mobilization: an in vitro study. J Hand Surg Am 1992;17A:559–566.
12. Jaibaji M. Advances in the biology of zone II flexor tendon healing and adhesion formation. Ann Plast Surg 2000;45:83–92.
13. Jupiter JB, Pess GM, Bour CJ. Results of flexor tendon tenolysis after replantation in the hand. J Hand Surg Am 1989;14A:35–44.
14. Kato H, Minami A, Suenaga N, et al. Long-term results after primary repairs of zone 2 flexor tendon lacerations in children younger than age 6 years. J Pediatr Orthop 2002;22:732–735.
15. Kirchhoff R, Jensen PB, Nielsen NS, et al. Repeated digital nerve block for pain control after tenolysis. Scand J Plast Reconstr Surg Hand Surg 2000;34:257–258.
16. Lilly SI, Messer TM. Complications after treatment of flexor tendon injuries. J Am Acad Orthop Surg 2006;14:387–396.
17. Mitsionis G, Fischer KJ, Bastidas JA, et al. Feasibility of partial A2 and A4 pulley excision: residual pulley strength. J Hand Surg Br 2000;25B:90–94.
18. Moran SL, Ryan CK, Orlando GS, et al. Effects of 5-fluorouracil on flexor tendon repair. J Hand Surg Am 2000;25A:242–251.
19. Schneider LH. Tenolysis and capsulectomy after hand fractures. Clin Orthop Relat Res 1996;327:72–78.
20. Strickland JW. Flexor tendon surgery, part 2: free tendon grafts and tenolysis. J Hand Surg Br 1989;14B:368–382.
21. Strickland JW, Glogovac SV. Digital function following flexor tendon repair in zone II: a comparison of immobilization and controlled passive motion techniques. J Hand Surg Am 1980;5A:537–543.
22. Swanson AB, Goran-Hagert C, de Groot Swanson G. Evaluation of impairment in the upper extremity. J Hand Surg Am 1987;12A:896–926.
23. Tang JB. Clinical outcomes associated with flexor tendon repair. Hand Clin 2005;21:199–210.
24. Taras JS, Kaufmann RA. Flexor tendon reconstruction. In: Green DP, Hotchkiss RN, Pederson WC, et al, eds. Green's Operative Hand Surgery. Philadelphia: Churchill-Livingstone Elsevier, 2005:241–276.
25. Trumble TE, Sailer SM. Flexor tendon injuries. In: Trumble TE, ed. Principles of Hand Surgery and Therapy. Philadelphia: WB Saunders Company, 2000:231–262.
26. Tsubone T, Moran SL, Amadio PC, et al. Expression of growth factors in canine flexor tendon after laceration in vivo. Ann Plast Surg 2004;53:393–397.
27. Tsubone T, Moran SL, Subramaniam M, et al. Effect of TGF-beta inducible early gene deficiency on flexor tendon healing. J Orthop Res 2006;24:569–575.
28. Verdan C. Tenolysis. In: Verdan C, ed. Tendon Surgery of the Hand. Edinburgh: Churchill Livingstone, 1979:137–142.
29. Wang H. Secondary surgery after digit replantation: its incidence and sequence. Microsurgery 2002;22:57–61.
30. Weinzweig N, Chin G, Mead M, Gonzalez M. "Spaghetti wrist": management and results. Plast Reconstr Surg 1998;102:96–102.
31. Whitaker JH, Strickland JW, Ellis RK. The role of flexor tenolysis in the palm and digits. J Hand Surg Am 1977;2A:462–470.
32. Zhang AY, Pham H, Ho F, et al. Inhibition of TGF-beta-induced collagen production in rabbit flexor tendons. J Hand Surg Am 2004;29A:230–235.
33. Zhao C, Amadio PC, Zobitz ME, et al. Resection of the flexor digitorum superficialis reduces gliding resistance after zone II flexor digitorum profundus repair in vitro. J Hand Surg Am 2002;27A:316–321.

Chapter 56

Staged Digital Flexor Tendon Reconstruction

Kevin J. Malone and Thomas Trumble

DEFINITION

- Staged flexor tendon reconstruction is required in the settings of delayed diagnosis of a flexor digitorum profundus (FDP) and flexor digitorum superficialis (FDS) disruption or failed previous attempt at primary repair within zone II of the digital tendon sheath.
- During the first stage of the reconstruction process, a silicone rod is placed within the flexor tendon sheath. The role of this implant is to help re-establish a frictionless inner lining of the sheath that will accommodate the placement of a tendon graft in the second stage.

ANATOMY

- Flexor tendons can be divided into five zones (**FIG 1A**).
- Bunnell originally described the region between the A1 pulley and the FDS insertion, zone II, as "no man's land" because the initial results after attempted primary tendon repair were so poor he felt that no one should attempt this procedure.
- In the limited confines of zone II the two flexor tendons function together and rely on the digital sheath and its frictionless synovial interface for gliding and proper function.
- Another complicating anatomic characteristic of zone II is the chiasm of Camper. Here FDP passes through the slips of FDS, creating another potential region for adhesions (**FIG 1B**).

PATHOGENESIS

- Zone II has the highest probability of developing adhesions and the poorest prognosis after repair.
- Violation of the sheath, the lining, or the blood supply to the tendons by trauma or infection may lead to dense scar and adhesion formation and can compromise the results after either a primary repair or an attempt at single-stage reconstruction with a tendon graft.

NATURAL HISTORY

- Flexor tendon injuries that are not reconstructed can progress to a stiff and sometimes painful digit.
- If both tendons are not functional, no active proximal (PIP) or distal (DIP) interphalangeal motion will be possible, but if only the FDP tendon is disrupted, active PIP flexion will be present.
- If a digit with incompetent flexor tendons is subjected to repeated extension stress, as in pinch, the volar supporting structures will become lax over time, leading to hyperextension and an unstable joint.

PATIENT HISTORY AND PHYSICAL FINDINGS

- The examiner should elicit information about the initial injury, such as when it occurred and if there were

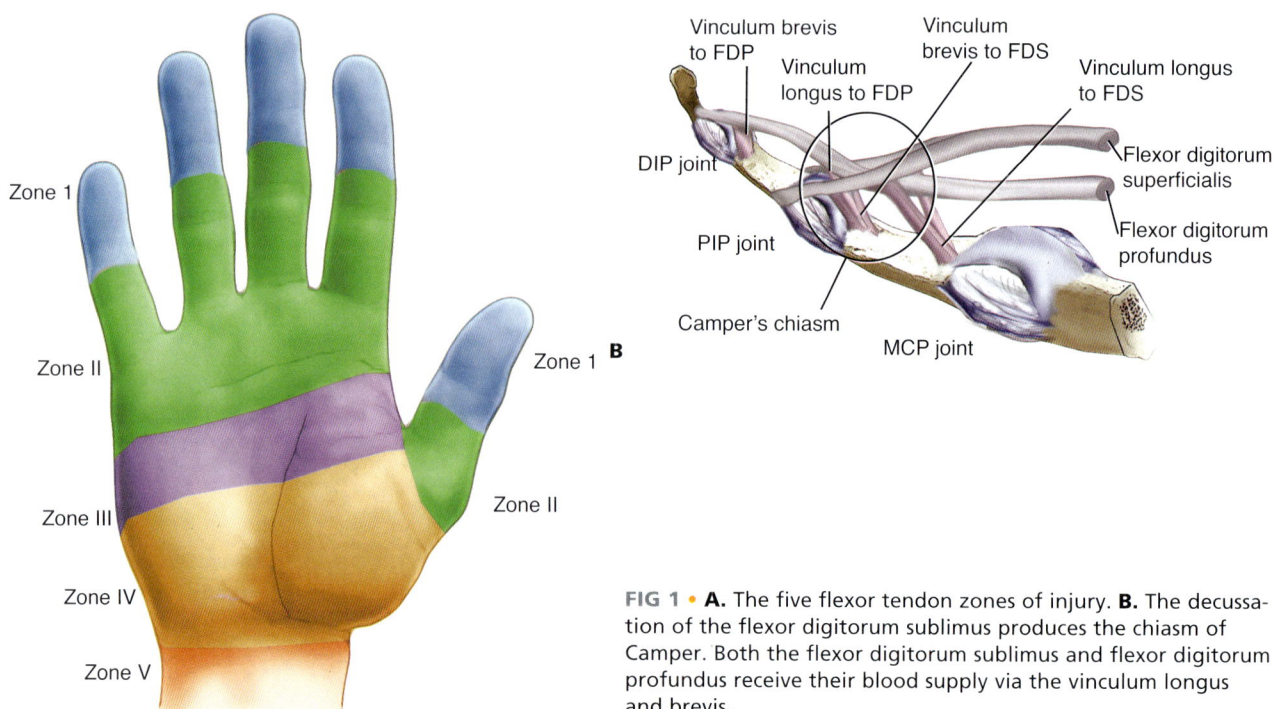

FIG 1 • **A.** The five flexor tendon zones of injury. **B.** The decussation of the flexor digitorum sublimus produces the chiasm of Camper. Both the flexor digitorum sublimus and flexor digitorum profundus receive their blood supply via the vinculum longus and brevis.

associated injuries (fractures, laceration of digital nerves or vessels).

- The examiner should determine when the patient first noticed a decrease in the function of the digit (if flexor tendon repair has already been attempted).
- Staged flexor tendon reconstruction is contraindicated in the setting of an active infection, and for that reason an infection history must be sought.
  - If an infection is identified, it should be treated aggressively with antibiotics and débridement to minimize the destruction of the flexor tendon sheath from the inflammatory process.
- Tests for tendon function include:
  - Finger cascade: Loss of the normal cascade suggests disruption or loss of function of the flexor tendons.
  - FDP examination: Loss of active DIP flexion suggests disruption or loss of FDP function.
  - FDS examination: Loss of active PIP flexion suggests disruption or loss of FDS function.
  - Tenodesis effect: Loss of the tenodesis effect suggests disruption of the flexor tendons.
- It is also important to assess the vascular supply and the digital sensation to determine if there is a concomitant injury to the digital neurovascular structures.
- Both active and passive range of motion must be recorded for the metacarpophalangeal (MP), PIP, and DIP joints.
  - If contractures are present, as evidenced by decreased passive joint motion, intensive therapy should be initiated before proceeding with staged flexor tendon reconstruction.

IMAGING AND OTHER DIAGNOSTIC STUDIES

- Radiographs should be obtained to rule out fractures or other associated injuries to the hand and digits.
- Ultrasound or MRI can be used to help localize the site of tendon rupture and position of the proximal stump if not clear by clinical examination.

DIFFERENTIAL DIAGNOSIS

- Fracture or dislocation of digits
- Proximal compression of anterior interosseous nerve, median nerve, or ulnar nerve
- Cervical radiculopathy
- Upper motor neuron lesion

NONOPERATIVE MANAGEMENT

- There is no acceptable nonoperative management for combined FDS and FDP tendon lacerations. Alternatives to staged flexor tendon reconstruction include arthrodesis and amputation.

- Isolated chronic disruption of the FDP tendon with an intact FDS tendon is best treated nonoperatively. Attempts at reconstruction of the FDP tendon risk function of the FDS tendon.
- Buddy taping or trapping of the injured finger by an adjacent figure during finger flexion may allow concealment of the functional deficit between stage 1 and stage 2 or in the patient who is not a candidate for staged-tendon reconstruction.

SURGICAL MANAGEMENT

- Indications for two-stage flexor tendon reconstruction include:
  - Loss of FDP and FDS
  - Protective sensation
  - Nearly full passive range of motion
  - Good quality skin in the region of zone II
  - A cooperative patient willing to participate fully in rehabilitation
- The patient will need to have access to a good hand therapist before and after each of the stages of this complex reconstructive process.

Preoperative Planning

- For the second stage of the procedure a tendon must be harvested to use for the reconstruction. Often, a palmaris longus graft is used. If the patient does not have a palmaris longus, then a long toe extensor or plantaris tendon can be used. In this situation, the lower extremity must also be prepared out into the surgical field.

Positioning

- For both stages of the procedure the patient is placed supine on the operating table with the arm abducted on a hand table. A nonsterile tourniquet is placed around the upper arm for hemostasis.

Approach

- Stage 1: A volar Brunner incision is made over the flexor tendon sheath and extended proximally into the palm. A second incision is made in the distal forearm to ensure placement of the rod within the carpal tunnel.
- Stage 2: A limited Brunner incision is made at the level of the distal junction of the repair. A separate incision is made at the level of the proximal junction of the repair. This can be the same incision in the distal forearm as in stage 1 if the tendon graft is long enough. Alternatively, the proximal junction will be in the palm with shorter tendon grafts. A third incision or set of incisions will be made for the tendon harvest.

STAGE 1

- A volar Brunner incision is made over the course of the flexor tendons.
- The flexor tendon sheath is incised, taking care to preserve the A2 and A4 pulleys. L-shaped flaps can be made within the flexor sheath to aid in access to the flexor tendons and protect the A2 and A4 pulleys (**TECH FIG 1A**).
- The scarred tendon is excised, leaving a portion of the distal stump of the FDP intact at its insertion.
  - This is useful in securing the tendon rod in stage 1 and the tendon graft in stage 2.

- If a digital nerve laceration is identified, it should be repaired at this stage.
- Release any adhesions within the sheath.
- Release any flexion contractures of the joints by releasing the volar plate and accessory collateral ligaments.
  - Be sure to preserve the proper collateral ligaments.
- If the A2 or A4 pulleys are absent or have been excised with the scar release, they need to be reconstructed. A tendon graft can be used to reconstruct the pulleys (**TECH FIG 1B**).

TECHNIQUES

TECHNIQUES

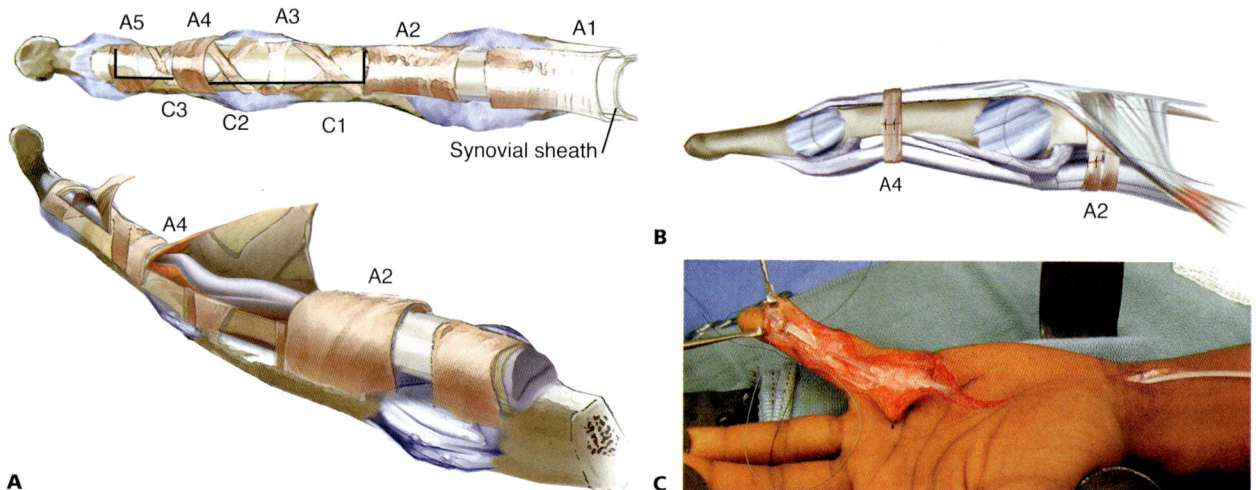

TECH FIG 1 • **A.** Creating a L-shaped flap can aid in accessing the underlying flexor sheath contents while preserving the important A2 and A4 pulleys. **B.** Tendon weaves for reconstruction of A2 and A4 pulleys. **C.** A "passive" silicone implant running under A2 and A4 pulleys is secured distally to the flexor digitorum profundus stump and extends proximally to the distal forearm.

- The tendon should be passed between the proximal phalanx and the extensor tendon for A2 reconstruction.
- For A4 reconstruction, the tendon can be passed dorsal to the extensor tendon.
- A silicone Hunter rod is inserted into the sheath. Distally, it is secured to the remnant of the FDP tendon with nonabsorbing suture.
  - If there is not enough of the tendon remnant, it can be secured to surrounding tissue at the base of the distal phalanx.
  - Some Hunter rods can be secured using a screw placed in the distal phalanx.

- Proximally, the silicone rod is passed through the carpal tunnel and allowed to glide free with the flexor tendons in the distal forearm (**TECH FIG 1C**).
- All skin incisions are closed with 4-0 nylon after ensuring hemostasis.
- The patient is then placed into a dorsal blocking splint holding the fingers into an intrinsic plus posture.
- Rehabilitation is started early after surgery, often within 1 week, to ensure that the patient regains full passive range of motion. The scar tissue must be soft and supple before the patient is scheduled for the second stage of tendon reconstruction. On average this takes 3 months.

STAGE 2

Incisions and Graft Harvest

- A limited Brunner incision is made distally at the level of the DIP joint so that the distal FDP stump can be located within the sheath. The sutures securing the silicone rod to the profundus stump are released.
  - Do not extend the incision or dissection into zone II, as this will compromise the re-established tendon sheath that has been created by the body's reaction to the silicone rod.
- A second incision is made in the distal forearm so that the proximal portion of the silicone rod can be localized.
- A third set of incisions is then made for tendon graft harvest. This is typically from the palmaris longus, long toe extensor, or plantaris tendon (**TECH FIG 2**).
  - Plantaris often makes the best donor if a long segment of tendon is needed.

Graft Placement

- The tendon graft is then sutured to the proximal end of the silicone rod. The silicone rod is then retrieved from

the distal wound, pulling the tendon graft into the tendon sheath (**TECH FIG 3A**).
- The distal end of the tendon graft is secured to the distal phalanx with bone anchors. The anchors should be inserted in the footprint of the FDP stump and angled slightly proximally. The proximal angle will ensure that the anchor stays within the bone rather than penetrating the dorsal cortex. It is important to ensure that the anchor does not penetrate the DIP.
  - Alternatively, the tendon graft can be secured to the distal phalanx with a pullout suture tied over the nail, as in a zone I flexor tendon repair. This has been associated with deformities to the nail after suture removal and has no proven biomechanical advantage over suture anchors.
  - Additional fixation can be provided by using the remaining FDP stump and securing this to the tendon graft with a nonabsorbable suture in figure 8 fashion.
- The distal incision is closed at this point. It will become difficult to gain access to this incision after graft tension is set.

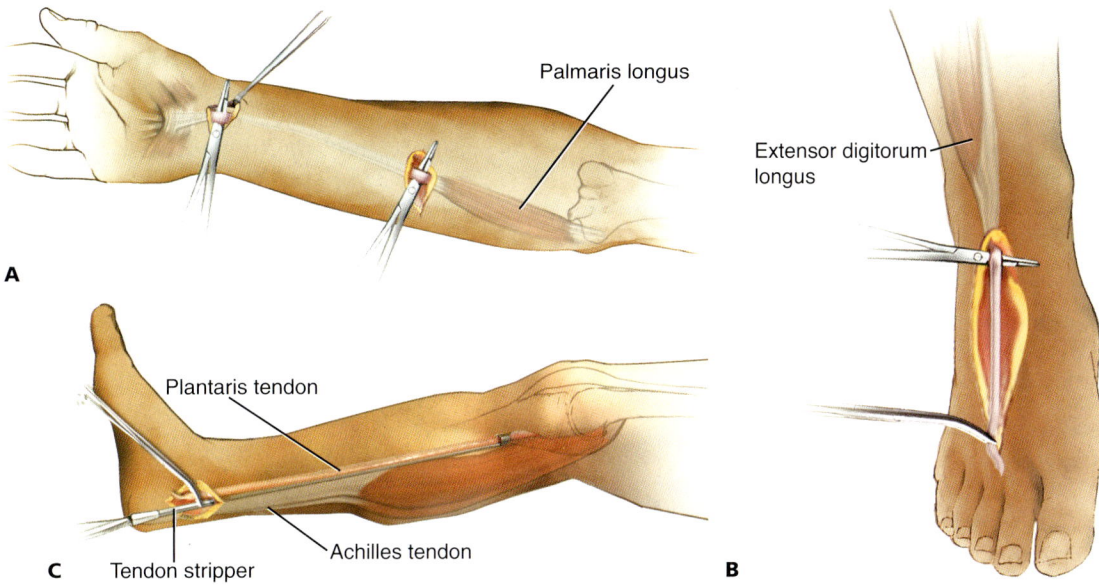

TECH FIG 2 • **A.** Technique for harvesting palmaris longus tendon graft. **B.** Technique for harvesting long toe extensor tendon graft. **C.** Technique for harvesting plantaris tendon graft.

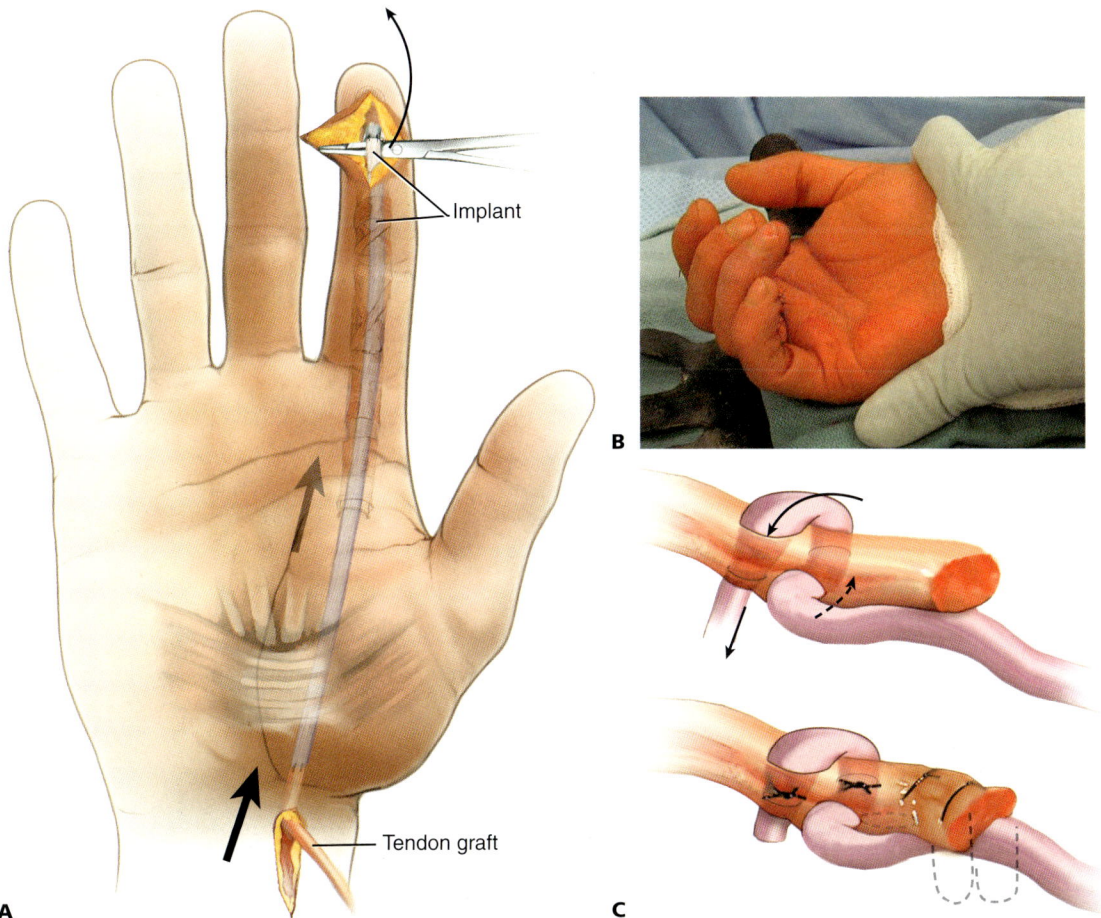

TECH FIG 3 • **A.** Technique for using the silicone rod to draw the tendon graft into the flexor tendon sheath and out through the distal incision. **B.** Re-creation of the normal finger cascade. **C.** A Pulvertaft weave is used for the proximal junction between the tendon graft and the flexor digitorum profundus or superficialis in the forearm.

TECHNIQUES

- Tendon graft tension is set from the proximal wound. The correct amount of tension is determined with the wrist in a neutral posture and is set by evaluating digital flexion cascade (**TECH FIG 3B**).
  - It may be wise to exaggerate the cascade slightly so that as the graft relaxes and lengthens, the normal flexion cascade is created.
  - If the cascade is significantly exaggerated, however, a quadriga effect will result.
- The proximal end of the tendon graft is then woven into the proximal recipient tendon stump with a Pulvertaft weave (**TECH FIG 3C**).

- The recipient stump proximally can be either the FDS or the FDP to the injured finger. If the initial injury is more than a few months old, the muscle belly of the injured FDP or FDS may be atrophic or scarred proximally in the forearm, which would limit postoperative results. In this setting, the recipient tendon can be a side-to-side anastomosis to the neighboring FDP, which will provide the appropriate excursion.
- All skin incisions are closed after ensuring hemostasis. The patient is then placed into a dorsal blocking splint with the wrist slightly flexed and the MP and IP joints flexed.
- Rehabilitation is started within a few days (see Postoperative Care).

TENOLYSIS

- This is often necessary after stage 2 of tendon reconstruction. Tenolysis is indicated when passive range of motion is greater than active range of motion. This surgery should not be performed until 3 to 6 months after stage 2.
- The tendon must be exposed within zone II of the tendon sheath and tenolysis performed within the flexor sheath, taking care to preserve the A2 and A4 pulleys. If

residual resistance is noted after tenolysis in the finger, an additional incision may be made at the level of the proximal junction to address any adhesions at that level.
- Immediate hand therapy must be initiated postoperatively and can be easier on the patient if a wrist block is performed with a long-acting local anesthetic to preserve motor function while producing an effective sensory block.

ALTERNATIVE TO STAGE 1

- The silicone rod that we use is considered "passive" and has no attachment to the proximal flexor motor.
- An "active" alternative exists in which the rod can be secured to the tendon proximally and function as a graft. This can eliminate the need for stage 2 (**TECH FIG 4**).
- These implants have been associated with a higher rate of complication in the limited number of studies that have examined them.

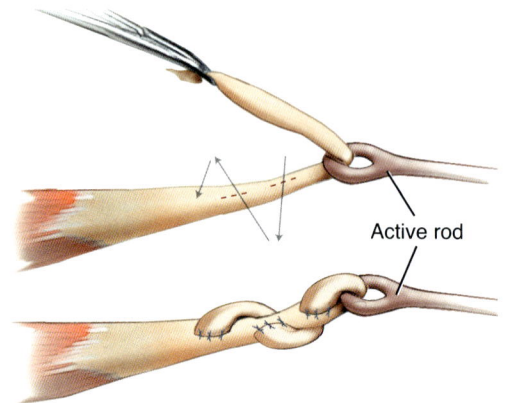

Active rod

TECH FIG 4 • In an active tendon rod, the motor tendon is looped through the ring in the proximal rod, woven through itself, and fixed with nonabsorbable suture so that active motion can be performed.

PEARLS AND PITFALLS

Pulley preservation	Both the A2 and A4 pulleys must be maintained or reconstructed at stage 1 to prevent bowstringing and maximize the amount of active flexion (**FIG 2**; see Tech Fig 1B).

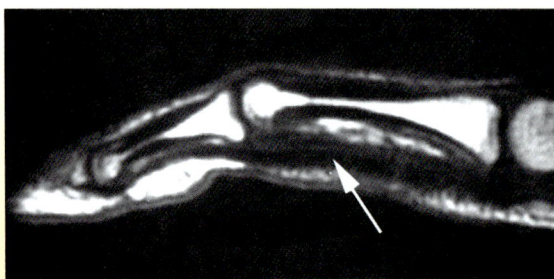

FIG 2 • Sagittal MRI showing bowstringing of a flexor tendon (*arrow*) over the proximal phalanx due to an incompetent A2 pulley.

Full passive range of motion	Full passive range of motion should be achieved before stage 1 and again before stage 2. Less than maximum passive range of motion preoperatively will markedly worsen the functional result after stage 2.
Finger cascade	Establishing the correct cascade with the appropriate amount of tension on the tendon graft in stage 2 is important. The graft will likely relax and lengthen as the patient goes through rehabilitation. A slight exaggeration of the cascade at the time of surgery may ultimately produce the normal cascade as the tendon graft lengthens. Gross exaggeration of the cascade, however, will produce a quadriga effect. The uninjured digits will be less than fully flexed when the injured digit has reached full flexion in the palm (**FIG 3**).
Hand therapy	A good therapist and a motivated patient are critical for a good outcome for this surgery.

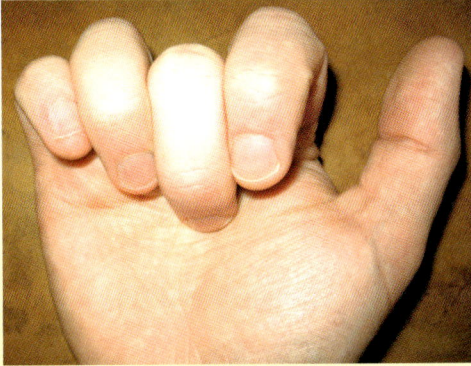

FIG 3 • Clinical photograph of the quadriga effect. The long finger, in which the flexor digitorum profundus has been repaired with too much tension, is maximally flexed into the palm and the adjacent fingers cannot be actively flexed further.

POSTOPERATIVE CARE

- The pre- and postoperative hand therapy is perhaps the most important component of this reconstruction procedure.
  - Patients must be motivated and compliant.
  - Therapists must be knowledgeable.
- Before stage 1 and stage 2, the patient must have nearly full passive range of motion and a soft tissue envelope that will accommodate the subsequent stages of the process.
- Stage 1 postoperative therapy is initiated within 48 hours and continues until the patient is ready for stage 2.
  - If pulley reconstruction was performed, the therapist can make ring splints for the patient to wear to protect the pulleys.
- In general, the patient needs to be monitored for signs of infection. Edema should be controlled with elevation and compressive dressings as needed.
- A custom splint is used when not exercising. This splint should hold the injured fingers in an intrinsic plus posture, with the MP joints in 70 degrees of flexion and the IP joints held in full extension. The wrist is held at neutral.
- Passive range of motion of all involved digits is initiated, with emphasis on obtaining full composite flexion and full PIP extension.
- Active range of motion exercises are also used to establish full active extension of all digits and full flexion of the uninvolved digits. Buddy-taping can be employed to facilitate motion of the operated digit.
- The protocol for postoperative therapy after stage 2 is as follows:
  - 0 to 3 weeks postoperatively
    - Precautions: No active finger flexion, no passive finger extension
    - The patient is splinted with a dorsal extension block splint holding the involved digits in an intrinsic plus posture and the wrist at neutral. The splint should be worn at all times.
    - Therapist-directed exercises begin with passive flexion and active extension in the splint. The PIP and DIP joints are secured to the splint in extension between exercise sessions.
    - Wound care and edema control are also incorporated and the patient must be observed for signs of infection.
  - 3 to 6 weeks postoperatively
    - Precautions: Monitor closely for PIP flexion contractures, no passive finger extension, no splint removal
    - Active range of motion is initiated with "place and hold" exercises and progressed to full active range-of-motion exercises by 4 weeks after surgery while still in the splint.
    - Once the surgical wounds have healed, soft tissue massage should be incorporated to soften the volar tissues.
  - 6 to 9 weeks postoperatively
    - Precautions: No resisted active motion, light functional activities only
    - Reliable patients can be weaned from the dorsal blocking splint.
    - The active flexion and extension exercises should be continued. Blocking exercises are initiated for PIP and DIP flexion to facilitate tendon glide and pull-through. Combined finger extension exercises are slowly initiated with the wrist in slight flexion. If the patient is a heavy scar former, this begins at 6 weeks; if average, at 7 weeks; if light, at 8 weeks.
  - 9 to 12 weeks postoperatively
    - Precautions: No lifting or uncontrolled use
    - Splinting should be modified to correct any residual joint contractures and increase soft tissue excursion.
    - The patient can be allowed to begin progressive strengthening and should continue active range-of-motion and tendon gliding exercises as well as scar management as needed.
  - 12 to 14 weeks postoperatively
    - Precautions: No heavy lifting

■ Splinting is continued as needed to address contractures.

■ Active range-of-motion and strengthening activities are continued. Resistance is gradually increased up to about 30 lbs by week 14.

■ 14 to 16 weeks postoperatively

■ The patient progresses to full resistive strengthening exercises and activities.

■ A work-hardening program is initiated if needed to prepare for return to work.

■ If the patient is less reliable, the above protocol is followed except that dorsal blocking splinting is continued for up to 9 weeks and active motion is delayed until at least 4 weeks.

OUTCOMES

■ Because there are few alternatives to this staged process of reconstruction, there are limited articles comparing this treatment to another. Most of the investigations in the literature are retrospective reviews documenting overall postoperative motion and outcome ratings based on objective and subjective rating systems.

■ The larger studies have shown good and excellent results in the 70% to 80% range, depending on the grading system used.[3–5]

■ Final total active motion is about 70% of the contralateral uninjured digit.

■ Typically a significant discrepancy exists between ultimate total passive motion and total active motion. A flexion contracture of about 20 degrees at the DIP joint is common.[3]

■ The most common reported complication, seen in 30% of patients, was the need for a tenolysis.[2–6]

■ Other common complications that resulted in the need for further surgery included infection, tendon rupture, pulley rupture with bowstringing, and incorrect tendon tensioning.[2–6]

COMPLICATIONS

■ The most common complication is the development of adhesions that limit active motion. This can be assessed by a discrepancy between the active and passive range of motion. If there are significant discrepancies after at least 3 months of therapy after stage 2, then a tenolysis is recommended. This is followed immediately by a rigorous course of therapy to regain active motion. By 3 months, the tendon graft and junction sites should be strong enough to allow for unrestricted active motion.

■ Bowstringing is common if the A2 and A4 pulleys are compromised by initial trauma or released with the scar and adhesions during stage 1. In this setting, these pulleys should be reconstructed during stage 1. If they are found to be incompetent during the stage 2, then pulley reconstruction must be performed and the tendon graft must be delayed until the patient has healed from the pulley reconstruction and once again demonstrated nearly full passive range of motion.

■ Infection should be monitored for closely, given the previous history of a penetrating wound that caused the tendon laceration in the first place and the implantation of a synthetic material during stage 1 of the procedure. Infections should be managed aggressively because the local inflammation can produce further contractures and adhesions.

REFERENCES

1. Amadio PC, Hunter JM, Jaeger SH, et al. The effect of vincular injury on the results of flexor tendon surgery in zone 2. J Hand Surg Am 1985;10A:626–632.
2. Beris AE, Darlis NA, Korompilias AV, et al. Two-stage flexor tendon reconstruction in zone II using a silicone rod and a pedicled intrasynovial graft. J Hand Surg Am 2003;28A:652–660.
3. Frakking TG, Depuydt KP, Kon M, et al. Retrospective outcome analysis of staged flexor tendon reconstruction. J Hand Surg Br 2000;25B:168–174.
4. Hunter JM, Singer DI, Jaeger SH, et al. Active tendon implants in flexor tendon reconstruction. J Hand Surg Am 1988;13A:849–859.
5. Hunter JM. Staged flexor tendon reconstruction. J Hand Surg Am 1983;8A:789–793.
6. Trumble TE, Sailer SM. Flexor tendon injuries. In: Trumble TE, ed. Principles of Hand Surgery and Therapy. Philadelphia: WB Saunders, 2000:231–262.

Chapter 57

Repair Following Traumatic Extensor Tendon Disruption in the Hand, Wrist, and Forearm

David B. Shapiro and Mark A. Krahe

DEFINITION

- Traumatic disruptions of the extensor mechanism represent a broad spectrum of injuries, frequently seen because of the tendons' superficial location, and frequently associated with concomitant injury to bone, skin, and joint.[15]
- Repair can be technically demanding. The extensor tendons are thin, have limited excursion, and are intolerant of shortening, especially in the digits.
- Reconstruction of subacute and chronic extensor tendon injuries are more challenging and less effective than early repair, underscoring the importance of appropriate treatment of an acute injury.

ANATOMY

- Extensor tendon zones of injury (Verdan) (**FIG 1A**)[13]
  - The extensor mechanism is divided into eight zones in the fingers and five in the thumb, numbered from distal to proximal.

- Even-numbered zones are over bones and odd-numbered ones are over joints.
- Extrinsic extensors (**FIG 1B** and Table 1)
  - Digital and wrist extensor muscles originate from the lateral epicondyle and condyle, with musculotendinous junctions 3 to 4 cm proximal to the wrist joint. The extensor indicis proprius (EIP), extensor pollicis longus (EPL), abductor pollicis longus (APL), and extensor pollicis brevis (EPB) all originate more distally from the ulna, the radius, or both and have more distal extension of muscle fibers.
  - The four extensor digitorum communis (EDC) tendons originate from a common muscle belly and have progressively limited independence moving from the index to small fingers.
  - The fascia over the extensor tendons thickens at the wrist to form the extensor retinaculum, with vertical septa separating the six extensor compartments (**FIG 1B**).
- Juncturae tendinum provide interconnections between the EDC tendons just proximal to the metacarpophalangeal (MCP) joints.

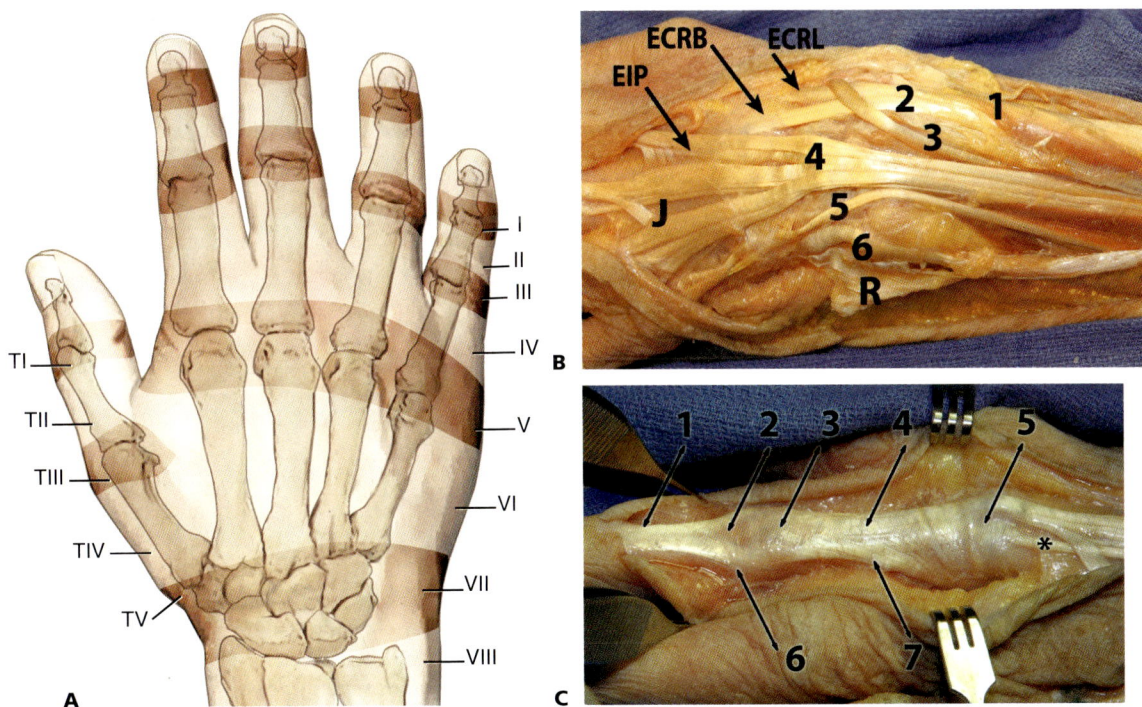

FIG 1 • **A.** Extensor tendon zones of injury. **B,C.** The digits are to the left and the wrist is to the right. **B.** The top of the figure is radial and the bottom is ulnar. Wrist and hand extensor tendon anatomy, with numbers to identify the extensor tendon compartments. *R* is the reflected extensor retinaculum and *J* is a junctura tendinum. Note the combined extensor digitorum communis (EDC) tendon to the ring and small finger. In the fourth compartment, the extensor indicis proprius (EIP) tendon is deep to the EDC tendons and has more distal muscle fibers. In the hand, it is just deep and ulnar to the index EDC tendon. See Table 1 for more details. **C.** The digital extensor mechanism. *1.* Terminal tendon. *2.* Triangular ligament. *3.* Proximal interphalangeal (PIP) joint. *4.* Central slip tendon. *5.* Sagittal band. *6.* Lateral band, which will become the terminal tendon distally. *7.* Conjoined lateral band, with fibers to base of middle phalanx and to the lateral band. This patient has an unusual proprius tendon to the long finger (*), passing ulnar to the EDC tendon and beneath the junctura.

Table 1	Extrinsic Extensor Tendons		
Compartment	**Muscle**	**Abbreviation**	**Comment**
1	Abductor pollicis longus	APL	Compartment is more palmar than others
	Extensor pollicis brevis	EPB	
2	Extensor carpi radialis longus	ECRL	Two wrist extensors
	Extensor carpi radialis brevis	ECRB	
3	Extensor pollicis longus	EPL	Third compartment tendon goes to the thumb
4	Extensor digitorum communis	EDC	Four EDC tendons and "fore" finger tendon
	Extensor indicis proprius	EIP	
5	Extensor digiti quinti (minimi)	EDQ or EDM	Fifth finger independent extensor tendon
6	Extensor carpi ulnaris	ECU	Most ulnar extensor tendon

- The EIP and extensor digiti minimi are ulnar and deep to the EDC in the hand and at the MCP joint.[15] The EIP passes beneath the junctura tendinum.
- There can be considerable variability of the extensor tendons on the dorsum of the hand, with less than 50% of people having a separate EDC tendon to the small finger.[19] Duplicated, interconnected tendons are common.[11]
- The sagittal band holds the extensor tendon over the metacarpal head at the MCP joint, and, through its connection to the volar plate, extends the joint.
- Intrinsic extensors (**FIG 1C**)
  - Intrinsic extensors originate in the hand and include the four dorsal interossei, three palmar interossei, and four lumbricals. The thenar and hypothenar muscles also contribute to interphalangeal extension.
  - The intrinsic tendons join to form the conjoined lateral bands volar to the axis of the MCP joint, and continue dorsal to the axis of the proximal (PIP) and distal (DIP) interphalangeal joints.[1,19] This allows them to simultaneously flex the MCP joint and extend the PIP and DIP joints, in addition to providing digital adduction and abduction.

PATHOGENESIS

- Zone I
  - Disruption of the extensor tendon over the DIP joint will result in a terminal extensor lag after an open or closed injury (**FIG 2**).
  - Sudden forced flexion of the extended DIP joint can lead to an avulsion of the tendon from its insertion on the distal phalanx (mallet finger), possibly with an associated distal phalanx fracture.
  - The long, ring, and small fingers are most frequently involved, although closed mallet injuries can also be seen in the index finger and thumb.[1]

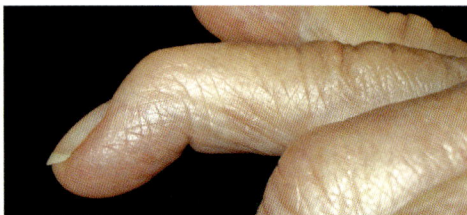

FIG 2 • Mallet finger. (Zone I extensor tendon injury.)

- Zone II
  - Laceration over the middle phalanx can give the clinical appearance of a zone I injury.
  - Injury to the periosteum and middle phalanx can lead to increased swelling, extensor tendon adherence, and DIP stiffness.
- Zone III
  - Disruption of the central slip at the PIP joint may occur as a closed rupture (with or without an associated bone injury) or be associated with traumatic arthrotomy.
    - Central slip avulsion is seen with volar PIP joint dislocations.
  - Early closed injuries may present with swelling, pain, and little extension loss but can progress to a boutonnière deformity as the lateral bands migrate palmarly and become flexors of the PIP joint in the weeks after injury.[19] Close follow-up is warranted for suspicious injuries.
- Zone IV
  - Injuries occur over the proximal phalanx and typically involve only a portion of the extensor mechanism.
    - Lacerations are usually partial as the extensor "hood" covers almost 75% of the circumference of the digit. With a complete central slip laceration, PIP extension may be maintained (through the lateral bands) initially, although a boutonnière deformity may develop later.
  - Differentiation between complete and incomplete injury can be difficult, but pain or weakness with resisted PIP extension (especially from an initially flexed position) can be suggestive. As above, close follow-up is warranted for suspicious injuries.
- Zone V
  - Tendon injury occurs over the MCP joint.
  - There may be an open laceration or a closed injury to the sagittal band with extensor tendon subluxation.
    - Most frequently, the radial sagittal band is disrupted in closed injuries allowing ulnar subluxation of the extensor tendon.
  - The surgeon should assume there is an open MCP joint injury with any tendon laceration around the joint.
- Zone VI
  - Disruption of extensor tendon is over the dorsum of the hand.
  - Single tendon and partial tendon lacerations may be difficult to identify due to maintenance of some digital extension though an intact junctura tendinum and EDC tendon from an adjacent digit (**FIG 3**).

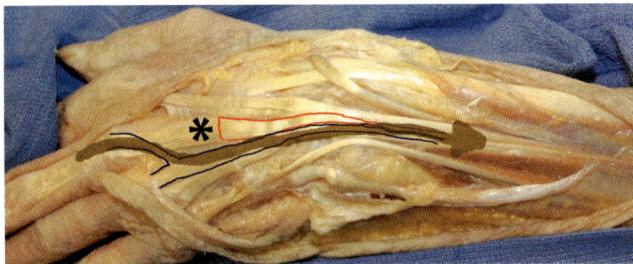

FIG 3 • Extensor digitorum communis laceration to the long finger at the *asterisk*. The long finger can still be extended by action of the ring extensor and junctura tendinum. This may be associated with long-term weakness, pain, or extensor lag.

- Zone VII
  - Lacerations occur over the wrist and through the extensor retinaculum.
- Zone VIII
  - Pathology is located in the forearm at the musculotendinous junction or muscle belly.
  - It may be difficult to detect concurrent posterior interosseous nerve injury in the presence of proximal extensor muscle lacerations.
- Thumb
  - The terminal extensor tendon is thicker than in other digits—mallet injury is rare.
  - Tendon lacerations at, and distal to, the MCP joint are not associated with retraction of tendon ends, and primary repair is straightforward. Lacerations proximal to the MCP joint are associated with EPL retraction (often to the wrist).

NATURAL HISTORY

- Untreated complete tendon lacerations at and distal to zone V will lead to persistent (and sometimes progressively worsening) digital deformity, often with continued pain and development of a flexion contracture.
  - Untreated terminal tendon injuries may lead to a swan-neck deformity due to proximal migration of the digital extensor mechanism and increased extension force at the PIP joint.
  - Delayed treatment of central slip injuries may lead to boutonnière deformity and PIP flexion contracture as the lateral bands migrate palmarly.
- Untreated tendon lacerations proximal to zone V will heal in lengthened fashion with pseudotendon formation. There may be a persistent extensor lag, weakness, or pain. Gradual loss of muscle length and elasticity (sometimes within as little as a week or two) can make delayed primary repair more difficult.
- EPL tendon lacerations proximal to the MCP joint may be difficult to primarily repair as little as 2 weeks after the injury, requiring tendon grafting or EIP transfer.
- Partial tendon lacerations involving less than 50% of the tendon width, longitudinal lacerations, and single lateral band lacerations will generally function well without repair.

PATIENT HISTORY AND PHYSICAL FINDINGS

- Assessment and documentation of skin and soft tissue injury is important to aid in planning for débridement and extension

of the skin incision for exposure and determining the need for soft tissue coverage.
- A complete neurologic and tendon examination is critical to rule out concurrent or remote injury that will alter treatment or outcome.
  - The EIP is examined. It is deep to other extensor tendons, with the most distal musculotendinous junction.
  - The extrinsic extensor tendons are examined with the wrist in neutral, testing MCP extension against resistance. (Isolated PIP extension can be performed by the intrinsic muscles even in the presence of complete extrinsic extensor tendon lacerations.)
  - Examination of the digits may identify extensor lag, weakness, or pain with resistance to extension at the PIP or DIP joints.
- Active and passive range of motion and strength are assessed. Active motion loss helps determine tendon deficits, while loss of passive motion may be pain-related or represent remote injury or arthritis. Lacerations proximal to the juncturae tendinum may have nearly full motion, but with weakness on strength testing (**FIG 3**).

IMAGING AND OTHER DIAGNOSTIC STUDIES

- Plain radiographs are necessary to evaluate for any fractures, foreign bodies, preexisting injury, or arthritis that may alter treatment or affect the final result.
- Ultrasound or MRI are occasionally useful for suspected radiolucent foreign bodies. While both studies can be used to more fully evaluate tendon injuries, treatment decisions are usually based on history and physical examination.

DIFFERENTIAL DIAGNOSIS

- Radial nerve or posterior interosseous nerve injury
- Extensor tendon subluxation at the MCP joint
- Chronic PIP flexion contracture and "pseudo-boutonnière" deformity
- Physiologic swan-neck deformity or DIP joint osteoarthritis with apparent mallet deformity
- Underlying joint deformity and arthrosis

NONOPERATIVE MANAGEMENT

- Disruption of the terminal extensor tendon (mallet finger)
  - Treatment consists of full-time static DIP splinting for 6 to 8 weeks, followed by an additional 6 weeks of protective splinting at night and with high-risk activities.
  - Patients must be counseled as to the importance of maintaining full DIP extension, even during splint changes.
  - A dorsal splint (**FIG 4A**) can allow the patient nearly full use and sensibility of the digit, although palmar or thermoplastic splints can be used in some cases (provided that full DIP extension can be ensured). A good fit without excessive DIP hyperextension which can cause skin injury is critical.
  - The PIP is generally left free and motion encouraged. For patients with moderate PIP hyperextension, the PIP may be flexed 30 degrees and incorporated in the splint for the first 3 weeks of treatment.
  - Treatment can be initiated as late as 4 months after the original injury and still lead to a good result, although a couple more weeks of full-time splinting may be necessary.[7]

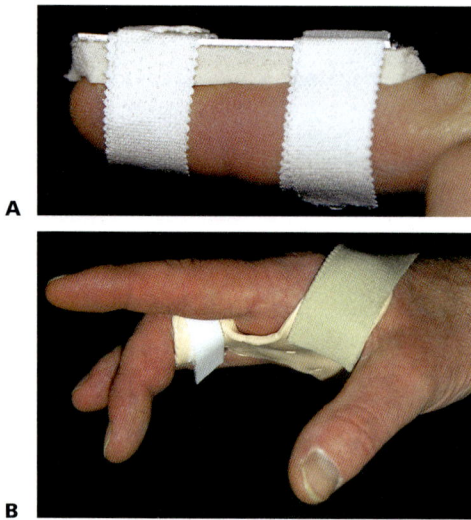

FIG 4 • **A.** Example of mallet finger splint. Any type of distal interphalangeal (DIP) joint splint will work, as long as the DIP is extended to neutral, and the splint is worn full time. **B.** Example of hand-based splint to support metacarpophalangeal joint.

▪ Final results: About 80% of patients should regain full flexion with less than a 10-degree extensor lag. Patients with a greater extension lag after 6 weeks may benefit from 2 or 3 more weeks of full-time splinting. Swelling around the DIP joint can persist for months.
- Central slip avulsion
  ▪ This is treated with full-time static PIP splinting in extension, with active and passive DIP flexion encouraged for 6 weeks, followed by 6 weeks of night splinting.
  ▪ Intermittent use of dynamic extension splint is warranted for PIP flexion contracture.
- Closed sagittal band rupture
  ▪ The patient is placed in a below-elbow cast with the MCP joints supported in full extension (to allow no more than 10 degrees of flexion) for 6 weeks.
  ▪ Compliant patients can be switched to a hand-based splint after 3 weeks of casting with the MCP joint supported in 30 degrees of flexion (**FIG 4B**).
  ▪ Surgical treatment is indicated for closed ruptures presenting more than 2 weeks after injury or those that do not respond to conservative treatment.
- Partial extensor tendon lacerations
  ▪ Conservative treatment is indicated if the laceration is known to involve less than 50% of the tendon width and in longitudinal tendon lacerations.
  ▪ If the degree of injury is unknown, conservative treatment should be considered in patients with full active extension, minimal or no pain with resisted extension, and good extension strength. Surgical exploration and repair is indicated if there is an extensor lag, weakness, or pain with resisted extension.
    ▪ Partial digital extensor tendon lacerations are treated in the manner described earlier, with splinting for 2 to

3 weeks, followed by a monitored gradual exercise program to ensure that an extensor lag does not develop.
  ▪ Partial hand and forearm extensor tendon injuries are treated similarly. A splint or cast is used for 3 weeks with mild wrist extension and 30 degrees of MCP flexion. The PIP joints are left free.

SURGICAL MANAGEMENT

Preoperative Planning

▪ A careful examination is performed to determine the structures that are injured or will need repair (eg, open joint injuries, fractures, flexor tendon or nerve injuries) and to inform the patient of the extent of the procedure, anticipated rehabilitation, need for occupational and non-occupational restrictions, and expected outcome.
▪ If the wound is infected at the time of presentation, irrigation and débridement should be followed by a course of antibiotics. Delayed primary tendon repair can be carried out 7 to 14 days later (sooner for EPL lacerations proximal to the MCP joint and EDC lacerations proximal to the juctura).
▪ The surgeon should anticipate the need for tendon graft or transfer for subacute injuries or those with tendon loss.
▪ Local anesthesia and a digital tourniquet can be used for injuries distal to the PIP joint. The need for an upper arm tourniquet for more proximal injuries may necessitate a general or regional anesthetic, unless the anticipated surgical time is less than 30 minutes. Regional anesthesia can offer extended postoperative pain relief and muscle relaxation during the initial recovery period.

Positioning

▪ Standard positioning is used with the hand on a hand table and the surgeon at the head.
▪ Preparation and draping is done above the elbow to allow dressing and splint application before removal of drapes.
▪ A carefully padded tourniquet is applied, set to 100 mm Hg above systolic blood pressure (sometimes more for obese patients, and less for children or those with small arms).

Approach

▪ Wound exploration and débridement are performed in a bloodless field, with appropriate light and magnification. Injuries over a joint usually require joint exploration and irrigation.
▪ The skin laceration can be extended to improve exposure, allow retrieval of retracted tendons, provide access to place sutures, and to decrease skin tension during retraction. Long, narrow skin flaps are avoided. Longitudinal incisions on the dorsum of the hand and fingers can cross over joints (unlike on the digital flexor surface).
▪ Bipolar electrocautery is used as needed, with care taken not to injure dorsal cutaneous nerves. If there is any doubt regarding hemostasis, the tourniquet is deflated before closure. Drains are seldom needed.
▪ Only the skin in the fingers, hand, and distal forearm is closed, with limited subcutaneous sutures more proximally if needed.

SUTURE TECHNIQUES

- Suture technique is determined by the thickness and shape of the tendon and the nature and character of the laceration (**TECH FIG 1**).
  - Thin tendons (eg, in digits) can be repaired with a horizontal cross-stitch suture (Silfverskiöld), simple running, figure 8, or horizontal mattress suture using 4-0 or 5-0 braided or monofilament nonabsorbable material.
  - Thicker tendons can support a two- or four-strand grasping repair with a 2-0, 3-0, or 4-0 nonabsorbable braided suture (eg, Ethibond, Ticron, or Fiberwire), optionally reinforced with a 5-0 or 6-0 monofilament epitendinous suture placed in a simple running or cross-stitch fashion.
- In general, repair strength is related to number of suture strands crossing the repair site, the thickness of the suture, and the locking style of the stitch.

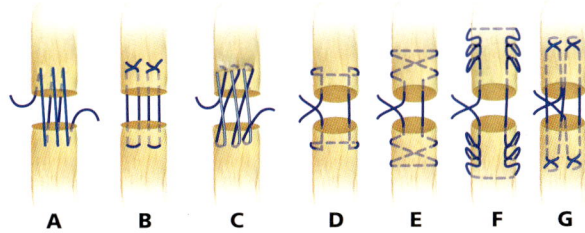

TECH FIG 1 • Some suture techniques for extensor tendon repair. The strongest repairs are the Silfverskiöld cross-stitch for flat tendons, and the four-strand cruciate suture for tendons able to accept a core suture. **A.** Running suture. **B.** Horizontal mattress. **C.** Silfverskiöld cross-stitch (which can also be used as a circumferential epitendinous tidying suture over a core suture). **D.** Modified Kessler. **E.** Modified Bunnell. **F.** Krackow. **G.** Four-strand cruciate suture.

REPAIR IN THE FINGERS

Zone I (DIP Joint)

Soft Tissue Mallet Treatment

- In patients with closed tendon disruptions who cannot tolerate a splint for occupational reasons, pinning across the DIP joint with a 0.045-inch Kirschner wire exposed at the tip or buried under the skin may be indicated. Pin removal is performed 6 weeks later, followed by motion exercises and 6 weeks of splinting at night and during vigorous activity.
- Lacerations in zone I are treated with primary surgical repair.
  - A figure 8 or running cross-stitch with a 5-0 nonabsorbable suture can be placed in the tendon, taking care to avoid shortening the tendon. This is supported with a 0.045-inch Kirschner wire across the DIP joint for 6 weeks. The DIP should be in neutral extension, without hyperextension.
  - An easier and often better alternative is use of a "tenodermodesis" stitch of 4-0 nylon through both the tendon and skin (**TECH FIG 2**).[4,10] This can be especially useful in cases treated in the emergency room, or in children, where the small tendon is difficult to accurately repair.
    - Full-time extension splinting (as in a closed mallet finger) or a 0.045-inch Kirschner wire across the extended DIP joint is required.
    - The suture can be removed in 2 to 3 weeks, but the splinting should continue for a total of 6 weeks full time and another 6 weeks at night.

Bony Mallet Treatment

- It remains controversial whether mallet fractures with greater than 50% of the distal phalanx involved or with DIP joint subluxation should be treated surgically or by splinting alone. Surgery is more likely warranted in younger patients and those with greater amounts of subluxation.[21] If conservative management is being con-

sidered, be sure to obtain a good lateral radiograph with the digit in the DIP splint, as DIP extension to neutral may demonstrate subluxation that was not apparent when the joint was flexed.

- A large bone fragment is present, with subluxation of the DIP joint (**TECH FIG 3A,B**).
- Place a 0.045-inch Kirschner wire down the shaft of the distal phalanx, almost to the DIP joint.
- Maximally flex the DIP and place a 0.035-inch Kirschner wire at the anticipated location of the reduced dorsal fragment of the distal phalanx. The skin entry point is

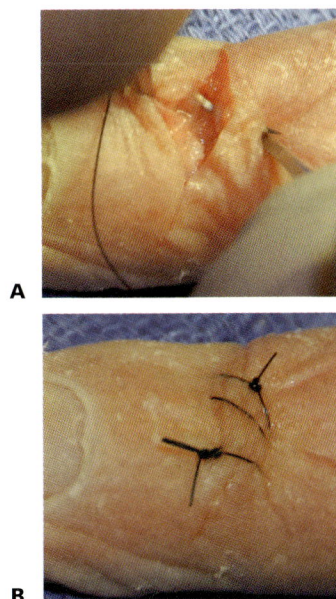

TECH FIG 2 • Tenodermodesis can be a useful way of suturing terminal tendon lacerations, especially in the emergency department or office. The suture (passing from left to right in **A**) goes through the skin and tendon proximally and distally.

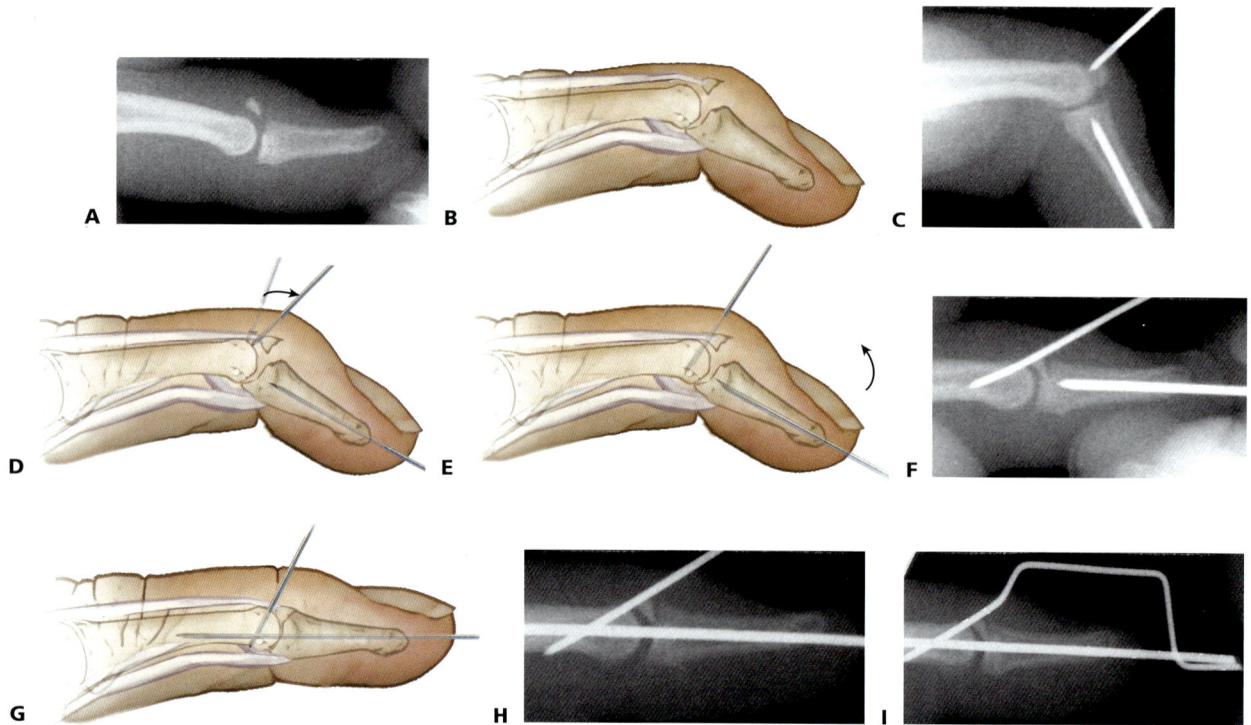

TECH FIG 3 • Technique for pinning a mallet fracture. **A,B.** Large bone fragment is present, frequently with subluxation of the distal interphalangeal (DIP) joint. **C.** A pin is placed in the distal phalanx. Maximally flex the DIP and place a 0.035-inch Kirschner wire where you would anticipate the dorsal edge of the distal phalanx to be. The skin entry point is relatively distal, to enable pin movement in the next step. **D,E.** Angle the wire distally, pushing the fragment and buttressing it. Advance the wire into the middle phalanx. **F,G.** Extend and reduce the distal phalanx, bringing it up to the fragment, and stabilizing it by advancing the 0.045-inch Kirschner wire across the DIP joint. If a significant articular step-off persists after a couple tries, leave the longitudinal wire and allow the fragment to heal where it lies. **H.** Dorsal pins buttress the fragment, and the longitudinal pin reduces the flexion and subluxation. **I.** Pins bent to fit in a single pin cap.

relatively distal to enable pin movement in the next step. Hold the pin against the middle phalanx (**TECH FIG 3C**).

- Angle the wire distally, pushing the fragment distally and buttressing it. Advance the wire into the middle phalanx (**TECH FIG 3D,E**).
- Extend and reduce the distal phalanx, bringing it up to the fragment. Drive the 0.045-inch wire across the DIP joint. Maintain full extension and correction of any subluxation (**TECH FIG 3F–H**).
- Bend the pins so they can be included in a single pin cap to prevent rotation or movement of the proximal pin (**TECH FIG 3I**).
- If an articular step-off persists after a couple of attempts, remove the dorsal wire but leave the longitudinal wire in place supporting the joint in neutral extension and correcting the subluxation. This may leave a dorsal prominence but will correct the subluxation.
- Pins can be removed in about 6 weeks with institution of a protected motion program and 4 to 6 weeks of additional night splinting.

Zone II (Over Middle Phalanx)

- Perform primary tendon repair with a running 4-0 or 5-0 cross-stitch suture.
- The DIP joint can be splinted or pinned extended for 6 weeks, followed by splinting for vigorous activity and at night for 6 weeks.

Zone III (Over PIP Joint)

- Use a running 4-0 or 5-0 suture to repair the central slip in the manner detailed earlier (**TECH FIG 4**).
- Repair the lateral band or bands with single 4-0 or 5-0 monofilament suture in a figure 8 fashion.

Reconstruction in Cases with Tendon Loss

- Consider V-Y advancement of the central tendon or a "turndown" of the central slip proximal to the laceration to cover the defect.[20]
- Extend the skin incision proximally, almost to the MCP joint.
- Incise a V in the central slip, with the apex just distal to the MCP joint, and the distal end the width of the tendon, taking care not to damage the overlying epitenon (**TECH FIG 5A**, red line).
- Advance the tendon distally. Disrupt the loose alveolar tissue between the tendon and periosteum as little as possible.
- Close the V into a Y with a 4-0 or 5-0 suture, and repair the distal end of the advanced central slip as described earlier (**TECH FIG 5B**).
- An alternative method involves creating a rectangular flap of central slip proximally and turning it up to attach distally (**TECH FIGS 5A,C,D**).[20]
- Suture anchors or small holes drilled in the middle phalanx are occasionally needed to secure the tendon to the

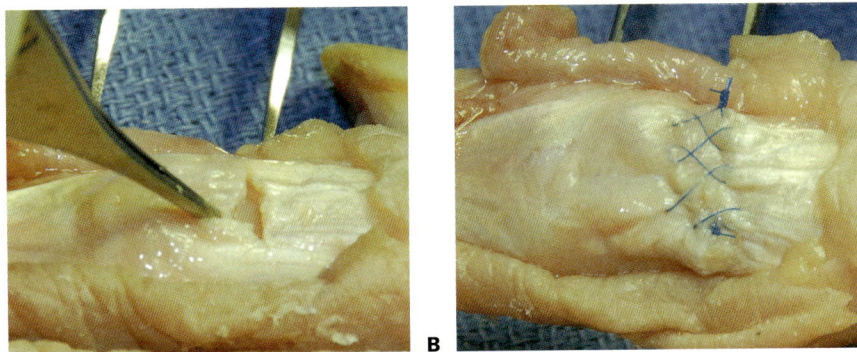

A

B

TECH FIG 4 • Simulated central slip laceration on a cadaver specimen. Note how difficult it would be for a laceration to cut all the way around the extensor mechanism. This example has been repaired with a running, cross-stitch suture (Silfverskiöld).

dorsal base of the middle phalanx, especially if the dorsal margin of the base of the phalanx is lost.

Postoperative Management

- Postoperative rehabilitation for children, less compliant adults, and cases with a tenuous repair involves static splinting or pinning of the PIP joint in full extension for 4 weeks, followed by a protected motion program.
- For compliant adults, an early motion protocol can be initiated.[6]
  - 0 to 30 degrees of active PIP flexion and extension is allowed starting a few days after surgery, using a palmar flexion block splint with a free wrist and MCP joint.
  - 10 to 20 repetitions are performed each hour, with a static PIP splint in full extension when not exercising.

- DIP flexion exercises are performed in the static PIP extension splint.
- If no extensor lag develops, PIP motion can be increased to 40 degrees after 2 weeks, 50 degrees after 3 weeks, and 70 degrees after 4 weeks. The splinting is discontinued at 6 weeks.
- Results are often less than perfect, especially in cases with tendon loss, where some loss of motion should be expected.

Zone IV (Over Proximal Phalanx)

- The tendon at this level may be thicker and support a grasping or locking core stitch with a 4-0 braided nonabsorbable suture, reinforced with a running 5-0 monofilament suture.
- If the tendon is too thin, repair as in zone III.
- Postoperative management is as in zone III.

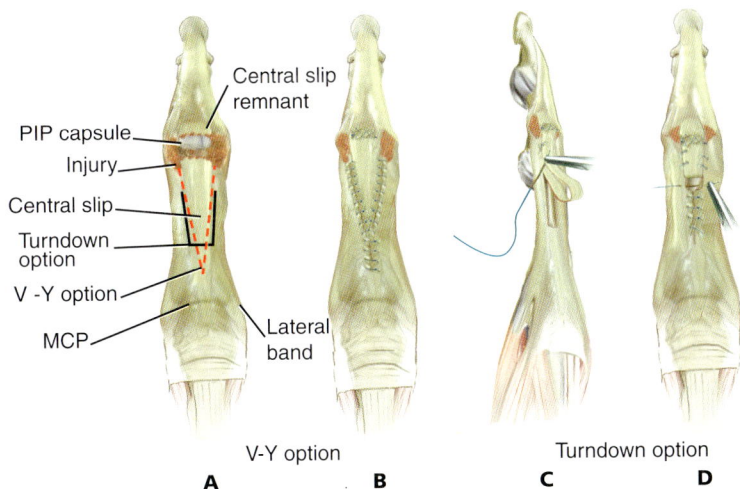

Central slip
remnant

PIP capsule

Injury

Central slip

Turndown
option

V -Y option

MCP

Lateral
band

V-Y option

Turndown option

A   **B**   **C**   **D**

TECH FIG 5 • **A.** Central slip loss (eg, abrasions, grinders) can lead to significant stiffness. **B.** V-Y advancement of the central tendon. **C,D.** "Turndown" of a portion of the central slip.

REPAIR IN THE HAND, WRIST, AND FOREARM

Zone V (Over the MCP Joint)

- The tendon is much thicker at this level and can sometimes support a 3-0 or 4-0 braided nonabsorbable core suture with a running simple or cross-stitch suture over the repair, incorporating any laceration of the sagittal band.
- An abnormal resting cascade of the digits suggest a tendon laceration (**TECH FIG 6A**).

- Lacerations over the MCP joint often extend into the joint. The skin laceration is extended and débrided and the wound explored. Large capsular rents (arrow in **TECH FIG 6B**) can be repaired with a simple running 5-0 absorbable monofilament suture. Small capsular lacerations are left open.
- The tendon end is retrieved, and a 3-0 nonabsorbable core suture is placed. The first loops of the cruciate stitch are shown (**TECH FIG 6C**).

TECHNIQUES

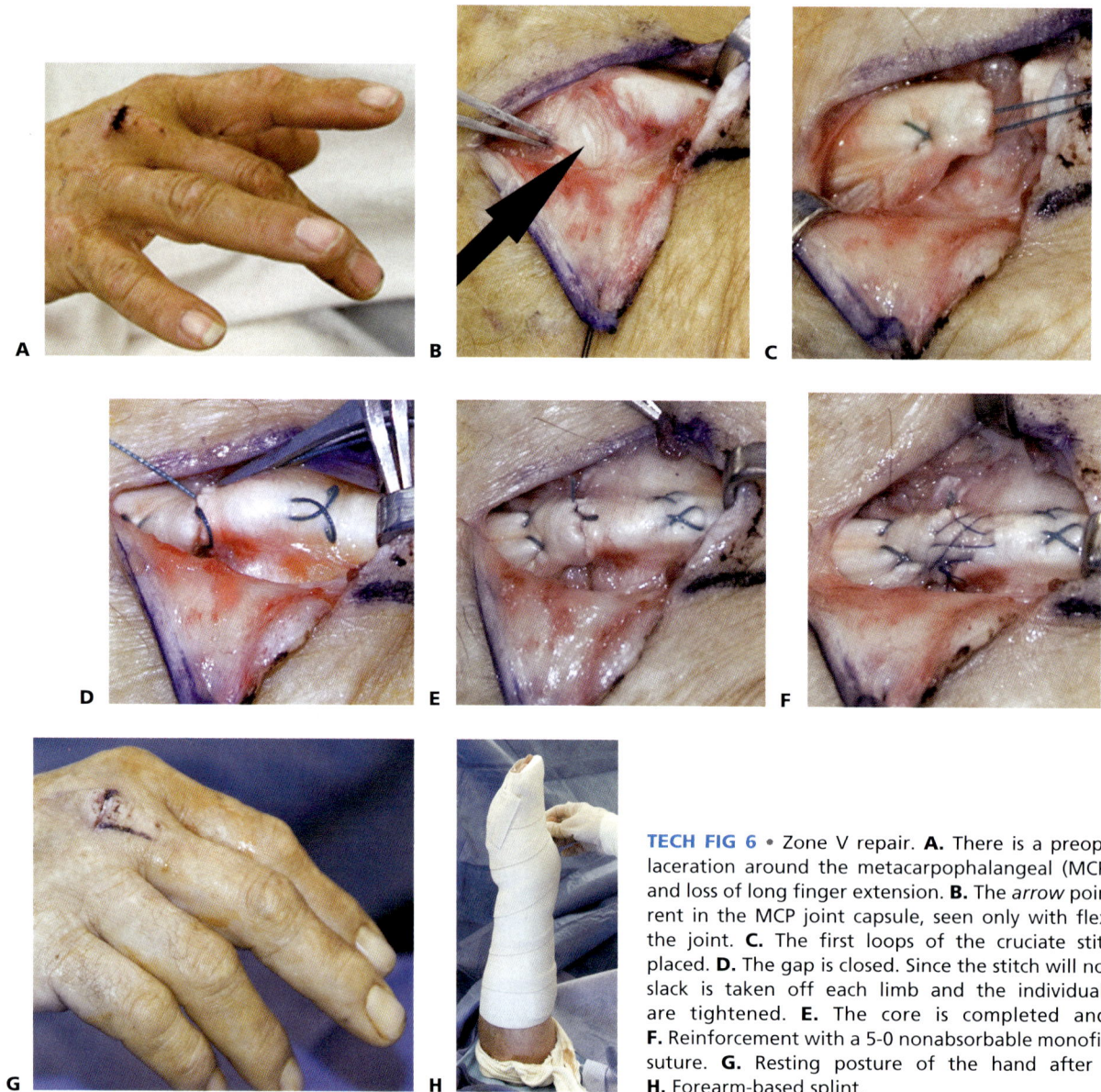

TECH FIG 6 • Zone V repair. **A.** There is a preoperative laceration around the metacarpophalangeal (MCP) joint and loss of long finger extension. **B.** The *arrow* points to a rent in the MCP joint capsule, seen only with flexion of the joint. **C.** The first loops of the cruciate stitch are placed. **D.** The gap is closed. Since the stitch will not slide, slack is taken off each limb and the individual loops are tightened. **E.** The core is completed and tied. **F.** Reinforcement with a 5-0 nonabsorbable monofilament suture. **G.** Resting posture of the hand after repair. **H.** Forearm-based splint.

- The distal locking stitch is placed on one side of the tendon but not pulled tight until the tendon ends are accurately approximated. The limbs of the X are individually tightened (**TECH FIG 6D**).
- The core suture is completed and will not slide (**TECH FIG 6E**).
- The repair is reinforced with a 5-0 nonabsorbable monofilament suture. This can be circumferential proximal to zone V, but only over the dorsal surface of the tendon distally (**TECH FIG 6F**).
- The resting cascade of the digits shows the repaired finger to be slightly "tighter" than normal immediately after the repair (**TECH FIG 6G**).
- A forearm-based splint is applied with 30 degrees of wrist extension, less than 30 degrees of MCP flexion, and fully extended PIP and DIP joints (**TECH FIG 6H**).
- After 8 to 10 days, this splint is converted to a short-arm cast supporting the MCP joints in extension (including all fingers for index lacerations and the ulnar three for other lacerations) but leaving the PIP joints free

for another 3 weeks before institution of a therapy program.
- Alternatively, an early protected motion program can be initiated.[3,9]

Repair of Distal "Compromised" Zone V Lacerations

- In this clinical situation a standard end-to-end repair may be tenuous or may not be possible secondary to contracted or lost tendon substance. A tendon interpositional graft may be required.
- Partially incise the distal tendon transversely 5 mm distal to the cut edge.
- Weave tendon graft in a volar to dorsal direction through this transverse incision in the distal stump.
- Sew the graft to the proximal stump to the distal tissue and back to itself using nonabsorbable material (**TECH FIG 7**).
- Sew the proximal stump to the tendon graft using a Polvertaft weave.

Zone VI (Metacarpal Level)

- The tendon is thicker and repair is similar but technically easier than in zone V.

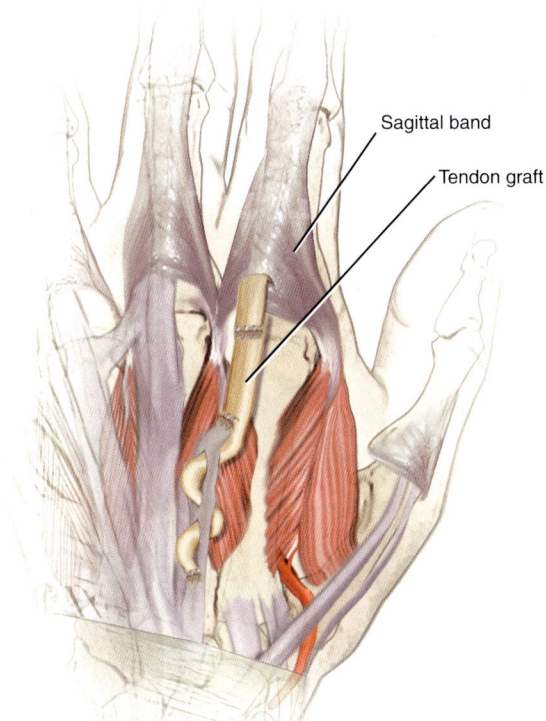

Sagittal band

Tendon graft

TECH FIG 7 • Tendon graft is woven volar to dorsal through the transverse incision in the distal tendon stump. A Polvertaft weave is used to secure the graft to the proximal tendon stump.

- Use a 3-0 or 4-0 braided nonabsorbable suture, reinforced with a circumferential running cross-stitch 5-0 or 6-0 monofilament suture.
- Rehabilitation is as for zone V.

Zone VII (Wrist and Extensor Retinaculum)

- Suture repair and postoperative management are as in zone VI.
- The extensor retinaculum is incised for repair and retrieval of the proximal tendon stump.
- Retinacular closure is performed with a 4-0 absorbable suture to prevent tendon bowstringing. A portion of the retinaculum may need to be excised to allow the repair site to glide smoothly.
- The EPL can be repaired outside of the retinaculum and left in the subcutaneous tissue.
- Postoperative management is the same as for Zone V injuries.

Zone VIII

- Make a generous incision to determine the resting orientation of the tendons before débridement and repair. It may be helpful to tag proximal tendon ends with labels to define them before further dissection changes their position.
- In the distal forearm, conventional repair with grasping sutures is possible. EDC tendons can be repaired as a group if necessary.
- Proximally, repair can be much more difficult. 3-0 interrupted absorbable sutures can be used in fibrous septa within muscle along with repair of epimysium.
- Postoperative management is as for zones V to VII.

PEARLS AND PITFALLS

Tetanus prophylaxis[16]	■ Tetanus toxoid "booster" should be given to patients with at least three previous doses, but last dose more than 5 years ago for tetanus-prone wounds (>1-cm laceration, crush, burn, high-energy injury, or with infection, devitalized tissue, or gross contamination) or more than 10 years ago for wounds not prone to tetanus. ■ Tetanus immune globulin should be given for tetanus-prone wounds in patients with unknown or incomplete vaccination history. It is not clear, however, that "tetanus-prone wounds" are more likely to cause tetanus. ■ The greatest protection against tetanus is a completed childhood vaccination series. ■ A tetanus booster at the time of injury does not change the likelihood of developing tetanus.
Lacerations proximal to juncturae tendinum	■ Extensor lag may be more subtle, sometimes noted only with lack of active MCP hyperextension, pain with resisted range of motion, or lack of palpable EDC tendon on dorsum of hand. ■ Full PIP extension may be possible through the lateral bands even in the presence of a complete tendon laceration.
Subacute lacerations	■ Be prepared for EIP transfer or free tendon graft for delayed treatment of EPL lacerations. ■ Side-to-side repair to adjacent extensor tendons or use of a free tendon graft is occasionally needed for treatment of chronic injuries involving other tendons.
Clenched-fist injuries	■ Extensor tendon injury may be well proximal to the skin injury. ■ Associated MCP joint injuries are common.
Shortened repair	■ Digital extensor mechanism is very sensitive to shortening, with resulting loss of flexion.
Distal forearm extensor tendon lacerations	■ Before exploring proximal injury, locate and label individual tendon ends (based on location). ■ Detailed exploration (for incision and drainage, foreign body removal, etc.) may distort tendon position, making it impossible to determine correct proximal motor to attach to each distal tendon end.
Proximal forearm lacerations	■ Associated nerve injury (especially the posterior interosseous nerve) can make diagnosis and treatment difficult.

TECHNIQUES

	▪ If the laceration is proximal and the EPL does not function, then the likelihood of nerve injury is greater (due to the EPL's more distal origin).
	▪ Lack of tenodesis effect suggests extensor tendon injury.
Suture techniques	▪ To most easily do the Silverskiöld cross-stitch, start on the side of the tendon closest to the surgeon.
	▪ After the first knot is tied, advance away across the tendon, keeping the needle pointed back at the surgeon for the horizontal component of the stitch.

POSTOPERATIVE CARE

▪ Postoperative care is detailed under the surgical technique for each individual location.

OUTCOMES

▪ Good or excellent results can be anticipated in most patients, with worse outcomes seen in the digits and with concomitant soft tissue or bone injury. Loss of digital flexion is a greater problem than small losses of extension.[2,16]

▪ Stronger suture techniques and early dynamic postoperative protocols may result in better functional outcomes earlier,[17] although few controlled studies show improvement in long-term results when compared to static splinting programs, which are easier, more predictable, and less expensive.[12,14] Early motion programs may be most beneficial in zones III and IV.

COMPLICATIONS

▪ Infection
▪ Rupture of repaired tendons
▪ Stiffness
  ▪ Primary joint stiffness after immobilization
  ▪ Adherence of repaired tendon to surrounding skin, bone
▪ Extensor lag

REFERENCES

1. Bendre AA, Hartigan BJ, Kalainov DM. Mallet finger. J Am Acad Orthop Surg 2005;13:336–344.
2. Carl HD, Forst R, Schaller P. Results of primary extensor tendon repair in relation to the zone of injury and pre-operative outcome estimation. Arch Orthop Trauma Surg 2007;127:115–119 [e-pub Sept. 30, 2006].
3. Crosby CA, Wehbe MA. Early protected motion after extensor tendon repair. J Hand Surg Am 1999;24A:1061–1070.
4. Doyle JR. Extensor tendons: Acute injuries. In Green DP, ed. Operative Hand Surgery, 4th ed. New York: Churchill Livingstone; 1999:1950–1987.
5. Elson RA. Rupture of the central slip of the extensor hood of the finger. A test for early diagnosis. J Bone Joint Surg Br 1986;68B:229–231.
6. Evans RB. Early active short arc motion for the repaired central slip. J Hand Surg Am 1994;19A:991–997.
7. Garberman SF, Diao E, Peimer CA. Mallet finger: results of early versus delayed closed treatment. J Hand Surg Am 1994;19A:850–852.
8. Hofmeister EP, Mazurek MT, Shin AY, et al. Extension block pinning for large mallet fractures. J Hand Surg Am 2003;28A:453–459.
9. Howell JW, Merritt WH, Robinson SJ. Immediate controlled active motion following zone 4-7 extensor tendon repair. J Hand Ther 2005;18:182–190.
10. Iselin F, Levame J, Godoy J. A simplified technique for treating mallet fingers: tenodermodesis. J Hand Surg Am 1977;2A:118–121.
11. Kaplan EB, Hunter JM. Extrinsic muscles of the fingers. In Spinner M, ed. Kaplan's Functional and Surgical Anatomy of the Hand, 3rd ed. Philadelphia: JB Lippincott Co, 1984:93–112.
12. Khandwala AR, Webb J, Harris SB, et al. A comparison of dynamic extension splinting and controlled active mobilization of complete divisions of extensor tendons in zones 5 and 6. J Hand Surg Br 2000;25B:140–146.
13. Kleinert HE, Verdan C. Report of the Committee on Tendon Injuries (International Federation of Societies for Surgery of the Hand). J Hand Surg Am 1983;8A:794–798.
14. Mowlavi A, Burns M, Brown RE. Dynamic versus static splinting of simple zone V and zone VI extensor tendon repairs: a prospective, randomized, controlled study. Plast Reconstr Surg 2005;115:482–487.
15. Newport ML. Extensor tendon injuries in the hand. J Am Acad Orthop Surg 1997;5:59–66.
16. Newport ML, Blair WF, Steyers CM Jr. Long-term results of extensor tendon repair. J Hand Surg Am 1990;15A:961–966.
17. Newport ML, Williams CD. Biomechanical characteristics of extensor tendon suture techniques. J Hand Surg Am 1992;17A:1117–1123.
18. Rhee P, Nunley MK, Demetriades D, et al. Tetanus and trauma: a review and recommendations. J Trauma 2005;58:1082–1088.
19. Rockwell WB, Butler PN, Byrne BA. Extensor tendon: anatomy, injury, and reconstruction. Plast Reconstr Surg 2000;106:1592–1603.
20. Snow JW. A method for reconstruction of the central slip of the extensor tendon of a finger. Plast Reconstr Surg 1976;57:455–459.
21. Wehbe MA, Schneider LH. Mallet fractures. J Bone Joint Surg Am 1984;66A:658–669.

Chapter 58

Tendon Transfer and Grafting for Traumatic Extensor Tendon Disruption

John S. Taras and Daniel J. Lee

DEFINITION

■ Traumatic injury to the extensor tendons of the hand and forearm results in the disruption of tendon substance, causing a loss of active wrist or digital extension.

■ Primary repair of the extensor tendon usually can be performed within 7 days after appropriate irrigation and débridement of wounds and stabilization of any fractures.[5]

■ Late reconstruction of extensor tendon injuries presents an operative challenge and often requires the use of tendon transfer and grafting techniques.

ANATOMY

■ The extensor mechanism of the hand and wrist is a complex system involving balanced interplay between extrinsic and intrinsic components (**FIG 1**).

■ The extrinsic extensor tendons are divided into superficial and deep groups in the forearm:
  ■ Superficial: extensor carpi radialis longus and brevis (ECRL and ECRB), extensor digitorum communis (EDC), extensor digiti minimi (EDM), extensor carpi ulnaris (ECU), and anconeus
  ■ Deep: abductor pollicis longus (APL), extensor pollicis brevis and longus (EPB and EPL), extensor indicis proprius (EIP), and supinator

■ Wrist extension is provided by the ECRB, ECRL, and ECU.

■ Finger and thumb extension is provided by the APL, EPB, EPL, EDC, EIP, and EDM.

■ The radial nerve innervates all extensor muscles of the hand, except the intrinsics, which are innervated by the median and ulnar nerves. The radial nerve's deep motor branch becomes the posterior interosseous nerve (PIN).

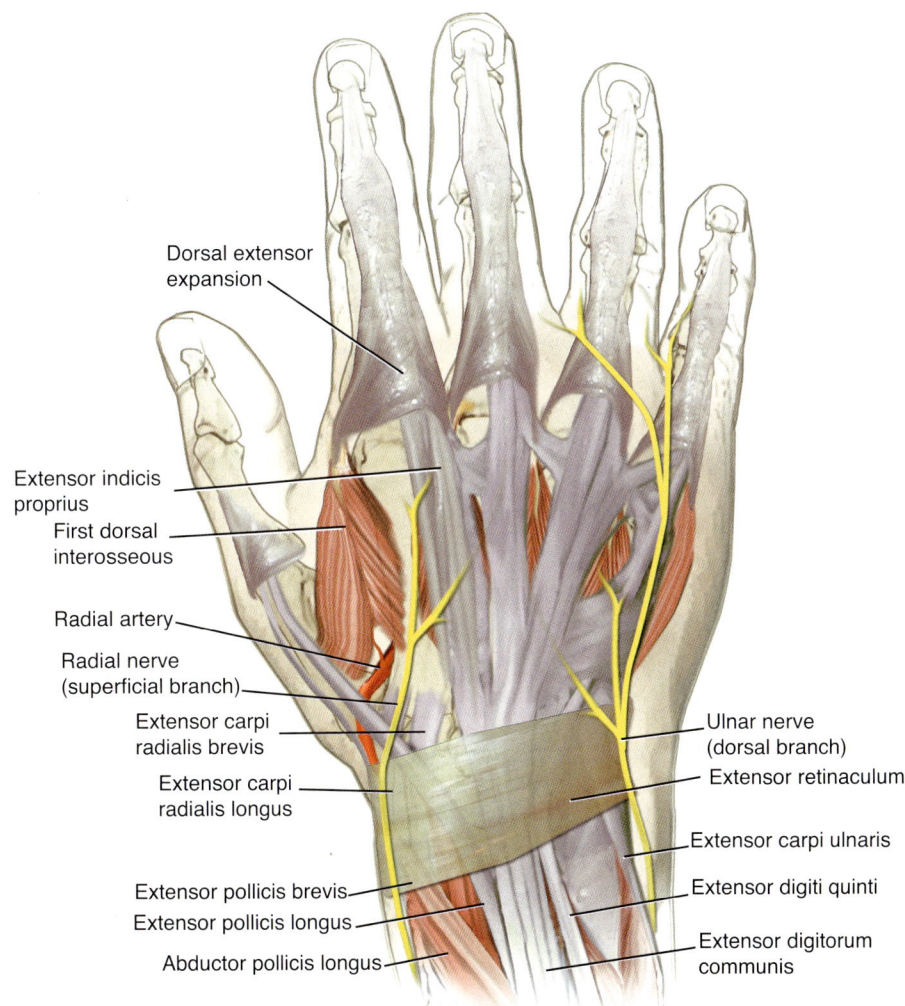

Dorsal extensor expansion

Extensor indicis proprius

First dorsal interosseous

Radial artery

Radial nerve (superficial branch)

Extensor carpi radialis brevis

Extensor carpi radialis longus

Extensor pollicis brevis

Extensor pollicis longus

Abductor pollicis longus

Ulnar nerve (dorsal branch)

Extensor retinaculum

Extensor carpi ulnaris

Extensor digiti quinti

Extensor digitorum communis

FIG 1 • Tendons on the dorsum of the hand, extensor retinaculum.

2587

- There are six fibro-osseous dorsal compartments at the level of the wrist covered by the extensor retinaculum. The contents of each compartment are as follows:
  - I: APL, EPB
  - II: ECRL, ECRB
  - III: EPL
  - IV: EDC, EIP
  - V: EDM
  - VI: ECU
- The intrinsic system of the hand consists of the seven interosseous muscles (three palmar and four dorsal) and four lumbrical muscles.
  - The intrinsic muscles pass volar to the axis of the metacarpophalangeal (MP) joints and dorsal to the interphalangeal (IP) joints; thus, the intrinsic system will flex the MP joints and extend the IP joints.
- On the dorsum on the hand, the fibrous bands of the juncturae tendinum connect the extensor digitorum tendons of the long, ring, and small fingers.
  - This interconnection is what allows grouped extension of the fingers.
  - The EIP and EDM are ulnar to their respective EDC tendons and function as independent extensors of the index and small fingers.
- Over the MP joints, tendons are held in a central position by the sagittal bands, which envelop the MP joint and attach to the volar plate.
- The dorsal extensor apparatus is formed distal to the MP joint from contributions of both extrinsic and intrinsic tendons.
  - The central slip, the continuation of the extrinsic extensor tendon, inserts into the dorsal base of the middle phalanx.
  - The lateral bands are formed from the intrinsic muscles on either side of the finger and send fibers to the middle phalanx as well as contributions to the central slip.
  - The lateral bands combine dorsally over the middle phalanx to form the terminal extensor tendon, which inserts on the dorsal base of the distal phalanx.
  - The transverse and oblique retinacular ligaments stabilize the tendons of the dorsal apparatus.
- Traumatic injuries to the extensor tendons can be described in terms of nine anatomic zones (Table 1).[3]
- Traumatic injuries to the extensor tendon of the thumb have a separate numbering system and are divided into five anatomic zones (Table 2).
  - Even-numbered zones overlie bones and odd-numbered zones overlie joints.

Table 1	Extensor Tendon Zones of Fingers	
Zone	**Location**	
I	Distal interphalangeal	
II	Middle phalanx	
III	Proximal interphalangeal	
IV	Proximal phalanx	
V	Metacarpophalangeal	
VI	Metacarpal	
VII	Wrist	
VIII	Distal forearm	
IX	Proximal forearm	

Table 2	Extensor Tendon Zones of Thumb	
Zone	**Location**	
T-I	Interphalangeal	
T-II	Proximal phalanx	
T-III	Metacarpophalangeal	
T-IV	First metacarpal	
T-V	Wrist	

- Vascular supply[5]
  - Forearm: nutrition via small arterial branches from the surrounding fascia
  - Wrist: derived from mesotenon; nutrition via diffusion
  - Hand: derived from paratenon; nutrition via perfusion

PATHOGENESIS

- Extensor tendons are susceptible to traumatic injury because of their relatively superficial location and thin tendon substance.
- Acute repair within 7 days is recommended, but direct repair of acute injuries is occasionally impractical in cases with extensive soft tissue damage or segmental tendon loss.
  - In these cases, skeletal stabilization is obtained first (**FIG 2**), followed by soft tissue coverage, and finally late reconstruction of the disrupted extensor mechanism.
- Also, late presentation of traumatic disruptions of an extensor tendon makes direct repair difficult because of tendon retraction and subsequent extrinsic tightness.
- Traumatic injury to the extensor tendons can also occur after upper extremity fractures.
  - Acute rupture of the EPL tendon has been associated with displaced distal radius fractures.
  - Delayed EPL rupture has been associated with minimally displaced distal radius fractures. These attritional ruptures are generally attributed to compromise of the tendon's vascular supply by soft tissue damage and hemorrhage after fracture with an intact third extensor compartment.[4]
- Delayed extensor tendon ruptures of the EPL, EDC, and EIP have been reported as a complication after volar and dorsal plate fixation of distal radius fractures.[2]

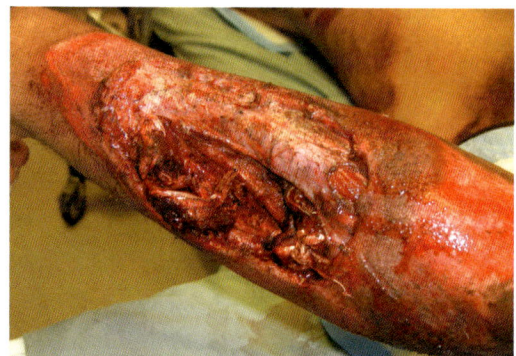

FIG 2 • Preoperative picture of a patient with severe soft tissue loss, including extensor muscle, after a motorcycle accident, which required extensor tendon reconstruction.

NATURAL HISTORY

- Without treatment, complete extensor tendon disruptions will result in a persistent loss of active extension or incomplete extension of the wrist or digits (or loss of active abduction and extension of the thumb, depending on which tendon or tendons are involved).
- A late tendon imbalance resulting from pull of the flexor tendons against a disrupted or weakened extensor mechanism with or without fixed joint contracture may develop if reconstruction is not performed.

PATIENT HISTORY AND PHYSICAL FINDINGS

- The patient most commonly has a history of penetrating or blunt trauma to the dorsal forearm or hand with resultant loss of active extension of the wrist, fingers, or thumb (**FIG 3**). Loss of soft tissue may be associated with the original injury.
- In cases of attritional rupture of the EPL tendon, the patient may have a recent or remote history of a distal radius fracture, usually only minimally displaced.
- Physical examination methods include the following:
  - MP extension. Incomplete MP extension indicates extensor tendon disruption in zones proximal to the MP. If the other fingers are not kept flexed, the patient may be able to fully extend the affected finger in the presence of a completely lacerated tendon.
  - EPL test. An EPL rupture manifests as a loss of extension of the thumb IP and MP joints.
  - Tenodesis test. A loss of extensor tendon continuity will result in loss of the tenodesis effect. Wrist flexion will have no effect on finger extension.
- A complete evaluation of the elbow, forearm, wrist, or hand begins with a thorough inspection of all open wounds and an assessment of the extent of soft tissue compromise.
  - Local or regional anesthesia can assist with patient comfort during the examination.
- A comprehensive neurovascular examination must be performed before using any anesthetic. Special attention is directed to the status of the radial nerve, specifically the PIN.
  - Compromise in PIN function may result from compression neuropathy, direct injury, or underlying elbow pathology.
- If there is a suspicion of joint violation, then injection of sterile saline with or without methylene blue into the joint can verify whether the joint capsule has been disrupted.

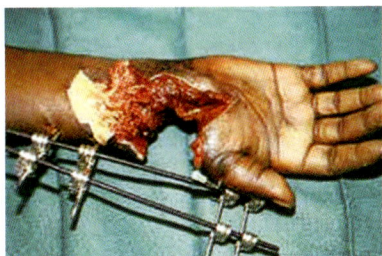

FIG 3 • Segmental loss of extensor and flexor tendons from a shotgun blast.

IMAGING AND OTHER DIAGNOSTIC STUDIES

- AP, lateral, and oblique plain radiographs of the affected area (elbow, forearm, wrist, or hand) are obtained to rule out the presence of a foreign body, underlying fracture, or bony deformity or pathology.
- In cases of late presentation of suspected extensor tendon rupture, MRI is occasionally useful to confirm the diagnosis and identify the location of the retracted tendon ends.

DIFFERENTIAL DIAGNOSIS

- Radial nerve or PIN palsy
- Flexor tendon injury
- Intrinsic tightness
- Tendon adhesions
- Tendon subluxation (MP joint level)
- Joint contracture, subluxation, or deformity
- Soft tissue contracture

NONOPERATIVE MANAGEMENT

- Conservative treatment of injuries proximal to the metacarpals usually is not possible because of tendon retraction and muscle contracture and will result in persistent loss of extension of the wrist or digits.[4]
- Chronic extensor mechanism disorders distal to the metacarpals without fixed deformity will respond to splinting and intensive therapy. Such conservative management may result in an acceptable functional outcome for select patients.

SURGICAL MANAGEMENT

- Most extensor tendon lacerations are amenable to direct primary repair if treated relatively early.
- Indications for reconstruction of extensor tendon injuries include loss of extension of the wrist, fingers, or thumb resulting in a functional deficit.
- When delay or loss of tendon substance precludes a direct repair, tendon grafting or transfer may restore function successfully.

Preoperative Planning

- The patient must be provided with a realistic assessment of the potential gains from surgery as well as details of the treatment plan.
- Any fixed joint contractures should be identified and treated with therapy and splinting before extensor tendon reconstruction to optimize outcomes.
- In cases of severe soft tissue loss, coverage must be obtained before proceeding with extensor system reconstruction.
  - This may include free or island muscle, fascial, or skin flaps in addition to full- or split-thickness skin grafts.

Positioning

- The patient is positioned supine with a hand table attached to the operative side.
- A tourniquet is usually used to operate in a bloodless field

Approach

- The approach depends on the tendon transfer or grafting technique required and is detailed in the Techniques section.

TECHNIQUES

END AND SIDE WEAVE JUNCTURES

- Tendon transfer or graft junctures are often best secured using an end weave technique (**TECH FIG 1**).
- The Pulvertaft method is a common weave used.
    - A pointed tendon-grasping and -passing instrument is invaluable and allows one tendon to be brought through the substance of the other tendon with minimal trauma.
    - The tendon weave is performed at right angles. For example, the first entry is horizontal, the next vertical, and then the third horizontal. At least three weaves are needed.

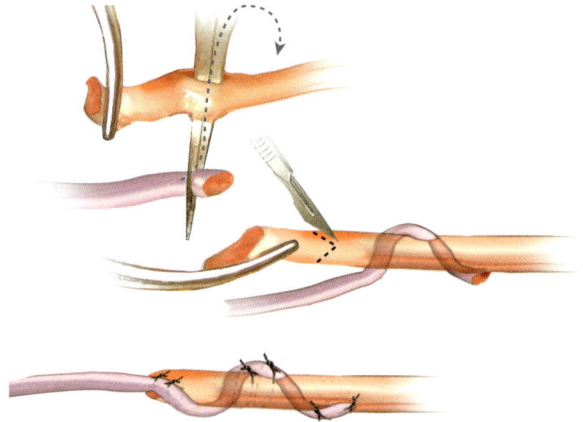

TECH FIG 1 • End weave technique. The smaller tendon is passed through and sutured.

EIP TO EPL TRANSFER

- The distal EIP tendon is identified through a 1-cm incision over the index finger MP joint. The EIP is ulnar to the EDC II.
- A second incision is made just distal to the extensor retinaculum at roughly the radiocarpal joint level, and the EIP tendon is identified in the radial aspect of the fourth extensor compartment.
    - The EIP is readily identified by its distal muscle belly.
- The EIP tendon is separated from the EDC II and transected through the incision over the MP joint.
- The tendon is then brought through to the proximal incision.
- A third incision is centered over the scaphotrapezial trapezoid joint and the distal stump of the disrupted EPL tendon is identified (**TECH FIG 2A**).

- A subcutaneous tunnel is created to connect the incision at the wrist and the incision near the base of the thumb.
- The EIP tendon is passed through the tunnel and attached to the distal stump of EPL using an end weave technique (**TECH FIG 2B**).
- Tension should be set so that when the wrist is extended, the thumb IP joint flexes, allowing the tip of the thumb to touch the tip of the index finger. The thumb IP joint should fully extend when the wrist is flexed (**TECH FIG 2C**).
- The thumb is immobilized with the wrist extended about 20 degrees and the thumb IP joint at 0 degrees for 4 weeks.

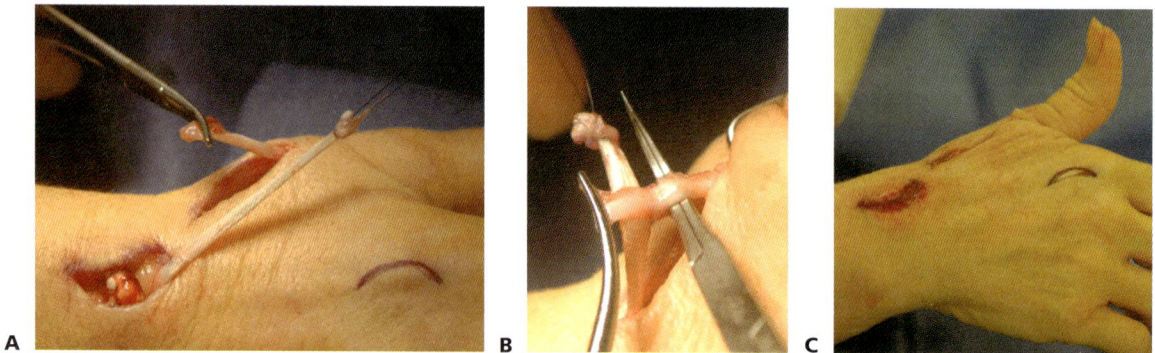

TECH FIG 2 • Extensor indicis proprius (EIP) to extensor pollicis longus (EPL) transfer. **A.** After the EIP tendon is identified, it is brought through the proximal incision. The distal stump of the EPL tendon is identified as well. **B.** The EIP tendon is passed through and is woven into the EPL tendon. **C.** After proper tensioning, the thumb should extend as the wrist flexes.

END-TO-SIDE SUTURING FOR EDC DISRUPTIONS

- A longitudinal incision is made on the dorsum of the hand over the appropriate area.
- The disrupted tendon end is identified and isolated.
- An end-to-side repair is performed to the adjacent intact tendon.

- Tension must be set so that the fingers are in extension when the wrist is flexed and the MP joints are flexed 20 to 30 degrees when the wrist is extended about 20 degrees. The normal flexion cascade must be re-established.

EIP TO EDC (FOURTH/FIFTH) TRANSFER

- The EIP tendon is isolated and freed in a manner similar to that described for the EIP-to-EPL transfer.
- An incision is made dorsally on the hand, over the disrupted extensor tendons of the ring and small fingers.
- The EIP is mobilized and inserted into the distal stump of the disrupted tendon of the small finger.
  - If disrupted, the extensor digiti quinti (EDQ) is sewn side to side to the transfer.
- The distal stump of the ring finger is attached to the adjacent intact common extensor tendon of the long finger. If the EDC to the long finger is also ruptured, it is sewn to the intact EDC to the index while the EDC to the ring is sewn to the EIP transfer (**TECH FIG 3**).

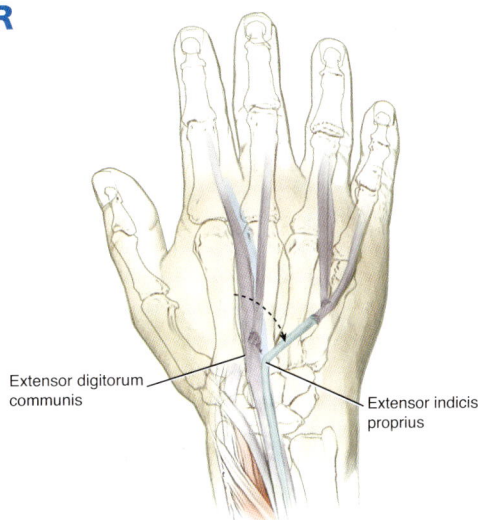

Extensor digitorum communis

Extensor indicis proprius

TECH FIG 3 • Extensor indicis proprius (EIP) to extensor digitorum communis IV/V tendon transfer.

FLEXOR CARPI ULNARIS TO EDC TRANSFER

- A longitudinal incision is made over the flexor carpi ulnaris (FCU) in the distal forearm.
- The FCU tendon is transected just proximal to the pisiform and is freed up proximally.
- A second oblique incision is made 5 cm below the medial epicondyle in the proximal forearm.
- The FCU fascial attachments are incised to free up the entire muscle belly.
- A third incision begins on the dorsal-ulnar mid-forearm and angles distally toward the tubercle of Lister to expose the disrupted EDC tendons.

- A tendon passer or Kelly clamp is passed subcutaneously around the ulnar border of the forearm to pull the FCU tendon into the dorsal wound.
- Muscle may be excised from the FCU to reduce bulk.
- The FCU tendon is woven through the EDC tendons at a 45-degree angle just proximal to the dorsal retinaculum.
- The FCU is secured under maximum tension, with the wrist and MP joints in neutral.

FLEXOR CARPI RADIALIS TO EDC TRANSFER

- A longitudinal incision is made over the flexor carpi radialis (FCR) in the distal forearm.
- The FCR tendon is identified and transected near its insertion.
- The tendon is freed up proximally to allow additional excursion.
- A second longitudinal incision is made on the dorsal forearm, extending from the mid-forearm to just distal to the dorsal retinaculum.

- The FCR is then passed subcutaneously around the radial border of forearm and delivered into the dorsal wound.
- The FCR tendon is then inserted into the EDC tendons and positioned superficial to the retinaculum.
- The transfer is secured with the FCR under maximum tension and wrist and MP joints in neutral (**TECH FIG 4**).

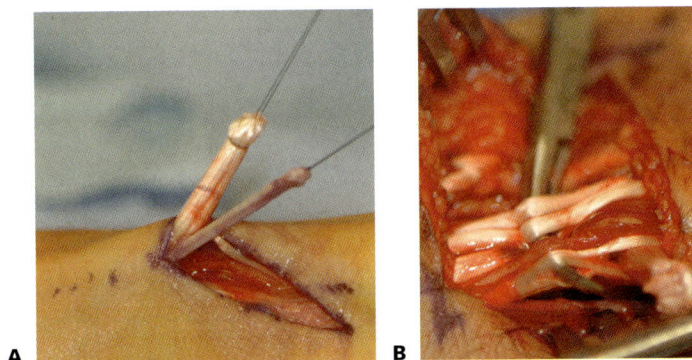

A

B

TECH FIG 4 • **A–F.** Flexor carpi radialis (FCR) and palmaris longus (PL) transfer for loss of thumb and digital extension. **A.** FCR and PL transected. **B.** FCR woven into extensor digitorum communis (EDC) II, III, IV, and V. *(continued)*

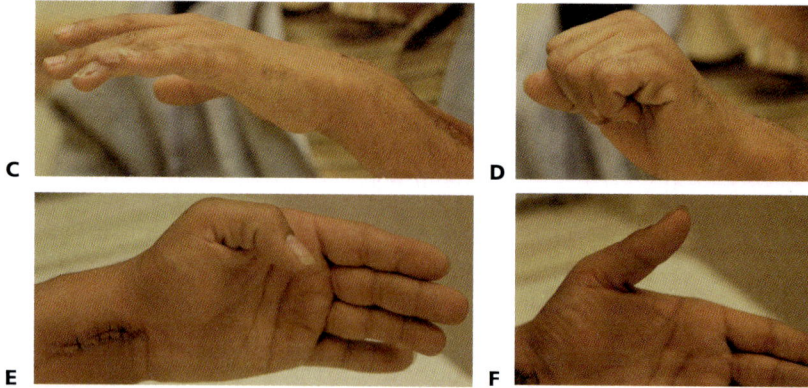

TECH FIG 4 • *(continued)* **C–F.** Patient demonstrating restored digital and hand extension.

Pronator Teres to ECRB Transfer

- An incision is made over the volar-radial aspect of the mid-forearm.
- The pronator teres (PT) tendon is identified and followed to its insertion into the radius.
- A strip of periosteum is kept intact when freeing up the insertion to ensure sufficient length of the transferred tendon.
- The PT muscle is freed up proximally to improve excursion.
- The PT muscle and tendon is then passed subcutaneously around the radial border of the forearm.
- The tendon is inserted into the ECRB just distal to the musculotendinous junction through a second incision if needed (**TECH FIG 5**).
- The transfer is secured with PT in maximum tension and the wrist in 45 degrees of extension.

Flexor Digitorum Superficialis Transfer for Multiple Extensor Disruption

- A transverse incision is made in the distal palm to expose the long and ring superficialis tendons.
- The flexor digitorum superficialis (FDS) tendons to III and IV in the distal palm are divided proximal to the chiasma.

- A longitudinal incision is made on the volar-radial mid-forearm and the interosseous membrane is exposed.
- The two tendons are then delivered into the proximal wound.
- Two openings are excised from the interosseous membrane, large enough to pass the muscle bellies through to minimize adhesions.

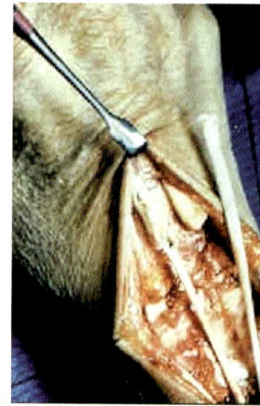

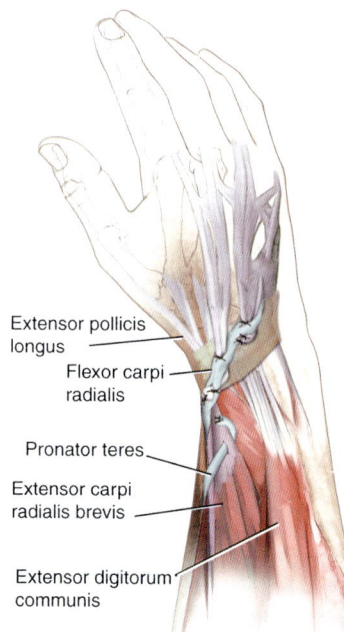

TECH FIG 5 • FCR to EDC and pronator teres to extensor carpi radialis brevis tendon transfer.

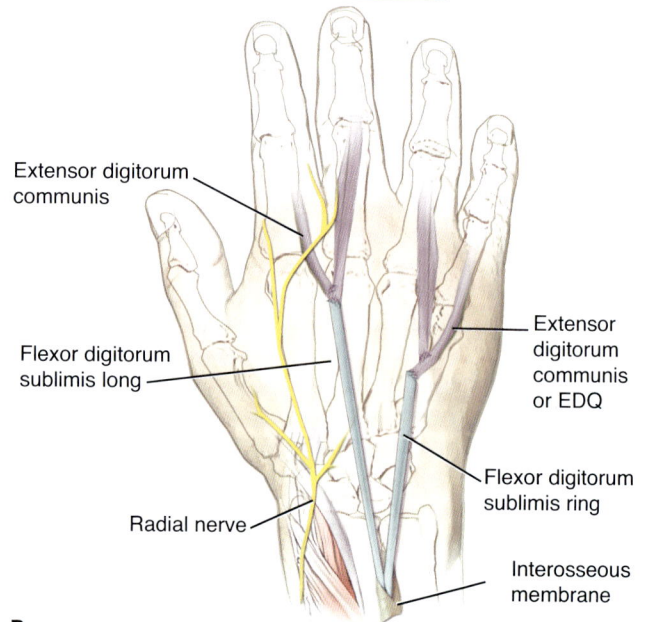

TECH FIG 6 • **A.** Flexor digitorum superficialis (FDS) III and IV transferred to reconstruct segmental injuries of extensor digitorum communis (EDC) II, III, IV, and V. **B.** FDS III and IV to EDC II–V tendon transfers. The FDS is transferred through a rent created in the interosseous membrane.

- A J-shaped incision is made on the dorsum of the distal forearm and the tendons are passed through the interosseous membrane.
- The FDS III is routed radially, and the FDS IV is routed ulnarly to the profundus muscle mass.

- The FDS III is interwoven into the tendons of the EIP and EDC II and III (**TECH FIG 6**).
- The FDS IV is interwoven into EDC IV and V.
- Tension is set with the FDS under maximum tension, the wrist in 20 degrees of extension, and the fingers and thumb held in a fist.

STAGED RECONSTRUCTION WITH SILICONE RODS

- In patients with loss of soft tissue over the dorsum of the hand and forearm, appropriate soft tissue coverage is obtained first.
- At the time of coverage, the proposed path of the tendon transfer or graft is preserved with the use of a silicone tendon rod.

- Once maturation of soft tissue has occurred, the appropriate tendon transfer or graft may be performed 2 to 3 months after silicone rod placement (**TECH FIG 7**).

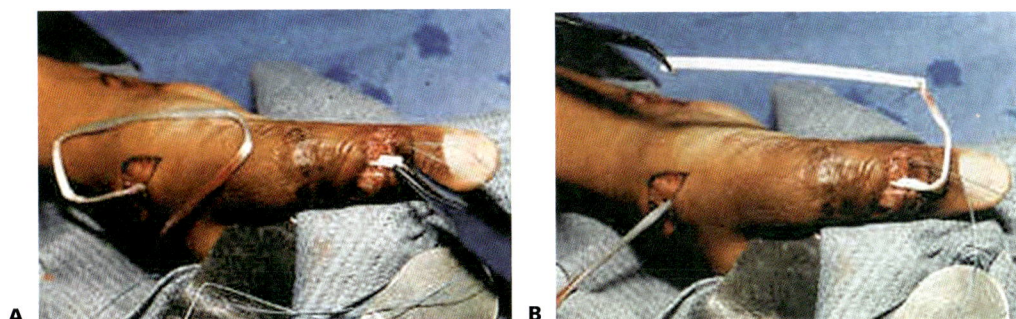

TECH FIG 7 • A. Silastic spacer (tendon rod) used to create adhesion-free bed. **B.** Silastic spacer replaced by tendon graft after soft tissue healing and remodeling.

PEARLS AND PITFALLS

Preoperative issues	• In patients with severe soft tissue compromise, skeletal stabilization is obtained first, followed by soft tissue coverage. Reconstruction of the extensor mechanism is addressed later. • Joint contractures should be addressed before surgery.
Selection of transfer	• The type of transfer performed depends on the tendon to be reconstructed and on surgeon preference. We generally prefer using the FCR.

POSTOPERATIVE CARE

- Initial splinting should immobilize the wrist in about 30 degrees of extension, the MP joints in about 15 degrees of flexion, and the IP joints in full extension.
- If transferred tendons originate proximal to the elbow, the elbow should be immobilized in 90 degrees of flexion with appropriate forearm rotation.
- The thumb IP and MP joints should be immobilized in full extension.
- After 4 weeks, active range of motion is started under the supervision of a certified hand therapist and with a protective splint. Active-assisted and passive range of motion follows 2 weeks later.

OUTCOMES

- Staged extensor tendon reconstruction using a silicone implant followed by tendon grafting for restoration of PIP joint extension was reported to have good results in six fingers with severe dorsal soft tissue injuries, improving hand function in all cases.[1]

COMPLICATIONS

- Extrinsic tightness
- Intrinsic tightness
- Rupture
- Donor deficits
- Joint stiffness

REFERENCES

1. Adams BD. Staged extensor tendon reconstruction in the finger. J Hand Surg Am 1997;22:833–837.
2. Al-Rachid M, Theivendran K, Craigen MAC. Delayed ruptures of the extensor tendon secondary to the use of volar locking compression played for distal radius fractures. J Bone Joint Surg Br 2006;88B: 1610–1612.
3. Baratz ME, Schmidt CC, Hughes TB. Extensor tendon injuries. In: Green DP, Hotchkiss RN, Pederson WC, eds. Green's Operative Hand Surgery, 5th ed. Philadelphia: Elsevier Churchill Livingstone, 2005:187–217.
4. Burton RI, Melchior JA. Extensor tendons—late reconstruction. In: Green DP, Hotchkiss RN, Pederson WC, eds. Green's Operative Hand Surgery, 4th ed. New York: Churchill Livingstone, 1999:1988–2021.
5. Newport ML. Extensor tendon injuries in the hand. J Acad Orthop Surg 1997;5:59–66.

TECHNIQUES

Extensor Tendon Centralization Following Traumatic Subluxation at the Metacarpophalangeal Joint

Ross J. Richer, Craig S. Phillips, and Leon S. Benson

DEFINITION

- Instability of the extensor digitorum tendons at the metacarpophalangeal (MCP) joint has been subdivided into two categories: subluxation and dislocation.
  - Subluxation of the extensor digitorum tendons at the MCP joint is defined as lateral displacement of the tendon with its border reaching beyond the midline, but remaining in contact with the condyle during full MCP joint flexion.
  - Dislocation describes the condition in which the extensor tendon is located in the groove between the metacarpal heads.[12]
- Instability of the extensor digitorum tendons at the MCP joint usually occurs in patients with underlying inflammatory conditions (ie, rheumatoid arthritis).
- Traumatic injury to the sagittal bands, particularly the radial sagittal band, can cause instability of the extensor tendon. Although ulnar-sided injuries have been reported, the overwhelming majority of injuries occur to the radial sagittal band.
- Instability of the extensor tendon is relatively rare in nonrheumatoid patients.
- The sagittal bands are sometimes referred to as the "shroud" ligament because of the way they cover, or wrap, the MCP joint.
- Sagittal band injuries are classified as type I, II, or III depending on the degree of extensor tendon instability.[12]

- Traumatic extensor tendon subluxation at the MCP joint level is classified as type II injury; dislocation is type III. These injuries have been given the eponym "boxer's knuckle."[5]
- Not all injuries to the sagittal bands result in extensor tendon subluxation. Clinical examination will identify those patients in which extensor tendon instability has occurred.
- Factors influencing treatment include symptoms and time elapsed since injury.

ANATOMY

- The digital extensor mechanism at the level of the MCP joint consists of the extensor tendon, sagittal bands, and volar plate. The sagittal bands are part of a complex extensor retinacular system that includes the triangular ligament between the lateral bands, the transverse retinacular ligament, and the oblique retinacular ligament at the proximal interphalangeal (PIP) joint level (**FIG 1A**).
- The sagittal bands are dynamic structures that envelop the extensor tendons, centering them over the MCP joint during flexion, preventing bowstringing during hyperextension, and controlling tendon excursion. The sagittal bands insert onto the volar plate overlying the MCP joint (**FIG 1B**).[13]
- The sagittal bands are the primary stabilizers of the extensor digitorum tendons at the MCP joints, and their integrity is essential for normal extensor tendon function.[10,13,15,18]

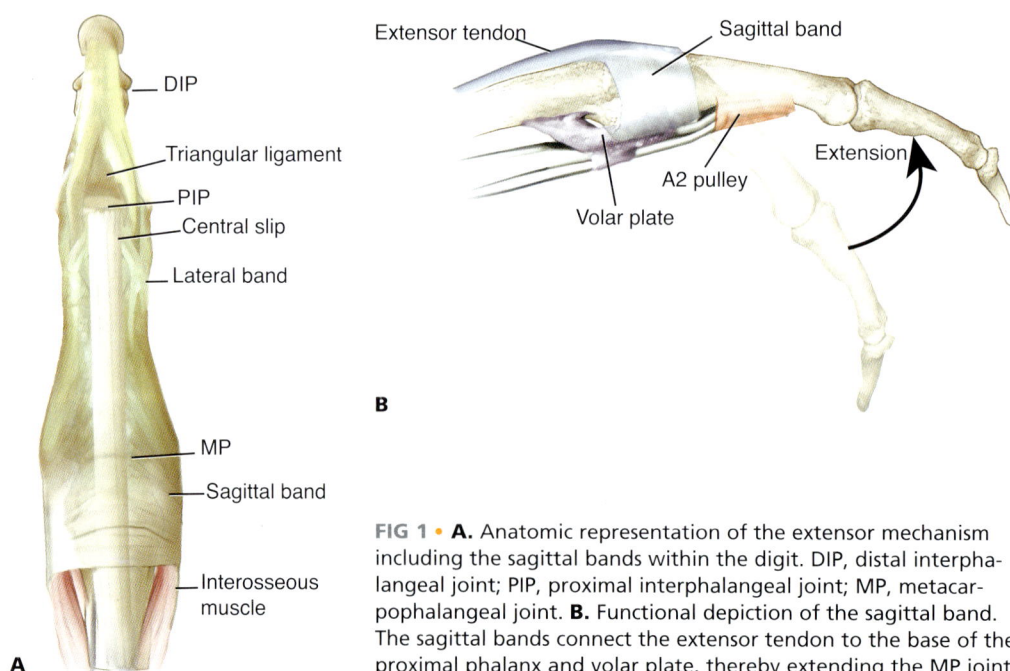

FIG 1 • **A.** Anatomic representation of the extensor mechanism including the sagittal bands within the digit. DIP, distal interphalangeal joint; PIP, proximal interphalangeal joint; MP, metacarpophalangeal joint. **B.** Functional depiction of the sagittal band. The sagittal bands connect the extensor tendon to the base of the proximal phalanx and volar plate, thereby extending the MP joint.

- When the MCP joint is maintained in neutral extension, the sagittal bands are oriented perpendicular to the tendon.
- The sagittal bands are anatomically and physiologically distinct from the deeper collateral ligaments.
- The radial sagittal band is often thinner and longer than its ulnar counterpart.
- The greatest tension on the sagittal bands occurs with wrist and MCP flexion and radioulnar deviation.
- The lumbrical muscles function to flex the MCP joint and extend the interphalangeal (IP) joint through the lateral bands. They originate on the flexor digitorum profundus (FDP) tendon and traverse on the radial aspect of the digit inserting into the extensor expansion.
- The intermetacarpal ligaments are stout ligaments that originate and insert on adjacent metacarpal necks. These ligaments pass dorsal to the lumbrical tendons and volar to the interosseous tendons.

PATHOGENESIS

- The mechanism of sagittal band injury commonly involves a direct blow to a flexed MCP joint.
- Injury may result indirectly from forced flexion or directly from shear forces across the sagittal band.
- Other described mechanisms include forceful deviation of the digit against resistance, usually with the MCP joint extended.
- In open injuries, the sagittal band is usually lacerated.
  - Sometimes laceration of the junctura tendinum can also lead to extensor tendon subluxation.
- Extensor tendon subluxation typically occurs with at least 50% disruption of the proximal sagittal band.[18] The extensor tendon no longer remains centralized over the MCP joint through flexion, but rather subluxates ulnarly.
- It has been suggested that frequency of injury among the digits is related to the cross-sectional diameter of the sagittal band, the extent of distal attachment, and the length of the sagittal band.[6,12,13] The long finger is most commonly injured.
- It has been suggested that traumatic subluxation occurs when there is tearing of both the superficial and deep layers of the sagittal band enveloping the extensor tendon.[7]
- When underlying inflammatory conditions are present, the sagittal bands become attenuated and atrophic, allowing for atraumatic subluxation of the extensor tendons into the troughs (usually ulnar) between metacarpal heads.

NATURAL HISTORY

- Symptoms from acute injuries typically resolve within 3 weeks with appropriate treatment. However, pain can persist for up to 9 months before fully dissipating.[5]
- When sagittal band injuries associated with discomfort, swelling, and subluxation are neglected, patients will experience ongoing symptoms that may worsen over time. The extensor tendon may become fixed in the valley between the metacarpal heads, leading to loss of extension and deviation of the digit. These patients will require surgical treatment for resolution of their symptoms.[6,12,14]

PATIENT HISTORY AND PHYSICAL FINDINGS

- This chapter deals with traumatic subluxation. Treatment protocols for inflammatory subluxation differ and are beyond the scope of this chapter.
- A critical aspect of treatment involves understanding the circumstances surrounding the injury. This information will help identify those at risk for infection in open injuries (eg, clean laceration, fight bite), or the possibility of underlying systemic disease contributing to closed injuries caused by low-energy trauma.
- Shortly after injury soft tissue swelling may obscure the alignment of the tendon over the MCP joint.
- Initially after traumatic injury to the sagittal bands with subsequent extensor tendon instability, symptoms and signs include the following:
  - Localized pain
  - Swelling over the involved MCP joint
  - Limited motion (**FIG 2A**)
  - Limited or deviated MCP joint extension, or both (**FIG 2B**)
  - Weak MCP extension
  - A potentially painful snapping of the tendon over the MCP joint with active flexion (**FIG 2C**)
  - Ulnar deviation deformity and difficulty adducting (or abducting in the case of the index) the affected finger early or late
- Chronic cases of tendon instability often exhibit pain during MCP joint flexion, such as during grip, along with localized tenderness and swelling over the injured sagittal band.[14]
- MCP extension can be actively maintained when the joint is passively placed into extension; however, difficulty is usually encountered when attempts are made to extend the MCP joint from flexion or when flexing the MCP joint from full extension.

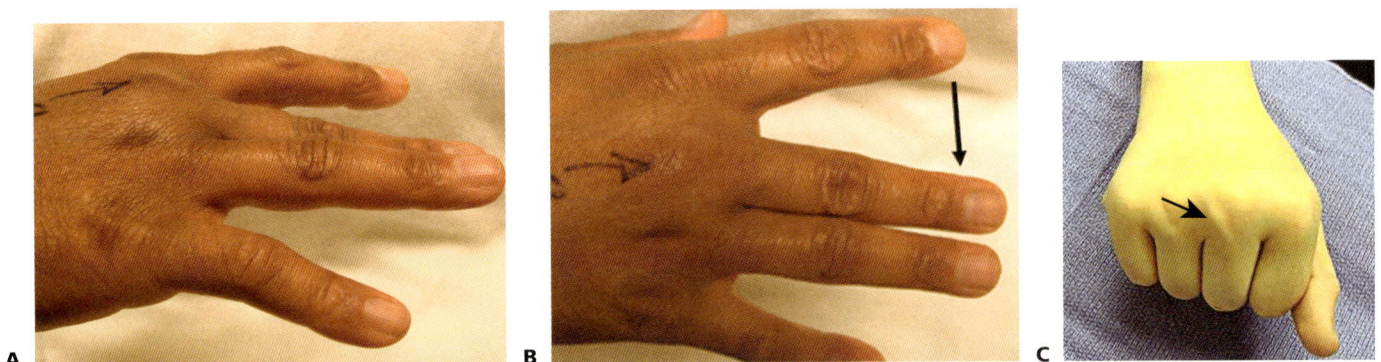

FIG 2 • **A.** Lack of complete active digital extension at the metacarpophalangeal joint associated with a sagittal band disruption. **B.** Ulnar deviation of the long finger associated with a radial sagittal band disruption. **C.** Dislocation of the long finger extensor tendon into the ulnar trough of the fourth web space (*arrow*). (**A,B:** Courtesy of Brian Hartigan.)

■ Methods for examining extensor tendon instability over the MCP joint include the following:

- Assess sagittal bands throughout MP range of motion.
- Assess swelling, open injuries, and so forth. Determine location of pathology.
- Palpate over the MCP joints and in the groove between the metacarpal heads.
  - Sagittal band injuries will exhibit pain with superficial palpation. In contrast, pain associated with collateral ligament injury is usually deeper, within the groove between the metacarpal heads.
- Perform tendon instability examination.
- Ask the patient to flex the MCP joint and wrist. This position places the maximum amount of ulnar force on the extensor tendon at the MCP joint. This will help to determine the amount of instability.
- Pain provocation test: With the distal and proximal IP joints extended and the MCP joint flexed, ask the patient to try to extend the MCP joint against resistance.

IMAGING AND OTHER DIAGNOSTIC STUDIES

■ A standard radiographic series, including posteroanterior, lateral, and oblique views of the MCP joints, is obtained.
  - These views will exclude any mechanical or bony pathology limiting extension of or predisposing the sagittal band to dislocate.
■ A Brewerton view (AP view with dorsal surface of the fingers touching the cassette and the MCP joints flexed 45 degrees) or stress views may be needed to rule out collateral ligament avulsion injury.
■ Magnetic resonance imaging (MRI) has been used with success to identify patients with sagittal band injuries, especially when the physical examination is obscured by swelling and patient discomfort. MRI with the injured MCP joint flexed facilitates the diagnosis.
  - Acute injuries demonstrate morphologic and signal intensity abnormalities within and around the sagittal bands on axial T1- and T2-weighted images, together with poor definition, focal discontinuity, and focal thickening.[4]
■ Dynamic ultrasound has been reported as a useful modality for diagnosis of extensor tendon subluxation when swelling obscures the physical examination.[9]

DIFFERENTIAL DIAGNOSIS

- MCP joint collateral ligament injury
- Trigger finger
- Ulnar nerve palsy
- Congenital sagittal band deficiency
- Extensor digitorum communis tendon rupture
- Radial nerve injury
- Junctura tendinum disruption
- MCP joint arthritis

NONOPERATIVE MANAGEMENT

■ In our experience, most symptomatic patients presenting within 3 weeks of injury with acute sagittal band disruptions and extensor tendon instability can be treated successfully nonoperatively with a splint.[12]
  - Success in the literature varies, however. Studies have shown that 44% to 100% of patients treated conservatively will be asymptomatic at an average of 13.5 months.[2,3,6,12]

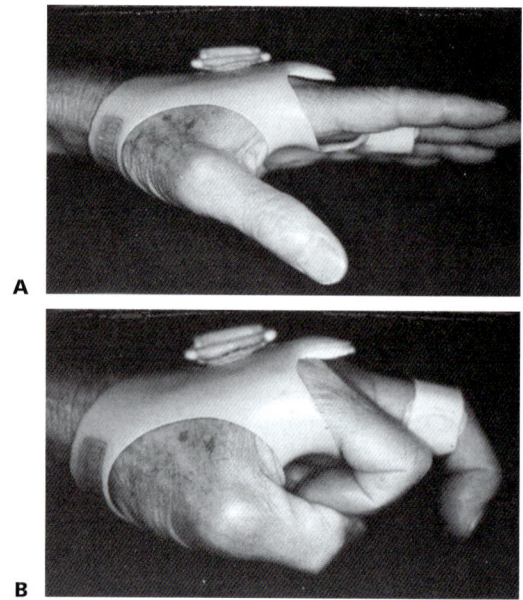

FIG 3 • Typical splint used for the conservative treatment of sagittal band disruption. The interphalangeal joints are free and no more than 30 degrees of metacarpophalangeal joint flexion is allowed.

■ Certainly, except in special circumstances such as the professional athlete, conservative therapy should initially be attempted.
■ Although several different protocols and splints have been described, most share one common objective: maintaining the MCP joint in neutral (full extension) for a period of weeks. In all situations, motion of the IP joint should be accommodated and encouraged.
  - A hand-based, custom orthoplast splint holding the involved digit in 0 to 20 degrees of MCP joint flexion (**FIG 3**) is worn for 4 to 6 weeks, depending on the patient's progress at the 2- and 4-week follow-up visits.
  - After 6 weeks of MCP immobilization in extension, the splint is weaned except for sporting endeavors and other heavy activities, in which case the splint is used for another 2 weeks. Buddy taping can provide long-term support as may be indicated.
  - Active range-of-motion activities are initiated and slowly progressed to gentle passive flexion of the involved MCP joint.
  - Thereafter, unrestricted use of the hand is promoted. It is unusual to need formal hand therapy; however, when excessive joint stiffness is present and radiographs fail to document any bony pathology, a short course of therapy along with modality use can be helpful.
  - If the injury clearly is not responding to immobilization, surgery is recommended.

SURGICAL MANAGEMENT

- Operative indications
  - Patients with painful extensor tendon instability more than 3 weeks after the injury
  - Patients whose injury has failed to respond to nonsurgical management and have persistent, painful tendon instability beyond 6 weeks of conservative care
  - Professional athletes[5] and other high-demand individuals

- When possible, direct repair of the sagittal band should be performed.
    - Although we believe that this is usually not possible more than 8 weeks after injury, Hame and Melone[5] reported on 11 direct repairs at an average of 3.3 months out from time of injury. No patient had prior splinting. All patients were asymptomatic with full recovery of range of motion and return to professional sports at an average of 5 months.
    - Carroll et al[2] reported on five patients who underwent reconstruction after failed conservative management. All patients regained full, asymptomatic range of motion.
- If tissue deficiency or scarring exists, reconstruction as opposed to primary repair will be required.

Preoperative Planning

- With open injuries, the surgeon should determine if the cause was related to a bite. In this situation, MCP joint contamination is likely and surgical irrigation and débridement as well as antibiotic treatment is warranted. When severe contamination is present, delayed sagittal band repair is indicated.
    - Concomitant MCP joint capsular injury is possible. Once surgically exposed, methylene blue injection into the joint, out of the zone of injury, can help to reveal any rents in the MCP joint capsule. These defects should be débrided with subsequent irrigation of the joint. Afterward, no capsular repair is necessary.[5]
- The surgeon should be prepared to perform either a repair or a reconstruction.
- Local anesthesia with sedation is preferred, but regional or general anesthesia is acceptable.

Positioning

- The patient is placed supine on the operating table with the affected hand outstretched onto a hand table.
- A tourniquet is applied to the arm and inflated to the appropriate pressure before starting the procedure.

EXPOSURE

- A curvilinear incision is placed dorsally over the ulnar aspect of the affected MCP joint.
    - This is used for primary sagittal band repair.
- A longitudinal incision is centered dorsally over the affected MCP joint.
    - This is used for reconstructive cases requiring greater exposure.
- Sensory branches of the radial or ulnar nerves, or both, are identified and protected.

- The extensor tendon is exposed, the tear identified, and scar tissue débrided.
- The MCP capsule, which is deep to the extensor tendon, is usually left undisturbed; however, when MCP joint pathology needs to be addressed, the capsule may be incised.

PRIMARY REPAIR

- The sagittal band disruption is identified and the extensor tendon centralized (**TECH FIG 1A,B**).
- Excess tissue is excised from the area between the torn sagittal band and the common extensor tendon.

- The sagittal fibers are then repaired using 4-0 or 5-0 nonabsorbable suture (Ethibond). The knots are buried where possible.
    - The repair is performed with the joint in 60 to 70 degrees of flexion to avoid tension on the repair and stiffness of the joint.
- The joint is flexed and extended to ensure midline stability (**TECH FIG 1C–E**).
- The wound is closed with interrupted 4-0 nylon sutures.

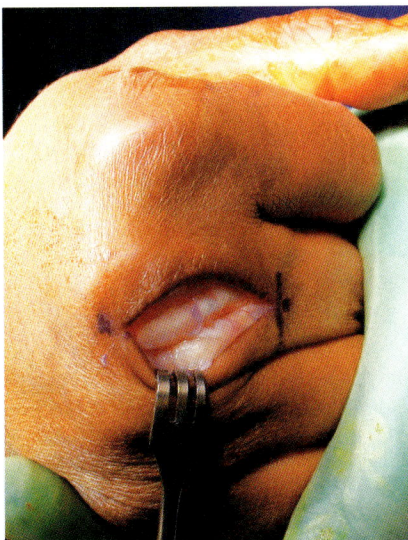

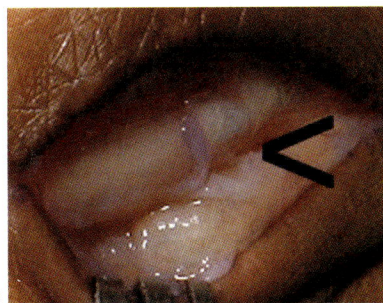

TECH FIG 1 • A. Traumatic extensor tendon dislocation (ulnar) over the metacarpophalangeal (MCP) joint (*arrowhead*) with the MCP joint extended. **B.** Extensor tendon subluxation over the MCP joint with the joint flexed. *(continued)*

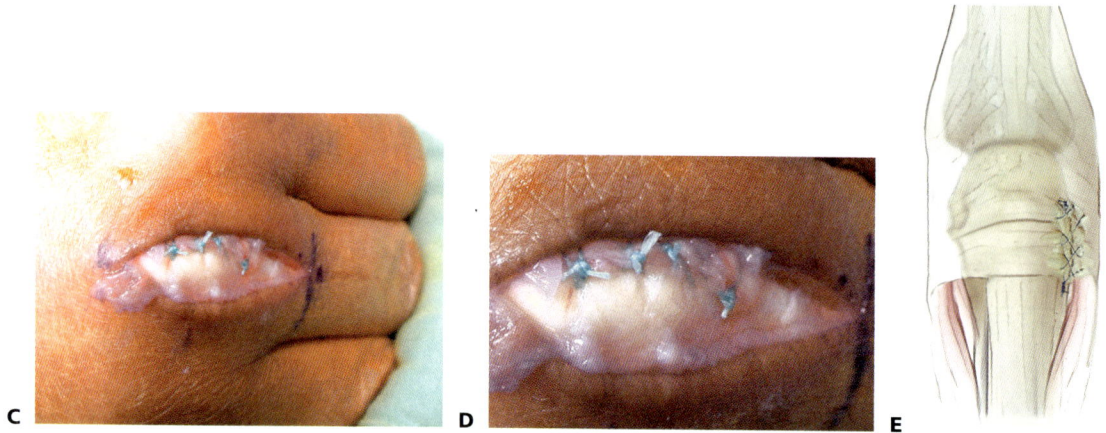

TECH FIG 1 • *(continued)* **C.** Primary repair of the sagittal band with the MCP joint extended. **D.** Primary sagittal band repair with the MCP joint flexed. The extensor tendon remains centralized dorsally with flexion. **E.** Primary repair of the deficient sagittal band. (**A–D:** Courtesy of Brian Hartigan.)

RECONSTRUCTION WITH EXTENSOR TENDON SLIP (CARROLL/KILGORE)[2,8] (AUTHORS' PREFERRED TECHNIQUE)

- Release of the ulnar sagittal band may be necessary to mobilize the scarred tendon dorsally and radially (**TECH FIG 2A,B**).
- A distally based radial or ulnar slip of extensor tendon (about one third) is fashioned and routed deep to the intact extensor tendon (**TECH FIG 2C**).
- In a distal-to-proximal direction, the tendon graft is then looped around the radial collateral ligament (if subluxed ulnarly) (**TECH FIG 2D**).
- Once proper tension is determined, the slip is then sutured back to the main tendon with interrupted, nonabsorbable suture or woven through the tendon in a Pulvertaft fashion (**TECH FIG 2E,F**).
  - As with all reconstruction techniques, tension is determined by taking the joint through a full range of motion and documenting stability dorsally.
- The wound is closed with interrupted 4-0 nylon sutures.

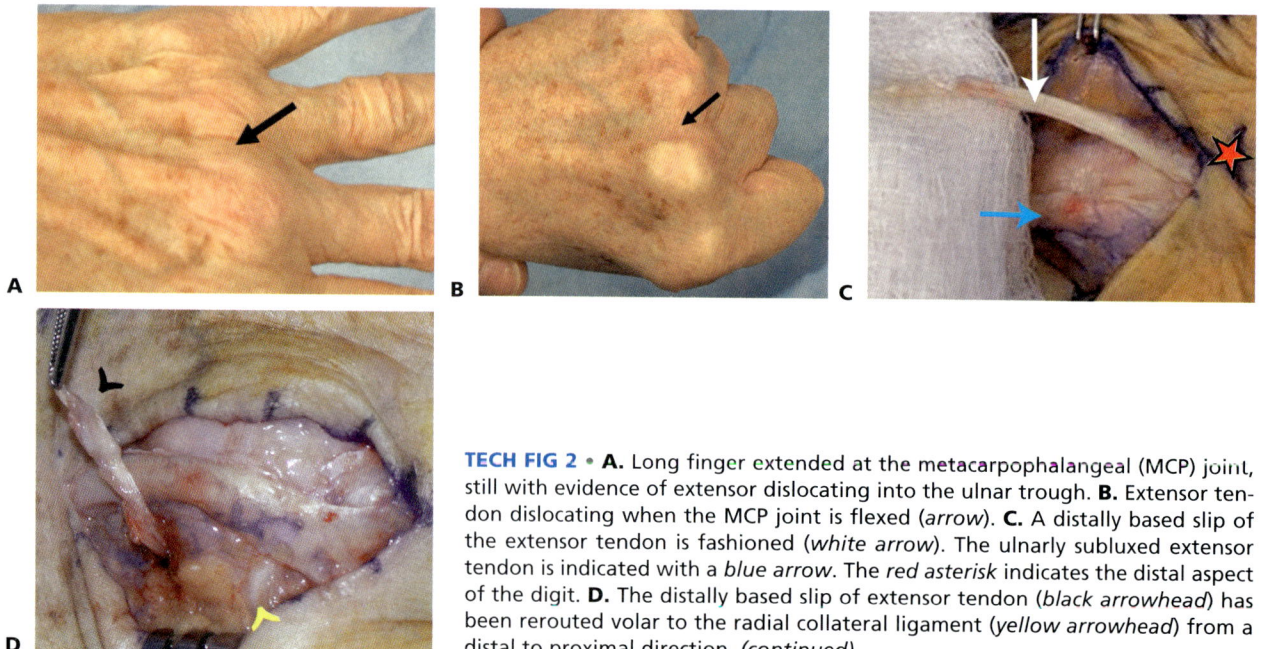

TECH FIG 2 • A. Long finger extended at the metacarpophalangeal (MCP) joint, still with evidence of extensor dislocating into the ulnar trough. **B.** Extensor tendon dislocating when the MCP joint is flexed (*arrow*). **C.** A distally based slip of the extensor tendon is fashioned (*white arrow*). The ulnarly subluxed extensor tendon is indicated with a *blue arrow*. The *red asterisk* indicates the distal aspect of the digit. **D.** The distally based slip of extensor tendon (*black arrowhead*) has been rerouted volar to the radial collateral ligament (*yellow arrowhead*) from a distal to proximal direction. *(continued)*

TECHNIQUES

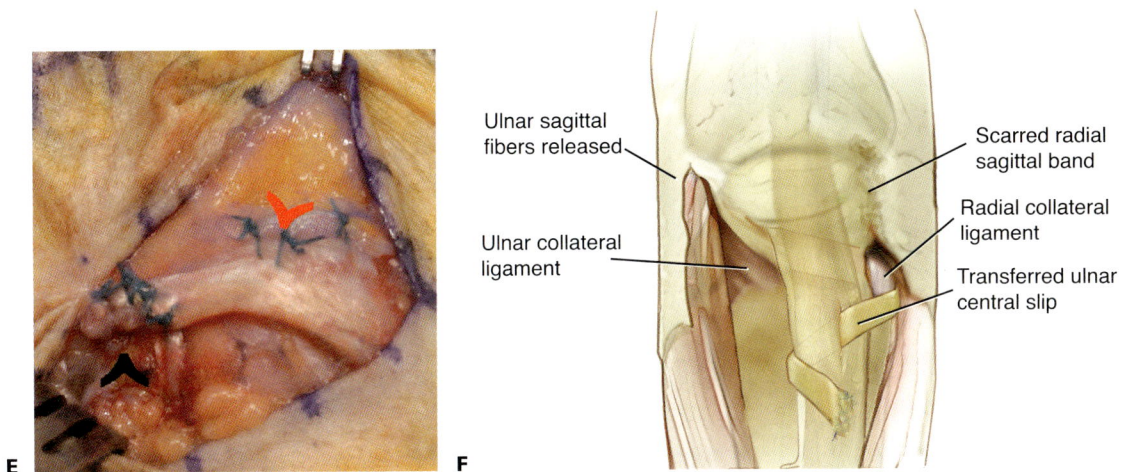

TECH FIG 2 • *(continued)* **E.** The distally based slip of extensor tendon has been secured to the extensor tendon proximal to the MCP joint (*black arrowhead*). The remaining ulnar sagittal band was repaired to prevent radial subluxation of the extensor tendon (*red arrowhead*). **F.** Reconstruction of the sagittal band using a distally based radial slip of extensor tendon wrapped around the radial collateral ligament (RCL) and reattached to the extensor tendon (with a weave).

DYNAMIC LUMBRICAL MUSCLE TRANSFER (SEGALMAN[16])

- The lumbrical muscle is identified on the radial side of the joint and mobilized (**TECH FIG 3A,B**).
- Begin proximally by separating the lumbrical muscle from the more dorsal interossei.
- Once the lumbrical muscle is separated, continue distally to identify its tendinous insertion.
- The lumbrical tendon is harvested just proximal to its insertion into the lateral band (**TECH FIG 3C**).
- With the extensor tendon reduced, an isometric point in the extensor tendon must be identified. This is achieved

by gently ranging the finger or asking the patient to flex. Once it is identified, a small longitudinal slit is made and the lumbrical tendon is passed through from volar to dorsal (**TECH FIG 3D**).

- Tension is set appropriately while gently ranging the finger to confirm the absence of subluxation. The tendon is sutured back to itself using interrupted, nonabsorbable suture.
- The wound is closed with interrupted 4-0 nylon sutures.

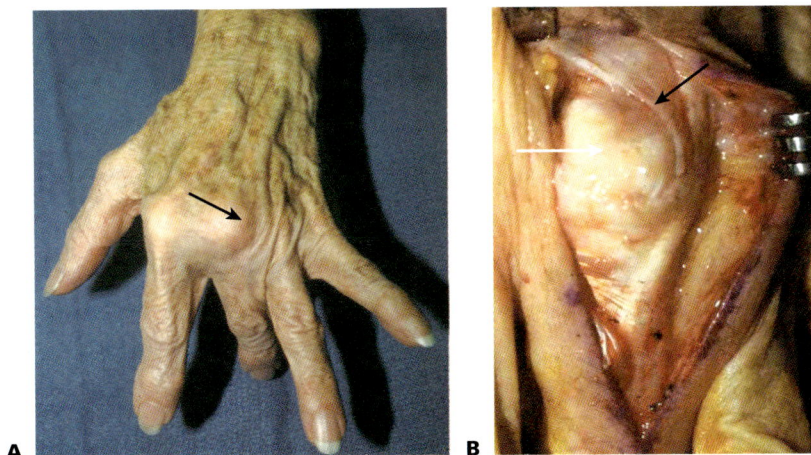

TECH FIG 3 • Technique using the lumbrical muscle for dynamic extensor tendon stabilization. **A.** Ulnar dislocation of the extensor tendon over the long finger metacarpophalangeal (MCP) joint (*arrow*). **B.** Surgical exposure identifying the extensor dislocation (*black arrow*) with a large chronic defect in the radial sagittal band (*white arrow*). *(continued)*

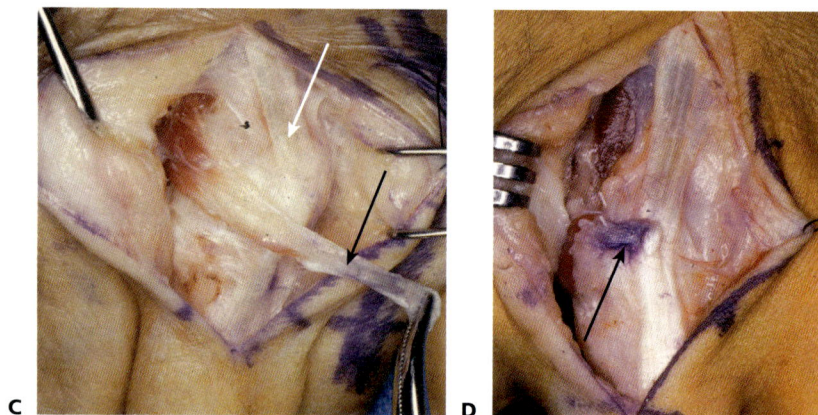

TECH FIG 3 • *(continued)* **C.** The lumbrical muscle–tendon unit is isolated and mobilized for transfer (*black arrow*). The extensor tendon is indicated by the *white arrow*. **D.** The lumbrical tendon is woven into the extensor tendon (*arrow*), now stabilizing the extensor tendon during MCP motion. (Courtesy of Keith Segalman, MD.)

SAGITTAL BAND RECONSTRUCTION TO THE DEEP TRANSVERSE INTERMETACARPAL LIGAMENT (WATSON)

- A 4-cm, distally based slip of extensor tendon consisting of no more than one-third the tendon width is harvested starting proximal to the MCP joint on the affected side (**TECH FIG 4A**).
- This segment of tendon is then passed through a small slit in the remaining tendon at the level of the deep transverse metacarpal ligament to prevent further propagation of the tendon split.

- The segment is then passed around or through the deep transverse intermetacarpal ligament using a curved clamp (**TECH FIG 4B**).
- The free end of the tendon graft is then woven through and sutured to the remaining extensor tendon once it has been centralized and properly tensioned using nonabsorbable suture (**TECH FIG 4C**).
- Wounds are closed with interrupted 4-0 nylon sutures.

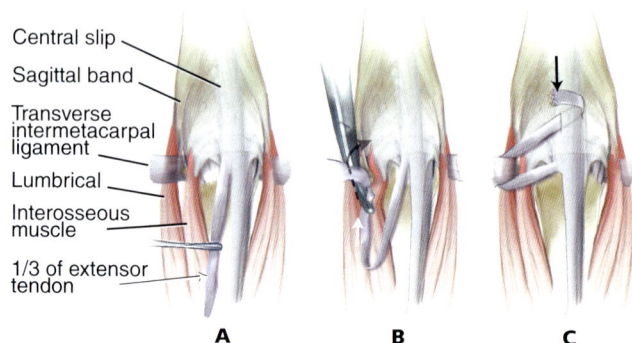

TECH FIG 4 • **A.** A distally based slip of extensor tendon constituting no more than one-third the width of the tendon is harvested. **B.** The slip of extensor tendon is rerouted from proximal to distal, around the deep intermetacarpal ligament. **C.** The tendon slip is then attached to the extensor tendon (usually radially) through a weave distal to the metacarpophalangeal joint.

CENTRALIZATION USING JUNCTURA TENDINUM

- A longitudinal incision is centered dorsally over the affected MCP joint.
- The extensor tendon is identified and held in a centralized position.
- The MCP joint is flexed to reveal the more proximal, ulnar-sided junctura tendinum to the adjacent tendon.
- The junctura tendinum is released from its ulnar-sided insertion into the adjacent tendon.

- It is then brought over to the radial side of the affected finger, still in continuity with the tendon, and sutured to the palmar portion of the remaining sagittal band after correct tension has been set to centralize the tendon.
- Wounds are closed with interrupted 4-0 nylon sutures.

PEARLS AND PITFALLS

Range of motion	■ Preoperatively, ensure that there is good passive range of motion of the MCP joint. ■ Avoid overtensioning and malpositioning of the repair or reconstruction. A reconstruction too proximal will limit extension. A reconstruction too distal will lead to recurrent subluxation.
Anesthesia	■ Local anesthesia will enable the patient to actively flex the MCP joint during the procedure, allowing the surgeon to intraoperatively assess centralization after the repair or reconstruction.
MCP joint capsule	■ Identify and débride rents in the MCP joint capsule. Repair is unnecessary.[5] Also be aware of any injury to the junctura tendinum; this should be repaired.
MCP flexion	■ Range the MCP joint once the tendon is exposed, both before and after repair or reconstruction. The repair or reconstruction should be performed with the MCP joint in 60 to 70 degrees of flexion.
Additional releases	■ Sometimes the sagittal band, as well as the junctura tendinum, on the uninjured side will require release to centralize the tendon.

POSTOPERATIVE CARE

■ Wounds are sterily dressed immediately after the procedure and a splint is applied.

  ■ A volar and dorsal splint is used with the wrist slightly extended, the MCP joints at 0 to 30 degrees flexion, and the IP joints extended.

■ On postoperative day 5, the patient is seen in the office. Sutures are removed and a short-arm cast is applied with the wrist slightly extended, the MCP joints at 0 to 30 degrees of extension, and the IP joints free.

  ■ Sometimes, in the compliant elderly patient, we favor a hand-based splint fabricated to include the MCP joints in 30 degrees of flexion and the IP joints free.

■ Several postoperative protocols have been described for nondynamic reconstructions.

  ■ Inoue and Yukihisa[6] placed the involved finger in a plaster cast for 3 weeks with the MCP joint in neutral or slightly flexed, allowing active IP joint motion.

  ■ Carroll et al[2] splinted the MCP joint neutral for 6 weeks. At 2 weeks after surgery they began PIP joint range of motion, and at 6 weeks active range of motion at the MCP was initiated.

  ■ Watson et al[17] used a splint and Kirschner wire to immobilize the MCP joint at 15 to 20 degrees of flexion for 3 weeks.

  ■ Hame and Melone[5] used cast immobilization of the MCP joint in 60 to 70 degrees of flexion for 6 weeks, with active flexion, but not extension, allowed.

■ For dynamic transfers, the patient is immobilized for 4 weeks in a short-arm cast with the wrist in neutral, MCP joints in extension, and the PIP joints free. Active motion is begun 4 weeks after surgery and strengthening at 6 weeks. Therapy is then continued for 6 to 8 weeks.

OUTCOMES

■ Rayan et al[13] treated three type II injuries nonoperatively with 3 weeks of splinting the MCP joint at 0 degrees of extension, followed by 2 to 3 weeks of protected range of motion out of the splint three times a day, with a final 4 weeks of buddy splinting. They reported full range of MCP joint motion and no tenderness or pain with resisted digital abduction in all three patients. However, one patient did experience residual painless subluxation.

■ Carroll et al[2] treated nine subluxed extensor tendons. Four were treated nonoperatively with 6 weeks of splinting the MCP joint in 0 degrees of extension, followed by range-of-motion therapy. Five were treated operatively using a slip of extensor tendon looped around the collateral ligament. After splinting and therapy, all patients were pain-free with full extension and active flexion to 90 degrees or more. There were no recurrences of symptoms in either group and no complications in the surgical group.

■ Watson et al[17] described 16 patients treated operatively with a slip of extensor tendon looped through the deep transverse metacarpal ligament. They reported an average MCP joint flexion of 90 degrees postoperatively, with no subluxation of the tendon. All patients were pain-free. There were no complications and no need for further surgery.

■ Hame and Melone[5] reported on eight professional athletes who underwent immediate repair of sagittal band injuries with subluxation of the extensor tendon. There were 11 injured fingers in total. Seven of the 11 had capsular injuries; they were all débrided but not repaired. Each athlete demonstrated full range of motion postoperatively and all returned to professional sport at 5 months on average. No additional intervention was necessary and there were no complications.

COMPLICATIONS

■ Complications are rare. Most series in the literature do not report any complications.

■ With nonoperative therapy, possible complications include joint stiffness, skin irritation from splinting, and failure of treatment.

■ With operative therapy, possible complications include infection, joint stiffness, injury to neurovascular structures, and failure of treatment with recurrent subluxation or dislocation either in a radial or ulnar direction.

REFERENCES

1. Araki S, Ohtani T, Tanaka T. Acute dislocation of the extensor digitorum communis tendon at the metacarpophalangeal joint. J Bone Joint Surg Am 1987;69A:616–619.
2. Carroll C, Moore JR, Weiland AJ. Posttraumatic ulnar subluxation of the extensor tendons: a reconstructive technique. J Hand Surg Am 1987;12A:227–231.

3. Catalano LW, Gupta S, Ragland R, et al. Closed treatment of non-rheumatoid extensor tendon dislocations at the metacarpophalangeal joint. J Hand Surg Am 2006;31A:242–245.

4. Drape JL, Dubert T, Silbermann P, et al. Acute trauma of the extensor hood of the metacarpophalangeal joint: MR imaging evaluation. Radiology 1994;192:469–476.

5. Hame S, Melone C. Boxer's knuckle in the professional athlete. Am J Sports Med 2000;28:879–882.

6. Inoue G, Yukihisa T. Dislocation of the extensor tendons over the metacarpophalangeal joints. J Hand Surg Am 1996;21A:464–469.

7. Ishizuki M. Traumatic and spontaneous dislocation of extensor tendon of the long finger. J Hand Surg Am 1990;15A:967–972.

8. Kilgore ES, Graham WP, Newmeyer WL, et al. Correction of ulnar subluxation of the extensor communis. Hand 1975;7:272–274.

9. Lopez-Ben R, Lee DH, Nicolodi DJ. Boxer knuckle (injury of the extensor hood with extensor tendon subluxation): diagnosis with dynamic US: report of three cases. Radiology 2003;228:642–646.

10. Milford LW Jr. Retaining Ligaments of the Digit of the Hand. Philadelphia: WB Saunders, 1968:26–27.

11. Pfirrmann CWA, Theumann NH, Botte MJ, et al. MRI Imaging of the metacarpophalangeal joints of the fingers. Radiology 2002;222:447–452.

12. Rayan GM, Murray D. Classification and treatment of closed sagittal band injuries. J Hand Surg Am 1994;19A:590–594.

13. Rayan GM, Murray D, Chung KW, et al. The extensor retinacular system at the metacarpophalangeal joint: an anatomical and histological study. J Hand Surg Br 1997;22B:585–590.

14. Saldana MJ, McGuire RA. Chronic painful subluxation of the metacarpophalangeal joint extensor tendons. J Hand Surg Am 1986;11A:420–423.

15. Scheweitzer T, Rayan G. The terminal tendon of the digital extensor mechanism, part I: anatomic study. J Hand Surg Am 2004;29A:898–902.

16. Segalman KA. Dynamic lumbrical muscle transfer for correction of posttraumatic extensor tendon subluxation. Tech Hand Up Ext Surg 2006;10:107–113.

17. Watson HK, Weinzweig J, Guidera PM. Sagittal band reconstruction. J Hand Surg Am 1997;22A:452–456.

18. Young CM, Rayan GM. The sagittal band: anatomic and biomechanical study. J Hand Surg Am 2000;25A:1107–1113.

Chapter 60

Flexor and Extensor Tenosynovectomy

Jay T. Bridgeman and Sanjiv Naidu

DEFINITION

- Synovium lines the joint spaces and tendon sheaths.
  - It secretes lubricant (synovial fluid) needed for tendon gliding and reduces friction in synovial joint motion.
- Tendons may be both extra- and intrasynovial.
- Flexor tendons in the carpal tunnel have the added feature of subsynovial connective tissue, which can become inflamed.
- Tenosynovitis is inflammation of the tendon sheath in extrasynovial tendons, and inflammation of the synovial lining in intrasynovial tendons.[3]

ANATOMY

- The extensor tendons lie under the dorsal retinaculum in six separate compartments. These may be divided into the extensor tendon zones. The portion of the extensor tendon that lies under the dorsal retinaculum is lined with a synovial sheath (**FIG 1A**).
- The first extensor tendons originate as outcropper muscles from the distal third of the forearm and cross over the second extensor compartment tendons—the extensor carpi radialis longus (ECRL) and the extensor carpi radialis brevis—distally at the level of the wrist about 4 cm proximal to the radial styloid.
- The extensor pollicis longus (EPL) in the third extensor compartment makes an acute angle at the Lister's tubercle at the level of the wrist.
- The fourth extensor compartment tendons—the extensor digitorum communis and the extensor indicis proprius—lie under a broad retinaculum. The deep branch of the posterior interosseous nerve courses deep to the fourth extensor compartment.
- The extensor digitorum quinti in the fifth extensor compartment often is the only tendon to motor the small finger metacarpophalangeal (MCP) joint in the act of extension.
- The extensor carpi ulnaris (ECU) tendon in the sixth compartment lies in a fibro-osseous tunnel and is intimately held in the ulnar groove by a subsheath that is critical for distal radioulnar joint stability.
- The wrist flexor tendons—the flexor carpi radialis (FCR), the palmaris longus, and the flexor carpi ulnaris—are extrasynovial tendons.
  - The FCR passes through a tight fibro-osseous tunnel in the trapezium before inserting on the base of the second metacarpal (**FIG 1B,C**).
- The digital flexor tendons lie under the transverse carpal ligament in the carpal tunnel. Unlike digital extensor tendons, flexor tendons are almost entirely intrasynovial.
- The flexor tendons in the digits lie in a fibro-osseous canal formed by the annular and cruciate ligaments.[2]

PATHOGENESIS

- Rheumatoid arthritis is a disease of synovial tissue that can lead to inflammatory tensosynovitis.
  - Flexor and extensor tenosynovitis is most commonly a sequlae of rheumatoid arthritis.
- Rheumatoid arthritis causes formation of hypertrophic synovium in the joint spaces, thereby destabilizing joints. The hypertrophic synovium invades the tendon sheaths and synovial lining of all tendons.[3]

NATURAL HISTORY

- Inflammatory tenosynovitis usually is painless and can be the first sign of rheumatoid arthritis.
- The dorsal and volar wrist, as well as the volar digits, are most commonly affected.

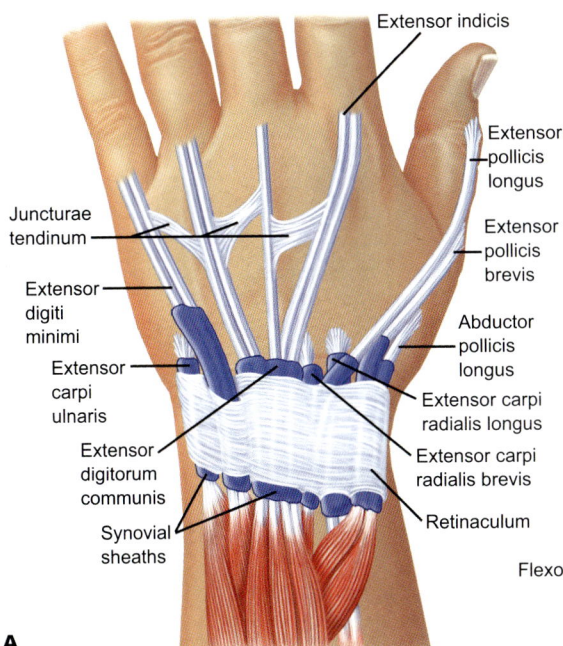

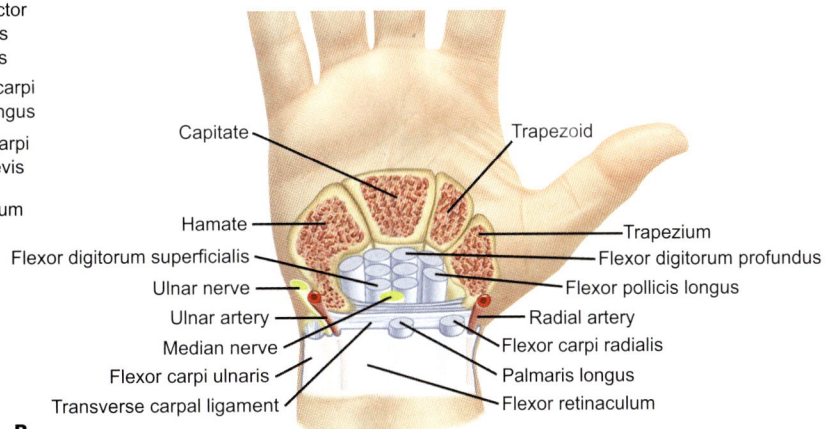

FIG 1 • A. Extensor compartments of the hand.
B. Flexor tendons. (*continued*)

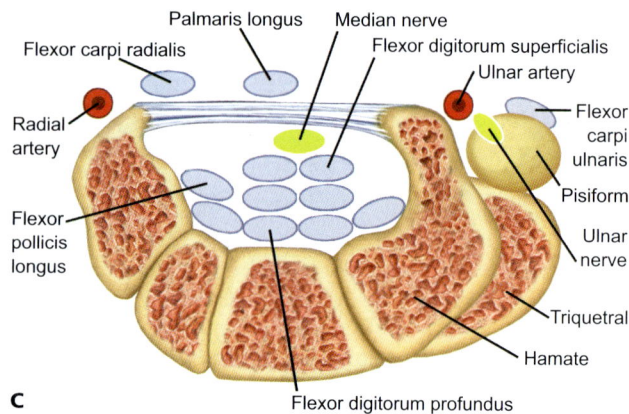

FIG 1 • (*continued*) **C.** Carpal tunnel.

- The synovial tissue proliferates in the tendon sheath and eventually may invade the tendon.
- The end result is weakening and rupture of the tendon.[3]

PATIENT HISTORY AND PHYSICAL FINDINGS

- Tenosynovitis of the first extensor compartment reveals thickening of the extensor pollicis brevis and abductor pollicis longus tendon sheaths at the radial styloid.
  - This thickening can produce a positive Finkelstein's test: ulnar wrist abduction of a hand in a fist position, causing pain along the first extensor compartment.
- Second compartment extensor tenosynovitis presents with painless swelling of the dorsum of the wrist 4 cm proximal to the radial styloid. There is focal tenderness to palpation with swelling and positive Tinel sign of the sensory branch of the radial nerve.
- Third extensor compartment tenosynovitis usually presents with rupture of the EPL tendon.
  - This results in inability to raise the thumb when the hand is placed flat on a table.
- Fourth extensor compartment tenosynovitis presents with focal swelling in extensor zone 7 along with multiple tendon ruptures (**FIG 2**).
- Fifth extensor compartment tenosynovitis usually is accompanied by dorsal distal ulna instability and tendon rupture.
- Sixth extensor compartment tenosynovitis is manifested as ECU instability in addition to significant intrasynovial inflammation at the level of the ulnar styloid.
- Pain at the wrist indicates that the radiocarpal or radioulnar joint is affected.
- Flexor tenosynovitis at the wrist can cause median nerve compression in the carpal tunnel, as well as decreased active and passive range of motion of the fingers.
- Flexor tenosynovitis of the digits can cause triggering.[2]
- The flexor tendon that most commonly ruptures due to rheumatoid arthritis is the flexor pollicis longus. This is termed the Mannerfelt lesion and results in loss of thumb interphalangeal joint flexion.
- The following examinations, all of which may detect weakness or rupture, are graded on a scale of 0 to 5:
  - First dorsal compartment (abductor pollicis longus and extensor pollicis brevis): abduct the thumb radially.

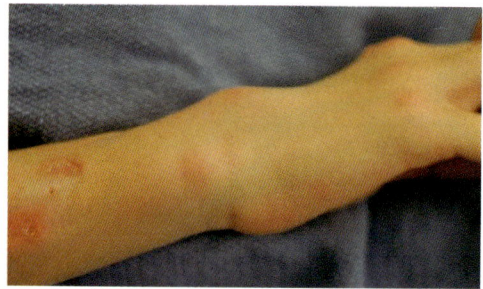

FIG 2 • Dorsal swelling secondary to extensor tenosynovitis.

- Second extensor compartment (extensor carpi radialis longus and extensor carpi radialis brevis): extend and radially deviate the wrist.
- Third extensor compartment (EPL): with the hand flat on table surface, extend the thumb.
- Fourth extensor compartment
  - Extensor digitorum communis: extend the fingers at the MCP joints.
  - Extensor indicis proprius: extend index finger at the MCP joint with other fingers flexed.
- Fifth extensor compartment (extensor digitorum quinti): extend the small finger at the MCP joints with other fingers flexed.
- Sixth extensor compartment (ECU): extend and ulnarly deviate the wrist.
- FCR: wrist flexion and radial deviation
- Flexor carpi ulnaris: wrist flexion and ulnar deviation
- Flexor digitorum superficialis: flex the proximal interphalangeal joint while holding adjacent fingers extended.
- Flexor digitorum profundus: block the proximal interphalangeal joint in extension and flex the distal interphalangeal joint.
- Flexor pollicis longus: flex the thumb interphalangeal joint against resistance.

IMAGING AND OTHER DIAGNOSTIC STUDIES

- MRI may be useful to evaluate low-grade tenosynovitis and mechanical dysfunction of the fibro-osseous digital pulley system.
- In general, flexor or extensor tenosynovitis is a clinical diagnosis made on physical findings.

DIFFERENTIAL DIAGNOSIS

- Extensor tendon weakness
  - Rupture of sagittal bands
  - Posterior interosseous nerve palsy
  - Intrinsic muscle tightness or contracture
  - Extensor tendon rupture
- Flexor tendon weakness
  - Flexor tendon rupture
- Nerve palsy (median nerve, anterior interosseous nerve, ulnar nerve)

NONOPERATIVE MANAGEMENT

- Medical control of rheumatoid arthritis
- Splinting
- Cortisone injections are only *very* rarely indicated due to the risk of tendon rupture.

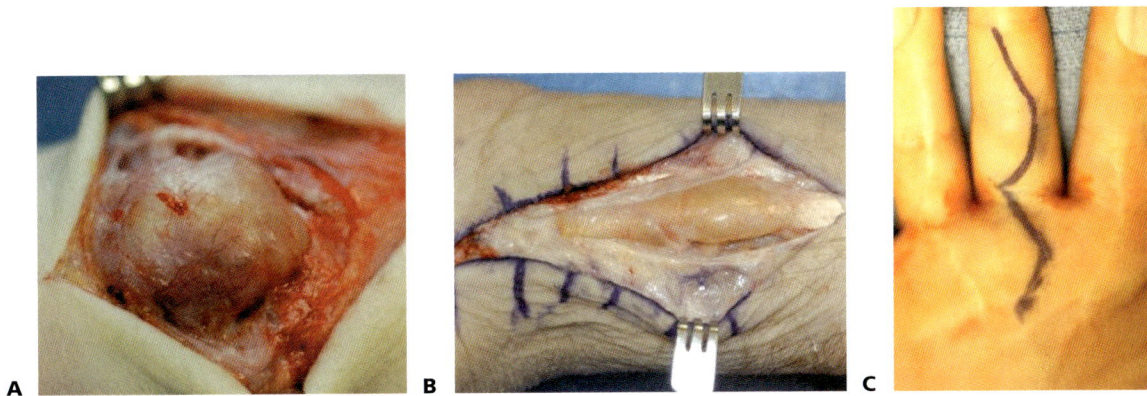

FIG 3 • **A.** Dorsal extensor tenosynovitis. **B.** Volar flexor tenosynovitis. **C.** Zigzag (Brunner) approach to digital flexor tendons.

SURGICAL MANAGEMENT

- Tenosynovectomy is indicated if no improvement is observed after 4 to 6 months of adequate medical treatment or if tendon ruptures are detected.[3]
- Flexor tenosynovectomy is relatively indicated if active digit motion becomes worse than passive motion.[3]

Preoperative Planning

- Consider withholding rheumatoid medications (eg, methotrexate, Etanercept, Imuran) 1 week before and 1 week after surgery.[3]

Positioning

- The patient is positioned supine with an armboard.

Approach

- For an extensor tenosynovectomy, the wrist dorsal midline approach is used (**FIG 3A**).
- For a flexor tenosynovectomy, the wrist volar approach to the carpal tunnel is chosen (**FIG 3B**).
- A digital tenosynovectomy is done using the volar zigzag approach to the digits (**FIG 3C**).

EXTENSOR TENOSYNOVECTOMY

- A straight longitudinal incision is made.
- Full-thickness skin flaps are created, exposing the extensor retinaculum (**TECH FIG 1A**).
- A straight longitudinal incision is made of the extensor retinaculum over the third compartment.
- Transverse incisions are made over the proximal and distal borders of the retinaculum, creating a radially based flap.
- Divide the vertical septum, opening each extensor compartment.
- Remove hypetrophic synovium from each tendon sheath with a rongeur or by sharp dissection (**TECH FIG 1B**).
- Frayed tendons are repaired with fine interrupted sutures.
- Tendons at risk for rupture are sutured to adjacent tendons.
- If synovitis of the wrist is encountered, wrist synovectomy is performed, and, if possible, the capsule is closed.
- The distal ulna is resected if it is prominent dorsally or if significant distal radioulnar joint arthrosis is noted.
- The retinaculum is passed deep to the extensor tendons and sutured (**TECH FIG 1C,D**).
  - Suturing a portion of the retinaculum over the extensor tendons prevents bowstringing.[2]

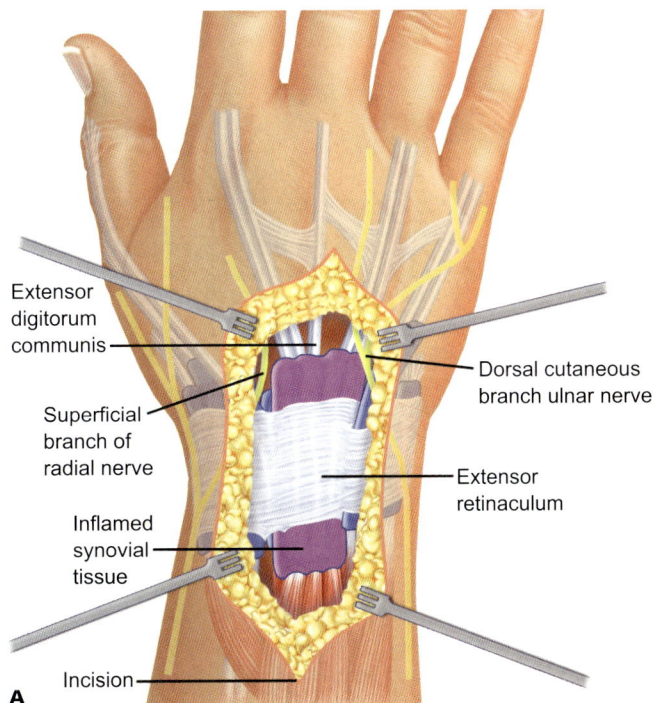

Extensor digitorum communis

Superficial branch of radial nerve

Inflamed synovial tissue

Dorsal cutaneous branch ulnar nerve

Extensor retinaculum

Incision

TECH FIG 1 • A. Dorsal midline approach. (*continued*)

TECHNIQUES

TECHNIQUES

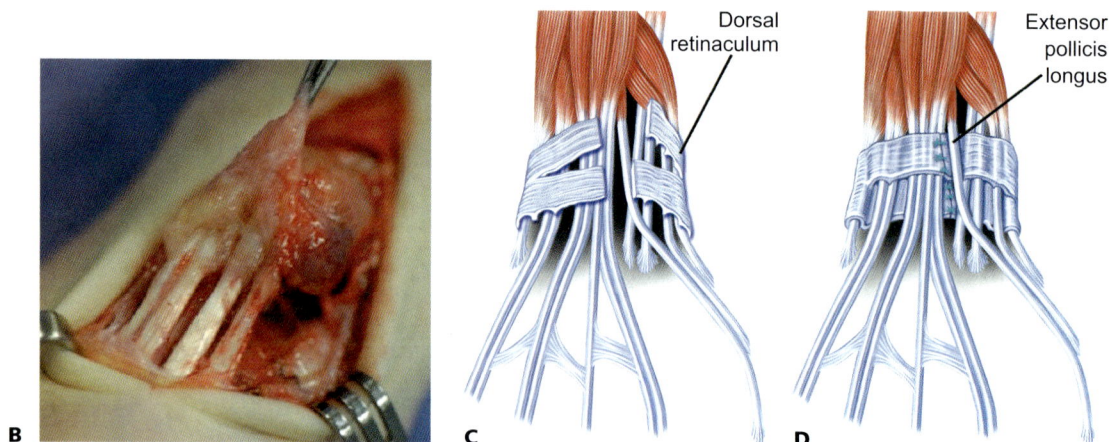

Dorsal retinaculum

Extensor pollicis longus

TECH FIG 1 • (*continued*) **B.** Débridement of dorsal tenosynovitis. **C.** Sharply elevating the dorsal retinaculum. **D.** Closing the dorsal retinaculum.

FLEXOR TENOSYNOVECTOMY

- Use a standard carpal tunnel approach with a mid-palm incision parallel to the thenar crease in line with the long finger.
- Extend the incision proximally 4 cm in a zigzag fashion when crossing the wrist crease.
- Protect the palmar cutaneous branch of the median nerve at the wrist flexion crease.
- Divide the volar antebrachial fascia and protect the median nerve in the forearm.
- Divide the palmar fascia and transverse carpal ligament longitudinally.
- Excise hypertrophic synovium surrounding the flexor tendons (**TECH FIG 2**).
  - A complete synovectomy is not required when the excess synovium involves more than half of the tendon diameter. Synovectomy in this case would lead to loss in function.

- Inspect the floor of the carpal tunnel. Any bony spicules (commonly originating from the scaphoid) are removed with a rongeur.
- Check flexor tendons for decreased excursion, indicating digit tenosynovitis.[2]

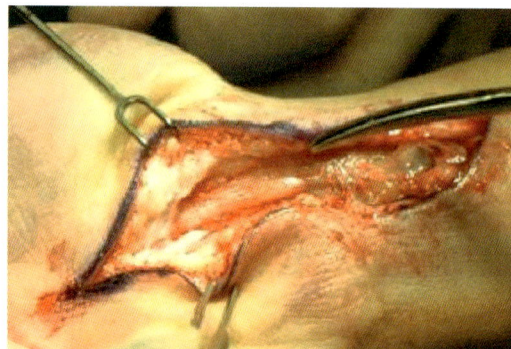

TECH FIG 2 • Carpal tunnel approach to flexor tendons.

DIGITAL FLEXOR TENOSYNOVECTOMY

- Use a volar zigzag incision to explore the flexor tendons in the digit.
  - Extend the incision proximally and distally for more exposure.
- Excise all hypertrophic synovium (**TECH FIG 3**).
- Carefully preserve the annular second and fourth pulleys to prevent bowstringing.
- Excise nodules in the tendon and close defects with fine suture.
- Check tendon excursion for smooth gliding.
- Passive flexion of the finger should equal the flexion obtained when pulling on the tendon (simulating active flexion).
  - If passive and active flexion are not equal, additional synovectomy is required.[2]

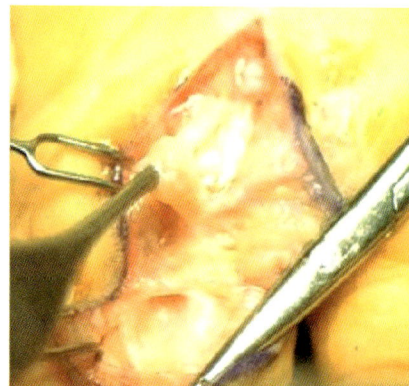

TECH FIG 3 • Débridement of digit flexor tenosynovitis.

PEARLS AND PITFALLS

Indications	▪ Failed adequate medical management for 4–6 months
Extensor tenosynovectomy	▪ Débride radiocarpal synovitis if present. ▪ Resect the distal ulna if prominent or dislocated.
Flexor tenosynovectomy	▪ Débride bony spicules on the carpal tunnel floor (ie, scaphoid).
Digital flexor tenosynovectomy	▪ Preserve annular pulleys to prevent bowstringing. ▪ Passive flexion of the finger should be the same as the flexion observed when the surgeon pulls on the tendon.

POSTOPERATIVE CARE

▪ Splint the wrist in neutral position.
▪ Early (within 48 hours) active and passive digit range of motion exercise is key to maintaining motion.[1]

OUTCOMES

▪ Long-term studies show less than 10% tendon rupture and recurrent tenosynovitis at 5 years.

COMPLICATIONS

▪ Wound dehiscence
▪ Tendon adhesions
▪ Tendon rupture[1]

REFERENCES

1. Brown FE, Brown ML. Long-term results after tenosynovectomy to treat the rheumatoid hand. J Hand Surg Am 1998;13:704–708.
2. Feldon P, Terrano A, Nalebuff E, et al: Rheumatoid arthritis and other connective tissue disease. In Green DP, Hotchkiss R, Pederson WC, eds. Green's Operative Hand Surgery, ed 5. New York: Churchill Livingstone, 2005:2060–2068.
3. Millender L, Nalebuff E, Albin R, et al. Dorsal tenosynovectomy and tendon transfer in the rheumatoid hand. J Bone Joint Surg Am 1974;56A:601–610.
4. Ryu J, Patel S. Rheumatoid arthritis: Soft tissue reconstruction. In: Trumble T, ed: Hand Surgery Update 3. Rosemont, IL: American Society for Surgery of the Hand, 2003:535–536.
5. Thirupathi R, Ferlic D, Clayton M. Dorsal wrist synovectomy in rheumatoid arthritis: A long-term study. J Hand Surg Am 1983;8:848–856.

Chapter 61

Tendon Transfers Used for Treatment of Rheumatoid Disorders

John D. Lubahn and D. Patrick Williams

DEFINITION

- Rheumatoid arthritis is a progressive disease that, if uncontrolled, leads to joint destruction, secondary to progressive synovitis, ligament instability, joint dislocation or subluxation, and attrition of adjacent tendons either by bony erosion or direct tenosynovial infiltration.
- When tendon rupture occurs on the dorsum of the hand or wrist, patients cannot extend their fingers and have difficulty grasping objects.
- The most common tendon ruptures on the dorsum of the hand begin on the ulnar side and usually are a result of subluxation of the distal radial ulnar joint (DRUJ), the so-called Vaughan-Jackson or caput ulnae syndrome.[6]
- On the volar side of the wrist, the most common tendons to rupture are the flexor pollicis longus and the adjacent flexor digitorum profundus (FDP) tendon to the index finger or possibly the long finger. This is referred to as Mannerfelt syndrome.[3]

ANATOMY

- The extensor tendons of the hand and forearm pass beneath the extensor retinaculum at the wrist. The retinaculum is divided into six separate compartments lined by tenosynovium, which can become involved in the pathology of rheumatoid arthritis.
  - The first compartment contains the tendons of the abductor pollicis longus and the extensor pollicis brevis. The former tendon often contains multiple slips, which can contribute to limited space in its respective compartment and secondary De Quervain tenosynovitis.
  - The second compartment consists of the extensor carpi radialis longus (ECRL) and brevis (ECRB), the former tendon inserting at the base of the index metacarpal and the latter at the base of the long finger.
  - The third compartment contains only the tendon of the extensor pollicis longus (EPL), which passes around the tubercle of Lister at a fairly sharp angle. While frequently involved in tendon ruptures in rheumatoid arthritis, the EPL may also present as an isolated tendon rupture after nondisplaced fractures of the distal radius.
  - The fourth compartment contains the extensor indicis proprius (EIP) and the extensor digitorum communis (EDC), sending tendons from the common extensor muscle in the forearm to each of the fingers. The EIP is a separate muscle tendon unit located within the fourth compartment. It can be differentiated by its distal muscle belly.
  - The fifth extensor compartment contains the extensor digiti quinti (EDQ), often consisting of two slips and passing almost directly over the DRUJ.
  - The sixth compartment contains only the extensor carpi ulnaris.
- On the palmar side of the wrist, the flexor pollicis longus is located most radially and passes over the radiocarpal joint adjacent to the trapeziometacarpal joint of the thumb. The flexor pollicis, along with the median nerve and the profundus and sublimis tendons to each digit, passes beneath the deep transverse carpal ligament and represents the contents of the carpal canal.
  - Tenosynovial proliferation can exist within the carpal tunnel, arising from the undersurface of the ligament but more commonly proliferating along the tendons themselves.

PATHOGENESIS

- Tendon rupture on the dorsum of the wrist is usually the result of instability in the DRUJ, leading to secondary subluxation and bony erosion through the capsule of the joint and then the tendon.
  - The tendon initially affected is the EDQ. As the carpus supinates and subluxates volarly, causing the distal ulna to be more dorsal, tendons typically rupture sequentially in an ulnar to radial direction.
  - The tendons may also be compromised by direct infiltration from the tenosynovium.
  - While the ulnar tendons are involved most commonly, it is possible for all of the tendons crossing the dorsum of the wrist to rupture, making reconstruction more difficult.
- On the volar side of the wrist, the flexor pollicis longus may become compromised through erosion by osteophytes and rough bony surfaces at the level of the trapeziometacarpal joint of the thumb or the scaphotrapezial articulation. The adjacent profundus tendon to the index and occasionally the long finger can rupture as well.
- Tendons of the flexor surface of the wrist and forearm are also subject to rupture via direct tenosynovial infiltration, but this is less common.

NATURAL HISTORY

- Before the advent of treatment for rheumatoid arthritis, the natural history was one of relentless progression. The disease would occasionally "burn itself out," however, with the radiocarpal joint subluxing in a volar and radial direction, leading to instability and loss of function.
- Also, before the development and routine use of antitumor necrosis factor drugs, patients were occasionally refractory to nonsteroidal medication, corticosteroids, and stronger anti-inflammatory drugs such as methotrexate. When these drug combinations failed, proliferative tenosynovitis occasionally occurred on the dorsum of the wrist, leading to direct tendon rupture as a result of tenosynovial ingrowth into the tendon and collagen destruction and rupture (**FIG 1**).
- The worst-case scenario is secondary rupture of all of the finger extensors, with subluxation of the extensor carpi ulnaris volar to the axis of wrist motion such that it becomes more of a wrist flexor and ulnar deviator than a wrist extensor. The radial wrist extensors may also rupture; however, in part as a result of the more robust nature of the tendons themselves, they tend to remain intact even with progressive disease.

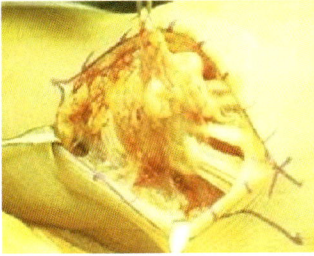

FIG 1 • Exposure of the extensor tendons of the wrist shows proliferative tenosynovitis originating from the tenosynovial lining of the extensor retinaculum. If left unchecked, such proliferative tenosynovitis can contribute to extensor tendon rupture at the level of the wrist.

■ The French Impressionist painter Pierre Auguste Renoir was said to have had such severe rheumatoid arthritis that in his later years he would tape a brush to his hand to paint.

PATIENT HISTORY AND PHYSICAL FINDINGS

■ Patients often note a spontaneous loss of finger motion, but there may be minimal swelling and discomfort. Patients occasionally report a snap or twinge of discomfort as the tendon ruptures.
■ With an extensor tendon rupture, patients cannot actively extend the metacarpophalangeal (MCP) joints of the involved digit.
  ■ In the case of isolated rupture of the extensor digiti quinti, an intact EDC to the small finger may make it difficult to confirm the diagnosis.
  ■ The proximal and distal interphalangeal joints of the finger may be extended through the intrinsics even when the extensors are ruptured.

■ Wrist flexion should result in MCP joint extension through tenodesis if the extensor tendons are intact. When the finger extensors are ruptured, this tenodesis effect is absent (**FIG 2A,B**).
■ On the volar side of the wrist, the examiner should check closely for the possibility of associated tenosynovial proliferation proximal and deep to the transverse carpal ligament.
  ■ Active digital motion may cause palpable crepitance at this level.
■ Such proliferation may result in coexisting carpal tunnel syndrome (CTS). The examiner should question the patient regarding symptoms of CTS and should assess for signs of CTS.
■ The patient should also be examined carefully for active flexion at the distal interphalangeal joints of the index and long fingers as well as the interphalangeal joint of the thumb.
  ■ Absence of flexion should alert the surgeon to the possibility of rupture of the flexor pollicis longus and the FDP to the index and occasionally the long finger.
  ■ These tendons are particularly vulnerable when subluxation and spur formation are present at the trapeziometacarpal or scaphotrapezial joints as well as the volar radiocarpal joint.
  ■ Tendon rupture at this level is referred to as Mannerfelt syndrome (**FIG 2C**) and needs to be differentiated from an anterior interosseous nerve palsy.
    ■ Direct pressure on the flexor pollicis longus muscle in the forearm should lead to passive flexion in the interphalangeal joint of the thumb if the tendon is intact.
    ■ The tenodesis test also is effective for the flexor pollicis longus and profundus and sublimis tendons to the fingers; however, in patients with progressive rheumatoid arthritis, the radiocarpal joint and the interphalangeal joints may become arthritic, making passive motion of the wrist and fingers somewhat more difficult and therefore the test more unreliable.

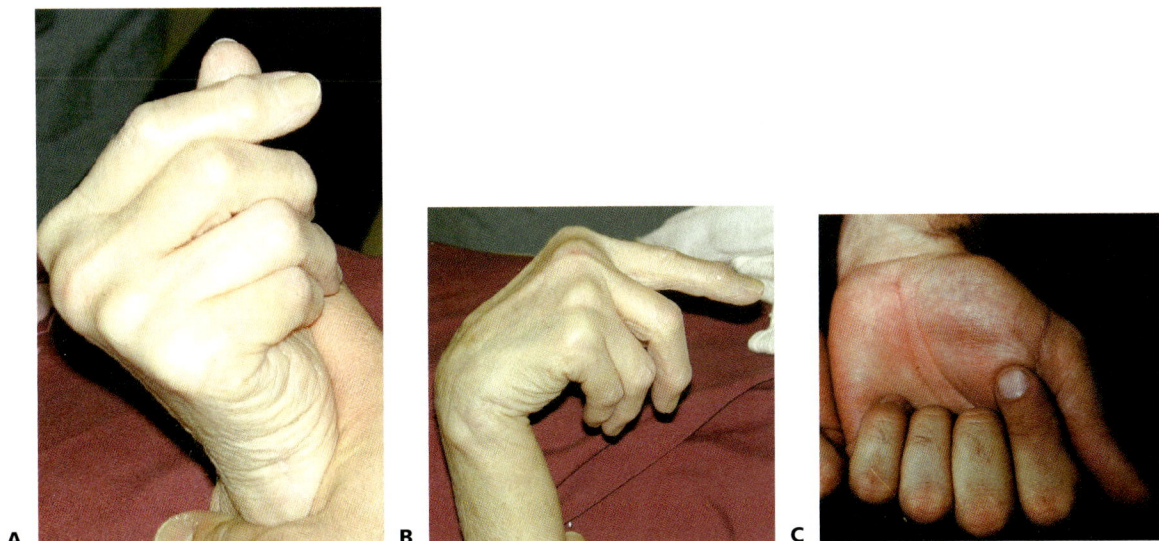

FIG 2 • **A.** Passive wrist extension results in passive finger flexion with intact finger flexors. **B.** Passive wrist flexion should result in passive finger extension when the finger extensor tendons are intact. In this situation, however, those tendons are not intact and passive wrist flexion results in the long, ring, and small extensor fingers remaining in a flexed position. **C.** In a patient with Mannerfelt syndrome, attempted active flexion of the thumb and fingers results in absent flexion of the interphalangeal joint of the thumb and in this situation the distal interphalangeal joint of the index finger. Clinically this is similar to anterior interosseous nerve syndrome and must be distinguished clinically and often by electromyography.

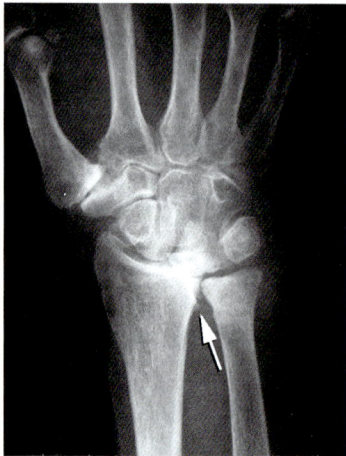

FIG 3 • AP radiograph of the wrist of the patient in Figure 4 shows osteophyte formation in the distal radioulnar joint (*arrow*). (From Lubahn JD, Wolfe TL. Surgical treatment and rehabilitation and tendon ruptures in the rheumatoid hand. In: Mackin EJ, Callahan AD, Skirven TM, et al, eds. Rehabilitation of the Hand and Upper Extremity, ed 5. St. Louis: Mosby, 2002:1598–1607.)

IMAGING AND OTHER DIAGNOSTIC STUDIES

■ AP and lateral radiographs of the hand and wrist should be obtained to look for subtle changes of the DRUJ, such as subluxation or a small osteophyte (**FIG 3**), which may be consistent with the physical findings of tendon rupture (**FIG 4**).
■ Similar attention should be paid to the volar surface of the radiocarpal joint and the trapeziometacarpal joint of the thumb as well as the scaphotrapezial and trapezoidal joints.
  ■ Radiographs may reveal arthrosis and deformity in the digits themselves responsible for motion loss.

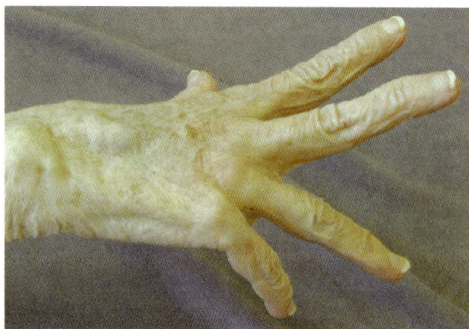

FIG 4 • The clinical consequences of a spur in the distal radioulnar joint: rupture of the extensor digiti quinti and extensor digitorum communis to the ring and small fingers. When the patient attempts to actively extend the fingers, the ring and small finger remain flexed. (From Lubahn JD, Wolfe TL. Surgical treatment and rehabilitation and tendon ruptures in the rheumatoid hand. In: Mackin EJ, Callahan AD, Skirven TM, et al, eds. Rehabilitation of the Hand and Upper Extremity, ed 5. St. Louis: Mosby, 2002:1598–1607.)

■ Radiographs of the cervical spine may reveal subluxation, possibly causing nerve compression and secondary digital motion loss or weakness.
■ CT and MRI are not routinely needed.
■ Electromyography and nerve conduction studies are crucial in the evaluation of the patient with potential tendon ruptures, particularly if tenodesis testing is normal in the face of a loss of active finger extension or flexion.
  ■ Compression of both the anterior interosseous and posterior interosseous nerves can occur in rheumatoid arthritis, usually secondary to ganglion cyst formation at the level of the elbow joint.

DIFFERENTIAL DIAGNOSIS

■ In the case of tendon ruptures on the dorsum of the hand and wrist, the differential diagnosis is primarily with that of posterior interosseous nerve compression or posterior interosseous nerve syndrome.
  ■ Compression of the posterior interosseous branch of the radial nerve, or the radial nerve itself more proximally, needs to be considered as the cause of the patient's inability to extend the fingers. Diagnosis can be suspected by history and clinical examination. Electrophysiologic testing may also prove helpful.
  ■ Cervical disc disease or rheumatoid arthritis of the cervical spine with subluxation or instability may also be the cause for weakness of the finger or wrist extensors, and the cervical spine should also be imaged.
■ With respect to Mannerfelt syndrome, absence of flexion at the interphalangeal joint of the thumb and the distal interphalangeal joints in the index and long fingers should be differentiated from the anterior interosseous nerve syndrome, which when present in rheumatoid arthritis is usually due to a large ganglion originating on the volar surface of the elbow.

NONOPERATIVE MANAGEMENT

■ Nonoperative management probably is more feasible with respect to Mannerfelt syndrome than with the Vaughn-Jackson or caput ulnae syndrome. While the functional deficit is generally greater with loss of finger extensors than loss of active flexion of the interphalangeal joint of the thumb and distal interphalangeal joints of the index and long fingers, some patients may still function remarkably well.
■ Supportive measures in patients who for one reason or another are not deemed suitable surgical candidates may be provided by a certified hand therapist or occupational therapist able to assist the patient with his or her activities of daily living.
■ With median nerve entrapment and compression from the proliferative tenosynovitis at the level of the radiocarpal joint, disability becomes more progressive and nonsurgical treatment more difficult. There may be a role for corticosteroid injection at the level of the radiocarpal joint, and certainly referral to a rheumatologist is crucial for the control and management of the disease before any surgical intervention.
■ In the case of wrist or finger extensor tendon rupture, nonsurgical treatment may be beneficial in terms of resting the radiocarpal joint and interphalangeal joints of the fingers to prevent further tendon rupture by attrition. Splinting the wrist or hand may prove beneficial, particularly if motion in the radiocarpal joint or fingers is painful.

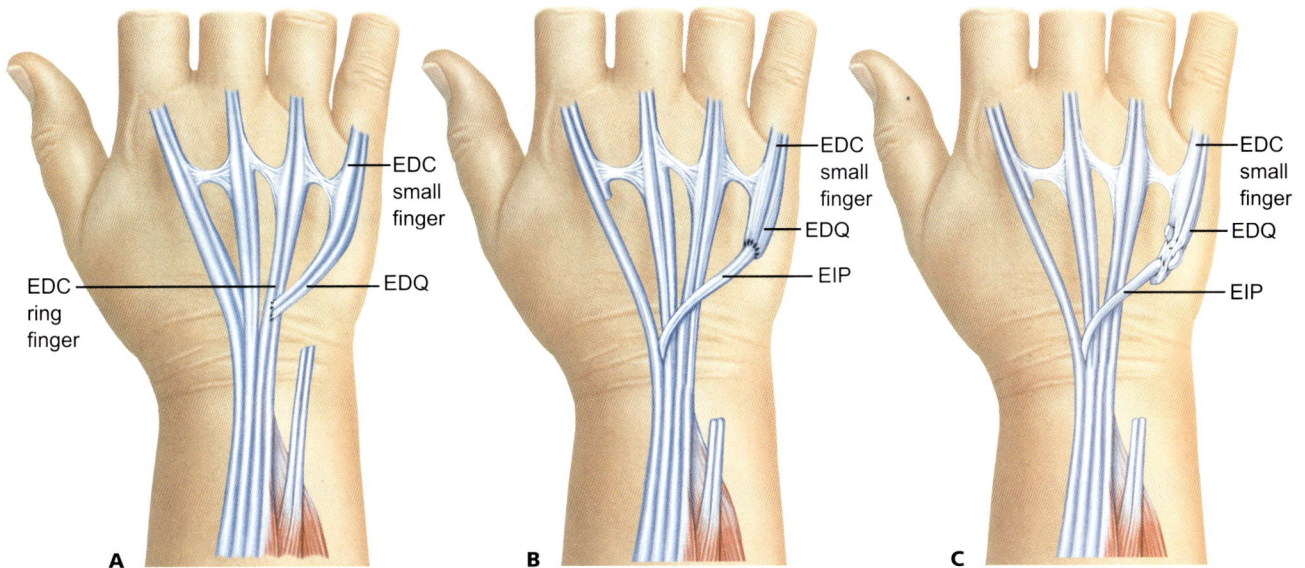

FIG 5 • **A.** When extensor tendon rupture leads to loss of extension in only one digit, such as the small finger, end-to-side transfer of the distal ruptured tendon to the more proximal, adjacent extensor digitorum communis tendon of the ring finger can be performed. **B.** If the ruptured end is distal to the mid-metacarpal region, this transfer may lead to abduction of the small finger metacarpal, and under these circumstances, tendon transfer of the extensor indicis proprius to the distal stump of the extensor digiti quinti is undertaken (depicted here as an end-to-end transfer). **C.** Extensor indicis proprius to extensor digiti quinti, depicted here as a Pulvertaft weave between the distal tendon and the proximal transferred extensor indicis proprius.

SURGICAL MANAGEMENT

Extensor Tendon Rupture

- A variety of tendon transfers are available for reconstruction of single and multiple extensor tendon ruptures.
- It is important for the surgeon to locate the site of tendon rupture, and identify as well as treat the cause.
  - Usually, rupture is secondary to the distal ulna subluxing dorsally through the attenuated fibers of the DRUJ. When subluxation occurs at this level, it erodes through the floor of the fourth and fifth extensor compartments.
  - Tendon reconstruction is therefore not complete unless it involves removal of the dorsal osteophyte by a modified Darrach procedure and coverage of the distal ulna with a flap of extensor retinaculum.
  - When the distal ulna is unstable, the pronator quadratus may be brought dorsal to stabilize the bone.
- Small finger extension loss
  - Single tendon rupture of the EDQ may go unnoticed, particularly if there is a strong EDC to the small finger. Often, however, this common extensor to the small finger is hypoplastic or absent and all that is present is a juctura tendinae from the small finger to the adjacent ring finger. Isolated loss of function in the EDQ is manifest by weakness or lack of extension of the small finger.
  - The distal stump of the ruptured tendon is sewn end to side to the intact ring finger EDC tendon. The risk of this transfer, however, is excessive abduction of the small finger when the distal tendon is short (**FIG 5A**).
  - Alternatively, an EIP transfer may be performed (**FIG 5B,C**).
- Ring and small finger extension loss (Fig 4)
  - In addition to the EDC tendons to the ring and small fingers, the EDQ usually will have ruptured.

- The EIP is transferred to the EDQ.
- The distal ring finger EDC tendon is transferred end to side to the adjacent intact long finger EDC tendon (**FIG 6**).
- Long and ring finger extension loss (**FIG 7A**)
  - Although two fingers are seemingly involved, the EDC tendon to the small finger is usually ruptured as well. The EDQ remains intact.

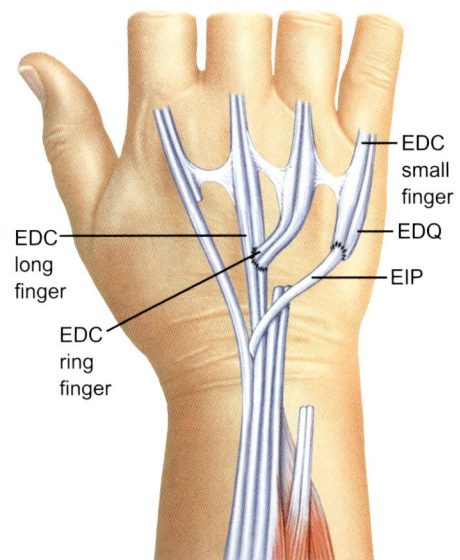

FIG 6 • In cases of double rupture in the ring and small fingers, transfer of the extensor indicis proprius to the distal extensor digiti quinti, with end-to-side transfer of the distal extensor digitorum communis of the ring finger to the adjacent extensor digitorum communis to the long finger, is a standard transfer.

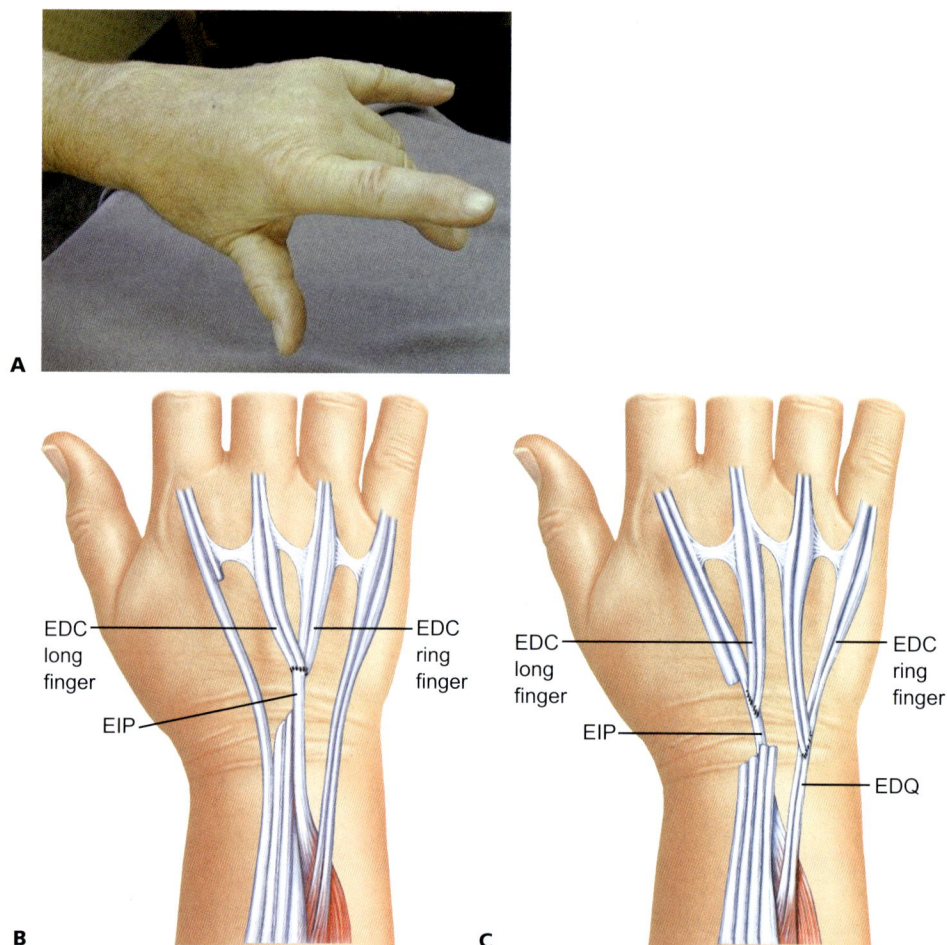

FIG 7 • A. Clinical appearance of a hand with rupture of the extensor digitorum communis (EDC) to the long and ring fingers. (From Lubahn JD, Wolfe TL. Surgical treatment and rehabilitation and tendon ruptures in the rheumatoid hand. In: Mackin EJ, Callahan AD, Skirven TM, et al, eds. Rehabilitation of the Hand and Upper Extremity, ed 5. St. Louis, Mosby, 2002:1598–1607.) **B.** Optional tendon transfer when the EDC to the index finger is intact is transfer of the extensor indicis proprius (EIP) to the distal stumps of the long and ring fingers. **C.** When the EDC to the index finger has been ruptured and EIP transfer is not an option, transfer of the distal EDC of the long finger to the adjacent EIP of the index, and transfer of the distal ring EDC to the adjacent small finger extensor, is shown here. (**B,C** from Williams DP, Lubahn JD. Reconstruction of extensor tendons. Atlas Hand Clin 2005;10:209–222.)

▪ If the index finger EDC tendon is intact, EIP transfer to the long and ring finger EDC tendons is performed (**FIG 7B**).
▪ If the EDC tendon to the index finger has ruptured, end-to-side transfer of the distal tendon of the long finger EDC to the adjacent intact EIP and transfer of the distal tendon of the ring finger EDC to the adjacent intact EDQ may be considered (**FIG 7C**).
▪ Long, ring, and small finger extension loss
  ▪ If the EIP and EDC tendons to the index finger are intact, the EIP can be transferred to the distal stumps of the ring and small finger EDC tendons using end-to-end or end-to-side techniques, depending on the length of the distal stumps.

▪ The EDC to the long finger is transferred end to side to the adjacent intact index EDC tendon (**FIG 8**).
▪ If only the EIP is intact and all remaining tendons on the dorsum of the wrist have ruptured, transfer of the flexor digitorum sublimis (FDS) of the ring finger around the radial or ulnar border of the forearm is the next logical choice.
▪ In patients with partial or complete wrist fusion, or in patients with limited wrist motion, transfer of the ECRL may be considered. Although not "in phase" with the finger extension, the line of pull matches reasonably well.
▪ Index, long, ring, and small finger extension loss
  ▪ The two most common transfers are the FDS around the radial and ulnar sides of the forearm or through the interosseous membrane (**FIG 9A,B**).

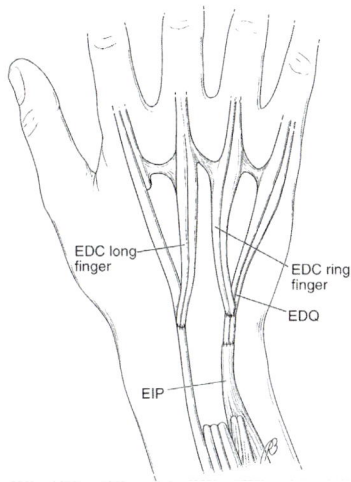

FIG 8 • Rupture of the common extensors to the long, ring, and small fingers with extensor digiti quinti rupture can be treated, as shown here, with transfer of the extensor indicis proprius to the distal stumps of the ring and small finger with distal end-to-side transfer from the extensor digitorum communis to the long finger to the adjacent index extensor digitorum communis.

- Transfer of one of the radial wrist extensors is a suitable alternative (**FIG 9C**).
- Loss of thumb extension
  - EPL rupture is common and often results in minimal loss of function.
    - If diagnosed early, an interposition graft may be used.[2] The palmaris tendon, a strip of the flexor carpi radialis, and a slip of the EDQ are suitable choices.

- Late or chronic ruptures require transfer of the EIP to the distal end of the EPL. The proximal muscle will usually begin to atrophy and become nonfunctional by 6 months after the injury.
- If the EIP is not available, transfer of the FDS from the long or ring finger can be considered. The FDS can be routed through the interosseous membrane or around the radial side of the forearm as described for transfer to restore finger extension.[7]
- Chronic synovitis at the thumb MCP joint may lead to attritional rupture of the dorsal capsule and the extensor pollicis brevis.
  - This boutonnière deformity of the thumb is a type I as described by Nalebuff[4] and Nalebuff and Millender[5] (**FIG 10**).
  - The deformity usually progresses after extensor pollicis brevis rupture. The EPL shifts ulnarward, the collateral ligaments weaken, and the thumb metacarpal becomes abducted radially. The interphalangeal joint hyperextends as a reciprocal response to the MCP joint flexion.
  - Transfer of the EPL to the extensor pollicis brevis and dorsal capsule is performed. Local anesthesia is typically adequate.

Flexor Tendon Rupture

- Tendon transfer for the treatment of flexor tendon disruption in the rheumatoid patient is much less common than for extensor tendon rupture.
- Mannerfelt syndrome should be treated by transfer of the brachioradialis tendon to the flexorpollicis longus.
  - Associated disruption of a FDP tendon is usually treated by transferring the distal stump end to side to the adjacent digit's FDP tendon.

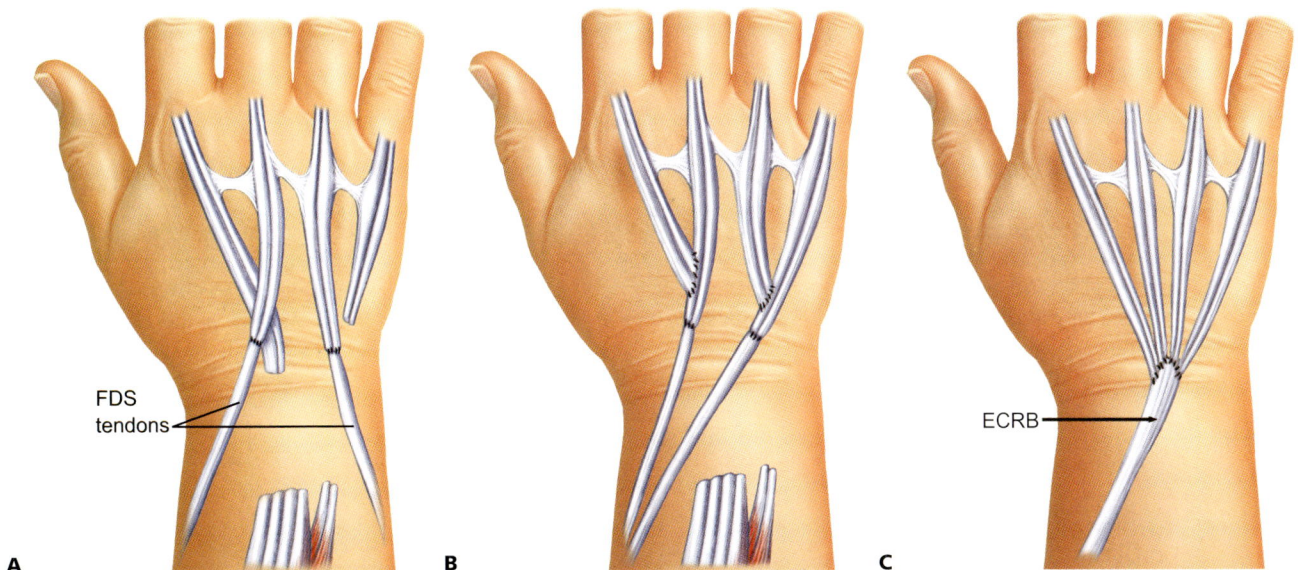

FIG 9 • **A.** Rupture of all four finger extensors may be treated alternatively with transfer of the flexor digitorum superficialis (FDS) to the long and ring fingers, harvested in the distal palm and transferred around the radius and ulna, with the two forearm bones serving as pulleys for the transferred tendon. **B.** Alternatively, both FDS tendons may be transferred around the radial side of the forearm and sutured to the distal stumps of the extensor digitorum communis tendons. **C.** With rupture of all common extensor tendons to the fingers as well as the extensor indicis proprius and the extensor digiti quinti, extension may be restored through transfer of one of the radial wrist extensors. This is ideal when a partial wrist fusion is being planned, as shown.

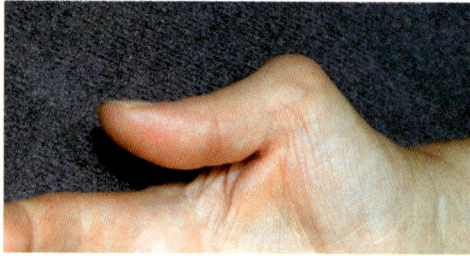

FIG 10 • Extensor pollicis brevis rupture. Boutonnière deformity of the thumb (Nalebuff type I).

Preoperative Planning

- All patients with rheumatoid arthritis require a thorough general physical examination as well as careful evaluation of their cervical spine, including posteroanterior and lateral radiographs, often with flexion and extension views to evaluate cervical spine instability.
- Limited joint mobility is a contraindication to tendon transfer.
  - Brachioradialis tendon transfer to the flexor pollicis longus is an ideal transfer and is likely to yield an excellent result, but only if there is adequate passive motion at the interphalangeal joint and MCP joint as well as the basal joint and the thumb. If these joints are stiff, the brachioradialis might be better saved for other needs as the patient's arthritis progresses.
- The carpus should be examined for stability. In particular, the DRUJ on the ulnar side of the wrist should be checked for dorsal instability and subluxation and the volar, radial side of the wrist for palmar subluxation.

- Planning needs to take into consideration the results of preoperative radiographs of the wrist, hand, and cervical spine as well as electromyographic tests.
  - If the findings on electromyography are negative and the surgeon is certain that tendon rupture is responsible for the lack of active finger motion, plans should be made to transfer expendable existing tendons to those that have ruptured. In the case of multiple extensor tendon ruptures to the fingers, the ECRL and the FDS from the long and ring fingers are two of the most common donor tendons.
  - If radiographs reveal significant joint destruction and instability, appropriate arthrodesis or arthroplasty should be considered rather than tendon transfer.
- Instruments and suture needed for tendon weaves and repairs are extremely valuable.
  - Sharp tendon passers facilitate a Pulvertaft weave. When sharp, pointed tendon passers are not available, a no. 11 blade can be passed through the tendon followed by a hemostat to grasp the knife and guide the hemostat through the tendon. The hemostat then grasps the transferred tendon, weaving it through the recipient tendon.
  - 3-0 and 4-0 braided nonabsorbable sutures on appropriate needles are required for tendon repairs.

Positioning

- Most tendon transfers are done with the patient in the supine position on the operating table.
- The contralateral arm or lower extremity may be sterilely draped in the event that a tendon graft is needed.
- Anesthesia may be either general or an axillary block, depending on the patient's preference and the stability of the cervical spine.

TECHNIQUES

EXTENSOR INDICIS PROPRIUS TENDON TRANSFER

- Isolate the EIP through a 1-cm longitudinal or curvilinear incision on the dorsal ulnar aspect of the index MCP joint.
  - The EIP is usually the ulnar tendon of the two located dorsal to the MCP joint of the index finger.
- Make a second 2- to 3-cm incision over the mid-dorsal wrist (unless a dorsal wrist incision has already been made for another procedure).
- Incise the retinaculum overlying the fourth extensor compartment and locate the EIP tendon ulnar and deep to the EDC tendons.
  - The EIP muscle belly is the most distal in the fourth extensor compartment.
- Once the identity of the EIP is confirmed proximally and distally, suture the index EIP and EDC tendons together as far distal as possible using 4-0 nonabsorbable, usually braided nylon, suture.
  - Invert or bury the knot to void prominence under thin rheumatoid skin.

- Incise the EIP just proximal to the stitch, then free any tendinous interconnections over the dorsum of the hand.
- Use a blunt instrument or Penrose drain to pull the EIP tendon into the wrist wound.
- Transfer the EIP to the exposed recipient tendon using a Pulvertaft weave.
  - A single weave, while usually sufficient for smaller tendons, should be supplemented with an additional one or two weaves if possible. This will significantly strengthen the repair site.
  - If insufficient distal tendon is present for a weave, either an end-to-end repair or a weave in which the transferred tendon is brought through a transverse incision in the distal recipient stump from volar to dorsal is an effective option.
- Skin incisions are closed and a splint is applied.

FLEXOR DIGITORUM SUPERFICIALIS TENDON TRANSFER

- In the case of rupture of all of the extensor tendons on the dorsum of the wrist, and when wrist motion is still intact, tendon transfer of the FDS, as suggested by Boyes,[1] is a reliable method to restore finger extension.

- The FDS and FDP to each of the donor fingers must be intact.
- Pre-existing swan-neck deformity in a donor digit may worsen after harvest of the FDS tendon.
- Long and ring FDS tendons are used most often.

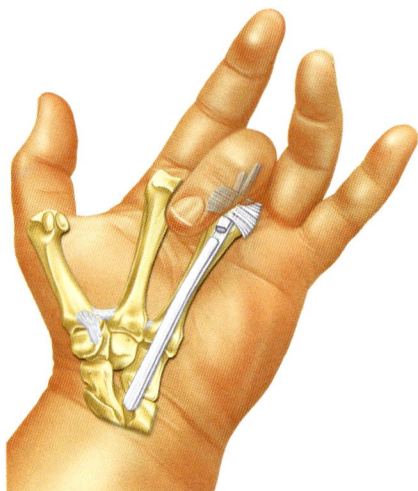

TECH FIG 1 • Transfer of the flexor digitorum sublimis to the long and ring fingers. The distal incision in the palm is used to isolate the sublimis tendon as far distal as possible by flexing the finger so that the chiasm of Camper is visible in the wound. The tendon is divided just proximal to the chiasm, leaving enough distal tendon to contribute to the stability of the proximal interphalangeal joint in extension and thereby avoiding a secondary instability of that joint and possible swan-neck deformity.

- Make a transverse incision in the distal palm and divide the FDS tendon proximal to the bifurcation, leaving the chiasm of Camper intact to provide proximal interphalangeal stability and help prevent development of a swan-neck deformity (**TECH FIG 1**).
  - Splinting the proximal interphalangeal joint in flexion postoperatively will also help to minimize the risk of developing a swan-neck deformity.
- Isolate the FDS tendon proximally through a Henry-type incision in the distal forearm and atraumatically deliver it into that incision.
- Pass the tendon deep to the median nerve, the FDP, the flexor carpi radialis, the flexor pollicis longus, and the radial artery and the nerve at the wrist with a blunt tendon passer, hemostat, or Kelly clamp.
  - The transferred tendon sits on the radius using the bone as a pulley to enhance the effectiveness of the transfer.

- If the FDS to the ring finger is too short to pass around the radial side of the wrist, an alternative route is beneath the FDP, flexor carpi ulnaris, and ulnar artery and nerve around the ulnar side of the forearm using the ulna as the pulley.
  - In general the radial path is preferred to minimize ulnar deviation of the digits.
- Alternatively, the FDS tendon is passed volar to dorsal though an incision in the interosseous membrane just proximal to the DRUJ.
  - The membrane functions as the pulley.
- Weave the smaller distal tendon stumps through the larger transferred FDS tendon in the manner described by Pulvertaft.
  - Adjust tension such that with slight wrist flexion, the fingers are maintained in full extension.
- Immobilize the hand and wrist with the wrist in 40 degrees of extension and the fingers flexed until tension is noted at the suture line (**TECH FIG 2**).
  - Ideally, this should be close to the "safe position" with slight MCP joint flexion and relative interphalangeal joint extension.

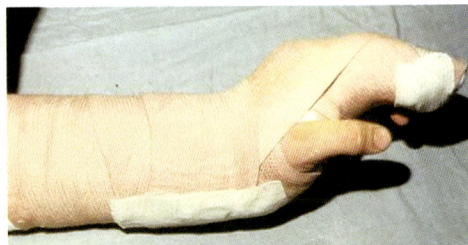

TECH FIG 2 • The ideal splint for transfer to the extensor tendons of the finger immobilizes the wrist in the so-called safe position. With wrist extension, tension at the site of transfer is usually minimal. Finger flexion at the metacarpophalangeal joint is ideal to prevent scarring of the collateral ligaments and secondary loss of finger flexion. The amount of flexion possible is judged in the operating room by passive flexion of the finger until a minimum amount of tension is seen at the repair site. (From Williams DP, Lubahn JD. Reconstruction of extensor tendons. Atlas Hand Clin 2005;10:209–222.)

EXTENSOR CARPI RADIALIS LONGUS OR BREVIS TRANSFER

- When all of the finger extensors have ruptured, wrist motion is severely limited (ie, after a partial or complete wrist fusion), and the radiocarpal joint is stable, the wrist extensors become potential muscles for use as transfers.
  - The ECRL and the ECRB are located in the second dorsal compartment of the wrist adjacent to the fourth compartment and are separated only by the tubercle of Lister and the EPL.

- Expose the ECRL or ECRB using a straight dorsal incision or a limited transverse incision over the base of the index and long metacarpals, at their respective insertion sites.
- Divide the tendon selected for transfer, usually the ECRL, at its insertion and transfer it ulnarward to the recipient tendon stump.

TECHNIQUES

BRACHIORADIALIS TENDON TRANSFER (RECONSTRUCTION OF MANNERFELT SYNDROME)

- Expose the forearm muscles and the brachioradialis tendon insertion on the distal radial aspect of the radius through a Henry-type incision.
- Confirm the tendon rupture by direct exposure of the slightly more distal and radial tendon of the flexor pollicis longus.
- Mobilize the distal tendon stump and perform a tenolysis to remove adhesions.
- Weave the distal flexor pollicis longus through the brachioradialis in a Pulvertaft fashion. Sharp tendon passers

facilitate this technique (**TECH FIG 3**).
- Adjust tension such that with wrist flexion, the MCP and interphalangeal joints of the thumb extend fully, and with wrist extension, they flex 30 to 40 degrees.
- Secure the weaves with 3-0 or 4-0 braided nonabsorbable sutures.
- If the index or long FDP tendons also are ruptured, isolate the distal tendon stumps and repair them end to side.

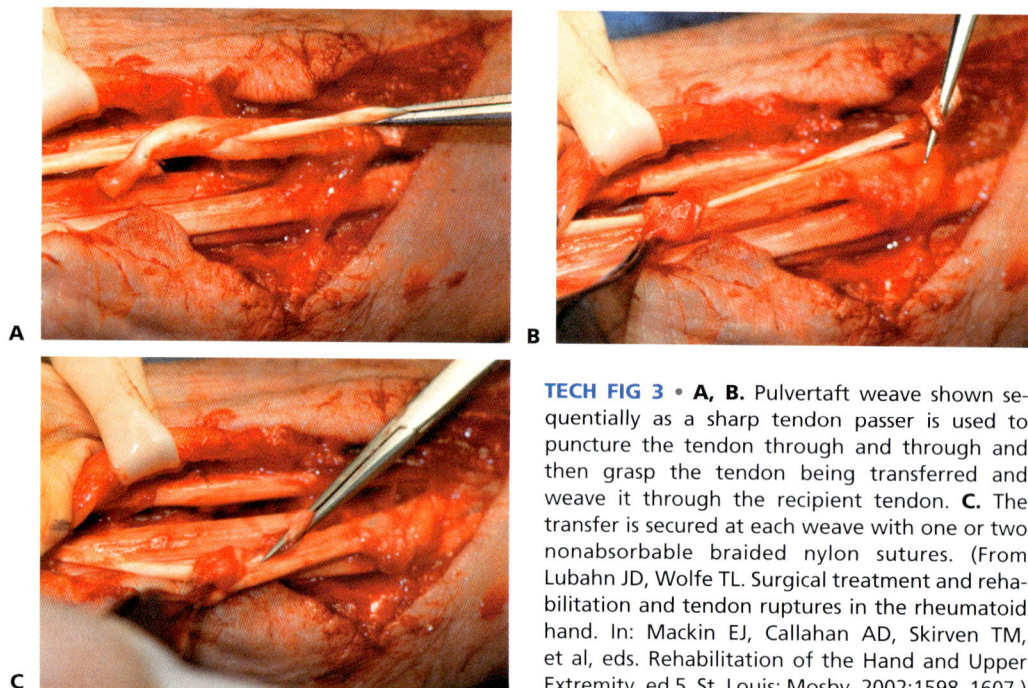

TECH FIG 3 • **A, B.** Pulvertaft weave shown sequentially as a sharp tendon passer is used to puncture the tendon through and through and then grasp the tendon being transferred and weave it through the recipient tendon. **C.** The transfer is secured at each weave with one or two nonabsorbable braided nylon sutures. (From Lubahn JD, Wolfe TL. Surgical treatment and rehabilitation and tendon ruptures in the rheumatoid hand. In: Mackin EJ, Callahan AD, Skirven TM, et al, eds. Rehabilitation of the Hand and Upper Extremity, ed 5. St. Louis: Mosby, 2002:1598–1607.)

EXTENSOR POLLICIS LONGUS TENDON TRANSFER (RECONSTRUCTION OF THUMB BOUTONNIÈRE DEFORMITY)

- Make a longitudinal incision to expose and identify the EPL tendon at its insertion onto the base of the distal phalanx.
- Incise the tendon at that level and mobilize it proximally (**TECH FIG 4A**).
  - Carefully protect the intrinsic tendon, which will now be the sole extensor for the thumb interphalangeal joint.
- Expose the dorsal base of the proximal phalanx and weave the EPL tendon through the dorsal capsule, securing it

using a 3-0 or 4-0 nonabsorbable braided suture (**TECH FIG 4B**).
- Alternatively, secure the EPL tendon in place using drill holes or a suture anchor in the proximal phalanx (**TECH FIG 4C,D**).
- The thumb is splinted or casted for 4 weeks and a protective splint is worn for strenuous activities for 6 to 8 weeks.

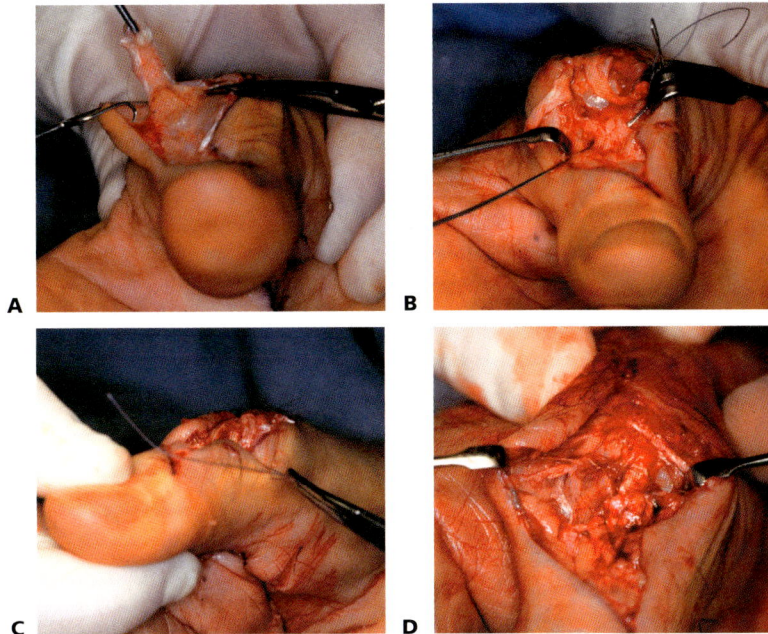

TECH FIG 4 • Extensor pollicis brevis rupture. **A,B.** Tendon transfer of the extensor pollicis longus proximally to the site of insertion of the extensor pollicis brevis, allowing the hyperextended interphalangeal joint to drop into a more flexed position and allowing active extension at the level of the metacarpophalangeal joint. **C,D.** Extensor pollicis longus is anchored through drill holes to the base of the proximal phalanx. (From Lubahn JD, Wolfe TL. Surgical treatment and rehabilitation and tendon ruptures in the rheumatoid hand. In: Mackin EJ, Callahan AD, Skirven TM, et al, eds. Rehabilitation of the Hand and Upper Extremity, ed 5. St. Louis: Mosby, 2002:1598–1607.)

PEARLS AND PITFALLS

EIP harvest	■ Obtain the EIP transfer by tracing the ulnarmost inserting tendon in the MCP joint region of the index finger proximally at the level of the wrist. In a certain percentage of patients, the ulnarmost tendon is in fact the EDC rather than the EIP. The EIP, however, is always the deeper, more volar tendon at the level of the wrist. Tracing this independent muscle tendon unit from the wrist to the index finger MPJ will help assure the surgeon that the correct tendon is being released for transfer.
	■ Distal repair of the dorsal apparatus at the site of EIP harvest is somewhat controversial. While some experts recommend repair, others feel confident that the defect can be left with no risk of extensor lag. The surgeon needs to be aware of the potential risk of extensor lag, and we recommend attention to the defect by suture repair.
EDQ transfers	■ Sufficient length of the distal segment of the EDQ should be available to allow tendon transfer to the adjacent EDC without abducting the small finger. If this transfer is tight, the side-to-side transfer of EDQ to the EDC of the ring finger should be abandoned and tendon transfer to the EIP or another suitable donor pursued.
Unstable DRUJ	■ At the time of tendon transfer, inspect the DRUJ to be certain that any osteophytes have been débrided and a localized flap rotated to cover the exposed bone created. If the DRUJ is deemed unstable, transfer of the pronator quadratus dorsally may be used to stabilize the distal ulna.
Suturing	■ When suturing tendon grafts at the site of tendon weave (ie, where a graft or transfer is passed through another tendon), one or two sutures should be sufficient. Take care that the needle does not pass through the tendon near the thread from another suture. If this occurs, the suture is weakened or possibly cut in two by the needle, and the graft or transfer is predisposed to rupture. Cutting needles should never be used as they place both the suture and the tendon at risk.

POSTOPERATIVE CARE

- Postoperative care for each of these tendon transfers is similar.
- In the case of tendon transfer to restore loss of finger extensors, the hand and wrist are immobilized with the wrist extended about 40 degrees. More may be desirable in certain instances, but too much extension could damage already fragile joints.
  - The MCP joints are brought into flexion until tension is noted at the suture line. Forty degrees or more is ideal to maintain the desired length of the collateral ligaments and prevent MCP joint extension contractures.
  - Immobilization is continued for 3.5 to 4 weeks, and gentle active motion is begun, maintaining the hand in a splint for protection.
  - At 6 weeks, some resistive exercises may be added to the program. By 12 weeks, the patient should be able to resume normal activities.
- In the case of flexor tendon rupture, the hand and wrist are immobilized with the wrist in 60 degrees of flexion, the MCP joints in 40 degrees of flexion, and the interphalangeal joints allowed to extend until tension is noted at the suture line. Immobilization is continued for 6 weeks, at which time a gentle active range-of-motion program is begun without resistance.
  - At 12 weeks resistive exercises are added and the patient is permitted to gradually resume normal activity.

OUTCOMES

- Outcomes in tendon transfer surgery in rheumatoid arthritis are highly dependent on the patient's medical condition and ability to cooperate with the postoperative splinting and rehabilitation program. Most patients who are supervised by a therapist achieve a better result than those who try to make it on their own.
  - With good medical management of rheumatoid arthritis, when the disease is well controlled, and in cooperative patients who are motivated to improve, good results should be expected.
- Tendon transfer should always be delayed in patients with active disease as results will be poor.
- The only surgical procedure to be performed in poorly controlled patients is synovectomy, and with the caveat that success hinges on eventual good medical control of the disease.

COMPLICATIONS

- Infection
- Skin or surgical wound breakdown
- Attenuation of the transferred tendon
- Rerupture of the tendons
- Loss of motion due to improper tensioning of the transferred tendon
- Joint stiffness

REFERENCES

1. Boyes JH, ed. In: Bunnell's Surgery of the Hand, 5th ed. Philadelphia: JB Lippincott, 1970.
2. Hamlin C, Littler JW. Restoration of the extensor pollicis longus tendon by an intercalated graft. J Bone Joint Surg Am 1977;59A: 412–414.
3. Mannerfelt L, Norman O. Attrition ruptures of flexor tendons in rheumatoid arthritis caused by bony spurs in the carpal tunnel: a clinical and radiological study. J Bone Joint Surg Br 1969;51B: 270–277.
4. Nalebuff EA. Diagnosis, classification and management of rheumatoid thumb deformities. Bull Hosp Joint Dis 1968;29:119–137.
5. Nalebuff EA, Millender LH. Surgical treatment of the boutonniere deformity in rheumatoid arthritis. Orthop Clin North Am 1975; 6:753–763.
6. Vaughan-Jackson OJ. Rupture of extensor tendons by attrition at the inferior radio-ulnar joint: report of two cases. J Bone Joint Surg Br 1948;30B:528–530.
7. Williamson SC, Feldon P. Extensor tendon ruptures in rheumatoid arthritis. Hand Clin 1995;11:449–459.

Mark Wilczynski, Martin I. Boyer, and Fraser J. Leversedge

DEFINITION

- Rheumatoid arthritis is a poorly understood systemic disease affecting the synovium of joints and tendon sheaths. The synovial tissue in rheumatoid arthritis is characterized by a proliferation of synovial lining cells, angiogenesis, and relative lymphocytosis.[14]
  - A combination of cartilage degeneration, synovial expansion and periarticular erosion, and ligamentous laxity creates an imbalance within the extrinsic and intrinsic tendon systems of the digit to cause progressive deformity.
- A boutonnière ("buttonhole") deformity involves disruption of the central slip. It results in a characteristic deformity involving hyperextension at the metacarpophalangeal (MCP) joint, flexion at the proximal interphalangeal (PIP) joint, and hyperextension at the distal interphalangeal (DIP) joint.
- Swan-neck deformity is characterized by hyperextension of the PIP joint and flexion of the DIP joint. MCP joint flexion may also be present.
  - In the posttraumatic setting, it results from laxity of the PIP joint volar plate and inability of the terminal slip to extend the DIP joint.
  - Chronic deformity may be associated with progressive digital contracture.

Classification

- Rheumatoid thumb deformity[26,33]
  - Type I: Boutonnière deformity: MCP joint flexion and interphalangeal joint hyperextension. Carpometacarpal (CMC) joint is not primarily involved.
  - Type II: Rare; a combination of types I and III involving MCP joint flexion and interphalangeal joint hyperextension and associated CMC joint subluxation or dislocation
  - Type III: Swan-neck deformity: MCP joint hyperextension, interphalangeal joint flexion, and thumb metacarpal adduction, resulting from progressive CMC joint pathology
  - Type IV: Gamekeeper's deformity. Attenuation of the ulnar collateral ligament of the thumb MCP joint results in radial deviation through the MCP joint and secondary metacarpal adduction deformity or contracture.
  - Type V: Results from attenuation of the MCP volar plate with progressive MCP joint hyperextension and secondary interphalangeal joint flexion. There is no metacarpal adduction deformity.
- Boutonnière deformity
  - Stage I—mild: PIP joint synovitis and a mild, fully correctable extension lag
  - Stage II—moderate: Marked flexion deformity of the PIP joint, either flexible or fixed
  - Stage III—severe: PIP joint articular destruction
- Swan-neck deformity
  - Type I: PIP joint is fully mobile and flexible.

- Type II: Active and passive motions of the PIP joint are limited, with the MCP joint held in extension due to intrinsic tightness.
- Type III: Decreased PIP joint motion in all positions of MCP joint flexion and extension
- Type IV: Fixed PIP joint hyperextension with advanced destruction of the PIP joint articular surfaces

ANATOMY

Bone and Joint

- The MCP joint is a condyloid joint with average range of motion from 15 degrees hyperextension to 90 degrees flexion.
  - A cam effect for collateral ligaments is due to the shape of the metacarpal head; collateral ligaments are taut with MCP joint flexion and lax with MCP joint extension.
- The PIP joint (**FIG 1A**) is a hinge joint with greater inherent osseous stability than the MCP joint due to the configuration of the two condyles of the head of the proximal phalanx, which articulates with the median ridge at the base of the middle phalanx.
  - The collateral ligaments are taut throughout the joint arc of motion.
  - The volar plate is a thick, fibrocartilage structure that serves to resist PIP joint hyperextension; the volar plate originates within the A2 pulley on the proximal phalanx and inserts into the "rough area" at the base of the middle phalanx.
- The DIP joint is stabilized by the collateral ligaments, the terminal extensor tendon insertion, the flexor digitorum profundus insertion, and the volar plate.

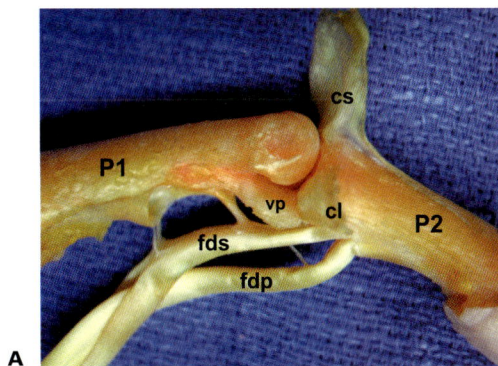

FIG 1 • A. Proximal interphalangeal (PIP) joint relationships. The flexor tendons (flexor digitorum superficialis [FDS] and profundus [FDP]) have been removed from the proximal digital flexor sheath at the A2 pulley. The FDP and FDS tendon orientation is demonstrated before they re-enter the flexor sheath at the A4 pulley. The PIP joint collateral ligament (*cl*) and the insertion of the central slip (*cs*) at the dorsal base of the middle phalanx have been reflected distally to highlight the volar plate (*vp*) and its proximity within the flexor sheath. *P1*, proximal phalanx; *P2*, middle phalanx. *(continued)*

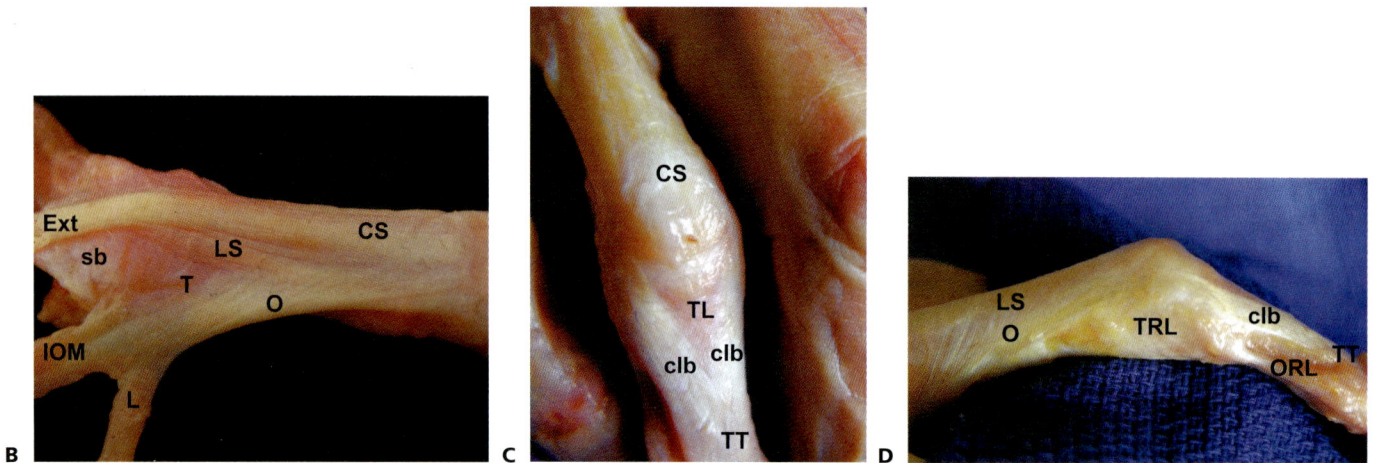

FIG 1 • B. *(continued)* The dorsal digital extensor apparatus is derived from contributions of the extrinsic extensor tendons and the intrinsic musculature of the hand. The extrinsic extensor tendon (*Ext*) is identified at the level of the distal hand and splits into two lateral slips (*LS*) and the central tendon slip (*CS*). At the dorsal metacarpophalangeal (MCP) joint the extensor tendon is stabilized by the vertically orientated fibers of the sagittal band (*sb*), which originate from the radial and ulnar sides of the volar plate of the MCP joint and the volar base of the proximal phalanx. The MCP joint is extended via a sling-like mechanism of the sagittal band as there is no direct fiber insertion from the extrinsic extensor tendon at the proximal phalanx. The deep head of the interosseous muscle (*IOM*) courses superficial to the sagittal band (*sb*) at the level of the MCP joint and runs parallel and distal to the sagittal band over the proximal phalanx to form the transverse fibers (*T*) of the extensor apparatus. The lumbrical muscle (*L*) on the radial aspect of the digit forms the oblique fibers (*O*) of the extensor apparatus, which join with the lateral slip of the extrinsic extensor tendon to form the conjoined lateral band. **C.** The extrinsic extensor tendon divides into a central slip (*CS*) and two lateral slips. The central slip inserts at the dorsal base of the middle phalanx to extend the PIP joint, and the two lateral slips receive contributory fibers from the lumbricals via oblique fibers of the extensor hood to form the conjoined lateral bands (*clb*). These conjoined lateral bands coalesce to form the terminal tendon (*TT*), which inserts at the dorsal base of the distal phalanx to extend the distal interphalangeal joint. The triangular ligament (*TL*) stabilizes the conjoined lateral bands from volar subluxation. **D.** Lateral view of the digit demonstrating the coalescing fibers of the lateral slip (*LS*) and oblique fibers of the extensor apparatus (*O*), which combine to form the conjoined lateral band (*clb*). The two conjoined lateral bands combine to form the terminal tendon (*TT*), which inserts into the dorsal base of the distal phalanx. The transverse retinacular ligament (*TRL*) prevents dorsal subluxation of the lateral bands. The oblique retinacular ligament (*ORL*) passively links the proximal and distal interphalangeal joints as it travels from volar to dorsal from the fibro-osseous gutter (middle third of the proximal phalanx and A2 pulley) to the proximal aspect of the distal phalanx through the extensor tendon. (Photographs © Copyright of Fraser J. Leversedge, Charles A. Goldfarb, and Martin Boyer.)

Dorsal Restraining Structures of the Digit (FIG 1B–D)

- The sagittal bands originate on both sides of the MCP joint, from the volar plate and the base of the proximal phalanx, and insert into the lateral margins of the extensor tendon over the dorsal MCP joint.
  - They stabilize the extrinsic extensor tendon over the MCP joint to prevent lateral subluxation.
  - They contribute indirectly to MCP joint extension and prevent extensor bowstringing.
- The triangular ligament stabilizes the two conjoined lateral bands over the dorsal aspect of the middle phalanx and prevents volar subluxation of the conjoined lateral bands.
- The transverse retinacular ligament is composed of fibers oriented in a volar–dorsal direction at the level of the PIP joint. It prevents dorsal subluxation of the conjoined lateral bands.
- The oblique retinacular ligament (ORL) is a static restraining ligament, linking the PIP and DIP joints. It runs from the fibro-osseous gutter at the A2 flexor pulley and the middle third of the proximal phalanx to insert into the terminal extensor tendon and couples PIP joint and DIP joint extension.

Flexor Tendon: Digit

- At the level of the A1 pulley, the flexor digitorum superficialis (FDS) tendon flattens and bifurcates to allow the more dorsal flexor digitorum profundus (FDP) tendon to pass distally within the flexor sheath to insert at the volar base of the distal phalanx.
- The FDS tendon slips rotate laterally and dorsally around the FDP and then divide again into medial and lateral slips. The medial slips rejoin dorsal to the FDP tendon and insert into the distal aspect of the proximal phalanx. The lateral slips continue distally to insert into the base of the middle phalanx.

Extensor Tendon: Digit

- At the base of the proximal phalanx, the extrinsic extensor tendon trifurcates with the central portion inserting into the dorsal base of the middle phalanx as the central slip.
- The lateral slips are joined by the oblique fibers of the lumbrical tendons to form the conjoined lateral band. The conjoined lateral bands converge over the middle phalanx to form the terminal tendon, which inserts at the dorsal base of the distal phalanx, where it functions to extend the DIP joint.
- The interosseous muscles contribute to the dorsal extensor apparatus through their deep muscle belly, which travels superficial to the sagittal band as the lateral tendon, becoming the transverse fibers of the extensor hood (MCP joint flexion).

PATHOGENESIS

Posttraumatic Boutonnière Deformity

- Disruption of the central slip is the inciting pathology in the development of the boutonnière deformity.
- Injury patterns can be grouped into two broad categories, closed and open.
  - Closed injuries: Forceful hyperflexion of the PIP joint may result in a detachment of the central slip from its insertion. An associated avulsion fracture involving the insertion of the central slip may be identified from the dorsal base of the middle phalanx.
    - Volar dislocations of the PIP joint or digital crush injuries may disrupt the central slip.
  - Open injuries: Dorsal laceration or deep abrasions over the PIP joint may disrupt the integrity of the central slip.
- Disruption of the central slip and attenuation of the triangular ligament allows for the migration of the lateral bands volar to the PIP joint axis of rotation. This results in flexion at the PIP joint and extension at the DIP joint through the action of the displaced lateral bands.
  - The displaced lateral band becomes a flexor of the PIP joint and an extensor of the DIP joint.

Posttraumatic Swan-Neck Deformity

- Unrecognized volar plate injury at the PIP joint may result in volar plate insufficiency. This leaves the action of the central slip unchecked by the volar plate, resulting in a progressive PIP joint hyperextension deformity.
  - Recurrent dorsal dislocation of the PIP joint is an example of an injury pattern that may result in volar plate incompetence.
- Avulsion of the terminal tendon from its insertion at the base of the dorsal distal phalanx results in an imbalance in the extensor mechanism. Extension forces are concentrated at the central slip, producing a progressive hyperextension deformity of the PIP joint.
  - Patients predisposed to volar plate laxity (such as from generalized ligamentous laxity, inflammatory conditions, and collagen vascular disorders) are particularly susceptible to the development of deformity.
- An extension malunion of the middle phalanx or peritendinous adhesions secondary to previous digital fracture or injury may contribute to the development of a swan-neck deformity.
- Hyperextension of the PIP joint and attenuation of the transverse retinacular ligament permits dorsal migration of the lateral bands relative to the PIP joint axis of rotation. The displaced lateral bands act to extend the PIP joint and to flex the DIP joint.

Rheumatoid Boutonnière Deformity

Fingers

- Boutonnière ("buttonhole") deformity results from pathologic synovitis of the PIP joint that causes progressive attenuation of the central slip, transverse retinacular ligaments, and triangular ligament. The PIP joint essentially "buttonholes" through the extensor mechanism.[30] Characteristic flexion of the PIP joint and hyperextension deformities of the MCP and DIP joint prevail due to the extensor imbalance[21] (**FIG 2A**).

- Subluxation of the lateral bands, volar to the axis of PIP joint rotation, occurs due to the loss of these restraints. The lateral bands become flexors of the PIP joint rather than extensors.
  - It is important to differentiate this pathologic involvement of the extensor mechanism from a flexion contracture of the PIP joint.
- Due to persisting PIP joint flexion, the volar plate, collateral ligaments, and oblique retinacular ligaments become increasingly contracted, resulting in a stiff and subsequently fixed boutonnière deformity.

Thumb

- Type I boutonnière deformity is the most common rheumatoid deformity of the thumb.[29,37] It is characterized by MCP joint flexion and interphalangeal joint hyperextension (**FIG 2B**).
- The pathologic changes affecting the thumb typically involve synovitis of the MCP joint with resulting attenuation of the extensor mechanism (dorsal joint capsule, extensor pollicis brevis tendon insertion, extensor hood). This relative extensor imbalance results in MCP joint flexion and possible joint subluxation.
  - Attenuation of the sagittal band permits ulnar and volar subluxation of the extensor pollicis longus (EPL) tendon, which accentuates MCP joint flexion and interphalangeal joint hyperextension as it translates volar to the axis of MCP joint rotation.
- The destructive influence of prolific MCP joint synovitis can cause progressive articular erosion and altered joint surface mechanics, resulting in progressive joint instability and deformity.

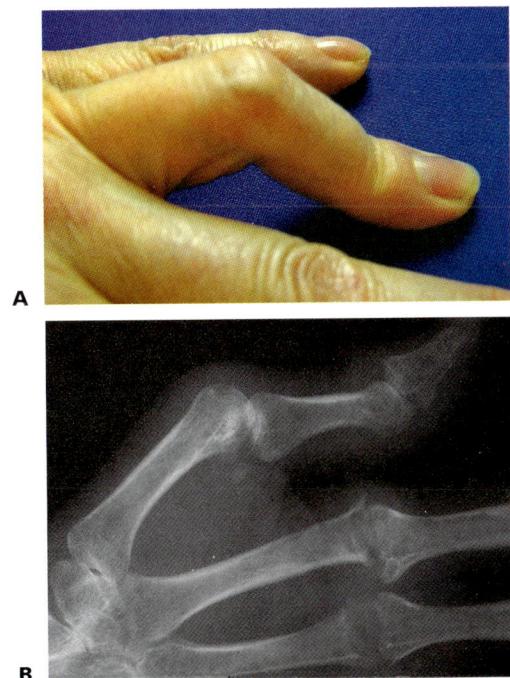

FIG 2 • **A.** Boutonnière deformity of the finger. Note the flexion posture of the proximal interphalangeal joint and hyperextension of the distal interphalangeal joint. **B.** Lateral radiograph of the thumb demonstrating a boutonnière deformity. (Photographs © Copyright of Fraser J. Leversedge, Charles A. Goldfarb, and Martin Boyer.)

- As the MCP joint flexion posturing increases in severity, compensatory radial abduction deviation of the thumb metacarpal ensues.
- Rupture of the EPL tendon at the wrist can result in a similar "extrinsic-minus" deformity of the thumb.[20,25]
- Boutonnière deformity can result, also, from a hyperextension deformity of the thumb interphalangeal joint secondary to joint synovitis with attenuation of the volar plate or to rupture of the flexor pollicis longus tendon.[19]
  - Generally, these primary interphalangeal joint etiologies present with less dramatic MCP joint flexion deformity.[33]

Rheumatoid Swan-Neck Deformity

Fingers

- Swan-neck deformity may result from pathologic rheumatoid synovitis of the MCP, PIP, or DIP joints and is characterized by PIP joint hyperextension and MCP and DIP flexion deformities.
  - Progressive attenuation of the volar plate, collateral ligaments, and insertion of the FDS tendon results in the development of a PIP hyperextension deformity.
  - Attenuation of the transverse retinacular ligaments may occur from synovitis, thereby resulting in a loss of the normal restraints to dorsal translocation of the lateral bands. As the lateral bands subluxate dorsal to the axis of PIP joint rotation, they become a constant hyperextension force on the PIP joint.
- The DIP joint may be the primary cause of swan-neck deformity where synovitis results in the attenuation and possible rupture of the terminal extensor tendon. This leads to a concentration of the extensor forces at the PIP joint and a resultant hyperextension deformity.
- Pathologic alterations in MCP joint mechanics may initiate the development of a swan-neck deformity. Progressive flexion deformity and ulnar drift of the digit results in an imbalance of the extensor mechanism whereby the lateral bands are drawn dorsally, concentrating an extension–hyperextension force at the PIP joint. Flexion deformity at the MCP joint may be secondary to several causes (**FIG 3A,B**):
  - Chronic synovitis and associated attenuation of the sagittal bands
  - Articular destruction with associated joint deformity and volar joint subluxation
  - The influence of intrinsic tightness or contracture
- Persisting PIP hyperextension results in contracture of the extensor apparatus, particularly the triangular ligament, as well as the skin. These progressive changes result in a stiff and subsequently fixed PIP joint hyperextension contracture.
- Digital flexor tenosynovitis may contribute to poor initiation of digital flexion and an increased extension imbalance at the PIP joint.
- Chronic synovitis of the PIP joint, combined with altered joint mechanics, may result in progressive articular destruction that leads to greater joint deformity, a progressively fixed contracture, and, potentially, painful dysfunction of the digit.

Thumb

- Type III rheumatoid thumb deformity is the second most common thumb deformity after boutonnière deformity.[25,29]
- The deformity occurs as the result of CMC joint synovitis and associated alterations in thumb mechanics.
  - Progressive dorsal and radial subluxation of the thumb CMC joint occurs with the deleterious effects of chronic synovitis, including capsular attenuation and articular erosions.
- The force vectors associated with pinch and grasp activities accentuate the CMC deformity and accentuate a progressive thumb metacarpal adduction contracture due to a loss of thumb abduction.
- As the adduction contracture worsens, hyperextension of the MCP joint (permitted by volar plate laxity) and interphalangeal joint flexion becomes a functional compensation (**FIG 3C,D**).

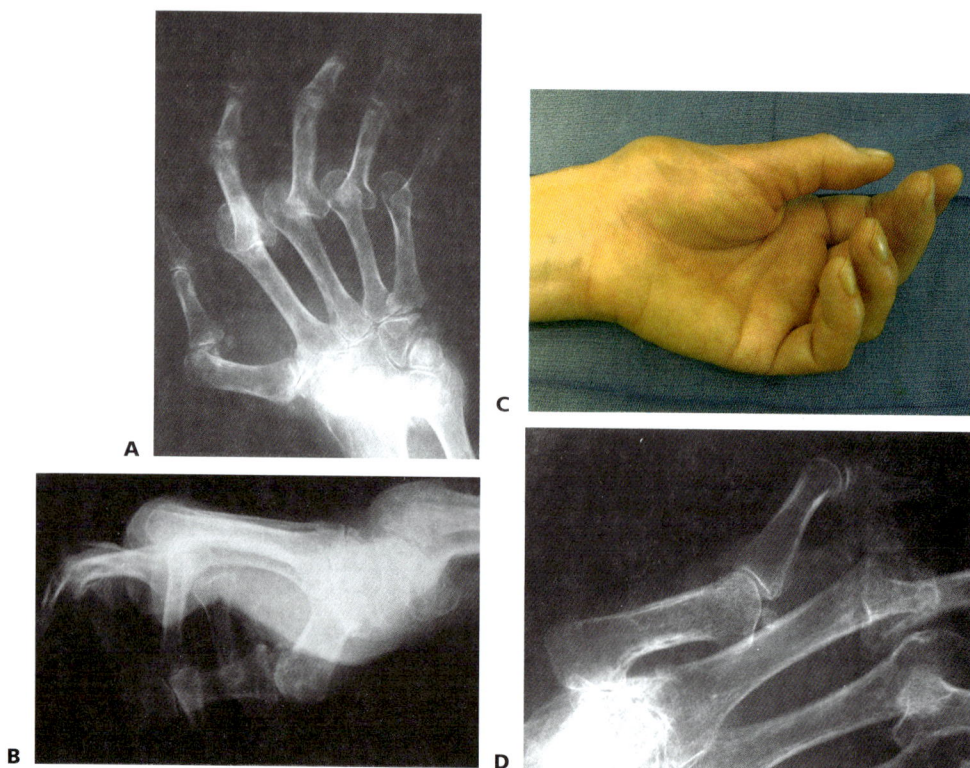

FIG 3 • **A,B.** AP and lateral radiographs demonstrating the volar dislocation and ulnar drift of the metacarpophalangeal joints of the fingers. **C.** Swan-neck deformity of the thumb. **D.** Lateral radiograph of the thumb demonstrating a swan-neck deformity involving carpometacarpal joint subluxation, metacarpal adduction contracture, hyperextension of the metacarpophalangeal joint, and thumb interphalangeal joint flexion. (Photographs © Copyright of Fraser J. Leversedge, Charles A. Goldfarb, and Martin Boyer.)

NATURAL HISTORY

Traumatic Injury

- Early diagnosis is critical for achieving satisfactory outcomes. Reconstructive options become limited as the deformity becomes rigid.

Boutonnière Deformity

- Deformity may not be evident immediately after injury but may develop over 2 to 3 weeks.
- The pathologic finger posture develops through five stages[7]:
  - Disruption of the central slip results in resting flexion of the PIP joint and weak extension of the middle phalanx via the lateral bands.
  - Attenuation of the triangular ligament and contracture of the transverse retinacular ligaments results in the volar migration of the lateral bands. Active PIP joint extension is absent.
  - Extension forces are transmitted through the lateral bands, causing hyperextension at the DIP joint.
  - Progressive contracture of the PIP joint volar plate and the oblique retinacular ligament results in fixed flexion contracture at the PIP joint.
  - Progressive articular degeneration occurs after prolonged and untreated pathology.

Swan-Neck Deformity

- The deformity may be subclassified into four groups that describe the natural history[24]:
  - Presence of full passive range of motion at the PIP joint
  - Prolonged hyperextension of the PIP joint results in intrinsic tightness. The PIP joint exhibits full range of motion when the MCP joint is flexed. However, with the MCP joint extended, PIP flexion becomes limited.
  - As the transverse retinacular ligament attenuates and the triangular ligament contracts, the subluxated lateral bands become fixed dorsal to the PIP joint axis of rotation. Hyperextension of the PIP joint becomes fixed regardless of MCP joint position.
  - Progressive PIP joint articular degeneration occurs with chronic, fixed deformity.

Rheumatoid Deformity

- The rate of progressive rheumatoid arthritis-related upper extremity deformity appears to be slowing due to improved medical management of this systemic disease process.
- The incidence of uncorrectable boutonnière and swan-neck deformities during the first 2 years after the onset of systemic disease is about 16% and 8%, respectively.[7]
- The prevalence of finger deformities in patients with established rheumatoid arthritis is about 36% for boutonnière and 14% for swan-neck deformities.[7]
- The wrist, MCP, and PIP joints are the most commonly affected joints of the upper extremity, and pathologic proliferation of the flexor and extensor tenosynovium may influence digital function and deformity.

PATIENT HISTORY AND PHYSICAL FINDINGS

Posttraumatic Injury

Boutonnière Deformity

- A history of blunt trauma to the digit with swelling and tenderness over the PIP joint should arouse suspicion as to the condition. Often, patients report "jamming" or spraining the digit. History of a dorsal digital laceration is similarly concerning.
- Deformity may not develop until 10 to 21 days after the injury, making early diagnosis challenging and diligent follow-up imperative. Laceration, ecchymosis, or tenderness over the dorsum of the PIP joint may be diagnostic when a PIP joint extension lag is present.
- If the examination is limited due to pain, a digital block should be considered to facilitate a comfortable examination.
- The following physical findings are supportive in confirming an early diagnosis:
  - 15- to 20-degree PIP joint extension lag with the wrist and MCP joint fully flexed[5]
  - Weak extension of the middle phalanx against resistance[18]
  - Elson test: Effort to extend the PIP joint accompanied by rigidity of the DIP joint suggests that the central slip is ruptured and forces are being transferred by the lateral bands.
    - The Elson test is most reliable in diagnosing early boutonnière deformities.[31]
  - Boyes test: When the central slip is disrupted, passive extension of the PIP joint causes tension across the lateral bands, resulting in loss of active flexion at the DIP joint. When flexion at the PIP joint is restored, motion at the DIP joint returns.

Swan-Neck Deformity

- A history of unrecognized or undertreated trauma or multiple dorsal PIP joint dislocations is common. A patient who presents with a longstanding "mallet" deformity should arouse suspicion, particularly if there is associated hypermobility in the PIP joint of unaffected digits.
- Physical examination begins with inspection of the involved digit.
  - Typically, the PIP joint is hyperextended and the DIP joint is flexed. MCP joint flexion may be present also.
- Active and passive range of motion of the PIP joint should be assessed.
- In the presence of a flexible deformity, a Bunnell test for intrinsic tightness should be performed.
  - This test assists the examiner in determining the relative contribution of intrinsic tightness to the deformity.
  - Increased resistance to passive PIP flexion with the MCP joint in extension compared with flexion indicates a relative shortening of the intrinsic muscle–tendon units.

Rheumatoid Deformity

- Diagnostic criteria for rheumatoid arthritis are based on the American College of Rheumatology's 1988 recommendations.[2]
- Current medications and medical comorbidities may influence decision making for treatment and the timing for surgical intervention.
- The evaluation of digital deformities associated with rheumatoid arthritis requires careful global assessment, including neurologic assessment (cervical spine, peripheral compressive neuropathy); appreciation for shoulder, elbow, and wrist involvement; and the awareness of lower extremity deformities that will need reconstructive surgery for which the use of ambulatory aids might be necessary.
- As progressive deformity of the wrist occurs, its pathologic influence on digital function and deformity should be recognized.
  - The carpus typically collapses into supination, with concomitant volar translation and ulnar translocation.[3]

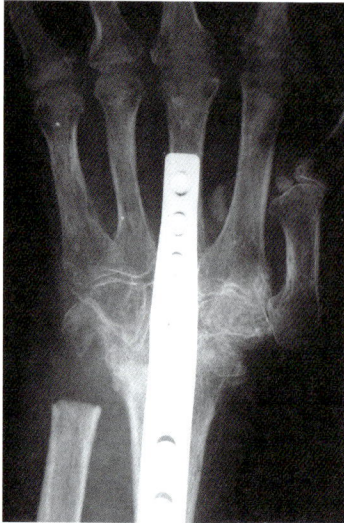

FIG 4 • Preoperative assessment of the digits should include evaluation of the wrist and metacarpophalangeal joints due to their influence on digital function. Wrist stabilization with total wrist arthrodesis and concomitant distal ulnar resection may include soft tissue reconstruction such as tendon repair or tenodesis; such reconstruction should occur before digital reconstructions due to its influence on the outcomes of swan-neck or boutonnière reconstructions. Reconstruction of the metacarpophalangeal joints should occur before or simultaneously with digital swan-neck or boutonnière reconstructions. (Photographs © Copyright of Fraser J. Leversedge, Charles A. Goldfarb, and Martin Boyer.)

- Relative dorsal prominence of the distal ulna may involve a loss of distal radioulnar joint (DRUJ) congruity and may be associated with ruptures of the extensor carpi ulnaris tendon and extensor tendons to the small and ring fingers (caput ulnae syndrome). Inspection of the extrinsic digital extensors, including the EPL,[20] should be done, particularly in the presence of active synovitis of the radiocarpal joint and DRUJ (**FIG 4**).

- The MCP joint should be assessed for active synovitis and for characteristic volar subluxation and ulnar drift.

- Just as pathologic changes to both the wrist and MCP joints may influence the development of swan-neck and boutonnière deformities of the digits, these changes may adversely affect the outcomes of digital reconstruction if they are not addressed.

- Evaluation of the digits should be performed individually with inspection of the resting posture of each digit, assessment of the active and passive motion of each digital joint, and inspection for joint synovitis or tenosynovitis. Skin integrity is assessed for attenuation and for its contribution to joint contracture.

- Flexor tenosynovitis may be identified by a palpable fullness in the distal volar forearm or along the digital flexor sheath. Swelling, palpable crepitus along the digital flexor sheath, and a discrepancy between active and passive digital motion are hallmarks of flexor tenosynovitis of the digit.

  - Flexor tendon rupture may be present, often secondary to attenuation at the volar carpus,[19] and should be addressed in the presence of a loss of active digital joint flexion.

- Extensor tenosynovitis at the wrist may be determined by palpable tenosynovial hypertrophy, or fullness, and crepitus along the dorsal extensor compartments, proximal and distal to the extensor retinaculum.

  - Tendon ruptures may be identified by a lack of active digital extension despite active muscular contraction, by palpable tendon deficit, and by a lack of digital extension through tenodesis with passive wrist flexion.

  - The adhesion of a ruptured tendon to the surrounding tissues and the influence of the junctura tendinea may limit the accuracy of these evaluations.

- As described above, the Bunnell intrinsic tightness test should be performed for all fingers of patients with rheumatoid arthritis, particularly for patients with swan-neck deformity of the digits. This test assists the examiner in determining the relative contribution of intrinsic tightness to the development of the deformity.

- Tightness of the oblique retinacular ligament, often appreciated in digits with early boutonnière deformity, is evaluated by assessing the relative degree of resistance to passive DIP joint flexion with the PIP joint held by the examiner in maximum extension.

IMAGING AND OTHER DIAGNOSTIC STUDIES

- Plain radiographs (three views) are the mainstay of hand and wrist evaluation in the patient with either a traumatic or rheumatoid cause for deformity.

  - Staging of arthritis-related joint pathology and identification of joint subluxation or dislocation, important for diagnostic and management considerations, is performed using plain radiographs (**FIG 5A**).

- Avulsion fractures from the dorsal base of the middle phalanx, volar subluxation of the PIP joint, or both suggest a central slip injury (**FIG 5B**).

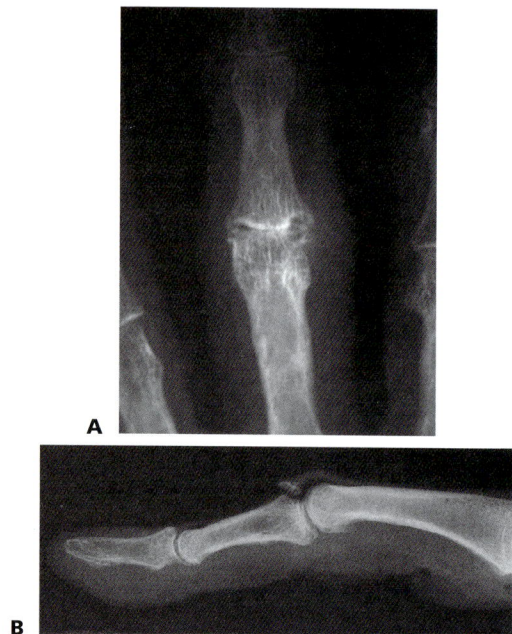

FIG 5 • **A.** Radiographic appearance of periarticular (proximal interphalangeal [PIP] joint) soft tissue swelling and synovitis and moderate articular erosions involving the PIP joint. **B.** Lateral radiograph of the finger demonstrating a central slip avulsion injury involving an avulsion fracture from the dorsal base of the middle phalanx. There is no volar subluxation of the PIP joint in this example. (Photographs © Copyright of Fraser J. Leversedge, Charles A. Goldfarb, and Martin Boyer.)

- In the presence of a fixed PIP joint flexion deformity, concomitant avulsion fracture of the volar plate suggests pseudo-boutonnière pathology.
- Fluoroscopic imaging or stress views may be helpful in differentiating collateral ligament injury from disruption of the central slip.
- Avulsion fractures from the dorsal base of the distal phalanx suggest terminal tendon injury.
- The presence of volar plate avulsion fractures in the setting of PIP joint hyperextension suggests volar plate incompetence.
- MRI may be useful in assessing for soft tissue pathology such as tenosynovitis and tendon rupture, especially in rheumatoid patients.

DIFFERENTIAL DIAGNOSIS
Posttraumatic Injury
- Pseudo-boutonnière deformity
- Collateral ligament injury
- Mallet finger
- Volar plate avulsion fracture

Rheumatoid Deformity
- Osteoarthritis
- Psoriatic arthritis
  - Similar deformities as seen in rheumatoid arthritis, but skin lesions are common and DIP joint "pencil-in-cup" deformities may be present
- Connective tissue disorders (scleroderma, systemic lupus erythematosus)
  - Systemic lupus erythematosus primarily affects soft tissue structures (ligamentous laxity, tendon subluxation) rather than joint destruction. Radiographs typically demonstrate joint deformities with well-preserved joint spaces. The thumb may be the first digit affected; lateral subluxation of the interphalangeal joint and flexion deformity of the MCP joint (secondary to extensor tendon subluxation) are common.
  - Patients with scleroderma often develop PIP joint flexion contractures and compensatory hyperextension posturing of the MCP joints.
- Crystal-induced arthropathy (gout, calcium pyrophosphate deposition disease)
- Hemochromatosis
- Remitting symmetric seronegative synovitis

NONOPERATIVE MANAGEMENT
Posttraumatic Injury
Boutonnière Deformity

- Nonoperative management is indicated if correction of the deformity restores the anatomic length relationship between the central slip and the lateral bands. It is most appropriate in those with closed injuries who present within 8 to 12 weeks of injury. It may be attempted in those with central slip avulsion fractures or volar dislocation if satisfactory reduction and PIP joint stability can be obtained.
- For patients with full passive extension of the PIP joint, PIP joint extension splinting is the treatment of choice.
  - A transarticular Kirschner wire maintaining the PIP joint in full extension is an alternative or adjunct to external splinting.
- For patients with a PIP joint flexion contracture without secondary joint degenerative changes, progressive static or dynamic extension splinting should be pursued.

- Full passive extension of the PIP joint should be sought before surgical intervention is considered.
- Active and passive DIP joint range of motion should be emphasized while the PIP joint is being treated. Restoration of active DIP joint flexion while the PIP joint is extended suggests successful treatment. Restoration of full active extension at the PIP joint is the goal.
- For most injuries, PIP joint extension splinting should be maintained for 6 to 8 weeks at all times, transitioning to protective buddy straps for daily activity and nighttime extension splinting for an additional 4 to 6 weeks.

Swan-Neck Deformity

- Once the deformity has developed, nonoperative treatment is rarely effective.
- Some patients with flexible deformities are capable of initiating PIP joint flexion with little impairment. They may complain of "snapping" or "cogwheeling" as the lateral bands relocate volarly during PIP joint flexion. These patients may benefit from a digital splint, such as a figure 8 ring splint, to prevent continued PIP joint hyperextension and to maintain the lateral bands in their anatomic position (**FIG 6**).

Rheumatoid Deformity
Boutonnière Deformity

- Nonoperative management of an early boutonnière deformity includes low-profile PIP joint extension splinting.
- Oral anti-inflammatory medications, intra-articular corticosteroid injection of the PIP joint, or both are used to minimize joint synovitis.

Type I Swan-Neck Deformity

- The goals of treatment for the flexible swan-neck deformity are prevention of PIP joint hyperextension and improvement in PIP joint flexion.
- In the presence of minimal PIP joint synovitis, use of digital splints, such as a figure 8 ring splint, is advocated to prevent PIP joint hyperextension (Fig 6).

SURGICAL MANAGEMENT
Posttraumatic Injury
Boutonnière Deformity

- Surgical intervention is indicated for patients who fail to respond to at least 3 months of extension splinting, patients with open injuries, and patients with fixed deformity with associated degenerative joint changes.

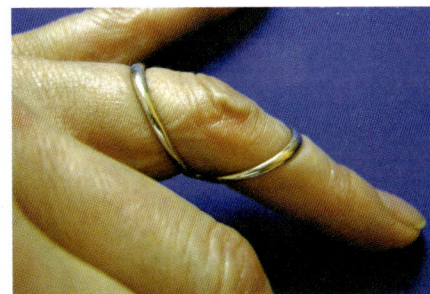

FIG 6 • A figure 8 ring splint (Silver Ring Splint; Charlottesville, VA) used to prevent proximal interphalangeal joint hyperextension in a mild, flexible swan-neck deformity. (Photographs © Copyright of Fraser J. Leversedge, Charles A. Goldfarb, and Martin Boyer.)

- Surgical decision making should be tempered by the observations of Burton and Melchior[4]:
  - Boutonnière reconstructions are most successful on supple joints. If necessary, joint contracture release can be performed as a first stage. If the release is followed by an intensive exercise and splinting program, the second stage may be avoided.
  - An arthritic joint usually precludes soft tissue reconstruction. The surgeon should consider either a PIP joint fusion or arthroplasty with extensor reconstruction.
  - Boutonnière deformities rarely compromise PIP joint flexion and grip strength. The surgeon should not trade extension at the PIP joint for a stiff finger and a weak hand.

Swan-Neck Deformity

- Surgery is indicated for patients with a flexible deformity who cannot actively initiate PIP joint flexion and in those with fixed deformities.
- Patients with flexible deformities benefit from volar mobilization of the lateral bands and tenodesis to prevent PIP joint hyperextension.
- Patients with fixed deformities have difficulty grasping objects. Often, functional contact is limited to the volar surface of the hyperextended PIP joint.
  - If the articular surfaces are well preserved, PIP joint release with concomitant procedures to restore flexion may be beneficial.
  - If the articular surfaces are damaged, PIP arthrodesis is a practical option.

Rheumatoid Deformity

- Principles of surgical correction of rheumatoid deformities in the hand should be guided by the relief of pain and the improvement of function.[28]

Boutonnière Finger Deformity

- Stage I—mild
  - For progressive boutonnière deformity associated with persistent PIP joint synovitis unresponsive to oral medication and intra-articular corticosteroid injection, PIP joint synovectomy may be considered. Concomitant central slip reconstruction and lateral band repositioning may be indicated due to soft tissue attenuation over the dorsal PIP joint.
  - Functional limitation due to DIP joint hyperextension may be treated by sectioning the terminal extensor tendon over the dorsal middle phalanx.
- Stage II—moderate
  - For patients with moderate boutonnière deformity and preservation of the articular cartilage of the PIP joint, central slip reconstruction and terminal extensor tendon release may be indicated.[12,44]
- Stage III—severe
  - If articular destruction is evident or if a severe fixed flexion contracture of the PIP joint is present, even without articular changes, then arthrodesis of the PIP joint is a reliable option for reducing pain and for improving function.
  - Implant arthroplasty of the PIP joint and concomitant terminal extensor tendon release is a less reliable option, particularly when there is attenuation of the dorsal extensor apparatus.

Swan-Neck Finger Deformity

- Type I
  - The primary cause of the flexible swan-neck deformity must be determined before proceeding with surgical inter-

vention. Although PIP synovitis and a resulting weakness of the volar PIP joint restraining structures are the most common findings, DIP joint synovitis may be a source of progressive deformity secondary to the transfer of extension forces to the PIP joint.
  - The potential influence of MCP joint pathology must be assessed. Extensor tendon subluxation at the level of the MCP joint or flexion contracture of the MCP joint should be addressed before, or concurrently with, surgical correction of the swan-neck deformity.
  - In a primary rheumatoid mallet finger where full PIP joint flexibility is preserved, DIP joint arthrodesis is a reasonable option. Postoperatively, the PIP joint is not immobilized, although the DIP joint is protected in a mallet-finger splint.
  - Frequently, patients with a flexible swan-neck deformity cannot initiate active PIP joint flexion from a resting, hyperextension position. Soft tissue reconstructive procedures that provide a check-rein to prevent PIP joint hyperextension may be considered, including volar skin dermodesis, oblique retinacular ligament reconstruction, lateral band tenodesis,[13,45] and PIP joint flexor tenodesis.[8]
- Type II
  - In type II swan-neck deformities, active and passive PIP joint motion is limited, with the MCP joint held in extension secondary to intrinsic tightness. MCP joint arthritis may be present. Therefore, MCP joint implant arthroplasty, intrinsic release, or both should be considered in planning for this swan-neck reconstruction.
  - Intrinsic release is accomplished via a dorsal approach to the MCP joint with exposure of the lateral band and extensor hood. A 1-cm segment of lateral band with attached sagittal band fibers is excised as described by Nalebuff.[24,27] Release of the ulnar intrinsic tendon, with or without tendon transfer, may reduce the deforming force on the digit and reduce ulnar drift at the MCP joint.
  - If intrinsic release or MCP joint arthroplasty is performed, concomitant flexor tenodesis of the PIP joint may be required.
- Type III
  - Type III swan-neck deformity is characterized by decreased active and passive PIP joint flexion irrespective of MCP joint positioning. The lateral bands are adherent dorsal to the PIP joint axis of rotation and a PIP joint soft tissue contracture is often present. Reconstruction involves lateral band release and volar translocation, combined with dorsal PIP joint capsulectomy, collateral ligament release, and extensor tenolysis.[3,15,34]
- Type IV
  - There is a fixed hyperextension deformity of the PIP joint as well as destructive changes to the articular cartilage of the PIP joint.
  - Soft tissue procedures will not reliably relieve pain nor restore joint motion or function, and definitive treatment is limited to arthrodesis or implant arthroplasty.[3]

Rheumatoid Thumb

- Type I: Boutonnière deformity
  - Mild: Passively correctable MCP and interphalangeal joints
    - Soft tissue reconstruction is indicated, as this may improve function despite a high incidence of deformity recurrence.[38]
    - Synovectomy of the MCP joint combined with EPL tendon rerouting will increase the extensor moment at the

MCP joint through EPL attachment to the dorsal MCP joint capsule.[26]

- Moderate: Fixed MCP joint deformity
  - The condition of the adjacent CMC and interphalangeal joints must be considered to determine whether to proceed with MCP arthrodesis or arthroplasty. Often, treatment at this stage of disease reduces the progression of thumb deformity.
  - If the extent of interphalangeal joint involvement warrants intervention, treatment of the interphalangeal joint is limited to arthrodesis. Therefore, preservation of motion at the MCP joint may be optimal through MCP implant arthroplasty, although function after MCP and interphalangeal arthrodesis is generally good.
  - Arthroplasty of the thumb MCP joint involves resection of the involved joint surfaces and prosthetic placement, most commonly with a flexible silicone implant. Extensor reconstruction, including EPL rerouting, is considered to augment extensor forces acting at the MCP joint. Postoperatively, the thumb MCP joint is splinted in extension for 4 to 6 weeks, allowing for controlled CMC and interphalangeal joint exercises. Good functional results with minimal progression of CMC or interphalangeal joint arthritis have been reported.[11]
  - Arthrodesis of the MCP joint is accomplished by one of several methods, including tension band wire fixation, crossing Kirschner wires, a headless compression screw, or plate and screw fixation. The joint is typically placed in 15 degrees of flexion and the arthrodesis site may be augmented with bone graft as needed to maximize bone surface contact area. The arthrodesis site is protected in a splint until radiographic union is confirmed. Early interphalangeal joint range of motion is encouraged to minimize extensor adhesions and stiffness.
- Severe: Fixed deformities of MCP and interphalangeal joints
  - In this advanced stage, the treatment rationale is similar to that for moderate deformity, except that interphalangeal joint contracture or joint deterioration requires intervention. Rarely, interphalangeal joint capsular release may be indicated to improve motion, in the absence of articular deterioration. For cases involving interphalangeal joint instability or progressive arthritis, interphalangeal arthrodesis is indicated.
- Carpometacarpal joint involvement
  - As rheumatoid arthritis has the potential to involve greater numbers of joints, motion-sparing procedures of the CMC joint are preferred compared to arthrodesis.
  - While total trapezial implant arthroplasty is relatively contraindicated in the rheumatoid patient due to the higher risk for implant failure or dislocation, resection or hemi-resection arthroplasty with ligament reconstruction and soft tissue interposition arthroplasty should be considered.[33]
- Type III: Swan-neck deformity
  - Mild: Isolated CMC joint involvement
    - In the absence of symptomatic relief from conservative treatment, CMC hemi-trapeziectomy or trapeziectomy and ligament reconstruction with soft tissue interposition arthroplasty is indicated.
  - Moderate: CMC joint pathology with mild MCP joint involvement (flexible deformity)
    - For CMC joint pathology with progressive MCP joint hyperextension deformity, CMC hemi-trapeziectomy or

trapeziectomy and ligament reconstruction with soft tissue interposition arthroplasty and simultaneous MCP joint volar plate capsulodesis, sesamoidesis, or volar tenodesis are considered. Temporary transarticular pin stabilization of the MCP joint in 20 degrees of flexion for 3 to 4 weeks postoperatively permits early motion of the interphalangeal joint.

- Severe: CMC joint dislocation with metacarpal adduction contracture and fixed MCP joint hyperextension deformity
  - Treatment for this advanced stage requires:
    - CMC joint reconstruction with resection arthroplasty and ligament reconstruction or tendon interposition arthroplasty
    - Correction of the metacarpal adduction contracture
    - MCP arthrodesis
  - Often, adduction contracture of the thumb metacarpal may be adequately treated with resection of the thumb metacarpal base and release of the restraining ligaments of the CMC joint during resection arthroplasty. If the adduction contracture persists, then fasciotomy of the first dorsal interosseous and adductor muscles may be completed.[33] Web space reconstruction with Z-plasties is rarely indicated.

Preoperative Planning

- The surgeon must plan ahead. Extended procedures associated with multiple digital reconstructions or the combined treatment of multiple joints should warrant careful and efficient use of tourniquet time.
- Regional anesthesia (axillary block, IV regional) may be preferred for the reconstruction of digital deformities. This form of anesthesia may provide a greater duration of postoperative pain control and may minimize the systemic effects of general anesthesia.
  - Avoidance of general anesthesia may minimize the potential risks of cervical spine positioning in patients with cervical instability secondary to rheumatoid arthritis.
- Procedures that may require the use of bone grafting should involve preoperative discussion with the patient to explain the potential need for bone grafting and to identify potential sources for the graft (ie, iliac crest, olecranon, distal radius, allograft or synthetic bone substitutes).

Posttraumatic Injury

- A detailed history and physical examination should be performed.
- Active and passive PIP joint range of motion should be assessed. Chronic, rigid deformities may require staged procedures with surgical release of the PIP joint before subsequent reconstructive procedures.
- Radiographs should be reviewed for fractures, joint subluxation or dislocation, and degenerative joint changes.
- Adjacent joint injuries and pre-existing degenerative changes should be considered during surgical planning.

Rheumatoid Deformity

- Before surgical reconstruction of rheumatoid swan-neck or boutonnière deformities of the digits, a global assessment is completed to characterize the systemic involvement of rheumatoid disease.
  - Coordination of medical clearance and perioperative care may be pertinent for patients with medical comorbidities and for patients taking perioperative medications such as corticosteroids.

- Preoperative cervical spine evaluation may be indicated to confirm stability of the spine for safe anesthesia administration.
- Timing of rheumatoid swan-neck or boutonnière reconstruction should account for other musculoskeletal pathology as reviewed above. Postoperative protocols and anticipated prognosis for recovery should be reviewed carefully with patients to minimize potential conflicts with other medical or surgical management.

Positioning

- Surgical reconstruction of the hand is performed typically in a supine position with the upper limb placed on a well-padded hand table.
- A brachial tourniquet is used.
- Preoperative shoulder and elbow assessment will minimize potential difficulties with surgical positioning, particularly for patients with severe limitations to joint mobility or joint instability.

Approach

- Careful soft tissue handling is observed to minimize the risk of wound or soft tissue complications. Full-thickness skin flaps are raised during operative exposure.

Dorsal Approach

- A longitudinal midline or curvilinear incision from the proximal phalanx to the DIP joint provides excellent visualization of the extensor mechanism.

- Sharp dissection through the subcutaneous tissue and careful elevation of full-thickness flaps are performed to expose the central slip and lateral bands.
- Exposure of volar structures is limited with this approach but can be enhanced by extending the incision proximally and distally.
- Volarly, the Cleland ligament is divided, taking care to protect the neurovascular bundle, which is volar to the plane of dissection. The underlying PIP joint collateral ligament, PIP joint volar plate, and flexor sheath are exposed.
- A small window can be made in the membranous flexor sheath between the A2 and A4 pulleys to improve exposure of the volar plate.

Volar Approach

- Access to volar structures may be necessary to release the PIP joint. This can be accomplished via a midlateral or a Brunner incision centered at the PIP joint.
- Dissection is carried down to the flexor sheath, elevating full-thickness flaps and preserving the digital neurovascular bundles.
- Between the A2 and A4 pulleys, the membranous portion of the flexor sheath can be elevated to expose the flexor tendons and the underlying volar plate of the PIP joint.
- Arthrodesis and arthroplasty techniques are detailed in separate chapters.

TECHNIQUES

BOUTONNIÈRE RECONSTRUCTION

Primary Central Slip Repair

- Primary repair is accomplished through a dorsal approach.
- After isolating the central slip, assess the redundant tissue with the PIP joint held in full extension.
  - Excise a chevron-shaped segment of redundant fibrous tissue, permitting repair of the free tendon edges with 4-0 braided suture using a multistrand, grasping or locking repair method.
- V-Y advancement may be necessary to facilitate repair.
- In the case of an avulsion fracture, identify and carefully elevate the fragment, preserving the attachment of the central slip.
  - For smaller fragments inappropriate for Kirschner wire or screw fixation, the fragment may be excised and the central slip repaired directly into the dorsal base of the middle phalanx using a pullout suture or suture anchor method.
  - If the fracture fragment is larger, reduce the fragment anatomically and stabilize it using appropriate fixation such as small screws or two small Kirschner wires.
- The lateral bands must be restored to their anatomic location, dorsal to the axis of rotation of the PIP joint. Mobilize them by excising the triangular ligament and incising both transverse retinacular ligaments as necessary.
  - Approximate the lateral bands distal and dorsal to the PIP joint and suture them together using 4-0 nonabsorbable, braided suture.
- The repair is protected and the PIP joint is held fully extended, usually using a transarticular Kirschner wire, for 6 weeks.

Central Slip Reconstruction Using Local Tissue

- Central slip reconstruction using local tissue may be considered for patients with a flexible deformity and insufficient central slip for direct primary repair. Several methods have been described using a dorsal approach to the extensor apparatus.

Snow's Technique[32]

- Identify the proximal stump of central slip and dissect it free of the surrounding tissues.
- Elevate a distally based flap of extensor tendon sharply, preserving sufficient length to span the tendinous defect.
- Turn the flap down on itself and suture it to any distal tissue as well as the lateral bands using 4-0 braided, nonabsorbable suture.
- After repair, passive PIP joint flexion of no less than 60 degrees must be possible without excessive tension across the repair site.

Aiche's Technique[1]

- Isolate the radial and ulnar lateral bands and divide them longitudinally from the trifurcation of the extrinsic tendon to the triangular ligament.
- Mobilize the dorsal half of each lateral band dorsally and suture them together using 5-0 nonabsorbable, braided suture.
- Lateral band relocation is recommended when the lateral bands are fixed volar to the PIP joint axis of rotation.

TECHNIQUES

Littler and Eatron's Technique[17]

- Carefully isolate the radial and ulnar lateral bands.
- Incise the lateral bands over the middle phalanx. Preserve at least one ORL; otherwise, DIP joint extension will be compromised.
- Mobilize the incised lateral bands dorsally and suture them into the insertion of the central slip.
- If excessive attenuation of the central slip precludes suture stabilization, this repair method is contraindicated.

Matev's Technique[22]

- After isolating the lateral bands from the surrounding soft tissue, incise the ulnar lateral band at the level of the DIP joint and incise the radial lateral band at the midpoint of the middle phalanx.
- Suture the proximal stump of the ulnar lateral band to the distal stump of the radial lateral band over the dorsal digit, thereby lengthening the terminal slip (**TECH FIG 1**).
- Weave the proximal stump of the radial lateral band into the remnants of the central slip and suture it to the base of the middle phalanx to restore PIP joint extension.
- Postoperatively, the PIP joint is held in full extension for 6 weeks. A temporary transarticular Kirschner wire may be placed to protect the repair.

Central Slip Reconstruction Using Tendon Graft

- When a flexible deformity is present but there is insufficient local tissue for use in central slip reconstruction, a tendon graft reconstruction may be considered.

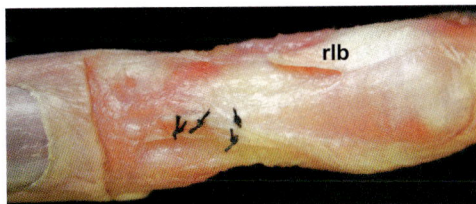

TECH FIG 1 • Boutonnière reconstruction using Matev's technique of lengthening the terminal tendon and reconstructing the central slip using the lateral bands. The ulnar lateral band is incised slightly proximal to the distal interphalangeal joint and the radial lateral band is incised more proximally, at the level of the mid-aspect of the middle phalanx. The proximal stump of the ulnar lateral band is then sutured into the distal stump of the radial lateral band as shown here. The free proximal stump of the radial lateral band (*rlb*) is then repaired into the dorsal base of the middle phalanx. (Photographs © Copyright of Fraser J. Leversedge, Charles A. Goldfarb, and Martin Boyer.)

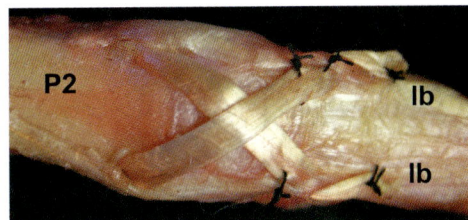

TECH FIG 2 • Boutonnière reconstruction using a tendon graft. The tendon graft is passed through a transverse osseous tunnel in the dorsal base of the middle phalanx (*P2*) and the limbs of the graft are woven into the lateral bands (*lb*). (Photographs © Copyright of Fraser J. Leversedge, Charles A. Goldfarb, and Martin Boyer.)

- Expose the extensor mechanism via a dorsal, curvilinear incision. Identify the proximal stump of the central slip and isolate it from the surrounding tissues.
- Harvest an autologous tendon graft, preferably the ipsilateral palmaris longus tendon (if present).
- Create a transverse bone tunnel through the dorsal base of the middle phalanx.
- Pass the palmaris longus tendon through the bone tunnel and weave the two limbs into the lateral bands with the digit held in neutral (**TECH FIG 2**).
- The repair is protected for 6 weeks by maintaining PIP joint extension with a transarticular Kirschner wire.

Extensor Tenotomy

- Hyperextension deformity of the DIP joint may be addressed with extensor tenotomy.[23]
- Tenotomy is indicated in the presence of mild, flexible deformities and for patients who have failed prior surgery directed at the PIP joint.
- Extensor tenotomy may be considered as an adjunct to PIP joint arthrodesis performed for chronic boutonnière deformity with associated PIP joint arthritis.
- Make a dorsal incision over the distal two thirds of the middle phalanx.
- Identify the terminal tendon and elevate it proximally over a distance of 1.5 cm from the underlying phalanx and DIP joint.
- Incise the terminal tendon distal to the triangular ligament.
- Preserve the radial ORL so that DIP joint extension is not compromised.
- Passively extend the PIP joint and passively flex the DIP joint to separate the incised tendon ends.

SWAN-NECK RECONSTRUCTION

Oblique Retinacular Ligament Reconstruction[16,39]

- Reconstruction of the ORL is indicated when a flexible swan-neck deformity develops secondary to an untreated mallet finger. This procedure is suited for patients with a well-preserved DIP joint.

- Make an incision from the ulnar margin of the MCP joint flexion crease and continue it volarly and distally along the radial midaxial line before curving it dorsally to end over the DIP joint.
- Isolate the radial neurovascular bundle from the surrounding tissue. Proximally, identify the A2 pulley. Distally, identify the terminal slip.

TECHNIQUES

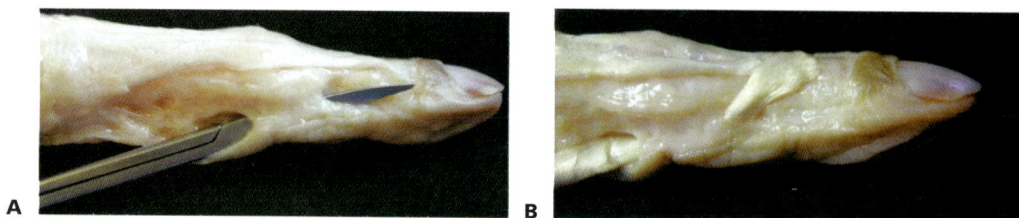

TECH FIG 3 • A. Oblique retinacular ligament reconstruction. The scissors illustrate the anatomic plane of dissection for the passage of a tendon graft for reconstruction. The plane extends from the A2 pulley volarly to the dorsal surface of the terminal extensor tendon. **B.** The palmaris tendon graft has been inserted, coursing from volar to the Cleland ligament to be secured to the dorsal aspect of the terminal extensor tendon insertion. The neurovascular bundle is carefully protected. (Photographs © Copyright of Fraser J. Leversedge, Charles A. Goldfarb, and Martin Boyer.)

- Harvest the ipsilateral palmaris longus tendon using a tendon stripper through a 1-cm transverse incision proximal to the wrist crease.
    - Alternatively, make a second transverse incision proximally, overlying the musculotendinous junction. Confirm the inserting muscular fibers at the musculotendinous junction before tendon harvest. If the palmaris longus is not present, obtain another suitable autologous tendon graft.
- The DIP joint is held in full extension and the PIP joint is held in 25 degrees of flexion with transarticular Kirschner wires.
- Suture the tendon graft to the terminal slip using nonabsorbable, braided suture.
- Pass the graft deep to the radial neurovascular bundle and bring it to the volar surface of the digit. Suture it to the distal edge of the A2 pulley after tensioning the graft appropriately (**TECH FIG 3**).

Proximal Interphalangeal Joint Flexor Tenodesis

- Creation of a check-rein to PIP joint hyperextension can be accomplished by PIP joint flexor tenodesis or by lateral band tenodesis (described below).
- Via a Brunner or midaxial incision, elevate full-thickness skin flaps to expose the digital flexor sheath, protecting the digital neurovascular bundles.
- Raise as a flap the membranous portion of the flexor sheath, from the distal aspect of the A2 pulley to the proximal edge of the A4 pulley, to expose the underlying flexor tendons.
- Identify one slip of the FDS tendon and divide it proximally at the level of the decussation, leaving its insertion into the base of the middle phalanx intact (**TECH FIG 4A,B**).
- Pass the divided tendon end from dorsal to volar through a transverse incision in the A2 pulley, about

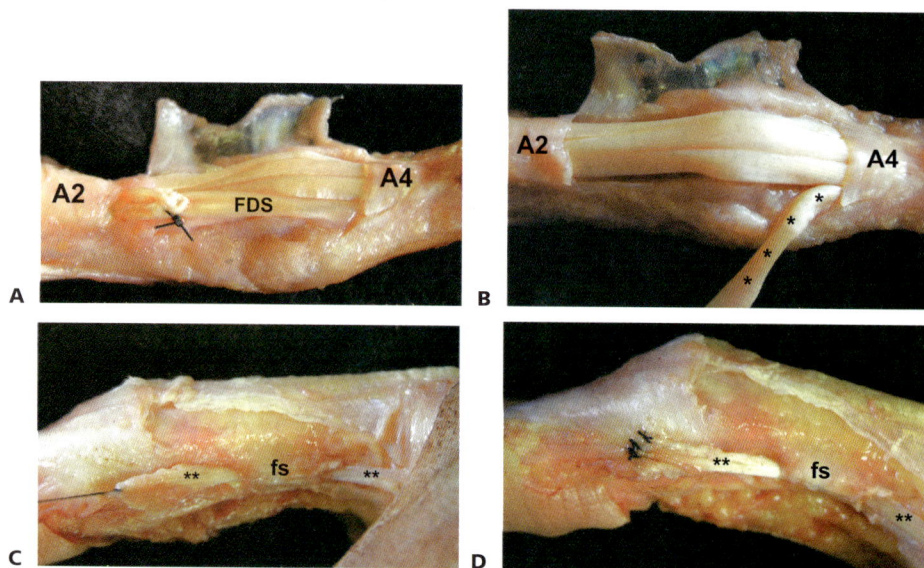

TECH FIG 4 • A. Proximal interphalangeal (PIP) joint flexor tenodesis with exposure of the flexor tendons between the A2 pulley and the A4 pulley. One slip of the flexor digitorum superficialis (*FDS*) tendon is divided at the level of the decussation, leaving its insertion intact. **B.** The harvested FDS tendon (****) is brought through an opening created in the distal aspect of the A2 pulley to be repaired to itself with the PIP joint held in 20 degrees of flexion. **C, D.** Lateral band tenodesis to provide a check-rein to PIP joint hyperextension. The lateral band (**) has been detached distally (**C**) and has been rerouted within the flexor sheath (*fs*) before repair distally (**D**). (Photographs © Copyright of Fraser J. Leversedge, Charles A. Goldfarb, and Martin Boyer.)

- 3 mm from the pulley's distal margin, and suture it back onto itself with the PIP joint held in about 20 degrees of flexion (**TECH FIG 4C,D**).
- Postoperative immobilization with a dorsal block splint maintains the joint in more than 20 degrees of flexion for 6 weeks. Flexion exercises for the PIP and DIP joints are started at 3 weeks postoperatively.

Lateral Band Tenodesis[42,45]

- The lateral band is rerouted so that it lies volar to the PIP joint axis of rotation and forms a restraint to PIP hyperextension.
- Approach the extensor apparatus via a dorsal curvilinear incision. Expose the Cleland ligament and divide it to access the flexor sheath with preservation of the digital neurovascular bundles.
- Leaving its proximal and distal attachments intact, dissect the dorsally subluxated lateral band free from the central slip and from its distal attachment to the triangular ligament overlying the base of the middle phalanx. Translocate the lateral band volar to the PIP joint axis of rotation, assisted by flexion of the PIP joint.
- At the level of the PIP joint, elevate a dorsally based flap of the flexor sheath 0.5 to 1 cm wide and place the mobilized lateral band volar to the flap. Repair the flap to its anatomic position, restraining the lateral band as an effective pulley.
- Alternatively, the lateral band may be detached from its insertion into the terminal tendon slip and rerouted within a roughly 0.5- to 1-cm segment of the flexor sheath at the A2 pulley before repairing it to the terminal tendon distally (Tech Fig 4A,B).
  - Confirm unimpeded gliding of the lateral band beneath the flexor sheath by gentle proximal and distal traction on the translocated lateral band.[45]

- Postoperatively, a dorsal block splint maintains the joint in more than 30 degrees of flexion. Digital flexion exercises are encouraged early in the postoperative period. Full active PIP joint extension is not allowed for 6 weeks.

Type III Swan-Neck Reconstruction

- Reconstruction of a type III swan-neck deformity must address the fixed translocation of the lateral bands dorsal to the PIP joint rotation axis and the associated PIP joint soft tissue contracture.
- Management of these pathologic changes includes lateral band release from the central tendon and from the triangular ligament; translocation of the lateral bands to a position volar to the PIP joint rotation axis; dorsal PIP joint contracture release, with dorsal capsulectomy and collateral ligament release; extensor tenolysis of the digit; and possible limited flexor tenolysis, as indicated, for flexor tenosynovitis.
- Via a dorsal curvilinear incision, raise full-thickness skin flaps to expose the underlying extensor apparatus.
- Release the lateral bands along their dorsal attachment to the central tendon, from the proximal phalanx to their confluence over the dorsal aspect of the middle phalanx.
- Complete a dorsal PIP joint capsulectomy and gradually release the radial and ulnar collateral ligaments, from dorsal to volar, until the PIP joint can be passively flexed to 90 degrees.
- Because the mobile lateral bands will passively translate volar to the PIP joint axis of rotation with passive joint flexion, the lateral bands do not require stabilization.
- After soft tissue releases, the PIP joint is stabilized in 20 degrees of flexion with a temporary transarticular Kirschner wire. The digital reconstructions are protected in a forearm-based splint, removed to permit MCP and DIP joint motion. The wire is removed 2 to 3 weeks postoperatively.

PEARLS AND PITFALLS

Patient selection	■ The PIP joint should be assessed for flexibility. ■ Reconstructive options are limited in the presence of PIP joint degenerative changes. Arthrodesis may be the only practical solution. ■ Assess for intrinsic tightness in all patients with digital deformity. ■ In rheumatoid patients, carefully evaluate the wrist and MCP joint before surgical reconstruction of the interphalangeal joints. ■ Tendon ruptures may not be clinically apparent in rheumatoid patients with severe deformity.
Boutonnière deformity	■ The deformity develops from injury to the central slip. ■ Delayed development of the deformity may occur after injury to the central slip. ■ Early diagnosis is important. The Elson test is useful in confirming early diagnosis. ■ Extension splinting is effective treatment in those who present within 2 to 3 months from the time of injury. A transarticular Kirschner wire holding the PIP joint in extension may serve as an effective internal splint. ■ It is important to differentiate boutonnière deformity from PIP joint contracture (pseudo-boutonnière deformity).
Swan-neck reconstruction	■ In rheumatoid patients a swan-neck deformity can arise from any of the MCP, PIP, or DIP joints. It is critical to identify which type of deformity is present in order to guide treatment.
Thumb CMC reconstruction	■ Implant interposition arthroplasty may have an increased failure rate due to poor soft tissue restraints and an increased risk of implant dislocation.
PIP joint implant arthroplasty	■ Avoid implant arthroplasty in patients with a severe PIP joint flexion contracture (more than 45 to 50 degrees). ■ Consider arthrodesis for the index PIP joint due to lateral stresses on the joint with pinch.

TECHNIQUES

- A volar approach, in the absence of extensor tendon attenuation, may preserve the extensor mechanism and minimize perioperative adhesions and stiffness.
- Care should be observed with implant broaching to reduce the risk of implant instability or iatrogenic fracture.

OUTCOMES

Traumatic Deformity Reconstruction

- Surgery for established boutonnière and swan-neck deformities is technically challenging.
- A variety of surgical options exist; there is little consensus regarding a preferred technique.
- There are relatively few studies evaluating the long-term results after surgery for posttraumatic boutonnière and swan-neck deformities. Direct comparisons may be difficult due to the variations in clinical stage at the time of presentation.

Boutonnière Deformity

- Towfigh and Gruber[43] reported on the results of surgical treatment of 114 flexible posttraumatic boutonnière deformities. The central slip was repaired directly, with local tissue, or reconstructed with a tendon graft. Follow-up averaged 40 months. Seventy-eight patients report good or excellent results. Satisfactory results were observed in 22 patients and poor results in 14 patients.
- Meadows et al[23] reported on the results of extensor tenotomy performed on 14 fingers with posttraumatic boutonnière deformity. The average preoperative PIP joint flexion contracture was 36 degrees. All the digits had DIP joint extension contractures with an average arc of motion from 6.5 degrees of hyperextension to 4.2 degrees of flexion. Postoperatively, DIP flexion improved to 44 degrees. Ten of the digits had an extension lag averaging 13 degrees. Seven digits had improved extension at the PIP joint by an average of 27 degrees.

Swan-Neck Deformity

- Tonkin et al[42] reported outcomes of lateral band tenodesis for swan-neck deformity. Thirty digits with swan-neck deformity of various causes were included. Preoperative PIP joint deformity averaged 16 degrees of hyperextension; this was improved to 11 degrees of flexion postoperatively.
- Reconstruction of the oblique retinacular ligament was first described by Thompson et al.[39] They reported improvement in PIP joint hyperextension and DIP joint flexion with this technique. Kleinman and Peterson[16] described similar results with reliable correction of DIP joint flexion and secondary PIP joint hyperextension.

Rheumatoid Deformity Reconstruction

- There is a relative lack of clinical outcomes studies evaluating the long-term results of surgical management for swan-neck and boutonnière deformities in patients with rheumatoid arthritis.
- Kiefhaber and Strickland[15] reported on the results of surgical treatment for type III swan-neck and stage II boutonnière deformities. In 92 patients undergoing lateral band release, extensor tenolysis, and PIP joint dorsal capsulectomy for type III swan-neck deformity, the authors reported an initial increase of 55 degrees flexion at the PIP joint; however, of 15 fingers assessed at 3 and 12 months postoperatively, there was a 17-degree loss of the early postoperative motion gains. Despite this deterioration

of postoperative results, the arc of PIP motion shifted toward flexion, improving functional grasp.

- In 19 patients undergoing central slip reconstruction for stage II boutonnière deformity, the authors found unpredictable results and reported that the deterioration of postoperative correction was greater with time. Four of 19 patients were able to extend the PIP joint beyond 20 degrees of flexion and 11 of 19 patients had a PIP joint extension deficit of greater than 45 degrees.
- Tonkin et al published two separate studies assessing the outcomes of treatment for swan-neck deformities with lateral band translocation[42] and with synovectomy and lateral band release and translocation.[41] While these studies are limited in their conclusions because of the varying stages of disease and their small patient populations, the trend toward positioning the arc of motion into flexion was observed, similar to the study results of Kiefhaber and Strickland.[15]
- Several long-term clinical outcomes studies of PIP and MCP joint implant arthroplasties have demonstrated poor correction of preoperative swan-neck or boutonnière deformities and in general have reported poorer results with respect to pain relief and range-of-motion recovery as compared to arthroplasties done for conditions of osteoarthritis or posttraumatic arthritis.[6,35,36]
- A review of surgical treatment of varying stages of thumb boutonnière deformity by Terrono et al[38] concluded that MCP joint synovectomy and EPL rerouting for early, correctable boutonnière deformity had a high rate of deformity recurrence (64%). The authors recommend MCP joint arthrodesis for cases of moderate severity with isolated joint involvement, but in severe cases, MCP joint arthroplasty and interphalangeal arthrodesis is considered.

COMPLICATIONS

- Perioperative complications in the treatment of posttraumatic boutonnière and swan-neck deformities can be avoided by careful patient selection, appropriate intervention, and adherence to proper surgical technique.
  - Thorough perioperative patient counseling and education is imperative to avoid unrealistic patient expectations and unanticipated outcomes.
- A successful operative result and the avoidance of perioperative complications in the treatment of a boutonnière or swan-neck deformity in the rheumatoid hand is largely dependent on a thorough preoperative evaluation, correct staging of the pathologic condition, and appropriate timing of operative intervention. While the goals of reducing pain and improving function are primary, patient education is critical for avoiding unrealistic expectations and unanticipated results.

REFERENCES

1. Aiche A, Barsky AJ, Weiner DL. Prevention of boutonniere deformity. Plast Reconst Surg 1970;46:164–167.
2. Arnett FC, Edworthy SM, Bloch DA, et al. The American Rheumatism Association 1987 revised criteria for classification of rheumatoid arthritis. Arthritis Rheum 1988;31:315–324.

3. Boyer MI, Gelberman RH. Operative correction of swan-neck and boutonniere deformities in the rheumatoid hand. J Am Acad Orthop Surg 1999;7:92–100.

4. Burton RI, Melchior JA. Extensor tendons: late reconstruction. In: Green DP, Hotchkiss RN, Pederson WC, eds. Green's Operative Hand Surgery, 4th ed. New York: Churchill Livingstone, 1999: 215–221.

5. Carducci T. Potential boutonniere deformity: its recognition and treatment. Orthopaedic Review 1981;10:121–123.

6. Cook SD, Beckenbaugh RD, Redondo J, et al. Long-term follow-up of pyrolytic carbon metacarpophalangeal implants. J Bone Joint Surg Am 1999;81A:635–648.

7. Coons MS, Green SM. Boutonniere deformity. Hand Clin 1995;11: 387–402.

8. Curtis R. Sublimis tenodesis. In: Edmonson AS, Crenshaw AH, eds. Campbell's Operative Orthopaedics, 6th ed. St. Louis: CV Mosby, 1980:319.

9. Eberhardt K, Johnson PM, Rydgren L. The occurrence and significance of hand deformities in early rheumatoid arthritis. Br J Rheumatol 1991;30:211–213.

10. Ferlic DC. Boutonniere deformities in rheumatoid arthritis. Hand Clin 1989;5:215–222.

11. Figgie MP, Inglis AE, Sobel M, et al. Metacarpal phalangeal joint arthroplasty of the rheumatoid thumb. J Hand Surg Am 1990;15A: 210–216.

12. Flatt AE. The Care of the Arthritic Hand. St. Louis: Quality Medical Publishing, 1995:263–264.

13. Gainor BJ, Hummel GL. Correction of rheumatoid swan-neck deformity by lateral band mobilization. J Hand Surg Am 1985;10A: 370–377.

14. Harris ED Jr. Rheumatoid arthritis: pathophysiology and implications for therapy. N Engl J Med 1990;18:1277–1289.

15. Kiefhaber TR, Strickland JW. Soft tissue reconstruction for rheumatoid swan-neck and boutonniere deformities: long-term results. J Hand Surg Am 1993;18A:984–989.

16. Kleinman WB, Peterson DP. Oblique retinacular ligament reconstruction for chronic mallet finger deformity. J Hand Surg Am 1984;9A: 399–404.

17. Littler JW, Eatron RG. Redistribution of forces in correction of boutonniere deformity. J Bone Joint Surg Am 1967;49A:1267–1274.

18. Lovett WL, McCalla MA. Management and rehabilitation of extensor tendon injuries. Orthop Clin North Am 1983;14:811–826.

19. Mannerfelt LG, Norman O. Attrition ruptures of flexor tendons in rheumatoid arthritis caused by bony spurs in the carpal tunnel: a clinical and radiological study. J Bone Joint Surg Br 1969;51B: 270–277.

20. Mannerfelt LG, Oetker R, Ostlunel B, et al. Rupture of the extensor pollicis longus tendon after Colles' fracture and by rheumatoid arthritis. J Hand Surg Br 1990;15B:49–50.

21. Massengill JB. The boutonniere deformity. Hand Clin 1992;8: 787–801.

22. Matev I. Transposition of the lateral slips of the aponeurosis in treatment of long-standing "boutonniere deformity" of the fingers. Br J Plast Surg 1964;17:281–286.

23. Meadows SE, Schneider LH, Sherwyn JH. Treatment of the chronic boutonniere deformity by extensor tenotomy. Hand Clin 1995;11: 441–447.

24. Nalebuff EA. The rheumatoid swan-neck deformity. Hand Clin 1989;5:203–214.

25. Nalebuff EA. The rheumatoid thumb. Clin Rheum Dis 1984;10: 589–607.

26. Nalebuff EA. Diagnosis, classification and management of rheumatoid thumb deformities. Bull Hosp Joint Dis 1968;29:119–137.

27. Nalebuff EA, Millender LH. Surgical treatment of the boutonniere deformity in rheumatoid arthritis. Orthop Clin North Am 1975;6:753–763.

28. O'Brien ET. Surgical principles and planning for the rheumatoid hand and wrist. Clin Plast Surg 1996;23:407–420.

29. Ratliff AHC. Deformities of the thumb in rheumatoid arthritis. Hand 1971;3:138–143.

30. Rizio L, Belsky MR. Finger deformities in rheumatoid arthritis. In: Ruby LK, Cassidy C, eds. Rheumatoid Arthritis of the Hand and Wrist. Hand Clin 1996;12:531–540.

31. Rubin J, Bozentha DJ, Bora FW. Diagnosis of closed central-slip injuries. J Hand Surg Br 1996;21B:614–616.

32. Snow JW. Use of a retrograde tendon flap in repairing a severed extensor at the PIP joint area. Plast Reconstr Surg 1973;51:555–558.

33. Stein AB, Terrono AL. The rheumatoid thumb. In: Ruby LK, Cassidy C, eds. Rheumatoid Arthritis of the Hand and Wrist. Hand Clin 1996;12:541–550.

34. Strickland JW, Boyer M. Swan neck deformity. In: Strickland JW, ed. The Hand. Master Techniques in Orthopaedic Surgery series. Philadelphia: Lippincott-Raven, 1998:459–470.

35. Swanson AB, Maupin BK, Gajjar NV, et al. Flexible implant arthroplasty in the proximal interphalangeal joint in the hand. J Hand Surg Am 1985;10A:796–805.

36. Takigawa S, Meletiou S, Sauerbier M, et al. Long-term assessment of Swanson implant arthroplasty in the proximal interphalangeal joint of the hand. J Hand Surg Am 2004;29A:785–795.

37. Terrono A, Millender L. Surgical treatment of the boutonniere rheumatoid thumb deformity. Hand Clin 1989;5:239–248.

38. Terrono A, Millender L, Nalebuff E. Boutonniere rheumatoid thumb deformity. J Hand Surg Am 1990;15A:999–1003.

39. Thompson JS, Littler JW, Upton J. The spiral oblique retinacular ligament (SORL). J Hand Surg Am 1978;3A:482–487.

40. Toledano B, Terrono A, Millender L. Reconstruction of the rheumatoid thumb. Hand Clin 1992;8:121–129.

41. Tonkin MA, Gianoutsos MP, Ryan D, et al. Synovectomy, joint release and lateral band translocation for stiff swan neck deformity. Hand Surg 1996;1:69–74.

42. Tonkin MA, Hughes J, Smith KL. Lateral band translocation for swan-neck deformity. J Hand Surg Am 1992;17A:260–267.

43. Towfigh H, Gruber P. Surgical treatment of the boutonniere deformity. Oper Orthop Traumatol 2005;17:66–78.

44. Urbaniak JR, Hayes MG. Chronic boutonniere deformity: an anatomic reconstruction. J Hand Surg Am 1981;6A:379–383.

45. Zancolli E. Structural and Dynamic Bases of Hand Surgery, 2nd ed. Philadelphia: JB Lippincott, 1979.

Chapter 63

Open Treatment of Medial Epicondylitis

Joseph E. Robison and Peter J. Evans

DEFINITION

- Medial epicondylitis involves tendinosis at the origin of the flexor–pronator mass.
- It is commonly referred to as "golfer's elbow," although there is a stronger association with racquet sports and manual labor.[4]

ANATOMY

- The common flexor–pronator origin is primarily on the anterior aspect of the medial epicondyle.
- The common flexor–pronator origin includes the humeral head of the pronator teres, the flexor carpi radialis (FCR), the flexor carpi ulnaris, and a small portion of the flexor digitorum superficialis.
- The palmaris longus also shares the origin, although this is not likely to be clinically relevant.

PATHOGENESIS

- Epicondylitis results from repetitive microtrauma followed by an incomplete reparative response that results in tendinosis, a pathologic state in which the degenerate tendon cannot heal itself effectively.
- Epicondylitis can be seen with medial collateral ligament instability whereby myotendinous overload occurs in an attempt to dynamically stabilize the ulnohumeral joint. In this scenario, ulnar neuropathy often is part of a trio of pathology.

NATURAL HISTORY

- Most patients improve with conservative treatment.
- However, a greater percentage of patients with medial epicondylitis go on to surgical treatment when compared to patients with lateral epicondylitis.[3]

PATIENT HISTORY AND PHYSICAL FINDINGS

- Patients commonly complain of forearm pain rather than elbow pain. At times the inflammation is significant enough to cause irritation of the ulnar nerve as it enters the flexor carpi ulnaris, causing ulnar nerve symptoms (eg, local irritability and distal numbness and tingling).
- Onset usually is insidious, but the patient may recall an inciting event.
- Medial epicondylitis can be present simultaneously with lateral epicondylitis.
- Examination methods include the following:
  - Palpation of the medial epicondyle for tenderness, a universal finding in medial epicondylitis
  - Resisted pronation is highly sensitive for medial epicondylitis.[1]
  - A decreased ROM suggests intra-articular pathology such as arthritis.

- If resisted wrist flexion reproduced symptoms, it supports a diagnosis of medial epicondylitis.
- Tap the ulnar nerve in the cubital tunnel and along its path into the ECU. Presence of a tingling sensation locally prompts further nerve investigation.

  Flex patient's elbow maximally, then compress the ulnar nerve just proximal to the cubital tunnel. Presence of hand numbness or tingling prompts further nerve investigation.

IMAGING AND OTHER DIAGNOSTIC STUDIES

- Plain radiographs may show calcifications at the flexor-pronator origin.
- MRI will reliably demonstrate increased intratendon signal on T2-weighted sequences. Most will also show increased intratendon signal and/or tendon thickening on T1-weighted sequences.
  - A small percentage of patients may show increased T2 signal in the medial epicondyle or anconeus edema.[2]
  - Periosteal reaction is *not* commonly seen on MRI.[2]
- Electrophysiologic testing (electromyography and nerve conduction studies) are warranted if patients have ulnar nerve symptoms, but with mild ulnar neuropathy these tests have a very low sensitivity.

DIFFERENTIAL DIAGNOSIS

- Pronator syndrome
- Medial collateral ligament injury
- Ulnar neuropathy
- Arthritis
- Cervical radiculopathy
- Malingering

NONOPERATIVE MANAGEMENT

- Appropriate initial treatment includes avoidance of painful activities and symptomatic relief with nonsteroidal anti-inflammatory drugs and ice.
- Daytime wrist bracing for exertional activities
- Physical or occupational therapy to supervise and instruct on stretching and strengthening protocol for patients not otherwise inclined to comply with those instructions
- Although corticosteroid injection at the medial epicondyle has been shown to provide temporary symptomatic relief, it does not affect the natural history.[5] Repeat injections should be avoided to avoid tendon weakening and rupture.
  - Ulnar nerve injury has been reported with injection, so careful attention should be paid to the location of the nerve and whether or not it is subluxed.

SURGICAL MANAGEMENT

- A minority of patients fail nonoperative management.
- Careful patient selection will ensure an excellent outcome with surgical management.

Preoperative Planning

■ Be prepared to address concurrent ulnar nerve pathology. If necessary, ulnar nerve decompression should be performed in situ, using subcutaneous or submuscular transposition.

■ In thin patients, and especially those who have lifestyles in which the inner elbow is struck frequently, we prefer submuscular transposition with flexor pronator lengthening, which definitively treats epicondylitis as well.

■ Be prepared to address flexor pronator tears or avulsion. These typically will present more abruptly, with acute or chronic pain, ecchymosis, and swelling.

■ It will be necessary to débride the ruptured degenerative tissue (**FIG 1**) and repair it by retensioning it close to the origin and closing the gap with healthier medial and lateral portions of the flexor pronator origin down to the medial epicondyle (as shown in Tech Fig 2D).

Positioning

■ The patient is placed in the supine position.

■ The arm is externally rotated at the shoulder and padding is placed under the elbow.

■ The arm should rest in a position allowing ready access to the medial aspect of the elbow without requiring constant holding by an assistant.

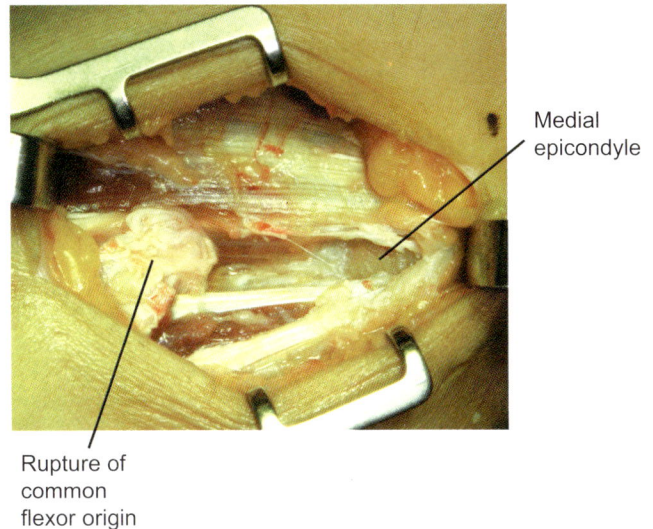

FIG 1 • The common flexors can be seen ruptured and retracted distal to the medial epicondyle.

Approach

■ The elbow should be examined after the administration of anesthesia to ensure stability, and the result documented in the operative note.

■ The goal of surgery is to débride the degenerative tissue at the flexor–pronator origin and create an environment conducive to proper healing of the tendon.

MEDIAL EPICONDYLAR FASCIECTOMY AND PARTIAL OSTECTOMY

Incision and Dissection

■ A 3- to 5-cm incision through the skin only is made beginning just proximal to and in the center of the medial epicondyle and extending distally along the axis of the forearm (**TECH FIG 1A**).

■ Blunt dissection with scissors is carried through the subcutaneous tissues, taking care to preserve medial antebrachial cutaneous nerve branches, which commonly cross the field (**TECH FIG 1B**).

■ The subcutaneous tissues are gently swept away, exposing the fascia of the flexor–pronator mass.

■ The ulnar nerve is palpated, and the elbow is put through a range of motion to check for ulnar nerve subluxation. The result is documented in the operative note.

■ The fascia overlying the interval between the pronator and FCR is then incised in line with the fibers to expose the tendon origin (**TECH FIG 1C**). The exact location can be altered depending on clinical examination and the point of maximal tenderness.

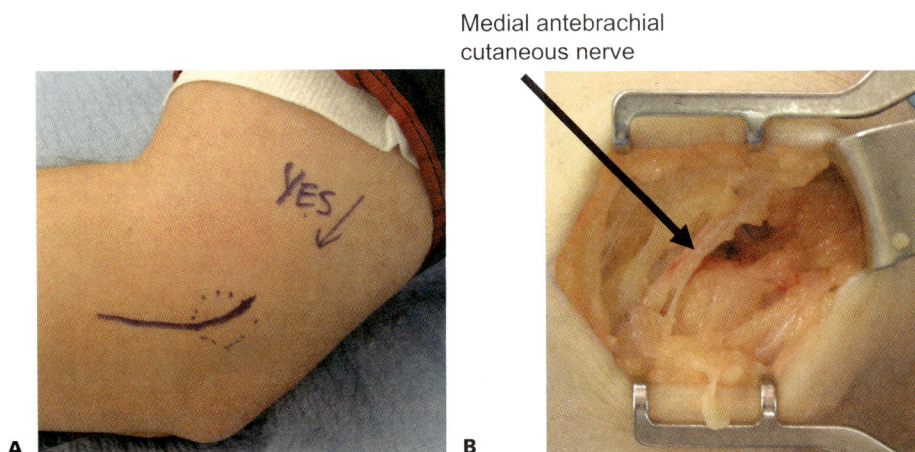

TECH FIG 1 • **A.** A 3- to 5-cm incision is started just proximal to the medial epicondyle. **B.** The medial antebrachial cutaneous nerve is identified and protected. *(continued)*

TECHNIQUES

TECHNIQUES

C

D

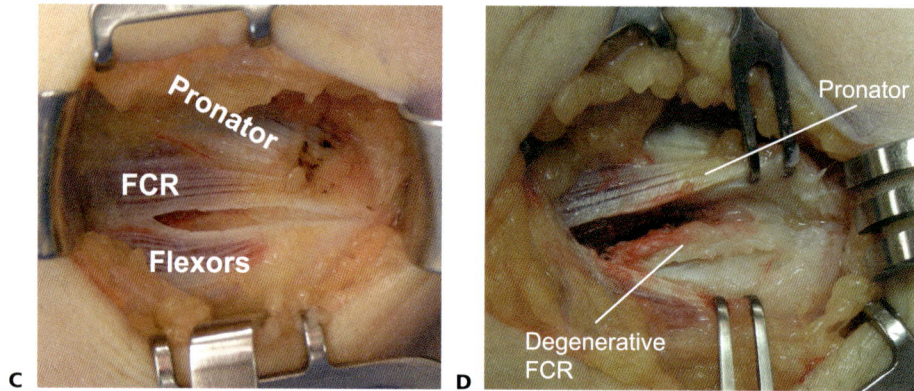

TECH FIG 1 • *(continued)* **C.** The interval between the FCR and common flexors is used and split in line with the fibers. **D.** The FCR is elevated, and the deeper degenerative tendon of the FCR and pronator is identified.

- The pronator is reflected anteriorly and the FCR posteriorly, exposing the abnormal, deeper tendon tissue (**TECH FIG 1D**).

Fasciectomy and Partial Ostectomy

- The abnormal tissue is excised. It can be identified by its grayish, unorganized mucoid appearance. Abnormal tissue will scrape away with a no. 15 blade, but normal tendon will remain attached (ie, Nirschl scratch test).
- The pathologic tissue is débrided to margins showing an organized, tendinous appearance.

- The area of excision usually is 1 to 1.5 cm long and 3 to 5 mm wide (**TECH FIG 2A**).
- A rongeur is used to roughen the anterior portion of the medial epicondyle to a bleeding surface without removing cortical bone (**TECH FIG 2B,C**).
- The defect in the tendon is closed with a running absorbable suture, using 0 or 1-0 suture material with a tapered needle (**TECH FIG 2D**).
- The subdermal layer is closed with buried, interrupted absorbable sutures, followed by a subcuticular skin closure and Steri-strips (**TECH FIG 2E**).

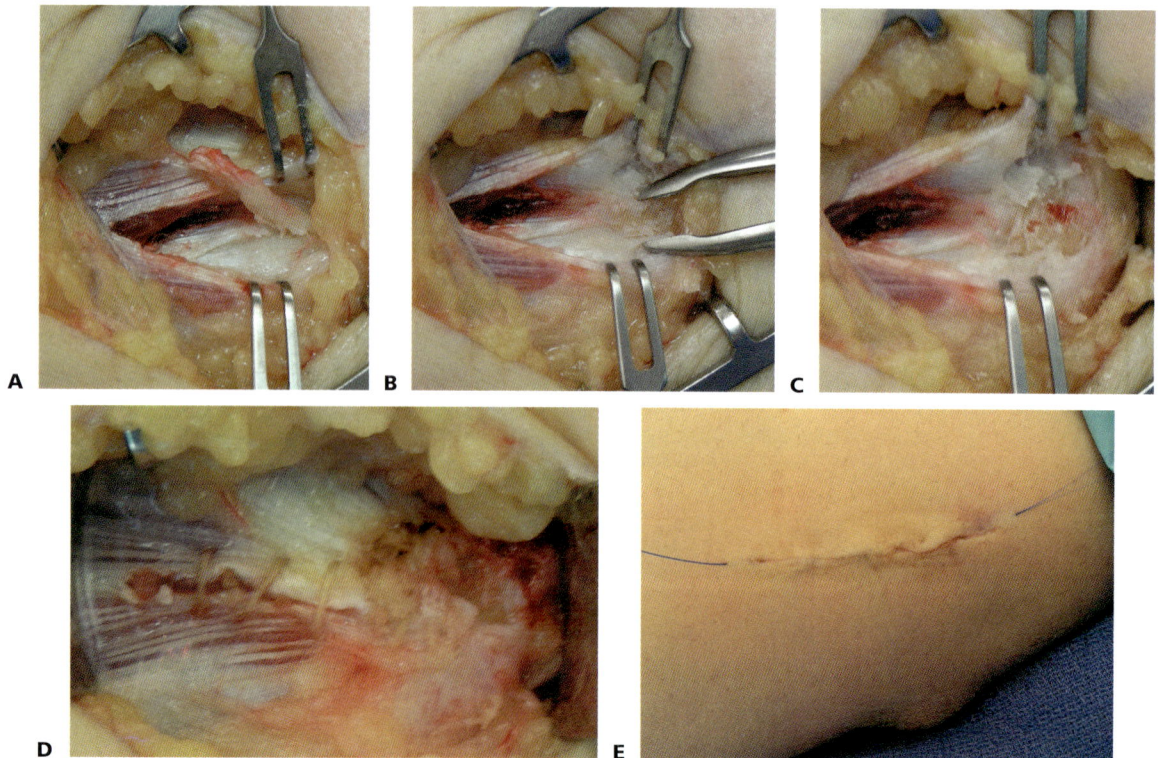

A

B

C

D

E

TECH FIG 2 • **A.** Degenerative tissue is excised. The remaining healthy tendon is stable and cannot be scraped away with a no. 15 blade. **B.** The anterior portion of the medial epicondyle is scraped or rongeured to remove any remaining degenerative tendon. **C.** The bony cortex is not violated, however. **D.** The muscle interval is closed with a running size 0 Vicryl suture and tied with inverted knots. **E.** Skin closure is done with a running 3-0 Prolene suture.

PEARLS AND PITFALLS

Indications	■ A minimum of 3 to 6 months of symptoms and failed nonoperative management
Coexisting conditions	■ Ulnar nerve irritation, neuropathy, and subluxation may require decompression and anterior transposition. ■ Flexor tendon origin rupture may require débridement and repair.
Failure to fully excise devitalized tendon	■ This will result in a poor result or recurrence; the rehabilitation protocol can be delayed in cases that require more significant débridement.
Injury to the medial collateral ligament	■ The ligament is deep to the tendon and lies on the anterior capsule, more posterior than the area of tendinosis, and can be distinguished from the rougher tendon origin.

POSTOPERATIVE CARE

■ Postoperatively, the patient is placed in a soft dressing and a removable cock-up wrist brace.

■ The elbow is not immobilized, and gentle ROM is allowed immediately.

■ The dressing is removed in 3 to 5 days. The patient may perform activities of daily living as tolerated with the wrist brace, removing the wrist brace several times daily for ROM.

■ Exertion is avoided.

■ A strengthening program is initiated in 6 weeks with a counterforce brace.

■ All restrictions are removed at 3 months, but impact activities are not allowed until 4 to 6 months postoperatively. Return of full, pain-free activity can take 6 to 24 months.

OUTCOMES

■ Over 85% of all patients will have return to full activities with no pain or only mild, occasional pain. Among high-level athletes, 75% to 85% will return to their previous level. In patients with mild or no ulnar nerve symptoms, the success rate is greater than 95%.[1,6]

■ In patients with more than moderate ulnar nerve symptoms, there is a trend toward less favorable and less predictable outcomes, although a satisfactory result still is possible.

■ It is uncommon for a patient to have absolutely no improvement in pain after surgery, even if the subjective outcome is unsatisfactory. Such a result should prompt consideration of incorrect diagnosis or the possibility of secondary gain issues.

COMPLICATIONS

■ Medial antebrachial cutaneous nerve injury
■ Grip weakness
■ Weakness with wrist flexion or pronation
■ Hematoma
■ Infection
■ Ulnar nerve injury
■ Medial collateral ligament injury

REFERENCES

1. Gabel GT, Morrey BF. Operative treatment of medial epicondylitis. Influence of concomitant ulnar neuropathy at the elbow. J Bone Joint Surg Am 1995;77A:1065–1069.
2. Martin CE, Schweitzer ME. MR imaging of epicondylitis. Skeletal Radiol 1998;27:133–138.
3. O'Dwyer KJ, Howie CR. Medial epicondylitis of the elbow. Int Orthop 1995;19:69–71.
4. Ollivierre CO, Nirschl RP, Pettrone FA. Resection and repair for medial tennis elbow: A prospective analysis. Am J Sports Med 1995;23:214–221.
5. Stahl S, Kaufman T. The efficacy of an injection of steroids for medial epicondylitis: A prospective study of sixty elbows. J Bone Joint Surg Am 1997;79:1648–1652.
6. Vangsness CT Jr, Jobe FW. Surgical treatment of medial epicondylitis: Results in 35 elbows. J Bone Joint Surg Br 1991;73:409–411.

Chapter 64

Open and Arthroscopic Treatment of Lateral Epicondylitis

Peter J. Evans

DEFINITION

- Lateral epicondylitis involves tendinosis at the origin of the common wrist extensors.
- It is commonly referred to as "tennis elbow" and is likely more correctly termed "lateral elbow tendinopathy."[6]

ANATOMY

- The common extensor origin is located on the lateral epicondyle.
- The common extensor origin includes the extensor carpi radialis brevis (ECRB), extensor digitorum communis (EDC), extensor digiti minimi, and extensor carpi ulnaris.
- The ECRB is the primary muscle–tendon unit affected, followed by the EDC, but an isolated origin does not exist.[1]

PATHOGENESIS

- Epicondylitis results from repetitive microtrauma followed by an incomplete reparative response, resulting in chronic tendinosis.[5]
- Functionally, this condition can more correctly be described as "gripper's elbow," as synergistic wrist extension increases finger flexion strength. Patients afflicted with lateral epicondylar tendinopathy commonly engage in repetitive forceful gripping activities as they lift, pull, twist, and push objects.

NATURAL HISTORY

- Lateral epicondylitis is a self-limiting condition that resolves in over 80% of patients over the course of 1 year.[2]
- Most patients receiving active treatment (eg, anti-inflammatory medication, orthotics, ultrasound, physical or occupational therapy, injections) improve with nonoperative treatment.
- Typically, fewer than 10% of patients require surgical intervention.

PATIENT HISTORY AND PHYSICAL FINDINGS

- Acute phase: lateral elbow pain or ache with activities that typically resolves with rest, ice, or anti-inflammatory medication
- Intermediate phase: lateral elbow pain or ache occurs at rest and may not resolve without prolonged activity restriction
- Chronic phase: pain or ache occurs with sleep and often is unresponsive to rest, medication, and injections.[5]
- Examination methods include the following:
  - Palpation of the lateral epicondyle for tenderness, a universal finding in lateral epicondylitis
  - Pain either at the epicondyle or radiating distally along the ECRB is a positive finding in any of these circumstances:
    - *Passive stretch test:* With the elbow in full extension, the wrist is flexed and the forearm is pronated.
    - *Mill's test:* With the elbow flexed, the forearm slightly pronated, and the wrist slightly dorsiflexed, the patient actively supinates against the examiner, who resists this rotation.
    - *Thompson test:* With the elbow extended, the wrist in slight dorsiflexion, and making a fist, the patient dorsiflexes against the examiner, who resists this motion.

IMAGING AND OTHER DIAGNOSTIC STUDIES

- Plain radiographs may show calcifications at the extensor origin.
- MRI
  - Increased intratendon signal is reliably demonstrated on T2-weighted sequences.
  - Most also show increased intratendon signal or tendon thickening on T1-weighted sequences.
  - A small percentage of patients may show increased T2 signal in the lateral epicondyle or anconeus edema.[3]
  - Periosteal reaction is *not* commonly seen on MRI.[3]
  - Lateral collateral ligament tears often are overcalled on MRI, but this possibility must be ruled out by an accurate history and pre- and intraoperative examinations.

DIFFERENTIAL DIAGNOSIS

- Synovial plica
- Lateral collateral ligament tear
- Radial tunnel syndrome
- Loose bodies
- Degenerative joint disease (typically early radiocapitellar joint)
- Avascular necrosis of the capitellum

NONOPERATIVE MANAGEMENT

- Appropriate initial treatment includes avoidance of painful activities and symptomatic relief with nonsteroidal anti-inflammatory drugs (NSAIDs) and ice.
- Daytime strapping is biomechanically and clinically effective.
- Nighttime wrist bracing to prevent palmar wrist flexion and prolonged tension on the extensor tendons
- Physical or occupational therapy to supervise and instruct on stretching and strengthening protocol for patients not otherwise inclined to perform these exercises
- Corticosteroid injection has had good response in the early stages of the condition.
- Platelet-rich plasma or blood clot tendon injection and botulinum toxin muscle injection currently are under investigation.

SURGICAL MANAGEMENT

- A minority of patients fail nonoperative management.
- Careful patient selection is critical to ensure an excellent outcome following surgical management.
- No prospective randomized studies have yet been done to examine the advantages of open versus arthroscopic techniques for the treatment of lateral epicondylitis. However, I choose arthroscopic treatment if there are any signs of a plica or synovial irritation (endpoint pain) that will allow direct examination and treatment.

Preoperative Planning

- Be prepared to address concurrent extensor tendon rupture.
- Be prepared to address lateral collateral ligament rupture.

Positioning

- The patient is placed in the supine position.
- The arm is internally rotated at the shoulder, and padding is placed under the elbow.

- The arm should rest in a position that allows ready access to the lateral aspect of the elbow without requiring constant holding by an assistant.
- The elbow should be examined after the administration of anesthesia to ensure stability, and the result documented in the operative note.
- The goal of surgery is to débride the degenerative tissue at the extensor origin and create an environment conducive to proper healing of the tendon.

OPEN LATERAL EPICONDYLAR FASCIECTOMY AND PARTIAL OSTECTOMY

- A 3- to 5-cm incision through skin only is made beginning at the proximal edge of the center of the lateral epicondyle and extending distally through the mid-radiocapitellar joint plane along the axis of the forearm (**TECH FIG 1A**).
- Blunt dissection with scissors is carried out through the subcutaneous tissues to expose the EDC aponeurosis and the ECRL.
- The more anterior and reddish ECRL and the more tendinous EDC originating on the epicondyle are identified (**TECH FIG 1B**).
  - The interval between the ECRL and the EDC aponeurosis is then split in line with the mid-radiocapitellar joint plane. Distally, a fat stripe along the aponeurosis typically is seen along this dissection plane.
  - A small posterior EDC flap is created for later closure and the ECRL is elevated anteriorly revealing the underlying ECRB origin. The origin may be obliterated by degenerative tissue.
- The abnormal tendon tissue to be excised can be identified by its grayish, unorganized mucoid appearance and should be sharply excised. Care is taken to dissect the ECRB off the underlying capsule.
  - Abnormal tissue typically will scrape away with a no. 15 blade, but normal tendon will not (Nirschl scratch test). Sometimes the ECRB tissue cannot be dissected free from the underlying capsule or it has already ruptured from its origin, and the underlying joint becomes exposed (**TECH FIG 1C**). This will not affect outcome.
  - If exposed, the joint should be inspected for degenerative change, which, if present, typically is found

beneath a plica. The plica should be removed (**TECH FIG 1D**).

- The pathologic tissue is débrided to margins showing an organized, tendinous appearance. Complete resection of the ECRB origin is not necessary if healthy viable portions remain (**TECH FIG 1E**).
  - The proximal stump of the ECRB should not be repaired, because it has ample attachments and will not retract significantly.
  - The area of excision usually is 1 to 2 cm long and 5 to 10 mm wide.
  - The undersurface of the EDC often is affected, and degenerative tissue should be similarly removed.
- A rongeur is used to roughen the anterior portion of the lateral epicondyle to a bleeding surface without removing cortical bone.
  - In some cases, patients have a significantly prominent epicondylar tip. This can be removed, especially if patients are focused on this finding and they are very thin, but the early recovery period will be more painful (**TECH FIG 1F**).
- The defect in the tendon is closed with a running absorbable suture, using 0 or 1-0 suture material with a tapered needle. If a capsular rent occurs, there is no need to make a separate capsular closure, but the proximal tendon repair should be close to the epicondyle and watertight to avoid a postoperative ganglion (**TECH FIG 1G**).
- The subdermal layer is closed with buried, interrupted absorbable sutures, followed by a subcuticular skin closure and Steri-strips.

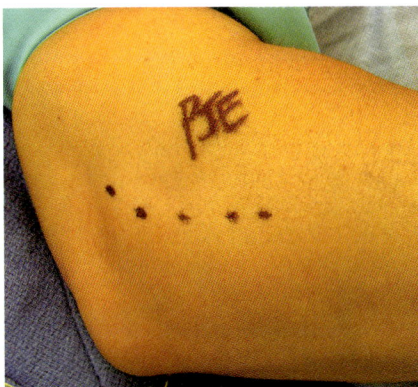

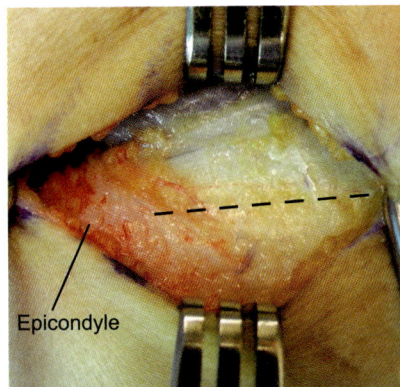

Epicondyle

TECH FIG 1 • A. Surgical approach uses a 3-cm incision over the lateral epicondyle and can be extended in line with the forearm axis to avoid injury to the lateral collateral ligament. **B.** The interval between the tendinous EDC aponeurosis and the darker muscle of the ECRL is entered, and the ECRL is elevated off the underlying ECRB. (The patient's hand is to the right.) *(continued)*

TECHNIQUES

C. Degenerative deep extensor — Plica

D. KW 25-45

E.

F. Intact deep extensor origin — Debrided epicondyle

G.

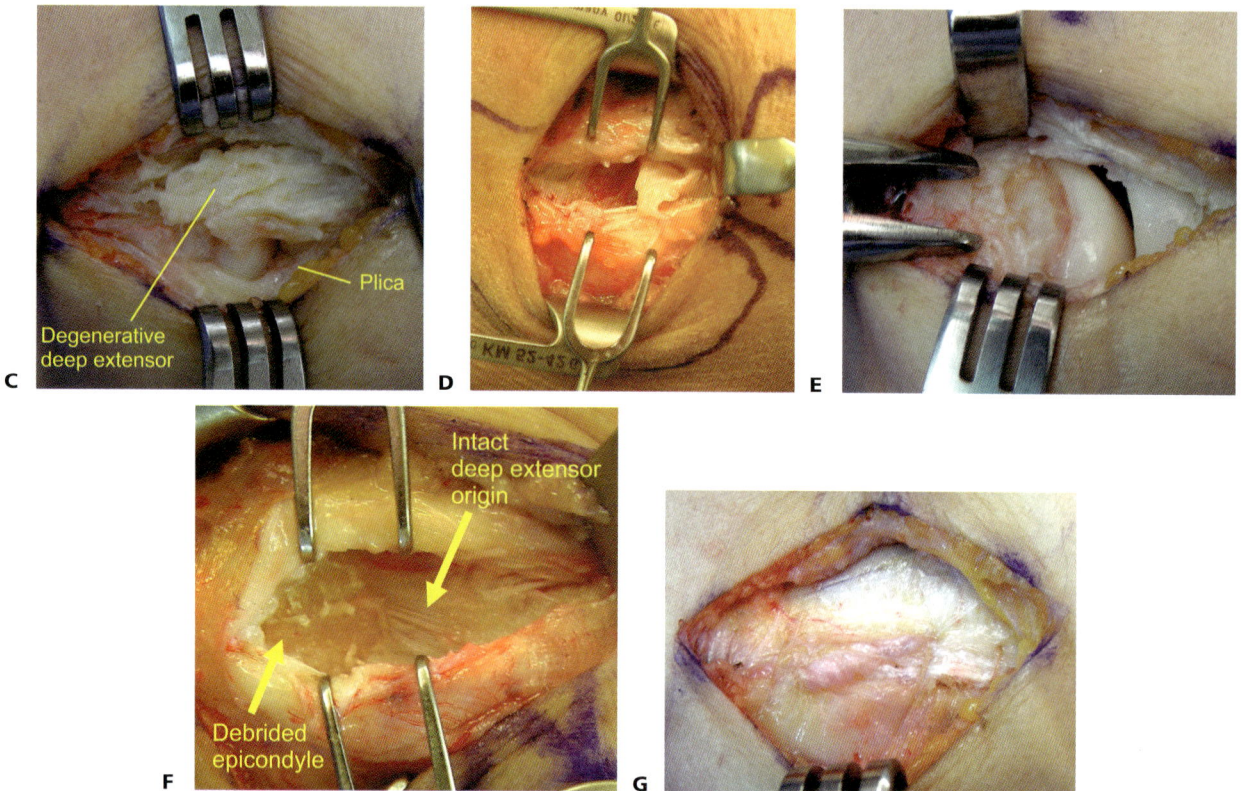

TECH FIG 1 • *(continued)* **C.** The degenerative ECRB is sharply excised. At times, as in this example, it is not possible to separate the ECRB and capsule, and a portion of the capsule also is excised. Neighboring tendon of the EDC is scraped with a no. 15 blade to remove loose degenerative tissue. **D.** In this example, it was possible to excise the degenerative portion of the ECRB without the underlying capsule. **E.** The anterior portion of the lateral epicondyle is scratched clean of degenerative tissue with a no. 15 blade or rongeur but not decorticated. **F.** Some intact, normal ECRB fibers are left if they are present. **G.** Closure is done with an inverted-stitch size 0 Vicryl suture on a tapered needle in a running fashion.

ARTHROSCOPIC LATERAL EPICONDYLAR FASCIECTOMY AND PARTIAL OSTECTOMY

- The patient is positioned according to surgeon preference for elbow arthroscopy.
  - We prefer the lateral decubitus position with the aid of the Tenet Spider Arm Holder (Smith & Nephew Inc., Andover, MA).
  - If prone or lateral, it is advantageous to keep the elbow well above the plane of the chest wall to optimize anterior superomedial portal camera positioning.
- The elbow is filled with 30 to 50 mL of irrigating solution until distended. An anterior superomedial portal is established.
  - A small longitudinal portal incision is made about 2 cm proximal to the medial epicondyle and just anterior to the medial intermuscular septum. A curved hemostat is used to spread underlying tissues and feel the medial intermuscular septum, and then is slid along its anterior surface to the lateral, then anterior humerus.
  - This is repeated with the scope trocar, which is then passed distally along the anterior humerus toward the radiocapitellar joint, piercing the capsule and entering the joint.
- Documentation of intra-articular (eg, loose bodies, plica [**TECH FIG 2A**], osteochondritis dissecans, arthritis) and

lateral capsular or tendon pathology (**TECH FIG 2B**) is made, and they are treated appropriately.

- A 25-gauge needle is placed from outside in to choose an optimal radiocapitellar portal at the upper rim of the radial head at or just proximal to the joint level (**TECH FIG 2C**).
- A shaver is used to débride the abnormal capsule lining the EDC origin. Abnormal ECRB is débrided until normal superficial tendon fibers are identified and protected. If ruptured, all degenerative portions of the ECRB are excised. Normal, shining ECRL fibers can be seen superficially as well as the dark muscular appearance (**TECH FIG 2D**).
- Débridement should not proceed posterior to the mid-radiocapitellar plane, to avoid injury to the lateral collateral ligament.
- A bone-cutting shaver or a less aggressive burr used in reverse will roughen, but not decorticate, the anterior aspect of the lateral epicondyle from the capitellum back to the portal entry site (**TECH FIG 2E**).
  - A hooked electrocautery probe is useful to divide a plica to facilitate its resection.
- Lateral and posterior portals are closed with 3-0 Prolene sutures, and the medial portal is left open for rapid resolution of fluid distention and pain relief.

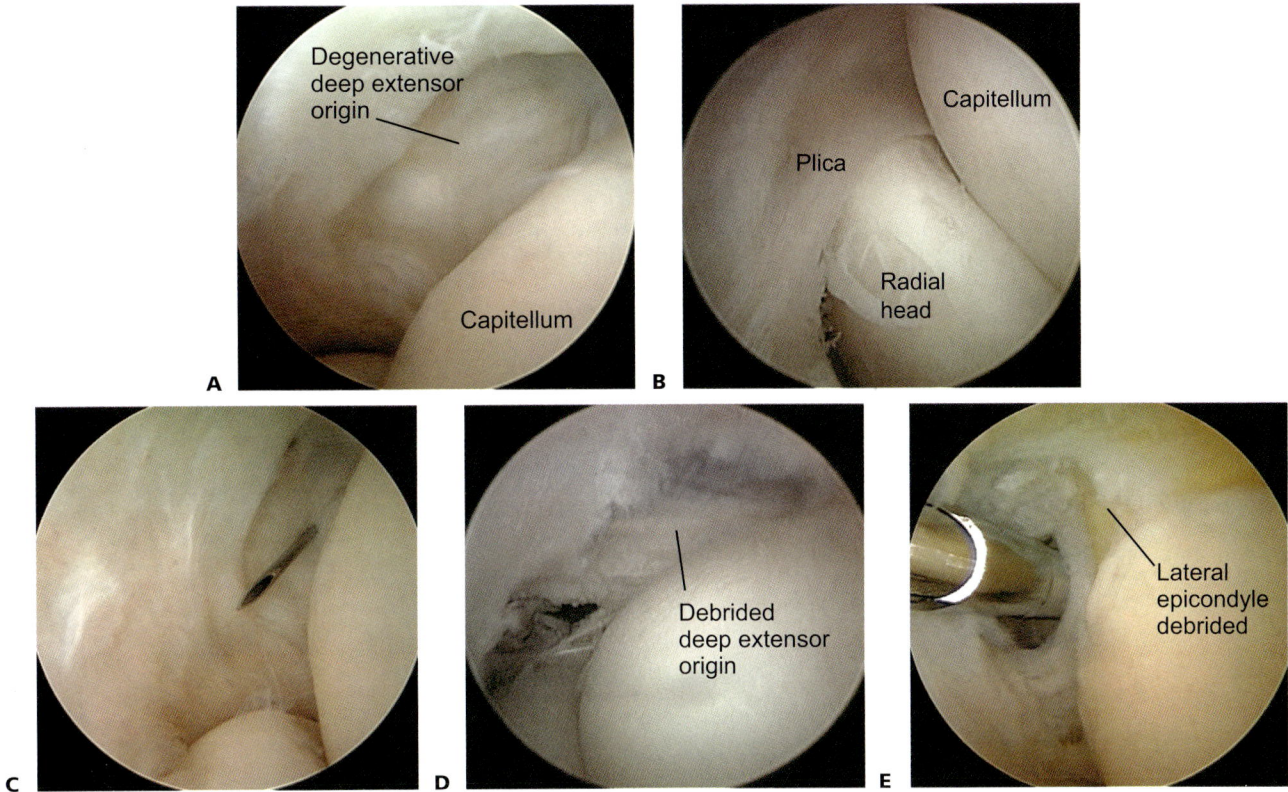

TECH FIG 2 • A. Arthroscopic view showing a capsular invagination lining a ruptured ECRB tendon. **B.** A radiocapitellar plica that is pathologic, causing degenerative changes on the radial head outer rim. **C.** A lateral portal is established at the anterior rim of the radial head, at or just proximal to the radiocapitellar joint, often directly through the primary pathology. **D.** A shaver is used to excise abnormal capsule and ECRB tendon, leaving intact, shiny ECRL tendon. **E.** The shaver or burr (in reverse) can be used to clear degenerative ECRB tendon of the anterior portion of the lateral epicondyle from the capitellum back to the portal.

PEARLS AND PITFALLS

Indications	▪ A minimum of 3 to 6 months of symptoms and failed nonoperative management
Coexisting conditions	▪ Extensor tendon origin rupture may require débridement and repair. ▪ Medial epicondylitis occurs in 30% of cases.
Failure to fully excise devitalized tendon	▪ This will result in a poor result or recurrence; the rehabilitation protocol can be delayed in cases that require more significant débridement.
Injury to the lateral collateral ligament	▪ The ligament is posterior to the mid-radiocapitellar joint, and dissection in this area should be avoided.
Extensor tendon rupture	▪ Rupture of the ECRB is of no consequence and should not be repaired. ▪ Rupture of the EDC mandates repair and can be achieved by advancing the ECRL posteriorly and the extensor carpi ulnaris anteriorly to close the gap. If this cannot be repaired, the anconeus muscle can be rotated to cover the defect.

POSTOPERATIVE CARE

▪ Postoperatively, the patient is placed in a soft dressing and a removable cock-up wrist brace.

▪ The elbow is not immobilized, and gentle range of motion is allowed immediately.

▪ The dressing is removed in 2 to 5 days. The patient may perform activities of daily living as tolerated with the wrist brace,

removing the wrist brace several times daily for range of motion exercises.

▪ Exertion is avoided.

▪ A strengthening program is initiated at 6 weeks.

▪ All restrictions are removed at 3 months, but impact activities are not allowed until 4 to 6 months postoperatively. Pain-free full activity may require 6 to 12 months.

OUTCOMES

■ Over 85% to 90% of all patients will have return to full activities with no pain. The remaining 10% to 15% have significant pain relief and strength, but do not return to normal preinjury levels. These outcomes hold true for both short follow-up and more than 10 years of follow-up.[4,5,7] Future prospective randomized trials will elucidate whether the reported more rapid recovery of the arthroscopic treatment is realized.

■ It is uncommon (<5% of cases) for a patient to have absolutely no improvement in pain after surgery, even if the subjective outcome is unsatisfactory. Such a result should prompt consideration of incorrect diagnosis or the possibility of secondary gain issues.

COMPLICATIONS

■ Hematoma
■ Infection
■ Lateral collateral ligament injury
■ Weakness in grip strength

REFERENCES

1. Greenbaum B, Itamura J, Vangsness CT, et al. Extensor carpi radialis brevis: An anatomical analysis of its origin. J Bone Joint Surg Br 1999;81B:926–929.
2. Hay EM, Paterson SM, Lewis M, et al. Pragmatic randomised controlled trial of local corticosteroid injection and naproxen for treatment of lateral epicondylitis of elbow in primary care. BMJ 1999;319:964–968.
3. Martin CE, Schweitzer ME. MR imaging of epicondylitis. Skel Radiol 1998;27:133–138.
4. Nirschl RP, Davis LD. Mini-open surgery for lateral epicondylitis. In: Yamaguchi K, King GJW, McKee M, et al, eds. Advanced Reconstruction—Elbow. Rosemont, IL: American Academy of Orthopaedic Surgeons, 2007:129–135.
5. Nirschl RP, Pettrone FA. The surgical treatment of lateral epicondylitis. J Bone Joint Surg Am 1979;61A:832–841.
6. Stasinopoulos D, Johnson MI. "Lateral elbow tendinopathy" is the most appropriate diagnostic term for the condition commonly referred-to as lateral epicondylitis. Med Hypotheses 2006;67:1400–1402.
7. Verhaar J, Walenkamp G, Kester A, et al. Lateral extensor release for tennis elbow: A prospective long-term follow-up study. J Bone Joint Surg Am 1993;75A:1034–1043.

Chapter 65

Surgical Treatment for Extensor Carpi Ulnaris Subluxation

David H. MacDonald and Thomas R. Hunt III

DEFINITION

- Extensor carpi ulnaris (ECU) subluxation occurs when the separate subsheath of the sixth dorsal compartment is torn or attenuated.
- Incompetence of the ECU subsheath permits subluxation or dislocation of the ECU tendon out of the ulnar groove of the ulna, with a painful click noted on resisted supination, ulnar deviation, and palmar flexion.

ANATOMY

- The dorsal extensor retinaculum of the wrist is composed of two primary layers (**FIG 1**).
  - The supratendinous retinaculum originates 2 to 3 cm proximal to the radiocarpal joint and ends distinctly at the carpometacarpal joints. The most radial attachment on the distal radius forms the radial septum for the first extensor compartment. The supratendinous retinaculum courses medially, surrounding the ulna.[10]
    - The supratendinous retinaculum participates as a block to tendon subluxation for the first through fifth extensor compartments but does not function to prevent subluxation of the ECU.
  - The infratendinous retinaculum runs from the radiocarpal to the carpometacarpal joints. It is found deep to the fourth and fifth extensor compartments on the radius. The ECU lies in its own separate fibro-osseous subsheath, which represents a duplication of the infratendinous retinaculum.
    - The ECU sheath is separated from the supratendinous retinaculum by loose areolar tissue.

- The fibro-osseous subsheath of the sixth dorsal compartment overlies 1.5 to 2.0 cm of the distal ulna and arcs from the radial to ulnar wall of the ECU osseous groove. It ensheathes the ECU and maintains the tendon tightly in the groove (**FIG 2**).
  - The ECU subsheath contributes to the dorsal portion of the triangular fibrocartilage complex (TFCC).

PATHOGENESIS

- The mechanism of a traumatic injury most commonly is active ECU contraction combined with forced supination, palmar flexion, and ulnar deviation.
  - Injuries resulting from trauma can range from simple attenuation to complete rupture of the ECU fibro-osseous sheath.
- Traumatic ECU subluxation is commonly reported in association with racket sports, baseball, and golf.

NATURAL HISTORY

- Chronic subluxation of the ECU tendon over the ulnar prominence of the groove in the distal ulna can lead to painful snapping of the tendon with supination and pronation. This can progress to ECU tendinopathy.
- An injury to the ECU sheath resulting in volar dislocation of the ECU tendon can result in distal radioulnar joint (DRUJ) instability. This joint laxity may cause pain and dysfunction, eventually leading to degenerative changes.
  - Dislocation of the ECU tendon removes a dynamic stabilizer of the DRUJ.

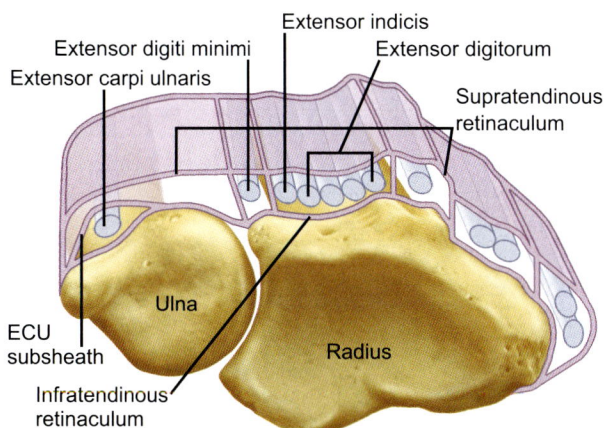

FIG 1 • Axial representation of dorsal extensor compartments. The ECU tendon has a separate compartment along the dorsum of the ulna. The supratendinous retinaculum courses ulnarward over the sixth compartment and does not communicate with the separate ECU fibro-osseous subsheath in any significant way.

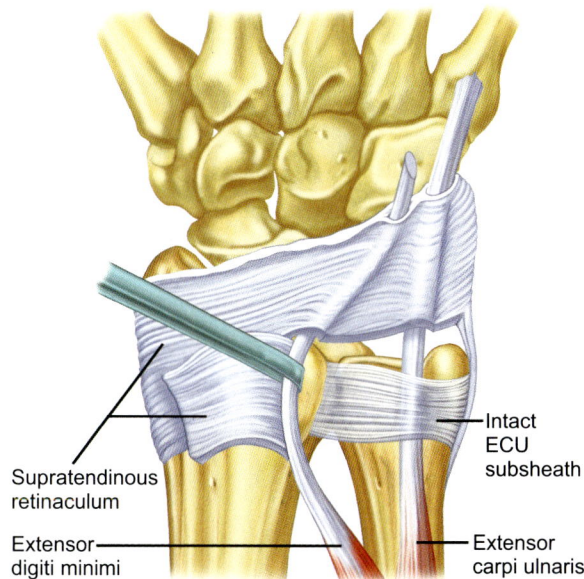

FIG 2 • Dorsal anatomic view of the sixth dorsal component. This representation shows the relation between the deep ECU subsheath and the superficial supratendinous extensor retinaculum.

- The subsheath of the sixth extensor compartment represents a component of the dorsal peripheral TFCC. Disruption can result in static instability of the DRUJ.
- Some patients may experience relatively minor ECU subluxation and related symptoms that do not progress and often improve with minimal intervention.

PATIENT HISTORY AND PHYSICAL FINDINGS

- Patients may present following an acute injury or, more commonly, in the subacute phase, complaining of persistent ulnar wrist pain aggravated by activities requiring pronation and supination. They may relate the sensation of a "click."
- A complete physical examination of the patient's ulnar-sided wrist complaints should be conducted to elucidate associated pathology and rule out confounding conditions in the differential diagnosis.
    - Palpation and inspection of sixth dorsal compartment and ECU tendon helps to localize the area of discomfort and focus the physical examination. Most acute sheath ruptures and tendinopathies will be tender to palpation at the level of the distal ulna and groove. Tenderness at the joint line may indicate an associated TFCC tear.
    - In range-of-motion testing, an inflamed ECU tendon usually will be most painful with full passive radial wrist flexion, although motion most often is full except in the acute setting.
    - If the tendon dislocates with passive supination, palmar flexion, and ulnar deviation, the ECU is grossly unstable. If the addition of ECU contraction is required for frank dislocation, some inherent stability remains. Pain with subluxation is a critical finding when contemplating surgical treatment.
    - In resisted finger abduction, pain over the wrist and ECU tendon signifies an inflammatory ECU condition, possibly due to subluxation or overuse.

IMAGING AND OTHER DIAGNOSTIC STUDIES

- Routine anteroposterior (AP), lateral, and oblique radiographs in neutral rotation are important.
- Pronated grip views and other specialized plain radiographs of the wrist can provide information on other pathologies that contribute to ulnar-sided wrist pain (see Differential Diagnosis).
- MRI is the most sensitive and specific imaging modality to detect ECU subluxation (**FIG 3A**).
    - The sensitivity increases in studies with both wrists positioned in pronation, neutral, and supination. This allows side-by-side comparison with the asymptomatic wrist and adequately shows the position of the ECU relative to the ulnar osseous groove in all three positions.
        - The actual subsheath tear may or may not be visualized.
        - Often, inflammation and partial interstitial tendon disruption are visualized.
- An MRI arthrogram may depict a subsheath tear and, therefore, an injury to the peripheral TFCC.
    - Contrast may extravasate into the sixth extensor compartment (**FIG 3B**).
    - The study will also provide additional information concerning the remainder of the TFCC and the integrity of the intercarpal ligaments.
- Ultrasound allows dynamic assessment of ECU stability and can be useful in quantifying the degree of ECU tendon subluxation.[8]

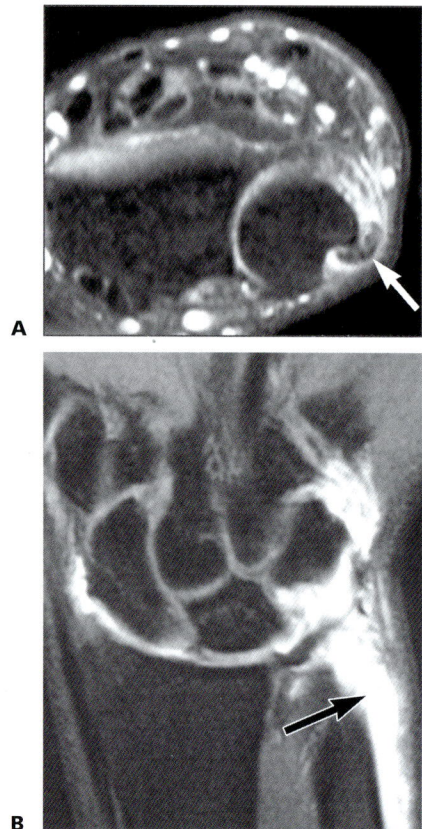

FIG 3 • **A.** This MRI scan shows a "perched" ECU tendon, out of the dorsal ulnar groove. Notice the increased signal in the tendon substance. **B.** The coronal MRI arthrogram projection illustrates leakage of the opaque dye into the ECU fibro-osseous subsheath.

DIFFERENTIAL DIAGNOSIS

- ECU tenosynovitis
    - Fullness and pain with palpation of the sixth dorsal compartment
    - The patient often can reproduce a painful snap or click with supination and ulnar deviation, even in the absence of ECU subluxation.
- TFCC injury
    - Tenderness with direct palpation of the TFCC
    - Pain with axial loading and rotation of the ulnar-deviated wrist (TFCC compression test)
    - Instability of the DRUJ with manual manipulation when compared to the contralateral wrist
- Lunotriquetral ligament injury
    - Tenderness to palpation over the dorsal lunotriquetral articulation
    - The patient may also describe pain and crepitance with ulnar deviation of the wrist.
    - Provocative maneuvers for lunotriquetral ligament injuries (ie, ballottement test, ulnar snuff box test) have sufficient sensitivity but poor specificity.
- Ulnocarpal impaction syndrome
    - More common in patients with ulna-positive variance
    - Usually a dynamic phenomenon occurring during forceful activity or pronated gripping

- The physical examination findings will be similar to those of TFCC injury, with pain on forced ulnar deviation of the wrist (TFCC stress test) that increases with rotation through the loaded ulnocarpal articulation.
  - Tenderness will be elicited along the ulnar border of the triquetrum and the distal ulna.
- Ulnar styloid nonunion
  - Uncommon; occurs more commonly with widely displaced styloid fractures at the time of injury
  - The intimate relationship with the ulnar TFCC attachment means that symptomatic nonunion can be associated with TFCC dysfunction and DRUJ instability.
- DRUJ arthrosis
  - Patients present with complaints of pain, swelling, and stiffness. The pain is exacerbated by forearm rotation, particularly when performed with manual compression of the DRUJ.

NONOPERATIVE MANAGEMENT

- In the acute setting (less than 3 weeks since injury), immobilize the patient in an above-elbow cast. The wrist should be in neutral to slight pronation, neutral to slight radial deviation, and neutral to slight extension.
  - The cast is removed about 4 to 5 weeks later, and therapy is initiated. A sugartong splint is fabricated with the forearm in slight pronation, and a progressive active and active-assisted ROM protocol is initiated.
  - Three weeks later, a forearm-based splint is provided and the patient slowly progresses back to activities.
  - Unprotected, full activity is allowed 3 to 4 months after the initiation of treatment.

- The literature does not agree on the efficacy of nonoperative treatment. Rowland[7] produced a compelling case report of surgical treatment in acute, traumatic ECU subluxation.
  - In this case, the intraoperative findings showed the edges of the ruptured subsheath to be separated by a minimum of 7 mm, regardless of the position of the wrist.
  - These findings suggest that nonoperative treatment could routinely lead to clinical ECU subluxation and persistent symptoms.

SURGICAL MANAGEMENT

- Surgical reconstruction of the ECU subsheath should be considered in patients with clinically significant symptoms related to painful subluxation of the ECU tendon, especially if the injury is more than 3 weeks old. Treatment must be individualized based on the needs and expectations of the patient.
- The guiding principles for surgical repair depend on the essential osteofibrous sheath lesion present at the time of surgery.
- Inoue and Tamura[5,6] classified three distinct patterns of injury (**TABLE 1**).
  - Treatment of type A and B lesions
    - In the acute setting, suture repair is sometimes possible and may be augmented using suture anchors.
    - When the fibro-osseous sheath is ruptured and deemed irreparable, reconstruction is accomplished using a retinacular sling or free retinacular graft (see Techniques box).
    - Because of its simplicity and the ability to place a gliding surface between the bone and tendon, the sling is preferred.

Table 1	Classification of ECU Subsheath Lesion with Recommended Surgical Treatment		
Lesion Type	**Illustration**	**Description of Pathology**	**Recommended Surgical Treatment**
A		The fibro-osseous sheath is disrupted from the ulnar wall. The tendon may lie beneath the disrupted sheath.	If injury is fairly acute and if adequate tissue is present, a direct repair may be attempted. If nonreconstructable, a sheath reconstruction with retinacular free graft or retinacular sling is employed.
B		The fibro-osseous sheath is disrupted from the radial wall. The tendon may rest on top of the sheath and prevent healing.	A sheath reconstruction with retinacular free graft or retinacular sling is suggested.
C		The fibro-osseous sheath is stripped from the periosteum but remains in continuity, forming a false pouch.	Imbrication of false pouch reinforced with suture anchors or drill holes.

- Treatment of type C lesions
  - Separation of the fibro-osseous sheath from bone necessitates repositioning of the tissue at the ulnar margin of the groove (see False Pouch Reconstruction and Imbrication for Type C Lesions).
    - Stretching and attenuation of the sheath without separation from bone may be effectively treated by suture imbrication, depending on the quality of the tissue.
- Although this chapter describes reconstruction of traumatic ECU subluxation, reconstruction also may be considered in the patient with inflammatory arthropathy and secondary volar dislocation of the ECU tendon. The opportunity to stabilize the ulnar wrist and DRUJ while forestalling progression of deformity may lead the patient and surgeon toward surgical care even in the absence of pain.

Preoperative Planning

- All preoperative information obtained from the history, the physical examination, and imaging studies should be thoroughly reviewed and synthesized into the operative plan. For example, a patient with joint line tenderness and an MRI indicating a TFCC injury might benefit from wrist arthroscopy before any open procedure is done.
  - Dorsal synovitis or tenosynovitis requiring débridement
  - The existence of a shallow ulnar osseous groove and the need to deepen the groove surgically for added stability
  - The paucity of soft tissue for reconstruction and the need for another graft choice for subsheath reconstruction. Graft options include the palmaris and flexor carpi ulnaris tendons.

Positioning

- The patient is positioned supine on the operating table with the injured extremity extended on an armboard in the usual manner.
- Initially, the procedure is performed with the arm extended and pronated. If the wrist must be placed in a neutral or supinated position, the elbow is flexed.

Approach

- A precise incision is chosen to allow for the predetermined method of reconstruction.
- Make a Brunner zigzag incision over the sixth extensor compartment.
  - The incision begins 1 to 2 cm distal to the ulnocarpal joint and is carried proximally 5 cm.
- Identify and protect the dorsal cutaneous branch of the ulnar nerve in the distal incision.
- Incise the extensor retinaculum on its far ulnar border and carefully separate it from the underlying sixth extensor compartment fibro-osseous sheath (see Fig 2).
  - Conservation of and planned incision in the extensor retinaculum is critical to allow for its use as a sling to stabilize the ECU tendon (see Retinacular Sling Reconstruction for Type A and B Lesions)
- Following exposure, inspect the separate fibro-osseous sheath of the ECU and note the position of the tendon through pronosupination.
- Perform a tenosynovectomy as indicated.

RETINACULAR SLING RECONSTRUCTION[2] FOR TYPE A AND B LESIONS

- Retinacular sling reconstruction[2] is performed when the sheath is ruptured and not repairable.
- At the level of the ulnar groove, create a rectangular flap of tissue, 2 to 3 cm wide, based on the septum separating the fifth and sixth extensor compartments (**TECH FIG 1A**).
- Pass this radially based sling in an ulnar direction, volar to the ECU tendon, then fold it back radially over the tendon and secure it to the ulnar portion of the fifth compartment (**TECH FIG 1B**).
  - This places the superficial surface of the retinaculum in contact with the ECU tendon.
- Avoid constricting the ECU tendon by ensuring that the sling is wide and loose, which still prevents subluxation of the tendon.
- The portion of the extensor retinaculum not used for the sling is repaired anatomically.

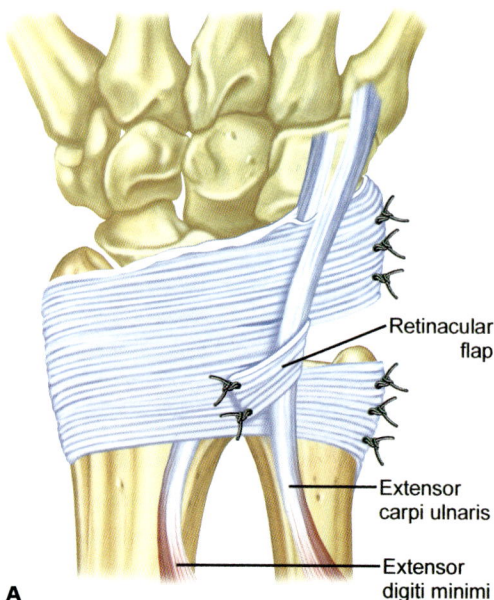

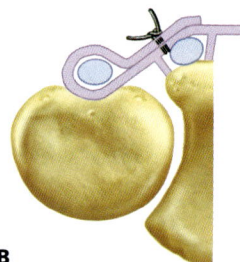

Retinacular flap

Extensor carpi ulnaris

Extensor digiti minimi

A

B

TECH FIG 1 • Retinacular sling reconstruction of type A and B lesions. **A.** Creation of a radially based extensor retinaculum sling. **B.** The retinacular flap is brought deep to the ECU tendon, then looped back over the tendon and sewn to the extensor retinaculum overlying the ulnar compartment. This places the superficial surface of the retinaculum in contact with the ECU tendon when the reconstruction is completed.

ALTERNATE RETINACULAR SLING RECONSTRUCTION FOR TYPE A AND B LESIONS

- An alternate retinacular sling reconstruction[9] requires the development of an ulnarly based, rectangular flap, 2 to 3 cm wide, of supratendinous retinacular tissue, beginning at Lister's tubercle or over the second extensor compartment if more length is required (**TECH FIG 2A**).
  - The flap is based on the ulnar septum of the fifth extensor compartment.

- Pass the tissue ulnarly, deep to the ECU tendon, then back over the tendon to create the sling.
  - This places the deep surface of the retinaculum in contact with the ECU tendon.
- Insert suture anchors on the radial and ulnar margins of the ulnar groove, and use this suture to stabilize the flap (**TECH FIG 2B**).
  - Avoid constricting the ECU tendon, as discussed previously.

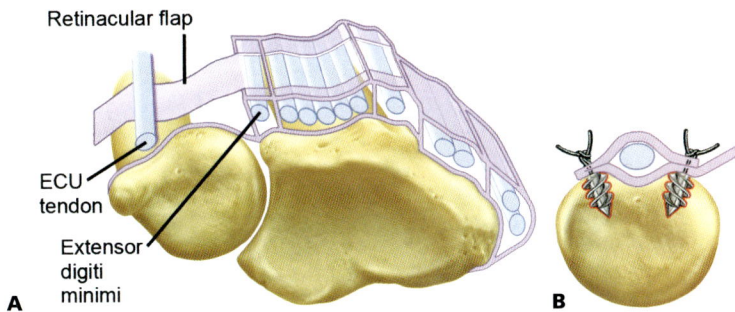

TECH FIG 2 • Alternate retinacular sling reconstruction of type A and B lesions. **A.** The ulnarly based extensor retinaculum flap is harvested, then swung ulnarward, deep to the ECU tendon. **B.** The tissue is then brought back over the tendon and secured to itself and the ulna, using bone anchors. The remaining retinaculum is repaired in an anatomic fashion. This places the deep surface of the retinacular flap in contact with the ECU tendon when the reconstruction is complete.

RETINACULAR GRAFT AUGMENTATION FOR TYPE A AND B LESIONS

- Retinacular graft augmentation[4] is performed when the sheath is ruptured and not repairable.
- Harvest a 2- × 2-cm square graft from the distal supratendinous retinaculum (**TECH FIG 3A**).
- Secure this graft to the periosteum on the ulnar and radial borders of the ulnar osseous groove to maintain the ECU tendon within the groove.
- Roughen the bone surface to encourage attachment, and place suture anchors at the anatomic attachment sites along the radial and ulnar borders of the ulnar osseous groove.
- Secure the harvested graft to the margins of the ulnar groove, allowing bony contact between the graft and the ulna (**TECH FIG 3B**).
  - Place the deep surface of the graft against the tendon.
  - This provides secure fixation and does not rely on questionable soft tissue for early fixation.

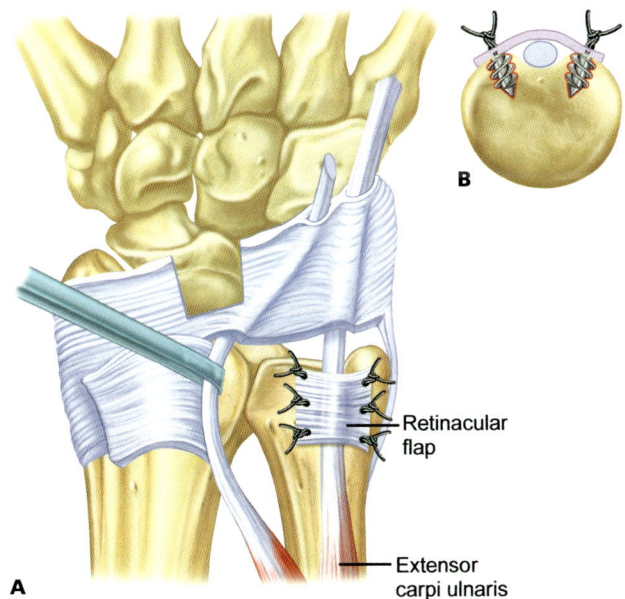

TECH FIG 3 • Free retinacular flap reconstruction of type A and B lesions. A 2- × 2-cm portion of distal extensor retinaculum is harvested and secured to the ulnar osseous groove using small bone anchors.

FALSE POUCH RECONSTRUCTION AND IMBRICATION FOR TYPE C LESIONS

- False pouch reconstruction and imbrication[6] is done when the fibro-osseous sheath of the ECU tendon is attenuated and stretched, but intact. The tendon subluxates out of the ulnar groove during forearm rotation (**TECH FIG 4A,B**).

- Incise the sheath on its ulnar margin (**TECH FIG 4C**).
- If the sheath has separated from the deep periosteum, roughen the medial surface of the ulna deep to the false pouch (**TECH FIG 4D**).

TECHNIQUES

- Insert suture anchors at the site of the true ulnar attachment of the sheath (**TECH FIG 4E**).
- Use suture from the bone anchors to capture and repair the fibro-osseous sheath, securing it to the prepared bone bed (**TECH FIG 4F**).

- The effect is to imbricate the attenuated sheath and obliterate the false pouch.
- Place additional permanent sutures to complete the repair (**TECH FIG 4G**).

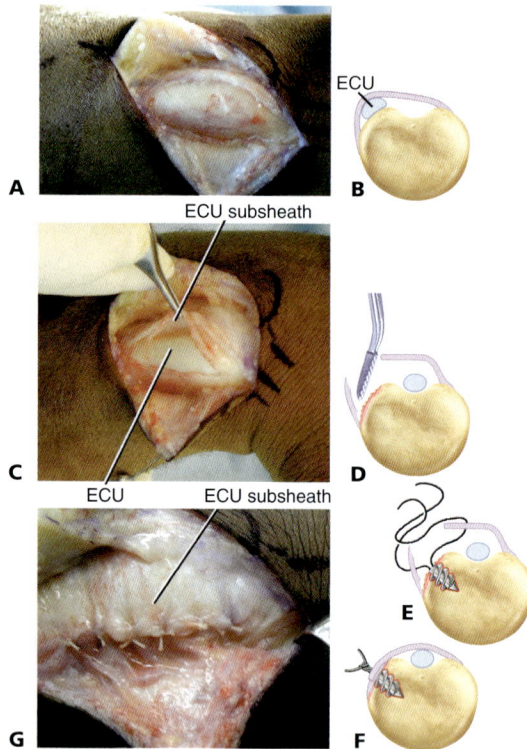

TECH FIG 4 • Type C lesion. **A.** The supratendinous retinaculum has been incised, revealing the ECU subsheath. The subsheath is inflamed, stretched, and attenuated, allowing tendon subluxation. **B.** Diagrammatic representation of a type C lesion in which the sheath has pulled away from the bone. **C.** An incision is made in the attenuated subsheath, allowing visualization of the tendon. Despite MRI findings that indicate potential intrasubstance injury (see Fig 3A), the tendon itself appears normal. **D.** The bone underlying the ulnar subsheath flap is roughened with a rasp. **E,F.** Mini–bone anchors are used to secure the tissue to the ulnar border of the groove and imbricate the subsheath. **G.** Additional permanent sutures complete the repair.

DEEPENING OF THE ULNAR OSSEOUS GROOVE

- Deepening of the ulnar osseous groove is an optional technique that may be used to address all lesion types.
- This technique is added to the reconstruction when preoperative studies or intraoperative findings suggest that a shallow ulnar osseous groove contributes significantly to subluxation of the ECU tendon (**TECH FIG 5A**).
- Retract the ECU tendon out of its groove.
- Carefully elevate the periosteum and a thin layer of bone along the ulnar 2 to 3 cm of the ulnar osseous groove using a sharp, curved osteotome (**TECH FIG 5B**).
  - The radial border is used as a hinge to expose the underlying cancellous bone.
  - Precise elevation of the osteoperiosteal flap ensures adequate coverage of the raw bony surfaces.
- Remove cancellous bone using a small curette (**TECH FIG 5C**), no deeper than 2 to 3 mm.
- The cortical bone flap is then returned to its position and tamped down using a small bone tamp (**TECH FIG 5D**). The periosteum is repaired (**TECH FIG 5E**).
- Treat any remaining exposed bony surface with bone wax.

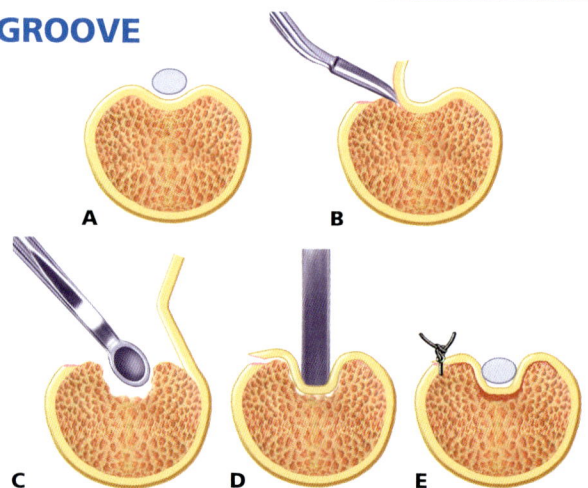

TECH FIG 5 • Deepening of the ulnar osseous groove. **A.** ECU tendon in a shallow ulnar groove. **B.** A sharp curved osteotome is used to create an osteoperiosteal "trapdoor" with a hinge of periosteum radially. **C.** A curette is used to remove cancellous bone. **D.** A bone tamp is used to close the trapdoor gently and deepen the osseous groove. **E.** The periosteum is then secured using 4-0 suture if feasible.

CLOSURE AND SPLINTING

- Perform passive motion testing to ensure that the ECU tendon is stable in its groove following reconstruction or repair.
- Close the extensor retinaculum in a side-to-side fashion using absorbable suture.
- Deflate the tourniquet and obtain hemostasis.
- Following routine skin closure and dressing placement, place a sugartong splint with the forearm mildly pronated and the wrist in mild extension and radial deviation.

PEARLS AND PITFALLS

Indications	▪ Symptomatic subluxation of the ECU tendon at the ulnar osseous groove ▪ Acute injuries often are effectively treated with immobilization.
Approach	▪ Protect against injury to the dorsal cutaneous branch of the ulnar nerve. ▪ Incise the supratendinous retinaculum along its ulnar border, remembering that the sixth extensor compartment is a separate, deeper structure. ▪ Carefully inspect the ECU subsheath for rupture or attenuation, and adjust the reconstruction based on those findings. ▪ Evaluate the ECU subsheath looking for a concomitant TFCC disruption.
Inspecting the ulnar osseous groove	▪ Consider deepening the ulnar groove to augment stability.
Subsheath repair versus reconstruction	▪ Repair the subsheath if the tissues appear substantial. ▪ Reconstruct the sheath if in doubt. ▪ Perform passive motion testing in the extremes of supination mild wrist flexion and ulnar deviation following the procedure to ensure that the problem has been addressed.
Pitfalls	▪ Avoid injury to the dorsal cutaneous branch of the ulnar nerve. ▪ Do not repair the supratendinous retinaculum to the ulna, because this will limit forearm rotation. ▪ If creation of an ulnar extensor retinaculum sling is required, avoid making it overly tight, inhibiting ECU tendon gliding. This can be easily accomplished by placing a pediatric feeding tube beside the ECU during the sling construction.
Return to activity	▪ Full activity is not considered until 3 to 4 months following surgery.

POSTOPERATIVE CARE

- The sutures are removed 2 weeks after surgery, and an above elbow cast is applied with the forearm and wrist positioned in the manner described.
- This cast is removed 2 weeks later, and therapy is initiated with use of a fabricated sugartong splint and progressive range of motion as described in Nonoperative Management.

OUTCOMES

- No large conclusive studies on which to base outcomes have yet been published.
- A few case reports and smaller series have reported good results following surgical treatment for ECU subluxation.[1–4,6,7,9] Our experience mirrors these reports.

COMPLICATIONS

- The uncommon nature of ECU subluxation, the uniformly acceptable surgical outcomes, and the lack of large surgical case series result in a sparse list of postoperative complications. Trends with which to define "routine" postsurgical complications are simply not present.
- Complications that have been reported in the literature include the following:
  - Complex regional pain syndrome[1]
  - Decreased wrist motion
  - Decreased grip strength

REFERENCES

1. Allende C, Le Viet D. Extensor carpi ulnaris problems at the wrist: Classification, surgical treatment and results. J Hand Surg Br 2005;30:3:265–272.
2. Burkhart S, Wood M, Linscheid RL. Posttraumatic recurrent subluxation of the extensor carpi ulnaris tendon. J Hand Surg Am 1982; 7:1:1–3.
3. Chun S, Palmer A. Chronic ulnar wrist pain secondary to partial rupture of the extensor carpi ulnaris tendon. J Hand Surg Am 1987; 12:1032–1035.
4. Eckhardt W, Palmer A. Recurrent dislocation of extensor carpi ulnaris tendon. J Hand Surg Am 1981;6:629–631.
5. Inoue G, Tamura Y. Recurrent dislocation of the extensor carpi ulnaris tendon. Br J Sports Med 1998;32:172–177.
6. Inoue G, Tamura Y. Surgical treatment for recurrent dislocation of the extensor carpi ulnaris tendon. J Hand Surg Br 2001;26:556–559.
7. Rowland S. Acute traumatic subluxation of the extensor carpi ulnaris tendon at the wrist. J Hand Surg Am 1986;11:809–811.
8. Pratt R, Hoy GA. Extensor carpi ulnaris subluxation or dislocation? Ultrasound measurement of tendon excursion and normal values. Hand Surg 2004;9:137–143.
9. Spinner M, Kaplan E. Extensor carpi ulnaris: Its relationship to the stability of the distal radio-ulnar joint. Clin Orthop Relat Res 1970;68:124–129.
10. Taleisnik J, Gelberman R, Miller BW, et al. The extensor retinaculum of the wrist. J Hand Surg Am 1984:9:495–501.

Chapter 66

A1 Pulley Release for Trigger Finger With and Without Flexor Digitorum Superficialis Ulnar Slip Excision

Alexander M. Marcus

DEFINITION

- Trigger finger is an entrapment of the digital flexor tendon(s) by the flexor tendon sheath.
- Trigger finger progressively causes inflammation, pain, catching, locking, and reduced range of motion (ROM).

ANATOMY

- The flexor digitorum profundus and superficialis (flexor pollicis longus in the thumb) pass under (dorsal to) the flexor sheath, which consists of annular and cruciate pulleys.
- The A1 pulley, which is volar to the metacarpophalangeal joint (MCP), is the most proximal pulley (except for a thickening known as the *palmar aponeurotic pulley*[6]), and is almost always the primary site of entrapment (**FIG 1**).

PATHOGENESIS

- High angular loads at the A1 pulley and often, other causes of local inflammation result in a flexor tendon sheath whose inner diameter is too narrow to accommodate the flexor tendon(s).

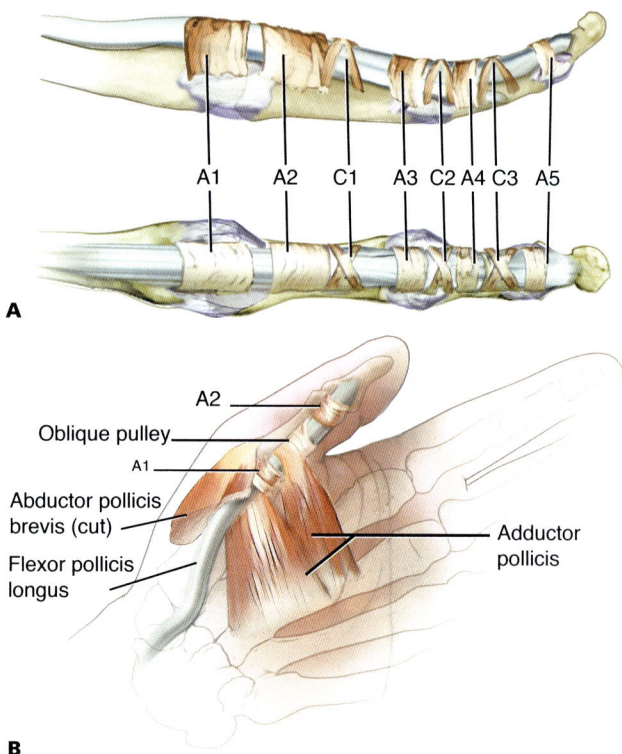

A

A1 A2 C1 A3 C2 A4 C3 A5

A2

Oblique pulley

A1

Abductor pollicis
brevis (cut)

Flexor pollicis
longus

Adductor
pollicis

B

FIG 1 • To understand trigger finger and its release, an appreciation of the flexor tendon pulley system of the finger (**A**) and thumb (**B**) is required.

- This size mismatch causes hypertrophy (thickening) of the A1 pulley and tendinous swelling.
- These changes exacerbate the size discrepancy, setting up a cycle in which entrapment causes hypertrophy and hypertrophy causes entrapment.

NATURAL HISTORY

- Trigger digits may develop spontaneously or may occur after swelling, from either trauma or a period of heavy use.
- Trigger digits may:
  - Resolve spontaneously (especially in mild cases)
  - Persist with the same level of symptoms
  - Advance to passively correctable locking
  - Become indefinitely locked in either flexion or extension

PATIENT HISTORY AND PHYSICAL FINDINGS

- The history may include any of the following:
  - Pain in the distal palm, often radiating proximally along the path of the flexor tendon
  - Pain occurring with use, and difficulty grasping objects or flexing the digit
  - Clicking or locking with digital flexion and extension, which is often perceived to be at the proximal interphalangeal joint (PIP)
  - The finger being stuck in flexion, often in the morning, requiring the other hand to straighten it
  - Being unable to flex or extend the digit fully, or at all (**FIG 2**)
- The history should elicit the following information:
  - Whether the patient has had a trigger finger before, in either the currently involved or any other digit
  - Previous treatments for trigger finger, and the extent and duration of the result

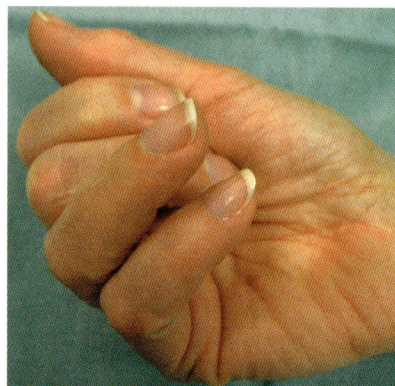

FIG 2 • Reduced flexion caused by ring finger triggering.

- Whether the condition began after a particular incident or period of increased hand use
- The patient's medical history should be evaluated for conditions that may cause trigger fingers and alter treatment, as well as commonly associated conditions, including:
  - Diabetes
  - Rheumatoid arthritis and other inflammatory arthropathies
  - Amyloidosis, most commonly secondary to renal disease requiring dialysis
  - Lysosomal storage diseases
  - Carpal tunnel syndrome (often seen in patients with trigger finger, but not causally related)
- The history and physical examination should exclude other conditions that cause overlapping symptoms, including:
  - Nerve compression
  - Muscle weakness
  - Tendon interruption from laceration (partial or complete) or rupture
  - Pulley rupture and bowstringing
  - Joint or soft tissue contracture or swelling, or both
  - Extensor tendon laceration or subluxation, especially at the MCP joint
  - Joint dislocation
- The physical examination should include the following:
  - ROM test, which is the most objective measure of severity. If the patient has absolutely no active motion at the PIP (or thumb IP), consider tendon interruption.
  - Palpation of the palm. If the A1 pulley is not tender, strongly consider other diagnoses. Examine for other causes of the patient's symptoms, including Dupuytren's contracture, tendon sheath ganglion, PIP joint injury, and A3 pulley triggering.
  - Examination of the extensor apparatus. Rule out extensor mechanism abnormalities that may cause overlapping signs or symptoms, including a popping sensation with ROM.
  - Perform a neurovascular examination. Carpal tunnel syndrome often is associated with trigger finger. Muscle weakness may cause similar findings. Any neurovascular deficit should be documented before treatment.

IMAGING AND OTHER DIAGNOSTIC STUDIES

- Radiographs can exclude some unusual causes of trigger finger symptoms and can assess for arthritis, but are not required to make the diagnosis of trigger finger.
- If other pathology is suspected, MRI can be useful.
- Nerve conduction studies can evaluate for anterior interosseous nerve (AIN) compression, which may mimic a trigger thumb or concomitant carpal tunnel syndrome.

DIFFERENTIAL DIAGNOSIS

- Extensor tendon subluxation at the MCP joint
- Joint contracture or injury, including MCP locking due to collateral ligaments and a swollen PIP joint
- Soft tissue swelling or contracture, including Dupuytren's contracture
- Partial tendon laceration
- Triggering at the A3 pulley (rare)
- Muscle weakness, including flexor pollicis longus weakness secondary to AIN palsy
- Masses (especially tendon sheath ganglions), which may cause A1 pulley tenderness

NONOPERATIVE MANAGEMENT

- Observation and splinting
  - Mild, early cases often resolve spontaneously or do not bother the patient significantly.
  - Use of a night extension splint may help alleviate swelling and morning locking.
  - Unless the PIP joint remains locked, in either flexion or extension, for several weeks, delayed treatment usually does not significantly change either the options available or their results.
- Injection
  - Long-term relief in most affected digits with one to three injections.[2]
  - Results in diabetic patients are not as good,[1,4] but it still is worth trying.
- Injection technique (**FIG 3**)
  - 1 mL of 2% plain (no epinephrine) lidocaine and 1 mL of a soluble corticosteroid solution (eg, betamethasone or

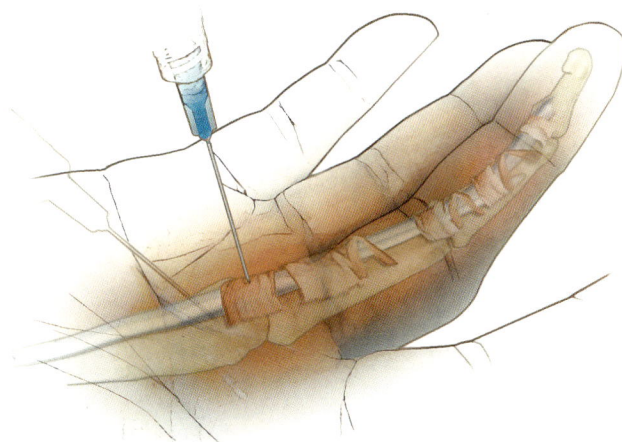

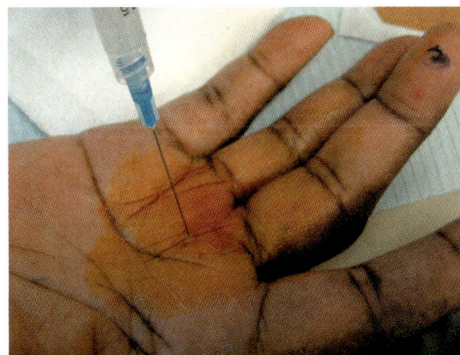

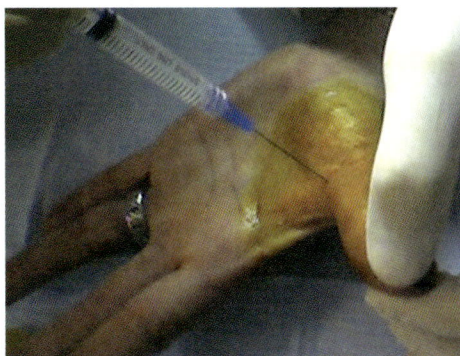

FIG 3 • Technique for trigger digit injection.

dexamethasone) in a single syringe with a 25-gauge needle is given.

- The A1 pulley area is prepped with an antiseptic solution such as alcohol or betadine.
- A topical spray may be used to reduce discomfort.
- 1 to 2 mL is injected in the sheath and subcutaneously.[11] Avoid injecting into the tendon itself; if increased resistance is encountered, this may be the cause.

SURGICAL MANAGEMENT

- Indications for surgical treatment include:
  - Symptoms that persist despite conservative management
  - Inability to flex or extend the finger even passively: this is an indication for earlier release to prevent secondary joint contracture.
- Open A1 pulley release is indicated for any routine trigger finger.
- Percutaneous trigger finger release:
  - Requires an actively triggering digit so the patient can flex to confirm needle placement and pulley release.
  - Is used primarily for the middle and ring fingers. Use in the other digits may place digital nerves in jeopardy.[13]
- In patients with very extensive synovitis, such as that seen in rheumatoid arthritis, lysosomal storage diseases, or amyloidosis associated with end-stage renal disease, releasing the A1 pulley percutaneously or through a routine, small incision is contraindicated. A more extensive tenosynovectomy and sometimes ulnar slip of the flexor digitorum superficialis (FDS) resection (USSR) is required.

Preoperative Planning

- Clinical notes and any studies obtained preoperatively should be reviewed.

- If procedures beyond an A1 pulley release are being considered (eg, possible resection of the ulnar slip of the flexor digitorum superficialis), they should be discussed with the patient preoperatively.

Positioning

- The patient is supine.
- The extremity is positioned so that the palm is facing up on a hand table.
  - For index, middle, ring, and small digits, a hand holder (eg, a "lead hand") is helpful.
  - For the thumb, it is more useful for the surgeon and assistant to position the hand and thumb throughout the procedure or to use a specialized thumb holder.
- Place a padded tourniquet and inflate it just before making the incision.

Approach

- Anesthesia is obtained by injecting 2% plain (no epinephrine) lidocaine subcutaneously around the incision and in the tendon sheath.
  - Sedation will mitigate the discomfort associated with the injection and the tourniquet. If sedation is used, the patient should be allowed to wake up in time to demonstrate complete active digital flexion and extension without locking, documenting successful pulley release.
- A standard volar approach to the A1 pulley is made with either an oblique, transverse, or longitudinal incision.
- For resection of the ulnar slip of the sublimis, a Bruner-type or midaxial longitudinal incision is used over the distal portion of the proximal phalanx.

TECHNIQUES

OPEN A1 PULLEY RELEASE

Incision and Exposure

- A 1-cm incision is placed over the A1 pulley.
  - Longitudinal (**TECH FIG 1A**)
  - If a transverse incision is used, it is placed in a palmar skin crease (**TECH FIG 1B**):
    - Distal palmar crease for small and ring fingers
    - Proximal palmar crease for index finger
    - An incision between creases may be required for middle finger release
  - Oblique or Bruner-type
- Avoid crossing palmar skin creases at a right angle with any incision type.
- Incise only the skin and dermis with a no. 15 blade.
- Bluntly spread subcutaneous tissue to avoid injury to the digital nerves.
- The digital neurovascular structures adjacent to the A1 pulley must be retracted and protected.
  - Extensive dissection and exposure of these structures is not required.
  - The radial digital nerve of the thumb is at the greatest risk because it typically crosses the surgical field (**TECH FIG 1C**).

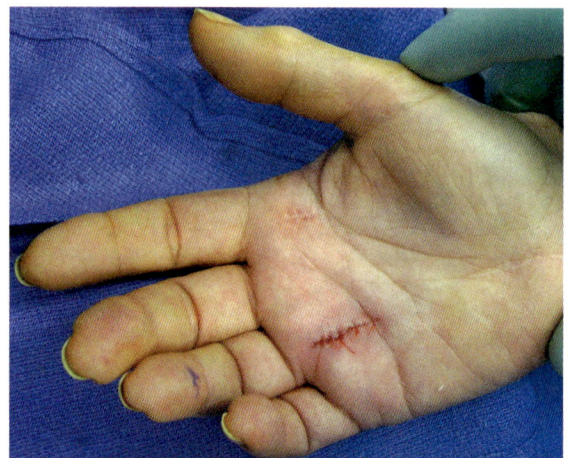

TECH FIG 1 • **A.** A longitudinal incision for ring finger A1 release. Index finger demonstrates a well-healed longitudinal incision without any contracture. *(continued)*

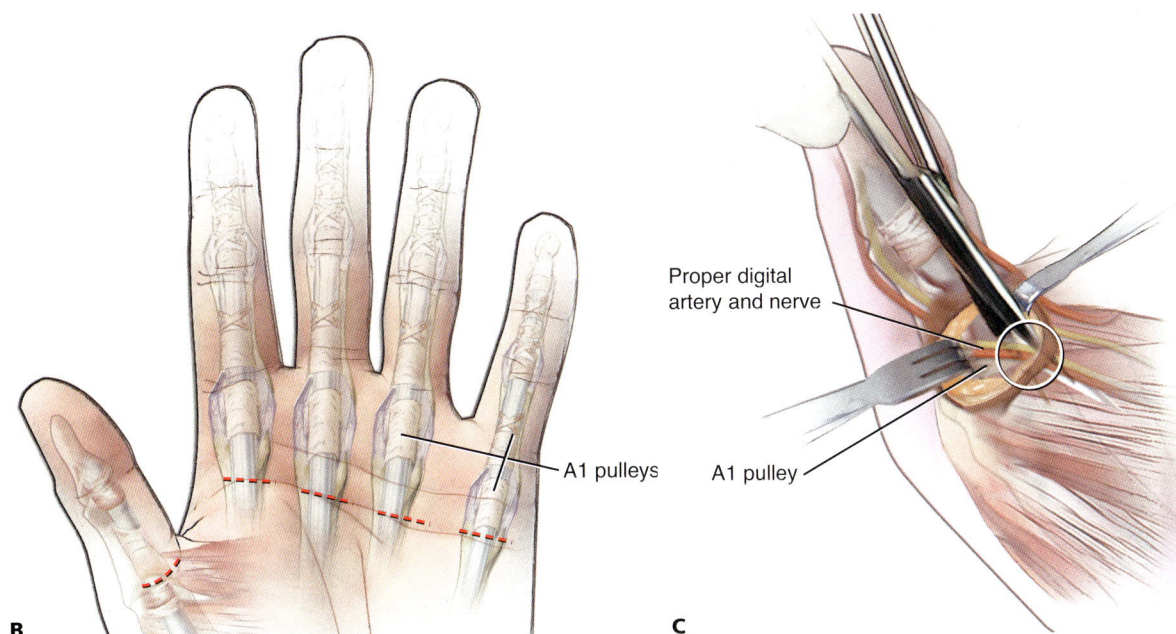

A1 pulleys

Proper digital artery and nerve

A1 pulley

B

C

TECH FIG 1 • *(continued)* B. Position of transverse incisions for trigger finger release in relation to the palmar skin creases and the A1 pulley. **C.** The digital neurovascular structures are right next to the A1 pulley and must be protected. This schematic demonstrates the proximity of the digital nerves and arteries. Because the radial digital nerve of the thumb may cross at the level of the A1 pulley, it is particularly vulnerable.

Performing the Release

- Clear off the A1 pulley with sponge dissection.
- The A1 pulley is not incised until it is clearly visualized (**TECH FIG 2A**).
  - Use of small right-angle retractors helps provide needed visualization.

- Begin the A1 pulley incision with a knife, taking care not to cut deep into the tendon.
- Complete the release with scissors until the pulley leaflets can be spread completely apart (**TECH FIG 2B**).
- Avoid cutting any significant portion of the A2 pulley (or the oblique pulley in the thumb).

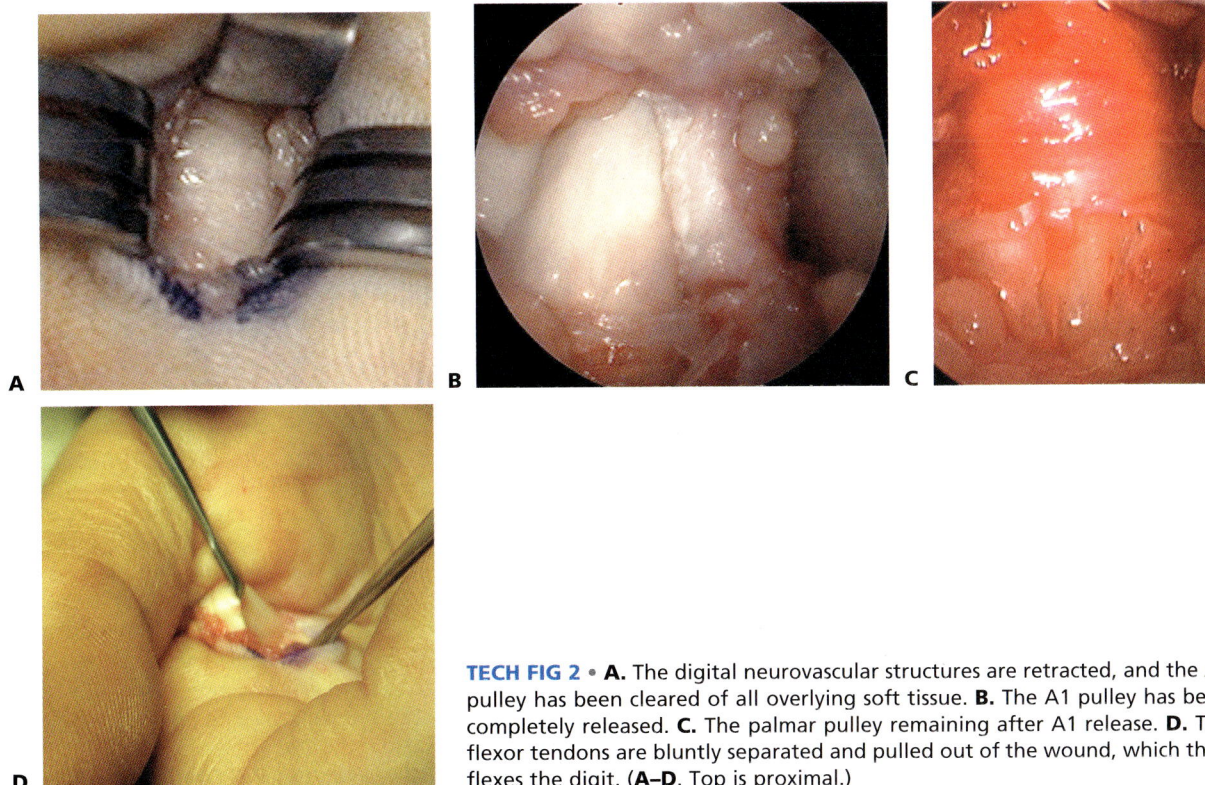

A

B

C

D

TECH FIG 2 • A. The digital neurovascular structures are retracted, and the A1 pulley has been cleared of all overlying soft tissue. **B.** The A1 pulley has been completely released. **C.** The palmar pulley remaining after A1 release. **D.** The flexor tendons are bluntly separated and pulled out of the wound, which then flexes the digit. (**A–D.** Top is proximal.)

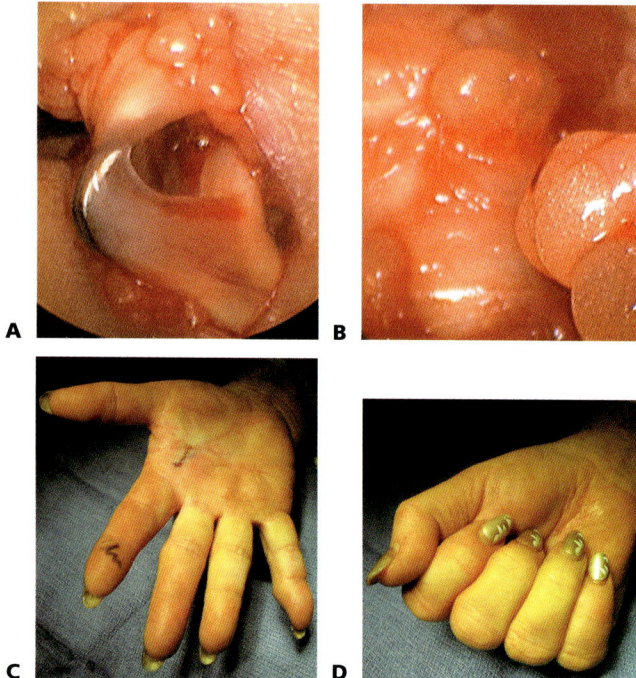

TECH FIG 3 • **A.** Tenosynovium between the tendons can be gently removed. **B.** A tendon sheath mass. Pathologic analysis confirmed it was a tendon sheath ganglion. **C,D.** Full active flexion and extension after release.

- The A2 pulley is separated from the A1 pulley either by a space (where there is no sheath) or a section of very thin sheath tissue.[9]
- If the tendons appear constricted by the palmar aponeurotic pulley[6] proximal to the A1 pulley, it should also be released (**TECH FIG 2C**).
- Bluntly separate the tendons (in the fingers) and pull the tendon(s) out of the wound (**TECH FIG 2D**). Minimize any direct handling of the tendons.

Completion

- A limited tenosynovectomy may be performed if required (**TECH FIG 3A**). Any unusual resected tissue or mass is sent to the pathology department for analysis (**TECH FIG 3B**).
- Confirm that the patient can actively flex and extend the finger (**TECH FIG 3C,D**). If the active ROM is not full or significantly improved, or if the tendons are not passing under the remaining pulleys, consider ulnar slip of the flexor digitorum superficilias resection (USSR) as well as etiologies other than standard trigger finger.[5,7,8,10]
- Release the tourniquet, and irrigate the wound.
- Obtain hemostasis, usually with manual compression. Reinspect the wound, check for any arterial bleeding, and confirm the finger has brisk capillary refill.
- Close the skin with interrupted sutures and place a mildly compressive dressing.

PERCUTANEOUS A1 PULLEY RELEASE

- The patient must have active triggering.
- The procedure is performed with a sterile prep in either the office or operating room.
- Hyperextend the MCP joints over a towel to help displace the neurovascular structures dorsally.
- Palpate the A1 pulley.
- Inject the local anesthetic (with or without corticosteroid) as described for nonoperative treatment.
- An 18- or 19-gauge needle is placed through the A1 pulley, centered radial to ulnar, and into the tendon (**TECH FIG 4**).

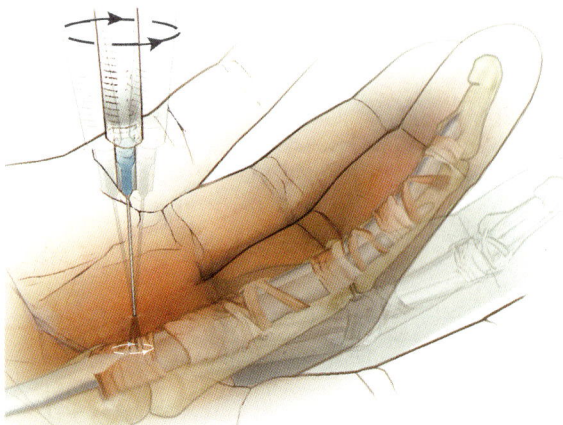

TECH FIG 4 • Percutaneous A1 release.

- The patient actively flexes the finger which moves the needle, confirming location.
- The needle is pulled back slightly so that it remains in the A1 pulley, but not the tendon.
- The needle is rotated so that the bevel is in line with the longitudinal axis of the pulley.
- Sweep the needle proximally and distally until grating is no longer felt.
- The patient should be able to actively flex and extend the finger without triggering, confirming release.

Open A1 Pulley Release With FDS Ulnar Slip Excision (USSR)

- The initial steps are performed in the same manner as described for an open A1 pulley release.
- A Bruner-type or ulnar midaxial incision is made over the proximal phalanx.
  - For a Bruner-type incision, a zigzag skin incision is made with the points over the finger flexion creases (**TECH FIG 5**).
  - The skin *only* is opened with a no. 15 blade, and blunt dissection is used to separate the neurovascular bundles as a unit. Formal dissection of the nerve and artery, or separating them from each other, is not required.
  - Care should be taken to stay more centrally as the incision proceeds distally (over the PIP and distal interphalangeal joints) because the neurovascular bundles can become less radial and ulnar on the digit.

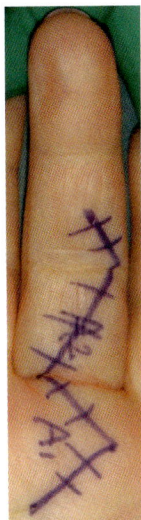

TECH FIG 5 • A Brunner-type incision. (Courtesy of Dominique Le Viet.)

- Inspect the tendon distal to the A2 pulley, confirming that there is no catching under the A3 pulley[8] and that an enlarged, bulbous flexor digitorum profundus is not catching under the distal end of the A2 pulley.[10] In either of these cases, USSR may or may not relieve the problem.
- Ulnar slip excision is then performed in either distal-to-proximal fashion[7] or with a proximal-to-distal technique.[5]

Distal-to-Proximal Ulnar Slip Excision

- Just distal to the A2 pulley, incise the tendon sheath, creating a radially based flap. This flap may be repaired later with 6-0 Prolene if desired.
- With the PIP joint maximally flexed, isolate and cut the ulnar slip of the flexor digitorum superficialis distally, taking care to preserve the vinculum brevis.
- Pull the tendon into the proximal wound and cut it as far proximal as can be reached safely.
- Confirm that the tendons now pass smoothly under the pulley system through a complete ROM.
- Release the tourniquet. Irrigate the wounds.
- Obtain hemostasis, usually with manual compression. Reinspect the wound, check for any arterial bleeding, and confirm the finger has brisk capillary refill.
- Close the skin with interrupted sutures and place a mildly compressive dressing.

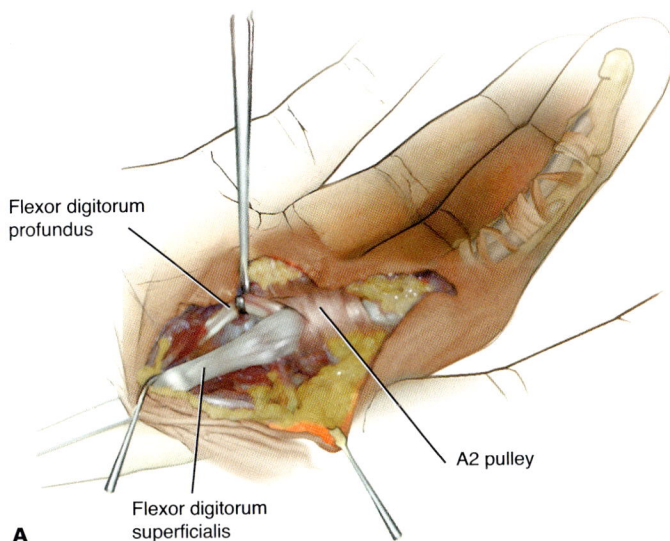

A

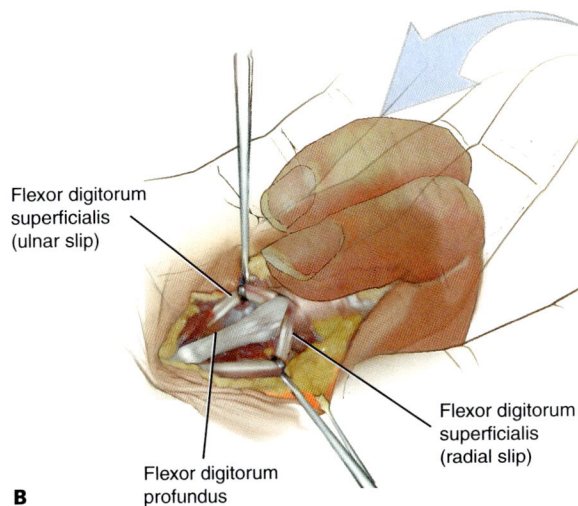

B

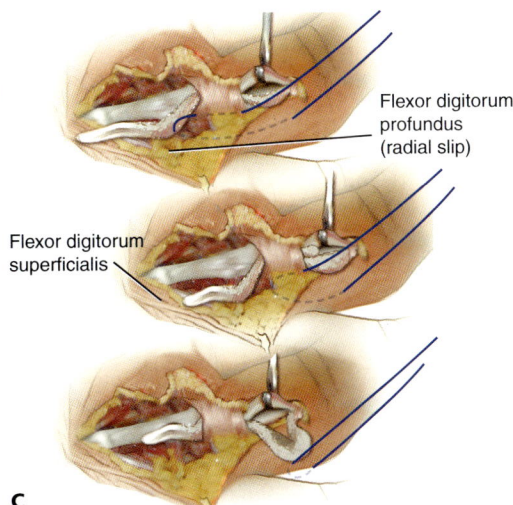

C

TECH FIG 6 • Open A-1 pulley release with FDS ulnar slip excision. **A.** Enlargement of tendon proximal to A-2 pulley (after A-1 release). **B.** Separating the FDS tendon slips. **C.** Use of a wire loop to separate tendon adhesions after cutting the FDS tendon proximally. (**A,B:** Modified from Le Viet D, Tsionos I, Boulouednine M, Hannouche D. Trigger finger treatment by ulnar superficialis slip resection [U.S.S.R.]. J Hand Surg 2004:29B:368–373.)

TECHNIQUES

Proximal to Distal Ulnar Slip Excision

- Examine the part of the tendon meant to glide under the A1 and A2 pulleys for enlargement, degeneration, longitudinal splitting, or loss of its smooth surface (**TECH FIG 6A**).
- Fully flex the finger, identify the ulnar and radial slips of the FDS distally, and split them longitudinally in a proximal direction (**TECH FIG 6B**).
- With the finger and wrist flexed, cut the ulnar slip of the FDS as far proximal as possible. Pull the ulnar slip distally,

carefully separating it through the chiasm, and, with the PIP joint flexed, cut it distally at the edge of the A3 pulley. The tendon slip is than removed from either direction; a loop of 3-0 wire can be used to separate adhesions if necessary (**TECH FIG 6C**).

- Release the tourniquet. Irrigate the wound.
- Obtain hemostasis, usually with manual compression. Reinspect the wound, check for any arterial bleeding, and confirm the finger has brisk capillary refill.
- Close the skin with interrupted sutures and place a mildly compressive dressing.

PEARLS AND PITFALLS

Satisfactory release	■ Confirm that the tendon glides freely after release. ■ If there was no joint contracture preoperatively, the patient should have significantly improved active (or passive, if the patient is under general anesthesia) ROM. ■ If not, assess the cause and correct.
Avoid injury to A2 pulley	■ Release of more than 25% of the A2 pulley may cause bowstringing, reducing flexion ROM, and require pulley reconstruction.

POSTOPERATIVE CARE

- A soft dressing is applied with all of the digits free (**FIG 4**). Active ROM as tolerated is encouraged. Minimize dressing bulk to avoid inhibiting motion.
- Formal therapy is required only if the patient has difficulty regaining ROM.
- Patients whose digits were locked preoperatively are more likely to need therapy. This may be started within the first week.
- Scar massage is encouraged after the wound is sealed.

OUTCOMES

- Surgical release of trigger digits has a high success rate with a low complication and recurrence rate.[3,12]

COMPLICATIONS

- Injury to digital nerve or artery
- Bowstringing
- Wound infection or dehiscence resulting in a flexor sheath infection

- Postoperative stiffness
- Incomplete release
- Recurrence
- Incisional tenderness

REFERENCES

1. Baumgarten KM, Gerlach D, Boyer MI. Corticosteroid injection in diabetic patients with trigger finger. A prospective, randomized, controlled double-blinded study. J Bone Joint Surg Am 2007;89A: 2604–2611.
2. Benson LS, Ptaszek AJ. Injection versus surgery in the treatment of trigger finger. J Hand Surg Am 1997;22:138–144.
3. Gilberts EC, Wereldsma JC. Long-term results of percutaneous and open surgery for trigger fingers and thumbs. Int Surg 2002;87:48–52.
4. Griggs SM, Weiss AC, Lane LB, et al. Treatment of trigger finger in patients with diabetes mellitus. J Hand Surg Am 1995;20:787–789.
5. Le Viet D, Tsionos I, Boulouednine M, et al. Trigger finger treatment by ulnar superficialis slip resection (U.S.S.R.). J Hand Surg Br 2004;29:368–373.
6. Manske PR, Lesker PA. Palmar aponeurosis pulley. J Hand Surg Am 1983:8:259–263.
7. Marcus AM, Culver J, Hunt TR. Treating trigger finger in diabetics using excision of the ulnar slip of the flexor digitorum superficialis with or without A1 pulley release. Hand 2007;2:227–231.
8. Rayan GM. Distal stenosing tenosynovitis. J Hand Surg Am 1990:15:973–975.
9. Ryzewicz M, Wolf JM. Trigger digits: Principles, management, and complications. J Hand Surg Am 2006;31:135–146.
10. Seradge H, Kleinert HE. Reduction flexor tenoplasty. J Hand Surg Am 1981:6:543–544.
11. Taras JS, Raphael JS, Pan WT, et al. Corticosteroid injections for trigger digits: Is intrasheath injection necessary? J Hand Surg Am 1998:23:717–722.
12. Turowski GA, Zdankiewicz PD, Thomson JG. The results of surgical treatment of trigger finger. J Hand Surg Am 1997:22:145–149.
13. Wilhelmi BJ, Mowlavi A, Neumeister MW, et al. Safe treatment of trigger finger with longitudinal and transverse landmarks: An anatomic study of the border finger for percutaneous release. Plast Reconstr Surg 2003:112:993–999.
14. Wolfe SW. Tenosynovitis. In: Green DP, Hotchkiss RN, Pederson WC, et al, eds. Green's Operative Hand Surgery, 5th ed. Philadelphia: Elsevier, 2005:2137–2158.

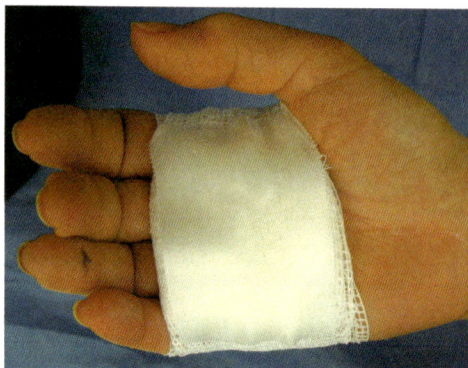

FIG 4 • A soft dressing is applied with all the digits free.

Chapter 67

Carpal Tunnel Release: Endoscopic, Open, and Revision

Edward Diao

DEFINITION

▪ Carpal tunnel syndrome (CTS) is the most common nerve compression condition in the upper extremity.

▪ Carpal tunnel release (CTR) is one of the most commonly performed procedures in the United States.

▪ CTS is a compressive neuropathy of the median nerve at the wrist.

▪ Early stages of CTS are reversible with treatment.

▪ Later or more severe stages of CTS may not be (fully) reversible.

ANATOMY

▪ The carpal tunnel or carpal canal is a space bounded by the carpal bones dorsally, the trapezium and scaphoid radially, the hook of the hamate ulnarly, and the transverse carpal ligament palmarly (**FIG 1A**).

▪ The carpal canal contains the median nerve and nine digital flexor tendons, along with the accompanying tenosynovium (**FIG 1C**).

▪ Anatomic anomalies include the following:
  ▪ A persistent median artery
  ▪ Muscle anomalies
  ▪ Median nerve branching anomalies (**FIG 1B**)

▪ Extraneous masses or structures may be found within the carpal canal, including sarcoid and ganglion cysts.

PATHOGENESIS

▪ Most cases of CTS are idiopathic.[9]

▪ Some cases are associated with systemic conditions, such as rheumatoid arthritis, diabetes, thyroid disease, chronic renal failure, and sarcoidosis. CTS is associated with pregnancy.

▪ There is an association of CTS with cumulative trauma and repetitive use.[9]

▪ Increased pressure within the carpal canal is associated with CTS.[2,6,11]

▪ Peripheral neuropathy and CTS have also been associated with shear forces on the nerve, such as with a traction injury.[7]

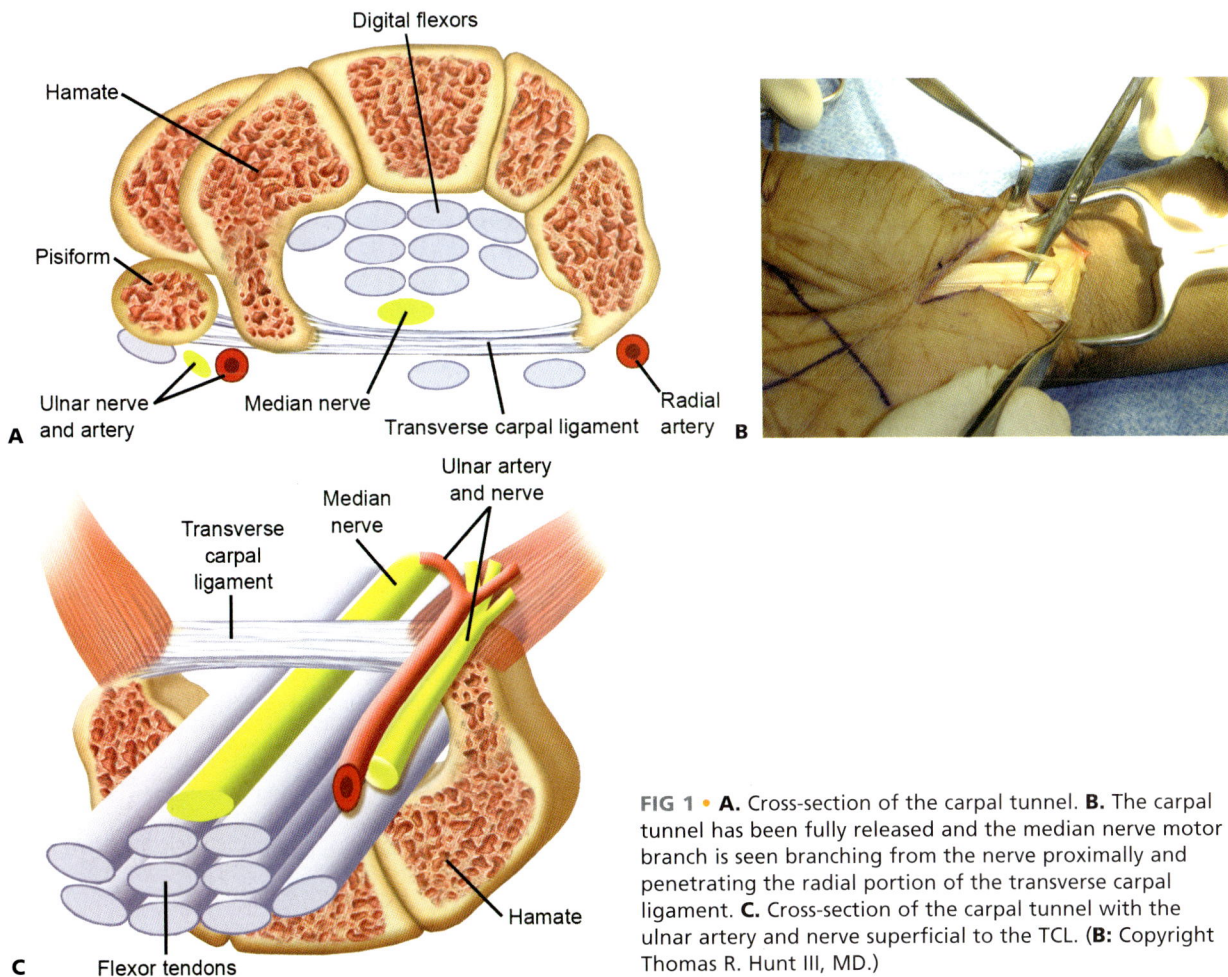

FIG 1 • **A.** Cross-section of the carpal tunnel. **B.** The carpal tunnel has been fully released and the median nerve motor branch is seen branching from the nerve proximally and penetrating the radial portion of the transverse carpal ligament. **C.** Cross-section of the carpal tunnel with the ulnar artery and nerve superficial to the TCL. (**B:** Copyright Thomas R. Hunt III, MD.)

NATURAL HISTORY

- CTS may have a variable course. It can improve, remain stable, or get more severe.
- Patients with severe CTS have motor and sensory changes and may have muscle weakness and atrophy.[9]
  - Patients with extremely advanced CTS frequently have little pain but constant numbness and weakness.

HISTORY AND PHYSICAL FINDINGS

- Presenting symptoms can be variable: some patients with mild CTS present with moderate to severe pain, numbness, and paresthesias, whereas other patients have minimal symptoms until their syndrome is severe and there is thenar muscle atrophy.
  - A common finding that drives patients toward a remedy is nocturnal waking.
- The surgeon should obtain a full medical history to identify for risk factors for CTS such as hypothyroidism and diabetes.
- The surgeon must understand the patient's occupational and recreational hand activities and any antecedent trauma that might contribute to symptoms.
  - The surgeon should inquire about activity triggers for the CTS.
- The surgeon should obtain a sense of symptom progression and severity.
  - Questions should be asked about sensory and motor function, pain pattern, and nocturnal waking.
- The physical examination includes the neck and shoulder girdle; the supraclavicular, infraclavicular, and axillary area; the humerus and elbow; the forearm; and the wrist and hand.
- It is important to generate a list of findings that may be responsible for the pain or paresthesias *other* than CTS.
- In addition to the standard joint evaluation with range of motion and assessments of stability, it is important to palpate the course of the nerves and elicit the Tinel sign along the course of the paracervical, brachial plexus, median, ulnar, and radial nerves.
  - The Tinel sign is mild, moderate, or severe subjective findings of radicular pain. The mechanical external stimulus threshold for depolarization–repolarization is lowered in a nerve that has a peripheral neuropathy. Anatomic distribution also is important.
  - Phalen's sign: Wrist flexion decreases the anatomic volume of the carpal canal and raises pressure in patients with CTS. The pattern of paresthesia can be important.
  - Carpal tunnel compression test: The mechanical external stimulus threshold for depolarization–repolarization is lowered in a nerve that has a peripheral neuropathy.
  - Two-point discrimination: In peripheral neuropathy the ability to distinguish one or two points is diminished.
  - Decreased range of motion and palmar wrist swelling can be indirect indications of tenosynovium in the carpal canal, and also any intra-articular wrist pathology.

IMAGING AND OTHER DIAGNOSTIC STUDIES

- AP, lateral, and oblique radiographs are not mandatory in the workup if the wrist examination is completely normal. If there is any possibility of wrist pathology, these studies should be obtained.
- Other imaging studies are not indicated in routine cases. In cases of recurrent CTS, MRI should be obtained to gain

further information regarding a complete versus incomplete release of the transverse carpal ligament (TCL) or evidence of median nerve compression, tenosynovitis, and scarring.[1]

- Electrodiagnostics: Nerve conduction studies (NCS) and electromyography (EMG) are important. CTS can be graded based on NCS and EMG findings:
  - CTS mild: Increased sensory or motor distal latency; may see decreased amplitude
  - CTS moderate: Increased nerve conduction velocity
  - CTS severe: EMG shows signs of chronic denervation with positive fibrillations and sharp waves or unobtainable recordings on the electrodes to median innervated muscles.
  - Although some experts believe the absence of any of the above electrodiagnostic findings means that there is no CTS, others believe that false-negatives exist due to sensitivity issues with NCS and EMG.[4]

DIFFERENTIAL DIAGNOSIS

- Cervical radiculitis
- Cervical pathology, joint disease, disc disease, facet disease with foramina stenosis
- Thoracic outlet syndrome
- Brachial plexopathy
- Syringomyelia, motor neuron disease, myelopathy
- "Double crush syndrome"
- Shoulder pain related to instability, intra-articular pathology, subacromial impingement
- Acromioclavicular joint pathology
- Medial epicondylitis
- Lateral epicondylitis
- Cubital tunnel syndrome
- Radial tunnel syndrome
- Pronator syndrome
- Elbow pathology instability or contracture
- Forearm or wrist tenosynovitis
- Wrist tenosynovitis, extensor, flexor, or De Quervain tenosynovitis
- Digital tenosynovitis (trigger finger)
- Guyon canal syndrome
- Hypothenar hammer syndrome
- Wrist or carpal fracture
- Intra-articular wrist pathology

NONOPERATIVE MANAGEMENT

- Mild CTS can often be modulated through conservative means.[5,16]
- Any systemic conditions should be identified and treated.[5,16]
- Activity modification can be attempted, especially if the activity includes highly repetitive loading of the hand, wrist, and upper extremity.
- Wrist splints can be introduced.
- The physician can recommend or prescribe nonsteroidal anti-inflammatory drugs (NSAIDs).
- Corticosteroid injection into the carpal canal can be considered (**FIG 2**).
  - Temporary relief from such an injection indicates that surgical decompression is likely to be successful.
- Hand therapy can be considered.
- Some believe oral vitamin B12 treatment can be helpful in some cases.

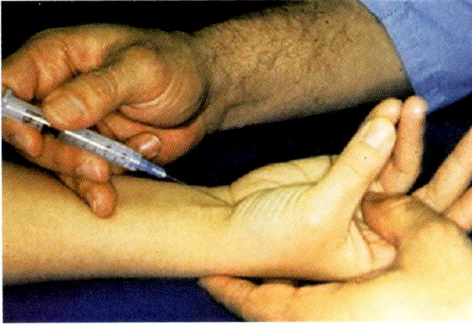

FIG 2 • Cortisone injection.

SURGICAL MANAGEMENT

- The diagnosis of CTS is confirmed by either the presence of classic clinical symptoms and signs or positive NCS or EMG studies.
  - If the NCS or EMG findings are negative, at least one trial of corticosteroid injection should be given to evaluate the clinical response.
- The surgeon should confirm that a trial of conservative treatment has been undertaken without a cure.
- The surgeon should confirm that differential diagnoses have been considered.
- The surgeon should understand that the presence of other diagnoses and conditions will affect the overall results of CTS treatment; this needs to be discussed with the patient before, not after, surgery. In fact, one should strongly consider delaying CTS treatment to control or improve other conditions that may be amenable to nonoperative treatment.
- If the above conditions are met, CTR should have good to excellent results in more than 90% of cases.[14]
- In the case of recurrent CTS, the key to success is patient selection. Although there are scant data to correlate the preoperative evaluation with results, the patient's clinical course, response to conservative treatment, and interpretation of electrodiagnostic studies and MRI should be carefully considered before revision surgery.

Positioning

- CTR surgery is performed with the arm outstretched on a hand table.
- Pneumatic tourniquet use facilitates accurate identification of critical anatomic structures.
- Loupe magnification is recommended.
- Anesthesia can be by general anesthesia or regional anesthesia such as an axillary block or Bier block.

- Experienced surgeons can perform CTS safely under wrist block or local infiltration.

Approach

- The goal of CTR surgery is to decompress the median nerve at the carpal canal by complete division of the TCL to allow the carpal tunnel to expand.
- A volar exposure is used, but incision position and length vary.
- The locations of critical deep structures are defined using superficial landmarks and a line drawn down the axis of the fourth ray and another drawn obliquely across the palm in line with the ulnar border of the abducted thumb (Kaplan cardinal line) (**FIG 3**).

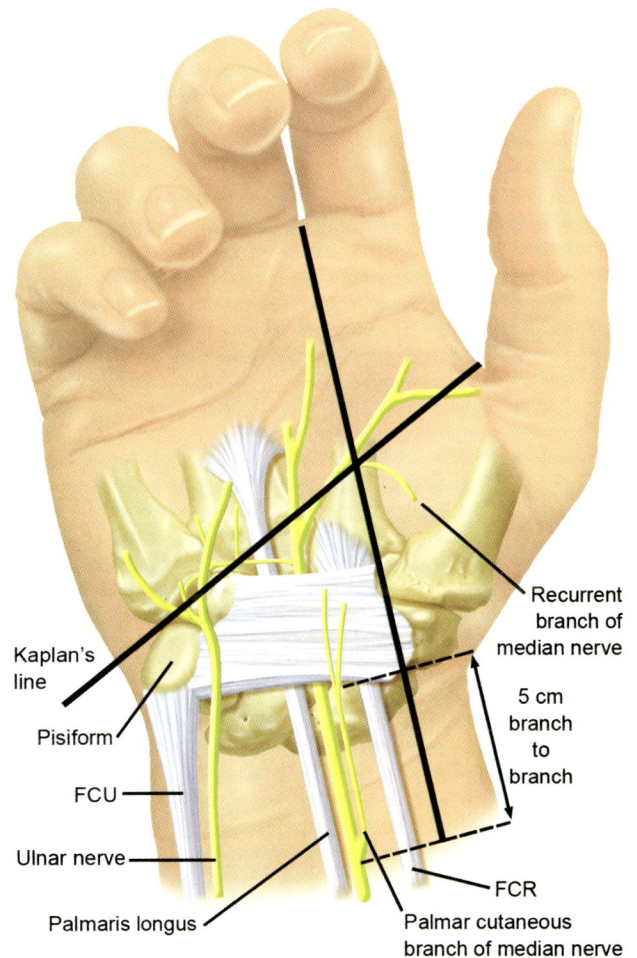

FIG 3 • Surface landmarks are critical when contemplating surgical release of the median nerve.

OPEN CARPAL TUNNEL RELEASE

Exposure

- Mark the skin incision location, beginning at the intersection of the Kaplan cardinal line and a line drawn along the radial border of the fourth ray, and ending at the wrist flexion crease (**TECH FIG 1A**).
  - Use a longitudinal hypothenar crease if available.
  - The incision may be placed anywhere along this mark (**TECH FIG 1B**), depending on the surgeon's

preference. I prefer the midpoint of the proximal third of the palm.
- The incision should be long enough to allow full access to the proximal to distal extent of the TCL to ensure full TCL division. This generally can be achieved without having the incision extend proximal to the wrist flexion crease.

TECHNIQUES

- Dissect in line with the incision using a scalpel or scissors, through the subcutaneous fat and the palmar fascia down to the TCL (**TECH FIG 1C**).
  - Frequently, the palmaris brevis muscle is encountered directly superficial to the TCL. It is incised and "feathered" from the ligament for adequate visualization of the TCL.

- Incise the TCL over a small segment, avoiding injury to deep structures (**TECH FIG 1D**).
  - Contents of the carpal canal will have a characteristic appearance due to the tenosynovium.
- Place an instrument such as a mosquito clamp or Carroll elevator into the carpal canal, just deep to the TCL (**TECH FIG 1E**).
  - This defines the undersurface of the TCL, the location of the hamate hook, and the proposed direction for release.
- Visualize the superficial surface of the TCL along its course and place a right-angle retractor to protect the critical structures located between the skin and the ligament (**TECH FIG 1F,G**).

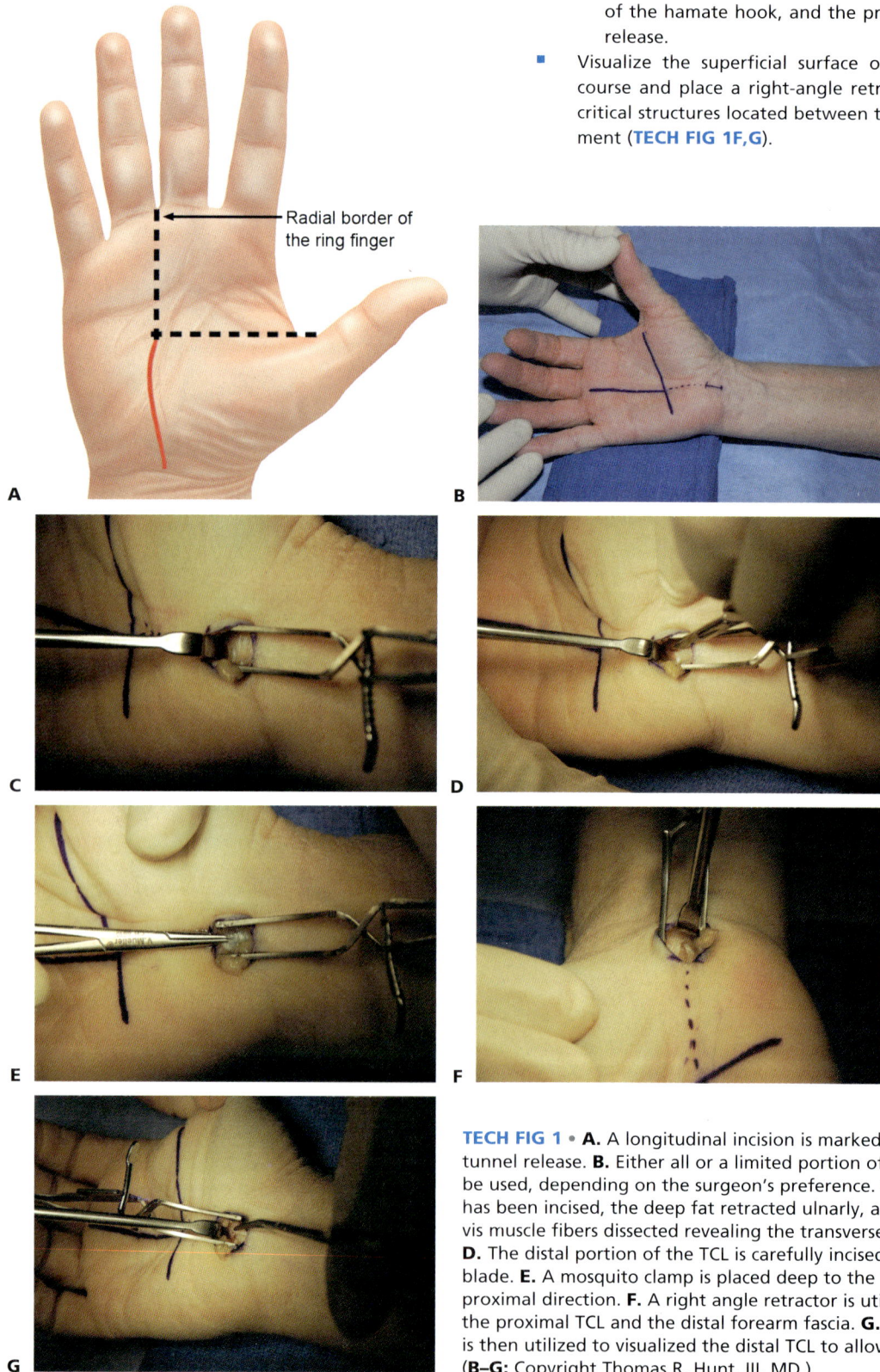

Radial border of the ring finger

A

B

C

D

E

F

G

TECH FIG 1 • **A.** A longitudinal incision is marked for an open carpal tunnel release. **B.** Either all or a limited portion of this incision may be used, depending on the surgeon's preference. **C.** The palmar fascia has been incised, the deep fat retracted ulnarly, and the palmaris brevis muscle fibers dissected revealing the transverse fibers of the TCL. **D.** The distal portion of the TCL is carefully incised with a no. 15 knife blade. **E.** A mosquito clamp is placed deep to the TCL in a distal to proximal direction. **F.** A right angle retractor is utilized to visualize the proximal TCL and the distal forearm fascia. **G.** The same retractor is then utilized to visualized the distal TCL to allow complete release. (**B–G:** Copyright Thomas R. Hunt, III, MD.)

Transverse Carpal Ligament Release

- Staying ulnar in the canal but still leaving a 2-mm cuff of TCL attached to the hamate hook, release the TCL under direct vision proximally and distally with a scalpel, scissors, or mini-meniscotome Beaver blade.
  - Keep a radially based TCL leaflet over the median nerve.
- Release the distal forearm fascia proximally (see Tech Fig 1F).
  - This tissue may be a secondary compression site, especially in patients with two wrist flexion creases.
- Completely divide the TCL and inspect the median nerve and canal contents (see Tech Fig 1G).
  - In rare instances a space-occupying lesion will require removal (ie, "billowing" synovium in a patient with rheumatoid arthritis).
  - In primary CTR procedures without systemic disease, there is no role for internal neurolysis or tenosynovectomy (**TECH FIG 2**).[3,8,10]
- The wound is closed and sterile dressings are applied.
- Use of a splint is based on the surgeon's preference.

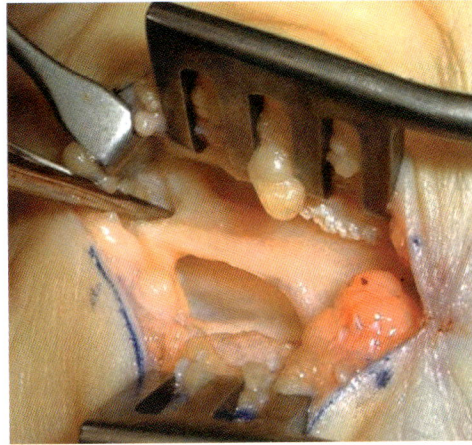

TECH FIG 2 • Open CTR with divided leaflets of the TCL retracted by the retractor jaws. The instrument is on the median nerve which is adherent to the undersurface of the TCL via tenosynovium.

SINGLE-INCISION ENDOSCOPIC CARPAL TUNNEL RELEASE (MODIFIED AGEE TECHNIQUE)[14]

Exposure

- Mark out the palmaris longus, the flexor carpi radialis, and the flexor carpi ulnaris.
- Make a transverse 1- to 2-cm incision in a wrist flexion crease centered over or just ulnar to the palmaris longus (**TECH FIG 3A**).
  - If the palmaris longus is not present, incise halfway between the flexor carpi radialis and the flexor carpi ulnaris.
- Expose the palmaris longus and retract it radially with a Ragnell retractor.
- Identify the flexor retinaculum deep to this structure (**TECH FIG 3B**).
- Incise the flexor retinaculum and create a distally based U-shaped flap 1 cm wide. Elevate and retract it with a mosquito clamp.
  - On the undersurface of the retinaculum adherent tenosynovium is frequently seen.
  - Visible deep to the opening should be the tenosynovium-covered digital flexor tendons and median nerve.
- Pass small and large hamate finders down the carpal canal in an antegrade manner to evaluate the space and the location of the hamate (**TECH FIG 3**).
- Palpate the tip of the instruments as they become subcutaneous distal to the distal edge of the TCL at the Kaplan cardinal line.
  - Make sure these instruments are not palpable subcutaneously in the proximal third of the palm, which would indicate incorrect placement superficial to the TCL and carpal canal and probably within the canal of Guyon.
- Use the tenosynovial elevator and pass it proximally and distally a dozen times along the axis of the fourth ray to dissect tenosynovium from the undersurface of the TCL.
  - A "washerboard effect" should be felt with this maneuver.

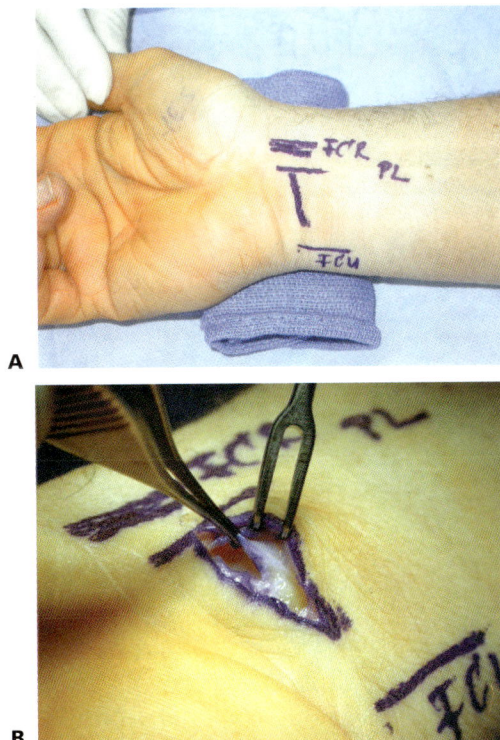

TECH FIG 3 • **A.** The key landmarks for ECTR are shown here: FCR, PL, FCU. The transverse incision is inscribed. **B.** The skin incision has been made and the fascia has also been incised. (Copyright Ekkehard Bonatz, MD.)

Device Insertion

- Introduce the assembled Agee endoscopic carpal tunnel release (ECTR) device into the carpal canal, with the scope directed palmarly.

TECHNIQUES

- The undersurface of the TCL with its characteristic transverse striations is visible.
- While viewing the monitor, advance the instrument until the distal edge of the TCL is identified.
  - The distal edge is noted by a transition from the white, transverse fibers of the TCL to the yellow amorphous midpalmar fat, which often contains visible vessels and nerves.
- Using your nondominant hand on the palm, perform a ballottement maneuver to help distinguish the transition between the midpalmar fat and the distal edge of the TCL while viewing the signal from the endoscope within the carpal canal on the monitor.
- In the palm, palpate the tip of the ECTR device as it emerges into the subcutaneous space just distal to the TCL. Drive the device with the other dominant hand (**TECH FIG 4**).
  - The transillumination pattern from the ECTR device light source changes from underneath the TCL to the midpalmar fat.

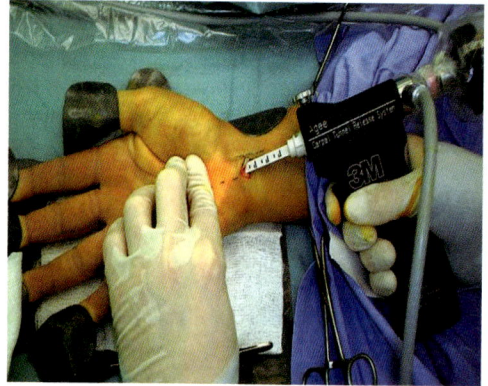

TECH FIG 4 • The surgeon's nondominant index and long digits palpate the tip of the endoscopic carpal tunnel release device as it emerges into the subcutaneous space just distal to the transverse carpal tunnel ligament. The transillumination pattern from the device light source changes from underneath the transverse carpal ligament to the midpalmar fat.

Transverse Carpal Ligament Release

- Elevate the blade and withdraw the device slowly, cutting the TCL from distal to proximal. Keep the device pressed up against the undersurface of the TCL so no structures come between the blade and the TCL; cut only the TCL (**TECH FIG 5**).
  - Cut only when visualization is excellent. If needed, withdraw the device and redefine the undersurface

of the TCL in the manner detailed above until visualization is ideal.
- Repeat the above step as needed until there is a full release of the TCL, with good separation of radial and ulnar leaflets from proximal to distal.
  - With a full release, it should not be possible to visualize the radial and ulnar leaflets simultaneously

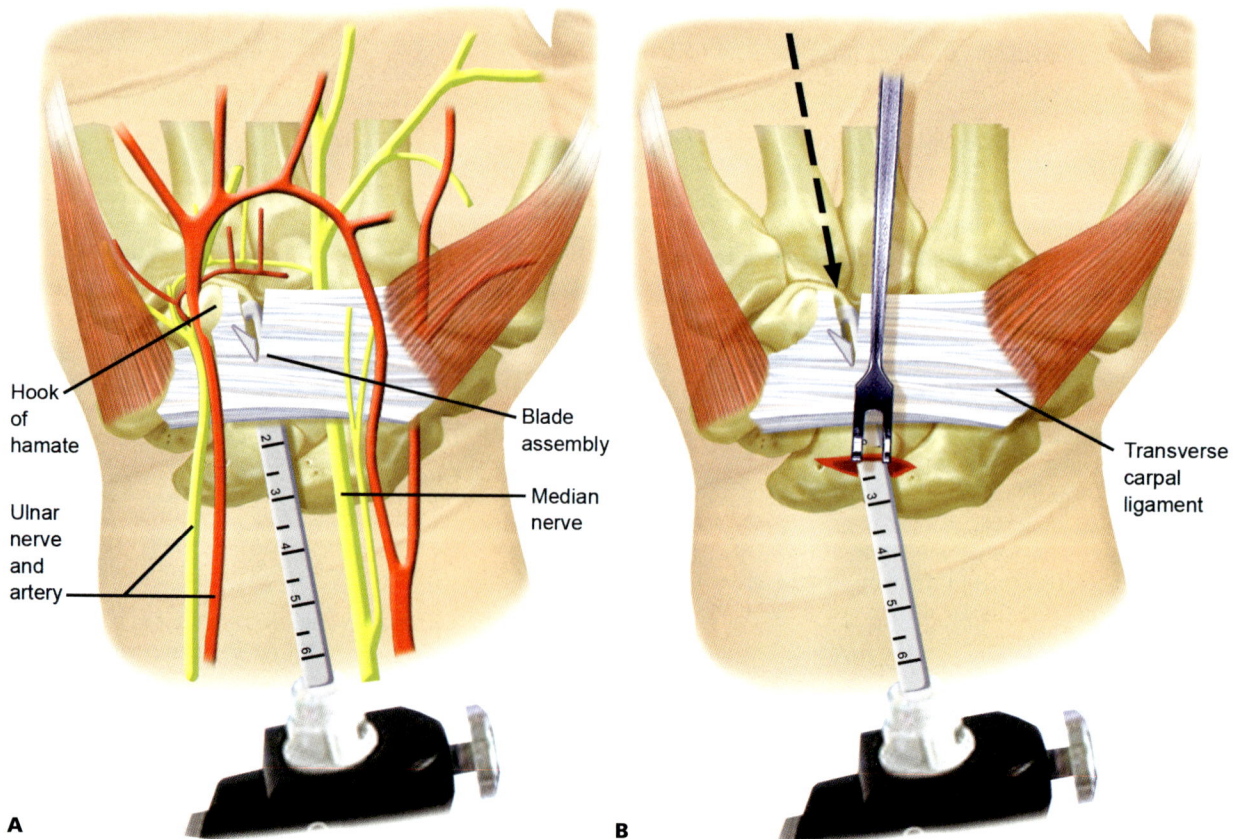

Hook of hamate

Ulnar nerve and artery

Blade assembly

Median nerve

Transverse carpal ligament

A

B

TECH FIG 5 • After careful identification of the distal edge of the transverse carpal ligament (**A**), the ligament is released from distal to proximal (**B**). *(continued)*

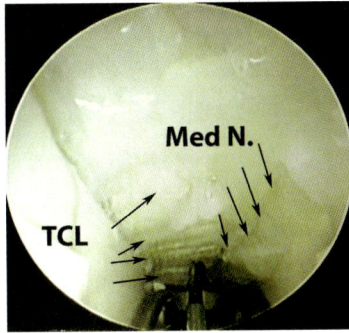

TECH FIG 5 • *(continued)* **C.** This is the start of the TCL division using the Agee device. The blade is elevated *(center)* and is shown starting to divide the TCL from distal to proximal. The median nerve is just seen radial to the blade. (Copyright Ekkehard Bonatz, MD.)

with the ECTR device up against the palmar tissues. Also, the ECTR device should be able to be placed within the trough between the radial and ulnar leaflets so neither leaflet is visible, just the fascia overlying the thenar muscles and the subcutaneous space.

- After full TCL release, withdraw the ECTR device.
- Confirm increased volume of the carpal canal by reintroducing the hamate finders down the carpal canal.
- Divide the proximal antebrachial fascia with long tenotomy scissors under direct vision.
  - Adson forceps help to deliver the tissue for cutting.
- The incision is closed and a soft dressing applied.
- If you cannot safely visualize the structures with the ECTR device, conversion to a two-incision or open CTR method is strongly suggested.

TWO-INCISION ENDOSCOPIC CARPAL TUNNEL RELEASE (CHOW TECHNIQUE)

- Make the proximal incision and create the distally based U-shaped flap of antebrachial fascia in the manner described for the single-incision ECTR technique.
- Introduce a clamp, elevator, or trocar under the TCL.
- Advance the instrument until it is palpable in the palm subcutaneously distal to the TCL.
- Make a second small incision to expose the tip of the instrument, usually at the junction of the middle and proximal thirds of the palm.
  - Take care to identify the superficial arch, common digital nerves, and fibers of the distal TCL in the area.
- A variety of techniques (open or scope-assisted) can be used at this point, including slotted trocars for two-incision endoscopic release, or use of a mini-meniscotome blade or scissor or other cutting instrument with a retractor or elevator to protect the median nerve and flexor tendons from the TCL cutting instrument.
- The complete distal TCL division can be ascertained by direct visualization, also taking note that the vessels and nerves have not been injured.
- A pitfall of the two incision techniques, aside from the potential injury to the palmar arterial arch and/or the branches of median or ulnar nerve, is incomplete release of the TCL distally. Therefore, inspection of the operative site with magnifying loupes at the distal incision is important.

REVISION RELEASE FOR RECURRENT OR RESIDUAL CARPAL TUNNEL SYNDROME

- If the recurrent CTS is due to prior incomplete release, revision surgery can be attempted using an ECTR technique; otherwise, open release is indicated (**TECH FIG. 6A,B**).
- Use a generous skin incision, incorporating previous incisions as needed.
- Perform the release using a similar technique to that described for primary open CTR.
  - Scarring often requires scalpel dissection, and separation of superficial tissues from the TCL is difficult.
- Carefully separate the TCL (in the area of its previous division) from the underlying median nerve.
  - Dense scarring of the median nerve to the TCL is expected and will place the nerve in jeopardy during this exposure.
- Completely release the TCL and the scarred median nerve, taking great care to protect the median nerve motor branch.
- Use an operating microscope to inspect the median nerve for signs of damage or scarring.

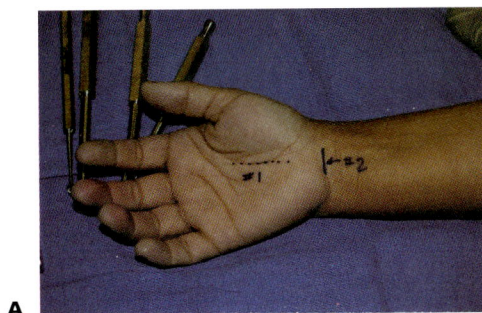

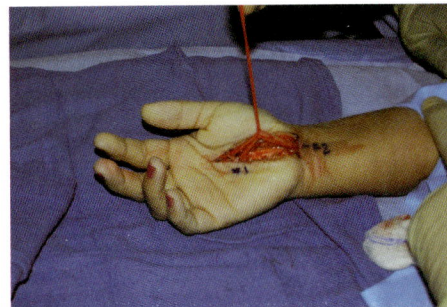

A

B

TECH FIG 6 • **A, B.** Revision of prior endoscopic carpal tunnel release with open technique. *(continued)*

TECHNIQUES

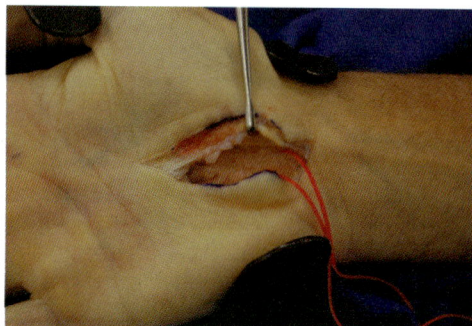

C

TECH FIG 6 • *(continued)* **C.** Revision carpal tunnel release with NeuraGen tube around scarred branch of median nerve.

- An external epineurotomy to expose the bands of Fontana on the surface fascicles of the median nerve is recommended in the case of significant nerve scarring.
- If there is minimal nerve scarring or damage, the wound can be closed in the usual manner.
- If nerve injury is dramatic and rescarring seems likely, cover the damaged nerve with a hypothenar fat pad flap, palmaris brevis muscle flap, vein wrapping, or neural conduit (**TECH FIG 6C**).

- Create a TCL flap through Z-lengthening and tissue rearrangement if flexor tendon prolapse or palmar migration of the median nerve seems likely.

Hypothenar Fat Pad

- When revision CTR reveals median nerve scarring, surgical tactics to improve the environment around the nerve after the neurolysis to reduce rescarring are attractive. Strickland[12] has described this technique in several publications. The tissue is readily available and has been shown to be of benefit. In a 1996 article,[12] 62 patients were reviewed. Results were good based on pre- and postoperative patient satisfaction scores, with only three transient minor complications.
- Dissect the fat pad to the level of the ulnar nerve and artery, and advance the radial edge to cover the median nerve.
- Sew this edge to the radial flap of the TCL.

Palmaris Brevis Flap

- Rose et al described this flap in 1991.
- Expose the thin palmaris brevis muscle on the ulnar side of the CTR incision.
- Divide it from its insertion in the subcutaneous space and transpose or rotate it into a position covering the median nerve.

PEARLS AND PITFALLS

Poor patient selection	■ Perform a full history and physical examination and contemplate the entire list of differential diagnoses.
Incomplete release of TCL	■ Whatever technique is used, make sure it is performed in a technically proficient manner. Confirm complete TCL division, especially distally.
Damage to median nerve	■ The surgeon must be able to identify the various anatomic structures and distinguish them. The median nerve must be protected during CTR. In techniques where the median nerve is visualized, inspection should be performed after TCL release and before skin closure.

POSTOPERATIVE CARE

■ Traditionally, CTR patients were managed in wrist splints for 1 to 3 weeks after surgery. However, multiple studies have shown that faster recovery occurs when the wrist is not splinted postoperatively.

　■ Temporary postoperative splints may still be indicated in specific clinical scenarios, such as open revision surgery.
■ Hand therapy is helpful in the postoperative period, especially if the patient is having difficulty with full digital active and passive motion.
■ Grip and pinch strength, subjective symptom measures, and functional evaluations are helpful to manage the postoperative course.
■ Some patients have prolonged periods of tenderness under the TCL, or pillar pain on the thenar or hypothenar side of the proximal palm, and require extended hand therapy and periods of time to gradually increase hand strength and endurance for hand activities.

OUTCOMES

■ There should be greater than 95% good or excellent results.[14] This randomized, double-blinded multicenter study compared open and single portal endoscopic CTR and showed statistically significant improvements in the endoscopic group between 6 weeks and 3 months postoperatively in terms of pain and hand strength compared to that of the open group, and equivalent good results in both groups at 1 year.
■ Stutz et al[13] reported on a retrospective series of 200 patients who underwent a secondary exploration during a 26-month period at a single institution for persistent or recurrent CTS symptoms after CTR. There were 108 cases of incomplete release of the TCL. Twelve patients had evidence of median nerve laceration during the index procedure. Forty-six patients had scarring of the nerve to surrounding tissues. In 13 patients the cause of their problem could not be determined.
■ Varitimidis et al[15] reviewed 22 patients (24 wrists) who underwent revision open CTR after an initial ECTR and who had

persistent CTS. Twenty-two patients had incomplete TCL release. One patient had a partial and another a complete median nerve transection. One patient had a Guyon canal release instead of a CTR. Twenty patients returned to work, 15 at the previous level and 5 at lighter duty. The two patients with nerve injuries continued to do poorly, one requiring a vein-wrapping procedure.

COMPLICATIONS

- Incomplete TCL release
- Median nerve scarring or damage (especially the common digital nerve to the third web space and the thenar motor branch)
- Ulnar nerve or artery damage
- Sympathetically mediated pain syndrome
- Damage to palmar arterial arch

REFERENCES

1. Ablove RH, Peimer CA, Diao E, et al. Morphologic changes following endoscopic and two-portal subcutaneous carpal tunnel release. J Hand Surg Am 1994;19A:821–826.
2. Diao E, Shao F, Liebenberg E, et al. Carpal tunnel pressure alters median nerve function in a dose-dependent manner: a rabbit model for carpal tunnel syndrome. J Orthop Res 2005;23:218–223.
3. Gelberman RH, Pfeffer GB, Galbraith RT, et al. Results of treatment of severe carpal-tunnel syndrome without internal neurolysis of the median nerve. J Bone Joint Surg Am 1987;69A:896–903.
4. Grundberg AB. Carpal tunnel decompression in spite of normal electromyography. J Hand Surg Am 1983;8A:348–349.
5. Kaplan SJ, Glickel SZ, Eaton RG. Predictive factors in the nonsurgical treatment of carpal tunnel syndrome. J Hand Surg Am 1990; 15:106–108.
6. Lundborg G, Gelberman RH, Minteer-Convery M, et al. Median nerve compression in the carpal tunnel: functional response to experimentally induced controlled pressure. J Hand Surg Am 1982;7A: 252–259.
7. Lundborg G, Rydevik B. Effects of stretching the tibial nerve of the rabbit: a preliminary study of the intraneural circulation and the barrier function of the perineurium. J Bone Joint Surg Br 1973;55B:390–401.
8. Mackinnon SE, McCabe S, Murray JF, et al. Internal neurolysis fails to improve the results of primary carpal tunnel decompression. J Hand Surg Am 1991;16A:211–218.
9. Rempel DM, Diao E. Entrapment neuropathies: pathophysiology and pathogenesis. J Electromyography Kinesiol 2004;14:71–75.
10. Rhoades CE, Mowery CA, Gelberman RH. Results of internal neurolysis of the median nerve for severe carpal tunnel syndrome. J Bone Joint Surg Am 1985;67A:253–256.
11. Rydevik B, Lundborg G, Bagge U. Effects of graded compression on intraneural blood flow: an in vivo study on rabbit tibial nerve. J Hand Surg Am 1981;6A:3–12.
12. Strickland JW, Idler RS, Lourie GM, et al. The hypothenar fat pad flap for management of recalcitrant carpal tunnel syndrome. J Hand Surg Am 1996;21A:840–848.
13. Stutz N, Gohritz A, Van Schoonhoven J, et al. Revision surgery after carpal tunnel release: analysis of the pathology in 200 cases during a 2-year period. J Hand Surg Br 2006;31B:68–71.
14. Trumble TE, Diao E, Abrams RA, et al. Single-portal endoscopic carpal tunnel release compared with open release: a prospective, randomized trial. J Bone Joint Surg Am 2002;84A:1107–1115.
15. Varitimidis SE, Herndon JH, Sotereanos DG. Failed endoscopic carpal tunnel release: operative findings and results of open revision surgery. J Hand Surg Br 1999;24B:465–467.
16. Weiss AP, Sachar K, Gendreau M. Conservative management of carpal tunnel syndrome: a reexamination of steroid injection and splinting. J Hand Surg Am 1994;19A:410–415.

Chapter 68

Decompression of Pronator and Anterior Interosseous Syndromes

E. Bruce Toby and Kyle P. Ritter

DEFINITION

- Pronator syndrome and anterior interosseous syndrome are compression neuropathies of the median nerve and its main branch, the anterior interosseous nerve (AIN), at the elbow and proximal forearm.

ANATOMY

- The median nerve passes in the distal upper arm between the brachialis and the medial intermuscular septum, with the brachial artery sitting lateral to it.
  - A rare supracondylar process may arise from the distal aspect of the humerus, giving origin to a fibrous band extending to the medial epicondyle. This is the ligament of Struthers.
  - If a ligament of Struthers is present, the median nerve passes underneath it.
- At the elbow, the median nerve sits underneath the lacertus fibrosus and then typically passes between the superficial (humeral) head and the deep (ulnar) head of the pronator teres.
  - In 20% of individuals, the deep head is absent or consists of a small fibrous band.
- Motor branches to the palmaris longus, flexor carpi radialis, flexor digitorum superficialis, and flexor digitorum profundus typically branch from the median nerve in an ulnar direction proximal to the pronator teres.
- Under the pronator teres, the AIN branches in a radial direction from the median nerve, and both pass underneath the fibrous arcade of the flexor digitorum superficialis.
- The surgeon should be cognizant of the cutaneous nerves passing over the antecubital and proximal forearm region. Damage to these nerves can result in numbness and paresthesia, as well as symptomatic neuromas in the forearm.
- Anomalous muscles and nerve branches may be present, the most common of which is the so-called Martin-Gruber anastomosis.
  - The surgeon should also be aware of more proximal or distal branching of the AIN from the median nerve.
  - The Martin-Gruber anastomosis, which occurs in about 15% of the population, consists of branches from either the median nerve or AIN to the ulnar nerve.

PATHOGENESIS

- Compression of the median nerve in the proximal forearm is rare compared with carpal tunnel syndrome.
- Median nerve compression in the proximal forearm has been labeled as either *pronator* or *anterior interosseous syndromes*.
- The true incidence of median nerve compression in the proximal forearm is difficult to ascertain, as is the relative contribution of the various potential impinging structures.
- Numerous studies have shown that the most common causes of median nerve compression in the region of the elbow and proximal forearm seem to be fascial bands and muscular anomalies of the pronator teres and the fibrous arcade of the flexor digitorum superficialis.[2,4]
  - Less common sites of nerve compression include the lacertus fibrosus and the ligament of Struthers (in cases with an existing supracondylar process).
  - A large number of additional structures have been identified as potential sources of compression of the median nerve. These include an accessory bicipital aponeurosis[5] and a variety of anomalous muscles, the most frequently cited of which is the accessory head of the flexor pollicis longus muscle, or *Gantzer's muscle*.
  - A persistent median artery penetrating the median nerve also has been described.[3]
  - Space-occupying lesions such as lipomas or scarring from trauma can result in nerve compression.
- Anterior interosseous syndrome caused by nerve compression must be differentiated from Parsonage-Turner syndrome, or mononeuritis.

NATURAL HISTORY

- Compression of the median nerve in the forearm often is transient, due to excessive physical activity or swelling from injury.
- Recovery from Parsonage-Turner syndrome can be prolonged, but the prognosis usually is good without surgical decompression.
- The natural history and prognosis of pronator syndrome is not well understood.

PATIENT HISTORY AND PHYSICAL FINDINGS

- Classically, pronator syndrome presents as paresthesia in the median nerve distribution with minimal or no weakness. The patient also may complain of pain localized to the proximal forearm that is increased with activities. There may be a focal area of increased pain localizing to the specific area of compression.
  - In severe cases, weakness of the anterior interosseous innervated muscles—the flexor pollicis longus, the index and long flexor digitorum profundus, and the pronator quadratus—might be seen, as well as select thenar muscles.
  - Theoretically, patients may have paresthesia in the distribution of the palmar cutaneous branch of the median nerve, in contrast to carpal tunnel syndrome.
- AIN syndrome presents as diminished motor function of the index (and long) flexor digitorum profundus, flexor pollicis longus, and pronator quadratus without injury or specific known cause.
  - The patient typically complains of spontaneous loss of dexterity and voices specific complaints related to flexion of the thumb IP joint and/or index DIP joint.

- Decreased sensation is not a common presenting symptom.
  - In cases of space-occupying lesions or scarring from trauma compressing the nerve, one would expect to see sensory symptoms as well as motor abnormalities.
- Patients suffering from Parsonage-Turner syndrome often will experience a prodromal viral-type illness together with significant pain for several days or weeks before the onset of weakness.
- Physical examinations to perform include:
  - *Pronator compression test.* Paresthesia in the median nerve distribution within 30 seconds is considered a positive test. The test is nonspecific and can be seen with carpal tunnel syndrome.
  - *Resisted PIP flexion of long finger.* Paresthesia in the median nerve distribution and pain in the forearm are considered a positive test. The test is thought to be consistent with compression of the median nerve at the fibrous arcade of the flexor digitorum superficialis.
  - *Resisted pronation test.* Paresthesia in the median nerve distribution and pain are considered a positive test. A positive finding is consistent with compression of the median nerve by the pronator teres.
  - Elbow flexion test. Paresthesia and pain are considered a positive test. A positive test is thought to be consistent with lacertus fibrosis compression of the median nerve.

IMAGING AND OTHER DIAGNOSTIC STUDIES

- Electrodiagnostic studies are often not helpful in pronator syndrome. Numerous studies have shown that symptoms and outcome of surgery do not correlate well with electrodiagnostic studies.
- In anterior interosseous syndrome, electrodiagnostic studies will confirm denervation of the anterior interosseous muscles.
- Electrodiagnostic studies are most valuable in the diagnosis of proximal median nerve compression for ruling out carpal tunnel syndrome.

- Ultrasonography and MRI are valuable tests for identifying space-occupying lesions such as lipomas or ganglions.
- Plain radiographs of the proximal forearm and elbow may reveal a supracondylar process or anatomic variation.

DIFFERENTIAL DIAGNOSIS

- Carpal tunnel syndrome
- Mononeuritis, or Parsonage-Turner syndrome
- Other form of neuritis

NONOPERATIVE MANAGEMENT

- In the acute phase, rest, immobilization, and avoidance of aggravating activities, such as repetitive pronation and heavy gripping, should be recommended.
- Forearm stretching exercises can be tried in chronic cases.
- Modalities such as ultrasound and electrostimulation have been advocated, although there is limited validation of their usefulness.
- Nerve gliding and nerve mobilization remain controversial.

SURGICAL MANAGEMENT

Approach

- The greatest variation in surgical technique concerns the skin incision.
- For decompression of both pronator and anterior interosseous syndromes, extensile exposures using a modification of Henry's approach allows for safe and thorough exposure of the median nerve and decompression of all sites of potential compression.
  - This incision sometimes is associated with unsightly scarring and injuries to the cutaneous nerves.
- Lesser incisions have been described, therefore; these include a lazy S-shape incision in the proximal volar forearm, as well as two longitudinal,[1] oblique,[4] and transverse[6] incisions.
  - Limited incisions require significant retraction to ensure decompression both proximally and distally.
- The surgeon's experience and comfort level may be the determining factors in deciding on the type of incision.

TECHNIQUES

EXTENSILE EXPOSURE

- The incision is made on the medial aspect of the distal arm proximal to the elbow flexion crease (**TECH FIG 1A**). It is brought across the elbow flexion crease and extended distally for approximately 10 cm.
- Cutaneous nerve branches, including branches of the lateral brachial and medial antebrachial cutaneous nerves, are identified and atraumatically mobilized.
- The median nerve is identified proximal to the elbow flexion crease and then is traced distally, releasing the lacertus fibrosus (**TECH FIG 1B**).
  - The existence of a ligament of Struthers and supracondylar process can then be ascertained.
- Motor branches of the median nerve to the muscles originating from the medial epicondyle must be protected throughout the operation. These include the palmaris longus; the flexor carpi radialis; and the flexor digitorum superficialis as well as the pronator teres (**TECH FIG 1C**).

- It will be necessary to ligate some vessels, but it will be possible to retract most of them.
- The radial artery lies radial to the nerve and must be protected throughout the procedure.
- The median nerve will be adherent to the pronator teres.
- Retracting the proximal portion of the pronator muscle mass identifies the median nerve and the pronator teres tendon (**TECH FIG 1D**).
- The larger, superficial pronator head is identified.
- It sometimes is possible to retract the entire muscle mass and follow the median nerve into the superficialis arcade. Frequently, however, it is necessary to release the tendinous portion of the pronator teres (**TECH FIG 1E**).
- Considerable variation exists within the pronator teres.
  - The median nerve can either pass between the superficial and deep pronator heads or, less commonly, pass underneath both heads.

TECHNIQUES

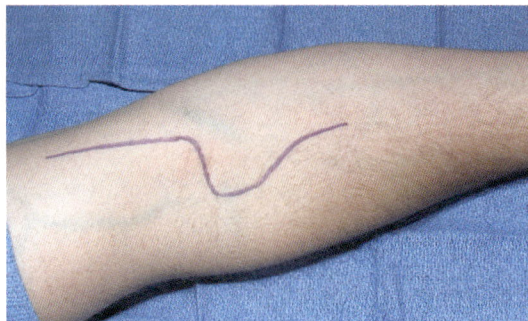

TECH FIG 1 • Extensile exposure. **A.** Skin incision. **B.** Incision with demonstrated lacertus fibrosis. **C.** Retracted but not released superficial pronator teres and intact flexor digitorum superficialis arch. **D.** Retracted pronator and released superficial arch. **E.** Z-lengthened superficial pronator teres tendon.

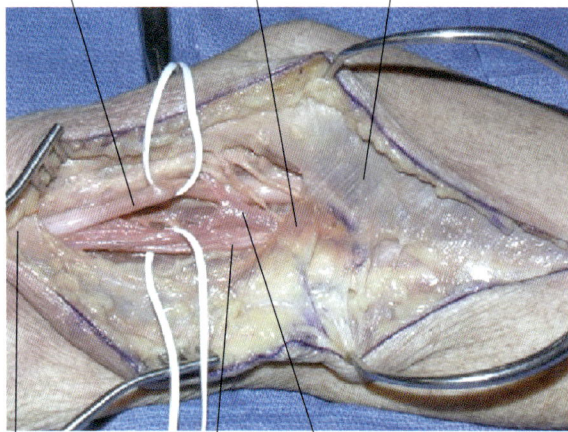

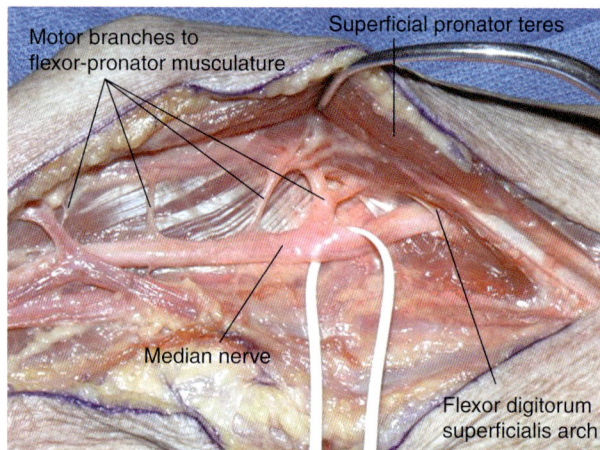

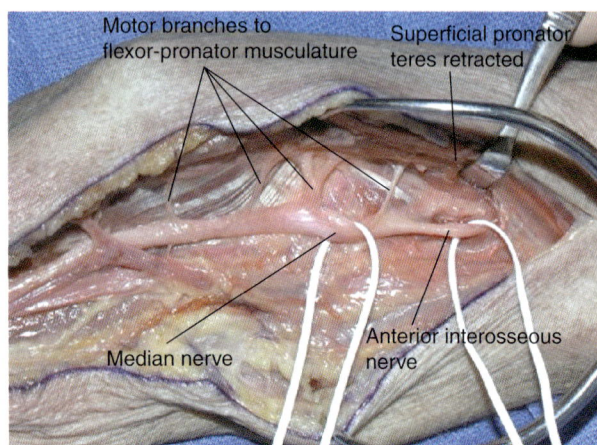

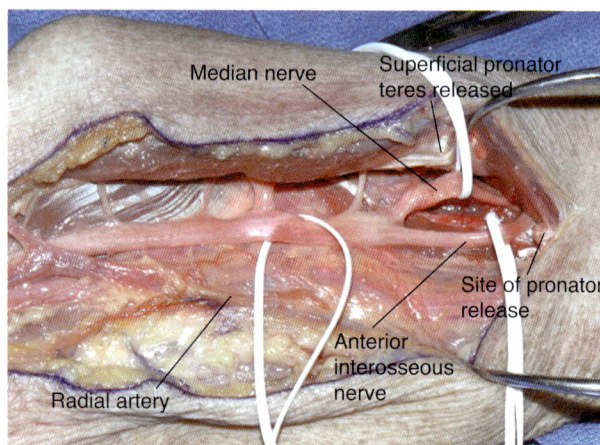

- Up to 20% of the time the deep head is absent.
- In the most uncommon variation, the median nerve pierces the humeral head.
- It is critical for all tendinous portions of the pronator teres potentially compressing the nerve to be released in the procedure.
- If scarring of the pronator teres is present as a result of trauma, a Z-lengthening of the pronator teres tendon is advisable.
  - This will improve exposure by allowing the humeral head to be reflected in an ulnar direction, exposing the AIN, the median nerve, and the flexor digitorum superficialis arcade (see Tech Fig 1E).

- The superficialis arcade can then be released, and the median nerve and AIN visualized distally by gentle retraction of the muscle fibers.
- Anterior interosseous nerve braches to the flexor pollicis longus and flexor digitorum profundus must be protected.
- Use of atraumatic technique with careful hemostasis is important to prevent postoperative scarring, with resultant pain and potential weakness.
- If the pronator teres tendon has been released, it should be repaired in a lengthened fashion.
- We prefer to use subcutaneous closure and subcuticular suturing.

LIMITED INCISION

- An oblique or transverse incision can be made in the proximal forearm just distal to the elbow flexion crease (**TECH FIG 2A**).
- Retractors are placed proximal and distal to identify the cutaneous nerve fibers.
- The lacertus fibrosus is released first, and then the median nerve is identified, as previously described.
- Retractors are placed to allow visualization and palpation of the median nerve proximally, to permit identifi-

cation of proximal lesions such as a ligament of Struthers (**TECH FIG 2B**).

- Distally, the pronator teres is identified and the muscle and tendon mobilized.
- If required, the superficial or deep tendons (or both) are released.
- Fascial impinging structures are identified and released as needed.
- The superficialis arcade is identified and released, protecting the median nerve and AIN.

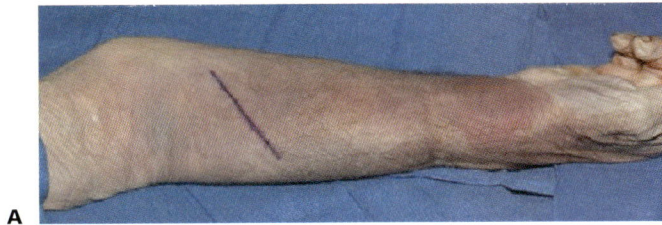

TECH FIG 2 • Oblique limited exposure. **A**. Skin incision. **B**. Retracted pronator teres with exposed superficialis arch.

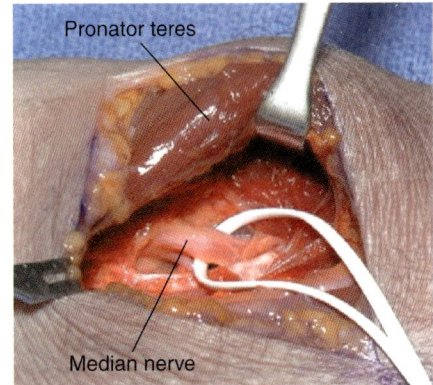

PEARLS AND PITFALLS

Anatomy	■ Tendinous portions of the pronator teres and the fibrous portions of the arcade of the flexor digitorum superficialis are the most common causes of compression. ■ Motor branches that go from the median nerve to the muscles originating from the medial epicondyle branch from the ulnar side of the nerve. ■ The AIN originates from the radial side of the median nerve and under the pronator teres. ■ Considerable variation occurs within the pronator teres. Tendinous portions of the pronator impinging on the median nerve should be released, with preservation of the muscle fibers when possible. ■ The humeral or superficial head of the pronator teres is the largest portion of the muscle. The ulnar head or deep head is far smaller, sometimes absent, and most commonly is deep to the median nerve. Both heads, however, have tendinous insertion sites, which may be sources of impingement. In addition, fascial connections between the heads may be present, impinging on the median nerve.
Surgical technique	■ The fibrous portion of the superficialis arcade can be released with preservation of the muscle. ■ Palpation and visualization proximally and distally can be obtained by appropriate retraction. ■ Extensile exposures result in easier surgery but at the expense of potential unsightly scarring and dysesthesia from cutaneous nerve injury. ■ Judicious release of the pronator teres limits the postoperative morbidity and decreases the recovery time.
Relation to carpal tunnel syndrome	■ Patients often may have both carpal tunnel syndrome and a more proximal compression, resulting in the so-called double crush phenomenon. ■ Some authors have implied that failed carpal tunnel syndrome is due to a misdiagnosis in which the more proximal compression of the median nerve in the forearm was not identified. ■ In cases, however, where electrodiagnostic studies clearly show carpal tunnel syndrome even when proximal forearm symptoms are present, it is wise to merely decompress the carpal canal, because the carpal tunnel procedure has a more predictable outcome with less morbidity than proximal forearm median nerve decompression.

POSTOPERATIVE CARE

- Splinting or casting is avoided.
- Early elbow range of motion is encouraged.
- If the pronator tendon has been released, lifting and forearm rotation are restricted for 4 weeks.

OUTCOMES

- Outcome following surgical treatment of proximal forearm median nerve compression has been inconsistent compared to the more uniformly good outcomes associated with carpal tunnel release.
- Many, if not most, patients continue to be at least somewhat symptomatic after surgical decompression.
  - This may reflect persistent compression due to inadequate release or scarring from the surgery itself.
  - It is more likely, however, that it reflects the difficulty in making the diagnosis due to the lack of objective criteria.
- Few studies have evaluated outcome following median nerve decompression in the forearm. Most such studies report results of decompression for pronator syndrome.
- Olehnik et al[4] and Hartz et al[2] both reported results for decompression of pronator syndrome.
  - Olehnik et al[4] showed surgery to be of benefit in 30 of 37 extremities, but 9 of 39 were unchanged and 20 had only partial relief.

- Hartz et al[2] showed 28 good or excellent results in 36 operations, but a majority of patients still had symptoms.

COMPLICATIONS

- Persistent symptoms due to incorrect diagnosis
- Damage to cutaneous nerve branches with subsequent dysesthesias
- Damage to or scarring of motor branches of median nerve or interosseous nerve
- Scarring of pronator teres and forearm musculature

REFERENCES

1. Gainor BJ. Modified exposure for pronator syndrome decompression: A preliminary experience. Orthopedics 1993;1612:1329–1331.
2. Hartz CR, Linscheid RL, Gramse RR, et al. The pronator teres syndrome: Compressive neuropathy of the median nerve. J Bone Joint Surg Am 1981;63A:885–890.
3. Jones NF, Ming NL. Persistent median artery as a cause of pronator syndrome. J Hand Surg Am 1988;13:728–732.
4. Olehnik WK, Manske PR, Sqerzinski J. Median nerve compression in the proximal forearm. J Hand Surg Am 1994;19:121–126.
5. Spinner RJ, Carmichael SW, Spinner W. Partial median nerve entrapment in the distal arm because of an accessory bicipital aponeurosis. J Hand Surg Am 1991;16:236–244.
6. Tsai TM, Syed SA. A transverse skin incision approach for decompression of pronator teres syndrome. J Hand Surg Br 1994;19:40–42.

DEFINITION

- The site of compression must be identified to determine the appropriate treatment for symptoms of ulnar nerve dysfunction. Guyon's canal at the wrist is the second most common site of ulnar nerve entrapment.
- Symptoms may be purely motor, purely sensory, or mixed, depending on the site and cause of compression.

ANATOMY

- In the distal half of the forearm, the ulnar nerve is joined on its lateral side by the ulnar artery. Proximal to the wrist, the nerve gives off a large dorsal sensory branch, which supplies sensation to the dorsum of the wrist and the ulnar side of the hand. The ulnar nerve continues into the hand through Guyon's canal.
- Guyon's canal is a triangular canal at the base of the ulnar side of the palm. It is 4 cm in length, extending from the proximal edge of the palmar carpal ligament to the fibrous edge of the hypothenar muscles.[4] The space functions as a physiologic tunnel with discrete anatomic landmarks (**FIG 1A**).
  - Both the ulnar nerve and artery pass through the canal to enter the hand.
  - The dorsal cutaneous branch of the ulnar nerve usually branches before the nerve enters Guyon's canal.
  - It is bordered laterally by the hook of the hamate and the transverse carpal ligament. The medial wall is formed by the pisiform and the attachments of the pisohamate ligament.
- Dividing the tunnel into three zones helps in correlating the clinical symptoms with the specific pathologic cause[4,13] (**FIG 1B**).
  - Zone 1, about 3 cm in length, is the area proximal to the bifurcation of the ulnar nerve into motor and sensory branches. Compression in zone 1 results in combined motor and sensory loss. It is most commonly caused by a fracture of the hook of the hamate or a ganglion cyst.
  - Zones 2 and 3 are located next to each other, from the point where the ulnar nerve divides into a superficial or sensory branch and a deep motor branch, to the region just beyond the fibrous arch of the hypothenar muscles.
  - Zone 2 encompasses the motor branch of the nerve, located in the dorsoradial portion of the tunnel. The deep motor branch, along with the deep branch of the ulnar artery, passes between the abductor digiti quinti and the flexor digiti quinti brevis, perforating the opponens digiti quinti. The motor branch then follows the deep volar arch across the palm to innervate the interossei.
    - The nerve supplies the three intrinsic muscles of the small finger, the third and fourth lumbricales, the volar and dorsal interossei, the adductor pollicis, and the deep head of the flexor pollicis brevis.
    - Compression in this area causes pure motor loss to all of the ulnar-innervated muscles in the hand. Ganglions

from the pisotriquetral joint and fractures of the hook of the hamate are the most common etiologic factors (**FIG 1C**). Due to the nerve's proximity to the hamate, it is unfortunately easy to damage the nerve while excising the hook of the hamate.
  - Zone 3, located ulnar to zone 2, encompasses the superficial or sensory branch of the bifurcated ulnar nerve. Compression here causes sensory loss to the hypothenar eminence, the small finger, and part of the ring finger, but does not usually cause motor deficits. Common causes are aneurysm of the ulnar artery, thrombosis, and synovial inflammation.
    - The superficial branch of the ulnar nerve in Guyon's canal supplies the palmaris brevis and the skin of the hypothenar eminence and forms the digital nerves to the small and ulnar side of the ring finger.
- Two specific nerve anomalies can confuse the diagnosis.
  - Martin-Gruber anastomosis in the forearm: fibers that supply the intrinsic muscles are carried in the median nerve to the middle of the forearm, where they leave the median nerve to join the ulnar nerve. Functioning intrinsic muscles can be observed when the ulnar nerve is injured proximal to this anastomosis.
  - Riche-Cannieu anastomosis: the median and ulnar nerves are connected in the palm. Even with an injury at the wrist, some intrinsic function remains.

PATHOGENESIS

- Causative factors of compression or injury of the ulnar nerve in Guyon's canal include repeated blunt trauma from power tools and gripping or hammering with the palm of the hand, which may result in thrombosis or aneurysm of the ulnar artery compressing the nerve (hypothenar hammer syndrome)[2,6,10] (**FIG 2A,B,** Table 1). Direct pressure on the ulnar nerve may occur during activities such as cycling.
- Fractures of the hook of the hamate can impinge on the nerve.
- Idiopathic compression may occur secondary to thickening of the proximal fibrous ligament at the entrance to the canal.
  - Compression also may occur as a result of swelling after distal radius fracture.
- Compression of the ulnar nerve at Guyon's canal also has been shown to occur in conjunction with carpal tunnel syndrome. It typically resolves after surgical decompression of the carpal canal.[9,16]
- Other etiologies include tumors, such as ganglia or lipomas (**FIG 2C,D**), anomalous muscle bellies,[8,15] or hypertrophy of the palmaris brevis.
  - Ganglia and other soft-tissue masses are responsible for 32% to 48% of cases of ulnar tunnel syndrome. Another 16% of cases are due to muscle anomalies.[12]
- Synovitis secondary to rheumatoid arthritis may encroach upon the canal and the nerve.

2671

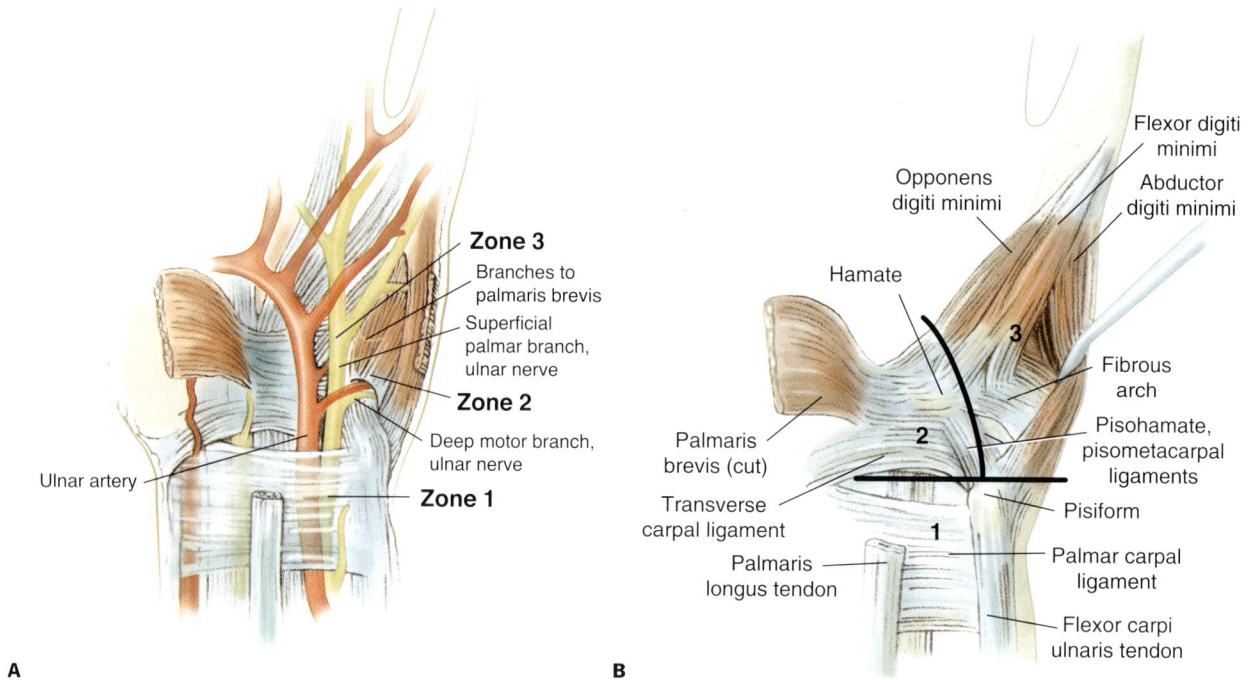

A

B

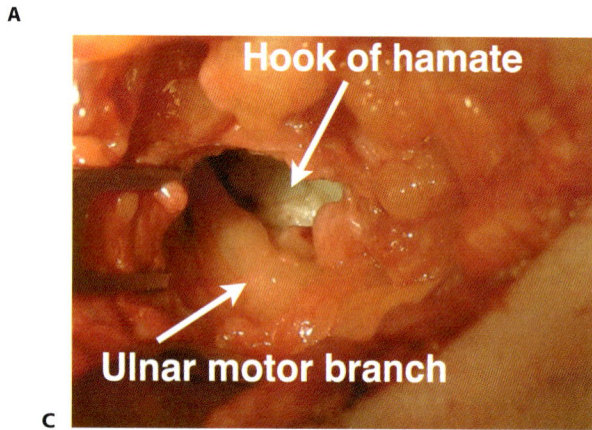

C

FIG 1 • **A.** Anatomic landmarks of the distal ulnar tunnel (Guyon's canal). *Zone 1:* Ulnar nerve in the region proximal to the bifurcation. *Zone 2:* Ulnar nerve motor segment, following bifurcation. *Zone 3:* Ulnar nerve sensory segment, distal to the bifurcation. **B.** Location of the three zones. Zone 1 is proximal to the bifurcation; zone 2 encompasses the motor branch; zone 3 is the region surrounding the sensory branch. **C.** The proximity of the motor branch of the ulnar nerve to the hook of the hamate as seen during excision of the hook.

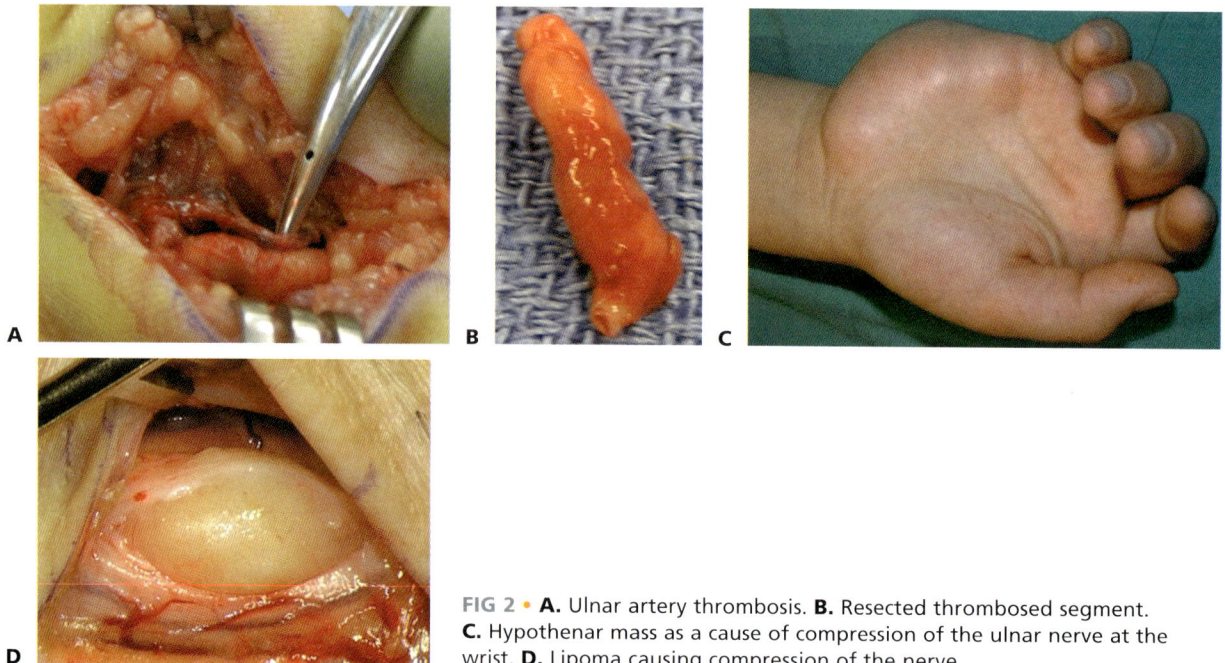

A

B

C

D

FIG 2 • **A.** Ulnar artery thrombosis. **B.** Resected thrombosed segment. **C.** Hypothenar mass as a cause of compression of the ulnar nerve at the wrist. **D.** Lipoma causing compression of the nerve.

Table 1	Causes of Compression or Injury of the Ulnar Nerve in Guyon's Canal

- Ganglia
- Soft tissue masses
- Abnormal muscle bellies
- Hook of hamate fracture
- Distal radial fracture
- Thickening of proximal fibrous hypothenar arch
- Hypertrophic synovium
- Iatrogenic (after opponensplasty)
- Physiology
- Inflammatory conditions
- Tenosynovitis
- Rheumatoid arthritis
- Edema secondary to burns
- Gout
- Coexistent carpal tunnel syndrome
- Vascular conditions
- Ulnar artery thrombosis
- Ulnar artery pseudoaneurysm
- Neuropathic conditions
- Diabetes
- Alcoholism
- Proximal lesion of ulnar nerve (double-crush syndrome)
- Occupation-related
- Vibration exposure
- Repetitive blunt trauma
- Direct pressure on ulnar nerve with wrist extended
- Typing
- Cycling

- Metabolic or infectious diseases such as diabetes, thyroid disease, or leprosy may also mimic the symptoms of nerve compression.
- Iatrogenic causes must also be recognized, such as compression by tendon or muscle transfer (Huber opponensplasty).[11]

NATURAL HISTORY

- Untreated compression may result in permanent dysfunction, weakness, and numbness.

PATIENT HISTORY AND PHYSICAL FINDINGS

Clinical History

- Presenting symptoms can vary from mild, transient paresthesias in the ring and small fingers to clawing of these digits and severe intrinsic muscle atrophy.
  - The patient may report severe pain at the elbow or wrist with radiation into the hand or up into the shoulder and neck.
  - Patients may report difficulty or clumsiness when opening jars or turning doorknobs.
  - Early fatigue or weakness may be noticed if work requires repetitive hand motions.
  - Depending on the climate and work conditions, cold intolerance in the ring and small fingers may be present.[5]
- A careful clinical history is imperative, noting the time of occurrence of symptoms. Determine whether symptoms are transient or continuous. Determine whether symptoms are related to work, sleep, or recreation. Elicit duration of symptoms and possible relation to trauma.

Physical Examination[7,17]

- It is important to determine the level of pathology of the ulnar nerve, because compression commonly occurs at four points: the cervical spine, the thoracic outlet, the elbow (cubital tunnel syndrome), or the wrist (Guyon's canal).
- Begin the clinical examination at the neck and shoulder and move down the affected extremity to the elbow.
  - Pain on neck movement mimicking the patient's symptoms could indicate cervical disc disease.
  - Pain on palpation of the plexus or with shoulder motion could indicate a pathologic condition in the brachial plexus or lung. Results of provocative maneuvers for thoracic outlet syndrome should be assessed.
  - Masses on the medial side of the arm could indicate a soft tissue tumor or hemorrhage compressing the nerve.
  - At the elbow, note any deformity, palpate the nerve, and determine whether abnormal mobility is present.
- The course of the nerve is palpated in the forearm all the way to the wrist.
  - A positive Tinel or Phalen's sign often is found at the wrist over the ulnar nerve.
  - Tenderness over the hook of the hamate is particularly important.
- Sensory function is assessed.
  - Semmes-Weinstein monofilament testing may be abnormal, but often is normal early in the course of the compression.
  - Two-point discrimination of the ring and small fingers usually becomes abnormal only late in the course of the disease.
- To help differentiate cubital tunnel syndrome from compression of the ulnar nerve at the wrist, assess flexor carpi ulnaris and flexor digitorum profundus strength.
- Intrinsic muscle function is tested by asking the patient to cross the long finger over the index finger (ie, crossed finger test).
- Only two muscles can be tested accurately in the hand—the abductor digiti quinti and the first dorsal interosseous. The tendons or bellies of these muscles can be palpated or visualized.
- Weakness of thumb pinch may be elicited by the Froment sign. Froment's sign is ruled positive if the person must flex the thumb interphalangeal joint to maintain grasp.

IMAGING AND OTHER DIAGNOSTIC STUDIES

- Radiographs of the elbow and wrist are mandatory in ulnar nerve compression, because entrapment of the ulnar nerve may occur at more than one level.
  - Radiographs of the hand and wrist should include carpal tunnel views as well as standard anteroposterior (AP), lateral, and oblique views. Radiographs of the wrist may reveal fractures of the hook of the hamate, dislocations of the carpal bones, or, less commonly, soft tissue masses and calcifications.
  - Radiographs of the elbow may reveal abnormal anatomy, such as a valgus deformity, bone spurs or bone fragments, a shallow olecranon groove, osteochondromas, or destructive lesions (eg, tumors, infections, abnormal calcifications).
- Radiographs of the neck should be obtained if cervical disc disease is suspected and to rule out cervical ribs.
- Obtain radiographs of the chest if a Pancoast tumor or tuberculosis is suspected.

- MRI is not usually necessary unless further delineation of soft tissue masses such as lipomas or ganglions[11] or visualization of fractures, aneurysms, congenital abnormality, or other abnormalities in the nerve is required. MRI also may detect structural abnormalities along the course of the ulnar nerve accounting for compression (eg, fibrous bands).
- Ultrasonography may be used to detect cysts or masses in Guyon's canal and to assess ulnar nerve diameter at the elbow.
- Electromyography (EMG) and nerve conduction studies are helpful to confirm the specific area(s) of entrapment as well as document the extent of the pathology.
  - Motor and sensory conduction velocities are more useful in a recent entrapment, whereas conduction velocities and EMG are useful in chronic neuropathies (EMG shows axonal degeneration).
  - Conduction velocity short-segment stimulation (also known as the *inching technique*) can increase the sensitivity of this method and can improve localization by helping the examiner determine exactly where a blockage is occurring.
  - EMG evaluation of motor unit morphology and recruitment patterns ascertains ongoing loss of muscle fibers via detection of abnormal spontaneous activity (eg, fibrillation potentials and fasciculations). It also checks the integrity of the muscle membrane to expand differential diagnosis (eg, myotonia, paramyotonia, periodic paralysis) as manifested by increased insertional activity such as complex repetitive discharges, myokymia, and (para)myotonic discharges.[1]

DIFFERENTIAL DIAGNOSIS[17]

- Cervical disc disease
- Brachial plexus abnormalities, thoracic outlet syndrome, Pancoast tumor
- Elbow abnormalities, epicondylitis
- Infections, tumors, diabetes mellitus, hypothyroidism, rheumatoid diseases, alcoholism
- Wrist fractures
- Ulnar artery aneurysms or thrombosis at the wrist

NONOPERATIVE MANAGEMENT

- Conservative treatment of ulnar nerve compression is most successful when paresthesias are transient. Patient education and insight are important.

- Flexing the wrist at work while typing for long periods, or resting the wrist on the handlebars of a bicycle or motorcycle while driving, are causes of paresthesia that can be corrected without surgical treatment.
- Avoiding the use of vibrating or power tools, wrist splinting in a neutral position, and correction of ergonomics at work should help alleviate transient palsies.
- Nonsteroidal anti-inflammatory medications also are useful adjuncts to relieve nerve irritation.
- Oral vitamin B_6 supplements may be helpful for mild symptoms. This treatment should be carried out for 6 to 12 weeks, depending on patient response.

SURGICAL MANAGEMENT

- Surgical intervention is indicated if paresthesia increases despite adequate conservative treatment combined with abnormal nerve conduction studies or EMGs, and at the first sign of motor changes.
- In a patient who sustains an immediate complete ulnar nerve injury as a result of a fracture of the wrist, the fracture should be reduced as soon as possible.
  - Elimination of any dorsal displacement of the distal radius or ulna should be achieved.
  - If ulnar nerve function does not improve within 24 to 36 hours following satisfactory reduction, the nerve should be explored and decompression carried out.[3,12]

Preoperative Planning

- The diagnosis should be confirmed with EMG and nerve conduction velocity or imaging studies (eg, MRI) before planning surgery.

Positioning

- Patients are operated on in the supine position with the arm extended on an armboard.
- A tourniquet is placed above the elbow and inflated to 250 to 265 mm Hg before the incision is made.

Approach

- Operative treatment is aimed at exploring and decompressing the nerve from the distal forearm into the hand throughout all three zones.

TECHNIQUES

ULNAR NERVE EXPLORATION AND DECOMPRESSION OF GUYON'S CANAL

- Palpate and mark the pisiform.
  - The hook of the hamate can be found 1 cm distal and lateral to the pisiform.
- Make a curvilinear incision beginning distally in the interval between the pisiform and the hook of the hamate. Cross the wrist, extending proximal to the distal wrist flexion crease, along the radial border of the flexor carpi ulnaris (**TECH FIG 1A**).
  - The wrist should be crossed in a zigzag fashion to prevent longitudinal contracture of the scar.
- Perform the dissection proximal to distal. Identify the ulnar nerve proximal to the distal wrist flexor retinaculum and follow it distally through Guyon's canal by reflecting the flexor carpi ulnaris and the pisohamate ligament.
  - The neurovascular bundle is traced distally to the point at which it enters Guyon's canal beneath the palmar carpal ligament.

- Incise the ligament, palmaris brevis muscle, and fibrous tissue, decompressing the nerve along its entire course through the canal.
  - The branches of the ulnar nerve to the hypothenar muscles and palmaris brevis, as well as the deep branch of the nerve, can be identified and protected with this approach.
- The incision should not be carried ulnarly over the hypothenar eminence, to avoid injury to the palmar cutaneous branch of the ulnar nerve.
- The ulnar artery should be examined for areas of thickening or thrombosis, and the ulnar nerve should be examined along its course for intra- or extraneural tumors (eg, schwannoma, neurolemmoma).
- Further exploration of the floor of the canal should be done to identify masses, ganglions, anomalous muscles,

TECHNIQUES

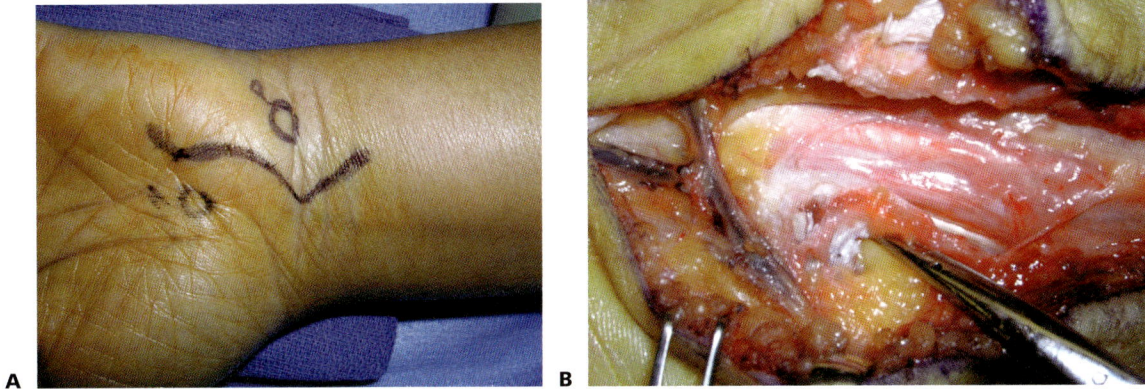

TECH FIG 1 • A. The skin incision is marked crossing the wrist at an angle to prevent scar contracture. **B.** The motor branch is followed into the interval between the flexor digiti minimi and abductor digiti minimi muscles.

- fibrous bands, osteophytes, or fracture fragments.
- The motor branch is followed into the interval between the flexor digiti minimi and abductor digiti minimi muscles and through the origin of the opponens digiti minimi (**TECH FIG 1B**).

- After exploration and decompression, release the tourniquet and coagulate all bleeders with a bipolar cautery before the wound is closed.
  - Hematoma in this area could potentially compress the nerve and artery.

PEARLS AND PITFALLS

Pearls	■ Differentiation between proximal and distal nerve compression: ■ Weakness of the small finger profundus points to ulnar nerve compression at the elbow. ■ Involvement of the dorsal sensory branch indicates compression proximal to Guyon's canal. ■ Clawing is seen more commonly in distal (wrist) than proximal (elbow) lesions.
Pitfalls	■ Inadequate preoperative evaluation, resulting in: ■ Inaccurate or incomplete diagnosis ■ Inadequate decompression

POSTOPERATIVE CARE

- Postoperatively, patients are placed into a protective splint for about 2 weeks to prevent excessive wrist flexion and extension.
- Sutures are removed at 10 to 14 days after surgery, at which time gentle active range of motion is started, as well as scar care.
- The wrist splint should be continued for 2 to 3 more weeks to prevent scar thickening, which is common in this area.
  - Silicone or otoform is helpful to prevent hard, firm scars.

OUTCOMES

- Symptoms can be expected to improve in all cases, with fewer than 20% of patients complaining of slight persistent numbness after the surgery.[14]
- The most common cause of failure of surgery is failure in diagnosis, followed by inadequate decompression of all of the branches of the ulnar nerve.

COMPLICATIONS

- Laceration of the ulnar nerve or artery (or both)
- Inadequate decompression
- Injury to the ulnar artery

REFERENCES

1. Agarwal SK, Schneider LB, Ahmad BK. Clinical usefulness of ulnar motor responses recording from first dorsal interosseous. Muscle Nerve 1995;18:1043.
2. Aguiar PH, Bor-Seng-Shu E, Gomes-Pinto F, et al. Surgical management of Guyon's canal syndrome, an ulnar nerve entrapment at the wrist: Report of two cases. Arq Neuropsiquiatr 2001;59:106–111.
3. Bartels RH, Grotenhuis JA, Kauer JM. The arcade of Struthers: An anatomical study. Acta Neurochir (Wien) 2003;145:295–300.
5. Beekman R, Schoemaker MC, Van Der Plas JP, et al. Diagnostic value of high-resolution sonography in ulnar neuropathy at the elbow. Neurology 2004;62:767–773.
6. Beekman R, Van Der Plas JP, Uitdehaag BM, et al. Clinical, electro-diagnostic, and sonographic studies in ulnar neuropathy at the elbow. Muscle Nerve 2004;30:202–208.
4. Beekman R, Wokke JH, Schoemaker MC, et al. Ulnar neuropathy at the elbow: Follow-up and prognostic factors determining outcome. Neurology 2004;63:1675–1680.
7. Bradshaw DY, Shefner JM. Ulnar neuropathy at the elbow. Neurol Clin 1999;17:447–461.
8. Buzzard EF. Some varieties of toxic and traumatic ulnar neuritis. Lancet 1922;1:317.
9. Campbell WW. Ulnar neuropathy at the elbow. Muscle Nerve 2000;23:450–452.
10. Cooke RA. Hypothenar hammer syndrome: A discrete syndrome to be distinguished from hand–arm vibration syndrome. Occup Med (Lond) 2003;53:320–324.

11. Feindel W, J Stratford J. Cubital tunnel compression in tardy ulnar palsy. Can Med Assoc J 1958;78:351–353.

12. Gelberman RH. Ulnar tunnel syndrome. In: Gelberman RH, ed. Operative Nerve Repair and Reconstruction. Philadelphia: JB Lippincott, 1991:1131–1143.

13. Gross MS, Gelberman RH. The anatomy of the distal ulnar tunnel. Clin Orthop Relat Res 1985;196:238–247.

14. Murata K, Shih JT, Tsai TM. Causes of ulnar tunnel syndrome: a retrospective study of 31 subjects. J Hand Surg Am 2003;28:647–651.

15. Pribyl CR, Moneim MS. Anomalous hand muscle found in Guyon's canal at exploration for ulnar artery thrombosis: a case report. Clin Orthop Relat Res 1994;306:120–123.

16. Silver MA, Gelberman RH, Gellman H, et al. Carpal tunnel syndrome: Associated abnormalities in ulnar nerve function and the effect of carpal tunnel release on these abnormalities. J Hand Surg Am 1985;10:710–713.

17. Szabo RM, Steinberg DR. Nerve entrapment syndromes in the wrist. J Am Acad Orthop Surg 1994;2:115–123.

Chapter 70

Surgical Treatment of Cubital Tunnel Syndrome

Catherine M. Curtin and Amy L. Ladd

DEFINITION

- Cubital tunnel syndrome is a compression neuropathy of the ulnar nerve that occurs at or around the level of the elbow (*cubis* is Latin for "elbow").
- Cubital tunnel syndrome is the second most common compression neuropathy of the upper limb requiring treatment, after carpal tunnel syndrome.

ANATOMY

- The ulnar nerve is the terminal branch of the medial cord of the brachial plexus, with contributions from C8 and T1 nerve roots.
- The ulnar nerve traverses the cubital tunnel, a fibro-osseous tunnel at the elbow. The medial epicondyle, the olecranon, the medial collateral ligament of the elbow (which forms the floor), and the fibrous retinaculum extending from the medial epicondyle to the olecranon make up the anatomic landmarks (**FIG 1**).[11]
- Any of several possible sites of compression of the ulnar nerve around the elbow can result in cubital tunnel syndrome. All of these sites should be considered when selecting the type of surgical decompression.
  - The arcade of Struthers is a controversial site of compression, because it is found in only a minority of patients. If present, it is found approximately 8 cm proximal to the medial epicondyle and consists of a fascial band running from the medial head of the triceps to the intermuscular septum.[15]
  - The medial intermuscular septum is a fascial band from the coracobrachialis to the medial humeral epicondyle, especially thick at its attachment to the epicondyle. The ulnar nerve may rest or scissor over the septum as it crosses from the anterior to the posterior compartment, as it approaches the medial epicondyle, or after an anterior transposition if it is not adequately excised.

- The arcuate ligament of Osborne at the cubital tunnel, which is the fibrous band extending from the medial epicondyle to the olecranon, can cause stenosis of the cubital tunnel and, thus, ulnar nerve compression.
- Distally, the nerve can be compressed as it passes between the two heads of the flexor carpi ulnaris, especially if each muscle head from the medial epicondyle and the olecranon converge close to the elbow joint.
- The presence of an anconeus epitrochlearis (**FIG 2**), an anomalous thin muscle extending from the triceps or olecranon to the medial epicondyle, also can cause ulnar nerve compression.
- The medial antebrachial cutaneous nerve and the medial brachial cutaneous nerve both emanate directly from the medial cord and are thus not ulnar nerve branches, but they importantly may lie in the surgical field. They are usually found deeper than expected, along the fascia of the triceps, brachialis, and flexor carpi ulnaris.

PATHOGENESIS

- Cubital tunnel syndrome is a compressive neuropathy. Several anatomic factors make the ulnar nerve susceptible to compression at the elbow.
  - The nerve is superficial at the level of the elbow, making it susceptible to minor and major trauma, ranging from mild repetitive contusion to high-energy injury.
  - The bony tunnel and its soft tissue support between the olecranon and medial epicondyle may be shallow, either inherently or traumatically, promoting subluxation, "perching" on the epicondyle, and microtrauma.
  - Elbow flexion increases pressure on the nerve and decreases the volume of the cubital tunnel, resulting in compression of the nerve.[5]

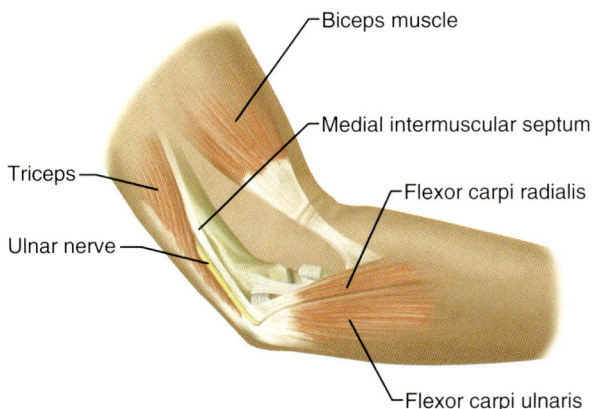

FIG 1 • Anatomy of the cubital tunnel.

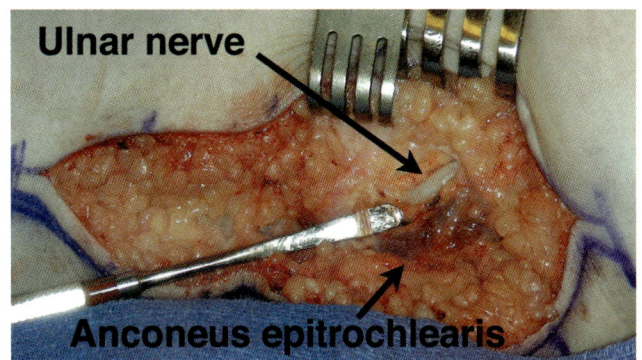

FIG 2 • An anomalous anconeus epitrochlearis encountered overlying the cubital tunnel. Anterior is at top and posterior at bottom; the forearm is to the left.

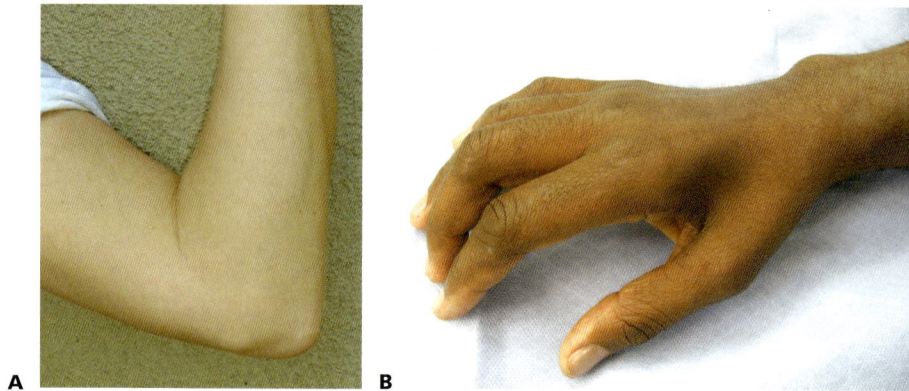

FIG 3 • **A.** "Perched" ulnar nerve. The nerve subluxates anteriorly, sitting on top of the medial epicondyle with the elbow in flexion. **B.** Wasting of first dorsal interosseous nerve. (**A:** Copyright Amy Ladd, MD.)

NATURAL HISTORY

▪ Without operative intervention, about half of mild cases can resolve with activity modification.[10]

▪ No long-term studies have been done of the natural history for severe disease.

PATIENT HISTORY AND PHYSICAL FINDINGS

▪ Subjective complaints include numbness in the small and ring fingers, often with accompanying burning pain around the medial epicondyle. Symptoms may be worse at night.

▪ As the disease progresses, patients may complain of weakness or clumsiness of their hands. More advanced disease will demonstrate wasting of the intrinsics and clawing of the ring and small fingers.

▪ Systemic diseases such as diabetes, amyloidosis, or alcoholism may cause peripheral neuropathy, which can mimic the symptoms of a compressive neuropathy.

▪ A smoking history is important, not only for impaired vascularity, but because it may point to the rare Pancoast tumor, an apical lung tumor, which causes plexus compression, mimicking the symptoms of cubital tunnel syndrome.

▪ Elbow trauma can create deformity, causing ulnar nerve compression. Deformities include a cubitus valgus, cubitus varus, or malunion. The elbow trauma can be remote and result in tardy ulnar nerve palsy.

▪ Look for atrophy of the intrinsic muscles of the hand or a clawed posture of the ring and small fingers. Check for masses around the elbow.

▪ Palpate the elbow and hand to evaluate for tender masses or other anomalous elbow anatomy.

▪ Put the elbow through its range of motion and assess whether the ulnar nerve subluxates or perches at the medial epicondyle with elbow flexion (**FIG 3A**).

▪ Visible atrophy of the first dorsal interosseous nerve correlates with significant ulnar nerve compression and can indicate significant motor impairment (**FIG 3B**).

▪ Perform a sensory examination of the hand, using Semmes-Weinstein monofilaments to obtain threshold measurements. Evaluate sensation on the ulnar dorsum of the hand. If sensation is normal, it suggests the problem may be distal, at the level of Guyon's canal.

▪ Clinical tests that can help with diagnosis include the following:
  ▪ Tinel's test. This test may not be specific, because many normal individuals will have a positive Tinel's response to percussion.
  ▪ Elbow flexion test. This test is sensitive for cubital tunnel syndrome.
  ▪ Crossed finger test. This test demonstrates weakness of dorsal and palmar interossei.
  ▪ Froment's sign. A positive Froment's sign indicates weakness of the adductor pollicis.
  ▪ Wartenberg's sign (in which the small finger assumes an abducted posture with finger extension). This sign is the result of weakness in the palmar interossei, resulting in unopposed ulnar pull of the extensor digiti quinti.

IMAGING AND OTHER DIAGNOSTIC STUDIES

▪ Radiographs of the elbow define the bony architecture and its alterations: masses, erosions, arthritis, and previous trauma. An axial view is helpful to evaluate the cubital canal (**FIG 4**).

▪ Normal results on electrodiagnostic studies (eg, nerve conduction and electromyography) do not exclude the diagnosis of cubital tunnel syndrome; the syndrome may be present but not severe.
  ▪ These tests localize the area of compression if the nerve conduction is measured at short segment intervals.
  ▪ Several positive electrodiagnostic findings suggest ulnar compression:
    ▫ Motor conduction across the elbow less than 50 m/sec.[13]
    ▫ Focal slowing of nerve velocity across the elbow

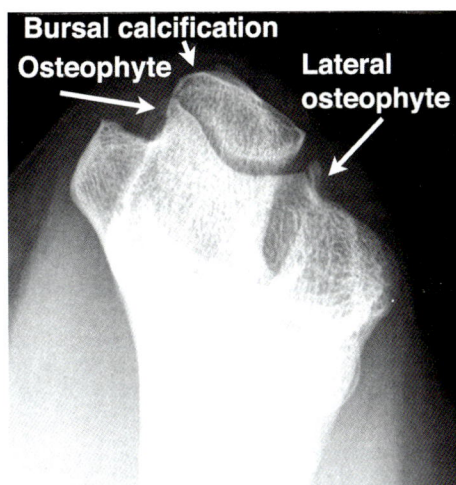

FIG 4 • Axial view of the elbow demonstrates a hooked osteophyte within the cubital tunnel, as well as calcification in the bursa and osteophyte. (Copyright Amy Ladd, MD.)

■ Fibrillation potentials or positive waves suggest axonal degeneration, representing a poorer prognosis for complete recovery.

■ MRI and CT may occasionally be helpful as ancillary imaging studies to define soft tissue aberrancies and localize bone abnormalities such as osteophytes in the cubital tunnel.

DIFFERENTIAL DIAGNOSIS

■ Cervical spine disease affecting C8 and T1
■ Compression of the inferior aspect of the brachial plexus from shoulder trauma
■ Apical lung tumor (Pancoast tumor)
■ Thoracic outlet syndrome
■ Entrapment of the ulnar nerve at the wrist (Guyon's canal)

NONOPERATIVE MANAGEMENT

■ Activity modification
 ■ Ulnar nerve protection limiting microtrauma to the nerve through elbow padding and limiting direct pressure on the nerve
 ■ Minimize prolonged elbow flexion, especially at night, through sleep modifications or splints.
■ Splinting
 ■ Splints to prevent elbow flexion; rigid splints are more effective but are less tolerated by patients. If persistent paresthesias exist, a trial of temporary full-time use is recommended. For milder cases, the splint is worn only at night.[2]
 ■ Nonoperative treatment requires a trial of several months before determining its success.

SURGICAL MANAGEMENT

■ Surgical intervention should be considered for patients presenting with motor involvement or permanent sensory changes, or for those who have failed nonoperative treatment.

Preoperative Planning

■ Review the history and physical examination.
■ Review plain radiographs for evidence of old trauma, valgus or varus deformity, or loose bodies.
■ Electrodiagnostic testing and examination may correlate with postoperative results.
■ Body habitus, especially the presence of abundant adipose tissue around the elbow, may help the surgeon select a subcutaneous transposition—a procedure with less dissection—rather than a more extensive but protective procedure such as an intra- or submuscular transposition.
■ A patient with a visible and symptomatic subluxating nerve may be considered for a medial epicondylectomy.
■ Patients with severe disease with muscle wasting are less likely to have complete recovery.[5]

Positioning

■ The patient usually is placed in the supine position.
■ If a sterile tourniquet is preferred, drape out the forequarter. A standard tourniquet may be used, but position it high in the axilla, with good padding. A proximally placed tourniquet can be challenging to position in the obese arm in either circumstance, because the tourniquet tends to gap distally. It is worth the extra time to position it properly, because adequate hemostasis and visualized proximal dissection are important aspects of ulnar nerve surgery.
■ The patient's shoulder is externally rotated and abducted on an arm table.
■ The tourniquet is inflated after exsanguination of the arm.
■ Folded towels stabilize and elevate the elbow (**FIG 5**).
■ An obese patient with sleep apnea under peripheral nerve block (most commonly supra- or infraclavicular block) may require slight truncal elevation, which may be vexing for the surgeon.

Approach

■ The choice of technique depends on the severity of symptoms, the patient's body habitus, the presence of elbow anatomic pathology, and the surgeon's preference.[9]
■ The three general types of release are in situ release, in situ release with medial epicondylectomy, and anterior transposition (subcutaneous, intramuscular, and submuscular).
■ Table 1 summarizes the surgical options for treating cubital tunnel syndrome.

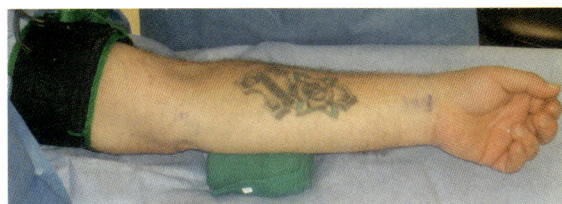

FIG 5 • The arm is draped, the sterile tourniquet is placed proximally, and a bump under the elbow assists visualization. Alternatively, a proximal tourniquet may be placed before the arm is draped.

Table 1	Techniques for Cubital Tunnel Release			
Technique	**Advantages**	**Disadvantages**	**Contraindications**	**Indications**
In situ release	Simplest dissection Does not devascularize the nerve with circumferential dissection Early mobilization	Keeps nerve in same tissue bed Does not address subluxation of the nerve	Subluxating ulnar nerve Abnormal elbow anatomy	Diabetic patient Frail patient Mild disease Patient with focal compression distal to medial epicondyle
In situ release with medial condylectomy	Preserves vascular supply to the nerve Early mobilization	Keeps nerve in same tissue bed Risk of destabilizing the medial elbow by damaging the medial collateral ligament of the elbow Tenderness at operative site	Abnormal elbow anatomy Not for throwing athletes	Patients with mild to moderate symptoms
Anterior subcutaneous transfer	Places the nerve in a fresh tissue bed	Nerve is superficial and may be more susceptible to trauma. Greater dissection More prolonged immobilization Possible creation of new point of compression	Very thin patient	Patient with a poor ulnar nerve bed from tumor, osteophyte, heterotopic bone Failed in situ release Throwing athlete
Anterior intermuscular transposition	Tension with elbow range of motion is minimized. Nerve is in fresh tissue bed.	Greater dissection Need for longer immobilization		
Anterior submuscular transposition	Tension with elbow range of motion is minimized. Nerve is well padded.	Greater dissection Need for longer immobilization		Thin patient Repeat cubital tunnel release Patients with severe compression

TECHNIQUES

IN SITU RELEASE

- Center the longitudinal incision just anterior to the medial epicondyle, making an incision about 8 cm long (**TECH FIG 1A**).
- Dissect through the fat, down to the level of the medial epicondyle.
- Preserve the branches of the medial brachial and antebrachial cutaneous nerves. Although the course is variable, branches can be found from 6 cm proximal to 6 cm distal to the medial epicondyle and often are at the level of the fascia[8] (**TECH FIG 1B,C**).
- Identify the ulnar nerve and dissect it free proximally until it pierces the medial intermuscular septum. Release any areas of constriction.
- Take the dissection distal to the level of the medial epicondyle and release the band spanning from the medial epicondyle to the olecranon.
- Preserve the branches of the ulnar nerve: the first is the articular sensory branch, followed by the motor branches to the flexor carpi ulnaris (FCU) and flexor digitorum profundus (FDP). The FCU branches are found proximally with appearance of the muscle.

TECH FIG 1 • A. The standard incision, centered just anterior or posterior to the medial epicondyle. **B,C.** Preservation of crossing medial brachial and antebrachial nerves. The cutaneous nerves lie deep in the fat, typically on the fascia. Here two branches are encountered before and after fasciotomies to expose the nerve. (Copyright Amy Ladd, MD.)

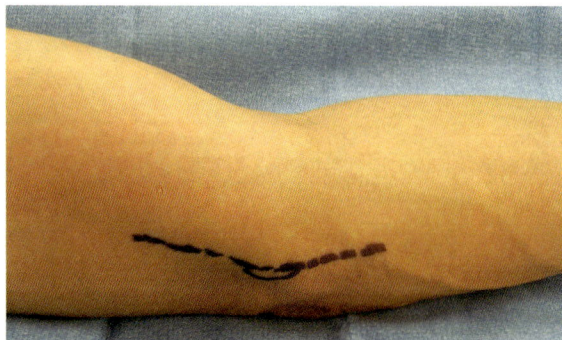

A

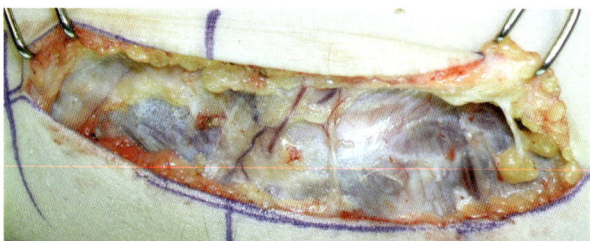

B

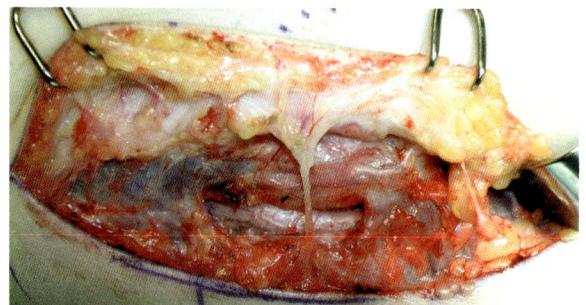

C

- The distal dissection proceeds through the thick arcade of fascia of the flexor pronator aponeurosis. Two layers exist: a superficial layer that covers both heads of the FCU, and a deeper one that overlies the nerve as it traverses between the two heads. Continue fascial release into the muscle for several centimeters to ensure that there are no areas of entrapment within the muscle belly, taking care to preserve nerve branches to the muscle.
- Gently palpate to ensure that the entire ulnar nerve is free from compressive bands.

- Range the elbow and check for smooth ulnar nerve excursion. If perching (snapping) over the medial epicondyle occurs, consider medial epicondylectomy. This is often a preclinical determination.
- Close the soft tissues using the surgeon's preferred technique.
- Typically, no drain is placed.
- Place the arm in a bulky supportive dressing or a posterior plaster elbow splint with flexion of about 60 degrees. Remove the splint according to wound care and the surgeon's mobilization preference.

IN SITU RELEASE WITH MEDIAL EPICONDYLECTOMY

- The incision and dissection are the same as the in situ release.
- Excise a strip of the tough fascial intermuscular septum as it attaches to the medial epicondyle to minimize the nerve "scissoring" over the firm edge.
- Once the nerve is free of all areas of entrapment, a longitudinal incision is made slightly anterior to the medial epicondyle with a knife or electrocautery, reflecting the periosteum to reveal the bony prominence of the epicondyle. Carefully protect the ulnar nerve; gentle retraction with a saline-lubricated ¼-inch Penrose drain on a short hemostat is sufficient.
- Expose the medial epicondyle subperiosteally.
- Remove the prominence of the epicondyle, which is most acute in its posterior position, removing 2 to 3 mm of

prominence and 6 to 8 mm in length. Use a small, sharp osteotome and smooth with a file while protecting the nerve (**TECH FIG 2A**).
- Place bone wax over the raw bone. This minimizes postoperative hematoma.
- The periosteum is closed with buried sutures, either braided absorbable or nonabsorbable, minimizing contact with the nerve.
- Check that the nerve glides, rather than perches, when the elbow is flexed and extended before closure of the skin (**TECH FIG 2B**).
- Because of potential bony bleeding, a drain is recommended.
- Apply a posterior plaster splint for 10 to 14 days, with protected mobilization thereafter.

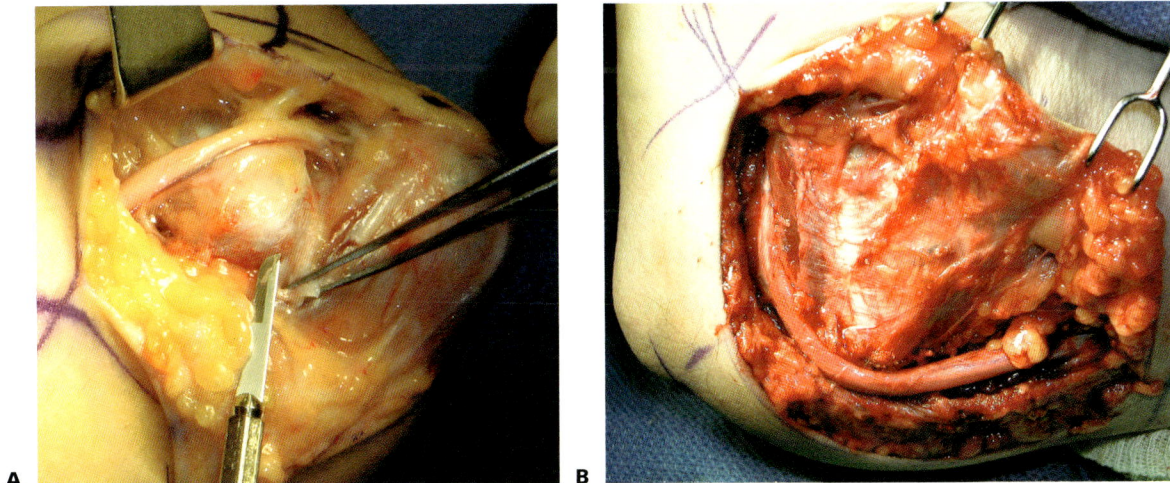

TECH FIG 2 • Medial epicondylectomy. **A.** The medial epicondyle is exposed, and the most prominent aspect is removed. We recommend removal of the most prominent and inferior portion, 2 to 3 mm in depth, to avoid disruption of the medial collateral ligament. **B.** Once the epicondylectomy is performed and the fascia closed, the elbow is flexed to visualize smooth movement of the nerve. The nerve no longer perches on the medial epicondyle. (Copyright Amy Ladd, MD.)

ANTERIOR SUBCUTANEOUS TRANSFER

- The incision and dissection are the same as for the in situ release, except that the incision may have to be slightly longer.
- Release the nerve at every potential level of entrapment.

- Circumferentially dissect the nerve to allow it to be moved anterior to the medial epicondyle. Free all posterior attachments to allow for maximal anterior excursion.

- Excise the intermuscular septum from the crossover of the ulnar nerve, anterior to posterior in the proximal dissection, all the way to its tough attachment at the medial epicondyle.
- Preserve the longitudinal vasculature accompanying the nerve to prevent devascularization of the nerve. Use caution around the medial epicondyle and the most fibrous part of the intermuscular septum, where lies an external but vulnerable large venous leash.
- Develop the interval between the skin and the fascia overlying the flexor pronator muscle mass anterior to the medial epicondyle, about 4 cm.
- Transpose the nerve to lie anterior to the medial epicondyle (**TECH FIG 3A**).

- The nerve should lie in its new position without any tension or areas of compression. An intraneural dissection to release the motor branches to the FCU may be required proximally.
- To prevent the nerve from subluxating, a 1-cm fasciodermal sling is constructed from the fascia overlying the flexor pronator mass (ie, the FCU, FCR, and the pronator teres)[3] (**TECH FIG 3B**). This flap is sutured to the skin. This flap prevents the nerve from sliding back to its old position.
- Care must be taken to ensure that this flap does not become a new area of compression.
- No drain is required.
- Apply a posterior plaster splint for 10 to 14 days, with protected mobilization thereafter.

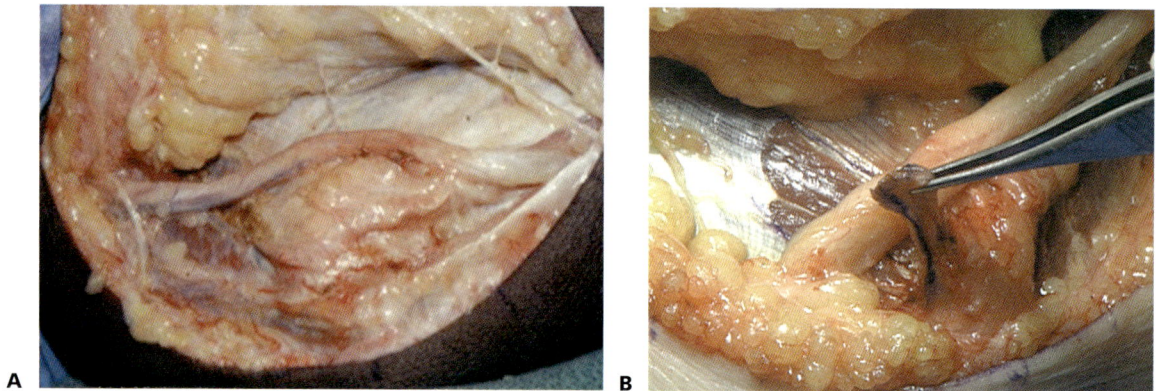

TECH FIG 3 • Anterior subcutaneous transposition. **A.** The subcutaneous flap at the level of the flexor pronator fascia has been developed and the nerve transposed anteriorly. **B.** A 1-cm fascial sling is developed from the flexor pronator mass to provide an inferior restraint for the transposed nerve. (**A:** Courtesy of Thomas R. Hunt, III, MD. **B:** From Glickel SZ, Barron OA, Eaton RG, et al. Stabilized subcutaneous ulnar nerve transposition with immediate range of motion. Video J Orthop 2000; www.vjortho.com/cgi/content/abstract/2511.)

ANTERIOR INTRAMUSCULAR TRANSPOSITION

- The nerve is fully released, as described for the subcutaneous transposition.
- The interval between the skin and the fascia is developed anterior to the medial epicondyle, to about 4 cm.
- Transpose the nerve so that its rests along the flexor pronator mass (ie, FCU, FCR, and the pronator teres).
- A trough slightly bigger than the nerve is carved out of the muscles along this anterior course (**TECH FIG 4**). Release any fascial bands found within the muscle substance.
  - Flex the elbow and place the nerve in the trough.
  - Suture fascia over the nerve, creating a tunnel.
- Range the elbow to ensure that there is no kinking or tethering of the transposed nerve.
- The arm is immobilized with a pronated forearm in an elbow splint for 2 to 3 weeks at 45 to 60 degrees of flexion with progressive protected mobilization.

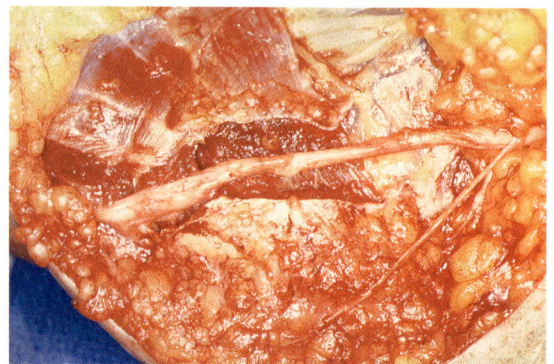

TECH FIG 4 • Intramuscular transposition. The nerve is placed in a tunnel in the muscle, and the fascia is closed. (Courtesy of William Kleinman, Indiana Hand Center.)

ANTERIOR SUBMUSCULAR TRANSPOSITION

- The nerve is fully released as described with the preceding procedures, and the skin flap is developed similarly to the intramuscular procedure.

- Divide the flexor pronator mass about 1 cm distal to its insertion on the medial epicondyle, either as a straight incision or in a V-Y fashion (**TECH FIG 5A**).

- Lift the flexor pronator mass distally at the level of the FDS muscle. There is a loose areolar plane between these muscle bellies.
- The median nerve and brachial artery lie in this plane. Transpose the ulnar nerve in the medial position (**TECH FIG 5B**).
  - Take care to avoid injury to the medial collateral ligament complex

- Flex the elbow and repair the flexor pronator mass with 3-0 Ethibond suture.
- Place a drain.
- The arm is immobilized with a pronated forearm in an elbow splint for 2 to 3 weeks at 45 to 60 degrees of flexion with progressive protected mobilization.

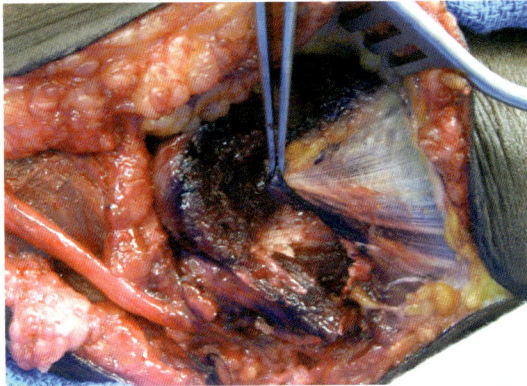

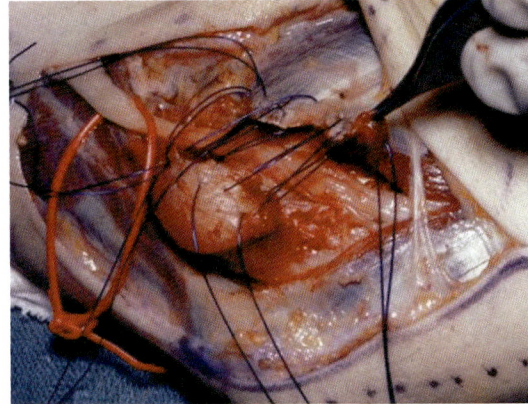

TECH FIG 5 • Submuscular transposition. The flexor pronator mass is incised (**A**), and the nerve is passed deep to the flexor pronator muscle mass (**B**). Sutures are in place to repair the muscle origin following use of a simple straight incision. (**A:** Copyright Amy Ladd, MD. **B:** Courtesy of Thomas R. Hunt, III, MD.)

PEARLS AND PITFALLS

Dissection	■ Avoid cutting the medial brachial and antebrachial nerve. Damage to this nerve is the most common cause of pain after cubital tunnel release.[8,14] ■ Make an adequate proximal dissection: follow the nerve to the crossover of the anterior-to-posterior compartment, where a thin or thick fascial band is present at the septum, or rarely, the arcade of Struthers. Make certain the tourniquet is high enough to reach this spot, usually 5 to 8 cm above the epicondyle. ■ Make an adequate distal dissection: follow the nerve several centimeters into the muscle bellies to ensure a full release, including the fascia of the FCU encasing its branches.
Transposition	■ Preserve the longitudinal blood supply to the nerve. ■ If transposing the nerve, ensure that a new point of compression is not created. Compression may be created at the following sites: proximally at the crossover from anterior to posterior; the intermuscular septum just proximal to the medial epicondyle; the flexor pronator mass if submuscular or intramuscular transposition is performed; and the entrance to the FCU muscle bellies.

POSTOPERATIVE CARE

- Postoperative care instructions are given individually with the discussion of each technique. In general, the more extensive the dissection, the more protected postoperative splinting and mobilization is required. Strengthening may begin a few weeks after an in situ decompression, for example, and 6 to 8 weeks following a submuscular transposition.

OUTCOMES

- Overall, all procedures have a success rate of about 90% for mild cases. The rate of total relief decreases as severity of disease increases.[9]
- Postoperative outcomes are proportional to disease severity: ie, severe disease is less likely to achieve full recovery.[5]
- Recent studies suggest that outcomes are similar for the different procedure types.[1,4,10]

COMPLICATIONS

- Pain at the elbow
- Decreased sensation around the scar
- Incomplete symptom relief
- Painful neuroma of cutaneous nerves
- Symptomatic subluxating nerve
- Injury to motor branches to the FCU

REFERENCES

1. Bartels R, Verhagen W, Gert J, et al. Prospective randomized controlled study comparing simple decompression versus anterior subcutaneous transposition for idiopathic neuropathy of the ulnar nerve at the elbow. Part 1. Neurosurgery 2005;56:522–530.
2. Dellon AL, Hament W, Gittelshon A. nonoperative management of cubital tunnel syndrome: An 8-year prospective study. Neurology 1993;43:1673–1677.

3. Eaton RG, Crowe JF, Parkes JC. Anterior transposition of the ulnar nerve using a noncompressing fasciodermal sling. J Bone Joint Surg Am 1980;62A:820–825.

4. Gervasio O, Gambardella G, Zaccone C, et al. Simple decompression versus anterior submuscular transposition of the ulnar nerve in severe cubital tunnel syndrome: A prospective randomized study. Neurosurgery 2005;56:108–117.

5. Hironori M, Yoshizu T, Maki Y, et al. Long-term clinical and neurologic recovery in the hand after surgery for severe cubital tunnel syndrome. J Hand Surg Am 2004;29;373–378.

6. Iba K, Wada T, Aoki M, et al. Intraoperative measurement of pressure adjacent to the ulnar nerve in patients with cubital tunnel syndrome. J Hand Surg Am 2006;31;553–558.

7. Kleinman WB, Bishop AT. Anterior intramuscular transposition of the ulnar nerve. J Hand Surg Am 1989;14:972–979.

8. Lowe JB, Maggi SP, Mackinnon SE. The position of crossing branches of the medial antebrachial cutaneous nerve during cubital tunnel surgery in humans. Plast Reconstr Surg 2004; 114:692–696.

9. Mowlavi A, Andrews K, Lille S, et al. The management of cubital tunnel syndrome: a meta analysis of clinical studies. Plast Reconstr Surg 2000;106:327–334.

10. Nabhan A, Ahlhelm F, Kelm J, et al. Simple decompression or subcutaneous anterior transposition of the ulnar nerve for cubital tunnel syndrome. J Hand Surg Am 2005;30:521–524.

11. O'Driscoll SW, Horii E, Carmichael SW, et al. The cubital tunnel and ulnar neuropathy. J Bone Joint Surg Br 1991;73B:613–617.

12. Padua L, Aprile I, Caliandro P, et al. Natural history of ulnar entrapment at elbow. Clin Neurophysiol 2002;113:1980–1984.

13. Practice parameter for electrodiagnostic studies in ulnar neuropathy at the elbow: summary statement. American Association of Electrodiagnostic Medicine, American Academy of Physical Medicine and Rehabilitation, American Academy of Neurology. Arch Phys Med Rehabil 1999;80:357–360.

14. Sarris I, Göbel F, Gainer M, et al. Medial brachial and antebrachial cutaneous nerve injuries: effect on outcome in revision cubital tunnel surgery. J Reconstr Microsurg 2002;18:665–670.

15. Siqueira MG, Martins RS. The controversial arcade of Struthers. Surg Neurol 2005;64S:S17–S20.

Chapter 71

Radial Nerve Decompression

Mark N. Awantang, Joseph M. Sherrill, Christopher J. Thomson, and Thomas R. Hunt III

DEFINITION

- Radial tunnel syndrome was first described by Michele and Krueger[7] in 1956 as *radial pronator syndrome.*
- It was described as a compression neuropathy involving primarily the posterior interosseous nerve (PIN), associated with a predominant symptom of pain.

ANATOMY

- The radial nerve pierces the lateral intermuscular septum 10 to 12 cm above the lateral epicondlye. It travels along the lateral border of the brachialis muscle and is covered laterally and anteriorly by the brachioradialis (BR), extensor carpi radialis longus (ECRL), and extensor carpi radialis brevis (ECRB) muscles (see Fig. 1B, Chap. 76).
- It divides into the PIN and the superficial radial sensory nerve 3 to 5 cm distal to the lateral epicondyle.
- The PIN then enters the "radial tunnel."
  - The floor of the tunnel begins at the anterior capsule of the radiocapitellar joint and continues as the deep head of the supinator.
  - The roof begins as inconstant fibrous bands between the brachialis and BR and then continues as the medial border of the ECRB. Distally, the roof of the tunnel consists of the superficial or oblique head of the supinator.
  - The radial tunnel ends with the distal edge of the supinator.
- Proximal to the supinator, the nerve often is crossed superficially by branches of the radial recurrent artery known as the *vascular leash of Henry.*

PATHOGENESIS

- Roles and Maudsley[11] described the concept of radial nerve compression in 1972, suggesting that it could result in a wide spectrum of symptoms. Radial tunnel syndrome, defined as localized pain over the mobile wad, is thought to be a result of compression of the PIN.
  - If the primary complaint is of weakness, the symptom complex is referred to as *posterior interosseous syndrome,* even though the pathogenesis in both conditions is thought to be due to a compression neuropathy.
- The compression may rarely be due to space-occupying lesions such as ganglion, neoplasm, or florid synovitis of the proximal radioulnar, radiocapitellar, or ulnotrochlear joints.
- The sites of compression of the PIN most often cited are the fibrous proximal border of the supinator (arcade of Frohse), the medial border of the ECRB, fibrous bands passing volar to the radial head, and the vascular leash of Henry.
  - The arcade of Frohse and the medial border of the ECRB are thought to be the most common sites of compression.
- Werner[17] recorded pressures from 40–50 mm Hg exerted on the nerve with passive stretch of the supinator muscle. Pressures exceeding 250 mm of Hg have been recorded on the nerve with stimulated tetanic contraction of the supinator muscle. Ischemia of the nerve has been demonstrated at 60–80 mm of Hg, and blockade of axonal transport at 50 mm of Hg.
- The documented changes in pressure due to positioning of the forearm in conjunction with the observation that symptoms often are associated with repetitive pronation and supination have led to the theory that the clinical syndrome may be provoked by dynamic and intermittent compression on the radial nerve.
- Although the PIN is considered a motor nerve, it has been well documented that afferent sensory fibers run within the nerve. The muscles innervated by the PIN contain nerve endings corresponding to group IIA fibers. These fibers are commonly thought to be responsible for the pain from muscle cramps, and, therefore, could likely be mediators of pain in radial tunnel syndrome.
- Because of the common association with (or difficulty in distinguishing it from) lateral epicondylitis, some authors have suggested that referred pain from lateral epicondylitis or intraarticular pathology may contribute to radial tunnel syndrome.
  - In 1984, Heyse-Moore[3] suggested that radial tunnel syndrome may be an analogue of a musculotendinous lesion of the common extensor tendon, causing lateral epicondylitis in the supinator.

PATIENT HISTORY AND PHYSICAL FINDINGS

- The diagnosis of radial tunnel syndrome is based on clinical findings. Historically, it was described as a cause of treatment-resistant lateral epicondylitis. The two disorders may have similar and overlapping symptoms.
- Symptoms can be variable, but the classic history described by the patient with radial tunnel syndrome is of pain over the lateral forearm musculature distal to the lateral epicondyle (along the course of the radial nerve) that is exacerbated by activity.
  - The pain is often described as a constant "aching" that is aggravated by or prevents activities.
  - Pain is most pronounced with active supination, and less severe with activities involving extension of the fingers.
- Lesser symptoms of weakness of the finger and wrist extensors also may be present, as may dysesthias over the distal lateral forearm and wrist.
- Other symptoms include writer's cramp, paresthesias, night cramps, and radiation of pain proximally and distally in the arm and forearm. Some patients complain of a "popping" sensation over the elbow during pronation.
- The most specific finding on physical examination is pain with digital pressure placed over the course of the radial nerve at the radial neck, or the proximal edge of the supinator.
- Two other pathognomonic signs (described by Lister et al[6]) are pain in the lateral forearm with resisted extension of the middle finger, and pain with resisted supination.

- These signs differ from those associated with lateral epicondylitis, which are tenderness over the lateral epicondyle and lateral epicondylar pain elicited by resisted wrist extension with the elbow in extension.
- The most sensitive examination for radial tunnel syndrome involves application of firm constant pressure over the mobile wad on to the radial neck to locate the point of maximum tenderness.
- The middle finger test—extension of the middle finger against resistance with the elbow extended—transmits pressure to the third metacarpal, indirectly tensioning the ERCB and causing increased pressure on the PIN.
- If pain is reproduced at the point of maximal tenderness with supination of the forearm against resistance, the supinator is implicated as the culprit in intermittently increasing pressure on PIN.

IMAGING AND OTHER DIAGNOSTIC STUDIES

- If the patient's clinical examination is suggestive of elbow arthritis or cervical radiculopathy, radiographs of the elbow and a cervical spine series may be helpful in elucidating associated pathology that may contribute to a neuropathy of the radial nerve caused by an anterior osteophyte of the elbow or degenerative disc disease of the cervical spine.
- MRI can be helpful in identifying possible cervical degenerative disc disease or elbow ganglia.
- Injection of lidocaine into the radial tunnel has been described as a diagnostic tool for radial tunnel syndrome.
  - Because it is difficult to reliably contain the anesthetic within the radial tunnel, the main criticism of this technique is the lack of specificity in differentiating pathology of the radial nerve from other sources of pain.
- Multiple studies using electromyography (EMG) and nerve conduction velocity have shown no consistent relation between symptoms of radial tunnel syndrome and the findings of either electromyographic or nerve conduction studies.
  - In 1980, Rosen and Werner[12] demonstrated that static motor nerve conduction at rest was not significantly different between symptomatic patients and a nonsymptomatic control group. They did find, however, that active supination of the forearm produced an increase in the conduction time of the PIN across the supinator muscle more often in patients with radial tunnel than in control subjects.
  - Verhaar and Spaans[16] tested patients while holding the forearm in active supination and found that 14 of 16 patients with radial tunnel syndrome had no abnormal latency on nerve conduction studies or abnormality of the EMG.
  - Kupfer et al[4] found that differential latency (ie, different latency measurements recorded in the same nerve in different positions) may be more significant in identifying "pathologic" latency than comparing a measured latency to a standard "normal " latency measurement. Differential latencies were higher in patients with radial tunnel syndrome than in the control group and improved after surgical decompression, correlating with clinical results.

DIFFERENTIAL DIAGNOSIS

- Lateral epicondylitis
- Posterior interosseous nerve palsy

- Cervical radiculopathy C5–6
- Neuritis of the lateral antebrachial cutaneous nerve
- Waardenburg syndrome
- Myofascial pain syndrome

NONOPERATIVE MANAGEMENT

- A course of nonoperative treatment should always be attempted.
- Activity modification may be helpful, particularly in patients whose vocation or avocation involves frequent repetitive supination and pronation of the forearm.
- The patient should attempt stretching exercises of the supinator and the ECRB, with pronation of the forearm and wrist flexion with the elbow in extension. Gentle strengthening exercise also may be helpful in improving symptoms.
- An injection of local anesthetic and corticosteroid in the radial tunnel may provide relief in some patients.

SURGICAL MANAGEMENT

- Surgical management should be considered in the patient who has failed nonoperative treatment. A 4- to 6-week trial of nonoperative treatment should be sufficient to determine whether there is any improvement.
- There is no consensus as to which anatomic structures should be released at the time of surgery. It is agreed, however, that this is typically a clinical decision. Electrodiagnostic studies have not been shown to locate the area of pathology reliably.
  - Most authors recommend releasing the PIN as it passes under the superficial head of the supinator by dividing the fibrous arcade of Frohse and the tendinous border of the ECRB, as needed.
  - Lister[6] and others emphasize release of the fibrous bands of the radial tunnel anterior to the radial head.
  - Sponseller[15] has reported cases where the PIN is compressed by the distal aspect of the supinator muscle.
  - Some surgeons advocate the release of the common extensors as well as structures compressing the PIN to address all potential causes of pain. Ritts et al[10] stated that the pathology of radial tunnel syndrome and that of lateral epicondylitis appear to be interrelated.
  - Little literature has been published supporting release of the superficial sensory branch of the radial nerve. It has been associated with neurapraxia and complex regional pain syndrome.[8]
  - The surgeon should remain mindful of less common causes of pain over the radial tunnel, including radial nerve compression proximal to the supinator.
- When the diagnosis is not clear on physical examination, and the patient has symptoms and examination findings suggestive of lateral epicondylitis, surgical treatment of lateral epicondylitis can be done concomitantly.

Preoperative Planning

- A tourniquet should be placed on the arm to facilitate visualization. If it is thought that more proximal release or exploration of the radial nerve into the arm may be necessary, a sterile tourniquet is used.

Positioning

- The patient is placed in the supine position, with the arm and forearm rotated as needed to facilitate the preferred approach.

Approach

- The most direct dissection path to the radial nerve may be established by palpating the radial nerve through the mobile wad and rolling the PIN under a thumb with enough force to cause an extension flicker of the digits.
- Multiple surgical approaches are possible. Determination of which structures require decompression may influence the approach chosen.
- Anterior approach
  - Advantages: it can easily be extended proximally to decompress the radial nerve in the arm if indicated. This exposure may be of benefit in cases of compression on the nerve by rarer causes such as elbow synovitis or ganglia.
  - Disadvantages: in muscular patients it can be difficult to retract the BR radially well enough to obtain adequate visualization of the radial tunnel. Distal compression sites often are difficult to release.

- Transbrachioradialis approach
  - Advantage: provides a more direct approach to the radial tunnel, improving exposure
  - Disadvantage: some surgeons find the intramuscular dissection unappealing given the relative paucity of definable landmarks.
- Posterior and posterolateral approaches (the author's favored approaches)
  - Advantage: dissection between the ECRB and the extensor digitorum communis (EDC), or between the BR and ECRL, allows direct exposure to the entire radial tunnel with relatively less dissection and a bloodless field.
  - Disadvantage: the ECRB–EDC interval is limited in that it does not allow easy extension of the incision to expose the radial nerve more proximally.

POSTERIOR APPROACH AND NERVE DECOMPRESSION (EDC–ERCB INTERVAL)

Exposure

- The forearm is held in pronation. The radial nerve is palpated just posterior to the mobile wad (**TECH FIG 1A**).
- A 5-cm longitudinal incision is made over the proximal lateral forearm along Thompson's cardinal line from Lister's tubercle to the lateral epicondyle (**TECH FIG 1B**).
  - The posterior cutaneous nerve of the forearm is identified and protected (**TECH FIG 1C**).

- The interval between the EDC and ERCB is located. The overlying fascia is first incised, beginning distally where the structures are better identified. The incision is extended proximally to the lateral epicondyle.
- The EDC and ERCB muscles are separated bluntly, using finger dissection, or with scissors, as required (**TECH FIG 1D**).
  - Opening of this interval will reveal the superficial fascia of the ERCB, to which the fibers of the EDC often are securely attached and from which they must be carefully released.

TECHNIQUES

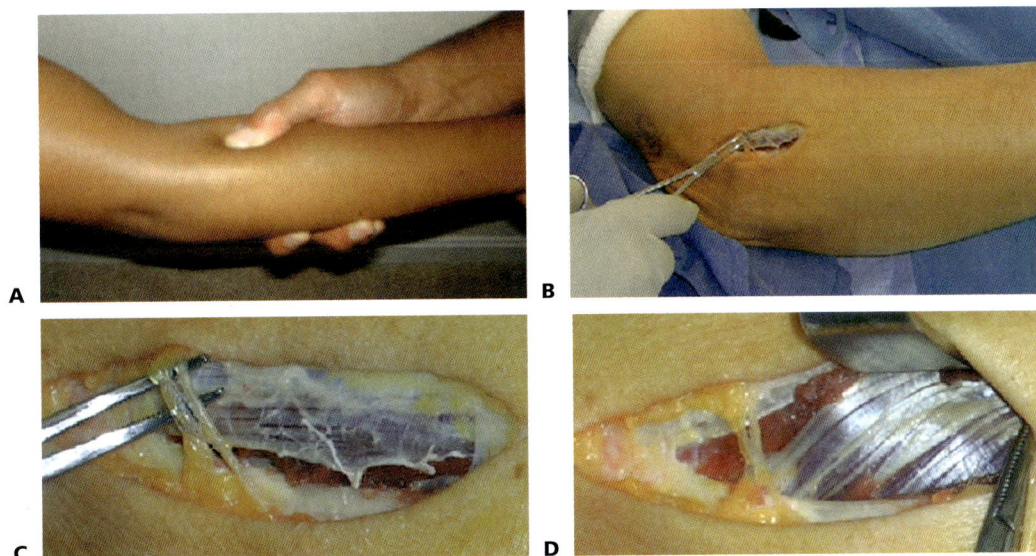

TECH FIG 1 • **A.** The points of maximal tenderness help delineate the course of the nerve and isolate areas of compression. **B.** Standard positioning, use of a sterile tourniquet, and placement of the 5-cm posterior proximal forearm incision. **C.** The posterior cutaneous nerve of the forearm is consistently seen crossing the proximal incision, superficial to the fascia. It must be protected. **D.** The fascia between the EDC and ECRB has been divided, and the supinator is exposed.

TECHNIQUES

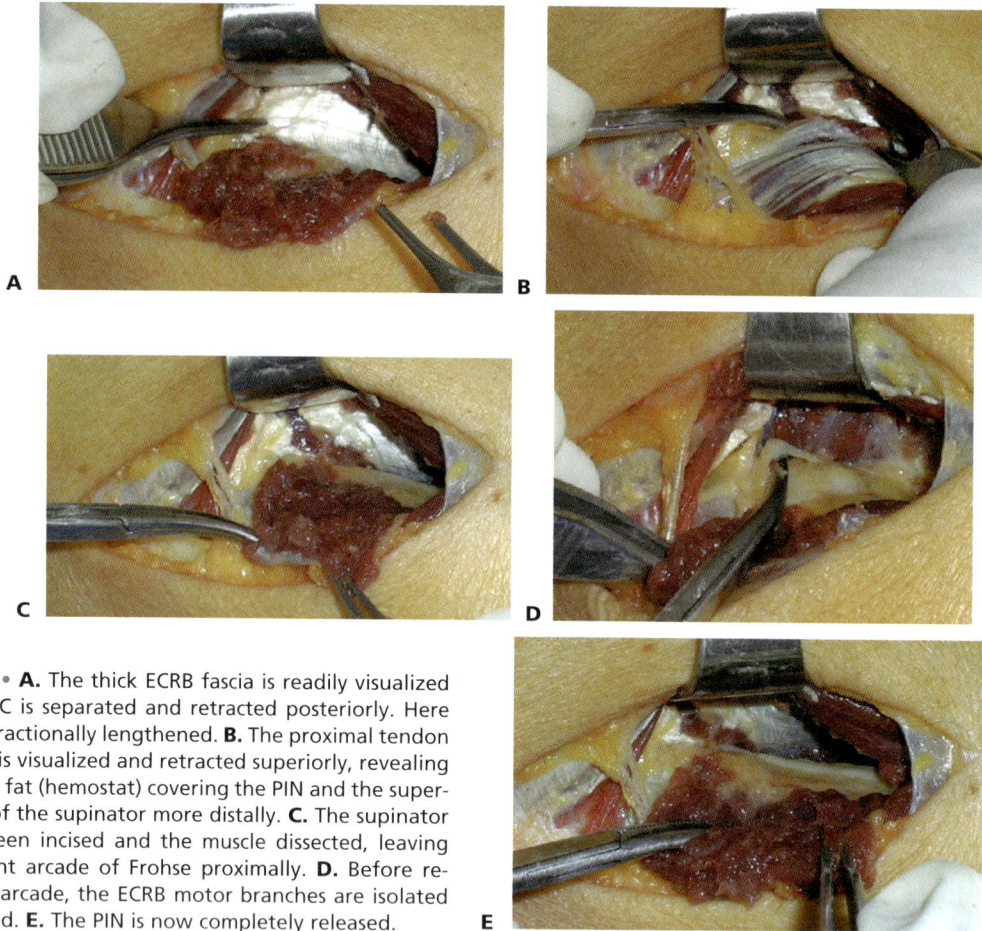

TECH FIG 2 • **A.** The thick ECRB fascia is readily visualized once the EDC is separated and retracted posteriorly. Here the ECRB is fractionally lengthened. **B.** The proximal tendon of the ECRB is visualized and retracted superiorly, revealing the proximal fat (hemostat) covering the PIN and the superficial fascia of the supinator more distally. **C.** The supinator fascia has been incised and the muscle dissected, leaving only the tight arcade of Frohse proximally. **D.** Before release of the arcade, the ECRB motor branches are isolated and protected. **E.** The PIN is now completely released.

Releasing the Compression

- The leading edge of the ECRB often is thickened and taut (**TECH FIG 2A**). This potential site of nerve compression is incised.
  - Release of the origin of the ECRB simultaneously treats coexisting lateral epicondylitis.
- Further blunt dissection in the EDC–ECRB interval reveals fibers of the superficial head of the supinator distally and fat more proximally over the radial neck (**TECH FIG 2B**).
  - The PIN will be found within this fat.
  - Gentle dissection of the nerve is performed through this proximal fat as necessary for complete visualization of the nerve.
- Proximally, the leash of Henry usually is seen running transversely, superficial to the nerve.
  - Typically the vessels are not large or obviously constricting.
  - If any of the vessels of the leash are substantial enough to appear to cause compression, or if they impede full decompression of the supinator, they are separated and coagulated with bipolar cautery.
- Once the nerve is well visualized proximally, the superficial fascia of the supinator is released in a proximal-to-distal direction to the most distal border of the supinator.

- A white crescent-shaped band of fibers represents the proximal border of the superficial head of the supinator; this is termed the *arcade of Frohse* (**TECH FIG 2C**).
  - This arcade can be observed to tighten over the PIN as the forearm is pronated.
- These fibers of the superficial head of the supinator are then carefully released. Protect the small motor branches to the ECRB (**TECH FIG 2D**).
  - This release generally results in significant stretching of the remaining underlying supinator muscle fibers and appears to reduce tension over the nerve.
- The nerve is inspected and palpated along its entire course for any other sites of compression.
  - During palpation, special attention is paid to the proximal nerve in the interval between the brachialis and BR.
- A thin fascial layer occasionally is present. This layer is confluent with the fascia of the superficial supinator that extends proximally, causing compression of the nerve. If this is present, it is carefully released.
- Before completion, visualize and palpate the nerve over its entire course to make sure there are no further sites of compression, especially proximally (**TECH FIG 2E**).
- The fascial layer between the ECRB and the EDC is closed with absorbable suture, the skin is closed in the usual manner, and an above-elbow splint is applied with the elbow at 90 degrees and the wrist extended 20 to 30 degrees.

POSTEROLATERAL APPROACH AND NERVE DECOMPRESSION (ERCL–BR INTERVAL)

- A 5- to 7-cm incision is made starting at the lateral epicondyle and heading distally along the posterior border of the BR with protection of the sensory nerve branches.
- The fascial interval between the BR and the ECRL is defined.
  - The BR is a deeper red compared with the ECRL due to its thinner overlying fascia.

- The interval is further developed using blunt finger dissection
  - Difficulty in dissection usually indicates that the muscular interval is not correct.
- The remainder of the procedure mirrors that detailed for the EDC–ERCB interval.

BRACHIORADIALIS MUSCLE-SPLITTING APPROACH AND NERVE DECOMPRESSION

- A 4- to 6-cm longitudinal incision is made over the proximal, anterolateral surface of the forearm, starting distal to the elbow flexion crease and 3 cm radial to the biceps tendon and extending over the radial head.
  - A 4-cm transverse incision just distal to the radial head also may be used.
- The deep fascia is divided in the line of the skin incision, and the BR is exposed. Its fibers are parted by blunt dissection.
- Immediately deep to this muscle, the vivid white of the superficial branch of the radial nerve is seen. Inspection at the level of the radial head reveals the fat overlying the PIN.
- The transverse branches of the radial recurrent artery and accompanying veins are divided as they pass between the PIN and radial sensory nerve.

- The radial nerve and its branches are now more fully exposed by dividing adhesions and fibrous bands overlying the nerve as well as the proximal fibrous edge of the ECRB.
- The superficial branch is followed distally anterior to the extensor carpi radialis brevis.
- The PIN is traced as it disappears beneath the fibrous edge of the superficial proximal border of the supinator, easily distinguished by its prominent oblique striations.
  - This fibrous edge and the muscle are divided longitudinally.
- The nerve is carefully inspected for untreated sites of compression before closure and splinting.

MODIFIED ANTERIOR APPROACH OF HENRY AND NERVE DECOMPRESSION

- A 5-cm longitudinal incision is made beginning at the antecubital flexion crease and proceeding distally along the medial border of the BR.
  - More proximal and extensile exposure may be obtained by extending the incision obliquely across the elbow flexion crease in the interval between the brachialis and the BR.
- The deep fascia is incised, and the BR is retracted radially. The proximal radial tunnel can be visualized over the capitellum.
- Any constricting vessels are ligated and divided.
- The superficial sensory branch of the radial nerve and the PIN are identified.

- The PIN is traced distally.
  - Significant retraction of the BR is required for adequate exposure.
  - The medial border of the ERCB is released to aid in exposure and to eliminate a potential site of compression.
- The arcade of Frohse is visualized, and the supinator muscle is divided to its distal border.
- The arm is supinated and pronated to identify constricting structures, and the course of the PIN is carefully inspected.
- Despite closure and splinting, as detailed previously, the scar often is conspicuous.

PEARLS AND PITFALLS

Surgical indications	■ Attempt a course of nonoperative treatment for at least 3 months. ■ Take care to differentiate radial tunnel syndrome from other pathology using a thorough history and multiple physical examinations.
Surgical approach	■ Dictated by inciting pathology, coexistent diagnoses, and surgeon comfort
Decompression	■ At the time of release, make sure that the PIN is released from the proximal radiocapitellar joint to the distal border of the supinator.

POSTOPERATIVE CARE

- Patients are splinted for 7 to 10 days.
- Gentle active range of motion exercises are initiated and progressively advanced. Nerve gliding exercises are emphasized.
- Patients are allowed to resume normal activities in a progressive and graded fashion over the next few weeks.

OUTCOMES

- The efficacy of surgical treatment for radial tunnel syndrome is widely variable.
  - This variability in results may be due to heterogeneous patient populations and varying diagnostic criteria.
- Lister et al,[6] Roles and Maudsley,[11] and Ritts et al[10] all reported high cure rates after release of the PIN.
- Sotereanos et al[14] reported more modest results (11 of 38 good or excellent), although their population did have a high proportion of worker's compensation patients.
- Verhaar and Spaans[16] reported even more modest results (1 of 10 patients had good results; 3 of 10 had fair results). Their diagnostic criterion was limited to tenderness over the radial nerve where it passes under the arcade of Frohse.

COMPLICATIONS

- The incidence of PIN palsy following the procedure is reported to be low.
- Sotereanos et al[14] reported a 31% incidence of paresthesias of the superficial radial nerve.
- Paresthesias of the lateral cutaneous nerve of the arm have also been reported.

REFERENCES

1. Eaton CJ, Lister GD. Radial nerve compression. Hand Clin 1992; 8:345–357.
2. Hall HC, MacKinnon SE, Gilbert RW. An approach to the posterior interosseous nerve. Plast Reconstr Surg 1984;74:435–437.
3. Heyse-Moore GH. Resistant tennis elbow. J Hand Surg Br 1984;9(1):64–66.
4. Kupfer DM, Bronson J, Gilber LW. Differential latency testing: a more sensitive test for radial tunnel syndrome. J Hand Surg Am 1998;23:859–864.
5. Lawrence T, Mobbs P, Fortems Y. Radial tunnel syndrome: a retrospective review of 30 decompressions of the radial nerve. J Hand Surg Br 1995;20:454–459.
6. Lister GD, Belsole RB, Kleinert HE. The radial tunnel syndrome. J Hand Surg Am 1979;4:52–59.
7. Michele AA, Kreuger FJ. Lateral epicondylitis of the elbow treated by fasciotomy. Surgery 1956;39(2):277–284.
8. Lawrence T, Mobbs P, Fortems Y, Stanley JK. Radial tunnel syndrome. A retrospective review of 30 decompressions of the radial nerve. J Hand Surg Br 1995;20(4):454–459.
9. Moss SH, Switzer HE. Radial tunnel syndrome: a spectrum of clinical presentations. J Hand Surg Am 1983;8:414–420.
10. Ritts GD, Wood MB, Linscheid RL. Radial tunnel syndrome: A ten-year surgical experience. Clin Orthop Relat Res 1987;219:201–205.
11. Roles NC, Maudsley R. Radial tunnel syndrome: resistant tennis elbow as a nerve entrapment. J Bone Joint Surg Br 1972;54:499–508.
12. Rosen I, Warren CO. Neurophysiological investigation of posterior interosseous nerve entrapment causing lateral elbow pain. Electroencephalogr Clin Neurophysiol 1980;50(1):125–133.
13. Sponseller PD, Engber WD. Double-entrapment radial tunnel syndrome. J Hand Surg Am 1983;8:420–423.
14. Sarhadi NS, Korday SN, Bainbridge LC. Radial tunnel syndrome: Diagnosis and management. J Hand Surg Br 1998;23:617–619.
15. Sotereanos DG, Sokratis VE, Giannakopoulos PN. Results of surgical treatment for radial tunnel syndrome. J Hand Surg Am 1999; 24:566–570.
16. Verhaar J, Spaans F. Radial tunnel syndrome: an investigation of compression neuropathy as a possible cause. J Bone Joint Surg Am 1991;73:539–544.
17. Werner CO, Haeffner F, Rosen I. Direct recording of local pressure in the radial tunnel during passive stretch and active contraction of the supinator muscle. Arch Ortho Trauma Surg 1980;96(4):299–301.

Chapter 72

Primary Repair and Nerve Grafting Following Complete Nerve Transection in the Hand, Wrist, and Forearm

Randy R. Bindra and Jeff W. Johnson

DEFINITION

- *Complete transection* of a peripheral nerve is defined as interruption of all of the axons within the nerve.
- *Primary nerve repair* is the tension-free reapproximation of severed nerve ends performed within a week of injury.
- *Delayed primary repair* is performed up to 3 weeks from injury when local soft tissue injuries do not permit primary wound closure.
- The healing of an injured peripheral nerve is different from the healing of other tissue types.
- Injury is followed by an immediate degeneration, followed by incomplete recovery.
- Irreversible changes in the motor and sensory end-organs make timing of repair critical to achieve useful recovery.

ANATOMY

- The anatomy of the peripheral nerve can be simplified by examining its component parts (**FIG 1**).
- *Axon.* The basic unit of a nerve is composed of a cell body, dendrites, and longer axons.
  - All axons are surrounded by Schwann cells, which produce the myelin sheath surrounding the axon.
  - Interruptions in the myelin sheath are referred to as *nodes of Ranvier.* Impulse propagation is faster in myelinated axons, because the depolarization potential "jumps" between nodes.
  - Myelinated fibers are between 2 and 22 μm in diameter. The larger the fiber, the faster the conduction speeds.
  - Axonal transport of cytoskeletal elements and neuronal factors is oxygen-dependent. Antegrade transport along the axon occurs at roughly 1 to 4 mm per day. The transport is the rate-limiting step in nerve regeneration.

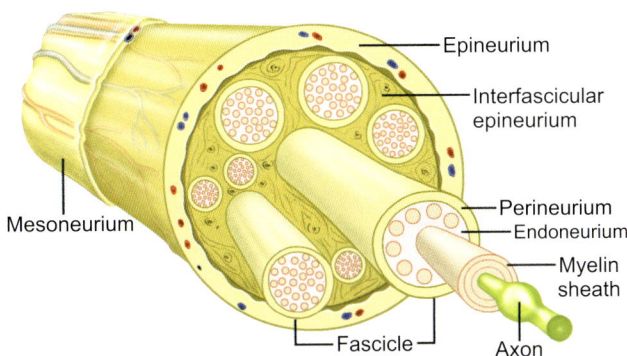

FIG 1 • Schematic of ultrastructure of the nerve. The smallest nerve unit visible to the naked eye is the nerve fascicle.

- *Endoneurium.* Delicate connective tissue that supports and surrounds each axonal fiber and associated Schwann cells
  - Consists of longitudinally arranged collagen fibrils and intrinsic blood vessels
- *Perineurium.* The connective tissue that surrounds groups of axons, creating bundles referred to as *fascicles.* The fascicle is the smallest visible unit of the nerve at surgery.
  - The fascicle is several layers thick and acts as a protective membrane and a barrier to diffusion.
- *Epineurium.* Surrounds groups of fascicles to form the superstructure of a peripheral nerve
  - Forms a sheath about the entire nerve and also supports the fascicular structure by passing between all the fascicles
  - Forms 60% to 85% of the cross-sectional area of a peripheral nerve
  - Composed on longitudinally oriented collagen fibers, fibroblasts, and intrinsic vessels
- *Paraneurium or mesoneurium.* Loose areolar tissue surrounding the epineurium
  - Limited to the outer surface of the nerve
  - Location for the extrinsic vascular supply of the nerve
  - Makes up the gliding apparatus of a peripheral nerve
- Fascicles have a definite topographic arrangement within a peripheral nerve.
  - Fascicular segregation into motor and sensory components is important when aligning a sectioned nerve before repair.
  - This concept of functional segregation allows for use of part of a donor healthy nerve for nerve transfer with minimal functional deficit.

PATHOGENESIS

- Injuries involving peripheral nerves can be simply classified as tidy or untidy.
- *Tidy wounds* involve sharp transections with minimal to no tissue loss:
  - Sharp lacerations from glass or knife wounds
  - Most iatrogenic nerve injuries
- *Untidy wounds* involve maceration of all tissues in the area:
  - Bony injury may be present.
  - Surrounding soft tissue may have been lost or rendered nonviable and is expected to heal with significant scarring.

NATURAL HISTORY

- Complete transection of a nerve results in retraction of the nerve ends. The nerve will not heal without surgical intervention to approximate the nerve ends.
- Wallerian degeneration occurs in the nerve segment distal to the level of transection.
  - The axon distal to the injury degenerates and does not directly contribute to repair. The axonal and myelin debris are

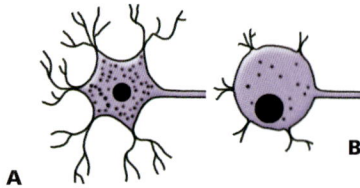

FIG 2 • Comparison of a normal neuron cell body (**A**) with that of a nerve after transection (**B**). Note cellular swelling, dissolution of Nissl granules in the cytoplasm, and retraction of the dendritic processes.

cleared by macrophages. Schwann cells proliferate, releasing nerve growth factors or neurotrophic factors. The distal stump does produce a complex protein, neurotropic factor, that attracts regenerating axons from the proximal stump.
▪ The cell body swells, Nissl granules in the cytoplasm diminish, and its dendritic processes retract. Several cells rupture and die, especially with more proximal nerve injuries (**FIG 2**).
▪ Regenerating axons sprout from the surviving axons and migrate toward the empty tubules in the degenerate distal stump at a rate of 1 to 3 mm/day.
  ▪ Proliferating Schwann cells myelinate the newly regenerated axons.
  ▪ In an unrepaired nerve, the random proliferation of axons from the proximal stump forms a tender mass or neuroma.

PATIENT HISTORY AND PHYSICAL FINDINGS

▪ History of trauma
  ▪ Penetrating, ballistic, burn, stretch, blunt, fracture, or previous surgery
  ▪ Timing of onset of symptoms: at initial presentation; after procedure, eg, manipulation and casting or internal fixation of a fracture
  ▪ Depth and location of the injury
  ▪ Severity of bleeding-associated blood vessel injury
▪ Patient reports
  ▪ Paresthesias (pins and needles) or absent sensation (numbness) in fingers
  ▪ Weakness
  ▪ Paralysis due to nerve or associated tendon injury
  ▪ Pain: neurogenic type; can be constant and severe
  ▪ Rarely, a sensation of warmth or anhydrosis
▪ Physical examination
  ▪ Note the distribution of sensory loss. The area of sensory loss varies with the nerve that is injured (**FIG 3**).
  ▪ Examine the skin for trophic changes or dry skin. Dry, warm skin implies sympathetic interruption.
  ▪ Perform thumb abduction test to check for paralysis of the abductor pollicis brevis from median nerve injury.
  ▪ Perform the Froment's sign test. The test is positive if paper is held by flexing the thumb interphalangeal joint (IP), indicating recruitment of the flexor pollicis longus, which implies paralysis of the adductor pollicis from ulnar nerve injury.
  ▪ The thumb IP hyperextension test may indicate paralysis of the extensor pollicis longus due to posterior interosseous palsy.

▪ Perform the Tinel sign test. The test is positive if the patient notes a tingling sensation in the sensory distribution of the nerve. Serial progression of Tinel sign distally is useful to monitor axon progression after repair.
▪ When performing physical examinations, it is helpful to use motor function grading according to the Medical Research Council system. This grading allows for quantitative measurement of function and allows the clinician to chart recovery objectively:
  ▪ M0: no contraction
  ▪ M1: palpable contraction with only a flicker of motion
  ▪ M2: movement of the part with gravity eliminated
  ▪ M3: muscle contraction against gravity
  ▪ M4: ability to contract against moderate resistance
  ▪ M5: normal function
▪ Sensory grading is also useful in evaluation. Sensory function is evaluated within the anatomic distribution of the nerve in question. Sensation is quantified using two complementary tests—(1) Semmes-Weinstein monofilaments, which measure innervation threshold, and (2) two-point discrimination, which measures innervation density. Vibratory, pain, and temperature sensation should also be evaluated. Semmes-Weinstein filaments demonstrate subtle and early sensory loss and are more useful in evaluation of compressive neuropathy. Two-point discrimination measurements help gauge the severity of nerve injury, with two-point discrimination of less than 12 mm indicating neurapraxic injury and readings greater than 15 mm suggesting complete disruption. Used together, the various sensory tests allow for quantitative measurement of function and allow for the clinician to objectively chart recovery:
  ▪ S0: lack of sensation
  ▪ S1: recovery of deep cutaneous pain sensibility within the autonomous area of the nerve
  ▪ S2: return of some degree of superficial cutaneous pain and tactile sensibility
  ▪ S3: Return of function (S2) without evidence of hypersensibility
  ▪ S3 plus: return of function (S3) with some return of two-point discrimination
  ▪ S4: normal function
▪ Sensory recovery classification on two-point discrimination alone:
  ▪ Normal: < 6 mm
  ▪ Fair: 6–10 mm
  ▪ Poor: 11–15 mm

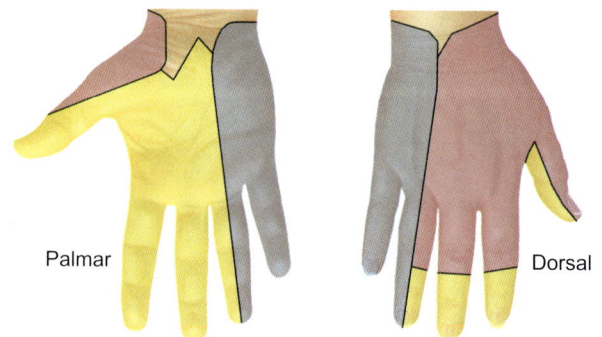

FIG 3 • Distribution of sensory loss with nerve injury. *Yellow*, median nerve; *blue*, ulnar nerve; *pink*, radial nerve.

IMAGING AND OTHER DIAGNOSTIC STUDIES

- Diagnosis in acute injuries is usually based on history and clinical examination alone without need for additional investigations.
- Plain radiographs are of little use in evaluation of the nerves themselves, but may be helpful in cases of injury from fracture or projectiles.
- CT myelography is useful for evaluation of injuries to the brachial plexus. The formation of a pseudomeningocele is indicative of root avulsion.
- MRI is useful for evaluation of peripheral injury but is not routinely indicated for peripheral nerve injuries.
  - Short tau inversion recovery (STIR) MRI may show enhancement of the nerve near the site of injury or interruption of the nerve trunk on T1- and T2-weighted images.
  - MRI provides visualization of pseudomeningoceles at the spinal cord levels in root avulsion injuries.
- Electrodiagnostic testing
  - Nerve conduction velocity (NCV) and electromyography (EMG) are useful in evaluation of closed nerve injuries, eg, after fracture or multiple nerve injuries such as brachial plexus injury.
  - If stimulation distal to the suspected injury elicits a motor response about 3 days after injury, then the lesion is likely a conduction block. However, muscle action may be present in the case of complete transection for up to 9 days.
  - Fibrillation potentials on EMG appear after 2 to 3 weeks and indicate muscle denervation and a severe grade nerve injury.
  - Recovery is best evaluated with serial examination of compound muscle action potentials. Early recovery of only a few motor units may indicate reinnervation from adjacent intact nerves and should not be used as an indicator of recovery of the repaired nerve.

DIFFERENTIAL DIAGNOSIS

- Muscle or tendon injury in open lacerations
- Parsonage-Turner syndrome (brachial plexus neuritis)
- Peripheral nerve entrapment

NONOPERATIVE MANAGEMENT

- Nonoperative management of a completely transected nerve after an open injury is doomed to failure, because cut ends retract and scar tissue forms in the gap.
- Pending recovery of the nerve, splinting of the paralyzed joint maintains functional position and prevents contractures.

- Serial clinical examination and electrodiagnostic testing are helpful to evaluate recovery.

SURGICAL MANAGEMENT

- Nerves that have been completely interrupted require surgical measures to restore continuity.
- All open injuries with neurologic impairment must be explored expeditiously.
- With closed injuries or delayed presentation, consider the overall functional capacity of the injured limb.
- In a largely motor nerve, eg, the radial nerve, tendon transfers may restore function more reliably than nerve repair.

Preoperative Planning

- The cause of the peripheral nerve injury must be identified. The repaired nerve must have a favorable local environment if the repair is to be successful.
- Underlying fractures must be stabilized.
- Adequate soft tissue coverage of the nerve repair must be planned.
- Repair should be delayed when multiple débridements are necessary until the bed for the repaired nerve is optimal and wound can be primarily closed.
- If segmental loss is suspected, as with a crushing injury, the patient must give informed consent for additional options such as conduit repair or nerve grafting.
- Injuries that present late should be evaluated with electrophysiologic studies to look for signs of recovery.
- If intraoperative nerve stimulation is to be used, muscle relaxants should be avoided at induction of general anesthesia.
- If associated muscle or tendon lacerations are present, muscle relaxation facilitates their repair.
- Regional anesthetics such as supraclavicular block provide excellent muscle relaxation, and a supraclavicular catheter will help in administering postoperative analgesia.

Positioning

- The patient is positioned supine, with the arm positioned on a hand table.
- Use of a tourniquet facilitates dissection but will interfere with intraoperative nerve stimulation, because it results in ischemic conduction blocks after 15 minutes.
- Use of intraoperative magnification (eg, loupes) for the dissection and a surgical microscope during nerve repair is essential.
- Microinstrumentation is needed for nerve handling and repair.
- Alcoholic solutions should be avoided for the preparation of open wounds to avoid chemical damage to nerve tissue.

APPROACH

- The area of injury should be exposed both proximally and distally to allow for visualization of the proximal and distal nerve stumps using extensile approaches.
- After all injured structures have been assessed, repair fractures and tendons first to take tension off the nerve repair.
- Mobilize nerve ends for about 1 to 2 cm at either end, avoiding unnecessary stripping of the mesoneurium over long distances.

- Preserve the common sheath of neurovascular bundles to maintain nerve vascularity and minimize tension on nerve repair.
- Nerve end preparation is critical. Crushing is present even after sharp lacerations.
- Under an operating microscope, the nerve end is stabilized over a sterile wooden spatula and a fresh no. 11 blade is used to progressively cut back 2-mm segments of the nerve end until sprouting fascicles are seen (**TECH FIG 1**).

TECHNIQUES

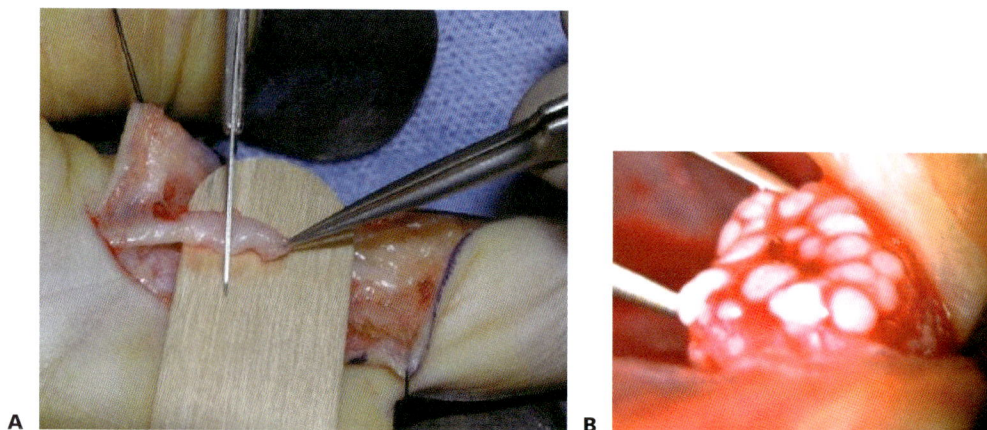

TECH FIG 1 • **A.** Freshening of a lacerated nerve end. The nerve is stretched over a sterile, moistened tongue depressor and cut using a sharp no. 11 scalpel. **B.** Sprouting fascicles must be seen at the cut surface of each nerve end before the repair.

- The distal and proximal joints are placed in minimal flexion. Excessive flexion is to be avoided, because it will result in flexion contractures or tension on healing nerve.
- Additional length can be gained by transposition of the proximal nerve, eg, ulnar nerve at the elbow, or bone shortening, eg, during replantation surgery.

- End-to-end repair should be attempted as long as this can be accomplished with minimal tension on the repair and with minimal mobilization of the nerve.
- If a single epineurial stitch of 8-0 suture fails to maintain nerve approximation, tension is excessive. Additional mobilization or alternative options such as conduit repair or nerve grafting must be considered.

EPINEURIAL REPAIR

- Epineurial repair, the most common type of nerve repair, consists of alignment and approximation of the nerve ends using sutures placed in the epineurium.
- After clean, pouting bundles of fascicles are exposed, the epineurium is identified circumferentially by resection or pushing back of the mesoneurium.
- Correct alignment of the nerve ends is critical. Line up blood vessels and other external markings in the epineurium, and match fascicular bundles in the two ends.
- Suture must be monofilament (eg, nylon) on an atraumatic needle to minimize trauma to the nerve ends. Suture size varies with the size of the nerve. Usually an 8-0 suture is used in the arm and 9-0 in the fingers. Repair with larger suture dimensions does not add strength to the repair: sutures fail by pull-out of the neural tissue.
- Two simple sutures are placed 180 degrees from one another. Care must be taken to avoid penetrating fascicles with the needle (**TECH FIG 2A**).
- One tail of each suture is left long to stabilize the nerve during repair.
- Three or four additional sutures are placed on the anterior face of the repair as necessary to approximate the epineurium and prevent fascicular extrusion.
- By flexing the limb further to relax the nerve, the nerve is turned over, using the suture tails, to expose the posterior wall. Each suture tail can be weighted down with a small vascular clip.

- Posterior wall repair is completed with three or four simple epineurial sutures, as needed.
- The long tails are then cut short, and the nerve is examined carefully to ensure that a complete epineurial seal is achieved (**TECH FIG 2B**).

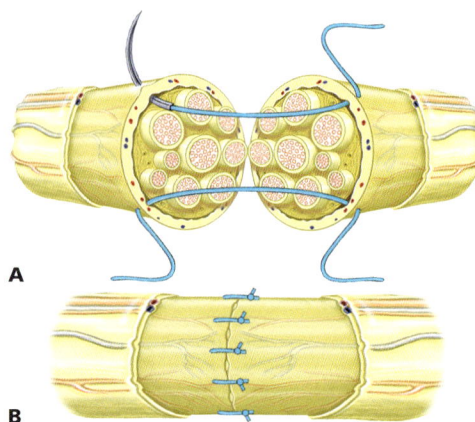

TECH FIG 2 • Steps of epineurial repair. **A.** The nerve ends are aligned, and two sutures are placed 180 degrees from each other. Tension across the repair is tested with two sutures. **B.** Additional sutures are placed in the epineurium.

GROUP FASCICULAR REPAIR

- Groups of nerve fascicles are approximated by perineurial sutures (**TECH FIG 3**).
- Group fascicular repair is indicated for partial nerve injury involving a few groups of fascicles or in a mixed nerve with distinct motor and sensory components, such as the median nerve proximal to the wrist.
- The advantage of improved fascicular alignment may be counteracted by increased intraneural scarring from the increased surgical dissection and manipulation of the group fascicular repair.
- After exposing clean, pouting bundles of fascicles, the epineurium is resected back for 5 mm to clearly exposed groups of fascicles surrounded by perineurium.
- The internal arrangement of the fascicles is noted, and similarly sized fascicular groups are aligned.
- For partial nerve injury with a few injured fascicles, repair individual fascicles with 10-0 nylon simple sutures placed in the perineurium. Usually, two sutures per fascicle are adequate.
- In the case of a complete nerve injury involving a larger nerve, a group fascicular repair that approximates groups of fascicles is faster and less traumatic.
- When approximating larger groups of fascicles, four to six sutures are placed per group in a circumferential pattern. For additional stability, sutures at the external surface of the fascicular group should be passed through both the epineurium and perineurium. (These sutures are known as *epi-perineurial sutures*.)
- After completion of fascicular repair, four additional sutures of 9-0 nylon are placed in the epineurium to take tension off the repair.

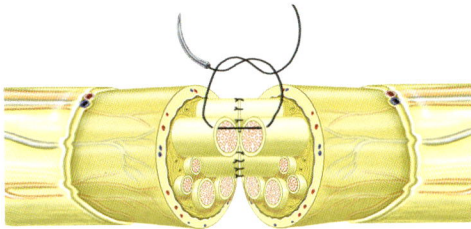

TECH FIG 3 • Technique of group fascicular repair. The epineurium is pulled back, and sutures are placed in the perineurium after fascicular groups have been aligned.

CABLE GRAFT REPAIR

- Nerve grafting is indicated when end-to-end approximation is not possible, eg, after crushing of the nerve ends, retraction of nerve ends after delay in surgical intervention, or after neuroma resection.
- After the nerve ends are prepared back to pouting bundles of fascicles, the epineurium is identified circumferentially.
- The internal arrangement of the fascicles is noted, and a quick sketch of the fascicular arrangement helps to plan graft alignment (**TECH FIG 4**).
- Epineurium is resected to expose the perineurium of the fascicles.
- The gap between the prepared nerve ends is measured.
- When grafting a larger-diameter nerve such as the median nerve using a smaller diameter nerve such as the sural nerve, several strands of donor nerve are interposed in the gap as a cable graft.
- The length of nerve graft needed is calculated as follows: gap + 15% × estimated number of strands.
- Donor nerves include the sural (located midway between the lateral border of the tendo achilles and the lateral malleolus), posterior interosseous (located in the floor of the fourth extensor compartment), and the medial antebrachial cutaneous nerve (located in the anteromedial forearm along branches of the basilic vein).
- Each segment of graft is reversed and attached to a similar-sized group of fascicles at the proximal stump using two sutures of 9-0 nylon, 180 degrees from one another.
- Although the donor nerve allows growth of regenerating axons in either direction, reversing the nerve graft helps to minimize the possibility of regenerating axons growing out along branches of the donor nerve.
- Place the limb in a neutral position; then lay the graft in the defect and align it with a similar fascicular group in the distal stump. The graft is cut and sutured to the distal stump fascicles.
- Follow the same sequence, laying segments of graft across the gap until the gap is filled.
- The repair can be reinforced with fibrin glue placed at the anastomosis and between segments of the graft.

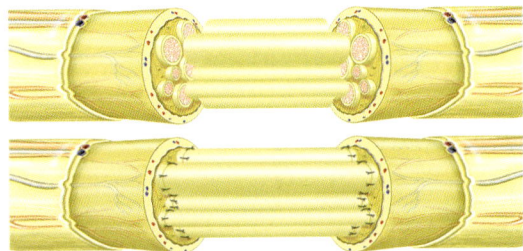

TECH FIG 4 • Nerve grafting using "cables" of nerve graft. After aligning the nerve ends, similar fascicular groups are bridged with segments of nerve graft.

TECHNIQUES

VASCULARIZED NERVE GRAFT REPAIR

- Vascularized nerve graft repair may be indicated in cases when the gap is 6 cm or more, or in a scarred tissue bed in large proximal nerve reconstruction after brachial plexus injuries.
- The most common vascularized nerve graft donor is the ulnar nerve (following C8 and T1 root avulsion), along with its mesoneurium, containing the superior ulnar collateral vessels.
- For local nerve defects, the ulnar nerve segment is divided, preserving the vascular pedicle. The segment is transposed with its intact pedicle, and epineurial repair is performed.
- If a more remote defect is to be grafted, the vascular pedicle and nerve segment are divided. The nerve is reversed and placed in the defect. Following epineurial repair, microvascular anastomosis is performed between the artery and vein in the vascular leash to a local arterial and venous recipient vessel.

CONDUIT REPAIR

- Conduit repair is indicated for clinical use in nerve gaps up to 2 cm.
- Advantages over conventional repair are that it is tension free, less traumatic, permits no axonal escape, and allows spontaneous axonal orientation.
- Two types are in clinical use: reversed autogenous vein or artificial conduits.
  - Artificial conduits may be either manufactured using absorbable materials such as polyglycolic acid or made of collagen engineered from natural xenograft sources such as bovine tendon. Artificial conduits have obvious advantages over a vein conduit in regard to shelf availability, size variation, no additional dissection for harvesting, and resilience and elasticity. Collagen tubes degrade over time with natural processes and without any inflammatory reaction.
  - After nerve end preparation, the nerve diameter is measured. A conduit that is oversized by 1 mm is chosen to avoid constriction of the regenerating nerve.
  - The conduit is rehydrated in saline for 5 minutes.
- The aim of repair is to invaginate each end of the nerve into the tube for a distance of 5 to 8 mm using a mattress suture followed by a single anchoring suture for stability (**TECH FIG 5**).
- The suture is first passed through the tube from the outside in and about 5 mm from the tube edge. The suture is then passed transversely across the epineurium 3 mm from the edge of the nerve stump and then back through the tube in an inside-to-outside direction.
- Gently ease the nerve into the tube as the knot is tightened.
- Place a simple suture between the epineurium and the edge of the tube at a diametrically opposite point to anchor the tube and prevent rotation.
- Repeat the same steps for the distal stump, and fill the tube with saline using a fine cannula.

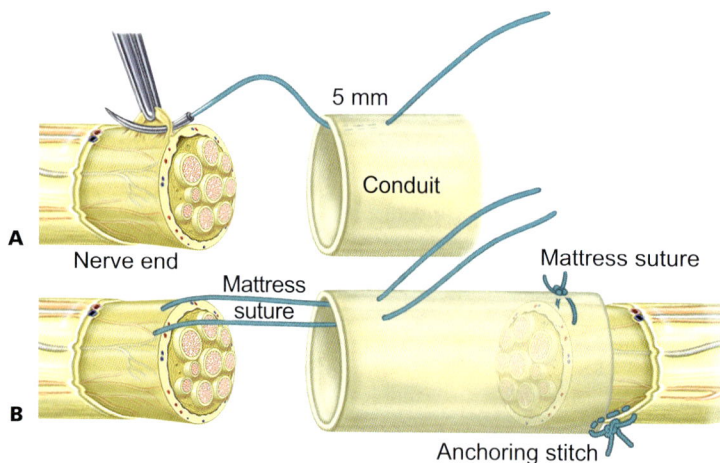

TECH FIG 5 • Technique of conduit repair. **A.** A horizontal mattress suture is placed between the conduit and the epineurium of the nerve. **B.** As the suture is tightened, the nerve is drawn into the conduit. A simple stitch is placed anchoring the epineurium to the tube opposite the location of the mattress suture.

PEARLS AND PITFALLS

Intraoperative precautions	■ If contemplating intraoperative nerve stimulation, avoid muscle relaxants and tourniquets. ■ Repair bones and tendons before undertaking fragile nerve repair. ■ Proceed with nerve repair only if the wound bed is clean and healthy and primary closure is possible. ■ If delayed repair is planned, place a marking suture in the epineurium to facilitate later identification.
Nerve precautions	■ Limit handling of nerve and use microsurgical instruments. ■ Use operating microscope to prepare nerve ends and for fascicular alignment. ■ Always be prepared to use graft or conduit rather than suture nerve under tension or with joints excessively flexed. ■ Keep nerves (including grafts) moist. ■ Repair should be tension-free. ■ Soft tissue coverage is a must.
Instrumentation	■ Make certain microinstrumentation is in good repair. ■ Forceps should be free of spurs and should approximate correctly. ■ Use 8-0 or 9-0 suture with atraumatic taper-point needles.

POSTOPERATIVE CARE

■ Consider use of a local anesthesia infusion pump for postoperative pain control.
■ Immobilization is very important to prevent tension across the repair:
  ■ The elbow should be held at 90 degrees of flexion.
  ■ Wrist flexion greater than 20 degrees should be avoided.
  ■ The metacarpophalangeal joints should be held at 70 degrees of flexion.
■ Mobilization varies with associated tendon repair. After isolated nerve repair, gentle finger flexion and shoulder range of motion are started soon after surgery to promote nerve gliding and prevent finger stiffness.
■ Remove skin sutures after 2 weeks and replace the splint.
■ For nerve repairs around the elbow, allow motion in an extension blocking splint. Full extension is permitted after 6 weeks.
■ For repairs in the distal forearm and wrist level, immobilize the wrist at 20 degrees flexion and block metacarpophalangeal hyperextension for 4 weeks. Allow active finger motion within the splint. Bring the wrist to neutral at 4 weeks, and then allow mobilization out of the splint at 6 weeks.
■ Nerve regeneration is followed at regular intervals with clinical examination of motor and sensory recovery and Tinel sign.
  ■ The distal-most point at which the Tinel sign is observed is recorded at each visit and its distance from the suture line noted.
  ■ Expect distal progression of Tinel sign at the rate of about 1 mm per day, with a delay of 1 month after the date of repair.
  ■ Failure of Tinel progression over serial visits may indicate repair failure: consider re-exploration and grafting.
■ Sensory re-education is initiated early in the postoperative phase with the goal of teaching recognition of new input in a useful manner.
■ Three stages to this process are introduced sequentially in the recovery period:
  ■ *Desensitization:* the patient is presented with graded stimuli to decrease unpleasant sensations.
  ■ *Early-phase discrimination and localization:* the patient works with static and moving touch, using visual reinforcement.
  ■ *Late-phase discrimination and tactile gnosis:* the patient works with varying shaped objects.

OUTCOMES

■ The outcome after nerve repair is generally less favorable than that of repair of other tissues, such as bone or tendon injury.
■ It is difficult to predict the outcome because of several variables, including type of nerve (pure sensory versus mixed), age of patient, type of injury—clean or crushed, associated soft tissue injuries.
■ The single most important factor that correlates with outcome is patient age. The best results are seen in children younger than 10 years of age.
■ Pure motor or pure sensory nerves fare better than mixed nerves.
■ The outcome also correlates with level of injury. Injuries closer to the end organs fare better, because there is less distance for the regenerating axons to cover.
■ Peripheral factors that are determined by the injury and cannot be modified by the treating surgeon include axonal cell death, end-organ atrophy, and extensive scarring from surrounding crush injury.
■ The surgeon can control, to a limited extent, the scarring in and around the nerve repair.
■ Central factors that account for poor results include cortical remapping and reorganization, with reduced and disorganized cortical representation of denervated areas.
■ Children recover greater function than their adult counterparts with primarily repaired lesions at similar levels due to a combination of better axonal regeneration and cortical plasticity.
■ Delayed repairs fare worse than those repaired acutely, with an estimated 1% decrease in performance for every 6 days of delay in the repair.
■ The nature of the injury often determines the likelihood of recovery. Massive soft tissue injury or burns involving a peripheral nerve are less likely to regain function than injuries involving sharp or limited transection of a nerve.
■ Median nerve outcome after high injuries usually is poor because of hand intrinsic atrophy. After low injuries, useful

motor function is regained in 40% to 90% of repairs, and useful sensation is restored in 53% to 100% of patients.

▪ Ulnar nerve injuries show similarly poor results for motor recovery, with functional restoration in 35% of cases and functional sensory recovery in 30% to 68% of cases.

▪ Because the ulnar nerve is largely a motor nerve, better results can be expected after acute radial nerve repairs, with functional return in 60% to 75% of patients. Poor results are noted with high injuries, however.

▪ After repair of digital nerves, about 50% of patients regain static two-point discrimination of less than 10 mm. Younger children demonstrate near-normal sensory recovery due to their cortical adaptability.

▪ Lingering symptoms of hypersensitivity and cold intolerance are common with sensory nerve injury in the upper extremity, resolving in most patients after 2 to 3 years. The cause is unclear.

▪ Complex regional pain syndrome is more likely to be present after untreated nerve injuries. If it does occur, significant joint contractures and atrophic changes can result, and the patient generally has a prolonged recovery period and a poor outcome.

COMPLICATIONS

▪ Causes for failure of repair include:
  ▪ Tension on the initial repair
  ▪ An unfavorable local tissue environment with excessive scarring
  ▪ Noncompliance with protective measures or therapy and consequent joint contractures

▪ Painful neuromas usually form in unrepaired or poorly repaired nerves close to the surface. These usually are treated with desensitization, local padding, etc. because surgical results are often disappointing.

▪ Altered sensation is a result of axonal misdirection and cortical misrepresentation and can present as loss of temperature sensation or cold intolerance, hyperesthesia, or neuropathic pain.

▪ Some amount of altered function is inevitable after all complete nerve injuries in the upper extremity except in young children. It is due to a combination of altered sensation and proprioception along with loss of motor strength.

▪ Complex regional pain syndrome type II can occur after nerve injury especially in untreated cases or after delayed treatment or failure to control pain. Typical features include dramatic changes in the color and temperature of the skin accompanied by intense burning pain, skin sensitivity, sweating, and swelling. Early recognition is the key with referral to a pain management specialist for stellate blocks along with steroids, antiepileptic drugs, and therapy.

SUGGESTED READING

Al-Ghazal SK, McKiernan M, Khan K, et al. Results of clinical assessment after primary digital nerve repair. J Hand Surg Br 1994;19:255–257.

Birch R. Nerve repair. In: Green D, Hotchkiss R, Pederson W, et al, eds. Green's Operative Hand Surgery. Philadelphia: Elsevier Churchill Livingstone, 2005.

Birch R, Bonney C, Wynn Parry CB. Surgical Disorders of the Peripheral Nerves. Edinburgh: Churchill Livingstone, 1998.

Birch R, Raji AR. Repair of median and ulnar nerves: Primary suture is best. J Bone Joint Surg Br 1991;73B:154–157.

Chaise F, Friol JP, Gaisne E. Results of emergency repair of wounds of palmar collateral nerves of the fingers. Rev Chir Orthop Reparatrice Appar Mot 1993;79:393–397.

Clark WL, Trumble TE, Swiontkowski MF, et al. Nerve tension and blood flow in a rat model of immediate and delayed repairs. J Hand Surg Am 1992;17:677–687.

de Medinaceli L, Prayon M, Merle M. Percentage of nerve injuries in which primary repair can be achieved by end-to-end approximation: Review of 2,181 nerve lesions. Microsurgery 1993;14:244–246.

Giddins GE, Wade PJ, Amis AA. Primary nerve repair: Strength of repair with different gauges of nylon suture material. J Hand Surg Am 1989;14:301–302.

Goldberg SH, Jobin CM, Hayes AG, et al. Biomechanics and histology of intact and repaired digital nerves: an in vitro study. J Hand Surg Am 2007;32:474–482.

Goldie BS, Coates CJ, Birch R. The long term result of digital nerve repair in no-man's land. J Hand Surg Br 1992;17:75–77.

Hudson DA, de Jager LT. The spaghetti wrist: Simultaneous laceration of the median and ulnar nerves with flexor tendons at the wrist. J Hand Surg Br 1993;18:171–173.

McAllister RM, Gilbert SE, Calder JS, et al. The epidemiology and management of upper limb peripheral nerve injuries in modern practice. J Hand Surg Br 1996;21:4–13.

Puckett CL, Meyer VH. Results of treatment of extensive volar wrist lacerations: The spaghetti wrist. Plast Reconstr Surg 1985;75:714–721.

Shergill G, Bonney G, Munshi P, et al. The radial and posterior interosseous nerves. Results of 260 repairs. J Bone Joint Surg Br 2001;83:646–649.

Sullivan DJ. Results of digital neurorrhaphy in adults. J Hand Surg Br 1985;10:41–44.

Wynn Parry CB, Salter M. Sensory re-education after median nerve lesions. Hand 1976;8:250–257.

Chapter 73

Surgical Treatment of Nerve Injuries in Continuity

Randy R. Bindra and Jeff W. Johnson

DEFINITION

- A *nerve injury in continuity* occurs when there is loss of axonal function with preserved structure of the supportive connective tissue.
  - By definition, the epineurium is preserved in a nerve injury in continuity.
- Because varying degrees of axonal interruption may occur, the extent of functional loss in terms of numbness and paralysis is variable.
- The severity of injury varies with degree of preservation of the endoneurium and the perineurium.

ANATOMY

- The cross-sectional anatomy of the peripheral nerve is discussed in detail in Chapter HA-72.
- Endoneurial tubes form the basic conduit for the Schwann cell–encased axon.

PATHOGENESIS

- Several mechanisms may cause a nerve injury in continuity, but the most common is nerve stretch.
  - When a nerve is subject to blunt injury or stretch, axonal disruption can occur without externally visible injury to the nerve.
  - Stromal elements are more resilient to stretch and remain preserved to a variable extent (**FIG 1**).
  - The type of recovery seen after an injury depends on preservation of the endoneurial tube.

- In the mildest forms of injury, with preserved endoneurial tubes, regenerating axons follow their original path. The destination is reached with good outcome. There is no axonal mismatch, and the recovery is termed *uncomplicated regeneration*.
- When the endoneurial tube is disrupted, axonal regeneration is disorganized. Axons sprout and grow in a different direction, and mismatch occurs. This form of repair, termed *complex regeneration*, is associated with a clinically less satisfactory outcome.
- With more severe forms of stretch injury, additional disruption of the perineurium occurs, resulting in a greater fibrotic response and resultant scarring of the nerve.
  - The nerve trunk, which externally appears uninterrupted due to the intact epineurium, demonstrates an injured segment that is enlarged due to intraneural fibrosis surrounding a mass of disorganized axons. This is referred to as a *neuroma in continuity* (**FIG 2**).

NATURAL HISTORY

- Pathoanatomy associated with the injury, pathologic changes resulting from this altered anatomy, and functional recovery are closely related.
- More anatomic disruption results in a stronger pathologic response and worse outcome.
- Sunderland's classification of injury severity is useful to categorize injury and plan treatment.
  - Type I
    - The mildest form of injury involves loss of axonal function without actual structural interruption: *neurapraxia* (**FIG 3A**).
    - Type I injury is seen after mild stretch injuries, tourniquet palsy, and external compression of a nerve, as in radial nerve compression in "Saturday night palsy."
    - Although structurally intact, axons fail to conduct impulses, secondary to malfunction of ion channels along the injured segment.
    - No visible change in the microscopic or macroscopic appearance of the nerve is present, and there is no wallerian degeneration of the distal segment.
    - Electrophysiologic testing does not reveal a conduction block or denervation potentials.

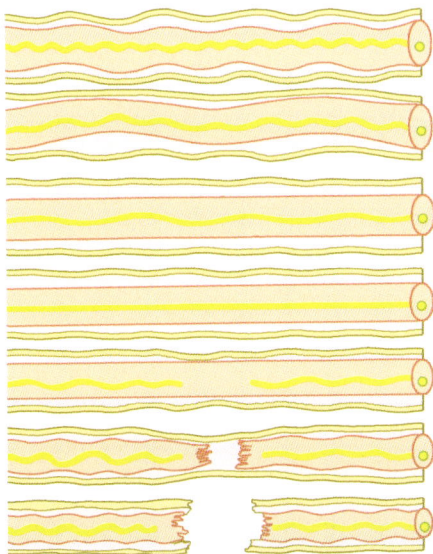

FIG 1 • Pathogenesis of a nerve injury in continuity. The effect of increasing stretch is seen, from normal nerve at the top to complete rupture at the bottom. Neural elements fail first in response to stretch; epineurium fails last.

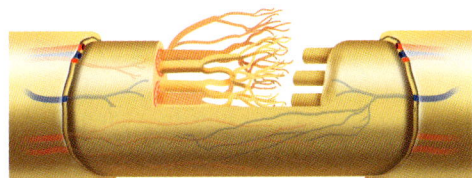

FIG 2 • Neuroma in continuity. The enlarged part of the nerve consists of a mixture of intact and damaged axons surrounded by scar tissue and regenerating axons.

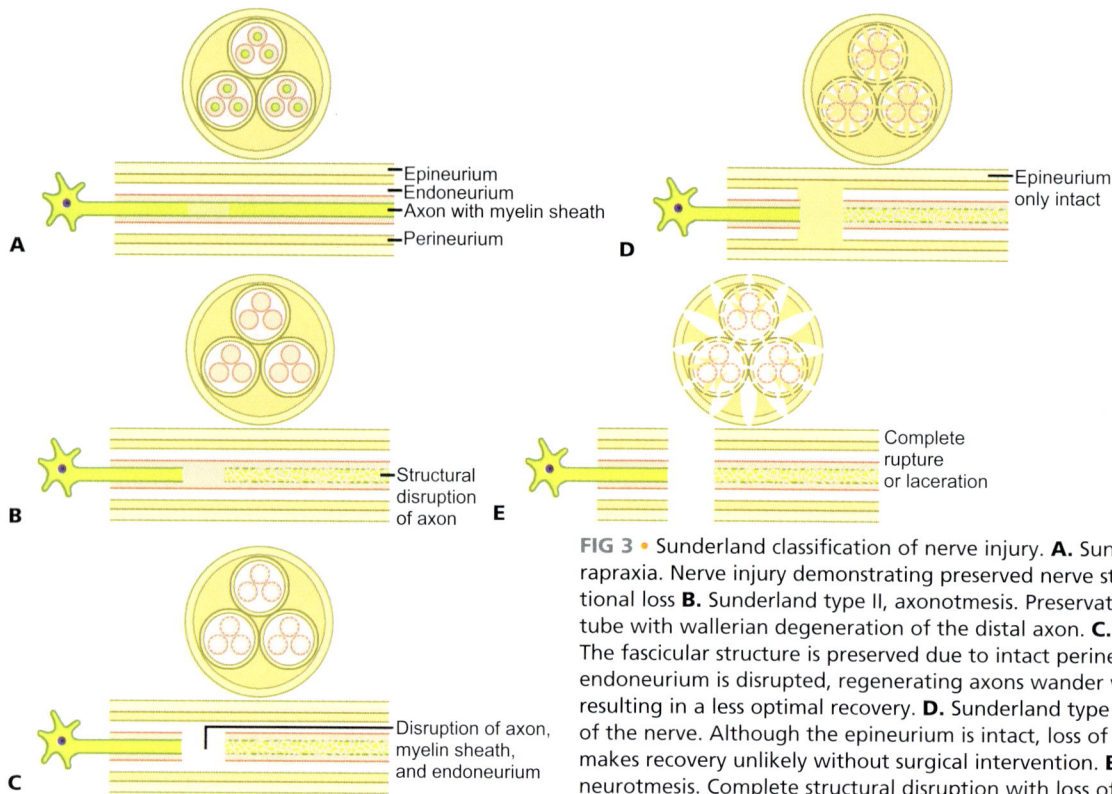

FIG 3 • Sunderland classification of nerve injury. **A.** Sunderland type I, neurapraxia. Nerve injury demonstrating preserved nerve structure with functional loss **B.** Sunderland type II, axonotmesis. Preservation of the endoneurial tube with wallerian degeneration of the distal axon. **C.** Sunderland type III. The fascicular structure is preserved due to intact perineurium. As the endoneurium is disrupted, regenerating axons wander within the fascicle, resulting in a less optimal recovery. **D.** Sunderland type IV. A severe disruption of the nerve. Although the epineurium is intact, loss of fascicular organization makes recovery unlikely without surgical intervention. **E.** Sunderland type V, neurotmesis. Complete structural disruption with loss of continuity.

■ Recovery starts within a few weeks and can be expected to be complete.

■ Because axons recover conductivity in a variable pattern, clinical recovery follows a random pattern.

■ Type II

■ There is structural disruption of the axon, but the endoneurium is preserved (**FIG 3B**).

■ Type II injury is seen after more severe stretch injuries, such as radial nerve palsy resulting from a closed humerus fracture.

■ Wallerian degeneration results and electrophysiologic tests reveal distal conduction block and denervation.

■ As regenerating axons progress distally, proximal muscles are reinnervated first. Clinically, recovery occurs in a proximal-to-distal direction.

■ Because there is no axonal mismatch, recovery usually is complete but takes longer, usually several months.

■ Type III

■ The axon, myelin sheath, and endoneurium are interrupted (**FIG 3C**).

■ Recovery is less predictable, because regenerating axons may not follow previous pathways (complicated regeneration).

■ With the perineurium preserved, recovery can take place without surgical intervention but usually is incomplete due to axonal misdirection.

■ Injury to small vessels within the endoneurium leads to an inflammatory response. Fibroblast activation results in a variable degree of interfascicular scarring that may impede nerve regeneration.

■ Type IV

■ In more severe stretch injuries, the internal nerve structure is completely disrupted, leaving only an intact epineurium (**FIG 3D**).

■ Retraction of fascicles and scarring within the nerve are present. Even though the nerve is in continuity, no clinically significant recovery can be expected without surgical intervention.

■ Type V

■ Complete rupture or laceration of the nerve with retraction of the nerve ends (see Chap. HA-93) (**FIG 3E**)

PATIENT HISTORY AND PHYSICAL FINDINGS

■ Stretch injuries that result in nerve injury in continuity usually are proximal. These injuries often take place as the nerve root exits the spinal cord or involve the brachial plexus in the neck or upper arm.

■ At more distal levels, nerve stretch injuries usually are the result of displaced fractures or dislocations.

■ There usually is a history of significant trauma, and patients complain of pain and paresthesias with a variable amount of functional loss distal to the site of injury.

■ Incomplete loss of function often indicates an incomplete nerve injury.

■ Severe pain or paresthesias after any closed fracture should alert the clinician to the possibility of an associated nerve injury.

■ Complete loss of function does not necessarily imply complete disruption of the nerve.

■ Documented lack of recovery on serial clinical examinations is essential to determine the severity of the injury and the need for surgical intervention.

■ Muscle strength is charted against a timeline at every visit. Progressive muscle recovery in a proximal-to-distal direction indicates spontaneous axonal regeneration.

■ Tinel sign and its gradual progression is also a useful measure of nerve recovery.

- Recovery within a few weeks of injury and with a random pattern usually suggests a Type I injury or neurapraxia.
- After incomplete injury to a peripheral nerve, function is lost in a predictable order: motor, proprioception, touch, temperature, pain, and sympathetic function.
  - Recovery usually occurs in the reverse order.
- In a closed injury without any obvious fractures, the site of nerve injury is not always obvious.
  - Careful mapping of the motor and sensory deficit will help to distinguish the level of injury.
  - The pattern of sensory loss is a reliable way to determine the level of injury. A more proximal injury usually follows a dermatomal pattern, whereas a distal injury follows the distribution of the nerve.

IMAGING AND OTHER DIAGNOSTIC STUDIES

- MRI done several weeks after injury may reveal an enlarged nerve segment, suggesting a neuroma in continuity.
- Neurophysiologic studies are useful in evaluating and monitoring an injured nerve when there is no external injury.
  - Conduction blocks usually reverse within 10 to 14 days; therefore, tests should be delayed until this time.
  - Complete loss of muscle action potentials does not necessarily indicate a complete interruption of all axons.
  - Electromyograms (EMGs) will show variable denervation of muscle groups innervated by the nerve in question.
  - Fibrillation potentials on EMG usually appear within 10 to 40 days, indicating complete denervation of a muscle group.
- Electromyographic evidence of reinnervation may precede voluntary muscle contraction by several weeks and may be of use in tracking the progress of nerve regeneration.
  - Return of a muscle action potential requires not only regeneration of the nerve to the level of the end organ but also re-establishment of a physiologic connection between the nerve and the target tissue. Re-establishment of the motor endplate is required before EMG provides evidence of functional return.
- Nerve conduction studies (NCSs) also are useful in the evaluation of a closed nerve injury.
  - In a closed injury, lesions may be localized using NCSs.
  - Continuity of the nerve also may be assessed, but should be undertaken at about 10 days after the injury to prevent erroneous results, because the axons distal to a complete transection may continue to conduct during this initial period after injury.
  - Parameters evaluated include amplitude and latency.

DIFFERENTIAL DIAGNOSIS

- Complete transection
- Conduction block
- Partial axonal injury
- Compressive injury

NONOPERATIVE MANAGEMENT

- Lesions in continuity may improve spontaneously, especially in types I and II, in which recovery is complete without any surgical intervention.
- Type I through III injuries can be watched closely with serial mapping of the sensory and motor recovery.
- Type IV and V injuries usually require surgical repair of the nerve to restore axonal continuity.

- Preservation of some function distal to the suspected level of the injury within the distribution of the injured nerve suggests a partial injury, and observation is appropriate.
- If there is a complete palsy of a nerve after a closed injury, an initial period of observation may be best until signs of denervation appear in end organs.
  - If signs of reinnervation appear, such as a Tinel sign distal to the level of injury, continued observation is prudent.
  - If no signs of innervation appear, one should strongly consider electrodiagnostic studies to evaluate the continuity of the axonal fibers.
- Physical therapy is very important to maintain mobility during the period of observation.

SURGICAL MANAGEMENT

- If no signs of recovery are present at 2 to 4 months, then surgical exploration may be indicated.
  - Electrodiagnostic testing should be used in this instance to define the level of injury.
  - Longer delays may compromise the efficacy of surgical repair, secondary to end organ degenerative changes.
- Focal injuries are usually observed for shorter periods, because the extent of the injured nerve segment usually is smaller.
- Blunt or blast injuries may be observed for up to 6 months given the often large segments of injured nerve undergoing repair.

Preoperative Planning

- Intraoperative nerve action potentials (NAPs) may provide information about lesions in continuity, including the degree and extent of interruption.
- If NAPs are not recordable across a lesion, then resection and direct repair rather than grafting will likely be required.
  - Resection is performed from the point at which NAPs are lost to the point where they return.
- If NAPs are present, external neurolysis or nerve decompression may be adequate treatment.

Positioning

- The patient is positioned supine, with a hand table.
- If nerve grafts may be required, the opposite leg is prepared to allow access to the sural nerve. Rarely, if bilateral sural nerves are to be harvested, the patient initially is placed prone.
- Use of a tourniquet may result in ischemic conduction blocks, which will render intraoperative nerve stimulation ineffective.
  - It generally is preferable to use a tourniquet for only the first 20 minutes of surgery, to facilitate initial dissection.
- The use of an operating microscope and fine soft tissue sets or microinstrumentation is necessary for nerve handling and repair.

Approach

- Surgical exposure should provide adequate access to the section of damaged nerve as well as proximal and distal to this site.
  - Mobilization should be minimized to prevent additional vascular insult to the nerve.
  - Sources of external compression should be identified and alleviated.
  - The bed for repair should be free of scar tissue. Nerve transposition may be required.

TECHNIQUES

EXTERNAL NEUROLYSIS

- External neurolysis is defined as the circumferential freeing of a peripheral nerve from surrounding scar tissue (**TECH FIG 1A**).
- Dissection proceeds from normal nerve (both proximal and distal) to the area of scarring (**TECH FIG 1B**).
- The nerve should be mobilized away from the scar tissue bed to prevent recurrence.

- Use of a xenograft nerve wrap or fat graft may be considered to prevent recurrence of scarring (**TECH FIG 1C**).
- External neurolysis may relieve neuropathic pain associated with compression, but results for sensory and motor recovery are variable.

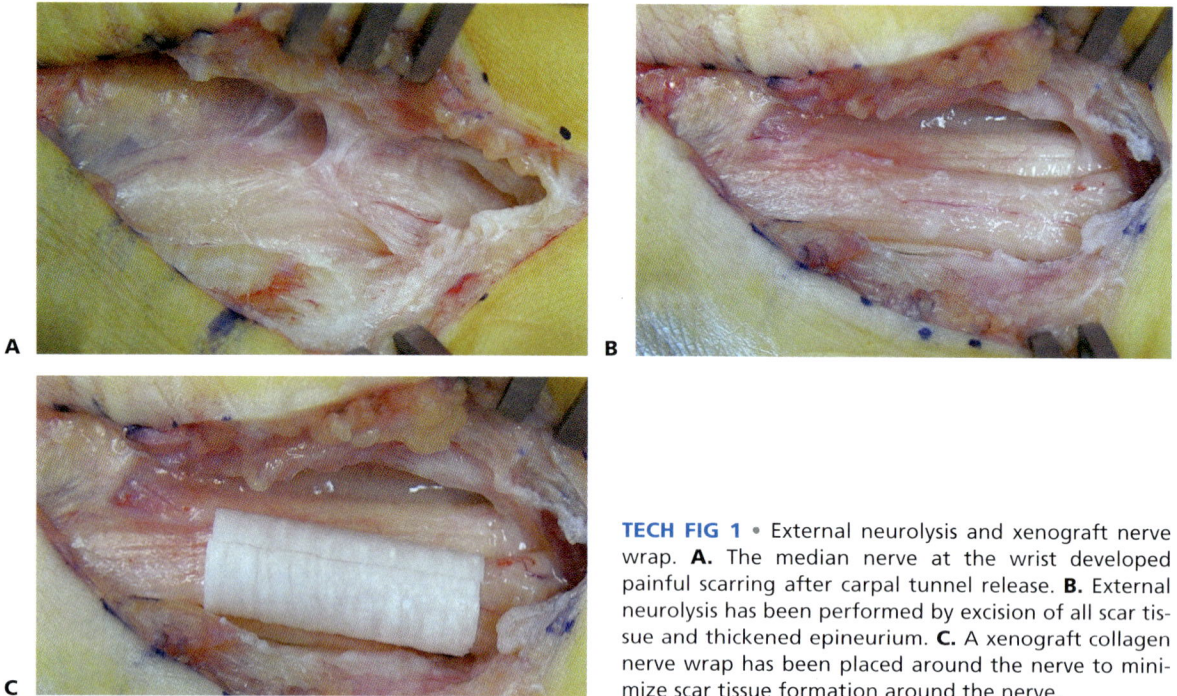

TECH FIG 1 • External neurolysis and xenograft nerve wrap. **A.** The median nerve at the wrist developed painful scarring after carpal tunnel release. **B.** External neurolysis has been performed by excision of all scar tissue and thickened epineurium. **C.** A xenograft collagen nerve wrap has been placed around the nerve to minimize scar tissue formation around the nerve.

INTERNAL NEUROLYSIS

- Internal neurolysis is defined as the resection of fibrotic tissue from within the structure of the nerve itself.
- This procedure is indicated for late management of incomplete injuries such as stretch injuries when the nerve has regained partial function that is clinically inadequate.

- Intraoperative recording of NAPs will indicate functioning fascicular groups and help guide the surgeon during this procedure.
- Internal neurolysis is performed along the fascicular segment that has lost NAPs (**TECH FIG 2**).

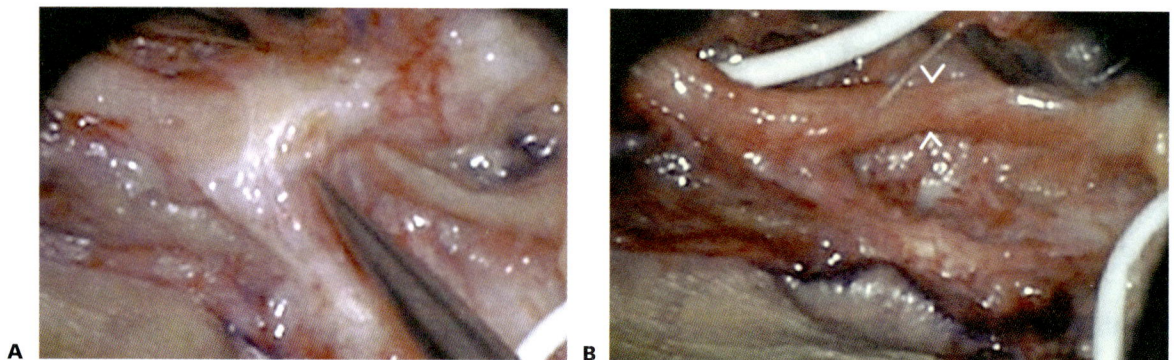

TECH FIG 2 • **A–C.** Intraoperative microscope images of internal neurolysis of the ulnar nerve at the wrist. **A.** The ulnar nerve is surrounded by dense scar tissue. **B.** After external neurolysis, there is a persistent area of narrowing of the nerve (*arrows*) requiring internal neurolysis. *(continued)*

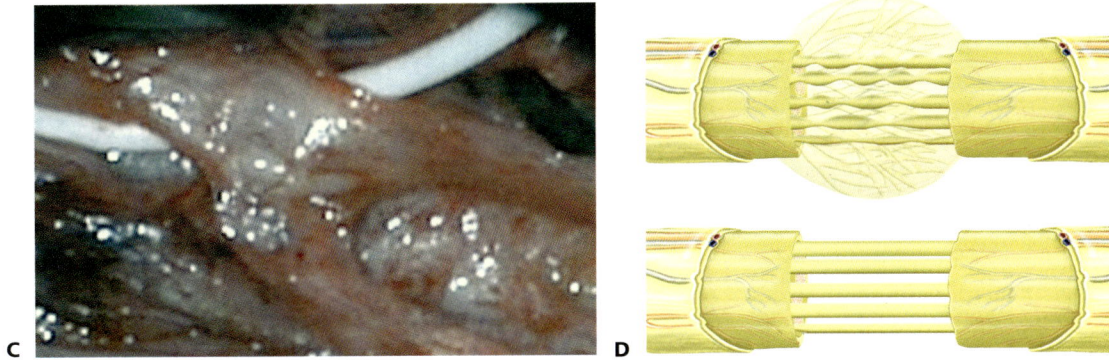

TECH FIG 2 • *(continued)* **C.** Appearance after internal neurolysis—the constricting epineurium and scar between fascicles has been excised. **D.** Illustration of a neuroma in continuity treated by internal neurolysis. The segment of scarred epineurium is excised, and all scar tissue between fascicles also is excised.

- This procedure is performed in cases of incomplete functional loss distal to the site of injury.
- Some loss of intact axons can be expected as a result of the dissection, so the patient should be advised that additional loss of function could be possible with this procedure.

SPLIT REPAIR

- *Split repair* is defined as a procedure in which intraoperative NAP recordings are used to guide the resection of individual nonconducting fascicles.
- First, external neurolysis is performed to expose the injured segment of the nerve.
- The epineurium is excised circumferentially to expose the injured fascicles (**TECH FIG 3A**).
- Intraoperative NAP recordings are made to identify the injured fascicular segments (**TECH FIG 3B**).
- Resection of the nonconducting segments is performed using either a blade or sharp microvascular scissors (**TECH FIG 3C**).
- Repair is performed either directly or with autogenous grafting.

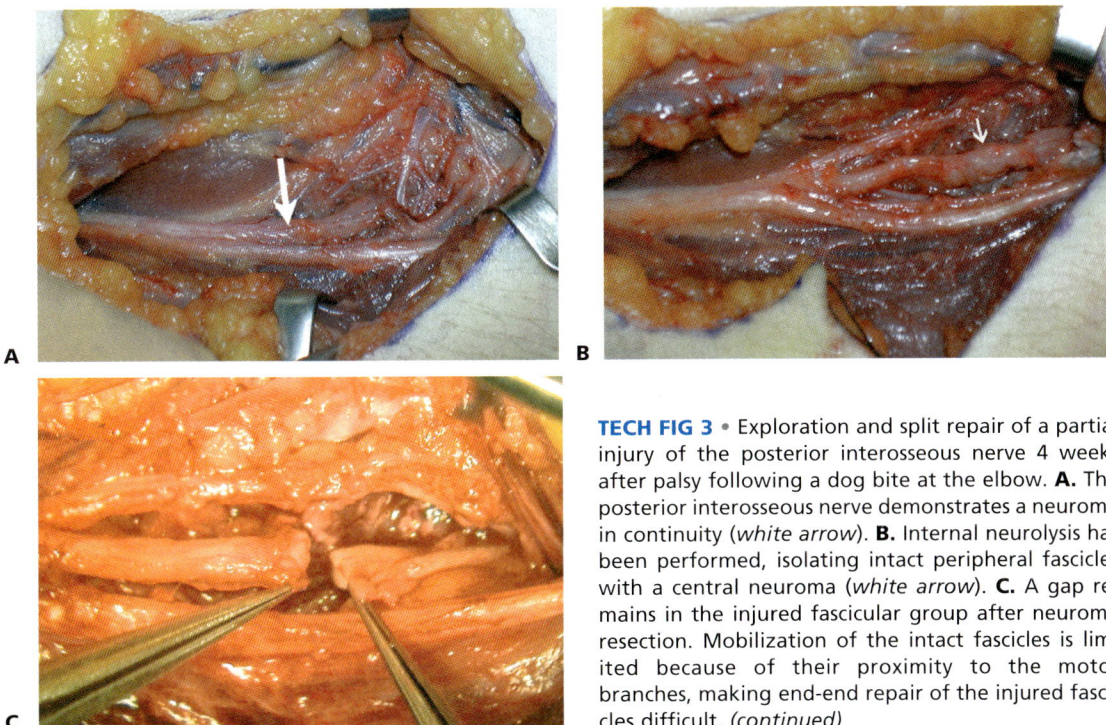

TECH FIG 3 • Exploration and split repair of a partial injury of the posterior interosseous nerve 4 weeks after palsy following a dog bite at the elbow. **A.** The posterior interosseous nerve demonstrates a neuroma in continuity (*white arrow*). **B.** Internal neurolysis has been performed, isolating intact peripheral fascicles with a central neuroma (*white arrow*). **C.** A gap remains in the injured fascicular group after neuroma resection. Mobilization of the intact fascicles is limited because of their proximity to the motor branches, making end-end repair of the injured fascicles difficult. *(continued)*

TECHNIQUES

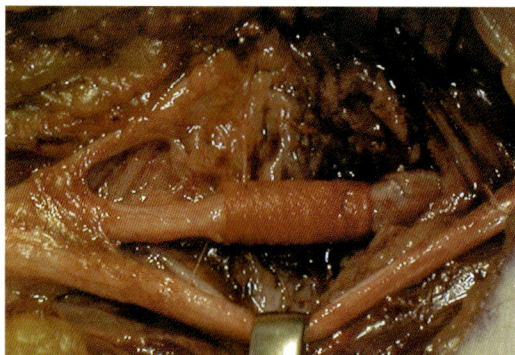

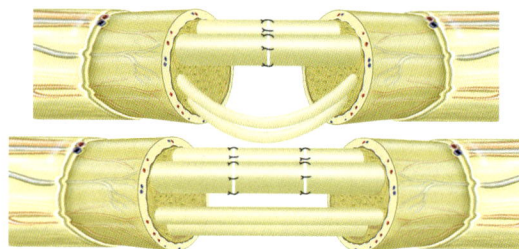

D

E,F

TECH FIG 3 • *(continued)* **D.** Conduit repair of the injured fascicles has been performed. **E, F.** Illustrations of split repair of a partially injured nerve. Nonconducting fascicular segments are excised and either repaired by end-to-end group fascicular repair (**E**) or by interposing nerve grafts (**F**).

- Cable grafting is the more common technique, using donor nerve from either the sural or antebrachial cutaneous nerve.
- Grouped fascicular repair is then performed (**TECH FIG 3D–F**).
  - The internal arrangement of the fascicles is noted, and a quick sketch of the fascicular arrangement is made to allow alignment of the nerve ends.
  - Nerve grafts will not match the exact fascicular pattern—the aim is to place graft "cables" between groups of fascicles.
  - The gap between nerve ends is measured, and the length of graft needed is calculated.

- Length = gap + 15% × estimated number of grafts
- Grafts are attached to a group of fascicles using two sutures of 9-0 or 10-0 nylon, 180 degrees from one another.
- Each graft is sutured to the proximal and distal stumps before moving on to the next graft, thus allowing for more accurate fascicular matching.
- Check the repair to ensure that no stitches have pulled out. The repair may be reinforced with fibrin glue
- Handling of the grafts should be minimized.
- Grafts should be kept moist from harvest to repair.

RESECTION OF THE NERVE LESION IN CONTINUITY

- If no conduction of NAPs is noted across a lesion after internal neurolysis is performed, then the entire lesion should be resected.
- The proximal and distal portions of the nerve flanking the lesion should be mobilized to prevent undue tension on the repair. During mobilization, longitudinal blood vessels within the epineurium must be preserved.
- The lesion is sharply excised using a fresh, sharp blade against a block (usually a moistened tongue depressor).

Epineurial Repair

- If the extent of the lesion is short, then direct end-to-end epineurial repair without tension often is possible.
- Direct epineurial repair is then performed as described in Chapter HA 93.

Cable Graft Repair

- Cable graft repair is useful when the extent of the lesion precludes direct repair because of either tension or a large gap (**TECH FIG 4A**).
- Cable graft repair is then performed as described in Chapter HA-93.
- Sural nerve graft can be harvested through a single longitudinal or multiple transverse incisions (**TECH FIG 4B**).

- The nerve is easily identified by careful spreading dissection in the subcutaneous tissue midway between the lateral malleolus and the tendo-achilles (**TECH FIG 4C**).
- Use of a tendon stripper to harvest the nerve is not recommended.
  - This technique can result in stretch or laceration of the sural nerve.
  - Additionally, the posterior tibial nerve may be inadvertently injured.

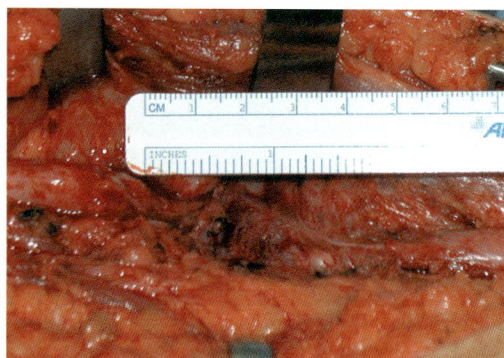

A

TECH FIG 4 • Cable grafting for reconstruction of a sciatic nerve laceration in the thigh. **A.** The ends of the sciatic nerve lie 6 cm apart. *(continued)*

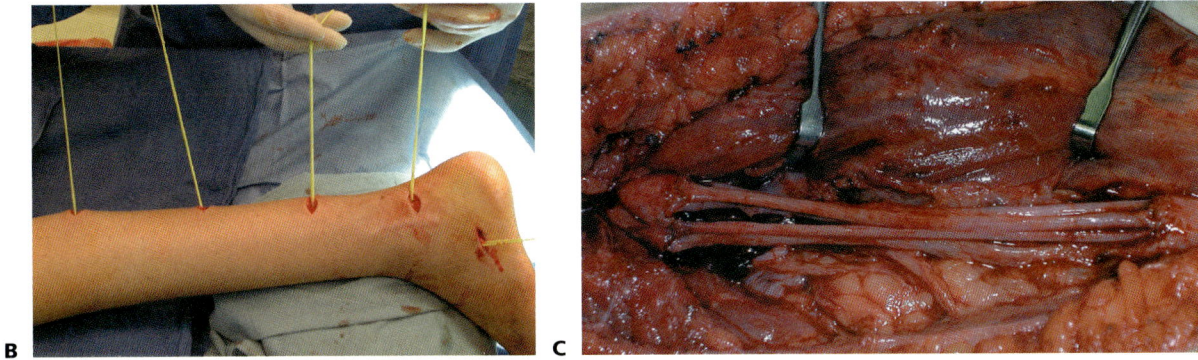

TECH FIG 4 • *(continued)* **B.** The ipsilateral sural nerve is harvested by multiple transverse incisions in the leg. Yellow rubber slings have been placed around the nerve at each incision for identification and gentle traction to facilitate dissection. **C.** Multiple segments of the sural nerve have been aligned and inserted in the nerve gap and fixed with group fascicular sutures.

PEARLS AND PITFALLS

Timing of surgical intervention	■ With lesions in continuity, function may return spontaneously, especially when there is distal functional sparing. Focal injuries can be observed for 2 to 3 months, while lengthy lesions may be observed for up to 5 months.
Is the lesion in continuity?	■ A combination of clinical and electrodiagnostic testing should be used to evaluate an injury. Serial examinations may provide valuable information about the return of function. Intraoperative measurement of NAPs may provide valuable and objective data of the injured nerve's ability to conduct electrical signals and may guide operative decisions.
Surgical delay	■ Avoid lengthy periods of observation in the absence of progressive signs of recovery as irreversible end organ damage may result.

POSTOPERATIVE CARE

■ General guidelines for splinting and postoperative care are detailed in Chapter HA-72.

■ Serial examination is important to follow the progress after surgical repair.

OUTCOMES

■ Neurolysis
  ■ If NAPs are recorded through a nerve segment, recovery is thought to be about 90%.
  ■ NAP recording and subsequent neurolysis without resection have been found to consistently result in better outcomes than direct or graft repair.
■ Split repair
  ■ Outcomes are superior to complete repair when NAPs are recorded through some portion of the nerve.
  ■ Direct and graft repair of the injured fascicles yield similar results.
■ Complete resection with direct repair or graft repair
  ■ The outcome of direct repairs appears to be superior to those requiring the use of a graft; however, injuries requiring a nerve graft often are more substantial and require regeneration along a greater distance.
  ■ In general, radial nerve repairs are more successful than median nerve repairs, and both are better than ulnar nerve repairs.
■ Children generally have better overall outcomes than adults.

■ Internal neurolysis or resection of any lesion in continuity may be related to a decrease in preoperative function as some intact axons may be transected.

COMPLICATIONS

■ Infection
■ Scarring
■ Loss of function
■ Increased neuropathic pain
  ■ Either distal to the lesion or in the form of a painful neuroma
■ Failure of recovery of function

SUGGESTED READINGS

Birch R, Bonney C, Wynn Parry CB. Surgical Disorders of the Peripheral Nerves. Edinburgh: Churchill Livingstone, 1998.

Kline DG. Surgical repair of peripheral nerve injury. Muscle Nerve 1990;13:843–852.

Lundborg G, Rosén B, Dahlin L, et al. Tubular versus conventional repair of median and ulnar nerves in the human forearm: Early results from a prospective, randomized, clinical study. J Hand Surg Am 1997;22:99–106.

Mackinnon SE, Novak CB. Nerve transfers: new options for reconstruction following nerve injury. Hand Clin 1999;15:643–666.

Mujadzic M, Ozyurekoglu T, Gupta A, et al. Intraoperative nerve recordings as a useful aid in the management of neuroma-in-continuity. J Reconstruct Microsurg 2005;21:341.

Seddon HJ. Nerve grafting. J Bone Joint Surg Br 1963;43B:447–461.

Sunderland S. A classification of peripheral nerve injuries producing loss of function. Brain 1951;74:491–516.

Chapter 74

Tendon Transfers for Median Nerve Palsy

Jeffrey B. Friedrich and Scott H. Kozin

DEFINITION

- The median nerve can be compromised by any number of causes, including trauma, tumor, chronic compression, or synovitis.
- Palsy of the median nerve can result in motor or sensory deficits, or both, within the distribution of this nerve.

ANATOMY

- The median nerve enters the forearm between the two heads of the pronator teres muscle.
- The median nerve travels down the forearm between the flexor digitorum superficialis and profundus muscles to enter the carpal tunnel.
- Along its course, the anterior interosseous nerve branches from the median nerve to provide innervation to the flexor pollicis longus, flexor digitorum profundus (FDP) to the index, and the pronator quadratus muscles.
- The median nerve proper provides innervation to the flexor carpi radialis, pronator teres, flexor digitorum superficialis (FDS), palmaris longus, and FDP to the long finger.
- The palmar cutaneous branch arises from the median nerve 5 cm proximal to the wrist joint, crosses the wrist volar to the transverse carpal ligament, and supplies sensibility to the thenar eminence.
- Just proximal to the wrist, the median nerve becomes superficial and travels within the carpal tunnel.
- The recurrent motor branch originates from the central or radial portion of the median nerve during its passage through the carpal tunnel. The recurrent branch usually passes distal to the transverse carpal ligament to innervate the thenar muscles. The nerve can also pass through the transverse carpal ligament (occurs in 5% to 7% of individuals).[6]
- The thenar muscles are the opponens pollicis, flexor pollicis brevis, and abductor pollicis brevis. The flexor pollicis brevis muscle receives dual innervation from both the recurrent branch and the deep motor branch of the ulnar nerve.
- The median nerve terminates into multiple sensory branches, which supply sensibility to the thumb, index, long, and ring (radial side) fingers. The sensory branches to the radial side of the index and radial side of the long fingers possess a minor motor component that sends a small branch that innervates the adjacent lumbrical muscle.

PATHOGENESIS

- Most injuries to the median nerve occur at the wrist and affect the thenar muscles. The resultant functional loss is lack of thumb opposition.
- Compression injuries are most common and are usually attributed to prolonged carpal tunnel syndrome.
- Carpal tunnel compression may also be secondary to tumor, adjacent synovitis, or fracture-dislocation.
- Penetrating or perforating injuries may directly damage the median nerve.

- Pediatric causes include lipofibrohamartoma of the median nerve or Charcot-Marie-Tooth disease, a demyelinating process that has a preference for the median and ulnar nerves (**FIG 1**).[6]
- High median nerve injuries are rare. Similar causes exist, including trauma and nerve compression.

NATURAL HISTORY

- With a median nerve compression neuropathy (ie, carpal tunnel syndrome), palsy of the median nerve is insidious in onset and manifestation. Over a period of months to years, patients can progress to decreased median nerve function as well as sensory changes in the dermatome of this nerve.
- Acute injuries to the median nerve at the wrist or elbow have a traumatic onset followed by sensory or motor changes, or both.

PATIENT HISTORY AND PHYSICAL FINDINGS

- Compressive neuropathy of the median nerve
    - Patients report pain, numbness, and tingling in the thumb, index, middle, and sometimes ring ringer of the affected hand. They frequently describe problems with fine coordination of the hand, notably problems with pinch. Patients often report pain and numbness that awakens them at night.
    - Physical examination findings include thenar muscle wasting and diminished thumb opposition (defined as the

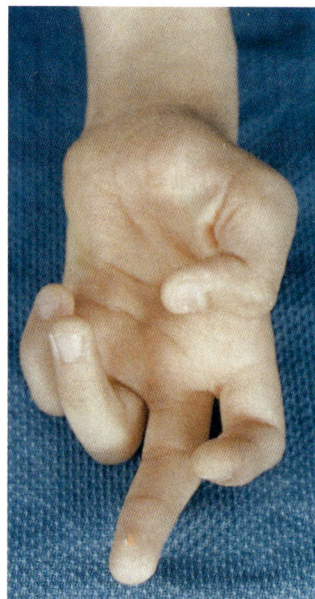

FIG 1 • Left hand of 16-year-old boy with Charcot-Marie-Tooth disorder resulting in median nerve palsy. Note inability to oppose thumb with attempt to touch small fingertip. (Courtesy of Shriners Hospital for Children, Philadelphia.)

combination of palmar abduction, metacarpophalangeal [MCP] joint flexion, and thumb pronation).
- Additional signs include the Tinel sign, the Phalen sign, the carpal tunnel compression sign, and increased two-point discrimination in the thumb, index, and long fingers.
- High median nerve neuropathies have similar findings, in addition to loss of forearm pronation and flexion of the thumb, index, and long fingers.
- Acute median nerve injury
  - There is nearly always a wound on the upper extremity, usually on the volar wrist.
  - Physical findings include diminished sensibility in the thumb, index, and long fingers; increased two-point discrimination in those fingers; and an inability to touch the thumb tip to the small finger (ie, loss of opposition).
  - Depending on the level of injury, patients may display diminished sensibility of the thenar eminence of the thumb, signifying an injury proximal to the palmar cutaneous branch of the median nerve, or a concomitant injury to the palmar cutaneous branch.
  - Higher median nerve neuropathies have similar findings, in addition to loss of forearm pronation and flexion of the thumb, index, and long fingers.
- Patients with median nerve palsy will not be able to oppose thumb to small finger. There may be some palmar abduction due to function of the abductor pollicis longus or extensor pollicis brevis muscles, but this will be minor. The ulnar-innervated deep head of the flexor pollicis brevis muscle will still function, creating MCP joint flexion but not true opposition.
- Inability to make an "OK" sign indicates anterior interosseous nerve injury and high median nerve pathology.
- The clinician should ask the patient to try to touch thumb to small finger with the wrist flexed. Due to median nerve palsy, the patient will likely not be able to fully touch the thumb to the small finger. However, if the palmaris longus is present, it will be visible as it tents up the skin over the volar wrist.
- The patient is asked to spread his or her fingers apart and hold them against adduction pressure on the small finger. The examiner feels for resistance and palpates the hypothenar eminence at the same time. There should be resistance to adduction force on the small finger, and firmness of the hypothenar eminence should be appreciated.

IMAGING AND OTHER DIAGNOSTIC STUDIES
- Radiographs
  - Plain radiographs are helpful in determining the nature of fractures or dislocations after acute trauma to the upper extremity.
  - Specific carpal tunnel radiographic views may demonstrate osteophytes within the carpal tunnel, but they are not routinely performed.
- Electrodiagnostic studies
  - In the setting of compressive neuropathy of the median nerve, nerve conduction studies typically show increased motor and sensory latencies in the median distribution.
  - In advanced stages of compressive neuropathy, electromyography demonstrates fibrillation potentials in various muscles tested, most commonly the abductor pollicis

brevis. These fibrillation potentials signify denervation of the tested muscle.
- Advanced high median nerve neuropathy reveals fibrillation potentials in more proximal muscles, such as the flexor carpi radialis and the pronator teres.

DIFFERENTIAL DIAGNOSIS
- Carpal tunnel syndrome
- Anterior interosseous syndrome
- Pronator syndrome
- Wrist synovitis
- Direct injury to the median nerve
- Tumor compression of the median nerve
- Charcot-Marie-Tooth disease
- Brachial plexus injury
- Stroke or other brain injury

NONOPERATIVE MANAGEMENT
- Patients with demonstrable carpal tunnel syndrome can undergo a trial of splinting, wrist corticosteroid injection, or both.
- Work modification is indicated in patients with compressive neuropathy as a result of overuse for both carpal tunnel and pronator syndromes.
- Anti-inflammatory and immunomodulatory medications are indicated in patients with wrist synovitis secondary to inflammatory arthropathy.

SURGICAL MANAGEMENT
- The chief surgical modality for a low or high median nerve palsy that has not responded to surgery or other interventions is tendon transfer.[3,6]
- Typically, in a low median nerve palsy, the only function that requires restoration via tendon transfer is thumb opposition, which is a combination of palmar abduction, MCP joint flexion, and thumb pronation.
- In a high median nerve palsy, the additional loss of flexion of the thumb, index, and long fingers requires tendon transfer. In addition, lack of pronation may require tendon transfer.

Preoperative Planning
- The surgeon must ensure that there is good passive range of motion of the joints to be mobilized.
  - In longstanding median nerve palsy, the thumb MCP and carpometacarpal joints can become quite stiff.
  - Physical therapy must be employed to loosen these joints and increase their range of motion.[3] This can usually be accomplished in 3 to 6 weeks.
- A thorough assessment of muscle function and strength is made before selecting a transfer, especially in the setting of combined nerve deficits.
- When performing an opponensplasty, the donor tendon and attachment site are individualized to the particular patient, his or her injury, his or her needs, and the donor muscle–tendon availability. As the attachment site moves more dorsal, the amount of pronation and thumb extension is increased.
- Donor options for opponensplasty include:
  - FDS
  - Abductor digiti minimi (Huber)
  - Extensor indicis proprius (EIP)

■ Palmaris longus (Camitz). The palmaris transfer is associated with more abduction and less opposition compared to other opposition transfers.[3]

■ Other less common donors include the extensor pollicis longus, extensor carpi ulnaris, extensor carpi radialis brevis, and extensor digitorum quinti.[4]

■ Opponensplasty attachment site options include the following:[3]

■ Abductor pollicis brevis tendon. This yields a lot of thumb abduction and some opposition.

■ Extensor pollicis brevis or longus tendons. This yields thumb abduction, pronation, and MCP joint extension.

■ Single attachment options

■ Riordan's technique involves interweaving the transferred tendon into the abductor pollicis brevis tendon, with continuation onto the extensor pollicis longus tendon distal to the MCP joint.

■ Littler's technique attaches the transferred tendon into the abductor pollicis brevis tendon.

■ Bunnell's method involves passing the tendon through a small drill hole made at the proximal phalanx base from the dorso-ulnar to palmar-radial direction to provide pronation of the thumb.

■ Dual attachment options

■ These are designed to rotate (pronate) the thumb and either passively stabilize the MCP joint or minimize interphalangeal joint flexion.

■ There is a theoretical benefit in patients with combined median and ulnar nerve deficits who lack all thumb intrinsic function.

■ Some authors question the utility of dual insertion techniques since the transfer will only function predominantly on the tighter of the two insertions.

■ In Brand's technique, one half is woven through the abductor pollicis brevis tendon and then passed distal to the MCP joint and attached to the extensor pollicis longus tendon.

■ In the Royle-Thompson method, a slip is passed through a drill hole made in the metacarpal neck, from radial to ulnar, with the metacarpal pulled into as much opposition as possible. This slip is tied to the other half that is initially passed dorsally over the extensor hood at the MCP joint and through a small tunnel in the fascia and periosteum at the base of the proximal phalanx.

■ High median nerve palsies require additional restoration of thumb, index, and long finger flexion. On occasion, re-establishment of pronation is required.

■ Flexion of the index and long fingers can be accomplished by side-to-side transfers of the FDP tendons of the index and long to the ring and small. We transect the recipient tendons proximal to the wrist and weave them into the donor tendons.

■ Thumb flexion can be restored by transfer of the brachioradialis to the flexor pollicis longus.

■ Loss of pronation can be overcome by rerouting the biceps around the radius, which converts the biceps from a supinator into a pronator.

Positioning

■ The patient is positioned supine on the operating table.

■ The affected limb is abducted at the shoulder and placed on an attached hand table or armboard.

Approach

■ The approach to opponensplasty for median nerve palsy depends on two factors: the donor tendon and the site of attachment.

LOW MEDIAN NERVE TRANSFERS

Flexor Digitorum Superficialis Transfer (Authors' Preferred Technique[6])

■ Make a palmar transverse skin incision over the first annular pulley of the ring finger.

■ Identify the A1 pulley and incise it longitudinally. Isolate the FDS tendon.

■ Apply traction to the FDS tendon to flex the proximal interphalangeal joint (**TECH FIG 1A**), and divide the FDS tendon transversely just proximal to its bifurcation while protecting the FDP tendon.

■ Make a second zigzag incision at the volar ulnar distal forearm in the region of the flexor carpi ulnaris (FCU) tendon insertion.

■ Isolate the FCU and the ring finger FDS tendons and protect the ulnar neurovascular bundle.

■ Divide the radial half of the FCU tendon transversely about 4 cm proximal to its insertion onto the pisiform.

■ Separate the radial half of the tendon longitudinally from the ulnar half, creating a distally based strip of tendon graft.

■ Loop the tendon graft distally and pass it through the distal portion of the FCU near the pisiform insertion to create a pulley.

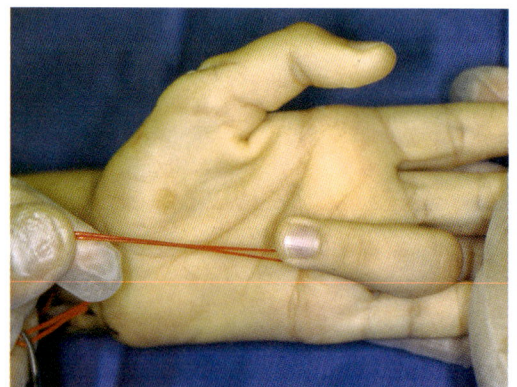

TECH FIG 1 • **A.** Isolation of ring finger flexor digitorum superficialis (FDS) to be transferred for thumb opposition. *(continued)*   **A**

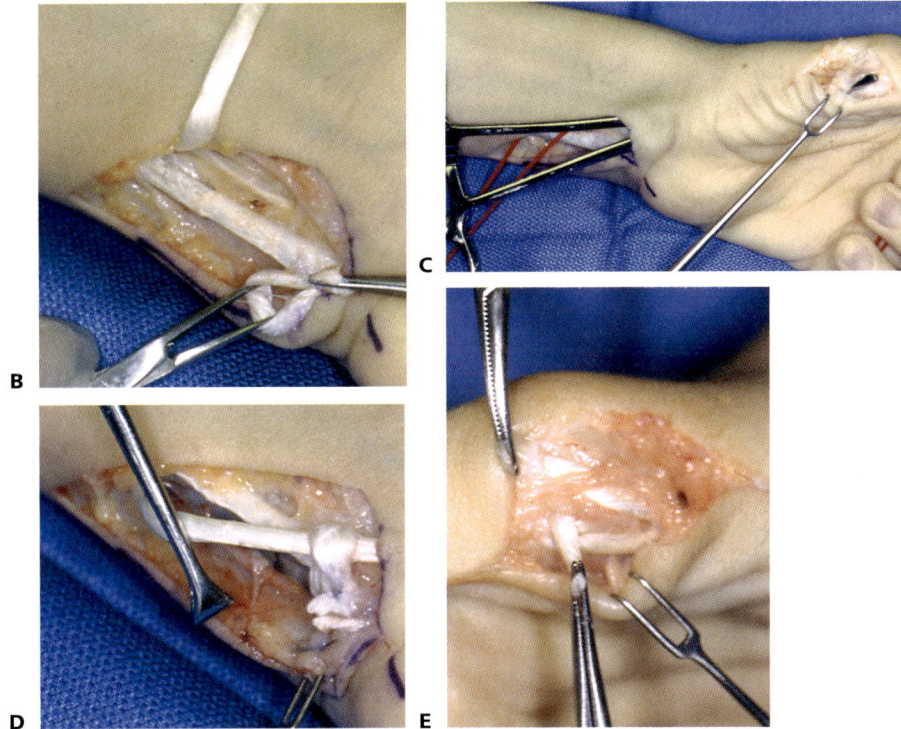

TECH FIG 1 • *(continued)* **B.** Ring finger FDS passed through the flexor carpi ulnaris, which now serves as the pulley for the transferred tendon. **C.** Creation of the subcutaneous tunnel between the ulnar wrist and thumb incisions, through which the FDS tendon will be passed. **D.** Ring finger FDS tendon shown passing through both the flexor carpi ulnaris tendon and the subcutaneous tunnel. **E.** Suture fixation of the FDS tendon to the abductor tendon and extensor hood of the thumb. (Courtesy of Shriners Hospital for Children, Philadelphia.)

- Pull the cut ring finger FDS tendon into the volar ulnar forearm incision and pass it through the constructed pulley (**TECH FIG 1B**).
- Make a third incision on the radial aspect of the thumb MCP joint.
- Create a subcutaneous tunnel between this incision and the wrist incision (**TECH FIG 1C**).
- Pass the ring FDS tendon through this tunnel to the thumb incision (**TECH FIG 1D**).
- Place the thumb into opposition with the small finger.
- Secure the FDS tendon to the thumb with a 3-0 or 4-0 braided polyester suture (**TECH FIG 1E**).
  - The attachment sites usually include the abductor tendon plus or minus the dorsal capsule and extensor pollicis brevis tendon.

Abductor Digiti Minimi Transfer (Huber)[4]

- Make an oblique or zigzag incision beginning distally on the ulnar border of the small finger proximal phalanx, curving radially along the radial border of the hypothenar eminence.
- Separate the abductor digiti minimi (ADM) muscle from the flexor digiti minimi. Dissect the ADM distally to its insertion into the proximal phalanx and lateral band.

- Protect the ulnar sensory nerve to the small finger.
- Divide the ADM insertion sites, including a portion of the lateral band to increase its overall length.
- Dissect the muscle proximally to the pisiform (**TECH FIG 2A**).
- Release the origin from the pisiform; identify and protect the neurovascular bundle (on the dorsoradial side).
- Make a longitudinal incision on the radial aspect of the thumb MCP joint.
- Use blunt dissection to create a subcutaneous tunnel in the palm.
- Pass the ADM through the tunnel to the thumb MCP joint (**TECH FIG 2B**).
- Secure the ADM tendon to the thumb using 3-0 or 4-0 braided polyester suture (**TECH FIG 2C**).

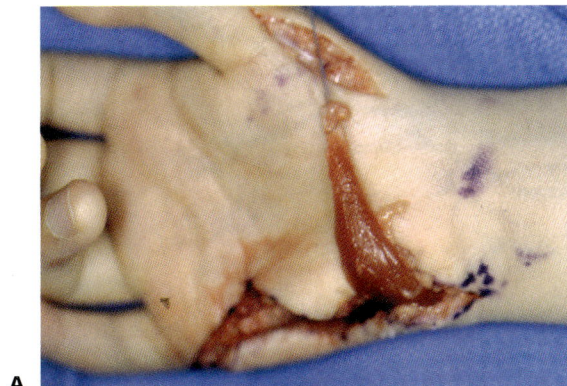

TECH FIG 2 • **A.** Isolated and dissected abductor digiti minimi (ADM) muscle–tendon unit, to be used for transfer for thumb opposition (Huber transfer). *(continued)*

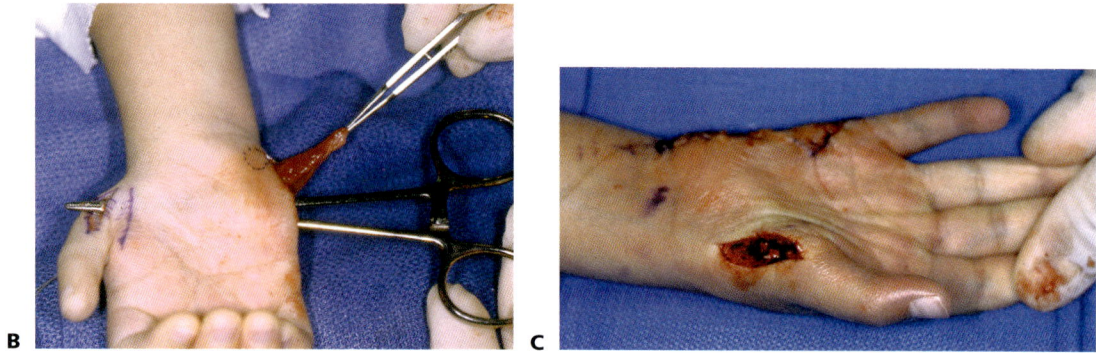

TECH FIG 2 • *(continued)* **B.** Passage of the ADM muscle–tendon unit through the previously created subcutaneous tunnel to the thumb. **C.** Final position of thumb after suture fixation of the ADM to the thumb. Note opposition and palmar abduction. (Courtesy of Shriners Hospital for Children, Philadelphia.)

Extensor Indicis Proprius Transfer[4]

- Make a longitudinal incision on the dorsum of the index finger MCP joint.
- Locate the EIP tendon deep and ulnar to the extensor digitorum communis tendon to the index finger (**TECH FIG 3A**).
- Identify the EIP tendon along with the extensor hood.
- Divide the EIP tendon on the proximal edge of the extensor hood. The EIP tendon can be elongated by taking a 3- to 4-mm slip of extensor mechanism along the proximal phalanx. Repair the rent in the extensor hood with interrupted 4-0 braided polyester suture.
- Make a longitudinal incision on the dorso-ulnar aspect of the wrist, just proximal to the point where the dorsal sensory branch of the ulnar nerve crosses near the ulnar styloid.

- Carry dissection from this incision radially until the proximal EIP tendon can be identified (just distal to the extensor retinaculum) (**TECH FIG 3B**).
- Divide the distal extensor retinaculum over the fourth compartment to release the EIP tendon.
- Bring the EIP tendon out through the ulnar wrist incision (**TECH FIG 3C**).
- Make another small longitudinal incision on the radial edge of the pisiform.
- Make a fourth incision over the thumb MCP joint.
- Create a subcutaneous tunnel from the ulnar wrist incision to the pisiform incision, then on to the thumb MCP joint incision, using blunt dissection.
- Pass the EIP tendon first through the pisiform incision, then on to the thumb incision (**TECH FIG 3D**).
- Suture the EIP tendon to the thumb using a 3-0 or 4-0 braided polyester suture.

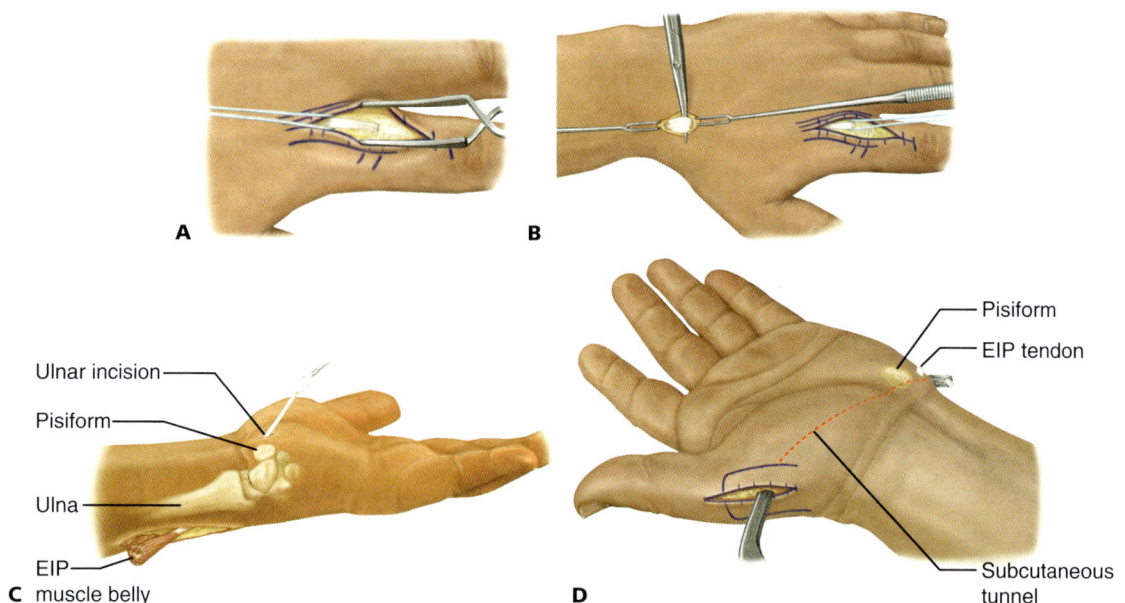

TECH FIG 3 • **A.** Isolation of extensor indicis proprius (EIP) tendon ulnar and deep to the extensor digitorum communis tendon to the index finger. **B.** Wrist incision through which the proximal aspect of the EIP is found and isolated. **C.** The EIP tendon is brought out through the previously created ulnar wrist incision. **D.** Passage of EIP tendon through the subcutaneous tunnel between ulnar wrist incision and thumb incision.

TECHNIQUES

Palmaris Longus Transfer (Camitz[10])

- Confirm the presence of a palmaris longus (PL) tendon by having the patient attempt to oppose the thumb to the small fingertip with the wrist flexed.
- Make a longitudinal incision beginning at the distal wrist crease and continuing distally to the proximal palmar crease. This incision may be "zigzagged" at the wrist to prevent scar contracture.
- Dissect the PL tendon proximally to distally.

- Take a small (about 1 cm square) patch of palmar aponeurosis along with the PL tendon.
- Make an incision over the dorsum of the thumb MCP joint.
- Create the subcutaneous tunnel between the PL tendon and the MCP joint with blunt dissection.
- Pass the PL tendon through the tunnel to the thumb incision.
- Finally, secure the PL tendon to the thumb with 3-0 or 4-0 braided polyester suture.

HIGH MEDIAN NERVE TRANSFERS

Brachioradialis Transfer

- Make a long radial incision from the radial styloid to the brachioradialis muscle belly.
- Release the brachioradialis tendon from the radial styloid and mobilize it along the forearm to optimize available excursion (**TECH FIG 4**).[7]
- Identify the flexor pollicis longus tendon deep to the flexor carpi radialis tendon.
- Weave the harvested brachioradialis tendon into the flexor pollicis longus using a tendon braider and multiple weaves.
- Determine proper tension of the transfer by placing the wrist in flexion and extension and judging tenodesis lateral pinch position and thumb release, respectively.

Biceps Rerouting

- Biceps rerouting is our preferred technique for supple supination deformities of the forearm to correct the forearm position and to apply a pronation moment.
- Surgery is performed under general anesthesia and an upper arm tourniquet is used. The upper extremity is prepared and draped in the usual sterile fashion. The limb is exsanguinated and the tourniquet inflated.
- Design a Z-incision with a horizontal limb across the antecubital fossa (**TECH FIG 5A**).
- Identify the lateral antebrachial cutaneous nerve lateral to the biceps tendon and protect it (**TECH FIG 5B**).
- Isolate the biceps tendon and incise the lacertus fibrosis while protecting the underlying median nerve and brachial artery.

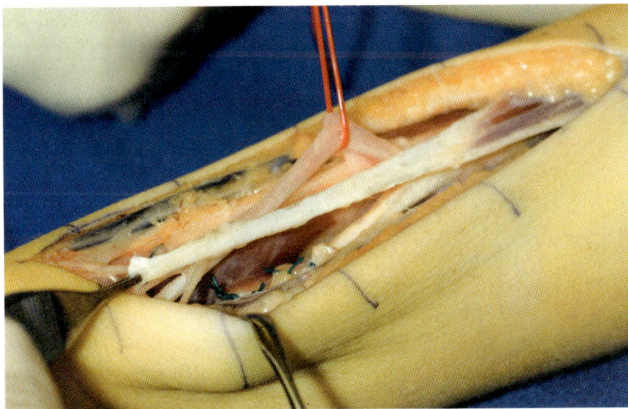

TECH FIG 4 • Brachioradialis harvested as donor for transfer to the flexor pollicis longus tendon (*red loop*) to restore lateral pinch. (Courtesy of Shriners Hospitals for Children, Philadelphia.)

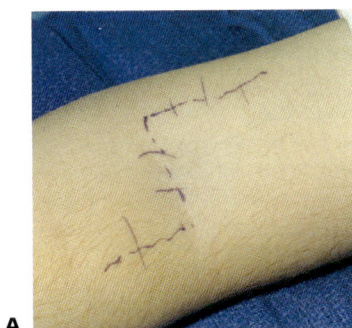

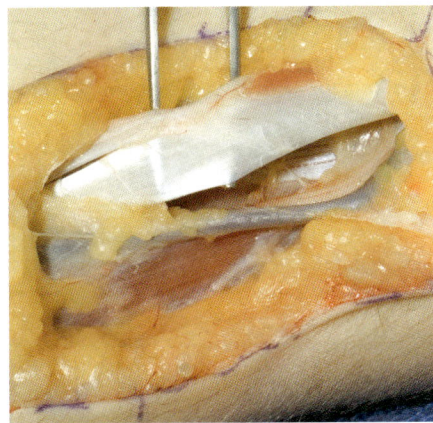

A   B

TECH FIG 5 • **A.** Skin incision for biceps rerouting. **B.** Isolation of the biceps tendon and lacertus fibrosis. The lateral antebrachial cutaneous nerve is just lateral to the tendon. *(continued)*

TECHNIQUES

C

D

E

F

G

H

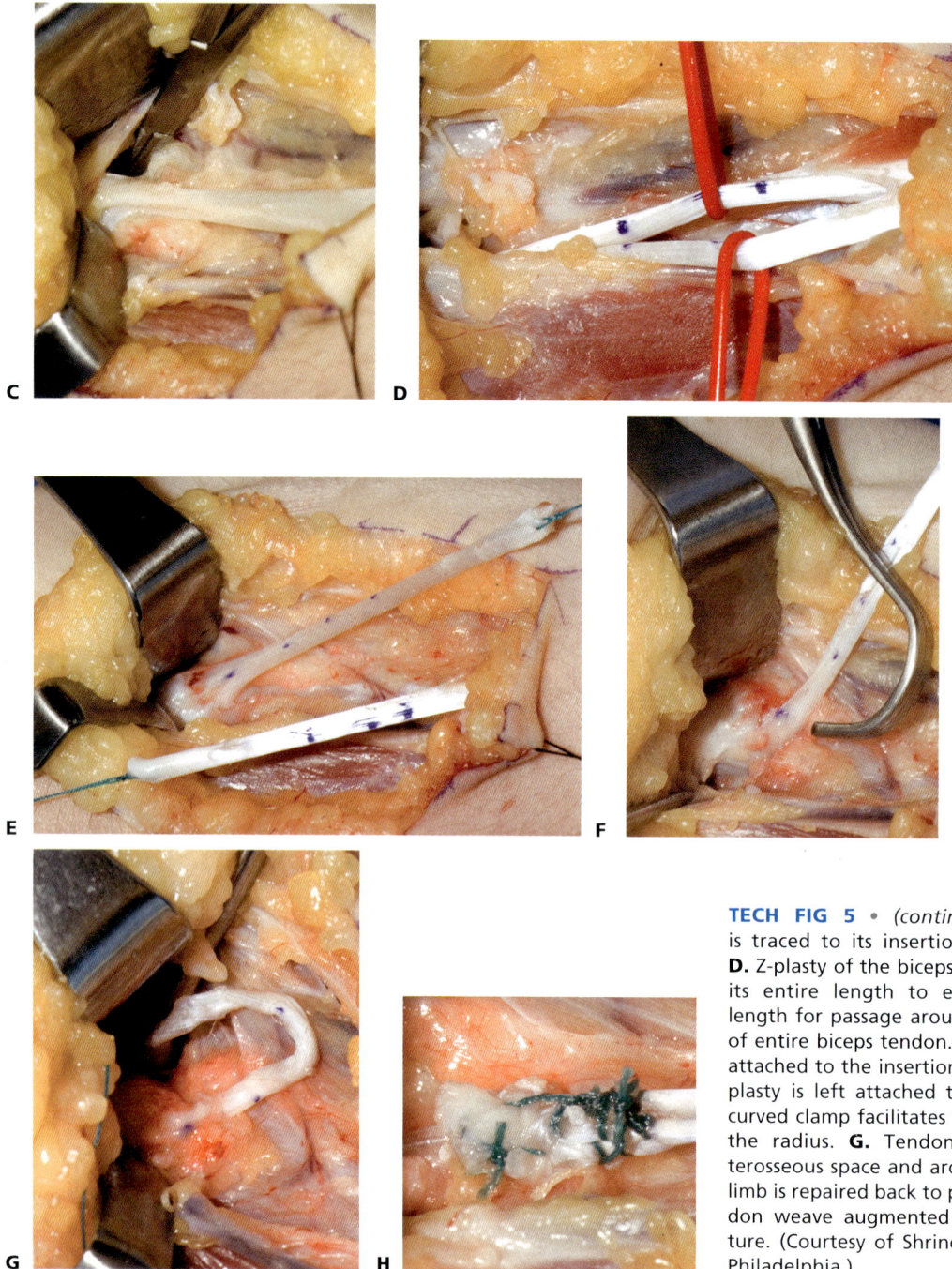

TECH FIG 5 • *(continued)* **C.** Biceps tendon is traced to its insertion into radial tuberosity. **D.** Z-plasty of the biceps tendon is planned along its entire length to ensure sufficient tendon length for passage around the radius. **E.** Z-plasty of entire biceps tendon. The distal Z-plasty is left attached to the insertion site and the proximal Z-plasty is left attached to the muscle belly. **F.** A curved clamp facilitates tendon rerouting around the radius. **G.** Tendon is passed through interosseous space and around the radius. **H.** Distal limb is repaired back to proximal limb using a tendon weave augmented with nonabsorbable suture. (Courtesy of Shriners Hospital for Children, Philadelphia.)

- Trace the biceps tendon to its insertion into the radial tuberosity by careful dissection and placement of the forearm into supination (**TECH FIG 5C**).
- Plan a Z-plasty of the biceps tendon along its entire length to ensure sufficient tendon length for passage around the radius (**TECH FIG 5D**).
- Leave the distal Z-plasty attached to the insertion site and leave the proximal Z-plasty attached to the muscle belly (**TECH FIG 5E**).
- Carefully reroute the distal attachment around the radius through the interosseous space to create a pronation force. A curved clamp, such as a Deborah cast clamp

or Castaneda pediatric clamp, facilitates tendon passage (**TECH FIG 5F,G**).
- Protect the supinator muscle and posterior interosseous nerve to prevent injury.
- Place the elbow in 90 degrees of flexion and the forearm in pronation. Repair the rerouted distal tendon back to the proximal tendon that is still attached to the biceps muscle using a tendon weave augmented by nonabsorbable suture (**TECH FIG 5H**).
- Close the subcutaneous tissue and skin in routine fashion. Apply a long-arm cast with the elbow in 90 degrees of flexion and the forearm in pronation. The cast is worn for 5 weeks.

PEARLS AND PITFALLS

Tendon transfer selection	▪ Patients should be carefully examined to determine which donor tendons are present and functioning, and what motions the patient needs to regain function for work and daily activities.
Pulley construction	▪ Use the FCU or the pisiform when transferring the FDS ring finger tendon.[3] ▪ Use the pisiform when transferring the EIP tendon. ▪ Palmaris longus transfer does not require a pulley, but it creates more of a palmar abduction motion than the other opposition transfers.
Attachment site	▪ Usually the abductor pollicis brevis tendon; however, if additional pronation and extension is necessary, then a more dorsal attachment is performed.
Subcutaneous tunnel creation	▪ Tunnels should be ample to allow easy passage of transferred tendons.
Tendon transfer tensioning	▪ After suturing the tendon transfer, the thumb should be in full opposition with the wrist in extension. In flexion, the thumb should relax out of the palm.[6]
Stiff joints before tendon transfer	▪ Affected joints, especially in the thumb, must have good passive range of motion before tendon transfer. Otherwise, transfer risks failure due to inability to motor the joints.

POSTOPERATIVE CARE

▪ A bulky hand dressing and short-arm plaster splint is placed with the wrist in flexion and the thumb in full opposition.

▪ Immediate hand therapy commences to maintain motion in the fingers, especially the ring finger after FDS harvest.

▪ If the ring finger tends to position into flexion, a proximal interphalangeal joint extension splint is fabricated for nighttime wear.

▪ In contrast, a ring finger that tends to swan-neck secondary to loss of the FDS tendon requires a silver ring splint to prevent deformity until the remaining FDS scars along the volar aspect of the proximal interphalangeal joint.

▪ After 2 to 3 weeks, the plaster splint is removed and therapy is initiated. Longer periods of immobilization may yield scarring of the FDS tendon within the reconstructed pulley.

▪ An Orthoplast splint is fabricated to maintain mild wrist flexion and thumb opposition. The splint is removed four to six times a day to encourage tendon gliding exercises and retraining of the transferred tendon.

▪ Similar occupational therapy principles are applied after other opposition transfers as described, including the palmaris longus, EIP, abductor digiti minimi, and other transfers.

▪ Patients are instructed in other modalities, including scar management, muscle–tendon re-education, and incorporation of the transfer into activities of daily living.

OUTCOMES

▪ In general, opposition transfers are successful: most patients regain opposition adequate to perform normal daily activities such as writing, buttoning clothes, and other fine manipulation tasks (**FIG 2**).[9]

▪ Burkhalter et al[2] reported excellent results in 57 of 65 cases of EIP opponensplasty; excellent results were defined as those with 75% function compared to the opposite normal thumb or those with less than a 20-degree difference between the plane of the opposite thumbnail and the plane of the palm with good power.

▪ Jacobs and Thompson,[5] using a variety of donor tendons (mainly FDS IV and FDS III tendons), pulley designs, and insertion techniques, reported 77 good or excellent, 9 fair, and 17 poor results. Similar results were obtained with the FDS IV and FDS III tendons.

▪ In a comparison of FDS versus EIP opponensplasty, Anderson et al[1] compared 50 EIP to 116 FDS ring finger opponensplasty cases. Their analysis demonstrated that the EIP opponensplasty was best in supple hands, while the FDS opponensplasty was more suitable in less pliable hands.

COMPLICATIONS

▪ Suboptimal transfer outcome due to stiff joints
▪ Selection of suboptimal or weak muscle–tendon unit for transfer
▪ Incorrect vector of pull due to lack of or poor selection of pulley
▪ Rupture of transferred tendon
▪ Tendon adhesions
▪ Loss of grip strength after FDS ring finger transfer
▪ Difficulty with muscle–tendon re-education, especially with tendon transfers that are not synergistic. For example, EIP transfer is more difficult to learn compared to FDS tendon transfer.

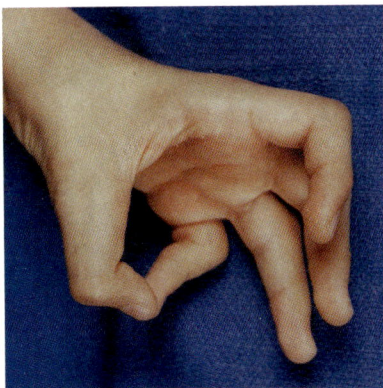

FIG 2 • Postoperative photo of patient from Figure 1. This demonstrates good thumb opposition after ring finger flexor digitorum superficialis transfer for thumb opposition. (Courtesy of Shriners Hospital for Children, Philadelphia.)

REFERENCES

1. Anderson GA, Lee V, Sundararaj GD. Opponensplasty by extensor indicis and flexor digitorum superficialis tendon transfer. J Hand Surg Br 1992;17B:611–614.

2. Burkhalter W, Christensen RC, Brown P. Extensor indicis proprius opponensplasty. J Bone Joint Surg Am 1973;55A:725–732.

3. Cooney WP. Tendon transfer for median nerve palsy. Hand Clin 1988;4:155–165.

4. Davis T. Median nerve palsy. In Green D, Hotchkiss R, Pederson W, et al, eds. Green's Operative Hand Surgery, 5th ed. Elsevier, 2005: 1131–1160.

5. Jacobs B, Thompson TC. Opposition of the thumb and its restoration. J Bone Joint Surg Am 1960;42A:1015–1026.

6. Kozin SH. Tendon transfers for radial and median nerve palsies. J Hand Ther 2005;18:208–215.

7. Kozin SH, Bednar M. The excursion of the brachioradialis muscle during tetraplegia reconstruction. J Hand Surg Am 2001; 26A:510–514.

8. Rath S. Immediate active mobilization versus immobilization for opposition tendon transfer in the hand. J Hand Surg Am 2006; 31A:754–759.

9. Sundararaj GD, Mani K. Surgical reconstruction of the hand with triple nerve palsy. J Bone Joint Surg Br 1984;66B: 260–264.

10. Trumble T. Tendon transfers. In Trumble T, ed. Principles of Hand Surgery and Therapy, 1st ed. Saunders, 2000:343–360.

Chapter 75

Tendon Transfers for Ulnar Nerve Palsy

Michael S. Bednar

DEFINITION

- Ulnar nerve palsy refers to loss of sensory and motor function after injury to the ulnar nerve above or below the wrist (high vs. low ulnar nerve palsy).

ANATOMY

- The ulnar nerve is the terminal branch of the medial cord (C8 and T1).
- The ulnar nerve consists of motor and sensory fibers. There are no muscles innervated by the ulnar nerve in the arm. In the forearm, the flexor carpi ulnaris receives its nerve branches after the ulnar nerve passes through the cubital tunnel. The other muscles innervated in the forearm are the flexor digitorum profundus of the ring and small fingers.
- The muscles innervated in the hand (by order of innervation) are:
  - Hypothenar muscles
    - Abductor digiti minimi
    - Flexor digiti minimi
    - Opponens digiti minimi
  - Ring and small lumbricals
  - Dorsal and palmar interosseous muscles
  - Adductor pollicis
  - Deep head of flexor pollicis brevis
  - First dorsal interosseous (last muscle innervated by the ulnar nerve)
- The sensory fibers of the ulnar nerve supply the small finger and the ulnar half of ring finger over the entire palmar surface and the dorsal surface distal to the proximal interphalangeal (PIP) joint. The dorsal surface proximal to the PIP joint of the small finger and the ulnar half of the ring finger and ulnar dorsum of the hand is innervated via the dorsal sensory branch of the ulnar nerve, which arises from the ulnar nerve 7 cm proximal to the wrist. The sensory branch crosses from volar to dorsal at the level of the ulnar styloid.

PATHOGENESIS

- Ulnar nerve palsy can arise from a laceration anywhere along its course. Proximal injuries to the medial cord may present with additional sensory loss in the distribution of the medial brachial or antebrachial cutaneous nerves. Nerve compression typically occurs either at the cubital tunnel at the elbow or the canal of Guyon at the wrist.
- A variety of systemic conditions may mimic ulnar neuropathy, including Charcot-Marie-Tooth disease, syringomyelia, and leprosy. In Charcot-Marie-Tooth disease and syringomyelia, there is weakness involving other nerves. In leprosy, there is a profound loss of sensation in the ulnar nerve distribution in addition to the claw deformity of the fingers.

NATURAL HISTORY

- The severity of the nerve palsy depends on the degree of the nerve lesion and the presence of anomalous innervation patterns (Martin-Gruber, Riche-Cannieu) in determining the number of muscles involved and the extent of palsy. Anomalous innervation patterns can confuse the examiner.
- Martin-Gruber anastomosis patterns are divided into four types:
  - Type I (60%): motor branches from the median nerve are sent to the ulnar nerve to innervated "median" muscles
  - Type II (35%): motor branches from the median nerve are sent to the ulnar nerve to innervated "ulnar" muscles
  - Type III (3%): motor branches from the ulnar nerve are sent to the median nerve to innervated "ulnar" muscles
  - Type IV (1%): motor branches from the ulnar nerve are sent to the median nerve to innervated "median" muscles
- With prolonged nerve palsy, secondary abnormalities of the hand occur, such as stretching of the central slip of the extensor mechanism at the PIP joint or fixed joint flexion contractures.

PATIENT HISTORY AND PHYSICAL FINDINGS

- An important point is to identify the cause and timing of palsy to determine whether the pathology can be reversed. Treatment is first addressed at improving nerve function by procedures such as decompression of a compressed nerve or acute repair of a lacerated nerve. Recovery can be gauged by progression of symptoms, such as advancing Tinel sign, return of muscle function, and return of sensation. Tendon transfers are indicated when nerve recovery is not expected or possible.
- Loss of sensation in the medial arm or forearm indicates a proximal lesion. Loss of sensation to the dorsal side of the ulnar hand indicates a lesion proximal to the wrist to affect the dorsal sensory branch.
- The following specific tests of motor dysfunction are used to determine the functional loss of the hand:
  - Froment sign: hyperflexion of thumb interphalangeal joint (**FIG 1A**); indicates substitution of flexor pollicis longus (median nerve) for adductor pollicis (ulnar nerve)
  - Jeanne sign: reciprocal hyperextension of thumb metacarpophalangeal (MCP) joint (Fig 1A); indicates substitution of flexor pollicis longus for adductor pollicis
  - Wartenberg sign: abduction of small finger at MCP joint; indicates paralyzed palmar intrinsic muscle (ulnar nerve) with abduction from extensor digiti minimi (radial nerve)
  - Duchenne sign: clawing of ring and small fingers, hyperextension of MCP joints, and flexion of PIP joints (**FIG 1B**); indicates paralysis of interosseous and lumbrical muscles of the ring and small fingers (low ulnar nerve), more pronounced in low rather than high ulnar nerve palsy secondary

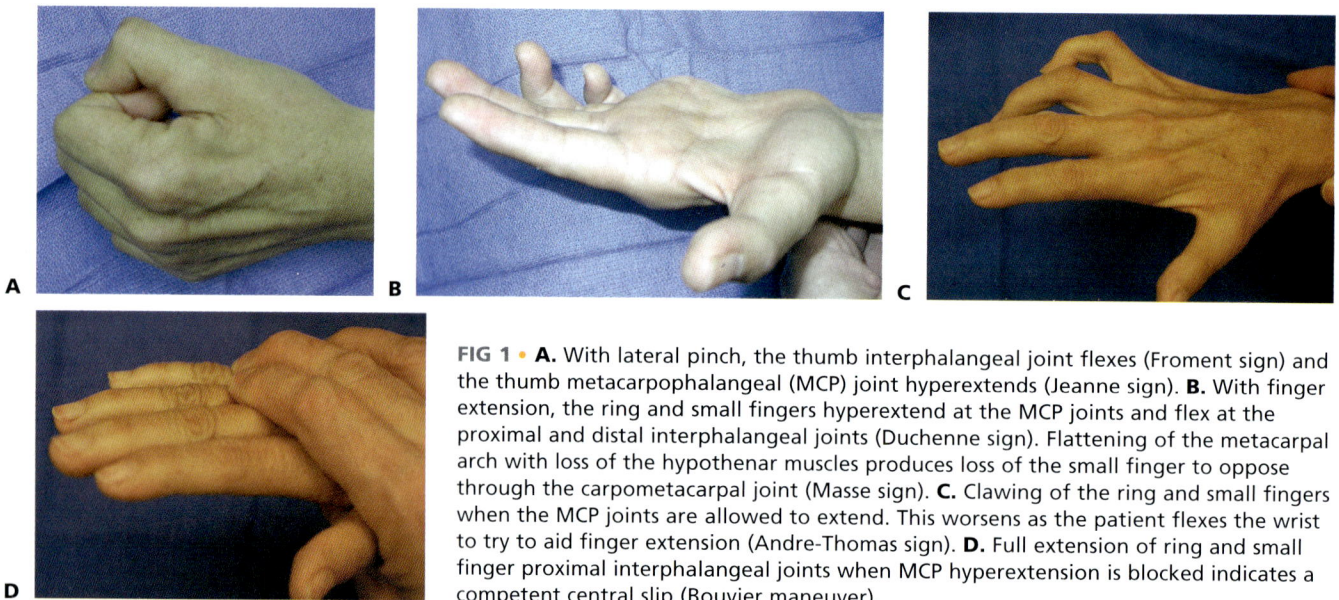

FIG 1 • **A.** With lateral pinch, the thumb interphalangeal joint flexes (Froment sign) and the thumb metacarpophalangeal (MCP) joint hyperextends (Jeanne sign). **B.** With finger extension, the ring and small fingers hyperextend at the MCP joints and flex at the proximal and distal interphalangeal joints (Duchenne sign). Flattening of the metacarpal arch with loss of the hypothenar muscles produces loss of the small finger to oppose through the carpometacarpal joint (Masse sign). **C.** Clawing of the ring and small fingers when the MCP joints are allowed to extend. This worsens as the patient flexes the wrist to try to aid finger extension (Andre-Thomas sign). **D.** Full extension of ring and small finger proximal interphalangeal joints when MCP hyperextension is blocked indicates a competent central slip (Bouvier maneuver).

to functioning flexor digitorum profundus of ring and small fingers (high ulnar nerve)

■ Bouvier maneuver: inability to actively extend PIP joint when MCP joints are hyperextended and ability to actively extend PIP joint when MCP joints are blocked from hyperextension (**FIG 1C,D**). When active PIP joint extension is possible with the MCP joints blocked, this indicates competence of the central slip (positive test). When PIP joints cannot actively extend (negative test), this implies central slip attenuation. In this case, tendon transfers will need to block MCP joint hyperextension and provide PIP joint extension.

■ Andre-Thomas sign: clawing of ring and small fingers, hyperextension of MCP joints and flexion of PIP joints, flexion of wrist (Fig 1C). An increase in the claw deformity as the patient tries to extend the fingers by flexing the wrist indicates a poor prognosis for tendon transfer surgery.

■ Masse sign: flattening of the metacarpal arch (Fig 1B); inability to oppose the small finger carpometacarpal joint

■ Pollack sign: inability to flex the distal interphalangeal joint of the ring and small fingers; used to differentiate high from low ulnar nerve palsy

■ In assessing for tendon transfers in ulnar nerve palsy, the primary functional concerns are:
  ■ Lack of thumb adduction and lateral pinch
  ■ Claw deformity of fingers that impairs object acquisition and grip
  ■ Loss of ring and small finger flexion (high palsy)

IMAGING AND OTHER DIAGNOSTIC STUDIES

■ Electromyographic and nerve conduction velocity studies are used to isolate the ulnar nerve pathology and rule out other diagnoses. Serial studies may demonstrate the potential for recovery.

DIFFERENTIAL DIAGNOSIS

■ Cervical radiculopathy
■ Lower brachial plexopathy
■ Charcot-Marie-Tooth disease

■ Syringomyelia
■ Leprosy

NONOPERATIVE MANAGEMENT

■ When the Bouvier test is positive (active PIP joint extension is possible when MCP joint hyperextension is prevented), a dorsal MCP blocking splint for the ring and small fingers is fabricated to preserve the integrity of the PIP joint central slips.

■ If a fixed flexion contracture of more than 45 degrees occurs at the PIP joint, a supervised hand therapy program consisting of serial casting is required.

■ If the fixed flexion contracture does not respond to therapy, preliminary surgical joint release is necessary before tendon transfers.

SURGICAL MANAGEMENT

■ Tendon transfers address the primary functional concerns listed above:
  ■ Lack of thumb adduction and lateral pinch
  ■ Claw deformity of the fingers that impairs object acquisition and grip
  ■ Loss of ring and small finger flexion (high palsy)

Considerations

Restoring Thumb Adduction

■ The first factor to consider in performing a transfer to restore thumb adduction is what donor muscle to use.
  ■ The extensor carpi radialis brevis (ECRB) and the flexor digitorum superficialis (FDS) are the most commonly used.
  ■ The FDS of the ring finger can be used in low ulnar nerve palsy when the flexor digitorum profundus of the ring finger is functioning.
  ■ In high ulnar nerve palsy, the FDS of the middle finger can be used instead of the FDS of the ring finger.
  ■ The brachioradialis can be used if the ECRB is required for an intrinsic reconstruction of the fingers.
  ■ Alternatively, the extensor indicis proprius or abductor pollicis longus can be used.

- The second factor to consider is placement of the pulley.
  - For transfers coming from the dorsum of the hand, the pulley is either the index or middle finger metacarpal. Passing the transfer through the third web space, using the middle metacarpal as the pulley, allows the transferred tendon to lie palmar to the adductor pollicis but dorsal to the flexor tendons and neurovascular bundles.
  - For transfers originating from the palm of the hand (FDS), the vertical septum of the palmar fascia attached to the third metacarpal forms the pulley.
- The third factor is attachment of the transfer to the thumb.
  - The transfer can be inserted directly into the thumb metacarpal, into the adductor pollicis tendon, or into the abductor pollicis brevis tendon.
  - This last technique, favored by Omer, allows the tendon to be sewn to the strong fascia abductor pollicis longus tendon and improves pronation of the thumb to aid in pinch.
- The last factor to address is stability of the MCP and interphalangeal joints.
  - For patients with a persistent Froment sign and mild hyperextension of the MCP joint, the split flexor pollicis longus to extensor pollicis longus tenodesis will stabilize the interphalangeal joint without fusion.
  - When the MCP joint shows substantial instability or arthritic changes, it should be fused.

Correcting Claw Deformity of Fingers

- Procedures to correct MCP hyperextension may be either static or dynamic.
  - A static procedure prevents hyperextension of the MCP joint, improving extension of the fingers. The Bouvier maneuver must be positive. The disadvantage of static procedures, either the MCP volar capsulodesis or tenodesis procedure, is that they tend to stretch with time.
  - A dynamic transfer uses the FDS, extensor carpi radialis longus, ECRB, or flexor carpi radialis as a donor muscle.
  - If the Bouvier maneuver is positive, there is no need to restore PIP joint extension.
  - If the Bouvier maneuver is negative, the procedure must address both MCP joint flexion and PIP joint extension. The insertion site of the tendon transfer determines which joints are affected by the transfer.
- FDS transfers for finger clawing
  - Advantages
    - No need for tendon graft
    - Not passing tendon through interosseous spaces or through carpal tunnel
  - Disadvantages
    - Does not increase grip strength
    - High incidence of swan-neck deformities
    - Cannot use FDS of ring and small fingers in high ulnar nerve palsy
- Wrist motors for transfers for finger clawing
  - Advantage: increases grip strength
  - Disadvantages
    - Requires tendon graft, either palmaris longus, plantaris, fascia lata, or toe extensor
    - Passes tendon through interosseous spaces or through carpal tunnel

Restoring Ring and Small Finger Extrinsic Muscle Function

- In patients with high ulnar nerve palsy, it is important to restore extrinsic flexion power before performing intrinsic transfers.
- Claw deformity of the ring and small fingers will worsen after these transfers.

Preoperative Planning

- Tendon transfers are indicated when no further nerve recovery is anticipated.
- In evaluating a patient for tendon transfer procedures, the examiner assesses the number of functions lost, determines the number of muscles available for transfer, and assesses the strength and excursion of each of the donor and recipient muscles.
- When there are insufficient donor muscles to substitute for all functions that are lost, tenodesis and arthrodesis procedures may partially substitute for the lost function.
- There should be no fixed flexion contractures of the joints affected by the transfers.
- The transferred tendons need to be placed in a smooth, scar-free bed to glide.
- The principle of "one muscle and one function" should apply to each tendon transfer.

Positioning

- The patient is supine with the arm abducted on an arm table.

Approach

- All transfers for thumb adduction must pass distal to the pisiform.
- All transfers for intrinsic reconstruction must pass palmar to the axis of rotation of the MCP joint and dorsal to the axis of the PIP joint.

TRANSFERS TO RESTORE THUMB ADDUCTION

Brachioradialis Extended With Tendon Graft, Through Third Web Space, Inserted into Abductor Pollicis Brevis Tendon

- Make an incision between the flexor carpi radialis tendon and the radial artery beginning at the wrist crease and extending to the proximal third of the forearm.
- Dissect free of fascia the brachioradialis tendon and its muscle 7 to 10 cm proximal to the musculotendinous junction.
- Extend the tendon with a palmaris longus graft. Use a three-pass Pulvertaft weave to secure the palmaris longus graft to the brachioradialis tendon (**TECH FIG 1A**).
- Make incisions over the radial thumb MCP joint and in the third web space, both palmar and dorsal.
- Sew a tendon graft, using one slip of the abductor pollicis longus tendon, in a three-pass Pulvertaft fashion into the abductor pollicis brevis tendon.

TECHNIQUES

TECHNIQUES

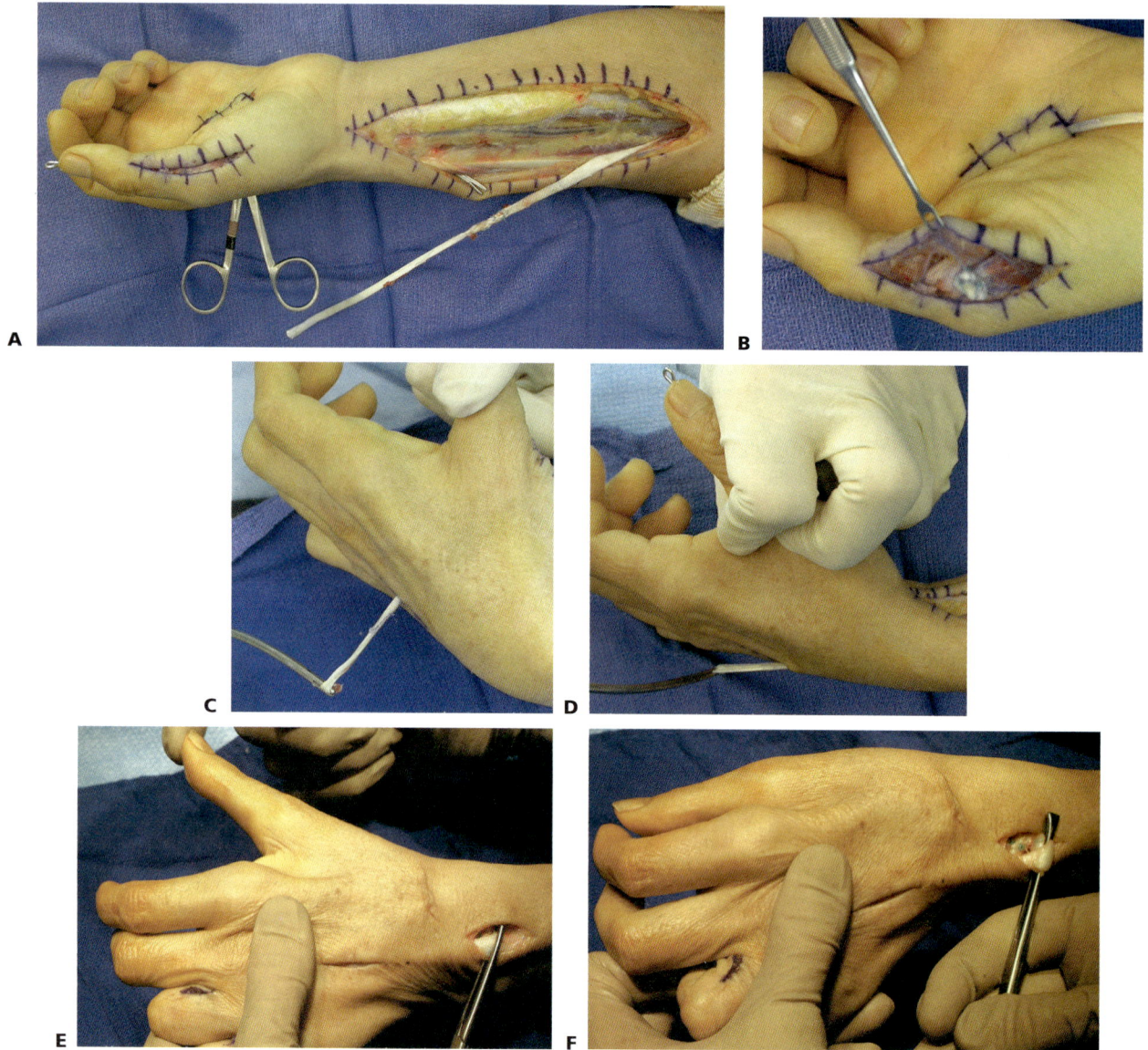

TECH FIG 1 • **A.** The brachioradialis muscle is freed into the proximal third of the forearm. The tendon is lengthened with a palmaris longus graft via a three-pass Pulvertaft method. **B.** Tendon graft taken from a slip of the abductor pollicis longus is sewn into the insertion of the abductor pollicis brevis tendon. The graft is passed palmar to the adductor pollicis muscle. The tendon is shown through the palmar incision before being passed dorsally through the third web space. **C.** Abductor pollicis longus tendon graft passed dorsally through the third web space. **D.** Brachioradialis with tendon graft passed into the incision over the dorsal hand. **E.** Tensioning of tendon transfer. With the wrist in neutral and no tension on the graft, the thumb should fully extend. **F.** Tensioning of tendon transfer. With the wrist in neutral and moderate tension on the tendon, the thumb strongly adducts to the index finger.

- Pass the tendon palmar to the adductor pollicis but dorsal to the flexor tendons and neurovascular bundles, as identified through the palmar incision over the third web space (**TECH FIG 1B**).
- Use the tendon passer to bring the graft from palmar to dorsal, using the proximal metaphysis of the third metacarpal as the pulley (**TECH FIG 1C**).
- Bring the tendon graft from the brachioradialis to the dorsum of the hand and perform the final Pulvertaft weave (**TECH FIG 1D**).
- Set tension to allow the thumb to rest palmar to the index finger when the wrist is in neutral.

- Take care to weave the tendons proximally enough on the hand such that the weave does not enter the third web space.
- Tension on the graft will pull the thumb into adduction (**TECH FIG 1E,F**).

Split Flexor Pollicis Longus to Extensor Pollicis Longus Tenodesis

- Make an incision along the radial proximal phalanx of the thumb. Identify the flexor pollicis longus (FPL) and extensor pollicis longus tendons. Take care to preserve the oblique pulley.

TECHNIQUES

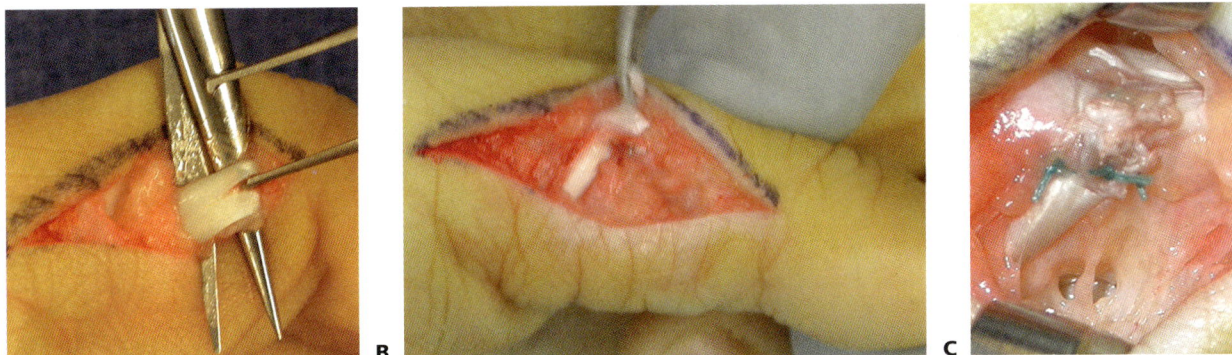

TECH FIG 2 • A. The flexor pollicis longus (FPL) tendon is split into radial and ulnar halves at its insertion into the distal phalanx. The radial half is transected at the level of the interphalangeal joint. **B.** The radial half of the FPL tendon is woven into the radial half of the extensor pollicis longus tendon. A pin is placed across the interphalangeal joint in full extension. **C.** FPL split tenodesis sewn into place.

- Identify the natural cleft between the radial and ulnar fibers of the FPL and split the tendon (**TECH FIG 2A**).
- Weave the radial half of the FPL tendon into the extensor pollicis longus tendon (**TECH FIG 2B,C**).

- Pin the interphalangeal joint in extension with a 0.045-inch smooth pin.

TENDON TRANSFERS FOR CLAW DEFORMITY OF FINGERS

Zancolli Lasso

- This operation is indicated when there is a positive Bouvier maneuver.
- Make a midpalm Bruner zigzag incision.
- Incise the tendon sheath between the A-1 and A-2 pulleys. Identify the FDS tendon and transect it just proximal to the bifurcation. Leaving the bifurcation intact will decrease the incidence of PIP hyperextension.
  - Zancolli recommends using the FDS of each finger, but Anderson recommends using the FDS of the middle finger, split into four tails, to control MCP flexion of all four fingers.
- Pull the FDS tendon out of the tendon sheath distal to the A-1 pulley, bring it palmar to the A-1 pulley, and sew it to itself proximal to the A-1 pulley. If insufficient MCP flexion is attained, the tendon exits the pulley sheath in the middle of the A-2 pulley to improve the lever arm of the transfer.
- Set tension so the MCP joint is in 40 to 50 degrees of flexion with the wrist in neutral.
- When one FDS tendon is used for all four fingers, transect the FDS middle tendon distal to the A-2 pulley through an oblique incision on the finger.
- Make a transverse midpalm incision, retrieve the tendon, and split it into four tails.
- Pass each tail down the lumbrical canal, palmar to the deep transverse metacarpal ligament and into the flexor sheath proximal to the A-1 pulley. Pass the tendon around the pulley and sew the distal end of the tendon back to itself proximal to the A-1 pulley, tensioning it while the MCP joint is in 40 to 50 degrees of flexion with the wrist in neutral.
- For either the Zancolli or Anderson technique, the tendon may be sewn to the proximal metaphyseal–diaphyseal junction of the proximal phalanx via suture anchors or pullout drill holes.

Stille Bunnel Transfer

- This technique is indicated when the Bouvier maneuver is negative.
- One FDS tendon is used to motor two digits. Make radial midaxial incisions over the proximal phalanges of the digits. Make a midpalmar incision to retrieve the tendon. Cut the FDS ring tendon just proximal to its bifurcation between the A-1 and A-2 pulleys.
- Split the tendon and pass each half down the lumbrical canal. Pass the tendon passer from distally to proximally, going palmar to the deep transverse intermetacarpal ligament.
- Sew the tendon to the lateral band to restore PIP extension. Set tension with the MCP joint in 40 to 50 degrees of flexion and the PIP joints in full extension with the wrist in neutral. Excessive tension will cause PIP hyperextension.

Dorsal Route Transfer of Extensor Carpi Radialis Brevis

- Make radial midaxial incisions over the proximal phalanges of the digits.
- Pass the tendon passer from distally to proximally, going palmar to the deep transverse intermetacarpal ligament.
- For the ring and small fingers, make an incision in the dorsal fourth web space to retrieve the tendon grafts (**TECH FIG 3A**).
- Sew the distal end of the tendon graft to the proximal metaphyseal–diaphyseal junction of the proximal phalanx via suture anchors or pullout drill holes if the Bouvier maneuver is positive. Tension on the tendon graft will produce MCP flexion (**TECH FIG 3B**).

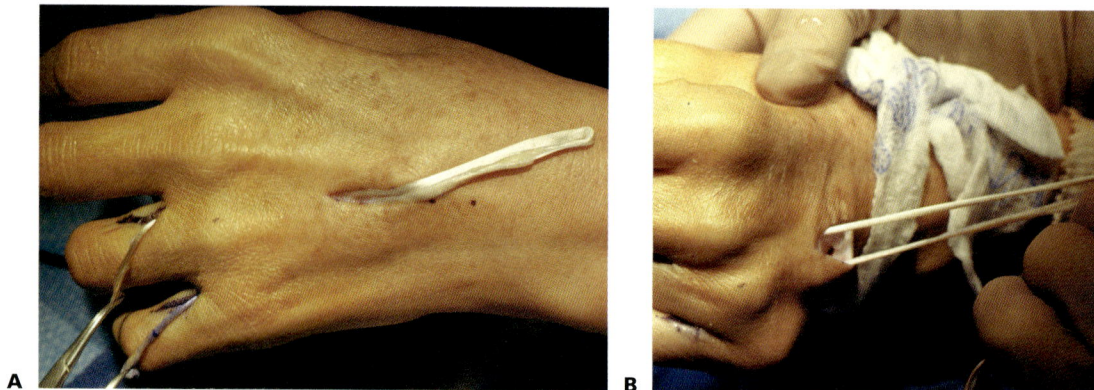

TECH FIG 3 • **A.** Tendon graft is passed from the dorsum of the hand over the fourth web space, palmar to the deep transverse intermetacarpal ligament, and through the lumbrical canals of the ring and small fingers to exit over the radial lateral bands of the fingers. **B.** Tendon grafts have been sewn to the proximal phalanges by suture anchors. Tension on the tendon grafts causes metacarpophalangeal flexion.

- If the Bouvier maneuver is negative, attach the graft to the radial lateral band of the middle, ring, and small fingers and the ulnar lateral band of the index finger.
- Retrieve the ECRB tendon through a dorsal incision. Bring the tendon grafts through the same wound.

First sew the grafts to each other, synchronized to obtain even pull through the grafts. Then sew the grafts to the ECRB tendon with the wrist in 30 degrees of extension and the MCP joints in 60 degrees of flexion.

TRANSFER OF FLEXOR DIGITORUM PROFUNDUS RING AND SMALL TO FLEXOR DIGITORUM PROFUNDUS MIDDLE (HIGH ULNAR NERVE PALSY)

- Make a longitudinal incision over the distal third of the forearm.
- Identify the flexor digitorum profundus tendons.
- After synchronizing the long, ring, and small tendons, place two rows of horizontal sutures between the three tendons.

PEARLS AND PITFALLS

Evaluation	▪ Differentiate high from low ulnar nerve palsy. ▪ Determine the potential for nerve and muscle recovery. ▪ Critically assess the strength of the donor muscles. ▪ Determine the integrity of the PIP central slip (Bouvier maneuver). ▪ Have the patient prioritize functional impairment.
Adductorplasty	▪ Assess both adduction and opposition. ▪ Dorsal transfers passed through the third web space allow for strong adduction using a wrist extensor or the brachioradialis muscle. ▪ Hyperextension of the MCP joint and hyperflexion of the interphalangeal joint must be addressed with either a capsulodesis and fusion of the MCP joint or a split FPL tenodesis. Both the MCP and interphalangeal joints should not be fused.
Claw finger deformities	▪ Determine the integrity of the PIP central slip (Bouvier maneuver). ▪ When the Bouvier maneuver shows that the PIP central slip is competent, the tendon transfer should be sewn to the proximal phalanx or the pulleys. If the central slip is not competent, the tendon transfer is sewn into the lateral band. ▪ Transfers need to pass palmar to the axis of rotation of the MCP joints.

POSTOPERATIVE CARE

- A knowledgeable hand therapist plays an important role in the postoperative care of tendon transfers for ulnar nerve palsy. Protecting the transfers with well-made splints while mobilizing uninvolved joints requires strict adherence to postoperative protocols.
- For most procedures, the hand is immobilized for 3 weeks, followed by a blocking splint to allow motion within the restraints of the splint for the next 3 weeks.

■ Passive exercises are begun at 6 weeks and strengthening at 8 weeks for the adductorplasty and at 10 to 12 weeks for the intrinsic tendon transfers.

OUTCOMES

■ After tendon transfers for thumb adduction, pinch strength usually improves to 25% to 50% of normal.

■ Tendon transfers to improve intrinsic function maintain good to excellent correction of the claw deformity in 80% to 90% of patients.

■ Only the ECRB transfer improves grip strength.

COMPLICATIONS

■ More complications occur after intrinsic muscle transfers than adductorplasty because of the delicate balance of the extensor hood mechanism.

■ Transfer not strong enough
  ■ Problems include choice of a muscle with insufficient strength or excursion, use of a soft tissue pulley that stretched, or elongation at the tendon transfer site.
  ■ Elongation is a particular problem with sewing the transfer into the lateral bands of the extensor hood.
  ■ Patients with this transfer must be instructed on not hyperextending the MCP joints.
  ■ Transfers that are not strong enough can be treated with a therapy program to strengthen the muscle but often require surgical revision.

■ Transfer too strong
  ■ Problems include choice of a muscle that is too strong or with too short of an excursion, or sewing the transfer in with too much tension.
  ■ When the transfer is sewn too tightly into the lateral band, it can produce a swan-neck deformity of the digit.

■ Transfers that are too tight can be treated with passive range of motion in therapy, trying to stretch the transfer.

REFERENCES

1. Anderson GA. Ulnar nerve palsy. In Green DP, Hotchkiss RN, Pederson WC, et al, eds. Green's Operative Hand Surgery. Philadelphia: Elsevier, 2005:1161–1196.
2. Brand PW, Beach RB, Thompson DE. Relative tension and potential excursion of muscles in the forearm and hand. J Hand Surg Am 1981;6A:209–219.
3. Fisher T, Nagy L. Buechler U. Restoration of pinch grip in ulnar nerve paralysis: extensor carpi radialis longus to adductor pollicis and abductor pollicis longus to first dorsal interosseous tendon transfers. J Hand Surg Br 2003;28B:28–32.
4. Hamlin C, Littler JW. Restoration of power pinch. J Hand Surg Am 1980;5A:498–501.
5. Hastings H II, Davidson S. Tendon transfers for ulnar nerve palsy: evaluation of results and practical treatment considerations. Hand Clin 1988;4:167–178.
6. Hastings H II, McCollam SM. Flexor digitorum superficialis lasso tendon transfer in isolated ulnar nerve palsy: a functional evaluation. J Hand Surg Am 1994;19A:275–280.
7. Ozkan T, Ozer K, Gulgonen A. Three tendon transfer methods in reconstruction of ulnar nerve palsy. J Hand Surg Am 2003; 28A:35–43.
8. Rath S. Immediate postoperative active mobilization versus immobilization following tendon transfer for claw deformity in the hand. J Hand Surg Am 2008;33A:232–240.
9. Sachar K. Reconstruction for ulnar nerve palsy. In Berger RA, Weiss APC, eds. Hand Surgery. Philadelphia: Lippincott Williams & Wilkins, 2004:979–990.
10. Smith RJ. Extenson carpi radialis brevis tendon transfer for thumb adduction: a study of power pinch. J Hand Surg Am 1983; 8A:4–15.
11. Zancolli EA. Claw hand caused by paralysis of the intrinsic muscles: a simple surgical procedure for its correction. J Bone Joint Surg Am 1957;37A:1076.

Chapter 76

Tendon Transfers for Radial Nerve Palsy

Harry A. Hoyen

DEFINITION

- Radial nerve palsy that is distal to the triceps innervation affects the forearm musculature. A lesion that does not recover results in predictable wrist, finger, and thumb extensor deficits.

ANATOMY

- The brachioradialis and forearm extensor musculature originate in the lateral humeral epicondyle and the interosseous membrane (**FIG 1A**).
  - Each of the extensor muscles has a relatively flat muscle belly before forming a flat, broad tendon.
  - The myotendinous junction for the wrist extensors is in the mid-forearm, whereas the myotendinous junction of the finger and wrist extensors is the distal forearm.
- The radial nerve arises from the posterior cord of the infraclavicular brachial plexus (**FIG 1B**). Multiple triceps motor branches are present as the nerve courses in the posterior compartment of the upper arm. The nerve traverses into the anterior compartment through the intramuscular septum. The nerve then lies between the brachialis and brachioradialis before it enters the forearm. The brachioradialis (BR), extensor carpi radialis longus (ECRL), and extensor carpi radialis brevis (ECRB) are innervated as the nerve divides into the deep radial nerve, the posterior interosseous nerve (PIN), and the superficial radial nerve. The PIN innervates the extrinsic extensors after exiting the supinator musculature.

  - The motor point for each nerve is fairly consistently located just proximal to the myotendinous junction. In most cases, there is one larger motor branch from the radial nerve or PIN to each muscle.
- The sequence of muscle innervation is an important distinction when considering the anatomy of the radial nerve. Whereas some nerves distribute their nerve branches in a tree-like fashion, the radial nerve innervates the extensor

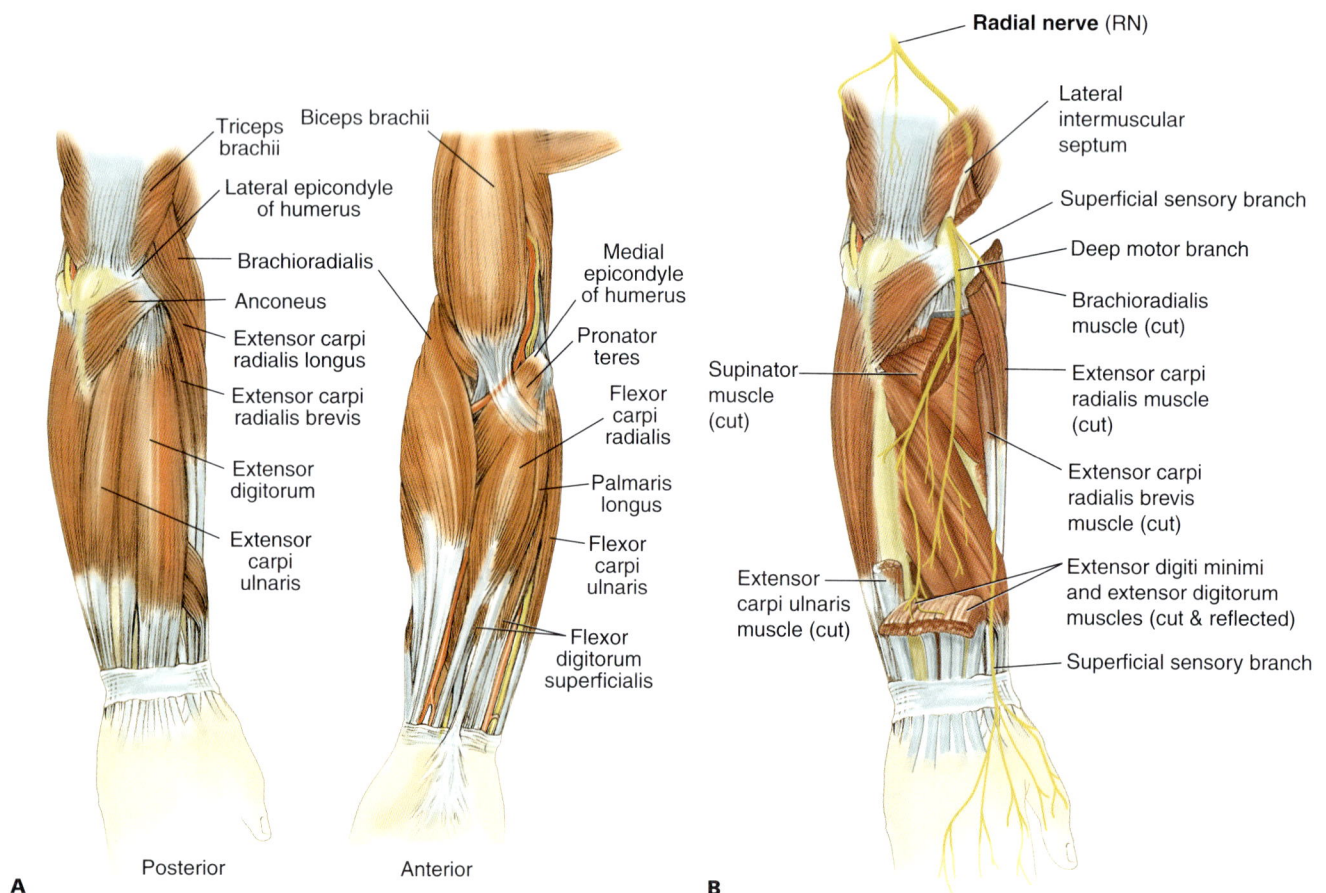

FIG 1 • **A.** Muscles of the forearm. **B.** Course of the radial nerve.

musculature in an orderly pattern, from proximal to distal. The proper radial nerve supplies the BR, the ECRL, and occasionally the ECRB. The PIN innervates the ECRB, the extensor digitorum communis (EDC), the extensor carpi ulnaris (ECU), the extensor indicis proprius (EIP), and the extensor pollicis longus (EPL).

- The order of innervation is important in differentiating a radial nerve injury from a mechanical myotendinous injury or muscle disruption after a forearm laceration.
- Understanding the innervation also is helpful while observing and assessing the clinical recovery after radial nerve injury or repair.

PATHOGENESIS

- Most radial nerve deficits result from traumatic injuries. Idiopathic and neoplastic etiologies are less common.
- Radial nerve injury is most commonly associated with mid- to distal shaft humerus fractures.[1,4,24,25,28]

NATURAL HISTORY

- The type of traumatic injury is an important predictor of recovery after humerus trauma.
  - Neurapraxic lesions typically result from low-energy injuries. Recovery can be expected over the course of 3 months. The clinical recovery can be followed by observing the advancing Tinel sign and the reinnervation sequence.
  - Conditions that persist after 3 months can be further evaluated with electrodiagnostic studies. In the clinical setting of a nonadvancing Tinel sign and electromyographic findings of axonal loss, exploration with intraoperative electrophysiologic testing is warranted. Nerve grafting across the injury is indicated in lesions that do not demonstrate improvement after external neurolysis.[18,24,25]
- Exploration of open and penetrating injuries is recommended. The choice of primary repair or nerve grafting depends on the injury zone. Recent evidence warrants exploration of high-energy injuries, because these lesions have not demonstrated recovery. It is difficult to determine the injury at the acute setting. Interposition nerve graft is often necessary.[18]

PATIENT HISTORY AND PHYSICAL FINDINGS

- A deficit in radial nerve innervation of the extrinsic wrist and finger extensors results in no active wrist, finger, and thumb extension.
- The clinical presentation of radial and PIN palsies is differentiated by the fact that the brachioradialis and ECRL are preserved in PIN palsies.
- The brachioradialis can be palpated during resisted, neutral position elbow flexion, and the wrist assumes a radial deviated position during attempted active extension.

IMAGING AND OTHER DIAGNOSTIC STUDIES

- Electrodiagnostic studies (eg, nerve conduction studies and electromyography) are used initially for assessment and for determining subsequent treatment.
  - Axonal loss injuries are evident about 4 weeks after the injury; therefore, the initial study is obtained 4 to 6 weeks after the injury.
  - The electrodiagnostic study also can identify other nerve injuries that were not as evident on the initial evaluation.

- Recovery can be followed by clinical examination or with supplemental studies.
- A final study is obtained before tendon transfer at 12 to 18 months.

DIFFERENTIAL DIAGNOSIS

- Muscle or tendon laceration
- Closed myotendinous rupture
- Cervical spinal disease
- Joint or tendon subluxation (especially if there is lost digital extension)

NONOPERATIVE MANAGEMENT

- Splint
- Active and passive motion exercises to maintain motion and prevent contracture[28]

SURGICAL MANAGEMENT

- Tendon transfer is the mainstay of treatment. Microvascular repair and nerve graft are discussed in another chapter.
- The goal of treatment is independent wrist, finger, and thumb extension with thumb abduction. Donor muscles include the pronator teres (PT), flexor carpi ulnaris (FCU), flexor carpi radialis (FCR), flexor digitorum superficialis (FDS) 3 and 4, and palmaris longus (PL).
- Timing of surgical intervention is controversial. Conventional surgical recommendations are to proceed after the patient has reached a documented clinical and electromyographic plateau of useful radial nerve regeneration. This typically occurs 1 year after the nerve lesion.[25]
- Tendon transfer primarily for wrist extension may be performed early, at the same setting as nerve surgery, to improve function and minimize brace reliance as the nerve regenerates.

Preoperative Planning

- Prerequisites
  - MHC grade 4+ or 5 median or ulnar nerve–innervated donor musculature
  - Maintained passive motion in wrist and finger extension with no contracture
  - Controlled systemic disease processes

Positioning

- The patient is positioned supine with arm table support and a tourniquet.

Approach

- Three general exposures are used:
  - Radial incision with volar exposure for FCR and PT and dorsal exposure for the ECRB and ECRL
  - Distal, dorsal incision for EDC exposure
  - Individual approaches for harvest of the FCU, FCR, and FDS
- The ideal tendon transfer tension is based on the individual muscle properties. In general, the optimal tension is established at the peak of the length–tension curve for the donor muscle, while the wrist and fingers are maintained in the ideal position. Because this donor muscle position is difficult to determine intraoperatively without specialized equipment, this point reasonably corresponds to the midpoint of the passive muscle excursion. The ideal joint position for each transfer is discussed with the individual transfers.

WRIST EXTENSION RESTORATION THROUGH PT TO ECRL AND ECRB[2,8,27]

- Make a longitudinal radial incision over the midshaft of the radius.
  - This allows exposure of the PT and the wrist extensors through a single incision.
- Identify and expose the PT volarly while protecting the radial artery and superficial radial nerve (**TECH FIG 1A**).
- Extend the pronator insertion by harvesting a strip of periosteum distally (**TECH FIG 1B**).

- Release the proximal muscle to improve its excursion (**TECH FIG 1C**).
- Develop the dorsal subcutaneous flap and identify the ECRB and ECRL.
- Deliver the PT dorsally, deep to the brachioradialis (**TECH FIG 1D**).
- Perform a Pulver-Taft weave into the ECRL and ECRB, and then secure the transfer with 2-0 or 3-0 nonabsorbable braided suture (**TECH FIG 1E,F**).

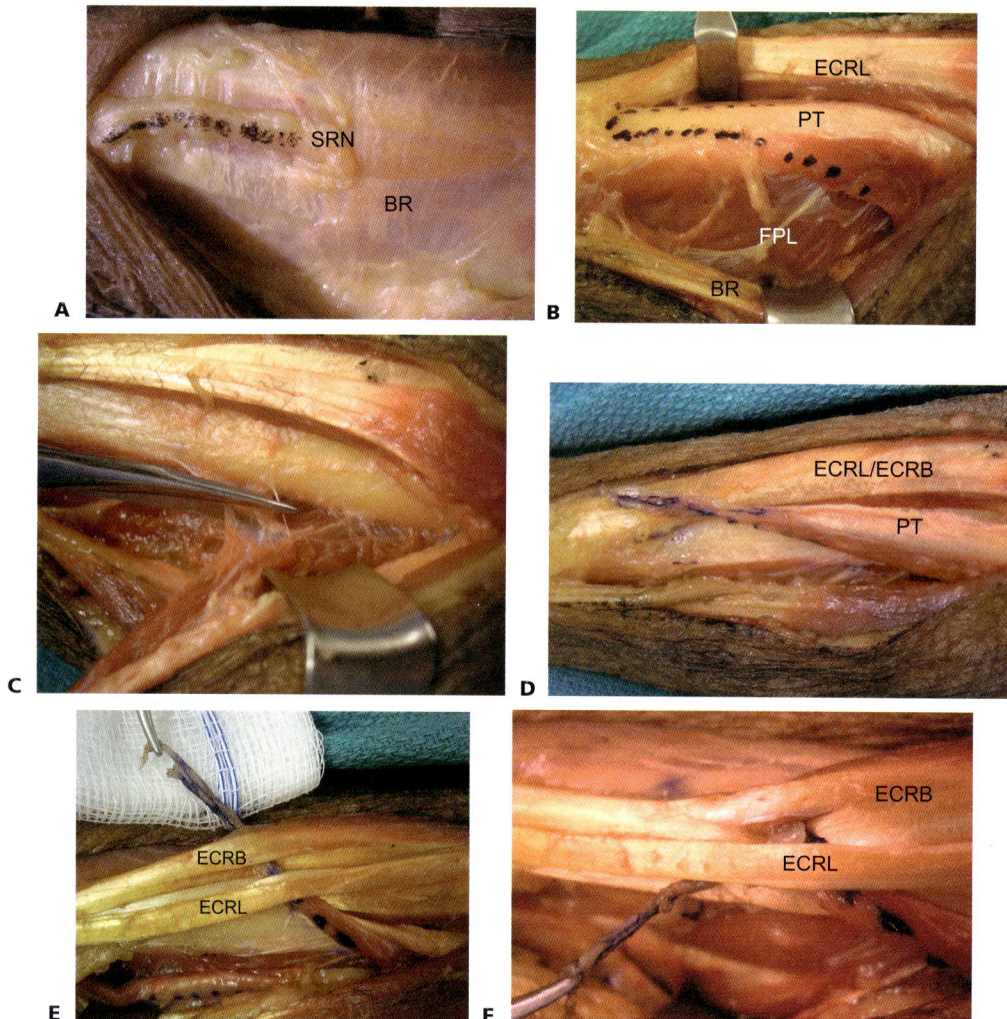

TECH FIG 1 • **A.** The PT is harvested through the volar-radial approach. The superficial radial nerve seen here is protected during the exposure between the FCR and BR or between the BR and ECRL. **B.** The PT tendon can be extended by carefully fashioning a distal periosteal sleeve. **C.** Muscle excursion can be improved by releasing the PT proximally. **D.** The tendon is transferred deep to the BR. **E,F.** The PT is then woven through the ECRL and ECRB tendons.

FINGER EXTENSION THROUGH FCU TO EDC TRANSFER[7,16,19,20]

- Make a distal, volar longitudinal incision to expose the FCU insertion at the pisiform (**TECH FIG 2A**).
- Extend the exposure proximal to a point 8 cm from the humeral insertion and release the FCU periosteal attachments as necessary to improve excursion (**TECH FIG 2B**).

- Identify the ulnar neurovascular structures.
- Develop a broad subcutaneous dorsal flap to improve the ECU line of pull to the EDC (**TECH FIG 2C**). The ECU may be placed beneath the most superficial subcutaneous fascial layer.

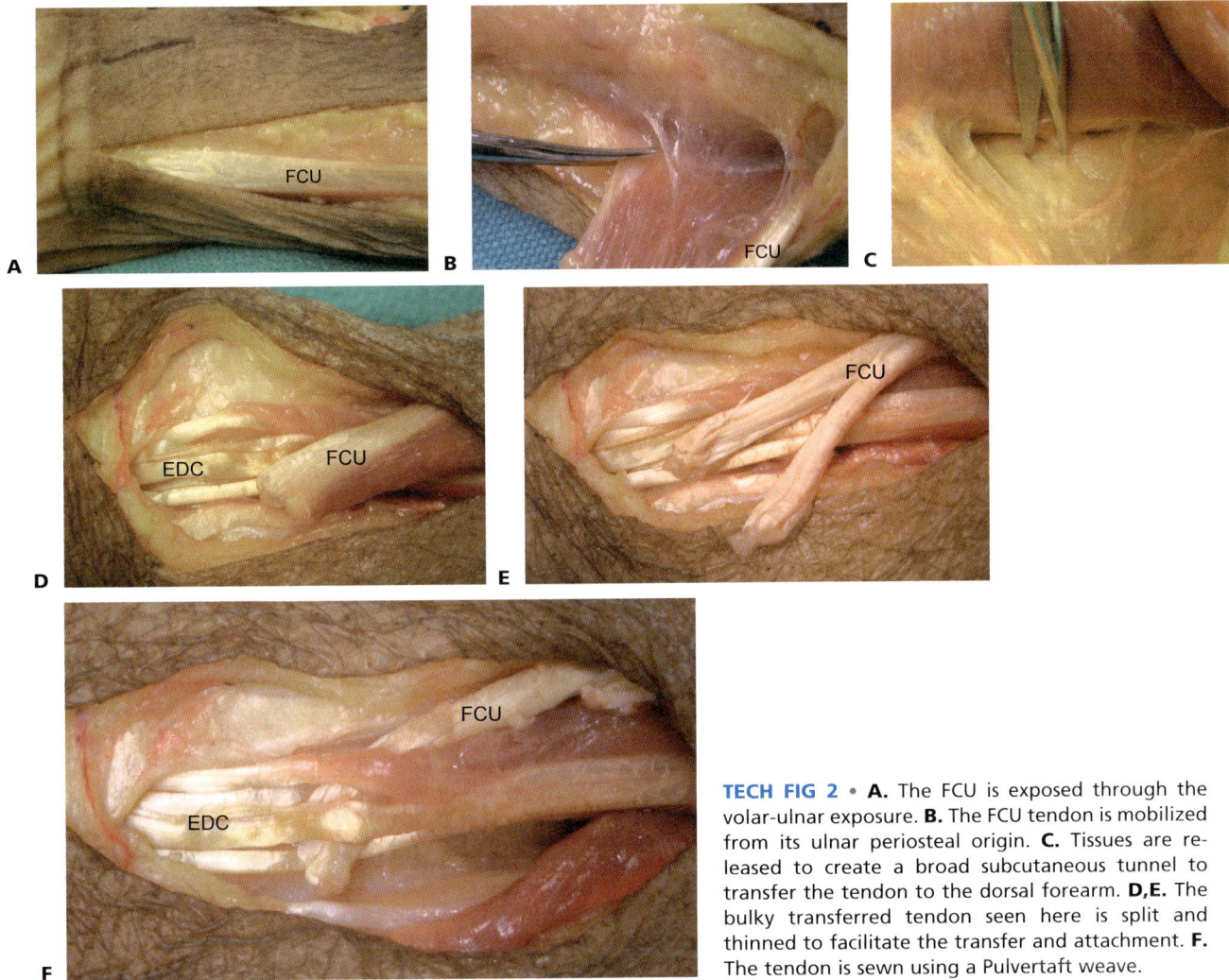

TECH FIG 2 • **A.** The FCU is exposed through the volar-ulnar exposure. **B.** The FCU tendon is mobilized from its ulnar periosteal origin. **C.** Tissues are released to create a broad subcutaneous tunnel to transfer the tendon to the dorsal forearm. **D,E.** The bulky transferred tendon seen here is split and thinned to facilitate the transfer and attachment. **F.** The tendon is sewn using a Pulvertaft weave.

- Trim distal muscle and, if necessary, the tendon to enable passage of tendon into the EDC (TECH FIG 2D,E).
- Make a dorsal longitudinal incision 5 to 7 cm long in the retinaculum of the distal forearm.
- Release the proximal extensor retinaculum to permit excursion after transfer.
- Perform a single or double weave into the EDC tendons.

- Locate the point of insertion into each slip that recreates the normal finger cascade (TECH FIG 2F).
- The final transfer tension is set with the metacarpophalangeal joints in full extension while the wrist is in 30 degrees of extension.
- Secure finger extensor transfers with 3-0 or 4-0 nonabsorbable braided sutures.

FINGER EXTENSION THROUGH FCR TO EDC TRANSFER[7,9,12]

- Use volar radial exposure to identify the radial artery and the FCR (TECH FIG 3A).
- Incise the FCR sheath and transect the tendon while maintaining the wrist in flexion.
- Two different passage techniques may be chosen.
  - In the first, a subcutaneous tunnel to the dorsal incision (similar to the FCU transfer) is developed (TECH FIG 3B,C), and the FCR is passed beneath the superficial radial nerve to the EDC.

- In the second, the FDS and median nerve are retracted ulnarly to identify the anterior interosseous nerve and the interosseous membrane proximal to the pronator quadratus (TECH FIG 3D–F), and the FCR tendon is passed volar-to-dorsal through an enlarged opening in the IOM (TECH FIG 3G,H).
  - Be cautious of the anterior interosseous nerve.
  - Do not violate the central band.
- Tension, weave, and suture into EDC, as with FCU transfer (TECH FIG 3I,J).

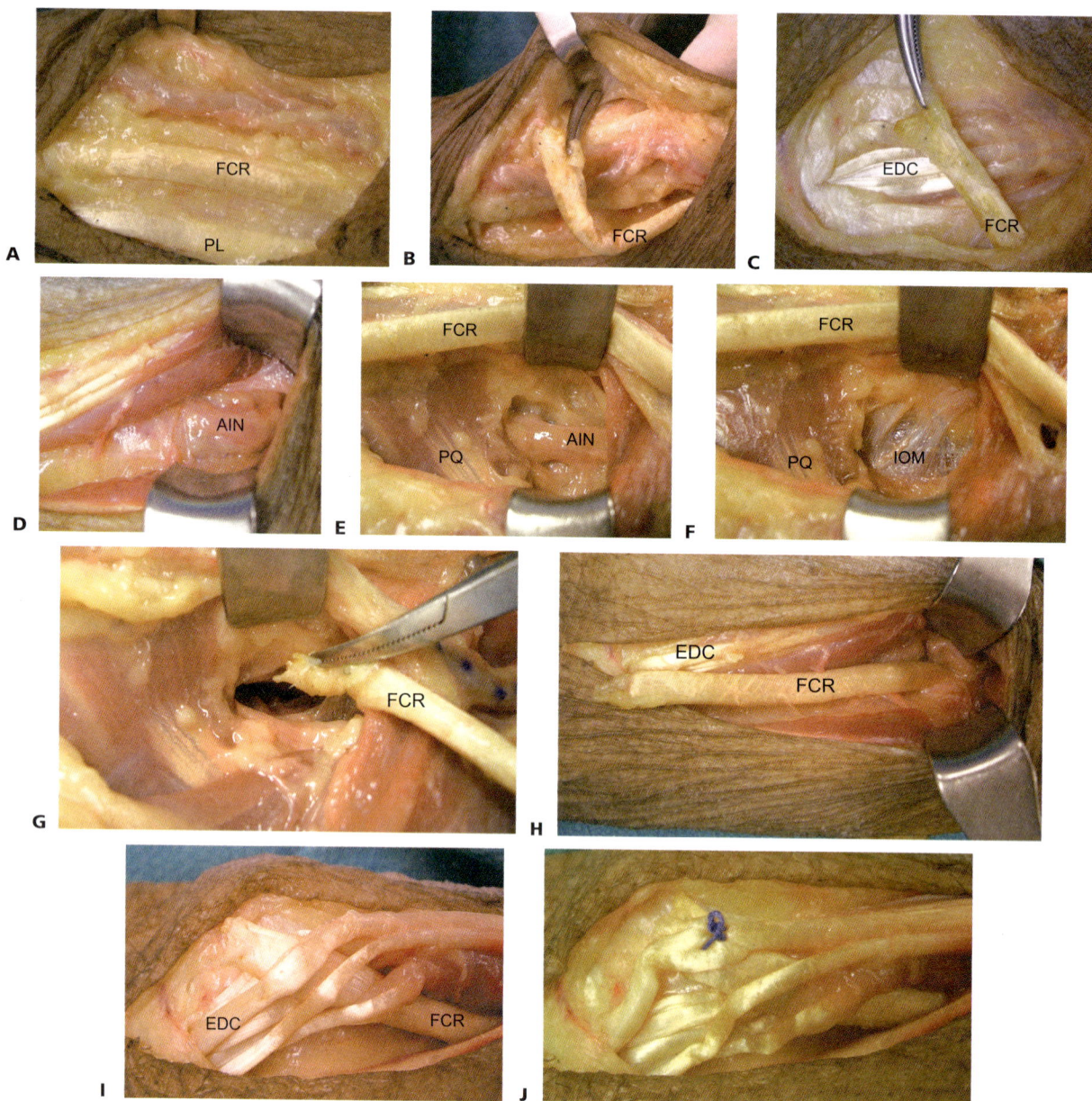

TECH FIG 3 • **A.** The FCR is identified and the tendon mobilized through a volar–radial exposure. **B,C.** A radial subcutaneous tunnel is developed, and the FCR tendon is passed deep to the radial sensory nerve, emerging dorsally. Alternatively, the FCR tendon may be passed through the IOM. **D,E.** The AIN is identified and protected. **F.** The IOM is exposed just proximal to the pronator. **G,H.** The FCR is transferred through the window in the IOM to the dorsal forearm quadratus. **I,J.** The transfer is secured with 3-0 nonabsorbable suture.

THUMB EXTENSION THROUGH PL TO EPL[2,17,21]

- Identify the palmaris longus at the wrist crease through the same incision described for exposure of the FCR (**TECH FIG 4A**).
- Dissect and divide the proximal fascial bands to facilitate harvest (**TECH FIG 4B**).
- Develop a subcutaneous tunnel to the dorsal thumb below the cutaneous nerves.
- The EPL may be addressed in either of two ways:
  - Release the EPL from the third compartment to facilitate transfer location. This technique permits the muscle–tendon connection to remain intact if radial nerve recovery is possible (**TECH FIG 4C**).
  - Divide the EPL proximally (only if recovery is not possible) and perform the transfer in a more volar location. The thumb extension vector is improved with the transfer in this location.
- Set the tension at the level of the thumb metacarpal with the wrist in neutral and close to maximum tension on the PL and EPL (**TECH FIG 4D,E**).
- Secure the weave with 3-0 or 4-0 nonabsorbable braided suture.

TECHNIQUES

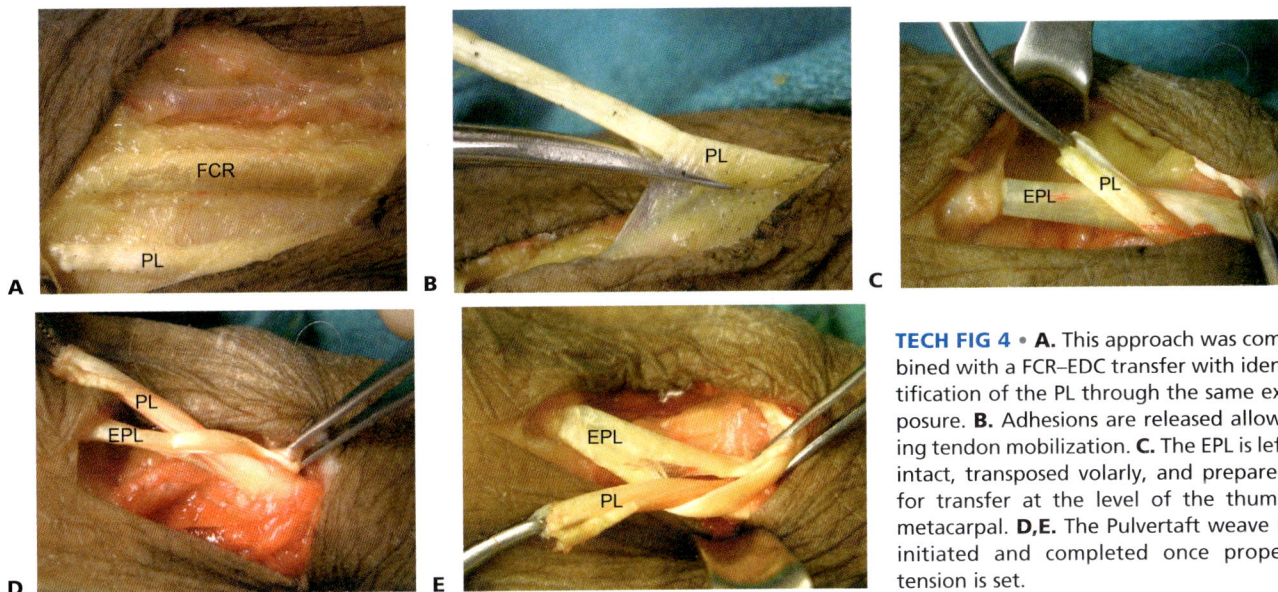

TECH FIG 4 • A. This approach was combined with a FCR–EDC transfer with identification of the PL through the same exposure. **B.** Adhesions are released allowing tendon mobilization. **C.** The EPL is left intact, transposed volarly, and prepared for transfer at the level of the thumb metacarpal. **D,E.** The Pulvertaft weave is initiated and completed once proper tension is set.

MODICATION: FINGER EXTENSION AND THUMB ABDUCTION THROUGH LONG FINGER FDS TO EIP/EPL; RING FINGER FDS TO LONG, RING, AND SMALL EDC; AND PL TO ABDUCTOR POLLICIS LONGUS[5,9]

- Perform oblique palmar incisions to harvest the FDS of the long and ring fingers.
  - Include both slips for transfer.
  - Suture the remaining distal tendon to the volar plate or soft tissue to prevent proximal interphalangeal hyperextension.
- Use the volar incision to retrieve the FDS tendons and to harvest the PL.
- Precisely expose the interosseous membrane (IOM) and make preparations for tendon transfer as discussed in the preceding section.
- Perform a dorsal incision and exposure similar to that detailed in the preceding section. Transfer the two FDS tendons dorsally through the IOM.

- The long finger FDS is transferred to the EIP and the EPL. The ring finger FDS is transferred to the long, ring, and small EDC tendons.
- Set tension at the wrist at 30 degrees and at the MP joint at full extension.
- Secure the transfer with 3-0 or 4-0 suture.
- The PL is harvested as detailed for the EPL transfer.
- The radial subcutaneous route also is used to transfer the PL to the abductor pollicis longus (APL), proximal to the retinaculum.
  - The location of this transfer is slightly more proximal to the PL than the EPL transfer due to the length available for the APL.
- Set tension in near-full thumb abduction at wrist 30 degrees; secure with 3-0 or 4-0 suture.

FINGER EXTENSION AND THUMB ABDUCTION THROUGH FCU TO EDC AND EPL, AND PL TO APL

- Although one donor muscle is not typically transferred to two recipients,[3] an FCU transfer to the EPL and EDC has been described. This may be combined with a wrist extension transfer.

- The technique is similar to that discussed for the FCU to EDC transfer along the ulnar subcutaneous route. The tension is such that the thumb and index metacarpal are parallel.

PEARLS AND PITFALLS

Donor muscle properties	■ In setting tendon transfer tension, the donor muscle length–tension properties are important to consider. A good clinical approximation of a muscle at the peak of the length–tension curve is to place the muscle near the 50% excursion point. The distal recipient tendon is then pulled proximally until the ideal position of the joints has been achieved.[11]
Pulvertaft weave	■ In performing a Pulvertaft weave, a curved tendon passer is very helpful. The weaves should be placed at 90 degrees to each other and secured with multiple mattress sutures. The sutures should have small purchase into the donor and recipient tendons to prevent necrosis. At least three weaves should be used.

Goals	■ With finger extension transfers, it is important to determine the preoperative goals for the FCU/FCR transfers, because they do not match the total EDC excursion. Preoperative assessments can determine whether the ideal working range of the transfer should be more in wrist extension or flexion, because the force will be less in the opposite position.[11]
Choice of transfer	■ The choice between the most common extensor transfers—FCR or FCU—is difficult. Usually, the FCU generates greater force and has longer sarcomere excursion and greater fiber length variability. It has better potential excursion than the FCR, but an extensive proximal release is necessary. Because of muscle bulk, the ulnar route is easier to do than the interosseous passage. There may be some loss of ulnar deviation and grip strength as compared to FCR, but it does not appear to have functional implications.[16,22]

POSTOPERATIVE CARE

■ Postoperative splint with wrist at 30 to 40 degrees and MP joints in 0 to 10 degrees of hyperextension

■ Proximal and distal interphalangeal active and passive motion at 3 to 5 days

■ Static immobilization for 3 weeks, then tenodesis motions with activation of wrist extension transfer

■ Integration of finger and thumb active extension as wrist motion improves

■ The most difficult motion to obtain is independent finger extension with the wrist in the extended position.

■ Passive wrist flexion exercises are determined by the recovery of wrist flexion after splint removal. The arc of flexion can be expected to be less than the preoperative level.

■ A dynamic splint may be applied so that finger extension may begin at 1 week postoperative. An articulated splint may be used to permit dynamic wrist motion, but the patient must be very adept and have a clear understanding of the therapy regimen.[23,28]

OUTCOMES

■ Wrist extension of 40 to 50 degrees (80% M4), wrist flexion 20 to 40 degrees

■ Finger extension: at wrist neutral, 0 to 10 degrees flexion; at wrist in 30 degrees of extension, 0 to 30 degrees

■ Functional scores: 80% excellent to good[21]; no reported disabilities of the arm, shoulder, or hand

COMPLICATIONS

■ If transfer adhesions occur, the therapy can be modified according to postoperative course. Tenolysis should be delayed until at least 9 to 12 months after surgery.

■ Transfer attenuation

REFERENCES

1. Amillo S, Barrios RH, Martínez-Peric R, et al. Surgical treatment of the radial nerve lesions associated with fractures of the humerus. J Orthop Trauma 1993;7:211–215.
2. Boyes JH. Selection of a donor muscle for tendon transfer. Bull Hosp Joint Dis 1962;23:1–4.
3. Brand PW. Biomechanics of tendon transfer. Orthop Clin North Am 1974;5:205–230.
4. Burkhalter WE. Early tendon transfer in upper extremity peripheral nerve injury. Clin Orthop Relat Res 1974;104:68–79.
5. Chuinard RG, Boyes JH, Stark HH, et al. Tendon transfers for radial nerve palsy: Use of superficialis tendons for digital extension. J Hand Surg Am 1978;3:560–570.
6. Gousheh J, Arasteh E. Transfer of a single flexor carpi ulnaris tendon for treatment of radial nerve palsy. J Hand Surg Br 2006;31:542–546.
7. Ishida O, Ikuta Y. Analysis of Tsuge's procedure for the treatment of radial nerve paralysis. Hand Surg 2003;8:17–20.
8. Kozin SH, Hines B. Anatomical approach to the pronator teres. Tech Hand Up Extrem Surg 2002;6:152–154.
9. Krishnan KG, Schakert G. An analysis of results after selective tendon transfers through the interosseous membrane to provide selective finger and thumb extension in chronic irreparable radial nerve lesions. J Hand Surg Am 2008;33:223–231.
10. Kruft S, von Heimburg D, Reill P. Treatment of irreversible lesion of the radial nerve by tendon transfer: Indication and long-term results of the Merle d'Aubigné procedure. Plast Reconstr Surg 1997;100:610–618.
11. Lieber RL, Pontén E, Burkholder TJ, et al. Sarcomere length changes after flexor carpi ulnaris to extensor digitorum communis tendon transfer. J Hand Surg Am 1996;21:612–618.
12. Lim AY, Lahiri A, Pereira BP, et al. Independent function in a split flexor carpi radialis transfer. J Hand Surg Am 2004;29:28–31.
13. Lowe JB, Sen SK, Mackinnon SE. Current approach to radial nerve paralysis. Plast Reconstr Surg 2002;110:1099–1113.
14. Omer GE. Tendon transfers in combined nerve lesions. Orthop Clin North Am 1974;5:377–387.
15. Omer GE. Tendon transfers for combined traumatic nerve palsies of the forearm and hand. J Hand Surg Br 1992;17:603–610.
16. Raskin KB, Wilgis EF. Flexor carpi ulnaris transfer for radial nerve palsy: Functional testing of long-term results. J Hand Surg Am 1995;20:737–742.
17. Reid RL. Radial nerve palsy. Hand Clin 1988;4:179–185.
18. Ring D, Chin K, Jupiter JB. Radial nerve palsy associated with high-energy humeral shaft fractures. J Hand Surg Am 2004;29:144–147.
19. Riordan DC. Radial nerve paralysis. Orthop Clin North Am 1974;5:283–287.
20. Riordan DC. Tendon transfers in hand surgery. J Hand Surg Am 1983;8:748–753.
21. Ropars M, Dreano T, Siret P, et al. Long-term results of tendon transfers in radial and posterior interosseous nerve paralysis. J Hand Surg Br 2006;31:502–506.
22. Skie MC, Parent TE, Mudge KM, et al. Functional deficit after transfer of the pronator teres for acquired radial nerve palsy. J Hand Surg Am 2007;32:526–530.
23. Skoll PJ, Hudson DA, de Jager W, et al. Long-term results of tendon transfers for radial nerve palsy in patients with limited rehabilitation. Ann Plast Surg 2000;45:122–126.
24. Sunderland S. Decision making in clinical management of nerve injury and repair. In: Sunderland S, ed. Nerve Injuries and Their Repair. Edinburgh: Churchill Livingstone, 1991:413–431.
25. Thomsen NO, Dahlin LB. Injury to the radial nerve caused by fracture of the humeral shaft: Timing and neurobiological aspects related to treatment and diagnosis. Scand J Plast Reconstr Surg Hand Surg 2007;41:153–157.
26. Tsuge K. Tendon transfer. In: Tsuge K, ed. Comprehensive Atlas of Hand Surgery. Chicago: Year Book Medical Publishers, 1989:485–544.
27. Tubiana R. Problems and solutions in palliative tendon transfer surgery for radial nerve palsy. Tech Hand Up Extrem Surg 2002;6:104–113.
28. Walczyk S, Pieniazek M, Pelczar-Pieniazek M, et al. Appropriateness and effectiveness of physiotherapeutic treatment procedure after tendon transfer in patients with irreversible radial nerve injury. Orthop Traumatol Rehabil 2005;7:187–197.

Chapter 77

Metacarpophalangeal Joint Synovectomy and Extensor Tendon Centralization in the Inflammatory Arthritis Patient

Andrew L. Terrono, Paul Feldon, and Hervey L. Kimball III

DEFINITION

- The finger metacarpophalangeal joint (MCP joint) is commonly and characteristically involved in inflammatory arthritis.
- The MCP joint is often involved early in inflammatory arthritis and usually presents with ulnar extensor tendon subluxation resulting in ulnar deviation of the fingers.
- Occasionally in systemic lupus erythematosus (SLE) radial subluxation of the extensor tendon is seen.

ANATOMY

- The normal MCP joint is a condylar joint that allows flexion and extension as well as radial and ulnar deviation and a combination of these movements. Normally there is 90 degrees of flexion, although hyperextension can vary.
- The stability of the MCP joint is provided by the radial and ulnar collateral ligaments, the accessory collateral ligaments, the volar plate, the dorsal capsule, and the extensor tendon (**FIG 1**).
- The metacarpal head diameter increases in both the transverse and sagittal planes and therefore has a cam effect, making the collateral ligaments tight in flexion and lax in extension. This allows more radial and ulnar deviation of the MCP joint in extension.
- The MCP joint collateral ligaments are asymmetric.
  - The ulnar collateral ligament is more parallel to the long axis of the fingers.

- The radial collateral ligament is more oblique.
- This causes supination of the MCP joint with MCP joint flexion.
- The collateral ligament also resists volar-directed forces.
- The volar plate is fibrocartilaginous distally and has a membranous portion proximally. It limits MCP joint extension.
- The transverse intermetacarpal ligament connects the volar plates to each other.
- The accessory collateral ligament connects the collateral ligament and volar plate and keeps the volar plate close to the volar aspect of the MCP joint throughout motion.
- The A-1 pulley of the flexor tendon sheath is attached to the volar plate.
- The extensor digitorum tendon is maintained centrally over the MCP joint by the transverse fibers of the sagittal band that attach volarly to the volar plate and the intermetacarpal ligament. This forms a sling mechanism. The ulnar sagittal band is felt to be stronger and denser than the radial sagittal band.
- There is usually no direct extensor tendon insertion into the proximal phalanx. The proximal phalanx is extended through the sling mechanism.
- The lumbrical muscle originates from the tendon of the flexor digitorum profundus and is volar to the intermetacarpal ligament. It inserts into the lateral band.
- There are three volar (which adduct) and four dorsal (which abduct) interossei that have tendons that all pass dorsal to the

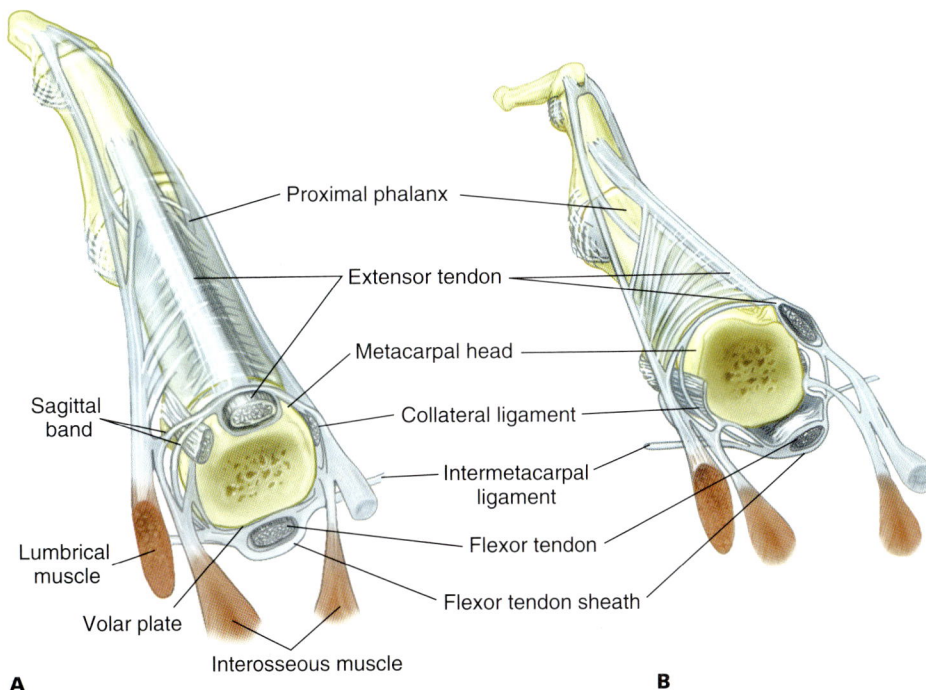

FIG 1 • **A.** Normal anatomy of the metacarpophangeal joint. **B.** Abnormal anatomy seen in inflammatory arthritis. The extensor tendon is subluxated ulnarly.

Labels (A): Proximal phalanx, Extensor tendon, Metacarpal head, Collateral ligament, Intermetacarpal ligament, Flexor tendon, Flexor tendon sheath, Sagittal band, Lumbrical muscle, Volar plate, Interosseous muscle

2729

transverse intermetacarpal ligament. They have variable insertions into the proximal phalanx and extensor mechanism.

■ The first dorsal interosseous almost always inserts completely into the radial side of the proximal phalanx of the index finger.

PATHOGENESIS

■ The pathology of inflammatory arthritis begins with proliferative synovitis.

■ Selective changes in static and dynamic stabilizers of the MCP joint occur, resulting in alteration in the equilibrium of the joint. The most common deformity produced is ulnar deviation of the fingers (**FIG 2A**).

   ■ Which comes first, the changes to the dynamic or static stabilizers, is unclear and may vary.

   ■ The capsule, radial collateral ligament, and radial sagittal band are stretched by the synovitis and allow the equilibrium to move toward ulnar deviation.

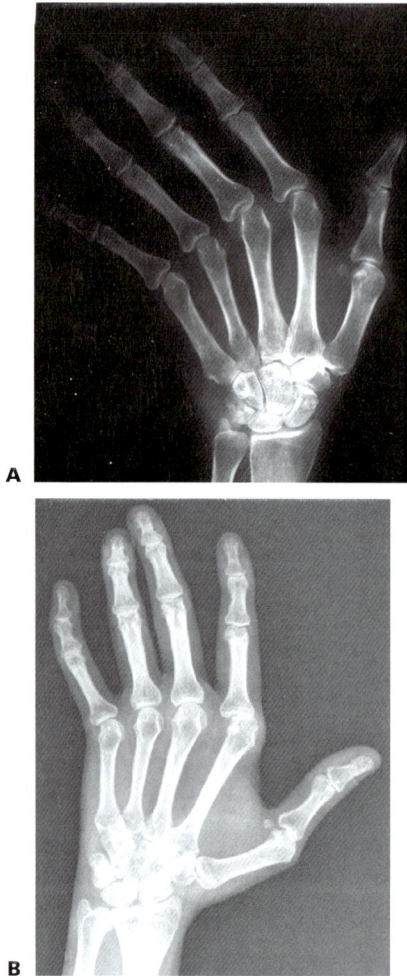

FIG 2 • **A.** Radiograph of a patient with extensor tendon subluxation and ulnar deviation of the metacarpophalangeal (MCP) joints. The joint spaces are maintained and the joints are not subluxated. **B.** Radiograph of a patient with extensor tendon subluxation and ulnar deviation of the MCP joints with reducible MCP joint subluxation involving the index and middle MCP joints.

■ The accessory collateral ligament and the membranous portion of the volar plate become lax.

■ The joint capsule becomes thinned and a defect in the dorsal capsule may occur.

■ With increasing ulnar deviation, the ulnar intrinsic muscle shortens.

■ The intrinsic muscle contribution to the deformity is unclear. It may be a primary or secondary change. There is a cycle that is set up as the MCP joint ulnarly deviates and the extensor tendon acts as an ulnar deviator and may even act as a flexor of the MCP joint.

■ The laxity of the volar plate and accessory collateral ligament causes the flexor tendons to develop a mechanical advantage and increased flexion force. This results in an increase in the deformity.

■ The combination of changes to the capsule, radial collateral ligament, radial sagittal band, accessory collateral ligament, and the membranous portion of the volar plate and the increased mechanical advantage of the flexor tendon is magnified by the normal ulnar and volar slope of the metacarpal condyles and allows ulnar deviation and volar displacement of the proximal phalanx (**FIG 2B**).

■ The wrist may be a contributing factor to the development of the MCP joint deformity, and this must be considered in each case before correcting the MCP joint.

   ■ Radial deviation of the wrist can be a compensatory position to the ulnar deviation of the MCP joints to allow the fingers to line up with the forearm.

   ■ Ulnar deviation of the digit is more common in patients with radial deviation of the wrist.

■ At first the deformity is correctable passively, but gradually this mobility is lost and the deformity becomes fixed.

■ Articular cartilage changes progress from softening of the cartilage to erosion with significant loss of cartilage and bone. This contributes to the deformity.

   ■ Once there are significant cartilage and bone changes, extensor tendon realignment alone, without joint resurfacing, is not indicated.

■ The changes seen in SLE are secondary not to synovitis but rather to alteration in the collagen that results in a change in the equilibrium of the MCP joint and subsequent deformity.

   ■ The finger deformity in SLE is often ulnar deviation, but radial deviation is not uncommon.

   ■ In SLE it is easy to change one deformity to another (ie, ulnar drift into a radial deviation deformity after surgery) because of the global changes to the supporting structures.

   ■ Despite the MCP deformity becoming fixed, the articular cartilage is usually preserved.

NATURAL HISTORY

■ The natural history of the MCP joint changes in inflammatory arthritis is not known and is probably highly variable and influenced by the new disease-modifying medications.

■ Mild ulnar deviation of the fingers is normal and increases with MCP joint flexion.

■ In inflammatory arthritis, such as rheumatoid arthritis, deformity is initially passively correctable.

■ Mild ulnar deviation of the fingers is seen in less than 10% of the patients in the first 5 years of having rheumatoid arthritis.[3]

- Ulnar deviation has been reported in 30% of patients with rheumatoid arthritis, with palmar subluxation in 20%.[3]
- Palmar subluxation almost always occurs with ulnar deviation.[3]

PATIENT HISTORY AND PHYSICAL FINDINGS

- In a patient with inflammatory arthritis who is being considered for MCP joint surgery, the entire upper extremity is evaluated. Involvement of the lower extremities must also be considered, given that the upper extremities may need to assist in ambulation.
  - The need to use the upper extremities for weight bearing can significantly affect the durability of the correction obtained after MCP joint surgery.
  - Ideally MCP joint surgery is performed when the upper extremity is not needed for such support.
- The wrist is evaluated for the presence of a static deformity at the time of MCP joint surgery. Presence of a static radial deviation deformity will negatively affect the results of MP joint surgery.
- The skin over the MCP joint is evaluated; it should be in good condition.
- Motion of the MCP joint is assessed. The surgeon should specifically ensure that ulnar deviation and flexion deformities can be easily corrected passively.
- Proximal interphalangeal (PIP) joint motion and alignment must be critically evaluated.
  - If there is a significant boutonnière deformity, this should be corrected before the MCP joint surgery since the PIP flexion will influence the amount of MCP joint flexion obtained postoperatively.
  - If there is a swan-neck deformity, this can be treated at the same time or after the MCP joint. A stiff PIP joint in extension will cause the patient to flex the finger at the MCP joint and can help obtain better flexion postoperatively.
  - Any radial or ulnar deformity at the PIP joint must be corrected before the MCP joint surgery.
- The flexor and extensor tendons must be intact before any MCP joint surgery.

IMAGING AND OTHER DIAGNOSTIC STUDIES

- Radiographs of the hand and wrist are essential before MCP joint surgery to evaluate alignment, congruence, and joint integrity.

DIFFERENTIAL DIAGNOSIS

- The most common cause of inflammatory arthritis that affects the MCP joint is rheumatoid arthritis.
- SLE is more common in black women, and the deformity is secondary to a collagen abnormality causing ligament and tendon imbalance. Articular cartilage loss is a much less common problem in SLE. Soft tissue realignment can be performed even after the condition has been present for a long time.
- Psoriatic arthritis is more common in men and has a characteristic skin rash, although patients may have joint involvement before a clinically obvious skin rash. The patient with psoriatic arthritis often has an asymmetric deformity and more stiffness. The cartilage and bone are also affected.

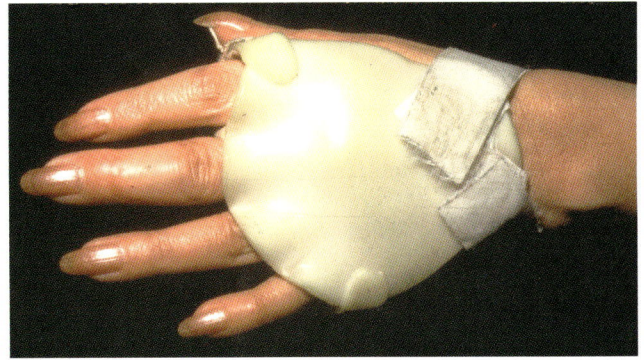

FIG 3 • A splint used to try to prevent progression of the ulnar deviation. Usually this is not successful and ulnar deviation eventually progresses.

NONOPERATIVE TREATMENT

- A team approach to patients with inflammatory arthritis is important.
- Splinting in a corrected position (**FIG 3**) and joint protection may decrease the forces that contribute to the deformity.
- This may be helpful, but the effect in the long term is unknown, and we have not noticed significant long-term benefit.

SURGICAL MANAGEMENT

- One the most difficult operations to decide to perform is MCP joint synovectomy and realignment.
  - This is usually best performed early when there is minimal deformity.
  - However, at this time the patient often has minimal pain and only slight loss of function.
  - With the use of disease-modifying medications, if the anatomy can be restored and the mechanical problems corrected, salvage procedures may be prevented or significantly delayed.
- The ideal patient for surgery is one with increasing deformity and good medical management with control of his or her synovitis.
- The deformity should be passively correctable with good active MCP joint motion.
  - Ideally the MCP joint is not volarly subluxated, since correction and maintenance of correction is more unreliable.
- There should be a well-aligned wrist with good PIP joint function without deformity.
  - If the deformity is passively correctable but cannot be actively corrected, obtaining active ulnar deviation such as by an extensor carpi ulnaris tendon relocation or transfer should be considered.
- The radiographs should reveal good preservation of the joint space without volar subluxation.
- If all of these criteria are met and the joints are not passively correctable or there is volar subluxation of the MCP joint, surgery can be performed, although the results may not be as reliable.[2]
- A firm diagnosis can help with establishing a prognosis for the maintenance of correction obtained at surgery.
  - The effect of the new disease-modifying medication is not known.

- It is possible that the soft tissue correction obtained at surgery may now last longer and therefore the procedure should be entertained earlier and more often.
- Ideally, earlier surgery will solve the correctable mechanical problem and will end the cycle of deformity.

Positioning

- The procedure is performed using tourniquet control. The hand is supported by a hand table.

Approach

- The procedure usually is performed on all four fingers through a transverse dorsal incision over the MCP joint (**FIG 4**).
  - If a single digit is involved, a longitudinal incision should be used.
- If not all of the fingers are going to be corrected, the fingers on the side of the deformity (ie, if there is ulnar deviation deformity, the radial involved digits) must be corrected first to limit recurrent deformity.

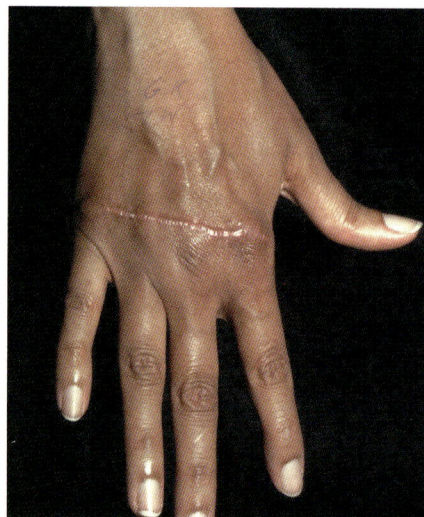

FIG 4 • A transverse incision is used to expose the metacarpophalangeal joints when performing an extensor tendon centralization.

EXPOSURE

- Expose the extensor mechanism at each joint (**TECH FIG 1A**).
- Release the juncture tendineae as needed (**TECH FIG 1B**).
- Develop the interval between the extensor hood and capsule.
- Try to relocate the extensor tendon to the midline.
  - Sometimes this can be done without releasing the ulnar sagittal band.
- If the extensor tendon can be relocated to the midline, expose the joint by incising the radial sagittal band.
  - The radial sagittal band will be reefed at the end of the procedure.
- If the extensor tendon cannot be relocated to the midline, release the ulnar sagittal band to expose the capsule.
- A central defect in the joint capsule is often present. Open the capsule through this defect using a distally based dorsal capsular flap (**TECH FIG 1C**).

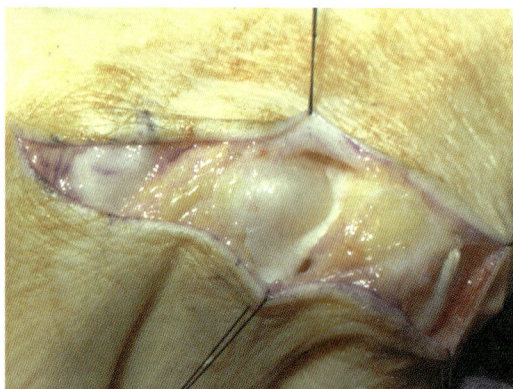

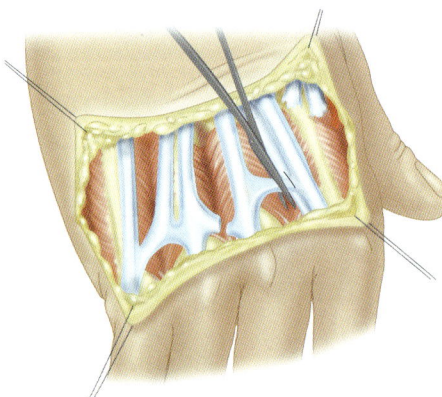

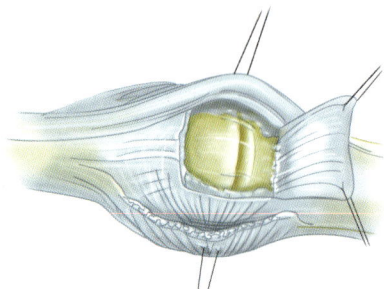

TECH FIG 1 • **A.** The extensor tendons are exposed through a transverse skin incision. The extensor tendons are subluxated ulnarly. **B.** The juncture tendineae are released as needed. **C.** The capsule is opened by creating a distally based dorsal capsular flap.

SYNOVECTOMY AND TENDON REALIGNMENT

- Perform a synovectomy using small rongeurs, curettes, and elevators (**TECH FIG 2A**).
- Evaluate the intrinsics after the extensor tendon is relocated and the joint is in neutral position. Perform an intrinsic tightness test. If positive and intrinsic tightness persists, release the ulnar intrinsics.
  - Incise the sagittal band and expose the intrinsic tendon on the ulnar side of the joint.
    - It is superficial to the collateral ligament and capsule.
  - Pass a curved hemostat beneath the ulnar intrinsic tendon as it inserts into the lateral band (see Fig 1) and divide the tendon.
    - A section of the oblique fibers may be excised.
  - If intrinsic tightness continues, release the proximal phalanx insertion by grasping the proximal portion of the tendon with a clamp and sectioning (**TECH FIG 2B**).
  - A step-cut lengthening of the ulnar intrinsics may be preferred to complete intrinsic release in patients with SLE to avoid late radial deviation.
- If the joint still cannot be corrected, release the ulnar collateral ligament.
- If the ulnar intrinsic has been released, an intrinsic transfer can be performed, usually attaching it to the radial collateral ligament (**TECH FIG 2C**).
  - The advantage of using the radial collateral ligament as the attachment site is that it does not increase the extensor force at the PIP joint, which could result in a swan-neck deformity.
- If the joint was subluxated volarly preoperatively, pin the MCP joint in extension with a Kirschner wire.
- After the proximal phalanx is reduced, reef or advance the radial collateral ligament as needed (**TECH FIG 2D**).
- Close the capsule in a pants-over-vest manner so that the MCP joint is in extension (**TECH FIG 2E**).
- The extensor tendon is relocated onto the dorsal midline of the joint.
- Strip the periosteum from the dorsum of the proximal phalanx base and tenodese the central tendon to the proximal phalanx using a suture anchor (**TECH FIG 2F,G**).
  - Alternatively, place two drill holes in the proximal phalanx to suture the tendon directly to the bone.
  - 2-0 PDS suture is used. Nonabsorbable suture may result in prominent knots in this patient population with thin skin.
- Reef the radial sagittal band fibers with a 4-0 nonabsorbable suture to rebalance and support the extensor tendon directly over the joint.
- Repair the juncture tendineae.
- Traction on the central tendon should result in full MCP joint extension.
- A bulky dressing with fluffs between the fingers is applied, followed by a volar splint supporting the MCP joints in extension and in a slightly overcorrected position.

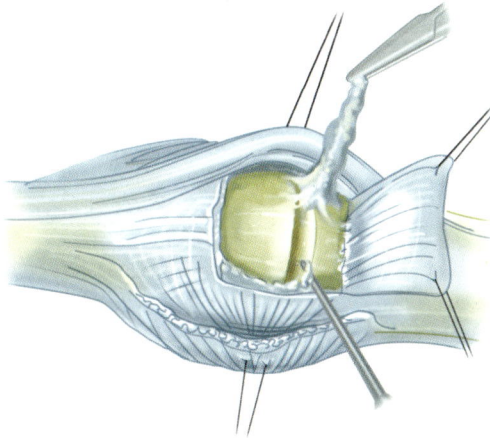

A

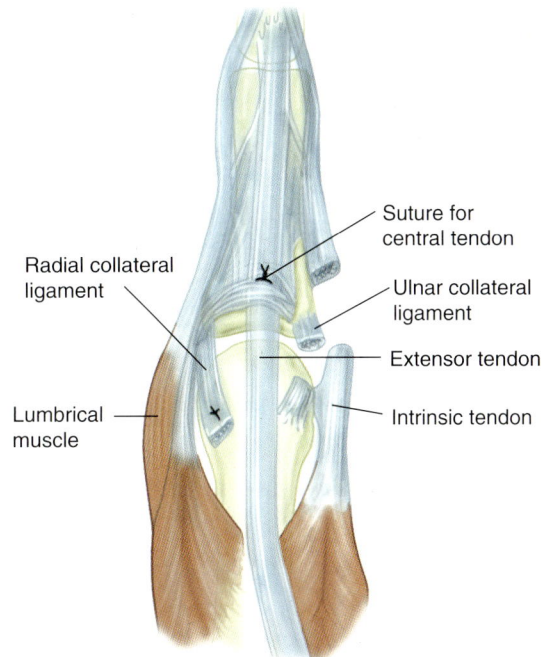

B

Radial collateral ligament

Lumbrical muscle

Suture for central tendon

Ulnar collateral ligament

Extensor tendon

Intrinsic tendon

TECH FIG 2 • **A.** A metacarpophalangeal joint synovectomy is performed. **B.** The ulnar intrinsic tendon is sectioned and the ulnar collateral ligament is released. The central tendon is centralized and sutured to the proximal phalanx. *(continued)*

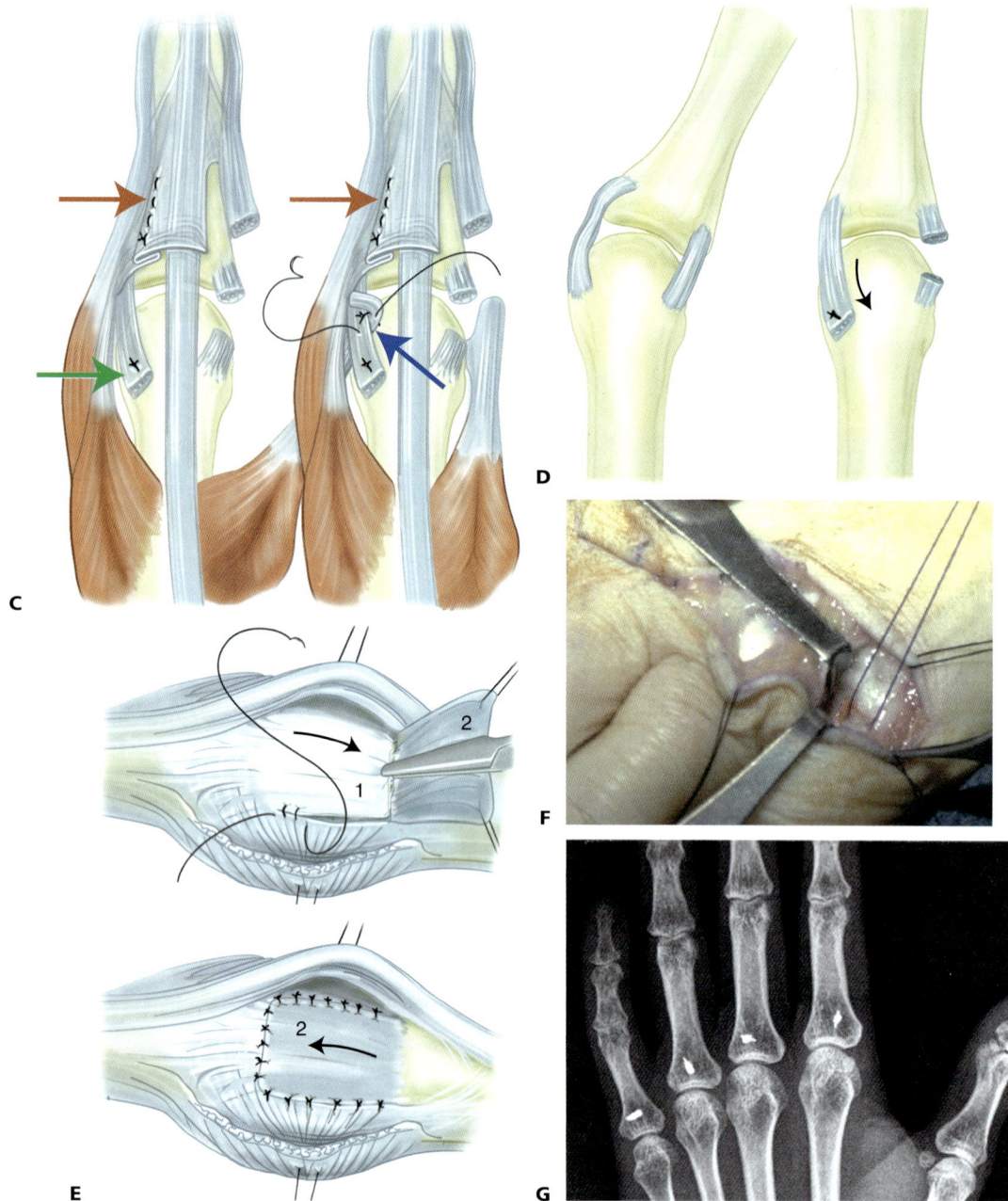

TECH FIG 2 • *(continued)* **C.** The contracted ulnar sagittal fibers are released and the radial sagittal fibers are reefed (*red arrows*) to rebalance and support the extensor tendon in the midline. The radial collateral ligament is advanced (*green arrow*) and the ulnar intrinsic muscle is transferred to the radial collateral ligament (*blue arrow*) of the adjacent digit. **D.** The radial collateral ligament is advanced, as in this case, or reefed. **E.** The capsule is closed in a pants-over-vest manner so that the metacarpophalangeal joint is supported in extension. **F.** The extensor tendon is sutured directly to the dorsal base of the proximal phalanx using absorbable suture. **G.** Postoperative radiograph of a patient showing suture anchors in place after extensor tendon centralization.

PEARLS AND PITFALLS

- Patient selection and control of the disease process are probably the most important factors.
- Joints with fixed deformities and cartilage loss are best treated with replacement arthroplasty.
- Proximal joint and distal joint correction must be performed before MCP joint surgery.
- Intrinsic transfers do not improve the long-term outcome of this procedure.
- Intrinsic lengthening is used only in patients with SLE.

POSTOPERATIVE CARE

- The postoperative dressing is removed at about 10 to 14 days and the sutures are removed.
- An Orthoplast splint with the MCP joints extended and slightly overcorrected, usually in slight radial deviation, is applied until 4 weeks postoperatively.
- At 4 weeks postoperatively, if Kirschner wires were inserted they are removed. Splinting is then continued for 2 additional weeks.
- At 6 weeks postoperatively, hand therapy is started, concentrating on active MCP joint extension. Active MCP flexion is also started. Protective splinting is continued for another 2 weeks in between exercises and at night.
- The fingers are splinted together as a unit to maintain alignment and concentrate flexion at the MCP level.
- To increase the postoperative flexion, the PIP joint is occasionally splinted in extension, concentrating the flexion force at the MCP joint.
- Dynamic splinting can be used to support extension and maintain digital alignment during the early healing stage but is usually not necessary.
- At 8 weeks postoperatively daytime splinting is decreased and gradual return to functional activities is encouraged.
- Nighttime extension splinting is continued for 3 months.

OUTCOMES

- MCP joint extension and ulnar drift are improved postoperatively.
- MCP flexion is usually slightly less than it was preoperatively.
- Strength is not significantly improved.

- Maintenance of correction is usually good with slight increase in ulnar drift, usually without recurrent subluxation.
- When the deformity is seen early and is still passively correctable with preserved joints, extensor tendon centralization and MCP joint synovectomy (as needed) is often beneficial, improving patient function.
- As with all joint procedures for deformities resulting from inflammatory arthritis, the procedure itself does not stop the progression of the disease. However, the new generation of disease-modifying medications combined with surgery may result in long-lasting correction of joint deformity.

COMPLICATIONS

- Infection
- Wound healing problems
- Loss of motion
- Recurrent ulnar drift with tendon subluxation
- Radial subluxation of the extensor tendon (seen in SLE)
- Progressive joint destruction from the arthritis and need for joint replacement

REFERENCES

1. Abboud JA, Beredjiklian PK, Bozentka DJ. Metacarpophalangeal joint arthroplasty and rheumatoid arthritis. J Am Acad Orthop Surg 2003;11:184–191.
2. Nalebuff EA. Surgery for systemic lupus erythematosus arthritis of the hand. Hand Clin 1996;12:591–602.
3. Wilson RL, Carlblom ER. The rheumatoid metacarpophalangeal joint. Hand Clin 1989;8:223–237.
4. Wood VE, Ichtertz DR, Yahiku H. Soft tissue metacarpophalangeal reconstruction for treatment of rheumatoid hand deformity. J Hand Surg Am 1989;14A:163–174.

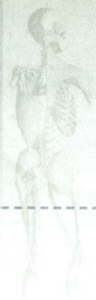

Chapter 78

Proximal Interphalangeal and Metacarpophalangeal Joint Silicone Implant Arthroplasty

Charles A. Goldfarb

DEFINITION

- Arthritis of the metacarpophalangeal (MCP) or proximal interphalangeal (PIP) joints may cause pain, deformity, and decreased motion. Rheumatoid arthritis (RA), osteoarthritis, and posttraumatic arthritis are common causes.
- Silicone implant arthroplasty may be considered as a surgical option after failure of nonoperative treatment in the patient with pain, functional disability, or both secondary to arthritis at the MCP or PIP joint.
- The primary function of the silicone implant is to serve as a dynamic spacer until the joint is encapsulated; thereafter, the joint can be expected to maintain alignment and provide a satisfactory range of motion.

ANATOMY

Metacarpophalangeal Joint

- The MCP joint is condyloid with motion in three planes: flexion–extension, abduction–adduction, and rotation.
- The head of the metacarpal is wider on its volar aspect, providing greater stability in flexion. The radial condyle is larger as well, contributing to the ulnar deviation posture most commonly seen in RA patients.
- Collateral ligaments arise dorsal to the center of rotation; this, together with the shape of the metacarpal head, contributes to the cam effect that is manifest by collateral ligament laxity in extension and tightness in flexion.
- Hyperextension of the MCP joints is common; however, the volar plate limits excessive motion.

Proximal Interphalangeal Joint

- The PIP joint is a hinge joint with an average arc of motion of 0 to 100 degrees of flexion.
- The bony anatomy is crucial to PIP joint stability in all positions; the base of the middle phalanx is wider volarly, thus helping to prevent dorsal dislocation. The PIP joint is more stable in all positions compared to the MCP joint.
- The proper collateral ligaments originate from the center of rotation of the proximal phalanx head and insert onto the volar base of the middle phalanx; they provide stability in all positions. The accessory collateral ligaments insert onto the volar plate and provide more stability in extension. There is no significant cam effect with the PIP joint.
- The volar plate resists hyperextension and is a key supporting structure of the joint.

PATHOGENESIS

- Arthritis of the MCP or PIP joints may be idiopathic, posttraumatic, or inflammatory (RA).
- Idiopathic osteoarthritis involves the distal interphalangeal joint most commonly, but the PIP joint is also affected; the MCP joint is less commonly involved.
- The PIP joint is the most frequently traumatized finger joint and, thus, has the highest incidence of posttraumatic arthritis.

Given the shortcomings of the salvage procedures for PIP joint arthritis, an anatomic joint reduction and aggressive restoration of the normal anatomy after trauma is critical as a means of prevention of arthritis.

- The bony congruity of the PIP joint makes it poorly tolerant of any loss of cartilage; deformity and loss of motion may progress quickly.
- Inflammatory arthritis (RA) most commonly affects the MCP joint but may also involve the PIP joint. In RA, a proliferative synovitis compromises the soft tissue support of the affected joint and may lead to the characteristic deformities at the MCP joint, including volar subluxation (and a flexed posture) and ulnar deviation. In the PIP joint, an attenuation of the volar supporting structures may lead to joint hyperextension, while compromise of the central slip insertion will lead to a joint flexion deformity.
- The efficacy of the disease-modifying antirheumatic drugs has dramatically decreased the need for joint arthroplasty in these patients.

NATURAL HISTORY

- The natural history of osteoarthritis or posttraumatic arthritis of the PIP joint is progression with loss of motion, pain, and in some patients deformity. The MCP joint is less commonly affected and is also more tolerant of arthritis, given its increased mobility in all planes.
- In the patient with severe RA not controllable by disease-modifying antirheumatic drugs, joint inflammation will lead to progression of the arthritis.
- The functional affect of the arthritis depends on both the degree of involvement of the specific joint and the involvement of the adjacent joints.

PATIENT HISTORY AND PHYSICAL FINDINGS

- It is vital that the surgeon understand how the arthritis specifically affects the function of a particular patient. This depends on many factors, including adjacent joint involvement, specific patient activities, and the degree of pain experienced.
- Physical examination methods include the following:
  - Palpation of the joint at the joint line: Confirms origin of the pain and allows evaluation for synovitis
  - Active and passive range of motion of the joint are measured with a goniometer. Joint motion is lost with arthritis. Pain with motion is noted.
  - Deformity of joint alignment is measured with a goniometer. Progressive arthritis leads to deformity.
  - Radial–ulnar stress testing: Evaluation of collateral ligaments. The MCP should be tested in flexion; the PIP joint may be tested in any position but is most commonly tested in extension. Attenuation of collateral ligaments may occur in RA or after trauma.

■ Integrity of tendon function: Most commonly abnormal in RA or after prior trauma

■ Intrinsic tightness (Bunnell) test: If the intrinsics are tight, therapy or surgical intervention may be needed.

■ Elsen test: Integrity of the central slip is important when contemplating PIP joint arthroplasty.

■ The alignment and function of the adjacent joints (including the wrist) should be assessed, given the intimate relationship between the joints.

■ A complete examination of the hand includes an examination of adjacent joints. The ligamentous stability of all joints of the hand and the functioning of the extrinsic and intrinsic flexor and extensor musculature are evaluated.

■ In inflammatory conditions, the proximal joints, most importantly the wrist, must be examined. If wrist deformity is not corrected before surgical correction of distal disease, surgical correction (such as MCP arthroplasty) will have a higher incidence of failure due to the uncorrected deforming forces.

■ In patients with posttraumatic arthritis (especially affecting the PIP joints), the functioning of the flexor and extensor tendons must be understood. The presence of tendon shortening or lengthening (for example, after repair of an open injury) and the presence of tendon adhesions should be sought.

■ Intrinsic or extrinsic contractures after hand trauma are assessed before surgical intervention.

IMAGING AND OTHER DIAGNOSTIC STUDIES

■ Plain radiographs provide sufficient diagnostic information. AP and lateral radiographs are usually sufficient, although oblique radiographs may be helpful (**FIG 1**).

■ MRI and CT are of limited utility in the evaluation of the MCP and PIP joints.

DIFFERENTIAL DIAGNOSIS

■ Acute fracture with or without joint subluxation
■ Collateral ligament injury
■ Joint infection
■ Flexor or extensor mechanism injury

NONOPERATIVE MANAGEMENT

■ Anti-inflammatory medications
■ Steroid injections
■ Splinting

SURGICAL MANAGEMENT

■ Surgery is considered if nonoperative management fails. Given the limitations of silicone implant arthroplasty as noted below, the decision for surgical intervention should be patient-driven.

■ The best outcome is expected in patients with a preserved arc of motion, minimal deformity, and pain. Patients without pain and presenting with deformity or a lack of motion are not ideal candidates for arthroplasty, especially if the adjacent joints are functioning well. Joint arthroplasty does not reliably increase motion at long-term follow-up.

■ In RA, an ulnar drift and volar subluxation of the MCP joints with a flexion posture of the joints may lead to weakness and a loss of the ability to grasp larger objects. These deformities are also unsightly. Surgical intervention in these patients can be expected to improve the aesthetic appearance and function of the hand.

Preoperative Planning

■ All imaging studies should be reviewed.
■ Involvement of adjacent joints should be assessed.
■ Multiple MCP or PIP joints can be treated with silicone arthroplasty at the same surgical setting, but we do not typically recommend MCP and PIP joint silicone arthroplasty in the same finger.

  ■ In patients with symptomatic disease at both the MCP joint and the PIP joint, the MCP is typically treated with silicone implant arthroplasty and the PIP joint is fused.

■ An assessment of the ligamentous stability of the MCP and PIP joints should be performed under anesthesia.

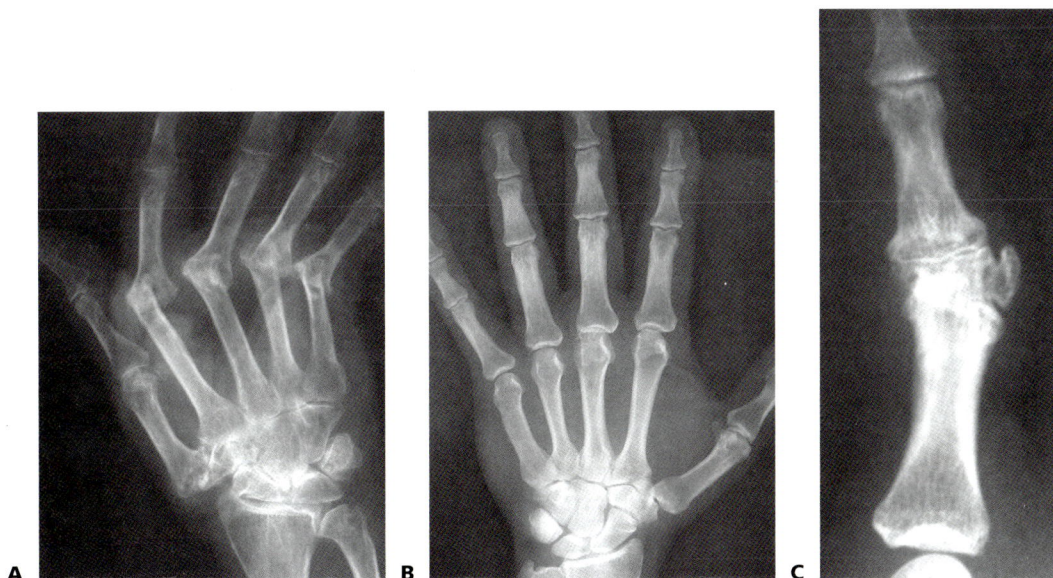

FIG 1 • A. Rheumatoid arthritis affecting hand, with most notable disease affecting metacarpophalangeal (MCP) joints. The wrist is also affected. **B.** Isolated osteoarthritis of the MCP joint of the long finger. **C.** Posttraumatic arthritis affecting the small finger proximal interphalangeal joint.

- MCP and PIP arthroplasty is performed cautiously in the index (or long) finger as pinch forces may be problematic for joint stability.
- Templating should be performed to ensure that appropriate-sized implants are available.

Positioning

- The patient is placed supine with the extremity on an arm table.

- A nonsterile arm tourniquet is used.
- General or axillary block anesthesia is used.

Approach

- The MCP joint is approached from dorsally with a midline incision.
- The PIP joint may be approached from either the dorsal or volar approach.

METACARPOPHALANGEAL JOINT SILICONE ARTHROPLASTY[2]

Incision and Dissection

- If a single joint is being addressed (osteoarthritis or post-traumatic arthritis), make a longitudinal incision over the MCP joint. If multiple joints are being addressed, make a transverse incision over the metacarpal necks (**TECH FIG 1A**).
- Protect the superficial veins (most importantly in RA patients).
- Identify and protect the extensor tendons.
- In RA, the tendons may be translocated in an ulnar direction. If so, divide the sagittal bands on the ulnar side to allow later centralization of the tendons.
  - If the tendons are centralized, the interval between tendons (index and small finger between extensor indicis proprius or extensor digit minimi and extensor digitorum communis) can be used to approach the joint (**TECH FIG 1B**).
- In RA, the ulnar intrinsic tendon is often a deforming force. In fingers with marked ulnar deviation, bring the tendon into the surgical field with a blunt hook and divide it.
- Divide the joint capsule longitudinally for later repair.
- Débride the joint (**TECH FIG 1C**).
- It may be necessary to recess the collateral ligaments off their origin from the metacarpal head. Carefully protect their insertion onto the base of the proximal phalanx.
  - In osteoarthritis or posttraumatic arthritis, the collateral ligaments need not be released if adequate exposure can be obtained.
- If the joint is volarly subluxated, it may exhibit a flexion contracture that must be released.

- Perform a soft tissue release using a Freer to elevate the volar plate off the volar distal metacarpal; this, together with bony resection, will allow joint reduction.
- Once the proximal phalanx can be mobilized dorsal to the metacarpal head, a sufficient release has been obtained.

Bone Preparation

- Using an oscillating saw, remove the metacarpal head just distal to the collateral ligament origin, staying perpendicular to the axis of the bone in the posteroanterior and lateral planes.
  - The amount of bone removed depends on the degree of deformity and contracture (**TECH FIG 2A**).
  - In severe cases it is necessary to elevate the collateral ligaments from their origins to resect more metacarpal. In these cases, radial collateral (and ulnar) ligaments are repaired during closure.
- Prepare the base of the proximal phalanx by removing the articular cartilage using osteotomes or a rongeur. Carefully protect the collateral ligament insertions.
- Use an awl to identify the metacarpal medullary canal first.
  - The awl typically enters the canal dorsal to the apparent center of the cut end of the metacarpal given the dorsal–volar bone curvature.
- Use hand reamers to prepare the bone.
  - Use progressive broaches, taking care to ensure correct broach alignment and integrity of the cortex (**TECH FIG 2B**).

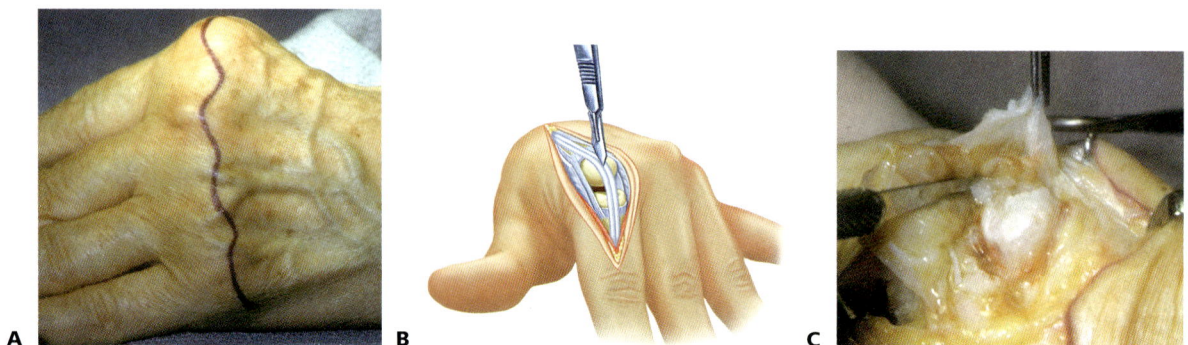

A   B   C

TECH FIG 1 • A. Transverse dorsal incision for metacarpophalangeal arthroplasty of all four fingers. The incision may be straight or undulating. **B.** The interval between the extensor tendons may be chosen to approach the joint for the index or small fingers. The interval between the extensor digitorum communis and the extensor indicis proprius is illustrated. **C.** The joint is débrided. This can be an extensive process in severe rheumatoid disease.

TECHNIQUES

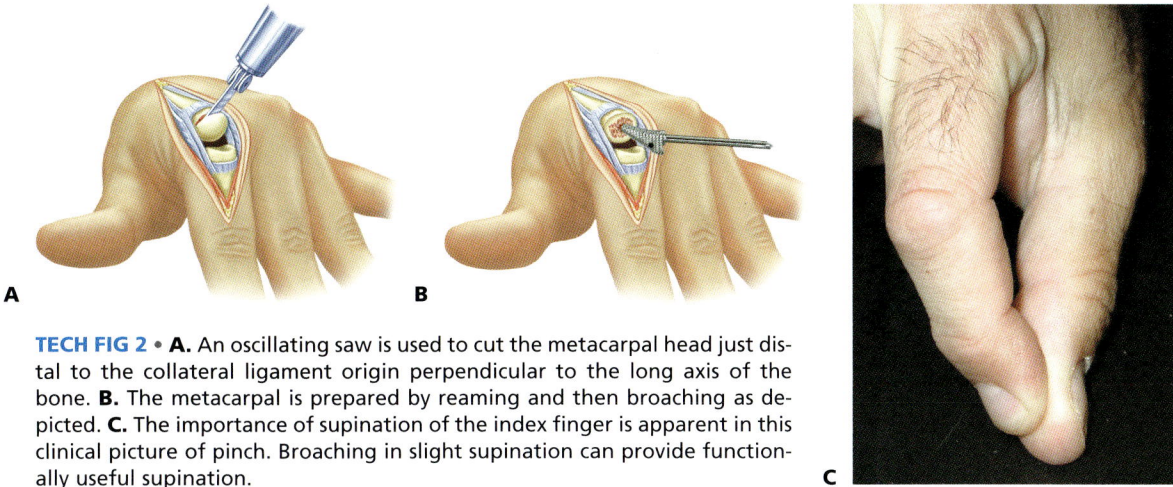

TECH FIG 2 • **A.** An oscillating saw is used to cut the metacarpal head just distal to the collateral ligament origin perpendicular to the long axis of the bone. **B.** The metacarpal is prepared by reaming and then broaching as depicted. **C.** The importance of supination of the index finger is apparent in this clinical picture of pinch. Broaching in slight supination can provide functionally useful supination.

- The ring finger metacarpal is frequently much narrower and may require more reaming, use of a burr, and potentially a smaller implant.
- Once the metacarpal is prepared, initiate the same procedure for the proximal phalanx.
  - The base of the proximal phalanx can be reamed in slight supination for the index finger to improve pinch (**TECH FIG 2C**).

Implant Placement and Closure

- Place a trial prosthesis, choosing the largest "comfortable" fit that allows full joint motion. Ensure proper clinical alignment (**TECH FIG 3A**).
  - If the prosthesis buckles, choose a smaller prosthesis or create more space through soft tissue release or additional bone resection.
  - If the prosthetic stem is too long and is contributing to buckling of the prosthesis, the stem may be trimmed using scissors.
- If the origins of the collateral ligaments were disturbed, drill holes in the dorsal radial and the dorsal ulnar (in the case of osteoarthritis or posttraumatic arthritis)

metacarpal and place 2-0 nonabsorbable suture for later repair of the collateral ligaments.
  - The radial collateral ligaments are typically attenuated in RA, especially if the joints have been ulnarly deviated. The ligaments are tightened when repaired through imbrication (**TECH FIG 3B**).
  - A distally based radial slip of the volar plate may be mobilized and integrated into the repair in the case of severely attenuated radial collateral ligaments.
- Place the final implants using a "no touch" technique.
  - To minimize the risk of a reaction between the silicone implant and the sterile gloves, do not directly handle the implants; instead, insert them using forceps.
  - Grommets are not routinely used.
- Insert the proximal stem first; then bend the implant and place the distal stem.
- Once the implant has been placed in a stable position, the collateral ligaments are repaired.
- The collateral ligaments are repaired, imbricated, or reconstructed as may be required to restore stability (especially against ulnar deviation).
- If the capsule is sufficiently robust, repair it with interrupted 3-0 absorbable suture.

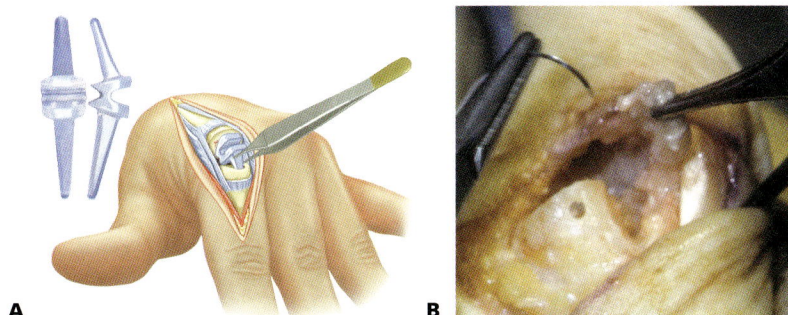

TECH FIG 3 • **A.** Trial implant is placed to test range of motion and implant fit. **B.** After final implant placement, the collateral ligaments are repaired through drill holes placed in the metacarpal. This is most important for the radial collateral ligament in rheumatoid arthritis.

TECHNIQUES

- Repair the extensor mechanism in a centralized position with nonabsorbable 2-0 suture. Use passive joint range of motion to ensure there is no tendon subluxation after repair.
    - If the radial sagittal band is attenuated, imbricate or incise it and advance it deep to the extensor digitorum communis tendon in a pants-over-vest manner.

- Additional release of the ulnar sagittal band may also be required to centralize the extensor mechanism.
- Obtain C-arm or standard radiographs to confirm clinical alignment.
- Close the skin with 4-0 nylon suture. Once the wound is closed, deflate the tourniquet.
    - A Penrose drain may be used if excessive bleeding is noted (uncommon). The drain is removed the next day.

PROXIMAL INTERPHALANGEAL JOINT SILICONE ARTHROPLASTY

Volar Approach for Proximal Interphalangeal Joint Arthroplasty[4,6]

Incision and Dissection

- Use a volar, Brunner incision centered at the PIP joint (**TECH FIG 4A**).
- Raise full-thickness flaps with careful protection of the neurovascular bundles.
- Divide the C1, A3, and C3 pulleys at their insertion on one side and elevate them to expose the flexor tendons (**TECH FIG 4B,C**).
    - Protect the A2 and A4 pulleys.
- Retract the flexor tendons to either side using a Penrose drain.
- Detach the volar plate proximally and divide the accessory collateral ligaments from their insertion onto the volar plate. Leave the volar plate attached distally (**TECH FIG 4D**).
- Detachment of the collateral ligaments at their insertion is required for optimal exposure and visualization (may be repaired back to volar plate at closure).
- Dislocate the joint in a "shotgun" manner to expose the articular surfaces.

Bone Preparation

- Using an oscillating saw, remove the condyles of the proximal phalanx head, staying perpendicular to the long axis of the bone in both the posteroanterior and lateral planes.
- Carefully prepare the base of the middle phalanx, taking great care not to injure the central slip insertion or proper collateral ligament insertion. Remove remaining cartilage with a rongeur or osteotome. Create a flat surface to accommodate the implant.
- Use awls, hand reamers, and broaches to prepare the medullary canals of the proximal and middle phalanges.
    - The proximal phalanx is typically prepared before the middle phalanx.
    - Use the rectangular shape of the broach base to ensure correct rotation of the final implant.

Implant Placement and Closure

- The trial should allow satisfactory joint range of motion without buckling or displacement.
    - The trial and final implant should remain flush against the cut ends of the bones.
    - The implant can be shortened or additional reaming can be performed as needed for the trial that buckles.

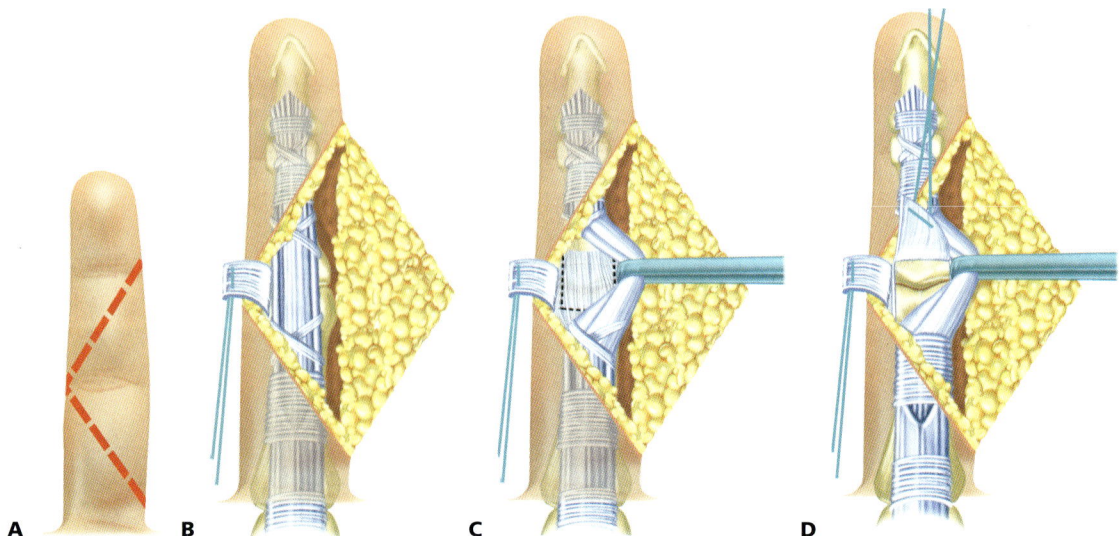

TECH FIG 4 • **A.** A volar skin incision is centered at the proximal interphalangeal joint in a Brunner fashion. **B, C.** The flexor tendon sheath is incised between the A2 and A4 pulleys to allow retraction of the tendons. **D.** The volar plate is released proximally for exposure.

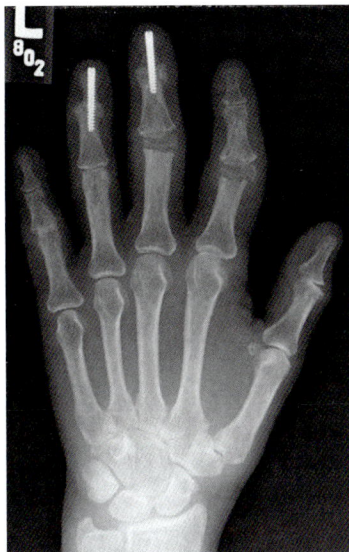

TECH FIG 5 • Postoperative radiograph of patient with diffuse osteoarthritis. Note the silicone implant arthroplasties for the proximal interphalangeal joints of the index and long fingers as well as the fusions of the distal interphalangeal joints of the long and ring fingers.

- Create small drill holes at the radial and ulnar bases of the proximal phalanx before final prosthesis fitting to allow volar plate repair.
- Create dorsal drill holes at the origin of the proper collateral ligaments to be used for repair.

- The volar plate can be divided longitudinally and used to reconstruct the collateral ligaments if needed.
- Obtain C-arm or standard radiographs to confirm clinical alignment (**TECH FIG 5**).
- The flexor sheath need not be repaired.
- Use 4-0 nylon sutures to close the skin.

Dorsal Approach for Proximal Interphalangeal Joint Arthroplasty

- Make a straight or gently curved longitudinal incision centered over the dorsal PIP joint.
- Raise full-thickness flaps at the level of the extensor mechanism.
- Split the central slip longitudinally and elevate it radially and ulnarly, taking care not to injure the central slip insertion and create an iatrogenic boutonnière deformity. Other alternatives are as follows:
    - The longitudinal split of the extensor mechanism may be carried to one or both sides of the central slip insertion for its protection (**TECH FIG 6A**).
    - The Chamay approach may be used. A distally based triangular flap of the extensor mechanism is created; this provides excellent joint exposure and the extensor mechanism is later repaired (**TECH FIG 6B**).[1]
- Recess the collateral ligaments off their origin from the proximal phalanx head for later repair. Before final implant placement, drill holes adjacent to the collateral ligament origin to allow suture passage for ligament repair (**TECH FIG 6C**).
- The volar plate is protected with the dorsal approach.
- The remaining portion of the procedure is similar to that described as part of the volar approach.

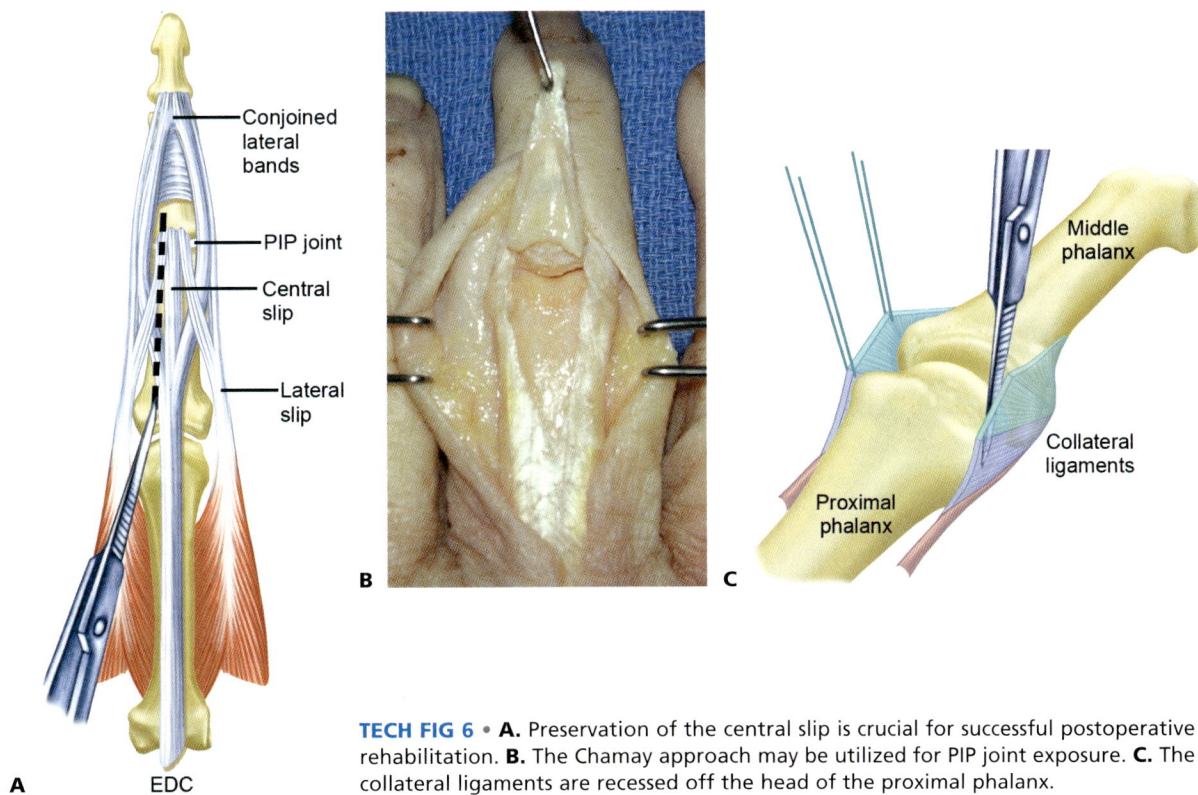

TECH FIG 6 • **A.** Preservation of the central slip is crucial for successful postoperative rehabilitation. **B.** The Chamay approach may be utilized for PIP joint exposure. **C.** The collateral ligaments are recessed off the head of the proximal phalanx.

PEARLS AND PITFALLS

Indications	■ Painless loss of motion is not an ideal indication; the operation does not reliably increase motion at long-term assessment.
	■ Osteoarthritis and posttraumatic arthritis are more common in the PIP joint than in the MCP joint. MCP arthroplasty has traditionally been performed for RA but has declined in frequency due to better control of disease in RA patients.
	■ PIP joint arthroplasty is helpful in maintaining motion in the ring and small fingers (for grip); PIP fusion is more acceptable in the index and long fingers (especially in workers).
	■ Avoid arthroplasty at both the MCP and PIP joints in one finger.
Technique	■ Broaching should be carefully performed to avoid penetration of the cortex and rotation of the implant.
	■ The central slip insertion must be carefully protected at the PIP joint.
	■ The implant fit must be carefully assessed; buckling of the implant requires bony or soft tissue adjustments before final implant placement.
Rehabilitation	■ Motion must be carefully allowed until joint encapsulation.
	■ Rotation or deformity after arthroplasty may be corrected with dynamic splinting.

POSTOPERATIVE CARE

■ The patient is placed in a plaster splint after surgery for 3 to 5 days. The MCP and PIP joints are immobilized in extension.

■ Some surgeons advocate 3 to 4 weeks of immobilization after MCP joint implant arthroplasty before the initiation of hand therapy.

■ Early joint motion is important for appropriate joint encapsulation.

■ An engaged hand therapist is crucial in obtaining a satisfactory surgical outcome.

■ Early therapy emphasizes edema control and patient comfort through splinting.

■ Subsequent therapy focuses on range of motion.

■ MCP joint arthroplasty, especially in the rheumatoid patient, requires meticulous postoperative hand therapy.

■ Dynamic extension (daytime) splints, static extension (nighttime) splints, or both are fabricated.

■ The alignment and motion of the fingers are carefully monitored. Adjustments to the splints are commonly required as the encapsulation process and the healing process progress.

■ Active and gentle passive motion are progressively allowed.

■ After PIP joint implant arthroplasty through a volar approach, the flexor and extensor mechanism need not be protected. Active and gentle passive motion may be initiated quickly, although the collateral ligament repairs should be protected for at least 6 weeks.

■ Dynamic extension splinting may be used during the first 6 weeks.

■ If the central slip was spared during a dorsal PIP joint approach and implant placement, early active motion is initiated with progression to gentle passive motion.

■ If the approach for PIP implant arthroplasty required central slip takedown and repair, the extensor mechanism should be carefully protected during the rehabilitation period.

OUTCOMES

■ Pain is reliably improved in patients with MCP or PIP joint arthroplasty.[2–7]

■ Most patients are improved functionally after silicone MCP arthroplasty. Patients with RA and a marked flexion and ulnar deviation posture of the MCP joints stand to benefit most.[2,3] While the arc of motion may be improved in the early postoperative period, at long-term follow-up the arc of motion is not dramatically increased; however, the arc is moved to a more extended and functional position.[2,3]

■ The ulnar drift of the MCP joints most commonly seen in RA is improved (although some recurrence in drift over time may also occur).[2,3]

■ MCP arthroplasty for osteoarthritis can be expected to maintain or somewhat improve MCP range of motion and strength while decreasing pain. In contrast to RA patients, MCP joint flexion may be increased in patients treated for osteoarthritis.[2,5]

■ PIP arthroplasty can be expected to place the PIP joint in a more extended and functional posture but should not be expected to increase range of motion at long-term follow-up. Total joint motion depends on the preoperative motion but typically averages about 45 degrees. Pain relief is reliable for most patients no matter what the diagnosis.[4,6,7]

■ PIP arthroplasty for RA may have a lesser outcome compared for PIP arthroplasty performed for posttraumatic arthritis or osteoarthritis. Patients with a boutonnière or swan-neck deformity are most likely to be unchanged or worse in regard to their deformity.[7]

■ PIP silicone implant survivorship decreases from 98% at 2 years to 80% at 10 years to 49% at 16 years (in a mixed population analysis).[7]

COMPLICATIONS

■ Infection

■ Implant fracture (which may or may not necessitate revision arthroplasty; if the encapsulated joint is stable, a fractured implant may not need to be addressed)

■ Rotational malalignment

■ Joint subluxation

■ Silicone synovitis

■ In RA patients, recurrent ulnar drift may occur.

REFERENCES

1. Chamay A. A distally based dorsal and triangular tendinous flap for direct access to the proximal interphalangeal joint. Ann Chir Main 1988;7:179–183.
2. Goldfarb CA, Stern PJ. Metacarpophalangeal joint arthroplasty in rheumatoid arthritis: a long- term assessment. J Bone Joint Surg Am 2003;85A:1869–1878.

3. Kirschenbaum D, Schneider LH, Adams DC, et al. Arthroplasty of the metacarpophalangeal joints with use of silicone-rubber implants in patients who have rheumatoid arthritis: long-term results. J Bone Joint Surg Am 1993;75A:3–12.

4. Lin HH, Wyrick JD, Stern PJ. Proximal interphalangeal joint silicone replacement arthroplasty: clinical results using an anterior approach. J Hand Surg Am 1995;20A:123–132.

5. Rettig LA, Luca L, Murphy MS. Silicone implant arthroplasty in patients with idiopathic osteoarthritis of the metacarpophalangeal joint. J Hand Surg Am 2005;30A:667–672.

6. Schneider LH. Proximal interphalangeal joint arthroplasty: the volar approach. Semin Arthroplasty 1991;2:139–147.

7. Takigawa S, Meletiou S, Sauerbier M, et al. Long-term assessment of Swanson implant arthroplasty in the proximal interphalangeal joint of the hand. J Hand Surg Am 2004;29:785–795.

Chapter 79

Proximal Interphalangeal and Metacarpophalangeal Joint Surface Replacement Arthroplasty

Peter M. Murray and Christopher R. Goll

DEFINITION

▪ Rheumatoid arthritis is a disorder that can affect the hands and can cause fatigue, muscle pain, loss of appetite, depression, weight loss, anemia, and immunocompromise. The effect on the hands is a combination of tenosynovitis and inflammation of the metacarpophalangeal (MCP) synovial lining of the joints (synovitis).[10,12]

▪ Rheumatoid arthritis less frequently involves the proximal interphalangeal (PIP) joints of the hand; more commonly, the PIP joints are affected by degenerative arthritis. Degenerative arthritis may occur after trauma or infection or may arise as an idiopathic process.[1]

ANATOMY

▪ Anatomy of the extensor tendon mechanism is shown in **FIG 1**.

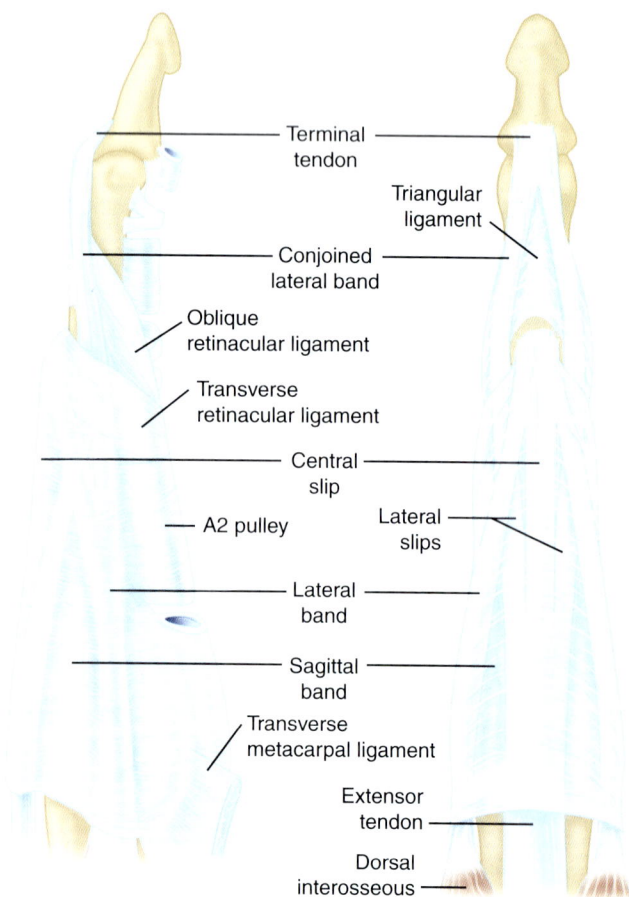

Terminal tendon
Triangular ligament
Conjoined lateral band
Oblique retinacular ligament
Transverse retinacular ligament
Central slip
A2 pulley
Lateral slips
Lateral band
Sagittal band
Transverse metacarpal ligament
Extensor tendon
Dorsal interosseous

FIG 1 • Anatomy of the extensor mechanism of the finger.

PATHOGENESIS

▪ Rheumatoid arthritis is a multifactorial entity and is poorly understood.

  ▪ The disease is autoimmune mediated and may occur after a bacterial or viral infection.

  ▪ There is a hereditary influence.

  ▪ The B lymphocytes, T lymphocytes, and macrophages lead to proliferation and hypertrophy of synovial cells. The enzymes released by these cells can cause bony erosions, ligamentous laxity, and tendon ruptures.[10]

▪ MCP joint deformities in rheumatoid patients include ulnar deviation and volar subluxation or dislocation of the proximal phalanx on the metacarpal head (**FIG 2**).[4,11]

  ▪ These deformities occur after synovial proliferation in the recesses between the collateral ligaments and the metacarpal head, attenuating the collateral ligaments.

  ▪ Radial inclinations of the metacarpals and wrist joint destruction often leads to an ulnar translation of the entire carpus. This translation can cause ulnar and volar extensor tendon subluxation between the metacarpal heads. Ulnar forces generated by the extensor apparatus and volar forces produced by the flexors lead to ulnar drift of the fingers and fixed MCP flexion deformities or volar dislocations of the MCP joints.

▪ Degenerative arthritis affecting the PIP joints of the hand is a process whereby the articular cartilage develops irreversible wear changes, caused by an incompletely understood mechanism. Subchondral bone stiffens and periarticular new bone formation occurs, which leads to restricted joint motion and pain.[9]

▪ Less commonly, degenerative arthritis can affect the MCP joints of the hand. This can occur after trauma, infection, or osteonecrosis.[9]

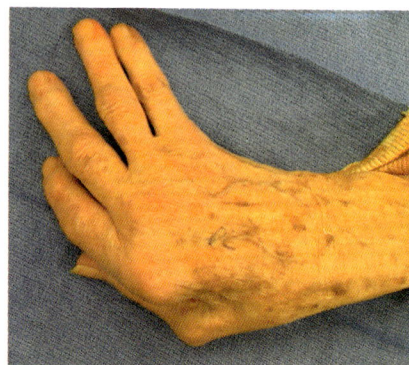

FIG 2 • Ulnar drift of the digits.

NATURAL HISTORY

- Rheumatoid arthritis has a variable prognosis based on the severity of the disease and the structures involved. Mild presentations may go undiagnosed for years, while severe presentations may progress to rapid joint destruction in the third or fourth decade of life.
- Three clinical stages of rheumatoid arthritis exist.
  - First, swelling of the synovial lining, which causes pain, warmth, stiffness, redness, and fullness around the joint
  - Second, synoviocyte hypertrophy and proliferation leading to synovial thickening
  - Third, enzymatic release causing bone and cartilage destruction, ligamentous laxity, and tendon ruptures
- Medical management as well as surgical synovectomy can halt or minimize progression of rheumatoid arthritis in the destructive stage.

PATIENT HISTORY AND PHYSICAL FINDINGS

- A thorough patient history and physical examination are important before implant arthroplasty of the fingers.
  - The surgeon should note the patient's occupation, hobbies, and expectations.
  - The history of the patient's condition is helpful in gauging the progression of the disease.
  - The primary indication for surface replacement arthroplasty of the MCP or PIP joints is pain relief. Correction of deformity and improvement in function are secondary considerations. Mild deformity may be painful for some, while profound deformity may be painless and functional for others.
- Examination of the entire upper extremity should be performed. Although the order of reconstruction is controversial, deficits of the shoulder, wrist, and elbow should be addressed before addressing hand conditions.
- Particular attention should be paid to elements of radiocarpal instability or ulnar translation of the carpus. In some situations a wrist arthrodesis may be necessary before performing MCP arthroplasties.
  - Failure to correct carpal collapse and radial deviation of the metacarpals can result in recurrence of ulnar drift deformity after MCP arthroplasty.
- Careful examination of flexor and extensor tendons of the hand and wrist should be performed. The extensor digiti quinti minimi, extensor pollicis longus, and flexor pollicis longus often rupture in more active forms of rheumatoid arthritis.
  - Extensor tendon or flexor tendon ruptures should be treated before considering implant arthroplasty of the hand.
- Examination of the PIP joint should include range-of-motion assessment of the joint, assessment of volar plate integrity, central slip integrity, and collateral ligament stability.
  - Normal range of motion of the PIP joint is 0 to 110 degrees.
  - Varus and valgus stability should be compared to the contralateral side.
  - Failure of volar plate integrity in rheumatoid arthritis can lead to swan-neck deformity, which is characterized by PIP joint hyperextension, dorsal subluxation of the lateral

bands, and flexion of the distal phalangeal joint. The swan-neck deformity is considered a relative contraindication for surface replacement arthroplasty of the PIP joint (**FIG 3A**).
  - A boutonnière deformity is caused by failure of the central slip mechanism. This can occur in rheumatoid arthritis or after trauma (**FIG 3B**). It is characterized by flexion of the PIP joint due to central slip incompetence, volar subluxation of the lateral bands, and hyperextension of the DIP joint.
- Normal MCP range of motion is between 0 and 90 degrees.
- Instability testing: The individual MCP or PIP joints are tested by the examiner grasping the patient's finger and then applying a valgus and then a varus stress. The resultant motion is compared to the contralateral side. Differences in laxity indicate ligamentous instability. Attempts at hyperextension of the digit at the PIP or the MCP joint can identify volar plate instability and the propensity of the digit to subluxate or dislocate. Surface replacement arthroplasty of either the MCP or the PIP joint is contraindicated in patients with ligamentous instability as these are minimally constrained devices.
  - Grade 1: No difference in joint line opening compared to the contralateral joint
  - Grade 2: Notable opening of the joint line compared to the contralateral joint, but a solid "endpoint" is reached
  - Grade 3: Complete opening of the radial or lateral joint line with valgus or varus stress. This can be demonstrated at either the MCP or the PIP joints. No endpoint can be discerned.
- Bunnell test of intrinsic tightness of the PIP joints: The resistance encountered with the MCP joint in this position is compared with the resistance encountered with the MCP joint

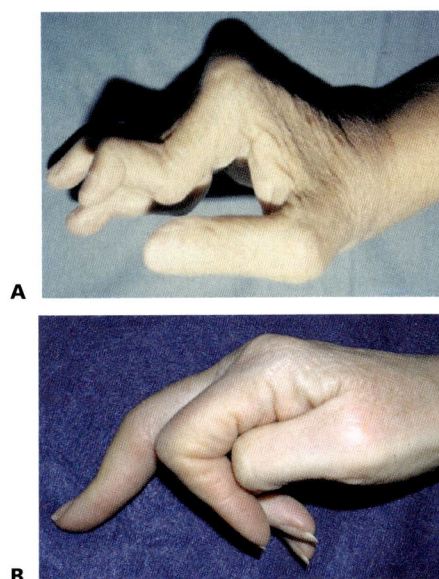

FIG 3 • **A.** Rheumatoid arthritis of the hand demonstrating swan-neck deformities and volar subluxation of the metacarpophalangeal joints. **B.** Boutonnière deformity of the digit.

in the flexed position. An increase of resistance with the MCP joint in the extended position indicates intrinsic tightness of that digit.

- It is important to distinguish intrinsic tightness from extrinsic tightness. Extrinsic tightness is encountered when the long extensors of the digits are adherent to either the surrounding soft tissues or the metacarpals. The result is increased resistance to flexion of the PIP joint with the MCP in flexion. In either instance, the limitation of motion is important to clarity as it can affect the outcome of implant arthroplasty of the MCP or the PIP joint.

IMAGING AND OTHER DIAGNOSTIC STUDIES

- Posteroanterior, lateral, and oblique views of the hands will adequately image the MCP joints. Brewerton views may add additional information.
- Posteroanterior and lateral views are sufficient to image the PIP joints.

DIFFERENTIAL DIAGNOSIS

- Psoriatic arthritis
- Chronic septic arthritis
- Osteomyelitis
- Gout
- Calcium pyrophosphate dihydrate arthropathy
- Articular malunions of the MCP and PIP joints
- Scleroderma
- Lupus

NONOPERATIVE MANAGEMENT

- Nonoperative management in rapidly progressing rheumatoid arthritis is largely ineffective.
- In the quiescent forms of rheumatoid arthritis, nighttime wrist and hand splinting in conjunction with medical management may provide pain relief. Various combinations of methotrexate, prednisone, remitting agents, and nonsteroidal anti-inflammatory agents may prove effective for extended periods in certain cases.
- During periods of active rheumatoid arthritis of the MCP joints, corticosteroid injections into the joint may provide acute pain relief and improve function in the short term.
- The symptoms of MCP and PIP joint degenerative arthritis may come and go, successfully responding to nighttime wrist and hand splinting and nonsteroidal anti-inflammatory agents.
- Corticosteroid injection into the MCP and PIP joints for advanced degenerative arthritis seldom provides long-term benefits.

SURGICAL MANAGEMENT

- The indications for surface replacement or pyrocarbon MCP arthroplasty are similar to those for flexible MCP implants. These include pain in the face of deformity and worsening function.
  - Surface replacement implants are designed to recreate the anatomy of a native joint, potentially resulting in greater stability than with flexible MCP implants.

- The enhanced stability of these implants is best demonstrated in the index and long fingers, where flexible MCP implants are prone to failure.
- Contraindications to surface replacement implant arthroplasty of the MCP joint include infection, lack of adequate bone stock, insufficient radial or ulnar collateral ligament support, lack of adequate soft tissue coverage, and excessively small metacarpal or proximal phalanx medullary canals.
  - These implants rely on intact soft tissue elements. This includes functioning flexors and extensors as well as intact radial and ulnar collateral ligaments.
- Indications for PIP joint surface replacement arthroplasty are pain and diminishing function in the context of advanced radiographic articular degeneration.[1,7]
- Contraindications to PIP joint surface replacement arthroplasty include inadequate bone stock of either the proximal or the middle phalanx, ulnar or radial collateral ligament insufficiency, acute or chronic infection, inadequate soft tissue coverage, insufficient digital flexor function, or disruption of the extensor central slip insertion on the middle phalanx.
  - Relative contraindications include the presence of a static swan-neck[8] or boutonnière deformity.
  - In general PIP joint surface replacement arthroplasty is not indicated in patients with rheumatoid arthritis.
- The importance of postoperative therapy should be emphasized. To ensure that the implants heal with a stable and a functional range of motion the patient must wear a combination of static and dynamic splints for several weeks to months after. Patients must also be aware that heavy lifting or gripping must be avoided indefinitely.

Preoperative Planning

- Sizing templates with a 3% parallax enlargement are available for MCP and PIP joint systems and should be used preoperatively to give the surgeon an idea of the size implant required.

Positioning

- The patient is positioned supine with the arm placed on an armboard for either MCP or PIP joint surface replacement arthroplasty.
- A nonsterile tourniquet is placed proximal to the drapes on the arm.
- The hand is pronated to allow access to the dorsum.

Approach

- For MCP surface replacement arthroplasty, two different incisions can be used.
  - A transverse incision across the dorsum of the hand, centered over the MCP joints, will facilitate access to multiple joints.
  - Alternatively, multiple longitudinal incisions can be used to address all four MCP joints.
  - If a single joint is being addressed, a longitudinal incision should be used.
- For PIP joint surface replacement arthroplasty, a midline longitudinal incision is preferred.
  - Alternative approaches include the lateral approach and the volar approach.

METACARPOPHALANGEAL JOINT SURFACE REPLACEMENT ARTHROPLASTY

Exposure

- Incise the extensor hood just ulnar to the extensor mechanism.
- Carry dissection down through the subcutaneous tissue to expose the extensor tendons.
  - Preserve the dorsal veins.
- Retract the extensor hood and extensor mechanism radialward.
- In the rheumatoid patient, the extensor tendon ulnarly translates with destruction of the radial sagittal band. If possible, dissect the sagittal bands from the capsule and preserve them so that the extensor tendon can be relocated and the sagittal bands imbricated at the end of the procedure in order to maintain a centralized extensor tendon position.
- Incise the remnants of the MCP joint capsule and use small Hohmann retractors to deliver the head of the metacarpal into the wound.
- After the joint is exposed, perform a synovectomy, carefully preserving the collateral ligaments.
- If the joint is irreducible, it may be necessary to release one or both collateral ligaments from their origins.
  - Tag the ends of the collateral ligaments for later repair to their tuberosity origins.

Joint Preparation and Trial Implant Insertion

- Use a metacarpal sizing template to identify the appropriate amount of metacarpal head to be resected.
- Remove the metacarpal head by first making a vertical saw cut distal to the collateral ligaments. A second cut oriented 45 degrees proximally and volarly removes the remainder of the metacarpal head, retaining the collateral ligament origins.
- Remove the articular surface along with a small portion of the base of the proximal phalanx, preserving the collateral ligaments (**TECH FIG 1A**).
  - Contracture of the ulnar capsule may require detaching the ulnar collateral ligament to achieve alignment of the finger in some circumstances.
- Insert an awl into the dorsal aspect of the intramedullary canal of the metacarpal (**TECH FIG 1B**).
- Perform sequential broaching for the metacarpal until a proper fit has been attained.
  - For the index and long finger, the broaching is slightly ulnarly displaced. This provides a better moment arm for the radial intrinsic and extrinsic tendons to compensate for ulnar drift.
- Repeat the broaching in a similar fashion for the proximal phalanx.
- A plastic impactor with a concave surface aids insertion of the metacarpal proximal trial component.
  - The tip of the prosthesis should pass the midpoint of the metacarpal.
  - Avoid forceful impaction in order to avoid fracture.
- A convex impactor aids insertion and seating of the distal component.
- Once the trial components are inserted and the joint is reduced, check component fit and position using an image intensifier. Then assess range of motion, component tracking, and stability.
  - Revisions of bone cuts may be necessary for soft tissue balancing and to ensure adequate range of motion.
- If release of the collateral ligaments was required, drill two holes through the tuberosity at the dorsal radial and dorsal ulnar aspect of the remaining metacarpal head for reattachment of the ligaments.

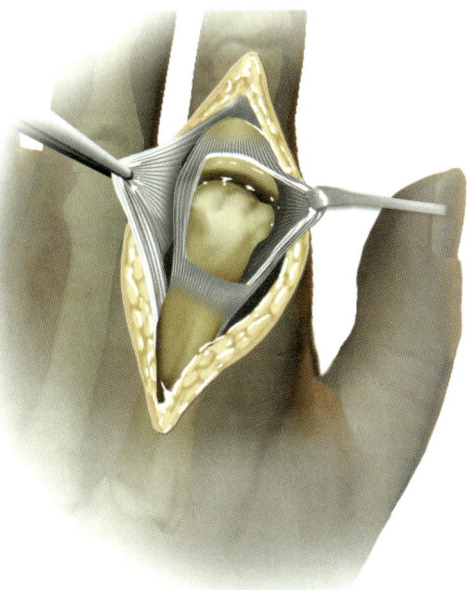

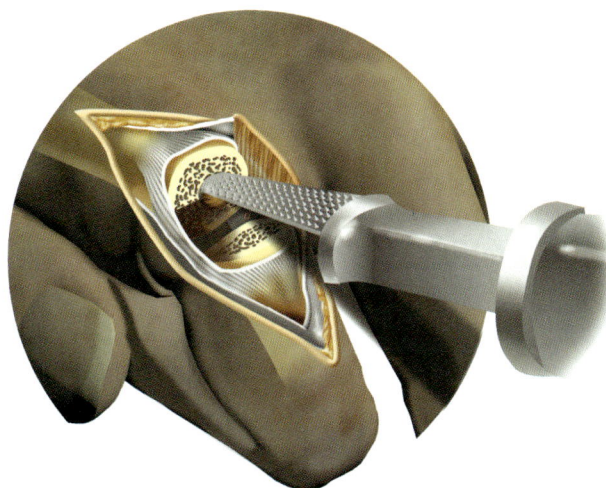

A   B

TECH FIG 1 • A. Exposure of the metacarpophalangeal (MCP) joint demonstrating the bone cuts for preparation of MCP surface replacement arthroplasty. **B.** Broaching of the metacarpal preparing for MCP surface replacement arthroplasty. (Courtesy of Small Bone Innovations, Morrisville, PA.)

TECHNIQUES

Insert sutures for repair of the collateral ligament (4-0 Ticron/Mersilene).

Final Implant Insertion

- Irrigate the intramedullary canal with saline and 0.5% neomycin solution, then dry it.
- Inject polymethylmethacrylate (PMMA) in a liquid state into the metacarpal and the proximal phalanx using a size no. 14 plastic angiocath catheter attached to a 10-cc syringe.
  - Under some circumstances "finger packing" may be necessary.
- Insert the distal component first. Convex and concave plastic impactors are provided to assist in implant insertion (**TECH FIG 2**).
  - Avoid impacting with metallic instruments, which can accelerate prosthetic wear.
- The joint is extended and viewed under the image intensifier before allowing the cement to harden so that last-minute corrections in alignment can be made.
- Cement fixation of one finger at a time is advisable if positioning is difficult.
  - If multiple MCP joints are to be implanted, it may be easier to do the distal components as a group, followed by the proximal components.
- After the cement has cured, check passive range of motion to ensure adequate range without impingement or prosthetic binding.

Closure and Soft Tissue Balancing

- After hardening of the cement, tighten the collateral ligaments or reattach them to the tuberosity of the metacarpal head with nonabsorbable suture.
  - Ensure proper radial and ulnar stability as well as rotational alignment before securing the sutures.
- Close any remaining capsule with absorbable suture before extensor apparatus closure.
- Centralize the extensor tendon and imbricate the radial sagittal bands in rheumatoid hands using nonabsorbable suture.
  - A pants-over-vest centralization of the sagittal bands may be required in moderate to severe ulnar drift along with intrinsic releases or crossed-intrinsic transfers (**TECH FIG 3**).
  - With the finger held in slight overcorrection, imbricate the radial sagittal band over the extensor tendon.
- The skin is closed in a routine manner and a splint is applied with the MCP joints in slight flexion.

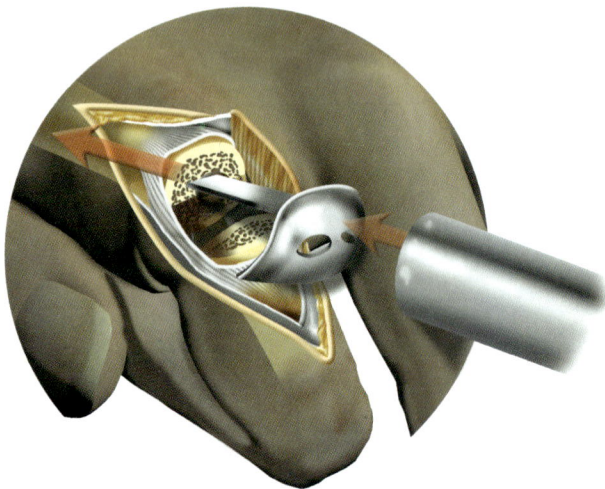

TECH FIG 2 • Insertion of the metacarpal component of the metacarpophalangeal surface replacement arthroplasty. (Courtesy of Small Bone Innovations, Morrisville, PA.)

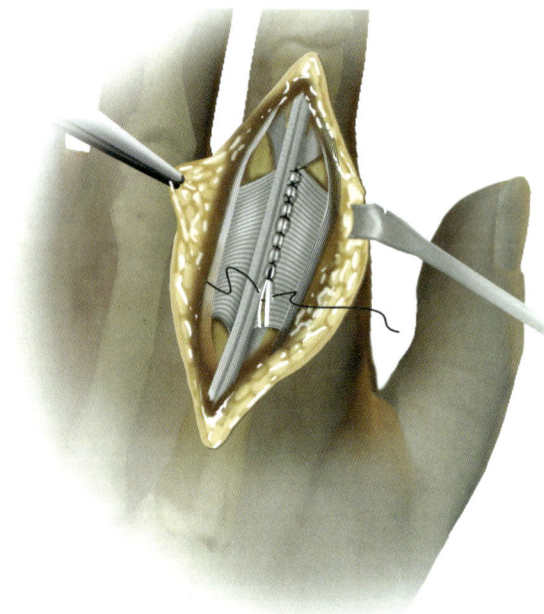

TECH FIG 3 • Radially directed "pants-over-vest" reefing of the extensor mechanism after metacarpophalangeal surface replacement arthroplasty. (Courtesy of Small Bone Innovations, Morrisville, PA.)

PROXIMAL INTERPHALANGEAL JOINT SURFACE REPLACEMENT ARTHROPLASTY

Exposure

- Through a midline longitudinal incision, reflect the extensor tendon distally by creating a distally based flap, as described by Chamay[2] (**TECH FIG 4A**).
- Identify and incise remnants of the dorsal PIP joint capsule.
- Protect the radial and ulnar collateral ligaments using small Hohmann retractors while bringing the articular surface of the middle phalanx into view.

Joint Preparation and Trial Implant Insertion

- Resect the proximal phalanx head by an osteotomy performed 90 degrees to the long axis of the proximal phalanx, just proximal to the most proximal extent of the articular surface (**TECH FIG 4A**).
- During the osteotomy, protect the origins of the radial and ulnar collateral ligaments by using small retractors or by hyperflexing the joint.
  - It may be necessary to release a small portion of the proximal phalangeal origin of the collateral ligaments to facilitate the proximal phalangeal osteotomy and prosthesis insertion.
  - Minamikawa et al[8] have shown that the PIP joint remains stable after removal of 50% of the collateral ligament substance.
- While protecting the volar plate with a small retractor, use a 2-mm burr to assist in making a small back cut (or chamfer cut) to accept the posterior aspect of the prosthetic condyles of the proximal phalangeal component.
  - This can also be accomplished with the oscillating saw, but that can place the volar plate at risk.
- Make a perpendicular osteotomy at the base of the middle phalanx with a small rongeur and remove no more than 1 to 2 mm of bone.
  - Protect the collateral ligament insertions with small retractors or by hyperflexing the digit.

- Broach the proximal and middle phalanges with specific and sequential instruments.
  - Broach the proximal and middle phalanges to the largest size possible (**TECH FIG 4B**).
  - Undersized components can result in limited motion due to bony impingement during flexion.
- Insert the trial components using proximal and middle phalanx-specific impactors.
  - The components are not modular and are generally not interchanged. Under certain circumstances, such as revision surgery, it is permissible to implant unmatched sizes, but no more than one size up or one size down should be used.
- After trial component insertion, examine the digit for implant position, range of motion, and stability as detailed for the MCP joint. Make appropriate adjustments.

Final Implant Insertion and Closure

- Implant the permanent components by "press-fit" using the "no-touch" technique.
  - Cementing is discouraged except perhaps in cases with capacious canals or in patients with substantial bone loss or articular erosion. In these circumstances, the prosthetic stems and flanges are simply coated with cement. Excessive cement packing into the medullary canal is not necessary.
  - Another technique is to pack the canal with morselized allograft bone. This is analogous to

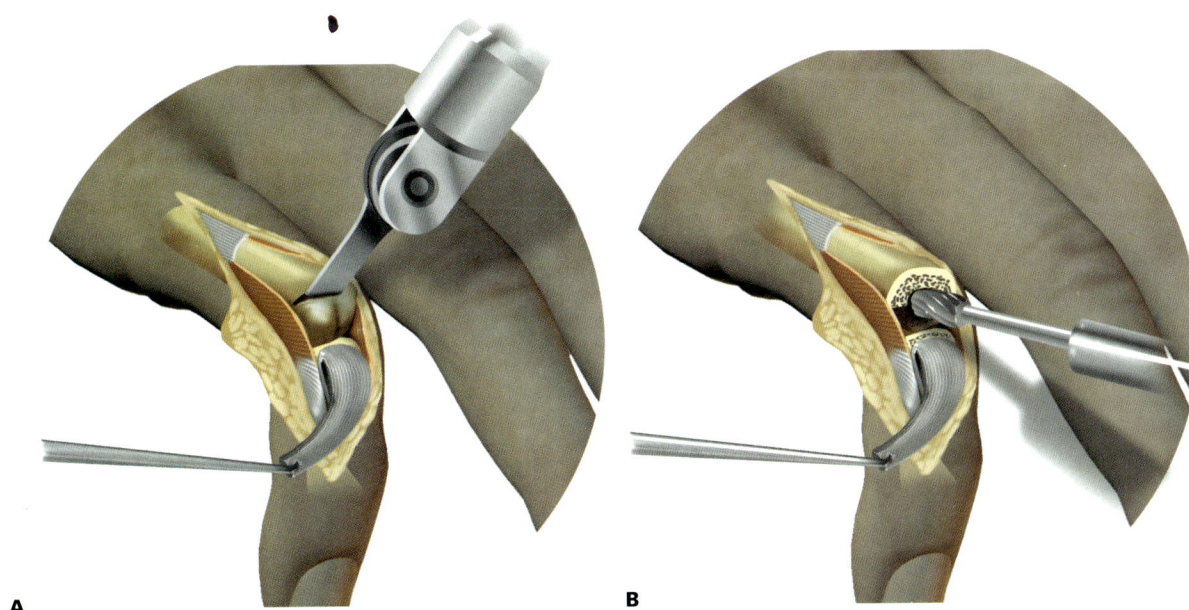

TECH FIG 4 • A. Proximal phalanx exposed using the Chamay approach. An oscillating saw is used to accomplish an osteotomy in preparation for the proximal interphalangeal joint surface replacement arthroplasty placement. **B.** Broaching of the proximal phalanx in preparation for proximal interphalangeal joint surface replacement arthroplasty.

the Ling technique described for revision total hip arthroplasty.[5]

- Using specific impactors, seat the permanent components (**TECH FIG 5**).
- Repair the extensor mechanism with 3-0 Surgilon suture.
- Release the tourniquet before skin closure.
- The patient leaves the operating room with a sterile dressing, splinted in extension.

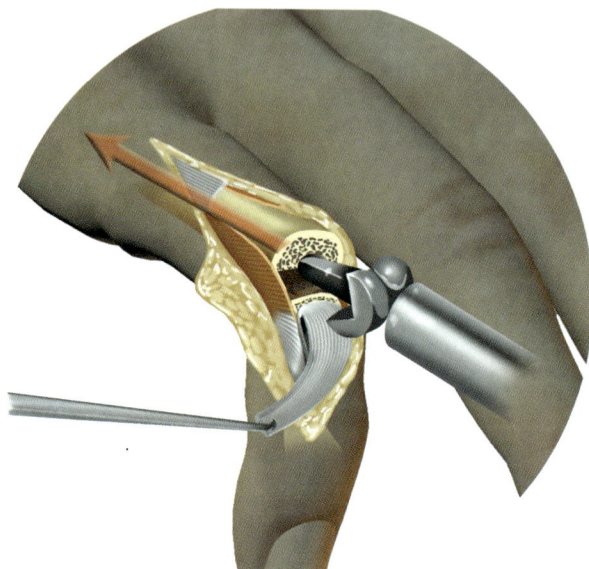

TECH FIG 5 • Insertion of the proximal phalangeal component of the proximal interphalangeal surface replacement arthroplasty. (Courtesy of Small Bone Innovations, Morrisville, PA.)

PEARLS AND PITFALLS

PIP joint surface replacement arthroplasty	■ Take care to preserve the insertion of the central slip. ■ Osteotomy of the proximal phalanx must avoid the origin of the PIP joint collateral ligaments. ■ Remove only a small amount of bone from the middle phalanx. ■ Broach the proximal phalanx to the largest size that can be accommodated. Failure to use appropriate-sized implants may result in subsidence of the implants and posterior cortical impingement of the phalanges.
MCP joint surface replacement arthroplasty	■ Contracture of the ulnar capsule may require detaching the ulnar collateral ligament. ■ Broaching of the index finger should be slightly ulnarly displaced. ■ Centralization of the extensor tendon is generally necessary in rheumatoid hands; it can be achieved by imbricating the radial sagittal bands. ■ Imbrication of the radial sagittal bands should be performed with the digit in radial deviation. ■ "Water-tight" closure of the extensor mechanism is necessary to prevent PIP joint flexion lag or contracture.

POSTOPERATIVE CARE

- Postoperatively the MCP joints should be placed in slight flexion and the PIP joints in about 45 degrees of flexion. If there was ulnar deviation before surgery, the fingers should be placed in 10 degrees of radial deviation.
- The dressing is removed 2 to 4 days after surgery and a dynamic splint is applied for daytime exercises. A static rest or nocturnal splint capable of holding the fingers in the corrected position is used for 4 to 6 weeks.
- The rehabilitation program is enhanced by the close supervision of a hand therapist. The first week of therapy is best carried out with daily supervision.
- Follow-up examinations should include range-of-motion assessment for all the joints of the hand and wrist. Static deformities, grip strength, and pinch strength should also be assessed and recorded.
- Follow-up radiographic examination includes posteroanterior, lateral, and oblique views of the hand. Any residual deformity should also be assessed and recorded.
- For the PIP joint surface replacement arthroplasty, a controlled rehabilitation protocol is needed to prevent central slip failure.

- Initiation of formal postoperative rehabilitation is encouraged by postoperative day 5. A dynamic extension splint permitting active flexion is applied at this time and used for about 6 weeks. A static forearm-based digital extension splint is used at bedtime.
  - During the first 2 weeks after surgery, PIP flexion is limited to 30 degrees.
  - Flexion to 60 degrees is allowed beginning at 4 weeks.
  - By 6 weeks, the extension outrigger splint is discontinued and unrestricted flexion and extension is permitted.
  - The static bedtime splint is used for an additional 6 weeks. Heavy lifting or gripping is not permitted.

OUTCOMES

- Initial results after 76 PIP joint surface replacement arthroplasties were published.[6]
  - At a mean follow-up of 4.5 years, 32 joints had good results, 19 fair, and 25 poor.
  - Better results were obtained with arthroplasties performed through a dorsal approach rather than the volar approach.
  - Range of motion at follow-up averaged −14 degrees of extension and 61 degrees of flexion. There was a 12-degree

improvement in the flexion–extension arc compared to the preoperative examination.

■ The MCP joint surface replacement arthroplasty (Small Bone Innovations, Morrisville, PA) has been available in Europe for 8 years and is under clinical trial in the United States. No series has been published reporting results of this implant. Although from a theoretical perspective there are advantages to the use of the MCPJ surface replacement arthroplasty, it currently cannot be considered a replacement for the Swanson Silastic MCP joint spacer.

■ Previous primate studies have shown no evidence of debris or inflammatory reaction after implantation of the pyrolytic carbon MCP joint arthroplasty. Good bone incorporation of the prosthesis was also observed.

■ In contrast to the Small Bone Innovations MCP joint surface replacement arthroplasty, a series of 151 pyrolytic carbon MCP prostheses (Ascension Orthopaedics, Austin, TX) implanted over an 8-year period, mostly in patients with rheumatoid arthritis, have been followed for an average of 11.7 years.[3]

■ The arc of MCP joint motion improved an average of 130 degrees.

■ The 10-year survivorship was 81.4%.

■ At follow-up, the degree of digital ulnar drift was the same as preoperative.

■ Complications led to 18 implant revisions (12%).

COMPLICATIONS

■ PIP

■ Failure of the central slip can occur, resulting in extensor lag or, more commonly, a flexion contracture or boutonnière deformity.

■ With the volar approach, failure of the volar plate may occur, leading to swan-neck deformity.

■ Tenodesis as well as joint instability and joint subluxation can occur.

■ Postoperative infection or prosthesis loosening is seldom seen.[6]

■ MCP

■ Stiffness

■ Loosening

■ Subluxation

■ Proliferative synovitis

REFERENCES

1. Amadio PC, Murray PM, Linscheid RL. PIP arthroplasty. In: Morrey BF, ed. Joint Replacement Arthroplasty, 3rd ed. Churchill Livingstone, 2003:163–174.
2. Chamay A. A distally based dorsal and triangular tendinous flap for direct access to the proximal interphalangeal joint. Ann Chir Main 1988;7:179–183.
3. Cook SD, Beckenbaugh RD, Redondo J, et al. Long-term follow-up of pyrolytic carbon metacarpophalangeal implants. J Bone Joint Surg Am 1999;81A:635–648.
4. Flatt AE. Some pathomechanics of ulnar drift. Plast Reconstr Surg 1966;37:295–303.
5. Halliday BR, English HW, Timperley AJ, et al. Femoral impaction grafting with cement in revision total hip replacement: evolution of the technique and results. J Bone Joint Surg Br 2003;85B:809–817.
6. Linscheid RL, Murray PM, Vidal MA, et al. Development of a surface replacement arthroplasty for proximal interphalangeal joints. J Hand Surg Am 1997;22A:286–298.
7. Linscheid RL. Implant arthroplasty of the hand: retrospective and prospective considerations. J Hand Surg Am 2000;25A:796–816.
8. Minamikawa Y, Horii E, Amadio PC, et al. Stability and constraint of the proximal interphalangeal joint. J Hand Surg Am 1993;18:198–204.
9. Murray PM. New-generation implant arthroplasties of the finger joints. J Am Acad Orthop Surg 2003;11:295–301.
10. Smith RJ, Kaplan EB. Rheumatoid deformities at the metacarpophalangeal joints of the fingers: a correlative study of anatomy and pathology. J Bone Joint Surg Am 1967;49A:31–37.
11. Stack HG, Vaughan-Jackson OJ. The zigzag deformity in the rheumatoid hand. Hand 1971;3:62–67.
12. Wilson RL, Carlblom ER. The rheumatoid metacarpophalangeal joint. Hand Clin 1989;5:223–237.

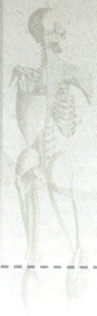

Chapter 80

Distal Interphalangeal, Proximal Interphalangeal, and Metacarpophalangeal Joint Arthrodesis

Charles Cassidy and Jennifer Green

DEFINITION

- Conditions resulting in the need for arthrodesis in the hand include arthritis, unreconstructable soft tissue problems, and certain neurologic conditions.

ANATOMY

- The proximal (PIP) and distal (DIP) interphalangeal joint configurations are quite similar.
  - The condylar heads are biconvex but slightly asymmetric, being about twice as wide volarly as dorsally.
  - The reciprocal bases of the distal segment are biconcave, having a central ridge.
- The volar plate extends from the neck of the phalanx to the volar base of the more distal phalanx, preventing joint hyperextension.
- Radial and ulnar collateral ligaments provide additional joint stability. The "true" collateral ligaments have bony attachments at both ends, whereas the accessory collateral ligaments extend from the condylar head to the volar plate.
- The axis of rotation and radius of curvature for a given interphalangeal joint are fairly constant. Consequently, the true collateral ligaments are effectively isometric, while the accessory collateral ligaments resist lateral translation when the joint is extended.
- As a result of the ligamentous and bony architecture, the PIP and DIP joints normally function as highly constrained hinge joints.
- The extensor tendon crosses the DIP joint dorsally as the terminal tendon, inserting slightly distal to the dorsal base of the distal phalanx.
  - The germinal matrix of the nailbed is close to the terminal tendon insertion (average of 1.3 mm distal).
- The flexor digitorum profundus (FDP) tendon inserts broadly on the volar aspect of the distal phalanx, extending from the base to the midshaft.
- Over the PIP joint, the extensor apparatus splits into thirds. Contributions from the extensor tendon, the interosseous tendons, and lumbricals form the central slip, which inserts onto the dorsal base of the middle phalanx. The lateral bands travel past the PIP joint along the lateral margins, and then combine to form the terminal tendon distally.
- The flexor digitorum superficialis (FDS) tendon splits to insert on the volar lateral margins of the proximal shaft of the middle phalanx.
- Unlike the interphalangeal joints, the metacarpophalangeal joints (MCP) are multiaxial, permitting motion in multiple planes.
- The metacarpal head has a complex, convex shape. Viewed end-on, the metacarpal head is pear-shaped, being wider volarly. In the sagittal plane, the radius of curvature increases progressively from dorsal to volar.
- The metacarpal attachment of the collateral ligaments is dorsal to the axis of rotation. The phalangeal and volar plate attachments are similar to the interphalangeal joint.
- As a consequence of the metacarpal head shape and ligament attachments, the MCP joints are typically more lax in extension and tight in flexion.
- Significant variability exists in the shape of the thumb metacarpal head. Some heads are more square than round, potentially limiting lateral translation and MCP flexion.
- In the thumb, the extensor pollicis brevis (EPB) tendon inserts onto the dorsal base of the proximal phalanx. The size of the EPB tendon is variable.
  - For some patients, the extensor pollicis longus (EPL) tendon assumes the major role in MCP joint extension.
  - In the other digits, no direct extensor attachment exists. MCP joint extension occurs through a sling effect of the sagittal hood fibers lifting the proximal phalanx through the pull of the extensor tendon.
- MCP joint flexion is produced through a combination of direct intrinsic tendon attachments to the volar-lateral phalangeal base and indirect actions of the intrinsics on the more distal transverse fibers of the extensor hood.

PATHOGENESIS

- Arthritis is the principal indication for small joint arthrodesis.
- Osteoarthritis (OA) most commonly affects the DIP joints. It is estimated that at least 60% of individuals over age 60 have DIP joint arthritis, which may not necessarily be symptomatic.
- In the early stages, the joints may be painful and swollen in spite of normal radiographs. As the arthritis progresses, osteophytes and mucous cysts may develop. Bony prominences (Heberden nodes) and angular deformities in both the coronal and sagittal planes (mallet appearance) may develop. In the final stages, DIP joint motion may be severely restricted.
- OA may also involve the PIP joints and the MCP joints, especially in the index and middle fingers.
- Inflammatory arthritis may also affect the small joints of the hand. About 70% of rheumatoid patients have hand involvement. Synovitis may result in deformity due to attenuation of supporting structures (collateral ligaments, extensor tendons) long before arthritic changes are evident.
  - At the DIP joint, terminal tendon incompetence may result in a secondary swan-neck deformity.
  - At the PIP joint, central slip attenuation results in a boutonnière deformity.
  - At the MCP joint, collateral ligament involvement may contribute to ulnar drift. Persistent synovitis produces cartilage loss.

- Hand involvement in systemic lupus erythematosus (SLE) may mimic rheumatoid arthritis. Supporting structures are affected principally in SLE, which may result in joint subluxation or dislocation with relatively normal-appearing articular cartilage. The capsuloligamentous problems may compromise attempts at joint salvage.
- In contrast, psoriatic arthritis may produce a remarkable degree of bone loss as the arthritis progresses. Pencil-in-cup deformity is a characteristic feature of psoriatic arthritis of the interphalangeal joints. Severe bone resorption is the characteristic feature of arthritis mutilans, most commonly seen in patients with psoriatic arthritis. Arthrodesis is the most reliable method for halting this destructive process.
- Scleroderma typically produces PIP flexion and MCP extension contractures. Impaired vascularity of the digits may result in dorsal PIP ulcer formation and central slip attenuation, compounding the PIP flexion deformity.
- Presentations of crystalline arthropathy in the small joints of the hand may be varied. The process may be indolent, presenting as gouty tophi over the DIP joint, or acute, presenting as an exquisitely painful, swollen, tender joint. Untreated, gout results in a resorptive arthritis.
- Infection is another cause of small joint arthritis.
  - A "fight bite" directly inoculates the MCP joint and, if undertreated, can result in rapid joint destruction.
  - Contiguous spread, for example, from a felon or a wound over the DIP or PIP joint, may destroy the adjacent joint.
  - Hematogenous spread is an uncommon cause of septic arthritis in the hand.
- Trauma is another cause of unreconstructable problems in the small joints of the hand.
  - Intra-articular fractures and fracture-dislocations may result in arthritis, particularly in cases of residual joint incongruity. The PIP joint does not tolerate injury well.
  - Severe periarticular soft tissue injuries may cause severe joint stiffness, even if the underlying joint surface is not initially involved. Certain soft tissue injuries, such as central slip disruptions, may confound attempts at reconstruction.
- Central or peripheral nerve injury may produce imbalances in the hand. Arthrodesis can potentially simplify reconstructions in an effort to improve function.

PATIENT HISTORY AND PHYSICAL FINDINGS

- Pain is the most common complaint of patients who are candidates for arthrodesis. Ideally, the location of the pain should correlate with the joint in question.
- In OA, multiple DIP joints may appear abnormal, although they may not necessarily be painful.
- Polyarticular involvement is common in rheumatoid arthritis. A priority list should be elicited from the patient.
- Handedness, occupation, and avocational activities should be documented.
- The functional impact of the problem should be clearly defined.
- When a single joint is involved, a history of trauma should be sought.
- In cases of acute, painful swelling, a history of penetrating injury, gout, or recent infection should be considered.
- The physical examination should include the appearance of joints and overlying skin, active and passive range of motion

of the affected joints, stability, grip and pinch strength, and sensibility.
- The status of adjacent joints should be evaluated.
  - For example, chronic DIP OA resulting in a DIP flexion deformity may produce a secondary hyperextension deformity of the PIP (swan-neck) that may be more disabling than the primary (DIP) problem.
- Multiple DIP joint bumps (Heberden nodes) are a characteristic feature of OA.
- Mucous cysts are suggestive of underlying DIP OA.
- Onycholysis and eczema are suggestive of psoriatic arthritis.
- Discrepancies between active and passive motion are indicative of an associated tendon problem.
- Stress examination may demonstrate collateral ligament incompetence.

IMAGING AND OTHER DIAGNOSTIC STUDIES

- Plain radiographs (posteroanterior [PA], lateral, oblique) of the affected digit are usually sufficient to make the diagnosis.
- In cases of suspected inflammatory arthritis, a collagen vascular screen is ordered. This blood panel includes a rheumatoid factor, ANA, complete blood count with differential, erythrocyte sedimentation rate (ESR), and C-reactive protein (CRP).
- A uric acid level may be drawn in cases of suspected gout.
- Blood tests are not generally helpful in the setting of an acute finger infection.
- MRI or ultrasound may rarely be ordered to evaluate tendon pathology if stiffness is associated with tendon abnormality.

DIFFERENTIAL DIAGNOSIS

- OA
- Inflammatory arthritis (rheumatoid, SLE, psoriatic arthritis)
- Crystal arthritis
- Posttraumatic arthritis
- Infection

NONOPERATIVE MANAGEMENT

- The mainstays of nonoperative treatment for unreconstructable small joint problems in the hand include oral medications, splints, and intra-articular corticosteroid injections.
- For OA and posttraumatic arthritis, oral anti-inflammatory agents may reduce pain and stiffness.
  - Glucosamine and chondroitin sulfate appear to be of limited value for hand arthritis.
- Rheumatoid patients can consider modifications in their medication regimen, supervised by a rheumatologist.
- Resting splints may reduce pain and inflammation.
  - At the DIP and PIP joints, a simple padded aluminum splint may suffice.
  - Corrective splints, such as the safety pin static progressive or LMB dynamic splint (DeRoyal), will not be tolerated when the joint is inflamed.
  - For the thumb MCP joint, a hand-based thermoplast splint may lessen discomfort and improve function.
  - Buddy taping to the adjacent digit may be appropriate for some MCP joint problems. Dynamic MCP joint splints are usually reserved for postoperative protection.
- Corticosteroid injections may provide temporary relief of pain and synovitis. The joint may be difficult to access and the joint capacity is quite small.

■ The surgeon should use a 27-gauge needle and inject 0.5 mL of Celestone Soluspan and 0.5 mL of 1% Xylocaine through a dorsal approach.

SURGICAL MANAGEMENT

Arthrodesis Versus Arthroplasty

■ Arthrodesis is a reliable procedure for managing arthritis and instability of the DIP joint. The functional impairment from loss of motion at the DIP joint is minimal.

■ At the PIP joint level, the surgeon and patient must weigh the potential benefits of stability and pain relief against the functional impairment resulting from the loss of PIP joint motion. For the index finger, PIP joint stability is critical for pinch. On the other hand, in the small finger, PIP joint mobility is necessary for grip.

■ As a general rule, for isolated unreconstructable PIP problems, the index finger gets arthrodesis, the middle finger gets arthrodesis or arthroplasty, and the ring and small fingers get arthroplasty.

■ Exceptions to the rule include associated unsalvageable tendon problems and soft tissue coverage issues, in which arthrodesis may be preferred.

■ The status of the adjacent joints is an important factor in deciding whether to perform arthrodesis or arthroplasty. In the rheumatoid patient with both MCP and PIP involvement, the temptation is to perform arthroplasties of all involved joints. So-called double-row arthroplasties tend to compromise the results at both the MCP and PIP joints. In such instances, the goal is stability at the PIP joint (arthrodesis) and motion at the MCP joint (arthroplasty).

■ Arthrodesis of the thumb MCP joint is a reliable procedure for managing arthritis and unreconstructable ligament problems. Arthrodesis is a far superior procedure to arthroplasty for the thumb. However, before undertaking this, it is important to ensure adequate motion and function of the adjacent joints (interphalangeal, carpometacarpal).

■ The chronic radial collateral ligament tear with static volar-ulnar subluxation is a good indication for thumb MCP fusion.

■ Arthrodesis of the digital MCP joints is not commonly performed. Indications include multiply failed arthroplasty or inadequate bone stock for arthroplasty, unrelenting infection, refractory instability of the index MCP, and an unreconstructable extensor mechanism.

■ Candidates for arthrodesis must understand that all motion in the affected joint will be eliminated, and that the principal goals are pain relief and stability.[19]

Arthrodesis Position

■ The fusion position varies with the digit and joint involved. Invariably, the decision is a compromise between appearance and function. The ideal posture should replicate the normal digital cascade (**FIG 1**).

■ In general, the DIP joints and thumb interphalangeal joint should be fused in 0 to 10 degrees of flexion.[14]

■ For the PIP joint, some authors recommend a uniform 40-degree flexion position for all digits,[6] while others recommend 40 degrees for the index finger, progressing ulnarward in 5-degree increments to 55 degrees in the small finger.[17]

■ Many prefer a slightly more extended position for the index PIP that will still allow functional tip-to-tip pinch.

■ The recommended fusion angle of the MP joints is a cascade from 25 degrees of flexion in the index digit, progressing

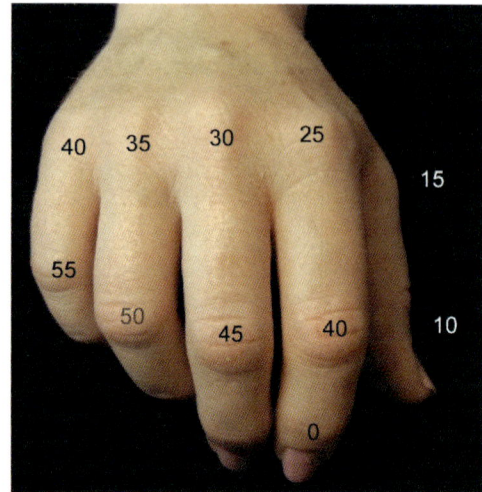

FIG 1 • Recommended positions for digital joint fusion.

ulnarward in 5-degree increments to 40 degrees in the small finger.[14]

■ The recommended fusion angle of the MP joint of the thumb is 10 to 15 degrees of flexion.[14]

Fixation Options

■ The choice of surgical technique depends on a number of factors, including the affected joint to be fused, the availability and cost of implants, the adequacy of bone stock, and the comfort of the surgeon. The goal is to achieve a solid fusion of the affected joint in a timely manner. Bone preparation is essential.

■ The specific method of fixation may be less important in obtaining union than specific patient factors such as bone quality. Certain constructs, such as the tension band, are more rigid but may be associated with more hardware-related problems.

■ The biomechanical issues must be weighed against potential soft tissue problems when deciding on a form of fixation. Maintenance of motion in the adjacent joints is critical.

■ Kirschner wire fixation has been associated with fusion rates of up to 99%.

■ Advantages

■ Simplicity of the technique

■ Ready availability of low-cost implants

■ Disadvantages

■ Infection risk, including superficial pin site and deep wound infections, osteomyelitis; pin migration; minimal compression across the fusion site

■ Less rigid fixation,[9] requiring additional external immobilization to enhance stability, possibly leading to stiffness of surrounding joints[8,15]

■ Interosseous wiring has been found to be biomechanically stronger than Kirschner wire fixation.[18] It is especially useful for PIP fusion and thumb interphalangeal fusion.

■ Advantages

■ Biomechanically stronger than Kirschner wire fixation[18]

■ Readily available low-cost implants

■ Disadvantages

■ Large amount of soft tissue stripping for appropriate placement of drill holes

■ Higher rate of nonunion, up to 9%[11]

- Tension band fixation is a biomechanically stable method of fixation[16] combining parallel Kirschner wires for rotational control and interosseous wiring for compression. This technique is especially useful for MCP, PIP, and thumb interphalangeal arthrodesis.
    - The tension band construct converts the strong distracting force created by the finger flexors to a compressive force across the arthrodesis interface.
    - This technique is relatively simple, with a high fusion rate and reliable outcomes,[1,16] especially when used for arthrodesis of the MCP and PIP joints.
    - Postoperative immobilization is necessary only in the immediate postoperative period to allow for healing of the incision.[1,8]
    - Advantages
        - Simplicity of the procedure
        - Low rate of infection[16]
        - High fusion rates, reportedly 97% to 100%[1,16]
        - Readily available, low-cost implants
        - Enhanced biomechanical stability and strength of the construct, allowing for early active range of motion[16] The tension band construct for small joint arthrodesis has been shown to be biomechanically superior compared to crossed Kirschner wire fixation and intraosseous wiring, especially in anteroposterior bending and in axial torsion.[9]
    - Disadvantages
        - Increased soft tissue dissection to place the drill holes, with resultant increased risk of soft tissue and tendon scarring
        - Difficult to remove fully internalized hardware if necessary
- Plate fixation provides biomechanically strong fixation, especially useful for PIP and MCP joint arthrodesis.[4,19]
    - Advantages
        - Excellent fusion rate by 6 weeks, 96% to 100%[16]
        - Ability to correct deformity
        - Useful in cases with segmental bone loss[4]
    - Disadvantages
        - Technically demanding
        - Time-consuming
        - Extensor tendon adhesions, possibly necessitating hardware removal and tenolysis[16]; stiffness in adjacent joints
        - Hardware prominence
- Compression screw fixation is a biomechanically strong fixation technique[20] that is especially useful for arthrodesis of the finger DIP and PIP joints, as well as the thumb interphalangeal joint.

- Using a headless screw keeps the fixation hardware low profile and prevents the problems associated with prominent hardware.
- PIP joint fusion uses the same principles but has a slightly different surgical technique.[2]
    - Advantages
        - Fusion rates 85% to 98%[2,3]
        - Hardware is buried and low profile.
    - Disadvantages
        - Risk of infection
        - Risk of penetration and fracture of the dorsal cortex,[3] especially with screw fixation of the PIP joint,[20] resulting in poor fixation
        - Risk of nail irregularities from disturbance of germinal matrix[3] in DIP fusion
    - Complications
        - Risk of infection, hardware complications, nail irregularities secondary to penetration of the dorsal cortex of the distal phalanx by the screw, and fractures of the dorsal cortex from screw breakthrough[3]
        - Easily avoided by maintaining adequate space between the dorsal proximal entry site and the arthrodesis site
        - For DIP arthrodesis, the nail-associated complications usually occurred in the small finger because of the large diameter of the screw used relative to the size of the small finger distal phalanx medullary canal.[20] This is less of a problem in the distal phalanges of the other fingers or thumb.[2,3]

Preoperative Planning

- Radiographs of the affected joint must be reviewed before operative management. Assessment of the bone stock, quality, and size is useful in helping to determine the optimal type of surgical fixation.
- Should a fusion screw be considered, templates may be used to determine the appropriate screw length and diameter.

Positioning

- The patient is placed in the supine position, with the affected limb resting on a hand table. Sterile preparation and draping is performed.
- For arthrodesis of the PIP and DIP joints, local anesthesia with or without sedation is adequate.
    - Two percent mepivacaine provides a rapid rate of onset and lasts about 1 hour.
    - For the PIP joint, a web space block is performed, including the dorsal cutaneous branches.
    - For the DIP joint, the flexor tendon sheath is injected.
    - For the MCP joint, either regional or general anesthesia is necessary.

DIP JOINT ARTHRODESIS

Exposure

- A digital tourniquet is used.
- Center a dorsal H-shaped incision over the DIP joint (**TECH FIG 1A**).
- Transect the terminal tendon (**TECH FIG 1B**).
- Release the collateral ligaments from the middle phalanx, using a no. 15 blade directed dorsally, parallel to the sides of the phalanx (**TECH FIG 1C**).

Preparation of the DIP Joint

- Hyperflex the DIP joint and remove peripheral osteophytes with a small rongeur.
- Remove the volar condyles of the head of the middle phalanx with the rongeur.
- Identify the periphery of the base of the distal phalanx with a no. 15 blade, protecting the germinal matrix and the neurovascular bundles.

TECHNIQUES

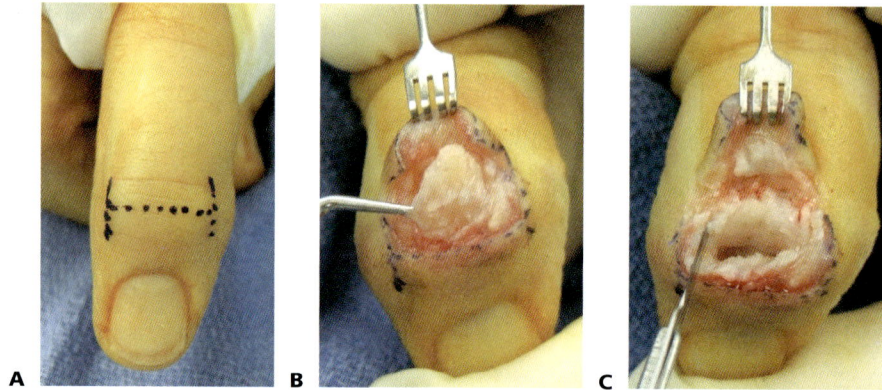

TECH FIG 1 • **A.** Dorsal H-shaped incision, centered over the distal interphalangeal joint. **B.** The terminal tendon is transected and flaps are elevated. The probe is under a large dorsal loose body. **C.** The collateral ligaments are released from the head of the middle phalanx by orienting a no. 15 blade upward and parallel to the ligament recesses.

- Remove bone necessary to correct any joint malalignment, but minimize loss of digital length.
- Dechondrify and decorticate the opposing surfaces until healthy-appearing bone is present.
- Contour the head of the middle phalanx into a transversely oriented cylindrical shape (**TECH FIG 2A**), and fashion the base of the distal phalanx into a reciprocal shape.
  - Alternatively, create flat opposing surfaces perpendicular to the shafts.
- On occasion, the base of the distal phalanx is eburnated. Multiple 0.035-inch drill holes may be placed ("pepperpot" technique), which may then be connected with a small rongeur to unveil subchondral bone (**TECH FIG 2B,C**).

Reduction and Fixation

- The type of fixation depends on the size of the bone. An Acutrak fusion screw (Acumed, Hillsboro, OR) is preferred when the diameter of the middle and distal phalanges is sufficient to accommodate the screw.
- Insert a 0.062-inch Kirschner wire antegrade beginning at the base of the distal phalanx and exiting the tip of the distal phalanx, just volar to the nail plate (**TECH FIG 3A**).
  - If the Kirschner wire penetrates the nail plate, discard it and use another to minimize the likelihood of contamination.

- Drive a smooth 0.062-inch Kirschner wire retrograde into the center of the middle phalanx to create a pilot hole, and then remove it (**TECH FIG 3B**).
- Reduce and compress the joint and then advance the wire retrograde across the DIP joint into the middle phalanx (**TECH FIG 3C**).
- Assess the reduction and Kirschner wire position clinically and fluoroscopically (**TECH FIG 3D**).
- While manually maintaining the joint position, remove the Kirschner wire and replace it with the appropriate drill bit.
  - Proper drill bit size is based on preoperative templating as well as an estimate of the available space based on the lateral fluoroscopic image with the 0.062-inch Kirschner wire in place.
- While maintaining compression across the joint, advance the drill retrograde by hand along the path created by the removed Kirschner wire (**TECH FIG 3E**).
- Determine the proper depth by fluoroscopy, using the external drill bit markings as a reference.
- Remove the drill bit and insert the appropriate-sized fusion screw (**TECH FIG 3F**) while maintaining manual compression across the joint.
  - Final seating of the screw is based on the external reference used for the drill bit.

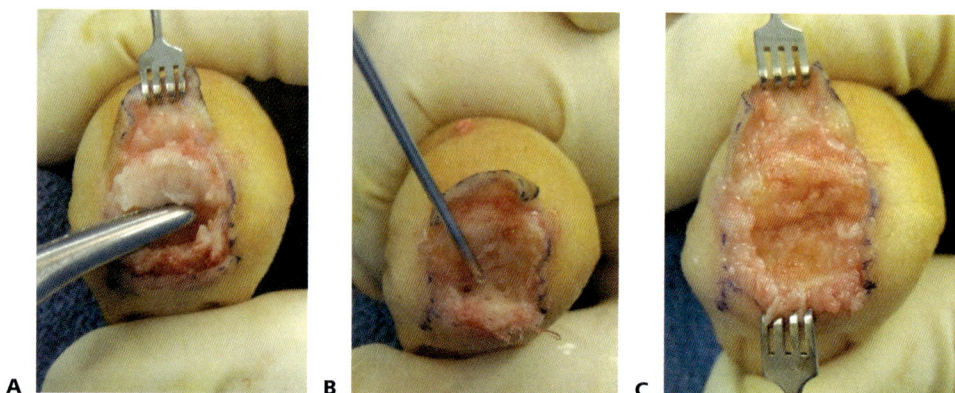

TECH FIG 2 • **A.** The distal interphalangeal joint is hyperflexed. Peripheral osteophytes and the volar condyles are removed. The remaining articular surface is dechondrified and decorticated with a rongeur, fashioning reciprocal surfaces. **B.** Placing multiple small drill holes facilitates débridement of eburnated bone at the base of the distal phalanx. **C.** Appearance after preparation of the distal interphalangeal joint.

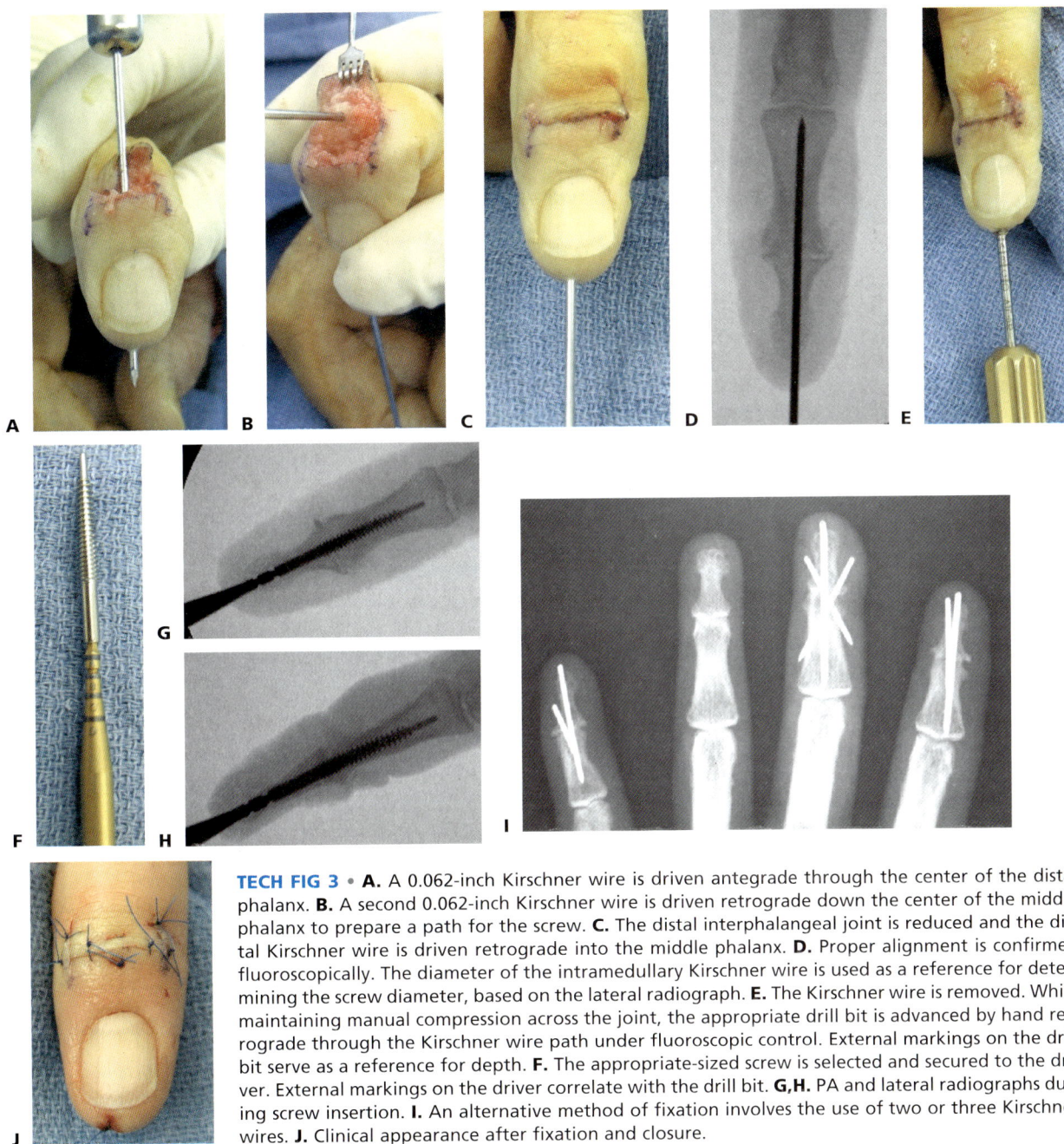

TECH FIG 3 • **A.** A 0.062-inch Kirschner wire is driven antegrade through the center of the distal phalanx. **B.** A second 0.062-inch Kirschner wire is driven retrograde down the center of the middle phalanx to prepare a path for the screw. **C.** The distal interphalangeal joint is reduced and the distal Kirschner wire is driven retrograde into the middle phalanx. **D.** Proper alignment is confirmed fluoroscopically. The diameter of the intramedullary Kirschner wire is used as a reference for determining the screw diameter, based on the lateral radiograph. **E.** The Kirschner wire is removed. While maintaining manual compression across the joint, the appropriate drill bit is advanced by hand retrograde through the Kirschner wire path under fluoroscopic control. External markings on the drill bit serve as a reference for depth. **F.** The appropriate-sized screw is selected and secured to the driver. External markings on the driver correlate with the drill bit. **G,H.** PA and lateral radiographs during screw insertion. **I.** An alternative method of fixation involves the use of two or three Kirschner wires. **J.** Clinical appearance after fixation and closure.

- Avoid inadvertent malrotation of the distal segment as the screw is tightened.
- Obtain final radiographs and evaluate the stability (**TECH FIG 3G,H**).
  - Insert a supplemental 0.035-inch oblique Kirschner wire if necessary for stability.
- If Kirschner wires are used as the sole form of fixation, drive an appropriate-diameter pin antegrade into the distal phalanx, reduce the joint, and advance the pin retrograde, preferably into the subchondral plate at the base of the middle phalanx.
  - One or two additional Kirschner wires are inserted obliquely in a retrograde fashion.

- Final radiographs are obtained, and the pins are cut beneath the skin (**TECH FIG 3I**).

Completion

- Remove the digital tourniquet and achieve hemostasis using bipolar electrocautery.
- Irrigate the wound copiously.
- Approximate the skin with 5-0 nylon interrupted sutures (**TECH FIG 3J**).
  - Repair of the terminal tendon is unnecessary.
- Apply a sterile dressing and dorsal aluminum DIP splint, leaving the PIP joint free.
- Instruct the patient on PIP exercises.

PIP JOINT ARTHRODESIS

Exposure

- Make a longitudinal dorsal incision.
  - The surgical approach is similar to the thumb MCP arthrodesis (discussed later).
  - In the multiply operated finger, a pre-existing mid-axial scar may be used.
- The central slip and capsule are split longitudinally and elevated subperiosteally.
- The collateral ligaments are released from the middle phalanx, using a no. 15 blade directed dorsally, parallel to the sides of the phalanx.

Preparation of the PIP Joint

- Hyperflex (shotgun) the PIP joint and prepare the joint in the manner detailed for the DIP joint.
- Correct joint malalignment but minimize loss of digital length.
- As for the DIP joint, contour the head of the proximal phalanx into a transversely oriented cylindrical shape, and fashion the base of the distal phalanx into a reciprocal shape.
- Alternatively, use a water-cooled sagittal saw to cut flat surfaces perpendicular to the phalangeal shafts in the coronal plane, and with an appropriate degree of flexion in the sagittal plane.
  - The flexion angle is built into the proximal phalanx saw cut. The middle phalanx cut is perpendicular to the axis of the phalanx in the sagittal plane.
  - There is little room for error with the bone cuts. Commitment to the final position of the arthrodesis is made when the bone cuts are made. Any change may result in excessive shortening of the bone.[7]
- On occasion, as with the DIP joint, the base of the middle phalanx is eburnated. Multiple 0.035-inch drill holes may be placed ("pepperpot" technique), which may then be connected with a small rongeur to unveil subchondral bone.

Kirschner Wire Fixation

- In patients with inflammatory arthritis, the overlying skin is quite thin and may not tolerate prominent hardware. In those instances, crossed 0.035- to 0.045-inch Kirschner wires are used.
- Preset the appropriately sized Kirschner wires into the sides of the middle phalanx.
- Reduce and compress the joint manually, then advance the Kirschner wires in a retrograde manner into the proximal phalanx.
- If the skin is very thin, it may be impossible to cut the Kirschner wires beneath the skin. In those instances, the Kirschner wires are simply bent and left exposed.

Tension Band Fixation

- A tension band technique is used for posttraumatic and OA cases, particularly those involving the index PIP joint (**TECH FIG 4A**).
- Use a 0.035-inch Kirschner wire to make a transverse hole in the middle phalanx, dorsal to the mid-axis, about 8 mm distal to the joint.
- Pass a 26-gauge surgical steel wire through the hole.
- With the joint manually reduced, drive parallel 0.035- to 0.045-inch Kirschner wires antegrade across the PIP joint into the subchondral head of the middle phalanx.
  - Begin the Kirschner wires on the dorsoradial and dorsoulnar margins of the proximal phalanx, about 10 mm proximal to the fusion site.
  - The Kirschner wires should remain intramedullary in the middle phalanx.
- Loop the 26-gauge wire into a figure 8 configuration around the Kirschner wires proximally and tighten carefully with a needle driver.
  - A gentle distraction force on the needle holder as the device is used to turn the wire and compress the fusion site helps avoid wire breakage.
- Remove the excess knot and impact the knot into bone.
- Withdraw the Kirschner wires slightly, bend them as close to the bone as possible so they can capture the 26-gauge wire, cut the Kirschner wires just distal to the bend, and advance them using the needle holder.
- Obtain final radiographs (**TECH FIG 4B**) and assess stability.
- Remove the tourniquet, achieve hemostasis, and irrigate the wound.
- Reapproximate the extensor tendon using interrupted inverted 4-0 nonabsorbable sutures. Close the skin with 5-0 nylon interrupted sutures.
- Place a sterile dressing and dorsal aluminum splint, leaving the DIP joint free. Instruct the patient on DIP joint exercises.

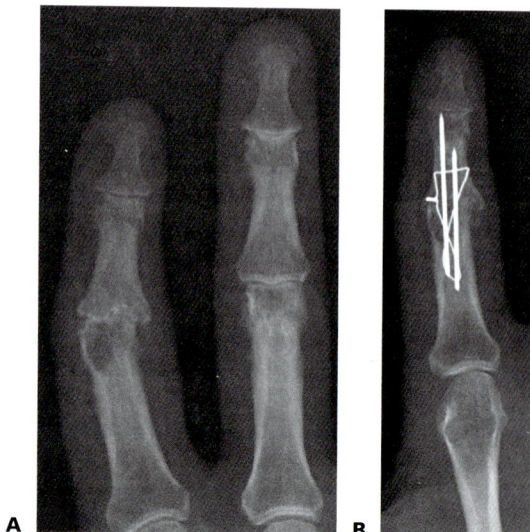

TECH FIG 4 • **A.** Preoperative PA radiograph demonstrating advanced osteoarthritis of the index proximal interphalangeal joint. Note the angular deformity, joint space loss, and large subchondral cyst. **B.** Postoperative PA radiograph demonstrating proximal interphalangeal arthrodesis with tension band fixation.

THUMB MCP JOINT ARTHRODESIS

Exposure

- Make a longitudinal dorsal incision over the MCP joint (**TECH FIG 5A**).
- Incise the extensor apparatus longitudinally between the EPB and EPL tendons (**TECH FIG 5B**). This will reveal the joint capsule (**TECH FIG 5C**).
- Perform a longitudinal capsulotomy and subperiosteally dissect around the dorsal base of the middle phalanx (**TECH FIG 5D**).
- Release the collateral ligaments from the metacarpal head (**TECH FIG 5E**), and hyperflex the MCP joint (**TECH FIG 5F**).

Joint Preparation

- Dechondrify the articular surfaces and remove peripheral osteophytes as well as the volar condyles of the metacarpal head with a rongeur (**TECH FIG 6A**).
- Decorticate and prepare the fusion surfaces in a "cup-and-cone" configuration[7,12] using Coughlin reamers (Howmedica, Rutherford, NJ) (**TECH FIG 6B,C**).
  - This method allows for maintenance of thumb length and subtle adjustments in joint position while still maintaining optimal bone contact.
  - The 14- and 16-mm sizes are most often appropriate. Size selection is usually based on the size of the metacarpal head in order to avoid notching.
  - The same dimensions must be used for both metacarpal and phalangeal reaming or the surfaces will be incongruent.

- Ream the base of the middle phalanx first to avoid iatrogenic injury to the metacarpal head.
- Place an elevator anterior to the base of the proximal phalanx to deliver the phalanx away from the metacarpal head and to protect the flexor pollicis longus.
- Advance a 0.062-inch Kirschner wire antegrade into the proximal phalanx, centered in the coronal plane (**TECH FIG 6D**) and slightly flexed (Kirschner wire tip dorsal) in the sagittal plane (**TECH FIG 6E**).
- Ream the base of the middle phalanx over the Kirschner wire using the selected phalangeal "cup" reamer until uniform cancellous bone is exposed (**TECH FIG 6F**). Remove the reamer and the pin.
- Prepare the metacarpal head by first advancing a 0.062-inch Kirschner wire retrograde from the center of the head, angled slightly radially (**TECH FIG 6G**) and dorsally (**TECH FIG 6H**).
- Ream the metacarpal head using the matching metacarpal "cone" reamer (**TECH FIG 6I**) until healthy subchondral bone is exposed (**TECH FIG 6J**). Then remove the reamer and the Kirschner wire.

Fixation and Reduction

- Tension band fixation is performed to stabilize the thumb MCP joint fusion in much the same manner as detailed for arthrodesis of the PIP joint.
  - Alternative methods of fixation include Kirschner wires alone, headed or headless screw fixation, and plate fixation.

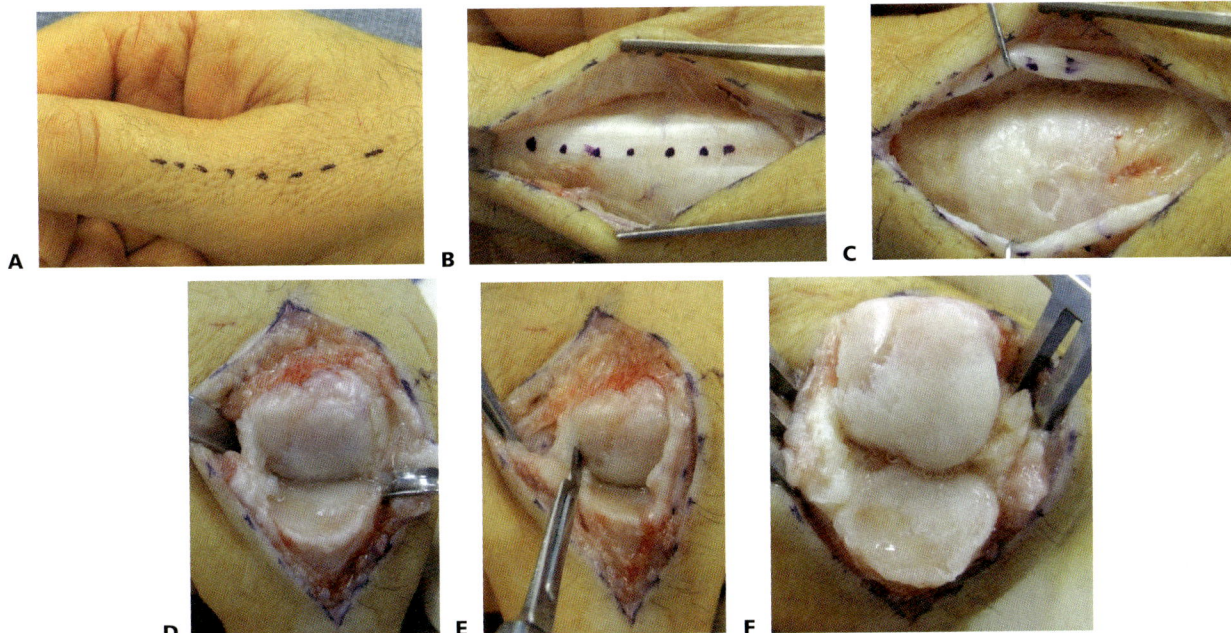

TECH FIG 5 • A. A longitudinal incision is centered over the metacarpophalangeal joint. **B.** The extensor hood is incised between the extensor pollicis longus and brevis tendons (*dotted line*). **C.** The hood has been split, revealing the dorsal joint capsule. **D.** The capsule has been incised longitudinally and reflected subperiosteally from the dorsal base of the proximal phalanx. Note the full-thickness cartilage loss along the ulnar aspect of the metacarpal head and dorsal base of the proximal phalanx secondary to volar-ulnar subluxation. **E.** The collateral ligaments are released from the metacarpal head. **F.** The metacarpophalangeal joint is now hyperflexed.

TECHNIQUES

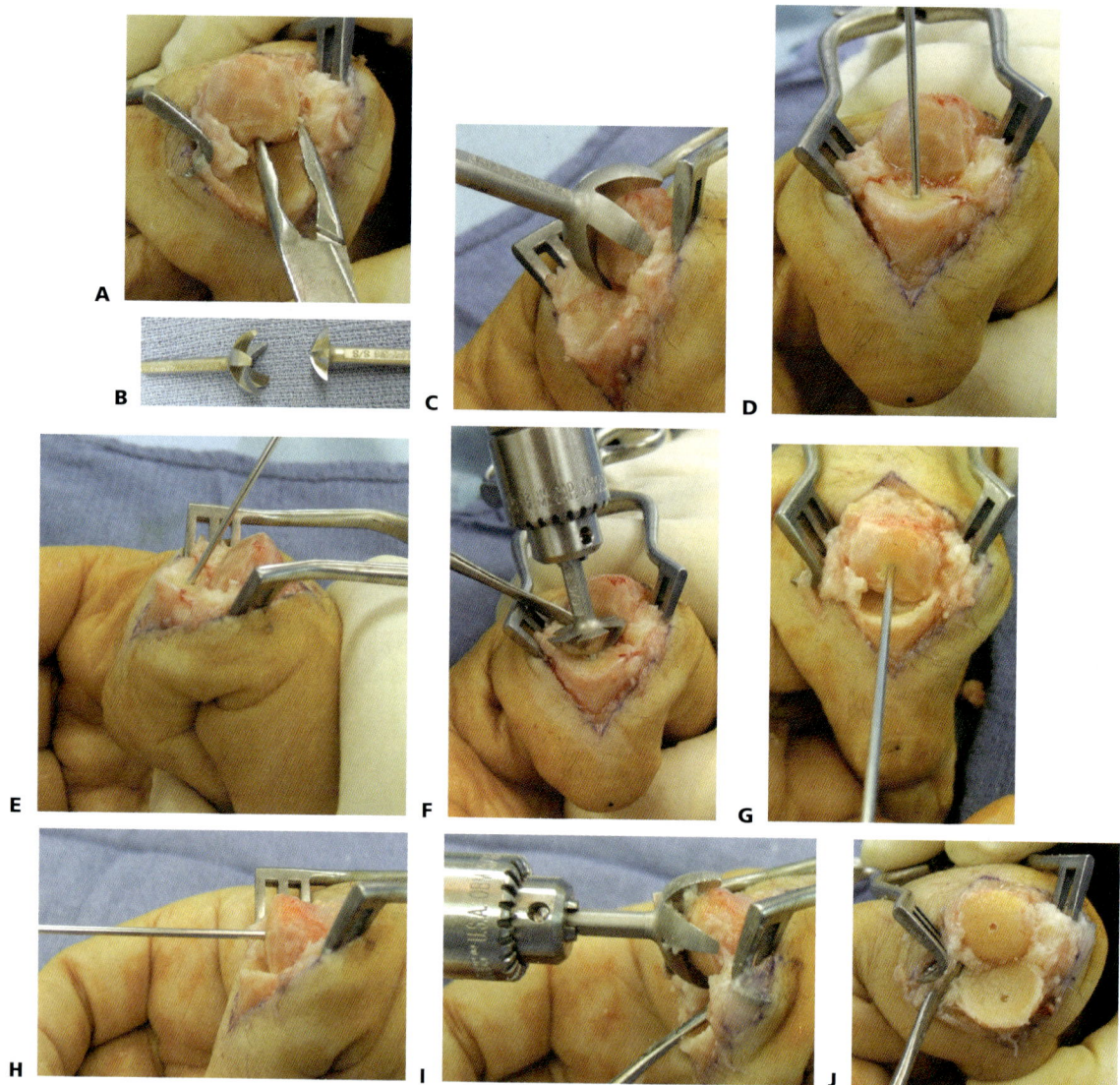

TECH FIG 6 • A. The remaining articular cartilage is removed. Peripheral osteophytes and the volar condyles are trimmed with a rongeur. **B.** Coughlin cup and cone reamers. Care must be taken to ensure that the same-sized reamer is used for both sides to maximize bone contact. **C.** The metacarpal head is used as a reference in determining reamer size. The smallest reamer that will not notch the cortex is selected. **D,E.** A 0.062-inch Kirschner wire is advanced antegrade in the proximal phalanx to be used as a guidewire. The pin is positioned in the center of the bone in the coronal plane (*dot* in the center of the interphalangeal joint) and in slight flexion in the sagittal plane. **F.** The "cup" reamer is placed over the Kirschner wire under power with frequent irrigation until bleeding subchondral bone is revealed. The asymmetry of the base of the proximal phalanx due to chronic subluxation is corrected. **G,H.** A 0.062-inch Kirschner wire is then inserted retrograde into the metacarpal head. The pin is positioned in slight flexion and slight ulnar deviation. **I.** The matching "cone" reamer is placed over the Kirschner wire under power with frequent irrigation until bleeding subchondral bone is apparent. **J.** Appearance of the surfaces after joint preparation.

- The tension band construct is strong enough to allow for early motion with a hand-based splint.
- Plate fixation is reserved for cases of bone loss requiring supplemental grafting.
- Use a 0.045-inch smooth Kirschner wire to create a transverse hole in the proximal phalanx, about 1 cm distal to the joint and dorsal to the midline.
- Pass a 24- or 26-gauge surgical steel wire though the tunnel (TECH FIG 7A).

- Anticipating the ultimate position of the thumb fusion, advance parallel 0.054- or 0.062-inch Kirschner wires retrograde, exiting dorsally along the metacarpal shaft (TECH FIG 7B).
- Reduce the MCP joint in slight (less than 25 degrees) flexion, abduction (5 degrees), and pronation (5 degrees), and drive the preset Kirschner wires antegrade.
  - Take care to avoid perforating the volar cortex into the flexor tendon sheath.

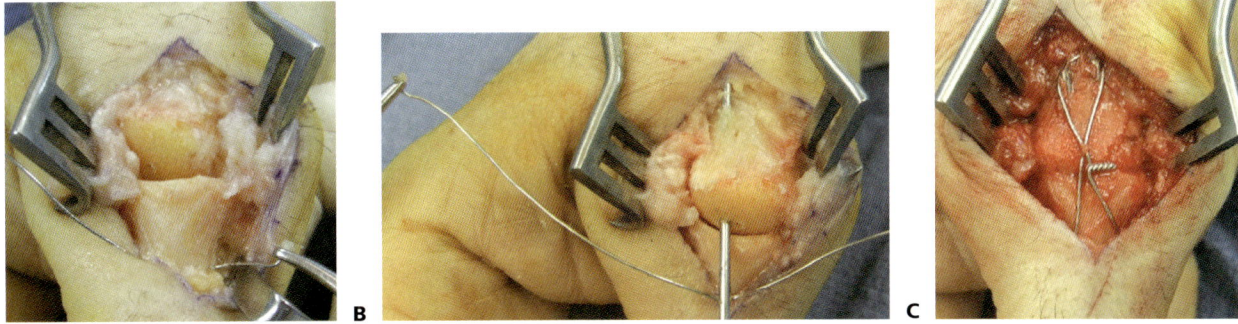

TECH FIG 7 • **A.** A 24-gauge wire is passed through a drill hole in the proximal shaft of the proximal phalanx, dorsal to the midline and parallel to the joint. **B.** A 0.062-inch Kirschner wire is then driven retrograde in the metacarpal head, exiting dorsally, anticipating the ultimate position of the metacarpophalangeal joint. **C.** The 24-gauge wire is looped around the base of the Kirschner wires in figure 8 fashion and tensioned. The Kirschner wires are cut short and the wire knot is tamped against the cortex.

- Loop the wire in a figure 8 configuration around the Kirschner wires, and tighten using a needle driver.
- Trim excess wire and impact the knot into the bone.
- Pull back, bend, cut, and advance the Kirschner wires (as detailed earlier) to secure the tension band wire (**TECH FIG 7C**).

Completion

- Remove the tourniquet, achieve hemostasis, and irrigate the wound.
- Close the capsule over the hardware using absorbable 4-0 suture and then close the extensor mechanism using 4-0 nonabsorbable interrupted inverted stitches (**TECH FIG 8A**).
- Approximate the skin using 5-0 nylon interrupted suture, and apply a sterile dressing and radial gutter splint.
  - The interphalangeal joint is left free, and the patient is instructed on interphalangeal motion exercises.
- Obtain final radiographs (**TECH FIG 8B,C**).

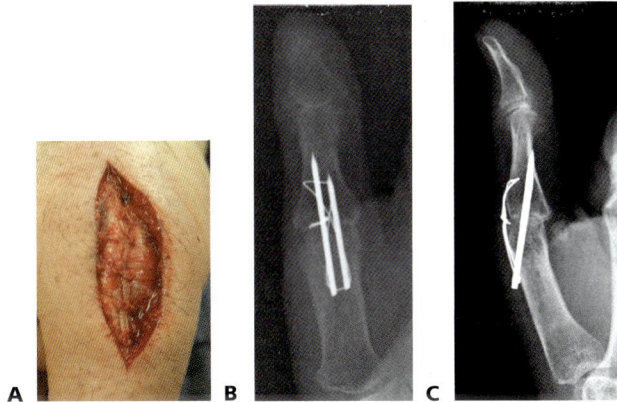

TECH FIG 8 • **A.** The capsule and extensor hood are repaired in layers. **B,C.** Postoperative PA and lateral radiographs demonstrate good joint apposition and alignment.

INDEX THROUGH SMALL FINGER MCP JOINT ARTHRODESIS

- The approach and bone preparation mirror those described for the thumb.
- Fixation may be achieved with Kirschner wires alone, a tension band construct, screws, or plates (**TECH FIG 9**).
  - Keep in mind the anticipated deforming forces, which may be out of plane with the fixation.
- Immobilization should protect the fused joint from stress, while simultaneously permitting motion of the PIP and DIP joints. We prefer to apply a short-arm cast extending out to the PIP joints, allowing PIP and DIP motion.

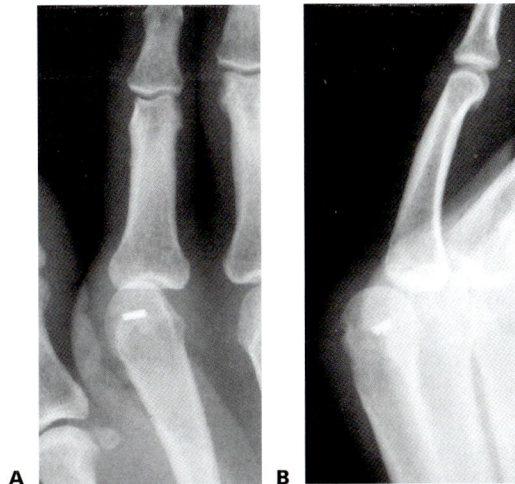

TECH FIG 9 • **A, B.** PA and lateral radiographs showing chronic right index metacarpophalangeal volar-ulnar subluxation in patient who had undergone two previous attempts at radial collateral ligament reconstruction. *(continued)*

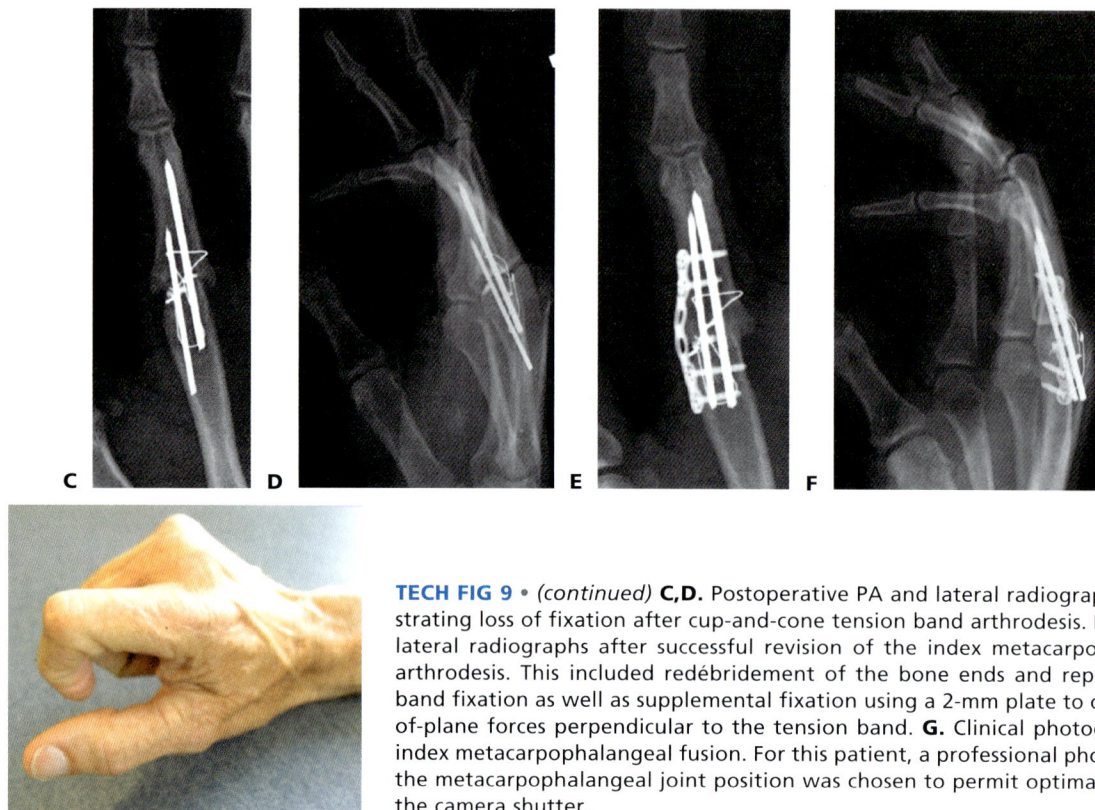

TECH FIG 9 • *(continued)* **C,D.** Postoperative PA and lateral radiographs demonstrating loss of fixation after cup-and-cone tension band arthrodesis. **E,F.** PA and lateral radiographs after successful revision of the index metacarpophalangeal arthrodesis. This included redébridement of the bone ends and repeat tension band fixation as well as supplemental fixation using a 2-mm plate to control out-of-plane forces perpendicular to the tension band. **G.** Clinical photograph after index metacarpophalangeal fusion. For this patient, a professional photographer, the metacarpophalangeal joint position was chosen to permit optimal control of the camera shutter.

ADDITIONAL FIXATION METHODS

- The surgical approach, bone preparation, and closure are performed as detailed earlier.
- Most frequently, flat bone cuts are used with these fixation techniques.

Interosseous Wiring

- Drill two parallel holes from dorsal to volar, each 3 to 4 mm away from the arthrodesis site, using a 0.035-inch Kirschner wire.
- Drill two additional holes, this time in the radioulnar plane, again about 3 to 4 mm on either side of the arthrodesis site.
- Thread two 26-gauge surgical steel wires through the drill holes.
  - A 20-gauge hypodermic needle may be used to facilitate wire placement.
- Pass one wire from dorsal to volar through one drill hole, and then volar to dorsal in the parallel drill hole, forming a loop.
- Pass the second 26-gauge steel wire through the drill holes in the coronal plane, forming a second loop.
- After the wires are placed, tighten the ends of the wires sequentially and shorten and bend them to decrease their profile.
- This configuration results in two perpendicular loops providing compression and fixation across the arthrodesis interface.

Plate Fixation

- Fill bone defects with intercalary grafts as needed (**TECH FIG 10A,B**).
- Select the largest compression plate that will not be prominent.
  - These range in size from 1.5 to 2.7 mm.
- The plate is precontoured to match the angle of the fusion.
  - A slight increase in concavity is created to allow compression of the volar cortex when the plate is applied (**TECH FIG 10C**).
- Insert a bicortical screw through the plate into the distal fragment.
  - Be certain that this and other screws do not penetrate the volar cortex and impair the function of the flexor tendons.
- Using AO compression technique, place a screw through the plate into the proximal fragment.
  - Drill as proximally and eccentrically as possible within the plate's screw hole so that when the screw is tightened, compression is obtained.
- Place the remaining screws (**TECH FIG 10D**).
  - Four to six cortices on either side of the fusion site provides adequate fixation.[14]

Compression Screw Fixation

- In much the same manner as described for placement of Kirschner wires for tension band fusion of the

TECHNIQUES

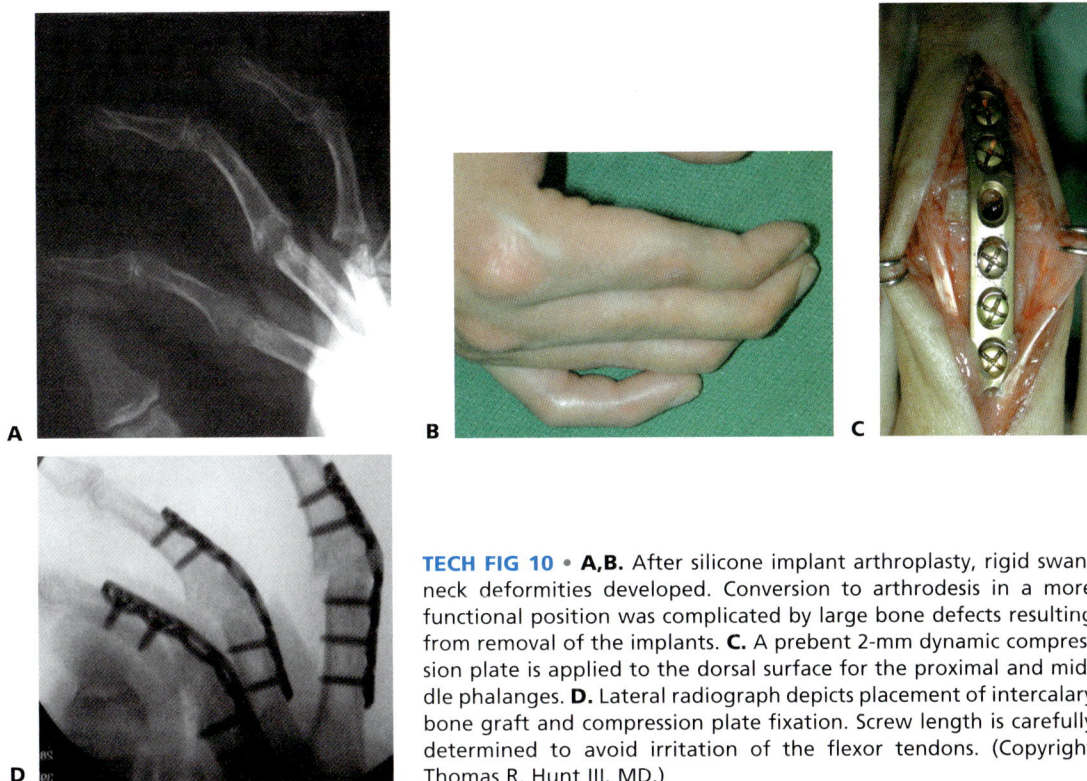

TECH FIG 10 • **A,B.** After silicone implant arthroplasty, rigid swan-neck deformities developed. Conversion to arthrodesis in a more functional position was complicated by large bone defects resulting from removal of the implants. **C.** A prebent 2-mm dynamic compression plate is applied to the dorsal surface for the proximal and middle phalanges. **D.** Lateral radiograph depicts placement of intercalary bone graft and compression plate fixation. Screw length is carefully determined to avoid irritation of the flexor tendons. (Copyright Thomas R. Hunt III, MD.)

thumb MCP joint, the guidewire is introduced into the proximal fragment in a retrograde manner, exiting the dorsal cortex at least 5 mm proximal to the arthrodesis site.

- This protects against inadvertent fracture of the dorsal cortex.
- Manually reduce and compress the prepared joint.
- It may be helpful to place a small (0.028- to 0.035-inch) provisional Kirschner wire away from the anticipated screw site to provide rotational stability.
- Advance the guidewire antegrade from proximal to dis-

tal, perpendicular to the fusion interface, and into the medullary canal of the distal segment.
- Advance the wire just beyond the mid-diaphyseal region of the distal fragment.
- Evaluate clinically and fluoroscopically to ensure proper position (**TECH FIG 11**).
- Measure the guidewire and choose the appropriate-length screw to ensure that after compression, the distal screw threads will engage the endosteal cortex and the proximal aspect of the screw will be buried.
- Remove the derotation Kirschner wire.

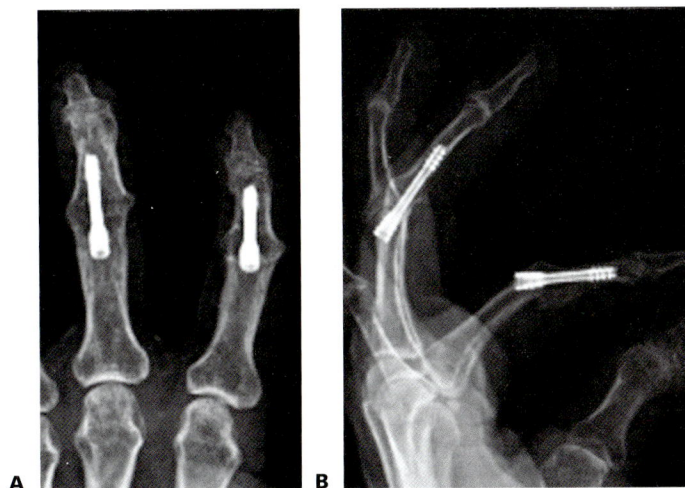

TECH FIG 11 • PA and lateral radiographs demonstrating arthrodesis of proximal interphalangeal joints with cannulated, headless compression screws. (Copyright Thomas R. Hunt III, MD.)

PEARLS AND PITFALLS

Bone end preparation	■ If flat bone cuts are to be used, predetermine and create accurate flexion angles for the joint fusion. There is little room for error with this technique. Inaccurate cuts will result in excessive bone shortening. ■ The cup-and-cone preparation technique is more forgiving, allowing for angular and rotational adjustments while maintaining bone contact. ■ Ensure that there is no malrotation of fusion interface.
Surgical approach	■ Preserve joint capsule for later repair to minimize extensor tendon adherence.
Tension band fixation	■ To minimize hardware problems, position the Kirschner wires within the intramedullary canal and advance them into the subchondral plate.
Compression screw fixation	■ In the PIP and MCP joints, ensure that the starting point is 5 mm from the bony end of the proximal fragment to prevent fracture of the dorsal cortex.

POSTOPERATIVE CARE

■ Postoperative management depends on the involved joint and method of fixation. Early motion of the adjacent joints is critical to minimize stiffness.

■ For DIP joint arthrodesis, protection with a simple aluminum splint is sufficient. PIP motion is encouraged. Splinting may be unnecessary if a fusion screw is used. Radiographs are taken at 6 weeks postoperatively. Buried pins may be removed once the fusion is radiographically solid (at least 8 weeks postoperatively).

■ For PIP joint arthrodesis, tension band, screw, and plate constructs are usually strong enough to obviate the need for supplemental splinting. Early MCP and DIP motion is encouraged; however, the patient is advised against lateral stress or forceful grip with the affected digit. With simple pin fixation, a supplemental dorsal aluminum or thermoplast PIP splint is used until radiographs demonstrate union.

■ For the thumb MCP joint treated with tension band fixation, a protective custom-molded thermoplast hand-based MCP splint is used for about 6 weeks. Early IP joint motion is encouraged.

■ In general, arthrodesis of the other MCP joints must be protected with a hand- or forearm-based splint, regardless of the type of fixation. Significant flexion and lateral stresses must be neutralized while simultaneously allowing for PIP and DIP motion. It may be necessary to splint the PIP joint in extension part-time to prevent an extensor lag from developing.

OUTCOMES

■ Multiple studies have evaluated the biomechanical advantages of one type of surgical technique versus another in order to establish the most rigid type of fixation that will allow a rapid and complete arthrodesis.

■ A comparison between the failure load of a Herbert screw and the failure load of a tension band construct showed no significant difference between the two[2]; the authors concluded that these two methods of fixation have similar biomechanical strength.

■ A comparison of multiple fixation techniques showed that arthrodesis by screw fixation had a better fusion rate than Kirschner wires, tension band construct, and plate fixation.[10]

■ A comparison of tension band constructs versus Kirschner wire fixation for PIP joint arthrodesis concluded that tension bands provide more rigid fixation.[9]

■ Biomechanical testing comparing the Herbert screw and tension band construct for DIP arthrodesis showed that the Herbert screw has significantly higher bending strength as well as more rigidity against axial torsion, although no difference was noted in the bending stiffness between these two methods of fixation.[20]

COMPLICATIONS

■ Pin tract infection
■ Nonunion
■ Malunion
■ Vascular insufficiency
■ Skin necrosis
■ Cold intolerance
■ Stiffness of adjacent digits
■ Painful hardware

REFERENCES

1. Allende B, Engelem JC. Tension-band arthrodesis in the finger joints. J Hand Surg Am 1980;5A:269–271.
2. Ayres JR, Goldstrohm GL, Miller GJ, et al. Proximal interphalangeal joint arthrodesis with the Herbert Screw. J Hand Surg Am 1988;13A:600–603.
3. Brutus JP, Palmer AK, Mosher JF, et al. Use of a headless compressive screw for distal interphalangeal joint arthrodesis in digits: clinical outcome and review of complications. J Hand Surg Am 2006;31A:85–89.
4. Buchler U, Aiken MA. Arthrodesis of the proximal interphalangeal joint by solid bone grafting and plate fixation in extensive injuries to the dorsal aspect of the finger. J Hand Surg Am 1988;13A:589–594.
5. Burton R, Margles SW, Lunseth PA. Small joint arthrodesis in the hand. J Hand Surg Am 1986;11A:678–682.
6. Carroll RE, Dick HM. Arthrodesis of the wrist for rheumatoid arthritis. J Bone Joint Surg Am 1971;53A:1365–1369.
7. Carroll RE, Hill NA. Small joint arthrodesis in hand reconstruction. J Bone Joint Surg Am 1969;51A:1219–1221.
8. Ijsselstein CB, van Egmond DB, Hovius SE, et al. Results of small-joint arthrodesis: comparison of Kirschner wire fixation with tension band wire technique. J Hand Surg Am 1992;17A:952–956.
9. Kovach JC, Werner FW, Palmer AK, et al. Biomechanical analysis of internal fixation techniques for proximal interphalangeal joint arthrodesis. J Hand Surg Am 1986;11A:562–566.
10. Leibovic SJ, Strickland JW. Arthrodesis of the proximal interphalangeal joint of the finger: comparison of the use of the Herbert screw with other fixation methods. J Hand Surg Am 1994;19A:181–188.
11. Lister G. Intraosseous wiring of the digital skeleton. J Hand Surg Am 1978;3A:427.
12. McGlynn J, Smith RA, Boqumill GP. Arthrodesis of small joint of the hand: a rapid and effective technique. J Hand Surg Am 1988;13A:595–599.

13. Moberg E. Arthrodesis of finger joints. Surg Clin North Am 1960;40: 465–470.
14. Shin A, Amadio P. Stiff finger joints. In: Green's Operative Hand Surgery. Philadelphia: Elsevier, 2006:417–457.
15. Stern PJ, Fulton DB. Distal interphalangeal joint arthrodesis: an analysis of complications. J Hand Surg Am 1992;17A: 1139–1145.
16. Stern PJ, Gates NT, Jones TB. Tension band arthrodesis of small joints in the hand. J Hand Surg Am 1993;18A:194–197.
17. Tubiana R. Arthrodesis of the fingers. In: Tubiana R, ed. The Hand, vol 2. Philadelphia: WB Saunders, 1985.
18. Vanik RK, Weber RC, Matloub HS, et al. The comparative strengths of internal fixation techniques. J Hand Surg Am 1984;9A:216–221.
19. Wright CS, McMurtry RY. AO arthrodesis in the hand. J Hand Surg Am 1983;8A:932–935.
20. Wyrsch B, Dawson J Aufranc S, et al. Distal interphalangeal joint arthrodesis comparing tension-band wire and Herbert screw: a biomechanical and dimensional analysis. J Hand Surg 1996;21A:438–443.

Chapter 81

Thumb Metacarpal Extension Osteotomy

Matthew M. Tomaino

DEFINITION

- When ligamentous restraint at the thumb carpometacarpal (CMC) joint is compromised, functional grip and pinch may result in painful synovitis and hypermobility long before the development of cartilage wear and arthritis.
- So-called Eaton stage 1 disease can be treated with an extension osteotomy at the base of the thumb metacarpal as an alternative to either ligament reconstruction or arthroscopic synovectomy and pinning.[7,8]

ANATOMY

- The thumb metacarpal (TM) joint is a biconcave-convex saddle joint with minimal bony constraints, so ligamentous support is extremely important, especially considering the compressive forces transmitted across the joint during functional pinch. Eaton and Littler identified the anterior oblique "beak" ligament, so called for its attachment on the palmar beak of the thumb metacarpal, as the primary stabilizer of the TM joint.
- With the assistance of TM joint arthroscopy, Bettinger et al[1] have further defined the anterior oblique ligament (AOL) into a superficial (sAOL) and deep ligament (dAOL). The dAOL, which is intracapsular, is, in fact, the beak ligament. The dAOL plays an important role in the kinematics of thumb opposition. It acts as a pivot point and becomes tight during pronation, opposition, and palmar abduction. The dAOL limits pronation in flexion and both pronation and supination in extension.
- In their comprehensive assessment of the ligamentous anatomy of the TM joint, Bettinger et al[1] described a total of 16 ligaments that stabilize the trapezium and TM. Seven of these ligaments, including the sAOL, dAOL "beak" ligament, dorsoradial (DRL), posterior oblique, ulnar collateral, intermetacarpal, and dorsal intermetacarpal, are responsible for directly stabilizing the TM joint.
- The DRL's role in joint stability has been debated, but Bettinger et al[1] showed that the DRL is an important joint stabilizer. The DRL, which covers a large percentage of the posterior aspect of the joint, is a wide thick ligament that attaches to the trapezium and inserts on the dorsum of the metacarpal base. This ligament tightens with dorsoradial and dorsal translational forces in all positions except full extension. It also tightens in supination and in pronation with joint flexion.

PATHOGENESIS

- Functional incompetence of the basal joint's AOL results in pathologic laxity, abnormal translation of the metacarpal on the trapezium, and generation of excessive shear forces between the joint surfaces, particularly within the palmar portion of the joint during grip and pinch activity. Histologic study has shown that attritional changes in the AOL at its attachment to the palmar lip of the metacarpal precede degeneration of cartilage.[2]

NATURAL HISTORY

- Because the AOL appears to be the primary stabilizer of the TM joint, and since its detachment results in dorsal translation of the metacarpal, its reconstruction has been recommended to restore thumb stability not only in cases of end-stage osteoarthritis but also for early-stage disease.
- Pellegrini et al[5] were the first to evaluate the biomechanical efficacy of extension osteotomy. Palmar contact area was unloaded with a concomitant shift in contact more dorsally so long as arthrosis did not extend more dorsal than the midpoint of the trapezium.
- Shrivastava et al[6] studied the effect of a simulated osteotomy on TM joint laxity by flexing the metacarpal base 30 degrees, thus placing the joint in the relationship it would assume if an extension osteotomy was performed.
  - The simulated extension osteotomy reduced laxity in all directions tested: dorsal-volar (40% reduction), radial-ulnar (23% reduction), distraction (15% reduction), and pronation-supination (29% reduction).
  - They hypothesized that the beneficial clinical effects of a TM extension osteotomy may be partially due to tightening of the DRL, which might reduce dorsal translation.

PATIENT HISTORY AND PHYSICAL FINDINGS

- Basal joint arthritis may present with mild symptoms beneath the thenar eminence at the level of the TM joint, particularly during pinch and grip. Ultimately, the greatest functional impairment occurs with advanced disease—limiting breadth of grasp and forceful lateral pinch activities such as brushing teeth, turning a key, opening a jar, or picking up a book.
- Complaints are directed toward the base of the thumb, and pain is frequently associated with a sensation of movement or "slipping" within the joint. An enlarging prominence, or "shoulder sign," inevitably develops at the base as the clinical manifestation of dorsal metacarpal subluxation on the trapezium and metacarpal adduction.
- Early presentation may result in only pain with TM stress and palpation beneath the thenar cone, without deformity, instability, subluxation, or crepitance.
- Methods for examining the thumb CMC joint for hypermobility (stage 1 disease) include the following:
  - Trapeziometacarpal stress test, which may cause pain or a slight shift or subluxation
  - Thenar CMC joint palpation test, which may cause pain

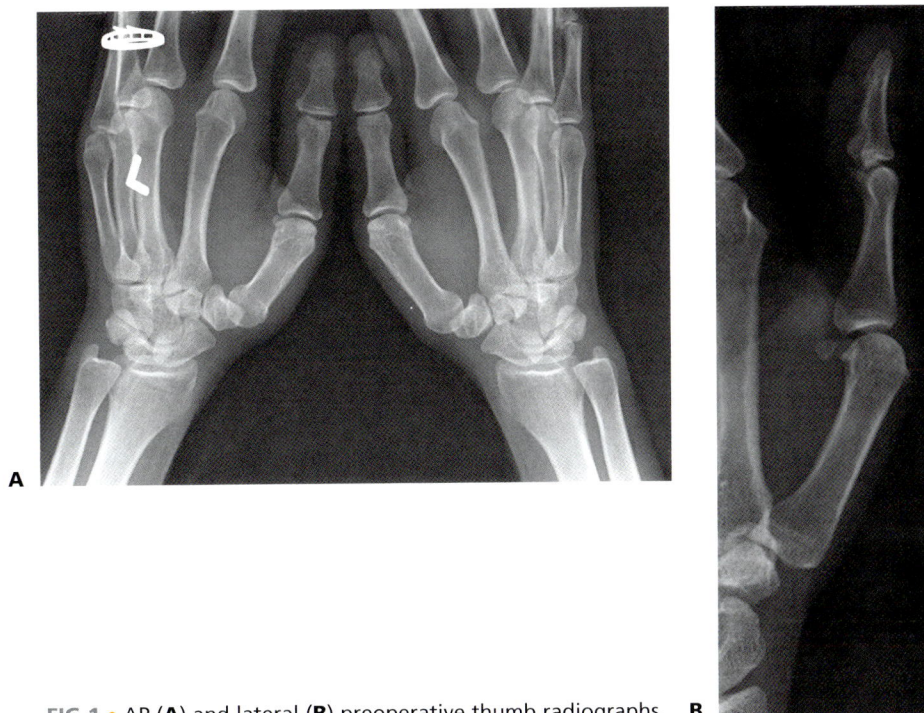

FIG 1 • AP (**A**) and lateral (**B**) preoperative thumb radiographs.

IMAGING AND OTHER DIAGNOSTIC STUDIES

▪ Radiographic evaluation includes a posteroanterior (PA) 30-degree oblique stress view, lateral view, and a Robert (pronated anteroposterior [AP]) view (**FIG 1**).

▪ Osteoarthritis may be confined to the TM joint, or it may involve the pan-trapezial joint complex. Indeed, the staging system described by Eaton and Littler describes four stages:

  ▪ Stage 1: a normal joint with the exception of possible widening from synovitis
  ▪ Stage 2: joint space narrowing with debris and osteophytes smaller than 2 mm
  ▪ Stage 3: joint space narrowing with debris and osteophytes larger than 2 mm
  ▪ Stage 4: scaphotrapezial joint space involvement in addition to narrowing of the TM joint

DIFFERENTIAL DIAGNOSIS

▪ CMC arthritis (stages 2 to 4)
▪ De Quervain tendonitis
▪ Flexor carpi radialis tendinitis

NONOPERATIVE MANAGEMENT

▪ Nonoperative treatment includes anti-inflammatory medication, intra-articular steroid injection, hand- or forearm-based thumb spica splint immobilization, and thenar muscle isometric conditioning.

▪ Although none of these measures may provide permanent or even long-lasting relief from symptoms, they may indeed provide temporary relief. This allows the patient to contemplate surgery, to gain acceptance, and to participate in the surgical decision-making process.

SURGICAL MANAGEMENT

▪ Until recently, surgical treatment has centered around reconstruction of the palmar beak ligament with a slip of flexor carpi radialis tendon, as described by Eaton and Littler.[3]

▪ The rationale for TM extension osteotomy involves dorsal load transfer and a shift in force vectors during pinch. Pellegrini et al[5] showed that a 30-degree closing wedge extension osteotomy effectively unloaded the palmar compartment when eburnation involved less than half, and optimally only one third, of the palmar joint surfaces. Osteotomy in this setting shifted the contact areas to the intact dorsal articular cartilage.

▪ The most recent biomechanical assessment of metacarpal osteotomy suggested that joint laxity is reduced in lateral pinch because of obligatory metacarpal flexion and resulting increased tightening of the dorsal radial ligament.[6]

Preoperative Planning

▪ Radiographs should show a normal joint or slight widening from synovitis. A trapeziometacarpal stress test should elicit pain along with palpation of the joint beneath the thenars. Obviously, other causes of discomfort in the region should be excluded.

Positioning

▪ The extremity is placed on a standard hand table.

Approach

▪ A dorsal approach is used and subperiosteal exposure of the base of the metacarpal is provided.

▪ The osteotomy is made 1 cm distal to the base and is 5 mm wide, so the incision should extend 4 cm distal to the base.

  ▪ The base of the wedge is therefore 5 mm wide and is dorsal. Its apex is palmar.

EXTENSION OSTEOTOMY WITH STAPLE FIXATION

- Regional, axillary block anesthesia is performed and a nonsterile tourniquet is placed.
- After exsanguination with an Esmarch bandage and inflation of the tourniquet to 250 mm Hg, make a dorsal incision from the base of the TM distally for about 3 cm.
- In the subcutaneous tissue, identify and protect the sensory branches of the radial and lateral antebrachial cutaneous nerves. Obtain subperiosteal exposure without injuring the extensor pollicis longus, and identify the TM joint with a 25-gauge needle.
  - One centimeter distal to the TM joint, obtain near-circumferential access around the metacarpal in anticipation of the osteotomy.
- Visualize the volar extent of the metacarpal at this location to facilitate accurate resection of a dorsally based 30-degree wedge of bone (**TECH FIG 1A**).

- Use a microsagittal saw to score the metacarpal 1 cm distal to its base transversely, but do not make a complete cut through the volar cortex.
  - Leave a new saw blade in that partial osteotomy site and use a second blade about 5 mm distal to the first cut at an angle of 30 degrees so that the two blades intersect at the volar cortex.
- Remove the wedge of bone, extend the distal metacarpal and compress it against the proximal fragment, and place one 11 × 8 staple (OSStaple™ BioMedical Enterprises, Inc., San Antonio, TX).
  - Typically, I maintain the reduced position of the metacarpal while my assistant predrills and then places the staple (**TECH FIG 1B,C**).
- Perform a layered closure of the periosteum and skin and place an overlying thumb spica splint.

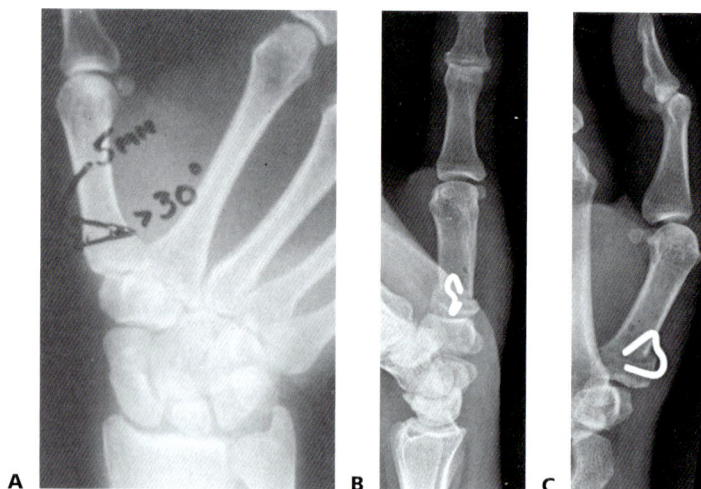

TECH FIG 1 • **A.** Radiograph showing planned osteotomy. **B,C.** AP and lateral postoperative thumb radiographs.

EXTENSION OSTEOTOMY WITH KIRSCHNER WIRE AND TENSION BAND FIXATION

- The technique is as described for staple fixation except for the use of Kirschner wires.
- Use a microsagittal saw to score the metacarpal 1 cm distal to its base transversely, but do not make a complete cut through the volar cortex.
  - Leave a new saw blade in that partial osteotomy site and use a second blade about 5 mm distal to the first cut at an angle of 30 degrees so that the two blades intersect at the volar cortex.
- Remove the wedge of bone and use a 0.045-inch Kirschner wire to place a transverse hole on either side of the osteotomy.

- Pass a 22-gauge wire radial to ulnar and ulnar to radial.
- Place a 0.045-inch Kirschner wire retrograde through the distal osteotomy site, exiting out the ulnar aspect of the thumb, and compress the osteotomy by extending the distal metacarpal.
- With an assistant maintaining compression, tighten the wire, cut it, and bend it beneath the thenar musculature. Then advance the Kirschner wire anterograde.
- Cut the Kirschner wire external to the skin to facilitate removal, and repair the periosteal origin of the thenar musculature with absorbable suture.

PEARLS AND PITFALLS

Intra-articular osteotomy	▪ Accurately locate the CMC joint with a 25-gauge needle so that the osteotomy is made 1 cm distal to the base.
Accurate execution of a 30-degree osteotomy	▪ Make the most proximal cut perpendicular to the metacarpal—with the metacarpal parallel to the table. ▪ Make the second cut at an angle of 30 degrees—5 mm distal to the first cut—such that the saw blade intersects the volar cortex at the location of the first blade.

POSTOPERATIVE CARE

- A thumb spica splint is placed for 10 days.
- At that time sutures are removed, and a thumb spica cast with the interphalangeal joint of the thumb left free is placed for an additional 4 weeks.
- About 6 weeks after surgery a forearm-based thumb spica Orthoplast splint is placed, and the patient is instructed to begin gentle TM motion.
- Grip and pinch exercises are started at about 8 weeks after surgery unless union is delayed.

OUTCOMES

- In light of Pellegrini et al's biomechanical data[5] and my own relative dissatisfaction with Eaton ligament reconstruction for stage 1 disease, primarily related to a prolonged recovery period (8 to 10 months) and a stiff TM joint, I prospectively evaluated the efficacy of a 30-degree extension osteotomy in 12 patients (12 thumbs) between 1995 and 1998.[8]
  - TM arthrotomy allowed accurate intra-articular assessment and verified AOL detachment from the metacarpal rim in each case.
  - Follow-up averaged 2.1 years (range 6 to 46 months).
  - All osteotomies healed at an average of 7 weeks. Eleven patients were satisfied with outcome. Grip and pinch strength increased an average of 8.5 and 3 kg, respectively.
- Since that study's publication, I have become even more impressed by the efficacy of the procedure and believe, as Koff et al[4] suggested, that osteotomy decreases laxity and shifts contact area more dorsally. It seems logical that the DRL participates in this effect, and this substantiates the contention that the DRL is an important stabilizer.

COMPLICATIONS

- Nonunion
- Persistent pain necessitating resection arthroplasty with trapezium excision
- Radial sensory nerve injury or dysethesia

REFERENCES

1. Bettinger P, Lindschied, Berger R, et al. An anatomic study of the stabilizing ligaments of the trapezium and trapeziometacarpal joint. J Hand Surg Am 1999;24A:786–798.
2. Doerschuk SH, Hicks DG, Chinchilli VM, et al. Histopathology of the palmar beak ligament in trapeziometacarpal osteoarthritis. J Hand Surg Am 1999;24A:496–504.
3. Eaton RG, Lane LB, Littler JW, et al. Ligament reconstruction for the painful thumb carpometacarpal joint: a long-term assessment. J Hand Surg 1984;9A:692–699.
4. Koff MF, Shrivastava N, Gardner TR, et al. An in vitro analysis of ligament reconstruction or extension osteotomy on trapeziometacarpal joint stability and contact area. J Hand Surg Am 2006;31A:429–439.
5. Pellegrini VD, Parentis M, Judkins A, et al. Extension metacarpal osteotomy in the treatment of trapeziometacarpal osteoarthritis: a biomechanical study. J Hand Surg 1996;21A:16–23.
6. Shrivastava N, Koff MF, Abbot AE, et al. Simulated extension osteotomy of the thumb metacarpal reduces carpometacarpal joint laxity in lateral pinch. J Hand Surg Am 2003;28A:733–738.
7. Tomaino MM. Thumb by metacarpal extension osteotomy: rationale and efficacy for Eaton stage disease. Hand Clin 2006;22:137–141.
8. Tomaino MM. Treatment of Eaton stage I trapeziometacarpal disease with thumb metacarpal extension osteotomy. J Hand Surg Am 2000;25A:1100–1106.

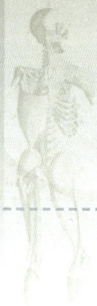

Warren C. Hammert and Matthew M. Tomaino

DEFINITION

- Osteoarthritis, or more appropriately termed osteoarthrosis, is a common problem in the hand.
- The trapeziometacarpal joint is frequently affected, second in frequency only to the distal interphalangeal joint, but much more disabling due to pain and weakness of grip and pinch strength.
- The surgical management of symptomatic basilar joint arthrosis depends on anatomy, radiographic staging, and patient requirements, followed by intraoperative confirmation of the stage of disease.
- Arthrodesis of the thumb carpometacarpal (CMC) joint was initially described by Muller over 50 years ago.[6] With refinements in arthroplasty procedures, arthrodesis of the basal joint of the thumb has become less popular, but the procedure still can provide an excellent result in the right circumstances; it is a valid treatment option for stage II or stage III disease only.

ANATOMY

- The thumb CMC joint is a biconcave joint, allowing for motion in three planes: flexion-extension, abduction-adduction, and pronation-supination.
- There are minimal osseous constraints, making the ligamentous structures extremely important stabilizers of the thumb base.
- A total of 16 ligaments have been described around the thumb CMC joint.
  - Seven are primary stabilizers of the thumb metacarpal:
    - Superficial and deep anterior oblique (sAOL and dAOL)
    - Dorsal radial
    - Posterior oblique
    - Ulnar collateral
    - Intermetacarpal
    - Dorsal intermetacarpal
  - The remainder stabilize the trapezium, providing a stable foundation for the thumb.[2]

PATHOGENESIS

- The pathogenesis of CMC joint arthrosis is multifactorial, involving biochemical and biomechanical influences. The synovial fluid within the joints contains cytokines, which invariably play a role in cartilage degradation and decreased ability to withstand the loads generated at the joint during daily activities.[10]
  - Although not clearly delineated, there probably is some protective role played by estrogen or estrogen-related compounds, which may explain the increased incidence of osteoarthritis in postmenopausal women (10 to 15:1).
- The anterior (palmar) oblique ligament, or so-called beak ligament, has been shown to be the most important stabilizing ligament of the thumb, and its degeneration or functional incompetence leads to laxity, followed by abnormal translation of the metacarpal on the trapezium, resulting in increased shear forces and abnormal wear patterns. This eventually leads to eburnation of the articular cartilage, initially along the palmar aspect of the joint.[9] With progression of disease, osteophytes develop and eburnation progresses throughout the entire joint surface.

- Osteoarthrosis can also develop from disruption of the articular cartilage. Any fracture involving the articular surfaces (most commonly the base of the thumb metacarpal) will predispose to or accelerate the development of arthrosis.
  - Anatomic restoration of the joint surface can minimize this progression but not eliminate it completely.
  - Paradoxically, a Bennett fracture may protect the joint from the development of osteoarthritis (assuming subluxation is not present) by virtue of consequential unloading of the volar aspect of the joint.

NATURAL HISTORY

- Arthrosis of the thumb CMC joint begins along the palmar aspect of the metacarpal secondary to laxity of the AOL.
- The entire base of the metacarpal and the distal trapezium experience eburnation of the cartilage, which progresses to develop osteophytes.
- The thumb metacarpal assumes an adducted position and the metacarpophalangeal (MCP) joint may compensate by becoming hyperextensile, resulting in hyperextension.
- Finally, the entire surface of the trapezium becomes involved, resulting in degeneration between the proximal trapezium and the distal scaphoid.
- Disease can involve all the trapezial articulations as well as the scaphotrapezoidal joint.[8,11]

PATIENT HISTORY AND PHYSICAL FINDINGS

- Thumb CMC joint arthrosis will often present with pain at the base of the metacarpal.
  - The pain will be exacerbated with activities involving loading the thumb metacarpal base, such as turning a doorknob, twisting a lid off a jar, or turning a key.
  - Pain at rest may or may not be present.
- Symptoms do not always correlate with the clinical or radiographic appearance. A patient may have advanced clinical and radiographic disease but be minimally symptomatic. Conversely, a patient may have significant symptoms with minimal radiographic changes and no clinical deformity at rest.
- Physical examination of the patient with advanced disease reveals deformity.
  - The thumb subluxates in a dorsal direction and becomes fixed in adduction, manifesting as a prominence at the base of the thumb and decreased ability to abduct the thumb away from the palm.
  - In an effort to compensate for this limitation, the MCP joint will often hyperextend, creating a zig-zag deformity.

- Asking the patient to place one finger on the point that is most symptomatic helps localize the point of maximal tenderness to the CMC joint or another area.
- CMC grind test: Reproduction of symptoms confirms the CMC joint as a site of disease.
- CMC distraction test: Reproduction of symptoms confirms the CMC joint as a site of disease.
- Finkelstein maneuver: Maximal tenderness indicates that DeQuervain disease may be a greater source of symptoms.
- Phalen test: Reproduction of symptoms indicates carpal tunnel syndrome as a more likely etiology.
- Carpal tunnel compression test: Reproduction of symptoms indicates carpal tunnel syndrome as a more likely etiology.
- Trigger evaluation: Reproduction of pain, triggering, or locking of the thumb indicates trigger thumb as an etiology.
- Allen test: The radial and ulnar arteries are compressed and the hand is exsanguinated. The ulnar artery is released and the circulation of the hand is assessed. The process is repeated, releasing the radial artery while the ulnar artery is occluded. Surgical procedures often involve mobilization of the radial artery in the snuffbox. Damage to this artery will require reconstruction if the ulnar artery cannot compensate.
- Other conditions causing pain at the base of the thumb must be eliminated, such as DeQuervain disease, trigger thumb, and carpal tunnel syndrome. Although more than one condition may exist, the physical examination can usually determine the most problematic area.

IMAGING AND OTHER DIAGNOSTIC STUDIES

- Plain radiographs are the imaging modality of choice for evaluation of thumb CMC joint arthrosis (**FIG 1**).
  - These include a pronated AP (Robert view), lateral, and a 30-degree posteroanterior stress view.
- Eaton and Littler[3] have described a radiographic staging system that is commonly used, but Tomaino et al[11] have emphasized routine assessment of the scaphotrapezoidal joint, both radiographically and intraoperatively, to rule out scaphotrapezoidal arthritis, or what they termed "stage V disease."

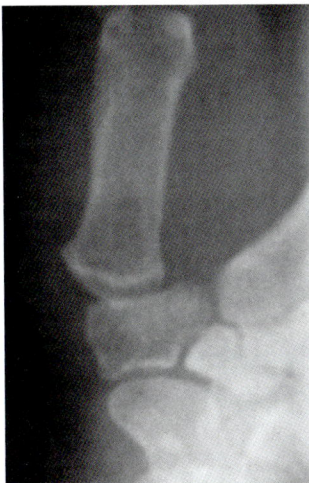

FIG 1 • AP radiograph of the thumb carpometacarpal joint.

- Stage I: normal-appearing or widened joint space secondary to synovitis
- Stage II: joint space narrowing and osteophyte formation smaller than 2 mm
- Stage III: joint space narrowing with osteophytes larger than 2 mm
- Stage IV: stage III appearance with the addition of narrowing or osteophytes in the scaphotrapezial joint
- The scaphotrapezoid joint is not specifically addressed in this system and may be difficult to assess radiographically, but this joint should always be assessed at the time of surgery because it may be a source of continued pain.

DIFFERENTIAL DIAGNOSIS

- Thumb CMC arthrosis
- DeQuervain disease
- Trigger thumb or stenosing tenosynovitis
- Carpal tunnel syndrome
- Intramuscular (thenar) processes, such as vascular or tumor etiologies

NONOPERATIVE MANAGEMENT

- Most patients with symptomatic thumb CMC joint arthrosis benefit from a trial of conservative therapy, which may include corticosteroid injection, thenar isometric strengthening exercises, and splinting.[1]
  - Although this will not eliminate the problem or alter the underlying disease process, it often reduces symptoms, at least transiently, allowing the patient the opportunity to plan for surgical treatment at the most opportune time.
- Steroid injections can also be helpful in determining how much of a patient's symptoms are coming from the thumb CMC joint versus other areas (carpal tunnel or De Quervain disease).

SURGICAL MANAGEMENT

- The indications for surgical intervention for symptomatic thumb basilar joint arthrosis include pain and weakness not responsive to conservative treatments.
- There are multiple procedures used to treat symptomatic CMC thumb arthritis, many of which have merit depending on several factors. Consideration should be given to the age of the patient and the demands placed on the thumb (specifically looking at the patient's occupation) as well as the radiographic stage and the condition of surrounding joints.
- The best candidates for thumb CMC arthrodesis are young, active patients who need to maintain power grip and pinch, and regularly place high demand on their thumb. These are typically young male manual laborers with stage II or III disease.
- Special consideration should be given to the thumb MCP joint. If hyperextension and laxity are present, arthrodesis of the CMC joint is not an appropriate option, because fusion of both the thumb CMC and MCP joints will result in significant functional impairment.
- Pan-trapezial involvement represents a contraindication for CMC arthrodesis because of the risk of incomplete pain relief.

Preoperative Planning

- The patient should be made aware of the decreased mobility, inability to flatten the palm on the table, potential difficulty in placing the hand in tight confined spaces, and possible difficulty placing the hand in a glove.

- Patients also should understand the risks of nonunion, potential for hardware complications, and potential for developing degenerative changes at adjacent joints.

Positioning

- The procedure is performed under regional or general anesthesia with the use of a pneumatic tourniquet.
- The patient is in supine position with the arm extended on an armboard.

Approach

- The procedure can be performed through a Wagner-type incision, along the junction of the glabrous and dorsal skin, or through a dorsal incision.
- The dorsal incision can be oriented in a longitudinal fashion, along the radial aspect of the first dorsal compartment tendons, or in a transverse direction, with the incision oriented in the resting skin tension lines centered over the trapeziometacarpal joint.

THUMB CMC (TRAPEZIOMETACARPAL) ARTHRODESIS

Incision and Dissection

- Make a dorsal longitudinal incision along the radial aspect of the first dorsal compartment tendons (TECH FIG 1A).
- Identify and protect sensory branches of the radial nerve and the lateral antebrachial cutaneous nerve (TECH FIG 1B).
- Identify the first dorsal compartment tendons and release the compartment along the ulnar aspect to allow for better exposure (TECH FIG 1C).
- Identify the dorsal branch of the radial artery deep to the abductor pollicis longus and extensor pollicis brevis tendons running in a dorsal and ulnar direction (TECH FIG 1D). Carefully mobilize and protect it.
- Identify the base of the metacarpal, and complete a longitudinal capsulotomy to expose the base of the metacarpal, the entire trapezium, and the distal aspect of the scaphoid.
- Fluoroscopy is used to confirm the location of the CMC joint if necessary.

Preparation of the Joint

- Inspect the scaphotrapeziotrapezoid joints (TECH FIG 2A).
  - If there is evidence of arthrosis, consideration is given to alternative procedures.

- Then inspect the CMC joint (TECH FIG 2B).
  - By freeing the surrounding capsular attachments, the base of the metacarpal can be flexed to allow better access to the joint.
- Use a rongeur to remove osteophytes (TECH FIG 2C), any remaining articular cartilage, and subchondral bone. Shape the metacarpal base in a cone fashion to provide a larger surface area and greater freedom for obtaining the ideal position for arthrodesis (TECH FIG 2D).
- Decorticate the distal aspect of the trapezium in a similar fashion, creating a cup for placement of the prepared metacarpal base.

Positioning and Fixation

- The position for arthrodesis should allow the tip of the thumb to rest against the radial aspect of the index middle phalanx when the hand is placed in the fisted position.
  - The exact angles to accomplish this position are debated, but in general there should be about 45 degrees of palmar abduction and adequate pronation to allow positioning.
- Place three 0.045-inch smooth Kirschner wires through the decorticated metacarpal base in a antegrade manner,

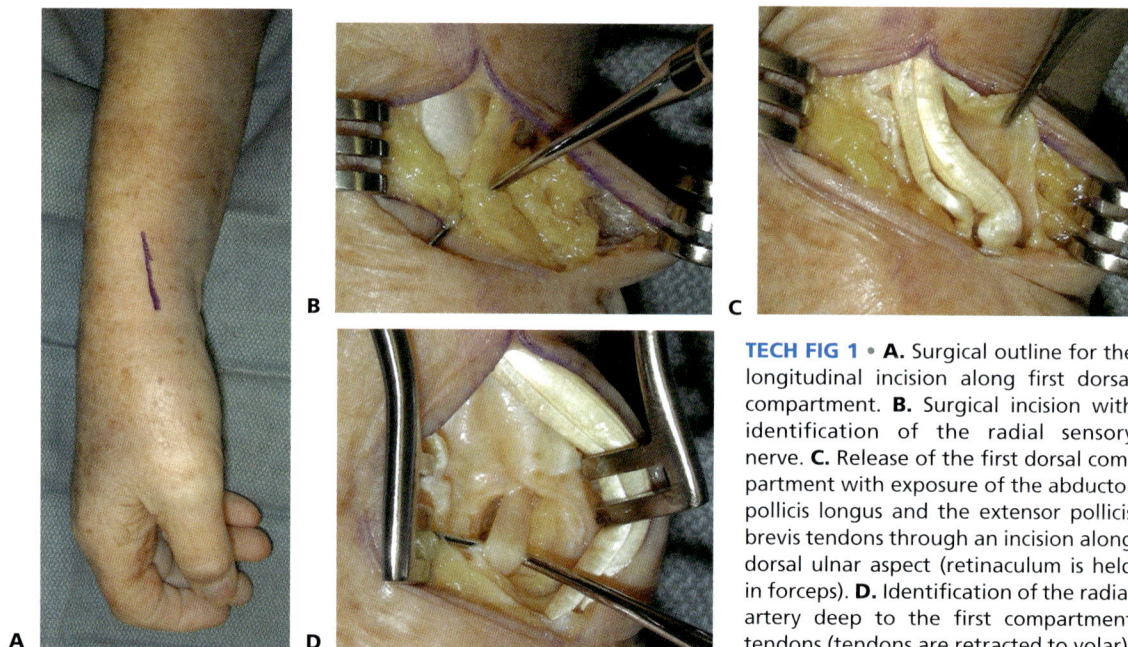

TECH FIG 1 • A. Surgical outline for the longitudinal incision along first dorsal compartment. B. Surgical incision with identification of the radial sensory nerve. C. Release of the first dorsal compartment with exposure of the abductor pollicis longus and the extensor pollicis brevis tendons through an incision along dorsal ulnar aspect (retinaculum is held in forceps). D. Identification of the radial artery deep to the first compartment tendons (tendons are retracted to volar).

TECHNIQUES

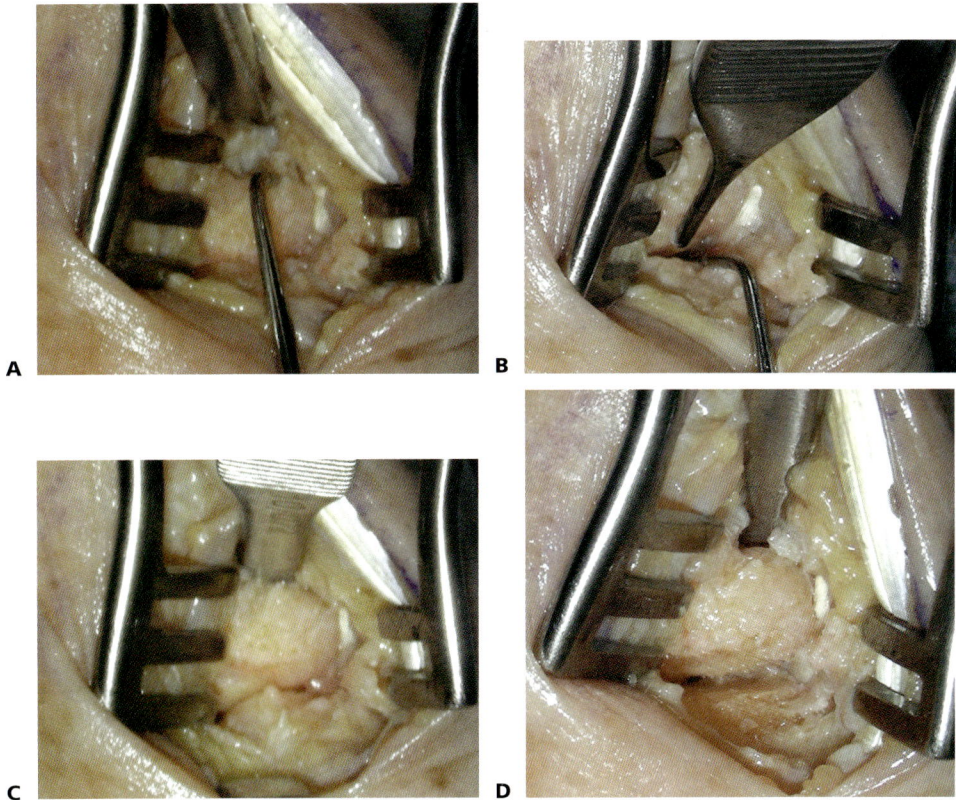

TECH FIG 2 • A. Inspection of the scaphotrapeziotrapezoid (STT) joint for arthrosis (probe is in the scaphotrapezial joint). **B.** Exposure of the carpometacarpal (CMC) joint (forceps are around trapezium and probe is in CMC joint). **C.** Close-up view of small dorsal osteophyte along base of thumb metacarpal. **D.** View of the CMC joint after removal of articular cartilage in preparation for arthrodesis.

exiting the dorsal aspect of the metacarpal until the tip of the wires are just beneath the prepared proximal metacarpal (**TECH FIG 3A**).

- The metacarpal is then aligned with the trapezium, properly positioned, and compressed with axially directed force (**TECH FIG 3B**).
- Advance the Kirschner wires retrograde across the joint into the trapezium, anchoring in the subchondral bone.
  - The wires can be advanced into the carpus (**TECH FIG 3C**).
- Fluoroscopy is used to confirm reduction and Kirschner wire placement (**TECH FIG 3D**). If there is inadequate

bony apposition, distal radius bone graft can be harvested and used to fill any voids.

- Close the capsule with a nonabsorbable suture and close the skin with buried absorbable sutures.
- Bend the Kirschner wires and cut them external to the skin.
- If mild thumb MCP joint hyperextension is noted at this juncture, pin the MCP joint in 20 degrees of flexion. If dynamic collapse accompanies pinch, then perform volar capsulodesis.
- Apply a well-padded short-arm thumb spica splint.

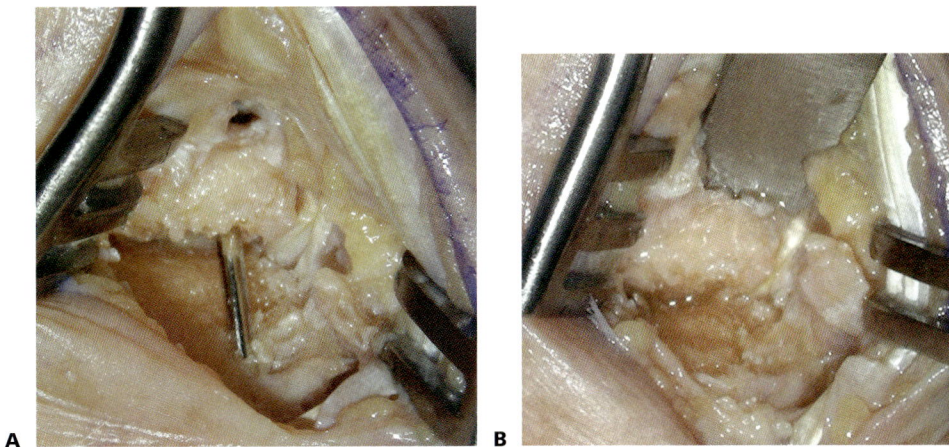

TECH FIG 3 • A. Preliminary placement of Kirschner wire to check alignment before compression of the arthrodesis site. **B.** Final inspection of the prepared surfaces before compression and advancement of the Kirschner wires across site of arthrodesis. *(continued)*

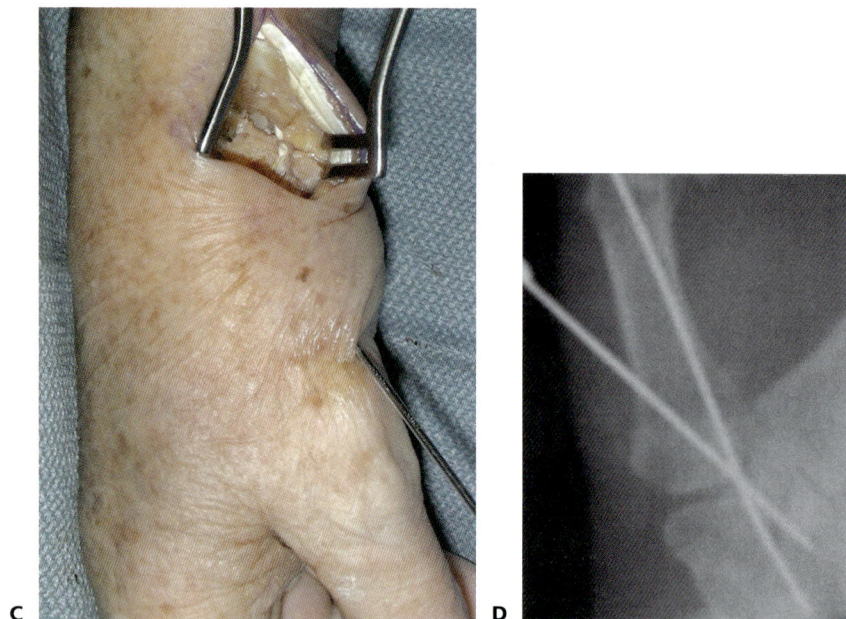

TECH FIG 3 • *(continued)* **C.** Appearance of the arthrodesis site after compression and advancement of the Kirschner wires. **D.** Radiograph of the thumb carpometacarpal arthrodesis with the Kirschner wires in place.

VARIATIONS

Bony Preparation

- Rather than the "cup and cone" technique, an oscillating saw can be used to create two flat surfaces that can be apposed, allowing a large contact area.
- Make the cuts in the exact plane desired, or the position of the thumb will be compromised.
- This is a much less forgiving technique than the cup and cone method, which allows for correction by rotation of the metacarpal while positioning it on the trapezium.

Fixation Devices

- Single or multiple smooth Kirschner wires, tension band wiring, cerclage wiring, staples, compression screws, and plates and screws have all been used with documented success.
- Union rates are comparable for Kirschner wires and more rigid fixation devices, but plates and screws result in a higher rate of additional procedures, typically due to hardware prominence or tendon irritation.
- Kirschner wires are associated with the fewest complications and are the simplest method of fixation.

PEARLS AND PITFALLS

Surgical approach	▪ Take care to protect the cutaneous branches of the radial sensory nerve and the lateral antebrachial cutaneous nerve throughout the entire procedure. ▪ Protect the radial artery located under the abductor pollicis longus and extensor pollicis brevis tendons.
Intraoperative joint inspection	▪ Carefully inspect the scaphotrapeziotrapezoid joints, as arthritic involvement at these joints will preclude success with CMC arthrodesis.
Judicious use of bone graft	▪ Make sure there is good apposition of the bony surfaces before closure. Use bone graft to fill any voids, which may lead to nonunion.
Treatment of MCP joint laxity	▪ Consider pinning the MCP joint in 20 degrees of flexion if mild hyperextension exists.
Radial sensory nerve injury	▪ If there is inadvertent injury to the radial sensory nerve and this is recognized, it should be repaired with fine epineurial suture.
Radial artery injury	▪ If there is inadvertent injury to the radial artery, it should be temporarily clipped with temporary vascular clamps. After the arthrodesis is completed and the capsule is closed, the tourniquet is deflated. If there is good perfusion to all the digits, the artery can be ligated. If the perfusion is inadequate, microvascular repair must be accomplished.
Nonunion or malunion	▪ Inadequate preparation of joint surfaces may lead to nonunion. ▪ Improper positioning of thumb metacarpal on the trapezium may lead to malunion.

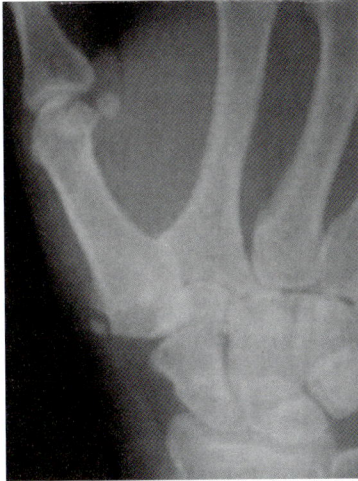

FIG 2 • Final radiograph, demonstrating fusion of the carpometacarpal joint.

POSTOPERATIVE CARE

■ The patient is seen in the office at 10 to 14 days to check the wound and the Kirschner wires and to obtain radiographs.

■ If fixation is secure and the Kirschner wires are not advanced through the trapezium, a well-molded short-arm thumb spica splint is applied and removed for hygiene purposes only. If the Kirschner wires are advanced into the carpus, the patient is placed in a thumb spica cast.

■ If there is any concern about fixation, a short-arm thumb spica cast is applied and the patient is seen at 2- to 3-week intervals until clinical tenderness subsides and there is radiographic evidence of fusion (**FIG 2**). This typically occurs by 6 to 8 weeks after surgery.

■ Once healing is documented, the pins are removed and range-of-motion exercises are begun under the direction of a hand therapist. The splint is continued for protection.

■ At 3 months, strengthening exercises are begun, the splint is discontinued, and the patient is allowed to return to unrestricted activities.

OUTCOMES

■ The outcomes of trapeziometacarpal arthrodesis are generally good, with predictable pain relief and patient satisfaction.

■ Hartigan et al[5] retrospectively reviewed patients who had arthrodesis and compared them to those having trapezial excision and ligament reconstruction. At 6 to 9 months there were no significant differences in pain, function, patient satisfaction, or grip strength. The arthrodesis group had greater key pinch and three-point pinch but more difficulty with opposition and the ability to flatten the hand, all of which were statistically significant. The arthrodesis group also had a higher complication rate, most of which was attributable to

nonunion. Interestingly, all patients with nonunion had improvement in their pain and were satisfied with their outcomes.

■ Forseth and Stern[4] compared the complication rate with Kirschner wire fixation to that with plates and screws and found similar nonunion rates (less than 10% in their small series), but there were higher rates of secondary procedures and lower patient satisfaction in the plate and screw group.

■ Despite Hartigan et al's report, which found that the ligament reconstruction and tendon interposition (LRTI) arthroplasty and arthrodesis resulted in high levels of patient satisfaction, Mureau et al[7] found less subjective improvement with arthrodesis in comparison to arthroplasty and no significant differences in pinch strength. They also found a higher incidence of complications in the arthrodesis group.

COMPLICATIONS

■ Complications from thumb CMC arthrodesis are generally related to nonunion or hardware problems, including malposition (screws in the trapeziotrapezoid joint), prominence and tendon irritation, and rupture.

■ The patient should be made aware of the possible need for secondary procedures.

REFERENCES

1. Berggren M, Joost-Davidsson A, Lindstrand J, et al. Reduction in the need for operation after conservative treatment of osteoarthritis of the first carpometacarpal joint: a seven year prospective study. Scand J Plastic Reconstr Surg Hand Surg 2001;35:415–417.
2. Bettinger P, Linscheid RL, Berger R, et al. An anatomical study of the stabilizing ligaments of the trapezium and trapeziometacarpal joint. J Hand Surg Am 1999;24A:786–798.
3. Eaton RG, Littler JW. Ligament reconstruction for the painful thumb carpometacarpal joint. J Bone Joint Surg Am 1973;55A:1655–1666.
4. Forseth MJ, Stern PJ. Complications of trapeziometacarpal arthrodesis using plate and screw fixation. J Hand Surg Am 2003;28A:342–345.
5. Hartigan BJ, Stern PJ, Kiefhaber TR. Thumb carpometacarpal osteoarthritis: arthrodesis compared with ligament reconstruction and tendon interposition. J Bone Joint Surg Am 2001;83A:1470–1478.
6. Muller GM. Arthrodesis of the trapeziometacarpal joint for osteoarthritis. J Bone Joint Surg Br 1949;31B:540–542.
7. Mureau M, Rademaker R, Verhaar J, et al. Tendon interposition arthroplasty versus arthrodesis for the treatment of trapeziometacarpal arthritis: a prospective comparative follow-up study. J Hand Surg Am 2001;26A:869–876.
8. North ER, Eaton RG. Degenerative arthritis of the trapezium: a comparative roentgenologic and anatomic study. J Hand Surg Am 1983;8A:160–166.
9. Pellegrini VD, Olcott CW, Hollenberg G. Contact patterns in the trapeziometacarpal joint: the role of the palmar oblique ligament. J Hand Surg Am 1993;18A:238–244.
10. Pellegrini VD, Smith RL, Ku CW. Pathobiology of articular cartilage in trapeziometacarpal osteoarthritis. I. Regional biochemical analysis. J Hand Surg Am 1994;19A:70–85.
11. Tomaino MM, Vogt M, Weiser R. Scaphotrapezoid arthritis: prevalence in thumbs undergoing trapezium excision arthroplasty and efficacy of proximal trapezoid excision. J Hand Surg 1999;24A:1220–1224.

Chapter 83

Thumb Carpometacarpal Joint Resection Arthroplasty

Matthew M. Tomaino

DEFINITION

▪ Osteoarthritis, or more appropriately osteoarthrosis, is a common problem in the hand. The trapeziometacarpal joint is commonly affected, second in frequency only to the distal interphalangeal joint. Trapeziometacarpal joint osteoarthritis, however, can be much more disabling secondary to pain and weakness of grip and pinch strength.

▪ The surgical management of symptomatic basilar joint arthrosis varies according to the anatomy, radiographic staging, intraoperative confirmation of disease stage, and patient requirements.

ANATOMY

▪ The thumb carpometacarpal (CMC) joint is a biconcave joint, allowing for motion in three planes: flexion-extension, abduction-adduction, and pronation-supination.

▪ There are minimal constraints from an osseous standpoint, making the ligamentous structures extremely important in providing stability to the base of the thumb. A total of 16 ligaments have been described around the thumb CMC joint, 7 of which are primary stabilizers of the thumb metacarpal (TM).

▪ The superficial and deep anterior oblique, dorsal radial, posterior oblique, ulnar collateral, intermetacarpal, and dorsal intermetacarpal ligaments directly stabilize the TM, while the remainder serve to stabilize the trapezium, allowing for a stable foundation for the thumb to rest on (**FIG 1**).[1]

PATHOGENESIS

▪ The pathogenesis of CMC joint arthrosis is multifactorial, involving biochemical and biomechanical influences. The synovial fluid within the joints contains cytokines that invariably play a role in cartilage degradation and decreased ability to withstand the loads generated at the joint during daily activities.[8] Although not clearly delineated, estrogen or estrogen-related compounds probably play some protective role, which may explain the increased incidence of osteoarthritis in postmenopausal women (10 to 15:1).

▪ The palmar or anterior oblique ligament (AOL), or so-called beak ligament, has been shown to be the most important stabilizing ligament of the thumb. Degeneration or functional incompetence of this ligament leads to laxity, abnormal translation of the metacarpal on the trapezium, increased shear forces, and resultant abnormal wear patterns. This eburnation of the articular cartilage initially occurs along the palmar aspect of the joint.[9] With progression of disease, osteophytes develop and eburnation progresses throughout the entire joint surface.

▪ Osteoarthrosis can also develop from damage and disruption of the articular cartilage. Any fracture through the metacarpal or trapezium joint surfaces yield arthrosis. Anatomic restoration of the joint surface can minimize this sequela but cannot eliminate the risk entirely. Paradoxically, however, a Bennett fracture may protect the joint from the development of osteoarthritis, assuming subluxation has been treated, by virtue of consequential unloading of the volar aspect of the joint.

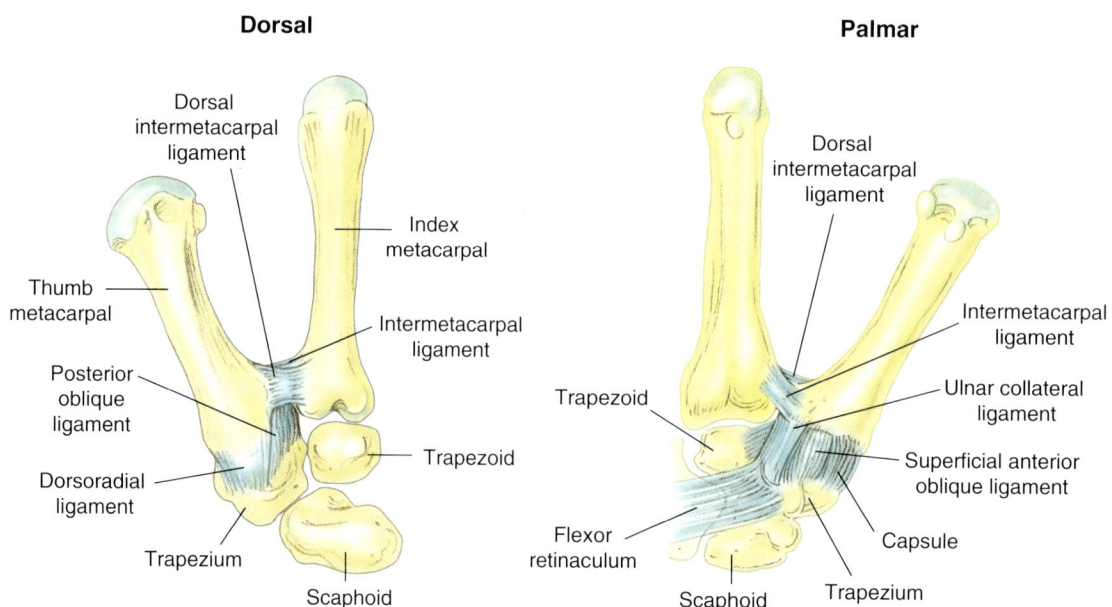

Dorsal

- Dorsal intermetacarpal ligament
- Index metacarpal
- Thumb metacarpal
- Intermetacarpal ligament
- Posterior oblique ligament
- Trapezoid
- Dorsoradial ligament
- Trapezium
- Scaphoid

Palmar

- Dorsal intermetacarpal ligament
- Intermetacarpal ligament
- Trapezoid
- Ulnar collateral ligament
- Superficial anterior oblique ligament
- Flexor retinaculum
- Capsule
- Scaphoid
- Trapezium

FIG 1 • Carpometacarpal thumb joint.

NATURAL HISTORY

▪ Arthrosis of the thumb CMC joint begins along the palmar aspect of the metacarpal secondary to laxity of the AOL. As the process progresses, the entire base of the metacarpal and distal trapezium becomes involved.

▪ There is initial eburnation of the cartilage, which progresses to osteophyte formation. As the disease continues, the TM assumes an adducted position and the metacarpophalangeal (MCP) joint may compensate by becoming hyperextensile, resulting in varying degrees of MCP joint hyperextension.

▪ The disease can involve all the trapezial articulations as well as the scaphotrapezoidal joint.[14]

PATIENT HISTORY AND PHYSICAL FINDINGS

▪ Thumb CMC joint arthrosis often presents with pain at the base of the metacarpal. The pain may or may not be present at rest. It will be exacerbated with activities involving loading the TM base, such as turning a doorknob, twisting a lid off a jar, or turning a key.

▪ With advanced disease, the thumb subluxes in a dorsal direction and becomes fixed in adduction. This manifests as a prominence at the base of the thumb and decreased ability to abduct the thumb away from the palm. In an effort to compensate for this, the MCP joint will often hyperextend, creating a zig-zag deformity.

▪ Symptoms do not always correlate with the clinical or radiographic appearance, meaning that a patient may have advanced clinical and radiographic disease but be minimally symptomatic. Conversely, a patient may have substantial symptoms with minimal radiographic changes and no clinical deformity at rest.

▪ Other conditions causing pain at the base of the thumb must be eliminated, such as De Quervain disease, trigger thumb, and carpal tunnel syndrome. Although more than one condition may exist, the physical examination can usually determine the most troubled area.

▪ Physical examination includes the following:
  ▪ Point tenderness assessment: With the TM adducted, the CMC joint is palpated beneath the thenars. Tenderness confirms the clinical significance of changes seen on radiographs.
  ▪ Reproduction of symptoms on the CMC grind test confirms the CMC joint as a site disease.
  ▪ Key pinch assessment: If dynamic collapse accompanies pinch, MCP joint fusion or capsulodesis is recommended (**FIG 2**).

IMAGING AND OTHER DIAGNOSTIC STUDIES

▪ Plain radiographs are the imaging modality of choice for evaluation of thumb CMC joint arthrosis. These include a pronated AP (Robert view), lateral, and a 30-degree posteroanterior stress view (**FIG 3**).

▪ Eaton and Littler have described a radiographic staging system, which is commonly used, but Tomaino et al[14] have emphasized routine assessment of the scaphotrapezoidal joint, both radiographically and intraoperatively, to rule out scaphotrapezoidal arthritis—what they termed stage V disease.

  ▪ Stage I: normal-appearing or widened joint space secondary to synovitis
  ▪ Stage II: joint space narrowing and osteophyte formation smaller than 2 mm
  ▪ Stage III: joint space narrowing with osteophytes larger than 2 mm
  ▪ Stage IV: scaphotrapezial joint space involvement in addition to narrowing of the TM joint

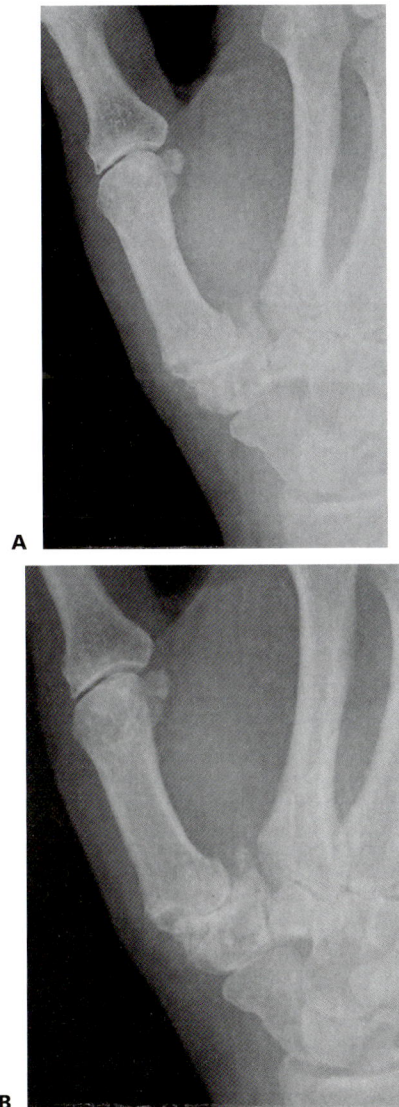

FIG 3 • Preoperative PA stress and lateral radiographs of the right thumb.

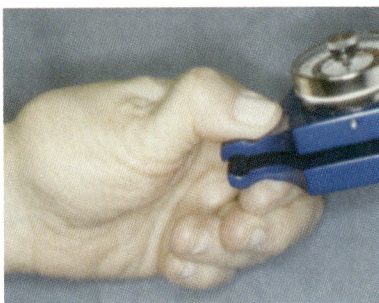

FIG 2 • Dynamic collapse of the thumb on key pinch testing.

■ Stage V: stage IV appearance with the addition of narrowing or osteophytes in the scaphotrapezoid joint
■ The scaphotrapezoid joint is not specifically addressed in this system and may be difficult to assess radiographically, but it should always be assessed clinically during operative intervention because it may be a source of continued pain.

DIFFERENTIAL DIAGNOSIS

■ De Quervain disease
■ Trigger thumb or stenosing tenosynovitis
■ Carpal tunnel syndrome

NONOPERATIVE MANAGEMENT

■ Most patients with symptomatic thumb CMC joint arthrosis benefit from a trial of conservative therapy, which may include corticosteroid injection, thenar isometric strengthening exercises, and splinting.
■ Although this will not eliminate the problem or alter the underlying disease process, conservative treatment often reduces symptoms, at least transiently, allowing the patient the opportunity to plan for surgical treatment at the most opportune time.
■ Differential injection of steroids can also be helpful to assess how much of a patient's symptoms are coming from the thumb CMC joint versus other areas (carpal tunnel or De Quervain disease).

SURGICAL MANAGEMENT

■ The indications for surgical intervention for symptomatic thumb basilar joint arthrosis include pain and weakness.
■ There are multiple procedures used to treat symptomatic CMC thumb arthritis, many of which have merit depending on the extent of arthritic involvement.
■ Pan-trapezial involvement contraindicates the use of arthrodesis or implant arthroplasty, in particular, because of the risk of incomplete pain relief.
■ Arthrodesis may be preferable in younger, high-demand patients such as laborers.
■ Resection arthroplasty can be performed with ligament reconstruction or without (hematoma distraction arthroplasty).[4,6]
■ The flexor carpi radialis (FCR) and abductor pollicis longus (APL) are most commonly used when performing "suspensionplasty."

Preoperative Planning

■ Consideration should be given to the age of the patient and the demands placed on the thumb.
■ Dynamic collapse of the MCP joint during key pinch necessitates MCP fusion or capsulodesis.
■ Intraoperative evaluation of the scaphotrapezotrapezoidal (STT) joint is critical to ensure adequate pain relief after surgery. Thus, hemitrapeziectomy is rarely performed once the decision to proceed with conventional resection arthroplasty is made. If retention of the proximal trapezium is elected because of the absence of STT disease, Artelon resurfacing or joint arthroplasty may be elected.
■ Intraoperative assessment of the scaphotrapezoidal joint is recommended, and if changes exist, a 2- to 3-mm resection of the proximal trapezoid is performed.[14] Care is taken not to injure the capitate.
■ Suspensionplasty ensures stability of the TM during pinch and grip, resisting the cantilever bending forces that will potentially lead to subluxation and proximal migration compared to trapeziectomy alone.
■ Intermediate-term outcome of the hematoma distraction arthroplasty suggests that this procedure may have a role in providing excellent pain relief in well-selected patients for whom grip strength is a less important issue.[4]

Positioning

■ The patient is supine and the involved hand and arm are supported by a hand table.

Approach

■ Trapezium excision and ligament reconstruction and suspensionplasty can be performed using the Wagner (volar) approach or a dorsal approach. I prefer the dorsal approach except when performing an Eaton ligament reconstruction, in which case a volar approach is used. I have modified my technique since performing the ligament reconstruction and tendon interposition (LRTI) arthroplasty exclusively during the first 10 years of practice.[11,12]
■ Over the past 5 years I have performed a suspensionplasty using a distally based slip of the APL tendon, which obviates the need for a bony channel. This is a variation of other suspensionplasty techniques.[7,10,15] In addition, I no longer pin the joint or interpose tissue into the space remaining after trapezial resection. The procedure is performed more expeditiously and seems to be associated with equivalent outcomes.[13]

LRTI ARTHROPLASTY USING THE FCR TENDON[11,12]

Incision and Superficial Dissection

■ A triradiate is drawn before the tourniquet is inflated to allow palpation of the radial pulse in the vicinity of the anatomic snuffbox; this typically identifies the scaphotrapezial joint.
■ When a substantial shoulder sign (prominence associated with dorsal subluxation of the proximal phalanx trapezium) exists, it can be difficult to identify the TM joint. In these cases, palpation of the scaphoid tuberosity is helpful to ensure that the incision is neither too distal nor too proximal.

■ The triradiate incision facilitates dissection of the radial artery off the dorsal capsule; when first extensor compartment release is planned, however, a longitudinal incision may be preferred.
■ At the outset, the radial sensory nerve must be identified and small branches must not be skeletonized or divided. This may cause postoperative radial sensory neuritis and even transient reflex sympathetic dystrophy.
■ Place blunt retractors beneath the extensor pollicis longus (EPL) in a dorsal and ulnar position and the APL radially and volarly.

TECHNIQUES

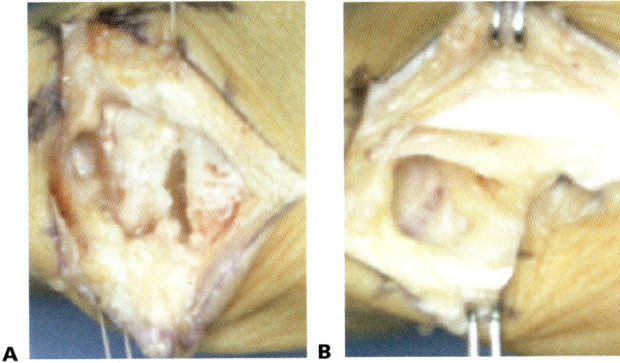

TECH FIG 1 • The base of the metacarpal is resected (**A**), and the trapezium is excised (**B**).

- ■ The radial artery courses within this interval, and deep perforators to the dorsal capsule must be coagulated and divided so the artery can be retracted dorsally and ulnarly.

Capsular Incision and Trapezial Excision

- ■ With gentle traction on the thumb, perform a longitudinal capsulotomy and obtain subperiosteal exposure of the trapezium and the base of the metacarpal (**TECH FIG 1A**). Extend the capsulotomy proximally so the scaphotrapezial joint is identified.
    - ■ Either retractors or tag sutures of 3-0 Vicryl can be used to retract the capsule.
- ■ Before the trapezium is excised, use a microsagittal saw to remove a thin sliver of bone at the base of the metacarpal. This facilitates exposure of the distal extent of the trapezium and, with further traction on the thumb, provides a safer window for sectioning of the trapezium.
- ■ Cut the trapezium into quadrants, beginning with the limb that parallels the expected course of the FCR tendon. Injury to the tendon during this portion of the procedure is unlikely if the saw is not brought completely through the trapezium.
- ■ After making perpendicular cuts in the trapezium, place an osteotome and twist it to break apart its four quadrants. Removal of the trapezium in pieces with a rongeur is facilitated by sharp dissection of the remaining capsule, particularly volarly and around loose bodies. Avoid inordinate ripping and pulling with the rongeurs because damage to the underlying capsule can increase postoperative discomfort, particularly where it abuts the carpal tunnel.
- ■ Remove osteophytic bone between the base of the thumb and index metacarpal so that pain does not accompany key pinch after the procedure. Identify the FCR tendon at the base of the arthroplasty space so it is not injured; remember that the trapezium may encircle the flexor carpi radialis tendon at its volar extent.
- ■ At this portion of the procedure, I routinely have an assistant place traction on the index and long finger to allow inspection of the scaphotrapezoidal joint. If there is cartilage fraying or eburnation, a motorized burr or rongeur is used to remove 2 to 3 mm of proximal trapezoid so that, with axial compression applied to the index

and long finger metacarpals, there is no contact between the remaining trapezoid and scaphoid (**TECH FIG 1B**). I do not interpose soft tissue or FCR tendon into the space. Take care not to remove bone from the capitate.

Creation of the Bony Channel Through the Metacarpal Base

- ■ One centimeter distal to the squared-off base of the metacarpal, in the plane of the nail, create a bone tunnel with a motorized 3-mm burr that exits at the volar base of the metacarpal (**TECH FIG 2**).
    - ■ This position is selected rather than central exit point in the metacarpal base because passage of the FCR tendon volarly more closely simulates the original attachment of the beak ligament.
- ■ Enlarge the bony channel with two curettes of increasing size, but do not make it large enough for the entire width of the leading edge of the FCR tendon. Rather, trim the full width of the FCR at its tip to facilitate passage with a Carroll tendon passer. In that light, the bony channel needs to be large enough only for the Carroll tendon passer to be used.

FCR Harvest

- ■ Palpate the FCR tendon at wrist level during passive flexion and extension of the wrist, where it is clearly tendinous. More proximally in the forearm the tendon becomes less discrete. This generally correlates with the proximal one third to half of the forearm. At that location make a 1.5-cm transverse incision.
- ■ Open the fascia, maximally flex the wrist, and identify the interval between the FCR tendon and muscle. Lift it into the wound via a curved clamp and divide it. Close this wound with 5-0 nylon sutures.
- ■ Retract the capsular flaps to protect the overlying radial artery dorsally and ulnarly. Place a curved snap beneath the FCR tendon and pull it. This typically delivers the entire tendon into the arthroplasty space.
- ■ Grasp the tendon at its tip and mobilize it to its insertion at the base of the index metacarpal without violating the small blood vessels that perfuse the tendon insertion itself.
    - ■ If adhesions between the FCR and the volar capsule are not released, the vector of the ligament reconstruction is based more proximally and will not closely

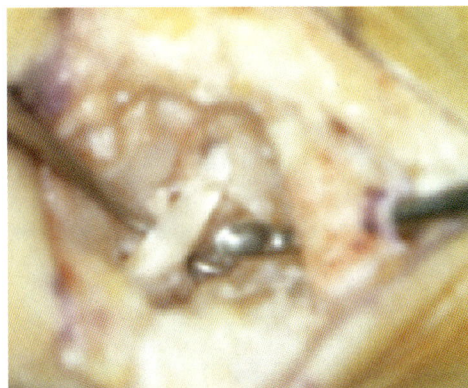

TECH FIG 2 • A tunnel is made at the base of the metacarpal.

simulate the original vector of the beak ligament. This, in my opinion, is a potential cause of early subsidence after ligament reconstruction.

- Taper the tendon for about 2 to 3 cm so the diameter of the tip of the tendon will easily fit through the bone tunnel via the Carroll tendon passer.
    - Use a 4-0 Vicryl suture on a small needle to purchase the volar capsule for subsequent stabilization of the tendon interposition.
    - If there are rents in the volar capsule, this same suture can be used to repair them, but I no longer am inordinately preoccupied with repairing small tears in the volar capsule because there is little risk of the tendon interposition extruding into the carpal canal or into the base of the metacarpal.

Stabilization of the Thumb Metacarpal (Optional) and FCR Tendon Tensioning

- Kirschner wire placement, when elected, is one of the more tedious parts of the procedure and must be performed skillfully so that the bony channel is not violated. If the Kirschner wire inadvertently purchases the FCR tendon within the bony channel in the metacarpal, it will impair the ability to pull it tight and properly tension the new ligament.
    - Usually a 0.045- or 0.054-inch wire is used. It begins obliquely at the dorsoradial aspect of the metacarpal and purchases the ulnar carpus.
- I place the thumb in the "fisted" position as if engaged in key pinch. The TM is suspended at the level of the index metacarpal. Its base should be colinear with the scaphoid articular surface and the thumb tip should rest on the index finger, neither too extended nor flexed at its base.
    - Ideally, this positions the thumb intrinsic muscles optimally on the Blix curve and ensures optimal restoration of pinch strength.
    - Bend the wire external to the skin and cut it.
- A hand probe or the like is used to take the FCR tendon at the base of the metacarpal and pull it proximally (**TECH FIG 3**).
    - When pinning has been performed, it should not prevent free excursion of the FCR through the bone

channel. Pull the tendon tightly as it exits the dorsum of the TM and suture it to adjacent periosteum and soft tissue with 3-0 Vicryl suture.
    - If pinning is not performed, at this point, ensure that you have suspended the metacarpal at the level of the index CMC joint.
- The extensor pollicis brevis (EPB) tendon is sutured more radially and divided distally. This completes the EPB tenodesis, rendering it an abductor of the metacarpal as opposed to a potential hyperextender of the MP joint.
- Place a second suture slightly more proximal to the tenodesis suture so that the ligament reconstruction is stabilized adequately, and perform tissue interposition.

Tissue Interposition (Optional)

- Although Burton's original technique continues to "resurface" the metacarpal base to minimize the chance that interposition material may extrude through the channel, this is unlikely. Studies have suggested that interposition is not a critical element of the procedure if suspension of the metacarpal has been effectively executed.[3] Furthermore, proximal migration, short of causing scaphometacarpal impingement, appears not to affect the functional outcome.[5]
- In a higher-demand patient, however, residual length of the FCR is available for interposition as follows. The tendon is folded into the volar aspect of the arthroplasty space to ensure that it will sink into its depth. From that point distally, the tendon is folded back and forth about four times on a single Keith needle, like ribbon candy.
- A 4-0 Vicryl suture is used to stabilize each corner of the tendon anchovy, and then a second Keith needle is placed through it, parallel to the first. Apertures in each needle should be volar, the tip of each needle dorsal, and, with the previously placed volar capsular suture, each limb is threaded and the anchovy is slid down and delivered into the arthroplasty space. The two Vicryl limbs are tied, securing the tissue interposition (**TECH FIG 4**).

Capsular Repair and Wound Closure

- Tightly repair the capsule using 3-0 Vicryl sutures. If redundant capsule is present, a pants-over-vest closure can be performed.

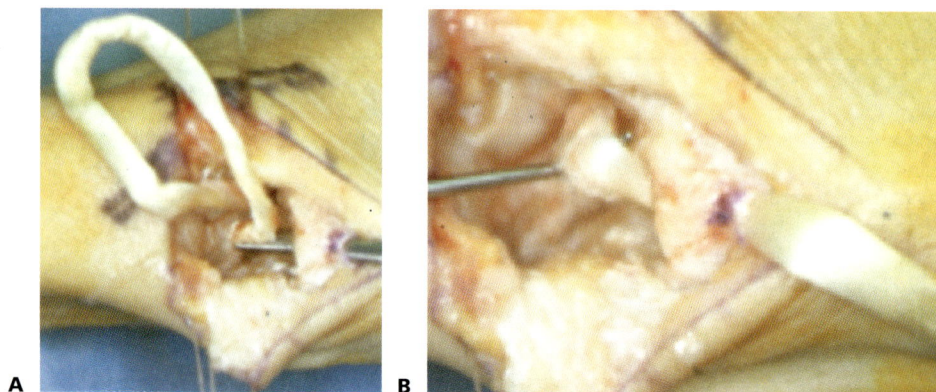

A   **B**

TECH FIG 3 • A. The flexor carpi radialis (FCR) is passed through bony tunnel. **B.** A hand probe indicates FCR suspensionplasty.

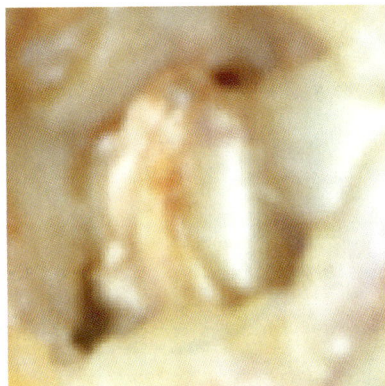

- When closing the capsule, protect radial artery and neighboring radial sensory nerve branches to avoid damage.
- Close the incisions with 4-0 nylon and repeat identification of underlying radial sensory nerve branches to avoid inadvertent injury during skin closure. This may be a cause of dystrophic pain after surgery.
- Place a bulky thumb spica dressing, followed by volar and thumb spica splints.
- The hand is elevated for 3 or 4 days after surgery.

TECH FIG 4 • The tendon anchovy held in place with Vicryl sutures.

APL SUSPENSIONPLASTY[13]

Incision and Deep Dissection

- Make a 6-cm curvilinear incision from two finger-breadths proximal to the radial styloid process to 1 cm distal to the base of the metacarpal (**TECH FIG 5A**). Expose and retract the radial artery and branches of the radial sensory nerve.
- Release the first extensor compartment retinaculum as would be performed for De Quervain disease, leaving the volar attachment intact.
- At the myotendinous junction of the APL, release the ulnarmost slip of APL and free it to the level of its insertion at the metacarpal base (**TECH FIG 5B**).
- Expose the EPL and APL tendons—in between is the capsule of the TM joint.
- Perform a capsulotomy to expose the trapezium (**TECH FIG 5C**), which is resected after being cut partially into four fragments with a saw and osteotome.
  - The base of the thumb metacarpal is not squared off; not resecting a small sliver from the metacarpal base may help to preserve the intermetacarpal ligament.
- The FCR tendon is visualized in the base of the arthro-

plasty space. With traction on the index and long fingers, inspect the scaphotrapezoidal joint; if it is arthritic, resect the proximal trapezoid.

Creation of the APL Suspensionplasty

- Poke the APL slip through the capsule to within the arthroplasty space. Using a right-angle clamp, pass it through a slit in the FCR tendon or around the FCR, while grabbing some local capsule as well (**TECH FIG 6**).
- Position the thumb so that it rests on the index finger in the fisted position—distracted so that the metacarpal base is at the level of the index CMC joint. A Kirschner wire is not placed.
- Pull the APL slip taut and place a 3-0 Vicryl suture between the APL slip, at the level of the metacarpal base, and the EPB (radially) and the tissue deep to the EPL (ulnarly).

Capsular Closure and Rehabilitation

- The capsule is closed and a thumb spica splint is placed for 14 days.

TECH FIG 5 • Abductor pollicis longus suspensionplasty technique. **A.** Skin incision. **B.** Distally based slip of abductor pollicis longus. **C.** Trapezium excision (*arrow* identifies the trapezium).

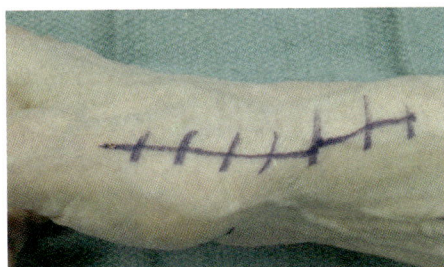

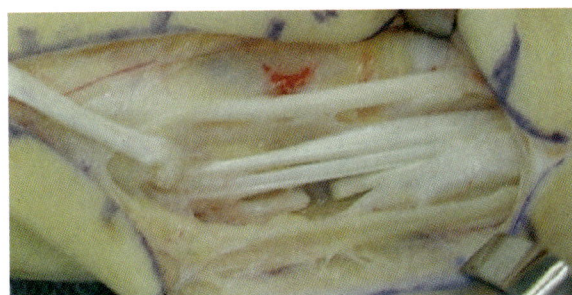

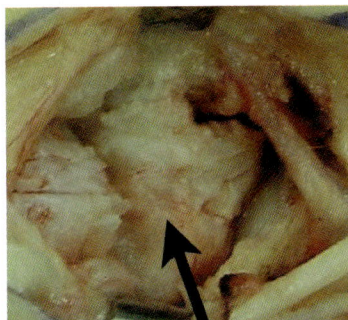

TECHNIQUES

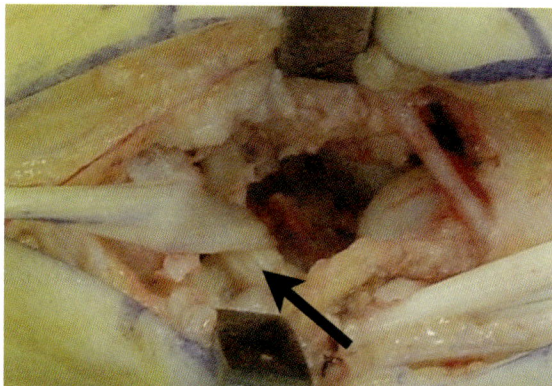

TECH FIG 6 • Abductor pollicis longus slip is passed through and around flexor carpi radialis (*arrow*).

PEARLS AND PITFALLS

Address MCP joint hyperextensibility	▪ Static laxity is no longer viewed as an absolute indication for capsulodesis or fusion. Rather, dynamic collapse during pinch is a relative indication.
Address scaphotrapezoidal disease	▪ If proximal trapezoid excision is not performed, pain at this articulation may persist.
Pinning is not essential; tissue interposition is not essential	▪ Neither pinning for 4 weeks nor tissue interposition is required. Outcomes appear not to be compromised by modest proximal metacarpal migration. However, these elements of the procedure do have a role if concern about any potential for scaphometacarpal impingement exists.
Ensure stability of the APL suspension	▪ The APL should be placed through the FCR or around it and should capture some capsule. This technical point will prevent the APL and thumb metacarpal from sliding proximally along the FCR.
Joint fusion timing	▪ When necessary, concomitant MCP joint fusion should be performed after tendon harvest and passage to avoid thumb manipulation after fusion.

POSTOPERATIVE CARE

- First month
  - At 2 weeks, the patient returns for suture removal, wound inspection, and placement of a fiberglass thumb spica cast that allows full motion of the thumb interphalangeal joint, unless MCP joint fusion has been performed.
  - At 4 weeks, the patient returns again, the Kirschner wire is pulled (if one has been placed), and a forearm-based thumb spica Orthoplast splint is fashioned by the hand therapist.
  - Gentle wrist and thumb MCP joint range-of-motion exercises are initiated, as well as thenar isometric exercises. The latter are performed with the thumb in the splint.
- Month 2
  - At 6 weeks, if the patient is comfortable, gentle pinch and grip strengthening exercises are initiated.
  - By 8 weeks, flexion-adduction and opposition exercises are begun.
- Month 3
  - By this time, the patient is usually doing well enough that the splint can be discarded.
  - Grip and pinch exercises are typically continued by the patient via a home program.

- No rigorous attempt is made for the thumb to reach the ring and small finger bases because there is no functional relevance to these activities and they risk stretching the ligament. In addition, passive range of motion is not a part of the postoperative regimen.
- During months 3 to 6, the patient is encouraged to use the hand and to push the exercises vigorously. Typically, patients return to normal activities, including golf and tennis.

OUTCOMES

LRTI Arthroplasty

- Improvements in grip strength typically exceed improvements in key pinch strength. In 1995, Tomaino et al[12] noted that key pinch strength took at least 6 years to equal preoperative measurements.
- At an average follow-up of 9 years (range 8 to 11), these authors[12] reported on 24 thumbs in 22 patients and found that average grip strength increased 93%, average key pinch strength increased 34%, and tip pinch strength increased 65% compared with preoperative values.
- In contrast to many other studies, stress radiographs showed an average subluxation of the metacarpal base of only 11%

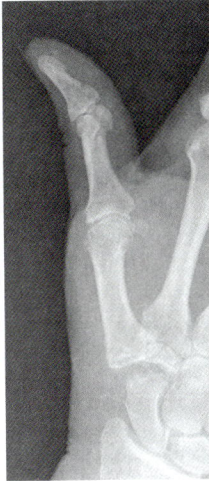

FIG 4 • Postoperative lateral radiograph shows arthroplasty space 1 year after surgery.

and subsidence of only 13%. This compares favorably with the radiographic outcomes after the hematoma distraction arthroplasty.[4,6]

■ Even in series in which proximal migration of the metacarpal base averaged greater than 20%, there has been no significant correlation between maintenance of arthroplasty space height and objective or subjective clinical outcome (**FIG 4**).[5]

APL Suspensionplasty

■ My evaluation of outcomes after the APL suspensionplasty found a satisfaction rate and functional return equivalent to the LRTI procedure.[13]

■ Evaluation of 23 thumbs in 22 patients at a minimum of 1 year after surgery showed that grip and key pinch strengths were 82% and 77%, respectively, compared to the opposite side. Proximal migration of the metacarpal averaged 50% of the preoperative trapezial height. Experience and the literature show that modest proximal migration does not correlate with outcome.[5]

■ In summary, APL suspensionplasty is a simple yet effective treatment alternative for basal joint arthritis. The suspensionplasty technique uses our current understanding of the forces involved during pinch and grip,[2] as well as the role of normal ligamentous anatomy.

COMPLICATIONS

■ One cause of unsatisfactory outcome after basal joint arthroplasty is residual pain because of failure to address scaphotrapezial or scaphotrapezoidal disease.[14] Routine complete excision of the trapezium certainly precludes the scaphotrapezial joint pain. Routine intraoperative observation and treatment of the scaphotrapezoidal disease by partial excision of the proximal trapezoid prevents scaphotrapezoidal joint pain.[14]

■ Unaddressed instability of the MCP joint can also impair functional outcome after ligament reconstruction. During lateral pinch, MCP joint hyperextension causes reciprocal deformity more proximally, imposing metacarpal adduction and stressing the reconstructed ligament. Accordingly, early identification of hyperextension in excess of 30 degrees during key pinch should prompt stabilization to protect the integrity of the basal joint ligament reconstruction. Even with a sound ligament reconstruction and appropriate stabilization of the MCP joint, it is theoretically possible to develop recurrent laxity at the basal joint due to stretching of the ligament reconstruction.

REFERENCES

1. Bettinger P, Lindschied, Berger R, et al. An anatomic study of the stabilizing ligaments of the trapezium and trapeziometacarpal joint. J Hand Surg Am 1999;24A:786–798.
2. Cooney WP, Chao EYS. Biomechanical analysis of static forces in the thumb during hand function. J Bone Joint Surg Am 1977;59A:27–36.
3. Gerwin M, Griffith A, Weiland AJ, et al. Ligament reconstruction basal joint arthroplasty without tendon interposition. Clin Orthop Relat Res 1997;342:42–45.
4. Gray KV, Meals RA. Hematoma and distraction arthroplasty for thumb basal joint osteoarthritis: minimum 6.5-year follow-up evaluation. J Hand Surg Am 2007;32A:23–29.
5. Kriegs-Au G, Petje G, Fojtl E, et al. Ligament reconstruction with or without tendon interposition to treat primary thumb carpometacarpal osteoarthritis. J Bone Joint Surg Am 2004;86A:209–218.
6. Kuhns CA, Emerson ET, Meals RA. Hematoma and distraction arthroplasty for thumb basal joint osteoarthritis: a prospective, single-surgeon study including outcomes measures. J Hand Surg Am 2003;28A:381–389.
7. Nylen S, Juhlin LJ, Lugnegard H. Weilby tendon interposition arthroplasty for osteoarthritis of the trapezial joints. J Hand Surg Br 1987;12B:68–72.
8. Pellegrini VD. Pathomechanics of the thumb trapeziometacarpal joint. Hand Clin 2001;17:175–184.
9. Pellegrini VD, Olcott CW, Hollenberg G. Contact patterns in the trapeziometacarpal joint: the role of the palmar beak ligament. J Hand Surg Am 1993;18A:238–244.
10. Sigfusson R, Lundborg G. Abductor pollicis longus tendon arthroplasty for treatment of arthrosis in the first carpometacarpal joint. Scand J Plast Reconst Hand Surg 1991;25:73–77.
11. Tomaino MM. Ligament reconstruction tendon interposition arthroplasty for basal joint arthritis. Hand Clinics 2001;17:207–221.
12. Tomaino MM, Pellegrini VD, Burton RI. Arthroplasty of the basal joint of the thumb: long-term follow up after ligament reconstruction with tendon interposition. J Bone Joint Surg Am 1995;77A:346–355.
13. Tomaino MM. Suspensionplasty for basal joint arthritis: why and how. Hand Clin 2006;22:171–175.
14. Tomaino MM, Vogt M, Weiser R. Scaphotrapezoid arthritis: prevalence in thumbs undergoing trapezium excision arthroplasty and efficacy of proximal trapezoid excision. J Hand Surg Am 1999;24A:1220–1224.
15. Weilby A. Tendon interposition arthroplasty of the first carpometacarpal joint. J Hand Surg Br 1988;13B:421–425.

Chapter 84

Thumb Carpometacarpal Joint Implant and Resurfacing Arthroplasty

Matthew J. Robon and Matthew M. Tomaino

DEFINITION

- Trapeziometacarpal joint (basal joint) arthritis is a debilitating condition that most commonly affects women in their 50s and 60s.[18,19] The stage of arthritis dictates the treatment for this disorder.[4,5,20]
- Ligament reconstruction and tendon interposition arthroplasty, fusion, and nonbiologic reconstruction of this joint are common techniques to treat this condition.[9,10,21,22]
- This chapter will discuss the role of resurfacing arthroplasty and total joint replacement.

ANATOMY

- The anatomy of the thumb metacarpal (TM) joint is extremely complex and has been well studied. The deep anterior oblique ligament ("beak ligament") is the primary stabilizer of the TM joint.[10] More recently, 16 ligaments have been described that stabilize the TM joint. Seven of these ligaments, including the superficial anterior oblique ligament (sAOL), deep anterior oblique (dAOL), dorsoradial, posterior oblique, ulnar collateral, intermetacarpal, and dorsal intermetacarpal directly stabilize the TM joint. The other nine ligaments indirectly stabilize the TM joint by directly stabilizing the trapezium.
- The TM joint is the most complex joint in the hand. It is a biconcave-convex saddle joint with minimal bony constraints. This joint allows flexion-extension, abduction-adduction, and pronation-supination of the thumb ray. For optimal treatment outcomes with joint replacement, normal kinematics—six degrees of freedom—should be restored as closely as possible.

PATHOGENESIS

- Degeneration of the AOL of the TM joint has been linked to the development of osteoarthritis.
- Pathologic laxity, abnormal translation of the metacarpal on the trapezium, and generation of abnormally high shear forces within the TM joint, especially on the palmar aspect of the joint during pinch and grip motions, occur when the AOL becomes incompetent.
- The base of the metacarpal tends to sublux dorsally with AOL detachment, emphasizing the importance of the AOL. In advanced osteoarthritis, adduction and flexion contractures tend to develop, producing further functional impairment and joint overload.

NATURAL HISTORY

- The vast number of described operations to treat osteoarthritis of the TM joint demonstrates the lack of consensus among treating surgeons as to the best way to approach this disorder. This chapter details the role of resurfacing and implant arthroplasty for the treatment of osteoarthritis of the TM joint.
- Various materials, techniques, and prostheses have been used in the past. Hemiarthroplasty and total joint arthroplasty of the TM joint have largely failed, with mediocre long-term results compared with soft tissue arthroplasty.[1,2,5,7,14,20] However, the appeal of a replacement may lie with quicker recovery and more normal kinematics.
- Obviously, the perils of this alternative revolve around durability, survivability, and complication rate. Joint resurfacing with the Artelon implant (SBI) may have the most potential in terms of a biologic resurfacing procedure that avoids the use of a semiconstrained device—which has been associated with trapezial component loosening and failure.

PATIENT HISTORY AND PHYSICAL FINDINGS

- Arthritis of the TM joint often presents with pain at the base of the thumb during pinch and grip (stressful activities for the TM joint). Women are 10 to 15 times more likely than men to develop this disorder. Asian and Caucasian populations have an increased prevalence as well.
- Common offending activities include brushing teeth, opening a jar, picking up a book, or turning a key. All of these activities involve increasing the breadth of grasp or forceful lateral pinch. Usually the pain is localized at the base of the thumb on the dorsal or volar radial aspect of the thenar cone. Patients often feel the joint slipping or subluxing radially.
  - A "shoulder sign" is an enlarging prominence (the result of a dorsally subluxing proximal metacarpal on the trapezium and metacarpal adduction) that develops with progressive disease.
- Other causes of pain in the hand should be evaluated (see differential diagnosis list) as well. This is important because any concomitant disease, such as a trigger thumb, may hamper the postoperative therapy regimen and negatively affect the patient's final outcome.
- The treating physician should also keep the diagnosis of carpal tunnel syndrome in mind, as it coexists in about 44% of patients with TM joint arthritis. Further, the postoperative swelling from a basal joint arthroplasty may exacerbate even mild cases of carpal tunnel syndrome.
- The Allen test should be performed on every patient who is undergoing surgery for basal joint arthroplasty, as the radial artery will be near or in the operative field and may need to be mobilized depending on the exact procedure performed. Any injury to the radial artery should be repaired immediately.
- The stability of the metacarpophalangeal (MCP) joint of the thumb is also critical, as this is a source of postoperative stress on the reconstructed beak ligament from either ligament reconstruction or suspensionplasty procedures.
  - MCP joint fusion or volar plate capsulodesis should be performed when the MCP joint hyperextends to greater than 20 degrees.[13]
- Methods for examining the carpometacarpal (CMC) joint of the thumb include the following:
  - CMC grind test: A positive test is suggestive of degenerative disease.

- CMC instability test: Laxity of the TM joint is common in early stages of degeneration, but as the joint degenerates, it usually becomes stiffer.
- MCP joint stability test: If the MCP joint is actively hyperextending, this could put undue stress on a reconstructed TM joint and lead to failure. This hyperextendable metacarpophalangeal joint (MPJ) should be stabilized.
- Metacarpal base compression test: Glickel[11] believed this is more commonly painful in advanced stages rather than milder stages of TM joint disease.
- Distraction test: A positive result from this maneuver is thought to be caused by traction on an inflamed TM joint capsule.

IMAGING AND OTHER DIAGNOSTIC STUDIES

- Imaging of the TM joint includes a true AP view of the TM joint (called a Robert view or pronated AP), lateral, and posteroanterior 30-degree oblique stress view (with thumb tips pressing against each other).
- The most common staging system was originally described by Eaton and Littler:[9,10] stage 1 shows slight widening of the joint, possibly from synovitis; stage 2 demonstrates some joint space narrowing and osteophytes smaller than 2 mm; stage 3, osteophytes larger than 2 mm; and stage 4 disease, scaphotrapezial joint space involvement along with TM joint narrowing.
- The senior author of this chapter has described a "fifth stage" in which the disease process is pan-trapezial and there is TM, scaphotrapezial, and scaphotrapezoidal joint degeneration. Scaphotrapezoidal arthritis can be a source of continued pain and this joint should be evaluated intraoperatively in every patient because, unfortunately, preoperative radiographs are only 44% sensitive and 86% specific for diagnosing arthritis at this joint.[23]

DIFFERENTIAL DIAGNOSIS

- Scaphotrapezial arthritis
- Scaphotrapezoidal arthritis
- Thumb sesamoid arthritis
- Carpal tunnel syndrome
- De Quervain tenosynovitis
- Stenosing flexor tenosynovitis (trigger finger)

NONOPERATIVE MANAGEMENT

- Initial management of TM joint arthritis is nonoperative and includes anti-inflammatory medication, thenar cone muscle isometric strengthening exercises, hand- or forearm-based thumb spica splint immobilization, steroid injections, and activity modification.
- These measures may not alleviate any or all of the patient's symptoms, but they may help enough to provide temporary relief, allowing the patient ample time to educate himself or herself and to contemplate the treatment alternatives.
- The time afforded by the nonoperative measures may also allow the patient to schedule the operation at a more convenient time.

SURGICAL MANAGEMENT

- There are several options for surgical treatment of TM joint arthritis. Ligament reconstruction and tendon interposition (LRTI), suspensionplasty, and CMC joint fusion are discussed in other chapters. This chapter focuses on the role of resurfacing and implant arthroplasty. Resurfacing is an increasingly attractive option in younger, more active patients in whom one might prefer to avoid trapeziectomy to eliminate the risk of metacarpal subsidence with time. Subsidence can result in recurrent pain and weakness.
- The Artelon (SBI) spacer is a bioabsorbable implant (**FIG 1A**) that degrades and is replaced with scar tissue that protects the base of the thumb metacarpal and the distal aspect of the trapezium. This implant is ideal for a younger laborer with TM arthritis in whom grip and pinch strength are of critical importance. The attraction of this alternative is that it is a potentially definitive procedure that does not "burn the bridge" of resection arthroplasty in the future.[17]
- Pyrocarbon resurfacing using the "saddle" implant (Ascension Orthopaedics, Austin, TX; **FIG 1B**) is an alternative to Artelon. Its design mimics the articular shape of the metacarpal articular surface, which may more closely restore CMC joint kinematics compared to Artelon implant use. Little information exists in the literature, however, regarding outcomes.
- Total joint arthroplasty, such as with the Avanta CMC implant (**FIG 1C**), is another option. This is designed to require less immobilization, leading to quicker return of functional abilities, and is ideal (theoretically) for an elderly, lower-demand patient. However, the literature is full of articles describing failures of innumerable prosthetic implants for the TM joint.

Preoperative Planning

- Many other hand pathologies can coexist with TM joint arthritis. These other diagnoses should be evaluated before the day of surgery.

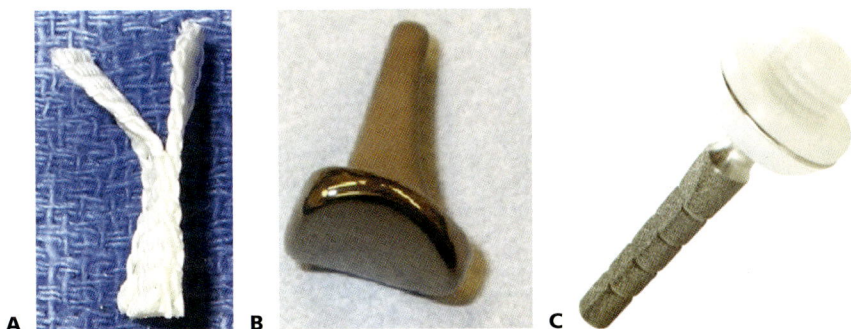

FIG 1 • **A.** Artelon implant demonstrating T shape with two dorsal wings. **B.** Pyrocarbon saddle implant. **C.** Avanta CMC implant. (**C**: Courtesy of Small Bone Innovations, Morrisville, PA.)

■ If an Allen test had not been performed previously, it should be performed before the surgery.

Positioning

■ The patient is positioned supine on the operating table with the affected hand placed on a hand table extension. A tourniquet is placed above the elbow.

■ When using a dorsal approach, we tend to keep the hand in neutral pronation–supination, with an assistant holding the hand stable and at times pulling traction or directly stabilizing the thumb with the nail plate parallel to the floor.

Approach

■ There are several different approaches for soft tissue arthroplasties, but for resurfacing or implant arthroplasties, a dorsal approach seems to work the best and to offer the best visualization.

TECHNIQUES

ARTELON RESURFACING ARTHROPLASTY

Exposure

■ A dorsal approach is needed for placement of the Artelon implant between the distal trapezium and the proximal metacarpal of the thumb.

■ Make a longitudinal incision centered over the CMC joint. Identify and protect branches of the superficial radial nerve throughout the case, along with the extensor pollicis longus (EPL) and extensor pollicis brevis (EPB).

■ After mobilizing and protecting the radial artery, mobilize the EPL and EPB tendons enough to facilitate a longitudinal incision through the capsule. Reflect the capsule enough to completely visualize the joint (**TECH FIG 1**).

■ Visualize the scaphotrapezoidal joint; if it is found to have substantial degeneration, this joint surface would need to be addressed as part of the procedure.

Joint Preparation

■ Use a high-speed sagittal saw to remove the distal facet of the trapezium. Take care not to injure the flexor carpi radialis (FCR) or flexor pollicis longus (FPL) tendons, which lie on the volar side of the bony cut. Alternatively, a burr can be used to decorticate the trapezial surface while maintaining its native contour.

■ Use a high-speed burr to slightly decorticate the dorsum of the proximal metacarpal to stimulate healing, but not enough to affect the suture anchor fixation (**TECH FIG 2**).

Implant Placement

■ The implant (Fig 1A) comes in two sizes; pick the appropriate size to fill the void from radial to ulnar as well as dorsal to volar between the trapezium and the base of the metacarpal. The larger size may be able to be trimmed down to fit more anatomically.

■ The Artelon implant is shaped similar to a T, with two wings for the dorsum of the trapezium and metacarpal, with the other part to be placed between the fresh bone edges of the trapezium and the base of the metacarpal.

■ Bioabsorbable suture anchors (with 2-0 fiberwire or equivalent) are used to hold the dorsal wings down to the bone (**TECH FIG 3**). Although cortical bone screws were recommended to secure the implant early on, experience has shown that screws are a frequent source of complication and may pull through the mesh. Screws should be avoided. Suture anchors are much easier and quicker and provide better fixation of the implant.

■ After this, close the capsule with absorbable suture and the skin with 3-0 nylon. At the end of the surgery, the patient is placed into a thumb spica splint and will follow up in 2 weeks for suture removal and placement into a thumb spica cast for 4 more weeks.

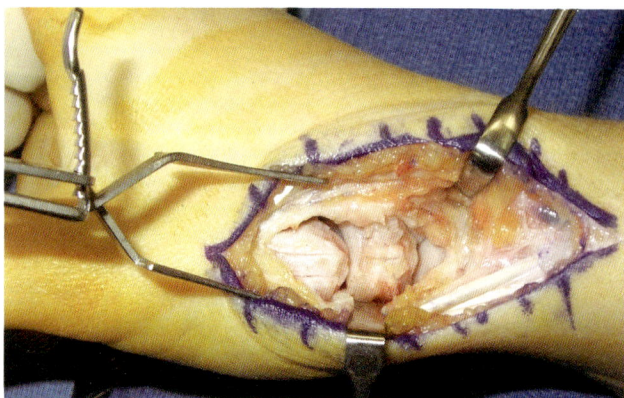

TECH FIG 1 • Dorsal approach to the thumb metacarpal joint after reflecting the joint capsule.

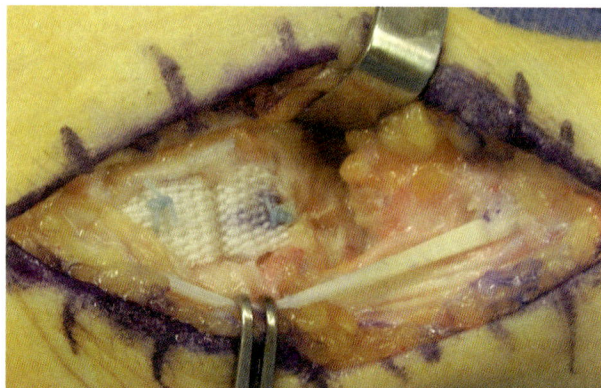

TECH FIG 2 • Appearance of the thumb metacarpal joint after bone cuts on trapezium, burring of proximal thumb metacarpal, and placement of bioabsorbable suture anchors.

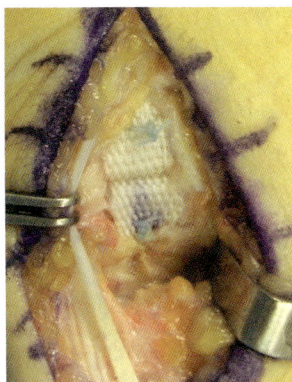

TECH FIG 3 • Appearance of the resurfacing arthroplasty after stabilization of the Artelon implant with suture anchors.

PYROCARBON RESURFACING ARTHROPLASTY

Exposure

- Make a dorsal longitudinal incision centered over the CMC joint. Identify and protect branches of the superficial radial nerve throughout the procedure, along with the EPL and EPB.
- After mobilizing and protecting the radial artery, mobilize the EPL and EPB tendons enough to facilitate a longitudinal incision through the capsule. Reflect the capsule enough to completely visualize the joint. Subperiosteal release allows the base of the metacarpal to be dislocated dorsal to the trapezium. Place a Hohmann retractor beneath the palmar surface to maintain exposure.

Joint Preparation

- First, place a sizing guide over the surface as a guide toward what the ultimate size implant is likely to be.
- Resect the base using the cutting guide, which is assembled after an intramedullary rod is inserted. Just the articular surface is removed.

- Start broaching. Ensure that the broach is started just volar to the central portion of the cut to ensure that the implant is not placed too dorsal (**TECH FIG 4**).

Implant Placement

- Check stability with the final implant in place (**TECH FIG 5A**). Gentle cross-palm pressure before capsular closure should not cause dislocation.
- The implant comes in four sizes. If the trial is not stable, upsizing the implant may be necessary.
- Close the capsule with absorbable suture and the skin with 4-0 nylon.
- At the end of the surgery, the patient is placed into a thumb spica splint and will follow up in 2 weeks for suture removal and placement into a thumb spica splint for 4 more weeks.
- Radiographs are checked at that time to ensure that the implant is reduced (**TECH FIG 5B**).

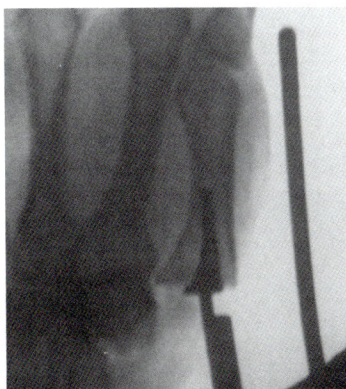

TECH FIG 4 • Extramedullary guide to plan placement of saddle implant.

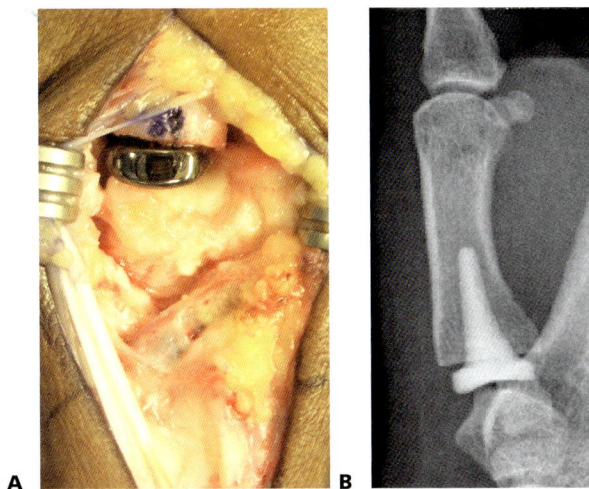

TECH FIG 5 • **A.** Saddle implant in place. **B.** Postoperative lateral radiograph showing implant in place.

TOTAL JOINT REPLACEMENT

Exposure

- We use a technique and surgical approach similar to that described by Badia and Sambandam[2] for implanting a Braun-Cutter trapeziometacarpal joint prosthesis (or Avanta CMC implant; Small Bone Innovations, Morrisville, PA; Fig 1C) using bone cement.

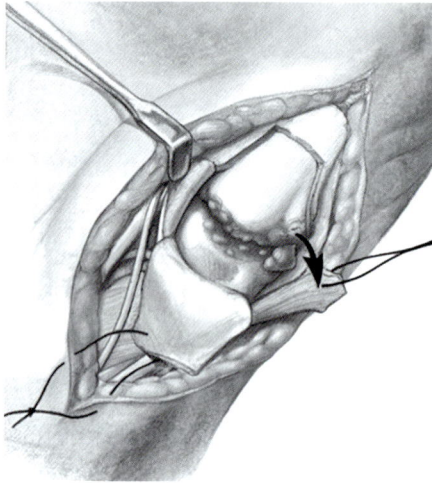

TECH FIG 6 • The first compartment is opened from the volar side and the strands of the abductor pollicis longus (APL) are inspected. A strand of the APL that inserts on the base of the metacarpal in the bone area that will be resected should be freed from its insertion and tagged for later repair. (Courtesy of Small Bone Innovations, Morrisville, PA.)

- Make a 4-cm longitudinal incision over the dorsal aspect of the base of the thumb. Identify and protect branches of the superficial sensory radial nerve. Perform further dissection between the EPL and EPB tendons, isolating and protecting the dorsal branch of the radial artery.
- Open the dorsal capsule of the trapeziometacarpal joint longitudinally. Reflect the periosteum and the dorsal capsule radially and ulnarly as a single flap to be repaired later (**TECH FIG 6**).

Joint Preparation

- Using a sagittal saw, remove about 8 mm of the thumb metacarpal base. This resection is necessary to provide enough exposure to the trapezium (**TECH FIG 7A,B**).
- Release the adductor pollicis if required to allow abduction of the thumb metacarpal away from the palm. At this point, longitudinal traction and flexion are applied to better expose the trapezial surface.
- Use a rongeur to remove the marginal osteophytes and flatten the joint surface of the trapezium.
- With imaging, identify the center of the trapezium with a small burr. Enlarge the center hole to create a deep channel within the trapezium where the polyethylene cup will be cemented (**TECH FIG 7C**).
- For the thumb metacarpal, use a guide to open the intramedullary canal, which is broached with a burr to allow for an ample cement mantle (**TECH FIG 7D**).

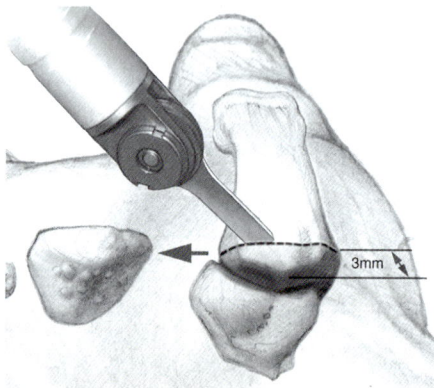

A

TECH FIG 7 • The capsule of the trapeziometacarpal joint is excised (**A**) and the joint is exposed (**B**). **C.** The alignment of the metacarpal component is parallel to the axis of the metacarpal shaft, with slight volar inclination. The trapezial joint surface is evaluated. If the surface is fairly intact, blocking volar, ulnar, and radial osteophytes are removed and the hole is burred for the trapezium component. **D.** The metacarpal canal is reamed and prepared for prosthetic insertion. (**A, C, D**: Courtesy of Small Bone Innovations, Morrisville, PA.)

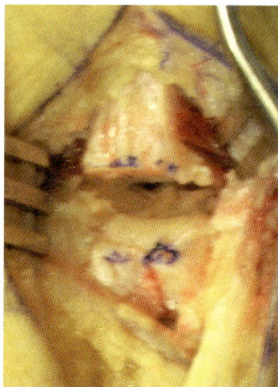

B

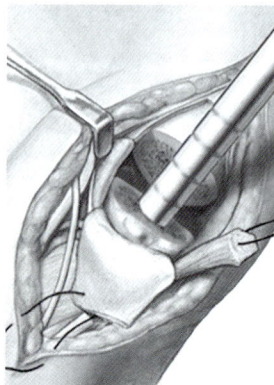

C

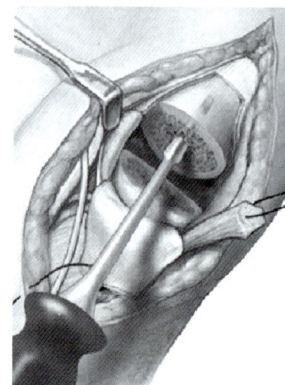

D

Implant Placement

- Place the implant and perform a trial reduction so that motion and fluoroscopic images can be assessed. If there is any bony impingement at the periphery of the residual trapezium, this can be addressed before placing the permanent prosthesis.
- For final placement, first cement the trapezial cup in the trapezium, taking care to impact the cement beneath the subcortical bone.
  - Once the cup has been inserted but before the cement has cured, insert the thumb metacarpal component with bone cement (**TECH FIG 8A**).
  - The two components are linked, but because this stem is collarless, it is important to maintain adequate neck length (to prevent subsidence) until the bone cement has cured. Make sure the stem neck does not impinge on the edge of the trapezium (**TECH FIG 8B**).
- Assess stability and circumferential motion to ensure there is no impingement on the implant.
- Close the capsule–periosteal flap with absorbable suture.
- After inserting the implant and before closure, use intraoperative fluoroscopy to check proper alignment and placement of the prosthesis (**TECH FIG 8C**).
- Close the skin and subcutaneous tissue with a resorbable suture and place a well-padded short-arm thumb spica splint.

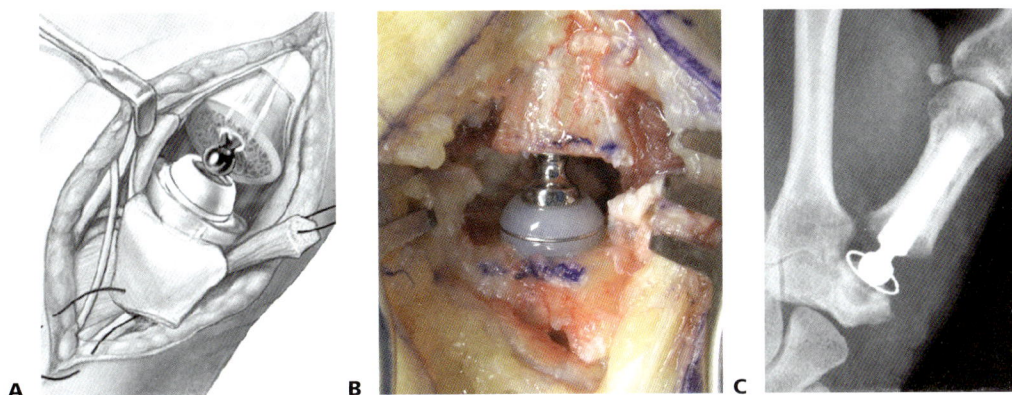

TECH FIG 8 • **A,B.** The components are cemented into place, the trapezium first and the metacarpal second. Compression should be maintained until the bone cement has completely set. **C.** Postoperative lateral radiograph showing implant in place. (**A**: Courtesy of Small Bone Innovations, Morrisville, PA.)

PEARLS AND PITFALLS

Preoperative	▪ Always do an Allen test before surgery.
	▪ Always evaluate the thumb MCP joint for active instability–hyperextension.
Intraoperative	▪ Use extreme caution mobilizing the radial artery. Often bipolar electrocautery facilitates mobilization, especially of the deep perforators at the volar base of the TM joint.
	▪ Evaluate the scaphotrapezoidal joint, as preoperative radiographs are not good at predicting disease.
	▪ Be careful when sawing or drilling not to injure structures deep to the bone.
	▪ After making the bone cuts on the trapezium and burring the proximal metacarpal, drill and place the suture anchors far enough away from the prepared bone to avoid inadvertent breakout in the fresh cancellous bone surfaces.
	▪ Once the implant has been secured and the capsule repaired, do not manipulate by the thumb, as this may put undue stress on the soft tissue repair.
	▪ After the procedure, before contaminating the sterile field, release the tourniquet and observe the reperfusion of the hand to ensure that no unexpected arterial injury occurred.
Postoperative	▪ Have a postoperative therapy protocol for patients to follow.

POSTOPERATIVE CARE

- At the end of the surgery, the patient is placed into a thumb spica splint to keep the thumb in opposition. At 2 weeks postoperatively, the sutures are removed and placement into a thumb spica cast continues for 2 more weeks.

- The cast immobilization is discontinued at 6 weeks postoperatively if Artelon resurfacing has been used and at 2 weeks if CMC replacement has been performed. A custom Orthoplast thumb-based spica splint (Johnson & Johnson, New Brunswick, NJ) is worn full time for protection, except during showers and therapy.

■ Formal therapy is usually not required after total joint replacement. In the case of resurfacing, therapy will focus on range-of-motion exercises only for postoperative weeks 4 to 6, advancing to thenar isometrics for weeks 6 to 8. At 8 weeks postoperatively, the patient will start grip and pinch strengthening exercises; the splint is also discontinued at this point.

OUTCOMES

■ Several long-term studies have shown better than 90% satisfaction and pain relief with soft tissue arthroplasties, but long-term outcome studies do not exist for the Artelon implant, and most of the literature for total joint arthroplasty for TM joint arthritis is not favorable.

COMPLICATIONS

■ Superficial branch of the radial nerve injury
■ Damage to flexor tendons during saw use
■ Radial artery injury
■ Dislocation or subsidence of total joint implant
■ Subluxation of TM joint
■ Continued pain or discomfort
■ Failure to recognize other sources of pathology in the hand and wrist

REFERENCES

1. Athwal GS, Chenkin J, King GJ, et al. Early failures with a spheric interposition arthroplasty of the thumb basal joint. J Hand Surg Am 2004;29A:1080–1084.
2. Badia A, Sambandam SN. Total joint arthroplasty in the treatment of advanced stages of thumb carpometacarpal joint osteoarthritis. J Hand Surg Am 2006;31A:1605–1614.
3. Bettinger P, Linschied RL, Berger R, et al. An anatomic study of the stabilizing ligaments of the trapezium and trapeziometacarpal joint. J Hand Surg Am 1999;24A:786–798.
4. Burton RI, Pellegrini VD Jr. Basal joint arthritis of thumb. J Hand Surg Am 1987;12A:645.
5. Burton RI, Pellegrini VD Jr. Surgical management of basal joint arthritis of the thumb, part II: ligament reconstruction with tendon interposition arthroplasty. J Hand Surg Am 1986;11A:324–332.
6. Cooney WP III, Chao EY. Biomechanical analysis of static forces in the thumb during hand function. J Bone Joint Surg Am 1977;59A:27.
7. De Smet L, Sioen W, Spaepen D, et al. Total joint arthroplasty for osteoarthritis of the thumb basal joint. Acta Orthop Belg 2004;70:19–24.
8. Doerschuk SH, Hicks DG, Chinchilli VM, et al. Histopathology of the palmar beak ligament in trapeziometacarpal osteoarthritis. J Hand Surg Am 1999;24A:496–504.
9. Eaton R, Littler J. A study of the basal joint of the thumb: treatment of its disabilities by fusion. J Bone Joint Surg Am 1969;51A:661–668.
10. Eaton R, Littler J. Ligament reconstruction for the painful thumb carpometacarpal joint. J Bone Joint Surg Am 1973;55A:1655–1666.
11. Glickel SZ. Clinical assessment of the thumb trapeziometacarpal joint. Hand Clinics 2001;17:185–195.
12. Haines RW. The mechanism of rotation at the first carpometacarpal joint. J Anat 1944;78:44–46.
13. Lourie GM. The role and implementation of metacarpophalangeal joint fusion and capsulodesis: indications and treatment alternatives. Hand Clinics 2001;17:255–260.
14. Naidu SH, Kulkarni N, Saunders M. Titanium basal joint arthroplasty: a finite element analysis and clinical study. J Hand Surg Am 2006;31A:760–765.
15. Nanno M, Buford WL, Patterson RM, et al. Three-dimensional analysis of the ligamentous attachments of the first carpometacarpal joint. J Hand Surg Am 2006;31A:1160–1170.
16. Napier J. The form and function of the carpometacarpal joint of the thumb. J Anat 1955;89:362.
17. Nilsson A, Liljensten E, Bergstrom C, et al. Results from a degradable TMC Joint Spacer (Artelon) compared with tendon arthroplasty. J Hand Surg Am 2005;30A:380–389.
18. Pellegrini V. Osteoarthritis of the trapeziometacarpal joint: the pathophysiology of articular cartilage degeneration, I: anatomy and pathology of the aging joint. J Hand Surg Am 1991;16A:967–974.
19. Pellegrini VD. Osteoarthritis of the trapeziometacarpal joint: the pathophysiology of articular cartilage degeneration, II: articular wear patterns in the osteoarthritic joint. J Hand Surg Am 1991;16A:975–982.
20. Pellegrini VD Jr, Burton RI. Surgical management of basal joint arthritis of the thumb, part I: long-term results of silicone implant arthroplasty. J Hand Surg Am 1986;11A:309–324.
21. Tomaino MM. Suspensionplasty for basal joint arthritis: why and how. Hand Clinics 2006;22:171–175.
22. Tomaino MM, Pellegrini VD Jr, Burton RI. Arthroplasty of the basal joint of the thumb: long-term follow-up after ligament reconstruction with tendon interposition. J Bone Joint Surg Am 1995;77A:346–355.
23. Tomaino MM, Vogt M, Weiser R. Scaphotrapezoid arthritis: prevalence in thumbs undergoing trapezium excision arthroplasty and efficacy of proximal trapezoid excision. J Hand Surg Am 1999;24:1220–1224.

Chapter 85

Wrist Denervation

Carlos Heras-Palou

DEFINITION

- Arthrosis of the wrist often presents with functional movement, but with substantial disability due to pain. The purpose of wrist denervation is to decrease pain by surgically dividing the nerves that transmit the afferent pain signal from the wrist.

ANATOMY

- The posterior interosseous nerve (PIN) is considered to be the most important nerve innervating the wrist joint.
- Other nerves involved are branches from the anterior interosseous nerve (AIN), the radial nerve, the dorsal branch of the ulnar nerve, the palmar branch of the median nerve, and recurrent intermetacarpal nerve branches.[1]

PATHOGENESIS

- Common causative conditions include scaphoid nonunion advanced collapse, scapholunate advanced collapse, degeneration secondary to crystalline arthropathy, inflammatory arthritis, and trauma.

NATURAL HISTORY

- The natural history of wrist arthrosis is slow progression, but the correlation between radiologic staging and symptoms is sometimes poor.

PATIENT HISTORY AND PHYSICAL FINDINGS

- Patients with wrist arthrosis present with wrist pain, weakness of the grip, swelling, and stiffness.
- Often there is a sensation of grating during wrist movement, and occasionally clicking or clunking.

- Some patients report a history of wrist injury years previously, but many do not recall any wrist trauma.
- It is important to inquire about neurologic symptoms to identify any associated compressive neuropathy at the carpal tunnel, the canal of Guyon, or both.
- Examination of the wrist usually reveals dorsoradial swelling, loss of movement, weak grip strength secondary to pain, and crepitation.

Local Anesthetic Blocks

- Although controversial in the literature, selective injection of a local anesthetic can be used to predict the results of wrist denervation.
- Local anesthetic is injected about 1 cm ulnar and 3 cm proximal to the tubercle of Lister, delivering 1 mL Marcaine 0.5% around the PIN (**FIG 1A**). The needle is pushed forward through the interosseous membrane to deliver 1 cc of local anesthetic adjacent to the AIN.
- One cc Marcaine is then injected under the branches of the radial nerve (**FIG 1B**), under the dorsal cutaneous branch of the ulnar nerve (**FIG 1C**), under the palmar branch of the median nerve (**FIG 1D**), and finally between the base of the second and third metacarpals to block the recurrent intermetacarpal branches.
- The wrist is examined before the injections and again 20 minutes afterward. Baltimore Therapeutic Equipment is used where available.
  - A decrease in pain rating by 90% and an increase in work output of more than 200% indicate a significant improvement.
  - Patients with these results are considered good candidates for surgical denervation.

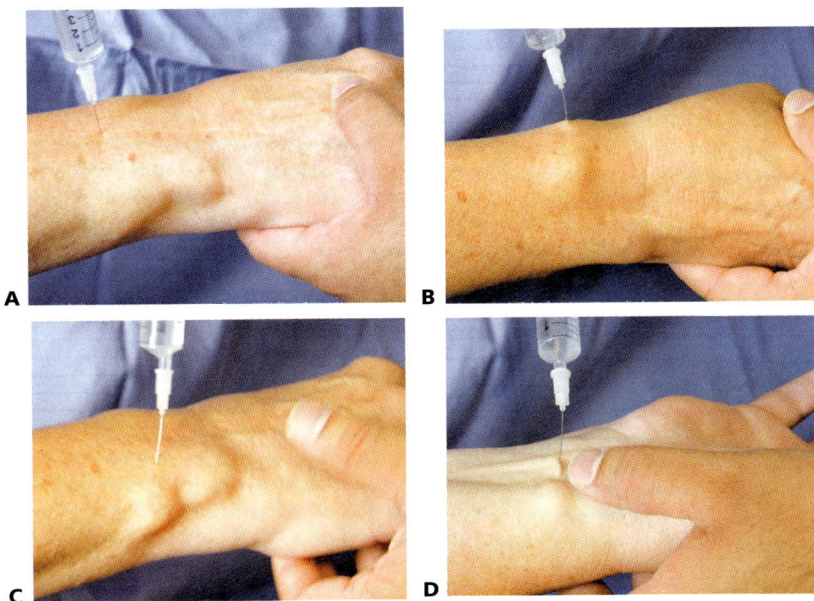

FIG 1 • One mL of 0.5% bupivacaine is injected to block the posterior and anterior interosseous nerves (**A**), the branches of the radial nerve (**B**), the branches of the dorsal cutaneous ulnar nerve (**C**), the palmar branch of the median nerve (**D**), and the branches of the intermetacarpal nerve. (Reprinted from Hunt T, Herlas-Palou C. Wrist denervation. In Chunk K. Operative Techniques: Hand and Wrist Surgery. Philadelphia: Elsevier, 2008:209–230.)

IMAGING AND OTHER DIAGNOSTIC STUDIES

- Posteroanterior and lateral radiographs of the wrist confirm the degenerative changes in the wrist joint.
- If there is any doubt about the degree of degeneration, an advanced imaging study (eg, MRI) or wrist arthroscopy can provide more precise information, but these are seldom required.

DIFFERENTIAL DIAGNOSIS

- Wrist denervation is a good option for patients with wrist pain secondary to degeneration. It is important to rule out other causes of pain, such as infection.
- Patients with frank wrist instability and patients with active inflammatory arthritis are unlikely to benefit from wrist denervation.

NONOPERATIVE MANAGEMENT

- For patients with wrist degeneration, conservative management, including anti-inflammatory drugs and splints, should be tried before considering surgery.

SURGICAL MANAGEMENT

- Wrist denervation is indicated in a patient with considerable pain due to wrist degeneration, recalcitrant to conservative measures.
- Alternatives to wrist denervation include open or arthroscopic wrist débridement, radial styloidectomy, partial carpal arthrodesis, proximal row carpectomy, and wrist arthrodesis. Some of these procedures can be combined with a denervation.

Positioning

- The patient is positioned supine with the affected arm on a hand table, under regional block, with a high arm tourniquet, and the procedure is carried out under loupe magnification.

Approach

- Standard denervation of the wrist is carried out through four incisions: dorsal, dorsal–ulnar, volar–radial, and dorsal, over the base of the metacarpals.
- A partial denervation is carried out through one dorsal incision.

PARTIAL DENERVATION OF THE WRIST

- Partial denervation involves excision of the PIN with or without excision of the AIN just proximal to the radio-carpal joint.
- Make a 2-cm transverse dorsal incision 3 to 5 cm proximal to the wrist.
- Incise the fourth extensor compartment in a longitudinal direction and retract the extensor tendons ulnarward.
- Isolate the PIN on the radial floor of the fourth extensor compartment.
  - The PIN travels with the posterior interosseous artery and veins.

- Excise a 1-cm segment of nerve.[2,3]
- Retract the fourth compartment extensor tendons radially and make a small window in the interosseous membrane.
- Excise a segment of AIN just deep to the interosseous membrane.
- Close the extensor retinaculum with absorbable suture and close the skin in a routine manner.
- Apply a soft dressing with or without a temporary splint.

FULL DENERVATION OF THE WRIST

- A full wrist denervation involves four separate incisions (**TECH FIG 1**).

Incision 1

- Make the same transverse incision described for a partial denervation 3 to 5 cm proximal to the wrist on the dorsal forearm.

  - If a more distal incision is used, some articular branches from the PIN may not be completely eliminated.
- Excise the PIN (**TECH FIG 2A**) and branches of the AIN (**TECH FIG 2B**) as discussed above.

Incision 2

- Make a 2- to 3-cm dorsal–ulnar incision over the wrist at the level of the ulnar head.

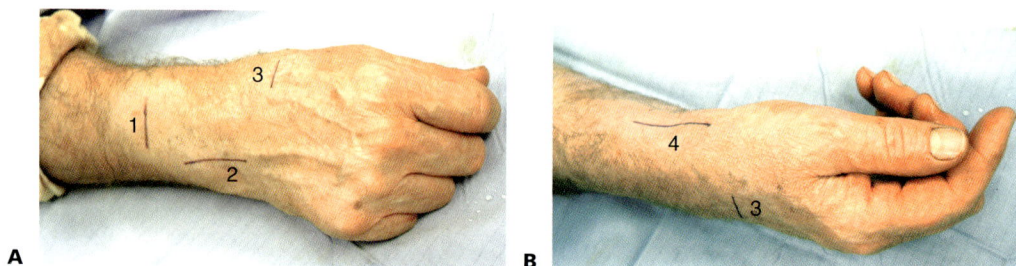

TECH FIG 1 • The four incisions for a complete wrist denervation are marked on the skin. (Reprinted from Hunt T, Herlas-Palou C. Wrist denervation. In Chunk K. Operative Techniques: Hand and Wrist Surgery. Philadelphia: Elsevier, 2008:209–230.)

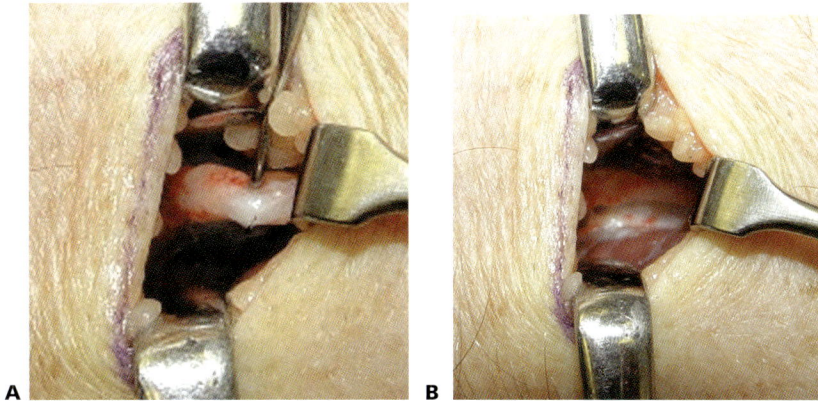

TECH FIG 2 • A. The posterior interosseous nerve is isolated on the radial floor of the fourth extensor compartment. **B.** A longitudinal incision in the interosseous membrane reveals the anterior interosseous nerve. (Reprinted from Hunt T, Herlas-Palou C. Wrist denervation. In Chunk K. Operative Techniques: Hand and Wrist Surgery. Philadelphia: Elsevier, 2008:209–230.)

- Dissect to the level of the extensor retinaculum.
- In the subcutaneous flap, isolate the dorsal branch of the ulnar nerve along with its small articular branches to the wrist joint (**TECH FIG 3**).
- Divide these small branches close to the point where they enter the extensor retinaculum.

Incision 3

- Make a 2- to 3-cm volar–radial incision centered over the radial artery at the level of the wrist and distal forearm.
- Resect a portion of perivascular tissue from around the radial artery.

- Eliminate sympathetic branches to the wrist by using finger dissection to develop planes deep to the vessel, deep to the palmar cutaneous branch of the median nerve, and deep to the radial sensory nerve.

Incision 4

- Make a 2-cm transverse incision over the dorsal base of the second and third metacarpals.
- Dissect through the fascia to expose and resect the recurrent intermetacarpal branches (**TECH FIG 4**).
- Close in standard fashion.
- Apply a soft dressing with or without a temporary splint.

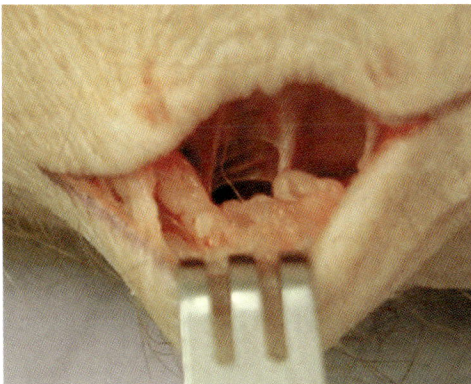

TECH FIG 3 • Through a dorsal–ulnar incision, a subcutaneous flap is raised containing the dorsal cutaneous branch of the ulnar nerve and its small branches, seen here heading toward the retinaculum. (Reprinted from Hunt T, Herlas-Palou C. Wrist denervation. In Chunk K. Operative Techniques: Hand and Wrist Surgery. Philadelphia: Elsevier, 2008:209–230.)

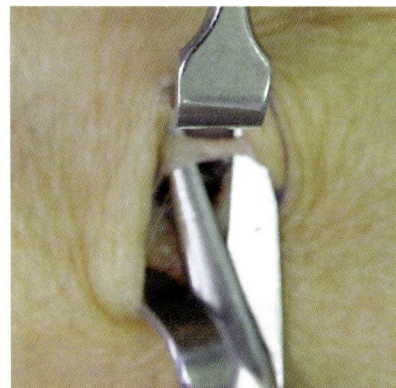

TECH FIG 4 • The recurrent intermetacarpal branch is exposed and resected between the bases of the second and third metacarpal. (Reprinted from Hunt T, Herlas-Palou C. Wrist denervation. In Chunk K. Operative Techniques: Hand and Wrist Surgery. Philadelphia: Elsevier, 2008:209–230.)

PEARLS AND PITFALLS

Indications	■ Patients with wrist degeneration and substantial pain but some useful wrist movement ■ Avoid denervation in patients with frank wrist instability or active inflammatory arthritis. ■ Use local anesthetic blocks to help in patient selection.
Options	■ Partial denervation ■ Full denervation ■ Denervation combined with other procedures
Alternatives to denervation	■ Arthroscopic or open wrist débridement ■ Radial styloidectomy ■ Partial carpal arthrodesis ■ Proximal row carpectomy ■ Wrist arthrodesis

POSTOPERATIVE CARE

■ Early range of motion is initiated but little formal therapy is required.

■ A removable splint may be provided for comfort initially.

■ Patients usually return to work 2 to 4 weeks after surgery.

OUTCOMES

■ Wrist denervation is successful in providing pain relief in the long term in two thirds of patients.

■ A partial wrist denervation seems to provide good results initially, but there is often deterioration after 12 months.

COMPLICATIONS

■ Although there is a theoretical risk of causing a neuropathic Charcot joint, to our knowledge this has never been reported.

This proves that a complete denervation of the wrist joint is never achieved.

■ Neuroma formation has been reported in 2% of patients.

REFERENCES

1. Buck-Gramcko D. Denervation of the wrist joint. J Hand Surg Am 1977;2A:54–61.
2. Ferreres A, Suso S, Foucher G. Wrist denervation: surgical considerations. J Hand Surg Br 1995;20B:769–772.
3. Weinstein LP, Berger RA. Analgesic benefit, functional outcome, and patient satisfaction after partial wrist denervation. J Hand Surg Am 2002;27A:833–839.

Chapter 86

Open and Arthroscopic Radial Styloidectomy

Bruce A. Monaghan

DEFINITION

- Arthritis between the radial styloid and the distal aspect of the scaphoid can lead to pain, weakness of grip, and limitation of motion. This arthritis can occur in the early stages of a variety of pathologic states of the radiocarpal joint.
- Radial styloidectomy is a technique that involves resection of the distalmost aspect of the articular surface of the distal radius.
- A radial styloidectomy can be performed as a distinct procedure via an open incision or by arthroscopic means. It is more commonly undertaken as an adjunct procedure with reconstructive or salvage procedures for scaphoid nonunions, carpal instabilities, Kienböck disease, or posttraumatic arthritis of the radiocarpal joint.[9,17]

ANATOMY

- The radial styloid is the distalmost projection on the lateral aspect of the terminal end of the radius (**FIG 1A,B**).
  - When viewed from the lateral aspect, the styloid has a gentle slope volarly, placing it below the midcoronal longitudinal axis of the radius.
  - The intra-articular component of the radial styloid encompasses part of the scaphoid facet.
  - The extra-articular aspect of the styloid serves as the origin of several dorsal, palmar, and radial extrinsic ligaments that are vital to normal carpal kinematics (**FIG 1C**).
- The palmar radiocarpal ligaments serve as a constraint to radiocarpal pronation, ulnar translation, and distal pole scaphoid stabilization. Global disruption of this complex has been implicated in perilunate dislocation. The palmar radiocarpal ligaments are composed of the following structures:
  - The radial collateral ligament (RCL) is a thin structure that originates from the tip of the radial styloid and inserts into the waist and distal aspect of the scaphoid. The integrity of the ligament is always sacrificed with a radial styloidectomy, but no untoward effects have been reported.[3,4]
  - The radioscaphocapitate (RSC) ligament originates from the palmar cortex of the distal radius coursing distally and ulnarly, attaching to the waist and proximal cortex of the distal pole of the scaphoid and the body of the capitate.[3,4]
  - The long radiolunate ligament (LRL) originates from the palmar cortical margin of the distal radius immediately adjacent and medial to the RSC ligament. It is separated from the RSC by a distinct sulcus that serves an arthroscopic landmark.[3,4]
- The dorsal radiocarpal (DRC) ligament originates broadly from the dorsal rim of the distal radius around the tubercle of Lister, coursing ulnarly, distally, and obliquely to insert on the dorsal tubercle of the triquetrum.
  - The radialmost fibers of this ligament also insert on the dorsal lunate.
  - The DRC ligament, in concert with the dorsal intercarpal ligament, has a crucial role in maintaining normal carpal kinematics and carpal stability and preventing ulnar translation of the carpus.[14,15]

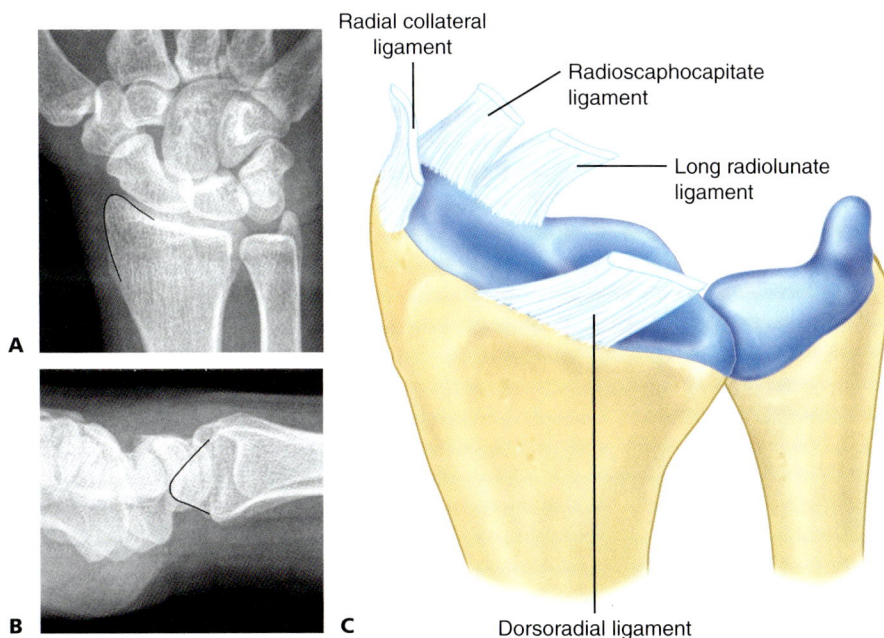

FIG 1 • A,B. The radial styloid outlined on a standard PA and lateral wrist radiograph. **C.** Palmar and dorsal extrinsic ligaments of the radiocarpal joint. Note the broad origin of the dorsoradial ligament. The radial collateral ligament originates from the tip of the styloid. The radioscaphocapitate and long radiolunate ligaments are separated by a well-defined sulcus readily seen arthroscopically.

Radial collateral ligament

Radioscaphocapitate ligament

Long radiolunate ligament

Dorsoradial ligament

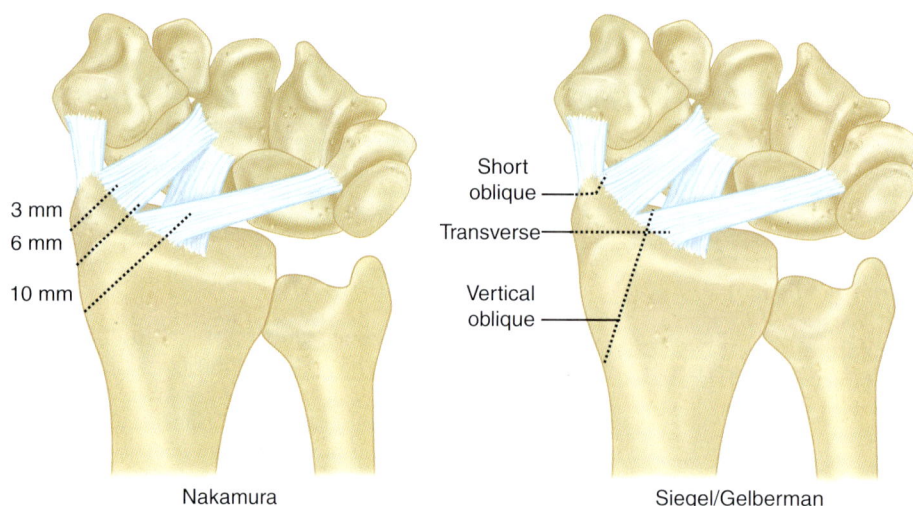

FIG 2 • Styloidectomies as described by Nakamura and Siegel and Gelberman.

■ Siegel and Gelberman[13] examined the effect of three different styloidectomy configurations on palmar radiocarpal ligament integrity in a cadaver model (**FIG 2**).

■ The most conservative osteotomy (short oblique) removed only 9% of the RSC and none of the LRL ligaments.

■ A vertical oblique osteotomy sacrificed 92% of the RSC and 21% of the LRL ligaments.

■ A transverse styloidectomy was the most aggressive and resulted in loss of 95% of the RSC and 42% loss of the LRL ligaments.

■ Nakamura et al[10] examined the effect of radial styloidectomy on carpal alignment and ulnar translation in cadaveric limbs. They demonstrated that as a larger segment of the radial styloid was resected (**FIG 2**), a greater tendency toward ulnar translation, as manifested by decreased stiffness, was observed. No frank ulnar translation with axial loading was observed.

■ Based on their analysis, they recommended that no more than 3 to 4 mm of radial styloid should be resected. This correlated with a short oblique styloidectomy as described by Siegel and Gelberman.

■ Although ulnar translation is a stated complication of overly vigorous styloidectomy, Viegas et al[14] demonstrated in a cadaver model that ulnar translation can occur only with resection of the DRC, RSC, LRL, and SRL ligaments.

PATHOGENESIS AND NATURAL HISTORY

Scapholunate Instability

■ Watson and Ballet[16] reviewed radiographs of individuals with scapholunate dissociation to establish the sequential progression of arthritis in the scapholunate advanced collapse (SLAC) wrist (**FIG 3**).

■ SLAC I: Degenerative changes are confined to the radial styloid area.

■ SLAC II: Changes are characterized by joint space narrowing involving the entire radioscaphoid articulation.

■ SLAC III: Changes involve additional arthritis between the capitate and lunate.

■ Several authors have examined the mechanics of scapholunate dissociation in cadaver models and have demonstrated that scapholunate instability leads to a shift in the contact pressures from the proximal pole of scaphoid articulation with the radial articular surface toward the distal pole of the scaphoid with the dorsal lip of the radial styloid.[6,7] The pathomechanics of these changes can occur even before the frank radiographic appearance of scapholunate diastasis is present (ie, static scapholunate instability). Prolonged exposure to these abnormal contact stresses leads to the predictable arthritic changes described above.

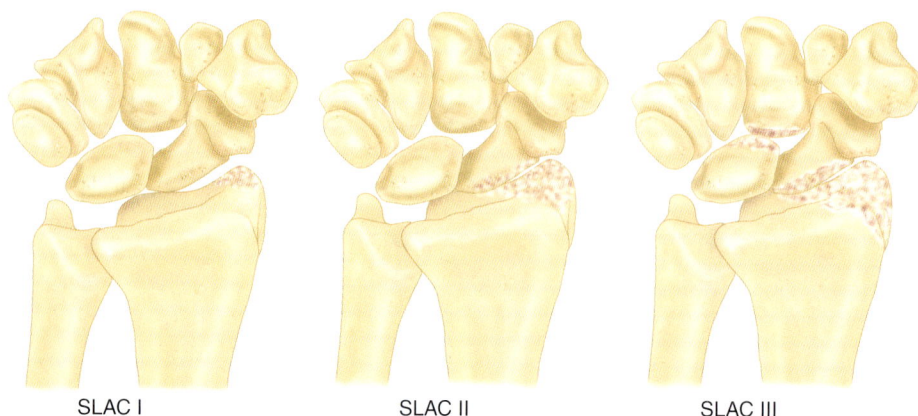

FIG 3 • Stages of arthritis with scapholunate advanced collapse (SLAC). SLAC I: degenerative changes are confined to the radial styloid. SLAC II: joint space narrowing of the entire radioscaphoid articulation. SLAC III: chondral changes in the radioscaphoid and capitolunate joint.

- Scaphoid nonunion
  - With an unstable scaphoid fracture, the proximal pole of the scaphoid remains firmly fixed to and extends with the lunate through an intact scapholunate interosseous ligament. The distal pole adopts a flexed posture, which can then impinge upon the radial styloid, leading to abnormal contact stresses and arthritic changes.
  - The natural history of scaphoid nonunion has not been established by rigorous prospective analysis. Nonetheless, most surgeons believe that unstable scaphoid fractures result in abnormal carpal kinematics with a dorsal intercalated segment instability (DISI) deformity and subsequent arthritis (scaphoid nonunion advanced collapse [SNAC] wrist).
  - Inoue and Sakuma[8] reviewed 102 patients with scaphoid nonunions clinically and radiographically; they found that arthritis initially developed at the scaphoid–radial styloid articulation and subsequently the midcarpal joint. All patients had radiographic arthritis within 10 years of injury. They also demonstrated that although radiographic progression did not correlate with wrist pain, it did correlate with a decrease in grip strength and range of motion.
- Impingement after triscaphe (scaphoid-trapezoid-trapezium) fusion
  - Rogers and Watson[12] reviewed 93 patients after triscaphe fusion and found a 33% incidence of painful impingement between the fusion mass and the radial styloid that resolved after limited radial styloidectomy. They hypothesized that the fixed scaphoid could no longer be accommodated in the fossa and impacted upon the radial styloid.
- Proximal row carpectomy
  - Although not all surgeons routinely perform a radial styloidectomy in the setting of a proximal row carpectomy, a recent cadaveric study demonstrated that radial deviation after proximal-row carpectomy was limited by impingement of the trapezoid on the radial styloid.[5]

PATIENT HISTORY AND PHYSICAL FINDINGS

- Patients with clinically significant radial styloid arthritis or impingement frequently complain of pain along the dorsal radial aspect of the wrist that is exacerbated by extension of the wrist or gripping activities. They may also note focal swelling or a decrease in the range of motion.
- A complete physical examination of the radiocarpal, the midcarpal, and the first carpometacarpal joints is necessary to assess for associated conditions and to rule out alternative diagnoses.
- Styloid impingement typically causes radial-sided wrist pain that is exacerbated by radial deviation, extension, and loading of the wrist.
- Physical findings of styloid impingement are centered around the anatomic snuffbox (**FIG 4**).
  - The anatomic snuffbox is triangular, with its radial border formed by the extensor pollicis brevis tendon, its ulnar border by the extensor pollicis longus tendon, and its proximal border by the dorsal rim of the distal radius at the level of the styloid. The waist of the scaphoid and a small segment of the trapezium are palpable in the floor of the snuffbox, more readily with ulnar deviation.

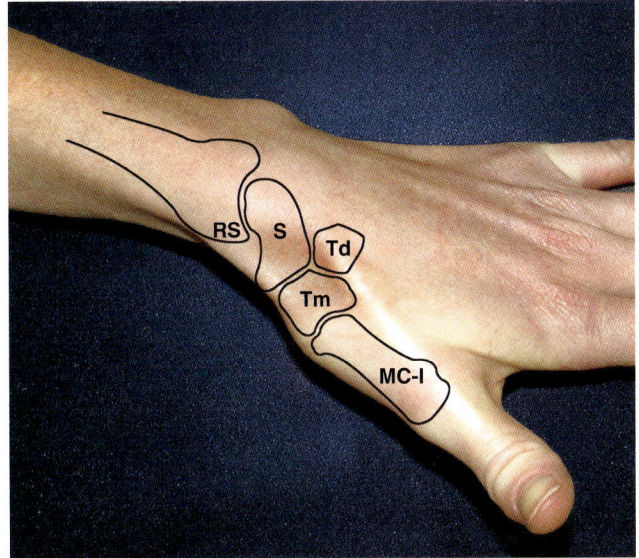

FIG 4 • Meticulous and systematic physical examination of this region can rule out diagnoses other than radial styloid impingement. *RS*, radial styloid; *S*, scaphoid; *Tm*, trapezium; *Td*, trapezoid; *MC-I*, thumb metacarpal.

  - Focal tenderness and synovitis along the proximal edge of the snuffbox made worse by forced radial deviation and extension may be indicative of styloid impingement.
- More diffuse tenderness, synovitis, and global limitations of motion may be indicative of a more advanced stage of posttraumatic arthritis or an inflammatory process (rheumatoid arthritis), which would preclude the success of a radial styloidectomy.

IMAGING AND OTHER DIAGNOSTIC STUDIES

- Plain radiographs of the wrist
  - To diagnosis and stage SNAC and SLAC (**FIG 5**)
  - To rule out scaphoid fracture or other acute injury
- Stress radiographs (clenched fist and radial–ulnar deviation posteroanterior) of the wrist can yield information concerning dynamic impingement between the scaphoid and the radial styloid.

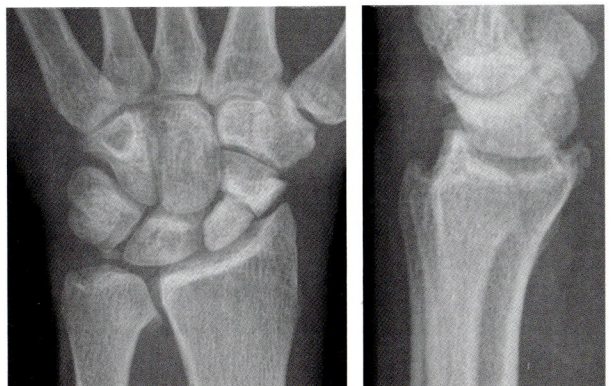

FIG 5 • Impingement of the flexed distal pole of the scaphoid nonunion against the radial styloid leading to arthritic changes.

DIFFERENTIAL DIAGNOSIS

■ DeQuervain stenosing tenosynovitis: Tenderness usually extends along the extra-articular component of the radial styloid, proximally and radially over the first dorsal compartment. A positive Finkelstein test is highly suggestive of this disorder.

■ Scapho-trapezoid-trapezial arthritis: focal tenderness in the distal-ulnar aspect of the snuffbox under the extensor pollicis long tendon along the axis of the second metacarpal

■ Thumb carpometacarpal instability or arthritis: tenderness distal to the anatomic snuffbox that is worsened by loading of the thumb ray (CMC grind test)

■ Scaphoid fracture: After an acute injury, special imaging (bone scan or MRI) may be required to rule out an acute scaphoid fracture.

■ Preiser disease

■ Inflammatory arthritis (ie, rheumatoid)

■ Radial sensory neuritis or neuroma

■ Tenosynovitis of the extensor carpi radialis longus and brevis

■ Not uncommonly, styloid impingement coexists with other diagnoses, especially basilar thumb arthritis and De Quervain stenosing tenosynovitis.

NONOPERATIVE MANAGEMENT

■ Individuals with chronic SLAC or SNAC wrist arthritis frequently present with acute pain after a recent injury. After obtaining an accurate medical history of prior injury and radiographic assessment, the chronicity of the problem is usually evident.

■ In this situation, a course of conservative treatment with activity modification, nonsteroidal anti-inflammatory drugs, rest in a forearm-based thumb spica splint, and selective corticosteroid injection in the radial styloid area is appropriate.

■ If the arthritic changes are truly isolated to the area of articulation between the scaphoid and the styloid, the surgeon may elect earlier operative intervention with the theoretical goal of slowing or preventing progressive arthrosis and the need for a more extensive reconstructive procedure.

SURGICAL MANAGEMENT

■ Isolated radial styloidectomy is a limited procedure to treat the early stage of progressive posttraumatic arthritis.

■ It cannot be expected to prevent its pathologic progression.

■ It can also be employed as a temporizing solution in a low-demand individual or in a patient unfit or unwilling to undertake a more extensive procedure and postoperative rehabilitative course.

■ In that instance, patient expectations with respect to motion and pain relief must be assiduously managed.

■ Arthroscopic radial styloidectomy has the theoretical advantages of being minimally invasive and allowing more precise control of the level of bony resection to minimize injury to the palmar radiocarpal ligaments. In addition, arthroscopic evaluation of the radiocarpal and midcarpal joints can allow for diagnosis and treatment of concomitant intra-articular pathology.[17]

Preoperative Planning

■ Precise radiographic assessment and patient selection are critical in ensuring a good outcome. The surgeon must review all radiographic studies and the severity, characteristics, and nature of the patient's symptoms and physical findings.

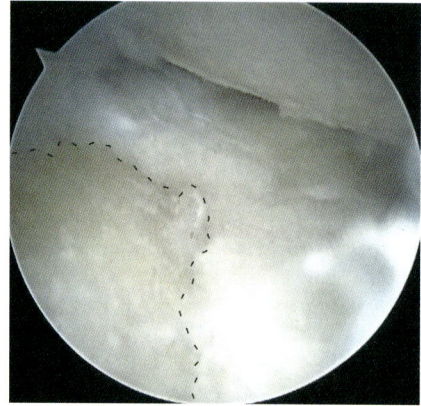

FIG 6 • Arthroscopic findings of full-thickness cartilage loss in the entire scaphoid facet (*dashed line*) and proximal pole of the scaphoid as viewed from the dorsal 3-4 portal. These degenerative changes were not readily apparent on plain radiographs. An isolated radial styloidectomy cannot be expected to confer pain relief in this instance.

■ In some cases, final staging of the severity of articular degeneration can be made only by direct visualization with diagnostic wrist arthroscopy (**FIG 6**). An isolated radial styloidectomy or a more extensive reconstructive procedure can be done at the time of arthroscopy or at a later time, after the implications of the arthroscopic findings are discussed with the patient.

Positioning

■ The patient is positioned supine on a stretcher with an attached hand table and the arm centered on the hand table with the shoulder abducted 90 degrees. A mini-fluoroscopy unit is draped in a sterile fashion and placed in a plane perpendicular to the hand table.

■ For arthroscopic procedures, the arm is stabilized to the hand table with a strap that allows countertraction.

■ The shoulder is abducted 90 degrees, the elbow is flexed 90 degrees, and finger traps are placed on the index and middle fingers.

■ The forearm is suspended in a standard wrist traction tower with 8 to 12 pounds of traction employed.

■ A mini-fluoroscopy unit is draped in a sterile fashion and placed in a plane parallel to and above the hand table.

■ Alternatively, the hand can be suspended via finger traps using a nonsterile overhead traction boom (ie, an arthroscopic shoulder holder); in this case, the wrist traction tower will not be an impediment to intraoperative fluoroscopic assessment.

Approach

■ A radial styloidectomy can be performed in conjunction with other reconstructive procedures such as proximal-row carpectomy, intercarpal fusion, or bone grafting for a scaphoid nonunion.

■ In these instances, the primary procedure usually requires wide exposure through a standard dorsal approach to the wrist.

■ An isolated styloidectomy can be performed through a limited radial incision.

■ An arthroscopic styloidectomy can be performed through standard arthroscopic portals.

OPEN RADIAL STYLOIDECTOMY

- Palpate the distalmost aspect of the radial styloid on the volar radial aspect of the wrist. Make an incision from that point for 2 or 3 cm proximally and obliquely between the first and second extensor compartments (**TECH FIG 1A**).
  - Alternatively, a transverse incision may provide a more cosmetically pleasing scar but also may limit exposure.
- At this level, there will be arborization of the terminal branches of the radial sensory and lateral antebrachial cutaneous nerves in the subcutaneous tissue.[2] Use blunt dissection and gentle retraction to expose the first and second compartments.
  - Distal placement of the incision may place the dorsal branch of the radial artery at risk and should be recognized.
- Incise the extensor retinaculum in the 1–2 interval and expose the radial styloid by subperiosteal dissection. Alternatively, the radius can be approached through the floor of the first compartment (**TECH FIG 1B**).

- Expose the radial styloid by sharp dissection (**TECH FIG 1C**).
- Using a sharp osteotome, remove the distal 3 to 4 mm of radial styloid. The plane of the cut should be perpendicular to the articular surface (**TECH FIG 1D**).
  - Fluoroscopic imaging of the level of resection can be useful at this point in the procedure.
- A narrow malleable retractor can be placed in the radiocarpal joint to prevent damage to the scaphoid as the styloid is being resected (**TECH FIG 1E**).
- After styloidectomy, fluoroscopic examination with the wrist in radial and ulnar deviation to assess for impingement confirms adequacy of the resection level (**TECH FIG 1F,G**).
- Loosely reapproximate the periosteum with resorbable suture, allow the extensor compartments to fall back into their anatomic position, and suture the skin. A bulky dressing and volar splint holding the wrist is applied.

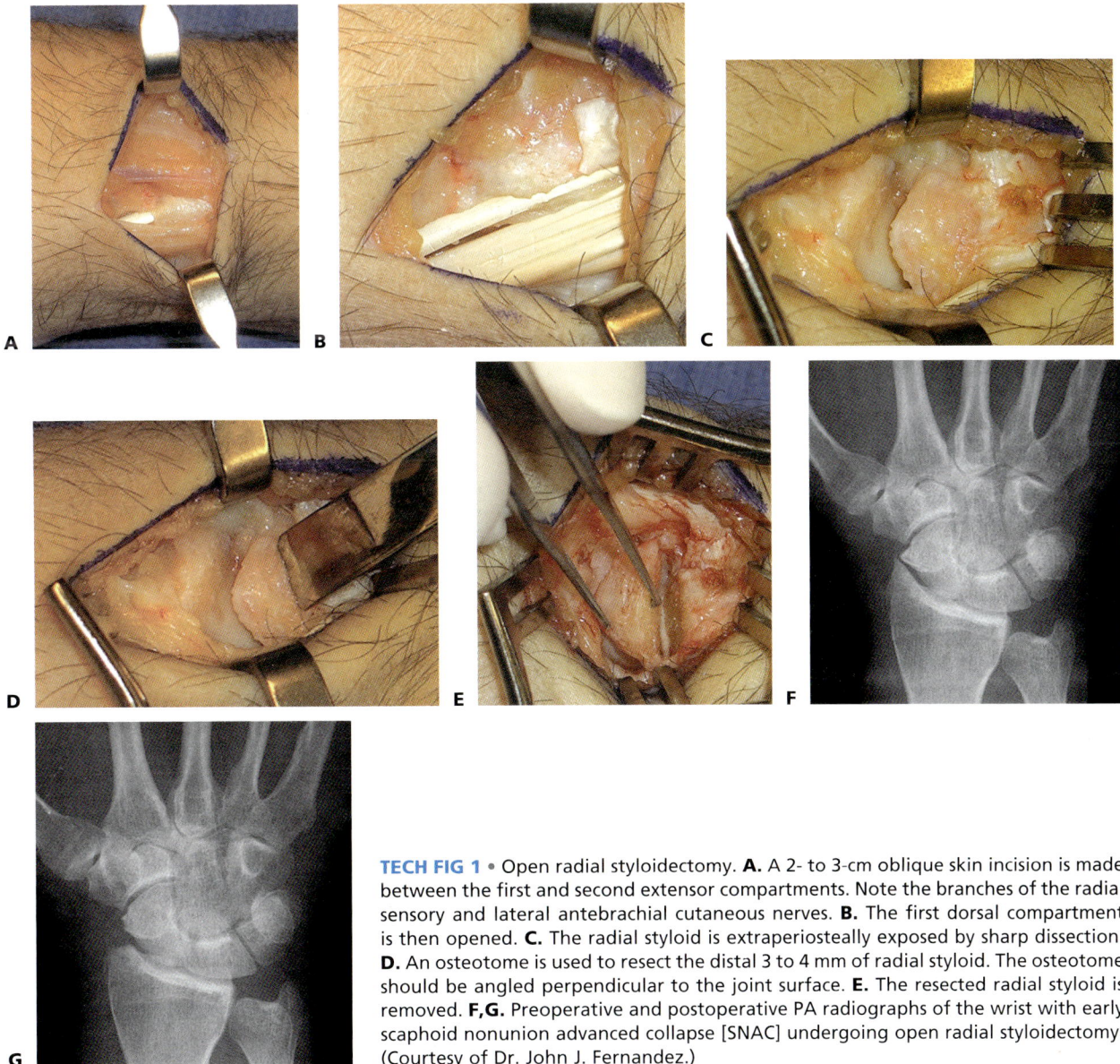

TECH FIG 1 • Open radial styloidectomy. **A.** A 2- to 3-cm oblique skin incision is made between the first and second extensor compartments. Note the branches of the radial sensory and lateral antebrachial cutaneous nerves. **B.** The first dorsal compartment is then opened. **C.** The radial styloid is extraperiosteally exposed by sharp dissection. **D.** An osteotome is used to resect the distal 3 to 4 mm of radial styloid. The osteotome should be angled perpendicular to the joint surface. **E.** The resected radial styloid is removed. **F,G.** Preoperative and postoperative PA radiographs of the wrist with early scaphoid nonunion advanced collapse [SNAC] undergoing open radial styloidectomy. (Courtesy of Dr. John J. Fernandez.)

ARTHROSCOPIC STYLOIDECTOMY

- After patient positioning as previously described, insufflate the joint with 5 to 10 mL of sterile saline and establish the 3-4 portal. Outflow is achieved by placing an 18-gauge needle in the 6U interval. Perform a complete arthroscopic evaluation of the radiocarpal joint.
- Establish the radial and ulnar midcarpal portals and perform an arthroscopic evaluation to confirm capitolunate joint preservation.
- Place a localization needle into the styloscaphoid joint space, in the interval between the first and second compartments.
  - Confirm the adequacy of the position of this working portal by arthroscopic evaluation from the 3–4 interval.
  - Develop the portal by sharp dissection through skin only and blunt dissection in the subcutaneous tissues

- to the capsule to prevent damage to the radial sensory nerve, the lateral antebrachial cutaneous nerve, and the radial artery.
- Resect the radial styloid with a 2.9-mm full-radius resector, an arthroscopic covered burr, or both (**TECH FIG 2A**). This is initiated at the radial margin of the radioscaphocapitate ligament and carried radially. The diameter of the burr can be used as a gauge for the amount of bone being resected.
- Intraoperative fluoroscopy is critical in the assessment of the resection level (**TECH FIG 2B**).
- After completing the styloidectomy, remove the arthroscopic instruments and suture the portals. Apply a sterile bulky dressing and volar splint to the wrist and forearm.

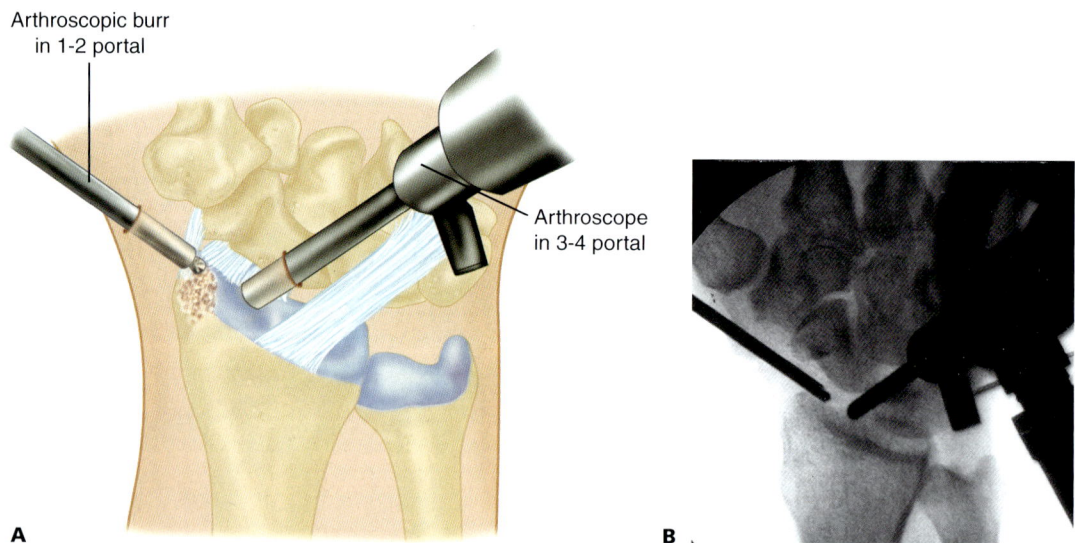

TECH FIG 2 • Arthroscopic radial styloidectomy. **A.** The arthroscopic burr is in the 1,2 portal and the arthroscope is in the 3,4 portal. **B.** Fluoroscopic image obtained during arthroscopic radial styloidectomy for scapholunate instability and secondary degeneration. Note the disruption of the line of Gilula in the proximal carpal row.

PEARLS AND PITFALLS

Indications	▪ A complete history and physical examination emphasizing clinical staging is essential. The final decision to proceed with styloidectomy may require staging arthroscopy.
Insufficient or excessive styloid resection	▪ Arthroscopic visualization of the RSC ligament to prevent significant injury ▪ Using the diameter of the burr as a gauge for the amount of bone resected ▪ Intraoperative fluoroscopic evaluation
Poor arthroscopic visualization	▪ Convert from arthroscopic to open procedure.

POSTOPERATIVE CARE

- If the radial styloidectomy is performed concomitantly with another reconstructive procedure (PRC, four-corner arthrodesis, scaphoid bone grafting and fixation), the rehabilitation is dictated by the requirements of that additional procedure.

- After either open or arthroscopic radial styloidectomy, the postoperative dressing and sutures are removed in 7 to 10 days. Early active, active-assisted, and passive motion is initiated under the guidance of a hand therapist. Usually a removable splint is used initially for patient comfort. As the patient's symptoms permit, graded strengthening and unrestricted activities are allowed.

OUTCOMES

- Stubbins and Barnard[1] first described a radial styloidectomy as part of an operative treatment strategy for scaphoid nonunion in 14 patients in 1948. They thought that the styloidectomy removed impingement, enhanced exposure of the scaphoid, and provided material for bone grafting from the same operative field. Since that time there have been no series of outcomes in the indexed English literature for outcomes after isolated open radial styloidectomy. Several reports of radial styloidectomy performed with open reduction and internal fixation of scaphoid nonunion or with triscaphe fusion have demonstrated good pain relief but no significant improvement in range of motion.[12,16]
- Page et al[11] presented their experience with the arthroscopic technique in 22 patients to the European Federation of National Associations of Orthopaedics and Traumatology in 2003. In short-term follow-up, they reported 75% good and satisfactory results.
- Radial styloidectomy is most often performed as a limited procedure to address posttraumatic arthritis of the wrist early in its pathogenesis. While it can provide long-lasting symptomatic relief, it cannot be expected to halt the progression of the arthritis. A successful radial styloidectomy could be one in which a more extensive reconstructive procedure was delayed by several years.

COMPLICATIONS

- Incomplete resection leading to persistent pain
- Excessive resection leading to extrinsic ligament incompetence and wrist instability with ulnar translation
- Nerve injury to the terminal branches of the radial sensory nerve or lateral antebrachial cutaneous nerve
- Arthrofibrosis
- Infection
- Complex regional pain syndrome

REFERENCES

1. Barnard L, Stubbins SG. Styloidectomy of the radius in the surgical treatment of non-union of the carpal navicular: a preliminary report. J Bone Joint Surg Am 1948;30A:98–102.
2. Beldner S, Zlotolow DA, Melone CP, et al. Anatomy of the lateral antebrachial cutaneous and superficial radial nerve in the forearm: a cadaver and clinical study. J Hand Surg Am 2005;30A:1226–1230.
3. Berger RA, Landsmeer JMF. The palmar radiocarpal ligaments: a study of adult and fetal human wrist joints. J Hand Surg Am 1990;15A:847–854.
4. Berger RA. The ligaments of the wrist: a current overview of anatomy with considerations of their potential functions. Hand Clin 1997;13:63–82.
5. Blankenhorn BD, Pfaeffle HJ, Tang P, et al. Carpal kinematics after proximal row carpectomy. J Hand Surg Am 2007;32A:37–46.
6. Blevens AD, Light TR, Jablonsky WS, et al. Radiocarpal articular contact characteristics with scaphoid instability. J Hand Surg Am 1989;14A:781–790.
7. Burgess RC. The effect of rotatory subluxation of the scaphoid on radio-scaphoid contact. J Hand Surg Am 1987;12A:771–774.
8. Inoue G, Sakuma M. The natural history of scaphoid non-union: radiologic and clinical analysis in 102 cases. Arch Orthop Trauma Surg 1996;115:1–4.
9. Kalainov DM, Cohen MS, Sweet S. Radial styloidectomy. In: Geissler WB, ed. Wrist Arthroscopy. New York: Springer-Verlag, 2005:134–138.
10. Nakamura T, Cooney WP, Lui W, et al. Radial styloidectomy: a biomechanical study on the stability of the wrist. J Hand Surg Am 2001;26A:85–93.
11. Page RS, Waseem M, Stanley JK. Clinical outcome of arthroscopic radial styloidectomy. J Bone Joint Surg Br 2004;86B:280.
12. Rogers WD, Watson HK. Radial styloid impingement after triscaphe fusion. J Hand Surg Am 1989;14A:297–301.
13. Siegel DB, Gelberman RH. Radial styloidectomy: an anatomical study with special reference to radiocarpal intracapsular ligamentous morphology. J Hand Surg Am 1991;16A:40–44.
14. Viegas SF, Patterson RM, Ward, K. Extrinsic wrist ligaments in the pathomechanics of ulnar translation instability. J Hand Surg Am 1995;20A:312–318.
15. Viegas SF, Yamaguchi S, Boyd NL, et al. The dorsal ligaments of the wrist: anatomy, mechanical properties and function. J Hand Surg Am 1999;24A:456–468.
16. Watson HK, Ballet FL. The SLAC wrist: scapholunate advanced collapse pattern of degenerative arthritis. J Hand Surg Am 1984;9A:358–365.
17. Yao J, Osterman AL. Arthroscopic techniques for wrist arthritis (radial styloidectomy and proximal pole hamate excision). Hand Clin 2005;21:519–526.

Chapter 87

Proximal Row Carpectomy

Alex M. Meyers, Mark E. Baratz, and Thomas Hughes

DEFINITION

- Proximal row carpectomy (PRC) involves removal of the proximal carpal row (scaphoid, lunate, and triquetrum).
- PRC has been described as a treatment option for a number of pathologic conditions:
  - Scaphoid nonunion advanced collapse (SNAC) wrist
  - Scapholunate advanced collapse (SLAC) wrist
  - Kienböck disease
  - Chronic or missed perilunate dislocation
  - Scaphoid osteonecrosis or Preiser disease
  - Wrist deformity or contracture

ANATOMY

- The proximal row of the wrist consists of three bones: scaphoid, lunate, and triquetrum.
- The proximal row moves as a single unit through intercarpal ligamentous attachments and bony congruity.
  - The proximal row flexes with radial deviation and extends with ulnar deviation.
- The capitate, in the distal row, articulates with the lunate.
  - The proximal capitate articular surface is relatively, although not completely, congruous with the lunate facet of the radius.

PATHOGENESIS

- A number of pathologies may eventually result in wrist degeneration requiring PRC. Patients experience progressive pain and limitation in motion, often requiring PRC to improve symptoms.
  - SNAC and SLAC
    Stage I: Degenerative changes along the radial half of the radioscaphoid articulation. In SNAC wrists, the degenerative changes are typically limited to the articulation between the distal scaphoid fragment and the radius.
    Stage II: Degenerative changes involving the entire radioscaphoid articulation (**FIG 1**). In SNAC wrists, the articulation between the proximal scaphoid fragment and the radius is preserved, and instead stage II degeneration occurs in the scaphocapitate joint.
    Stage III: Degenerative changes at the capitolunate joint. The radiolunate joint is spared.
  - Kienböck disease
    Stage I: Normal plain radiographs with wrist pain and positive MRI finding
    Stage II: Sclerosis without collapse of the lunate
    Stage IIIa: Lunate collapse without instability
    Stage IIIb: Lunate collapse with carpal instability
    Stage IV: Fixed carpal instability with pan-carpal degenerative changes
  - Missed perilunate dislocation
  - Scaphoid osteonecrosis (Preiser disease)

- Congenital or spastic wrist and hand flexion contractures may be so severe that a PRC allows deformity correction that tendon-lengthening procedures alone would be unable to correct.

PATIENT HISTORY AND PHYSICAL FINDINGS

- It is important to seek the cause of the wrist degeneration.
- Mechanical wrist pain is aggravated by use and relieved by rest. The history must support this for the proposed treatment to be successful.
- The history defines the patient's symptoms, level of severity, and progression over time, as well as any previous attempts at treatment.
- Limited and painful wrist motion with diminished grip strength tends to be a common denominator regardless of the initial source of pathology.
  - Normal range of motion: wrist extension, 70 degrees; wrist flexion, 75 degrees; radial deviation, 20 degrees; ulnar deviation, 35 degrees
  - Normal grip strength: Mean grip for males is 103 to 104 for the dominant extremity and 92 to 99 for the nondominant extremity. Mean grip for females is 62 to 63 for the dominant extremity and 53 to 55 for the nondominant extremity.
- Radioscaphoid joint line tenderness on palpation implies radioscaphoid arthritis.
- Swelling over the dorsal and dorsoradial aspects of the wrist can be associated with radiocarpal and intercarpal arthritis. Most often dorsoradial wrist swelling will be visible and palpable in cases of SLAC and SNAC.

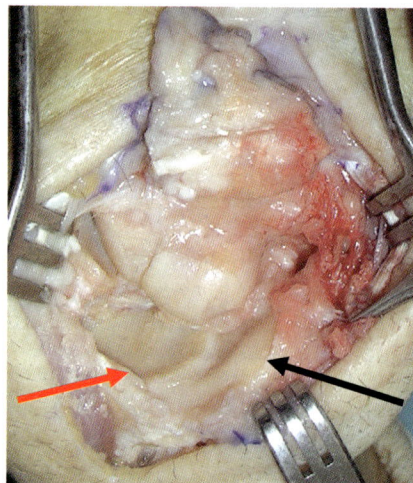

FIG 1 • Intraoperative photograph showing wear at the dorsal half of the scaphoid fossa seen with SLAC wrist, as indicated by the *black arrow*. Cartilage integrity is preserved in the lunate fossa, as indicated by the *red arrow*.

IMAGING AND OTHER DIAGNOSTIC STUDIES

- Plain radiographs assist with making the underlying diagnosis (eg, SNAC wrist, SLAC wrist, Kienböck disease).
  - The surgeon should evaluate the articular facets and surfaces, specifically of the proximal capitate and lunate facet of the radius.
  - The surgeon should evaluate for other sources of limited wrist motion, diminished grip strength, and pain (eg, thumb carpometacarpal arthritis, scapholunate instability without degenerative changes, fracture).
- Although MRI may assist in making the underlying diagnosis (eg, Kienböck disease, Preiser disease, scaphoid avascular necrosis) and evaluating the joint surfaces, it is rarely used.

DIFFERENTIAL DIAGNOSIS

- Triangular fibrocartilage complex or distal radioulnar joint pathology
- Extensor carpi ulnaris, flexor carpi ulnaris, flexor carpi radialis tendinitis
- De Quervain tenosynovitis
- First carpometacarpal arthritis
- Scapholunate or lunotriquetral instability without degenerative changes
- Midcarpal arthritis

SURGICAL MANAGEMENT

- Regardless of the initial source of pathology when considering treatment via PRC, the integrity of the articular cartilage and the congruity between the proximal capitate and the lunate facet of the radius are critical. This determination is often made intraoperatively.
- Indications
  - SLAC and SNAC wrist degeneration: stage I, II, or III (only if the degenerative changes at proximal capitate are limited to thinning or minor fissuring)
  - Kienböck disease (stage III and IV)
  - Chronic or missed perilunate dislocations
  - Scaphoid osteonecrosis (Preiser disease)
  - Wrist deformity or contracture
- Contraindications
  - Active inflammatory arthritis (rheumatoid arthritis). PRC may be used for inflammatory arthritis patients with "burnt-out" disease (those without active tenosynovitis).
  - Advanced degenerative changes at the proximal articular surface of the capitate or lunate facet of the radius
  - Ulnar carpal translation or subluxation of the radiocarpal joint
- Relative contraindications
  - Heavy laborers
  - Young (less than 35 years) active patients (controversial)[7]

Preoperative Planning

- Plain radiographs of the wrist should be reviewed. The surgeon should scrutinize the location of degenerative changes, should know the amount of radial styloid beaking (and potential need for radial styloidectomy), and should note any previous fractures or hardware (may need to be removed).
- The surgeon should discuss and obtain consent for alternative procedures from the patient (ie, if one should find excessive degenerative changes at the capitate, one might proceed with intercarpal arthrodesis).
- Regional anesthesia, general anesthesia, or a combination of the two (for postoperative analgesia) is suitable.

Positioning

- The patient is supine with the arm on a radiolucent armboard.
- A nonsterile tourniquet preset at 250 mm Hg is on the upper arm.
- The shoulder, elbow, and hand are positioned such that the hand rests in pronation at the center of the armboard (if a dorsal approach is planned).

INCISION AND EXPOSURE

- Make a dorsal longitudinal skin incision over the fourth dorsal compartment or a transverse incision across the dorsal wrist crease just distal to the tubercle of Lister.
  - The longitudinal incision is more extensile and versatile.
  - The transverse incision tends to be more cosmetic.
- Expose the extensor retinaculum.
  - Maintain full-thickness flaps when elevating soft tissues off the extensor retinaculum to minimize the risk of damage to the radial and ulnar sensory nerves (**TECH FIG 1A**).
- Incise the extensor retinaculum in line with extensor pollicis longus (EPL) with scissors and transpose the EPL radially, dorsal to the retinaculum.
- Incise the radial septum of the fourth dorsal compartment and expose the wrist capsule by retracting the fourth compartment extensor tendons ulnarly and the EPL and radial wrist extensor tendons radially.
- Look for the distal extent of the posterior interosseous nerve (PIN) in the proximal portion of the incision on the radial floor of the fourth compartment. Perform a PIN neurectomy after coagulating the accompanying vessels.
- Create a distally based "inverted-U" capsular flap by first incising the wrist capsule transversely over the radiocarpal joint (from radial to ulnar) and then, at the margins, extending the incision distally (**TECH FIG 1B**).
  - Making a U-shaped capsular hood provides flexibility should one elect to add a dorsal capsular interposition arthroplasty in the setting of mild midcarpal arthrosis.
  - The dorsal branch of the radial artery is radial to the second compartment, so take care at the radial aspect of the capsulotomy.
- Inspect the articular cartilage on the proximal capitate and lunate facet of the radius for any degenerative changes.
  - If the cartilage is in good condition, proceed with PRC; if not, consider alternative procedures (**TECH FIG 1C**).

TECHNIQUES

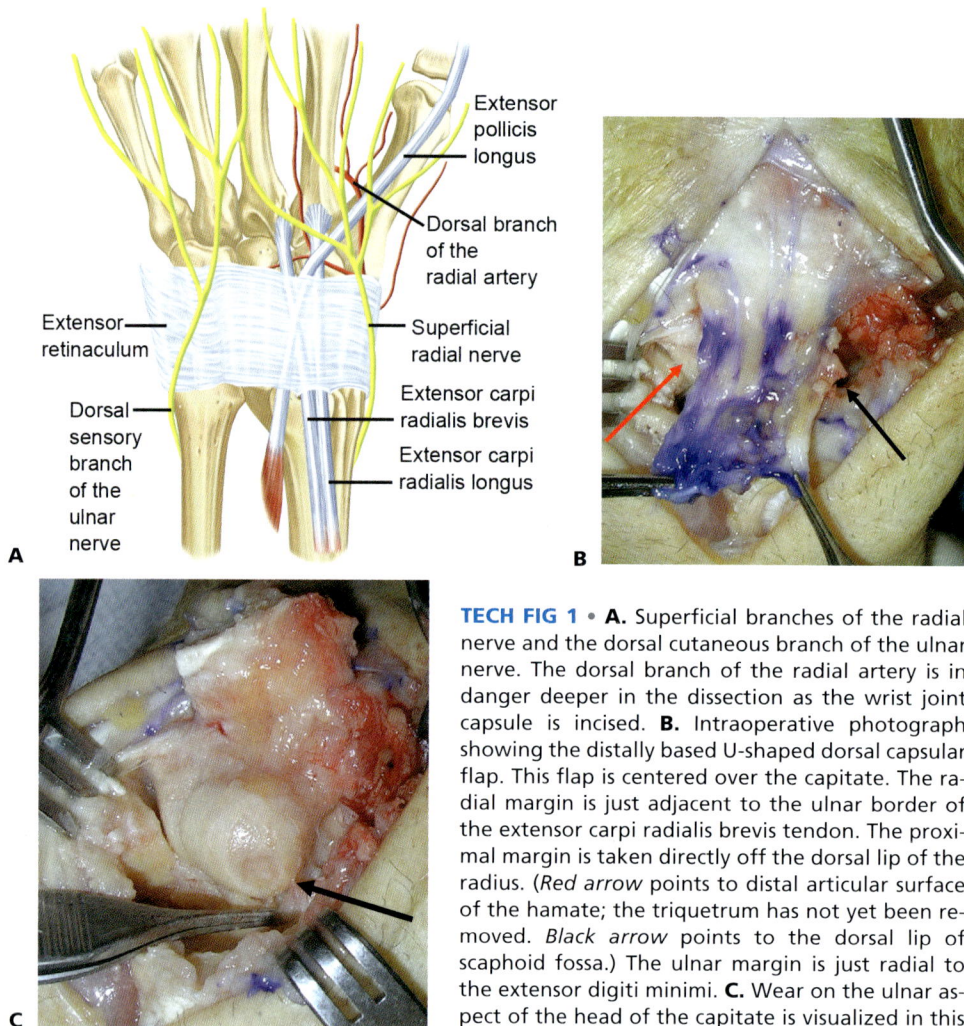

TECH FIG 1 • **A.** Superficial branches of the radial nerve and the dorsal cutaneous branch of the ulnar nerve. The dorsal branch of the radial artery is in danger deeper in the dissection as the wrist joint capsule is incised. **B.** Intraoperative photograph showing the distally based U-shaped dorsal capsular flap. This flap is centered over the capitate. The radial margin is just adjacent to the ulnar border of the extensor carpi radialis brevis tendon. The proximal margin is taken directly off the dorsal lip of the radius. (*Red arrow* points to distal articular surface of the hamate; the triquetrum has not yet been removed. *Black arrow* points to the dorsal lip of scaphoid fossa.) The ulnar margin is just radial to the extensor digiti minimi. **C.** Wear on the ulnar aspect of the head of the capitate is visualized in this case. (*Arrow* points to a cartilage defect on the capitate head.) Arthrosis affecting the non-weight-bearing portion of the capitate does not preclude the use of a proximal row carpectomy but one may want to include a capsular interposition. This is usually employed in older, lower-demand individuals.

CARPECTOMY

- Precisely ensure the anatomy and which bones are to be removed.
  - Consider intraoperative fluoroscopy if there is any question.
- Note the location of the radioscaphocapitate ligament at the waist of the scaphoid. Protect it and the other volar extrinsic ligaments while removing the proximal carpal row.
- Avoid iatrogenic injury to the cartilaginous surfaces of the capitate head and lunate facet of the radius.
- Osteotomize the scaphoid at its waist with a straight osteotome to facilitate scaphoid excision.
  - Place the osteotome such that it parallels the flexor carpi radialis tendon to minimize the risk of transection (**TECH FIG 2A,B**).

- The distal pole of the scaphoid is particularly difficult to remove (especially with SNAC wrist deformities).
- Consider using a threaded Kirschner wire (0.062 inch) or a large threaded Steinmann pin (5/32 inch) as a joystick to control the bone to be removed (**TECH FIG 2C**). Try to create tension between the proximal carpal bones during dissection (a combination of no. 15 blade; Beaver blade; periosteal, Freer, or Carroll elevator; and small straight or curved curettes is valuable; **TECH FIG 2D**).
- If possible, remove the carpal bones whole rather than piecemeal. This facilitates removal when possible and ensures that no portions are left behind (**TECH FIG 2E**).

TECH FIG 2 • **A,B.** The appropriate location for the scaphoid osteotomy. **C.** A large threaded pin inserted into the lunate is used to facilitate resection. **D.** An elevator placed in the lunotriquetral joint and then levered against the triquetrum helps strip the volar capsule off the lunate. **E.** Resected lunate.

Labels in figures: Osteotome; Scaphoid; Placement of osteotome; Flexor carpi radialis; Scaphoid base excision; Flexor carpi radialis

A   B   C   D   E

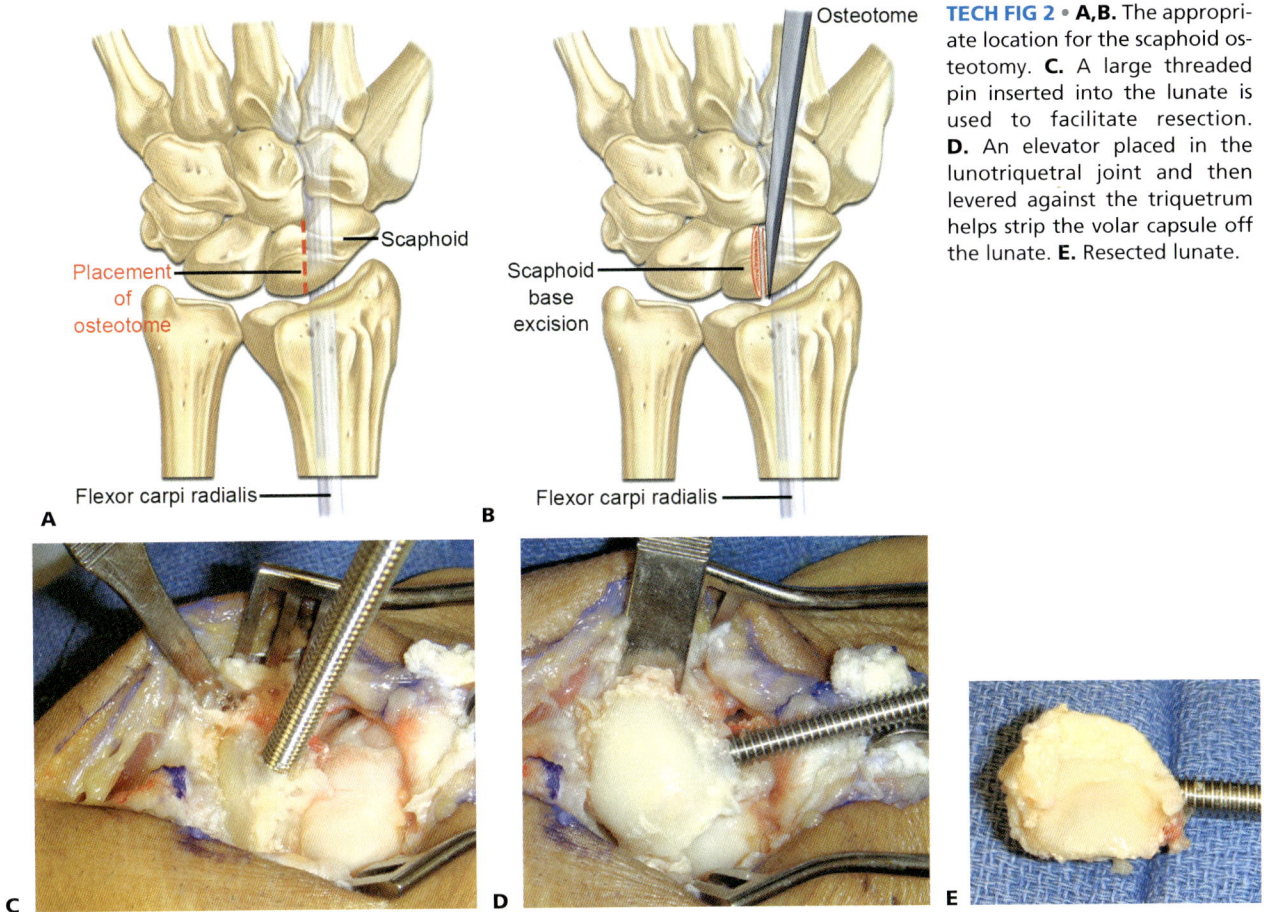

ASSESSMENT OF REDUCTION AND IMPINGEMENT

- Once the proximal row is removed, seat the capitate into the lunate facet on the radius to evaluate congruity.
- Check for impingement between the trapezium and radial styloid with extreme radial deviation.
- The trapezium has been shown to be volar to the styloid, making impingement less common than once thought.
- If radial-sided impingement is a concern, proceed with a radial styloidectomy.

RADIAL STYLOIDECTOMY

- See Chapter HA-86.
- Elevate the tendons of the second and then the first extensor compartments off the radial styloid through the same dorsal incision.
  - Take care to avoid injuring the dorsal branch of the radial artery just radial to the second dorsal compartment.
- The styloidectomy can be performed from proximal-radial to distal-ulnar with a straight osteotome (remove no more than 5 to 7 mm) (**TECH FIG 3**).

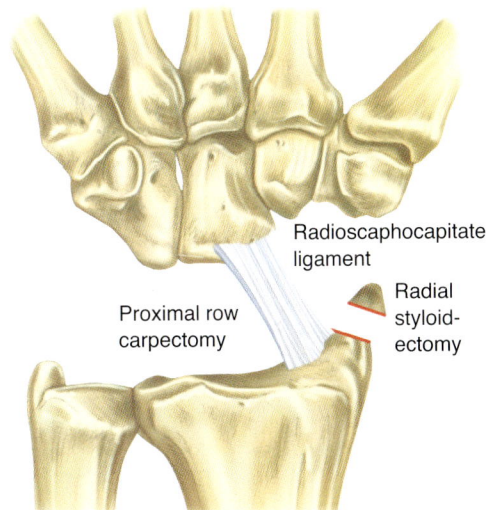

Labels in figure: Radioscaphocapitate ligament; Radial styloidectomy; Proximal row carpectomy

TECH FIG 3 • The amount of radial styloid that is removed and the direction of the osteotomy. The origin of the radioscaphocapitate ligament is carefully preserved.

TECHNIQUES

WOUND CLOSURE

- Close the capsule with nonabsorbable 2-0 suture.
- Plain radiographs or fluoroscopic images should be obtained in AP and lateral planes to ensure that the capitate is seated in the lunate fossae.
  - While uncommon, radiocarpal subluxation is possible with a PRC.
  - Maintenance of the volar ligaments (especially the radioscaphocapitate, which is most at risk during removal of the scaphoid) minimizes any risk of radiocarpal instability after PRC.
- Close the retinaculum with nonabsorbable 3-0 suture, leaving the EPL superficial to the retinaculum.

- Consider placing a drain in the subcutaneous tissues, to be removed in 24 to 48 hours.
- Close the skin with a 3-0 nonabsorbable running subcuticular Prolene stitch with "rescue loops" to facilitate removal at 10 to 14 days.
- Cover the incision with nonadherent gauze.
- Fashion a sugar-tong splint over a bulky dressing.
  - Keep the fingers and the thumb free proximal to the metacarpophalangeal joints.
  - Hold the wrist at neutral or slight extension (10 degrees).

PROXIMAL ROW CARPECTOMY WITH INTERPOSITION ARTHROPLASTY

- If mild to moderate chondral changes are noted on the capitate head, a PRC may still be indicated with the addition of an interpositional arthroplasty between the capitate head and lunate fossae.
- Use the previously created distally based inverted U-shaped capsular flap as the interpositional material.
- Place three simple stitches (2-0 PDS) connecting the dorsal capsular flap to the palmar capsule.

- Place and tag all stitches into the dorsal capsule (passing from deep to superficial) and into the palmar capsule (passing from proximal to distal) before tying them down to the palmar capsule (**TECH FIG 4A**).
- Loosely reapproximate the lateral margins of the dorsal flap to the residual dorsal capsule after interposing the dorsal capsule (**TECH FIG 4B**).
- Postoperative management is not altered.

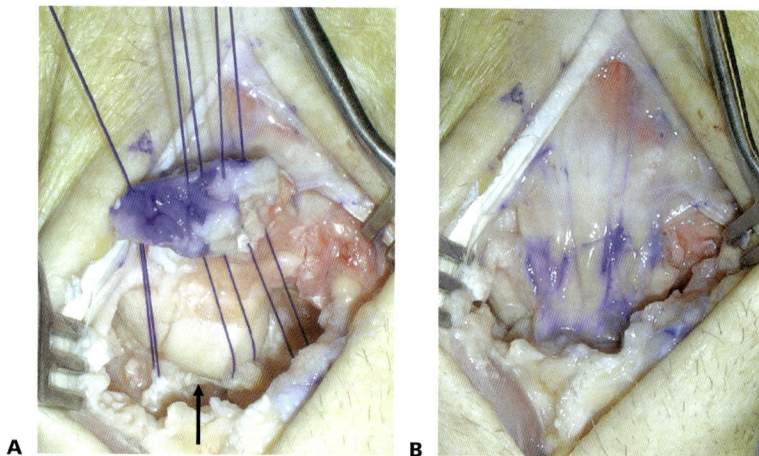

TECH FIG 4 • A. Sutures are passed in a mattress fashion through dorsal capsule, volar capsule, and then dorsal capsule to interpose the dorsal capsular flap between the capitate and lunate fossa. (*Arrow* points to the head of the capitate.) **B.** The dorsal capsule interposed between the capitate (shown above) and the radius (shown below) after the PDS sutures have been tied down.

PEARLS AND PITFALLS

Intraoperative pearls	▪ Consider using finger traps with weights (or assistant traction) to open the radial carpal joint during proximal row excision. Mastisol can be used on the fingers to assist in holding the traps. ▪ Threaded Kirschner wires (0.062 inch) or large threaded Steinmann pins (5/32 inch) in the scaphoid, lunate, or triquetrum can serve as a joystick or fulcrum to assist in removing the carpal bones.
Excessive styloidectomy	▪ Removing more than 5 to 7 mm of the radial styloid has been associated with compromise of the radioscaphocapitate ligament, with resultant ulnar carpal translation and radiocarpal instability.
Reflex sympathetic dystrophy	▪ Associated with prolonged immobilization (more than 2 weeks) ▪ Thought to be minimized by accelerated rehabilitation (immediate finger and thumb passive range of motion and wrist motion at 2 to 3 weeks)
Damage to the radial sensory and dorsal ulnar sensory branches	▪ Dissect directly down to the extensor retinaculum and elevate subcutaneous fat in full-thickness flaps off the extensor retinaculum to minimize the risk of nerve injury.

POSTOPERATIVE CARE

- PRC tends to be an outpatient procedure; an overnight stay may be necessary for postoperative pain or nausea.
- A short splint is applied in the operating room with the wrist in neutral and the fingers and thumb free at the metacarpophalangeal joints.
- Passive thumb and finger motion is encouraged immediately postoperatively, along with elevation and ice for the first 48 hours.
- At the first postoperative follow-up visit (in 10 to 14 days) the splint is removed, plain wrist AP and lateral radiographs are obtained to ensure the capitate is located in the radial lunate facet, and sutures are removed.
- At 2 weeks postoperatively, gentle active wrist extension and flexion and radioulnar deviation are added and a removable cock-up wrist splint or custom Orthoplast wrist splint is worn between exercises.
- Scar massage can begin once the incision is healed.
- Edema control may be necessary with compressive dressings.
- The removable splint can be removed as the patient feels comfortable (typically in 3 to 4 weeks).
- At 6 weeks, objective measurements of wrist extension, flexion, radioulnar deviation arcs, grip and pinch strength should be obtained.
- Therapy is initiated if the patient seems to be struggling to regain wrist or finger motion.
- At 3 months, full activities are encouraged.

OUTCOMES

- A broad range in grip strength outcome has been reported postoperatively.
  - 60% to 100% grip strength of the contralateral wrist (and a 20% to 30% increase in postoperative grip versus preoperative grip) can be expected.[3,7]
  - A decrease in postoperative wrist motion can be expected, as well as a decrease in flexion–extension by 20%, a decrease in radioulnar deviation by 10%,[3] and a 72- to 75-degree arc of motion in flexion and extension.[2,7]
- Satisfactory pain relief can be expected in 80% to 100% of patients.[3,5]

- Return to work for manual laborers after PRC has been unpredictable, varying from 20% in one series[3] to 85% in another.[5]
- Age less than 35 years has been shown to be predictive of early failure with PRC.

COMPLICATIONS

- Incomplete removal of the carpal bones (typically distal scaphoid)
- Use of pins has been associated with pin site infections and rapid degenerative changes when placed through the radiocapitate articulation (because of this, pins are not routinely recommended as they once were).
- Reflex sympathetic dystrophy
- Excessive styloidectomy and compromise of the radioscaphocapitate ligament
  - Compromise of the radioscaphocapitate ligament can lead to ulnar carpal subluxation.
  - Conversely, failure to check intraoperatively for radial-sided impingement may lead to radial-sided wrist pain postoperatively.
- Damage to sensory nerves (radial sensory and dorsal ulnar branches)
- Progressive arthritis

REFERENCES

1. Begley BW, Engber WD. Proximal row carpectomy in advanced Kienböck's disease. J Hand Surg Am 1994;19A:1016–1018.
2. Calandruccio JH. Proximal row carpectomy. J Am Soc Surg Hand 2001;1:112–122.
3. Culp RW. Proximal row carpectomy: a multicenter study. J Hand Surg Am 1993;18:19–25.
4. Nakamura R, Horii E, Watanabe K, et al. PRC vs. limited wrist arthrodesis for advanced Kienböck's disease. J Hand Surg Br 1998; 23:741–745.
5. Imbriglia JE, Broudy AS, Hagberg WC, et al. Proximal row carpectomy: clinical evaluation. J Hand Surg Am 1990;15:426–430.
6. Mathiowetz V, Kashman N, Volland G, et al. Grip and pinch strength: normative data for adults. Arch Phys Med Rehabil 1985;66: 69–74.
7. Stern PJ, Agabegi SA, Kiefhaber TR, et al. Proximal row carpectomy. J Bone Joint Surg Am 2004;86A:2359–2365.

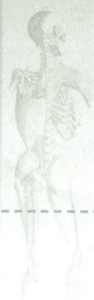

Chapter 88 Limited Wrist Arthrodesis

Andrew W. Cross and Mark E. Baratz

DEFINITION

- Limited wrist arthrodeses are salvage procedures for post-traumatic and degenerative conditions of the wrist as well as symptomatic instabilities.
- The goal is to reduce pain by selected fusion of the affected joints, thereby sparing motion, and improving the function of the remaining joints.

ANATOMY

- The carpus consists of four bones in the proximal row (scaphoid, lunate, triquetrum, pisiform) and four bones in the distal row (trapezium, trapezoid, capitate, hamate).
- The scaphoid and lunate bones are intimately joined by the scapholunate ligament both dorsally and volarly. This ligament is the keystone to the motion of the wrist.
- Numerous other named ligaments hold the carpal bones stable as the wrist moves through its five planes of motion (flexion, extension, radial and ulnar deviation, and circumduction).
- Most reconstructive wrist procedures require a dorsal approach to the wrist. The wrist and finger extensor tendons are separated into six compartments by the dorsal extensor retinaculum. The most common interval for exposure of the wrist is the 3–4 interval between the extensor pollicis longus and extensor digitorum communis tendons.

PATHOGENESIS

- Distraction forces across the joint and twisting motions while the wrist joint is being loaded can lead to a ligament injury.
- Failure of the scapholunate interosseous ligament, either by trauma or inflammatory arthritis, allows the scaphoid to flex and the lunate to extend, leading to dorsal intercalated segment instability.[17,30] When this occurs, abnormal loading of the carpal bones results. This leads to degenerative arthritis, particularly at the radioscaphoid joint due to the abnormal distribution of force across this elliptical joint.[7] This has been termed scapholunate advanced collapse (SLAC).
  - Scaphoid nonunion advanced collapse (SNAC), perilunate dislocations, calcium pyrophosphate dihydrate deposition, and rheumatoid arthritis can also lead to this pattern of arthritis.
- Other ligament injuries, Kienböck disease, and localized arthritis can lead to wrist pain, instability, and deformity.

NATURAL HISTORY

- Much of our knowledge of the natural history of scaphoid nonunion was reported by Mack et al.[18] We have learned that most ununited fractures of the scaphoid and SLAC wrists develop progressive osteoarthritis in a predictable pattern.
- Cyst formation and bony resorption are the hallmarks of arthritis and are usually seen 5 to 10 years after injury.
- Arthritis of the radioscaphoid joint can appear within a year after scaphoid nonunion. At that point most patients become symptomatic.[12,28]

PATIENT HISTORY AND PHYSICAL FINDINGS

- Typically, the patient describes a traumatic injury to the wrist. The absence of trauma should not exclude traumatic causes.
- Painful wrist motion and a limited arc of motion are common findings.
- Methods for examining the wrist include the following:
  - Finger extension test.[27] The wrist is passively flexed while the examiner resists active finger extension. A positive test yields pain and may represent periscaphoid inflammatory changes, radiocarpal or midcarpal instability, or Kienböck disease. A negative test essentially excludes dorsal wrist syndrome, Kienböck disease, midcarpal instability, and SLAC as the cause of pain.
  - Anatomic snuffbox palpation.[27] The examiner palpates the anatomic snuffbox with the index finger while moving the wrist from radial to ulnar deviation. A positive test yields severe pain at the articular–nonarticular junction of the scaphoid. Periscaphoid synovitis, scaphoid instability, and radial styloid arthrosis from SLAC are possible causes.
  - Triscaphe (scaphoid–trapezium–trapezoid [STT]) joint palpation.[27] The examiner palpates the second metacarpal proximally until it falls into a recess, the triscaphe joint. Pain with palpation indicates pathology of the distal scaphoid or the triscaphe joint.

IMAGING AND OTHER DIAGNOSTIC STUDIES

- Plain radiographs, including AP, lateral, oblique, and scaphoid views, should be obtained.
- The stage of wrist arthritis, as seen on plain radiographs, helps to determine the treatment options. Watson and Ballet[26] classified the radiographic findings into stages I–III.
  - Stage IV, not originally described, demonstrates arthritis in most all joints of the wrist. Fortunately, the radiolunate joint is rarely involved and serves as the basis for several treatment options.
  - Arthritis involving the radiolunate joint is usually seen only in patients with inflammatory wrist arthritis.

DIFFERENTIAL DIAGNOSIS

- SNAC
- SLAC
- Arthritis after perilunate dislocation
- Gout
- Pseudogout
- Rheumatoid arthritis
- Infectious arthritis
- Kienböck disease

NONOPERATIVE MANAGEMENT

- Nonoperative measures include rest, anti-inflammatory medications, splinting, occasional casting for flare-ups of arthritis, and cortisone injections.

SURGICAL MANAGEMENT

- Indications
  - Four-corner (capitate–hamate–lunate–triquetral [CHLT]) arthrodesis
    - Stage II or III SLAC wrist arthritis
    - Chronic symptomatic volar intercalated segmental instability (VISI) deformity or midcarpal instability
  - STT arthrodesis
    - Chronic static or dynamic scapholunate instability
    - Scapho–trapezium–trapezoid arthritis
    - Kienböck disease
    - Radiocarpal instability
  - Lunotriquetral arthrodesis
    - Lunotriquetral ligament tears
    - Posttraumatic instability
  - Scapholunate arthrodesis
    - Posttraumatic instability
    - Scapholunate instability
    - Dorsal intercalated segmental instability (DISI) deformity
  - Scaphocapitate arthrodesis
    - Scaphoid nonunion
    - Chronic DISI deformity with rotatory scaphoid instability
    - Kienböck disease
    - Lunate nonunion
  - Radiolunate arthrodesis
    - Rheumatoid arthritis primarily involving the radiolunate joint
    - Ulnar translocation of the carpus (relative indication)

Preoperative Planning

- The patient's history and pertinent physical examination findings are reviewed.
- Any prior surgical scars are noted.

- All radiographs are reviewed, noting any associated pathology that might need to be simultaneously addressed to yield the best outcome.
- Postoperative pain control should be discussed with the patient and the anesthesia team, and a local or axillary block should be considered for prolonged pain relief after surgery.

Positioning

- The patient is placed in the supine position on the operating table with the arm draped to the side on a radiolucent armboard.
- A tourniquet is used to control bleeding during the procedure.

Approach

- The wrist is approached through a dorsal longitudinal incision between the third and fourth extensor compartments.
  - Alternatively, the 4–5 extensor compartment interval may be used to better visualize the lunate–triquetrum–capitate–hamate articulations.
- The extensor pollicis longus (EPL) tendon sheath is opened and it is released both proximally and distally. The tendon is allowed to be transposed out of its compartment in a radial direction.
  - Although the EPL tendon is typically exposed and subsequently transposed, a more limited incision beginning just distal to the tubercle of Lister and proceeding distally may avoid significant exposure of the EPL tendon altogether.
- All joints are exposed fully and a precise decortication is performed down to bleeding bone.
- In almost every case, bone graft is harvested from the distal radius and used to augment the fusion.
  - Iliac crest graft may be substituted but is associated with higher morbidity.

FOUR-CORNER (CHLT) ARTHRODESIS USING KIRSCHNER WIRE FIXATION[1]

- Make a standard dorsal longitudinal incision between the third and fourth extensor compartments using the tubercle of Lister as a landmark (**TECH FIG 1A**).
- Incise the retinaculum over the third extensor compartment.
- Incise the radial septum of the fourth extensor compartment and retract the tendons ulnarly.

- Perform a ligament-splitting dorsal approach to the carpus as described by Berger et al.[4]
  - This capsular incision allows access to the carpus while preserving the dorsal intercarpal ligament and dorsal radiotriquetral ligament (see Chap. HA-44).
- Inspect the radiolunate joint for articular cartilage wear (**TECH FIG 1B**).

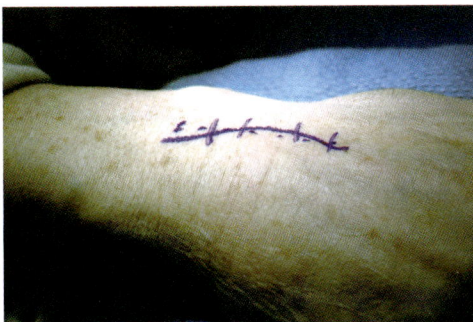

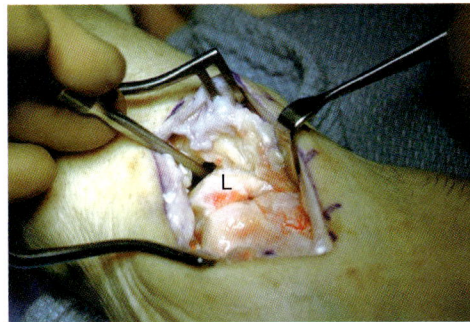

A   **B**

TECH FIG 1 • A. Skin incision is centered just ulnar to the tubercle of Lister. (Fingers are to the right or bottom in all intraoperative photos.) **B.** The radiolunate joint should be inspected for arthritis. If lunate cartilage is not preserved, a total wrist fusion may be required. *(continued)*

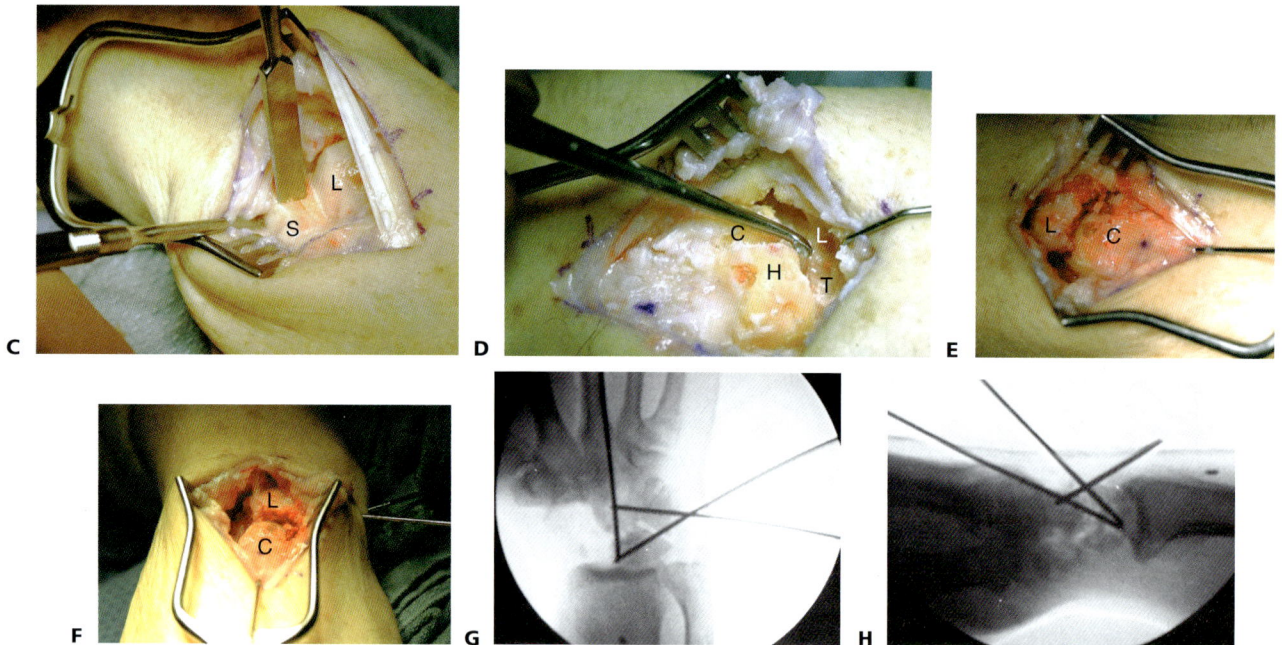

TECH FIG 1 • (continued) **C.** The scaphoid is excised with an osteotome and a rongeur. The volar ligaments are carefully protected to prevent iatrogenic ulnar shift of the carpus. **D.** The articulating surfaces of the lunate, triquetrum, capitate, and hamate are decorticated. **E.** The capitate is secured to the lunate (L) with a retrograde 0.062 Kirschner wire. **F.** Remaining joints are secured with Kirschner wires in a triangular pattern. **G,H.** AP and lateral radiographs showing Kirschner wires properly positioned. S, scaphoid; L, lunate; T, triquetrum; C, capitate; H, hamate.

- Identify and excise the scaphoid either piecemeal with a rongeur or sharply using a scalpel (**TECH FIG 1C**).
  - Kirschner wires and tenaculum clamps facilitate the visualization and excision of the distal volar scaphoid.
  - Take care to protect the volar radioscaphocapitate ligament.
- Once the scaphoid is excised, decorticate the opposing joint surfaces of the lunate, triquetrum, capitate, and hamate (**TECH FIG 1D**).
  - Longitudinal traction with fingertraps helps to distract these joints, making decortication easier.
  - Thorough removal of the volar-third cartilage from the lunate and capitate facilitates correction of the pre-existing DISI deformity but shortens the intercarpal bone distances. This may restrict final wrist range of motion.
- Once these joint surfaces are denuded, harvest distal radius bone graft and place it into the fusion bed.

- Use a 0.062 Kirschner wire to joystick the lunate into a more flexed position, and apply dorsal pressure to volarly translate the capitate on the lunate. Place one or two 0.062 Kirschner wires across this joint (**TECH FIG 1E**).
- Verify correction of the DISI deformity using fluoroscopy.
- Pin the lunotriquetral joint and the capitohamate joint with two 0.062 Kirschner wires (**TECH FIG 1F**).
  - Intraoperative fluoroscopic images should reveal a stable triangular construct of Kirschner wires traversing the four bones (**TECH FIG 1G,H**).
- The Kirschner wires may be cut under the skin or left external, depending on the surgeon's preference.
- After irrigation, close the capsule with absorbable suture, and repair the extensor retinaculum, leaving the EPL tendon transposed subcutaneously.
- Close the skin in a routine manner.
- Apply a large bulky dressing including a dorsal and volar forearm-based splint.

FOUR-CORNER ARTHRODESIS USING A CIRCULAR PLATE[9,13,29]

- The approach, scaphoid excision, and joint preparation are analogous to those described above.
- Place a 0.062 Kirschner wire through the distal radius articular surface. Use a separate 0.062 Kirschner wire as a joystick to hold the lunate reduced in neutral alignment while advancing the Kirschner wire across the radiolunate joint in a dorsal to volar direction.
  - Obtain fluoroscopic images to verify correction of the dorsally tilted lunate.

- After volarly translating the capitate (as described above) and fully correcting the DISI deformity, secure the triquetrum to the hamate and the lunate to the capitate with two additional Kirschner wires.
  - Place these Kirschner wires as volar as possible to avoid interference during rasping and plate placement.
- Center the power rasp over the four bones in the AP and lateral planes and bury the rasp down to subchondral bone.

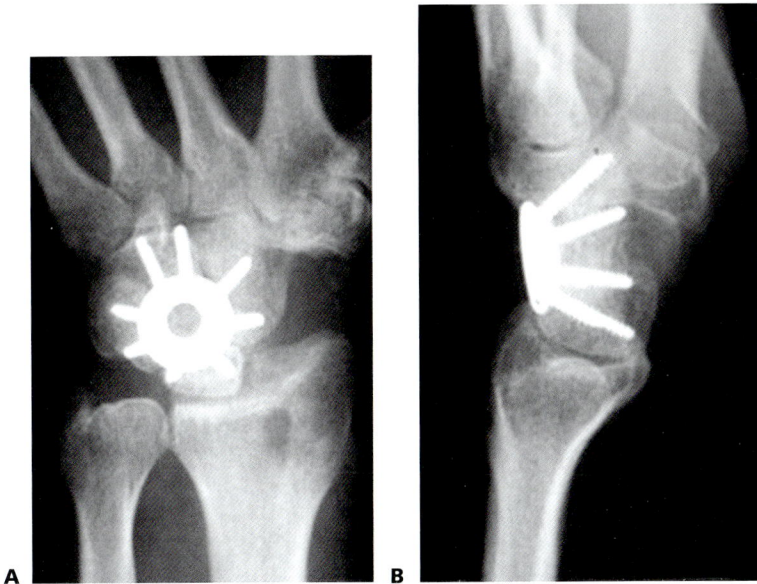

TECH FIG 2 • AP and lateral radiographs showing a circular plate fusion construct. On the lateral view, the plate is nicely seated to prevent dorsal impingement.

- Ideal rasp placement does not always coincide with the central point between the four bones.
- Pack bone graft, obtained preferably from the distal radius or iliac crest, between the four prepared bones.
- Center the plate over the four bones in the AP and lateral planes and place the circular plate into the bony crater created by the rasp.
- Rotate the plate to maximize screw purchase into each of the four bones. Two screws should be planned for each of the four carpal bones.
  - All screws must be placed in a unicortical fashion.
- Place the first screw through the plate into the lunate. Do not tighten this screw completely or it will cause the circular plate to tilt up and compromise screw fixation in the remaining bones.
- Place a second screw into the hole opposite the first screw. This sets the plate position.
- Check a lateral fluoroscopic image to ensure the plate is well seated and there is no impingement with wrist extension.
- Fill in the remainder of the holes with screws.
  - Placing the screws opposite one another and tightening them sequentially helps prevent malpositioning of the plate.
- Obtain final images to check screw length and position, carpal reduction, and construct stability (**TECH FIG 2**).
- Close the wound as described above. Apply the dressing and splint.

SCAPHOID–TRAPEZIUM–TRAPEZOID (STT) FUSION[2,6]

- Make a transverse or dorsoradial incision centered over the STT joint.
- Protect the superficial radial nerve branches, and coagulate the small perforators from the dorsal branch of the radial artery (**TECH FIG 3A**).
- Make a longitudinal capsulotomy over the STT joint, and reflect the capsule to expose the bone surfaces (**TECH FIG 3B**).
- Verify scaphoid alignment with fluoroscopy. The ideal scapholunate angle is 41 to 60 degrees.

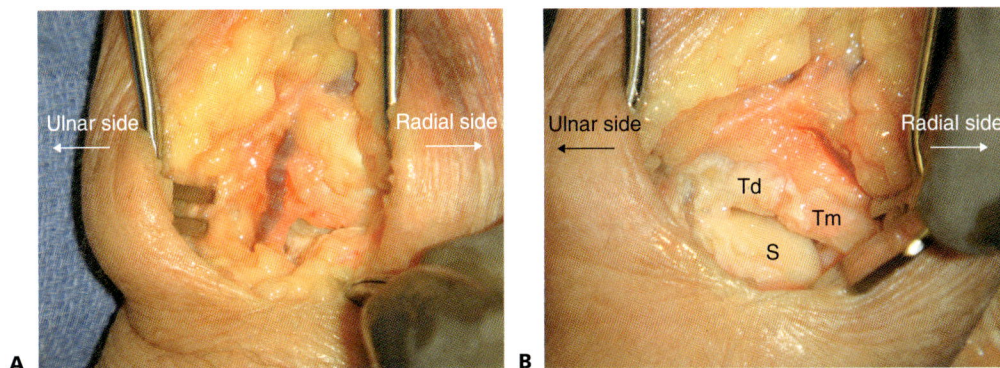

TECH FIG 3 • **A.** Location of the dorsal branch of the radial artery as it crosses the scaphoid–trapezium–trapezoid (STT) joints. (Fingers are at top in all images.) **B.** Exposed STT joints. *(continued)*

TECHNIQUES

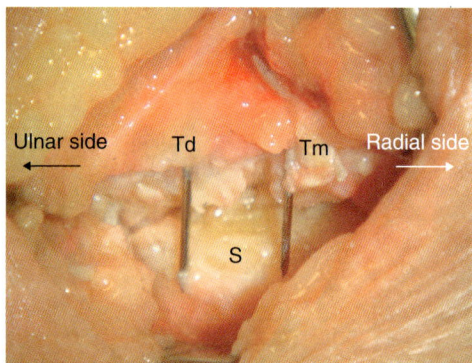

C

TECH FIG 3 • *(continued)* **C.** Kirschner wire position in the trapezium and trapezoid bones before advancement into the scaphoid bone. A separate pin traversing the trapezio–trapezoidal joint is added for stability.

- Failure to correct this malalignment could lead to persistent pain.
- Overcorrection of an increased scapholunate angle may limit postoperative motion.

- Remove only the dorsal 70% of the articular cartilage from the three bones.
  - Preserving the volar 30% maintains the intercarpal bone distances but still ensures successful fusion.
- Perform a radial styloidectomy.
  - Resect no more than 3 or 4 mm of the styloid to avoid iatrogenic injury to the origin of the radioscaphocapitate and long radiolunate ligaments.
- Fixation may be accomplished with Kirschner wires or a circular plate.
- Place two 0.045 Kirschner wires anterograde into the trapezium and trapezoid (**TECH FIG 3C**). Add a third 0.045 Kirschner wire in an ulnar to radial direction from the trapezoid toward the trapezium.
  - The above wires are preset in place and should be advanced across the joints after bone graft placement.
- Harvest cancellous bone graft from the distal radius and pack it into the interstices of the STT joints.
- Reduce the joints and advance the preset Kirschner wires.
- The Kirschner wires can be cut and buried under the skin or left out of the skin to facilitate removal.
- Perform a routine closure and apply a well-padded forearm-based thumb spica splint.

LUNOTRIQUETRAL FUSION[27]

- Make a transverse incision over the dorsal and ulnar aspect of the radiocarpal joint.
- Retract the extensor tendons and incise the capsule transversely to expose the lunotriquetral joint.
- Remove any remaining lunotriquetral ligament with a small rongeur.
- Decorticate the lunotriquetral articulation, leaving the volar 25% of the joint surface intact to maintain intercarpal distances (**TECH FIG 4A**).
- Harvest distal radius bone graft and pack it into the void created.

- Place two cannulated screw guidewires through the triquetrum, and after reducing the joint, advance the pins across the lunotriquetral joint into the lunate.
  - Verify pin position using fluoroscopy.
- Advance two partially threaded cannulated screws over the guide pins across the lunotriquetral joint (**TECH FIG 4B**).
  - Make sure the thread length on the screw is short enough to allow compression across the lunotriquetral joint.
  - Alternatively, headless screws, staples, or Kirschner wires may be used for fixation.
- Perform routine wound closure and apply a wrist splint.

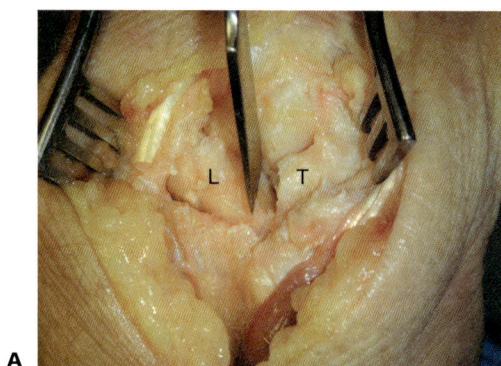

A

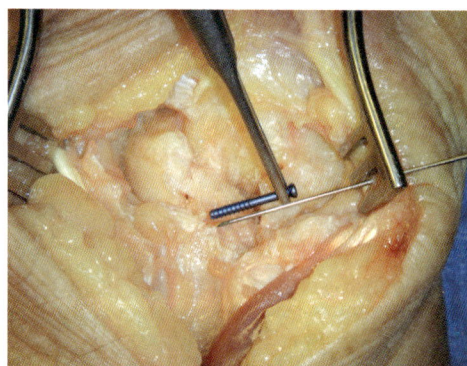

B

TECH FIG 4 • **A.** Lunotriquetral joint during decortication. (Fingers are at top in all images.) **B.** Lunotriquetral joint fusion construct with a partially threaded cannulated screw and a derotation pin.

SCAPHOLUNATE FUSION[27]

- Use a standard dorsal incision ulnar to the tubercle of Lister and perform a longitudinal capsular incision.
- Place two dorsal joystick Kirschner wires, one into the palmar-flexed scaphoid distally, directed proximally and

ulnarly, and a second into the dorsiflexed lunate proximally, directed distally.
  - When these two wires are brought together the joint is reduced.

- Decorticate the bone surfaces and obtain bone graft from the distal radius.
- Reduce the scaphoid and lunate with the Kirschner wires and hold them in place with a Köcher clamp.
- Verify scapholunate reduction via fluoroscopy before proceeding.

- Stabilize the scapholunate joint with headless cannulated screws, multiple 0.045 to 0.062 Kirschner wires, or staples.
- Perform routine closure and apply a standard dressing and thumb spica splint.

SCAPHOCAPITATE FUSION[3,27]

- Use the 3–4 extensor compartment approach followed by a longitudinal capsulotomy directly over the scaphocapitate interval between the second and fourth compartments.
- Denude the articulating scaphoid and capitate surfaces of articular cartilage down to bleeding cancellous bone.
- For cannulated screw fixation, make a V-shaped incision on the radial aspect of the wrist superficial to the radial styloid. A styloidectomy performed through this incision creates a superior view of the lateral aspect of the scaphoid. Preset two guidewires in the scaphoid, aimed toward the capitate (radial to ulnar).
  - A radial styloidectomy is an option to facilitate accurate positioning of the Kirschner wires.
  - Compression screws (our preference), Kirschner wires, or staples may be used for fixation.
- Harvest distal radius cancellous bone graft and place it between the two prepared bones.
- Reduce the articulation, advance the guidewires, and verify pin placement with fluoroscopy.
  - Obtain a scapholunate angle of about 45 degrees.
- Advance the threaded compression screws across the scaphocapitate joint (**TECH FIG 5**).

- Perform a routine closure and apply the dressing and splint as above.

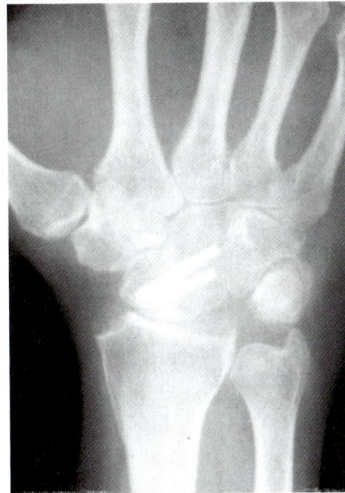

TECH FIG 5 • Scaphocapitate fusion construct using two headless, cannulated compression screws. Note the addition of a radial styloidectomy. (Fingers are at top.)

RADIOCARPAL (RADIOLUNATE) ARTHRODESIS[15,22]

- Use the 3–4 extensor compartment approach followed by a ligament-sparing incision to the wrist capsule as described above.
- Remove the dorsal lip of the radius over the lunate to facilitate visualization.
- Maintaining general bony contours, decorticate the lunate facet of the radius and the proximal lunate articular surface using curettes, rongeurs, and curved osteotomes.
- Under fluoroscopy, correct any preoperative VISI or DISI deformity.

  - A Kirschner wire inserted into the dorsal lunate may be used as a joystick to effect correction.
- Stabilize the lunate in the reduced position with provisional Kirschner wires from the radius into the lunate.
- Harvest bone graft from the distal radius or iliac crest and pack the graft tightly into the palmar radiolunate joint.
- Secure the lunate to the radius with Kirschner wires, headless screws, staples, or small blade plates.
- Pack the remaining bone graft into the dorsal radiolunate joint.
- Perform a routine closure and apply a splint.

PEARLS AND PITFALLS

Pearls	
CHLT Kirschner wire arthrodesis	■ For excellent visualization of the wrist capsule, incise the distalmost aspect of the extensor retinaculum between the third and fourth compartments to the level of the tubercle of Lister.[1]
	■ Protect the volar radioscaphocapitate ligament when excising the scaphoid to prevent iatrogenic ulnar translocation of the carpus.[1]
	■ Preserve the dorsal intercarpal and radiotriquetral ligament during the capsulotomy.[1]
CHLT circular plate	■ Place the screws opposite one another in the circular plate and tighten them sequentially to help prevent plate malpositioning.[13]

CHLT circular plate and STT arthrodesis	■ The bones here are extremely hard, and a high-speed burr may be needed for adequate decortication.[1]
Lunotriquetral arthrodesis	■ Leave the volar 25% of the articular surface intact during decortication to maintain proper intercarpal distances.
Scapholunate arthrodesis	■ Use Kirschner wires as joysticks and clamp the Kirschner wires together with a Köcher clamp to maintain the reduction during fixation.
Scaphocapitate arthrodesis	■ Correct intercarpal alignment is between 45 and 60 degrees.
Radiolunate fusion	■ Maintaining the normal joint space distance between the radius and lunate is desired to preserve as much wrist motion as possible at the surrounding joints.
Pitfalls	
CHLT Kirschner wire arthrodesis	■ Expect less predictable pain relief and poorer recovery of motion in elderly individuals and in patients with severe wrist stiffness.[1] ■ One common mistake is not completely correcting the DISI deformity of the wrist before fusion.[1] This will limit wrist motion postoperatively.
CHLT circular plate	■ Dorsal placement of the Kirschner wires will interfere with bone rasping and plate application.[13] ■ Optimal rasp placement does not always coincide with the central point between the four bones. ■ A plate that is not adequately seated will result in dorsal impingement of the plate against the distal radius.[13]
STT arthrodesis	■ Headless screws may cause midcarpal compression and alter joint kinematics. ■ Overcorrection of an increased SL angle may decrease motion postoperatively.
STT arthrodesis and scaphocapitate arthrodesis	■ The radial sensory and lateral antebrachial cutaneous nerves may be injured during exposure and Kirschner wire placement.
Scapholunate arthrodesis	■ There is an extremely high nonunion rate with this procedure, likely due to the high degree of motion between these bones and the relatively small area of contact between them.
Radiolunate arthrodesis	■ Inadvertent bone graft placement in the adjacent joints may be a cause of persistent wrist pain. A small osteotome can be used to block the passage of bone graft into the adjacent joints. ■ Avoid Kirschner wire penetration into the carpal tunnel.

POSTOPERATIVE CARE

■ The sutures are removed from the wound in 10 to 14 days and a short-arm cast is applied.

■ Immobilization is typically 8 to 12 weeks, but this period may be shortened if stable fixation is obtained with screws.

■ Plain radiographs are taken at the first postoperative visit and at all subsequent visits until signs of consolidation at the fusion site are noted.

■ At this time, the pins are removed and a functional brace is applied to support the wrist but still allow controlled range of motion of the wrist during supervised therapy.

■ Strengthening begins about 12 to 16 weeks after surgery.

OUTCOMES

■ Nonunion rates range from 4% to 63%, depending on the joints being fused and the stresses placed across the joints before fusion.[5,11,16,20]

■ For limited wrist fusions, a loss of grip strength on the order of 25% can be expected.[5,11,16,20]

■ About 50% of patients will have some chronic wrist pain.[5,11,16,20]

■ For stage I and II SLAC arthritis, four-corner arthrodesis yields clinical results comparable to those of proximal row carpectomy (**FIG 1**).[10,23,30]

■ Stage III SLAC arthritis can be managed with either a four-corner fusion or a proximal row carpectomy with dorsal capsular interposition.[23]

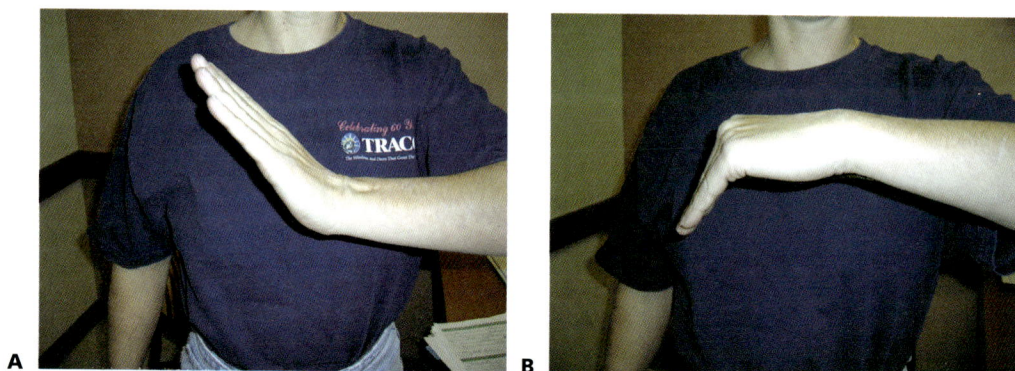

FIG 1 • Nine-year follow-up of four-corner fusion. **A,B.** Maximal active wrist extension and flexion. *(continued)*

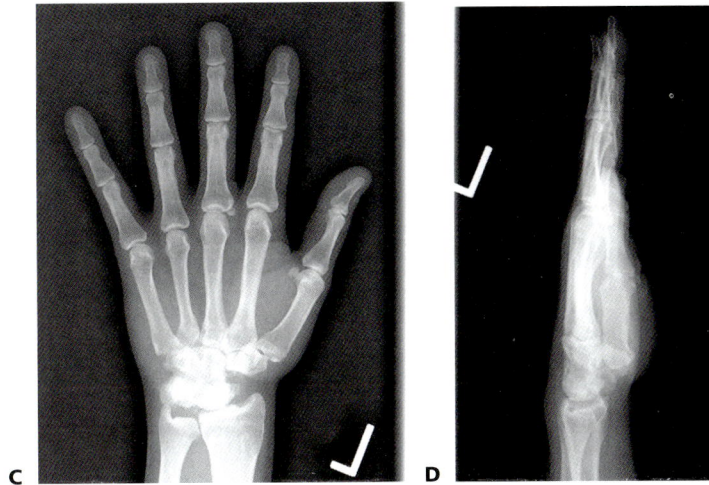

FIG 1 • *(continued)* **C,D.** AP and lateral radiographs.

- In patients 35 years of age or younger at the time of proximal row carpectomy, subjective and objective function may decline over time, and they may eventually require a wrist fusion.[23]
- Circular plate fixation for capitate–lunate–triquetrum–hamate fusion is a newer trend. Weiss et al reported a union rate approaching 100% and high patient satisfaction.[13] However, several subsequent studies have documented higher nonunion rates, higher hardware failure rates, higher pain scores, and an overall lower rate of patient satisfaction compared to other traditional methods of fixation.[8,14,19,24]

COMPLICATIONS

- Pin tract infections
- Osteomyelitis
- Avascular necrosis of the lunate
- Radiolunate arthritis
- Reflex sympathetic dystrophy
- Tendon ruptures
- Persistent wrist pain
- Nonunion
- Fracture through fusion
- Neurapraxia
- Hardware failure
- Neuroma
- Pseudarthrosis

REFERENCES

1. Baratz ME, Rosenwasser, MP, Adams BD, et al. Wrist Surgery: Tricks of the Trade. New York: Thieme, 2006:133–134.
2. Baratz ME, Rosenwasser, MP, Adams BD, et al. Wrist Surgery: Tricks of the Trade. New York: Thieme, 2006:138–140.
3. Baratz ME, Rosenwasser, MP, Adams BD, et al. Wrist Surgery: Tricks of the Trade. New York: Thieme, 2006:167–169.
4. Berger RA, Bishop AT, Bettinger PC. New dorsal capsulotomy for the surgical exposure of the wrist. Ann Plast Surg 1995;35:54–59.
5. Brown RE, Erdmann D. Complications of 50 consecutive limited wrist fusions by a single surgeon. Ann Plast Surg 1995;35:46–53.
6. Burge PD. Scaphotrapeziotrapezoid and scaphocapitate fusions. In: Berger RA, Weiss AP, eds. Hand Surgery. Philadelphia: Lippincott Williams & Wilkins, 2004:1299–1308.
7. Burgess RC. The effect of a simulated scaphoid malunion on wrist motion. J Hand Surg Am 1987;12A:771–774.
8. Chung KC, Watt AJ, Kotsis SV. A prospective outcomes study of four-corner wrist arthrodesis using a circular limited wrist fusion plate for stage II scapholunate advanced collapse wrist deformity. Plast Reconstr Surg 2006;118:433–442.
9. Cohen MS. Four-corner fusions. In: Berger RA, Weiss AP, eds. Hand Surgery. Philadelphia: Lippincott Williams & Wilkins, 2004:1309–1318.
10. Cohen MS, Kozin SH. Degenerative arthritis of the wrist: proximal row carpectomy versus scaphoid excision and four-corner arthrodesis. J Hand Surg Am 2001;26A:94–104.
11. Dacho A, Grudel J, Holle G, et al. Long-term results of midcarpal arthrodesis in the treatment of scaphoid nonunion advanced collapse (SNAC-wrist) and scapholunate advanced collapse (SLAC-wrist). Ann Plast Surg 2006;56:139–144.
12. Duppe H, Johnell O, Lundborg G, et al. Long-term results of fracture of the scaphoid: a follow-up study of more than thirty years. J Bone Joint Surg Am 1994;76A:249–252.
13. Enna M, Hoepfner P, Weiss AP. Scaphoid excision with four-corner fusion. Hand Clin 2005;21:531–538.
14. Kendall CB, Brown TR, Millon SJ, et al. Results of four-corner arthrodesis using dorsal circular plate fixation. J Hand Surg Am 2005;30A:903–907.
15. Krimmer H. In: Weiss AP-C, Berger RA, eds. Hand Surgery. Philadelphia: Lippincott Williams & Wilkins, 2004:1319–1329.
16. Larsen CF, Jacoby RA, McCabe SJ. Nonunion rates of limited carpal arthrodesis: a meta-analysis of the literature. J Hand Surg Am 1997;28A:66–73.
17. Linscheid RL, Dobyns JH, Beaubout JW, et al. Traumatic instability of the wrist: diagnosis, classification, and pathomechanics. J Bone Joint Surg Am 1972;54A:1612–1632.
18. Mack GR, Bosse MJ, Gelberman RH, et al. The natural history of scaphoid non-union. J Bone Joint Surg Am 1984;66A:504–509.
19. Shindle MK, Burton KJ, Weiland AJ, et al. Complications of circular plate fixation for four-corner arthrodesis. J Hand Surg Br 2007;32B:50–53.
20. Siegel JM, Ruby LK. A critical look at intercarpal arthrodesis: review of the literature. J Hand Surg Am 1996;21A:717–723.
21. Stern PJ, Agabegi SS, Kiefhaber TR, et al. Proximal row carpectomy. J Bone Joint Surg Am 2005;87A:166–174.
22. Taliesnik J. In: Blair WF, ed. Techniques in Hand Surgery. Baltimore: Williams & Wilkins, 1996:879–886.
23. Tomaino MM, Miller RJ, Cole I, et al. Scapholunate advanced collapse wrist: proximal row carpectomy or limited wrist arthrodesis with scaphoid excision? J Hand Surg Am 1994;19A:134–142.

24. Vance MC, Hernandez JD, DiDonna ML, et al. Complications and outcome of four-corner arthrodesis: circular plate fixation versus traditional techniques. J Hand Surg Am 2005;30A:1122–1127.

25. Watson HK, Ashmeade D 4th, Makhlouf MV. Examination of the scaphoid. J Hand Surg Am 1988;13A:657–660.

26. Watson HK, Ballet FL. The SLAC wrist: scapholunate advanced collapse pattern of degenerative arthritis. J Hand Surg Am 1984;9A: 358–365.

27. Watson HK, Weinzweig J. Intercarpal arthrodesis. In: Green DP, ed. Operative Hand Surgery, 4th ed. Philadelphia: Churchill Livingstone, 1999:108–130.

28. Watson HK, Weinzweig J, Zeppieri J. The natural progression of scaphoid instability. Hand Clin 1997;13:17–34.

29. Weiss AP. Principles of limited wrist arthrodesis. In: Berger RA, Weiss AP, eds. Hand Surgery. Philadelphia: Lippincott Williams & Wilkins, 2004:1289–1298.

30. Wyrick JD. Proximal row carpectomy and intercarpal arthrodesis for the management of wrist arthritis. J Am Acad Orthop Surg 2003;11:277–281.

31. Young VL, Higgs, PE. The injured wrist. In: Martin DS, Collins ED, eds. Manual of Acute Hand Injuries. Mosby-Year Book, 1998:404–496.

Chapter 89

Complete Wrist Arthrodesis

John C. Elfar and Andrew D. Markiewitz

DEFINITION

- Wrist arthritis occurs when the codependent joints of the wrist lose the ability to rotate, thereby impairing normal wrist kinematics.
- Wrist arthritis can originate from many causes, including osteoarthritis, degenerative arthritis, and inflammatory arthritis.
- While sacrificing motion at the wrist, arthrodesis has been shown to reliably relieve pain.

ANATOMY

- The wrist is perhaps the most complex set of joints in the body.
- The eight bones of the wrist work together to provide motion in multiple planes, governed by the complex array of soft tissue ligaments that unite them.
  - Single ligament disruptions can cause degenerative change in nonadjacent bones and at times unlikely sites.
- In broad terms, the wrist is divided into two distinct rows of bones.
  - The distal row, including the trapezium, trapezoid, capitate, and hamate, is united to the hand and shows little gross motion relative to the metacarpals.
  - As such, the most significant articulations in the wrist occur in the proximal row bones, which are the scaphoid, lunate, and triquetrum. These proximal row bones allow the wrist to flex, extend, deviate both radially and ulnarly, and pronosupinate.

PATHOGENESIS

- Because of the many possible routes to the eventual destruction of the wrist joint, it is difficult to describe a single chain of events that leads to end-stage arthritis, most suitably treated by complete wrist fusion.

NATURAL HISTORY

- Causes of wrist degeneration and the often-predictable pattern and pace of wear are detailed in other chapters.

PATIENT HISTORY AND PHYSICAL FINDINGS

- Patients describe pain and stiffness as their major reasons for presentation. Pain limits their function and their strength.
  - Most patients are less concerned with motion loss if their dominant extremity is not involved.
  - If their dominant wrist is involved, patients prefer to preserve some motion even if faced with low-grade persistent pain after treatment. In this clinical setting complete wrist fusions are less often performed as the index operation.
- Physical examination findings include tenderness, soft tissue swelling, loss of motion, and pain with motion. Pinch and grip strength are reduced compared with age-matched peers and the uninvolved contralateral extremity.

IMAGING AND OTHER DIAGNOSTIC STUDIES

- Wrist arthritis is best studied with standard posteroanterior and lateral radiographs of the wrist.
  - These images often reveal the cause of the degeneration together with its pattern and progression.
  - Special attention is paid to the alignment of the wrist and the bone stock available for fusion and fixation.
- Computed tomography helps plan limited fusions or salvage procedures when arthritis may have spared areas of the midcarpal or proximal carpal rows.

DIFFERENTIAL DIAGNOSIS

- Limited wrist arthritis
- Extrinsic joint contracture (including calcific tendinitis)
- Inflammatory arthritis and synovitis (ie, rheumatoid, gout, or pseudogout)
- Infection
- Connective tissue diseases

NONOPERATIVE MANAGEMENT

- In most every case, the first form of treatment for wrist arthritis is nonoperative:
  - Nonsteroidal anti-inflammatory medications (NSAIDs)
  - Disease-modifying medications (if the cause of the degenerative process can be identified and is appropriate)
  - Splinting
    - A custom-made thumb spica splint allows interphalangeal motion of the thumb but limits painful wrist motion.
  - Local steroid injections placed in the wrist

SURGICAL MANAGEMENT

- Alternative motion-sparing procedures, including partial wrist fusions and proximal row carpectomy, should be considered before performing a complete wrist fusion, especially in patients who have at least 60 degrees of wrist flexion–extension and have isolated articular degeneration.
- Wrist arthroplasty remains in its infancy and is associated with high revision rates and frequent implant design changes.
  - Wrist arthrodesis after arthroplasty is more difficult due to bone stock loss.
- Wrist arthrodesis is the final treatment method for end-stage wrist degeneration due to multiple causes or as a salvage procedure in patients who have failed the more limited procedures mentioned above.
  - Arthrodesis can be obtained reliably and provides a stable wrist in a high-demand patient.[1,2,11,13]
  - In patients who have undergone lower extremity joint replacements and therefore require support for ambulation, fusion of the wrist is generally regarded as a reliable procedure.

- The two most popular methods used to fuse a wrist are plate osteosynthesis and rod osteosynthesis.[2,8,13]
- The chief considerations when choosing between these two options are the desired position of fusion, the quality of the bone and available soft tissue coverage, and the possibility of future infection.
  - The strongest grip is achieved when the wrist is fused in 20 to 30 degrees of extension. Advocates of fusion in this position favor the use of a plate and screw construct that is fabricated to reproduce this position.[2,4,14] Straight wrist fusion plates are also available, and all these devices include screws and plates that match the size of the radius and the metacarpal.
  - A neutral wrist position obtained with rod osteosynthesis may be more favorable for activities of daily living, including perineal care.[2,3,5,11]
  - Plate and screw constructs rely on solid screw purchase and stable soft tissue coverage. If good-quality bone and viable soft tissues are not present, as might be the case in a patient with severe rheumatoid disease, intramedullary rod fixation may be a more effective means of fixation.
  - In patients taking aggressive disease-remitting medications, the possibility of late infection should be considered. These patients may benefit from metal removal, which is often more easily accomplished after rod osteosynthesis.

Preoperative Planning

- While the use of aspirin may be continued, warfarin (Coumadin) and clopidogrel (Plavix) should be discontinued to avoid bleeding and flap complications.

- Radiographs should be reviewed before performing a wrist arthrodesis. Specific attention should be paid to the amount of available bone stock and the bony alignment.
- Intraoperative evaluation will require a fluoroscopic device. Appropriate alignment, reduction, and implant length should be confirmed before closure.

Positioning

- Patients are placed supine with the operative hand extended on a hand table extension.
- A tourniquet is applied to the proximal arm over padding.
- Before anesthesia is induced, the patient's comfortable shoulder position should be assessed. The armboard should not place the shoulder above this position. This test is especially important in rheumatoid patients with limited joint mobility.

Approach

- Both arthrodesis procedures are performed through a standard dorsal approach to the wrist.[12–14] A longitudinal midline dorsal incision ulnar to the tubercle of Lister is used.
- The extensor pollicis longus tendon is released from its sheath and retracted radially.[12]
- The fourth extensor compartment is subperiosteally elevated from the dorsum of the distal radius and retracted ulnarly.
  - The posterior interosseous nerve can be dissected free and excised.
- The dorsal capsule is incised in line with the skin incision and elevated off the carpus.[12]
- This exposure allows for performance of concomitant procedures such as a distal ulna excision and dorsal tenosynovectomy.

PLATE AND SCREW OSTEOSYNTHESIS

- In addition to the approach described above, the proximal portion of the third metacarpal is exposed subperiosteally.
- Expose the radioscaphoid, radiolunate, scaphocapitate, capitolunate, and third carpometacarpal joints (**TECH FIG 1A**), clean them of any remaining cartilage and soft tissue, and then fully denude them to below the subchondral bone.
  - Maintain the general bony geometry to allow the prepared carpal bones to interdigitate effectively.
  - A combination of a no. 15 blade, small curettes, and rongeurs is usually adequate for preparing the joint surfaces. Use of a water-cooled power burr and repeated penetration of the articular surfaces with a 0.045-inch smooth Kirschner wire are sometimes helpful.
  - The triquetrolunate, triquetrohamate, scaphotrapezial-trapezoid, and capitohamate joints may be left undisturbed if not arthritic.
  - If one expects to remove the plate at a second surgery, the second and third carpometacarpal joints can be left intact. This limits the fusion mass to the radiocarpal and midcarpal joints, preserving motion at the carpometacarpal level.
- Obtain autologous bone graft from the distal radius in two forms, a corticocancellous graft and cancellous bone chips.
- Measure the distance from the base of the third metacarpal to the radius platform and harvest a cortico-

cancellous bone graft of equal length from the dorsal radial surface of the distal radius.
- Take care to avoid disrupting the radial cortex of the distal radius (and thereby destabilizing the bone) and removing the cortex on which the plate will eventually sit.
- Outline the graft using a wire driver and a 0.045-inch Kirschner wire, and then harvest it with a sharp osteotome and mallet.
- After removing this graft, harvest cancellous bone from the site and tightly pack it between the prepared bony surfaces.
  - In cases of severe deformity, the carpus may be held in general alignment with temporary Kirschner wires.
- Key the corticocancellous graft into the space between the third metacarpal base and the radius platform.
  - This graft will be located directly under the plate (**TECH FIG 1B**).
- Choose the desired wrist fusion plate and secure it distally to the third metacarpal with appropriately sized screws.
  - Plate options include a long bend, a short bend, and a straight plate (Synthes USA).
  - In selected instances, the second metacarpal may be used rather than the third metacarpal.
- With the carpus aligned and the prepared joints reduced and grafted, apply the plate to the distal radius in a com-

TECHNIQUES

TECHNIQUES

pression mode using appropriately sized screws. Complete the fixation with additional screws (**TECH FIG 1C,D**).

■ Any remaining bone graft is added in and around the prepared joints.

■ Close the capsule with absorbable suture. If needed, the extensor retinaculum may be split, with one portion repaired deep to the extensor tendons to allow coverage of prominent portions of the plate. The other portion is repaired superficial to the tendons to resist "bowstringing." Transpose the extensor pollicis longus tendon into the subcutaneous space. Close the skin in the usual manner.

■ Strongly consider using a drain.

■ A sterile dressing and below-elbow volar splint are applied.

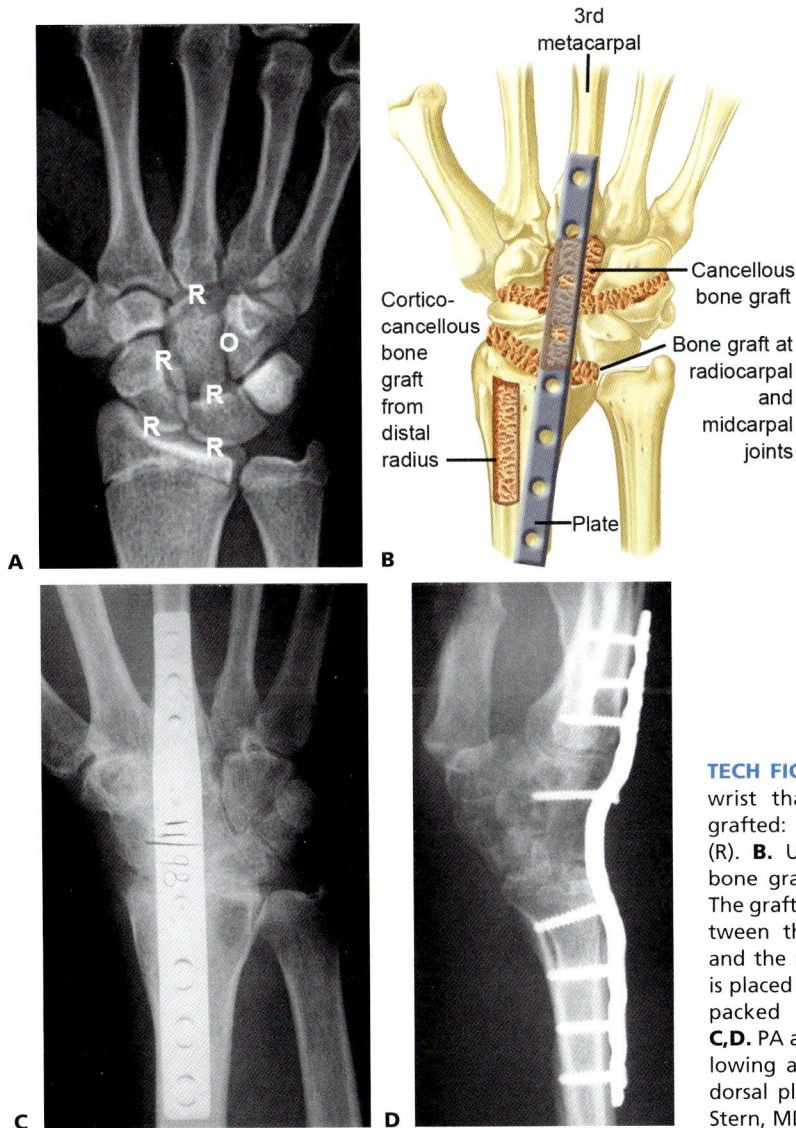

TECH FIG 1 • **A.** Joints within the wrist that are decorticated and grafted: optional (O) or required (R). **B.** Use of a corticocancellous bone graft from the distal radius. The graft is keyed into the space between the third metacarpal base and the radius platform. The plate is placed on top. Cancellous graft is packed into prepared joints. **C,D.** PA and lateral radiographs following a wrist arthrodesis using a dorsal plate. (**C,D**: Courtesy of P.J. Stern, MD.)

FUSION WITH STEINMANN RODS

■ Fusion with Steinmann rods is performed using a technique similar to that described above, typically in patients with advanced inflammatory arthritis.

■ Because bone loss and deformity are substantive, precise joint preparation and reduction is not possible and the goal is generation of a fusion mass.

■ Typically, cancellous autograft taken from the distal radius is used between the prepared bony surfaces.

■ Fixation may be accomplished using an intramedullary rod inserted through the head of the third metacarpal (**TECH FIG 2A–D**).

■ As an alternative, two rods can be inserted between the second and third, and third and forth metacarpals (**TECH FIG 2E,F**). These are usually smaller pins that produce an interference fit in the radius shaft.

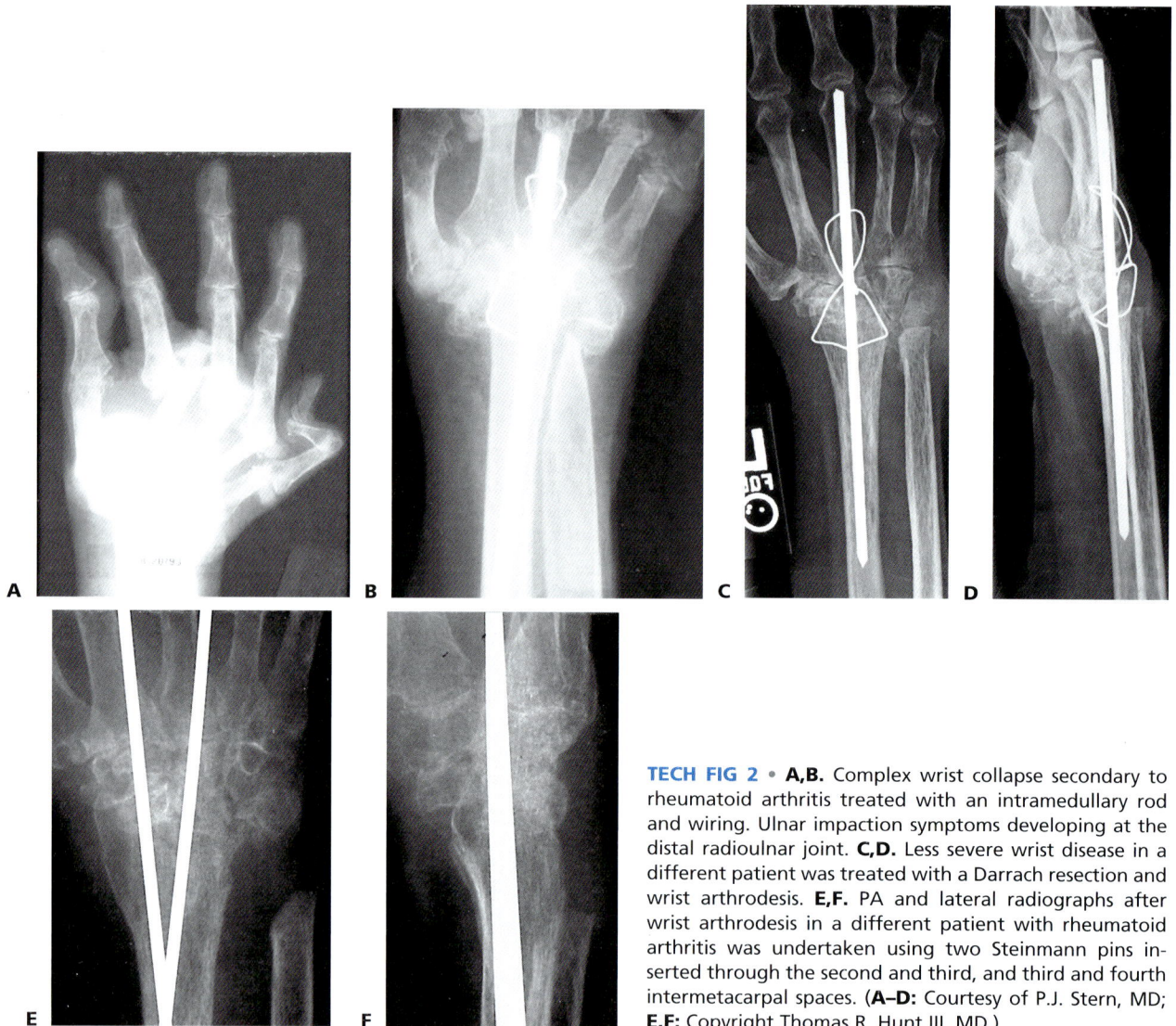

TECH FIG 2 • A,B. Complex wrist collapse secondary to rheumatoid arthritis treated with an intramedullary rod and wiring. Ulnar impaction symptoms developing at the distal radioulnar joint. **C,D.** Less severe wrist disease in a different patient was treated with a Darrach resection and wrist arthrodesis. **E,F.** PA and lateral radiographs after wrist arthrodesis in a different patient with rheumatoid arthritis was undertaken using two Steinmann pins inserted through the second and third, and third and fourth intermetacarpal spaces. (**A–D:** Courtesy of P.J. Stern, MD; **E,F:** Copyright Thomas R. Hunt III, MD.)

- Placing an intramedullary rod through the third metacarpal head necessitates an incision in the dorsal web space and in the sagittal band.
  - Metacarpophalangeal joint replacement may eventually be required.
- Choose the largest pin that will fit within the metacarpal and advance it retrograde through the reduced carpus and into the radius.
  - A second smaller derotation pin can be placed through the radial styloid into the carpus and metacarpals to prevent rotation.
- Alternatively, a figure 8 wire can be placed around the third metacarpal and through the radius to compress the construct.
- If the metacarpophalangeal joints have already been replaced, two Steinmann pins through the second and third web spaces may be effective.
- Closure is similar to that described above.

PEARLS AND PITFALLS

- The third metacarpal should be aligned with the radius. This alignment is essential when applying a plate.
- Patients prefer to be in slight wrist extension without significant radial or ulnar deviation; significant deviation into flexion or radial deviation leads to problems and weakness. Patients already stiff at neutral may prefer a neutral position.
- Bilateral fusions may not be preferred but rarely affect function.[2]
- If the proximal row has displaced, proximal row carpectomy and fusion has been shown to be successful.[4]
- If the ulnar head appears arthritic or prominent, it will need to be addressed using a Darrach procedure, hemiresection techniques, or head replacement. If not addressed, it may be a source of pain postoperatively.

POSTOPERATIVE CARE

▪ Patients are placed into a removable brace 2 weeks after surgery and started on active finger flexion–extension exercises as well as pronation and supination.

▪ Patients with an extensor lag due to dorsal swelling are started on a program of dynamic extension with an outrigger splint until full active extension is regained.

▪ Strengthening is reserved for when the radiographs demonstrate union. Union usually takes 6 to 8 weeks but is prolonged in smokers. Comorbidities may also affect healing rates.

▪ If patient compliance is an issue, a cast may be used for the first 4 weeks to protect the construct with plate osteosynthesis.

▪ A cast is recommended for 4 to 6 weeks when using Steinmann rods until the patient's wrist is nontender.

▪ Therapy may also need to be modified depending on any additional procedures performed.

COMPLICATIONS

▪ Infection
▪ Nonunion, delayed union, and malunion
▪ Dorsal wrist tenderness
▪ Tendon adhesions and ruptures
▪ Neuromas and complex regional pain syndromes
▪ Pin migration
▪ Wound breakdown

OUTCOMES

▪ Wrist arthrodesis boasts a high fusion rate, a high satisfaction rate, and a low complication rate.[1,5,7,8,9,13] It is for this reason that fusion of the wrist is selected in patients who can tolerate fewer trips to the operating room for secondary procedures.

▪ While more satisfying than rod stabilization in rheumatoid patients (74% vs. 37%), plate fixation may require tenolysis or plate removal after arthrodesis.[1,11] Satisfaction may be affected by the patient's underlying disease.

▪ Housian and Schroder[6] found that plate removal was common (15%) due to the complications listed above but was successful in relieving symptoms.

REFERENCES

1. Barbier O, Saels P, Rombouts JJ, et al. Long-term functional results of wrist arthrodesis in rheumatoid arthritis. J Hand Surg Br 1999; 24B:27–31.
2. Calundruccio JH. Osteoarthritis of the wrist. In: Trumble TE, ed. Hand Surgery Update 3. Rosemont, IL: ASSH, 2003:528–529.
3. Clendenin MP, Green DP. Arthrodesis of the wrist: complications and their management. J Hand Surg Am 1981;6:253–257.
4. Hartigan BJ, Nagle DJ, Foley MJ. Wrist arthrodesis with excision of the proximal carpal bones using the AO/ASIF wrist fusion plate and local bone graft. J Hand Surg Br 2001;26B:247–251.
5. Hayden RJ, Jebson PJ. Wrist arthrodesis. Hand Clin 2005;21:631–640.
6. Housian S, Schroder HA. Wrist arthrodesis with the AO titanium wrist fusion plate: a consecutive series of 42 cases. J Hand Surg Br 2001;26B:355–359.
7. Jebsen PJ, Adams BD. Wrist arthrodesis: review of current techniques. J Am Acad Orthop Surg 2001;9:53–60.
8. Krimmer H. Radiocarpal and total wrist arthrodesis. In: Berger RA, Weiss AP, eds. Hand Surgery. Philadelphia: Lippincott Williams & Wilkins, 2004:1319–1337.
9. Mack GR, Bosse MJ, Gelberman RH, et al. The natural history of scaphoid non-union. J Bone Joint Surg Am 1984;66A:504–509.
10. Ruby LK, Stinson J, Belsky MR. The natural history of scaphoid non-union: a review of fifty-three cases. J Bone Joint Surg Am 1985;67A: 428–432.
11. Toma CD, Machacek P, Bitzan P, et al. Fusion of the wrist in rheumatoid arthritis: a clinical and functional evaluation of two surgical techniques. J Bone Joint Surg Br 2007;89B:1620–1626.
12. Weil C, Ruby LK. The dorsal approach to the wrist revisited. J Hand Surg Am 1986;11A:911–912.
13. Weiss AC, Wiedeman G Jr, Quenzer D, et al. Upper extremity function after wrist arthrodesis. J Hand Surg Am 1995;25A:813–817.
14. Weiss AP, Hastings H. Wrist arthrodesis for traumatic conditions: a study of plate and local graft application. J Hand Surg Am 1995;20A: 50–56.

Chapter 90

Wrist Implant Arthroplasty

Joel C. Klena, Andrew K. Palmer, and James W. Strickland

DEFINITION

- In the past, the gold standard for the treatment of end-stage wrist degeneration and debilitating pain was fusion of the wrist joint. As a salvage procedure, arthrodesis can provide reasonable pain relief and relative preservation of upper extremity function. Unfortunately, fusion of the painful wrist does not guarantee pain relief, nor does it come without functional impairment.[7,9,12,17,18]

- In contrast, total wrist arthroplasty provides an attractive motion- and function-sparing alternative to wrist arthrodesis. Pain relief is achieved, along with preservation of wrist motion and function.[2,10,11]
  - Multiple studies have demonstrated that patients consistently prefer motion-sparing procedures over arthrodesis.[1,5,8,16]

- In much the same vein as arthroplasty efforts in the other major joints, early wrist replacement designs were successful in both relieving pain and maintaining function. Unfortunately, early wrist prostheses failed to achieve the long-term survivorship results provided by joint replacements in the shoulder, hip, and knee joints.

- Early prosthetic designs suffered from significant biomechanical design flaws. Difficulties arose with implant centering, balance, and fixation.
  - Significant improvements in implant design have capitalized on modularity, better material considerations, and improved anatomic designs to provide improved longevity.

- Current designs strive to achieve the following:
  - A more anatomic wrist joint than previous wrist designs, either through component design or implant instrumentation
  - Stable distal fixation by using screw fixation into the carpus while at the same time avoiding the lever arm created by a stem inserted into the third metacarpal

- The three most popular wrist designs in the United States today are the Universal 2 (KMI/Integra), the Re-Motion (Small Bone Innovations [SBI]), and the Maestro (Biomet) (**FIG 1**).
  - The Universal 2 Total Wrist prosthesis is an improved version of the original wrist of the late Dr. Jay Menon (**FIG 1A**). A great debt of gratitude is owed to Dr. Menon for popularizing distal screw fixation to the carpus.
    - The Uni2 design uses a flat carpal cut, screw fixation distally into both the second metacarpal and hamate, and a modular, distally based polyethylene cap that articulates with a proximal cobalt chrome radial component. The improved design attempts to preserve the distal radioulnar joint (DRUJ).
    - The Uni2 wrist is the prosthesis with which there is the greatest clinical experience to date. The results are encouraging.[4]

- The Re-Motion Total Wrist is essentially the prosthesis marketed initially by Avanta and then SBI with new and improved instrumentation (**FIG 1B**). It is fundamentally a prosthesis designed to resurface the distal radius.
  - A concave, cobalt chrome radial component articulates with a convex, distally based, polyethylene cap snapped over a flat carpal plate. The carpal plate is anchored to the carpus with a radial screw that does not penetrate the second metacarpal, and a second screw placed ulnarly. About 15 degrees of "wiggle" or intended motion is built into the

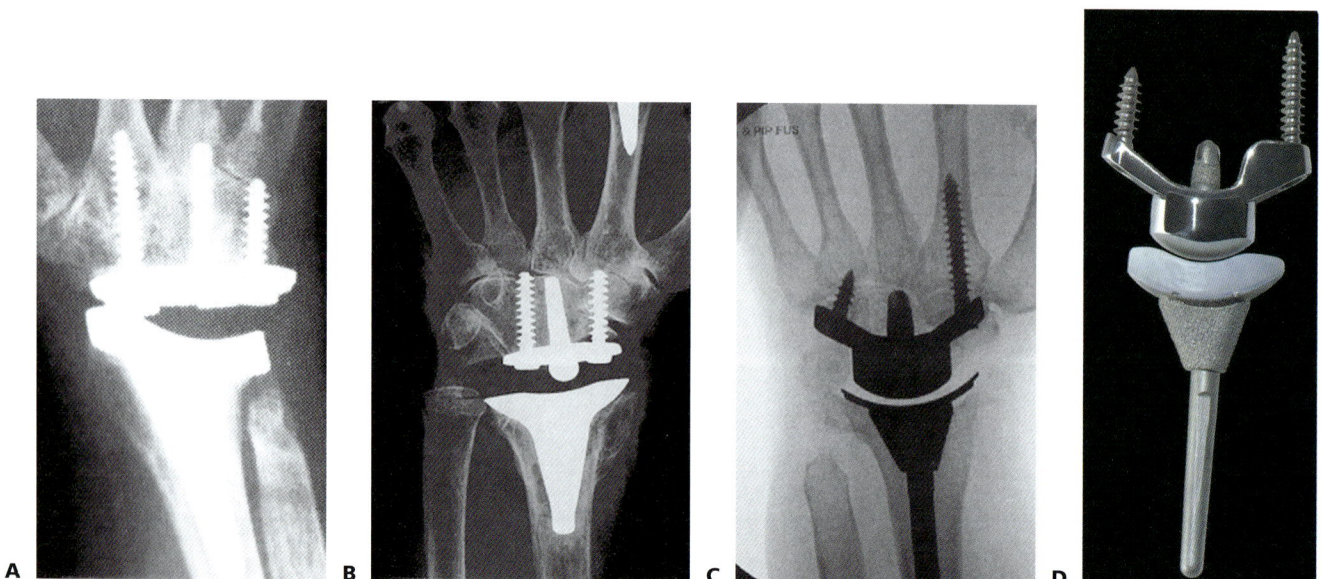

FIG 1 • **A.** Universal 2 total wrist replacement. **B.** Re-Motion total wrist replacement. **C,D.** Maestro (Biomet) wrist replacement.

snap fit of the polyethylene cap with the carpal plate. No attempt is made to preserve the DRUJ with this implant.

■ Many Re-Motion wrist replacements have been performed in conjunction with ulnar head replacement arthroplasty. Preliminary results with the Re-Motion wrist are encouraging.[3]

■ The Maestro Wrist is the most recent implant to enter the wrist joint replacement market (**FIG 1C,D**). It differs significantly in design from the Uni2 and the Re-Motion wrists, having been conceived to resemble successful total hip, knee, and shoulder designs, which use a metal convex component articulating with a concave polyethylene component.

   ■ The convex metallic distal component articulates with the proximally based, concave polyethylene body. This UPMWPE body is direct compression molded onto a cobalt chrome (CoCr) alloy radial body with a modular titanium stem. The distal component is composed of a CoCr alloy carpal plate (with or without scaphoid augment) and carpal body and a titanium capitate stem. All components are modular.

   ■ Unlike the Uni2 and the Re-Motion wrists, it is not always necessary to attempt fusion of the distal pole of the scaphoid to the surrounding carpus. The Maestro Wrist has a provision to replace the entire scaphoid using a carpal plate incorporating a modular radial augment.

   ■ The modular radial stem component is designed to fill the distal radius canal to prevent loosening and provide stability. The instrumentation used to prepare the distal radius is designed to preserve the DRUJ.

■ The excitement over these three wrist replacement systems has stimulated other investigators to work with companies in producing a total wrist replacement. These other wrist replacement systems are in various stages of design but offer promise for even further advancement of the technology.

ANATOMY

■ The wrist joint consists of the distal radial articular surface, the distal ulna and triangular fibrocartilage complex, eight carpal bones arranged into proximal and distal rows, and five metacarpal bases.

■ Four significant articulations exist: the radiocarpal joint, the midcarpal joint, the carpometacarpal joints, and the DRUJ. A combination of interosseous, intrinsic, and extrinsic ligaments provides stabilization (**FIG 2**).

■ The proximal row of the carpus articulates with the distal radius to form the radiocarpal joint. The distal carpal row articulations with the metacarpal bases form the carpometacarpal joints. Within the distal carpal row, the center of wrist motion is located at the head of the capitate, slightly palmar to the center of the head. This center of rotation may or may not be colinear with the third metacarpal shaft, depending on each patient's anatomy.

■ Proximally, the center of wrist motion lies ulnar to the radial intramedullary canal. Normal anatomic parameters of the distal radial articular surface include a volar tilt of 11 degrees and a radial inclination of 22 degrees.

■ The sigmoid notch of the distal radius provides the articulation for the DRUJ. Strong dorsal and palmar radioulnar ligaments provide DRUJ stability.

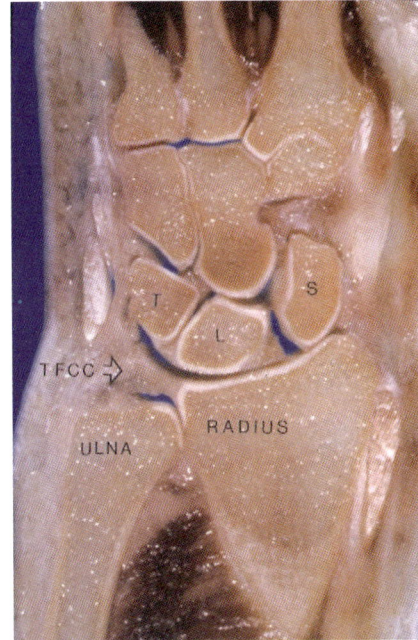

FIG 2 • Anatomy of the carpus. **L**, lunate; **S**, scaphoid; **T**, triquetrum.

PATHOGENESIS

■ End-stage wrist degeneration, a common endpoint of multiple pathways, involves loss of joint space and carpal collapse. The primary indication for total wrist arthroplasty is joint destruction secondary to the effects of rheumatoid arthritis.

■ The classic pattern of deformity and destruction involves the radiocarpal and midcarpal joints and the DRUJ. Attenuation of the extrinsic wrist ligaments destabilizes the carpus, often resulting in an ulnar and volar translation of the wrist (**FIG 3**).[6]

■ Joint replacement is also indicated to manage the pain, deformity, and loss of motion coincident with end-stage arthritis resulting from osteoarthritis, posttraumatic arthritis, or avascular necrosis. Total wrist arthroplasty can provide a salvage option for functional deformities such as scapholunate advanced collapse (SLAC) or irreparable trauma to the distal radius or carpus.

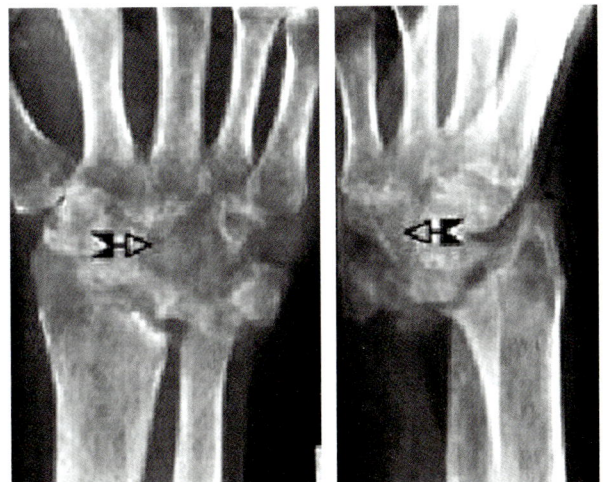

FIG 3 • AP and lateral radiographs showing end-stage rheumatoid wrist arthritis.

NATURAL HISTORY

▪ Irrespective of the pathway taken to end-stage wrist joint destruction, the result is a painful wrist with significant limitation of motion and function.

▪ Instability and misalignment are often present, particularly in the presence of rheumatoid arthritis or functional deformities such as SLAC wrist.

PATIENT HISTORY AND PHYSICAL FINDINGS

▪ Preoperative examination reveals decreased range of motion, decreased grip strength, and difficulties with normal activities. Pain is seen throughout the arc of motion as well as at the endpoint of motion.

▪ In patients with rheumatoid arthritis, the gross alignment of the wrist can be dramatic due to carpal collapse, ulnar translation, or volar subluxation.

▪ The ideal patient for wrist implant arthroplasty is one with significant wrist pain and loss of a functional range of wrist motion with preservation of adequate bone stock, a balanced wrist, and intact tendons.

IMAGING AND OTHER DIAGNOSTIC STUDIES

▪ Standard posteroanterior and lateral wrist radiographs provide sufficient imaging for preoperative planning and templating.

DIFFERENTIAL DIAGNOSIS

▪ Sources of end-stage wrist arthritis
  ▪ Rheumatoid arthritis
  ▪ Osteoarthritis
  ▪ Posttraumatic arthritis
  ▪ Avascular necrosis
  ▪ Functional deformities (eg, SLAC wrist)
  ▪ Trauma to the distal radius and carpus

NONOPERATIVE MANAGEMENT

▪ Nonoperative management consists of activity modification, anti-inflammatory medications, and corticosteroid injections.

▪ Supportive bracing may be a useful adjunct at the expense of decreased motion and function.

▪ Persistent pain and loss of function despite conservative measures can be considered a failure of nonoperative treatment and an indication for arthroplasty.

SURGICAL MANAGEMENT

▪ Absolute contraindications to wrist replacement are ongoing or deep infection and septic arthritis of the wrist.
  ▪ Patients considered for arthroplasty must be capable of understanding the risks and potential benefits of the procedure and be capable of complying with the postoperative protocol.

▪ Relative contraindications to wrist replacement are unstable and markedly collapsed wrists, lack of adequate wrist motors, and significant bone loss.
  ▪ If instability, deformity, motor power, or bone loss can be corrected, wrist replacement can be successfully performed.
  ▪ Previous proximal row carpectomy and even previous arthrodesis are not contraindications to wrist replacement, but one should not expect the same postoperative range of motion of the wrist.

Preoperative Planning

▪ Preoperative radiographs are used for templating.

▪ A determination of size can be made for the radial body and stem, the capitate stem, the carpal plate and body, the scaphoid augment, and the radial and ulnar screws.

▪ A gross estimate of the amount of distal radius to be resected can also be made.

Positioning

▪ The procedure is performed on a hand table using a tourniquet, with either general or regional anesthesia.

Approach

▪ A dorsal incision, slightly radial to midline, is made from 4 cm proximal to the radiocarpal joint to the midpoint of the third metacarpal.
  ▪ Dissection is carried down to the extensor retinaculum.

▪ The third dorsal compartment is opened and the extensor pollicis longus (EPL) tendon is exposed and mobilized radially.
  ▪ The radial wrist extensors are also exposed and mobilized radially.
  ▪ The first compartment tendons are mobilized from the distal radius and protected.
  ▪ The tendons of the fourth and fifth compartments are mobilized ulnarly, without opening their respective compartments.

▪ With the extensor tendons mobilized and retracted radially and ulnarly, the capsule is opened longitudinally and reflected radially and ulnarly, exposing the distal radius and entire carpus to the base of the third metacarpal.

TECHNIQUES

MAESTRO PROSTHESIS

▪ The senior author's personal experience is primarily with the Maestro prosthesis, and thus the technique of the Maestro total wrist arthroplasty is presented here.

▪ Although approved for implantation with cement, most wrists are implanted without cement fixation.

▪ Cement is usually preferred in cases of significant absent bone stock and in revision situations.

Carpal Preparation

▪ Position the carpal resection guide to allow resection of 2 to 3 mm of the capitate head. It is held in position with two 0.062-inch Kirschner wires (**TECH FIG 1A,B**).
  ▪ Place the first wire into the capitate neck and the second into the metaphysis of the third metacarpal, ensuring that the guide is parallel to the third metacarpal axis.

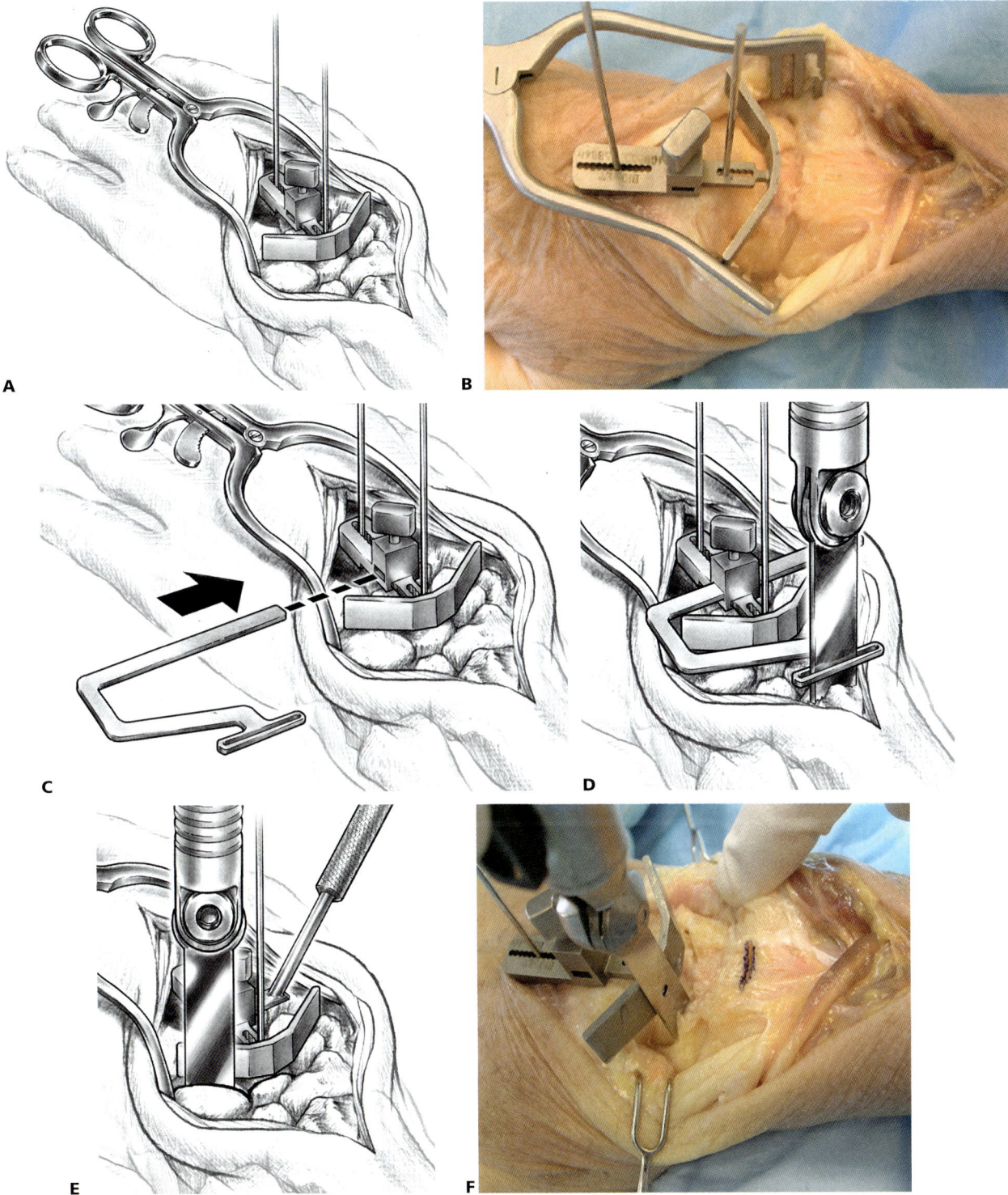

TECH FIG 1 • A,B. Carpal resection guide in place. Kirschner wires in the capitate head and third metacarpal metaphysis.
C. Insertion of the radial resection guide. **D.** Scoring of the distal radius resection reference line. **E,F.** Proximal carpal resection.
(**A,C–E:** Courtesy of Biomet, Warsaw, IN.)

- With proper placement, the ulnar guide wing will lie close to the triquetrum–hamate articulation and the radial wing will bisect the scaphoid at its distal third.
- Loosen the thumbscrew on the carpal resection guide to allow insertion of the radial resection guide boom (**TECH FIG 1C**).

- With the wrist in neutral, score the radius through the cutting slot in the guide to provide a reference for the distal radial resection (**TECH FIG 1D**).
- Remove the radius resection guide and use the carpal resection guide handle to stabilize the carpal guide during carpal resection.

- Cut the scaphoid, capitate head, hamate edge, and triquetrum at a 90-degree angle to the axis of the forearm–jig (**TECH FIG 1E,F**).
- As an alternative, the scaphoid can be completely removed and a carpal plate incorporating a scaphoid augment used.

Capitate Reaming and Selection of Carpal Plate

- After removing the carpal resection guide and Kirschner wires, remove the proximal carpus.
- Place a guidewire into the capitate at the apex of the resection, directly into the center of the capitate (**TECH FIG 2A**). This may or may not coincide with the center of the third metacarpal. Attention is focused on the capitate and not the capitate–third metacarpal relation.
- Ream the capitate (**TECH FIG 2B**).
- The depth of reaming can be verified under fluoroscopy. A direct indication of the trial stem size is indicated by depth marks on the reamer.

- Provisionally determine the trial carpal plate by the curvature and width of the remaining proximal carpal surface. The plate should lie flush with the hamate and proximal capitate surfaces.
  - Three separate scaphoid augments are available (**TECH FIG 2C**).
  - Assemble the plate and stem and insert them into the reamed capitate and onto the resected carpal surface. (**TECH FIG 2D**).
  - With adequate plate fitting, alignment is such that a radial screw will easily be inserted into the second metacarpal and an ulnar screw inserted into the hamate.

Radius Resection

- Insert a 0.062-inch Kirschner wire directly into the center of the medullary canal of the radius (**TECH FIG 3A**).
  - The correct insertion point is in the lower corner of the dorsal-ulnar quadrant of the radius articular surface (**TECH FIG 3B**). This corresponds to a point near

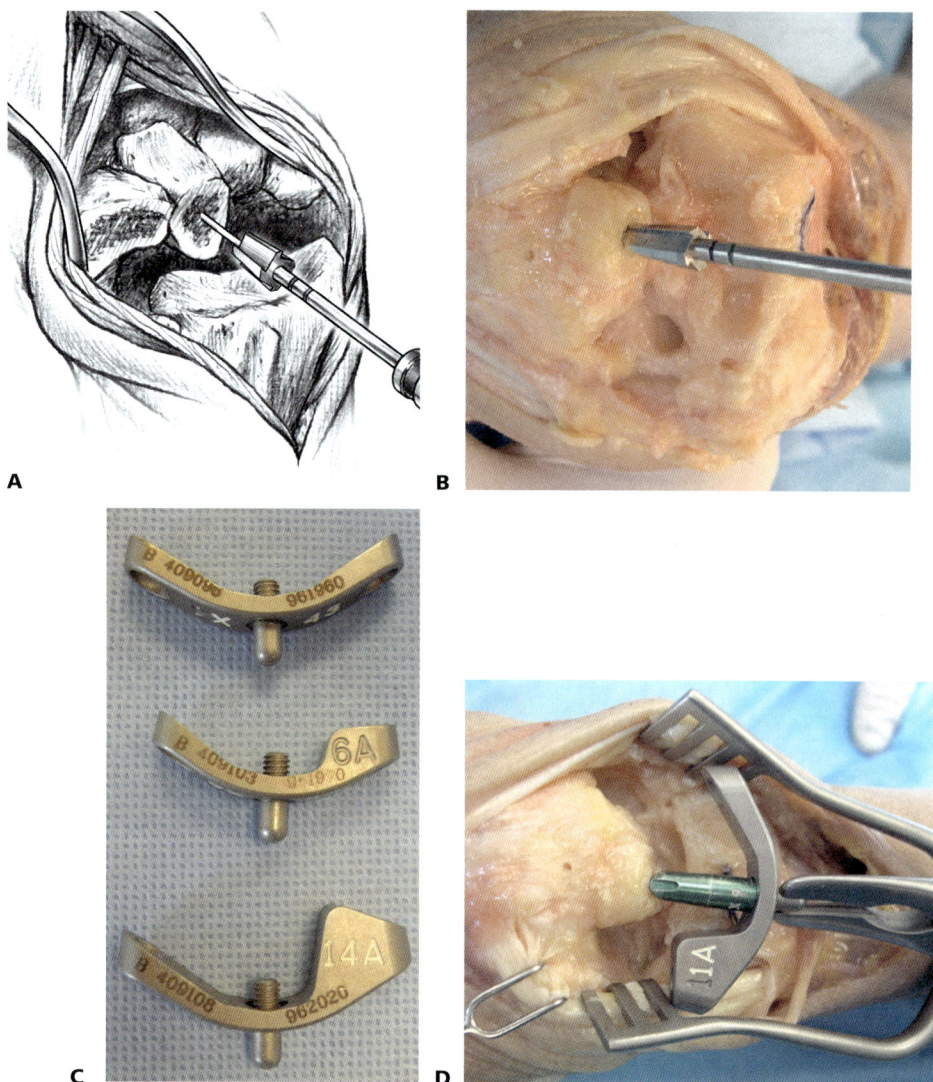

TECH FIG 2 • **A,B.** Capitate reaming over the previously placed guidewire. **C.** Scaphoid augments. **D.** Insertion of the trial carpal plate and stem. (**A:** Courtesy of Biomet, Warsaw, IN.)

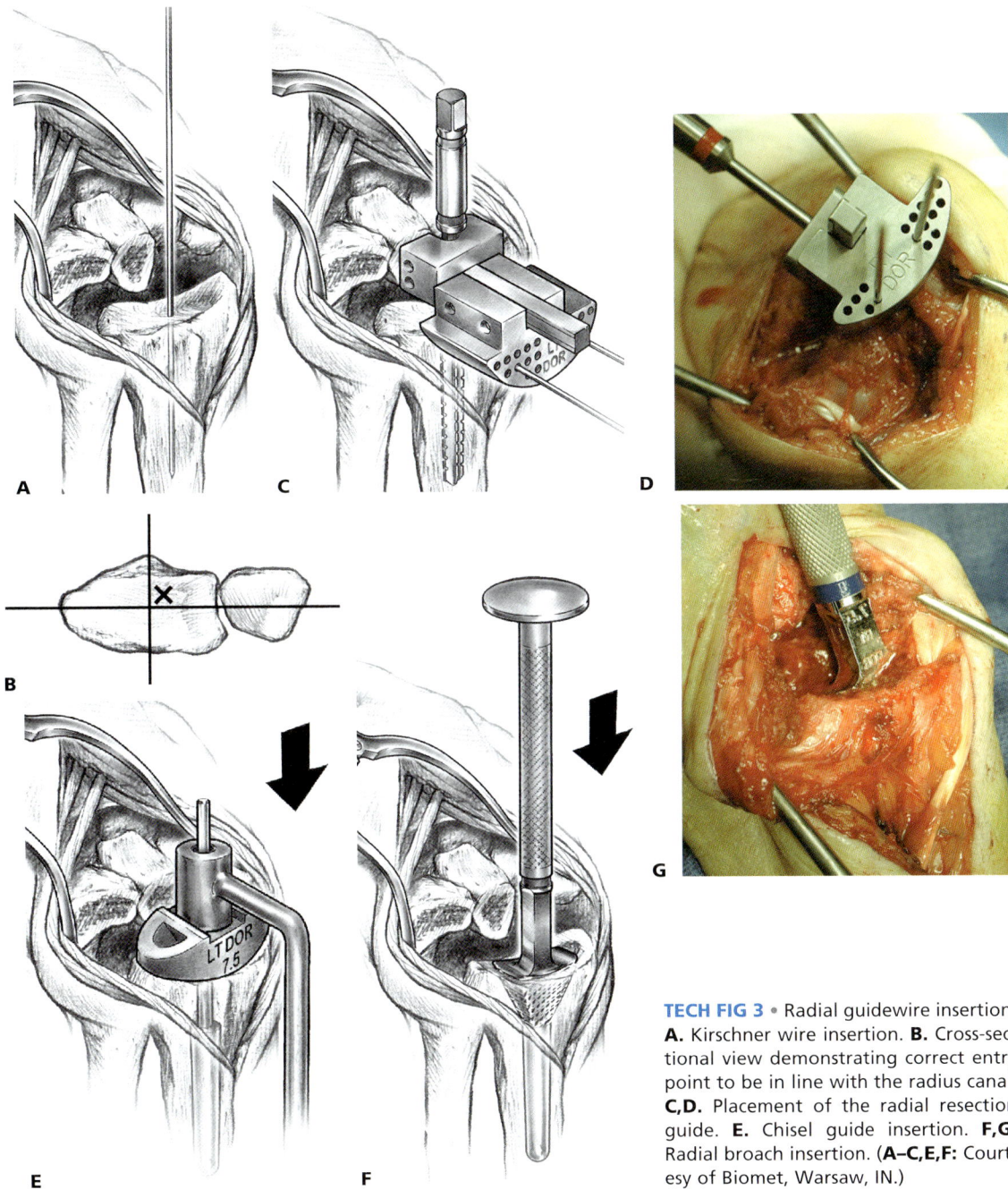

TECH FIG 3 • Radial guidewire insertion. **A.** Kirschner wire insertion. **B.** Cross-sectional view demonstrating correct entry point to be in line with the radius canal. **C,D.** Placement of the radial resection guide. **E.** Chisel guide insertion. **F,G.** Radial broach insertion. (**A–C,E,F:** Courtesy of Biomet, Warsaw, IN.)

the center of the radius and immediately below the groove of the tubercle of Lister. Correct wire placement is confirmed under fluoroscopy.
- The perfectly placed Kirschner wire is overdrilled with the cannulated drill bit to a minimum depth of 40 mm.
- Remove the Kirschner wire and successively ream the radius by hand until the reamer chatters on the intramedullary canal.
  - The final reamer is left in the canal and the radius resection guide boom and guide are attached (**TECH FIG 3C,D**).

- Align the proximal portion of the guide over the score mark made on the dorsal cortex and secure it with Kirschner wires.
- After removing the reamer and guide boom from the medullary canal, cut the radius.
  - The saw cut should follow exactly the contour of the resection guide and should not enter the DRUJ, thus maintaining its normal anatomy.
- Place the appropriate radius intramedullary guide into the canal and insert the chisel guide until flush with the resected surface (**TECH FIG 3E**).

- Insert the chisel into each side of the guide in sequence and gently tap it until fully seated.
- After removing the chisel and guide, remove the chiseled bone from the distal radius. Reinsert the intermedullary guide, and over this, broach the distal radius to the templated size desired (**TECH FIG 3F,G**).

Trial of Carpal and Radial Components

- Insert the previously assembled trial components for the carpal and the radial stem–body assembly (**TECH FIG 4A**).
  - With the wrist in full flexion, a standard-size carpal head is snap fit to the carpal plate (**TECH FIG 4B**).
  - The wrist is distracted and extended for reduction (**TECH FIG 4C**). About 2 to 3 mm of joint separation with distraction indicates appropriate tension. The carpal head may be adjusted to a +2 or +4 size until tension is appropriate. Satisfactory radial and ulnar deviation should be demonstrated.
- Excessive tissue tension can be remedied with additional radial resection. Distal ulnar impingement can be addressed with a Darrach-type resection of the distal ulna.
  - Remove the trial components; if the proper tension has been achieved, perform final irrigation.

Carpal Body Insertion and Fixation

- Assemble the carpal implant and inject bone cement, if indicated, into the capitate. Insert the stem of the assembled prosthesis into the capitate and impact it.

- Insert a single 0.062-inch Kirschner wire into the ulnar screw hole using the drill guide. Verify under fluoroscopy that the wire is directed centrally into the central portion of the hamate.
- Insert a second Kirschner wire through the radial screw hole and verify that it is through the trapezoid into the intermedullary canal of the second metacarpal.
- Overdrill both Kirschner wires with the cannulated drill bit (**TECH FIG 5**). Screw depth can be measured directly from the score marks on the drill bit.
  - Place the appropriate-size screws and verify placement fluoroscopically if needed.

Radial Body Insertion and Fixation

- Assemble the radial stem to the radial body. If indicated, inject bone cement into the radius, and impact the stem until fully seated.
  - Reduce the wrist components and take final radiographs (see Fig 1C).

Closure

- Close the wrist capsule and dorsal retinaculum with nonabsorbable sutures.
  - If the distal ulna was resected, the capsular closure should include a secure closure of the DRUJ.
- The placement of a drain before closure is at the surgeon's preference.
- Close the skin and place a sterile bulky dressing and palmar splint.

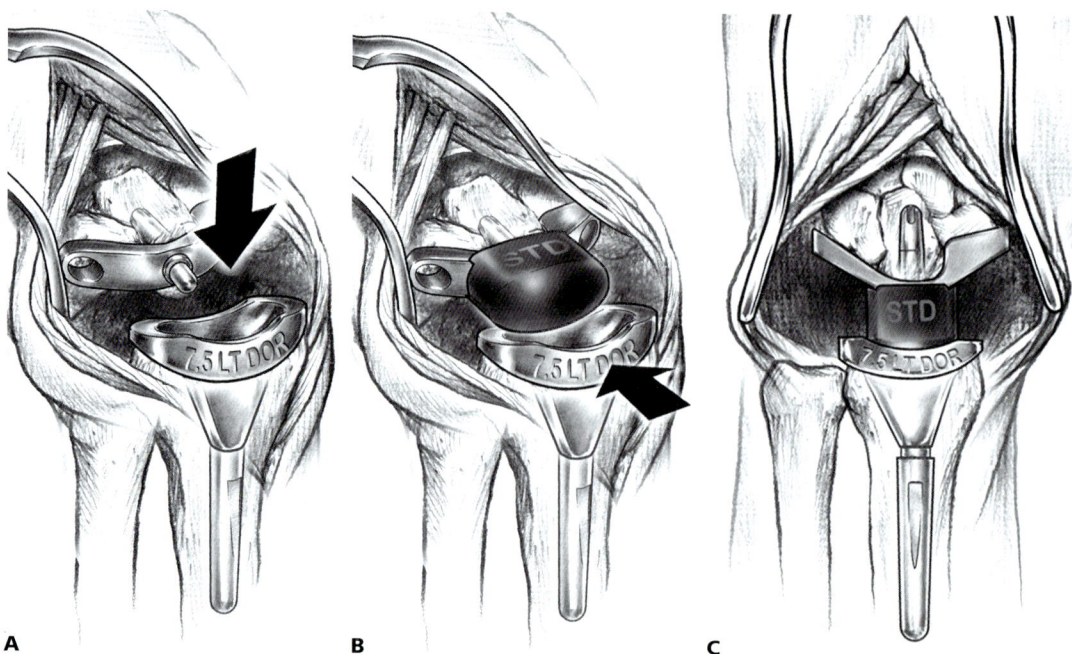

TECH FIG 4 • **A.** Trial component placement. **B.** Carpal head attached to carpal plate. **C.** Reduction of trial components. (Courtesy of Biomet, Warsaw, IN.)

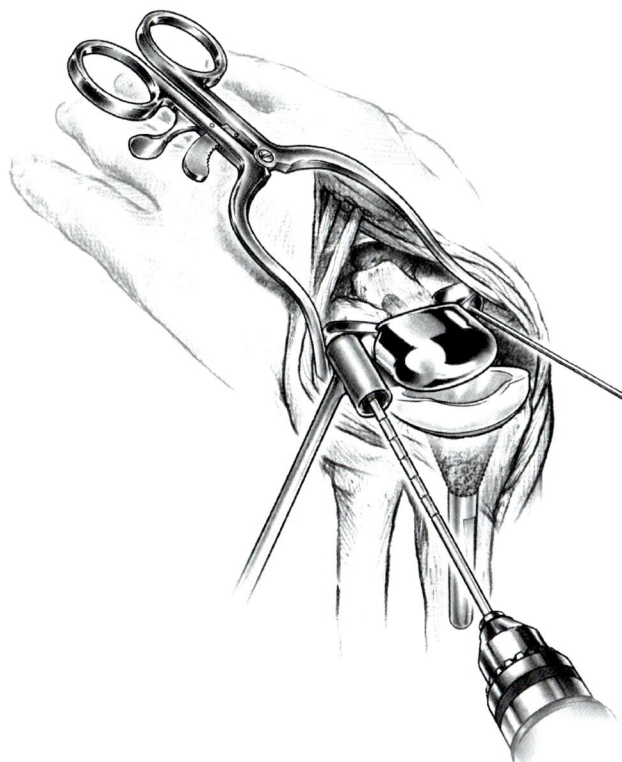

TECH FIG 5 • Drilling for ulnar screw placement. The first screw is placed into the central portion of the hamate. (Courtesy of Biomet, Warsaw, IN.)

PEARLS AND PITFALLS

Approach	▪ Careful preservation of the wrist capsule and dorsal retinaculum ensures that adequate tissue will be available for closure.
Radius resection	▪ Radius resection sets the tension on the implant. Close attention should be given to placing the radial guidewire into the absolute center of the medullary canal of the radius, as confirmed by radiographs. Guidewire placement is a key component of overall alignment.
Scaphoid excision	▪ The distal pole of the scaphoid can be routinely removed as part of the carpal resection. Excision of the distal pole of the scaphoid and replacement with a radially augmented carpal plate significantly decreases the difficulty of the operative procedure in regard to insertion of the distal component.
Center of wrist motion	▪ The center of motion is located at the head of the capitate. This may or may not coincide with the center of the third metacarpal, depending on individual patient anatomy. Attention should be focused on the capitate and not the capitate–third metacarpal relationship.

POSTOPERATIVE CARE

▪ Early finger motion is begun as allowed by the bulky postoperative bandage. Any drains placed are removed within 24 hours.
▪ The splint is removed at the 1-week follow-up visit and a cast or splint is placed for an additional 1 to 3 weeks.
▪ Splint removal with gentle active motion several times daily is permitted at 2 weeks after surgery.
  ▪ If a distal ulna resection was performed, the forearm is splinted in neutral rotation for at least 3 weeks before starting forearm rotation exercises.
▪ More vigorous active and passive range of motion is begun at 4 weeks postoperatively.

OUTCOMES

▪ The results of a prospective study evaluating the use of the Universal 2 total wrist replacement in rheumatoid patients showed that this wrist provides good early outcomes in this cohort of patients if severe preoperative wrist laxity is not present.[4]
  ▪ The authors reported significant improvement in range of motion and an improvement in the DASH score (Disabilities of the Arm, Shoulder and Hand) of 14 points at 1 year and 24 points at 2 years.
  ▪ Three prostheses were unstable and required further treatment.

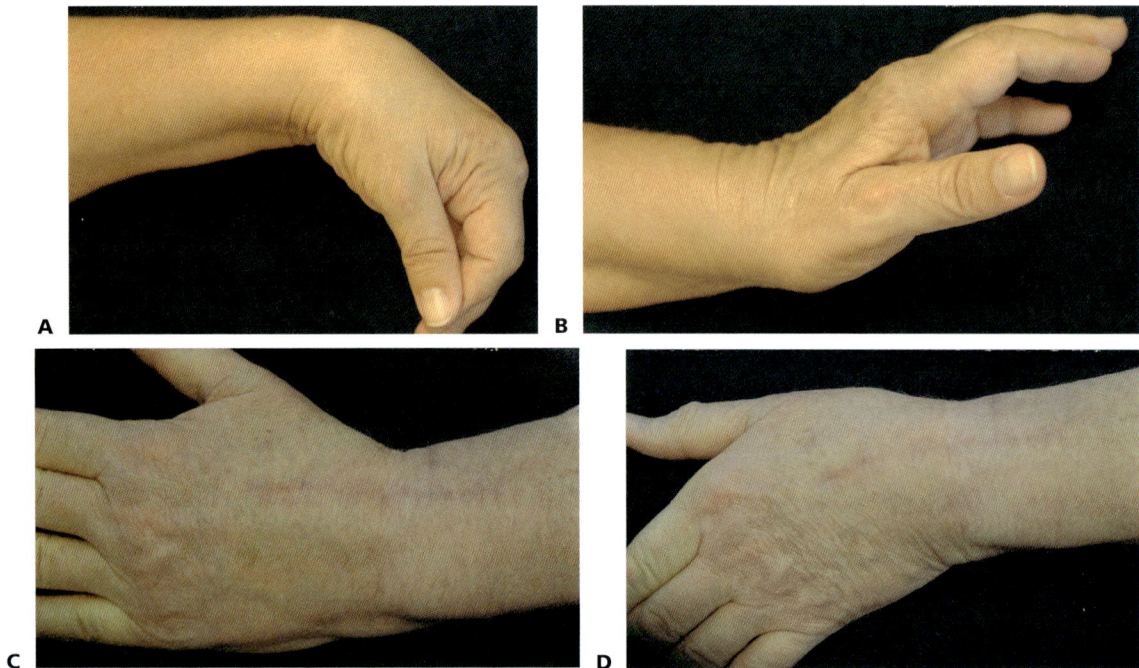

FIG 4 • Postoperative range of motion. **A.** Flexion. **B.** Extension. **C.** Radial deviation. **D.** Ulnar deviation.

■ Early results of the Maestro wrist replacement have been encouraging. A recent series of 14 patients with a minimum follow-up of 24 months (average 28 months) revealed that all patients had satisfactory pain relief postoperatively.

■ Motion (**FIG 4**) improved from an average of 28 degrees flexion and 27 degrees extension before surgery to 41 and 43 degrees, respectively, postoperatively. Radial and ulnar deviation averaged 19 and 23 degrees, respectively.

■ No significant complications were noted.[15]

COMPLICATIONS

■ Short-term complications include early postoperative wound concerns, superficial infections, and deep infections.

■ The most significant long-term complication encountered is implant loosening. Loosening is not an immediate indication for revision but does necessitate close clinical and radiographic monitoring for progression.

■ Implant instability may result from poor component placement, implant loosening, ligamentous instability, or component wear. Each case must be dealt with individually after determining the cause of such instability.

■ Periprosthetic fracture is also an infrequently seen complication. Two options are available for salvage of loose or fractured prostheses: component revision or wrist arthrodesis.[13,14]

REFERENCES

1. Adey L, Ring D, Jupiter J. Health status after total wrist arthrodesis for posttraumatic arthritis. J Hand Surg Am 2005;30A:932–936.
2. Cobb TK, Beckenbaugh RD. Biaxial total-wrist arthroplasty. J Hand Surg Am 1996;21A:1011–1021.
3. Cooney W. SBI Breakfast Symposium on TWA, Meeting of the ASSH, Washington, DC, 2006.
4. Divelbiss BJ, Sollerman C, Adams BD. Early results of the Universal total wrist arthroplasty in rheumatoid arthritis. J Hand Surg Am 2002;27A:195–204.
5. Goodman MJ, Millender LH, Nalebuff ED, et al. Arthroplasty of the rheumatoid wrist with silicone rubber: an early evaluation. J Hand Surg Am 1980;5A:114–121.
6. Herren DB, Simmen BR. Limited and complete fusion of the rheumatoid wrist. J Am Soc Surg Hand 2002;2:21–32.
7. Houshian S, Schroder H. Wrist arthrodesis with the AO titanium wrist fusion plate. J Hand Surg Br 2001;26B:355–359.
8. Kobus RJ, Turner RH. Wrist arthrodesis for treatment of rheumatoid arthritis. J Hand Surg Am 1990;15A:541–546.
9. Meads BM, Scougall PJ, Hargreaves IC. Wrist arthrodesis using a Synthes wrist fusion plate. J Hand Surg Br 2003;28B:571–574.
10. Menon J. Universal total wrist implant: experience with a carpal component fixed with three screws. J Arthroplasty 1998;13:515–523.
11. Meuli HC. Total wrist arthroplasty: experience with a noncemented wrist prosthesis. Clin Orthop Relat Res 1997;342:77–83.
12. Murphy DM, Khoury JG, Imbriglia JE, et al. Comparison of arthroplasty and arthrodesis for the rheumatoid wrist. J Hand Surg Am 2003;28A:570–576.
13. Rettig ME, Beckenbaugh RD. Revision total wrist arthroplasty. J Hand Surg Am 1993;18A:798–804.
14. Sagerman SD, Palmer AK. Wrist arthrodesis using a dynamic compression plate. J Hand Surg Br 1996;21B:437–441.
15. Strickland J. Abstract: early results of the Maestro Total Wrist Arthroplasty, submitted to the 2008 ASSH annual meeting.
16. Vicar AJ, Burton RI. Surgical management of the rheumatoid wrist—fusion or arthroplasty. J Hand Surg Am 1986;11A:790–797.
17. Weiss AC, Hastings H. Wrist arthrodesis for traumatic conditions. J Hand Surg Am 1995;20A:50–56.
18. Zachary SV, Stern PJ: Complications following AO/ASIF wrist arthrodesis. J Hand Surg Am 1995;20:339–344.

Chapter 91

Resection Arthroplasty of the Distal Radioulnar Joint

Jeffrey A. Greenberg

DEFINITION

- Dr. William Darrach described the distal ulna resection that bears his name in the early 1900s for the treatment of a post-traumatic volar distal radioulnar joint (DRUJ) dislocation. This operation continues to have a place for the treatment of a variety of afflictions of the DRUJ.
- In an effort to preserve some of the critical stabilizing soft tissue elements of the distal ulna, alternative treatments to complete ablation of the distal ulna have been developed.
  - Bowers[3] published his results of the hemiresection-interposition technique (HIT). This procedure differs from the Darrach in that the weight-bearing seat and pole are resected, preserving the styloid and soft tissue elements of the triangular fibrocartilage (TFC).
  - Watson et al[21,22] advocated the matched resection procedure.
  - The essential element is matching the profile of the resected distal ulna to the medial side of the radius.

ANATOMY

- The DRUJ is formed by the articulation between the sigmoid notch and the head of the ulna (**FIG 1A,B**). The sigmoid notch is the articular cartilage surface on the medial aspect of the distal radius. This concave surface matches the corresponding convex surface or "seat" of the distal ulna. The arc of curvature of the sigmoid notch ranges between 47 and 80 degrees, with an average radius of 12 to 18 mm.
- The articulation is constrained loosely, allowing both forearm rotation through a 150-degree arc and proximal and distal migration as well as dorsal and palmar translation of the ulna relative to the radius during forearm rotation. The articular cartilage-covered "cap" of the distal ulna can be divided into two functional regions. The seat of the ulna is the concave portion that articulates with the sigmoid notch. The arc

of curvature ranges between 90 and 135 degrees, with an average radius of 8 to 13 mm. This region is covered by articular cartilage around 270 degrees of its surface. This is the region that supports the compressive loads of the distal radius during most activities of daily living and can be considered the fulcrum for load support.

- The pole is the distal portion of the ulna that lies deep to the cartilaginous TFC. This region supports the centrum of the TFC as compressive loads pass from the ulnar carpus to the bony elements of the forearm. The medial-distal portion of the ulna projects as the ulnar styloid. The base of the styloid contains the critical attachment of the deep layer of the TFC, the ligamentum subcruentum (**FIG 1C**).
  - Distal to this, and in a more peripheral location, is the attachment of the superficial layer of the TFC. The dorsal and volar portions of the TFC are thickened, forming the limbi of the TFC, the volar and dorsal radioulnar ligaments. These ligaments play critical roles in stabilizing the DRUJ.

PATHOGENESIS

- Conditions that cause DRUJ degenerative change or altered DRUJ mechanics can lead to pain and DRUJ dysfunction. Most commonly, distal ulna resection is performed in patients with inflammatory arthropathy, usually rheumatoid arthritis. Frequently, treatment of the DRUJ is performed in conjunction with other bone or soft tissue reconstructions.
- DRUJ instability secondary to trauma or attritional changes of the supporting soft tissue elements can lead to degenerative change of this articulation.
- Malunions of the distal radius can negatively affect the sigmoid notch by alterations in angulation or length and can disrupt DRUJ kinematics.
- A less common cause of DRUJ arthritis is primary osteoarthritis, which may also lead to osteophytes and loose bodies.

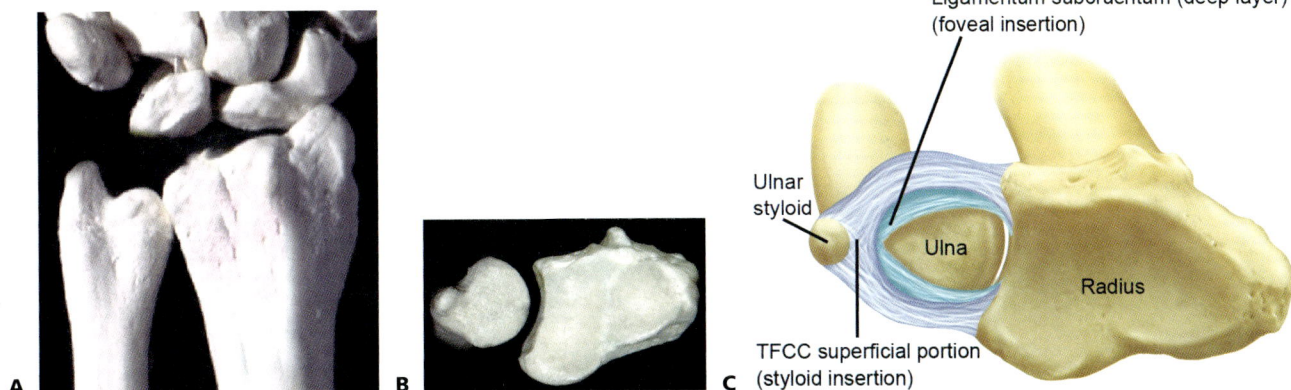

FIG 1 • Diagrammatic representations of the bony anatomy (**A**) and relationship of the radius and ulna at the distal radioulnar joint (DRUJ) (**B**). **C.** Soft tissue elements of the DRUJ, including the deep (ligamentum subcruentum) and superficial peripheral attachments of the triangular fibrocartilage.

■ Developmental conditions, such as Madelung deformity, can alter DRUJ joint mechanics. Painful forearm rotation and degenerative changes as well as ulnar impaction can develop.

PATIENT HISTORY AND PHYSICAL FINDINGS

■ Patients with DRUJ problems present with pain and limited forearm rotation.

■ In isolated DRUJ arthrosis, the patients usually localize their pain at the DRUJ articulation.

■ In patients with concomitant associated pathology of the soft tissue elements and DRUJ stabilizers, the ulnar-sided pain is more diffuse.

■ Pain occurs with activities that require forearm rotation, such as turning doorknobs, turning keys in locks, starting a car, and opening jars. Lifting activities with the arm away from the body are difficult since the DRUJ is loaded in this position.

■ Limited forearm motion may be secondary to an arthritic DRUJ; however, other conditions (eg, capsular contracture) must be considered.

■ Prominence and deformity of the distal ulna is common in patients with inflammatory changes and in patients with distal radial fracture malunions.

■ Inspection is usually unremarkable in patients with isolated DRUJ osteoarthritis. In contrast, DRUJ deformity and prominence is common in patients with rheumatoid arthritis. Fullness due to synovial proliferation may be visible and secondary attritional changes of surrounding soft tissue elements, such as extensor tendon rupture, can lead to abnormal hand posture.

■ Radial malunions with shortening and angulation produce visible prominence of the distal ulna (**FIG 2**).

■ Tenderness with pressure on the dorsal aspect of the DRUJ is frequently elicited. In patients with associated impaction or TFC pathology, tenderness may be more diffuse. Palpable crepitance with rotation is often present. Compressing the distal ulna into the sigmoid notch while rotating the forearm elicits painful crepitation and is suggestive of arthrosis.

■ Pain on the ulnocarpal stress test is indicative of TFC pathology.

■ Pain on application of pressure in the interval between the ulnar styloid and flexor carpi ulnaris tendon is indicative of TFC or capsuloligamentous pathology (foveal sign).[2]

■ Piano key maneuver: Visible dorsal winging or instability of the distal ulna is noted. If the ulna is dorsally prominent, the examiner can manually reduce the ulna into the sigmoid notch. The ulna spontaneously dorsally subluxates when pressure is removed. Winging is associated with loss of structural support of the DRUJ.

■ Grip strength is frequently limited secondary to painful compressive loading of the DRUJ.

IMAGING AND OTHER DIAGNOSTIC STUDIES

■ Plain radiographs are usually sufficient to supplement physical examination findings. It is essential to obtain a neutral forearm rotation, posteroanterior (PA) lateral view (**FIG 3A**) to accurately assess ulnar variance, styloid morphology, inclination of the sigmoid notch, and position of the ulnar styloid. These factors are important in selecting the appropriate surgical management for disorders of the distal ulna.

■ Thin-section CT scanning can provide useful additional information about DRUJ articular surfaces and subluxation.

■ MRI evaluation is rarely necessary to diagnose arthritic disorders of the DRUJ but can be useful when detailed information about the radioulnar ligaments or surrounding bony ligaments of the TFC is necessary (**FIG 3B**).

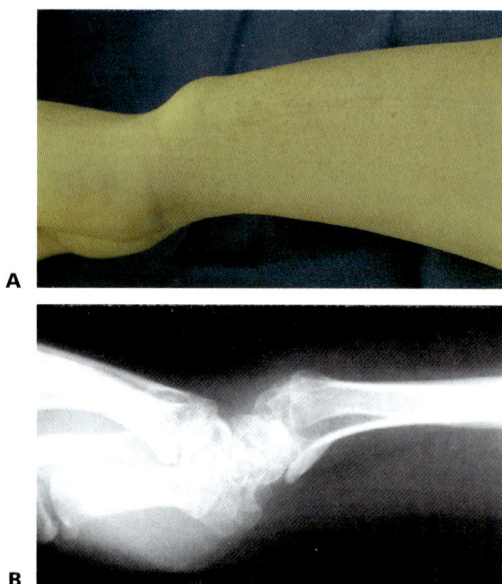

FIG 2 • Loss of the soft tissue support with or without associated degenerative change or malunion of the radius with resultant sigmoid notch incongruity leads to dorsal prominence and winging of the ulna relative to the radius. **A.** Dorsal prominence of the ulna relative to the radius is seen in a patient with a radial malunion. **B.** Radiograph of a wrist of a patient with rheumatoid arthritis shows the volar translation and secondary changes in the carpus that are associated with dorsal ulna prominence.

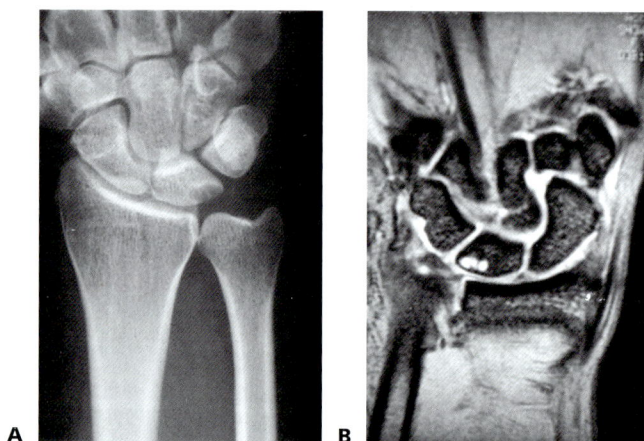

FIG 3 • **A.** The zero-rotation view is taken with the patient's shoulder abducted at 90 degrees, the elbow flexed 90 degrees, and the wrist pronated in the PA position. The ulnar styloid is seen in full profile in this view. This view is the standard radiographic view used to determine ulnar variance. **B.** While not part of the routine imaging evaluation for the triangular fibrocartilage, MRI can confirm the diagnosis for related conditions. This MRI in a patient with an ulnar-positive wrist shows a discrete intense lesion at the ulnar base of the lunate consistent with ulnar impaction.

DIFFERENTIAL DIAGNOSIS

- DRUJ arthritis
  - Inflammatory
  - Osteoarthritis
  - Traumatic
  - Iatrogenic (eg, altered joint mechanics after ulnar shortening)
- DRUJ instability
- TFC tears
- Ulnar impaction
- Lunotriquetral ligament tears or instability
- Extensor carpi ulnaris tendinitis
- Extensor carpi ulnaris instability
- Pisotriquetral disorders
- Nerve entrapment (canal of Guyon)
- Nerve injury (eg, neuromas of dorsal ulnar sensory nerve)
- Madelung deformity with DRUJ dysfunction

NONOPERATIVE MANAGEMENT

- Patients with mild symptoms and minimal functional impairment may be managed with oral anti-inflammatories, intra-articular injections, or splinting.
- Splinting must include the elbow to eliminate forearm rotation.

SURGICAL MANAGEMENT

- Maintaining the distal ulna has gained recent popularity as resection can be associated with considerable postoperative complications and functional disability. Meticulous attention to preoperative, intraoperative, and postoperative detail is essential for a successful result.

Adjunctive Procedures

- After complete or partial resection of the distal ulna, convergence between the radius and ulna can develop.[13] Loss of the weight-bearing fulcrum of the ulna seat can yield convergence with grip or loaded lifting with the arm extended and the forearm in neutral rotation (**FIG 4**).

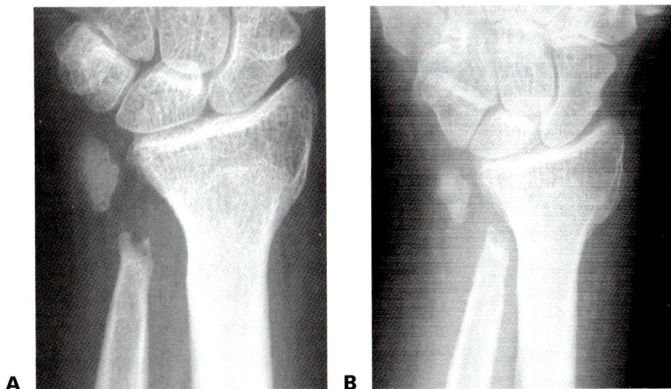

FIG 4 • Impingement of the resected distal ulna against the medial wall of the radius is common after distal ulna resection. It can be demonstrated radiographically even in patients who may be asymptomatic after distal ulna resection. Convergence is demonstrated with a weighted PA radiograph. **A.** Radiograph of a patient who has undergone Darrach resection shows a wide separation between the ulna and radius without external load. **B.** Significant convergence is noted on a weighted, loaded view.

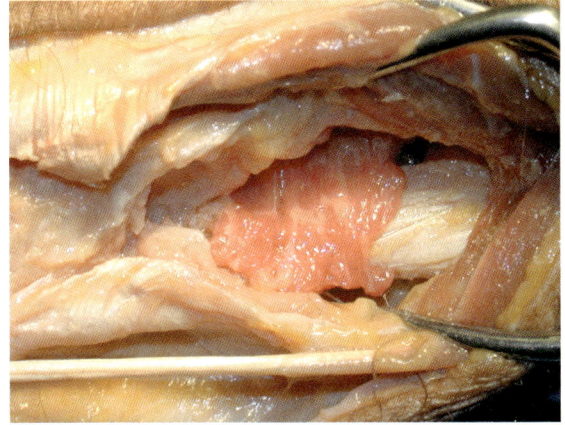

FIG 5 • After resection of the distal ulna, the pronator quadratus muscle has been transferred dorsally through the interosseous space, providing a dynamic interpositional material to help mitigate impingement and dorsal translation of the ulna relative to the radius.

- Adjunctive procedures incorporate some type of tendon transfer or interpositional material to stabilize the resected ulnar stump (**FIG 5**). The pronator quadratus, extensor carpi ulnaris, and flexor carpi ulnaris tendons have been used alone and in combination.
- In addition to tendon transfer, some authors have recommended suturing the ulnar capsule to the dorsal ulnar stump to help stabilize the remaining ulna.[19] Kleinman and Greenberg[10] advocated use of a dynamic pronator quadratus interosseous transfer in conjunction with an extensor carpi ulnaris distal tenodesis for failed distal ulna resections. More recently, allograft soft tissue interposition has been advocated,[11] as well as distal ulna implant arthroplasty.[24]
- Most adjunctive procedures have been described for treatment of a failed symptomatic Darrach procedure; however, they can be incorporated during the initial surgery. Symptomatic convergence tends to develop in a relatively younger, higher-demand patient. If distal ulna resection is necessary in this patient population, use of an adjunctive procedure is recommended.

Preoperative Planning

- The ideal candidate for a Darrach resection is a patient with a relatively low-demand upper extremity that does not require the load-bearing DRUJ.
- Coexisting pathology is frequently present in patients with distal ulna dysfunction, especially in patients with inflammatory arthropathy. Assessing for associated tenosynovitis and tendon ruptures is necessary.
  - The status of the radiocarpal joint is critical. Patients with loss of radial-sided carpal support due to tenosynovitis often have ulnar translation. In advanced cases, the carpus may abut the distal ulna and isolated Darrach resection without carpal stabilization is contraindicated to avoid exacerbating ulnar translation.
- If a limited resection of the distal ulna is considered, one must evaluate the length of the ulna, ulna variance, and position of the styloid. If stylocarpal abutment exists, it will persist after limited resection. Therefore, consideration needs to be

given to a joint leveling procedure or styloid recession in conjunction with limited resection.

- Alternatively, a complete distal ulna resection that addresses the ulna head as well as the styloid or a Sauvé-Kapandji DRUJ arthrodesis may be considered.

Positioning

- The patient is positioned supine. The operative arm is extended with the shoulder abducted at 90 degrees. The arm is supported on a standard table used for upper extremity surgery.
- A tourniquet is used.
- The motion of the elbow and shoulder should be noted before surgery. Limited passive motion can create awkward arm positioning.

Approach

- The incision used for distal ulna resection is based on whether the resection is performed alone or in conjunction with other procedures (**FIG 6**).
- The recommended approach for distal ulna resections is dorsal, deep to the fifth extensor compartment.
- A medial approach between the extensor carpi ulnaris and flexor carpi ulnaris tendons is not recommended. This approach has greater potential for disrupting the linea jugata, with resultant potential extensor carpi ulnaris destabilization.

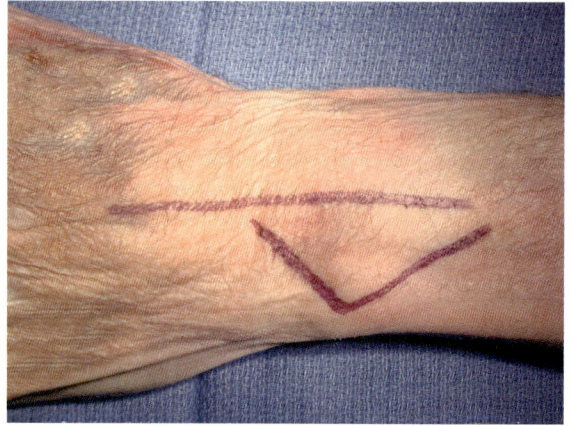

FIG 6 • Options for incisions when approaching the distal radioulnar joint and triangular fibrocartilage. The longitudinal incision is frequently used in patients undergoing complex reconstructions involving the distal radioulnar joint and radiocarpal or midcarpal joint. This incision is also recommended in patients requiring extensor tendon reconstruction in conjunction with treatment of the distal radioulnar joint. The chevron incision, with its distal limb paralleling the dorsal sensory branch of the ulnar nerve, is recommended for isolated arthroplasty of the distal radioulnar joint.

TECHNIQUES

COMPLETE DISTAL ULNA RESECTION: THE DARRACH PROCEDURE

Incision and Dissection

- Frequently, Darrach resection is performed in conjunction with other procedures, especially in patients with inflammatory arthropathies. In this situation, the surgical incision is usually dorsal midline longitudinal, which enables all aspects of the wrist reconstruction (wrist fusion, arthroplasty, tenosynovectomy, tendon transfer, etc.) to be completed via a single approach.
- If the Darrach procedure is to be performed independently, a single oblique or chevron dorsal approach is made (Fig 6) overlying the fifth dorsal compartment.
- During the dissection to the retinacular layer, take care to avoid injury to the transverse retinacular branch and dorsal sensory branch of the ulnar nerve that pass from the medial forearm to the dorsal hand between the ulnar styloid and pisiform (**TECH FIG 1A**).
  - Keep the oblique incision or distal limb of the chevron approach parallel to this nerve to minimize this complication.
- Frequently, dorsal capsular reinforcement is necessary after distal ulna resection. This is especially true in patients with inflammatory arthropathies and multiple extensor tendon ruptures.
  - When performed in conjunction with other procedures, raise opposing extensor retinacular flaps so that one of the flaps can be used to reinforce the dorsal capsule and create a stabilizing extensor carpi ulnaris sling during closure (**TECH FIG 1B,C**).
  - When performed as an isolated procedure, raise a retinacular flap from the margin of the fourth dorsal compartment (**TECH FIG 1D**).

Capsulotomy and Osteotomy

- Perform a longitudinal capsulotomy deep to the fifth dorsal compartment (**TECH FIG 2A**). This capsular approach starts proximal to the dorsal radioulnar ligament and proceeds in a proximal direction.
  - Extend the capsular release parallel and just proximal to the dorsal radioulnar ligament to facilitate exposure. Take care during the deep periosteal dissection

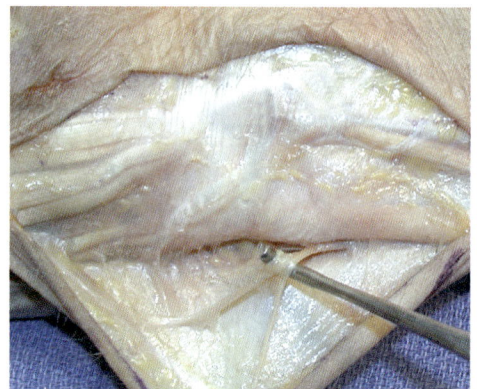

A

TECH FIG 1 • **A.** The dorsal sensory branch of the ulnar nerve, held in the retractor, passes from volar to dorsal just distal to the head of the ulna. It is vulnerable in all approaches to the distal radioulnar joint and triangular fibrocartilage and should be protected. *(continued)*

B

C

D

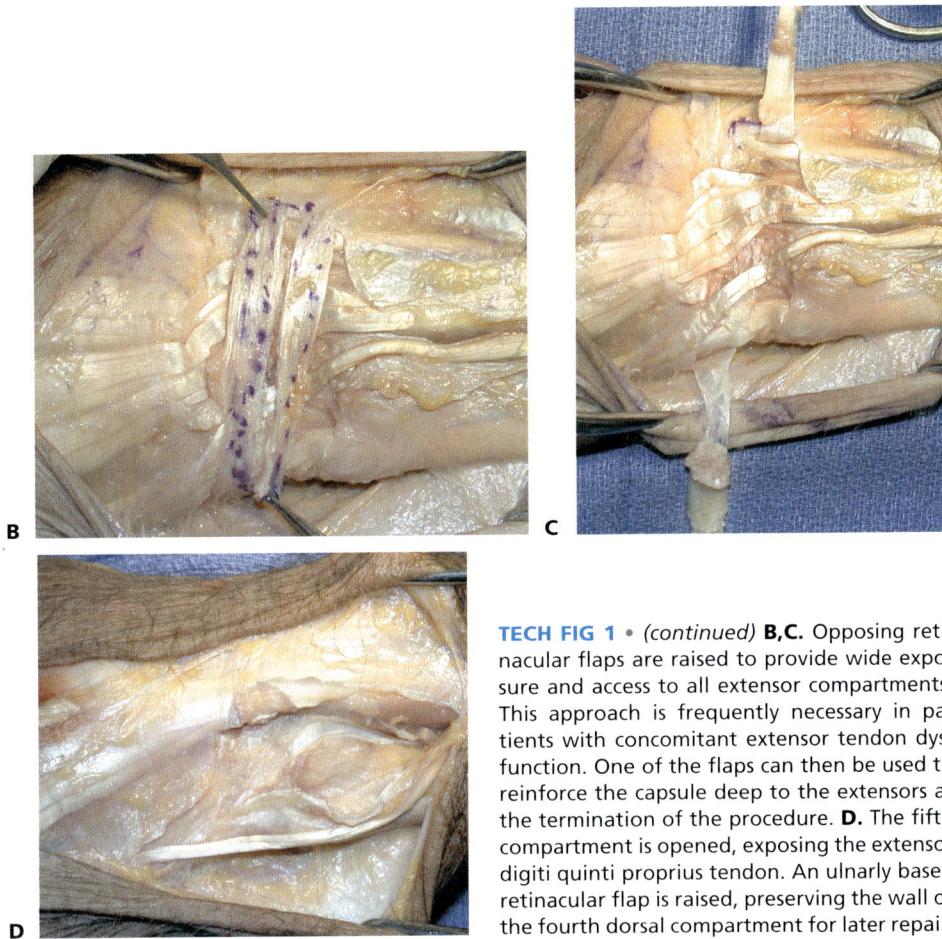

TECH FIG 1 • *(continued)* **B,C.** Opposing retinacular flaps are raised to provide wide exposure and access to all extensor compartments. This approach is frequently necessary in patients with concomitant extensor tendon dysfunction. One of the flaps can then be used to reinforce the capsule deep to the extensors at the termination of the procedure. **D.** The fifth compartment is opened, exposing the extensor digiti quinti proprius tendon. An ulnarly based retinacular flap is raised, preserving the wall of the fourth dorsal compartment for later repair.

to elevate and maintain as thick a periosteal sleeve as possible.

- Osteotomize the distal ulna using a power oscillating saw just proximal to the sigmoid notch (**TECH FIG 2B**). Enough ulna is sacrificed to completely decompress the DRUJ. Keep resection to 2 cm or less.

- Intraoperative fluoroscopic guidance is frequently helpful to assist with the location of the osteotomy.
- Once the distal pole and seat are resected, there is no advantage to preserving the ulnar styloid, and the entire styloid should be removed with the distal ulna.

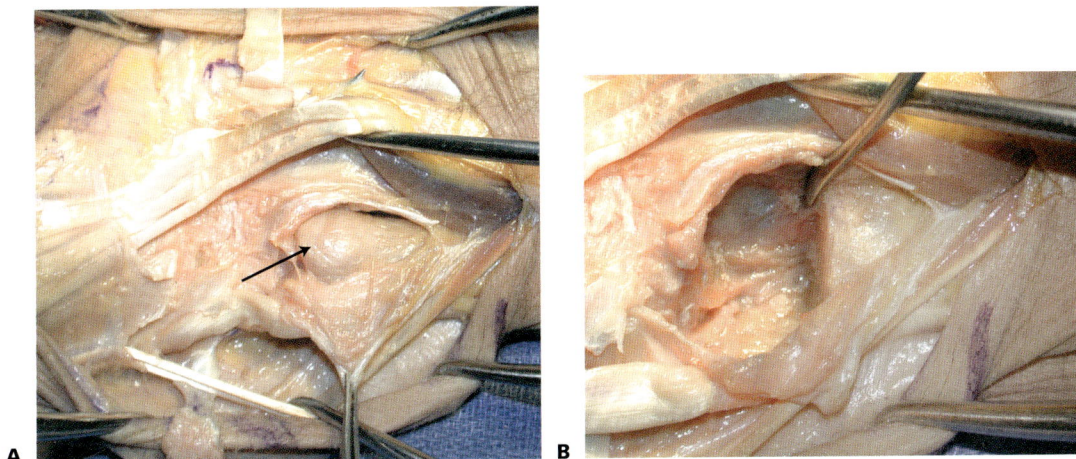

A

B

TECH FIG 2 • **A.** A longitudinal capsulotomy exposes the distal ulna (*arrow*) and allows access to the distal metaphysis, depending on the reconstruction being performed. **B.** The distal ulna has been osteotomized just proximal to the sigmoid notch. The resection should be less than 2 cm and should clear all abnormal bony elements that may affect rotation from within the sigmoid notch.

TECHNIQUES

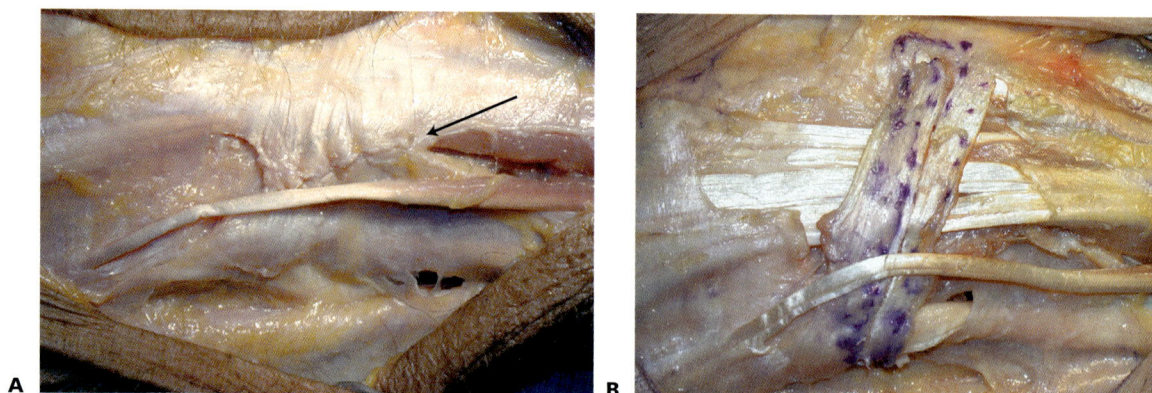

TECH FIG 3 • **A.** Closure is performed (*arrow*), leaving the extensor digiti quinti proprius (EDQP) superficial to the retinaculum. **B.** In another example, both retinacular flaps have been closed deep to the EDQP but superficial to the other extensors. If capsular reinforcement is necessary, the distal flap can be closed deep to the extensors. The ulnar portion of the proximal radially based flap is used to reinforce the sixth dorsal compartment.

Wound Closure

- Meticulous attention to closure is imperative.
- Perform a secure multilayered closure. Perform separate closure of the periosteal and capsular layers with nonabsorbable sutures.

- Suture the retinacular flaps for capsular reinforcement.
  - Transpose the EDQP tendon dorsal to the extensor retinaculum. This does not create any functional disability (**TECH FIG 3**).
- Routine skin closure follows.

DISTAL ULNA HEMIRESECTION-INTERPOSITION TECHNIQUE

- The surgical approach for the HIT procedure as developed by Bowers is identical to the Darrach resection. The difference lies in the treatment of the bone and soft tissue interposition after bone resection.
- Instead of resecting the distal ulna at the proximal margin of the sigmoid notch, the osteotomy removes the seat and pole of the ulnar head (**TECH FIG 4A,B**). The entire shaft and the styloid are left intact.
- After resection, the forearm is rotated through a full arc. This ensures that prominent osteophytes or bone that may interfere with forearm rotation have been removed.

- The resected shaft should be round in cross-section and should taper distally. The resection is lateral to the insertion of the deep portion of the TFC, so the integrity of both the deep and superficial components of the TFC is maintained. If the TFC is incompetent or cannot be made functionally competent by reconstruction, then there are no advantages over the Darrach complete distal ulna resection.
- Convergence of the radius and ulna develops after ulnar head resection. To mitigate this, the ulnarly based capsular flap raised during the approach is interposed between the radius and resected ulna. Interposition bulk may be increased by using a free tendon graft (**TECH FIG 4C**).

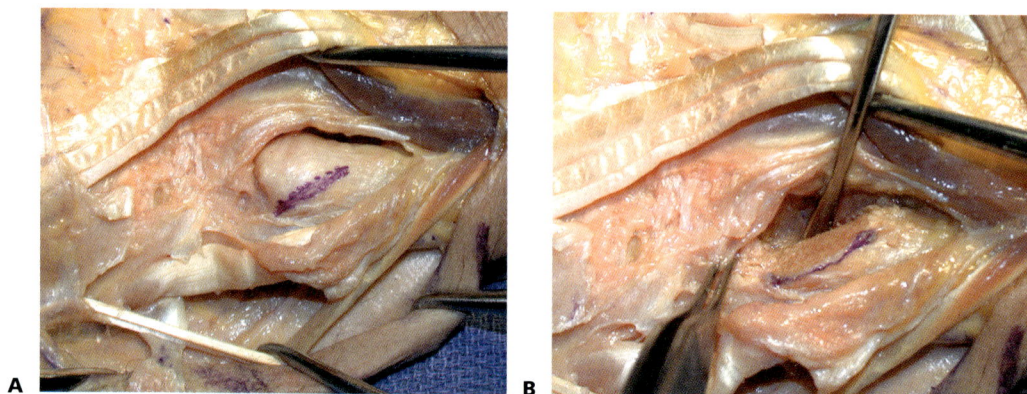

TECH FIG 4 • **A.** The level of osteotomy for the hemiresection-interposition technique (HIT) procedure is marked before osteotomy. **B.** This osteotomy eliminates the entire ulnar head but leaves the attachments of the triangular fibrocartilage intact. *(continued)*

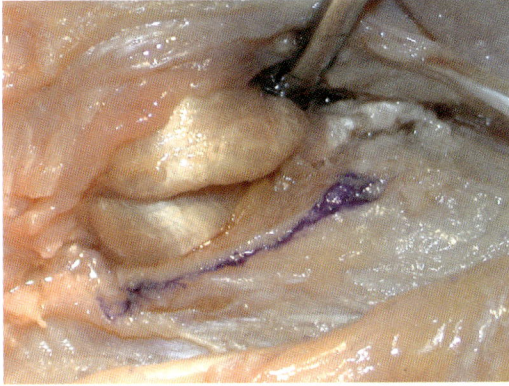

TECH FIG 4 • *(continued)* **C.** After osteotomy and removal of the ulnar head, the space is filled with a free tendon graft that provides bulky tissue and mitigates impingement of the resected ulna against the medial wall of the distal radius.

Modification

- In an effort to avoid an interpositional tendon graft, Adams[1] advocates a modification of the HIT procedure.
- In this technique, an ulnar-based retinacular flap is raised from the radial margin of the extensor carpi ulnaris sheath.
- Only 3 to 7 mm of bone is resected, and the ulna is tapered distally in a dowel shape. The fovea is not violated, thereby preserving all TFC attachments.
- The retinacular flap is then interposed and sutured to the volar DRUJ capsule. As in other procedures, attention is paid to avoid stylocarpal impingement.

MATCHED DISTAL ULNA RESECTION

- In this modification, developed by Watson, the distal ulna is resected in a long, sloping convex curve that matches the opposing concave radius (**TECH FIG 5**).
- The surgical approach is identical to the approaches listed for prior procedures. Although Watson advocated a transverse incision just proximal to the DRUJ, I prefer a more utilitarian longitudinal or chevron incision as previously described.
- The entire 270-degree arc of the ulna is addressed. Similar to the HIT procedure, great care is taken after bone resection to ensure full, unimpeded forearm rotation. Any osteophytes or prominent bone that may interfere with rotation must be removed.
- This technique differs from the HIT procedure since the ulna is reshaped over a longer distance and no interposition material is used. While this technique is advocated to preserve the ulnar sling, by necessity the resection sacrifices both the deep and superficial insertions of the TFC. Any resultant stability of the residual stump of the ulna is generated only by soft tissue scarring.

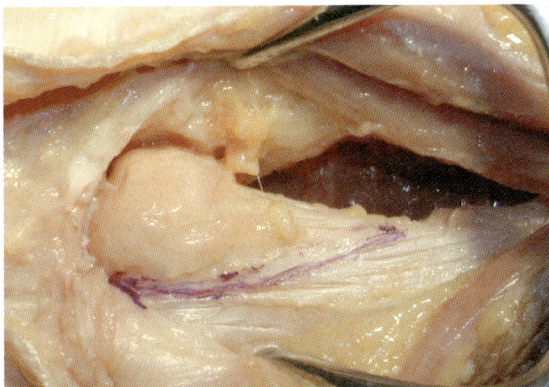

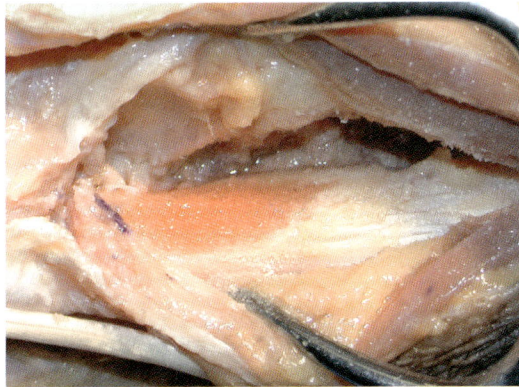

TECH FIG 5 • The matched resection osteotomy is more proximal than the Bowers osteotomy (**A**) and is resected in a long, sloping curve matching the opposite concave surface of the radius through a complete 270-degree arc (**B**).

PEARLS AND PITFALLS

Indications	■ Consider distal ulna resection as a final salvage procedure. Consider alternative procedures that will preserve the load-bearing fulcrum of the DRUJ. Distal ulna resections are tolerated in a relatively older, lower-demand patient.
Associated conditions	■ Diagnose and treat associated bone and soft tissue pathology. Consider the effects of distal resection on the radiocarpal joint.
Approach	■ Meticulous attention to soft tissue handling and avoiding injury to cutaneous nerves is essential. Raise retinacular and capsular flaps carefully so they can be used for stabilization or interposition if necessary. Avoid destabilizing the extensor carpi ulnaris. If the extensor carpi ulnaris sheath is violated and stability needs to be restored, reconstruct the sheath using retinacular flaps.
Bone resection	■ Decompress the entire length of the sigmoid notch when performing a Darrach resection. Avoid removing the insertions of the TFC during the HIT procedure. Ensure that full forearm rotation is possible after bone resection. Similarly, after partial distal ulna resection, eliminate any remaining osteophytes or bony prominences to ensure full range of motion. Assess for postresection stylocarpal impingement, and correct length if impingement is present.
Convergence and instability	■ Consider additional procedures that may stabilize or prevent symptomatic convergence and impingement, especially in the younger, more active, higher-demand patient.
Aftercare	■ Maintain neutral forearm rotation with a long-arm or Munster-type splint for the first 3 postoperative weeks. Allow gentle forearm rotation until 6 weeks postoperatively. Full activity is allowed at 3 months postoperatively.

POSTOPERATIVE CARE

■ Postoperatively, the extremity is maintained in a long-arm bulky dressing with the elbow at 90 degrees and the forearm supinated for 3 weeks. At 3 weeks postoperatively, long-arm splintage between exercises and at night begins and persists until 6 to 8 weeks postoperatively. Strengthening without splint immobilization can begin at that time.

OUTCOMES

■ In general, distal ulna resections are associated with relief of pain and restoration of function. Elderly patients with lower demands on the upper extremities tend to have more favorable results than younger, active, higher-demand patients.

■ Good results regarding relief of pain and recovery of function can be expected in 60% to 95% of patients with rheumatoid arthritis.[5] Early clinical reports on the Darrach resection demonstrated marked improvement in pain and range of motion in greater than 80% of patients; however, other series do not present such optimistic clinical results.

■ Leslie et al[12] in 1990 and Melone and Taras[14] in 1991 demonstrated 85% and 86% favorable results, respectively. Fraser et al's 1999 study[6] supported the use of the Darrach resection in patients with rheumatoid arthritis, finding 85% good to excellent results in 23 patients with rheumatoid arthritis versus only 36% satisfactory results in 27 patients with posttraumatic arthritis.

■ George et al[7] demonstrated satisfactory results in 21 patients treated with Darrach resections compared to a group who underwent Sauvé-Kapandji resection. They concluded that results were comparable and unpredictable. Despite reported complications, authors have advocated the use of the Darrach resection for patients with rheumatoid arthritis, emphasizing attention to correct technique as a critical factor in the procedure's success.[9,16]

■ Compiled results using the HIT procedure for a variety of afflictions indicate that 76% of patients are pain-free and 24% report mild pain.[4,8,15,25]

■ Minami et al[16] demonstrated better clinical outcomes using the HIT or Sauvé-Kapandji procedure than the Darrach procedure in 61 patients with osteoarthritis. This study supports the use of the Darrach procedure for the lower-demand, elderly patient. Van Schoonhoven and Lanz[20] advocate use of partial resection of the ulnar head in cases of instability or radial malunion associated with arthrosis. These authors feel that maintaining the remaining contact of the TFC adds a biomechanical advantage to prevent secondary problems after resection.

■ Two publications on the matched resection report good to excellent results in 24 of 32 patients with posttraumatic or mechanical disorders of the DRUJ[10] and no or mild pain in 44 patients, most with rheumatoid arthritis.[22] Weinzweig and Watson[23] report excellent results in their entire series of 97 wrists over 21 years. Pain was improved in 14 of 15 patients with rheumatoid arthritis in Srikanth et al's clinical study.[18]

COMPLICATIONS

■ Persistent pain
■ Distal ulnar stump instability (coronal, sagittal)
■ Radioulnar impingement
■ Loss of forearm rotation
■ Ulnar translation due to loss of ulnar support in rheumatoid arthritis
■ Extensor tendon rupture
■ Soft tissue irritation
■ Cutaneous nerve injury
■ Stylocarpal impingement
■ Complex regional pain syndrome
■ Extensor carpi ulnaris tendinitis or instability

REFERENCES

1. Adams BD. Distal radioulnar joint instability. In: Green DP et al, eds. Green's Operative Hand Surgery. Philadelphia: Churchill Livingstone, 2005.
2. Berger RA, Tay SC, Tomita K. The "ulna fovea sign" for defining ulna wrist pain: an analysis of sensitivity and specificity. J Hand Surg Am 2007;32A:438–444.

3. Bowers WH. Distal radioulnar joint arthroplasty: the hemiresection-interposition technique. J Hand Surg Am 1985;10A:169–178.

4. Bowers WH, Zelouf DS. Treatment of chronic disorders of the distal radioulnar joint. In: Lichtman DM, ed. The Wrist and its Disorders, 2nd ed. Philadelphia: WB Saunders, 1997.

5. DeSmet L. The distal radioulnar joint in rheumatoid arthritis. Acta Orthop Belgica 2006;72:381–386.

6. Fraser KE, Diao E, Peimer CA, et al. Comparative results of resection of the distal ulna in rheumatoid arthritis and post-traumatic conditions. J Hand Surg Br 1999;24B:667–670.

7. George MS, Kiefhaber TR, Stern PJ. The Sauvé-Kapandji procedure and the Darrach procedure for distal radioulnar joint dysfunction after Colles' fracture. J Hand Surg Br 2004;29B:608–613.

8. Glowacki KA. Hemiresection arthroplasty of the distal radioulnar joint. Hand Clin 2005;21:591–601.

9. Greenberg JA. Resection of the distal ulna: the Darrach procedure. Hand Clin 2000;5:19–30.

10. Greenberg JA, Kleinman WB. Salvage of the failed Darrach procedure. In: Gelberman RH, ed. The Wrist. Philadelphia: Lippincott Williams & Wilkins, 2002.

11. Greenberg JA, Sotereanos D. Achilles allograft interposition for failed Darrach distal ulna resections. Tech Hand Upper Extrem Surg 2008; 12:121–125.

12. Leslie BM, Carlson G, Ruby LK. Results of extensor carpi ulnaris tenodesis in the rheumatoid wrist undergoing a distal ulnar excision. J Hand Surg Am 1990;15A:547–551.

13. McKee M, Richards R. Dynamic radio-ulnar convergence after the Darrach procedure. J Bone Joint Surg Br 1996;78B:413–418.

14. Melone CP, Taras JS. Distal ulna resection, extensor carpi ulnaris tenodesis, and dorsal synovectomy for the rheumatoid wrist. Hand Clin 1991;7:335–343.

15. Minami A, Kaneda K, Itoga H. Hemiresection-interposition arthroplasty of the distal radioulnar joint associated with repair of triangular fibrocartilage complex lesions. J Hand Surg Am 1991;16A:1120–1125.

16. Minami A, Iwasaki N, Ishikawsa JI, et al. Treatments of osteoarthritis of the distal radioulnar joint: long-term results of three procedures. Hand Surg 2005;10:243–248.

17. Papp SR, Athwal GS, Pichora DR. The rheumatoid wrist. J Am Assoc Orthop Surg 2006;14:65–77.

18. Srikanth KN, Shahane SA, Stilwell JH. Modified matched ulnar resection for arthrosis of distal radioulnar joint in rheumatoid arthritis. Hand Surg 2006;11:15–19.

19. Syed AA, Lam WL, Agarwal M, et al. Stabilization of the ulna stump after Darrach's procedure at the wrist. Int Orthop 2003;27:235–239.

20. Van Schoonhoven J, Lanz U. Salvage operations and their differential indications for the DRUJ. Orthopade 2004;33:704–714.

21. Watson HK, Gabuzda GM. Matched distal ulna resection for post-traumatic disorders of the distal radioulnar joint. J Hand Surg Am 1992;17A:724–730.

22. Watson HK, Ryu J, Burgess RC. Matched distal ulnar resection. J Hand Surg Am 1986;11A:812–817.

23. Weinzweig J, Watson HK: Matched ulnar resection arthroplasty. In: Gelberman RH, ed. The Wrist. Philadelphia: Lippincott Williams & Wilkins, 2002.

24. Willis AA, Berger RA, Cooney WP. Arthroplasty of the distal radioulnar joint using a new ulnar head endoprosthesis: preliminary report. J Hand Surg Am 2007;32A:177–189.

25. Zelouf DS, Bowers WH, Osterman AL. Distal radioulnar joint reconstruction: hemiresection-interposition technique and Sauvé-Kapandji. In: Osterman AL, Katzman B, and Feldon P, eds. Atlas of the Hand Clinics: Rheumatoid Arthritis of the Wrist. Philadelphia: WB Saunders, 2005.

Chapter 92

Sauvé-Kapandji Procedure for Distal Radioulnar Joint Arthritis

Robert M. Szabo

DEFINITION

- Disorders of the distal radioulnar joint (DRUJ) are a significant source of wrist pain for patients.
- The etiology of symptoms referable to this joint includes displaced fractures or malunions of the distal radius, which cause pain with forearm pronation–supination, and tears of the triangular fibrocartilage complex (TFC), which result in DRUJ instability, mechanical symptoms, and pain.
- Both Madelung deformity[23] and rheumatoid arthritis (RA) can display secondary incongruity of the DRUJ, causing pain and loss of forearm rotation. Radial head fracture treated by resection and subsequent shortening of the radius (Essex-Lopresti lesion) also can result in painful incongruity or instability of the DRUJ.
- Management of DRUJ pain, incongruity, or instability alone is challenging, but the Sauvé-Kapandji procedure is one solution that treats all three disorders.[11,20]

ANATOMY

- The DRUJ is a distal articulation in the biarticulate rotational arrangement of the forearm that allows one degree of motion: pronation and supination. The sigmoid notch of the radius is concave, with a 15-mm radius of curvature.
    - The ulnar head is semicylindrical, with a radius of curvature of 10 mm, and has an articulate convexity of 220 degrees. It is surrounded by the ulnolunate and ulnotriquetral ligaments, which originate from the palmar radioulnar ligament near the ulnar styloid.
    - The TFC is a fibrocartilaginous disc originating at the junction of the lunate fossa and the sigmoid notch inserting at the base of the ulnar styloid. Its central portion is cartilaginous and avascular and is designed for weight bearing.
    - The peripheral margins, the dorsal and palmar radioulnar ligaments, are thick lamellar cartilage designed for tensile loading. They are well vascularized from the palmar and dorsal branches of the anterior interosseous artery and from the ulnar artery.
    - The ulnar styloid acts as a strut on the end of the ulna to stabilize the ulnar soft tissues of the wrist. The sheath of the extensor carpi ulnaris (ECU), the ulnocarpal ligaments, and the TFC attach at the base of the ulnar styloid and together are known as the TFCS.
- The radius of curvature of the head of the ulna does not equal that of the sigmoid notch. In the extremes of pronation–supination, less than 10% of the ulnar head may be in contact with the notch. In pronation, the ulnar head translates 2.8 mm dorsally from a neutral position and in supination the ulnar head translates 5.4 mm volarly from a neutral position.
    - The stability of the DRUJ comes from the joint surface morphology, the joint capsule, the dorsal and palmar radioulnar ligaments, the interosseous membrane, and the musculotendinous units that cross the joint, primarily the ECU and pronator quadratus (PQ). The PQ actively stabilizes the joint by coapting the ulnar head in the sigmoid notch in pronation and passively by viscoelastic forces in supination. The ECU is retained over the dorsal distal ulna by a separate fibro-osseous tunnel deep to and separate from the extensor retinaculum, allowing unrestricted rotation of the radius and ulna.[18]

PATHOGENESIS

- Traumatic injury to the wrist can lead to derangement of the DRUJ, which can result in instability and eventually painful degenerative changes.
- Distal radial malunions with dorsal or volar subluxations or dislocations of the DRUJ produce secondary rupture, elongation, or functional shortening of the distal radioulnar ligaments.
- Arthritis of the DRUJ is a common complication of Colles fractures, particularly when fractures involve the sigmoid notch.
- Congenital disorders such as Madelung disease as well as traumatic epiphyseal closures of the distal radius can produce marked positive ulnar variance with dorsal dislocation of the DRUJ.
- In the rheumatoid wrist, progression of distal radioulnar synovitis typically results in the "caput ulnae syndrome" as described by Backdahl, which consists of the following:
    - Wrist weakness with pain on pronation and supination
    - Dorsal prominence of the ulnar head
    - Limitation of pronation and supination
    - Swelling of the distal radioulnar area
    - Secondary tendon changes with possible extensor tendon rupture and ECU subluxation[1]
    - If allowed to progress without intervention, the carpus will eventually fall in a more ulnarward and palmarward direction, with strength, mobility, and function all suffering.[21]
- A chronically unstable DRUJ without degenerative changes can be treated with various soft tissue reconstructions, depending on the abnormalities and underlying pathology.
    - As a group, many of these reconstructions fail to restore stability; even if stability is restored, limitation of forearm motion persists.

NATURAL HISTORY

- The natural history of DRUJ derangement is painful limitation of forearm rotation, often with additional functional deficits.
    - When positive ulnar variance exceeds a few millimeters, additional limitations of wrist flexion–extension as well as radial–ulnar deviation movements can occur.

PATIENT HISTORY AND PHYSICAL FINDINGS

- Clinical evaluation begins with a detailed and accurate history.
  - A history of fracture involving the forearm or wrist is clearly important. Patients may recall a specific injury involving damaging forces of torque with axial load applied to the involved wrist and forearm.
  - The patient's occupation or hobbies may give insight into the mechanism of injury as well as the most important functional deficits currently experienced by the patient.
  - A complete medical history is important, including questions about inflammatory arthritis or osteoarthritis.
- DRUJ pathology most often causes ulnar-sided wrist pain, diminished grip strength, limited forearm pronation and supination, and limited wrist ulnar deviation.
  - Pain is exacerbated with activity and increases with resisted rotation of the forearm.
  - With large ulnar length discrepancy (positive ulnar variance), limited flexion–extension also can be seen.
- During the physical examination, the clinician should determine whether loss of forearm rotation is solely due to DRUJ pathology or if there is a concurrent problem at the proximal radioulnar joint or interosseous membrane. Other sources of wrist pain and dysfunction must be ruled out.
  - The clinician should check for instability or chronic dislocation of the joint, comparing the injured with the uninjured wrist.
  - The patient's normal and affected wrist and forearm ranges of motion, both active and passive, should be measured. A rigid endpoint with loss of motion suggests bony pathology such as fracture malunion, whereas a soft endpoint with limited motion suggests soft tissue contractures.
  - The clinician should carefully palpate, ballote, and compress around the DRUJ and compare the findings to the opposite side. Grip strength measurements should be checked bilaterally.
  - When evaluating patients with RA, the clinician should try to distinguish the pain and instability of the DRUJ from radiocarpal and midcarpal joint symptoms by careful palpation, ballottement, and compression of areas around the DRUJ, comparing the degree of symptoms elicited by forearm rotation versus wrist flexion–extension.
- Examinations to perform include:
  - Piano key test. The test, which isolates DRUJ disorders, is positive if it causes pain and/or crepitus.
  - Selective anesthetic injections. The test is positive when precise, selective injection of anesthetic into the area eliminates pain and improves function. Injections help to confirm pathologic changes and can be used to distinguish intra-articular from extra-articular lesions.
  - Ulnocarpal compression test. A positive test reproduces the ulnar-sided wrist pain and grinding by translating force across the TFC. It also isolates pathologic changes in the TFC.
  - Lunotriquetral (Regan) shuck test. Pain, sometimes with increased joint mobility and grinding, represents a positive test. This test detects and assesses abnormalities or pathologic conditions associated with the lunotriquetral joint.

IMAGING AND OTHER DIAGNOSTIC STUDIES

- Standard neutral rotation posteroanterior (PA), lateral, and ulnar variance radiographs of the wrist should be obtained and compared with the normal side. The clinician should look for evidence of fractures, arthritic changes, bone lesions, and distal ulna position relative to the radius.
- Forearm and elbow radiographs are obtained if there is a history of an elbow injury (especially a radial head fracture) or forearm injury.
- If ulnocarpal abutment is suspected, a PA radiograph is obtained with the forearm in pronation and the fist clenched. This will increase ulnar variance and potentially reveal ulna impaction.
- CT is best to evaluate subluxation and articular congruity of the distal radioulnar joint.[4,18] To assess the distal radioulnar articular surfaces, simultaneous views are obtained of both extremities with the forearms in neutral rotation, full supination, and full pronation.
- MRI with single-injection gadolinium arthrography (MRA) is a good way to evaluate TFC lesions as well as the integrity of the scapholunate and lunotriquetral interosseous ligaments.

DIFFERENTIAL DIAGNOSIS

- Extensor carpi ulnaris tendinitis or subluxation
- Flexor carpi ulnaris tendinitis
- Pisotriquetral arthritis
- Lunotriquetral ligament tear
- TFC tear
- Acute DRUJ dislocation

NONOPERATIVE MANAGEMENT

- A trial of nonoperative management is helpful for some patients with DRUJ disorders.
- Minor strains of the DRUJ capsule or sprains of other ulnar-sided wrist ligaments may respond to rest, ice after activity, wrist splints, and oral anti-inflammatory medications.
- Easily reducible dislocations of the DRUJ can be treated by immobilization in a rigid splint or cast for 6 weeks.
- Inflammation of the ulnar-sided wrist tendons often accompanies DRUJ problems.
  - Tendinitis should be treated first with stretching exercises, other physical therapy modalities, and sometimes a steroid injection before addressing the DRUJ surgically.

SURGICAL MANAGEMENT

- The Sauvé-Kapandji procedure is especially useful for patients with RA. Despite advanced radiographic findings of radiocarpal or midcarpal arthritis, complaints of wrist pain can be relieved in many RA patients by addressing the DRUJ pathology with a Sauvé-Kapandji procedure.
  - Commonly, resection of the distal end of the ulna, the Darrach procedure, is recommended for patients with RA and ulnar-sided wrist pain. However, the inflammatory changes and deforming forces acting on the hand and wrist in RA tend to cause palmar and ulnar translocation of the wrist, resulting in decreased mobility, strength, and function. Removal of the distal ulna exacerbates and accelerates the problem.

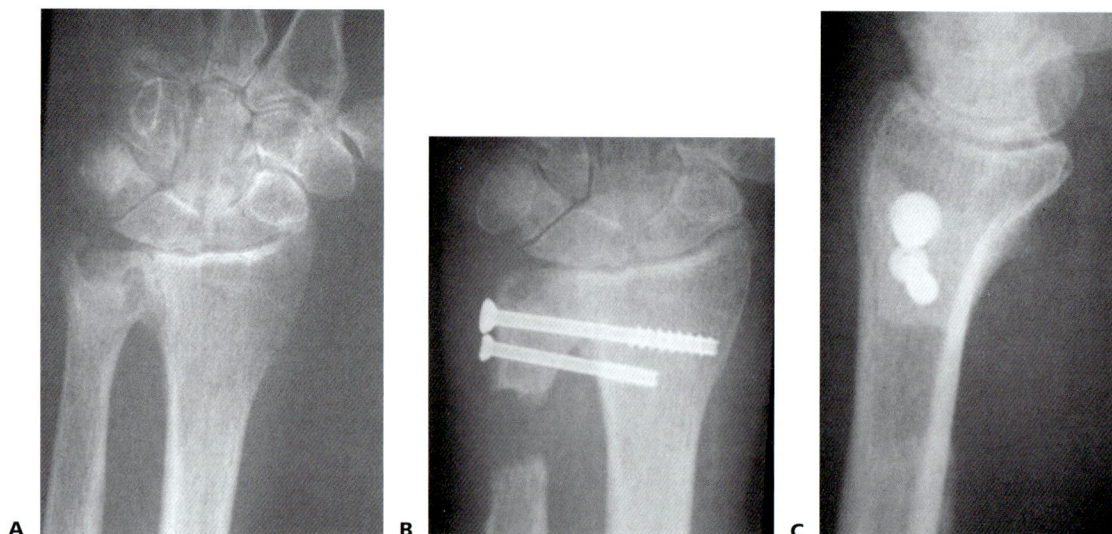

FIG 1 • Radiographs from a patient with rheumatoid arthritis before (**A**) and after (**B,C**) a Sauvé-Kapandji procedure.

■ With the Sauvé-Kapandji procedure, the retained distal ulna provides bony support for the ulnar corner of the wrist to help stabilize against the palmar–ulnar slide of the carpus (**FIG 1**). In addition, the important attachments of the ulno-carpal complex are preserved.[21]

■ The Sauvé-Kapandji procedure is also beneficial in the treatment of DRUJ disorders resulting from trauma.

■ In cases of wrist trauma with ulnar-sided ligamentous injury and incompetence, retaining the ulnar head, as is performed with a Sauvé-Kapandji reconstruction, maintains the ulnocarpal buttress and the TFC to allow a more physiologic transmission of load from the hand to the forearm.

■ The osteotomy made in the ulna in the Sauvé-Kapandji procedure allows as much shortening as is needed to match the level of the radius while retaining supination and pronation.

■ Other surgical options include hemiresection and interposition arthroplasty, matched resection of the distal part of the ulna, Darrach resection, and more recently prosthetic replacement.[2]

Preoperative Planning

■ The clinician should review preoperative radiographs and carefully assess whether fixation of the ulna head can be performed before any osteotomy or if an osteotomy and excision of the ulna segment needs to be done first to restore proper length and head position into the sigmoid fossa.

Positioning

■ The patient is positioned supine with the upper extremity on a hand table.

■ A pneumatic tourniquet is placed on the arm.

■ An intraoperative fluoroscope is draped sterile and made available throughout the procedure.

TECHNIQUES

AUTHOR'S PREFERRED TECHNIQUE FOR THE SAUVÉ-KAPANDJI PROCEDURE

Incision and Dissection

■ Make a straight longitudinal incision, 6 to 8 cm long, along the ulnar border of the distal forearm.

■ An alternative incision may be used if additional procedures are planned at the same sitting. For example, in patients with RA, often the Sauvé-Kapandji procedure needs to be combined with another soft tissue procedure such as a dorsal wrist synovectomy, tenosynovectomy, or tendon transfer to treat extensor tendon ruptures that result from the caput ulnae syndrome. If that is the case, start the incision more dorsally to facilitate exposure for the additional procedure, and then extend it proximally and obliquely to expose the distal ulna.

■ Identify the dorsal cutaneous branch of the ulnar nerve and protect it throughout the case (**TECH FIG 1**).

■ Expose the distal 4 to 6 cm of the ulna extraperiosteally through the interval between the ECU and flexor carpi ulnaris (FCU).

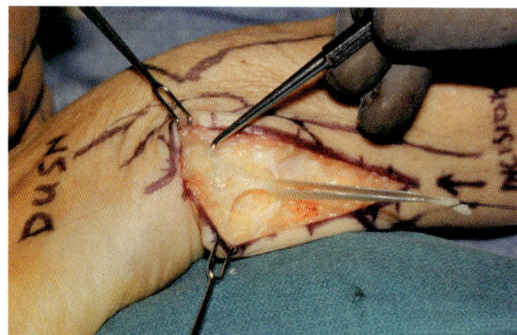

TECH FIG 1 • Identification and mobilization of the dorsal sensory ulnar nerve, which is tagged with a rubber dam. Notice a dorsal branch under the probe.

Osteotomy of the Ulnar Diaphysis

- Select the appropriate level for an osteotomy of the ulnar diaphysis (**TECH FIG 2A**).
- Cut the bone just proximal to the flare of the ulnar head; this will leave enough of the distal ulna to accommodate two fixation screws.
- Confirm with fluoroscopy that the proposed osteotomy site is appropriate.
- Make a second cut proximal and parallel to the first (**TECH FIG 2B**), and remove a 10- to 14-mm segment of ulna (**TECH FIG 2C**). Resect the periosteum in the region of the gap and irrigate thoroughly to remove bone debris.
  - If there is a positive ulnar variance, remove a correspondingly longer segment of the ulna so that when the ulnar head is recessed to neutral ulnar variance, the resulting gap will be adequate.
- Save the removed bone for subsequent grafting into the DRUJ arthrodesis site (**TECH FIG 2D**).

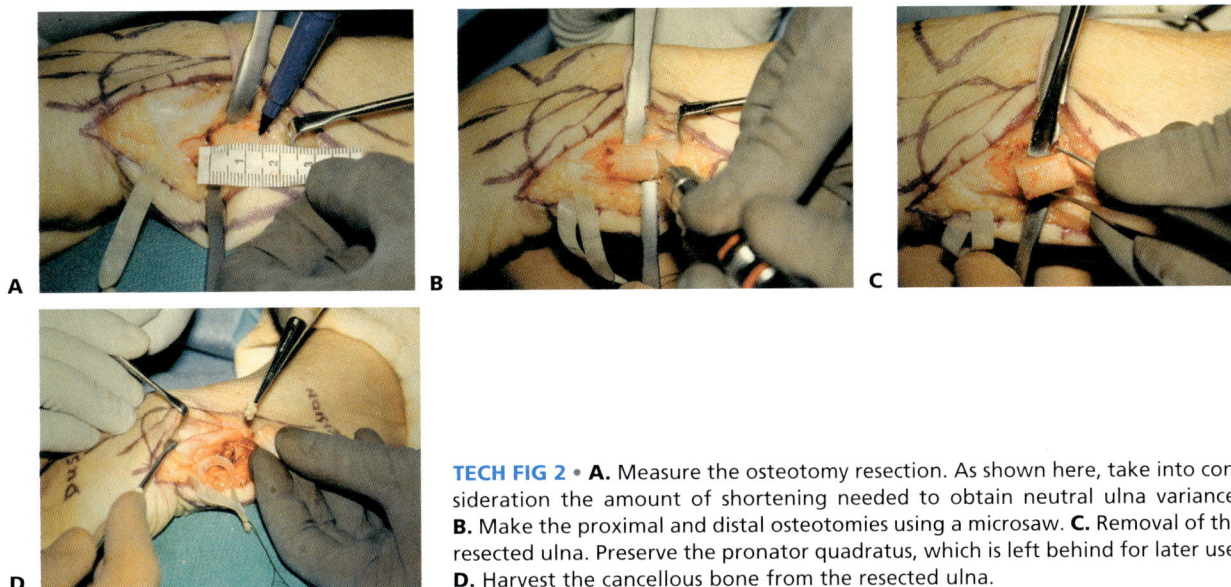

TECH FIG 2 • A. Measure the osteotomy resection. As shown here, take into consideration the amount of shortening needed to obtain neutral ulna variance. **B.** Make the proximal and distal osteotomies using a microsaw. **C.** Removal of the resected ulna. Preserve the pronator quadratus, which is left behind for later use. **D.** Harvest the cancellous bone from the resected ulna.

Distal Radioulnar Joint Exposure and Preparation

- Expose the DRUJ with a dorsoulnar capsulotomy just radial to the ECU tendon.
- Denude both the ulnar head and sigmoid fossa of the radius of all remaining cartilage to create flush surfaces of cancellous bone on each side of the arthrodesis site, and pack the harvested cancellous bone from the removed ulna segment (**TECH FIG 3**).
  - In patients with severe bone loss, after decortication of the corresponding articular surfaces of the DRUJ, sculpt the resected segment of the ulna to fit into the space between the ulnar head and sigmoid notch as a corticocancellous bone graft.

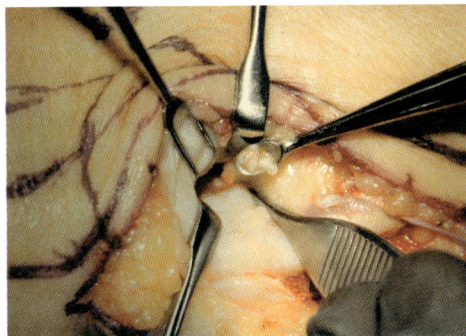

TECH FIG 3 • Curette the sigmoid notch of any remaining cartilage and then pack in the bone graft from the resected ulna.

Fixation

- Cannulated self-tapping screws are preferable to K-wires for fixation of the arthrodesis site.
  - K-wires can irritate cutaneous nerves when buried or can cause wound problems when placed percutaneously.
  - There is usually no need to remove hardware when screws are used, and rehabilitation can begin sooner because of secure fixation.
  - Cannulated screws over guidewires allow accurate screw placement and facilitate the alignment of the cortices of the distal ulna and radius.
- Establish ulnar neutral variance by moving the ulnar head proximally or distally to bring its distal surface parallel with the distal radius surface; confirm correct placement fluoroscopically.
  - Do this while holding the forearm in neutral rotation with the patient's elbow resting on the operating table while supporting the forearm perpendicular to the table in neutral rotation.
  - Temporarily fix the ulnar head to the sigmoid notch of the distal part of the radius with a single K-wire, and ensure proper position with fluoroscopy.
- While maintaining neutral forearm rotation, drill two guidewires across the DRUJ to stabilize the ulnar head in proper position.
  - Place one wire a few millimeters proximal to the subchondral bone of the distal ulna, and position the second wire proximal enough to allow for seat-

TECHNIQUES

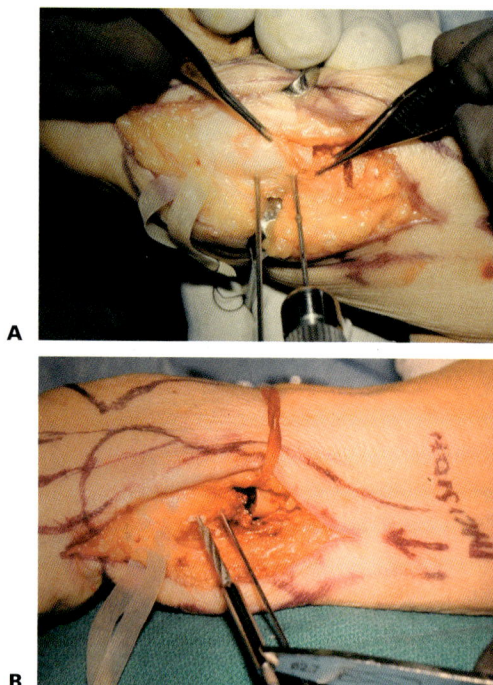

TECH FIG 4 • **A.** Placement of the two K-wires to stabilize the ulna head. **B.** Drill over the K-wires, measure, and put in the screws.

ing of both screw heads without impingement (**TECH FIG 4A**).

- Confirm correct placement of the guidewires with fluoroscopy.

- Advance the distal wire into the far (radial) cortex of the radius and measure for screw length.

  - The proximal screw provides rotational control and needs only tricortical fixation. It can be 5 mm shorter than the distal screw.

- After the screw lengths are measured, advance the wires through the skin to the radial side of the forearm with a mallet and grasp them with a clamp to avoid having the wire come out during drilling and screw placement.

  - With a mallet, the chances of injuring a branch of the radial sensory nerve branch are less than those with a power driver.

- Drill over the guidewires with a cannulated drill bit (**TECH FIG 4B**).

- Pack additional cancellous bone harvested from the excised ulnar segment into the DRUJ space.

- Insert the selected screws over the guidewires while manually compressing the ulnar head against the radius.

- Tighten the distal screw first to avoid compressing the radial and ulnar shafts together and levering the ulnar head out of position.

- Do not use lag-screw technique on the proximal screw, and avoid tilting the head of the ulna; it must remain parallel to the long axis of the ulnar shaft.

Extensor Carpi Ulnaris Stabilization of the Proximal Ulna Stump[14,15]

- After fixation of the DRUJ, drill a 3.5-mm hole from the dorsoulnar aspect of the ulnar shaft proximal stump into its intramedullary cavity.

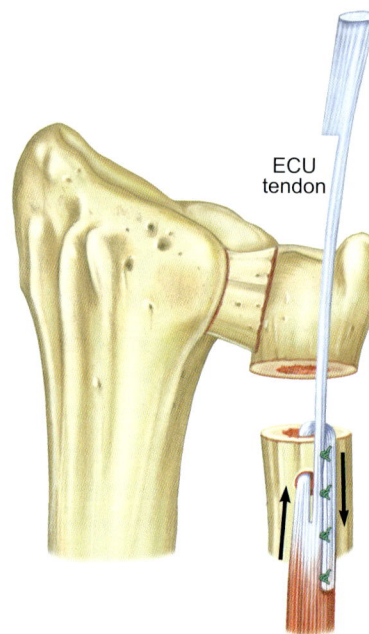

TECH FIG 5 • Modification of the Sauvé-Kapandji procedure with ECU tenodesis as described by Minami et al.[14] After the Sauvé-Kapandji procedure, a 3.5-mm hole was drilled from the dorsoulnar aspect of the ulnar shaft into the intramedullary cavity. The ECU tendon was then split in the central sulcus and the radial half released at the ulnocarpal level. It was then reflected proximally, leaving it attached at the musculotendinous junction. This proximally based strip was then passed into the medullary canal through the drill hole, retrieved at the distal stump of the ulna, and then sutured back on itself in an interlacing fashion.

- Split the ECU tendon in the central sulcus and release the radial half at the ulnocarpal level.

- Reflect this half of the ECU proximally, leaving it attached at the musculotendinous junction.

- Pass this proximally based strip, approximately 6 to 8 cm long, into the medullary canal through the drill hole, and retrieve it at the distal stump of the ulna, pulling it distally under moderate tension, and then suture it back onto itself in an interlacing fashion (**TECH FIG 5**).

Flexor Carpi Ulnaris Stabilization of the Proximal Ulna Stump[12]

- Over a distance of 8 to 10 cm through the volar aspect of the incision, isolate a distally based slip of FCU tendon (measuring about half the width of the tendon) attached to the pisiform.

- Drill a 4- to 4.5-mm hole on the volar cortex, 1 cm proximal to the end of the osteotomized surface of the proximal ulnar segment.

  - This is facilitated by inserting the drill bit obliquely through the medullary cavity in a dorsal to volar direction.

- Pass the slip of FCU tendon deep to the FCU muscle through the distal end of the ulnar stump, and loop it back on itself, securing it with nonabsorbable suture (**TECH FIG 6**).

- Suture the tendon under moderate tension, keeping the forearm in neutral rotation and the wrist in neutral flexion–extension and neutral radioulnar deviation.

Extensor carpi ulnaris

Flexor carpi ulnaris

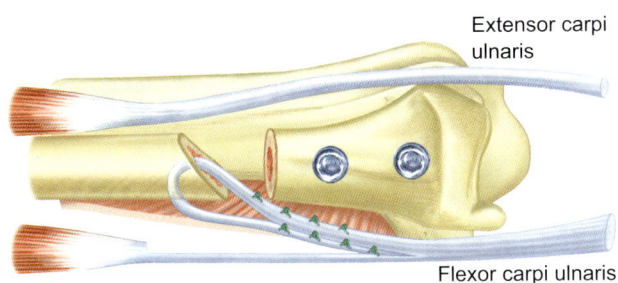

TECH FIG 6 • Modification of the Sauvé-Kapandji procedure with FCU tenodesis as described by Lamey and Fernandez.[12] Lateral aspect of the wrist, showing stabilization of the proximal ulnar segment with use of a distally based slip of the FCU tendon.

- Pull the pronator quadratus muscle into the gap in the ulna and suture it to the volar aspect of the tendon sheath of the ECU.
- Reattach the sixth dorsal compartment within the groove on the ulnar head and close the wound.

Wound Closure

- Make sure that there is a gap of 10 to 12 mm between the proximal and distal ulnar segments.
- Suture the fascia of the underlying pronator quadratus into the gap to prevent reossification across the pseudarthrosis site and stabilize the stump of the ulnar shaft (**TECH FIG 7A**).
- Repair the retinacular compartments (**TECH FIG 7B**) and close the skin in routine fashion.

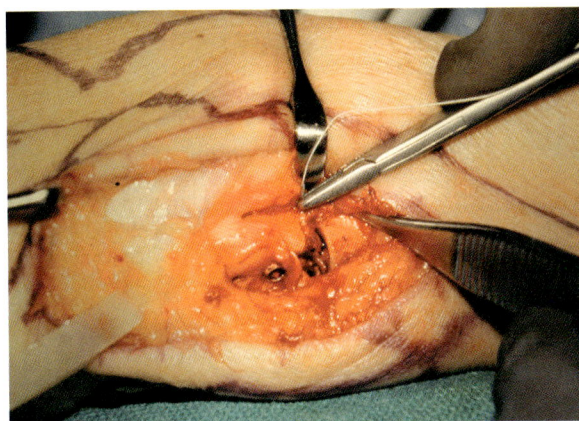

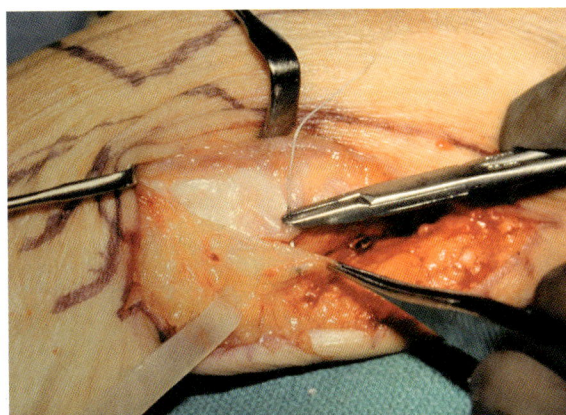

TECH FIG 7 • **A.** Suturing the pronator quadratus into the gap. **B.** Closure of the retinaculum.

TECHNIQUE FOR CASES CHARACTERIZED BY POOR BONE QUALITY (FUJITA TECHNIQUE[8,9])

- Make a 7-cm longitudinal skin incision on the dorsal aspect of the wrist centered on the ulna head (**TECH FIG 8A**).
- Open the fourth dorsal compartment. Divide the septum between the fourth and fifth compartments and reflect the retinaculum ulnarly to preserve a single common retinacular flap.
- Retract the extensor digitorum communis and extensor digiti minimi tendons radially and perform a neurectomy of the terminal branch of the posterior interosseous nerve.
- Incise the capsule of the DRUJ and dissect the distal part of the ulna subperiosteally.
- Perform an oblique osteotomy with an oscillating saw 30 mm proximal to the distal end of the ulna and excise the ulna head (**TECH FIG 8B**).
- Perform a synovectomy of the DRUJ and remove the periosteum of the resected portion of the ulna.
- Interpose the pronator quadratus muscle at the osteotomy site.
- Drill a hole 10 mm in diameter at the sigmoid notch of the radius while viewing the distal articular surface of

the radius through the TFC, which is usually ruptured. Do not penetrate the subchondral bone (**TECH FIG 8C**).
- Remove all soft tissue from the resected portion of the ulna and then rotate it 90 degrees and insert the cut end of the ulnar graft into the hole in the radius, creating a shelf 12 to 15 mm long.
- Impact the ulnar graft into the subchondral and cancellous bone of the distal part of the radius without penetrating the radial cortex, and fix it in the drill hole with a cancellous bone screw (**TECH FIG 8D**). Do not overtighten the screw.
- Cover the graft with the joint capsule contiguous with a periosteal flap.
- Mobilize and relocate the ECU tendon by dissecting the septum between the fifth and sixth compartments.
- If subluxation of the ECU tendon is evident during rotation of the forearm, reflect the distal portion of the periosteal flap ulnarly beneath the ECU tendon to act as a sling, and suture it to the adjacent soft tissue to restrain the ECU in a dorsal and radial position over the graft.
- Close in the fashion previously outlined.

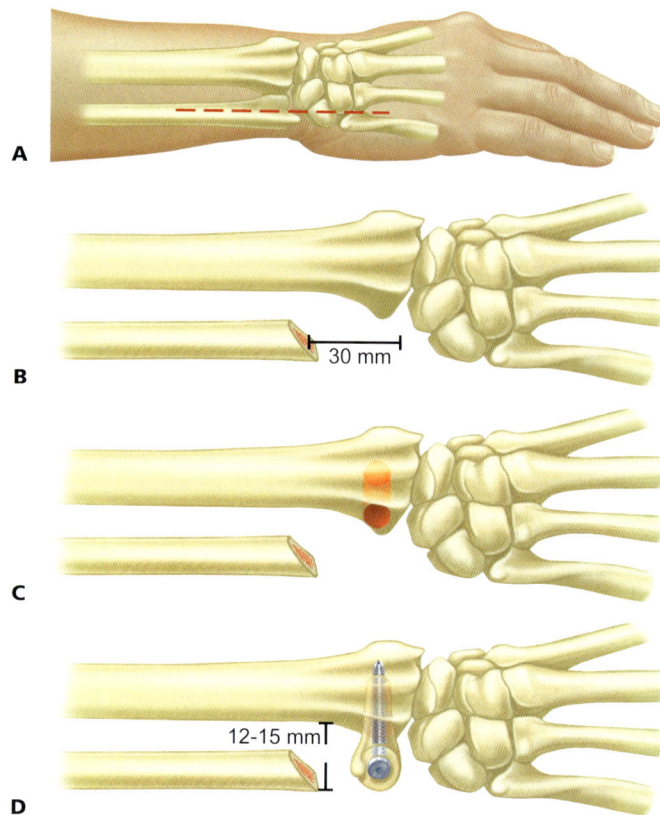

TECH FIG 8 • Modification of the Sauvé-Kapandji procedure with the distal ulna used as a bone peg as described by Fujita et al.[9] **A.** Make a 7-cm longitudinal skin incision on the dorsal aspect of the wrist centered on the ulna head. **B.** Perform an oblique osteotomy with an oscillating saw 30 mm proximal to the distal end of the ulna and excise the ulna head. **C.** Drill a hole 10 mm in diameter at the sigmoid notch of the radius while viewing the distal articular surface of the radius through the TFC, which is usually ruptured. Do not penetrate the subchondral bone. **D.** Remove all soft tissue from the resected portion of the ulna and then rotate it 90 degrees and insert the cut end of the ulnar graft into the hole in the radius, creating a shelf 12 to 15 mm long. Impact the ulnar graft into the subchondral and cancellous bone of the distal part of the radius without penetrating the radial cortex, and fix it in the drill hole with a cancellous bone screw.

PEARLS AND PITFALLS

Indications	■ Ulnocarpal pain should be distinguished from DRUJ pain. This procedure should not be done for a pain-free, stable DRUJ.
	■ If the DRUJ is unstable and arthritic, use of either the FCU or ECU tenodesis of the proximal ulna stump should be strongly considered.
	■ In patients with rheumatoid arthritis, DRUJ symptoms should be distinguished clinically, not radiographically, from radiocarpal symptoms. Many patients can be treated with the Sauvé-Kapandji procedure successfully despite radiocarpal changes on radiographs.
Technical details	■ The dorsal sensory branch of the ulnar nerve should be identified and protected to avoid neuromas and stretch injuries.
	■ Osteotomy of the ulna should be performed as distal as possible. To avoid stump instability, no more than 1 cm of ulna should be excised.

POSTOPERATIVE CARE

■ Rehabilitation after the Sauvé-Kapandji procedure follows guidelines published by Skirven.[16]

■ Postoperatively, a bulky dressing with plaster splints extending above the elbow, maintaining the forearm in neutral position, is applied for 7 to 10 days.

■ Sutures are then removed and the patient is given a removable, lightweight splint to support the wrist.

■ Hand therapy is initiated with an emphasis on gentle active wrist, digit, and forearm rotation exercises.

■ Except for exercise sessions and bathing, the splint is worn at all times.

■ In the postoperative period, the goal is to allow adequate healing by supporting and protecting the arthrodesis site from stress, followed by gradual restoration of functional mobility without sacrificing the stability of the ulnar shaft or the arthrodesis.

■ The arthrodesis is protected from loading forces for 4 to 6 weeks.

■ When the arthrodesis appears healed radiographically, usually 8 weeks postoperatively, light strengthening exercises are initiated. Heavy lifting and forearm torque are avoided until 3 months postoperatively.

■ For conservative management of postoperative instability of the ulnar shaft, Skirven has recommended a small, cuff-style splint to support the pseudarthrosis site and help stabilize the ulnar shaft.[16]

■ The splint, which is made of thermoplastic material, extends from the distal radius ulnarly to a few centimeters proximal to the pseudarthrosis site.

■ An adjustable strap allows the patient to set the tension on the splint to provide comfort and the level of stability required for specific activities.

OUTCOMES

- There is a broad international experience with this operation on many patients.
- Zimmermann in Austria retrospectively reported on 43 patients' clinical results and DASH questionnaires 8 years (range 5 to 12 years) after a Sauvé-Kapandji operation.[24] Forearm rotation improved in all patients. Ulnar wrist pain was diminished in 97% of the patients, and 9% had mild pain at the proximal ulnar stump. Grip strength compared to the contralateral side improved from a preoperative mean of 38% to a postoperative mean of 55%. The mean DASH score was 28 points (range 0 to 53 points). In all cases the arthrodesis fused within 8 weeks.
- In Australia, Millroy reported on 81 procedures in 71 patients and found that "almost all patients were pain free during normal activity, although 7 experienced discomfort with overuse."[13]
- In Belgium, De Smet conducted a prospective survey on 84 patients treated for posttraumatic arthritis of the DRUJ with the procedure.[7] According to the Mayo wrist score, there were 20 excellent, 34 good, 18 fair, and 12 poor results, with an overall satisfaction rate of 74%.
- In Denmark, Jacobsen found that 15 of 17 employed patients returned to work.[10]
- In England, Carter found that 86% of his patients would have the operation again.[3]
- In Germany, Daecke looked at the functional outcomes of 56 patients with the DASH and Mayo wrist scores as well as clinical results.[5] Although only 50% of patients were free of symptoms during heavy labor, 95% had excellent results. The postoperative DASH score was 24.2 ± 22.5 and the Mayo wrist score was 76.1 ± 17.6.
- In Switzerland, Lamey reported on 18 patients who underwent the Sauvé-Kapandji procedure with the FCU tenodesis of the ulna stump.[12] There were 6 excellent, 7 good, 4 fair, and 1 poor Mayo wrist scores. Eight of the patients who had performed heavy manual labor before the injury were able to return to work full-time without restrictions.
- Many other studies report similar outcomes, confirming the utility and broad appeal of this operation.

COMPLICATIONS

- The main source of complications from the Sauvé-Kapandji procedure is the distal stump of the ulna.
- Pain, ulnar impingement syndrome, and a feeling of instability of the ulnar shaft have been reported, but these symptoms are usually transient and resolve by 3 months postoperatively.
- Significant instability of the ulnar shaft is more commonly reported after the Darrach procedure, but it can also occur if too much bone is resected during the described procedure.[6]
  - To prevent instability, the surgeon should carefully stabilize the ulnar stump with pronator quadratus fascia advancement, should place the osteotomies as far distally as possible, and should not resect too much bone.
  - The surgeon should also avoid excessive stripping of the interosseous membrane. A soft tissue tube should surround the pseudarthrosis site to connect and stabilize the proximal and distal ulnar segments.

- Despite these precautions, painful instability of the distal ulnar stump can occur. In this scenario, the stump can be stabilized by using a strip of the ECU or FCU tendon based on its distal attachment.
- Another complication from the Sauvé-Kapandji procedure is ossification of the pseudarthrosis site.[6]
  - The pronator quadratus should be interposed in the ulnar gap after the osteotomy is complete and the ulnar segment should be removed extraperiosteally to minimize the occurrence of this complication.
  - If ossification does occur, the bone may be resected when mature. The patient should then immediately begin forearm rotation exercises.
- Injury of the dorsal cutaneous branch of the ulnar nerve is a potential problem and can be avoided with careful dissection.
- Wada and Ishii reported closed rupture of a finger extensor tendon after the Sauvé-Kapandji procedure. They postulated that this was due to the ulnar shaft stump's being left distal to the edge of the extensor retinaculum, causing attritional rupture of the tendon trapped between the bone edge and the retinaculum.[22]
  - This could be avoided by contouring the ulnar shaft edge to a smooth edge and covering the stump with the interposed pronator quadratus.
- Painful neuromas of the dorsal sensory branch of the ulna nerve have also been reported.
  - Lamey and Fernandez noted that this may be more common when harvesting a distally based slip of the FCU from one incision. They recommend this be done from a second incision.[12]
- Some patients develop hardware pain from palpable screw heads. These screws can be removed.

REFERENCES

1. Backdahl M. The caput ulnae syndrome in rheumatoid arthritis: a study of the morphology, abnormal anatomy and clinical picture. Acta Rheum Scand 1963;(Suppl)5:1–75.
2. Bowers WH. Distal radioulnar joint arthroplasty: current concepts. Clin Orthop Relat Res 1992;275:104–109.
3. Carter PB, Stuart PR. The Sauvé-Kapandji procedure for posttraumatic disorders of the distal radio-ulnar joint. J Bone Joint Surg Br 2000;82B:1013–1018.
4. Cone RO, Szabo R, Resnick D, et al. Computed tomography of the normal radioulnar joints. Invest Radiol 1983;18:541–545.
5. Daecke W, Martini AK, Streich NA. Kapandji-Sauvé procedure for chronic disorders of the distal radioulnar joint with special regard to the long-term results. Handchir Mikrochir Plast Chir 2003;35:164–169.
6. Daecke W, Martini AK, Schneider S, et al. Amount of ulnar resection is a predictive factor for ulnar instability problems after the Sauvé-Kapandji procedure: a retrospective study of 44 patients followed for 1–13 years. Acta Orthop 2006;77:290–297.
7. De Smet LA, Van Ransbeeck H. The Sauvé-Kapandji procedure for posttraumatic wrist disorders: further experience. Acta Orthop Belg 2000;66:251–254.
8. Fujita S, Masada K, Takeuchi E, et al. Modified Sauvé-Kapandji procedure for disorders of the distal radioulnar joint in patients with rheumatoid arthritis. J Bone Joint Surg Am 2005;87A:134–139.
9. Fujita S, Masada K, Takeuchi E, et al. Modified Sauvé-Kapandji procedure for disorders of the distal radioulnar joint in patients with rheumatoid arthritis. Surgical technique. J Bone Joint Surg Am 2006;88A(Suppl 1 Pt 1):24–28.

10. Jacobsen TW, Leicht P. The Sauvé-Kapandji procedure for posttraumatic disorders of the distal radioulnar joint. Acta Orthop Belg 2004; 70:226–230.

11. Kapandji IA. The Kapandji-Sauvé operation. Its techniques and indications in nonrheumatoid diseases. Ann Chir Main 1986;5:181–193.

12. Lamey DM, Fernandez DL. Results of the modified Sauvé-Kapandji procedure in the treatment of chronic posttraumatic derangement of the distal radioulnar joint. J Bone Joint Surg Am 1998;80A:1758–1769.

13. Millroy P, Coleman S, Ivers R. The Sauvé-Kapandji operation. Technique and results. J Hand Surg Br 1992;17B:411–414.

14. Minami A, Kato H, Iwasaki N. Modification of the Sauvé-Kapandji procedure with extensor carpi ulnaris tenodesis. J Hand Surg Am 2000;25A:1080–1084.

15. Minami A, Suzuki K, Suenaga N, et al. The Sauvé-Kapandji procedure for osteoarthritis of the distal radioulnar joint. J Hand Surg Am 1995;20A:602–608.

16. Skirven T. Rehabilitation following surgery for the distal radioulnar joint. Tech Hand Upper Extrem Surg 1997;1:219–225.

17. Slater RR Jr, Szabo RM. The Sauvé-Kapandji procedure. Tech Hand Upper Extrem Surg 1998;2:148–157.

18. Szabo RM. Distal radioulnar joint instability. J Bone Joint Surg Am 2006;88A:884–894.

19. Szabo RM, Anderson KA, Chen JL. Functional outcome of en bloc excision and osteoarticular allograft replacement with the Sauvé-Kapandji procedure for Campanacci grade 3 giant-cell tumor of the distal radius. J Hand Surg Am 2006;31A:1340–1348.

20. Taleisnik J. The Sauvé-Kapandji procedure. Clin Orthop Relat Res 1992;275:110–123.

21. Vincent KA, Szabo RM, Agee JM. The Sauvé-Kapandji procedure for reconstruction of the rheumatoid distal radioulnar joint. J Hand Surg Am 1993;18A:978–983.

22. Wada T, Ogino T, Ishii S. Closed rupture of a finger extensor following the Sauvé-Kapandji procedure: a case report. J Hand Surg Am 1997;22A:705–707.

23. White GM, Weiland AJ. Madelung's deformity: treatment by osteotomy of the radius and Lauenstein procedure. J Hand Surg Am 1987;12A:202–204.

24. Zimmermann R, Gschwentner M, Arora R, et al. Treatment of distal radioulnar joint disorders with a modified Sauvé-Kapandji procedure: long-term outcome with special attention to the DASH Questionnaire. Arch Orthop Trauma Surg 2003;123:293–298.

Chapter 93

Ulnar Head Implant Arthroplasty

Cari Cordell and Randy R. Bindra

DEFINITION

- As with any synovial joint, the distal radioulnar joint (DRUJ) can degenerate due to osteoarthritis, inflammatory arthritis, chronic instability, infection, and trauma.
- Standard treatments such as partial ("matched resection") or complete (Darrach procedure) distal ulnar resection have the potential to destabilize the forearm axis and cause painful forearm rotation.
  - The normal compressive muscle forces acting between the radius and ulna help stabilize the DRUJ.
  - When the distal ulna has been resected and the forearm is rotated under such a compressive load, a palpable grinding between the ulnar stump and the radius may develop; this is referred to as ulnar impingement. This may progress from minor irritation to painful erosion of the radius. These patients present with pain on stress loading of the upper extremity, weakness in grip strength, decreased forearm rotation, and difficulty with lifting.[1]
- Ulnar head implant arthroplasty is designed to maintain the DRUJ, thereby avoiding ulnar impingement. An adequate soft tissue envelope repaired over the implant provides stability.
  - The first prosthesis used was a silicone cap designed to provide a soft end to the ulnar stump. These prostheses understandably failed under loading.
  - Newer designs aim to restore the ulnar head using a metallic prosthesis to articulate with the sigmoid notch.

ANATOMY

- See Chapters HA-5, HA-49, HA-50, HA-51, HA-91, HA-92, and HA-95.

PATHOGENESIS

- See Chapters HA-91 and HA-92.

NATURAL HISTORY

- See Chapters HA-91 and HA-92.

PATIENT HISTORY AND PHYSICAL FINDINGS

- Patients who have had an ulnar head resection complain of painful forearm rotation, often associated with instability of the forearm axis, decreased strength, and joint grinding.
- In addition to recording the range and fluidity of DRUJ motion, the examiner must determine the stability of the joint and the contribution of ulnar impingement to the patient's pain.
- Radioulnar compression creates radioulnar impingement by external passive compression.
  - The examiner should encircle the patient's distal forearm with his or her hands and apply firm compression.
  - A positive sign is reproduction of the patient's pain.
- Active radioulnar impingement is reproduced by active muscle contraction, specifically the brachialis.
  - The patient has pain lifting a load of 2 lbs with the forearm in neutral position.
- Ulnar stump instability results from compromised soft tissue stabilizers of the distal stump, which tends to fall away from the radius as the forearm is rotated.
  - The patient is asked to actively rotate the forearm. Dorsal and palmar subluxation of the ulnar stump is visible.

IMAGING AND OTHER DIAGNOSTIC STUDIES

- Standard posteroanterior, lateral, and oblique radiographs of the wrist
  - These x-rays demonstrate scalloping of the ulnar cortex of the radial metaphysis and some corresponding pencilling of the distal ulnar stump.
- Posteroanterior stress-loaded radiographs
  - May demonstrate impingement between the radius and ulna
  - The patient stands with the involved forearm facing the x-ray tube. The wrist is stress-loaded by asking the patient to hold a 2.2-kg lead cylinder with the shoulder adducted, the elbow flexed to 90 degrees, and the forearm in the position of neutral rotation.
  - The forearm rests on the x-ray cassette and the radiograph is then taken with the beam aligned in the coronal plane, creating a posteroanterior view of the neutral forearm.
  - Radiographs are obtained before and after stress-loading.
- CT scanning
  - In patients with osteoarthritis of the DRUJ, axial scans are essential for evaluation of the extent of degenerative changes in the ulnar head and the need for total or partial replacement.
  - CT scanning is also essential for evaluation of the sigmoid notch for osteophytes and erosion in patients with painful ulnar head replacement.
  - CT scanning with forearm in pronation and supination is also useful in detecting radioulnar instability if clinical examination is equivocal.

DIFFERENTIAL DIAGNOSIS

- In addition to radioulnar impingement, a patient who has pain at the DRUJ after resection of the ulnar head may have pain due to the following conditions:
  - Ulnar neuropathy
  - Painful surgical scar due to sensory nerve injury or scarring
  - Radiocarpal or midcarpal arthritis

NONOPERATIVE MANAGEMENT

- Activity modification to minimize forearm rotatory movements will diminish pain.
- A Russe splint is partially helpful for patients with instability of the distal ulna stump but is of no help in preventing radioulnar impingement pain.

SURGICAL MANAGEMENT

- The most common indication for distal ulnar implant arthroplasty is to relieve impingement symptoms in patients who have undergone previous ulnar head resection.
- Other less common indications include:
  - Treatment of patients with primary degenerative arthritis of the DRUJ who have failed to respond to splinting and steroid injections
  - Reconstruction of the ulna after excision of a tumor involving the ulnar head
  - After unreconstructable fractures of the ulnar head as either a primary or delayed procedure
  - Relative indication: patients with well-controlled inflammatory arthritis but well-preserved bone stock
- The amount of the DRUJ that is replaced may vary for any given case.
  - Partial ulnar head replacement
  - Unconstrained replacement of the entire distal ulna with or without sigmoid notch resurfacing
  - Constrained total DRUJ replacement, including the sigmoid fossa of the distal radius
- Partial ulnar head replacement preserves the styloid process and the attachment of the triangular fibrocartilage.
  - This procedure is indicated when the disease process, typically arthritis, is limited to the distal ulnar articular surface.
  - Contraindications include instability of the distal ulna, excessive ulnar positive variance, and degeneration at the sigmoid notch.
  - Two types of implants are available: a one-piece stemmed metal prosthesis and a two-piece prosthesis with a titanium stem and an articulating pyrolytic carbon disc that replaces the head (**FIG 1**).
  - The long-term results of partial ulnar head replacement are not known. The articulating two-piece prosthesis has the theoretical advantage of less radius erosion from articulation with the pyrocarbon head.
- Unconstrained complete ulnar head replacement is indicated for reconstruction of ulnar impingement after resection or replacement of an arthritic DRUJ associated with insta-

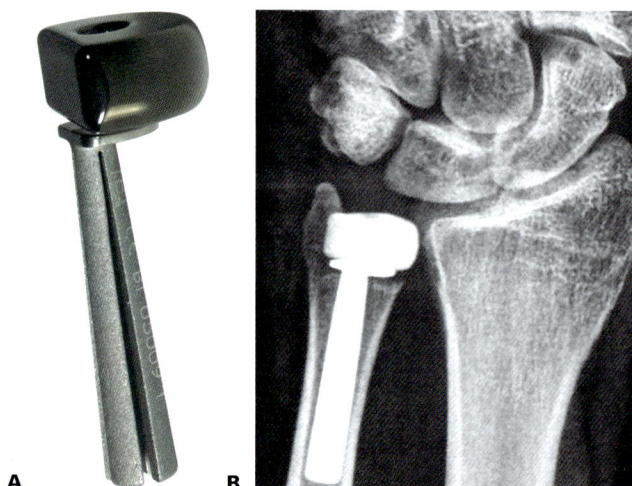

FIG 1 • The Eclypse partial ulnar head replacement (Tornier Surgical Implants, FR) consists of an expandable titanium stem with a mobile pyrocarbon spacer (*left*). When implanted, the prosthesis preserves the ulnar styloid and attachment of the triangular fibrocartilage complex (*right*).

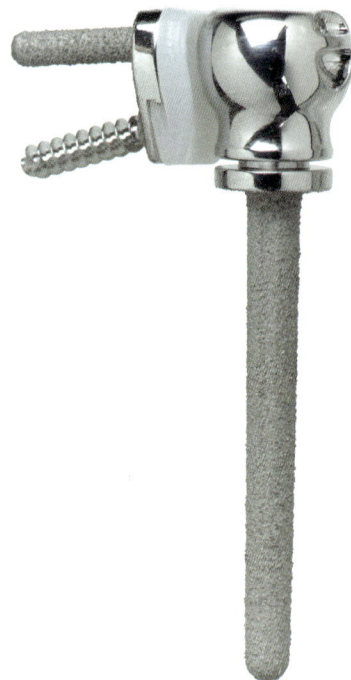

FIG 2 • The Stability total ulnar head arthroplasty system (Small Bone Innovations, Inc.) consists of a metal ulnar head component that articulates with a metal-backed polyethylene sigmoid notch. The ulnar head component can be used individually as a hemiarthroplasty.

bility of the distal ulna. With mild instability, repair of the soft tissue envelope is adequate to restore stability. In cases with more obvious instability, an additional soft tissue procedure is indicated along with ulnar head replacement.

- Ulnar head prostheses are generally spherical and made of metal or ceramic. An eccentric-shaped metallic head has been designed to more closely approximate the shape of the normal head. However, biomechanical studies have demonstrated normal tracking patterns of the distal ulna around the radius, closely simulating the normal joint, even with the use of spherical heads.
- Ulnar head prostheses may articulate with a metal-backed polyethylene resurfacing of the sigmoid notch in an unconstrained manner (**FIG 2**).
- An adequate soft tissue envelope is essential to prevent subluxation of a complete ulnar head replacement. The triangular fibrocartilage complex (TFCC) is no longer attached to the distal ulna, making the prosthesis prone to dislocation. Thus, an essential part of the surgical technique is reconstructing the capsuloligamentous envelope surrounding the ulnar prosthesis.
- Other contraindications include previous open fracture, infection in or around the joint, skeletal immaturity, and known sensitivity to the implant materials.
- In cases of marked instability, with lack of an adequate soft tissue stabilizing envelope and ablation of the DRUJ after trauma or tumor resection, a constrained total DRUJ replacement should be used (**FIG 3**).
  - The radial component consists of a plate with a polyethylene-lined metal sphere affixed to the interosseous surface of the radius.
  - The ulnar stem has a protruding peg that is captured and rotates within the polyethylene liner. The stem has limited

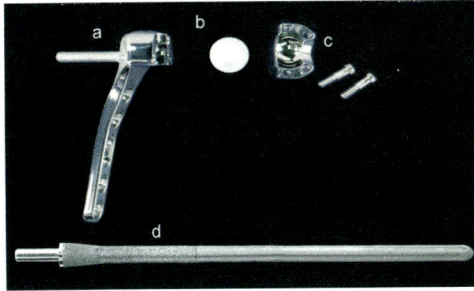

FIG 3 • The Aptis system (Aptis Medical) replaces the entire distal radioulnar joint with a constrained articulation. The components include (*a*) radial plate with socket, (*b*) polyethylene ball, (*c*) hemi-socket with screws, and (*d*) ulnar stem with peg.

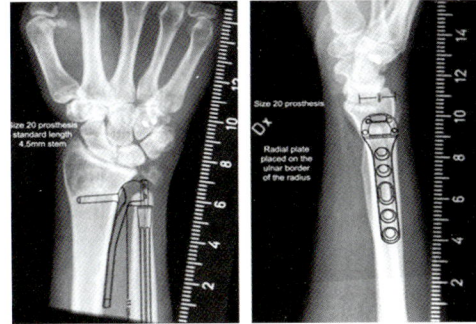

FIG 4 • Preoperative templating for the Aptis system is done in the frontal and lateral planes to determine the appropriate size of implants to be used at surgery.

freedom of proximodistal and limited dorsopalmar motion, simulating normal DRUJ mechanics.

Preoperative Planning

- Preoperative radiographs of both sides are used for templating (**FIG 4**).
  - Normal anatomy and ulnar variance are reproduced to the extent possible.
  - The appropriate implant size is chosen.

Positioning

- Standard positioning and tourniquet application are used.

Approach

- An incision is made along the ulnar border of the shaft of the distal ulna in line with the ulnar styloid. The interval between the flexor carpi ulnaris (FCU) and extensor carpi ulnaris (ECU) tendons is developed for access to the ulna.
- A dorsal approach is an alternative and is indicated for partial head replacement. Access to the articular portion of the ulnar head is gained through the floor of the fifth extensor compartment.

PARTIAL ULNAR HEAD REPLACEMENT ARTHROPLASTY

- Make a longitudinal incision in line with the fourth metacarpal.
- Divide the extensor retinaculum over the fourth compartment and reflect it ulnarly.
- Retract the two slips of the extensor digiti minimi tendon and elevate a large ulnar-based triquetral flap of capsule.
  - The flap includes the dorsal radiotriquetral ligament distally.
  - The TFCC should be repaired back to bone if foveal detachment is detected.
- Leave in place the ECU subsheath and ECU tendon.
- Resect the articular portion of the ulnar head using a customized jig specific to the implant system to be used.
- Ream the ulnar medullary canal and place a trial prosthesis of the appropriate size. Obtain intraoperative radiographs to confirm correct sizing of head and ulnar variance.

- Ascertain range of motion and stability and insert a definitive prosthesis. Restore the capsular flap and imbricate it if necessary for stability (**TECH FIG 1**).

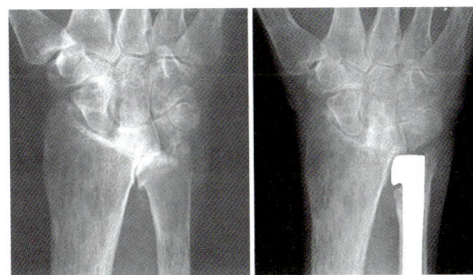

TECH FIG 1 • Pre- and postoperative radiographs of a patient with monoarticular rheumatoid arthritis treated with First Choice partial ulnar head arthroplasty (Ascension Inc).

ULNAR HEAD HEMIARTHROPLASTY (WITHOUT SIGMOID NOTCH RESURFACING)

- Make a longitudinal skin incision on the ulnar border of the distal forearm (**TECH FIG 2A**).
- Incise the extensor retinaculum along the medial border of the distal ulna between the ECU and FCU.
  - Identify and protect the dorsal cutaneous branch of the ulnar nerve as it crosses from volar to dorsal across the most distal part of the incision.

- Elevate the ECU tendon subsheath subperiosteally off the distal ulna along with the TFCC and ulnar collateral ligament distally.
- Determine the resection level of the distal ulna using a template and mark it with a pen or osteotome (**TECH FIG 2B**).

TECHNIQUES

TECHNIQUES

- The aim is to create ulnar neutral variance after the implant is in place.
- When the distal ulna has been previously excised, use the distal end of the sigmoid fossa of the distal radius as a landmark to determine the ulnar osteotomy level.
- With soft tissue retractors in place, use an oscillating saw to osteotomize the distal ulna (**TECH FIG 2C**).
  - Take care to ensure that the cut is perpendicular to the long axis of the ulna.
- Remove and size the ulnar head.
  - To allow for easy identification for soft tissue repair, place a tagging suture into the TFCC attachment in the fovea before releasing it from the ulna.
- Inspect the sigmoid notch of the distal radius for incongruity. Remove osteophytes.
- Define the intramedullary canal of the distal ulna using an awl or sharp broach. Gently enlarge the canal to the appropriate stem size using broaches of increasing diameter (**TECH FIG 2D**).
- Gently impact the appropriate trial stem into the shaft of the distal ulna (**TECH FIG 2E**). The collar should seat firmly against the resected surface of the distal ulna.
  - In cases with previous excessive ulnar resection, a prosthesis with an extended collar may be indicated.
  - To ascertain the need for an extended collar, place a trial spacer on the neck of the trial stem before placing the trial head.

- Place the trial head of the appropriate size onto the neck of the trial stem and reduce the DRUJ.
  - Supination and pronation should be full and smooth, with no instability at the articulation.
- Obtain intraoperative radiographs to evaluate the size of the ulnar head and the ulnar variance.
  - If the prosthesis is too distal, resection of more distal ulna is necessary.
- Remove the trial implant by gently applying anteriorly directed pressure on the distal ulna to dislodge the ulnar head from the sigmoid notch.
- If a firm fit is obtained with the trial, a press-fit technique may be used with the final implant. In patients with osteopenia or previous wrist fusion, use cement to secure the ulnar stem.
- Prepare the appropriately sized head for soft tissue stabilization before the stem is fully impacted. Pass two 3-0 nonabsorbable sutures with curved double needles through each row of holes in the prosthesis head. Pass the needles from the deeper suture through the TFCC at its previous foveal insertion, and insert the needles from the superficial suture into the ECU subsheath. Leave the sutures untied (**TECH FIG 2F**).
- Insert and impact the final stem (with or without cement) using the stem impactor.

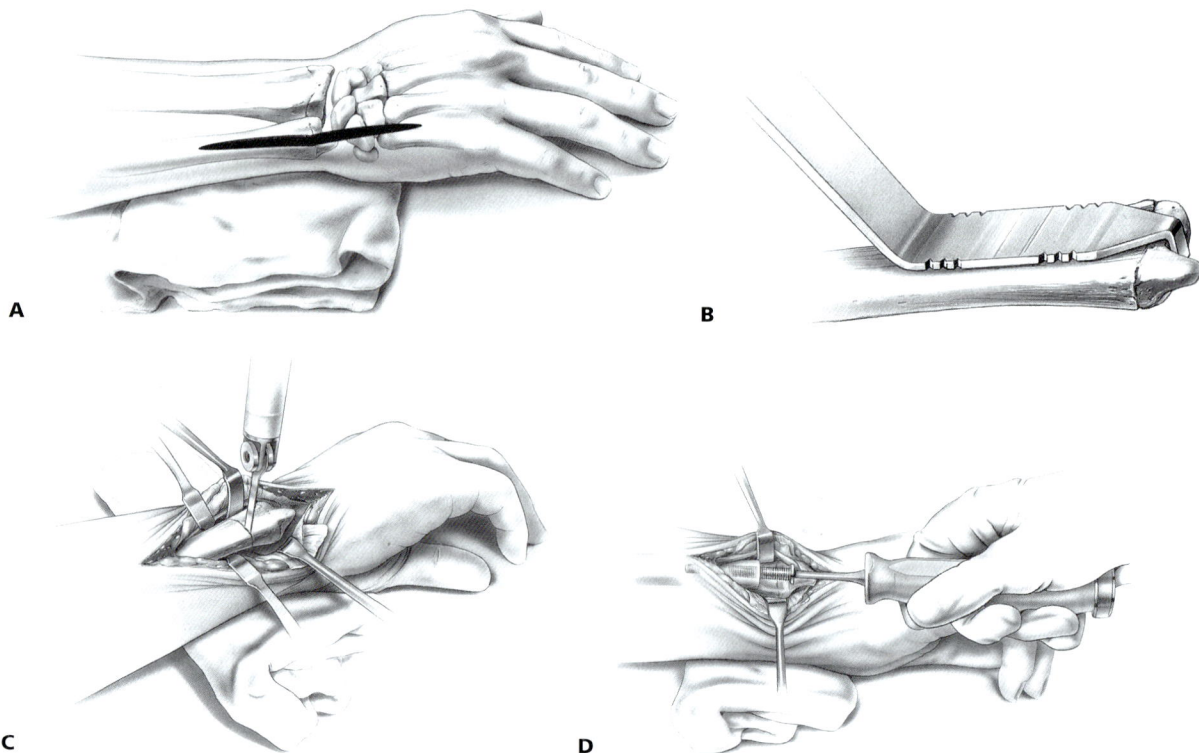

TECH FIG 2 • **A.** A longitudinal incision is made between the flexor and extensor carpi ulnar tendons on the ulnar border of the distal forearm and wrist. **B.** The cutting guide helps determine the level of resection of the ulnar head. The distal notches are for use with the three head sizes and standard stem, and the proximal notches are for use with a collared stem in cases of previous resection or resorption of the distal ulna. **C.** An oscillating saw is used to resect the ulnar head at the determined level. **D.** The ulnar medullary cavity is reamed using broaches. *(continued)*

E

F

G

H

I

J

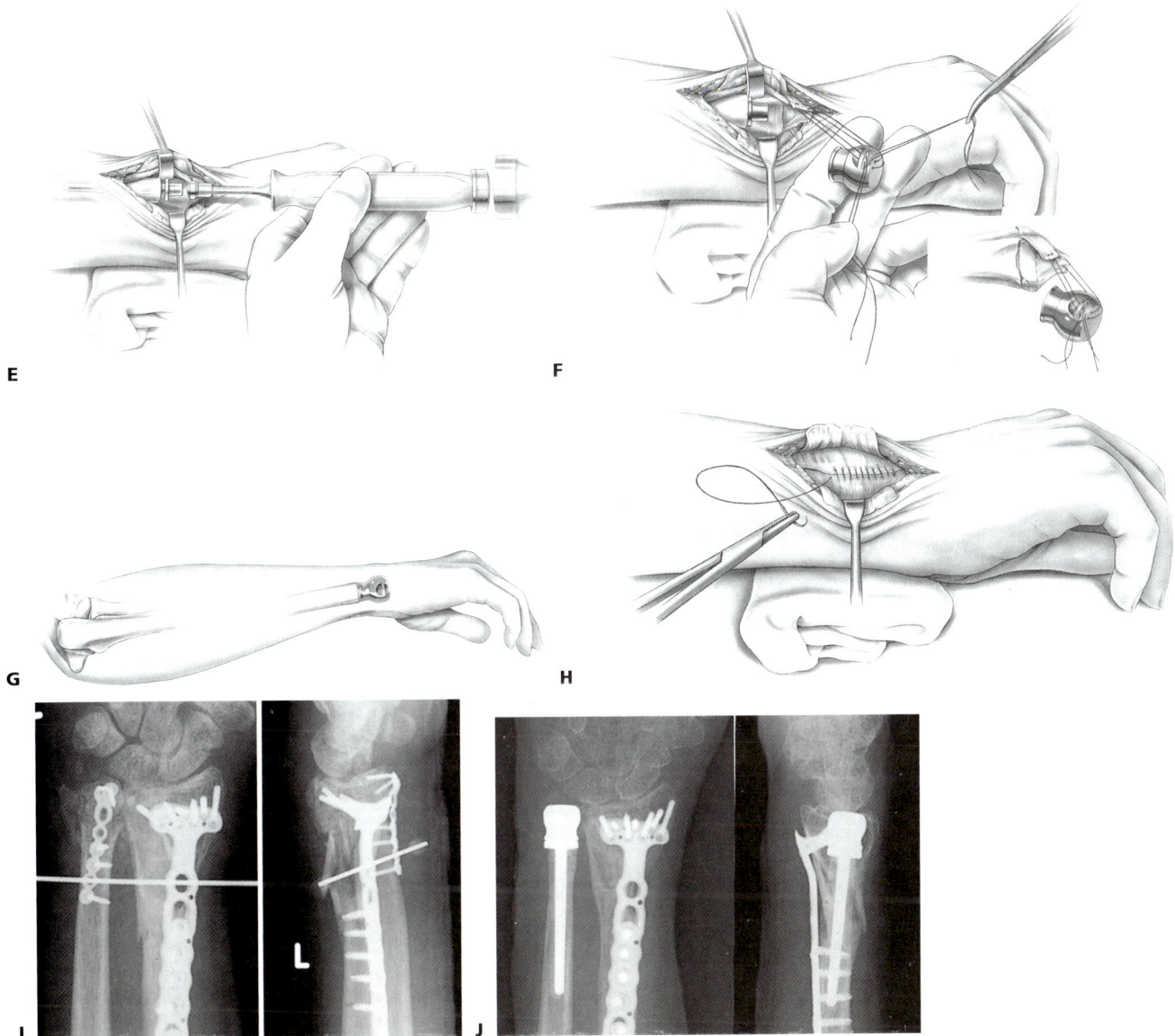

TECH FIG 2 • *(continued)* **E.** The appropriate trial stem is inserted into the ulnar shaft using an impactor and gentle taps with a mallet. **F.** Soft tissue-stabilizing sutures are placed in holes in the definitive head implant before impaction onto the stem. (*Inset*) The triangular fibrocartilage complex sutures are passed through holes in the deeper distal row of holes corresponding to the fovea of the native head. Sutures from the extensor carpi ulnaris subsheath are passed through the proximal superficial row of holes. The sutures are left untied until final closure. **G.** Because the head does not freely rotate on the stem, it is essential to align the head before impaction onto the stem. The holes on the head are lined up with the subcutaneous border of the ulna. **H.** After the pull-through sutures of the prosthesis are tied down, the remaining soft tissue envelope deep to the extensor retinaculum is approximated with the forearm in neutral position. **I.** Preoperative radiographs of an unstable and incongruous ulnar head after comminuted fracture of the distal radius and ulna. **J.** Ulnar head replacement and soft tissue imbrication restored congruity and stability to the articulation.

- Align the head of the prosthesis such that the two rows of suture holes are along the subcutaneous border of the ulna (**TECH FIG 2G**). Then place it onto the tapered neck of the stem and gently impact it.
- Advance the soft tissues ulnarly over the head of the prosthesis as it is reduced into the sigmoid notch. With the forearm in midrotation, tie down the sutures placed in the head, closing the ECU subsheath over the top of the prosthesis.

- Imbricate the remaining soft tissue envelope over the distal ulna while approximating the FCU–ECU interface (**TECH FIG 2H**).
- Check the stability of the prosthesis in supination and pronation.
- Close the extensor retinaculum over the capsule.
- Obtain final radiographs (**TECH FIG 2I, J**).
- Obtain hemostasis after the tourniquet is deflated.

TECHNIQUES

CONSTRAINED DISTAL RADIOULNAR JOINT ARTHROPLASTY

- Make an 8-cm longitudinal incision in the shape of a hockey stick along the ulnar border of the distal forearm between the fifth and sixth dorsal extensor compartments (**TECH FIG 3A**).
- Create a rectangular ulnarly based fascia flap (**TECH FIG 3B**). Use the flap to create a barrier between the prosthesis and the ECU at closure.
  - The width of the flap should cover the head of the implant and may include the most proximal part of the extensor retinaculum.
- Expose the distal ulna through the floor of the fifth extensor compartment and mobilize the tendons of the extensor digiti minimi proximally for a distance of 8 cm.
- Divide the sensory branch of the posterior interosseous nerve to avoid avulsion of the nerve from the thumb extensors when placing an elevator between the extensor mass and the radius.
- Incise the ECU sheath to its insertion at the base of the fifth metacarpal.
  - This is to avoid pressure against the distal end of the implant.
- Excise the remaining head of the ulna at a level just proximal to the cartilage, or where the DRUJ would have been.
- Leave the radial attachment of the TFCC undisturbed to provide a barrier between the prosthesis and the carpal bones.
- Displace the ulnar shaft in a volar direction to expose the radius and sigmoid notch (**TECH FIG 3C**).
- Elevate the interosseous membrane along the distal 8 cm of the radius.

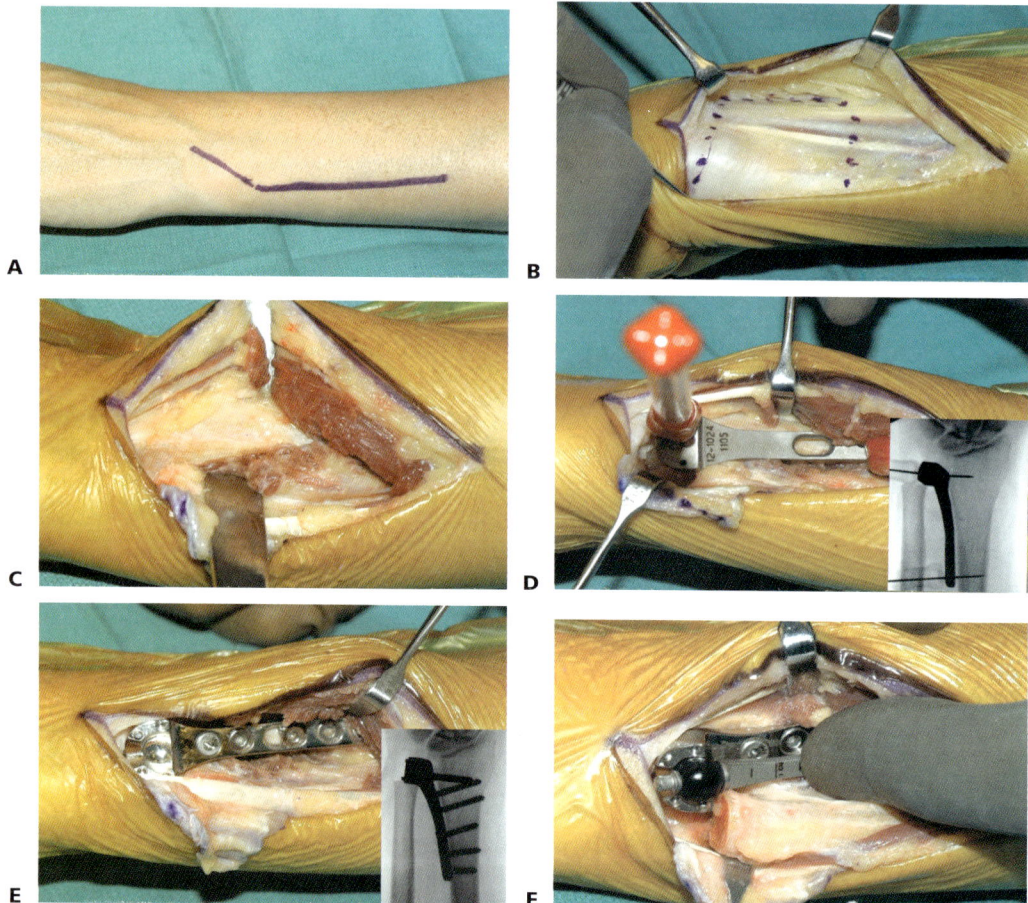

TECH FIG 3 • **A.** Intraoperative photograph of implantation with the Aptis system. The dorsoulnar skin incision is placed between the fifth and sixth extensor compartments. **B.** A large ulnar-based flap of retinaculum is raised for later interposition between the extensor carpi ulnaris tendon and the implant. **C.** The ulna is displaced volarly with retractors to expose the interosseous surface of the radius and the sigmoid notch. **D.** The radial plate template is positioned and temporarily fixed to the radius. The plate's position is checked with radiographs (*inset*). **E.** Operative photograph demonstrating completion of fixation of the radial component. Radiographs confirm correct placement of implant and screw length (*inset*). **F.** A sizer with an attached ball is used to determine the level of ulnar resection. This ensures that the ulnar implant with seated polyethylene ball will be level with the radial socket. (*continued*)

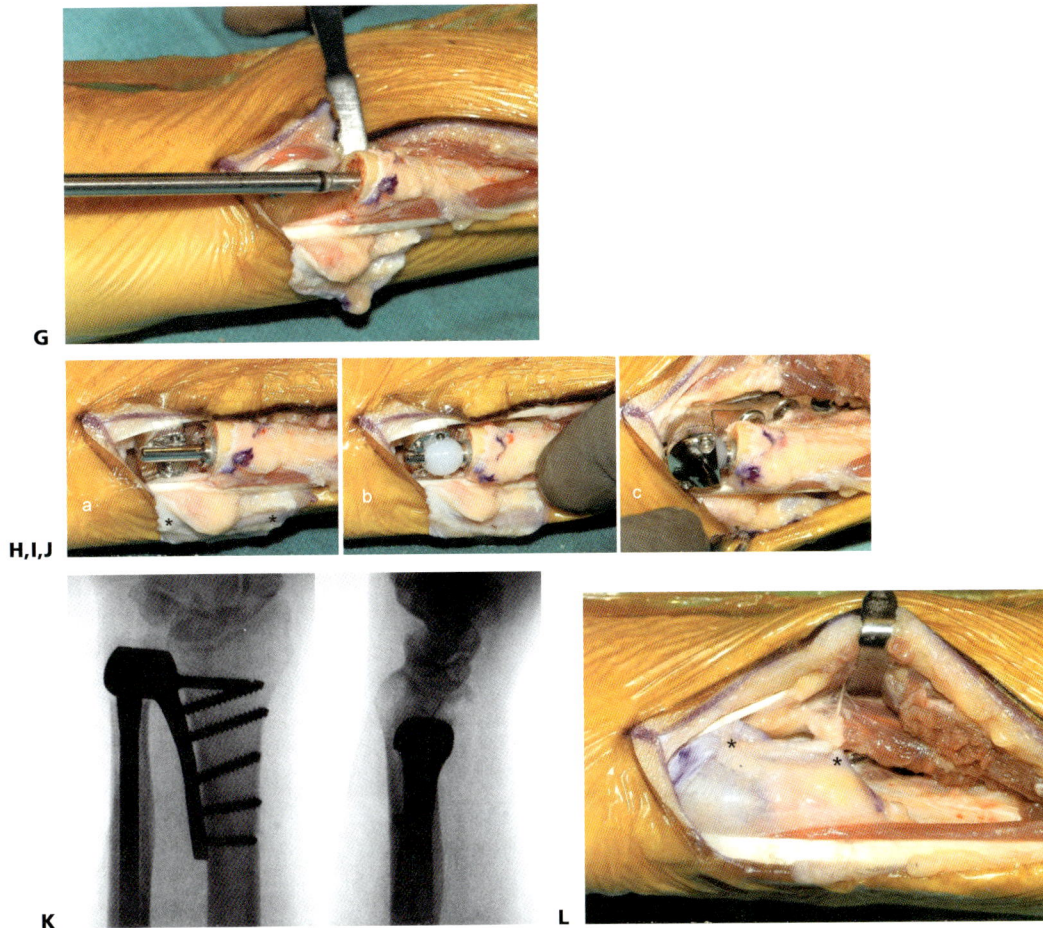

TECH FIG 3 • *(continued)* **G.** Medullary broaches are used to enlarge the medullary canal of the distal ulna. **H, I, J.** Steps for final assembly of the system. After the ulnar stem is inserted, the polyethylene ball is placed over the peg. The ball is then aligned with the radial socket and the cap is placed over it and secured with two screws. **K.** Final radiographs demonstrate correct placement of the implant. **L.** The previously raised retinacular flap (*marked by asterisks*) is then placed over the prosthesis and beneath the extensor carpi ulnaris tendon.

- Place the radial trial plate over the interosseous crest of the radius with the volar border aligned with the volar surface of the radius (**TECH FIG 3D**).
    - The plate should lie at least 3 mm proximal to the distal end of the sigmoid notch of the radius to avoid impaction with the carpus.
- Use a burr to contour the distal radius as necessary to accommodate the plate. Position the plate and hold it temporarily with Kirschner wires passed through the plate.
- Use intraoperative imaging to check the position of the plate.
- After drilling the hole for the radial peg, remove the trial and gently impact the final radial component in place. Insert fixation screws into the radius to secure the implant and take radiographs (**TECH FIG 3E**). Remove the Kirschner wires.
- With the forearm fully pronated, seat a sizer with attached ball into the hemi-socket of the radius and align it with the ulna (**TECH FIG 3F**). Determine the level of ulnar resection.

- After resecting the distal ulna, insert a 1.6-mm guidewire into the medullary canal and use a cannulated drill to ream the canal.
- Insert a medullary broach of the appropriate size into the canal to bevel the distal ulna and plane its distal end (**TECH FIG 3G**).
- Irrigate the medullary canal and insert the stem of the ulnar component (**TECH FIG 3H**). Place the ultra-high-molecular-weight polyethylene ball over the distal peg and position the ulnar component within the hemi-socket of the radial component (**TECH FIG 3I**).
- Position the cover of the socket over the ball and secure it with two small screws (**TECH FIG 3J**).
- Obtain radiographs to confirm satisfactory positioning of the prosthesis (**TECH FIG 3K**).
- Position the fascia and retinacular flap between the prosthesis and the ECU tendon and suture them to the radius before doing a layered closure (**TECH FIG 3L**).

PEARLS AND PITFALLS

Scar sensitivity or tenderness	▪ Identify and protect the sensory branch of the ulnar nerve.
Intraoperative fracture of the distal ulna	▪ Broach the distal ulna with caution. In hard cortical bone, use a drill to enlarge the cavity before impacting a broach in the ulna.
Incorrect ulnar variance	▪ Before making the ulnar osteotomy, identify the correct level of the DRUJ using radiographs or along the distal edge of the sigmoid notch.
Instability of the prosthesis	▪ Raise a thick and large flap of soft tissue when exposing the distal ulna. This tissue can be imbricated to stabilize the prosthesis if needed. Alternatively, a distally based strip of the FCU can be wound around the prosthesis to provide volar stability.

POSTOPERATIVE CARE

▪ The forearm is immobilized in neutral rotation and held in a supportive long-arm or Muenster-type splint or cast for 3 weeks.

▪ Active range of motion of the wrist and forearm is initiated at 3 weeks.

  ▪ A removable splint is required between therapy sessions for 3 weeks.

▪ Therapy is advanced as tolerated after 6 weeks, with strengthening starting only after functional wrist and forearm motion has been obtained.

▪ For a patient with rheumatoid arthritis, poor-quality soft tissue coverage, or mild instability intraoperatively, immobilization in supination for up to 6 weeks must be considered.

▪ Postoperative radiographs should be obtained at 6 weeks, 6 months, and then yearly.

OUTCOMES

▪ Outcomes vary with the indication and type of prosthesis used.

▪ The pain of radioulnar impingement is relieved in patients with previous excision arthroplasty and stability is restored.

▪ The range of motion of the forearm after prosthetic replacement remains largely unchanged, as it depends on previous scarring.

▪ Grip strength recovered depends on the underlying problem, but in patients with severe pain and weakness preoperatively, final grip averages about 60% of the opposite side.

▪ The long-term results and the incidence of prosthetic loosening, failure, and radius erosion are not known.

COMPLICATIONS

▪ Immediate or short-term complications
  ▪ Infection and wound breakdown, especially in revision cases with poor soft tissue cover
  ▪ Injury to the dorsal sensory branch of the ulnar nerve, leading to tender neuroma
  ▪ Fracture of the distal ulna during reaming or impaction of the prosthesis
  ▪ Dislocation of the prosthesis from the DRUJ postoperatively
▪ Long-term complications
  ▪ Progressive degeneration of the sigmoid notch
  ▪ Implant loosening
  ▪ Tenosynovitis of the ECU tendon
  ▪ Erosion of the radius sigmoid notch with pain
  ▪ Ectopic bone formation around the distal ulna
  ▪ Stress shielding and resorption of distal ulna
  ▪ Prosthetic fracture

ACKNOWLEDGMENTS

The authors thank Small Bone Innovations for permission to use their illustrations for demonstration of operative technique, Dr. Luis Scheker for the images of the Aptis system, Dr. Marc Garcia-Elias for the images of the Eclypse prosthesis, and Dr. Brian D. Adams for the images of the First Choice partial ulnar head replacement.

REFERENCES

1. Berger RA, Cooney WP. Use of an ulnar head endoprosthesis for treatment of an unstable distal ulnar resection: review of mechanics, indications, and surgical technique. Hand Clin 2005;21:603–620.
2. Conaway DA, Kuhl TL, Adams B. Comparison of the native ulnar head and a partial ulnar head resurfacing implant. J Hand Surg Am 2009;34A:1056–1062.
3. Garcia-Elias M. Eclypse: Partial ulnar head replacement for isolated DRUJ arthrosis. Tech Hand Upper Ext Surg 2007;11:121–128.
4. Gordon KD, Roth SE, Dunning CE, et al. An anthropometric study of the distal ulna: Implications for implant design. J Hand Surg Am 2002;27A:57–60.
5. Scheker LR, Babb BA, Killion PE. Distal ulnar prosthetic replacement. Orthop Clin North Am 2001;32:365–376.
6. Van Schoonhoven J, Fernandez DL, Bowers WH, et al. Salvage of failed resection arthroplasties of the distal radioulnar joint using a new ulnar head prosthesis. J Hand Surg Am 2000;25A:438–446.

Chapter 94

Arthroscopically Assisted Triangular Fibrocartilage Complex Débridement and Ulnar Shortening

Daniel J. Nagle

DEFINITION

- A tear of the triangular fibrocartilage complex (TFCC) is one of the most common causes of ulnar wrist pain. The treatment of TFCC tears and the associated synovitis is one of the primary indications for operative wrist arthroscopy.
- Ulnar-sided wrist pain associated with a TFCC tear in the presence of ulnar-neutral or ulnar-plus variance constitutes ulnar abutment syndrome. Successful treatment of an ulnar abutment syndrome requires not only the débridement of the TFCC tear but also shortening of the ulna.
  - Patients with Palmer type IA[8] TFCC tears are prime candidates for TFCC débridement.
  - Patients with Palmer type II (degenerative central tears) can also benefit from TFCC débridement. For the more advanced degenerative tears associated with lunatotriquetral ligament tears (Palmer type IID and E), other procedures such as an ulnar shortening osteotomy must be considered.

ANATOMY

- The triangular fibrocartilage is the primary stabilizer of the distal radioulnar joint. It attaches radially on the distal lip of the sigmoid notch (**FIG 1**). Ulnarly, the triangular fibrocartilage inserts at the base of the ulnar styloid via a continuation of the dorsal and palmar radioulnar ligaments and the fibers of the ligamentum subcruentum.[4]

PATHOGENESIS

- Tears of the triangular fibrocartilage are typically the result of a fall on the outstretched upper extremity. The ulna is driven distally and compresses the TFCC between itself and the lunate, producing a central or radial tear of the articular disc. This same mechanism can result in lunatotriquetral tears and peripheral TFCC tears (reviewed elsewhere).
- Forceful ulnar deviation, such as noted in racquet sports and golf, can lead to TFCC tears. Gymnastics, with its significant axial loading of the wrist, can also lead to a TFCC tear.
  - The combination of ulnar axial load and torque noted during these sports can be sufficient to tear the triangular fibrocartilage.
- At least 50% of intra-articular distal radius fractures are associated with tears of the triangular fibrocartilage.[1] Many of these tears remain asymptomatic and require no surgical treatment.
- An ulnar abutment (impaction) syndrome can develop as a result of shortening after a distal radius fracture (**FIG 2**). Radial collapse of the articular platform leads to a relative lengthening of the ulna.
  - Palmer et al[9] have demonstrated an increase in the ulnocarpal load with increasing ulnar variance.
- Repetitive axial loading of the wrist in a patient with an ulnar-zero or ulnar-plus variance can lead to an attritional tear of the triangular fibrocartilage and ulnar abutment syndrome.

NATURAL HISTORY

- The natural history of TFCC tears is not well established. Many asymptomatic TFCC tears are noted on routine wrist arthroscopy. If left untreated one could assume that a TFCC

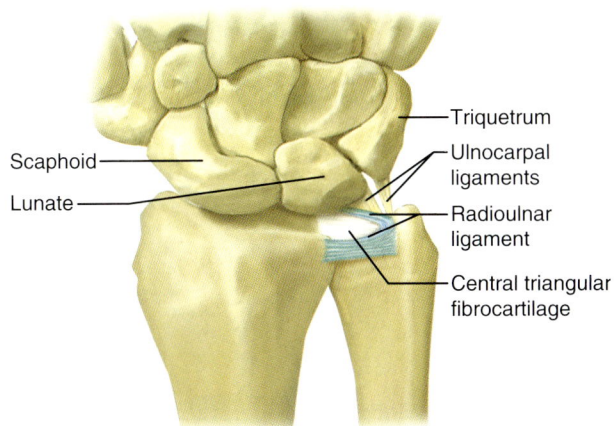

FIG 1 • Triangular fibrocartilage anatomy.

Scaphoid
Lunate
Triquetrum
Ulnocarpal ligaments
Radioulnar ligament
Central triangular fibrocartilage

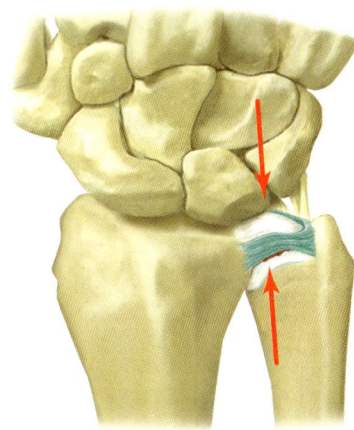

FIG 2 • Ulnar abutment. The triangular fibrocartilage complex is compressed between the proximal ulnar lunate and the distal ulnar head.

tear could lead to chondromalacia of the lunate, triquetrum, and distal ulnar head. This in turn could lead to painful ulno-carpal synovitis.

- The increase in the force transmitted through the ulnocarpal joint noted in an ulnar abutment syndrome can lead to a degenerative tear of the triangular fibrocartilage, chondromalacia of the lunate, triquetrum, and distal ulna, and a triquetrolunate ligament tear.

PATIENT HISTORY AND PHYSICAL EXAMINATION

- Physical examination includes the following:
  - Ulnocarpal compression test: Pain at the ulnocarpal joint with or without popping and grinding is suggestive of a TFCC tear and possible ulnar abutment syndrome.
  - Lester press test: Pain at the ulnocarpal joint is suggestive of a TFCC tear and possible ulnar abutment syndrome.
  - Ulnocarpal palpation: Pain at the ulnocarpal joint suggests the presence of TFCC pathology as well as ulnocarpal synovitis.

IMAGING AND OTHER DIAGNOSTIC STUDIES

- The radiographic evaluation of a patient with an ulnar abutment should include a standard wrist series and a Palmer 90 × 90 neutral rotation view.[10]
  - The Palmer 90 × 90 view places the forearm in neutral rotation while the elbow is flexed to 90 degrees and the shoulder is abducted to 90 degrees. The ulnar variance is calculated from this view (**FIG 3A**). Ulnar abutment is suspected in a patient with an ulnar-zero or ulnar-plus variance.
  - The ulnar aspect of the lunate should be carefully examined for subchondral cysts.
- An MRI should be considered when evaluating the patient for ulnar abutment syndrome. The MRI will demonstrate increased signal in the lunate on the T2 images (**FIG 3B,C**). This corresponds to either a cyst or intraosseous edema.
  - The triangular fibrocartilage can also be evaluated on the MR images. Whether an MR arthrogram is needed is a function of the MR resolution. The accuracy of lower-resolution MR is increased with the addition of an intra-articular gadolinium injection.

DIFFERENTIAL DIAGNOSIS

- TFCC tear
- Distal radioulnar ligament injury
- Distal radioulnar joint instability
- Ulnocarpal ligament injury
- Lunotriquetral joint instability
- Ulnocarpal synovitis
- Lunate chondromalacia
- Triquetral chondromalacia
- Distal ulnar chondromalacia
- Kienböck disease

NONOPERATIVE TREATMENT

- Immobilization of the involved wrist with either a Munster splint or long-arm cast for 4 weeks, combined with a course of nonsteroidal anti-inflammatories or an intra-articular steroid injection (or both), can be helpful in patients who present acutely.
- A TFCC tear that is exacerbated by specific activities can occasionally respond to activity modification.

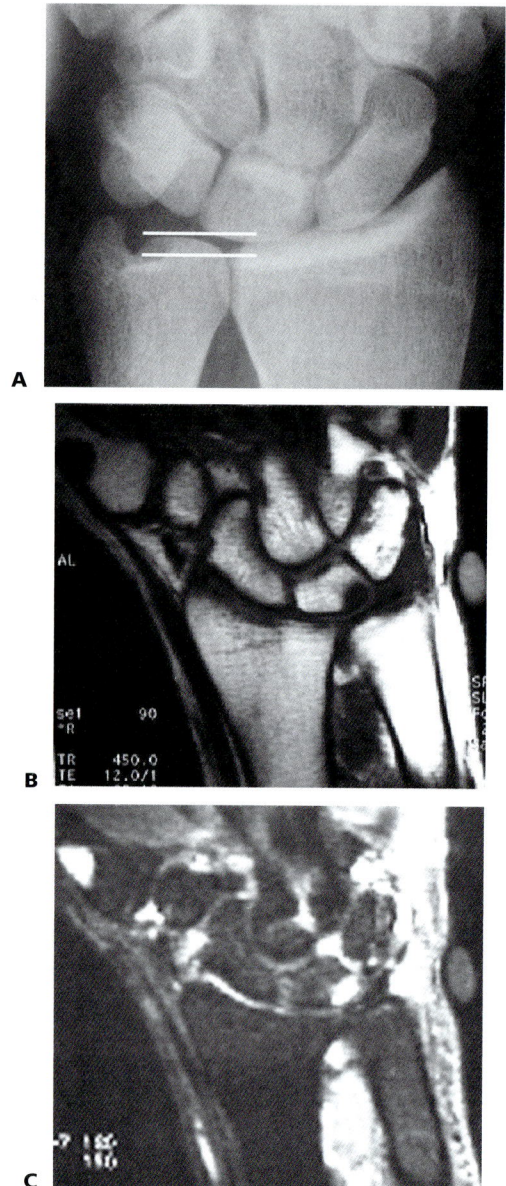

FIG 3 • **A.** Ulnar-plus variance noted on 90 × 90 neutral rotation view. **B,C.** T1- and T2-weighted MRIs of a wrist with an ulnar abutment demonstrating the change in signal at the ulnar proximal lunate.

SURGICAL MANAGEMENT

- The failure of nonoperative treatment (splinting, rest, nonsteroidal anti-inflammatory medications, activity modification, and therapy) leads the surgeon and patient to choose surgical débridement of a TFCC tear.
- Mechanical débridement of the triangular fibrocartilage has been successful although it can be challenging, particularly in regard to the débridement of the ulnar and dorsal aspects of the triangular fibrocartilage tear.
  - There are two potential problems with mechanical TFCC débridement:
    - Passage of the instruments across the radiocarpal joint places those joints at risk of scuffing.

The proximity of the scope to the operative site (TFCC) can distort the operator's perception of the ulnocarpal joint.

■ Radiofrequency devices have become increasingly popular for TFCC débridement because of the small probe size and relatively low cost. Monopolar and bipolar radiofrequency devices are currently in use. The instrument settings vary with the device.

■ Arthroscopic ulnar shortening is indicated in patients with a TFCC tear who have longstanding or acute exacerbation of ulnar abutment syndrome and who do not respond to nonoperative treatment.

■ It is generally thought that an arthroscopically assisted ulnar shortening is indicated if the ulnar-plus variance is less than 4 mm.

■ The goal of the surgery is to create an ulnar-minus variance of 2 mm.

Preoperative Planning

■ TFCC débridement: Preoperative evaluation should include wrist radiographs: a "wrist series" and a "90 × 90" view described by Palmer.[10] An MRI with or without an arthrogram can also be helpful.

■ Arthroscopic ulnar shortening

■ The patient must be informed that an arthroscopically assisted ulnar shortening may not be possible should there be laxity of the ulnocarpal ligaments, a peripheral TFCC tear, or lunatotriquetral laxity.

■ The amount of shortening should be calculated preoperatively.

■ The surgeon should verify that the operating room is equipped with a mini C-arm to permit intraoperative assessment of the amount of ulna resected.

Positioning

■ The patient is placed in the supine position.
■ A pneumatic tourniquet is placed on the proximal arm.
■ The involved extremity is prepared and draped in the usual fashion.
■ The wrist is distracted using a commercially available wrist traction device.

TECHNIQUES

MECHANICAL TFCC DÉBRIDEMENT

Portals and Arthroscopic Examination

■ The standard dorsal 3-4 and 4-5 or 6R wrist arthroscopy portals are used for TFCC débridement (**TECH FIG 1**). These portals should be wide enough to permit the easy passage of instruments.

■ Before débriding the TFCC, perform a thorough and systematic arthroscopic examination of the radiocarpal, ulnocarpal, and midcarpal joints because associated intrinsic and extrinsic ligament injury and articular and synovial pathology could affect the treatment plan.

■ Perform ulnocarpal synovectomy to ensure clear visualization of that joint.

Radial and Palmar Débridement

■ The initial débridement of the radial and palmar and a portion of the dorsal aspects of the TFCC tear is accomplished with a scope in the 3-4 portal while the instruments enter through the 4-5 portal.

■ Use small joint punches (straight and angled), graspers, mini-banana blades, and mini-hook knives to débride the TFCC. The suction punch is particularly useful.

■ Take care not to injure the underlying ulnar head and overhanging lunate and triquetrum (**TECH FIG 2**).

Ulnar Débridement

■ Once the radial and palmar aspects of the TFCC have been débrided, move the arthroscope to the 4-5 portal.

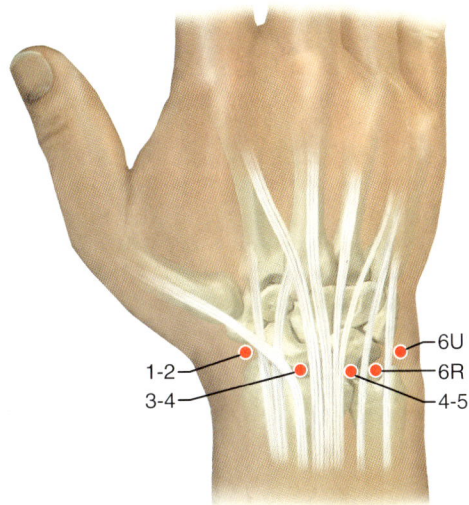

TECH FIG 1 • Wrist arthroscopy portals.

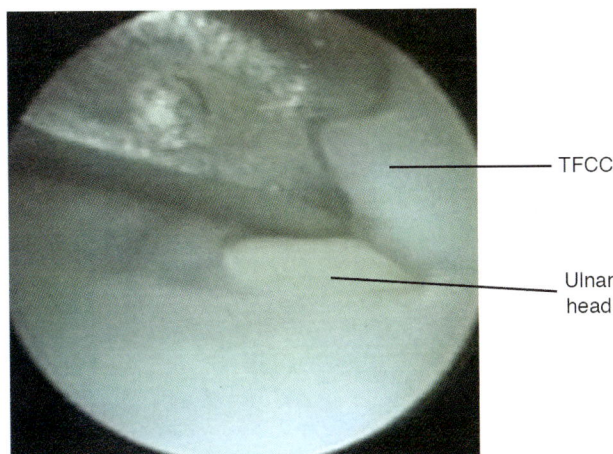

TECH FIG 2 • Mechanical débridement of the TFCC. The arthroscope is in the 3-4 portal looking ulnar, while the suction punch enters through the 4-5 portal to débride the palmar aspect of the TFCC.

TECHNIQUES

- Débride the ulnar aspect of the triangular fibrocartilage by passing the instruments through the 3-4 portal.
- Keep three points in mind while débriding the ulnar aspect of the TFCC:
  - Avoid injuring the attachment of the triangular fibrocartilage at its insertion at the base of the ulnar styloid.
  - Avoid injuring the dorsal or palmar radioulnar ligaments. If the ulnar attachment of the TFCC is transected, or if the dorsal and palmar radioulnar ligaments are injured, distal radioulnar joint instability will result.
  - Avoid scuffing the articular surfaces while passing the cutting and grasping instruments from the 3-4 portal across the radiocarpal joint into the ulnocarpal joint.

Dorsal Débridement

- The dorsal aspect of the TFCC tear can usually be débrided using the 3-4 and 4-5 portals. Occasionally, however, the instruments need to be passed through the 6U portal while the scope is placed in the 3-4 portal.
  - Injury to the dorsal sensory branch of the ulnar nerve is avoided when establishing the 6U portal by using a longitudinal portal incision and blunt dissection to reach the ulnocarpal joint capsule.

Completion

- Once the TFCC has been débrided with the punches and knives, smooth the rough edges of the débrided TFCC using a full radius cutter.
  - The 2.0-mm cutters are small but relatively ineffective, while the 2.9-mm cutters are effective but must be controlled so as to avoid collateral damage to the adjacent articular surfaces (**TECH FIG 3A**).
- The end point of the TFCC débridement is reached when the ulnar head is visible through the TFCC and a stable TFCC perimeter is created (**TECH FIG 3B**).
  - Typically, a central defect measuring at least 1 cm in diameter is created.
- Before declaring the surgery complete, remove the instruments from the wrist, release the traction, and ulnarly deviate, axially load, and repeatedly supinate and pronate the wrist.
  - The presence of popping or clicking is a sign that further débridement might be needed or that some other pathology is causing the popping and clicking.
  - One source of such post-débridement popping is thickened synovium in the distal radioulnar joint just proximal to the TFCC.
- Close wounds using subcuticular sutures of 4-0 Prolene and apply a volar splint.

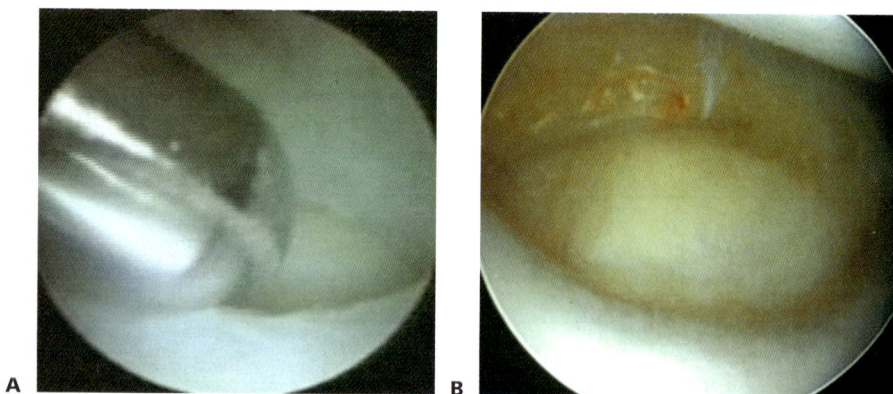

TECH FIG 3 • **A.** The arthroscope is in the 3-4 portal and the full radius cutter is passed through the 4-5 portal to smooth the edges of the débrided central TFCC tear. **B.** The débridement of the TFCC is complete. The ulnar head is clearly visible and ready for shortening.

LASER- OR RADIOFREQUENCY-ASSISTED TFCC DÉBRIDEMENT

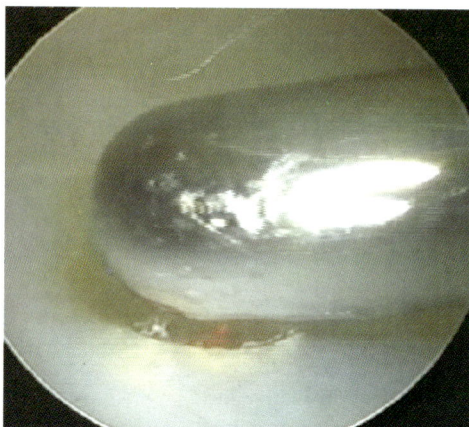

TECH FIG 4 • Laser-assisted débridement of a TFCC tear. The laser probe is placed 1 mm from the TFCC.

- The technique of laser-assisted TFCC débridement is similar to that of mechanical débridement, with the exception that the arthroscope can be left in the 3-4 portal while the laser probe is kept in the 4-5 portal.
- The laser is set to 1.4 to 1.6 joules at a frequency of 15 pulses per second. With the help of a side-firing 70-degree laser tip, the triangular fibrocartilage can be rapidly and precisely débrided.
  - The 70-degree laser tip permits ablation of not only the radial and palmar portions of the TFCC tear but also the ulnar and dorsal components.
  - There is no need to bring the laser probe in through the 3-4 portal.
- During the débridement, take care not to injure the ulnar head. This is avoided by firing the laser tangentially to the head of the ulna or passing the probe beneath the triangular fibrocartilage and firing distally (**TECH FIG 4**).

TECHNIQUES

- This latter technique presents minimal danger to the lunate or triquetrum as the fluid used to expand the joint acts as a heat sink and absorbs the laser energy as it emerges from beneath the triangular fibrocartilage.
- Radiofrequency-assisted débridement is similar to laser-assisted débridement.
  - Monopolar probes have a theoretical disadvantage compared to bipolar probes in that the energy imparted to the TFCC flows through the adjacent tissue in the direction of the grounding pad. This could lead to tissue damage beyond the TFCC.
  - The flow of irrigation fluid must be sufficient to cool the joint when using the radiofrequency devices.

ARTHROSCOPIC ULNAR SHORTENING

- The goal of the surgery is to create an ulnar-minus variance of 2 mm without any irregularities of the remaining distal ulna.
  - Small irregularities, however, tend to flatten out with the passage of time.
- Arthroscopic ulnar shortening is accomplished by placing the scope in the 3-4 portal and introducing the instruments through the 4-5 portal.
  - Occasionally the 6U portal can be used, as can the distal distal radioulnar joint portal.
- While the holmium:YAG laser is useful for ulnar shortening, the barrel abrader can also be used alone or in combination with the laser.
  - If the holmium:YAG laser is used, it is introduced through the 4-5 portal and the cartilage and subchondral bone of the ulnar seat of the distal ulna are rapidly vaporized (**TECH FIG 5A,B**).

- The laser becomes less efficient once the trabeculae of the distal ulna are visible (**TECH FIG 5C**). At that point, the 2.9-mm barrel abrader is brought in to finish the shortening (**TECH FIG 5D**).
- It is important to avoid injury to the sigmoid notch, and frequent fluoroscopic monitoring of the amount of bone resected is mandatory.
- Take care to fully supinate and pronate the wrist to adequately débride the ulnar head.
- Remove all instruments at the end of the procedure, and ulnarly deviate, axially load, and supinate and pronate the wrist to be sure no clicking or popping is noted. If any clicking or popping is noted and it appears to be emanating from the area of the surgery, further ulnar leveling may be required.
- Close wounds using subcuticular sutures of 4-0 Prolene and apply a volar splint.

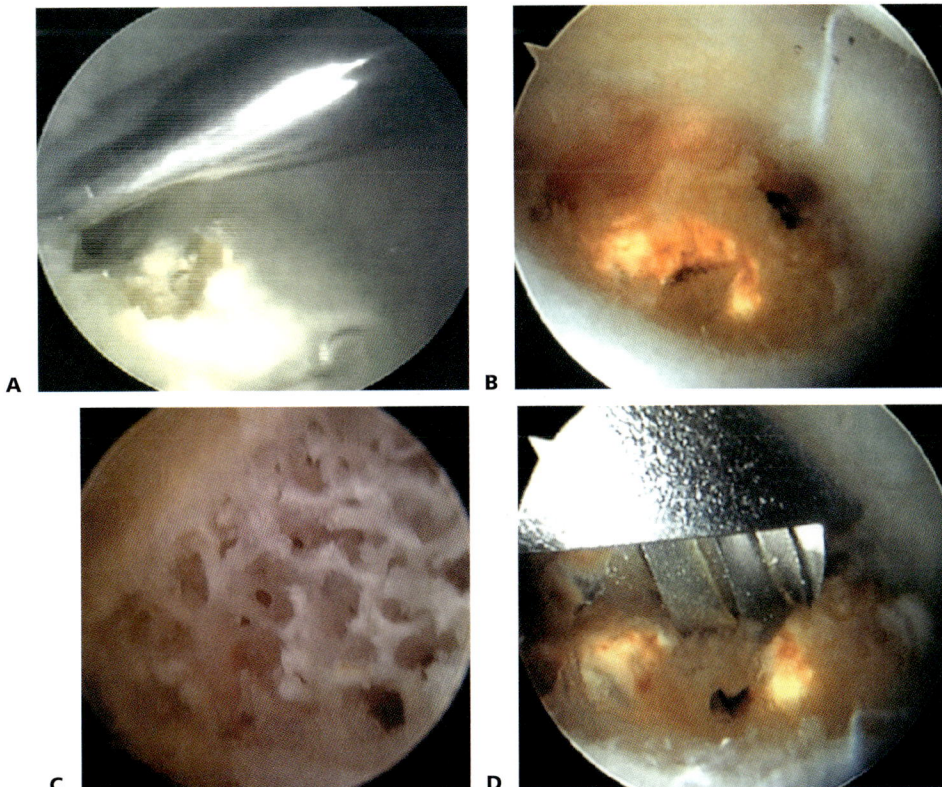

TECH FIG 5 • A. The 70-degree side-firing laser probe easily vaporizes the hyaline cartilage and subchondral bone of the ulnar head. **B.** The laser has cleared the ulnar head of its cartilage and subchondral plate. **C.** The spacing of the bony trabeculae of the ulnar head decreases the laser's efficiency. The final leveling of the ulnar head is achieved with the small joint burr. **D.** The small joint burr is brought in through the 4-5 or 6R portal to finish the ulnar shortening.

PEARLS AND PITFALLS

TFCC débridement Portal complications	▪ The 4-5 and 6R portals should be placed just distal to the distal surface of the TFCC. ▪ Inappropriate distal placement of the portals can lead to scuffing of the lunate and triquetrum.
Nerve injury	▪ The dorsal branch of the ulnar nerve is at risk during the creation of all ulnar portals. ▪ All portals should be made by incising the skin with a no. 15 blade (avoid plunging a no. 11 blade into the joint). Once the skin is cut, a Hartmann hemostat should be used to bluntly dissect through the subcutaneous tissue and penetrate the wrist joint capsule.
Débridement	▪ Avoid injury to the peripheral attachments of the TFCC and the dorsal and palmar radioulnar ligaments.
Incision orientation	▪ Small transverse incisions in Langer lines closed with a subcuticular Prolene produce a superior cosmetic result.
Scope	▪ The 1.9-mm arthroscopes are less likely to scuff the wrist joint articular surfaces.
Rehabilitation	▪ Avoid early (before 4 weeks) heavy loading of the wrist.
Arthroscopic ulnar shortening Indications	▪ Arthroscopically assisted ulnar shortening should not be combined with other procedures that require postoperative wrist immobilization.
Excision of ulnar head	▪ A systematic approach to the excision of the ulnar head is critical. The assistant must take the wrist from full supination to full pronation while the operator maintains the arthroscope in the 3-4 portal and the instruments in the ulnar portals. The ulnar head is débrided as it is presented to the surgeon by the assistant during the rotation of the distal radioulnar joint.

POSTOPERATIVE CARE

▪ Postoperative care includes early range of motion and suture removal at 2 weeks.
  ▪ Early range of motion is critical as it leads to a more supple scar and a better range of motion.
▪ Strengthening exercises are initiated at 6 weeks if needed.
  ▪ Premature resumption of heavy lifting or repetitive activities will lead to ulnocarpal synovitis.
  ▪ Some patients are pain-free after as little as 2 weeks, and the surgeon must temper the patient's desire to return to full activity.
▪ The patient is instructed to avoid heavy lifting for 3 months.
▪ Typically patients are able to return to unrestricted activities in 12 weeks, although they may experience some discomfort for 6 to 12 months.
  ▪ Patients who undergo a simple TFCC débridement will recover more rapidly than those who undergo an arthroscopic ulnar shortening.

OUTCOMES

▪ The results of arthroscopic débridement of traumatic triangular fibrocartilage tears have been very good.[2,3]
▪ Minami et al[5] noted, however, that degenerative tears (Palmer type II) have a less favorable prognosis due to the associated ulnar wrist pathology noted in these patients.
▪ Our results[11] and those reported by Osterman[7] and Palmer[8] suggest that arthroscopically assisted ulnar shortening in properly selected patients provides excellent and good results in over 80% of patients (**FIG 4**).

COMPLICATIONS

▪ TFCC débridement
  ▪ Infection and injury to the dorsal branch of the ulnar nerve are rare.

▪ Excessive débridement of the TFCC (dorsal and palmar radioulnar ligaments, attachment in the ulnar fovea) can lead to instability.
  ▪ Formation of portal site cysts (very rare)
▪ Arthroscopic ulnar shortening
  ▪ Inadequate bony resection can lead to a nonresolution of the patient's symptoms.
  ▪ Uneven resection of the distal ulna can lead to catching of any significant residual bony prominence on the overlying triangular fibrocartilage.
  ▪ We have seen one patient reconstitute his triangular fibrocartilage and require repeat débridement. This phenomenon has been anecdotally reported by others.
  ▪ The surgeon must remain vigilant and avoid injury to the sigmoid notch.
  ▪ The surgeon must avoid excessive ulnar débridement, which could lead to the detachment of the triangular fibrocartilage from the fovea.

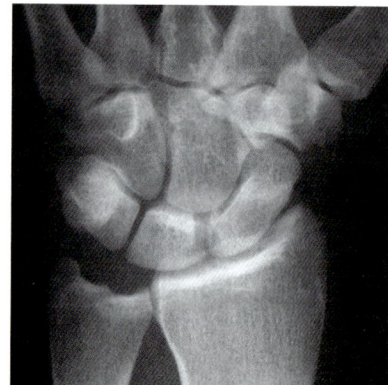

FIG 4 • Six-month postoperative radiograph after arthroscopic ulnar shortening in patient in Techniques Figure 5.

REFERENCES

1. Bombaci H, Polat A, Deniz G, et al. The value of plain X-rays in predicting TFCC injury after distal radial fractures. J Hand Surg Br 2008;33B:322–326.
2. Husby T, Haugstvedt JR. Long-term results after arthroscopic resection of lesions of the triangular fibrocartilage complex. Scand J Plast Reconstr Surg Hand Surg 2001;35:79–83.
3. Infanger M, Grimm D. Meniscus and discus lesions of triangular fibrocartilage complex (TFCC): treatment by laser-assisted wrist arthroscopy. J Plast Reconstr Aesthet Surg 2009;62:466–471 [Epub 2008 May 12].
4. Kleinman WB. Stability of the distal radioulnar joint: biomechanics, pathophysiology, physical diagnosis, and restoration of function what we have learned in 25 years. J Hand Surg Am 2007;32A: 1086–1106.
5. Minami A, Ishikawa J, Suenaga N, et al. Clinical results of treatment of triangular fibrocartilage complex tears by arthroscopic debridement. J Hand Surg Am 1996;21A:406–411.
6. Nagle DJ, Bernstein MA. Laser-assisted arthroscopic ulnar shortening. Arthroscopy 2002;18:1046–1051.
7. Osterman AL. Arthroscopic debridement of triangular fibrocartilage complex tears. Arthroscopy 1990;6:120–124.
8. Palmer AK. Triangular fibrocartilage disorders: injury patterns and treatment. Arthroscopy 1990;6:125–132.
9. Palmer AK, Glisson RR, Werner FW. Relationship between ulnar variance and triangular fibrocartilage complex thickness. J Hand Surg Am 1984;9A:681–682.
10. Palmer AK, Glisson RR, Werner FW. Ulnar variance determination. J Hand Surg Am 1982;7A:376–379.
11. Wnorowski DC, Palmer AK, Werner FW, et al. Anatomic and biomechanical analysis of the arthroscopic wafer procedure. Arthroscopy 1992;8:204–212.

Chapter 95

Ulnar Shortening Osteotomy

Lance G. Warhold and Nelson L. Jenkins

DEFINITION

- Ulnar impaction syndrome (ulnocarpal abutment) results from a chronic compressive overloading of the ulnocarpal articulation secondary to static or dynamic ulnar-positive variance.
- Ulnar variance defines the relationship of the length of the ulna to that of the radius.
- Ulnar-positive variance can be the result of a congenital anomaly; traumatic radial shortening from a distal radius, Essex-Lopresti, or Galeazzi fracture; injury to the distal radius physis; or a variant of normal anatomy.
- An ulnar shortening osteotomy is designed to decompress the ulnocarpal joint while simultaneously tightening the ulnocarpal and radioulnar marginal ligaments of the triangular fibrocartilage complex (TFCC).[14]

ANATOMY

- The distal radius has three articular surfaces: the scaphoid fossa, the lunate fossa, and the sigmoid notch.
- The radius articulates with and rotates around the ulnar head via the sigmoid notch. The sigmoid notch has well-defined dorsal, palmar, and distal margins, while the proximal margin is indistinct.
- The distal radioulnar joint (DRUJ) and ulnocarpal relationships are maintained by numerous ligamentous structures (**FIG 1A**).

- The interosseous membrane is a complex structure with a thickened central portion. It almost completely spans the radius and ulna, acting as a hinge for forearm rotation.
- The diaphysis of the distal half of the ulna is supplied by small segmental branches from the anterior and posterior interosseous arteries. These enter the ulna in 1- to 3-cm intervals from the direction of the interosseous membrane and must be protected during the surgical approach.[22]
- The dorsal capsule of the DRUJ contains two ligaments: the proximal metaphyseal arcuate ligament and the distal radioulnar ligament. The palmar capsule is composed of a single radioulnar ligament.[1]
- The TFCC spans the ulnocarpal joint and connects the distal radius to the distal ulna (**FIG 1B**). The TFCC functions to cover the distal ulna, to partially dampen and transmit a portion of the axial load of the wrist through the ulna, to stabilize the DRUJ, and to provide support for the ulnar side of the carpus.
- The TFCC contains a central avascular articular disc composed of types I and II collagen. It is of variable thickness

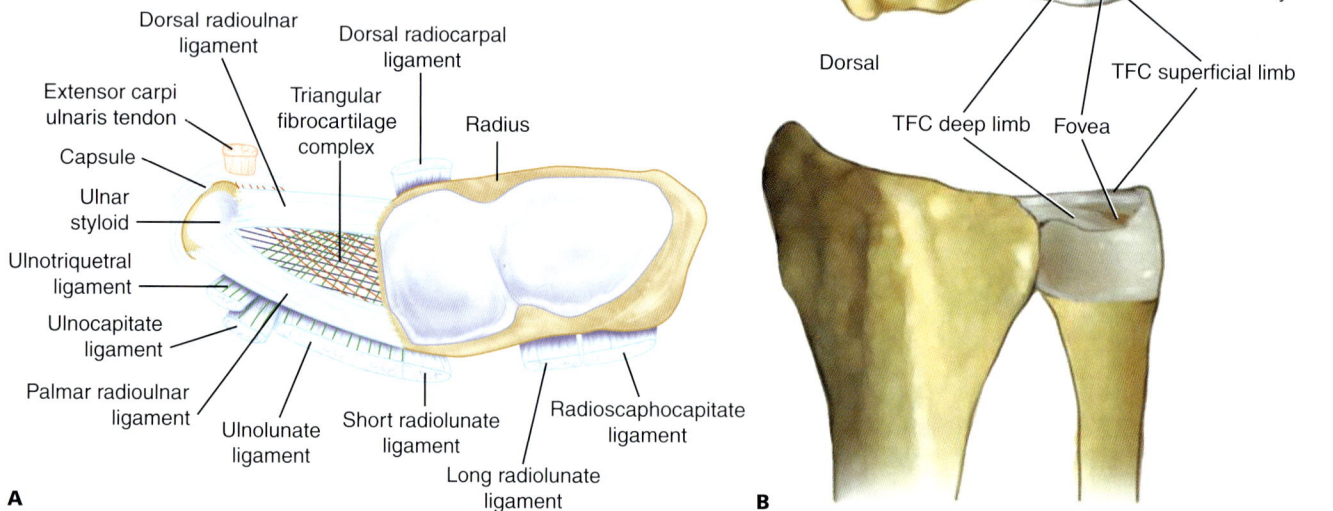

FIG 1 • **A.** The soft tissue structures encompassing the triangular fibrocartilage complex (TFCC) of the wrist stabilizing the radioulnocarpal unit. The TFC proper originates from the radius medially and attaches to the base of the ulnar styloid. Fibers originating from the subsheath of the extensor carpi ulnaris dorsally cross path with fibers originating from the ulnocarpal ligaments volarly and blend with the TFC proper. **B.** Distal radioulnar joint (DRUJ) ligaments. (The disc component of the TFCC has been removed to show the deep limbs of the radioulnar ligaments.) The volar and dorsal radioulnar ligaments are the major soft tissue stabilizers of the DRUJ and insert onto the base of the ulnar styloid.

(average, 2 mm) and chiefly functions in load transmission between the ulnar head and ulnar carpus.

- The articular disc is connected to the peripheral palmar and dorsal radioulnar (marginal) ligaments, which originate on the medial border of the distal radius and insert into the base of the ulnar styloid at the fovea. These ligaments are composed of linear type I collagen and are stabilizers of the DRUJ.
- The ulnolunate and ulnotriquetral ligaments originate from the ulnar fovea and pass palmar to the palmar radioulnar ligament. They traverse the palmar surface of the TFCC to insert on their respective carpal bones. These ulnocarpal ligaments stabilize the ulnar side of the carpus relative to the ulna and resist carpal supination.
- The periphery of the TFCC is supplied by dorsal and palmar branches of the anterior interosseous artery and the ulnar artery. Because of this vascular distribution, injuries to the periphery of the TFCC are capable of healing and are often amenable to repair. Injuries to the central avascular portion of the articular disc do not heal in a predictable manner and are often treated with débridement.

PATHOGENESIS

- Normal ulnar variance ranges from neutral to plus or minus 2 mm. The average axial load transmitted across the TFCC and subsequently the ulna is 20% if ulnar variance is neutral. An ulnar-positive variance of 2.5 mm increases the load across the distal ulna 42.7%, while an ulnar variance of −2.5 mm decreases the ulnar load to 3.1% (Table 1).[15]
- Congenital or acquired ulnar-positive variance (**FIG 2**) can lead to degenerative wear of the TFCC and surrounding structures.
- The Palmer classification divides TFCC lesions into traumatic (type I) or degenerative (type II).[16] Type II lesions are associated with ulnocarpal impaction and are further subdivided based on the severity and the other structures involved. Type II TFCC tears are generally not amenable to direct repair.
  - Type IIA: TFCC wear
  - Type IIB: TFCC wear plus lunate or ulnar head chondromalacia
  - Type IIC: TFCC perforation plus lunate or ulnar head chondromalacia
  - Type IID: TFCC perforation plus lunate or ulnar head chondromalacia plus lunotriquetral ligament perforation

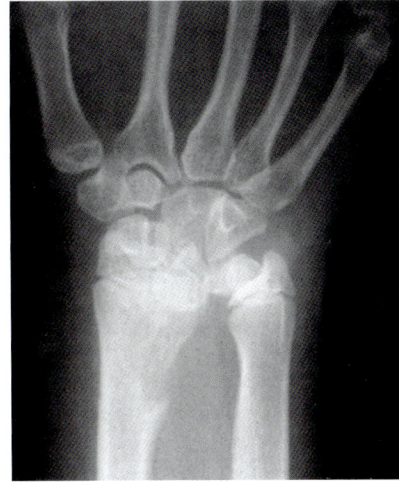

FIG 2 • Radiograph of Madelung deformity showing congenital ulnar-positive variance.

  - Type IIE: TFCC perforation plus lunate or ulnar head chondromalacia plus lunotriquetral ligament perforation plus ulnocarpal arthritis

NATURAL HISTORY

- Defining the natural history of ulnocarpal impaction syndrome is at best challenging.
- The Palmer classification provides an accurate anatomic description of the degenerative changes seen in the ulnocarpal structures, but it does not dictate treatment, suggest prognosis, or indicate timing of progression.
- Deterioration of the ulnocarpal structures is very common regardless of ulnar variance. Numerous cadaveric studies have found TFCC perforations and chondromalacia of the ulnar head, lunate, and triquetrum in up to 70% of "normal specimens."[11,15]
- Ulnar-positive variance and persistent heavy demand across the ulnocarpal joint can hasten the development of the disease.
- An individual's ability to unload the ulnar side of the wrist with conservative measures and change of lifestyle may slow or even prevent progression.

PATIENT HISTORY AND PHYSICAL FINDINGS

- The patient history must be detailed and must include:
  - Medical history
  - Description of previous surgical procedures involving not only the wrist but also the elbow
  - Analysis of whether the pain was caused by an acute injury or brought on by repetitive motion activities
    - A distal radius or radial head fracture can lead to ulnocarpal impaction, as can a chronic distal radius physeal injury (ie, the gymnast's wrist).
  - Characterization of the pain
    - Description of the location, duration, and radiation of the pain as well as any associated swelling, burning or tingling sensations, or sounds (clicks, etc.)
    - Aggravating and alleviating factors
- The physical examination should always begin with inspection.

Table 1	Percentage of Force Transmitted Through the Ulna (Nine Arms)			
Ulnar Length (mm)	Amount removed of the articular disk of the triangular fibrocartilage complex			
	None	1/3	2/3*	All*
Neutral	17.6%	16.1%	13.4%	8.0%
−2.5	3.1%	2.7%	2.4%	2.3%
+2.5	42.7%	41.9%	36.1%	26.3%

*Removal of two thirds or more of the horizontal portion of the triangular fibrocartilage complex statistically decreased the percentage of force through the nine ulnas tested.
(Adapted from Palmer AK, Werner FW. The triangular fibrocartilage complex of the wrist: anatomy and function. J Hand Surg Am 1981;6A:153–162.)

- The wrist and elbow should be examined for surgical scars.
- Prominence of the ulna either palmarly or dorsally may indicate instability of the DRUJ. A palmar sag and a supination posture of the wrist may indicate the capsuloligamentous instability that occurs in rheumatoid arthritis.
- Swelling, bruising, perforations of the skin, or obvious dislocations may indicate trauma.
- Intrinsic atrophy and clawing may indicate ulnar nerve pathology.
- Splinter hemorrhages beneath the nails and decreased turgor in the volar digital pads suggests vascular insufficiency.
- Single-finger palpation should proceed in a systematic fashion by isolating anatomic structures. The examination should be performed with the patient's elbow resting on a table, the hand pointing toward the ceiling, and the forearm in a neutral position.
  - Tenderness over any anatomic structure suggests a specific clinical diagnosis.
- Active and passive range-of-motion (ROM) maneuvers may illicit pain, suggesting pathology. Limitations of ROM may be the result of swelling or obstruction (blocking). The examiner should listen for sounds of pathology throughout ROM.
- Specific provocative tests should be performed in an attempt to further define the injured structure(s).
  - Piano key test: A positive result is characterized by painful laxity in the affected wrist compared with the contralateral wrist, suggesting DRUJ synovitis.
  - Ulnar compression test: A positive test is exacerbation of pain, which suggests arthritis or instability; dorsal or palmar subluxation may be noted.
  - Lunotriquetral ballottement test: Used to elicit laxity associated with pain and crepitus in the presence of lunotriquetral instability
  - Reagan shuck test: Positive if pain and clicking at the lunotriquetral joint is present, suggesting lunotriquetral ligament perforation or disruption

IMAGING AND OTHER DIAGNOSTIC STUDIES

- Plain radiographic views should include neutral rotation posteroanterior and lateral projections of both wrists. These are obtained with the patient seated and the elbow flexed at 90 degrees and the shoulder abducted at 90 degrees.
  - The contralateral wrist films may be used as a template for reconstruction.
  - Radiographic assessment of ulnar variance has used a neutral rotation radiographic view of the wrist that provides an image of the radioulnar length with the wrist unloaded. Such views may underestimate variance in wrists in which power grip and pronation result in significant proximal migration of the radius. Tomaino[21] found that ulnar variance increased an average of 2.5 mm using the pronated grip view and ranged from an increase of 1 to 4 mm (**FIG 3A**).
- Other plain views may be obtained based on clinical suspicion.
  - The carpal tunnel (**FIG 3B**) view visualizes the hook of the hamate and the pisotriquetral joint.
  - An oblique view in 30 degrees of pronation (**FIG 3C**) allows evaluation of the dorsal ulnar wrist.
  - The reverse oblique view (30 degrees of supination) (**FIG 3D**) allows evaluation of the palmar ulnar wrist with a profile of the pisotriquetral joint.
  - An ulnar deviation posteroanterior view (**FIG 3E**) may reveal lunotriquetral instability or evidence of ulnocarpal abutment. If ulnocarpal abutment is suspected, it is often useful to obtain a posteroanterior radiograph with the forearm in pronation and the fist clenched (Fig 3A), which increases ulnar variance.
- Videofluoroscopy is useful for evaluating dynamic ligament instabilities. The wrist should be examined through an entire active and passive ROM as well as with provocative maneuvers in an attempt to demonstrate pathology while reproducing symptoms.
- Arthrography may demonstrate a TFCC defect or interosseous ligament disruption if contrast material injected into one compartment leaks into an adjacent space.
- MRI can aid in the detection of soft tissue and osseous lesions, including interosseous and extrinsic ligament tears, TFCC defects, tumors, avascular necrosis, and occult fractures (**FIG 3F**).
  - Sensitivity of the MRI increases if it is combined with arthrography. The ability to show marrow changes in the

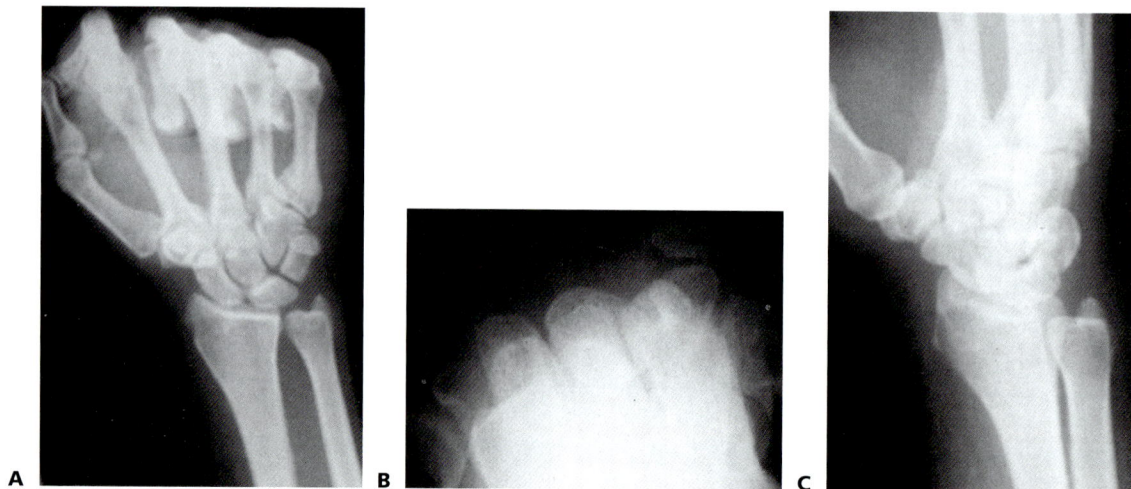

FIG 3 • **A.** Clenched fist view. **B.** Carpal tunnel view. **C.** Oblique view in 30 degrees of pronation. *(continued)*

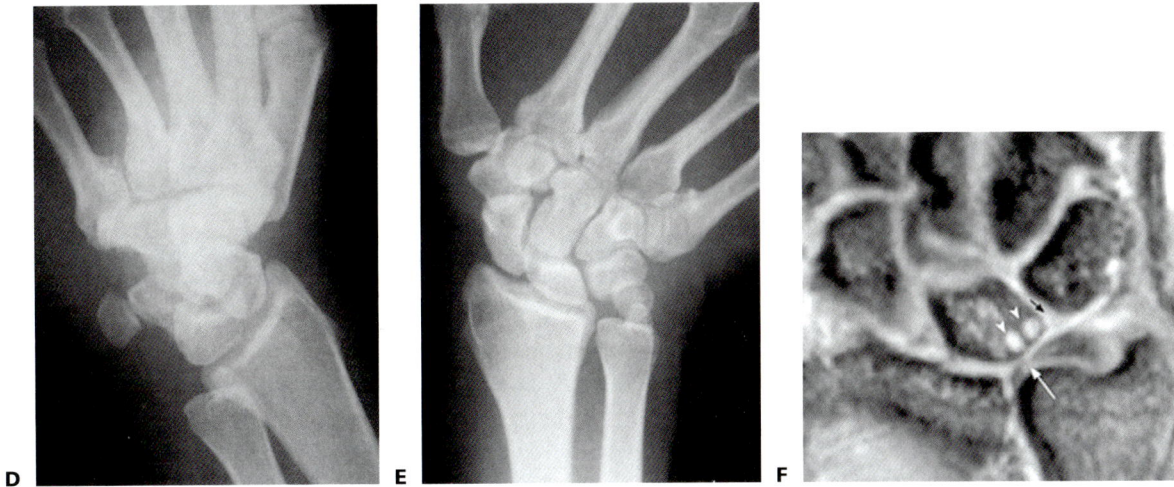

FIG 3 • *(continued)* **D.** Oblique view in 30 degrees of supination. **E.** Ulnar deviation view. **F.** Coronal gradient-echo MR image reveals a central triangular fibrocartilage perforation (*white arrow*), subchondral cystic changes in the lunate bone (*arrowheads*), and a lunotriquetral ligament tear (*black arrow*) in a 41-year-old man with ulnar impaction syndrome with positive variance and chronic ulnar-sided wrist pain (Palmer class IID lesion).

ulnar portion of the lunate and simultaneous central TFCC pathology is very helpful in confirming a diagnosis of ulnocarpal impaction.
- Arthroscopy can confirm a diagnosis suggested by findings from other diagnostic modalities.
  - This is the most sensitive tool for diagnosis of chondral and ligamentous pathology.
  - It has therapeutic applications in the management of ulnar abutment, TFCC defects, interosseous ligament tears, chondral defects, loose bodies, synovitis, and degenerative arthritis.
- Bone scan, ultrasonography, and computed tomography serve a very limited role in the diagnosis of ulnar impaction syndrome.

DIFFERENTIAL DIAGNOSIS

- Extensor carpi ulnaris (ECU) subluxation or tenosynovitis
- DRUJ arthritis (degenerative or inflammatory), incongruity, intra-articular pathology, instability
- Ulnar styloid fracture nonunion
- Isolated TFCC tears
- Lunate and triquetrum lesions: chondromalacia, cyst, or interosseous ganglion (lunate/capitate), intraosseous pathology (enchondroma, osteoid osteoma)
- Kienböck disease
- Lunotriquetral instability (trauma or impaction)
- Midcarpal joint arthritis or chondromalacia
- Hamate hook, triquetral, or pisiform fractures
- Flexor carpi ulnaris tendinitis
- Pisotriquetral arthritis
- Guyon canal pathology: ganglion, tunnel syndrome, ulnar artery thrombosis
- Ulnar neuritis

NONOPERATIVE MANAGEMENT

- Rest and avoidance of any aggravating maneuvers are the mainstay of nonoperative management for ulnar impaction syndrome.

- The success of this treatment lies with the patient's ability to change the way he or she does any number of routine tasks and may involve a change of employment.
- Ice and elevation may help to reduce any swelling associated with overuse or aggravation of a previous injury.
- Nonsteroidal anti-inflammatory medications will also reduce swelling and provide some analgesia.
- Neutral splinting provides support for the wrist and may help to prevent aggravating maneuvers.
- Injection of a steroid and local anesthetic mixture into the wrist may provide some temporary relief of symptoms and decrease swelling.
  - An intra-articular injection may also help differentiate intra- and extra-articular disorders.
- A combination of hand therapy modalities (ie, ultrasound, iontophoresis) and patient education may alleviate some symptoms.

SURGICAL MANAGEMENT

- Surgical treatment of ulnar impaction syndrome is indicated for patients who fail to respond to conservative modalities or those who cannot avoid aggravating maneuvers.
- Patients undergoing ulnar shortening osteotomy must be good surgical candidates, with a high likelihood of healing the osteotomy site.
  - Otherwise, an alternative surgical procedure, such as a wafer resection osteotomy, should be considered.
- Wrist arthroscopy is frequently used to document physical findings consistent with ulna impaction syndrome before performing a shortening osteotomy, especially in cases of diagnostic uncertainty even after nonoperative management and injections discussed above.

Commercial Devices for Ulnar Shortening Osteotomy

- Plates and jigs to assist with ulnar osteotomy are commercially available. These offer features such as low-profile plate design, locking screws, simplicity of use, decreased surgical time, and improved accuracy of the osteotomy cuts.

- The surgeon must consider whether the potential advantages of these systems justify the additional expense.[18]

Preoperative Planning

- Neutral rotation posteroanterior and lateral radiographs of both wrists demonstrate ulnar variance and the morphology of the DRUJ, helping to determine the degree of shortening required to unload the joint and still provide a congruent articulation.
- In principle, a long ulna should be shortened to neutral or 1 mm of negative variance. If there is ulnar-neutral variance as a baseline, 2 mm of bone should be removed.[7]
- Care must be taken to prevent excessive shortening of the ulna, as this has the potential to increase pressures across the DRUJ articular surface[11] and can lead to limitation of forearm rotation.
- The absolute amount of shortening possible is limited by the marginal ligaments of an intact TFCC.
  - This is reportedly 15 mm in the setting of posttraumatic ulna impaction syndrome.[8]
- DRUJ anomalies, congenital disorders, or arthritis should be ruled out.
- DRUJ stability is best assessed with examination under anesthesia.

Positioning

- Preoperative antibiotics with a coverage spectrum for skin flora are given intravenously about 30 minutes before the skin incision.
- The patient is positioned supine on the operating table with the upper extremity on an armboard.

- A single-bladder brachial tourniquet is placed over Webril in the upper brachial region and the arm is prepared and draped to the midbrachial level.
  - Extremity exsanguination is achieved with an elastic bandage wrap from the distal fingertips to midbrachial region, and then the tourniquet is inflated to about 250 mm Hg (the pressure may have to be increased in hypertensive patients).
- Unobstructed access to the elbow during the procedure is crucial to accurately evaluate pronation and supination.
- Intraoperative fluoroscopy helps the surgeon to discern the degree of correction in ulnar variance after the osteotomy.

Approach

- An 8- to 10-cm midaxial incision is made over the distal third of the ulnar diaphysis, ending at, or just proximal to, the distal ulnar metaphysis.
- The interval between the ECU and the flexor carpi ulnaris is developed to expose the ulnar periosteum.
- Although it is unlikely to be encountered, the location of the dorsal sensory branch of the ulnar nerve must be considered and protected.
  - It takes off from the ulnar nerve an average of 6.4 cm proximal to the distal aspect of the head of the ulna and runs along the subcutaneous border of the ulna for about 5 cm proximal to the pisiform.
  - The dorsal sensory branch typically courses along the medial border of the ulnar head with the forearm supinated and runs in a more palmar position with the forearm pronated.[2]
- Circumferential subperiosteal dissection is avoided to prevent injury to the segmental blood supply to the distal ulnar diaphysis, with the exception of a 1-cm zone at the site of the planned osteotomy.[22]

TECHNIQUES

AUTHORS' PREFERRED TECHNIQUE FOR ULNAR SHORTENING OSTEOTOMY

Exposure

- Make an 8- to 10-cm incision over the subcutaneous border of the ulna as previously described (**TECH FIG 1A**).
- Elevate the ECU muscle–tendon from the distal, dorsal aspect of the ulna to allow sufficient room for a six- or seven-hole AO dynamic compression plate (Synthes LC-DCP, Synthes USA, Paoli, PA) (**TECH FIG 1B**).
  - Take care to avoid disrupting the ECU subsheath distally.

Osteotomy

- Position the LC-DCP plate along the distal dorsal ulnar shaft to ensure fit, and prebend it into a very slightly concave configuration to ensure compression of the volar cortex with plate application.
  - A 3.5-mm plate is appropriate for most individuals, although a 2.7-mm plate may be used for smaller patients.
- Draw the proposed oblique osteotomy site beneath the third (for a six-hole plate) or fourth (for a seven-hole plate) hole in the plate.

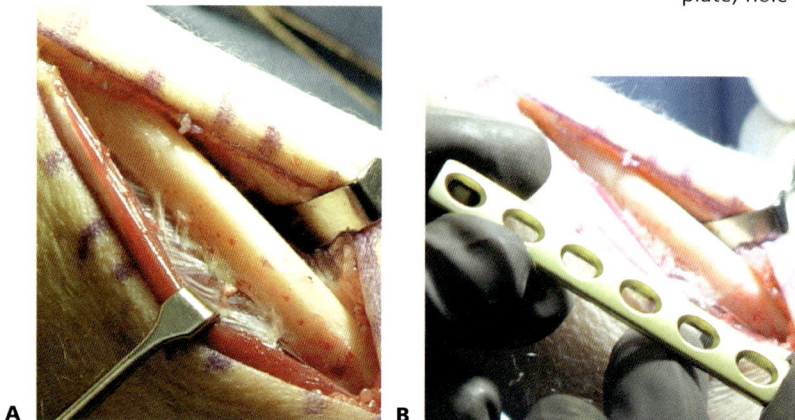

A   **B**

TECH FIG 1 • **A.** 8- to 10-cm incision over the subcutaneous border of the ulna. **B.** Six-hole AO-type dynamic compression plate (DCP) (Synthes USA, Paoli, PA).

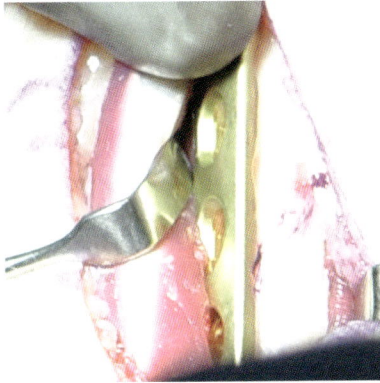

TECH FIG 2 • **A.** Dorsal compression plate in dorsal position. Proposed osteotomy drawn. The oblique osteotomy angle is about 45 to 60 degrees, and it is typically 5 to 6 cm proximal to the ulnar styloid. **B.** Synthes small distractor apparatus secured along the ulnarmost border with four 2.5-mm threaded Kirschner wires.

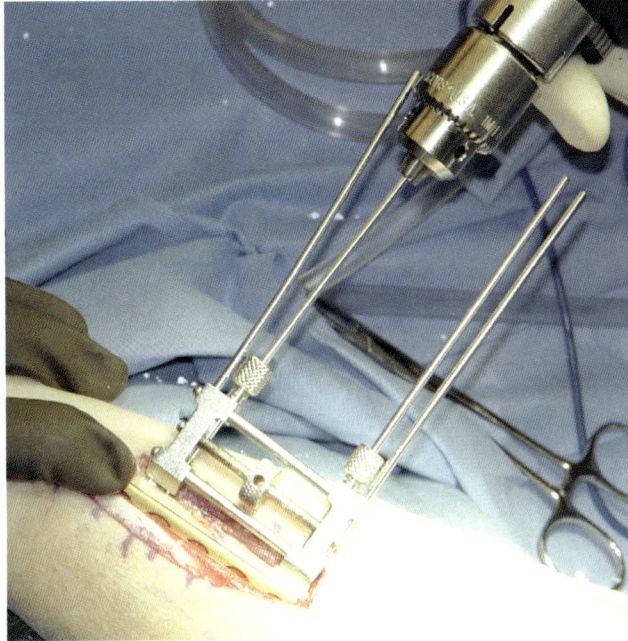

- The osteotomy is made obliquely in a dorsal to palmar direction so that the osteotomy site can later be secured with an interfragmentary screw applied through the dorsal plate.
- The oblique osteotomy angle is about 45 to 60 degrees, and it is typically 5 to 6 cm proximal to the ulnar styloid (**TECH FIG 2A**).
- The orientation of the osteotomy (either distal dorsal to proximal palmar or vice versa) is designed such that the acute angle (point) of the cut bone is adjacent to the plate on the side of the fragment to be compressed. This technique compresses the bone to the plate, avoiding displacement of the osteotomy.
- Secure the Synthes small distractor–compressor apparatus over the proposed osteotomy site (along the ulnar border) with four 2.5-mm threaded Kirschner wires (**TECH FIG 2B**).
  - Place the pins into the ulna in a region that will later be spanned by the plate to avoid creating unprotected stress risers after removal.
  - Avoid interfering with the osteotomy when placing the pins by referring to the line drawn at the proposed osteotomy site.
  - Place the pins palmar enough to allow the plate to be securely seated over the dorsal surface of the ulna.

Ulna Osteotomy

- Remove the plate from the operative field and complete the first osteotomy cut using a precise oscillating blade (**TECH FIG 3**).
  - It may be helpful to complete the distal cut first to avoid removing too much distal bone, forcing distal placement of the plate and poor fixation.
  - Take care to continuously irrigate the bone edges while sawing to avoid thermal necrosis of the bone and periosteum.
- The kerf (amount of bone resected by the saw blade itself) must be taken into account when planning the site of the second osteotomy cut to determine accurately the total amount of bone removed.

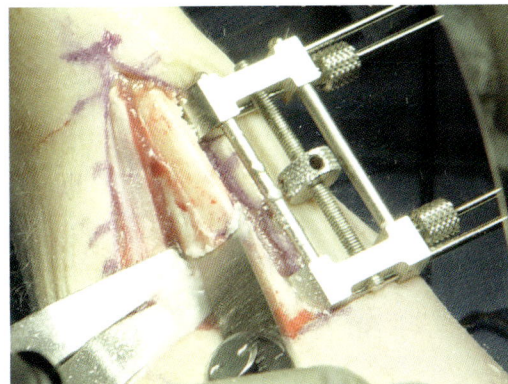

- Kerf thickness varies based on the specific blade used and can be obtained from the manufacturer.[8]
- Make the second parallel osteotomy cut proximal to the first, using a freehand technique, and remove the wafer of bone.
- Distract the osteotomy site and inspect it to ensure that there are no bony excrescences or residual uncut bone margins, which could interfere with apposition of the fragments.

Alternative Osteotomy Technique

- Perform a single osteotomy cut using stacked saw blades. This theoretically removes some of the "human element" and provides a more precise cut with improved apposition of the fragments.
- Using a single cut technique, reproducible ulnar shortening with precision within 0.2 mm of the exact desired ulnar variance has been reported.
- A relatively steep angled cut (60 degrees) using stacked blades with a kerf thickness of 4.45 mm can allow for up to 9 mm of shortening with a single cut.
- Cuts may be made at lesser angles and with lesser kerf thicknesses to allow for lesser degrees of shortening.[8]

TECH FIG 3 • Oblique osteotomy created.

TECHNIQUES

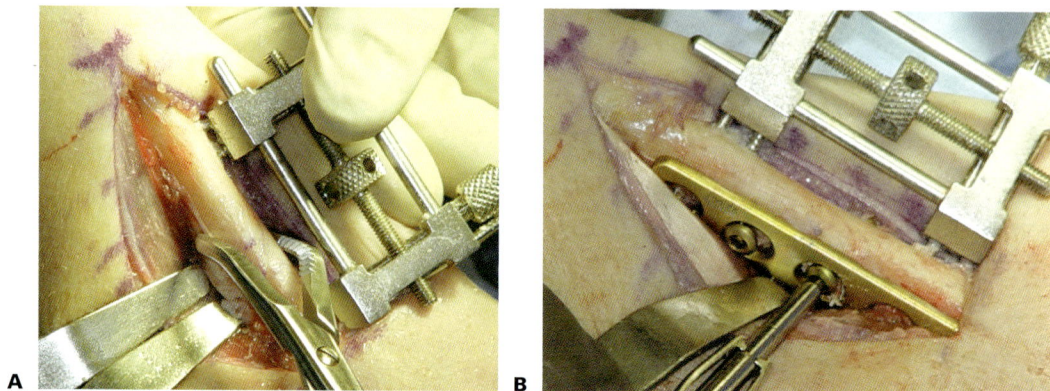

TECH FIG 4 • A. Osteotomy compression. **B.** An interfragmentary lag screw is placed through the plate.

Reduction and Stabilization

- Dial down the small distractor apparatus to achieve compression at the osteotomy site and bone-to-bone abutment (**TECH FIG 4A**).
  - A reduction clamp is valuable in guiding and then securing the fragments as compression is applied.
- Examine the radioulnar relationship under fluoroscopy to ensure adequate correction of ulnar variance and DRUJ congruence.
  - Additional bone resection followed by repeat reduction and compression can be easily achieved if necessary.
- Again place the Synthes nonlocking LC-DCP plate on the dorsum of the ulna, and drill screw holes using a compression or neutral drill guide.
  - With the exception of the interfragmentary lag screw hole, directly over the osteotomy site, all screw holes in the plate are drilled using a 2.5-mm drill followed by a 3.5-mm tap (unless self-tapping screws are used).
- First secure the plate with static screws to the fragment with the acute angle (point) on the side away from the plate (palmar in this case, using a dorsal plate).
- Reduce and secure the osteotomy, and then place compression screws in the other fragment, the one with the acute angle (point) adjacent to the plate.
  - Place the first compression screw in the second hole away from the osteotomy.

- Fill the remaining more proximal holes with either compression or static screws.
- As a final step, insert an interfragmentary lag screw through the osteotomy via the hole in the plate directly over the osteotomy (**TECH FIG 4B**).
  - Pass a 3.5-mm drill only through the near cortex, followed by a 2.5-mm drill through the far cortex. Tap this hole and fill it with a 3.5-mm bone screw.
  - Once proximal and distal stabilization has been achieved, it may be necessary to remove the 2.5-mm pins to fill the remaining screw holes.

Completion

- Again examine the bone under fluoroscopy to ensure good plate-to-bone and osteotomy site apposition and to assess screw lengths. Make a final assessment of the radioulnar relationship using standard posteroanterior and lateral neutral rotation views (**TECH FIG 5**).
- Irrigate the wound with normal saline. Close the deep subcutaneous layer with 3-0 Vicryl and approximate the skin edges with interrupted horizontal mattress 4-0 nylon.
- Apply a palmar, forearm-based plaster wrist splint after the tourniquet is deflated and sterile dressings have been applied.
- The arm is protected in a cast or splint until bony union has occurred.

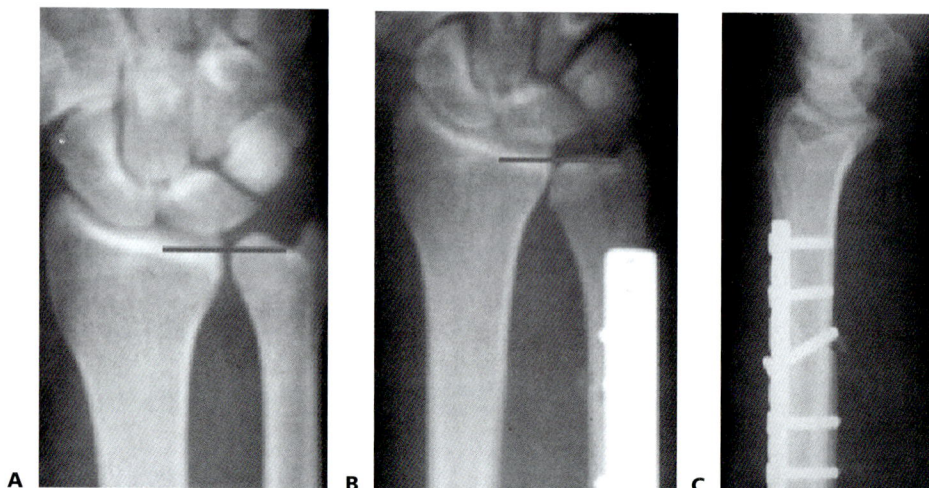

TECH FIG 5 • A. PA wrist radiograph showing ulnar-positive variance. **B,C.** PA and lateral radiographs after ulnar shortening osteotomy. The interfragmentary lag screw compresses the osteotomy site.

ULNAR SHORTENING OSTEOTOMY USING AN AO COMPRESSION DEVICE[5]

- Expose the ulna in the manner previously described and plan the osteotomy about 5 to 6 cm proximal to the ulnar styloid.
- Place a five- or six-hole 3.5-mm LC-DCP plate on the flat surface of the distal ulna, centered about the planned osteotomy site, with two or three holes distal, one hole across, and two or three holes proximal to the osteotomy.
  - Although the plate may be placed dorsal or volar, palmar positioning of the plate may be preferable to avoid subcutaneous prominence of the hardware after surgery.
  - Contour the plate in the manner described above.
- Fix the plate distally with two or three 3.5-mm cortical screws placed in a static mode.
- For a dorsal plate, draw the planned osteotomy on the bone with a marking pen at an angle of about 45 degrees distal dorsal to proximal palmar so that the proximal fragment will compress into the plate (**TECH FIG 6**).
- Fix the standard AO compression device to the ulna proximally with one unicortical screw and engage the mobile arm in the most proximal plate hole.

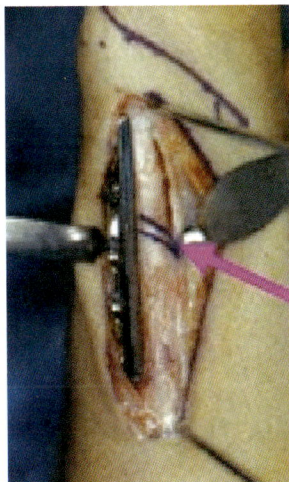

TECH FIG 6 • The proposed site of the osteotomy is marked on the ulna. This will allow for compression of the osteotomy when using a dynamic compression plate and placement of an interfragmentary lag screw. (Courtesy of Thomas R. Hunt III, MD.)

- Place the unicortical screw far enough proximal that adequate compression can be obtained. This distance will vary based on the amount of bone to be removed.
- Once shortening is complete and the compression device removed, the empty screw hole must not be too close to the proximal margin of the plate in order to avoid a stress riser.
- Remove the compression device and one distal screw, and loosen the most distal screw slightly, allowing the plate to be rotated away.
- Using a water-cooled oscillating saw, make the distal cut first using the freehand technique.
  - Interrupt the osteotomy cut after it is two thirds complete.
  - The saw blade may be left in this initial cut to act as a planar guide for the second parallel and proximal osteotomy cut.
- Place a new blade into the saw and make the proximal cut two thirds of the way through the bone.
- Complete the initial distal cut, followed by the proximal cut, and remove the perfectly round wafer of bone.
- Replace the previously removed distal screw and tighten both screws.
- Reapply the compression device and compress the osteotomy.
- Place the screw just proximal to the interfragmentary compression hole in a compression mode using the compression guide.
- Place the interfragmentary compression screw by first drilling a gliding hole through the near cortex with a 3.5-mm drill bit.
- Then, using a drill guide ("top hat"), drill the far cortex with a 2.5-mm drill bit. Measure the hole, tap the far cortex with a 3.5-mm tap, and place the interfragmentary compression screw.
- Remove the compression device and fill the remaining proximal screw hole(s) using the static drill guide.
- Irrigate and close the wound and apply a splint as previously described.

OSTEOCHONDRAL SHORTENING OSTEOTOMY[19]

- Wrist arthroscopy is performed to both stage and treat any ulnocarpal arthrosis or TFCC tear that may require débridement or repair.
- After arthroscopy, make a longitudinal incision over the fifth dorsal compartment.
  - Take care to identify and protect the dorsal sensory branch of the ulnar nerve.
- Incise the fifth extensor compartment, retract the extensor digiti quinti tendon, and create a capsulotomy through the floor of this fifth compartment.
  - Complete the capsulotomy in an L-shaped fashion by extending the incision transversely just proximal to the dorsal radioulnar ligament of the TFCC, thus preserving its stabilizing function for the DRUJ.

- Based on preoperative determinations, resect a 3- to 5-mm wafer of bone using a microsagittal saw at the level of the proximal margin of the DRUJ.
  - Leave the distal ulna articular surface and the TFCC foveal attachments intact (**TECH FIG 7A–C**).
- Reduce and compress the osteotomy with a hemostat and a Kirschner wire placed for temporary stabilization.
- Intraoperative fluoroscopy is used to confirm the adequacy of resection and osteotomy reduction.
- More bone can be removed if necessary, up to 5 mm total.
  - Excessive bony resection could lead to DRUJ instability or impingement.

TECHNIQUES

- Thread a cannulated headless compression screw over the previously inserted Kirschner wire while manual compression is maintained (**TECH FIG 7D,E**).
- Remove the Kirschner wire and irrigate the wounds.
- Repair the dorsal capsule with interrupted nonabsorbable sutures.

- Transpose the extensor digiti quinti tendon out of the fifth compartment as the capsule is repaired.
- Close the skin incision with a nonabsorbable monofilament suture, and inject all incisions, as well as the wrist, with a local anesthetic.
- Place the wrist in a bulky dressing with a volar splint.

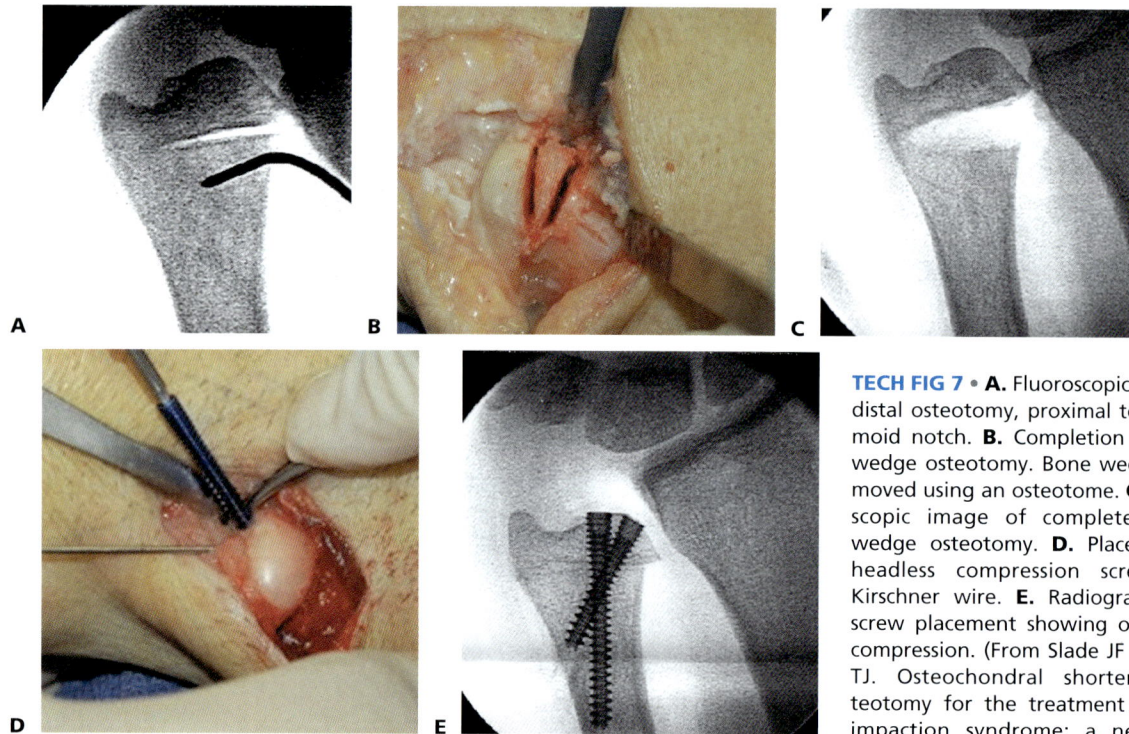

TECH FIG 7 • **A.** Fluoroscopic image of distal osteotomy, proximal to the sigmoid notch. **B.** Completion of radial wedge osteotomy. Bone wedge is removed using an osteotome. **C.** Fluoroscopic image of completed radial wedge osteotomy. **D.** Placement of headless compression screw over Kirschner wire. **E.** Radiograph after screw placement showing osteotomy compression. (From Slade JF III, Gillon TJ. Osteochondral shortening osteotomy for the treatment of ulnar impaction syndrome: a new technique. Tech Hand Up Extrem Surg 2007;11:74–82.)

PEARLS AND PITFALLS

- In very osteopenic bone, the surgeon should consider using a longer plate or locking hardware to achieve better bony purchase (**FIG 4**).
- Smokers, malnourished patients, and patients with poorly controlled diabetes or vascular compromise have a higher risk of osteotomy nonunion. The surgeon should consider a procedure that does not require bone healing (Darrach or wafer osteotomy).

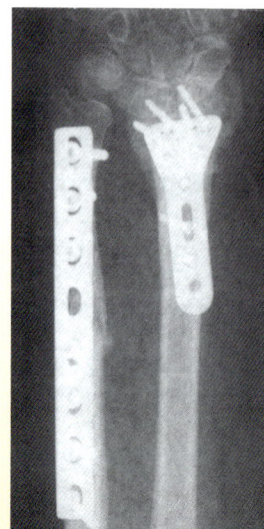

FIG 4 • Ulnar impaction syndrome in a 73-year-old woman after distal radius fracture nonunion and subsequent collapse. She underwent open reduction and internal fixation of the radius fracture as well as ulnar shortening osteotomy to correct the posttraumatic ulnar-positive variance. Severe osteopenia prevented stable fixation of the ulnar osteotomy with the standard plate and necessitated a longer eight-hole dynamic compression plate.

- Ulnar shortening osteotomy should be avoided in patients with DRUJ arthritis. The surgeon should consider unloading the ulno-carpal axis with a Sauvé-Kapandji or Darrach procedure.
- The dorsal sensory branch of the ulnar nerve should be protected during the surgical exposure. It runs medial to the ulnar head with the forearm supinated and more palmar with the forearm pronated.[2]
- The surgeon should avoid circumferential exposure of the ulna to avoid injury to the segmental blood supply to the ulnar diaphysis, which typically enters the bone from the region of the interosseous membrane.[22]
- The ECU subsheath should not be disrupted during the surgical approach.
- In smaller patients, the surgeon should consider using a 2.7-mm AO dynamic compression plate.
- The Kirschner wires used in the Synthes distractor apparatus should be inserted far enough away from the osteotomy site such that they will not interfere with the osteotomy cuts. They should be biased palmarly in the ulna if dorsal plating is planned. The four pins should be inserted in the region that will be spanned by the plate to prevent creation of an unprotected stress riser. The surgeon should avoid passing the distal pins through the ulna into the radius, as this will prevent shortening of the ulna.
- Making the distal cut first may help to avoid placing the plate too distally on the ulna.
- The osteotomy site should be continuously irrigated while the bone is being cut to avoid thermal necrosis of the bone and periosteum.
- The surgeon should avoid overshortening the ulna, as this can lead to DRUJ instability, loss of forearm rotation, and increased DRUJ contact pressures. Failure to consider the kerf thickness when planning the osteotomy can lead to excessive shortening.
- After the cuts are made, the surgeon should distract the osteotomy and inspect for bony excrescences or residual uncut bone margins, which can interfere with apposition of the proximal and distal fragments.
- Although the plate may be placed on the dorsal or palmar surface of the ulna, palmar positioning of the plate may be preferable to avoid a subcutaneous prominence of the hardware after surgery in thin or smaller patients.

POSTOPERATIVE CARE

- Short-arm below-elbow splint immediately postoperatively
- Ice and elevation to assist with swelling control
- Elbow and finger range of motion is encouraged immediately.
- Sutures are removed at 10 to 14 days.
- A removable splint is applied and protected range of motion is started at 6 to 8 weeks, depending on the radiographic appearance of healing.
- More aggressive range-of-motion exercises are started with hand therapy after 8 to 10 weeks if necessary.

OUTCOMES

- Chun and Palmer[6] reviewed their series of 30 wrists in 27 patients with an average follow-up of 51 months. Wrists were graded preoperatively and postoperatively according to the Gartland and Werley wrist system. Preoperative wrists graded as poor (28) and fair (2) improved to excellent (24), good (4), fair (1), and poor (1) after ulnar shortening osteotomy. They reported no ulnar nonunions, and complications were rare.
- Loh et al[10] evaluated 23 wrists at a mean follow-up of 33 months. A statistically significant reduction in pain intensity by visual analogue scale assessment was seen in 77% of patients. Preoperative versus postoperative change in range of motion was not statistically significant, and postoperative wrist function and grip strength also failed to show a statistically significant improvement. Sixty-eight percent of patients complained of local irritation secondary to prominent hardware and 32% eventually had the implant removed.
- We do not think that the use of specialized equipment is necessary to achieve accurate cuts and stable fixation for an ulnar shortening osteotomy.
  - Sunil et al[20] reported no significant differences in duration of surgery, relief of pain, return to work, postoperative complications, time elapsed between surgery and return to work, or osteotomy union in patients undergoing ulnar shortening osteotomy using the Rayhack device versus those undergoing freehand osteotomies.

- Braun[3] reported a $650 increase in cost with use of the Rayhack device compared to performing the technique freehand.
- Our preferred technique is simple, it does not require specialized equipment (Synthes Small External Fixation and Small Fragment Bone Fixation Systems), it provides for rotational control of the distal segment, it provides compression of the osteotomy site, and it uses only one size of drill bit, tap, and screw except for the single interfragmentary hole at the osteotomy site.

COMPLICATIONS

- Wound infection and osteomyelitis (rare)
- Hardware fracture (rare with 3.5-mm plate)
- Hardware failure with very osteopenic bone
- Delayed union rates in smokers (7.1 months for smokers versus 4.1 months for nonsmokers)[4]
- Painful, prominent hardware: It is generally not necessary to remove hardware, but 3.5-mm compression plates seem to be removable at 6 to 9 months in symptomatic patients with a low risk for refracture when sequential sets of radiographs confirm healing of the osteotomy site.[17]

REFERENCES

1. Berger RA. The ligaments of the wrist: a current overview of anatomy with considerations of their potential functions. Hand Clin 1997; 13:63–82.
2. Botte MJ, Cohen MS, Lavernia CJ, et al. The dorsal branch of the ulnar nerve: an anatomic study. J Hand Surg Am 1990;15A: 603–607.
3. Braun RM. A comparative study of ulnar-shortening osteotomy by the freehand technique versus the Rayhack technique. [Letter to the editor.] J Hand Surg Am 2006;31A:1411.
4. Chen F, Osterman AL, Mahony K. Smoking and bony union after ulna-shortening osteotomy. Am J Orthop 2001;30:486–489.
5. Chen NC, Wolfe SW. Ulna shortening osteotomy using a compression device. J Hand Surg Am 2003;28A:88–93.
6. Chun S, Palmer AK. The ulnar impaction syndrome: follow-up of ulnar shortening osteotomy. J Hand Surg Am 1993;18A:46–53.

7. Friedman SL, Palmer AK. The ulnar impaction syndrome. Hand Clin 1991;7:295–310.

8. Fricker R, Pfeiffer KM, Troeger H. Ulnar shortening osteotomy in posttraumatic ulnar impaction syndrome. Arch Orthop Trauma Surg 1996;115:158–161.

9. Labosky DA, Waggy CA. Oblique ulnar shortening osteotomy by a single saw cut. J Hand Surg Am 1996;21A:48–59.

10. Loh YC, Van Den Abbeele K, Stanley JK, et al. The results of ulnar shortening for ulnar impaction syndrome. J Hand Surg Br 1999;24B: 316–320.

11. Mikic ZD. Age changes in the triangular fibrocartilage of the wrist joint. J Anat 1978;126:367–384.

12. Miura T, Firoozbakhsh K, Cheema T, et al. Dynamic effects of joint-leveling procedure on pressure at the distal radioulnar joint. J Hand Surg Am 2005;30A:711–718.

13. Mizuseki T, Tsuge K, Yoshikazu I. Precise ulna-shortening osteotomy with a new device. J Hand Surg Am 2001;26A:931–939.

14. Nishiwaki M, Nakamura T, Nakao Y, et al. Effect on distal radioulnar joint stability: a biomechanical study. J Hand Surg Am 2005; 30A:719–726.

15. Palmer AK, Werner FW, Glisson RR, et al. Partial excision of the triangular fibrocartilage complex. J Hand Surg Am 1988;13A: 391–394.

16. Palmer AK, Werner FW. The triangular fibrocartilage complex of the wrist: anatomy and function. J Hand Surg Am 1981;6A:153–162.

17. Pomerance J. Plate removal after ulnar-shortening osteotomy. J Hand Surg Am 2005;30A:949–953.

18. Rayhack JM. Ulnar shortening. Tech Hand Up Extrem Surg 2003;7:52–60.

19. Slade JF III, Gillon TJ. Osteochondral shortening osteotomy for the treatment of ulnar impaction syndrome: a new technique. Tech Hand Up Extrem Surg 2007;11:74–82.

20. Sunil TM, Orth MS, Wolff TW, et al. A comparative study of ulnar-shortening osteotomy by the freehand technique versus the Rayhack technique. J Hand Surg Am 2006;31A:252–257.

21. Tomaino MM. The importance of the pronated grip x-ray view in evaluating ulnar variance. J Hand Surg Am 2000;25A:352–357.

22. Wright TW, Glowczeskie F. Vascular anatomy of the ulna. J Hand Surg Am 1998;23A:800–804.

Chapter 96

Surgical Decompression of the Forearm, Hand, and Digits for Compartment Syndrome

Marci D. Jones, Rodrigo Santamarina, and Lance G. Warhold

DEFINITION

- Acute compartment syndrome is a condition in which increased tissue pressure compromises the circulation within the enclosed space of fascial compartments. As a result of this elevated interstitial pressure, the blood supply to the soft tissues is impaired. If left untreated, elevated pressures can cause irreversible muscle and nerve damage resulting in fibrosis and contracture.

ANATOMY

- Compartment syndrome is most common in the forearm and hand but can occur in the arm and in the finger.
- The arm is divided into two fascial compartments, the forearm into three compartments, the hand into ten compartments, and the finger into two compartments.
- The two arm compartments are the anterior and posterior, separated by the medial and lateral intermuscular septa (**FIG 1A**).

- The anterior arm compartment contains the biceps brachii, brachialis, and coracobrachialis.
- The posterior arm compartment contains the triceps brachii.
- The forearm consists of three compartments: the volar, the dorsal, and the mobile wad of three (**FIG 1B**).
  - The contents of the volar compartment include the flexor muscles and can be subdivided into superficial and deep components. The superficial muscles are the flexor carpi ulnaris, palmaris longus, pronator teres, and flexor carpi radialis. The deep muscles are the flexor digitorum superficialis and profundus, and the flexor pollicis longus.
  - The dorsal compartment of the forearm contains the extensor muscles. The superficial extensors include the extensor digitorum communis, extensor digiti minimi, and extensor carpi ulnaris. The deep layer includes the supinator, abductor pollicis longus, extensor pollicis longus, extensor pollicis brevis, and extensor indicis.

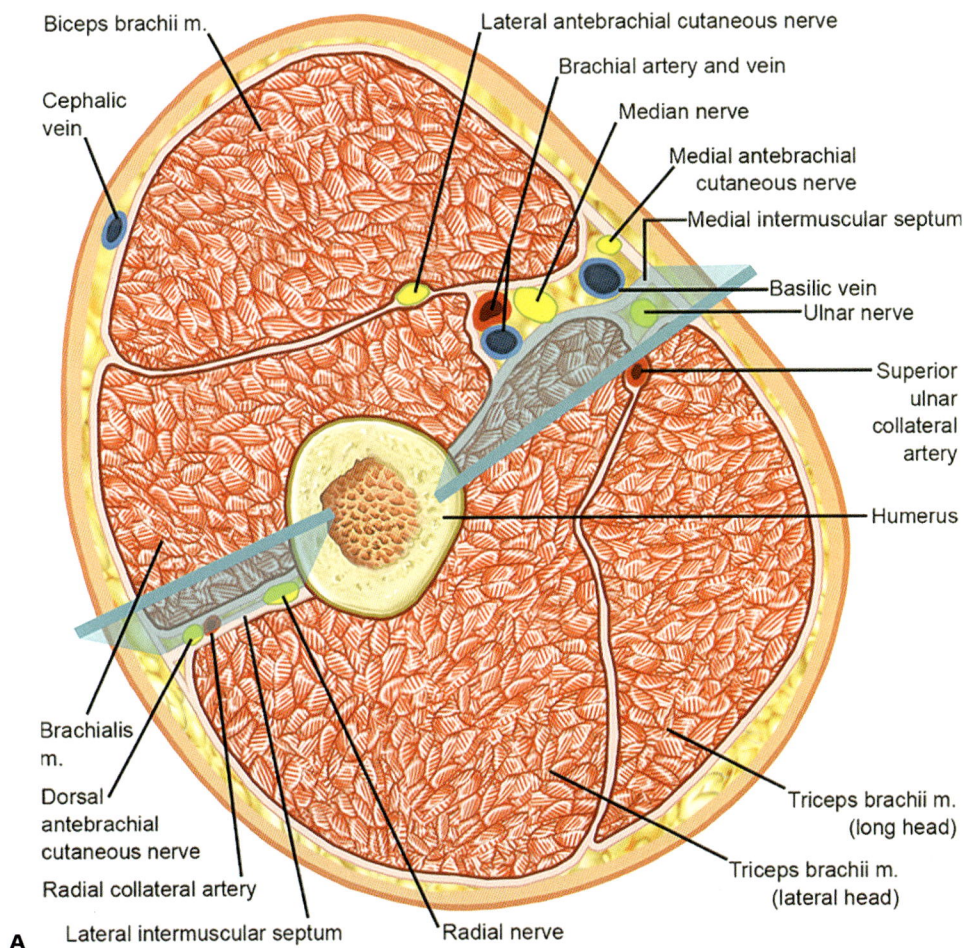

FIG 1 • A. Compartments of the arm. *(continued)*

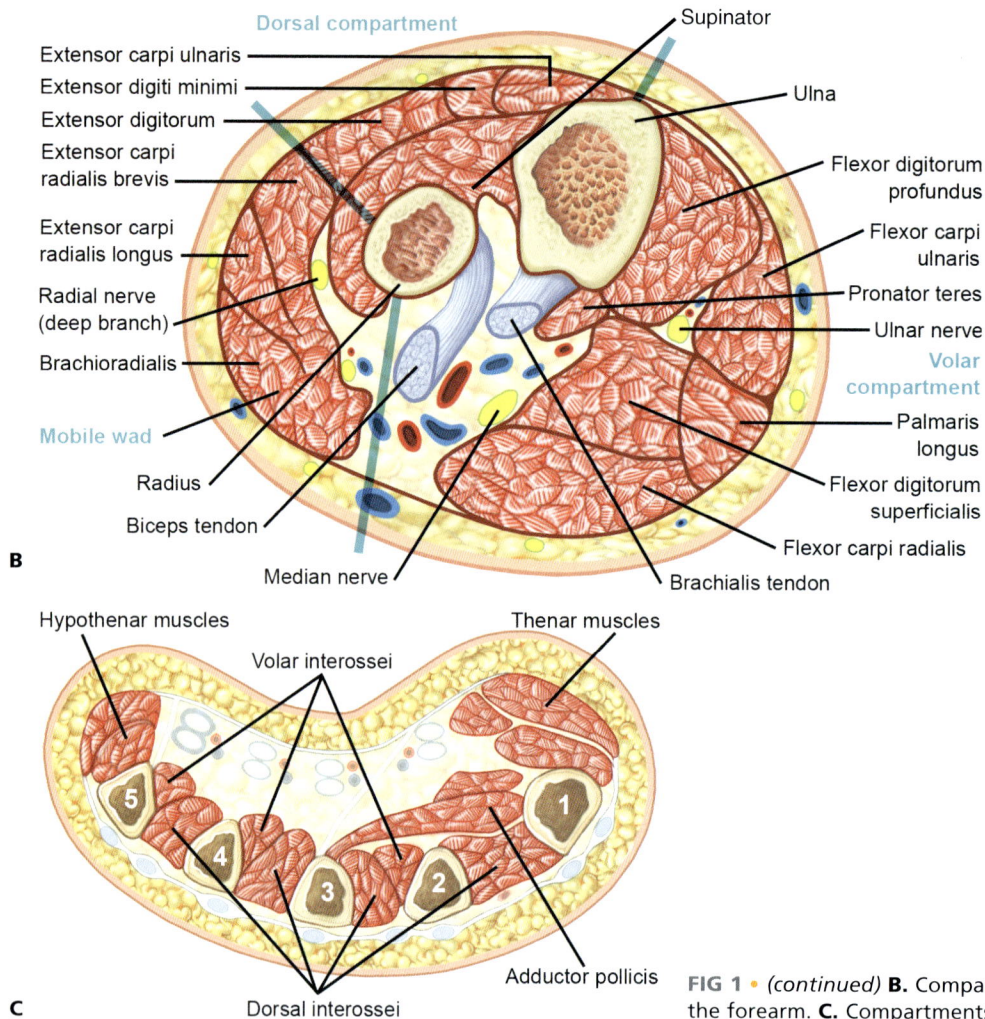

FIG 1 • (continued) **B.** Compartments of the forearm. **C.** Compartments of the hand.

- The mobile wad of three is a distinct muscle compartment that contains the brachioradialis, extensor carpi radialis longus, and extensor carpi radialis brevis.
- The wrist has one significant closed space, the carpal tunnel. Although not a compartment in the strictest sense, increased pressure in this tunnel can be detrimental to the median nerve.
- The hand contains ten distinct compartments (**FIG 1C**).
    - There are seven compartments for the interossei. Each of the four dorsal and three palmar interossei has a separate compartment.
    - The adductor compartment contains the adductor pollicis.
    - The thenar compartment contains the abductor pollicis brevis, the opponens pollicis, and the flexor pollicis brevis.
    - The hypothenar compartment contains the abductor digiti minimi, flexor digiti minimi, and opponens digiti minimi.
- Compartment syndrome can also occur in the finger due to the limited skin compliance from the multiple fascial attachments.

PATHOGENESIS

- Increased pressure within a compartment decreases the blood supply to the soft tissues and can result in tissue ischemia and ultimately necrosis. The blood flow to a compartment is determined by several factors, including venous pressure, arterial pressure, and local interstitial pressure. Increased capillary permeability results from muscle ischemia. This increased permeability leads to intramuscular edema, increases the tissue pressure, decreases blood flow and oxygen transport, and leads to more tissue damage. It is easy to appreciate the vicious cycle that escalates the pathophysiology of the compartment syndrome.
- Many conditions are associated with compartment syndrome. These can be divided into two major categories[3]:
    - Conditions that decrease compartment volume (tight casts or dressings, burn eschar, limb lengthening or application of traction, increased external pressure on limb from prolonged weight [lying on limb or entrapment under a weight])
    - Conditions that increase compartment contents (bleeding—arterial or venous injury, anticoagulation, trauma, reperfusion injury, edema, infiltrated infusion, snakebite, infection, high-pressure injection)

NATURAL HISTORY

- Compartment syndrome results in hypoxic cell damage and ultimately anoxic cell death. Functional changes occur in muscle after 2 to 4 hours of total ischemia. Hypoxia to nerves causes paresthesia and hypoesthesia within 30 minutes of ischemia, but irreversible nerve damage may not occur until 12 hours or more of total ischemia.

- An untreated compartment syndrome can result in permanent neural deficit, tissue necrosis, growth arrest, Volkmann contracture, and even wet gangrene.

PATIENT HISTORY AND PHYSICAL FINDINGS

- It is important to elicit a detailed history and evaluate the possible causes of compartment syndrome (discussed above).
- Pain out of proportion to physical findings is the most important finding. For patients with this finding, one must have a high clinical suspicion regardless of the presumed severity of the inciting event.
- Most commonly, patients will present with a history of trauma or a crushing injury; however, other causes must not be overlooked.
- Compartment syndrome may involve single or multiple compartments in the extremity.
- Physical examination findings include:
  - A tense, swollen, and tender compartment (**FIG 2**)
  - Pain with passive stretch of the muscles within the compartment
  - Paresthesias or sensory disturbances in the nerve distribution of the compressed nerve are intermediate findings. This can be accompanied by motor weakness. Motor paralysis is a later finding.
  - Pallor and pulselessness are late findings.
- The findings of pain out of proportion to physical examination, a tense compartment, and pain with passive stretch are sufficient to warrant intracompartmental pressure measurements. One should not delay definitive diagnosis and treatment until later findings are present.

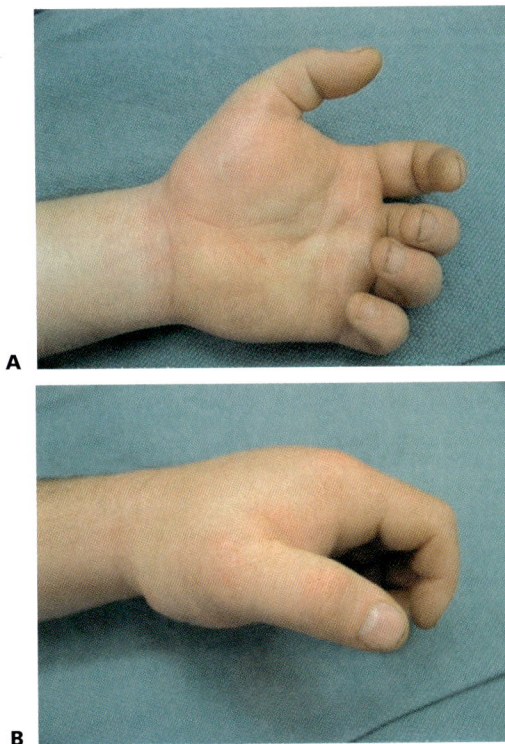

FIG 2 • Diffuse, tense swelling of the hand. **A.** Palmar view with loss of palmar concavity. **B.** Radial view.

- In obtunded or sedated patients, a tense, swollen compartment is sufficient to warrant intracompartmental pressure measurements.

IMAGING AND OTHER DIAGNOSTIC STUDIES

- Clinical examination is the cornerstone of the diagnosis, and it is important to have a high degree of suspicion for compartment syndrome.
- Immediate fasciotomy is indicated in patients with unequivocal symptoms and signs of compartment syndrome. Direct measurement of compartment pressures is indicated in all cases when the patient's symptoms and physical examination signs are indicative of compartment syndrome, and it is especially important in patients who are obtunded or sedated.
- Diagnosis of compartment syndrome of the finger is made clinically and not through the use of pressure measurement.
- Pressure measurement in the arm is made in both anterior and posterior compartments. Anteriorly, the pressure is measured over the biceps muscle, and posteriorly over the triceps muscle.
  - The physician must be careful not to injure the radial nerve when measuring the arm compartment pressure. The nerve courses deep to the triceps in the spiral groove of the humerus. Ten centimeters proximal to the lateral epicondyle, it passes through the lateral intermuscular septum to the anterior compartment.
- In the forearm, the pressure is measured over the palmar, mobile wad, and dorsal compartments.
  - The median and ulnar nerves are at risk during measurement of the palmar compartment. The ulnar nerve courses deep to the flexor carpi ulnaris in the ulnar forearm; the median nerve is between the flexor digitorum superficialis and profundus muscles.
  - When measuring the mobile wad, the superficial branch of the radial nerve is deep to the brachioradialis in the forearm but emerges between the brachioradialis and extensor carpi radialis longus tendons about 8 cm proximal to the radial styloid.
    - The posterior interosseous nerve courses around the radial neck in the proximal radial forearm and should be avoided when measuring the mobile wad and dorsal compartments.
- In the hand, pressure measurements should be made in the affected compartments; measurements are generally made in the area of the planned incisions.
- There is not an absolute increased compartment pressure that warrants fasciotomy. When the pressure approaches 30 to 45 mm Hg, or 30 mm Hg less than the diastolic pressure, with concordant physical examination findings, decompressive fasciotomy should be performed.[4] In the hand, lower pressures (15 to 20 mm Hg) may indicate compartment syndrome.
- Plain radiographs should be performed to evaluate any underlying bony abnormality. Fractures and dislocations should be reduced as anatomically as possible.
- Arterial injury can lead to ischemia and can present similarly. Arteriography is indicated if the history may be significant for arterial injury (fracture, avulsion, or laceration).

DIFFERENTIAL DIAGNOSIS

- Arterial injury
- Nerve injury

NONOPERATIVE MANAGEMENT

▪ There is no role for nonoperative management of an acute compartment syndrome. In acute cases of compartment syndrome with elevated compartment pressure, prompt decompressive fasciotomies are required to relieve tissue ischemia.

▪ In patients with early symptoms and signs of compartment syndrome, but without elevated compartment pressures, removal of all compressive dressings and casts, and elevation of the affected extremity to the level of the heart is indicated.

  ▪ Frequent close monitoring by physical examination and repeated pressure measurements as necessary are critical.

▪ In patients presenting late with aseptic muscle necrosis, acute fasciotomy and débridement may not be indicated.

SURGICAL MANAGEMENT

Preoperative Planning

▪ The surgeon should review radiographs and plan for surgical stabilization as necessary.

Positioning

▪ The patient is positioned supine on the operating table with the upper extremity on an armboard.

▪ Tourniquets are not routinely used during decompressive fasciotomy.

▪ If the arm is affected, the shoulder and axilla are included in the sterile field to allow exposure to the entire extremity.

Approach

▪ Skin is considered a significant compressive structure, and it is important to create a skin incision of sufficient length to allow complete decompression. Cosmesis is not a concern.

▪ Incisions are planned to afford complete and rapid decompression of the compartments while maintaining coverage of vital structures and avoiding joint contractures due to scarring.

▪ The viability of muscles is determined by muscle tone and color, contractility, and bleeding.

  ▪ If the viability is still unclear, the muscle should be left alone and reinspected in 24 to 48 hours.

▪ The skin is left open and the wounds are copiously irrigated and covered with wet saline dressings. Occasionally, a wound vacuum dressing can be applied to facilitate care and reduce edema and pain associated with frequent dressing changes.

▪ Once the wound is considered to be stable and clean, the skin can be closed if under no tension. If tension is present, split-thickness skin grafts are usually applied.

TECHNIQUES

DECOMPRESSION OF THE ARM

▪ Compartment syndrome of the arm is rare. It can be approached from the lateral, posterior, or anteromedial approach.

  ▪ The choice of incision may be based on the need for fracture fixation.[1,2]

▪ The lateral approach begins at the deltoid insertion and extends to the lateral epicondyle. The fascia overlying the biceps anteriorly and triceps posteriorly is split through the incision (TECH FIG 1A).

▪ The anteromedial approach extends from the medial epicondyle toward the axilla, and the fascia overlying the biceps and triceps is split (TECH FIG 1B). This incision can be continued from the forearm skin incisions.

  ▪ The ulnar nerve must be protected in this approach.

▪ For isolated posterior compartment syndrome, a posterior incision can be made from 8 cm distal to the acromion to the olecranon[6] (TECH FIG 1C). The triceps fascia is directly exposed and incised.

  ▪ The radial nerve runs between the long and lateral heads of the triceps and is at risk during muscle débridement.

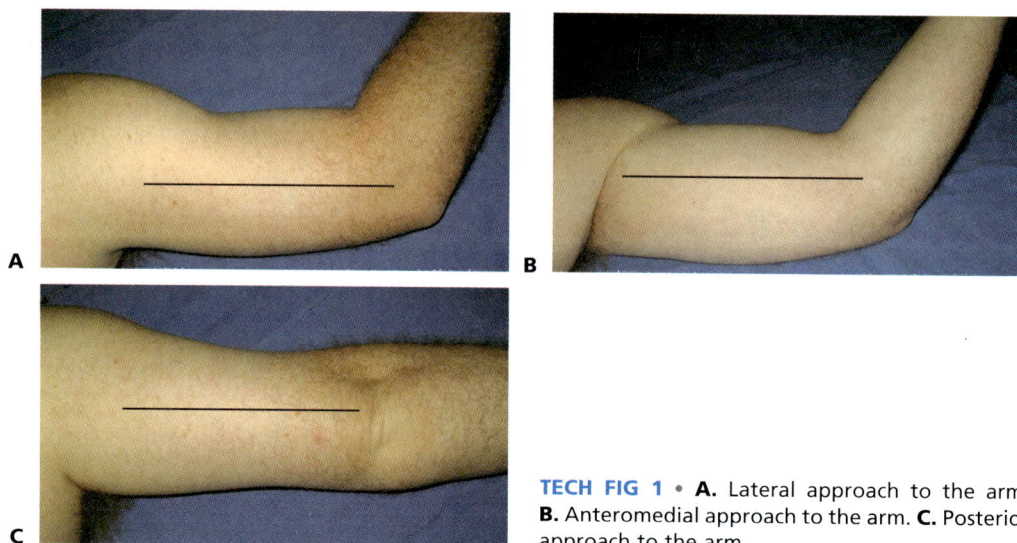

TECH FIG 1 • **A.** Lateral approach to the arm. **B.** Anteromedial approach to the arm. **C.** Posterior approach to the arm.

DECOMPRESSION OF THE VOLAR FOREARM

- Design a curvilinear incision from the carpal tunnel to the antecubital fossa. A complete carpal tunnel release is indicated if symptoms of median nerve compression are present (TECH FIG 2).
- Start the incision distally between the thenar and hypothenar eminences in line with the radial border of the ring finger. Release the skin, palmar fascia, and transverse carpal ligament.
- Continue the incision proximally to the distal wrist crease, then curve it ulnarly to the pisiform and extend it proximally along the ulnar side of the distal forearm.
    - This prevents exposure of the flexor tendons and median nerve and protects the palmar cutaneous branch of the median nerve.
- Curve the incision radially in the mid-forearm and then just anterior to the medial epicondyle at the elbow.
    - Creation of this flap provides coverage of the median nerve.
- At the antecubital fossa, curve the incision slightly anteriorly to meet the incision of the arm, if necessary.
    - This prevents a linear incision at the level of the elbow and provides coverage for the brachial artery.

- Release the fascia covering the superficial and deep compartment of the forearm, as well as the mobile wad, through this incision. Release the lacertus fibrosis at the elbow. Release individual muscle fascia if release of the compartment fascia does not relieve the pressure within each muscle.
- Loosely close the wound over the carpal tunnel; it is generally left open over the forearm.
    - If the swelling is mild, the fascia may be left open and the skin closed, or the skin edges may be approximated with a vessel loop-stapling technique.
    - If the wound is left open, it is covered with a sterile nonocclusive dressing. Alternatively, a VAC dressing may be applied.
- An alternative incision uses the Henry approach between the brachioradialis and the flexor carpi radialis, connecting to the carpal tunnel distally and proximally crossing the antecubital fossa obliquely from radial to ulnar.
    - If this approach is used, take care not to injure the palmar cutaneous branch of the median nerve at the wrist.

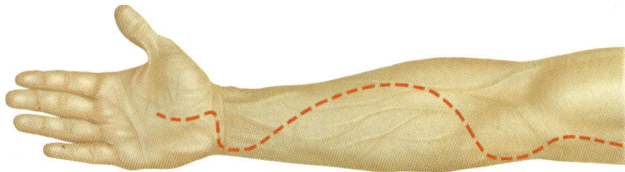

TECH FIG 2 • Incision for decompression of the palmar forearm. Note the incision in the hand used here for release of the thenar compartment.

DECOMPRESSION OF THE DORSAL FOREARM

- In the forearm, release of the volar compartment and mobile wad may decrease the pressure in the dorsal compartment. Once the palmar fasciotomy has been performed, the dorsal compartment should be re-evaluated for the need for fasciotomy.
- Make a longitudinal dorsal incision just ulnar to the tubercle of Lister and extending proximally toward the lateral epicondyle. Release the fascia over the dorsal compartment (TECH FIG 3).
- Release individual muscle fascia if necessary.
- If posterior interosseous nerve involvement is suspected, separate the extensor carpi ulnaris and extensor digitorum communis muscles to expose and release the fascia overlying the supinator.

- The wound is managed in a similar way to that described for the volar forearm fasciotomy.

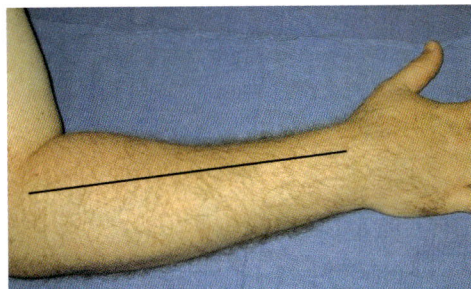

TECH FIG 3 • Incision for approach to the dorsal forearm.

DECOMPRESSION OF THE HAND COMPARTMENTS

- To release the four dorsal and three palmar interosseous compartments and the adductor compartment, make two dorsal longitudinal incisions over the second and fourth metacarpals (TECH FIG 4A).

- Take the incisions to the level of the extensor tendons. Avoid the sensory branches of the radial and ulnar nerves, and preserve dorsal veins to minimize postoperative edema.

TECHNIQUES

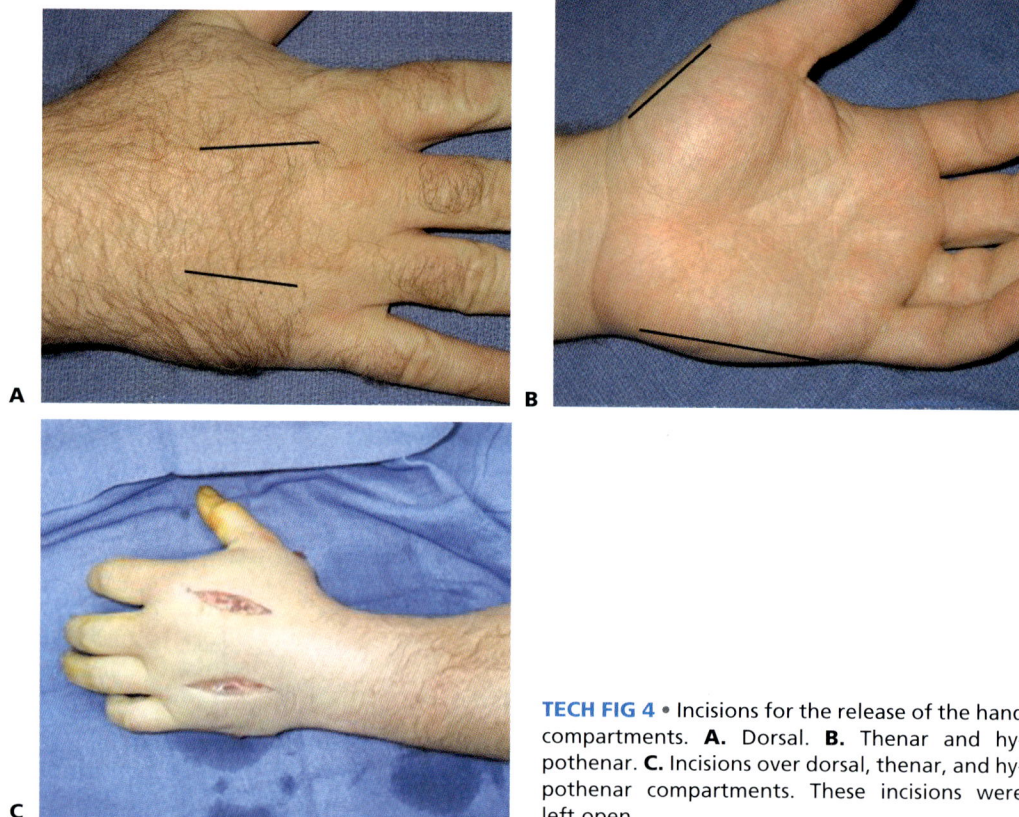

A

B

C

TECH FIG 4 • Incisions for the release of the hand compartments. **A.** Dorsal. **B.** Thenar and hypothenar. **C.** Incisions over dorsal, thenar, and hypothenar compartments. These incisions were left open.

■ Retract the extensor tendons and the dorsal surface of the metacarpal. Release the dorsal compartments on each side of the metacarpal (the first and second dorsal compartments are reached on either side of the second metacarpal, and the third and fourth dorsal compartments are found on either side of the fourth metacarpal). Continue blunt dissection palmarly through the dorsal interosseous to release the three palmar interosseous compartments.

■ Release the adductor compartment through the incision over the second metacarpal.

■ Release the thenar compartment through a longitudinal incision along the radial border of the thumb metacarpal, and release the hypothenar compartment through an incision along the ulnar border of the fifth metacarpal (**TECH FIG 4B**). Split the underlying fascia longitudinally.

■ The wounds are left open (**TECH FIG 4C**) and the hand is placed in a bulky splint in intrinsic-plus position (metacarpophalangeal joints flexed 70 degrees and interphalangeal joints extended).

DECOMPRESSION OF THE FINGER

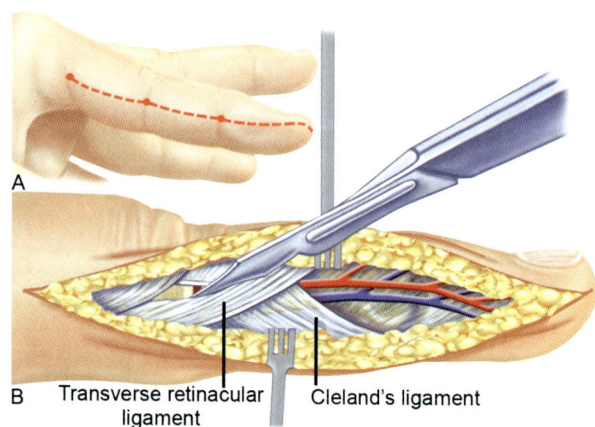

A

B   Transverse retinacular   Cleland's ligament
     ligament

■ Make longitudinal midaxial incisions along the finger. These incisions are made by connecting the most dorsal portions of the joint flexion creases (**TECH FIG 5A**). These are more easily seen with the finger in flexion.

■ Avoid making a more palmar, midlateral incision to prevent postoperative flexion contracture.

■ Carefully divide the transverse retinacular ligament and Cleland's ligament to release the neurovascular bundles on both radial and ulnar sides (**TECH FIG 5B**).

■ If possible, loosely approximate the skin.

TECH FIG 5 • **A.** Incision for the release of the finger. Dots are placed at the apex of each flexion crease, and connecting the dots provides the midaxial line. **B.** Division of the transverse retinacular ligament and Cleland's ligament.

PEARLS AND PITFALLS

Indications	■ Have a low threshold for measurement of compartment pressures. Perform pressure measurements if clinical examination findings are equivocal.
Surgical management	■ Take care to completely decompress the skin and fascia. ■ Do not injure superficial nerves. ■ Débride any devitalized muscle. ■ Do not close the fascia. ■ Close the skin loosely or leave it open at the initial procedure.
Postoperative management	■ Return to the operating room for a second look if there is muscle of questionable viability. ■ Base closure of the wounds on the skin tension and viability. Choose delayed primary closure, split-thickness skin grafting, or flaps as appropriate.

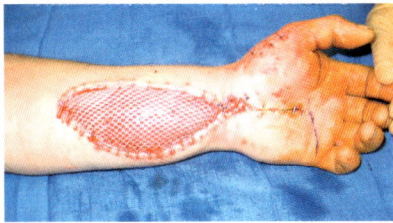

FIG 3 • Wound coverage after second look with delayed primary closure and split-thickness skin grafting.

POSTOPERATIVE CARE

■ A second look is planned 48 to 72 hours after the index procedure.

  ■ Additional débridement of devitalized tissue is performed. Serial débridements are performed until no devitalized tissue remains.

  ■ Delayed primary closure of the skin (not fascia) may be possible. More frequently, split-thickness skin grafting is performed to cover the wounds (**FIG 3**). If significant soft tissue has been lost with exposed tendon, nerve, or bone, flap coverage is planned.

■ Wound coverage should be performed as soon as possible to minimize complications such as infection, desiccation, and amputation.

■ The upper extremity should be elevated and splinted in an intrinsic-plus position. Gentle active and active assisted range of motion of the hand, wrist, and elbow should be initiated as soon as swelling begins to subside, generally within 2 to 3 days after wound closure. Placement of a flap or skin graft may preclude motion at certain joints, but unaffected joints should be ranged.

OUTCOMES

■ The outcome after compartment release depends both on the severity of the initial injury and the time elapsed before release.

■ Patients with prompt diagnosis and treatment and limited devitalized tissues generally have favorable outcomes.

■ Patients with severe initial injuries, delayed treatment, or extensive tissue necrosis have a more guarded prognosis for functional recovery of the upper extremity.

COMPLICATIONS

■ Volkmann ischemic contracture is the result of untreated acute compartment syndrome.

■ Necrosis and fibrosis of the muscle occur, with a resultant claw hand deformity. This deformity is due to extrinsic flexor and extensor contracture with concomitant intrinsic muscle dysfunction.

■ Nerve dysfunction results either from the initial ischemic injury or from subsequent compressive neuropathy due to the dense scarring of the tissues surrounding the nerves.

■ The deeper compartments are more severely compromised, with the flexor digitorum profundus alone affected in milder cases, and fibrosis of all muscles in the most severe.

REFERENCES

1. Antebi E, Herscovici D Jr. Acute compartment syndrome of the upper arm: a report of 2 cases. Am J Orthop 2005;34:498–500.
2. Diminick M, Shapiro G, Cornell C. Acute compartment syndrome of the triceps and deltoid. J Orthop Trauma 1999;13:225–227.
3. Gulgonen A. Compartment syndrome. In: Green DP, Pederson WC, Hotchkiss RN, et al, eds. Green's Operative Hand Surgery, 5th ed. New York: Elsevier Churchill Livingstone, 2005:1985–2006.
4. Whitesides E, Heckman MW. Acute compartment syndrome: update on diagnosis and treatment. J Am Acad Orthop Surg 1996;4:209–218.
5. Yabuki S, Kikuchi S. Dorsal compartment syndrome of the upper arm: a case report. Clin Orthop Relat Res 1999;366:107–109.

Chapter 97

Surgical Treatment of Injection Injuries in the Hand

Rimma Finkel, Emese Kalnoki-Kis, and Morton Kasdan

DEFINITION

- Since the beginning of the Industrial Revolution and the advent of industrial machinery, high-pressure injuries have been reported in the literature.
  - The force needed to break the skin is 100 pounds per square inch (psi). In general, high-pressure injuries are forced into the tissues at a pressure of 141 to 703 kg/cm^2 (2000 to 12,000 psi)[8] (**FIG 1**).
- The substances typically injected include grease, paint, paint thinners, diesel fuel, oil, water, and cement. Cases involving molten metal,[4] dry cleaning solvents,[10] and veterinary vaccines[6] also have been documented.

ANATOMY

- The site of injection and pressure helps to determine the extent of injury.
  - Kaufman[14,15] found that fingers that were injected with wax experienced tissue injury until a point of resistance was encountered. In the digits, the limiting factors to the extent of injury are the pulleys. He noted that the cruciate pulleys are pliable and thin, whereas the annular pulleys are rigid.
- If the injection occurs at the level of the proximal or distal interphalangeal joints (PIP or DIP joints), the substance injected will dissect through the tendon sheath.[14]
  - The synovial sheaths of the index, long, and ring fingers extend to the metacarpophalangeal joint; the synovial sheaths of the thumb and little finger extend into the proximal palm at the radial and ulnar bursae.[9]
- Any injections that occur over the middle segments of the fingers, away from the joints, will be diverted around the digit and spread laterally in the superficial tissues.[14]
  - Based on this information, the proximal spread of material can be predicted.
- Injections into the palm, thenar, and hypothenar eminences are generally contained in those myofascial spaces and lead to less permanent impairment.[18]
- The morbidity is determined by the volume, pressure, viscosity, resistance of the tissues, location of injection, anatomy of the compartment, and toxicity of the material injected.

PATHOGENESIS

- High-pressure injuries are divided into three stages.
- The *acute stage* occurs immediately.
  - The injection causes compression and spasm of the vessels, leading to compromised blood flow. This is manifested by white, mottled tissue; numbness; severe pain; or a combination of these findings.
  - Any initial paresthesias that occur are due to local compression or chemical irritation of the digital nerves.

- During this stage, the site of injection is key in determining where the material has spread. Very high pressures can overcome tissue resistance.
- The volume of material injected also determines the degree of tissue distention and impairment in blood flow.
  - In several studies by Gelberman,[8] Schoo,[25] and Hayes,[12] patients with hands that had higher-volume injections and longer time to decompression had higher morbidity rates.
- During the *intermediate stage*, a foreign body reaction induces oleogranuloma formation and fibrosis.
  - The inflammation that occurs is determined by the volume and type of substance.
  - The injection of paint solvent has a significantly higher morbidity due to its low viscosity, allowing diffusion through the soft tissues. Its corrosive effects cause severe tissue necrosis.[9]
  - Patients with grease injections have more chronic inflammatory reactions, leading to prolonged sequelae (foreign body granulomas).[12,26]
  - Schoo[25] reported that amputation rates associated with various injection injuries were as follows: paint thinner, 80%; paint (soya alkyl base), 58%; automotive grease, 23%; and hydraulic fluid, 14%.
- The late stage of injury occurs when the granulomas break open, resulting in draining sinuses and cutaneous lesions.
  - Chronic sinuses may degenerate into malignancies (squamous epithelioma).[7,25]
  - Secondary infections may occur in this stage; these may be due to *Staphylococcus aureus, Streptococcus epidermidis, Pseudomonas* spp., or a variety of polymicrobial flora.[23,24]

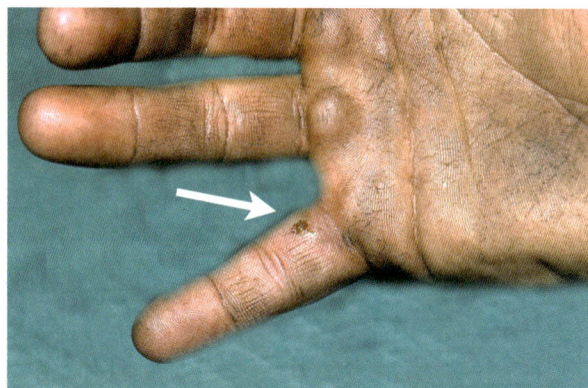

FIG 1 • An innocuous-appearing puncture of the volar radial surface of the right small finger. This may be the only visible point of injury in a high-pressure injection injury.

NATURAL HISTORY

- Most patients with high-pressure injection injuries are young men. These injuries occur more commonly among manual laborers (**FIG 2**).
  - Previously it was thought that most of these injuries occurred to people who had been on the job for less than 6 months, but more recent studies show that the mean time on the job was 11 years.[11,31]
- The nondominant hand (58%–76%)[7,11] is injured more often than the dominant hand.
  - The index finger, thumb, palm, and small finger are affected in descending order.
- Controversy continues as to what induces the inflammatory response in these injuries.
  - Some authors have suggested that the injury overwhelms the patient, leading to morbidity, whereas others believe that the injury induces a significant inflammatory response.
  - Most agree that surgery should be done within the first 3 hours after injury to decrease the morbidity. [27,28]

PATIENT HISTORY AND PHYSICAL FINDINGS

- Important factors to discover include the patient's hand dominance and occupation; the sequence of events post-injury; and the type of injector and pressure, as well as the substance injected.
- Comorbidities, including vascular disease, diabetes, and smoking history, are relevant risk factors that influence healing and post-treatment function.[18]
- If possible, the material safety data sheet (MSDS) for the substance injected should be obtained from the company.
- Physical examination should include:
  - Determining the location of the puncture site to determine the spread of the injectate. It is not uncommon for the site of injury to be small and difficult to find.
  - Observing range of motion when the patient attempts to form a fist
  - Palpation of the digit, hand, and arm to help determine the extent of débridement that will be required

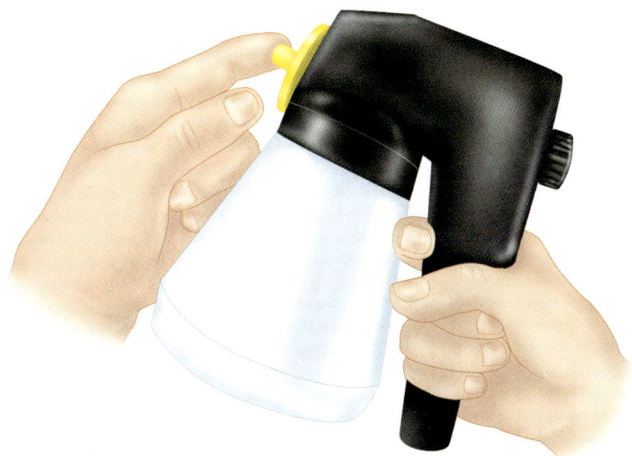

FIG 2 • Injury commonly occurs while attempting to clean a clogged high-pressure gun. Note that the guard has been removed.

IMAGING AND OTHER DIAGNOSTIC STUDIES

- Radiographs of the hand and forearm are helpful in evaluating the extent of injury.
- Although not all injected substances are radiopaque, air may be present in the compartments of the hand and forearm, which may help in determining how far the substance has traveled.[20,23,30]
- It may be necessary to obtain radiographs of the arm and chest. Extension into the arm, chest wall, and mediastinum from injuries to the hand has been reported.[29]
- Imaging studies also document pre-existing pathology.

DIFFERENTIAL DIAGNOSIS

- Snake bite
- Spider bite
- Crush injury
- Suppurative tenosynovitis
- Black thorn tenosynovitis
- *Mycobacterium marina* infection (chronic)

NONOPERATIVE MANAGEMENT

- Most injuries require surgical débridement, and there are only few case reports of nonoperative management for such injuries.
- Cases that are managed without surgery include air injection into the hand, which leads to subcutaneous emphysema that resolves within hours to days[17] or, occasionally, water injection that is managed conservatively.[16]

SURGICAL MANAGEMENT

- Early and aggressive decompression and débridement of all tissues is the cornerstone of treatment.
- The time from injury to surgery is the major determinant of morbidity and prognosis in high-pressure injection injuries.[27,28]

Preoperative Planning

- Radiographic studies should be reviewed.
  - Attention should be paid to radiopaque areas of the hand and forearm.
  - Air in the soft tissue should be evaluated.
  - The bones should be evaluated for any possible fractures or pre-existing lesions.
- Any intravenous lines should be placed in the patient's noninjured extremity, and manipulation of the injured extremity should be limited.

Positioning

- The patient should be placed supine with the arm abducted.
- The arm should not be exsanguinated with an Esmarch bandage, to avoid proximal spread of the injected material and further trauma to the tissues.
- Regional anesthesia can be used to avoid general anesthesia, if necessary, but local blocks and injections should not be performed.
  - If the IV regional (Bier) block is selected, gravity exsanguination is performed without a compression wrap but with 4 minutes of elevation.

Approach

- Two basic techniques are used to approach high-pressure injection injuries. Both are based on the idea of wide débridement, limited by scar formation over joint areas.

BRUNER'S INCISIONS

- The hand is prepped and exsanguinated by elevation.
- For longitudinal exposure of the digits, it is important to avoid crossing the joint creases in a straight line. This is accomplished by creating Bruner zigzag incisions at the joint creases.
    - The digit is incised to avoid crossing the flexion creases so that no longitudinal incisions are made through the crease itself (**TECH FIG 1A**).
- The injectate is removed, avoiding the neurovascular bundles located on the volar radial and volar ulnar surfaces of the digits.

- The incision is continued across the palm, if necessary. The palmar incisions also are placed in such a manner as to avoid postoperative contracture of the crease (**TECH FIG 1B**).
- If extension is necessary proximal to the wrist crease, the incision should be angled with the point toward the ulnar surface to avoid injury of the palmar sensory branch of the median nerve (**TECH FIG 1C**).
- Extension onto the forearm may be longitudinal or in an S curve, if compartment decompression is necessary[1-3] (**TECH FIG 1D**).

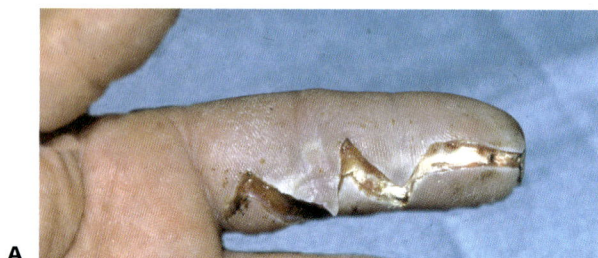

A

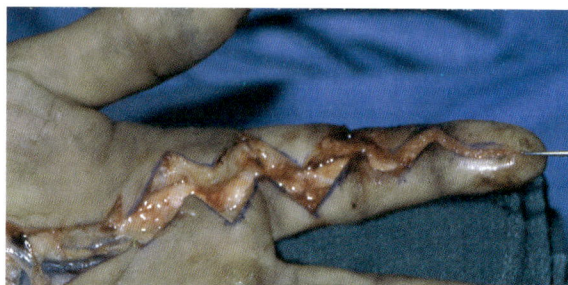

B

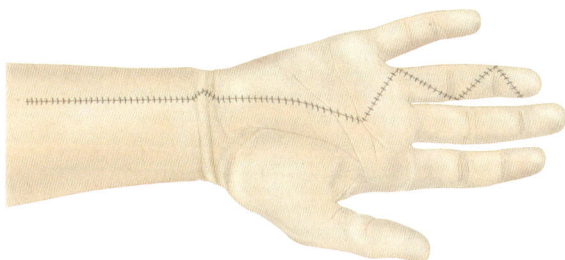

C

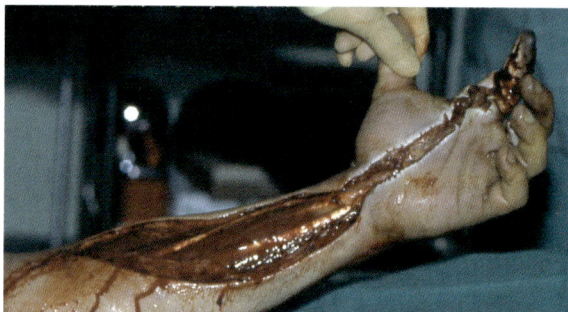

D

TECH FIG 1 • Bruner's incision of the right index finger. **A.** The incision was made for adequate exposure to remove grease debris in the finger while avoiding crossing the joint creases. **B.** The incision is extended to the palm to allow for visualization of affected tissues and further débridement. **C.** Incision across the wrist crease. Crossing the crease is avoided by creating a Bruner's incision or a curvilinear incision at the wrist crease. **D.** Longitudinal extension of the incision into the forearm. High-pressure injectate was pushed into the forearm tissues.

MIDAXIAL INCISIONS

- Longitudinal midaxial incisions are made on the digit, radially and ulnarly.
    - These incisions are made dorsal to the neurovascular bundles (**TECH FIG. 2**).

- If extension onto the palm is necessary, then it may be necessary to cross the web space, including the neurovascular bundles, but it must not be divided.
- Incision across the palm continues as described for Bruner's incision.[3]

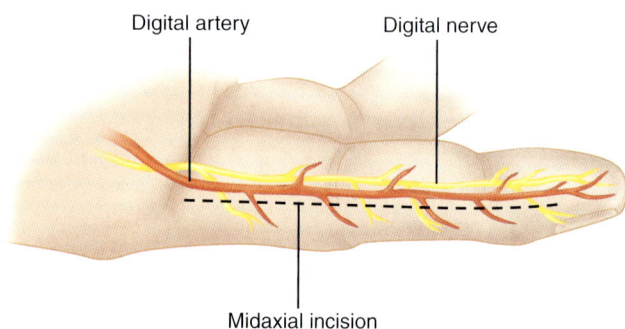

Digital artery   Digital nerve

Midaxial incision

TECH FIG 2 • Midaxial incision of the finger. This will sacrifice the dorsal branches of the neurovascular bundle, but the digital nerve and artery are protected in the volar tissues.

MODIFIED BRUNER'S INCISION

- The digit is incised with a Bruner's incision distal to the flexion crease, extending to the lateral aspect of the skin on the volar digital skin (**TECH FIG 3A**).
- At the flexion crease, a transverse incision is made through the flexion crease, and the next interphalangeal

incision is another oblique Bruner's incision (**TECH FIG 3B**).

- This is continued along the length of the digit onto the palm.

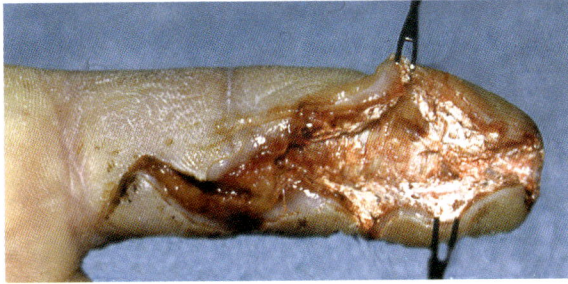

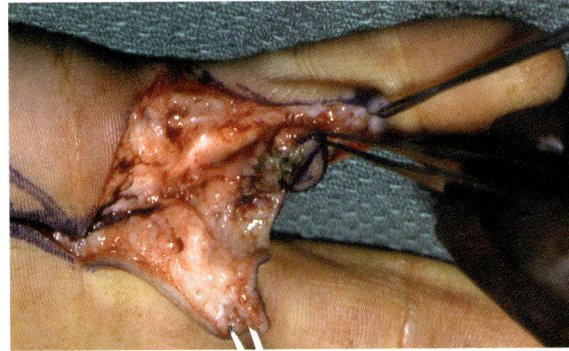

TECH FIG 3 • **A.** Modified Bruner's incision with transverse extensions at the interphalangeal flexion creases allows for a widened visual field and more complete débridement. **B.** Modified Bruner's incision at the metacarpophalangeal joint crease allows for visualization of the A1 pulley system, the neurovascular bundles, and the surrounding soft tissues.

PEARLS AND PITFALLS

- Understand that the underlying pathology usually will be worse than the external wound.
- Comorbidities are critically important in management of patients with injection injuries.
- Obtain the Material Safety Data Sheet (MSDS) to understand the toxic effects of the injected material.
- Exploration should extend to clearly healthy tissue. Avoid "minimally invasive" treatment.
- Leave the wound open or very loosely closed.

POSTOPERATIVE CARE

- The wound should be left open and packed, or very loosely closed. The hand should then be splinted in the "safe" position (**FIG 3A,B**).
- Any additional débridement should be performed at 48-hour intervals, as necessary, until the wound can be primarily closed or covered (**FIG 3C**).
  - Less involved injuries often are allowed to heal by secondary intention, especially if critical structures are covered.
  - Occasionally, free tissue transfer may be necessary for coverage.[5,22]
- Parenteral corticosteroids have been advocated to decrease the inflammatory response postoperatively.
  - The possibility of increasing the infection rate with corticosteroids does exist, although neither animal data nor human clinical findings show such an increase.
  - Animal studies have suggested that corticosteroids may be beneficial for patients sustaining injections of organic solvents.
  - No convincing human data have been published that show that corticosteroids are effective in limiting tissue loss, and they should be used cautiously.[13,21]

OUTCOMES

- Outcomes of high-pressure injection injuries are based on the volume, pressure, viscosity, resistance of the tissues, location of injection, anatomy of the compartment, and toxicity of the material.
- Morbidity includes cold intolerance, hypersensitivity, paresthesias, constant pain, impairment of the activities of daily living, infection, oleoma formation (**FIG 4A**), squamous degeneration,[25] and amputation.
- Amputation rates ranging from 14% to 88% have been reported in the literature.[12,19,25]
  - The highest amputation rates are associated with organic solvent injection into the fingers.[13]
  - In this subset of patients, the time to débridement also had a significant impact on the amputation rate.
    - If surgery occurs within 6 hours of injury, the amputation rate is 40%.
    - If the surgery is delayed for more than 6 hours, the amputation rate increases to 57%.
    - If débridement is delayed to more than 1 week after injury the amputation rate is 88%.[13]
- Metacarpophalangeal range of motion decreases an average of 8.1%, proximal interphalangeal range of motion decreases

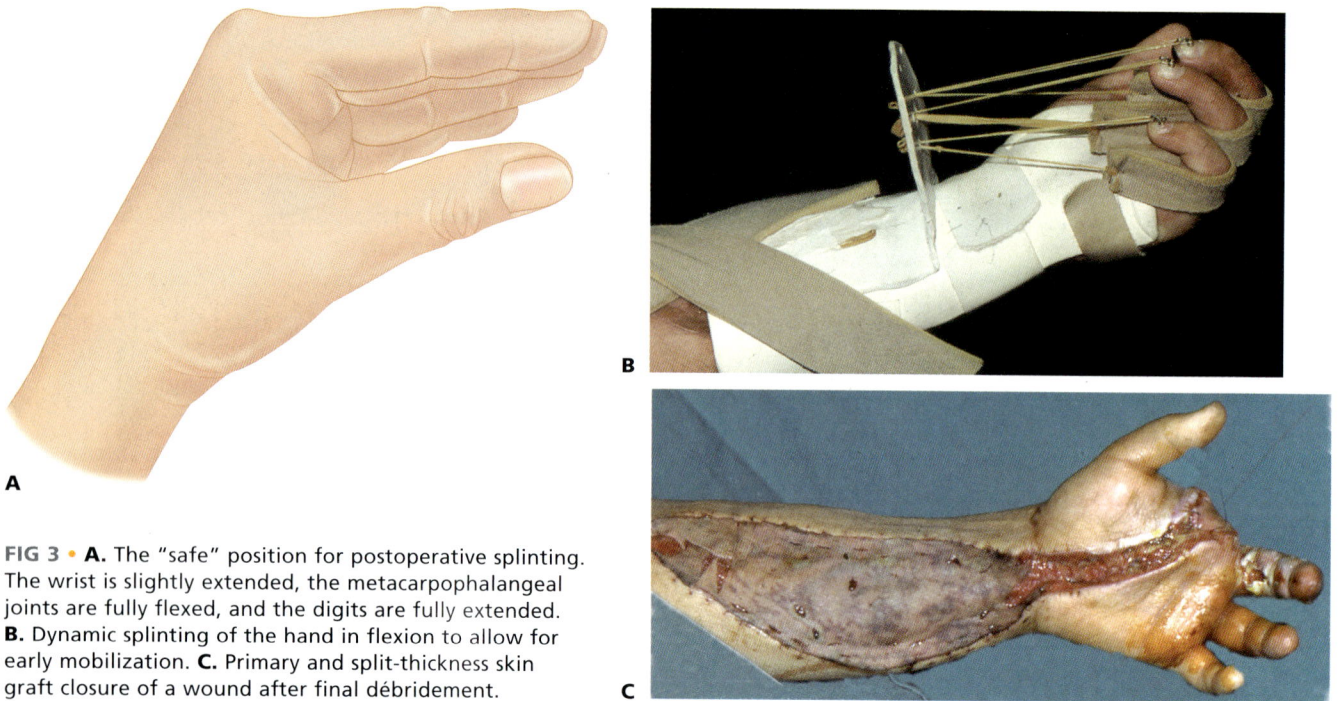

FIG 3 • A. The "safe" position for postoperative splinting. The wrist is slightly extended, the metacarpophalangeal joints are fully flexed, and the digits are fully extended. **B.** Dynamic splinting of the hand in flexion to allow for early mobilization. **C.** Primary and split-thickness skin graft closure of a wound after final débridement.

23.9%, and distal interphalangeal range of motion decreases by 29.7%.

- Maximum grip strength diminishes by 12%, and pinch strength decreases by 35%.
- Two-point discrimination increases by 49%[31] (**FIG 4B,C**).
- Permanent partial impairment of the injured hand depends on the mechanism of injury and the time to treatment.

- The average impairment for injuries caused by spray guns is 15%, by pneumatic hoses less than 2%, and by hydraulic fluid 6%.[30]
- If treatment is delayed more than 6 hours after injury, then the permanent impairment rate is approximately 17%; however, if treatment is obtained in under 6 hours, that rate is only 4%.[30]
- Loss of work related to these injuries also varies, from 6 to 26 weeks, with about 92% of patients returning to their previous jobs.[12]

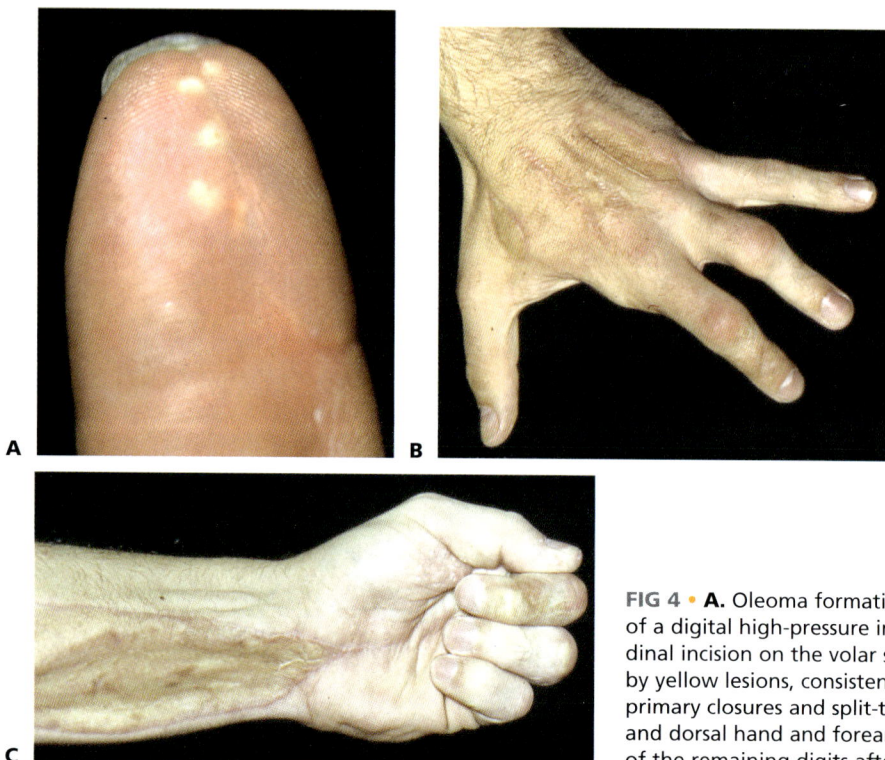

FIG 4 • A. Oleoma formation after débridement and closure of a digital high-pressure injection. The well-healed longitudinal incision on the volar surface of the digit is surrounded by yellow lesions, consistent with oleomas. **B,C.** Well-healed primary closures and split-thickness skin grafts of the volar and dorsal hand and forearm. There is full range of motion of the remaining digits after amputation of the index finger.

COMPLICATIONS

- Infection
- Cold intolerance
- Hypersensitivity
- Oleoma formation
- Malignant degeneration
- Decreased range of motion and function
- Paresthesias
- Diminished two-point discrimination
- Amputation

REFERENCES

1. Bruner JM. Incisions for plastic and reconstructive (non-septic) surgery of the hand. Br J Plast Surg 1951;4:48–51.
2. Bruner JM. Optimum skin incisions for the surgical relief of stenosing tenosynovitis in the hand. Plast Reconstr Surg 1966;38:197–201.
3. Bruner JM. The zig-zag volar-digital incision for flexor-tendon surgery. Plast Reconstr Surg 1967;40:571–574.
4. Caddick JF, Rickard RF. A molten metal, high-pressure injection injury of the hand. J Hand Surg Br 2004;29:87–89.
5. Chan BK, Tham SKY, Leung M. Free toe pulp transfer for digital reconstruction after high-pressure injection injury. J Hand Surg Br 1999;24:534–538.
6. Couzens G, Burke FD. Veterinary high pressure injection injuries with inoculations for larger animals. J Hand Surg Br 1995;20:497–499.
7. Fialkov JA, Freiberg A. High pressure injection injuries: an overview. J Emerg Med 1991;9:367–371.
8. Gelberman RH, Madison JL, Posch JL, et al. High-pressure injection injuries of the hand. J Bone Joint Surg Am 1975;57A:935–937.
9. Gonzalez R, Kasdan ML. High pressure injuries of the hand. Clin Occup Environ Med 2006;5:407–411.
10. Gutowski KA, Chu J, Choi M, et al. High-pressure hand injection injuries caused by dry cleaning solvents: case reports, review of the literature, and treatment guidelines. Plast Reconstr Surg 2003;111:174–177.
11. Hart RG, Smth GD, Haq A. Prevention of high-pressure injection injuries to the hand. Am J Emerg Med 2006;24:73–76.
12. Hayes CW, Pan HC. High-pressure injection injuries to the hand. South Med J 1982;75:1491–1498, 1516.
13. Hogan CJ, Ruland RT. High-pressure injection injuries to the upper extremity: A review of the literature. J Orthop Trauma 2006;20:503–511.
14. Kaufman HD. The anatomy of experimentally produced high-pressure injection injuries of the hand. Br J Surg 1968;55:340–344.
15. Kaufman HD. The clinicopathological correlation of high-pressure injection injuries. Br J Surg 1968;55:214–218.
16. Kon M, Sagi A. High-pressure water jet injury of the hand. J Hand Surg Am 1985;10:412–414.
17. Lo SJ, Hughes J, Armstrong A. Non-infective subcutaneous emphysema of the hand secondary to a minor webspace injury. J Hand Surg Br 2005;30:482–483.
18. Luber KT, Rehm JP, Freeland AE. High-pressure injection injuries of the hand. Orthopedics 2005;28:129–132.
19. Neal NC, Burke FD. High-pressure injection injuries. Injury 1991;22:467–470.
20. O'Reilly RJ, Blatt G. Accidental high-pressure injection-gun injuries of the hand: The role of the emergency radiologic examination. J Trauma 1975;15:24–31.
21. Phelps DB, Hastings H, Boswick JA. Systemic corticosteroid therapy for high-pressure injection injuries of the hand. J Trauma 1976;17:206–210.
22. Pinal F, Herrero F, Jado E, et al. Acute thumb ischemia secondary to high-pressure injection injury: salvage by emergency decompression, radical debridement, and free hallus hemipulp transfer. J Trauma 2001;20:571–574.
23. Pinto MR, Turkula-Pinto LD, Cooney WP, et al. High-pressure injection injuries of the hand: review of 25 patients managed by open wound technique. J Hand Surg Am 1993;18:125–130.
24. Schnall SB, Mirzayan R. High-pressure injection injuries to the hand. Hand Clin 1999;15:245–248.
25. Schoo MJ, Scott FA, Boswick JA. High-pressure injection injuries of the hand. J Trauma 1980;20:229–238.
26. Sirio CA, Smith JS Jr, Graham WP III. Related articles, links high-pressure injection injuries of the hand: A review. Am Surg 1989;55:714–718.
27. Stark HH, Wilson JN, Boyes JH. Grease-gun injuries of the hand. J Bone Joint Surg Am 1961;43:485–491.
28. Stark HH, Ashworth CR, Boyes JH. Paint-gun injuries of the hand. J Bone Joint Surg Am 1967;49:637–647.
29. Temple CLF, Richards RS, Dawson WB. Pneumomediastinum after injection injury to the hand. Ann Plast Surg 2000;45:64–66.
30. Vasilevski D, Noorbergen M, Depierreux M. High-pressure injection injuries to the hand. Am J Emerg Med 2000;18:820–824.
31. Wieder A, Lapid O, Plakht Y, et al. Long-term follow-up of high-pressure injection injuries to the hand. Plast Reconstr Surg 2006;117:186–189.

Chapter 98

Revascularization and Replantation of the Digits

Marc Richard, R. Gordon Lewis, Jr., and L. Scott Levin

DEFINITION

- *Replantation* is the reattachment of a completely amputated body part.
- *Revascularization* is the restoration of circulation and repair of all injured structures in an incompletely amputated, dysvascular body part. Revascularization always includes repair of the arteries to re-establish blood flow to the part.
- *Revision amputation* is the procedure performed at the site of amputation to gain soft tissue coverage and to address concomitant injuries to the digit.
- The decision of whether to perform replantation or revascularization and revision amputation of a digit is multifactorial. The relative indications and contraindications for each are discussed later in the chapter.

ANATOMY

- An understanding of the anatomy over the complete length of the digit is essential for successful replantation. The anatomy of the thumb is different from that of the four fingers.
- Palmar and dorsal cutaneous ligaments maintain the position of the neurovascular bundle during range of motion of the digit.
  - Grayson's ligament is palmar to the neurovascular bundle, originates from the flexor tendon sheath, and inserts on the skin.
  - Cleland's ligament travels dorsal to the neurovascular bundle from the phalanx to the overlying skin.
- A radial and ulnar proper digital artery supplies each digit. Each vessel travels with a respective radial and ulnar proper digital nerve. At the level of the digit, the artery lies dorsal to the nerve.
- The ulnar digital artery is typically larger in the thumb and index finger. The radial digital artery usually is larger in the small finger.
  - Three major palmar arches arise from the digital arteries. The proximal, middle, and distal arches are consistently located at the level of the C1 pulley, C3 pulley, and just distal to the flexor digitorum profundus (FDP) insertion, respectively.
  - Four palmar and four dorsal branches usually extend from each digital artery.
- Injection studies have demonstrated that the venous system of the digit consists of a series of arcades on the dorsal and palmar surfaces, with connecting oblique and transverse anastomotic veins.[14] The dorsal veins have a larger caliber than the palmar veins, which do not consistently travel with the digital artery and nerve.
- A radial and ulnar proper digital nerve travels with each proper digital artery. The digital nerve is sensory only and typically contains one to three fascicles. It trifurcates at the level of the distal interphalangeal (DIP) joint.
- Each finger has two flexor tendons within the flexor tendon sheath.

- The FDP tendon inserts at the proximal base of the distal phalanx.
- The flexor digitorum superficialis (FDS) tendon inserts as two slips into the midportion of the middle phalanx. The FDS tendon splits into two slips, and its relative position to the FDP tendon switches from palmar to dorsal at Camper's chiasm. This allows the deeper FDP tendon to continue to its more distal insertion.
- There are a series of five annular and three cruciform pulleys, which are discrete thickenings of the fibro-osseous sheath. The annular pulleys prevent bowstringing of the flexor tendons during flexion, whereas the cruciate pulleys are collapsible, accommodating flexion.
  - The odd-numbered annular pulleys are located over the joints of the finger, and the even-numbered annular pulleys are over the proximal and middle phalanx, respectively.
  - The A2 and A4 pulleys are most important in preventing bowstringing and should be preserved if possible.
- Each lesser digit receives a tendon from the extensor digitorum communis (EDC). The index and small fingers each have a second extensor tendon, the extensor indicis proprius (EIP) and extensor digiti minimi (EDM), respectively. Both of these tendons are ulnar to the EDC tendons.

PATHOGENESIS

- The mechanism of injury has a considerable effect on the potential for replantation.
- Sharp amputations are ideal for replantation because of the narrow zone of injury.
- The degree of tissue injury increases substantially with crush and avulsion mechanisms and may prohibit successful replantation (**FIG 1**).
- Most digit amputations occur as an isolated injury. When amputations occur in the multiply injured patient, consideration of other systemic injuries and adherence to ATLS (Advanced Trauma Life Support) protocols may prevent replantation.

NATURAL HISTORY

- Replantation of an amputated digit results in longer hospital stays and more prolonged rehabilitation than revision amputation. Patient satisfaction, however, usually is higher with replantation than with revision amputation or a prosthesis.[11,15,16]
- Functionally, the expected range of motion in a replanted digit is 50% of normal.
- Secondary procedures, such as tenolysis, are common.
- The literature reports rates of reoperation ranging from 3% to 93%. In a series of more than 1000 replants and revascularizations, 35% of patients required at least one secondary surgery.[22] The incidence is higher for replantations than for revascularizations.
- Expected survival rates of replanted digits are 80% or higher, with even higher survival rates in revascularized digits.

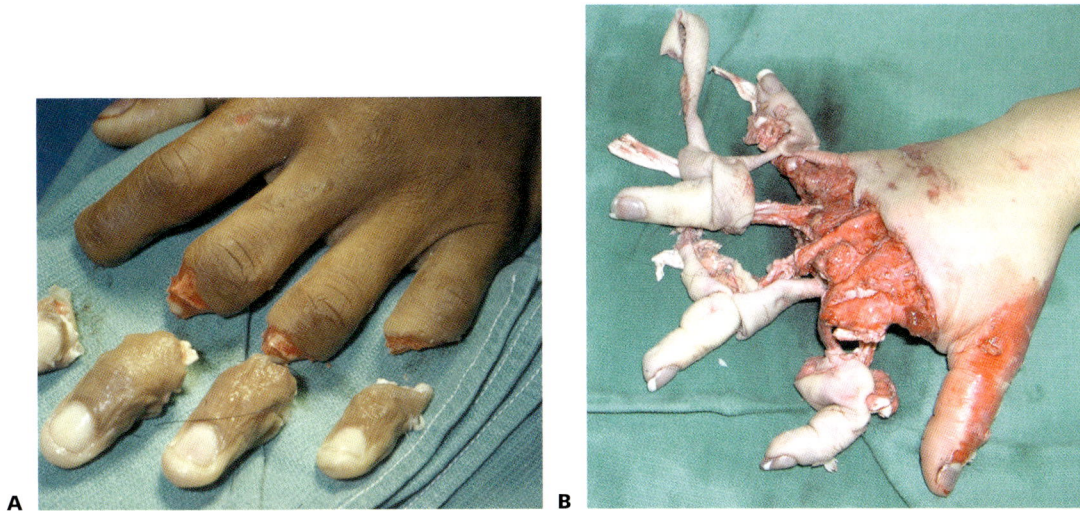

FIG 1 • **A.** This hand sustained sharp amputation of the digits from a table saw. The narrow zone of injury made the digits ideal for replantation. **B.** This hand sustained a crush injury. The resultant wide zone of injury prohibited successful replantation.

PATIENT HISTORY AND PHYSICAL FINDINGS

- The surgeon must evaluate the patient in the emergency room immediately on arrival. A complete history and physical examination are performed.
- The history should include specific details regarding the mechanism and timing of the injury. Identification of the specific machinery involved often reveals valuable information about potential contamination and the pattern of injury sustained by the amputated part.
- A history of mental instability is relevant, because rehabilitation protocols require significant patient compliance to maximize functional outcomes. Furthermore, self-inflicted amputations are unlikely to yield the same functional results after replantation as accidental amputations.
- A history of medical comorbidities should be thoroughly evaluated. Conditions such as diabetes, peripheral vascular disease, hypercoaguability, and tobacco use are not absolute contraindications to replantation but must be considered.
- Similarly, the surgeon must evaluate for medical conditions that prevent the patient from tolerating the blood volume changes associated with major limb replantation. Revision amputation may be the best choice if the patient has a history of previous trauma or arthritis in the amputated part.
- Ischemia time and method of transport should be evaluated for appropriateness. In the digits, a warm ischemia time of less than 6 hours is desired. In more proximal amputations containing muscle, ischemia time is more critical.
  - Cooling the amputated part reduces metabolic acidosis, bacterial growth, and muscle necrosis. Cold ischemia times of up to 12 hours are tolerated for replantation of digits. There are reports of successful replantation of digits with warm ischemia times of 42 hours and cold ischemia times of 96 hours.[3,24]
- Proper transportation of the amputated part is essential. Never place the part directly on ice. The part should be wrapped in a sterile gauze moistened with Ringer's lactate or normal saline. The gauze is then placed in a leak-proof plastic

bag and the bag is placed on ice (**FIG 2**). The goal temperature is 4°C.
  - Alternatively, the part may be immersed in Ringer's lactate or normal saline in a plastic bag with the bag then placed on ice.
- The surgeon examines the part and the injured extremity to evaluate suitability for replantation. The number of digits, level of injury, and type of injury are assessed.
- Specifically, the surgeon evaluates the injured parts for the red-line sign and the ribbon sign.
  - The *red-line sign* refers to a red streak of ecchymosis along the lateral border of the digit, which is the result of hemorrhage from avulsed branches of the digital artery after a traction injury (**FIG 3**).
  - The *ribbon sign* also represents an avulsion injury. Coiling of the artery at the amputation site results from

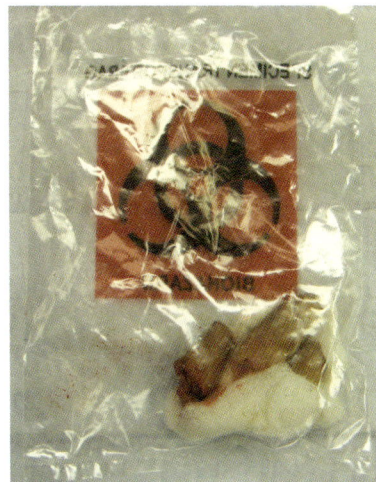

FIG 2 • The amputated part should be wrapped in a sterile gauze moistened with Ringer's lactate or normal saline. The gauze is then placed in a leak-proof plastic bag, which is placed on ice. The part should never be placed directly on ice.

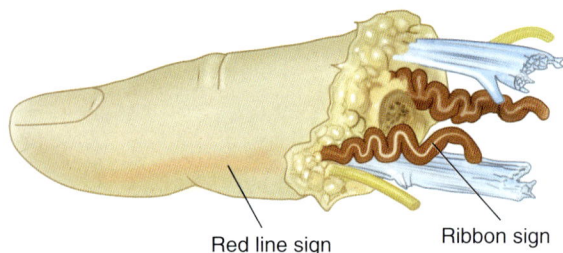

Red line sign   Ribbon sign

FIG 3 • The red-line sign, which represents an avulsion injury, is seen clinically as a red streak of ecchymosis along the lateral border of the digit. This ecchymosis is the result of hemorrhage from avulsed branches of the digital artery after a traction injury. The ribbon sign, which also represents an avulsion injury, refers to the corkscrew appearance of the digital artery resulting from disruption of the vessel wall layers. When these clinical signs are present, the zone of injury must be bypassed with vein grafts if replantation is attempted.

disruption of the vessel wall layers from traction.[21] If replantation is attempted, vein grafting is required.

IMAGING AND OTHER DIAGNOSTIC STUDIES

▪ When the patient arrives in the emergency department, standard radiographs of the amputated parts and the injured limb are obtained (**FIG 4**).
▪ Laboratory evaluations should include a complete blood count, basic metabolic panel, coagulation panel, drug screen, and blood type and crossmatch. Other preoperative tests are ordered as indicated by the patient's age and comorbidities.

NONOPERATIVE MANAGEMENT

▪ There is no role for nonoperative management of these injuries.
▪ Some surgeons advocate performing revision amputations in the emergency department under local anesthesia. It has been our experience that these procedures are best performed in the

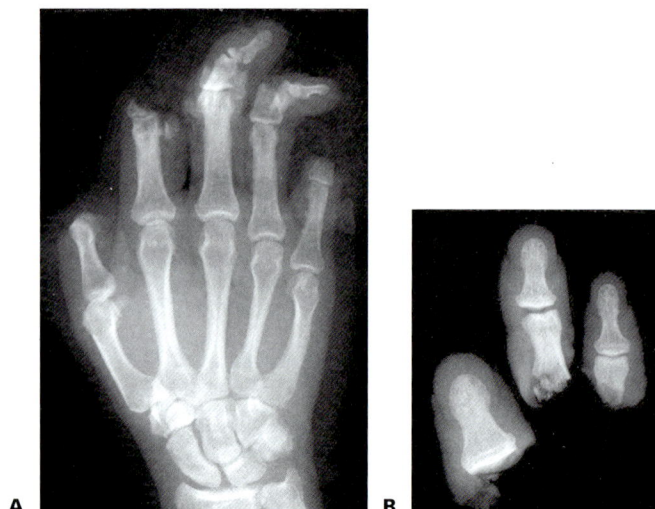

FIG 4 • **A.** Standard PA radiograph of the injured hand. **B.** A radiograph of the amputated parts is also obtained by placing the bag containing the parts directly on the x-ray cassette.

operating room with appropriate anesthesia, hemostasis, sterile conditions, lighting, and equipment.

SURGICAL MANAGEMENT

▪ The decision to replant a digit is predicated on the determination that the anticipated function after replantation will be better than that of a revision amputation. This determination is made after careful consideration of the factors influencing the predicted survival of the replanted digit, morbidity to the patient, and functional outcome.
▪ Specific factors related to the status of the amputated part and the status of the patient include:
  ▪ Mechanism of injury (eg, sharp, crush, avulsion)
  ▪ Level of amputation
  ▪ Ischemia time (warm or cold)
  ▪ Health of patient
  ▪ Age of patient
  ▪ Presence of segmental injury
  ▪ Predicted rehabilitation
  ▪ Vocation and hobbies
▪ Informed consent for replantation versus revision amputation must reference the postoperative care differences.
  ▪ Patients undergoing revision amputation typically are discharged from the hospital much quicker and have much shorter, less intensive rehabilitation protocols.
  ▪ Patients treated by replantation typically require a 5- to 7-day hospital course, avoidance of smoking and caffeine, possible blood transfusions, and prolonged rehabilitation. Furthermore, these patients must be advised about the likelihood of cold intolerance.
▪ The techniques we use for replantation of amputated digits are described in detail in the following sections. The same techniques and sequence of repair are followed for the revascularization of partially amputated parts.
  ▪ In partial amputations, not all structures will be injured, so it may be that only some structures require repair. For example, if the dorsal skin and its veins remain intact, the procedure does not require venous anastomosis for outflow.
  ▪ Each case should be examined individually, and all structures should be carefully evaluated for injury.

Preoperative Planning

▪ Broad-spectrum antibiotics and tetanus prophylaxis are administered on presentation in the emergency department.
▪ The patient, hand, and amputated parts are examined to confirm suitability for possible replantation.
▪ A urethral catheter should be placed for long procedures.
▪ Regional anesthesia is preferred due to the autonomic block, which yields increased peripheral vasodilation. Ideally, an indwelling catheter is placed to allow for continuous postoperative pain relief and sympathetic block. General anesthesia is required for children.
▪ If an attempt at replantation is determined to be appropriate and desired, the parts are brought to the operating room as soon as possible. Initial preparation of the parts can begin while the anesthesia team evaluates the patient.
▪ The operating room and patient must be kept warm to prevent peripheral vasoconstriction.
▪ The sequence of repair is as follows:
  1. Débridement and identification of structures
  2. Bone shortening and fixation

3. Extensor tendon repair
4. Flexor tendon repair
5. Arterial repair
6. Nerve repair
7. Vein repair
8. Skin closure/coverage

Positioning

■ The patient is positioned supine on a standard operating room table with a hand table attachment. The table is rotated 90 degrees to allow access for the operating microscope and fluoroscopy.

Approach

■ Slightly dorsal midaxial incisions are made on both the radial and ulnar sides of the digits. These incisions allow for rapid identification of both the neurovascular bundles and the dorsal veins. Both the palmar and dorsal flaps can be reflected as needed (**FIG 5**).

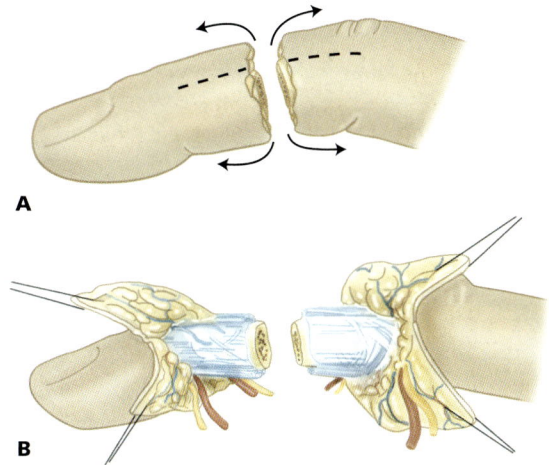

FIG 5 • Bilateral longitudinal midaxial incisions allow for easy exposure of the neurovascular bundles and dorsal veins.

PREPARATION OF THE AMPUTATED PART

■ A two-team approach is used. One team prepares the amputated part while the other team prepares the patient.
■ The parts should continue to be kept cool until they are reattached. A sterile prep table and a sterile covered ice-filled basin are required for preparation of the parts (**TECH FIG 1**).
   ■ A sterile metal irrigation basin is filled with ice and covered with a sterile adhesive drape.

■ A moist sterile towel is placed over the drape as a working surface.
■ The basin should be filled such that the ice forms a mound above its rim.
■ The parts are brought to the operating room and cleaned on the sterile prep table with Hibiclens and sterile Ringer's lactate.

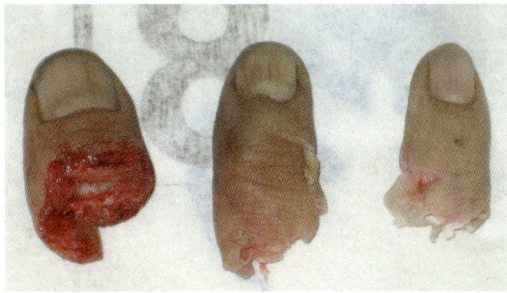

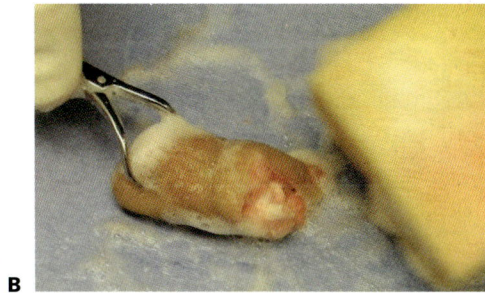

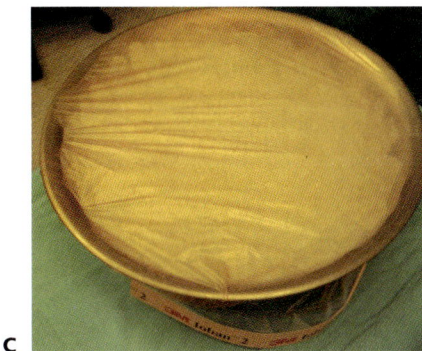

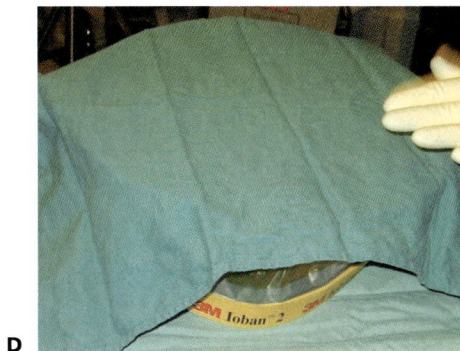

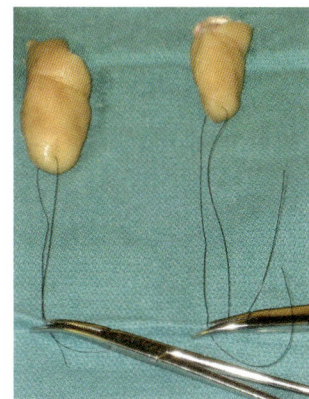

TECH FIG 1 • **A,B.** The amputated parts are removed from the bag, and a sterile prep is performed on a separate table. **C.** A sterile metal irrigation basin is filled with ice and covered with a sterile adhesive drape. Use as much ice as can be placed without disruption of the sterile environment to maximize contact with the amputated parts. **D.** A sterile surgical towel is then placed over the drape and used as a working surface. **E.** Nylon sutures placed through the amputated parts are secured to the surgical towel. The amputated parts are now ready for débridement and preparation.

TECHNIQUES

TECHNIQUES

- A nylon suture is passed through the tip of each amputated part and secured to the towel with a small hemostat.
- Under loupe magnification, the contaminated skin edges and subcutaneous tissues are débrided.
- Slightly dorsal midlateral incisions are made on the radial and ulnar sides of the digit. Arteries, nerves, and veins are identified and tagged for later with small hemoclips. The hemoclips should be placed as close to the vessel and nerve ends as possible to avoid damaging the structures.
- The nerves and vessels are exposed for a length of 1.5 to 2 cm. The veins lie in the subdermal plane and can be identified by elevating the dorsal skin flap. If the veins are difficult to isolate, the surgeon may defer their identification until after the anastomosis of one artery when engorgement makes them more prominent.
- The flexor tendons are identified, and a 4-0 nonabsorbable braided suture is placed in each tendon in a Tajima fashion. The crossing limb of the Tajima suture should be placed 1.0 to 1.2 cm from the free end of the tendon.

- The bone is then shortened appropriately. Consideration of the level and geometry of amputation is required. It is necessary to reference the recipient site to match the orientation of the bone ends.
- In general, 4 to 10 mm of total digit shortening allows for appropriate débridement of nerves and vessels to healthy tissue and subsequent primary repair without tension. Shortening also eases skin coverage of the repair site. The amount of shortening depends partly on the mechanism of injury. Crush injuries typically require more resection than sharp injuries.
- Two 0.045-inch K-wires are placed longitudinally down the long axis of the bone in a retrograde fashion. The K-wires should exit through the tip of the digit just palmar to the nail. The K-wires are advanced until the tips are showing through the bone so that the amputated digit is now ready for immediate attachment.
- The parts should continue to be kept cool under ice packs until they are reattached.

PREPARATION OF THE STUMP

- The second surgical team initiates preparation of the injured extremity while the amputated parts are being prepared.
- Under tourniquet ischemia and loupe magnification, débridement of the skin and subcutaneous tissues is performed.
- In an identical manner to the amputated parts, the arteries, nerves, and veins are identified, tagged, and exposed through slightly dorsal midlateral incisions. The veins are the most difficult structures to identify on the stump.

Once a vein is located, continue the dissection in the same subdermal plane to identify others. If possible, two veins are repaired for each artery.

- Flexor tendons are identified, and a Tajima suture is placed in each (**TECH FIG 2**). If the tendons have retracted proximally, atraumatic retrieval is necessary to avoid inducing spasm or damaging the proximal vessels. If required, a separate proximal incision is made to retrieve the tendons safely.

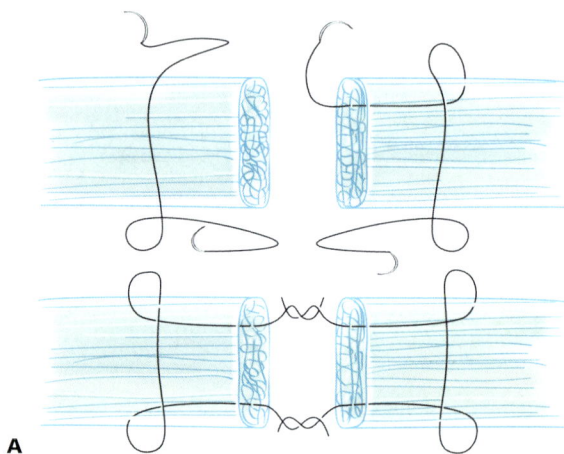

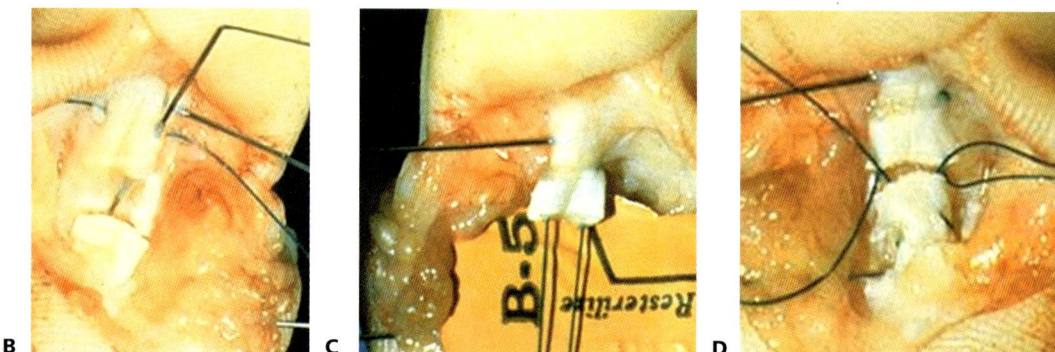

TECH FIG 2 • **A.** A Tajima-type suture repair is used so that the flexor tendons can be opposed and secured at the ideal time. **B,C.** The suture is placed in the proximal and distal ends of the tendon. **D.** The sutures are then tied in the repair site at the appropriate time.

- After identifying all structures, evaluate the need for grafts. Every attempt should be made to repair all structures primarily. Delayed reconstructions are much more difficult, place the repaired vessels at risk, and subject the patient to additional surgery and rehabilitation.

- Any amputated parts that are not being replanted should not be discarded, because these are an excellent source for donor grafts.

BONE FIXATION

- Bone shortening has already been performed at the time of débridement. If shortening was limited by the proximity of joints, the use of vein grafts should be entertained at the time of vessel anastomosis. When shortening the bone in a thumb amputation, the resection should be maximized on the amputated part so that if the replant fails, thumb length is maintained.
- Numerous methods of bone fixation are available, including longitudinal K-wires, crossed K-wires, intraosseous wiring, tension band, intramedullary screw, and plate and screws.
    - Parallel longitudinal K-wires are quick, easy, and have low nonunion and complication rates.[10] When possible, this is my preferred technique (**TECH FIG 3A–D**).
    - Crossed K-wires are also relatively quick and easy to use. The drawback to crossed K-wires is potential risk

to the neurovascular bundles, either directly or by tethering (**TECH FIG 3E–H**).
- Intraosseous wiring takes more time and exposure to perform, but allows for early range of motion. Drill holes accepting of a 24-gauge wire are placed in a dorsal-to-palmar and radial-to-ulnar orientation at each bone end. Two loops of 24-gauge wire are then passed perpendicular to each other through the analogous drill holes at each bone end and tightened in standard cerclage fashion.
- The tension band technique is a useful option for arthrodesis, because it allows the surgeon to set the desired amount of flexion. Two parallel 0.045-inch K-wires are placed across the fusion site, and a figure-8 loop of 24-gauge wire is used over the dorsum of the finger to complete the construct.

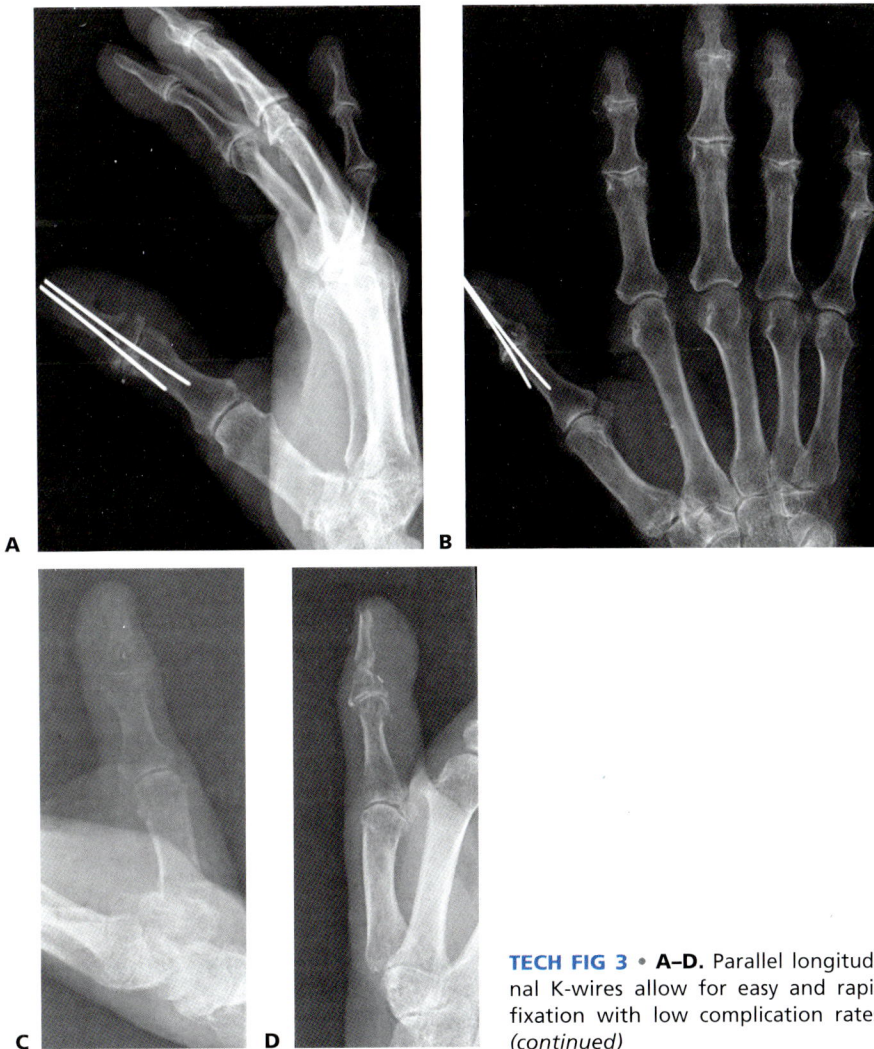

TECH FIG 3 • A–D. Parallel longitudinal K-wires allow for easy and rapid fixation with low complication rates. *(continued)*

TECHNIQUES

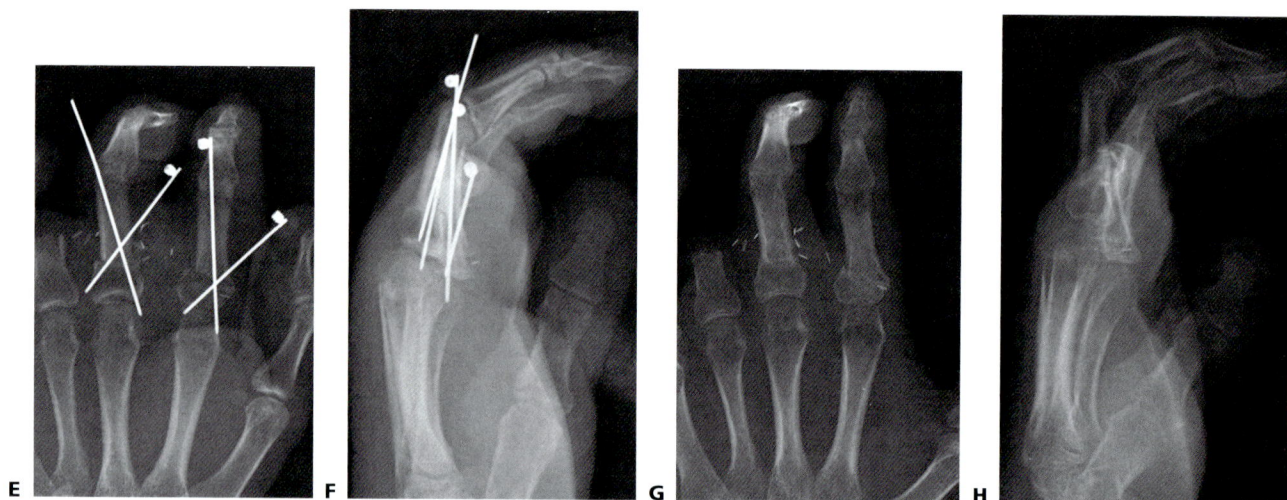

TECH FIG 3 • *(continued)* **E–H.** In more proximal amputations, longitudinal K-wires may not be possible. Crossed K-wires can be used successfully in these injuries.

- The intramedullary screw is most useful in thumb amputations at the metacarpal level. Removal of this hardware is difficult, so its use should be avoided in highly contaminated wounds where the risk of infection is high.
- Lag screw fixation is appropriate to treat long oblique fractures. However, because most amputations do not result in this fracture pattern, this technique is seldom used in replantation surgery.

- Plate-and-screw fixation is generally not required in digit replantation because nonunion is rare. While it provides rigid fixation, the hardware is bulky, increases tendon adhesions, and requires more time and exposure.
- Regardless of the method of fixation, the surgeon must constantly evaluate alignment and rotation of the digit in both flexion and extension. The flexed fingertips should point toward the distal pole of the scaphoid.

EXTENSOR TENDON REPAIR

- After bone stabilization, the extensor mechanism is repaired.
- In the digit, the tendon is repaired with two horizontal mattress sutures using a 4-0 nonabsorbable suture.

- It is imperative to repair the entire extensor mechanism. If the amputation is through the proximal phalanx, repair of the lateral bands will optimize functional outcomes.

FLEXOR TENDON REPAIR

- Because the Tajima sutures have already been placed, they are now ready to be tied in the repair site. The two strands of the repair should be tied simultaneously to achieve a symmetric repair.
- In certain circumstances, the surgeon may choose to delay tying the sutures until after the microsurgical portion of the case. Specifically, in very proximal amputations, the ability to position the digit in slight hyperextension may facilitate the vessel and nerve repair.

- Both the FDS and FDP are repaired when feasible. If the amputation is in zone 2 and the tendons are not cleanly cut, repair of only the FDP tendon is reasonable.
- If the amputation level is distal to the FDS insertion, but proximal to the DIP joint, we typically do not repair the FDP or extensor tendon. We favor arthrodesis of the DIP joint with K-wires and direct rehabilitation toward early active and passive range of motion of the proximal interphalangeal (PIP) joint.

ARTERIAL REPAIR

- We have found that both digital arteries should be repaired, when feasible, to maximize survival rates.
- The operating microscope and microsurgical instrument set are used.
- The most important factor affecting survival is achieving a tension-free anastomosis of normal intima to normal intima (**TECH FIG 4A–C**).

- Débridement of damaged arteries is performed under the operating microscope. The surgeon must resect until normal intima is identified. The liberal use of vein grafts is advocated for resulting defects.
- The tourniquet is released to ensure good blood flow from the proximal stumps.

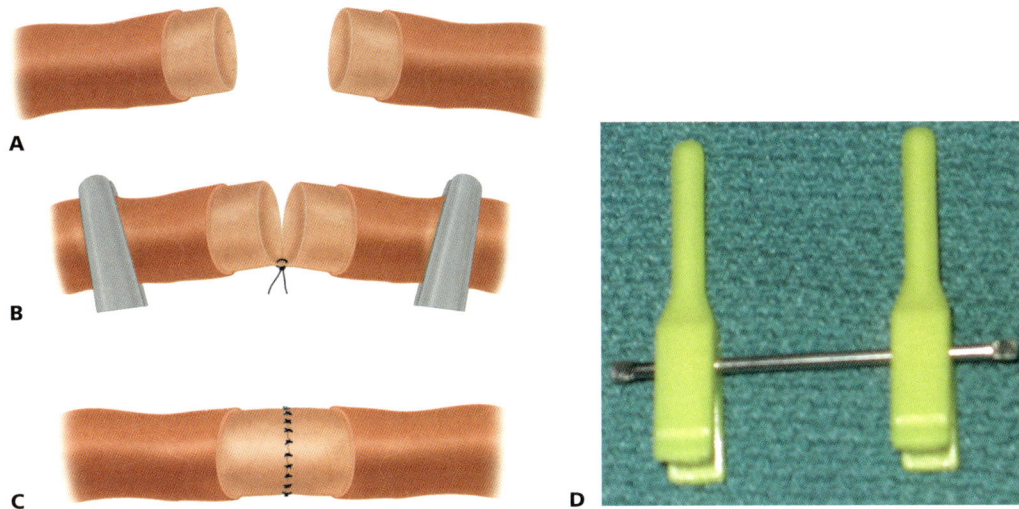

TECH FIG 4 • A–C. Arterial repair is performed using the operating microscope. A tension-free anastomosis of normal intima to normal intima is essential for survival of the replanted part. **D.** The vascular approximating clamp should have less than 30 g of closing pressure. Two clamps on a sliding bar allow for tension-free positioning of the vessel ends.

- Sharply trim the proximal stump with angled Potts scissors and dilate the lumen with jeweler's forceps or a lacrimal duct dilator.
- If adequate blood flow is not obtained, evaluate for all reversible causes of vasospasm, including hypotension, hypovolemia, acidosis, pain, or cold. Double check that the tourniquet was deflated.
- Evaluate the proximal vessel for mechanical constriction.
- Thoroughly irrigate the lumen with warm heparinized Ringer's lactate through a 30-gauge blunt-tipped needle on a 10-mL syringe.
- If vasospasm persists, irrigate the proximal vessel with papaverine solution (diluted 1:20 with sterile normal saline).
- After appropriate blood flow is established, the proximal and distal stumps are placed within the vascular approximators. Several types of approximating devices are available. We favor two clamps on a sliding bar. The clamps should have less than 30 g of closing pressure and should be limited to no more than 30 minutes of application time due to the potential for vessel damage (TECH FIG 4D).
- Place a microsurgical background deep to the repair site.
- A bolus of 3000 to 5000 U of intravenous heparin is given just before the anastomosis. After the bolus, we typically initiate a heparin drip at 1000 U/hr.
- Repeat inspection of the intima is performed proximally and distally to confirm its integrity. Verify that the anastomosis is tension-free and that no adventitia overhangs the lumen.

- Appropriately sized monofilament nylon sutures (Table 1) are used, and initial sutures are placed 180 degrees apart.
- The size of each "bite" should be about one to two times the thickness of the arterial wall.
- Care must be taken to avoid damaging the intima of the vessel.
- One limb each of the initial sutures should be cut long for use in manipulating the vessel without directly handling it.
- Suture the front wall of the artery sequentially between stay sutures.
- Irrigate the lumen after each suture is tied, and inspect the repair site to confirm that the back wall was not captured.
- Flip the approximating clamp to expose the back wall and complete the anastomosis.
- Remove the vessel from the approximating clips and repeat the procedure on the other digital artery.

Table 1	Needle and Suture Sizes	
Site of Repair	**Suture Size**	**Needle Size (μm)**
Palm	9-0	100
Proximal digit	10-0	75
Distal digit	11-0	50

NERVE REPAIR

- The proximal and distal nerve ends are examined under the operating microscope.
- The ends are cut sharply with a no. 11 blade against a wooden tongue depressor. The nerve is resected until pouting fascicles are visualized.
- The fascicles are aligned, and an epineurial repair is performed using two or three 9-0 or 10-0 sutures (TECH FIG 5).

- If a tension-free repair is not possible, primary nerve grafting is performed. The medial antebrachial cutaneous nerve is the ideal caliber for digital nerves and can be obtained from the ipsilateral extremity. Similarly, any amputated digits that are not candidates for replantation provide an excellent source for grafts.

TECHNIQUES

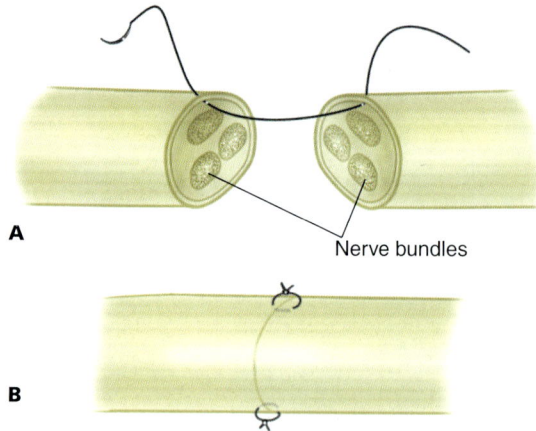

A

Nerve bundles

B

TECH FIG 5 • The digital nerve is approximated using an epineurial repair consisting of two or three sutures.

VEIN REPAIR

- Ideally, a minimum of two veins are repaired for each artery.[1,10] The largest veins identified should be repaired.
- When performing the anastomosis, each "bite" should be about two to three times the thickness of the vein wall.
- Constant irrigation with heparinized Ringer's lactate helps to "float" the lumen of the vein open.
- Due to the low pressure flow, the venous anastomosis can be performed with fewer sutures than are required for the arterial anastomosis (**TECH FIG 6**).
- Familiarity with alternatives to venous anastomosis is necessary in the event suitable veins cannot be located.

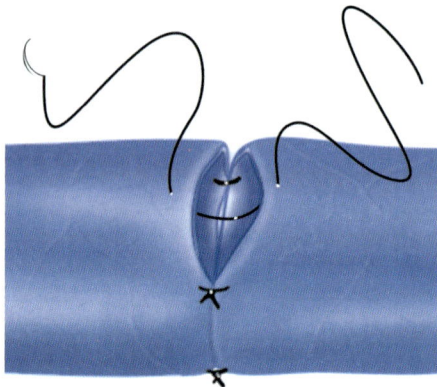

TECH FIG 6 • The venous anastomosis is performed with fewer sutures than the arterial repair due to the low pressure flow.

- Continuous venous oozing can be encouraged by removal of the nail with subsequent scraping of the matrix. This scraping is performed every 2 hours with a cotton-tipped applicator and is followed by the application of heparin-soaked pledgets.
- If proximal veins are present but distal veins are not, creation of either an arteriovenous or venous-cutaneous fistula may facilitate outflow to reduce congestion. This scenario is most common in very distal amputations just proximal to the nail. An arteriovenous fistula may be created possibly if one artery has been successfully repaired and back-bleeding is present from the other distal artery. This artery can be anastomosed to the proximal vein. Alternatively, a vein graft can be used to create a temporary shunt from the skin of the pulp to the proximal vein.
- Medicinal leeches (*Hirudo medicinalis*) can be placed on the engorged part if venous congestion occurs. They should be changed every few hours and should be used for a minimum of 7 days to allow for the establishment of collateral circulation. Although the leeches may fall off after engorgement, they secrete hirudin, a local anticoagulant that keeps the digit bleeding for 8 to 12 hours. While using leech therapy, the patient should be treated with a third-generation cephalosporin as prophylaxis against *Aeromonas hydrophilia* infection, a symbiotic gram-negative rod in the leech gut.

SKIN COVERAGE AND WOUND CLOSURE

- Before the wound is closed, meticulous hemostasis must be achieved. Even small postoperative hematomas can compress the vascular repairs and result in failure of the replant.
- Interrupted nylon sutures are used to close the wounds, avoiding constriction of underlying structures. The midlateral incisions can be left open without concern for healing difficulties. If the repaired dorsal veins lack local coverage, a split- or full-thickness graft should be applied.

- No part of the postoperative dressing should be circumferential. Small strips of petroleum-impregnated gauze are applied to the incisions. A bulky dressing is constructed with a plaster splint extending above the elbow. The tips of all digits must remain exposed, and a temperature probe is taped to the pulp of the replanted digit for monitoring.
- The limb is elevated in a foam pillow.

PEARLS AND PITFALLS

Amputated parts	■ Take the amputated parts to the operating room to begin débridement and identification of structures as soon as the room is ready.
Heterotopic replantation	■ Prioritize the functional goals for replantation. If multiple digits are amputated, but not all parts are suitable for replantation, put the salvageable digits in the most functional position (eg, replant a finger in the thumb position if the thumb cannot be saved).
Vein grafts	■ If there is concern for intimal damage, resection and the liberal use of vein grafts saves time and frustration. Always reverse the vein graft in case valves are present in the segment. The volar aspect of the wrist contains numerous veins 1 to 2 mm in diameter.
Spare-parts surgery	■ Never discard any amputated parts until the conclusion of the case. Amputated parts that are not suitable for replantation are an ideal source of autologous grafts.
Vascular anastomosis	■ Never perform an anastomosis under tension. Either additional bone shortening or vein grafting should be performed.
Multiple digit replantations	■ The overall duration of surgery is decreased by performing a structure-by-structure repair instead of a digit-by-digit repair (ie, repair the same anatomic structure in all digits before repairing the next structure).[6]

POSTOPERATIVE CARE

■ Usually, the hand is elevated, with the level of elevation adjusted for changes in vascular status. If arterial inflow becomes problematic, the hand is lowered. If venous congestion is present, the hand is raised.

■ Color, warmth, turgor, and capillary refill are monitored by the surgeon.

■ The patient's room should be kept warm, preferably above 22° C (72°F). The temperature probe is monitored by the nursing staff, and the surgeon is notified if the digital temperature is less than 30°C or if the temperature drops 2°C over 1 hour.

■ The patient is maintained on bed rest for the first 2 or 3 days, and the room is kept dark with minimal stimulation. Visitors are limited to two at a time.

■ The patient is restricted from nicotine and caffeine products.

■ The intravenous heparin drip is continued at 1000 U/hr. The rate is adjusted for a goal activated partial thromboplastin time (aPTT) of 1.5 times normal. It is maintained for 5 days, then weaned by 100 U/hr until off.

■ Dextran 40 is given as a 50-mL bolus and then maintained at a rate of 20 mL/hr while the patient is in the hospital.

■ Enteric-coated aspirin (325 mg daily) and dipyridamole (50 mg tid) are initiated and maintained for 6 weeks postoperatively.

■ Chlorpromazine (25 mg orally q 8 h) is useful as both an anxiolytic and a peripheral vasodilator. We generally use it for the duration of the patient's hospital stay.

■ Appropriate antibiotics are maintained for 7 days.

■ We prefer to leave the operative dressing in place for 7 days to avoid causing vasospasm. Excessive bleeding with formation of a blood cast that would restrict venous outflow should prompt an earlier dressing change.

■ Gentle active motion is started on postoperative day 3 within the confines of the splint. Formal hand therapy is initiated after the splint is removed.

OUTCOMES

■ A survival rate greater than 80% is expected for replantation surgery.

■ Functional outcomes are greatest for replantation of the thumb, proximal hand, and single digit distal to the FDS insertion (**FIG 6A–D**).[8,9,17,20]

■ Recovery of sensation is correlated with function. As in other peripheral nerve injuries, age is the most important

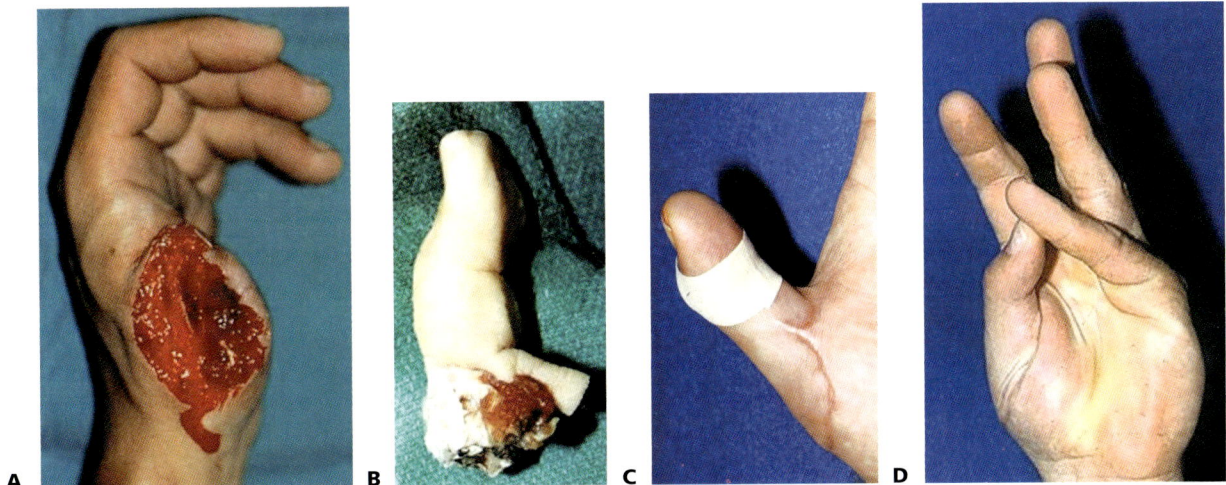

FIG 6 • A–D. This patient sustained an amputated thumb, which was successfully replanted with good cosmetic and functional results. *(continued)*

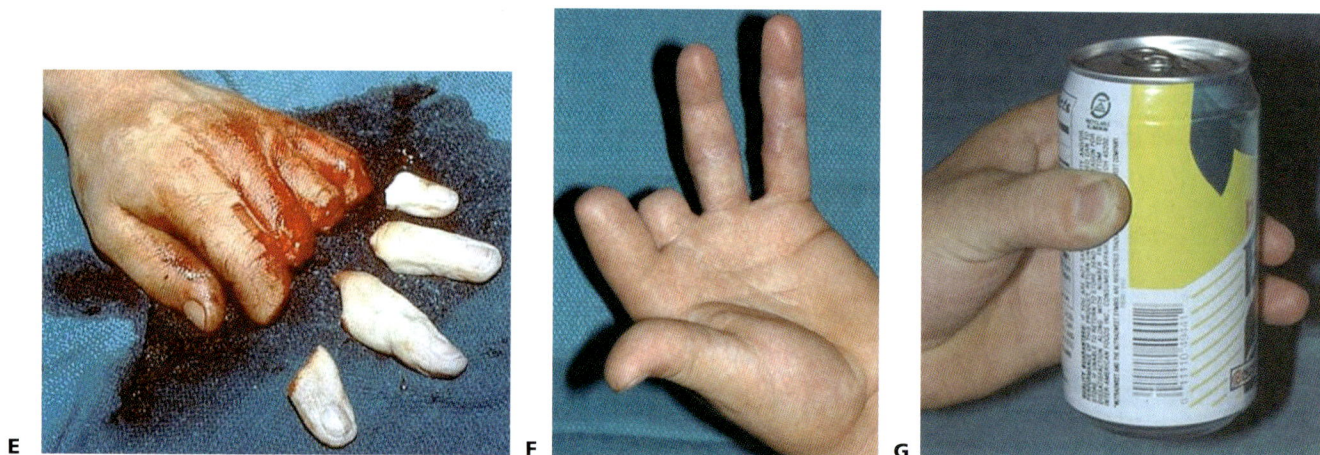

FIG 6 • *(continued)* **E–G.** Successful replantation of the ring and small fingers resulted in a functional hand capable of holding common objects.

factor for recovery, with better results in younger patients. The average two-point discrimination in replanted thumbs is 11 mm and in fingers is 8 mm.[7] These values represent the average recovery for sharp amputation. Crush and avulsion mechanisms result in poorer two-point discrimination.

■ Range of motion is related to level of amputation. Active PIP joint motion in replantations proximal to the FDS insertion average 35 degrees, whereas replantations distal to the FDS insertion result in 82 degrees of PIP joint motion (**FIG 6E–G**).[10]

COMPLICATIONS

Immediate Complications

■ Immediate complications affect the survival of the replanted digit and typically relate to the vascular status.

■ Arterial insufficiency may result from unrecognized vessel injury away from the anastomosis, which causes thrombosis or vasospasm.

 ■ A check for reversible causes is initiated to ensure that the patient is warm, comfortable, hydrated, and calm.

 ■ Check the dressings to confirm that there is no mechanical constriction.

 ■ Confirm that the patient's hematocrit is near normal and that all ordered medications are being given appropriately.

 ■ The hand should be lowered to increase inflow, and an intravenous bolus of heparin (3000–5000 U) is given. If the patient has not been anticoagulated or has not achieved therapeutic levels, a regional sympathetic block will aid peripheral vasodilation.

 ■ Vigilant re-examination of color, warmth, turgor, and capillary refill is necessary to decide whether exploration in the operating room is indicated. Revisions after 4 to 6 hours of reduced perfusion seldom result in digit salvage.[10]

■ If venous engorgement occurs postoperatively, elevate the hand and remove constrictive dressings (including sutures that are too tight).

 ■ Consideration for return to the operating room is based on intraoperative findings affecting the possibility of revising the venous anastomosis.

 ■ If this is not possible, leeches or nail removal are used to alleviate venous congestion. These methods typically are used to bridge the first 4 to 6 days until adequate outflow is established.

Long-term Complications

■ Long-term complications include pin tract infections, cold intolerance, stiffness, malunion, and nonunion.

■ Pin tract infections usually occur more than 4 weeks after surgery. They are easily treated by pin removal and a course of oral antibiotics.

■ Cold intolerance is almost universal. (This also is a problem in revision amputations.) Cold intolerance is expected to improve over the first 2 years but it remains debatable whether it completely resolves.[3,18]

■ Digital stiffness is common, because both the flexor and extensor tendons are repaired. Tenolysis should be delayed for at least 3 months post-replantation but has demonstrated good results.[12]

■ Malunion usually results from malalignment at the time of bone fixation. Intraoperatively, rotational alignment is the most difficult to assess. Malunion is more common in proximal amputations, because even slight malalignment at the amputation level is greatly accentuated at the fingertip.

■ Nonunion is not common after replantation of the digit. It has been reported in fewer than 10% of digit replantations and rarely requires reoperation.[19,20]

REFERENCES

1. Allen DM, Levin LS. Digital replantation including postoperative care. Tech Hand Up Extrem Surg 2002;6:171–177.
2. Al-Shammari S, Gupta A. Revascularization of the digits and palm. Hand Clin 2001;17:411–417.
3. Backman C, Nystrom A, Backman C, et al. Arterial spasticity and cold intolerance in relation to time after digital replantation. J Hand Surg Br 1993;18:551–555.
4. Baek SM, Kim SS. Successful digital replantation after 42 hours of warm ischemia. J Reconstr Microsurg 1992;8:455–458.
5. Boulas HJ. Amputations of the fingers and hand: indications for replantation. J Am Acad Orthop Surg 1998;6:100–105.
6. Camacho FJ, Wood MB. Polydigit replantation. Hand Clin 1992;8:409–412.
7. Glickman LT, MacKinnon SE. Sensory recovery following digital replantation. Microsurgery 1990;11:236–242.
8. Goldner RD, Howson MP, Nunley JA, et al. One hundred eleven thumb amputations: replantation versus revision. Microsurgery 1990;11:243–250.

9. Goldner RD, Stevanovic MV, Nunley JA, et al. Digital replantation at the level of the distal interphalangeal joint and the distal phalanx. J Hand Surg Am 1989;14:214–220.

10. Goldner RD, Urbaniak JR. Replantation. In: Green D, Hotchkiss RN, Pederson WC, et al, eds. Green's Operative Hand Surgery, ed 5. Philadelphia: Elsevier Churchill Livingstone, 2005:1569.

11. Hattori Y, Doi K, Ikeda K, et al. A retrospective study of functional outcomes after successful replantation versus amputation closure for single fingertip amputations. J Hand Surg Am 2006;31:811–818.

12. Jupiter JB, Pess GM, Bour CJ. Results of flexor tendon tenolysis after replantation in the hand. J Hand Surg Am 1989;14:35–44.

13. Lim BH, Tan BK, Peng YP. Digital replantations including fingertip and ring avulsion. Hand Clin 2001;17:419–431.

14. Lucas GL. The pattern of venous drainage of the digits. J Hand Surg Am 1984;9:448–450.

15. Matsuzaki H, Yoshizu T, Maki Y, et al. Functional and cosmetic results of fingertip replantation: Anastomosing only the digital artery. Ann Plast Surg 2004;53:353–359.

16. Ozkan O, Ozgentas HE, Safak T, et al. Unique superiority of microsurgical repair technique with its functional and aesthetic outcomes in ring avulsion injuries. J Plast Reconstr Aesthet Surg 2006;59:451–459.

17. Patradul A, Ngarmukos C, Parkpian V. Major limb replantation: a Thai experience. Ann Acad Med Singapore 1995;24(4 Suppl):82–88.

18. Povlsen B, Nylander G, Nylander E. Cold-induced vasospasm after digital replantation does not improve with time: a 12-year prospective study. J Hand Surg Br 1995;20:237–239.

19. Urbaniak JR, Hayes MG, Bright DS. Management of bone in digital replantation: Free vascularized and composite bone grafts. Clin Orthop 1978;133:184–194.

20. Urbaniak JR, Roth JH, Nunley JA, et al. The results of replantation after amputation of a single finger. J Bone Joint Surg Am 1985; 67A:611–619.

21. Van Beek AL, Kutz JE, Zook EG. Importance of the ribbon sign, indicating unsuitability of the vessel, in replanting a finger. Plast Reconstr Surg 1978;61:32–35.

22. Waikakul S, Sakkarnkosol S, Vanadurongwan V, et al. Results of 1018 digital replantations in 552 patients. Injury 2000;31:33–40.

23. Wang H. Secondary surgery after digital replantation: Its incidence and sequence. Microsurgery 2002;22:57–61.

24. Wei FC, Chang YL, Chen HC, et al. Three successful digital replantations in a patient after 84, 86 and 94 hours of cold ischemia. Plast Reconstr Surg 1988;82:346–350.

Chapter 99

Surgical Treatment of Vasospastic and Vaso-occlusive Diseases of the Hand

Scott L. Hansen, Neil F. Jones, and Charles K. Lee

DEFINITION

- Vasospastic and vaso-occlusive diseases of the hands include a wide range of disorders that cause decreased or limited blood flow to the digits, resulting in chronic ulcerations and even loss of digits.
- Vasospastic disorders result from constriction of the microvasculature, resulting in decreased blood flow.
  - The most common vasospastic disorder is Raynaud syndrome.
    - Raynaud syndrome may also have an obstructive component.
- Vaso-occlusive disorders produce disruption of blood flow due to a reduction in cross-sectional area of the vessel lumen.

ANATOMY

- The right common carotid artery and right subclavian artery originate from the brachiocephalic trunk, whereas the left subclavian artery branches directly from the aorta.
- The subclavian artery becomes the axillary artery at the distal edge of the first rib and ends at the distal edge of the teres major tendon.
- The brachial artery is a continuation of the axillary artery, beginning at the distal margin of the teres major.
- The hand is supplied by the radial and ulnar arteries, which originate from the brachial artery at the level of the antecubital fossa.
- The radial artery becomes the deep palmar arch; the ulnar artery becomes the superficial palmar arch (**FIG 1**).

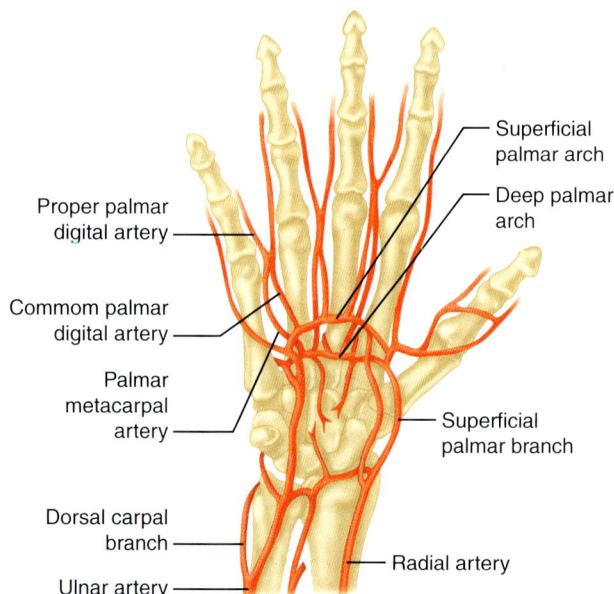

Proper palmar digital artery

Commom palmar digital artery

Palmar metacarpal artery

Dorsal carpal branch

Ulnar artery

Superficial palmar arch

Deep palmar arch

Superficial palmar branch

Radial artery

FIG 1 • Vascular anatomy of the hand.

- The superficial palmar arch is the major arterial inflow to the fingers on the ulnar aspect of the hand, whereas the deep palmar arch supplies blood to the digits on the radial aspect of the hand.
  - The superficial palmar arch lies more distal in the palm than the deep palmar arch.
- In about 80% of patients, the deep and superficial palmar arches are in continuity, a configuration described as a *complete palmar arch*.[3]
- In a small subset of patients, a persistent median artery also can contribute blood supply to the hand.
- Sympathetic nerves exit the spinal cord along with the ventral roots of the second and third thoracic nerves, passing via the brachial plexus into the forearm and hand.
  - The sympathetic nerve fibers innervate the blood vessel walls, controlling the tone of the vascular smooth muscle.

PATHOGENESIS

- Raynaud's syndrome, a vasospastic disorder, is characterized by significant structural narrowing of the arterial lumen due to intimal hyperplasia. Vasospasm can occur from increased sympathetic tone in response to temperature, vibratory stimuli, and sometimes emotional stress, causing further ischemia and the clinical manifestation of color changes.
- Vasospasm can also be associated with pheochromocytoma, carcinoid syndrome, and cryoglobulinemia.
- Emboli can shower from a cardiac source (eg, chronic atrial fibrillation) or from microemboli in ulcerated, atherosclerotic plaques, either spontaneously or from iatrogenic cannulation of vessels during vascular procedures.
- Thrombosis may occur spontaneously from atherosclerotic disease or from repetitive blunt trauma to the vessels, as in hypothenar hammer syndrome.
- Low-flow states can occur in sepsis, malignant disease, hypercoagulable states (eg, polycythemia, lupus anticoagulant antibody), and after intra-arterial drug injections.
  - These states predispose end organs to global thrombosis.
- Focal stenosis and segmental occlusion of vessels may result from intimal proliferation secondary to connective tissue disorders, atherosclerosis, and renal vascular disease.
- Vasospastic disorders may result from increased sympathetic tone.
- Vaso-occlusive disorders result in ischemia distal to the site of occlusion.

NATURAL HISTORY

- Clinical manifestations of vasospastic disorders range from episodic digital vasospasm and pain, to severe hand and digit ischemia, progressing to gangrene.
- The classic triphasic attack in Raynaud's syndrome consists of sudden onset of digital pallor or blanching after cold exposure

or emotional stress, followed by a period of cyanosis and then redness with rewarming, resulting in the classic white-blue-red sequence of color changes.[1]

- The typical Raynaud's attack lasts for 15 to 45 minutes.
- Vaso-occlusive disorders follow a more predictable clinical course in that they usually result from fixed lesions that are progressive.
- Cold intolerance and vasomotor color changes in the hand develop, forcing patients to seek treatment.

PATIENT HISTORY AND PHYSICAL FINDINGS

- A complete history and physical examination must be done on each patient, focusing on evidence of connective tissue or cardiovascular disease.
  - Does the patient describe paresthesias, pallor, cold intolerance, pain, digit ulceration?
- The entire upper extremity is examined for range of motion, skin color and turgor, capillary refill, radial and ulnar pulses, temperature, and presence of ulcerations.
- The distal fingertips and nails of each finger are examined closely.
- The radial and ulnar pulses are palpated and examined by Doppler probe if necessary.
- The palmar arch is assessed with the Doppler probe as well as the radial and ulnar digital arteries to each finger.
- Allen's test is performed.
  - The radial and ulnar arteries are occluded at the level of the wrist.
  - The arterial flow is then re-established to the hand sequentially by releasing the radial and ulnar arteries, and capillary refill is assessed.
  - This test evaluates the patency of arterial inflow to the hand through the radial and ulnar arteries.
- Any pulsatile masses are noted and evaluated.

IMAGING AND OTHER DIAGNOSTIC STUDIES

- Posteroanterior (PA), lateral, and oblique radiographs to evaluate bone architecture and the presence of any calcification in the radial and ulnar arteries, palmar arches, or digital arteries
- Doppler examination
- Echocardiogram to evaluate potential sources of emboli
- Digital photoplethysmography, which measures digital volume changes over time, can be used to differentiate vasospastic from vaso-occlusive disease.
- Segmental arterial pressure measurements
- Nielsen digital hypothermic challenge test[14]
- Ultrasonography[7]
- Angiography: remains the gold standard to evaluate blood flow to the hand
- MR angiography[4]
- Laboratory tests: complete blood cell count (CBC) with platelet count, coagulation studies, markers for collagen vascular diseases

DIFFERENTIAL DIAGNOSIS

- Raynaud's disease
- Hypothenar hammer syndrome
- Malignancy
- Trauma

- Buerger disease (thromboangiitis obliterans): an inflammatory occlusive disease of the small and medium-sized vessels of the limbs
- Arteritis: a group of disorders characterized by acute or chronic inflammation in the walls of small, medium, and large arteries. Patients with these conditions often present with concurrent fever, malaise, weight loss, cutaneous lesions, and arthralgias.
- Diabetes
- Peripheral vascular disease, atherosclerosis
- Thoracic outlet syndrome
- Connective tissue disorders (eg, scleroderma, systemic lupus erythematosus, rheumatoid arthritis)
- Illicit drug use
- Vascular tumors
- Pseudoaneurysm
- Iatrogenic injury

NONOPERATIVE MANAGEMENT

- Pharmacologic therapy is the mainstay of treatment of vasospastic disorders of the hand.
- Avoidance of smoking and exposure to cold temperatures may control vasospastic episodes.
- Biofeedback
  - Patients are trained to control certain bodily processes that occur involuntarily.
  - Electrodes are attached to the skin of the patient and physiologic responses monitored.
  - The biofeedback therapist then leads the patient through exercises that bring about desired physical changes.
- Occlusive dressings may be helpful both to protect areas from recurrent trauma and to promote healing of lesions.
- Calcium channel blockers, eg, nifedipine
- Pentoxifylline decreases blood viscosity and may result in relaxing vascular smooth muscle.
- Prostacyclins[22]
- Nitrates
- Local anesthetic blockade
- Botulinum toxin A[21]
- Thrombolytic therapy

SURGICAL MANAGEMENT

- The surgical management of vasospastic and vaso-occlusive diseases should proceed in a systematic fashion.
- Indications for operative management are progressive symptoms (eg, Raynaud's syndrome, ulcers, pain, cold intolerance) despite optimal medical management and with angiographically defined occlusion of one or both inflow arteries (ie, radial, ulnar).
- Indications for a digital sympathectomy are progressive symptoms of Raynaud syndrome or ulcerations refractory to medical management with no evidence of major occlusion of the radial or ulnar arteries and with good visualization of three common digital arteries in the palm.
- Cold challenges are very painful for patients with scleroderma and systemic lupus erythematosus and are used on a case-by-case basis.
- The patient should be educated on the outcomes of the various procedures and realize the limitations of each one.

Preoperative Planning

- The preoperative history and physical examination are reviewed.

- The site of operative intervention is determined primarily by the preoperative imaging studies (eg, angiogram).
- If vascular grafting is indicated, the donor vessels are identified and marked.

Positioning

- The patient is placed in the supine position on the operating room table with the extremity on an appropriately padded hand table.
- An upper arm tourniquet is placed, because a bloodless field is essential.
- If a vein graft is anticipated, another extremity (usually a leg) is prepped and a proximal tourniquet applied.

Approach

- Usually, the hand surgeon must access proximal arterial inflow vessels when treating either vasospastic or vaso-occlusive disorders of the hand.

- The brachial artery in the upper arm is approached via an incision on the medial aspect of the arm.
- The distal brachial artery and proximal radial and ulnar arteries are approached through a lazy S incision in the antecubital fossa.
  - Care is taken to avoid making a straight line incision across the antecubital fossa.
- The radial and ulnar arteries in the forearm are approached through a longitudinal incision over the specific vessel.
- The palmar arches are accessed via Bruner incisions extending proximally from the proximal phalanges, using natural creases in the palm where possible, or through an inverted J-shaped incision in the palm.
- The digital arteries are approached through Bruner incisions on the palmar aspect of the finger or through a midlateral incision on the digit.

FLATT DIGITAL SYMPATHECTOMY[5]

- Flatt digital sympathectomy is used for patients with vasospastic disorders such as Raynaud phenomenon.
- Proximal or cervical sympathectomy has largely fallen out of favor due to the high recurrence rates.
- Peripheral sympathectomy has gained popularity since Pick[17] identified sympathetic nerve fibers innervating the arteries from the wrist to the fingers.
  - Sympathectomy is performed at the level of the digital arteries.
- Make Bruner incisions in the distal palm and expose the digital arteries.
- Disrupt all connections between the digital nerves and digital arteries.

- Strip the adventitia from the digital arteries over a distance of 0.5 to 2.0 cm using the operating microscope (**TECH FIG 1A,B**).
  - This must be performed very carefully to avoid damaging the digital arteries themselves.
- In cases of more widespread vasospasm, when more radical digital sympathectomy is required, strip the adventitia from the distal radial and ulnar arteries, the superficial palmar arch, and the common digital arteries in the palm[8,9,15] (**TECH FIG 1C,D**).

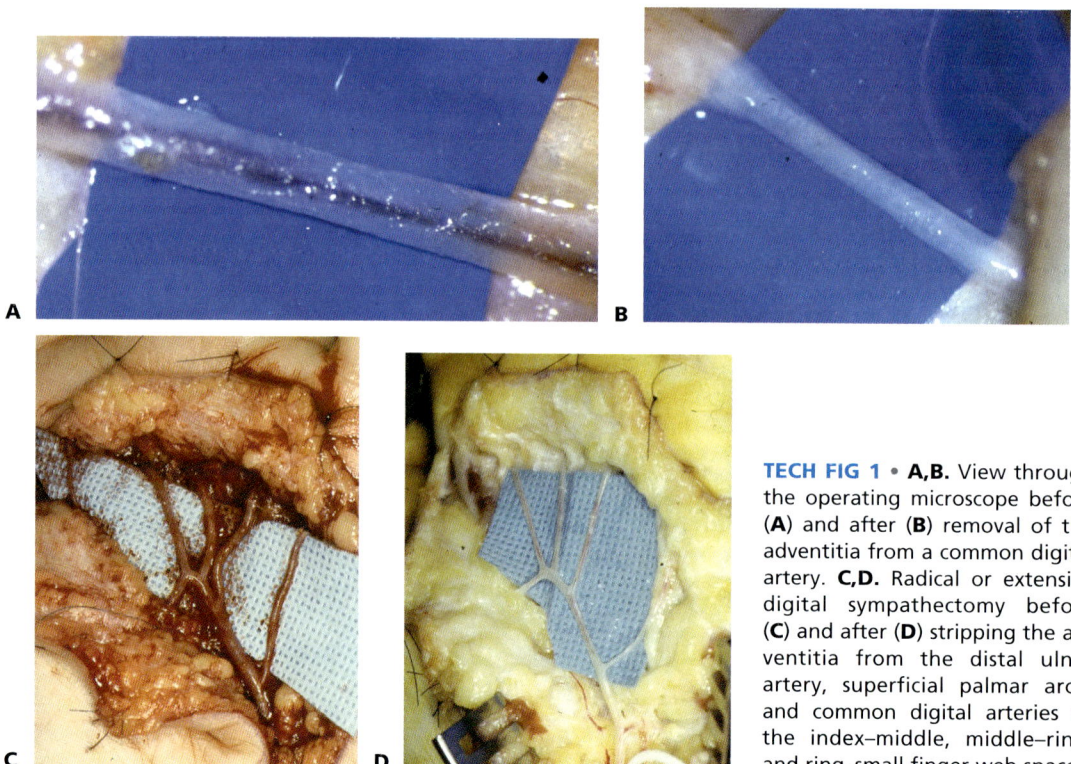

TECH FIG 1 • **A,B.** View through the operating microscope before (**A**) and after (**B**) removal of the adventitia from a common digital artery. **C,D.** Radical or extensive digital sympathectomy before (**C**) and after (**D**) stripping the adventitia from the distal ulnar artery, superficial palmar arch, and common digital arteries to the index–middle, middle–ring, and ring–small finger web spaces.

LERICHE SYMPATHECTOMY[12]

- If adequate collateral flow is present, consider excision of a segment of thrombosed or occluded artery.[12]
- This is thought to reduce the sympathetic discharge from the diseased artery that is producing vasospasm in the more distal vessels.

- It also occasionally is used to treat a thrombosed or occluded ulnar artery in hypothenar hammer syndrome.

MICROSURGICAL REVASCULARIZATION

- Reconstruction of a thrombosed or occluded artery is considered if:
  - A discrete segment of artery can be resected and bypassed.
  - Adequate arterial inflow and patent distal arteries with adequate distal "run-off" are present.
- Resect the arterial segment and measure the defect.
- Reverse vein grafts (eg, cephalic, saphenous) or arterial grafts (eg, deep inferior epigastric artery, lateral circumflex artery, thoracodorsal artery) are harvested in the standard fashion.
- Draw an axial line down the length of the vessel to be harvested while it is still in situ.
  - This helps prevent inadvertent "twisting" of the graft during the anastomoses.
- Perform standard microsurgical anastomoses using 9-0 or 10-0 nylon sutures and the operating microscope between the distal radial or ulnar arteries and the

deep or superficial palmar arches respectively, or directly to one or more common digital arteries (**TECH FIG 2**).
- An end-to-side anastomosis of the graft to the inflow artery is preferable to maximize any remaining circulation to the hand, but end-to-end anastomoses are technically easier.
- The distal anastomosis usually is end-to-end to the superficial or deep palmar arches or end-to-side to the common digital arteries.
- After the anastomoses have been completed, the tourniquet is deflated, and vascular inflow through the other artery is occluded by manual compression for a few minutes to maximize flow across the anastomoses.
- Restoration of arterial flow into the hand is assessed either by using a pencil Doppler probe or by performing an Acland "adventitial strip test" distal to the distal anastomosis.

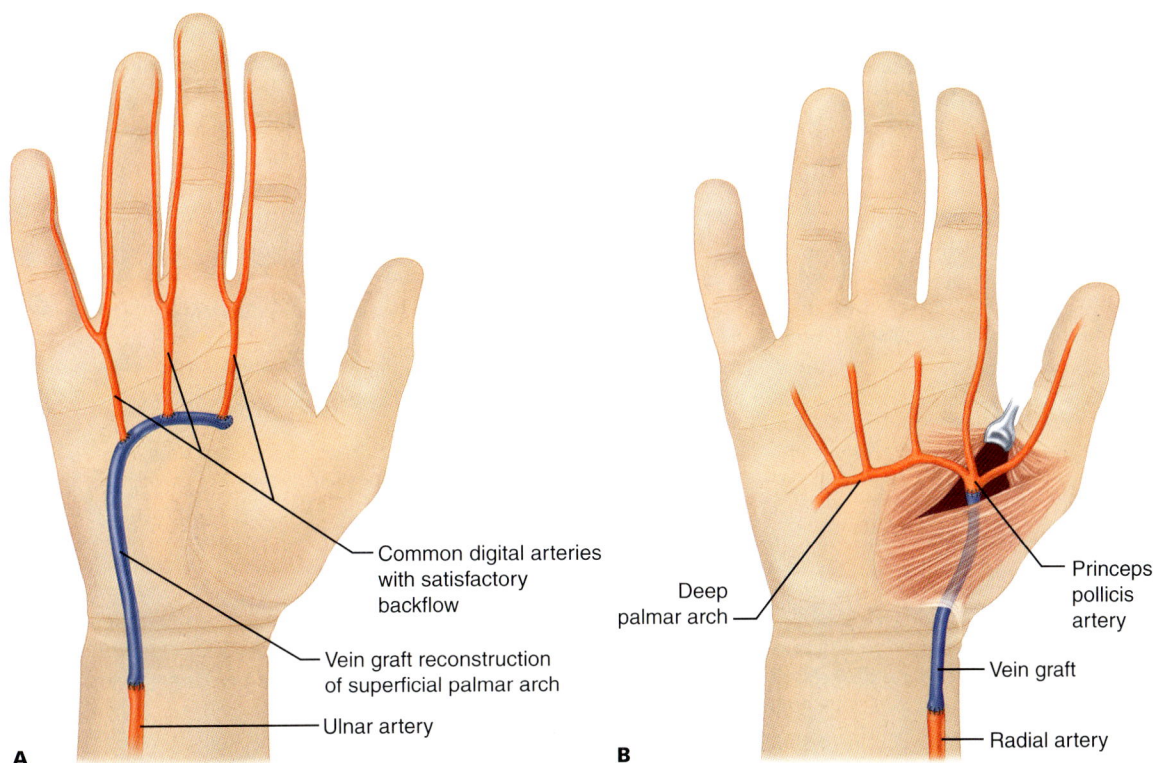

TECH FIG 2 • A. Microsurgical revascularization for thrombosis or occlusive disease of the distal ulnar artery and superficial palmar arch, using an interposition vein graft from the ulnar artery to the common digital arteries. **B.** Microvascular revascularization for thrombosis or occlusive disease of the distal radial artery and deep palmar arch, using an interposition vein graft from the radial artery to the princeps pollicis artery.

TECHNIQUES

EMBOLECTOMY

- An acute embolus is treated by immediate heparinization to prevent propagation of the embolus more distally into the digits.
- Small Fogarty embolectomy catheters may be used selectively at the arm, elbow, forearm, and wrist levels, but use of embolectomy catheters in the hand and digits is difficult and can itself lead to vascular injury.
- After identification of the segment involved by the embolus, control the affected artery both proximal and distal to the embolus.
- Make a longitudinal arteriotomy proximally to access the vessel lumen.
  - A side branch may be chosen if available.

- Insert the Fogarty catheter into the artery, and pass it down the lumen beyond the area of occlusion; then inflate the balloon.
- Gently withdraw the catheter to retrieve any thrombus.
  - This is repeated until the lumen is completely cleared of the embolus, as demonstrated by improved backbleeding from the distal vessel.
- Suture the arteriotomy and release arterial inflow.
- Assess the restoration of arterial flow into the hand either by using a pencil Doppler probe on the artery more distally or by performing an Acland "adventitial strip test" distal to the site of embolism.

ARTERIALIZATION OF THE VENOUS SYSTEM

- Choose a suitable vein on the dorsum of the hand, that is, one that will lie in a straight line following anastomosis to the radial or ulnar artery near the palmar wrist.[16]
- Mobilize the vein and ligate the multiple side branches of the vein with small hemoclips to maximize flow to the fingers.
- Perform valvulotomies in the vein to prevent valvular obstruction.
- Ligate the vein proximally and perform an end-to-side microsurgical anastomosis between the vein and the radial or ulnar artery at the wrist.

- After the anastomosis has been performed, assess arterial flow through the distal vein.
  - Any remaining obstruction due to a valve should be relieved by an open valvulotomy and excision of the valve leaflets, followed by microsurgical closure of the vein.
- Postoperative monitoring is performed using a pencil Doppler probe over the distal arterialized vein to the fingers.

PEARLS AND PITFALLS

Indications	■ A thorough history and physical examination must be performed. ■ Preoperative studies must be reviewed before surgical intervention.
Sympathectomy	■ The adventitia of the artery must be stripped over a distance of 0.5 to 2.0 cm.
Microsurgical revascularization	■ A discrete segment of thrombosed or occluded artery must be identified for this to be effective. ■ Adequate arterial inflow and distal runoff is essential.
Embolectomy	■ Identification of an embolus must be treated with heparinization immediately to prevent propagation of the clot. ■ The use of embolectomy catheters in the hand and digits should be done selectively and with caution.
Arterialization of the venous system	■ Generally used for unreconstructable vascular lesions ■ Valvulotomies must be performed to prevent vascular obstruction when flow is established. ■ All venous side branches should be ligated to maximize flow distally.

POSTOPERATIVE CARE

- The hand is immobilized in a lightweight splint to protect the operative site, with care taken to avoid any pressure on the underlying anastomoses or vulnerable mobilized arteries.
- The fingertips are observed for color and capillary refill, temperature using small temperature probes or oxygen saturation using a pulse oximeter.
- Microvascular reconstruction with interposition grafts can be monitored using a pencil Doppler probe.
- Relative anticoagulation can be achieved using a continuous infusion of dextran 40 or low-dose aspirin.

OUTCOMES

- Calcium channel blockers have been shown to be moderately effective in patients with Raynaud's phenomenon, with 35% reporting improvement in severity of their symptoms.[19]
- The results of sympathectomy remain variable, although surgeons have reported improvements in pain, ulcer healing, cold intolerance, and quality of life.[8,11,18,20]
- Long-term patency rates for vascular bypass grafting secondary to occlusive disease have been reported to range between 53% and 94%.[2,8,10,13]

■ Combining sympathectomy with arterial reconstruction may offer improved outcomes versus sympathectomy alone.[6]

COMPLICATIONS

■ Bleeding and hematoma
■ Infection
■ Thrombosis of the interposition graft
■ Progression of the underlying systemic disease

REFERENCES

1. Allen E. Raynaud's disease: A review of minimal requisites for diagnosis. Am J Med Sci 1932:83:187–200.
2. Barral X, Favre JP, Gournier JP, et al. Late results of palmar arch bypass in the treatment of digital trophic disorders. Ann Vasc Surg 1992:6:418–424.
3. Coleman SS, Anson BJ. Arterial patterns in the hand based upon a study of 650 specimens. Surg Gynecol Obstet 1961:113:409–424.
4. Dalinka MK, Meyer S, Kricun ME, et al. Magnetic resonance imaging of the wrist. Hand Clin 1991:7:87–98.
5. Flatt AE. Digital artery sympathectomy. J Hand Surg Am 1980:5:550–556.
6. Given KS, Puckett CL, Klienert HE. Ulnar artery thrombosis. Plast Reconstr Surg 1978:61:405–411.
7. Hutchinson DT. Color duplex imaging: Applications to upper extremity and microvascular surgery. Hand Clin 1993:9:47–51.
8. Jones NF. Acute and chronic ischemia of the hand: pathophysiology, treatment, and prognosis. J Hand Surg Am 1991:16:1074–1083.
9. Jones NF. Ischemia of the hand in systemic disease: the potential role of microsurgical revascularization and digital sympathectomy. Clin Plast Surg 1989:16:547–556.
10. Koman LA, Ruch DS, Aldridge M, et al. Arterial reconstruction in the ischemic hand and wrist: effects on microvascular physiology and health-related quality of life. J Hand Surg Am 1998:23:773–782.
11. Koman LA, Smith BP, Pollack FE. The microcirculatory effect of peripheral sympathectomy. J Hand Surg Am 1999:20:709–717.
12. Leriche R, Fontaine R, Dupertius SM. Arterectomy with follow-up studies on 78 operations. Surg Gynecol Obstet 1937:64:149–155.
13. McCarthy WJ, Flinn WR, Yao JST, et al. Result of bypass grafting for upper limb ischemia. J Vasc Surg 1986:3:741–746.
14. Nielsen SL, Lassen NA. Measurement of digital blood pressure after local cooling. J Appl Physiol 1977:43:907–910.
15. O'Brien BM, Kumar PA, Mellow CG, et al. Radical microarteriolysis in the treatment of vasospastic disorders of the hand, especially scleroderma. J Hand Surg Br 1992:17:447–452.
16. Pederson WC, Woodward C, Hermansdorfer J. Arterialization of the venous system for the treatment of end-stage ischemia of the upper extremity. J Reconstr Microsurg 1996:12:414.
17. Pick J. The Autonomic Nervous System. Philadelphia JB Lippincott, 1970.
18. Ruch DS, Koman LA, Smith TL. Chronic vascular disorders of the upper extremity. J Am Soc Surg Hand 2001:1:73–80.
19. Thompson A, Shea B, Welch V, et al. Calcium channel blockers for Raynaud's phenomenon in systemic sclerosis. Arthritis Rheum 2001:44:1841–1847.
20. Tomaino MW, Goitz RJ, Medsger TA. Surgery for ischemic pain and Raynaud's phenomenon in scleroderma: a description of treatment protocol and evaluation of results. Microsurgery 2001:21:75–79.
21. Van Beek AL, Lim PK, Gear AJL, et al. Management of vasospastic disorders with botulinum toxin A. Plast Reconstr Surg 2007:119:217–226.
22. Wigley F, Wise R, Seibold J, et al. Intravenous iloprost infusion in patients with Raynaud's phenomenon secondary to systemic sclerosis. Ann Intern Med 1994:120:199–206.

Chapter 100

Surgical Treatment of Acute and Chronic Paronychia and Felons

Eric Stuffmann and Jeffrey Yao

DEFINITION

- An *acute paronychia* is an infection of the soft tissue fold around the fingernail.
  - It is the most common soft tissue infection of the hand.
  - The most common infecting organism is *Staphylococcus aureus*, although these infections are commonly mixed infections.
- A *chronic paronychia* is characterized by repeated infection and inflammation of the eponychium.
  - The eponychium becomes thickened and rounded.
  - This problem often occurs in the setting of repeated and prolonged exposure to water.
  - The most commonly isolated organisms are *Candida albicans*, gram-positive cocci, gram-negative rods, and *Mycobacterium* spp.
- *Herpetic whitlow* is caused by an outbreak of herpes simplex virus in the skin of the finger and can be confused with acute paronychia or felon.
  - Herpetic whitlow is common in children and medical personnel who come into contact with oral secretions.
- A *felon* is a tense abscess of the distal pulp of the finger or thumb that involves multiple septal compartments (**FIG 1**).

ANATOMY

- The nail complex consists of the nail bed, nail plate, and perionychium (**FIG 2**).
- The nail plate sits below the proximal nail fold.
- The *perionychium* is the border tissue which surrounds the nail.
- The *eponychium* is the tissue that attaches closely to the nail plate proximally, commonly referred to as the *cuticle*.
- The nail folds consist of skin, which continues underneath the visible edges to form a protective barrier.
- The pulp of each digit consists of multiple compartments separated by fibrous septa.
  - These vertical septa extend from the periosteum of the distal phalanx to the epidermis, lending structural support to the fingertip.

PATHOGENESIS

- Acute paronychia results from the introduction of bacteria into the space between the nail fold and the nail plate, either proximally or laterally.
  - This commonly occurs as a result of a hangnail, nail biting, or an overzealous manicure.
- Chronic paronychia results from colonization and infection by organisms that enter the space between the nail plate and the cuticle, eponychium, and nail fold.
  - This chronic infection and inflammation lead to fibrosis of the eponychium, which, in turn, leads to decreased vascularity of the dorsal nail fold.
  - This decreased vascularity predisposes to repeated bacterial insults, resulting in the characteristic clinical exacerbations.
- Felons often result from penetrating trauma, or from bacterial inoculation through the exocrine sweat glands contained within the pulp.
  - Cellulitis and local inflammation lead to local ischemia, which, in the setting of the closed spaces defined by septa, leads to increased pressure.
  - Fat necrosis and abscess formation result from the increased pressure, which, in turn, causes a further increase in pressure, and, in effect, a compartment syndrome.

NATURAL HISTORY

- If acute paronychia is left untreated, an early infection will turn into an abscess along the nail fold.
  - The abscess may then extend into the pulp space or into the eponychium and then to the opposite side of the nail.
  - Purulence at the base of the nail may cause ischemia of the germinal matrix, which then may lead to temporary or permanent nail growth arrest.
- Herpetic whitlow improves without any intervention in approximately 3 weeks.
  - Many cases of herpetic whitlow are misdiagnosed as acute paronychia or felon.

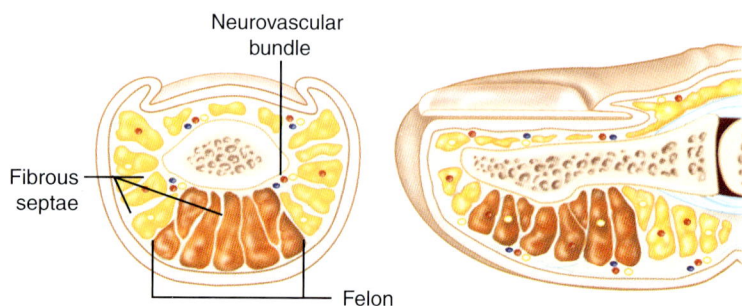

FIG 1 • Felon in coronal and sagittal section.

Neurovascular bundle

Fibrous septae

Felon

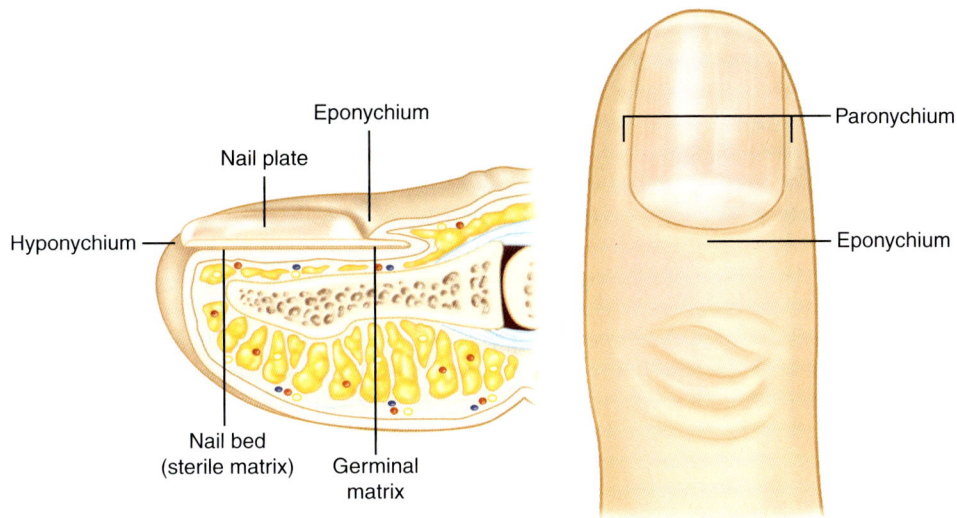

FIG 2 • Anatomy of the nail complex.

- Subsequent incision and drainage may lead to secondary bacterial infection.
- Chronic paronychia are characterized by induration of the eponychium punctuated by episodes of swelling and drainage.
- A felon, if left untreated, may lead to osteomyelitis or septic flexor tenosynovitis.

PATIENT HISTORY AND PHYSICAL FINDINGS

- In acute paronychia, the patient will complain of swelling and pain immediately adjacent to the nail.
  - If an abscess has formed, there may be purulent drainage.
- In chronic paronychia, the patient will present with a chronically indurated and rounded eponychium characterized by repeated episodes of inflammation and drainage.
- Herpetic whitlow is characterized by pain and swelling followed by the appearance of multiple vesicular lesions.
  - The pain typically is out of proportion to the physical findings, and the fingertip is not tense (in contrast to a felon).
- A patient with a felon will present with severe throbbing pain, swelling, and a tense fingertip pad.
  - A felon will not extend proximal to the distal interphalangeal (DIP) joint flexion crease unless it is associated with septic flexor tenosynovitis.

IMAGING AND OTHER DIAGNOSTIC STUDIES

- Radiographs are indicated to rule out osteomyelitis or if a foreign body is suspected.
- The diagnosis of herpetic whitlow is confirmed by Tzanck smear, which will show multinucleated giant cells.
- Patients suspected of having a systemic illness should have the appropriate laboratory workup.

DIFFERENTIAL DIAGNOSIS

- Acute paronychia
- Chronic paronychia
- Herpetic whitlow

- Felon
- Osteomyelitis
- Septic arthritis of the DIP joint

NONOPERATIVE MANAGEMENT

- Acute paronychia may be treated with warm soaks and oral antibiotics if infection is caught early and if no significant abscess is present.
- Herpetic whitlow is managed by keeping the hands clean to prevent bacterial superinfections; these lesions will resolve on their own.
  - Some recommend treatment with oral acyclovir, but multiple clinical trials have failed to show any definite benefit.
- Nonoperative treatment has no role in the treatment of chronic paronychia unless there is a concomitant fungal infection that may benefit from medical therapy.
- Given the rapid clinical progression of a felon, nonoperative treatment with antibiotics rarely will be successful, except in very early cases.

SURGICAL MANAGEMENT

- If the abscess is superficial, drainage may sometimes be performed without anesthesia.
- If the infection is more extensive or involves both sides of the nail, incision and drainage should be performed under digital nerve block.
  - Use lidocaine or a mixture of lidocaine and bupivacaine without epinephrine.
  - Instillation of the medication at the level of the distal metacarpal from dorsal to volar is the safest and best tolerated technique.
- Chronic paronychia usually are treated with eponychial marsupialization.
  - Chronic paronychia associated with underlying fungal infections may be amenable to more standard surgical treatments as performed for acute paronychia after the fungal infection has been successfully treated medically.
- Herpetic whitlow is treated with incision and drainage *only* if a bacterial superinfection has occurred.

Positioning

■ The patient is placed in the supine position with a standard hand table and either digital or forearm tourniquet.

Approach

■ The surgical approach is dictated by the location of the infection.

■ Infection under the nail plate will require elevation of part of the nail.

■ Infection under the eponychial fold will require elevation of the eponychium.

■ Infection into the pulp will require incision deep into the pulp space.

INCISION AND DRAINAGE OF AN ACUTE PARONYCHIA

Single Incision

■ Use a no. 15 scalpel to incise into the paronychial sulcus, keeping the blade directed away from the nail bed (**TECH FIG 1A**).

■ If the abscess extends below the nail plate, then that portion of the nail is freed from the underlying bed, a longitudinal incision is made in the nail, and that section of the nail is removed in an atraumatic manner (**TECH FIG 1B,C**).

■ Alternatively, if the purulence extends into the pulp space, the perionychium may be incised peripheral and parallel to the nail sulcus (**TECH FIG 1D,E**).

■ If the abscess extends to the eponychium, the incision may be carried as far proximally as necessary; a portion of nail may then be removed if necessary.

Parallel Incisions

■ If the abscess involves the eponychium and is not completely decompressed with a single incision, a parallel incision may be made on the opposite paronychial sulcus. The entire eponychial fold is elevated, and the proximal third of the nail is excised (**TECH FIG 2**).

■ This is then irrigated and packed with gauze to prevent premature closure.

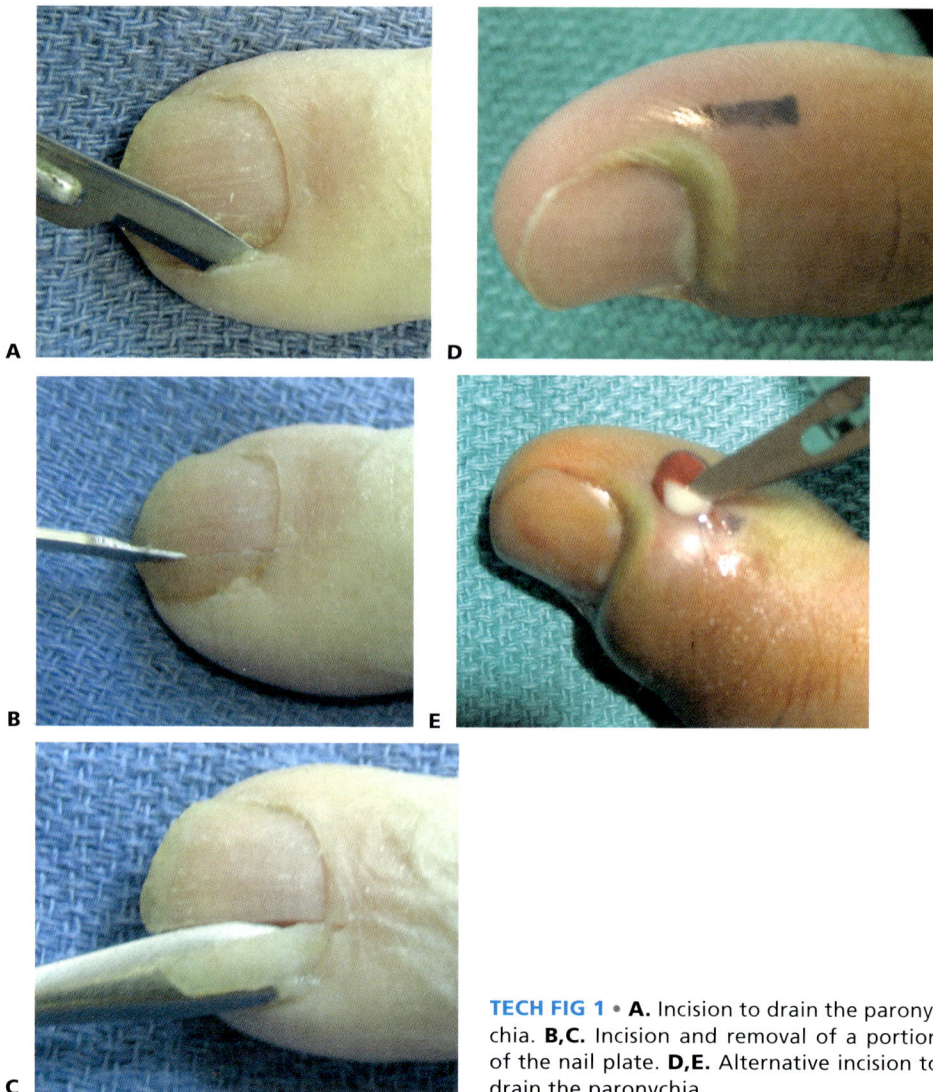

TECH FIG 1 • **A.** Incision to drain the paronychia. **B,C.** Incision and removal of a portion of the nail plate. **D,E.** Alternative incision to drain the paronychia.

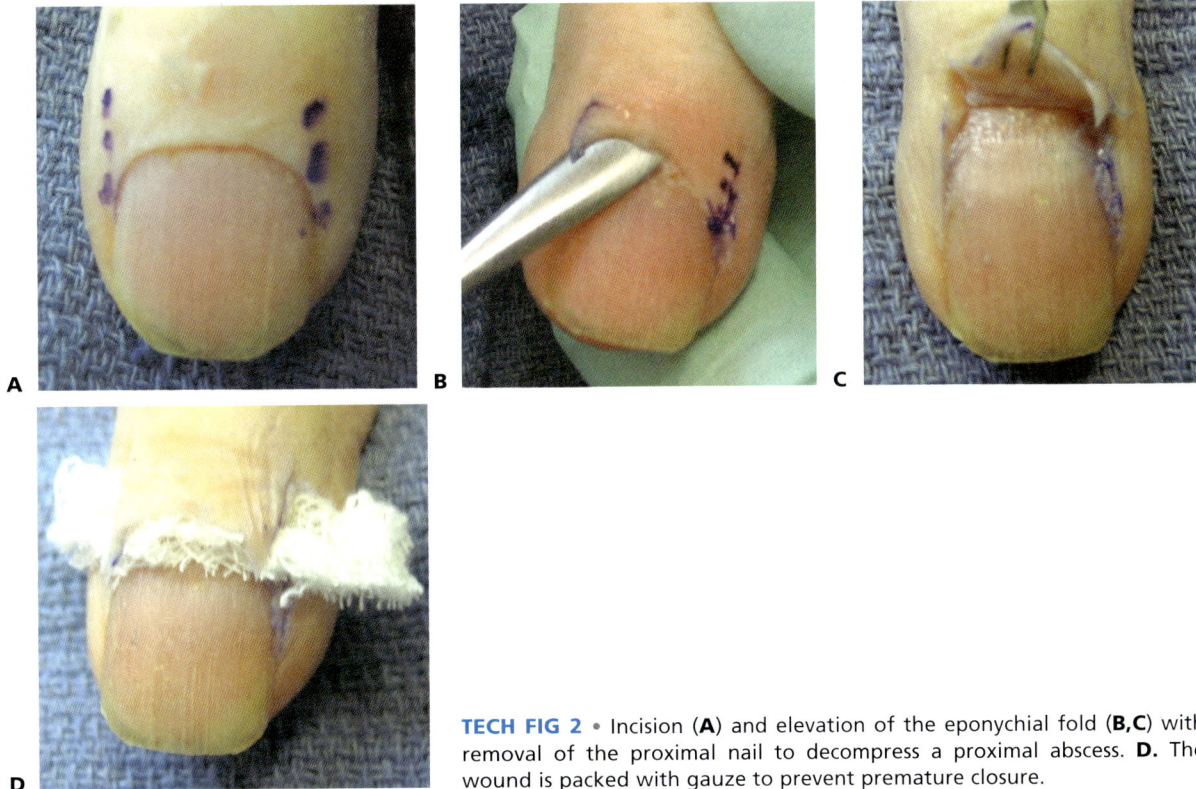

TECH FIG 2 • Incision (**A**) and elevation of the eponychial fold (**B,C**) with removal of the proximal nail to decompress a proximal abscess. **D.** The wound is packed with gauze to prevent premature closure.

EPONYCHIAL MARSUPIALIZATION FOR A CHRONIC PARONYCHIA

- Make a crescent-shaped incision 1 to 3 mm proximal to the eponychial fold, extending 3 to 5 mm proximally and extending to the edge of each nail fold (**TECH FIG 3A,B**).

- Excise this tissue, taking care not to damage the underlying germinal matrix (**TECH FIG 3C**).
- Irrigate and dress the wound appropriately.
- Allow the wound to heal by secondary intention.

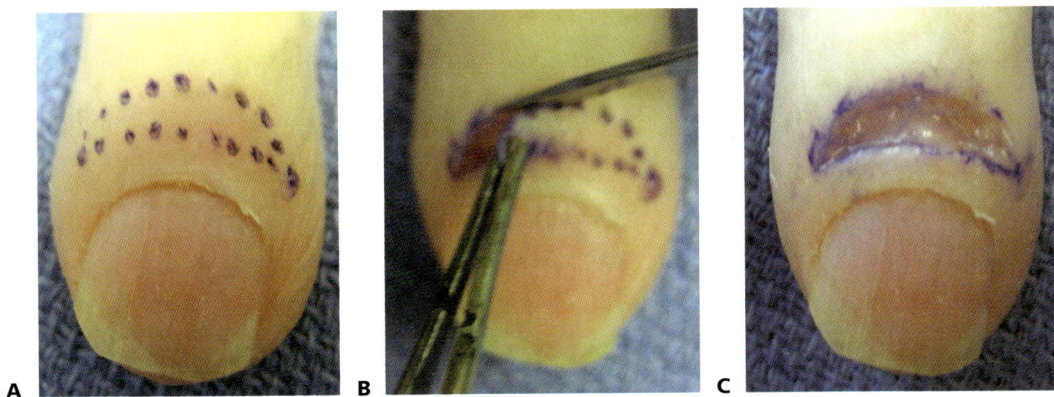

TECH FIG 3 • **A,B.** Incision for marsupialization of chronic paronychia. **C.** Tissue removed with the underlying germinal matrix exposed.

INCISION AND DRAINAGE OF A FELON

- Base the incision over the point of maximal tenderness. Be aware that an incision on the pulp can result in a tender scar.
  - For a volarly oriented abscess, make an incision precisely in the midline distal to the DIP joint flexion crease (**TECH FIG 4A,B**).

- When the point of maximal tenderness is on the side of the finger pulp, make the incision longitudinally, dorsal to the tactile surface of the finger, not more than 3 mm from the edge of the nail. A more volar incision risks damage to the digital nerve branches (**TECH FIG 4C**).

TECHNIQUES

- Carry the incision deep enough to disrupt all involved septa, or spread with a hemostat (TECH FIG 4D,E).
- Irrigate the wound with normal saline.

- Place a strip of gauze into the open wound to allow for drainage, and dress appropriately.

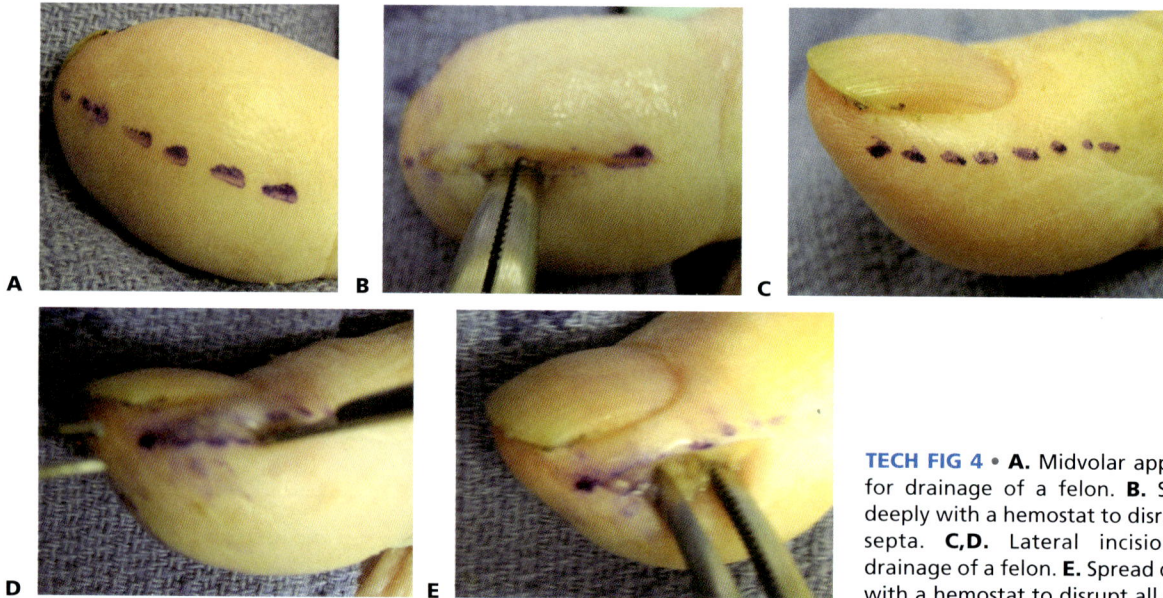

TECH FIG 4 • **A.** Midvolar approach for drainage of a felon. **B.** Spread deeply with a hemostat to disrupt all septa. **C,D.** Lateral incision for drainage of a felon. **E.** Spread deeply with a hemostat to disrupt all septa.

PEARLS AND PITFALLS

Misdiagnosis	▪ Avoid misdiagnosis of herpetic whitlow as an acute paronychia with concomitant overtreatment of this problem resulting in a secondary bacterial infection and no improvement in the herpetic whitlow. ▪ Recognize underlying osteomyelitis in longstanding cases. ▪ Recognize any systemic illness that may hinder resolution of the infection. ▪ Chronic paronychia: avoid missing a cyst, tumor, or associated fungal infection.
Technique	▪ *Acute paronychia:* Determine whether purulence is present under the nail plate or extending into the pulp. Avoid incising into the sterile matrix by keeping the blade turned away from the nail bed. ▪ *Chronic paronychia:* Excise tissue superficial to the germinal matrix; avoid damaging the germinal matrix. ▪ *Felon:* Base the incision on the location of maximal tenderness. With a lateral incision, avoid damaging the digital nerve branches by remaining within 3 mm of the lateral edge of the nail. With a volar incision, do not cross the DIP joint flexion crease and avoid incising the flexor tendon sheath. Such incisions may lead to septic tenosynovitis.
Postoperative care	▪ *Acute paronychia and felons:* Treat with 10 days of oral antibiotics. Use of a removable splint over the distal digit is valuable early in recovery for patient comfort. Encourage early digital range of motion exercises during daily soaks. ▪ *Chronic paronychia:* Failure to modify environmental factors and treat systemic disease may lead to recurrence.

POSTOPERATIVE CARE

- Acute paronychia and felons
  - Oral antibiotics should be started postoperatively.
  - Soaks in a dilute solution of either chlorhexidine or povidone-iodine may be started on postoperative day 2 and continued until wound healing is completed. The packing is removed when the soaks begin.
  - Begin early range-of-motion exercises to avoid stiffness.
- Chronic paronychia
  - Oral antibiotics usually are not necessary.
  - Soaks in a dilute solution of either chlorhexidine or povidone-iodine may be started on postoperative day 2 and continued until wound healing is completed.

- Correction of environmental factors or systemic illness is critical.
- Begin early range-of-motion exercises to avoid stiffness.

COMPLICATIONS

- Recurrent infection (systemic spread of the infection)
- Incisional tenderness (pulp)
- Digital nerve injury
  - Decreased sensation
  - Neuroma
- Osteomyelitis
- Nail plate deformity

REFERENCES

1. Kesson AM. Use of acyclovir in herpes simplex virus infections. J Paediatr Child Health 1998;34:9

2. Bednar M, Lane L. Eponychial marsupialization and nail removal for surgical treatment of chronic paronychia. J Hand Surg Am 1991;16:314–317.

3. Gill J, Arlette J, Buchan K. Herpes simplex virus infection of the hand. Am J Med 1988; 84:89–93.

4. Jebson PJ. Infections of the fingertip: Paronychias and felons. Hand Clin 1998;12:547.

5. Canales FL, Newmeyer WL III, Kilgore ES Jr. The treatment of felons and paronychias. Hand Clin 1989;5:515–523.

6. Hausman MR, Lisser SP. Hand infections. Orthop Clin North Am 1992;23:171–185.

Chapter 101

Surgical Treatment of Deep Space Infections of the Hand

Eric Stuffmann and Jeffrey Yao

DEFINITION

- Deep space infections occur in one of three anatomically defined potential spaces within the hand—the thenar, midpalmar, and hypothenar spaces—or in one forearm potential space, Parona's space.
- Thenar space infections are the most common deep space infections. Midpalmar and hypothenar space infections are much more rare.
- Deep space infections usually result from direct penetrating trauma or spread from an adjacent infection such as a superficial abscess or a flexor tenosynovitis (in the case of thenar and midpalmar space infections).
- The single most common infecting organism is *Staphylococcus aureus*, although most of these infections are mixed.

ANATOMY

- The thenar space (**FIG 1**) is defined by the fascia of the adductor pollicis muscle dorsally and the tendon sheath of the index finger and palmar fascia volarly.
  - The radial border is defined by the insertion of the adductor pollicis tendon and fascia on the thumb proximal phalanx.
  - The ulnar border is the midpalmar (oblique) septum, which extends from the third metacarpal to the palmar fascia.
- The midpalmar space (see **FIG 1**) is bordered radially by the midpalmar septum and bordered ulnarly by the hypothenar septum, which extends from the fifth metacarpal to the palmar fascia.
  - The dorsal border of the midpalmar space is the fascia of the second and third palmar interosseous muscles, and the volar border is the flexor sheaths of the long, ring, and small fingers and the palmar fascia.

- The hypothenar space (**FIG 1**) is bordered radially by the hypothenar septum and dorsally by the periosteum of the fifth metacarpal. The fascia of the hypothenar muscles forms the ulnar and palmar borders.
- Parona's space is a deep potential space in the distal forearm superficial to pronator quadratus and deep to the flexor digitorum profundus tendons. It is continuous with the midpalmar space.

PATHOGENESIS

- Thenar space infections may result from penetrating injury or local spread from adjacent flexor tenosynovitis or a subcutaneous abscess.
  - If not treated early, the infection may spread to the dorsal side of the hand after destroying the fascia of the adductor pollicis muscles and traveling between the transverse and oblique heads.
- Midpalmar space infections usually result from direct penetrating trauma, but may also result from spread of an adjacent flexor tenosynovitis or superficial abscess.
- Hypothenar space infections usually result from direct penetrating trauma, but may also result from spread of a superficial abscess.
- Parona's space infection may result from direct penetrating trauma, in which case the infection may be isolated to Parona's space.
  - Infection involving Parona's space may also result from contiguous spread from a ruptured radial or ulnar bursae (**FIG 2**). The end result will be involvement of the midpalmer space and a horseshoe abscess (**FIG 3**).

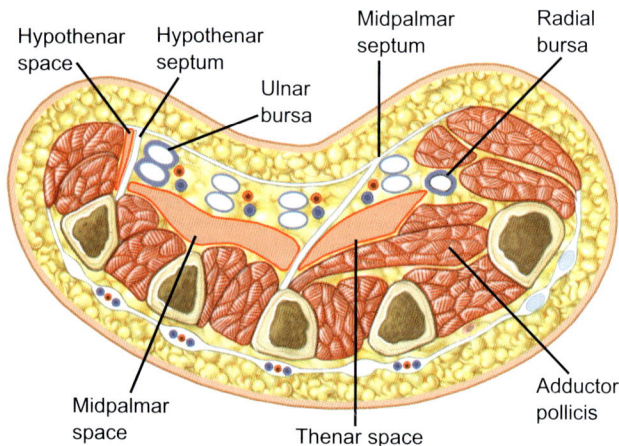

FIG 1 • Cross-sectional anatomy of the hand demonstrating the deep spaces.

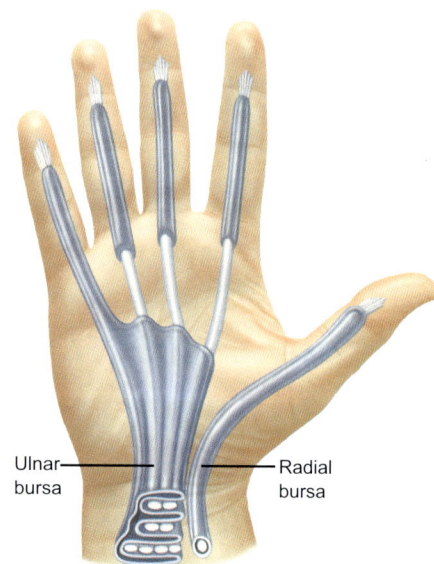

FIG 2 • Radial and ulnar bursae may communicate in the distal volar forearm (Parona's space).

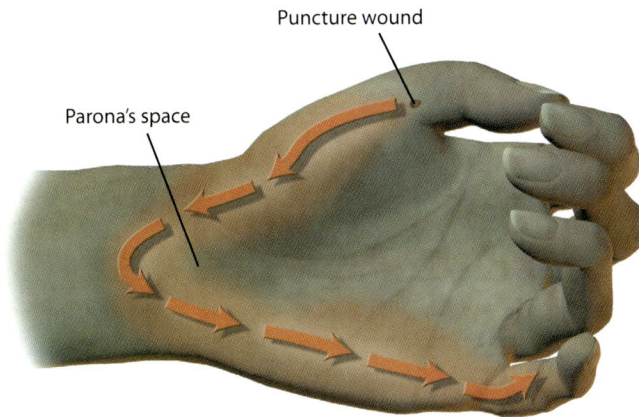

FIG 3 • Drawing representing the clinical appearance of a horseshoe abscess.

PATIENT HISTORY AND PHYSICAL FINDINGS

- The patient may recall a history of a penetrating injury in the vicinity of the involved deep space.
- In the case of a thenar space infection, the patient will present with swelling and tenderness in the thenar region.
  - The patient will hold the thumb in an abducted position to minimize the pressure for comfort.
  - If the infection has been present for some time, it may have spread dorsally, in which case swelling and tenderness will be found dorsally in the first web space.
- In the case of a midpalmar space infection there will be tenderness and swelling in the midpalm, although dorsal swelling may be more impressive due to the strength of the palmar aponeurosis.
  - The fingers will be held in a semiflexed posture.
  - This condition is distinguished from flexor tenosynovitis by relative lack of pain with passive motion of the fingers and with direct palpation of the flexor sheath along the digit.
- Infection of Parona's space is characterized by swelling in the distal volar forearm and pain with digital flexion.

IMAGING AND OTHER DIAGNOSTIC STUDIES

- Radiographs should be obtained in all cases to rule out the presence of foreign bodies.
- Radiographs also may reveal underlying osteomyelitis in the setting of more chronic infections.
- Patients suspected to have systemic illness should have an appropriate laboratory workup.

DIFFERENTIAL DIAGNOSIS

- Thenar space infection
- Midpalmar space infection
- Hypothenar space infection

- Flexor tenosynovitis
- Superficial abscess
- Osteomyelitis

NONOPERATIVE MANAGEMENT

- There is no role for nonoperative treatment in the setting of deep space infections.
- Antibiotics should be avoided until adequate cultures can be obtained, unless the patient is systemically ill and there will be a forced delay in operative treatment.

SURGICAL MANAGEMENT

- Drainage of deep space infections should be carried out in the operating room under general anesthesia.
- Gram stain and cultures for aerobes, anaerobes, mycobacteria, and fungi should be obtained intraoperatively just before IV antibiotics are administered.
- Thorough irrigation with 6 to 9 L of normal saline should be performed.
- All nonviable tissue must be débrided sharply.
- Surgical wounds may be closed very loosely over a drain if all necrotic tissue has been thoroughly débrided.
  - If there is any doubt, the wound should be left open to heal by secondary intention using wet-to-dry dressing changes and soaks.
  - In very severe cases, a second irrigation 48 to 72 hours later may be required.

Positioning

- The patient is positioned supine with a standard hand table and nonsterile tourniquet.

Approach

- Drainage of thenar space infections can be performed through a volar incision or a dorsal longitudinal incision (or, sometimes, both).
  - A volar incision involves risk to the recurrent motor branch of the median nerve, the digital nerves to the thumb and index finger, the princeps pollicis artery, and the proper digital arteries.
  - A volar incision also allows concomitant treatment of a thumb septic flexor tenosynovitis.
  - A dorsal longitudinal incision avoids the painful scar associated with a volar incision.
- Drainage of midpalmar space infections may be performed through a transverse skin incision in, or parallel to, the distal palmar crease over the third and fourth metacarpals.
  - Alternatively, a curved longitudinal incision may be used.
- Hypothenar space infections are approached through an incision in line with the ulnar border of the ring finger extending from 3 cm distal to the wrist crease to just proximal to the midpalmar crease.
- Parona's space may be approached through a longitudinal incision just ulnar to the palmaris longus.
  - Alternatively, a trans–flexor carpi radialis approach may be used.

TECHNIQUES

INCISION AND DRAINAGE OF THENAR SPACE INFECTIONS

- In the case of a volar approach, make an incision just adjacent and parallel to the thenar crease, beginning 1 cm proximal to the web space and extending 3 to 4 cm proximally (**TECH FIG 1A**).
- After blunt dissection through the palmar fascia, the digital nerves to the thumb and index finger, the princeps pollicis artery, the proper digital arteries, and the recurrent motor branch of the median nerve are encountered (**TECH FIG 1B,C**).
- The abscess will lie superficial to the adductor pollicis muscle.
- Dissection should then continue dorsally over the distal edge of the adductor muscle to decompress any dorsal extension of the abscess.

- Alternatively, a thenar space infection may be approached dorsally through a longitudinal incision (**TECH FIG 1D**).
- The dorsal incision may be straight or slightly curved and should bisect the space between the first and second metacarpals.
  - Dissection should be carried down to the interval between the first dorsal interosseous muscle and adductor pollicis muscle, where the purulence will be encountered.
- Thoroughly débride all necrotic tissue, and irrigate copiously with sterile saline.
- Place a strip of packing strip gauze into the open wound to allow for drainage, and dress the wound appropriately.

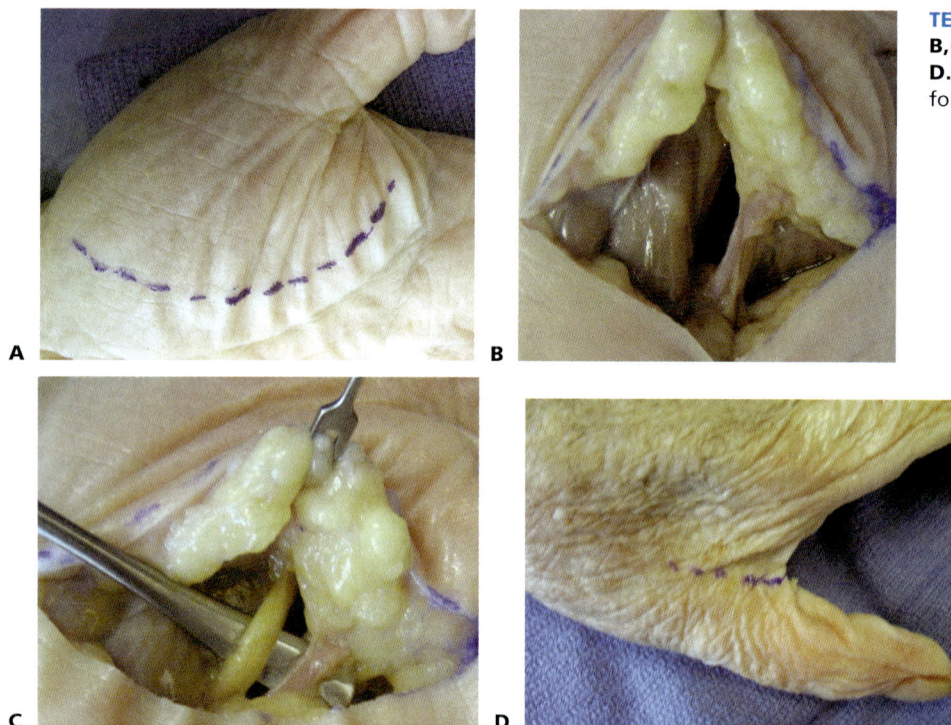

TECH FIG 1 • **A.** Thenar incision. **B,C.** Neurovascular bundle. **D.** Alternative dorsal incision for drainage of thenar abscess.

INCISION AND DRAINAGE OF MIDPALMAR SPACE INFECTIONS

- Make a transverse incision parallel to or in the distal palmar crease over the third and fourth metacarpals (**TECH FIG 2A**).
  - Alternatively, a curved longitudinal incision may be used (**TECH FIG 2B**).
- Bluntly dissect to either side of the flexor tendons to the ring or middle finger, where the abscess will be encountered.

- Protect the neurovascular bundles, which lie on either side of the tendons (**TECH FIG 2C**).
- Thoroughly débride all necrotic tissue, and irrigate copiously with sterile saline.
- Place a strip of packing strip gauze into the open wound to allow for drainage, and dress the wound appropriately.

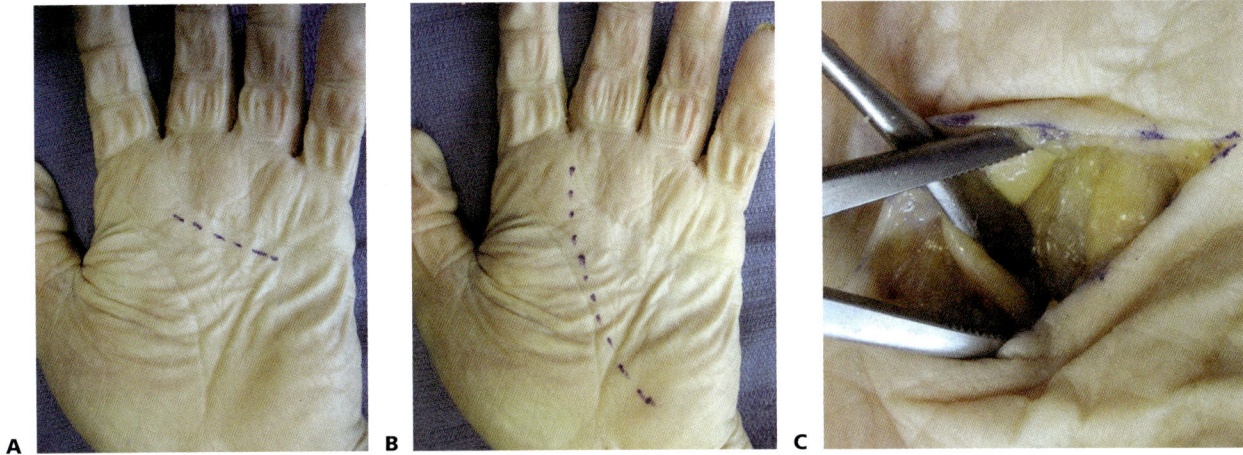

TECH FIG 2 • **A.** Transverse incision for drainage of midpalmar abscess. **B.** Curved longitudinal incision for drainage of midpalmar abscess. **C.** Drainage of midplanar abscess (neurovascular bundle protected by freer).

INCISION AND DRAINAGE OF HYPOTHENAR SPACE INFECTIONS

- Make an incision in line with the ulnar border of the ring finger extending from just proximal to the midpalmar crease to 3 cm distal to the wrist crease (**TECH FIG 3A**).
- Incise the hypothenar fascia in line with the skin incision, and the purulence will be encountered (**TECH FIG 3B**).

- Thoroughly débride all necrotic tissue, and irrigate copiously with sterile saline.
- Place a strip of packing strip gauze into the open wound to allow for drainage, and dress the wound appropriately.

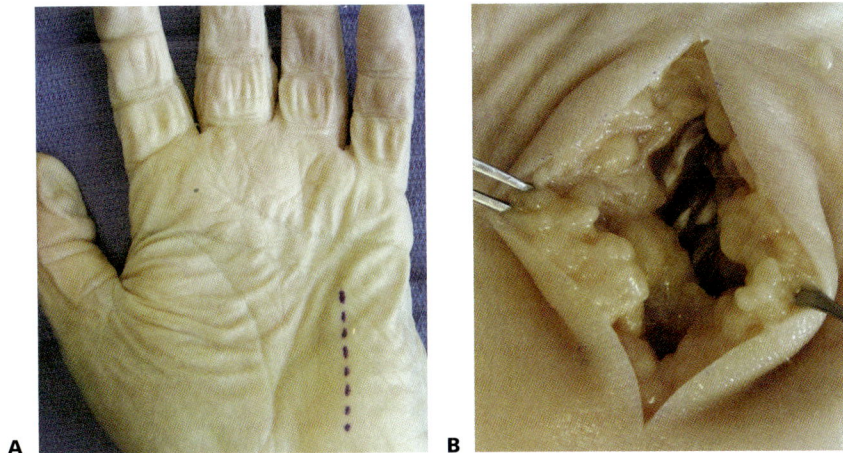

TECH FIG 3 • Incision (**A**) and drainage (**B**) of a hypothenar abscess.

INCISION AND DRAINAGE OF PARONA'S SPACE INFECTIONS

- Approach Parona's space with a longitudinal incision in the distal forearm just ulnar to the palmaris longus.
- If the infection is isolated to Parona's space, keep the incision proximal to the wrist flexion crease.

- If the infection is contiguous with a midpalmar space abscess, the incision is carried across the wrist in Brunner fashion.

PEARLS AND PITFALLS

Misdiagnosis	■ Recognize underlying osteomyelitis in longstanding cases. ■ Recognize any systemic illness that may hinder resolution of the infection.
Presurgical planning	■ Always obtain radiographs to evaluate for osteomyelitis or a foreign body.
Technique	■ When approaching the thenar space, protect the digital nerves to the thumb and index finger, the princeps pollicis artery, the proper digital arteries, and the recurrent motor branch of the median nerve. ■ In the midpalmar space, protect the superficial palmar arch and the digital nerves and arteries. ■ In the hypothenar space, protect the ulnar nerve and its branches, together with the ulnar artery. ■ Obtain Gram stain and cultures for anaerobes, aerobes, mycobacteria, and fungi. ■ Administer IV antibiotics intraoperatively once cultures have been obtained. ■ May close over Penrose drain if débridement is adequate ■ If there is the possibility of remaining necrotic tissue, the wound should be left open to close by secondary intention.
Postoperative care	■ Allow open wounds to heal by secondary intention with wet-to-dry dressing changes. ■ IV oral antibiotics for 7 to 14 days ■ Infectious disease consultation, if necessary ■ Maintain elevation. ■ Use of a removable splint will rest soft tissues and improve patient comfort. ■ Perform soaks in warm water three times per day ■ Begin early digital range-of-motion exercises. ■ Be prepared to repeat irrigation and débridement if there is no clinical improvement after 48 hours.

POSTOPERATIVE CARE

■ Intravenous antibiotics, initially given intraoperatively, are continued postoperatively.

■ The patient may be switched to oral antibiotics once cultures and sensitivities return from the microbiology laboratory and if he or she is responding to IV antibiotic therapy.

■ Let open wounds heal by secondary intention using wet-to-dry dressing changes and soaks or whirlpools.

■ Remove drains after 24 to 48 hours, depending on the condition of the wound and particulars associated with surgery.

■ Begin early range-of-motion exercises during soaks or whirlpool treatments to minimize digital stiffness.

■ Treatment of systemic illness is critical.

COMPLICATIONS

■ Persistent abscess formation if irrigation and débridement is inadequate or the wound is closed tightly and not allowed to drain

■ Systemic spread of the infection if appropriate treatment is delayed

SUGGESTED READING

Burkhalter WE. Deep space infections. Hand Clin 1989;5:553–559.

Hausman MR, Lisser SP. Hand infections. Orthop Clin North Am 1992;23:171–185.

Leddy JP. Infections of the upper extremity. J Hand Surg Am 1986;11:294–297.

Siegel DB, Gelberman RH. Infections of the hand. Orthop Clin North Am 1988;19:779–789.

Chapter 102

Surgical Treatment of Septic Arthritis in the Hand and Wrist

Asif M. Ilyas

DEFINITION

- *Septic arthritis* is defined as an infection within the closed space of a joint.
- It is usually acute and purulent secondary to a pyogenic bacterial infection.
- It causes irreversible damage to articular cartilage and therefore warrants prompt treatment with adequate drainage and an appropriate antibiotic regimen.
- Delay in making the diagnosis and initiating treatment has serious implications for prognosis.

ANATOMY

- The interphalangeal (IP) and metacarpophalangeal (MP) joints of the hand are hinge joints (**FIG 1**).
- The IP joint space is maximized in slight flexion and the MP joint in extension.
- The wrist joint includes the radiocarpal, midcarpal, and radioulnar joints. Septic arthritis may be present in all of these wrist joint spaces, concomitantly or separately, if there are no interosseous ligament perforations, as is the case in younger patients (see Fig 1).

PATHOGENESIS

- Septic arthritis may affect any joint of the hand or wrist.
- Septic arthritis does not have a gender or race predilection, but it is more common in adults than in children.

- The inoculation of the joint is most likely due to a penetrating injury (ie, lacerations, puncture wounds, and bites). Other causes include hematogenous seeding or contiguous spread.[10]
  - At the distal IP joint, septic arthritis is common from penetrating trauma as well as contiguous infection from a mucous cyst, felon, paronychia, or suppurative flexor tenosynovitis.
  - At the proximal IP joint, contiguous infection is most commonly related to a suppurative flexor tenosynovitis.
  - At the MP joint, septic arthritis is most common after direct inoculation from a clenched fist injury or fight bite.
- Hematogenous spread can result from any concomitant or preceding infection of the body, including oral, upper respiratory, gastrointestinal, and genitourinary infections.
  - The synovium is highly vascular and contains no limiting basement membrane, promoting easy access of blood contents to the synovial space.[3]
- The presence of bacteria within the joint induces a cellular and immunologic response that is detrimental to the joint. Bacteria rapidly replicate, producing toxins. The presence of bacteria stimulates an immunogenic response, resulting in the arrival of leukocytes, which produce proteolytic enzymes. Both the bacterial toxins and leukocytic enzymes destroy the articular cartilage of the joint by degrading proteoglycans and eventually injuring the underlying chondrocytes.
- Multiple risk factors can predispose a patient to septic arthritis[6] (Table 1).
  - Any disorder that results in an immunocompromised state can predispose to septic arthritis.
  - Rheumatoid arthritis, in particular, poses a high risk. This risk is related to a variety of factors including general debilitation, immunosuppressive medication, tumor necrosis factor blockers (eg, infliximab or etanercept) and chronic joint injury.

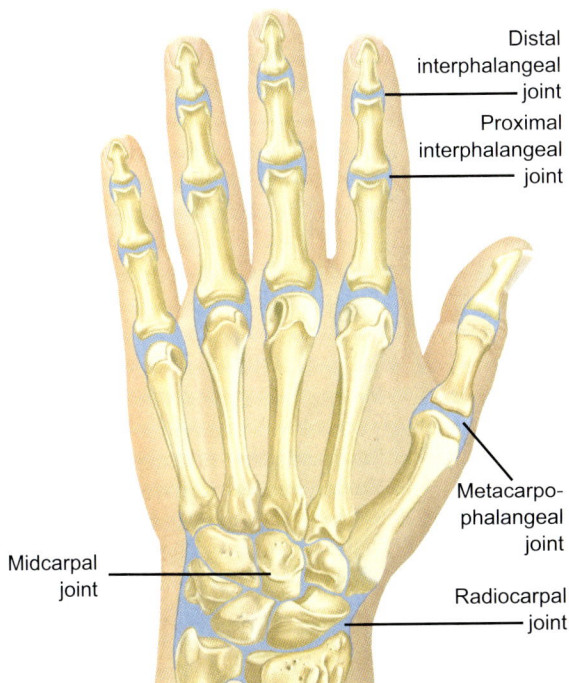

FIG 1 • Anatomy of the interphalangeal, metacarpophalangeal, and wrist joints.

Table 1	Common Risk Factors Predisposing to Septic Arthritis	
Local Factors		**Systemic Disorders**
Penetrating joint trauma		Rheumatoid arthritis
Recent joint surgery		Diabetes mellitus
Open reduction of intra-articular fractures		Liver diseases, alcoholism
Osteoarthritis		Chronic renal failure, hemodialysis
Prosthetic joints		Malignancies
Social Factors		Acquired immunodeficiency syndrome
Newborns		Immunosuppressive medication
Elderly		IV drug abusers
Occupational exposure to animals		
Low socioeconomic status		

Table 2	Common Microorganisms Causing Septic Arthritis

Gram-positive aerobes	**Anaerobes**
Staphylococcus aureus	Eikenella corodens
Streptococcus pyogenes	Borrelia burgdorferi
Streptococcus pneumoniae	Mycobacterial species
Gram-negative aerobes	**Fungus**
Haemophilus influenzae	Sporotrichosis
Escherichia coli	Cryptococcus
Pasteurella multocida	Blastomycosis
Neisseria gonorrhoeae	

- In patients with rheumatoid arthritis, a diagnosis of septic arthritis may be delayed because of misinterpretation of a rheumatoid flare. A high index of suspicion must be maintained when evaluating for septic arthritis in patients with rheumatoid arthritis.[9]
- Virtually any microbial pathogen is capable of causing pyogenic septic arthritis (Table 2).
  - *Staphylococcus aureus* and *Streptococcus* spp. are the most common offending organisms.
  - Gram-negative, anaerobic, and polymicrobial infections also are possible, especially in IV drug abusers and immunocompromised patients.
  - Specific bacterial pathogens are related to certain circumstances, eg, *Eikenella corrodens* in human bite wounds, *Pasteurella multocida* after domestic animal bites, *Neisseria gonorrhoeae* infections in sexually active young patients, and fungal and mycobacterial infections in immunocompromised patients.

NATURAL HISTORY

- The combination of the growing bacterial load and the ensuing inflammatory response results in a growing effusion that causes synovial ischemia, pressure necrosis of the cartilage, and infiltration of the bacteria into both the subchondral bone and overlying skin.
- Bacterial infiltration out of the joint can result in secondary osteomyelitis, suppurative flexor tenosynovitis, and skin breakdown with spontaneous drainage.

PATIENT HISTORY AND PHYSICAL FINDINGS

- Patients will complain of pain and swelling.
- Systemic signs of joint infection may include fevers, chills, malaise, and tachycardia.
- The patient should be asked about a history of penetrating trauma; human, animal, or insect bites; recent joint aspirations; recent infections elsewhere; and the presence of an immunocompromising condition.
- On examination, patients will manifest a painful swollen joint, with overlying erythema and warmth.
- The most important physical examination finding is exquisite pain with motion, in contrast to a noninfectious effusion or overlying cellulitis.
  - Medical professionals at the triage level may attempt to perform a regional block for pain relief. This must be prevented, because it will mask the condition.

- Attempted active digital motion will result in significant guarding, and passive flexion and extension should induce exquisite tenderness.
- Physical examination of the wrist often is less dramatic than that of the digits. The joint typically is held in a neutral position.
- Active wrist motion also will induce guarding and passive flexion, and extension should induce exquisite tenderness.
  - Passive pronation and supination may help evaluate involvement of the distal radioulnar joint.

IMAGING AND OTHER DIAGNOSTIC STUDIES

- Laboratory studies should include white blood cell count (WBC), erythrocyte sedimentation rate, C-reactive protein, and blood cultures.
  - The WBC usually is not elevated, but the erythrocyte sedimentation rate and C-reactive protein levels are consistently elevated (unless the patient is immunocompromised).
- Diagnosis of a septic arthritis is best accomplished by joint aspiration and analysis.
  - If infection is present, increased fluid will be present in the joint.
  - Joint aspirates should be sent for a cell count with differentiation, Gram stain, crystal analysis, glucose, and cultures (aerobic, anaerobic, fungal, and mycobacterial; Table 3).
  - Diagnosis can be made most reliably with a joint fluid WBC count greater than 50,000 (and a differential of 75% or more segmented neutrophils); a Gram stain confirming the presence of bacteria; or positive cultures.[5]
  - A low WBC count with a high percentage of neutrophils (>90%) may indicate an early septic arthritis.[11]
  - A joint glucose of 40 mg/dL or less compared with the fasting blood glucose level also suggests a septic process.[7]
- Crystal analysis is necessary to rule out the presence of gout or pseudogout, because they also can present similarly, including an elevated WBC count in the aspirate.
- The role of imaging studies early in the course of the septic process is limited. Radiographs may reveal joint distention, presence of foreign bodies, osteomyelitis, air in the soft tissues, and chondrocalcinosis—characteristic of both gout and pseudogout (**FIG 2A**). Later radiographs will reveal joint destruction.
- MRI is effective in diagnosing early septic arthritis and in differentiating it from osteomyelitis or overlying tenosynovitis (**FIG 2B**).

Table 3	Differential Diagnosis of Synovial Fluid Analysis		
Test	**Normal**	**Septic**	**Inflammatory**
Clarity	Transparent	Opaque	Straw
Color	Clear	Yellow-green	Yellow
Viscosity	High	Variable	High
WBC count	< 200	> 50,000	2000–10,000
PMN (%)	< 25	> 75	> 50
Culture	Negative	Often positive	Negative
Glucose (mg/dL)	Equivalent to plasma	−25 < plasma	−40 < plasma

PMN, polymorphonuclear leukocyte; WBC, white blood cell.

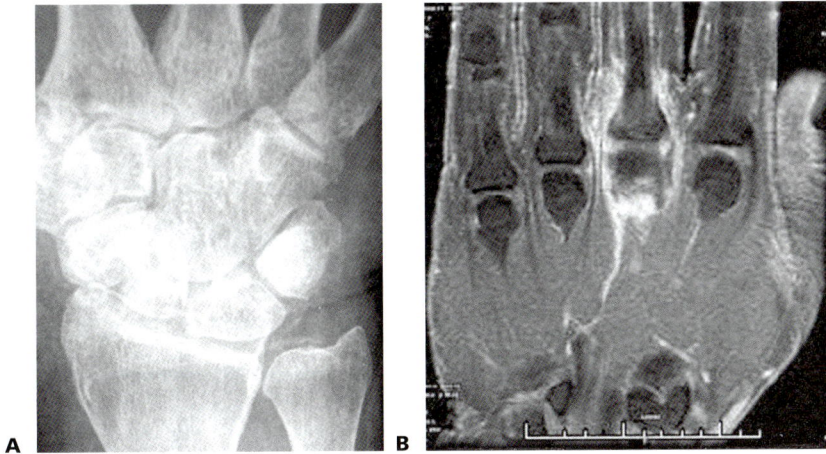

FIG 2 • **A.** Radiograph showing chondrocalcinosis of the triangular fibrocartilage complex from chronic pseudogout. **B.** Coronal T2-weighted MRI of a metacarpophalangeal joint with underlying septic arthritis. Note the normal bone signal but the presence of high signal within the joint from the fluid and surrounding soft tissue inflammation.

DIFFERENTIAL DIAGNOSIS

- Rheumatoid arthritis
- Crystalline arthropathies: gout, pseudogout
- Seronegative arthropathies: systemic lupus erythematosus, psoriatic arthritis, Reiter syndrome, ankylosing spondylitis, rheumatic fever
- Lyme disease
- Cellulitis
- Osteomyelitis
- Suppurative flexor tenosynovitis

NONOPERATIVE MANAGEMENT

- If septic arthritis is detected or suspected early enough, antibiotics alone have been suggested in the medical literature to be sufficient to eradicate the infection.[3]
- In cases where comorbid conditions contraindicate surgery, serial aspiration of the involved joint can be done to decrease the bacterial load, decompress the joint, and allow medical management with antibiotics to treat the infection.
  - This technique has been shown to be less effective than open surgical drainage in large joints and, therefore, would be even less reliable in small joints.[4]

SURGICAL MANAGEMENT

- Septic arthritis usually is considered a surgical pathology that warrants prompt treatment.
- Open and arthroscopic techniques are available for surgical drainage of the wrist.

Preoperative Planning

- Arrangements for instruments, irrigation fluid, drains, sutures, and assistants should be made in advance of surgery.

Positioning

- Approaches to the hand and wrist can be accomplished with the patient supine and the operative extremity extended on a hand table with the surgeon and assistants seated.
- The hand table should be stable and well-secured, and should allow adequate space for both the operative limb and the surgeon's elbow and forearm, to minimize surgeon fatigue and enhance stability.
- Tourniquet use is advised to obtain a bloodless field and clear visualization of anatomic structures.
  - The limb usually is exsanguinated via gravity with elevation before inflating the tourniquet to avoid proximal spread of the bacteria.
- A small-joint wrist arthroscopy tower should be used. This will provide positioning and application of traction during arthroscopy and also facilitate conversion to an open procedure if necessary. Additionally, small-joint arthroscopy equipment, including a 30-degree 2.7-mm camera, should be used.

Approach

- Multiple approaches to a joint are available. The choice of which approach to use should be based on ease of the approach while still allowing adequate joint exposure for débridement and minimizing contiguous spread of infection.
- All surgical approaches of the hand and wrist warrant a sound understanding of surface anatomy, surgical anatomy, internervous planes, and surgical technique.

ASPIRATION OF INTERPHALANGEAL OR METACARPOPHALANGEAL JOINTS

- Prepare the skin with an antiseptic wash, but avoid placing local anesthesia before the aspiration, because it may mask the location of the joint space.
- As large a needle as possible should be used, preferably 18- or 20-gauge.
- A syringe no larger than 3 or 5 mL should be used, because larger syringes cause too great a vacuum aspiration and collapse the joint, making them, therefore, less effective for aspiration.

- The joint space can be identified just radial or ulnar to the extensor mechanism on the dorsal surface.
  - The needle should be inserted in a dorsal-to-volar direction with a 30- to 45-degree angle toward the midline.
  - A palpable "pop" or sensation of entering the joint should be felt, and the joint should be aspirated.
  - Distraction of the joint can sometimes aid entry.
  - If there is resistance to aspiration, the needle should be redirected while maintaining suction on the syringe.

TECHNIQUES

SURGICAL DRAINAGE OF INTERPHALANGEAL OR METACARPOPHALANGEAL JOINTS

- For the MP joint, a dorsal longitudinal incision is made (**TECH FIG 1A**). The extensor mechanism is exposed and also incised longitudinally to expose the capsule.
  - Alternatively, the capsule can be exposed by incising the ulnar sagittal band.
- The joint is exposed by incising the capsule dorsal to the collateral ligaments.
- For the proximal IP joint, a midaxial incision is preferred to avoid injury to the central slip and creation of a septic boutonniere deformity (**TECH FIG 1B**).

- The neurovascular bundle may be identified and retracted volarly. The dorsal sensory branches are at risk and should be retracted with the dorsal flap.
- The extensor mechanism, including the lateral bands, is identified and retracted dorsally, thereby exposing the capsule laterally. The accessory collaterals (volar to the proper collaterals) are released to allow entry into the joint.
- The distal IP joint can be approached through a midaxial incision or through a dorsal "H" incision and the terminal tendon retracted laterally, exposing the joint dorsal to the collateral ligaments.
  - Injury to the terminal tendon can result in a mallet finger and possible late swan-neck deformity.
- Obtain cultures and thoroughly irrigate and débride the joint with gravity cystoscopy tubing or a bulb syringe.
  - In-line traction on the digit will help expose the joint space.
- Inspect the joint surfaces for articular damage.
- Leave a small wick in the joint to prevent premature closure of the joint capsule, and reapproximate the extensor mechanism using a monofilament suture. Avoid using deep braided sutures in the face of an infection.
- Loosely close the skin around the wick with one or two 4-0 nylon sutures.
- Place the hand in a volar splint for comfort and emphasize that the patient should keep it elevated.

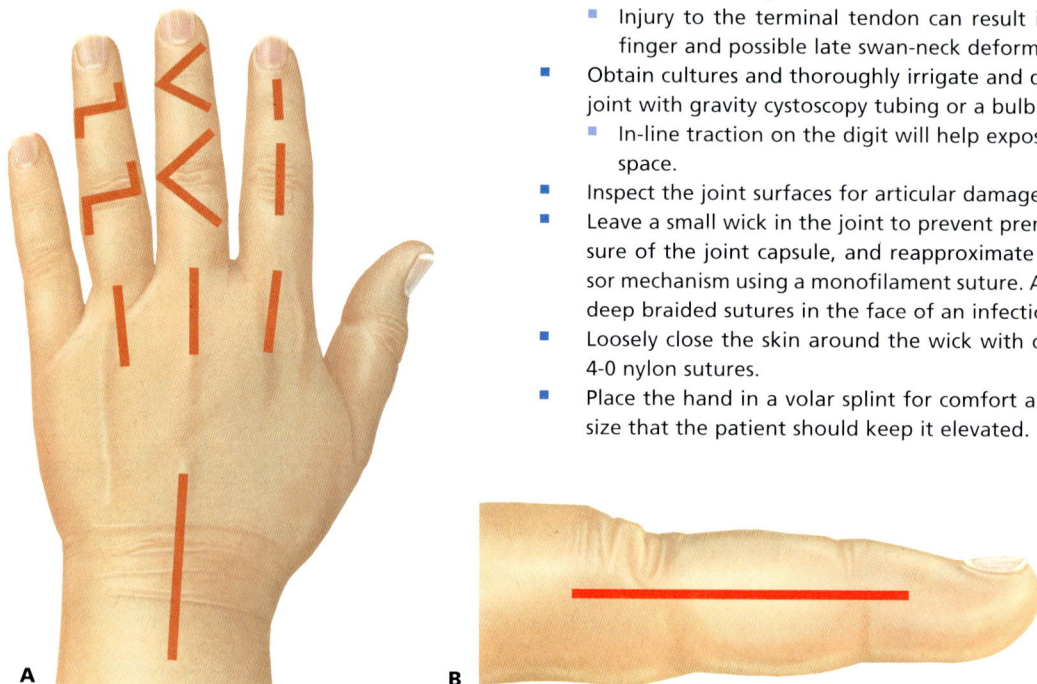

TECH FIG 1 • **A.** Sample incisions for open dorsal drainage of the interphalangeal, metacarpophalangeal, and radiocarpal joints. **B.** Sample midaxial incision for open drainage of the interphalangeal joints.

ASPIRATION OF THE WRIST

- Prepare the skin with an antiseptic wash but avoid placing local anesthesia pre-aspiration, because it may mask the location of the joint space.
- As large a needle as possible should be used, preferably 18-gauge.
- A syringe no larger than 5 or 10 mL should be used.
  - Larger syringes cause too great a vacuum on aspiration and collapse the joint, and are, therefore, less effective for aspiration.
- The joint space can be identified just distal to Lister's tubercle on the dorsum of the wrist. The needle should be

angled approximately 10 degrees volar to accommodate for the normal volar tilt of the radius.
  - Alternatively, the joint may be easily entered through the dorsal ulnocarpal space, just distal to the triangular fibrocartilage complex.
- A palpable pop or sensation of entering the joint should be felt and the joint should be aspirated. If there is resistance to aspiration then the needle should be redirected while maintaining suction on the syringe.

TECHNIQUES

ARTHROSCOPIC DÉBRIDEMENT OF THE WRIST

- Secure the hand and wrist in a sterile small-joint arthroscopy tower. Apply 5 to 10 pounds of traction.
- Identify and mark the dorsal surface anatomy of the wrist. Specifically, palpate the dorsal and distal surface of the radius, ulna, distal radioulnar joint, and Lister's tubercle. These landmarks will guide safe establishment of portals and maximize visualization (**TECH FIG 2**).
- The 3–4 portal is the main "viewing" portal and should be established first to visualize the radiocarpal joint. Begin by identifying the soft spot just distal to Lister's tubercle. The portal is bordered by the third and fourth dorsal compartments.
  - An 18-gauge needle is directed just distal to Lister's tubercle and should be angled about 10 degrees volar to accommodate for the normal volar tilt of the radius. The joint is then insufflated with 5 to 10 mL of normal saline.
  - Create the portal with a 3-mm longitudinal skin incision using a no. 11 blade directed superiorly. Spread the soft tissue bluntly with a curved hemostat down to the joint, avoiding inadvertent penetration of the capsule.
  - Direct a blunt-tipped cannula and trocar into the joint, again angling about 10 degrees volar just distal

to Lister's tubercle. Avoid plunging the cannula uncontrolled into the joint, because this may cause iatrogenic articular cartilage injury.
  - Replace the trocar with the camera.
- Cultures can be taken through the cannula.
- Systematically explore the radioscaphoid, radiolunate, and ulnocarpal joints for turbid fluid.
  - In addition, evaluate the scapholunate ligament and triangular fibrocartilage complex for tears that may allow the infection to communicate with the midcarpal and distal radioulnar joints, respectively.
- Establish a second "working" portal. Arthroscopic equipment such as the shaver and probe will be used through this portal. A 25-gauge needle is directed into the proposed site under direct arthroscopic visualization before making the skin incision.
  - The 4–5 portal is identified just ulnar to the fourth dorsal compartment and just distal to the distal radioulnar joint (see Tech Fig 2).
  - Alternatively, a 6-R or 6-U portal can be used and can be identified just radial or ulnar, respectively, to the sixth dorsal compartment. Diligent blunt dissection with a curved hemostat must be performed before inserting the blunt cannula and trocar to avoid inadvertent injury to the dorsal ulnar sensory nerve.
- The joint can be both visualized and washed through the camera cannula in the viewing portal and drained through the working portal with a cannula. Drainage can be applied to gravity or suction.
- The joint can be further débrided with the aid of a shaver with suction placed through the working cannula.
  - Devitalized tissues and synovial shavings can be taken through the shaver.
- Thorough arthroscopic débridement of the wrist should include visualization and irrigation of the midcarpal joint as well.
  - Palpate a soft spot about 1 cm distal to the 3–4 portal.
  - Place a 25-gauge needle first, and insufflate the joint with 5 mL of normal saline.
  - Direct a blunt cannula and trocar into the midcarpal joint just radial to the base of the capitate.
- After thorough visualization, irrigation, and débridement of the wrist, insert a small Hemovac drain through the working portal cannula.
- Remove the arthroscopic equipment. Close the portals with 4-0 nylon stitches.
- Place the wrist in a volar splint for comfort, and encourage limb elevation and active finger motion.

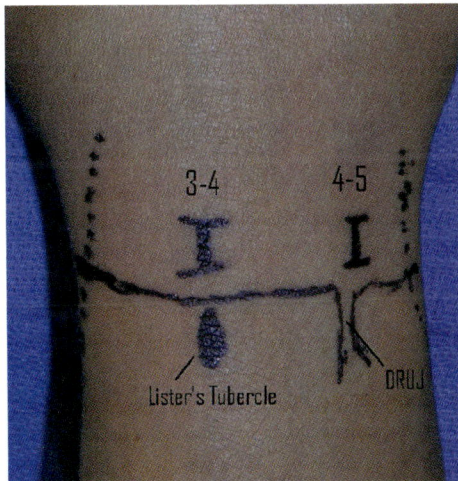

TECH FIG 2 • Dorsal surface anatomy of the wrist. The 3–4 and 4–5 portals are marked. The dashed lines represent approximate location of the radial sensory nerve on the radial side and the dorsal ulnar sensory nerve on the ulnar side.

OPEN SURGICAL DRAINAGE OF THE WRIST

- A dorsal longitudinal incision should be placed just ulnar to Lister's tubercle (**TECH FIG 3A**). The incision should be approximately 4 cm in length, with about two thirds distal to the tubercle.
  - Alternatively, a transverse incision may be used. Although more cosmetic, it may not provide adequate exposure.

TECHNIQUES

- Once the extensor retinaculum is exposed with blunt dissection, the distal third is released perpendicular to the fibers and ulnar to the third dorsal compartment.
- The interval between the third and fourth extensor compartments is bluntly dissected, and the joint capsule is exposed (**TECH FIG 3B**).
- The joint capsule is incised longitudinally, and limited flaps are raised subperiosteally off the dorsal distal radius, like an inverted T (**TECH FIG 3C**).
- Cultures are taken, and synovial tissue should be sent for culture and histology.

- The joint should be thoroughly débrided and irrigated with gravity cystoscopy tubing or a bulb syringe.
  - Pulse lavage should be avoided due to its potential to cause additional soft tissue injury.
  - The joint should be ranged during irrigation to maximize the effect of the lavage.
- The joint surfaces are inspected for articular damage.
- Leave a small wick or drain in the joint and loosely close the skin around the wick.
  - Primary closure of the joint risks reaccumulation of pus.
  - Typically, two to three loosely placed 4-0 nylon sutures will be sufficient.
- Place the wrist in a volar splint for comfort and encourage limb elevation.

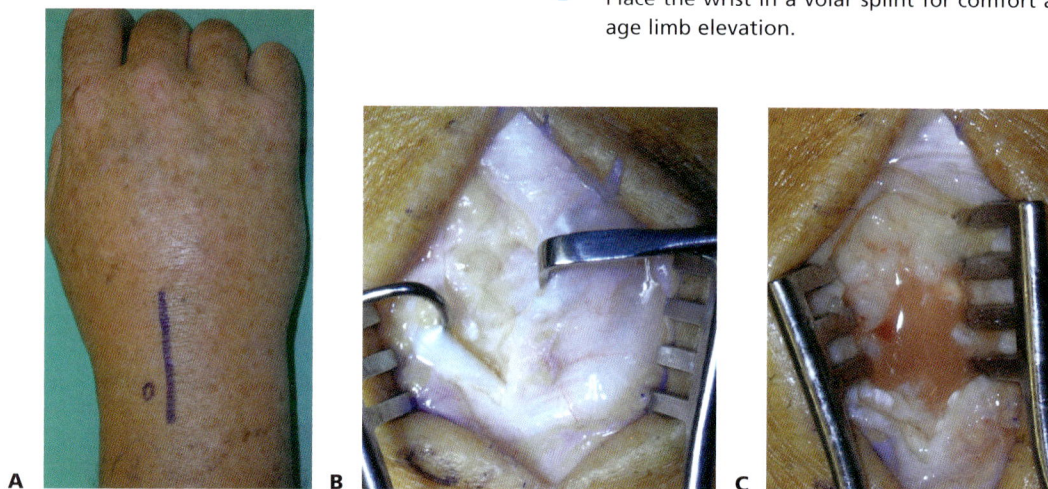

TECH FIG 3 • A. Incision for open drainage of the wrist. **B.** The distal third of the extensor retinaculum is released and the interval between the third and fourth dorsal compartment developed. **C.** The capsule is arthrotomized with an inverted T.

PEARLS AND PITFALLS

Diagnosis	▪ Diagnosis is best accomplished by joint aspiration and analysis.
Antibiotics	▪ Obtain cultures before beginning antibiotics. ▪ Empiric antibiotics should be tailored to the most likely organism based on mechanism of injury and patient factors.
Aspiration	▪ Avoid using larger syringes, because the vacuum created can collapse the joint and may be less effective for aspiration.
Arthroscopic drainage	▪ Identify the surface landmarks of the joint and avoid inadvertent injury to the dorsal tendons and cutaneous nerve. ▪ Be prepared to convert to an open procedure if adequate exposure and débridement are not possible.
Open surgical drainage	▪ Be prepared to perform a second open surgical débridement if symptoms do not improve.

POSTOPERATIVE CARE

- Empiric IV antibiotics are initiated immediately after obtaining cultures and then later tailored to the results of laboratory cultures and sensitivities.
- IV antibiotics should be continued for 2 weeks or at least through symptom resolution, followed by oral antibiotics.[8]
- The duration of antibiotics is the subject of some controversy. This should be determined on a case-by-case basis, with

consideration of surgical findings, virulence of the offending bacterial pathogen, and the response to treatment.
- Early range of motion (active and active-assisted) in diluted povidone-iodine soaks is initiated three times daily to provide mechanical lavage of the joint and to prevent premature wound closure.
- The wick or drain is removed 1 or 2 days postoperatively.

■ As symptoms resolve, the soaks are discontinued to allow the wound to heal, and progressive range of motion exercises are initiated.

■ If symptoms do not improve within 2 days, then a repeat surgical drainage should be considered.

OUTCOMES

■ The results of surgical treatment of septic arthritis are not well-documented in the literature, and it is difficult to predict the outcome even during the course of treatment.

■ Functional outcome is most closely correlated to the duration of symptoms before treatment is initiated.[10]

■ Some loss of motion and joint stiffness are expected, even in cases treated with early surgical drainage and rehabilitation.[1,10,12–14]

■ Some joint space narrowing usually is seen following treatment, and significant arthrosis and ankylosis may occur in severe cases or when treatment has been delayed.

COMPLICATIONS

■ Joint stiffness, arthrosis, osteomyelitis, and secondary tendon adhesions

■ Salvage options for postseptic arthritis include arthrodesis, resection arthroplasty, or amputation.

■ Implant arthroplasty is controversial and is not generally recommended for a previously infected joint.

REFERENCES

1. Boustred AM, Singer M, Hudson DA, Bolitho GE. Septic arthritis of the metacarpophalangeal and interphalangeal joints of the hand. Ann Plast Surg 1999;42:623–628.
2. Glass K. Factors related to the resolution of treated hand infections. J Hand Surg Am 1982;7:388–394.
3. Goldenberg DL, Reed JI. Bacterial arthritis. N Engl J Med 1985; 312:764–771.
4. Leslie B, Harris J III, Driscoll D. Septic arthritis of the shoulder in adults. J Bone Joint Surg Am 1989;71:1516–1522.
5. Li SF, Cassidy C, Chang C, et al. Diagnostic utility of laboratory tests in septic arthritis. Emerg Med J 2007;24:75–77.
6. Linscheid R, Dobyns J. Common and uncommon infections of the hand. Orthop Clin North Am 1975;6:1063–1104.
7. Moran G, Talan D. Hand infections. Emerg Med Clin North Am 1993;11:601–619.
8. Murray P. Septic arthritis of the hand and wrist. Hand Clin 1998; 14:579–587.
9. O'Dell JR. Anticytokine therapy: a new era in the treatment of rheumatoid arthritis. N Engl J Med 1999;340:310–312.
10. Rashkoff E, Burkhalter W, Mann R. Septic arthritis of the wrist. J Bone Joint Surg Am 1983;65:824–828.
11. Shmerling RH, Delbanco TL, Tosteson ANA, et al. Synovial fluid tests: What should be ordered? JAMA 1990;264:1009–1014.
12. Sinha M, Jain S, Woods DA. Septic arthritis of the small joints of the hand. J Hand Surg Br 2006;31:665–672.
13. Willems C. Treatment of purulent arthritis by wide arthrotomy followed by immediate active mobilization. Surg Gynecol Obstet 1919; 28:546–554.
14. Wittels N, Donley J, Burkhalter W. A functional treatment method for interphalangeal pyogenic arthritis. J Hand Surg Am 1984;9:894–898.

Chapter 103

Nail Matrix Repair, Reconstruction, and Ablation

Reuben A. Bueno, Jr. and Elvin G. Zook

DEFINITION

▪ Injury to the nail usually occurs in the traumatic setting. Because of its location at the distal end of the digits, the perionychium is the most frequently injured part of the hand.[9]

  ▪ Restoration of normal nail appearance is best achieved by acute treatment of the nail matrix.

  ▪ Reconstructive techniques may be used to provide a more normal-appearing nail.

▪ Excision of benign and malignant tumors involving the nail bed matrix may require techniques of nail bed repair and reconstruction also used in the traumatic setting.

▪ Optimal treatment depends on thorough understanding of the components of the perionychium—skin, sterile matrix, germinal matrix, eponychial fold, and distal phalanx—and their anatomic relationship with each other.

ANATOMY

▪ The nail serves multiple functions: protecting the fingertip, regulating peripheral circulation, and contributing to sensory feedback of the fingertip.[9]

▪ The perionychium includes the nail plate, nail bed, hyponychium, eponychium and fold, and paronychium (**FIG 1**).

▪ The proximal portion of the nail matrix is the germinal matrix, and the distal portion is the sterile matrix. The germinal matrix produces about 90% of the nail, while the sterile matrix produces the remaining 10% of the nail and produces the cells on the undersurface of the nail responsible for nail adherence.

▪ The hyponychium is the skin distal to the nail bed, the paronychium is the skin on each side of the nail, and the eponychium is the skin over the nail fold.

▪ The nail bed is adherent to the distal phalanx.

PATHOGENESIS

▪ The main causes of nail deformity are trauma and tumor.

▪ The middle finger is the most commonly injured finger.[13]

▪ Inadequate treatment in the acute setting often leads to a nail deformity.

▪ There is an associated distal phalanx fracture in 50% of nail bed injuries. This type of injury should be considered an open fracture and treated as such, with irrigation and débridement, reduction of the fracture and fixation if necessary, and repair of the nail bed (**FIG 2**).[1,4]

▪ Scarring can lead to a split nail deformity.

▪ Absence of nail matrix can lead to detachment of the nail.

▪ Lack of support from the distal phalanx leads to the hook nail deformity.

▪ Benign tumors (glomus tumor, distal interphalangeal joint ganglion), and malignant tumors (squamous cell carcinoma, melanoma) can affect nail appearance.

NATURAL HISTORY

▪ Repair in the acute period provides the best chance for normal appearance of the nail.

▪ The nail plate grows at about 0.1 mm per day or 2 to 3 mm per month. When the nail plate is removed for nail bed repair, new nail growth is delayed for 3 to 4 weeks.[9]

▪ If placed back on after repair, the old nail will remain adherent for 1 to 3 months and then fall off as a new nail pushes out the old nail.[12]

▪ After nail repair, it will take about 12 months for the nail to achieve its final appearance. Thickening of the nail proximal to the level of injury is seen for about 50 days (**FIG 3**).[9,12,13]

PATIENT HISTORY AND PHYSICAL FINDINGS

▪ Traumatic injury to the perionychium is usually caused by a crush injury.[1,4]

▪ In the acute setting, the status of the entire fingertip must be assessed: quality of the skin, presence of a subungual hematoma, quality of the nail matrix, capillary refill, sensory

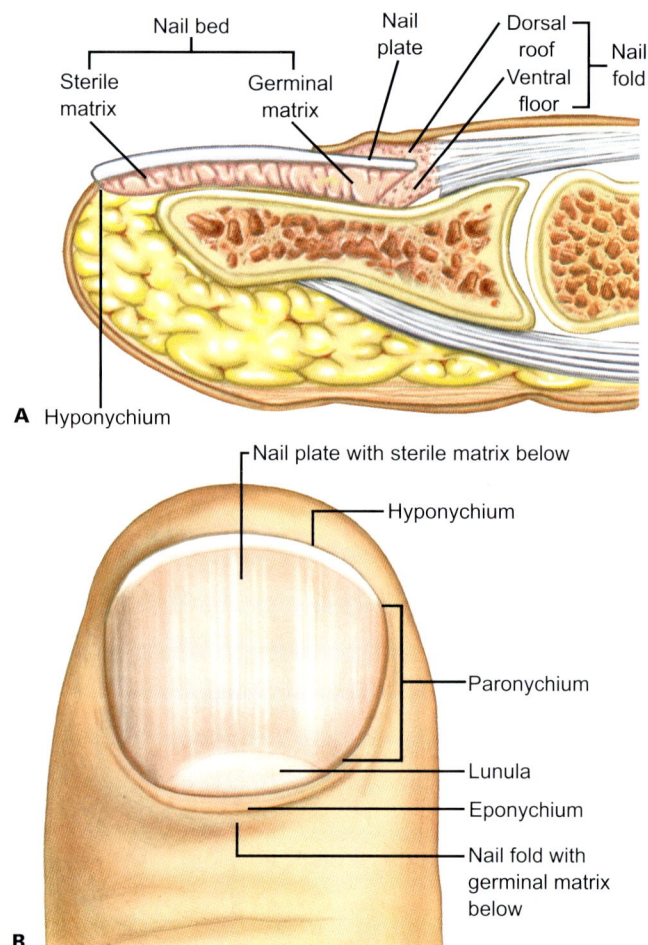

FIG 1 • The perionychium and its associated structures.

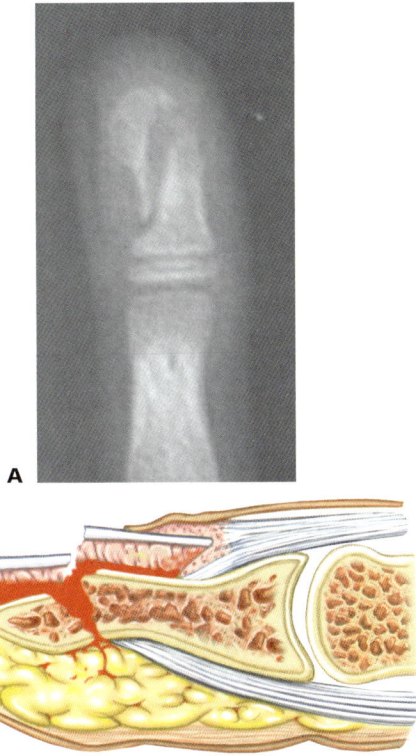

FIG 2 • A. Radiograph showing distal phalanx fracture associated with a nail bed crush injury. **B.** Nail bed injury with concomitant distal phalanx fracture. With a break in the periosteum, there is communication of the distal phalanx with the outside environment. There is a risk for osteomyelitis if not treated appropriately.

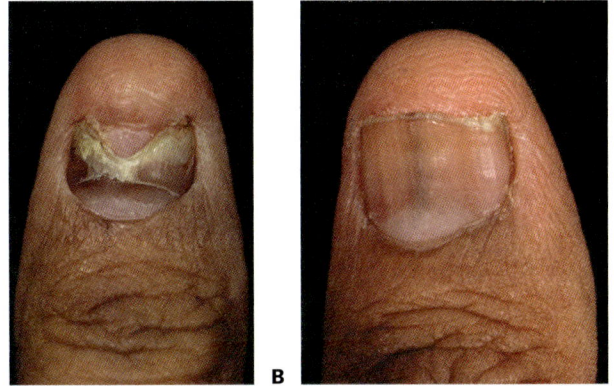

FIG 3 • A. Nail appearance at 3 months after repair. Patients should be aware of the heaped-up appearance as the nail grows distally. **B.** Nail appearance at 1 year after repair.

function, flexion and extension at the distal interphalangeal joint, presence of a distal phalanx fracture.
- Features of acute nail bed injury
  - Subungual hematoma (**FIG 4A,B**): bleeding beneath the nail from laceration of the nail bed
    - Pain secondary to pressure in the space between the nail plate and the nail bed
    - Treated with evacuation of hematoma by trephination
  - Laceration of nail bed (**FIG 4C,D**)
    - Mechanism of injury usually is crush.
    - Concomitant injury to fingertip skin or distal phalanx fracture may be present.
    - Nail lacerations can be described in one of four ways: simple laceration, stellate laceration, severe crush, and avulsion.
    - Repair of nail bed laceration and Kirschner wire fixation of distal phalanx fracture if unstable
  - Nail bed avulsion (**FIG 4E**)
    - Quality of avulsed nail matrix and size of defect will determine treatment.
    - Treatment options include returning avulsed piece back on defect or harvesting a split nail graft from the adjacent matrix or from the great toe.
- Posttraumatic nail deformities
  - Nail nonadherence or split nail (**FIG 4F**)
    - Usually due to injury to the sterile matrix, which produces the cells responsible for adherence

  - Excision of scar and primary closure or nail matrix reconstruction with a split graft from the great toe
  - Hook nail deformity (**FIG 4G**)
    - Due to excessive tension at junction of nail bed and hyponychial skin and loss of support of distal phalanx
    - Revision amputation or reconstruction of nail bed and bone graft to the distal tip of the distal phalanx
  - Nail remnant (**FIG 4H**)
    - Due to presence of residual germinal matrix not completely ablated at the time of initial repair or revision amputation
    - Complete nail matrix ablation or revision amputation
  - Pincer nail deformity (**FIG 4I**): characterized by excessive transverse curvature of the nail and progressive pinching off of the distal fingertip, causing pain and abnormal appearance
    - Partial or complete nail ablation
    - Reconstruction of nail bed with elevation of the lateral nail bed using dermal graft or AlloDerm

IMAGING AND OTHER DIAGNOSTIC STUDIES

- AP and lateral radiographs of the distal phalanx are recommended to rule out a fracture.
  - Depending on the level of injury, the following fractures are seen: distal tuft fracture, comminuted fracture, and a transverse or oblique fracture of the midshaft.
  - Intra-articular fractures at the distal interphalangeal joint are rare with an associated nail bed injury.

DIFFERENTIAL DIAGNOSIS

- Trauma
- Benign tumor
  - Glomus tumor
  - Distal interphalangeal joint ganglion cyst
- Malignant tumor
  - Squamous cell carcinoma
  - Melanoma

NONOPERATIVE MANAGEMENT

- Left untreated, traumatic injury to the nail matrix may result in an abnormal appearance of the nail.

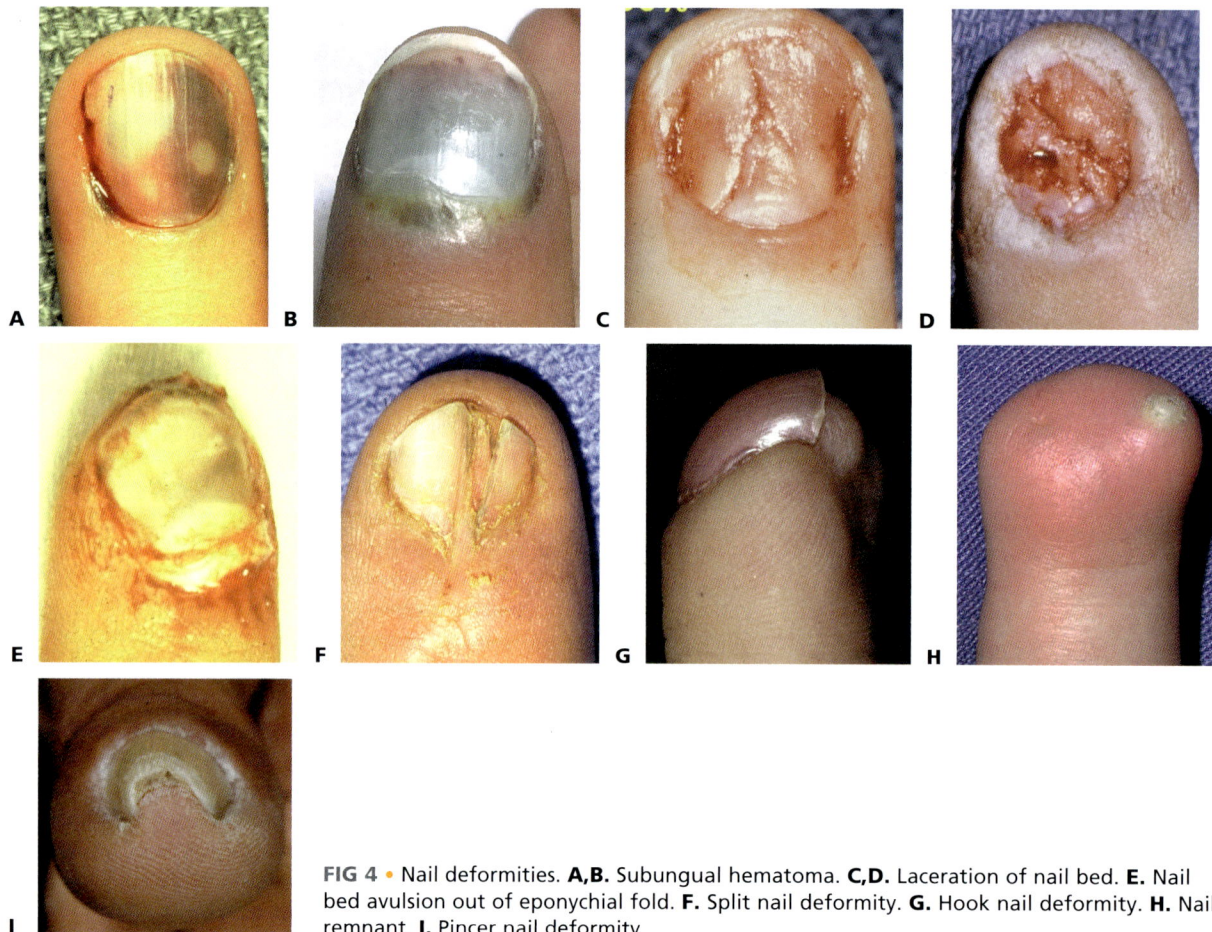

FIG 4 • Nail deformities. **A,B.** Subungual hematoma. **C,D.** Laceration of nail bed. **E.** Nail bed avulsion out of eponychial fold. **F.** Split nail deformity. **G.** Hook nail deformity. **H.** Nail remnant. **I.** Pincer nail deformity.

SURGICAL MANAGEMENT

■ Repair in the acute period increases the chance of a normal-appearing nail.

■ Both surgeon and patient should be aware of the stages of nail growth and characteristic appearance at different points in the healing process as the nail grows out.

■ Reconstruction of the nail matrix in a chronic injury should be approached with realistic expectations.

■ Reconstruction of the nail matrix after tumor excision will depend on the amount of nail bed excised and the amount remaining.[2,6–8]

Preoperative Planning

■ Management of malignant tumors involving the nail bed requires an understanding of the safe level of amputation (usually to the level of the more proximal joint) and the need for sentinel node biopsy.

Positioning

■ To provide a bloodless field, use of a Penrose drain tourniquet at the base of the digit secured with a clamp is recommended (**FIG 5**).

■ Use of a portion of a surgical glove as a tourniquet is discouraged because of the risk of leaving the tourniquet at the base of the digit after repair and placement of the dressing.

The dressing may then hide the tourniquet, and vascular compromise and subsequent necrosis of the finger is possible in the postoperative period.

Approach

■ Sterile preparation and draping is done.

■ A digital block with 1% plain lidocaine (maximum dose 7 mg/kg) is administered.

■ Use of surgical loupes (2.5× magnification is sufficient) is recommended for the most accurate repair.

■ A Kleinert elevator is used to separate the nail plate from the nail matrix.

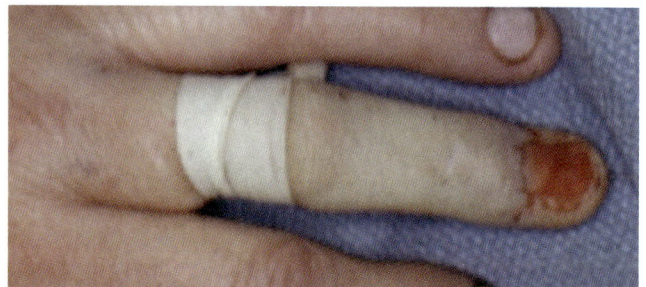

FIG 5 • Use of Penrose drain tourniquet at base of digit.

■ The nail plate is cleaned and soaked in povidone–iodine (Betadine) as nail bed repair is done. If the nail plate is not available, a silicone sheet or nonadherent gauze can be used to maintain the eponychial fold after repair.

■ Minimal débridement of the nail matrix is performed to preserve as much of the nail bed as possible.

■ Incisions perpendicular to the eponychial fold may be necessary for adequate exposure of the germinal matrix (**FIG 6**).

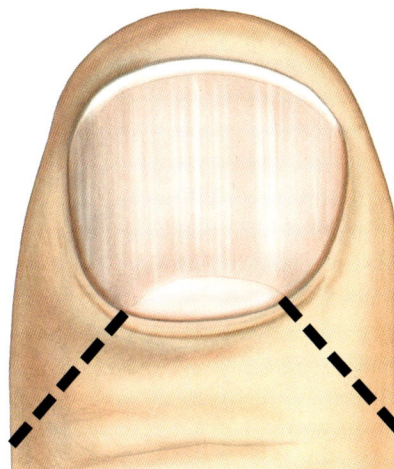

FIG 6 • Incisions made perpendicular to eponychial fold for exposure of the germinal matrix.

DRAINAGE OF SUBUNGUAL HEMATOMA

■ A standard surgical preparation is performed to prevent introducing bacteria into the subungual space.

■ Trephination of the nail can be accomplished using a heated paper clip, needle, or handheld battery-powered cautery (**TECH FIG 1**).

■ Nail removal and repair is recommended if more than 50% of the nail is lifted up by the underlying hematoma or if the nail edges are not intact.

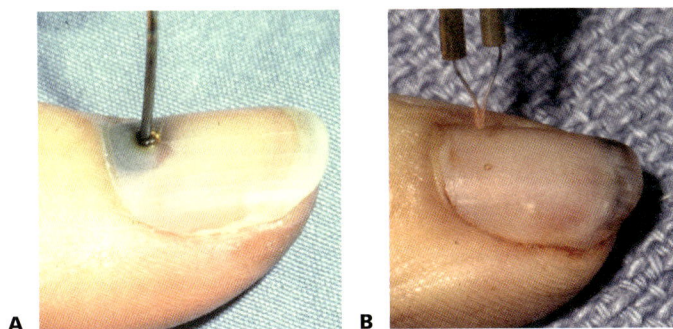

TECH FIG 1 • Trephination of the nail to drain a subungual hematoma using a heated paper clip (**A**) or battery-powered cautery (**B**).

REPAIR OF NAIL BED LACERATION

■ Use a digital block, standard surgical preparation, and a Penrose drain at the base of the digit to serve as tourniquet.

■ Use the Kleinert elevator to separate the nail plate from the nail bed for adequate exposure (**TECH FIG 2A**).

■ Repair the laceration under loupe magnification using simple sutures of 7-0 chromic (**TECH FIG 2B**).
  ■ Avoid aggressive débridement of the nail bed.
■ Clean the nail plate, soak it in Betadine, and rinse it with normal saline; then place it back into the proximal fold

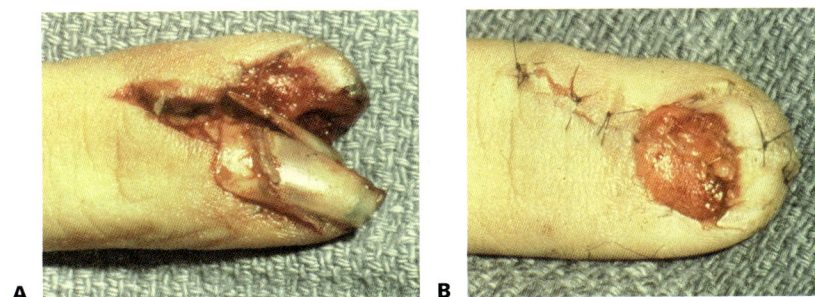

TECH FIG 2 • Repair of nail bed laceration. **A.** Laceration with nail plate present. The nail plate is cleaned and will be used later as a splint to maintain the eponychial fold. **B.** Repair of nail bed and surrounding skin after débridement. *(continued)*

TECHNIQUES

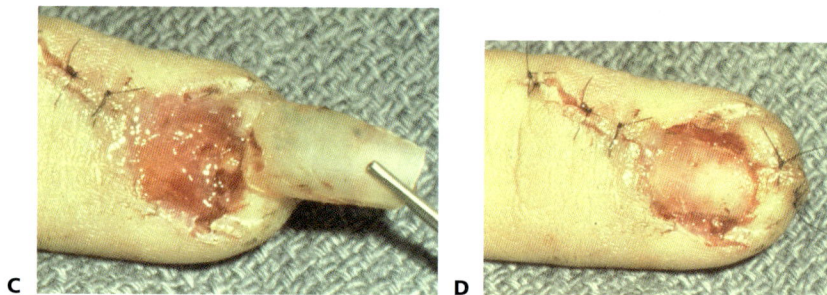

TECH FIG 2 • (continued) **C.** Nail plate being placed back into fold. **D.** Completed nail bed laceration repair.

to maintain this space and to serve as a splint for a distal phalanx fracture (**TECH FIG 2C**).

- A figure 8 suture of 5-0 nylon or a simple stitch from nail to hyponychium can be used to hold the nail in place if desired (**TECH FIG 2D**).
  - A silicone sheet may be used if the nail plate is not available.

- Repair of a nail bed avulsion and resultant proximal germinal matrix disruption may require incisions perpendicular to the curved portion of the eponychial fold for exposure.

TREATMENT OF NAIL BED DEFECTS

- A defect amenable to reconstruction may be present after excision of scar (causing nonadherence or a split nail deformity) from prior injury to the nail bed (**TECH FIG 3A**).
  - Small areas (less than 5 mm) can be left to heal by secondary intention but may result in recurrent scarring and nail deformity.
  - Defects larger than 5 mm can be treated with split-thickness nail bed grafts from the adjacent noninjured nail bed, the nail bed from another digit, or the nail bed from a toe (**TECH FIG 3B**).[2,6,9,13]
- Prepare and drape the recipient and donor sites in standard surgical fashion and perform a digital block.
- Exsanguinate the digit and place a Penrose drain tourniquet at its base.
- Expose both nail beds and measure the defect.

- Harvest split-thickness nail bed graft from the sterile matrix of the donor digit using a no. 15 scalpel (**TECH FIG 3C,D**).
  - To reduce the risk of donor-site nail deformity, the germinal matrix should not be used as a graft for a defect of the sterile matrix.
  - Graft is carefully harvested by placing the blade parallel to the nail bed and taking it thin enough so that the blade can be seen through the graft.
- Suture the split-thickness nail bed graft in place using 7-0 chromic, as is done in a laceration repair (**TECH FIG 3E**).
- Reconstruction of the germinal matrix with subsequent nail growth on the recipient digit requires harvest of a full-thickness germinal matrix graft from a toe (preferably the second toe) (**TECH FIG 3F**).[10]

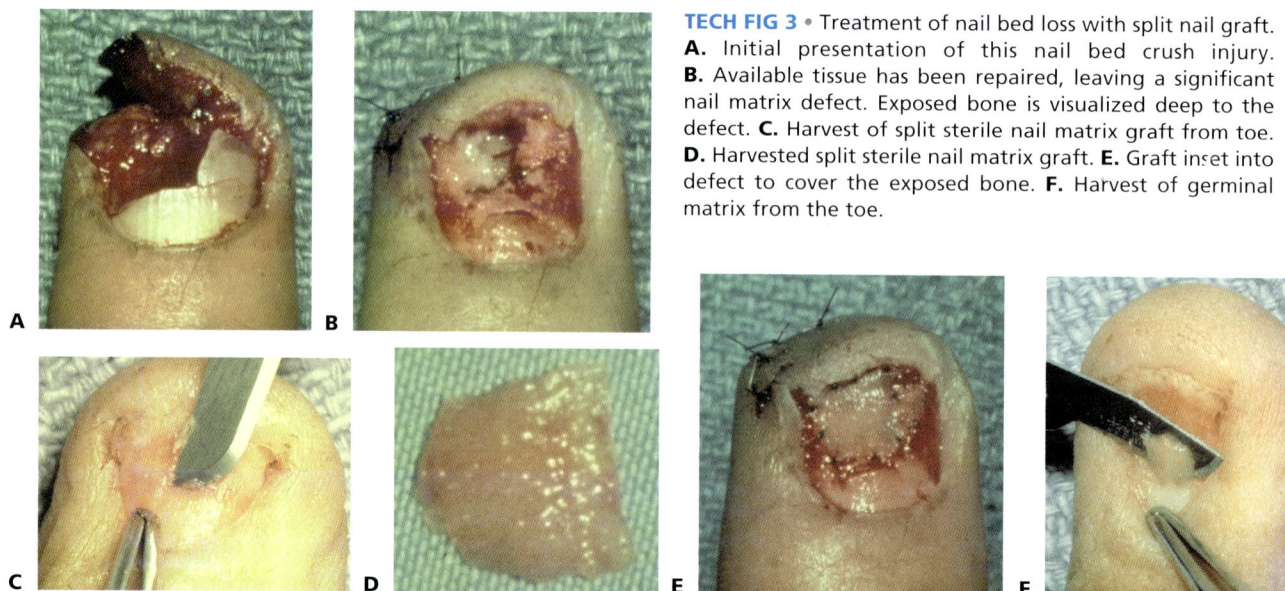

TECH FIG 3 • Treatment of nail bed loss with split nail graft. **A.** Initial presentation of this nail bed crush injury. **B.** Available tissue has been repaired, leaving a significant nail matrix defect. Exposed bone is visualized deep to the defect. **C.** Harvest of split sterile nail matrix graft from toe. **D.** Harvested split sterile nail matrix graft. **E.** Graft inset into defect to cover the exposed bone. **F.** Harvest of germinal matrix from the toe.

NAIL MATRIX ABLATION

- A nail remnant may grow at the site of a previous nail ablation (**TECH FIG 4A**). It may grow in a dorsal direction, catching on clothes and requiring frequent clipping. This remnant may be a source of persistent pain, irritation, or infection.
  - A cyst may form from a nail remnant after a revision amputation and become a source for a subcutaneous abscess (**TECH FIG 4B**).
  - Complete excision of the residual germinal matrix is the goal of treatment.
  - It is important to tell the patient that a nail will no longer grow at the fingertip.
- Re-enter the old incision, preserving skin to allow adequate primary closure.

- Dissect to the proximal portion of the distal phalanx at the expected location of germinal matrix.
  - The distal interphalangeal joint is used as a landmark to guide dissection to the level of the germinal matrix. It may be difficult to distinguish scar from residual germinal matrix after traumatic injury.
- Use a scalpel, curette, or rongeur (or some combination) to ablate the residual nail bed germinal matrix (**TECH FIG 4C,D**).
- To preserve length yet fully ablate the nail, a full-thickness skin graft can be used to cover the distal phalanx.
- The distal phalanx is a unique area where a skin graft may survive even after being placed directly on bone without the presence of periosteum.

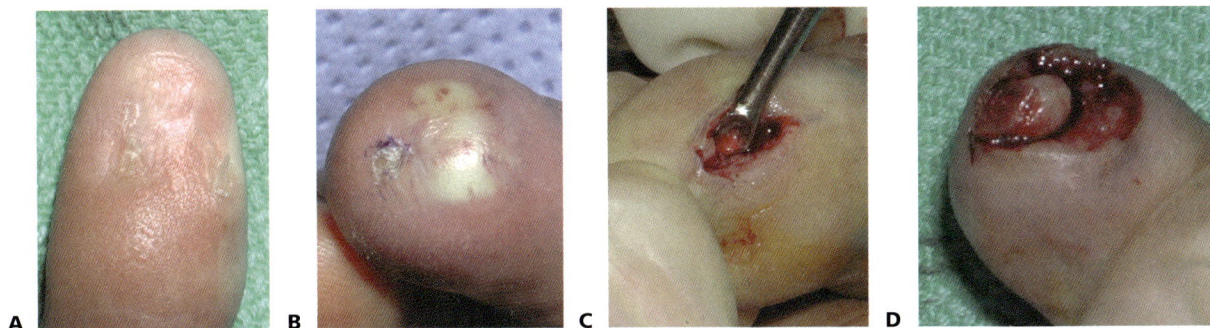

TECH FIG 4 • A. Right small finger after nail bed avulsion from fingertip trauma treated with nail bed ablation. Full-thickness skin graft was placed directly on the distal phalanx to preserve length and avoid revision amputation. Good take of skin graft was seen, but a nail remnant appeared on the proximal ulnar aspect of the fingertip, causing pain. **B.** Subcutaneous abscess from a nail remnant after revision amputation. **C.** Ablation of symptomatic nail remnant shown in **A.** An elliptical incision was made and all residual germinal matrix was removed with a scalpel. A curette was used to scrape the distal phalanx. **D.** A nail cyst is seen after incision and drainage of the abscess shown in **B.** The nail remnant was found within the cyst. Cyst and nail remnant were removed, and symptoms resolved.

TREATMENT OF HOOK NAIL DEFORMITY

- Hook nail deformity can be caused by overaggressive débridement of the distal phalanx, resulting in lack of support, or by too much tension on the closure at the tip, creating an unnatural, curved appearance of the nail.
  - If the germinal matrix is still present, the nail will continue to grow but will hook without adequate bony support.
- Three treatment options exist: doing nothing, reconstruction of the nail to produce a flatter nail with or without bone graft, and revision amputation.

- Additional soft tissue bulk to the volar pad may be required to support the reconstructed nail.
  - A thenar flap is available for reconstruction of the index or middle fingertips.
- Bone graft can be used for support, but there is a high rate of resorption.
- A favorable cosmetic result is often difficult to achieve.

TREATMENT OF PINCER NAIL DEFORMITY

- The goal of treatment is to flatten out the excessive curvature of the nail and correct the "pinched-in" appearance of the nail (**TECH FIG 5A**).

- Elevate the lateral margins of the nail bed from the distal phalanx using a Kleinert-Kutz elevator (**TECH FIG 5B**).
  - Avoid injuring the paronychium as the nail bed is elevated.

- Make stab incisions on the ulnar and radial fingertip.
- Through these stab incisions, create subcutaneous tunnels to the radial and ulnar eponychium using the elevator. Make a second set of stab incisions at that proximal location (**TECH FIG 5C**).
- Cut dermal graft or AlloDerm to the appropriate length and place it through each tunnel.

- Pull the graft through the tunnel, distal to proximal, with the aid of a suture. This positions the graft in the desired location (**TECH FIG 5D**).
- Close the stab incisions with 6-0 nylon and replace the nail (**TECH FIG 5E,F**).

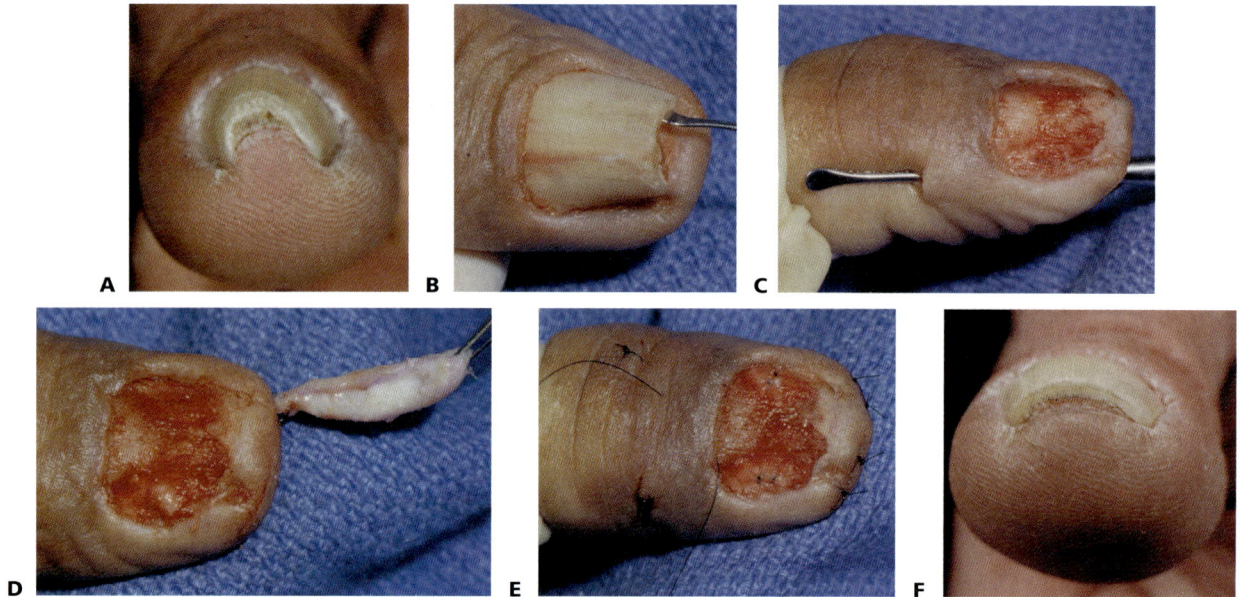

TECH FIG 5 • Treatment of pincer nail deformity. **A.** Pincer nail deformity with characteristic "pinched-in" appearance. **B.** The lateral borders of the nail are lifted from the distal phalanx in an atraumatic manner with a Kleinert-Kutz elevator. **C.** Creation of subcutaneous tunnels through stab incisions on the radial and ulnar sides. **D.** Placement of AlloDerm or dermal graft in subcutaneous tunnel. The graft is pulled into the tunnels with the aid of a suture in a distal-to-proximal direction. **E.** The wounds are closed and the stitch is placed to hold the nail under the proximal nail fold. **F.** Postoperative appearance.

PEARLS AND PITFALLS

Traumatic injury	▪ With prompt treatment of nail bed injury, subacute and chronic problems can be avoided and a more complex reconstruction may be avoided. ▪ Failure to treat a nail bed laceration and concomitant distal phalanx fracture as an open fracture may result in osteomyelitis. ▪ Too much tension at the site of nail bed repair or a lack of support from the distal phalanx may result in a hook nail deformity.
Nail growth	▪ An accurate repair of the nail matrix allows the nail plate to grow out with a smooth, flat appearance. ▪ The germinal matrix produces about 90% of the nail. ▪ The sterile matrix contributes cells that are responsible for nail adherence to the underlying nail bed. ▪ The nail grows at 0.1 mm a day. ▪ New nail growth is completed by 6 to 9 months.
Nail bed reconstruction	▪ The goal of reconstruction is to restore the nail bed after loss due to trauma, scarring, or excision to allow more normal growth. ▪ Reconstruction of the sterile matrix can be accomplished with a split nail bed graft from the adjacent nail bed, an adjacent digit, or a toe. ▪ Reconstruction of the germinal matrix and sterile matrix can be accomplished with a germinal matrix and sterile matrix graft from the second toe.

POSTOPERATIVE CARE

- The postoperative dressing is left on for 5 to 7 days and may need to be soaked in a mixture of hydrogen peroxide and water for removal. The repaired nail is checked for signs of infection, seroma, and hematoma.
- Nonadherent gauze placed to maintain the eponychial fold should be removed. Any suture used to hold the nail or silicone sheet within the fold should also be removed at 5 to 7 days postoperatively.
- Sutures placed in the skin of the hyponychium or paronychium should be removed at 10 to 14 days after repair.
- A fingertip splint that does not include the proximal interphalangeal joint can be used for the first 3 to 5 weeks after injury to protect the nail bed repair and immobilize a distal phalanx fracture if present.
  - Early motion of the proximal interphalangeal joint should be encouraged. The fingertip splint provides protection of the tip and will allow earlier motion of the injured digit.
- Hypersensitivity of the tip may be present for 1 to 3 months after injury, and desensitization exercises may be necessary to promote use of the affected digit.

OUTCOMES

- While repair in the acute period provides the best chance for a normal-appearing nail (**FIG 7**), scarring at the site of injury may produce a nail deformity, and patients should be reminded of this possibility at the time of repair.[10,13,14]
- Results of nail bed repair are adversely affected by avulsion or crush injury of the fingertip, presence of a distal phalanx fracture, three or more sites injured, and the need to use a silicone sheet for replacement of the nail.[1,4,13]
- Late reconstruction of the nail bed is often not as successful as surgeon or patient would desire.[9]
- Management plans must be individualized and realistic expectations must be discussed when treating patients with nail bed injuries.

COMPLICATIONS

- Complications in the acute or subacute setting include soft tissue infection, osteomyelitis of the distal phalanx, nonunion of the distal phalanx fracture, and posttraumatic stiffness and loss of motion at the distal interphalangeal joint.
- Complications or unfavorable outcomes in the chronic setting include scarring in the sterile matrix, leading to a split nail or nonadherent nail; scarring at the eponychial fold, which may interfere with nail plate growth; and persistent nail growth after an unsuccessful attempt at nail ablation.

REFERENCES

1. Brown RE, Acute nail bed injuries. Hand Clin 2002;18:561–575.
2. Brown RE, Zook EG, Russell RC. Reconstruction of fingertips with combination of local flaps and nail bed grafts. J Hand Surg Am 1999;24A:345–351.
3. Brown RE, Zook EG, Williams J. Correction of pincer-nail deformities using dermal grafting. Plast Reconstr Surg 2000;105:1658.
4. Guy RJ. The etiologies and mechanisms of the nail bed injuries. Hand Clin 1990;6:9–21.
5. Kumar VP, Satku K. Treatment and prevention of "hook nail" deformity with anatomic correlation. J Hand Surg Am 1993;18A:617–620.
6. Shepard GH. Nail grafts for reconstruction. Hand Clin 1990;6:79–102.
7. Shepard GH. Perionychial grafts in trauma and reconstruction. Hand Clin 2002;18:595–614.
8. Shepard GH. Treatment of nail bed avulsions with split thickness nail bed grafts. J Hand Surg 1983;8:49–54.
9. Van Beek AL, Kassan MA, Adson MH, et al. Management of acute fingernail injuries. Hand Clin 1990;6:23–35.
10. Zook EG. Reconstruction of a functional and aesthetic nail. Hand Clin 2002;18:577–594.
11. Zook EG. The perionychium: anatomy, physiology and care of injuries. Clin Plast Surg 1981;8:21–31.
12. Zook EG, Brown RE. The perionychium. In Green DP, ed. Operative Hand Surgery, 3rd ed. New York: Churchill Livingstone, 1993.
13. Zook EG, Guy RJ, Russell RC. A study of nail bed injuries: causes, treatment and prognosis. J Hand Surg Am 1984;9A:247–252.
14. Zook EG, Van Beek AL, Russell RC, et al. Anatomy and physiology of the perionychium: a review of the literature and anatomic study. J Hand Surg Am 1980;5:528–536.

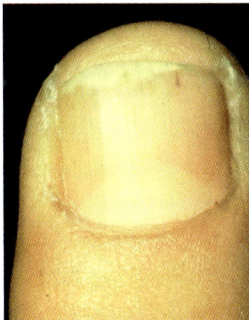

FIG 7 • Appearance of the nail in Techniques Figure 3, 1 year after nail matrix reconstruction with a split graft from the toe.

Chapter 104

Soft Tissue Coverage of Fingertip Amputations

Christian Ford and Jeffrey Yao

DEFINITION

▪ A fingertip injury or amputation involves trauma to the finger distal to the distal interphalangeal (DIP) crease.

▪ The fingertip is the most sensitive area of the hand.

▪ Fingertip injuries are common, accounting for 45% of emergency room hand injuries.

ANATOMY

▪ **FIGURE 1** depicts the anatomy of the fingertip.

▪ Eponychium: the cuticle or the thin membrane over the dorsum of the nail at the nail fold

▪ Perionychium: the skin at the lateral nail margin

▪ Hyponychium: the skin below the distal aspect of the nail plate, consisting of a mass of keratin with a high concentration of lymphocytes and polymorphonuclear cells; serves as a barrier to infection

▪ Nail root: portion of the nail plate proximal to the eponychial fold

▪ Lunula: the curved white opacity representing the distal, visible portion of the germinal matrix

▪ Germinal matrix: produces 90% of the nail plate volume

▪ Sterile matrix: contributes to nail plate adherence

▪ Nail plate: consists of flattened sheets of anuclear keratinized epithelium

▪ Nail bed: the floor of the nail plate, comprising proximal germinal matrix and distal sterile matrix

▪ Distal phalanx: lies deep to the nail bed

▪ Pulp: composed of fibrous septa

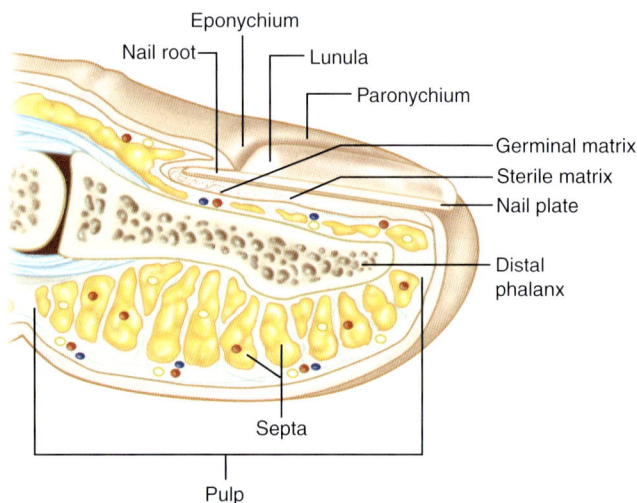

FIG 1 • Cross-section of a fingertip depicting key anatomic structures.

PATHOGENESIS

▪ Various mechanisms of trauma
  ▪ Avulsion
  ▪ Crush
  ▪ Compression
  ▪ Sharp
  ▪ Dull

NATURAL HISTORY

▪ Fingertip injuries with no bone exposed will ultimately heal by secondary intention.

▪ In the setting of wounds less than 1 cm^2, secondary-intention healing aided by daily dressing changes actually allows for increased recovery of sensation.

▪ The use of secondary-intention healing for larger injuries involves a prolonged period of dressing changes with associated risk of infection and unfavorable scarring.

PATIENT HISTORY AND PHYSICAL FINDINGS

▪ Full history and physical examination
  ▪ Mechanism of injury
  ▪ Age
  ▪ Handedness
  ▪ Occupation
  ▪ Level of cooperation and understanding
▪ Injury assessment
  ▪ Digit or digits involved: thumb versus finger
  ▪ Transverse versus dorsal oblique–volar oblique versus radial–ulnar
  ▪ Damage to nail or nail bed
  ▪ Exposure of bone
  ▪ Static and moving two-point discrimination: There is decreased density of innervation with increased two-point discrimination.
  ▪ Terminal flexion and extension: Injury to tendons will require more significant flap coverage.
  ▪ Vascularity: Prolonged capillary refill is suggestive of arterial injury.

IMAGING AND OTHER DIAGNOSTIC STUDIES

▪ Plain radiographs in orthogonal planes (posteroanterior, lateral)

NONOPERATIVE MANAGEMENT

▪ Most fingertip amputations can be treated at the bedside using sterile technique and employing a metacarpal block, finger tourniquet, and loupe magnification.

- There should be a low threshold for operative management.
- If no bone is exposed, options include healing by secondary intention, primary closure, or skin grafting.
- Secondary-intention healing aided by daily dressing changes provides the best recovery of sensation and is appropriate for wounds less than 1 cm^2.
- Primary closure is an option only if there is minimal skin loss.
  - Tight closures should be avoided. This can minimize function by causing joint contracture and distal tip tenderness due to poor soft tissue coverage of the bony prominences.
    - Sewing the volar skin tightly to the distal nail can result in a cosmetically displeasing "hook nail."
- If a nail bed laceration is suspected, the nail plate should be removed with a Freer elevator, allowing repair of the nail bed with either 6-0 or 7-0 simple interrupted absorbable sutures (chromic gut). Loupe magnification is extremely helpful.
- The eponychial fold should be stented open with either trimmed and carefully cleansed nail or other material (e.g., foil from a suture pack) to prevent abnormal growth of the future nail.
- With amputations through the germinal matrix, any remaining unrepairable matrix should be removed to prevent formation of a painful nail remnant.

SURGICAL MANAGEMENT

- The decision to take a patient with a fingertip injury to the operating room depends on the size of the defect, presence of exposed bone, angle of amputation, willingness of the patient to do dressing changes, and surgeon experience.
- The goals are to preserve function and sensation and allow early return to activity.

- In terms of functional outcome, healing by secondary intention provides equal or better results for defects less than 1 cm in diameter.
- Full-thickness grafts are preferable to split-thickness grafts.
  - Split-thickness grafts should be used only on the ulnar side of the index, middle, and ring fingers.
  - Donor site options include the volar wrist skin (should be avoided as it can mimic a suicide attempt laceration), antecubital skin, medial upper arm skin, and hypothenar skin.
    - These donor sites can be closed primarily.
- If salvageable, the original skin from the amputated segment can be defatted and applied as a graft–biologic dressing.
- If bone is exposed, options include bone shortening and primary closure and bone shortening and healing by secondary intention or fingertip flaps.

Preoperative Planning

- Preliminary irrigation and débridement, exploration
- Antibiotics
- Patient comorbidities
  - Is the patient a diabetic? Smoker? Recreational drug user?
  - Is the tetanus status up to date?
- Anesthesia assessment

Positioning

- Supine with standard hand table. An arm, forearm, or digital tourniquet is used. The arm is placed in the center of the hand table for equal access by the surgeon and assistant.

Approach

- Once the decision to perform a flap has been made, the angle of amputation, patient age, and patient gender determines whether an advancement or regional flap is appropriate.

SKIN GRAFTING

- Measure the size of the defect carefully and create a template.
  - This template is used to draw a corresponding defect on the donor site (**TECH FIG 1A**).
- Harvest the full-thickness graft with a no. 15 blade. Take great care to defat the graft down to dermis (**TECH FIG 1B,C**).
- Sew the graft into place and secure it using absorbable suture (**TECH FIG 1D**).
  - At four corners the suture is left long so that later it may be tied over a bolster.
- Cover the skin graft with Xeroform dressing and mineral oil-soaked sterile cotton balls.
- Tie down the four long sutures over the cotton balls to create a bolster, placing gentle pressure on the graft to minimize shear.
- The finger is padded with gauze and protected with a finger splint, leaving the proximal interphalangeal (PIP) joint free for 5 to 7 days.
- After 5 to 7 days, the splint and dressing should be carefully removed, the graft inspected, and daily Xeroform dressing changes instituted until the graft is fully healed.

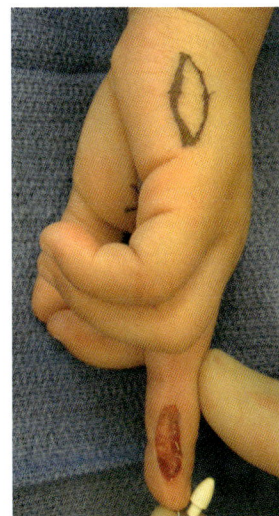

TECH FIG 1 • A. Ulnar defect of the long finger with the proposed hypothenar graft drawn out. *(continued)*

TECHNIQUES

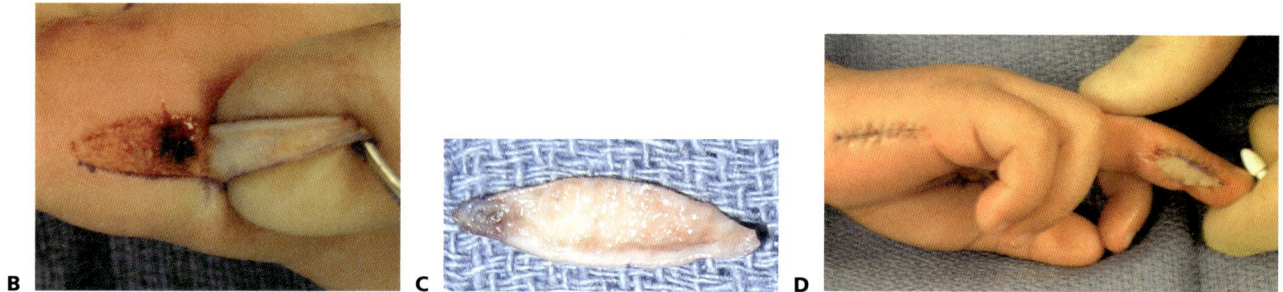

TECH FIG 1 • *(continued)* **B.** The hypothenar full-thickness skin graft is harvested, taking great care to defat the graft; only the dermis and epidermis are harvested. **C.** The hypothenar full-thickness skin graft ex vivo. Note a paucity of fat. **D.** The skin graft is inset using absorbable sutures. Four bolster sutures are then tied over a mineral oil-soaked cotton ball placed on top of the graft (not pictured). A dry dressing is applied. The bolster is left in place for 5 to 7 days.

MOBERG ADVANCEMENT FLAP

- Indication: thumb tip amputation less than 1.5 cm; preserves sensation and length (**TECH FIG 2A,B**)
- Make a longitudinal incision just dorsal to the neurovascular bundles, based at the metacarpophalangeal joint flexion crease (**TECH FIG 2C**).
- Elevate a flap elevated from the flexor sheath (**TECH FIG 2D**).
- If the flap is difficult to advance, consider the following (**TECH FIG 2E**):

- Flexing the interphalangeal joint
- Extending the lateral incisions toward the palm with excision of skin at base to create an island flap; skin grafting of the secondary defect
- Excise a triangle of skin at the bilateral flap base (ie, triangle of Burow).
- Carefully preserve bridging vessels.
- Close with permanent suture under minimal tension (**TECH FIG 2F**).

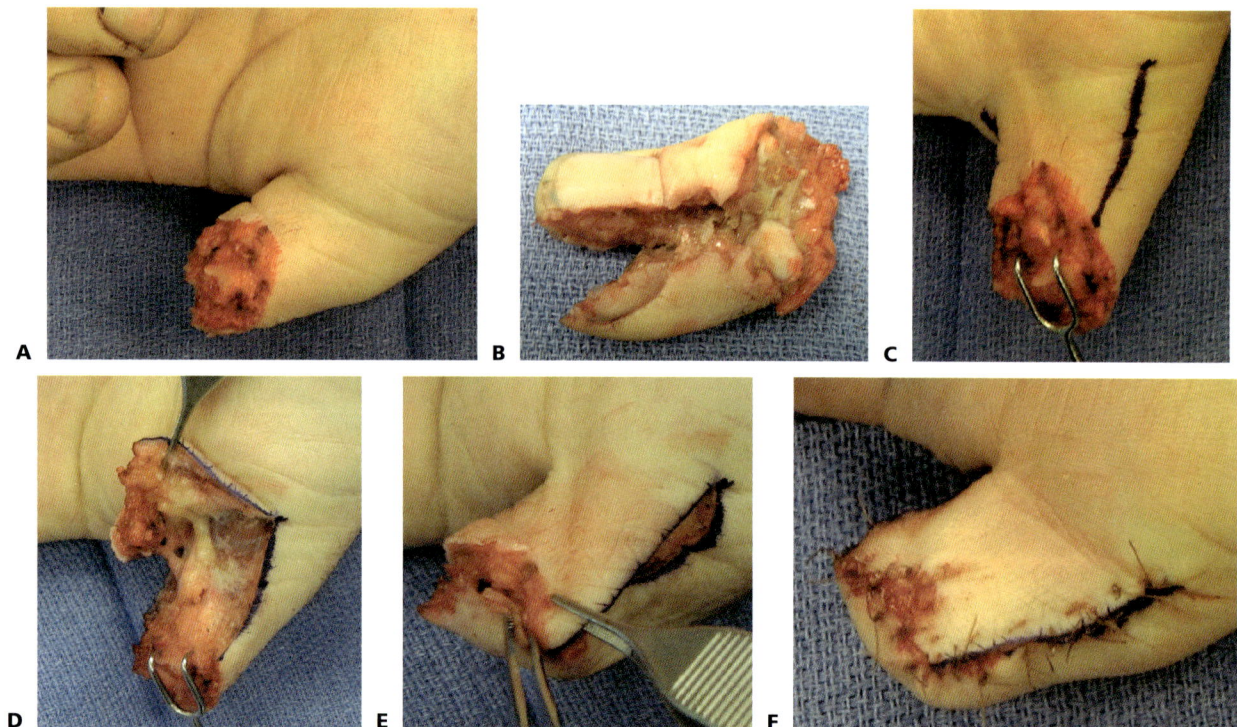

TECH FIG 2 • **A.** Distal thumb defect with exposed proximal phalanx. **B.** Nonreplantable distal phalanx. **C.** Intraoperative photograph indicating planned Moberg flap with longitudinal incisions just dorsal to neurovascular bundles and based at metacarpophalangeal joint flexion crease. **D.** Moberg flap elevation from flexor sheath. **E.** Advancement of Moberg flap was possible without creation of an island flap or use of a triangle of Burow. **F.** Closure of the defect after advancement of Moberg flap. (Courtesy of James Chang, MD.)

LATERAL V–Y ADVANCEMENT FLAPS (KUTLER)

- Indication: transverse fingertip amputation with exposed bone
- The apex of the V is located at the lateral distal digital crease (TECH FIG 3).
- Adequately mobilize the flap: only nerves and vessels need to be kept intact.
- Bilateral triangles are advanced and sutured together distal to the nail bed.

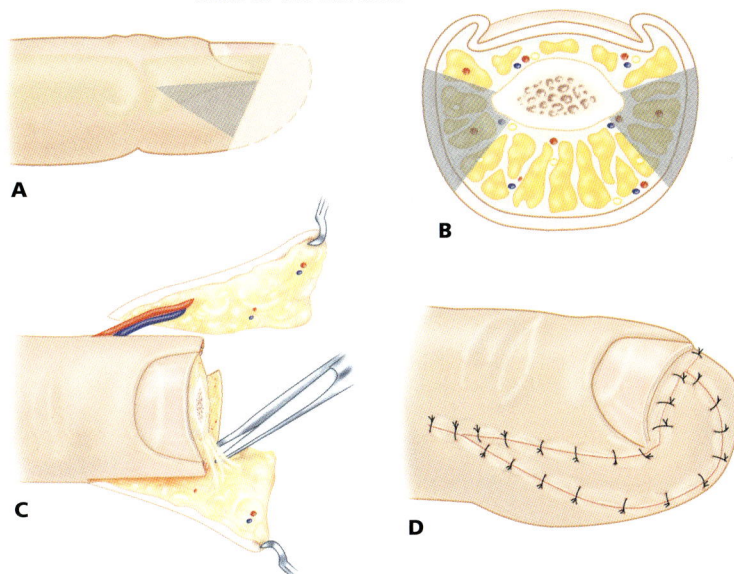

TECH FIG 3 • **A.** Lateral view of the digit with triangular flaps raised along the midlateral line. **B.** Flaps raised on both the radial and ulnar neurovascular bundles. **C.** Adventitia is released and the flaps are advanced distally to cover the defect. **D.** The flaps are sewn together to cover the defect and the donor area is closed primarily in a lateral V–Y fashion.

VOLAR V–Y ADVANCEMENT FLAP (ATASOY-KLEINERT)

- Indication: dorsal oblique fingertip amputation (ie, more dorsal than palmar skin loss) with exposed bone
- The apex of the V is at the volar midpoint of the distal digital crease (TECH FIG 4).
- The base of the triangle should be as wide as the nail bed.
- Adequately mobilize the flap.

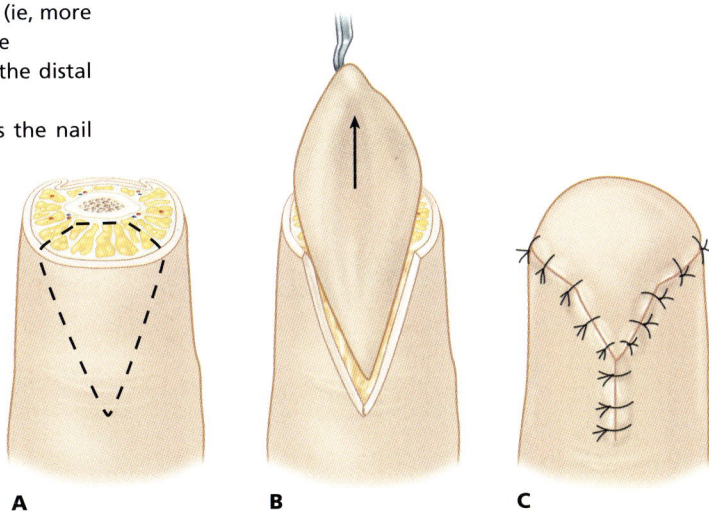

TECH FIG 4 • **A.** Volar-based V is incised. **B.** The volar flap is advanced distally to cover the distal defect. **C.** The flap is secured distally, and the donor area is closed primarily in a volar V–Y fashion.

CROSS-FINGER FLAP

- Indication: volar fingertip defects up to 1.5 × 2.5 cm with an uninjured adjacent digit present (TECH FIG 5A–C)
- The donor area is the dorsal aspect of the middle phalanx skin of the adjacent finger.
  - The middle finger is used for an index finger tip amputation; otherwise the donor skin is derived from the radial digit.
- Make two transverse midaxial to midaxial incisions on the donor area at roughly the DIP and PIP extension

creases. Make one longitudinal midaxial incision on the side of the donor digit away from the injured digit to connect these two transverse incisions.
- Dissection is carried out in the loose areolar plane above the extensor paratenon.
  - The graft is mobilized to the midaxial line adjacent to the injured digit (TECH FIG 5D).
- Apply a full-thickness skin graft to the secondary defect.

- The full-thickness graft should be first sewn to the hinge margin of the primary defect.
- The flap and full-thickness graft are then each rotated 180 degrees, allowing the flap to cover the primary de-

fect and the full-thickness graft to cover the secondary defect (**TECH FIG 5E**).
- The flap is divided 2 to 3 weeks after the index procedure (**TECH FIG 5F,G**).

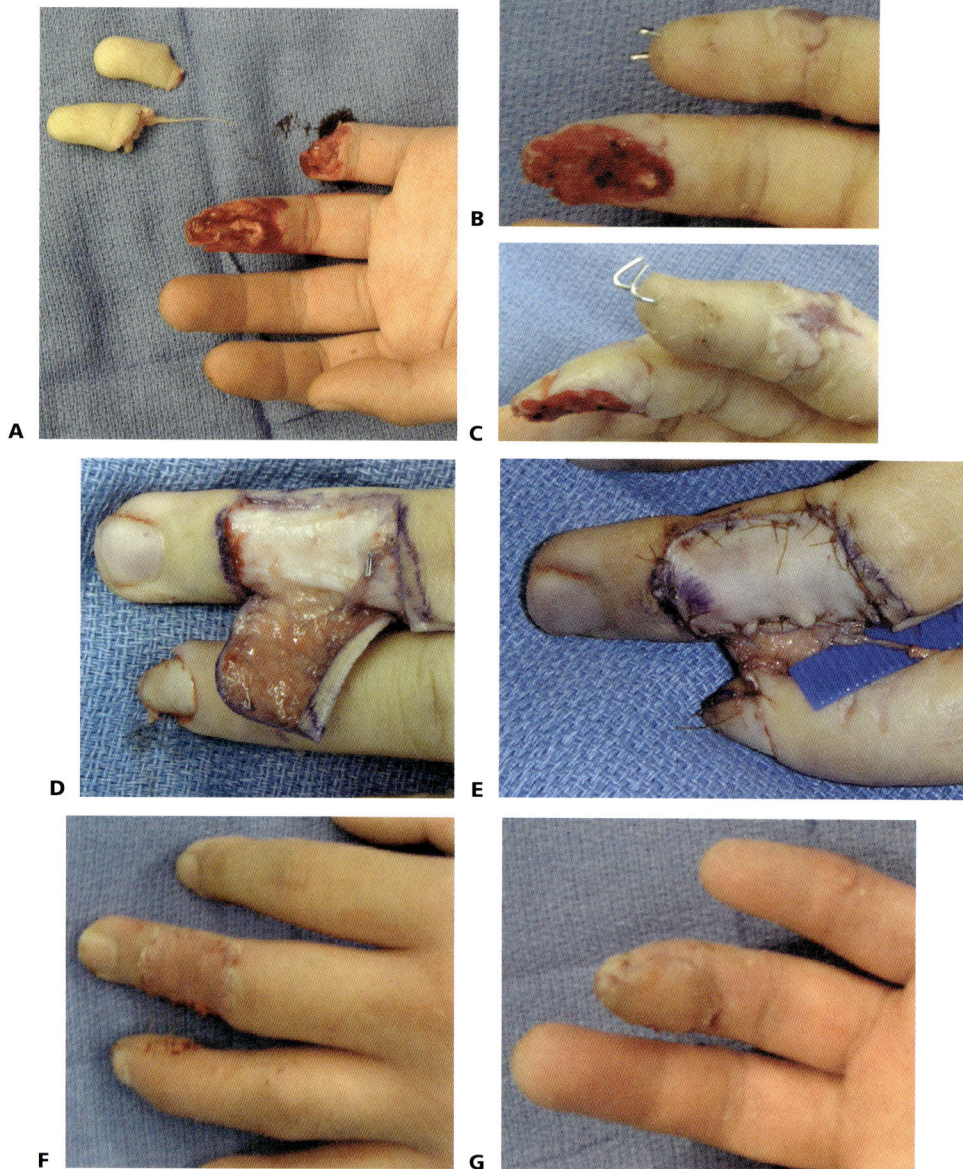

TECH FIG 5 • A. Intraoperative photograph depicting ring finger volar fingertip avulsion with exposed flexor tendon and small finger amputation at middle phalanx level. **B,C.** Two weeks after successful replantation of small finger with continued problem of ring finger wound, which had been treated with daily dressing changes. **D.** Intraoperative photograph after elevation of cross-finger flap from dorsal aspect of middle phalanx skin of adjacent finger. **E.** Intraoperative photograph after cross-finger flap from middle finger for coverage of volar ring finger defect. Donor site was covered with a full-thickness skin graft. Blue background indicates preservation of sensory branch. **F,G.** Intraoperative photographs after cross-finger flap division at 3 weeks.

REVERSE CROSS-FINGER FLAP

- Indication: dorsal fingertip injury
- Raise a de-epithelialized full-thickness flap from the dorsal middle phalanx skin (**TECH FIG 6A,B**).
- Elevate the subcutaneous tissues underlying the raised graft (**TECH FIG 6C,D**).

- Cover the primary defect with the elevated deep tissue and then with a full-thickness graft (**TECH FIG 6E**).
- Cover the secondary defect with the previously described native full-thickness flap (**TECH FIG 6F**).
- The subcutaneous flap is divided in 2 to 3 weeks (**TECH FIG 6G**).

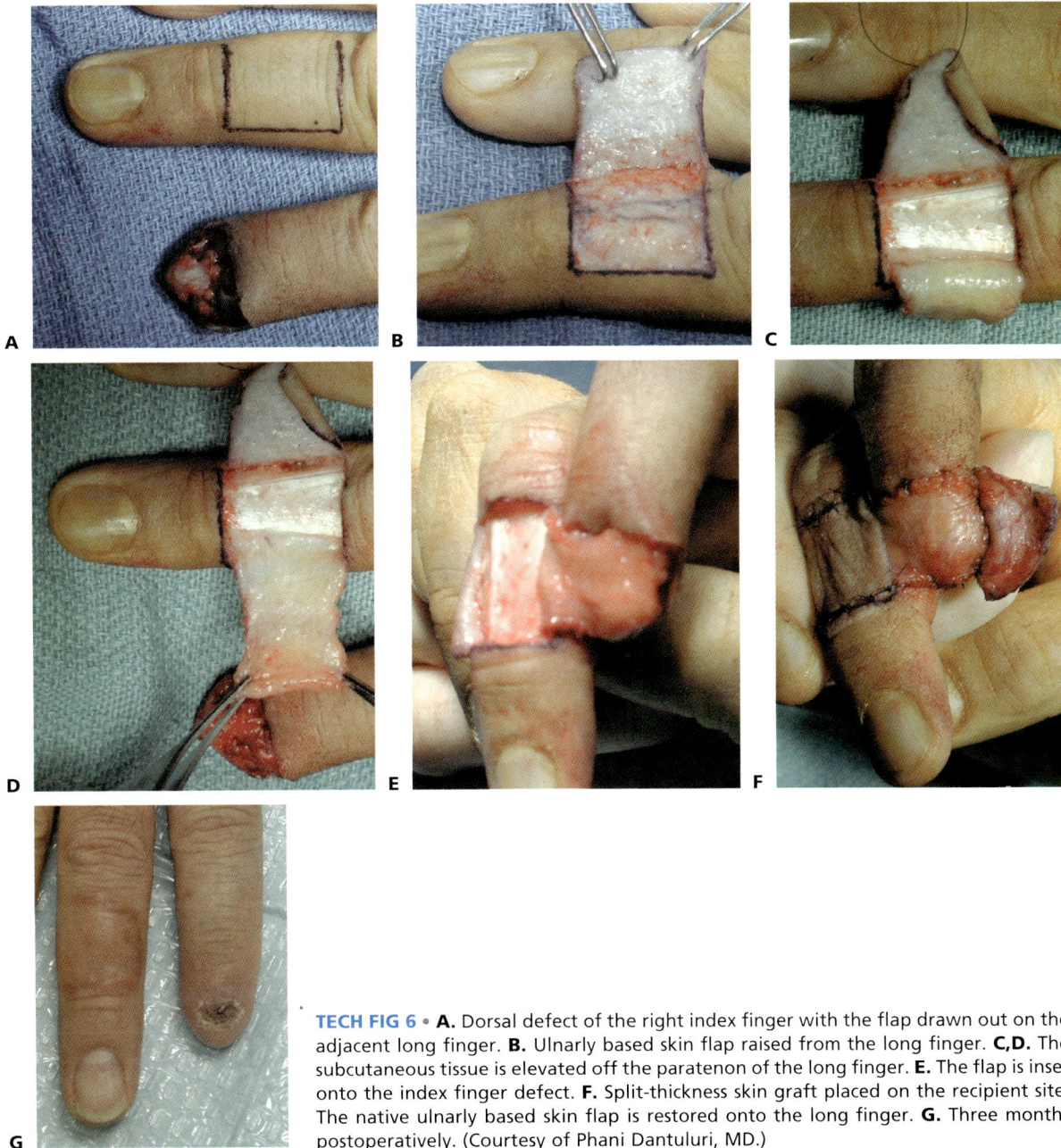

TECH FIG 6 • **A.** Dorsal defect of the right index finger with the flap drawn out on the adjacent long finger. **B.** Ulnarly based skin flap raised from the long finger. **C,D.** The subcutaneous tissue is elevated off the paratenon of the long finger. **E.** The flap is inset onto the index finger defect. **F.** Split-thickness skin graft placed on the recipient site. The native ulnarly based skin flap is restored onto the long finger. **G.** Three months postoperatively. (Courtesy of Phani Dantuluri, MD.)

THENAR FLAP

- Indication: index or middle fingertip injury with exposed bone and more palmar than dorsal skin loss (defects roughly 1 × 1.5 cm in size) in patients younger than 35 years of age who are less likely to develop PIP joint contractures
  - Women are better candidates for this flap than men.
- Press the amputated tip against the thenar eminence with the digit in the position of least PIP flexion (**TECH FIG 7A**).
- The position of the H-flap is indicated by the bloody imprint from the amputation site (**TECH FIG 7B**).

- The designed H-flap should be 50% wider than the defect to fully cover the pulp's semicircular contour.
- Raise the flap at the level of the thenar muscles with as much subcutaneous tissue as possible (**TECH FIG 7C**).
  - Take care to avoid injury to the digital nerves to the thumb.
- The H-flaps may either be "tubed" around the defect or one flap may be advanced to fill the defect of the other flap that is sewn to the amputation site (**TECH FIG 7D**).
- The flaps are divided at 3 weeks.
- One or both H-flaps can be used to close the donor defect primarily.

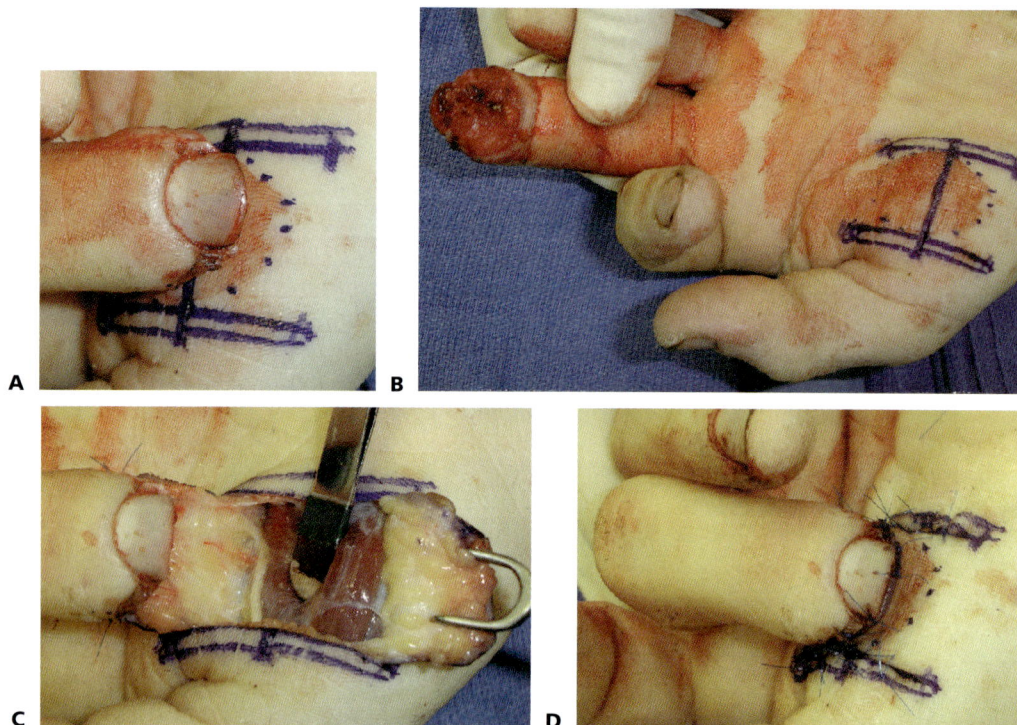

TECH FIG 7 • **A.** The middle digit is passively flexed to the thenar eminence and the thenar H-flap outlined. **B.** The outside pen lines reveal that the flap is widened past the bloody impression to accommodate for the contour of the pulp. Note the volar oblique fingertip amputation of the middle digit. **C.** Dissection of the flap is performed at the level of the thenar musculature. Note the digital nerve present in the field of dissection. **D.** The flap is sewn in position. (Courtesy of Thomas R. Hunt III, MD.)

NEUROVASCULAR ISLAND PEDICLE FLAP (LITTLER)

- Indication: volar distal thumb defect as well as volar radial index or volar ulnar small finger defects sufficient to produce a scarred pulp and an anesthetic tip (**TECH FIG 8A,B**)
- Use Doppler to ensure that flow is present in the ulnar digital artery of the ring finger and the radial digital artery of the middle finger.
- Create a template of the defect on the ulnar aspect of the donor digit.

- Apply the pattern to the distal ulnar aspect of the middle finger with small V-shaped indentations at the DIP joint creases.
  - The flap may be continued posteriorly, beyond the midaxial line.
- Make a Bruner incision to the distal flexor retinaculum.
  - Dissection is commenced in the palm to ensure normal anatomy.
- Isolate and ligate the radial digital artery to the ring finger.

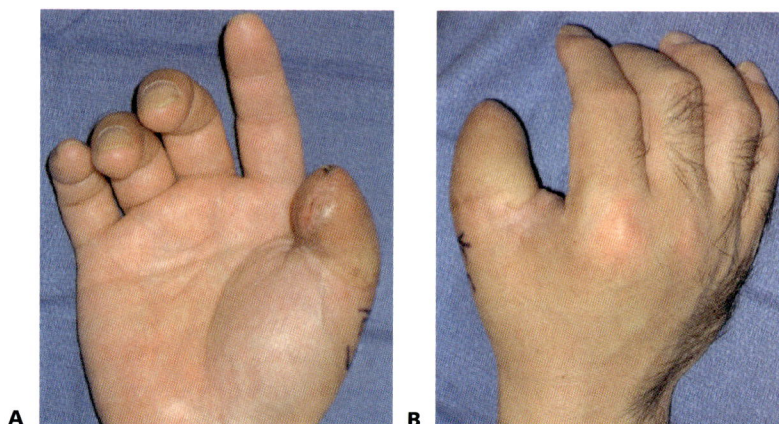

TECH FIG 8 • **A,B.** Insensate volar distal thumb after coverage of amputation site with free flap. (*continued*)

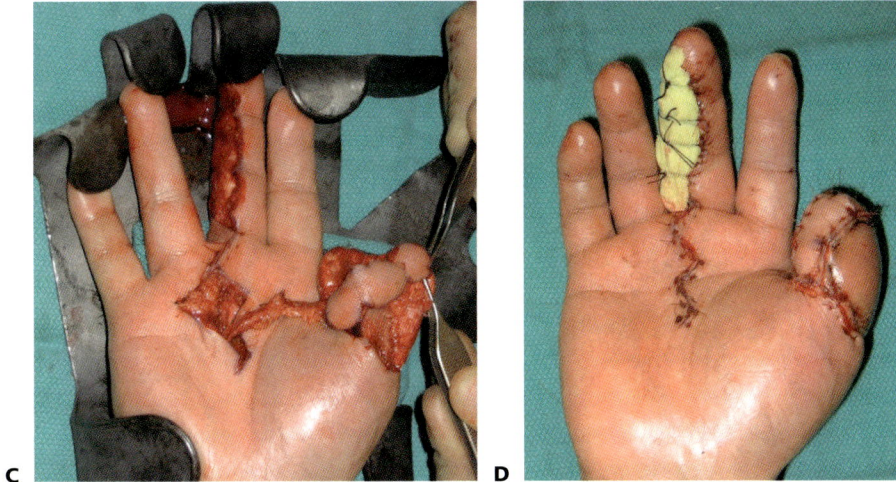

TECH FIG 8 • (continued) **C.** Intraoperative photograph depicting neurovascular island pedicle flap (Littler) harvested from ulnar aspect of middle finger. **D.** Intraoperative photograph after tunneling of neurovascular island pedicle flap (Littler) to volar distal thumb, closure of wounds, full-thickness skin grafting of donor site, and application of a bolster dressing. (Courtesy of James Chang, MD.)

- Mobilize the vessel to the level of the superficial palmar arch to allow maximum pedicle length (**TECH FIG 8C**).
- Pass the entire pedicle beneath the digital nerve if it causes tension.
- Create a subcutaneous tunnel to the thumb using blunt scissor dissection.
- The tourniquet is released and flap viability assessed.
- The flap is then gently placed into a Penrose drain and secured in place with a 4-0 nylon suture to the tip of the flap skin.
  - The Penrose drain is used to avoid kinking and twisting of the pedicle as the flap is passed through the subcutaneous tunnel to the recipient site.
- The flap is sutured in place under minimal tension and the donor site is closed primarily or with a full-thickness graft (**TECH FIG 8D**).

PEARLS AND PITFALLS

- Fingertip injuries less than 1 cm² can generally be treated with dressing changes with equal or better results than flap closure.
- The bridging vessels should be carefully preserved when performing a Moberg flap to prevent skin necrosis.
- V–Y advancement flaps may lead to scarring and hypersensitivity at the fingertip.
- The radial digital nerve should be carefully preserved and protected when performing a thenar flap.
- Cross-finger flaps (nonglabrous skin) may lead to hair growth on the fingertip and deficiency of pulp.
- Thenar flaps (glabrous skin) allow good sensibility in the flap but may be complicated by development of PIP joint contractures, especially in older male patients.
- Poor sensory outcome in neurovascular island flaps can be minimized by use of the most distal portion of donor skin, preservation of as much subcutaneous skin on the pedicle as possible, and avoidance of tension and kinking in the pedicle.

POSTOPERATIVE CARE

- When possible, the patient should meet the hand therapist preoperatively.
- Active and passive range of motion
- Sensory re-education
- Scar massage
- Moberg advancement flap: thumb spica splint for 10 days to 2 weeks followed by range-of-motion exercises
- Lateral V–Y advancement and volar V–Y advancement flaps: finger splintage of only the involved joint for 10 days to 2 weeks, followed by range-of-motion exercises
- Cross-finger flap and reverse-cross finger flap: A nonadherent bolster dressing is applied to the skin graft site and a splint is applied. PIP joints and the DIP joint of the donor finger can be gently ranged 2 weeks after flap inset, taking care to avoid tension on the flap. After flap division at 3 weeks, range-of-motion exercises are directed toward extending the PIP joints. Severe contractures may be treated with static progressive splinting.
- Thenar flap: A splint is applied postoperatively. Gentle range of motion of unaffected digits is started 2 weeks after flap inset, with care taken to avoid tension on the flap. Full range-of-motion exercises are started after flap division at 3 weeks. Severe contractures may be treated with static progressive splinting.
- Neurovascular island flap: The splint is changed 10 days after surgery, when sutures can be removed; gentle active range of motion is started, with full range of motion delayed until 3 weeks after surgery. Sensory re-education is necessary to help differentiate thumb from middle finger sensation.

OUTCOMES

- Moberg flaps consistently provide return of normal two-point discrimination or within 2 mm of the contralateral digit and may result in a decrease in the hyperextensibility of the interphalangeal joint with no functional impairment.[3]
- V–Y advancement flaps result in return of sensation to within 2.75 mm of the contralateral digit but may also result in paresthesia, hypersensitivity, and cold intolerance (50%).[3]
- Patients who undergo a cross-finger flap have a return of protective sensation (8 mm of two-point discrimination), most predictably in younger patients, but the sensation remains less than the normal pulp.[3]
- Hematoma or seroma significantly impairs the return of sensation.[8]
- Thenar flaps provide superior return of sensation compared to cross-finger flaps, but still less than normal.[3]
- Neurovascular island flaps may result in hyperesthesia (23%) and cold intolerance (32%), which can be minimized by proper attention to detail and technique.[3]

COMPLICATIONS

- Moberg flap: interphalangeal joint flexion contracture and skin necrosis[19]
- Lateral V–Y advancement flaps (Kutler): scarring at the fingertip, which may be insensate or painful[3]
- Volar V–Y advancement flap (Atasoy-Kleinert): hook nail or hypersensitivity[3]
- Cross-finger flap: deficiency of fingertip pulp and hair growth on the fingertip[8]
- Thenar flap: PIP joint flexion contracture of recipient finger[8]
- Hematoma[8]
- Seroma[8]
- Infection[8]
- Skin necrosis[8]
- Dysesthesia or altered sensation[8]
- Flexion contractures[8]
- Loss of flap[8]
- Epidermal inclusion cysts[8]
- Nail deformities[8]
- Symptomatic neuromas[8]

REFERENCES

1. Atasoy E. Reversed cross-finger subcutaneous flap. J Hand Surg Am 1982;7A:481–483.
2. Barvato BD, Guelmi K, Nomani SJ, et al. Thenar flap rehabilitation: a review of 20 cases. Ann Plast Surg 1996;37:135.
3. Blair WF, ed. Techniques in Hand Surgery. Baltimore: Williams & Wilkins, 1996:19–25, 39–67.
4. Baumeister S, Menke H, Wittemann M, et al. Functional outcome after Moberg advancement flaps in the thumb. J Hand Surg Am 2002;27A:105–114.
5. Fitoussi F, Ghobani A, Jehanno P, et al. Thenar flap for severe finger-tip injuries in children. J Hand Surg Br 2004;29B:108–112.
6. Foucher G, Delaere O, Citron N, et al. Long-term outcome of neurovascular palmar advancement flaps for distal thumb injuries. Br J Plast Surg 1999;52:64–68.
7. Goitz RJ, Westkaemper JG, Tomaine MM, et al. Soft tissue defects of the digits: coverage considerations. Hand Clin 1997;13:189–205.
8. Green DP, Hotchkiss RN, Pederson WC, eds. Green's Operative Hand Surgery, 4th edition, vol. 2. Philadelphia: Churchill Livingstone, 1999:1798–1816.
9. Henderson HP, Reed DA. Long-term follow-up of neurovascular island flaps. Hand 1980;72:113–122.
10. Koch H, Kielnhofer A, Hubmer M, et al. Donor site morbidity in cross-finger flaps. Br J Plast Surg 2005;58:1131–1135.
11. Koppel DA, Bureck JG. The cross-finger flap: an established reconstruction procedure. Hand Clin 1985;1:677–683.
12. Lav C, Knutson GH, Brown WA. A thenar and palmar flap repair in fingertip amputation. Can J Surg 1969;17:294.
13. Melone CP Jr, Beasley RW, Carstens JH Jr. The thenar flap: an analysis of its use in 150 cases. J Hand Surg Am 1982;7A:791.
14. Nicolai JP, Hentennav G. Sensation in cross-finger flaps. Hand 1981;13:12–16.
15. Nishikawa H, Smith PJ. The recovery of sensation and function after cross-finger flaps for fingertip injury. J Hand Surg Br 1992;17B:102–107.
16. Nomura S, Kurakata M, Sekiya S, et al. The modified thenar flap and its usefulness. J Jpn Soc Hand Surg 2000;16:707.
17. Okazaki M, Hasegawa H, Kano M, et al. A different method of fingertip reconstruction with the thenar flap. Plast Reconstr Surg 2005;115:885–888.
18. Shepard GH. The use of lateral V-Y advancement flaps for fingertip reconstruction. J Hand Surg Am 1983;8A:254–259.
19. Trumble TE. Principles of Hand Surgery and Therapy. Philadelphia: WB Saunders, 2000:192–200.

Chapter 105

Skin Grafts and Skin Graft Substitutes in the Distal Upper Extremity

James N. Long, Jorge de la Torre, and Luis O. Vasconez

DEFINITION

- Upper extremity wounds that are candidates for skin grafting very closely parallel wounds suitable for skin grafting in other areas of the body. Certain wound conditions must be adhered to, and the principles of grafting remain constant, no matter the location of a wound.

Terminology

- *Autograft* refers to skin that is harvested from the same individual to whom it will be applied at a different location.
- *Isograft* refers to skin harvested from an identical twin of the recipient individual. Isograft behaves like autograft.
- *Allograft* refers to skin harvested from an individual of the same species as the recipient individual. Due to histocompatibility mismatch, these grafts eventually separate from the wound, except in immunosuppressed patients, and so provide only temporary coverage.
- *Xenograft* refers to the use of skin grafts from a species different from the recipient individual. Due to histocompatibility mismatch, these eventually separate from the wound, except in the immunosuppressed patient, and so provide only temporary coverage. Xenograft use is associated with an elevated rate of wound bed infection.
- *Split-thickness skin grafts* contain epidermis, along with a varying thickness of dermis that represents less than the full thickness of the dermis.
- *Full-thickness skin grafts* incorporate the full thickness of dermis and epidermis.
- *Donor site* refers to an area from which either a split- or full-thickness skin graft is harvested. Depending on the thickness of the graft, donor site treatment varies, from topical dressings, which typically are used for split-thickness skin graft donor sites, to direct closure, which is the usual method for addressing full-thickness skin donor defects.
- *Skin substitutes* are semisynthetic or purely synthetic constructs designed to act as replacements for lost skin structures. Ideally, they will be incorporated into the host to act as durable long-term replacements for lost tissue. In 1984, Pruitt and Levine[11] described the characteristics of ideal biologic dressings and skin substitutes. Their list of qualities considered to be ideal for skin substitutes still holds true more than 20 years later:
  - Little or no antigenicity
  - Tissue compatibility
  - Lack of toxicity
  - Permeability to water vapor, as would be seen in normal skin
  - Impenetrability to microorganisms
  - Rapid and long-term adherence to the wound bed
  - Capacity for ingrowth of fibrovascular tissue from the wound bed
  - Malleability, which would allow the construct to conform to the wound bed
  - Inherent elasticity that would not impede motion
  - Structural stability against linear and shear forces
  - Smooth surface to hinder bacterial proliferation
  - Good to tensile strength that would allow it resist fragmentation
  - Biodegradability
  - Low cost
  - Ease of storage
  - An indefinite shelf life

Wound Bed

- Before making a decision about using skin grafts or a substitute, it is important to be familiar with the characteristics of a wound bed that make it suitable for grafting.
  - Graft beds should be properly débrided so that they are free of dead tissue and made as clean as possible to help minimize the risk of graft loss from infection.
  - Beds that are being considered for grafting must have an appropriate substrate from which the graft can derive its blood supply. In the context of upper extremity wounds, the bed specifically should contain no areas of denuded tendon or bone, as these denuded areas will not support inosculation (ie, neovascularization of the graft).
  - A further requirement, once débridement is complete, is the reduction of bacteria in the wound, which usually is effected through the use of a pulse lavage system. Enhanced skin graft survival by means of reducing bacterial counts is supported by studies published by Perry[10] in 1989.
- A useful tool in maturing a wound bed for grafting is the vacuum-assisted closure device (VAC). This device provides microdébridement of the wound bed and can help to promote the development of healthy granulation tissue, an ideal substrate for the support of skin graft adherence. Moreover, the vacuum-assisted closure device can be used over the top of a skin graft applied to a wound and, through its negative pressure effect, limit fluid collection beneath the graft, also helping to ensure contact between graft and bed through an even distribution of pressure across the interface.
- Elements key to the development of an adequate graft bed are:
  - Débridement of all nonviable tissue
  - Minimization of bacterial colonization within the wound bed
  - Ensuring that there exists an appropriate substrate for adherence of graft
  - Microdébridement and maturation of the graft bed using appropriate dressings, which may include myriad measures ranging from the use of wet-to-moist saline gauze dressings to use of the VAC device.

ANATOMY

- The decision-making process in choosing split- versus full-thickness graft in the distal upper extremity involves both gross and microanatomic considerations.
- The lack of secondary contraction seen in full-thickness skin grafts supports their use on surfaces that overlie or are juxtaposed to joints. This lack of secondary contraction helps minimize the risk of unwanted joint contracture as the grafts mature.
- Over broad flat surfaces, such as the dorsal or volar aspect of the forearm, split-thickness skin grafts perform well.
- Wounds that involve the glabrous surface of the hand ideally are replaced with skin that possesses the same characteristics as the adjacent skin.
  - Harvest of glabrous skin from the sole of the foot or from the contralateral uninjured hand should be considered for such use.
  - In some cases, the wound may be so large that it is not possible to harvest sufficient donor skin while still permitting primary closure of the donor site. When this is the case, the arch within the sole of the foot may yield a full-thickness glabrous skin graft sufficient to cover the area of the original wound; however, the donor site then may require a skin graft itself. The donor site from the arch of the foot can be grafted with nonglabrous, meshed split-thickness graft with minimal morbidity due to its minimal weight-bearing requirement.

Microanatomy

- As suggested earlier, the surgeon must be concerned with the microanatomic conditions of the wound bed.
  - An appropriately vascular substrate is required to ensure proper graft take. Healthy fat, muscle, paratenon, or periosteum must be present within the base of the wound to ensure success.
  - Additional considerations include proper débridement of nonviable tissues from the wound bed as well as the minimization of bacterial contamination.

Donor Sites

- Glabrous skin
  - The sole of foot within the arch, beginning at the junction of glabrous and nonglabrous skin along the medial aspect of the arch
  - The ulnar aspect of the hand, beginning at the junction of the glabrous and the nonglabrous skin along the ulnar aspect of the palm
- Full-thickness skin
- Redundant areas of full-thickness skin available for harvest that maintain ease of primary closure of the donor defect include the lower abdomen, running from the anterior superior iliac spine in a gentle arc around the lower portion of the abdomen to the contralateral anterior superior iliac spine.
  - Skin harvested from this area may be hair-bearing. Depending on requirements of the recipient site, selection of full-thickness skin graft can range from the relatively hairless portions found laterally to the hirsute areas found centrally.
- Smaller areas of satisfactory full-thickness skin can be harvested from the upper inner arm. This skin, located at the junction of the medial biceps and triceps muscle groups, is thin and usually hairless.

- Split-thickness skin graft
  - Traditionally preferred sites have included the anterior thighs due to the ease of harvest and postoperative care of these areas.
  - Another site that has favorable characteristics in terms of quality of graft donor, as well as healing of donor site, includes the scalp.
  - Harvest of split-thickness skin graft from the scalp requires shaving of the head and the injection of epinephrine-containing wetting solution, eg, Pitkin's solution or Klein's solution, which is directed via puncture into a subgaleal plane to help minimize blood loss from the harvest.
  - The very rich vascular supply to the scalp makes split-thickness skin grafts from this site quite robust.
  - If the harvest is kept within the hair-bearing portions of the scalp, little to no donor defect can be detected once hair has grown back. Moreover, because of the high density of epidermal appendages in the scalp, re-epithelialization of this area is more rapid than at other sites on the body. This rapid re-epithelialization helps to minimize the potential for donor deformity (ie, scarring and dyspigmentation).

Harvest

- Skin harvest is greatly facilitated by proper preparation of the chosen site.
- First, a template of the bed to be grafted should be transferred to the donor site to ensure an adequate harvest. This is easily done with gentian violet and a sterile glove wrapper.
- Limiting blood loss from the harvest site is desirable and is easily achieved by pre-injecting the hypodermis of the planned harvest area with an epinephrine-containing local anesthetic.
- If a long-acting local anesthetic such as Marcaine with epinephrine is used, the patient will have the additional benefit of prolonged donor site anesthesia postoperatively.
  - As split-thickness donor sites are typically quite painful, this is a real benefit and is appreciated by the patient.
- When a large area is planned for harvest, attention must be paid to the appropriate maximum dosage for the local anesthetic selected. Dilute solutions in these cases can provide the benefits sought for these larger surface areas while still respecting the maximum allowed dosages.

PATHOGENESIS

- Wounds in the distal upper extremity requiring coverage arise from a host of different mechanisms. Among the most common are traumatic injuries, which commonly result in avulsive loss of skin. Other causes include burn injury to the upper extremity, as well as defects created by tumor removal.
- Any one of these mechanisms may result in a wide range of injuries, from simple skin loss to injuries of deeper structures, including loss of paratenon or periosteum.

NATURAL HISTORY

- Skin graft healing varies from site to site on the body, and each location will vary from person to person.
- Skin in young adults is thick and healthy; however, in about the fourth decade the skin begins to thin.
- Despite differences in skin thickness at differing anatomic locations, the overall dermal-to-epidermal ratio remains relatively constant: about 95% dermis to 5% epidermis.
- Blood vessels form arborizations into the dermis of the skin through access portals in the dermal papillae.

How Do Grafts Work?

- After application to an appropriately prepared wound bed, both split- and full-thickness grafts undergo a process that has been commonly termed "take."
- The process involved in adherence of skin graft to wound bed is complex and involves an initial hypermetabolic condition within the graft, supported by plasmatic imbibition. Plasmatic imbibition is the process whereby nutrients and oxygen are drawn into the graft by absorption and capillary action. During this time, the graft remains adherent by a thin and friable film of fibrin between wound bed and graft.
- This early phase of graft support is followed by inosculation and capillary ingrowth. Before inosculation, there is a period during which ischemia and, therefore, hypoxia within the graft, with attendant histologic findings, are present.
- Once capillary ingrowth occurs and makes contact with the vascular network inherently present within the graft, blood flow is re-established, and the skin graft takes on a pinkish hue. This process likely involves both the use of the inherent network of vessels within the graft and new vascular proliferation.
- Secondary adherence is mediated through fibrovascular ingrowth. The new vascular connections between graft and bed, as well as the new fibrous connections, solidify graft adherence.

Properties of Skin Grafts

- Skin grafts have been used to provide both temporary and permanent coverage, offering the inherent benefit of protection of the host bed from additional trauma while also providing an important barrier to infection.
- Split-thickness grafts tend to adhere to wound beds more easily and under adverse conditions that would not typically support full-thickness graft viability. This characteristic of split-thickness skin grafts provides a considerable advantage in managing difficult wounds; however, certain disadvantages can arise from their use. Once healed, split-thickness skin grafts undergo secondary contraction which, under uncontrolled conditions, can lead to pathologic contracture.
  - *Contracture* refers to a disability in function that arises from secondary contraction.
  - Additional disadvantages arising from the use of split-thickness skin grafts include dyschromia, poor elasticity, and reduced durability when referenced against their full-thickness counterparts.
- Full-thickness skin grafts include the full thickness of the dermis, along with the epidermis. In the initial phases, full-thickness skin grafts tend not to show the hardy "take" often seen with split-thickness skin grafts. To ensure full-thickness graft success, their use should be limited to well-vascularized recipient beds only.
  - Once established, full-thickness grafts offer distinct advantages; specifically, secondary contraction is far less problematic. Their thickness offers more resistance to external trauma and tends to be less likely to experience the dyspigmentation often associated with split-thickness grafts. They have much better inherent elasticity than split-thickness grafts, and for this reason they are the graft of choice for use over and around joints.

Contraction

- As mentioned earlier, split-thickness skin can undergo a process of secondary contraction that ultimately may lead to pathologic contracture. Immediately on harvest, full- and split-thickness skin grafts behave differently.
  - The phenomenon of *primary contraction* refers to the tendency of a graft to shrink on elevation from the donor site. Substantial primary contraction is more often associated with full-thickness skin grafts than with split-thickness skin grafts.
  - It is clinically important to remember that the immediate and long-term elasticity of full-thickness skin grafts is much greater that in split grafts. It is this elastic property that makes full-thickness skin grafts an ideal choice for use around joints.
  - Once skin grafts have healed in place, the secondary process of contraction occurs more than in split-thickness grafts.
  - Full-thickness grafts tend to remain about the same size and, for practical purposes, show little to no secondary contraction. Full-thickness skin grafts have the capacity to increase their surface area with limb growth over time, whereas split-thickness grafts tend to decrease in size by a process of contraction, or, alternatively, their size remains static.

Reinnervation

- The restoration of sensation in skin grafts is mediated through both peripheral ingrowth and direct growth into the graft from the bed.
- Factors affecting reinnervation of skin grafts include the location and quality of the recipient bed, as well as the choice of full- versus split-thickness skin graft.
- Timing of recovery is variable, with some sensory recovery at between 4 and 6 weeks post grafting. The return of normal sensation occurs between 12 and 24 months.
- The speed with which sensory recovery is realized depends on the accessibility of graft neural sheaths to wound bed nerve fibers. Accessibility of neural sheaths is improved in full-thickness grafts over their split-thickness counterparts, and, therefore, sensory recovery in full-thickness grafts is both more rapid and more complete.

Dyspigmentation

- The harvest of a graft disrupts its normal circulation, causing a loss of melanoblast content. This reduction results in a significant decrease in the number of pigment-producing cells within the graft.
- After graft revascularization, the initial hypoxia is corrected, and the melanocyte population recovers to a normal level.

Skin Substitutes

- The use of skin substitutes for wound coverage in the distal upper extremity typically is considered when the surface area involved is greater than that which could be reasonably covered with a full-thickness skin graft, but for which a split-thickness skin graft is suboptimal, for cosmetic or functional reasons.
- Of the several skin substitutes on the market, the most clinically relevant are AlloDerm (LifeCell Corporation, Branchburg, NJ) and Integra Dermal Regeneration Template (Integra LifeSciences Corporation, Plainsboro, NJ). AlloDerm is a de-antigenized human cadaveric acellular dermal construct. Integra consists of a bovine collagen dermal matrix sheathed with a silicone top membrane creating a bilaminar structure.

Prognosis

- For beds that have been prepared using proper technique with an appropriate choice of graft type, a high degree of successful take with excellent functional results can be obtained.
- It is important to bear in mind the process whereby the graft becomes mated with the bed to achieve good end results. Improperly prepared beds will not provide the vascularity required to ensure graft take.
- Excessive bacterial colonization of the wound also can lead to graft loss.
- Graft immobilization on the wound bed after placement is key to successful adherence.
    - Additional agents that act to prevent successful adherence include the accumulation of subgraft hematoma or seroma as well as shearing forces acting across the graft–wound interface.
    - Immobilization strategies must be directed toward the prevention of unwanted shear while providing pressure adequate to minimize the accumulation of fluid between graft and bed.
- All efforts should be made to minimize the risk of infection before graft application by means of débridement, lavage, and the use of both topical and systemic antibiotics, as directed by culture results.
- The rigid application of these principles produces high success rates.

PATIENT HISTORY AND PHYSICAL FINDINGS

- When considering a patient for skin grafting, along with the normal complete history and physical examination, special attention should be given to inspection of the wound bed.
- The surgeon should ascertain that all tissues within the prospective graft bed are viable and that bacterial growth within the wound is addressed through both wound débridement and treatment with appropriate antimicrobials. Areas of denuded tendon or bone are not acceptable for graft adherence.
- Other factors that negatively impact graft take are factors known to be responsible for impaired wound healing. The most common of these are cigarette smoking, diabetes mellitus, and malnourished states. It is important to elicit this information before proceeding with the operative plan.

IMAGING AND OTHER DIAGNOSTIC STUDIES

- Wounds with a bacterial content greater than 10^5 colony-forming units (CFUs) have significantly reduced successful graft take. A quantitative culture can be performed to assess this variable before skin grafting.
    - A punch biopsy is used to obtain a portion of vascularized wound bed, and this tissue sample is sent to the laboratory, where it is homogenized and then plated. CFUs on the culture plate are counted and then referenced against the initial sample weight. A concentration of more than 10^5 CFUs per gram of sample tissue is a negative predictor of successful graft adherence.
    - The area of tissue biopsied must be delivered from the viable portions of the tissue bed and not from devitalized tissues, which will show very high colony counts and are not representative of the graftable bed.

DIFFERENTIAL DIAGNOSIS

- Superficial or partial thickness skin loss
- Full-thickness skin loss
- Full-thickness skin loss concomitant with deep tissue injury
- Loss of paratenon or periosteum
- Wound over or adjacent to joints
- Wound over broad, flat surface that does not overlie a joint

NONOPERATIVE MANAGEMENT

- Superficial abrasions or burns over broad surfaces with maintained viability of the dermal and hypodermal structures can be treated by local wound care without the use of grafting. Areas of skin with abundant epidermal appendages (sebaceous glands, sweat glands, and hair follicles) have inherent source tissue for re-epithelialization of these superficial wounds.
    - Conservative management ideally includes a moist wound-healing environment that limits bacterial growth and does not inhibit the process of neoepithelialization, such as the petrolatum-based antimicrobial ointments (eg, Neosporin [Johnson & Johnson, New Brunswick, NJ] and Xeroform gauze [Covidien, Mansfield, MA).
    - When conservative wound management is being employed, serial observation is advised to ensure that the process of neoepithelialization is underway and is not hindered by the development of local infection or other unforeseen factors.
    - If the process of re-epithelialization is complete by the end of 2 weeks after the event of the initial injury, scarring at the site of injury will be minimized.
- Smaller wounds that are deeper and penetrate through dermis into the hypodermis may be treated conservatively as well.
    - Local wound care, with serial wet-to-moist changes or by use of the Vacuum-Assisted Closure (VAC) Device (KCI, Inc., San Antonio, TX) can help facilitate healing by secondary intention.
- Larger areas of skin loss allowed to heal by secondary intention can result in a substantial delay in wound healing. In addition, functionally limiting contractures can develop as a byproduct of secondary intention healing.
- Larger, superficial dermal wounds such as second-degree burns can be managed nonoperatively by use of synthetic membrane dressings such as Biobrane (Smith & Nephew, Hull, UK, **FIG 1**) or TransCyte (Smith & Nephew). These dressings are applied immediately after débridement of nonviable skin.
    - This class of dressing is effective for superficial wounds that penetrate only to middermal levels. They depend on retained epidermal appendages (ie, hair follicles, sebaceous and sweat glands) to accomplish the task of re-epithelialization.
- Deeper, full-dermal thickness areas of wounding require deeper débridements that typically are followed by skin grafting or skin graft substitutes.

SURGICAL MANAGEMENT

Preoperative Planning

- Once appropriate débridement has been performed, and the wound is deemed clean and the wound bed is appropriately vascularized, the surgeon can proceed with skin grafting.
- Before beginning in the operating room, the surgeon should have discussed the proposed donor site with the patient and also should have decided whether a full- or split-thickness graft is most appropriate.

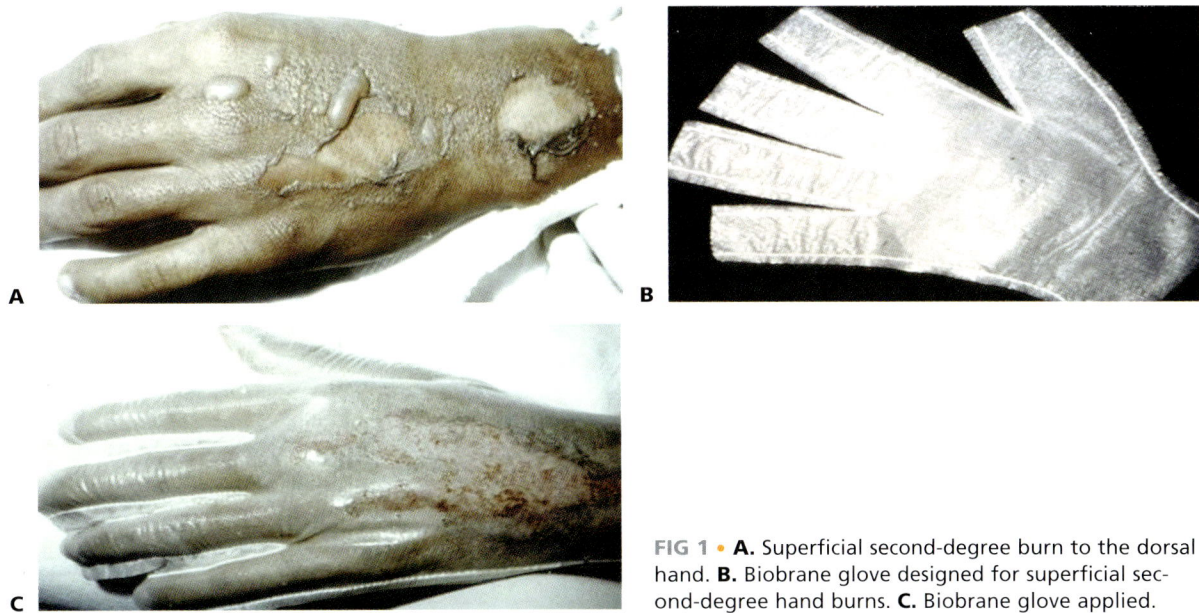

FIG 1 • **A.** Superficial second-degree burn to the dorsal hand. **B.** Biobrane glove designed for superficial second-degree hand burns. **C.** Biobrane glove applied.

Positioning

■ The volar and dorsal aspects of the distal upper extremity can be accessed easily with the patient in a supine position with the arm placed on an arm table.

■ Occasionally, patients who have limited range of motion in their joints at the shoulder or elbow must be placed prone to facilitate access to certain areas.

■ Decisions about positioning should be made well in advance of initiation of the procedure.

Approach

■ Wounds that are being considered for placement of skin graft or skin graft substitutes are, by definition, vascularized wound beds with direct superficial access.

■ Logical preoperative planning determines the approach.

SPLIT-THICKNESS SKIN GRAFT

Determining Wound Size and Making a Template

■ To begin the procedure, a sterile ruler is used to measure the size of the wound to be addressed with skin grafting.

■ A simple and effective way to determine the shape of a wound bed is to place a sheet of sterile glove paper within the wound. The mark left on the paper by the wound is a close match of the wound bed. (This technique is not as accurate for wounds with markedly irregular contours.)

■ Once the wound has transferred moisture onto the glove paper, the paper can be trimmed with scissors to provide a template of the wound bed. This template then can be transferred to the area of planned skin harvest.

■ The shape of the template is marked with a dashed line, using a gentian violet marker, on the skin that is to be harvested.

Harvesting the Graft

■ Most modern dermatomes are designed to harvest skin in a quadrangular pattern.

■ To ensure that the harvested graft is capable of proper wound coverage, it should be larger than the gentian violet marks on all sides, both to offset shrinkage from primary graft contraction and to compensate for the difficulties in harvesting amorphous shapes with an instrument designed to cut quadrangular patterns.

■ The degree of primary contraction is a function of the depth of dermis harvested. For very thin split-thickness grafts, primary contraction is virtually absent.

■ Grafts usually are harvested with either nitrogen- or electric-powered dermatomes (**TECH FIG 1**), which can be adjusted for depth of harvest as well as the desired harvest width.

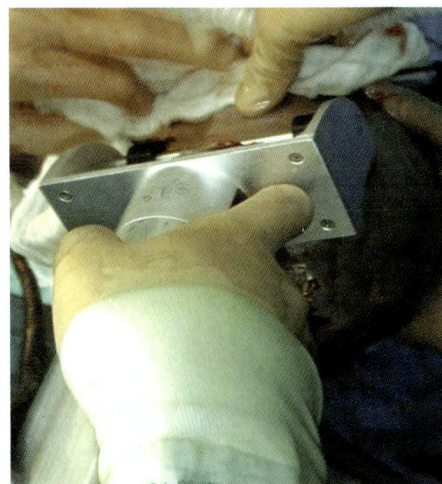

TECH FIG 1 • Technique of split-thickness skin graft harvest.

- The usual appropriate depth for harvesting skin to be applied to a wound bed in the distal upper extremity is between 0.012 and 0.014 inch.

Unmeshed versus Meshed Grafts

- Once a graft of appropriate size has been harvested, it must be decided whether to use the graft as a sheet graft (unmeshed) versus an expanded graft (meshed) (TECH FIG 2).
- Sheet grafts, because of their contiguous nature, have a greater tendency to develop subgraft seromas and hematomas.
  - This complication can lead to graft loss; for this reason, it is worth considering the use of meshed grafts.
- Under ideal circumstances, a meshed graft can be used in its nonexpanded state.
  - To do this, simply mesh the graft using the appropriate device, and after placing it in the wound bed, close the small fenestrations made by meshing.
  - This closure will give a final healed appearance very close to that of a sheet graft but without the complication of accumulated fluid beneath the graft, which can lead to graft loss.

Placing the Graft

- Once the graft has been placed in the wound with the dermis side down, the graft can be secured in place using either staples or sutures around the periphery.
- As this is done, excess peripheral graft may develop. This is the byproduct of the quadrangular shape of the harvest versus the amorphous shape of the typical wound.
  - Excesses are easily trimmed by holding the graft in place and using thin, sharp scissors to skirt just outside the periphery of the wound.
- Once excess has been removed and the entire peripheral edge of the skin graft has been secured, any surface irregularity leading to noncontact with the undersurface of the graft can be addressed by placement of quilting sutures.
  - These sutures are placed through the surface of the graft into the depth of the contour irregularity and then back out of the graft.
  - When tied, the sutures draw the deep surface of the graft into contact with the wound bed.
  - A suitable suture for this purpose is 4-0 chromic.
- A nonadherent interface (eg, Xeroform [Kendall, Mansfield, MA] or Aquaphor [Beiersdorf AG, Hamburg, Germany] gauze) should be placed over the graft to prevent the graft from adhering to the bolster that will further secure the graft in position.
  - If Aquaphor gauze is used and the patient is not allergic to bacitracin ointment, a triple antibiotic ointment

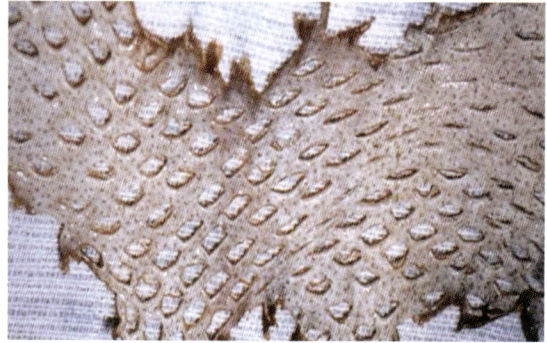

TECH FIG 2 • Meshed graft. Appearance of meshed split-thickness graft, dermis side up.

doping of the Aquaphor further inures the graft from injury when the overlying bolster is removed.
- In the upper extremity, lightly applied circumferential dressings work well as bolsters.
- Tie-over bolsters typically are not required, but they can be used if preferred. Reston foam (3M, St. Paul, MN) or saline- and mineral oil–doped cotton batting secured in place with light gauze and an elastic overwrap from the tips of the fingers to a point several centimeters beyond the most proximal aspect of the grafted site is sufficient.
- A sugar-tong splint should then be applied to help prevent the shear stress created between the wound bed and the undersurface of the graft, which occurs as a byproduct of pronation and supination, as well as wrist and finger flexion and extension.
- The patient's arm should be elevated to help minimize accumulation of edema at the graft site.

Postoperative Care

- On postoperative day 5, dressings should be removed and the graft examined. Typically, at this time, the graft will have acquired a pink coloration, and although most of the fenestrated areas may not have fully epithelialized, it should be clear that graft take is underway. If this is not the case, the wound should be inspected to determine why the graft is not taking.
- For fenestrated grafts, it is unusual for either hematoma or seroma to be a cause of graft failure. The more common cause for graft failure with fenestrated split-thickness grafts is wound infection.
  - Quantitative cultures obtained preoperatively will help guide the surgeon in appropriate antibiotic treatment for these patients pre-, intra-, and postoperatively.
- Once early graft healing has occurred, wound infection is unlikely, and the application of a hypoallergenic emollient cream helps keep the graft supple and moisturized while at the same time promoting slough of scaling stratum corneum and eschar.

FULL-THICKNESS SKIN GRAFT

Donor Site

- If the area of the wound is over or in proximity to a joint, it may be decided to use a full-thickness graft. Again, a

template can be made using sterile glove paper, with this glove-paper template then transferred to the area desired for harvest of the full-thickness graft.

- There are limitations on the surface area that can be obtained from full-thickness skin graft donor sites, and, therefore, consideration should be given to the recipient bed surface area when deciding on the type of graft.
- Typical donor sites include the lower abdomen and the inner aspect of the upper arm.

Graft Harvest

- Once the template has been transferred to the skin, harvest can be facilitated by injection of 1% lidocaine with epinephrine into the subcutaneous fat directly beneath the area planned for harvest.
  - Allow approximately 7 minutes for the epinephrine to take effect and help minimize bleeding during harvest.
- A no.15 scalpel blade can be used to accurately incise the periphery of the planned graft harvest, followed by elevation of the full-thickness graft in the plane directly beneath the undersurface of the full thickness of dermis, directly above the subdermal fat and below dermal papillae.
  - In most cases, some fat is adherent to the underlying dermis after elevation.
    - The full-thickness skin graft can be stretched over the finger and curved scissors used to directly excise fat from the undersurface of the full-thickness graft.
    - The removal of unwanted fat maximizes the surface area of deep dermis in direct contact with the wound bed, which helps to facilitate the inosculation and revascularization process.
- Full-thickness grafts have a greater degree of primary contraction than do split-thickness grafts; therefore, upon immediate harvest the graft will appear much smaller than it did when in situ. Once sewn in place around the periphery, however, the graft will return to the actual size of the template with little effort.
  - This ability to return to the template size, and even extend beyond it, means that when harvesting full-thickness graft, the harvest should not be extended much beyond the periphery of the template, as is done with split-thickness grafts.

Graft Preparation

- To minimize the accumulation of hematoma or seroma beneath the graft, a well-prepared bed is required.

- One measure to help prevent subgraft fluid accumulation is "pie-crusting," a technique in which the surgeon simply makes random perforations through the full thickness of the graft using a no.11 scalpel blade.
  - These perforations provide avenues of egress for accumulated subgraft fluid in much the same way that meshing does for split-thickness grafts.

Graft Placement

- To improve the precision of dermal edge contact of the graft in the wound, suture fixation is preferred over staple fixation. Again, an ideal suture for this purpose is 4-0 chromic.
- The process for dressing this graft is the same as that for a split-thickness graft: the use of either Aquaphor or Xeroform gauze dressings with an overlying bolster of Reston foam or cotton batting secured with gauze and an elastic wrap, followed by appropriate immobilization of the area.
- The VAC is not recommended for unmeshed grafts and so should not be used for full-thickness skin grafts even if pie-crusted (**TECH FIG 3**).

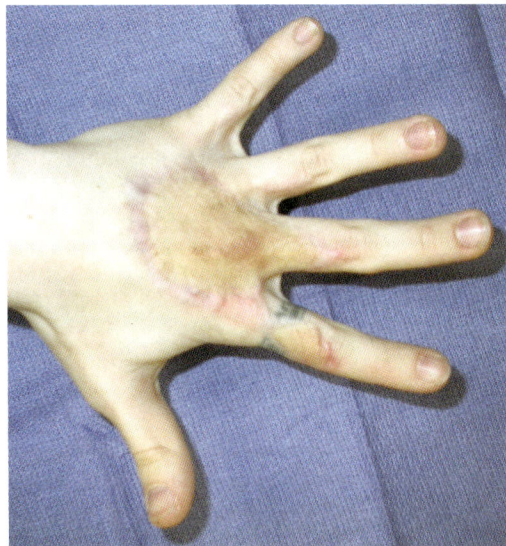

TECH FIG 3 • Full-thickness graft to dorsal hand. Appearance of mature full-thickness skin graft applied over joint.

SKIN SUBSTITUTES

- The goal with skin substitutes is to place within the wound bed a biosynthetic dermal construct that will offer the advantages of a full-thickness skin graft, but without the physical cost of obtaining such a large full-thickness skin graft harvest from the patient.
- The dermal constructs are placed within the wound in much the same manner as a full-thickness graft. They become fibrovascularly integrated into the wound bed as a synthetic neodermis. After maturity, application of a thin split-thickness skin graft (0.008 to 0.010 inch) converts these nonepithelialized constructs to closed wounds.

- The technical application of AlloDerm and Integra is the same as placement of a full-thickness skin graft.
  - AlloDerm and Integra usually are secured in place around the periphery with either 4-0 chromic or staples (**TECH FIG 4A**).
- Once a split-thickness skin graft is applied to a site treated with either AlloDerm or Integra, these split-thickness grafts should be treated in just the same manner as split-thickness skin grafts on any wound bed, observing the postoperative technical requirements of such grafts (**TECH FIG 4B**).

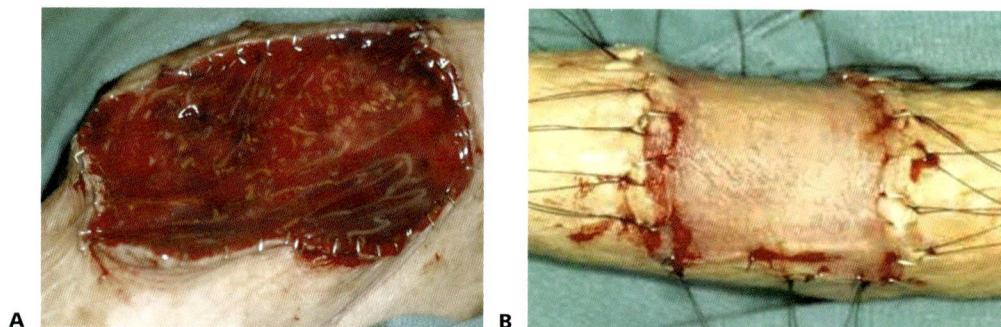

TECH FIG 4 • **A.** Appearance of mature Integra applied over open forearm wound. **B.** Very thin split-thickness graft applied and now adherent to mature Integra bed.

AlloDerm

- When using AlloDerm, bolstering dressings are applied over a petrolatum-doped nonadherent gauze interface, and the dermal construct is observed periodically at twice-weekly intervals.
- AlloDerm will demonstrate granulation tissue issuing through the pores of the dermal construct, typically at about 2 to 3 weeks after graft placement.
- Once this has occurred, the AlloDerm is ready for split-thickness skin grafting.

Integra

- On initial placement, Integra appears white, with a transition over the succeeding 2 to 3 weeks to a rosy color, the byproduct of neovascularization. At this point the Silastic layer of the Integra can be separated and the vascularized dermal construct grafted with a thin split-thickness skin graft.
- If desired, Integra can be meshed 1:1 with a specialized mesher designed not to crush the construct (eg, Brennen Medical Skin Graft Mesher, Brennen Medical, LLC, St. Paul, MN).
  - Meshing may help the construct conform to the wound bed and also help limit subgraft fluid accumulations.
- The meshed construct should not be expanded on the wound bed, since its purpose is to replace absent dermis. Its expansion thins the Integra construct and diminishes its benefits.
- Fenestrations in Integra are made only for the purpose of creating an avenue for fluid escape. Integra has a Silastic membrane that acts as an external barrier.
- Integra's Silastic membrane obviates the need for petrolatum-doped dressing and is transparent, which allows direct observation of the process of maturation of the dermal construct beneath.

Biobrane

- Biobrane is appropriate for use only in wounds that have some retained dermis and, because of this distinction, acts as an advanced wound dressing rather than a skin substitute. For wounds with full-thickness loss of skin, Biobrane is not an appropriate choice, because epidermal appendages, which are required to act as the source of cells needed for re-epithelialization, must be present.
- Biobrane acts as a protective barrier and a scaffold for the healing process. It notably decreases pain; allows for the retention of moisture within the wound, improving the healing environment; acts as a barrier to infection; and promotes more rapid healing.
- Its clinical use is most evident in treatment of burn injuries, but it also may be used to treat split-thickness skin graft donor sites to minimize morbidity in these areas.
- The application of Biobrane includes tangential excision of nonviable tissues or rough débridement with an antibiotic solution–doped lap sponge, followed by drying and then application of the Biobrane to the wound surface.
  - It is secured in place around the periphery using staples.
  - This is followed by application of a nonadherent gauze dressing with placement of an absorbent dressing, such as a sterile absorbent gauze pad held in place with gauze and an elastic wrap.
- The site is immobilized for 24 hours, after which all dressings are removed, leaving Biobrane in place.
  - At this stage, the Biobrane should be adherent to the wound bed.
- Biobrane is observed over time and allowed to separate from the wound without disturbance.
- Small abscesses below the Silastic layer, if they develop, can be treated by simple incision and drainage. As edges release they are trimmed.

PEARLS AND PITFALLS

Primary contraction	■ Full-thickness grafts tend to shrink immediately on harvest. This primary contraction is easily overcome by application of peripheral sutures to draw the elastic full-thickness graft back out to its original surface area when applied to the wound.
Secondary contraction	■ Split-thickness grafts tend to shrink over time as a function of harvesting less than the full thickness of dermis. This problem is exacerbated by meshed graft expansion. Secondary contraction can lead to functional contracture, especially when grafts are used over or near joints.

Graft meshing	▪ Meshing of split-thickness graft to provide fenestrations that will allow subgraft fluid accumulations to be expelled. This will help to keep the dermal surface of the graft in apposition to the wound bed, thereby enhancing the opportunity for inosculation and ultimately revascularization to occur.
Wound bed preparation	▪ Preparation requires débridement of nonviable tissue and bacteria. Quantitative culture can assist the surgeon in defining the species and number of bacterial colonies within the wound. More than 10^5 colony-forming units per gram of harvested tissue increases the likelihood of graft loss secondary to infection.
Enhancing graft adherence	▪ Proper immobilization to prevent shear stress across the wound-graft interface cannot be overemphasized.
Vacuum-assisted closure device	▪ The VAC device may be used as a skin graft bolster over fenestrated grafts. Its negative pressure serves to effectively immobilize graft on the wound bed, as well as draw interstitial fluid from the wound, preventing its accumulation beneath the graft.

POSTOPERATIVE CARE

▪ On admission to the postanesthesia care unit, the patient's operated extremity should be placed in elevation and kept relatively immobile until time to take down dressings and evaluate the graft.

▪ Examination of the graft can be done as early as 3 days postoperatively; however, the graft at this point is very sensitive to manipulation.

▪ If takedown of the dressings is done on postoperative day 5 or 6, allowing time for additional graft maturation, the risk of disturbing the graft is reduced.

▪ Once maturation of the graft has been noted to be underway, application of a nonadherent dressing such as Xeroform or Aquaphor gauze should be continued, with light overpressure provided by an absorbable gauze dressing held in place by gauze and a light elastic wrap and splinting.

▪ After the graft has more fully matured, with all interstices fully epithelialized, at between 2 and 3 weeks postoperatively, the graft will require no further application of nonadherent dressings. Instead, light application of a hypoallergenic emollient cream such as Eucerin (Beiersdorf North America Inc., Wilton, CT) is preferred. This helps to keep the graft hydrated while maturation continues without the restrictions of constant compression and splinting.

▪ An occupational therapist should be consulted to help develop a program of appropriate splinting in tandem with an exercise regimen that will provide the foundation for maximizing the patient's final functional range of motion.

OUTCOMES

▪ Because of the disparate nature of wounds and the significant variation that exists in patient physiology, it is impossible to provide standardized outcome measures for skin grafting.

▪ The goal of the general principles defined in this chapter is to assist the surgeon in optimizing outcomes for all cases. Collectively, they will work to help limit complications while maximizing functional outcomes.

COMPLICATIONS

▪ Wound or graft infection with loss
▪ Subgraft seroma or hematoma
▪ Hypertrophic or keloid scarring
▪ Contractures
▪ Loss of functional range of motion

▪ Tendon adherence to graft
▪ Poor durability
▪ Hyperpigmentation

REFERENCES

1. Birch J, Branemark PI. The vascularization of a free full-thickness skin graft. I. A vital microscopic study. Scand J Plast Reconstr Surg 1969;3:1.
2. Brown D, Garner W, Young VL. Skin grafting: Dermal components in inhibition of wound contraction. South Med J 1990;83:789.
3. Burleson R, Eiseman B. Nature of the bond between partial-thickness skin and wound granulations. Am Surg 1973;177:181.
4. Caldwell RK, Giles WC, Davis PT. Use of foam bolsters for securing facial skin grafts. Ear Nose Throat J 1998;77:490.
5. Conway H, Sedar J. Report of the loss of pigment in full thickness autoplastic skin grafts in the mouse. Plast Reconstr Surg 1956;18:30.
6. Davison PM, Batchelor AG, Lewis-Smith PA. The properties and uses of non-expanded machine-meshed skin grafts. Br J Plast Surg 1986;39:462.
7. Hauben DJ, Baruchin A, Mahler D. On the history of the free skin graft. Ann Plast Surg 1982;9:242.
8. Jeschke MG, Rose C, Angele P, et al. Development of new reconstructive techniques: Use of Integra in combination with fibrin glue and negative-pressure therapy for reconstruction of acute and chronic wounds. Plast Reconstr Surg 2004;113:525.
9. Molnar JA, DeFranzo AJ, Hadaegh A, et al. Acceleration of Integra incorporation in complex tissue defects with subatmospheric pressure. Plast Reconstr Surg 2004;113:1339.
10. Perry AW, et al. Skin graft survival—the bacterial answer. Ann Plast Surg 1989;22:479.
11. Pruitt BA Jr, Levine NS. Characteristics and uses of biologic dressings and skin substitutes. Arch Surg 1984;119:312.
12. Ratner D. Skin grafting. From here to there. Dermatol Clin 1998;16:75–90.
13. Robson MC, Krizek TJ. Predicting skin graft survival. J Trauma 1973;13:213.
14. Rudolph R, Klein L. Healing processes in skin grafts. Surg Gynecol Obstet 1973;136:641.
15. Saltz R, Bowles BJ. Reston: An alternate method of skin graft fixation (letter). Plast Reconstr Surg 1997;99:601.
16. Schneider AM, Morykwas MJ, Argenta LC. A new and reliable method of securing skin grafts to the difficult recipient bed. Plast Reconstr Surg 1998;102:1195.
17. Smahel J. The healing of skin grafts. Clin Plast Surg 1977;4:409.
18. Smoot EC. A rapid method for splinting skin grafts and securing wound dressings (letter). Plast Reconstr Surg 1997;100:1622.
19. Waris T, et al. Regeneration of cold, warmth and heat-pain sensibility in human skin grafts. Br J Plast Surg 1989;42:576.
20. Wolter TP, Noah EM, Pallua N. The use of Integra in an upper extremity avulsion injury. Br Assoc Plast Surgeons 2005;58:416–418.

Chapter 106

Rotational and Pedicle Flaps for Coverage of Distal Upper Extremity Injuries

R. Gordon Lewis, Jr., Marc Richard, and L. Scott Levin

DEFINITION

- A *flap* is a composite collection of tissue (ie, skin, fascia, muscle, bone) that is moved from its original location to another location in or on the body.[5]
- Several different types of flaps exist, defined by their blood supply.
  - *Random flaps* (eg, Z-plasty, V-Y, cross-finger) depend on preserving enough of the subcutaneous and subdermal vascular plexus for flap survival (**FIG 1A**).
  - *Axial flaps* depend on the blood supply from a single consistent (usually named) blood vessel; this includes radial forearm and dorsal metacarpal artery flaps (**FIG 1B**).

- *Free flaps* depend on the division and microscopic reanastomosis of the artery and vein to re-establish blood flow to the flap.
- Flaps also can be defined by how the tissue is moved.
  - *Advancement flaps* are elevated and advanced in a linear direction away from the base of the pedicle (**FIG 1C**).
  - *Rotational flaps* are elevated adjacent to the defect and re-inset within the same bed[10] (**FIG 1D**).
  - *Transpositional flaps* are elevated and moved across normal tissue to a new defect site (**FIG 1E**).
  - *Island flaps* are elevated, then moved within a subcutaneous tunnel to the defect site.

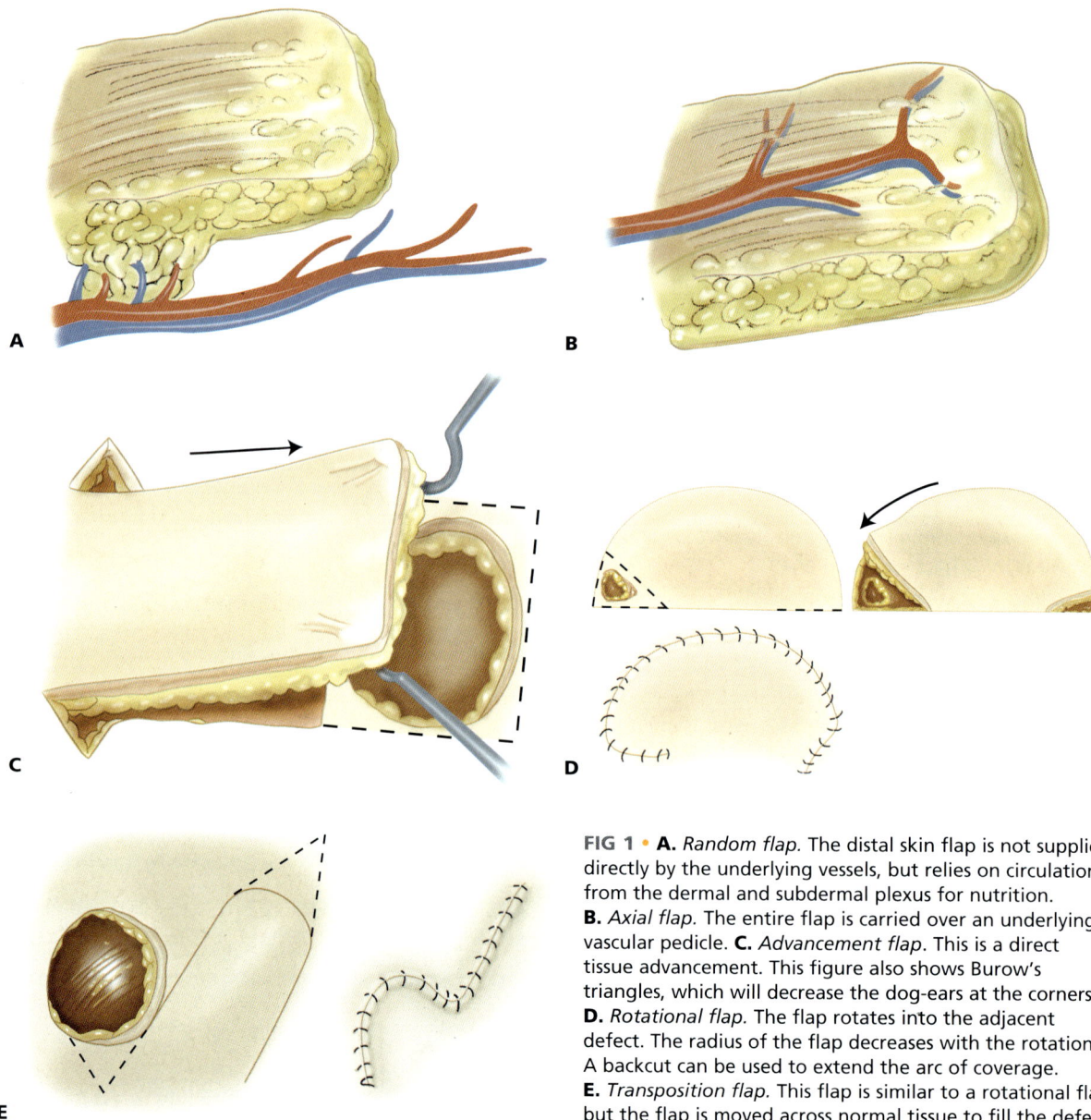

FIG 1 • A. *Random flap.* The distal skin flap is not supplied directly by the underlying vessels, but relies on circulation from the dermal and subdermal plexus for nutrition. **B.** *Axial flap.* The entire flap is carried over an underlying vascular pedicle. **C.** *Advancement flap.* This is a direct tissue advancement. This figure also shows Burow's triangles, which will decrease the dog-ears at the corners. **D.** *Rotational flap.* The flap rotates into the adjacent defect. The radius of the flap decreases with the rotation. A backcut can be used to extend the arc of coverage. **E.** *Transposition flap.* This flap is similar to a rotational flap, but the flap is moved across normal tissue to fill the defect.

- Grafts are differentiated from flaps in that there is no native blood supply to the tissue. A skin graft survives initially by osmosis (imbibition) before it obtains vascular ingrowth into the graft. This process works only for fairly thin tissue grafts.[3,4]

ANATOMY

- A thorough understanding of the anatomy of the area injured and the donor area of the flap is necessary for safe elevation and insetting of these flaps.
- A full description of the anatomy of the forearm and hand is beyond the scope of this chapter, but the key points of the relevant anatomy will be addressed in the separate sections.
- The skin and soft tissue covering the forearm and hand vary by location, and this variation must be accounted for when considering coverage.
- The palm (volar surface) of the hand consists of very thick dermis and epidermis that is structurally anchored to the underlying tissues by numerous vertical fascial connections.
  - The glabrous skin of the palm should be used to cover palmar defects, if possible.
- The dorsum of the hand has thin dermis and subcutaneous fat covering gliding extensor tendons.
  - Coverage here should be as thin as possible, to match the lost tissue.
- Fingertip sensation and durability should be of high consideration when deciding on type of coverage.
- The forearm has thin soft-tissue coverage.
  - Proximally there is muscle, which often can be covered with a skin graft.
  - Distally there is tendon on the palmar and dorsal surfaces. Trauma to the soft tissue often disrupts the paratenon and will require flap coverage.

PATHOGENESIS

- The mechanism of injury has a considerable effect on the need for flap coverage.
  - Sharp injuries can usually be closed primarily, without the need for flap coverage.
  - Abrasive injuries commonly occur as a result of motor vehicle accidents. These usually involve one surface of the hand, and the extent of injury is usually relatively apparent. However, the level of contamination often is high, and extensive débridement of contaminated and devitalized tissue is necessary.
  - Crush injuries can lead to necrosis of skin, tendon, bone, and muscle. The zone of injury often is large and can be underestimated on initial inspection.
- Other systemic injuries may delay treatment of extremity injuries. However, treatment for compartment syndrome and gross contamination must not be delayed any longer than necessary.

NATURAL HISTORY

- The natural history of a wound depends greatly on the type of injury. The degree of original injury is the primary factor contributing to the prognosis for function of the hand.
- A large wound involving the bones, tendons, or joints often has a profound negative affect on future function of the hand.
- Early coverage can decrease total inflammation of the injured area and can limit the detrimental effect of the injury on the return to function.

- Many wounds will heal secondarily without coverage. Secondary healing can lead to acceptable results in some locations, but also may lead to very poor results in others. These factors must be taken into account when deciding type of coverage.
  - Small wounds (< 1 cm) on the fingertips, without exposed bone or tendon, will likely heal well on their own. This secondary healing often gives the strongest soft tissue coverage with the best sensibility and is the preferred treatment for most wounds of this type.
  - If dorsal hand wounds secondarily heal or "granulate" over tendons, the tendons tend to scar, which limits gliding and impairs finger motion.
  - Exposed bones, tendons, nerves, or vessels usually should be covered with a flap. Secondary healing or skin grafts will result in more scarring or unstable coverage.
  - Skin grafts are best for wounds that have no exposure of tendons, nerves, or vessels. However, in dire circumstances, a skin graft can provide temporary coverage over most viable tissue. Skin grafts will not survive on bone or tendon when the periosteum or paratenon is not viable.
  - A well-performed flap will provide stable, durable coverage over any viable wound bed. This will allow earlier therapy and motion.

PATIENT HISTORY AND PHYSICAL FINDINGS

- After a traumatic injury, a complete history and physical examination are performed.
- The mechanism of the injury is important. Contaminated or crush injuries often require more than one procedure for adequate irrigation and débridement.
- Any past medical history of diabetes, smoking, heart disease, peripheral vascular disease, or hypercoagulability will impact the healing of any flap, but none of these is an absolute contraindication.
- Examination of the wound and extremity should be comprehensive:
  - Assessment of vascular status
  - Imaging for fracture
  - Motor and sensory examination to evaluate for nerve, tendon, or muscle injury
  - Examination for compartment syndrome in severe injuries

IMAGING AND OTHER DIAGNOSTIC STUDIES

- Radiographs of the hand should be obtained to evaluate for bony injury.
- Advanced imaging, such as CT scan or MRI, may be warranted for fracture pattern delineation, but these studies rarely are needed to assess the indications for flap coverage.
- Questionable blood flow or limb perfusion warrants further evaluation, such as angiography.
  - Adequate blood flow to the extremity must be restored before considering flap coverage.

TYPES OF FLAPS

Radial Forearm Flap

- Workhorse flap to cover upper extremity wounds. This flap can be a pedicle or free flap and provides excellent thin soft tissue coverage.[9]

- The donor site is the major area of morbidity.
  - The volar forearm donor site is relatively conspicuous.
  - If a skin graft is needed to close the donor site, the appearance is poor.
- The radial artery is divided during movement of the flap. Therefore, ulnar artery patency is critical. This must be confirmed with an Allen's test, or with direct Doppler evaluation of the hand with the radial artery occluded with manual pressure.
- The flap can be elevated with a proximal (anterograde) or distal (retrograde or reversed) pedicle.
- The anterograde flap is useful for coverage of the elbow, as either a pedicled flap or a free flap.
- The reversed radial forearm flap can cover the volar and dorsal hand to near the tips of the fingers.
- The reversed radial forearm flap has arterial flow through the ulnar artery and palmar arches and back through the radial artery. The venous return is compromised due to valves in the vein, but occurs through interconnections in the vena comitans that bypass the valves.
- Advantages
  - Thin pliable tissue
  - Reliable anatomy
  - Fair color match
  - Can be elevated under tourniquet control
- Disadvantages
  - Poor donor site
  - Requires patent ulnar artery
  - Reversed flap can often appear congested (but loss of flap is rare)
- Relevant anatomy
  - The brachial artery divides in the proximal forearm to form the radial and ulnar arteries. The ulnar artery is the dominant arterial blood supply to the hand in most people.
  - The radial artery courses distally just deep to the interval between the brachioradialis (BR) and the flexor carpi radialis (FCR) muscles. In the proximal forearm, the superficial branch of the radial nerve is adjacent to the radial artery.
  - The radial artery has paired venae comitantes that are important for venous egress from the flap once it is elevated.
  - There is a loose tissue septum between the FCR and BR. Within this septum, there are perforating branches of the radial artery to the skin that provide blood supply to the overlying skin. These are meticulously preserved to perfuse the flap (**FIG 2**).

Groin Flap

- The groin flap is another workhorse pedicled flap for coverage of larger soft tissue avulsions of the hand.
- This fasciocutaneous flap is based on the superficial circumflex iliac artery (SCIA) and is located on the anterior thigh, just below the inguinal ligament.[8]
- It can be taken as a free flap, but more commonly is used as a pedicled flap and a two-stage operation.
  - In the first stage, the flap is elevated laterally and inset onto the injured area. It is still attached medially to its pedicle coming off the femoral vessels.
  - In the second stage (2 to 3 weeks later), the pedicle is divided, freeing the arm from its connection to the groin.
- Advantages
  - The flap is thin.
  - It is nearly hairless, which may or may not be an advantage, depending on the recipient site.
  - It is very reliable.
  - Flap elevation is relatively quick.
  - The donor site can be closed primarily with widths up to about 10 cm.
- Disadvantages
  - Mandatory two-stage operation
  - The injured hand is connected to the patient's groin for 2 to 3 weeks while waiting for vascular ingrowth.
  - Poor color match
  - Postoperative numbness in the lateral femoral cutaneous nerve is common.
- Relevant anatomy
  - The SCIA arises off the femoral artery about 3 cm inferior to the inguinal ligament and deep to the deep fascia of the thigh (**FIG 3**).
  - SCIA travels superolaterally beneath the deep fascia.

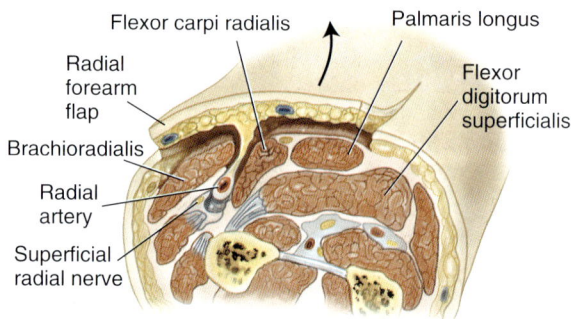

FIG 2 • Cross-section showing the relevant forearm anatomy for a radial forearm flap. The septum lies between the brachioradialis and the flexor carpi radialis. The skin and subcutaneous tissue and fascia above the volar forearm musculature are elevated as a unit with the radial artery and septum with perforating vessels.

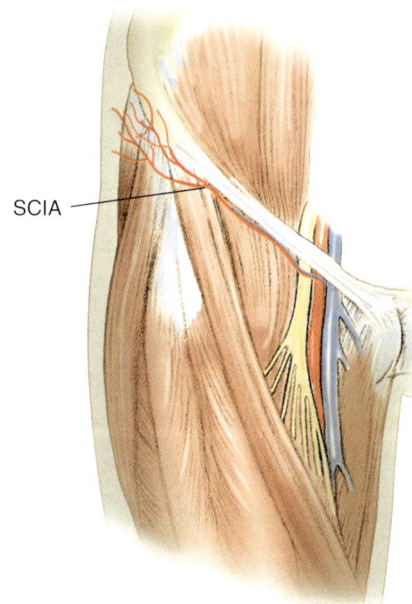

FIG 3 • Relevant groin flap anatomy. The superficial circumflex iliac artery (SCIA) arises from the femoral artery 3 cm distal to the inguinal ligament. It then travels laterally, anterior to the thigh musculature, parallel and inferior to the inguinal ligament.

- As the SCIA crosses the sartorius, it supplies branches to the muscle.
- About 6 cm from the femoral artery, the SCIA travels superficial to Scarpa's fascia.

Kite Flap

- The kite flap, or first dorsal metacarpal artery flap, is a reliable flap taken from the dorsum of the index finger over the proximal phalanx.
- Its most common use is for reconstruction of palmar thumb defects. Both soft tissue coverage and sensibility can be provided if the dorsal branches of the radial nerve are moved with the flap.[1]
- It also can be used for web space reconstruction or covering smaller defects on the dorsum of the hand or wrist.
- The flap can be 2 × 4 cm in size.
- Relevant anatomy
  - The radial artery travels through the anatomic "snuffbox," then onto the dorsum of the thumb, before diving between the two heads of the first dorsal interosseous muscle. This artery has three main branches:
    - The dorsal carpal arch
    - The princeps pollicis artery to the thumb
    - The first dorsal metacarpal artery

- The first dorsal metacarpal artery extends dorsally out along the surface of the first dorsal interosseous muscle to the dorsum on the index finger (**FIG 4**).
- The venous drainage of the flap is from the dorsal venous system of the finger.
- The radial nerve provides sensation to the dorsum of the radial hand and fingers distally. These small branches can be preserved and brought with the flap, if desired.

Posterior Interosseous Flap[11]

- The posterior interosseous flap, a fasciocutaneous flap, is a less-used flap on the dorsum of the forearm. This flap can be based proximally to cover the elbow or distally to cover the dorsum of the hand, or can be harvested as a free flap.
- The reversed flap, as used to cover the hand or wrist, relies on retrograde venous and arterial flow. The valves within the veins are bypassed by interconnections between the paired venae comitantes.
- The donor site on the dorsal forearm is more visible and subsequently less desirable than even the radial forearm flap.
- The flap is based on the perforating arteries coming from the posterior interosseous artery.
  - The posterior interosseous artery travels on the posterior side of the interosseous membrane and arises from either a common interosseous artery or the ulnar artery.
- Septocutaneous perforators travel in the septum between the extensor digiti quinti (EDQ) and extensor carpi ulnaris (ECU) to the skin.
- The posterior interosseous artery connects with the anterior interosseous artery near the distal radioulnar joint (DRUJ), and also will get retrograde flow through the dorsal carpal arch. This site is the location of the distal pivot point of the flap.
- Proximally, the posterior interosseous artery enters the posterior compartment of the forearm at the junction of the proximal and middle thirds of the forearm (**FIG 5**).
  - Advantages
    - Thin pliable tissue with good match to dorsal hand tissue
    - Preservation of both the ulnar and radial arteries
    - Can be closed primarily if flap width is less than 5 cm

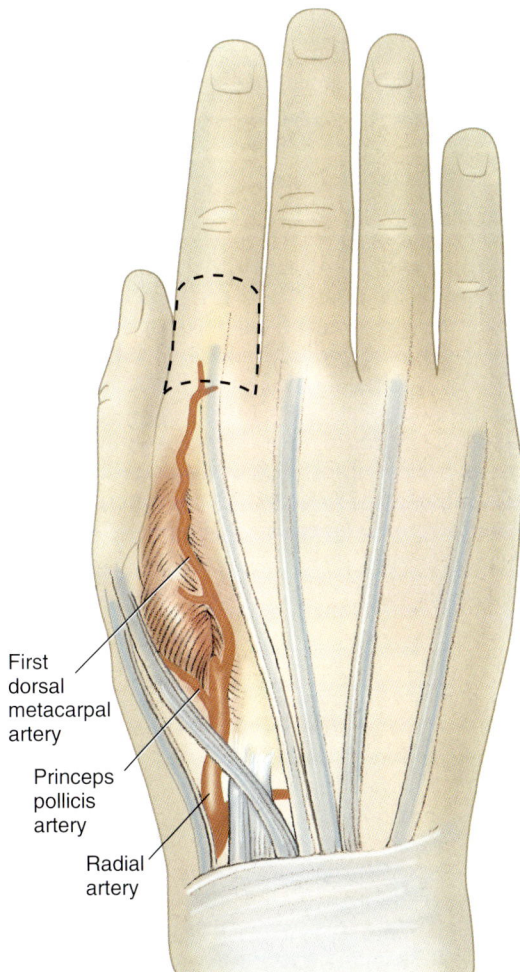

First dorsal metacarpal artery

Princeps pollicis artery

Radial artery

FIG 4 • Anatomy of the dorsal metacarpal artery.

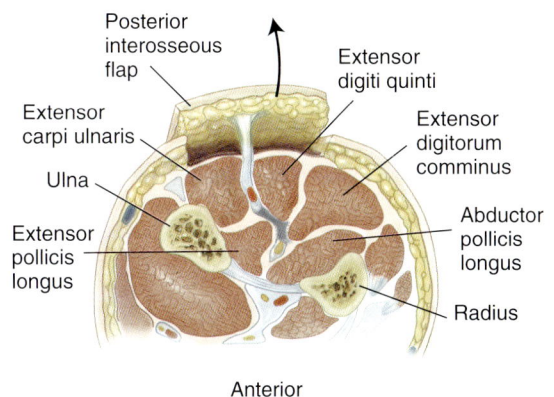

Posterior interosseous flap

Extensor carpi ulnaris

Ulna

Extensor pollicis longus

Extensor digiti quinti

Extensor digitorum comminus

Abductor pollicis longus

Radius

Anterior

FIG 5 • The posterior interosseous flap is elevated with the posterior interosseous artery in a retrograde fashion. Perforating vessels are present within a septum that lies between the extensor digitorum quinti (EDQ) and extensor carpi ulnaris (ECU). The skin, subcutaneous tissue, fascia, and septum are all elevated with the artery.

- Disadvantages
  - Technically difficult dissection due to the proximity of the posterior interosseous nerve
  - The anatomy does not always allow safe dissection of the flap, and the surgeon should have a plan for an alternate flap if necessary.
  - Flap repair is contraindicated with wrist trauma due to disruption of the dorsal wrist vascular arcade.

Z-Plasty

- Although Z-plasty is not often used during immediate reconstruction, it is a useful adjunct for secondary reconstruction due to scar contracture.
- This method lengthens or redirects a scar by transposing two triangular flaps to bring normal tissue within a scarred area.
- A prerequisite is good tissue on either side of the area to be lengthened, because this tissue is interposed in the place of the original scar.

NONOPERATIVE MANAGEMENT

- As with all reconstructive procedures, if nonoperative management is possible, it should be considered and may be preferred.
- Small wounds often will heal secondarily with good results.
  - Fingertip injuries that do not expose bone or tendon usually heal with good results and with good sensibility. These wounds should be débrided and cleaned, then dressed appropriately and allowed to heal over 2 to 3 weeks.
- Wounds on the distal forearm and hand often have exposure of tendon, bone, nerve, or vessel. Except in rare circumstances, these should all be covered with good tissue.
  - Primary closure is the ideal, but with tissue loss this may not be possible.
  - Skin grafts provide good coverage for muscle or clean wounds of the hand, but often do not offer the best coverage for future function of the hand.
    - A skin graft will heal on bone or tendon if the periosteum or paratenon is intact, but this may create a thin, unstable wound. Skin grafting over tendons is prone to scarring and may decrease tendon excursion.
    - Skin grafts will heal over nerves or vessels, but can result in hypersensitivity with nerves or thin coverage over vessels increasing the chance of bleeding.
- In many cases, early flap closure with a good gliding surface (for tendon movement) may be better than delayed healing with increased scar tissue.

SURGICAL MANAGEMENT

- The wound should be débrided back to viable tissue before it is covered.
- If there is gross contamination, the débridement often can be done in several stages to obtain a clean wound.
- The wound depth and size must be taken into consideration.

Preoperative Planning

- If there is tendon or bone involvement of the injury site, the selected reconstruction should consider these factors.
- The affected area should be well perfused when the patient is brought to the operating room for flap coverage.
- Only rarely should flaps be performed on an emergent basis in an unhealthy patient.
- Flap coverage should be performed over a stable skeleton, and devitalized or contaminated tissue should not be covered.

Positioning

- The arm usually is placed on an armboard at a 90-degree angle. The operating table is positioned to allow the surgeon and the assistant to sit on either side of the arm.
- This positioning gives excellent access to the palmar and dorsal forearm, arm, and hand.
- If a skin graft is considered, the ipsilateral groin or thigh is prepped to allow for full- or split-thickness grafting, respectively.
- Small full-thickness grafts can be obtained from the antecubital fossa, the ulnar forearm, or the ulnar side of the palm (for thick glabrous skin).

Approach

- For all procedures, a padded tourniquet is used on the patient's arm and inflated for the duration of the débridement of the wound and for flap elevation.
  - At the end of the flap elevation, the tourniquet is released and bleeding controlled with bipolar electrocautery.
  - Easily visible vessels are divided with clips or ties while the tourniquet is inflated.
- The wound site is always well débrided back to good tissue. Any foreign material is removed, and the wound irrigated with saline. Pulse lavage irrigation is used for heavily contaminated wounds.
- Careful handling of the tissue is imperative. Avoid handling the skin edges with pickups because the corners of flaps are particularly susceptible to trauma. Use retention sutures and skin hooks as much as possible.

TECHNIQUES

RADIAL FOREARM FLAP[2]

- A template of the defect is made (**TECH FIG 1A**).
- The position of the radial artery is established using Doppler ultrasound and marked on the forearm (**TECH FIG 1B**).
- The template is placed over the radial artery on the volar forearm and marked in place.
  - If a reversed flap is to be used for hand coverage, it usually is obtained from the proximal forearm.
  - If antegrade flap is to be used, it is obtained from the distal forearm.
  - The proximally based flap can pivot at the bifurcation of the radial and ulnar arteries. The distally based flap will pivot at the level of the radial styloid.

- An incision is made distal to the flap to identify the radial artery.
- Then, starting on the ulnar aspect, the skin and subsequently the forearm fascia are incised.
- The flap is elevated deep to the forearm fascia.
- Care must be taken when approaching the radial artery not to cross and divide the septum between the FCR and BR (see Fig 2).
  - The perforating vessels that perfuse the skin paddle lie within this septum.
- Once the radial artery is identified along the course of the flap on the ulnar aspect, the radial aspect of the flap is elevated in a similar fashion.

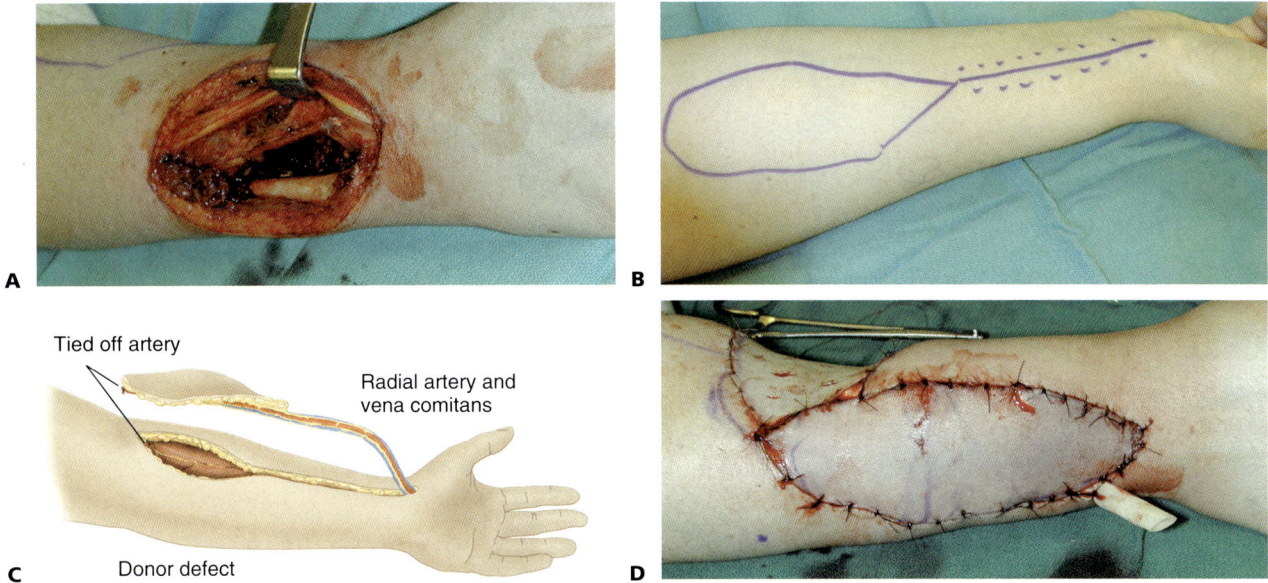

TECH FIG 1 • **A.** After resection of a recurrent sarcoma, this patient had a large dorsal defect with exposure of bone and tendon. **B.** The radial forearm flap is planned on the proximal forearm overlying the radial artery. Distal to the flap, the incision is drawn over the radial artery to extend the pedicle length. **C.** The flap is elevated from the proximal forearm, and once freed from its bed, the pedicle dissection is completed to the wrist. **D.** After the flap is elevated, it is inset in the excised wound. The flap defect is covered with a split-thickness skin graft.

- The radial artery exposure is facilitated by lateral opposing traction on FCR and BR, which can be provided by a self-retaining retractor.
- The radial artery is then divided proximally (or distally) and the flap elevated (**TECH FIG 1C**).
- It is imperative that the venae comitantes be preserved with the flap during the dissection and elevation of the radial artery. These will provide venous outflow for the flap.

- As the flap is elevated over the tendons of the FCR and palmaris longus, the paratenon must be preserved, because this will provide the vascular bed for the skin graft that will cover the donor site.
- Once flap elevation is complete, the flap is inset in the defect, and the donor defect covered with a skin graft (**TECH FIG 1D**).

GROIN FLAP[6]

- A template of the defect is made (**TECH FIG 2A**).
- The inguinal ligament is marked from the anterior superior iliac spine to the pubic tubercle (see Fig 3).
- The origin of the SCIA is about 3 cm below the inguinal ligament, and off the femoral artery.

- A second line is drawn parallel to the first, 3 cm inferior to it, indicating the SCIA.
- The flap can be as large as needed up to the following guidelines—any larger and the donor site may not close primarily. The flap margins are marked as follows:

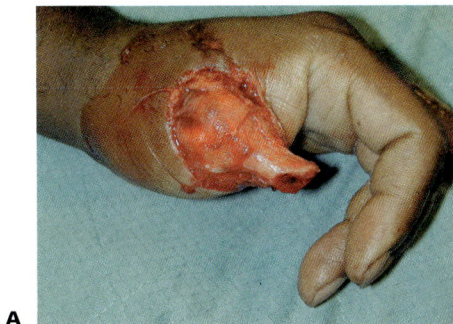

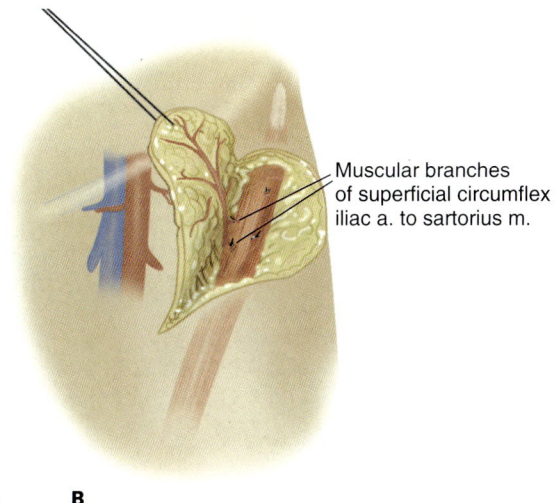

TECH FIG 2 • **A.** This patient had a traumatic amputation of his thumb, leaving reasonable bony length, but no soft tissue coverage. **B.** The groin flap is elevated from lateral to medial. Lateral to the sartorius, the superficial fascia is elevated with the flap. At the lateral border of the sartorius, the deep fascia is elevated, and the perforating branches are ligated. Elevation stops at the medial border. *(continued)*

TECHNIQUES

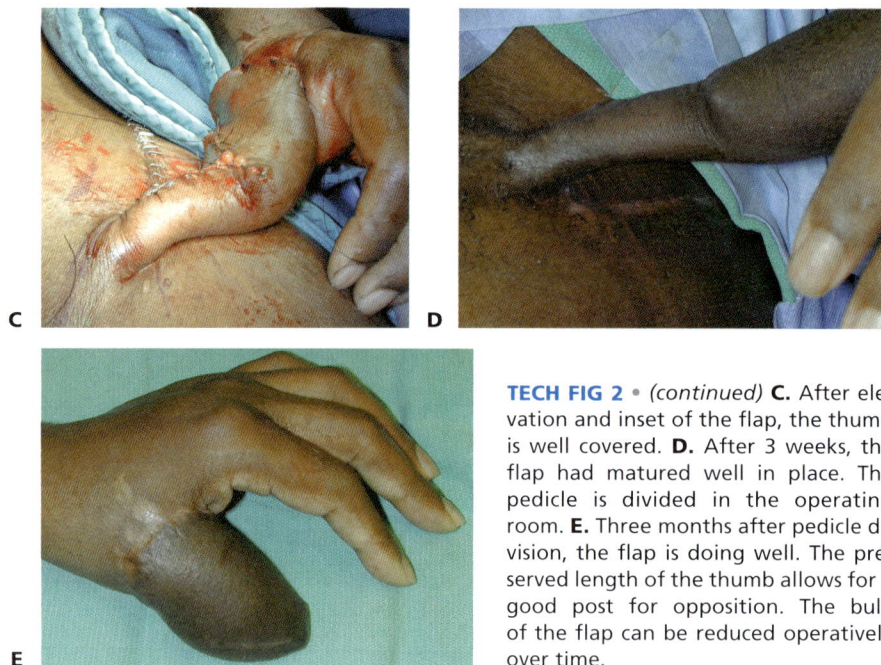

TECH FIG 2 • *(continued)* **C.** After elevation and inset of the flap, the thumb is well covered. **D.** After 3 weeks, the flap had matured well in place. The pedicle is divided in the operating room. **E.** Three months after pedicle division, the flap is doing well. The preserved length of the thumb allows for a good post for opposition. The bulk of the flap can be reduced operatively over time.

- Superior margin: 2 to 3 cm above the inguinal ligament
- Inferior margin: 7 to 8 cm below the inguinal ligament
- Lateral margin: 8 to 10 cm lateral to the anterior superior iliac spine
- The flap is then elevated from lateral to medial (**TECH FIG 2B**).
- The skin is incised laterally, and the flap elevated at the level below the superficial fascia (Scarpa's fascia).
- When the lateral border of the sartorius is encountered, the dissection proceeds beneath the deep fascia, just on top of the muscle fascia.
- The penetrating branches to the sartorius are ligated and divided.

- When the medial border of the sartorius is encountered, the dissection stops (for the pedicled flap).
- The donor site is then closed over a drain. Near the origin of the flap, care is taken not to strangulate the flap with the closure.
- The proximal portion of the flap is then tubed if possible; however, there cannot be any tension on the tube.
- The flap is then inset on the hand, usually over a Penrose drain (**TECH FIG 2C**).
- The flap may then be divided 2 to 3 weeks later (**TECH FIG 2D,E**). Perfusion of the flap can be tested before division by temporarily occluding the pedicle with a circumferential Penrose drain and assessing flap perfusion.

KITE FLAP: FIRST DORSAL METACARPAL ARTERY FLAP[1,11]

- A template of the defect is made (**TECH FIG 3A**).
- The template is transferred to the dorsum of the index finger overlying the proximal phalanx, on the radial aspect.
- The flap is marked, then a proximal incision is marked in a zigzag or curvilinear fashion to extend to the takeoff of the first dorsal metacarpal artery (**TECH FIG 3B**).

- The flap is incised along the sides and distally down to the level of the extensor apparatus. Care is taken to preserve the paratenon of the extensors.
- The first dorsal interosseous artery will be elevated, with the subcutaneous tissue lying above it. The skin above the artery is left in its original location.

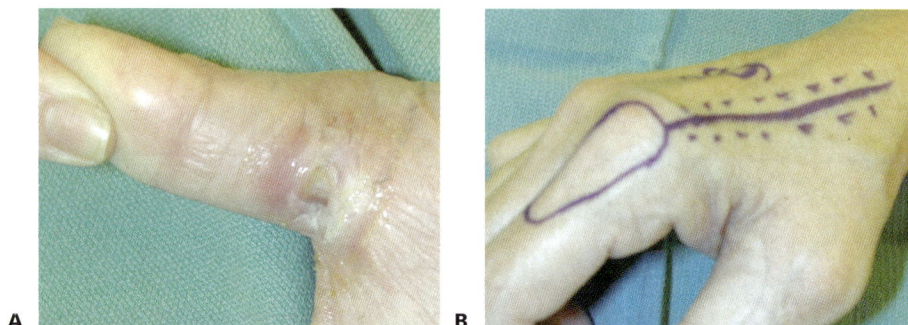

TECH FIG 3 • **A.** This wound of the volar thumb has exposed tendon and will not heal without a vascularized skin flap. **B.** The flap is planned on the dorsoradial aspect of the index finger. The proximal incision is for pedicle dissection. *(continued)*

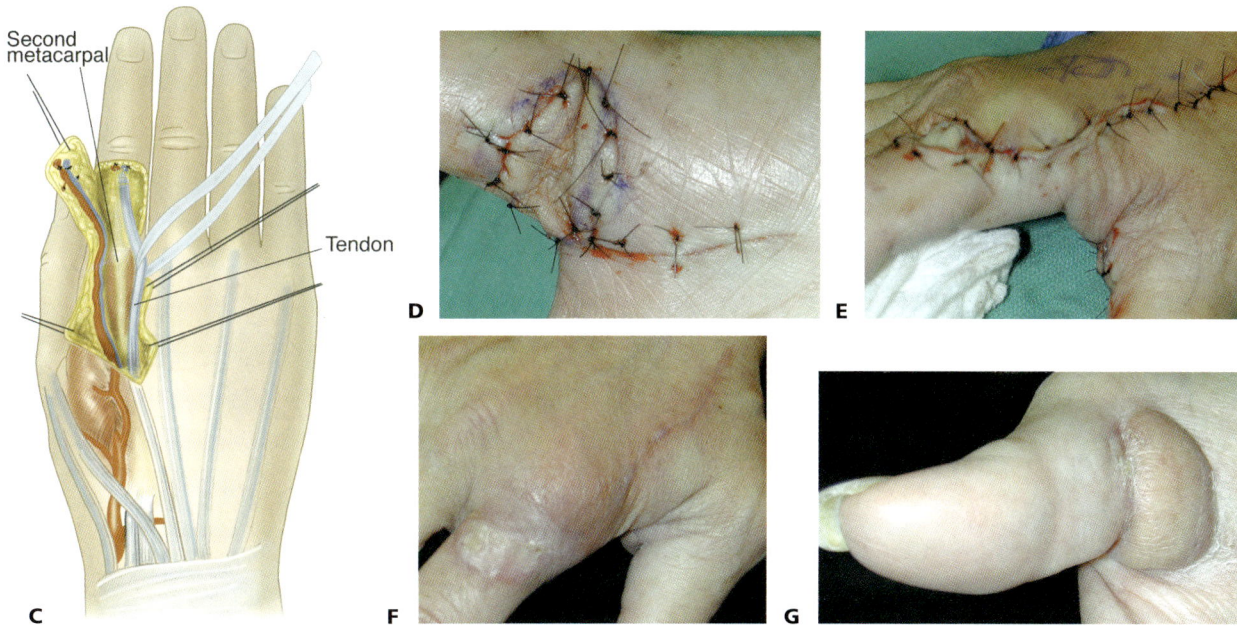

TECH FIG 3 • *(continued)* **C.** The first dorsal metacarpal artery flap is a vascularized skin flap from the dorsum of the index finger over the proximal phalanx. The dissection will give a flap that is good for small dorsal defects of the volar thumb. **D.** The flap is inset on the wound. **E.** The defect is closed. A small skin graft is needed to assist in closure. **F.** At 3 weeks postoperatively, the donor defect is healed. **G.** At 6 months postoperatively, the flap is well healed and allows for full tendon excursion.

- The skin incision is made proximal to the flap. The incision around the proximal border of the flap needs to remain shallow, at the subdermal level as the venous drainage is through the small veins in the subcutaneous tissue.
- The skin proximal to the flap is elevated on the radial and ulnar side of the artery. The skin is elevated off the fat at the subdermal level.
- The pedicle should be elevated, with a total width of about 1 cm. On the ulnar side the pedicle border is the middle of the metacarpal. On the radial side, the pedicle border is 5 to 10 mm radial to the artery (**TECH FIG 3C**).

- The artery lies on top of the fascia of the first dorsal interosseous muscle. To help preserve the artery and subcutaneous tissue, the muscle fascia is elevated with the pedicle.
- Once the dissection of the pedicle has reached the radial artery proper, as it dives palmar to the deep palmar arch, the elevation typically ends.
- This should allow enough pedicle length for coverage of many volar thumb defects and some dorsal hand defects (**TECH FIG 3D–G**).

POSTERIOR INTEROSSEOUS FLAP

- The operation is performed under tourniquet control, but without Esmarch exsanguination, to maintain visibility of the small vessels.
- The wound is débrided and irrigated, and then a template is made (**TECH FIG 4A**).
- A line is drawn from the lateral epicondyle to the DRUJ. The line approximates the position of the posterior interosseous artery (**TECH FIG 4B,C**).
- The template is placed over the line marking the pedicle. It can be placed proximally as close as 6 cm from the lateral epicondyle of the humerus.
- An incision is made along the flap outline proximal to the pivot point. Dissection is carried between the EDQ and ECU to look for the posterior interosseous artery (see Fig 4).
- If the artery is found at this location, it is generally consistent with favorable anatomy. If the artery is not satisfactory, the operation is aborted.
- Once the artery has been determined to be acceptable, the radial incision is made. The skin flap is elevated below the level of the muscular fascia. The EDC, extensor

indicis proprius, and EDQ muscles are all retracted radially to facilitate exposure of the septum.
- The muscular branches of the posterior interosseous artery (PIA) are carefully divided, exposing the PIA along the septum.
- Once one good septocutaneous perforator is located, the PIA is divided proximal to this branch. Further dissection to obtain more perforators is discouraged because of the proximity to the posterior interosseous nerve and potential damage to this nerve.
- After locating the major perforator and dividing the PIA proximally, the ulnar incision around the flap is made. This side is also elevated at a subfascial level.
- The flap is then elevated from proximal to distal. This dissection is facilitated with ulnar retraction of the ECU. A generous cuff of surrounding tissue is taken with the PIA to help preserve its vena comitans.
- A superficial vein may be preserved in the elevation for distal reanastomosis to help with venous drainage (**TECH FIG 4D,E**).

TECHNIQUES

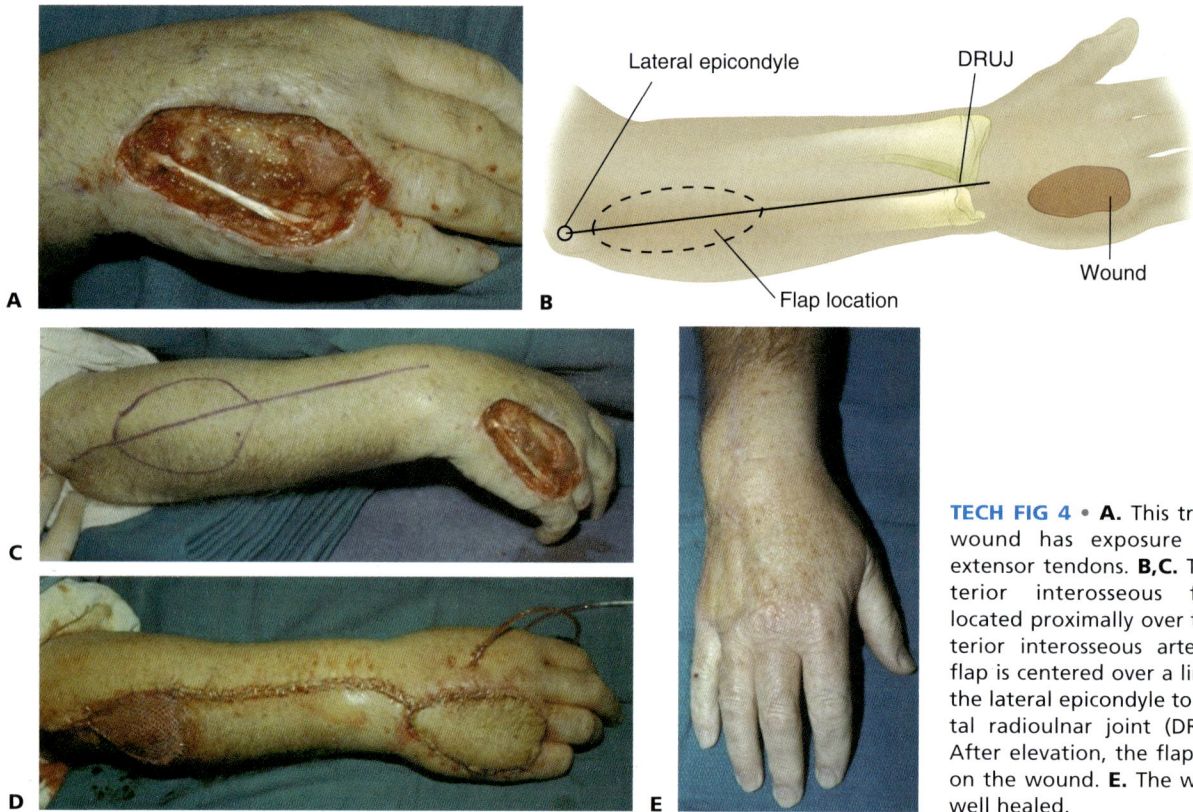

TECH FIG 4 • A. This traumatic wound has exposure of the extensor tendons. **B,C.** The posterior interosseous flap is located proximally over the posterior interosseous artery. The flap is centered over a line from the lateral epicondyle to the distal radioulnar joint (DRUJ). **D.** After elevation, the flap is inset on the wound. **E.** The wound is well healed.

Z-PLASTY

- The angle of the flaps in Z-plasty is most commonly 60 degrees (**TECH FIG 5A**), but it can be varied to give more or less lengthening, depending on the quality of the adjacent tissue. Theoretically, 60-degree flaps will provide a lengthening of 75%.
- The central incision is designed along the tight scar. This scar often is excised during this part of the procedure (**TECH FIG 5B**).
- The two limbs are designed at opposing ends of the scar on opposite sides of the central member. These limbs are

placed at about 60 degrees from the central incision (**TECH FIG 5C**).
- The flaps created are then elevated at a subcutaneous level. Then the two triangular flaps are transposed and sutured into place.
- Once the two flaps are elevated, they often "fall" into the correct position and are easily sutured in place.
- This usually gives an obvious and considerable lengthening immediately after flap transposition and insetting (**TECH FIG 5D**).

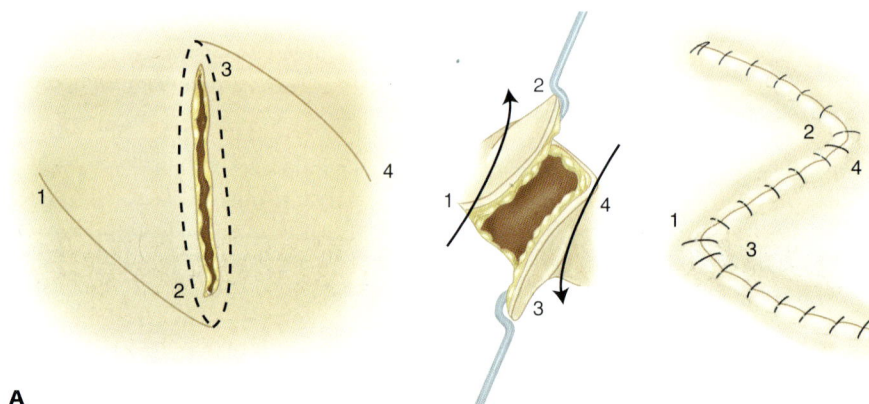

TECH FIG 5 • A. With a Z-plasty, two triangular flaps are elevated and transposed, to interpose normal tissue into a contracted scar. The angle of the flaps usually is 60 degrees. *(continued)*

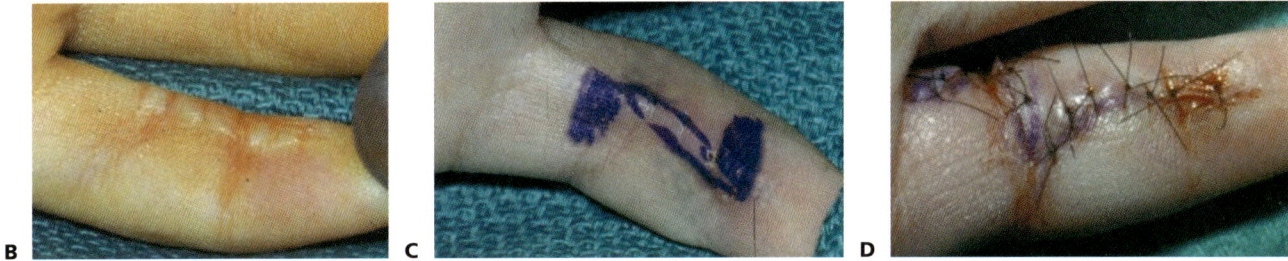

TECH FIG 5 • *(continued)* **B.** This small finger has a contracted scar on the volar radial border. As it crosses both interphalangeal joints, the scar decreases the finger's ability to extend fully. **C.** The Z-plasty is designed. **D.** After the flaps are elevated and transposed, the scar is lengthened, allowing full extension of the finger.

PEARLS AND PITFALLS

Indications	▪ A thorough physical examination must be completed before reconstruction of any defect. ▪ The choice of reconstruction is guided by the reconstructive ladder. Less invasive operations should be considered before more invasive procedures, but, ultimately, the expected outcome of the type of operation will direct the choice. ▪ Before any wound is covered, it must be clean, with no foreign material or dead tissue. Delaying reconstruction a few days until these goals are met is worthwhile.
Flap elevation	▪ Flap elevation must be done with care and precision, with attention to preservation of the feeding blood vessels. The small vessels perfusing the flaps are vital to flap survival. ▪ Frequent use of Doppler ultrasound facilitates vessel identification.
Radial forearm flap	▪ The dissection is safest when the fascia is elevated first from the ulnar side. The septum rises obliquely under the BR. ▪ Preservation of the paired venae comitantes and the septal perforators is critical to survival of the flap. ▪ The reversed flap needs a patent palmar vascular arch.
Groin flap	▪ The patient must be prepared to have the hand connected to the groin and must understand that a second operation is mandatory. ▪ This flap and the radial forearm flap are the workhorse flaps for large soft tissue flaps of the hand.
First dorsal metacarpal artery flap	▪ Reliable coverage for volar thumb or small dorsal hand defects ▪ Sensation can also be preserved with this flap through branches of the superficial radial nerve. ▪ The dissection is somewhat complex due to the small caliber of the vessels.
Posterior interosseous flap	▪ This flap is not typically a first choice. ▪ It is used when there is not a patent palmar arch (ie, when a radial forearm flap is contraindicated) and when there is a reason not to use a groin flap.

POSTOPERATIVE CARE

▪ The postoperative care largely depends on the flap that has been used.

▪ For all of the operations, some of the same principles are followed.

▪ Postoperative antibiotics often are indicated, because the wounds have been open for some time, have been contaminated, or have associated open fractures. The choice of antibiotic is individualized for each patient.

▪ The operative site usually is splinted to allow for healing of the flap without movement. If there is no bony injury, this is usually for 7 to 10 days, but the length of time may vary.

▪ The arm should be elevated above the level of the heart as much as possible. This will help decrease both edema within the flap and patient discomfort.

▪ The radial forearm flap should be monitored in the hospital for 2 or 3 days.

▪ When distally based, this flap may be susceptible to venous congestion.

▪ Care should be taken during the operation to meticulously preserve the vena comitans.

▪ If the cephalic vein has been preserved with the flap, it can be anastomosed to a vein in the field of the flap, but this is rarely necessary with the reversed flap.

▪ Care should be taken not to make the splint or dressing too tight.

▪ If a skin graft is placed during the operation, the bolster dressing is removed at 5 to 7 days, and the skin graft is dressed daily with petrolatum-infused gauze or a nonadhering dressing until fully healed.

▪ Sutures around the flap are removed at 10 to 14 days.

▪ Early active motion of the fingers is encouraged to promote tendon gliding and lessen edema, unless contraindicated after coverage.

▪ Hand therapy is initiated in most patients at 1 to 2 weeks following surgery.

COMPLICATIONS

- Short-term complications include those related to flap survival and healing of the wound.
- Long-term complications result from undesirable scarring relating to both the primary injury and the method of closure.
- Complete flap loss due to flap ischemia is uncommon. More often, a small area of the flap margin may not heal to the native skin margin, due to inadequate débridement of the skin edges or rough handling of the flap skin.
- As the flaps heal, the function of the hand depends on subsequent scarring, which, if it occurs, leads to poor tendon gliding. Persistent tendon scarring requires later tenolysis. After 3 months, loss of the flap by inadvertent pedicle division is rare, but late flap loss has been reported.
- If scarring from the flap margin creates a contracture across a joint, a Z-plasty may be necessary.
- Overall, the complications related to flap closure are less than complications related to secondary healing. The long-term outcome will be better with flap coverage compared to secondary healing, because secondary intention creates an abundance of scar tissue, which can impair function of the hand.

REFERENCES

1. Foucher G, Baun JB. A new island flap transfer from the dorsum of the index to the thumb. Plast Reconstr Surg 1979;63:344–349.
2. Foucher G, van Genechten N, Merle M, et al. A compound radial artery flap in hand surgery: an original modification of the Chinese forearm flap. Br J Plast Surg 1984;37:139–148.
3. Mathes SJ, Nahai F. Reconstructive Surgery: Principles, Anatomy, and Technique. New York: Churchill Livingstone, 1997:37–161, 775–803, 1005–1020.
4. Pederson WC, Lister GD. Skin flaps. In Green DP, Pederson WC, Hotchkiss RN, et al, eds. Green's Operative Hand Surgery. Philadelphia: Elsevier, 2005:1648–1703.
5. Place MJ, Herber SC, Hardesty RA. Basic techniques and principles in plastic surgery. In: Aston SJ, Beasley RW, Thorne CH, eds. Grabb and Smith's Textbook of Plastic Surgery. Philadelphia: Lippincott Williams & Wilkins 1997:13–16.
6. Serafin D. The groin flap. In: Serafin D, ed. Atlas of Microsurgical Composite Tissue Transplantation. Philadelphia: WB Saunders, 1996:57–65.
7. Sherif MM. First dorsal metacarpal artery flap in hand reconstruction: I. Anatomical study. J Hand Surg Am 1994;19:26–31.
8. Smith PJ, Foley B, Mcgreggor IA, et al. The anatomic basis of the groin flap. Plast Reconstr Surg 1972;49:41–47.
9. Song R, Gao Y, Song Y, et al. The forearm flap. Clin Plast Surg 1982;9:21–26.
10. Spector JA, Levine JP. Cutaneous defects: flaps, grafts, and expansion. In: McCarthy JG, Galiano RD, Boutros SG, eds. Current Therapy in Plastic Surgery. Philadelphia: WB Saunders, 2006:11–21.
11. Zancoli EA, Angrigiani C. Posterior interosseous island flap. J Hand Surg Br 1988;13:130–135.

Chapter 107

Surgical Treatment of Thermal and Electrical Injury and Contracture Involving the Distal Upper Extremity

Edwin Y. Chang and Kevin C. Chung

DEFINITION

- Burns and electrical injuries of the hand and forearm can present as both acute and long-term surgical problems.
- High-voltage electrical injury is defined as involving a power source with a voltage greater than 600 volts.
- Electrical burns constitute a unique type of injury, because "hidden" local and regional deep tissue damage exists beyond the confines of the cutaneous burn.
- Acutely, circumferential or near-circumferential full-thickness burns of the extremity may require escharotomy, in which the unyielding burned tissue is released to reduce soft tissue tension.
- Compartment syndrome is a serious sequela that warrants immediate surgical attention.
- Contractures are common in burn patients, resulting from loss of normal skin pliability when the skin is replaced by scar tissue after second- and third-degree burns.
- Despite aggressive acute care, splinting, and therapy, long-term hand and wrist deformities are common.[6]

ANATOMY

- *Compartments* are anatomic spaces enveloped by fascia, bones, and interosseous membrane.
- The forearm is divided into three compartments: volar, dorsal, and the mobile wad (**FIG 1A**).
- The hand has compartments housing four dorsal interosseous muscles, three volar interosseous muscles, thenar muscle, and hypothenar muscle (**FIG 1B**).
- Postburn scarring and contracture tend to produce the "classic" clawing deformity with flexed wrist and proximal interphalangeal (PIP) joints, extended distal interphalangeal (DIP) and metacarpophalangeal (MCP) joints, and adducted web spaces[1] (**FIG 1C,D**).

PATHOGENESIS

Electrical Burns

- Electrical shock produces a complex pattern of injury in which the severity of injury depends on the intensity of the current and the duration of contact.
- Tissue damage occurs predominantly by two mechanisms: thermal injury and electroporation.[7]
- As an electrical current travels, heat is generated along its path, leading to thermal damage.
  - Tissues with high electrical resistance, such as the skin and bone, generate more heat, causing more damage to both themselves and the surrounding tissues.
- *Electroporation* is cellular damage induced by the electric field. The severity of injury is determined by the cell's size and its transmembrane potential.
  - Cells with larger surface area, such as myocytes, are more prone to electroporation injury.
  - In addition, it has been suggested that due to the architecture and orientation, myocytes near a bone may experience increased transmembrane potential compared to those further from the bone.
- Secondary to these mechanisms, patients with high-voltage electric burns often sustain extensive deep tissue and muscle injuries that predispose the patient to developing acute compartment syndrome.

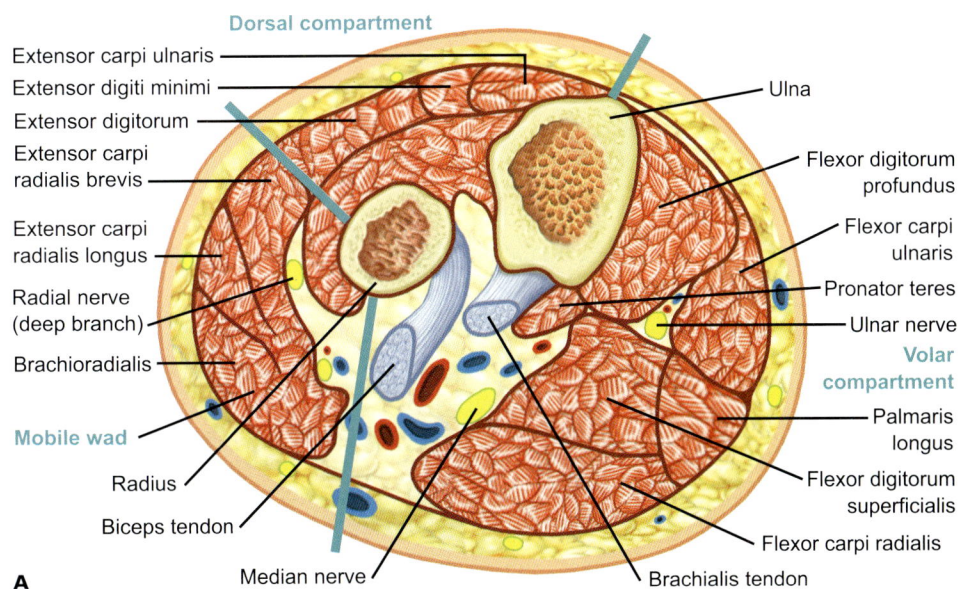

FIG 1 • A. Cross-section of midforearm depicting the fascial compartments. *(continued)*

Labels (left, top to bottom): Dorsal compartment; Extensor carpi ulnaris; Extensor digiti minimi; Extensor digitorum; Extensor carpi radialis brevis; Extensor carpi radialis longus; Radial nerve (deep branch); Brachioradialis; Mobile wad; Radius; Biceps tendon; Median nerve

Labels (right, top to bottom): Ulna; Flexor digitorum profundus; Flexor carpi ulnaris; Pronator teres; Ulnar nerve; Volar compartment; Palmaris longus; Flexor digitorum superficialis; Flexor carpi radialis; Brachialis tendon

A

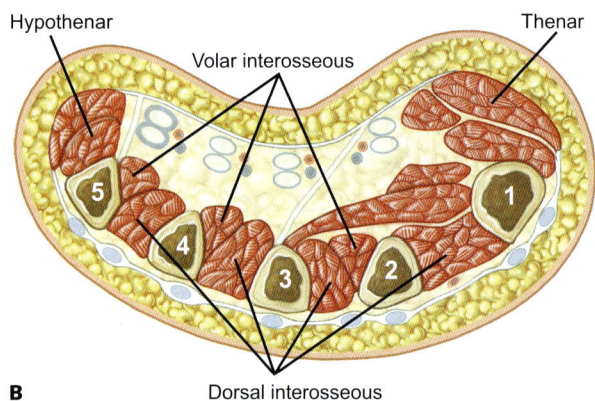

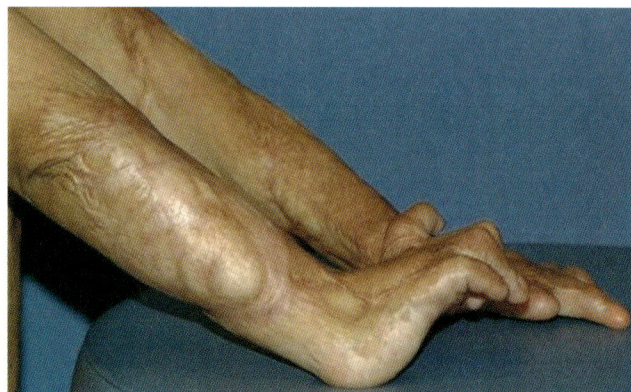

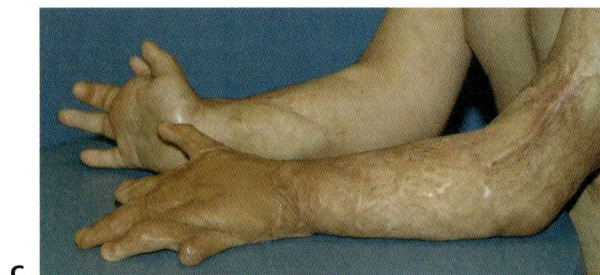

FIG 1 • *(continued)* **B.** Cross-section of the hand showing the intrinsic fascial compartments. **C, D.** Classic deformities associated with severe hand burn, with flexed proximal interphalangeal (PIP) joint and extended metacarpophalangeal (MCP) and distal interphalangeal (DIP) joints.

Compartment Syndrome

■ Arteriovenous gradient theory is commonly accepted as describing the relation between increasing soft tissue pressure and decreasing arterial inflow.

■ In burns, vascular permeability leads to swelling of the soft tissues and, in particular, the muscles.

■ The inelastic fascia housing each compartment does not allow the edematous muscles to expand. The increased pressure within the compartments eventually interrupts arterial inflow to the muscles.

■ Although compartment syndrome most often is discussed in relation to fascial compartments, it can occur in full- or near–full-thickness burns because the inelastic skin limits the ability of underlying soft tissue to expand.

   ■ The inelastic skin in a circumferential burn acts as a tourniquet, compromising venous return and capillary perfusion, and leading to tissue ischemia distal to the burns.[8]

Burn Contractures

■ Increased and disorganized deposition of collagen fibers has been observed in burn wounds, forming compact and shortened scars.[6]

■ The amount and severity of hypertrophic scarring and contracture is directly related to the depth of the burn and the time required for wound healing.

■ Inflammation, pain, and edema from burn injuries promote immobility (in the position of comfort) and cause wound contracture.[1]

■ Immobility and abnormal scarring lead to rapid formation of contractures in the pattern described under Anatomy.

NATURAL HISTORY

Evolution of Compartment Syndrome

■ Acute burn management for large body surface area burns requires aggressive fluid resuscitation. Massive edema is seen within 36 hours of injury.

■ Intracompartmental pressure can, in turn, elevate rapidly in the early postburn period.

■ Classic studies have shown that myonecrosis occurs after 6 hours of ischemia. Once tissue is ischemic for longer than 8 to 12 hours, irreversible functional damage occurs.[5,8]

■ Prompt fasciotomy minimizes functional loss and promotes recovery.

■ If compartment syndrome is left untreated, the result is Volkmann's ischemic contracture, a late sequela in which muscles and nerves die and are replaced by fibrous tissue.[12]

Natural Progression of Burn Injury

■ Proper management of burn injuries includes early excision and grafting, followed by appropriate therapy programs.

■ Even with splinting, range-of-motion exercises, compression, and positioning, 80% of patients will have decreased joint motion, and up to 10% will have difficulties with activities of daily living.[3]

PATIENT HISTORY AND PHYSICAL EXAMINATION

Acute Burn Injuries

■ In addition to routine medical history, it is imperative to obtain the mechanism of the burn injury.

   ■ High-voltage electrical burns, burns that occurred in an enclosed space, or burns associated with explosions require trauma and critical care consultation to evaluate for other life-threatening injuries.

■ Thermal and electrical burns are evaluated for depth.

   ■ First-degree burns involve only the epidermis and appear as a painful, erythematous plaque that blanches with pressure.

   ■ Second-degree burns involve the epidermis as well as partial thickness of the dermis. Second-degree burns invariably are associated with blistering of the skin that evolve into moist, weepy, and painful wounds after sloughing of the epidermis.

■ Third-degree burns involve the entire thickness of the skin and are characterized by charred, painless, leathery skin with visible coagulated vessels.

Acute Compartment Syndrome

■ Clinically, elevated soft tissue pressure presents with severe edema and tightness of the hand, wrist, and forearm distal to the burn.

■ Treatment for fascial compartment syndrome of the forearm and hand should be initiated based on clinical suspicion.

■ Compartment syndrome can present with a constellation of symptoms:
  ■ Pain with passive muscle stretch
  ■ Progressive pain despite immobilization
  ■ Nerve ischemia symptoms such as diminished sensation and muscle weakness
  ■ Compartments tender and firm to palpation

■ Compartment and soft tissue pressures can be measured using a pressure transducer (**FIG 2**).
  ■ A simple device for measuring pressure can be made with an 18- or 20-gauge needle attached to a syringe containing saline and a pressure transducer, all connected via a three-way stopcock.
  ■ The transducer is set to zero at the level of the soft tissue or compartment to be measured.
  ■ After the needle is inserted into the subcutaneous tissue, a small amount (0.2–0.5 mL) of saline is injected to establish a water column.
  ■ The transducer is then opened to the needle for pressure monitoring.

■ Compartment and soft tissue pressures can also be measured using a commercially available device.

■ The recommended threshold for performing fasciotomy is pressure higher than 30 mm Hg for normotensive patients.
  ■ In patients with hypotension, when the compartment pressure rises to within 20 mm Hg of the diastolic pressure, fasciotomy is indicated.[9]

Secondary Burn Reconstruction and Contracture Release

■ Preoperative examination for patients undergoing secondary burn reconstruction should include a complete hand examination, focusing on range of motion of the affected joints.

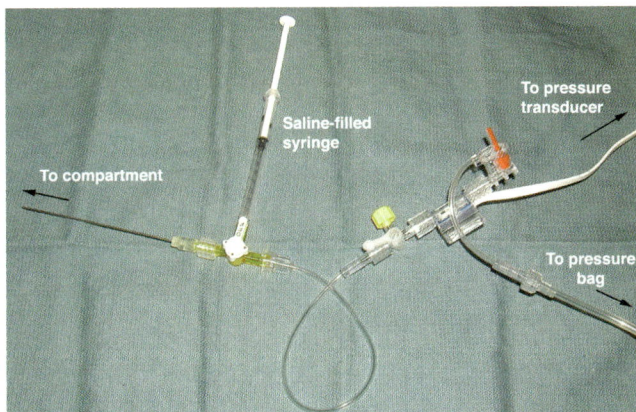

FIG 2 • Pressure transducer adapted for measurement of compartment pressure.

■ Substantial limitation of active and passive joint motion in the PIP and MCP indicates contracture of underlying joint tissues.[4,11]

■ Examination should also focus on the scar and skin quality, because immature scars may still be amenable to nonoperative management.

■ Poor or unstable skin coverage may limit local tissue rearrangement options and necessitate coverage with a distant flap.

Physical Examination

■ Vascular examination includes checking pulse and capillary refill.
  ■ Pulse is graded as normal, diminished, or absent compared to the contralateral side.
  ■ Capillary refill is graded as delayed, normal (2–3 second), or quickened.
    ■ Absent or diminished pulse is a late finding in compartment syndrome.
    ■ Quickened capillary refill is suggestive of venous congestion.
    ■ Delayed capillary refill may suggest increased soft tissue or compartment pressure.

■ The neurologic examination includes light touch, two-point discrimination, and motor function testing.
  ■ Sensibility to light touch is graded as normal, diminished, significantly diminished, and absent.
  ■ Two-point discrimination is graded as normal (< 6 mm static, < 3 mm moving), and abnormal.
  ■ Motor examination is graded from 0 to 5, with 0 being absent, and 5 normal.
  ■ Altered neurologic finding compared to the contralateral limb is an indication of increased compartment pressure.

■ A passive stretch test should be performed.
  ■ Pain with passive stretch is an abnormal finding.
  ■ A positive passive stretch test is indicative of muscle ischemia and injury.

■ Measure subeschar and compartment pressure. Elevated pressure is confirmed if the measured pressure is greater than 30 mm Hg or within 20 mm Hg of the diastolic pressure. Persistently or worsening elevated pressure is an indication for escharotomy or fasciotomy.

■ Examine MCP range of motion:
  ■ Type I: mild limitation in MCP flexion with wrist flexion, more than 30 degrees of flexion with wrist in extension
  ■ Type II: severe limitation in MCP flexion with wrist in flexion, less than 30 degrees of flexion with wrist in extension
  ■ Type III: severe limitation in MCP flexion with wrist in extension
  ■ Type II and III contractures signify underlying joint and ligamentous pathology that cannot be corrected with soft tissue release alone.

■ Examine PIP range of motion:
  ■ Type I: near-normal PIP extension with MCP in flexion
  ■ Type II: moderately limited PIP extension with MCP in flexion
  ■ Type III: fixed PIP flexion regardless of MCP position
  ■ Type II and III contractures signify underlying joint and ligamentous pathology that cannot be corrected with soft tissue release.

IMAGING AND OTHER DIAGNOSTIC STUDIES

- Currently, no available imaging modality can detect acute increases in compartment pressure.
- For secondary reconstruction of the contracted hand and fingers, plain radiographs should be obtained to evaluate the condition of the joint and determine whether heterotrophic ossification is present, because that requires alternative treatment options.

DIFFERENTIAL DIAGNOSIS

- The differential diagnosis for compartment syndrome includes:
  - Nerve injury
  - Arterial insufficiency or injury
  - Venous thrombosis
- Burn contractures should be differentiated from:
  - Intrinsic joint disease
  - Other scarring or contracture phenomena (eg, Dupuytren disease)

NONOPERATIVE MANAGEMENT

- Early in the healing process (usually within 6 months of injury), immature scars are hyperemic in appearance and amenable to conservative measures.
- Conservative management includes the use of pressure garments, silicone dressing, and physical therapy.
- Pressure garments and silicone have been shown to control hypertrophic scars and must be worn for several months.[6]
- Therapy should focus on aggressive range-of-motion exercises and splinting in an antideforming posture (**FIG 3**).

SURGICAL MANAGEMENT

- Burn débridement, escharotomy, fasciotomy, local tissue rearrangement for linear and web space contracture, and pedicled groin flap coverage for soft tissue defects are discussed in the Techniques section.

Indications for Surgical Management of Acute Burns and Acute Compartment Syndrome

- High-voltage injury is an indication for immediate fasciotomy and burn débridement because it is difficult to assess the extent of deep thermal damage.
- Patients with thermal burns and low-voltage electric injury require closed monitoring by experienced personnel to assess potential increased soft tissue or compartment pressure, but may otherwise be débrided in 48 to 72 hours to allow for demarcation of burned areas.

- Elevated soft tissue pressure and fascial compartment pressure are indications for emergent surgical intervention.
- Despite the potential utility of pressure monitors, diagnosis of the pathology still relies on clinical judgment.
- If there is any doubt regarding the diagnosis, escharotomy and fasciotomy should be undertaken expeditiously.
- Fascial compartment syndrome may be masked by elevated pressure of the overlying soft tissue, and it is of the utmost importance to check muscle compartment pressures after an escharotomy.
- If elevated compartment pressure is not relieved by escharotomy of the overlying burned tissue, a full fasciotomy is necessary.
- After escharotomy or fasciotomy, patients must be observed closely for signs and symptoms of inadequate release, which will require urgent reoperation.

Considerations in Contracture Release and Secondary Burn Reconstruction

- Burn injuries cause soft tissue contracture and result in tissue deficiency. The secondary effects of soft tissue contracture are joint and tendon changes that also require release.
- Mild volar and dorsal linear scar bands, as well as web space contractures, can be corrected with scar release and local tissue rearrangement.
- Basic Z-plasty is a technique of local tissue rearrangement in which two equal triangular skin flaps are transposed (**FIG 4A**). Z-plasty is ideally suited for linear scar release because it lengthens and interrupts a scar, and also redirects the line of tension.
  - The theoretical gain in length is proportional to the angle of the Z-plasty. A larger angle provides more lengthening but is more difficult to transpose (Table 1).
  - However, an adequately sized Z-plasty flap often is difficult to fit into a contracted web space.
- For web space contracture release we prefer a five-flap "jumping man" Z-plasty, which is a combination of two Z-plasty flaps with a Y-to-V advancement flap (**FIG 4B**).

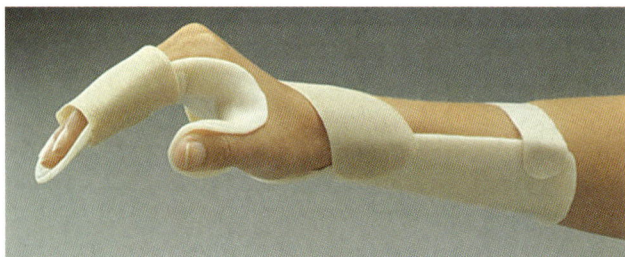

FIG 3 • Immature burn scars that are amenable to conservative treatment. A volar intrinsic-plus splint with the thumb in palmar abduction to prevent debilitating postburn contractures.

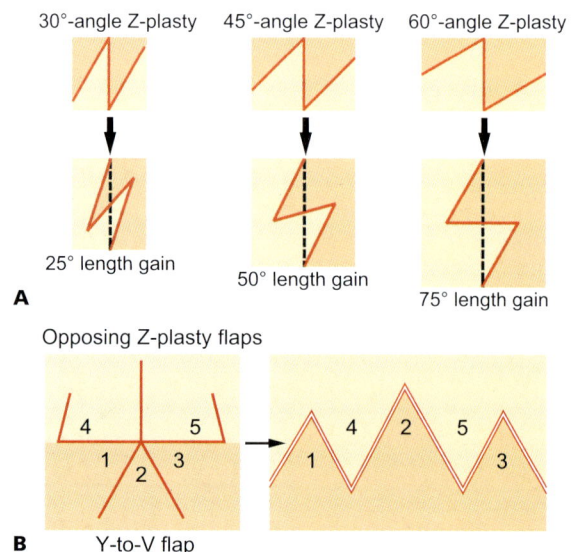

FIG 4 • **A.** Basic Z-plasty flaps and their theoretical gain in length. **B.** Five-flap jumping man Z-plasty, which is made up of two opposing Z-plasty flaps and a Y-to-V flap.

Table 1	Z-plasty Angles and Corresponding Theoretical Gains in Length	
Z-plasty angle (degrees)	Theoretical gain in length (%)	
30	25	
45	50	
60	75	
75	100	

- Compared to a basic Z-plasty, the additional flaps maximize gain in length. In addition, the Y-to-V flap introduces unscarred skin into the reconstruction, providing more pliability and elasticity to the reconstructed web space.
- Even without scar resection, surgical release of burn scars often result in a large soft tissue defect due to tissue deficiency.
  - Thick split- or full-thickness skin grafts can be used to resurface the soft tissue defect.
- Flap coverage may be necessary if contracture release or scar excision leads to exposure of joint structures, tendons, or neurovascular bundles.

- Pedicled groin flaps are versatile flaps based on the superficial circumflex iliac artery, useful for coverage of large soft tissue defects in the hand and forearm.

Preoperative Planning

- If hand and forearm burns are part of a larger insult, the ABCs (airway, breathing, and circulation) of trauma resuscitation and patient stabilization cannot be overlooked.
- Burn débridements may incur a significant amount of blood loss, and blood products should be made available intra- and perioperatively.
- For secondary burn reconstruction, one must appreciate the structure involved in the deformity.
- If tightness of the deep tissue is present, capsulotomy and ligamentous release should be addressed simultaneously.

Positioning

- Supine positioning with the affected arm extended on an arm table is adequate for most described procedures.
- For secondary reconstruction, an upper arm tourniquet is used.
- The ipsilateral upper thigh and lower abdominal quadrant is prepped and draped if a groin flap is planned for soft tissue coverage.

ESCHAROTOMY FOR FULL OR DEEP PARTIAL-THICKNESS BURNS

- Escharotomy can be performed at the bedside using electrocautery with the patient under sedation.
- A full-thickness skin incision is made the length of the full-thickness burn on the radial aspect of the forearm, along the line connecting the lateral end of the antecubital flexion crease and radial styloid (**TECH FIG 1**).
- The incision is deepened until viable tissue is encountered. The length of the incision spans the entire burn, from normal skin to normal skin.
- If the hand and the forearm are still tight after a radial release, a second escharotomy incision can be made along a line just volar to the ulna, spanning the entire burn (see Tech Fig 1).
- To perform escharotomy of the hand, one can extend the radial incision onto the hand with the radial incision at the midaxial line over the thenar eminence. The radial sensory nerve will lie along this incision and must be protected.
- The ulnar incision can be carried onto the hypothenar eminence as needed.

- Circumferential finger burns are treated with a digital escharotomy. A midlateral incision down into subcutaneous fat is made along one side of the finger, from the MCP joint to the fingertip.
- If the compartment pressure is still high after escharotomy, fasciotomy should be carried out as described in the following section.
- Escharotomy wounds are dressed with a moist dressing.

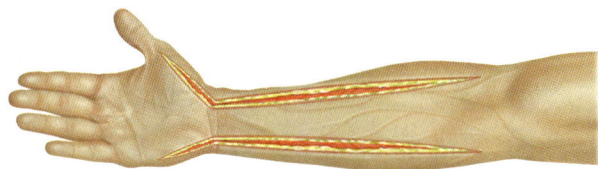

TECH FIG 1 • Location for radial and ulnar escharotomy incisions. If necessary, the incisions can be carried onto the thenar and hypothenar eminences.

FASCIOTOMY OF HAND AND FOREARM

Intrinsic Compartment Release

- Two dorsal incisions centered over the index and ring metacarpals are used to release the interosseous muscle and the thumb adductor muscle compartments (**TECH FIG 2A**).
- Incisions are carried down ulnar and radial to the index and ring extensors. Dissection is continued until the fascia of the dorsal interosseous muscles is encountered. The fascia is opened sharply.

- Blunt dissection is performed along the ulnar and radial side of the index finger metacarpal to open the first volar interosseous and adductor pollicis muscles.
- The second volar interosseous muscle is opened with deep blunt dissection along the radial border of the ring finger metacarpal.
- Finally, through the ring finger metacarpal incision, deep blunt dissection along the radial border of the small finger metacarpal releases the third volar interosseous muscle.

TECHNIQUES

TECHNIQUES

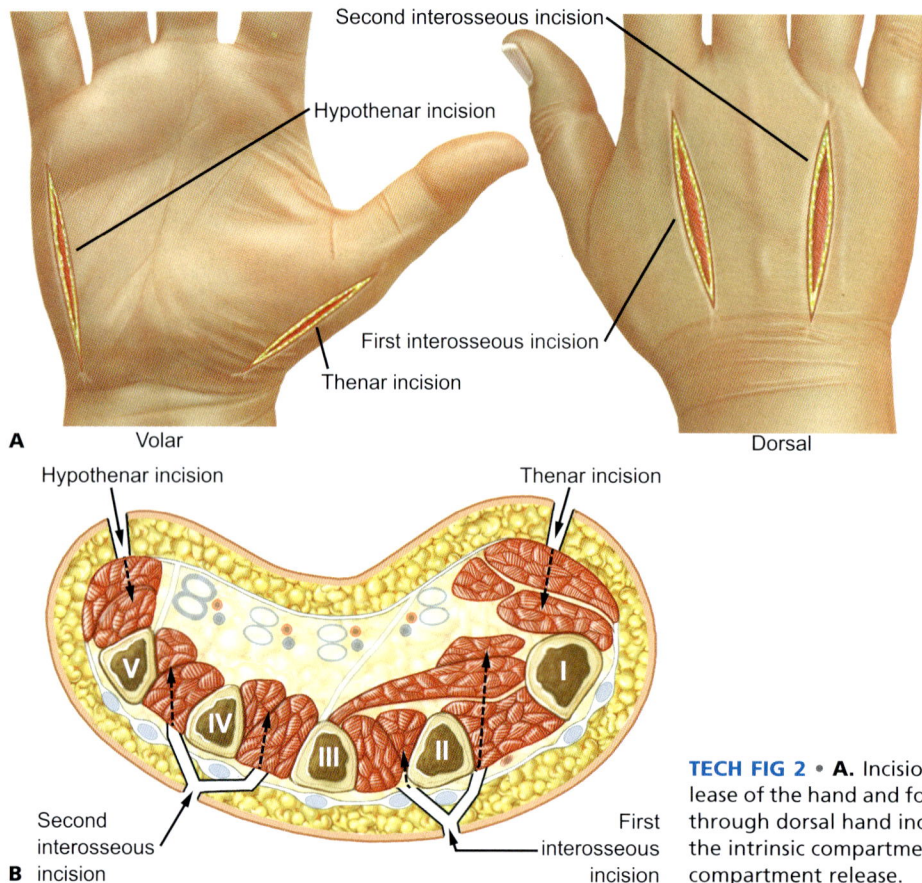

TECH FIG 2 • **A.** Incisions for intrinsic compartment release of the hand and for release of interosseous muscles through dorsal hand incisions. **B.** Cross-sectional view of the intrinsic compartments of the hand and incisions for compartment release.

- Thenar muscles are released through an incision on the radial border of the thumb metacarpal between the volar glabrous and dorsal pliable skin. The dissection is volar to the metacarpal to expose the fascia of the thenar muscles, which is sharply opened.
- The hypothenar muscles are released similarly with an incision on the ulnar aspect of the small finger metacarpal (**TECH FIG 2B**).

Carpal Tunnel Release

- The carpal tunnel is released through a standard incision over the palm, along the ring metacarpal.
- Incision begins at the Kaplan's cardinal line (the line connecting the apex of the first web space to the hook of the hamate), and extends 2 to 3 cm proximally (**TECH FIG 3**).
- We prefer to avoid an incision across the wrist joint, to protect the median nerve from exposure.
- The palmar fascia is divided sharply to expose the transverse carpal ligament.
- The transverse carpal ligament is divided under direct visualization.

Forearm Fasciotomy

- We prefer to perform fasciotomy of all three forearm compartments at the same time to avoid lingering doubts regarding inadequate release. Two incisions are used (**TECH FIG 4A**).

- A straight-line incision is made over the first third of the ulnar aspect of the volar forearm, beginning just proximal to the wrist crease and extending to just distal to the ulnar aspect of the elbow flexion crease (**TECH FIG 4B**).
- The incision is carried down through the fascia, into the volar compartment. The fascia is opened along the length of the compartment.
  - The superficial and deep muscles are examined.

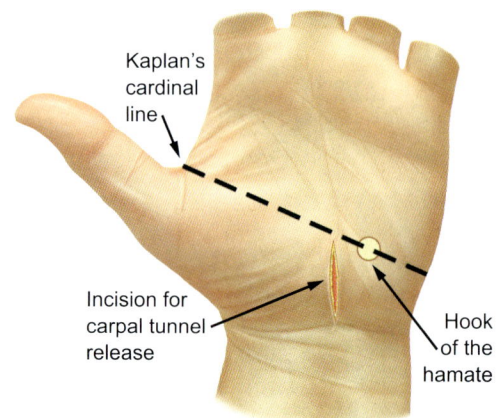

TECH FIG 3 • Incision for carpal tunnel release. Kaplan's cardinal line is used as a guide for the incision for carpal tunnel release.

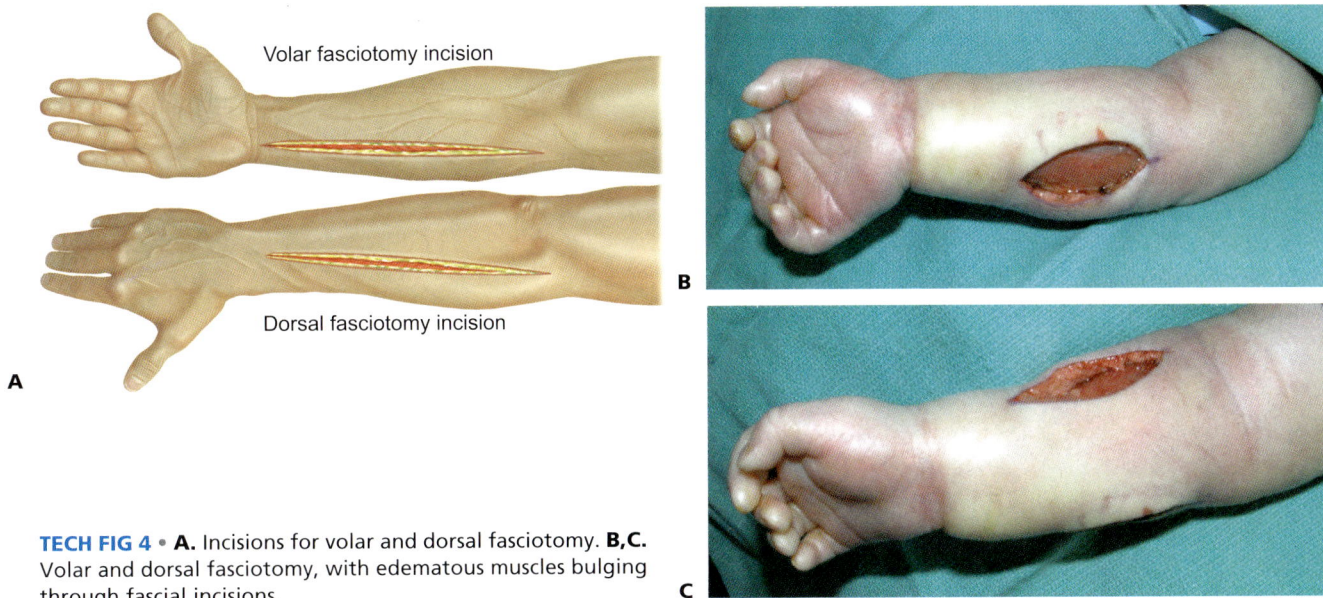

Volar fasciotomy incision

Dorsal fasciotomy incision

A

B

C

TECH FIG 4 • **A.** Incisions for volar and dorsal fasciotomy. **B,C.** Volar and dorsal fasciotomy, with edematous muscles bulging through fascial incisions.

- The mobile wad and dorsal compartment release is accomplished by placing a middorsal straight line incision beginning 3 to 4 cm proximal to the wrist crease and extending to the radial aspect of the flexion crease at the elbow (**TECH FIG 4C**).
- The compartmental fascia for both compartments are incised over their entire length and the muscles are examined.
- After release, the muscles should bulge out over the incision.
- The muscles are not débrided until a second-look procedure at 48 hours, because some muscles with questionable viability may recover after fascial release.
- The open wounds are packed with moist dressing until the second-look procedure.

Burn Débridement

- Burn débridement is performed without a tourniquet and can be carried out with escharotomy or fasciotomy.
- Sharp débridement is used to removed partial- and full-thickness burns.
  - For small areas or areas with irregular contour, a no. 15 or no. 10 blade is used to remove burnt tissue, layer by layer, until bleeding tissue is encountered.
  - For larger areas, a Weck blade with a no. 8 or no. 10 guard is used to tangentially remove burn tissue until punctate bleeding is encountered.

- For uncomplicated thermal burns, immediate coverage can be accomplished.
  - For uncomplicated wounds, a .012-inch split-thickness skin graft can be placed. We typically use unmeshed graft for the hand and over the wrist joint. Forearm burns can be covered with a graft meshed 1 to 1½ expansion.
  - For deeper wounds with small areas of exposed deep structures (eg, tendons or joints), a dermal substitute such as Integra is used to provide a revascularized dermal foundation. Delayed split-thickness skin grafting is done in 2 weeks.
- Large burn wounds with exposed deep structures or exposed neurovascular bundles are temporarily covered with moist dressing changes, and will require local flap, distant flap, or free tissue coverage within 48 to 72 hours.
- Electrical burns often have injuries to subcutaneous tissues and muscles in addition to cutaneous burns. After débridement of the cutaneous portion of the burns, as described in Burn Débridement, the subcutaneous tissue and muscles are sharply débrided with a no. 10 blade in a layered manner until bleeding tissue is encountered.
- Patients with electrical burns are managed with moist dressing changes and taken back to the operating room for a second look procedure in 48 hours.

SECOND-LOOK PROCEDURE

- The second-look procedure is performed without the use of a tourniquet.
- Necrotic tissues are aggressively débrided with a no. 10 blade in a tangential manner until bleeding tissue is encountered.

- Electrical burns may require multiple débridements every 48 hours until the area of injury is demarcated and all necrotic tissues are removed.
- Large wounds with exposed deep structures or exposed neurovascular structures are temporarily covered with

TECHNIQUES

moist dressing changes and will require local flap, distant flap, or free tissue transfer coverage within 48 to 72 hours.

■ For uncomplicated fasciotomy wounds, once adequate débridement has been achieved, moist dressing changes are performed for 7 to 14 days in preparation for primary closure or skin grafting.

■ With increasing frequency, a negative-pressure dressing is being used for fasciotomy defects as an alternative to traditional wound care.

■ Edema often subsides and allows for primary wound closure (**TECH FIG 5**).

■ Open defects are covered with a .012-inch split-thickness skin graft.

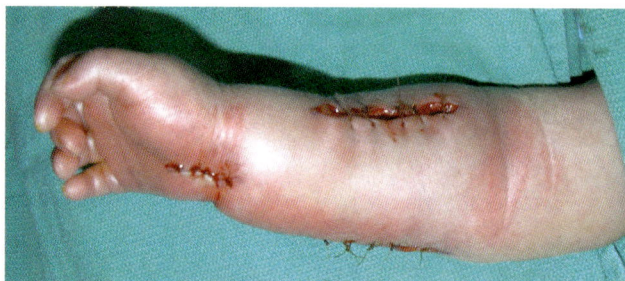

TECH FIG 5 • Immediate postoperative photograph of a forearm fasciotomy with carpal tunnel release. The skin has been loosely reapproximated.

LOCAL TISSUE REARRANGEMENT FOR RELEASE OF CONTRACTURE BANDS

Basic Z-Plasty

■ One or multiple Z-plasty flaps are used to break up mild to moderate linear contractures.

■ The central limb of the Z is planned along the axis of the scar band, and the angle of the Z-plasty can be varied, with a larger angle providing more release. We prefer 45-degree flaps (**TECH FIG 6A**).

■ The Z-plasty flaps are elevated just below the dermis, preserving a small cuff of subcutaneous fat on the underside of the flaps.

■ Foreshortened fibrous bands that require release with scissors or a knife often are present in the underlying soft tissue.

■ Care is taken to protect the neurovascular bundle.

■ After release of underlying tissue and extension of the joint, the Z-plasty flaps should fall naturally into a transposed position.

■ The flaps are sutured in place with nonabsorbable sutures (**TECH FIG 6B**).

■ Xeroform (Covidien, Mansfield, MA) strips and bacitracin are applied to the incision, followed by a gauze dressing. A gentle elastic bandage is applied.

■ The bandage is removed in 2 days, and patients are allowed progressive gentle range of motion. Stretching and scar massage are encouraged to begin 2 to 3 weeks postoperatively.

Five-Flap Z-Plasty for Release of Web Space Contractures

■ The central limb of the five-flap Z-plasty is designed to lie on the axis of the web space contracture.

■ The Z-plasty is oriented with the Y-to-V flap occupying normal skin, to maximize advancement of unburned skin into scar tissue (**TECH FIG 7**).

■ Skin incisions are made in the central limb as well as the Y-to-V flap. The lateral limbs of the Z-plasty flaps are not incised initially.

■ The Y-to-V flaps and the skin around the central limb are elevated just below the dermal fat junction.

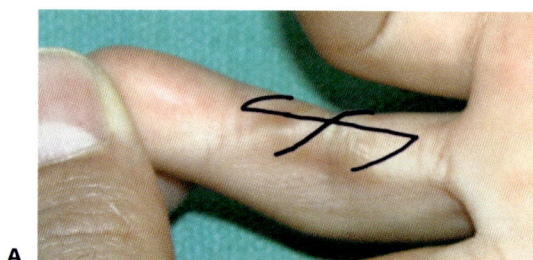
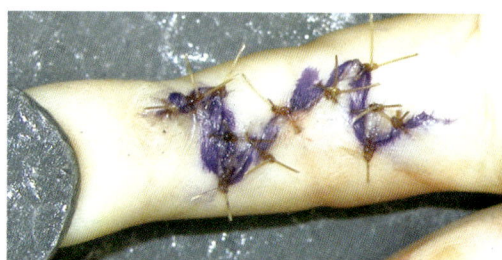

TECH FIG 6 • **A.** Design of two Z-plasty flaps for release of a flexion contracture. **B.** Same flexion contracture after release and flap transposition.

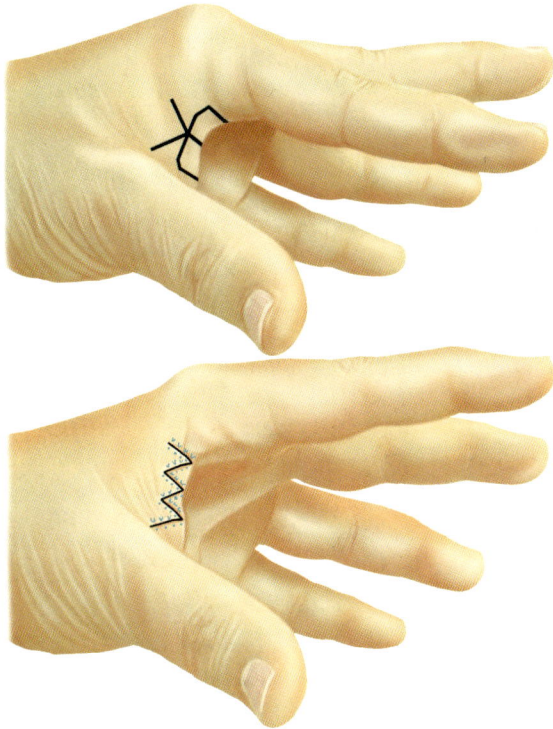

TECH FIG 7 • Design of a five-flap Z-plasty for release of a first web space contracture.

- The underlying fibrous tissues are released using a combination of blunt and sharp dissection.
- At this point, the Y-to-V flap is advanced into place.
- More advancement can be achieved by lengthening the Y-to-V limbs and enlarging the flap. The central limb is lengthened accordingly. Flap size is limited by the size of the web space.
- The lateral limbs of the Z-plasty flaps are now incised corresponding to the length of the enlarged Y-to-V flap (now a V-flap).
- The flaps are then secured in their transposed position with nonabsorbable sutures.
- Xeroform and bacitracin are applied, followed by gauze dressing and a gentle elastic bandage.
- The bandage is removed in 2 days, and the patient is allowed progressive gentle range of motion. Stretching and scar massage are encouraged to begin 2 to 3 weeks postoperatively.

Groin Flap for Extensive Burn Contracture

Scar Excision

- An incision is made around the contracted scar into the subcutaneous fat and underlying structures. Often, the scar is adherent to underlying fascia, tendons, and joints.
- Traction is applied to assist in identifying the areolar plane between scar and normal tissue.
- The scar is lifted in its entirety. Tight underlying fibrous bands are broken up with blunt and sharp dissection.

- After complete excision of the scar, the affected joints are put under stretched to evaluate the need for capsulotomy or ligamentous release.

Flap Harvest

- Attention is then paid to harvest of the ipsilateral groin flap.
- Doppler ultrasound is used to identify the superficial circumflex iliac artery.
- At the ipsilateral groin, a line between the anterior superior iliac spine (ASIS) and pubic tubercle is drawn, identifying the inguinal ligament. A second parallel line is drawn 2 to 3 cm below as the midaxis of the flap, which should correspond to the course of the superficial circumflex iliac artery.
- Using a pattern of the defect, a flap is designed inferior to the ASIS to lie along the previously marked midaxis. If necessary, the flap can be extended lateral to the ASIS for additional length (**TECH FIG 8A**).
- A flap up to 20 × 10 cm can be closed primarily and is sufficient for most hand and wrist defects.
- It is important to keep in mind that a small portion of the flap will be tubularized near the pedicle and will have to be included in the design.
- The flap is oriented to minimize kinking and twisting of the pedicle after inset.
- The flap is incised down to the underlying fascia. Inferiorly, the fascia lata and sartorius muscle fascia are identified.
- The flap is elevated tangentially off the fascia in a lateral-to-medial fashion until the lateral aspect of the sartorius fascia is encountered (**TECH FIG 8B**).
- The sartorius fascia is incised at its lateral margin and elevated from the underlying muscle, with care taken to avoid injuring the lateral femoral cutaneous nerve.
- At this point, scissor dissection is used to identify the vascular pedicle as it traverses out of the femoral triangle and through the sartorius fascia.
- A cuff of sartorius fascia is incised superior and inferior to the pedicle to untether the pedicle from the muscle (see Tech Fig 8B).
- The proximal portion of the flap is tubularized around the pedicle.
- The donor defect is closed primarily. The standing cutaneous deformity at the lateral aspect is excised. A small open area may be left at the base of the flap.

Completion of the Groin Flap

- The flap is gently thinned along the margins.
- The defect is then brought into the field, and the flap is inset using nonabsorbable sutures (**TECH FIG 8C**).
- The forearm is then secured to the abdominal skin with several large nonabsorbable sutures.
- Xeroform and bacitracin are applied, followed by fluffed gauze dressing.
- An elastic bandage is wrapped around the hip to further stabilize the reconstruction.
- Members of the surgical team must be present at the time of recovery from anesthesia to mitigate the chance of accidental flap avulsion.

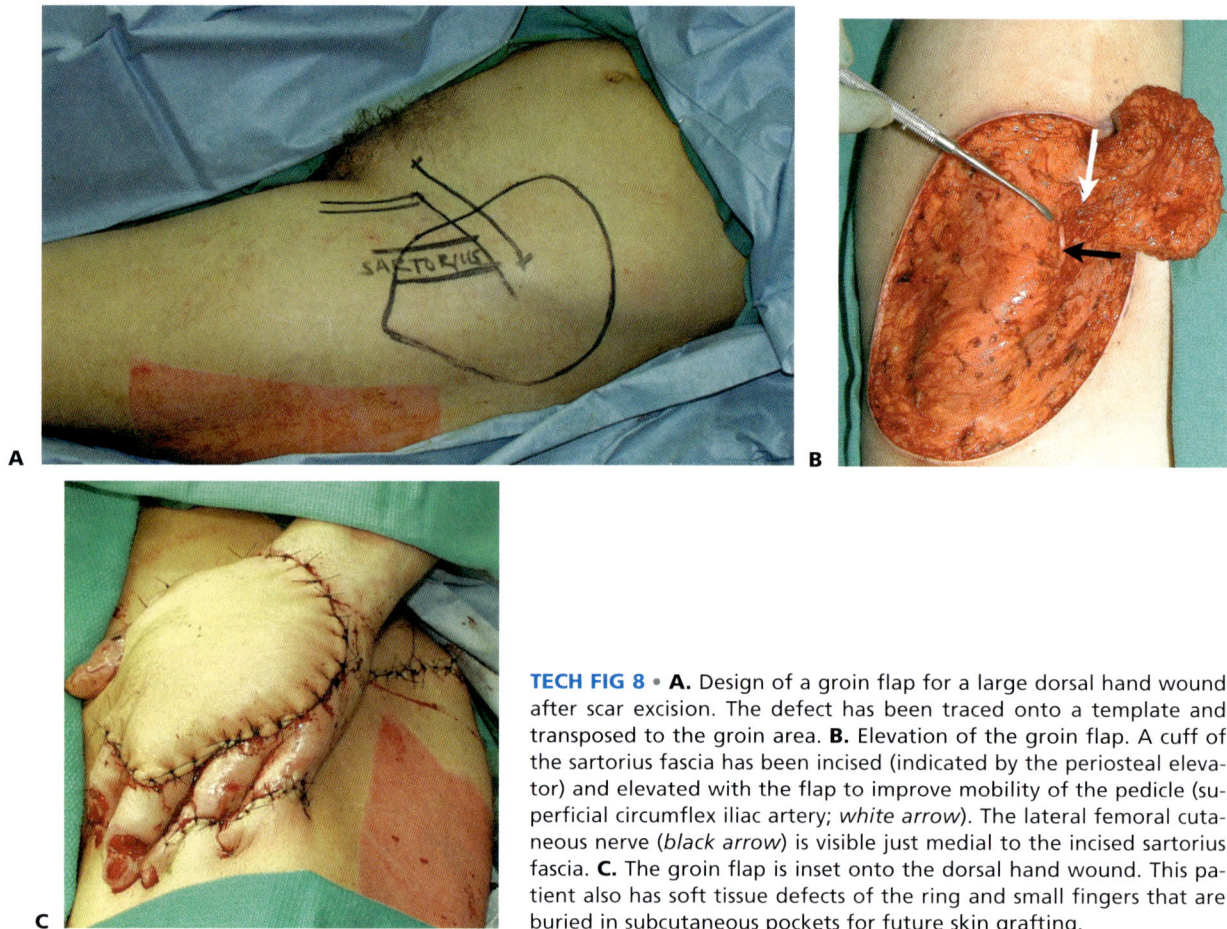

TECH FIG 8 • A. Design of a groin flap for a large dorsal hand wound after scar excision. The defect has been traced onto a template and transposed to the groin area. **B.** Elevation of the groin flap. A cuff of the sartorius fascia has been incised (indicated by the periosteal elevator) and elevated with the flap to improve mobility of the pedicle (superficial circumflex iliac artery; *white arrow*). The lateral femoral cutaneous nerve (*black arrow*) is visible just medial to the incised sartorius fascia. **C.** The groin flap is inset onto the dorsal hand wound. This patient also has soft tissue defects of the ring and small fingers that are buried in subcutaneous pockets for future skin grafting.

PEARLS AND PITFALLS

Fasciotomy and escharotomy	▪ Blood products should be made available before escharotomy, because significant bleeding can occur. ▪ Early recognition and intervention for compartment syndrome are key to prevent irreversible damage, and the threshold for pressure measurement should be low. ▪ The patient must be monitored closely after the procedure for evidence of inadequate release, especially with ongoing resuscitation.
Web space release	▪ The Y-to-V advancement of the five-flap Z-plasty provides most of the elongation. ▪ The five-flap Z-plasty should be designed to maximize the amount of unburned tissue in the Y-to-V flap.
Groin flap	▪ Flap orientation must be carefully designed. ▪ A template of the upper extremity defect can be made with an extension to simulate the pedicle to test various flap configurations and orientations. ▪ Postoperative congestion or ischemia is likely, secondary to kinking of the pedicle, and should resolve with proper positioning of the arm.

POSTOPERATIVE CARE

▪ After acute burn and wound management, the affected upper extremity will require appropriate splinting (intrinsic-plus with thumb in palmar abduction), elevation, and early range of motion to prevent secondary complications.

▪ A soft dressing consisting of gauze and an elastic bandage is applied after scar release and local tissue rearrangement. Sutures are removed in 2 weeks.

▪ Early mobilization and therapy are initiated about 2 weeks postoperatively to maintain release.

▪ Abduction or extension splints may be used at night to maintain posture.

▪ Upon completion of the groin flap, elastic bandages are used to strap the arm to the torso for 3 to 4 days. Care is taken to avoid kinking of the pedicle.

▪ During the immediate postoperative period, the flap is monitored for arterial insufficiency or congestion. A kinked pedicle necessitates repositioning of hand or patient. Suture release near the pedicle may be needed for congestion.

- If present, the small open area at the base of the flap is cared for with daily Xeroform dressing changes.
- Range-of-motion exercises for the nonaffected joint can start immediately postoperatively. Exercises for the affected joints can resume 2 weeks postoperatively.
- Before flap division, the pedicle is gently occluded to check for viability.
- The flap is divided, thinned, and inset 3 to 4 weeks after the index procedure.

OUTCOMES

- When adequately done, the outcome after fasciotomy, in any location, is closely related to its timing. In fasciotomy performed within 12 hours of onset of compartment syndrome, normal function has been reported in 68% of patients. The number decreases sharply, to 8%, if fasciotomy is delayed beyond 12 hours.[10]
- Approximately 30% of fasciotomy wounds can be closed primarily. The rest require skin grafting.[2]
- Several articles describing various local tissue rearrangement procedures for contracture release document low complication rates and good results.
- Our experience agrees with published series that pedicled groin flaps provide stable soft tissue coverage of upper extremity defects with low complication rates.

COMPLICATIONS

- Complications for escharotomy and fasciotomy include:
  - Bleeding
  - Inadequate release
- Complications for local tissue rearrangement for contracture release include:
  - Partial skin necrosis
  - Dehiscence

- Recurrence
- Injury to neurovascular bundle
- Complications for groin flap include:
  - Flap necrosis
  - Avulsion
  - Excessive bulk requiring revisions

REFERENCES

1. Beasley RW. Secondary repair of burned hands. Clin Plast Surg 1981; 8:141–162.
2. Dente CJ, Feliciano DV, Rozycki GS, et al. A review of upper extremity fasciotomies in a level I trauma center. Am Surg 2004;70:1088–1093.
3. Esselman PC, Thombs BD, Magyar-Russell G, et al. Burn rehabilitation: State of the science. Am J Phys Med Rehabil 2006;85:383–413.
4. Graham TJ, Stern PJ, True MS. Classification and treatment of postburn metacarpophalangeal joint extension contractures in children. J Hand Surg Am 1990;15:450–456.
5. Hargens AR, Romine JS, Sipe JC, et al. Peripheral nerve-conduction block by high muscle-compartment pressure. J Bone Joint Surg Am 1979;61A:192–200.
6. Larson DL, Abston S, Willis B, et al. Contracture and scar formation in the burn patient. Clin Plast Surg 1974;1:653–666.
7. Lee RC, Zhang D, Hannig J. Biophysical injury mechanism in electrical shock trauma. Annu Rev Biomed Eng 2000;2:477–509.
8. Matsen FA III. Compartmental syndrome: an unified concept. Clin Orthop Relat Res 1975;113:8–14.
9. Mubarak SJ, Owen CA, Hargens AR, et al. Acute compartment syndromes: Diagnosis and treatment with the aid of the wick catheter. J Bone Joint Surg Am 1978;60:1091–1095.
10. Sheridan GW, Matsen FA 3rd. Fasciotomy in the treatment of the acute compartment syndrome. J Bone Joint Surg Am 1976;58:112–115.
11. Stern PJ, Neale HW, et al. Classification and treatment of postburn proximal interphalangeal joint flexion contractures in children. J Hand Surg Am 1987;12:450–457.
12. von Volkmann R. Ischaemic muscle paralyses and contractures. Clin Orthop Relat Res 1967;50:5–6.

Chapter 108

Release of Posttraumatic Metacarpophalangeal and Proximal Interphalangeal Joint Contractures

Christopher L. Forthman and Keith A. Segalman

DEFINITION

- Post-traumatic metacarpophalangeal (MCP) joint and proximal interphalangeal (PIP) contractures may develop directly as a result of injury to the joints and adjacent tissues or indirectly as a result of excessive immobilization or poor splinting of the hand.
- The circumstances precipitating the contracture determine the structures most involved:
  - Joint capsule and collateral ligament contracture
  - Flexor tendon adhesions
  - Intrinsic musculature contracture
  - Extensor tendon adhesions
  - Skin and subcutaneous tissue scarring
- The MCP joint generally becomes stiff in the extended position. Flexion contractures are uncommon and, when present, generally do not cause significant disability.
- The PIP joint often becomes contracted in the flexed position, although extension and combined contractures are not uncommon.
- The key to successfully mobilizing a stiff MCP or PIP joint is anticipating the pathologic causes before surgery.

ANATOMY

- MCP joint osteology allows biaxial motion, including circumduction. The articular surface of the metacarpal head is asymmetrical, with a relatively flat mediolateral convex arc (abduction–adduction) and a large anteroposterior convex arc (flexion–extension) that extends more volarly (**FIG 1A**).
- The MCP joint is enveloped by a relatively loose capsule inserting onto ridges surrounding the articular cartilage.
- Proper collateral ligaments originate from a dorsolateral tubercle on the metacarpal head and insert on the lateropalmar edge of the phalangeal base (**FIG 1B**).
- The volar plate of the MCP joint is an extension of the phalangeal articular surface. Unlike the volar plate of the PIP joint, the volar plate of the MCP joint is collapsible and there is little tendency to produce check reins.
  - This is one reason why MCP joint flexion contractures are much less common than those in the PIP joint.
- The flexor and extensor mechanisms surround the MCP joint.
  - Volarly, the flexor sheath lies directly on the palmar plate and is thick, forming the first annular pulley.
  - Dorsally, the extensor tendon gives rise to fibroaponeurotic sagittal bands that wrap around to insert on the palmar plate. The tendons of the lumbricals and interossei join the dorsal expansion of the extensor. A slip of the dorsal interossei inserts on the dorsolateral aspect of the phalangeal base.
- The PIP joint is stabilized by a boxlike arrangement of structures consisting of the proper and accessory collateral ligaments, the volar plate, and the dorsal capsule (**FIG 1C,D**).

PATHOGENESIS

- The irregular contour of the MCP joint functions as a cam, transforming joint flexion into translation (or elongation) of the collateral ligaments. When flexed, the MCP joint has minimal capsular volume and is maximally constrained. Conversely, extension allows maximal capsular volume and joint laxity.
- Direct trauma to the MCP joint causes joint effusions and hemarthrosis. Hand trauma elsewhere results in edema, which also collects within the MCP joints. In both cases, as the capsule fills with fluid the MCP joint is hydraulically pushed into a nearly fully extended position.
- With time the dorsal capsule becomes thick and noncompliant, leading to an extension contracture. The overlying extensor mechanism may become adherent to the capsule. The underlying collateral ligaments shorten and scar laterally to the metacarpal head. The volar recess may fill with adhesions between the volar plate and condyles.
- The extended MCP joint increases flexor tone and relaxes the extensor mechanism, leading to interphalangeal joint flexion, and may *indirectly* result in a fixed flexion contracture of the PIP joint.
  - The combination of extended MCP joints and flexed interphalangeal joints defines the intrinsic-minus hand.
- Injury, infection, excess immobilization, and inappropriate splinting may *directly* result in fixed flexion or extension contracture of the PIP joint.
  - An accumulation of fluid or blood within the capsule leads to stiffness, as does articular damage.
- Curtis[3,4] has reported that a contracture of the PIP joint can be due to:
  - Contracture of the volar plate or the capsular structures
  - Collateral ligament contracture
  - Scar contracture over the joint
  - Volar skin contracture
  - Flexor sheath contracture
  - Extensor tendon contracture or adhesions
  - Interosseous contracture or adhesions
  - A bony block or exostosis
- Additional causes not pertinent to this chapter include fascia contracture, as in Dupuytren disease.
- Watson et al[11] reported that a flexion contracture of the PIP joint is due to contracture of the check reins on the proximal surface of the volar plate.

NATURAL HISTORY

- Longstanding scarring and contracture of the MCP or PIP joint capsule almost invariably leads to adhesions to the adjacent extensor mechanism.
- Residual joint kinetics is often altered with joint motion occurring through incongruous articular motions such as pivoting.

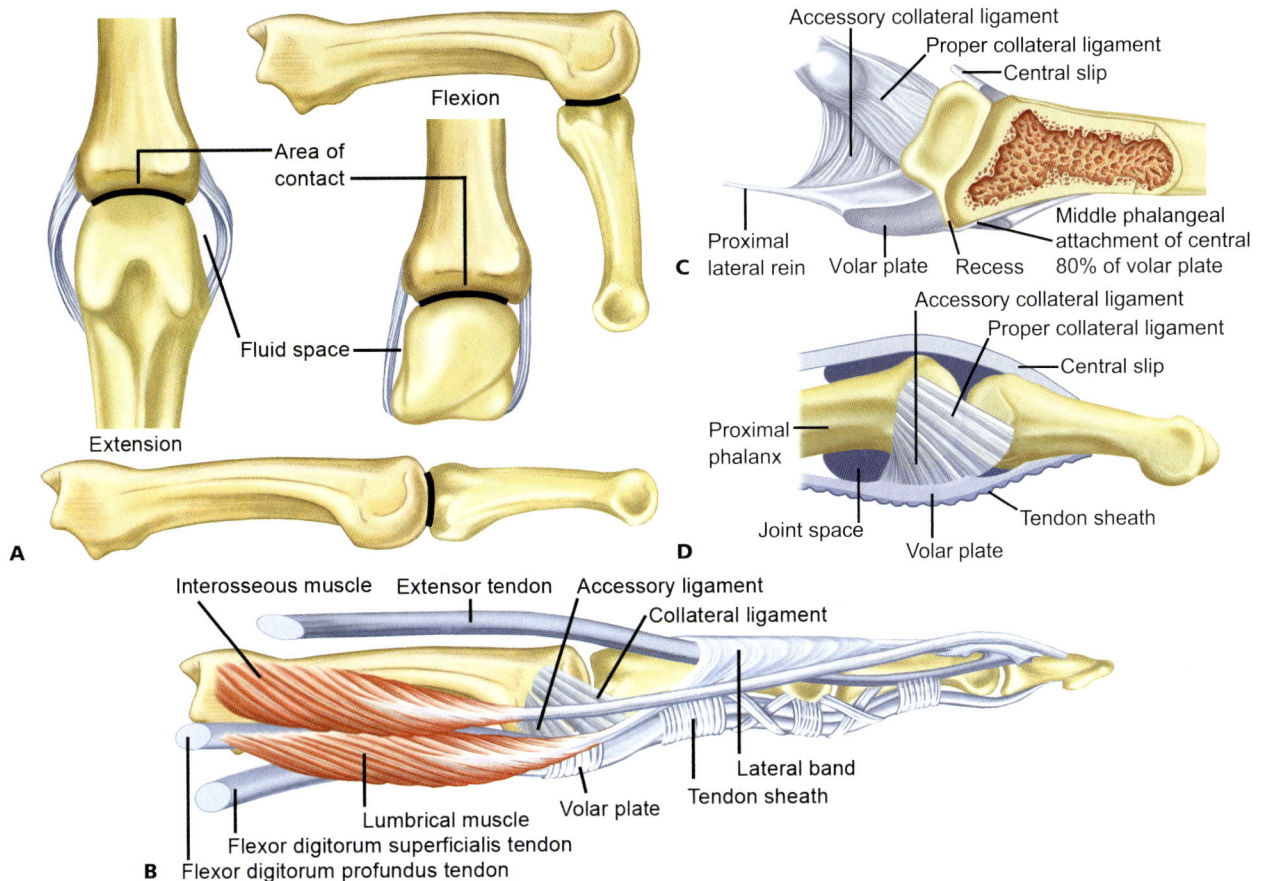

FIG 1 • A. The articular surface of the metacarpal head protrudes volarly, making the capsule (and proper collateral ligaments) taut with flexion. **B.** Metacarpophalangeal joint anatomy can be considered in two layers: the capsule and collateral ligaments, which lie immediately adjacent to the articular surfaces, and the flexor and extensor mechanisms, which envelop the joint. **C.** Normal anatomy of the proximal interphalangeal joint showing the arrangement of the collateral ligaments and the volar plate. **D.** Normal proximal interphalangeal anatomy showing the arrangement of the proper and accessory collateral ligaments.

■ Cartilage gradually atrophies and softens with disuse. Surface irregularities may develop.

PATIENT HISTORY AND PHYSICAL FINDINGS

■ The history should identify:
  ■ The inciting cause of the joint contracture
  ■ The time of the insult
  ■ Efforts made to mobilize the digit
■ The hand is evaluated for edema and the return of normal skin creases.
  ■ Ongoing swelling and inflammation (**FIG 2A**) must subside before surgery.
■ The dorsal soft tissues are assessed for mobility and compliance.
  ■ Capsulectomy after burns and crush injuries may fail due to inadequate dorsal coverage.
  ■ Skin contracture can also be an original inciting cause for digital stiffness.
■ The MCP and interphalangeal joints are assessed for differences in active and passive motion. Passive motion is always greater than active; however, a large difference suggests extrinsic tendon adhesions.
■ Bunnell intrinsic tightness test: Intrinsic release may be necessary to mobilize a PIP joint with extension contracture.

■ Finger threshold sensitivity is checked, along with overall sensitivity to percussion and cold. Vascularity is assessed by checking capillary refill. The painful and insensate stiff finger may be a better candidate for amputation than capsulectomy. Poor vascularity is a relative contraindication to capsulectomy.
■ Concomitant PIP flexion and distal interphalangeal hyperextension mark a boutonnière deformity (**FIG 2B**), whereas hyperextension at the PIP joint is a sign of a swan-neck deformity (**FIG 2C**).

IMAGING AND OTHER DIAGNOSTIC STUDIES

■ Plain radiographs of the hand are made to evaluate for extrinsic and intrinsic causes of joint stiffness.
  ■ Extrinsic
    ▪ Metacarpal neck or shaft fracture: Extensor tendon adhesions at the fracture site may restrict MCP joint flexion (passive and active).
    ▪ Proximal phalangeal fracture: Flexor and extensor tendon adhesions at the fracture site may limit active PIP (and sometime MCP) joint motion; passive motion may be maintained.
  ■ Intrinsic
    ▪ Intra-articular fracture: Articular incongruity may serve as a bony restraint to joint motion.

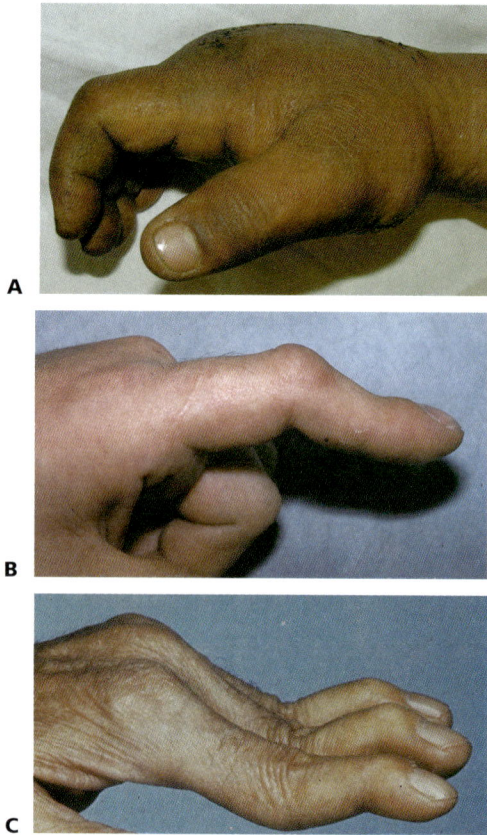

FIG 2 • A. Swollen hand. **B.** Boutonnière deformity. **C.** Swan-neck deformity.

- Arthritic changes: Cartilage softening and erosion often result in some degree of radiographically apparent arthritis.
- A "true" lateral radiograph of the involved joint must be closely examined for significant arthritic changes or any subluxation.
- There is little role for CT scanning or MRI of the digits.

DIFFERENTIAL DIAGNOSIS

- MCP extension contracture from extrinsic extensor muscle spasticity or intrinsic muscle paralysis or denervation
- PIP contracture from tendon imbalances, including boutonnière deformity and swan-neck deformity
- Skin contracture
- Dupuytren disease

NONOPERATIVE MANAGEMENT

- Nonoperative efforts to improve joint motion must be tried until motion has plateaued and the soft tissues are absolutely quiescent.
- As a general rule, inflammation and edema will subside and range of motion will improve for a minimum of 3 to 4 months after a traumatic or surgical insult to the hand.
- During this time a supervised hand therapy program is essential.
  - Most MCP contractures occur in extension. In addition to regular exercises, dynamic flexion splints (daytime) and static extension splints (nighttime) are useful.

- Most PIP contractures occur in flexion. Treatment begins with application of a nonelastic extension force across the PIP joint for an extended time. This can be done with serial finger casts or commercially available splints such as the Joint-Jack (Joint-Jack Company, Wetherfield, CT) or wire-foam splints. Once the contracture is corrected, elastic splints such as the Joint-Spring or clock-spring splints can be used.
- Prosser[8] presented one of the few studies to follow patients treated conservatively. Using a Capener splint to be worn for 8 to 12 hours per day over an 8-week period, there was an average improvement in the flexion contracture from 39 to 21 degrees. There was no association between time in the splint with final extension or with final stiffness.
- PIP extension contractures are treated conservatively with serial static splints such as a joint-strap system.
  - Curtis[3,4] has reported that these joints do not require surgery if the joint can be passively flexed more than 75 degrees.
  - The only study in the literature on the results of conservative treatment comes from Weeks et al.[12] In a review of 212 patients with 415 stiff PIP joints, 87% responded favorably to nonoperative treatment. The average improvement in total active motion was 36 degrees.

SURGICAL MANAGEMENT

- A capsulectomy is indicated only for a contracture not associated with articular incongruity or persistent subluxation of the joint.
- A stiff MCP or PIP joint in the face of articular incongruity or subluxation is best treated as an arthritic joint with a salvage type of surgery such as arthroplasty or arthrodesis.
  - Mild to moderate joint wear is not a contraindication to capsulectomy, particularly in younger patients. Focal areas of articular cartilage irregularity and dorsal osteophytes may be débrided at the time of surgery.
- The literature does not give any specifics as to when to recommend surgery. We usually make this decision when a "functional arc of motion" has not been achieved after 3 months of therapy.
- There is no absolute functional arc of motion for the MCP joint. In the absence of interphalangeal contractures, we have found that index, middle, ring, and small finger MCP flexion of 30, 35, 40, and 45 degrees, respectively, is generally satisfactory. When the interphalangeal joints have limited flexion, greater degrees of MCP flexion may be useful.
- Similarly, 45 degrees or more of total PIP motion is usually satisfactory. Flexion contractures greater than 45 degrees are poorly tolerated and may benefit from surgical release.
  - Extreme flexion contractures (more than 60 or 70 degrees) may be best managed with arthrodesis.
  - Extension contractures are better tolerated, especially if there is flexion to at least 75 degrees.
- When a patient has exhausted nonoperative management options and joint stiffness exceeds the preceding guidelines, surgery for contracture release is considered.

Preoperative Planning

- The patient is required to demonstrate a commitment to therapy before surgery is undertaken. A preoperative meeting between the patient and the therapist is arranged to plan the first postoperative visit and to fabricate a dynamic flexion splint.

- If possible, surgery is planned under a form of anesthesia that will allow patient cooperation and active motion during the procedure.
  - A wrist block with sedation is optimal; however, a Bier block may be used and reversed with deflation of the tourniquet.
- In severely scarred hands (eg, massive crush injuries and burn patients), the surgeon must anticipate inadequate dorsal soft tissue and extensor tendon excursion. A transverse incision and extensor tenotomy is indicated and coverage of the residual soft tissue defect is planned and discussed with the patient. Kirschner wire fixation of the MCP joints in flexion may be necessary to maintain a flexed joint and protect the dorsal soft tissue reconstruction.

Positioning

- Patients are positioned supine with the affected extremity on a hand table. A brachial tourniquet is applied that allows access to the forearm should a full-thickness skin graft be necessary.

Approach

- The approach for MCP contracture depends on three factors:
  - The number of involved MCP joints
  - The need to operate on the PIP joint
  - The quality of the dorsal soft tissues
- A single MCP joint is approached with a dorsal longitudinal incision. If the PIP joint has an extension contracture, the incision is carried over the PIP in the midline. If the PIP has a flexion contracture, the incision may be extended distally in the midaxial line (**FIG 3A**).
- Multiple MCP joint extension contractures are approached using separate dorsal longitudinal incisions.
  - This is the most extensile method and facilitates management of associated extensor tendon adhesions and PIP contractures (**FIG 3B**).
- Two adjacent MCP joints may also be approached by making a dorsal longitudinal incision centered in the web between affected rays.
  - If necessary, it is safe to extend this incision as a Y onto each digit to complete a tenolysis or operate on the PIP joints.
- Multiple MCP joints may be also approached by making a

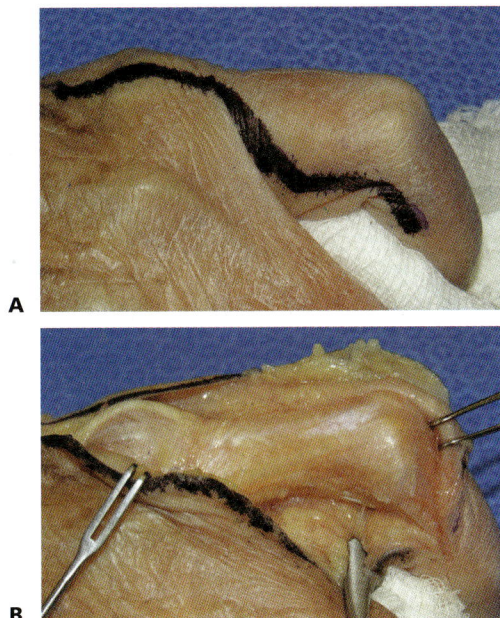

FIG 3 • **A.** A combined metacarpophalangeal extension contracture and proximal interphalangeal flexion contracture of the index finger is approached by extending the dorsal incision distally in the midaxial line. **B.** Excellent exposure of the finger extensor mechanism is coupled with visualization of the volar aspect of the proximal interphalangeal joint.

single transverse incision lying just proximal to the metacarpal heads.

- This approach is preferred only when the dorsal soft tissues are fibrotic and noncompliant. In this situation, the surgeon should plan for skin graft or flap coverage of the anticipated defect.
- The surgical approach for *isolated* PIP joint contractures varies with the procedure used.
  - A capsulectomy for a flexion contracture is performed through a lateral approach, a check-rein release through a volar approach, and percutaneous release laterally.
  - A dorsal skin incision could be used with a capsulectomy for an extension contracture or when there is a previous dorsal incision or specific hardware to remove.

MCP JOINT CONTRACTURES
Dorsal Capsulectomy of the Joint

- Make the skin incision based on the aforementioned considerations (**TECH FIG 1A**).
- Carry dissection down sharply to the extensor mechanism, preserving small dorsal nerves.
  - If the soft tissues about the MCP joint are excessively scarred, identify the extensor mechanism proximally and distally with careful development of soft tissue planes in between.
- Raise full-thickness soft tissue flaps over the length of the extensor mechanism (**TECH FIG 1B**).

- Use a Freer elevator to lyse adhesions beneath the extensor mechanism, especially over the metacarpal proximally (**TECH FIG 1C**).
- As described by Curtis[3,4] and later Tsuge,[10] the extensor tendon is bisected sharply over the MCP joint (**TECH FIG 1D**); the sagittal fibers are preserved. Do not carry the extensor split into the transverse fibers of the extensor hood.
  - In the index or small finger, the split is made between the extensor communis and the extensor proprius tendons.

TECHNIQUES

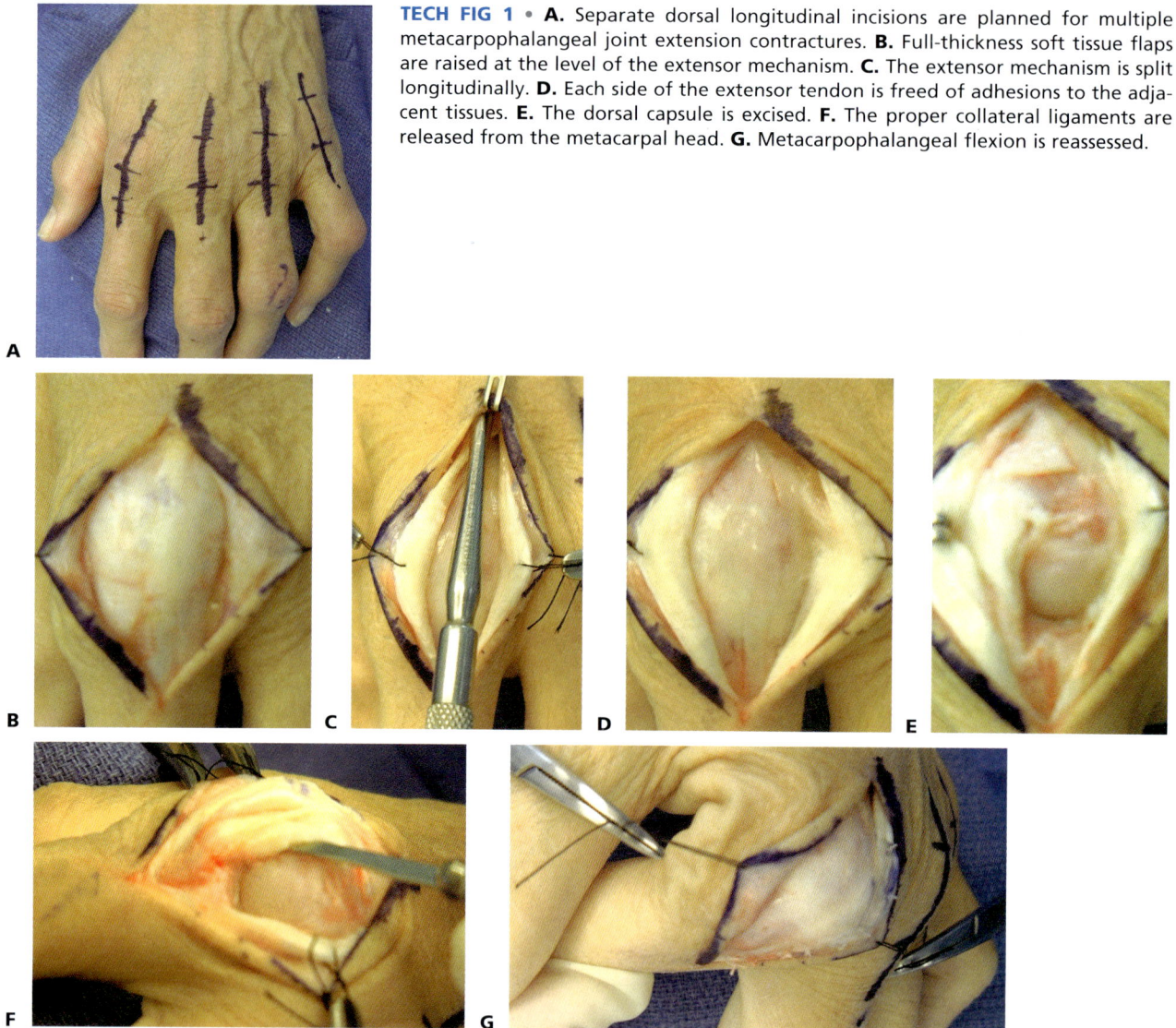

TECH FIG 1 • **A.** Separate dorsal longitudinal incisions are planned for multiple metacarpophalangeal joint extension contractures. **B.** Full-thickness soft tissue flaps are raised at the level of the extensor mechanism. **C.** The extensor mechanism is split longitudinally. **D.** Each side of the extensor tendon is freed of adhesions to the adjacent tissues. **E.** The dorsal capsule is excised. **F.** The proper collateral ligaments are released from the metacarpal head. **G.** Metacarpophalangeal flexion is reassessed.

- Retract each half of the extensor tendon and attached sagittal band to expose the joint capsule.
- At times it may be painstakingly difficult to develop the interval between the extensor mechanism and capsule, and a combination of both sharp and blunt dissection is necessary.
- The capsule is usually quite thick and generally should be excised rather than released (**TECH FIG 1E**).
- Attempt passive finger flexion; it usually is limited, necessitating release or excision of the collateral ligaments (**TECH FIG 1F**).
  - Start dorsally and release the proper collateral ligaments from the collateral recess and from any adhesions to the metacarpal head. Often, the collateral origin may be gently pried away from the metacarpal head with a Freer elevator.
  - Dense adhesions and excessively thick collateral ligament tissue may need to be incised at the metacarpal origin and removed.
- Reassess passive MCP flexion (**TECH FIG 1G**). If flexion remains inadequate or the joint "jumps" or "snaps"

when reaching full extension, then the accessory collaterals may need to be released as well.
  - The goal is an incremental collateral ligament release—enough to restore joint motion but not compromise stability, especially on the radial (pinch) side.
- Assess the volar recess and release any adhesions between the volar plate and condyle with a Freer elevator.
  - Failure to release the volar adhesion can result in joint "hinging" with dorsal gapping of the joint during flexion.
- The joint should now have a smooth arc of passive motion without any hinging during flexion or snapping into extension. Ninety degrees of flexion can usually be achieved.
- If the patient is under a wrist or Bier block anesthesia, check active flexion.
  - Alternatively, a short incision may be made on the volar ulnar aspect of the forearm and traction applied to the appropriate extrinsic flexor tendons.

TECHNIQUES

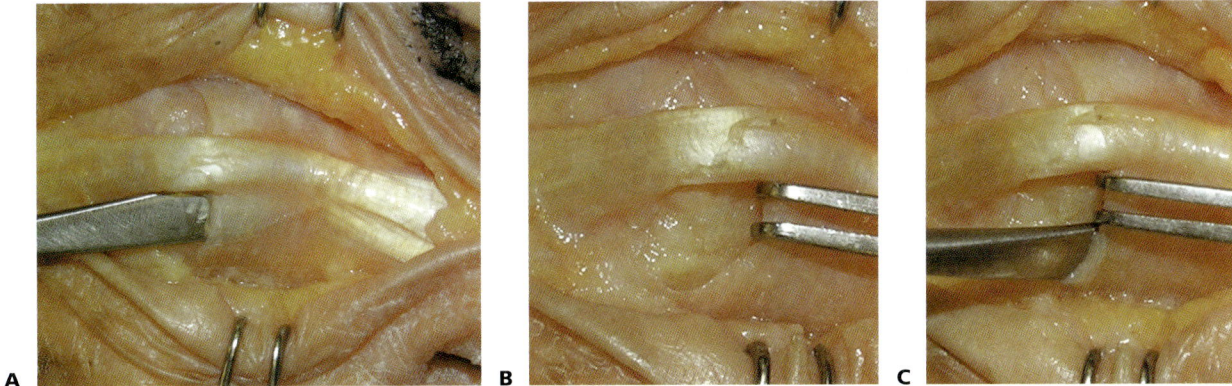

TECH FIG 2 • A–C. The wrist is located to the left and the finger to the right in each figure. **A.** The leading edges of the sagittal fibers are identified and liberated from the underlying dorsal capsule. **B.** Sagittal fibers are retracted distally and the capsule is incised transversely. **C.** A Freer elevator is used to release the proper collateral ligament origins.

- If active flexion is limited, consider performing a flexor tenolysis.
  - We prefer to release the flexor at the same sitting, although the tenolysis may be staged, emphasizing passive motion between surgeries.
- Release the tourniquet and achieve hemostasis with bipolar electrocautery.
- While keeping the MCP joint flexed, close the extensor mechanism with 4-0 interrupted inverted nonabsorbable braided suture and close the skin with nonabsorbable interrupted sutures.
- If bleeding from scar is excessive, then use a small rubber vascular loop or a quarter-inch Penrose drain to stent open the wound to allow drainage for the first 24 hours.
- A dorsal splint is applied to maintain the MCP joints in 70 degrees of flexion.

Limited Dorsal Capsulotomy of the MCP Joint

- In mild contractures, a dorsal capsulectomy may not be necessary. Bode and Gottlieb[1] have described a limited capsulotomy.
- Expose the extensor mechanism as described earlier (Tech Fig 1).
- Use a Freer elevator to release the extensor mechanism and sagittal bands from the dorsal capsule (**TECH FIG 2A**).

- Retract the dorsal capsule distally.
- Incise the capsule transversely at the distal dorsal aspect of the metacarpal head (**TECH FIG 2B**).
  - The incision extends from one collateral recess to the other.
- Using a Beaver blade or Freer elevator directed to the periphery of the capsulotomy, perform a stepwise release of the collateral ligaments off the metacarpal head (**TECH FIG 2C**).

Extensor Tenotomy of the MCP Joint

- In longstanding densely scarred multidigit MCP contractures, the extensor communis tendon may need to be tenotomized to achieve flexion (**TECH FIG 3A**).
- Make a tenotomy at the distal margin of the sagittal bands.
- Capsulectomy and collateral ligament release follow as described earlier.
- At closure, sew the proximal tendon to the sagittal bands; close the extensor hood upon itself in the midline dorsally.
- Given the chronicity of these contractures, consider temporary Kirschner wire fixation of the MCP joints in flexion (**TECH FIG 3B**).
  - Kirschner wire fixation is especially useful for protection of skin grafts or flaps when the dorsal soft tissues are deficient (**TECH FIG 3C**).

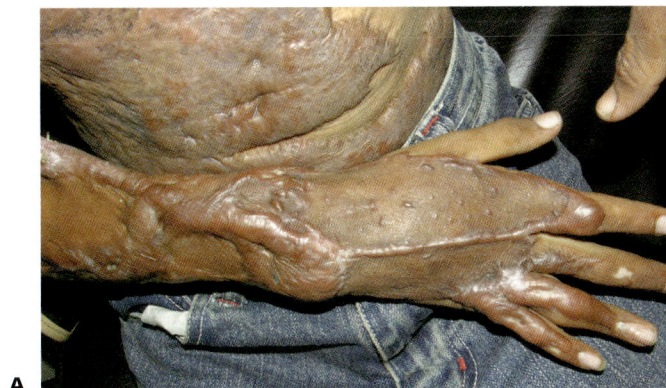

TECH FIG 3 • A. Release of metacarpophalangeal extension contractures in the severely burned hand is accomplished through a transverse skin incision and extensor tenotomy. *(continued)*

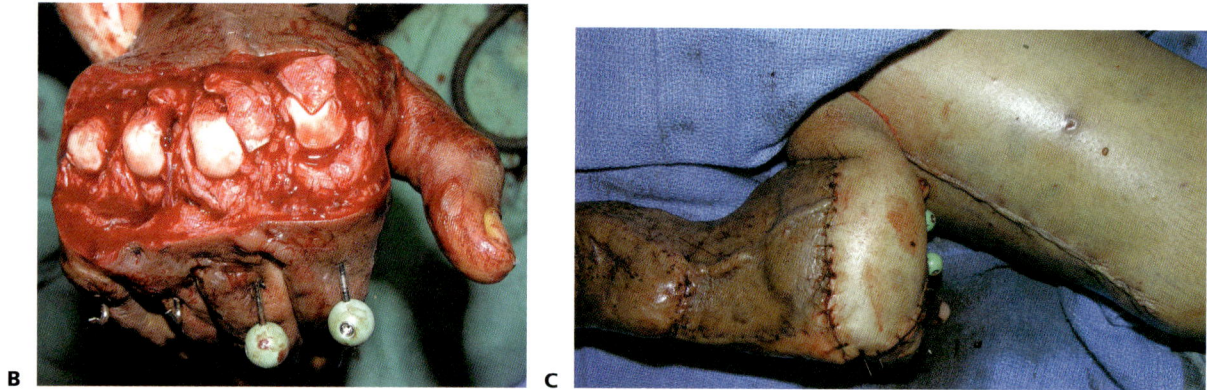

TECH FIG 3 • (continued) **B.** The metacarpophalangeal joints are maintained in flexion with Kirschner wires. **C.** The dorsal soft tissue defect is covered with a pedicled tensor fascia lata flap.

PIP JOINT CONTRACTURE

Capsulectomy for PIP Joint Flexion Contracture

- If there is an adequate skin envelope, the finger is approached through a midaxial incision (**TECH FIG 4A**).
- Make a radial incision centered over the PIP joint; it is usually 4 cm long.
- Retract the neurovascular structures volarly and protect them. Take care to preserve the dorsal branch of the digital nerve, which typically crosses the proximal aspect of the incision.
- Open the flexor sheath just distal to the A2 pulley.
    - Excise a segment of pulley if it is contracted.
- Perform a formal flexor tenolysis as necessary.

- If a more extensive tenolysis is required, the incision can be extended volarly over the flexor sheath. Take care to avoid injury to the digital nerve and artery that cross the operative field at the level of the web space.
- Excise a volar segment of collateral ligament (including the underlying capsule) using a no. 69 Beaver blade while carefully protecting the transverse retinacular fibers (**TECH FIG 4B**). Excise the entire accessory collateral ligament as necessary.
    - Isolate and preserve the transverse retinacular fibers by bluntly dissecting perpendicular to the fibers (**TECH FIG 4C**).
- Do not excise the volar plate (joint capsule), but expand the volar pouch by lifting the volar plate from the phalanges with a Freer elevator. Lengthen the interossei as needed.

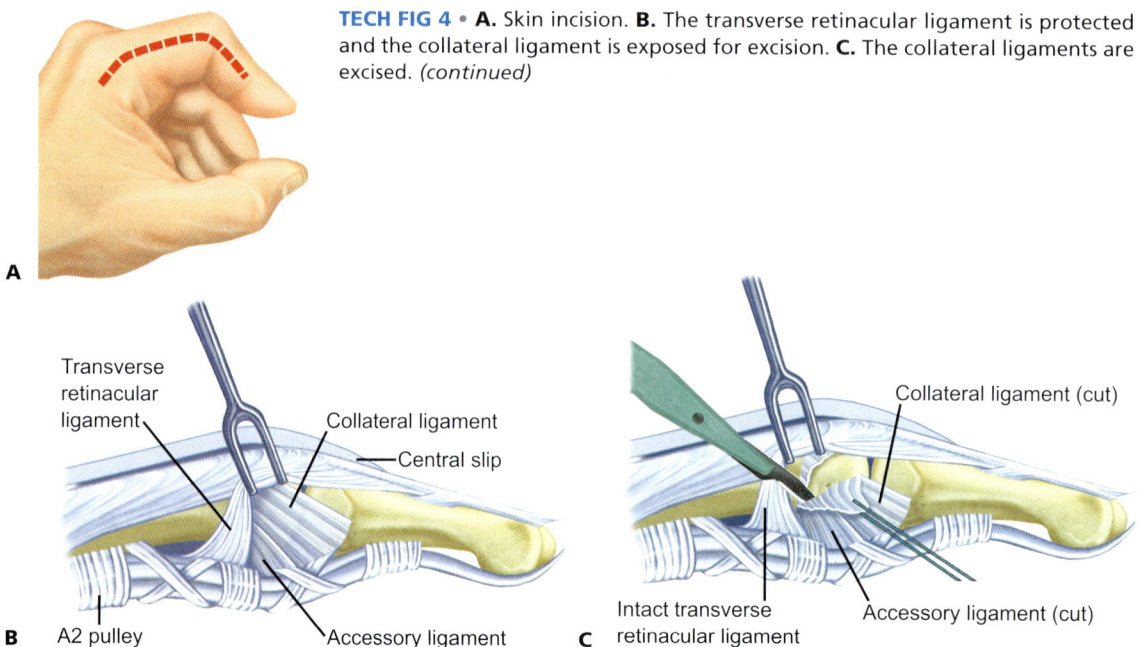

TECH FIG 4 • **A.** Skin incision. **B.** The transverse retinacular ligament is protected and the collateral ligament is exposed for excision. **C.** The collateral ligaments are excised. (continued)

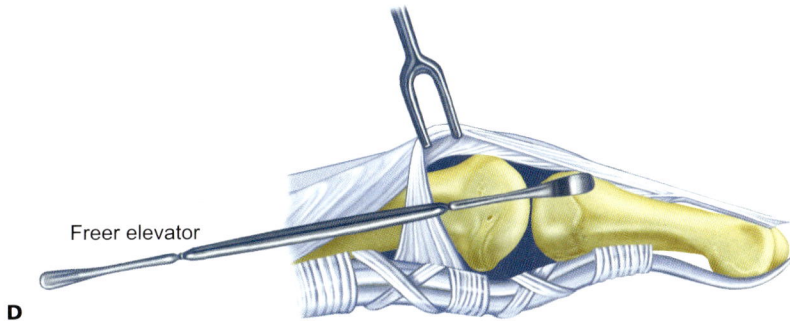

TECH FIG 4 • *(continued)* **D.** Extensor tenolysis is done if required.

- If there is still stiffness after completing the dissection on the radial side of the finger, then make a similar incision on the ulnar side of the digit.
- The ulnar incision is usually only 3 cm long, as the flexor and extensor tendon disorders have already been addressed. If there is concern that extensor tendon adhesions may limit active extension after release of the flexion contracture, then an extensor tenolysis is performed by elevating the dorsal skin. During the extensor tenolysis, protect the central slip insertion (**TECH FIG 4D**).
- A skin graft or local flap may be required if there is inadequate soft tissue coverage after joint mobilization.
  - If there is insufficient volar skin or unstable volar skin, then raise a cross-finger flap from the adjacent finger. When a cross-finger flap is used, make a transverse incision over the volar aspect of the PIP joint and extend it with a radial midaxial incision.
- Curtis[3,4] originally described pinning the joint in extension for 1 week, but most surgeons do not follow this recommendation.

Check-Rein Ligament Release for PIP Flexion Contracture

- According to Watson et al,[11] the volar plate does not flex but rather slides proximally and distally with flexion and extension. PIP joint adhesions causing contracture occur proximal to the volar plate and involve the check-rein ligaments.
  - Excision of the volar plate or division of the collateral ligaments is rarely required to achieve full extension.
- The joint is approached volarly, often with a V–Y incision to address palmar skin contracture.
- Open the theca between the A2 and A4 pulleys and retract the flexor tendons (**TECH FIG 5A**).
- Release the check-rein ligaments, preserving the nutrient vessel (**TECH FIG 5B**).
- If there is still a contracture after release of the check reins, release the dorsal portion of the collaterals or the oblique retinacular ligament of Landsmeer.
- This technique is helpful if a palmar exposure is required for excision of Dupuytren disease or during flexor tendon reconstruction.

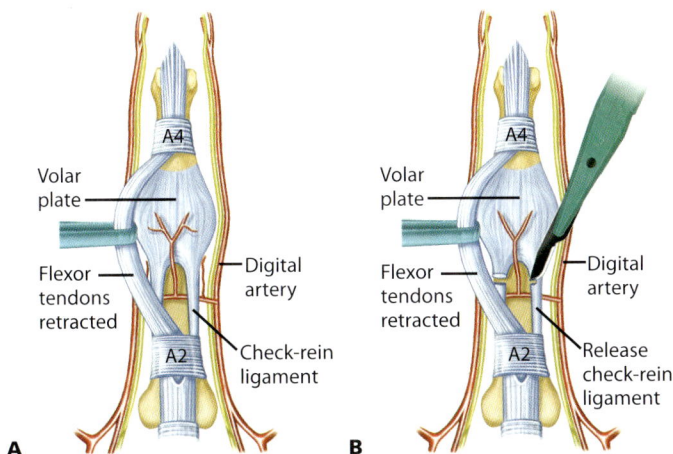

TECH FIG 5 • **A.** The flexor sheath is exposed and the check-rein ligament on the proximal edge of the volar plate is exposed. **B.** Watson's technique for release of the check-rein ligaments to correct a proximal interphalangeal flexion contracture.

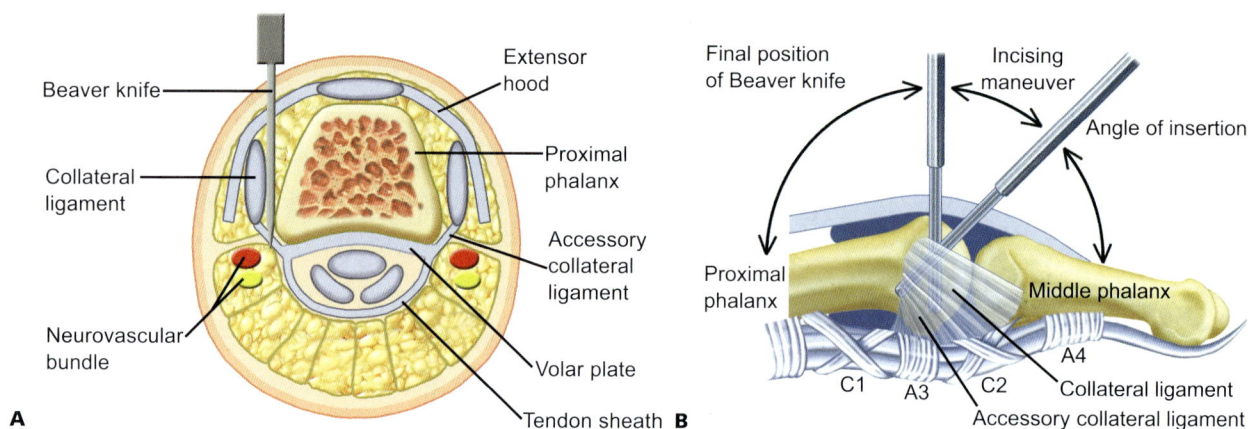

TECH FIG 6 • **A.** Cross-section shows placement of the no. 69 Beaver blade parallel to the proximal phalanx and adjacent to the proximal interphalangeal collateral ligament origin. **B.** Sagittal view demonstrates the technique of "sweeping" the Beaver blade and detaching the collateral ligament from its origin.

Percutaneous Collateral Ligament Release for PIP Flexion Contracture

- Stanley et al[9] described a percutaneous release of the collateral ligaments for persistent PIP flexion contractures.
- Place a no. 69 Beaver blade percutaneously adjacent to the proximal phalangeal head (**TECH FIG 6A**).
- Disinsert the proper collateral ligaments with a sweeping-type motion (**TECH FIG 6B**).
- Gently manipulate the finger into extension.

Use of an External Fixator for PIP Flexion Contracture

- Two types of distractors have been used.
  - Kasabian et al[7] described the use of a multiplanar distractor used for mandible reconstruction.
  - The use of a Digit Widget (Hand Biomechanics Lab, Inc., Sacramento, CA) has become popular (**TECH FIG 7**).

- An external frame is applied without any soft tissue release.
- The frame is left in place for about 6 weeks.
- There are no outcomes reported in the literature. In several of our patients we have noted initial favorable results followed by contracture recurrence.

Capsulectomy for PIP Joint Extension Contracture

- Make a dorsal curvilinear incision.
- Preserve the transverse retinacular ligament by blunt dissection and excise the proper collateral ligaments with a no. 69 Beaver blade as described earlier (**TECH FIG 8**).
- Perform a dorsal capsulectomy and an extensor tenolysis. If there is intrinsic tightness, perform a lengthening or release.

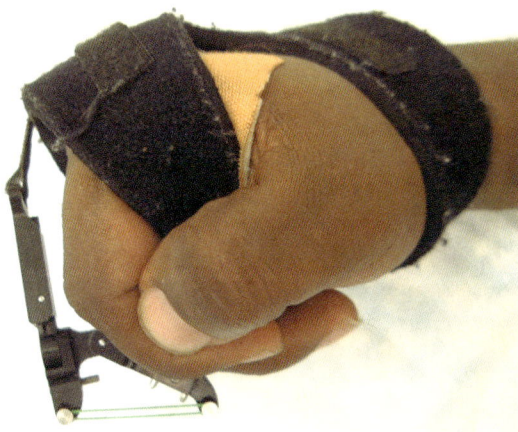

TECH FIG 7 • Application of the Digit Widget for proximal interphalangeal flexion contractures.

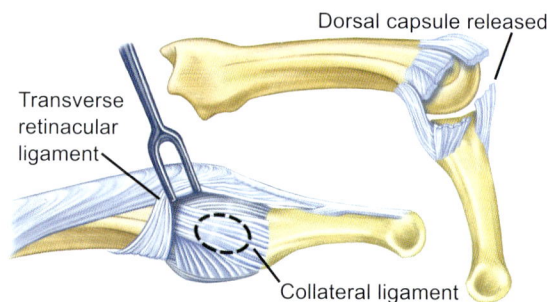

TECH FIG 8 • Through a dorsal incision, the transverse retinacular ligament is protected and the collateral ligament is excised. The dorsal capsule is also released.

PEARLS AND PITFALLS

MCP Joint	
Indications	■ The patient must have participated in a well-supervised rehabilitation protocol AND be committed to another 8 to 12 weeks of therapy.
Approach	■ A transverse skin incision is more likely to restrict flexion and more prone to breakdown in the postoperative period; however, a transverse skin incision facilitates soft tissue coverage of multiple MCP joints when operative release of the severely crushed or burned hand is undertaken.
Capsulectomy and collateral release	■ Adhesions between the volar plate and condyles may be responsible for limited flexion after release of the proper collateral ligaments. ■ Accessory collateral ligament release may be necessary to achieve full extension without catching.
Associated pathology	■ Intraoperative attempts at active flexion by the patient will identify associated flexor tendon adhesions in a surprisingly large number of patients. ■ Flexor tenolysis may be made by extending the dorsal incision in the midaxial line or by making a separate Brunner-type volar approach.
PIP Joint	
Persistent stiffness	■ Failure to recognize intrinsic contracture, inadequate skin envelope, flexor sheath contracture. Unrecognized reflex sympathetic dystrophy.
Postoperative instability	■ Failure to preserve transverse retinacular fibers or excessive release of the soft tissues
Preoperative flexion contracture more than 75 degrees	■ Consider an arthrodesis rather than soft tissue release.
Best patients for a release	■ Younger patient, without a crush injury, reflex sympathetic dystrophy, or revascularization. Preoperative flexion contracture of less than 43 degrees.

POSTOPERATIVE CARE

■ Patients are instructed in strict elevation until the first postoperative visit.

■ The wounds are assessed 48 to 72 hours after surgery and, if stable, immediate active-assisted range of motion is begun.

■ Wound care and edema control measures are also instituted. A nonadherent gauze should be applied until the wound is watertight. A Coban wrap and gauze finger sleeve limit swelling. Once the wound is healed, compression gloves or elastic finger sleeves further decrease swelling.

■ Therapy may quickly advance to include active and passive range of motion as the status of the extensor mechanism allows.

■ For MCP extension contractures:

■ Patients are maintained in a static splint full time to keep the MCP joints in 70 degrees of flexion. A daytime dynamic flexion splint is applied at about 1 week once the initial postoperative swelling has subsided (**FIG 4**).

■ If Kirschner wire fixation was performed, then only interphalangeal joint motion is begun immediately and MCP therapy is delayed until wire removal at 7 to 10 days.

■ Patients are reassessed 2 to 3 weeks after surgery. If there is a significant extensor lag (as may follow an extensive extensor tenolysis), a dynamic extension splint can be alternated with the dynamic flexion splint during the day.

■ Nighttime static splinting is continued for a minimum of 6 to 8 weeks.

■ Therapy is usually continued for about 3 months.

■ PIP release often benefits from early dynamic splinting during the day and passive splinting at night.

OUTCOMES

■ Final motion is often much less than that obtained at surgery but often makes a substantial difference in hand function.

■ Motion plateaus 3 to 6 months after surgery.

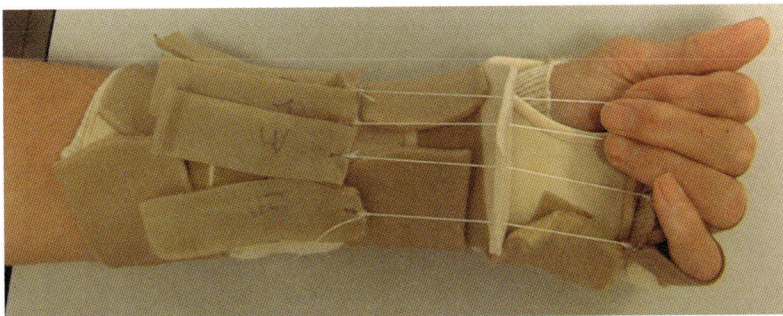

FIG 4 • Dynamic flexion splinting is instituted after surgery for correction of metacarpophalangeal joint extension contracture.

■ Results are best when the joint can be mobilized with capsulectomy alone. Each additional procedure, such as tenolysis, increases postoperative swelling and scar formation, limiting long-term gains.[4]

■ In some cases, an improvement in MCP or PIP joint motion of 30 to 45 degrees is a reasonable expectation.[2,13]

■ According to Gould and Nicholson,[6] improvement in MCP and PIP motion depends on the cause of the contracture. In a study of 105 MCP capsulectomies and 112 PIP capsulectomies, patients with direct joint trauma (fractures or crush injuries) gained an average of about 20 degrees of active motion, slightly more for the MCP and less for the PIP. Patients with indirect causes of capsular contracture (nerve injury, stroke, or skin burns) did better.

■ Ghidella et al[5] reported on the results of 68 PIP capsulectomies. The average overall improvement was a disappointing 7 degrees. The best results occurred in young patients without a history of crush injury, pain syndrome, or revascularization. The average improvement measured 17 degrees in this group compared with 0 degrees when there was a "complex diagnosis."

COMPLICATIONS

■ Wound dehiscence and infection
■ Persistent or recurrent contracture
■ Extensor rupture
■ Ulnar deviation of the finger at the MCP joint
■ Postoperative subluxation or dislocation
■ Injury to the dorsal branch of the digital nerve

REFERENCES

1. Bode L, Gottlieb M. Dorsal capsulectomy of the metacarpophalangeal joint. In Blair WF, ed. Techniques in Hand Surgery. Baltimore: Williams & Wilkins, 1996:923–929.
2. Buch VI. Clinical and functional assessment of the hand after metacarpophalangeal capsulotomy. Plast Reconstr Surg 1974;53:452–457.
3. Curtis R. Stiff finger joints. In Grabb W, Smith J, eds. Plastic Surgery. Boston: Little, Brown, 1979:598–603.
4. Curtis RM. Capsulectomy of the interphalangeal joints of the fingers. J Bone Joint Surg Am 1954;36A:1219–1232.
5. Ghidella SD, Segalman KA, Murphey MS. Long-term results of surgical management of proximal interphalangeal joint contracture. J Hand Surg Am 2002;27A:799–805.
6. Gould JS, Nicholson BG. Capsulectomy of the metacarpophalangeal and proximal interphalangeal joints. J Hand Surg Am 1979; 4:482–486.
7. Kasabian A, McCarthy J, Karp N. Use of a multiplanar distracter for the correction of a proximal interphalangeal joint contracture. Ann Plast Surg 1998;40:378–381.
8. Prosser R. Splinting in the management of proximal interphalangeal joint flexion contracture. J Hand Ther 1996;9:378–386.
9. Stanley J, Jones W, Lynch MC. Percutaneous accessory collateral ligament release in the treatment of proximal interphalangeal joint flexion contracture. J Hand Surg Br 1986;11B:360–363.
10. Tsuge K. Contractures. In: Tsuge K, ed. Comprehensive Atlas of Hand Surgery. Chicago: Year Book Medical Publishers, 1989:239–241.
11. Watson HK, Light TR, Johnson TR. Check-rein resection for flexion contracture of the middle joint. J Hand Surg Br 1979;4B:67–71.
12. Weeks PM, Wray RC, Kuxhause M. The results of non-operative management of stiff joints in the hand. Plast Reconstr Surg 1978;61:58–63.
13. Young VL, Wray RC Jr, Weeks PM. The surgical management of stiff joints in the hand. Plast Reconstr Surg 1978;62:835–841.

Chapter 109

Surgical Treatment of Dupuytren's Disease

Ghazi Rayan

DEFINITION

- Dupuytren disease (DD) is a fibroproliferative disorder that affects primarily the palmar fascial complex of the hand, with occasional secondary involvement of other areas of the hand as well as remote tissues.
- It is an unparalleled condition that clinically and pathophysiologically resembles no other known ailment.
- Although physiologically DD bears a resemblance to the processes associated with normal wound healing, the perpetual and progressive proliferation and abnormal collagen deposition with resultant tissue contracture is astonishing.
- There have been attempts to classify DD under other headings such as inflammatory and neoplastic disorders; however, its uniqueness places it in a class of its own.

ANATOMY

- The radial, ulnar, and central aponeuroses, palmodigital fascia, and digital fascia are elements of the palmar fascial complex.[14]
- The radial aponeurosis has four components:
  - The thenar fascia, which is an extension of the central aponeuroses
  - The thumb pretendinous band, which is small or absent
  - The distal and the proximal commissural ligaments
- The ulnar aponeurosis has three components:
  - The hypothenar muscle fascia, which is an extension of the central aponeurosis
  - The pretendinous band to the small finger, which is consistent and substantial
  - The abductor digiti minimi confluence
- The central aponeurosis is the core of DD activity and has a triangular shape with a proximal apex (**FIG 1A**).

- Its fibers are oriented longitudinal, transverse, and vertical.
- The longitudinal fibers fan out as the pretendinous bands to the three central digits. Each pretendinous band bifurcates distally and each bifurcation has three layers. The superficial layer inserts into the dermis, the middle layer continues to the digit as the spiral band, and the deep layer passes almost vertically dorsally toward the flexor tendon and its digital sheath.
- The transverse fibers make up the natatory ligament (NL) located in the distal palm and the transverse ligament of the palmar aponeurosis (TLPA). The TLPA is proximal and parallel to the NL (**FIG 1B**) and lies deep to the pretendinous bands. Its distal, radial extent is the proximal commissural ligament. The TLPA gives origin to the septa of Legueu and Juvara, which protect the neurovascular structures and provide an additional proximal pulley to the flexor tendons.
- The vertical fibers of the central aponeurosis are the minute but strong vertical bands of Grapow and the septa of Legueu and Juvara (**FIG 1C,D**), which lie deep to the palmar fascia. There are eight septa that form seven fibro-osseous compartments[3] of two types: four flexor septal canals that contain the flexor tendons and three web space canals that contain common digital nerves and arteries, and lumbrical muscles. These septa are inserted in a soft tissue confluence that consists of five structures: A1 pulley, palmar plate, sagittal band, inter-palmar plate ligament (IPPL; **FIG 1D,E**), and septum of Legueu and Juvara.
- The palmodigital fascia encompasses a number of fascial structures, including the terminal fibers of the pretendinous bands, the spiral bands, the beginning of the lateral digital sheet, and the NL. The middle layer of the bifurcated pretendinous band spirals about 90 degrees and the peripheral fibers run vertically adjacent to the metacarpophalangeal (MCP) joint.

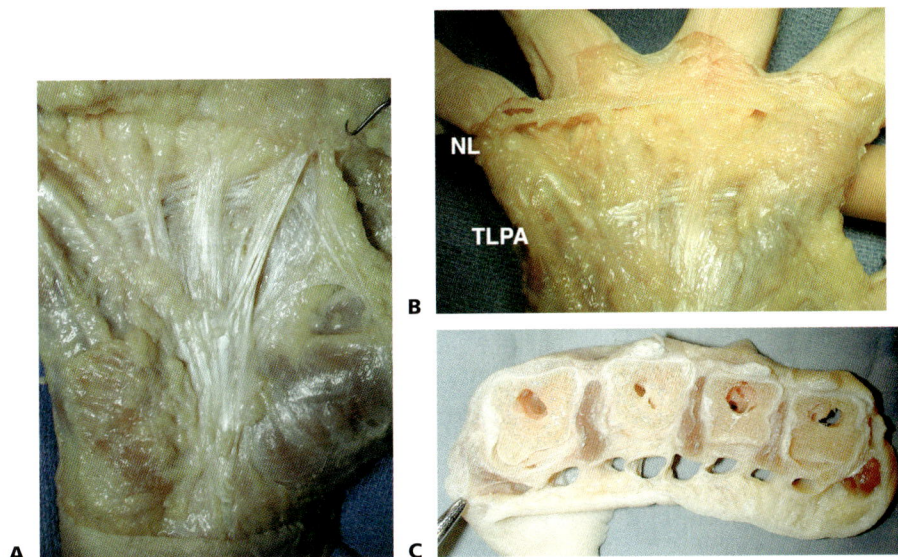

FIG 1 • A. The central aponeurosis is the core of Dupuytren disease activity and has a triangular shape with a proximal apex. **B.** The transverse fibers make up the natatory ligament (NL) located in the distal palm and the transverse ligament of the palmar aponeurosis (TLPA). **C.** There are eight septa of Legueu and Juvara that form seven fibro-osseous compartments of two types: four flexor septal canals that contain the flexor tendons and three web space canals that contain common digital nerves and arteries, and lumbrical muscles. *(continued)*

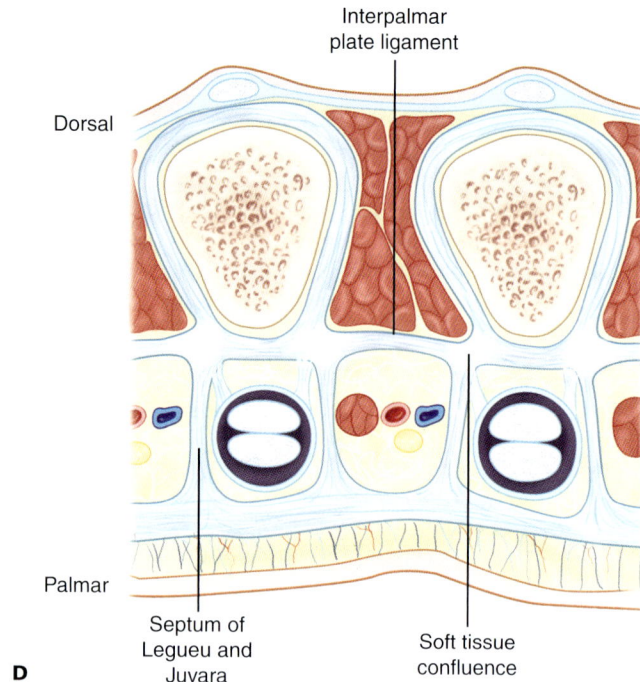

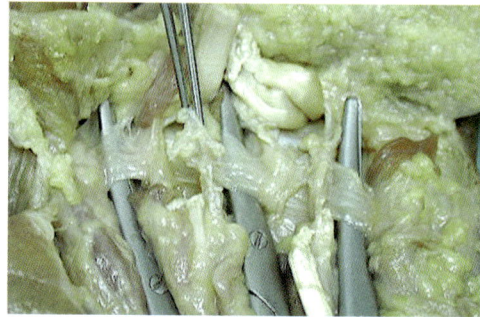

FIG 1 • *(continued)* **D.** Interpalmar plate ligament and septum of Legueu and Juvara. **E.** There are three interpalmar plate ligaments radial (to the left), central, and ulnar (to the right). These form the floor of the three web space canals.

They continue distally deep to the neurovascular bundle and NL and emerge distal to this ligament and contribute to the formation of the lateral digital sheet. The proximal fibers of the NL run in a transverse plane, but the distal fibers form a U that continues longitudinally along both sides of the digit, forming the lateral digital sheet. The lateral digital sheet therefore has deep and superficial contributions from the spiral band and NL.

- The digital fascia surrounds the neurovascular bundle in the digit, and this includes the Grayson ligament (palmar), the Cleland ligaments (dorsal), the Gosset lateral digital sheet laterally, and possibly fibers from the check-rein ligaments medially and dorsally that were described previously as Thomaine retrovascular fascia.

PATHOGENESIS

- In DD normal bands become diseased cords,[11] and Dupuytren nodules and cords are pathognomonic of the disease.[12]
- A nodule usually appears first, followed by the cord.
- The cords involve the palmar, palmodigital, or digital regions and progressively shorten, leading to joint and soft tissue contracture.
- The Grapow vertical bands become microcords, leading to thickening of the skin, which is one of the earliest manifestations of DD.
- Skin pits develop from the first layer of the split pretendinous band.
- The pretendinous cord develops from the pretendinous band and is the most common cord in DD. It leads to MCP joint flexion deformity and often extends distally, contributing to the digital cords. The pretendinous cord may bifurcate distally with each branch extending into a different digit, forming a commissural Y cord (**FIG 2**).
- The vertical cords, or diseased septa of Legueu and Juvara,[2] are short and thick. They are connected to the pretendinous cord and extend deeply in between the neurovascular bundle and flexor tendon fibrous sheath.

- Extensive palmar fascial disease is encountered in severe conditions and affects larger areas of the palm, leading to diffuse thickening of many components of the palmar fascial complex.
- The spiral cord has four components: the pretendinous band, the spiral band, the lateral digital sheet, and the Grayson ligament. It is encountered most often in the small finger.
  - In the palm, this cord is located superficial to the neurovascular bundle. Distal to the MCP joint, it passes deep to the neurovascular bundle and in the digit it runs lateral to the neurovascular bundle as it involves the lateral digital sheet and again becomes superficial to the neurovascular bundle as it involves the Grayson ligament.
  - Initially the cord spirals around the neurovascular bundle, but as it contracts, the cord straightens and the neurovascular bundle spirals around the cord.
  - The distorted anatomy of the neurovascular bundle, which is displaced medially and centrally, becomes at risk of injury during surgery.[19]
- The natatory cord develops from the NL, converting the U-shaped web space fibers into a V shape, resulting in contracture of the second, third, and fourth web spaces.
  - This cord extends along the dorsal lateral aspect of the adjacent digits and is best detected by passively abducting the digits and at the same time flexing one digit and extending the other at the MCP joints.
- The most commonly encountered digital cord is the lateral cord, followed by the central and spiral cords. These are responsible for proximal interphalangeal (PIP) joint flexion deformity.
  - The central cord is an extension of the pretendinous cord in the palm.
  - The lateral cord originates from the lateral digital sheet and attaches to the skin or to the flexor tendon sheath near the Grayson ligament. The lateral cord leads to contracture of the PIP joint but can also cause a distal interphalangeal joint contracture.

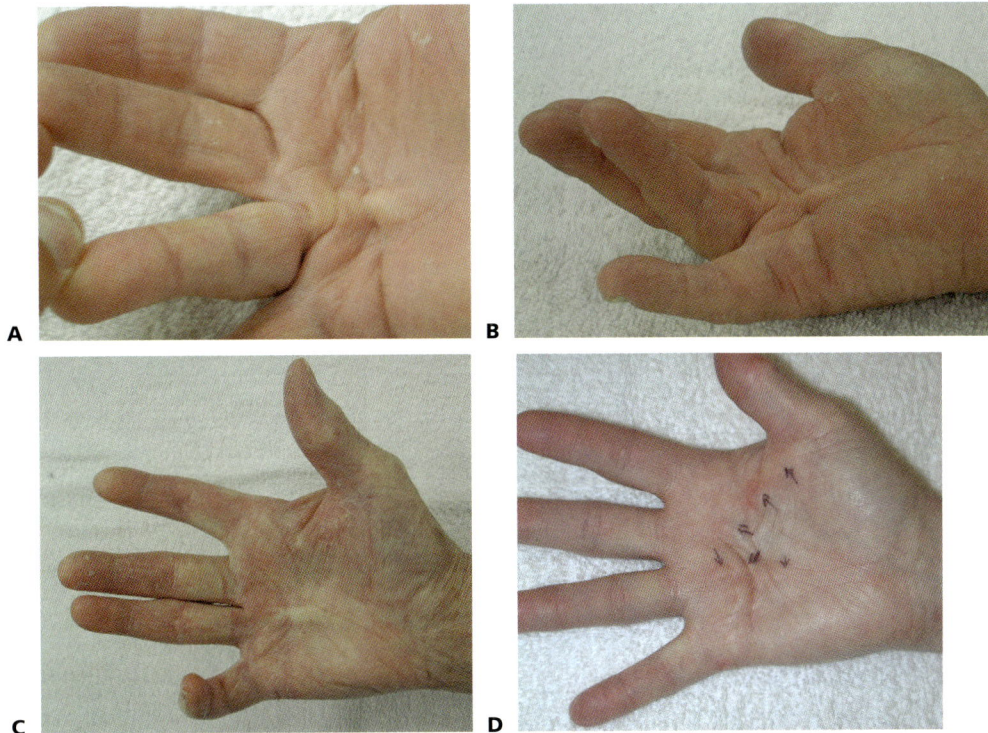

FIG 2 • A,B. Pretendinous cord and a nodule in the palm in line with the ring finger causing metacarpophalangeal flexion contracture. **C.** Two pretendinous cords in the palm in line with the small and ring fingers causing metacarpophalangeal and proximal interphalangeal flexion contracture of the small finger. A small proximal commissural cord in the first web space is also present. **D.** Diffuse Dupuytren palmar fascial disease is present with nodular thickening in the entire palm.

■ The abductor digiti minimi cord, also known as the isolated digital cord, takes origin from the abductor digiti minimi tendon, but may also arise from adjacent muscle fascia at the base of the proximal phalanx.

■ It courses superficial to the neurovascular bundle, and infrequently entraps and displaces the bundle toward the midline.

■ It inserts on the ulnar side of the base of the middle phalanx but may attach on the radial side or have an additional insertion in the base of the distal phalanx, causing a distal interphalangeal joint contracture.

■ The distal commissural cord develops from the diseased distal commissural ligament, which is the radial extension of the NL. The proximal commissural cord originates from the proximal commissural ligament, which is the radial extension of the TLPA.

■ Both of these cords cause first web space contracture.

■ The thumb pretendinous cord originates from the thumb pretendinous band and causes thumb MCP joint flexion deformity, which is uncommon.

NATURAL HISTORY

■ DD has three clinical phases: early, intermediate, and late.[13]

■ Skin changes with loss of normal architecture and skin pitting characterize the early phase.

■ Nodules and cords form during the intermediate phase.

■ Contractures mark the late phase, with the MCP joint most frequently affected, followed by the PIP joint.

PATIENT HISTORY AND PHYSICAL FINDINGS

■ The classic DD patient is a Caucasian man with a positive family history. The condition is bilateral and progressive and may extend to the digits, leading to their contracture.

■ Palmar involvement usually precedes disease extension into the digits, but the disease may begin and remain in the digits.

■ The ring finger is the most commonly involved digit, followed in order of frequency by the small, middle, and index finger and last by the thumb.

■ DD may affect areas outside the palmar surface of the hand.

■ Ectopic disease can be either regional in the upper extremity or distant in other parts of the body.

■ Garrod nodes are different from knuckle pads, occur on the dorsum of the hand, and are almost always limited to the finger (**FIG 3**).

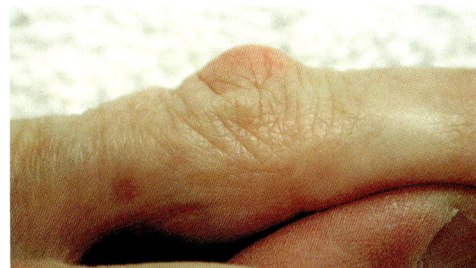

FIG 3 • A Garrod node over the dorsum of the proximal interphalangeal joint.

- Distant ectopic DD affects the plantar fascia and male genitals.
- Patients said to express a Dupuytren diathesis or genetic predisposition typically have faster and more severe development of the condition.
  - Positive family history
  - Young age of onset
  - Ectopic sites of fibromatosis such as the dorsal digital area (Garrod nodes), plantar fascia (Ledderhose disease), and male genitals (Peyronie disease)

DIFFERENTIAL DIAGNOSIS

- Non-Dupuytren disease[15]
  - Occurs in a diverse ethnic group, is unilateral and non-progressive, usually involves a single digit, and frequently follows trauma or surgery
  - Patients with this disease rarely require surgical treatment. Confusing this with DD will produce contrasting epidemiologic data.
- Epithelioid sarcoma
- Occupational thickening and callus formation that mimic Dupuytren nodules
- Palmar subcutaneous soft tissue lesions, such as localized pigmented villonodular synovitis, palmar ganglions, and inclusion cysts
- Stenosing tenosynovitis without triggering can be associated with thickening and adherence of the skin to the underlying flexor tendon sheath.
- Prominent flexor tendons can be confused with pretendinous cords because of attenuation of annular pulleys, as seen in rheumatoid arthritis.

NONOPERATIVE MANAGEMENT

- No treatment is necessary for non-Dupuytren disease.
- Observation is appropriate for nonprogressive DD with minimal contracture and without compromise of function.
  - Surgical treatment for minor disease or pitting can result in a disease flare and must be avoided.
- Basic science research has shown the potential of certain local agents in the treatment of DD. These include calcium channel blockers, nifedipine, and verapamil[16] for early stages and collagenase[1] for advanced stages of the disease.
- Steroid injection of nodules has been used to suppress the disease.

SURGICAL MANAGEMENT

- Surgery is the most widely used treatment method for symptomatic and severe DD.
  - Outpatient surgery offers substantial savings and should be used in an otherwise healthy patient with moderate hand involvement.
  - Local, regional, or general anesthesia can be used depending on the procedure performed.
- Flexion contractures of the MCP joint of greater than 30 degrees and PIP flexion contractures of 15 degrees interfere with function and, in the presence of a well-developed cord, are indications for surgical treatment.
- The outcome after surgery for MCP joint contracture is more successful than that for PIP joint contracture.
  - PIP joint check-rein release is indicated if 40 degrees of residual flexion is present after conventional fasciectomy.

Procedures

Percutaneous Fasciotomy

- Percutaneous fasciotomy is indicated for palmar cords in elderly unhealthy patients.
  - This technique carries a higher risk for complications when performed in the thumb than in the digits.
- In severe cases, this technique may be useful as a preliminary procedure before definitive removal of diseased tissue.
- Injuries to flexor tendons and digital nerves as well as chronic regional pain syndromes have been reported after percutaneous releases.

Open Palm Fasciectomy

- This method was first used by Dupuytren, who left the transverse palmar incision wound open after fasciotomy.
- This method is indicated for extensive involvement of the palmar fascia and if primary closure is not possible and skin grafting is not desired.
- Satisfactory results with this method continue to be reported in the literature,[7,10,20] including less pain, better motion, and low rates of complication. The primary disadvantage is prolonged postoperative wound healing.

Partial Fasciectomy

- Partial fasciectomy is the excision of the diseased tissue with preservation of normal-appearing fascia.
  - Other terms for this procedure are selective, regional, or limited fasciectomy.
- Partial fasciectomy remains the most widely used technique for treatment of DD among hand surgeons today. It is associated with a lower recurrence rate than fasciotomy.

Dermofasciectomy

- Dermofasciectomy involves excision of skin and diseased tissue simultaneously followed by grafting of the skin defect.[8]
- Dermofasciectomy is the procedure of choice for recurrent or aggressive disease with marked adherence of skin to underlying diseased cords. It was reported to have lower recurrence rates compared to other surgical techniques even for recurrent disease.[9]

Extensive Fasciectomy

- Extensive fasciectomy involves a wide, generous fasciectomy of diseased tissue involving most of the palmar fascial complex.
  - This can be combined if necessary with partial fasciectomy in the digits.
  - This technique is indicated when broad involvement of the palmar fascial complex is present.
  - The NL and TLPA may be involved in severe DD and these can be included in the extensive fasciectomy.
  - After extensive fasciectomy, the skin sometimes can be closed primarily. If a defect is present, the wound can be skin grafted or left open.
- Total or radical fasciectomy entails removal of the entire diseased and normal palmar fascia with or without excision of the overlying skin.
  - This highly morbid, radical approach is not warranted.

Positioning

- The patient is positioned supine and the hand is placed on a hand table with the shoulder abducted 90 degrees.

■ A padded pneumatic tourniquet is placed on the arm as proximally as possible. The upper extremity is exsanguinated and the tourniquet is inflated to 250 mm Hg.

Approach

■ The most commonly used incision is the Brunner zigzag incision (**FIG 4A**).

■ A midline longitudinal incision that is closed with multiple Z-plasties can be also used (**FIG 4B**).

■ Transverse palmar incisions can be used for the open palm method or for removal of extensive palmar fascial complex disease.

■ Local rotation flaps sometimes should be used to cover exposed flexor tendons or neurovascular structures, and the remaining secondary defect can be grafted with full-thickness skin.

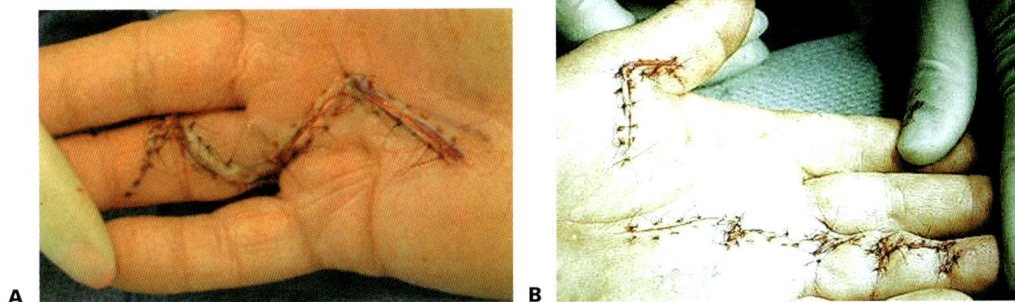

FIG 4 • **A.** Partial fasciectomy through a zigzag Brunner incision. **B.** A longitudinal incision closed with multiple Z-plasties.

PERCUTANEOUS FASCIOTOMY

- Local anesthesia is used.
- A tourniquet is not necessary.
- Select the point of fasciotomy adjacent to the cord.
- Use a no. 11 blade held vertically (**TECH FIG 1**).

- Make a stab wound and turn the blade horizontally to cut the cord while the digit is manually extended.
- A gratifying snap is felt and the finger should extend.

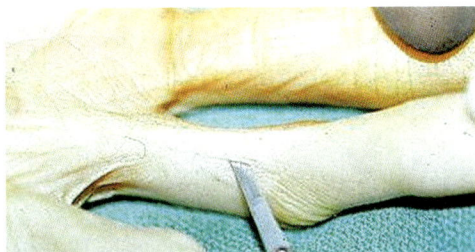

TECH FIG 1 • The no. 11 blade is used to incise the midline cord to improve the proximal interphalangeal joint contracture in this elderly patient.

OPEN PALM FASCIECTOMY

- Make a transverse incision in the middle of the palm and extend it if necessary to the digits as a zigzag Brunner incision.
- Undermine the skin flaps and identify the diseased tissue.
- Carry the dissection proximally until a transition between normal and diseased fascia is identified.
  - Isolate the neurovascular structures from the diseased tissue and protect them.

- Release the diseased tissue proximally; dissection is followed distally and excised.
- Leave the transverse incision open to heal by secondary intention but close any extensions of the original incision into the fingers.
- Apply nonadherent gauze to the wound and immobilize the hand in a forearm-based splint with the fingers in extension.

PARTIAL FASCIECTOMY

- Make a zigzag Bruner incision; it may extend from the proximal palm to the digital pulp in cases of palmar and digital disease.
- Undermine the skin flaps by careful dissection to separate relatively normal dermis from the diseased tissue.

This can be difficult in recurrent cases. Make every effort not to buttonhole the flaps.

- It is better to leave diseased tissue in the dermal flap rather than thinning the flap too much and running the risk of buttonholing the flap.

TECHNIQUES

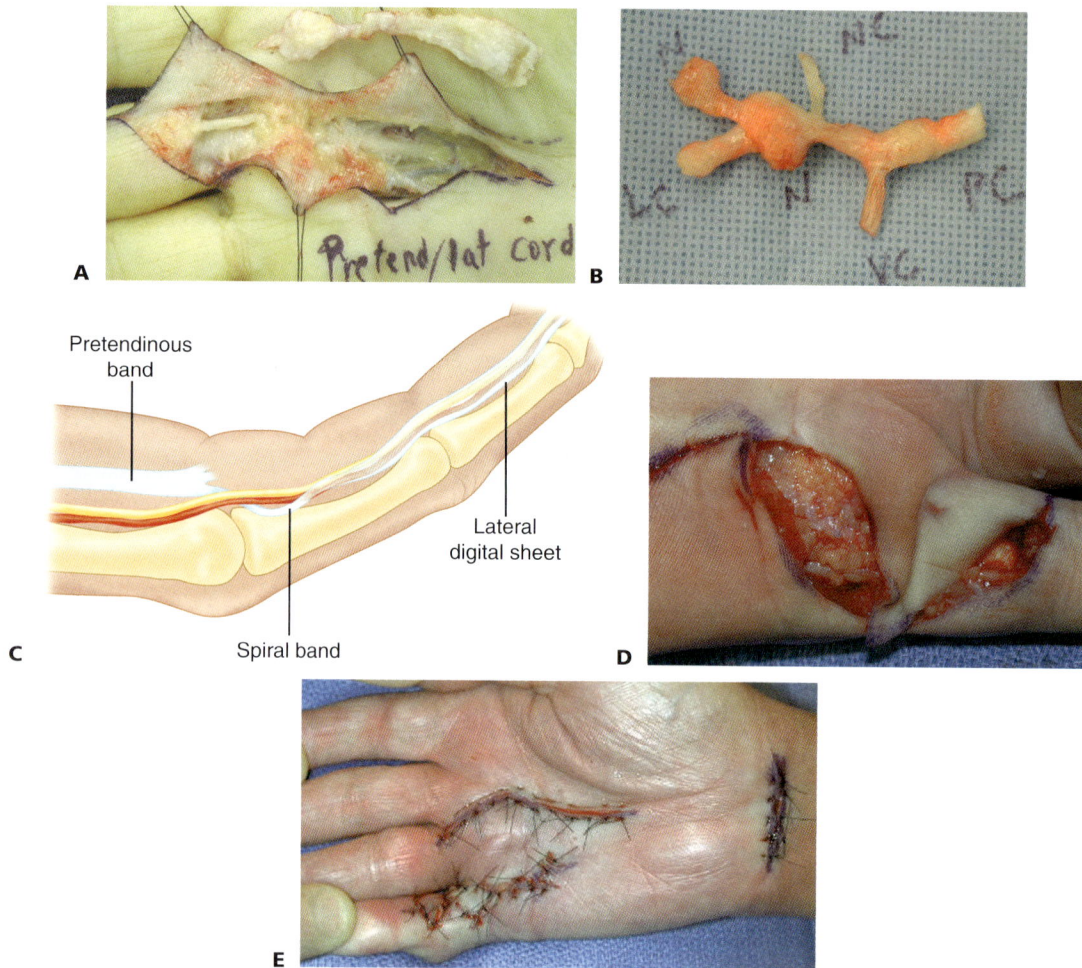

TECH FIG 2 • **A.** The neurovascular structures are dissected and protected during surgery. **B.** An excised specimen showing pretendinous (*PC*), vertical (*VC*), natatory (*NC*), nodule (*N*), and lateral (*LC*) cords. **C.** With a spiral cord, care must be taken to prevent injury to the digital nerve and vessel, which are intertwined with and spiraled around the diseased cord. **D.** A local flap is rotated to cover neurovascular structures. **E.** Skin shortage in the small finger was covered with a full-thickness skin graft from the volar wrist.

- Identify the neurovascular structures, dissect them from the diseased cords, retract them, and protect them during the entire procedure (**TECH FIG 2A**).
- Begin the dissection proximally in the palm until a transition between relatively normal and diseased fascia is identified.
- Carry the dissection in a proximal-to-distal direction.
- Transect the pretendinous cord proximally and follow the cord distally, dividing all connections to adjacent normal fascia.
- If present, include in the excised specimen a vertical cord from the diseased septa of Legueu and Juvara and a natatory cord from the diseased NL (**TECH FIG 2B**).
- Special attention must be given to a spiral cord (**TECH FIG 2C**) to prevent injury to the digital nerve and vessel, which are intertwined with and spiraled around the diseased cord.
- If the diseased tissue is confined to the palm in the form of a pretendinous cord, the distal end of the cord can be seen inserted in the flexor tendon sheath distal to the MCP joint. The cord can be excised at this level.

- If the diseased tissue extends to the digit, follow the digital cord into the finger.
  - Pretendinous cord extension in the digit can be in the form of lateral, central, or spiral cord.
  - The digital cord must be dissected in the finger with great care because of its proximity to the neurovascular bundle.
  - Identify and release the distal insertion of the digital cord.
- Release the tourniquet and coagulate bleeders with a bipolar forceps.
- After adequate hemostasis is achieved, close the wound without a drain.
- If skin shortage is present, perform full-thickness skin grafting.
- If the neurovascular bundle or flexor tendons are exposed, a flap may be rotated to cover these structures, and skin grafting is done for the secondary defect (**TECH FIG 2D,E**).
- A palmar plaster splint with the digits in the corrected extended position is used for 1 week or less.

DERMOFASCIECTOMY

- Plan the incision by mapping the area of diseased tissue and skin with a marker. The remaining exposure is done through a zigzag Brunner incision that extends from the dermofascial island (**TECH FIG 3**).

- Remove the diseased fascia and adherent overlying skin as one component.
- Close the zigzag Bruner incision and cover the skin defect with full-thickness skin graft from the volar wrist.

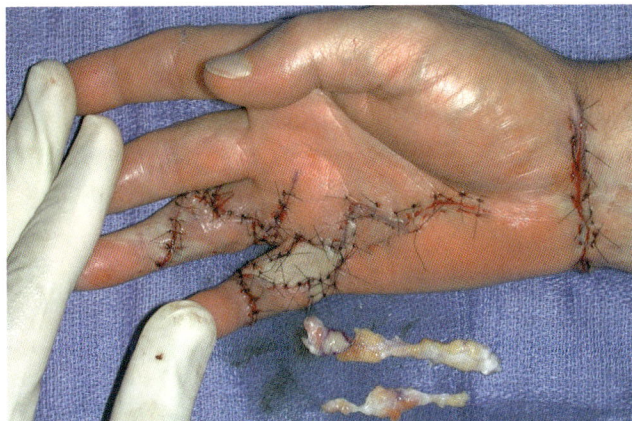

TECH FIG 3 • In a patient with recurrent Dupuytren disease with two pretendinous cords in the palm in line with the small and ring fingers causing severe metacarpophalangeal and proximal interphalangeal flexion contracture of the small finger, dermofasciectomy was done for the small finger and partial fasciectomy through a zigzag Brunner incision was done for the ring finger. Correction of the contractures was achieved. Skin shortage in the small finger was covered with a full-thickness skin graft from the volar wrist.

EXTENSIVE FASCIECTOMY

- Make either a transverse incision in the middle of the palm or a U-shaped incision in the distal palm (**TECH FIG 4A**).
- The incision has two limbs extending proximally on the ulnar and radial aspect of the digits, forming a broad proximally based skin flap. These can be continued if necessary to the digits with zigzag Brunner incisions.

- Undermine the proximal skin flap and distal skin margin by separating the skin from the extensive diseased palmar fascial complex. Retract the flap proximally to expose the deeper structures (**TECH FIG 4B**).
- Carry the dissection proximally and distally to expose the majority of the palmar fascia. A transition between normal and diseased fascia may not be identified. Leave

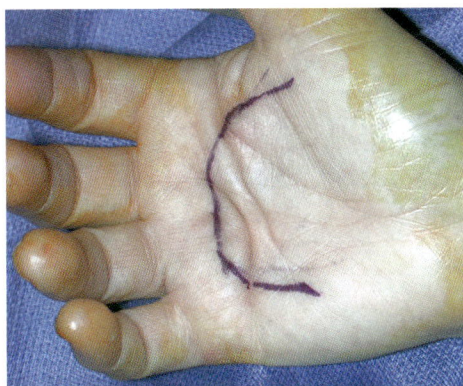

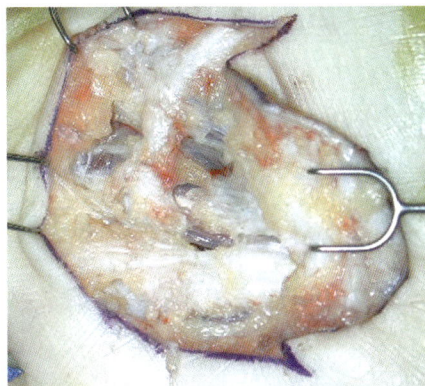

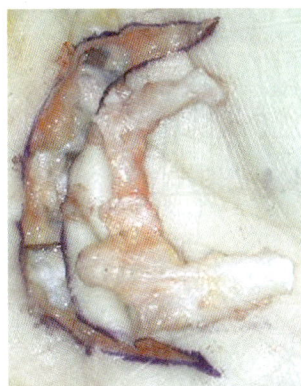

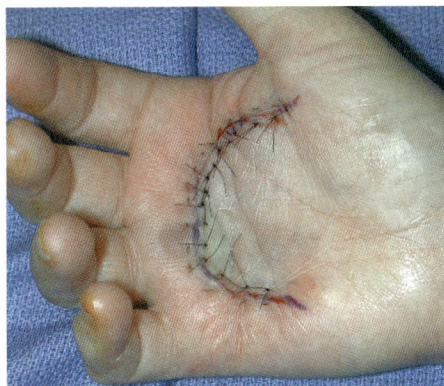

TECH FIG 4 • **A.** A U-shaped incision is planned in a patient with diffuse Dupuytren palmar fascial disease with nodular thickening in the entire palm. **B.** The diseased fascia is exposed after reflection of the proximally based skin flap. **C.** The excised specimen includes a pretendinous cord from the ring finger and diseased transverse ligament of the palmar aponeurosis. **D.** The surgical wound after skin closure.

behind any normal-appearing fascial tissue and excise the entire diseased pretendinous cords and adjacent thick nodular structures (**TECH FIG 4C**).

- Keep the neurovascular structures in sight and protected all the time.
- The TLPA is usually involved, forming a transverse cord that extends from the ulnar to the radial aspect of the palm.
  - This should be removed with the diseased tissue, along with any natatory cords.
  - Divide all the septa of Legueu and Juvara to remove most of the diseased fascial carpet.

- If these septa are diseased, they will form vertical cords that should be incorporated in the mass of excised tissue.
- Release the tourniquet and achieve adequate hemostasis.
- Close the wound if possible (**TECH FIG 4D**), leaving a Penrose drain; it is removed the second postoperative day.
- If skin shortage is present, perform full-thickness skin grafting.
- Alternatively, the wound can be left open as in the open palm method.

PEARLS AND PITFALLS

- Injury to digital nerves is more common in cases with severe MCP and PIP joint contracture and altered nerve anatomy by a spiral cord. Such a complication is especially common in previously operated cases with an exuberant amount of scar tissue. Preventive measures include isolation of the neurovascular bundle by careful dissection, using loupe magnification, and knowledge of pathoanatomy. The dissection is carried out in a proximal-to-distal direction and is sometimes combined with distal-to-proximal dissection before removal of the diseased cord. If the nerve is transected, a primary repair should be performed.
- Vascular injury can be in the form of an arterial laceration, arterial spasm, intimal hemorrhage, or vessel rupture from vigorous correction of severe digital joint contracture. Arterial laceration that results in vascular compromise requires immediate repair or interposition vein graft. Arterial spasm and intimal hemorrhage are treated first by repositioning the digit in flexion, then irrigating with warm saline, applying topical lidocaine, even using intravenous heparin, and, if all else fails, vascular reconstruction.
- Separating diseased tissue from adherent skin is difficult, especially in recurrent cases. To reduce the risk of buttonholing the skin, using a no. 15C scalpel and the back of the knife as a dissector will allow precise separation of diseased tissue from normal skin. In addition, using an operating room light to transilluminate from the epidermal side of the skin allows visualization of the thickness of the flap and can alert the surgeon when the dissection is too superficial.

POSTOPERATIVE CARE

Open Palm Fasciectomy

- The surgical wound is covered with sterile nonadhesive gauze, which can be changed daily. By 4 weeks no dressings should be necessary.
- Forty-eight to 72 hours after surgery the patient begins active range of motion every 2 to 3 hours but maintains nocturnal extension splint immobilization.
- Whirlpool therapy can be used early in the postoperative period if unwarranted or excessive bleeding occurred.
- Wound healing takes place within 6 to 8 weeks, depending on the extent of the incision.

Partial Fasciectomy and Dermofasciectomy

- Range-of-motion exercises are encouraged out of the splint after 1 week. The sutures are removed and splint use is discontinued 2 weeks after surgery in uncomplicated cases.
- Formal hand therapy is used after surgery for extensive disease, especially if residual flexion deformity is present. Range of motion alternating with extension splinting is emphasized.

COMPLICATIONS

- Complications related to patient physiology include postoperative stiffness, chronic regional pain syndromes, recurrence, loss of digital flexion, and reflex symptomatic dystrophy. The surgeon has little influence in preventing these complications.
- Early postoperative complications
  - Hematoma is prevented by tourniquet deflation and adequate hemostasis before wound closure. Deflating the tourniquet and assessing the skin vascularity before closure to ensure adequate circulation is the best way to prevent skin necrosis.
  - Closure under tension should be avoided and consideration should be given to grafting or the open palm method if a primary closure is too tight.
  - Skin necrosis develops after excessive thinning of skin flaps and tight skin closure. Small areas of skin necrosis may be allowed to heal by secondary intention, but large areas of necrotic tissue should be excised, and skin graft or flap coverage is done.
  - Reflex sympathetic dystrophy, also referred to as a "flare" reaction, may occur after surgery. The patient presents with swelling, hyperemia, dysesthesias, and pain out of proportion to that expected. Direct trauma to the nerve and excessive dissection or stretch of the nerves are thought to be predisposing factors. A simultaneous carpal tunnel release with DD surgery, especially in women, is a predisposing factor. Atraumatic technique and gentle handling of nerves and tissues during surgery should minimize the risk of this complication. If no cause can be identified, the treatment is therapy for pain control. In recalcitrant cases a series of stellate sympathetic ganglion blocks can be helpful.
- Late postoperative complications
  - Inclusion cysts can occur near the scar due to dermal tissue entrapment in the subcutaneous space. This can be prevented by careful attention to skin approximation during wound closure. The risk of hypertrophic scar formation is lessened by careful attention to placement of the skin incisions.

OUTCOMES

- The recurrence rate varies between 2% and 60%, with an average of 33%. This may be a true recurrence (recurrent disease at the operated site) or disease extension (disease outside the area of prior surgery). Recurrence is more common in patients with PIP joint involvement, disease in the small finger, more than one digit affected, a longer time since surgery, and a secondary fasciectomy.

- Roush and Stern[17] reported that the postoperative total range of motion of recurrent DD was better after fasciectomy and flap converge compared to skin grafting or arthrodesis.

- DD has intrigued basic scientists and clinicians for centuries. Both ancient[6] and current publications[5,18] underscore the interest in and the advances toward understanding the pathophysiology of this disease and improving its treatment.

REFERENCES

1. Badalamente M, Hurst L. Enzyme injection as nonsurgical treatment of Dupuytren disease. J Hand Surg Am 2000;25A:629–636.
2. Bilderback K, Rayan G. Dupuytren's cord involving the septa of Legueu and Juvara: a case report. J Hand Surg Am 2002;27A:344–346.
3. Bilderback K, Rayan G. The septa of Legueu and Juvara: an anatomic study. J Hand Surg Am 2004;29A:494–499.
4. Boyer M, Gelberman R Complications of the operative treatment of Dupuytren disease. Hand Clin 1999;15:161–166.
5. Brenner P, Rayan G. Dupuytren's Disease: A Concept of Surgical Treatment. Vienna: Springer, 2002.
6. Elliot D. The early history of Dupuytren disease. Hand Clin 1999; 15:1–19.
7. Gelberman R, Panagis J, Hergenroder P, et al. Wound complications in the surgical management of Dupuytren's contracture: a comparison of operative incisions. Hand 1982;14:248–253.
8. Hueston J. The control of recurrent Dupuytren's contracture by skin replacement. Br J Plast Surg 1969;22:152–156.
9. Ketchum L, Hixon F. Treatment of Dupuytren's contracture with dermofasciectomy and full thickness skin graft. J Hand Surg Am 1987;12A:659–663.
10. Lubahn J. Open palm technique and soft tissue coverage in Dupuytren disease. Hand Clin 1999;15:127–136.
11. Luck JV. Dupuytren's contracture: a new concept of the pathogenesis correlated with surgical management. J Bone Joint Surg Am 1959; 41A:635.
12. McFarlane RM. Patterns of the diseased fascia in the fingers of Dupuytren's contracture. Plast Reconst Surg 1974;54:31–44.
13. Rayan G. Dupuytren disease: anatomy, pathology, presentation and treatment. J Bone Joint Surg Am 2007;89A:190–198.
14. Rayan G. Palmar fascial complex anatomy and pathology in Dupuytren disease. Hand Clin 1999;15:73–86.
15. Rayan G, Moore J, Non-Dupuytren's disease of the palmar fascia. J Hand Surg Br 2005;30B:551–556.
16. Rayan G, Parizi M, Tomasek J. Pharmacologic regulation of Dupuytren's fibroblast contraction in vitro. J Hand Surg Am 1996; 21A:1065–1070.
17. Roush T, Stern P. Results following surgery for recurrent Dupuytren disease. J Hand Surg Am 2000;25A:291–296.
18. Tubiana R, Leclercq C, Hurst L, et al. Dupuytren's Disease. London: Martin Dunitz, 2000.
19. Ulmas M, Bischoff R, Gelberman R. Predictors of neurovascular displacement in hands with Dupuytren's contracture. J Hand Surg Br 1994;19B:644–666.
20. Zachariae L. Operation for Dupuytren's contracture by the method of McCash. Acta Orthop Scand 1970;41:433–438.

Chapter 110

Surgical Treatment of Vascular Tumors of the Hand

Rimma Finkel and Morton Kasdan

DEFINITION

- Vascular tumors are diverse, ranging from benign vascular malformations to malignant lesions.
- The incidence of vascular tumors is about 2% to 6%.[14,16]
- About 26% of vascular and lymphatic tumors are found in the extremities.[17]
  - When found in the upper extremity, they are more common in the hand and forearm.
  - Vascular tumors are fourth in frequency of upper extremity tumors, after ganglions, giant cell tumors, and inclusion cysts.
- Most vascular tumors are congenital, and 10% of pediatric tumors involve the upper extremity. Of these, 90% can be classified as hemangiomas or vascular malformations.[23]
- Benign vascular tumors can be congenital or acquired and include hemangiomas, lymphangiomas, congenital arteriovenous fistulas, aneurysms, vascular leiomyomas, glomus tumors, and pyogenic granulomas.
- Malignant vascular tumors include hemangioendotheliomas, hemangiosarcomas, glomangiosarcomas, and malignant hemangiopericytomas.

ANATOMY

- The ulnar and radial arteries form the superficial and deep arches of the hand, which then branch into the common digital arteries. There are multiple anatomic variants.[5] The common digital arteries then branch into the proper digital arteries that course along the midlateral aspect of each digit, slightly volar to midline.
- The arteries terminate at either a capillary bed or a glomus body. The glomus is a neuromyoarterial mechanoreceptor—that is, a specialized arteriovenous shunt. It lies in the stratum reticulum of the skin, especially in the subungual region and distal pads of the digits. The glomus body acts as a thermoregulator, and it regulates peripheral blood flow in the digits and possibly controls peripheral blood pressure. It contains the glomus cells surrounding the Sucquet-Hoyer canals, which are narrow vascular anastomotic channels.

PATHOGENESIS

- The theory is that vascular tumors occur as a failure of differentiation of the common embryonic vascular channels, which results in the congenital lesions.[17] These are more commonly seen in the pediatric population, but they may be discovered late, in adults.
- Acquired vascular tumors are usually due to trauma that induces aneurysms or fistulas.

NATURAL HISTORY

Congenital Lesions

Hemangiomas

- Thirty percent of hemangiomas are visible at birth, but this increases to 70% to 90% before the infant is 4 weeks old.

- These lesions show rapid growth, then slower growth that is proportional to the child. Next a slow involutional process occurs.[29] Fifty percent of hemangiomas will involute by the time the child is 5 years old and 70% will involute by the age of 7.
- Hemangiomas consist of plump endothelial cells with high turnover rates.[14] They may be classified by histology, location (superficial, subcutaneous, or intramuscular), or involutional status.[17] Thirty percent of upper extremity hemangiomas will ulcerate. This becomes a problem with these hand and finger tumors that may present with acute or chronic paronychia, especially in children who suck their fingers.[23]
- They present as reddish lesions that become raised during the growth phase.

Congenital Aneurysms

- The histologic classification of congenital aneurysms includes capillary hemangiomas, sclerosing hemangiomas, and venous or cavernous hemangiomas (**FIG 1**).[17]
- Capillary hemangiomas consist primarily of proliferated capillaries. There is a compact mass of endothelial cells where

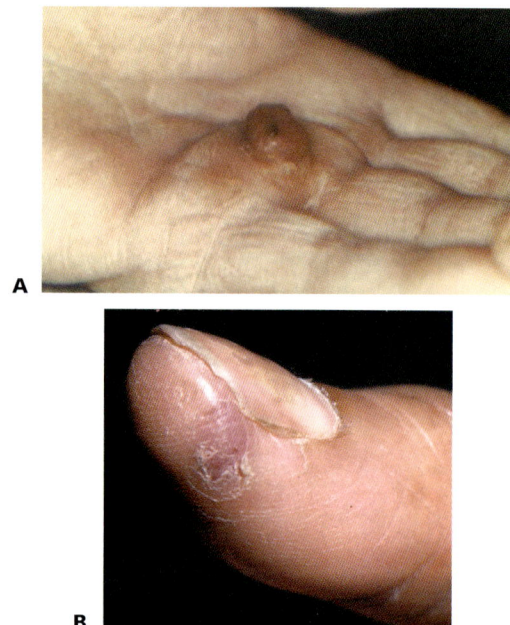

FIG 1 • A. Hemangioma of the volar fourth web space of the left hand. This patient had a raised, ulcerated lesion and pathology showing a polypoid lesion with central capillary and slightly larger vascular spaces. **B.** Cavernous hemangioma of the thumb. There is a pinkish hue to the skin without any raised tissue. Although the lesion appears ulcerated, on pathologic examination there were no ulcerations and large vascular spaces were found immediately beneath the epidermis.

there are small or no capillary lumina. These extend from the dermis into the subcutaneous tissue and make up about 57% of subcutaneous hemangiomas.[18]

■ If the hemangioma is associated with thrombocytopenia and consumptive coagulopathy, it is termed Kasabach-Merritt syndrome. This is unrelated to the size of the hemangioma and may be life-threatening if untreated.

■ If there are thin-walled sinuses secondary to widely dilated thin-walled spaces with little stroma, they become cavernous or venous hemangiomas. These make up about 23% of hemangiomas.

■ Sclerosing hemangiomas contain a perivascular thickening of the lymphatic cells. There is a fibrous, not hematogenous, origin to these lesions. This type represents 10% of all hemangiomas.[17]

Lymphangioma

■ Lymphangiomas are rare and classified as simple, cavernous, and cystic. The most common variety is cavernous lymphangiomas. These present at birth or soon thereafter and they are composed of dilated lymphatic sinuses.

Congenital Arteriovenous Fistula

■ Congenital arteriovenous fistulas (AVFs) develop early in the embryo. The upper extremity is the second most common location for these lesions after the head and neck. They have several arteriovenous communications at birth and are associated with syndromes such as Parkes-Weber syndrome and Klippel-Trenaunay syndrome.[9]

■ Parkes-Weber syndrome is a combination of multiple AVFs, vascular malformations, and skeletal hypertrophy of the affected limb.

■ Klippel-Trenaunay syndrome is characterized by a combined type of vascular malformation and limb enlargement due to hypertrophy of soft tissue and bone.

■ Both of these syndromes may have significant medical sequelae, including congestive heart failure, pulmonary embolism, venous thrombosis, bleeding, and cellulitis.

Vascular Malformations

■ Vascular malformations are uniformly present at birth but may not be visible until childhood, adolescence, or adulthood. Most appear by ages 2 to 5 years.[29] They enlarge proportionately with the child unless they are stimulated by trauma, hormones, infection, or surgery.[2] These lesions have an equal sex distribution. Malformations generally have flat, slowly dividing endothelial cells.

■ They can be categorized as low-flow or high-flow lesions based on their hemodynamic features at the time of angiography.

  ■ High-flow lesions have an arterial component. Marked enlargement and increased number of arteries, small vessels, and veins are consistent findings.[3]

  ■ Low-flow malformations have large channels without intervening parenchyma and often with associated phleboliths. These lesions are more common than high-flow lesions. They are subdivided into capillary, venous, lymphatic, and combined.

■ Capillary malformations (port wine stain, nevus flammeus) show dilated capillaries and postcapillary venules in the upper dermis. They are dark red to purple and may have another associated vascular lesion. Over time, they become darker and have a cobblestone appearance. They may be associated with limb or digit overgrowth.[23]

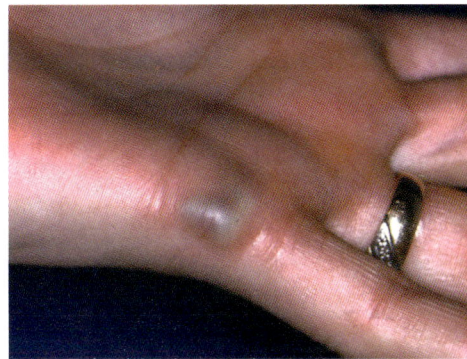

FIG 2 • Venous malformation of the ulnar side of the left hand. Notice the blue color and slightly raised appearance.

■ Seventy-five percent of venous malformations are recognized at birth. They are the most common anomaly of the low-flow group (40%).[14] It is important to differentiate them from hemangiomas because venous malformations do not involute. They, like lymphatic malformations, present with a mass or skin discoloration. They enlarge shortly after birth and grow with the child.[23] Slow commensurate growth, compressibility, and phleboliths are pathognomonic for venous malformation (**FIG 2**).[14]

■ Patients with vascular malformations will complain of the mass effect of the lesion, increased size with exercise, or pain due to thrombosis. Elevation of the extremity eases symptoms. They may lead to nerve compression at the forearm and wrist, and digital compression may be seen with localized thrombosis.[23]

■ Lymphatic malformations enlarge secondary to fluid accumulation, cellulitis, or inadequate drainage of lymphatic channels.[14] They can limit hand motion, and infections are common.[23] They can cause bone hypertrophy.

■ Mixed vascular malformations share the characteristics of their combination of vascular malformations.

■ High-flow malformations present early as a painless mass. They have a bimodal occurrence: 40% show up at birth and another 34% after 10 years old.[23] They are not compressible. These lesions can lead to distal ischemia or even high-output heart failure if large and untreated. They have been divided into three types (**FIG 3**):

  ■ Type A lesions have single or multiple arteriovenous fistulas, aneurysms, or ectasias of the arterial side.[24,29]

  ■ Type B lesions consist of arteriovenous anomalies with microfistulas or macrofistulas that are localized to a single limb, hand, or digit. They have stable flow characteristics and provoke minimal to no distal symptoms. As with type A lesions, they remain localized to a specific anatomic region.[23,24,29]

  ■ Type C lesions enlarge slowly. They are diffuse, with microfistulas and macrofistulas involving all limb tissues. With increasing size, vascular steal occurs. The lesions and associated symptoms worsen with pregnancy and do not reverse with delivery. They can cause distal ischemic pain, tachycardia, and congestive heart failure. Compartment syndrome, compression neuropathies, and ulceration secondary to ischemia or attempted surgical interventions can also occur. The result can be unrelenting, progressive pain, eventually leading to amputation.[23,24]

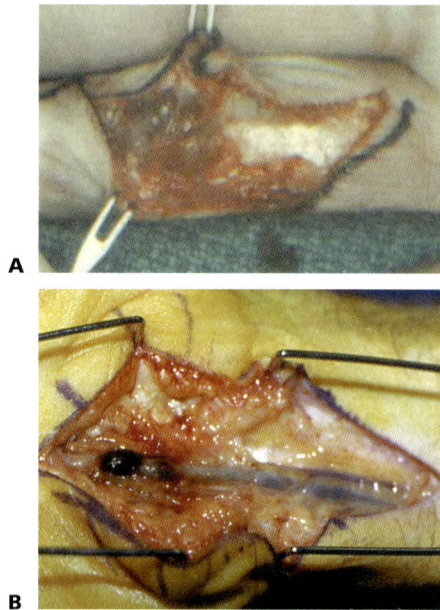

FIG 3 • **A.** Arteriovenous malformation of the digit. The margins are indistinct and it is difficult to dissect from the surrounding tissues. **B.** Arteriovenous malformation of the palm at the ulnar artery. There is a bulbous region where the malformation has occurred.

Acquired Lesions

▪ Acquired lesions comprise both true and false aneurysms of the vessels, glomus tumors, pyogenic granulomas, fistulas, and vascular leiomyomas.

▪ True aneurysms contain all three layers of the vessel wall: intima, media, and adventitia. False or pseudoaneurysms do not contain all three layers of the vessel wall.

True Aneurysms

▪ True aneurysms account for 6% of all tumors of the hand.[17]
▪ True aneurysms, most notably hypothenar hammer syndrome, usually follow blunt trauma in the area of the vessel. The trauma may be a single event or repeated injury. The vessel dilates in response to injury to the arterial media, leading to a fusiform vessel.
▪ Aneurysms occur secondary to other disease processes such as arteriosclerosis, metabolic disorders, Kawasaki disease, Buerger disease, hemophilia, osteogenesis imperfecta tarda, granulomatous arteritis, and cystic adventitial disease (**FIG 4**).[14]

Pseudoaneurysms

▪ False or pseudoaneurysms account for most (83%) aneurysms of the hand and generally occur on the palmar surface of the hand.
▪ They may be secondary to a puncture wound (such as from a knife or pencil lead) or complete rupture of the vessel wall with continuity maintained by the surrounding soft tissues.[14,17]
▪ Pseudoaneurysms occur slowly over time and are usually not evident for weeks to months after the injury.
▪ A bruit may be noted on examination. Like true aneurysms, the most common site is in the ulnar artery.

Acquired Arteriovenous Fistulas

▪ Acquired AVFs occur secondary to trauma or surgical intervention. AVFs consist of a communication between an artery and a vein that shunts away from the higher-resistance capillary system.

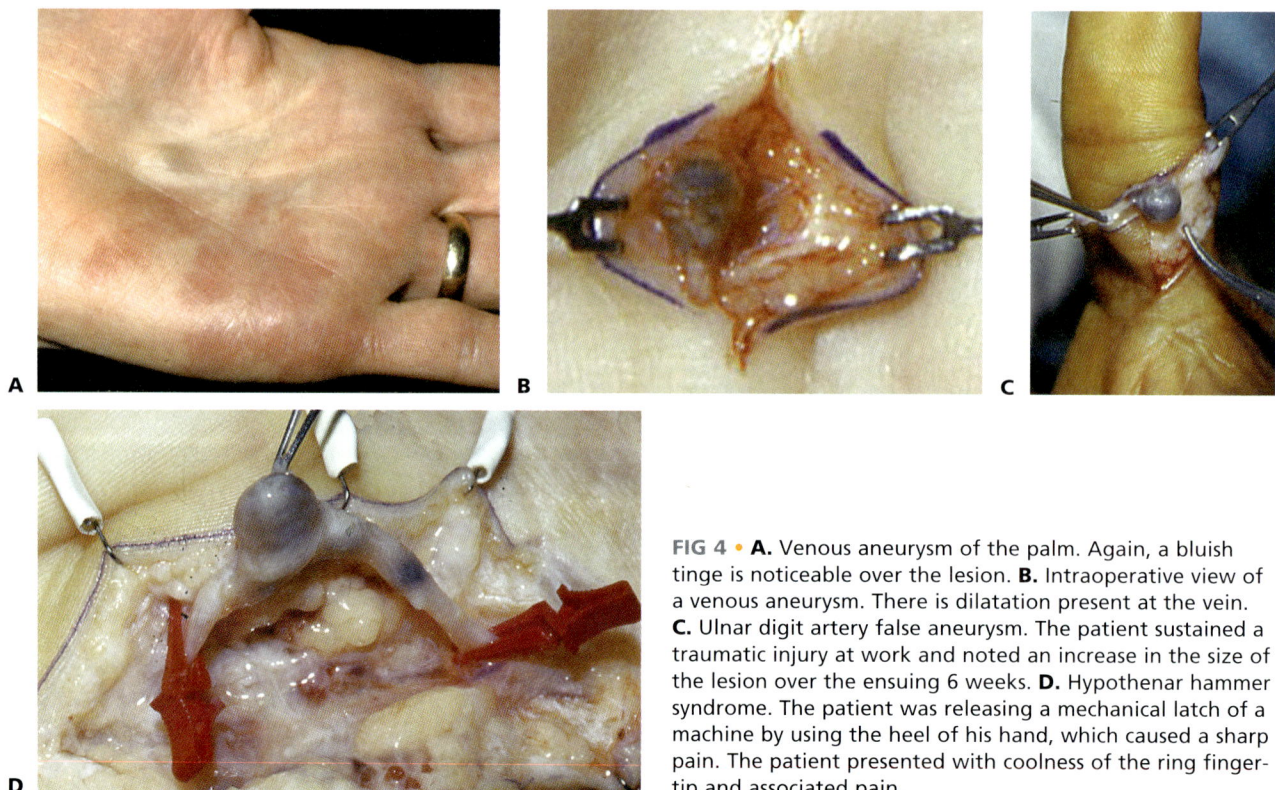

FIG 4 • **A.** Venous aneurysm of the palm. Again, a bluish tinge is noticeable over the lesion. **B.** Intraoperative view of a venous aneurysm. There is dilatation present at the vein. **C.** Ulnar digit artery false aneurysm. The patient sustained a traumatic injury at work and noted an increase in the size of the lesion over the ensuing 6 weeks. **D.** Hypothenar hammer syndrome. The patient was releasing a mechanical latch of a machine by using the heel of his hand, which caused a sharp pain. The patient presented with coolness of the ring fingertip and associated pain.

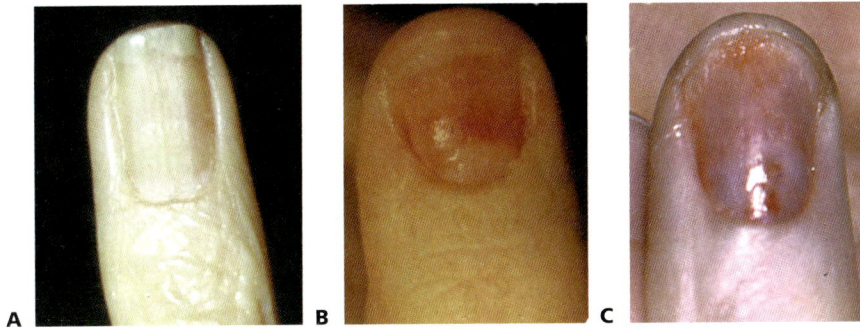

FIG 5 • **A.** Glomus tumor of the left ring finger, subungual region. The patient presented with minimal discoloration and sensitivity to heat and cold. **B.** Glomus tumor of the left thumb. The patient had more significant discoloration of the subungual region consistent with a glomus tumor. **C.** Glomus tumor of the left ring finger after removal of the nail plate. Although the patient had minimal discoloration with the nail plate on, the bluish hue becomes more discernible after the nail is off.

- Traumatic AVFs occur when there is penetrating injury to an artery and the adjacent vein, leading to a hematoma and shunting. This may occur secondary to injury with such objects as small knives or pencils, but it may also be due to venipuncture, arterial cannulation, or catheterization procedures. AVFs secondary to iatrogenic vascular injuries tend to occur slowly, while those that occur secondary to trauma are usually rapid in onset. This may be secondary to the size of the puncture that occurs; iatrogenic injuries tend to be smaller punctures than traumatic ones.[25] Patients with intrinsic coagulation deficiencies are more vulnerable to this complication.
- Surgical AVFs are formed for dialysis access in renal failure patients and can cause similar symptoms, including steal, ischemia, venous arterialization, and hand edema.

Glomus Tumors

- Glomus tumors make up 8% of the vascular tumors of the hand and 1% to 4.5% of all hand tumors.[17,27] They arise in the neuromyoarterial apparatus that was first described by Wood[30] in 1812 and then again by Masson[13] in 1924. These lesions have been found in the stomach, trachea, and retina but are most commonly found in the digits. Glomus tumors are more consistent with a hamartoma than a true tumor.[14] Sixty-five percent of these lesions are found in women 30 to 50 years old.
- Between 26% and 90% of solitary glomus tumors are located in the subungual region.[14,17,27] These lesions tend to be small—normally 5 mm and usually less than 1 cm. They are encapsulated and contain numerous small lumina when found as single tumors. Multiple tumors tend to be unencapsulated, rarely subungual, with larger-shaped vascular spaces.
- Multiple glomus tumors tend to be asymptomatic and present earlier in life, whereas solitary tumors often go undiagnosed or misdiagnosed for years because the lesions are small and not palpable and with varying presentations (**FIG 5**).[15]

Vascular Leiomyomas

- Vascular leiomyomas are very rare tumors of the hand. They arise in the smooth muscle of the tunica media of veins in 50% of cases. These masses are typically well encapsulated, small, round, firm, colorless, and curable (**FIG 6**).[10]

Pyogenic Granulomas

- Pyogenic granulomas make up 20% of the vascular tumors of the hand and may be a variation of a capillary hemangioma. They appear as a circumscribed lesion.
- They develop rapidly and become a pedunculated, friable lesion that is easily traumatized and bleeds. In children, these lesions are more commonly found on the glabrous portion of the palm and digits as well as in the mouth and around the lips and face. In adults, these are more commonly found on the fingers and toes.
- They may occur spontaneously but are more frequently present as an overgrowth of granulation tissue in an area of previous penetrating trauma (**FIG 7**).[6,17,23,29]

Malignant Tumors

- Malignant vascular tumors account for less than 1% of all vascular hand and forearm tumors.[17] There are several types of malignant vascular tumors: hemangioendothelioma, glomangiosarcoma (malignant glomus tumors), angiosarcoma, Kaposi sarcoma, lymphangiosarcoma, and hemangiopericytoma.
- Hemangioendotheliomas tend to arise adjacent to or within veins. They extend centrifugally from the vessel. They are slow-growing tumors, and tumors that show more than one mitosis per high-power field on histology are more likely to metastasize. Metastasis may occur locally to nodes or be distant to the lungs, liver, or bone.[29]
- Glomangiosarcomas are extremely rare and were first described in 1972 by Lumley and Stansfield. They tend to be

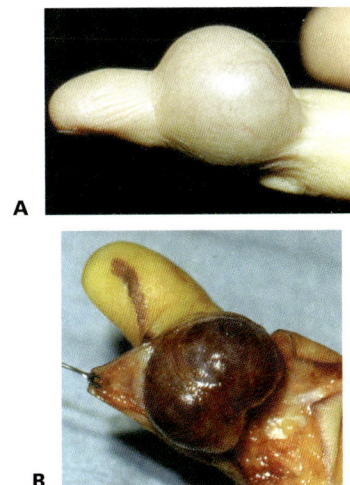

FIG 6 • **A.** Vascular leiomyoma of the right index finger. The patient presented after a 7-month history of having a trauma at work. She stated that the growth appeared 3 months later and had increased in size since then. **B.** Intraoperative photograph of the above vascular leiomyoma. It is a well-circumscribed lesion that is difficult to differentiate from an aneurysm except on pathology.

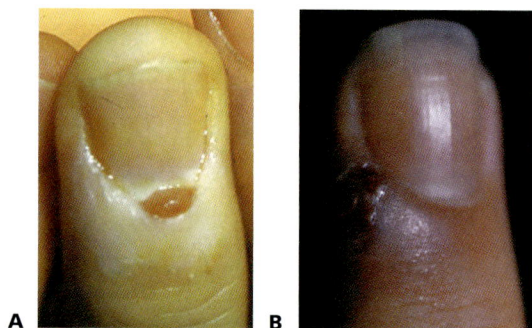

FIG 7 • **A.** Pyogenic granuloma of the left ring finger. The patient developed an open lesion of the cuticle that progressively swelled and then blistered over the nail bed. **B.** Pyogenic granuloma of the left index finger. Notice the granular, raised appearance.

low-grade tumors that are locally invasive. They occur in adults ages 20 to 89 years. There are three categories of glomangiosarcoma: locally infiltrative glomus tumor (LIGT), glomangiosarcoma arising in a benign glomus tumor (GABG), and de novo glomangiosarcoma (GADN).

- LIGT is identical to solitary glomus tumors except that it has infiltrating growth and tends to recur with resection.
- GABG is a sarcomatous tumor in association with a benign glomus tumor.
- GADN is a sarcoma with round cells and features of a benign glomus tumor.[12,19,20]
- Angiosarcomas are rare and aggressive and metastasize early. They may occur after radiation therapy or long-term exposure to polyvinyl chloride. They are sometimes mistaken for hemangioendotheliomas on histology. The prognosis is extremely poor with these tumors, with survival times averaging 2.5 years.[14,17,29]
- First described by Kaposi in 1872 in elderly men of Jewish and Mediterranean heritage, Kaposi sarcoma present as small, purple macules. They are a malignant degeneration of the reticuloendothelial system. These lesions tend to start on the hands or lower extremities, progress onto the trunk, and coalesce into large papules. In this patient population, the disease has an indolent course and may be treatable with surgery and radiation. In the age of HIV/AIDS, however, the disease is much more aggressive, with a larger number of lesions. In these patients, it is associated with human herpes virus 8.[14,17,29]
- Lymphangiosarcoma is a rare cancer that occurs after longstanding lymphedema, as seen in some postmastectomy patients. These lesions metastasize rapidly.
- Hemangiopericytoma is a diffuse proliferation of capillaries, encased in connective tissue and surrounded by pericytes. They have no nerve elements and are generally painless. Patients tend to delay treatment secondary to lack of pain. They may present as a nonpigmented bleeding mole, an ulceration with prominent telangiectasia, or a dark blue, hemorrhagic swelling. Histologically, they have sheets of spindle cells surrounding capillaries, regular oval nuclei without anaplasia, indistinct cytoplasmic borders, and a reticulin sheath surrounding each cell on silver stain.[11,28] Pathologists have described three histologic grades based on the above criteria: benign, borderline malignant, and malignant. It has an unpredictable behavior and may metastasize years after excision; therefore, long-term (5 to 10 years) follow-up is recommended (**FIG 8**).

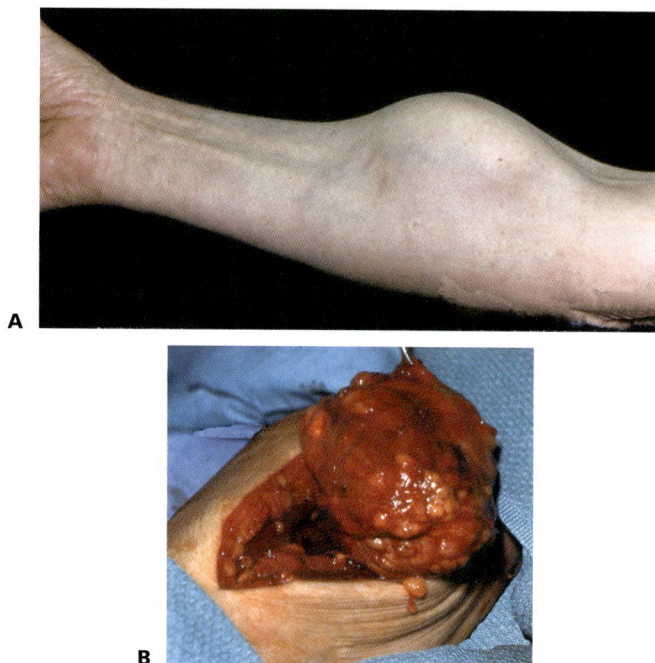

FIG 8 • **A.** Hemangiopericytoma of the right forearm. The patient presented with a large mass of the forearm that had been present for 46 years. **B.** Intraoperative view of hemangiopericytoma. The lesion was 9 × 6.6 × 5 cm and weighed 168 g.

PATIENT HISTORY AND PHYSICAL FINDINGS

- It is imperative to get a complete history and physical examination of the patient and family.
  - Determine whether the lesion was present at birth or infancy or whether it appeared later in adolescence or adulthood.
  - Rate of growth should be sought. This may help to differentiate between a hemangioma and an arteriovenous malformation in early childhood. Hemangiomas grow out of proportion to the growth of the child.
- Hemangiomas
  - Hemangiomas will appear as a reddish lesion that becomes raised. Lesions of the axilla or interdigital region will be chronically macerated. Fingertip hemangiomas may present with findings similar to an acute or chronic paronychial infection, especially in children who suck on their fingers.[23]
- Vascular malformations
  - Low-flow malformations most commonly present as a mass or skin discoloration. If a capillary component is present, there may be a reddish stain of the skin. The physician should ascertain whether there are any compressive symptoms from the lesion consistent with a mass effect, distention, or pain with exercise that would indicate a venous malformation.
    - Ulceration is uncommon in these lesions.
    - If there is a lymphatic component, patients may present with intralesional infections secondary to ruptured vesicles and maceration of large lesions.
    - They may also be found in association with syndromes such as Parkes-Weber, Klippel-Trenaunay, proteus (capillary malformations, venous malformations, macrodactyly, hemihypertrophy, lipomas, scoliosis, and pigmented

nevi), and Mafucci (lymphaticovenous malformations and enchondromas).[23]

- High-flow malformations tend to be painless early on but then progress to be warm, painful masses with palpable thrills and bruits as the child grows.
  - Asking the patient if he or she gets relief of the pain with elevation, if there is increased pain with exercise, and increased warmth in the lesion may help to distinguish these from low-flow lesions.
  - It is also important to ask about any symptoms of congestive heart failure, which may occur as sequelae of an untreated high-flow malformation.[23]
- Any patient evaluated in the office for a suspected arteriovenous malformation should be evaluated for other lesions, Nicoldani sign (decrease in pulse with occlusion of the fistula), and any evidence of distal ischemia.[14]
- Aneurysms and pyogenic granulomas
  - For evaluation of possible aneurysms and pyogenic granulomas, it is important to know whether there is a history of trauma in the region, how long the lesion has been present, whether it is a pulsatile mass, and whether it has bled.
- Glomus tumors
  - The classic triad of paroxysmal pain, pinpoint tenderness, and temperature intolerance, especially cold, should be elicited if glomus tumors are in the differential.
  - On physical examination, the physician should look for a bluish discoloration (found in 28% of patients) and a pulp nodule or nail deformity (found in 33% of patients).[15]
  - The length of time that the patient has had symptoms can assist in differentiating glomus tumors from other tumors of the upper extremities, since most patients tend to have symptoms for more than 10 years. If the patient has had previous excisions of glomus tumors, it is necessary to find out the amount of time between resection and recurrence. This can help to determine whether the lesion is an incomplete excision or a new tumor.[26]
  - During the physical examination, the patient should also be evaluated for multiple glomus tumors, which tend to be less symptomatic.
- Patients with lesions of the hand, wrist, or distal forearm should have an Allen's test performed.
  - The hand is elevated and the patient is asked to make a tight fist for about 30 seconds. The ulnar and radial arteries are occluded and the patient opens his or her hand slowly. The ulnar artery is then released and the color should return in 5 seconds. If color returns to the radial aspect of the hand within 5 seconds, the superficial arch is complete and the radial artery may be ligated.
- A thorough evaluation of the rest of the patient's medical history, including a history of axillary dissections, HIV/AIDS status, and irradiation, is also necessary if the patient presents with a lesion that may be cancerous.
- Methods for examining the vascular lesions of the hand
  - The examiner should look at the hand to check for blue spots, nail ridging, reddish, raised lesions, pulsatile masses, or traumatic injury, which helps to differentiate between malformations, aneurysms, pyogenic granulomas, and glomus tumors.
  - A stethoscope is gently placed over the lesion to listen for bruits or thrills. In fast-flow arteriovenous malformations, a bruit or thrill may be heard, which would not be found in other vascular lesions.

- The mass is gently palpated. If a pulsatile mass is felt, the examiner should ascertain whether the lesion is compressible and whether there is associated pain.
- Love pin test: The head of a pin or paperclip is gently pressed against the tender area to localize the pain. This locates a glomus tumor. In subungual tumors, the pin is placed on the nail plate at various locations to find the tumor.[15]
- Hildreth test: The digit is exsanguinated by placing a tourniquet at its base or the hand is exsanguinated by elevating it and making a tight fist. The point of tenderness located by the Love pin test is then repalpated. If the patient has diminished or resolved pain with this maneuver, then the test is considered positive for a glomus tumor.[8]

IMAGING AND OTHER DIAGNOSTIC STUDIES

- Plain radiographs of the digits and hands
  - Phleboliths (in 6%) and bony hypertrophy may be noted.[14,17]
  - There may be evidence of a soft tissue mass or signs of bone erosion or destruction of the cortical surface, which is seen in about 6% of patients with hemangiomas.[17]
- Doppler ultrasonic flow detection is a noninvasive study that does not require the use of contrast.
  - It has been used to confirm high-flow anomalies and to help differentiate between hemangiomas and malformations.[24] Doppler ultrasonography will show these lesions to be monophasic with low-flow velocity averaging 0.22 kHz.[22]
- Computed tomography with contrast enhancement may show bony involvement of the tumor, especially in type A high-flow malformations.[24]
- MRI can be used to evaluate the site, size, flow rate, and characteristics of the lesion as well as involvement of contiguous structures.[24]
  - It may be used to determine whether a malformation is low-flow or high-flow and can also distinguish between dense parenchymal lesions and malformations with large vascular channels.[14]
  - It can also be used to evaluate glomus tumors, which have a high signal intensity on T2-weighted spin-echo MRI or after gadolinium injection.[15]
  - MRI has a sensitivity of 90% and a specificity of 50% for glomus tumors, so that it cannot be used as the single diagnostic study for glomus tumors, especially if they are less than 2 to 3 mm in size.[1]
  - Hemangiomas will appear as well-circumscribed mass lesions that enhance with gadolinium and will have a high T1 signal secondary to infiltrative margins and fatty tissue overgrowth as well an extremely high, heterogeneous T2 signal. A serpentine pattern in the mass may also be seen on MRI.[29]
- MR angiography may be performed at the time of MRI to evaluate lesions in patients who are unable to undergo angiography secondary to renal problems or contrast allergies. It can be used to define the anatomic extent of lesions and their relationship with the surrounding tissue. It can be used to evaluate for both arterial and venous tumors without contrast enhancement.[7]
- Technetium-99m red blood cell perfusion and blood pool scintigraphy will show increased activity on early and late blood pool images with increased perfusion in hemangiomas and may be useful in their diagnosis.[29]
- Angiography is the gold-standard evaluation of certain tumors, including vascular malformations. No longer routinely used for diagnosis of a lesion, it is used as an evaluation for

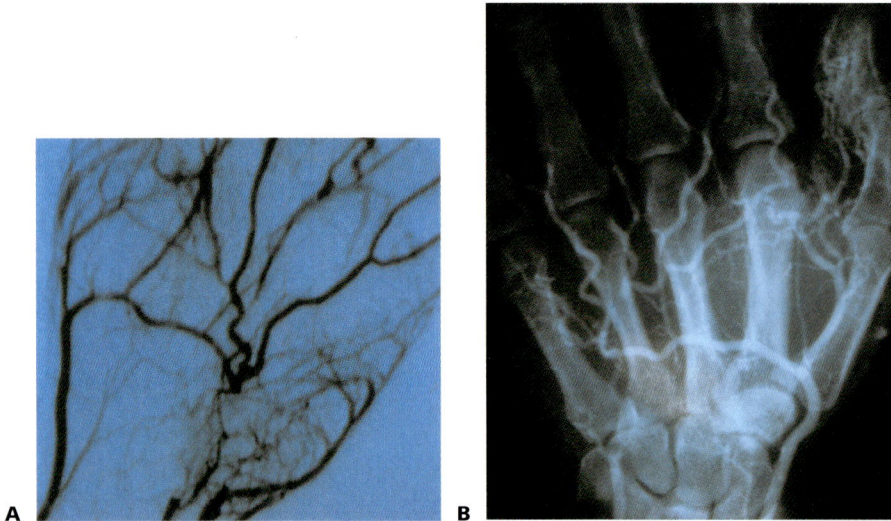

FIG 9 • **A.** Angiogram of hypothenar hammer syndrome. The ulnar artery flow is absent and collaterals have formed to allow for flow in the palmar arch. This patient was relatively asymptomatic until a trauma to the hand. **B.** Angiogram of a second patient with hypothenar hammer syndrome. In this patient, there are no collaterals present, and he presented with coldness of the ulnar distribution digits.

operation or embolization.[24] It may show a cluster of anomalous arterial branches with multiple communications with venous trunks draining the site of involvement.[16]

■ Closed venous angiography uses contrast injected into the venous system distal to a proximal arterial tourniquet applied on the upper arm. Dye is injected into the exsanguinated extremity distal to the tumor and radiographs are taken as the vascular tumor fills to get an accurate assessment of the anatomy.[14] Arterial angiography is performed through a stick into the femoral artery with a catheter that is fed into the involved extremity. Dye is then injected and both the arterial and venous phases of circulation are evaluated. This can be used to evaluate the size of the tumor, locate the feeding vessels, and embolize feeding vessels before operation (**FIG 9**).[14]

DIFFERENTIAL DIAGNOSIS

- Foreign body
- Bacillary angiomatosis
- Pyogenic granuloma
- Glomus tumor
- Hemangioma
- Arteriovenous or lymphatic malformation
- AVFs (traumatic, congenital, iatrogenic)
- Traumatic aneurysm (true or false)
- Mycotic aneurysm (hematogenous or exogenous)
- Arteriosclerotic aneurysm
- Congenital aneurysm
- Metabolic aneurysm (eg, osteogenesis imperfecta, granulomatous arteritis, Buerger disease)
- Vascular leiomyomas
- Glomangiosarcoma
- Angiosarcoma
- Hemangioendothelioma
- Hemangiopericytoma
- Kaposi sarcoma
- Lymphangiosarcoma

NONOPERATIVE MANAGEMENT

- Observation is important for hemangiomas. Up to 70% of these lesions will involute by the age of 7.

- Large venous or capillary malformations should be observed for limb growth disturbances and a possible underlying high-flow lesion.
- Limb compression garments can be used to compress massive congenital arteriovenous fistulas that are inoperable, giant venous malformations, lymphatic malformations, or large hemangiomas in the arm and forearm.[17,23] For larger lymphatic lesions, home compression pumps can be used to decrease edema at night.[23]
- Antibiotic prophylaxis is indicated in patients who have recurrent infections in lymphatic malformations. The bacteria most commonly responsible for these infections is penicillin-sensitive beta-hemolytic streptococcus.[23]
- If a patient with venous malformations or capillary-venolymphatic malformation has recurrent intralesional thrombosis, then low-dose aspirin may be added to the compression garments for effective therapy.[23]
- Local wound care and dressings may be required if ulcerations occur in the periungual regions or the central portions of large lesions during the involutional phase.[23]
- Pulsed-dye laser or argon laser may be used with some hemangiomas to treat the pigmented lesion without damaging the overlying skin, sweat glands, and hair follicles. Lasers of 585-nm wavelength work well on vascular lesions, such as hemangiomas, which are rich in hemoglobin. The laser heats the hemoglobin, causing coagulation of the vessels in the dermis. Scar formation ensues and replaces the damaged blood vessels.[17]
- Sclerotherapy with 1% sodium tetradecylsulfate, for small superficial lesions, or 100% ethanol, for large, deep saccular lesions, may be used in treating venous malformations.
  - With the larger lesions, there is a possibility of skin ulceration, necrosis, inflammatory changes, and contracture due to the treatment, and patients should be warned to watch for these sequelae.[23]
- In arteriovenous malformations interventional radiology may be used for embolization of selectively catheterized vessels with polyvinyl alcohol foam or tissue adhesive. This may be helpful if surgical resection is performed 24 to 48 hours later. If the lesion is small, this may completely occlude the malformation and destroy the lesion, eliminating the need for surgical resection. Several embolizations may be necessary to fully destroy small lesions.[14]

■ Embolization may lead to residual tissue loss, neurologic deficit, and enlargement of the malformation if the lesion is large and not excised promptly.[9,16]

■ Either intralesional or systemic steroids may be useful for the treatment of hemangiomas, and a 6-week course may help to treat life-threatening or tissue-threatening lesions. This is also true for interferon alpha-2a or 2b. However, neither of these medications has been shown to have any effects on malformations, and the morbidity (neutropenia, elevation of liver enzymes, and spastic diparesis) of interferon must be considered before its use.[24,29]

■ Radiation therapy was used in the past for sclerosis of hemangiomas; however, it leads to atrophic changes in the skin and subcutaneous tissue as well as arrest of skeletal growth.[17]

SURGICAL MANAGEMENT

■ Indications for surgery include pain, intralesional thrombi, episodic bleeding or ulceration, recurrent infection, or functional problems related to the size or weight of the extremity. It is important to consider whether the extremity will be functional after the proposed surgical treatment; in many cases amputation may be a better option.[23]

■ Lymphatic malformations have the added difficulties of beta-hemolytic streptococcal septicemia, skin maceration, and vesicular eruptions. This makes the planning of surgical resection complex. Complications occur in 25% of all procedures. The surgeon should be aware that tumor-free tissues, such as grafts or flaps, may be necessary for coverage.[23]

Preoperative Planning

■ Radiographic studies should be reviewed carefully to plan resection of large or complex lesions.

■ An Allen's test should be performed on the patient to evaluate for the patency of the superficial palmar arch and to see if the patient has an adequate ulnar artery.

■ If the Allen's test is positive, reconstruction of the radial artery is necessary if it is to be resected.

Positioning

■ The patient should be placed in supine position with the arm abducted.

■ A proximal arm tourniquet is used, but the arm should not be exsanguinated with an Esmarch bandage to avoid the proximal spread or localized compression of the tumor. Exsanguination with the Esmarch bandage may also obscure the margins of hemangiomas and malformations.

■ Injections around the tumor should also be avoided to reduce the risk of local spread and compression of the mass, which could cause incomplete resection.

Approach

■ The technique chosen is based on the location of the lesion and the access necessary for excision.

Ligation of Feeding Vessel

■ For lesions that are small, with few feeder vessels, direct exploration and ligation of the feeding vessels can lead to involution of the lesion without significant tissue loss.

■ If tissue loss occurs, excision of the area and either primary closure, skin grafting, or flap reconstruction can be performed.

Staged Excision

■ Staged excision is useful for venous malformations, lymphatic malformations, combined malformations, and types A and B high-flow malformations.[24]

■ For larger lesions, the interventional radiologist may be helpful in embolizing feeding vessels. This will decrease or limit the amount of open exposure necessary in the first stage.

■ In this approach, the extremity is not exsanguinated completely to allow identification of the vessels more readily.

■ In the first stage, the tributary and exiting vessels are ligated proximal and distal to the tumor. It is possible that ligation of the vessels may induce distal ischemia. If this occurs, the surgeon should be prepared to bypass the anatomic defect with autogenous vein grafts.

■ At a second stage, the lesion is removed after the above procedure and depending on the condition of the patient. If necessary, the second procedure may be delayed. If the tumor is adherent to the skin, that portion of tissue is excised as well and the area is covered with grafts or flaps.[17]

Amputation

■ Amputation is the treatment choice for highly aggressive malignancies such as hemangiosarcoma, lymphangiosarcoma, aggressive hemangioendothelioma, and massive arteriovenous malformations that have created a nonfunctional extremity.

■ This should be performed with a proximal tourniquet for operative hemostasis.

■ If the lesion is too proximal for a tourniquet, an internal vascular balloon can be used to occlude the feeding vessel or vessels.

■ Guillotine amputation is an option if infection is present; otherwise, closure should be performed at the time of amputation.

■ The most common error we have seen after amputation of a digit or hand is failure to obtain adequate, tension-free soft tissue coverage.

■ Wide local excision may be considered for less aggressive hemangioendothelioma, hemangiopericytomas, malformations, and hemangiomas that have not involuted.

TRANSUNGUAL EXCISION

■ Transungual excision is an approach to subungual lesions, such as glomus tumors.

■ Make small radial and ulnar corner incisions over the nail fold (**TECH FIG 1A,B**).

■ Half the nail is then elevated and folded over, allowing for visualization of the nail matrix (**TECH FIG 1C**).

■ The nail can be completely removed with a Freer elevator if necessary for access to the tumor (**TECH FIG 1D**).

■ Make a longitudinal incision with a no. 15 blade into the nail matrix, directly over the tumor, and excise the lesion circumferentially down to the phalanx (**TECH FIG 1E,F**).

■ Curette the bone before the nail bed is closed with 6-0 plain gut.

■ Replace the nail into the eponychial fold as a dressing for the nail bed and suture the corner incision closed (**TECH FIG 1G**).[15,21]

TECHNIQUES

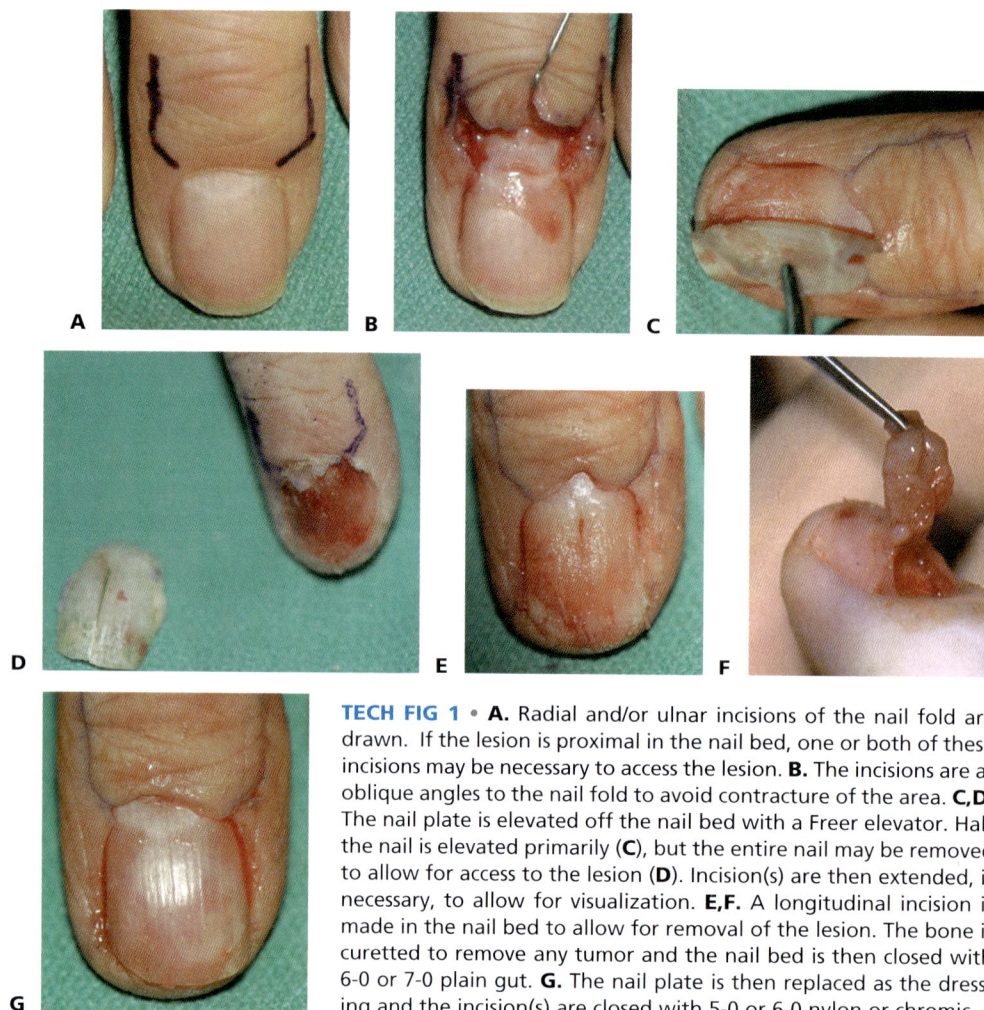

TECH FIG 1 • **A.** Radial and/or ulnar incisions of the nail fold are drawn. If the lesion is proximal in the nail bed, one or both of these incisions may be necessary to access the lesion. **B.** The incisions are at oblique angles to the nail fold to avoid contracture of the area. **C,D.** The nail plate is elevated off the nail bed with a Freer elevator. Half the nail is elevated primarily (**C**), but the entire nail may be removed to allow for access to the lesion (**D**). Incision(s) are then extended, if necessary, to allow for visualization. **E,F.** A longitudinal incision is made in the nail bed to allow for removal of the lesion. The bone is curetted to remove any tumor and the nail bed is then closed with 6-0 or 7-0 plain gut. **G.** The nail plate is then replaced as the dressing and the incision(s) are closed with 5-0 or 6-0 nylon or chromic.

LATERAL INCISION

- This is an alternative to the transungual excision and allows exposure of the dorsal distal phalanx without violating the nail matrix. Because the view of the tumor is narrower, we do not recommend this approach.[15]
- If this approach is to be used, then a longitudinal midaxial incision slightly dorsal to the neurovascular bundle is used (**TECH FIG 2A**).
  - The incision is placed on the radial or ulnar surface of the digit, based on the location of the lesion.
- Sharp dissection is carried out to the distal phalanx without manipulating the surrounding soft tissue.

- A small, sharp elevator is used to create a subperiosteal dorsal flap (**TECH FIG 2B**).
- A small curette or elevator is used to excise the lesion.
- The flap is replaced and the incision is closed with interrupted or running nylon suture.[21,27]

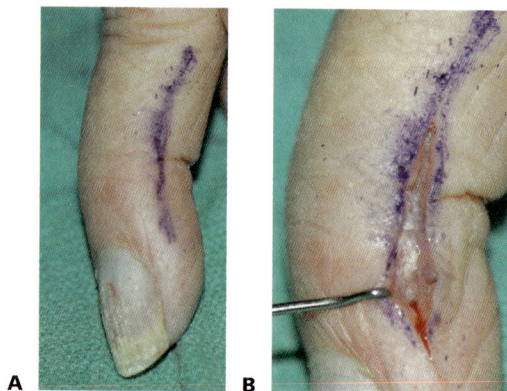

TECH FIG 2 • **A.** A midlateral incision is drawn just dorsal to the midaxial line. The incision is carried sharply down to the bone, keeping the neurovascular bundle volar to the incision and dissection. **B.** A Freer elevator is then used to create a subperiosteal flap to allow removal of the lesion. The incision is then closed with 5-0 or 6-0 nylon.

EPIPHYSIODESIS

- Epiphysiodesis, destroying the growth plate by scraping or drilling, may help to diminish hypertrophy in patients whose digits have reached adult size.
- Make a midaxial incision sharply, with dissection continued to the bone.
  - Retract the neurovascular bundle volarly to avoid injury (**TECH FIG 3A**).
- The dorsal branches may be transected if it is necessary to gain access to the dorsal aspect of the phalanx.
- Use a drill to destroy the growth plate of the phalanx (**TECH FIG 3B**).
- Close the incision with 5-0 or 6-0 nylon.

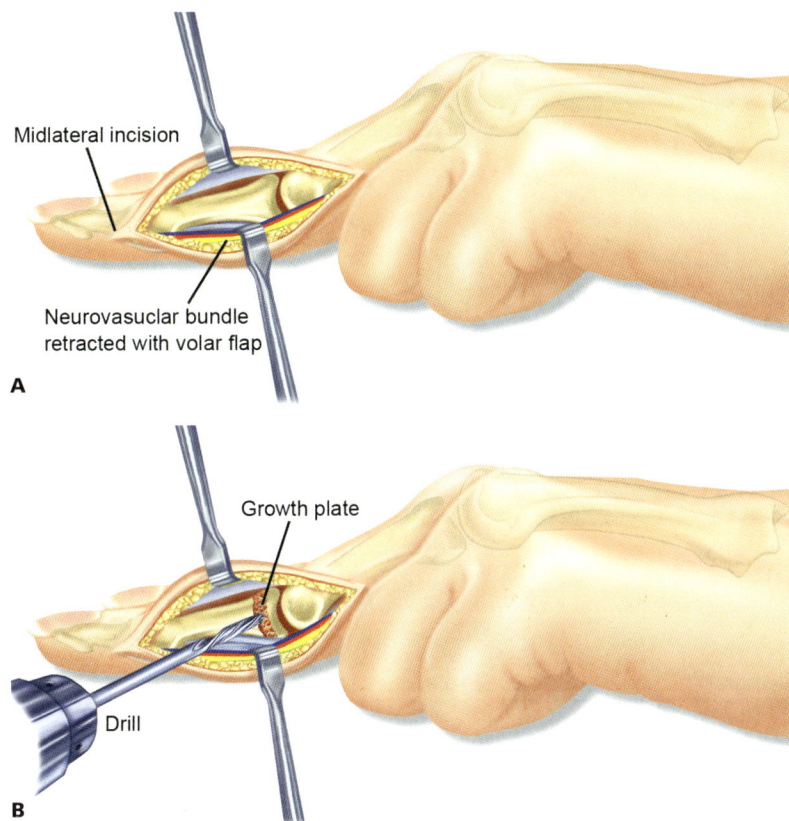

TECH FIG 3 • A. A midlateral incision is made sharply and dissection continues to the level of the bone. The neurovascular bundle is retracted with the volar flap to ensure that it is not injured during dissection. The dorsal branches may be ligated or left intact, if it does not interfere with the exposure of the phalanx. **B.** A drill is used to annihilate the growth plate of the phalanx to halt its growth. The incision is then closed with 5-0 or 6-0 nylon.

PEARLS AND PITFALLS

Have a tourniquet on the extremity before the incision for arteriovenous malformations.	▪ Avoid overly aggressive resection of lesions.
Make the family aware of the guarded prognosis for complete removal of arteriovenous malformations and the possibility of overgrowth or recurrence of the lesions.	▪ Exsanguination of an arteriovenous malformation may lead to incomplete excision.
Insist on multiple high-quality imaging studies to evaluate the lesions	▪ For small lesions, imaging may not fully show the lesion.
Check patient for associated syndromic abnormalities.	

POSTOPERATIVE CARE

- After excision of the lesion, most patients will require a bulky dressing, and most will be able to return to their normal activity within 1 to 2 weeks.
  - Patients with partial resection of arteriovenous malformations may need to continue wearing compressive garments postoperatively when the dressings are removed.
- If patients required skin grafts or flaps, dressings and splints can be left in place to keep the patient from shearing the graft or pulling at the flap until the incisions are healed.
  - Graft bolsters or splints should be left in place for about 3 to 5 days to allow the graft to adhere well.
- For patients who require amputations, prosthetics may be formed, depending on the level of the amputation. These are

more readily available for patients who have below- or above-elbow amputations, although patients who have forequarter amputations may also be candidates for specialized prosthetics.

▪ Patients will require physical therapy to teach them how to use prosthetics or to relearn hand function, if wide excisions were necessary.

OUTCOMES

▪ The prognosis of hemangiomas is not affected by race, gender, tumor site, size, or presence at birth.[16]

▪ Attempts to excise arteriovenous malformations may lead to serious complications.

▪ Complications are seen in about 22% of slow-flow lesions and 28% of fast-flow lesions. Wound dehiscence, seromas, and hematomas are noted early on. Partial skin loss and incision site infection are seen in the late postoperative period.

▪ In fast-flow malformations, episodic bleeding and wound breakdown are more common.[23]

▪ After resection of venous malformations and lymphatic malformations, persistent edema and swelling are more frequent. Patients with type C malformations more consistently require multiple operative procedures due to complications.

▪ Disseminated intravascular coagulation has been reported, and coagulation studies should be obtained before any intervention.

▪ In the study by Mendel and Louis,[16] 13 of 17 lesions persisted after excision through extension or recurrence. Ten of these lesions were diffuse. Thus, two fifths of lesions that are thought to be localized are diffuse and will require more than one procedure for complete excision.

▪ In view of the high recurrence rate, excision should be considered in specific situations. Partial resection might be chosen to provide relief of symptoms, but as a balance between aggressive resection and preservation of function.[16]

▪ Patients who had wide local excision of venous malformations were found to have a 2% recurrence rate.[14]

▪ It is generally accepted that primary tumor excision is the treatment of choice in all adults with venous malformations and children who have been observed for 1 year without regression of the lesion.

▪ Glomus tumors recur in 15% to 24% of patients, with an average time before recurrence of 2.9 years.

▪ Late presentation of recurrence is thought to be due to a new tumor near the site of excision. Patients who had incomplete excisions had recurrence of the tumor within weeks of surgery.

▪ In patients who had transungual excisions, nail deformities were noted in 26% of patients postoperatively.

▪ The prognosis of hemangioendothelioma depends on the grade of the tumor. Patients with low-grade lesions have a good long-term survival rate, and those with aggressive tumors may not survive longer than 2 years.[11]

▪ Kaposi sarcoma in elderly non-HIV patients may be cured with wide-local excision; however, the accepted treatment for these patients is chemoradiation and alpha-interferon therapy. The 5-year survival rate of these patients is only 19%. In patients with HIV/AIDS, the mortality rate of Kaposi sarcoma was 80% at 2 years, but this has improved with highly active antiretroviral therapy (HAART).[17]

▪ For patients with hemangiosarcoma, early radical amputation is the treatment of choice. Palliative radiation has also been used. The average survival is 2.5 years, and the 5-year survival rate is less than 20%. One third of patients with hemangiosarcoma have hemorrhage or coagulopathy, and 45% have nodal metastases.[4,17]

▪ Glomangiosarcomas are believed to be low-grade malignancies; however, more than 25% of reported cases develop metastases.[12] Wide local excision is the treatment of choice for these lesions, and close long-term follow-up is necessary.

COMPLICATIONS

▪ High-output cardiac failure
▪ Consumptive coagulopathy
▪ Bacterial endocarditis
▪ Distal ischemia
▪ Tissue loss
▪ Local infection
▪ Compartment syndrome
▪ Arterial steal
▪ Hematoma
▪ Seroma
▪ Partial wound dehiscence
▪ Cellulitis at the operative site
▪ Hypertrophic scarring
▪ Joint contracture
▪ Neuromas
▪ Reflex sympathetic dystrophy
▪ Pain
▪ Partial or total extremity gangrene
▪ Vesicle formation
▪ Recurrence
▪ Amputation

REFERENCES

1. Al-Qattan MM, Al-Namla A, Al-Thunayan A, et al. Magnetic resonance imaging in the diagnosis of glomus tumours of the hand. J Hand Surg Br 2005;30B:535–540.
2. Boyd JB, Mulliken JB, Kaban LB, et al. Skeletal changes associated with vascular malformations. Plast Reconstr Surg 1984;74:789–797.
3. Burrows PE, Mulliken JB, Fellows KE, et al. Childhood hemangiomas and vascular malformations: angiographic differentiation. AJR Am J Roentgenol 1983;141:483–488.
4. Carsi B, Sim F. Angiosarcoma. January 2006. http://www.emedicine.com/med/ topic138.htm
5. Coleman SS, Anson BJ. Arterial patterns in the hand based upon a study of 650 specimens. Surg Gynecol Obstet 1961;113:409–424.
6. DiFazio F, Mogan J. Intravenous pyogenic granuloma of the hand. J Hand Surg Am 1989;14A:310–312.
7. Disa JJ, Chung KC, Gellad FE, et al. Efficacy of magnetic resonance angiography in the evaluation of vascular malformations of the hand. Plast Reconstr Surg 1997;99:136–147.
8. Giele H. Hildreth's test is a reliable clinical sign for the diagnosis of glomus tumours. J Hand Surg Br 2002;27B:157–158.
9. Griffin JM, Vasconez LO, Schatten WE. Congenital arteriovenous malformations of the upper extremity. Plast Reconstr Surg 1978;62:49–58.
10. Hauswald KR, Kasdan ML, Weiss DL. Vascular leiomyoma of the hand: case report. Plast Reconstr Surg 1975;55:89–91.
11. Kasdan ML, Stallings SP. Malignant hemangiopericytoma of the forearm. Plast Reconstr Surg 1993;91:533–536.
12. Khoury T, Balos L, McGrath B, et al. Malignant glomus tumor: a case report and review of literature, focusing on its clinicopathologic features and immunohistochemical profile. Am J Dermatopathol 2005;27:428–431.
13. Masson P. Le glomus neuromyo-arteriel des regions tactiles et ses tumeurs. Lyon Chir 1924;21:257–280.
14. McClinton MA. Tumors and aneurysms of the upper extremity. Hand Clin 1993;9:151–169.

15. McDermott EM, Weiss AP. Glomus tumors. J Hand Surg Am 2006; 31A:1397–1400.

16. Mendel T, Louis DS. Major vascular malformations of the upper extremity: long-term observation. J Hand Surg Am 1997;22A:302–306.

17. Palmieri TJ. Vascular tumors of the hand and forearm. Hand Clin 1987;3:225–240.

18. Palmieri TJ. Subcutaneous hemangiomas of the hand. J Hand Surg Am 1983;8A:201–204.

19. Park JH, Oh SH, Yang MH, et al. Glomangiosarcoma of the hand: a case report and review of the literature. J Dermatol 2003;30:827–833.

20. Perez de la Fuente T, Vega C, Gutierrez Palacios A, et al. Glomangiosarcoma of the hypothenar eminence: a case report. Chir Main 2005;24:199–202.

21. Takata H, Ikuta Y, Ishida O, et al. Treatment of subungual glomus tumour. Hand Surg 2001;6:25–27.

22. Trop I, Dubois J, Guibaud L, et al. Soft-tissue venous malformations in pediatric and young adult patients: diagnosis with Doppler US. Radiology 1999;212:841–845.

23. Upton J, Coombs C. Vascular tumors in children. Hand Clin 1995; 11:307–337.

24. Upton J, Coombs CJ, Mulliken JB, et al. Vascular malformations of the upper limb: a review of 270 patients. J Hand Surg Am 1999;24A:1019–1035.

25. Upton J, Sampson C, Havlik R, et al. Acquired arteriovenous fistulas in children. J Hand Surg Am 1994;19A:656–658.

26. Van Geertruyden J, Lorea P, Goldschmidt D, et al. Glomus tumours of the hand: a retrospective study of 51 cases. J Hand Surg Br 1996; 21B:257–260.

27. Vasisht B, Watson HK, Joseph E, et al. Digital glomus tumors: a 29-year experience with a lateral subperiosteal approach. Plast Reconstr Surg 2004;114:1486–1489.

28. Vathana P. Primary hemangiopericytoma of bone in the hand: a case report. J Hand Surg Am 1984;9A:761–764.

29. Walsh JJ IV, Eady JL. Vascular tumors. Hand Clin 2004;20:261–268.

30. Wood W. On painful subcutaneous tubercle. Edinburgh Med J 1812;8:283.

Chapter 111

Excision and Coverage of Squamous Cell Carcinoma and Melanoma of the Hand

Mark F. Hendrickson and Benjamin J. Boudreaux

DEFINITION

■ Squamous cell carcinoma and melanoma represent malignant transformation of specific cells in either cutaneous or noncutaneous regions of the body.

■ Both squamous cell carcinoma and melanoma demonstrate ability to extend locally, involve regional lymph node basins, and metastasize to distant sites.

■ In the upper extremity, the nail matrix is the noncutaneous location for these malignancies (**FIG 1**).

■ In 1886, Hutchinson first described subungual melanoma and initially termed it melanotic whitlow, because it often resembled an infection. Subungual melanoma is rare, accounting for only 1% to 3% of all cases of melanoma.

■ Critical to management of squamous cell carcinoma and melanoma of the hand and upper extremity are early diagnosis, accurate histopathologic evaluation, detailed staging, appropriate surgical, medical, and radiation management, and appropriate follow-up.

ANATOMY

■ Both squamous cell carcinoma and melanoma develop from different skin layers. Intact skin demonstrates histologic features of the epidermis and dermis that act as physiologic barriers to infection and malignancy.

■ Squamous cell carcinomas develop from epidermal keratinocyte cell layers but can develop in the nail matrix complex.

■ Melanoma cells derive from the dendritic cells of the epidermis; they originate from neural crest cells. These neural crest cell–derived melanocytes migrate to both cutaneous and noncutaneous locations. For the hand and upper extremity, the nail apparatus is a significant migration site. Melanomas are not always pigmented (amelanotic melanomas). However, melanomas are typically pigmented and reflect irregular color, surface, and perimeter.

PATHOGENESIS

■ Squamous cell carcinomas develop from epidermal keratinocyte cell layers. Risk factors include the following:
  ■ Damage from sun, heat, and wind
  ■ Severe burns and chronic ulcers
  ■ Increasing age
  ■ Immune compromise (organ transplantation and AIDS)

■ The typical squamous cell carcinoma lesion is a rapidly growing, firm, scaly papule or nodule that develops a central ulcer and an indurated raised border with some surrounding inflammation (**FIG 2A–D**).
  ■ In contrast to basal cell carcinomas, there is no pearly telangiectatic perimeter.

■ Major risks for melanoma include:
  ■ Personal or family history of melanoma. Patients with a history of melanoma have a 3.5% chance of developing a second melanoma.
  ■ The presence of a mole that has changed over time

■ Other general risk factors for skin cancer, including sun sensitivity; excessive sun exposure; immune compromise; prior basal cell or squamous cell cancers; or exposure to coal tar, pitch, arsenical compounds, x-radiation, or radium

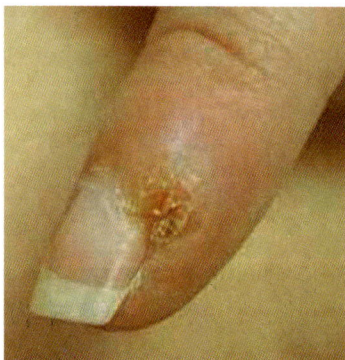

FIG 1 • Thumb eponychial lesion treated as both an infection and mucous cyst. Histopathology demonstrated invasive squamous cell carcinoma. Treatment included amputation at the IP joint level and selective lymph node sampling.

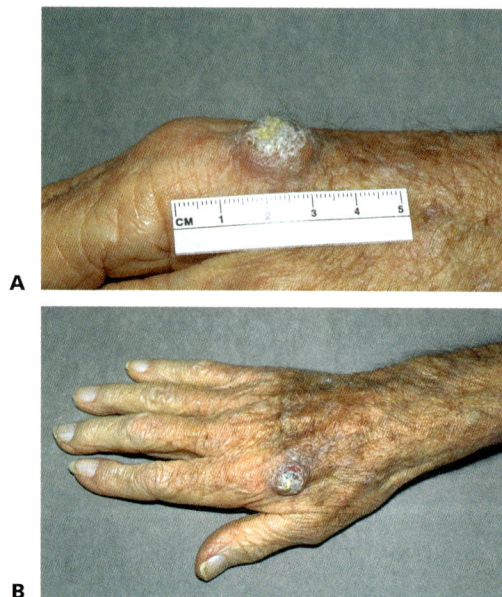

FIG 2 • A. Radial view of invasive squamous cell carcinoma of right second MP joint area in a kidney-pancreas transplant patient. **B.** Dorsal view of invasive squamous cell carcinoma of right second MP joint area in a kidney-pancreas transplant patient. *(continued)*

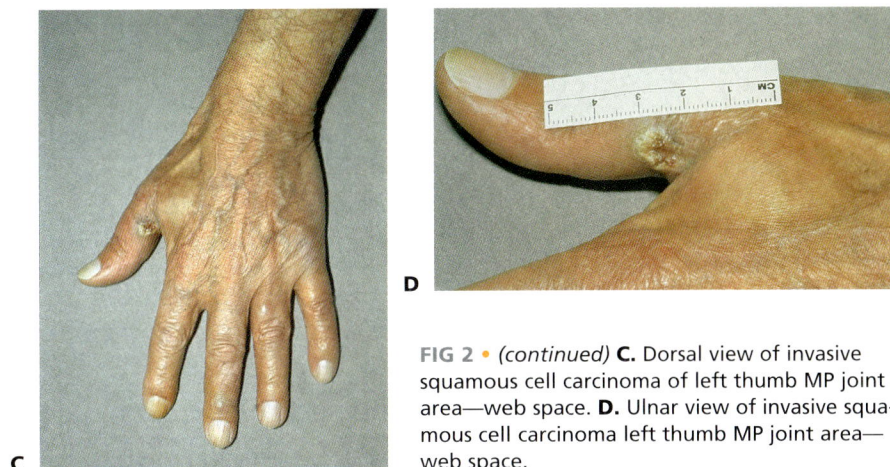

FIG 2 • *(continued)* **C.** Dorsal view of invasive squamous cell carcinoma of left thumb MP joint area—web space. **D.** Ulnar view of invasive squamous cell carcinoma left thumb MP joint area—web space.

NATURAL HISTORY

- In 2007, the American Cancer Society estimated 59,940 new cases of melanoma for both sexes, with an estimated 8110 deaths. Additionally, an estimated 48,290 cases of melanoma in situ were diagnosed.
- The probability of developing melanoma from birth to death is 2.04 (1 in 49) in males and 1.38 (1 in 73) in females. Neither basal cell carcinoma nor squamous cell carcinoma is a reportable disease. Basal cell carcinoma is the most common form of skin cancer and squamous cell carcinoma is the second most common type.
- For 2007, the American Cancer Society estimated more than 1 million new diagnoses of basal and squamous cell carcinomas of the skin. However, basal and squamous cell skin cancers account for less than 0.1% of patient deaths caused by all cancers.
- Nail matrix and nail bed squamous cell carcinoma or melanoma account for less than 1% of respective cutaneous malignancies. The histologic features of the epidermis and dermis, including physiologic barriers, are absent in the nail complex. In the nail complex, the matrix is adherent to the underlying phalanx.

PATIENT HISTORY AND PHYSICAL FINDINGS

- Patients typically present for evaluation of skin findings or after noting a change.
- Change or variation in an existing lesion and the presence of other risk factors are the important components of patient history.
  - Changes in size, shape, or color of a skin or matrix lesion or the development of a new skin or matrix lesion over a limited time should be monitored.
  - Such changes over a limited time must be diagnosed by histopathology.
- The lesion should be precisely characterized on physical examination. Critical findings include:
  - Irregularity or asymmetry
  - Diameter more than 6 mm
  - Presence of satellite lesions
- Regional lymph nodes (epitrochlear and axillary) should be routinely examined in all suspected cases of squamous cell carcinoma and melanoma.

- Close regional lymph node examination is required in cases of squamous cell carcinoma arising in sites of chronic ulceration or inflammation, burn scars, or sites of previous radiation therapy, especially for high-risk areas of the hand.
- Melanoma and squamous cell carcinoma can metastasize. A full local, regional, and metastatic workup is necessary.
- Nail matrix and nail bed squamous cell carcinoma or melanoma requires specific consideration during the physical examination.
- The presence of the Hutchinson sign (extension of brown-black pigment from the nail bed, matrix, and nail plate onto the adjacent cuticle and proximal or lateral nail folds) is consistent with a subungual melanoma.
  - Subungual melanoma is also suspected when the nail bed contains a new or enlarging pigmented streak wider than 3 mm.
- The absence of periungual pigmentation does not preclude the diagnosis of subungual melanoma.
  - Although there have been reports of amelanotic melanoma of the nail bed, the actual incidence is unknown and has never been reported in the literature.

IMAGING AND OTHER DIAGNOSTIC STUDIES

- Radiographic evaluation with plain views can reveal bone involvement, especially for matrix lesions.
- For both squamous cell carcinoma and melanoma, a chest radiograph, complete blood count, and liver panel should be obtained.
- More detailed imaging studies (CT, MRI, and PET) are performed to evaluate specific organ systems (central nervous system, pulmonary, gastrointestinal, and others) as indicated.
- Diagnosis of these pathologies requires adequate histopathologic evaluation. Full-thickness (surface to full depth) perimeter and core samples are required. Suspicious lesions must never be shaved, cauterized, or vaporized.
  - If the initial surgical pathologist is uncertain of the histopathology, the specimen slides and appropriate imaging studies must be forwarded to an independent qualified pathologist for review.
  - There is significant discordance among pathologists in the histologic diagnosis regarding melanoma and benign pigmented lesions. One study noted discordance in 37 of 140 cases examined by a panel of experienced dermatopathologists

on melanoma versus benign lesions. Another study noted a 38% discordance rate in cases examined by an expert pathologist panel.

- Squamous cell carcinoma is graded 1 to 4 based on the proportion of differentiating cells present, the degree of atypicality of tumor cells, and the depth of tumor penetration.
- The clinicopathologic cellular malignant melanoma subtypes are (these are descriptive, not prognostic or therapeutic):
  - Superficial spreading: most common, 70%
  - Nodular: 15% to 30%, more aggressive
  - Lentigo maligna: most common subtype among Asians and African-Americans
  - Acral lentiginous (palmar–plantar and subungual)
  - Miscellaneous unusual types:
    - Mucosal lentiginous (oral and genital)
    - Desmoplastic
    - Verrucous
- Malignant melanoma microstage is determined by histopathologic evaluation of the vertical thickness of the lesion in millimeters (Breslow classification) or the anatomic level of local invasion (Clark classification).
  - The Breslow thickness is more reproducible and more accurately predicts subsequent behavior of malignant melanoma in lesions thicker than 1.5 mm. Estimates of prognosis should be modified by sex and anatomic site in coordination with clinical and histologic evaluation.
  - For cutaneous melanoma, Breslow thickness and presence of ulceration demonstrated the highest concordance. Discordance was significant for Clark level of invasion, presence of regression, and lymphocytic infiltration.
  - The Clark classification ranges from level I (in situ lesions involving only the epidermis) to level V (invasion through the reticular dermis into the subcutaneous tissue).
- Micrometastases are diagnosed by elective sentinel lymphadenectomy; macrometastases are defined as clinically detectable lymph node metastases confirmed by therapeutic lymphadenectomy, or when any lymph node metastasis exhibits gross extracapsular extension.
- Clinical staging includes microstaging of the primary melanoma and clinical or radiologic (or both) evaluation for metastases. By convention, AFCC stage should be assigned after complete excision of the primary melanoma with clinical assessment for regional and distant metastases.
- With the exception of clinical stage 0 or stage IA patients (who have a low risk of lymphatic involvement and do not require pathologic evaluation of the lymph nodes), pathologic staging includes microstaging of the primary melanoma and pathologic information about the regional lymph nodes after sentinel node biopsy and, if indicated, complete lymphadenectomy.

DIFFERENTIAL DIAGNOSIS

- Seborrheic keratosis
- Pigmented actinic keratosis
- Hemangioma
- Dermatofibroma
- Blue nevus
- Basal cell carcinoma
- Cutaneous T-cell lymphomas (eg, mycosis fungoides)
- Kaposi sarcoma
- Extramammary Paget disease

- Apocrine carcinoma of the skin
- Metastatic malignancies from various primary sites
- The differential diagnosis of subungual melanoma includes chronic paronychia and onychomycosis, subungual hematoma, pyogenic granuloma, and glomus tumor.

NONOPERATIVE MANAGEMENT

Squamous Cell Carcinoma

- Electrodesiccation and curettage, and cryosurgery may be useful for small, well-defined in situ tumors in patients with medical conditions limiting excisional surgery.
  - Depth of treatment may not correlate with depth of tumor and therefore may be inadequate.
  - Cryosurgery should not be used for carcinomas fixed to the underlying bone, cartilage, or tendons.
  - Proximity of nerves limits cryosurgery use, such as in tumors situated on the lateral margins of the digits and at the cubital tunnel.
  - Cryosurgery is complicated by significant morbidity, particularly edema, which is common after treatment. Permanent depigmentation and atrophy are common.
- Radiation therapy is a logical treatment choice, particularly for medically compromised patients with primary lesions requiring difficult or extensive surgery.
  - Radiation therapy can be used for recurrent lesions after a primary surgical removal.
  - Radiation therapy is contraindicated for patients with xeroderma pigmentosum, epidermodysplasia verruciformis, or the basal cell nevus syndrome.
- Topical fluorouracil (5-FU) may be helpful in the management of selected in situ squamous cell carcinomas (Bowen disease).
  - Deep follicular tumors may not be reached by topical 5-FU. In these instances, recurrence or progression can occur. Close follow-up over time is required.
- Carbon dioxide laser treatment may be useful in a subset of medically compromised patients with small squamous cell carcinoma in situ.
  - Since the CO_2 laser coagulates, this technique is valuable for patients with a bleeding diathesis.
- Malignant melanoma can spontaneously regress, but the incidence of spontaneous, complete regressions is less than 1%.

SURGICAL MANAGEMENT

- The fundamental oncologic principle of tumor clearance first and then reconstruction second should be followed without compromising tumor ablation.
- Lymph node management is directed by clinical involvement or selective lymph node sampling results.
- Wide local excision is recommended for melanomas.

Cutaneous Squamous Cell Carcinoma

- The two primary methods of treatment are surgical excision with frozen or permanent histopathologic sections and Mohs micrographic surgery.
- When surgically excising these lesions, the surgeon should maintain a 3- to 10-mm margin of disease-free tissue (depending on the diameter).
- Surgical excision without Mohs technique, using either frozen or permanent histopathologic control, is associated with a significant recurrence rate.

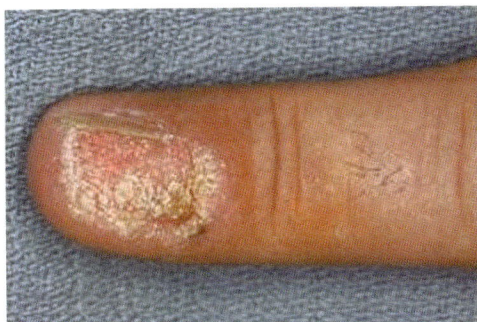

FIG 3 • Chronic matrix lesion treated for 2 years with oral and topical antibiotics and antifungals. Matrix biopsy demonstrated invasive squamous cell carcinoma.

▪ The Mohs technique to microscopically track subclinical tumor extensions results in the highest cure rate with maximal preservation of normal tissue.

Nail Matrix Squamous Cell Carcinoma

▪ For invasive squamous cell carcinoma of the nail matrix (**FIG 3**), the appropriate technique is amputation at the distal joint level for that digit.
▪ However, Mohs technique with grafting has been reported in small series of invasive squamous cell carcinoma of the nail matrix with limited follow-up.
▪ For noninvasive nail matrix squamous cell carcinoma, Mohs technique with grafting is performed.

Cutaneous Melanoma

▪ Melanomas of the hands and feet less than 1.5 mm thick have a low incidence of nodal metastases and are treated effectively with wide excision of the primary tumor with a 1-cm margin.

▪ Thicker melanomas are associated with a more than 50% rate of regional or systemic failure. In the absence of metastatic disease, these individuals should undergo local excision with a 2-cm margin and intraoperative lymphatic mapping followed by lymphadenectomy if the sentinel node is positive (**FIG 4A,B**).
▪ Specific recommendations are individualized for each patient. Factors that affect these recommendations include the primary tumor's anatomic location, specific tumor features, healing ability, and medical risk factors.
▪ The surgical goal is to minimize local and regional recurrence and metastasis while maintaining acceptable risks to minimize morbidity and mortality.

Nail Matrix Melanoma

▪ Melanomas of the nail complex (**FIG 5**) are unique because of the lack of the biologic barriers of skin and the proximity of the underlying phalanx and tendons.
  ▪ These features cause Breslow thickness and Clark level to be less useful.
▪ Complete digital or ray amputations of the thumb or fingers result in significant functional deficits without significant survival benefit.
▪ The respective digit is amputated proximal to the distal interphalangeal joint of the fingers and the interphalangeal joint of the thumb if the extent of nail apparatus involvement allows.
▪ For more proximal digital melanoma with bone involvement or perineural invasion, either complete digital amputation or ray amputation is indicated for more proximal phalangeal or metacarpal bony involvement respectively or nerve invasion.
▪ Without bony involvement or perineural invasion, the area of wide local excision is directed by the Breslow thickness.

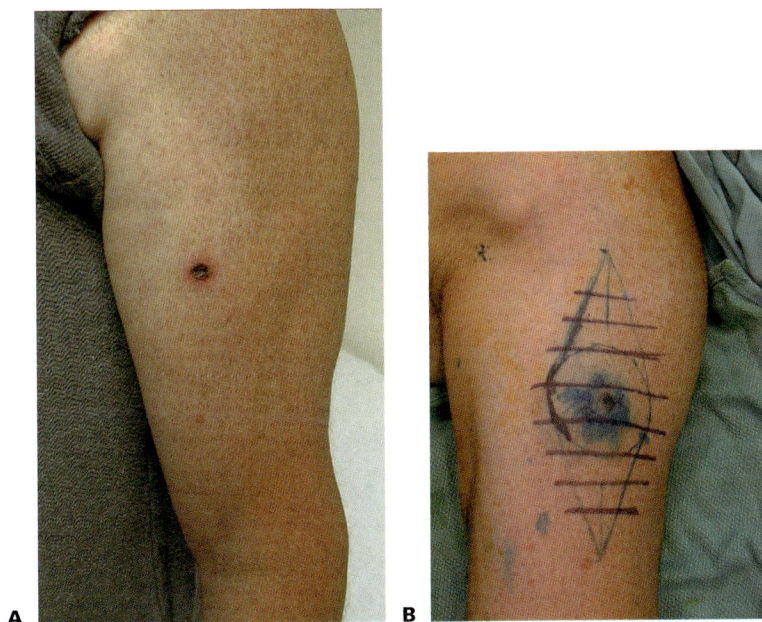

FIG 4 • A. Invasive melanoma treated initially with cutaneous laser ablation. **B.** Intraoperative invasive melanoma lesion with margins marked out and after injection of isosulfan blue. Note visible adenopathy in anterior superior axilla.

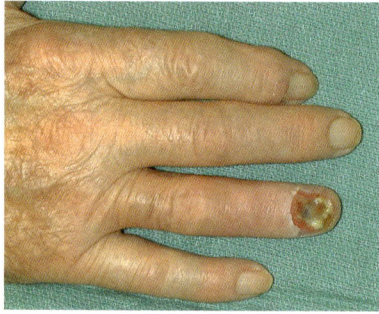

FIG 5 • Invasive matrix melanoma with delayed presentation.

■ Specific recommendations are individualized for each patient. Other significant factors, such as the primary tumor anatomic location, specific tumor features, healing ability, and medical risk factors, must be considered. The surgical goal is to minimize local and regional recurrence and metastasis while maintaining acceptable risks to minimize morbidity and mortality.

Coverage and Reconstruction

■ After wide local excision, most wounds can be closed primarily without tension using minimal perimeter undermining and layered closure.
■ If time is required to establish final histopathology, a temporary negative-pressure wound system can be used.
■ Coverage and reconstruction must match requirements at the ablation site.
■ The coverage options progress from less to more complex: closure, skin graft, local flap, regional flap, then microsurgically transplanted flap.
  ■ Exposed vessels, nerves, tendons, and bone often necessitate flap coverage.
  ■ Surgical flaps benefit poorly vascularized and chronic (more than 3 weeks) wounds.
  ■ Skin grafting can be either split or full thickness depending on the wound bed vascularity, anatomic area, and aesthetics.

■ Digital V-Y flaps, cross-finger flaps, flag flaps, dorsal metacarpal artery flaps, and radial forearm flaps are commonly used local and regional flaps.

Preoperative Planning

■ To direct management of local tumor, regional lymph nodes, and metastatic disease, the patient must be staged for both squamous cell carcinoma and melanoma. The histopathology of the primary tumor is determined by an accurate histopathologic diagnosis.
■ Mohs micrographic surgery requires the assistance of a trained dermatologist.
■ Before resection, plans must be made for coverage.

Positioning

■ Positioning is supine with the upper extremity supported on an arm table.
■ Positioning should allow approach to the primary tumor and the regional lymph node basin.
■ A sterile tourniquet is used. When access to the axillary lymph nodes is required, the tourniquet is removed.

Approach

■ For wide local excision, the primary lesion is marked and the indicated margin is measured around the lesion using calipers.
  ■ Wide local excision includes the intact tumor or biopsy site en bloc with a defined perimeter of normal skin and underlying subcutaneous tissue. The underlying muscular fascia is not typically included.
  ■ Inadequate, narrow excisions increase the risk of local and regional failure and affect survival.
■ For primary closure, an ellipse is marked out incorporating the required margins for wide local excision.
  ■ The excised length-to-lesion-diameter is at least 3:1.
■ For amputation, the distal joint level is marked, along with the fish-mouth dorsal and volar flaps.
■ For selective lymph node sampling, a grid is marked over the axillary area. The point of highest radioactivity is marked on the grid.

MOHS MICROGRAPHIC SURGERY

■ Remove all gross tumor.
■ Excise a thin layer of tissue with 2- to 3-mm margins. Flatten the specimen with the beveled peripheral skin edge positioned in the same horizontal plane with the deep margin.
■ Map the tissue with color-coded three-dimensional orientation.

■ Send the specimen for frozen-section processing.
  ■ Both the deep and peripheral margins are examined in one horizontal plane by frozen-section analysis with total (theoretically 100%) margin control.
■ After histologic interpretation of the frozen-section specimens, the precise anatomic location of any residual tumor is identified and re-excised until tumor-free three-dimensional margins are obtained.

PEARLS AND PITFALLS

Chronic or nonhealing skin or matrix lesion	■ Send tissue biopsy for histopathologic evaluation and culture (bacterial, fungal, and tuberculosis).
Patient referred for treatment with histopathologic report	■ Obtain and review original histopathologic slides before treatment.
Nonpigmented chronic or nonhealing skin or matrix lesion	■ Remember amelanotic melanoma. Send tissue biopsy for histopathologic evaluation and culture (bacterial, fungal, and tuberculosis).

TECHNIQUES

POSTOPERATIVE CARE

- Initial postoperative care focuses on pain control and protection of the operated part.
- Occupational therapy is by protocol, depending primarily on the coverage performed.
- Patients must be monitored.
  - Squamous cell carcinoma has metastatic potential. Depending on the relative risk for recurrence and invasion, patients should be re-examined every 3 months for the first several years, then every 6 months for 3 years, and then yearly indefinitely. Evaluation is for local recurrence, lymph node involvement, metastasis, additional nonmelanoma skin cancers, and melanomas. Laboratory evaluation, blood count, and liver enzymes may be useful for monitoring particularly aggressive squamous cell tumors.
  - For melanoma, the follow-up schedule for patients who have surgically resected disease is based on the primary lesion's Breslow thickness and the nodal involvement. Patients with thin primary melanoma and negative nodes are followed with clinical examination for evidence of occurrence every 6 months for the first 2 to 3 years and then yearly for 2 to 3 years beyond that. Patients with intermediate or thick melanomas and negative regional nodes are followed every 3 to 6 months for the first 2 to 3 years and every 6 to 12 months for the next 2 to 3 years. Patients with resected regional disease require follow-up every 3 to 4 months for the first 2 years, then every 6 months up to year 5, and yearly beyond that. All patients must maintain routine lifelong dermatologic screening. Patients with one melanoma remain at higher-than-average risk for a second primary melanoma and are at risk for basal cell and squamous cell carcinomas.

OUTCOMES

- Squamous cell carcinoma is the second most common type of skin malignancy. Although the basal cell and squamous types of skin cancer are the most common of all malignancies, they account for less than 0.1% of cancer deaths.
- The overall cure rate for squamous cell carcinoma is directly related to the stage of the disease and the type of treatment used. Since squamous cell carcinoma is not a reportable disease, precise 5-year cure rates are not known.
- Melanoma 5-year survival rates are related to stage and range from 18% for stage IV to 99% for stage IA.

COMPLICATIONS

- Sentinel lymph node biopsy is not without complications. The most common complications are hematoma and seroma. The rate of lymphedema after sentinel lymph node biopsy has been reported to be 0.7% to 1.7%, compared with 4.6% (axillary) and 31.5% (inguinal) with completion lymphadenectomy.
- Inadequate margin for squamous cell carcinoma on final pathology is corrected by re-excision using the Mohs technique.
- Inadequate margin for melanoma on final pathology is corrected by appropriate increase or expansion of the surgical margins.
- Excessive tension on wound closure is corrected by skin graft or appropriate flap coverage.

REFERENCES

1. Abide JM, Nahai F, Bennett RG. The meaning of surgical margins. Plast Reconstr Surg 1984;73:492–497.
2. Balch CM, Urist MM, Karakousis CP, et al. Efficacy of 2-cm surgical margins for intermediate-thickness melanomas (1 to 4 mm): results of a multi-institutional randomized surgical trial. Ann Surg 1993;218:262–269.
3. Cottel WI. Perineural invasion by squamous-cell carcinoma. J Dermatol Surg Oncol 1982;8:589–600.
4. Essner R, Conforti A, Kelley MC, et al. Efficacy of lymphatic mapping, sentinel lymphadenectomy, and selective complete lymph node dissection as a therapeutic procedure for early-stage melanoma. Ann Surg Oncol 1999;6:442–449.
5. Gershenwald JE, Thompson W, Mansfield PF, et al. Multi-institutional melanoma lymphatic mapping experience: the prognostic value of sentinel lymph node status in 612 stage I or II melanoma patients. J Clin Oncol 1999;17:976–983.
6. Hochwald SN, Coit DG. Role of elective lymph node dissection in melanoma. Semin Surg Oncol 1998;14:276–282.
7. Lee ML, Tomsu K, Von Eschen KB. Duration of survival for disseminated malignant melanoma: results of a meta-analysis. Melanoma Res 2000;10:81–92.
8. Leo F, Cagini L, Rocmans P, et al. Lung metastases from melanoma: when is surgical treatment warranted? Br J Cancer 2000;83:569–572.
9. Morton DL, Cochran AJ, Thompson JF, et al. Sentinel node biopsy for early-stage melanoma: accuracy and morbidity in MSLT-I, an international multicenter trial. Ann Surg 2005;242:302–313.
10. Mraz-Gernhard S, Sagebiel RW, Kashani-Sabet M, et al. Prediction of sentinel lymph node micrometastasis by histological features in primary cutaneous malignant melanoma. Arch Dermatol 1998;134:983–987.
11. Ollila DW, Hsueh EC, Stern SL, et al. Metastasectomy for recurrent stage IV melanoma. J Surg Oncol 1999;71:209–213.
12. Preston DS, Stern RS. Nonmelanoma cancers of the skin. N Engl J Med 1992;327:1649–1662.
13. Thomas RM, Amonette RA. Mohs micrographic surgery. Am Fam Physician 1988;37:135–142.
14. Thomas JM, Newton-Bishop J, A'Hern R, et al. Excision margins in high-risk malignant melanoma. N Engl J Med 2004;350:757–766.
15. Veronesi U, Cascinelli N. Narrow excision (1-cm margin): a safe procedure for thin cutaneous melanoma. Arch Surg 1991;126:438–441.
16. Veronesi U, Cascinelli N, Adamus J, et al. Thin stage I primary cutaneous malignant melanoma: comparison of excision with margins of 1 or 3 cm. N Engl J Med 1988;318:1159–1162.
17. Wagner JD, Gordon MS, Chuang TY, et al. Current therapy of cutaneous melanoma. Plast Reconstr Surg 2000;105:1774–1801.

Chapter 112

Open and Arthroscopic Excision of Ganglion Cysts and Related Tumors

Mitchell E. Nahra and John S. Bucchieri

DEFINITION

Ganglion Cysts

- Ganglion cysts, although not true cysts, are the most common tumors of the hand and wrist.
- These fluid-filled cysts are a frequent cause of hand and wrist pain.
- Ganglion cysts typically arise from either a joint or tendon sheath.
- Most ganglion cysts occur in the wrist. Dorsal wrist ganglion cysts account for 60% to 70% of all ganglion cysts, with volar wrist ganglion cysts accounting for about 18% to 20%.[1]
- Ganglion cysts may also arise from a tendon sheath (volar retinacular cyst), or occur in association with arthritis (degenerative mucous cyst).

Giant Cell Tumors

- Giant cell tumors of the tendon sheath—also referred to as localized nodular synovitis,[11] fibrous xanthoma, and pigmented villonodular synovitis—are benign, slow-growing soft tissue tumors.
- After ganglion cyst cysts, these lesions are the second most common tumor in the hand.[6]

Epidermal Inclusion Cysts

- Epidermal inclusion cysts are benign, slow-growing soft tissue tumors.
- They are the third most common type of hand tumor.

ANATOMY

Ganglion Cysts

- Ganglion cysts typically consist of a cyst sac that communicates through a stalk to an underlying joint or tendon sheath (**FIG 1**).

- The cyst sac may have a single cavity or be multilobulated.
- Although not a true cyst, lacking an epithelial lining, ganglion cysts are typically filled with a clear, viscous, jelly-like mucinous fluid made up of glucosamine, albumin, globulin, and a high concentration of hyaluronic acid.[17]

Giant Cell Tumors

- The tumor is usually a multilobular, well-circumscribed mass, ranging in size from 0.5 to 7 cm.[6]
- The color ranges from yellow to deep brown depending on the amount of hemosiderin, histiocytes, and collagen present in the lesion.
- These lesions have a thin pseudocapsule. Aggressive lesions may invade adjacent soft tissue, tendon, and capsular structures and can envelop neurovascular bundles. A large study showed joint involvement in one fifth of all cases.[7] Longstanding lesions may erode into cortical bone but will not involve cartilage or the medullary canal of bone. Satellite lesions may occur.
- Histologically, giant cell tumors contain collagen-producing polyhedral-shaped histiocytes, scattered multinucleated giant cells, and hemosiderin deposits.[6]

Epidermal Inclusion Cysts

- Epidermal inclusion cysts are well-circumscribed, firm, and slightly mobile lesions.
- They are often superficial and adherent to overlying skin.
- They may be flesh-colored, yellow, or white.
- They contain a thick white keratinous material.
- Cysts in the fingertip may erode into the distal phalanx, causing a lytic lesion.
- Histologically, they are cysts filled with keratin and lined with epithelial cells.

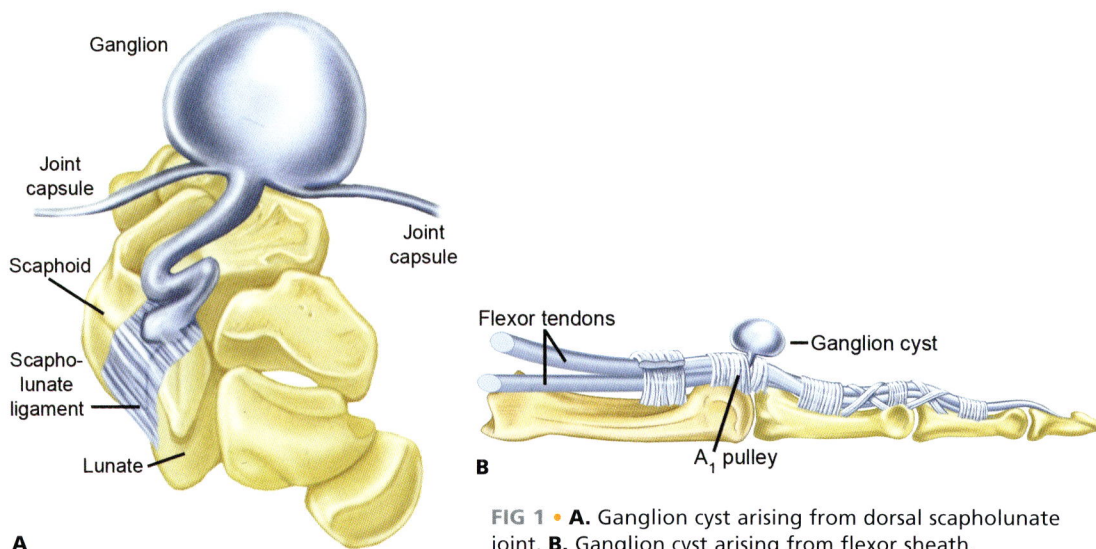

FIG 1 • **A.** Ganglion cyst arising from dorsal scapholunate joint. **B.** Ganglion cyst arising from flexor sheath.

PATHOGENESIS

Ganglion Cysts

- The true causes of ganglion cysts remain unclear, although multiple theories have been proposed.
- Some early investigators theorized that ganglion cysts occurred as the result of synovial herniation, and others felt that ganglion cysts resulted from mucoid degeneration.
- A more recent theory proposes that ganglion cysts arise from stress at the synovial capsular interface. This stress, such as stretching of the capsular and ligamentous structures, stimulates the production of mucin from modified synovial, mesenchymal, and fibroblast cells, all of which have been shown to produce hyaluronic acid. The mucin then dissects through the capsular and ligamentous tissues, forming the main cyst. The fluid may enter the cyst from the capsular ligamentous interface via a one-way valve type of mechanism and then decrease as the water component is resorbed, accounting for the often-fluctuating cyst size.[1]

Giant Cell Tumors

- The cause of giant cell tumors is not known. There is a strong association of giant cell tumors with rheumatoid arthritis. There are no clinical studies associating these tumors with trauma.[6]
- Although these tumors are histologically similar to the pigmented villonodular synovitis seen in large joints in the lower extremity, they are thought to be clinically distinct lesions.

Epidermal Inclusion Cysts

- Epidermal inclusion cysts occur as a result of trauma when epithelial cells are introduced into the underlying subcutaneous tissues or bone. These cells slowly grow to produce a cyst lined with epithelial cells and filled with keratin.

NATURAL HISTORY

Ganglion Cysts

- Ganglion cysts typically arise spontaneously and are most common in the second through the fourth decade but may arise in the pediatric population[20] as well as the aged.
- Once present, ganglion cysts tend to fluctuate in size depending on the amount of fluid present in the cyst at any given time. Patients often note that the cyst becomes larger after increased periods of activity and decreases in size with inactivity.
- Ganglion cysts tend to be self-limiting and do not typically continue to expand in size.
- If left untreated, ganglion cysts can persist for years. They may resolve or rupture spontaneously. One cannot predict how long that they will persist or if and when they will resolve.
  - Resolution is far more common in the pediatric population.

Giant Cell Tumors

- The lesion begins as a single nodule, becoming multinodular as it enlarges.
- Malignant transformation of giant cell tumor of the tendon sheath in the hand has not been reported.[6]

Epidermal Inclusion Cysts

- These lesions occur months to years after a traumatic event. They grow slowly to produce a painless mass, most commonly seen in the fingertip.
- Malignant transformation of these lesions in the hand has not been reported.[12]

PATIENT HISTORY AND PHYSICAL FINDINGS

Ganglion Cysts

- Patients often present with an asymptomatic mass that has been present for weeks to years.
- A history of trauma is often absent.
- Pain if present is often described as a dull ache. Nocturnal pain is uncommon and pain is more common with active hand use.
- Paresthesias are rare but can occur if the ganglion cyst compresses any local nerves.
- Patients often report that the mass tends to fluctuate in size, a characteristic typical of ganglion cysts and not typical of other types of soft tissue tumors.
- Patients with wrist ganglion cysts—particularly dorsal wrist cysts—will often complain of weakness of grip.
- Patients with dorsal wrist ganglion cysts most commonly note a mass over the dorsum of the wrist, typically over the dorsal scapholunate region. In contrast, patients with volar wrist ganglion cysts typically note a mass over the volar aspect of the wrist in the interval between the flexor carpi radialis and first extensor compartment tendons.
- Volar retinacular cysts or ganglion cysts of tendon sheath usually present as a mass in the palm in the region of the first and second annular pulleys. The cyst is typically fluctuant but may feel like a firm nodule. The cyst is usually slightly mobile but does not often glide with flexor tendon movement.
  - These types of cysts are often painless at rest but become painful when patients perform activities that involve forceful grip.
- Degenerative mucous cysts are ganglion cysts that arise from the distal interphalangeal joint, usually in association with underlying osteoarthritis.[4] Patients often note a painless soft tissue mass that arises from the dorsal surface of the joint, radially or ulnarly (less commonly in the midline), often extending into the eponychial fold region.
  - Commonly, the cyst will thin the overlying dermis, resulting in rupture of the skin, and the patient often reports drainage.
- Physical examination begins with inspection (**FIG 2**).
  - Being fluid-filled, ganglion cysts will often transilluminate, whereas other more solid soft tissue lesions will not.
  - Ganglion cysts usually occur in specific locations in the hand and wrist. Swelling or masses in these locations are diagnostic clues that a ganglion cyst may be present.
- The examiner should palpate the mass for fluctuance and mobility and assess tenderness.
  - Ganglion cysts are generally fluctuant and slightly mobile. When they become more distended with fluid they may feel more firm and less fluctuant. Firm, less mobile masses suggest the possibility of other soft tissue lesions.
  - Ganglion cysts of tendon sheath do not usually glide with tendon motion, but less common ganglion cysts, such as those that arise in the fourth extensor compartment, are often adherent and do glide with tendon motion.
- The examiner should assess joint mobility through the range of motion. With the exception of dorsal wrist ganglion cysts, which may cause some loss of wrist dorsiflexion secondary to impingement, loss of joint range of motion suggests the possibility of an underlying joint abnormality.

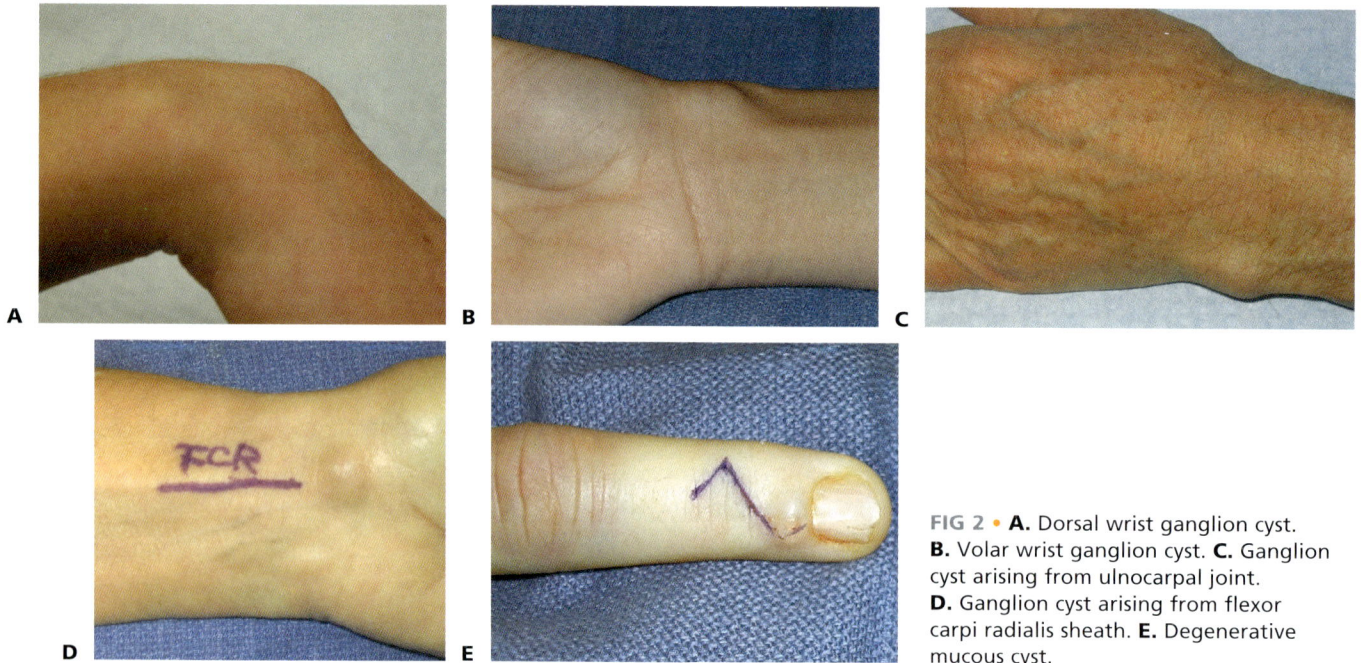

FIG 2 • **A.** Dorsal wrist ganglion cyst. **B.** Volar wrist ganglion cyst. **C.** Ganglion cyst arising from ulnocarpal joint. **D.** Ganglion cyst arising from flexor carpi radialis sheath. **E.** Degenerative mucous cyst.

Giant Cell Tumors

■ Giant cell tumors are most common in the fourth to sixth decade, with a slight predominance in women.

■ Patients typically present with a slow-growing, multilobulated, firm, painless mass present for several months to years.

■ Lesions usually occur in the radial three digits of the hand on the volar surface. Dorsal involvement, particularly around the distal interphalangeal joint, is not uncommon.[7]

■ These lesions are typically firmer than ganglion cysts and do not transilluminate.

■ Large lesions may limit range of motion or result in neuropathic symptoms as a result of compression of digital nerves.

■ Direct palpation typically reveals a firm, multinodular, nontender lesion.

■ Loss of range of motion may occur when large lesions occur near the interphalangeal joints.

■ Patients may have sensory deficits secondary to digital nerve compression. These can be revealed by testing two-point discrimination.

Epidermal Inclusion Cysts

■ Epidermal inclusion cysts are more common in men than in women and occur in the third to fourth decade.[2]

■ Patients commonly present with a painless, slow-growing mass after a laceration, puncture wound, or traumatic amputation of the finger.[2]

■ These lesions should be suspected in laborers who have a painless mass in the palm.[12]

■ Erythematous and painful lesions have been reported. One study reported two cases mimicking a collar button abscess resulting from rupture of the cyst in the palmar soft tissues.[21]

■ These lesions are typically firmer than ganglion cysts and do not transilluminate.

■ Direct palpation will reveal a lesion that is firm, nontender, superficial, and mobile.

■ Loss of range of motion may occur when large lesions occur near the interphalangeal joints.

■ Two-point discrimination testing may reveal sensory deficits secondary to digital nerve compression.

IMAGING AND OTHER DIAGNOSTIC STUDIES

Ganglion Cysts

■ Radiographs are obtained if there is clinical suspicion of an underlying bony abnormality noted on physical examination, such as joint crepitation, swelling, carpal instability, or a history of trauma.

■ Radiographs are also useful in identifying an intraosseous ganglion cyst in patients with wrist pain of uncertain cause (**FIG 3A**).

■ Radiographs are also often obtained in patients with a degenerative mucous cyst of the digit since the cysts typically arise as the result of degenerative arthritis of the distal interphalangeal joint.

■ If the clinical findings suggest the possibility of an occult ganglion cyst, or if there is suspicion that the patient may have a symptomatic intraosseous ganglion cyst, magnetic resonance imaging (MRI) can be a useful tool to confirm the diagnosis (**FIG 3B**).

■ MRI can also be used to better localize the site of origin as part of preoperative planning in ganglion cysts that occur in atypical locations (**FIG 3C,D**).

■ Ultrasound can also be used to diagnose ganglion cysts, but this test is examiner-dependent and less sensitive and specific than MRI.

■ Computed tomography scans are generally obtained only for preoperative planning to better localize and evaluate the bony architecture of intraosseous ganglion cysts.

Giant Cell Tumors

■ Plain radiographs show a soft tissue mass. Juxtacortical lesions may show bony erosion.

■ MRI demonstrates a benign-appearing encapsulated mass, with decreased signal on T1- and T2-weighted images.

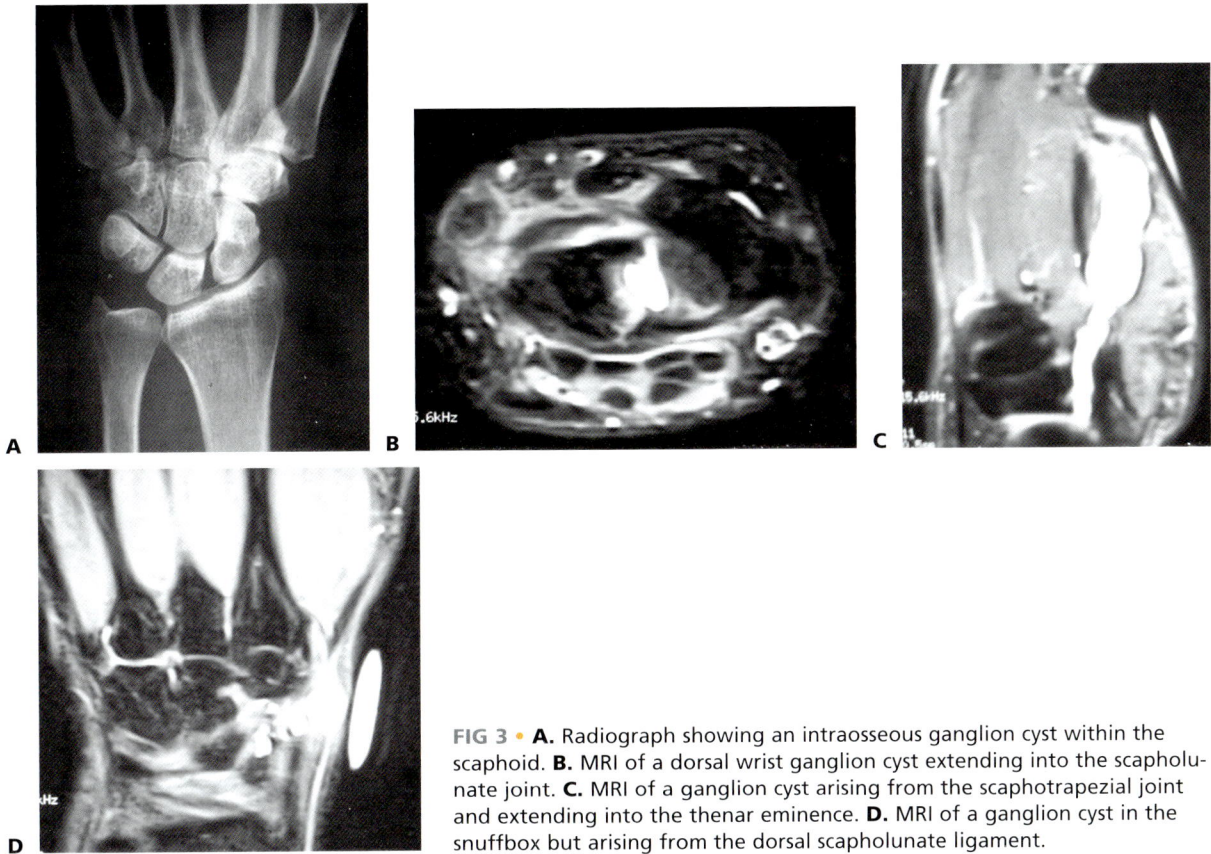

FIG 3 • A. Radiograph showing an intraosseous ganglion cyst within the scaphoid. **B.** MRI of a dorsal wrist ganglion cyst extending into the scapholunate joint. **C.** MRI of a ganglion cyst arising from the scaphotrapezial joint and extending into the thenar eminence. **D.** MRI of a ganglion cyst in the snuffbox but arising from the dorsal scapholunate ligament.

Epidermal Inclusion Cysts

▪ Plain radiographs show a soft tissue mass.
▪ A lytic lesion may be seen in the distal phalanx if it erodes into bone.

DIFFERENTIAL DIAGNOSIS

Ganglion Cysts

▪ Epidermoid inclusion cyst
▪ Giant cell tumor of tendon sheath
▪ Lipoma
▪ Synovial cyst

Giant Cell Tumors

▪ Fibroma of the tendon sheath, synovial chondromatosis, synovial hemangioma, tophaceous gout, foreign body granuloma, periosteal chondroma

Epidermal Inclusion Cysts

▪ Tophaceous gout, foreign body granuloma, giant cell tumor, ganglion cyst, sebaceous cyst
▪ Bony destruction may mimic a malignant or infectious process.[11] Some patients with these lesions have been treated with primary amputation before pathologic diagnosis.[6]

NONOPERATIVE MANAGEMENT

▪ Of the three tumors discussed in this chapter, only ganglion cysts can be managed without surgery.
▪ Ganglion cysts are benign cysts that may resolve spontaneously. Treatment often depends on the level of a patient's symptoms. Many patients seek medical care because they are concerned about the presence of a soft tissue mass and possibility of malignancy.[23] Once a diagnosis of a ganglion cyst is made, with proper counseling as to the nature of these lesions, many patients will be satisfied with a course of observation.
▪ In patients who are symptomatic, typical nonoperative treatments include rest and immobilization, oral analgesics such as nonsteroidal anti-inflammatories and acetaminophen, and aspiration of the cyst with or without injection.[3,13,14,23]
▪ In wrist ganglion cysts, the results of aspiration have variable cure rates in the literature, ranging from 15% to 89%.[12] Various agents have been injected into the ganglion cyst after aspiration, including hyaluronidase and methylprednisolone.[15]
  ▪ On average, injection does not seem to increase the cure rate after aspiration, and we now typically perform aspiration alone. We generally inform patients that aspiration has about a 50% cure rate. The use of sclerosing agents is frowned on since these agents may cause articular damage.[10]
▪ Traditional methods of traumatic rupture of the cyst from a direct blow with an object such as a large book (hence the term "Bible cyst") are mostly of historical significance.
▪ Ganglion cysts of tendon sheath (volar retinacular cysts) when symptomatic often respond to aspiration and injection and rarely require surgery when not associated with stenosing tenosynovitis. When they occur in association with stenosing tenosynovitis (trigger finger, De Quervain tendinitis), they often resolve with successful treatment of the underlying tendinitis.
  ▪ We typically do not aspirate ganglion cysts of tendon sheath but have had great success by injecting these cysts with local anesthetic and a small amount of corticosteroid (1.5 to 2 mL of 1% lidocaine and 10 mg of Depo-Medrol). The cyst is entered with a 25-gauge needle and then distended

to the point of rupture. The remaining fluid in the syringe is then injected into the tendon sheath. If necessary, gentle digital massage can be used to rupture the cyst after injection if the cyst fails to rupture with distention.

SURGICAL MANAGEMENT

Indications

Ganglion Cysts

■ Surgery is generally indicated in patients who have symptoms and who either have failed nonoperative treatment or choose to proceed directly with surgery.

■ In patients who have been diagnosed with a symptomatic wrist ganglion cyst, we generally describe the nature of the condition and outline the available forms of treatment, allowing the patient to decide which treatment is best for him or her. Some patients will choose observation, others will elect to undergo an aspiration, and some will chose to proceed directly with surgical excision.

■ In the case of symptomatic ganglion cysts of tendon sheath, most of these will resolve with a corticosteroid injection, and surgery is reserved for cysts that continue to recur.

■ Degenerative mucous cysts that are draining or have a history of draining should be treated operatively, since these cysts are at risk for infection that may extend into the distal interphalangeal joint and result in septic arthritis. If not draining, these cysts can be treated nonoperatively or surgically, depending on the patient's symptoms and choice of treatment.

■ Intraosseous ganglion cysts that are symptomatic or have resulted in pathologic fracture or may exhibit an impending pathologic fracture are often treated operatively.

Giant Cell Tumors

■ Indications for surgery include appearance, neuropathic symptoms, or loss of function.

■ Careful, meticulous marginal excision of the lesion is the treatment of choice.

■ Care must be taken to protect the neurovascular structures.

■ Satellite lesions must be identified and carefully removed to minimize the chance of recurrence.

Epidermal Inclusion Cysts

■ Indications for surgery include appearance, diagnosis, pain, and loss of function.

■ Marginal excision of the lesion is the treatment of choice.

Preoperative Planning

Ganglion Cysts

■ When removing ganglion cysts arising in atypical locations, MRI studies can help to identify the cyst origin and plan appropriate surgical exposure.

■ MRI and CT scans, along with plain radiographs, are valuable to determine the ideal exposure and for treating intraosseous ganglion cysts with curettage and bone grafting.

■ Plain radiographs are reviewed before excising degenerative mucous cysts to determine the extent of underlying osteophytes that may need to be addressed.

Giant Cell Tumors

■ While the diagnosis of giant cell tumor is primarily made based on history and clinical examination, radiographic studies should be reviewed to rule out other conditions.

■ The patient should be advised that even with careful surgical techniques, the recurrence rate can be as high as 5% to 50%. Risk factors for local recurrence include proximity to the distal interphalangeal joint, degenerative joint disease, and bony erosion.[16]

■ Temporary digital nerve neurapraxias may also occur after extrication of these tumors during surgery.

Epidermal Inclusion Cysts

■ While the diagnosis of epidermal inclusion cyst is primarily made based on history and clinical examination, radiographic studies should be reviewed to rule out other conditions.

■ If a lytic lesion is present in the distal phalanx, a biopsy should be considered before surgical removal.

■ The recurrence rate after marginal excision is low.

Positioning

■ Patients undergoing hand or wrist surgery are positioned supine on the operating table with the operative extremity resting on a hand table. This position allows for circumferential access to the hand and wrist.

■ The procedure is performed under regional anesthesia with a tourniquet applied to the upper arm, or under a digital block with a tourniquet applied to the digit.

■ For arthroscopic procedures, a traction tower or longitudinal fingertrap traction is used (**FIG 4**).

Approach

Ganglion Cysts

■ Standard approaches to the hand and wrist are used, depending on the location of the cyst.

■ It is important to have a good understanding of the anatomy and the most likely origin of the cyst to best plan the incision and dissection to avoid injury to important neurovascular structures.

■ When treating ganglion cysts in atypical locations, preoperative studies can aid in determining the best surgical

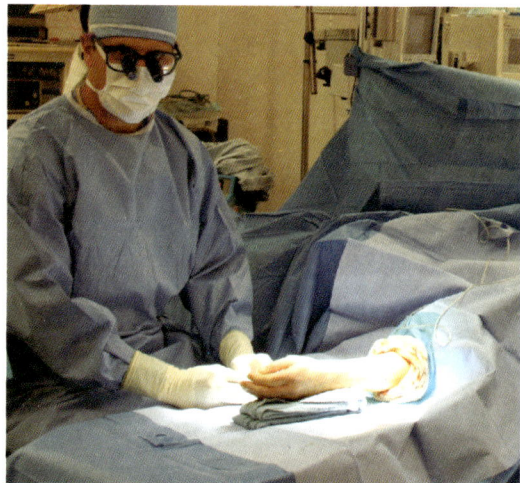

FIG 4 • The patient is positioned supine with an armboard attached to the operating table, and the upper extremity is prepared and draped in a standard manner. The surgeon is generally seated in the axilla with full access to the hand and wrist.

approach, since the origin of the cyst can be remote from the cyst (Fig 3D).

- Volar giant cell tumors and epidermal inclusion cysts are approached through Brunner zigzag incisions (**FIG 5A**).
- Dorsal giant cell tumors require dorsal midline or curvilinear incisions, whereas dorsal epidermal inclusion cysts can be approached through small longitudinal incisions directly over the lesion (**FIG 5B**).
- Incisions should be designed for a possible extensile exposure, which may be necessary for complete excision of the lesion.

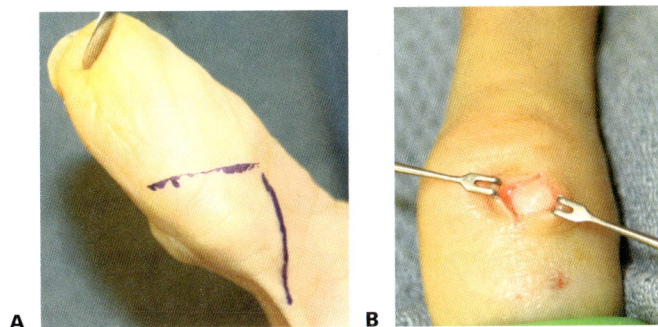

FIG 5 • **A.** A Brunner incision is made for a volar multilobular mass. **B.** A dorsal epidermal inclusion cyst is approached through a small longitudinal incision directly over the lesion.

OPEN EXCISION OF A DORSAL WRIST GANGLION CYST

- The location of the cyst is typically dorsal to the scapholunate interosseous ligament. The incision needs to provide access to this ligament. The scapholunate ligament is found just distal to the tubercle of Lister in the third and fourth extensor compartment interval (**TECH FIG 1A**).
- We generally perform a transverse skin incision centered over the scapholunate ligament region and cyst. This incision heals with the best appearance (**TECH FIG 1B**).
- Dissect the subcutaneous tissues with blunt dissection, taking care to protect and preserve any branches of the dorsal radial and ulnar sensory nerves. Loupe magnification is often helpful.
- The extensor retinaculum is generally not well developed at this level and is incised transversely as the cyst is dissected from the surrounding soft tissues (**TECH FIG 1C**).

- The cyst is identified typically in the interval between the third and fourth extensor compartments. Retract the second and third extensor compartment tendons radially and the fourth extensor compartment tendons ulnarly (**TECH FIG 1D**).
- The dorsal wrist capsule is also incised transversely as the cyst is traced to a stalk, which usually arises from the dorsal aspect of the scapholunate interosseous membrane, just proximal to the dorsal scapholunate ligament (**TECH FIG 1E**).
- Excise the cyst at the base of the stalk and send it for pathologic examination (**TECH FIG 1F**).
- Although excision of a small window of tissue at the site of cyst origin has been previously recommended, we have concern that overzealous excision may lead to injury to the scapholunate ligamentous complex. We

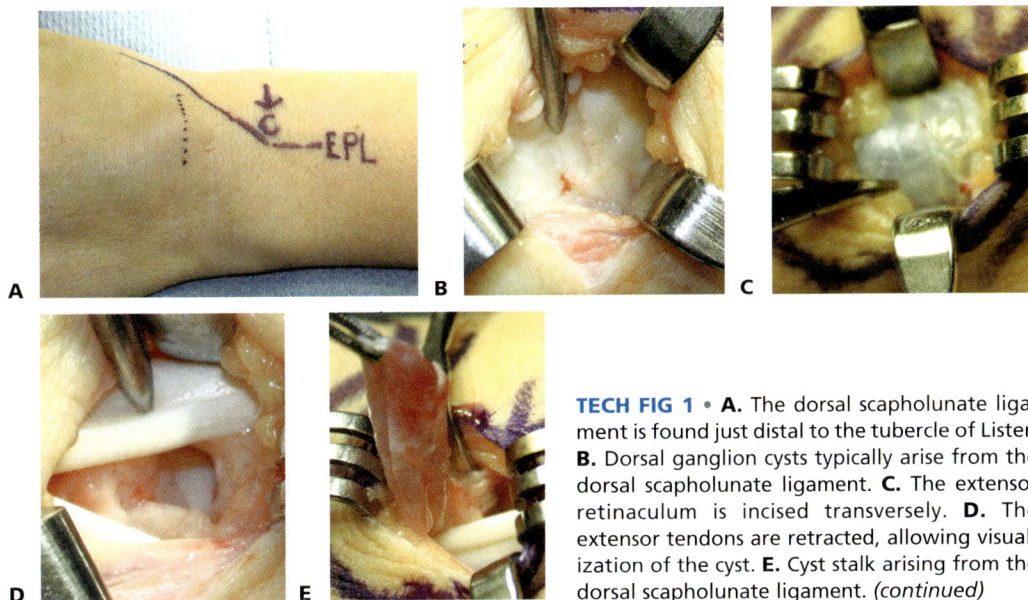

TECH FIG 1 • **A.** The dorsal scapholunate ligament is found just distal to the tubercle of Lister. **B.** Dorsal ganglion cysts typically arise from the dorsal scapholunate ligament. **C.** The extensor retinaculum is incised transversely. **D.** The extensor tendons are retracted, allowing visualization of the cyst. **E.** Cyst stalk arising from the dorsal scapholunate ligament. *(continued)*

TECHNIQUES

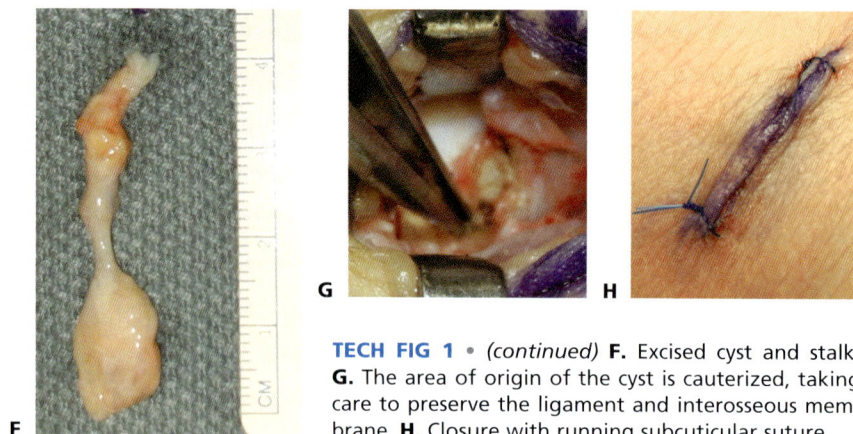

TECH FIG 1 • *(continued)* **F.** Excised cyst and stalk. **G.** The area of origin of the cyst is cauterized, taking care to preserve the ligament and interosseous membrane. **H.** Closure with running subcuticular suture.

recommend the use of a bipolar cautery to precisely cauterize the site of origin (**TECH FIG 1G**).

- After excision of the cyst, inspect the joint for any abnormalities.
- Allow the capsular tissues and tendons to return to their anatomic position. Avoid capsular closure, as this may lead to joint stiffness.
- Skin closure is usually accomplished with a running subcuticular nonabsorbable monofilament suture (**TECH FIG 1H**).

- We prefer to dress the wound with an antibiotic ointment and petroleum gauze, and a bulky hand dressing is applied with a plaster palmar splint maintaining the wrist in a neutral position.
  - The dressing is removed along with the sutures at about 1 week postoperatively and Steri-Strips are applied to the wound.

OPEN EXCISION OF A VOLAR WRIST GANGLION CYST

- Volar wrist ganglion cysts most often arise from the volar radiocarpal ligaments. They may also arise from the scaphotrapezial joint or at times from the flexor carpi radialis (FCR) sheath. The cysts are typically located in the interval between the FCR sheath and first extensor compartment tendons, just proximal to the wrist flexion crease.
- Under tourniquet control, we prefer to use a zigzag type of incision that begins at the wrist flexion crease and extends proximally over the cyst in the FCR and first extensor compartment interval. This incision provides access in both the longitudinal and transverse planes. A longitudinal incision may heal with scar contracture, whereas a transverse incision may not provide adequate exposure in the longitudinal plane (**TECH FIG 2A**).

- Under loupe magnification, the subcutaneous tissues are carefully dissected and branches of the lateral antebrachial cutaneous nerve and dorsal radial sensory nerve are carefully protected. If dissection ulnar to the FCR tendon is required, the palmar cutaneous branch of the median nerve must also be identified and protected.
- Ganglion cysts in this location are commonly adherent to the radial artery and its venae comitantes (**TECH FIG 2B**). Take care to avoid injury to the artery. If the cyst cannot be freely dissected from the artery, a small cuff of cyst wall can be left adherent to the artery without a significant increase in recurrence.
- The cyst is traced to a stalk that most often arises from the volar radial carpal ligaments (**TECH FIG 2C**). The cyst

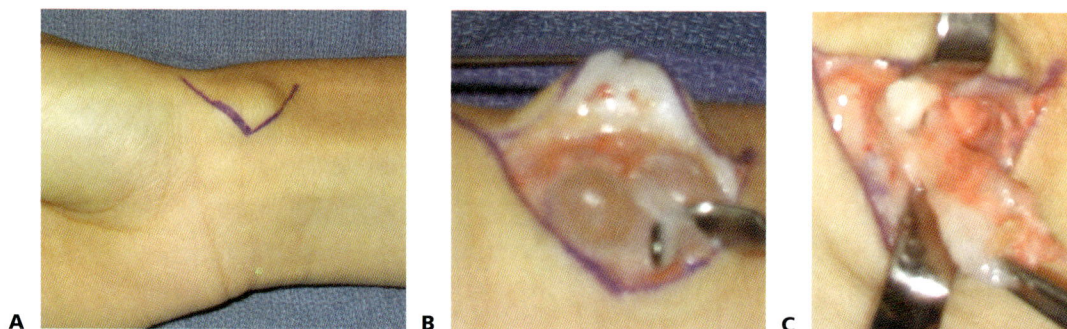

TECH FIG 2 • **A.** A Brunner type of incision allows for more exposure and avoids contracture associated with straight longitudinal incisions in this location. **B.** A volar cyst adherent to the radial artery and venae comitantes. **C.** A volar wrist ganglion stalk arising from the volar radial carpal ligaments.

- is excised at the base of the stalk. We routinely send the cyst for pathologic evaluation.
- As with dorsal ganglion cysts, we cauterize the site of origin of the cyst with a bipolar electrocautery.
- After excision of the cyst, the tourniquet is deflated to ensure that the radial artery is uninjured. Satisfactory hemostasis is achieved.
- We generally close the wound with a running subcuticular suture, removed about 7 to 10 days after surgery.

- We prefer to dress the wound with antibiotic ointment and petroleum gauze, and a bulky hand dressing is applied with a plaster palmar splint maintaining the wrist in a neutral position.
  - The dressing is removed along with the sutures at about 1 week postoperatively and Steri-Strips are applied to the wound.

OPEN CURETTAGE AND BONE GRAFTING OF AN INTRAOSSEOUS GANGLION CYST

- The patient is positioned supine on the operating table with the operative hand resting on a hand table.
- Symptomatic intraosseous ganglion cysts most often involve the carpal bones. Surgical incisions are planned according to the preoperative studies (MRI and CT scans) to identify the best location for creating a cortical window and avoiding injury to cartilaginous surfaces.
- Under tourniquet control, make an appropriate incision and carry dissection to the level of the wrist capsule. Loupe magnification is often helpful during the dissection. Enter the wrist capsule, preserving important capsular ligaments.
- The bony cortex is generally weakened in the area of the cyst and access is easily accomplished with a handheld

curette. If the cortex is not weak, a small cortical window can be created using 0.045-inch Kirschner wires to create small drill holes to create a cortical window.
- Curette the cyst cavity along with any mucinous material. Remove the cyst membrane.
- Pack the cyst cavity with bone graft or a bone graft substitute.
- Wound closure is accomplished in the usual manner.
- We usually immobilize the patient in a plaster splint for 1 week and then a cast for 3 to 5 weeks, depending on the cyst size and bone integrity.
- Obtain postoperative radiographs to monitor and ensure incorporation of the bone graft.

EXCISION OF A DEGENERATIVE MUCOUS CYST

- Mucous cysts can be excised under local digital block anesthesia.
- The hand is prepared in the standard fashion.
- A finger tourniquet is applied to the involved digit.
- We usually use a Brunner type of incision or a simple transverse incision incorporating the cyst and allowing access to the origin of the cyst, which arises from the distal interphalangeal joint capsule between the terminal extensor tendon and collateral ligament (**TECH FIG 3A**).
- During the dissection, take care to avoid injury to the germinal matrix of the nail bed (**TECH FIG 3B**).
- Excise the cyst at the base of its stalk along with a portion of the joint capsule (**TECH FIG 3C**).

- Excising underlying osteophytes and hypertrophic synovial tissue is the key to preventing recurrence of the cyst (**TECH FIG 3D**).
- The wound is irrigated, the tourniquet is removed, and hemostasis is achieved with bipolar cautery.
- Wound closure is accomplished with nonabsorbable monofilament sutures.
- I dress the wound with antibiotic ointment, petroleum gauze, gauze fluff, and tube gauze dressing.
- The patient is instructed to remove the dressing in 3 to 5 days and then cleanse the wound daily with antibacterial soap and water.
- Sutures are removed at 7 to 10 days.

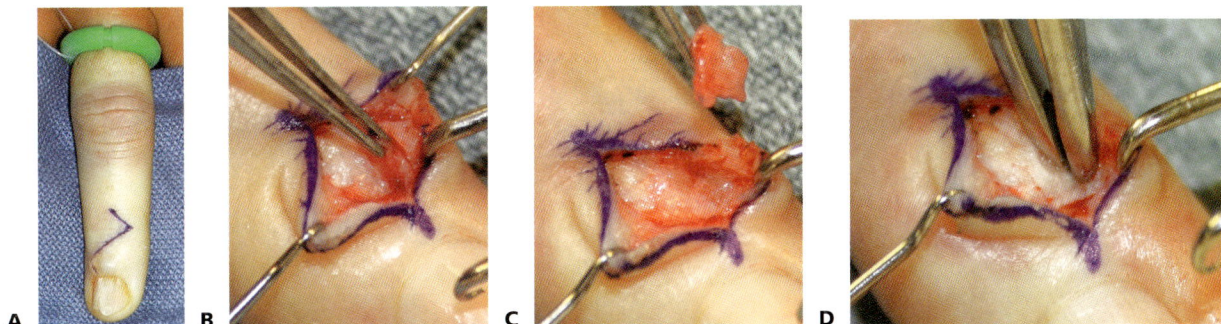

TECH FIG 3 • A. Degenerative mucous cyst in the eponychial region resulting in nail plate deformity. **B.** Aggressive dissection is avoided distally to protect the nail germinal matrix. The cyst is traced proximally to its origin at the distal interphalangeal joint. **C.** The cyst is excised along with a portion of the joint capsule at its point of origin between the central tendon and collateral ligament. **D.** A rongeur is used to débride underlying osteophytes.

TECHNIQUES

EXCISION OF A GANGLION CYST OF TENDON SHEATH (VOLAR RETINACULAR CYST)

- The patient is supine on the operating table with the involved upper extremity resting on a hand table.
- Anesthesia is usually accomplished with local anesthetic.
- Under tourniquet control (well tolerated by most awake patients for the 10 to 15 minutes required), a skin incision is made over the suspected ganglion cyst.
- Loupe magnification aids in limiting the size of the incision and identifying important anatomic structures. Retract the soft tissues and the digital neurovascular bundles.

- The ganglion cyst is commonly identified arising from the first or second annular pulley region.
- Dissect the ganglion cyst from the surrounding soft tissues and excise it at its base. We usually cauterize the site of origin with the bipolar cautery, which lowers the chance of a recurrence.
- The tourniquet is released, hemostasis is achieved, and wound closure is performed.
- A light hand dressing is applied for 7 to 10 days.

ARTHROSCOPIC EXCISION OF A DORSAL WRIST GANGLION CYST

- The patient is positioned supine on the operating room table with the operative upper extremity positioned in an arthroscopic traction tower (**TECH FIG 4**).
- Identify the standard wrist arthroscopic and anatomic landmarks.
- The 3–4, 4–5, 6R, and 6U portals are typically used.
- Under tourniquet control, insert a 2.7-mm small joint arthroscope into the 3–4 or 4–5 portal sites to inspect the joint and identify the ganglion stalk. The stalk in the typical dorsal wrist ganglion cysts is found arising from the dorsal distal margin of the scapholunate intraosseous membrane just proximal to the dorsal scapholunate intraosseous ligament. The stalk is not always identifiable or visualized.[17]
- Introduce a 2.9-mm resector shaver into the joint and excise the stalk (when visible) along with a 1-cm portion of dorsal wrist capsule and ganglion cyst.
- Use extreme caution when resecting the ganglion stalk and capsule to avoid injury to the scapholunate ligament and intraosseous membrane as well as the overlying extensor carpi radialis brevis and extensor digitorum communis tendons.
- Midcarpal arthroscopy is performed if indicated, but routine inspection is not necessary when treating a dorsal wrist ganglion cyst.
- The portal sites are typically closed with a removable monofilament suture.
- A light hand dressing is applied with a plaster palmar splint, which is left in place for about 5 to 7 days.

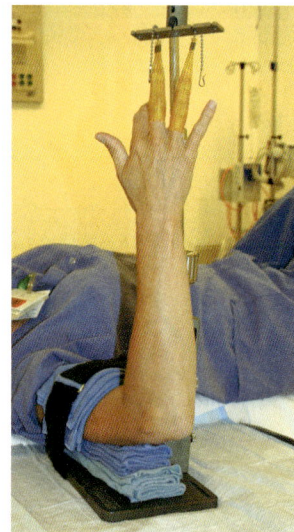

TECH FIG 4 • Standard arthroscopic setup using a traction tower. The traction tower, which can be sterilized, is typically positioned in this manner on a hand table after standard preparation and draping.

EXCISION OF A GIANT CELL TUMOR OF THE TENDON SHEATH

- The standard treatment is complete surgical removal.
- Careful surgical dissection is performed under loupe magnification (**TECH FIG 5A**).
- After initial exposure, isolate the neurovascular bundle proximal and distal to the lesion (**TECH FIG 5B**).
- Once the pseudocapsule is identified, it can be bluntly dissected or teased away from underlying structures with a Freer elevator, with care taken not to seed the surrounding tissues.[6] Alternatively, a small portion of the tendon sheath may be excised with the tumor origin and the area cauterized with bipolar electrocautery[12] (**TECH FIG 5C,D**).

- Carefully examine the local tissues for satellite lesions, which may be only a few millimeters in size. These lesions need to be completely excised (**TECH FIG 5E**).
- If the extensor tendon is involved, surgical excision of a portion of the tendon may be required. In rare cases, tendon reconstruction may be necessary. Lesions eroding into bone may require local curettage.
- If the tumor appears to arise from an underlying joint, it is important to perform a capsulotomy to inspect the joint and débride any pigmented tissue.[11]
- Arthrodesis of the distal interphalangeal joint may be necessary to completely excise some lesions.

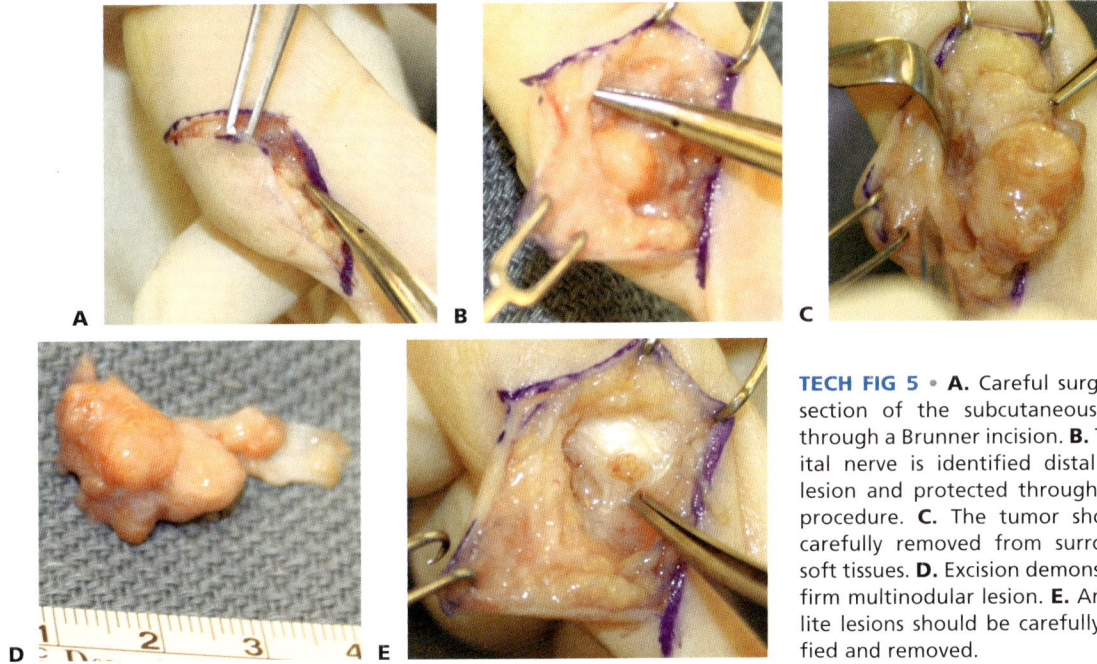

TECH FIG 5 • A. Careful surgical dissection of the subcutaneous tissues through a Brunner incision. **B.** The digital nerve is identified distal to the lesion and protected throughout the procedure. **C.** The tumor should be carefully removed from surrounding soft tissues. **D.** Excision demonstrates a firm multinodular lesion. **E.** Any satellite lesions should be carefully identified and removed.

MARGINAL EXCISION OF AN EPIDERMAL INCLUSION CYST

- Careful surgical dissection is undertaken under loupe magnification.
- After initial exposure, isolate the neurovascular bundles in the area of the lesion.
- Once the capsule is identified, it can be sharply dissected from overlying skin and bluntly dissected from deeper soft tissues (**TECH FIG 6**).

- Take care to remove the entire capsule.
- Lesions eroding into bone may require local curettage and bone graft.
- In rare cases with advanced bony destruction, amputation is an alternative.

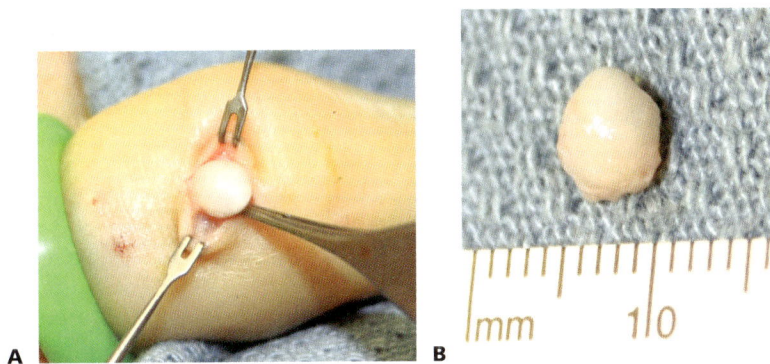

TECH FIG 6 • A. Through a small longitudinal incision directly over the lesion, the cyst is bluntly excised from surrounding soft tissues. **B.** Excision of the lesion demonstrates a firm, white, encapsulated mass.

PEARLS AND PITFALLS

Dorsal ganglion cysts	■ The scapholunate ligament is just distal to the tubercle of Lister. Dorsal ganglion cysts almost always arise from the distal margin of the dorsal scapholunate intraosseous membrane, just proximal to the dorsal scapholunate ligament.
	■ Excise the cyst at the base of the stalk, which is the site of origin.
	■ Cauterize the site of origin with a bipolar cautery to decrease the chances of recurrence.
	■ Take care to avoid injury to the dorsal scapholunate ligament.
	■ If the ganglion cyst recedes in size before surgery, dissect to identify the scapholunate ligament, which will often reveal the cyst.

Volar wrist ganglion cysts	▪ Always identify both superficial and deep branches of the radial artery when excising these cysts. These vessels are often adherent to the artery. ▪ Take care to avoid injury to branches of the lateral antebrachial cutaneous and dorsal radial sensory nerves when exposing the cysts.
Degenerative mucous cysts	▪ Perform a small capsulectomy at the site of cyst origin and débride underlying osteophytes and hypertrophic synovium to prevent recurrence. ▪ Take care to avoid injury to the extensor origin and germinal matrix of the nail bed. ▪ Even when the cyst thins the overlying dermis, preserve the skin for closure. Rarely, skin grafts are required. A portion of the cyst wall attached to the skin can be left behind as long as the cyst origin is excised and osteophytes are débrided.
Giant cell tumors	▪ The patient should be advised of the high recurrence rate after excision. ▪ Neurovascular structures should be carefully isolated. ▪ Satellite lesions should be completely excised. ▪ An arthrotomy should be performed for suspected joint involvement.
Epidermal inclusion cysts	▪ Biopsy should be considered for cases where a lytic bony lesion is present to rule out neoplasm or infection. ▪ Neurovascular structures should be carefully protected. ▪ Bony lesions may require curettage and bone graft.

POSTOPERATIVE CARE

Ganglion Cysts of the Wrist

▪ The splint and sutures are removed about 1 week postoperatively and Steri-Strips applied to the wound.

▪ Range-of-motion exercises and light use of the hand are initiated at 1 week, with gradual advancement of activities as tolerated.

▪ Scar massage is encouraged at 2 weeks.

Ganglion Cyst of Tendon Sheath and Degenerative Mucous Cyst

▪ Patients are instructed to remove their postoperative dressing 4 to 5 days after surgery. We prefer to have the patients clean their wound at least twice daily with antibacterial soap and water. The wound is redressed with light gauze or an adhesive bandage.

▪ Sutures are generally removed at 1 week and Steri-Strips applied to the wound.

▪ Range-of-motion exercises and light use of the hand are initiated, with gradual advancement of activities as tolerated.

▪ Scar massage is encouraged at 2 weeks.

Intraosseous Ganglion Cysts

▪ Postoperative dressing and sutures are removed at 1 week and Steri-Strips applied to the wound.

▪ We generally apply a short-arm cast for 3 to 5 weeks. The cast is removed and range-of-motion exercises and light hand use are initiated.

▪ Incorporation of the bone graft is monitored with use of serial radiographs. If the intraosseous ganglion cyst has weakened the bone, a protective splint may be used once the cast is removed until incorporation of the bone graft.

Giant Cell Tumors and Epidermal Inclusion Cysts

▪ Patients should be instructed about the high rate of recurrence of giant cell tumors.

▪ Range-of-motion exercises and antiedema techniques should be started immediately after surgery.

▪ Sutures can be removed at 8 to 10 days.

OUTCOMES

Ganglion Cysts

▪ Symptomatic relief is often accomplished after excision of most ganglion cysts.

▪ Recurrence rates after ganglion cyst surgery have been reported to range from 4% to 40%.[19] With adherence to the above principles, however, the recurrence rate in our experience is less than 5%.

▪ Complications of ganglion cyst removal are infrequent.

▪ The recurrence rate of giant cell tumors has varied from 5% to 50%. The high rate of recurrence is due to incomplete excision or satellite lesions.[6]

▪ Recurrence rates are even higher after excision of a recurrent tumor.[16]

▪ In contrast, the recurrence rate after epidermal inclusion cyst excision, even with bony involvement, is low.

COMPLICATIONS

▪ Wound complications (eg, painful or unsightly scar), infection, digital neurapraxia, or recurrence can occur.

▪ Ganglion cyst excision can result in a neurovascular injury. This complication is rare with adherence to good surgical technique and a good understanding of the local anatomy. Volar wrist ganglion cysts are adherent to the radial artery and can be difficult to dissect free from the artery. If necessary, a cuff of the cyst is left attached to the artery. If injury to the artery does occur, a repair should be performed.

▪ Stiffness is a complication of ganglion cyst excision. Avoiding direct capsular closure reduces the risk of this complication.

▪ Complications associated with degenerative mucous cysts include extensor lag, joint stiffness, infection, nail plate deformity, and distal interphalangeal joint deformity.[5]

REFERENCES

1. Angelides AC. Ganglions of the hand and wrist. In: Green DP, Hotchkiss RN, Pederson WC, eds. Operative Hand Surgery, vol. 2, 4th ed. New York: Churchill Livingstone, 1999:2171–2183.

2. Athanasian EA. Bone and soft tissue tumors. In: Green DP, Hotchkiss RN, Pederson WC, et al., eds. Operative Hand Surgery, vol. 2, 5th ed. New York: Churchill Livingstone, 2005:2211–2264.

3. Burge P. Aspiration of ganglia. J Hand Surg Br 1993;8B:409–410.

4. Dodge LD, Brown RL, Niebauer JJ, et al. The treatment of mucous cysts: long-term followup in sixty-two cases. J Hand Surg Am 1984;9A:901–904.

5. Fritz GR, Stern PJ, Dickey M. Complications following mucous cyst excision. J Hand Surg Br 1997;22B:222–225.

6. Glowacki KA. Giant cell tumors of the tendon sheath. J Am Soc Surg Hand 2003;3:100–107.

7. Glowacki KA, Weiss APC. Giant cell tumor of the tendon sheath. Hand Clin 1995;II:245–253.

8. Greendyke SD, WIlson M, Shepier TR. Anterior wrist ganglia from the scaphotrapezial joint. J Hand Surg Am 1992;17A:487–490.

9. Lister GD, Smith RR. Protection of the radial artery in the resection of adherent ganglions of the wrist. Plast Reconstr Surg 1978; 61:127–129.

10. Mackie IG, Howard CB, Wilkins P. The dangers of sclerotherapy in the treatment of ganglia. J Hand Surg Br 1984;9B:181–184.

11. Moore JR, Weiland AJ, Curtis RM. Localized nodular tenosynovitis: experience with 115 cases. J Hand Surg Am 1982;9A:412–417.

12. Nahra ME, Bucchieri JS. Ganglion cysts and other tumor related conditions of the hand and wrist. Hand Clin 2004;20:249–260.

13. Nield DV, Evans DM. Aspiration of ganglia. J Hand Surg Br 1986; 11B:264.

14. Oni JA. Treatment of ganglia by aspiration alone. J Hand Surg Br 1992;17B:660.

15. Paul AS, Sochart DH. Improving the results of ganglion aspiration by the use of hyaluronidase. J Hand Surg Br 1997;22B:219–221.

16. Reilly KE, Stern PJ, Dale A. Recurrent giant cell tumors of the tendon sheath. J Hand Surg 1999;24A:1298–1302.

17. Rizzo M, Berger RA, Steinman SP, Bishop AT. Arthroscopic resection in the management of dorsal wrist ganglions: results with a minimum 2-year follow-up period. J Hand Surg Am 2004;29A:59–62.

18. Soren A. Pathogenesis and treatment of ganglion. Clin Orthop Relat Res 1996;48:173–179.

19. Thornburg LE. Ganglions of the hand and wrist. J Am Acad Orthop Surg 1999;7:231–238.

20. Wang AA, Hutchinson DT. Longitudinal observation of pediatric hand and wrist ganglia. J Hand Surg Am 2001;26A:599–602.

21. Ward WA, Labosky DA. Ruptured epidermal inclusion cyst in the palm presenting as a collar-button abscess. J Hand Surg Am 1985;10A:899–901.

22. Westbrook AP, Stephen AB, Oni J, et al. Ganglia: the patient's perception. J Hand Surg Br 2000;25B:566–567.

23. Zubowicz VN, Ishii CH. Management of ganglion cysts of the hand by simple aspiration. J Hand Surg Am 1987;12A:618–620.

Chapter 113

Surgical Treatment of Nerve Tumors in the Distal Upper Extremity

Christopher L. Forthman and Philip E. Blazar

DEFINITION

- Nerve tumors make up less than 5% of tumors about the hand and wrist.[11]
- Most nerve tumors are benign and grow without causing neural dysfunction. As a result, the neural origin of a mass is often not anticipated and unexpected loss of function may occur after surgery.
- The key is to prepare for excision of any mass by discussing the possibility of a nerve tumor with the patient, by recognizing patients and masses with a high likelihood of a nerve tumor, and by being familiar with surgical techniques that allow preservation or, if necessary, reconstruction of the affected nerve.

ANATOMY

- Peripheral nerves consists of axons surrounded by a nerve sheath (**FIG 1**).
- The epineurium is a thin outer layer of connective tissue containing blood vessels that supply the nerve.
- Perineural cells form a strong cellular layer, the perineurium, surrounding each fascicle (bundle) of axons.
- An endoneurial layer of protective Schwann cells surrounds each individual axon.

PATHOGENESIS

- Tumors of the peripheral nerve arise from and resemble components of the nerve sheath.
- Most nerve tumors arise from the Schwann cell and are informally called schwannomas (or neurilemomas) and neurofibromas, depending on the pattern of growth and histology.
- Other benign peripheral nerve sheath tumors (BPNSTs) include the granular cell tumor, neurothekeoma, nerve sheath myxoma, and perineurioma. Electron microscopy and immunohistochemistry may be necessary to determine the type of tumor and cell of origin in some cases.[3]

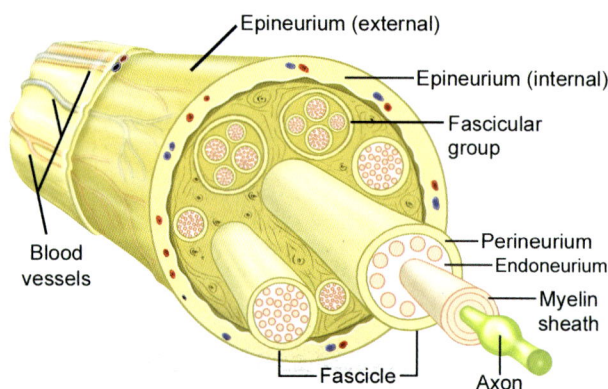

FIG 1 • Peripheral nerve anatomy. Individual axons travel together within a well-organized nerve sheath. The cells of the nerve sheath (not the axons) form the nerve tumor.

- Malignant peripheral nerve sheath tumors (MPNSTs) arise de novo or from malignant change within a BPNST.
  - About half of MPNSTs occur in patients with neurofibromatosis (NF) type I (von Recklinghausen disease).
  - The incidence of a MPNST in patients with NF type I is 2%,[7] although the lifetime risk rises to 13%.[2]

NATURAL HISTORY

- Upper extremity BPNSTs are usually solitary, and most occur in middle-aged adults.[4,6]
  - Pediatric nerve tumors are uncommon.[1]
- BPNSTs are typically painless and slow-growing, with malignant degeneration being exceedingly rare. Most tumors are relatively small (less than 2.5 cm), although they may cause nerve dysfunction due to focal impingement on the adjacent axons.
- Patients with NF type I often have multiple schwannomas, neurofibromas, or both of major upper extremity nerves. Thick tortuous "plexiform" neurofibromas are common in NF type I and have a high risk of progression to malignancy.

PATIENT HISTORY AND PHYSICAL FINDINGS

- The history should include the duration, growth characteristics, and local effects of the mass. Mild discomfort is common with nerve tumors but paresthesias are the exception rather than the rule. Hence, the possibility of a nerve tumor must often be entertained for the sake of completeness alone. Similarly, physical examination may suggest but cannot definitively diagnose a nerve tumor.
- A complete examination of a distal upper extremity soft tissue mass should evaluate other nonneural possibilities within the differential diagnosis.
  - Ganglia: Arise from joint and tendon sheaths in characteristic locations. The mass will typically transilluminate and the diagnosis can be confirmed by aspiration of highly viscous mucinoid material. Ganglia may mimic nerve tumors by causing compression of an adjacent nerve (eg, a ganglion in the canal of Guyon may cause ulnar neuropathy) (**FIG 2**).
  - Giant cell tumors (GCTs) of the tendon sheath: Reactive lesions of synovium that occur about the palm and fingers in similar locations to nerve tumors. GCTs are often palpably nodular, compared to the smooth margins of a nerve tumor.
  - Lipomas: These fatty tumors are usually more superficial and mobile than a nerve tumor. Rarely, lipomas grow in the carpal canal, causing median neuropathy.
  - Epidermal inclusion cysts: Should be suspected when examination reveals evidence of prior penetrating trauma. Unlike neuromas, these cysts do not cause nerve symptoms and a Tinel sign is not present.
  - Nodular fasciitis: A firm, reactive soft tissue proliferation that may grow rapidly on the volar surface of the forearm

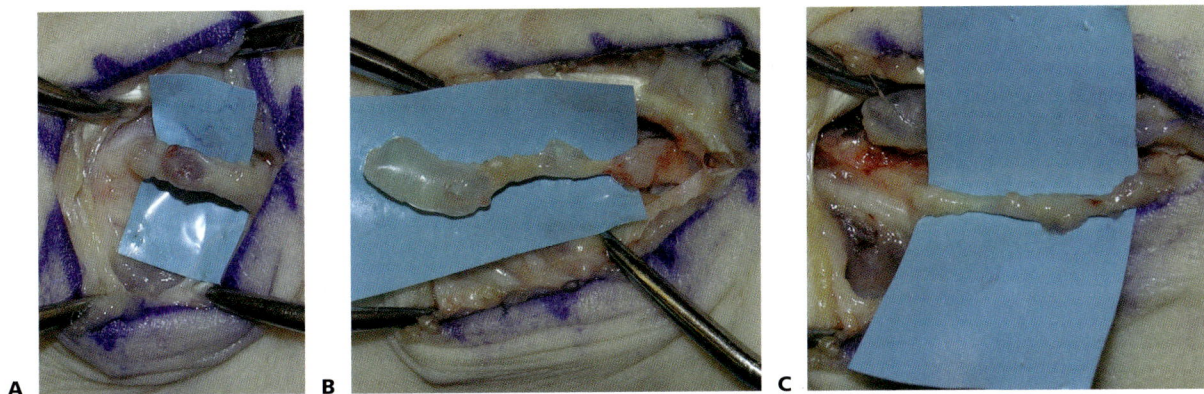

FIG 2 • A. Hypesthesia of the thenar eminence caused by an apparent tumor of the palmar cutaneous branch (PCB) of the median nerve. **B.** Careful dissection reveals a ganglion arising from the radioscaphoid articulation. **C.** The PCB is freed from the compressive mass.

or hand. The location may suggest a nerve tumor and the aggressive spread mimics sarcoma. While most nerve tumors are mobile in the transverse plane, palpation of nodular fasciitis reveals dense adhesions to the adjacent subcutaneous tissue.

- Patients with NF type I may have multiple nerve tumors, along with features such as café-au-lait spots, freckling in the axilla or groin, optic pathway tumors, iris hamartomas, and bone dysplasias. In patients with NF type 1, rapid growth of a neurofibroma, severe pain, and a new neurologic deficit often herald malignant degeneration.
- Examination techniques include the following:
  - Palpation: The examiner moves the mass transversely and longitudinally. Nerve tumors may be translated transversely but are tethered in the longitudinal plane.
  - Sensory testing using Semmes-Weinstein monofilament. Early nerve compression increases threshold while innervation density (two-point) remains normal. In a busy clinical practice, light moving touch may be as reliable (Stauch).
  - The examiner assesses visible atrophy and weakness in motor units innervated by the affected nerve. Manual strength testing is usually normal.
  - Direct pressure is applied over the nerve just proximal to the mass. Nerves under compression by a mass are sometimes sensitive to touch and may produce paresthesias when manipulated.
  - The nerve is percussed immediately adjacent to the mass. A positive result is paresthesias in the cutaneous distribution of the nerve. The Tinel sign is positive only when an injured nerve is attempting to regenerate. Most nerve tumors do not have a positive Tinel sign.

IMAGING AND OTHER DIAGNOSTIC STUDIES

- Plain radiographs should be obtained to look for intralesional calcification or invasion of adjacent bony architecture.
  - Intralesional calcification is rarely seen in BPNST and should alert the surgeon to the more likely possibility of a lipoma, hemangioma, giant cell tumor of tendon sheath, synovial chondromatosis, calcific tendonitis, myositis ossificans, or synovial sarcoma.

- A malignant nerve tumor may invade nearby osseous structures.
- An MRI is useful for evaluating tumor characteristics, delineating the surrounding anatomy, and planning a surgical approach.
  - Localization of the tumor to the vicinity of a large nerve trunk suggests a peripheral nerve tumor (**FIG 3A**).
  - MRI may also occasionally demonstrate subtle muscle atrophy of the distally innervated musculature. Tumor margins are smooth and there is mild intralesional inhomogeneity.
  - Nerve tumors have intermediate signal intensity on T1-weighted images secondary to intermingled adipose tissue (**FIG 3B**).
  - BPNSTs are bright on T2-weighted images.[12] These MRI features are similar to those of other soft tissue neoplasms and are not diagnostic.[8]
  - Irregular margins may be seen with plexiform neurofibromas or malignant tumors.
  - Other characteristics of a malignant neoplasm include size more than 5 cm, invasion into adjacent tissues, and tumor necrosis.
- Electrodiagnostic studies are most useful in the rare case of a clinically significant preoperative nerve deficit. Slowing of the nerve conduction velocity at the site of the tumor manifests as increases in the distal motor and sensory latencies, while electromyography will detect subtle muscle denervation.

DIFFERENTIAL DIAGNOSIS

- Neuroma
- Lipofibromatous hamartoma (fibrofatty infiltration)
- Nerve sheath ganglion
- Intraneural tumors of nonneural origin
  - Intraneural lipoma
  - Intraneural hemangioma

NONOPERATIVE MANAGEMENT

- In the absence of rapid growth, pain, or nerve dysfunction it is reasonable to observe a distal upper extremity mass. An MRI may be obtained to identify features consistent with a BPNST and to exclude signs of malignancy (see above).

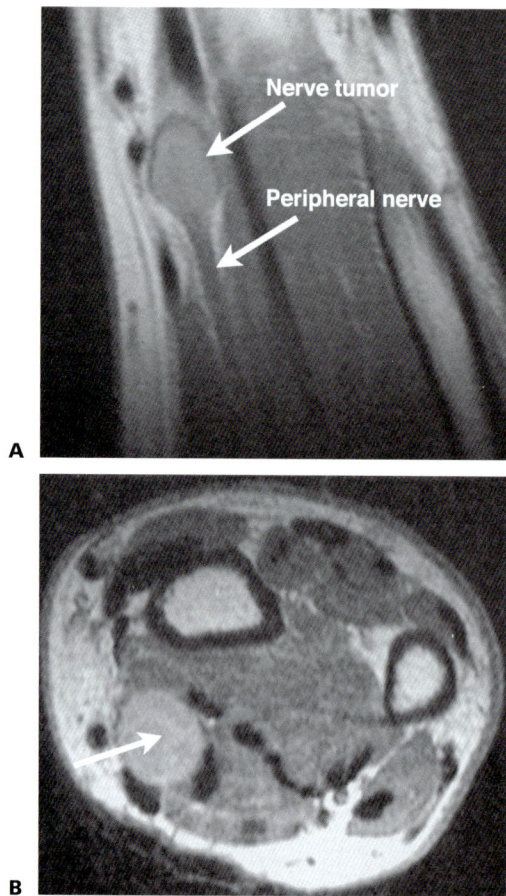

FIG 3 • **A.** Cross-sectional imaging of a benign peripheral nerve sheath tumor reveals the mass to be contiguous with normal axons proximally. **B.** MRI of a benign nerve sheath tumor (*arrow*) often demonstrates a high fat content, seen best on T1-weighted images.

- Patients with NF type I often have multiple neurofibromas, including dermal and plexiform types.
  - Dermal neurofibromas grow through the dermis and subcutaneous tissue to form plaque-like swellings. While sometimes unsightly, these tumors are routinely observed as the surgical defects are no more cosmetically pleasing.
  - Plexiform neurofibromas are visible as nodular masses lying longitudinally along the course of peripheral nerves. These tumors must be carefully followed as progression to a MPNST (neurofibrosarcoma) is common.
  - Pain is the most predictive symptom of malignant change. If there is no concern for malignancy, surgical excision is generally avoided as it frequently results in nerve deficits postoperatively.
- Children and young adults may develop masses of fibrofatty tissue infiltrating major nerves and their branches, particularly the median nerve.
  - These lipofibromatous hamartomas cause slow progressive nodular swelling and, at times, distal soft tissue overgrowth (macrodactyly).

- When asymptomatic, nonoperative management may be preferred, particularly if MRI shows pathognomonic features of this lesion.[13]
- Carpal tunnel symptoms may be treated with limited surgery, including an open carpal tunnel release and a definitive biopsy of a small cutaneous branch of the nerve.

SURGICAL MANAGEMENT

- An isolated distal upper extremity mass is treated surgically for definitive diagnosis, to control symptoms, or to exclude malignancy.

Preoperative Planning

- MRI is reviewed to confirm characteristics of a BPNST and to plan a surgical approach.
- Nerve reconstruction options are discussed with the patient.
- We consider synthetic absorbable nerve conduits for defects of up to 2 cm, particularly in the palm.
  - We avoid conduits when there is any concern of extrusion (eg, about joints in the digits) or in superficial sites where foreign body reaction may be confused with a tumor recurrence.
  - The medial antebrachial cutaneous nerve (MABC) is a suitable graft for the common and proper digital nerves.
  - A sural nerve cable graft may be necessary for major peripheral nerve defects.
- If significant nerve dysfunction is present before surgery (or is expected afterward), consideration should be given to performing concomitant tendon transfers, particularly in adults.

Positioning

- The patient is positioned supine with the affected extremity placed on a hand table. A brachial tourniquet is applied proximally, allowing access to the medial elbow for MABC nerve harvest if necessary.
- If sural nerve harvest is considered a possibility, we place a proximal thigh tourniquet and prepare and drape the contralateral lower extremity so that a second team may operate unencumbered.

Approach

- The surgical approach varies with tumor location.
  - A midlateral approach to digital nerve lesions allows excellent visualization of the tumor, protection of the adjacent digital artery, and good soft tissue coverage of the adjacent flexor tendon sheath.
  - Lesions in the palm are approached with a Brunner zigzag type of skin incision, which provides excellent visualization and minimizes restrictive postoperative longitudinal scar formation.
  - An open carpal tunnel approach is included for tumors close to the median nerve to decrease nerve compression from postoperative edema.
- Any suspected malignancy is managed according to the principles described in the oncology section of this text: a biopsy incision must allow optimal definitive resection options later. For example, a biopsy of a possible neurofibrosarcoma of the radial sensory nerve should be made through the mobile wad compartment as opposed to the more familiar Henry approach to this region.

TECHNIQUES

ENUCLEATION

- Most isolated BPNSTs are schwannomas and arise eccentrically from the nerve sheath (**TECH FIG 1A**). The tumor is encapsulated and can be safely enucleated without removing nerve fascicles.
- The nerve is exposed and fascicles are seen to drape over the mass, sometimes with a pedicled or multilobulated appearance. Inspect the nerve circumferentially for the window of splayed fascicles that affords the best resection plane (**TECH FIG 1B**).
- Incise the nerve sheath longitudinally, preserving the vessels running in the epineurium. Expand the window by carefully peeling away the fascicles and, ultimately, delivering the tumor out of the nerve (**TECH FIG 1C**).
- The resected specimen contains no nerve fascicles (**TECH FIG 1D**).

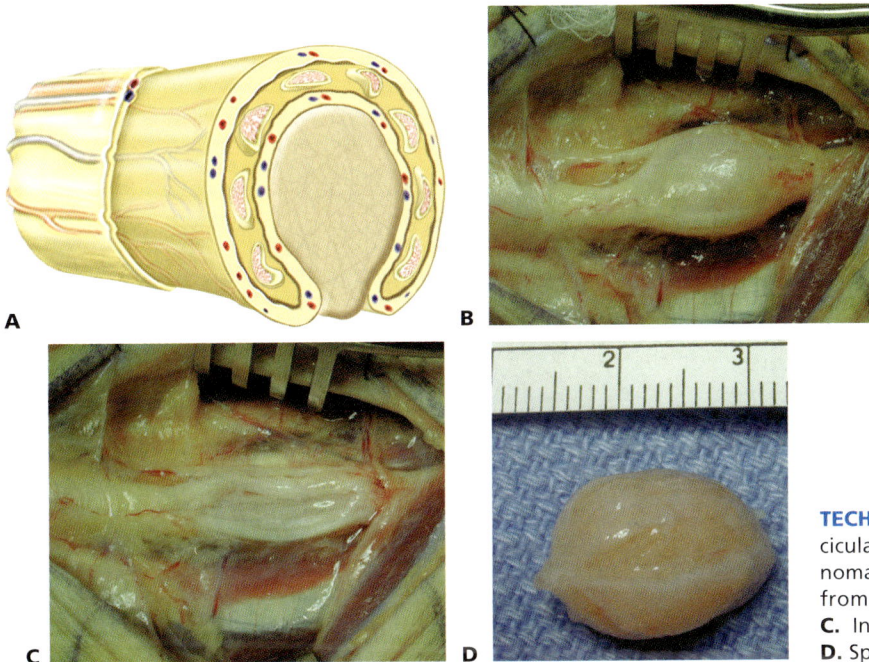

TECH FIG 1 • **A.** Nerve fascicles and fascicular groups are displaced by a schwannoma. **B.** The tumor may be "shelled out" from between the splayed fascicles. **C.** Intact fascicles after tumor resection. **D.** Specimen.

NERVE REPAIRS, GRAFTS, AND CONDUITS

- Surgical exploration of a nerve tumor may reveal a centrally placed expansile lesion with characteristic incorporation of nerve fascicles within the mass—the neurofibroma (**TECH FIG 2A**). While poorly encapsulated within the nerve, these tumors are typically free of adhesions to the adjacent soft tissues. Complete excision may require resection of the involved section of the nerve.
- The neurofibroma is exposed similar to the schwannoma. In this case, fusiform expansion of the posterior interosseous nerve is identified. Fascicles are seen entering the lesion at its proximal and distal extent, confirming the diagnosis of a neurofibroma (**TECH FIG 2B**).
- A microscope may allow identification of a prominent fascicular group that can be microdissected from the adjacent normal fascicles. If no prominent fascicular group or groups can be identified, then tumor resection will require nerve transection through normal fascicles at each end of the mass.
  - Direct reapproximation of the nerve ends is optimal but should be done only with minimal joint flexion and tension. Direct repairs done with significant joint flexion or high tension have poor results.
- The MABC is harvested if an autologous nerve graft is required (**TECH FIG 2C**). The nerve exits the brachial fascia adjacent to the basilic vein at the junction of the middle and distal third of the forearm.
  - The length of the nerve may be harvested for a nerve cable graft if a major peripheral nerve has been sacrificed.
- The small anterior branch of the MABC may be harvested an inch anterior and distal to the medial epicondyle. The anterior branch is generally a good size match for a digital nerve, as seen in this case of a nerve tumor with iatrogenic soft tissue loss (**TECH FIG 2D**).
  - Alternatively, a nerve tube may be used to bridge an intercalary nerve defect (**TECH FIG 2E**).
- A digital neurofibroma can be resected and the defect bridged with a nerve tube (**TECH FIG 2F**). Studies suggest that nerve conduits are best suited for defects of 2 cm or less.

TECHNIQUES

A

B

Basilic vein
Medial antebrachial cutaneous nerve
Anterior branch
Posterior branch
Cephalic vein
Lateral antebrachial cutaneous nerve

C

D

Nerve guide

E

F

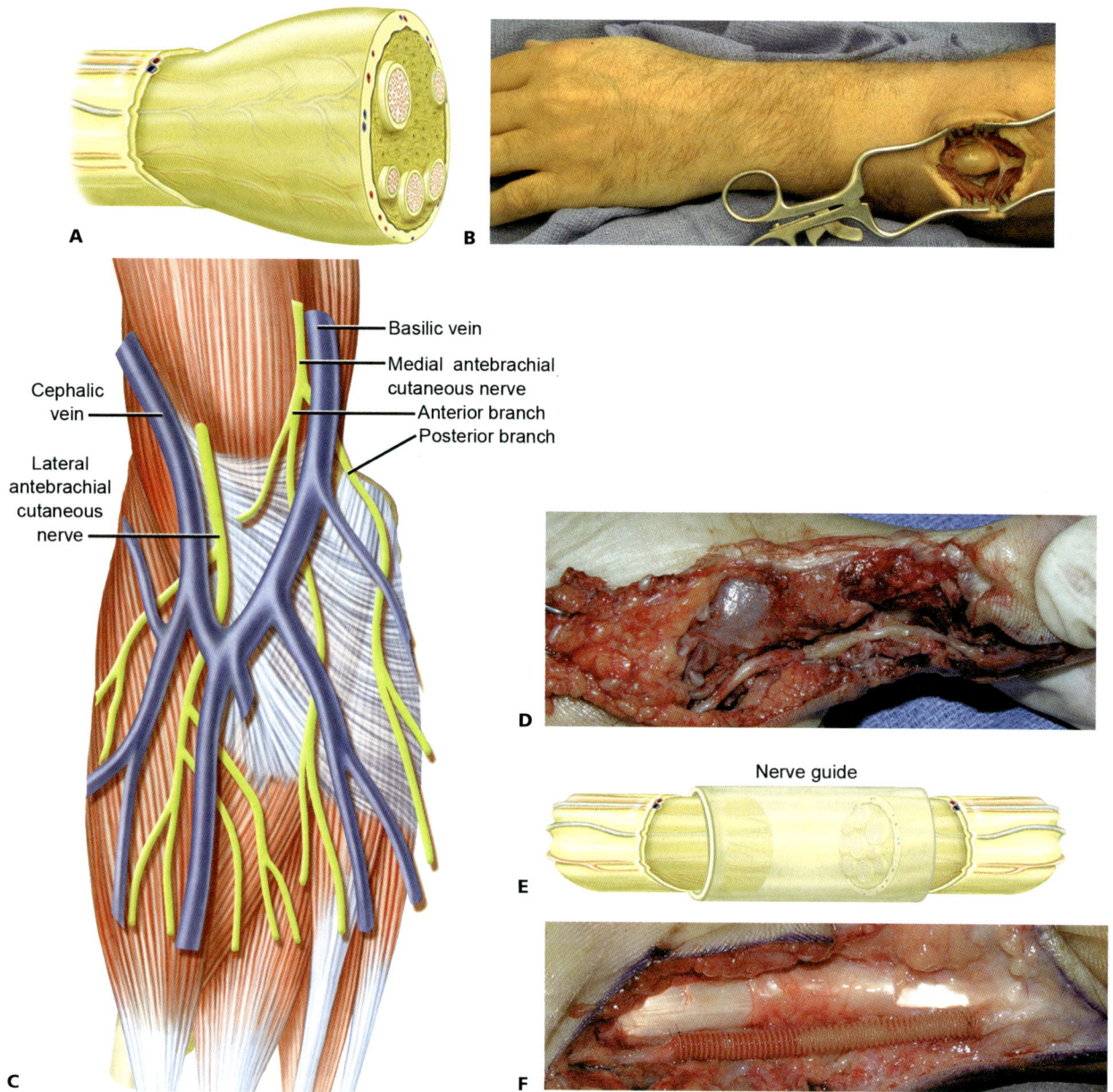

TECH FIG 2 • **A.** Fascicles are intertwined with tumor cells in a neurofibroma; tumor resection often requires excising a segment of nerve. **B.** A neurofibroma of the posterior interosseous nerve (PIN). This tumor was inseparable from normal nerve fascicles and excision resulted in permanent loss of finger extension. **C.** Branches of the medial antebrachial cutaneous nerve (MABC) run with the basilic vein. The anterior branch is a good match for a digital nerve and can be harvested near the elbow. **D.** The ulnar digital nerve of the thumb has been grafted with the MABC in this patient with prior nerve tumor resection and iatrogenic soft tissue loss. **E.** Nerve conduits provide an environment for nerve regeneration and have been shown to be as good as or better than nerve grafts in many situations. **F.** A digital neurofibroma was resected and a nerve conduit placed to bridge the intercalary defect. The soft tissues were slow to heal due to motion about the conduit at the metacarpophalangeal joint. Newer, less rigid collagen nerve guides may be better suited for use around the finger joints; however, human trials are lacking.

MICRODISSECTION

- Digital nerve schwannomas may sometimes require microdissection to preserve axons.
- The nerve is isolated under loupe magnification.
- The operating microscope facilitates identification of normal nerve fibers proximally. These axon bundles are traced distally and carefully dissected free of the mass.
- Occasionally, microdissection will allow the surgeon to identify and preserve normal fascicles from a neurofibroma of a large peripheral nerve.[11]

TECHNIQUES

LIPOFIBROMATOUS HAMARTOMA: LIMITED RESECTION AND SURAL NERVE GRAFTING

- A lipofibromatous hamartoma of the median nerve is most apparent about the proximal and distal extent of the transverse carpal ligament (**TECH FIG 3A**). The contained space of the carpal canal limits outward expansion of the hamartoma causing compression of nerve fascicles. Open carpal tunnel release may improve pain and nerve dysfunction. However, a mass that continues to grow, causing pain and nerve dysfunction, may need to be resected. Nerve grafts should be considered, especially in young patients.[5] Management in adults is controversial.

- Sagittal-plane MRI images will show the extent of the lesion (**TECH FIG 3B**).
- Surgical exposure begins with an open carpal tunnel release to identify the transition zone between normal and abnormal nerve. The incision is carried distally in a Brunner zigzag type of fashion to find the end of the lesion (**TECH FIG 3C**).
- The hamartoma is excised en bloc at healthy-appearing fascicular margins (**TECH FIG 3D**).
- A sural nerve is harvested and interposed as a cable graft (**TECH FIG 3E**).

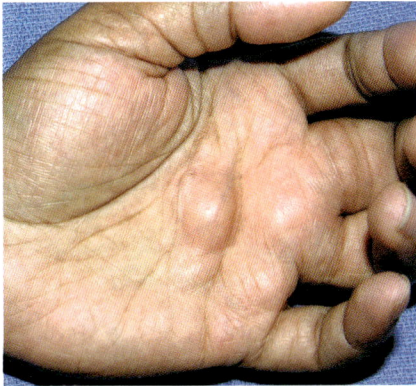

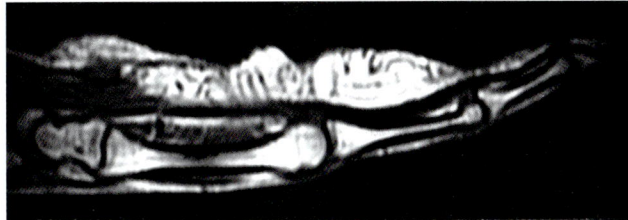

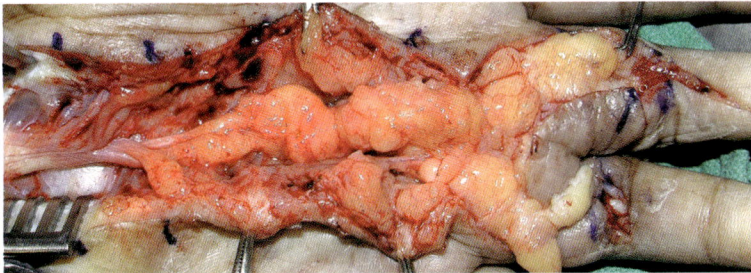

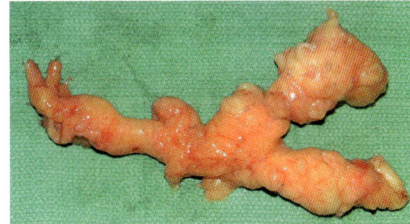

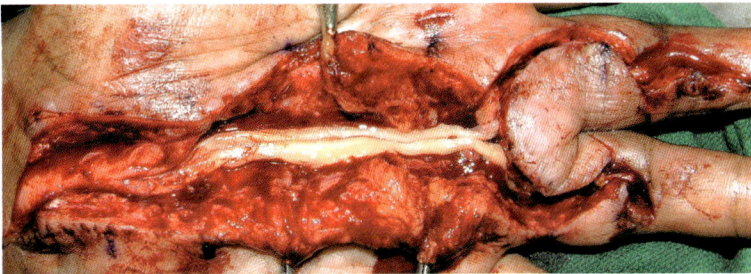

TECH FIG 3 • **A.** Painful expanding soft tissue mass along the common digital nerve to the third web space. The middle and ring fingers had slowly lost sensibility on the affected sides. **B.** MRI shows that the mass originates from the median nerve and extends to the proximal interphalangeal joint. Low-intensity normal nerve fascicles are seen coursing through the high-intensity fatty mass. **C.** At surgery, normal fascicles cannot be distinguished from the fibrofatty proliferation. **D.** Specimen. **E.** Sural nerve graft to the middle and ring finger proper digital nerves.

PEARLS AND PITFALLS

Diagnosis	▪ A nerve tumor must be part of the differential diagnosis for any distal upper extremity mass. ▪ Anticipation allows for appropriate preoperative planning and discussions with the patient.
Nonsurgical management	▪ Watch for signs of malignancy, including increasing nerve dysfunction, rapid growth, and pain. ▪ Plexiform neurofibromas seen in patients with NF type 1 have a high risk for malignant change.
Surgical approach	▪ Masses should be resected through an extensile approach; avoid transverse incisions. ▪ Tumors that are invasive into the adjacent tissue are likely malignant. An incisional biopsy should be performed and the wound closed.
Tumor resection	▪ Loupe magnification and microinstruments facilitate enucleation of a tumor (schwannoma). ▪ A microscope should be available should microdissection or nerve resection and reconstruction become necessary (neurofibroma).

POSTOPERATIVE CARE

▪ At a minimum, short arcs of joint motion are initiated early to discourage adhesion formation between the cutaneous scar and the underlying nerve.

▪ If necessary, the end range of motion may be avoided for up to 1 month to protect nerve repairs or reconstructions.

▪ When axons have been injured, a hand therapist may assist with desensitization or sensory re-education.

▪ A Tinel sign may be followed for renervation along the course of the affected nerve.

▪ Late changes in nerve function or swelling suggest the possibility of recurrence.

OUTCOMES

▪ Transient paresthesias are common after enucleation of a schwannoma; however, long-term nerve function is generally the same as or improved compared to the preoperative state. Tumor recurrence is rare.

▪ Permanent neurologic deficits follow en bloc resection of a neurofibroma, thus limiting the surgical indications for this procedure. Microdissection preserves nerve function[11] but likely has an increased risk of recurrence.

▪ Resection of a lipofibromatous hamartoma of the median nerve (including partial excision or interfascicular dissection) often results in permanent nerve deficits. There is limited long-term follow-up for nerve grafting of these lesions.

COMPLICATIONS

▪ Loss of nerve function after tumor resection
▪ Loss of motion due to prolonged immobilization

▪ Neuroma formation at a nerve donor site (eg, MABC neuroma)
▪ Wound breakdown over a nerve conduit, especially in the digits

REFERENCES

1. Colon F, Upton J. Pediatric hand tumors: a review of 349 cases. Hand Clin 1995;11:223–243.
2. Evans DG, Baser ME, McGaughran J, et al. Malignant peripheral nerve sheath tumours in neurofibromatosis 1. J Med Genet 2002;39:311–314.
3. Forthman CL, Blazar PE. Nerve tumors of the hand and upper extremity. Hand Clin 2004;20:233–242.
4. Holdsworth BJ. Nerve tumours in the upper limb: a clinical review. J Hand Surg Br 1985;10B:236–238.
5. Houpt P, Storm van Leeuwen JB, van den Bergen HA. Intraneural lipofibroma of the median nerve. J Hand Surg Am 1989;14A:706–709.
6. Kehoe NJ, Reid RP, Semple JC. Solitary benign peripheral-nerve tumours: review of 32 years' experience. J Bone Joint Surg Br 1995;77B:497–500.
7. King AA, Debaun MR, Riccardi VM, et al. Malignant peripheral nerve sheath tumors in neurofibromatosis 1. Am J Med Genet 2000;93:388–392.
8. Kransdorf MJ, Jelinek JS, Moser RP Jr. Imaging of soft tissue tumors. Radiol Clin North Am 1993;31:359–372.
9. Rinaldi E. Neurilemomas and neurofibromas of the upper limb. J Hand Surg Am 1983;8A:590–593.
10. Strauch B, Lang A, Ferder M, et al. The ten test. Plast Reconstr Surg 1997;99:1074–1078.
11. Strickland JW, Steichen JB. Nerve tumors of the hand and forearm. J Hand Surg Am 1977;2A:285–291.
12. Stull MA, Moser RP Jr, Kransdorf MJ, et al. Magnetic resonance appearance of peripheral nerve sheath tumors. Skeletal Radiol 1991;20:9–14.
13. Toms AP, Anastakis D, Bleakney RR, et al. Lipofibromatous hamartoma of the upper extremity: a review of the radiologic findings for 15 patients. AJR Am J Roentgenol 2006;186:805–811.

Chapter 114

Treatment of Enchondroma, Bone Cyst, and Giant Cell Tumor of the Distal Upper Extremity

Edward A. Athanasian

DEFINITION

- Enchondromas are benign cartilaginous neoplasms that are commonly seen in the medullary cavity of phalanges and metacarpals and less commonly the radius and ulna. Enchondroma is the most common neoplasm of bone arising in the hand.
- Unicameral bone cysts are benign endothelial-lined fluid-filled cavities arising in metaphyseal bone; they are occasionally seen in the distal radius and rarely seen in the hand.
- Giant cell tumor of bone is an uncommon benign neoplasm of bone, which is locally aggressive and can metastasize. While its histology suggests a benign process, is behaves as a low-grade malignancy.

ANATOMY

- Enchondroma most commonly arises in the proximal phalanx or metacarpal when seen in the hand (**FIG 1A**). It can be seen in metaphyseal and epiphyseal regions and is typically confined to the bone. The enchondroma may distend the bone and pathologic fracture may be seen.
- Unicameral bone cysts are rarely seen in the hand. When presenting in the radius they are often metaphyseal and may be in continuity with the distal radial physis (**FIG 1B**). Unicameral bone cysts are typically confined to bone and pathologic fracture may be seen.
- Giant cell tumor of bone most commonly arises in the epiphyseal region except in the skeletally immature patient, in whom it may arise in the metaphysis. The distal radius is the third most frequent location for these tumors (**FIG 1C**), after the distal femur and the proximal tibia. Hand lesions account for 2% of giant cell tumors of bone.

PATHOGENESIS

- The pathogenesis of enchondroma, unicameral bone cyst, and giant cell tumor of bone is uncertain. Enchondroma and unicameral bone cysts may be associated with bone development and growth.
- Enchondroma, unicameral bone cyst, and giant cell tumor of bone can weaken the bone and predispose the patient to pathologic fracture.

NATURAL HISTORY

- Enchondromas are most commonly identified incidentally during unrelated evaluation. They also can present after pathologic fracture. On occasion, a patient may complain of painful swelling in the bone.
  - Enchondromas found incidentally and not causing considerable mechanical weakness may be observed if typical radiographic findings are seen.
  - Enchondromas causing substantial fracture risk and those presenting after pathologic fracture can be treated surgically with a low risk of recurrence.[6]
  - Enchondroma can extremely rarely transform to chondrosarcoma.
- Unicameral bone cysts are most commonly seen during adolescence or childhood. They are most commonly identified after pathologic fracture. Proximal humerus lesions may be seen.
  - Unicameral bone cysts with a low risk of fracture may be observed with activity modification.
  - Unicameral bone cysts causing substantial weakness and fracture risk may be treated with surgery or injection.
  - Suspected unicameral bone cysts in the bones of the hand are sufficiently rare that strong consideration should be given to biopsy when this lesion is suspected.

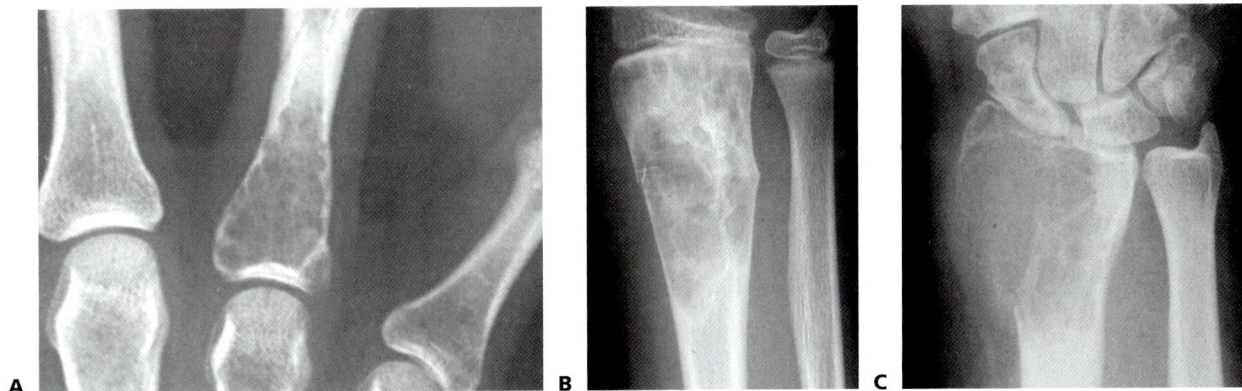

FIG 1 • **A.** Enchondroma of the proximal phalanx. **B.** Unicameral bone cyst of the distal radius. **C.** Giant cell tumor of the distal radius.

- Giant cell tumor of bone is locally aggressive. Patients may present with pain and swelling or after pathologic fracture.
  - Giant cell tumor of bone metastasizes 2% to 10% of the time, with metastasis more frequently seen with distal radius and hand lesions.[1,2,4,5] Metastasis most frequently occurs concurrent with or after a local recurrence.
  - Patients with giant cell tumor of bone require systemic staging, treatment, and long-term surveillance, as recurrence may be seen late.

PATIENT HISTORY AND PHYSICAL FINDINGS

- Enchondroma is most often an incidental finding and is asymptomatic. Pain and deformity can be seen after pathologic fracture. On occasion there will be bone distention and tenderness with palpation.
- Unicameral bone cysts are most commonly seen after pathologic fracture. On occasion there will be swelling and tenderness.
- Giant cell tumor of bone may cause swelling, pain, tenderness, and a sense of weakness. Loss of range of motion is common as these lesions are typically periarticular. Pathologic fracture may be seen.

IMAGING AND OTHER DIAGNOSTIC STUDIES

- Plain radiographs are indispensable in the initial evaluation of primary bone tumors (**FIG 2A**).

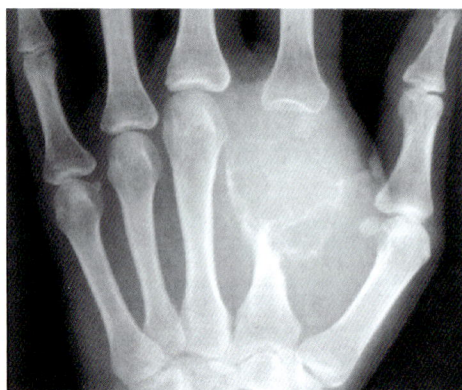

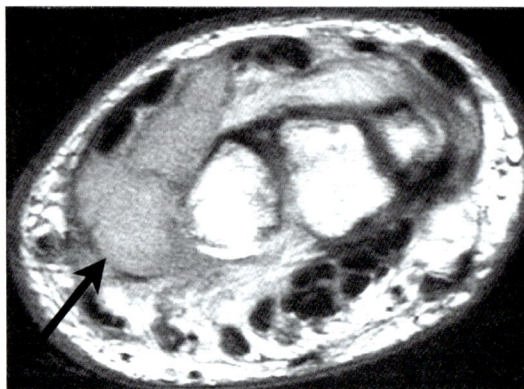

FIG 2 • **A.** Radiograph showing giant cell tumor of the metacarpal. **B.** MRI axial image of grade 3 giant cell tumor of the distal radius (*arrow*).

- MRI is useful when an aggressive lesion or soft tissue extension is suspected. MRI may allow better identification of the local extent of disease and may assist in operative planning (**FIG 2B**).
  - Campanacci et al's[3] grading system may be used:
    - Grade 1 lesions are confined to the intramedullary cavity without distention or distortion of the cortex.
    - Grade 2 lesions distend the cortex but do not extend into the surrounding soft tissues.
    - Grade 3 lesions destroy the cortex and extend into the surrounding soft tissues.
- Total body bone scan and lung CT scan are required for staging patients with giant cell tumor of bone.
- Incision or needle biopsy may be required when radiographs and MRI are not diagnostic.

DIFFERENTIAL DIAGNOSIS

- Enchondroma
- Chondromyxoid fibroma
- Chondrosarcoma
- Unicameral bone cyst
- Infection
- Aneurysmal bone cyst
- Giant cell tumor of bone
- Primary malignant bone neoplasms
- Acrometastasis

NONOPERATIVE MANAGEMENT

- Enchondroma and unicameral bone cyst may be observed provided radiographic assessment is diagnostic or the differential is limited to benign, nonaggressive lesions with an indolent natural history. The assessment of risk of pathologic fracture is paramount. Lesions with a substantial risk of pathologic fracture in the context of the patient's activity level are best treated operatively.
- The rare risk of malignant degeneration of enchondromas should be considered and discussed with the patient.
- Suspected giant cell tumor of bone requires biopsy. Rarely these can be treated with radiation alone; however, this approach is the exception and should not be considered first-line treatment. Radiation is associated with a risk of subsequent true malignant degeneration to a highly malignant giant cell tumor of bone.

SURGICAL MANAGEMENT

- All suspected giant cell tumors of bone and those enchondromas and unicameral bone cysts with a high risk of fracture are best treated surgically.

Preoperative Planning

- The radiographic extent of disease must be assessed.
- The approach will vary depending on the anatomic location.
- Bone graft source (autologous or allograft) must be considered.
- Precautions to prevent donor-site cross-contamination must be considered and reviewed with the operating room team.
- The surgeon must determine the anticipated need for frozen section and discuss this with the pathologist and review radiographs before any anticipated frozen section.

- The surgeon must secure and confirm the availability of any necessary grafting materials, instruments, implants, or adjuvants (ie, liquid nitrogen).
- The surgeon must confirm the availability of intraoperative imaging. Radiographs will give better resolution than fluoroscopy.

Positioning

- Surgery is typically done in the supine position with the arm extended on a radiolucent armboard.
- Proximal humerus lesions may be approached in a modified beach-chair position.

Approach

- Phalanx lesions may be approached from the dorsal or lateral approach.

- Metacarpal lesions are best approached dorsally in most instances.
- Carpal lesions are usually best approached dorsally.
- Distal radius lesions may be approached at the tubercle of Lister or at the interval between the radial border of the pronator quadratus and the first dorsal compartment, proximal to the radial styloid.
- Ulna lesions are usually best approached dorsally or ulnarly.
- Proximal humerus lesions are best approached just lateral to the deltopectoral interval.
- Biopsy must always take into consideration the potential for malignancy. It must be done in a way that does not compromise the potential need for a subsequent limb-sparing procedure.

CURETTAGE AND EXCISION OF PROXIMAL PHALANGEAL ENCHONDROMA

- The mid-axial approach from the ulnar side is preferred whenever possible (**TECH FIG 1A**).
- After making the incision under tourniquet control, identify the lateral band and retract it dorsally.
- Reflect the periosteum and create a bone window using curettes, rongeur, or drill (**TECH FIG 1B**).

- Curette the lesion in its entirety. The use of flexible fiberoptic lights may improve visualization.
- Pack the cavity with preferred bone grafting material.
- Obtain plain radiographs in the operating room to confirm complete excision and appropriate grafting.

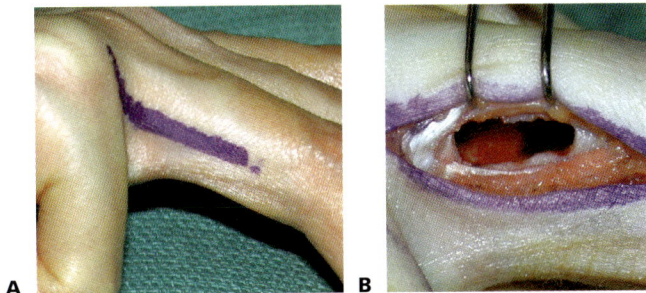

TECH FIG 1 • A. Mid-axial approach to proximal phalanx enchondroma. **B.** The lateral band is retracted and a bone window is created before curettage.

CURETTAGE AND EXCISION OF METACARPAL ENCHONDROMA

- Metacarpal lesions are approached dorsally through longitudinal incisions.
- Reflect the periosteum and create a bone window using curettes, rongeur, or drill.

- Curette the lesion in its entirety. Ensure adequate visualization through a longitudinal bone trough.
- Pack the cavity with preferred bone grafting material.
- Obtain plain radiographs in the operating room to confirm complete excision and appropriate grafting.

CURETTAGE, CRYOSURGERY, AND CEMENTATION OF DISTAL RADIUS GIANT CELL TUMOR OF BONE

- Preoperative preparation includes confirming the availability of liquid nitrogen, proper storage containers, cryosurgery instruments, and trained operative staff.
- Grade 1, 2, or 3 lesions with a single plane of palmar perforation can be approached from a palmar radial incision between the first dorsal compartment and the radial artery (TECH FIG 2A,B).
  - A branch of the superficial radial nerve may be encountered and should be retracted and protected. The radial 50% of the pronator quadratus is exposed.
- When palmar soft tissue perforation is present it will commonly be contained by the pronator quadratus. The pronator overlying the region of perforation should be excised en bloc with the bone window, effectively converting a grade 3 lesion to a grade 2 lesion with a palmar bone window.

- Wide exteriorization of the lesion with a window roughly two-thirds the maximum dimension of the lesion is needed to ensure adequate visualization.
- Thoroughly curette the lesion. Fiberoptic lighting may assist in viewing the extent of radial styloid involvement.
- Burr the endosteal surface if it is sufficiently thick. Irrigate and dry the cavity.
- The argon beam coagulator may be used to achieve hemostasis in the cavity and may have a beneficial effect as an adjuvant causing surface necrosis.
- Perform cryosurgery using three separate freeze–thaw cycles with either the direct pour technique or the spray gun (TECH FIG 2C).
- Fill the cavity with polymethylmethacrylate bone cement. Reinforcing Rush pins (Rush Pin, Meridian, MS) may be used (TECH FIG 2D).
- Apply a bulky compressive bandage and volar splint.

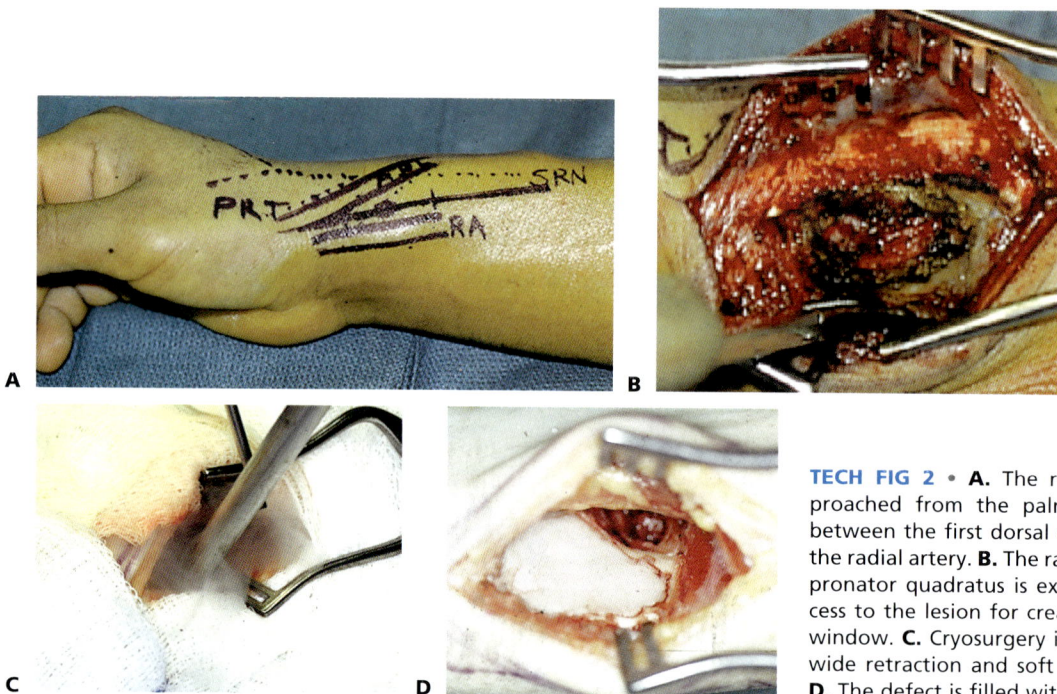

TECH FIG 2 • **A.** The right radius is approached from the palmar radial aspect between the first dorsal compartment and the radial artery. **B.** The radial border of the pronator quadratus is exposed to gain access to the lesion for creation of the bone window. **C.** Cryosurgery is performed after wide retraction and soft tissue protection. **D.** The defect is filled with bone cement.

WIDE EN BLOC EXTRA-ARTICULAR DISTAL RADIUS RESECTION

- Wide extra-articular excision of the distal radius may be indicated for grade 3 giant cell tumors with extensive cortical destruction, recurrent lesions, and those with pathologic fracture into the radiocarpal articulation.
- A dorsal approach maximizes exposure and facilitates subsequent intercalary arthrodesis.
- Finger extensors are released from the retinaculum while wrist extensors and often thumb extensors or abductors may need to be sacrificed.
- Cut the radius proximal to the tumor. Cut the ulna proximal to the distal radioulnar joint, away from the ulnar extent of the lesion (TECH FIG 3A).
- "Evert" the radius and ulna into the wound while the interosseous membrane is transected (TECH FIG 3B).

- Dissect the flexor pollicis longus and the radial artery away from the tumor-bearing segment.
- Mobilize the flexor tendons, median nerve, and ulnar nerve away from the tumor-bearing segment.
- The midcarpal articulation can be disarticulated initially from a dorsal approach and then circumferentially to complete the resection (TECH FIG 3C).
- Alternatively, the midcarpal articulation can be excised en bloc with the tumor-bearing segment by cutting with an oscillating saw from dorsal to palmar through the distal aspect of the distal carpal row bones.
- Reconstruction is readily accomplished by means of a vascularized or nonvascularized fibula graft (TECH FIG 3D).
- Spanning rigid internal fixation with a 3.5-mm dynamic compression plate lowers the risk of nonunion.

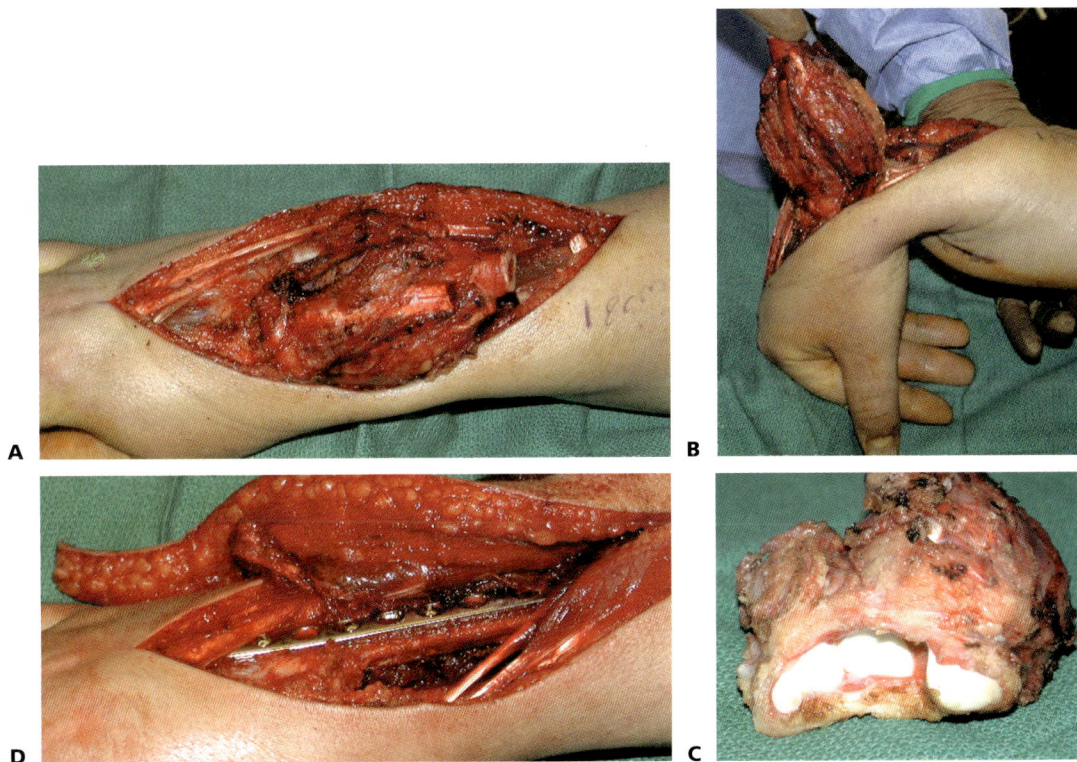

TECH FIG 3 • **A.** Dorsal exposure of the distal radius and ulna with transection of the radius and ulna proximally. **B.** The radius and ulna are everted into the dorsal wound to allow palmar exposure and dissection of palmar soft tissues. **C.** The resection specimen, demonstrating the midcarpal articulation of the proximal carpal row. **D.** Reconstruction is by means of an osteoseptocutaneous vascularized fibula graft for intercalary arthrodesis. A spanning 3.5-mm compression plate is used for fixation.

PEARLS AND PITFALLS

"Exteriorization"	■ Make the bone window to the lesion two-thirds the greatest dimension of the lesion to allow adequate visualization of the cavity.
Pathology consultation	■ Consult the pathologist in advance. Frozen section analysis of cartilaginous lesions is notoriously difficult.
Approach	■ A lateral approach to phalanx lesions provides more rapid return to normal motion and a better appearance. A volar radial approach for distal radius grade 1 and 2 giant cell tumors of bone allows excellent visualization and limits local contamination risk. ■ The dorsal approach for large grade 3 giant cell tumor distal radius lesions is best when wide excision and reconstruction or arthrodesis is anticipated.
Monitoring	■ Surveillance monitoring is mandatory, particularly for giant cell tumor of bone, which can recur late and metastasize.

POSTOPERATIVE CARE

■ Phalanx or metacarpal enchondroma
  ■ Bulky protective dressings are applied and range of motion is initiated at the first dressing change, usually 8 to 10 days postoperatively.
  ■ Protective splinting is continued for 6 weeks after surgery. High-risk activities are restricted for 12 to 16 weeks.
  ■ Periodic surveillance continues for 3 to 5 years.
■ Curettage, cryosurgery, and cementation of distal radius giant cell tumor of bone
  ■ Dressings are changed 10 days postoperatively. Sutures are removed and the patient is fitted with a removable splint.
  ■ Active range-of-motion exercises are initiated. Active-assisted and passive range-of-motion exercises are added at week 6.
  ■ Activities are gradually increased, with high-risk activities being restricted for up to 2 years due to cryonecrosis of bone caused by cryosurgery.
■ Wide en bloc extra-articular distal radius resection
  ■ Patients are dressed in a bulky compressive dressing, most commonly with a volar splint.
  ■ Elevation is encouraged for the first 48 hours and digit range of motion is encouraged.
  ■ Formal supervised therapy is initiated at the first dressing change, typically 8 to 10 days after surgery.
    ■ At that time bandages are removed and sutures can be removed.
  ■ Most commonly, active and active-assisted range-of-motion exercises are initiated. When not exercising, patients are asked to use a protective splint for an additional month. Activities are progressively increased as soft tissue and bone healing allows.
  ■ Range-of-motion exercises are initiated no later than 10 days after surgery.
  ■ Protective splinting continues a total of 6 weeks minimum after intralesional procedures and until bone healing is confirmed after arthrodesis.
  ■ Sporting activities are typically restricted for 12 to 18 weeks. High-risk activities are avoided for longer periods.
  ■ Surveillance for local recurrence should continue for 5 years for benign lesions and 10 years for giant cell tumor of bone.

OUTCOMES

■ Local recurrence
  ■ The local recurrence rate after curettage and bone grafting of enchondromas is about 5%. When recurrence is seen, the question of malignant transformation should be considered.[6]
  ■ The local recurrence rate after curettage and bone grafting of giant cell tumor of bone in the distal radius is about 50%, and adjuvants such as liquid nitrogen can lower this to about 20%. Intralesional treatment (curettage) is best reserved for lesions without soft tissue extension (grade 1 and 2 lesions).[4,5]
  ■ Wide excision of distal radius lesions is associated with local recurrence rates of less than 10%; however, reconstruction in the form of articular allograft or intercalary arthrodesis results in inferior function, motion, and strength and higher levels of pain.[4,5,8]
  ■ The local recurrence rate after curettage and bone grafting of giant cell tumor of bones of the hand is about 80%. Isolated curettage without the use of adjuvants cannot be advocated in this setting. There are several successful examples of curettage cryosurgery and cementation of giant cell tumor of the small bones of the hand. This type of procedure is best done at a tumor referral center.[1,2]
  ■ Wide excision or amputation has been advocated for giant cell tumor of bone when it arises in the phalanges or metacarpals. Local recurrence may still be seen, but the rate is probably less than 10%.[1,2]
  ■ The local recurrence rate after curettage of enchondromas arising in the hand is about 5%.[6]
  ■ The local recurrence rate after wide excision or amputation for giant cell tumor of the bones of the hand is less than 10%.
  ■ The local recurrence rate after curettage, cryosurgery, and cementation of distal radius giant cell tumor of bone is about 20% to 25% and correlates with soft tissue extension.[5]
  ■ The local recurrence rate after wide excision of distal radius giant cell tumor of bone is likely less than 10%.[8]
■ Metastasis
  ■ Benign giant cell tumor of bone metastasizes in 2% to 8% in general case series.[1,2,4]
■ Motion and strength
  ■ Range of digit motion is typically excellent after curettage for enchondroma.
  ■ Range of motion of the wrist may be slightly diminished after curettage of enchondromas in the distal radius.
  ■ Grip strength is reduced to 60% of normal after wide excision of the distal radius for giant cell tumor with intercalary segmental arthrodesis. Forearm rotation is typically preserved.

COMPLICATIONS

▪ Infection, hematoma, nerve injury, intraoperative fracture, postoperative fracture, nonunion, limited range of motion, and tendon gliding problems may be seen after treatment of enchondroma or giant cell tumor of bone when arising in the upper extremity.

▪ Delayed complications include extensor tendon rupture due to prominent residual ulna, nonunion, and fracture after hardware removal.

REFERENCES

1. Athanasian EA, Wold LE, Amadio PC. Giant cell tumors of the bones of the hand. J Hand Surg Am 1997;22A:91–98.
2. Averill RA, Smith RJ, Campbell CJ. Giant-cell tumors of the bones of the hand. J Hand Surg Am 1980;5A:39–50.
3. Campanacci M, Laus M, Boriani S. Resection of the distal end of the radius. Ital J Orthop Traumatol 1979;5:145–152.
4. O'Donnell RJ, Springfield DS, Motwani HK, et al. Recurrence of giant-cell tumors of the long bones after curettage and packing with cement. J Bone Joint Surg Am 1994;76A:1827–1833.
5. Sheth DS, Healey JH, Sobel M, et al. Giant cell tumor of the distal radius. J Hand Surg Am 1995;20A:432–440.
6. Takigawa K. Chondroma of the bones of the hand: a review of 110 cases. J Bone Joint Surg Am 1971;53A:1591–1600.
7. Vander Griend RA, Funderburk CH. The treatment of giant-cell tumors of the distal part of the radius. J Bone Joint Surg Am 1993;75A:899–908.
8. Weiland AJ, Kleinert HE, Kutz JE, et al. Free vascularized bone grafts in surgery of the upper extremity. J Hand Surg Am 1979;4A:129–144.

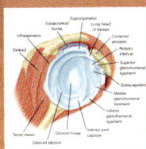

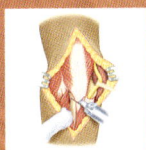

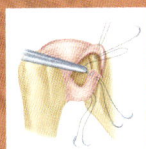

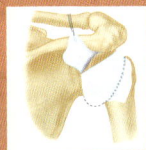

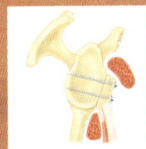

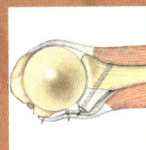

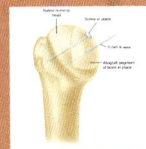

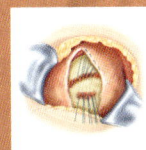

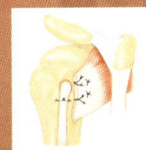

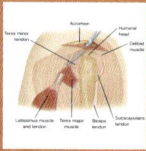

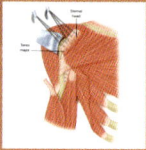

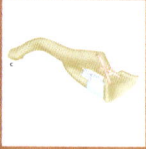

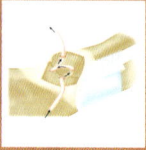

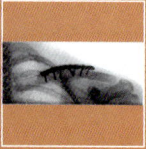

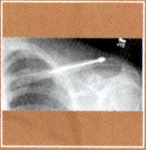

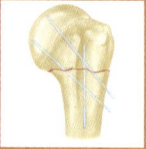

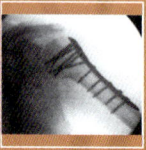

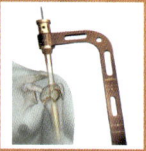

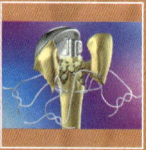

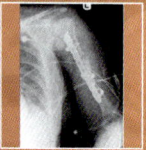

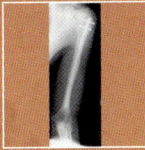

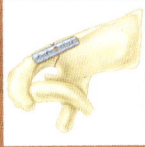

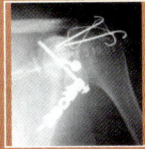

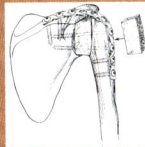

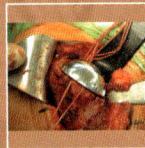

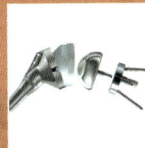

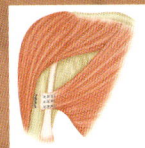

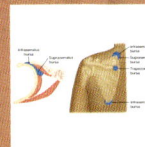

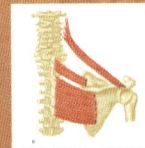

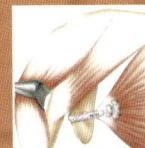

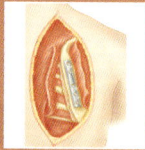

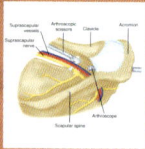

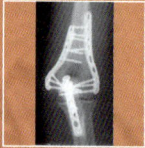

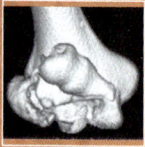

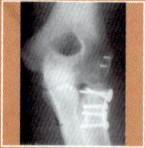

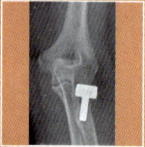

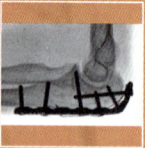

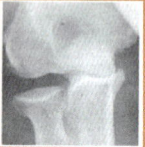

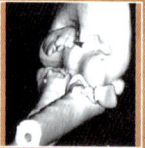

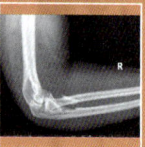

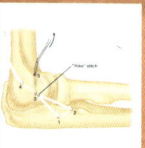

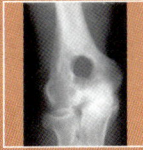

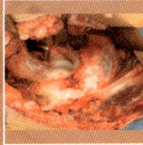

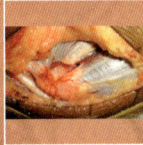

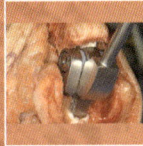

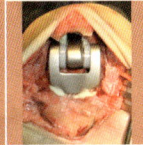

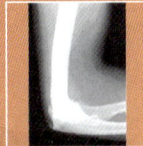

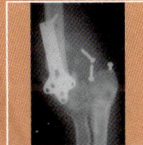

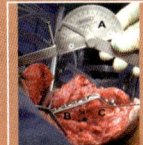

Anatomy of the Shoulder and Elbow

Joseph A. Abboud, Matthew L. Ramsey, and Gerald R. Williams

OVERVIEW OF SHOULDER AND ELBOW SURGERY

- In order to diagnose and treat problems of the shoulder and elbow, one must fully understand the anatomy of the region and appreciate how this translates to functional derrangements.
- There is no line of demarcation between the shoulder and elbow regions. Pain in the arm may originate at the neck or shoulder and refer down the arm. Less often pain noted by patients at the elbow or forearm have local origin. If the slightest doubt exists as to the etiology of the pain, the patient is examined from neck to fingers.
- The upper extremity functions to position and move the hand in space. The upper extremities are attached to the body by the sternoclavicular joint. Otherwise, they are suspended from the neck and held fast to the torso by soft tissues (muscles and fascia).
  - The upper extremity gains leverage against the posterior aspect of the thorax by virtue of the broad, flat body of the scapula.
  - The elbow along the upper extremity is a complex modified hinge articulation. Unlike the shoulder, the elbow has a much more intrinsic stability based on its bony architecture. The primary purpose of the elbow is to position the hands in space. The elbow joint is perhaps the main joint responsible for communicating the actions of the hand to the trunk.
- The surgical management of major shoulder and elbow conditions has rapidly progressed over the last 30 years as our understanding of the pathoanatomy and biomechanics has greatly enhanced our ability to treat certain problems. Consequently, new surgical techniques have allowed the surgeon to more effectively treat many disorders.
  - Arthroscopic surgery in particular has significantly increased our ability to surgically manage conditions and reduce morbidity. The sports medicine portion of this textbook handles the arthroscopic management of shoulder and elbow disorders.
- The art of any surgery lies in the reconstruction of diseased or injured tissues with minimal additional destruction. Skillful handling of the soft tissues is the hallmark of all upper extremity surgery, including the shoulder and elbow. Knowledge of anatomy defines the precision and safety of surgery. Approaches to any joint in the body are developed on this foundation, with particular emphasis on the exploitation of internervous planes. Familiarity with the intricate anatomy and multiple approaches to the shoulder and elbow allows the surgeon to confidently embark on the repair or reconstruction of the injury or disorder of the joint.

ANATOMY OF THE SHOULDER

- The shoulder has the greatest mobility of any joint in the body and therefore the greatest predisposition to dislocation.

- This great range of motion is distributed to three diarthrodial joints: the glenohumeral, the acromioclavicular, and the sternoclavicular.
- The last two joints, in combination with the fascial spaces between the scapula and the chest, are known collectively as the scapulothoracic articulation.

OSTEOLOGY

Clavicle

- This is a relatively straight bone when viewed anteriorly, whereas in the transverse plane, it resembles an italic S (**FIG 1**).
- There are three bony impressions for ligament attachment to the clavicle:
  - On the medial side is an impression for the costoclavicular ligament, which at times may be a rhomboid fossa.
  - At the lateral end of the bone is the conoid tubercle.
  - Just lateral to the conoid tubercle is the trapezoid tubercle.
- Muscles that insert on the clavicle are the trapezius on the posterosuperior surface of the distal end and the subclavius muscle, which has an insertion on the inferior surface of the middle third of the clavicle.
- Functionally, the clavicle acts mainly as a point of muscle attachment.
  - Some of the literature suggests that with good repair of the muscle, the only functional consequences of surgical removal of the clavicle are with heavy overhead and that, therefore, its function as a strut is less important.
- Four muscles take origin from the clavicle: deltoid, pectoralis major, sternocleidomastoid, and sternohyoid.
- Important relations to the clavicle are the subclavian vein and artery and the brachial plexus posteriorly.

Scapula

- This is a thin sheet of bone that functions mainly as a site of muscle attachment (**FIG 2A**).
- It is thicker at its superior and inferior angles in its lateral border, where some of the more powerful muscles are attached.

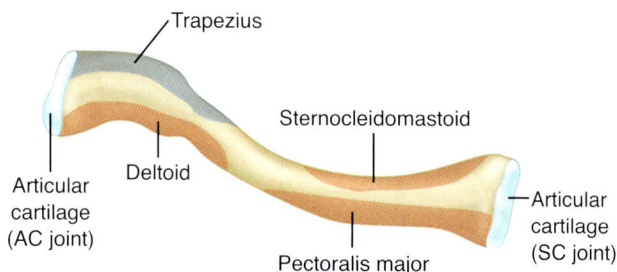

FIG 1 • The clavicle.

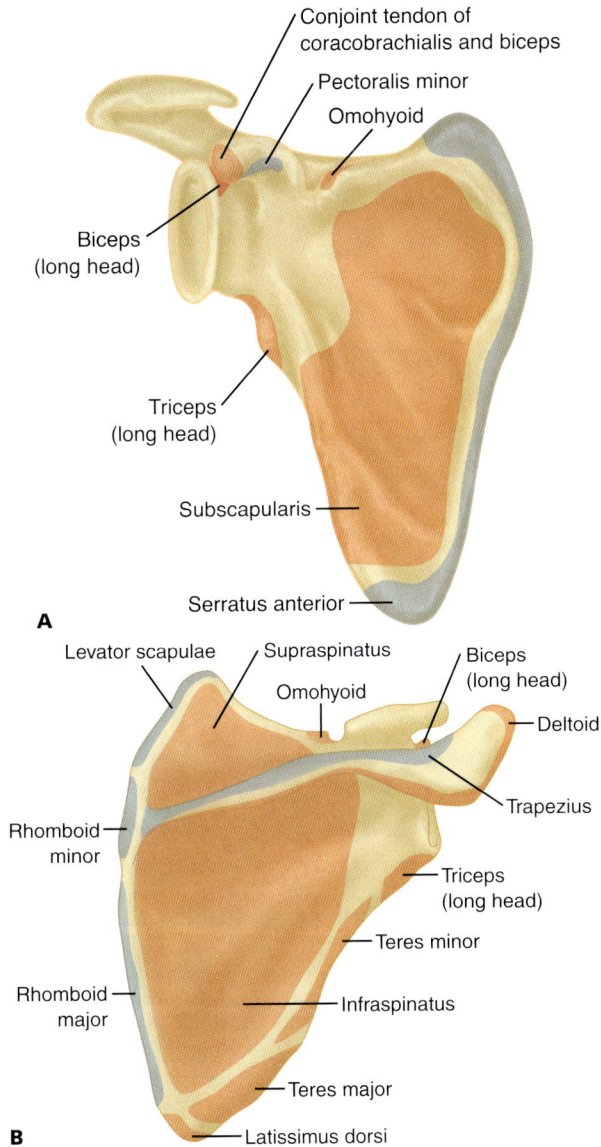

FIG 2 • A. The scapula. **B.** The supraspinatus and infraspinatus fossa.

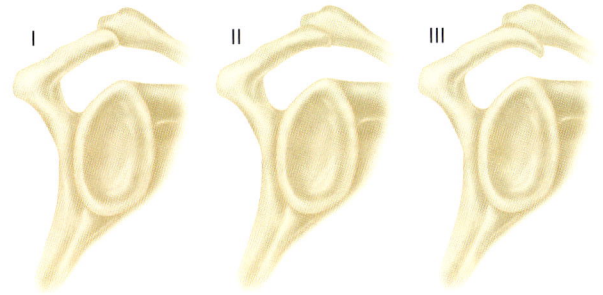

FIG 3 • Acromion morphologies.

- The acromion is the most studied process of the scapula because of the amount of pathology involving the acromion and the rotator cuff.
  - Three types of acromion morphologies have been defined by Bigliani and Morrison (**FIG 3**).
  - Type 1, with its flat surface, provided the least compromise of the supraspinatus outlet, whereas type 3, which has a hook, was associated with the highest rate of rotator cuff pathology in a series of cadaver dissections.
- The glenoid articular surface is within 10 degrees of being perpendicular to the blade of the scapula, with the mean being 6 degrees of retroversion.
  - More caudad portions face more anteriorly than cephalad.
- Three processes—the spine, the coracoid, and the glenoid—create two notches in the scapula.
  - Suprascapular notch is at the base of the coracoid.
  - Spinoglenoid, or greater scapular notch, is at the base of the spine.
- Major ligaments that take origin from the scapula are:
  - Coracoclavicular
  - Coracoacromial
  - Acromioclavicular
  - Glenohumeral
  - Coracohumeral
- Blood supply to the scapula derives from vessels in the muscles that take fleshy origin from the scapula.
  - Vessels cross these indirect insertions and communicate with bony vessels.

Humerus

- The articular surface of the humerus at the shoulder is spheroid, with a radius of curvature of about 2.25 cm.
- With the arm in the anatomic position (ie, with the epicondyles of the humerus in the coronal plane), the head of humerus has retroversion of about 30 degrees, with a wide range of normal values.
- The intertubercular groove lies about 1 cm lateral to the midline of the humerus (**FIG 4**).
- The axis of the humeral head crosses the greater tuberosity at about 9 mm posterior to the bicipital groove.
- The lesser tuberosity lies directly anterior, and the greater tuberosity lines up on the lateral side.
  - The lesser tuberosity is the insertion for the subscapularis tendon.
  - The greater tuberosity bears the insertion of the supraspinatus, infraspinatus, and teres minor in a superior to inferior order.

- It is also thick in forming its processes: coracoid, spine, acromion, and glenoid.
- The coracoid process comes off the scapula at the upper base of the neck of the glenoid and passes anteriorly before hooking to a more lateral position.
  - Functions as the origin of the short head of the biceps and the coracobrachialis tendons
  - Serves as the insertion of the pectoralis minor muscle and the coracoacromial, coracohumeral, and coracoclavicular ligaments
- The spine of the scapula functions as part of the insertion of the trapezius on the scapula as well as the origin of the posterior deltoid.
  - Also serves to suspend the acromion in the lateral and anterior directions to serve as a prominent lever arm for function of the deltoid
- The posterior surface of the scapula and the presence of the spine create the supraspinatus and infraspinatus fossa (**FIG 2B**).

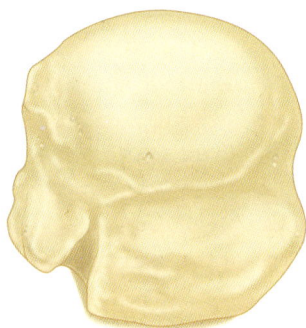

FIG 4 • The humerus.

- Greater and lesser tuberosities make up the boundaries of the intertubercular groove through which the long head of the biceps passes from its origin on the superior lip of the glenoid.
    - The intertubercular groove has a peripheral roof referred to as the intertubercular ligament or the transverse humeral ligament, which has varying degrees of strength.
- In the coronal plane, the head–shaft angle is about 135 degrees.
- The space between the articular cartilage and the ligamentous and tendon attachments is referred to as the anatomic neck of the humerus.
- Below the level of the tuberosities, the humerus narrows in a region that is referred to as the surgical neck of the humerus because of the frequent occurrence of fractures at this level.

STERNOCLAVICULAR JOINT

- This is the only skeletal articulation between the upper limb and the axial skeleton.

Ligaments

- The major ligaments of the sternoclavicular joint are the anterior and posterior sternoclavicular ligaments.
- The most important ligament of this group, the posterior sternoclavicular ligament, is the strongest.

Blood Supply

- Blood supply of the sternoclavicular joint derives from the clavicular branch of the thoracoacromial artery, with additional contributions from the internal mammary and the suprascapular arteries.

Nerve Supply

- Arises from the nerve to the subclavius, with some contribution from the medial suprascapular artery

ACROMIOCLAVICULAR JOINT

- Only articulation between the clavicle and the scapula

Ligaments

- Ligaments about the acromioclavicular articulation are the trapezoid and the conoid ligaments (**FIG 5**).
    - The anteroposterior stability of the acromioclavicular joint is controlled by the acromioclavicular ligaments, and the vertical stability is controlled by the coracoclavicular ligaments.

Blood Supply

- Blood supply derives mainly from the acromial artery, a branch of the deltoid artery of the thoracoacromial axis.

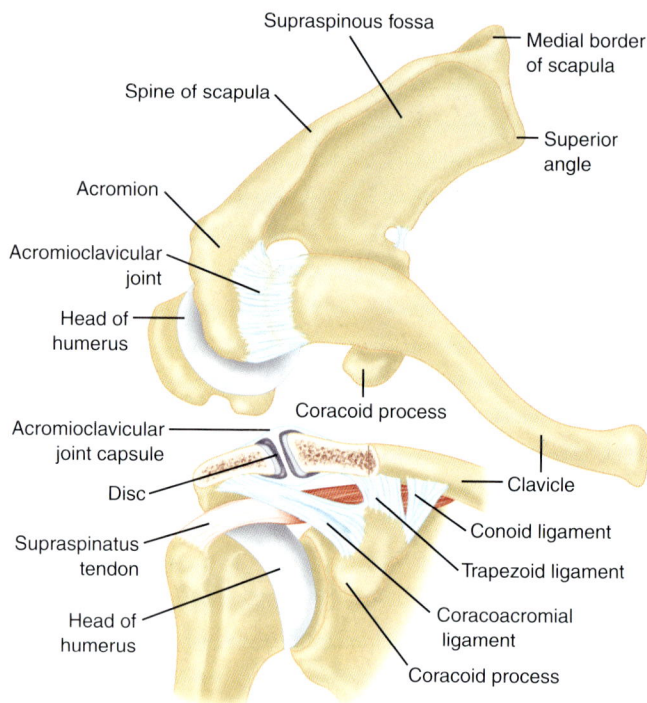

FIG 5 • Acromioclavicular joint.

- There are rich anastomoses between the thoracoacromial artery, suprascapular artery, and posterior humeral circumflex artery.
- The acromial artery comes on to the thoracoacromial axis anterior to the clavipectoral fascia and perforates back through the clavipectoral fascia to supply the joint.

Nerve Supply

- Innervation of the joint is supplied by the lateral pectoral, axillary, and suprascapular nerves.

SHOULDER LIGAMENTS: CAPSULOLIGAMENTOUS AND LABRAL ANATOMY (FIG 6)

Superior Glenohumeral Ligament (SGHL)

- Arises near the origin of the long head of the biceps brachii
- If the glenoid had the markings of a clock, with the 12-o'clock position superiorly and the 3-o'clock position anteriorly, the origin of the superior glenohumeral ligament would correspond to the area from the 12-o'clock to the 2-o'clock positions.
- SGHL runs inferiorly and laterally to insert on the humerus, superior to the lesser tuberosity.

Middle Glenohumeral Ligament (MGHL)

- Usually arises from the neck of the glenoid just inferior to the origin of the SGHL and inserts into the humerus just medial to the lesser tuberosity
- Presence of the MGHL most variable of any shoulder ligament

Inferior Glenohumeral Ligament (IGHL)

- Most important ligament for providing anterior and posterior shoulder stability
- IGHL has been described as having an anterior and posterior band, with an axillary pouch between the bands.

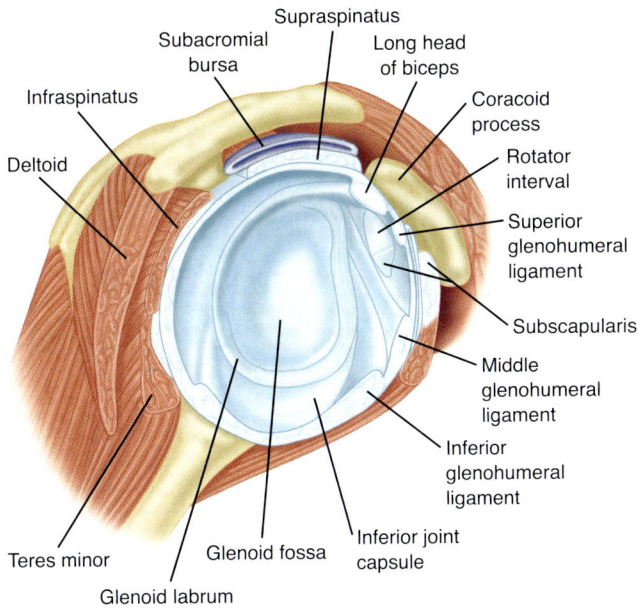

FIG 6 • Shoulder ligaments

■ With abduction and external rotation, the anterior band fans out and the posterior band becomes cordlike.
　■ Likewise, with internal rotation, the posterior band fans out and the anterior band appears cordlike.
■ Anterior band of the IGHL arises from various areas corresponding to the 2- to 4-o'clock positions on the glenoid.
　■ Insertion site of this ligament has two attachments, one to the glenoid labrum and the other directly to the anterior neck of the glenoid.
■ Posterior band originates at the 7-o'clock to 9-o'clock positions.
■ With the arm at the side, both the anterior and the posterior bands pass through a 90-degree arc and insert on the humerus.

Labrum

■ Surrounds the periphery of the glenoid and is a site of attachment of the capsuloligamentous structures
■ It is composed of dense fibrous connective tissue, with a small fibrocartilaginous transition zone at the anteroinferior attachment of the osseous glenoid rim.
■ The labrum acts as a load-bearing structure for the humeral head and serves to increase the surface area of the glenoid.
■ Howell and Galinat showed that the labrum deepened the glenoid socket by nearly 50%.
■ Lippett and coworkers have shown that removal of the labrum decreases the joint's stability to sheer stress by 20%.
　■ Triangular cross-section of the labrum allows it to act as a chock-block to help prevent subluxation.

SCAPULOTHORACIC MUSCLES

Trapezius

■ Largest and most superficial of scapulothoracic muscles
■ Takes origin from spinous process of C7 through T12 vertebrae
■ Insertion of the upper fibers is over the distal one third of the clavicle.

■ Lower cervical and upper thoracic fibers of the trapezius have their insertion over the acromion and spinous scapula.
■ Lower portion of the muscle takes insertion at the base of the scapular spine.
■ Acts as a scapular retractor, with the upper fibers used mostly for elevation of the lateral angle
■ Spinal accessory nerve is the motor supply.
■ Arterial supply is derived from transverse cervical artery.

Rhomboids

■ Similar in function to the midportion of the trapezius, with origin from the lower ligamentum nuchae, C7 and T1 for the rhomboid minor and T2 through T5 for the rhomboid major
■ Rhomboid minor inserts on the posterior portion of the medial base of the spine of the scapula.
■ Rhomboid major inserts to the posterior surface of the medial border, from where the minor leaves off down to the inferior angle of the scapula.
■ Action of the rhomboids is retraction of the scapula, and because of their oblique course they also participate in elevation of the scapula.
■ Innervation is the dorsal scapular nerve (C5), which may arise off the brachial plexus in common with the nerve to the subclavius or with the C5 branches of the long thoracic nerve.
■ Dorsal scapular artery provides arterial supply to the muscles through their deep surfaces.

Levator Scapula and Serratus Anterior

■ The levator scapula and the serratus anterior are often discussed together because of their close relationship anatomically and functionally.
■ The levator scapula takes origin from the posterior tubercles of the transverse process from C1 through C3 and sometimes C4.
　■ Inserts on the superior angle of the scapula
　■ Acts to elevate the superior angle of the scapula
　■ In conjunction with the serratus anterior, produces upward rotation of the scapula
　■ Innervation is from the deep branches of C3 and C4.
■ Serratus anterior takes origin from the ribs on the anterior lateral wall of the thoracic cage.
　■ Bounded medially by the ribs and intercostal muscles and laterally by the axillary space
　■ Protracts the scapula and participates in upward rotation of the scapula
　■ More active in flexion than in abduction because straight abduction requires some retraction of the scapula
　■ Absence of serratus activity, usually because of paralysis, produces a winging of the scapula with forward flexion of the arm and loss of strength in that motion.
　■ Innervation is supplied by the long thoracic nerve (C5, C6, and C7).
　■ Blood supply is from the lateral thoracic artery, with a large contribution from the thoracodorsal artery.

Pectoralis Minor

■ Takes fleshy origin anteriorly on the chest wall, and second through fifth ribs, and has its insertion onto the base of the medial side of the coracoid

- Function is protraction of the scapula if the scapula is retracted and depression of the lateral angle or downward rotation of the scapula if the scapula is upwardly rotated.
- Innervation is from the medial pectoral nerve (C8 and T1).
- Blood supply is through the pectoral branch of the thoracoacromial artery.

GLENOHUMERAL MUSCLES (FIG 7)

Deltoid

- Largest and most important of the glenohumeral muscles, consisting of three major sections:
  - Anterior deltoid takes origin off the lateral third of the clavicle, middle third of the deltoid takes origin off the acromion, and posterior deltoid takes origin from the spine of the scapula.
- The deltoid is supplied by the axillary nerve (C5 and C6), which enters the posterior portion of the shoulder through the quadrilateral space and innervates the teres minor in this position.
  - Nerves to the posterior third of the deltoid enter the muscle very close to their exit from the quadrilateral space, traveling in the deltoid muscle along the medial and inferior borders of the posterior deltoid.
  - Branch of the axillary nerve that supplies the anterior two thirds of the deltoid ascends superiorly and then travels anteriorly, about 2 inches inferior to the rim of the acromion.
- Vascular supply to the deltoid is largely derived from the posterior humeral circumflex artery, which travels with the axillary nerve through the quadrilateral space of the deep surface of the muscle.
  - Deltoid is also supplied by the deltoid branch of the thoracoacromial artery.

Supraspinatus

- Lies on the superior portion of the scapula
- It takes origin from the supraspinatus fossa and overlying fascia and inserts into the greater tuberosity.
- Its tendinous insertion is in common with the infraspinatus posteriorly.
- It is active in any motion involving elevation.
- It exerts maximum effort at about 30 degrees of elevation.
- Innervation of the supraspinatus is supplied by the suprascapular nerve (C5, C6).
- Arterial supply is the suprascapular artery.
- Nerve comes through the suprascapular notch and is bound above by the transverse scapular ligament.
  - Artery travels above this ligament.
- Suprascapular vessels and nerve supply the deep surface of the muscle.

Infraspinatus

- Second most active rotator cuff muscle
- Its tendinous insertion is in common with the supraspinatus anterosuperiorly and the teres minor inferiorly at the greater tuberosity.
- One of the two main external rotators of the humerus and accounts for as much as 60% of external rotation force
- Also functions as a depressor of the humeral head
- Even in a passive state, it is an important stabilizer against posterior subluxation.
- Innervated by the suprascapular nerve
- Blood supply is from two large branches of the suprascapular artery.

Teres Minor

- One of the few external rotators of the humerus
- It provides up to 45% of the external rotation force.

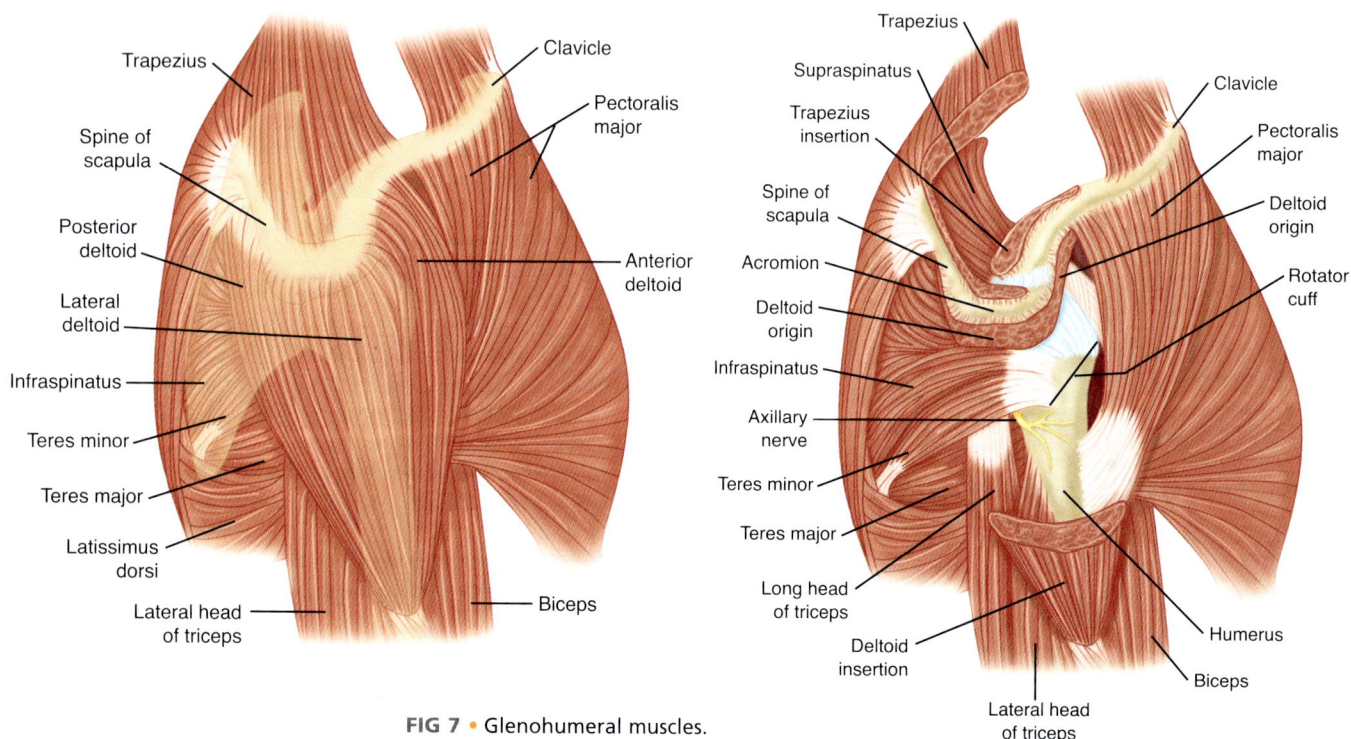

FIG 7 • Glenohumeral muscles.

■ It is important in controlling stability in the anterior direction.
■ Innervated by the posterior branch of the axillary nerve (C5 and C6)
■ Blood supply is derived from several vessels in the area, especially the posterior humeral scapular circumflex artery.

Subscapularis

■ Makes up the anterior portion of the rotator cuff
■ Takes origin from the subscapularis fossa, which covers most of the anterior surface of the scapula
■ Its upper 60% inserts through a cartilaginous tendon into the lesser tuberosity of the humerus, and its lower 40% has a fleshy insertion into the humerus below the lesser tuberosity cupping the head and neck.
■ Functions as an internal rotator and passive stabilizer to anterior subluxation and serves in its lower fibers to depress the humeral head
■ Innervation usually supplied by two sources:
  ■ Upper subscapular nerve (C5) and lower subscapular nerves (C5 and C6)
  ■ Upper subscapular nerves usually come off the posterior cord.
■ Blood supply originates from the axillary and subscapular arteries.

Teres Major

■ Takes origin from the posterior surface of the scapula along the inferior portion of the lateral border
■ It has a muscular origin and a common tendinous insertion with the latissimus dorsi into the humerus along the medial lip of the bicipital groove.
■ In their course, both the latissimus dorsi and the teres major undergo a 180-degree spiral; thus, the formerly posterior surface of the muscle is represented by fibers on the anterior surface of the tendon.
■ Function is internal rotation, adduction, and extension of the arm.
■ Innervation is supplied by the lower subscapular nerve C5 and C6.
■ Blood supply is derived from the subscapular artery.

Coracobrachialis

■ Originates from the coracoid process, in common with and medial to the short head of the biceps, and inserts onto the anteromedial surface in the midportion of the humerus
■ Action is flexion and adduction of the glenohumeral joint.
■ Innervation supplied by small branches from the lateral cord and the musculocutaneous nerve
■ Because the larger musculocutaneous nerve's entrance to the muscle may be situated as high as 1.5 cm from the tip of the coracoid to as low as 7 to 8 cm, it must be protected during certain types of repair.
■ Major blood supply is usually off the axillary.

MULTIPLE JOINT MUSCLES

Pectoralis Major

■ Consists of three portions:
  ■ Upper portion takes origin from the medial one half to two thirds of the clavicle and inserts along the lateral lip of the bicipital groove.
■ Middle portion takes origin from the manubrium and upper two thirds of the body of the sternum and ribs 2 through 4.
  ■ It inserts directly behind the clavicular portion and maintains a parallel fiber arrangement.
■ Inferior portion of the pectoralis major takes origin from the distal body of the sternum, the fifth and sixth ribs, and the external oblique muscle fascia.
■ Action
  ■ Clavicular portion participates somewhat in flexion with the anterior portion of the deltoid while the lower fibers are antagonistic.
  ■ Is active in internal rotation against resistance and will extend the shoulder from flexion until the neutral position is reached
  ■ Powerful adductor of the glenohumeral joint
■ Innervation is supplied by two sources:
  ■ Lateral pectoral nerve (C5, C6, and C7) innervates the clavicular portion of the muscle.
  ■ Loop contribution from the lateral to the medial pectoral nerve carrying C7 fibers into the upper sternal portion
■ Major blood supply derives from two sources:
  ■ The deltoid branch of the thoracoacromial artery supplies the clavicular portion and the pectoral artery supplies the sternocostal portion of the muscle.

Latissimus Dorsi

■ Takes origin by the large and broad aponeurosis from the dorsal spines of T7 through L5, a portion of the sacrum, and the crest of the ilium
■ Wraps around the teres major and inserts into the medial crest and floor of the bicipital or intertubercular groove
■ Actions are inward rotation and abduction of the humerus, shoulder extension, and indirectly through its pull on the humerus downward rotation of the scapula.
■ Innervation is through the thoracodorsal nerve (C6 and C7).
■ Major blood supply is derived from the thoracodorsal artery.

Biceps Brachii

■ There are two origins of the biceps muscle in the shoulder:
  ■ The long head takes origin from the bicipital tubercle at the superior rim of the glenoid.
  ■ The short head takes origin from the coracoid tip lateral.
■ Has two distal tendinous insertions:
  ■ Lateral insertion is to the posterior part of the tuberosity of the radius
  ■ Medial insertion is aponeurotic (lacertus fibrosus), passing medially across and into the deep fascia of the muscles of the volar forearm.
■ Loss of the long head attachment expresses itself mainly as loss of supination strength (20%), with a smaller loss (8%) of elbow flexion strength.
■ Actions of the biceps are flexion and supination at the elbow.
■ Main action is at the elbow rather than the shoulder.
■ Innervation is supplied by branches of the musculocutaneous nerve (C5 and C6).
■ Blood supply derives from a single large bicipital artery from the brachial artery (35%), multiple very small arteries (40%), or combination of two types.

Triceps Brachii

■ Long head takes origin from the infraglenoid tubercle.
■ Major action of the muscle is extension at the elbow.

- Innervation is supplied by the radial nerve with root innervation C6 to C8.
- Arterial supply is derived mainly from the profunda brachial artery and the superior ulnar collateral artery.

BRACHIAL PLEXUS

- The standard brachial plexus is made up of distal distribution of the anterior rami of spinal nerve roots C5, C6, C7, C8, and T1. The plexus has contributions from C4 and T1 (**FIG 8**).

Trunks, Divisions, and Cords

- The roots combine to form trunks: C5 and C6 form the superior trunk; C7 forms the middle trunk; and C8 and T1 form the inferior trunk.
- The trunks then separate into anterior and posterior divisions.
- The posterior divisions combine to form the posterior cord, the anterior division of the inferior trunk forms the medial cord, and the anterior division of the superior and middle trunks forms the lateral cord.
- These cords give off the remaining largest number of the terminal nerves of the brachial plexus, and roots from the lateral and medial cords come together to form the median nerve.
- The brachial plexus leaves the cervical spine and progresses into the arm through the interval between the anterior and middle scalene muscles.
- The subclavian artery follows the same course. The plexus splits into cords at or before it passes below the clavicle.
- As the cords enter the axilla, they become closely related to the axillary artery, attaining positions relative to the artery indicated by their names: lateral, posterior, and medial.

Terminal Branches

- Plexus gives off some terminal branches above the clavicle.
- The dorsal scapular nerve comes off C5 with some C4 fibers and penetrates the scalenus medius and the levator scapulae, sometimes contributing with C4 fibers to the latter.
- The dorsal scapular nerve accompanies the deep branch of the transverse cervical artery or the dorsal scapular artery on the undersurface of the rhomboids and innervates them.
- Rootlets of the nerves C5, C6, and C7 immediately adjacent to the intravertebral foramina contribute to the formation of the long thoracic nerve, which immediately passes between the middle and posterior scalene muscles or penetrates the middle scalene.
- Next most proximal nerve is the suprascapular nerve.
  - It arises from the superolateral aspect of the upper trunk shortly after its formation at Erb's point.
- The lateral cord generally contains fibers of C5, C6, and C7 and gives off three terminal branches:
  - Musculocutaneous
  - Lateral pectoral
  - Lateral root of the median nerve
- Posterior cord supplies most of the innervations of the muscles of the shoulder, in this order:
  - Upper subscapularis, thoracodorsal, lower subscapular, axillary, and radial
- Medial cord has five branches, in the following order:
  - Medial pectoral nerve, medial brachial cutaneous, medial antebrachial cutaneous, medial root of the median nerve, and ulnar nerve

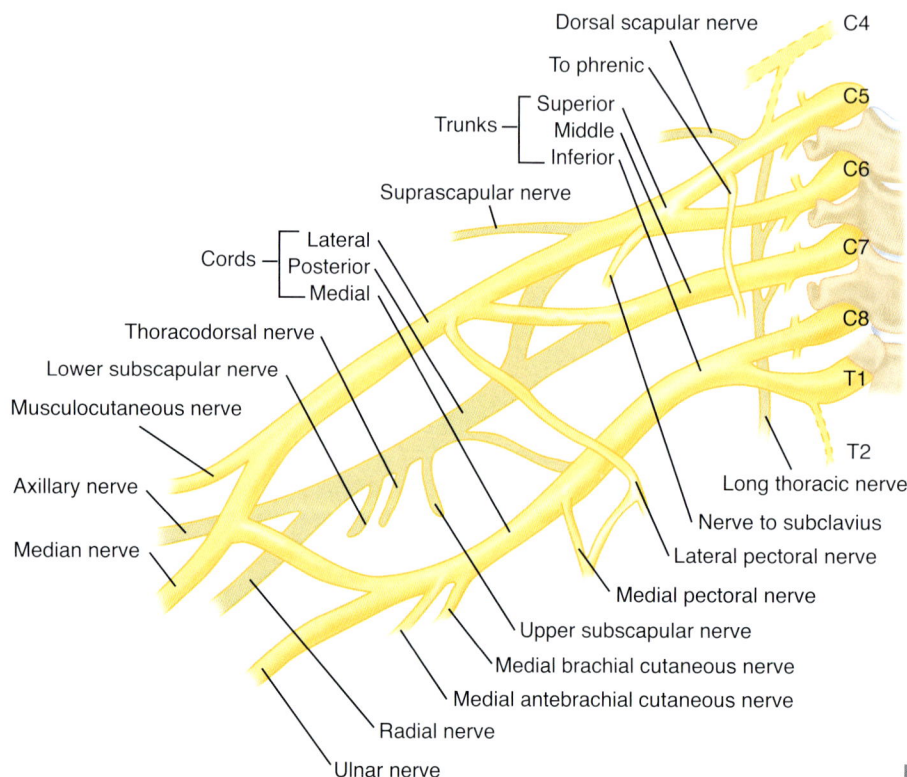

FIG 8 • The brachial plexus.

ARTERIES

Subclavian Artery

- Blood supply to limb begins with the subclavian artery, which ends at the lateral border of the first rib.
- Divided into three portions in relation to the insertion of the scalenus anterior muscle
- Vertebral artery takes origin in the first portion, and the costocervical trunk and thyrocervical trunk take origin in the second portion.
- There are usually no branches in the third portion of the artery.
- Two vessels encountered more frequently by the shoulder surgeon are the transverse cervical artery and the suprascapular artery.
  - Come off the thyrocervical trunk in 70% of dissections
  - In the remaining cases, they come off directly, or in common from the subclavian artery.

Axillary

- Is the continuation of the subclavian artery
- It begins at the lateral border of the first rib and continues along the inferior border of the latissimus dorsi, at which point it becomes the brachial artery.
- This artery is traditionally divided into three portions:
  - First portion is above the superior border of the pectoralis minor.
  - Second portion is deep to the pectoralis minor.
  - Third portion is distal to lateral border of the pectoralis minor.
- Usual number of branches for each of the three sections corresponds to the name of the section: one branch in the first portion, two in the second, and three in the third.
  - First section gives off the superior thoracic artery.
  - Second portion gives off the thoracoacromial artery and the lateral thoracic artery.
  - Third portion gives off the following:
    - Largest branch is the subscapular artery, and this is the largest branch of the axillary.
    - Next branch is the posterior humeral circumflex artery, and the third branch is the anterior humeral circumflex artery.
    - Anterior humeral circumflex artery is an important surgical landmark because it travels laterally at the inferior border of the subscapularis tendon, marking the border between the upper tendinous insertion of the subscapularis and the lower muscular insertion.

VEINS

Axillary Vein

- Begins at the inferior border of the latissimus dorsi as the continuation of the basilic vein, continues along the lateral border of the first rib, and becomes the subclavian vein

Cephalic

- Cephalic vein is the superficial vein in the arm that lies deep to the deep fascia after reaching the deltopectoral groove and finally pierces the clavipectoral fascia, emptying into the axillary vein.

ANATOMY OF THE ELBOW

OSTEOLOGY

Distal Humerus

- The distal humerus consists of two condyles, which form the articular surfaces of the trochlea and capitellum (**FIG 9A**).

Trochlea

- Hyperbolic, pulley-like surface that articulates with the semilunar notch of the ulna, covered by articular cartilage over an arc of 300 degrees
- Medial margin is large and projects more distally than does the lateral margin.
- The prominent medial and lateral margins are separated by a groove that courses in a helical manner from an anterolateral to the posteromedial direction.

Capitellum

- Capitellum is almost spheroidal in shape and is covered with hyaline cartilage, which is about 2 mm thick anteriorly.
- Posteromedial limit of the capitellum is marked by a prominent tubercle.
- A groove separates the capitellum from the trochlea, and the rim of the radial head articulates with this groove throughout the arc of flexion and during pronation and supination.

Joint Surface Orientation

- In the lateral plane, the orientation of the articular surface of the distal humerus is located anteriorly about 30 degrees with respect to the long axis of the humerus (**FIG 9B**).
- The center of the concentric arc formed by the trochlea and capitellum is on a line that is coplanar with the anterior and distal cortex of the humerus.
- In the transverse plane, the articular surface is rotated inwardly about 5 degrees, and in the frontal plane, it is tilted about 6 degrees in valgus (**FIG 9C**).

Epicondyles of Humerus

- Medial epicondyle serves as the source of attachment of the ulnar collateral ligament and the flexor pronator group of muscles.
- Lateral epicondyle is located just above the capitellum and is much less prominent than the medial epicondyle.
- The lateral collateral ligament and the supinator extensor muscle group originate from the flat, irregular surfaces of the lateral epicondyle.

Anterior Surface of Humerus

- Anteriorly, the radial and coronoid fossae accommodate the radial head and coronoid, respectively, during flexion.

Posterior Surface of Humerus

- Posteriorly, the olecranon fossa receives the tip of the olecranon in extension (**FIG 9D**).

Radius

- The proximal radius includes the radial head, which articulates with the capitellum and exhibits a cylindrical depression in the midportion to accommodate the capitellum.

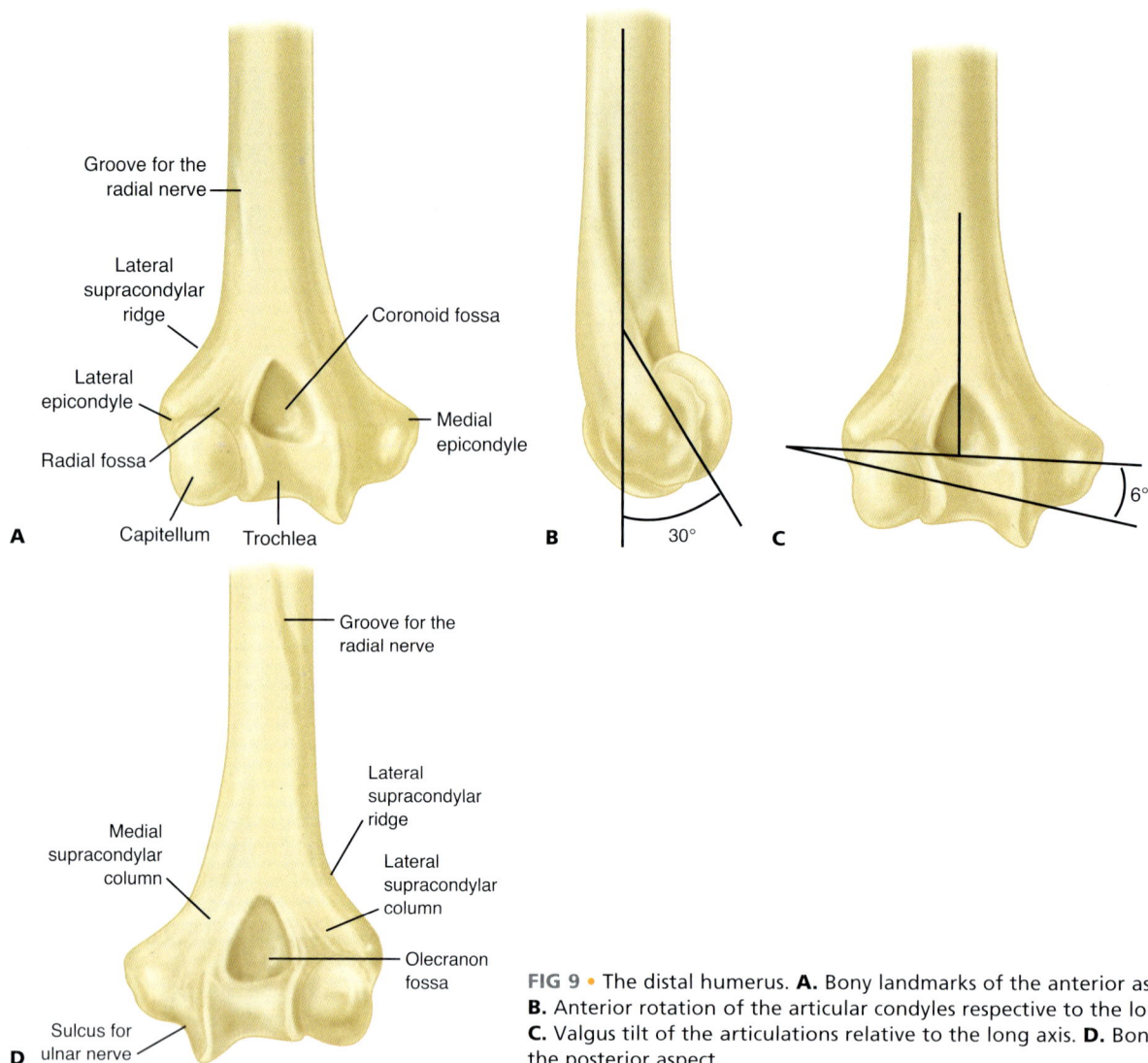

FIG 9 • The distal humerus. **A.** Bony landmarks of the anterior aspect. **B.** Anterior rotation of the articular condyles respective to the long axis. **C.** Valgus tilt of the articulations relative to the long axis. **D.** Bony landmarks of the posterior aspect.

■ Hyaline cartilage covers the depression of the radial head. The outside circumference of the radial head articulates with the ulna at the lesser sigmoid notch.

  ■ About 240 degrees of the circumference of the radial head is covered with cartilage. With the arm in neutral rotation, the anterolateral third of the circumference of the radial head is void of cartilage.

  ■ This part of the radial head lacks subchondral bone, and thus is not as strong as the part that supports the articular cartilage.

  ■ This part has been demonstrated to be the portion most often fractured.

■ The disc-shaped head is held against the ulna by the annular ligament distal to the radial head.

■ The head and neck of the radius are not colinear with the rest of the bone. The head and neck are offset by an angle of about 15 degrees with respect to the shaft of the radius opposite to the radial tuberosity (**FIG 10**).

■ The neck of the radius is tapered, and the angular relationship between the head and neck has been implicated in the etiology of radial neck fractures.

Ulna

■ The proximal ulna provides the major articulation of the elbow that is responsible for its inherent stability (**FIG 11A,B**).

■ The broad, thick proximal aspect of the ulna consists of the greater sigmoid notch (incisura semilunaris), which articulates with the trochlea of the humerus.

■ The sloped cortical surface of the coronoid process serves as the site of insertion of the brachialis muscle.

■ The olecranon comprises the posterior portion of the articulation of the ulnohumeral joint and is the site of attachment for the triceps tendon.

■ On the lateral aspect of the coronoid process, the lesser sigmoid or radial notch articulates with the radial head and is oriented roughly perpendicular to the long axis of the bone.

■ On the lateral aspect of the proximal ulna, a tuberosity, the crista supinatoris, is the site of the insertion of the lateral ulnar collateral ligament (**FIG 11C**).

  ■ This stabilizes the humeroulnar joint to resist varus and rotational stresses.

■ The medial aspect of the coronoid process (sublime tubercle) serves as the site of attachment of the anterior bundle of the medial collateral ligament.

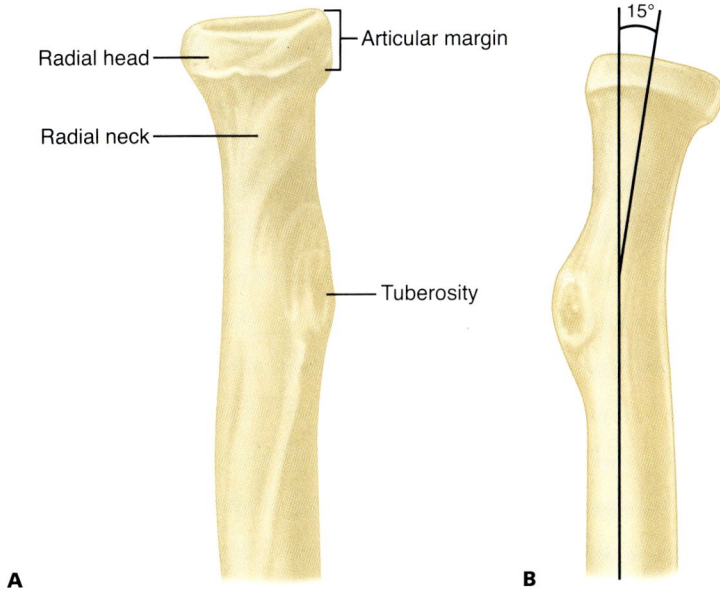

FIG 10 • The proximal radius. **A.** Bony landmarks. **B.** Angle of the radial neck relative to long axis.

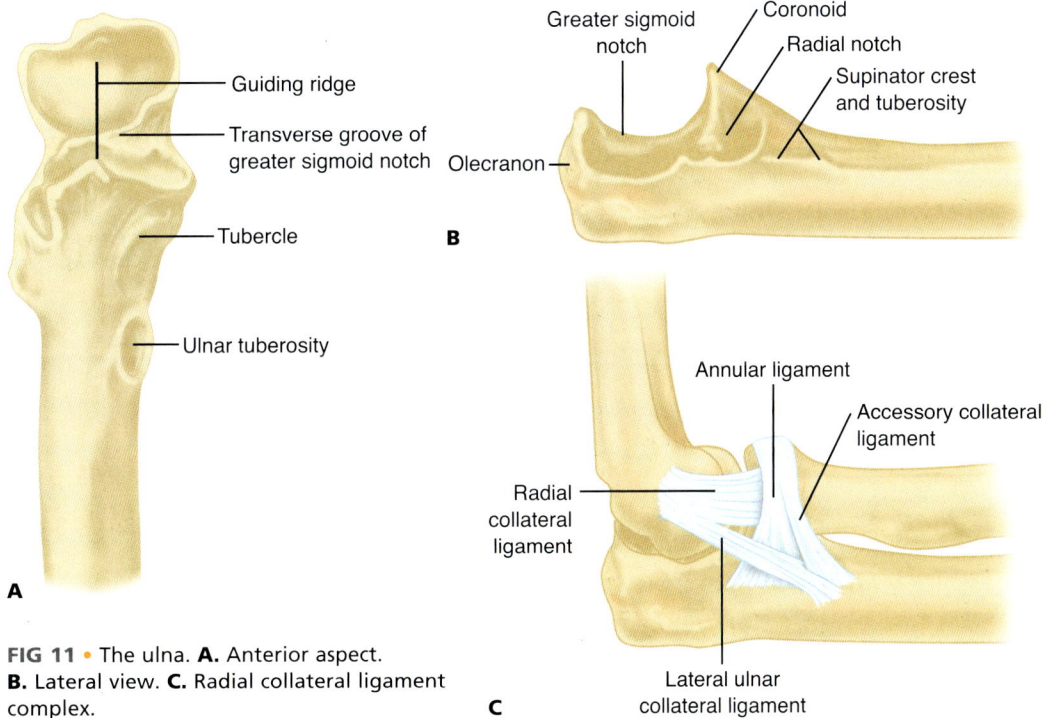

FIG 11 • The ulna. **A.** Anterior aspect. **B.** Lateral view. **C.** Radial collateral ligament complex.

SURVEY OF TOPICAL ANATOMY

Landmarks

Lateral Landmark

■ The tip of the olecranon, the lateral epicondyle, and the radial head form an equilateral triangle, providing an important landmark for entry into the elbow for such things as joint aspiration.

Flexion Crease

■ The flexion crease of the elbow is in line with the medial and lateral epicondyles. It is actually 1 to 2 cm proximal to the joint line when the elbow is extended.

Antecubital Fossa

■ Inverted triangular depression on the anterior aspect of the elbow that is just distal to the epicondyles

Topographical Regions of the Elbow and Corresponding Musculature

Lateral Margin of Antecubital Fossa

■ Extensor forearm musculature originates from the lateral epicondyle and has been termed the mobile wad.
■ This forms the lateral margin of the antecubital fossa and the lateral contour of the forearm and comprises the brachioradialis and the extensor carpi radialis longus and brevis muscles.

Medial Margin of the Antecubital Fossa

■ Muscles making up the contour of the medial anterior forearm include the pronator teres, flexor carpi radialis, palmaris longus, and flexor carpi ulnaris.

Dorsum

■ The dorsum of the forearm is contoured by the extensor musculature, consisting of the anconeus, extensor carpi ulnaris, extensor digitorum quinti, and extensor digitorum communis.

Cutaneous Innervation

Proximal Elbow

■ Skin about the proximal elbow is innervated by the lower lateral cutaneous (C5, C6) and the medial cutaneous (radial nerve, C8, T1, and T2) nerves of the arm.

Forearm

■ Forearm skin is innervated by the medial (C8, T1), lateral (musculocutaneous, C5, C6), and posterior (radial nerve, C6 through C8) cutaneous nerves of the forearm.

Elbow Joint Structure

Joint Articulation

■ The elbow joint consists of two types of articulations:
■ The ulnohumeral joint resembles a hinge (ginglymus), allowing flexion and extension.
■ The radiohumeral and the proximal radioulnar joint allow actual rotation or pivoting type of motion.
■ Because of this joint articulation, the elbow is classified as a trochoginglymoid joint and is one of the most congruent joints of the body.

Carrying Angle

■ Angle formed by the long axis of the humerus and the ulna with the elbow fully extended
  ■ In males, mean carrying angle is 11 to 14 degrees.
  ■ In females, mean carrying angle 13 to 16 degrees.

Joint Capsule

■ The anterior capsule inserts proximally above the coronoid and radial fossae.
■ Distally, the capsule attaches to the anterior margin of the coronoid medially as well as to the annular ligament laterally.
■ Posteriorly, the capsule attaches just above the olecranon fossa, distally along the supracondylar bony columns, and then down along the medial and lateral margins of the trochlea.
■ Distally, the attachment is along the medial and lateral articular margin of the sigmoid notch; laterally, it occurs along the lateral aspect of the sigmoid notch and blends with the annular ligament.
■ Normal capacity of the fully extended joint capsule is 25 to 30 mL.
■ The joint capsule is innervated by branches from all major nerves crossing the joint, including contributions from the musculocutaneous nerve.

LIGAMENTS OF THE ELBOW

■ Ligaments of the elbow consist of specialized thickening of the medial and lateral capsule that forms medial and lateral collateral ligament complexes.

Medial Collateral Ligament Complex

■ The medial collateral ligament consists of three parts: anterior, posterior, and transverse segments.
■ Anterior bundle is the most discrete component.
■ The posterior portion, being a thickening of the posterior capsule, is well defined only in about 90 degrees of flexion.
■ The transverse component appears to contribute a little or nothing to elbow stability.
■ Clinically and experimentally, the anterior bundle is clearly the major portion of the medial ligament complex.

Lateral Collateral Ligament Complex

■ Unlike the medial collateral ligament complex, with a rather consistent pattern, the lateral ligaments of the elbow joint are less discrete and some individual variation is common.
■ Several components make up the lateral ligament complex: radial collateral ligament, the annular ligament, a variably present accessory lateral collateral ligament, and the lateral ulnar collateral ligament.

Lateral Ulnar Collateral Ligament

■ This structure originates from the lateral epicondyle and blends with the fibers of the annular ligament, but arching superficial and distal to it.
■ Insertion is through the tubercle of the crest of the supinator on the ulna.
■ The function of this ligament is to provide stability to the ulnohumeral joint; it was shown to be deficient in posterolateral rotary instability of the joint.
■ This ligament represents the primary lateral stabilizer of the elbow and is taut on flexion and extension.

Accessory Lateral Collateral Ligament

■ Its function is to further stabilize the annular ligament during varus stress.

VESSELS

Brachial Artery and Its Branches

■ The brachial artery descends in the arm, crossing in front of the intramuscular septum to lie anterior to the medial aspect of the brachialis muscle.
■ The median nerve crosses in front of and medial to the artery at this point, near the middle of the arm. The artery continues distally at the medial margin of the biceps muscle and enters the antecubital space medial to the biceps tendon and lateral to the nerve.
■ At the level of the radial head, it gives off its terminal branches, the ulnar and radial arteries, which continue into the forearm.

Radial Artery

■ Usually the radial artery originates at the level of the radial head, emerges from the antecubital fossa between the brachioradialis and the pronator teres muscle, and continues down the forearm under the brachioradialis muscle.

Ulnar Artery

■ The ulnar artery is the larger of the two terminal branches of the brachial artery.
■ The artery traverses the pronator teres between its two heads and continues distally and medially behind the flexor digitorum superficialis muscle.

■ It emerges medially to continue down the medial aspect of the forearm under the cover of the flexor carpi ulnaris.

NERVES

Musculocutaneous Nerve

■ Originates from C5 through C8 nerve roots and is a continuation of the lateral cord

■ Innervates the major elbow flexors and the biceps and brachialis and continues through the brachial fascia lateral to the biceps tendon, terminating as the lateral antebrachial cutaneous nerve

■ Motor branch enters the biceps about 15 cm distal to the acromion; it enters the brachialis about 20 cm below the tip of the acromion.

Median Nerve

■ Median nerve arises from C5 through C8 and T1 nerve roots.

■ The nerve enters the anterior aspect of the brachium, crossing in front of the brachial artery as it passes across the intramuscular septum.

  ■ It follows a straight course into the medial aspect of the antecubital fossa, medial to the biceps tendon and the brachial artery.

  ■ It then passes under the bicipital aponeurosis.

  ■ There are no branches of the median nerve in the arm.

■ The first motor branch is given to the pronator teres, through which it passes.

■ In the antecubital fossa, a few small articular branches are given off before the motor branches to the pronator teres, the flexor carpi radialis, the palmaris longus, and the flexor digitorum superficialis.

Anterior Interosseous Nerve

■ Arises from the median nerve near the inferior border of the pronator teres and travels along the anterior aspect of the interosseous membrane in the company of the anterior interosseous artery

■ Innervates the flexor pollicis longus and the lateral portion of the flexor digitorum profundus

Radial Nerve

■ Is a continuation of the posterior cord and originates from the C6, C7, and C8 nerve roots, with variable contributions of the C5 and T1 roots

■ In the midportion of the arm, the nerve courses laterally just distal to the deltoid insertion to occupy the groove in the humerus that bears its name.

■ It then emerges in a spiral path inferiorly and laterally to penetrate the lateral intramuscular septum.

■ Before entering the anterior aspect of the arm, it gives off the motor branches to the medial and lateral heads of the triceps, accompanied by the deep branch of the brachial artery.

■ After penetrating the lateral intramuscular septum in the distal third of the arm, it descends anterior to the lateral epicondyle behind the brachioradialis.

■ It innervates the brachioradialis with a single branch to this muscle.

■ In the antecubital space, the nerve divides into the superficial and deep branches. The superficial branch is the continuation of the radial nerve and extends into the forearm to innervate the mid-dorsal cutaneous aspect of the forearm.

■ Motor branches of the radial nerve are given off to the triceps above the spiral groove, except for the branch to the medial head of the triceps, which originates at the entry to the spiral groove.

■ This branch continues distally through the medial head to terminate as a muscular branch to the anconeus.

■ In the antecubital space, the recurrent radial nerve curves around the posterolateral aspect of the radius, passing deep through supinator muscle, which it innervates. During its course through the supinator muscle, the nerve lies over the bare area, which is distal to and opposite to the radial tuberosity. The nerve is believed to be at risk at this site with fractures of the proximal radius. It emerges from the muscle as the posterior interosseous nerve, and the recurrent branch innervates the extensor digitorum minimi, the extensor carpi ulnaris, and occasionally the anconeus.

■ The posterior interosseous nerve is accompanied by the posterior interosseous artery and sends further muscle branches distally to supply the abductor pollicis longus, the extensor pollicis longus, the extensor pollicis brevis, and the extensor indicis on the dorsum of the forearm.

Ulnar Nerve

■ The ulnar nerve is derived from the medial cord of the brachial plexus from roots C8 and T1. In the mid-arm, it passes posteriorly through the medial intramuscular septum and continues distally along the medial margin of the triceps in the company of the superior ulnar collateral branch of the brachial artery and the ulnar collateral branch of the radial artery.

■ There are no branches of this nerve in the brachium.

■ The ulnar nerve may undergo compression as it passes behind the medial epicondyle, emerging into the forearm through the cubital tunnel.

■ The roof of the cubital tunnel has been defined by a structure termed the cubital tunnel retinaculum.

■ The first motor branch is the single nerve to the ulnar origin of the pronator and another one to the epicondylar head of the flexor carpi ulnaris. Distally, the nerve sends a motor branch to the ulnar half of the flexor digitorum profundus.

■ Two cutaneous nerves arise from the ulnar nerve in the distal half of the forearm to innervate the skin of the wrist and the hand.

MUSCLES

Elbow Flexors

Biceps

■ Covers the brachialis muscle in the distal arm and passes into the cubital fossa as the biceps tendon, which attaches to the posterior aspect of the radial tuberosity

■ Bicipital aponeurosis or lacertus fibrosus is a broad, thin band of tissue that is a continuation of the anterior, medial, and distal muscle fascia. It runs obliquely to cover the median nerve and the brachial artery and inserts into the deep fascia of the forearm and possibly into the ulna as well.

■ The biceps is a flexor of the elbow that has a large cross-sectional area but an intermediate mechanical advantage because it passes relatively close to the axis of rotation.

■ In the pronated position, the biceps is a strong supinator of the forearm.

Brachialis

- Largest cross-sectional area of any of the elbow flexors but suffers from a poor mechanical advantage because it crosses so close to the axis of rotation
- Origin consists of the entire anterior distal half of the humerus, and it extends medially and laterally to the respective intermuscular septa.
- Crosses the anterior capsule, with some fibers inserting into the capsule that are said to help retract the capsule during elbow flexion
- Insertion of the brachialis is along the base of the coronoid and into the tuberosity of the ulna.
- More than 95% of the cross-sectional area is muscle tissue at the elbow joint, a relationship that may account for high incidence of trauma to this muscle with elbow dislocation.

Brachioradialis

- Has a lengthy origin along the lateral supracondylar column that extends proximally to the level of the junction of the middle and distal humerus
- Origin separates the lateral head of the triceps and the brachialis muscle
- Lateral border of the cubital fossa is formed by this muscle, which crosses the elbow joint with the greatest mechanical advantage of any elbow flexor. It progresses distally to insert into the base of the radial styloid.
- Protects and is innervated by radial nerve (C5 and C6) as it emerges from the spiral groove
- Major function is elbow flexion.

Extensor Carpi Radialis Longus

- Originates from the supracondylar bony column joint just below the origin of the brachioradialis
- As it continues into the midportion of the dorsum of the forearm, it becomes largely tendinous and inserts to the dorsal base of the second metacarpal.
- Innervated by the radial nerve
- Functions as wrist extensor, and possibly an elbow flexor

Extensor Carpi Radialis Brevis

- Originates from the lateral superior aspect of the lateral epicondyle
- Its origin is the most lateral of the extensor group and is covered by the extensor carpi radialis longus.
- This relationship is important as the most commonly implicated site of lateral epicondylitis.
- Extensor carpi radialis brevis shares the same extensor compartment as the longus as it crosses the wrist under the extensor retinaculum and inserts into the dorsal base of the third metacarpal.
- Function of the extensor carpi radialis brevis is pure wrist extension, with little or no radial or ulnar deviation.

Extensor Digitorum Communis

- Originating from the anterior distal aspect of the lateral epicondyle, the extensor digitorum communis accounts for most of the contour of the extensor surface of the forearm.
- Extends and abducts fingers
- Innervation is from the deep branch of the radial nerve, with contributions from the sixth through eighth cervical nerves.

Supinator

- This flat muscle is characterized by the virtual absence of tendinous tissue and has a complex origin and insertion.
- It originates from three sites above and below the elbow joint: the lateral anterior aspect of the lateral epicondyle; the lateral collateral ligament; and the proximal anterior crest of the ulna along the crista supinatoris, which is just anterior to the depression for the insertion of the anconeus.
- Form of the muscle is roughly that of a rhomboid as it runs obliquely, distally, and radially to wrap around and insert diffusely on the proximal radius, beginning lateral and proximal to the radial tuberosity and continuing distal to the insertion of the pronator teres at the junction of the proximal middle third of the radius.
- The radial nerve passes through the supinator to gain access to the extensor surface of the forearm.
  - This anatomic feature is clinically significant with regard to exposure of the lateral aspect of the elbow joint and the proximal radius and in certain entrapment syndromes.
- Functions as a supinator of the forearm, but it is a weaker supinator than the biceps.
  - Unlike the biceps, however, the effectiveness of the supinator is not altered by the position of the elbow flexion.
- Innervation is derived from the muscular branch given off by the radial nerve just before and during its course through the muscle.

Elbow Extensors

Triceps Brachii

- Comprises the entire musculature of the arm posteriorly
- Two of its three heads originate from the posterior aspect of the humerus.
- The long head has a discrete origin from the infraglenoid tuberosity of the scapula.
- The lateral head originates in a linear fashion from the proximal lateral intramuscular septum on the posterior surface of the humerus.
- The medial head originates from the entire distal half of the posteromedial surface of the humerus, bounded laterally by the radial groove and medially by the intramuscular septum.
- Each head originates distal to the other with progressively larger areas of origin.
- The long and lateral heads are superficial to the deep medial head, blending in the midline of the humerus to form a common muscle that then tapers into the triceps tendon and attaches to the tip of the olecranon with Sharpey fibers.
  - The tendon is usually separated from the olecranon by the subtendinous olecranon bursa.
- Innervated by the radial nerve, the long and lateral heads are supplied by branches that arise proximal to the entrance of the radial nerve into the groove.
  - The medial head is innervated distal to the groove with a branch that enters proximally and passes through the entire medial head to terminate by innervating the anconeus.

Anconeus

- This muscle has little tendinous tissue because it originates from a rather broad site on the posterior aspect of the lateral epicondyle and from the lateral triceps fascia and inserts into the lateral dorsal surface of the proximal ulna.

- Innervated by the terminal branch of the nerve to the medial head of the triceps
- Function of this muscle has been the subject of considerable speculation.
- Some suggest that the primary role is that of a joint stabilizer.
- Covers the lateral portion of the annular ligament and the radial head
- For the surgeon, the major significance of this muscle is its position as a key landmark in various lateral and posterolateral exposures, and it is used for some reconstructive procedures.

Flexor Pronator Muscle Group

Pronator Teres

- This is the most proximal of the flexor pronator group.
- There are usually two heads of origin; the larger arises from the anterosuperior aspect of the medial epicondyle and the second from the coronoid process of the ulna, which is absent in about 10% of individuals.
  - Two origins of the pronator muscle provide an arch through which the median nerve typically passes to gain access to the forearm.
  - This anatomic characteristic is a significant feature in the etiology of median nerve entrapment syndrome.
- The common muscle belly proceeds radially and distally under the brachioradialis, inserting at the junction of the proximal middle portion of the radius by a discrete broad tendinous insertion into a tuberosity on the lateral aspect of the bone.
- A strong pronator of the forearm, it also is considered a weak flexor of the elbow.
- Innervated by two motor branches from the median nerve

Flexor Carpi Radialis

- The flexor carpi radialis originates inferior to the origin of the pronator teres and the common flexor tendon at the anteroinferior aspect of the medial epicondyle.
- It continues distally and radially to the wrist, where it can be easily palpated before it inserts into the base of the second and sometimes third metacarpal.
- Chief function is as a wrist flexor
- Innervation is from one or two branches of the median nerve.

Palmaris Longus

- When present, it arises from the medial epicondyle and from the septa it shares with the flexor carpi radialis and flexor carpi ulnaris.

- It becomes tendinous in the proximal portion of the forearm and inserts into and becomes continuous with the palmar aponeurosis.
- Absent in about 10% of the extremities
- Innervated by a branch of the median nerve

Flexor Carpi Ulnaris

- Most posterior of the common flexor tendons originating from the medial epicondyle
- Second and largest source of origin is from the medial border of the coronoid and the proximal aspect of the ulna.
- Ulnar nerve enters and innervates the muscle between these two sites of origin with two or three motor branches given off just after the nerve has entered the muscle. The muscle continues distally to insert into the pisiform, where the tendon is easily palpable, because it serves as a wrist flexor and ulnar deviator.
- With an origin posterior to the axis of rotation, weak elbow extension may also be provided by the flexor carpi ulnaris.

Flexor Digitorum Superficialis

- The flexor digitorum superficialis muscle is deep to those originating from the common flexor tendon but superficial to the flexor digitorum profundus; thus it is considered the intermediate muscle layer.
- This broad muscle has a complex origin.
  - Medially, it arises from the medial epicondyle by way of the common flexor tendon and possibly from the ulnar collateral ligament and medial aspect of the coronoid.
  - The lateral head is smaller and thinner and arises from the proximal two thirds of the radius.
- The unique origin of the muscle forms a fibrous margin under which the median nerve and ulnar artery emerge as they exit from the cubital fossa.
- The muscle is innervated by the median nerve with branches that originate before the median nerve enters the pronator teres.
- Action of the flexor digitorum superficialis is flexion of the proximal interphalangeal joints.

Flexor Digitorum Profundus

- Originates from the proximal ulna distal to the elbow joint and is involved in flexion of the distal interphalangeal joints

Chapter 2

Surgical Approaches to the Shoulder and Elbow

Joseph A. Abboud, Matthew L. Ramsey, and Gerald R. Williams

SHOULDER APPROACHES

ANTERIOR APPROACH TO THE SHOULDER

Indications

- Surgical stabilization for recurrent dislocations
- Subscapularis and biceps tendon repair
- Shoulder arthroplasty
- Fracture fixation

Incisions

- Anterior shoulder can be approached through two different incisions.
- Anterior incision:
  - 10- to 15-cm incision along the deltopectoral interval (**FIG 1A**)
  - Incision begins just above the coracoid process and progresses toward the deltoid tuberosity.
- Axillary incision
  - Vertical incision 8 to 10 cm long (**FIG 1B**)
  - Incision begins inferior to the tip of the coracoid and progresses toward the anterior axillary fold.

Internervous Plane

- Deltoid muscle is supplied by the axillary nerve.
- Pectoralis major muscle is supplied by medial and lateral pectoral nerves.

Surgical Dissection

- Skin flaps are developed around the deltopectoral interval.
- The deltopectoral interval, with its cephalic vein, is identified.
- The deltopectoral interval is developed by retracting the pectoralis major medially and the deltoid laterally.
  - Vein may be retracted either medially or laterally.
  - We prefer to take it laterally, as fewer tributaries are disrupted.
- The lateral border of the conjoint tendon is identified and the short head of the biceps (supplied by the musculocutaneous nerve) and coracobrachialis (supplied by the musculocutaneous nerve) are displaced medially to allow access to the anterior aspect of the shoulder joint.
  - Simple medial retraction of the conjoined tendon may be enough for a procedure such as subscapularis repair or capsular repair.
  - If more exposure is necessary, the conjoint tendon can be detached with the tip of the coracoid process.
- The axillary artery is surrounded by cords of brachial plexus, which lie behind the pectoralis minor muscle.
  - To minimize risk for nerve injury, the arm should be kept adducted while work is being done around the coracoid process.
  - Remember, the musculocutaneous nerve enters the coracobrachialis on its medial side.

- Overly aggressive retraction can cause a neurapraxia of the musculocutaneous nerve.
- Behind the conjoined tendon of the coracobrachialis and the short head of biceps lies the subscapularis muscle.
- Externally rotating the arm brings the subscapularis further into the operative field.
  - This maneuver increases the distance between the subscapularis and axillary nerve as it disappears below the lower border of the muscle.
- Identifiable landmarks on the inferior border of the subscapularis are three small vessels (from the anterior humeral circumflex artery) that run transversely and often require ligation or cauterization.
  - These vessels run as a triad (often called the "three sisters"): a small artery with its two surrounding venae comitantes.
- The superior border of the subscapularis muscle blends in with the fibers of the supraspinatus muscle in the rotator interval (**FIG 1C**).
  - The tendon of the subscapularis is tagged with stay sutures.
  - There are various ways of taking down the subscapularis as per surgeon preference.
    - Some divide the subscapularis 1 to 2 cm from its insertion onto the lesser tuberosity.
    - Some detach this insertion with a small flake of bone using an osteotome.
- Inferior border of the subscapularis is the easiest location to allow separation between the subscapularis and capsule.
- The capsule is incised longitudinally to enter the joint wherever the selected repair must be performed.

ANTEROSUPERIOR APPROACH TO THE SHOULDER

Indications

- Rotator cuff repair
- Subacromial decompression of the shoulder
- Acromioclavicular reconstructions
- Greater tuberosity fractures
- Removal of calcific deposits from the subacromial bursa
- Reverse shoulder replacement

Incision

- An incision is made paralleling the lateral acromion that begins at the anterolateral corner of the acromion and ends just lateral to the tip of the coracoid (**FIG 2A**).

Internervous Plane

- The deltoid muscle is detached proximal to its nerve supply; therefore, there is no internervous plane with this approach.

Surgical Dissection

- The incision is deepened to the deep deltoid fascia.
- Subcutaneous flaps are raised.

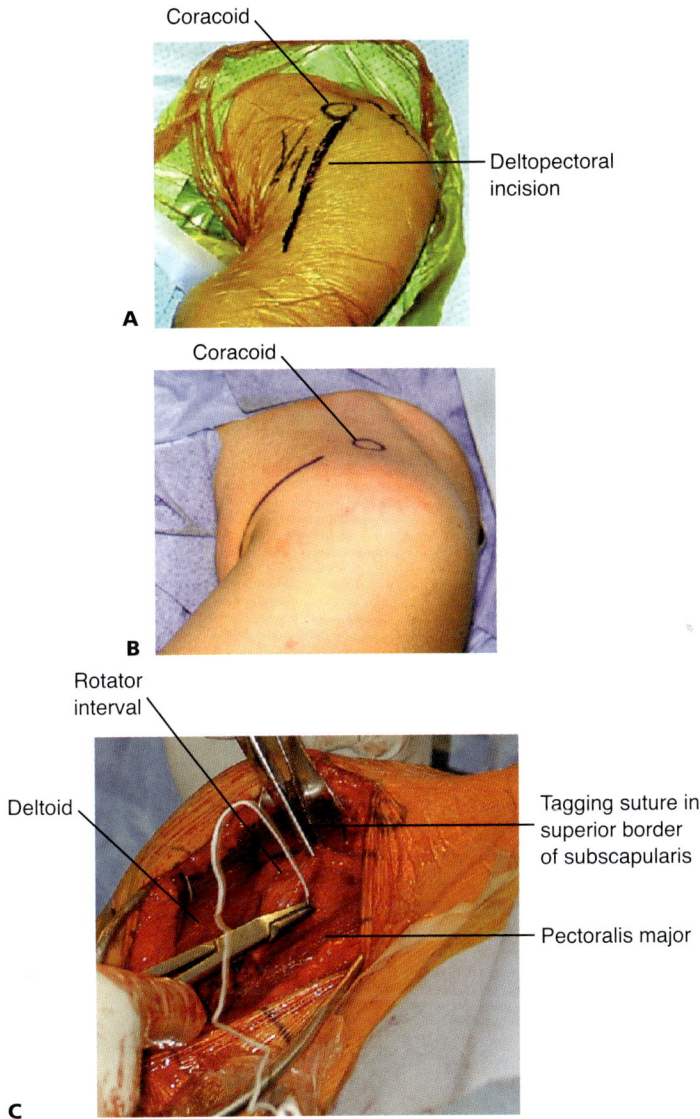

FIG 1 • **A.** Deltopectoral incision. **B.** Axillary incision beginning inferior to the tip of the coracoid and progressing toward the anterior axillary fold. **C.** In this dissection, the subscapularis tendon is being tagged at the superior border of the rotator interval.

- The location of the deltoid split depends on the pathology being managed. When the pathology requires more exposure, moving the deltoid split posteriorly will improve exposure (**FIG 2B**).
- Subperiosteally, the anterior deltoid is elevated from the acromion and the acromioclavicular joint. Continue the detachment by sharp dissection laterally to expose the anterior aspect of the acromion.
  - Bleeding will be encountered during this dissection as a result of the division of the acromial branch of the coracoacromial artery.
  - The surgeon should not detach more of the deltoid than is necessary.
- The deltoid split is extended 2 to 3 cm distal to the acromion.
  - Stay sutures are inserted in the apex of the split to prevent the muscle from inadvertently splitting distally during retraction and damaging the axillary nerve.

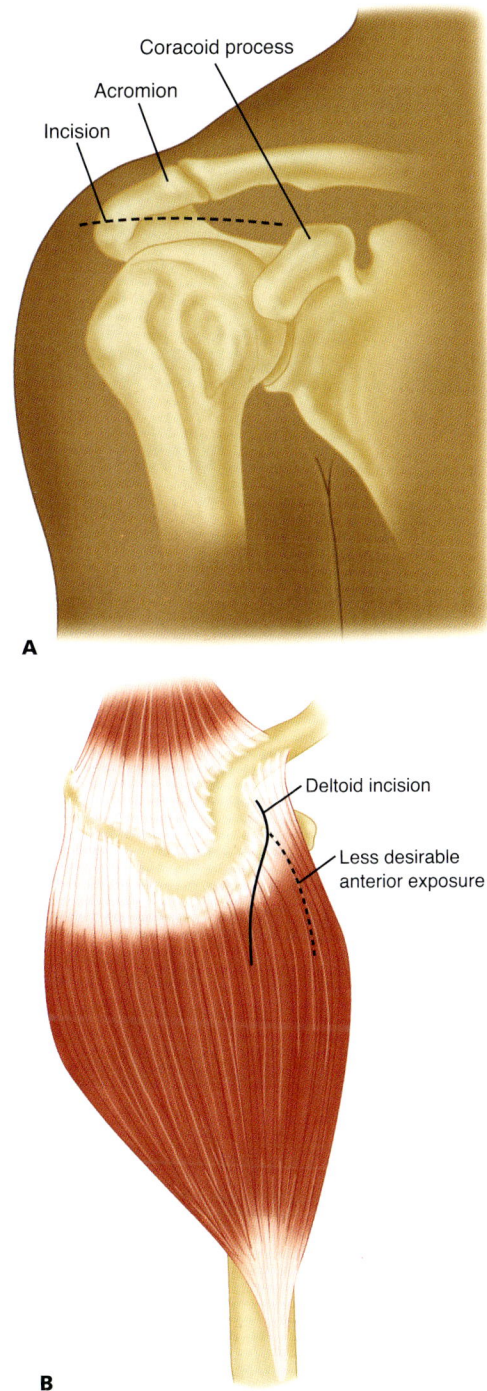

FIG 2 • **A.** Anterosuperior approach to the shoulder. A transverse incision begins at the anterolateral corner of the acromion and ends just lateral to the coracoid. **B.** The posterior curve of the deltoid incision can be moved more posteriorly, as depicted here, to allow necessary exposure as dictated by the pathology.

- The split edges of the deltoid muscle are retracted to reveal the underlying coracoacromial ligament.
- The coracoacromial ligament is detached from the acromion by sharp dissection.
- The supraspinatus tendon with its overlying subacromial bursa now can be visualized.
- The head of the humerus is rotated to expose different portions of the rotator cuff.

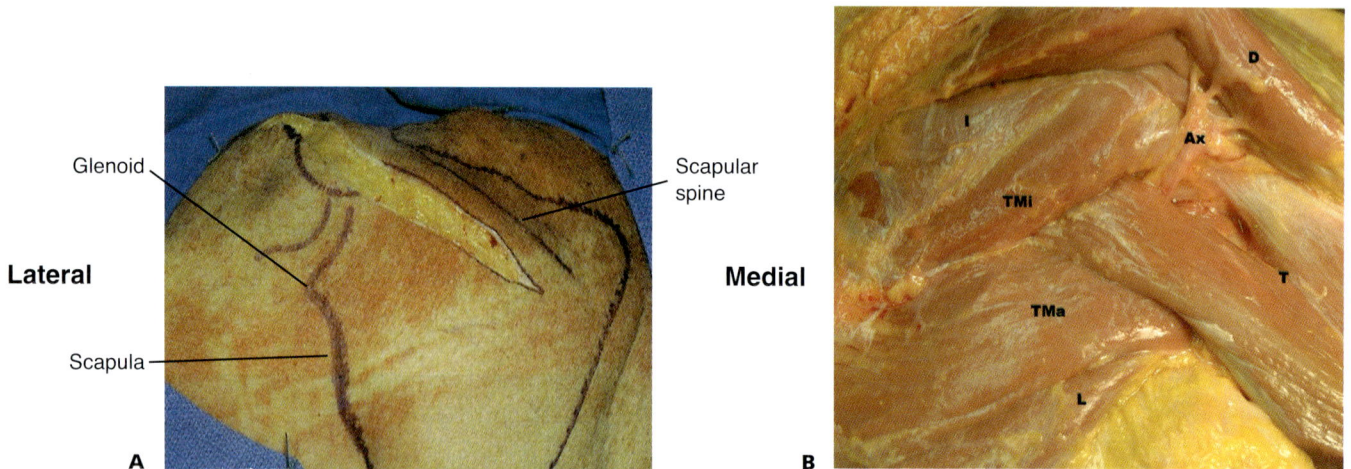

FIG 3 • A. Horizontal incision along the scapular spine allowing for the posterior approach to the shoulder. **B.** Cadaveric specimen depicting the internervous plane between the infraspinatus and teres minor as well as the axillary nerve in the quadrangular space. (**A:** From Goss TP. Glenoid fractures: open reduction and internal fixation. In: Widd, DA, ed. Master Techniques in Orthopaedic Surgery: Fractures, ed 2. Philadelphia: Lippincott Williams & Wilkins, 1998:3–17; **B:** Courtesy of Jesse A. McCarron, MD, Michael Codsi, MD, and Joseph P. Iannotti, MD.)

POSTERIOR APPROACH TO THE SHOULDER

Indications

▪ Repair in cases of recurrent posterior dislocation or subluxation of the shoulder
▪ Glenoid osteotomy
▪ Treatment of fractures of the scapular neck
▪ Treatment of posterior fracture and dislocations of the proximal humerus
▪ Spinoglenoid notch cyst drainage

Incision

▪ A horizontal incision is made along the scapular spine extending to the posterolateral corner of the acromion (**FIG 3A**)

Internervous Plane

▪ Between teres minor (axillary nerve) and infraspinatus (suprascapular nerve)
▪ The suprascapular nerve passes around the base of the spine of the scapula as it runs from the supraspinatus fossa to the infraspinatus fossa.

Surgical Dissection

▪ The origin of the deltoid is identified on the scapular spine. There are three ways to manage the deltoid during posterior exposures:
  ▪ Detach the origin on the scapular spine
  ▪ Split the deltoid muscle along the length of its fibers
  ▪ Elevate the deltoid from the inferior margin
▪ The plane between the deltoid muscle and the underlying infraspinatus muscle is identified.
  ▪ The plane is easier to locate at the lateral end of the incision.
▪ The internervous plane between the infraspinatus and teres minor muscles is identified (**FIG 3B**).
  ▪ The axillary nerve runs longitudinally in the quadrangular space beneath the teres minor.
  ▪ The posterior circumflex humeral artery runs with the axillary nerve in the quadrangular space between the inferior borders of the teres minor muscle.

▪ The infraspinatus is retracted superiorly and the teres minor inferiorly to reach the posterior regions of the glenoid cavity and the neck of the scapula.
▪ The posteroinferior corner of the shoulder joint capsule should be visible.

HUMERUS APPROACHES

ANTERIOR APPROACH TO THE HUMERUS

Indications

▪ Internal fixation of fractures of the humerus
▪ Management of humeral nonunions
▪ Osteotomy of the humerus

Incision

▪ A longitudinal incision is made over the tip of the coracoid process of the scapula; it runs distally and laterally in the line of the deltopectoral interval to the insertion of the deltoid muscle on the lateral aspect of the humerus, about halfway down its shaft.
▪ The incision should be continued distally as far as necessary, following the lateral border of the biceps muscle (**FIG 4A**).

Internervous Plane

▪ The anterior approach uses two different internervous planes.
▪ Proximally, the plane lies between the deltoid muscle (supplied by axillary nerve) and the pectoralis major muscle (supplied by medial and lateral pectoral nerves) (**FIG 4B**).
▪ Distally, the plane lies between the medial fibers of the brachialis muscle (musculocutaneous nerve) and the lateral fibers of the brachialis muscle (radial nerve) (**FIG 4C**).

Surgical Dissection

Proximal Humeral Shaft

▪ The deltopectoral interval is identified using the cephalic vein as a guide and the two muscles are separated, retracting the cephalic vein either medially with the pectoralis major or laterally with the deltoid.

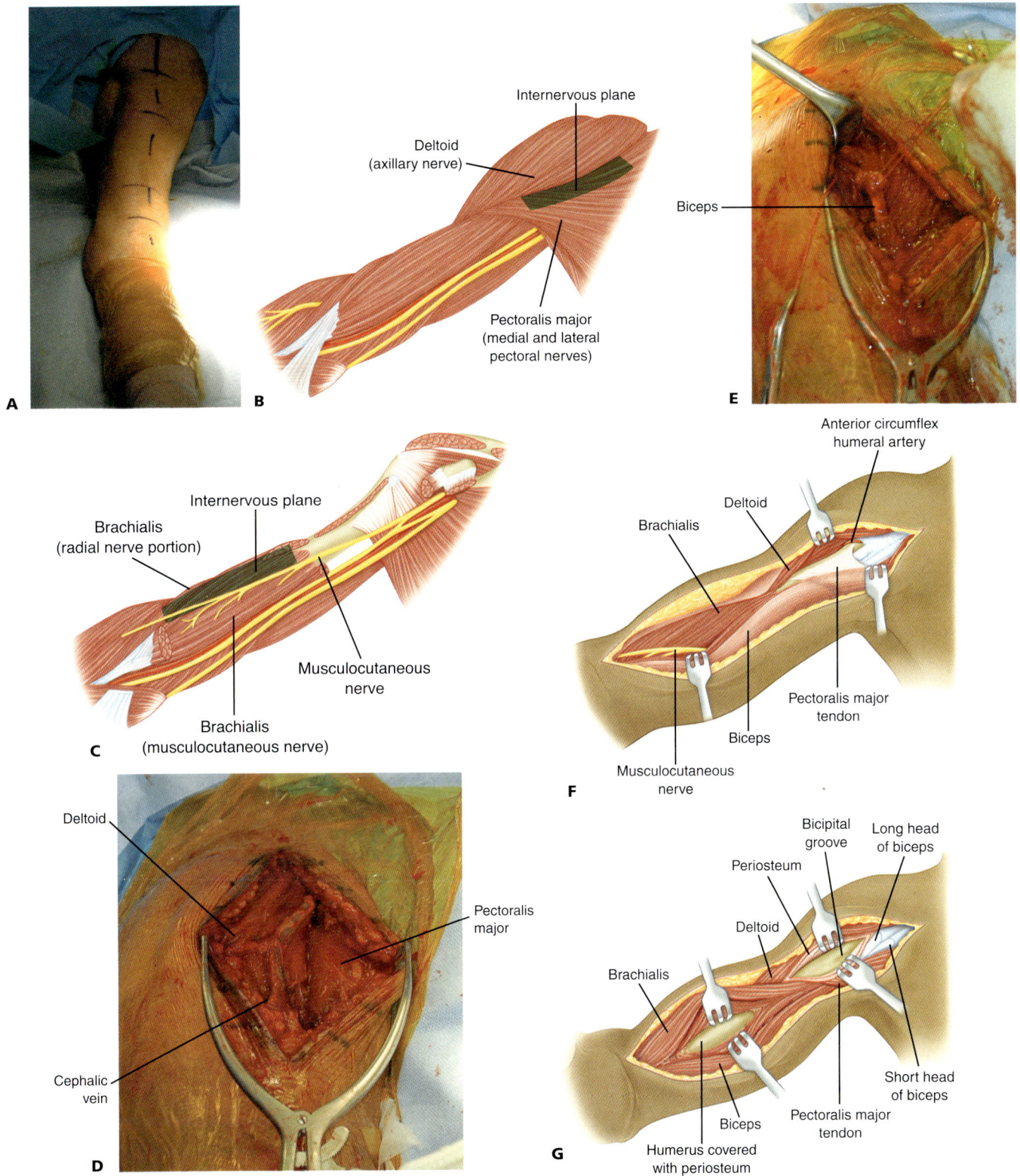

FIG 4 • A. Patient prepared for an anterior approach to the humerus. **B.** The internervous plane between the deltoid muscle and the pectoralis major muscle. **C.** Further distally, one can appreciate the internervous plane between the medial fibers of the brachialis (musculocutaneous nerve) medially and the lateral fibers of the brachialis (radial nerve) laterally. **D.** Deltopectoral incision: developing the interval between the deltoid and pectoralis major. The cephalic vein can be seen separating these two structures. **E.** With deeper dissection, the biceps tendon is seen running in the rotator interval. **F.** Further distal dissection reveals the musculocutaneous nerve passing along the medial border of the biceps muscle. **G.** To expose the distal third of the humerus, the fibers of the brachialis are split. Flexion of the elbow will relieve the tension off the brachialis, making the exposure easier. (**A**: Courtesy of Matthew J. Garberina, MD, and Charles L. Getz, MD.)

- The muscular interval is developed distally down to the insertion of the deltoid into the deltoid tuberosity and the insertion of the pectoralis major into the lateral lip of the bicipital groove (**FIG 4D,E**).
- To expose the bone fully, the surgeon may need to detach part or all of the insertion of pectoralis major muscle.
- The minimum amount of soft tissue should be detached to allow adequate visualization and reduction of the fracture.
- If further exposure is needed, the surgeon dissects medially in a subperiosteal manner to avoid damage to the radial nerve, which lies in the spiral groove of the humerus and crosses the back of the middle third of the bone in a medial to lateral direction.

Distal Humeral Shaft

- The surgeon identifies the muscular interval between the biceps brachii and brachialis.
- The interval is developed by retracting the biceps medially (**FIG 4F**).
- Beneath it lies the brachialis muscle, which covers the humeral shaft.
- The fibers of the brachialis are split longitudinally in the interval between the medial 2/3 and the lateral 1/3 to expose the periosteum on the anterior surface of the humeral shaft.
- The periosteum is incised longitudinally in line with the muscle dissection, and the brachialis is stripped off the anterior surface of the bone (**FIG 4G**).
- In the anterior compartment of the distal third of the arm, the radial nerve pierces the lateral intermuscular septum and lies between the brachioradialis and brachialis muscles.

POSTERIOR APPROACH TO THE HUMERUS

Indications

- Open reduction and internal fixation of a fracture of the humerus
- Treatment of nonunion
- Exploration of the radial nerve in the spiral groove

Incision

- A longitudinal incision is made in the midline of the posterior aspect of the arm, from 8 cm below the acromion to the olecranon fossa (**FIG 5A**).

Internervous Plane

- There is no true internervous plane; dissection involves separating the heads of the triceps brachii muscles, all of which are supplied by the radial nerve.
- The medial head, which is the deepest, has a dual nerve supply (radial and ulnar nerves).

Surgical Dissection

- The surgeon incises the deep fascia of the arm in line with the skin incision.
- The triceps muscle has two layers:
- The outer layer consists of two heads: the lateral head arises from the lateral lip of the spiral groove, and the long head arises from the infraglenoid tubercle of the scapula (**FIG 5B**).
- The inner layer consists of the medial head, which arises from the whole width of the posterior aspect of the humerus

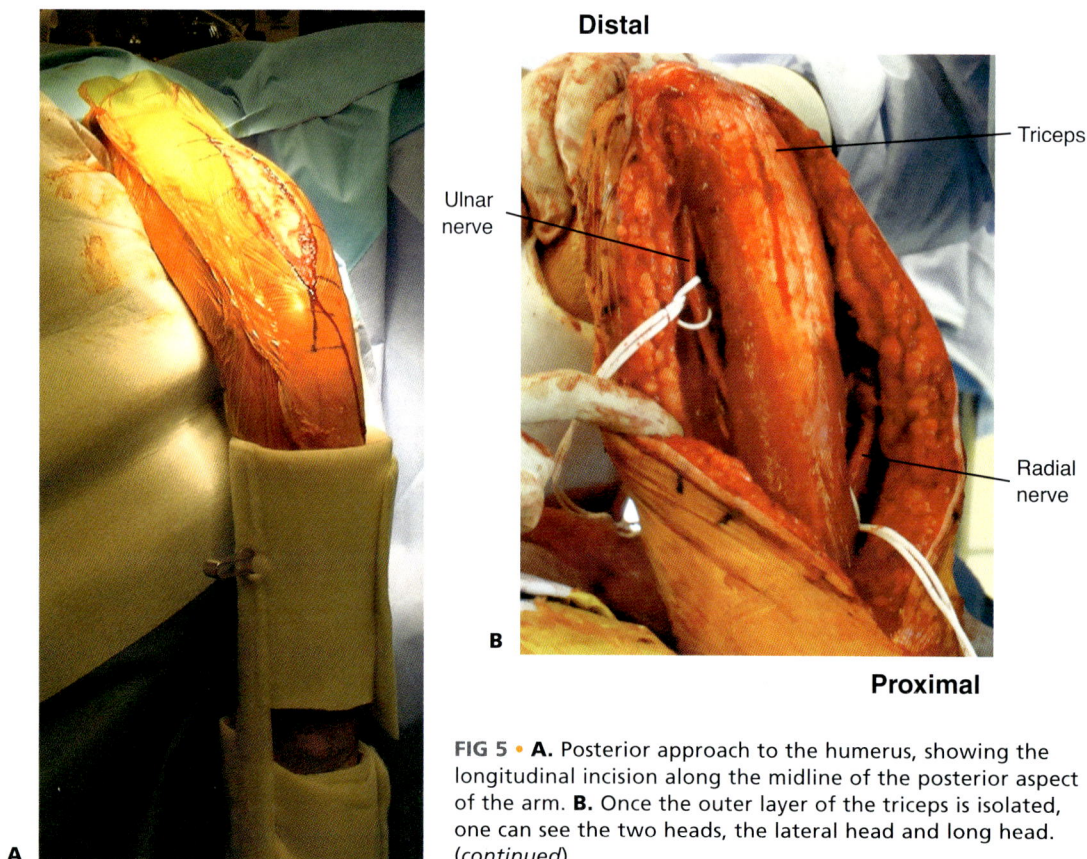

FIG 5 • **A.** Posterior approach to the humerus, showing the longitudinal incision along the midline of the posterior aspect of the arm. **B.** Once the outer layer of the triceps is isolated, one can see the two heads, the lateral head and long head. (*continued*)

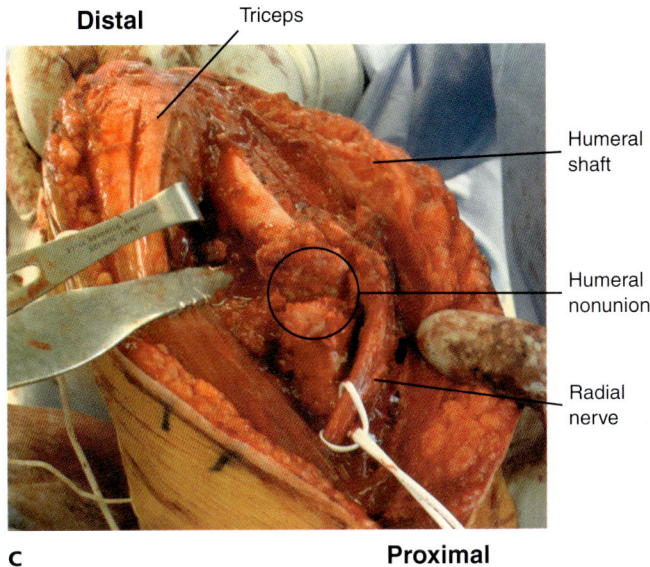

Distal Triceps

Humeral shaft

Humeral nonunion

Radial nerve

C **Proximal**

FIG 5 • (*continued*) **C.** In this humeral shaft nonunion, the triceps is reflected medially and the radial nerve can be seen passing through the spiral groove. (**A**: Courtesy of Matthew J. Garberina, MD, and Charles L. Getz, MD.)

below the spiral groove all the way down to the distal fourth of the bone.

▪ The spiral groove contains the radial nerve; the radial nerve separates the origins of the lateral and medial heads (**FIG 5C**).

▪ To avoid iatrogenic nerve injury, the surgeon should never continue dissection down to bone in the proximal two thirds of the arm until the radial nerve has been identified.

MODIFIED POSTERIOR APPROACH TO THE HUMERUS

Indications

▪ Open reduction and internal fixation of humeral shaft fractures

▪ Open reduction and internal fixation of lateral condyle fractures

▪ Treatment of humeral nonunion

▪ Exploration of the radial nerve in the spiral groove

Incision

▪ The surgeon makes a straight incision along a line between the posterolateral aspect of the acromion and the lateral edge of the olecranon.

▪ The length of the incision is dictated by the requirement for exposure.

▪ Extensile exposure is limited proximally by the axillary nerve.

Internervous Plane

▪ There is no true internervous plane, because both the medial and lateral heads of the triceps are supplied by the radial nerve.

Surgical Dissection

▪ The deep fascia is incised in line with the skin incision along the lateral aspect of the triceps.

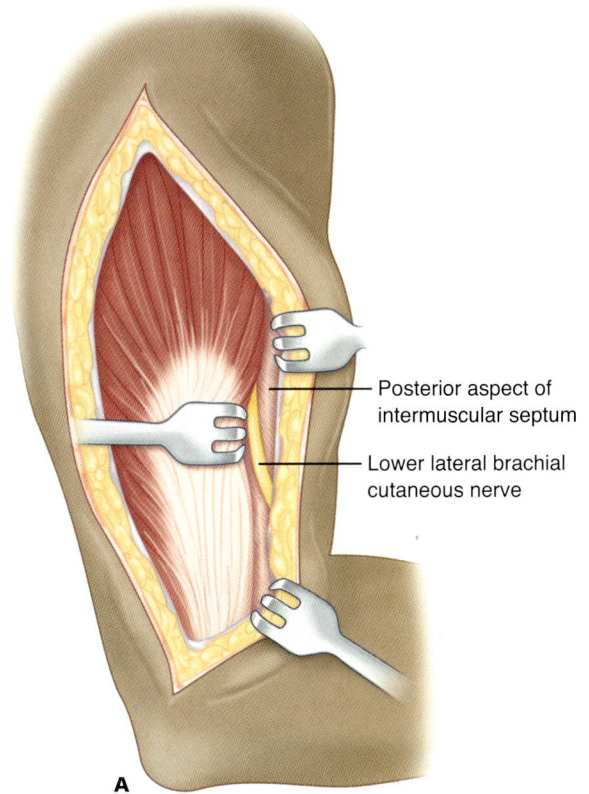

Posterior aspect of intermuscular septum

Lower lateral brachial cutaneous nerve

A

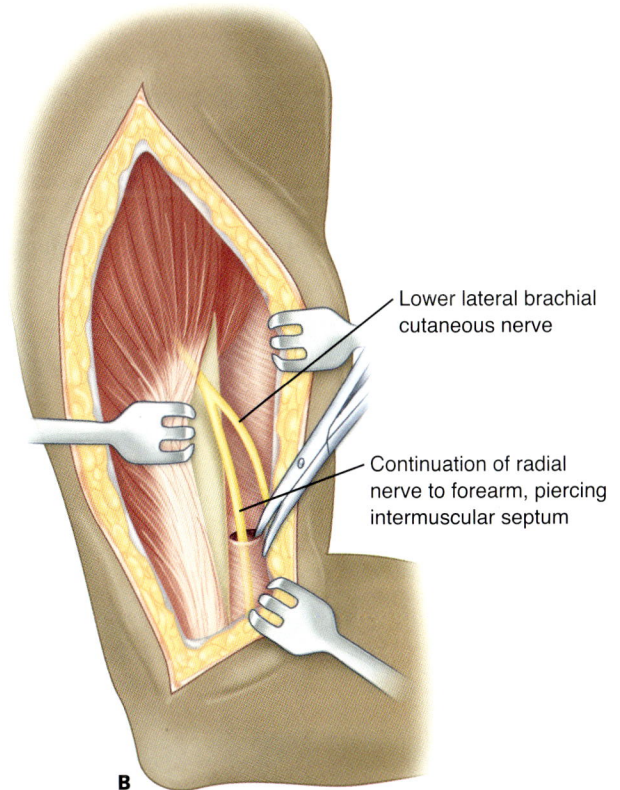

Lower lateral brachial cutaneous nerve

Continuation of radial nerve to forearm, piercing intermuscular septum

B

FIG 6 • A. The lower lateral brachial cutaneous nerve, which branches off the radial nerve, is identified along the posterior aspect of the intermuscular septum. The entire triceps here is retracted slightly medially. **B.** The intermuscular septum is divided deep to the lower lateral brachial cutaneous nerve for 3 cm to expose the radial nerve distally. (*continued*)

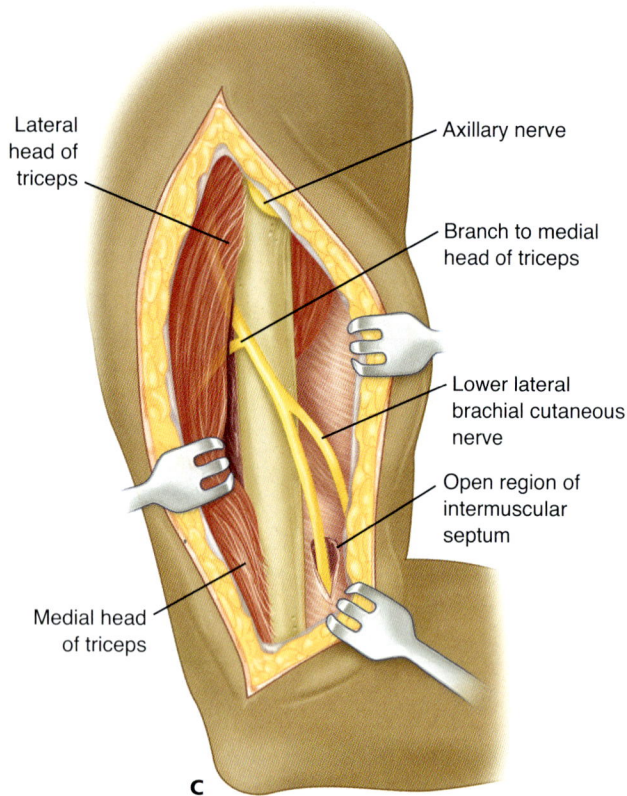

Lateral
head of
triceps

Axillary nerve

Branch to medial
head of triceps

Lower lateral
brachial cutaneous
nerve

Open region of
intermuscular
septum

Medial head
of triceps

c

FIG 6 • (continued) **C.** The medial and lateral heads of the triceps are retracted subperiosteally in a medial direction to expose the posterior aspect of the humeral diaphysis.

■ The triceps is retracted medially and the lower lateral brachial cutaneous nerve branch from the radial nerve is identified. This nerve is traced proximally to the main trunk of the radial nerve (**FIG 6A**).
■ The intermuscular septum is divided distally to allow the radial nerve to be mobilized (**FIG 6B**).
■ Subperiosteally, the medial and lateral heads of the triceps are reflected medially to expose the humeral shaft (**FIG 6C**).

ELBOW APPROACHES

■ The surgical exposures described for the elbow are divided into posterior, medial, and lateral approaches. These descriptions denote the deep surgical interval employed.
■ Often, these deep approaches can be performed through a direct medial or lateral skin incision or a more versatile posterior incision.

POSTERIOR APPROACH TO THE ELBOW

■ Releasing the triceps attachment to the olecranon is not advisable, owing to the difficulty of adequate repair and possible disruption during rehabilitation. Today, there are four choices of posterior exposure:
  ■ Triceps splitting
  ■ Triceps reflecting
  ■ Triceps preserving
  ■ Olecranon osteotomy

Triceps-Splitting Approaches

Posterior Triceps-Splitting Approach (Campbell)

■ Care must be exercised to maintain the medial portion of the triceps expansion over the forearm fascia in continuity with the flexor carpi ulnaris.
■ Laterally, the anconeus and triceps are more stable, with less chance of disruption.

INDICATIONS

■ Total elbow arthroplasty
■ Distal humerus fracture
■ Removal of loose bodies
■ Capsulectomies
■ Posterior exposure of the joint for ankylosis, sepsis, synovectomy, and ulnohumeral arthroplasty

APPROACH

■ Skin incision begins in the midline over the triceps, about 10 cm above the joint line, and is generally placed laterally or medially across the tip of the olecranon. It continues distally over the lateral aspect of the subcutaneous border of the proximal ulna for about 5 to 6 cm (**FIG 7A**).
■ Triceps is exposed, along with the proximal 4 cm of the ulna.
■ A midline incision is made through the triceps fascia and tendon as it is continued distally across the insertion of the triceps tendon at the tip of the olecranon and down the subcutaneous crest of the ulna (**FIG 7B**).
■ Triceps tendon and muscle are split longitudinally, exposing the distal humerus.
■ Anconeus is then reflected subperiosteally laterally, while the flexor carpi ulnaris is similarly retracted medially.
■ Insertion of the triceps is carefully released from the olecranon, leaving the extensor mechanism in continuity with the forearm fascia and muscles medially and laterally (**FIG 7C**).
■ Ulnar nerve is visualized and protected in the cubital tunnel.
■ Closure of the triceps fascia is required only proximal to the olecranon, but the insertion should be repaired to the olecranon with a suture passed through the ulna.
■ The incision is then closed in layers.

Triceps-Splitting, Tendon-Reflecting Approach (Van Gorder)

■ A variation of the technique described earlier
■ Allows lengthening of the triceps if necessary
■ Has been largely abandoned in favor of the triceps-reflecting techniques

INDICATIONS

■ Same as those for midline-splitting approach described earlier

APPROACH

■ A posterior midline incision begins 10 cm proximal to the olecranon and extends distally onto the subcutaneous border of the ulna between the anconeus and the flexor carpi ulnaris.
■ Triceps fascia and aponeurosis are exposed along the tendinous insertion into the ulna.

Proximal

Forearm

Olecranon

A **Distal** **C**

Triceps tendon
being elevated

Shoulder

B Triceps tendon   Ulnar nerve

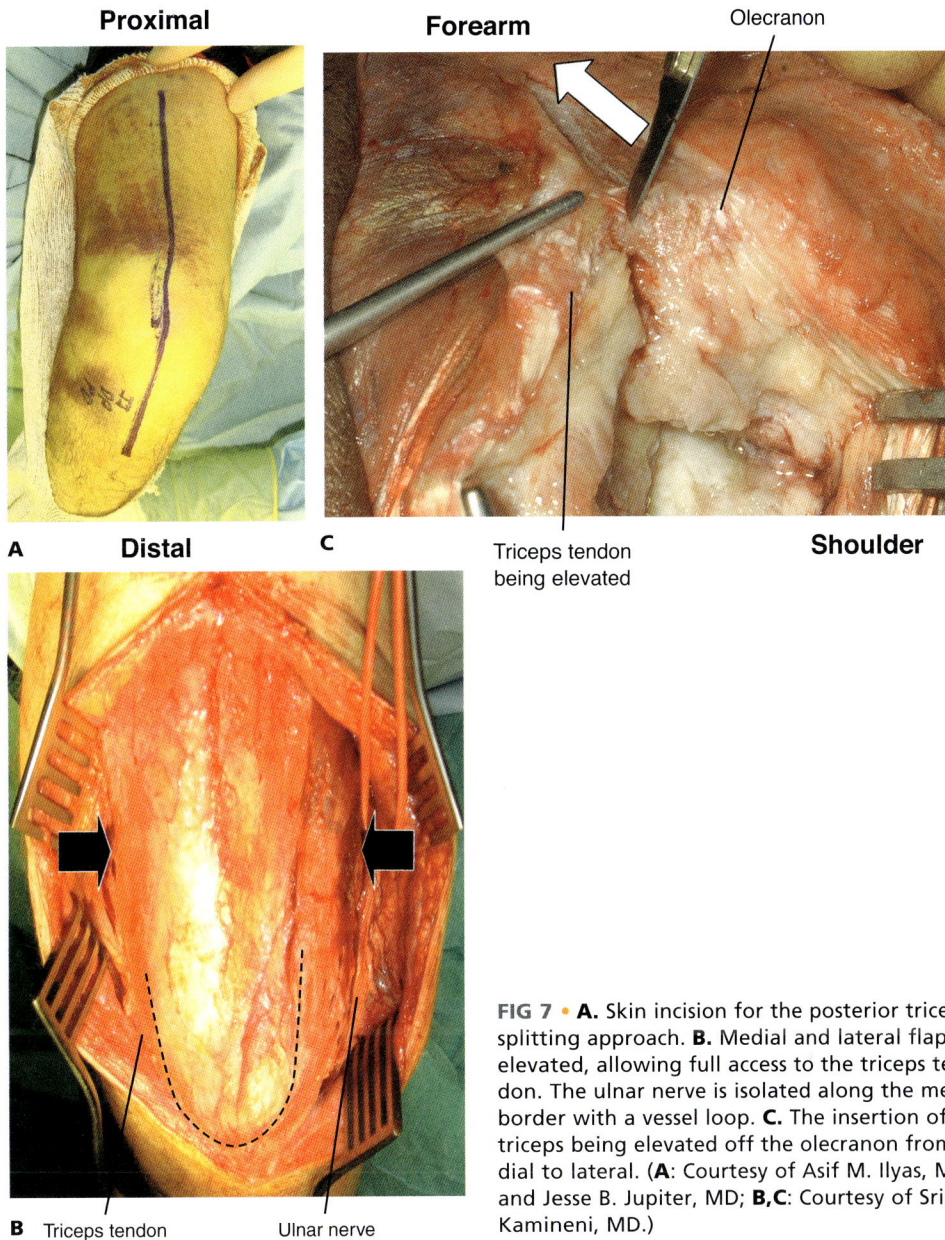

FIG 7 • A. Skin incision for the posterior triceps-splitting approach. **B.** Medial and lateral flaps are elevated, allowing full access to the triceps tendon. The ulnar nerve is isolated along the medial border with a vessel loop. **C.** The insertion of the triceps being elevated off the olecranon from medial to lateral. (**A**: Courtesy of Asif M. Ilyas, MD, and Jesse B. Jupiter, MD; **B,C**: Courtesy of Srinath Kamineni, MD.)

- Tendon is reflected from the muscle in a proximal to distal direction, freeing the underlying muscle fibers while preserving the tendinous attachment to the olecranon (**FIG 8**).
- Triceps muscle is then split in midline, and the distal humerus is exposed subperiosteally.
- Periosteum and triceps are elevated for a distance of about 5 cm proximal to the olecranon fossa, exposing the posterior aspect of the joint.
- If more extensive exposure is desired, the subperiosteal dissection is extended to the level of the joint, exposing the condyles both medially and laterally.
- Ulnar nerve should be identified and protected.
- After the procedure, if an elbow contracture has been corrected, the joint should be maximally flexed.
- The tendon slides distally from its initial position, and the proximal muscle and tendon are reapproximated in the lengthened relationship.

- The distal part of the triceps is then securely sutured to the fascia of the triceps expansion, and the remainder of the wound is closed in layers.

Triceps-Reflecting Approaches

- The triceps mechanism may be preserved in continuity with the anconeus and simply reflected to one side or the other.
- Three surgical approaches have been described that preserve the triceps muscle and tendon in continuity with the distal musculature of the forearm fascia and expose the entire joint.

Bryan-Morrey Posteromedial Triceps-Reflecting Approach

- Developed to preserve the continuity of the triceps with the anconeus

INDICATIONS

- Total elbow arthroplasty
- Interposition arthroplasty

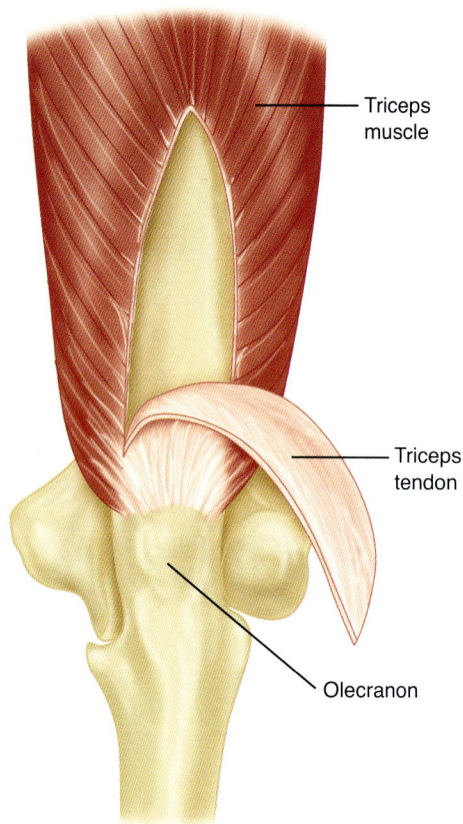

FIG 8 • Triceps-splitting, tendon-reflecting approach. The tendon is reflected from the muscle in a proximal to distal direction.

- Elbow dislocation
- Distal humerus fracture
- Synovial disease
- Infection

APPROACH

- A straight posterior incision is made medial to the midline, about 9 cm proximal and 8 cm distal to the tip of the olecranon (**FIG 9A**).
- The ulnar nerve is identified proximally at the margin of the medial head of the triceps and, depending on the procedure, is either protected or carefully dissected to its first motor branch and transposed anteriorly.
- The medial aspect of the triceps is elevated from the posterior capsule.
- The fascia of the forearm between the anconeus and the flexor carpi ulnaris is incised distally for about 6 cm.
- The triceps and the anconeus are elevated as one flap from medial to lateral, skeletonizing the olecranon and subcutaneous border of the ulna (**FIG 9B**). This should be performed at 20 to 30 degrees of flexion to relieve tension on the insertion, thereby facilitating dissection.
- The collateral ligaments may be released from the humerus for exposure as needed (**FIG 9C**).
  - If stability is important, these ligaments should be preserved or anatomically repaired at the conclusion of the surgery.
  - When performing a linked total elbow replacement, it is not necessary to preserve or repair the collateral ligaments.

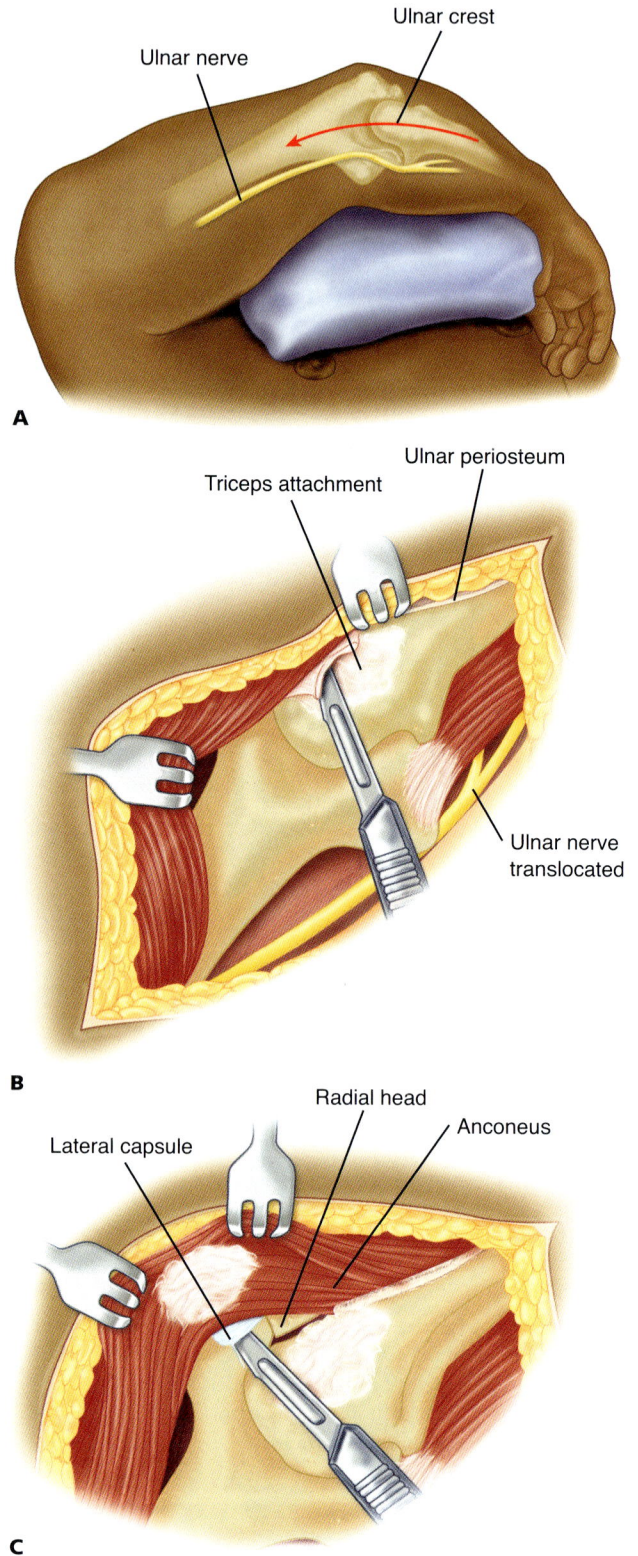

FIG 9 • The Bryan-Morrey posterior approach. **A.** Straight posterior skin incision. **B.** The ulnar nerve has been translocated anteriorly. The medial border of the triceps is identified and released and the superficial forearm fascia is sharply incised to allow reflection of the fascia and periosteum from the proximal ulna. **C.** The extensor mechanism has been reflected laterally and the collateral ligaments have been released.

■ The triceps attachment can be thin at the attachment to the ulna and it is not uncommon for a buttonhole to be created when reflecting the triceps.
　■ To prevent this, the flap can be raised as an osteoperiosteal flap (see osteocutaneous flap approach).
　■ A small osteotome is used to elevate the fascia with the petals of bone.
　■ The flap is mobilized laterally, elevating the anconeus origin from the distal humerus until it can be folded over the lateral humeral condyle.
　■ At this point, the radial head can be visualized.
■ The tip of the olecranon can be excised to help expose the trochlea.

Osteoanconeus Flap Approach

■ This provides excellent extension and reliable healing of the osseous attachment to the olecranon.
■ This approach exposes only the ulnar nerve, whereas the Mayo approach translocates the nerve.

INDICATIONS

■ This is a triceps-reflecting approach similar in concept to the Bryan-Morrey triceps-reflecting approach.
■ Most often used for joint replacement or distal humeral fractures

APPROACH

■ A straight posterior incision is made medial to the midline, about 9 cm proximal and 8 cm distal to the tip of the olecranon.
■ The ulnar nerve is identified and protected, but not translocated.
■ The triceps attachment is released from the ulna by osteotomizing the attachment with a thin wafer of bone.
　■ This is the essential difference from the Bryan-Morrey approach.
■ The medial aspect of the triceps, in continuity with the anconeus, is elevated from the ulna (**FIG 10A,B**).
■ The collateral ligaments are either maintained or released, depending on the pathology being addressed and the need for stability.
■ After the surgical procedure, the wafer of bone is secured to its bed by nonabsorbable sutures placed through bone holes (**FIG 10C**).
■ Interrupted sutures are used to repair the remaining distal portion of the extensor mechanism.

Extensile Kocher Posterolateral Triceps-Reflecting Approach

INDICATIONS

■ Joint arthroplasty
■ Ankylosis
■ Distal humerus fractures
■ Synovectomy
■ Radial head excision
■ Infection

APPROACH

■ Extensile exposure from the Kocher approach
■ Skin incision begins 8 cm proximal to the joint just posterior to the supracondylar ridge and continues distally over the Kocher interval between the anconeus and extensor carpi ulnaris about 6 cm distal to the tip of the olecranon

■ Proximally, the triceps is identified and freed from the brachioradialis and extensor carpi radialis longus along the intramuscular septum to the level of the joint capsule.
■ The interval between the extensor carpi ulnaris and the anconeus is identified distally.
■ The triceps in continuity with the anconeus is subperiosteally reflected. Sharp dissection frees the bony attachment of the triceps expansion to the anconeus from the lateral epicondyle.
■ The triceps remains attached to the tip of the olecranon.
■ The lateral collateral ligament complex is released from the humerus.
■ The joint may be dislocated with varus stress. If additional exposure is necessary, the anterior and posterior capsule can be released.
■ Routine closure of layers is performed, but the radial collateral ligament should be reattached to the bone through holes placed in the lateral epicondyle.

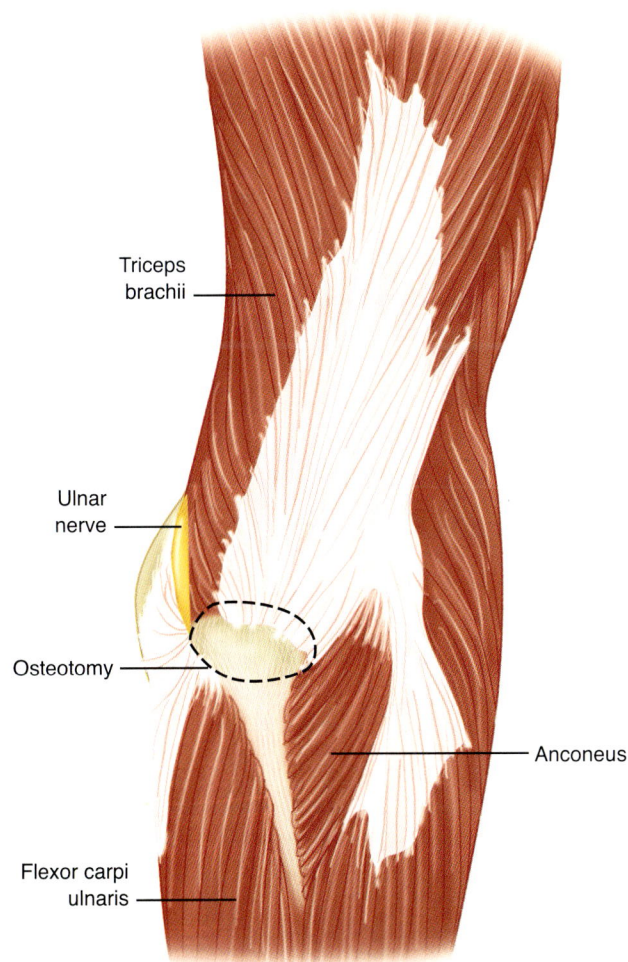

A

FIG 10 • Posterior view of the right elbow demonstrates a straight fascial incision to the lateral aspect of the tip of the olecranon. **A.** The line of release after the ulnar nerve has been identified and protected. *(continued)*

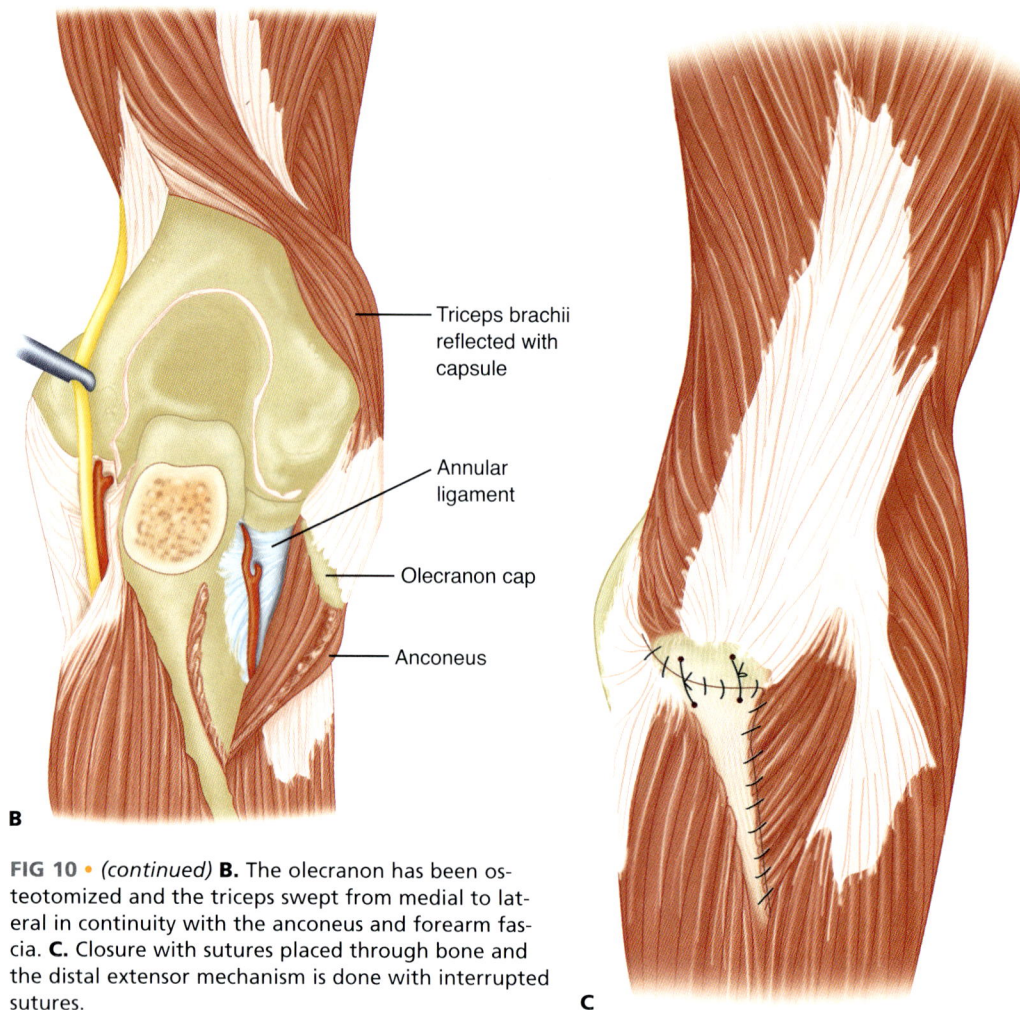

Triceps brachii
reflected with
capsule

Annular
ligament

Olecranon cap

Anconeus

B

FIG 10 • *(continued)* B. The olecranon has been osteotomized and the triceps swept from medial to lateral in continuity with the anconeus and forearm fascia. **C.** Closure with sutures placed through bone and
the distal extensor mechanism is done with interrupted
sutures.

C

Mayo Modified Extensile Kocher Approach

▪ The extensile Kocher approach and the Mayo modification
of the extensile Kocher approach provide sequentially greater
exposure from the initial Kocher approach.

INDICATIONS

▪ Release of ankylosed joint
▪ Interposition arthroplasty
▪ Replacement arthroplasty

APPROACH

▪ A modification of the extensile Kocher approach consists of
reflecting the anconeus and triceps expansion from the tip of
the olecranon by sharp dissection.
▪ The extensor mechanism (triceps in continuity with the anconeus) may be reflected from lateral to medial.
▪ The ulnar nerve should be decompressed or transposed if an
extensile lateral approach is used.
▪ The triceps is reattached in a fashion identical to that described for the Mayo approach.

Triceps-Preserving Approaches

Posterior Triceps-Sparing Approach

▪ Because the triceps is not elevated from the tip of the olecranon, rapid rehabilitation is possible.

INDICATIONS

▪ Tumor resection
▪ Joint reconstruction for resection of humeral nonunion
▪ Joint replacement

APPROACH

▪ A posterior incision is made medial to the tip of the
olecranon.
▪ Medial and lateral subcutaneous skin flaps are elevated.
▪ The ulnar nerve is identified and transposed anteriorly.
▪ The medial and lateral aspects of the triceps are identified
and developed distally to the triceps attachment on the ulna.
▪ For distal humerus fractures fixation:
  ▪ The common flexors and common extensors are partially
  released from the distal humerus to expose the supracondy-
  lar column for plate fixation.
▪ For total elbow arthroplasty or tumor resection:
  ▪ The common flexors and extensors are fully released
  from the medial and lateral epicondyle. The collateral
  ligaments and capsule are released and the distal humerus
  is excised.
  ▪ The distal humerus is exposed by bringing it through the
  defect along the lateral margin of the triceps.
  ▪ The ulna is exposed by supinating the forearm.
  ▪ After the implant has been inserted, the joint is articulated.

- There is no need to close or repair the extensor mechanism with this approach.

Olecranon Osteotomy

- Worldwide, the transosseous approach is probably the exposure most often used, especially for distal humeral fractures. The oblique osteotomy has almost been abandoned, and the transverse osteotomy has largely been replaced by the chevron.

Chevron Transolecranon Osteotomy

- Intra-articular osteotomy, first described by MacAusland, was originally recommended for ankylosed joints.
- It has been adapted by some for radial head excision and synovectomy and used or modified by others for T and Y condylar fractures.
- The chevron osteotomy enhances rotational stability compared to a transverse osteotomy.

INDICATIONS

- Ankylosed joints
- T or Y condylar fractures

APPROACH

- A posterior incision is made medial to the tip of the olecranon.
- Medial and lateral subcutaneous skin flaps are elevated.
- The ulnar nerve is identified and transposed anteriorly.
- The medial and lateral aspects of the triceps are identified and developed distally to the triceps attachment on the ulna.
- An apex-distal chevron or V osteotomy is performed with a thin oscillating saw but not completed through the subchondral bone. An osteotome completes the osteotomy, creating irregular surfaces that interdigitate increasing stability (**FIG 11A,B**).
- The triceps tendon, along with the osteotomized portion of the olecranon, may then be retracted proximally, and by flexing the elbow joint, the joint can be exposed (**FIG 11C**).

- Occasionally the medial or lateral collateral ligaments are released for better exposure.
    - These ligaments are then repaired at the end of the procedure.
- At the completion of the procedure, the tip of the olecranon is secured via tension-band or plate fixation.

LATERAL APPROACH TO THE ELBOW

- Lateral exposures to the elbow are widely used to treat a variety of elbow pathologies. The exposures differ according to the deep interval used.
- With any of the lateral exposures to the joint or to the proximal radius, the surgeon must be constantly aware of the possibility of injury to the posterior interosseous or recurrent branch of the radial nerve.

Anterolateral Approach to the Elbow (Kaplan)

Indications

- Anterior capsular release
- Posterior interosseous nerve exposure
- Capitellar/lateral column fractures

Approach

- Deep interval for the anterolateral approach lies between the extensor digitorum communis and the extensor carpi radialis longus muscles. (Intermuscular interval is best found by observing where vessels penetrate the fascia along the anterior margin of the extensor digitorum communis aponeurosis.)
- Fascia is split longitudinally between the extensor digitorum communis and the extensor carpi radialis longus. (As the dissection is carried deep through the extensor carpi radialis longus, the extensor carpi radialis brevis is encountered.)
- Deep to the extensor carpi radialis brevis, the transversely oriented fibers of the supinator are encountered, along with the posterior interosseous nerve. The posterior interosseous

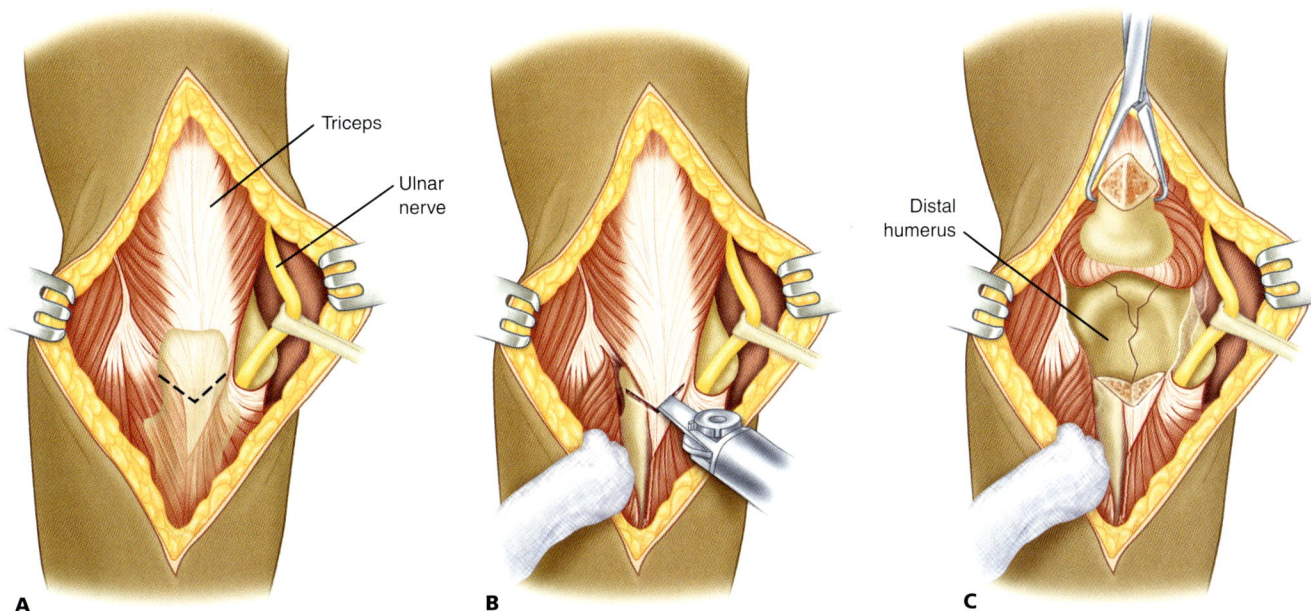

FIG 11 • Olecranon osteotomy. **A.** The triceps is released medially and laterally, while the ulnar nerve is protected. **B.** A chevron osteotomy with a distal apex is initiated with an oscillating saw. **C.** The proximal portion containing the olecranon osteotomy and triceps tendon is retracted proximally, exposing the elbow joint.

nerve defines the distal extent of the exposure. Pronation moves the radial nerve away from the surgical field.

- If required, proximal dissection with elevation of the extensor carpi radialis longus, extensor carpi radialis brevis, and brachioradialis anteriorly from the lateral supracondylar ridge of the humerus provides exposure of the anterior joint capsule.

Modified Distal Kocher Approach

Indications

- Reconstruction of the lateral ulnar collateral ligament

Approach

- The skin incision begins just proximal to the lateral epicondyle of the humerus and extends obliquely for about 6 cm in line with the fascia of the anconeus and extensor carpi ulnaris muscles (**FIG 12A**).
- The Kocher interval between the anconeus and flexor carpi ulnaris is incised (**FIG 12B**).
- Development of the Kocher interval reveals the lateral joint capsule.

- The anconeus is then reflected posteriorly off the joint capsule distally to expose the crista supinatoris.
- The extensor carpi ulnaris and the common extensor tendon are released from the lateral epicondyle and reflected anteriorly, exposing the lateral capsule. The radial nerve is at a safe distance from the dissection, and it is protected by the extensor carpi ulnaris and extensor digitorum communis muscle mass (**FIG 12C**).
- A longitudinal incision is made through the capsules to expose the radiocapitellar joint.

Boyd (Posterolateral) Approach

- Radioulnar synostosis may occur as the proximal radius and ulna are exposed subperiosteally.

Indications

- Monteggia fracture-dislocations
- Radial head fractures
- Radioulnar synostosis

Approach

- The incision begins just posterior to the lateral epicondyle lateral to the triceps tendon and continues distally to the lat-

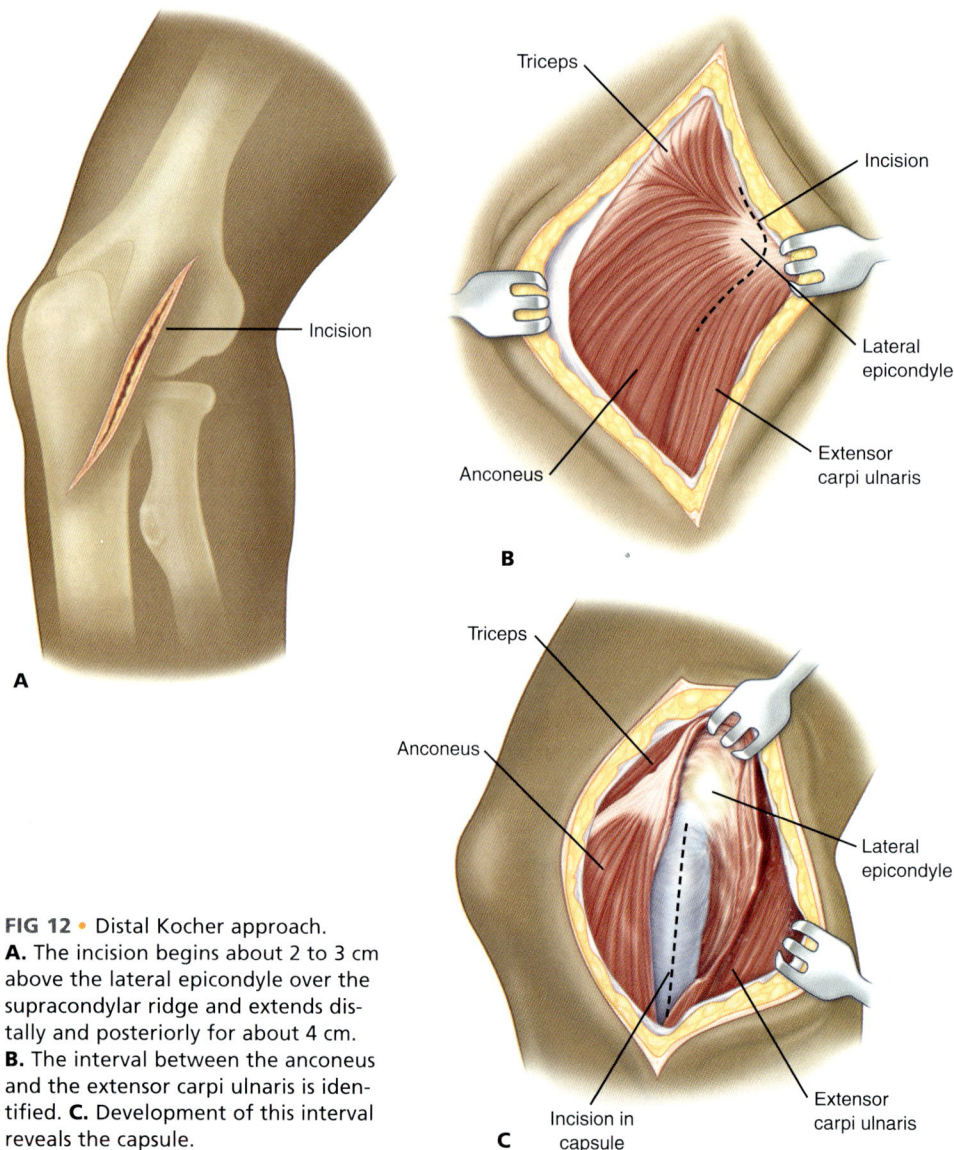

FIG 12 • Distal Kocher approach. **A.** The incision begins about 2 to 3 cm above the lateral epicondyle over the supracondylar ridge and extends distally and posteriorly for about 4 cm. **B.** The interval between the anconeus and the extensor carpi ulnaris is identified. **C.** Development of this interval reveals the capsule.

eral tip of the olecranon and then down to the subcutaneous border of the ulna.

- The anconeus and supinator are subperiosteally elevated from the subcutaneous border of the ulna (anconeus and supinator) (**FIG 13A,B**).
- Retraction of the anconeus and supinator exposes the joint capsule overlying the radial head and neck.
- The supinator muscle protects the posterior interosseous nerve.
- This lateral capsule contains the lateral ulnar collateral ligament, and its division can lead to posterolateral rotatory instability.
- To expose the radial shaft, the incision may be continued along the subcutaneous ulnar border, elevating the muscles off the lateral aspect of the ulna (extensor carpi ulnaris, abductor pollicis longus, and extensor pollicis longus).
- The posterior interosseous and recurrent interosseous arteries may need ligation.

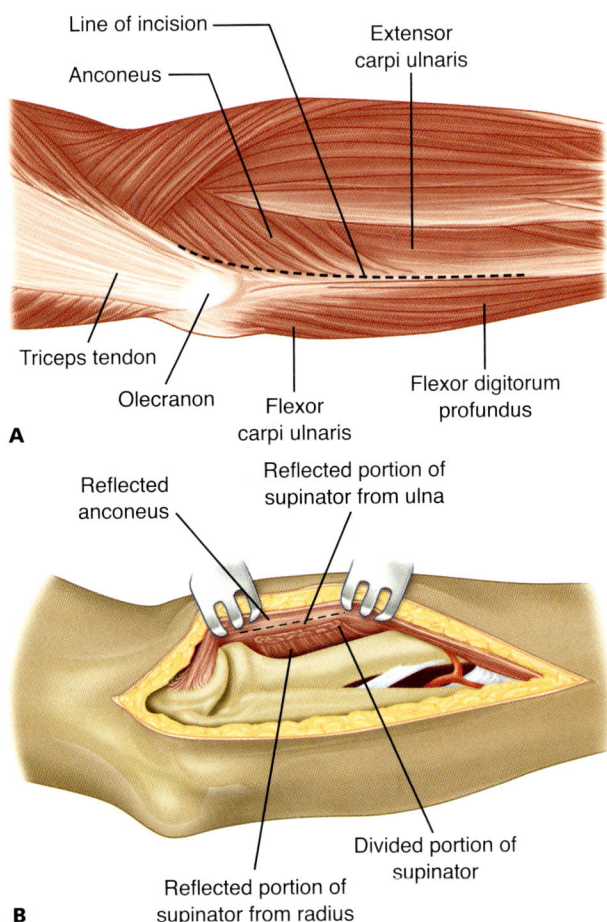

FIG 13 • The Boyd approach. **A.** The incision begins along the lateral border of the triceps about 2 to 3 cm above the epicondyle and extends distally over the lateral subcutaneous border of the ulna about 6 to 8 cm past the tip of the olecranon. The ulnar insertion of the anconeus and the origin of the supinator muscle are elevated subperiosteally. More distally, the subperiosteal reflection includes the abductor pollicis longus, the extensor carpi ulnaris, and the extensor pollicis longus muscles. The origin of the supinator at the crista supinatorus of the ulna is released, and the entire muscle flap is retracted radially, exposing the radiohumeral joint. **B.** The posterior interosseous nerve is protected in the substance of the supinator.

MEDIAL APPROACH TO THE ELBOW

- There are relatively few indications for medial exposure of the elbow joint. This has been superseded by arthroscopic approaches.
- The most valuable contribution to medial joint exposure is that described by Hotchkiss. This extensile exposure provides greater flexibility, particularly for exposure of the coronoid and for contracture release.

Extensile Medial Over-the-Top Approach

- Excellent visualization of the anteromedial and posteromedial elbow
- Not a sufficient approach for excision of heterotopic bone on the lateral side of the joint
- Does not provide adequate access to the radial head

Indications

- Coronoid fractures
- Contracture release (when ulnar nerve exploration required)
- Anterior and posterior access to the joint
- May be converted to a triceps-reflecting exposure of Bryan-Morrey

Approach

- Superficial dissection
  - Skin incision can vary between the boundaries of a pure posterior skin incision and midline medial incision (**FIG 14A**).
  - Subcutaneous skin is elevated.
  - The medial supracondylar ridge of the humerus, the medial intramuscular septum, the origin of the flexor pronator mass, and the ulnar nerve are identified.
  - Anterior to the septum, running just on top of the fascia (not in the subdermal tissue), the medial antebrachial cutaneous nerve is identified and protected.
  - The ulnar nerve is identified. If the patient previously had surgery, the ulnar nerve should be identified proximally before the surgeon proceeds distally.
    - If anterior transposition was performed previously, the nerve should be mobilized carefully before the operation proceeds.
  - The surface of the flexor pronator muscle mass origin is found by sweeping the subcutaneous tissue laterally with the medial antebrachial cutaneous nerve in this flap of subcutaneous tissue.
  - The medial intramuscular septum divides the anterior and posterior compartments of the elbow. The medial intramuscular septum is ultimately excised from the medial epicondyle to 5 cm proximal to it (**FIG 14B**).
  - The ulnar nerve is protected and the veins at the base of the septum are cauterized.
- Deep anterior exposure
  - The flexor pronator mass origin is identified and totally or partially released from the medial epicondyle.
    - If extensile exposure is needed, the entire flexor pronator mass is elevated from the medial epicondyle (**FIG 14C,D**).
    - If less extensile exposure is needed, the flexor pronator mass is divided parallel to the fibers, leaving about 1.5 cm of flexor carpi ulnaris tendon attached to the epicondyle.
    - A small cuff of fibrous tissue of the origin can be left on the supracondylar ridge as the muscle is elevated; this facilitates reattachment when closing.
  - The flexor pronator origin should be dissected down to the level of bone but superficial to the joint capsule. As this

plane is developed, the brachialis muscle is encountered from the underside.

■ The brachialis muscle is identified along the supracondylar ridge and released in continuity with the flexor pronator mass.

■ These muscles should be kept anterior and elevated from the capsule and anterior surface of the distal humerus.

■ The median nerve and the brachial vein and artery are superficial to the brachialis muscle and protected with the subperiosteal release of the brachialis.

■ Dissection of the capsule proceeds laterally and distally to separate it from the brachialis.

■ In the case of contracture, the capsule, once separated from the overlying brachialis and brachioradialis, can be sharply excised (**FIG 14E**).

■ Deep posterior capsule exposure

■ The ulnar nerve is mobilized to permit anterior transposition with a dissection carried distally to the first motor branch to allow the nerve to rest in the anterior position without being sharply angled as it enters the flexor carpi ulnaris.

■ With the Cobb elevator, the triceps is elevated from the posterior distal surface of the humerus.

■ The posterior capsule can be separated from the triceps as the elevator sweeps from the proximal to distal.

■ Closure

■ The flexor pronator mass should be reattached to the supracondylar ridge.

■ The ulnar nerve should be transposed and secured with a fascial sling to prevent posterior subluxation.

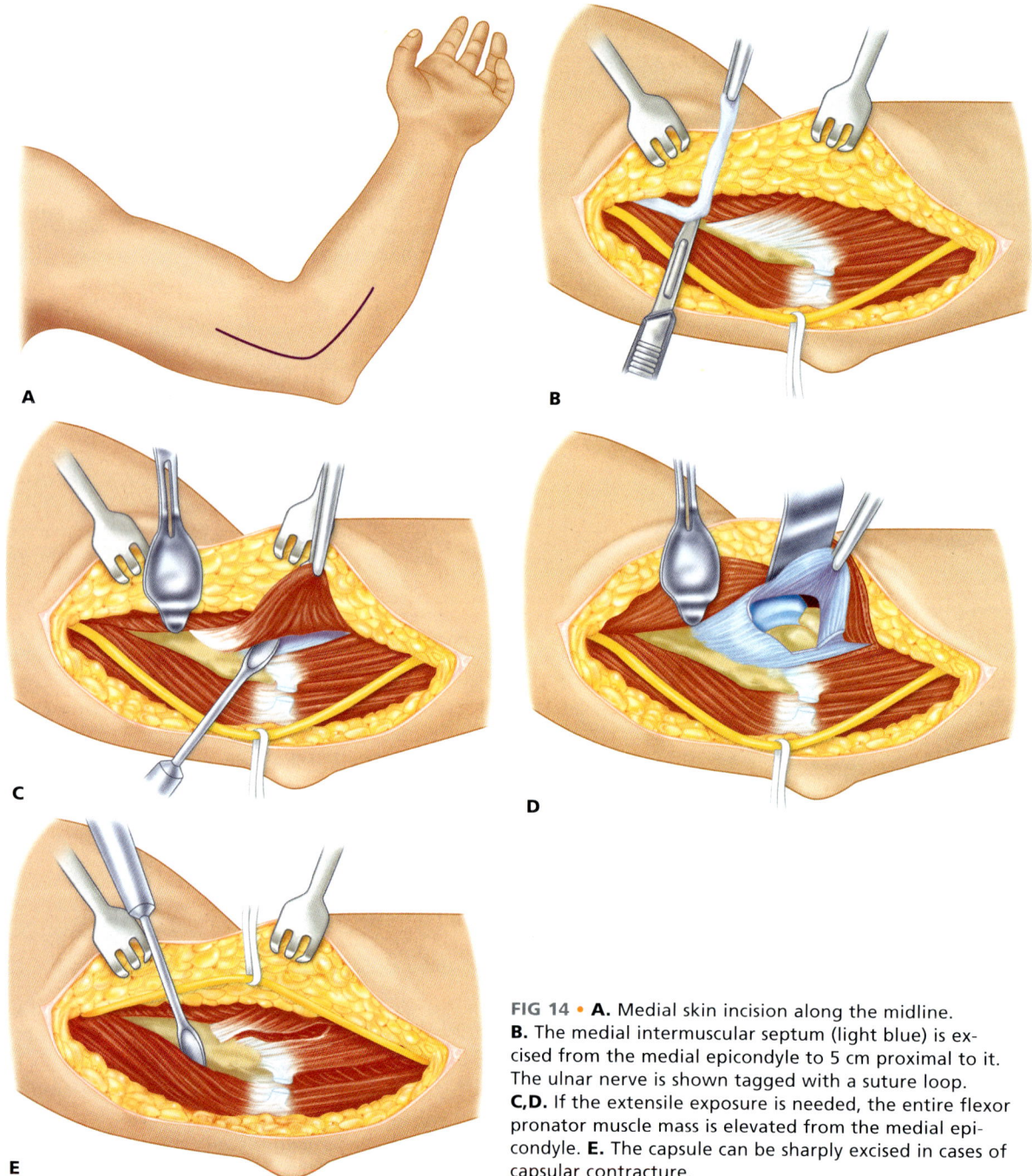

FIG 14 • **A.** Medial skin incision along the midline. **B.** The medial intermuscular septum (light blue) is excised from the medial epicondyle to 5 cm proximal to it. The ulnar nerve is shown tagged with a suture loop. **C,D.** If the extensile exposure is needed, the entire flexor pronator muscle mass is elevated from the medial epicondyle. **E.** The capsule can be sharply excised in cases of capsular contracture.

Table 1	**Indications and Recommended and Alternative Surgical Approaches**	
Indication	**Recommended Approach**	**Alternative Approach**
Total elbow arthroplasty	Bryan-Morrey, extended Kocher	Gschwend et al, Campbell, and Wadsworth
Soft tissue reconstruction	Global	Kocher, Bryan-Morrey, and Hotchkiss
T intercondylar fracture	MacAusland with chevron olecranon osteotomy	Alonso-Llames
Radial head fracture	Kocher	Kaplan
Capitellum fracture	Kaplan extended lateral approach	Kocher with or without Kaplan
Coronoid fracture	Taylor and Scham	Hotchkiss
Extra-articular distal humerus fracture	Alonso-Llames	Bryan-Morrey, Campbell
Monteggia fracture-dislocation	Gordon	Boyd
Radioulnar synostosis excision	Kocher or Gordon	Boyd or Henry

ANTERIOR APPROACH TO THE ELBOW

- Because of the vulnerability of the brachial artery and median nerve, the anterior medial approach to the elbow is not recommended.
- The extensile exposure described by Henry, and modified by Fiolle and Delmas, is best known and is the most useful for anterior exposure of the joint. Minor modifications of the Henry approach have been described, and a limited anterolateral exposure has been described by Darrach.

Modified Anterior Henry Approach

Indications

- Anteriorly displaced fracture fragments
- Excision of tumors in this region
- Reattachment of the biceps tendon to the radial tuberosity
- Exploration of nerve entrapment syndromes
- Anterior capsular release for contracture

Approach

- The skin incision begins about 5 cm proximal to the flexor crease of the elbow joint and extends distally along the anterior margin of the brachioradialis muscle to the flexion crease.
- At the elbow flexion crease, the incision turns medially to avoid crossing the flexor crease at a right angle. The incision continues transversely to the biceps tendon and then turns distally over the medial volar aspect of the forearm (**FIG 15A**).
- The fascia is released distally between the brachioradialis and pronator teres (**FIG 15B**).
- The interval between the brachioradialis laterally and the biceps and brachialis medially is identified. This interval is entered proximally, and gentle, blunt dissection demonstrates the radial nerve coursing on the inner surface of the brachioradialis muscle (**FIG 15C**).
- Care is taken to avoid injury to the superficial sensory branch of the radial nerve.

- Because the radial nerve gives off its branches laterally, it can safely be retracted with the brachioradialis muscle.
- At the level of the elbow joint, as the brachioradialis is retracted laterally and the pronator teres is gently retracted medially, the radial artery can be observed where it emerges from the medial aspect of the biceps tendon, giving off its muscular and recurrent branches in a mediolateral direction.
- The muscle branch is ligated, but the recurrent radial artery should be sacrificed only if the lesion warrants an extensive exposure.
- The posterior interosseous nerve enters the supinator and continues along the dorsum of the forearm distally.
- Dissection continues distally, exposing the supinator muscle, which covers the proximal aspect of the radius and the anterolateral aspect of the capsule (**FIG 15C**).
- Muscle attachments to the anterior aspect of the radius and those distal to the supinator include the discrete tendinous insertion of the pronator teres and the origins of the flexor digitorum sublimis and the flexor pollicis longus.
- The brachialis muscle is identified, elevated, and retracted medially to expose the proximal capsule.
- If more distal exposure is needed, the forearm is fully supinated, demonstrating the insertion of the supinator muscle along the proximal radius.
  - This insertion is incised and the supinator is subperiosteally retracted laterally (**FIG 15D**).
- The supinator serves as a protection to the deep interosseous branch of the radial nerve, but excessive retraction of the muscle should be avoided.
- The proximal aspect of the radius and the capitellum are thus exposed.
- Additional visualization may be obtained both proximally and distally, because the radial nerve has been identified and can be avoided proximally.
- The posterior interosseous nerve is protected distally by the supinator muscle, and the radial artery is visualized and protected medially if a more extensile exposure is required.

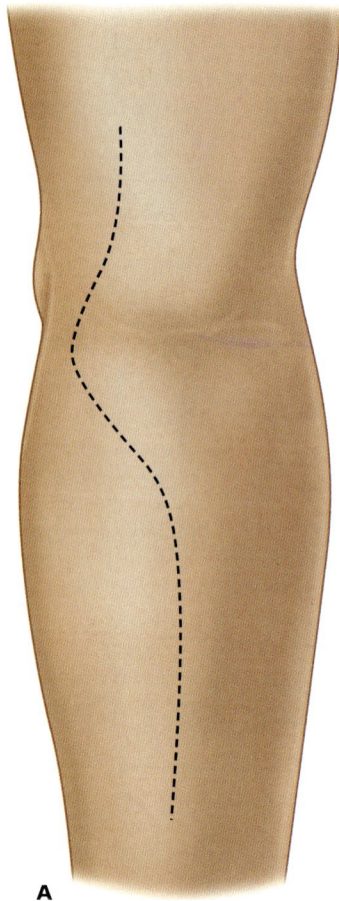

A

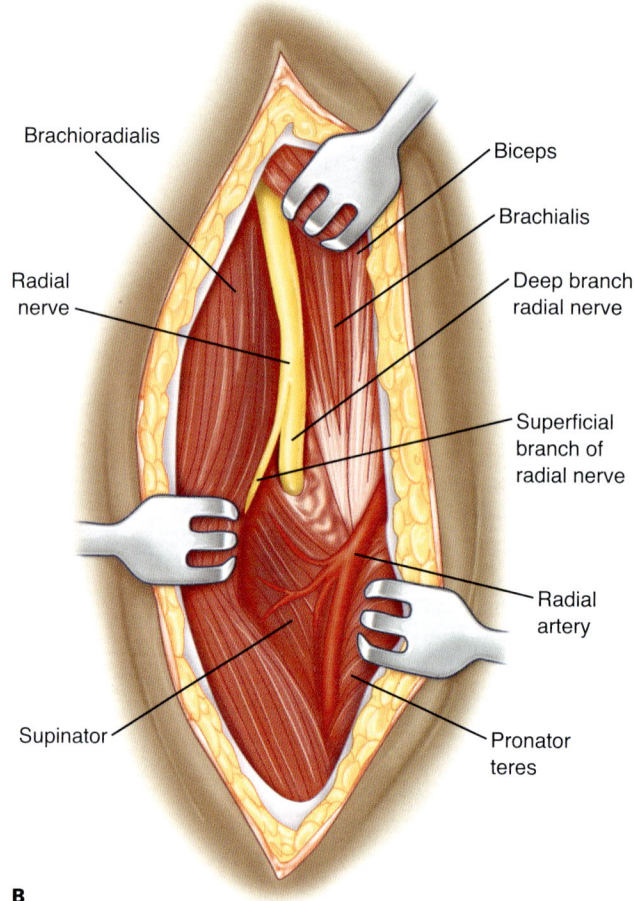

Brachioradialis

Radial nerve

Supinator

Biceps

Brachialis

Deep branch radial nerve

Superficial branch of radial nerve

Radial artery

Pronator teres

B

FIG 15 • The anterior Henry approach. **A.** An incision is made about 5 cm proximal to the elbow crease on the lateral margin of the biceps tendon. It extends transversely across the joint line and curves distally over the medial aspect of the forearm. The interval between the brachioradialis and brachialis proximally and the biceps tendon and pronator teres in the distal portion of the wound is identified. The radial nerve is protected and retracted along with the brachialis. **B.** The supinator muscle is released from the anterior aspect of the radius, which is fully supinated. **C.** The radial recurrent branches of the radial artery and its muscular branches are identified and sacrificed if more extensive exposure is required. The biceps tendon is retracted medially along with the brachialis muscle. **D.** This interval may now be developed to expose the anterior aspect of the elbow joint.

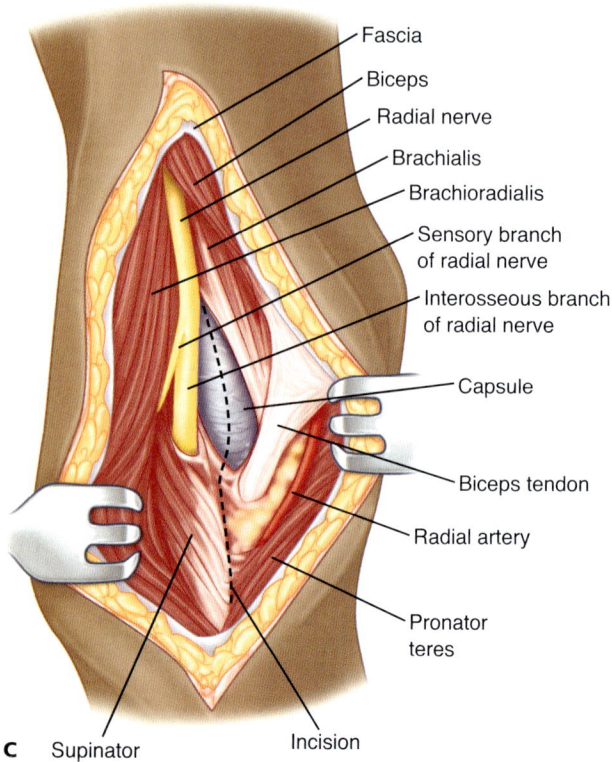

Fascia

Biceps

Radial nerve

Brachialis

Brachioradialis

Sensory branch of radial nerve

Interosseous branch of radial nerve

Capsule

Biceps tendon

Radial artery

Pronator teres

C Supinator Incision

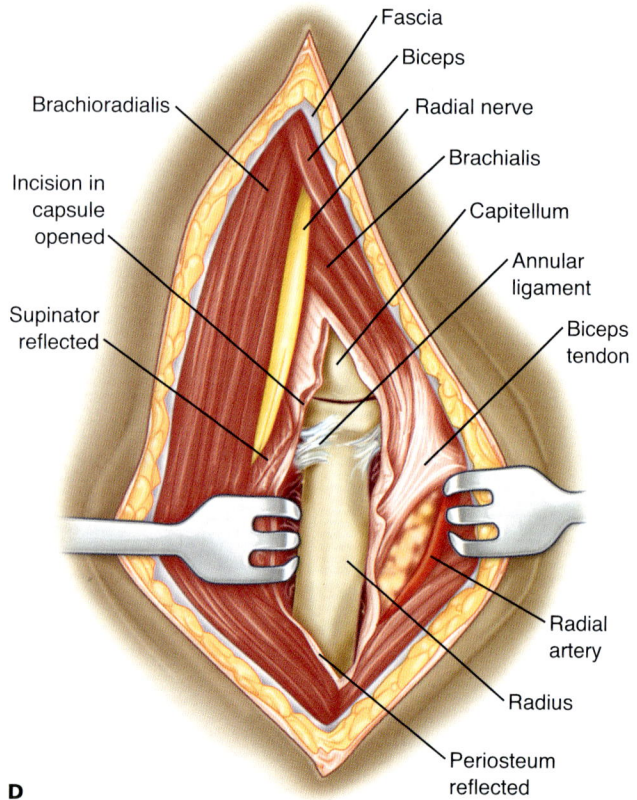

Fascia

Biceps

Radial nerve

Brachialis

Capitellum

Annular ligament

Biceps tendon

Radial artery

Radius

Periosteum reflected

Brachioradialis

Incision in capsule opened

Supinator reflected

D

Chapter 3

Bankart Repair and Inferior Capsular Shift

Theodore A. Blaine, Andrew Green, and Louis U. Bigliani

DEFINITION

▪ Shoulder instability is caused by a disruption of the normal stabilizing anatomic structures of the shoulder, leading to recurrent dislocation or subluxation of the glenohumeral joint.

ANATOMY

▪ Glenohumeral stability depends on the integrity of static and dynamic components.

▪ Dynamic stabilizers include the rotator cuff muscles, which provide a concavity compression effect, the scapular stabilizers, and the biceps tendon, which contributes to anterior stability when the arm is in an abducted and externally rotated position (**FIG 1A,B**).

▪ Static stabilizers consist of the bony and articular anatomy of the glenoid and humeral head, the negative intra-articular pressure supplied by the intact glenohumeral capsule, and the capsule–labral complex, which contains the glenoid labrum and anterior, middle, and superior glenohumeral ligaments (**FIG 1C**).

▪ The glenoid labrum plays an important role in deepening the glenoid socket and as an attachment site for the glenohumeral ligaments (**FIG 1D**).

▪ The primary restraint to anterior inferior translation of the humeral head in 90 degrees of abduction and external rotation is the inferior glenohumeral ligament (IGHL).

▪ The middle glenohumeral ligament (MGHL) has a variable attachment site into the glenoid labrum, glenoid neck, and biceps tendon origin. The MGHL is important in resisting anterior subluxation of the humeral head in the middle range of shoulder abduction (45 degrees).

▪ The superior glenohumeral ligament (SGHL) is located in the rotator interval capsule, and prevents inferior and posterior subluxation of the humeral head with the arm in an ad-

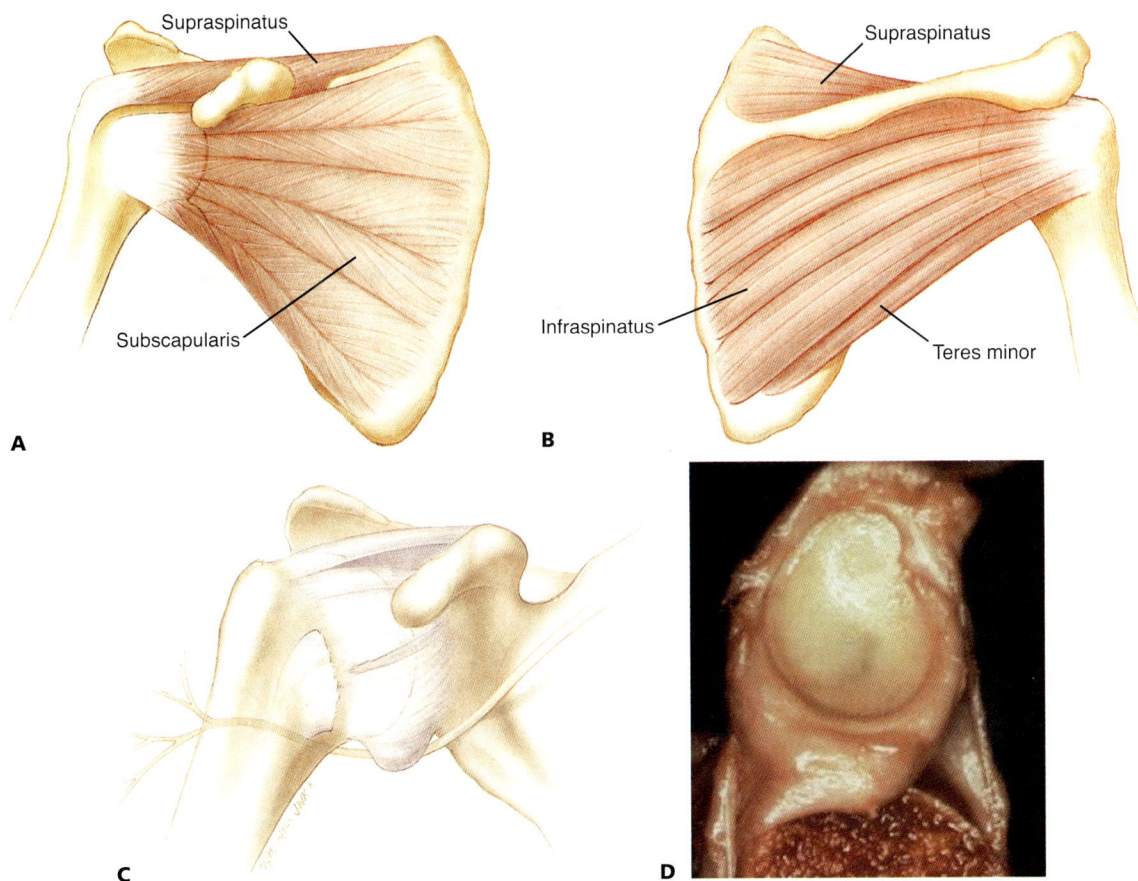

FIG 1 ▪ Dynamic stabilizers of the glenohumeral joint include the rotator cuff muscles (supraspinatus, infraspinatus, teres minor, subscapularis; **A,B**). The static stabilizers of the glenohumeral joint include the glenohumeral ligaments of the capsule (**C**), and the glenoid labrum (**D**), which deepens the socket and serves as an attachment for the glenohumeral ligaments and biceps tendon.

ducted and neutral or internally rotated position. The SGHL is important in inferior and posterior translation of the humeral head.

PATHOGENESIS

- Glenohumeral instability (subluxation or dislocation) occurs when the static or dynamic stabilizers of the glenohumeral joint are disrupted, either from acute rupture or repetitive microtrauma.
- The "essential anatomical defect," or Bankart lesion, was first described by a British pathologist, A. Blundell Bankart, in 1923, and the operative procedure was first described in 1938 (**FIG 2A**).[3,20]
  - The Bankart lesion is present in at least 40% of shoulders undergoing anterior instability procedures.
  - The "essential" nature of the Bankart lesion has been challenged, since a simulated Bankart lesion without capsular stretching does not lead to significant increases in glenohumeral translation.
- In addition to tearing of the glenoid labrum, the labrum may also be avulsed from the glenoid rim as a sleeve of tissue (anterior labral periosteal sleeve avulsion [ALPSA]) (**FIG 2B**).[17]
- Recurrent major trauma and repetitive microtrauma creates substantial deformation to the IGHL, producing subsequent episodes of symptomatic subluxation.
  - Biomechanical studies of this ligament have demonstrated that failure typically occurs at the glenoid insertion (40%), followed by the ligament substance (35%) and the humeral attachment (25%). Significant capsular stretching can occur (23% to 34%) before failure.
- Osseous deficiency on the anterior rim (bony Bankart) may contribute to glenohumeral instability (**FIG 2C**).
  - Significant defects accounting for instability occur when 30% of the glenoid is involved, and the glenoid acquires an "inverted pear" appearance (**FIG 2D**).

NATURAL HISTORY

- The incidence of glenohumeral instability has been estimated at 8.2 to 23.9 per 100,000 person-years.[23]
- The incidence in at-risk populations is significantly higher (military population, 1.69 per 1000 person-years; NCAA athletes, 0.12 injuries/1000 athletic exposures).[19]
- Overhead athletes are prone to this repeat injury as their motions in the abducted, externally rotated position put stress on the capsulolabral structures. Contact athletes (football players and wrestlers) have the highest incidence of shoulder dislocations as compared to other sports.
- Depending on the patient's age and activity level, redislocation rates in active patients may be as high as 92% with nonoperative treatment.[13,19,24]

PATIENT HISTORY AND PHYSICAL FINDINGS

- Evaluation of the patient with suspected instability begins with a thorough history.
- Arm dominance, sport, position, and level of competition should be noted, as well as associated factors, including other sporting activities, training modalities, and past history of injuries.
- Traumatic causes of instability should be determined, as these are more likely to be associated with Bankart lesions.
- The character of the problem should be elicited.
  - Does the athlete complain of pain or instability?
  - Does the shoulder subluxate or dislocate?
  - What arm positions reproduce symptoms?
- Any prior treatments (physical therapy, training modifications, medication, and surgery) should be noted.
- Physical examination should include assessment of both shoulders.
- Inspection should be performed to identify any skin incisions, evidence of wasting in the deltoid, rotator cuff, or periscapular

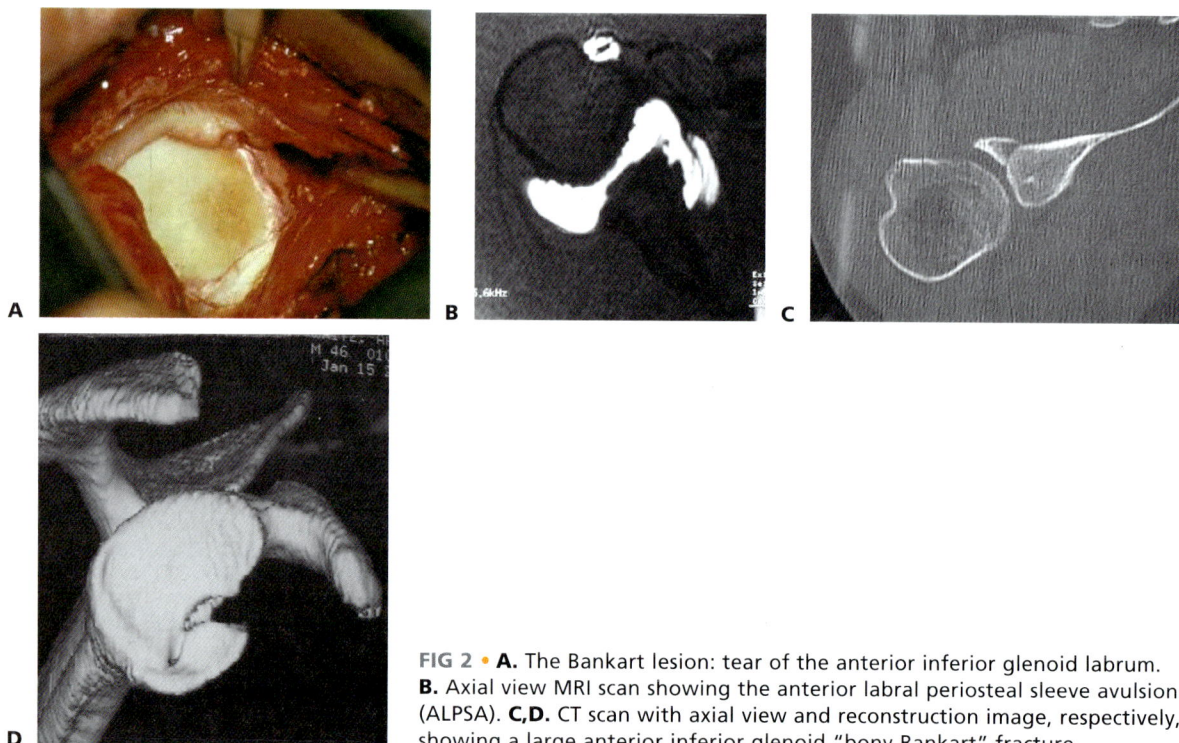

FIG 2 • **A.** The Bankart lesion: tear of the anterior inferior glenoid labrum. **B.** Axial view MRI scan showing the anterior labral periosteal sleeve avulsion (ALPSA). **C,D.** CT scan with axial view and reconstruction image, respectively, showing a large anterior inferior glenoid "bony Bankart" fracture.

musculature, and gross evidence of laxity, including sulcus signs or signs of generalized ligamentous laxity.

- Palpation is performed to identify point tenderness; anterior joint line tenderness may be present in acute anterior dislocations; subacromial tenderness may be present with impingement secondary to subtle instability.

- Active and passive motion tests are an important part of the instability examination. Significant variations in motion are encountered in throwing athletes, with increased external rotation and decreased internal rotation common in the affected shoulder.

- Provocative testing is perhaps the most important aspect in the clinical evaluation of shoulder instability.

  - The sulcus sign is often elicited in patients with inferior instability.

  - Anterior translation and posterior translation are similarly graded with the patient supine and with an anterior or posterior load and shift test, although this test is performed only in the anesthetized patient.

- In the awake patient, signs of instability can be more subtle. The apprehension test is routinely performed with the arm abducted, extended, and externally rotated. A sensation of impending subluxation or dislocation in the patient is diagnostic of instability. Pain is less specific and may instead indicate internal impingement of the articular surface of the rotator cuff or functional impingement of the bursal side of the rotator cuff on a prominent coracoacromial ligament.

  - A posterior-directed force on the arm by the examiner that relieves the apprehension in this position (Jobe relocation test) suggests an unstable shoulder.

- Subscapularis integrity and strength should be evaluated in patients with glenohumeral instability.

  - Inability to press the hand to the belly is a positive result of the belly press test and indicates subscapularis muscle weakness or tear.

  - Inability to lift the hand from the back is a positive result in the lift-off test and indicates subscapularis muscle weakness or tear.

IMAGING AND OTHER DIAGNOSTIC STUDIES

- Radiographs include anteroposterior (AP), lateral, and axillary views (**FIG 3A,B**).

  - The axillary view is particularly important for assessing anterior glenoid rim defects.

- The Hill-Sachs lesion of the posterosuperior humeral head is best seen on the AP internal rotation or Stryker notch views.

- CT scan is not necessary in all cases but may be helpful in patients with bony defects (see Fig 2C,D).

- MRI scan is not necessary in all cases but can be useful in identifying labral lesions as well as subscapularis tears (**FIG 3C**).

  - MRI arthrogram is more sensitive in identifying labral pathology and may be necessary when superior or posterior labral pathology is suspected.

DIFFERENTIAL DIAGNOSIS

- External impingement, subacromial bursitis, rotator cuff tendinitis
- Internal impingement
- SLAP (superior labral tear)
- Voluntary instability
- Collagen disorder (Ehlers-Danlos syndrome, Marfan syndrome)
- Subscapularis insufficiency, tear

NONOPERATIVE MANAGEMENT

- After reduction of an acute dislocation, a sling is used for immobilization. The duration of immobilization has been controversial, but 3 to 6 weeks is recommended.[21]

- Some surgeons recommend immobilization in a position of abduction and external rotation to improve healing. However, many patients will not tolerate this position, and a position of adduction and internal rotation therefore is more commonly used.

- For treatment of acute injuries, rotational and scapular strengthening exercises of the affected shoulder are started after the initial immobilization period. The program is progressed toward normalization of strength and motion through increased resistance training.

  - Return to sports is allowed when the patient has a full and pain-free range of motion, normal strength, and little or no apprehension.[21]

- For chronic and recurrent instability, strengthening is focused on the rotator cuff and scapular stabilizers, as well as core strengthening of the abdominal and trunk musculature. Resistive exercises of the rotator cuff are begun with the arm in neutral below 90 degrees and are progressed gradually. Strengthening of scapular stabilizers is particularly important.

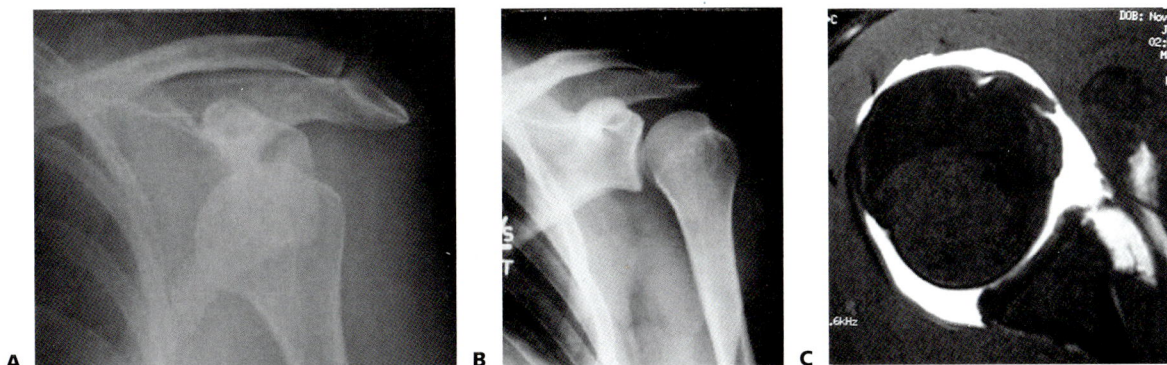

FIG 3 • AP radiographs of the left shoulder showing a dislocated shoulder (**A**) and subsequent reduction (**B**). There is a Hill-Sachs fracture of the posterolateral humeral head. **C.** Axial MRI scan in a patient with deficient glenoid labrum and subscapularis tendon tear.

- The rate of redislocation after nonoperative treatment depends on the patient's age and activity level. In young patients participating in high-risk activities (eg, military cadets), the rate of redislocation is as high as 92%.[24]
- In a meta-analysis comparing operative to nonoperative treatment for first-time dislocators, 50% of the conservatively treated patients eventually opted for surgery.[19]

SURGICAL MANAGEMENT

- Surgical treatment options are generally categorized into anatomic and nonanatomic procedures.
- Nonanatomic procedures (Putti-Platt, Magnuson-Stack) are aimed at tightening the anterior structures and preventing at-risk arm positions (ie, abduction and external rotation). These procedures have largely been abandoned after it was discovered that overtightening the anterior structures could lead to posterior subluxation and glenohumeral arthritis.[11,18]
  - The Putti-Platt procedure consists of a vertical incision through both the subscapularis tendon and capsule followed by repair of the lateral flap to the soft tissue at the glenoid rim.[18]
  - The Magnuson-Stack procedure is a transfer of the subscapularis tendon lateral to the bicipital groove (**FIG 4A**).
- Coracoid transfer procedures are other nonanatomic procedures where the coracoid process, with its attached short head of the biceps and coracobrachialis tendons, is transferred to the anterior glenoid rim and secured with screws.[1]
  - The Bristow procedure uses the tip of the coracoid and typically a single bicortical cancellous screw.
  - The Laterjet procedure lays the coracoid on its side and is typically secured with two screws (**FIG 4B**).
  - Although several authors have achieved excellent success with these procedures, the concern for hardware migration and late resorption of the bone block have made these procedures less popular than the anatomic procedures. They are used mainly for revision procedures and in cases where there is deficient glenoid bone stock.
- Anatomic reconstruction procedures have been aimed at reconstructing the anterior labrum using sutures, staples, or tacks.[2,8,9,12,22] These anatomic procedures have had excellent success, with minimal (less than 5%) recurrence rates, and therefore are the procedure of choice in the surgical treatment of glenohumeral instability.
- The Bankart repair and inferior capsular shift procedures are the most commonly used anatomic reconstruction procedures.

- Although recurrence rates for arthroscopic Bankart repair and capsular shift were initially higher than open procedures, these rates have become comparable to open as the arthroscopic techniques have evolved.
- Open treatment, however, is recommended over arthroscopic treatment in the following situations:
  - Significant bony Bankart lesions (over 30%)
  - Significant Hill-Sachs defects where the defect "engages" the glenoid rim with external rotation as visualized during diagnostic arthroscopy
  - Revision procedures
  - Some contact athletes (football) and extreme sports, where a slightly lower recurrence rate can be expected in comparison to the arthroscopic procedure

Preoperative Planning

- A careful assessment of the patient's expectations of the surgery and postoperative care, including thorough discussions with the patient and family, are required as part of the preoperative plan.
  - Noncompliance with the postoperative restrictions will increase the risk of redislocation after surgical repair.
- It is important to assess mental status and any secondary gain issues in patients with multidirectional instability. Patients with voluntary dislocations and malingering (Munchausen syndrome) patients have a high rate of failure and should be identified before surgery.
- It is important to identify before surgery any glenoid bony deficiency that may require bony augmentation via coracoid transfer or allograft reconstruction. Special equipment (allograft bone and instrumentation to perform ORIF) may be required and should be arranged before surgery.

Positioning

- Interscalene block anesthesia is preferred because of the excellent muscle relaxation and postoperative pain relief it offers. If an adequate block cannot be performed, however, general anesthesia can also be used.
- The patient is positioned in the beach-chair position with the back elevated. The patient should be moved to the edge of the table or the shoulder cut-out removed to allow access to the anterior and posterior shoulder as required.
- A hydraulic arm positioner (Tenet Spider) is particularly helpful and can obviate the need for an additional assistant to hold the arm (**FIG 5**).

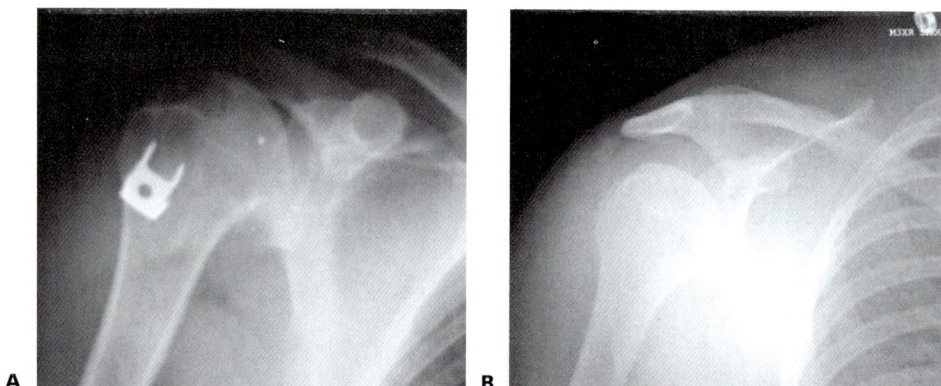

FIG 4 • A. AP radiograph of the right shoulder in a patient with previous Magnuson-Stack procedure (the subscapularis tendon has been stapled laterally to the bicipital groove). **B.** AP radiograph of the right shoulder in a patient with a Laterjet procedure. There are two screws securing the coracoid bone block to the glenoid.

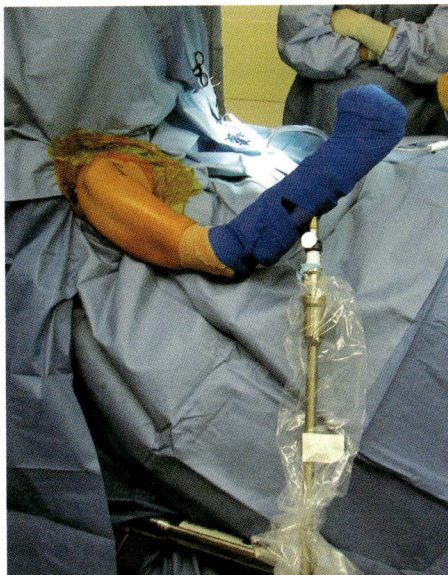

FIG 5 • Hydraulic arm positioner (Spider, Tenet Medical Engineering, Calgary, Alberta, Canada) used to position the arm during surgery.

Approach

- The bony landmarks of the shoulder are identified, including the acromion, clavicle, and coracoid process.
- Approaches to the shoulder that may be used include the deltopectoral, the concealed axillary incision, and the mini-incision approach. All of these are variations of the standard deltopectoral approach.
- Standard deltopectoral approach
  - This is the utility approach to the shoulder.
  - A 7- to 15-cm incision is made lateral to the coracoid process beginning below the clavicle and extending toward the anterior humeral shaft at the deltoid insertion. Skin flaps are elevated and the deltopectoral interval is identified.
  - The remainder of this approach is described in detail below.
- Concealed axillary incision
  - Whereas the traditional deltopectoral approach is about 15 cm in length, the concealed axillary incision begins 3 cm inferior to the coracoid and extends only 7 cm into the

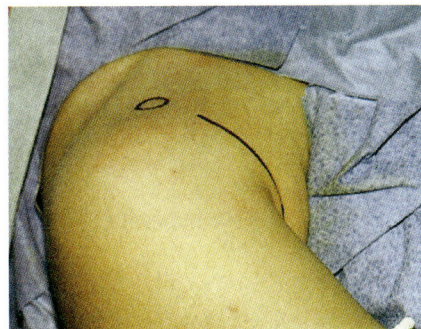

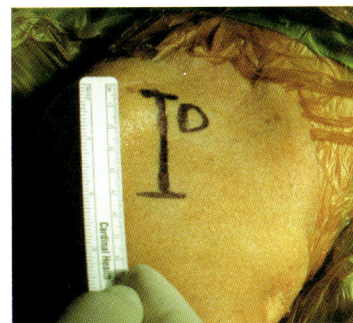

FIG 6 • **A.** The concealed axillary incision is made from below the coracoid process toward the axillary fold. **B.** The mini-incision is made in line with the deltopectoral interval and is centered one-third above and two-thirds below the coracoid process.

axillary crease (**FIG 6A**). Skin flaps are widely elevated and the deltopectoral interval is identified.
  - This incision is cosmetically appealing and is useful in patients where cosmesis is important.
- Mini-incision approach
  - A 5-cm incision just lateral to the coracoid process can be used in shoulder stabilization procedures (**FIG 6B**). Wide subcutaneous flaps are created and the deltopectoral interval is identified. The remainder of the exposure is similar to the standard deltopectoral approach.
  - The location of this incision is important to achieve direct access to the glenoid without extending the incision: one third of the incision should be above and two thirds below the coracoid process.

BANKART PROCEDURE

- The skin incision is based on surgeon preference as described above. The concealed axillary incision is the most commonly used.
- Skin flaps are elevated and the deltopectoral interval is identified (**TECH FIG 1A**).
- The cephalic vein is taken laterally with the deltoid muscle, and the clavipectoral fascia overlying the subscapularis tendon and strap muscles is exposed.
- When additional exposure is needed, it is helpful to incise and tag with a suture the upper third of the pectoralis major insertion into the humerus. Great care should be taken not to injure the biceps tendon, which lies just underneath the pectoralis major insertion.

- The clavipectoral fascia is incised lateral to the strap muscles, and a retractor is placed between them to expose the subscapularis muscle and tendon.
- A small wedge of the coracoacromial ligament can be removed to increase superior exposure (**TECH FIG 1B**).
- The branches of the anterior circumflex humeral vessels at the inferior margin of the subscapularis muscle should be cauterized at this time to control bleeding.
- The subscapularis tendon is exposed and incised vertically just medial to its insertion. The tendon can be peeled off the underlying capsule with a combination of the periosteal elevator for blunt dissection and the needle-tip Bovie cautery for sharp dissection (**TECH FIG 1C,D**).

TECHNIQUES

- The anterior capsule is then incised vertically at the level of the glenoid rim (TECH FIG 1E,F).
- With a curette or osteotome, the anterior glenoid rim is roughened and any soft tissue removed to allow for healing of the repair (TECH FIG 1G).
- Transosseous sutures are passed through holes made with pointed forceps or a drill.
    - Alternatively, suture anchors may be placed at the margin of remaining articular cartilage. Often, two

and sometimes three anchors are used between the 2:30 and 6:00 positions (TECH FIG 1H).

- The capsule is shifted or repaired anatomically as required. Typically, an inferior capsular shift procedure is performed in combination with the Bankart procedure as described below.
- The subscapularis tendon is repaired anatomically at its insertion.

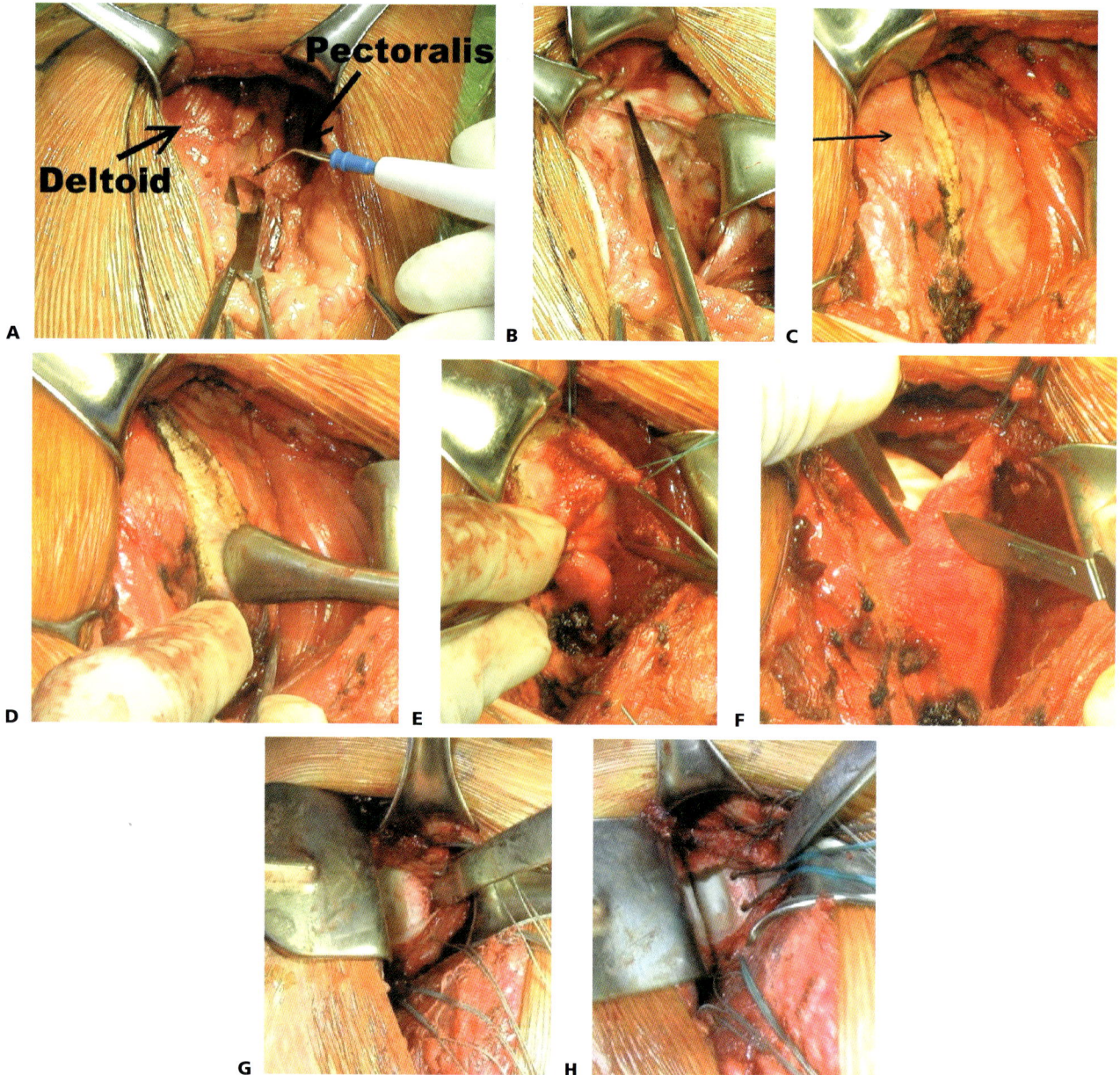

TECH FIG 1 • Bankart procedure. **A.** The deltopectoral interval is identified and incised using a needle-tip Bovie. The cephalic vein is retracted laterally with the deltoid. **B.** The anterolateral leading edge of the coracoacromial ligament (indicated by the clamp) is resected for improved superior exposure. **C.** The subscapularis is incised about 1 cm medial to its insertion, leaving a stout cuff of tissue laterally (*arrow*) for subsequent repair. **D.** Blunt dissection inferiorly, where the subscapularis muscle is not adherent to the capsule, facilitates finding the plane of separation between the subscapularis and anterior capsule. **E.** The capsule is sharply incised, taking care not to damage the humeral head cartilage below. **F.** An adequate cuff of tissue is left behind for subsequent repair. **G.** The glenoid rim is prepared using an osteotome or curette. **H.** Suture anchors are placed at the apex of the glenoid rim.

T-PLASTY MODIFICATION OF THE BANKART PROCEDURE

- To address capsular laxity in addition to the Bankart lesion, Altchek and Warren[2] described a modification of the Bankart procedure by performing a T incision in the capsule.
- The approach is the same as in the Bankart procedure described and involves dissection of the subscapularis from the anterior glenohumeral capsule.
- Unlike the inferior capsular shift procedure, the T-plasty involves a medially based capsular incision at the glenoid margin.
  - The T capsulotomy is made two thirds from the top of the capsule, with the vertical component adjacent to the glenoid rim (**TECH FIG 2**).
- The Bankart lesion is repaired using suture anchors or transosseous sutures.
- The laterally based inferior flap of capsule is advanced superiorly and medially and secured to the glenoid rim.
- The superior flap is then advanced medially and oversewn to the inferior flap.
- The subscapularis tendon is repaired anatomically at its insertion.

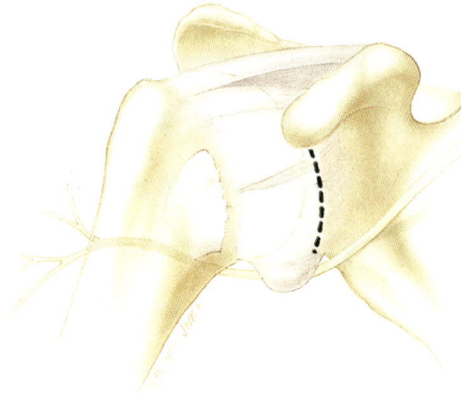

TECH FIG 2 • T-plasty modification of the Bankart procedure. The T capsulotomy is made two thirds from the top of the capsule, with the vertical component adjacent to the glenoid rim.

ANTERIOR CAPSULOLABRAL RECONSTRUCTION

- Because of the loss of strength and velocity in throwing athletes undergoing anterior stabilization procedures, Jobe[12] in 1991 proposed a subscapularis-sparing procedure in which the tendon is split in line with its fibers and its humeral attachment left intact.
- A deltopectoral approach to the shoulder is used and the strap muscles are retracted medially to expose the subscapularis tendon.

- The subscapularis is then divided horizontally in line with its fibers at the junction of the upper two thirds and lower one third (**TECH FIG 3A,B**).
- A horizontal capsulotomy is now made in the middle of the capsule extending medial to the glenoid rim. The capsule is elevated off the glenoid subperiosteally to allow for superior and inferior capsular advancement (**TECH FIG 3C**).

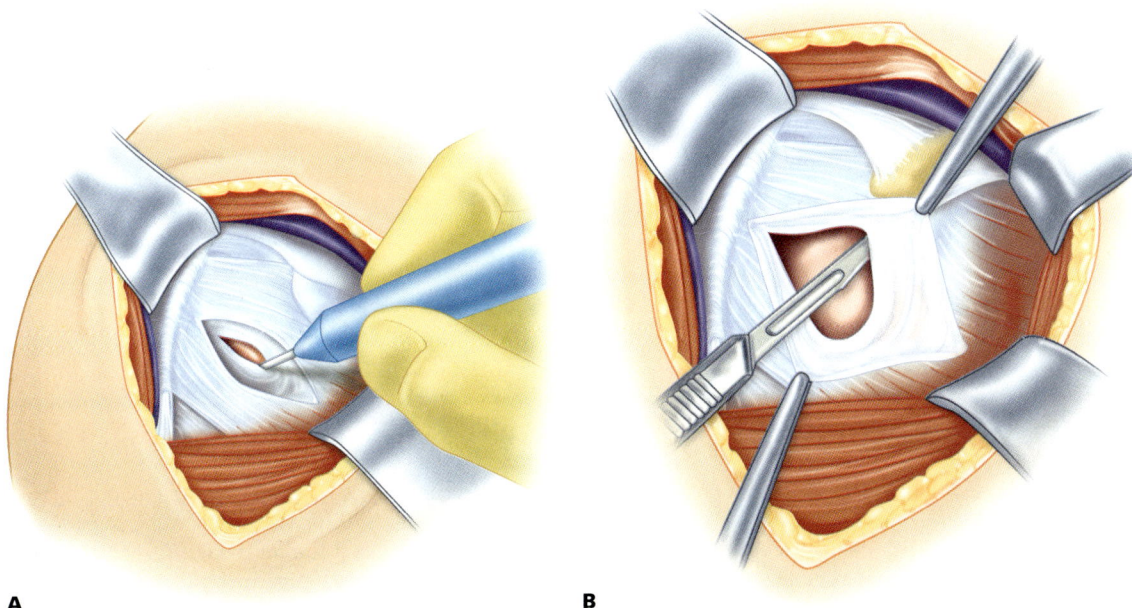

A

B

TECH FIG 3 • The anterior capsulolabral reconstruction procedure. **A.** The subscapularis is divided horizontally in line with its fibers at the junction of the upper two thirds and lower one third. **B.** A horizontal capsulotomy is now made in the middle of the capsule extending medial to the glenoid rim. *(continued)*

TECHNIQUES

C

D

E

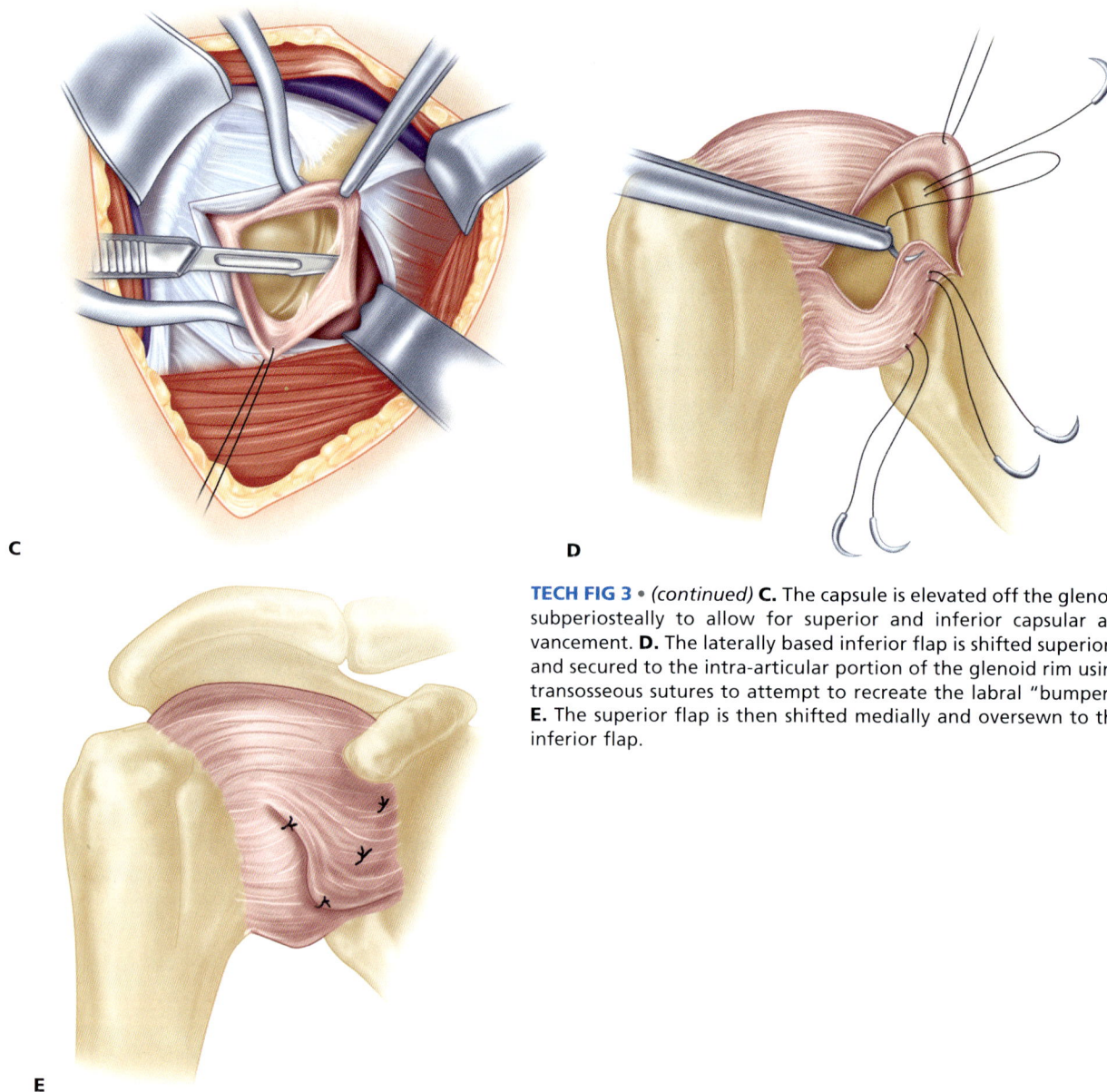

TECH FIG 3 • *(continued)* C. The capsule is elevated off the glenoid subperiosteally to allow for superior and inferior capsular advancement. **D.** The laterally based inferior flap is shifted superiorly and secured to the intra-articular portion of the glenoid rim using transosseous sutures to attempt to recreate the labral "bumper." **E.** The superior flap is then shifted medially and oversewn to the inferior flap.

- The laterally based inferior flap is then shifted superiorly and secured to the intra-articular portion of the glenoid rim using transosseous sutures to attempt to recreate the labral "bumper" (**TECH FIG 3D,E**).
- The superior flap is then shifted medially and oversewn to the inferior flap.

- Because the subscapularis tendon is not detached, active assistive rehabilitation exercises are begun immediately on postoperative day 1, and rehabilitation is progressed more rapidly.

ANTERIOR INFERIOR CAPSULAR SHIFT

- The anterior inferior capsular shift operation was first described by Charles Neer[16] in 1980.
  - The procedure was designed to treat involuntary inferior and multidirectional instability of the shoulder that could not be addressed by repair of the anterior glenoid labrum alone (the Bankart procedure).
- The skin incision may be chosen based on the desired approach.

- The subscapularis tendon is incised about 1 to 2 cm medial to its insertion at the lesser tuberosity, leaving an adequate cuff of tissue for repair.
- The subscapularis consists of both a superior tendinous portion (two thirds) and inferior muscular (one third) portion.[14]
  - To expose the inferior portion of the glenohumeral joint capsule, it is important to carefully separate the

muscle fibers' insertion from the underlying anterior capsule using a combination of sharp and blunt dissection. The arm should be in a position of adduction and external rotation during this inferior dissection, and great care is taken to protect the axillary nerve.

- A laterally based capsular shift is then performed by incising the capsule vertically about 5 to 10 mm medial to its insertion on the humeral neck (see Tech Fig 1E,F).
- The medial leaf of the capsule is tagged sequentially with nonabsorbable sutures as the capsular incision is continued inferiorly to at least the 6 o'clock position (**TECH FIG 4A**).
- By placing traction on the capsular tag sutures in a superior and lateral direction, the axillary pouch should be obliterated when an adequate amount of capsular dissection has been performed.
- It is important to release the inferior capsular attachments to the humerus, which have a broad insertion inferior to the articular surface. This is typically done with blunt subperiosteal dissection with the periosteal elevator and needle-tip Bovie cautery (**TECH FIG 4B,C**).
- The medial insertion of the glenohumeral ligaments and glenoid labrum should then be assessed for avulsion or tear. Bankart lesion and ALPSA both describe a disrup-

tion of the medial capsulolabral complex that must be repaired.
- This technique is described in the Bankart repair technique section.
- Once secure fixation to bone is achieved, the capsule is shifted superiorly and laterally and the nonabsorbable sutures are passed through the capsule from an intra-articular to extra-articular location.
- It is important to place the sutures as close to the glenoid rim as possible so that the capsule is not shortened by medial plication.
- A bimanual technique can be used in which one needle driver is used to pass the suture and a second to "catch" the needle on the extra-articular side.
- The sutures are then tied on the extra-articular side to secure the capsule to the glenoid rim.
- If excess anteromedial capsular redundancy (AMCR) exists after the Bankart repair, a "barrel stitch" technique has been described in which a nonabsorbable pursestring suture is placed to imbricate the anterior capsule.[7]
- The barrel stitch is placed vertically at the level of the glenoid rim and tied on the extra-articular side. Its size is titrated to the amount of AMCR encountered (**TECH FIG 4D,E**).

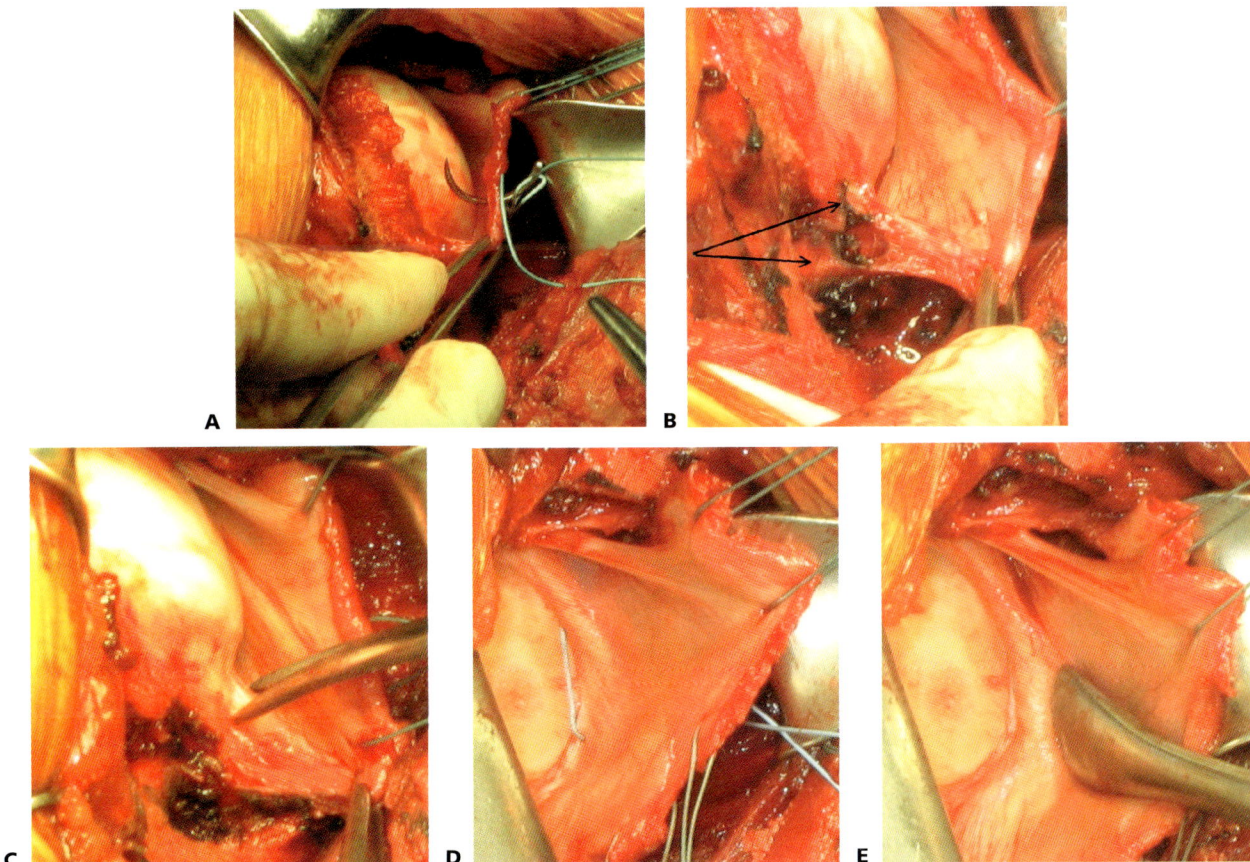

TECH FIG 4 • **A.** In the inferior capsule shift procedure, the laterally based capsular incision is continued inferiorly using tag stitches on the released anterior capsule to apply traction. **B.** There is a dual attachment of the inferior capsule on the humeral neck. **C.** Release of the dual inferior capsular attachment, allowing a complete shift of the capsule. **D.** An anterior crimping (barrel) stitch is used to decrease the redundancy of the anteroinferior capsule. This is a mattress stitch started on the superficial side of the capsule. **E.** Once tied, the barrel stitch reduces anterior medial capsular redundancy and an anterior inferior bolster is created. *(continued)*

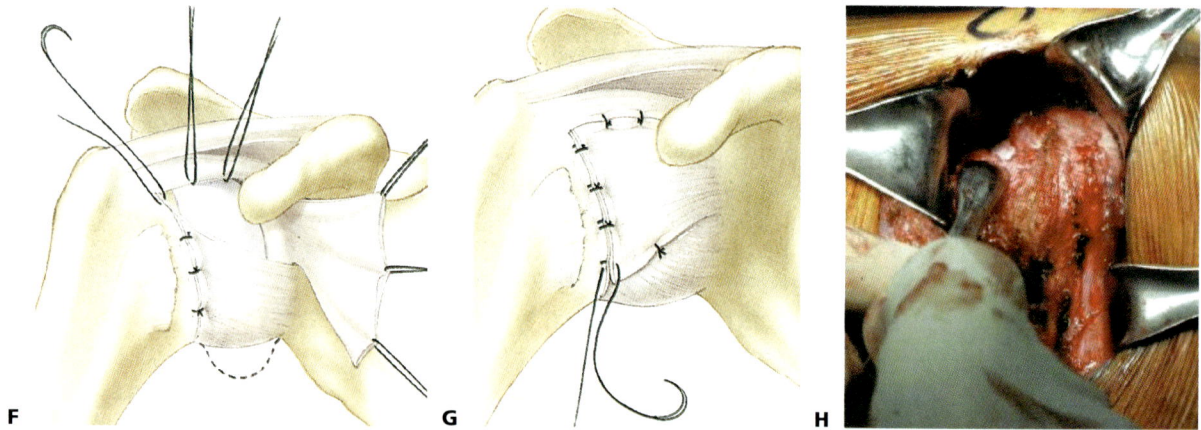

TECH FIG 4 • *(continued)* **F.** The anteroinferior capsule is advanced superiorly and reattached to the capsular sleeve preserved on the humeral neck. **G.** The superior flap is sewn to the inferior flap to reduce volume and increase strength. **H.** The rotator interval capsule is palpated between the subscapularis and supraspinatus tendons.

- Once the medial instability repair is complete, attention is directed to lateral repair of the capsule to the remaining cuff of tissue at the humeral neck.
- The capsule is shifted superiorly and laterally (**TECH FIG 4F**).
- The amount of external rotation should be titrated to the patient and should be based on the patient's age, quality of tissue, the presence of the generalized or local ligamentous laxity, sport, level of competition, arm dominance, and expected level of compliance with the prescribed rehabilitation program.
  - A good general guideline is to repair the shifted anterior capsule with the arm in 20 degrees of abduction and 30 degrees of external rotation.
- Throwers require an increased amount of external rotation in abduction and may require more laxity than a patient who is noncompliant or not involved in throwing sports.
- Excess tightening of the anterior capsule should be avoided to prevent the development of postcapsulorrhaphy arthropathy.[11]
- As the capsule is shifted superiorly and laterally, a lax capsule will have an abundance of capsular tissue remaining superiorly. In these shoulders, the capsular incision can be converted to a laterally based T capsulorrhaphy by incising the capsule between the inferior and middle glenohumeral ligaments down to the glenoid rim.
  - The inferior limb of the capsule is first repaired to its lateral insertion on the humerus.
  - The superior limb is folded down in a pants-over-vest fashion and repaired laterally to the insertion point (**TECH FIG 4G**). This will both reduce capsular volume and reinforce the anterior capsuloligamentous tissues.
- In addition to assessing residual capsular laxity, the rotator interval should also be assessed (**TECH FIG 4H**).
- If the rotator interval is widened or attenuated, it should be imbricated and closed using interrupted nonabsorbable sutures.
  - The amount of interval closure should also be titrated to the patient as mentioned previously, because excess tightening of the rotator interval can lead to restriction of external rotation.[10]
  - It may be preferable to close only the lateral portion of the rotator interval to preserve glenohumeral motion in competitive athletes.
- The subscapularis tendon is repaired anatomically at its insertion.

PEARLS AND PITFALLS

Voluntary instability	• Patients with voluntary instability should be carefully screened before surgery. If there are significant issues of secondary gain, surgical treatment will not be successful and should be discouraged. Preoperative psychiatric evaluation has been suggested but is seldom helpful in screening these patients.
Humeral bone defects (Hill-Sachs lesions)	• It is important to recognize and quantitate humeral bone defects, which are best seen on the radiograph (AP in internal rotation or Stryker notch view), CT scan, or MRI, or by diagnostic arthroscopy. With "engaging" defects, open treatment is favored over arthroscopic, and filling of the defect (autograft, allograft) may be considered.
Glenoid bone defects (bony Bankart)	• Glenoid defects can be assessed with preoperative imaging (radiographs, CT scan, MRI) and diagnostic arthroscopy. Significant defects (more than 30% of the glenoid) require a coracoid transfer (Bristow or Laterjet) procedure.

Posterior instability	■ The direction of instability should be assessed with preoperative examination and examination under anesthesia. If there is a significant posterior component, stability may be restored with a thorough inferior capsular shift. However, in some cases, an additional posterior approach may be required.
Associated SLAP (superior labral) tears	■ Additional labral pathology may be present in some patients with Bankart lesions. These injuries are often best managed arthroscopically, and if suspected, may require diagnostic arthroscopy to confirm and repair before an open incision.

POSTOPERATIVE CARE

- The rehabilitation protocol must be planned individually.
- The patient remains in a sling for 4 weeks postoperatively.
- Passive forward elevation to 110 degrees and external rotation to 15 degrees is begun at 10 days to 2 weeks, and is gradually increased to 140 degrees forward elevation and 30 degrees external rotation by 4 weeks. During this period, isometric strengthening exercises are begun.
- From 4 to 6 weeks, elevation is increased to about 160 degrees and external rotation to 40 degrees.
- After 6 weeks, motion is increased to achieve a normal range.
- Exercises should be progressed slowly to avoid apprehension and resubluxation.
- Resistive exercises are begun with the arm in neutral below 90 degrees and progressed gradually.
- Strengthening of scapular stabilizers is particularly important.
- Full motion and strength should be regained before contact sports are resumed, usually between 6 and 9 months, depending on the sport and the patient.

OUTCOMES

- The first long-term follow-up study of the Bankart procedure was reported by Carter Rowe[22] in 1978, with only a 3.5% rate of redislocation.
- Neer[16] reported on 40 unstable shoulders that were repaired with the anterior inferior capsular shift between 1974 and 1979, 11 of which had undergone prior procedures for glenohumeral instability. Satisfactory results were achieved in all except one patient, who had postoperative subluxation of the shoulder.
- Since Neer's initial report, multiple series have been published that have used the anterior inferior capsular shift procedure for anteroinferior instability. Although the surgical technique and the extent of capsular shift may vary with different surgeons, recurrence rates have ranged from 1.5% to 9%.[5,6,9,16,25]

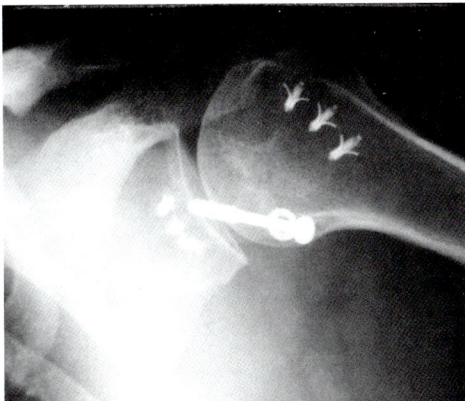

FIG 7 • AP radiograph of a left shoulder showing loose hardware after a prior coracoid transfer procedure.

- T-plasty results: In 42 shoulders with an average of 3 years of follow-up in this initial series, 95% of the patients were satisfied and there were four recurrences (10%).[2]
- A report on the results of anterior capsulolabral reconstruction at an average of 39 months of follow-up in 25 throwing athletes found excellent or good results in 92% of patients, and 17 (68%) returned to their prior level of competition.
  - A subsequent series of 22 subluxators and 9 dislocators found 97% good to excellent results and 94% return to sport.[15]
- Return-to-sport rates of 32% to 94% have been reported for open surgical treatment of anteroinferior instability in various series.[2,5,12]

COMPLICATIONS

- Injury to the axillary nerve can occur as it travels an average of only 2.5 mm deep to the IGHL and lies only 12 mm from the glenoid at the 6 o'clock position.
  - Nerve injury typically involves sensory function only, and function usually recovers spontaneously.
- Recurrent dislocations may occur in up to 5% of patients. However, this rate may be higher when appropriate indications for surgery are not strictly followed.
- Hardware-related complications may occur owing to loosening, bending or breakage of screws, anchors, or tacks (**FIG 7**).[26]
- Synovitis in response to PLLA absorbable implants has also been described.
- Misplacement of labral tacks or suture anchors, both metallic and absorbable, may lead to early arthrosis or arthritis.
- Complications due to positioning have been described including deep venous thrombosis and compression neurapraxia. Bony prominences should be well padded and constrictive bandaging avoided during and after surgery.
- Infection in shoulder surgery is uncommon. When it occurs, however, *Propionibacterium acnes* is a common organism, and specific cultures should be requested.

REFERENCES

1. Allain J, Goutallier D, Glorion C. Long-term results of the Latarjet procedure for the treatment of anterior instability of the shoulder. J Bone Joint Surg Am 1998;80A:841–852.
2. Altchek DW, Warren RF, Skyhar MJ, et al. T-plasty modification of the Bankart procedure for multidirectional instability of the anterior and inferior types. J Bone Joint Surg Am 1991;73A:105–112.
3. Bankart AS. The pathology and treatment of recurrent dislocation of the shoulder joint. Br J Surg 1938;26:23–29.
4. Bigliani LU, Kelkar R, Flatow EL, et al. Glenohumeral stability: biomechanical properties of passive and active stabilizers. Clin Orthop Relat Res 1996;330:13–30.
5. Bigliani LU, Kurzweil PR, Schwartzbach CC, et al. Inferior capsular shift procedure for anterior-inferior shoulder instability in athletes. Am J Sports Med 1994;22:578–584.
6. Cooper RA, Brems JJ. The inferior capsular-shift procedure for multidirectional instability of the shoulder. J Bone Joint Surg Am 1992;74A:1516–1522.

7. Flatow EL. Glenohumeral instability. In: Bigliani LU, Flatow EL, Pollock RG, et al., eds. The Shoulder: Operative Technique. Baltimore: Williams & Wilkins, 1998:183–184.

8. Gill TJ, Micheli LJ, Gebhard F, et al. Bankart repair for anterior instability of the shoulder: long-term outcome. J Bone Joint Surg Am 1997;79A:850–857.

9. Hamada K, Fukuda H, Nakajima T, et al. The inferior capsular shift operation for instability of the shoulder: long-term results in 34 shoulders. J Bone Joint Surg Br 1999;81B:218–225.

10. Harryman DT, Sidles JA, Harris SL, et al. The role of the rotator interval capsule in passive motion and stability of the shoulder. J Bone Joint Surg Am 1992;74A:53–66.

11. Hawkins RJ, Angelo RL. Glenohumeral osteoarthrosis: a late complication of the Putti-Platt repair. J Bone Joint Surg Am 1990;72A:1193–1197.

12. Jobe FW, Giangarra CE, Kvitne RS, et al. Anterior capsulolabral reconstruction of the shoulder in athletes in overhand sports. Am J Sports Med 1991;19:428–434.

13. Kirkley A, Griffin S, Richards C, et al. Prospective randomized clinical trial comparing the effectiveness of immediate arthroscopic stabilization versus immobilization and rehabilitation in first traumatic anterior dislocations of the shoulder. Arthroscopy 1999;15:507–514.

14. Klapper RJ, Jobe FW, Matsuura P. The subscapularis muscle and its glenohumeral ligament like bands: a histomorphologic study. Am J Sports Med 1992;20:307–310.

15. Montgomery WH III, Jobe FW. Functional outcomes in athletes after modified anterior capsulolabral reconstruction. Am J Sports Med 1994;22:352–358.

16. Neer CS II, Foster CR. Inferior capsular shift for involuntary inferior and multidirectional instability of the shoulder: a preliminary report. J Bone Joint Surg Am 1980;62A:897–908.

17. Neviaser TJ. The anterior labroligamentous periosteal sleeve avulsion lesion: a cause of anterior instability of the shoulder. Arthroscopy 1993;9:17–21.

18. Osmond-Clarke H. Habitual dislocation of the shoulder: the Putti-Platt operation. J Bone Joint Surg Br 1948;30B:19–25.

19. Owens BD, Dawson L, Burks R, et al. The incidence of shoulder dislocation in the United States military: demographic considerations from a high-risk population. J Bone Joint Surg [Am] 2009;91:791-796.

20. Perthes G. Uber Operationen bei habitueller Schulterluxation. Deutsche Zeitschr Chir 1906;85:199–227.

21. Pollock RG, Bigliani LU. Glenohumeral instability: evaluation and treatment. J Acad Orthop Surg 1993;1:24–32.

22. Rowe C, Patel D, Southmayd WW. The Bankart procedure, a long-term end result study. J Bone Joint Surg Am 1978;60A:1–16.

23. Simonet WT, Melton LJ, Cofield RH, et al. Incidence of anterior shoulder dislocation in Olmstead County, Minnesota. Clin Orthop Relat Res 1984;186:186–191.

24. Wheeler JH, Ryan JB, Arciero RA, et al. Arthroscopic versus non-operative treatment of acute shoulder dislocation in young athletes. Arthroscopy 1989;5:513–517.

25. Wirth MA, Groh GI, Rockwood CA Jr. Capsulorrhaphy through an anterior approach for the treatment of atraumatic posterior glenohumeral instability with multidirectional laxity of the shoulder. J Bone Joint Surg Am 1998;80A:1570–1578.

26. Zuckerman J, Matsen F. Complications about the shoulder related to the use of screws and staples. J Bone Joint Surg Am 1984;66A:175–180.

DEFINITION

- Symptomatic recurrent posterior instability represents up to 12% of all cases of shoulder instability and is subdivided into two discrete entities.[28,35]
- The first, true posterior dislocation is acute in nature and often related to trauma. It is readily managed with shoulder reduction and carries a low recurrence rate if not associated with a large engaging humeral head defect or a primary uncontrolled seizure disorder.
  - If the primary dislocation is overlooked, this condition can manifest itself as a chronic locked posterior dislocation with its pathognomonic internally rotated position and loss of external rotation on physical examination.
- The second entity is recurrent unidirectional posterior subluxation, which often represents the more challenging dilemma confronting the orthopaedic surgeon and will be the principal topic of this chapter.
  - Whether due to an increase in awareness by physicians or a more active athletic population, recurrent unidirectional posterior instability is being recognized, diagnosed, and treated more frequently.
  - Patients with recurrent posterior subluxation complain primarily of pain and weakness. As time progresses, symptoms of posterior subluxation become a secondary complaint. Eventually patients often learn the selected muscular contractions, scapular winging, and arm position (forward elevation, adduction, and internal rotation) needed to demonstrate their instability.
- See Table 1 for the classification of posterior instability.

ANATOMY

- Posterior instability may be secondary to a tear of the posteroinferior labrum or a patulous posterior capsule.

Table 1	Classification of Posterior Instability

Acute posterior dislocation
Without impression defect
With impression defect

Chronic posterior dislocation
Locked (missed) with impression defect

Recurrent posterior subluxation
Voluntary
   Habitual (willful)
   Muscular control (not willful)
Involuntary
   Positional (demonstrable)
   Nonpositional (not demonstrable)

- Rarely it can involve a posterior labrocapsular periosteal sleeve avulsion or an avulsion of the posterior glenohumeral ligaments as they insert on the humerus (posterior HAGL lesion).
- Recently Kim described a concealed and incomplete avulsion of the posteroinferior labrum (type II marginal crack or Kim lesion).[20]
- Pathology may also be bony in nature and secondary to posterior glenoid avulsions, erosions, increased glenoid retroversion or large engaging reverse Hill-Sachs impression defects.

PATHOGENESIS

- A significant percentage of patients (40% to 50%) with recurrent posterior subluxation relate a history of trauma. Usually athletes, these individuals are 18 to 30 years of age and are involved in competitive contact sports.
- Traumatic cases are often associated with the arm in a straight and locked position such as in weight lifting or during football while line blocking. A fall or collision with the individual's arm in at-risk position (forward elevation, adduction, internal rotation) can also be the cause.
- Frequently, instead of a traumatic event, subluxation episodes with a poorly defined onset are clearly documented.
- In many cases, especially with repetitive overhead endeavors such as swimming, gymnastics, baseball, and volleyball, the athlete recalls first the gradual onset of discomfort, with subluxation episodes occurring later. Such an onset is thought to be atraumatic and involves repetitive "microtrauma" with resultant stretching of the capsular restraints.

PATIENT HISTORY AND PHYSICAL FINDINGS

- Whether the patient presents with a clear traumatic episode or a longer atraumatic course, he or she often has a feeling of the shoulder "coming out." Such instability episodes occur when the arm is in the at-risk position of forward elevation, adduction, and internal rotation.
- Patients often describe a vague discomfort, pain, or weakness as their principal complaint. This actually may lead to misdiagnosis at first.
- True apprehension or a feeling of "impending doom" when the extremity is placed in the provocative position is less common but can be present.
- Overhead throwers may complain of a loss of velocity, fatigue, or aching over the posterior shoulder.
- Usually there is no obvious asymmetry of the muscles on inspection.
- Palpation may elicit some tenderness along the posterior glenohumeral joint line.
- Crepitation or a click along the posterior joint line due to labral pathology may be noted.
- The range of motion is full, often with a decrease in internal rotation and an excess of external rotation.

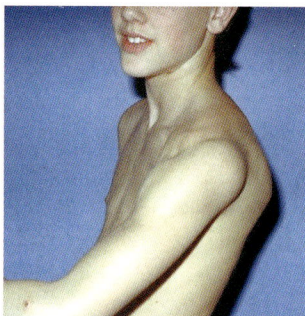

FIG 1 • Younger patient able to voluntarily demonstrate, with muscular contraction and positioning of the upper extremity, his posterior instability.

- Often patients, if voluntary subluxators, can reproduce the subluxation episode on command with arm position and selective muscular contraction (**FIG 1**).
- Physical examination should include the following:
  - Modified load shift test: documents direction and degree of instability
  - Supine load shift test (Gerber and Ganz)[13]: documents direction and degree of instability
  - Seated load shift test: documents direction and degree of instability
  - Posterior stress test: documents direction and degree of instability
  - Sulcus sign: evaluates for an inferior component of the posterior instability (bidirectional) or a more global instability (ie, multidirectional instability)
  - Scapular compression test: verifies the importance of scapular winging in the patient's ability to reproduce the instability and proves to the patient the need to strengthen the periscapular musculature to control instability
  - Jerk test: to document instability. A painful jerk test suggests a posteroinferior labral lesion and is a predictor of the success of nonoperative treatment.
  - Kim test: evaluates for the presence of a labral tear posteriorly
  - Pivot shift of the shoulder: documents direction of the instability

IMAGING AND OTHER DIAGNOSTIC STUDIES

- Radiographic evaluation includes a three-view trauma series of the shoulder, including a true anteroposterior (AP) view of the shoulder, a scapular lateral, and, more importantly, an axillary view.
  - A Velpeau axillary view can be substituted if the attempted axillary view is impossible because of painful abduction of the shoulder.
  - Axillary radiographs of patients with a voluntary component to their instability can be taken while the patient reproduces and maintains the subluxation episode to document the direction (**FIG 2A**).
  - A computed tomography (CT) scan is rarely needed but can be helpful to evaluate humeral head defects and associated fractures of the tuberosities, humeral shaft, and posterior glenoid rim. Significant posterior glenoid retroversion can also be demonstrated on CT scanning (**FIG 2B**).

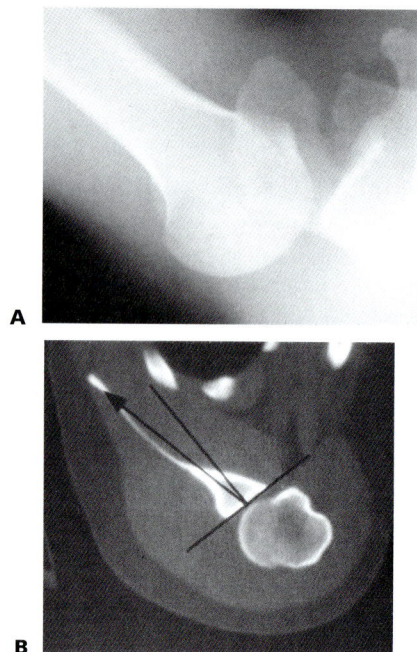

FIG 2 • **A.** Axillary radiograph of patient with voluntary posterior instability, reproducing the instability while taking the radiograph. **B.** CT scan demonstrating significant posterior glenoid retroversion in a patient with posterior instability.

- MRI is the imaging modality of choice after plain radiographs to evaluate the posterior capsule and labrum for tears and associated pathology.
- In certain situations a MRI arthrogram can help diagnose a posteroinferior labral tear.

DIFFERENTIAL DIAGNOSIS

- Superior labrum anterior from posterior tear (SLAP)
- Anterior instability
- Multidirectional instability
- Internal impingement
- Posterior Bennett lesion

NONOPERATIVE MANAGEMENT

- Nonsurgical treatment of posterior unidirectional instability is reportedly successful in up to 80% of the patients.[9,18]
  - The physical therapy program consists of concentric and eccentric resistive band exercises that strengthen the external rotators, the deltoid, and the important periscapular musculature.
    - Resistive upright and seated rows, with an emphasis on trying to pinch the medial scapular borders together during the exercise, are key, especially in patients whose scapular winging contributes to their instability.
  - A strengthening program as well as a sport-specific attempt to decrease those activities that place the arm at risk is key.
- The length of nonoperative treatment must be individualized.
  - Patients who have lower physical demands, are younger, and have an atraumatic history are treated 6 months or more.
  - Higher-level athletes or those who have a traumatic cause with an associated labral tear are more likely to respond to surgical treatment. Despite their associated labral tears, such

elite athletes are often treated with an exercise strengthening program for at least 3 months.

SURGICAL MANAGEMENT

■ Although open procedures have been the mainstay and gold standard in the treatment of patients with recurrent unidirectional posterior subluxation, when nonoperative care has failed, arthroscopic treatment has become common.

■ As with anterior instability 20 years ago, arthroscopic evaluation in posterior instability patients has led to the diagnosis and treatment of an increasing number of associated soft tissue and articular injuries. Obviously, arthroscopic treatment of posterior capsular avulsions or redundancy in the absence of soft tissue deficiencies or bony abnormalities can have similar success rates without the morbidity of more extensive open surgery.[2,6,20,33]

■ Surgical treatment is considered only after an adequate trial of strengthening has failed and the patient remains significantly symptomatic.

■ The ideal surgical candidates are those with recurrent posterior unidirectional subluxation secondary to a traumatic episode. These patients often have an associated traumatic posterior labral tear, which is optimal for arthroscopic repair.

■ Patients with atraumatic subluxation due to capsular redundancy can be managed either through an open procedure or an arthroscopic capsular shift or plication procedure.

■ Patients who have multifactorial causes for their instability or are revision situations are better treated with an open approach.

Preoperative Planning

■ An extensive history and physical examination are key to establishing the direction and degree of the patient's instability.

■ All imaging studies are reviewed. Plain films and MRI studies are reviewed for the presence of old fractures, loose bodies, and hardware from previous procedures. More importantly, the MRI establishes whether the instability is due to an associated traumatic posterior labral tear or capsular redundancy.

■ Associated bony pathology (traumatic glenoid avulsions, glenoid retroversion) and soft tissue deficiencies (from previous procedures) should be addressed concurrently.

■ Examination, this time under anesthesia, should be accomplished before positioning to confirm the direction and degree of the instability.

ARTHROSCOPIC POSTERIOR RECONSTRUCTION (AUTHORS' PREFERRED TECHNIQUE)

TECHNIQUES

Positioning

■ The patient is positioned in a lateral decubitus position with the operative arm placed in about 40 degrees of abduction and no more than 10 pounds of longitudinal traction.

■ All pressure points are carefully identified and an axillary roll is placed under the down axilla.

■ The patient's body is placed close to the operating surgeon and tipped posteriorly 15 to 20 degrees.

■ We do not employ a double traction set-up, as we do in anterior instability, because increased adduction tends to close down visualization of the posteroinferior joint line, and we have found optimal visualization with 40 degrees of abduction when viewing from the anterior portal.

Portal Placement

■ Most posterior reconstructions are performed using only two portals.

■ The first is a posterior portal established just lateral to the posterior lateral corner of the acromion.

■ This differs from the traditional posterior viewing portal, which is 1 cm medial and 2 cm inferior from the posterior lateral corner of the acromion.

■ Lateralization of this portal and moving it somewhat superiorly provides an optimal angle of attack to the posterior and inferior portion of the posterior glenoid.

■ The anterior portal is established in the rotator interval under direct visualization using needle localization.

■ A 6.5-mm cannula is established to allow insertion of the arthroscope and an 8-mm cannula is placed in the posterior portal to allow the passage of the Spectrum crescent suture-passing devices (ConMed Linvatec, Largo, FL).

Site Preparation

■ Repair is begun by assessing the posterior labral construct for the presence of labral displacement and tearing (**TECH FIG 1A**).

■ A grasper is used to capture the posterior band of the inferior glenohumeral ligament (IGHL), attempting to mobilize it superiorly to determine the amount of capsular laxity and ultimate position for repair.

■ If a posterior Bankart lesion is identified, a Liberator knife (ConMed Linvatec, Largo, FL) is used to mobilize the labrum (**TECH FIG 1B**), while a shaver or burr is used to débride the posterior face of the glenoid in preparation for anchor placement (**TECH FIG 1C**).

■ This is a critical step so that a freely mobile labrum can be placed up on the glenoid, thereby restoring its bumper effect. Anchor placement begins at the most inferior aspect of the glenoid, usually the 5:30 or 6:30 position, depending on the side involved (**TECH FIG 1D**).

■ This position allows secure placement of an anchor while allowing optimal inferior capsular plication. Bioabsorbable anchors are employed for this reconstruction (**TECH FIG 1E**).

TECHNIQUES

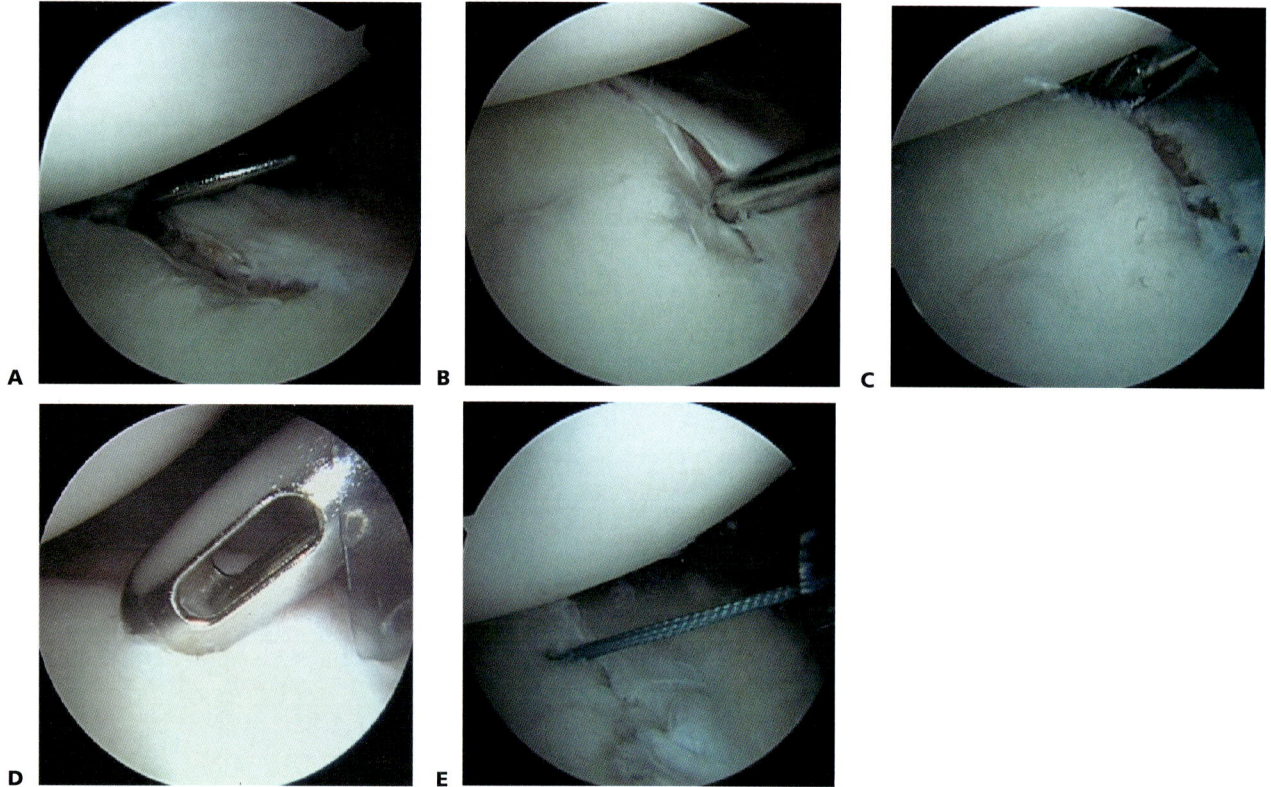

A   B   C

D   E

TECH FIG 1 • A. Probe entering the posterior cannula is demonstrating mobility of posterior Bankart lesion with evidence of granulation tissue in the defect. **B.** After the lesion is defined, a Liberator knife is introduced to take down the fibrous interface in the posterior Bankart lesion. **C.** After preparation using a high-speed burr, the posterior inferior aspect of the glenoid is lightly decorticated in preparation for anchor placement. **D.** Initial anchor placement begins at the inferior extent of the glenoid with the use of a guide. **E.** First anchor in place 2 mm up on the articular surface.

Suturing

- A Spectrum 45-degree-offset suture passer, preloaded with a number 0 polydioxanone (PDS) monofilament suture (Ethicon, Somerville NJ), is passed through the posterior cannula, capturing the inferior capsule in the area of the posterior band of the IGHL (**TECH FIG 2A**).
  - This tissue is brought superiorly and the second pass comes deep, exiting at the posterior labral defect.
- The PDS suture is reeled into the joint through the passer

and retrieved in the posterior cannula using a ring grasper (**TECH FIG 2B,C**).

- The deep limb of the PDS is tied to one limb of the anchor suture, and using a pulling technique, the PDS is drawn in a retrograde fashion, with the anchor suture attached, through the capsule and labral tissue, thereby creating a simple stitch (**TECH FIG 2D**).
  - This allows the inferior capsule to be drawn superiorly and medially while at the same time closing the posterior Bankart lesion.

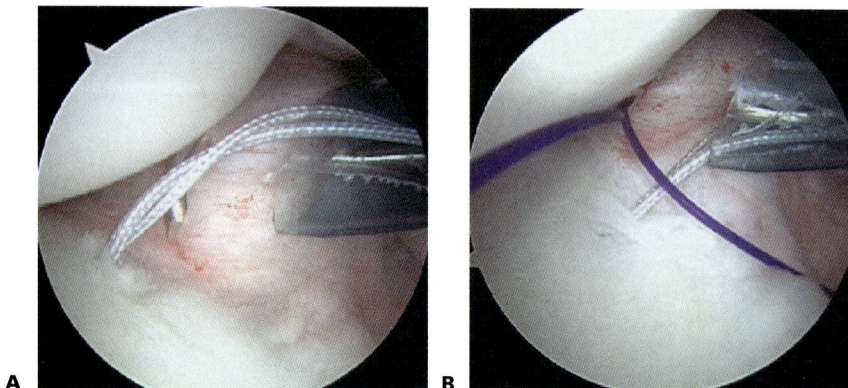

A   B

TECH FIG 2 • A. The Spectrum suture passer is used to capture inferior capsular tissue and the posterior band of the inferior glenohumeral ligament. **B.** After anchor placement, stability is assessed with gentle traction on the anchor sutures and a monofilament suture is passed through the suture passer. *(continued)*

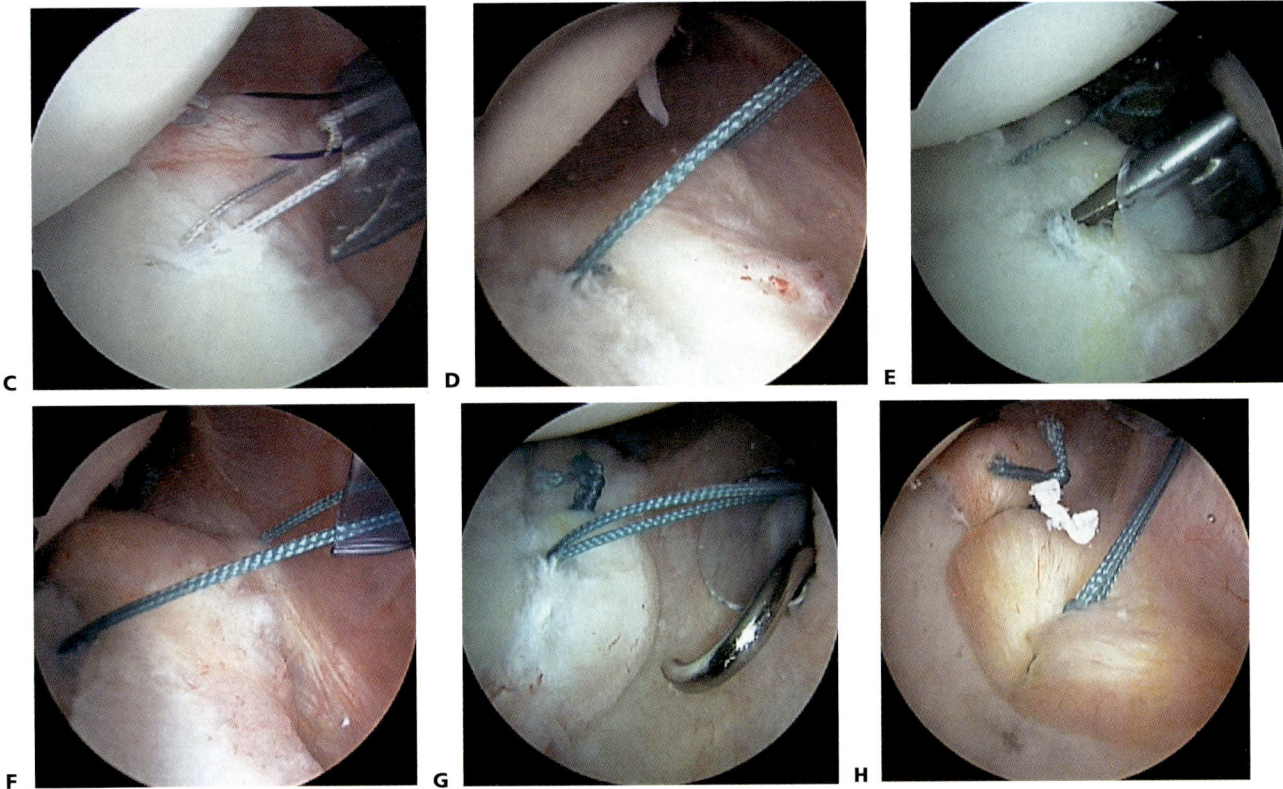

TECH FIG 2 • *(continued)* **C.** The monofilament suture, having been passed through a capsule inferiorly, is drawn up to assess capsular mobility and determine the amount of translation. **D.** One limb of the anchor suture is tied to the monofilament suture, which is then drawn back out the posterior cannula, thus creating a simple stitch. **E.** Having tied the suture on the first anchor, a drill hole is created 7 to 8 mm superiorly for the second anchor. **F.** A second anchor suture has been passed, demonstrating the purchase of additional posterior capsule. **G.** With the final superior anchor in position, the suture passer is directed superiorly to capture additional posteromedial capsule and superior labrum. **H.** Final anchor sutures are tied, demonstrating excellent reconstruction of the posterolabral defect, recreating the posterior labrum bumper effect.

- A second suture is placed after tying the first suture in a similar fashion, again incorporating the capsule as well as labrum (**TECH FIG 2E,F**).
- This process is repeated as many times as is necessary, moving superiorly at 6-mm to 8-mm increments, thereby obliterating any labral defect and capsular redundancy (**TECH FIG 2G,H**).

Capsular Plication

- Alternatively, if no labral detachment is identified and only excessive capsular redundancy exists, a posterior superior capsular shift without anchors is performed.
- The posterior capsule is lightly abraded with a synovial shaver or rasp to promote healing.
- A Spectrum suture passer is used again to pierce the capsule 1 cm lateral to the labrum at the 6:30 position on the glenoid.
- The capsule is then advanced superiorly and medially, with the suture passer re-entering the joint at the junction between the intact labrum and the glenoid rim articular cartilage.

- This is repeated at least two or three times, depending on amount of laxity.
- With each suture the capsule is advanced about one hour's position on the glenoid face (ie, 6:30 capsular stitch to the 7:30 labral position, 7:30 to 8:30, and so on).

Rotator Interval Plication

- In individuals with a significant component of ligamentous laxity, additional closure of the rotator interval is accomplished by moving the arthroscope back to the posterior portal.
- Through the anterior portal, a number 0 PDS suture is passed through the upper border of the middle glenohumeral ligament, capturing the superior glenohumeral ligament and rotator interval capsule.
  - This suture is used as a pulling stitch for a number 2 braided polyester fiber (TI•CRON) suture (Tyco, United States Surgical, Norwalk, CT).
- This is repeated again and sutures are tied just outside the capsule.

TECHNIQUES

OPEN POSTERIOR HUMERAL-BASED CAPSULAR SHIFT (AUTHORS' PREFERRED TECHNIQUE)

Positioning

- Under general anesthesia the patient is positioned in the lateral decubitus position using a full-length beanbag.
- A large axillary roll is placed under the down nonsurgical axilla.
- The operative arm and shoulder are draped free.

Incision and Dissection

- A longitudinal incision in the posterior axillary fold is made beginning at a point 2 cm medial to the posterolateral corner of the acromion and extending distally, following the posterior axillary line (**TECH FIG 3**).
- The underlying deltoid muscle is split along its fibers bluntly, and a self-retaining retractor is placed.[34]
  - Caution should be exercised as to not split the deltoid distally greater than 4 to 5 cm to avoid injuring the axillary nerve.[8,34]
  - If the individual is larger and more exposure is needed, the deltoid can be detached from its scapular origin for a short distance, leaving a small tendinous attachment to repair later.
- Repair of the deltoid origin can also be accomplished by placing drill holes along the scapular spine for suture passage.

- The underlying infraspinatus is identified by its bipennate nature, a central fatty raphe dividing the muscle, and the fiber direction change compared with the teres minor inferiorly.
- The infraspinatus can be handled in three ways:
  - It can be split horizontally to expose the underlying capsule.[32] Care is taken with this technique not to extend the split farther than 1.5 to 2 cm medial to the glenoid rim, as the infraspinatus branches of the suprascapular nerve are coursing along the inferior fascia of the infraspinatus directly on the scapular surface. Extension of the split into the branches or elevation of the fascia off the scapula will injure a number of, if not all, the branches to the infraspinatus.
  - The second method is to identify the interval between the infraspinatus and teres minor. This interval is developed with the muscle being worked superiorly, thereby exposing underlying capsule.
  - Third, the infraspinatus may be completely detached, leaving a 2-cm remnant of the tendon still attached for later repair (**TECH FIG 4**). It is tagged and carefully released from the underlying thin capsule.

Capsulotomy

- A vertical capsulotomy is made on the humeral side with the arm in neutral rotation (**TECH FIG 5A**).

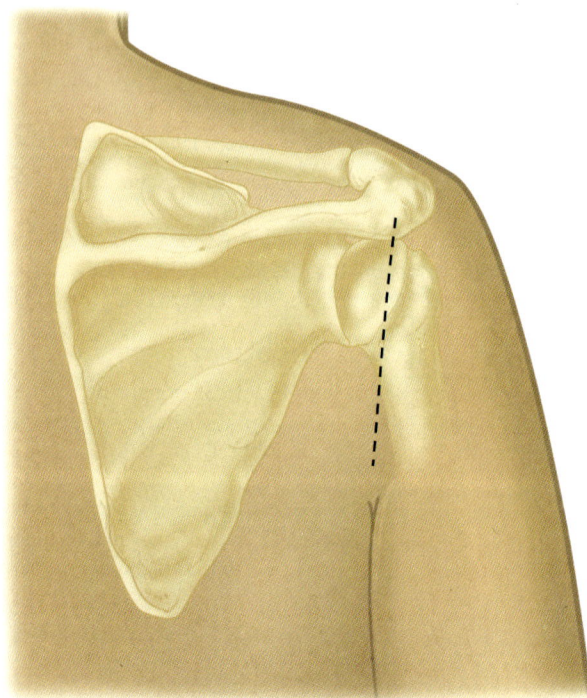

TECH FIG 3 • The posterior longitudinal incision begins about 2 cm medial to the posterolateral corner of the acromion and extends into the axillary crease.

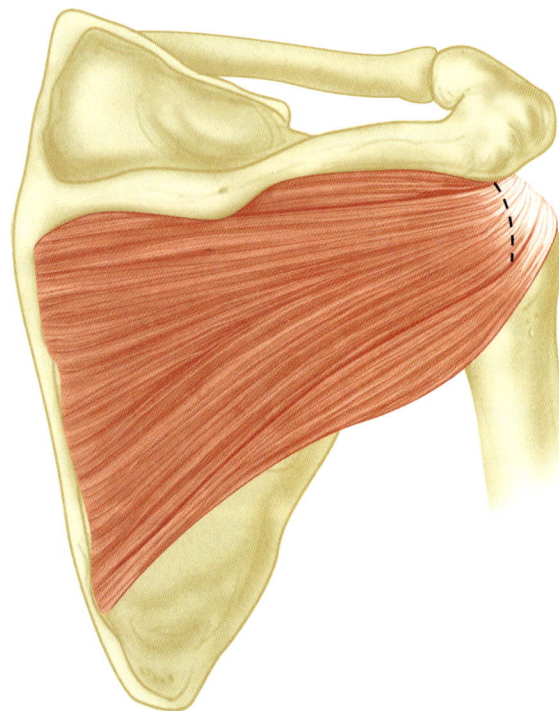

TECH FIG 4 • With the deltoid fibers bluntly split, a vertical incision is made directly through the infraspinatus while keeping a small stump of infraspinatus tendon attached laterally for reattachment later.

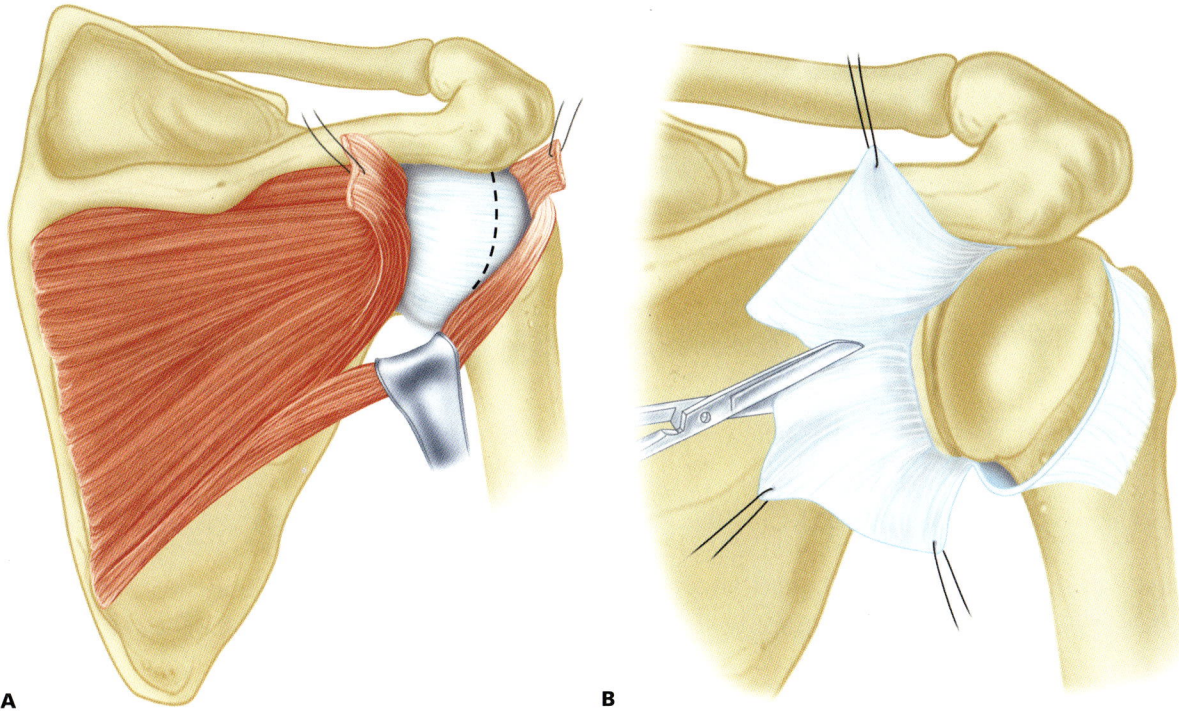

A

B

TECH FIG 5 • A. The infraspinatus is elevated as a single layer, exposing the underlying posterior capsule. A vertical cap-sulotomy is then made based on the humeral side from the 12 o'clock to the 6 o'clock position. **B.** Traction stitches are then placed as the medial capsule is divided horizontally, between the sutures, toward but not through the glenoid labrum.

- A small amount of capsule, 3 to 4 mm, can be left on its humeral attachment to aid in repair of the capsu-lar flaps laterally during the shift.
- Care is taken to protect the axillary nerve inferiorly from retractors as it is traversing from anterior to pos-terior to exit in the quadrangular space inferiorly.
- With the vertical capsulotomy completed, two traction stitches are placed at the midposition and the capsule is horizontally divided, between the stitches, toward the middle of the glenoid rim, stopping 1 to 2 mm from the posterior glenoid labrum (**TECH FIG 5B**).

T Capsulorrhaphy

- Although both medial and lateral capsular shifts have been described, we prefer a humeral-based T capsulor-rhaphy because we believe tensioning of the capsular flaps is easier to control and a larger volume reduction can be achieved, if desired.
- Those who prefer a glenoid-based T-capsular shift cite ad-vantages of a muscle-splitting approach and ease of repair if an associated reverse Bankart lesion is encountered.
  - If a glenoid-based shift is selected, most authors posi-tion the arm in 20 degrees of abduction and neutral to 20 degrees of external rotation while doing the capsular repair.

Posterior Inferior Capsular Shift

- The posterior glenoid labrum is inspected and if there is a small detachment, it is repaired before completing the capsular shift procedure.

- The inferior flap of the capsule is carefully mobilized past the 6-o'clock position, inferiorly on the humerus.
  - This step is critical as an inadequate release of the in-ferior capsule will prevent correction of the pos-teroinferior capsular redundancy and volume.
- The nonarticular sulcus, medial to the capsular remnant left behind, is then decorticated with a high-speed burr to facilitate healing (**TECH FIG 6A**).
- The inferior capsular flap is brought superiorly and slightly laterally with the arm held in 40 to 45 degrees of abduction and 15 to 20 degrees of external rotation.
- This inferior flap is sutured in place with multiple figure eight nonabsorbable sutures.
  - If the capsular remnant to suture to is of poor quality, suture anchors are used for repair. In a similar fashion, the superior capsular flap is shifted inferiorly down over the inferior flap and sutured (**TECH FIG 6B,C**).
- The horizontal portion of the T capsulorrhaphy is then closed and reinforced with nonabsorbable sutures.
  - The degree of closure of this horizontal portion can further tighten the posterior capsule if desired.
- If the infraspinatus was released with a small remnant left attached to the humeral side, the infraspinatus is su-tured back to its tendinous stump anatomically with nonabsorbable suture.
- If the infraspinatus was split, it is allowed to fall back in position and the fascia is closed with absorbable suture.
- Routine closure is performed, and the arm is placed into a shoulder orthosis or spica cast depending on patient compliance, incorporating 20 degrees of abduction and 20 degrees of external rotation.

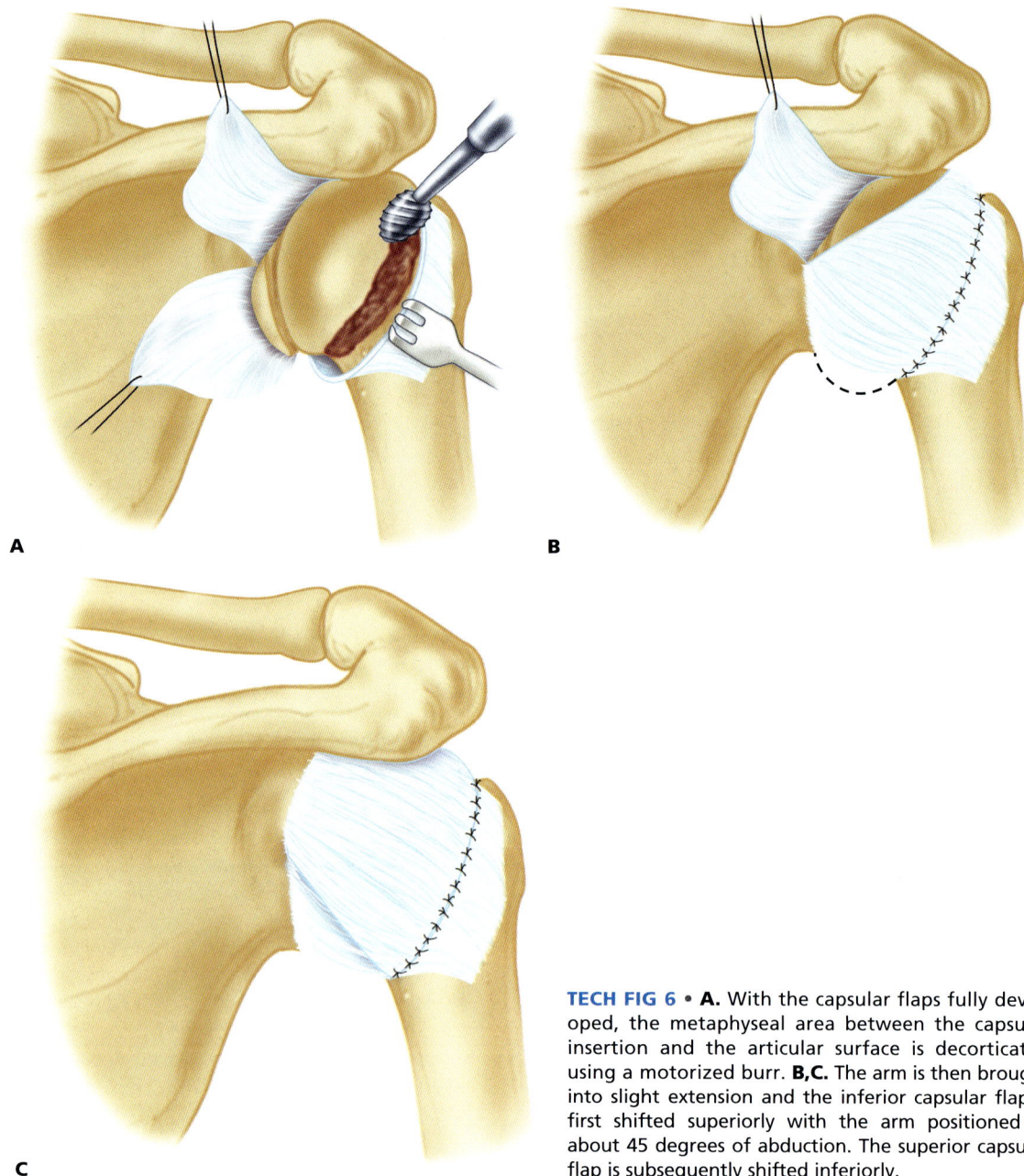

TECH FIG 6 • A. With the capsular flaps fully developed, the metaphyseal area between the capsular insertion and the articular surface is decorticated using a motorized burr. **B,C.** The arm is then brought into slight extension and the inferior capsular flap is first shifted superiorly with the arm positioned in about 45 degrees of abduction. The superior capsular flap is subsequently shifted inferiorly.

OPEN POSTERIOR LABRAL REPAIR (REVERSE BANKART REPAIR)

- The patient positioning and surgical exposure are similar down to the infraspinatus musculature.
- The infraspinatus can be split, as is our preference, or a horizontal incision can be made 2 cm lateral to the glenoid rim through both the infraspinatus and capsule as one layer.
- The posterior capsulolabral tissue is freely mobilized from the glenoid neck.
- The scapular neck is then decorticated with a motorized burr to promote healing and the labrum is reattached using the surgeon's preferred commercially available absorbable suture anchors or through transosseous tunnels.

- Again, the goal is to roll the labrum up onto the posterior glenoid rim, restoring the capsulolabral bumper effect.
- Although this procedure is usually done as a primary procedure, it may be combined with a humeral or glenoid based posterior-inferior T-capsular shift in patients with excessive laxity or instability on clinical examination.
- Care must be taken not to overtighten the repair when both procedures are used, since postoperative stiffness and loss of motion, especially internal rotation, can occur.

TECHNIQUES

OPEN POSTERIOR INFRASPINATUS CAPSULAR TENODESIS

- The posterior infraspinatus and capsular tenodesis, as described by Hawkins, is reproducible and takes advantage of the thick quality of the infraspinatus tendon and underlying capsule layer.[4,16]
- It is extremely useful, in our opinion, in situations of poor-quality capsular tissue, since often the posterior capsule is only 1 to 2 mm thick, and in revision cases in which multiple posterior procedures have failed (**TECH FIG 7**).

Positioning

- This technique is performed using the same positioning and exposure as described earlier down to the infraspinatus musculature.
- Preoperatively the patient can be placed into an outrigger shoulder spica cast with a fiberglass long-arm component and a detachable spica bar or a shoulder orthosis.
- Preparation and draping are done with the involved arm free.

Incision and Approach

- The same posterior axillary incision and split of the underlying deltoid muscle described earlier are used.
- With the arm in neutral position, the glenoid rim is located under the infraspinatus using a spinal needle, starting medially and walking the needle laterally over the glenoid rim until the exact location of the joint is identified.
- This position is then marked to confirm the lateral extent of the glenoid rim.
  - This is a crucial step because if the vertical incision to be made through both the infraspinatus and capsule is made too far laterally, severe overtightening will result.

Vertical Arthrotomy

- A single vertical incision is made through the infraspinatus tendon and underlying capsule parallel to and 1.0 to

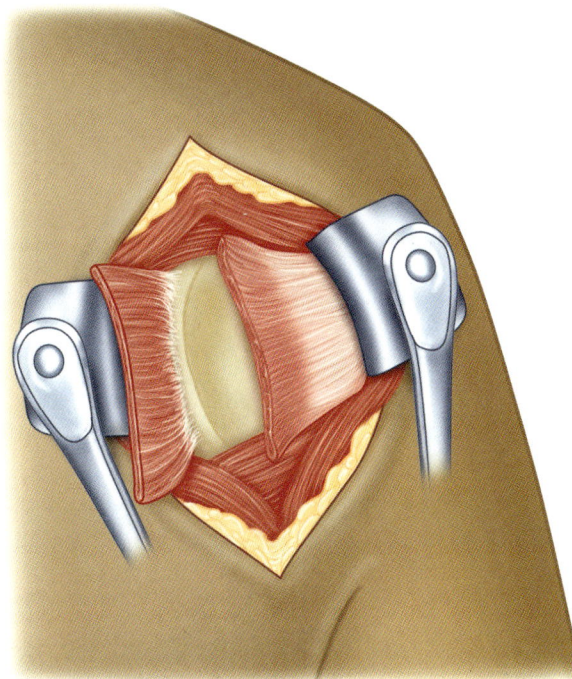

TECH FIG 8 • The arm is positioned in neutral rotation and the infraspinatus and underlying posterior capsule are incised together and parallel to the glenoid rim.

1.5 cm lateral to the joint line with the arm in neutral rotation (**TECH FIG 8**).
  - Most of the infraspinatus tendon runs on its inferior surface, with visible overlying muscle. This anatomic situation leads to a feeling of uneasiness as the surgeon begins to incise through the fleshy infraspinatus musculature portion posteriorly.
  - However, one should not worry, since the thicker tendinous portion of the infraspinatus will be encountered deeper during the vertical incision.
- With the capsulotomy complete, a Fukuda retractor is placed in the joint and the posterior labrum is inspected.

Posterior Repair

- The retractor is then removed and the arm is externally rotated 20 degrees (**TECH FIG 9A**).
- The lateral stump of the infraspinatus and capsule (one layer) is sutured to the intact posterior labrum using nonabsorbable sutures (**TECH FIG 9B**).
- The remaining medial portion of the infraspinatus and capsule is then reflected laterally overlapping the primary repair and sutured, again with nonabsorbable sutures (**TECH FIG 9C**).
- The deltoid is allowed to fall back together and the fascia is closed. Routine wound closure is performed.

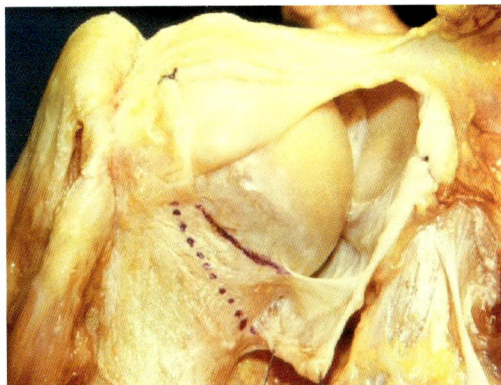

TECH FIG 7 • Anatomic dissection with the posterior rotator cuff musculature reflected, revealing the often thin posterior capsular structures.

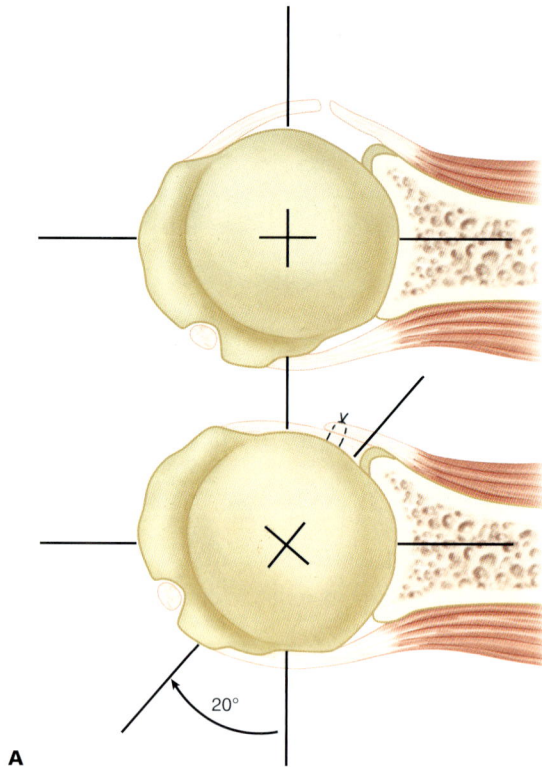

TECH FIG 9 • **A.** After completing the posterior capsulotomy, the arm is positioned in about 20 degrees of external rotation and the lateral tendon portion of the infraspinatus and capsule are sutured to the intact posterior labrum. **B.** The arm is then externally rotated 20 degrees and the lateral flap of infraspinatus and capsule is sutured to the posterior glenoid labrum. **C.** The medial flap of the infraspinatus is then overlapped and sutured to its lateral tendon.

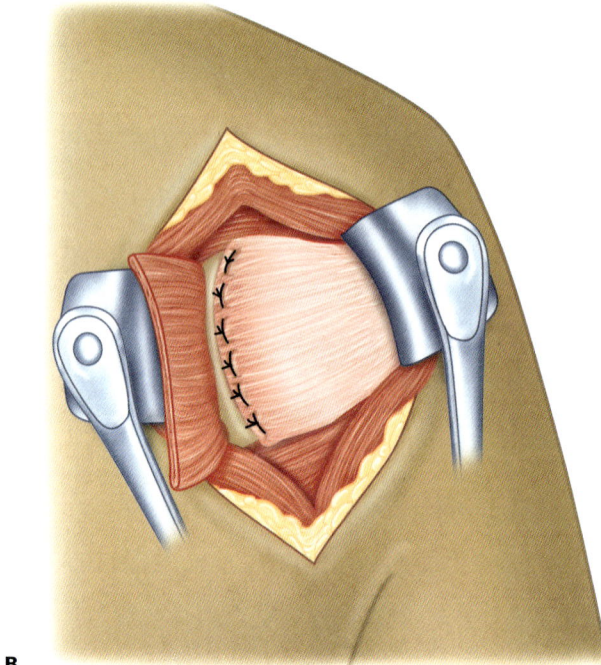

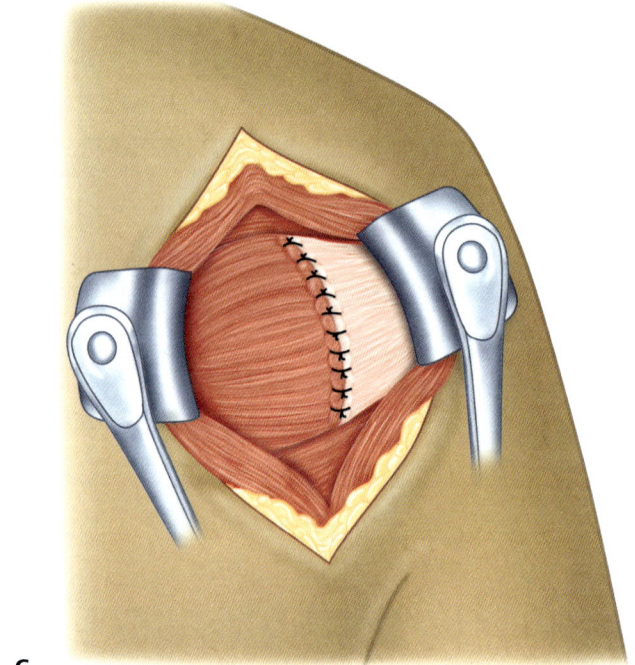

OPEN POSTERIOR GLENOID OSTEOTOMY

- Preoperative evaluation will rarely identify a patient who demonstrates excessive glenoid retroversion in excess of 20 degrees.[30,31]
  - In these situations, the surgeon may need to consider a posterior glenoid osteotomy as the primary procedure or in combination with a posterior capsulorrhaphy or shift.[17]
- This procedure is rarely needed, however, and is reserved for those special circumstances. This procedure is technically demanding and should be performed by a surgeon with previous exposure to the procedure.

Positioning and Approach

- The initial steps, including preoperative spica application and positioning, are repeated.
- The standard approach down to the infraspinatus is used, with the infraspinatus released from its lateral insertion.

Vertical Capsulotomy

- A vertical capsulotomy is made 1 cm lateral to the glenoid rim.
- The medial capsule is detached sharply from the posterior aspect of the glenoid, with the labrum left attached to the posterior glenoid rim.
  - Caution is again exercised because the suprascapular nerve is running superiorly around the spine of the scapula about 2 to 3 cm from the glenoid rim.
- The Fukuda retractor is placed into the joint to permit visualization of the glenoid retroversion and orientation of the plane of the glenoid.

Glenoid Osteotomy

- With the orientation determined and the line of the osteotomy marked, drill holes are made through both anterior and posterior cortices.
  - These holes should be no closer than 1 cm from the glenoid articular surface.
- The concavity of the glenohumeral joint as well as its superior to inferior and anterior to posterior orientation is kept in mind to avoid accidental intra-articular penetration and fracture.

- A depth gauge is used to measure each hole to get an idea of the depth of the glenoid neck.
- The oscillating saw blade is marked just short of this glenoid depth, thus decreasing the potential for traversing both the anterior and posterior cortices with the saw blade, which would result in creation of a free-floating glenoid (**TECH FIG 10A**).
- With the osteotomy complete, a 1-inch osteotome is gently tapped into place and the osteotomy is opened by moving the osteotome and glenoid laterally.
  - The partially intact anterior periosteum and cortex maintain the appropriate position of the glenoid fragment.
- The osteotomy is then opened with a 1-inch osteotome and a quarter-inch osteotome is placed perpendicular to the osteotomy at either the superior or inferior margin to hold the osteotomy in the open position (**TECH FIG 10B**).
- A tricortical graft harvested from the posterior acromion or iliac crest is placed into the osteotomy and its position and stability are checked.
  - Usually the humeral head against the glenoid will provide an adequate compressive force to close down the osteotomy and stabilize its position without hardware or internal fixation (**TECH FIG 10C**). If fixation is required, small fascial or hand set plates are ideal.
- This procedure can be combined, depending on how the infraspinatus is handled, with a humeral-based posteroinferior capsular shift or infraspinatus capsular tenodesis.
- The arm is placed in a shoulder spica postoperatively and held for 4 to 6 weeks to allow consolidation of the posterior bone graft.

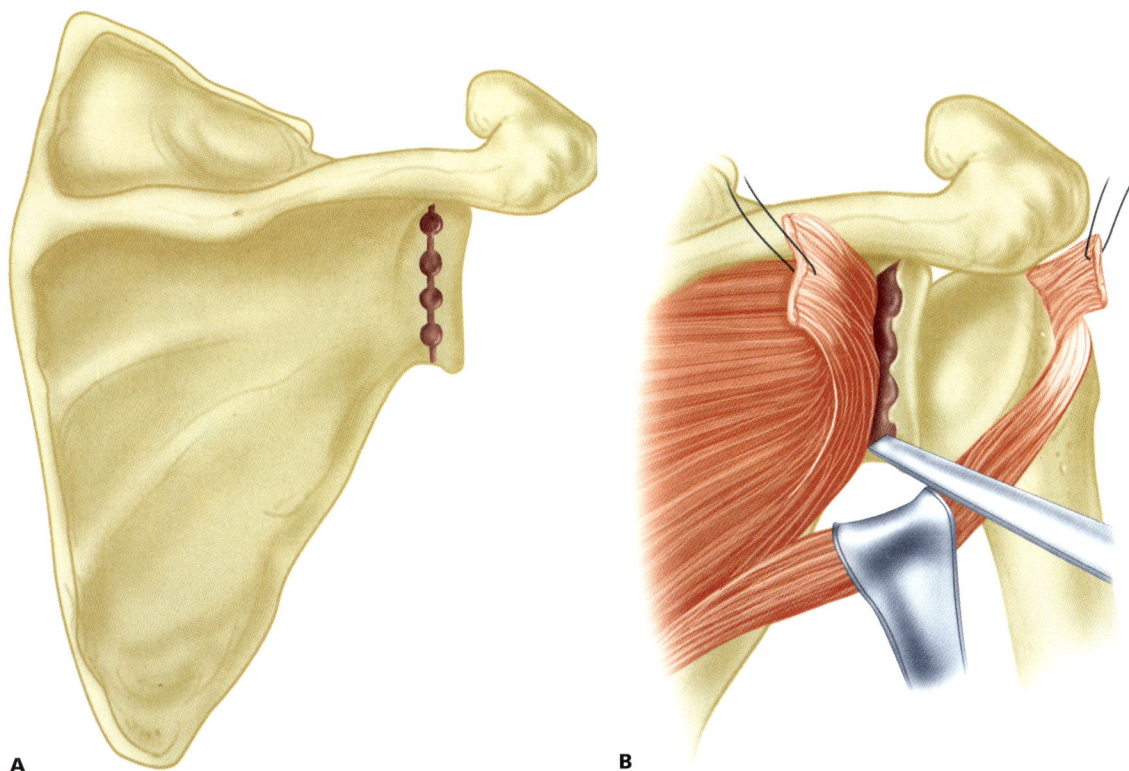

A **B**

TECH FIG 10 • A. Bicortical drill holes are created about 1 cm medial and parallel to the posterior glenoid rim. An oscillating saw then completes the osteotomy posteriorly. **B.** A small osteotome is used to gently hinge open the osteotomy site laterally, thus preserving somewhat the integrity of the anterior cortex and its periosteal and soft tissue attachments. *(continued)*

TECHNIQUES

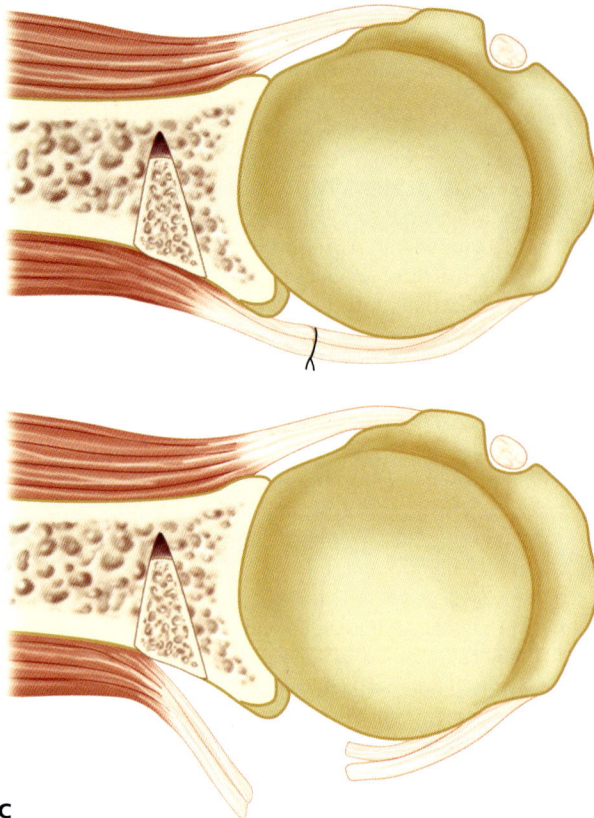

TECH FIG 10 • *(continued)* **C.** A tricortical graft is harvested from the posterior acromion or iliac spine and inserted into the osteotomy site. This procedure can be also combined with a posteroinferior capsular shift or also infraspinatus tenodesis.

OPEN POSTERIOR BONE BLOCK GRAFT AUGMENTATION

- A posterior-placed bone block may be selected as the primary procedure but is usually needed as an additional augmentation procedure to back up a soft tissue procedure in revision situations with inadequate capsular tissue.
  - This technique has been used only twice in 10 years as an augmentation procedure by the authors.
- We prefer a bone block placed extra-articularly in those often-difficult patients with soft tissue deficiencies, such as seen in Ehlers-Danlos syndrome.
  - Using the bone block extra-articularly allows the capsular repair anterior to the graft to act as a soft tissue interposition.
- The positioning and exposure down to the capsule are as earlier described.

- After the posterior capsule has been shifted, a 3 × 2-cm, 8- to 10-mm-thick bone graft is obtained either from the posterior acromial spine or iliac crest.
- After the glenoid neck is exposed and the glenoid neck decorticated, the cancellous side of the graft is placed posterior and inferior and fixated with two cancellous screws.
- The graft is tailored to its final desired shape using a motorized burr.
- Care must be used such that the graft is not placed excessively lateral to the glenoid rim with secondary impingement on the humeral head or too medial to the glenoid rim, rendering it ineffective. The goal is to increase the width and depth of the glenoid without contacting the humeral head.

PEARLS AND PITFALLS

Indications	■ Failure to make an accurate diagnosis of the direction or degree of instability ■ A complete history and physical examination is crucial and must be performed. If needed, an examination under anesthesia to rule out a more global instability is useful. ■ Patient selection is key for each planned procedure. ■ Failure to identify the habitual "pathologic" voluntary dislocator[29]
Soft tissue management	■ Failure to address associated ligamentous laxity ■ It is imperative to rule out a more global instability (multidirectional instability). ■ Beware of patients with previous failure from an extensive thermal capsulorrhaphy procedure.[36]

Bony deficiency management	▪ Significant glenoid rim deficiencies need to be addressed with reconstruction. Soft tissue procedures will not be sufficient. ▪ Rarely, excessive glenoid retroversion needs to be addressed.
Operative technique	▪ Proficiency in each procedure is key. A suboptimal attempt arthroscopically or open will doom the repair to failure. ▪ Capsular plication in conjunction with arthroscopic posterior labral repair may be required in patients with more ligamentous laxity. ▪ Care must be taken not to close down the rotator cuff interval too much, especially close to the glenoid, as a loss of external rotation can occur. It is important to close the interval based on the individual's clinical laxity. ▪ During arthroscopic repair it is crucial to place the suture anchors 1 to 2 mm over the glenoid rim onto the articular surface. This ensures that the capsulolabral tissue will be rolled up and onto the glenoid rim, restoring the bumper effect of the labrum. ▪ In patients with large capsular redundancy, inadequate release of the capsule past the 6 o'clock position on the humeral metaphysis, while performing a capsular shift, will lead to residual inferior symptomatic instability and failure. ▪ During the open infraspinatus tenodesis, the step of identifying the exact location of the glenoid rim is critical since a misplaced vertical incision through the infraspinatus and capsule, if done far laterally, will lead to overtightening, increased loss of internal rotation, and a risk of eventual secondary arthritis. ▪ Again, only rarely is glenoid osteotomy needed in those cases of excessive glenoid retroversion. Predrilling to the anterior cortex will decrease the risk of a free-floating glenoid or accidental intra-articular fracture. ▪ Postoperative loss of motion and stiffness, especially in open procedures, is often overlooked and most likely underreported. Although loss of internal rotation may be acceptable in revision cases to achieve stability, even insignificant losses of internal rotation and forward elevation in high-performance elite athletes, such as swimmers or overhead throwers, can be devastating. Thus, swimmers and elite overhead athletes are addressed arthroscopically if possible.

POSTOPERATIVE CARE

▪ Using these techniques, the procedure can be tailored to meet the patient's clinical instability; however, the rehabilitation is similar in all patients regardless of technique.

▪ After completion of the repair, the arm can be removed from traction and posterior translation reassessed.

▪ The patient is then placed in a 30-degree external rotation brace and held in this position for 3 to 4 weeks postoperatively (Ultra-Sling, DonJoy, Carlsbad, CA).

▪ At that point, gentle active-assisted range-of-motion exercises are begun, avoiding all internal rotation posterior to the coronal plane for the first 6 weeks.

▪ At the 6-week mark postoperatively, a gentle isometric strengthening program is started.

▪ Throwing activities are not started until the fourth month, with resumption of athletic endeavors anticipated at 6 months.

▪ While the surgical approach may vary, all posterior reconstructions are treated similarly in their postoperative regimen.

COMPLICATIONS

▪ Recurrent or residual instability
▪ Postoperative loss of motion or stiffness
▪ Neurovascular injury, especially posterior cord or axillary or suprascapular nerve
▪ Anchor pullout or hardware failure
▪ Infection
▪ Post–instability repair arthritis (capsulorrhaphy arthropathy)
▪ Chondral injury
▪ Chondrolysis secondary to thermal capsular shrinkage[36]
▪ Hematoma
▪ Postoperative rotator cuff atrophy or weakness

▪ Subcoracoid impingement (obligate anterior humeral head shift due to posterior capsular tightness or glenoid osteotomy)

OUTCOMES

▪ Posterior instability encompasses a continuum from acute and chronic posterior dislocation to the more frequently encountered recurrent posterior subluxation. Earlier reports in the literature have often involved small patient populations and isolated case reports with minimal follow-up.

   ▪ Past surgical treatment options included a number of nonanatomic reconstruction procedures to indirectly control posterior subluxation or dislocation.

   ▪ Eventually, a more anatomic approach developed, with procedures designed to openly repair the detached labrum (reverse Bankart repair)[3,27] or address the patient's excessive capsular redundancy (posteroinferior capsular shift).[5,12,15,21,26]

▪ Preliminary results, published in 1980 by Neer and Foster, described a humeral-based posterior and inferior capsular shift with early good results.[27] Since then, multiple authors have advocated the use of Neer's posteroinferior capsular shift with excellent results. Other authors have modified this concept by using a glenoid-based posterior T-capsular shift to similarly tighten the posterior capsule.[24]

▪ More recently, Misamore and Facibene[25] reported promising results in unidirectional posterior instability patients using such an open posterior glenoid-based capsular shift. Excellent results were achieved, with 12 of 14 returning to competitive sports.

   ▪ Fronek and colleagues,[11] using a similar capsular shift, reported on 10 of 11 patients without further episodes of instability and overall good results. However, only 3 patients were able to return to their preinjury ability level during sports. If the capsular laxity was not eliminated by this medial-based shift, then an additional lateral incision in the capsule and an H-type repair was used.

▪ Osseous reconstructions, including a posterior opening wedge glenoid osteotomy[4,7,14,23,32] and posterior bone block procedures,[1,10,11,19,26] to augment or address bony deficiencies have been described and although rarely used still have a place under certain circumstances. Hernandez and Drez[17] combined glenoplasty with a capsulorrhaphy and infraspinatus advancement.

▪ The posterior infraspinatus tenodesis, as illustrated, remains a valuable procedure, especially in cases of poor posterior capsular tissue or in revision cases. Hawkins and colleagues[16] reported an 85% success rate using such a tenodesis as a primary procedure. Even when including revision cases, Pollock and Bigliani[29] reported an 80% success rate using the same technique.

▪ Papendick and Savoie,[28] followed by McIntyre and associates,[24] were among the first of many to describe their arthroscopic techniques in the treatment of unidirectional posterior subluxation with encouraging results.

▪ Further improvements in arthroscopic suture repair techniques and instruments have led to the effective and reproducible arthroscopic treatment of recurrent posterior subluxation. The most promising arthroscopic repair techniques include posterior labral repair using suture anchor fixation, posterior capsulolabral plication, and the increasing role of rotator cuff interval plication as an augmentation to the primary repair.

　▪ Kim and colleagues[21] prospectively reported on 27 athletes with unidirectional recurrent posterior subluxation due to a distinct traumatic event. All were treated with an arthroscopic posterior Bankart repair and capsular shifting superiorly. Suture anchors were used in all cases and, if an incomplete labral lesion was encountered, it was converted to a complete detachment before repair. At a mean of 39 months postoperatively, patients had improved functional scores and only 1 patient out of 27 (4%) had a recurrence.

▪ Recently, Bradley and colleagues,[6] in the largest prospective study to date, reviewed 91 athletes (100 shoulders) with unidirectional, recurrent posterior instability. Three types of capsulolabral repairs were performed based on preoperative clinical examination and arthroscopic findings: capsulolabral plication without suture anchors, capsulolabral plication with suture anchors and additional plication sutures, and capsulolabral plication with suture anchors.

　▪ The capsulolabral repair without suture anchors was used in cases of significant posterior capsular laxity even though the labrum was not detached. The labrum was advanced superiorly and medially. Patients with acute traumatic injuries with minimal capsular stretching underwent minimal capsular advancement during the repair. Patients with chronic capsular redundancy required more advancement.[6]

　▪ The mean follow-up in the study was 27 months. All were involved in athletics, and 51% were involved in contact sports. Of these, 66% had an isolated posterior labral tear. Of the eight failures due to recurrent instability, pain, or decreased function, only one had a traumatic reinjuring event. All failures had a patulous capsule and 25% had a recurrent labral tear. Twenty-five percent of the failures had a previous thermal capsulorrhaphy before being referred for treatment. Only 11% of the patients in the study group did not return to their sport, and 33% returned but were unable to perform at the same level of competition.[6]

REFERENCES

1. Ahlgren S, Hedlund T, Nistor L. Idiopathic posterior instability of the shoulder joint: results of operation with posterior bone graft. Acta Orthop Scand 1978;49:600–603.
2. Antoniou J, Duckworth DT, Harryman DT II. Capsulolabral augmentation for the management of posteroinferior instability of the shoulder. J Bone Joint Surg Am 2000;82A:1220–1230.
3. Arciero RA, Mazzocca AD. Traumatic posterior shoulder subluxation with labral injury: suture anchor technique. Tech Shoulder Elbow Surg 2004;5:13–24.
4. Bell RH, Noble JS. An appreciation of posterior instability of the shoulder. Clin Sports Med 1991;4:887–899.
5. Bigliani LU, Pollock RG, McIlveen SJ, et al. Shift of the posteroinferior aspect of the capsule for recurrent posterior glenohumeral instability. J Bone Joint Surg Am 1995;77A:1101–1120.
6. Bradley JP, Baker CL, Kline AJ, et al. Arthroscopic capsulolabral reconstruction for posterior instability of the shoulder. Am J Sports Med 2006;34:1061–1071.
7. Brewer B, Wubben RC, Carrera GF. Excessive retroversion of the glenoid cavity: a cause of non-traumatic posterior instability of the shoulder. J Bone Joint Surg Am 1986;68A:724–731.
8. Bryan WJ, Schauder K, Tullos HS. The axillary nerve and its relationship to common sports medicine shoulder procedures. Am J Sports Med 1986;14:113–116.
9. Burkhead WZ Jr, Rockwood CA Jr. Treatment of instability of the shoulder with an exercise program. J Bone Joint Surg Am 1992;74A:890–896.
10. Fried A. Habitual posterior dislocation of the shoulder joint: a case report on 5 operated cases. Acta Orthop Scand 1949;18:329.
11. Fronek J, Warren RF, Bowen M. Posterior subluxation of the glenohumeral joint. J Bone Joint Surg Am 1989;71A:205–216.
12. Fuchs B, Jose B, Gerber C. Posterior-inferior capsular shift for the treatment of recurrent, voluntary posterior subluxation of the shoulder. J Bone Joint Surg Am 2000;82:16–25.
13. Gerber C, Ganz R. Clinical assessment of instability of the shoulder; with special reference to the anterior and posterior drawer tests. J Bone Joint Surg Br 1984;66B:551–556.
14. Gerber C, Ganz R, Vinh TS. Glenoplasty for recurrent posterior shoulder instability: an anatomic reappraisal. Clin Orthop Relat Res 1987;216:70–79.
15. Goss TP, Costello G. Recurrent symptomatic posterior glenohumeral subluxation. Orthop Rev 17;1988:1024–1032.
16. Hawkins RJ, Janda DH. Posterior instability of the glenohumeral joint: a technique of repair. Am J Sports Med 1996;24:275–278.
17. Hernandez A, Drez D. Operative treatment of posterior shoulder dislocations by posterior glenoidplasty, capsulorrhaphy, and infraspinatus advancement. Am J Sports Med 1986;14:187–191.
18. Hurley JA, Anderson TE, Dear W, et al. Posterior shoulder instability: surgical versus conservative results with evaluation of glenoid version. Am J Sports Med 1992;20:396–400.
19. Jones V. Recurrent posterior dislocation of the shoulder: report of a case treated by posterior bone block. J Bone Joint Surg Br 1958;40:203–207.
20. Kim SH, Ha KI, Yoo JC, et al. Kim's lesion: an incomplete and concealed avulsion of the posteroinferior labrum in posterior or multidirectional posteroinferior instability of the shoulder. Arthroscopy 2004;20:712–720.
21. Kim SH, Ha KI, Park JH, et al. Arthroscopic posterior labral repair and capsular shift for traumatic unidirectional recurrent posterior subluxation of the shoulder. J Bone Joint Surg Am 2003;85A:1479–1487.
22. Kim SH, Kim HK, Sun JI, et al. Arthroscopic capsulolabroplasty for posteroinferior multidirectional instability of the shoulder. Am J Sports Med 2004;32:594–607.
23. Kretzler HH. Scapular osteotomy for posterior shoulder dislocation. J Bone Joint Surg Am 1974;56A:197.
24. McIntyre LF, Caspari RB, Savoie FH III. The arthroscopic treatment of posterior instability: two-year results of a multiple suture technique. Arthroscopy 1997;13:426–432.
25. Misamore GW, Facibene WA. Posterior capsulorrhaphy for the treatment of traumatic recurrent posterior subluxations of the shoulder in athletes. J Shoulder Elbow Surg 2000;9:403–408.

26. Mowery CA, Garfin SR, Booth R, et al. Recurrent posterior dislocation of the shoulder: treatment using a bone block. J Bone Joint Surg Am 1958;67:777–781.

27. Neer CS II, Foster CR. Inferior capsular shift for involuntary inferior and multidirectional instability of the shoulder. J Bone Joint Surg Am 1980;62A:897–908.

28. Papendick LW, Savoie FH III. Anatomy specific repair techniques for posterior shoulder instability. J South Orthop Assoc 1995;4: 169–176.

29. Pollock RG, Bigliani LU. Recurrent posterior shoulder instability: diagnosis and treatment. Clin Orthop Relat Res 1993;291:85–96.

30. Rowe CR, Pierce DS, Clark JG. Voluntary dislocation of the shoulder: a preliminary report on a clinical, electromyographic, and psychiatric study of 26 patients. J Bone Joint Surg Am 1973;55A:445–460.

31. Schutte JP, Lafayette LA, Hawkins RJ, et al. The use of computerized tomography in determining humeral retroversion. Orthop Trans 1988;12:727.

32. Scott DJ Jr. Treatment of recurrent posterior dislocations of the shoulder by glenoplasty. J Bone Joint Surg Am 1967;49: 471–476.

33. Shaffer BS, Conway J, Jobe FW, et al. Infraspinatus muscle-splitting incision in posterior shoulder surgery. Am J Sports Med 1994;22: 113–120.

34. Williams RJ, Strickland S, Cohen M, et al. Arthroscopic repair for traumatic posterior instability. Am J Sports Med 2003;31: 203–209.

35. Wirth MA, Butters KP, Rockwood CA. The posterior deltoid splitting approach to the shoulder. Clin Orthop Relat Res 1993;296: 92–96.

36. Wolf EM, Eakin CL. Arthroscopic capsular plication for posterior shoulder instability. Arthroscopy 1998;14:153–163.

37. Wong KL, Williams GR. Complications of thermal capsulorrhaphy of the shoulder. J Bone Joint Surg Am 2001;83:151–155.

Chapter 5

Latarjet Procedure for Instability With Bone Loss

John Lunn, Juan Castellanos-Rosas, and Gilles Walch

DEFINITION

- Glenoid bone loss after anterior dislocation is the loss of bone due to fracture, abrasion, or compression at the anteroinferior glenoid.
- This bone loss is frequently seen after anterior dislocation and varies greatly in its extent and significance.[4,6]
- The use of a coracoid bone block to prevent anterior dislocation was first proposed by Latarjet[7] in 1954.
- In 1958 Helfet[5] described the Bristow technique, in which the tip of the coracoid is sutured to the capsuloperiosteal elements of the anterior glenoid. This was later modified to screw fixation.
- Patte[9] described the effectiveness of the Latarjet procedure as being due to the "triple blocking effect":
  - The effect of the conjoint tendon when the arm is in the abducted and externally rotated position, where it acts as a sling on the inferior subscapularis and the inferior capsule (**FIG 1**).
  - The effect of the anterior bone block
  - The effect of repairing the capsule to the stump of the conjoint tendon
- The original technique described by Latarjet involved cutting the subscapularis tendon, but this has been modified to a subscapularis split, thus preserving the integrity of its fibers.

ANATOMY

- The glenoid has a pear shape, with an average height of 35 mm and an average width of 25 mm.
- The fibrous glenoid labrum provides attachment for the glenohumeral ligaments to the bony glenoid and increases the depth of the glenoid by 50%.
- The inferior glenohumeral ligament (IGHL) attaches to the glenoid between the 2 o'clock and 4 o'clock positions in a right shoulder.

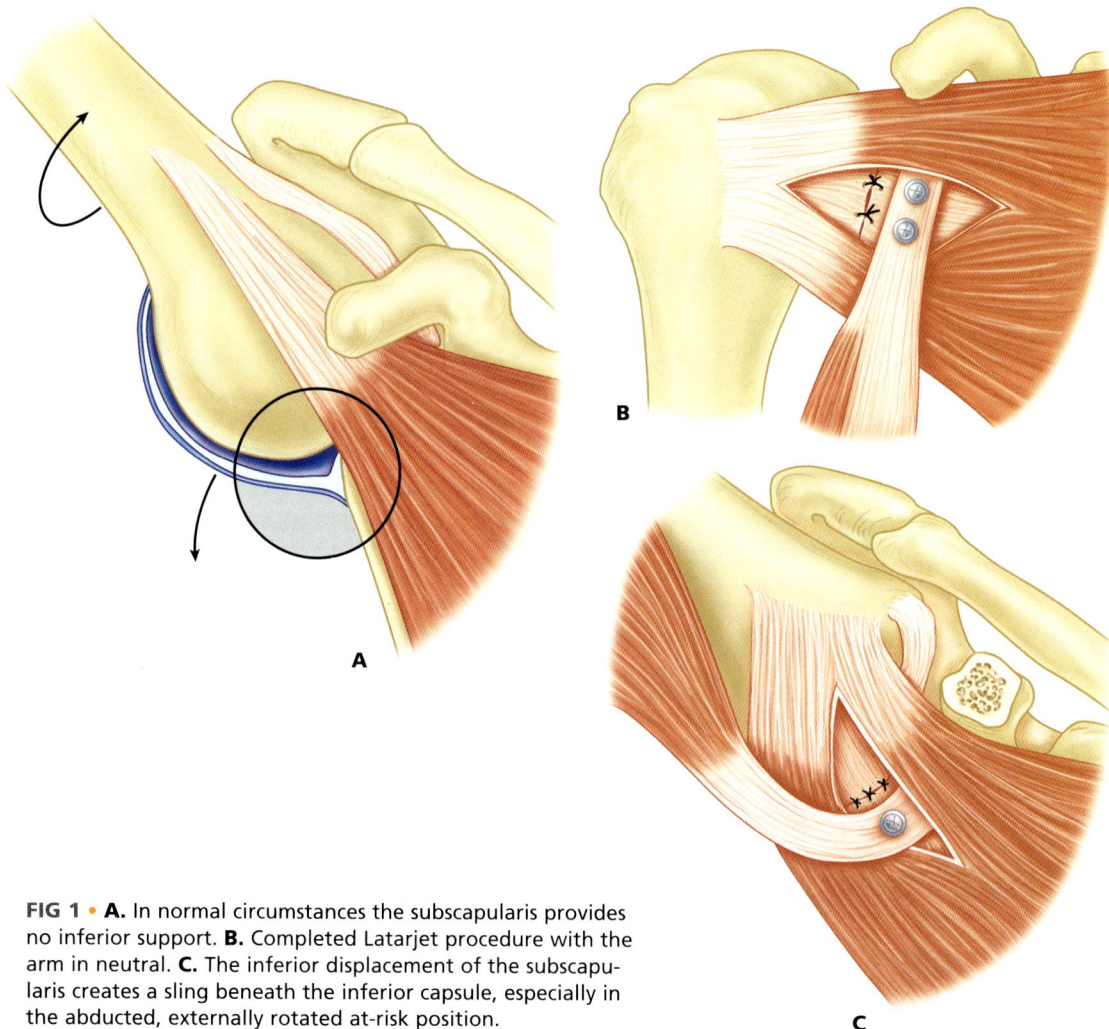

FIG 1 • A. In normal circumstances the subscapularis provides no inferior support. **B.** Completed Latarjet procedure with the arm in neutral. **C.** The inferior displacement of the subscapularis creates a sling beneath the inferior capsule, especially in the abducted, externally rotated at-risk position.

- The coracoid is directed anteriorly and then hooks laterally and inferiorly from its origin on the anterior scapular neck.
- The distal and lateral coracoid is the portion osteotomized for the Latarjet procedure. It is the origin for the short head of biceps and the coracobrachialis tendons (conjoint tendon) at its tip. Medially the pectoralis minor is attached, and laterally there is the insertion of the coracoacromial and the coracohumeral ligaments.
- Proximal to the "knee" of the coracoid and untouched by the osteotomy are the conoid and trapezoid ligaments.
- The musculocutaneous nerve enters the conjoint tendon from the medial aspect on its deep surface at an average of 5 cm from the tip of the coracoid (range 1.5 to 9 cm).
- The axillary nerve runs on the anterior surface of the subscapularis muscle lateral to the axillary artery before it enters the quadrilateral space at the inferior portion of the subscapularis.
- The anterior inferior glenohumeral ligament lies deep to the middle and lower portions of the subscapularis muscle.

PATHOGENESIS

- Anterior glenoid bone loss occurs because of either impaction of the humeral head on the anterior glenoid at the moment of dislocation or recurrent subluxation or dislocation.
- Acute impaction may result in anteroinferior glenoid fractures, the so-called bony Bankart lesions.
- Recurrent subluxation or dislocation may also result in erosion or impaction of the glenoid rim.
- Recurrent dislocation occurs owing to multiple factors, one of which is the presence of a bony lesion.
- Following Bankart repair, loss of external rotation is 25 degrees per centimeter of anterior glenoid defect. This is due to anterior capsular tightness.[6]
- An osseous defect with a width that is at least 21% of the glenoid length may cause instability.[6]
- The normally pear-shaped glenoid assumes the shape of an inverted pear.
- Redislocation in contact athletes after arthroscopic anterior stabilization occurs more frequently in those with anterior bone loss.[3]

NATURAL HISTORY

- Bone loss of varying degrees is seen in 90% to 95% of individuals with anterior shoulder instability.[4,10]

- This bone loss occurs more frequently with recurrent dislocation than subluxation.[4]
- A bony fragment was seen in 50% of 100 cases in a series using CT reconstruction, of which only one fragment was greater than 20% of the glenoid surface area.[10]

PATIENT HISTORY AND PHYSICAL FINDINGS

- The history should include the mechanism of dislocation (although this is often not clear), the site of the pain, maneuvers required for reduction, recurrence, and associated injuries.
- Recurrent anterior subluxation may be difficult to diagnose. A history of pain in the abducted externally rotated arm, pain resulting in a temporarily useless arm (dead arm syndrome), and more subtle variations can occur. Diagnosis is aided by a good clinical examination and imaging showing lesions of passage.
- The clinician should always assess for axillary nerve injury by checking sensation in the regimental badge area and motor power in the deltoid.
- Clinical examination should include:
  - Sulcus sign: presence suggests multidirectional hyperlaxity
  - External rotation with elbow at side: more than 90 degrees suggests multidirectional hyperlaxity
  - Anterior and posterior drawer tests: positive results suggests multidirectional hyperlaxity
  - Anterior apprehension test: apprehension anterior instability
  - Posterior apprehension test: positive apprehension suggests posterior instability
  - Gagey sign: Asymmetric difference in abduction of more than 30 degrees implies severe IGHL distention.

IMAGING AND DIAGNOSTIC STUDIES

- Plain radiographs should include anteroposterior (AP) views in neutral, internal and external rotation, and a profile view of the glenoid (ie, as per Bernageau[2]) of the normal and abnormal sides (**FIG 2A,B**).
- Radiographic accuracy and quality are improved when images are taken with fluoroscopic assistance.
- CT scanning may supplement radiographs (**FIG 2C**).

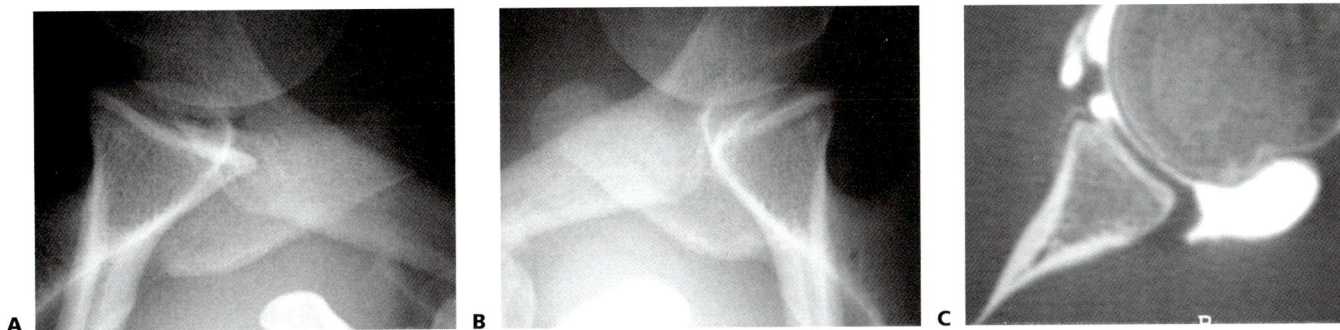

FIG 2 • **A.** This patient had recurrent dislocation of his shoulder; note the normal contour of the anterior glenoid on the unaffected side. **B.** The bone loss at the anterior border of the glenoid on the side with recurrent dislocation is clearly seen (Cliff sign). **C.** The CT scan also illustrates the bone loss.

DIFFERENTIAL DIAGNOSIS

▪ Posterior dislocation
▪ Posterosuperior cuff pathology in throwers
▪ Voluntary subluxation or dislocation
▪ Recurrent subluxation or dislocation

SURGICAL MANAGEMENT

Preoperative Planning

▪ Preoperative radiographs are analyzed to establish the presence and size of any bony glenoid defect.
▪ We use the Latarjet procedure for all individuals with anterior instability requiring surgery. The size of the glenoid defect does not change our operative technique.
▪ MRI or CT scans are not part of the standard preoperative planning but may assist in the diagnosis in cases of subtle instability.
▪ The presence of large Hill-Sachs lesions, SLAP lesions (superior labrum, from anterior to posterior), or other intra-articular pathology has no influence on outcome after the Latarjet procedure and hence does not influence the operative technique.

Positioning

▪ Under general anesthesia in association with an interscalene block for postoperative pain control, the patient is placed in the beach-chair position.
▪ A folded sheet is placed under the scapula to reduce scapula protraction and enable better access to the coracoid and glenoid (**FIG 3**).
▪ The arm is draped free to allow intraoperative abduction and external rotation.

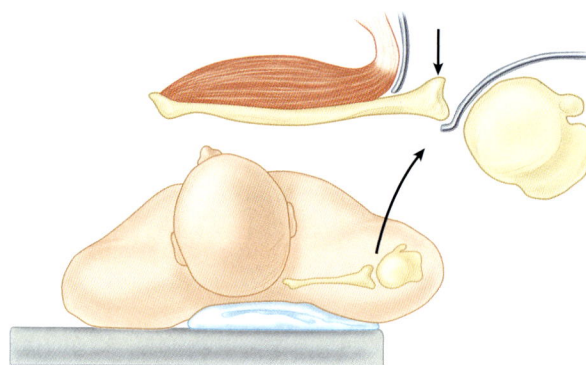

FIG 3 • Placement of the folded sheet on the medial border of the scapula reduces scapula protraction, making it easier to place your drill holes in the glenoid parallel to the articular surface.

Approach

▪ A deltopectoral approach is used.
▪ The skin incision is from the tip of the coracoid extending 4 to 5 cm toward the axillary crease.
▪ The cephalic vein is taken laterally and its large medial branch is ligated.
▪ A self-retaining retractor is used to maintain exposure between the deltoid and pectoralis major.
▪ The arm is placed in abduction and external rotation and a Hohmann retractor is placed over the top of the coracoid process.

TECHNIQUES

CORACOID OSTEOTOMY AND PREPARATION

▪ Maintain the arm in abduction and external rotation to tension the coracoacromial ligament, which is incised 1 cm from its coracoid attachment.
▪ Partially incise at the same time the coracohumeral ligament lying deep to the coracoacromial ligament and free the upper lateral aspect of the superior conjoint tendon (**TECH FIG 1A**).
▪ Now adduct and internally rotate the arm to allow exposure of the medial side of the coracoid process. The pectoralis minor is released from this attachment with electrocautery, taking care not to go past the tip of the coracoid and damage its blood supply.
▪ A periosteal elevator is then used to remove any soft tissue from the undersurface of the coracoid. This elevator also aids visualization of the "knee" of the coracoid, which is the site of the osteotomy.
▪ Using a 90-degree oscillating saw, the osteotomy is made from medial to lateral.
▪ The arm is then placed in abduction and external rotation for the second time. The coracoid is grasped with a toothed forceps and any remnants of the coracohumeral ligament are released.

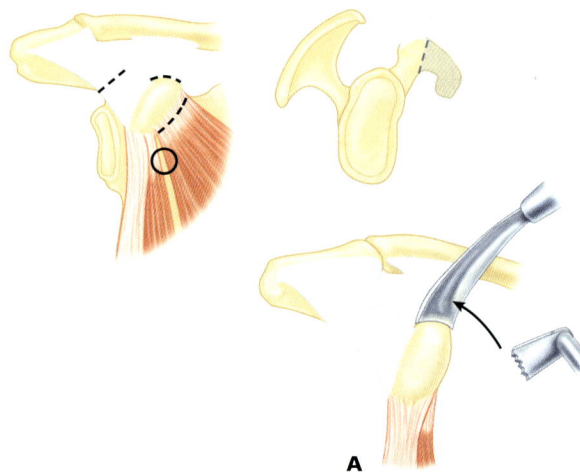

TECH FIG 1 • **A.** After release of the pectoralis minor and division of the coracoacromial ligament, the osteotomy is made distal to the coracoclavicular ligaments. *(continued)*

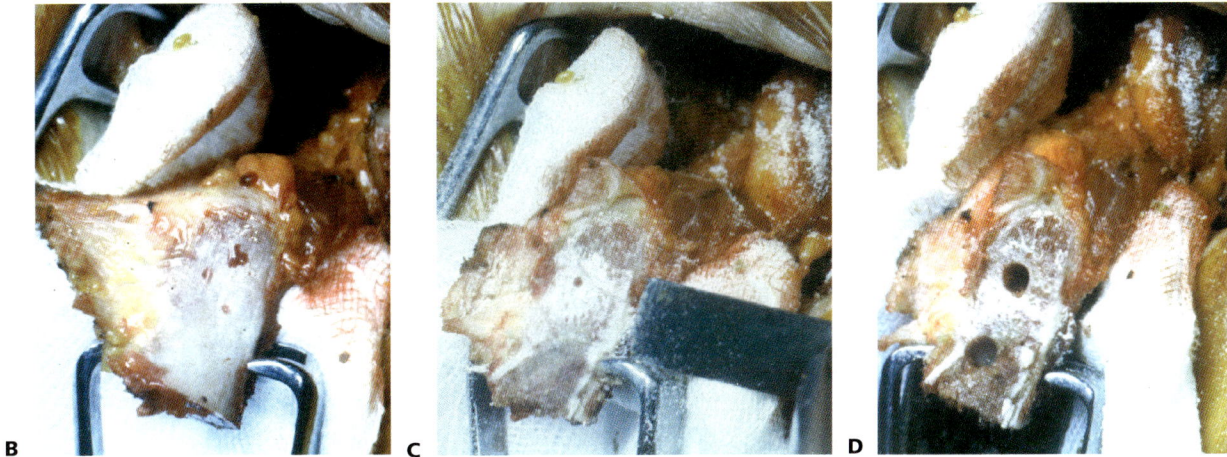

TECH FIG 1 • *(continued)* **B.** The coracoid is delivered onto a swab at the inferior part of the wound and held with a pointed grasping forceps. **C.** All cortical bone must be removed from this surface. **D.** A 3.2-mm drill is used to drill the holes.

- The arm is then returned to a neutral position and the coracoid is delivered onto a swab at the inferior aspect of the wound (**TECH FIG 1B**).
- Preparation of the bed of the coracoid is important to avoid a pseudarthrosis. Soft tissue is removed with a scalpel and then the oscillating saw is used to remove the cortical bone, exposing a cancellous bed for graft healing (**TECH FIG 1C**).
- An osteotome is placed beneath the coracoid to protect the skin and two drill holes are made using a 3.2-mm drill (**TECH FIG 1D**). The holes are in the central axis of the coracoid and about 1 cm apart.
- The swab protecting the skin is removed, the arm is externally rotated, keeping the elbow by the side, and the lateral border of the conjoint tendon is released for about 5 cm using a Mayo scissors.
- The coracoid is then pushed beneath the pectoralis major, exposing the underlying subscapularis muscle.

GLENOID EXPOSURE

- Identify the superior and inferior margins of the subscapularis; the location for the subscapularis split is at the junction of its superior two thirds and inferior one third (**TECH FIG 2A**).
- A Mayo scissors is used to create the split. It is pushed between the fibers as far as the capsule, then opened perpendicular to the plane of the muscle fibers. Keeping the scissors open, push a small swab into the subscapular fossa in a superomedial direction and then place a Hohmann retractor on the swab in the subscapularis fossa (**TECH FIG 2B**).
- Using a curved retractor such as a Bennett retractor on the inferior part of the subscapularis, extend the lateral part of the split with a scalpel to the lesser

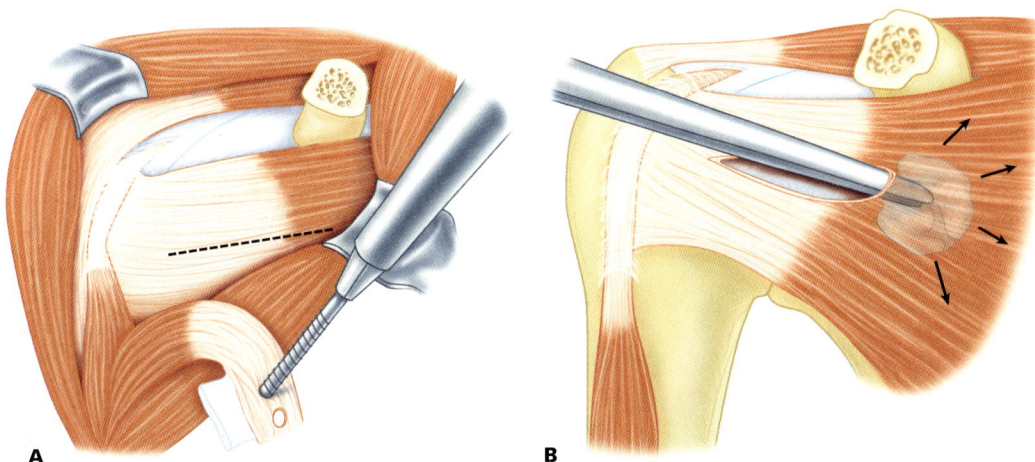

TECH FIG 2 • **A.** After drilling the holes in the coracoid, the subscapularis is split at the junction between its superior two thirds and its inferior one third. **B.** A small sponge is placed superomedially between the capsule and the subscapularis muscle. *(continued)*

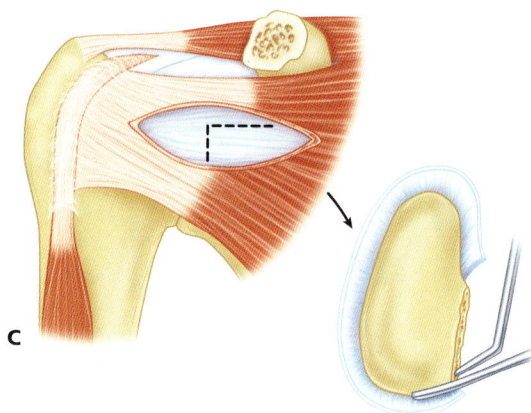

TECH FIG 2 • *(continued)* **C.** It is important to ensure the subscapularis split has been carried sufficiently laterally to allow easy visualization of the joint line.

tuberosity. The joint line is then more easily visualized and incised for about 1.5 to 2 cm, allowing a retractor to be placed in the joint (Trillat or Fukuda retractor; **TECH FIG 2C**).

- Superior exposure is created when a Steinmann pin is hammered into the superior scapular neck as high as possible.
- The medial Hohmann retractor is now exchanged for a link retractor and placed as medial as possible on the scapula neck.
- A small Hohmann retractor is placed inferiorly between the capsule on the inferior neck and the inferior part of the subscapularis.
- The anteroinferior part of the glenoid should now be easily visualized.

PREPARATION OF THE GLENOID AND CORACOID FIXATION

- The anteroinferior labrum and periosteum are incised with the electrocautery, exposing the glenoid 2 cm medially and from about 5 o'clock to 2 o'clock in a right shoulder (a vertical distance of 2 to 3 cm).
- An osteotome is then used to elevate this labral–periosteal flap from lateral to medial (**TECH FIG 3A**). The frequent presence of a Bankart lesion makes this quite simple.
- The osteotome is then used to decorticate this anteroinferior surface of the glenoid. We aim to create a flat surface on which to place our graft.
- The use of bone graft (excepting the coracoid process) is not required.
- Using the 3.2-mm drill, drill the inferior hole in the glenoid (**TECH FIG 3B**). This is at the 5 o'clock position, parallel to the plane of the glenoid and sufficiently medial that the coracoid will not overhang the glenoid (generally 7 mm, but depends on coracoid morphology). Both anterior and posterior cortices are drilled.

- The coracoid is now retrieved from its position under the pectoralis major and grasped at the cut end in a medial–lateral fashion.
- A 4.5-mm partially threaded malleolar screw is fully inserted into the inferior hole (tendinous end). The length of this screw is typically 35 mm but can be verified by adding together the depth of the coracoid and the depth of the glenoid hole (**TECH FIG 3C**).
- The screw is then placed into the already drilled inferior hole and tightened into position, ensuring that the coracoid comes to lie parallel to the anterior border of the glenoid with no overhang. A slightly medial position (2 to 3 mm) is acceptable. Rotation of the coracoid is adjusted using a heavy forceps.
- When the position of the coracoid is parallel to the glenoid, the second drill hole is made through the superior hole already drilled in the coracoid (**TECH FIG 3D**). It is important to avoid rotation of the coracoid at this stage.

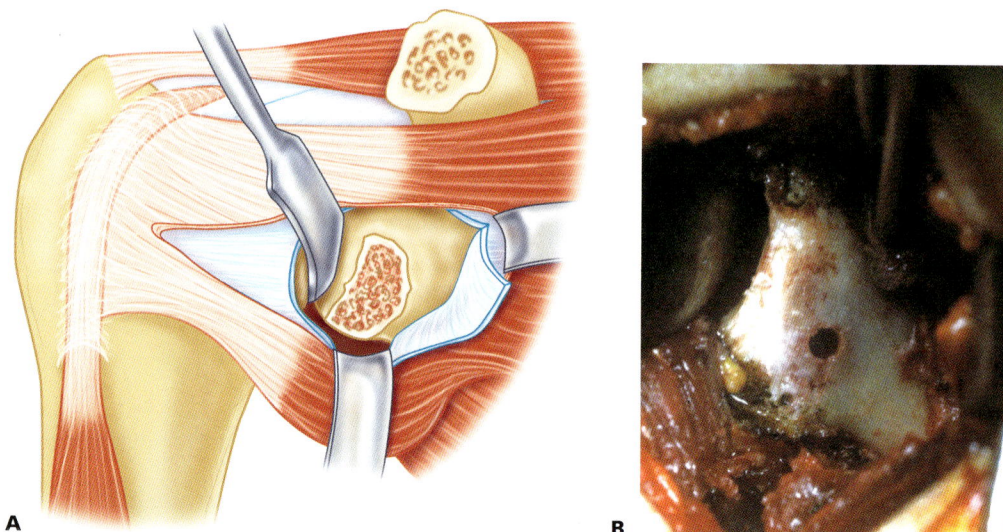

TECH FIG 3 • **A.** With an osteotome, cancellous bone is exposed on the glenoid neck. **B.** First glenoid drill hole. *(continued)*

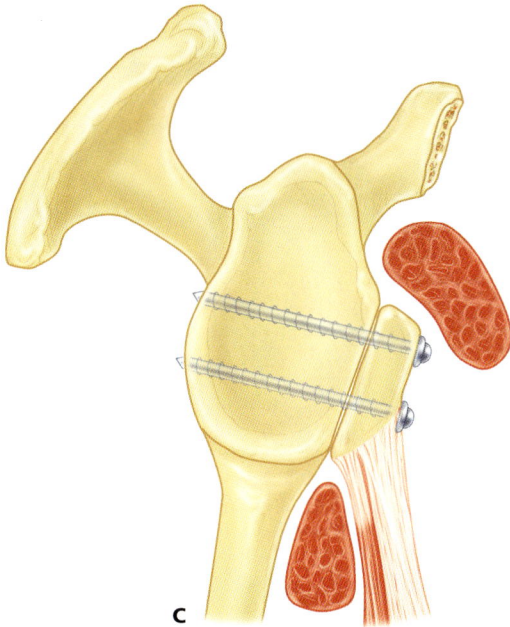

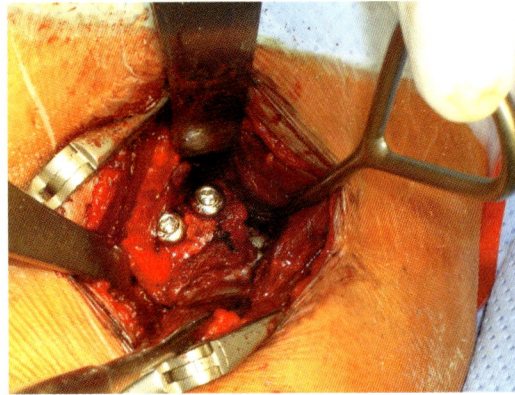

TECH FIG 3 • *(continued)* **C.** The coracoid increases the width of the anteroinferior bony glenoid. **D.** View after fixation of the coracoid to the glenoid neck.

- The hole is measured and the correct-sized malleolar screw is inserted into position.
- Repair of the capsule is then carried out by suturing the capsule to the stump of the coracoacromial ligament using a number 1 Dexon suture with the arm in external rotation, after removing the intra-articular retractor.

- The retractors are removed, as is the sponge that was on the medial scapula neck.
- There is no need to close the split in the subscapularis muscle.

PEARLS AND PITFALLS

- Dissection on the medial side of the coracoid is not necessary and risks nerve injury.
- The surgeon should not cut the subscapularis to gain access to the glenoid; the subscapularis split is used instead.
- The surgeon should decorticate the undersurface of the coracoid and the anterior glenoid to bleeding bone to avoid coracoid pseudarthrosis.
- Coracoid fracture can be avoided by using the two-fingers technique when tightening screws.
- Screws must be bicortical.
- Placing the coracoid in the "lying" position increases the coracoid–glenoid contact and decreases the risk of pseudarthrosis.
- If the coracoid fractures longitudinally, it should be turned 90 degrees. If it fractures transversely, the tip should be placed in a standing position.
- The coracoid must never overhang the glenoid, as this leads to arthritis[1] (**FIG 4**).

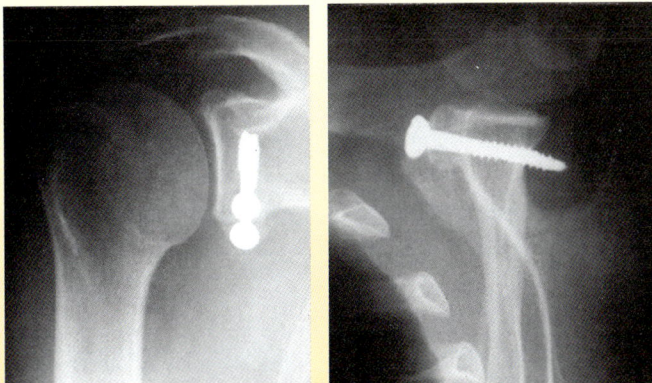

FIG 4 • Postoperative AP and lateral views showing correct placement of screws and no overhanging of the coracoid.

POSTOPERATIVE CARE

- A simple sling is used for 2 weeks.
- Rehabilitation begins on the first postoperative day with gentle active range-of-motion exercises.
- Full activities of daily living are allowed at 6 weeks and a return to all sports is permitted at 3 months.

OUTCOMES

- In a study of 160 Latarjet procedures, we had a recurrence rate of 1%. Of those who played sports, 83% returned to their preinjury level or better. Overall, 98% rated their result as excellent or good and 76% had excellent or good results using the modified Rowe score.[11]
- The occurrence of postoperative shoulder arthritis is related to preventable factors (ie, lateral overhang of the coracoid) and pre-existing factors (eg, increased age at the time of first dislocation, increased age at the time of surgery and the presence of arthritis before to surgery).

COMPLICATIONS

- Intraoperative fracture of the coracoid
- Infection
- Hematoma formation
- Pseudarthrosis (not associated with poor outcome)
- Pain related to screws (2% incidence of screw removal)
- Recurrence
- Arthritis (if graft overhangs the anterior glenoid)

REFERENCES

1. Allain J, Goutallier D, Glorion C. Long-term results of the Latarjet procedure for the treatment of anterior instability of the shoulder. J Bone Joint Surg Am 1998;80A:841–852.
2. Bernageau J, Patte D, Bebeyre J, et al. Interet du profile glenoidien dans les luxations recidivantes de l'epaule. Rev Chir Orthop 1976; 62:142–147.
3. Burkhart SS, De Beer JF. Traumatic glenohumeral bone defects and their relationship to failure of arthroscopic Bankart repairs: significance of the inverted-pear glenoid and the humeral engaging Hill-Sachs lesion. Arthroscopy 2000;16:677–694.
4. Edwards TB, Boulahia A, Walch G. Radiographic analysis of bone defects in chronic anterior shoulder instability. Arthroscopy 2003;19:732–739.
5. Helfet AJ. Coracoid transplantation for recurring dislocation of the shoulder. J Bone Joint Surg Br 1958;40B:198–202.
6. Itoi E, Lee SB, Berglund LJ, et al. The effect of a glenoid defect on anteroinferior stability of the shoulder after Bankart repair: a cadaveric study. J Bone Joint Surg Am 2000;82A:35–46.
7. Latarjet M. A propos du traitement des luxations recidivantes de l'epaule. Lyon Chir 1954;49:994–1003.
8. May VR Jr. A modified Bristow operation for anterior recurrent dislocation of the shoulder. J Bone Joint Surg Am 1970;52A: 1010–1016.
9. Patte D, Debeyre J. Luxations recidivantes de l'epaule. Encycl Med Chir. Paris-Technique chirurgicale. Orthopedie 1980;44265:4.4-02.
10. Sugaya H, Moriishi J, Dohi M, et al. Glenoid rim morphology in recurrent anterior glenohumeral instability. J Bone Joint Surg Am 200385A:878–884.
11. Walch G, Boileau P. Latarjet-Bristow procedure for recurrent anterior instability. Tech Shoulder Elbow Surg 2000;1:256–261.

Chapter 6

Glenoid Bone Graft for Instability With Bone Loss

Ryan W. Simovitch, Laurence D. Higgins, and Jon J.P. Warner

DEFINITION

- Anterior shoulder instability typically results from an injury to the capsule, ligaments, and labrum that stabilize the glenohumeral joint.
- In cases of higher-energy trauma or recurrent dislocation, however, there can be significant bone loss or erosion of the anterior glenoid rim.
- The key to correctly treating anterior shoulder instability is recognizing whether the lesion involves injury to only capsulolabroligamentous structures or if it also involves the anteroinferior glenoid bone.

ANATOMY

- Shoulder stability is provided by both dynamic and static stabilizers (**FIG 1**).
- Dynamic stabilizers include:
  - Rotator cuff
  - Biceps
  - Coordinated scapulothoracic motion
  - Proprioception
- Static stabilizers include:
  - Bony anatomy of the glenoid and humeral head
  - Labrum
  - Glenohumeral capsule and ligaments
  - Negative intra-articular pressure
- The inferior glenohumeral ligament (IGHL) complex limits anterior translation of the humeral head on the glenoid in abduction. It takes origin from the labrum on the glenoid inferiorly. The complex consists of an anterior band, posterior band, and intervening pouch. The anterior band is responsible for anterior restraint with the arm in high degrees of abduction with external rotation.
- Normal glenoid morphology is the shape of a pear. There is normally a surface area mismatch of the glenohumeral joint whereby only 20% to 30% of the humeral head contacts the glenoid surface at any point in time (Fig 1).
- The synchronized contraction of the rotator cuff and biceps provides a compressive force directing the convex humeral head into the concave glenoid and labrum unit. This is known as concavity compression.[7]

PATHOGENESIS

- Anterior shoulder instability typically follows a dislocation event that results from a fall or collision with the arm in external rotation and abduction.
- First-time dislocators typically require a closed reduction of their shoulder after muscle relaxation and sedation, while recurrent dislocators can often reduce their shoulders with minimal effort.
- An injury to the labrum in the anteroinferior quadrant of the glenoid destabilizing the IGHL complex as well as stretching or a tear of the anteroinferior capsule can result in anterior shoulder instability.
- A rotator cuff tear should be suspected in patients greater than 40 years old who suffer from a dislocation episode.
- Recurrent anterior glenohumeral instability can also occur in the setting of anterior glenoid bone loss due to glenoid fracture after a single dislocation event or erosion as a result of recurrent subluxations or dislocations.

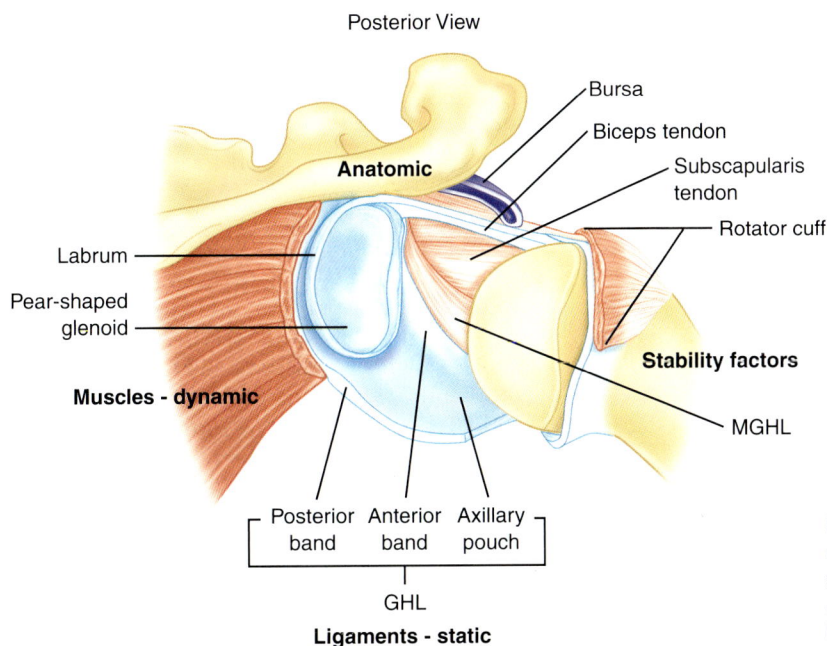

FIG 1 • Shoulder stability depends on the interaction of dynamic and static soft tissue restraints. The bony architecture of the glenoid and humerus also plays a critical role.

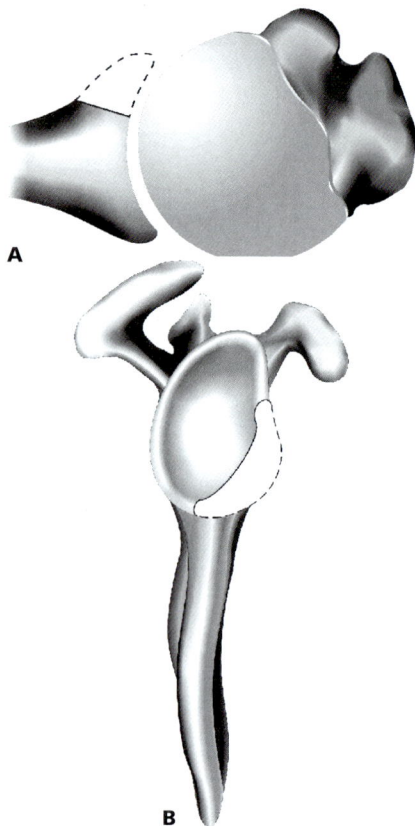

FIG 2 • Loss of anterior glenoid bone (*dashed line*) due to erosion or fracture results in loss of glenoid width (**A**) and depth (**B**). The result is an inverted-pear morphology that cannot resist displacement of the humeral head anteriorly as effectively as a normal pear-shaped glenoid.

- Deficiency of the anterior glenoid rim disrupts the normal mechanism of concavity–compression as a result of a decrease in width and depth of the socket (**FIG 2**).
- Anterior glenoid bone loss or fracture should be suspected in cases of recurrent anterior instability or acute dislocations from a high-energy mechanism.
- In cases of anterior glenoid bony deficiency, patients often report recurrent dislocation in their sleep and with minimal trauma.

NATURAL HISTORY

- In the context of anterior glenoid bone loss, both open and arthroscopic soft tissue management of anterior shoulder instability have demonstrated increased failure rates compared to the results in patients with normal bony glenoid anatomy.
- Burkhart and DeBeer[1] have shown that contact athletes with substantial bony glenoid defects, noted as an "inverted pear" morphology at arthroscopy, had an 87% recurrent instability rate compared to 6.5% in contact athletes with a normal bony glenoid who underwent an arthroscopic capsulolabral repair only.
- Given the high failure rate in patients with significant anterior glenoid bone loss, a comprehensive evaluation of the glenoid bony anatomy is imperative before treating recurrent anterior shoulder instability with a capsulolabral reconstruction alone.

PATIENT HISTORY AND PHYSICAL FINDINGS

- A complete examination of the shoulder should also include the evaluation of other concomitant injuries and ruling out differential diagnoses. A thorough examination includes but is not limited to the following:
  - Apprehension test: Apprehension, not simply pain, is required for a positive apprehension test.
  - Relocation test: Relief of apprehension with posterior pressure is necessary for a positive relocation maneuver.
  - Load and shift test: The examiner should note the degree of displacement of the humeral head on the glenoid rim.
  - Belly press: A positive belly press test is when the patient must flex the wrist and extend the arm to maintain the palm of the hand on the abdomen.
  - Assessment for generalized ligamentous laxity: Specifically, hyperextension of the elbows and knees as well as the ability to oppose the thumb to the forearm should be noted.
  - Rotator cuff: Manual strength testing of the subscapularis, supraspinatus, infraspinatus, and teres minor muscles must be done. Rotator cuff tears can contribute to instability.
  - Subscapularis insufficiency: Weakness of internal rotation with the shoulder adducted to the side suggests a subscapularis injury but is not specific. Increased external rotation of the injured side with the shoulder adducted compared to the contralateral shoulder, pain with external rotation of the shoulder, a positive belly press sign, or positive lift-off sign should raise suspicion for subscapularis insufficiency.
  - Axillary nerve injury: Both the deltoid motor strength and sensation in the distribution of the axillary nerve should be assessed. Atrophy of the deltoid muscle should be noted.

IMAGING AND OTHER DIAGNOSTIC STUDIES

- Plain radiographs are useful to detect Hill-Sachs lesion, glenoid dysplasia, and anterior glenoid fractures or erosion. Standard images should include a true anteroposterior (AP) view of the glenoid, an axillary view, and a Stryker notch view. Fractures and erosions of the glenoid as well as the position of the humerus on the glenoid should be noted.
- If a significant anterior bony glenoid lesion is suspected owing to plain film findings or a history of recurrent dislocations, a CT arthrogram should be obtained. This allows an evaluation of the subscapularis tendon, bony architecture of the glenoid, humeral head, and tuberosities as well the degree of capsulolabral injury and redundancy.
- Both Itoi[5,6] and Gerber[3] have described techniques to assess anterior glenoid bone quantitatively that serve as a guide for when bony augmentation is indicated for recurrent anterior shoulder instability. Gerber's method[3] is easily performed on oblique sagittal or 3D reconstructions of the glenoid surface (**FIG 3**). Cadaveric studies have shown that the force required for anterior dislocation is reduced by 70% from an intact glenoid if the length of the glenoid defect exceeds the maximum radius of the glenoid.

DIFFERENTIAL DIAGNOSIS

- Bankart lesion
- Multidirectional instability
- Hill-Sachs lesion
- Tuberosity fracture

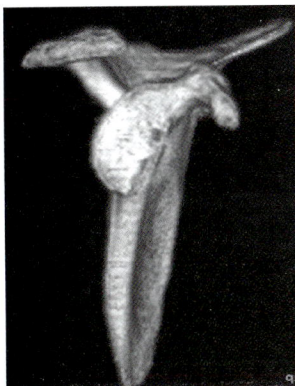

FIG 3 • A 3D CT reconstruction effectively demonstrates the degree of anterior glenoid bone loss.

- Rotator cuff tear (especially subscapularis)
- Scapular winging (especially serratus anterior dysfunction)
- Axillary nerve injury

NONOPERATIVE MANAGEMENT

- Conservative therapy for recurrent anterior shoulder dislocation includes strengthening of the rotator cuff musculature as well as the periscapular stabilizers. Deltoid muscle strengthening should be incorporated into a rotator cuff strengthening protocol. Periscapular strengthening should focus on the rhomboids, trapezius, serratus, and latissimus dorsi muscles.
- Conservative treatment of recurrent shoulder dislocation in the setting of a bony glenoid defect, however, is rarely successful.

SURGICAL MANAGEMENT

Preoperative Planning

- All imaging studies, including plain radiographs (true AP glenoid view, axillary view, Stryker notch view) and CT scan with intra-articular gadolinium, are reviewed. Additional radiographic views can be helpful. The apical oblique can demonstrate anterior glenoid lip defects as well as posterolateral impression fractures of the humeral head. Both the West Point and Bernageau views are useful to note defects of the anteroinferior glenoid rim.
- The CT arthrogram is examined for evidence of anterior glenoid bone loss:
  - The degree of bone loss is assessed on oblique sagittal reconstruction or a 3D reconstruction of the glenoid face (**FIG 4**).
  - The length of the anterior glenoid defect is measured.
  - If the length of the glenoid defect exceeds half of the maximum diameter of the glenoid, an anatomic glenoid reconstruction of the anterior glenoid with autologous iliac crest bone graft is considered.[3]
- Often, the anterior erosion is extensive, making it difficult to accurately measure the glenoid diameter. In these instances, the superoinferior axis of the glenoid should be drawn on the glenoid face image and the maximum radius determined from this line to the posterior aspect of the glenoid (Fig 4).
- Associated superior labral tears, biceps pathology, rotator cuff tears, and the presence of articular erosion and osteoarthritis should be noted preoperatively and treated appropriately at the index operation.
- An examination under anesthesia should assess passive range of motion, noting any restrictions as well as excessive motion,

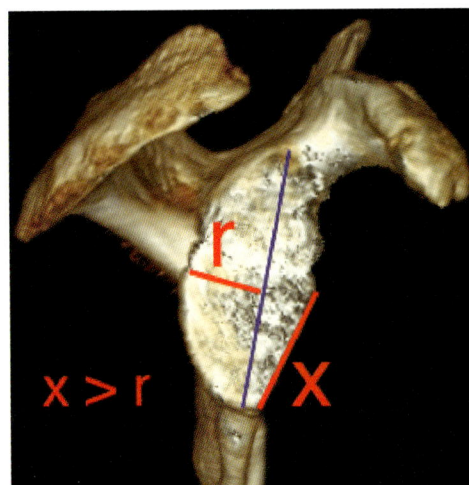

FIG 4 • Gerber's method for evaluating the degree of glenoid erosion. x is the length of the glenoid defect. Half of the maximum diameter of the glenoid, r, can be measured from a vertical line (*blue*) connecting the superior glenoid rim to the inferior glenoid rim in cases of significant erosion. If $x > r$, then the force for dislocation is decreased by 70%.

which may indicate subscapularis insufficiency. In addition, the glenohumeral joint should be assessed for laxity to ensure there is not a bidirectional or multidirectional component.

Positioning

- Although some surgeons choose to use a bean bag, we prefer to use a beach chair with an attachable hydraulic articulated arm holder (Spider Limb Positioner, Tenet Medical Engineering, Calgary, Canada) (**FIG 5**).
- The head of the beach chair is elevated 30 to 45 degrees to allow access to the ipsilateral iliac crest.

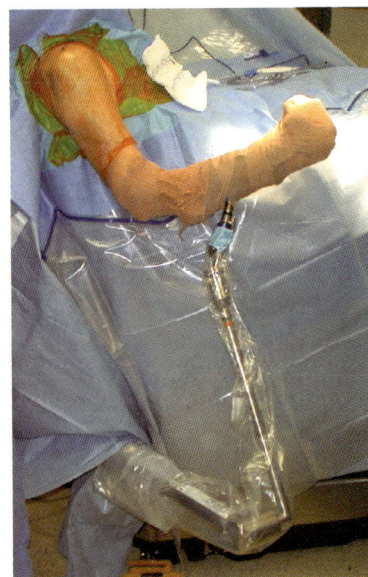

FIG 5 • The patient is secured into a beach chair with an attachable hydraulic articulated arm holder (Spider Limb Positioner, Tenet Medical Engineering, Calgary, Canada). The upper body is positioned at 30 to 45 degrees to allow access to the ipsilateral iliac crest.

TECHNIQUES

■ A well-padded bump is placed behind the ipsilateral buttock and hip to ensure that the iliac crest is prominent for ease of dissection.

■ The shoulder and iliac crest are prepared and draped in the standard sterile fashion.

Approach

■ Anterior glenoid reconstruction with iliac crest bone graft requires two approaches:
  ■ Deltopectoral approach for glenoid preparation
  ■ Tricortical anterior iliac crest bone graft harvesting

EXPOSURE OF GLENOID

■ A 5- to 7-cm incision is made in the anterior axillary fold beginning at the inferior border of the pectoralis major tendon and extended superiorly to the coracoid.

■ Once the initial incision is carried through the subcutaneous tissue down to the fascia investing the pectoralis and deltoid muscles, full-thickness skin flaps are sharply developed using a no. 15 blade superiorly to the level of the coracoid as well as medially and laterally at least 1 cm to allow identification of the cephalic vein and dissection of the interval between the deltoid and pectoralis major muscles.

■ Typically, there are more crossing vessels emanating from the lateral side of the cephalic vein. Thus, the investing fascia on the medial side of the vein is incised sharply while an assistant places countertraction on the pectoralis major using a two-pronged skin hook. This allows a clean dissection and medially based crossing vessels to be coagulated in a step-by-step fashion.

■ The deep surfaces of the deltoid and pectoralis are sharply dissected using a no. 15 blade to free up adhesions and broaden the ultimate exposure.

■ A four-quadrant self-retaining retractor is positioned to retract the pectoralis major medially and the deltoid laterally (**TECH FIG 1A**).

■ There is often a leash of vessels superficial to the clavipectoral fascia at the level of the coracoid. These should be coagulated if present.

■ The clavipectoral fascia is sharply incised lateral to the conjoint tendon, making sure to stay lateral to any muscle of the short head of the biceps.

■ The musculocutaneous nerve can then be palpated on the deep surface of the conjoint tendon. The conjoint tendon is retracted medially, exposing the subscapularis tendon and muscle.

■ The coracoacromial ligament can be released if additional exposure is needed superiorly.

■ The circumflex vessels are then identified and ligated or coagulated (**TECH FIG 1B**).

■ The axillary nerve can be palpated as it passes over the inferior portion of the subscapularis and loops under the inferior capsule. A blunt retractor can be placed lateral and deep to the axillary nerve, thus retracting it gently medially away from the subscapularis musculotendinous junction.

■ The subscapularis tendon is then incised from bone off the lesser tuberosity to avoid disrupting the long head of the biceps tendon in the bicipital groove (**TECH FIG 1C**).

■ Through sharp dissection, an interval between the subscapularis tendon and capsule is developed, leaving the capsule intact. It is often easier to start inferiorly and use a blunt elevator to dissect the interval.

■ The subscapularis tendon and muscle are retracted medially using an anterior glenoid neck retractor.

■ A blunt retractor is repositioned deep to the axillary nerve to retract away from the capsule, which should be widely exposed at this point.

■ An inverted L-shaped capsulotomy is then created based on the humeral neck and extending horizontally across the rotator interval region (**TECH FIG 1D**).

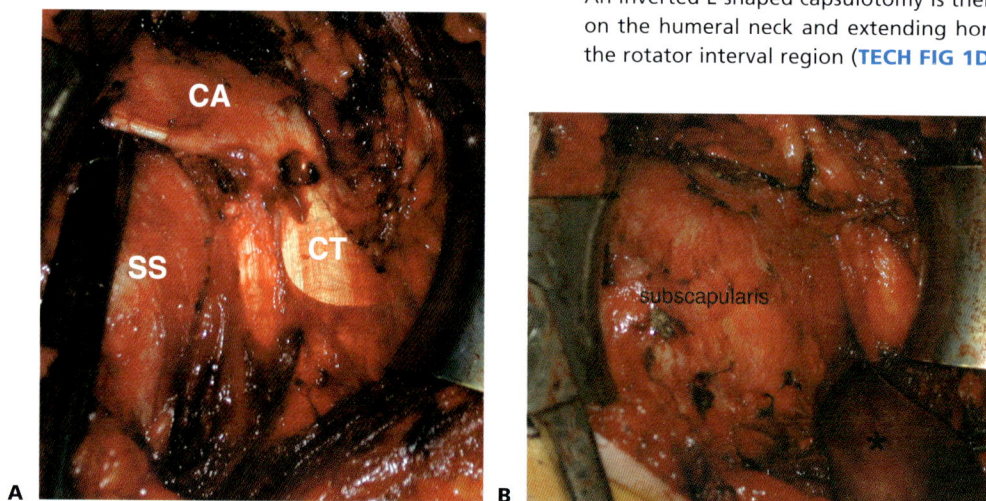

TECH FIG 1 • A. The pectoralis major and deltoid muscles are retracted to reveal a broad exposure of the conjoint tendon (*CT*) and muscle belly passing over the subscapularis muscle (*SS*). The coracoacromial ligament (*CA*) can be released if needed for additional exposure. **B.** A blunt curved retractor can be placed inferiorly along the subscapularis to protect the axillary nerve. *(continued)*

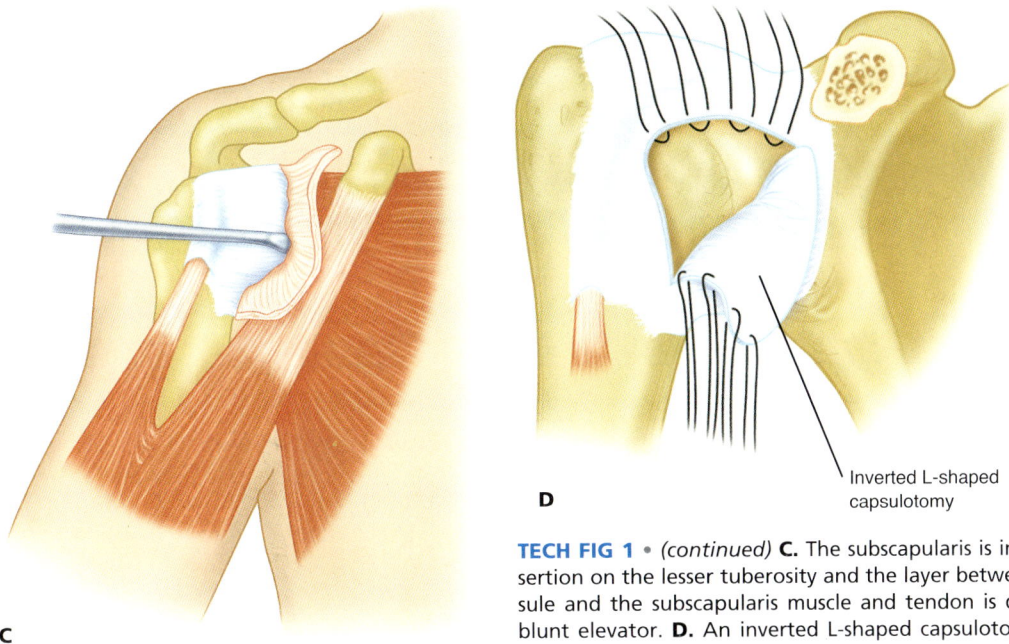

TECH FIG 1 • (continued) C. The subscapularis is incised from its insertion on the lesser tuberosity and the layer between the deep capsule and the subscapularis muscle and tendon is developed with a blunt elevator. **D.** An inverted L-shaped capsulotomy based on the humeral neck and extending across the rotator interval region allows access to the glenohumeral joint and leaves tissue for later repair.

GLENOID PREPARATION

- The anterior glenoid and scapular neck are then exposed (**TECH FIG 2**).
- After the L-shaped capsulotomy, a periosteal elevator is used to strip the periosteal sleeve from the anterior scapular neck.
- An anterior glenoid neck retractor is positioned to retract the capsule medially.

- A Fukuda retractor or similar blunt retractor is used to retract the humeral head posteriorly, thus exposing the face of the glenoid.
- The length of the osseous defect is measured and compared to the width of the maximum AP radius of the glenoid. The measured defect length will be the basis for the size of the iliac crest bone graft harvested.
- Soft tissue and scar tissue are removed from the anterior glenoid, and this bone and the adjacent scapular neck are roughened with a high-speed burr to create punctate bleeding and a smooth surface for bone grafting.

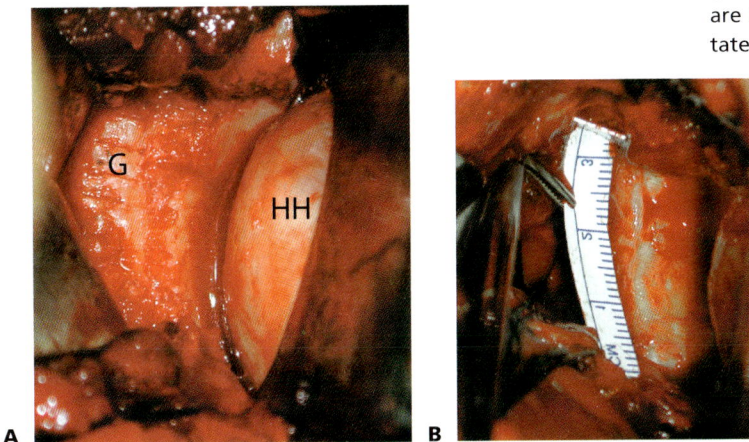

TECH FIG 2 • Glenoid preparation. **A.** The humeral head (*HH*) is retracted laterally and posteriorly using a Fukuda retractor or curved blunt retractor. The medial capsule and soft tissue are retracted medially, thus exposing the anterior scapular neck and eroded glenoid (*G*) surface. **B.** A malleable ruler is used to measure the length of the anterior glenoid defect.

HARVESTING AND PREPARING TRICORTICAL ILIAC CREST BONE GRAFT

- The iliac crest is harvested as a tricortical bone graft (**TECH FIG 3**).
- A 2- to 3-cm curved incision is made overlying the iliac crest and posterior to the anterosuperior iliac spine.

- The incision is carried sharply through subcutaneous tissue down to the periosteum, which is incised sharply and superiosteally elevated to expose the inner and outer tables. Self-retaining retractors are placed be-

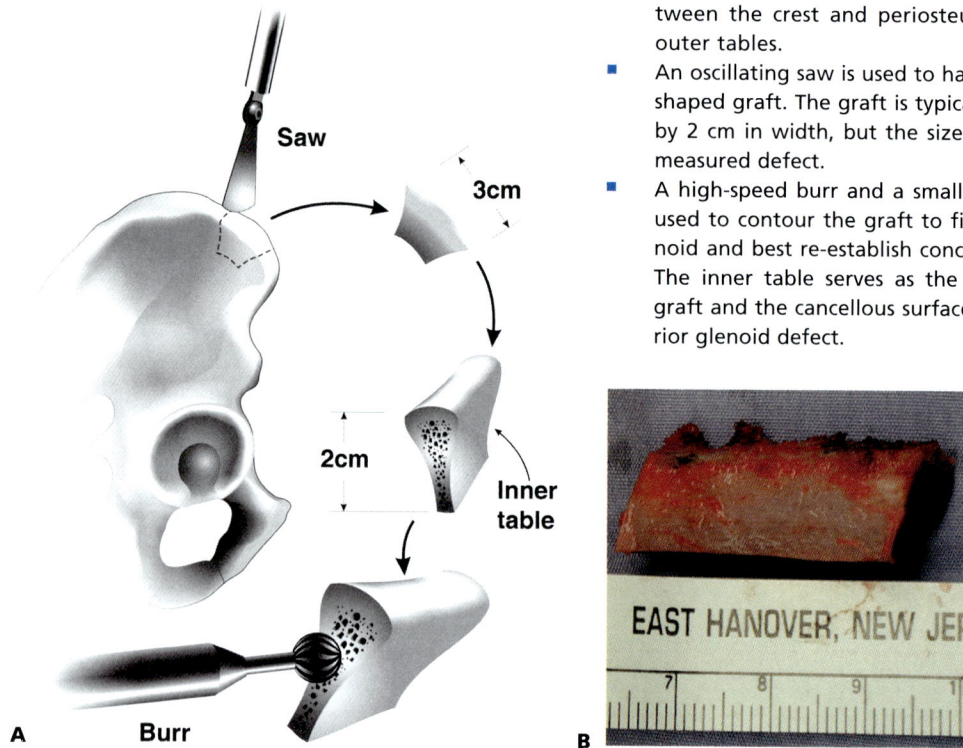

- tween the crest and periosteum along the inner and outer tables.
- An oscillating saw is used to harvest a tricortical wedge-shaped graft. The graft is typically about 3 cm in length by 2 cm in width, but the size should be based on the measured defect.
- A high-speed burr and a small oscillating saw are then used to contour the graft to fit along the anterior glenoid and best re-establish concavity, depth, and length. The inner table serves as the articular portion of the graft and the cancellous surface is opposed to the anterior glenoid defect.

TECH FIG 3 • Tricortical iliac crest bone graft. **A.** Bone graft is harvested from the iliac crest using an oscillating saw and preserving both the inner and outer tables. A high-speed burr is used to contour the graft. **B.** The size of the graft is typically 3 cm in length and 2 cm in width but should be based on the measured size of the defect.

FIXATION OF TRICORTICAL GRAFT TO GLENOID

- The tricortical iliac crest graft is secured to the glenoid (**TECH FIG 4**).
- The contoured graft is then positioned onto the anterior glenoid with the inner table of the iliac crest facing laterally as the articular surface.

- Positioning of the graft is critical. Glenoid concavity should be established but impingement or articular step-off should be avoided. This can be done by avoiding too vertical or too horizontal of an angle between the graft and glenoid.

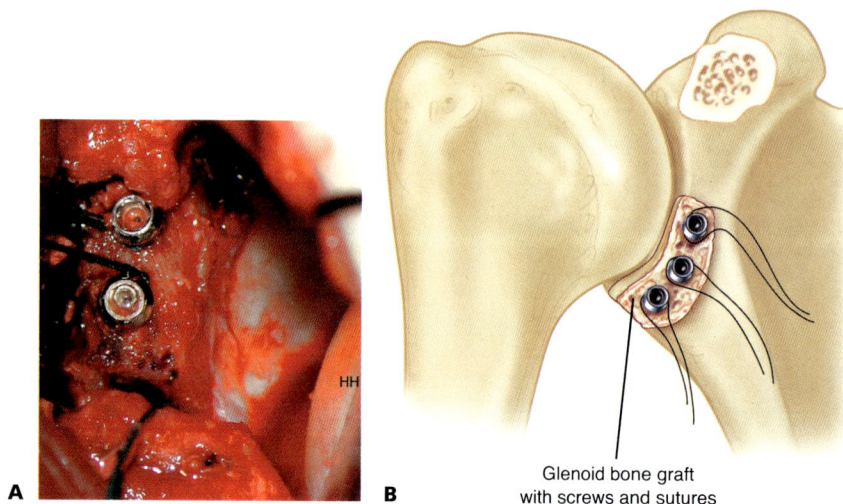

Glenoid bone graft with screws and sutures

TECH FIG 4 • Fixation of graft to the glenoid. **A.** The graft is positioned to establish concavity to the glenoid as well as a smooth transition between the graft and native glenoid to avoid an articular step-off. **B.** A number 2 braided polyethylene suture is placed around each 4.0-mm screw before it is fully tightened to assist in later capsular repair. (*continued*)

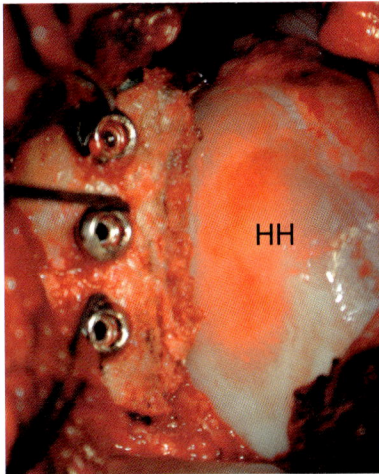

TECH FIG 4 • (continued) **C.** Once the graft is secured with screws, the glenohumeral retractor is removed and the position of the humeral head (*HH*) on the glenoid is noted.

- Avoid too vertical of an angle, as this may result in humeral impingement.
- Avoid too horizontal of an angle, as this may fail to re-establish glenoid concavity.
- With the graft correctly positioned, it can be temporarily secured to the anterior glenoid using two or three terminally threaded Kirschner wires from the stainless steel AO 4.0-mm cannulated screw set (AO/Synthes, Paoli, PA).
- Two or three partially threaded 4.0-mm cannulated screws are then placed over the Kirschner wires to secure the graft.
- A number 2 braided polyethylene suture is placed around the shaft of each screw before the screw is fully seated and compressing the graft. These sutures may be used for later capsular repair.
- The Fukuda retractor is gently removed and the position of the humeral head is noted. The glenohumeral joint is ranged and any incongruity or instability noted should prompt a change in graft position.

REPAIR OF CAPSULE AND SUBSCAPULARIS

- The capsulotomy and subscapularis are then repaired (**TECH FIG 5**).
- The sutures from the graft fixation screws are passed through the capsule–periosteal sleeve as horizontal mattress stitches and tied.
- The capsulotomy can be further repaired in one of two ways:
  - If the L-shaped capsulotomy can be repaired primarily, it is reapproximated using number 2 braided polyethylene suture. Often, though, the graft occupies enough space and the capsule is contracted so that a primary repair of the capsulotomy is not possible.
  - If the L-shaped capsulotomy cannot be repaired primarily to the neck of the humerus with the arm in at least 30 degrees of external rotation, then the capsule is repaired to the lateral portion of the subscapularis tendon. This will tension the anterior capsule as the subscapularis becomes more taut with external rotation.
- The lesser tuberosity is gently abraded with a high-speed burr to cause punctate bleeding.
- The subscapularis is then meticulously repaired to the lesser tuberosity with two or three suture anchors using a modified Mason-Allen stitch.
- The shoulder incision is closed in layers.

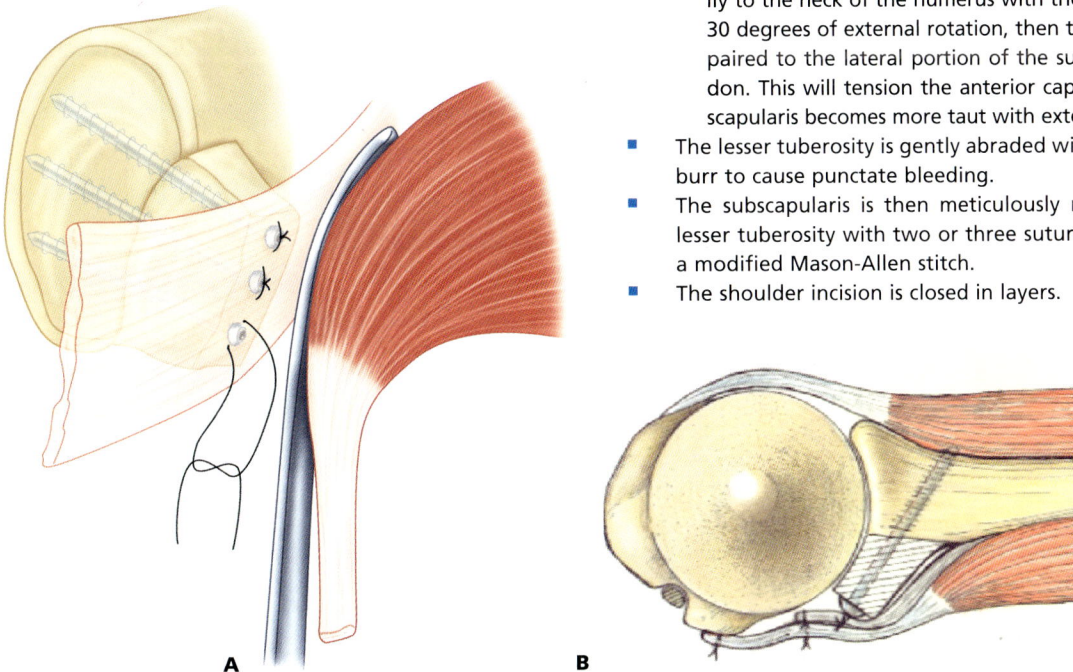

TECH FIG 5 • Repair of capsulotomy and subscapularis. **A.** The sutures around the screws are secured through the capsule with horizontal mattress stitches. **B.** If the capsule cannot be repaired back to the humeral neck without being excessively tight and restrictive of external rotation, it is secured to the deep surface of the subscapularis tendon with horizontal mattress sutures. The subscapularis is then repaired to the lesser tuberosity with suture anchors.

PEARLS AND PITFALLS

Indications	■ A complete history and physical should be performed.
	■ Associated pathology must be recognized and addressed:
	  ■ The glenohumeral joint must be assessed for osteoarthrosis.
	  ■ The humeral head must be assessed for a significant engaging Hill-Sachs lesion. It is rare for the lesion to be engaging after reconstruction of the width of the glenoid.

Tricortical graft harvest	■ Care should be exercised to avoid disrupting the anterosuperior iliac spine. ■ The lateral femoral cutaneous and ilioinguinal nerves are at risk during dissection of the anterior ilium.
Tricortical graft placement	■ Placement of the graft in too vertical of a position may result in impingement of the humeral head and articular erosion. ■ Placement of the graft in too horizontal of a position does not recreate concavity of the glenoid. ■ There must be a smooth transition between the native glenoid and bone graft. This is ensured by proper positioning. A burr can be used to remove any prominences from the graft that remain after fixation.
Stiffness	■ Patients should be counseled to expect some limitation of external rotation postoperatively. ■ The goal is to achieve a stable joint with no more than 20 degrees loss of external rotation to limit the risk of capsulorrhaphy arthropathy. This should be considered during capsular repair.

POSTOPERATIVE CARE

■ Radiographs are obtained to judge graft placement and screw position. A CT scan is helpful to estimate graft incorporation (**FIG 6**).

■ The shoulder is maintained in a sling immobilizer for 4 weeks.

■ Pendulum exercises are allowed after the first week.

■ At 4 weeks, the sling is removed to allow:
  ■ Activities of daily living
  ■ Passive range of motion, active assisted range of motion, water therapy

■ At 3 months, strengthening is initiated.

■ Participation in overhead recreational sport (golf, tennis, swimming) is allowed at 4 months.

■ Participation in contact or collision sports is allowed at 6 months.

OUTCOMES

■ With appropriate preoperative workup, diagnosis, and surgical technique, anatomic reconstruction of the glenoid with tricortical iliac crest bone graft is very effective at treating recurrent dislocations in the setting of a bony glenoid defect.

■ Hutchinson and colleagues[4] demonstrated no recurrent dislocations after tricortical iliac crest bone grafting in a population of epileptics who continued to have seizures postoperatively.

■ Warner and associates[8] reported no recurrent dislocations or subluxations after anterior glenoid bone grafting in a population of athletes with traumatic recurrent anterior instability. There was a mean loss of external rotation in abduction of 14 degrees.

COMPLICATIONS

■ Subscapularis insufficiency
■ Hardware failure and migration
■ Stiffness
■ Brachial plexus injury

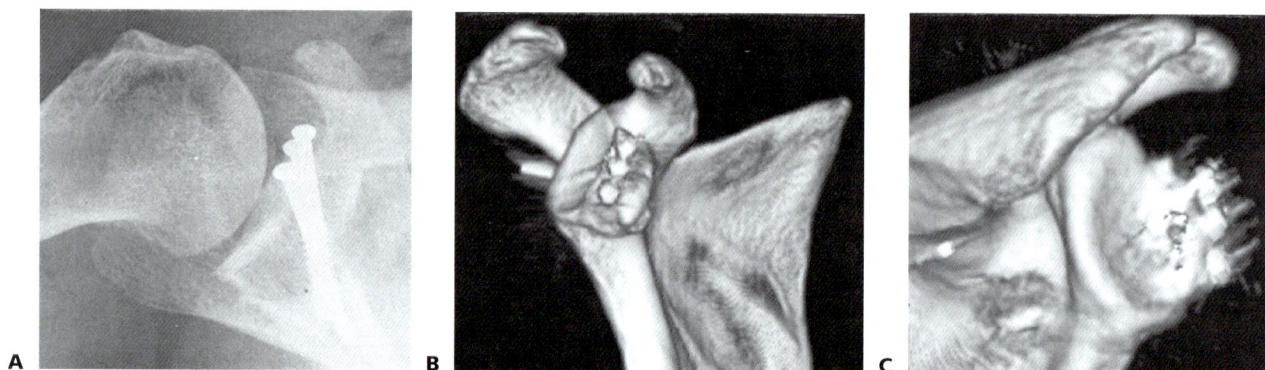

FIG 6 • Postoperative imaging of glenoid reconstruction with tricortical iliac crest bone graft. **A.** Axillary lateral. **B.** Anterior view of 3D CT reconstruction demonstrating position and incorporation of graft. **C.** Posterior view of 3D CT reconstruction demonstrating restored glenoid width, depth, and concavity.

REFERENCES

1. Burkhart SS, DeBeer JF. Traumatic glenohumeral bone defects and their relationship to failure of arthroscopic Bankart repairs: significance of the inverted-pear glenoid and the humeral enaging Hill-Sachs lesion. Arthroscopy 2000;16:677–694.
2. Farber AJ, Castillo R, Clough M, et al. Clinical assessment of three common tests for traumatic anterior shoulder instability. J Bone Joint Surg Am 2006;88A:1467–1474.
3. Gerber C, Nyffeler RW. Classification of glenohumeral joint instability. Clin Orthop Relat Res 2002;400:65–76.
4. Hutchinson JW, Neumann L, Wallace WA. Bone buttress operation for recurrent anterior shoulder dislocation in epilepsy. J Bone Joint Surg Br 1995;77B:928–932.
5. Itoi E, Lee SB, Berglund LJ, et al. The effect of glenoid defect on anteroinferior stability of the shoulder after Bankart repair: a cadaver study. J Bone Joint Surg Am 2000;82A:35–46.
6. Itoi E, Lee SB, Amrami KK, et al. Quantitative assessment of classic anteroinferior bony Bankart lesions by radiography and computed tomography. Am J Sports Med 2003;31:112–118.
7. Lippitt SB, Vanderhooft JE, Harris SL, et al. Glenohumeral stability from concavity-compression: a quantitative analysis. J Shoulder Elbow Surg 1993;2:27–35.
8. Warner JP, Gill TJ, O'Hollerhan JD, et al. Anatomical glenoid reconstruction for recurrent anterior glenohumeral instability with glenoid deficiency using an autogenous tricortical iliac crest bone graft. Am J Sports Med 2006;34:205–212.

Chapter 7

Management of Glenohumeral Instability With Humeral Bone Loss

Michael A. Rauh and Anthony Miniaci

DEFINITION

- The glenohumeral joint is one of the most commonly dislocated joints in the body.
- With anterior dislocations, bony defects of the anterior glenoid and posterosuperior aspect of the humeral head occur with relative frequency.
- One of the first descriptions of the lesions found on the humeral head was by Flower[4] in 1861, with many subsequent investigators reporting on these bony defects.[13]
- In 1940, two radiologists, Hill and Sachs,[6] reported that these defects were actually compression fractures produced when the posterolateral humeral head impinged against the anterior rim of the glenoid.
- Since then, Hill-Sachs lesions have been found to occur with an incidence between 32% and 51% at the time of initial anterior glenohumeral dislocation.
- In shoulders sustaining a Hill-Sachs lesion at the initial dislocation, there exists a statistically significant association with recurrent dislocation.[7,8]
- Although Hill-Sachs lesions are common after anterior glenohumeral dislocations, there are relatively few publications describing specific treatments for these humeral head defects.[14,19]
- In general, specific surgical procedures to address Hill-Sachs lesions have not been recommended in the initial surgical management of recurrent anterior dislocations because the majority of these lesions are small to moderate in size and do not routinely cause significant symptoms of instability.
- Certain subsets of patients exist with more significant bony defects and ongoing symptoms of "instability" or painful clicking, catching, or popping. This occurs even after surgical procedures directed at treating their anterior instability.

ANATOMY

- With an anterior shoulder dislocation, the humeral head is positioned anterior to the glenoid rim.
- The posterosuperior aspect of the humeral head then impacts upon the anterior aspect of the glenoid rim and creates the Hill-Sachs lesion (**FIG 1A**).
- Only after the shoulder joint is relocated can the influence of the size and shape of the Hill-Sachs lesion on overall shoulder stability be determined (**FIG 1B,C**).
- Although there is not scientific proof, our clinical experience suggests that lesions representing 25% to 30% of the articulating surface arc of the humeral head often lead to symptoms.

PATHOGENESIS

- The concept of "articular arc length mismatch" has been recently put forth by Burkhart to "explain the ongoing sensation of catching or popping" arising in the shoulder with a large Hill-Sachs lesion alone or in combination with glenoid defects."[1,2]
- Patients with these symptoms have often undergone previous anterior stabilization procedures and reconstruction of damaged glenohumeral ligaments at that time.

- This phenomenon, debatably referred to as "instability," occurs mainly in a position of abduction and external rotation of the shoulder.
  - In this position, a large "engaging" Hill-Sachs lesion encounters the anterior glenoid rim, resulting in the rim "dropping into" the Hill-Sachs lesion.
- The sudden loss of smooth articular surface on the humeral side of the joint presents an irregularly contoured area to the glenoid, causing an uneasy sensation in the patient that feels much like subluxation.
- As Burkhart and DeBeer pointed out, for every "Hill-Sachs lesion, there is a position of the shoulder at which the humeral bone defect will engage the anterior glenoid."
- Clinically, it is important to differentiate between "engaging" and "nonengaging" Hill-Sachs lesions.[1,2]
  - An *engaging* Hill-Sachs lesion is one that presents the long axis of its defect parallel to the anterior glenoid with the shoulder in a functional position of abduction and external rotation, such that the Hill-Sachs lesion encounters the rim of the glenoid.
    - Lesions can be considered engaging even in positions that are considered "nonfunctional," such as in some degree of extension, or in lesser degrees of abduction.
    - Apprehension and instability in lesser degrees of shoulder abduction often indicate a significant bony defect that is leading to the perceived instability.[14]
  - A *nonengaging* Hill-Sachs lesion is one that either fails to engage the glenoid or engages the glenoid only in a nonfunctional arm position. For example, the Hill-Sachs defect can pass diagonally across the anterior glenoid with external rotation; therefore, there is continual contact of the articulating surfaces and no engagement of the Hill-Sachs lesion by the anterior glenoid.[14]
- Hence, when a patient has symptomatic anterior instability associated with an engaging Hill-Sachs lesion with an articular arc deficit, treatment must be directed at both repairing the Bankart lesion, if present, and preventing the Hill-Sachs lesion from engaging the anterior glenoid.
- We believe that the treatment of symptomatic anterior glenohumeral instability, involving an engaging Hill-Sachs lesion with an articular arc deficit, can be accomplished satisfactorily with a technique of anatomic allograft reconstruction of the humeral head using a side- and size-matched humeral head osteoarticular allograft.
- This technique involves an anatomic reconstruction that eliminates the structural pathology while maintaining the range of motion of the glenohumeral joint.

NATURAL HISTORY

- One of the most clearly documented series of nonoperatively treated shoulder dislocations placed into immobilization is that of Hovelius and associates.[8]

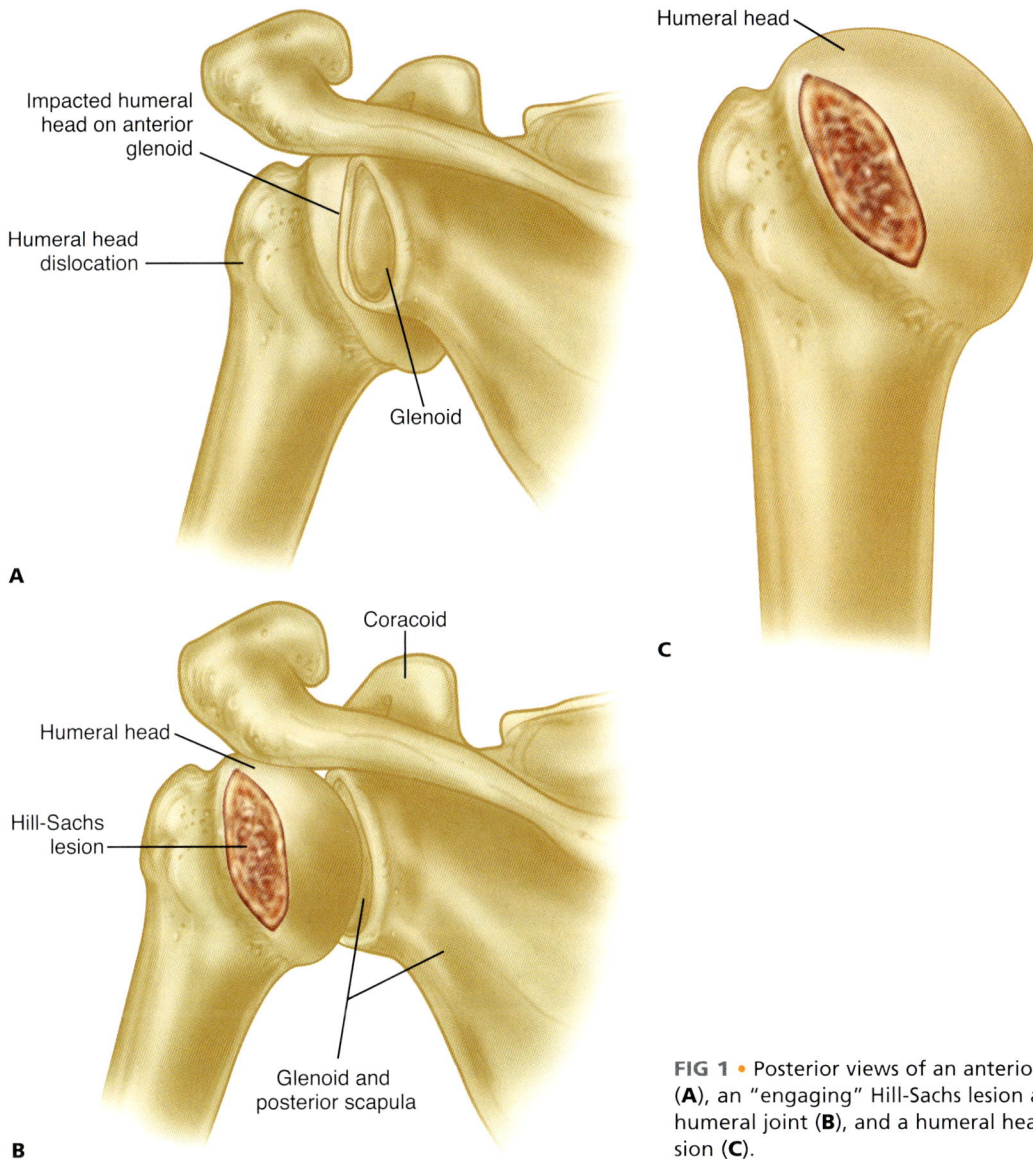

FIG 1 • Posterior views of an anterior glenohumeral dislocation (**A**), an "engaging" Hill-Sachs lesion after relocation of the glenohumeral joint (**B**), and a humeral head with a large Hill-Sachs lesion (**C**).

- They determined that the "type and duration of the initial treatment had no effect on the rate of recurrence; with a higher rate of recurrence the younger the patient."
- Overall, 52% of 247 primary anterior dislocations had no further dislocations.
- Patients who were 12 to 22 years old had a 34% redislocation rate, while those who were 30 to 40 years had a rate of 9%.
- Ninety-nine of 185 shoulders that were evaluated with radiographs had evidence of a Hill-Sachs lesion; and of these 99 shoulders, 60 redislocated at least once and 51 redislocated at least twice during the 10-year follow-up.
- This compares with 38 (44%) of the 86 shoulders that did not have such a lesion documented (P < 0.04).
- Acute first-time shoulder dislocations have traditionally been treated nonoperatively with reduction followed by a form of immobilization.
- Currently recommended types of immobilization after shoulder dislocations are as follows:
  - Simple sling immobilization with the arm in internal rotation[11]

- Immobilization in external rotation[9,10]
- No clear evidence has quieted this discussion.

PATIENT HISTORY AND PHYSICAL FINDINGS

- All patients are initially evaluated with complete history and physical examination.
  - Specifics of the history include questioning for the mode of onset and timing of initial symptoms, and for the details of present symptoms, including pain, frequency, instability, and level of function.
  - All previous surgical procedures performed on the shoulder should be noted.
- Most patients will give a history of recurrent dislocations or multiple surgical attempts to correct the instability.
- Although thought to be a procedure for failed attempts at shoulder stabilization after dislocation, there are other situations that might lead the surgeon to consider this procedure initially.
  - Significant traumatic mechanism with an extensive Hill-Sachs lesion (more than 25% to 30% of the articulating surface of the humeral head)

- Patients with a history of grand mal seizures often have fairly large Hill-Sachs defects and significant apprehension about the use of their arm. Also, as a result of the violence of the dislocations, the amount of bone pathology present, and the inability to predict the onset of epileptic events, it is worth considering treating this group of patients with an allograft reconstruction of the humeral head defect at the index procedure, as soft tissue repairs alone may not be enough to prevent recurrent injury.
- Physical examination should focus on inspection for previous scars, a thorough determination of active and passive range of motion, and evaluation of the integrity and strength of the rotator cuff.
- The clinician should perform a detailed examination for glenohumeral laxity in the anterior, posterior, and inferior directions.
- Examination for apprehension should be performed in multiple positions, as patients with large Hill-Sachs lesions usually exhibit apprehension that often occurs with the arm in significantly less than 90 degrees abduction and 90 degrees external rotation.[13,14]
- A comprehensive examination should include but is not limited to:
  - Anterior apprehension test: Positive apprehension can be associated with anterior labral injuries.
  - Bony apprehension test: Apprehension with fewer degrees of abduction may indicate a significant and symptomatic bony contribution to the instability.

IMAGING AND OTHER DIAGNOSTIC STUDIES

- Preoperative imaging includes a comprehensive plain film evaluation with anteroposterior (AP), true AP, axillary, and Stryker notch views of the involved shoulder (**FIG 2A**).
- All patients require a preoperative axial imaging study (CT or MRI) to more fully define the bony architecture of the glenoid and humeral head and specifically the details of the Hill-Sachs lesion (**FIG 2B**).
- One must be careful when interpreting these studies, since the plane of the Hill-Sachs defect is oblique to the plane of the axial image. Therefore, the size of these defects is often underestimated in standard axial imaging.
- Three-dimensional reconstruction can be a useful tool to more clearly define the size and location of the defect and to estimate the amount of the articular surface involved.
- While the volume and depth of the lesion certainly affect the stability of the shoulder, even more important may be the size of the defect in the articular arc.

DIFFERENTIAL DIAGNOSIS

- Anterior shoulder dislocation with or without:
  - Bankart lesion
  - "Bony Bankart" or an anterior glenoid lesion
  - Hill-Sachs lesion
  - Combination of the above
- Posterior shoulder dislocation with or without associated soft tissue and bony lesions
- Inferior shoulder dislocation with or without associated soft tissue and bony lesions

NONOPERATIVE MANAGEMENT

- Given a mechanism of shoulder dislocation, the presence of significant bony defects to the glenoid or the humeral head, and associated functional instability, there are not anticipated gains through nonoperative management.

SURGICAL MANAGEMENT

- Several techniques have been described in the literature to address symptomatic engaging Hill-Sachs lesions.
  - Open anterior procedures, such as an East–West plication to limit external rotation, designed to limit external rotation such that the humeral head defect is kept from engaging[1,2]
  - Rotational proximal humeral osteotomy as described by Weber and colleagues[17]
  - Transfer of the infraspinatus into the defect to render the lesion essentially extra-articular[3,18]
  - Filling in of the Hill-Sachs defect so that it can no longer engage, using either a corticocancellous iliac graft or a femoral head osteoarticular allograft
- If the defect is severe, prosthetic replacement using a hemiarthroplasty may become necessary.[16]
- In the case of posterior glenohumeral dislocation, Gerber and coworkers[5] have reported on the successful reconstruction of the humeral head by elevation of the depressed cartilage and subchondral buttressing with cancellous bone graft, as well as femoral head osteoarticular allograft reconstruction of the humeral head defect.
- The indications for anatomic allograft reconstruction of the humeral head are as follows:
  - Ongoing symptomatic anterior glenohumeral instability or painful clicking, catching, or popping in a patient with a large engaging Hill-Sachs lesion in patients who have failed to respond to previous soft-tissue stabilization procedures
  - A large engaging Hill-Sachs lesion is identified before undergoing initial surgical treatment. Clinical experience suggests that lesions involving more than 25% to 30% of the articular surface may be significant.[14]

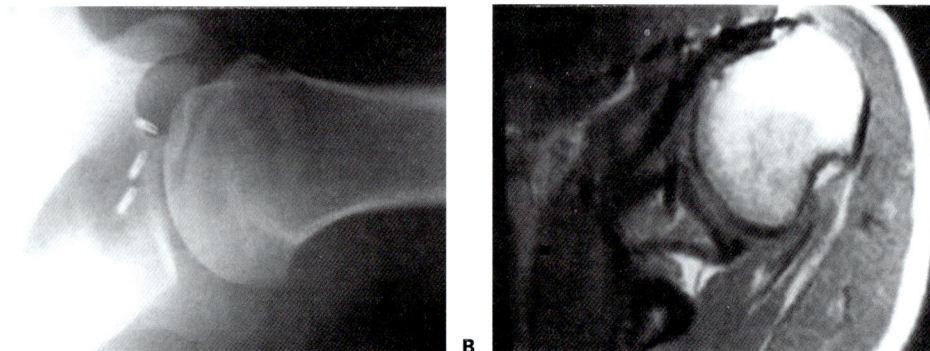

FIG 2 • **A.** AP radiograph of shoulder demonstrating a large Hill-Sachs lesion. **B.** Axial MRI image demonstrating large engaging Hill-Sachs lesion.

- Patients at high risk of redislocation (eg, epilepsy with recurrent anterior instability and large Hill-Sachs defects, or contact athletes with combined bony defects to the glenoid and humeral head) can consider this procedure as a primary treatment option.
  - Contact athletes can be considered in this group, as time lost from an activity can be a significant issue. Thus, treatment focused on all bony and soft tissue lesions might lessen the likelihood that they would sustain a failed procedure and the associated delay in returning to full competition.
- Contraindications to this procedure include routine medical comorbidities precluding an elective surgical procedure with general anesthetic, existing infection, or presence of a nonengaging or functionally nonengaging Hill-Sachs lesion.

Preoperative Planning

- A fresh-frozen cryopreserved osteoarticular humeral head allograft is obtained from a reputable, certified tissue bank.
  - It is important to obtain a side- and size-matched graft as this allows for an optimal recreation of the radius of curvature of the humeral head.
  - The details regarding treatment, preservation, and storage then differ depending on the type of sample and the preference of the surgeon.
  - The graft serves mainly a structural function, and cartilage viability is probably not essential for success.
  - The availability of fresh-frozen tissue can be problematic, and therefore we have sometimes performed the procedure using irradiated grafts.
  - In 2 of 20 cases using irradiated grafts, however, we observed partial collapse of the grafts, which required reoperation and screw removal. Fortunately, this did not lead to recurrent instability.
  - As a result, our present protocol favors the use of fresh-frozen tissue.
- Allograft sizing of the humeral head is performed by sending copies of your patient's films to the chosen bone bank for measurement.

- Plain radiographs can be used as long as they were obtained with magnification markers. Acceptable markers include some form of recognizable currency, such as a United States quarter or dime, or a standard magnification marker obtained from your tissue bank.
- CT or MRI scan of the proximal humerus would allow for direct sizing from the scan since the magnification effect is factored into the resulting images.
- Whichever way one chooses, the tissue bank should search for a match that has a side and size match to within about ±2 mm. Clinically, we have found that this tolerance yields acceptable results for this procedure.
- Specific details should be arranged between the surgeon and the tissue bank.
- Nevertheless, availability of an allograft is sometimes a problem.
  - If waiting is not an option, one may choose to use nonmatched humeral grafts or femoral head allograft.
  - The problem with this is that femoral heads often have evidence of osteoarthritis and loss of articular cartilage. This is a suboptimal situation and should be avoided.
- If different-sized grafts or femoral head grafts are used, they may not match the curvature of the native humeral head exactly and would need to be trimmed to obtain an optimal fit.
- It is important to discuss and understand the details of allograft use as it may have direct implications to your patient.

Positioning

- The patient is positioned in a modified beach chair position, inclined about 45 degrees, with the upper extremity draped free.

Approach

- An extended deltopectoral approach is used.
- The lateral border of the conjoined tendon is identified and gently retracted medially to expose the underlying subscapularis tendon.

RELEASE OF THE SUBSCAPULARIS MUSCLE AND CAPSULOTOMY

- The entire tendon is transected vertically about 0.5 cm medial to its insertion onto the lesser tuberosity.
- Tag sutures of number 2 Control Release Ethibond Excel (#DC494, Ethicon, Somerville, NJ) are placed in the lateral aspect of the subscapularis tendon as it is released from the lesser tuberosity.
- The interval between the subscapularis and the anterior capsule is then carefully developed using sharp dissection, continuing medially to the neck of the glenoid.

- The inferior capsule is then further isolated using careful blunt dissection.
- A laterally based capsulotomy is made with the vertical limb in line with the subscapularis incision and continuing superiorly.
- The anteroinferior capsule is then released off the surgical neck of the humerus with intra-articular dissection using a periosteal elevator.

TECHNIQUES

ANTERIOR LABRAL INSPECTION AND BANKART RECONSTRUCTION

- A standard humeral head retractor is placed into the glenohumeral joint, allowing inspection of the glenoid and anteroinferior capsulolabral structures for any pathology.

- If a Bankart lesion is found, it is repaired in the usual fashion using either bony drill holes or suture anchors. The sutures can be left untied until completion of the allograft reconstruction.

TECHNIQUES

EXPOSURE OF THE HILL-SACHS LESION

- The humeral head retractor is withdrawn and the humerus is brought into maximal external rotation to expose the Hill-Sachs lesion.
- Unroof the synovial expansion of the supraspinatus to allow the humerus to be more fully externally rotated, allowing better visualization and access to the Hill-Sachs lesion.
- A flat narrow retractor (eg, Darach) is then placed over the reflected undersurface of the subscapularis tendon and behind the neck of the humerus on the posterior rotator cuff in order to lever out the humeral head (**TECH FIG 1**).

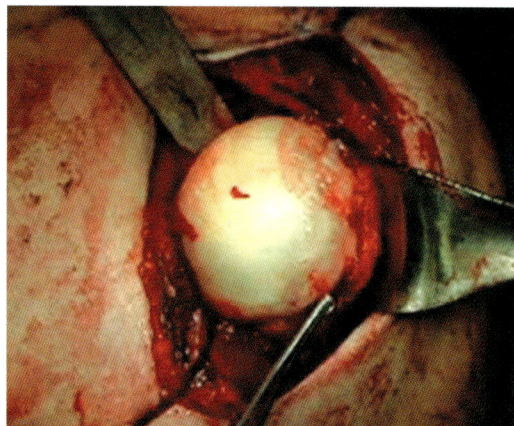

TECH FIG 1 • Intraoperative exposure of large Hill-Sachs lesion to be reconstructed.

HUMERAL HEAD OSTEOTOMY

- With the Hill-Sachs lesion adequately exposed, a micro-sagittal saw is used to smooth and reshape the defect into a chevron-type configuration.
- The piece of matching allograft humeral head to be inserted should resemble a deep-dish slice of pie (**TECH FIG 2A,B**).

- The base and side of the defect can then be further smoothed using a hand rasp to achieve precise, flat surfaces.
- The base (X), height (Y), length (Z), and rough outside partial circumference (C) of the defect are then measured to the nearest millimeter (**TECH FIG 2C**).

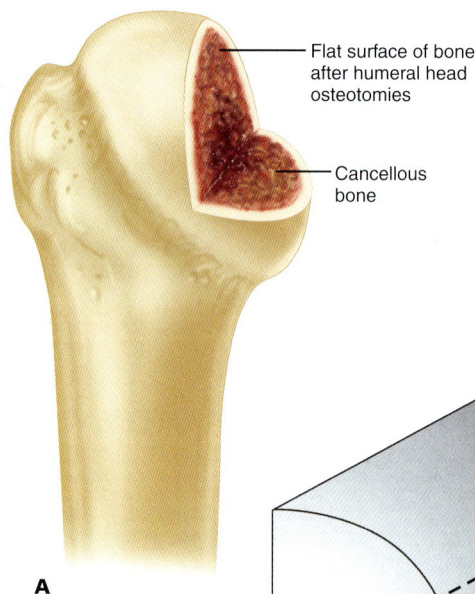

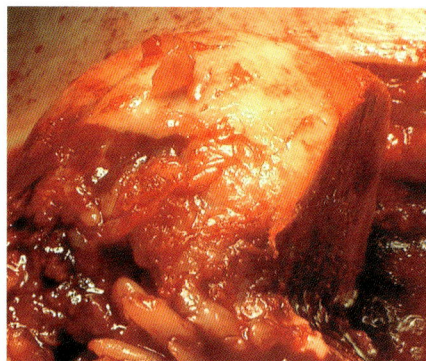

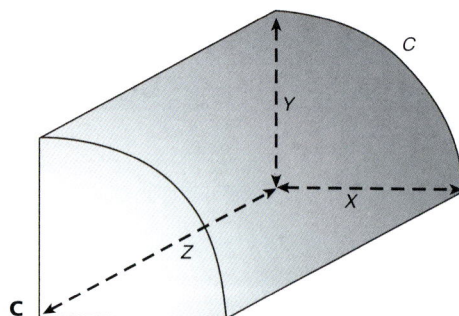

TECH FIG 2 • **A.** Diagram of the humeral head after osteotomies. **B.** Reshaping of Hill-Sachs lesion to prepare to receive allograft. **C.** Schematic representation of required measurements of the defect and graft. Base (X), height (Y), length (Z), and rough outside partial circumference (C) of the defect are then measured to the nearest millimeter.

OSTEOTOMY OF THE HUMERAL HEAD ALLOGRAFT

- A corresponding piece is cut from the matched humeral head allograft that is 2 to 3 mm larger in all dimensions than the measured defect.
- The allograft segment is then provisionally placed into the Hill-Sachs defect and resized in all three planes.

- Excess graft is then carefully trimmed with the micro-sagittal saw and is reshaped in the other two planes as well.
- Fine-tuning of graft size is then continued in one plane at a time until a perfect size match is achieved in all planes, including base (X), height (Y), length (Z), and outside partial circumference (C).

TECHNIQUES

FIXATION OF THE HUMERAL HEAD ALLOGRAFT

- The allograft segment is placed into the defect and aligned so as to achieve a congruent articular surface.
- It is provisionally secured in place with two or three smooth 0.045-inch Kirschner wires (**TECH FIG 3A,B**).
- The wires are then sequentially replaced with 3.5-mm fully threaded cortical or 4.0-mm cancellous screws placed in a lag fashion (**TECH FIG 3C,D**).

- Ensure that the screw heads are countersunk so that they are below the level of the articular surface.
- The joint is irrigated and taken through a range of motion to ensure that the reconstructed humeral head provides a smooth congruent articulating surface.

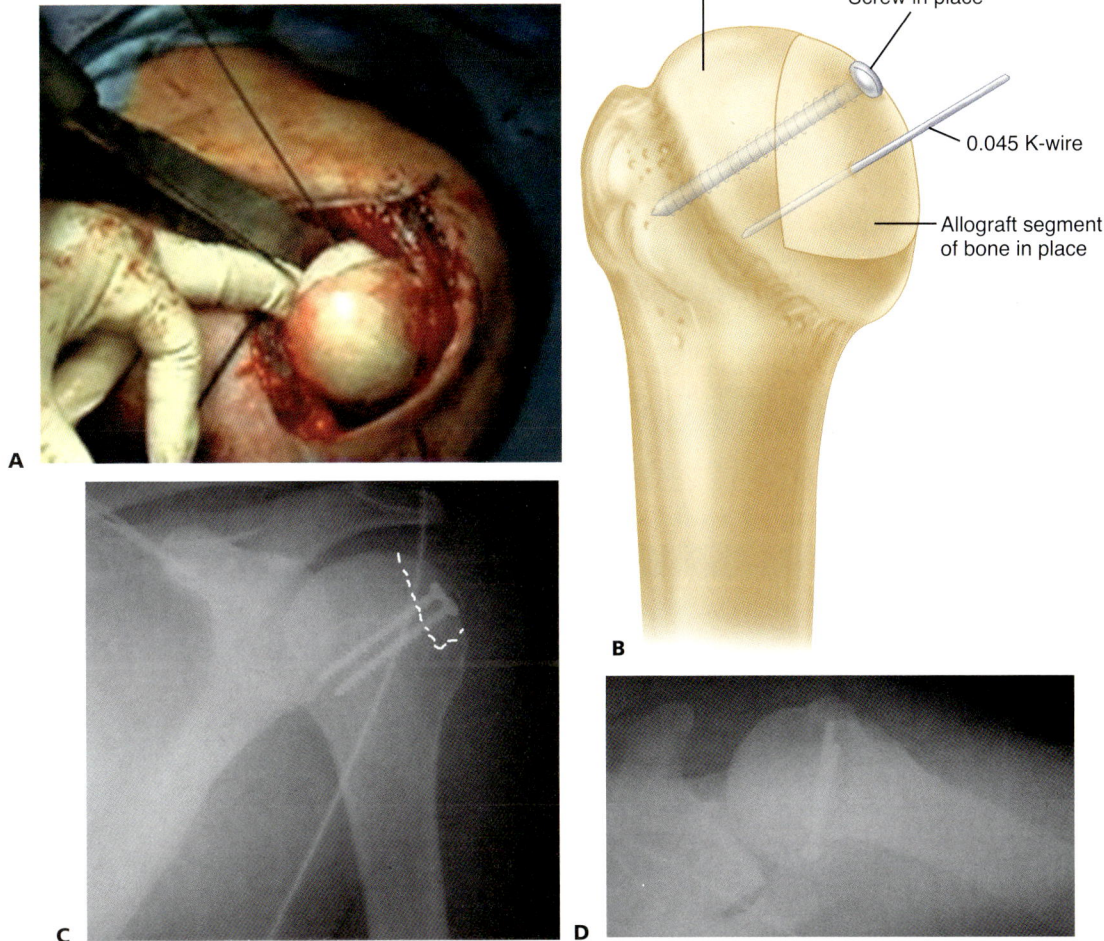

TECH FIG 3 • **A.** Anatomic allograft reconstruction of Hill-Sachs defect with humeral allograft provisionally held in place with two Kirschner wires. **B.** Diagram of allograft reconstruction of Hill-Sachs defect with humeral allograft held in place with a Kirschner wire and an AO screw. **C.** AP radiograph of shoulder demonstrating anatomic allograft reconstruction of Hill-Sachs defect fixed with two countersunk cortical screws. (*Dashed line* represents the area filled by the allograft.) **D.** Axillary view of shoulder demonstrating anatomic allograft reconstruction of Hill-Sachs defect fixed with two countersunk cortical screws.

LABRAL REPAIR AND SUBSCAPULARIS REAPPROXIMATION

- The capsulotomy is closed with absorbable suture, tying any previously placed sutures used to repair the capsulolabral pathology if present.
- The subscapularis tendon is then reapproximated to its stump anatomically, without shortening, using suture anchors or a soft tissue repair with nonabsorbable suture.

- Allow the conjoined tendon, deltoid, and pectoralis major muscles to return to their normal anatomic positions.
- A routine subcutaneous and skin closure is then performed.
- Sterile dressing is applied.
- The arm is placed into a shoulder immobilizer.

PEARLS AND PITFALLS

Anterior labral injury	▪ The surgeon should ensure this injury pattern is identified early after exposure of the joint. Anchors or sutures are placed in the anterior glenoid for later labral repair after reconstruction of the Hill-Sachs lesion.
Exposure of the posterior superior humeral head	▪ This area of the humeral head can be accessed through external rotation and forward flexion of the upper extremity. Appropriately placed retractors assist in this exposure.
Allograft sizing	▪ The surgeon should ensure the allograft obtained is larger in dimension by 2 to 3 mm than the actual defect. This allows for in situ sizing.
Screw placement	▪ It is easier to initially place two 0.045-inch Kirschner wires for fixation and then replace them with two 3.5-mm stainless steel AO screws lagged into position. ▪ Screw heads are countersunk beneath the surface of the allograft articular surface to prevent hardware penetration.

POSTOPERATIVE CARE

▪ After surgery, patients are given a sling for comfort and allowed full passive range of motion immediately as tolerated.

▪ Because of the subscapularis detachment, we protect against active and resisted internal rotation for 6 weeks.

▪ After the initial 6-week period, patients are allowed terminal stretching and strengthening exercises.

▪ The shoulders are imaged with repeat radiographs at 6 weeks and 6 months, and with CT scans at 6 months to assess for consolidation and incorporation of the graft.

OUTCOMES

▪ Between 1995 and 2001, we performed and reviewed this procedure in 18 patients who had failed previous attempts at surgical stabilization.[13,14]

▪ Fifteen patients had a history of traumatic anterior glenohumeral instability related to sports, and three patients had instability related to seizures or other trauma.

▪ All had posterolateral humeral head defects (Hill-Sachs lesions) that represented greater than about 25% to 30% of the humeral head.

▪ One patient had both anterior and posterior humeral head defects from bidirectional shoulder instability sustained as a result of a seizure disorder.

▪ No patients had true multidirectional instability.

▪ Patients in the formal review were assessed preoperatively and postoperatively with:
  ▪ Detailed history
  ▪ Physical examination
  ▪ Radiographic evaluation (plain films and axial imaging [CT, MRI, or both])
  ▪ Validated clinical evaluation measures (Constant-Murley shoulder scale, Western Ontario Shoulder Instability Index [WOSII], and SF-36)

▪ Findings at the time of surgery included:
  ▪ Nine patients with recurrent Bankart lesions
  ▪ Nine patients with capsular redundancy only
  ▪ No patients with subscapularis tears
  ▪ One patient with posterior glenoid erosion
  ▪ Three patients with anterior glenoid deficiency (less than 20%), which was not reconstructed

▪ Mean length of follow-up was 50 months (range 24 to 96 months).

▪ There were no episodes of recurrent instability. Sixteen of 18 (89%) patients returned to work.

▪ The average Constant-Murley score postoperatively was 78.5. The WOSII, which is a validated quality-of-life scale specific to shoulder instability using a visual analog scale response format, decreased and patients were significantly improved.

▪ Overall, this represents the first reported series of anatomic allograft reconstruction of Hill-Sachs defects for recurrent traumatic anterior instability after failed repairs.

▪ This technique has been shown to be effective for a difficult problem with few available treatment options.

▪ The patients demonstrated improvement in stability, loss of apprehension, and high subjective approval, allowing return to near-normal function with no further episodes of instability.

▪ Although infrequently a cause for clinical concern, Hill-Sachs defects can be the source of significant disability and recurrent instability in a subset of patients.

▪ One should consider anatomic allograft reconstruction of these defects as a viable treatment alternative.

COMPLICATIONS

▪ Complications that occurred in our series of humeral osteoarticular allograft reconstruction of the Hill-Sachs lesions included radiographic follow-up evidence of partial graft collapse in 2 of 18 patients, early evidence of osteoarthritis in 3 patients (marginal osteophytes), and 1 mild subluxation (posterior).[12-14]

▪ Hardware complications developed in two patients, who complained of pain with extreme external rotation.
  ▪ The screws were removed at about 2 years postoperatively in both patients, thereby relieving their symptoms.

▪ One must weigh the risks of continued shoulder dysfunction versus the risk associated with the use of fresh osteoarticular allografts.

REFERENCES

1. Burkhart SS, Danaceau SM. Articular arc length mismatch as a cause of failed Bankart repair. Arthroscopy 2000;16:740–744.
2. Burkhart SS, De Beer JF. Traumatic glenohumeral bone defects and their relationship to failure of arthroscopic Bankart repairs: significance of the inverted-pear glenoid and the humeral engaging Hill-Sachs lesion. Arthroscopy 2000;16:677–694.
3. Connolly J. Humeral head defects associated with shoulder dislocations: their diagnostic and surgical significance. AAOS Instr Course Lect 1972;1972:42–54.
4. Flower WH. On the pathological changes produced in the shoulder-joint by traumatic dislocations, as derived from an examination of all specimens illustrating this injury in the museums of London. Trans Pathol Soc London 1861;12:179.

5. Gerber C, Lambert SM. Allograft reconstruction of segmental defects of the humeral head for the treatment of chronic locked posterior dislocation of the shoulder. J Bone Joint Surg Am 1996;78A: 376–382.

6. Hill HA, Sachs MD. The groove defect of the humeral head: a frequently unrecognized complication of dislocations of the shoulder joint. Radiology 1940;35:690–700.

7. Hovelius L. Anterior dislocation of the shoulder in teen-agers and young adults: five-year prognosis. J Bone Joint Surg Am 1987;69: 393–399.

8. Hovelius L, Augustini BG, Fredin H, et al. Primary anterior dislocation of the shoulder in young patients: a ten-year prospective study. J Bone Joint Surg Am 1996;78A:1677–1684.

9. Itoi E, Hatakeyama Y, Kido T, et al. A new method of immobilization after traumatic anterior dislocation of the shoulder: a preliminary study. J Shoulder Elbow Surg 2003;12:413–415.

10. Itoi E, Sashi R, Minagawa H, et al., Position of immobilization after dislocation of the shoulder: a cadaveric study. J Bone Joint Surg Am 1999;81A:385–390.

11. Matsen FA, Thomas SC, Rockwood CA. Glenohumeral instability. In Rockwood CA, ed. The Shoulder. Philadelphia: Elsevier, 2004:655–780.

12. Miniaci A. Reconstruction of large humeral head defects in patients with failed instability surgery. In Norris TR, ed. Surgery of the Shoulder and Elbow: An International Perspective. Rosemont, IL: American Academy of Orthopaedic Surgeons, 2006.

13. Miniaci A, Gish MW. Management of anterior glenohumeral instability associated with large Hill-Sachs defects. Tech Should Elbow Surg 2004;5:170–175.

14. Miniaci A, Martineau PA. Humeral head bony deficiency (large Hill-Sachs). In El Attrache NS, ed. Surgical Techniques in Sports Medicine. Philadelphia: Lippincott Williams & Wilkins, 2006.

15. Neer CS II, Foster CR. Inferior capsular shift for involuntary inferior and multidirectional instability of the shoulder: a preliminary report. J Bone Joint Surg Am 1980;62A:897–908.

16. Pritchett JW, Clark JM. Prosthetic replacement for chronic unreduced dislocations of the shoulder. Clin Orthop Relat Res 1987;216: 89–93.

17. Weber BG, Simpson AL, Hardegger F. Rotational humeral osteotomy for recurrent anterior dislocation of the shoulder associated with a large Hill-Sachs lesion. J Bone Joint Surg Am 1984;66A:1443–1450.

18. Wolf E, Pollack ME, Smalley C. Hill-Sachs "remplissage": an arthroscopic solution for the engaging Hill-Sachs lesion. Arthroscopy Association of North America, San Francisco, CA, 2007.

19. Yagishita K, Thomas BJ. Use of allograft for large Hill-Sachs lesion associated with anterior glenohumeral dislocation: a case report. Injury 2002;33:791–794.

Acromioplasty, Distal Clavicle Excision, and Posterosuperior Rotator Cuff Repair

Robert J. Neviaser and Andrew S. Neviaser

DEFINITION

- Posterosuperior tears of the rotator cuff involve the supraspinatus, infraspinatus, and occasionally the teres minor.
- Some of the surgical techniques to be described here are not commonly used currently, as most tears can be repaired by arthroscopic approaches, either with mini-open or all-arthroscopic techniques.
- These approaches, however, are still useful for treating those massive tears that may need special procedures to accomplish the repair.

ANATOMY

- The rotator cuff is a group of four musculotendinous structures arising from the scapula: the supraspinatus, the infraspinatus, the teres minor, and the subscapularis. The first three insert on the greater tuberosity of the humerus, while the subscapularis inserts on the lesser tuberosity. The cuff muscles not only rotate the humerus at the glenohumeral joint but also act to keep the humeral head centered in the glenoid fossa, providing a fixed fulcrum for the arm to be elevated, primarily by the deltoid. The subacromial bursa overlies the tendons.
- These structures, in turn, sit under the coracoacromial arch, which consists of the acromion, the coracoacromial ligament, and the outer end of the clavicle at the acromioclavicular joint.
- The three parts of the deltoid arise from the acromion and lateral clavicle, and this muscle lies over the cuff and bursa. It acts to elevate, abduct, and extend the humerus at the shoulder joint.

PATHOGENESIS

- Rotator cuff tears have a multifactorial pathogenesis.
- Among the factors are tendon insertional degeneration (enthesopathy), shear (the inferior third of the cuff tendons being more susceptible to shear failure than the superior two thirds), hypovascularity, impingement, and microtrauma.
- Although impingement was felt to be the sole underlying cause of cuff disease for some time, it is now felt to be a secondary factor, in that it likely comes into play once the cuff is weakened and is unable to balance the upward pull of the deltoid. This then brings the cuff into contact with the undersurface of the anteroinferior acromion and the rest of the coracoacromial arch.
- Major injury is uncommonly a factor and usually involves an already degenerative tendon. A common major injury, which can result in a rotator cuff tear, is a primary, or a first-time, anterior dislocation of the shoulder in a patient over age 40. The older the patient, the more likely there is a cuff tear.

NATURAL HISTORY

- The natural history of rotator cuff tears is unknown. There have been several studies in cadavers and by MRI that have confirmed that the incidence of asymptomatic cuff tears over the age of 60 is around 33%. These subjects have been pain-free and fully functional.
- Any study that has tried to follow asymptomatic tears prospectively over time has suffered from an unacceptably high loss of patients being followed, thereby negating any conclusions.
- Even the condition of cuff tear arthropathy does not occur regularly with known cuff tears, even massive ones.
- It has been shown that after a traumatic tear, the outcome is influenced by the time interval to repair—in other words, those repaired within the first 3 weeks do better then those repaired between 3 and 6 weeks, and those older than 6 weeks do even worse. These outcomes apply only to the uncommon traumatic tear, not to the far more common degenerative type.
- Therefore, treatment should be based purely on the presenting symptoms of pain and functional limitation, not on the possibility that a tear may progress in size or develop into cuff tear arthropathy, since the latter possibilities cannot be predicted.

PATIENT HISTORY AND PHYSICAL FINDINGS

- Barring the unusual history of a significant injury, such as a primary anterior glenohumeral dislocation over the age of 40 resulting in a traumatic tear, most patients will present with a complaint of pain of indeterminate onset.
- The pain is often worse at night and with use, especially overhead.
- Use of nonsteroidal anti-inflammatories (NSAIDs) may provide some temporary relief, as might stretching.
- The pain can radiate, but not to below the elbow or into the neck and occiput.
- There rarely will be significant motion loss (ie, motion will be unaffected) nor will the patient often notice weakness.
- The first step in the physical examination is to examine the neck to eliminate that as a source of the pain.
- One should inspect the shoulder for atrophy of the supraspinatus and infraspinatus or rupture of the tendon of the long head of the biceps, which usually occurs with a large or massive tear. One should also palpate the region of the greater tuberosity and the bicipital groove for tenderness. In thin patients, it is possible to feel the cuff defect through the skin and deltoid.
- Motion is assessed by having the patient elevate the arms actively and comparing this to passive motion and by placing the arms in 90 degrees of abduction and maximal external rotation, as well as maximal external rotation with the arm at the side.
  - The inability to hold the arm in maximum active external rotation in abduction or at the side, causing the arm to drift toward internal rotation, is a positive lag sign, indicating a major defect in the musculotendinous unit.

- Internal rotation is evaluated by having the patient reach up the back to the highest point possible. Further testing for this (subscapularis function) is discussed in another chapter.
- Strength of the external rotators is tested with the arm at the side and in maximal external rotation, having the patient resist a force directed toward the body. Strength in elevation is assessed by resisting the patient's attempt to raise the arm.
- Provocative signs for cuff and biceps disease include the following:
  - Impingement sign: Forcing the fully forward elevated arm against the fixed scapula helps to localize the finding to the rotator cuff when the patient experiences pain.
  - Palm-down abduction test: By internally rotating the arm, the supraspinatus and anterior infraspinatus tendons are placed directly under the coracoacromial arch. Elevating the arm in the scapular plane when it is in internal rotation compresses these tendons against the undersurface of the acromion.
  - Biceps resistance test (Speed's test): Pain during this maneuver indicates involvement of the long head of the biceps tendon.

IMAGING AND OTHER DIAGNOSTIC STUDIES

- Standard radiographs, including anteroposterior (AP) views in internal and external rotation, an axillary view, and an outlet view at minimum, should always be taken to look for the type of acromion (**FIG 1A**), acromioclavicular joint changes, and narrowing of the acromial–humeral interval (**FIG 1B**) and to rule out other conditions.
- Additional preoperative studies include MRI, ultrasound, and arthrography.
- Ultrasound is institutional-specific and operator-dependent, so it is not widely used.
- Arthrography once was the gold standard but now is used only under rare circumstances (ie, when an MRI cannot be done). It can show a full-thickness cuff tear (**FIG 1C**) but requires an intra-articular injection with fluoroscopy and radiography.
- The most commonly used study is an MRI. It not only shows the integrity of the tendons but also provides a three-dimensional view of it (**FIG 1D–G**). This capacity makes the MRI a versatile preoperative planning tool.

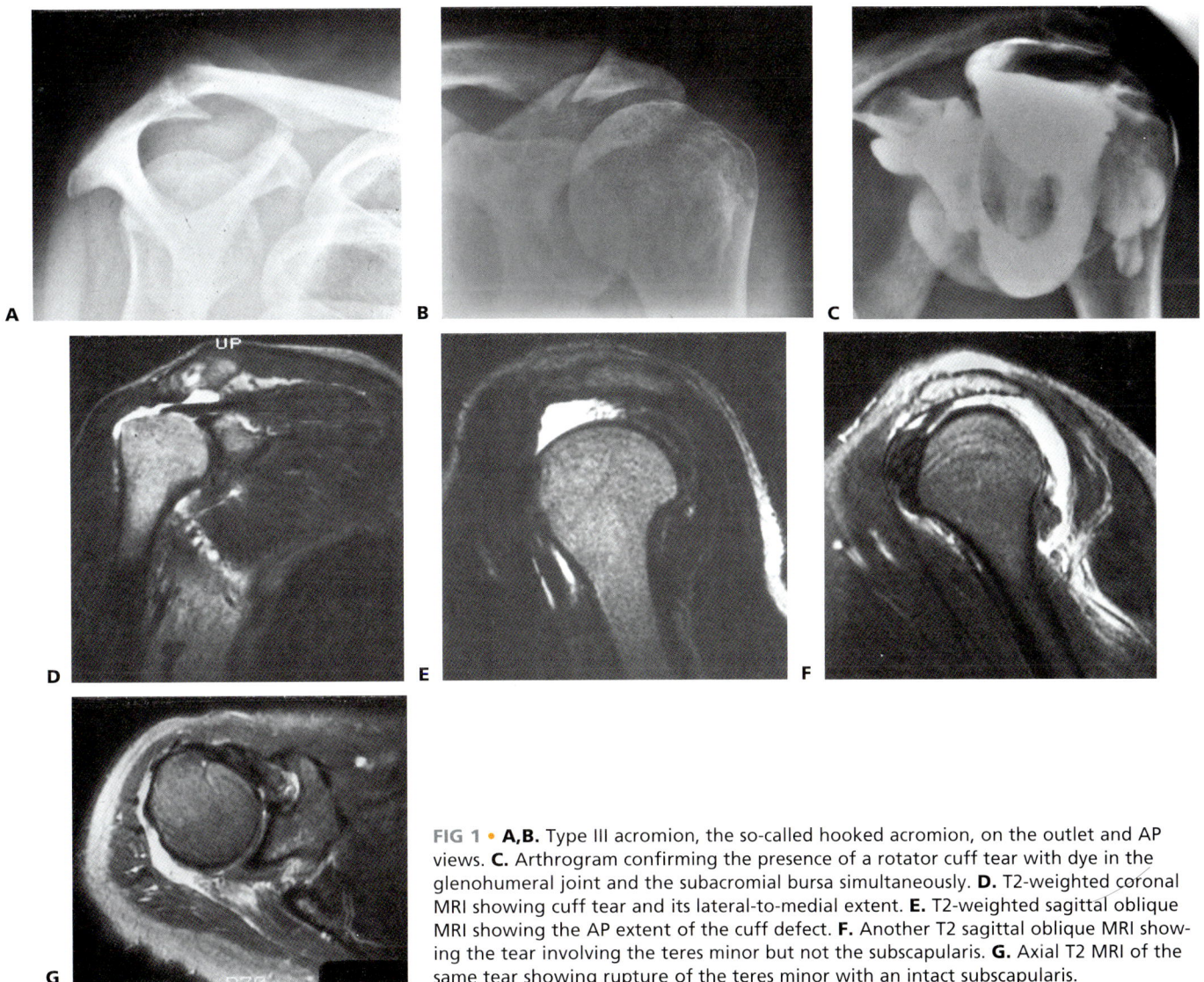

FIG 1 • A,B. Type III acromion, the so-called hooked acromion, on the outlet and AP views. **C.** Arthrogram confirming the presence of a rotator cuff tear with dye in the glenohumeral joint and the subacromial bursa simultaneously. **D.** T2-weighted coronal MRI showing cuff tear and its lateral-to-medial extent. **E.** T2-weighted sagittal oblique MRI showing the AP extent of the cuff defect. **F.** Another T2 sagittal oblique MRI showing the tear involving the teres minor but not the subscapularis. **G.** Axial T2 MRI of the same tear showing rupture of the teres minor with an intact subscapularis.

DIFFERENTIAL DIAGNOSIS

- Cuff tendinitis without tear
- Incomplete rotator cuff tear
- Bicipital tendinitis
- Calcific tendinitis
- Suprascapular neuropathy

NONOPERATIVE MANAGEMENT

- If there is a history of an acute injury with immediate inability to raise the arm, the patient can be treated symptomatically and followed every 5 to 7 days for the first 2 weeks. If the ability to raise the arm does not recover, then nonoperative treatment should be abandoned and surgery undertaken.
- The objective of treating rotator cuff disorders, in the absence of an acute injury with immediate loss of elevation, is primarily to relieve pain and secondarily to restore function or strength. Pain relief is a more predictable outcome of treatment than is restoration of function or strength. Therefore, nonoperative treatment should be directed at relieving pain.
- Although NSAIDs can help with pain, a subacromial steroid injection is often more effective and immediate in its relief.
- Once the pain is improved, physical therapy should be instituted. This involves two aspects: stretching and strengthening of the rotators and elevators.

SURGICAL MANAGEMENT

- As noted earlier, in the unusual case in which there is an acute injury resulting in an immediate loss of elevation of the arm, if symptomatic treatment fails to restore the ability to raise the arm, surgical repair should be undertaken before the 3-week mark.
- For the more common chronic attritional tear, surgery is considered if the injection, NSAIDs, and physical therapy fail to produce a level of pain relief and function that is acceptable to the patient.
- Patients make the decision to have surgery based on whether they can live with the pain and functional limitation that they have. They need to understand that the operation can help them but can also leave them unchanged or worse.

Preoperative Planning

- The radiographs and MRI should be reviewed preoperatively.
- The radiographs will help in planning the need for and extent of acromioplasty.
- The MRI will show which tendons are torn and the degree to which they are torn. It will also show the presence or absence of fatty infiltration of the muscles.

Positioning

- The patient is positioned in a sitting position, even more upright than the so-called beach chair position (**FIG 2A**). The arm is draped free to allow uninhibited mobility of the extremity (**FIG 2B**).
- This allows the surgeon to look down on the cuff from above, therefore, being able to see posterosuperiorly as well as superiorly and anteriorly. It also permits better access to the posterior part of the infraspinatus and the teres minor.

Approach

- There are basically three approaches to cuff repair:
  - The all-arthroscopic approach (discussed in another chapter)
  - Arthroscopic decompression and mini-open repair of the cuff
  - Open repair of the cuff: includes direct repair, grafting, and tendon transfers

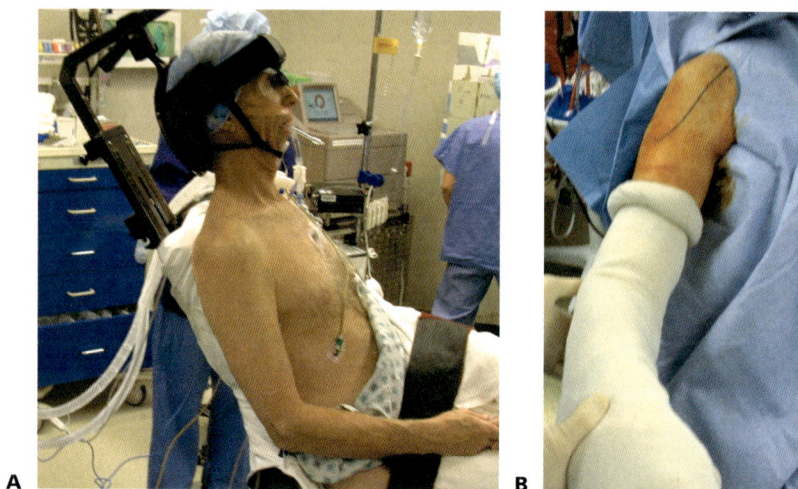

FIG 2 • **A.** Sitting position for surgery allows the surgeon to look down on the cuff and see posterior superior. **B.** The arm is draped free, giving extensive access to the entire shoulder.

ARTHROSCOPIC SUBACROMIAL DECOMPRESSION AND MINI-OPEN CUFF REPAIR

- The standard posterior viewing portal is established, and the glenohumeral joint is evaluated. The defect in the cuff is viewed from the articular side, and the long head of the biceps is assessed.
  - Any débridement or other intra-articular procedures deemed necessary can be carried out at this time.
- The arthroscope is then redirected into the subacromial space and enough bursa resected to allow adequate visualization of the cuff tear, the anterior inferior surface of the acromion, and the coracoacromial ligament. If deemed appropriate (as discussed later), the ligament is released and the anterior and anterolateral margins of the acromion are defined.
  - A burr is used to perform an acromioplasty to the same degree that is done in the open technique. This is an important point. Although the means of accomplishing the decompression differ, the ultimate result is the same: an adequate decompression.
- Through a small lateral portal, a suture punch is used to pass several traction sutures through the leading edge of the torn tendons. Using these sutures as handles to control and apply traction to the cuff, a small elevator is introduced through the same lateral portal and used to free the surrounding adhesions on both surfaces of the cuff. The degree of mobility achieved can be assessed by applying traction through the previously placed sutures.

- Once enough mobility of the cuff has been restored, an incision is made at the anterolateral corner of the acromion for about 1.5 to 2 cm (**TECH FIG 1**). The deltoid is split in the same line as the skin, and additional subdeltoid freeing is done. Narrow retractors are placed under the acromion and anteriorly to expose the tear.
- The procedure at this point is the same as described in the next section.

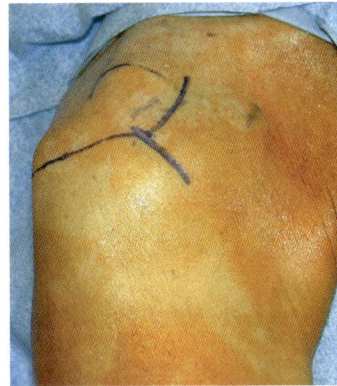

TECH FIG 1 • Skin incision for the mini-open repair technique.

OPEN REPAIR OF THE CUFF

Incision and Dissection

- With the patient in the position described above and the arm draped free, an incision is made beginning superiorly at the posterior aspect of the acromioclavicular joint, continuing over the top of the joint, and ending at a point at the lateral tip of the coracoid (**TECH FIG 2A**).
- After mobilization of the skin flaps, the deltotrapezial aponeurosis and the superior acromioclavicular ligament are incised into the acromioclavicular joint.
- The deltoid muscle is split in line with its fibers only as far distally as the tip of the coracoid.

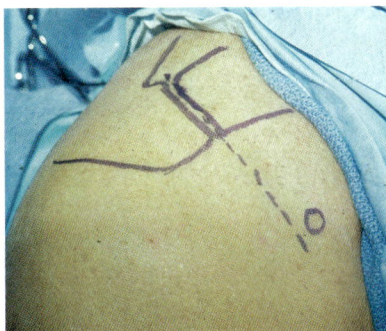

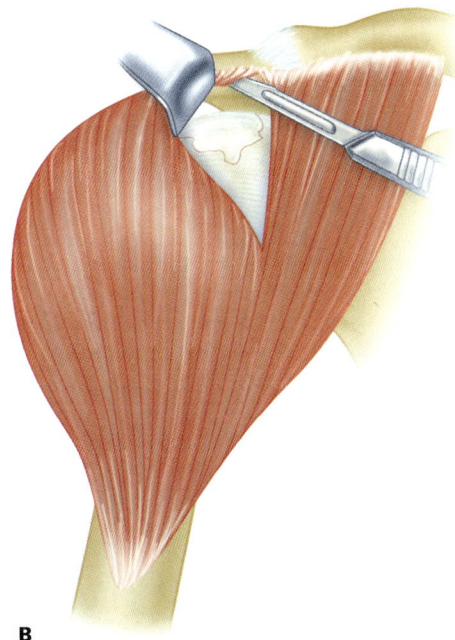

A   B

TECH FIG 2 • **A.** Skin incision for the standard anterosuperior approach. **B.** Subperiosteal dissection of deltoid origin from superior aspect of the lateral clavicle, acromioclavicular joint, and anterior acromion, without cutting across the deltoid origin. *(continued)*

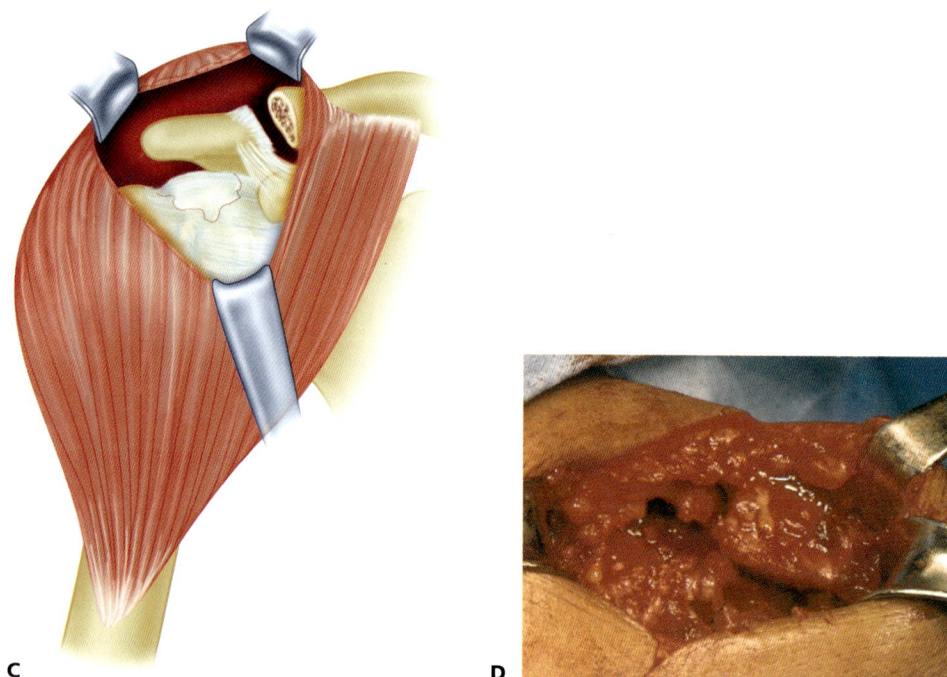

TECH FIG 2 • *(continued)* **C.** Completed elevation of the anterior deltoid origin. **D.** The completed dissection. (**A**: From Neviaser R, Neviaser AS. Open repair of massive rotator cuff tears: tissue mobilization techniques. In: Zuckerman J, ed. Advanced Reconstruction: Shoulder. Chicago, American Academy of Orthopaedic Surgery, 2007:177–184.)

- Using a sharp knife blade, the deltoid origin is dissected subperiosteally from the lateral clavicle for about 1 cm. It is also dissected from the anterior, superior, and undersurface of the acromion out to the anterolateral corner of the acromion (**TECH FIG 2B–D**).
  - No incision is made across the tendon of origin of the deltoid on the acromion; that is, the deltoid is not detached from the acromion.

Clavicular Resection and Acromioplasty

- The coracoacromial ligament is identified and isolated. If, in the judgment of the surgeon, the cuff can be securely repaired, the ligament is released from its attachment on the acromion. If the repair is tenuous, the ligament is not released, or if it is, it is dissected from the undersurface of the acromion to achieve maximal length and repaired back to the acromion through drill holes in the acromion at the end of the procedure.
  - This is necessary to prevent anterosuperior escape of the humerus, which occurs when the cuff is deficient and there is no coracoacromial arch to contain the humeral head, which is being pulled upward by the unopposed deltoid.
- Using a reciprocating saw, the lateral 7 to 8 mm of the lateral end of the clavicle are removed without damaging the periosteum or posterior capsule. The portion removed is trapezoidal in shape, with the larger base being posterior, to prevent contact of the clavicle with the acromion posteriorly.

- The clavicular resection allows the acromion and scapula to be rotated posteriorly more easily and gives greater access to the posterior cuff.
- Using the same instrument, an acromioplasty is performed by removing the anteroinferior surface of the acromion from the medial articular margin out to the anterolateral corner. The anterior edge is not recessed beyond its normal anatomy, and it is not the removal of the full thickness of the acromion, creating a type I acromion (**TECH FIG 3**). The portion removed is a triangular piece, with its base being the anterior edge.

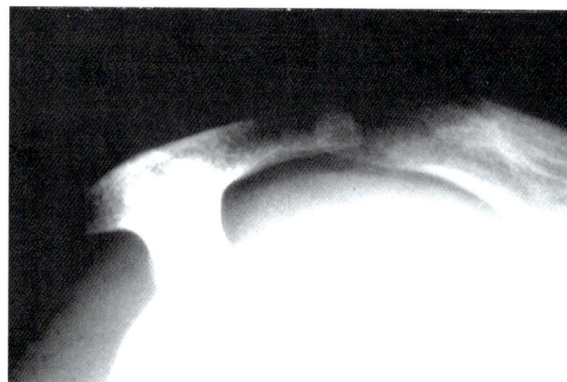

TECH FIG 3 • Type I acromion on outlet view.

- The entire subacromial space is freed bluntly of adhesions between the bursa and the undersurface of the deltoid. Retractors are placed into the subacromial space under the acromion to avoid tension on the deltoid.

Tear Repair

- The bursa is incised, undermined, and reflected. The tear in the cuff can now be seen. The friable, avascular edges are trimmed with a sharp knife. This resection is minimal—only until healthy tendon is seen (**TECH FIG 4A**), not to bleeding tendon. This usually requires the removal of only a few millimeters.
- Number 1 nonabsorbable traction sutures are placed in the edges of the freshened cuff. Applying traction through these sutures, blunt mobilization is done using an elevator, dissecting scissors, or the surgeon's finger.
  - This step of mobilization is critical, and as the musculotendinous unit becomes free, additional sutures are placed successively medially until the apex of the tear is identified (**TECH FIG 4B**).
- If the cuff edge cannot be brought sufficiently far to reach its original insertion, interval releases are done by incising between the supraspinatus and the subscapularis and between the infraspinatus and the teres minor. This restores the differential gliding between these adjacent tendons.
- When the leading edge of the cuff can be brought to its insertion on the greater tuberosity, a shallow trough is made in the anatomic neck at the greater tuberosity (**TECH FIG 4A**).
- Drill holes are made in the trough and the lateral side of the tuberosity and connected with a punch. Locking horizontal mattress sutures or modified Mason-Allen sutures are placed in the cuff and passed through the bone tunnels created by connecting the drill holes (**TECH FIG 4C**). Suture anchors can also be used in the trough and the tuberosity in a double-row fashion instead of the bone tunnels.
- With the arm in some internal rotation and slight abduction, the sutures are tied securely to bring the free edge of the cuff into the trough.
- This leaves a longitudinal split, which is sutured side to side, not only closing the split but also helping to relieve tension on the cuff advanced into the trough (**TECH FIG 4D**).

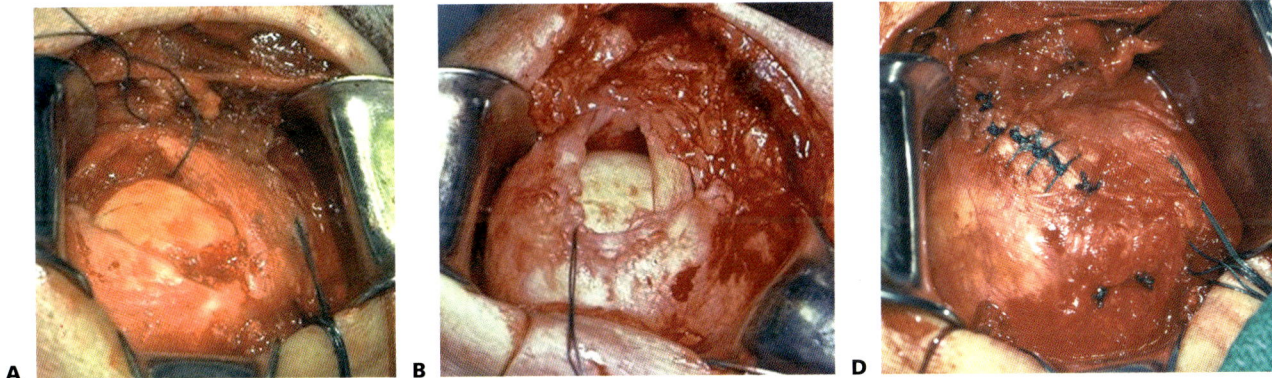

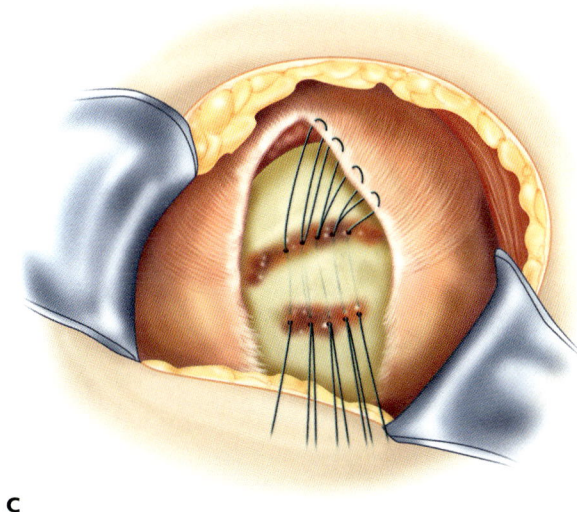

TECH FIG 4 • **A.** Intraoperative photograph showing freshened edges of tear. Healthy tendon is seen but not bleeding edges. Note cancellous trough at the anatomic neck and the greater tuberosity. **B.** Triangular tear with apex medially. **C.** Drawing of sutures passed through bone tunnels in the trough and greater tuberosity, pulling the edge of the cuff into the trough. Anchors can be used instead. **D.** Completed L-shaped repair. (**D:** From Neviaser R, Neviaser AS. Open repair of massive rotator cuff tears: tissue mobilization techniques. In: Zuckerman J, ed. Advanced Reconstruction: Shoulder. Chicago, American Academy of Orthopaedic Surgery, 2007:177–184.)

TECHNIQUES

BICEPS GRAFT

- If the cuff cannot be brought to the greater tuberosity and there is a residual defect of modest size, an interpositional graft of the tendon of the long head of the biceps can be used. The critical requirement to use this or any graft is that the musculotendinous motor must be functional, not fixed and immobile. If there is no springy give when traction is applied to the tendon, no graft should be done.

- First, the tendon of the long head is tenodesed to the transverse humeral ligament in the bicipital groove

using three figure 8 nonabsorbable number 1 sutures. The tendon is transected just above the most proximal suture and then released from its origin at the supraglenoid tubercle.

- This segment of tendon is filleted (**TECH FIG 5A**) and placed into the cuff defect. It is trimmed to fit the defect and contoured to accommodate it.

- It is sutured side to side to the cuff and to a trough in the anatomic neck at the greater tuberosity, as described above (**TECH FIG 5B**).

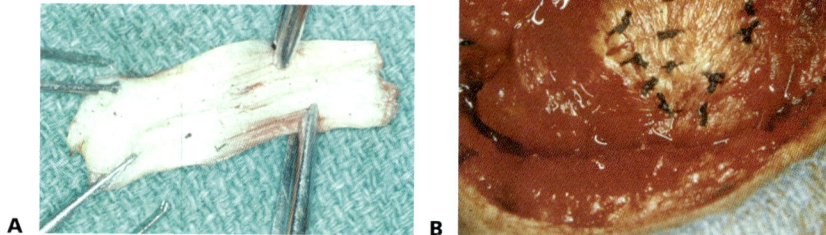

TECH FIG 5 • A. Filleted intra-articular portion of the tendon of the long head of the biceps. **B.** Biceps graft in place. (**A**: From Neviaser RJ. Tears of the rotator cuff. Orthop Clin North Am 1980;11:295–306. **B**: From Neviaser JS. Ruptures of the rotator cuff of the shoulder: new concepts in the diagnosis and treatment of chronic ruptures. Arch Surg 1971;102:483–485.)

FREEZE-DRIED CADAVER ROTATOR CUFF GRAFT

- If the residual defect is too large for a biceps graft to cover, a larger graft is needed. The best choice is a freeze-dried graft of human rotator cuff. As with every graft, the musculotendinous motor (ie, the native rotator cuff) must be a functional unit, as noted above.

- After the described mobilization techniques have reduced the size of the defect as much as possible, the graft is reconstituted in sterile saline for 30 minutes so that it becomes soft and pliable (**TECH FIG 6A**).

- It is then trimmed and contoured to accommodate the free edge of the native cuff and then sutured to it with nonabsorbable number 1 sutures.

- It is also trimmed to reach a trough in the anatomic neck adjacent to the greater tuberosity and secured in the same fashion as the direct repair through drill holes in the bone or by anchors, as previously described (**TECH FIG 6B**).

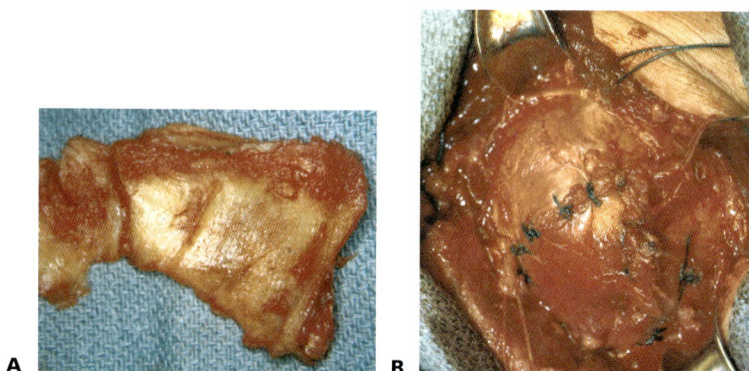

TECH FIG 6 • A. Reconstituted freeze-dried cadaver rotator cuff graft. **B.** Reconstituted freeze-dried cadaver rotator cuff graft sutures in place. (**A**: From Neviaser JS, Neviaser RJ, Neviaser TJ. The repair of chronic massive ruptures of the rotator cuff by use of a freeze-dried rotator cuff. J Bone Joint Surg Am 1978;60A:681–684. **B**: From Neviaser R, Neviaser AS. Open repair of massive rotator cuff tears: tissue mobilization techniques. In: Zuckerman J, ed. Advanced Reconstruction: Shoulder. Chicago, American Academy of Orthopaedic Surgery, 2007:177–184.)

LOCAL TENDON TRANSFERS

- When the cuff cannot be closed by direct repair and the proximal native cuff is not mobile, the subscapularis and teres minor can be used as local tendon transfers.
- The interval between the subscapularis and the anterior capsule is identified near the musculotendinous junction and traced laterally toward the insertion on the lesser tuberosity.
- The tendon is separated from the capsule and released from the insertion. A traction suture is placed in the tendon, and the subscapularis is mobilized so that it can be shifted superiorly.
- The subscapularis is then transferred superiorly (**TECH FIG 7A**) to close the residual defect. Its superior border is sutured to the intact portion of the cuff, its distal end to the greater tuberosity, and its inferior border to the superior edge of the undisturbed anterior capsule (**TECH FIG 7B,C**).
- If the subscapularis alone does not provide adequate closure of the tear, the teres minor can also be trans-

ferred from posterior to superior. The interval between the tendon of the teres minor and the posterior capsule is developed (**TECH FIG 7D**), starting medially at the musculotendinous junction, and freed laterally to its insertion on the greater tuberosity. It is detached from the tuberosity.

- The muscle–tendon unit is mobilized bluntly and transferred superiorly to meet the transposed subscapularis (**TECH FIG 7E**).
- The two tendons are sutured together to form a new broad tendon, which is inserted into a trough at the greater tuberosity, as described earlier.
- The inferior borders of the respective tendons are sutured to the superior edges of the undisturbed capsules (teres minor to the posterior capsule and the subscapularis to the anterior capsule) (**TECH FIG 7F,G**).
- If none of these techniques allows the cuff to be reconstructed satisfactorily, a latissimus dorsi transfer is undertaken; this is described elsewhere.

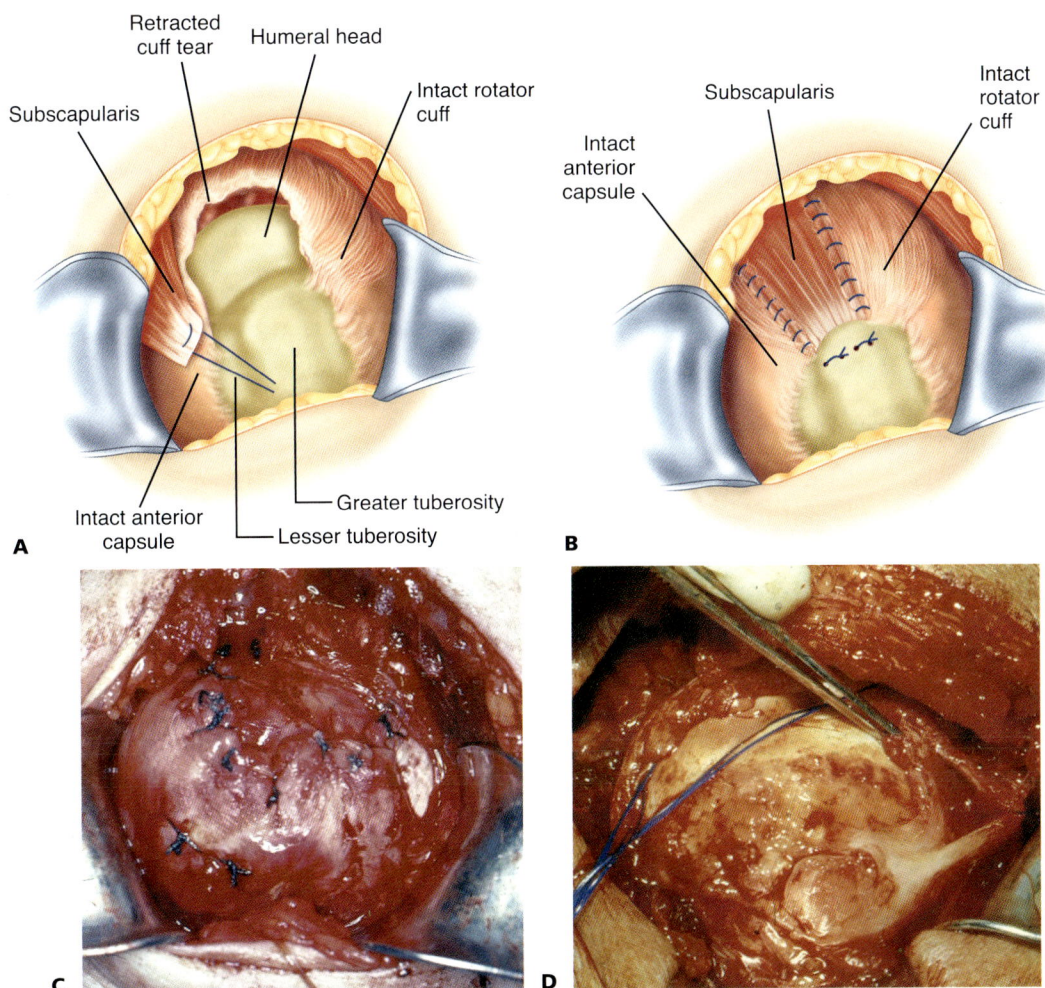

TECH FIG 7 • **A.** Detached subscapularis mobilized and moved superiorly. **B.** Subscapularis transferred and sutured to residual cuff, the greater tuberosity, and the superior border of the undisturbed anterior capsule. **C.** Subscapularis transferred and sutured. **D.** Interval between the teres minor and posterior capsule developed. (*continued*)

TECHNIQUES

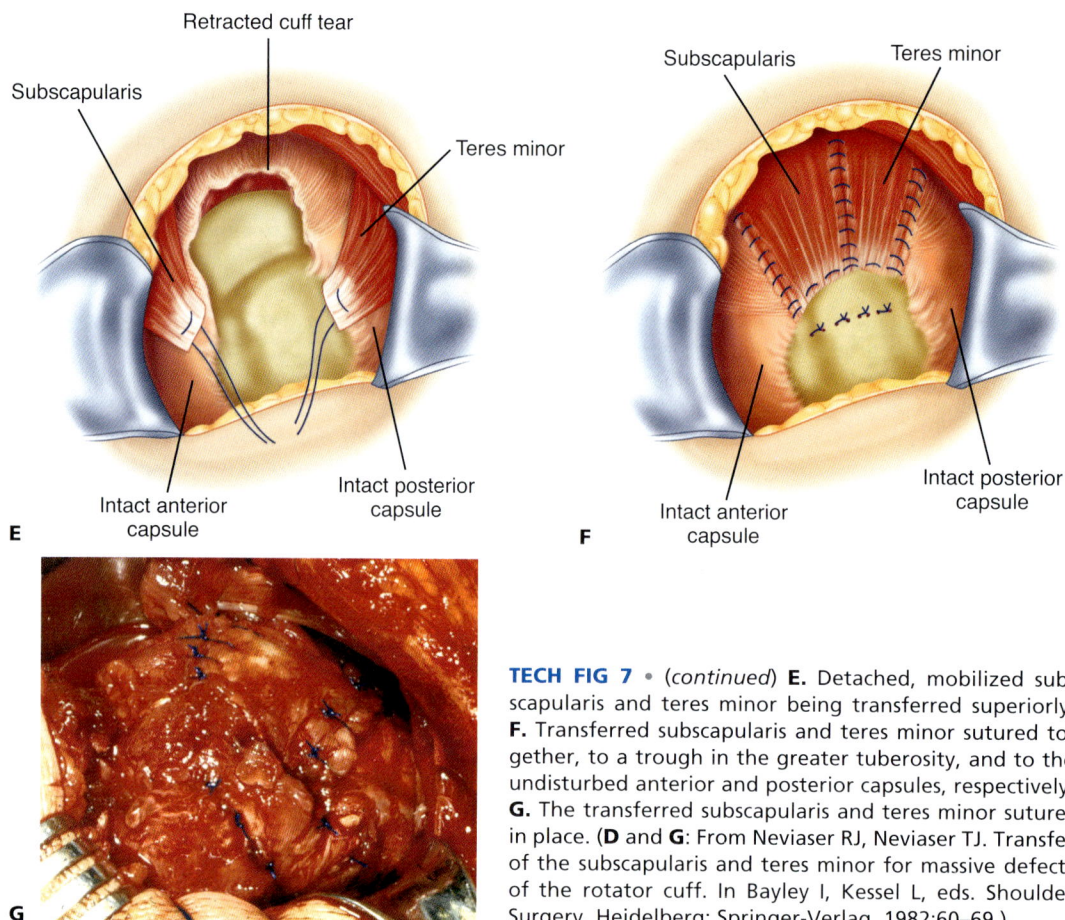

TECH FIG 7 • (*continued*) **E.** Detached, mobilized subscapularis and teres minor being transferred superiorly. **F.** Transferred subscapularis and teres minor sutured together, to a trough in the greater tuberosity, and to the undisturbed anterior and posterior capsules, respectively. **G.** The transferred subscapularis and teres minor sutures in place. (**D** and **G**: From Neviaser RJ, Neviaser TJ. Transfer of the subscapularis and teres minor for massive defects of the rotator cuff. In Bayley I, Kessel L, eds. Shoulder Surgery. Heidelberg: Springer-Verlag, 1982:60–69.)

CLOSURE

- The closure is the same for all procedures.
- Since the deltoid has not been detached from its origin, it is allowed to fall back to its normal anatomic position or brought back by the surgeon. Simple sutures with the knots buried under the deltoid are placed to repair the side-to-side split, being sure to pass the suture through the external muscle fascia, the muscle itself, and the internal muscle fascia.
- If the deltotrapezial aponeurosis and superior acromioclavicular ligament have been incised, they are repaired side to side with figure 8 sutures.
- The skin is closed with a subcuticular 3-0 nylon suture and Steri-Strips. A sterile dressing is applied, and the extremity is immobilized in an immobilizer with the elbow forward of the midline of the body and the shoulder in internal rotation.

PEARLS AND PITFALLS

Postoperative deltoid detachment	■ This can be avoided by subperiosteally elevating the origin and not incising across it.
Axillary nerve injury with deltoid split	■ This can be avoided by not splitting the deltoid beyond the tip of the coracoid. Exposure is achieved by superior access, not distally.
Excessive tendon resection	■ Friable, poor-quality tendon should be trimmed only to healthy fibers, not to bleeding tendon.
Postoperative repair failure	■ Tendons should be repaired to bone under only normal resting tension. If this is not possible, the described grafts or tendon transfers should be used. ■ The early postoperative rehabilitation program is used to regain motion; strengthening is avoided until at least 3 weeks.

POSTOPERATIVE CARE

- Within 24 to 72 hours of the surgery, the dressing is changed. The patient is instructed in passive-only forward elevation and external rotation at the side while lying supine. The operative arm must be completely relaxed with no muscle activity at all, and the arm is elevated to at least 90 degrees forward and external rotation to neutral only.

- Over the next 4 to 6 weeks the amount of passive forward elevation is slowly increased, as is the external rotation at the side, but the latter should not go beyond 10 to 15 degrees of external rotation at most.

- The extremity is kept in the immobilizer at all other times during this period. At 4 to 6 weeks postoperatively, depending on the security of the repair and the technique used, formal active and assisted exercises are permitted, along with continued passive stretching. Strengthening, weights, or resistive exercises are avoided until at least 3 months.

OUTCOMES

- Repairs of small and medium-sized tears have a high rate of success in relieving pain and recovering motion and function while remaining structurally intact, regardless of whether repaired by arthroscopic, mini-open, or open techniques.

- Repairs of large and massive tears also have resulted in good pain relief and functional recovery but have a much lower incidence of remaining intact structurally.

COMPLICATIONS

- Deltoid origin detachment
- Cuff repair dehiscence
- Anterosuperior instability or escape
- Infection
- Loss of motion
- Cuff tear arthropathy

REFERENCES

1. Cofield RH. Subscapularis muscle transposition for repair of chronic rotator cuff tears. Surg Gynecol Obstet 1982;154:667–672.
2. Karas SE, Giacello TL. Subscapularis transfer for reconstruction of massive tears of the rotator cuff. J Bone Joint Surg Am 1996;78A:239–245.
3. Neviaser JS. Ruptures of the rotator cuff: new concepts in the diagnosis and operative treatment for chronic tears. Arch Surg 1971;102:483–485.
4. Neviaser JS, Neviaser RJ, Neviaser TJ. The repair of chronic massive ruptures of the rotator cuff by use of a freeze-dried rotator cuff graft. J Bone Joint Surg Am 1978;60A:681–684.
5. Neviaser RJ, Neviaser TJ. Transfer of the subscapularis and teres minor for massive defects of the rotator cuff. In Bayley I, Kessel L, eds. Shoulder Surgery. Heidelberg: Springer-Verlag, 1982:60–69.
6. Neviaser RJ, Neviaser TJ. Major ruptures of the rotator cuff. In Watson M, ed. Practical Shoulder Surgery. London: Grune & Stratton, 1985:171–224.

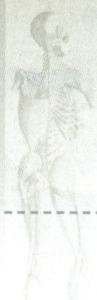

DEFINITION

- Subscapularis tears are less common than supraspinatus or infraspinatus tears. They occur in 2% to 8% of rotator cuff tears and are often missed.[5,12]
- Subscapularis tears can be:
  - Isolated tears (partial or complete)
  - Partial-thickness tears
  - Anterosuperior (involving the supraspinatus)
  - Rotator interval lesions (with associated biceps tendon injury)
- There is a high association of concomitant biceps tendon pathology.[12,18]

ANATOMY

- The subscapularis is innervated by the upper and lower subscapular nerves (C5–C8). Its origin is at the subscapularis fossa, and the upper two thirds inserts onto the lesser tuberosity, while the inferior third inserts onto the humeral metaphysis.
- The subscapularis is the strongest of the rotator cuff muscles. It acts to internally rotate the humerus along with the teres major, latissimus dorsi, and pectoralis major muscles. It resists anterior and inferior translation of the humeral head.[10,17]
- The upper fibers of the subscapularis and the anterior fibers of the supraspinatus contribute to the rotator interval as well as the transverse humeral ligament.
- The coracohumeral ligament is the roof of the rotator interval and blends with the supraspinatus and subscapularis. The coracohumeral ligament and the superior glenohumeral ligament are the primary stabilizers of the biceps.[2]
- The biceps muscle is innervated by the musculocutaneous nerve (C5–C6). It is composed of a long head, which originates from the supraglenoid tubercle, and a short head, which originates from the coracoid process. Both heads insert onto the bicipital tuberosity of the radius and the ulnar fascia of the forearm.
- The long head of the biceps tendon provides superior shoulder stability when the arm is abducted. It also provides posterior shoulder stability when the arm is in midranges of elevation.[14,21]
- The coracoid is located just anterior to the superior border of the subscapularis. It projects laterally, anteriorly, and inferiorly toward the glenoid.
  - The subcoracoid bursa does not communicate with the glenohumeral joint but can communicate with the subacromial bursa.

PATHOGENESIS

- In the young patient, subscapularis tears occur as a result of trauma. The typical mechanisms include hyperextension of an externally rotated arm or forced external rotation of an adducted arm.[5,8]
- In older patients a tear is typically degenerative in nature, although it may be the result of a glenohumeral dislocation or other trauma.[13,15,16]

- Frequently, there is associated long head of the biceps pathology. This may include tenosynovitis, subluxation, dislocation, degeneration, or complete rupture.[12,19]
- Subcoracoid impingement may also be a cause of subscapularis tendon tears.

NATURAL HISTORY

- Isolated subscapularis tendon ruptures are relatively rare. Subscapularis tears are often associated with tears of the supraspinatus and infraspinatus.
- One study found that subscapularis tears occur in 8% of rotator cuff tears.[7]
- An MRI study was performed on 2167 patients with rotator cuff tears.[12]
  - 2% of the patients had subscapularis tendon tears.
  - 27% of those tears were partial-thickness tears and 73% were full-thickness tears.
- One study found a high correlation between subscapularis tendon tears and medial biceps subluxation, biceps tendinopathy, superior labral pathology, and fluid within the subscapular recess or the subcoracoid space.[12,18]
- The above-listed MRI study found that 25 of the 45 patients with subscapularis tendon tears had associated biceps pathology.

PHYSICAL FINDINGS

- Patients with complete tears of the subscapularis have increased passive external rotation compared with the unaffected shoulder.
- Several muscles contribute to internal rotation of the shoulder, including the pectoralis major, latissimus dorsi, and teres major, and can compensate for loss of the subscapularis.
  - Passive external rotation: Increased passive external rotation may indicate a complete rupture of the subscapularis.
  - Passive forward flexion, external rotation, and internal rotation: Limited passive range of motion is indicative of adhesive capsulitis.
  - Active forward flexion: Limited active forward flexion is indicative of a possible large rotator cuff tear.
- The lift-off test isolates the subscapularis muscle. Inability to lift the hand off the back is a positive test.
- Internal rotation lag sign[11]: The examiner measures the lag between maximal internal rotation and the amount the patient can maintain. A positive sign shows increased sensitivity over the classic lift-off test.
- Belly press (Napoleon test)[8]: A positive test is the inability to bring the elbow forward. An intermediate test is the ability to bring the elbow forward partially. A positive test indicates a complete rupture, while an intermediate test indicates a partial tear of the subscapularis.
- The bear hug test[1]: If the examiner is able to lift the hand off the shoulder, then the patient likely has a partial or complete

tear of the upper subscapularis tendon. This is perhaps the most sensitive test for a subscapularis tear.

■ Coracoid impingement[6]: Reproduction of pain or a painful click indicates a positive test. A positive test indicates impingement of the coracoid onto the subscapularis.

■ Speed's test[4]: If the maneuver produces pain or tenderness, the test is positive, which may indicate bicipital pathology, although the test is not specific.

■ Yerguson test[22]: The patient will experience pain as the biceps tendon subluxes out of the groove with a positive test; this indicates biceps instability.

■ Pain may inhibit a patient from maneuvering the arm behind the body into the lift-off position, thereby preventing assessment.

■ A complete rupture of the long head of the biceps tendon will result in an obvious cosmetic deformity in the anterior arm as the muscle retracts distally.

■ Tests used to diagnose superior labral lesions will be discussed in a separate section.

IMAGING AND DIAGNOSTIC STUDIES

■ Anteroposterior (AP), outlet, and axillary view radiographs should be obtained to rule out any fractures or associated injuries.

■ In chronic cases of subscapularis tears, anterior subluxation of the humeral head may be noted on the axillary view.[18]

■ MRI is the modality of choice for diagnosing subscapularis tears (**FIG 1**).

■ MR arthrography improves the study accuracy to detect partial-thickness tears.

■ Fatty degeneration of the subscapularis correlates with poor tendon quality.[20]

■ Although not sensitive, these signs are highly specific for subscapularis tears[15]:

■ Leakage of contrast material onto the lesser tuberosity

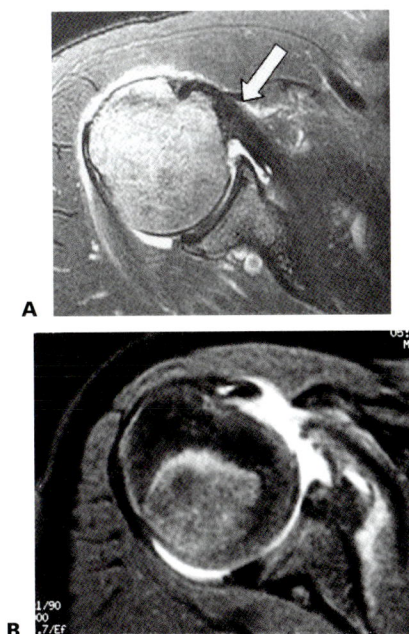

FIG 1 • Axial T2-weighted MR images of right shoulders with an intact subscapularis tendon (**A**; *arrow*) and a complete rupture of the subscapularis tendon.

■ Fatty degeneration of the subscapularis muscle

■ Abnormalities in the course of the long biceps tendon

■ Biceps dislocation deep to the subscapularis tendon is pathognomonic for a subscapularis tear.

■ Ultrasound is a noninvasive method for assessing the subscapularis and can be performed in the office. It is less expensive than MRI, but results are operator-dependent.

DIFFERENTIAL DIAGNOSIS

■ Impingement syndrome
■ Subscapularis tendinitis
■ Bicipital tendinitis
■ Posterosuperior rotator cuff tear (supraspinatus, infraspinatus, teres minor)
■ Biceps pathology
■ Coracoid impingement
■ Labral tear
■ Glenoid fracture
■ Glenohumeral instability
■ Glenohumeral arthritis
■ Pectoralis major injury
■ Contusion
■ Cervical radiculopathy

NONOPERATIVE MANAGEMENT

■ For subscapularis tears, nonoperative management is reserved for some chronic and atraumatic, degenerative, and asymptomatic tears.

■ Treatment includes activity modification, anti-inflammatory medications, and physical therapy.

■ Corticosteroid injections may be performed in the bicipital groove or subcoracoid bursa to treat biceps tendinitis and coracoid impingement.

■ It is likely that some degenerative subscapularis tendon tears are successfully treated nonsurgically without ever being diagnosed.

■ In most cases, an acute symptomatic subscapularis tear should be managed operatively and whenever possible within the first 6 to 8 weeks, when retraction and scarring are minimal, to reduce the risks of dissection in the axillary recess.

■ In young, active patients, attempts are made to repair acute biceps ruptures.

■ In older, less active patients and in cases of chronic biceps ruptures more than 8 weeks old, biceps repair is discouraged.

SURGICAL MANAGEMENT

Preoperative Planning

■ Physical therapy or a home exercise program emphasizing range of motion may be used to prevent stiffness and improve range of motion before surgery.

■ All imaging studies are reviewed.

■ An examination under anesthesia is performed before beginning surgery to evaluate for instability, increased external rotation, or decreased range of motion.

Positioning

■ The patient is placed in a low beach chair position with the arm draped free.

■ A McConnell arm holder (McConnell Orthopedic Manufacturing Co., Greenville, TX) is useful for maintaining arm positions throughout the case (**FIG 2**).

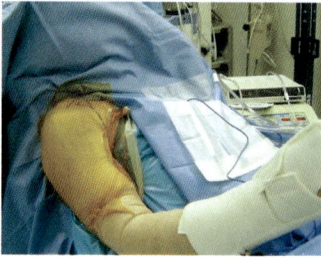

FIG 2 • Positioning for a subscapularis repair. The patient is placed in a beach chair position with the arm stabilized in a McConnell holder.

Approach

- Both the deltopectoral and anterolateral deltoid-splitting approaches have been described.[20]
- The anterolateral deltoid-splitting approach is useful for partial tears of the upper subscapularis and tears associated with supraspinatus tears. It is not recommended for large, retracted full-thickness subscapularis tears.
- The deltopectoral approach provides greater visualization and access to the inferior portion of the subscapularis. It also allows for concomitant biceps tenodesis and coracoplasty.

TECHNIQUES

INCISION AND DISSECTION

- The deltopectoral approach is started just proximal to the coracoid process and extended distally 8 to 10 cm.
- Adducting the arm identifies the major axillary crease.
- The cephalic vein and deltoid muscle are carefully retracted laterally and the pectoralis muscle is retracted medially to facilitate exposure (**TECH FIG 1A**).
- Once the deltopectoral interval is developed, the clavipectoral fascia is identified.
- The clavipectoral fascia is divided at the lateral aspect of the conjoined tendon.
- Avoid excessive retraction on the conjoined tendon to avoid injuring the musculocutaneous nerve.
- The tendon of the subscapularis is often retracted inferiorly and medially and requires mobilization.
- A layer of scar tissue may be seen overlying the lesser tuberosity, which can mimic the subscapularis tendon.

- If the subscapularis tendon cannot be brought back to the lesser tuberosity easily, then the subscapularis requires systematic release from the glenohumeral ligaments.
- Begin by releasing the superior aspect of the tendon from the coracohumeral ligament. The rotator interval is opened from the glenoid to the bicipital groove to facilitate the release.
- Next release the inferior portion of the tendon from the capsular attachments. Care must be taken to identify and protect the axillary nerve and vascular supply inferiorly.
- Finally, release the remaining capsular attachments on the undersurface of the subscapularis (**TECH FIG 1B**).

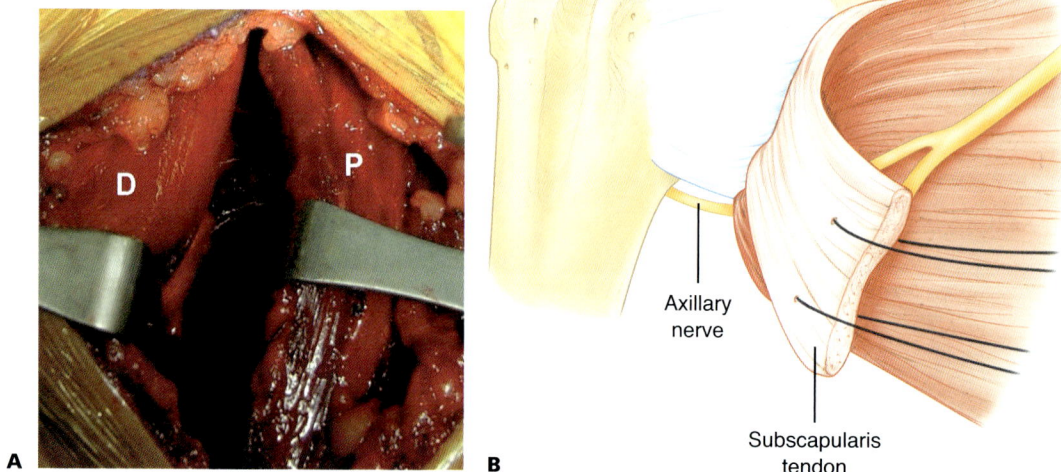

TECH FIG 1 • A. Deltopectoral interval in a right shoulder. The deltoid muscle (*D*) and cephalic vein are retracted laterally and the pectoralis muscle (*P*) is retracted medially. B. The subscapularis is released from the capsule to facilitate mobilization of the tendon. Note the proximity of the axillary nerve inferiorly.

BICEPS TENODESIS

- If a biceps tenotomy is performed, it is important to warn the patient of the resultant cosmetic deformity when the biceps retracts distally.
- Indications for biceps tenodesis include the following:
  - Tears involving more than 50% of the biceps tendon
  - Medial subluxation of the biceps tendon
- Open the bicipital groove from the medial side to expose the biceps tendon.

- The biceps tendon is released from the superior glenoid with curved scissors.
- The tendon is retracted distally from the bicipital groove.
- To ensure proper tensioning of the biceps tendon, the proximal portion of the tendon is resected to leave about 20 to 25 mm of tendon proximal to the musculotendinous junction.
- Running locking Krakow or whipstitches are placed up and down the proximal 15 mm of the biceps tendon.
- Abrade the bicipital groove to develop a bleeding surface.
- A burr hole the size of the biceps tendon is made in the bicipital groove about 15 mm from the articular surface. Two smaller 3.2-mm holes are made 15 mm distal to the burr hole in a triangular configuration.
- The tendon end is passed into the proximal hole by pulling the sutures out the distal holes. The sutures are then passed through and tied over the overlying biceps tendon (**TECH FIG 2A,B**).
- Another fixation option is to use a biotenodesis screw for the biceps tendon.
  - The tendon is prepared as above.
  - An 8-mm reamer is used to make a 25-mm-deep bone tunnel about 15 mm from the articular surface.
  - An 8 × 23-mm Arthrex Bio-Tenodesis screw is used for fixation.
  - One end of the suture is passed through the biotenodesis screw while the other suture passes outside of the screw. This ensures that the tendon will be pulled into the hole as the screw is advanced.
  - When the screw is flush with the bone tunnel, the sutures are tied over the screw (**TECH FIG 2C**). This provides both an interference fit and suture anchor stability.

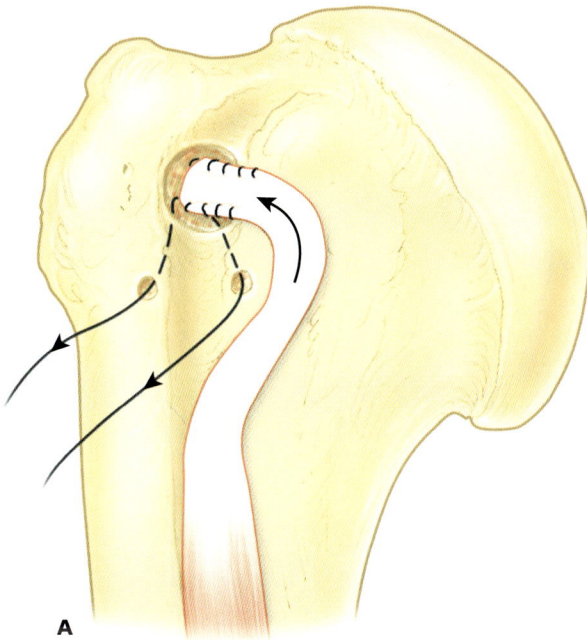

A

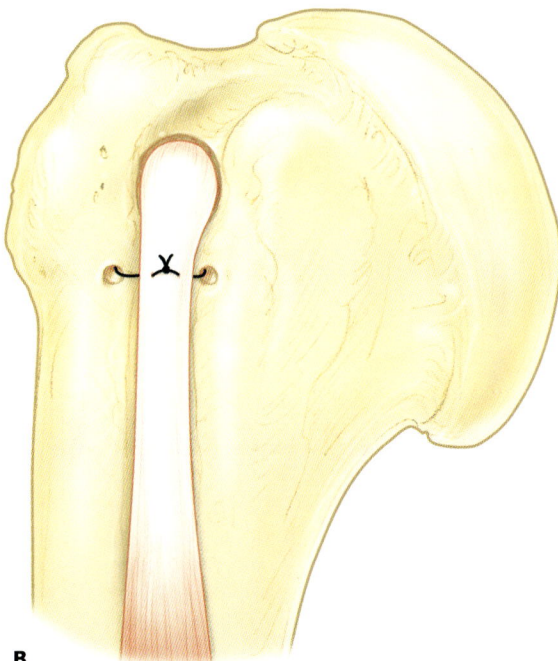

B

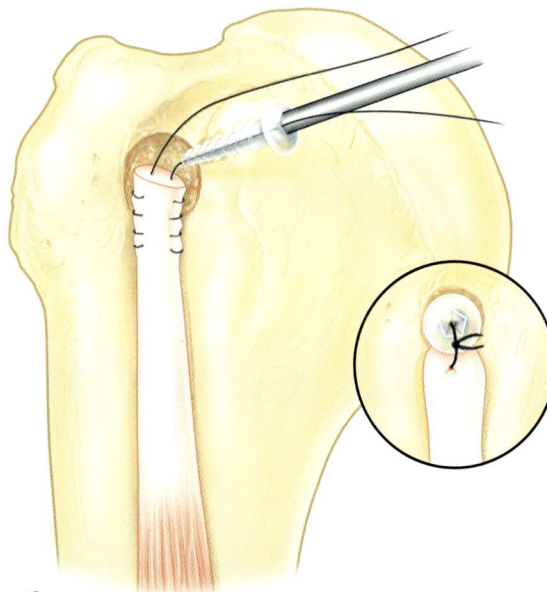

C

TECH FIG 2 • A,B. The tunnel technique uses bone tunnels to fix the biceps tendon upon itself. **C.** A biceps tenodesis with interference screw fixation.

CORACOPLASTY

- The conjoined tendons are identified.
- Care is taken not to retract vigorously on the conjoined tendons to avoid injury to the musculocutaneous nerve.
- The coracoacromial ligament is released from the coracoid.
- The posterior aspect of the coracoid is exposed by removing the overlying soft tissue. The posterolateral portion is then resected in line with the subscapularis muscle with an osteotome (**TECH FIG 3**). Alternatively, a burr may be used to accomplish the same resection. Protect the neurovascular structures by placing a retractor on the posterior aspect of the coracoid.
- A rasp is then used to smooth out the bony surface.
- The goal is a 7- to 10-mm clearance between the coracoid and subscapularis.

- Confirmation of adequate decompression can be determined by manipulating the arm into the impingement position and confirming that there is adequate clearance for the subscapularis.

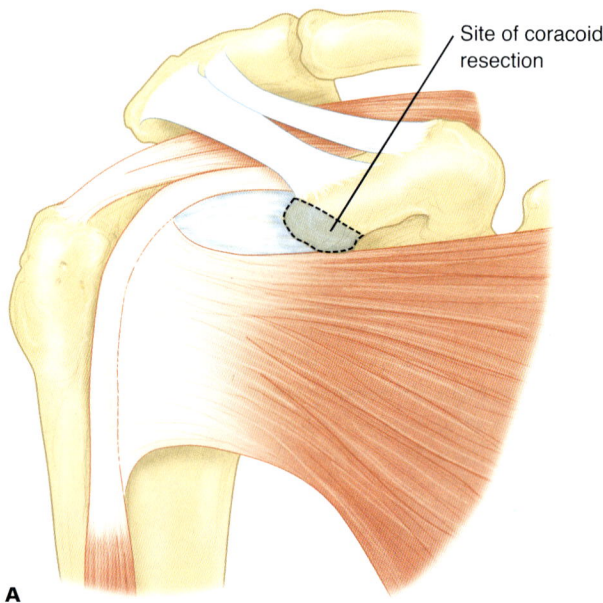

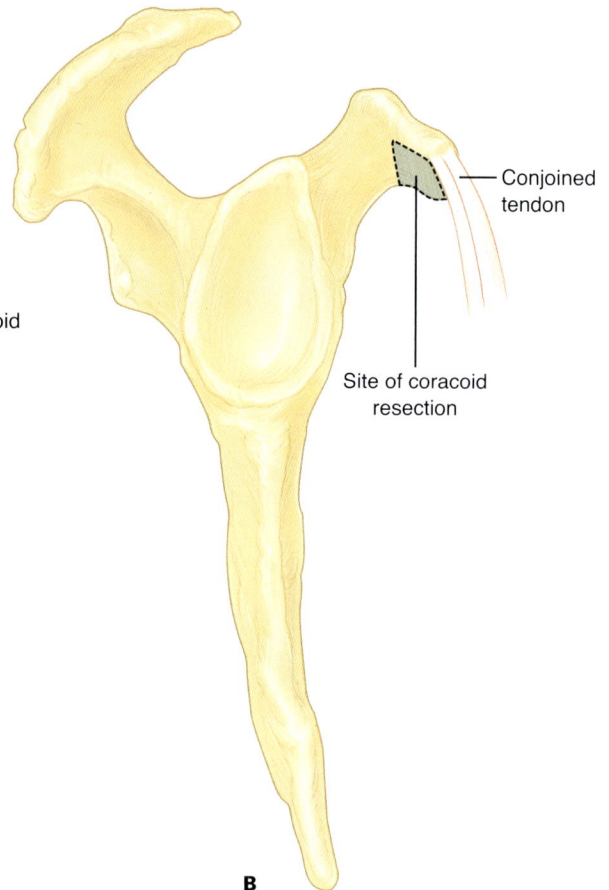

TECH FIG 3 • The posterolateral portion of the coracoid is resected, leaving the conjoined tendon attached. The goal is a 7- to 10-mm clearance space for the subscapularis.

SUBSCAPULARIS REPAIR

- The residual soft tissue is cleaned from the lesser tuberosity. A burr is then used to expose bleeding bone for the tendon to heal to.
- To recreate the anatomic footprint of the subscapularis insertion, four suture anchors are used for the repair.
- Two anchors are placed at 1-cm intervals along the medial aspect of the lesser tuberosity and two are placed at the lateral aspect of the lesser tuberosity (**TECH FIG 4A**).
- The sutures from the medial anchors are passed in a mattress fashion near the musculotendinous junction of the subscapularis (**TECH FIG 4B**).

- The sutures from the lateral anchor are passed through the lateral edge of the tendon in a simple fashion and tied down to the lesser tuberosity.
- After repair of the subscapularis tendon, the shoulder is taken through a gentle range of motion to determine the safe arcs for postoperative rehabilitation.
- The lateral aspect of the rotator interval is closed while maintaining about 30 degrees of external rotation of the arm to prevent overtightening of the subscapularis repair.

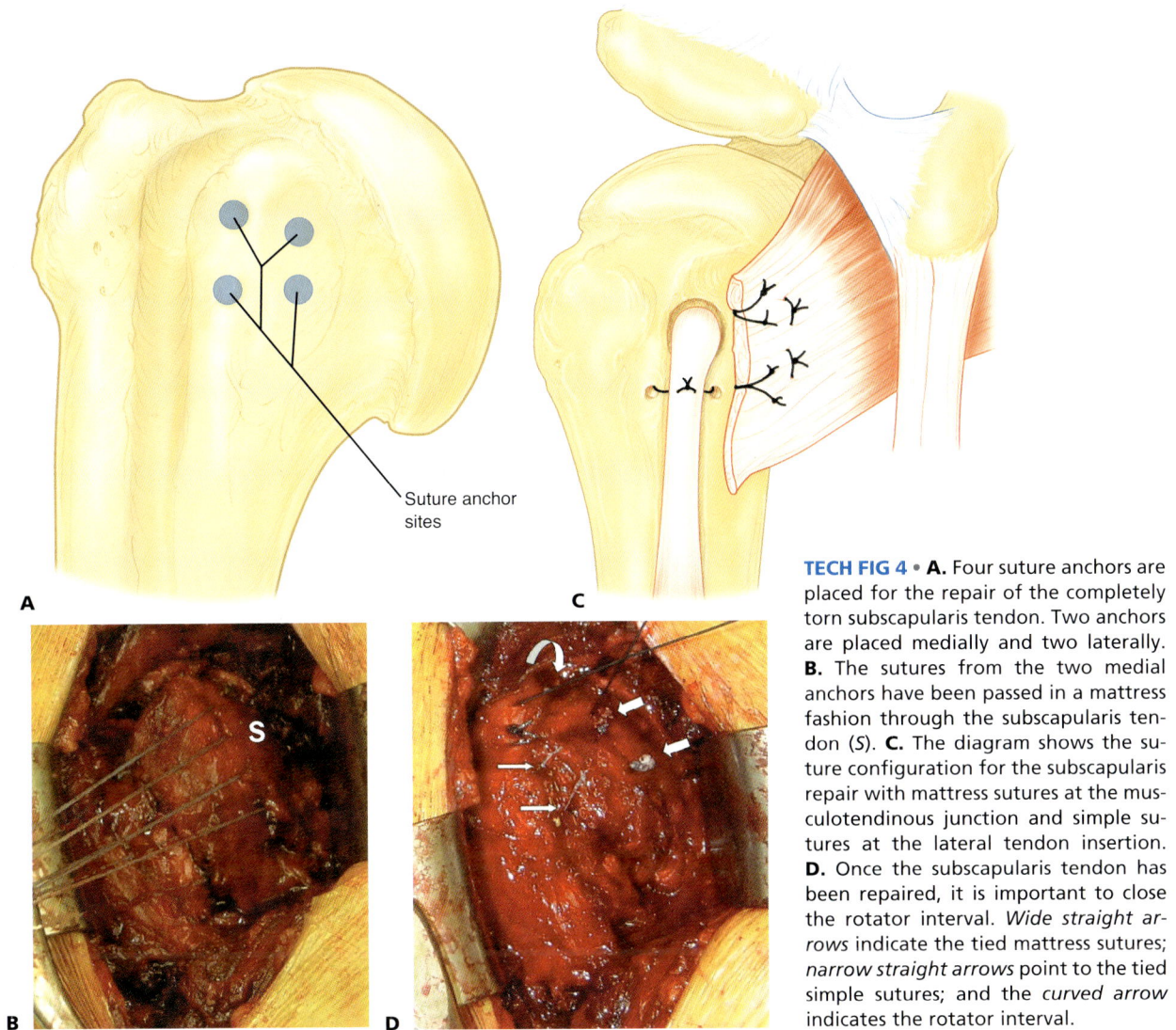

A

B

C

D

TECH FIG 4 • A. Four suture anchors are placed for the repair of the completely torn subscapularis tendon. Two anchors are placed medially and two laterally. **B.** The sutures from the two medial anchors have been passed in a mattress fashion through the subscapularis tendon (*S*). **C.** The diagram shows the suture configuration for the subscapularis repair with mattress sutures at the musculotendinous junction and simple sutures at the lateral tendon insertion. **D.** Once the subscapularis tendon has been repaired, it is important to close the rotator interval. *Wide straight arrows* indicate the tied mattress sutures; *narrow straight arrows* point to the tied simple sutures; and the *curved arrow* indicates the rotator interval.

PEARLS AND PITFALLS

Indications	■ A complete history and physical examination should be performed. ■ The surgeon should identify and address all associated pathology. ■ Any limitations of motion should be addressed before surgery.
Coracoplasty	■ The surgeon should take care to protect the musculocutaneous nerve. ■ A 7- to 10-mm clearance should be achieved for the subscapularis.
Biceps tenodesis	■ Tears in the biceps tendon of over 50% and subluxing tendons should be tenodesed. ■ The surgeon should maintain proper tension of the biceps muscle; typically, 20 to 25 mm of tendon should be maintained proximal to the musculotendinous junction. ■ A "hidden lesion" describes the presence of a partial undersurface subscapularis tear with a medially dislocated or subluxed biceps. This injury can be missed at the time of open surgery because the bursal surface of the subscapularis remains intact. Diagnostic arthroscopy or proper imaging will prevent missing this lesion.
Subscapularis repair	■ In chronic cases, a scar layer covers the lesser tuberosity and is usually attached at its medial extent to the retracted and scarred subscapularis tendon. The presence of this scar layer may lead to the misdiagnosis of an intact subscapularis. ■ The surgeon should prepare a bleeding bony surface for the tendon to heal to. ■ The rotator interval is closed in external rotation to avoid loss of motion. ■ External rotation is limited for 6 weeks postoperatively to protect the repair.

POSTOPERATIVE CARE

- The most important postoperative management for subscapularis tears is limitation of external rotation for 6 weeks to avoid stressing the repair.
  - Complete tears are not allowed to externally rotate past 0 degrees.
  - Partial tears are allowed to externally rotate 20 to 30 degrees.
- At 6 weeks the patient may begin active and active-assisted external rotation exercises, as well as overhead stretching.
- At 12 weeks strengthening exercises are initiated for partial tears. At 16 weeks strengthening exercises are initiated for complete tears.

OUTCOMES

- Isolated subscapularis tears have favorable surgical outcomes.
  - At 2 years of follow-up, good or excellent results were reported in 13 of 14 isolated subscapularis tears.[4]
  - Another study demonstrated good or excellent results in 13 of 16 patients with acute traumatic subscapularis tears at 43 months of follow-up. The Constant scores were 82% of age-matched controls.[8]
- Poor prognostic factors include chronic tears (symptoms for more than 6 months), fatty degeneration of the subscapularis muscle, and anterosuperior tears (combination of subscapularis and supraspinatus tears).[19]
- Comparative outcomes between open and arthroscopic techniques remain to be determined.

COMPLICATIONS

- Repair failure
- Infection
- Loss of motion
- Axillary nerve injury
- Vascular injury

REFERENCES

1. Barth JRH, Burkhart SS, DeBeer JF. The bear hug test: the most sensitive test for diagnosing a subscapularis tear. Arthroscopy 2006;22:1076–1084.
2. Burkhead WZ Jr, Arcand MA, Zeman C, et al. The biceps tendon. In: Rockwood CA Jr, Matsen FA III, Wirth MA, Lippitt SB, eds. The Shoulder, 3rd ed. Philadelphia: Saunders, 2004;1059–1119.
3. Constant CR, Murley AH. A clinical method of functional assessment of the shoulder. Clin Orthop Relat Res 1987;214:160–164.
4. Crenshaw AH, Kilgore WE. Surgical treatment of bicipital tenosynovitis. J Bone Joint Surg Am 1966;48A:1496–1502.
5. Deutsch A, Altchek DW, Veltri DM, et al. Traumatic tears of the subscapularis tendon: clinical diagnosis, magnetic resonance imaging findings, and operative treatment. Am J Sports Med 1997;25:13–22.
6. Dines DM, Warren RF, Inglis AE, et al. The coracoid impingement syndrome. J Bone Joint Surg Br 1990;72B:314–316.
7. Frankle MA, Cofield RH. Rotator cuff tears including the subscapularis [abstract]. Fifth International Conference of Surgery of the Shoulder, Paris, France, 1992:52.
8. Gerber C, Krushell RJ. Isolated rupture of the tendon of the subscapularis muscle: clinical features in 16 cases. J Bone Joint Surg Br 1991;73B:389–394.
9. Gerber C, Rippstein R. Combined lesions of the subscapularis and supraspinatous tendons: a multi-center analysis of 56 cases [abstract]. Fifth International Congress of Surgery of the Shoulder, Paris, France, 1992:51.
10. Halder AM, Itoi E, An KN. Anatomy and biomechanics of the shoulder. Orthop Clin North Am 2000;31:159–176.
11. Hertel R, Ballmer F, Lombert SM, et al. Lag signs in the diagnosis of rotator cuff rupture. J Shoulder Elbow Surg 1996;5:307–313.
12. Li XX, Schweitzer ME, Bifano JA, et al. MR evaluation of subscapularis tears. J Comput Assist Tomogr 1999;23:713–717.
13. Neviaser RJ, Neviaser TJ. Recurrent instability of the shoulder after age 40. J Shoulder Elbow Surg 1995;4:416–418.
14. Pagnani MJ, Deng XH, Warren RF, et al. Role of the long head of the biceps brachii in glenohumeral stability: a biomechanical study in cadavers. J Shoulder Elbow Surg 1996;5:255–262.
15. Pfirrmann CW, Zanetti M, Weishaupt D, et al. Subscapularis tendon tears: detection and grading at MR arthrography. Radiology 1999;213:709–714.
16. Symeonides PP. The significance of the subscapularis muscle in the pathogenesis of recurrent anterior dislocations of the shoulder. J Bone Joint Surg Br 1972;54B:276–283.
17. Tillett F, Smith M, Fulcher M, et al. Anatomic determination of humeral head retroversion: the relationship of the central axis of the humeral head to the bicipital groove. J Shoulder Elbow Surg 1993;2:255–256.
18. Travis RD, Burkhead WZ, Doane R. Technique for repair of the subscapularis tendon. Orthop Clin North Am 2001;32:495–500.
19. Tung GA, Yoo DC, Levine SM, et al. Subscapularis tendon tear: primary and associated signs on MRI. J Comput Assist Tomogr 2001;25:417–424.
20. Warner JJ, Higgins L, Parsons IM, et al. Diagnosis and treatment of anterosuperior rotator cuff tears. J Shoulder Elbow Surg 2001;10:37–46.
21. Warner JJ, McMahon PJ. The role of the long head of the biceps brachii in superior stability of the glenohumeral joint. J Bone Joint Surg Am 1995;77A:366–372.
22. Yergason RM. Supination sign. J Bone Joint Surg Am 1931;13A:60.

Chapter 10

Latissimus Transfer for Irreparable Posterosuperior Rotator Cuff Tear

Jesse A. McCarron, Michael J. Codsi, and Joseph P. Iannotti

DEFINITION

- Irreparable posterosuperior rotator cuff tears are tears that involve the supraspinatus and infraspinatus tendons, where there is an inability to repair the tendons back to the anatomic footprint of the greater tuberosity with the arm at the side.
- Some tears can be determined to be irreparable preoperatively, if the MRI or CT scans demonstrate severe muscle atrophy of the supraspinatus or infraspinatus muscles.
  - This may help indicate that a patient has an irreparable tear and may be a candidate for muscle transfer, but the final determination of whether a tear is reparable is made at the time of surgery.

ANATOMY

- The latissimus dorsi is normally an adductor and internal rotator of the humerus however, after transfer it is expected to act as an abductor and external rotator of the humerus.
  - The ability of the patient to retrain his or her neural pathways to achieve this active in-phase function varies dramatically.
  - In some cases, the latissimus dorsi transfer has only a tenodesis effect.
- Originating from the supraspinatus and infraspinatus fossa respectively, the supraspinatus and infraspinatus muscle–tendon units become confluent and insert as a common tendon on the greater tuberosity of the humerus immediately lateral to the humeral head articular margin.
  - Their combined footprint area averages 4.02 cm^2.
  - The insertion of the supraspinatus averages 1.27 cm from medial to lateral and 1.63 cm from anterior to posterior.
  - The infraspinatus insertion averages 1.34 cm medial to lateral and 1.64 cm anterior to posterior.[6]
- Over the superior aspect of the glenohumeral joint, the deepest fibers of the supraspinatus and infraspinatus tendons are intimately interwoven with the joint capsule such that the rotator cuff tendons and joint capsule function as a single unit. As a result, rotator cuff tears involving the supraspinatus or infraspinatus tendons result in direct communication between the glenohumeral and subacromial spaces.
- The latissimus dorsi muscle has a broad origin from the aponeurosis of spinous processes T7 through L5, the sacrum, the iliac wing, ribs 9 through 12, and the inferior border of the scapula.
- The latissimus dorsi tendon averages 3.1 cm wide and 8.4 cm long at its insertion between the pectoralis major and teres major tendons on the proximal, medial humerus.[13]
- The fibers of the latissimus dorsi twist 180 degrees from origin to insertion, allowing the latissimus dorsi muscle to originate posterior to the teres major muscle on the posterior chest wall but insert immediately anterior to the teres major tendon on the proximal humerus.

- The latissimus dorsi humeral insertion never extends more distal along the shaft than that of the teres major.
- In most patients, the latissimus dorsi and teres major tendons insert separately onto the proximal humerus; however, 30% of patients have conjoined latissimus dorsi and teres major tendons that cannot be separated without sharp dissection.[13]
- The neurovascular pedicle to the latissimus dorsi is the thoracodorsal artery and nerve (posterior cord, C6 and C7). The thoracodorsal artery and nerve enter the anterior, inferior surface of the latissimus dorsi, about 13 cm from the humeral insertion site.
  - Anatomic studies have shown that this neurovascular pedicle is of adequate length to allow transfer and excursion of the latissimus dorsi without risk of undue tension, once any adhesions and fibrous bands have been released from the anterior surface of the muscle belly.[14]
- Several important neurovascular structures lie close to the latissimus dorsi insertion, and careful attention to these structures must be given at the time of its release from the humerus to avoid injury.
  - Anterior to the latissimus, the radial nerve passes an average of 2.4 cm medial to the humeral shaft at the superior border of the tendon.
    - This distance increases with external rotation and abduction and decreases with internal rotation and adduction[2] (**FIG 1A,B**).

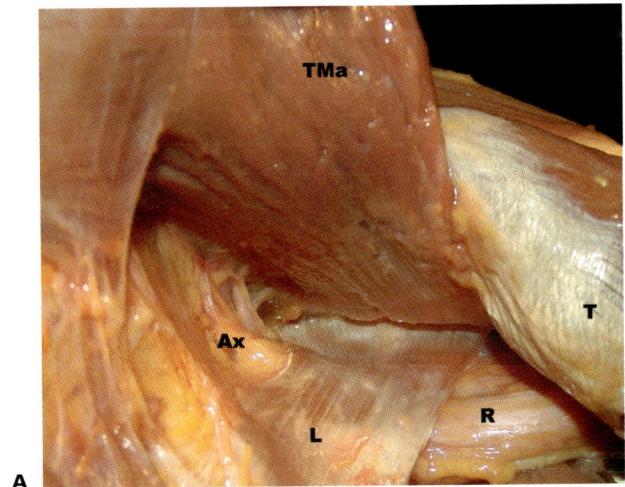

FIG 1 • A. Cadaveric dissection of the interval between the teres major (*TMa*) and latissimus dorsi (*L*) tendons running deep to the long head of the triceps (*T*) near their humeral insertion. The view is from a posterior approach to the right shoulder. Note the proximity of the radial nerve (*R*) lying deep to the latissimus tendon, and the axillary nerve (*Ax*) running with the posterior humeral circumflex artery over the superior border of the latissimus and teres major as it passes through the quadrilateral space. *(continued)*

3141

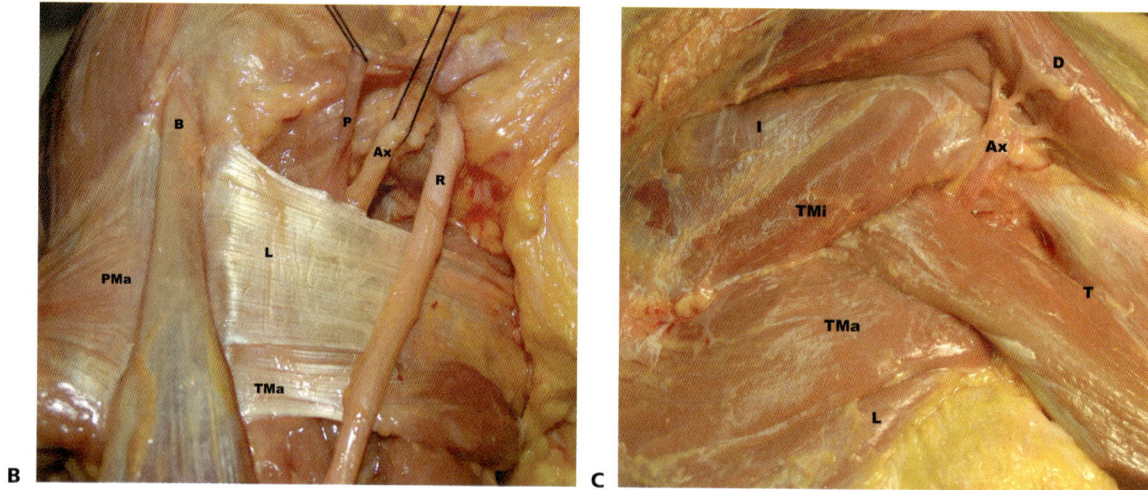

FIG 1 • *(continued)* **B.** Cadaveric dissection demonstrating the insertion of the latissimus dorsi (*L*) and teres major (*TMa*) tendons viewed from an anterior exposure. The pectoralis major (*PMa*) tendon has been reflected laterally and the long head of the biceps (*B*) tendon remains in the bicipital groove. Note the more distal insertion of the teres major relative to the latissimus dorsi. *Ax,* axillary nerve; *P,* posterior humeral circumflex vessel; *R,* radial nerve. **C.** Cadaveric dissection of the superficial muscular anatomy of the posterior shoulder. The axillary nerve (*Ax*) and posterior humeral circumflex artery are seen exiting the quadrilateral space before entering the posterior deltoid (*D*). *L,* latissimus dorsi; *TMa,* teres major; *TMi,* teres minor; *I,* infraspinatus; *T,* triceps.

- The axillary nerve runs superior to the latissimus dorsi tendon before exiting the quadrangular space (**FIG 1C**). In neural rotation and adduction, the average distance between the nerve and the superior border of the tendon is 1.9 cm.
  - This distance increases with external rotation and abduction and decreases with internal rotation.[2]
- The anterior humeral circumflex artery runs along the superior border of the latissimus dorsi tendon.

PATHOGENESIS

- Multiple causes have been proposed for the development of rotator cuff tears, including decreased vascular supply, mechanical compression between the humeral head and the coracoacromial ligament or the undersurface of the acromion, and traumatic causes such as humeral head dislocation, or rapid or repetitive eccentric loading of the rotator cuff muscle–tendon units.
- Isolated, acute traumatic events may cause massive rotator cuff tears, the majority of which can be repaired open or arthroscopically if diagnosis and surgical intervention are timely.
- Alternatively, most degenerative tendon tears start small and progressively get larger until the muscle retraction, muscle atrophy, and tendon loss prevent primary repair.
- Tear size may not predict reparability at the time of surgery, but it does influence healing postoperatively, with larger tears having a lower incidence of healing.
- Tissue quality and tendon retraction are the major determinants intraoperatively of whether a repair is possible. These factors also influence healing of a primary repair.
- Increased size and duration of a tear lead to retraction of the rotator cuff and fatty infiltration of the muscle belly within weeks to months of developing a tear. These changes result in decreased tendon excursion and tissue compliance that is often irreversible (**FIG 2**).

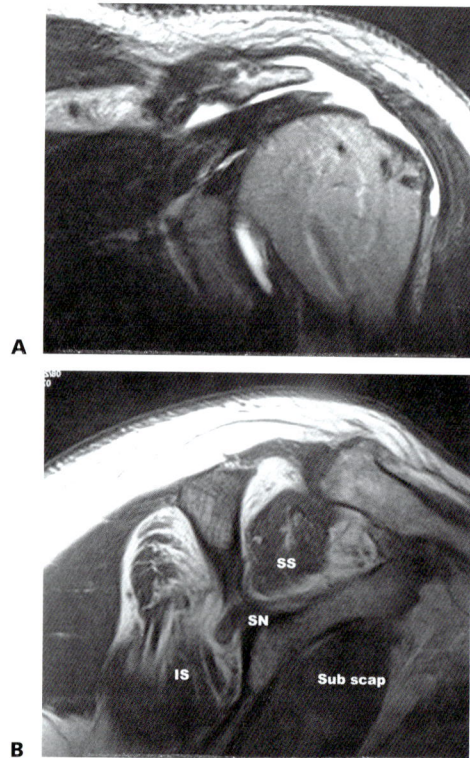

FIG 2 • **A.** Coronal MRI of a massive cuff tear showing tendon retraction to the midhumeral head. **B.** Sagittal MRI through lateral supraspinatus and infraspinatus fossae showing fatty degeneration and muscle wasting consistent with decreased muscle compliance and increased risk of repair failure at the time of surgery. The suprascapular nerve (*SN*) can be seen crossing through the spinoglenoid notch. *SS,* supraspinatus; *IS,* infraspinatus; *Sub scap,* subscapularis.

■ As a result, the longer these massive tears go untreated, the higher the likelihood that the tear will be irreparable at the time of surgery.

■ Presentation of the patient with a massive irreparable cuff tear is often precipitated by a minor traumatic event such as a fall onto an outstretched hand, resulting in an acute-on-chronic tear and functional decompensation of the shoulder. Others present with a history of longstanding, worsening symptoms that finally reach a point that is no longer tolerable to the patient.

NATURAL HISTORY

■ Massive posterosuperior rotator cuff tears are uncommon, representing less than one third of all rotator cuff tears even in practices limited to the treatment of shoulder pathology.[15]

■ Not all patients with large posterosuperior cuff tears experience enough loss of function or pain to require surgery or even seek treatment.

■ It can be difficult to predict who will have significant shoulder dysfunction based on radiographic or MRI findings or direct inspection of a torn rotator cuff.

■ Some patients with large tears can still use their arm for many activities, and some even retain the ability to perform overhead activities.

■ Others with smaller tears may have significant difficulty or an inability to use their arm for anything above chest level.

■ Regardless of tear size, it is loss of the rotator cuff muscles' ability to perform their role as humeral head stabilizers that eventually leads to functional decompensation.

■ As the tear progresses in size, behavioral and biomechanical compensation will allow maintenance of function to a point. However, once the rotator cuff can no longer stabilize the humeral head to create a fulcrum around which the deltoid can act to forward flex and abduct the arm, rapid decompensation, loss of function, and increased pain ensue.

PATIENT HISTORY AND PHYSICAL FINDINGS

■ The patient history should elicit the mechanism and duration of the current symptoms with the intent of determining if there was a specific traumatic event leading to the rotator cuff tear and whether symptoms of rotator cuff pathology were present before any such event.

■ Determining if the tear is a result of an acute injury as opposed to an acute-on-chronic process will help in estimating the quality of the tissues and whether they will be amenable to repair at the time of surgery.

■ The duration of dysfunction is also important in determining the likelihood of being able to repair any rotator cuff tear, since fatty degeneration of the supraspinatus and infraspinatus muscle bellies may start within weeks of the injury and will greatly decrease tissue compliance and increase tension placed on a potential repair.[9,16]

■ A careful neurologic examination, starting with the neck, must be performed to rule out neurologic causes of shoulder symptoms.

■ An understanding of the patient's current functional limitations as well as expectations for postoperative function is necessary to elicit whether the patient's disability is significant enough to benefit from the procedure.

■ A focused examination for the rotator cuff-deficient shoulder includes but is not limited to:

■ Active forward flexion examination: Patients with function at or above shoulder level are more likely to have improved active forward flexion postoperatively.

■ Active external rotation examination: Decreased external rotation on the affected side indicates partial or complete loss of infraspinatus function due to tear involvement or muscle dysfunction.

■ External rotation lag sign: Inability to maintain maximal external rotation (greater than or equal to a 20-degree lag sign) suggests tear extension well into the infraspinatus.

■ Passive range of motion should be compared to the contralateral limb. Decreased range of motion suggests joint contracture, which requires treatment before consideration for muscle transfer.

■ Modified belly press test: Inability to perform this action demonstrates a dysfunctional or torn subscapularis tendon, and these patients will have a higher rate of clinical failure with muscle transfer.

■ Abduction strength testing: This tests deltoid muscle strength. A weak deltoid suggests less postoperative active range of motion secondary to inadequate strength.

■ External rotation strength testing: Full strength suggests no infraspinatus tear involvement, whereas weakness suggests progressive infraspinatus involvement or dysfunction.

■ Evaluation for superior escape: Superior escape suggests an incompetent coracoacromial arch and a high likelihood of failure to improve with muscle transfer.

IMAGING AND OTHER DIAGNOSTIC STUDIES

■ A true anteroposterior (AP) radiographic view of the shoulder in the plane of the scapula and axillary view is obtained (**FIG 3A,B**).

■ This allows evaluation of glenohumeral arthritis, superior migration of the humeral head, and identification of any abnormal bony anatomy (**FIG 3C,D**).

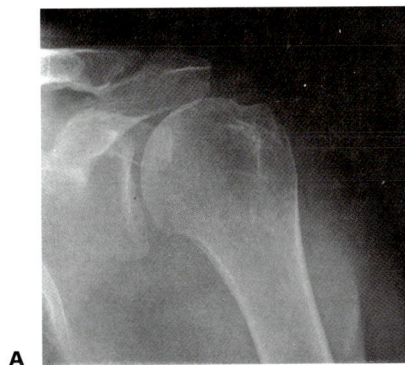

FIG 3 • A. True AP radiographic view of the glenohumeral joint showing minimal superior migration of the humeral head and preservation of the joint space. *(continued)*

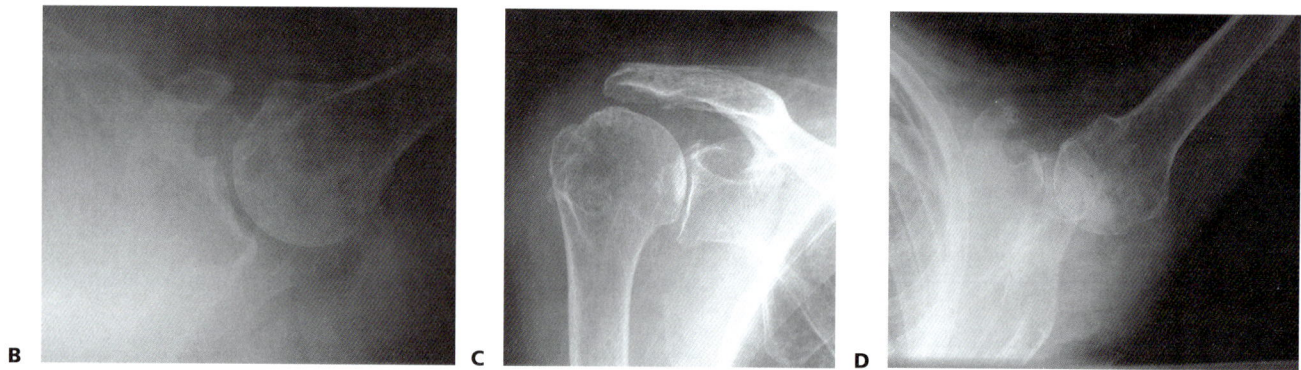

FIG 3 • *(continued)* **B.** Axillary lateral view of the glenohumeral joint demonstrating joint space preservation and the absence of osteophytes with a centered humeral head. **C,D.** Radiographic findings of degenerative arthritis, suggestive of a poor surgical candidate for a latissimus dorsi transfer. **C.** True AP radiographic view of the glenohumeral joint showing osteoarthritic changes, osteophyte formation, and superior migration of the humeral head. **D.** Axillary lateral view of the glenohumeral joint showing osteoarthritis with early posterior glenoid wear.

- MRI allows evaluation of the rotator cuff, biceps tendon, and labral and capsular pathology (see Fig 2):
  - The size of the rotator cuff tear, especially the extent of subscapularis and infraspinatus involvement
  - Distance of tendon retraction from the greater tuberosity
  - Extent of fatty degeneration seen in involved muscle bellies
- Electromyography is used to evaluate nerve function around the shoulder girdle.
  - It is necessary when nerve pathology is suspected as a cause of shoulder dysfunction.

DIFFERENTIAL DIAGNOSIS

- Frozen shoulder
- Adhesive capsulitis
- Massive rotator cuff tear that can be repaired
- Cervical nerve root compression
- Suprascapular nerve palsy
- Deltoid dysfunction

NONOPERATIVE MANAGEMENT

- Nonoperative management is directed toward optimizing the patient's current function, managing pain, and modifying activities and expectations.
- Treatment of irreparable cuff tears begins with physical therapy focused on maintaining motion and strengthening the deltoid and scapular stabilizers.
  - Physical therapy includes strengthening of the periscapular muscles and internal and external rotators, and stretching to prevent stiffness and further loss of motion.
  - Cortisone injection: Forty to 80 mg triamcinolone with 5 to 10 mL 1% Xylocaine is placed in the subacromial–glenohumeral space to decrease synovitis and bursitis, improve pain, and facilitate physical therapy.
  - Activity and expectation modification: The physician should explain avoidance of inciting activities that increase pain and discuss realistic functional goals for patients with irreparable cuff tears.
- Most patients with irreparable cuff tears who fail to gain adequate improvement from physical therapy and activity modification are still not good candidates for latissimus dorsi muscle transfers. For these patients, alternative surgical inter-

ventions such as limited-goals arthroscopic débridement or reverse total shoulder arthroplasty in low-demand patients, versus shoulder fusion in young, high-demand manual laborers, may be options.

- Limited-goals arthroscopy: If nonoperative management has failed but the patient is not a good candidate for latissimus transfer, an arthroscopic glenohumeral and subacromial débridement may be an option.
  - The ideal patient is over the age of 65 and retired, has low functional demands, and has an irreparable tear, and the primary indication for surgery is pain (not weakness).
  - These patients should have at least shoulder-level active elevation with an improvement in active elevation after having a positive injection test (10 cc lidocaine into the glenohumeral joint) and without shoulder arthritis.
  - This débridement can include synovial débridement, bursectomy, abrasion chondroplasty, acromioplasty–greater tuberosity-plasty, and biceps tenotomy or tenodesis to decrease mechanical symptoms and remove inflamed and painful tissues.
  - Successful results are characterized by a decrease in pain followed by a fairly aggressive postoperative strengthening program.

SURGICAL MANAGEMENT

- The treatment decisions regarding management of massive irreparable rotator cuff tears must be made in the context of the patient's current functional deficits, level of pain and its suspected cause, and physical examination findings.
- What the patient should expect in terms of postoperative pain relief and functional improvement must be clearly delineated before surgery, since return of full (normal) strength, active range of motion, and complete resolution of pain are not realistic goals for even the best latissimus transfer candidates.
- Only a carefully selected subset of patients with irreparable rotator cuff tears are good candidates for latissimus dorsi transfers.
  - Ideal patients are younger and have good deltoid and subscapularis muscle strength, limited glenohumeral arthritis, and the ability to get shoulder-level active forward flexion preoperatively.
- Table 1 lists specific prognostic factors.

| Table 1 | **Prognostic Factors for Latissimus Dorsi Transfers** |

Parameter	Better Prognosis	Worse Prognosis
Age	<60 years	>60 years
Gender	Male	Female
Function	Chest level or better	Below chest level
Subscapularis condition	Intact, functional	Torn, dysfunctional
Deltoid condition	Intact	Detached, dysfunctional
Previous surgery	No	Yes

Preoperative Planning

- Before surgery, plain radiographs and MRI must be reviewed to rule out other sources of pathology.
- Glenohumeral osteoarthritis should be ruled out as a predominant cause of the patient's current pain.
- An estimate should be made of the likelihood of successful primary repair based on the degree of cuff retraction and tissue quality.
- The equipment needed for both an attempted cuff repair and for muscle transfer should be available at the time of surgery.

- The possibility of needing to use autograft or allograft tendon to augment the length of the latissimus dorsi transfer should be discussed with the patient and the site for autograft harvest must be draped appropriately at the time of surgery, or allograft tissue must be available.

Positioning

- The patient is placed in the lateral decubitus position and secured with a bean-bag or hip positioner posts (**FIG 4A**).
- The patient is draped to keep the affected arm free during the case and allow access to the back, the superior aspect of the shoulder, and the arm down to the elbow (**FIG 4B,C**).
- An arm holder attached to the opposite side of the table will allow abduction, flexion, and rotation for positioning of the arm during the case.

Approach

- The surgical approach must allow wide access to the rotator cuff and to the muscle belly of the latissimus dorsi and its insertion.
- Although a single-incision technique has been described,[11] most authors prefer a two-incision technique—one incision for exposure and preparation of the rotator cuff and a second for dissection and release of the latissimus dorsi.[3,5,8,12,15]

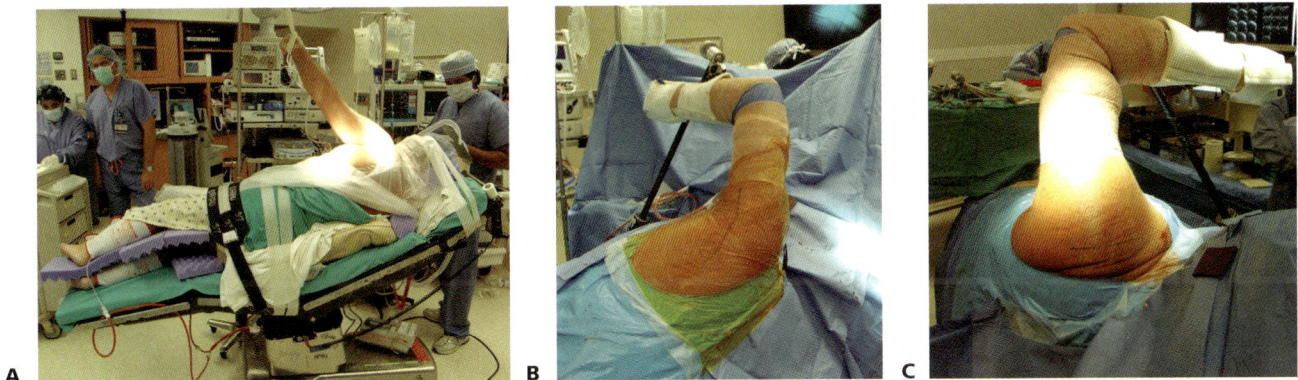

FIG 4 • Lateral decubitus positioning of the patient with a bean-bag, viewed from the back (**A**) and from the foot of the bed (**B**). Slight reverse Trendelenburg positioning of the table facilitates superior exposure of the subacromial space. **C.** Lateral decubitus positioning of the patient with a bean-bag after draping with the arm placed in an arm holder, viewed from the head of the table.

SUPERIOR APPROACH TO THE ROTATOR CUFF

- An incision is made at the lateral edge of the acromion parallel to the acromion's lateral border (**TECH FIG 1A**).
- Subcutaneous flaps are raised just superficial to the deltoid fascia.
- The anterior deltoid is taken off the acromion from the acromioclavicular joint to the midpoint between the anterior and posterior borders of the acromion.
  - This dissection is done in the subperiosteal plane to ensure strong fascial and periosteal tissue for later closure.
- The deltoid is split distally in line with its muscle fibers at the mid-lateral or posterolateral corner of the acromion (depending on the amount of deltoid released), and a stay suture is placed in the deltoid about 5 cm distal to the lateral edge of the acromion to prevent propagation of the split distally, which may result in injury to the axillary nerve (**TECH FIG 1B**).

- This exposure removes at least half and in some cases all of the middle deltoid origin. This extensive exposure helps in repair of the cuff as well as for transfer and repair of the latissimus dorsi tendon.
- A complete bursectomy is performed, the size and pattern of the rotator cuff tear are delineated, and the leading edge of the cuff tear is débrided (**TECH FIG 1C**).
- Inspection of the subscapularis tendon should be performed at this stage and partial detachments should be repaired.
  - Irreparable subscapularis tears should be considered for concomitant pectoralis major transfers.
  - Double muscle transfers are rarely performed and have a worse prognosis than single muscle transfers.

TECHNIQUES

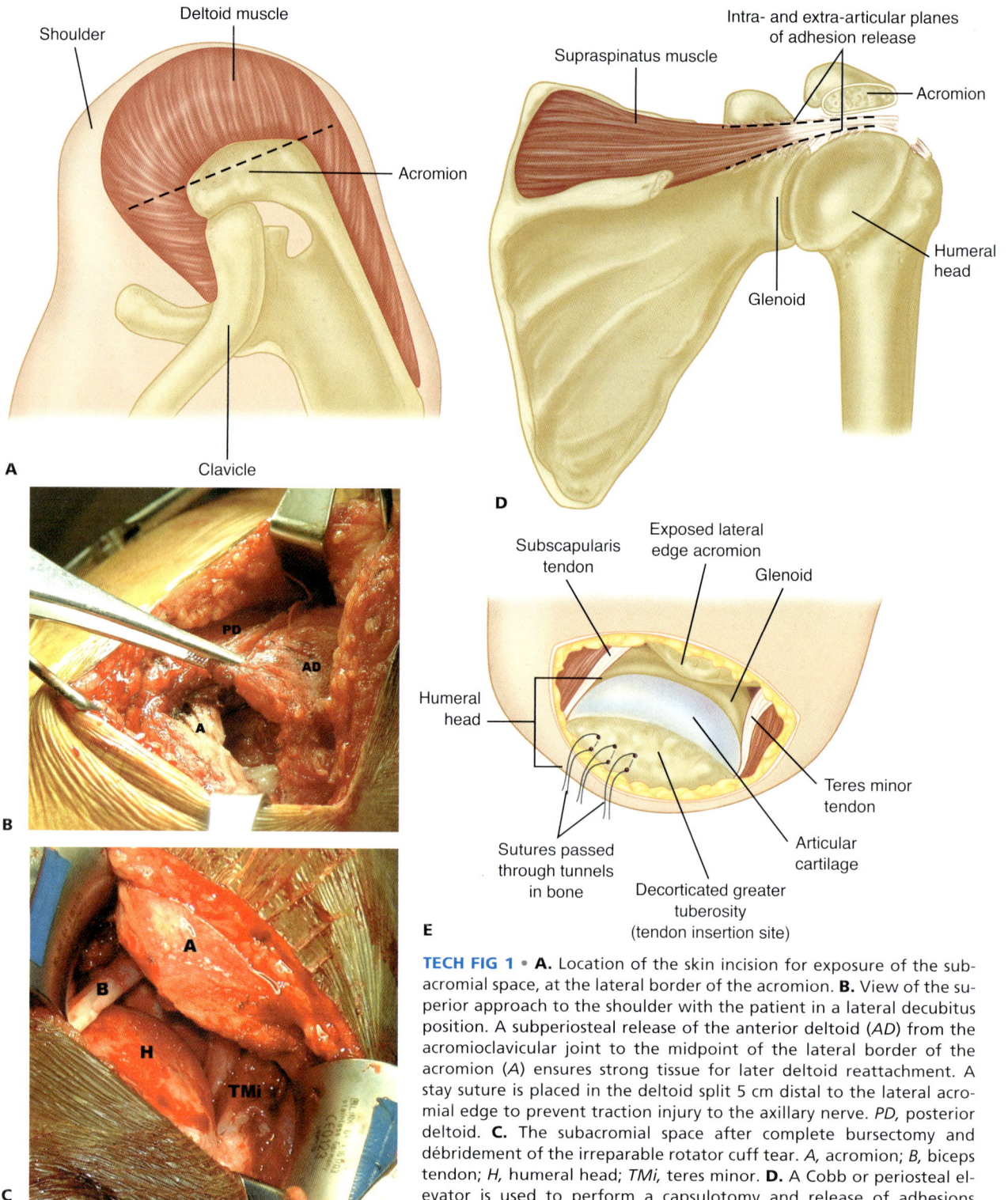

TECH FIG 1 • A. Location of the skin incision for exposure of the subacromial space, at the lateral border of the acromion. **B.** View of the superior approach to the shoulder with the patient in a lateral decubitus position. A subperiosteal release of the anterior deltoid (*AD*) from the acromioclavicular joint to the midpoint of the lateral border of the acromion (*A*) ensures strong tissue for later deltoid reattachment. A stay suture is placed in the deltoid split 5 cm distal to the lateral acromial edge to prevent traction injury to the axillary nerve. *PD*, posterior deltoid. **C.** The subacromial space after complete bursectomy and débridement of the irreparable rotator cuff tear. *A*, acromion; *B*, biceps tendon; *H*, humeral head; *TMi*, teres minor. **D.** A Cobb or periosteal elevator is used to perform a capsulotomy and release of adhesions around the superior glenoid rim. Articular and subacromial-sided release of adhesions from the retracted rotator cuff allows full mobilization of the torn tendons for an attempted primary repair. **E.** The prepared greater tuberosity, lightly decorticated, with sutures in place to allow tendon fixation.

- An acromioplasty is performed as needed.
  - Remove only that portion of the acromion that extends inferior to the plane of the posterior acromion.
  - Avoid decreasing the anteroposterior dimension of the acromion, which can increase the risk of superior escape of the humeral head.
- Keep the coracoacromial ligament at its maximum length and attached to the deep surface of the deltoid.
- At wound closure, place sutures in the acromial end of the coracoacromial ligament and suture this back to the anterior acromion to reconstruct the coracoacromial arch.

- ■ Reconstruction of the coracoacromial arch also helps minimize the risk of postoperative superior subluxation of the humeral head.
- ■ If degenerative changes are seen in the biceps tendon, it can be tenodesed in the bicipital groove and the intra-articular portion excised to remove it as a potential pain generator.
- ■ Complete mobilization of the retracted rotator cuff should be performed on both the intra-articular and extra-articular sides of the tendon.
  - ■ This is best performed with a scalpel, Cobb or periosteal elevator, and use of electrocautery where necessary on the intra-articular side of the tendons.
  - ■ Do not exceed 1.5 to 2.0 cm of medial dissection of the rotator cuff muscles within the fossa. Excessive medial dissection could injure the suprascapular nerve (**TECH FIG 1D**).
- ■ Débridement of remaining tissue and light decortication of the greater tuberosity with a rongeur or burr is per-

formed to prepare the site for rotator cuff reattachment or muscle transfer.
  - ■ Any portion of the cuff that is reparable to the tuberosity should be attached with number 2 or larger nonabsorbable suture to bone.
  - ■ Bone tunnels or suture anchors are placed in the lateral edge of the greater tuberosity (**TECH FIG 1E**).
- ■ If full mobilization of the rotator cuff will not allow solid repair of the tendon back to the greater tuberosity with the arm at the side, then the decision is made to proceed with the latissimus dorsi transfer.
  - ■ If a full repair is achieved but the quality of the repair or the tissue quality is fair or poor, we still prefer to perform the latissimus transfer when the likelihood for healing of the primary repair is low and the need for postoperative strength is high and of primary importance to the patient.

SURGICAL APPROACH TO THE LATISSIMUS DORSI

- ■ A 15-cm incision is made along the posterolateral border of the latissimus dorsi, extending proximally to the posterior axillary fold (**TECH FIG 2A**).
- ■ The incision can be extended proximally as needed for exposure, being careful to change directions when crossing skin creases in the axilla to avoid webbing and excessive scarring in the skin of the posterior axillary crease.
- ■ Skin flaps are raised just superficial to the muscular fascia of the latissimus dorsi, and the upper and lower borders of the muscle are defined (**TECH FIG 2B,C**).
  - ■ Identification of the inferior (lateral) border of the latissimus is the most reliable method for correctly identifying the muscle belly, as there is no large muscle inferior (lateral) to the latissimus on the posterior chest wall.

- ■ Blunt dissection is used to define and trace the tendon proximally toward its insertion on the proximal humerus (**TECH FIG 2D**).
- ■ Abduction and internal rotation of the arm provides the best visualization of the tendon at its insertion.[13]
- ■ Careful attention to neurovascular structures is critical at this stage, as the axillary and radial nerves, brachial plexus, and humeral circumflex vessels are all in proximity to the surgical field during this phase of the procedure.
  - ■ Internal rotation of the arm in abduction is necessary for adequate exposure but also brings the radial nerve closer to the latissimus dorsi tendon along its anterior, medial surface.[2]
  - ■ The axillary nerve and posterior humeral circumflex artery run along the superior border of the teres

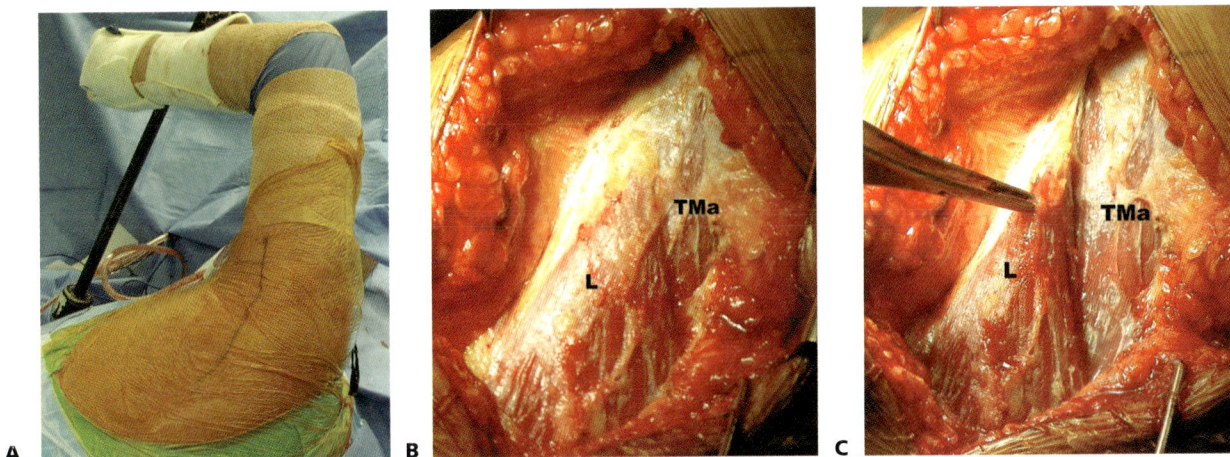

TECH FIG 2 • A. The posterior incision for harvest of the latissimus dorsi runs along the posterolateral border of the latissimus muscle belly, extending to the posterior axillary fold. It may be extended proximally to improve exposure, crossing skin creases at an angle to avoid postoperative contracture. **B.** Subcutaneous flaps are raised superficial to the muscular fascia of the latissimus dorsi (*L*) and teres major (*TMa*). **C.** The latissimus dorsi is the most inferior muscle belly running along the posterior and lateral chest wall. *(continued)*

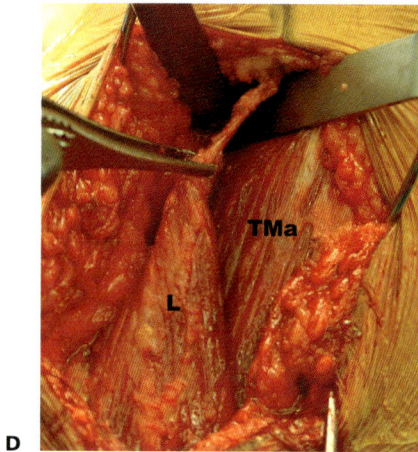

TECH FIG 2 • *(continued)* **D.** Exposure of the tendinous insertion of the latissimus dorsi (*L*) and teres major (*TMa*) on the proximal, medial humerus is facilitated by abduction and internal rotation of the arm.

major just proximal to the latissimus dorsi before exiting the quadrangular space.

- The anterior humeral circumflex vessels run along the superior border of the latissimus dorsi tendon and can be a source of significant bleeding if inadvertently cut.
- Dissection and release of the tendon should be carried out by working from the posterior surface of the tendon, as this keeps all important neurovascular structures anterior (deep) to the tendon.
- A significant number of patients will have latissimus dorsi and teres major tendons that fuse into one tendon along their superior border where they insert on the humerus, a condition that requires sharp dissection to separate the two.
- Once the humeral insertion of the latissimus dorsi has been identified, it should be released directly off the bone on the humeral shaft to ensure adequate tendon length for transfer.

TRANSFER AND FIXATION OF THE LATISSIMUS DORSI TO THE HUMERAL HEAD

- Once released from its insertion, the latissimus dorsi tendon is prepared by weaving number 2 fiberwire (Arthrex, Naples FL) through the tendon with a locking Krackow technique along both its superior and inferior borders (**TECH FIG 3A,B**).
- These locking sutures should be placed as soon as the tendon is released to minimize extensive handling of the tendon itself, which is easily frayed because it has few crossing fibers.
- These sutures can now be used as traction stitches, and the latissimus is freed from any adhesions on its anterior surface.
  - Be sure to pull the sutures in line with the long axis of the tendon.
  - Do not pull the locking sutures in divergent directions as it will separate the parallel fibers of the tendon.

- The neurovascular pedicle is identified and freed as well to prevent traction and damage to these structures during the transfer.
  - The pedicle is located on the deep surface of the muscle about 13 cm from the musculotendinous junction.
  - It is best seen and dissected after the tendon is released from its insertion and the muscle is flipped posteriorly, thereby exposing the undersurface of the muscle.
- Mobilization of the latissimus dorsi for transfer requires dissection of the deep fascial investments of the muscle from surrounding tissues into the chest wall.
  - If this is not performed, maximum excursion of the transfer will not be achieved and the tendon will not be long enough to reach the top of the humeral head.

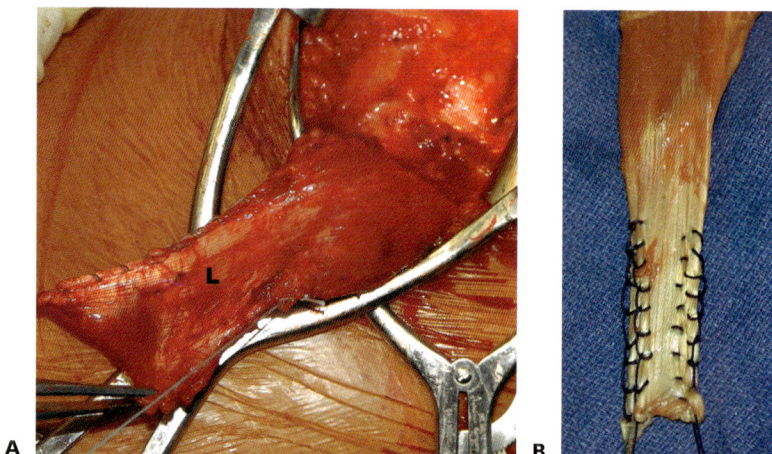

TECH FIG 3 • A single-strand (**A**) or double-strand (**B**) locking Krackow stitch is run along the upper and lower borders of the released latissimus tendon (*L*). This minimizes the risk of damage to the tendon fibers and facilitates passage of the latissimus into the subacromial space. *(continued)*

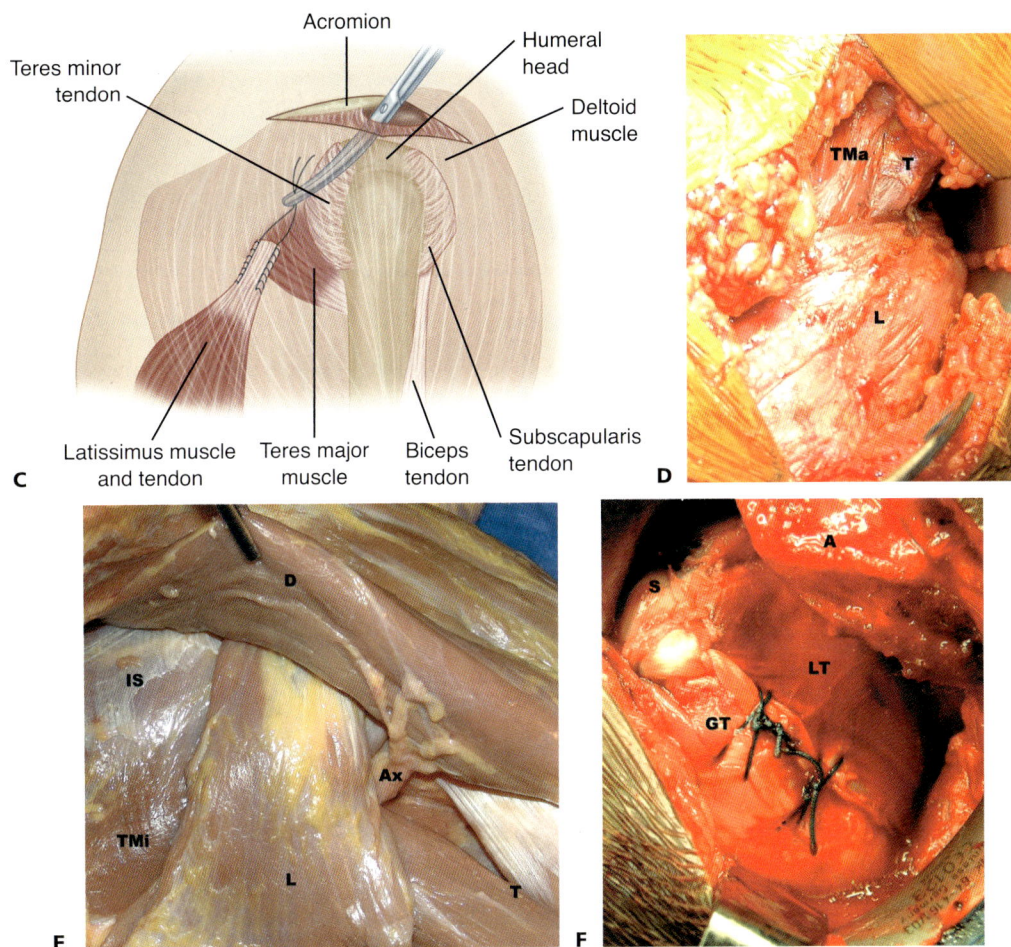

TECH FIG 3 • *(continued)* **C.** Using a large Kelly clamp, the latissimus dorsi is passed deep to the deltoid over the posterior surface of the rotator cuff muscles into the subacromial space. **D.** Intraoperative photo showing the transferred latissimus dorsi (*L*) viewed from the posterior chest wall incision on the left shoulder. **E.** Cadaveric dissection showing the subdeltoid passage of the released latissimus tendon in the right shoulder. Note the proximity of the axillary nerve (*Ax*) to the latissimus during this stage of the procedure. *D*, deltoid; *T*, triceps; *TMa*, teres major; *TMi*, teres minor; *IS*, infraspinatus. **F.** The latissimus dorsi tendon (*LT*) is anchored to the greater tuberosity (*GT*) laterally and sutured to the upper border of the subscapularis (*S*) anteriorly and to the leading edge of the torn, retracted rotator cuff tendons medially.

- Using sharp and scissor dissection and some blunt dissection, the plane underneath the deltoid and superficial to the rotator cuff muscles across the back of the shoulder is developed (about 4 to 6 cm wide) to connect the superior (rotator cuff exposure) and the posterior (latissimus exposure) wounds.
  - A large Kelly clamp is passed in this plane from the superior to the posterior wounds.
- Attention must be paid to enlarging this plane (4 to 6 cm) to prevent binding of the latissimus muscle belly within the tunnel, compromising its excursion.
- Grasping the previously placed traction sutures with the large curved Kelly clamp, the surgeon then passes the latissimus dorsi deep to the deltoid and into the subacromial space with the arm in adduction and neutral rotation (**TECH FIG 3C**).
- The effectiveness of this transfer depends on achieving a tenodesis effect of the transfer, thereby creating a passive humeral head depressor effect.

- To accomplish this, the arm is positioned in 45 degrees of abduction and at least 30 degrees of external rotation.
- In this position the transferred tendon is pulled to its maximum length over the top of the humeral head, and the traction sutures placed along the sides of the tendon are passed through the leading edge of the subscapularis tendon and tied. This step establishes the tendon transfer tension and places the tendon over the top of the humeral head (**TECH FIG 3D,E**).
- When the arm is brought to the patient's side and in internal rotation, the transfer is tensioned further, bringing the humeral head lower within the glenoid fossa.
  - We believe that this is one of the most important steps in the surgery to achieve proper transfer function.
- The lateral border of the latissimus dorsi tendon is now fixed to the greater tuberosity with three number 2 fiberwires passed through bone tunnels or with 5.5-mm biocorkscrew suture anchors (**TECH FIG 3F**).

TECHNIQUES

- The medial edge of the latissimus tendon is sutured to the retracted edge of the supraspinatus and infraspinatus tendons with several nonabsorbable sutures.
- Although some authors believe that the latissimus tendon should be attached only to the greater tuberosity to act as an external rotator of the humerus, we believe that repair of the leading edge to the upper border of the subscapularis allows the transfer to act as a humeral head depressor (either passively by a tenodesis effect or actively if the patient can learn how to fire the muscle actively [isotonically] in phase with external rotation or forward elevation).
- This suturing of the latissimus to the subscapularis can be done with two heavy, nonabsorbable sutures.

WOUND CLOSURE

- The anterior deltoid and middle deltoid are reattached to the acromion with nonabsorbable sutures placed through bone tunnels in the acromion as well as to the intact fascia (**TECH FIG 4A**).
- A drain is placed in the latissimus dorsi harvest site as needed, and both skin incisions are closed without closure of any deep fascial layers.
- Before emergence from general anesthesia, the patient is placed in a brace with 20 degrees of abduction and neutral rotation (**TECH FIG 4B**).

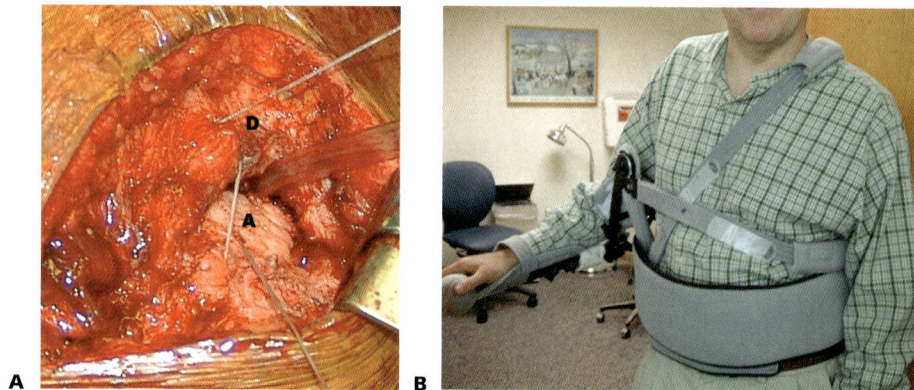

TECH FIG 4 • A. The deltoid (*D*) is reattached to the anterior and lateral edges of the acromion (*A*) with heavy, nonabsorbable sutures placed through bone tunnels. **B.** Patients are placed into an abduction brace in 20 degrees abduction and neutral rotation before extubation.

PEARLS AND PITFALLS

Indications and patient selection	■ Ideal candidates: physiologically young, thin, male gender, minimal muscle wasting, shoulder level function, minimal glenohumeral arthritis ■ Poor candidates: older, obese (big heavy arm), female gender, deltoid weakness, moderate arthritis, poorly compliant patient, subscapularis involvement, more limited preoperative function (less than shoulder-level active elevation), superior humeral head escape
Preoperative assessment of whether cuff can be repaired	■ Duration: Within weeks to months, rotator cuff muscle–tendon units demonstrate decreased compliance and inferior mechanical properties. ■ Cuff retraction: Retraction of torn tendons medial to the midpoint of the humeral head on MRI suggests the need for significant mobilization at the time of surgery to attempt a primary repair. ■ Muscle degeneration: MRI or CT imaging showing fatty degeneration of the rotator cuff muscle bellies suggests tendons will have limited excursion and inferior mechanical properties at the time of attempted repair.
Surgical	■ The surgeon should internally rotate the arm to fully visualize the latissimus insertion on the humerus. Inadequate exposure limits the ability to harvest the entire length of tendon, necessitating additional tendon graft. ■ The released latissimus tendon should be handled carefully to prevent fraying. ■ Release and mobilization of the latissimus dorsi muscle belly along the chest wall ■ The surgeon should ensure that the tunnel for the latissimus rerouting is large enough to prevent constriction of the latissimus muscle belly in the subdeltoid space.
Postoperative	■ Retraining of the latissimus to work in phase with forward flexion and external rotation of the arm

POSTOPERATIVE CARE

- The patient is placed into a brace postoperatively for 4 to 6 weeks to prevent internal rotation.
- During this time the brace can be removed for dressing and bathing, keeping the arm in neutral rotation.
- Passive forward flexion and external rotation is performed during the first 4 weeks to prevent shoulder stiffness.
- At 4 weeks, bracing is discontinued and passive range of motion in all planes is performed.
- At 7 to 9 weeks, active range of motion is started and physical therapy is begun, focused on retraining the latissimus dorsi to function as an abductor and external rotator of the arm.
  - External rotation training: A pillow is placed between the arm and chest wall holding the arm abducted 30 degrees. The patient is told to actively externally rotate the arm while adducting the arm against the pillow.
  - Forward elevation training: The patient squeezes a large rubber ball between the palms of the hands while raising both arms forward over the head.
  - Biofeedback can also be used to show the patient when he or she is actively contracting the latissimus during external rotation and forward elevation.

OUTCOMES

- Significant improvement in pain scores postoperatively is a consistent finding (80% to 100% of patients) across outcome studies, even for patients less satisfied with their final results.[7,11]
- Sixty-six to 81% of patients report satisfaction postoperatively. Patient satisfaction tends to be associated more with improved active shoulder function than pain relief.[7,11]
- Patients with better preoperative function tend to have greater postoperative improvements in range of motion and strength compared to patients starting with greater shoulder dysfunction.
- Based on our experience and that reported in the literature, postoperative range of motion improves by an average of 35 to 50 degrees in forward flexion and 9 to 40 degrees of external rotation.[1,7,11,16]
- Patients undergoing latissimus transfer as the first procedure to treat their rotator cuff pathology can expect better outcomes with regard to satisfaction, pain relief, and active range of motion compared to patients undergoing latissimus transfer who have had prior failed surgery for treatment of their rotator cuff.[16]
- Electromyographic studies show that about 40% to 50% of patients can be retrained to use in-phase latissimus dorsi contraction with active forward flexion or external rotation.[7,11]
- Female gender and advanced age are associated with worse outcomes.
- Subscapularis tendon tears and superior escape of the humeral head are associated with a higher failure rate.

- Patients with multiple negative preoperative prognostic factors should not undergo isolated latissimus muscle transfer, and other options should be considered either alone or in conjunction with a latissimus transfer.

COMPLICATIONS

- Deltoid detachment
- Wound infection
- Rupture of the transferred tendon
- Decreased active forward flexion

REFERENCES

1. Aoki M, Okamura K, Fukushima S, et al. Transfer of latissimus dorsi for irreparable rotator-cuff tears. J Bone Joint Surg Br 1996;78B: 761–766.
2. Cleeman E, Hazrati Y, Auerbach JD, et al. Latissimus dorsi transfers for massive rotator cuff tears: a cadaveric study. J Shoulder Elbow Surg 2003;12:539–543.
3. Codsi MJ, Hennigan S, Herzog R, et al. Latissimus dorsi tendon transfer for irreparable posterosuperior rotator cuff tears: factors affecting outcomes. J Bone Joint Surg Am 2007;89A(Suppl 2):1–9.
4. Cofield RH. Rotator cuff disease of the shoulder. J Bone Joint Surg Am 1985;67A:974–979.
5. Costouros JG, Gerber C, Warner JP. Management of irreparable rotator cuff tears: the role of tendon transfer. In: Iannotti JP, Williams GR, ed. Disorders of the Shoulder: Diagnosis and Management, 2nd ed. Philadelphia: Lippincott-Raven, 1999.
6. Dugas JR, Campbell DA, Warren RF, et al. Anatomy and dimensions of rotator cuff insertions. J Shoulder Elbow Surg 2002;11:498–503.
7. Gerber C. Latissimus dorsi transfer for the treatment of irreparable tears of the rotator cuff. Clin Orthop Relat Res 1992;275:152–160.
8. Gerber C, Vinh TS, Hertel R, et al. Latissimus dorsi transfer for the treatment of massive tears of the rotator cuff: a preliminary report. Clin Orthop Relat Res 1988;232:51–60.
9. Goutallier D, Postel JM, Bernageau J, et al. Fatty muscle degeneration in cuff ruptures: pre- and postoperative evaluation by CT scan. Clin Orthop Relat Res 1994;304:78–83.
10. Habermeyer P, Magosch P, Rudolph T, et al. Transfer of the tendon of latissimus dorsi for the treatment of massive tears of the rotator cuff: a new single incision technique. J Bone Joint Surg Br 2006;88B:208–212.
11. Iannotti JP, Hennigan S, Herzog R, et al. Latissimus dorsi tendon transfer for irreparable posterosuperior rotator cuff tears. J Bone Joint Surg Am 2006;88A:342–348.
12. Miniaci A, MacLeod M. Transfer of the latissimus dorsi muscle after failed repair of a massive tear of the rotator cuff: a two- to five-year review. J Bone Joint Surg Am 1999;81A:1120–1127.
13. Pearle AD, Kelly BT, Voos JE, et al. Surgical techniques and anatomic study of latissimus dorsi and teres major transfers. J Bone Joint Surg Am 2006;88A:1524–1531.
14. Schoierer O, Herzberg G, Berthonnaud E, et al. Anatomical basis of latissimus dorsi and teres major transfers on rotator cuff tear surgery with particular reference to the neurovascular pedicles. Surg Radiol Anat 2001;23:75–80.
15. Warner JP. Management of massive irreparable rotator cuff tears: the role of tendon transfers. AAOS Instr Course Lect 2001;50:63–71.
16. Warner PJ, Parsons IM. Latissimus dorsi tendon transfer: a comparative analysis of primary and salvage reconstruction of massive, irreparable rotator cuff tears. J Shoulder Elbow Surg 2001;10:514–521.

Chapter 11

Pectoralis Major Transfer for Irreparable Subscapularis Tears

Leesa M. Galatz

DEFINITION

- The subscapularis is one of four muscles making up the rotator cuff. Tears can result from chronic attenuation secondary to age or overuse, but more commonly they result from trauma.
- Subscapularis tears commonly occur after a fall on the outstretched arm, traction injuries resulting in a strong external rotation force applied to the arm, or an anterior shoulder dislocation.
- Many tears affect only the upper tendinous portion of the insertion. Other tears result in a complete tear of the tendinous and muscular portions of the insertion.
- Subscapularis tears are often missed early in the course of treatment. Tears older than about 6 months are usually not reparable because of atrophy and degeneration of the muscle, necessitating a pectoralis major muscle transfer.

ANATOMY

- The subscapularis muscle (**FIG 1A**) arises from the deep, volar surface of the scapular body (the subscapular fossa) and inserts on the lesser tuberosity. The upper two thirds of the insertion is tendinous and the lower third is a muscular insertion.
  - The anterior humeral circumflex artery courses laterally along the demarcation between the tendinous and muscular portions of the muscle.
  - Tears of the subscapularis differ from tears of the other rotator cuff muscles in that there is often an intact soft tissue sleeve across the front of the shoulder with the torn tendon retracted medially within this "sheath." In contrast, the supraspinatus and infraspinatus tear leaving exposed humeral head. The remaining soft tissue over the anterior humeral head after a subscapularis tear can be mistaken for an intact or partially torn tendon.
- The pectoralis major muscle is composed of two major heads (**FIG 1B**).
  - The clavicular head originates from the medial third of the clavicle. The sternal head originates from the manubrium, the upper two thirds of the sternum, and ribs 2 to 4. The muscle courses laterally to insert on the lateral lip of the biceps groove.
  - The sternal head lies deep to the clavicular head, forming the posterior lamina, and inserts slightly superior to the clavicular head. The clavicular head forms the anterior lamina. The laminae are usually continuous inferiorly.
- Some of the deep muscular fibers from the inferior aspect of the pectoralis major muscle course toward and insert on the more proximal or superior aspect of the muscle insertion. These inferior-to-superior–directed fibers tend to make the muscle "flip" when it is released. The superior corner should be tagged to assist with orientation if used for the transfer.
- The mean width of the pectoralis major insertion is 5.7 cm (range, 4.8 to 6.5 cm).[6] The undersurface of the insertion has a broad tendinous insertion, whereas the anterior surface is primarily muscular; only the most distal insertion is tendinous.
- The pectoralis major muscle is innervated by the medial and lateral pectoral nerves, which arise from the medial and lateral cords of the brachial plexus, respectively.
  - The medial pectoral nerve enters the pectoralis major muscle about 11.9 cm (range, 9.0 to 14.5 cm) from the

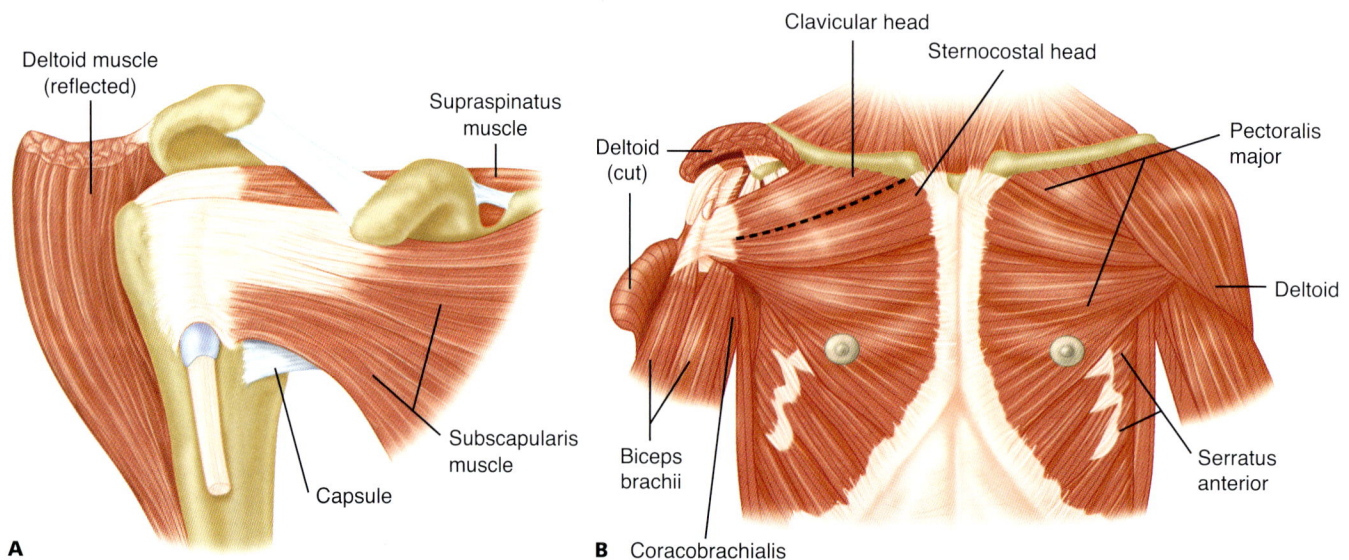

FIG 1 • A. Anterior view of the subscapularis muscle. **B.** Clavicular and sternal heads of the pectoralis muscle.

humeral insertion and 2.0 cm from the inferior edge of the muscle.[6]
- The lateral pectoral nerve enters the pectoralis major muscle at a mean of 12.5 cm (range, 10.0 to 14.9 cm) from the insertion.[6]
- The musculocutaneous nerve arises from the lateral cord of the brachial plexus and enters the conjoint tendon an average of 6.1 cm (range, 3.5 to 10 cm) from the coracoid (95% confidence interval, 3.1 to 9.1 cm).[6]
  - In some patients, a proximal branch enters the conjoint tendon proximal to the main branch of the musculocutaneous nerve. The function of this proximal branch is not known. It is likely innervation to the coracobrachialis, and its release has little clinical effect.

PATHOGENESIS

- Subscapularis tears result from:
  - Anterior shoulder dislocations
  - Traction injuries to the arm with extension and external rotation forces to the arm
  - Rarely, chronic attenuation from age and overuse
  - Possible relationship to coracoid impingement
- The subscapularis muscle is particularly prone to atrophy and degeneration after a tear. With complete, retracted tears of the muscle, there is a window of opportunity for about 6 months when a primary repair can be performed. Beyond that time point, the muscle is increasingly difficult to mobilize and repair is under substantial tension, leading to early failure.

NATURAL HISTORY

- Subscapularis tears can result in pain, loss of motion, and loss of strength in the affected shoulder.
- Failure to recognize the injury can result in a delay in treatment and possibly an irreparable tear.
- An untreated rotator cuff tear can lead to progressive loss of function, stiffness, and possibly arthritis. Loss of the subscapularis may result in dynamic proximal migration of the humeral head with arm elevation that can eventually become static elevation.

PATIENT HISTORY AND PHYSICAL FINDINGS

- Lift-off test: The patient will not be able to lift the hand off the back if the subscapularis is deficient.
- Abdominal compression test: With a tear, the patient will not be able to maintain this position and will flex wrist or hand will release from the belly if positive.
- Range-of-motion testing: A subscapularis tear will result in increased external rotation at the side, with a "softer" endpoint.

IMAGING AND OTHER DIAGNOSTIC STUDIES

- A standard shoulder series of radiographs comprising a shoulder anteroposterior (AP) view, a true scapular AP view, an axillary view, and a scapular Y view is obtained to rule out fractures, arthritis, or other injury.
  - A subscapularis tear may result in proximal migration of the humeral head relative to the glenoid, depending on the degree of tear and involvement of other rotator cuff muscles.

- In the absence of a subscapularis tear, slight anterior subluxation of the humeral head may be noted on the axillary view.
- An MRI will reveal the tear and also is helpful in assessing the degree of retraction, atrophy, and fatty degeneration of the subscapularis muscle. The proximal portion of the long head of the biceps tendon becomes unstable from the intertubercular groove when the subscapularis tears. An MRI can demonstrate a dislocated or subluxed biceps tendon.
- A CT arthrogram is an alternative to an MRI.
- Subscapularis tears can be diagnosed with ultrasound if performed by a competent, experienced ultrasonographer. Ultrasound is very sensitive for biceps tendon subluxation or dislocation from the groove.[1]

DIFFERENTIAL DIAGNOSIS

- Supraspinatus tears
- Infraspinatus tears
- Biceps tendon pathology
- Anterior instability
- Rotator cuff insufficiency secondary to neurologic etiology

NONOPERATIVE MANAGEMENT

- Physical therapy focusing on strengthening the intact rotator cuff muscles can be beneficial to maximize the function of remaining musculature.
  - Range-of-motion exercises focus on any areas of loss of motion or capsular contracture.
  - Rotator cuff strengthening with the use of light-resistance Therabands at waist level is an effective initial exercise. Progression to higher-resistance exercises is as tolerated.
- Cortisone injections may give some temporary pain relief but are unlikely to result in permanent resolution of symptoms.
- Nonsteroidal anti-inflammatory medication may be helpful for pain relief of mild to moderate pain.

SURGICAL MANAGEMENT

- An attempt is made at the time of surgery to repair the native subscapularis. Within reasonable limits, the subscapularis is mobilized by releasing surrounding soft tissues. Even a partial repair is recommended in conjunction with a pectoralis major transfer.
  - Surrounding soft tissues include the rotator interval and coracohumeral ligament, the anterior capsule of the shoulder (middle and inferior glenohumeral ligaments), and superficial soft tissue adhesions deep to the coracoid and conjoint tendon.
- The subscapularis differs from the other rotator cuff muscles in that it has a fascial sleeve that remains attached to the lesser tuberosity and covers the anterior humeral head. This is in contrast to the other rotator cuff muscles, which leave exposed greater tuberosity and cartilage without soft tissue coverage. This material is easily mistaken for an intact subscapularis, emphasizing the significance of preoperative evaluation.

Preoperative Planning

- Patient history, physical examination, and all imaging studies are reviewed. A soft tissue imaging study such as MRI or ultrasound of the rotator cuff is a necessity.

- Plain films should be assessed for proximal migration, anterior subluxation, and deformity secondary to trauma and arthritis. An MRI is useful for assessing the condition of the subscapularis. A high degree of retraction and degeneration of the muscle is highly suggestive of a chronic, irreparable tear that will necessitate a pectoralis major muscle transfer.
- Subscapularis tears result in instability of the long head of the biceps tendon with medial subluxation into the joint. The surgeon should be prepared to perform a biceps tenotomy or tenodesis of the tendon if it has not already ruptured from chronic, attritional changes.
- Associated tears of the other rotator cuff muscles are addressed concurrently. Isolated arthritic lesions are débrided, as is degenerative labral fraying or tear.

Positioning

- The pectoralis major transfer is most easily performed with the patient in the beach chair position. The head of the bed or positioning device is elevated about 60 degrees. The head is secured to avoid cervical injury. The arm is prepared and draped free and held in a commercially available arm holder that allows flexible arm positioning.[5]

Approach

- Several different variations of the pectoralis major transfer have been described.
  - Wirth and Rockwood[8] described a split pectoralis major muscle transfer superficial to the coracoid.
  - Resch and colleagues[7] described a split pectoralis major transfer deep to the coracoid.
  - Jost and colleagues[4] and Gerber and associates[3] recommended transfer of the whole pectoralis major muscle superficial to the coracoid.
  - Gerber and associates[3] described transfer of the sternal head of the pectoralis major with or without the teres major tendon.
- The procedure can be performed through a deltopectoral or anterior axillary incision.
  - The deltopectoral incision allows a more extensile approach and is recommended in revision cases.
  - The anterior axillary incision from the coracoid to the anterior axillary crease is useful in primary cases in smaller patients.
  - Both incisions use the deltopectoral interval for deep exposure.

TECHNIQUES

SPLIT PECTORALIS MAJOR MUSCLE TRANSFER

- The deltopectoral interval is identified. The cephalic vein is usually retracted laterally with the deltoid. The subdeltoid and subacromial spaces are released of adhesions.
- Regardless of technique, the native subscapularis is examined and mobilized to its full extent. If repair is not possible, a muscle transfer is performed.
- The superior 2.5 to 3 cm of the pectoralis major insertion is identified along the lateral edge of the biceps groove. This contains portions of both the anterior and posterior laminae. The identified portion of the pectoralis major insertion is released sharply from its insertion. Care is taken to avoid injury to the long head of the biceps tendon, which lies directly under the insertion in this case. The distal tendon is tagged with three or four stay sutures.
- Tension is applied to the stay sutures to facilitate the muscle split of the pectoralis major muscle. Muscle dissection is performed bluntly in a medial direction at the inferior portion of the split to mobilize the superior muscle for transfer. Dissection should be limited to 6 to 8 cm to preserve the medial pectoral nerve (**TECH FIG 1A**).

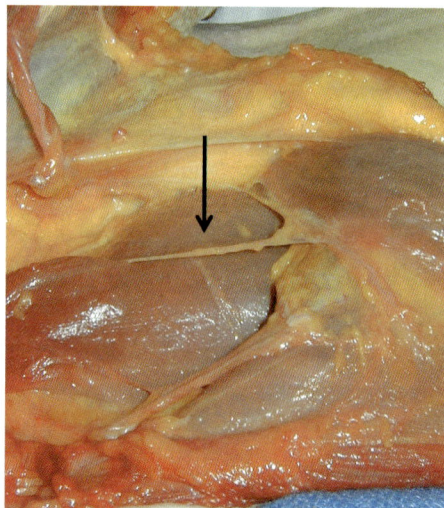

TECH FIG 1 • A. The medial pectoral nerve (*arrow*) arises from the medial cord of the brachial plexus and enters the pectoralis major muscle 6 to 8 cm medial to the muscle insertion. Thus, medial dissection and mobilization is limited to 6 to 8 cm to avoid denervating the muscle. **B.** The superior half of the pectoralis major insertion is freed from the humerus and mobilized. This half is transferred to the humeral head and secured in a small bone trough with drill holes for the sutures.

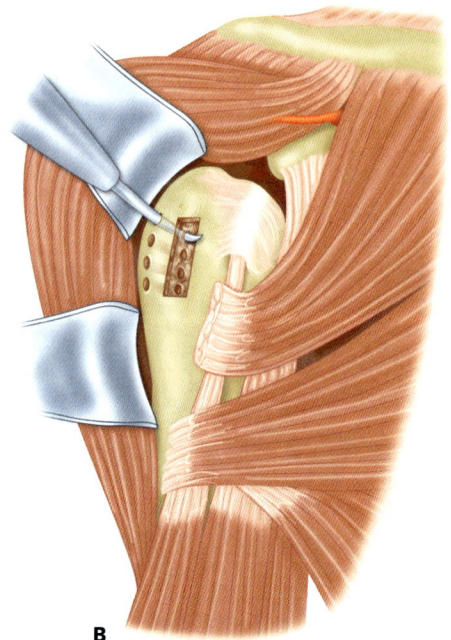

- The humerus is rotated internally to expose the greater tuberosity and humeral shaft lateral to the biceps groove. An osteotome or burr is used to make a bone trough measuring 5 × 25 mm oriented in a vertical position for reinsertion of the transferred pectoralis muscle.
- Three or four holes are drilled just lateral to the edge of the trough and a curved awl is used to connect the drill holes to the trough (**TECH FIG 1B**).

- The sutures in the tendon are passed into the trough and out through the drill holes. Tension is placed on the sutures, bringing the tendon into the trough. The sutures are then tied over the bone bridges between the holes, securing the tendon.
- A biceps tenotomy or tenodesis is performed as needed.

SUBCORACOID MUSCLE TRANSFER OF THE CLAVICULAR HEAD

- A deltopectoral incision and approach are used (**TECH FIG 2A**).
- The tendon of the pectoralis major insertion is exposed along its full length (**TECH FIG 2B**).
- The superior half to two thirds of the clavicular head is detached from the humerus. The muscle fibers corresponding to the detached section of the tendon are split or separated from the remaining muscle using blunt dissection in a medial direction. The blunt dissection is performed between the sternal and clavicular heads so that only the clavicular head muscle is released and preserved

for the transfer (**TECH FIG 2C**). The muscle fibers of the sternal portion that course into the proximal portion of the muscle are transected.
- The space between the medial border of the conjoint tendon and the pectoralis minor is gently dissected bluntly. The musculocutaneous nerve and its entry into the conjoint tendon are identified. The space deep to the conjoint tendon and superficial to the musculocutaneous nerve is developed for the muscle transfer (**TECH FIG 2D**).
- Stay sutures are attached to the distal pectoralis major tendon. The sutures are grasped with a curved forceps

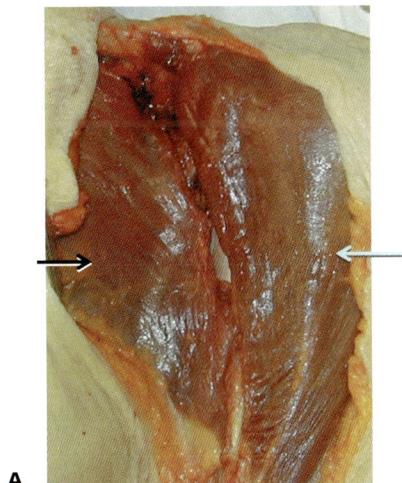

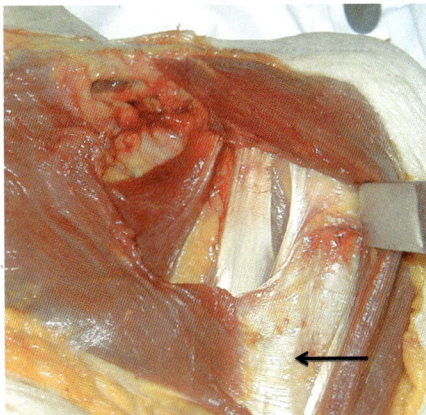

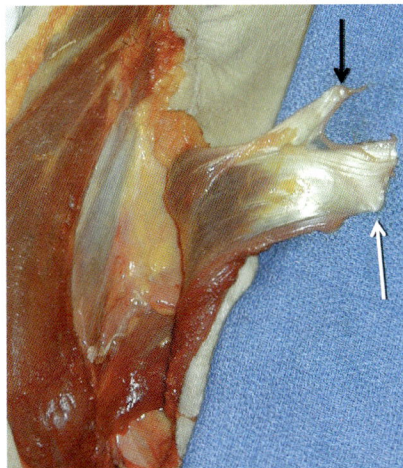

TECH FIG 2 • A. This cadaveric dissection illustrates the deltopectoral approach (*black arrow*, pectoralis major; *white arrow*, deltoid). The incision should be long enough to allow adequate exposure of the pectoralis major and the proximal humerus for reattachment. **B.** Cadaveric dissection illustrating the pectoralis major and its insertion (*arrow*). **C.** The pectoralis major has two heads, the superficial clavicular head (*white arrow*) and the deeper sternal head (*black arrow*). In this photo, the insertion has been released and is reflected medially. *(continued)*

A

B

C

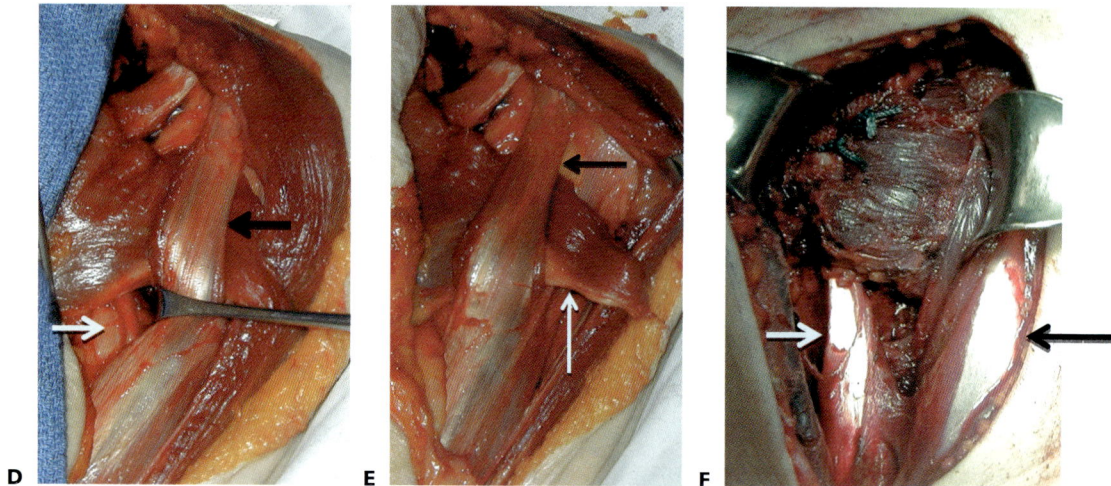

TECH FIG 2 • *(continued)* **D.** To avoid injury to the musculocutaneous nerve, it should be identified as part of the surgical procedure for a subcoracoid transfer. The muscle should be transferred deep to the conjoint tendon (*black arrow*) and superficial to the nerve (*white arrow*). **E.** The pectoralis major muscle (*white arrow*) is transferred deep to the conjoint tendon (*black arrow*), laterally to the greater tuberosity. **F.** Intraoperative photo of a right shoulder with a pectoralis major transfer secured to the greater tuberosity. *White arrow*, biceps; *black arrow*, conjoint tendon.

and passed deep to the conjoint tendon and superficial to the musculocutaneous nerve, advancing the muscle to the greater tuberosity (**TECH FIG 2E**).

■ The tendon is attached to the lesser tuberosity with transosseous nonabsorbable sutures. In very large individuals with substantial muscle mass, the muscle may need to be debulked to facilitate tension-free passage deep to the coracoid (**TECH FIG 2F**).

■ The transferred muscle is reattached using anchors or transosseous sutures.

WHOLE PECTORALIS MUSCLE TRANSFER

■ The deltopectoral approach is identical to that described above.

■ An attempt is made to mobilize and repair the subscapularis. Releases are performed at the rotator interval, the base of the coracoid, the brachial plexus, and the subscapularis fossa. A partial repair is performed if possible.

■ The entire tendon of the pectoralis major tendon is exposed and released from its insertion of the humerus.

■ Three nonabsorbable sutures are passed through the tendon using a modified Mason-Allen technique.

■ The muscle and tendon is mobilized and brought over (superficial) the coracoid to the medial aspect of the greater tuberosity, where it is secured using anchor fixation or to a bone trough (**TECH FIG 3**).

  ■ If a bone trough is used, the sutures are routed through the trough and the knots are tied over a small titanium plate to prevent suture pullout. The uppermost corner of the tendon is sutured to the anterolateral supraspinatus. Care is taken not to overtighten the rotator interval.

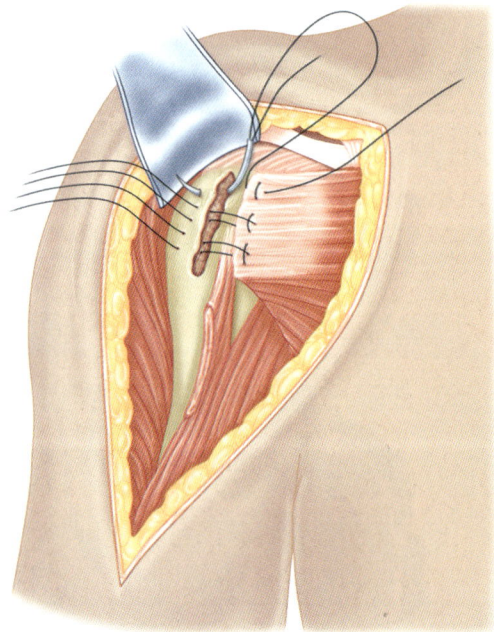

TECH FIG 3 • The whole pectoralis major muscle is released from its insertion on the humerus and transferred and secured to the humeral head using anchor fixation or a bone trough with tunnels.

SPLIT PECTORALIS MAJOR AND TERES MAJOR TENDON TRANSFER

- Setup and exposure are as described above.
- The plane between the sternal and clavicular heads is located and developed. The sternal head is sharply released from the humerus. Nonabsorbable sutures (no. 2) are placed in the tendon in Mason-Allen fashion.
- The sternal head is mobilized and pulled underneath the clavicular head to the lesser tuberosity, where it is secured (TECH FIG 4A). The transfer is superficial to the coracoid process and should be tight but allow 30 degrees of external rotation.
- If the subscapularis tear is completely irreparable, the authors recommend combining this transfer with the teres major muscle.
- To expose the teres major, the arm is externally rotated.

- The latissimus dorsi insertion is located and the superior and inferior aspects are demarcated. The latissimus is released, leaving a cuff of tissue laterally for repair.
- The teres major insertion is deep to the latissimus. The teres major is tagged and released. Often, the muscle must be released from confluence with the latissimus.
  - The axillary nerve and posterior humeral circumflex artery lie at the superior border of the teres major muscle. The radial nerve and brachial artery are in close approximation to the inferior border of the teres major.
- Finally, the teres major is transferred to the inferior portion of the lesser tuberosity, where it is secured with nonabsorbable sutures (TECH FIG 4B).

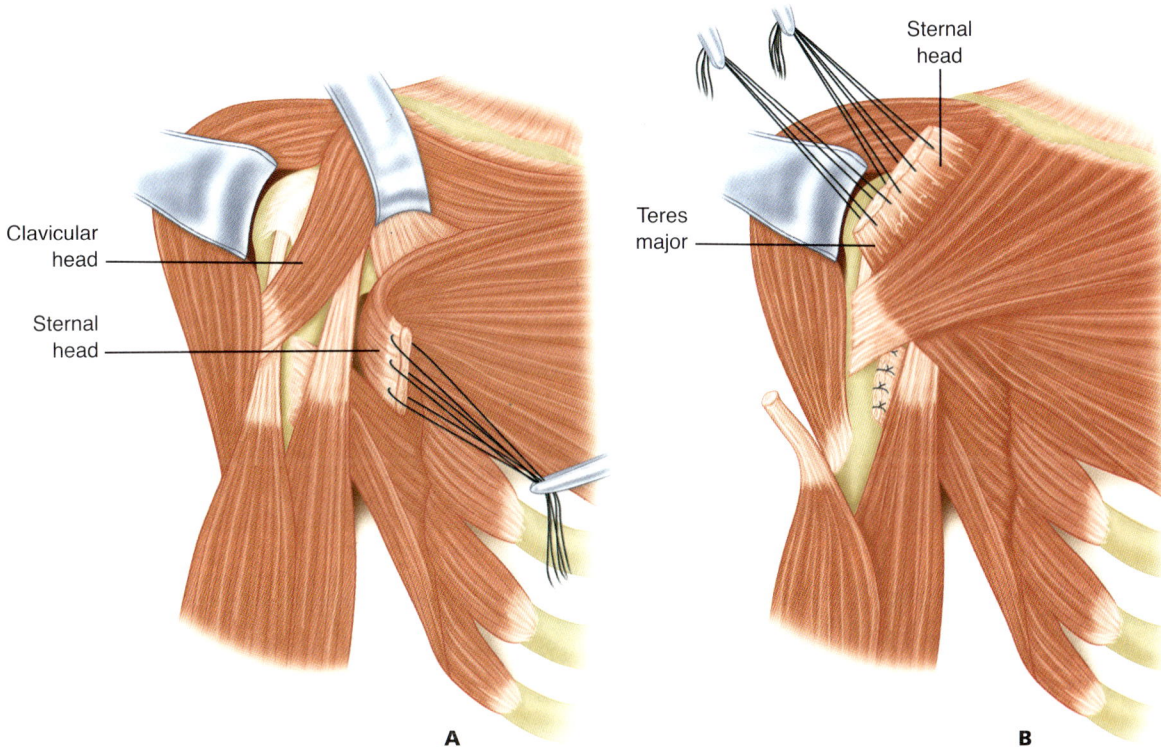

TECH FIG 4 • **A.** This transfer uses the sternal head of the pectoralis major muscle. It is released and mobilized underneath the clavicular head to the lesser tuberosity. **B.** The teres major muscle is released from its insertion on the humerus and transferred along with the sternal head of the pectoralis major to the lesser tuberosity. The teres major inserts deep to the latissimus dorsi, which is reattached in its anatomic position.

PEARLS AND PITFALLS

Indications	▪ Subscapularis tears are often missed, resulting in a delayed diagnosis. ▪ Elderly patients with generalized atrophy should be considered for a whole muscle transfer, whereas more muscular individuals are better candidates for split or sternal head transfers.
Pectoralis major muscle detachment and mobilization	▪ Mobilization of the muscle should not proceed greater than 8 cm from the insertion in order to protect the pectoral nerves. ▪ In whole muscle transfers, the medial pectoral nerve can enter the muscle within 1.2 cm of the inferior edge. ▪ Muscle split is performed bluntly.

Subcoracoid transfer of the pectoralis major muscle	■ The musculocutaneous nerve and its proximal branches are at risk. ■ The musculocutaneous nerve is identified. ■ Transferred muscle should course deep to the conjoint tendon and superficial to the nerve to avoid excessive traction and neurapraxia. ■ Scar in revision cases can make this dissection difficult; an intraoperative nerve stimulator may help identify structures of the brachial plexus if necessary.
Fixation problems	■ Mason-Allen or Krackow sutures are used to grasp the tendon securely.
Orientation	■ Before release of the muscle, the superior corner is tagged to keep muscle in its anatomic orientation (some inferior muscle fibers course to the superior insertion, so the muscle tends to flip after release).

POSTOPERATIVE CARE

■ A drain should always be used because release and transfer of the pectoralis major muscle[5] results in dead space, and hematoma formation is common.

■ The operative arm is placed in a sling postoperatively. Passive exercises are started on postoperative day 1.

■ The surgeon should evaluate tension on the transfer intraoperatively before closure to determine the limits of external rotation during early rehabilitation.

■ Forward elevation is performed in internal rotation or neutral rotation to minimize tension on the transfer.

■ Active internal rotation and extension are avoided for 6 weeks.

■ Active assisted and active range-of-motion exercises are started 6 weeks after surgery. Resistance exercises commence as tolerated thereafter. No internal rotation resistance exercises are recommended until 12 weeks postoperatively.

OUTCOMES

■ Jost and associates[4] reported a series of 30 transfers in 28 patients. Twelve had isolated subscapularis tears and 18 had concomitant supraspinatus–infraspinatus tears. The mean relative Constant score improved from 47% to 70% at an average of 32 months of follow-up. Thirteen patients were very satisfied, 10 patients were satisfied, 2 patients were disappointed, and 3 patients were dissatisfied.

■ Resch and colleagues[7] reported on a series of 12 patients with a subcoracoid transfer. The Constant score increased from 26.9% to 67.1%. Nine assessed their final result as good or excellent, three as fair, and none as poor. Four unstable shoulders were stable at the average of 28 months of follow-up.

■ Rockwood[8] reported a series of 13 patients. Seven had a pectoralis major transfer and six had a pectoralis minor transfer. Ten of the 13 were satisfied, but the results were not separated between the patients with the pectoralis major and minor transfers.

■ Galatz and associates[2] reported on the subcoracoid pectoralis major transfer in 14 patients as a salvage procedure for iatrogenic anterior superior instability. Nine of the 14 had satisfactory results in terms of pain relief, but the functional results are not as predictable for this particular indication.

■ Gerber and colleagues[3] reported a combination of sternal head and sternal head plus teres major transfers. In the sternal head patients, 9 of 11 had pain relief. Two had a rupture that required revision. In the sternal head plus teres major group, seven of nine patients had pain relief. One had a rupture discovered at the time of revision surgery (fusion). Final ASES scores were 61 in the sternal group and 55 in the sternal plus teres group.

■ In all series, most of the patients had had surgery before the transfer, and in most cases a pectoralis major transfer was performed for revision purposes. This has dramatic implications on outcome.

COMPLICATIONS

■ Musculocutaneous nerve injury
■ Pectoral nerve injury
■ Fixation failure
■ Mechanical impingement with the coracoid, either deep or superficial to the conjoint tendon

REFERENCES

1. Armstrong A, Teefey SA, Wu T, et al. The efficacy of ultrasound in the diagnosis of long head of the biceps tendon pathology. J Shoulder Elbow Surg 2006;15:7–11.
2. Galatz LM, Connor PM, Calfee RP, et al. Pectoralis major transfer for anterior-superior subluxation in massive rotator cuff insufficiency. J Shoulder Elbow Surg 2003;12:1–5.
3. Gerber A, Clavert P, Millett PJ, et al. Split pectoralis major and teres major tendon transfers for reconstruction of irreparable tears of the subscapularis. Tech Shoulder Elbow Surg 2004;5:5–12.
4. Jost B, Puskas GJ, Lustenberger A, et al. Outcome of pectoralis major transfer for the treatment of irreparable subscapularis tears. J Bone Joint Surg Am 2003;85A:1944–1951.
5. Klepps S, Galatz LM, Yamaguchi K. Subcoracoid pectoralis major transfer: a salvage procedure for irreparable subscapularis deficiency. Tech Shoulder Elbow Surg 2001;2:92–99.
6. Klepps SJ, Goldfarb C, Flatow E, et al. Anatomic evaluation of the subcoracoid pectoralis major transfer in human cadavers. J Shoulder Elbow Surg 2001;10:453–459.
7. Resch H, Povacz P, Ritter E, et al. Transfer of the pectoralis major muscle for the treatment of irreparable rupture of the subscapularis tendon. J Bone Joint Surg Am 2000;82:372–382.
8. Wirth MA, Rockwood CA Jr. Operative treatment of irreparable rupture of the subscapularis. J Bone Joint Surg Am 1997;79A:722–731.

Chapter 12

Acute Repair and Reconstruction of Sternoclavicular Dislocation

Steven P. Kalandiak, Edwin E. Spencer, Jr., Michael A. Wirth, and Charles A. Rockwood

DEFINITION

- Sternoclavicular dislocation is one of the rarest dislocations, but one most shoulder surgeons will encounter several times during a career (more in a practice with significant exposure to high-energy trauma).
- Sternoclavicular dislocations represented 3% of a series of 1603 injuries of the shoulder girdle reported by Cave et al.[6]
- The true ratio of anterior to posterior dislocations is unknown, since most reports focus on the rarer posterior type. Estimates range from a ratio of 20 anterior dislocations to each posterior by Nettles and Linscheid,[19] in a series of 60 patients (57 anterior and 3 posterior), to a ratio of approximately three to one (135 anterior and 50 posterior) in our series[23] of 185 traumatic sternoclavicular injuries.
- Not all sternoclavicular dislocations require surgery. Avoiding inappropriate patient selection, preventing hardware-related complications, and repairing or reconstructing the capsule and the rhomboid ligament if the medial clavicle has been resected require special emphasis.
- Although this region can be an intimidating one because of the surrounding anatomic structures, a knowledgeable and careful surgeon can treat this joint safely and reliably produce good results.

ANATOMY

- The epiphysis of the medial clavicle is the last epiphysis of the long bones to appear and the last to close. It does not ossify until the 18th to 20th year, and it generally fuses with the shaft of the clavicle around age 23 to 25.[14,15] For this reason, many sternoclavicular "dislocations" in young adults are in fact physeal fractures.
- The articular surface of the medial clavicle is much larger than that of the sternum. It is bulbous and concave front to back and convex vertically, creating a saddle-type joint with the curved clavicular notch of the sternum.[14,15]
- A small facet on the inferior aspect of the medial clavicle articulates with the superior aspect of the first rib in 2.5% of subjects.[5]
- There is little congruence and the least bony stability of any major joint in the body. Almost all of its integrity comes from the surrounding ligaments.

Ligaments

- The intra-articular disc ligament is dense and fibrous, arises from the synchondral junction of the first rib to the sternum, passes through the sternoclavicular joint, and divides it into two separate spaces[14,15] (**FIG 1**). It attaches on the superior and posterior medial clavicle and acts as a checkrein against medial displacement of the inner clavicle.
- The costoclavicular (rhomboid) ligament attaches the upper surface of the medial first rib to the rhomboid fossa on the inferior surface of the medial end of the clavicle.[14,15] It averages 1.3 cm long, 1.9 cm wide, and 1.3 cm thick.[5]

- The anterior fasciculus arises anteromedially, runs upward and laterally, and resists lateral displacement and upward rotation of the clavicle.
- The posterior fasciculus is shorter, arises laterally, runs upward and medially, and resists medial displacement and excessive downward rotation[1,5,15] (**FIGS 1 AND 2**).
- The interclavicular ligament (see Fig 1) connects the superomedial aspects of each clavicle with the capsular ligaments and the upper sternum. Comparable to the wishbone of birds, it helps the capsular ligaments to produce "shoulder poise"; that is, to hold up the lateral aspect of the clavicle.[14]
- The capsular ligaments cover the anterosuperior and posterior aspects of the joint and represent thickenings of the joint capsule (Figs 1 and 2). The clavicular attachment of the ligament is primarily onto the epiphysis of the medial clavicle, with some blending of the fibers into the metaphysis.[3,8]
- In sectioning studies, the capsular ligaments are the most important structures in preventing upward displacement of the medial clavicle caused by a downward force on the distal end of the shoulder.[1]
  - This lateral poise of the shoulder (ie, the force that holds the shoulder up) is attributed to a locking mechanism of the ligaments of the sternoclavicular joint.
- Other single ligament sectioning studies[26] have shown that the posterior capsule is the most important primary stabilizer to anterior and posterior translation. The anterior capsule is an important restraint to anterior translation. The costoclavicular ligament is unimportant if the capsule remains intact,[26] although it may be an important secondary restraint if the capsular ligaments are torn, much like the coracoclavicular ligament laterally.

Applied Surgical Anatomy

- A "curtain" of muscles—the sternohyoid, sternothyroid, and scaleni—lies posterior to the sternoclavicular joint and the inner third of the clavicle and blocks the view of vital structures—the innominate artery, innominate vein, vagus nerve, phrenic nerve, internal jugular vein, trachea, and esophagus.
- The anterior jugular vein lies between the clavicle and the curtain of muscles. Variable in size and as large as 1.5 cm in diameter, it has no valves and bleeds like someone has opened a floodgate when nicked.
- The surgeon who is considering stabilizing the sternoclavicular joint by running a pin down from the clavicle into the sternum should not do it and should remember that the arch of the aorta, the superior vena cava, and the right pulmonary artery are also very close at hand.

PATHOGENESIS

- Most sternoclavicular joint dislocations result from high-energy trauma, usually a motor vehicle accident. They occasionally result from contact sports.

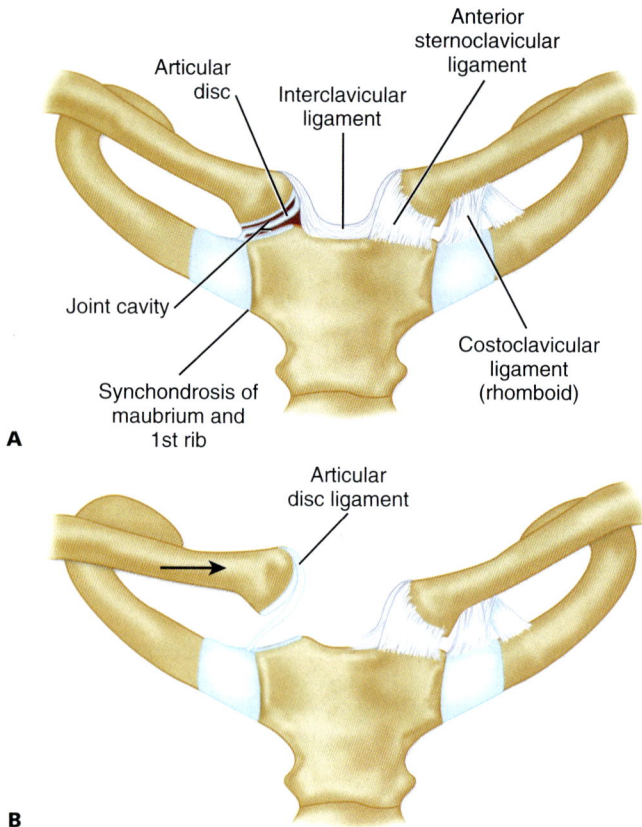

FIG 1 • **A.** Normal anatomy around the sternoclavicular joint. The articular disc ligament divides the sternoclavicular joint cavity into two separate spaces and inserts onto the superior and posterior aspects of the medial clavicle. **B.** The articular disc ligament acts as a checkrein for medial displacement of the proximal clavicle.

- A force applied directly to the anteromedial aspect of the clavicle can push the medial clavicle back behind the sternum and into the mediastinum.
- More commonly, a force is applied indirectly, from the lateral aspect of the shoulder. If the shoulder is compressed and rolled forward, a posterior dislocation results; if the shoulder is compressed and rolled backward, an anterior dislocation results.
- As noted above, many injuries of the sternoclavicular joint in patients under 25 years of age are, in fact, fractures through the medial physis of the clavicle.

NATURAL HISTORY

- Mild or moderate sprain
  - The mildly sprained sternoclavicular joint is stable but painful.
  - The moderately sprained joint may be slightly subluxated anteriorly or posteriorly, and may often be reduced by drawing the shoulders backward as if reducing and holding a fracture of the clavicle.
- Anterior dislocation
  - Although most anterior dislocations are unstable after closed reduction, we still recommend an attempt to reduce the dislocation closed.
  - Occasionally the clavicle remains reduced, but typically the clavicle remains unstable after closed reduction. We usually accept the deformity, because an anteriorly dislocated sternoclavicular joint typically becomes asymptomatic, and

we believe that the deformity is less of a problem than the potential complications of operative fixation.
- When the entire medial clavicle is stripped out of the deltotrapezial fascia, the deformity can be so severe that it may be poorly tolerated, so we consider primary fixation. In those rare cases when a chronic anterior dislocation is symptomatic, one may perform a capsular reconstruction or a medial clavicle resection and costoclavicular ligament reconstruction.
- Posterior dislocation
  - In contrast to anterior dislocations, the complications of an unreduced posterior dislocation are numerous: thoracic outlet syndrome, vascular compromise, and erosion of the medial clavicle into any of the vital structures that lie posterior to the sternoclavicular joint.
  - Closed reduction for acute posterior sternoclavicular dislocation can usually be obtained, and the reduction is generally stable. Often, general anesthesia is necessary. However, when a posterior dislocation is irreducible or the reduction is unstable, an open reduction should be performed.
  - When chronic posterior dislocation is present, late complications may arise from mediastinal impingement, so we recommend medial clavicle resection and ligament reconstruction.
- Physeal injuries
  - The typical history for physeal injuries is the same as for other traumatic dislocations. The difference between these injuries and pure dislocations is that most of these injuries will heal with time, without surgical intervention.
  - In very young patients, the remodeling process can eliminate deformity because of the osteogenic potential of an intact periosteal tube. Zaslav,[31] Rockwood,[23] and Hsu et al[16] have all reported successful treatment of displaced medial clavicle physeal injury in adolescents and provided radiographic evidence of remodeling.
  - Anterior physeal injuries may be reduced, but if reduction cannot be obtained, they can be left alone without problem. Posterior physeal injuries should likewise undergo an attempt at reduction. If a posterior dislocation cannot be reduced closed and the patient is having no significant symptoms, the displacement can be observed while remod-

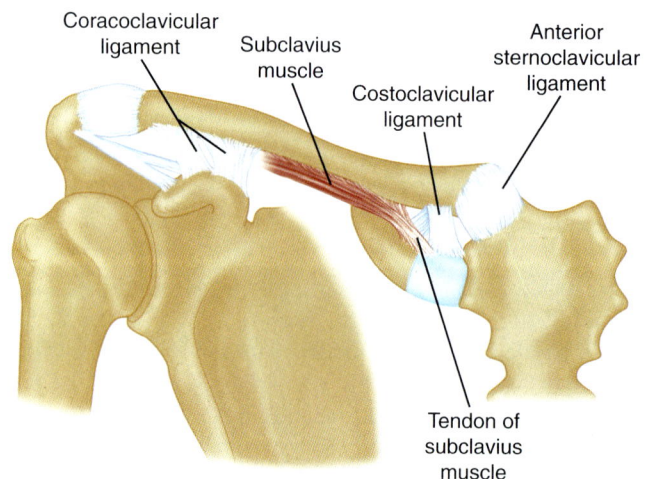

FIG 2 • Normal anatomy around the sternoclavicular and acromioclavicular joints. The tendon of the subclavius muscle arises in the vicinity of the costoclavicular ligament from the first rib and has a long tendon structure.

eling occurs. Even in older individuals, a posteriorly displaced fracture with moderate displacement and no mediastinal symptoms may be observed, as it usually becomes asymptomatic with fracture healing.

- However, as with severely displaced dislocations, one may wish to consider operative repair for severely displaced physeal fractures. Suture repair through the medial shaft and the epiphysis and Balser plate fixation have both been successfully used in this situation.[13,27,28]

PATIENT HISTORY AND PHYSICAL FINDINGS

- A history of high-energy trauma is almost a requirement for the diagnosis. Most cases will be due to a motor vehicle accident, a fall from a significant height, or a sports injury.
  - The absence of such a history suggests either an atraumatic instability or some other atraumatic condition of the joint.
- Posterior displacement may be obvious, but anterior fullness can represent either anterior displacement or swelling overlying posterior displacement.
- Careful examination is extremely important. Mediastinal injuries may occur when a traumatic dislocation is posterior, and the physician should seek evidence of damage to the pulmonary and vascular systems, such as hoarseness, venous congestion, and difficulty breathing or swallowing.
- Evaluation should also include the remainder of the thorax, shoulder girdle, and upper extremity, as well as the contralateral sternoclavicular joint.

IMAGING AND OTHER DIAGNOSTIC STUDIES

- Plain radiographs
  - Occasionally, routine anteroposterior chest radiographs suggest displacement compared with the normal side. However, these are difficult to interpret.
  - Serendipity view: A 45-degree cephalic tilt view is the most useful and reproducible plain radiograph for the sternoclavicular joint. The tube is centered directly on the sternum and a nongrid 11 × 14 cassette is placed on the table under the patient's upper shoulders and neck, so the beam will project the

medial half of both clavicles onto the film (**FIG 3**). The technique is the same as a posteroanterior view of the chest.
  - An anteriorly dislocated medial clavicle will appear to ride higher compared to the normal side. The reverse is true if the sternoclavicular joint is dislocated posteriorly (**FIG 4**).
- In the past, tomograms were useful in distinguishing a sternoclavicular dislocation from a fracture of the medial clavicle and defining questionable anterior and posterior injuries of the sternoclavicular joint. Although they provide more information than plain films, at present they have been replaced with CT scans.
- Without question, CT scanning is the best technique to study the sternoclavicular joint. It distinguishes dislocations of the joint from fractures of the medial clavicle and clearly defines minor subluxations (**FIG 5**).
  - The patient should lie supine. The scan should include both sternoclavicular joints and the medial halves of both clavicles so that the injured side can be compared with the normal.
  - If symptoms of mediastinal compression are present or displacement of the medial clavicle is severe, the use of intravenous contrast will aid in the imaging of the vascular structures in the mediastinum.

DIFFERENTIAL DIAGNOSIS

- Arthritic conditions: sternocostoclavicular hyperostosis, osteitis condensans, Friedrich disease, Tietze syndrome, and osteoarthritis
- Atraumatic (spontaneous) subluxation or dislocation: One or both of the sternoclavicular joints may spontaneously subluxate or dislocate during abduction or flexion during overhead motion. Typically seen in ligamentously lax females in their late teens or early 20s, it is not painful, it is almost always anterior, and it should almost always be managed nonoperatively.[22]
- Congenital or developmental or acquired subluxation or dislocation: Birth trauma, congenital defects with loss of bone substance on either side of the joint, or neuromuscular or other developmental disorders can predispose the patient to subluxation or dislocation.
- Iatrogenic instability may be due to failure to reconstruct the ligaments of the sternoclavicular joint adequately or to an excessive medial clavicle resection. History is significant for a prior procedure on the sternoclavicular joint.

NONOPERATIVE MANAGEMENT

- A mild sprain is stable but painful. We treat mild sprains with a sling, cold packs, and resumption of activity as comfort dictates.

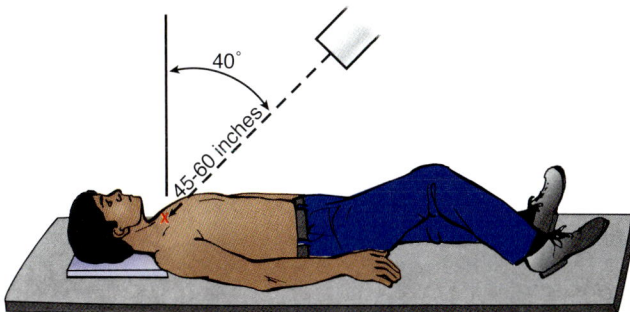

FIG 3 • Serendipity view. Positioning of the patient to take the serendipity view of the sternoclavicular joints. The x-ray tube is tilted 40 degrees from the vertical position and aimed directly at the manubrium. The nongrid cassette should be large enough to receive the projected images of the medial halves of both clavicles. In children the tube distance from the patient should be 45 inches; in thicker-chested adults the distance should be 60 inches.

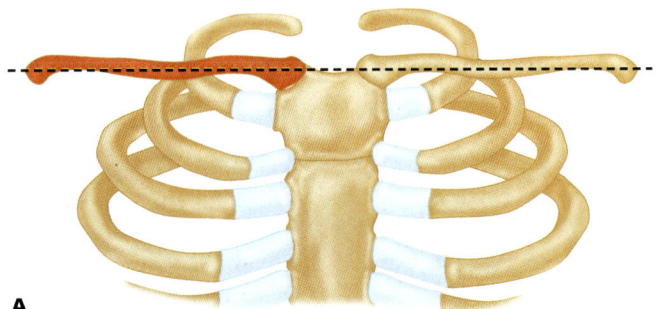

FIG 4 • Interpretation of the cephalic tilt films of the sternoclavicular joints. **A.** In a normal person, both clavicles appear on the same imaginary line drawn horizontally across the film. *(continued)*

B

C

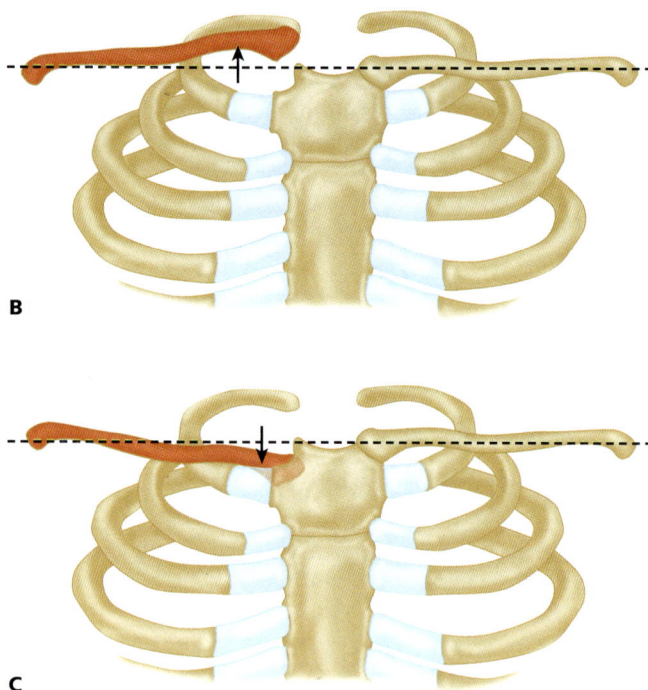

FIG 4 • (*continued*) **B.** In a patient with anterior dislocation of the right sternoclavicular joint, the medial half of the right clavicle is projected above the imaginary line drawn through the level of the normal left clavicle. **C.** If the patient has a posterior dislocation of the right sternoclavicular joint, the medial half of the right clavicle is displaced below the imaginary line drawn through the normal left clavicle.

■ A moderate sprain may be slightly subluxated anteriorly or posteriorly. Moderate sprains may be reduced by drawing the shoulders backward as if reducing a fracture of the clavicle. This is followed by cold packs and immobilization in a padded figure 8 strap for 4 to 6 weeks, then gradual resumption of activity as comfort dictates.

■ Anterior dislocations may undergo closed reduction with either local or general anesthesia, narcotics, or muscle relaxants.
  ■ The patient is supine on the table, with a 3- to 4-inch-thick pad between the shoulders. Direct gentle pressure over the anteriorly displaced clavicle or traction on the outstretched

arm combined with pressure on the medial clavicle will generally reduce the dislocation.

■ Posterior dislocation in a stoic patient may possibly be reducible under intravenous narcotics and muscle relaxation. However, general anesthesia is usually required for reduction of a posterior dislocation, because of pain and muscle spasm.
  ■ Our preferred method is the abduction traction technique.
    ▪ The patient is placed supine, with the dislocated side near the edge of the table. A 3- to 4-inch-thick sandbag is placed between the scapulae (**FIG 6**). Lateral traction is applied to the abducted arm, which is then gradually brought back into extension. The clavicle usually reduces with an audible snap or pop, and it is almost always stable. Too much extension can bind the anterior surface of the dislocated medial clavicle on the back of the manubrium.
    ▪ Occasionally it is necessary to grasp the medial clavicle with one's fingers to dislodge it from behind the sternum. If this fails, the skin is prepared, and a sterile towel clip is used to grasp the medial clavicle to apply lateral and anterior traction (see Fig 6C). If the joint is stable after reduction, the shoulders should be held back for 4 to 6 weeks with a figure 8 dressing to allow ligament healing.
  ■ Many investigators have reported that closed reduction usually cannot be accomplished after 48 hours. However, others have reported closed reductions as late as 4 and 5 days after the injury.[4]
■ Physeal fractures are reduced in the same manner as dislocations, with immobilization in a figure 8 strap for 4 weeks to protect stable reductions. Fractures that cannot be reduced and are being managed nonoperatively are treated with a figure 8 strap or a sling for comfort and mobilized as symptoms permit.

SURGICAL MANAGEMENT

■ A posterior displacement of the medial clavicle that is irreducible or redislocates after closed reduction is a well-accepted surgical indication.
■ More controversial is anterior displacement that fails to maintain a stable reduction.
  ■ Although the traditional treatment for persistent anterior displacement is nonoperative, extreme displacement can result in abundant heterotopic bone formation with accompanying pain, limited motion, and extraordinary deformity.

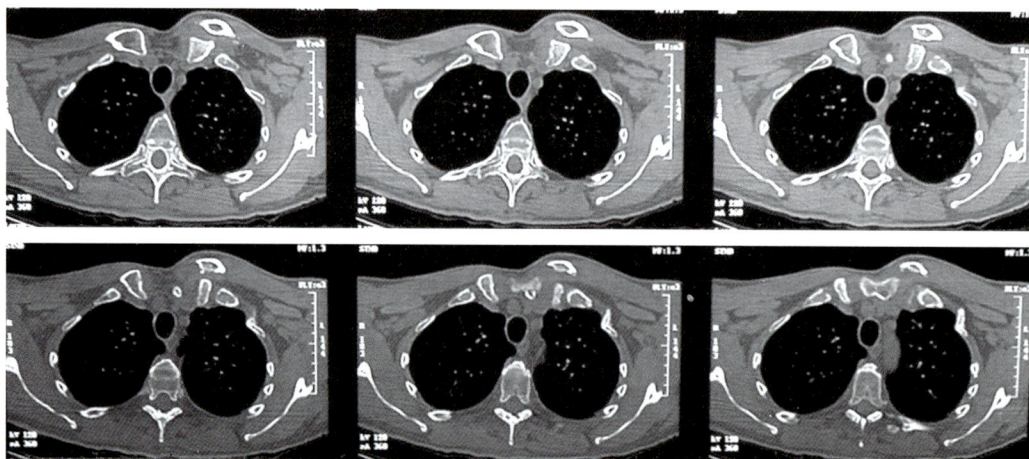

FIG 5 • CT scans of a 6-month-old medial clavicle fracture demonstrate anterior displacement without significant healing.

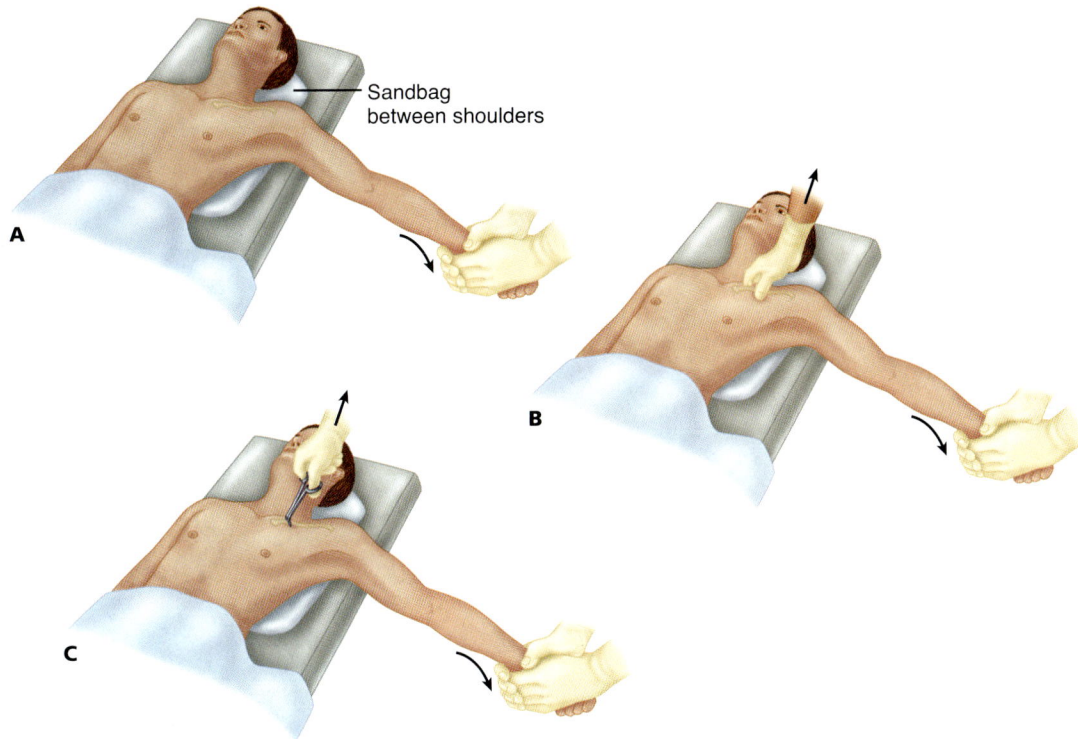

FIG 6 • Technique for closed reduction of the sternoclavicular joint. **A.** The patient is positioned supine with a sandbag placed between the two shoulders. Traction is then applied to the arm against countertraction in an abducted and slightly extended position. In anterior dislocations, direct pressure over the medial end of the clavicle may reduce the joint. **B.** In posterior dislocations, in addition to the traction it may be necessary to manipulate the medial end of the clavicle with the fingers to dislodge the clavicle from behind the manubrium. **C.** In stubborn posterior dislocations, it may be necessary to prepare the medial end of the clavicle sterilely and use a towel clip to grasp around the medial clavicle to lift it back into position.

■ We now consider operative treatment when the entire medial clavicle is torn out of the deltotrapezial sleeve.

Preoperative Planning

■ Careful review of the history and examination for symptoms of mediastinal compression is crucial.
■ Review of the CT scan for the direction and degree of displacement and determination of a very medial fracture versus pure dislocation follows.
■ If history or radiographic evidence of mediastinal compromise or potential compromise is present, a cardiothoracic surgeon should be either present or readily available.
■ Very medial fractures can occasionally be repaired with independent small-fragment lag screws or orthogonal minifragment plates. For pure dislocations, heavy nonabsorbable suture will sometimes suffice. Suture anchors are useful for augmenting ligament repairs. Allograft tendons may be used if the capsule is irreparable and must be reconstructed.
■ Closed reduction under anesthesia is then attempted and the stability of the joint is evaluated after reduction.

Positioning

■ To begin, the patient is positioned supine on the table, and three or four towels or a sandbag placed between the scapulae.
■ The upper extremity should be draped free so that lateral traction can be applied during the open reduction.

■ A folded sheet may be left in place around the patient's thorax so that it can be used for countertraction.
■ If there is concern regarding the mediastinum, the entire sternum should be draped into the field.

Approach

■ An anterior incision that parallels the superior border of the medial 3 to 4 inches of the clavicle and then extends downward over the sternum just medial to the involved sternoclavicular joint is used (**FIG 7A**).
  ■ As an alternative, a necklace-type incision may be created in Langer's lines, beginning at the midline and sweeping lateral and up along the clavicle.
■ Careful subperiosteal dissection around the medial clavicle and onto the surface of the manubrium allows exposure of the articular surfaces.
  ■ If the medial clavicle is resting posteriorly, it is safer to identify the shaft more laterally and then trace it back medially along the subperiosteal plane (**FIG 7B**).
■ Traction and blunt retractors can then be used to lever the medial clavicle back up into its anatomic location (**FIG 7C**). These retractors may be used behind the medial clavicle and manubrium to protect the posterior structures.
■ If one has chosen to operate on an anterior medial clavicle because of extreme displacement, it may generally be simply pushed back into place.

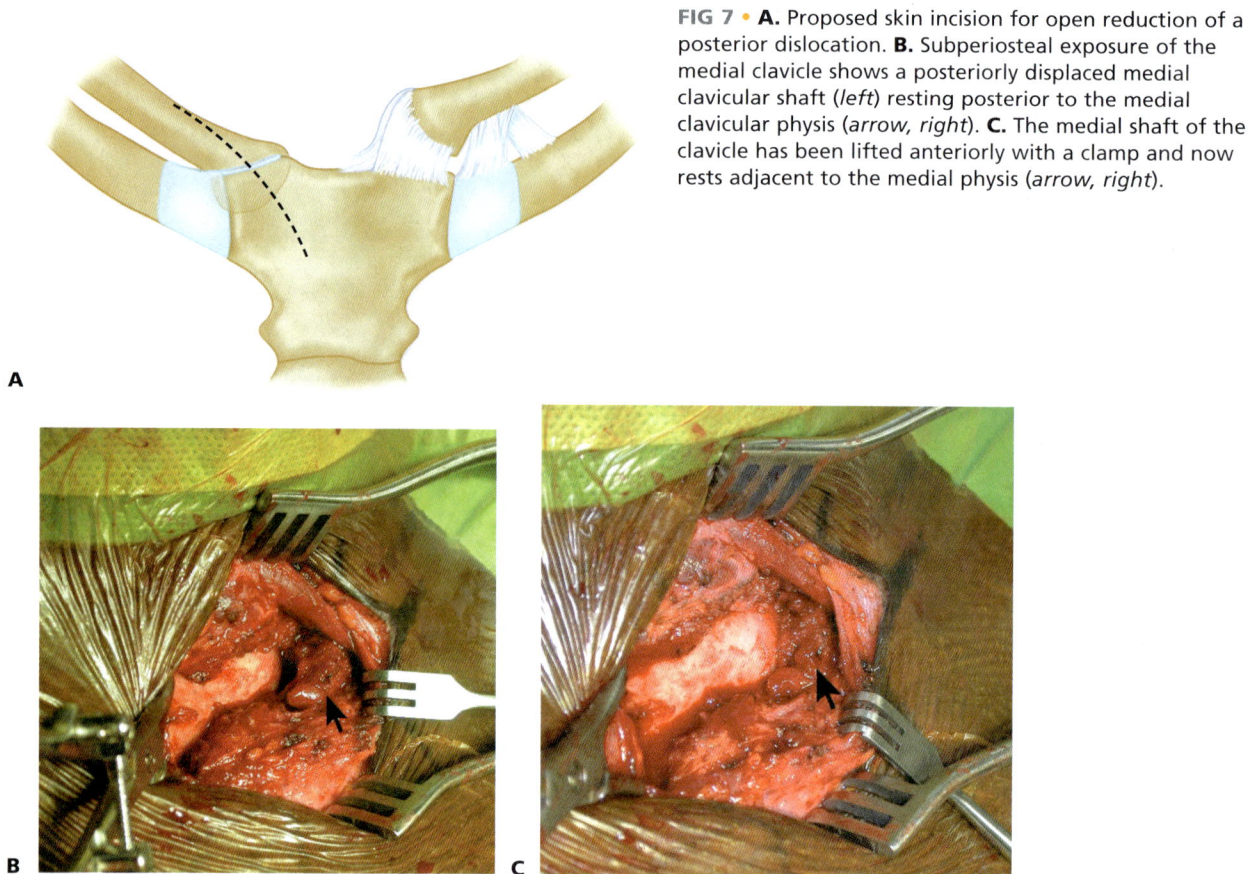

FIG 7 • A. Proposed skin incision for open reduction of a posterior dislocation. **B.** Subperiosteal exposure of the medial clavicle shows a posteriorly displaced medial clavicular shaft (*left*) resting posterior to the medial clavicular physis (*arrow, right*). **C.** The medial shaft of the clavicle has been lifted anteriorly with a clamp and now rests adjacent to the medial physis (*arrow, right*).

TECHNIQUES

PRIMARY REPAIR: MEDIAL FRACTURE

- In children and in young adults, the dislocation of the medial clavicle may occur through the medial physis or as a fracture, leaving a small amount of bone articulating with the manubrium.
- Because much of the capsule remains intact to this medial fragment, it can serve as an anchor for internal fixation of the medial clavicle shaft. Depending on the amount of bone, the type of fixation will vary.

- The smallest fragments will permit only osseous suture fixation, but the medial clavicle is cancellous bone and heals very quickly (**TECH FIG 1A**).
- As the fragment gets larger, independent lag screw fixation may be possible (**TECH FIG 1B,C**).
- For very medial shaft fractures, it may even be possible to use two orthogonal minifragment plates.

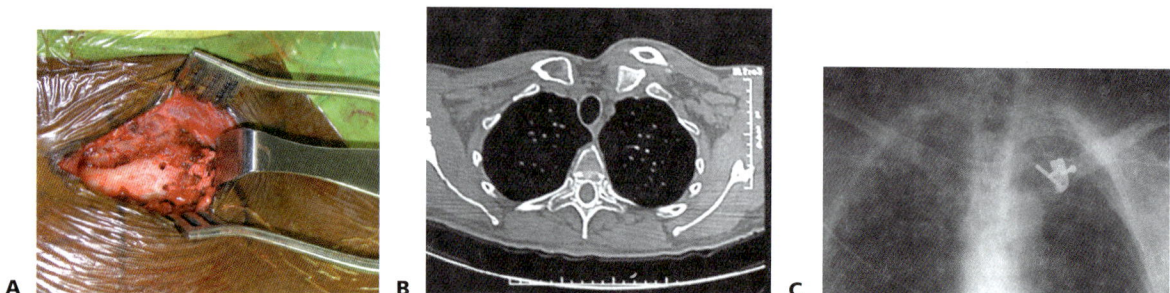

TECH FIG 1 • A. Heavy nonabsorbable suture has been placed through drill holes in the medial clavicle and through the physis to secure the fracture shown in Figure 7B,C. **B,C.** A symptomatic medial clavicle nonunion had a medial fragment large enough to allow fixation with three cortical lag screws.

PRIMARY REPAIR: CAPSULAR LIGAMENTS AND SUTURE AUGMENTATION

- After reduction, the ligaments may be repaired primarily with heavy nonabsorbable suture. This usually allows repair of the anterior and superior capsule, but, for obvious reasons, does not allow repair of the important posterior capsule.
- The reduction is often reinforced with either simple osseous sutures through drill holes in the medial clavicle and manubrium[27,28] or with suture anchors[18] (**TECH FIG 2**). The costoclavicular ligament may also occasionally be repaired primarily.
- This technique has generally been employed in children but may also be used in adults.

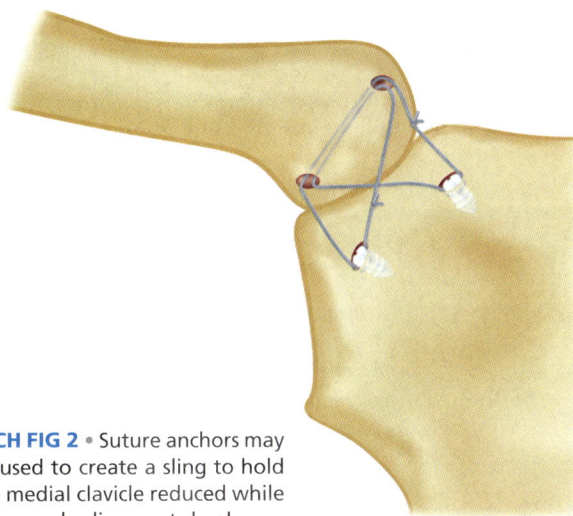

TECH FIG 2 • Suture anchors may be used to create a sling to hold the medial clavicle reduced while the capsular ligaments heal.

IMMEDIATE RECONSTRUCTION: CAPSULAR LIGAMENTS

- At times the joint may be reducible but the ligaments are damaged to the point where primary repair is not feasible. In this circumstance, the ligaments may be immediately reconstructed using tendon graft.
- This may be done by passing a tendon from the front of the sternum, through the articular surfaces and intra-articular disc, and out the front of the medial clavicle and tying the tendon to itself anteriorly.[20] Autograft or allograft tendon may be used.
- The capsule may also be reconstructed in the manner described by Spencer and Kuhn[25] (**TECH FIG 3**).
  - Drill holes 4 mm in diameter are created from anterior to posterior through the medial clavicle and the adjacent manubrium.
  - A free semitendinosus tendon graft is woven through the drill holes so the tendon strands are parallel to each other posterior to the joint and cross each other anterior to it.
  - The tendon is tied in a square knot and secured with no. 2 Ethibond suture.
  - This technique has the advantage of reconstructing both the anterior and the posterior ligament in a very strong and secure manner.

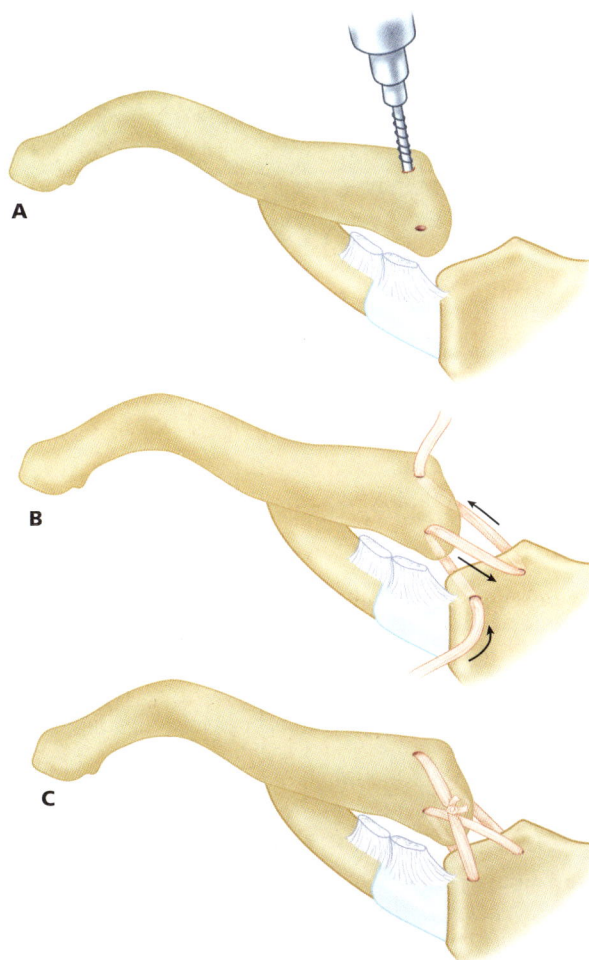

TECH FIG 3 • **A.** Semitendinosus may be used to reconstruct the capsular ligaments. **B,C.** The allograft tendon is pulled through the medial clavicle (*left*) and manubrium (*right*) and tied. *(continued)*

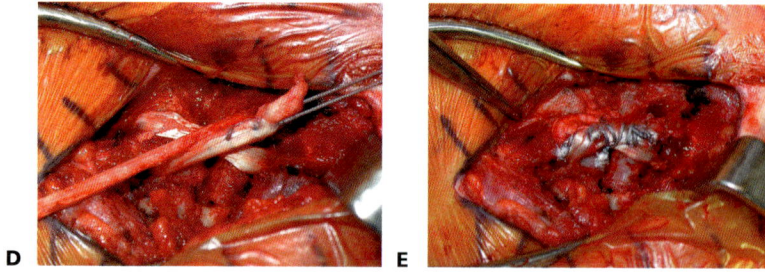

TECH FIG 3 • (continued) **D,E.** Intraoperative images showing the technique illustrated in **B** and **C.** (**A–C**, After Spencer EE Jr, Kuhn JE. Biomechanical analysis of reconstructions for sternoclavicular joint instability. J Bone Joint Surg Am 2004;86A:98–105.)

MEDIAL CLAVICLE RESECTION AND LIGAMENT RECONSTRUCTION

- If there is concern about the stability of a reconstruction or repair, if the dislocation is subacute and posterior, or if there is a question of impingement on the mediastinal structures, one may elect to resect the medial clavicle entirely. In this situation, it is important to repair or reconstruct the costoclavicular ligament (akin to a modified Weaver-Dunn procedure).

- The medullary canal can also be used to create an attachment point for an additional medial tether. We prefer to use the patient's own tissue, such as the sternoclavicular ligament, whenever possible (**TECH FIG 4**).

- The medial clavicle is resected and the canal curetted and prepared with drill holes on the superior surface.

- Grasping suture is woven through the remaining ligament, pulled through the superior drill holes, and tied over bone.

- Heavy nonabsorbable sutures are then passed through the remaining costoclavicular ligament and around the clavicle, and the periosteal tube is closed.

- If adequate local tissue is not present, an allograft such as Achilles tendon may also be used.[2]

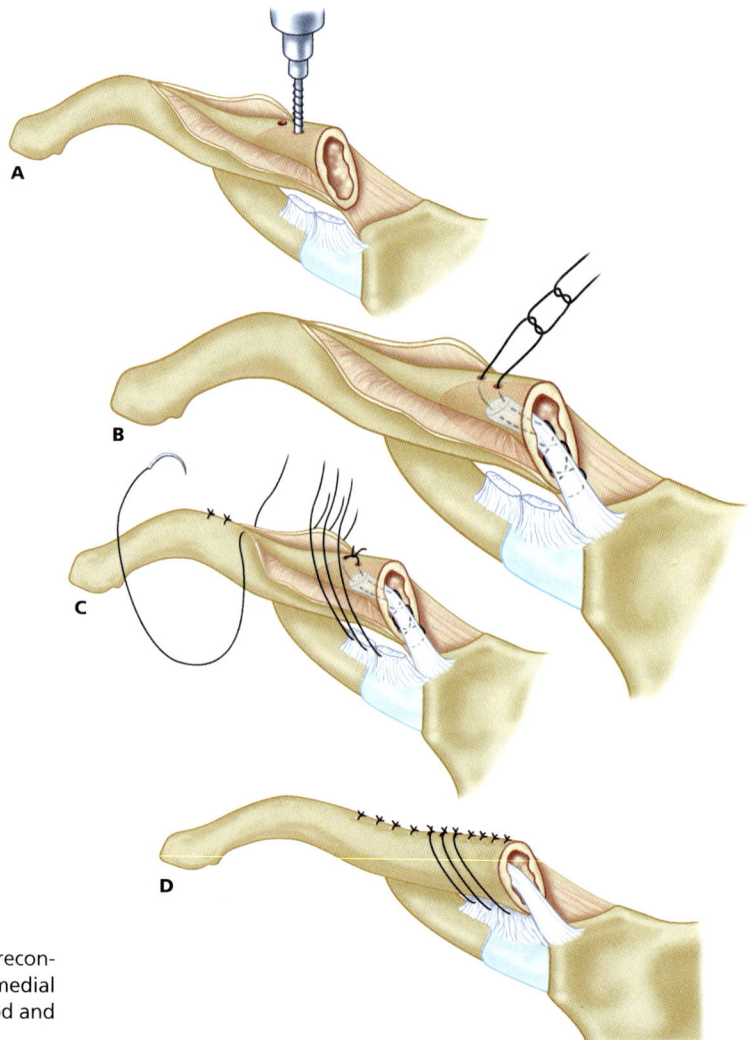

TECH FIG 4 • The residual capsule may be used to reconstruct a medial clavicular restraint, akin to a medial Weaver-Dunn procedure, as described by Rockwood and Wirth.[23]

REDUCTION AND BALSER PLATE FIXATION

- The use of K-wires around the sternoclavicular joint has been routinely condemned, and they should not be used.
  - There are reports, however, of temporary plate fixation from the medial clavicle to the sternum to maintain a reduced joint while the soft tissues heal.
- The Balser plate is a hook plate used in Europe for treatment of acromioclavicular joint separations and distal clavicle fractures. It has been used for sternoclavicular dislocations by placing the hook into the sternum and using screws to fix the plate onto the medial clavicle (**TECH FIG 5**).
  - Franck et al[12] published good results for 10 patients treated with Balser plates. They thought that the stability of this construct allowed a more rapid rehabilitation. The implant is quite bulky and removal is generally required.

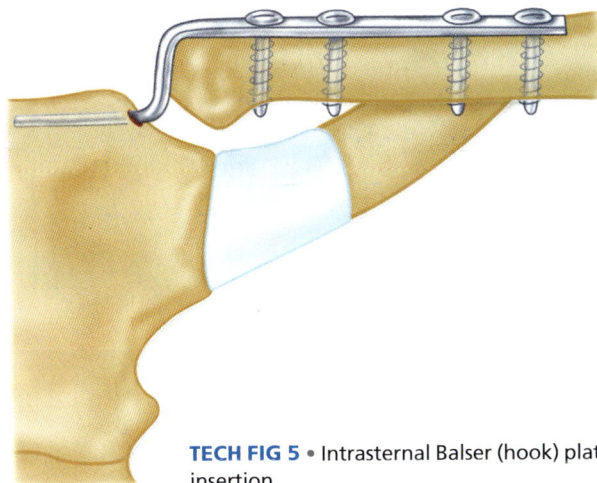

TECH FIG 5 • Intrasternal Balser (hook) plate insertion.

PEARLS AND PITFALLS

Diagnosis	■ Conventional studies are unreliable. A high index of suspicion, a thorough examination, and a prompt CT scan will ensure correct diagnosis.
Individualize treatment when necessary	■ Although anterior dislocations are generally treated nonoperatively, a severely anteriorly displaced medial clavicle may be reduced and fixed acutely, with a low risk of complications, in a reliable patient. ■ Posterior dislocations generally mandate surgery because delayed impingement on mediastinal contents may occur. However, there may be situations where displacement is mild and chronic and the risks of surgery may outweigh the benefits.
Prepare for complications	■ Although complications are uncommon, they are spectacular, and not in a good way. The surgeon needs to be ready for both pneumothorax and the unlikely possibility of a vascular injury. A cardiothoracic surgeon should be immediately available.
Use the medial clavicle	■ Even a medial epiphysis or a tiny piece of medial clavicle in its anatomic location provides an excellent anchor for heavy suture or lag screws for primary fracture repair.
Be flexible intraoperatively	■ Preserving the native joint is an admirable goal, but poor ligament and bone quality sometimes precludes primary repair, especially in the subacute dislocation. If the stability of the joint cannot be ensured, medial clavicle resection and costoclavicular reconstruction should be strongly considered.

POSTOPERATIVE CARE

- For sternoclavicular strains and anteriorly dislocated medial clavicles accepted in this position, a sling or figure 8 strap is prescribed and the patient is allowed to mobilize the extremity as function permits.
- Medial clavicle fractures that are stable after reduction are immobilized in a figure 8 strap for 4 to 6 weeks and then mobilized as comfort allows.
- Acute dislocations that have been reduced and are stable or have been surgically repaired receive a sling or figure 8 strap for 6 weeks to protect the reduction and allow ligament healing.
- Patients in the figure 8 strap are allowed use of the elbow and hand with the arm at the side for light activities of daily living, but the strap is conscientiously maintained.
- At 4 to 6 weeks they move to a sling and perform their own mobilization. Because the glenohumeral joint is unaffected, motion usually returns quickly to near full range.

- When full range of motion has been obtained, gentle progressive strengthening and resumption of normal activities commence.
- In general, patients treated with joint preservation can return to all activities, including heavy labor, but we have seen traumatic failure of costoclavicular reconstructions and do ask patients who have undergone medial clavicle resection and ligament reconstruction to avoid heavy overhead labor for their lifetimes.

OUTCOMES

- A recent Medline search for "sternoclavicular" and "dislocation" yielded 320 citations, most dealing with sternoclavicular instability and its sequelae. Most were case reports, a series of three or four patients, or a discussion of the complications of the injury or its treatment. There are very few large series, which makes discussing outcomes difficult. However, several themes do emerge.

- The need for proper patient selection becomes evident when one considers that some forms of sternoclavicular instability generally do well when treated without surgery.
  - Sadr and Swann[24] and Rockwood and Odor[22] have both documented the good long-term results obtained with nonoperative treatment of atraumatic sternoclavicular instability.
  - De Jong[7] has documented good long-term results in 13 patients with anterior dislocations treated nonoperatively.
- Several larger series[9,11,29] have reported on about a dozen patients treated with open reduction, ligament repair or reconstruction, and fixation with pins or sternoclavicular wiring. Good results were obtained when the medial clavicle was successfully stabilized.
  - Eskola,[10] however, noted a high failure rate if the remaining medial clavicle was not successfully stabilized to the first rib.
  - In a separate study, Rockwood et al[21] reported on seven patients who had previously undergone medial clavicle resection without ligament reconstruction. Six of the seven had worse symptoms than before their index procedure.

COMPLICATIONS

- Complications of injury
  - Anterior dislocation: cosmetic "bump" (which may occasionally be pronounced) and late degenerative changes
  - Posterior dislocation: Great vessel injuries, including laceration, compression, and occlusion, pneumothorax, rupture of the esophagus with abscess and osteomyelitis of the clavicle, fatal tracheoesophageal fistula, brachial plexus compression, stridor and dysphagia, hoarseness of the voice, onset of snoring, and voice changes from normal to falsetto with movement of the arm have all been reported. These all may occur acutely or in a delayed fashion.
  - Worman and Leagus[30] reported that 16 of 60 patients with posterior dislocations had suffered complications of the trachea, esophagus, or great vessels.
- Errors of patient selection
  - Operating in unindicated circumstances introduces another set of complications. Rockwood and Odor[22] reviewed 37 patients with spontaneous atraumatic subluxation.
  - Twenty-nine managed without surgery had no limitations of activity or lifestyle at over 8 years average follow-up. Eight treated (elsewhere) with surgical reconstruction had increased pain, limitation of activity, alteration of lifestyle, persistent instability, and significant scars.
  - Before surgery, most of these patients had minimal discomfort and excellent motion and complained only of a "bump" that slipped in and out of place with certain motions.
- Intraoperative complications
  - Little has been written about these, but a veritable jungle of vitally important structures lurks immediately behind the sternoclavicular joint. We always perform these operations with an available, in-house cardiothoracic surgeon on notice and request his or her presence in the operating suite for all but the most routine cases.
- Postoperative complications
  - Hardware migration: Because of the motion at the sternoclavicular joint, tremendous leverage is applied to pins that cross it; fatigue breakage of the pins is common. Numerous authors have reported deaths and many near-deaths from K-wires and Steinmann pins migrating into the heart, pulmonary artery, innominate artery, aorta, and elsewhere in the mediastinum. Despite numerous admonitions in the literature regarding the use of sternoclavicular pins, there have been continued reports of intrathoracic K-wire migration, most recently in 2005.[17]
  - For this reason, we do not recommend the use of any transfixing pins—large or small, smooth or threaded, bent or straight—across the sternoclavicular joint.
- Iatrogenic instability: Failure to preserve the costoclavicular ligament when it is intact and failure to reconstruct it when it is deficient both severely compromise the surgical result. As noted above, both Rockwood[21] and Eskola[10] noted vastly inferior results when the residual medial clavicle was not stabilized to the first rib, and an inability to obtain equivalent results when the costoclavicular ligament was reconstructed in a delayed fashion.
- Iatrogenic instability: An excessive resection that removes bone to a point lateral to the costoclavicular ligament is an extremely difficult problem that is best avoided because there is no reconstructive option. In these difficult cases, we have occasionally performed a subtotal claviculectomy to a point just medial to the coracoclavicular ligaments. This leaves the extremity without a "strut" connecting it to the thorax but can produce substantial relief of pain and improvement in motion and activity.

REFERENCES

1. Bearn JG. Direct observations on the function of the capsule of the sternoclavicular joint in the clavicular support. J Anat 1967;101:159–170.
2. Battaglia TC, Pannunzio ME, Chhabra AB, et al. Interposition arthroplasty with bone-tendon allograft: a technique for treatment of the unstable sternoclavicular joint. J Orthop Trauma 2005;19:124–129.
3. Brooks AL, Henning CD. Injury to the proximal clavicular epiphysis [abstract]. J Bone Joint Surg Am 1972;54A:1347–1348.
4. Buckerfield CT, Castle ME. Acute traumatic retrosternal dislocation of the clavicle. J Bone Joint Surg Am 1984;66A:379–385.
5. Cave AJE. The nature and morphology of the costoclavicular ligament. J Anat 1961;95:170–179.
6. Cave EF. Fractures and Other Injuries. Chicago: Year Book Medical Publishers, 1958.
7. De Jong KP, Sukul DM. Anterior sternoclavicular dislocation: a long-term follow-up study. J Orthop Trauma 1990;4:420–423.
8. Denham RH Jr, Dingley AF Jr. Epiphyseal separation of the medial end of the clavicle. J Bone Joint Surg Am 1967;49A:1179–1183.
9. Eskola A, Vainionpaa S, Vastamki M, et al. Operation of old sternoclavicular dislocation: results in 12 cases. J Bone Joint Surg Br 1989;71B:63–65.
10. Eskola A. Sternoclavicular dislocations: a plea for open treatment. Acta Orthop Scand 1986;57:227–228.
11. Ferrandez L, Yubero J, Usabiaga J, et al. Sternoclavicular dislocation, treatment and complications. Ital J Orthop Traumatol 1988;14:349–355.
12. Franck WM, Jannasch O, Siassi M, et al. Balser plate stabilization: an alternate therapy for traumatic sternoclavicular instability. J Shoulder Elbow Surg 2003;12:276–281.
13. Franck WM, Siassi RM, Hennig FF. Treatment of posterior epiphyseal disruption of the medial clavicle with a modified Balser plate. J Trauma 2003;55:966–968.
14. Gray H. Osteology. In: Goss CM, ed. Anatomy of the Human Body, ed 28. Philadelphia: Lea & Febiger, 1966:324–326.
15. Grant JCB. Method of Anatomy, ed 7. Baltimore: Williams & Wilkins, 1965.
16. Hsu HC, Wu JJ, Lo WH, et al. Epiphyseal fracture–retrosternal dislocation of the medial end of the clavicle: a case report. Chinese Med J 1993;52:198–202.
17. Kamiyoshihara M, Kakegawa S, Otani Y, et al. Video-assisted thoracoscopic surgery for migration of an orthopedic fixation wire in the

mediastinum: report of a case [in Japanese]. Kyobu Geka 2005; 58:403–405.

18. Mirza AH, Alam K, Ali A. Posterior sternoclavicular dislocation in a rugby player as a cause of silent vascular compromise: a case report. Br J Sports Med 2005;39:e28.

19. Nettles JL, Linscheid R. Sternoclavicular dislocations. J Trauma 1968;8:158–164.

20. Qureshi SA, Shah AK, Pruzansky ME. Using the semitendinosus tendon to stabilize sternoclavicular joints in a patient with Ehlers-Danlos syndrome: a case report. Am J Orthop 2005;34:315–318.

21. Rockwood CA Jr, Groh GI, Wirth MA, et al. Resection-arthroplasty of the sternoclavicular joint. J Bone Joint Surg Am 1997;79A:387.

22. Rockwood CA Jr, Odor JM. Spontaneous atraumatic anterior subluxation of the sternoclavicular joint. J Bone Joint Surg Am 1989; 71A:1280–1288.

23. Rockwood CA, Wirth MA. Disorders of the sternoclavicular joint. In: Rockwood CA, Matsen FA, eds. The Shoulder, ed 2. Philadelphia: WB Saunders, 1998:555–609.

24. Sadr B, Swann M. Spontaneous dislocation of the sternoclavicular joint. Acta Orthop Scand 1979;50:269–274.

25. Spencer EE Jr, Kuhn JE. Biomechanical analysis of reconstructions for sternoclavicular joint instability. J Bone Joint Surg Am 2004; 86A:98–105.

26. Spencer EE, Kuhn JE, Huston LJ, Carpenter JE, et al. Ligamentous restraints to anterior and posterior translation of the sternoclavicular joint. J Shoulder Elbow Surg 2002;11:43–47.

27. Thacker MM, Patankar JV, Goregaonkar AB. A safe technique for sternoclavicular stabilization. Am J Orthop 2006;35:64–66.

28. Waters PM, Bae DS, Kadiyala RK. Short-term outcomes after surgical treatment of traumatic posterior sternoclavicular fracture-dislocations in children and adolescents. J Pediatr Orthop 2003;23: 464–469.

29. Witvoet J, Martinez B. Treatment of anterior sternoclavicular dislocations: apropos of 18 cases. Rev Chir Orthop Reparatrice Appar Mot 1982;68:311–316.

30. Worman LW, Leagus C. Intrathoracic injury following retrosternal dislocation of the clavicle. J Trauma 1967;7:416–423.

31. Zaslav KR, Ray S, Neer CS. Conservative management of a displaced medial clavicular physeal injury in an adolescent athlete. Am J Sports Med 1989;17:833–836.

Chapter 13

Medial Clavicle Excision and Sternoclavicular Joint Reconstruction

John E. Kuhn

DEFINITION

- Many pathologic disorders affect the medial clavicle, the most common of which is osteoarthritis.
  - Other conditions include rheumatoid arthritis, seronegative spondyloarthropathies, crystal deposition disease, sternoclavicular hyperostosis, condensing osteitis, and avascular necrosis.[6]
- Infection, while rare, must be considered. When suspected, the sternoclavicular joint should be aspirated for culture, Gram stain, and cell counts and then treated with irrigation and débridement.
- Instability of the sternoclavicular joint is rare but potentially fatal.
- Traumatic instability is defined by the direction of displacement of the clavicular head and is superior, anterior, or posterior.
- Posterior instability has been associated with a variety of potentially fatal comorbidities.
- Atraumatic instability is usually anterior and is often seen in people with generalized ligamentous laxity.
- Symptomatic traumatic instability is best treated with closed reduction and possible reconstruction of the joint, not resection of the clavicle head.

ANATOMY

- The sternoclavicular joint is a saddle-shaped joint that is the most unconstrained joint in the human body.
- Important ligamentous restraints to motion include the anterior capsule (restrains anterior and posterior translation), the posterior capsule (restrains posterior translation),[10] and the costoclavicular ligament (which is the pivot point for motion in the axial plane).[2]
  - The interclavicular ligament seems to provide little function (**FIG 1**).

PATHOGENESIS

- Osteoarthritis is the most common disorder affecting the medial clavicle that may require surgical excision.
- Osteoarthritis is most commonly seen in male laborers, in women in the perimenopausal years, and after radical neck dissection.
- Rheumatologic disorders can affect the sternoclavicular joint as part of the systemic disease. Involvement of the sternoclavicular joint is usually late.
- Other atraumatic conditions are less common and the pathogenesis is largely unknown.
- Traumatic instability typically develops from a blow to the shoulder girdle.
  - If the force impacts the anterior shoulder, it will push the shoulder girdle posteriorly. The clavicle pivots over the first rib, forcing the head of the clavicle anteriorly.

- If the force impacts the posterior shoulder, it will push the shoulder girdle anteriorly. The clavicle pivots over the first rib, dislocating the head of the clavicle posteriorly.
- Direct blows to the sternoclavicular joint can also dislocate the clavicle head posteriorly.
- Atraumatic instability develops insidiously without a history of trauma.

NATURAL HISTORY

- Many people have asymptomatic sternoclavicular joint arthritis.
- Patients with symptoms may find relief with activity modification and time. This is particularly true with the pain and swelling seen in perimenopausal women.
- Infection may present with a relatively benign clinical picture but will progress and may become serious.
- It is rare for the sternoclavicular joint to be the primary joint involved in rheumatologic conditions or crystal deposition disease.

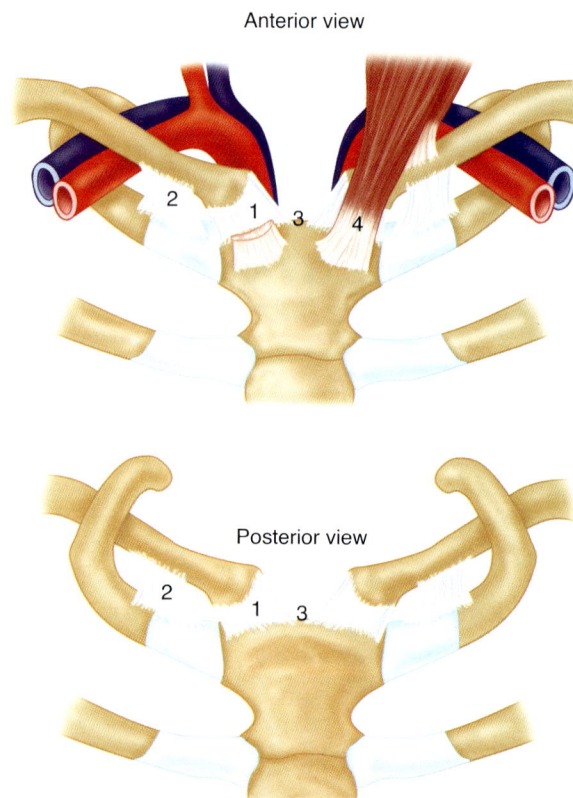

Anterior view

Posterior view

FIG 1 • Anterior and posterior anatomy of sternoclavicular joint. *1*, capsule; *2*, costoclavicular ligament; *3*, interclavicular ligament; *4*, sternocleidomastoid tendon.

Table 1	Clinical Features of Atraumatic Disorders of the Sternoclavicular Joint

Disorder	Age (yr)	Gender	Side	Pain	Erythema	Associated Conditions and Risk Factors
Osteoarthritis	>40	M=F	B	+	Rare	Manual labor, radical neck dissection, postmenopausal women
Rheumatoid arthritis	Any	F>M	B	+	+	Symmetric polyarthritis
Seronegative spondyloarthropathies	<40	M>F	B	Occasional	−	Urethritis, uveitis, nail pitting
Septic arthritis	Any	M=F	U	+++	+++	HIV, IVDA, DM
Crystal deposition disease	>40	M>F	U	+++ during flare	++	Other joint involvement
Sternoclavicular hyperostosis	30–60	M>F	B	+	−	Synovitis, acne, pustulosis, hyperostosis, osteitis
Condensing osteitis	25–40	F>M	U	+	−	None
Friedreich's disease	Any	F>M	U	+	−	None
Atraumatic subluxation	10–30	F>M	U	Infrequent	−	Generalized ligamentous laxity

DM, diabetes mellitus; F, female; IVDA, intravenous drug abuse; M, male.

- Traumatic instability may result from high-energy injuries (eg, motor vehicle collision) or may be related to contact in athletics.
- Posterior instability may be life-threatening as the clavicular head may compress vascular structures, the trachea, or the esophagus.
- Atraumatic instability may have an insidious onset and is often associated with other signs of generalized ligamentous laxity (eg, patellar subluxation, glenohumeral subluxation).

PATIENT HISTORY AND PHYSICAL FINDINGS

- Atraumatic disorders
  - Pain at the sternoclavicular joint is localized to the joint and may be referred up the sternocleidomastoid and trapezius.[5]
  - Infection typically is unilateral and has significant pain and erythema (Table 1).
  - Osteoarthritis, rheumatoid arthritis, seronegative spondyloarthropathies, and sternoclavicular hyperostosis are typically bilateral, with mild pain, and rare erythema.
  - Crystal deposition diseases, condensing osteitis, and Friedreich's disease are typically unilateral, and mildly painful.
- Traumatic disorders
  - With acute traumatic injuries, patients will have significant pain and will be unwilling to raise the arm. They may describe difficulty with swallowing or breathing in posterior dislocations.
  - The sternoclavicular joint is often swollen and tender.
  - The affected arm may demonstrate circulatory changes with arm swelling.
  - Physical examination may not be helpful in determining if the instability is anterior or posterior.

IMAGING AND OTHER DIAGNOSTIC STUDIES

- Special radiographic projections include the Rockwood (serendipity), Hobbs, Heinig, and Kattan views but are somewhat difficult to interpret (Table 2).[4]
- Computed tomography is particularly useful in trauma as it demonstrates displacement of the joint and bony anatomy.[4]

It very useful to determine whether a dislocation is anterior or posterior.

- Arteriography should be considered in posterior dislocations if vascular injury is suspected.
- MRI is helpful in atraumatic disorders to evaluate the soft tissues and can delineate marrow abnormalities, joint effusions, and disc and cartilage injury.[4]
- Laboratory findings in atraumatic disorders of the sternoclavicular joint are covered in Table 3.

DIFFERENTIAL DIAGNOSIS

- Atraumatic disorders
  - Osteoarthritis
  - Rheumatoid or other serologic arthritis
  - Seronegative spondyloarthropathies
  - Crystal deposition disease
  - Sternoclavicular hyperostosis
  - Condensing osteitis
  - Avascular necrosis
  - Septic arthritis
  - Instability

Table 2	Radiographic Features of Atraumatic Disorders of the Sternoclavicular Joint

Disorder	Radiographic Findings
Osteoarthritis	Sclerosis, osteophytes
Rheumatoid arthritis	Minimal change
Seronegative spondyloarthropathies	Marginal erosions, cysts
Septic arthritis	Sclerotic, lytic, or mixed lesions
Crystal deposition disease	Calcification of soft tissue
Sternoclavicular hyperostosis	Hyperostosis, ossification of intercostal ligaments
Condensing osteitis	Medial clavicle enlargement, preserved joint space, marrow obliteration
Friedreich's disease	Irregular end of medial clavicle
Atraumatic subluxation	Normal

Table 3	Laboratory Features of Atraumatic Disorders of the Sternoclavicular Joint	
Disorder	**Laboratory Findings**	
Osteoarthritis	Normal	
Rheumatoid arthritis	May have +RF, +ANA,	
Seronegative sponyloarthropathies	+HLA-B27	
Septic arthritis	WBC, ESR, CRP elevated	
Crystal deposition disease	+BRFC, -BRFC	
Sternoclavicular Hyperostosis	ESR elevated, other markers of rheumatologic disease normal	
Condensing osteitis	Normal	
Friedrich's disease	Normal	
Atraumatic subluxation	Normal	

ANA, antinuclear antibodies; BRFC, birefringement crystals; CRP, C-reactive protein; ESR, sedimentation rate; RF, rheumatoid factor; WBC, white blood cell count.

- Traumatic disorders
  - Medial-third clavicle fracture
  - Sternal fracture
  - First rib fracture

NONOPERATIVE MANAGEMENT

- Most atraumatic conditions can be managed nonoperatively.
- Nonoperative management includes nonsteroidal anti-inflammatories (NSAIDs) and rest. Sometimes topical lidocaine patches can help with pain.
- Acute dislocations should undergo closed reduction.
- In posterior dislocations, open reduction and possible reconstruction of the joint is indicated if closed reduction fails.

SURGICAL MANAGEMENT

- Surgery is indicated for atraumatic disorders of the sternoclavicular joint in every case of septic arthritis and when nonoperative management fails for the other conditions listed in the differential diagnosis.
- When infection is suspected, surgeons should perform incision and drainage quickly to prevent late osteomyelitis.
- Contraindications for resection of the medial clavicle include atraumatic instability of the joint.
- Acute dislocations should undergo closed reduction.
- In posterior dislocations, open reduction and possible reconstruction of the joint is indicated if closed reduction fails.

Preoperative Planning

- Due to the vital structures that lie behind the sternoclavicular joint, it is important to have a thoracic surgeon available should complications develop.

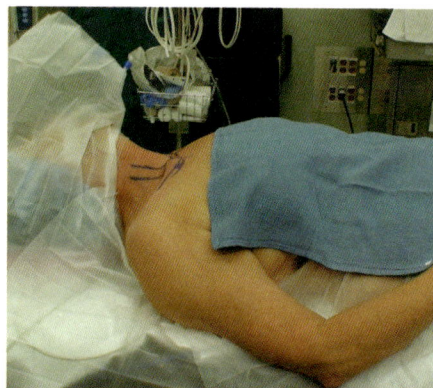

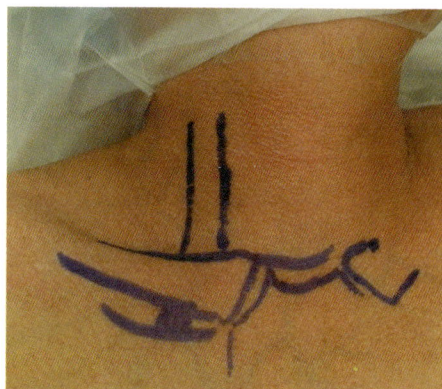

FIG 2 • **A.** Patient positioning. **B.** Anatomy is identified and marked.

Positioning

- The patient is positioned supine on the operating room table with a small rolled towel behind the middle of the back (**FIG 2A**).
- The entire chest is exposed for treatment of complications should they occur.
- Important structures, including the clavicle, manubrium, sternocleidomastoid, and costoclavicular ligament, are marked (**FIG 2B**).
- The ipsilateral hand is prepared and draped as well if the surgeon desires to use palmaris as an interposition graft.
- For reconstructions of the sternoclavicular joint, an ipsilateral hamstring may be used; as such, the knee should be prepared and draped.

Approach

- The approach is anterior. Care is taken to protect important structures during dissection, particularly the origin of the sternocleidomastoid muscle and the costoclavicular ligament.

INCISION AND DISSECTION

- The incision is made in the lines of Langer, which follow a necklace pattern over the head of the clavicle and manubrium (**TECH FIG 1A**).
- After undermining in the subcutaneous plane, the platysma is incised in line with the skin incision, exposing the joint capsule and sternocleidomastoid origin (**TECH FIG 1B**).
- The capsule of the joint is marked. Care must be taken to avoid incising the entire sternal head of the sternocleidomastoid tendon (**TECH FIG 1C**).

TECHNIQUES

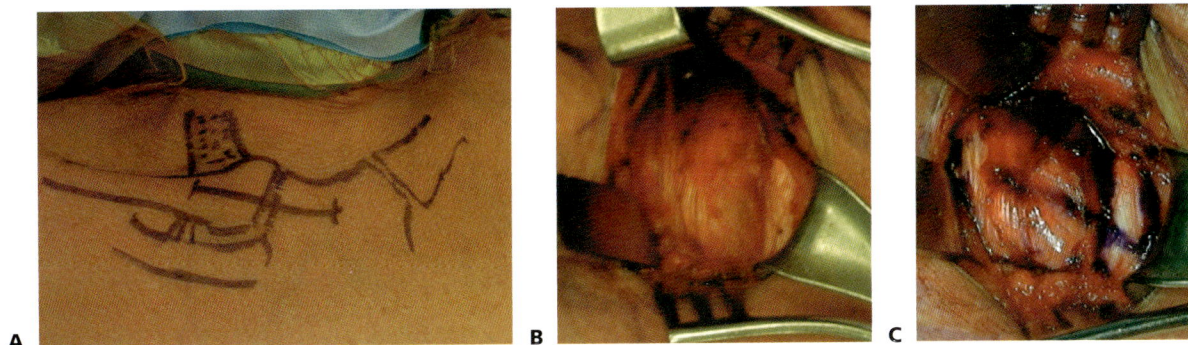

TECH FIG 1 • **A.** Location of incision. **B.** Incision of platysma. **C.** Incision in joint capsule.

ATRAUMATIC DISORDERS: REMOVING THE BONE

- Electrocautery can be used to carefully elevate the capsule from the clavicular head. It is important to avoid straying too far laterally to avoid detaching the capsule and injuring the costoclavicular ligament (**TECH FIG 2A**).
- The intra-articular disc is removed and the capsule is carefully dissected around the cartilaginous margin of the head of the clavicle (**TECH FIG 2B**).
- A self-retaining retractor is placed on the capsule, a blunt retractor is placed next to the articular surface, and

a small oscillating saw is used to remove between 0.5 and 1.0 cm of the medial clavicle (**TECH FIG 2C**).
- An osteotome may be used to lever the medial clavicle head out of the joint (**TECH FIG 2D**).
- Electrocautery is used to carefully dissect the posterior capsule from the back of the clavicular head (**TECH FIG 2E**).
- The resected head should be between 0.5 and 1.0 cm in size to preserve the costoclavicular ligaments (**TECH FIG 2F**).[3]

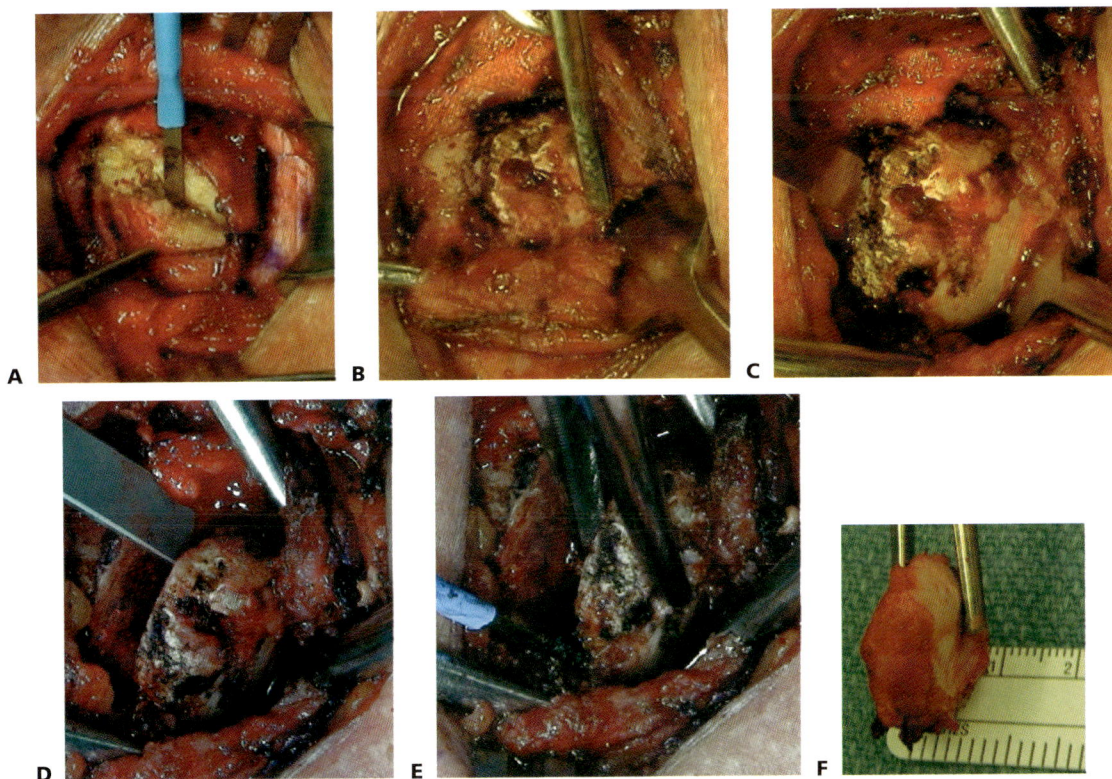

TECH FIG 2 • **A.** Elevating the capsule from the clavicle. **B.** Removing the intra-articular disc. **C.** Using an oscillating saw to remove the medial clavicle. **D.** Levering the medial clavicle from the joint. **E.** Removing the posterior soft tissue attachments. **F.** The excised medial clavicle.

TECHNIQUES

HARVESTING THE TENDON

- The palmaris tendon is isolated with a small incision in the wrist crease (**TECH FIG 3A**).
- After sutures are passed in the end of the palmaris, the tendon is removed percutaneously with a tendon stripper (**TECH FIG 3B**).
- The harvested tendon is rolled over a small spool and sutured to itself to create a rolled tendon (**TECH FIG 3C,D**).

- When resecting the clavicular head for atraumatic disorders, the rolled palmaris tendon is inserted into the defect to create a soft tissue interposition between the cut surface of the clavicle and the manubrial joint surface (**TECH FIG 3E**).
- Alternatively, the palmaris can be used to augment a reconstruction of an unstable sternoclavicular joint by passing it around the clavicle and first rib (see below).

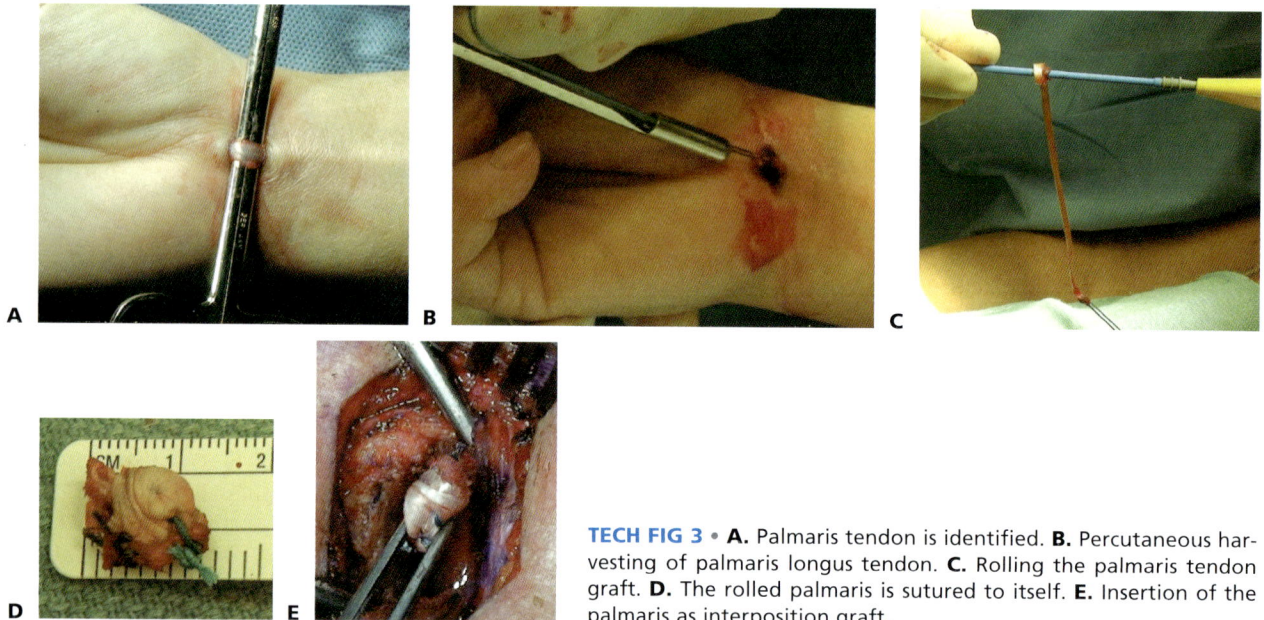

TECH FIG 3 • **A.** Palmaris tendon is identified. **B.** Percutaneous harvesting of palmaris longus tendon. **C.** Rolling the palmaris tendon graft. **D.** The rolled palmaris is sutured to itself. **E.** Insertion of the palmaris as interposition graft.

RECONSTRUCTION OF THE STERNOCLAVICULAR JOINT IN INSTABILITY

- A variety of techniques have been described. A figure 8 reconstruction has the best biomechanical properties.[11]
- With the assistance of a thoracic surgeon, the plane behind the manubrium is developed by dissecting above the sternal notch (**TECH FIG 4A**).
- With a ribbon retractor behind the manubrium, two drill holes are made in the manubrium and sutures are passed (**TECH FIG 4B**).

- Two drill holes are placed in the medial clavicle from anterior to posterior (**TECH FIG 4C**).
- The semitendinosus autograft is passed in figure 8 fashion and secured to itself (**TECH FIG 4D–F**).
- Additionally, the palmaris tendon may be passed around the first rib. This dissection behind the first rib should be performed by the thoracic surgeon to avoid injury to the internal mammary artery (**TECH FIG 4G**).

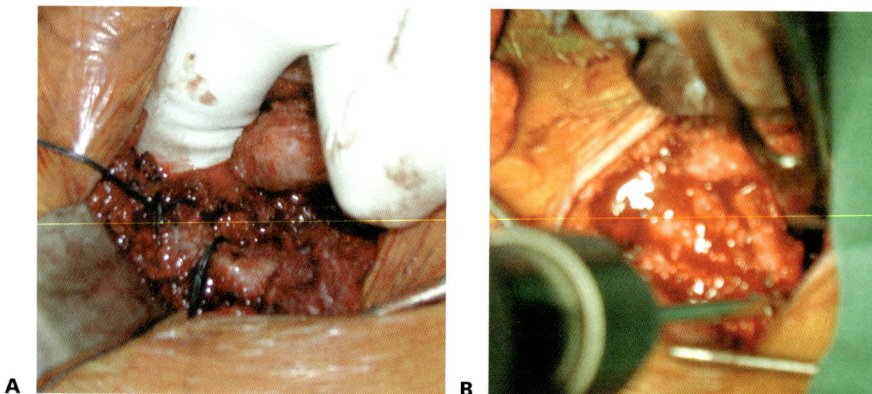

TECH FIG 4 • **A.** Development of the surgical plane behind manubrium. **B.** Drill holes are in manubrium with protection of mediastinal structures with an Army-Navy retractor. (continued)

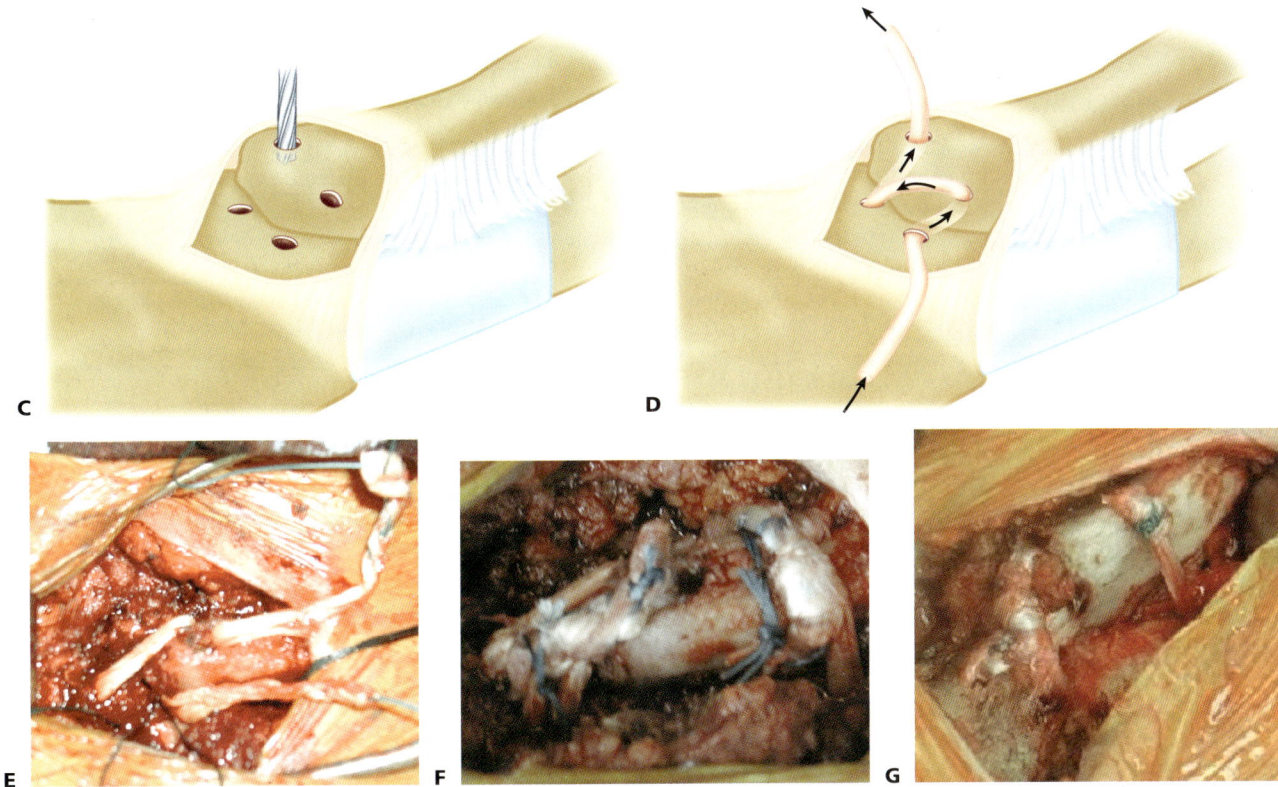

TECH FIG 4 • *(continued)* **C.** Drill holes in clavicle. **D–F.** Semitendinosus graft is passed in figure 8 fashion. **G.** Palmaris is passed around clavicle and first rib for augmentation. (**C** and **D**, Adapted from Kuhn JE. Sternoclavicular joint reconstruction for anterior and posterior sternoclavicular joint instability. In Zuckerman J, ed. Advanced Reconstruction of the Shoulder. Rosemont, IL: American Academy of Orthopaedic Surgeons, 2007:255–264.)

WOUND CLOSURE

- The capsule is closed with figure 8 interrupted permanent number 2 suture, and the sternal head of the sternocleidomastoid falls into place (**TECH FIG 5A**).

- The wound is closed in layers with 0 Vicryl in the platysma (**TECH FIG 5B**), 2-0 Vicryl in the subcutaneous layer, and 3-0 Monocryl in the skin (**TECH FIG 5C**).

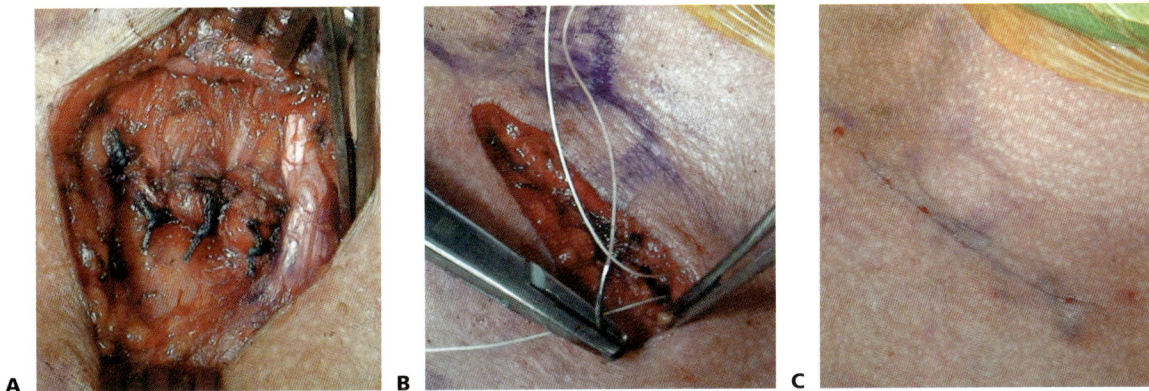

TECH FIG 5 • A. Repair of the joint capsule. **B.** Repair of the platysma. **C.** Surgical wound is closed.

PEARLS AND PITFALLS

Diagnosis	▪ CT and MRI imaging will help differentiate arthritis from other less common conditions. ▪ The surgeon must always be diligent for infection, which may have a relatively benign appearance. ▪ If it is unclear whether the sternoclavicular joint is the source of pain, a diagnostic injection with lidocaine can be helpful. ▪ CT is extremely helpful to determine if a dislocation is anterior or posterior.
Removing bone	▪ Great care must be taken to avoid perforating the posterior capsule and entering the mediastinum. It is better to do a partial resection and remove residual bone with a burr. ▪ Preserving the clavicular head is important for reconstructions of unstable sternoclavicular joints.
Preserving capsule	▪ Maintaining the integrity of the joint capsule is of critical importance. If the capsule is stripped completely off the clavicle, suture anchors in the clavicle can help restore stability.
Costoclavicular ligament	▪ If the costoclavicular ligament is sacrificed, the intra-articular disc and disc ligament can be passed into the intramedullary canal.
General surgery	▪ It is wise to have a thoracic surgeon available should complications develop in the mediastinum.

POSTOPERATIVE CARE

▪ Patients are typically admitted overnight for observation.

▪ Patients wear a sling with pillow support to support the arm when upright for 6 weeks.

▪ Patients are instructed to avoid moving the arm for 6 weeks to allow for capsular healing and preventing instability.

▪ After 6 weeks, patients gradually increase range of motion.

▪ After 12 weeks, patients can begin strengthening activities.

▪ After 16 weeks, patients have unrestricted activity.

OUTCOMES

▪ There is little reported on the outcomes after this procedure. All reports are level 4 case series.

▪ Rockwood and colleagues[9] reported that outcomes were improved if the costoclavicular ligament remained intact (eight of eight excellent with complete satisfaction). If the costoclavicular ligament was disrupted, however, the results were less predictable (three of five excellent).

▪ Arcus and associates[1] reported on 15 patients with a variety of pathologies. Sixty percent were graded as good to excellent, and 93% had significant pain relief and would have the procedure again.

▪ Pingsmann and colleagues[8] found seven of eight women with sternoclavicular joint arthritis had good to excellent results with medial clavicle excision after 31 months of follow-up.

▪ Meis and coworkers[7] modified the technique by interposing the sternal head of the sternocleidomastoid into the defect. Ten of 14 patients reported good to excellent outcomes; however, two patients reported incisional pain with head turning, and three patients had cosmesis concerns.

▪ A variety of case reports exist for other sternoclavicular joint reconstructions. To date, no reports are in the peer-reviewed literature for the figure 8 reconstruction.

COMPLICATIONS

▪ Rockwood and colleagues[9] report that patients may have severe discomfort if instability persists or develops. Consequently, it is imperative to preserve the costoclavicular ligament. If the costoclavicular ligament is disrupted, the intra-articular disc and ligament can be transferred into the intramedullary canal of the resected clavicle. In addition, reconstructing the costoclavicular ligament with a tendon graft around the first rib should be considered.

▪ Heterotopic ossification has been reported in about half of the patients but seems to be asymptomatic.[1]

▪ Although not reported to date, complications involving the great vessels, trachea, and other mediastinal contents are possible. A thoracic surgeon should be available for assistance if required.

REFERENCES

1. Acus RW III, Bell RH, Fisher DL. Proximal clavicle excision: an analysis of results. J Shoulder Elbow Surg 1995;4:182–187.
2. Bearn JG. Direct observations on the function of the capsule of the sternoclavicular joint in clavicular support. J Anat 1967;101:159–170.
3. Bisson LJ, Dauphin N, Marzo JM. A safe zone for resection of the medial end of the clavicle. J Shoulder Elbow Surg 2003;12:592–594.
4. Ernberg LA, Potter HG. Radiographic evaluation of the acromioclavicular and sternoclavicular joints. Clin Sports Med 2003;22:255–275.
5. Hassett G, Barnsley L. Pain referral from the sternoclavicular joint: a study in normal volunteers. Rheumatology 2001;40:859–862.
6. Higgenbotham TO, Kuhn JE. Atraumatic disorders of the sternoclavicular joint. J Am Acad Orthop Surg 2005;13:138–145.
7. Meis RC, Love RB, Keene JS, et al. Operative treatment of the painful sternoclavicular joint: a new technique using interpositional arthroplasty. J Shoulder Elbow Surg 2006;15:60–66.
8. Pingsmann A, Patsalis T, Michiels I. Resection arthroplasty of the sternoclavicular joint for the treatment of primary degenerative sternoclavicular arthritis. J Bone Joint Surg Br 2002;84B:513–517.
9. Rockwood CA Jr, Groh GI, Wirth MA, et al. Resection arthroplasty of the sternoclavicular joint. J Bone Joint Surg Am 1997;79A:387–393.
10. Spencer EE, Kuhn JE, Huston LJ, et al. Ligamentous restraints to anterior and posterior translation of the sternoclavicular joint. J Shoulder Elbow Surg 2002;11:43–47.
11. Spencer EE, Kuhn JE. Biomechanical analysis of reconstructions for sternoclavicular joint instability. J Bone Joint Surg Am 2004;86A:98–108.

Chapter 14

Plate Fixation of Clavicle Fractures

David Ring and Jesse B. Jupiter

DEFINITION

- Displaced, comminuted fractures of the clavicle are at risk for nonunion and malunion[3–5,7–9] and can be considered for open reduction and internal fixation with a plate and screws.

ANATOMY

- The clavicle and scapula are tightly linked through the strong coracoclavicular and acromioclavicular ligaments and link the axial skeleton to the upper extremity.
- Clavicles are present only in brachiating animals and apparently serve to help hold the upper limb away from the trunk to enhance more global positioning and use of the limb.
- The clavicle is named for its S-shaped curvature, with an apex anteromedially and an apex posterolaterally, similar to the musical symbol clavicula. The larger medial curvature widens the space for passage of neurovascular structures from the neck into the upper extremity through the costoclavicular interval.
- The clavicle is made up of very dense trabecular bone lacking a well-defined medullary canal. In cross section, the clavicle changes gradually between a flat lateral aspect, a tubular midportion, and an expanded prismatic medial end.
- The clavicle is subcutaneous throughout its length and makes a prominent aesthetic contribution to the contour of the neck and upper part of the chest.
- The supraclavicular nerves run obliquely across the clavicle just superior to the platysma muscle and should be identified and protected during operative exposure to offset the development of hyperesthesia or dysesthesia over the chest wall.

PATHOGENESIS

- Clavicle fractures usually result from a direct blow to the point of the shoulder.
- This is usually a moderate- to high-energy injury in younger adults but can result from a low-energy fall from a standing height in an older individual.

NATURAL HISTORY

- The overall nonunion rate for diaphyseal clavicle fractures is 4.5%.[7]
- The risk of nonunion increases with age, female gender, displacement, and comminution.[7]
- The risk of nonunion for completely displaced (no apposition) and comminuted fractures is between 10% and 20% (**FIG 1**).[9]
- Malunion of the clavicle can result in shoulder girdle deformity and weakness.[3–5,9]
- Malunion and nonunion of the clavicle can result in brachial plexus compression.

PATIENT HISTORY AND PHYSICAL FINDINGS

- The mechanism and date of injury should be elicited.
- A careful neurologic examination should be performed.

- In contrast to late dysfunction of the brachial plexus after clavicular fracture, a situation in which medial cord structures are typically involved, acute injury to the brachial plexus at the time of clavicular fracture usually takes the form of a traction injury to the upper cervical roots. Such root traction injuries generally occur in the setting of high-energy trauma and have a relatively poor prognosis.
- "Tenting" of the skin by a fracture fragment is dangerous only in patients who cannot protect their skin (eg, patients who are comatose).

IMAGING AND OTHER DIAGNOSTIC STUDIES

- An anteroposterior (AP) radiograph can be supplemented by a 20- to 60-degree cephalad-tilted view.
- The so-called apical oblique view (tilted 45 degrees anterior and 20 degrees cephalad) may facilitate the diagnosis of minimally displaced fractures (eg, birth fractures, fractures in children).
- The abduction lordotic view taken with the shoulder abducted above 135 degrees and the central ray angled 25 degrees cephalad is useful in evaluating the clavicle after internal fixation. Abduction of the shoulder results in rotation of the clavicle on its longitudinal axis, which causes the plate to rotate superiorly and thereby expose the shaft of the clavicle and the fracture site under the plate.
- Computed tomography with 3D reconstructions can help understand 3D deformity.

DIFFERENTIAL DIAGNOSIS

- Lateral or medial clavicle fracture
- Acromioclavicular or sternoclavicular dislocation

NONOPERATIVE MANAGEMENT

- Closed reduction of clavicular fractures is rarely attempted because the reduction is usually unstable and no reliable means of providing external support is available.
- A simple sling provides comfort and limits activity during healing. A figure 8 bandage leaves the arm free, but it cannot improve alignment.

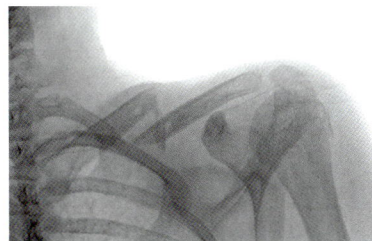

FIG 1 • An AP radiograph shows greater than 100% displacement and comminution with a vertical fracture fragment. The clavicle is shortened. (Copyright David Ring, MD.)

■ There is no need to be concerned about shoulder stiffness, and patients should be encouraged keep the arm at the side and limit activity for the first 4 to 6 weeks.

SURGICAL MANAGEMENT

■ Intramedullary fixation is an option when comminution is limited, but otherwise plate-and-screw fixation is preferred.
■ The plate can be placed on either the superior or the anterior[1,2] aspect of the clavicle.

Preoperative Planning

■ Planning of the surgery using tracings of radiographs helps limit intraoperative decision making and helps the surgeon anticipate problems and contingencies.

Positioning

■ The patient is supine with a variable amount of flexion of the trunk according to surgeon preference (**FIG 2**).

Approach

■ A longitudinal incision is made in line with the clavicle.

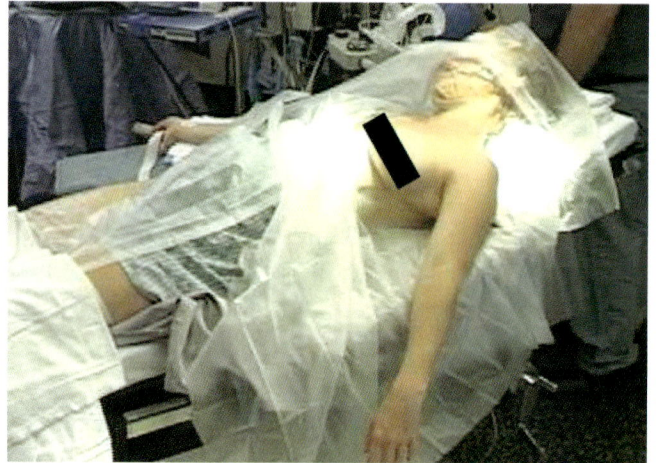

FIG 2 • The patient is positioned supine with the head and trunk elevated slightly. (Copyright David Ring, MD.)

SUPERIOR PLATE-AND-SCREW FIXATION

■ An incision is made parallel and just inferior to the long axis of the clavicle (**TECH FIG 1A**). Infiltration with dilute epinephrine can help limit bleeding.
■ The crossing supraclavicular nerves are identified under loupe magnification and preserved (**TECH FIG 1B**).
■ Muscle attachments and periosteum are preserved as much as possible.
■ Realignment and provisional fixation may be facilitated by the use of a small distractor or temporary external fixator (**TECH FIG 1C**).

■ A 3.5-mm limited-contact dynamic compression plate (LCDC plate, Synthes) or a precontoured plate is applied to the superior aspect of the clavicle (**TECH FIG 1D**). A minimum of three screws should be placed in each major fragment. If the fracture pattern is amenable, placement of an interfragmentary screw greatly enhances the stability of the construct.
■ When the vascularity of the fragments has been preserved, no bone graft is needed (**TECH FIG 1E**). When extensive stripping or gaps have occurred in the cortex

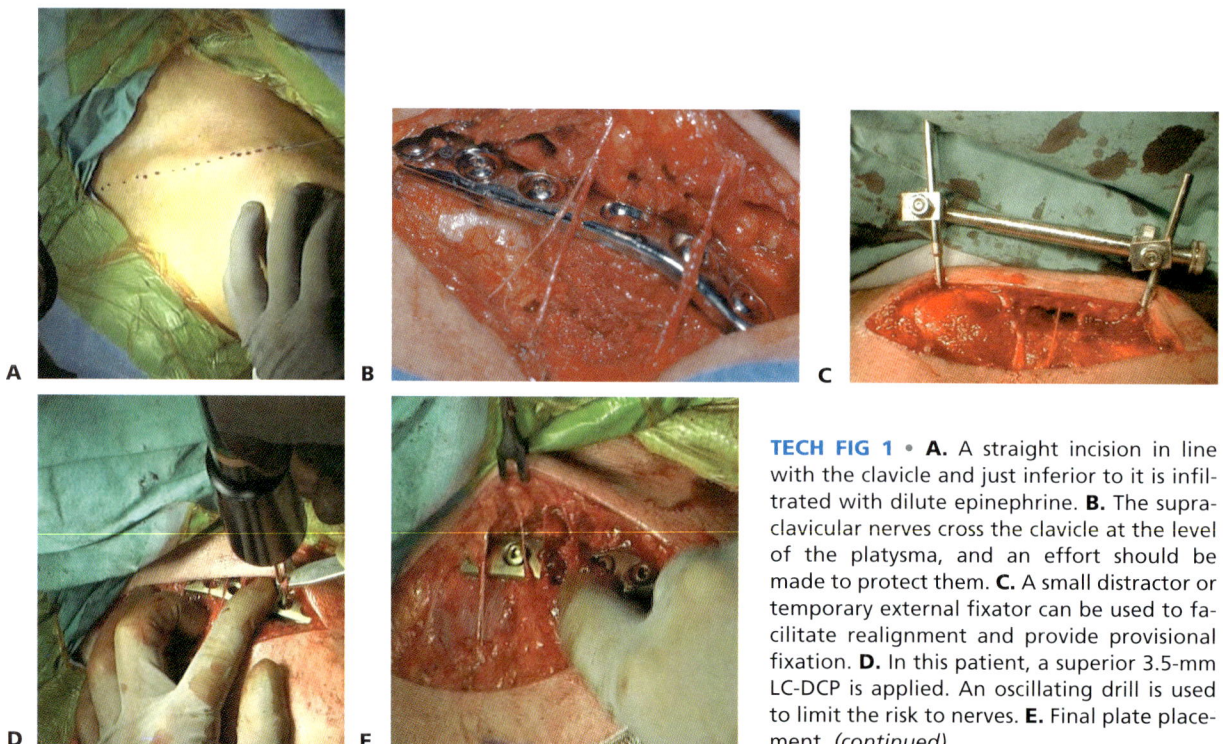

TECH FIG 1 • **A.** A straight incision in line with the clavicle and just inferior to it is infiltrated with dilute epinephrine. **B.** The supraclavicular nerves cross the clavicle at the level of the platysma, and an effort should be made to protect them. **C.** A small distractor or temporary external fixator can be used to facilitate realignment and provide provisional fixation. **D.** In this patient, a superior 3.5-mm LC-DCP is applied. An oscillating drill is used to limit the risk to nerves. **E.** Final plate placement. *(continued)*

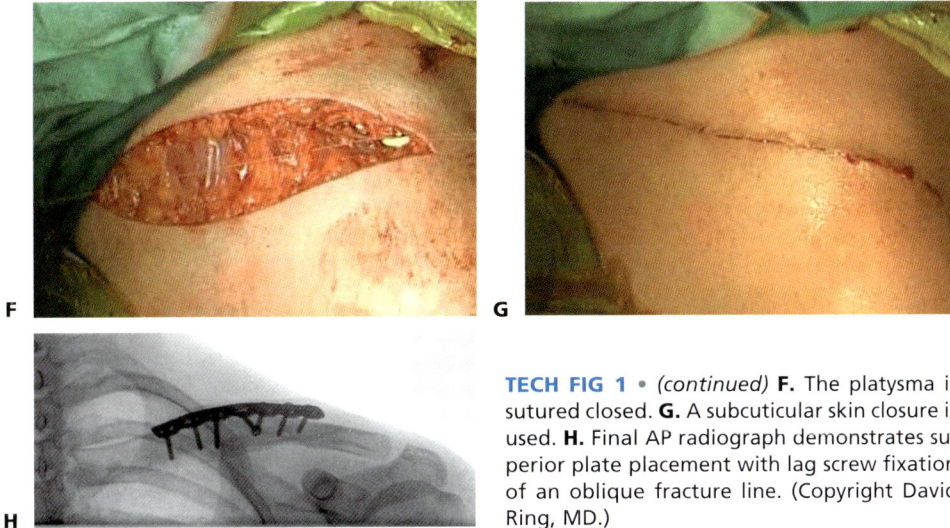

TECH FIG 1 • *(continued)* **F.** The platysma is sutured closed. **G.** A subcuticular skin closure is used. **H.** Final AP radiograph demonstrates superior plate placement with lag screw fixation of an oblique fracture line. (Copyright David Ring, MD.)

opposite the plate, one might consider adding a small amount of autogenous iliac crest cancellous bone graft.
- Close the platysma (**TECH FIG 1F**).

- If the skin condition is suitable, wound closure is accomplished in atraumatic fashion with a subcuticular suture (**TECH FIG 1G,H**).

ANTERIOR PLATE-AND-SCREW FIXATION

- The technique is identical for an anterior plate placement with the exception that the origins of the pectoralis major and deltoid are partially extraperiosteally elevated off the anterior clavicle (**TECH FIG 2**).
- The anterior plate placement may help to decrease hardware prominence, and the drill and screws are directed posterior rather than directly inferior to the clavicle, which may increase the margin of safety.

TECH FIG 2 • An alternative is to place the plate on the anterior surface of the clavicle. This limits plate prominence but requires greater stripping and muscle elevation. (Copyright David Ring, MD.)

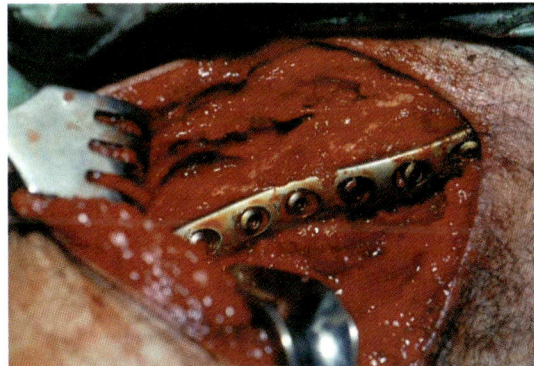

PEARLS AND PITFALLS

Supraclavicular nerve neuroma	■ Attempts to identify and protect these nerves are worthwhile.
Brachial plexus stretch injury	■ Realignment should be done gradually and can be facilitated by temporary external fixation. Pulling fragments out of the wound should be limited.
Loosening of fixation	■ At least three good bicortical screws should be placed on each side of the fracture.
Axial pull-out of locked screws	■ Locking screws may be troublesome when used on the lateral fragment with the plate in a superior position.
Plate prominence	■ Anterior plate placement may diminish plate prominence.

POSTOPERATIVE CARE

- Confident use of the hand at the side is encouraged immediately.
- Shoulder abduction and handling of more than 15 pounds is delayed until early healing is established.
- Shoulder stiffness is unusual and usually responds quickly to exercises. Shoulder exercises can therefore be delayed until healing is established.

OUTCOMES

- Plate loosening and nonunion occur in 3% to 5% of cases.[6]
- Healing leads to good function.

COMPLICATIONS

- Infection and wound complications occur but are uncommon.
- Neurovascular injury is very uncommon and pneumothorax has not been described.

REFERENCES

1. Collinge C, Devinney S, Herscovici D, et al. Anterior-inferior plate fixation of middle-third fractures and nonunions of the clavicle. J Orthop Trauma 2006;20:680–686.
2. Kloen P, Sorkin AT, Rubel IF, et al. Anteroinferior plating of midshaft clavicular nonunions. J Orthop Trauma 2002;16:425–430.
3. McKee MD, Pedersen EM, Jones C, et al. Deficits following nonoperative treatment of displaced midshaft clavicular fractures. J Bone Joint Surg Am 2006;88A:35–40.
4. McKee MD, Wild LM, Schemitsch EH. Midshaft malunions of the clavicle. J Bone Joint Surg Am 2003;85A:790–797.
5. Nowak J, Holgersson M, Larsson S. Can we predict long-term sequelae after fractures of the clavicle based on initial findings? A prospective study with nine to ten years of follow-up. J Shoulder Elbow Surg 2004;13:479–486.
6. Poigenfurst J, Rappold G, Fischer W. Plating of fresh clavicular fractures: results of 122 operations. Injury 1992;23:237–241.
7. Robinson CM, Court-Brown CM, McQueen MM, et al. Estimating the risk of nonunion following nonoperative treatment of a clavicular fracture. J Bone Joint Surg Am 2004;86A:1359–1365.
8. Robinson CM. Fractures of the clavicle in the adult: epidemiology and classification. J Bone Joint Surg Br 1998;80B:476–484.
9. Zlowodzki M, Zelle BA, Cole PA, et al. Treatment of acute midshaft clavicle fractures: systematic review of 2144 fractures: on behalf of the Evidence-Based Orthopaedic Trauma Working Group. J Orthop Trauma 2005;19:504–507.

Chapter 15

Intramedullary Fixation of Clavicle Fractures

Bradford S. Tucker, Carl Basamania, and Matthew D. Pepe

DEFINITION

- The clavicle is one of the most commonly fractured bones.
- The site on the clavicle most often fractured is the middle third.[9]
  - The midclavicular region is the thinnest and narrowest portion of the bone.
  - It is the only area not supported by ligament or muscle attachments.
  - It represents a transitional region of both cross-sectional anatomy and curvature.
    - It is the transition point between the lateral part, with a flatter cross section, and the more tubular medial.
- Because of the clavicle's S shape, an axial load creates a very high tensile force along the anterior midcortex. (Axial load makes a virtual right angle at midclavicle.)

ANATOMY

- The clavicle is the only long bone to ossify by a combination of intramembranous and endochondral ossification.[6]
- Its configuration is S-shaped, a double curve; the medial curve is apex anterior and the lateral curve is apex posterior (**FIG 1A**).
- The larger medial curvature widens the space for the neurovascular structures, providing bony protection.
- The clavicle is made up of very dense trabecular bone, lacking a well-defined medullary canal.

- The cross-sectional anatomy gradually changes from flat laterally, to tubular in the midportion, to expanded prismatic medially.
- The clavicle is subcutaneous throughout, covered by the thin platysma muscle.
- The supraclavicular nerves that provide sensation to the overlying skin of the clavicle are found deep to the platysma muscle.
- Very strong capsular and extracapsular ligaments attach the medial end to the sternum and first rib and the lateral end to the acromion and coracoid.
- Proximal muscle attachments include the sternocleidomastoid, pectoralis major, and subclavius. Distal muscle attachments include the deltoid and trapezius (**FIG 1B**).
- The clavicle functions by providing a fixed-length strut through which the muscles attached to the shoulder girdle can generate and transmit large forces to the upper extremity.

PATHOGENESIS

- The mechanism of clavicle fractures in the vast majority is a direct injury to the shoulder.[10] Stanley and associates studied 106 injured patients; 87% had fallen onto the shoulder, 7% were injured by a direct blow on the point of the shoulder, and only 6% reported falling onto an outstretched hand.
- Stanley suggests that in the patients who described hitting the ground with an outstretched hand, the shoulder became the next contact point with the ground, causing the fracture. Stanley

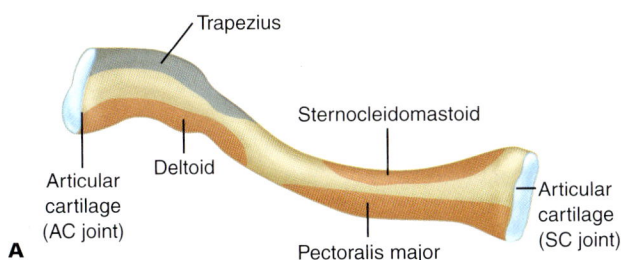

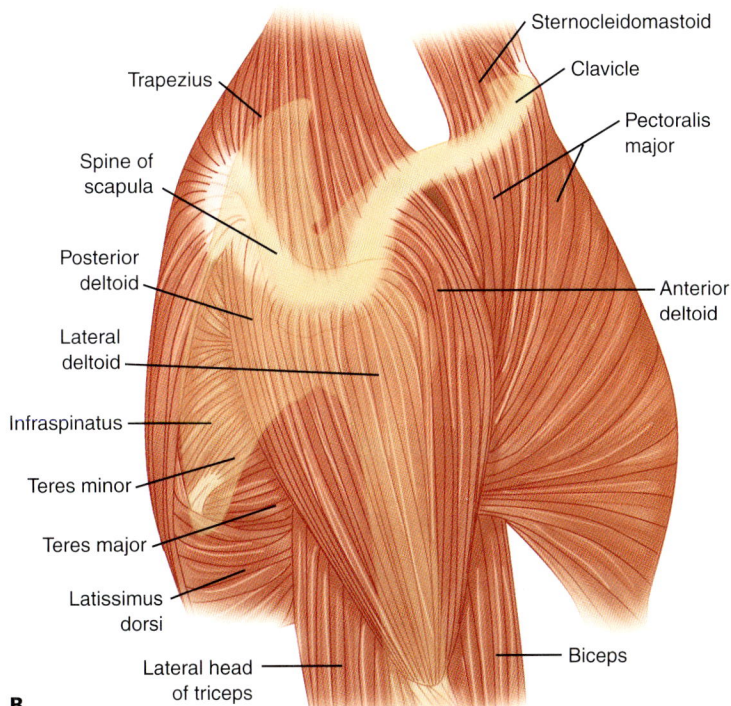

FIG 1 • **A.** The clavicle is S-shaped and has a double curve. The medial curve is apex anterior and the lateral curve is apex posterior. **B.** Proximal muscle attachments to the clavicle include the sternocleidomastoid, pectoralis major, and subclavius. Distal muscle attachments to the clavicle include the deltoid and trapezius.

stated that a compressive force equivalent to body weight would exceed the critical buckling load to cause the clavicle fracture.

NATURAL HISTORY

- In the 1960s, both Neer[7] and Rowe[9] published large series of midclavicle fractures, showing very low nonunion rate (0.1% and 0.8%) with closed treatment and a higher nonunion rate (4.6% and 3.7%) with operative treatment.
- More recent studies have shown that nonunion is more common then previously recognized and that a significant percentage of patients with nonunion are symptomatic.
- Malunion with shortening greater than 15 to 20 mm has also been shown to be associated with significant shoulder dysfunction.
- McKee and colleagues[5] identified 15 patients with malunion of the midclavicle after closed treatment. All patients had shortening of more than 15 mm, all were symptomatic and unsatisfied, and all underwent corrective osteotomy. Postoperatively all 15 patients improved in terms of function and satisfaction.
- Hill and associates[4] reviewed 52 completely displaced midshaft clavicle fractures and found that shortening of more than 20 mm had a significant association with nonunion and unsatisfactory results.
- Eskola and coworkers[3] reported on 89 malunions of the midclavicle, showing that shortening of more than 15 mm was associated with shoulder discomfort and dysfunction.

PATIENT HISTORY AND PHYSICAL FINDINGS

- The diagnosis is usually straightforward and is based on obtaining the mechanism of injury from a good history.
- On visual inspection the examiner will frequently see notable swelling or ecchymosis at the fracture site and possibly deformity of the clavicle, with drooping of the shoulder downward and forward if the fracture is significantly displaced. The skin is inspected for tenting at the fracture site and characteristic bruising and abrasions that might suggest a direct blow or seatbelt shoulder strap injury (**FIG 2A,B**).
- Palpation over the fracture site will reveal tenderness, and gentle manipulation of the upper extremity or clavicle itself may reveal crepitus and motion at the fracture site.
- The amount of shortening is identified by clinically measuring the distance of a straight line (in centimeters) from both acromioclavicular joints to the sternal notch and noting the difference (**FIG 2C**).
- It is important to perform a complete musculoskeletal and neurovascular examination of the upper extremity and auscul-

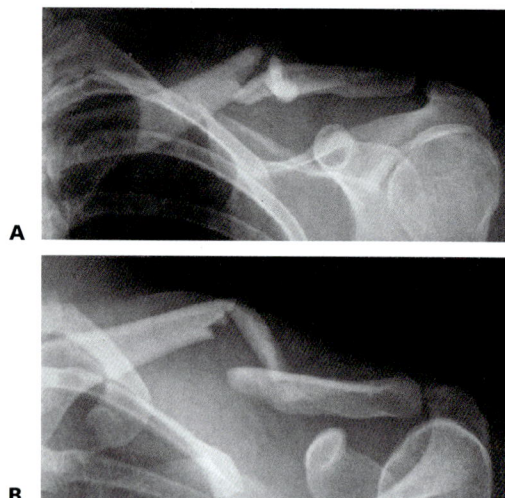

FIG 3 • Radiographs of the same displaced left clavicle fracture viewed from a standard AP projection (**A**) and a 45-degree cephalic tilt projection (**B**).

tation of the chest to identify the rare associated injuries; these are more closely related to high-energy injuries.

- Rib and scapula fracture
- Brachial plexus injury (usually traction to upper cervical root)
- Vascular injury (subclavian artery or vein injury associated with scapulothoracic dissociation)
- Pneumothorax and hemothorax

IMAGING AND OTHER DIAGNOSTIC STUDIES

- Two orthogonal radiographic projections are necessary to determine the fracture pattern and displacement, ideally 45-degree cephalic tilt and 45-degree caudad tilt views.
- Usually a standard anteroposterior (AP) view and a 45-degree cephalic tilt (**FIG 3**) view are adequate.
  - In practice, a 20- to 60-degree cephalic tilt view will minimize interference of thoracic structures.
- The film should be large enough to include the acromioclavicular and sternoclavicular joints, the scapula, and the upper lung fields to evaluate for associated injuries.
- An AP view of bilateral clavicles on a wide cassette to include the acromioclavicular joints and sternum is fairly helpful in determining the amount of shortening; however, this is a multiplanar deformity and a CT scan would have greater accuracy, although it is rarely required.

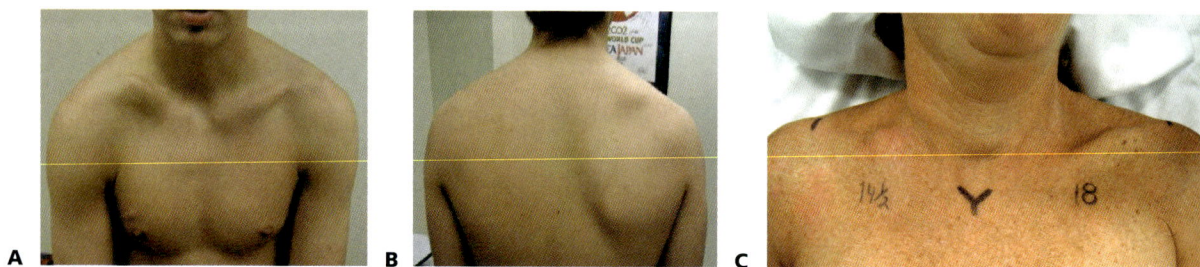

FIG 2 • **A,B.** Anterior and posterior photographs of a displaced right clavicle fracture showing deformity of the clavicle and drooping of the shoulder girdle downward and forward. **C.** Clinical picture of a displaced right clavicle fracture, showing 3.5 cm of shortening, measured from the sternal notch to the acromioclavicular joint.

DIFFERENTIAL DIAGNOSIS

- Sprain of acromioclavicular joint
- Sprain of sternoclavicular joint
- Rib fracture
- Muscle injury
- Contusion
- Hematoma
- Kehr sign: referred pain to the left shoulder from irritation of the diaphragm, signaled by the phrenic nerve. Irritation may be caused by diaphragmatic or peridiaphragmatic lesions, renal calculi, splenic injury, or ectopic pregnancy.

NONOPERATIVE MANAGEMENT

- If the clavicle fracture alignment is acceptable, generally a simple configuration with less than 15 mm of shortening, then any of a number of methods of supporting the upper extremity are adequate, including a figure 8 bandage, sling, sling and swathe, Sayre bandage, Velpeau dressing, and benign neglect, just to name a few.
- Nordqvist and colleagues[8] reported on 35 clavicle fracture malunions with shortening of less than 15 mm. They were all treated nonoperatively in a sling. All 35 had normal mobility, strength, and function compared to the normal shoulder.
- A prospective, randomized study[2] comparing sling versus figure 8 bandage showed that a greater percentage of patients were dissatisfied with the figure 8 bandage, and there was no difference in overall healing and alignment. The study concluded that the figure 8 bandage does little to obtain reduction.

SURGICAL MANAGEMENT

- Indications for operative treatment of acute midshaft clavicle fractures are as follows:
  - Open fractures
  - Fractures with neurovascular injury
  - Fractures with severe associated chest injury or multiple trauma: patients who require their upper extremity for transfer and ambulation
  - "Floating shoulder"
  - Impending skin necrosis
  - Severe displacement: possibly 15 to 20 mm of shortening

- In a multicenter, randomized, prospective clinical trial of displaced midshaft clavicle fractures, Altamimi and McKee[1] showed that operative fixation compared to nonoperative treatment improved functional outcome and had a lower rate of both malunion and nonunion.
- Potential advantages of intramedullary fixation of the clavicle are as follows:
  - Less soft tissue stripping and therefore potentially better healing
  - Smaller incision
  - Better cosmesis
  - Easier hardware removal
  - Less weakness of bone after hardware removal
- Potential disadvantages of intramedullary fixation of the clavicle are as follows:
  - Less ability to resist torsional forces
  - Skin breakdown from prominence distally
  - Pin breakage
  - Pin migration
- Newer designs and techniques prevent pin migration by placing a locking nut on the lateral end and technically avoiding penetration of the medial fragment cortex.

Preoperative Planning

- After the decision has been made to fix a clavicle fracture, one must evaluate whether the fracture pattern is amenable to intramedullary pin fixation.
- A simple fracture pattern in the middle third of the bone is ideal.
- The fracture should not extend past the middle third of the bone.
- Comminution and butterfly fragments (usually anterior) are common and do not preclude intramedullary fixation as long as the medial and distal main fragments have cortical contact.

Positioning

- There are two good options for patient positioning that facilitate use of an image intensifier or C-arm device, which will aid you during pin placement.
- The patient can be placed supine on a Jackson radiolucent surgical table so the C-arm can be brought in perpendicular from the opposite side of the table, which is out of the way of the surgeon (**FIG 4A,B**).

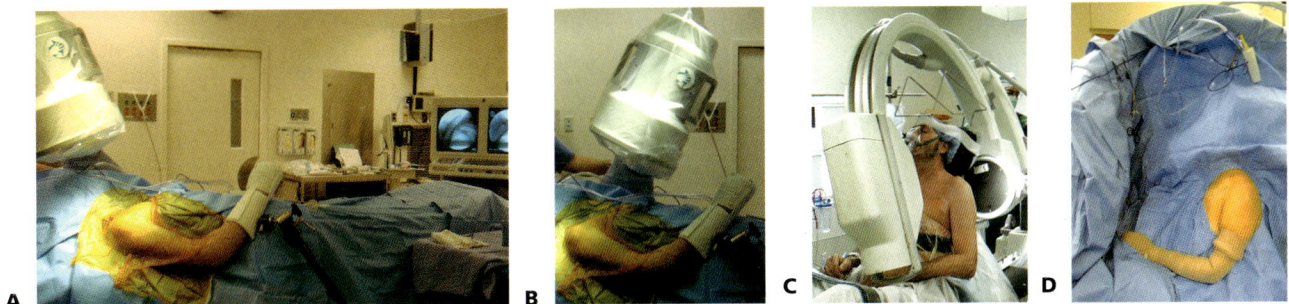

FIG 4 • A,B. The patient is placed supine on a Jackson radiolucent surgical table. A 1-L bag is placed under the affected shoulder, medial to the scapula, and the arm is prepared free and placed in an arm holder to aid in fracture reduction. The C-arm can be brought in perpendicular from the opposite side of the table, which is out of the way of the surgeon and facilitates getting orthogonal radiographic views of the fracture: 45-degree caudad tilt view (**A**) and 45-degree cephalic tilt view (**B**). **C,D.** Alternatively, the patient is placed in the beach chair position on the OR table, using a radiolucent shoulder-positioning device. **C.** The arm is prepared free and placed in an arm holder to facilitate fracture reduction. The C-arm is brought in from the head of the bed with the gantry rotated upside down and slightly away from the operative shoulder and oriented with a cephalic tilt. **D.** The same beach chair positioning shown sterilely draped.

■ A 1-L bag is placed under the affected shoulder, medial to the scapula, to aid in fracture reduction.

■ The arm is also prepared free and placed in an arm holder to facilitate fracture reduction.

■ This is our preferred method due to the ease and speed of the set-up and the ease of getting orthogonal radiographic views of the fracture (45-degree cephalic and caudad tilt views).

■ The other option is placing the patient in the beach chair position on the OR table, using a radiolucent shoulder-positioning device (**FIG 4C,D**).

■ The C-arm is brought in from the head of the bed with the gantry rotated upside down and slightly away from the operative shoulder and oriented with a cephalic tilt.

■ The arm is also prepared free and placed in an arm holder to facilitate fracture reduction.

INCISION AND DISSECTION

■ Mark out the clavicle, fracture site, and surrounding anatomy (**TECH FIG 1A**).

■ Use the C-arm to identify the appropriate position for the incision, which should be over the distal end of the medial fragment, in the Langer lines of the normal skin crease around the neck (**TECH FIG 1B**).

■ Make an incision of about 2 to 3 cm over the fracture site.

■ Divide the subcutaneous fat down to the platysma muscle using electrocautery (**TECH FIG 1C**).

■ Although there is usually very little subcutaneous fat, gently make full-thickness flaps to include skin and subcutaneous tissue around the entire incision to facilitate exposure.

■ Bluntly split the platysma muscle in line of its fibers to identify, protect, and retract the underlying supraclavic-

ular nerves; its middle branches are frequently found near the midclavicle (**TECH FIG 1D,E**).

■ The fracture site is then usually easily identifiable in acute injuries because the periosteum is disrupted and usually requires no further division.

■ Remove any debris, hematoma, or interposed muscle from the fracture site.

■ If there are butterfly fragments, be careful to keep any soft tissue attachments.

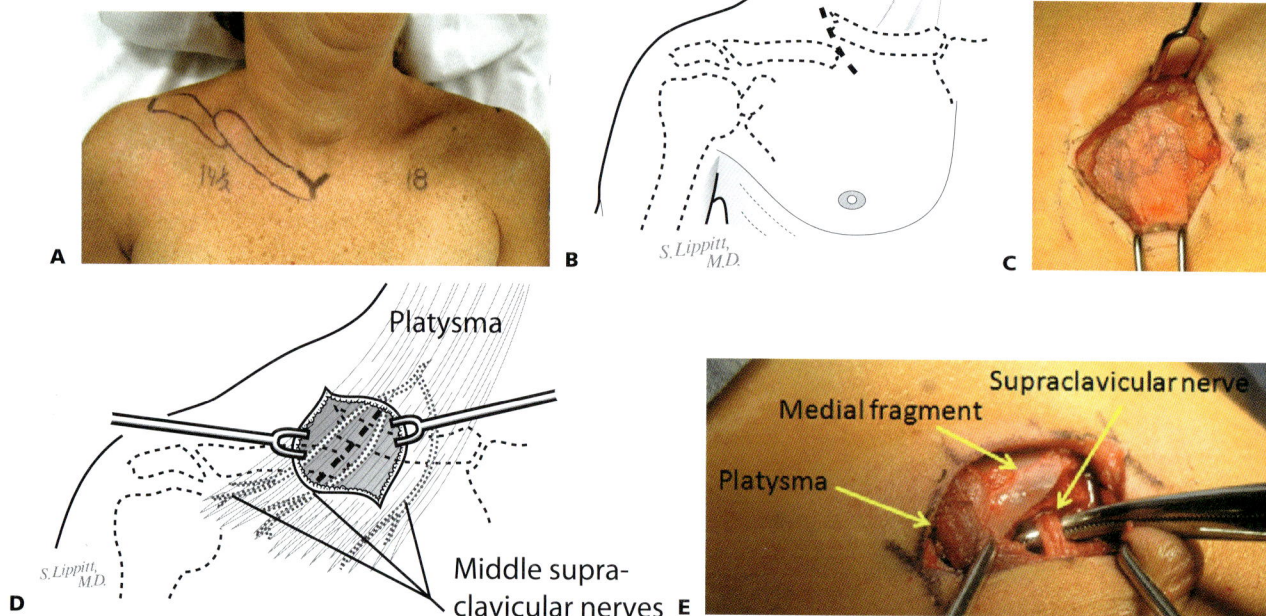

TECH FIG 1 • **A.** Displaced right clavicle fracture, showing the clavicle and fracture site marked out. **B.** A skin incision of about 2 to 3 cm is made over the distal end of the medial clavicular fragment, in the Langer lines of normal skin creases around the neck. **C.** Incision over a clavicle fracture site, showing full-thickness flaps to include skin and subcutaneous tissue around the entire incision. This exposes the fascia that covers the platysma muscle. **D.** Skin incision over a displaced clavicle fracture, with underlying platysma muscle and the middle supraclavicular nerves. **E.** Intraoperative photo showing the platysma muscle bluntly split in the line of its fibers to identify an underlying supraclavicular nerve, which is under the clamp. The fracture site is usually easily identifiable in acute injuries because the periosteum is disrupted and usually requires no further division; as shown here, the medial clavicular fragment is easily seen. (**B,D:** Courtesy of Steven B. Lippitt, MD.)

CLAVICLE PREPARATION

- The following technique uses a modified Hagie pin called the Rockwood Clavicle Pin (DePuy Orthopaedics, Warsaw, IN) (**TECH FIG 2A**).
- Use a bone-reducing clamp or towel clip to grab and elevate the medial clavicular fragment through the incision (**TECH FIG 2B**).
- Size the diameter of the canal with the appropriate-size drill bit; the C-arm can be useful to judge canal fill and orientation of the drill.
  - The fit should be snug to maximize fixation, but not too tight, to prevent splitting the bone.
- Attach the chosen drill to the T-handle and ream out the intramedullary canal without penetrating the anterior cortex (**TECH FIG 2C–E**).
- Next, attach the appropriate-sized tap (that corresponds to the drill size) to the T-handle and tap the intramedullary canal to the anterior cortex (**TECH FIG 2F,G**).
- Elevate the lateral clavicular fragment through the incision; this can be facilitated by externally rotating the arm.
- Use the same drill bit attached to the T-handle to ream out the lateral fragment, but this time, under C-arm guidance, penetrate the posterolateral cortex of the clavicle (**TECH FIG 2H,I**).
  - The drill should exit posterior and medial to the acromioclavicular joint capsule (**TECH FIG 2J**).
  - To prevent the pin nuts from being too prominent, make sure the drill does not exit in the upper half of the posterolateral clavicle.
- Attach the appropriate-sized tap to the T-handle and tap the intramedullary canal of the lateral fragment (**TECH FIG 2K**).

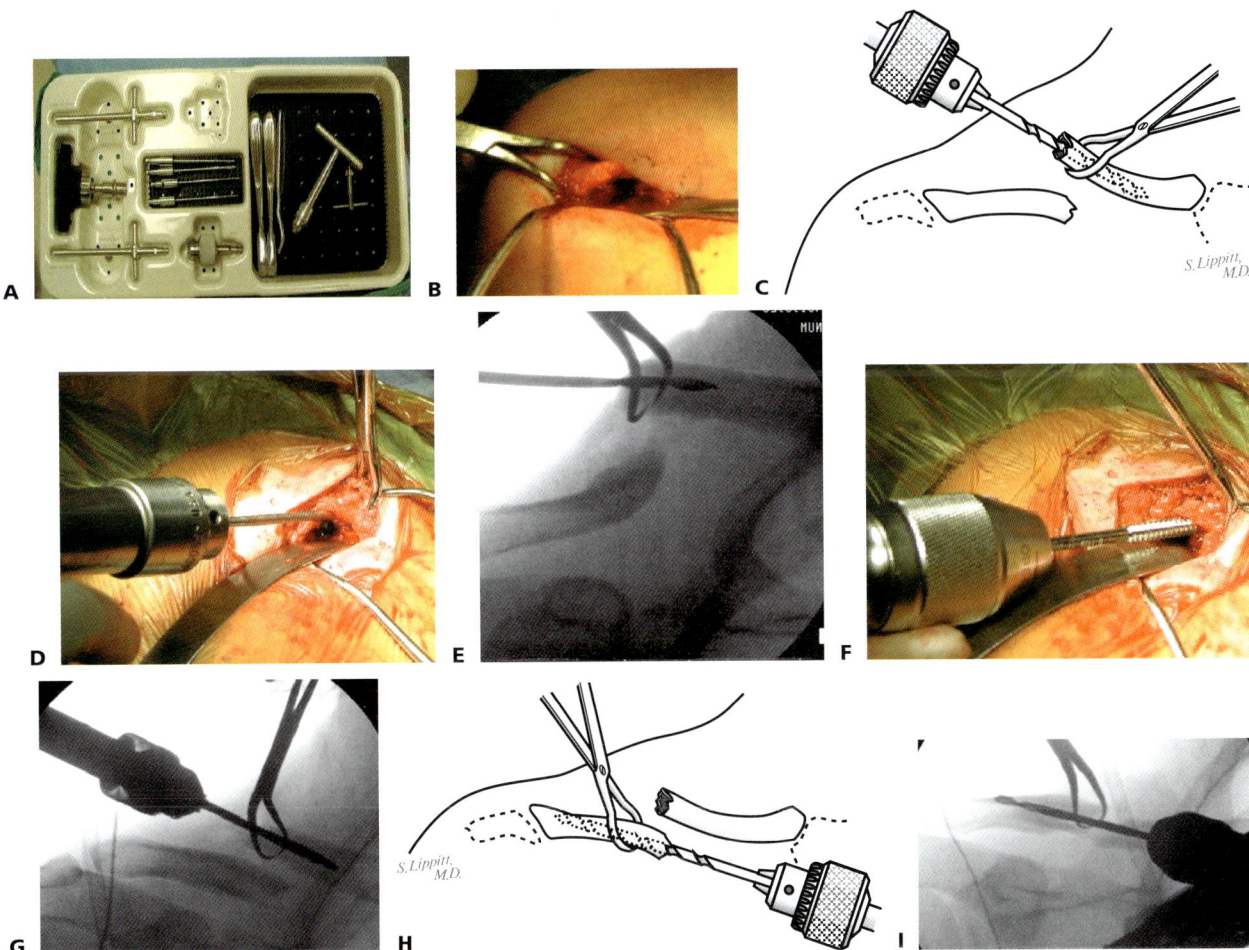

TECH FIG 2 • A. The Rockwood Clavicle Pin instrument set by DePuy Orthopaedics, Warsaw, IN, which is a modified Hagie pin. **B.** A bone-reducing clamp is used to elevate the medial clavicular fragment through the incision. **C–E.** The chosen drill is attached to a T-handle and the intramedullary canal of the medial clavicular fragment is reamed without penetrating the anterior cortex. **F,G.** An appropriate-sized tap is attached to a T-handle and the intramedullary canal of the medial clavicular fragment is tapped to the anterior cortex. **H,I.** The chosen drill is attached to a T-handle and the intramedullary canal of the lateral clavicular fragment is reamed out, penetrating the posterolateral cortex under direct C-arm guidance. *(continued)*

TECHNIQUES

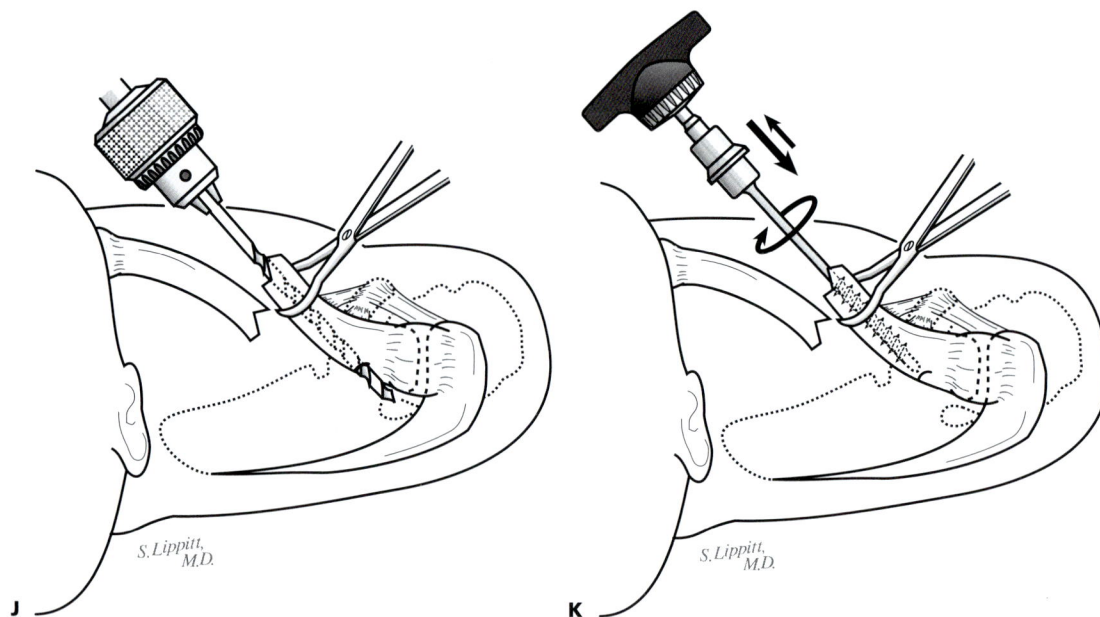

TECH FIG 2 • *(continued)* **J.** When drilling out the posterolateral cortex of the lateral clavicular fragment, the drill should exit posterior and medial to the acromioclavicular joint capsule. To prevent the pin nuts from being too prominent, the drill should not exit in the upper half of the posterolateral clavicle. **K.** The appropriate-sized tap is attached to the T-handle and the intramedullary canal of the lateral fragment is tapped. (**C,H,J,K:** Courtesy of Steven B. Lippitt, MD.)

PIN INSERTION AND FRACTURE REDUCTION

- Remove the nuts from the pin assembly and attach the T-handle using a Jacobs chuck to the medial end of the clavicle pin.
  - This is the end with the large threads.
  - Never tighten the chuck over the machined threads at either end.
- Continue firmly holding the lateral fragment while passing the trocar end (lateral end) of the clavicle pin into the intramedullary canal, out the previously drilled hole in the posterolateral cortex (**TECH FIG 3A**).
- Once you are just through the cortex, make a small incision over the palpable tip.
- Bluntly dissect the subcutaneous tissue with a hemostat until the tip of the pin can be felt, and then place the hemostat or a small elevator under the tip of the pin to facilitate the pin's passage through the incision (**TECH FIG 3B**).
  - Drill the pin out laterally until the large medial threads engage the lateral fragment.
- Now switch the T-handle to the lateral end of the pin and retract the pin into the lateral fragment (**TECH FIG 3C,D**).
- Reduce the fracture by lifting the arm, and pass the pin into the medial fragment.
  - Use the C-arm to ensure that the pin advances correctly down the line of the medial fragment and that all the medial threads cross the fracture site.

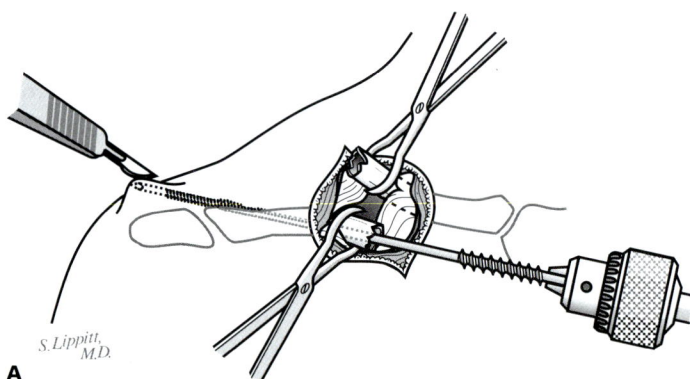

TECH FIG 3 • **A.** The surgeon continues firmly holding the lateral fragment while passing the trocar end (lateral end) of the clavicle pin into the intramedullary canal, out the previously drilled hole in the posterolateral cortex. Once just through the cortex, the surgeon makes a small incision over the palpable tip. *(continued)*

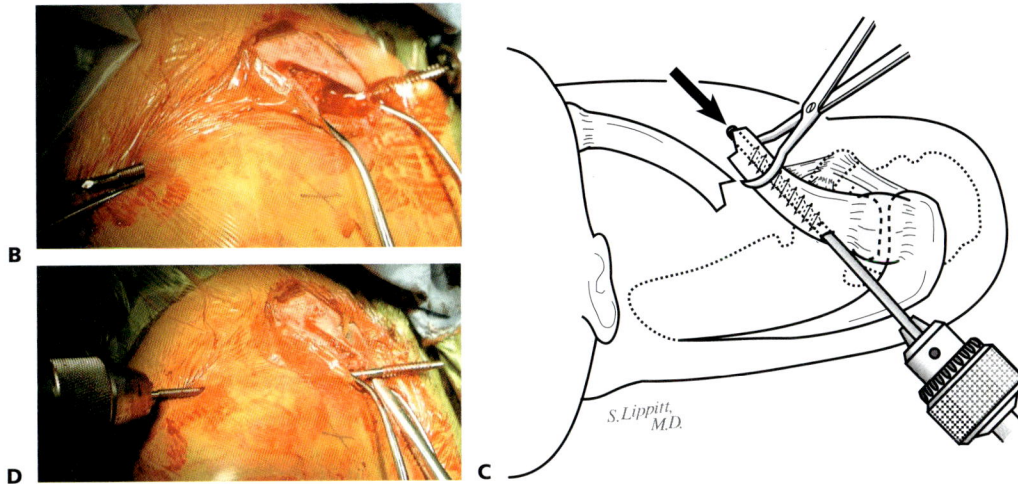

TECH FIG 3 • *(continued)* **B.** The subcutaneous tissue is bluntly dissected with a hemostat until the tip of the pin can be felt, and then the hemostat or a small elevator is placed under the tip of the pin to facilitate the pin's passage through the incision. **C,D.** The T-handle is switched to the lateral end of the pin and the pin is retracted into the lateral fragment. (**A,C:** Courtesy of Steven B. Lippitt, MD.)

FINAL POSITIONING OF PIN AND FRACTURE COMPRESSION

- Cold-weld the two nuts onto the lateral end of the pin.
  - First place the medial nut onto the pin, followed by the smaller lateral nut.
  - Grasp the medial nut with a needle-nose pliers and then tighten the lateral nut against the medial nut using the lateral nut wrench (**TECH FIG 4A,B**).
- Using the lateral nut wrench and C-arm guidance, now advance the pin assembly into the medial fragment until it contacts the anterior cortex (**TECH FIG 4C**).
- Break the cold weld by grasping the medial nut with needle-nose pliers and then loosen the lateral nut by turning it counterclockwise using the lateral nut wrench.

- Advance the medial nut against the posterolateral cortex of the clavicle to get desired compression across the fracture site.
- Cold-weld the lateral nut back onto the medial nut again.
- Use the medial nut wrench to back the pin assembly out of the soft tissues far enough to expose the nuts, usually about 1 cm. This will enable the pin to be cut flush to the lateral nut (**TECH FIG 4D,E**).
- Finally, use the lateral nut wrench to advance the pin assembly back into the medial fragment with the same desired fracture site compression (**TECH FIG 4F,G**).

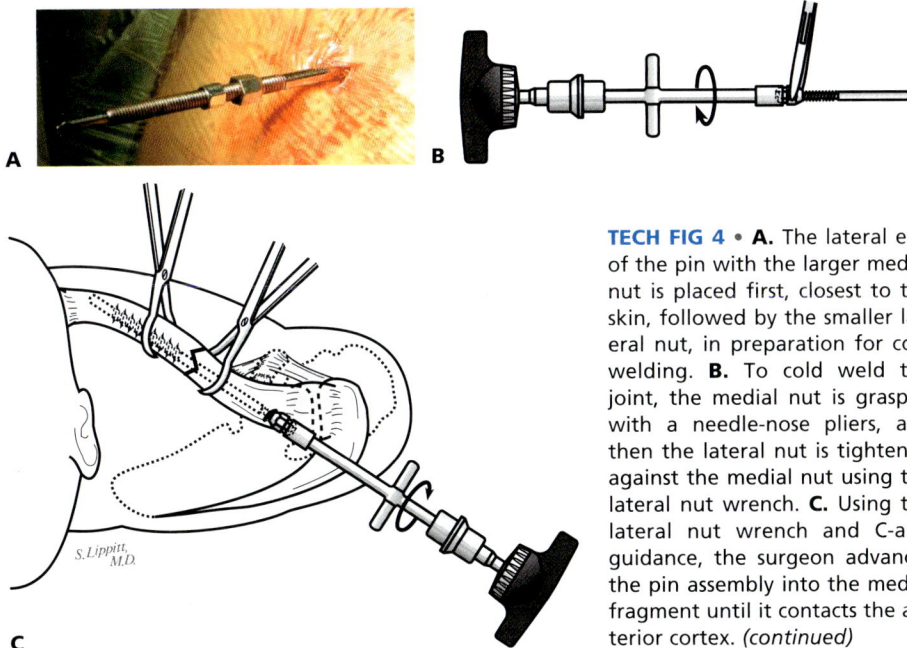

TECH FIG 4 • **A.** The lateral end of the pin with the larger medial nut is placed first, closest to the skin, followed by the smaller lateral nut, in preparation for cold welding. **B.** To cold weld the joint, the medial nut is grasped with a needle-nose pliers, and then the lateral nut is tightened against the medial nut using the lateral nut wrench. **C.** Using the lateral nut wrench and C-arm guidance, the surgeon advances the pin assembly into the medial fragment until it contacts the anterior cortex. *(continued)*

D

F

E

G

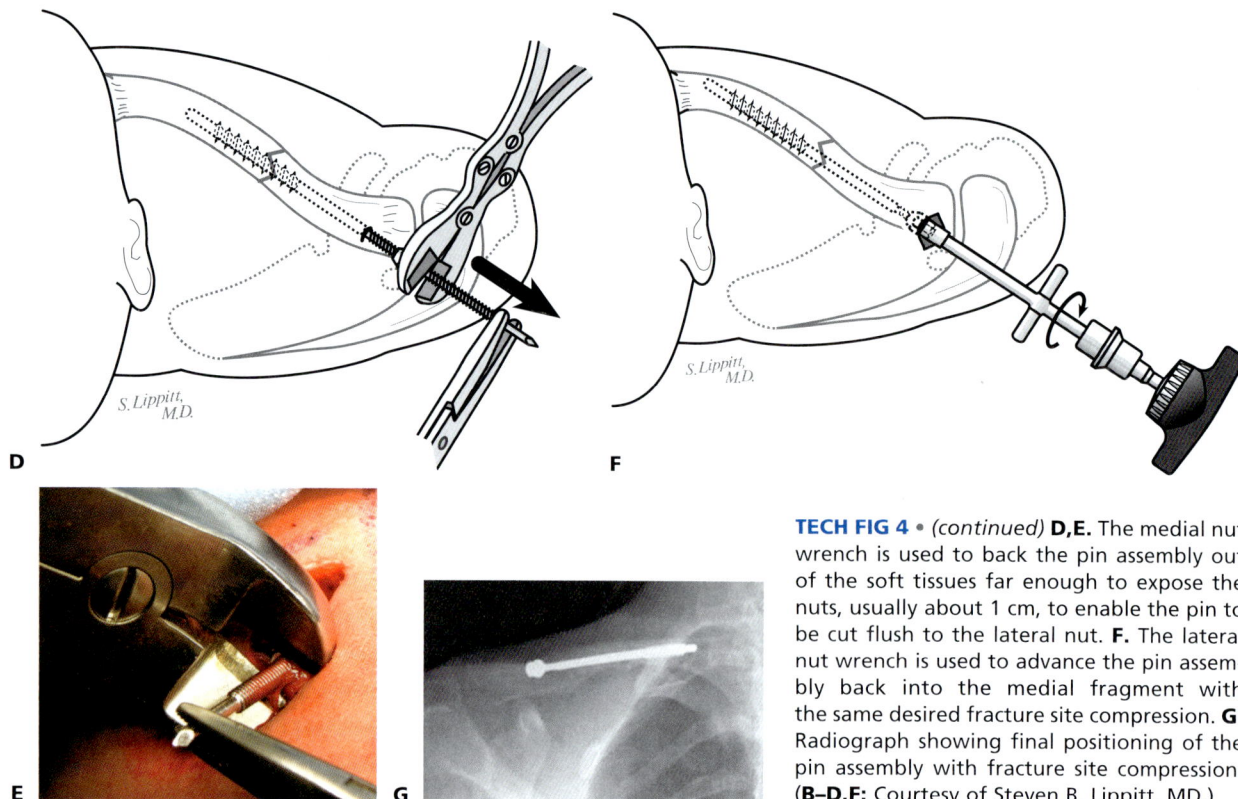

TECH FIG 4 • *(continued)* **D,E.** The medial nut wrench is used to back the pin assembly out of the soft tissues far enough to expose the nuts, usually about 1 cm, to enable the pin to be cut flush to the lateral nut. **F.** The lateral nut wrench is used to advance the pin assembly back into the medial fragment with the same desired fracture site compression. **G.** Radiograph showing final positioning of the pin assembly with fracture site compression. (**B–D,F:** Courtesy of Steven B. Lippitt, MD.)

BUTTERFLY FRAGMENT MANAGEMENT AND WOUND CLOSURE

- If an anterior butterfly fragment exists, cerclage is done using no. 0 or no. 1 absorbable suture.
  - Pass an elevator under the clavicle to deflect the sutures (**TECH FIG 5A**).

- Then pass the suture in a figure 8 manner through the periosteum of the butterfly fragment and around the fragment and the clavicle (**TECH FIG 5B**).
- Close the periosteum overlying the fracture site with no. 0 absorbable suture in an interrupted figure 8 manner.
- Reapproximate the fascia of the platysma muscle using 2-0 absorbable suture in an interrupted figure 8 manner.
- Close the subcutaneous tissue and skin of both incisions.

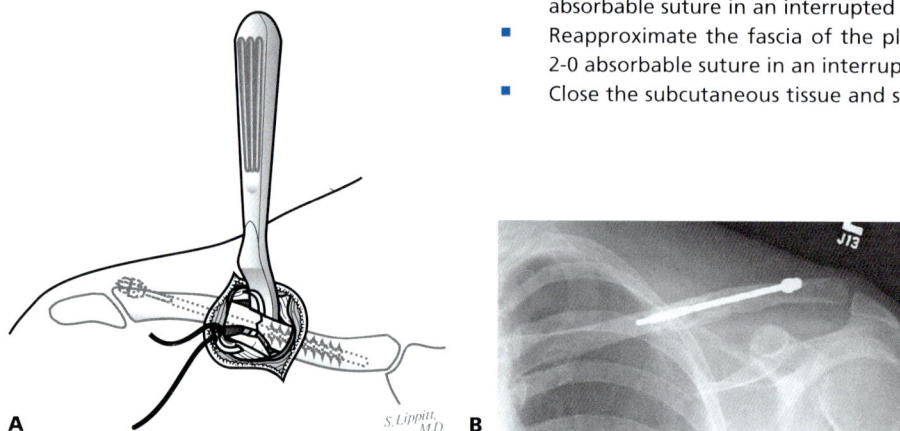

A

B

TECH FIG 5 • **A.** Cerclage of an anterior butterfly fragment is accomplished by first passing an elevator under the clavicle to deflect the sutures and then passing the suture, in a figure 8 manner, through the periosteum of the butterfly fragment and around the fragment and the clavicle. **B.** Radiograph showing an adequate reduction of a butterfly fragment. (**A:** Courtesy of Steven B. Lippitt, MD.)

PIN REMOVAL

- The pin is removed at 10 to 12 weeks if the fracture has healed.
- The patient is positioned on his or her side and a local anesthetic is delivered (**TECH FIG 6A**).

- An incision is made over the same previous lateral incision and the subcutaneous tissue is dissected using the hemostat until the medial nut is identified.
- The medial nut wrench is used to extract the pin assembly (**TECH FIG 6B,C**).
- If the nut is stripped, the T-handle and chuck can be used to extract the pin assembly.

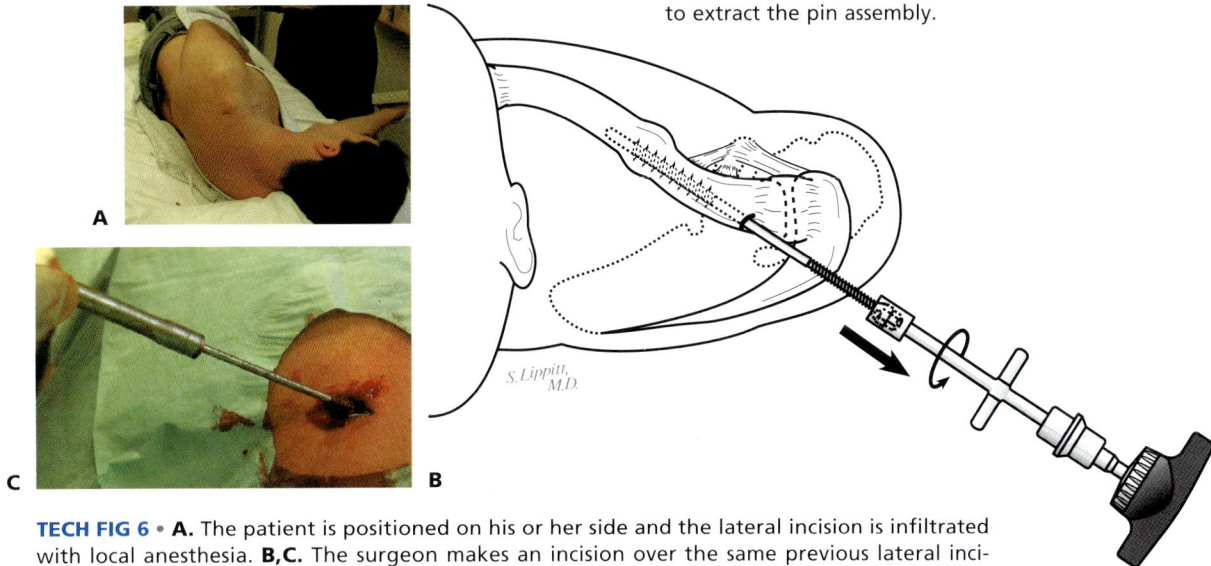

TECH FIG 6 • **A.** The patient is positioned on his or her side and the lateral incision is infiltrated with local anesthesia. **B,C.** The surgeon makes an incision over the same previous lateral incision, dissecting through the subcutaneous tissue using the hemostat until the medial nut is identified and freed up. The medial nut wrench is then used to extract the pin assembly. (**B:** Courtesy of Steven B. Lippitt, MD.)

PEARLS AND PITFALLS

Avoid splitting the clavicular fragments and aid in pin insertion	■ If tapping the medial or lateral clavicular fragments is too tight, the surgeon should redrill with the next larger drill size.
Achieve a more anatomic fracture reduction	■ When advancing the pin into the medial clavicular fragment, the surgeon should avoid starting too superior and anterior, which can lead to malreduction. Instead, the pin should be inserted more inferior and posterior to achieve a more anatomic reduction.

POSTOPERATIVE CARE

- A sling is worn for 4 weeks. During this time the sling is removed at least five times a day for active range of motion of the elbow and active assisted range of motion of the shoulder to 90 degrees of forward flexion.
- The sling is discontinued and full active range of motion of the shoulder is started at 4 weeks.
- Progressive resistance exercises are started at 6 weeks if the patient achieved full range of motion and there is clinical and radiographic evidence of healing.
- Once the clavicle fracture has healed, the pin is removed at 10 to 12 weeks, as described in the Techniques section (**FIG 5**).

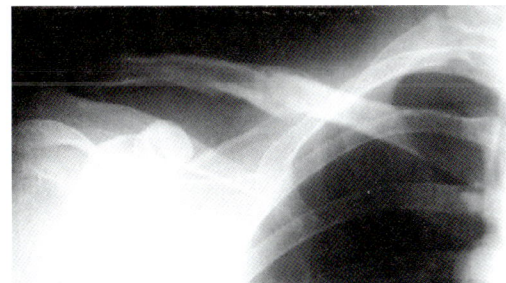

FIG 5 • Radiograph showing a healed clavicle fracture after pin assembly removal.

OUTCOMES

- One of the authors (C.B.) has performed intramedullary fixation of some 300 acute fractures; there have been 60 malunions and 30 nonunions of the clavicle, with a nonunion rate of 1.2%.
- Most of the nonunions occurred in older, sick patients with polytrauma.

COMPLICATIONS

- Pin migration is rare with this technique because of the locking nut on the lateral end of the pin, the blunt tip on the medial end of the pin, and technically avoiding penetration of the medial fragment cortex.
- The risk of skin breakdown from pin prominence laterally can be minimized by making sure the drill exits the posterolateral clavicle in the lower half.
- Neurovascular complications are rare.
  - There is no drilling toward the neurovascular structures with this technique.
  - When exposing the fracture site, the surgeon should stay on bone at all times.
- Nonunion rates are low as long as general fracture principles are maintained, soft tissue stripping of the fracture site is minimized, the technique is followed to get adequate fracture site compression and alignment, and the patient is compliant with the postoperative protocol.
- Malunion can rarely occur, especially in fractures with large butterfly fragments. Good imaging with the C-arm allows the surgeon to start inserting the pin more inferior and posterior down the line of the medial clavicular fragment to achieve a more anatomic reduction.
- Infection is rare, especially with this technique, which has a relatively short surgical time and small exposure. Preoperative antibiotics, meticulous handling of the soft tissues, and adequate irrigation should be part of any surgical technique.

REFERENCES

1. Altamimi S, McKee M. Nonoperative treatment compared with plate fixation of displaced midshaft clavicle fractures. J Bone Joint Surg Am 2008;90A:1–8.
2. Andersen K, Jensen PO, Lauritzen J. Treatment of clavicular fractures: figure-of-eight versus a simple sling. Acta Orthop Scand 1987;58:71–74.
3. Eskola A, Vainionpaa S, Myllynen P, et al. Outcome of clavicular fractures in 89 patients. Arch Orthop Trauma Surg 1986;105:337–338.
4. Hill J, McGuire M, Crosby L. Closed treatment of displaced middle-third fractures of the clavicle gives poor results. J Bone Joint Surg Br 1997;79B:537–539.
5. McKee M, Wild L, Schemitsch E. Midshaft malunions of the clavicle. J Bone Joint Surg Am 2003;85A:790–797.
6. Moseley HF. The clavicle: its anatomy and function. Clin Orthop Relat Res 1968;58:17–27.
7. Neer C. Nonunion of the clavicle. JAMA 1960;172:96–101.
8. Nordqvist A, Redlund-Johnell I, Von Scheele A, et al. Shortening of clavicle after fracture, incidence and clinical significance, a 5-year follow-up of 85 patients. Acta Orthop Scand 1997;68:349–351.
9. Rowe C. An atlas of anatomy and treatment of midclavicular fractures. Clin Orthop Relat Res 1968;58:29–42.
10. Stanley D, Trowbridge EA, Norris SH. The mechanism of clavicle fracture: a clinical and biomechanical analysis. J Bone Joint Surg Br 1988;70B:461–464.

Chapter 16

Percutaneous Pinning for Proximal Humerus Fractures

Leesa M. Galatz

DEFINITION

- *Proximal humerus fractures* are defined as those of the proximal portion of the humerus involving the shoulder joint.
- *Fracture lines* divide the proximal humerus into parts defined by anatomic structures that arise from early centers of ossification.
  - These "parts" first were described by Codman, and led to development of the Neer classification,[6] which is commonly used today.
  - The parts refer to the head of the humerus, the greater tuberosity, the lesser tuberosity, and the shaft (**FIG 1**).
  - Proximal humerus fractures are classified as two-, three-, or four-part fractures according to the Neer classfication.[6]
- Displacement of a "part" is classically defined as 1 cm of displacement or 45 degrees of angulation. Importantly, displacement is not necessarily an indication for surgery, but only a criterion for classification.
  - The type of fracture and degree of displacement, as well as patient considerations, all factor into surgical decision-making.

ANATOMY

- The proximal humerus arises from four distinct centers of ossification: the humeral head, the greater tuberosity, the lesser tuberosity, and the shaft.
  - The greater tuberosity has three distinct facets for the insertion of the supraspinatus, the infraspinatus, and the teres minor muscles of the rotator cuff.
- The lesser tuberosity is the insertion site for the subscapularis muscle.
- The rotator interval lies between the upper subscapularis and the anterior border of the supraspinatus.
  - The long head of the biceps tendon lies in a shallow groove on the anterior proximal humerus and enters the glenohumeral joint at the rotator interval.
  - The proximal 3 cm of the long head of the biceps tendon lies deep to the interval tissue intra-articularly.
- The anterior humeral circumflex artery (**FIG 2**) courses laterally along the inferior subscapularis.
  - The anterolateral branch of the anterior humeral circumflex artery travels superiorly along the lateral aspect of the biceps groove and enters the humeral head at the proximal-most aspect of the groove, providing about 85% of the blood supply to the humeral head.[1]
- The posterior humeral circumflex artery gives off several small branches that run adjacent to the inferior capsule of the shoulder, providing most of the remaining blood supply.
- The pectoralis major muscle inserts on the proximal shaft of the humerus lateral to the long head of the biceps tendon. The latissimus dorsi muscle inserts onto the proximal shaft medial to the biceps groove.

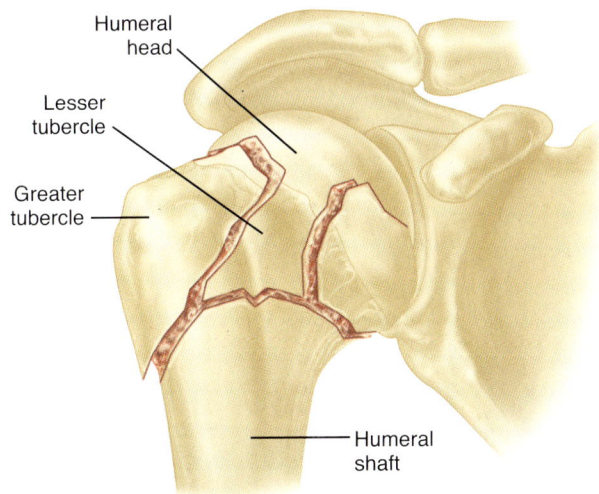

FIG 1 • Fractures of the proximal humerus are classified as two-, three-, or four-part fractures based on fracture and degree of displacement of the greater tuberosity, the lesser tuberosity, the humeral head, and the humeral shaft.

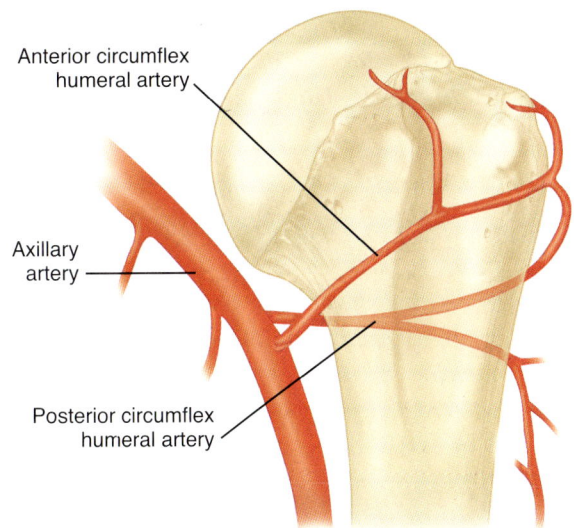

FIG 2 • The rotator interval lies between the upper border of the subscapularis and the anterior border of the supraspinatus. The biceps tendon runs deep to the rotator interval tissue. Importantly, the fracture line between the greater and lesser tuberosities lies just posterior to the biceps groove. The ascending branch of the anterior humeral circumflex artery provides 85% of the blood supply to the humeral head.

PATHOGENESIS

- Proximal humerus fractures occur in a bimodal distribution.
  - Most proximal humerus fractures are "fractures of senescence" in older individuals with age-related osteopenia. They commonly result from low-energy injures such as tripping and falling.
  - They also occur in younger individuals as the result of high-energy injuries such as motorcycle or automobile accidents.
- Associated nerve injuries can occur and usually resolve spontaneously. Axillary nerve neurapraxia is the most common.

NATURAL HISTORY

- Eighty-five percent of proximal humerus fractures can be treated nonoperatively.[6]
- Displacement at the surgical neck is better tolerated than displacement at the greater tuberosity.
  - Because of the vast range of motion (ROM) of the shoulder in multiple planes, the arm can compensate for translational displacement or angulation at the surgical neck.
  - Displacement of the tuberosities, however, affects the mechanics of the rotator cuff and is very poorly tolerated.
- Four-part fractures have an extremely high incidence of avascular necrosis—45% in Neer's classic series—with the exception of valgus impacted four-part fractures, in which the incidence is only 11%.[7]
  - In most four-part fractures, the blood supply from the anterior humeral circumflex artery is disrupted, contributing to the high incidence of avascular necrosis.
  - The blood supply is maintained in most valgus impacted fractures by the branches from the posterior humeral circumflex artery along the intact medial periosteal hinge (**FIG 3**), making this particular fracture configuration very amenable to fixation.

PATIENT HISTORY AND PHYSICAL FINDINGS

- A complete history of injury is important to determine the mechanism of injury. It is helpful to differentiate low-energy from high-energy injuries.
  - Elderly individuals often sustain proximal humerus fractures as the result of low-energy injuries such as slipping and falling. These injuries often are very amenable to minimally invasive fixation techniques, because the displacement is manageable and the periosteal sleeve between fracture fragments often is intact. The rotator cuff often is intact as

a sleeve. All these qualities facilitate minimally invasive reduction and fixation techniques.
  - In younger individuals, proximal humerus fractures often result from higher-energy injuries. These fractures commonly have greater fracture fragment displacement, rotator cuff tears between the tuberosities, and disruption of the periosteal sleeve. These factors do not necessarily preclude percutaneous pinning, but make it more challenging and should be considered in preoperative planning.
- Other important aspects of the history include:
  - Previous history of injury to the affected shoulder
  - Previous shoulder function
  - History of numbness or tingling in the affected extremity
- Rule out elbow and wrist fractures, especially in osteoporotic patients with injuries resulting from a fall on an outstretched arm.
- Patients often hold the shoulder inferior on the affected side.
- Examination should include skin integrity, presence of ecchymosis, downward carriage of shoulder girdle, and deformity consistent with shoulder dislocation or acromioclavicular joint separation.
- Examine for possible associated nerve injury (usually neurapraxia) by testing sensation to light touch in individual nerve distribution, two-point discrimination, and muscle strength (testing is limited to isometric at shoulder because of limited ROM and pain).
- Possible associated vascular injury can be determined by testing radial pulse and capillary refill.

IMAGING AND OTHER DIAGNOSTIC STUDIES

- A trauma series of radiographs of the shoulder should be obtained (**FIG 4**).
  - The series includes an AP view of the shoulder, a scapular AP view, a scapular Y view, and an axillary view.
  - A complete series with these views allows the fracture configuration to be determined in sufficient detail.
- A CT scan is helpful in many cases and should be obtained if there is any question regarding the extent of fracture involvement or the level of displacement of the fragments. It also is helpful if there is any question of joint dislocation or glenoid fracture.
- Radiographs are used to determine whether the fracture is a two-, three-, or four-part fracture and to assess the degree of displacement.

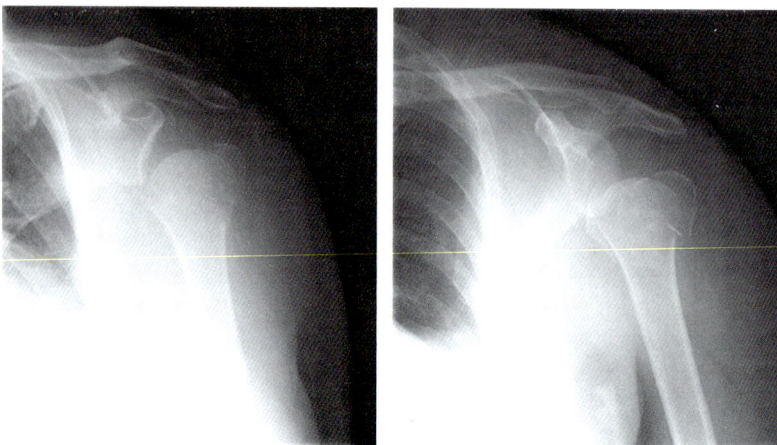

FIG 3 • Valgus impacted fractures maintain blood supply to the articular surface via ascending branches off the posterior humeral circumflex artery along the intact medial periosteal hinge.

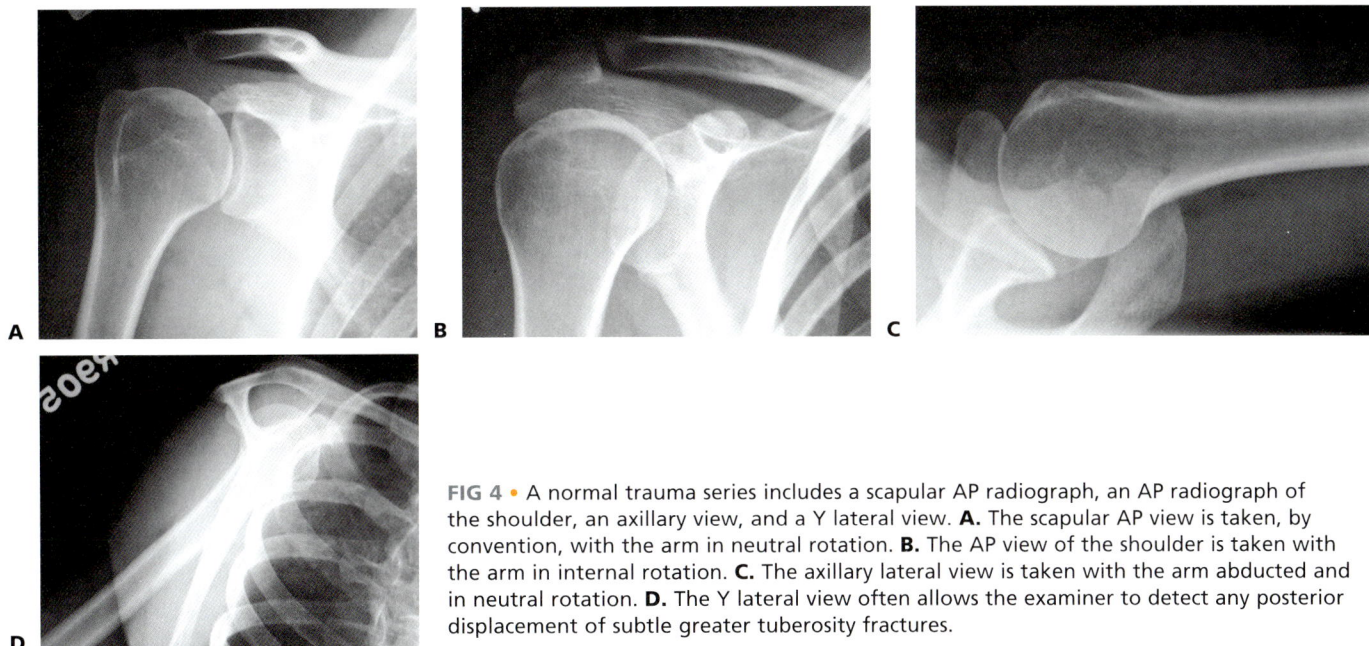

FIG 4 • A normal trauma series includes a scapular AP radiograph, an AP radiograph of the shoulder, an axillary view, and a Y lateral view. **A.** The scapular AP view is taken, by convention, with the arm in neutral rotation. **B.** The AP view of the shoulder is taken with the arm in internal rotation. **C.** The axillary lateral view is taken with the arm abducted and in neutral rotation. **D.** The Y lateral view often allows the examiner to detect any posterior displacement of subtle greater tuberosity fractures.

■ Three-dimensional reconstructions of the CT scan can be helpful in fracture evaluation, but are not routinely required.

DIFFERENTIAL DIAGNOSIS

■ Acromioclavicular joint separation
■ Glenohumeral joint dislocation
■ Humeral shaft fracture
■ Scapulothoracic dissociation
■ Elbow and wrist fractures (may coexist)

NONOPERATIVE MANAGEMENT

■ Minimally displaced fractures can be treated nonoperatively.
■ Displacement at the surgical neck is well tolerated.
  ■ An AP view of the shoulder can be misleading in the case of a surgical neck fracture.
    ■ The pectoralis major muscle exerts an anterior force on the shaft, resulting in anterior displacement of the shaft relative to the humeral head.
  ■ A scapular Y or axillary view can exhibit this angular deformity.
■ Displacement of the greater tuberosity is less well tolerated.
  ■ Historically, 1 cm of displacement has been used as the criterion for clinically significant tuberosity displacement.
  ■ Recently, however, even 5 mm of displacement has been considered an operative indication.
■ Patients wear a sling for 2 to 3 weeks or until the proximal humerus feels stable with gentle internal or external rotation of the arm.
  ■ Patients should be instructed to remove the sling for elbow and hand ROM to avoid stiffness of these joints.
  ■ Early signs of healing (eg, callus formation) also are helpful indicators of when it is safe to commence ROM exercises.
■ In borderline instances, it is better to err toward a longer period of immobilization to ensure healing, because shoulder stiffness is easier to address than a nonunion.
■ Therapy begins with passive stretching until 6 weeks when active ROM and strengthening can be started, progressing as tolerated.

SURGICAL MANAGEMENT
Preoperative Planning

■ All imaging studies should be reviewed carefully to determine the type of fracture, the degree of displacement, fracture configuration, and bone quality.
■ Certain radiographic findings that can suggest that minimally invasive fracture fixation is not appropriate for a given fracture are as follows:
  ■ *Poor bone quality.* The bone may not hold the pins and screws well and may be better treated with a more stable construct.
  ■ *Comminution of the greater tuberosity.* A comminuted bone fragment is not amenable to fixation with screws. Fractures with a comminuted greater tuberosity require suture fixation through the tendon–bone junction (required open approach).
  ■ *Comminution of the medial calcar region* leads to unstable reduction of the head onto the shaft.
■ Fractures amenable to minimally invasive fixation are two-part, three-part, and valgus impacted four-part fractures with:
  ■ Good bone quality
  ■ Substantial fracture fragments with minimal comminution of the tuberosities
  ■ Minimal or no comminution at the medial calcar region
■ Minimally invasive fixation is not appropriate for noncompliant or unreliable patients. This procedure should be performed only in patients committed to consistent follow-up in the postoperative period.
  ■ The pins require close surveillance in the early postoperative period.
  ■ Pin migration is possible and must be caught early in order to avoid potential injury to thoracic structures.

Positioning

■ Percutaneous pinning is performed with the patient in the straight supine or 10- to 15-degree beach chair position (**FIG 5**).
  ■ This allows easy intraoperative evaluation with C-arm fluoroscopy.

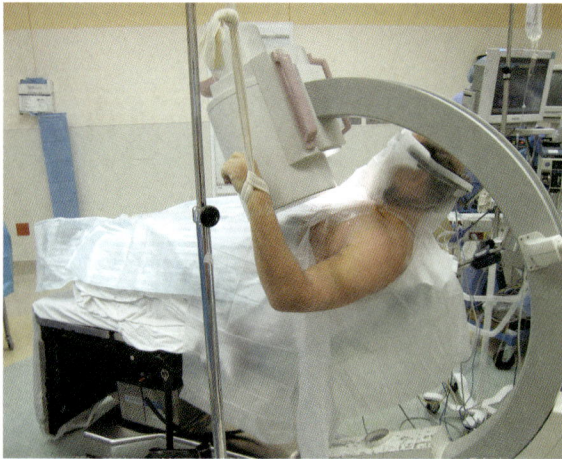

FIG 5 • The patient is placed in the supine or gently upright position. The C-arm is brought in parallel to the patient, leaving the lateral aspect of the arm free for instrumentation. The patient should be positioned laterally on the table such that an adequate fluoroscopic view can be obtained.

- The C-arm fluoroscope is placed parallel to the patient, extending over the shoulder from the cephalad direction.
  - This position leaves the lateral shoulder completely accessible for instrumentation and pin fixation.
- The patient must be positioned far lateral on the table or on a specialized shoulder surgery positioning device such that the shoulder can be imaged in the anteroposterior plane without the table obstructing the view.
  - This image should be checked before prepping and draping to confirm adequate visualization.
- The entire upper extremity is draped free.

Approach

- Closed fracture reductions are performed with the aid of a "reduction portal" (**FIG 6**).[2]
  - The reduction portal is a portal (analogous to that of an arthroscopic portal) or small incision used to access the fracture fragments.
  - Instruments can be introduced through this portal to lever fracture fragments or pull fragments into reduced position.
  - The surgeon also can insert a finger through this portal to palpate fragments.
    - Medially, the biceps tendon can be palpated.
    - The surgical neck fracture is located just deep to the portal.
    - By sweeping posterior and superior, the greater tuberosity and its extent of displacement can be palpated.
- The location of the reduction portal is critical (**FIG 6B**).
  - In three- and four-part fractures, the fracture line of the greater tuberosity is reliably 0.5 to 1 cm posterior and lateral to the biceps groove.
  - Therefore, the reduction portal is located at the level of the surgical neck and 1 cm posterior to the biceps groove.

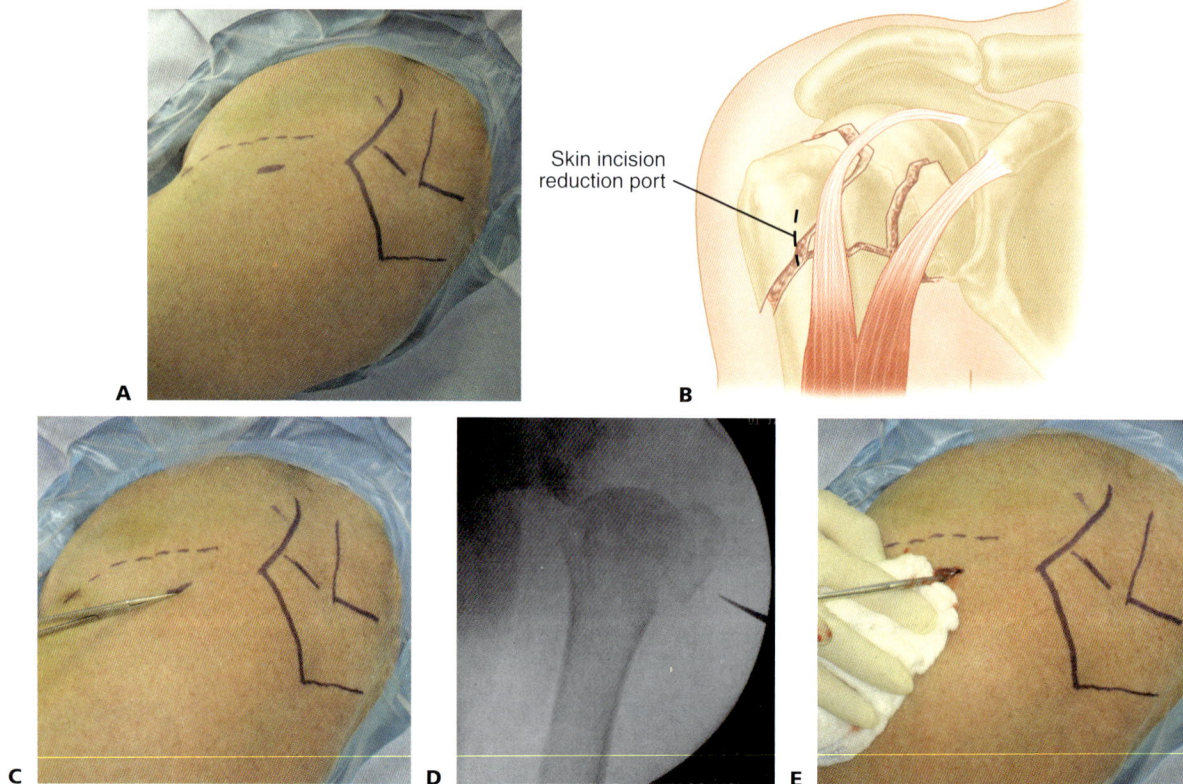

Skin incision reduction port

FIG 6 • **A.** The reduction portal is established off the anterolateral corner of the acromion. Instruments can be introduced through this portal to help reduce the fracture. **B.** The reduction portal is located at the level of the surgical neck fracture approximately 0.5 to 1 cm posterior to the biceps groove. The reduction portal is definitively localized using C-arm imagery. A hemostat is applied to the skin (**C**) and then imaged (**D**) to confirm that this portal will be directly at the level of the surgical neck fracture. **E.** A small incision is made in the skin, and the deltoid is spread bluntly to avoid injury to the underlying axillary nerve.

- The arm is held in neutral rotation.
  - The level of the surgical neck is located using fluoroscopic imagery (**FIG 6C,D**).
  - The location of the biceps tendon is estimated based on surface anatomic landmarks.

- A 2-cm incision is made in the skin (**FIG 6E**).
  - Subcutaneous tissues and the deltoid muscle are spread bluntly using a straight hemostat to avoid injury to the axillary nerve on the deep surface of the deltoid. Subdeltoid adhesions are gently released by sweeping finger if necessary.

TECHNIQUES

SURGICAL NECK FRACTURE

Reduction

- The pectoralis major muscle provides the major deforming force resulting in displacement of surgical neck fractures. The shaft usually is displaced anteriorly and medially with respect to the head.
  - An axillary or scapular Y radiograph is necessary to evaluate the extent of this displacement.
- The reduction maneuver involves flexion, adduction, and possibly some slight internal rotation to relax the pull of the pectoralis major muscle[3] (**TECH FIG 1**).
  - Longitudinal traction is applied to the arm, and a posteriorly directed force is applied to the proximal shaft of the humerus.
- A blunt instrument can be inserted into the fracture at the surgical neck to lever the head back onto the shaft. This maneuver can be a powerful reduction tool, but care should be used to avoid further damage or fracture to the humeral head during this maneuver, especially on osteopenic patients.
  - The long head of the biceps tendon can become interposed between the fracture fragments, precluding reduction. Therefore, if reduction is not achieved, check the biceps tendon through the reduction portal (or consider open reduction).

Fixation

- Two or three retrograde pins are placed from the shaft into the humeral head (**TECH FIG 2**).
  - The starting point for the pins is approximately 5 to 6 cm distal to the surgical neck fracture line.

- The pins must angle steeply to enter the head fragment and not cut out posteriorly (**TECH FIG 2B,C**).
- Pins should be smooth to avoid injury to soft tissue upon insertion, and terminally threaded to avoid backing out.
- 2.5- or 2.7-mm smooth, terminally threaded pins commonly are found in external fixation or 7.3-mm cannulated screw sets of instruments.
- The pins should enter at different directions to enhance stability of fixation construct.
  - One pin should enter lateral to the biceps in a primarily anterior-to-posterior direction.
  - Another pin should enter further laterally in a primarily lateral-to-medial direction.
- Stability should be checked under fluoroscopic imaging with live, gentle internal and external rotation.

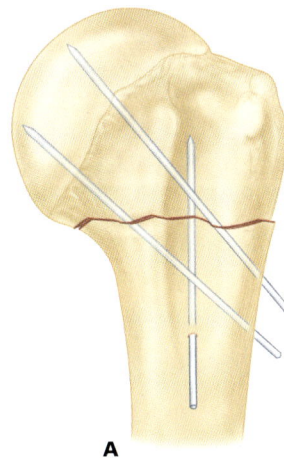

A

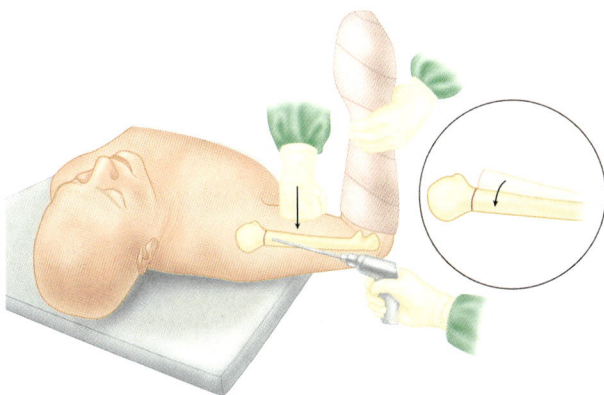

TECH FIG 1 • The reduction maneuver for surgical neck fractures involves flexion and internal rotation of the arm to negate the effect of the pectoralis major fragment on the proximal aspect of the shaft. Often a posterior vector must be applied to the shaft or an instrument can be introduced through the reduction portal to lever the head back onto the shaft.

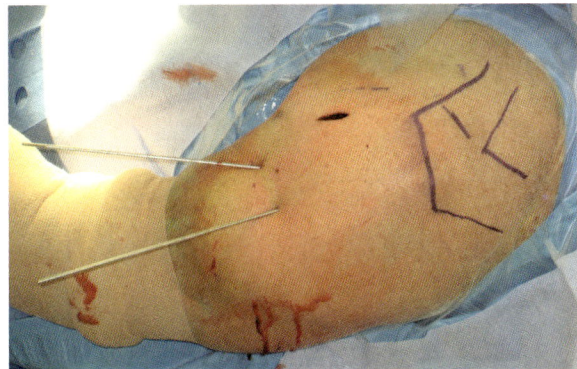

B

TECH FIG 2 • A. Retrograde pins are introduced several centimeters below the level of the surgical neck fracture into the head. The pins should be placed in different directions to provide stability to the construct. **B.** Placement of two pins. *(continued)*

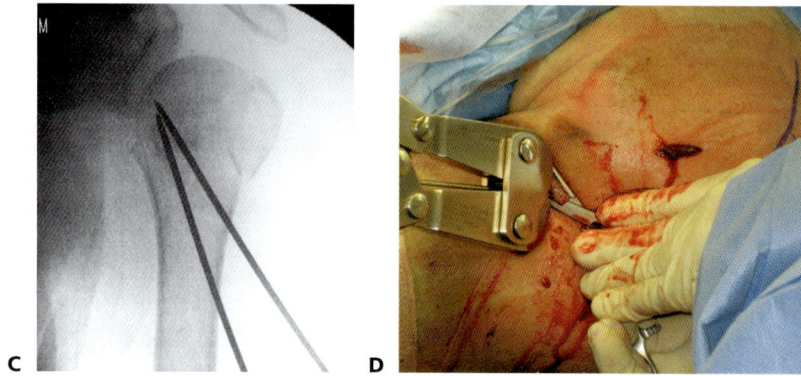

TECH FIG 2 • *(continued)* **C.** Fluoroscopic view of two retrograde pins in place. **D.** The pins should be cut below the skin after insertion to prevent pin site infection. They are easily removed a couple of weeks later with a small procedure in the office or operating room.

- Any suggestion of instability or motion at the fracture is an indication for open reduction and plate fixation at that point.
- Pins are cut below the skin to prevent pin site infection (**TECH FIG 2D**).

- The reduction portal is closed with interrupted nylon sutures.
- A soft dressing and sling are applied.

THREE-PART GREATER TUBEROSITY FRACTURES

Reduction

- Deforming forces influencing displacement of three-part fractures include the pectoralis major, as described earlier, and the rotator cuff muscles. The rotator cuff pulls the tuberosity medially (to a certain extent) and posteriorly. Posterior displacement and rotation often are underappreciated and must be considered.
- The surgical neck component is addressed first. (See Surgical Neck Fractures earlier in this section).
- The greater tuberosity fracture is reduced using the "reduction portal." A dental pick or small hooked instrument is inserted through the portal to engage the tuberosity and pull it inferior and anterior into a reduced position.

Fixation

- 4.5-mm cannulated screws are used to fix the tuberosity fragment.
  - The screw is placed through the tuberosity fragment distal to the cuff insertion through bone on the lateral cortex (**TECH FIG 3A**).
  - The proper location is confirmed with fluoroscopic imaging.
- The guidewire is first passed through a small incision in the skin just large enough to pass the drill guide and screw through the deltoid (**TECH FIG 3B,C**).
  - The guidewire is passed through the tuberosity, across the surgical neck fracture, and engages the medial cortex of the proximal humeral shaft.

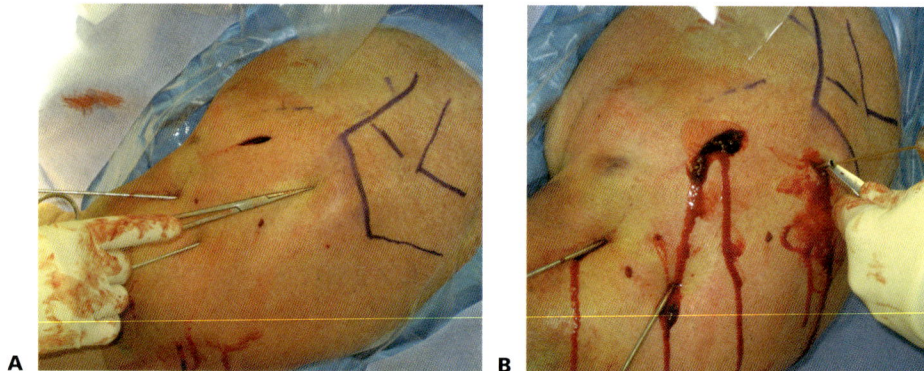

TECH FIG 3 • **A.** The greater tuberosity is localized under fluoroscopy using a hemostat. **B.** A small incision is made over the greater tuberosity, and a cannulated screw is used for fixation. This photograph demonstrates the drill guide used for soft tissue protection. *(continued)*

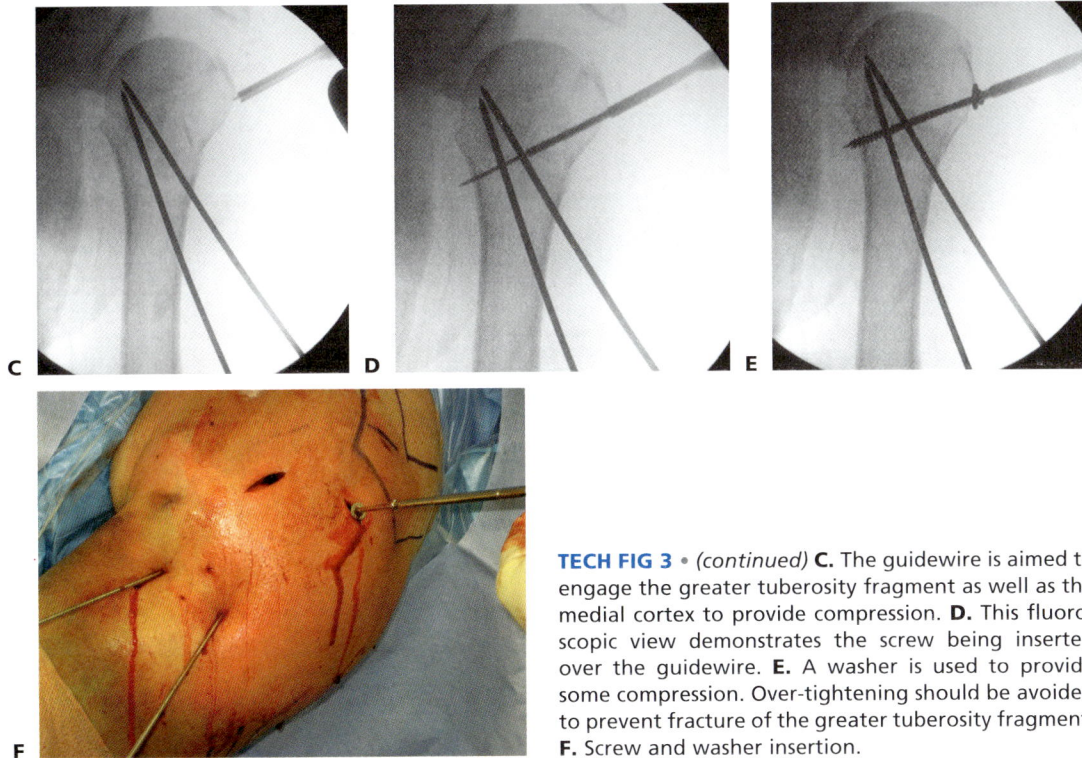

TECH FIG 3 • *(continued)* **C.** The guidewire is aimed to engage the greater tuberosity fragment as well as the medial cortex to provide compression. **D.** This fluoroscopic view demonstrates the screw being inserted over the guidewire. **E.** A washer is used to provide some compression. Over-tightening should be avoided to prevent fracture of the greater tuberosity fragment. **F.** Screw and washer insertion.

- After the guidewire is overdrilled, the screw is passed over the guidewire. We use a partially threaded screw with a washer (**TECH FIG 3D–F**).
- If the greater tuberosity fragment is large enough, a second cancellous screw is directed through the tuberosity fragment, engaging cancellous bone of the humeral head.
- Pins are cut beneath the skin.
- Incisions are closed with nylon interrupted sutures.
- A dressing and sling are applied.

VALGUS IMPACTED FOUR-PART PROXIMAL HUMERUS FRACTURES

- Valgus impacted fractures are recognized by the 90-degree angle between the long axis of the humeral shaft and the articular surface of the humeral head with loss of the normal neck shaft angle.[4] The tuberosities are displaced laterally from the head of the humerus and slightly proximally.
  - This fracture configuration results in a low incidence of avascular necrosis compared to that of other four-part fractures, because the medial periosteal hinge of soft tissues is intact along the medial and posterior anatomic neck, preserving the blood supply provided by the posterior humeral circumflex artery and its ascending vessels.
- The reduction maneuver for this fracture requires raising the humeral head back into its anatomic position.
  - The reduction portal described previously is created, and an instrument such as a blunt elevator or small bone tamp is inserted beneath the humeral head (**TECH FIG 4A,B**).
  - The instrument passes through the surgical neck fracture and through the fracture line between the tuberosities, which reliably exists 0.5 to 1 cm posterior and lateral to the biceps groove.

- The instrument is tapped with a mallet in a distal-to-proximal direction, lifting the head fragment into anatomic position (**TECH FIG 4C**).
- The surgical neck fractures and tuberosity fractures are then fixed using the techniques described earlier.

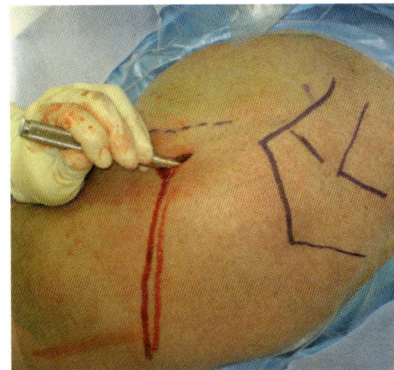

TECH FIG 4 • **A.** Valgus impacted proximal humerus fractures are reduced using a small bone tamp or other blunt-tipped instrument. *(continued)*

TECHNIQUES

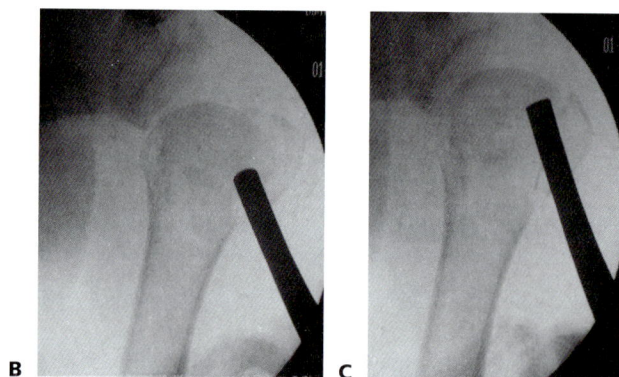

TECH FIG 4 • *(continued)* **B.** The instrument is inserted through the fracture line between the greater tuberosity and the lesser tuberosity, which lies posterior to the biceps groove. Position is confirmed with fluoroscopic imaging. **C.** The bone tamp is impacted in a superior direction, bringing the humeral head into a reduced position. The greater and lesser tuberosities fall naturally into a reduced position after this reduction maneuver.

- In some cases, there may be significant medial displacement of the lesser tuberosity. In these cases, the lesser tuberosity is reduced using the hook through the reduction portal and fixed with a screw placed in the anterior-to-posterior direction through the tuberosity into the head.

- In most cases, minimal medial displacement of the lesser tuberosity is well tolerated and no fixation is required.
- Pins are cut beneath the skin.
- Incisions are closed with nylon sutures.
- A dressing and sling are applied.

PEARLS AND PITFALLS

Indications	▪ Successful percutaneous pinning depends on appropriate patient selection. Criteria include good bone stock, minimal to no comminution at the greater tuberosity fragment, minimal to no comminution at the medial calcar and proximal shaft, and patient compliance. ▪ Contraindications include poor bone stock that will not hold pins, comminution of greater tuberosity or proximal shaft fragments, and a noncompliant patient with poor follow-up potential.
Positioning	▪ The patient must be lateral enough on the table to obtain unencumbered access to the shoulder and clear fluoroscopic images.
Reduction technique	▪ The location of the reduction portal is critical for maximizing its usefulness during the procedure. ▪ The surgeon must have a thorough understanding of three-dimensional anatomy, as well as interpretation and application of two-dimensional fluoroscopic images.
Pin placement	▪ Pins should engage the humerus distal to the axillary nerve, but proximal to the deltoid insertion to avoid nerve injury. ▪ The angle of insertion is steep to enter the humeral head and avoid cutting out posteriorly. ▪ At least two fluoroscopic images in different planes are necessary to confirm successful pin placement. ▪ A drill guide can be used to protect the soft tissues during pin insertion.
Screw placement	▪ The deltoid should be spread bluntly and a drill guide used to prevent injury to the axillary nerve in this location. In most cases, insertion will be proximal to the nerve, but precautionary measures should be taken. ▪ Overtightening the screw with a washer may result in fracture of the greater tuberosity. ▪ Engaging medial cortex of the proximal shaft gives stability to the screw construct.
Intraoperative assessment of stability	▪ The arm should be internally and externally rotated gently under continuous fluoroscopic imagery after completion of hardware placement. Any motion or suggestion of instability is an indication for open reduction and fixation.

POSTOPERATIVE CARE

- The operative arm is immobilized in a sling.
- The patient is instructed to begin active elbow, wrist, and hand ROM exercises.
- Radiographs are checked weekly to monitor for pin migration or loss of fixation.
  - Pins are removed as a short procedure in the office or operating room about 3 to 4 weeks postoperatively or when early signs of healing are evident radiographically.
- Pendulum exercises are initiated 2 to 3 weeks postoperatively, and passive stretching (forward elevation in scapular plane), external rotation, and internal rotation (all in supine position) is initiated when pins are removed.
  - Ideally, pins should be out and motion started no later than 4 weeks postoperatively.
- Active ROM progressing as tolerated to resistance exercises commences at 6 weeks postoperatively.

OUTCOMES

- Jaberg et al[3] reported good to excellent results in 38 of 48 fractures. There were 29 surgical neck, 3 anatomic neck, 8 three-part, and 5 four-part fractures.

- Resch et al[8] reported results of 9 three-part fractures and 18 four-part fractures. In the four-part fractures, the incidence of avascular necrosis was 11%. Good results correlated with anatomic reconstruction.

- Keener et al[5] reported a multicenter study of 35 patients—7 two-part, 8 three-part, and 12 valgus impacted fractures. Average duration of follow-up was 35 months. All fractures healed. American Shoulder and Elbow Surgeons and Constant scores were 83.4 and 73.9, respectively. Four patients had some residual malunion, and four developed posttraumatic arthritis. Neither of these affected outcome at this early follow-up period, however.

- Most studies report very satisfactory results with this procedure. Patient selection is critical. In published studies, patients are not randomized to percutaneous pinning, but, rather, careful patient selection is left to the treating surgeon. Therefore, it can be concluded that this is an appropriate technique in certain patients who meet the outlined criteria.

COMPLICATIONS

- Nerve injury[9]
- Pin migration
- Loss of fixation
- Malunion
- Nonunion
- Infection
- Glenohumeral joint stiffness

REFERENCES

1. Gerber C, Schneeberger AG, Vinh TS. The arterial vascularization of the humeral head. An anatomical study. J Bone Joint Surg Am 1990; 72A:1486–1494.
2. Hsu J, Galatz LM. Mini-incision fixation of proximal humeral four-part fractures. In Scuderi GR, Tria A, Berger RA, eds. MIS Techniques in Orthopedics. New York: Springer, 2006:32–44.
3. Jaberg H, Warner JJ, Jakob RP. Percutaneous stabilization of unstable fractures of the humerus. J Bone Joint Surg Am 1992;74A: 508–515.
4. Jakob RP, Miniaci A, Anson PS, et al. Four-part valgus impacted fractures of the proximal humerus. J Bone Joint Surg Br 1991;73B: 295–298.
5. Keener J, Parsons BO, Flatow EL, et al. Outcomes after percutaneous reduction and fixation of proximal humeral fractures. J Shoulder Elbow Surg 2007;16:330–338. Epub 2007 Feb 22.
6. Neer CS II. Displaced proximal humerus fractures. I. Classification and evaluation. J Bone Joint Surg Am 1970;52A:1077–1089.
7. Resch H, Beck A, Bayley I. Reconstruction of the valgus impacted humeral head fracture. J Shoulder Elbow Surg 1995;4:73–80.
8. Resch H, Povacz P, Frohlich R, et al. Percutaneous fixation of three- and four-part fractures of the proximal humerus. J Bone Joint Surg Br 1997;79B:295–300.
9. Rowles DJ, McGrory JE. Percutaneous pinning of the proximal humerus: An anatomic study. J Bone Joint Surg Am 2001;83A: 1695–1699.

Chapter 17

Open Reduction and Internal Fixation of Proximal Humerus Fractures

Mark T. Dillon and David L. Glaser

DEFINITION

- Proximal humerus fractures may involve the surgical neck, the greater tuberosity, or the lesser tuberosity.
- The Neer classification, which is most commonly used, categorizes fractures based on the number of displaced parts (**FIG 1**). This classification system involves four segments: the articular surface, the greater tuberosity, the lesser tuberosity, and the humeral shaft. Fracture fragments displaced 1 cm or angulated 45 degrees are considered displaced.[17,18]
- The AO/ASIF (Arbeitsgemeinschaft fuer Osteosynthesefragen–Association for the Study of Internal Fixation) broadly classifies fractures into three types: type 1, unifocal extra-articular; type 2, bifocal extra-articular, and type 3, intra-articular.
  - Each type is then further divided into groups and subgroups.[16]
  - This system places more emphasis on the vascular supply to the humerus, with intra-articular fracture patterns having the highest risk of avascular necrosis.[26]
- Studies have demonstrated that interobserver reliability for both classification systems is not high.[1,23,24]

- Although not included in Neer's original classification, valgus impacted fractures are a unique entity that is important to recognize:
  - Four-part fractures in which the humeral articular surface is impacted upon the shaft segment
  - Often minimally displaced owing to an intact rotator cuff[5]
  - Have a lower incidence of avascular necrosis, because the blood supply to the head is less likely to be disrupted

ANATOMY

- The osseous anatomy of the proximal humerus consists of the greater tuberosity, the lesser tuberosity, and the articular surface.
  - The subscapularis inserts onto the lesser tuberosity, whereas the supraspinatus, infraspinatus, and teres minor insert onto the greater tuberosity.
- Knowledge of deforming forces associated with humerus fracture allows the surgeon to better treat proximal humerus fractures by both operative and nonoperative means.
  - In a two-part surgical neck fracture, the pectoralis major pulls the humeral shaft anteromedial.
  - In a two-part greater tuberosity fracture, the pull of the supraspinatus, infraspinatus, and teres minor tendons displaces the greater tuberosity superiorly and/or posteriorly.

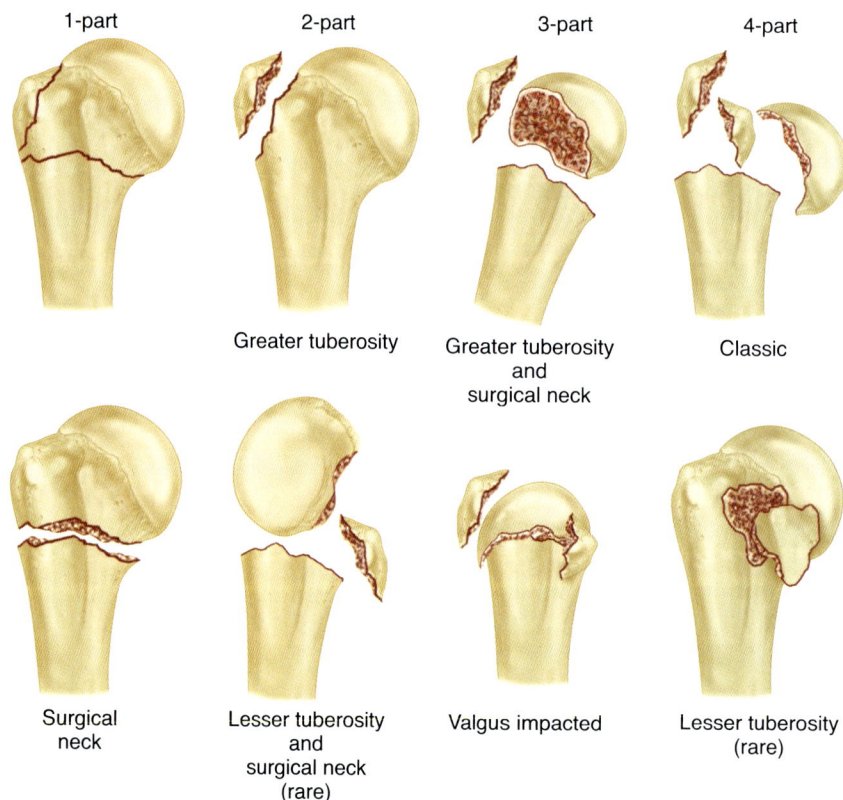

1-part	2-part	3-part	4-part
	Greater tuberosity	Greater tuberosity and surgical neck	Classic
Surgical neck	Lesser tuberosity and surgical neck (rare)	Valgus impacted	Lesser tuberosity (rare)

FIG 1 • Simplified Neer classification for fractures of the proximal humerus.

- With a three-part fracture involving the lesser tuberosity, the attachment site of these tendons into the greater tuberosity is intact, and the articular surface of the humeral head rotates externally to face anteriorly.
- Three-part fractures involving the greater tuberosity result in unopposed subscapularis function, and the humeral articular surface rotates posteriorly.
- Four-part fractures result in displacement of the shaft and both tuberosities, leaving a free head fragment with little soft tissue attachment.
- An understanding of the vascular anatomy is crucial to treat fractures of the proximal humerus effectively.
  - The main blood supply to the humeral head is the anterolateral ascending branch of the anterior circumflex artery.
  - This branch of the axillary artery runs just lateral to the bicipital groove, entering the humeral head at the proximal portion of the transition from bicipital groove to greater tuberosity.[9]
  - The intraosseous portion of this vessel, known as the *arcuate artery*, has been shown to supply the entire epiphyseal portion of the proximal humerus except for a small portion of the greater tuberosity and the posteroinferior humeral head, which is supplied by the posterior humeral circumflex artery.[9]

PATHOGENESIS

- In older patients, proximal humerus fractures usually result from a ground-level fall. Younger patients may sustain such an injury from a higher-energy mechanism such as an automobile collision or from sports.
- The presence of an associated glenohumeral dislocation also must be determined.

PATIENT HISTORY AND PHYSICAL FINDINGS

- On presentation, patients with proximal humerus fractures complain of pain in the shoulder that is made worse with attempted movement. Palpation of the proximal humerus results in diffuse pain.
- Visual inspection reveals ecchymosis and swelling of the arm.
- It is necessary to determine the stability of the fracture. If the shaft and the proximal portion move as a unit when taken through internal and external rotation, the fracture usually is stable. Unstable fractures will not move as a unit, and crepitus often is appreciated.
- If there is an associated dislocation, it may be possible to palpate the humeral head as an anterior fullness.
- It is crucial to perform a thorough neurovascular examination to determine the presence of associated injuries.
  - Patients over 50 years of age are more prone to nerve injuries. One study demonstrated nerve injury, usually of the axillary nerve, in nearly 40% of patients in this age group who sustained shoulder dislocations or surgical neck fractures.[2]

IMAGING AND OTHER DIAGNOSTIC STUDIES

- Initial imaging studies consist of anteroposterior, scapular Y, and axillary views.
  - Additional views also may include internal and external rotation views if the fracture pattern is stable. Internal rotation views help to visualize the lesser tuberosity, whereas external rotation shows the greater tuberosity.
  - Traction views also may prove helpful if tolerated by the patient.
- A CT scan may be helpful if radiographs do not demonstrate the fracture pattern adequately.
  - Studies have shown that the addition of a CT scan improves intraobserver reproducibility only minimally and does not affect interobserver reliability.[1]
  - However, CT scanning may prove valuable in determining the method of fixation as well as identifying associated injuries such as Hill-Sachs fractures and bony Bankart lesions.
- Indications for MRI are limited, although it may prove useful if there is any concern regarding soft tissue injuries, including the glenoid labrum and rotator cuff.

DIFFERENTIAL DIAGNOSIS

- Glenohumeral dislocation
- Scapula fracture
- Head-splitting fracture
- Clavicle fracture
- Humeral shaft fracture
- Neurovascular injury
- Neuropathic arthropathy

NONOPERATIVE MANAGEMENT

- Historically, conservative treatment usually is recommended for fractures with less than 1 cm of displacement and 45 degrees of angulation.[17] About 85% of proximal humerus fractures can be treated nonoperatively.[15] With newer fixation devices, however, indications for surgical management have been expanded. Whether a more aggressive approach leads to improved outcomes remains to be seen.
- There is less tolerance for displacement in isolated greater tuberosity fractures. It has been suggested that more than 5 mm of displacement leads to poor functional results.[14]
- For proximal humerus fractures not involving the humeral shaft, patients initially are immobilized in a simple sling.
  - When pain improves and the fracture moves as a unit, passive range of motion (ROM) is started. Patients begin with pendulum exercises, usually 2 to 3 weeks after injury, then progress to ROM in all planes.
  - Between 6 and 10 weeks, the fracture usually has healed enough that strengthening exercises may be started.[13]
- Physical therapy is very important when treating proximal humerus fractures conservatively. Koval et al[11] showed significant improvement with one-part fractures when physical therapy was initiated before 2 weeks.
- Several studies have shown that nonoperative management can lead to acceptable results with proximal humerus fractures.[22,25,28]
- Studies comparing patients treated surgically and nonsurgically have shown no difference in outcome with two-part surgical neck fractures[4] and displaced three- and four-part fractures,[27] although these studies were done before the advent of anatomic proximal humeral plating.

SURGICAL MANAGEMENT

- It is imperative that patients have reasonable expectations of their outcome following surgery. Patients also must be aware of the importance of physical therapy postoperatively.

Preoperative Planning

■ Acceptable imaging studies, either plain radiographs or a CT scan, are necessary before proceeding to surgery.

■ Each proximal humerus fracture is unique, and in most cases a planned method of fixation is chosen before entering the operating room. However, the definitive choice of fixation is not made until the fracture is visualized at surgery. Consequently, the surgeon should be prepared with an arsenal of different fixation techniques.

■ If the fracture is not deemed suitable for internal fixation intraoperatively, the surgeon must be prepared to perform a hemiarthoplasty.

■ Multiple techniques can be employed for surgical fixation of the proximal humerus. In this chapter, we describe several current techniques. The final choice of appropriate manner of fixation should be based on the individual patient, the fracture pattern, and the surgeon's own comfort level.

Positioning

■ The techniques discussed in this section are easiest to perform with the patient in the beach chair position. With the patient nearly seated, the hips and knees are flexed. The patient is moved as far laterally as possible on the table to allow full ROM of the shoulder. A lateral buttress is used to help keep the patient in position on the table.

■ C-arm fluoroscopy is helpful in determining the quality of reduction. The C-arm is best positioned with the intensifier posterior to the shoulder and the arm over the patient (**FIG 2**).

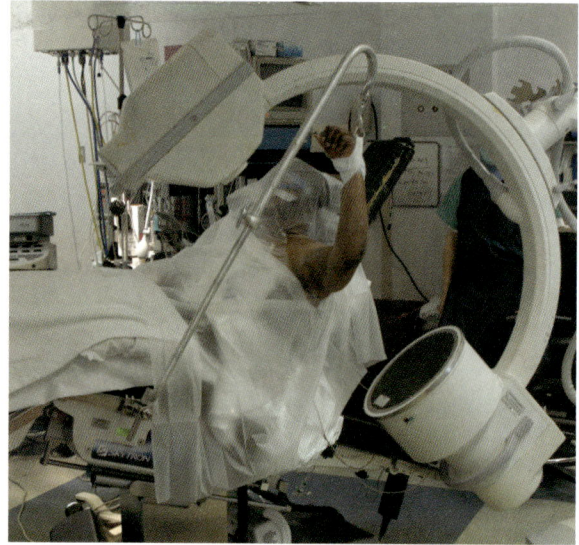

FIG 2 • Positioning of the patient in the beach chair position with fluoroscopic imaging. The C-arm intensifier should be posterior to allow for ideal visualization.

Approach

■ The approach depends on the surgical technique to be used and is discussed further in the Techniques section.

■ The deltopectoral approach is most commonly employed.

TECHNIQUES

FIXATION OF ISOLATED TUBEROSITY FRACTURES

■ The patient is placed in the beach chair position.

■ An incision is made from the tip of the acromion extending laterally down the arm.

■ Alternatively, an incision can be made parallel to the lateral border of the acromion, as used in open rotator cuff repair.

■ Skin flaps are then raised.

■ The deltoid is split in line with its fibers, and the anterior portion of the deltoid may be detached from the acromion.

■ A deltopectoral approach also could be used.

■ The deltoid fibers should not be split further than 5 cm below the acromion, to prevent damage to the axillary nerve. A suture at the distal aspect of the split can help prevent inadvertent extension.[10]

■ As with all open procedures described in this chapter, the fracture should be cleaned of hematoma to facilitate reduction.

■ The greater tuberosity usually is displaced posteriorly or superiorly. Abducting and externally rotating the shoulder will take tension off the posterosuperior rotator cuff, allowing the greater tuberosity fragment to be more easily reduced.

■ Traction sutures in the rotator cuff may prove valuable in obtaining reduction.

■ Provisional fixation can then be obtained with a K-wire (**TECH FIG 1A,B**).

■ Cannulated screws placed over the wire may then be used for definitive fixation if placed in an acceptable location.

■ Screws should be of the appropriate length to gain adequate purchase (**TECH FIG 1C,D**) but not so long that they are symptomatic.

■ The use of washers may prove beneficial.

■ Alternatively, suture fixation of the greater tuberosity back to the humerus may provide better fixation than cannulated screws in those patients with poor bone quality.

■ This can be accomplished by placing two suture anchors into the fracture bed (**TECH FIG 1E**).

■ Both limbs of each anchor can then be brought through drill holes in the fragment and tied over the top (**TECH FIG 1F**).

■ Suture also can be placed at the bone–tendon interface of the tuberosity fragment and then through bone tunnels in the shaft, as discussed later in this section.

■ If the anterior deltoid was detached during the approach, it must be repaired back to the acromion using nonabsorbable sutures.

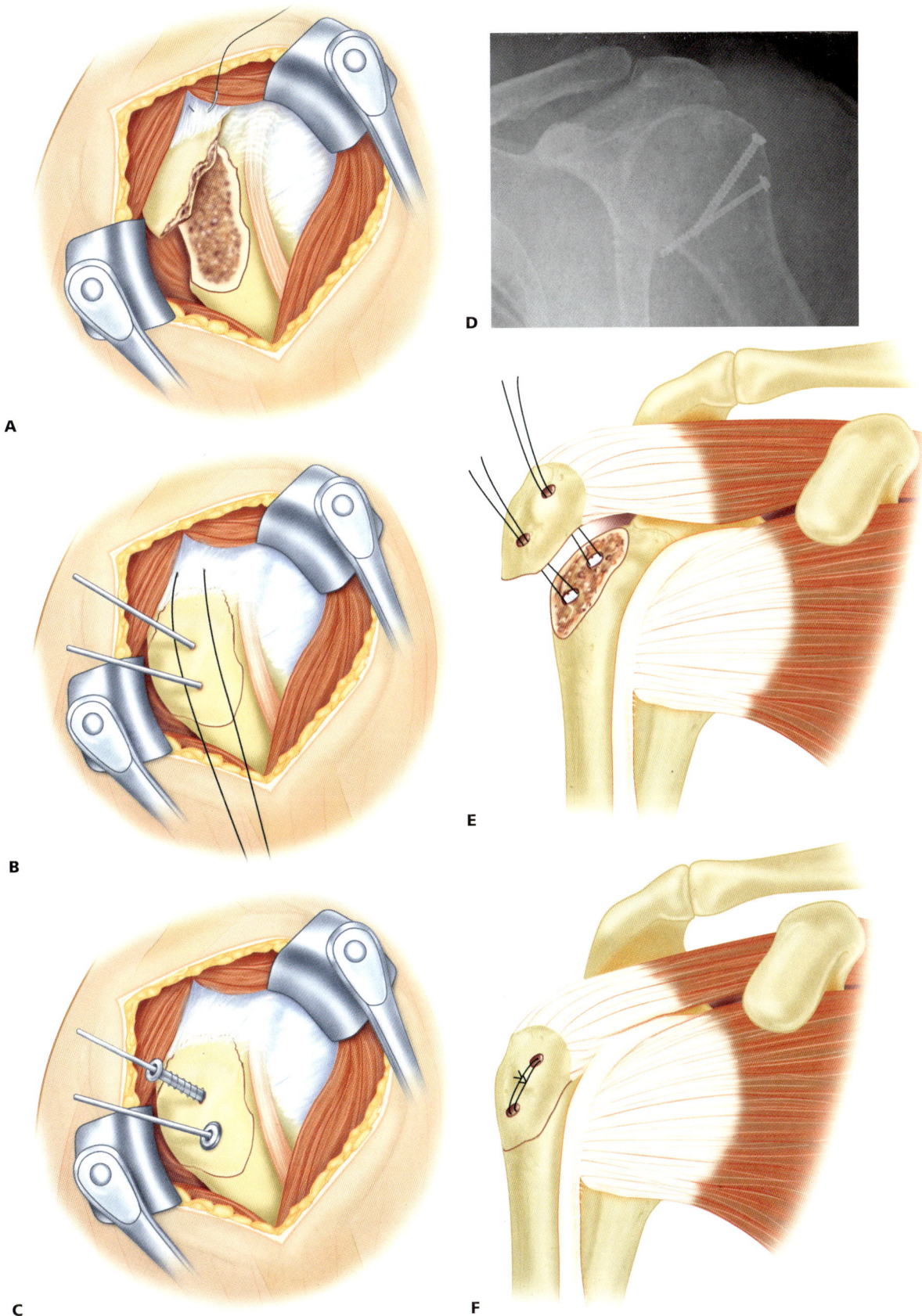

TECH FIG 1 • **A.** Traction sutures are placed through the rotator cuff tendon to aid in reduction of the displaced greater tuberosity. **B.** Wires may be used to maintain reduction of the tuberosity. **C.** Screw fixation with 4.5-mm cannulated screws. **D.** Final fixation. Screws should obtain purchase in the far cortex, but they must not be long enough to damage the axillary nerve. **E.** Placement of suture anchors into the fracture bed. **F.** Reduced fracture with sutures tied over the greater tuberosity.

TECHNIQUES

OPEN REDUCTION AND SUTURE FIXATION

- The patient is placed in the beach chair position. Depending on the pattern, the fracture may be approached via the deltopectoral interval or a deltoid-splitting approach.
- The rotator interval tissue may be incised. This "interval split" allows visualization of the humeral head articular surface, if needed, in the setting of intact tuberosities and rotator cuff, as with head split patterns.
- Multiple sutures are placed through the tendons of the rotator cuff, preferably no. 5 nonabsorbable sutures or 1-mm tapes.
  - Both the subscapularis tendon and the posterosuperior cuff tendons should be incorporated[20] (**TECH FIG 2A**).

- Drill holes should be placed distal to the fracture site. The bone on either side of the bicipital groove is of excellent quality and should hold sutures well (**TECH FIG 2B,C**).
- In most cases, anatomic reduction is desired.
- With three-part fractures involving the greater tuberosity, the head fragment should first be secured to the shaft, followed by reduction of the greater tuberosity.[20]
- For high surgical neck fractures, sutures should be placed into any remaining tuberosity on the head fragment to help maintain fixation.

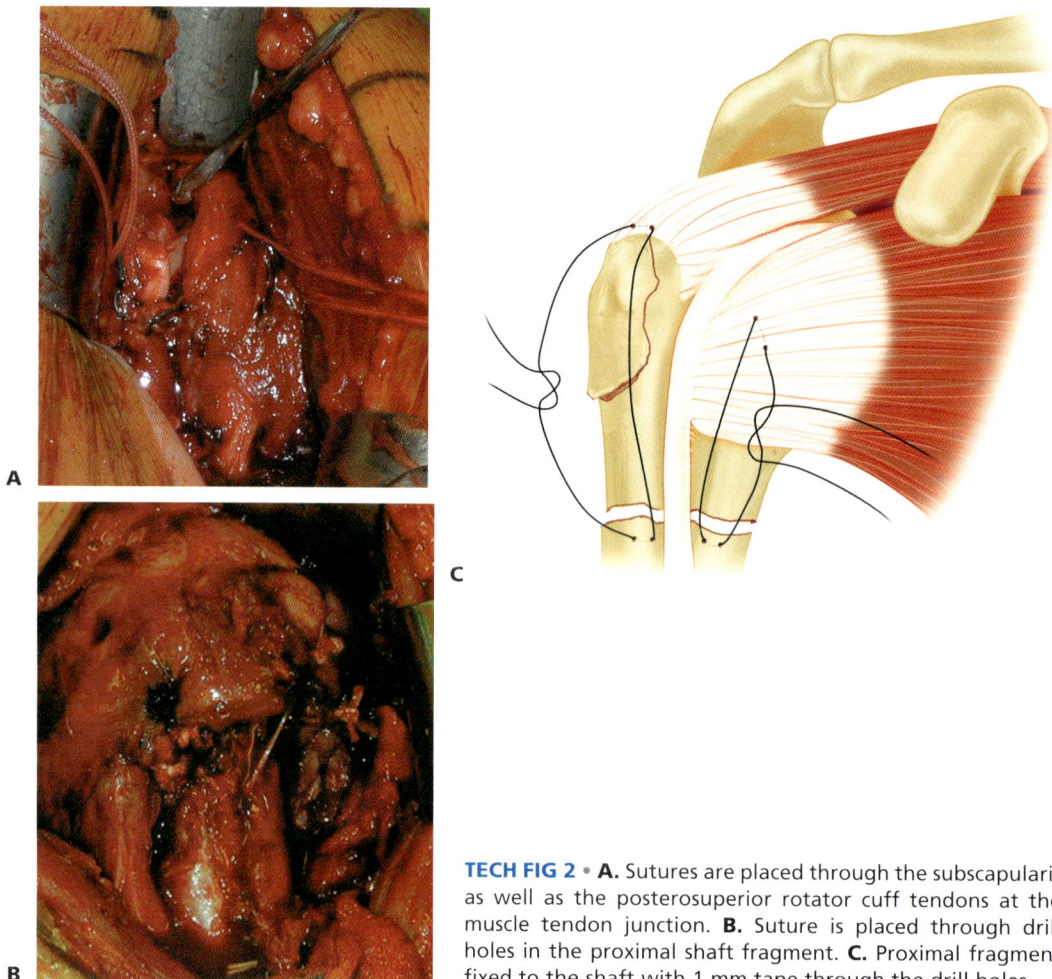

TECH FIG 2 • A. Sutures are placed through the subscapularis as well as the posterosuperior rotator cuff tendons at the muscle tendon junction. **B.** Suture is placed through drill holes in the proximal shaft fragment. **C.** Proximal fragment fixed to the shaft with 1 mm tape through the drill holes.

OPEN REDUCTION AND INTERNAL FIXATION USING ANATOMIC PLATING

Exposure

- Anatomic plating of the proximal humerus commonly is performed through the deltopectoral interval.
- With the patient in the beach chair position, an incision is made starting from above the coracoid process and

extending distally as needed along the deltopectoral groove (**TECH FIG 3A**).
- The plane between the deltoid and pectoralis major is developed, mobilizing the cephalic vein.
  - Cobb elevators can be used to develop this plane, making it easier for the surgeon to identify

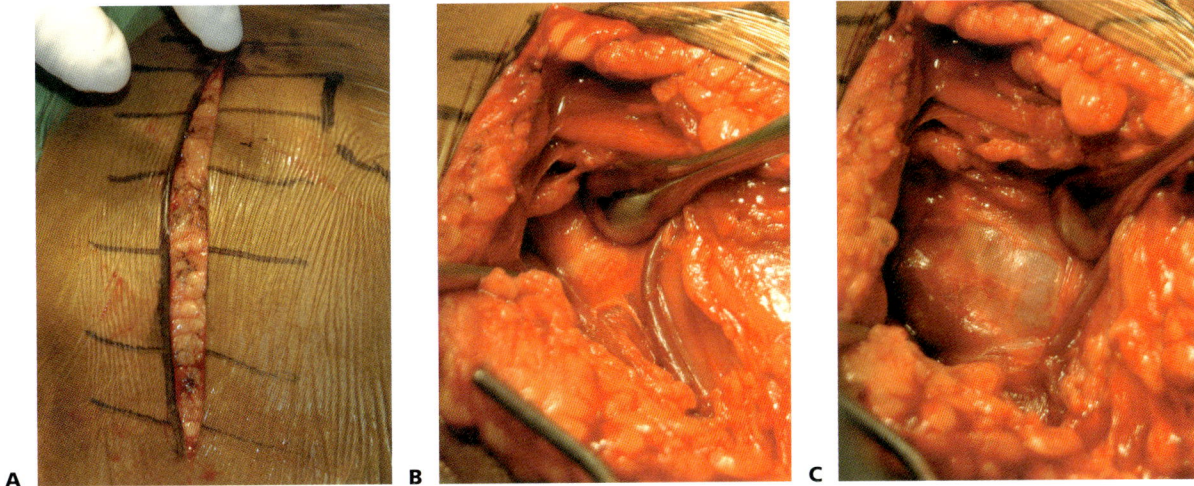

TECH FIG 3 • **A.** The incision is made extending from the coracoid process distally along the deltopectoral groove. **B.** Identifying the interval between the deltoid and pectoralis major. **C.** Using two Cobb elevators to develop the interval, bringing the cephalic vein laterally.

and ligate branches of the cephalic vein (**TECH FIG 3B,C**).

- The underlying clavipectoral fascia is identified and incised laterally to the conjoined tendon.[10]
  - The conjoined tendon is carefully retracted medially with the pectoralis major and the deltoid retracted laterally.

Reduction

- The fracture and rotator cuff are now visible. With fractures involving displaced tuberosities, we recommend obtaining control of the tuberosities with sutures placed at the bone–tendon interface (**TECH FIG 4A**).
  - Heavy sutures may be placed through the insertions of the cuff tendons and later used as supplemental fixation if necessary.
  - For fractures with minimally displaced tuberosities, sutures may not be needed before a reduction maneuver.

- A Cobb elevator placed in the fracture site will aid in reducing the fracture (**TECH FIG 4B**).
  - The pectoralis major insertion is elevated in a subperiosteal fashion if necessary. The plate should be placed lateral to the biceps tendon so as not to disrupt the blood supply to the humeral head (**TECH FIG 4C**).
  - Often, it may be necessary to release a small portion of the anterior deltoid insertion before placing the plate.

Plate Fixation

- Fluoroscopy should be used to confirm the reduction before placement of the plate, especially in regard to the superior aspect of the plate.
  - A plate positioned too high or a fracture fixed in varus may result in the plate impinging on the undersurface of the acromion. K-wires may be used to temporarily maintain fixation proximally and distally.
  - Alternatively, multiple guidewires may be placed into drill sleeves (**TECH FIG 5A**). Confirm plate location

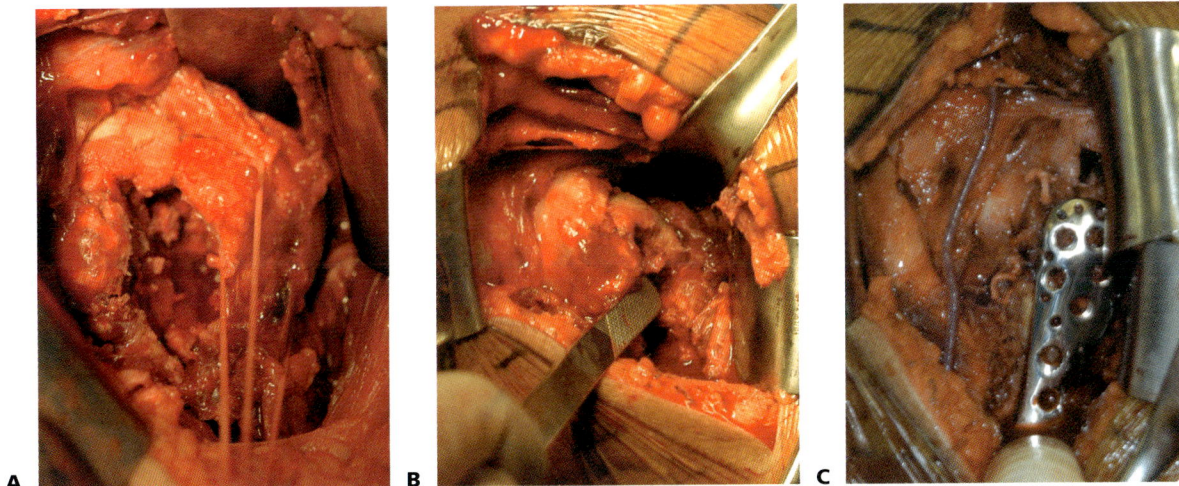

TECH FIG 4 • **A.** Traction sutures through the tendinous attachments of the rotator cuff may be helpful in correcting varus deformity. **B.** Reducing the fracture by elevating the proximal fragment. **C.** Correct placement of the plate is lateral to the biceps tendon (not seen here). Suture fixation has been used to help maintain fixation and supplement the plate.

TECHNIQUES

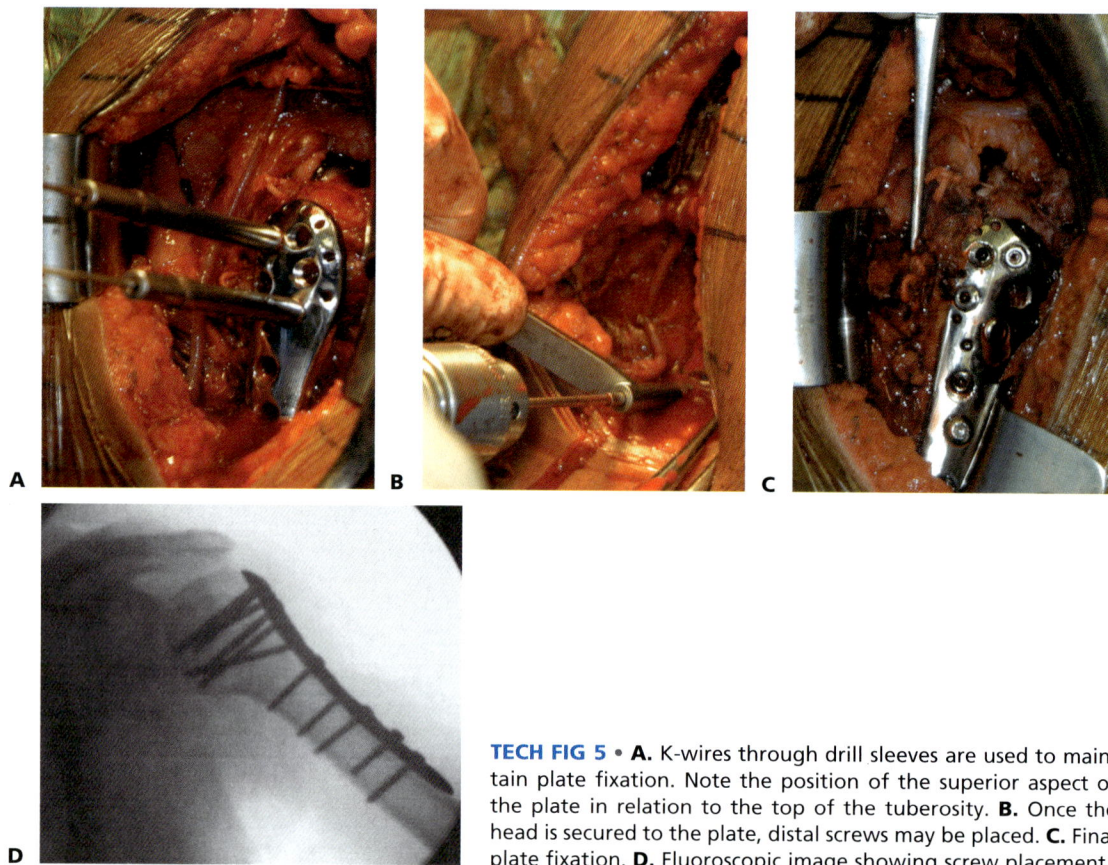

TECH FIG 5 • A. K-wires through drill sleeves are used to maintain plate fixation. Note the position of the superior aspect of the plate in relation to the top of the tuberosity. **B.** Once the head is secured to the plate, distal screws may be placed. **C.** Final plate fixation. **D.** Fluoroscopic image showing screw placement.

again, both proximally and distally, before placing screws.

- Locking screws usually are placed proximally into the head first, and multiple configurations of screws are possible.
  - Once the head is secured to the shaft, distal screws can be placed (**TECH FIG 5B**).
  - Final plate placement should be confirmed fluoroscopically (**TECH FIG 5C,D**).
- Sutures placed through the cuff tendons also may be secured to the plate, shaft, or other tuberosity.
  - At the completion of the procedure, the pectoralis major may be secured with sutures through holes in the plate.

- In osteoporotic bone, the tuberosities can first be attached to the shaft with sutures, following which a locking plate may be placed along the lateral aspect of the proximal humerus.
- Fixation of displaced two-part proximal humerus fractures also can be performed using a locking plate in a percutaneous fashion. With this technique, great care must be taken to prevent injury to the axillary nerve.
  - A recent cadaveric study[8] demonstrated that the axillary nerve was an average of 3 mm from the second most proximal diaphyseal screw hole, and an average of 7 mm from the third most proximal screw hole. All other screw holes were more than 1 cm from the nerve.

PEARLS AND PITFALLS

Indications	■ An understanding of the neurovascular anatomy as well as the deforming forces present in proximal humerus fractures is vital to treating these injuries effectively.
Exposure	■ Avoid devascularizing fracture fragments by stripping pieces minimally. ■ Development of the "interval split" aids in fracture visualization and reduction and does not require detachment of the rotator cuff tendons. This is especially helpful when trying to fix a head-splitting fracture in a young patient.
Maintaining fixation	■ K-wires are useful for maintaining initial fixation. ■ With suture fixation, the strong bone along the bicipital groove of the distal fragment will hold sutures the best.
Poor bone quality	■ With osteoporotic three-part fractures, consider suture fixation first, followed by a proximal humeral locking plate. ■ Anatomic plating is very helpful when medial comminution is present.
Superior impingement	■ Avoid placing the locking plate too high on greater tuberosity.

POSTOPERATIVE CARE

- Stable fixation must be obtained to allow for immediate ROM.
  - A physical therapy regimen should be established based on the stability of fixation, the fracture pattern, the quality of the bone, and individual patient factors.
  - Ideally, the fixation should allow pendulum exercises on the first postoperative day and 130 degrees of passive forward flexion and 30 degrees of passive external rotation.
  - Between 4 and 6 weeks after surgery, an overhead pulley can be added, with stretching and active motion added at 6 to 8 weeks.
  - Formal strengthening with elastic bands is not started until 10 to 12 weeks after surgery.[3]
- As with nonoperative treatment, participation in physical therapy is key to a successful outcome.
  - In a recent study looking at fixation of two- and three-part fractures, the only patients with unsatisfactory outcomes were those who were noncompliant with physical therapy.[20]

OUTCOMES

- Neer's original description called for fixation of greater tuberosity fractures when there was more than 1 cm of displacement.[17]
- One recent study had excellent or good results in 12 of 16 patients with fixation of greater tuberosity fractures displaced more than 1 cm.[7] Forward elevation averaged 170 degrees, and external rotation averaged 63 degrees.
- Some authors believe that greater tuberosity displacement of greater than 5 mm may lead to poor outcomes.
  - McLauglin[14] first suggested that patients in whom a greater tuberosity healed with residual displacement of more than 5 mm had longstanding pain with poor function. Displacement of less than 5 mm does not appear to warrant surgery.
  - Platzer et al[21] looked at minimally displaced fractures of the greater tuberosity and found no statistical significance with varying degrees of displacement less than 5 mm.
- Open reduction with suture or wire fixation can achieve acceptable fixation, especially in older patients with osteoporotic bone. The technique can be used reliably in two- and three-part fractures.
  - One study showed nearly 80% excellent results with average motion of 155 degrees of average forward flexion, 46 degrees average external rotation, and internal rotation to T11. Furthermore, there were no reported cases of osteonecrosis of the humeral head.[20]
- Early open reduction and internal fixation with a laterally placed T-plate failed to yield consistently good results, especially for four-part fractures.[12,19] Other early osteosynthesis techniques include the cloverleaf and the blade–plate, but the current trend is toward anatomic plating technology.
  - Recent studies show promise with the use of such locking plates, although this technique is not without complications.[6]

COMPLICATIONS

- Infection
- Nonunion
- Malunion
- Avascular necrosis
- Nerve injury
- Impingement secondary to fixation or residual tuberosity displacement
- Failure of fixation, including varus malposition and plate fracture with proximal humeral anatomic plating[6]

REFERENCES

1. Bernstein J, Adler LM, Blank JE, et al. Evaluation of the Neer system of classification of proximal humeral fractures with computed tomographic scans and plain radiographs. J Bone Joint Surg Am 1996; 78A:1371–1375.
2. Blom S, Dahlback LO. Nerve injuries in dislocations of the shoulder joint and fractures of the neck of the humerus. Acta Chir Scand 1970;136:461–466.
3. Cameron BD, Williams GR. Operative fixation of three-part proximal humerus fractures. Tech Shoulder Elbow Surg 2002;3:111–123.
4. Court-Brown CM, Garg A, McQueen MM. The translated two-part fracture of the proximal humerus: Epidemiology and outcome in the older patient. J Bone Joint Surg Br 2001;83B:799–804.
5. DeFranco MJ, Brems JJ, Williams GR Jr, et al. Evaluation and management of valgus impacted four-part proximal humerus fractures. Clin Orthop Relat Res 2006;442:109–114.
6. Fankhauser F, Boldin C, Schippinger G, et al. A new locking plate for unstable fractures of the proximal humerus. Clin Orthop Relat Res 2005;430:176–181.
7. Flatow EL, Cuomo F, Maday MG, et al. Open reduction and internal fixation of two-part displaced fractures of the greater tuberosity of the proximal part of the humerus. J Bone Joint Surg Am 1991;73A:1213–1218.
8. Gallo RA, Altman GT. A cadaveric study to evaluate the safety of percutaneous plating of the proximal humerus. Pennsylvania Orthopaedic Society 2006 Spring Scientific Meeting, Paradise Island, The Bahamas, May 4–6, 2006.
9. Gerber C, Schneeberger AG, Vinh T. The arterial vascularization of the humeral head. J Bone Joint Surg Am 1990;72A:1486–1494.
10. Hoppenfeld S, deBoer P. Surgical Exposures in Orthopaedics, ed 3. Philadelphia: Lippincott Williams & Wilkins, 2003.
11. Koval KJ, Gallagher MA, Marsicano JG, et al. Functional outcome after minimally displaced fractures of the proximal part of the humerus. J Bone Joint Surg Am 1997;79A:203–207.
12. Kristiansen B, Christensen SW. Plate fixation of proximal humeral fractures. Acta Orthop Scand 1986;57:320–323.
13. McKoy BE, Bensen CV, Hartsock LA. Fractures about the shoulder: Conservative management. Orthop Clin North Am 2000;31: 205–216.
14. McLauglin HL. Dislocation of the shoulder with tuberosity fractures. Surg Clin North Am 1963;43:1615–1620.
15. Moriber LA, Patterson RL Jr. Fractures of the proximal end of the humerus. J Bone Joint Surg Am 1967;49A:1018.
16. Muller ME, Nazarian S, Koch P, et al. The Comprehensive Classification of Fractures of Long Bones. Berlin: Springer-Verlag, 1990.
17. Neer CS II. Displaced proximal humeral fractures. Part I. Classification and evaluation. J Bone Joint Surg Am 1970;52A:1077–1089.
18. Neer CS II. Displaced proximal humeral fractures. Part II. Treatment of three-part and four-part displacement. J Bone and J Surg Am 1970;52A:1090–1103.
19. Paavolainen P, Bjorkenheim J, Slatis P, Paukku P. Operative treatment of severe proximal humeral fractures. Acta Orthop Scand 1983; 54:374–379.
20. Park MC, Murthi AM, Roth NS, et al. Two-part and three-part fractures of the proximal humerus treated with suture fixation. J Orthop Trauma 2003;17:319–325.
21. Platzer P, Kutscha-Lissberg F, Lehr S, et al. The influence of displacement on shoulder function in patients with minimally displaced fractures of the greater tuberosity. Injury 2005;36:1185–1189.
22. Rasmussen S, Hvass I, Dalsgaard J, et al. Displaced proximal humeral fractures: Results of conservative treatment. Injury 1992;23:41–43.

23. Sidor ML, Zuckerman JD, Lyon T, et al. The Neer Classification system for proximal humeral fractures. J Bone Joint Surg Am 1993; 75A:1745–1750.

24. Siebenrock KA, Gerber C. The reproducibility of classification of fractures of the proximal end of the humerus. J Bone Joint Surg Am 1993;75A:1751–1755.

25. Young TB, Wallace WA. Conservative treatment of fractures and fracture-dislocations of the upper end of the humerus. J Bone Joint Surg Br 1985;67B:373–377.

26. Zuckerman JD, Checroun AJ. Fractures of the proximal humerus: Diagnosis and management. In: Iannotti JP, Williams JR, eds. Disorders of the Shoulder: Diagnosis and Management. Philadelphia: Lippincott Williams & Wilkins, 1999;639–685.

27. Zyto K, Ahrengart L, Sperber A, et al. Treatment of displaced proximal humeral fractures in elderly patients. J Bone Joint Surg Br 1997;79B:412–417.

28. Zyto K. Non-operative treatment of comminuted fractures of the proximal humerus in elderly patients. Injury 1998;29:349–352.

J. Dean Cole

DEFINITION

- From 50% to 80% of proximal humerus fractures are nondisplaced or minimally displaced and stable.[12] Early range of motion after a short period of immobilization usually is sufficient to treat these fractures and has been shown to result in satisfactory outcomes.[1] The remaining 20% to 50% of patients with proximal humerus fractures may benefit from operative management.
- Numerous techniques of internal fixation for proximal humerus fractures have been described and reported, including cloverleaf and blade plating,[1] Rush pinning,[15,19] spiral pinning,[18] Kirschner wire and tension band fixation,[3] suture and external fixation,[7] and intramedullary nail fixation.[8]
- Extensive dissection and inadequate biomechanical fixation in the context of the severe soft tissue injury and devascularization associated with these complex fracture types are the commonly cited reasons for failure of internal fixation devices.[2]
- Prosthetic arthroplasty traditionally has been the recommended treatment for three-part fractures with osteoporosis, four-part fractures, head-splitting fractures, and articular compression fractures that involve more than 40% of the articular surface.[1,2,11]
- Recently, several authors have reported satisfactory results with various types of osteosynthesis for four-part fractures, leading them to recommend an attempt at internal fixation in younger patients.[3,4,7,16] The basis of this recommendation is that subsequent published series have been unable to reproduce Neer's results with early hemiarthroplasty for four-part fractures.
- Various reports have been made on the use of intramedullary nails in the proximal humerus. We prefer to use an intramedullary nail that permits stable fixation of the head to the shaft of the humerus using a minimally invasive rotator cuff–splitting approach (DePuy Inc., Warsaw, IN).
  - The method for treatment of proximal humeral fractures described in this chapter involves a minimally invasive anterior acromial surgical approach, an indirect method of reduction, and a unique intramedullary rod designed to permit a variety of proximal interlocking configurations.

ANATOMY

Osteology

- The proximal humerus includes the humeral head, the lesser tuberosity, the greater tuberosity, and the proximal humeral metaphysis.
- The position of the head is higher than the tuberosities, and changes in this relationship will cause impingement. The humeral head is slightly medial (3 mm) and posterior (7 mm) in relation to the humeral shaft (**FIG 1**).
- The humeral head is retroverted approximately 30 degrees (range 20 to 60 degrees).

- Minor losses in the humeral length between the head and the deltoid insertion can alter the deltoid length–tension ratio.
- Avulsion of the greater tuberosity indicates injury to the rotator cuff.

Vascular Supply of the Proximal Humerus

- The anterior and posterior humeral circumflex arteries are branches of the axillary artery.
  - The arcuate artery, the terminal vessel of the ascending branch of the anterior humeral circumflex artery, supplies most of the humeral head.
    - Avascularity of the humeral head can occur if this vessel is disrupted during a fracture of the anatomic neck.
  - The posterior circumflex artery becomes important in patients with proximal humerus fractures.
    - It may be the primary source of blood supply to the fractured head, so care should be taken to prevent additional devascularization.
- Traumatic and iatrogenic vascular insult may lead to devascularization of the fracture fragments, resulting in delayed union, nonunion, and avascular necrosis. Traumatic injury cannot be predicted; well-planned minimally invasive procedures should reduce the risk of further damage, however.

Innervation

- The brachial plexus is at risk in patients with upper extremity injury, and thorough neurologic evaluation is mandatory.

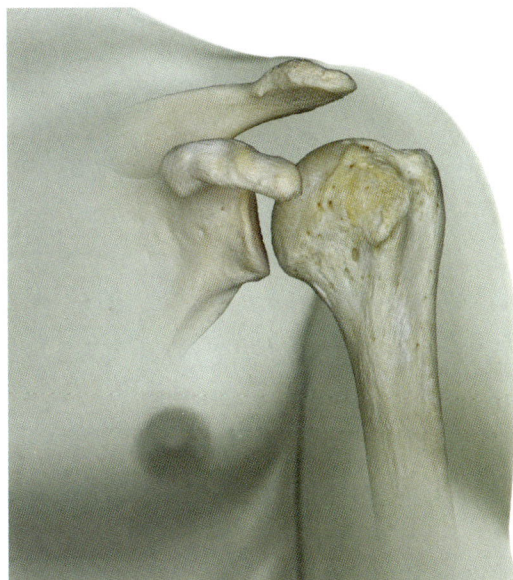

FIG 1 · Normal shoulder anatomy. The head is slightly higher than the tuberosities, slightly medial and posterior to the humeral shaft, retroverted 30 degrees. (Copyright J. Dean Cole, MD.)

- The axillary nerve courses through the quadrilateral space, where it is at risk during fracture dislocation.
- The lateral entry site for locking screw fixation (4–5 cm distal to the tip of the acromion) places the axillary nerve at risk.

PATHOGENESIS

- A blow to the anterior, lateral, or posterolateral aspect of the humerus typically is the cause.
- Axial load transmitted to the humerus may cause impacted fracture in osteoporotic bone.
- Violent muscle contractures, as in grand mal seizures and electric shock, are associated with posterior dislocation due to overpowering internal rotators and adductors.
- Pathologic causes include tumor, multiple myeloma, and metastatic or metabolic disorders.
- Osteoporosis is associated with fractures of the proximal humerus (more than any other fracture).
- In a three-part fracture with intact greater tuberosity, the humeral head is pulled by the supraspinatus and infraspinatus tendons; if the tendons are intact, the humeral head is externally rotated. The inverse is seen when the greater tuberosity is avulsed: the intact subscapularis internally rotates the humeral head (**FIG 2**).

NATURAL HISTORY

Epidemiology

- 4% to 5% of all fractures
- Increased incidence in osteoporosis, older middle-aged and elderly persons (third most common fracture in elderly)
- In persons older than 50 years of age, the female:male ratio is 4:1 (osteoporosis). Minor falls and trauma may cause comminuted fracture.
- In patients younger than 50 years of age, violent trauma, contact sports, and falls from heights are responsible for fractures.
- Surgical neck fracture is common.

Consequences of Injury

- Nondisplaced fractures may heal without major consequences.
- Acute, recurrent, or chronic dislocation

- Rotator cuff tears
- Neurovascular injury: axillary nerve, brachial plexus
- Avascular necrosis of the humeral head often results from disruption of the arcuate artery. The axillary artery also may be damaged, but less commonly, in fracture-dislocations.
- Malunion: loss of humeral length may cause deltoid weakness
- Posttraumatic arthrosis
- Adhesive capsulitis
- Chronic pain

PATIENT HISTORY AND PHYSICAL FINDINGS

- Associated injuries:
  - Rotator cuff tears
  - Dislocation
  - Forearm fractures
  - Brachial plexus, axillary, radial and ulnar nerve injuries (5%–30% of complex proximal humerus fractures)

IMAGING AND OTHER DIAGNOSTIC STUDIES

- Trauma series
  - Scapular anteroposterior (glenoid view)
  - Trans-scapular
  - Axillary
- Rotational views
- CT scan

SURGICAL MANAGEMENT

- Indications
  - Two-part proximal humerus fracture
  - Three-part proximal humerus fracture
  - Certain four-part proximal humerus fractures
- Prerequisites
  - Shoulder table, image intensification, and experienced radiology technician
  - Be aware of the learning curve (do not attempt nailing of a four-part fracture before acquiring adequate experience with two- and three-part fractures).

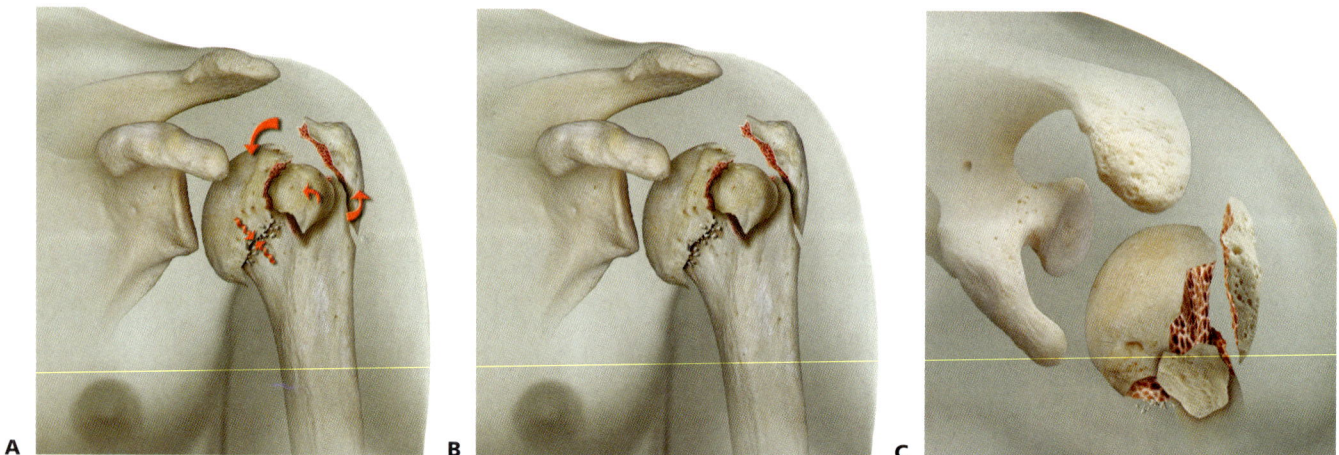

FIG 2 • A. Fracture pattern and deforming forces. The muscular attachments of the greater and lesser tuberosities will cause abduction, external rotation, and internal rotation, respectively. The head will follow whichever tuberosity is intact. **B,C.** In four-part fractures, the head often is in a neutrally rotated position. (Copyright J. Dean Cole, MD.)

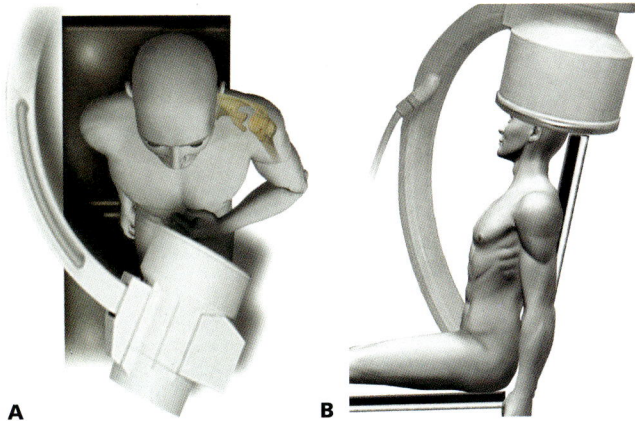

FIG 3 • Patient positioning should allow access of the C-arm to obtain orthogonal radiographs, which are critical in fracture reduction and fixation. **A.** Lateral view. **B.** Axial view. (Copyright J. Dean Cole, MD.)

- When treating patients with complex fractures, obtain the patient's consent for a hemiarthroplasty if that is determined to be the best treatment, and have the implant available in case it is found to be necessary.
- Contraindication: head-splitting, comminuted displaced humeral head fragment devoid of soft tissue attachment

Preoperative Planning

- Successful intramedullary nailing of the proximal humerus fracture depends on consistent integration between image intensification and the surgical steps.
- Patient positioning on a radiolucent table will allow the surgeon to use a minimally invasive approach.
- Any error on the entry site will cause inevitable problems with the rest of the procedure.
- It is crucial that the surgeon follow the surgical technique precisely.

Positioning

- Positioning on the table must allow orthogonal and overhead axillary views.

- The patient is placed supine in the beach chair position on a radiolucent table tilted at 60 to 70 degrees. The C-arm should be positioned on the opposite side of the table to allow the surgeon easy access to the proximal humerus (**FIG 3**).
- A bolster is used to elevate the shoulder from the table and to allow shoulder extension. Extension of the shoulder is necessary to expose the entry site in the humeral head. Flexion of the shoulder will result in the acromion overlying the center of the humeral head in the sagittal plane, obscuring the entry site or errantly directing an entry angle. Anterior cutout of the nail in the head fragment can easily occur in an osteoporotic humeral head with an associated greater tuberosity fracture.

Approach

- Intramedullary nailing for isolated surgical neck fractures may be performed completely percutaneously using most of the techniques described in the following paragraphs. However, when tuberosity reduction and fixation are required, a wider approach often is necessary.
- The timing of the open approach depends on the sequencing of head, shaft, and tuberosity fixation. In the technique we describe in this chapter, head–shaft fixation is accomplished percutaneously using nailing and interlocking screws before tuberosity fixation. Alternatively, an open approach with tuberosity reduction and fixation can be performed before nail insertion.
- The surgical approach for viewing tuberosity fractures that require fixation is a lateral deltoid-splitting approach made just below the acromion, approximately 4 cm long, that does not extend distally, to avoid injury to the axillary nerve (**FIG 4A**).
- For a lesser tuberosity approach, a separate, small deltopectoral incision is centered just over the lesser tuberosity, and the lesser tuberosity fixation or fixation to the subscapularis tendon is performed in that plane (**FIG 4B**).
- The rotator cuff is incised longitudinally away from the lateral watershed area of the rotator cuff and away from Sharpey's fibers and the connection of the tendon to the bone.
  - Significant rotator cuff defect is not created with this approach, as confirmed in cadaver dissection. The longitudinal incision on the rotator cuff does not weaken the cuff.

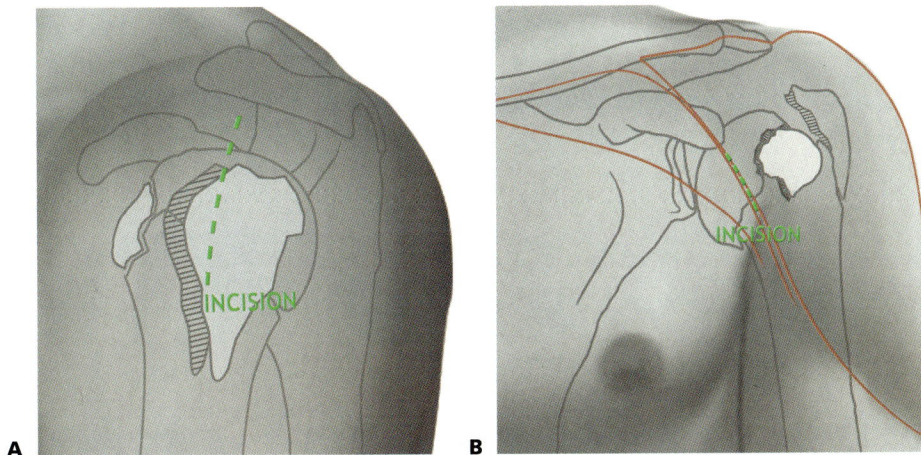

FIG 4 • Skin incisions. **A.** Deltoid-splitting incision specifically for greater tuberosity fixation. **B.** Deltopectoral incision specifically for lesser tuberosity fixation. (Copyright J. Dean Cole, MD.)

K-WIRE PLACEMENT

- Placement of K-wires allows fragment reduction and helps dictate placement of the skin incision and surgical approach. Hence, the first step involves placement of a K-wire in the subacromial space; it is inserted through the anterolateral aspect of the shoulder using the image intensifier (C-arm) and directed posteromedial toward the glenoid (**TECH FIG 1A,B**).
  - This initial pin will serve as a guide for the retroversion of the humeral head.
- Next, two K-wires are placed in the humeral head, directed lateral to medial, one anterior and one posterior to the central aspect of the head (**TECH FIG 1C,D**). The wires should be separated by enough distance to allow insertion of the nail between them (1.5 cm).

- The K-wires should be directed in the longest axis of the humeral head in the axial plane. Allowing for retroversion is important.
- Confirmation of the correct placement in the axial plane is done by the overhead axillary view. Then the C-arm is positioned to view the advancement of the pins in the coronal plane projection.
  - With longer K-wires, the surgeon's hand can be kept out of radiographs. Unfortunately, with internal rotation, extension also occurs in the humerus and the humeral head, depending on the soft tissue attachments.

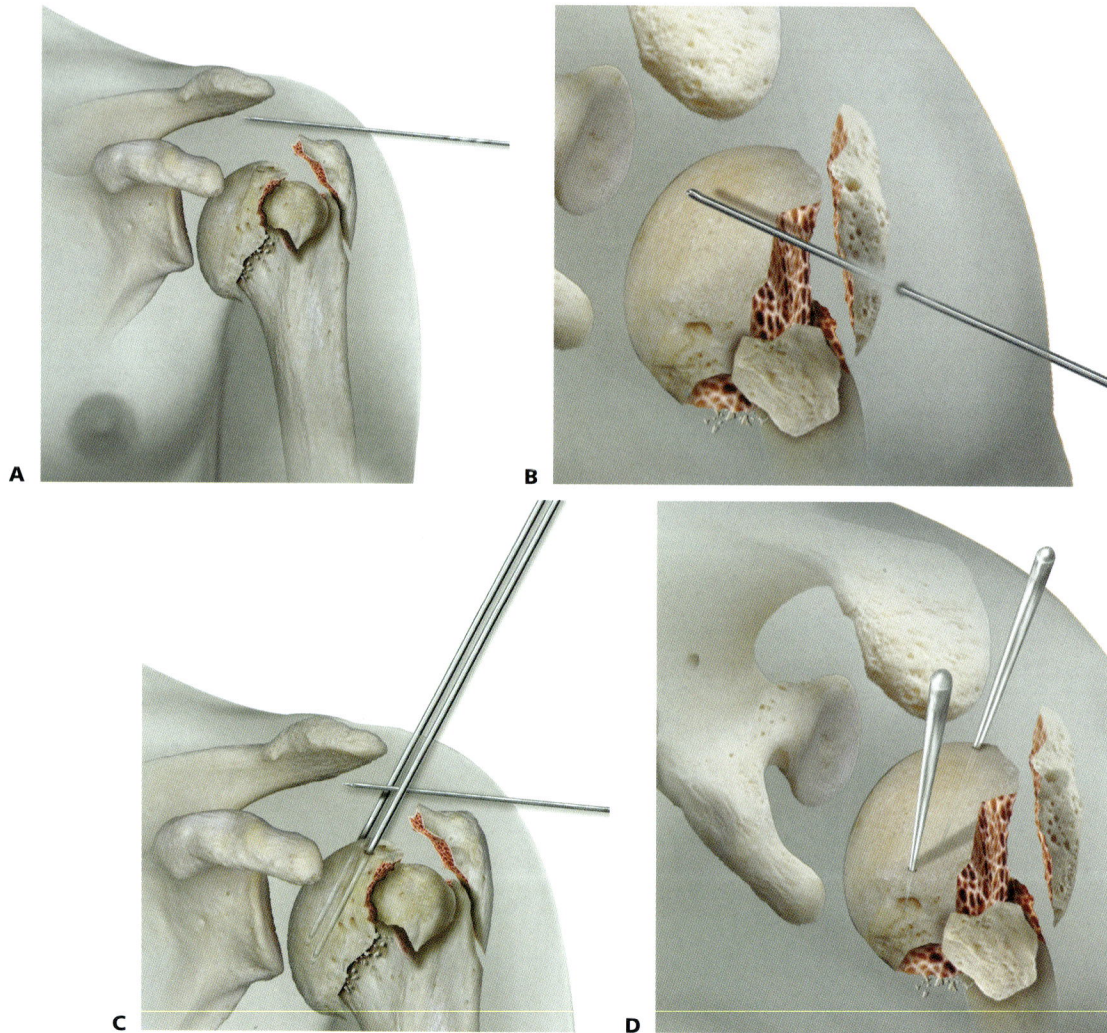

TECH FIG 1 • A,B. AP and axial views of initial K-wire insertion:. This initial pin will serve to orient the humeral head, specifically the desired degree of retroversion. **C,D.** AP and axial views of pins to control head fragment. These pins are inserted to control the head fragment in a joystick fashion. (Copyright J. Dean Cole, MD.)

FRAGMENT REDUCTION

- The K-wires can then be used in a joystick fashion to adduct and extend the head, exposing the supraspinatus tendon and optimal entry site in the head from beneath the anterior edge of the acromion (**TECH FIG 2A,B**).
- Image intensification can be used to place a K-wire through the head in line with intramedullary axis of the humerus. This maneuver includes two important aspects:
  - The first is to use the joysticks to extend and adduct the proximal humeral head, exposing the anterolateral portion of the head from under the acromion while simultaneously distracting the distal shaft,

thereby aligning the longitudinal intramedullary axis of the proximal and distal fragments (**TECH FIG 2C,D**).
  - The second is to drive the K-wire into the head in a central position with reference to the medullary canal in the sagittal plane and lateral to central in reference to the canal in the frontal or coronal plane (**TECH FIG 2E**).
- To achieve fracture reduction, the joysticks in the proximal fragment must be used to rotate the head while simultaneously rotating the distal shaft manually to obtain true orthogonal views of the head in reference to the shaft.

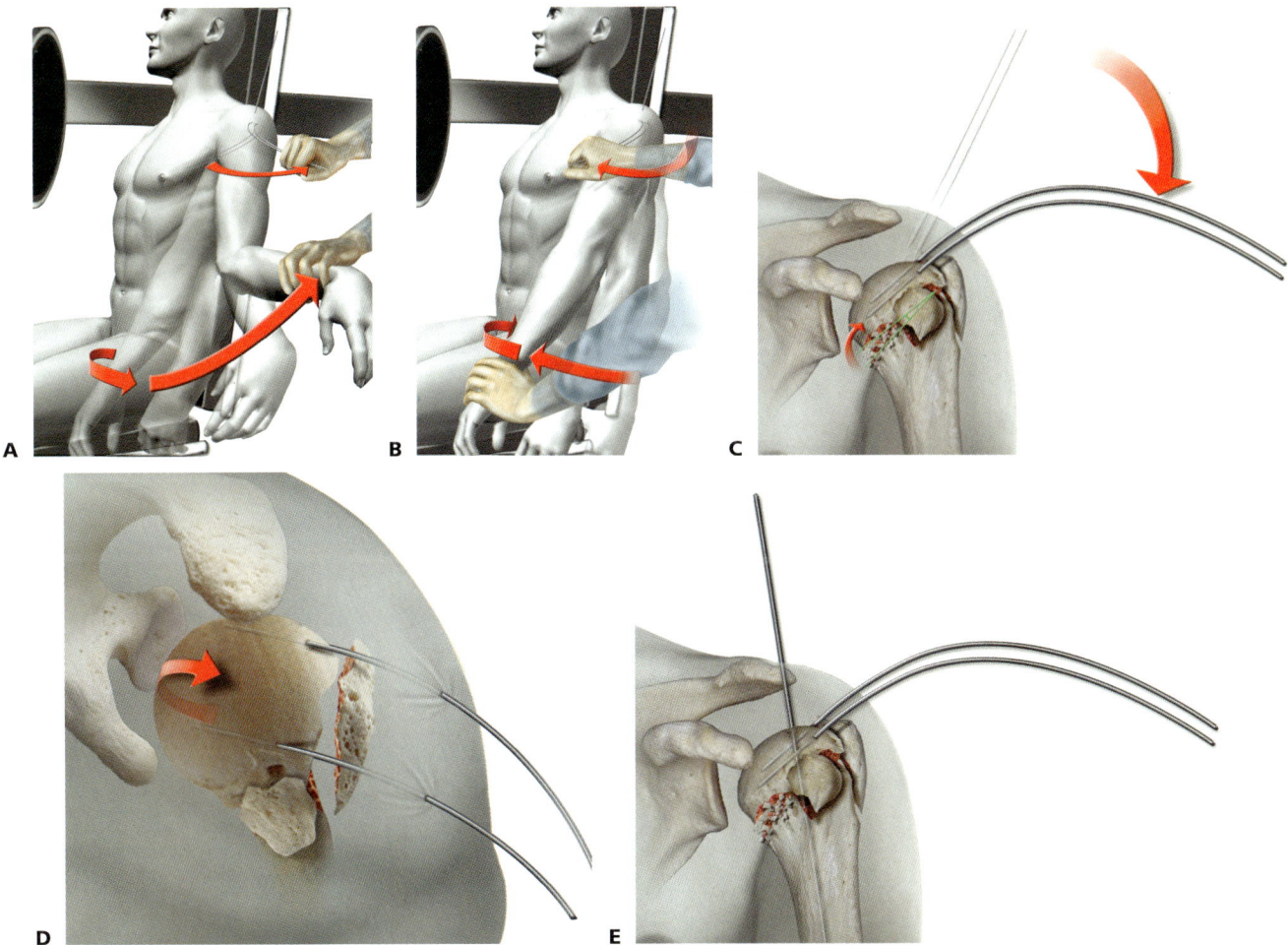

TECH FIG 2 • Fragment reduction maneuver. **A,B.** Combining rotation of the head fragment (K-wires) with the shaft (arm) is used to assist in fracture reduction. **C,D.** AP and axial views of humeral head reduction maneuver. Manipulation of the fracture fragments with the K-wires allows disimpaction of the fracture, improving the varus or valgus alignment. **E.** Pin entry site in humeral head. (Copyright J. Dean Cole, MD.)

GUIDEWIRE PLACEMENT

- The nail can be placed percutaneous just anterior to the anterior edge of the acromion.
- The anterior edge may be difficult to palpate and to differentiate from the humeral head because of edema and

hematoma from the fracture. Therefore, it is helpful to locate the anterior edge of the angle of the acromion under image intensification with a K-wire where it intersects the longitudinal axis of the humerus.

TECHNIQUES

- Correct placement of the guidewire is crucial; it should be centered in both frontal and sagittal planes.
- Manipulation of the proximal fragment has been the only reliable way to identify correct placement.

- This is easily accomplished in the coronal plane, but it is more difficult in the sagittal plane. Attention should be directed at the rotational alignment.

ENTRY SITE REAMING

- Reaming of the entry site should be performed carefully, as the percutaneous incision is small.
- The reamer is inserted over the guidewire, and the soft tissues are retracted and protected. The reamer is advanced through the rotator cuff in "reverse" until bone contact, then on "forward" through the humeral head. The reamer is left in place.
- The guidewire that was used to initiate the entry site is removed, and a longer guidewire is passed to the shaft

fragment. Manipulation of the shaft fragment sometimes is necessary. The reamer's sound must be used to gauge the canal diameter. It is necessary to ream 1 mm greater than the anticipated nail size.
- On some occasions, even external fixator placement from the scapular spine to the distal humerus is necessary. The external fixator is applied and distraction accomplished with manipulation of the proximal aspect of the shaft; guidewire passage usually is simple.

NAIL INSERTION

- Once the nail is inserted, confirm the rotation of the humerus in the axial plane; it is necessary to ensure proper alignment before impaction (**TECH FIG 3**).
- Usually, impaction of the distal fragment by blows against the olecranon, while supporting the proximal

humeral head indirectly through the soft tissues, is adequate.
- Large gaps are not acceptable, and it may be necessary to use filler substance.

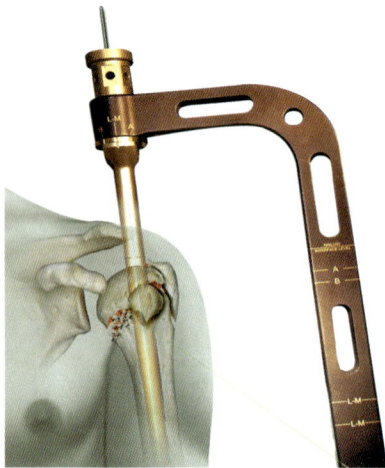

TECH FIG 3 • Nail insertion. (Copyright J. Dean Cole, MD.)

INTERLOCKING SCREW FIXATION

- We recommend that the oblique distal screw be the initial locking screw (**TECH FIG 4**). The goal of this screw is to attach the head to the shaft before fixation of the tuberosities.
- Screw placement puts the axillary nerve at risk. Careful blunt dissection to bone, drilling within the sheath, and placing the screw within the confines of the sheath are necessary. Drilling should be done very carefully, although it certainly does not completely negate the risk of drilling through the humeral head. Careful observation is important.

- It is occasionally helpful to remove the drill and then use a blunt guidewire and assure good humeral head subchondral bone contact before further drilling or screw placement.
- Central placement of the distal oblique screw in the humeral head is important. This step should flow very smoothly if the initial K-wires have been placed in the correct axial plane alignment.
  - Errant placement or acceptance of poorly positioned K-wires will result only in further deviation. If the distal oblique screw is not placed at the appropriate

- angle, the radiographs may be deceptive and may result in screw penetration.
- Screw placement on the subchondral bone is important for fixation. However, patients with osteoporosis do have a risk of the fracture fragment settling.

- A and B screws are placed depending on goals of fixation.
  - Overdrilling to countersink the more proximal screw usually is necessary to avoid impingement.
  - These screws rarely are helpful in tuberosity fixation.

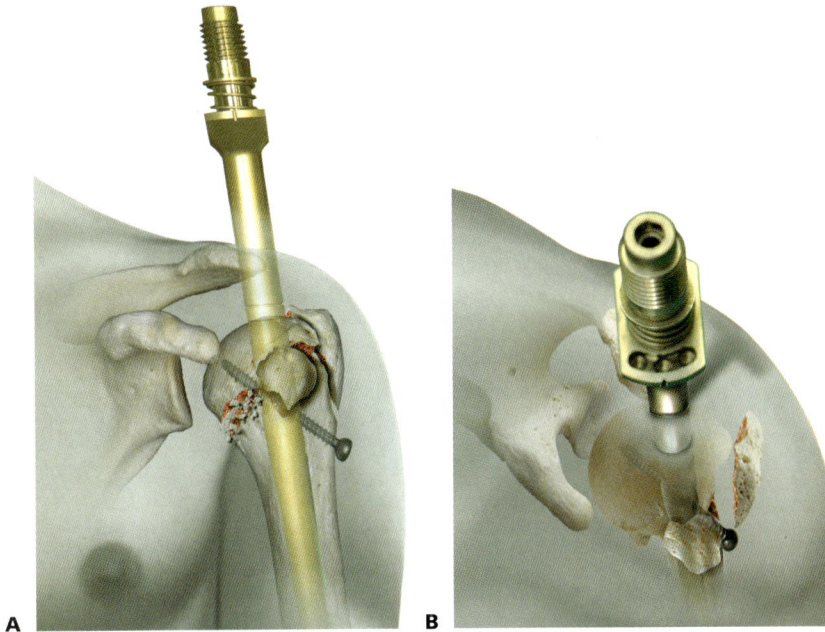

TECH FIG 4 • AP and axial views of intramedullary nail and proximal locking screw. (Copyright J. Dean Cole, MD.)

TUBEROSITY FIXATION

- The tuberosity fixation sequence is somewhat variable.
- With very displaced tuberosity fractures, if shaft-to-head fixation is performed initially with the tuberosities displaced, the guide will perforate the cuff and pin the cuff in a nonanatomic position, resulting in inability to perform reduction of the tuberosities. Therefore, if tuberosity fixation is going to be aided with the nail, the tuberosity alignment must be performed before nailing.
- Another sequence involves fixation of the head and shaft followed by later fixation of the tuberosity. Anchors can be passed through the nail with sutures used later to fix the tuberosities.

- The sequence of fixation should involve passing sutures through the musculotendinous junction of the subscapularis, infraspinatus, and supraspinatus. Sutures passed over the superior aspect of the head from the infraspinatus and subscapularis and sutures passed laterally around the head provide helpful, reliable fixation points. With practice, these maneuvers can be performed in a minimally invasive manner.
- Comminuted tuberosity fixation is challenging. It is difficult to achieve consistent fixation with screws. A headless screw has been used with some success in limited cases.

PEARLS AND PITFALLS

Indications	■ Two-part proximal humerus fracture ■ Three-part proximal humerus fracture ■ Select four-part proximal humerus fracture
Prerequisites	■ Shoulder table, image intensification, and *experienced* radiology technician ■ Be aware of the learning curve. ■ Plan B: for complex fractures, obtain consent for a hemiarthroplasty and have an implant available.
Contraindication	■ Head-splitting, comminuted displaced humeral head fragment devoid of soft tissue attachment
Positioning	■ Beach chair position to allow clear fluoroscopic images. Chair with metal extensions positioned to allow overhead axillary C-arm views.

Reduction technique	■ Humeral head is adducted; use K-wire as guide. ■ Percutaneously drill K-wires in the head fragment and use them as a "joystick" to rotate the head fragment. ■ Orthogonal views of the shoulder
Nail entry site	■ Erring at the entry site inevitably will cause problems with the rest of the procedure.
Screw placement	■ A drill guide is used to prevent injury to the axillary nerve.

POSTOPERATIVE CARE

■ The postoperative regimen depends on the stability of the fixation and the soft tissues.
  ■ Sling with abduction pillow that allows the proximal humerus to rest in neutral rotation and slight abduction (relax the rotator cuff and decrease tension on the greater tuberosity)
  ■ Gentle passive, pendulum, and active-assisted exercises of the shoulder
  ■ Active elbow and wrist exercises
  ■ Once fracture healing is detected on radiographic imaging, range of motion can be increased; weight lifting restrictions must be maintained until healing is complete.

COMPLICATIONS

■ Early
  ■ Injury to axillary nerve
  ■ Joint penetration
  ■ Loss of reduction
  ■ Infection
■ Late
  ■ Nonunion
  ■ Posttraumatic arthrosis
  ■ Avascular necrosis of humeral head
  ■ Prominent hardware

REFERENCES

1. Bigliani LU, Flatow EL, Pollock RG. Fractures of the proximal humerus: In: Rockwood CA, Green DP, Bucholz RW, et al, eds. Fractures in Adults. Philadelphia: Lippincott-Raven, 1996:1055–1107.
2. Connor PM, Flatow EL. Complications of internal fixation of proximal humeral fractures. Instr Course Lect 1997;46:25–37.
3. Darder A, Darder A Jr, Sanchis V, et al. Four-part displaced proximal humerus fractures: Operative treatment using Kirchner wires and a tension band. J Orthop Trauma 1993;7:497–505.
4. Esser RD. Open reduction and fixation of three- and four part fractures of the proximal humerus. Clin Orthop Relat Res 1994;299:244–251.
5. Goldman RT, Koval KJ, Cuomo F, et al. Functional outcome after humeral head replacement for acute three- and four-part proximal humeral fractures. J Shoulder Elbow Surg 1995;4:81–86.
6. Hawkins RJ, Switlyk P. Acute prosthetic replacement for severe fractures of the proximal humerus. Clin Orthop Relat Res 1993; 289:156–160.
7. Ko J, Yamamoto R. Surgical treatment of complex fracture of the proximal humerus. Clin Orthop Relat Res 1996;327:225–237.
8. Mouradian WI. Displaced proximal humeral fractures: seven years' experience with a modified Zickel supracondylar device. Clin Orthop Relat Res 1986;212:209–218.
9. Nayak NK, Schickendantz MS, Regan WD, et al. Operative treatment of nonunion of surgical neck fractures of the humerus. Clin Orthop Relat Res 1995;313:200–205.
10. Neer CS. Displaced proximal humeral fractures. Part I. Classification and evaluation. J Bone Joint Surg Am 1970;52A:1077–1089.
11. Neer CS. Displaced proximal humeral fractures. Part II. Treatment of three and four part displacement. J Bone Joint Surg Am 1970; 52A:1090–1103.
12. Norris TR. Fractures of the proximal humerus and dislocations of the shoulder. In: Browner BD, Jupiter JB, Levine AM, et al, eds. Skeletal Trauma: Fractures–Dislocations–Ligamentous Injuries. Philadelphia: WB Saunders, 1992:120–129.
13. Riemer BL, D'Ambrosia RD, Kellam JF, et al. The anterior acromial approach for antegrade intramedullary nailing of the humeral diaphysis. Orthopaedics 1993;16:1219–1223.
14. Robinson CM, Christie J. The two-part proximal humeral fracture: a review of operative treatment using two techniques. Injury 1993; 24:123–125.
15. Rush LV. Atlas of Rush Pin Technique: A System of Fracture Treatment. Meridian, MI: Bervion, 1955:166–167.
16. Szyszkowitz R, Seggl W, Schleifer P, et al. Proximal humeral fractures: management techniques and expected results. Clin Orthop Relat Res 1993;292:13–25.
17. Wheeler DL, Colville MR. Biomechanical comparison of intramedullary and percutaneous pin fixation for proximal humeral fracture fixation. J Orthop Trauma 1997;11:363–367.
18. Yano S, Takamura S, Kobayashi I, et al. Use of the spiral pin for fracture of the humeral neck. J Orthop Science 1981;55:1607–1619.
19. Weseley, MS, Barenfeld PA, Eisenstein AL. Rush pin intramedullary fixation for fractures of the proximal humerus. J Trauma 1977; 17:29–37.

Chapter 19

Hemiarthroplasty for Proximal Humerus Fractures

Kamal I. Bohsali, Michael A. Wirth, and Steven B. Lippitt

DEFINITION

- Proximal humerus fractures involve isolated or combined injuries to the greater tuberosity, lesser tuberosity, articular segment, and proximal humeral shaft.
- Overall, proximal humerus fractures account for 4% to 5% of all fractures.[8,13]

ANATOMY

- The proximal humerus consists of four segments: the greater tuberosity, lesser tuberosity, articular segment, and humeral shaft (**FIG 1**).
- The most cephalad surface of the articular segment is, on average, 8 mm above the greater tuberosity.[16] Humeral version averages 29.8 degrees (range 10 to 55 degrees).[23]
- The intertubercular groove lies between the tuberosities and forms the passageway for the long head of the biceps as it traverses from the intra-articular origin into the distal arm.
- The tuberosities attach to the articular segment at the anatomic neck. The greater tuberosity has three facets for the corresponding insertions of the supraspinatus, infraspinatus, and teres minor tendons; the lesser tuberosity has a single facet for the subscapularis.
- The deltoid, pectoralis major, and latissimus dorsi all insert on the humerus distal to the surgical neck. These soft tissue attachments contribute to the deforming forces sustained with proximal humerus fractures.

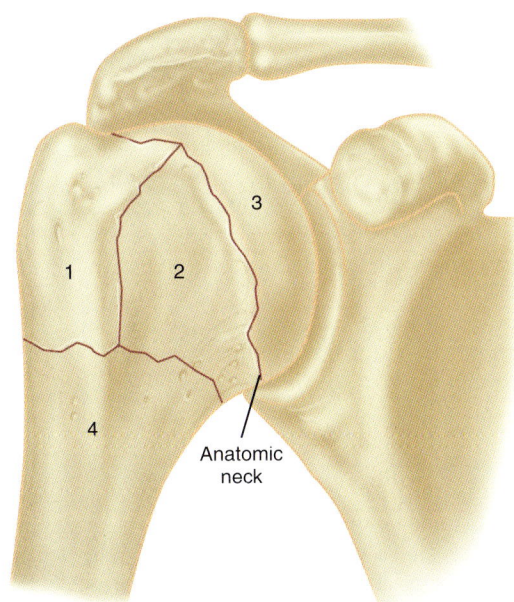

FIG 1 • Neer classification of proximal humerus fractures: *1*, greater tuberosity; *2*, lesser tuberosity; *3*, articular surface; *4*, shaft.

- The anterolateral branch of the anterior humeral circumflex artery (the arcuate artery of Laing) is the major blood supply to the humeral head. This vessel courses parallel to the lateral aspect of the long head of the biceps and enters the humeral head at the interface between the intertubercular groove and the greater tuberosity. Injury to the arcuate artery can result in osteonecrosis of the articular segment.[10,18]

PATHOGENESIS

- The incidence of proximal humerus fractures is increasing with an aging population and associated osteoporosis.
- The mechanism of injury may be indirect or direct and secondary to high-energy collisions in younger patients (eg, motor vehicle accidents, athletic injuries) or falls from standing height in elderly patients.
- Pathologic fractures from primary or metastatic disease should be included in the differential diagnosis.
- Risk factors for the development of proximal humerus fractures in the elderly patient population include low bone density, lack of hormone replacement therapy, previous fracture history, three or more chronic illnesses, and smoking.[15]

NATURAL HISTORY

- Neer's classic study in 1970 compared the results of nonoperative treatment with hemiarthroplasty for three- and four-part displaced proximal humerus fractures. No satisfactory results were found in the nonoperative group owing to inadequate reduction, nonunion, malunion, and humeral head osteonecrosis with collapse.[20]
- Stableforth[24] reaffirmed this in a study in which patients were randomized to nonoperative management or prosthetic replacement. The patients with displaced fractures treated nonoperatively had worse overall results for pain, range of motion, and activities of daily living.

PATIENT HISTORY AND PHYSICAL FINDINGS

- A thorough history and complete physical examination should be performed. History should include mechanism of injury, pre-morbid level of function, occupation, hand dominance, history of malignancy, and ability to participate in a structured rehabilitation program.[14]
- A review of systems should involve queries regarding loss of consciousness, paresthesias, and ipsilateral elbow or wrist pain.
- On physical examination, the orthopaedic surgeon should look for swelling, soft tissue injuries, ecchymosis, and deformity. Posterior fracture-dislocations will demonstrate flattening of the anterior aspect of the shoulder with an associated posterior prominence. Anterior fracture-dislocations present with opposite findings.[14]

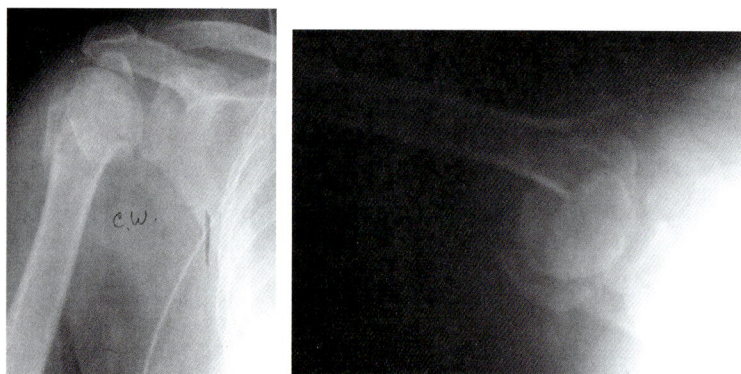

FIG 2 • AP and axillary views of a displaced three-part proximal humerus fracture without evidence of concomitant dislocation.

IMAGING AND OTHER DIAGNOSTIC STUDIES

- Appropriate radiographs include anteroposterior and axillary views of the shoulder[14] (**FIG 2**). If the axillary view cannot be obtained because of patient discomfort, alternate views such as the Velpeau trauma axillary view can be used to evaluate and classify the glenohumeral articulation.[2]
  - The Neer classification is based on the four anatomic segments of the proximal humerus: the humeral head, the greater and lesser tuberosities, and the humeral shaft (see Fig 1).[11] Number of parts is based on 45 degrees of angulation or 1 cm of displacement from neighboring segments.
  - The AO/ASIF/OTA Comprehensive Long Bone Classification system distinguishes the valgus impacted four-part proximal humerus fracture from other four-part fractures with partial preservation of the vascular inflow to the articular segment through an intact medial capsule.[17,22]
  - The current fracture classification systems have fair interobserver reliability, even with the addition of CT scans. Despite the limitations of these systems, they remain clinically useful when deciding on nonoperative versus operative treatment.[2,11]
- CT scans may be helpful in evaluating tuberosity displacement and articular surface involvement.[14]

DIFFERENTIAL DIAGNOSIS

- Acute hemorrhagic bursitis
- Traumatic rotator cuff tear
- Simple dislocation
- Acromioclavicular separation
- Calcific tendinitis [2]

NONOPERATIVE MANAGEMENT

- Nonoperative treatment usually is reserved for minimally displaced fractures of the proximal humerus, which account for nearly 80% of these injuries.
- The characteristics of the fracture (ie, bone quality, fracture orientation, concurrent soft tissue injuries), the personality of the patient (eg, compliant, realistic expectations, mental status), and surgeon experience all affect the decision to proceed with operative intervention.

- Moribund individuals and patients unable to cooperate with a postoperative rehabilitation program (eg, closed head injury) are not appropriate candidates for operative intervention.
- In general, nonoperative management of complex, displaced proximal humerus fractures has not proven as successful.
- Initial immobilization with a sling and axillary pad may be helpful. Gentle range-of-motion exercises may be started by 7 to 10 days after the fracture when pain has decreased and the patient is less apprehensive.[2]
- Intermittent biplanar radiographs are essential to determine additional displacement and the interval stage of healing.[2]
- Active and active assisted range-of-motion exercises are initiated with evidence of radiographic union. Inform the patient that he or she may never attain symmetric range of motion or strength when comparing the affected versus the uninjured side.

SURGICAL MANAGEMENT

- The goal of surgery is to anatomically reconstruct the glenohumeral joint with restoration of humeral length, placement of appropriate prosthetic retroversion, and establishment of secure tuberosity fixation.
- Prosthetic replacement is the preferred treatment of most four-part fractures, three-part fractures and dislocations in elderly patients with osteoporotic bone, head-splitting articular segment fractures, and chronic anterior or posterior humeral head dislocations with more than 40% of the articular surface involved.[25]
- Several studies have indicated that the outcome of primary hemiarthroplasty for acute proximal humerus fractures is superior to that from late reconstruction.[6,21]

Preoperative Planning

- Although some studies have suggested urgent intervention (ie, within less than 48 hours), most authors recommend preoperative planning with a careful neurovascular assessment of the injured shoulder, medical optimization of the patient, and preoperative templating with standard radiographs of the contralateral uninjured shoulder.[12]
- An interscalene block (regional anesthesia) may be used to supplement general anesthesia.
- Endotracheal intubation is recommended to allow for intraoperative muscle relaxation, but laryngeal mask intubation may be used.[12,14]

Positioning

- The patient is placed on an operating table in the beach chair position with the arm positioned in a sterile articulating arm holder or draped free if an appropriate number of assistants are available (**FIG 3**).

Approach

- The surgical prep site should include the entire upper extremity and shoulder region, including the scapular and pectoral regions.
- Appropriate prophylactic intravenous antibiotics are given to the patient before skin incision.
- A standard deltopectoral incision is used. Care is taken to minimize injury (eg, surgical detachment, contusion secondary to retractors) to the deltoid muscle. The musculocutaneous and axillary nerves are identified and protected during the procedure.

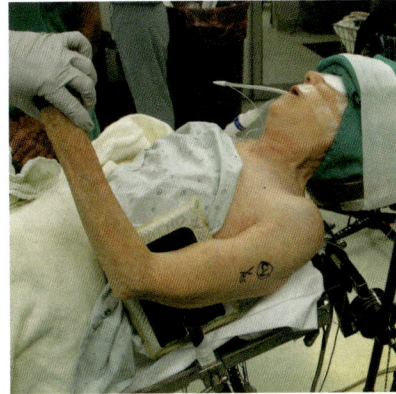

FIG 3 • Beach chair position. The patient is placed with the thorax at the end of the table. A kidney post and McConnell head holder are used to allow free and unencumbered access to the medullary canal of the humerus.

DELTOPECTORAL APPROACH

- The incision begins superior and medial to the coracoid process and extends toward the anterior aspect of the deltoid insertion (**TECH FIG 1A**).
- The cephalic vein is identified, preserved, and retracted laterally with the deltoid muscle. The pectoralis major is mobilized medially. If additional exposure is necessary, the proximal 1 cm of the pectoralis major insertion is released (**TECH FIG 1B**).

- Fracture hematoma usually is encountered once the clavipectoral fascia is incised. At this time, fracture fragments and the rotator cuff musculature become evident.
- The axillary and musculocutaneous nerves can be identified through digital palpation of the anteroinferior aspect of the subscapularis muscle and the posterior aspect of the coracoid muscles respectively. External rotation of the humerus results in reduced tension on the axillary nerve.

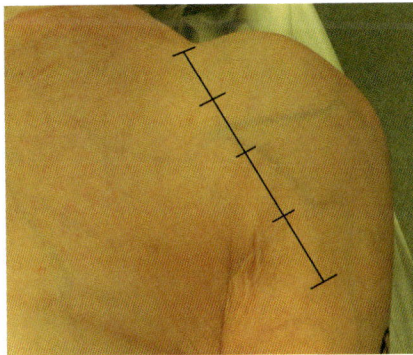

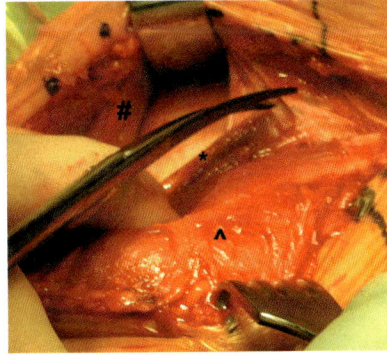

TECH FIG 1 • Skin incision and deltopectoral approach. **A.** The skin incision is centered over the anterior deltoid. The deltopectoral interval is developed with lateral retraction of the cephalic vein. **B.** For more exposure, the superior 1 cm of the pectoralis major tendon may be incised. (^, pectoralis major; #, deltoid; *, cephalic vein.)

TUBEROSITY MOBILIZATION

- The tendon of the long head of the biceps is identified as it courses in the bicipital groove toward the rotator interval. The tendon serves as a key landmark when re-establishing the anatomic relationship between the greater and lesser tuberosities.
  - The rotator interval and coracohumeral ligament are both released to allow for mobilization of the tuberosities (**TECH FIG 2A,B**).
- If the fracture does not involve the bicipital groove, an osteotome or saw may be used to create a cleavage

plane for tuberosity mobilization. Preservation of the coracoacromial ligament is advisable to maintain the coracoacromial arch.

- Heavy, nonabsorbable traction sutures (eg, 1-mm cottony Dacron) are placed through the rotator cuff insertions on the tuberosities. Two or three sutures should be placed through the subscapularis tendon, and three or four sutures through the supraspinatus.
- Tuberosity fragments vary in size and may require trimming for reduction and repair (**TECH FIG 2C,D**).

TECHNIQUES

TECHNIQUES

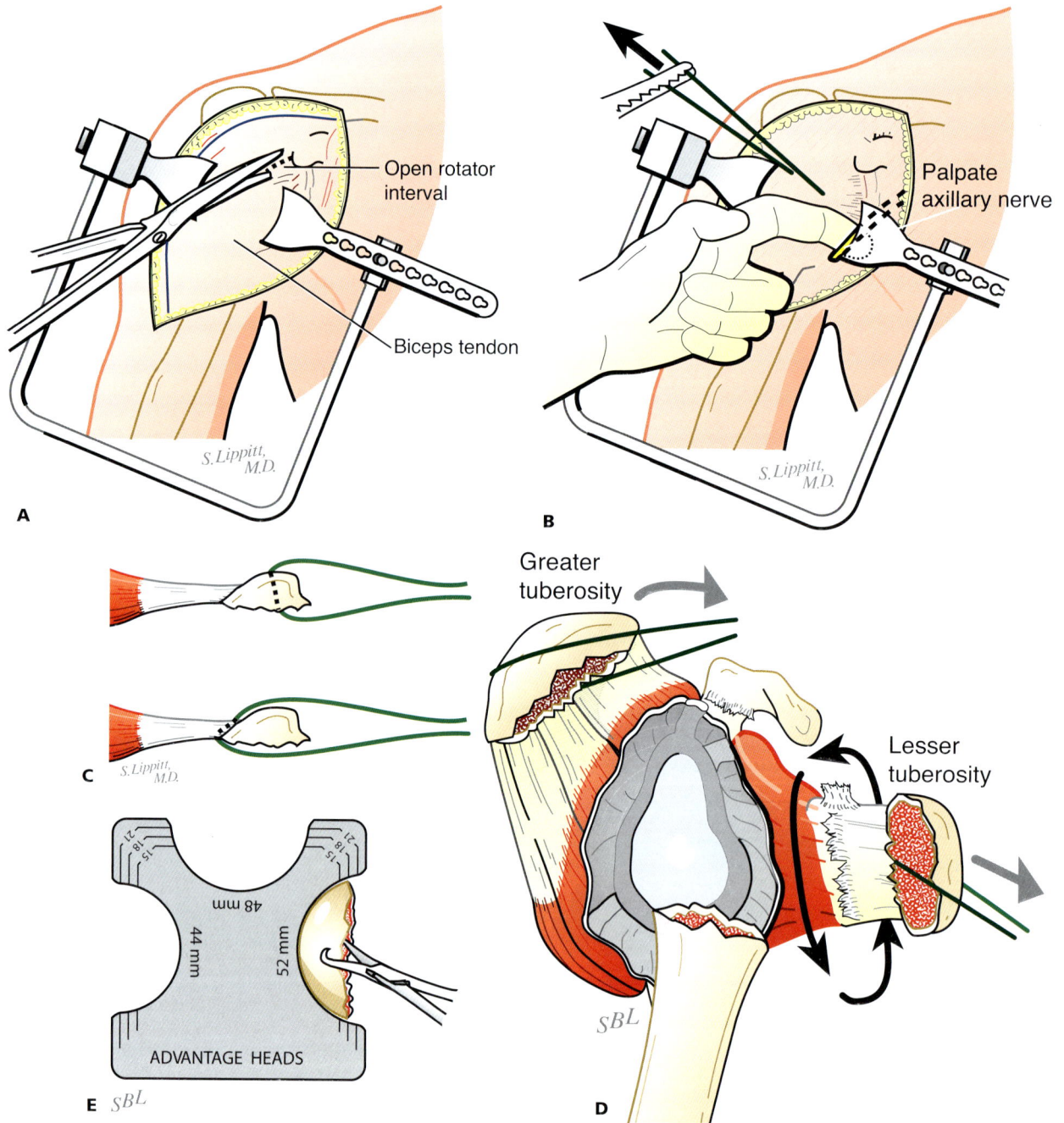

TECH FIG 2 • A. The long head of the biceps is identified and traced superiorly to the rotator interval. The tendon serves as a key landmark when re-establishing the anatomic relation between the greater and lesser tuberosities. **B.** The axillary nerve is identified at the anteroinferior border of the subscapularis. **C.** Nonabsorbable sutures are placed at the junction of the tendon–tuberosity interface and not through the tuberosities. **D.** Once the native humeral head is removed, the tuberosities with their respective rotator cuff attachments are mobilized for humeral canal preparation and later repair. **E.** Humeral head sizing. The extracted native humeral head is sized with the use of a commercially available template guide. (Copyright Steven B. Lippitt, MD.)

- With the tuberosities retracted on their muscular insertions, the humeral head and shaft fragments are removed.
- The native articular surface is removed and sized with a template for trial humeral head replacement (**TECH FIG 2E**).

- The glenoid must be examined for concomitant pathology. Hematoma and cartilaginous or bony fragments are removed with sterile saline irrigation.
- Glenoid fractures should be stabilized with internal fixation. If the glenoid exhibits significant degenerative wear or irreparable damage, a glenoid component must be used.

HUMERAL SHAFT PREPARATION

- The proximal end of the humeral shaft is delivered into the incisional wound. Loose endosteal bone fragments and hematoma are removed from the canal of the humeral shaft.
- Axial reamers, preferably without power, are used to prepare the humeral shaft for trial implantation.
- The trial humeral implant is placed with the lateral fin slightly posterior to the bicipital groove, and with the medial aspect of the trial head at least at the height of the medial calcar.
- Formerly, we used a sponge to anchor the trial stem within the intramedullary canal of the humerus. We currently use a commercially available fracture jig that can maintain the height and retroversion of the trial component through a functional range of motion (**TECH FIG 3**).[12,14]

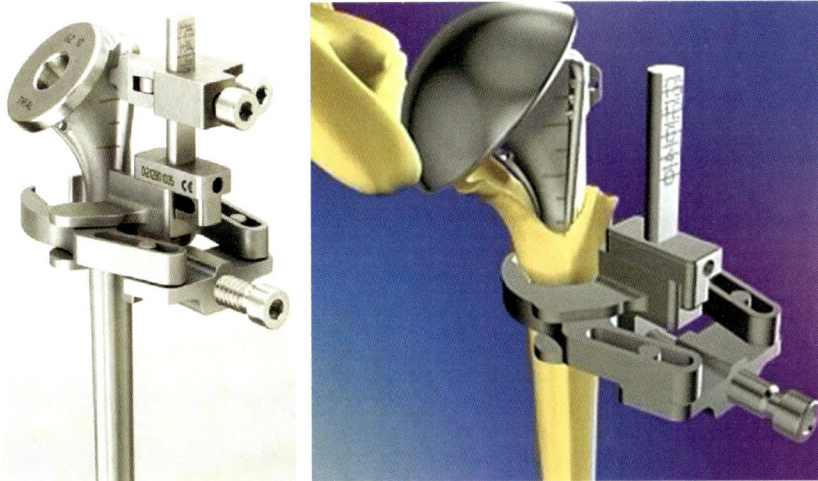

TECH FIG 3 • A commercially available fracture jig stably situates the implant at appropriate height and retroversion. (Courtesy of DePuy Orthopaedics, Warsaw, IN.)

DETERMINATION OF HUMERAL RETROVERSION

- Correct humeral retroversion is critical when recreating the glenohumeral articulation. Most techniques suggest 30 degrees as a guide during reconstruction, although native retroversion may vary from 10 to 50 degrees.
- Several methods are employed to gauge this angle:
  - External rotation of the humerus to 30 degrees from the sagittal plane of the body with the humeral head component facing straight medially
  - An imaginary line from the distal humeral epicondylar axis that bisects the axis of the prosthesis
  - Positioning of the lateral fin of the prosthesis about 8 mm posterior to the biceps groove (**TECH FIG 4**).

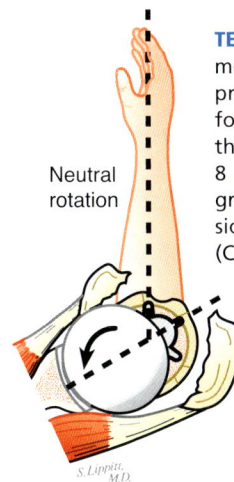

Neutral rotation

TECH FIG 4 • Retroversion assessment. The anterior fin of the prosthesis is aligned with the forearm in neutral rotation, and the lateral fin is positioned about 8 mm posterior to the biceps groove, establishing a retroversion angle of about 30 degrees. (Copyright Steven B. Lippitt, MD.)

DETERMINATION OF PROSTHETIC HEIGHT

- The prosthetic height also is critical in re-establishing appropriate muscle tension and shoulder mechanics.
- Preoperative templating may be helpful.
- Intraoperative examination of soft tissue tension, including the deltoid, rotator cuff, and the long head of the biceps, combined with fluoroscopic imaging aids in prosthetic height placement.
- Common errors involve placing the prosthesis too low, resulting in poor deltoid muscle tension and no room for the tuberosities (**TECH FIG 5**).

Align to notch
at anterior fin

1-2 cm

S. Lippitt,
M.D.

S. Lippitt,
M.D.

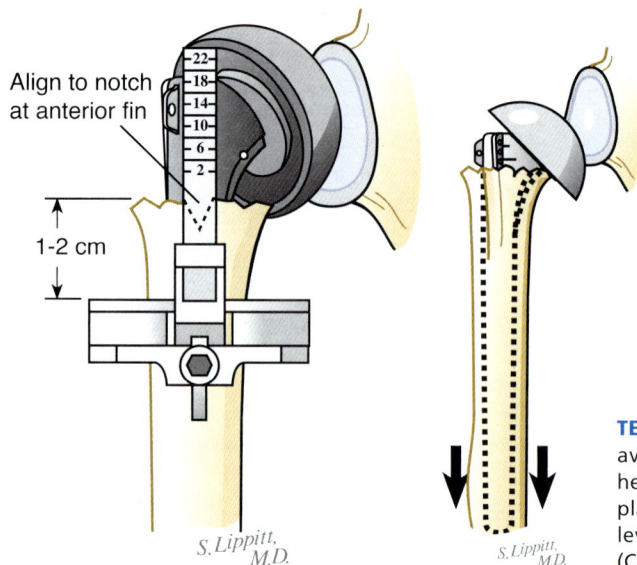

TECH FIG 5 • Height adjustment. A commercially available fracture jig permits intraoperative height adjustment. Similarly, a sponge may be placed holding the trial stem at a determined level, allowing for intraoperative assessment. (Copyright Steven B. Lippitt, MD.)

TRIAL REDUCTION

- Drill holes are placed in the proximal humerus medial and lateral to the bicipital groove, with 1-mm cottony Dacron sutures subsequently passed for fixation of the tuberosity to the shaft (**TECH FIG 6A**).
- A trial reduction is then performed with the mobilized tuberosities fitted below the head of the modular prosthesis.

- A towel clip can be used to hold the tuberosities for fluoroscopic examination and assessment of glenohumeral stability.
- Intraoperative fluoroscopy is helpful in confirming appropriate implant height and glenohumeral stability (**TECH FIG 6B**).
- The humeral head should not subluxate more than 25% to 30% of the glenoid height inferiorly.

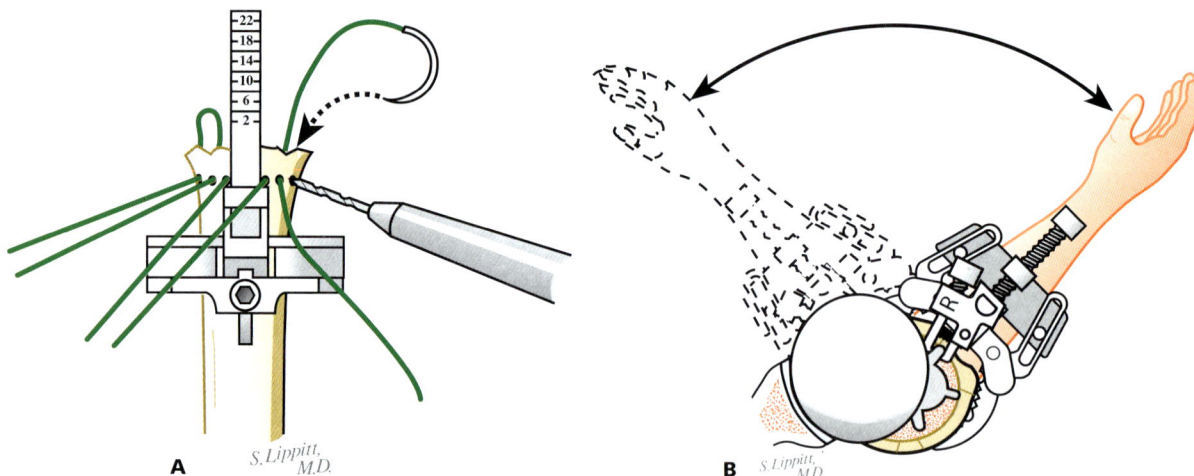

A

S. Lippitt,
M.D.

B

S. Lippitt,
M.D.

TECH FIG 6 • **A.** Humeral shaft preparation. Drill holes are placed in the proximal humerus medial and lateral to the bicipital groove with 1-mm cottony Dacron sutures. **B.** Trial reduction. A trial reduction may be performed with the fracture jig in place, allowing assessment of the functional range of motion. (Copyright Steven B. Lippitt, MD.)

FINAL IMPLANT PLACEMENT

- The final humeral component should be cemented in all fracture patients.
  - A cement restrictor is placed to prevent cement extravasation distally.

- Pulsatile lavage and retrograde injection of cement with suction pressurization also is used (**TECH FIG 7A**). Excess cement is removed during the curing phase.

- Spaces between the tuberosities, prosthesis, and shaft are packed with autogenous cancellous bone graft from the resected humeral head (**TECH FIG 7B**).
- A second trial reduction may be performed with a trial head after cement fixation of the humeral stem.
- The final head may be impacted before stem implantation or after the repeat trial reduction.
- A cerclage suture is placed circumferentially around the greater tuberosity and through the supraspinatus insertion, and then medial to the prosthesis and through the subscapularis insertion (lesser tuberosity). Several authors have indicated superior fixation with the cerclage

suture when compared to tuberosity-to-tuberosity and tuberosity-to-fin fixation alone.[23]

- Overreduction of the tuberosities should be avoided to prevent limitations in external (lesser tuberosity) and internal (greater tuberosity) rotation.
- Sutures are then tied, beginning with tuberosity-to-shaft reapproximation, followed by tuberosity-to-tuberosity closure using the previously placed suture limbs (**TECH FIG 7C**).
- The lateral portion of the rotator interval is closed with the arm in approximately 30 degrees of external rotation with no. 2 nonabsorbable suture (**TECH FIG 7D**).

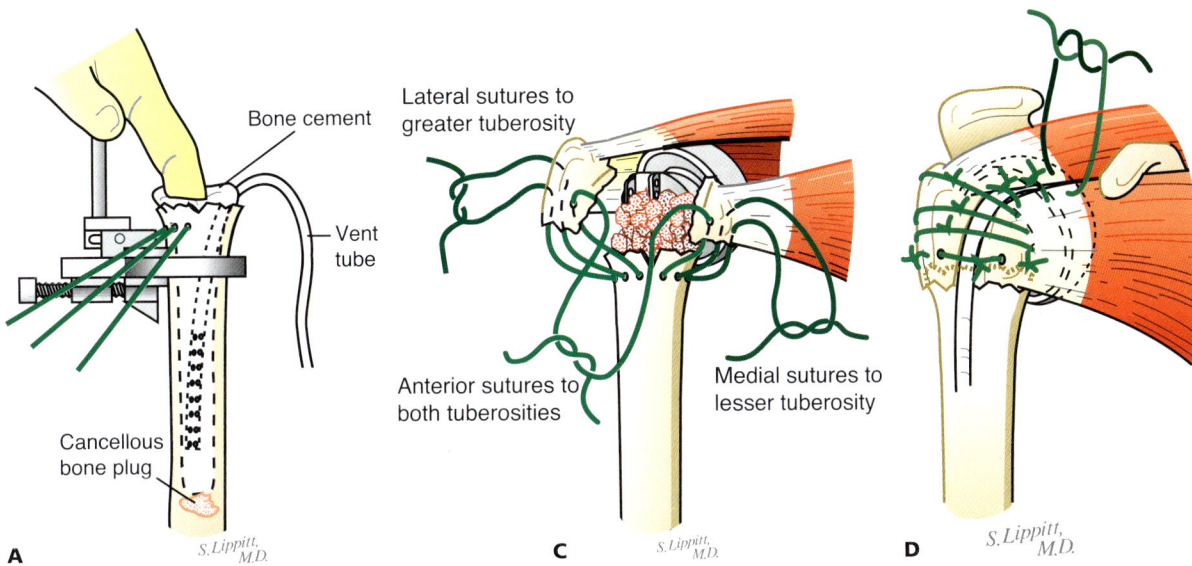

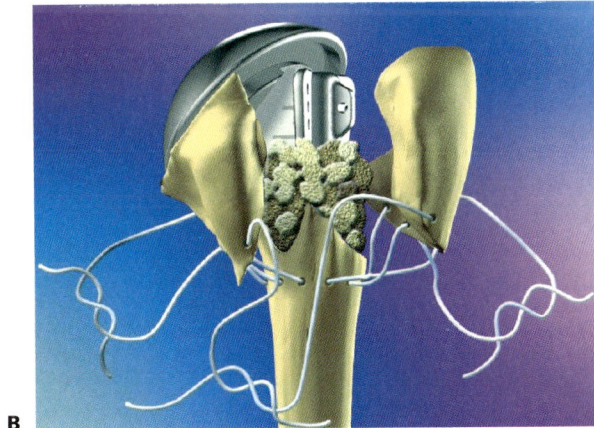

TECH FIG 7 • A. A cement restrictor is placed to prevent cement extravasation distally. Pulsatile lavage and retrograde injection of cement with suction pressurization is also used. **B.** Morselized cancellous bone graft is placed between the tuberosities and shaft. **C.** Tuberosity fixation. Previously placed suture limbs through the tuberosities and shaft are reapproximated. Not shown: a medial cerclage suture is placed circumferentially around the greater tuberosity and through the supraspinatus insertion, and then medial to the prosthesis and through the subscapularis insertion (lesser tuberosity) and tied. **D.** The rotator interval is closed with no. 2 nonabsorbable suture with the arm in about 30 degrees of external rotation. (**A,C,D:** Copyright Steven B. Lippitt, MD. **B:** Courtesy of DePuy Orthopaedics.)

SURGICAL WOUND CLOSURE

- The deltopectoral interval usually is not closed. Drain suction is recommended in both acute and chronic injuries to prevent hematoma formation.
- A commercially available pain pump may be used to augment postoperative analgesia and to reduce narcotic medication use.
- The subcutaneous tissues are reapproximated with 2-0 absorbable suture. Subcuticular closure is performed with 2-0 monofilament suture.
- The patient is then placed in a sling or shoulder immobilizer with 45 degrees of abduction for comfort.

PEARLS AND PITFALLS

Indications	■ A complete history and physical examination should be performed, with particular attention paid to the neurovascular status.
Imaging studies	■ Appropriate plain radiographs with possible CT scan supplementation aid in the surgical decision-making.
Tuberosity identification	■ Use the long head of the biceps to define the tuberosities for mobilization. ■ Tag this for later tenodesis before wound closure.
Implant placement	■ Know the specifics of the implant system, including its limitations. ■ Place the implant in appropriate retroversion (approximately 20 to 30 degrees). ■ Check the height of the trial stem before performing cement fixation, using a fracture jig or sponge for provisional fixation. ■ Intraoperative fluoroscopy can be used to assess appropriate implant height.
Tuberosity fixation	■ Avoid loss of external rotation or internal rotation with overreduction of the lesser and greater tuberosities, respectively.
Postoperative rehabilitation	■ On postoperative day 1, initiate gentle pendulum exercises, with passive forward flexion and external rotation (at 0 degrees of abduction). Always modify rehabilitation protocol based on intraoperative assessment of soft tissue compromise and patient neurologic status.

POSTOPERATIVE CARE

■ Physician-directed therapy is initiated on postoperative day 1 with gentle, gravity-assisted pendulum exercises, as well as passive pulley-and-stick exercises to maintain forward flexion and external rotation (motion limits placed by surgeon based upon intraoperative stability).

■ After discharge, the patient's wound is re-examined and sutures removed at 10 to 14 days. Gentle range-of-motion exercises are continued.

■ At 6 weeks, repeat radiographs are obtained to evaluate tuberosity healing. When tuberosity healing is evident, phase 2 exercises are initiated with isometric rotator cuff exercises and active assisted elevation with the pulley.

■ At 3 months, strength training with graduated rubber bands (phase 3) is implemented. Maximal motion and function are obtained at about 12 months from date of surgery.

OUTCOMES

■ About 90% of patients treated with hemiarthroplasty demonstrate minimal pain, despite a wide range of function, motion, and strength.

■ Factors that portend a poor outcome after hemiarthroplasty for fractures include tuberosity malposition, superior migration of the humeral prosthesis, stiffness, persistent pain, poor initial positioning of the implant (excessive retroversion, decreased height), and age over 75 years in women.[4]

■ When comparing acute intervention versus late reconstruction, most authors report poorer outcomes with delayed surgical intervention (more than 2 weeks), particularly with functional results.[20,25,26]

COMPLICATIONS

■ Complications include delays in wound healing, infection, nerve injury, humeral fracture, component malposition, instability, nonunion of the tuberosities, rotator cuff tearing, regional pain syndrome, periarticular fibrosis, heterotopic bone formation, component loosening, and glenoid arthritis.[3,7,19]

■ The most common problems in acute fracture treatment involve stiffness, nonunion, malunion or resorption of the tuberosities.[7,19]

■ In patients with chronic fractures treated with hemiarthroplasty, the most common problems encountered were instability, heterotopic ossification, tuberosity malunion or nonunion, and rotator cuff tears.[19]

REFERENCES

1. Beredjiklian PK, Iannotti JP, Norris TR, et al. Operative treatment of malunion of a fracture of the proximal aspect of the humerus. J Bone Joint Surg Am 1998;80:1484–1497.
2. Blaine TA, Bigliani LU, Levine WN. Fractures of the proximal humerus. In: Rockwood CA Jr, Masten FA III, Wirth MA, et al, eds. The Shoulder, ed 3. Philadelphia: Elsevier, 2004:355–412.
3. Bohsali KI, Wirth MA, Rockwood CA Jr. Current concepts review: complications of total shoulder arthroplasty. J Bone Joint Surg Am 2006;88A:2279–2292.
4. Boileau P, Krishnan SG, Tinsi L, et al. Tuberosity malposition and migration: reason for poor outcomes after hemiarthroplasty for displaced fractures of the proximal humerus. J Shoulder Elbow Surg 2002;11:401–412.
5. Boileau P, Walch G, Trojani C, et al. Surgical classification and limits of shoulder arthroplasty. In Walch G, Boileau P, eds. Shoulder Arthroplasty. Berlin: Springer-Verlag, 1999:349–358.
6. Bosch U, Skurek M, Fremery RW, et al. Outcome after primary and secondary hemiarthroplasty in elderly patients with fractures of the proximal humerus. J Shoulder Elbow Surg 1998;7:479–484.
7. Compito CA, Self EB, Bigliani LU. Arthroplasty and acute shoulder trauma. Clin. Orthop Relat Res 1994;307:27–36.
8. DeFranco MJ, Brems JJ, Williams GR Jr, et al. Evaluation and management of valgus impacted four-part proximal humerus fractures. Clin Orthop Relat Res 2006;442:109–114.
9. Frankle MA, Ondrovic LE, Markee BA, et al. Stability of tuberosity attachment in proximal humeral arthroplasty. J Shoulder Elbow Surg 2002;11:413–420.
10. Gerber C, Schneeberger A, Vinh T. The arterial vascularization of the humeral head: An anatomical study. J Bone Joint Surg Am 1990; 72:1486–1494.
11. Green A. Proximal humerus fractures. In: Norris T, ed. Orthopaedic Knowledge Update: Shoulder and Elbow 2. Rosemont, IL: AAOS; 2002:209–217.
12. Green A, Lippitt SB, Wirth MA. Humeral head replacement arthroplasty. In: Wirth MA, ed. Proximal Humerus Fractures. Rosemont, IL: AAOS, 2005:39–48.
13. Green A, Norris T. Proximal humerus fractures and fracture-dislocations. In: Jupiter J, ed. Skeletal Trauma, ed 3. Philadelphia: WB Saunders; 2003:1532–1624.

14. Hartsock LA, Estes WJ, Murray CA, et al. Shoulder hemiarthroplasty for proximal humeral fractures. Orthop Clin North Am 1998; 467–475.

15. Huopio J, Kroger H, Honkanen R, et al. Risk factors for perimenopausal fractures: A prospective study. Osteoporos Int 2000; 11:219–227.

16. Iannotti JP, Gabriel JP, Schneck SL, et al. The normal glenohumeral relationships: An anatomical study of one hundred and forty shoulders. J Bone Joint Surg Am 1992;74A:491–500.

17. Jakob R, Miniaci A, Anson P, et al. Four-part valgus impacted fractures of the proximal humerus. J Bone Joint Surg Br 1991;73B: 295–298.

18. Laing P. The arterial supply of the adult humerus. J Bone Joint Surg Am 1956;38A:1105–1116.

19. Muldoon MP, Cofield RH. Complications of humeral head replacement for proximal humerus fractures. Instr Course Lect 1997: 46:15–24.

20. Neer CS. Displaced proximal humeral fractures. Part II: Treatment of 3-part and 4-part displacment. J Bone Joint Surg Am 1970;52A: 1090–1103.

21. Norris TR, Green A, McGuigan FX. Late prosthetic shoulder arthroplasty for displaced proximal humerus fractures. J Shoulder Elbow Surg 1995;4:271–280.

22. Orthopaedic Trauma Association Committee for Coding and Classification: Fracture and Dislocation Compendium. J Orthop Trauma 1996;10(suppl):1–155.

23. Pearl ML, Volk AG. Retroversion of the proximal humerus in relationship to the prosthetic replacement arthroplasty. J Shoulder Elbow Surg 1995;4:286–289.

24. Stablebforth PG. Four part fractures of the neck of the humerus. J Bone Joint Surg Br 1984;66B:104–108.

25. Zuckerman JD, Cuomo F, Koval KJ. Proximal humeral replacement for complex fractures: Indications and surgical technique. Instr Course Lect 1997;46:7–14.

Chapter 20

Plate Fixation of Humeral Shaft Fractures

Matthew J. Garberina and Charles L. Getz

DEFINITION

- Humeral shaft fractures, which account for about 3% of adult fractures, usually result from a direct blow or indirect twisting injury to the brachium.
- These injuries are most commonly treated nonoperatively with a prefabricated fracture brace. The humerus is the most freely movable long bone, and anatomic reduction is not required.
- Patients often can tolerate up to 20 degrees of anterior angulation, 30 degrees of varus angulation, and 3 cm of shortening without significant functional loss.
- There are, however, several indications for surgical treatment of humeral shaft fractures:
  - Open fracture
  - Bilateral humeral shaft fractures or polytrauma; floating elbow
  - Segmental fracture
  - Inability to maintain acceptable alignment with closed treatment (ie, angulation greater than 15 degrees)—seen more commonly with transverse fractures
  - Humeral shaft nonunion
  - Pathologic fractures
  - Arterial or brachial plexus injury
- Open reduction with internal plate fixation requires extensive dissection and operative skill. However, it offers advantages over intramedullary fixation because the rotator cuff is not violated, which leads to improved postoperative shoulder function.[3]

ANATOMY

- The humeral shaft is defined using Key's landmarks: the area between the upper margin of the pectoralis major tendon and the supracondylar ridge.[7]
- The blood supply of the humeral shaft comes from the posterior humeral circumflex vessels and branches of the brachial and profunda brachial arteries.
- The radial nerve and profunda brachial artery pass through the triangular interval (bordered superiorly by the teres major, medially by the medial head of the triceps, and laterally by the humeral shaft). The nerve then transverses from medial to lateral behind the humeral shaft and travels distally to a location between the brachialis and brachioradialis muscles.
- The musculocutaneous nerve lies on the undersurface of the biceps muscle and terminates distally as the lateral antebrachial cutaneous nerve.
- The humeral shaft has anteromedial, anterolateral, and posterior surfaces. Proximal and midshaft fractures are more amenable to plating on the anterolateral surface, whereas distal fractures often require posterior plate fixation.

PATHOGENESIS

- Humeral shaft fractures occur after both direct and indirect injuries. Direct blows to the brachium can fracture the humeral shaft in a transverse pattern, often with a butterfly fragment. Injuries with high degrees of energy often result in a greater degree of fracture comminution.
- Indirect injuries, such as those that can occur with activities such as arm wrestling, often involve a twisting mechanism and result in a spiral fracture pattern. Higher-energy injuries may result in muscle interposition between the fracture fragments, which can inhibit reduction and healing.
- A study of 240 humeral shaft fractures revealed radial nerve palsies in 42 patients, for an overall rate of 18% (17% in closed injuries). Fractures in the midshaft were more likely to have concomitant radial nerve palsy. Twenty-five of these patients had complete recovery in a range of 1 day to 10 months. Ten patients did not have radial nerve recovery. Median and ulnar nerve palsies were seen very rarely in patients with open fractures.[7]
- Concomitant vascular injuries are present in about 3% of patients with humeral shaft fractures.

NATURAL HISTORY

- Almost all humeral shaft fractures heal with nonoperative management. The most common treatment method is initial splinting from shoulder to wrist, followed by application of a prefabricated fracture brace when the patient is comfortable, usually within 2 weeks of the injury.
- Studies by Sarmiento and coauthors[10,11] have shown the effectiveness of functional bracing in the treatment of humeral shaft fractures. Nonunion rates with this method of treatment are in the 4% range, lower than seen when treating with external fixators, plates, or intramedullary nails.
- Closed fractures with initial radial nerve palsy can be observed, with expected recovery over a period of 3 to 6 months. Late-developing radial nerve palsies require surgical exploration.
- Angulation of the humeral shaft after fracture healing is expected and is well tolerated when it is less than 20 degrees. Varus deformity is most common.[10]
- Adjacent joint stiffness of the shoulder and elbow also is common. If the situation dictates treatment, physical therapy reliably restores joint motion in these patients.
- Relative contraindications to closed treatment include bilateral humeral shaft fractures or patients with polytrauma who require an intact brachium to ambulate. Transverse fractures and those with significant muscle imposition also are more amenable to operative fixation.[11]

PATIENT HISTORY AND PHYSICAL FINDINGS

- The examining physician must perform a complete examination of the affected limb to rule out concomitant injuries.
- The skin should be thoroughly evaluated for evidence of an open fracture. This includes examination of the axilla. Entry

and exit wounds are sought in gunshot victims. Swelling is common, and the patient may have an obvious deformity.

- The patient often braces the affected limb to his or her side, making evaluation of shoulder and elbow range of motion difficult. Bony prominences should be gently palpated to evaluate for other injuries, such as an olecranon fracture.
- Evaluate the appearance and skeletal stability of the forearm to rule out the presence of a co-existing both-bone forearm fracture ("floating elbow"). This finding necessitates operative fixation of humeral, radial, and ulnar fractures.
- Determine the vascular status of the upper extremity by palpating the radial and ulnar pulses at the wrist. Compare these findings with the unaffected limb. Selected cases may require Doppler arterial examination.[2]
- A complete neurologic assessment is necessary, with particular attention focused on the status of the radial nerve. This structure is at risk proximally as it passes posterior to the humeral shaft after emerging from the triangular interval, as well as distally, as it lies adjacent to the supracondylar ridge (near the location of the Holstein-Lewis distal one-third spiral humeral shaft fracture).
- Examine sensory function in the first dorsal web space, wrist extension, and thumb interphalangeal joint extension to determine the functional status of the radial nerve.

IMAGING AND OTHER DIAGNOSTIC STUDIES

- At least two plain radiographs at 90-degree angles to each other are necessary to evaluate the displacement, shortening, and comminution of the humeral shaft fracture.
- Radiographic views of the shoulder and elbow are necessary to rule out proximal extension of the shaft fracture or concomitant elbow injury (ie, olecranon fracture). This is especially important in high-energy injuries
- If swelling or evidence of skeletal instability about the forearm is present, dedicated forearm radiographs can determine the presence of a floating elbow (ie, ipsilateral humeral shaft fracture plus both-bone forearm fractures).

DIFFERENTIAL DIAGNOSIS

- Distal humerus fracture
- Proximal humerus fracture
- Elbow dislocation
- Shoulder dislocation

NONOPERATIVE MANAGEMENT

- Most isolated humeral shaft fractures can be treated nonoperatively. Initial treatment can vary with fracture location and involves splinting in either a posterior elbow or coaptation splint. The elbow is positioned in 90 degrees of flexion. An isolated humeral shaft fracture rarely necessitates an overnight hospital stay.
- In the past, definitive nonoperative treatment involved coaptation splinting or the use of hanging arm casts. Currently, functional fracture bracing provides adequate bony alignment, while local muscle compression and fracture motion promote osteogenesis. These braces provide soft tissue compression and allow functional use of the extremity.[11]
- Timing of brace application depends on the degree of swelling and patient discomfort. On average, the brace is applied about 2 weeks after the injury. A collar and cuff help

with initial patient comfort and should be worn during recumbency until the fracture heals.

- The brace often requires frequent retightening over the first 2 weeks as swelling subsides. Elbow and wrist range-of-motion exercises out of the sling are encouraged.
- Functional bracing requires that the patient be able to sit erect, and weight bearing on the humerus is not allowed. The level of humeral shaft fracture does not preclude the use of functional bracing, even if the fracture line extends above or below the brace.
- Anatomic alignment of the humerus rarely is achieved, with varus deformity most common. However, patients often are able to tolerate the bony angulation and still perform activities of daily living after injury. A cosmetic deformity rarely exists.
- Pendulum exercises are encouraged as soon as possible post-injury. Active elevation and abduction are avoided until bony healing has occurred, to prevent fracture angulation. The surgeon obtains radiographs after brace application and again 1 week later. If alignment is acceptable, repeat radiographs are obtained at 3- to 4- week intervals until fracture healing occurs.[10,11]

SURGICAL MANAGEMENT

- Certain humeral shaft fractures are not amenable to conservative treatment. Open fractures or high-energy injuries with significant axial distraction are treated with open reduction and internal fixation. Patients with polytrauma, bilateral humeral shaft fractures, vascular injury, or an inability to sit erect are best treated with operative fixation. Unacceptable fracture alignment requires abandonment of nonoperative treatment. Finally, humeral shaft nonunion is a clear indication for open reduction and internal fixation with bone grafting.[4,9]

Preoperative Planning

- The surgeon must review all radiographic images and must rule out ipsilateral elbow or shoulder injury.
- Preoperative radiographs help the surgeon estimate the required plate length. Higher-energy injuries with comminution may benefit from plating and supplemental bone grafting. The surgeon must plan for various scenarios based on these studies: moderate comminution or bone loss can be addressed with cancellous allograft or autograft bone, whereas more extensive bone defects may require strut grafting.
- Proximal and middle-third humeral shaft fractures are addressed using an anterolateral approach. Distal-third humeral shaft fractures often are treated via a posterior approach, because the distal humeral shaft is flat posteriorly, making it an ideal location for plate placement.
- Fracture patterns with extension into the proximal humerus can be exposed with a deltopectoral extension to the anterolateral humeral dissection.
- The surgeon notes any pre-existing scars that may affect the desired surgical approach, and neurovascular status is documented, with particular attention to radial nerve function.

Positioning

- Positioning depends on the intended surgical approach. For an anterolateral or medial approach, the patient is brought to the edge of the bed in the supine position. A hand table is attached to the bed and the patient's injured arm is placed on the hand table in slight abduction (**FIG 1A**).

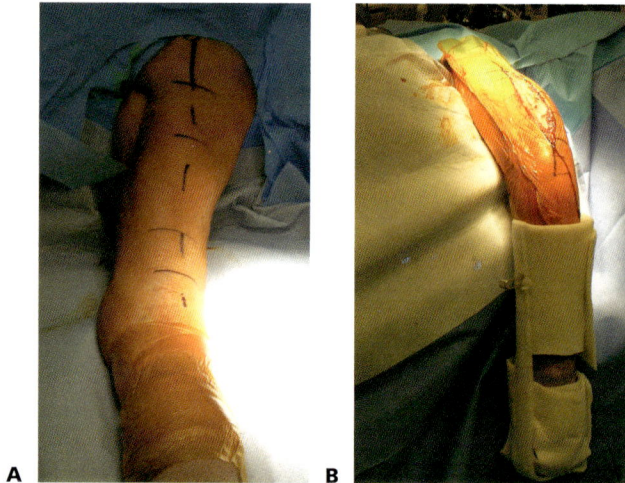

FIG 1 • **A.** Positioning for the anterolateral approach to the humeral shaft with the shoulder abducted and the arm on a hand table. **B.** Positioning for the posterior approach to the humeral shaft with the patient in the lateral decubitus position.

■ For a posterior approach, the patient can be placed prone or in the lateral decubitus position. A stack of pillows can support the brachium during the procedure (**FIG 1B**).

Approach

■ The approach depends on fracture location and the presence of any previous surgical incisions. The anterolateral and posterior approaches to the humerus are used most commonly, for proximal two-third and distal third fractures, respectively.

■ In patients who have already undergone multiple procedures to the affected extremity, Jupiter[6] recommends consideration of a medial approach to take advantage of virgin tissue planes.

TECHNIQUES

ANTEROLATERAL APPROACH TO THE HUMERUS

■ The incision courses over the lateral aspect of the biceps, beginning proximally at the deltoid tubercle and terminating just proximal to the antecubital crease (**TECH FIG 1**).

■ A tourniquet rarely is used, because it often limits proximal exposure.

■ The lateral antebrachial cutaneous nerve lies in the distal aspect of the incision and must be protected during exposure.

■ Bluntly enter the interval between the biceps and brachialis by sweeping a finger from proximal to distal.

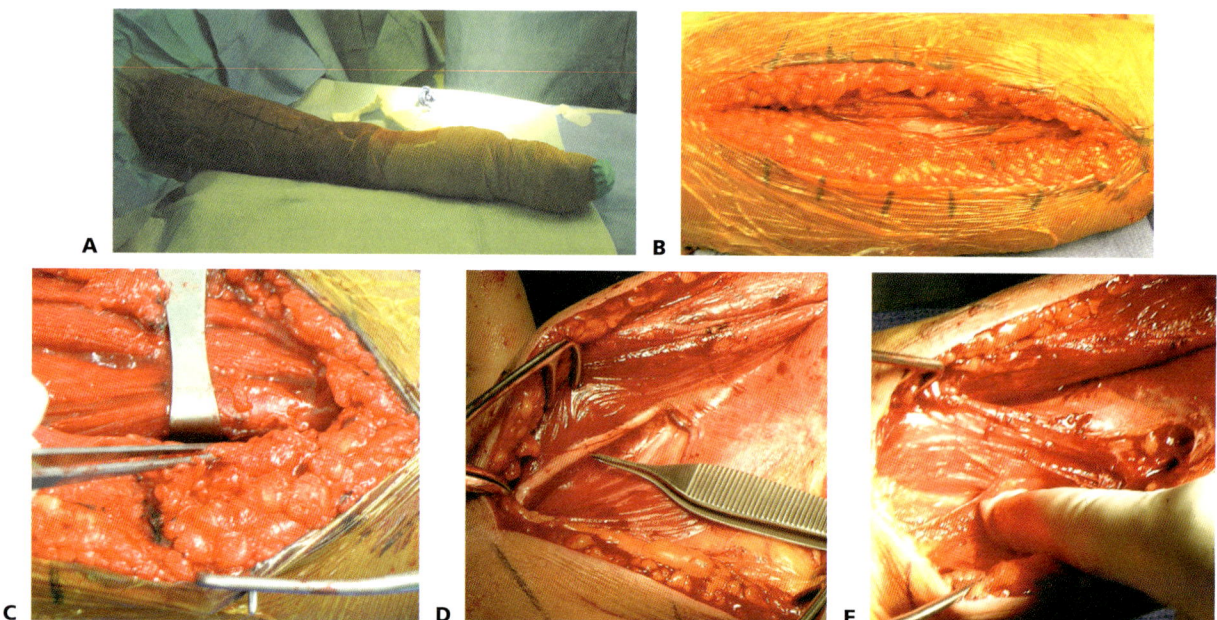

TECH FIG 1 • **A.** Anterolateral incision. **B.** Skin and subcutaneous tissue incised. **C.** Retractor on brachialis muscle, forceps on brachioradialis. **D.** Musculocutaneous nerve on undersurface of biceps muscle. **E.** Radial nerve in interval between brachialis and brachioradialis. *(continued)*

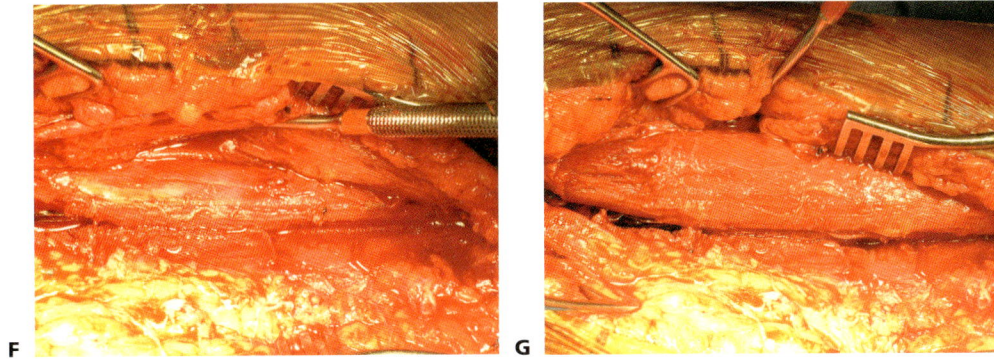

TECH FIG 1 • *(continued)* **F.** Biceps lifted to reveal brachialis muscle. **G.** Brachialis muscle split in its lateral third.

- At the level of the midhumerus, identify the musculocutaneous nerve on the undersurface of the biceps muscle. Trace this nerve out distally to protect its terminal branch, which forms the lateral antebrachial cutaneous nerve.
- Distally, the interval between the brachialis and brachioradialis is dissected to expose the radial nerve. Protect the radial nerve with a vessel loop so that it can be identified at all times.

- The brachialis is split in line with its fibers between the medial two thirds and lateral one third. This is an internervous plane between the radial nerve medially and the musculocutaneous nerve laterally.
- Identify the fracture site and proceed with reduction and fixation.

POSTERIOR APPROACH TO THE HUMERUS

- Make a generous incision over the midline of the posterior arm extending to the olecranon fossa (**TECH FIG 2**).
- Identify the interval between the long and lateral heads of the triceps proximally. Bluntly dissect this interval, taking the long head medially and the lateral head laterally.

- Distally, several blood vessels cross this plane; they require coagulation before transection.
- Identify the radial nerve proximal to the medial head of the triceps in the spiral groove. Protect the radial nerve throughout the case.
- Split the medial head of the triceps in its midline from proximal to distal to expose the fracture site.

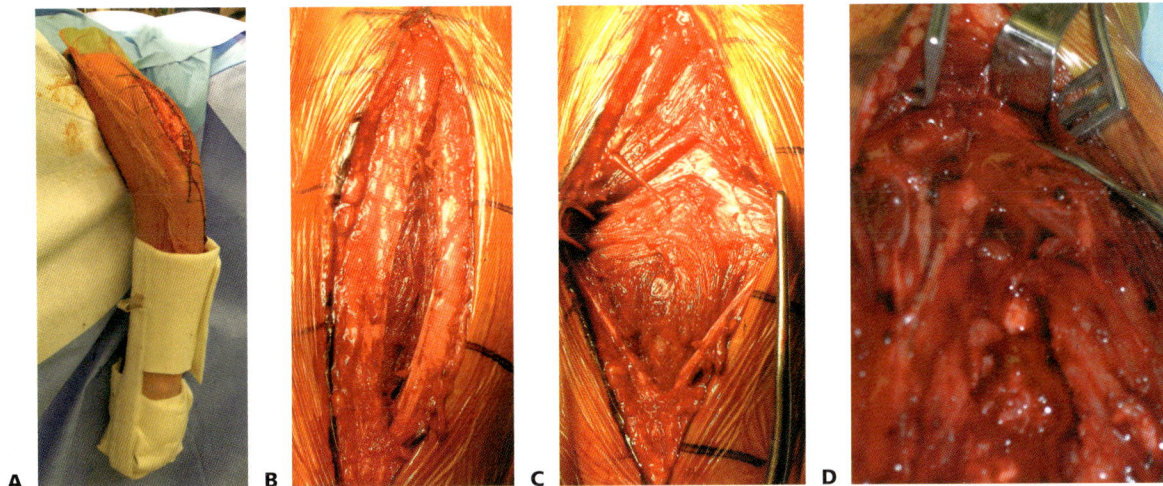

TECH FIG 2 • **A.** Incision for posterior approach. **B.** Superficial triceps split. **C.** Deep triceps split. **D.** The probe points to the radial nerve as it exits the spiral groove from medial to lateral; the fracture site is seen distally.

FRACTURE REDUCTION

- Sharp periosteal dissection exposes the fracture site. Evaluate the degree, if any, of comminution.
- Limit periosteal stripping to adequately expose the fracture. Make every attempt to leave some soft tissue attached to each fragment so as not to devascularize the fragments.
- Gentle traction and rotation often can bring the fracture fragments into better alignment.
- Anatomically reduce the fracture with one or more reduction clamps. It is advisable to reduce the fracture completely before definitive fixation, and this often requires the use of multiple reduction clamps (**TECH FIG 3**).
- After the fracture is reduced, the fragments can be provisionally fixed with Kirschner wires. Place the wires so as not to interfere with plate fixation.
- Alternatively, 3.5- or 4.5-mm interfragmentary screws can be used to hold the fracture aligned until plate fixation.
- Transverse fractures with minimal comminution often can be directly reduced with the plate and Faberge clamps.

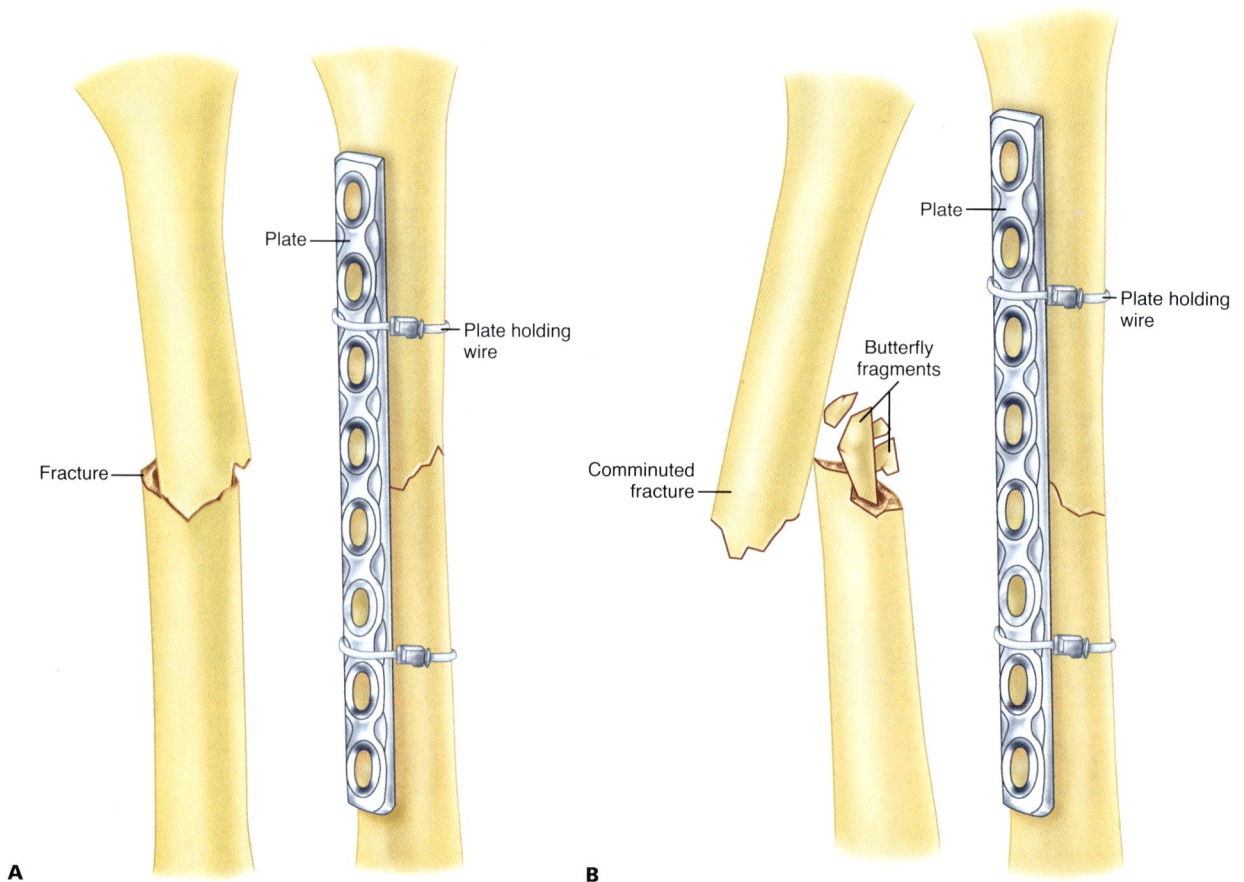

TECH FIG 3 • **A.** Fracture reduction maintained temporarily. **B.** Hold the plate over the reduced fracture with a plate-holding clamp.

EXPOSURE OF FRACTURE NONUNION

- Exposure of the radial nerve is more challenging, but it is very important in this situation. In many cases it is best to dissect out the nerve distally in the interval between the brachialis and brachioradialis and proximally medial to the spiral groove. The nerve is then carefully dissected free from the nonunion site.
- Pinpoint the exact location of the nonunion with a no. 15 scalpel.
- The ends of the nonunion can be brought out through the wound, and all fibrous material is extracted.
- After thorough fracture débridement, the amount of bone loss becomes clear. The surgeon can now determine whether standard cancellous bone grafting or strut grafting is necessary.

PLATE APPLICATION

- After fracture reduction, the plate length is determined.
- Humeral shaft fractures require at least six cortices of fixation above and below the fracture site.
- In larger bones, a broad 4.5-mm dynamic compression plate can provide optimal fixation. In smaller bones, a 4.5-mm limited contour dynamic compression plate often provides a better fit.
- Provisionally place the plate on a flat surface of the humerus and hold it in place with a plate-holding clamp.
- 4.5-mm cortical screws are placed through the plate holes proximal and distal to the fracture. Compression techniques can be used, where appropriate.
- Ensure that no soft tissue, especially nerve, is trapped between the plate and the bone.
- Make sure to obtain screw purchase in at least six cortices above and below the fracture (**TECH FIG 4**).
- Cerclage wiring over the plate can add supplemental fixation, especially in weak bone.
- Rotate the arm and flex and extend the elbow to evaluate fracture stability.
- Apply cancellous bone graft into defects as needed.

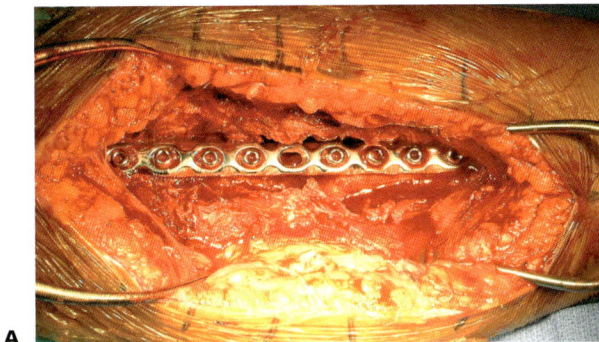

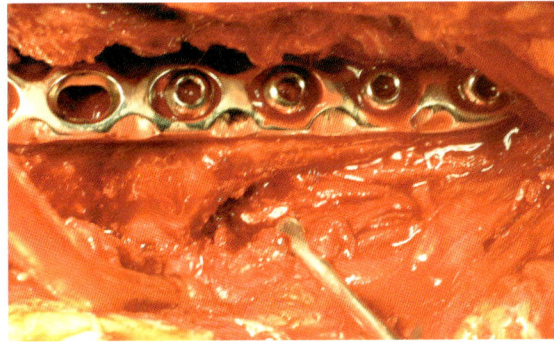

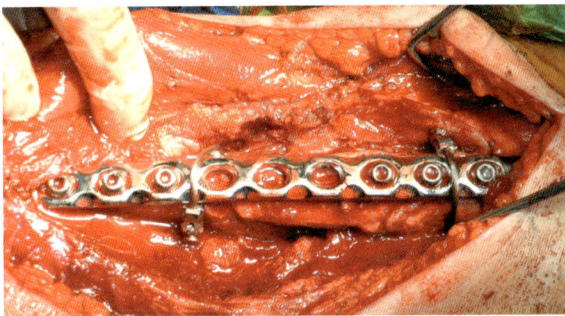

TECH FIG 4 • **A.** Plate spanning the fracture site with at least six cortices of fixation proximally and distally. **B.** Anterior plate with a probe pointing to the radial nerve as it exits the spiral groove posteriorly (proximal is to the right, distal to the left). **C.** Supplemental cerclage wire fixation can augment stability in weak bone.

MEDIAL APPROACH

- Positioning is similar to the anterolateral approach.
- Make an incision over the medial intermuscular septum from the axilla to 5 cm proximal to the medial epicondyle (**TECH FIG 5**).
- Mobilize the ulnar nerve.
- Resect the medial intermuscular septum; identify and coagulate the adjacent venous plexus with bipolar electrocautery.
- Mobilize the triceps posteriorly and the biceps/brachialis anteriorly.
- Expose the fracture site.
- The axillary incision raises concern for infection; there is also concern that the ulnar nerve can scar to the plate.

TECH FIG 5 • **A.** Incision for the medial approach. *(continued)*

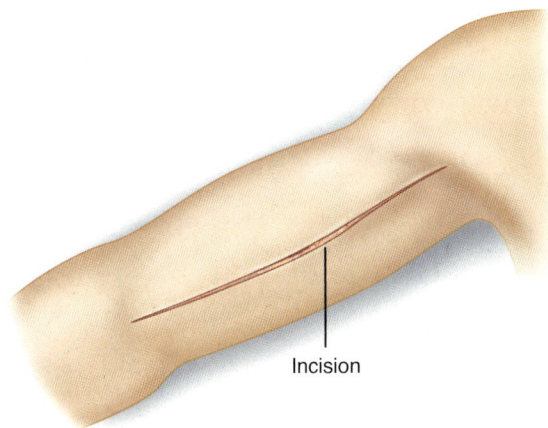

Incision

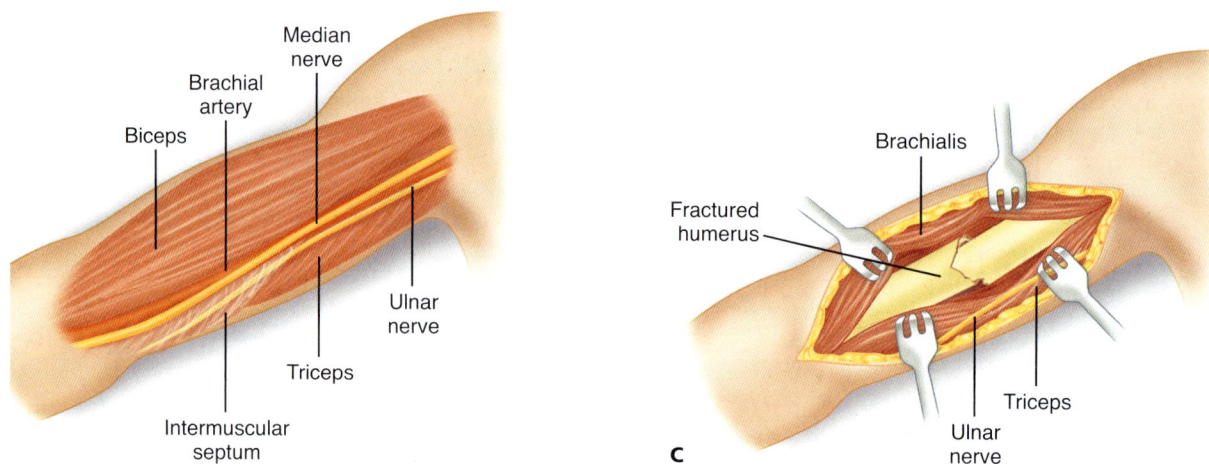

TECH FIG 5 • *(continued)* **B,C.** The brachialis and biceps are raised anteriorly, and the triceps is raised posteriorly for fracture exposure.

PEARLS AND PITFALLS

Indications	▪ Operative treatment is reserved for open fractures, patients with multiple fractures, and fractures with inadequate reduction.
Preoperative planning	▪ Review all radiographs and determine the best surgical approach. ▪ Estimate potential plate length and prepare for possible bone grafting.
Surgical exposure	▪ Locate and protect the radial nerve. ▪ Expose and reduce fracture fragments and temporarily hold them in place with pins or clamps. ▪ Alternatively, fix larger fragments with interfragmentary screws.
Plate fixation	▪ Ensure that plate length allows six cortices of fixation proximal and distal to the fracture. ▪ Use 4.5-mm dynamic compression plates or limited contact dynamic compression plates. ▪ Use compressive techniques when indicated.
Radial nerve function	▪ Preoperatively, document a detailed neurovascular examination. ▪ Ensure that the radial nerve is not trapped within the plate before closure.

POSTOPERATIVE CARE

▪ Postoperative radiographs ensure proper fracture alignment and plate placement (**FIG 2**).

▪ Initially, the patient can be placed in a sling or posterior elbow splint. This is removed and range-of-motion exercises are started when patient comfort allows (usually 1 to 2 days postoperative).

▪ Weight bearing on the affected upper extremity is allowed based on patient comfort.[12]

▪ Initial therapy consists of elbow range-of-motion and shoulder pendulum and passive self-assist exercises.

▪ The patient can come out of the sling after 2 weeks and start waist-level activities with the operative arm.

▪ At 6 weeks, elbow motion should be near normal range, and shoulder strengthening is added to the patient's physical therapy.

▪ At 3 months, radiographs should reveal some callus formation. If no callus is evident, radiographs are repeated every 6 weeks until evidence of healing appears.

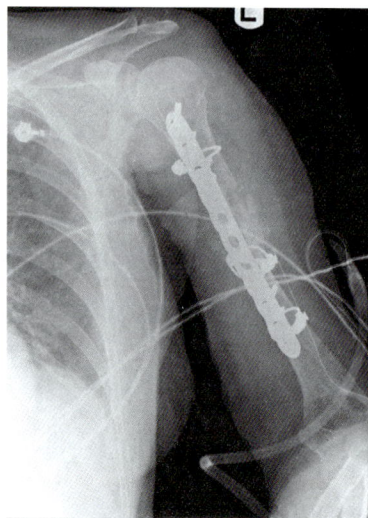

FIG 2 • Postoperative radiograph.

OUTCOMES

- Plate fixation leads to union in 90% to 98% of cases.
- Plating offers decreased complication rates compared to intramedullary nailing, especially in terms of shoulder dysfunction.[8]
- Iatrogenic radial nerve palsy occurs in about 2% to 5% of cases and usually resolves in 3 to 6 months. Electromyography helps monitor return of nerve function in patients with prolonged palsy. Radial nerve exploration is indicated when no nerve function returns by 6 months.
- Elbow and shoulder range of motion usually return to normal postoperatively.

COMPLICATIONS

- Infection
- Nonunion
- Malunion
- Hardware failure
- Radial nerve palsy
- Shoulder impingement
- Elbow stiffness

REFERENCES

1. Garberina MJ, Getz CL, Beredjiklian P, et al. Open reduction and internal fixation of humeral shaft nonunions. Tech Shoulder Elbow Surg 2006;7:131–138.
2. Gregory PR. Fractures of the shaft of the humerus. In Bucholz RW, Heckman JD, eds. Rockwood and Green's Fractures in Adults, ed 5, vol 1. Philadelphia: Lippincott Williams & Wilkins, 2001:973–996.
3. Gregory PR, Sanders RW. Compression plating versus intramedullary fixation of humeral shaft fractures. J Am Acad Orthop Surg 1997;5:215–223.
4. Healy WL, White GM, Mick CA, et al. Nonunion of the humeral shaft. Clin Orthop Relat Res 1987;219:206–213.
5. Hoppenfeld S, deBoer P. Surgical Exposures in Orthopaedics: The Anatomic Approach. Philadelphia: Lippincott Williams & Wilkins, 1994:51–82.
6. Jupiter JB. Complex non-union of the humeral diaphysis: Treatment with a medial approach, an anterior plate, and a vascularized fibular graft. J Bone Joint Surg Am 1990;72A:701–707.
7. Mast JW, Spiegel PG, Harvey JP Jr, et al. Fractures of the humeral shaft: A retrospective study of 240 adult fractures. Clin Orthop Relat Res 1975;112:254–262.
8. McCormack RG, Brien D, Buckley RE, et al. Fixation of fractures of the shaft of the humerus by dynamic compression plate or intramedullary nail: a prospective randomized trial. J Bone Joint Surg Br 2000;82B:336–339.
9. Ring D, Perey BH, Jupiter JB. The functional outcome of operative treatment of ununited fractures of the humeral diaphysis in older patients. J Bone Joint Surg Am 1999;81A:177–190.
10. Sarmiento A, Latta LL. Functional fracture bracing. J Am Acad Orthop Surg 1999;7:66–75.
11. Sarmiento A, Waddell JP, Latta LL. Diaphyseal humeral fractures: Treatment options. J Bone Joint Surg Am 2001;83A:1566–1579.
12. Tingstad EM, Wolinsky PR, Shyr Y, et al. Effect of immediate weightbearing on plated fractures of the humeral shaft. J Trauma 2000;49:278–280.

Chapter 21

Intramedullary Fixation of Humeral Shaft Fractures

Phillip Langer and Christopher T. Born

DEFINITION

- Incidence: 3% to 5% of all fractures[12]
- The AO/ASIF classification of humeral shaft fractures is based on increasing fracture comminution and is divided into three types according to the contact between the two main fragments:
  - Type A: simple (contact > 90%)
  - Type B: wedge/butterfly fragment (some contact)
  - Type C: complex/comminuted (no contact)
- Intramedullary nailing (IMN) can be used to stabilize fractures 2 cm distal to the surgical neck to 3 cm proximal to the olecranon fossa.[12]
- The precise role of IMN is not defined. Proponents offer the following benefits over formal open reduction with internal fixation (ORIF): it is minimally invasive, causing limited soft tissue damage and no periosteal stripping (preservation of vascular innervation); it is biomechanically superior; it is cosmetically advantageous (smaller incision); it is capable of indirect diaphyseal fracture reduction and metaphyseal fracture approximation.
  - Complications such as shoulder pain, delayed union or nonunion, fracture about the implant, iatrogenic fracture comminution, and difficulty in the reconstruction of failures, raise questions regarding the usefulness of intramedullary nailing over ORIF.
- Biomechanically, intramedullary nails are closer to the normal mechanical axis; consequently they act as a load-sharing device if there is cortical contact.
  - Unlike plate-and-screw fixation, a load-bearing construct, intramedullary nails are subjected to lower bending forces, making fatigue failure and cortical osteopenia secondary to stress shielding less likely.

ANATOMY

- Comparatively, there are several anatomic differences between the long bones of the upper extremity versus the long bones of the lower extremity (femur, tibia):
  - The medullary canal terminates at the metaphysis (versus diaphysis).
  - Isthmus: junction is at the middle–distal third (versus proximal–middle third).
  - Trumpet shape: the proximal two thirds of the humeral canal is cylindrical; distally. the medullary canal rapidly tapers to a prismatic end at the diaphysis (hard cortical bone) versus the wide flare of the metaphysis (soft cancellous bone).
- Because of the funnel shape of the humeral shaft, a true interference fit is difficult to obtain; therefore, proximal and distal static locking has become the standard of care for IMN of humeral fractures.
- Neurovascular considerations include average distances of key structures from notable bony landmarks:
  - Axillary nerve to proximal humerus, 6.1 ± 0.7 cm (range 4.5 to 6.9 cm)
  - Axillary nerve to surgical neck, 1.7 ± 0.8 cm (range 0.7 to 4.0 cm)
  - Axillary nerve to greater tuberosity, 45.6 mm
  - Axillary nerve to distal edge acromion, 5 to 6 cm
  - Crossing of radial nerve at lateral intermuscular septum to proximal humerus, 17.0 ± 2.3 cm (range 13 to 22 cm)
  - Crossing of radial nerve at lateral intermuscular septum to olecranon fossa, 12.0 ± 2.3 cm (range 7.4 to 16.6 cm)
  - Crossing of radial nerve at lateral intermuscular septum to distal humerus, 16.0 ± 0.4 cm (range 9.0 to 20.5 cm)[1,5,9]

PATHOGENESIS

- Biomodal distribution[17]
  - Young, male 21 to 30 years old: high-energy trauma
  - Older, female 60 to 80 years old: simple fall/rotational injury
- 5% open[17]
- 63% AO/ASIF type A fracture patterns[17]
- Various loading modes and the characteristic fracture patterns they create
  - Tension: transverse
  - Compression: oblique
  - Torsion: spiral
  - Bending: butterfly
  - High-energy: comminuted
- Red flags:
  - Minimal trauma indicates a pathologic process
  - Disconnect between history and fracture type suggests domestic abuse.

NATURAL HISTORY

- The humerus is well enveloped in muscle and soft tissue, hence its good prognosis for healing in most uncomplicated fractures.

PATIENT HISTORY AND PHYSICAL FINDINGS

- Patients with humeral shaft fractures present with arm pain, deformity, and swelling.
- Demographics, medical history, and information regarding the circumstance and mechanism of injury should be obtained.
- Particularly significant in upper extremity trauma: hand dominance, occupation, age, and pertinent comorbidities must be solicited from the patient. All of these factors play a major role in determining whether to pursue surgical versus nonsurgical treatment.
- On physical examination, the arm is typically shortened, angulated, or grossly deformed, with motion and crepitus on manipulation.
- Document the status of the skin (open versus closed fracture) and perform a careful neurovascular evaluation of the limb.

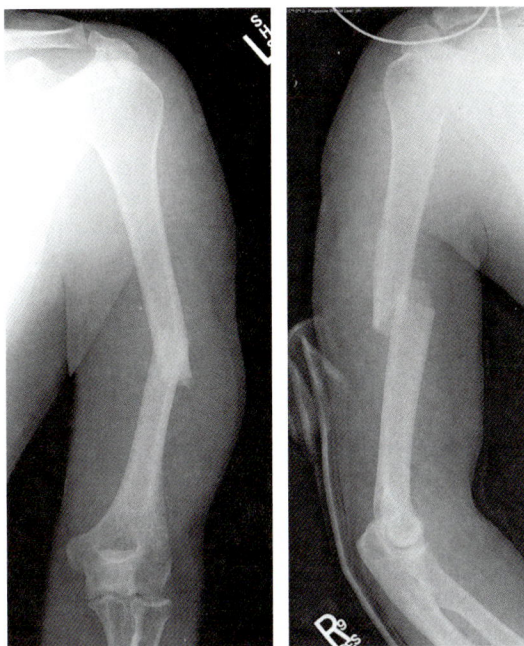

FIG 1 • AP and lateral radiographs of a displaced humeral shaft fracture, shortened and in varus angulation.

- If indicated, Doppler pulse and compartment pressures should be checked.
- Always examine the shoulder and elbow joint for possible associated musculoskeletal pathology.
- Examine the radial nerve for evidence of injury by testing resistance.

IMAGING AND OTHER DIAGNOSTIC STUDIES

- Initial studies must always include orthogonal views (anteroposterior [AP] and lateral radiographs) of the fracture site, shoulder, and elbow (**FIG 1**). To obtain these radiographs, move the patient rather than rotating the injured limb through the fracture site.
  - Traction radiographs may be helpful with comminuted or severely displaced fractures, and comparison radiographs of the contralateral side may be helpful for determining preoperative length.
- CT scans rarely are indicated. Rare situations in which they should be obtained include significant rotational abnormality, precluding accurate orthogonal radiographs, and suspicion of possible intra-articular extension or an additional fracture or fractures at a different level.
- Doppler pulse and compartment pressures should be checked if indicated following a thorough physical examination.
- Suspicion of vascular injuries warrants an angiogram.

DIFFERENTIAL DIAGNOSIS

- Osteoporosis
- Pathologic fractures
- High- or low-energy trauma
- Open or closed fractures
- Domestic abuse

NONOPERATIVE MANAGEMENT

- Most non- or minimally displaced humeral shaft fractures can be successfully treated nonoperatively, with union rates of more than 90% often reported.[12]
- Common closed techniques include hanging arm cast; coaptation splint; Velpeau dressing; abduction humeral/shoulder spica cast; functional brace; and traction.
  - Each of these modalities has been successfully employed, but most commonly either a hanging arm cast or coaptation splint is used for 1 to 2 weeks, followed by a functional brace, tightened as the swelling decreases.
  - Hanging arm casts are a very good option for displaced, midshaft humeral fractures with shortening, especially oblique or spiral fracture patterns, if the cast is able to extend 2 cm or more proximal to the fracture site.
- For nonoperative treatment to be effective, the patient should remain upright, either standing or sitting, and avoid leaning on the elbow for support. This allows for gravitational force to assist in fracture reduction.
  - As soon as possible, the patient should begin range-of-motion exercises of the fingers, wrist, elbow, and shoulder to minimize dependent swelling and joint stiffness.
- Acceptable alignment of humeral shaft fractures is considered to be 3 cm of shortening, 30 degrees of varus/valgus angulation, and 20 degrees of anterior/posterior angulation.[10]
  - Varus/valgus angulation is tolerated better proximally, and more angulation may be tolerated better in patients with obesity.
  - Patients with large pendulous breasts are at increased risk for varus angulation if treated nonsurgically.
  - No set values for acceptable malrotation exist, but compensatory shoulder motion allows for considerable tolerance of rotational deformity.[10]
- Low-velocity gunshot wounds act as closed injuries after initial treatment. Following irrigation and débridement of skin at entry and exit sites, tetanus status confirmation, and prophylactic antibiotic initiation, nonoperative treatment modalities are commonly employed.[10]

SURGICAL MANAGEMENT

- Successful nonoperative management may be impossible for various reasons:
  - Fracture pattern (eg, displaced, comminuted, segmental [segmental fractures are at risk of nonunion of one or both fracture sites])
  - Prolonged recumbency
  - Morbid obesity
  - Large, pendulous breasts (in women)
  - Patient's inability to maintain a semisitting or reclined position owing to polytraumatic injuries or patient noncompliance
- Operative indications include:
  - Proximal humeral fractures with diaphyseal extension
  - Massive bone loss
  - Displaced transverse diaphyseal fractures
  - Segmental fractures
  - Floating elbow
  - Pathologic or impending pathologic fractures
  - Open fractures
  - Associated vascular injury
  - Intra-articular extension

- Polytrauma
- Spinal cord or brachial plexus injuries
- Poor soft tissue over the fracture site(s), such as thermal burns
- The most commonly cited overall best indication for IMN from this extensive list is a pathologic or impending pathologic fracture.
- The need for operative intervention secondary to radial nerve dysfunction after closed manipulation is controversial.
  - There are advocates for both early nerve exploration and observation.
  - This condition was once thought to be an automatic indication for surgery; however, this assumption has since been called into question.[12]
- Isolated comminution is not an indication for operative treatment.[12] However, if surgical fixation is chosen over nonoperative management, antegrade IMN currently is favored over plate fixation for comminuted fractures.[2]
- Relative contraindications include:
  - Open epiphyses
  - Narrow intramedullary canal (ie, < 9 mm)
  - Prefracture deformity of the humeral shaft
  - Open fractures with obvious radial nerve palsy and neurologic loss after penetrating stab injuries
    - The last two conditions require nerve exploration with subsequent plate-and-screw fixation.
- Chronically displaced fractures should be treated with ORIF rather than IMN to prevent traction-induced brachial plexus palsy and radial nerve injury.

Preoperative Planning

- When selecting implant size, consider canal diameter, fracture pattern, patient anatomy, and postoperative protocol.
  - Nail length and diameter should take into account the distal narrowing of the humerus.
- Estimations of the nail diameter, length, and necessity of reaming can be made using preoperative roentgenograms of the uninjured humerus.
- Alternatively, the length and diameter of the medullary canal can be ascertained intraoperatively using a radiopaque gauge and C-arm imaging of the intact humerus. Use of a radiolucent table top will substantially improve the quality of the image as well as the ability to obtain accurate C-arm images.
  - Position the gauge anterior to the unaffected humerus with its distal end 2.5 cm or more proximal to the superior edge of the olecranon fossa and 1 cm distal to the superior edge of the articular surface.
  - Move the C-arm to the proximal end of the humerus and read the correct length directly from the stamped measurements on the nail length gauge. The IMN should end approximately 1 to 2 cm proximal to the olecranon fossa.
- Measure the length of the IMN to allow the proximal end to be buried. This will reduce the incidence of subacromial impingement if an antegrade technique is used, or encroachment on the olecranon fossa and blocked elbow extension if a retrograde approach is chosen.
  - In comminuted fractures, carefully chose the length to avoid distracting the humerus, which predisposes the patient to delayed union or nonunion.
- Measure the diameter of the medullary canal at the narrowest part that will contain the nail.

- In retrograde nailing, it is important to determine the relation between alignment of the humeral canal and the entry point of the nail by measuring the anterior deviation/distal humeral offset of the distal canal on the preoperative lateral radiograph.
  - Based on these calculations, if the deviation is small, make a distal, long entry portal that includes the superior border of the olecranon fossa.
  - If the anterior deviation is large, however, make the entry portal more proximal and shorter in length.

Positioning

- The patient's position for surgery is determined based on the method chosen for fixation.

Antegrade Intramedullary Nailing

- Place the patient in either a beach chair or supine position on a radiolucent table with the head of the bed elevated 30 to 40 degrees (**FIG 2**).
- Put a small roll between the medial borders of the scapula and rotate the head to the contralateral side to increase exposure of the shoulder.
- Certain fracture patterns may call for skeletal traction.
  - If it is used, place an olecranon pin and apply intermittent traction to avoid brachial plexus palsy.
- Clinically assess the rotational alignment by placing the shoulder in an anatomic position and rotating the distal fragment of the fracture humerus so that the arm and hand point toward the ceiling and the elbow is flexed 90 degrees.
- Prepare the affected extremity and drape the arm free in the typical manner. The operative area should encompass the shoulder proximal to the nipple line, the midline of the chest to the nape of the neck, and the entire affected extremity to the fingertips.
- Bring the patient to the edge of the radiolucent table to improve the ability to obtain orthogonal C-arm images of the affected extremity.
  - It may be necessary to have the patient lying partially off the table on a radiolucent support.
- Cover the C-arm imager with a sterile isolation drape. Most commonly, the C-arm is brought in directly lateral on the injured side, although some surgeons favor coming in from the contralateral side.
  - Regardless of which direction the C-arm is brought into the field, it is imperative to obtain orthogonal views of the entire humerus before the first incision is made.

Retrograde Intramedullary Nailing

- Put the patient in the lateral decubitus or prone position with dorsum placed near the edge of the operating table.
  - If the patient is in the prone position, the affected arm may be supported on a radiolucent arm board, or placed over a bolster or paint roller upper extremity support. The latter two options facilitate access to the olecranon fossa and prevent a traction injury to the brachial plexus. The arm should be positioned in 80 degrees of abduction with the elbow flexed at least 90 degrees.
  - If the lateral decubitus position is used, suspend the fractured extremity, taking care not to distract the fracture site or cause neurovascular compromise. Suspension can be aided by an olecranon pin.

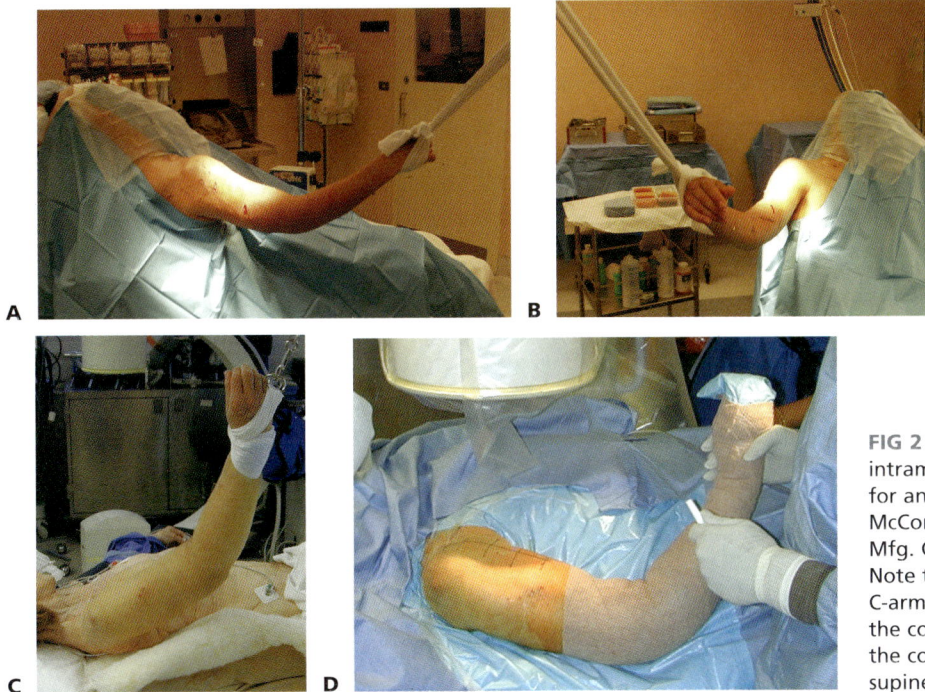

FIG 2 • **A.** Beach chair position for antegrade intramedullary nailing. **B.** Beach chair position for antegrade intramedullary nailing using a McConnell positioner (McConnell Orthopedic Mfg. Co, Greenville, TX). **C.** Supine position. Note the bump under the scapula and the C-arm image intensifier ready to come in from the contralateral side. **D.** C-arm imaging from the contralateral side. The patient is in the supine position.

■ Prepare the affected extremity and drape the arm free in the typical manner. Include the distal clavicle, the acromion, the medial scapula, and the entire arm and hand in the operative field.

■ Cover the C-arm imager with a sterile isolation drape. Bring the C-arm from the ipsilateral side and make sure that adequate orthogonal C-arm images are possible before making the surgical approach.

Approach

■ Standard locked intramedullary humeral nails can be inserted either antegrade or retrograde.

ANTEGRADE INTRAMEDULLARY NAILING

Approach

■ The antegrade approach, which has been the traditional method of IMN, typically involves a starting point at the proximal humerus—either through the rotator cuff, where the tissue is less vascular, or just lateral to the articular surface, where the blood supply is higher (**TECH FIG 1**).

■ Palpate and outline the surface anatomy of the acromion, clavicle, and humeral head.

  ■ Feel the anterior and posterior borders of the humeral head to locate and mark the midline.

  ■ Make a small longitudinal incision at the anterolateral corner of the acromion centered over the top of the greater tuberosity. Extend it distally 3 cm.

■ The C-arm can be used to locate the exact entry point before performing the anterior acromial approach.

  ■ Place a K-wire into the ideal entry point under C-arm imaging guidance. Confirm the location on orthogonal images.

  ■ Leave the K-wire intact while making an anterior acromial approach.

■ Split the deltoid fibers in line with the longitudinal cutaneous incision.

  ■ Do not extend the incision distally more than 4 or 5 cm in the deltoid muscle, to avoid damage to the axillary nerve.

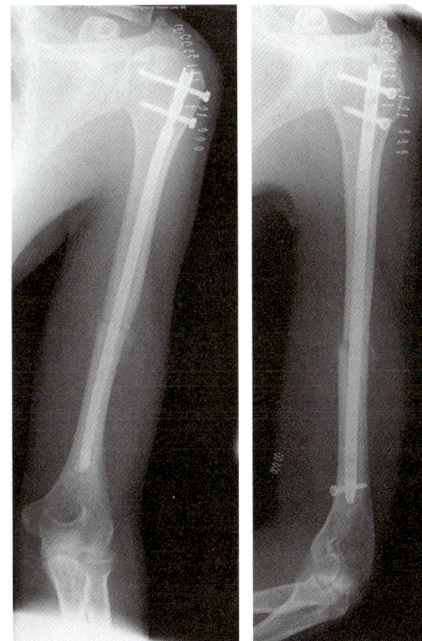

TECH FIG 1 • Postoperative AP and lateral radiographs of antegrade intramedullary nailing for a midshaft humerus fracture.

TECHNIQUES

- Excise any visible subdeltoid bursae to improve your visualization of the rotator cuff.
- Longitudinally incise the supraspinatus in line with the deltoid/cutaneous incision for 1 to 2 cm, just posterior to the bicipital tuberosity.
  - Placing suture tags at the margins of the supraspinatus will help retract its edges during the remainder of the procedure and assist in achieving an optimal rotator cuff repair during wound closure.
- There is insufficient evidence to indicate that a larger incision, in cases in which the rotator cuff is identified and purposely incised, is superior to a smaller incision made with the aid of C-arm imaging.[13]

Entry Hole

- Make the entry hole medial to the tip of the greater tuberosity, just lateral to the articular margin and approximately 0.5 cm posterior to the bicipital groove to minimize damage to the supraspinatus.
  - Linear access to the humeral medullary canal is possible only though an entry portal made in this sulcus between the greater tuberosity and the articular surface.
  - Make sure the entry portal is centered on AP and lateral C-arm images to ensure the nail will be in the midplane of the humerus.
  - If the entry hole is too medial, it will violate the supraspinatus; if the entry portal is too lateral, it will cause some degree of varus angulation (in proximal fractures) or substantially increase the risk of an iatrogenic fracture during nail insertion.
  - Proximal third fractures may require a more medially located entry hole to avoid varus angulation at the fracture site.

Entrance into Medullary Canal

- After establishing the entry hole, insert a K-wire through the portal into the medullary canal to the level of the lesser tuberosity.
- Next, to open the medullary canal, either use a cannulated awl or pass a cannulated drill bit over the K-wire, through a protection sleeve, and drill to the depth of the lesser tuberosity.
  - Adduct the proximal component of the fractured humerus and extend the shoulder to improve clearance of the acromion and facilitate awl or starter reamer access to the correct portal location.
- Once the medullary canal has been opened, remove the guidewire and insert a long, ball-tipped guidewire. Bending the tip of the guidewire may aid in its passage across the fracture site.

Provisional Reduction/ Guidewire Passage

- Manipulate the extremity to reduce the fracture. In many cases, reduction is obtained through a combination of adduction, neutral forearm rotation, and longitudinal traction.
- While advancing the guidewire down the canal, rotate the arm about its longitudinal axis and take several C-arm images to confirm that the guidewire remains contained in the canal.

- This is especially important if the humerus is substantially comminuted.
- Slowly and deliberately pass the guidewire across the fracture site.
  - Difficult passage may be a tip-off that soft tissue may be interposed (possibly the radial nerve).
  - An open fracture is advantageous in this situation because it provides the opportunity to directly visualize and clear the fracture site of any problematic soft tissue.
- After crossing the fracture site, advance the ball-tipped guidewire into the center of the distal fragment until the tip is 1 to 2 cm proximal to the olecranon fossa.
- Avoid shortening or distracting the fracture site while firmly securing the guidewire into the distal fragment.

Determining Nail Length

- Determine the correct nail length by one of two methods:
  - Guide rod method: with the distal end of the rod 1 to 2 cm proximal to the olecranon fossa, overlap a second guide rod extending proximally from the humeral entry portal. Subtract the length in mm of the overlapped guide rod from the total length of an identical guidewire to determine the correct nail length.
  - Nail length gauge: position the radiopaque gauge anterior to the fractured humerus. Move the C-arm to the proximal end of the humerus and read the length from the stamped measurements on the gauge.
- The ideal length of an IMN should be measured 1 cm distal to the articular surface of the humeral head to a point 1 to 2 cm proximal to the olecranon fossa.
  - If the calculated length falls between two standardized nail lengths of the chosen implant, always choose the smaller size.
  - Long nails are a risk factor for subacromial impingement and fracture site distraction.
    - Burying a long nail proximally below the subchondral surface has the potential to iatrogenically split the distal humerus or create a supracondylar fracture when the tip of the nail is wedged too close to the olecranon fossa.

Reaming the Humeral Shaft

- Reaming the humeral shaft usually is avoided, especially in comminuted fractures, to avoid reaming injury to the radial nerve or the rotator cuff.
- If it is warranted, slowly ream the entire humerus over the ball-tipped reamer guidewire in 0.5-mm increments.
  - Exercise greater caution when reaming the humerus than when reaming the long bones of the lower extremity, because the cortical thickness of the humerus is substantially less than that of the tibia or femur.
- Ream 0.5 mm to 1 mm larger than the selected nail diameter. Ream minimally until the sound of cortical chatter becomes audible.
- Choose a nail 1 mm smaller in diameter than the last reamer used.
- Some implant systems require that the ball-tipped guidewire be replaced with a rod that does not have a tip.
  - Use the medullary exchange tube when replacing the guidewire to maintain fracture reduction.

Inserting the Nail

- Once the correct nail length and the diameter of the selected implant have been verified, attach the nail adapter, place the nail-holding screw through the nail adapter, and then attach the radiolucent targeting device onto the nail adapter.
- Verify that this assembly is locked in the appropriate position and that its alignment is correct by inserting a drill bit through the assembled tissue protection/drill sleeve placed in the required holes of the targeting device.
- Insert the nail with sustained manual pressure.
  - Aggressive placement can result in iatrogenic fractures or displacement of the fracture fragments.
  - Use the C-arm image intensifier to identify the source of the problem if the IMN does not easily advance.
- Insert the nail at least to the first circumferential groove on the nail adapter but no deeper than the second groove.
  - Ideally, the IMN should be countersunk about 5 mm below the articular surface to avoid subacromial impingement.
  - Sinking the nail more than 1 cm below the articular surface may place the proximal interlocking screws at the level of the axillary nerve.
  - If the proximal end of the nail is properly countersunk, the incidence of shoulder pain is reportedly less than 2%.[4]
- Attach a strike plate to the targeting device and use a mallet to impact the proximal jig assembly to eliminate any fracture gap or advance the IMN.
  - Do not hit the targeting device or the nail-holding screw directly.
- The distal end of the IMN should come to lie about 2 cm proximal to the olecranon fossa.
- Remove the guidewire.

Compression

- Before proximal interlock insertion, make sure that optimal fracture site compression is present.
- Proximal compression locking can be used for transverse or short oblique fracture patterns. Severe osteopenia is a contraindication to its use.
  - Explore the radial nerve before compression locking if any possibility of radial nerve entrapment exists.
  - The nail must be overinserted by the same distance of anticipated interfragmentary travel because otherwise, during compression, the nail will back out and cause subacromial impingement.
  - Additionally, if the fracture is suitable for compression, the chosen implant should be 6 to 10 mm shorter than the calculated measurement to avoid proximal migration of the nail beyond the insertion site.
- Proximal locking screw placement
  - Oblique proximal locking screws are preferred because their insertion point is cephalad to axillary nerve.
  - Only lateral-to-medial placement is recommended for proximal interlocking screws.
  - It is important to make sure that these screws are inserted above the level of the humeral neck to avoid axillary nerve injury.

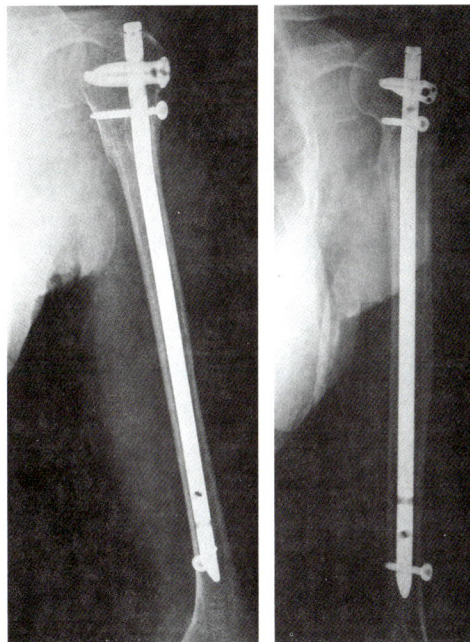

TECH FIG 2 • Postoperative AP and lateral radiographs of antegrade intramedullary nailing for a midshaft humerus fracture. A spiral blade has been used for proximal interlock fixation.

- Lateral screws placed too proximal can produce subacromial impingement with terminal arm elevation.
- Some implant systems may offer a spiral blade fixation as an option for proximal interlocking. In theory, it creates a fixed angle construct and has a higher resistance (versus screws) against loosening (ie, "windshield wiper" effect; **TECH FIG 2**).

Determining Rotation

- Confirm rotational alignment before placing distal interlock screws. Rotational alignment can be ascertained clinically and radiographically.
  - Magnified C-arm AP images of the fracture site can be used to judge the medial and lateral cortical width of the most proximal and most distal aspects of the fracture site.
  - Proper rotation is achieved when these widths are identical.

Distal Locking Screws

- Place anterior, then posterior and/or lateral, then medial directed distal interlocking screws.
- Insert distal interlocking screws using a freehand technique.
  - To place AP-directed screws, advance the C-arm over the distal humerus until the oval slot is seen to be in maximal relief—that is, "perfect circle."
  - Under C-arm imaging, place a scalpel over the skin to precisely determine the location of the incision. Make every attempt to keep this incision just lateral to the biceps tendon. This will decrease the risk to brachial artery, median nerve, and musculocutaneous nerve.

TECHNIQUES

- Carefully make the incision though the skin and use a blunt hemostat to spread under the brachialis muscle down to the bone.
- Insert a short drill bit through a soft tissue protector.
  - Center the drill bit in the locking hole and then position it perpendicular to the nail.
  - Ideally, place the drill bit distally in the oval hole to allow axial compression to occur postoperatively.
- Attach the drill and penetrate the near cortex. Then detach the drill bit from the drill and use a mallet to gently advance the drill bit through the nail up to the far cortex.
  - An orthogonal C-arm image may be used to verify that the position of the drill bit is satisfactory.
- Reattach the drill and penetrate the far cortex.
- A depth gauge can now be inserted to ascertain the length of the interlock screw.
  - The distal screws usually are 24 mm in length.
- Use C-arm image intensification to confirm screw position through the nail as well as screw length.
  - Avoid articular penetration into the glenohumeral joint.
- Lateral-to-medial directed distal locking screws
  - Either in combination with or as an alternative to anterior-to-posterior screws, insert lateral-to-medial screws.

- Make a generous 5 cm incision to decrease the risk to the radial nerve.
- Use the same technique employed when placing AP-directed screws: blunt dissection, a protecting drill/screw insertion sleeve, and perfect circle freehand technique.
- Finally, confirm the IMN position, fracture reduction, and interlocking screw(s) placement with multiple orthogonal C-arm images.
- After orthogonal C-arm images demonstrate satisfactory reduction and hardware implantation, remove the proximal targeting device and place an end cap (this last step is optional, depending on surgeon preference).
  - Carefully select the length of the end cap to avoid impingement.

Wound Closure

- Copiously irrigate all wounds before they are closed.
- During closure of the proximal insertion site, formally repair the surgically incised rotator cuff and deltoid raphe; side-to-side nonabsorbable sutures commonly are recommended.

RETROGRADE INTRAMEDULLARY NAILING

Approach

- Make a limited posterior approach centered over the distal humerus, starting at the olecranon tip to a point 6 cm proximal.
- Longitudinally split the triceps in line with its fibers to the cortical surface of the humerus and identify the olecranon fossa.
- Make every attempt to avoid entering the elbow joint, to decrease the possibility of periarticular scarring.

Starting or Entry Portals

- As previously discussed in the Approach section, the coronal deviation of the distal humerus is variable, and, therefore, two potential starting portals exist:
  - Traditional metaphyseal entry portal: created by reaming in the midline of the distal metaphyseal triangle 2.5 cm proximal to the olecranon fossa.
  - Olecranon fossa entry portal: established by reaming the proximal slope of the olecranon at the superior border of the olecranon fossa.
- The more distal location of the nontraditional olecranon fossa entry portal increases the effective working length of the distal segment and provides a straighter alignment with the medullary canal.
  - However, biomechanical investigation has found that the olecranon fossa entry portal provides greater reduction in torque resistance and load to failure, which may increase the probability of an iatrogenic or postoperative fracture.[16]
- When making either entry portal, pay careful attention to the relation between the olecranon fossa and the

longitudinal axis of the humerus in order to place the entry portal in line with the humeral shaft. The axis of the humerus usually is colinear with the lateral aspect of the olecranon fossa.
- Make the initial entry portal in one of two ways:
  - Open the near cortex with a 4.5-mm drill bit. Continue drilling while progressively lowering the drill toward the arm until the drill bit is in line with the medullary canal on the lateral C-arm images.
  - Drill three small pilot holes in a triangular configuration perpendicular to the cortical surface. Connect these holes with a large drill bit and small rongeur or enlarge the triangular site with a small curved awl to create a long, oval hole 1 cm wide × 2 cm long that leads directly into the medullary canal.
- Undercut the internal aspect of the posterior cortex in addition to the medial and lateral walls of the entry portal to create a distal bevel along the path of nail insertion.
  - This will facilitate easy passage of the guidewire, optional reamer, and final implant.

Provisional Reduction and Guidewire Passage

- Now follow the same steps outlined in the antegrade IMN technique section to pass the guidewire, reduce the fracture, ream (optional), measure the desired nail length and diameter, and insert the chosen implant.
  - Reduction of the fracture usually involves gentle longitudinal traction on the distal humerus and correction of the varus–valgus displacement.

Reaming (Optional)

- If it is necessary to ream, carefully select the reamer size to avoid damage to the posterior cortex. In addition, slowly advance the reamer under C-arm image guidance to avoid excessive reaming of the anterior humeral cortex.
  - Both of these steps decrease the risk of possible iatrogenically induced fractures.

Distal Locking Screws

- Next, distally lock the nail to prevent backing out, that is, blocked elbow extension.
  - Place the distal locking screws from posterior to anterior using a guide.
  - Make an indentation with the guide, incise the cutaneous layer, and then use a blunt hemostat to spread down to the bone.
  - Follow the remaining steps unique to the chosen implant.

- After distal interlocking, gently tap the insertion bolt with a mallet to compress the fracture site. Assess the reduction with C-arm images.

Proximal Locking Screws

- Next, place a proximal interlocking screw, either anterior to posterior, posterior to anterior, or lateral to medial.
- Incise the skin and use a blunt hemostat to spread down to bone to protect the biceps tendon (anterior-to-posterior directed screws) or axillary nerve (posterior-to-anterior and lateral-to-medial directed screws).
- Use C-arm image intensification to confirm screw position through the nail as well as screw length.

Wound Closure

- Copiously irrigate each wound before closing it. Close triceps split with interrupted nonabsorable sutures.

PEARLS AND PITFALLS

IMN contraindications	■ Pre-existing shoulder pathology (eg, impingement, rotator cuff) ■ Permanent upper extremity weight bearers (eg, para- or tetraplegics) ■ Narrow-diameter (<9 mm) canals: excessive reaming is not desirable in the humerus because of the risk of thermal necrosis or radial nerve injury.
Antegrade IMN entry site	■ If the entry portal is too far lateral, the lateral wall of the proximal humerus can be reamed out or fractured during nail insertion. ■ Pushing the reamer shaft medially may prevent this complication.
Nail insertion	■ If any resistance is met while attempting to pass the nail, either antegrade or retrograde, make a small incision to ensure that the radial nerve is not entrapped in the fracture site.
Interlock screws	■ In most cases, soft tissues should be bluntly spread down to the bone with a hemostat before holes are drilled for any interlocking screw, to minimize neurovascular injury. ■ Antegrade IMN distal interlock screws: An alternate and possibly safer method involves placing the screw posteroanteriorly to avoid neurovascular risk when AP (musculocutaneous nerve, brachial artery) or LM (radial nerve) direction is used. When placing interlock screws using the freehand technique, tie an absorbable suture to the screw so that if the screw becomes dislodged from the screwdriver, it will not be displaced in the soft tissues. ■ Antegrade IMN: rotate the C-arm 180 degrees, so the top can be used as a table to support the arm for placing the distal locking screws.
Nail length	■ Always err on the side of a shorter nail: do not distract the fracture site or cause iatrogenic fractures by trying to impact a nail that is excessively long. ■ The retrograde IMN must be long enough to engage the cancellous part of the humeral head; the wide medullary flare of the proximal one third of the shaft does not provide sufficient stability to the inserted nail.
Open fractures: reaming	■ After a thorough irrigation and débridement is performed and the guidewire is successfully passed across the fracture site, close the deep muscle layer around the fracture site to keep the osteogenic reaming debris from washing away.

POSTOPERATIVE CARE

- Tailor the postoperative rehabilitation regimen to the method of nailing (antegrade versus retrograde), stability of the fracture, overall patient health, and preinjury level of activity/workplace demands.
  - Antegrade IMN
    - Place the affected arm in a sling or shoulder immobilizer at the end of surgery.

- Postoperative day 2: remove the dressing and begin gentle shoulder pendulum and elbow ROM exercises.
- Postoperative days 10 to 14: remove the sutures. Institute a structured, supervised physical therapy program. Close patient monitoring and formal therapy are key components to achieving maximum postoperative function.
- Subsequently, schedule follow-up visits at 4- to 6-week intervals, depending on the patient's clinical and radiographic progression. Healing often takes 12 weeks or longer.

- As union progresses, the therapist may begin supervised exercises to recover upper extremity strength. Caution the therapist against instituting programs or exercises that create large rotational stresses to the arm until radiographic healing becomes evident.
- Retrograde IMN
  - Initial postoperative management is identical to treatment following antegrade nailing, unless weight bearing is necessary for wheelchair transfers, walkers, or crutch ambulation. Use a posterior splint and platform attachment if crutches are necessary.
  - It is important to institute early elbow active ROM or gentle passive ROM by the patient to prevent elbow stiffness.
- Avoid
  - Aggressive PROM or stretching to decrease the risk of myositis ossificans formation
  - Resisted elbow extension for the first 6 weeks after surgery to protect the repair of the triceps split.

OUTCOMES

- Randomized clinical trials comparing IMN to compression plating show a higher reoperation rate and greater shoulder morbidity with the use of nails.[11]
- Locked antegrade IMN has resulted in loss of shoulder motion in 6% to 37% of cases.[13]
- Recent antegrade nails designed to eliminate insertion site shoulder morbidity though an extra-articular start point have been introduced, and prospective randomized trials are pending.
- Retrograde IMN union rates range from 91% to 98%, and the mean healing time is 13.7 weeks.[15]
- Retrospective reviews of retrograde IMN have found shoulder function to be excellent in 92.3% of patients and elbow function excellent in 87.2% of patients after fracture consolidation.[15]
  - Functional end results were excellent in 84.6% of patients, moderate in 10.3% of patients, and bad in 5.1% of patients.
- Biomechanical studies have shown that, for midshaft fractures, both antegrade and retrograde nailing showed similar initial stability and bending and torsional stiffness—20% to 30% of normal humeral shafts.[8]
  - In proximal fractures (ie, 10 cm distal to the greater tuberosity tip), antegrade nails demonstrated significantly more initial stability and higher bending and torsional stiffness, as was true for distal fractures with retrograde nailing.

COMPLICATIONS

- Nonunion[3]
  - Antegrade IMN: 11.6%
  - Retrograde IMN: 4.5%
- Infection: 1% to 2%
- Insertion site morbidity
  - Antegrade IMN: shoulder pain, impingement, stiffness, and weakness
  - Retrograde IMN: elbow pain, stiffness, and triceps weakness
- Iatrogenic fractures[3]
  - Antegrade IMN: 5.1%
  - Retrograde IMN: 7.1%
- Iatrogenic comminution and distraction at the fracture site
- Neurovascular risk
  - Risk to the radial nerve in the spiral groove from canal preparation and nail insertion
  - Risk to the axillary nerve from proximal interlocking
  - Risk to the radial, musculocutaneous, and median nerves or brachial artery from distal interlocking
- Heat-induced segmental avascularity after reaming

REFERENCES

1. Bono CM, Grossman MG, Hochwald N, et al. Radial and axillary nerves. Anatomic considerations for humeral fixation. Clin Orthop Relat Res 2000;373:259–264.
2. Chen AL, Joseph TN, Wolinsky PR, et al. Fixation stability of comminuted humeral shaft fractures: locked intramedullary nailing versus plate fixation. J Trauma 2002;53:733–737.
3. Court-Brown C. Paper presented at the Orthopaedic Trauma Association Specialty Day Meeting; February 26, 2005; Washington, DC.
4. Crates J, Whittle AP. Antegrade interlocking nailing of acute humeral shaft fractures. Clin Orthop Relat Res 1998;350:40–50.
5. Farragos AF, Schemitsch EH, McKee MD. Complications of intramedullary nailing for fractures of the humeral shaft: a review. J Orthop Trauma 1999;13:258–267.
6. Foster RJ, Swiontowski MF, Back AW, et al. Radial nerve palsy caused by open humeral shaft fractures. J Hand Surg Am 1993;18: 121–124.
7. Green AG, Reid JS, Carlson DA. Fractures of the humerus. In: Baumgaertner MR, Tornetta P, eds. Orthopaedic Knowledge Update: Trauma. Rosemont, IL: American Academy of Orthopaedic Surgeons, 2005:163–180.
8. Lin J, Inoue N, Valdevit A, et al. Biomechanical comparison of antegrade and retrograde nailing of humeral shaft fracture. Clin Orthop Relat Res 1998;351:203–213.
9. Lin J, Hou SM, Inoue N, et al. Anatomic considerations of locked humeral nailing. Clin Orthop Relat Res 1999;368:247–254.
10. Lyons RP, Lazarus MD. Shoulder and arm trauma: bone. In: Orthopaedic Knowledge Update 8. Rosemont, IL: American Academy of Orthopaedic Surgeons, 2005:275–277.
11. McCormack RG, Brien D, Buckley RE, et al. Fixation of fractures of the shaft of the humerus by dynamic compression plate or intramedullary nail: A prospective randomized trial. J Bone Joint Surg Br 2000;82B:336–339.
12. McKee MD. Fractures of the shaft of the humerus. In: Bucholz RW, Heckman JD, Court-Brown C, eds. Rockwood and Green's Fractures in Adults, ed 6. Philadelphia: Lippincott Williams & Wilkins, 2006: 1117–1157.
13. Riemer BL, Foglesong ME, Burke CJ. Complications of Seidel intramedullary nailing of narrow diameter humeral diaphyseal fractures. Orthopedics 1994;17:19–29.
14. Roberts CS, Walz BM, Yerasimides JG. Humeral shaft fractures: Intramedullary nailing. In: Wiss D, ed. Master Techniques in Orthopaedic Surgery: Fractures, ed 2. Philadelphia: Lippincott Williams & Wilkins, 2006:81–95.
15. Rommens PM, Verbruggen J, Broos PL. Retrograde locked nailing of humeral shaft fractures. A review of 39 patients. J Bone Joint Surg Br 1995;77B: 84–89.
16. Strothman D, Templeman DC, Varecka T, et al. Retrograde nailing of humeral shaft fractures: a biomechanical study of its effects on strength of the distal humerus. J Orthop Trauma 2000;14:101.
17. Tytherleigh-Strong G, Walls N, McQueen MM. The epidemiology of humeral shaft fractures. J Bone Joint Surg Br 1998;80B:249–253.

Chapter 22

Open Reduction and Internal Fixation of Nonarticular Scapular Fractures

Brett D. Owens and Thomas P. Goss

DEFINITION

- Nonarticular scapular fractures include fractures of the glenoid neck, scapular spine and body, acromial process, and coracoid process. They account for 90% of scapular fractures.[6]
- Most nonarticular scapular fractures can be treated nonoperatively, including all isloated scapular body–spine fractures.
- Significant displacement at one or more of these sites, alone or in conjunction with ligamentous disruptions of the superior shoulder suspensory complex, require evaluation for surgical intervention.[1,10]

ANATOMY

- The scapula is a flat triangular bone with three processes laterally: the glenoid process, the acromial process, and the coracoid process.
- The glenoid proocess consists of the glenoid fossa, the glenoid rim, and the glenoid neck.
- The superior shoulder suspensory complex is a bone and soft tissue ring at the end of a superior and an inferior bony strut (**FIG 1**). This ring is composed of the glenoid process, the coracoid process, the coracoclavicular ligament, the distal clavicle, the acromioclavicular joint, and the acromial process. The superior strut is the middle third of the clavicle, whereas the inferior strut is the junction of the most lateral portion of the scapular body and the most medial portion of the glenoid neck.[1]

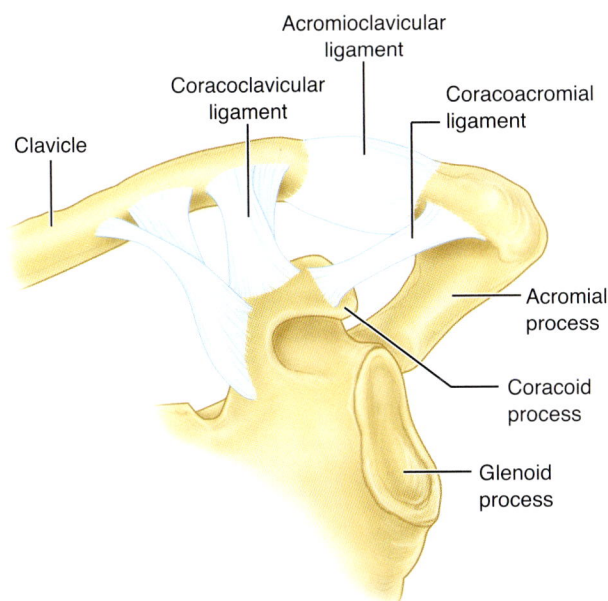

Acromioclavicular ligament

Coracoclavicular ligament

Coracoacromial ligament

Clavicle

Acromial process

Coracoid process

Glenoid process

FIG 1 • Superior shoulder suspensory complex.

PATHOGENESIS

- Scapular fractures usually are the result of high-energy trauma and have a high rate of associated musculoskeletal and underlying thoracic injuries.[3]
- Fractures of the acromion process may be the result of direct trauma due to its subdermal location, whereas coracoid process fractures may be due to a sudden muscular contraction.[4]

NATURAL HISTORY

- The results of nonoperative treatment of nonarticular scapular fractures generally are good. Nonunion is rare because the area has a rich blood supply. Angular deformities often are well compensated for by the wide range of motion of the glenohumeral joint and scapulothoracic articulation.

PATIENT HISTORY AND PHYSICAL FINDINGS

- In addition to the specifics of the injury, it is helpful to obtain an understanding of the functional demands on the extremity. Hand dominance, occupation, and sports participation are all relevant.
- A thorough neurovascular examination must be performed and deficits evaluated with angiography and electromyography, as necessary.
- A thorough soft tissue examination also is warranted, as wounds may represent an open fracture and warrant exploration. Blisters or swelling may delay surgery.

IMAGING AND OTHER DIAGNOSTIC STUDIES

- Nonarticular scapular fractures usually are identified on routine shoulder trauma series radiographs: a true anteroposterior (AP) view of the shoulder with the arm in neutral rotation, a true axillary view of the glenohumeral joint, and a true lateral scapular view. An AP weight-bearing view may be indicated.
- CT scans and three-dimensional reconstructions can be helpful for identification and classification of fractures owing to the complex bony anatomy in this region. In addition, the bony relationships should be evaluated for evidence of any ligamentous disruption.

DIFFERENTIAL DIAGNOSIS

- Nonarticular scapular fractures
- Intra-articular scapular fractures
- Double disruptions of the superior shoulder suspensory complex including a floating shoulder (ie, glenoid neck fracture with ipsilateral middle third clavicle fracture)
- Scapulothoracic dissociation

NONOPERATIVE MANAGEMENT

▪ Most (over 90%) scapular fractures can be treated nonoperatively.

▪ Glenoid fossa and rim fractures may require operative management and are discussed in Chapter SE-23.

▪ Glenoid neck fractures with more than 40 degrees of angulation in the coronal or sagittal plane or translational displacement of 1 cm or more require surgical management. Anatomic neck fractures (lateral to the coracoid process) are inherently unstable and should also be considered for operative intervention.[2]

▪ Isolated acromial and coracoid process fractures usually are minimally displaced and can be managed nonoperatively. Significant displacement or fractures in conjunction with other bony and soft tissue injuries to the shoulder girdle may require surgical stabilization.[4]

SURGICAL MANAGEMENT

Preoperative Planning

▪ Imaging studies should be reviewed and available for reference in the operating room. A draped fluoroscopy unit and competent technician should be available during the surgery.

Positioning

▪ Open reduction with internal fixation (ORIF) of scapular fractures requires wide access to the entire shoulder girdle. The patient may be placed in either the lateral decubitus position (**FIG 2A**) or in the beach chair position (**FIG 2B**), but care must be taken to allow adequate exposure of the entire scapula and clavicle.

▪ The shoulder girdle is prepped and draped widely, and the entire upper extremity is prepped and draped "free."

▪ Alternatively, a staged procedure can be performed using separate positions, sterile preparations, and separate exposures.[9]

Approach

▪ Glenoid neck fractures are approached posteriorly.

▪ A superior approach can added for control and positioning of a difficult-to-control glenoid fragment.

▪ An anterior approach is used for coracoid process fractures.

▪ A superior approach is used for access to acromial process fractures.

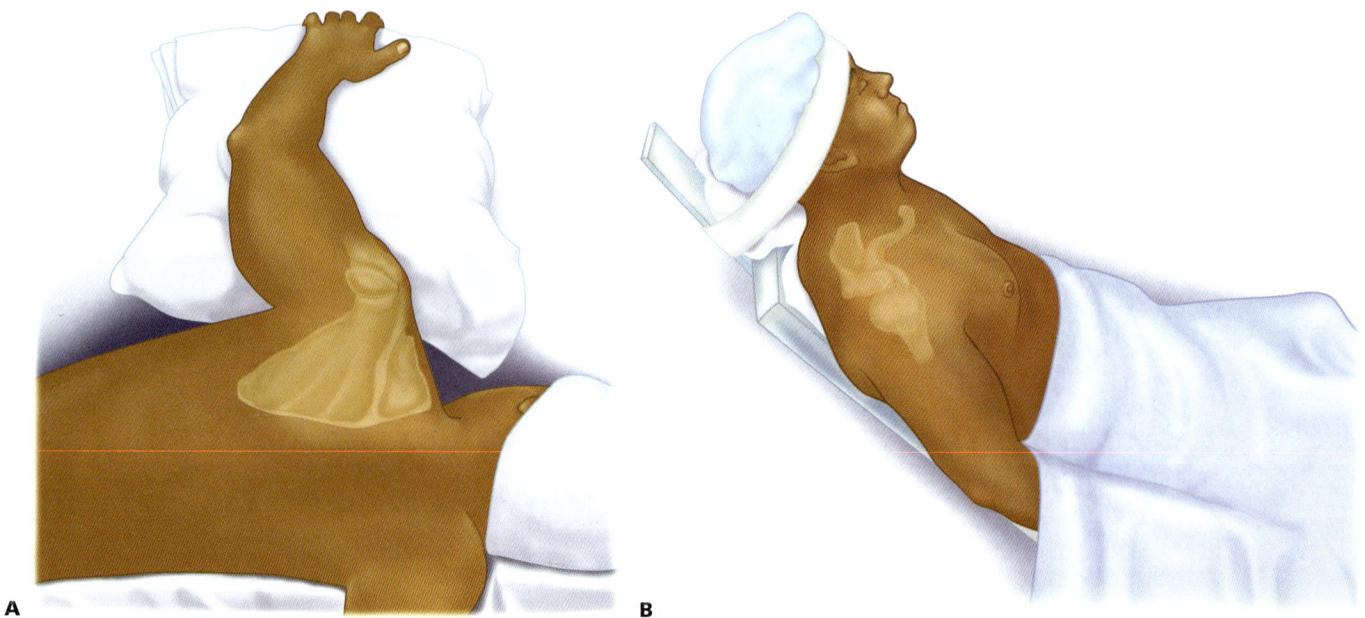

FIG 2 • A. The lateral decubitus position is used for posterior and posterosuperior approaches to the glenoid process. **B.** The beach chair position.

TECHNIQUES

POSTERIOR APPROACH TO GLENOID NECK

▪ Bony landmarks are outlined with marking pen (**TECH FIG 1A**).

▪ An incision is made along the scapular spine and acromion and down the lateral aspect of the shoulder, as needed.

▪ The origins of the posterior and middle heads of the deltoid muscle are sharply detached from the scapular spine–acromial process and retracted distally (**TECH FIG 1B**).

▪ The interval between infraspinatus and teres minor is developed.

　▪ If access to the glenoid fossa is necessary, the infraspinatus tendon and underlying posterior glenohumeral joint capsule are incised 2 cm lateral to their insertion on the greater tuberosity and reflected laterally (**TECH FIG 1C,D**).

▪ Mobilization of the teres minor muscle allows access to the lateral scapular border.

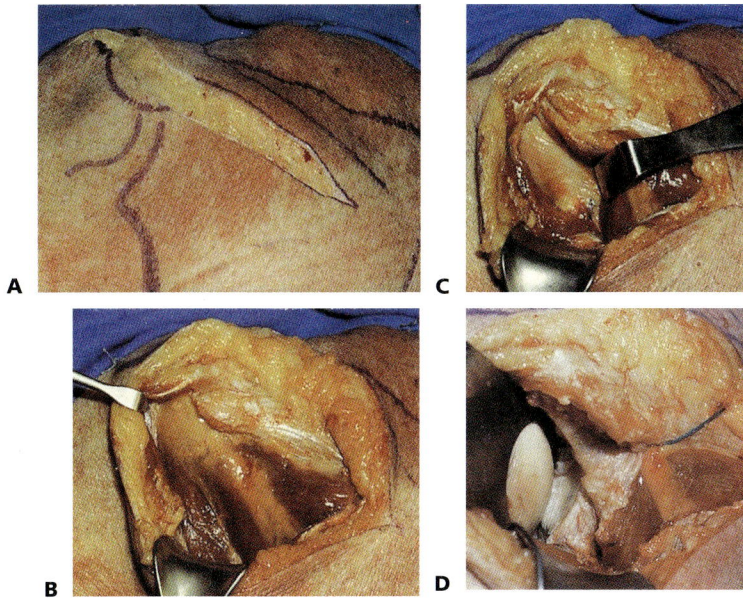

TECH FIG 1 • A. The standard posterior incision extends along the inferior margin of the scapular spine and the acromion. At the lateral tip of the acromion, the incision continues in the midlateral line for 2.5 cm. **B.** The posterior and middle heads of the deltoid muscle have been detached from the scapular spine–posterior acromial process and retracted distally to expose the infraspinatus musculotendinous unit. **C.** The infraspinatus–teres minor interval has been developed, with the infraspinatus retracted superiorly and the teres minor retracted inferiorly to expose the posterior glenohumeral joint capsule (the inferior portion of the infraspinatus insertion has been released). **D.** The infraspinatus tendon and underlying posterior glenohumeral joint capsule are incised 2 cm from insertion on the greater tuberosity to allow access to the glenohumeral joint. (From Goss TP. Glenoid fractures: Open reduction and internal fixation. In Wiss DA, ed. Master Techniques in Orthopaedic Surgery: Fractures. Philadelphia: Lippincott–Raven, 1998.)

- Reduction of the fracture is performed with lateral traction on the draped arm and manipulation of the fracture site.
- Temporary fixation may be obtained with K-wires.
- Rigid fixation may be obtained with a contoured reconstruction plate and 3.5-mm cortical screws (**TECH FIG 1D**).

- Care must be taken to avoid violating the glenoid fossa with the screws in the glenoid fragment.
- Meticulous repair of the deltoid origin to the scapular spine–acromion should be performed with permanent sutures through drill holes.

SUPERIOR APPROACH TO GLENOID NECK

- The superior approach to the glenoid neck is made in an extensile fashion by extending the posterior incision superiorly.
- The trapezius and underlying supraspinatus muscles are split in the line of their fibers (**TECH FIG 2**).

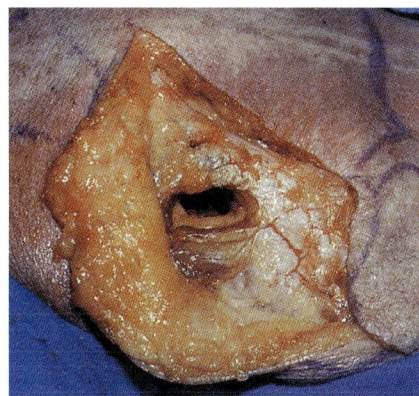

TECH FIG 2 • In the interval between the clavicle and the scapular spine–acromial process, the trapezius and supraspinatus tendon have been split in line of their fibers for exposure. (From Goss TP. Glenoid fractures: Open reduction and internal fixation. In Wiss DA, ed. Master Techniques in Orthopaedic Surgery: Fractures. Philadelphia: Lippincott–Raven, 1998.)

ORIF OF ACROMIAL PROCESS FRACTURE

- Incision directly over the acromial process
- Subperiosteal dissection to expose the superior surface of the acromion
- Anatomic fracture reduction under direct visualization

- Proximal fractures: fixation with a contoured 3.5-mm reconstruction plate (**TECH FIG 3A**)
- Distal fractures: fixation with a tension band construct (**TECH FIG 3B**)

TECHNIQUES

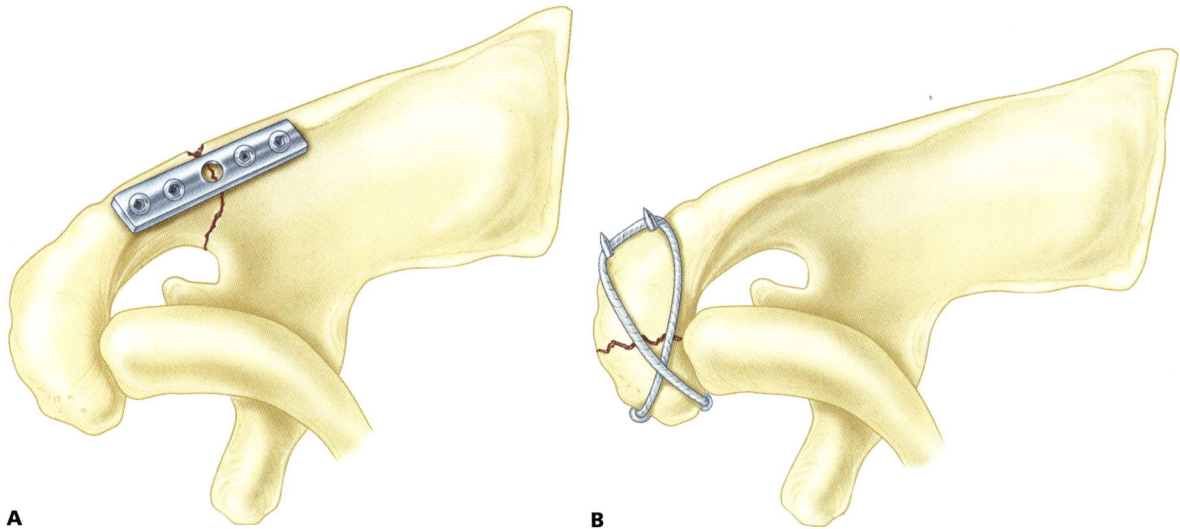

A

B

TECH FIG 3 • Fixation techniques for acromion process fractures. **A.** Plate-and-screw construct for a fracture of the base of the acromion. **B.** Tension band wire construct.

ORIF OF CORACOID PROCESS FRACTURE

- Vertical incision 1 cm lateral to coracoid process (**TECH FIG 4A**)
- Development of deltopectoral interval or split of the deltoid muscle in line with its fibers directly over the coracoid process
- Exposure of the fracture site (may need to open the rotator interval)
- If coracoid tip has sufficient stock, cannulated screw fixation can be performed (**TECH FIG 4B**).
- If not, fragment excision and suture fixation of conjoint tendon to remaining coracoid is performed (**TECH FIG 4C**).
- Coracoid base fractures are fixed with a single cannulated cortical screw (**TECH FIG 4D**).

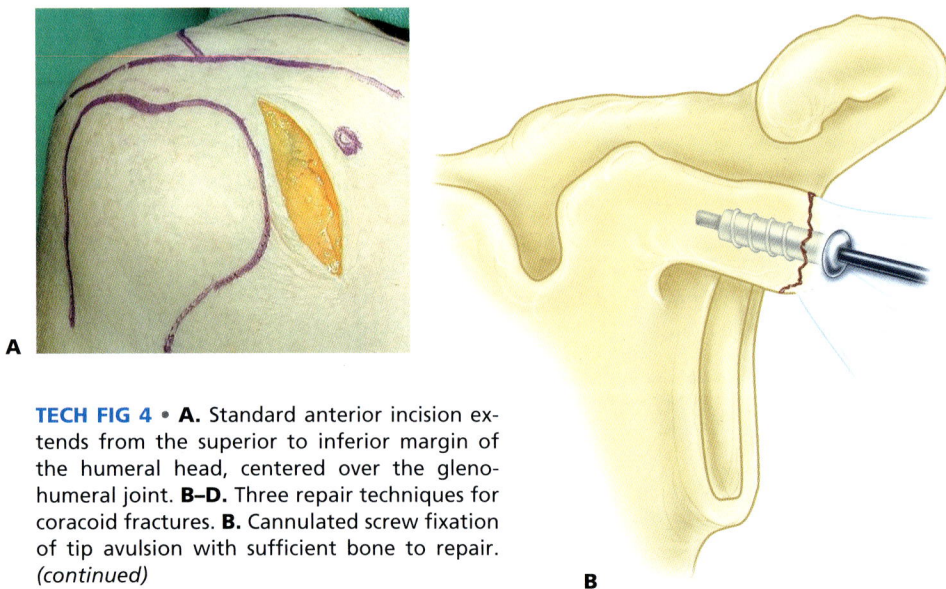

A

B

TECH FIG 4 • **A.** Standard anterior incision extends from the superior to inferior margin of the humeral head, centered over the glenohumeral joint. **B–D.** Three repair techniques for coracoid fractures. **B.** Cannulated screw fixation of tip avulsion with sufficient bone to repair. *(continued)*

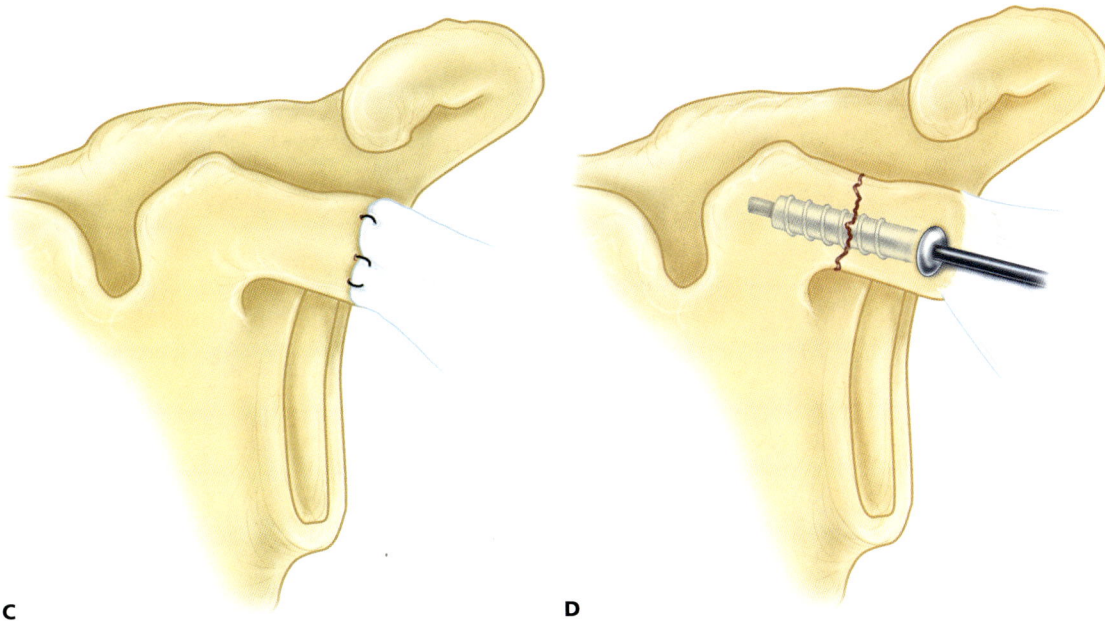

C   **D**

TECH FIG 4 • *(continued)* **C.** Suture fixation of conjoint tendon when insufficient bone is available to repair. **D.** Cannulated screw fixation for proximal fracture. (**A:** From Goss TP. Open reduction and internal fixation of glenoid fractures. In: Craig EV, ed. Master Techniques in Orthopaedic Surgery: The Shoulder, 2nd ed. Philadelphia: Lippincott Williams & Wilkins, 2004.)

PEARLS AND PITFALLS

Indications	▪ CT can help define the fracture, assess possible intra-articular involvement, and identify concomitant injuries. ▪ Most nonarticular injuries and all scapular body–spine fractures are treated nonoperatively.
Approach	▪ Deltoid detachment and reflection provides maximal visualization and is recommended for surgeons unfamiliar with the posterior approach. ▪ During the posterior approach, the internervous plane is between the infraspinatus (a bipennate muscle) superiorly and the teres minor inferiorly.
Reduction	▪ K-wires can be placed to serve as "joysticks" to assist with fracture reduction.
Fixation	▪ K-wires should be avoided for permanent fixation. However, they can be placed percutaneously and used for temporary or supplemental fixation, being removed at 4 to 6 weeks. ▪ Reconstruction plates may be pre-contoured using a scapula model.
Closure	▪ Meticulous repair of the deltoid to the scapular spine–acromial process is necessary, using nonabsorbable sutures placed through drill holes.

POSTOPERATIVE CARE

▪ How aggressive the rehabilitation program following ORIF of nonarticular scapular fractures must be is determined by the rigidity of the fixation construct and the adequacy of the soft tissue repair.[5]

▪ Patients are immobilized in a sling and swathe binder and started on gentle pendulum exercises during the first 2 weeks.

▪ Progressive passive and active-assisted range of motion exercises are emphasized during weeks 2 through 6 postoperatively.

▪ All protection is discontinued by 6 weeks postoperatively.

▪ Strengthening is begun after 6 weeks postoperatively and after range of motion is satisfactory.

▪ Return to sports or labor is restricted until 4 to 6 months postoperatively.

OUTCOMES

▪ Relatively few outcome studies detailing the results of scapular fractures treated operatively are available.

▪ While most nonarticular scapular fractures are treated nonoperatively, those that warrant surgical intervention appear to benefit from this treatment.[7,8]

COMPLICATIONS

▪ When neurologic complications occur, they most commonly are caused by overly aggressive retraction or misdirected dissection.

▪ The musculocutaneous and axillary nerves are vulnerable in the anterior approach, the suprascapular nerve in the superior approach, and the axillary and suprascapular nerves in the posterior approach.[9]

REFERENCES

1. Goss TP. Double disruptions of the superior shoulder complex. J Orthop Trauma 1993;7:99.
2. Goss TP. Fractures of the glenoid neck. J Shoulder Elbow Surg 1994;3:42–61.
3. Goss TP. Scapular fractures and dislocation: diagnosis and treatment. J Am Acad Orthop Surg 1995;3:22.
4. Goss TP. The scapula: Coracoid, acromial and avulsion fractures. Am J Orthop 1996;25:106.
5. Goss TP. Glenoid fractures: Open reduction and internal fixation. In: Wiss DA, ed. Master Techniques in Orthopaedic Surgery: Fractures, 2nd ed. Philadelphia: Lippincott Williams & Wilkins, 2006.
6. Goss TP, Owens BD. Fractures of the scapula: Diagnosis and treatment. In: Iannotti JP, Williams GR, eds. Disorders of the Shoulder: Diagnosis and Management, 2nd ed. Philadelphia: Lippincott Williams & Wilkins, 2007.
7. Hardegger FH, Simpson LA, Weber BG. The operative treatment of scapular fractures. J Bone Joint Surg Br 1984;66B:725.
8. Kavanagh BF, Bradway JK, Cofield RH. Open reduction of displaced intra-articular fractures of the glenoid fossa. J Bone Joint Surg Am 1993;75A:479.
9. Owens BD, Goss TP. Surgical approaches for glenoid fractures. Tech Shoulder Elbow Surg 2004;5:103–115.
10. Owens BD, Goss TP. The floating shoulder. J Bone Joint Surg Br 2006;88(11):1419–1424.

Open Reduction and Internal Fixation of Intra-articular Scapular Fractures

Brett D. Owens, Joanna G. Branstetter, and Thomas P. Goss

DEFINITION

- Intra-articular scapular fractures include fractures of the glenoid cavity, which includes the glenoid rim and the glenoid fossa. They account for 10% of scapular fractures.[6] Most scapular fractures are extra-articular, and 50% involve the body and spine.
- Over 90% of fractures of the glenoid cavity are insignificantly displaced and are managed nonoperatively.[3]
- Significant displacement requires evaluation for surgical intervention to achieve the best possible outcome.

ANATOMY

- The scapula is a flat triangular bone with three processes: the glenoid process, the acromial process, and the coracoid process.
- The glenoid process consists of the glenoid cavity (the glenoid rim and glenoid fossa) and the glenoid neck.
- The glenoid cavity provides a firm concave surface with which the convex humeral head articulates. The average depth of the articular cartilage is 5 mm.
- Glenoid cavity fractures are classified according to whether they involve the glenoid rim or the glenoid fossa and the direction of the fracture line (**FIG 1**).

PATHOGENESIS

- Scapular fractures usually are the result of high-energy trauma and have a high rate (90%) of associated bony and soft tissue injuries, both local and distant.[5]
- Fractures of the glenoid rim occur when the humeral head strikes the periphery of the glenoid cavity. They are true fractures, not avulsion injuries caused by indirect forces applied to the periarticular soft tissues by the humeral head.
- Fractures of the glenoid fossa occur when the humeral head is driven into the center of the concavity. The fracture then promulgates in a number of different directions, depending on the characteristics of the humeral head force.

NATURAL HISTORY

- The results of nonoperative treatment of intra-articular scapular fractures usually are good if the fracture displacement is minimal and the humeral head lies concentrically within the glenoid cavity.
- Significant displacement can result in posttraumatic degenerative joint disease, glenohumeral instability, and even nonunion.[2]

PATIENT HISTORY AND PHYSICAL FINDINGS

- In addition to the specifics of the injury, it is helpful to obtain an understanding of the functional demands on the extremity. Hand dominance, occupation, and sports participation are all relevant.
- A thorough neurovascular examination must be performed. Deficits are evaluated with angiography and electromyography, as necessary.
- A thorough soft tissue examination also is warranted. Wounds may represent an open fracture and warrant exploration. Blisters or swelling may delay surgery.

IMAGING AND OTHER DIAGNOSTIC STUDIES

- Intra-articular scapular fractures initially are evaluated with a routine scapula trauma radiographic series (a true anteroposterior view of the shoulder with the arm in neutral rotation, a true axillary view of the glenohumeral joint, and a true lateral scapular view; **FIG 2A**).
- CT scans and three-dimensional studies with reconstructions can be helpful in evaluating articular congruity and fracture displacement (**FIG 2B–D**). In addition, the bony relationships should be evaluated for evidence of ligamentous disruption(s) or instability.

DIFFERENTIAL DIAGNOSIS

- Intra-articular scapular fractures
- Nonarticular scapular fractures
- Scapulothoracic dissociation
- Double disruptions of the superior shoulder suspensory complex, including a floating shoulder (a glenoid neck fracture with an ipsilateral middle third clavicle fracture)

NONOPERATIVE MANAGEMENT

- Most (over 90%) intra-articular scapular fractures are insignificantly displaced and are managed nonoperatively.
- Significantly displaced glenoid fossa and glenoid rim fractures require operative management.

SURGICAL MANAGEMENT

- Surgical indications are as follows:
  - Rim fractures: 25% or more of the glenoid cavity anteriorly or 33% or more of the glenoid cavity posteriorly and displacement of the fragment 10 mm or more
  - Fossa fractures: an articular step-off of 5 mm or more, significant separation of the fracture fragments, or failure of the humeral head to lie in the center of the glenoid cavity

Preoperative Planning

- Imaging studies should be reviewed before the surgery and should be available for reference in the operating room. A draped fluoroscopy unit and a competent technician should be available. An examination for instability can be performed while under anesthesia.

Positioning

- Open reduction with internal fixation (ORIF) of intra-articular scapular fractures requires wide access to the entire

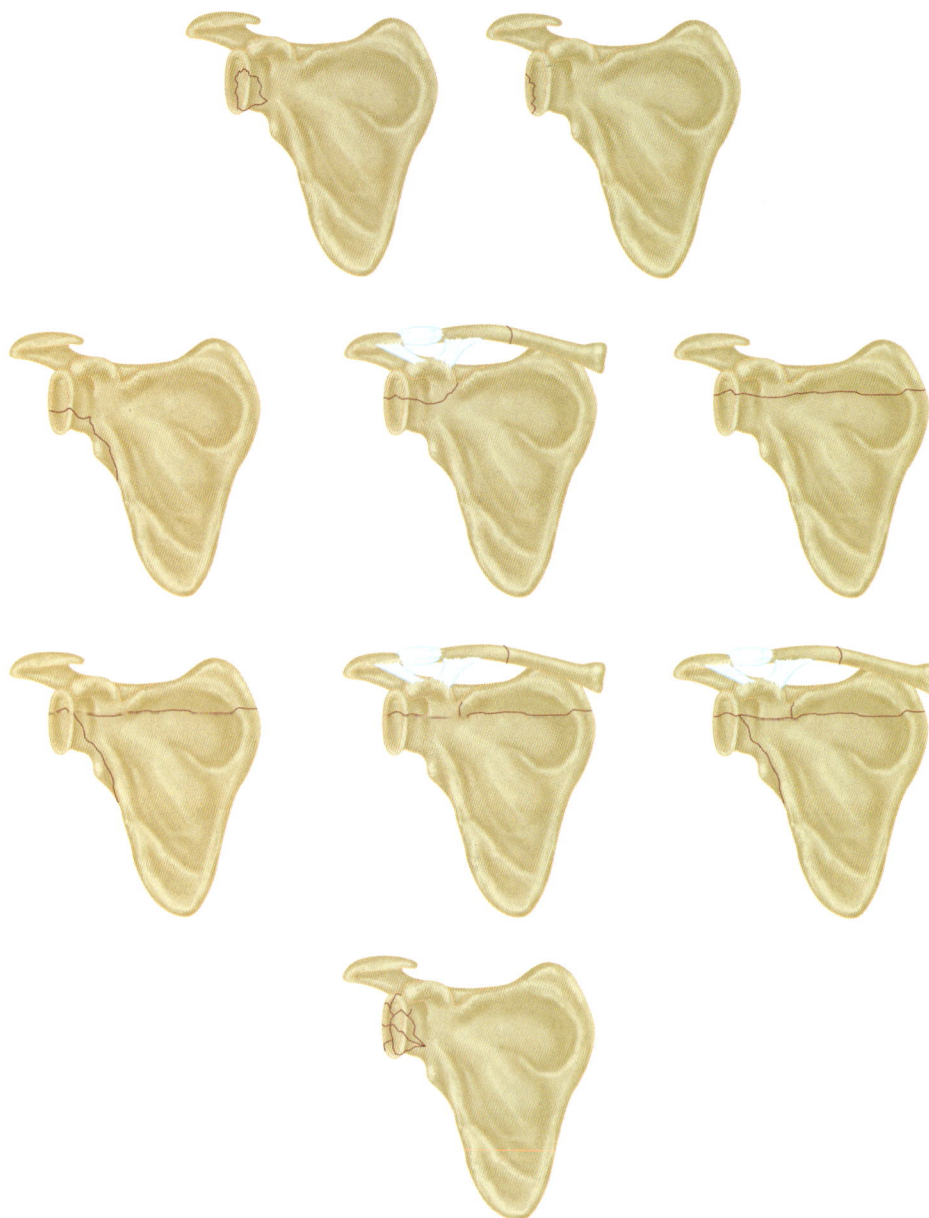

FIG 1 • Goss-Ideberg classification of glenoid cavity fractures. Ia, anterior rim; Ib, posterior rim; II, inferior glenoid; III, superior glenoid; IV, transverse through the body; V; combination II-IV; VI, comminuted.

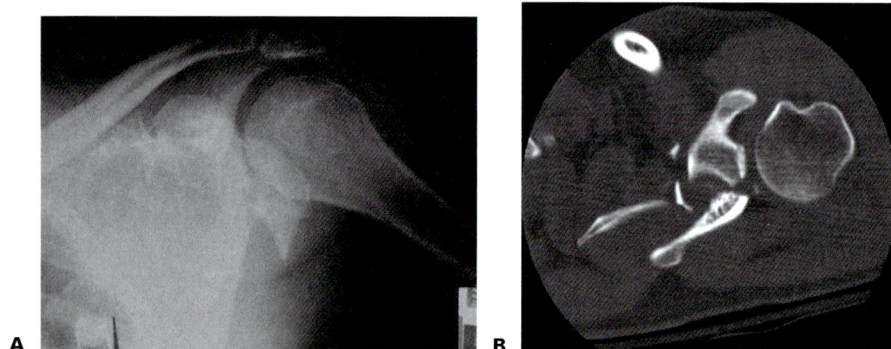

FIG 2 • **A.** The AP radiograph shows a type Vc glenoid cavity fracture. **B.** Axillary CT image shows a large anterosuperior glenoid cavity fragment including the coracoid process. *(continued)*

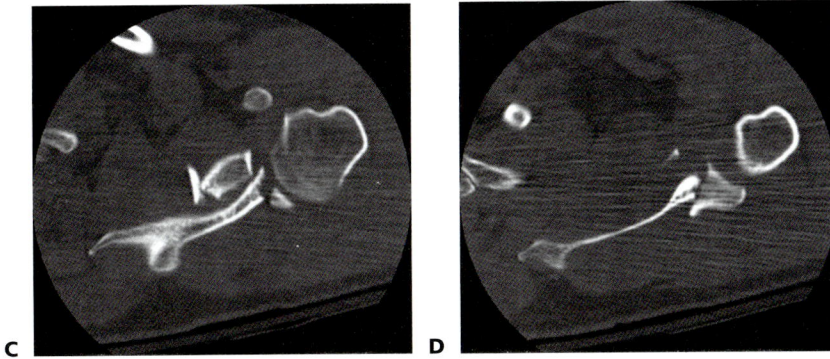

FIG 2 • *(continued)* **C.** Axillary CT image shows the lateral aspect of the scapular body lying between the two glenoid cavity fragments and abutting the humeral head. **D.** Axillary CT image shows a large posteroinferior cavity fragment. (From Goss TP, Owens BD. Fractures of the scapula: Diagnosis and treatment. In: Iannotti JP, Williams GR, eds. Disorders of the Shoulder: Diagnosis and Management, 2nd ed. Philadelphia: Lippincott Williams & Wilkins, 2007:793–840.)

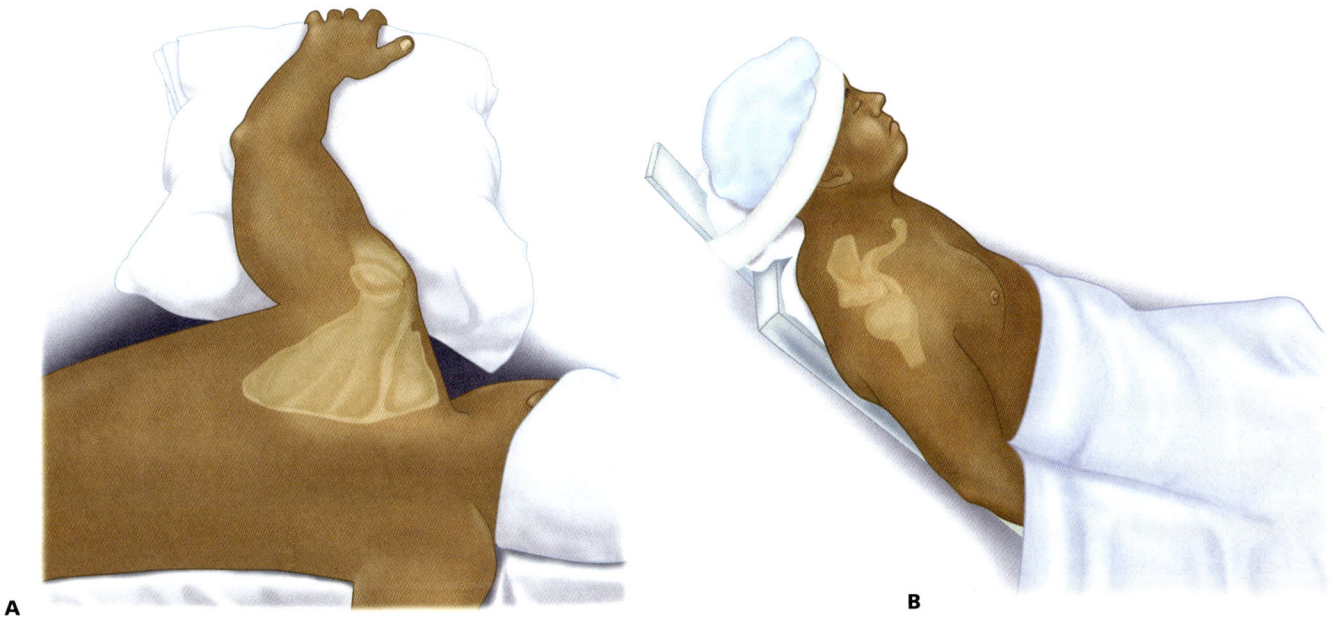

FIG 3 • Patient position: lateral decubitus (**A**) and beach chair (**B**).

shoulder girdle. Depending on the particular fracture, the patient is placed in either the lateral decubitus position (**FIG 3A**) or the beach chair position (**FIG 3B**).

▪ Care must be taken to allow adequate exposure of the entire scapula and clavicle. The shoulder girdle is prepped and draped widely, and the entire upper extremity is prepped and draped "free."

▪ In some cases, a staged procedure may be necessary using separate positions, sterile preparations, and exposures.[10]

Approach

▪ The posterior approach is used for fractures of the posterior glenoid rim and most fractures of the glenoid fossa.

▪ The superior approach is used, in conjunction with a posterior approach, for fractures of the glenoid fossa with a difficult-to-control superior fragment.

▪ The anterior approach is used for fractures of the anterior glenoid rim and some fractures involving the superior aspect of the glenoid fossa.

POSTERIOR APPROACH TO THE GLENOID CAVITY

▪ Bony landmarks are outlined with a marking pen.

▪ An incision is made along the scapular spine and acromion and down the midlateral aspect of the shoulder, as needed (**TECH FIG 1A**).

▪ Origins of the posterior and middle heads of the deltoid muscle are sharply detached from the scapular spine–acromial process, and the deltoid muscle is split in the line of its fibers for 2.5 cm in the midlateral line. It is then retracted distally (**TECH FIG 1B**).

▪ The interval between infraspinatus and teres minor is developed (**TECH FIG 1C**). To gain access to the glenoid fossa, the infraspinatus tendon and underlying posterior glenohumeral joint capsule are incised 2 cm lateral to their insertion on the greater tuberosity and reflected posteriorly (**TECH FIG 1D**).

▪ Subperiosteal mobilization of the teres minor muscle allows access to the lateral scapular border.

TECHNIQUES

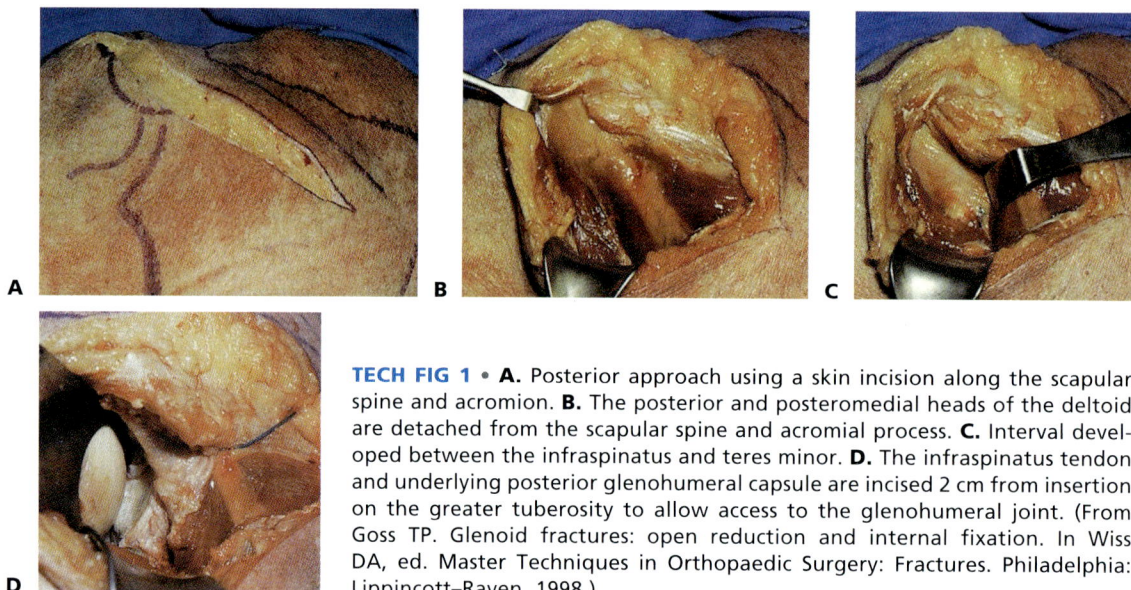

TECH FIG 1 • A. Posterior approach using a skin incision along the scapular spine and acromion. **B.** The posterior and posteromedial heads of the deltoid are detached from the scapular spine and acromial process. **C.** Interval developed between the infraspinatus and teres minor. **D.** The infraspinatus tendon and underlying posterior glenohumeral capsule are incised 2 cm from insertion on the greater tuberosity to allow access to the glenohumeral joint. (From Goss TP. Glenoid fractures: open reduction and internal fixation. In Wiss DA, ed. Master Techniques in Orthopaedic Surgery: Fractures. Philadelphia: Lippincott–Raven, 1998.)

SUPERIOR APPROACH TO THE GLENOID CAVITY

- The superior approach to the glenoid cavity is made by extending the posterior incision superiorly.
- The trapezius and underlying supraspinatus muscles are split in the line of their fibers (**TECH FIG 2**).

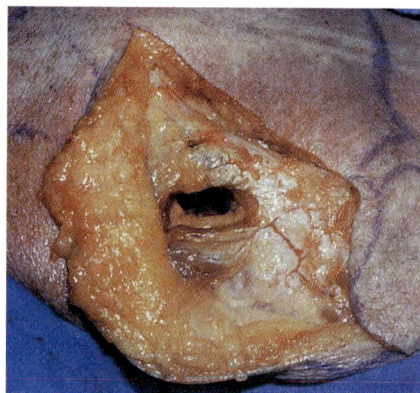

TECH FIG 2 • Superior approach. The trapezius and underlying supraspinatus muscles are split in line with their fibers. (From Goss TP. Glenoid fractures: open reduction and internal fixation. In Wiss DA, ed. Master Techniques in Orthopaedic Surgery: Fractures. Philadelphia: Lippincott–Raven, 1998.)

ANTERIOR APPROACH TO THE GLENOID CAVITY

- The incision is made in Langer's lines and centered over the glenohumeral joint from the superior to inferior level of the humeral head (**TECH FIG 3A**).
- The deltoid muscle is split in the line of its fibers over the palpable coracoid process and retracted medially and laterally.
- The conjoined tendon is retracted medially after division of the overlying fascia along its medial border (**TECH FIG 3B**).
- Care must be taken to protect all neurovascular structures from injury.

- Incise the subscapularis tendon vertically 2.5 cm medial to its insertion on the lesser tuberosity and along its superior and inferior borders.
  - Dissect it off the underlying anterior glenohumeral capsule.
- Tag the corners of the subscapularis unit and turn it back medially (**TECH FIG 3C**).
- Incise the anterior glenohumeral capsule in the same fashion, tag its corners, and turn it back medially to gain access to the glenohumeral joint.

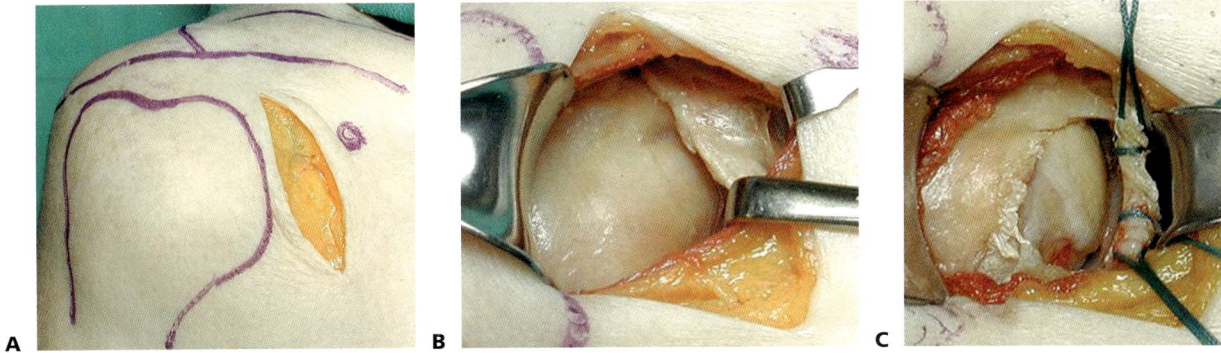

TECH FIG 3 • **A.** Anterior approach using a skin incision made in Langer's lines and centered over the glenohumeral joint. **B.** The conjoined tendon is retracted medially. **C.** Incise the subscapularis tendon 2 cm from its insertion on the lesser tuberosity, dissect it off the glenohumeral capsule, incise the capsule similarly, and turn both of them back medially to gain access to the glenohumeral joint. (From Goss TP. Open reduction and internal fixation of glenoid fractures. In: Craig EV, ed. Master Techniques in Orthopaedic Surgery: The Shoulder, 2nd ed. Philadelphia: Lippincott Williams & Wilkins, 2004.)

FIXATION TECHNIQUES

- The fracture is reduced as anatomically as possible.
- Temporary fixation may be obtained with K-wires.
- Rigid fixation may be obtained with a contoured reconstruction plate and 3.5-mm cortical screws or with cannulated interfragmentary compression screws, depending on the characteristics of the fracture.
- Care must be taken to avoid violating the glenoid fossa with any screws placed in the glenoid fragment (**TECH FIG 4A,B**).

- If severe comminution is present, an iliac crest tricortical bone graft is an option (**TECH FIG 4C**).
- All soft tissues divided to gain access to the fracture site must be meticulously repaired. With posterior approaches, the deltoid must be securely reattached to the acromion and scapular spine with permanent sutures through drill holes.

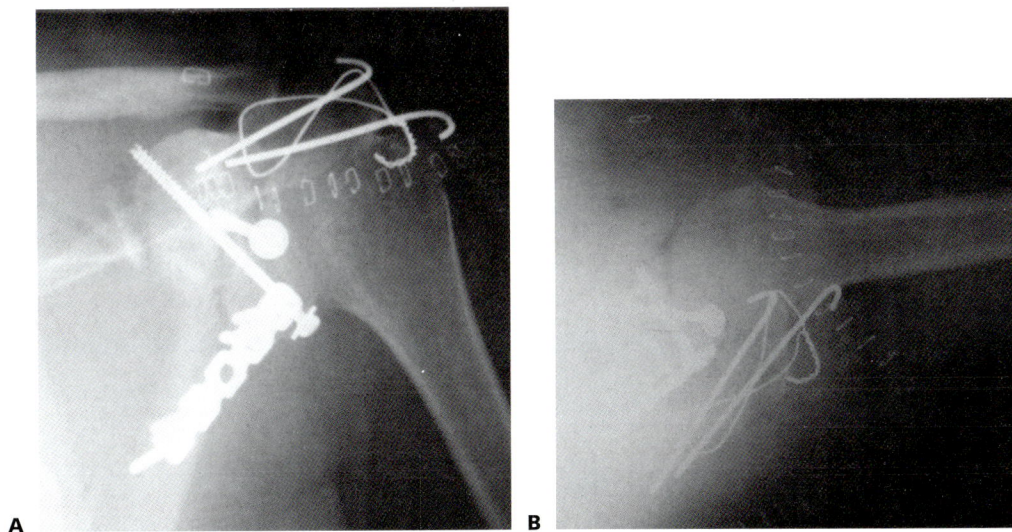

TECH FIG 4 • **A.** Postoperative AP image of the patient shown in Tech Fig 1. **B.** Axillary radiograph showing the glenoid cavity fragments secured together with cannulated screws and the glenoid unit secured to the scapular body with a malleable reconstruction plate (the acromial fracture was reduced and stabilized with a tension band construct). *(continued)*

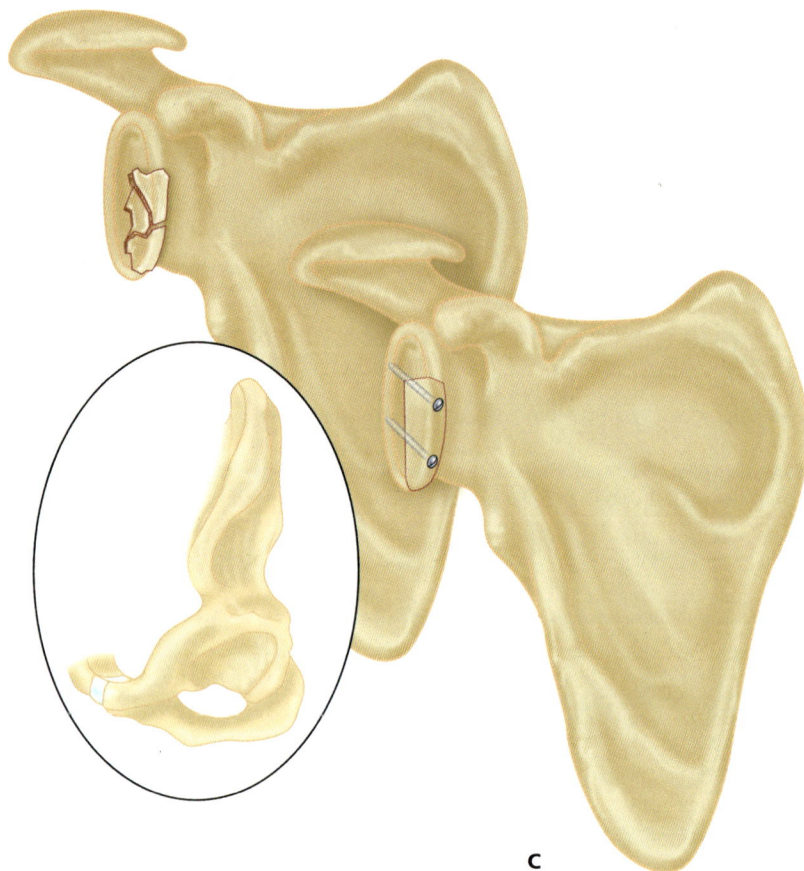

TECH FIG 4 • *(continued)* **C.** If severe comminution is present, an iliac crest tricortical bone graft is an option. (**A,B:** From Goss TP, Owens BD. Fractures of the scapula: diagnosis and treatment. In: Iannotti JP, Williams GR, eds. Disorders of the Shoulder: Diagnosis and Management, 2nd ed. Philadelphia: Lippincott Williams & Wilkins, 2007:793–840.)

PEARLS AND PITFALLS

Indications	■ Rim fractures: 25% or more of the glenoid cavity anteriorly or 33% or more of the glenoid cavity posteriorly and displacement of the fragment 10 mm or more ■ Fossa fractures: an articular step-off of 5 mm or more, significant separation of the fracture fragments, or failure of the humeral head to lie in the center of the glenoid cavity
Approach	■ Incising the rotator interval and leaving the subscapularis unit intact may allow adequate exposure for injuries involving a displaced superior glenoid fragment. ■ Some injuries require combined anteroposterior or posterosuperior approaches. ■ Deltoid detachment and retraction provide maximal posterior exposure and access. ■ During the posterior approach, develop the internervous plane in between the infraspinatus (a bipennate muscle) superiorly and the teres minor inferiorly.
Reduction	■ K-wires can be placed to serve as "joysticks" to assist with fracture reduction. They also can be driven across the fracture site to provide temporary or permanent fixation.
Fixation	■ Bone stock capable of allowing internal fixation is at a premium in the scapula. The four satisfactory areas include the glenoid neck, the acromion–scapular spine, the lateral scapular border, and the coracoid process. Reconstruction plates may be pre-contoured using a scapula model and flash-sterilized. If severe comminution is present, an iliac crest tricortical bone graft is an option. Cannulated interfragmentary screws can be inserted using previously placed K-wires as guidewires.
Closure	■ If the deltoid muscle is detached, meticulous repair to the scapular spine–acromial process is necessary using nonabsorbable sutures placed through drill holes.

POSTOPERATIVE CARE

■ The aggressiveness of the rehabilitation program following ORIF of intra-articular scapular fractures is determined by the rigidity of the fixation construct and the adequacy of the soft tissue repair.[4]

■ Patients are immobilized in a sling and swathe binder and started on gentle pendulum exercises during the first 2 weeks.
■ Progressive passive and active-assisted range-of-motion exercises emphasizing forward flexion and internal–external rotation are prescribed during weeks 2 through 6 postoperatively.

- All protection is discontinued at 6 weeks postoperatively.
- Strengthening is begun after 6 weeks postoperatively and when range of motion is satisfactory.
- Return to sports or physical labor is restricted until 3 to 6 months postoperatively.
- Close outpatient follow-up with radiographs, especially early in recovery, and a well-defined, closely monitored physical therapy program are extremely important.

OUTCOMES

- Good results have been reported for the operative management of glenoid rim fractures.[9,12]
- Bauer et al[1] reviewed six patients treated surgically for glenoid cavity fractures. Four patients with an anatomic reduction had good results; two patients with nonanatomic reductions developed arthritic changes.
- Kavanaugh and colleagues[7] presented their experience at the Mayo Clinic in which 10 displaced intra-articular fractures of the glenoid cavity were treated with ORIF. They found ORIF to be "a useful and safe technique" that "can restore excellent function of the shoulder." In their series, the major articular fragments were displaced 4 to 8 mm.
- Schandelmaier and coauthors[11] reported a series of 22 fractures of the glenoid fossa treated with ORIF with good results.
- Leung and colleagues[8] reviewed 14 displaced intra-articular fractures of the glenoid treated with ORIF (30.5-year average follow-up) and reported 9 excellent and 5 good results.
- On the basis of these reports, it seems reasonable to conclude that there is a definite role for surgical management in the treatment of glenoid cavity fractures.

COMPLICATIONS

- Neurologic complications most commonly are caused by overly aggressive retraction or misdirected dissection.
  - The musculocutaneous and axillary nerves are vulnerable in the anterior approach.
  - The suprascapular nerve is at risk in the superior approach, and the axillary and suprascapular nerves are vulnerable in the posterior approach.[10]
- A variety of other complications can occur as a result of poor surgical technique, inadequately directed or managed rehabilitation, and poor patient compliance.

REFERENCES

1. Bauer G, Fleischmann W, DuBler E. Displaced scapular fractures: Indication and long term results of open reduction and internal fixation. Arch Orthop Trauma Surg 1995;14:215.
2. DePalma AF. Surgery of the Shoulder, 3rd ed. Philadelphia: JB Lippincott, 1983.
3. Goss TP. Fractures of the glenoid cavity. J Bone Joint Surg Am 1992; 74:299–305.
4. Goss TP. Glenoid fractures—open reduction and internal fixation. In Wiss DA, ed: Master Techniques in Orthopaedic Surgery: Fractures. Philadelphia: Lippincott-Raven, 1998.
5. Goss TP. Scapular fractures and dislocation: diagnosis and treatment. J Am Acad Orthop Surg 1995;25:106.
6. Goss TP, Owens BD. Fractures of the scapula: Diagnosis and treatment. In: Iannotti JP, Williams GR, eds. Disorders of the Shoulder: Diagnosis and Management, 2nd ed. Philadelphia: Lippincott Williams & Wilkins, 2007:793–840.
7. Kavanagh BF, Bradway JK, Cofield RH. Open reduction of displaced intra-articular fractures of the glenoid fossa. J Bone Joint Surg Am 1993;75A:479.
8. Leung KS, Lam TB, Poon KM. Operative treatment of displaced intra-articular glenoid fractures. Injury 1993;24:324.
9. Niggebrugge AHP, van Heusden HA, Bode PJ, van Vugt AB. Dislocated intra-articular fracture of the anterior rim of glenoid treated by open reduction and internal fixation. Injury 1993;24:130.
10. Owens BD, Goss TP. Surgical approaches for glenoid fractures. Tech Shoulder Elbow Surg 2004;5:103–115.
11. Schandelmaier P, Blauth M, Schneider C, Krethek C. Fractures of the glenoid treated by operation. A 5- to 23-year follow-up of 22 cases. J Bone Joint Surg Br 2002;84B:173–177.
12. Sinha J, Miller AJ. Fixation of fractures of the glenoid rim. Injury 1992;23:418.

Brent B. Wiesel and Robin R. Richards

DEFINITION

- Despite significant advances in shoulder arthroplasty and other reconstructive procedures, glenohumeral arthrodesis remains an important treatment option in appropriately selected patients.
- The goal of glenohumeral arthrodesis is to provide a stable base for the upper extremity to optimize elbow and hand function.
- Given the tremendous normal range of motion of the glenohumeral joint and the relatively small amount of surface area available for fusion, particularly on the scapular side, successful arthrodesis is technically demanding and requires meticulous surgical technique.

ANATOMY

- The surface area of the glenoid is too small to allow for predictable fusion. Therefore, to increase the area available for fusion, the glenohumeral articular surface and the articulation between the humeral head and undersurface of the acromion are decorticated (**FIG 1**).

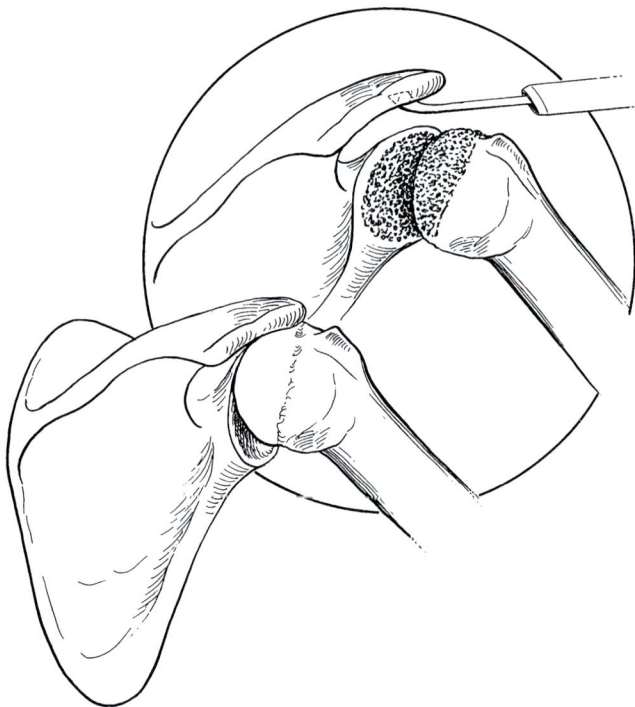

FIG 1 • The glenohumeral joint and the articulation between the humeral head and acromion are decorticated to increase the area available for fusion. (From Iannotti JP, Williams GR, eds. Disorders of the Shoulder: Diagnosis and Management, ed 2. Philadelphia: Lippincott Williams & Wilkins, 2007:684.)

- The bone of the scapula is extremely thin, with only the glenoid fossa and base of the coracoid providing sufficient strength for fixation.
- The optimal position for glenohumeral arthrodesis has been controversial.[1,4]
  - We use a position of 30 degrees of abduction, 30 degrees of forward flexion, and 30 degrees of internal rotation.
  - This position brings the hand to the midline anteriorly, allowing the patient to reach his or her mouth with elbow flexion.

PATIENT HISTORY AND PHYSICAL FINDINGS

- The history and physical findings are specific to the underlying condition requiring arthrodesis.
- All patients will exhibit symptomatic dysfunction at the glenohumeral joint that prevents them from effectively using the involved extremity.

IMAGING AND OTHER DIAGNOSTIC STUDIES

- Standard radiographs, including an anteroposterior, lateral, and axillary view, are used to assess any deformities as well as the bone stock available for fusion.
- If there is concern regarding bone loss on the glenoid side, especially in the setting of failed arthroplasty, this is better evaluated with a CT scan.
- When the neurologic condition of the shoulder girdle muscles is unclear, an electromyelogram of the scapular muscles is indicated.

SURGICAL MANAGEMENT

Indications

- The presence of a flail shoulder is an indication for glenohumeral arthrodesis.
  - Paralysis in patients with a flail shoulder can be the result of anterior poliomyelitis, severe proximal root or irreparable upper trunk brachial plexus lesions, or isolated axillary nerve paralysis.
  - Many patients with flail shoulders develop a painful inferior subluxation that responds well to arthrodesis.
  - The need for fusion following isolated axillary nerve injury depends on the level of impairment. Many patients, especially those with partial paralysis, have reasonable function; however, complete injury often leads to significant limitation of shoulder function.
- Glenohumeral arthrodesis is useful following en bloc resection of periarticular malignant tumors requiring resection of the deltoid, rotator cuff, or both.
- Fusion is useful for the treatment of joint destruction following septic arthritis of the shoulder, particularly in young patients.

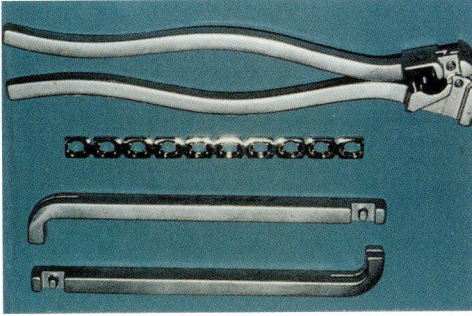

FIG 2 • Handheld bending irons and a plate press are needed to contour the 4.5-mm pelvic reconstruction plate. (From Iannotti JP, Williams GR, eds. Disorders of the Shoulder: Diagnosis and Management, ed 2. Philadelphia: Lippincott Williams & Wilkins, 2007:684.)

- Arthrodesis is a salvage option for patients with multiple failed total shoulder arthroplasties who have insufficient bone stock or soft tissue for revision arthroplasty.
- Symptomatic, uncontrolled shoulder instability that is recalcitrant to soft tissue or bony reconstructive procedures can be managed with fusion.
- Rarely, arthrodesis is indicated in young laborers with severe osteoarthritis who are poor candidates for arthroplasty because of their young age and high activity levels.

Contraindications

- The primary contraindication to glenohumeral arthrodesis is weakness or paralysis of the periscapular muscles, especially the trapezius, levator scapula, and serratus anterior.
  - Progressive neurologic disorders that are likely to lead to paralysis of these muscles also are a contraindication.
- Arthrodesis of the opposite shoulder is a contraindication to fusion.
- Shoulder fusion requires a significant effort by the patient to rehabilitate the shoulder and is contraindicated in patients unwilling or unable to participate in such a program.

Preoperative Planning

- Preoperative radiographs should be evaluated for any bone defects that may require bone grafting.

- The surgeon should make sure that the pelvic reconstruction plate and a set of handheld bending irons are available (**FIG 2**).

Positioning

- The patient is placed in the beach chair position with the back of the table elevated 30 to 45 degrees.
- A folded sheet is placed medial to the scapula to elevate it from the table.
- The drapes are applied as medial as possible, allowing access to the scapula and the anterior chest wall. The arm is draped free (**FIG 3**).
- We do not routinely use intraoperative fluoroscopy; however, early in their experience with this procedure, surgeons may find fluoroscopy useful to confirm the position of the hardware.

Approach

- We perform glenohumeral arthrodesis using a 10-hole, 4.5-mm pelvic reconstruction plate.
- Compression across the glenohumeral articular surface is achieved by placing the initial screws from the plate through the proximal humerus and into the glenoid fossa.
- The plate is then anchored to the spine of the scapula by a screw directed into the base of the coracoid.

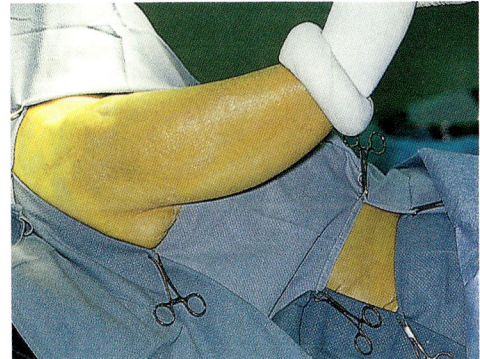

FIG 3 • The drapes are applied, taking care to allow sufficient access to the scapula spine. (From Craig EV, ed. Master Techniques in Orthopaedic Surgery: The Shoulder, ed 2. Philadelphia: Lippincott Williams & Wilkins, 2007:647.)

EXPOSURE

- An S-shaped skin incision begins over the scapular spine, transverses anteriorly over the acromion, and extends down the anterolateral aspect of the arm (**TECH FIG 1A**).
- The skin and subcutaneous tissue are incised down to the fascia along the entire length of the incision.
- The spine of the scapula and acromion are exposed first by electrocautery, and then by subperiosteal dissection (**TECH FIG 1B**).
- Anteriorly, the deltopectoral interval is developed, and the deltoid is subperiosteally elevated off the acromion, beginning at the medial aspect of the anterior head and progressing laterally and posteriorly to the posterolateral corner of the acromion.
  - Alternatively, if the deltoid is de-innervated, as may occur following brachial plexus injury, it can be split between the anterior and lateral heads. The anterior head is then elevated medially and the lateral head laterally to provide wide exposure of the proximal humerus.
- Distally, the biceps tendon is identified and tenodesed to the upper border of the pectoralis major tendon.

TECHNIQUES

TECHNIQUES

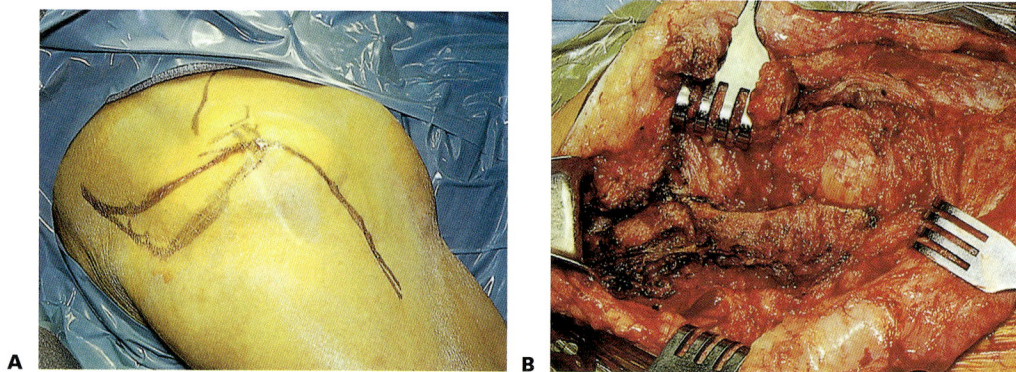

TECH FIG 1 • **A.** An S-shaped skin incision begins over the spine of the scapula. **B.** The spine of the scapula and acromion are exposed by subperiosteal dissection. (From Craig EV, ed. Master Techniques in Orthopaedic Surgery: The Shoulder, ed 2. Philadelphia: Lippincott Williams & Wilkins, 2007:647, 648.)

PERFORMING THE GLENOHUMERAL ARTHRODESIS

- The rotator cuff is resected from the proximal humerus, beginning at the inferior border of the subscapularis and proceeding superiorly and then posteriorly and inferiorly to the level of the teres minor.
- A ring or Hohmann retractor is placed on the posterior lip of the glenoid, and the humeral head is retracted posteriorly to expose the glenoid.
- The glenoid cartilage is removed using a ⅜-inch curved osteotome or burr (**TECH FIG 2A**). The glenoid labrum also is removed.
- The retractors are then removed, and the arm is extended, adducted, and externally rotated to expose the humeral head.
- A ½-inch curved osteotome or burr is used to remove the articular surface of the humerus in its entirety.
- The undersurface of the acromion is decorticated with a ¾-inch curved osteotome or burr.
- The arm is placed in 30 degrees of flexion, 30 degrees of abduction, and 30 degrees of internal rotation, and the humerus is brought proximally to appose the decorticated surface of the acromion (**TECH FIG 2B**).
  - The arm is maintained in this position by placing folded sheets between the thorax and the extremity and having an assistant stand on the opposite side of the table to support the forearm and hand.
- The 4.5-mm, 10-hole pelvic reconstruction plate is contoured to run along the spine of the scapula,

over the acromion and down the shaft of the humerus (**TECH FIG 2C**).
- The plate is bent 60 degrees between the third and fourth holes and then twisted 20 to 25 degrees just distal to the bend so it apposes the shaft of the humerus.
- With the arm supported in the appropriate position and the plate held against the scapula and humerus, a hole is drilled through the plate, through the humerus, and into the glenoid using a 3.2-mm drill bit.
- The screw length is measured; usually it is between 65 and 75 mm.
- The humeral cortex is tapped with a 6.5-mm tap.
- A short-thread 6.5-mm cancellous screw is inserted as a lag screw into the glenoid.
- Depending on glenoid bone stock, one or two more screws are placed in a similar manner.
- The plate is then anchored to the scapula by placing one or two fully threaded cancellous screws from the plate through the spine of the scapula and into the base of the coracoid.
- Another cancellous screw is placed across the acromiohumeral fusion site.
- Distally, the remaining holes are filled with cortical screws (**TECH FIG 2D**).
- The wound is closed in standard fashion over two ⅛ inch suction drains. Care is taken to reattach the deltoid to the acromion in an effort to cover as much of the plate as possible.

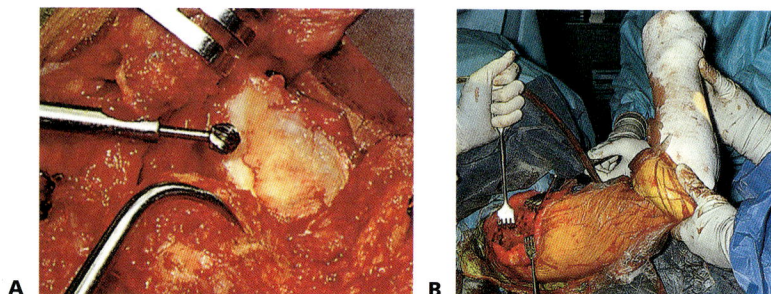

TECH FIG 2 • **A.** The glenoid articular surface is removed using a burr or 3/8-inch curved osteotome. **B.** The arm is placed in the arthrodesis position: 30 degrees of flexion, 30 degrees of abduction, and 30 degrees of internal rotation. This position allows the patient to reach his or her mouth with elbow flexion. (continued)

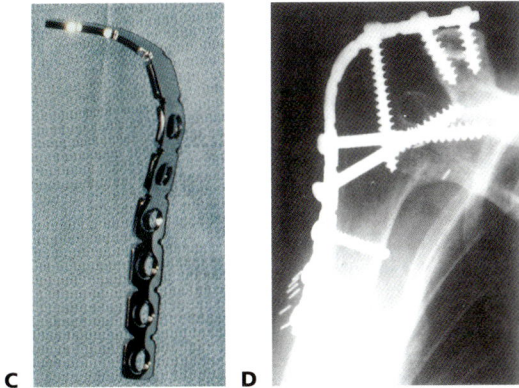

C   D

TECH FIG 2 • (continued) **C.** The 10-hole, 4.5-mm pelvic reconstruction plate is bent 60 degrees between the third and fourth holes and then twisted 20 to 25 degrees in the sagittal plane. **D.** AP radiograph following glenohumeral arthrodesis with a 10-hole, 4.5-mm pelvic reconstruction plate. The two 6.5-mm partially threaded screws are placed first to achieve compression at the glenohumeral joint. (**A,B:** From Craig EV, ed. Master Techniques in Orthopaedic Surgery: The Shoulder, ed 2. Philadelphia: Lippincott Williams & Wilkins, 2007:648, 649. **C,D:** From Iannotti JP, Williams GR, eds. Disorders of the Shoulder: Diagnosis and Management, ed 2. Philadelphia: Lippincott Williams & Wilkins, 2007:683, 685.)

BONE GRAFTING

- We do not routinely use bone graft when performing glenohumeral arthrodesis.
- Bone grafting is indicated to fill large defects in patients who are undergoing arthrodesis for complex and revision problems as well as following tumor resection.
- Nonstructural autogenous bone graft can be obtained from the ipsilateral iliac crest and is combined with revision of the internal fixation for the treatment of nonunited fusions.
- Tricortical iliac crest graft can be placed between the humerus and glenoid when structural bone graft is needed (**TECH FIG 3A**).
  - This type of graft commonly is needed to treat bone deficiency following failed shoulder arthroplasty.
  - The graft is placed underneath the plate so that the compression screws pass first through the plate and

any remaining proximal humerus and then through the graft and into the glenoid.
- When an intercalary defect larger than 6 cm is present, the surgeon should consider a vascularized fibular bone graft (**TECH FIG 3B**).
  - The vascularized graft should be fixed at each end with minimal internal fixation.
  - The entire defect is then spanned with a very long plate.
  - The vascular anastomosis is performed between the peroneal artery and its vena comitantes and a branch of either the axillary or brachial artery.
  - Nonstructural autogenous graft is placed at each end of the vascularized graft to maximize the likelihood of fusion occurring.

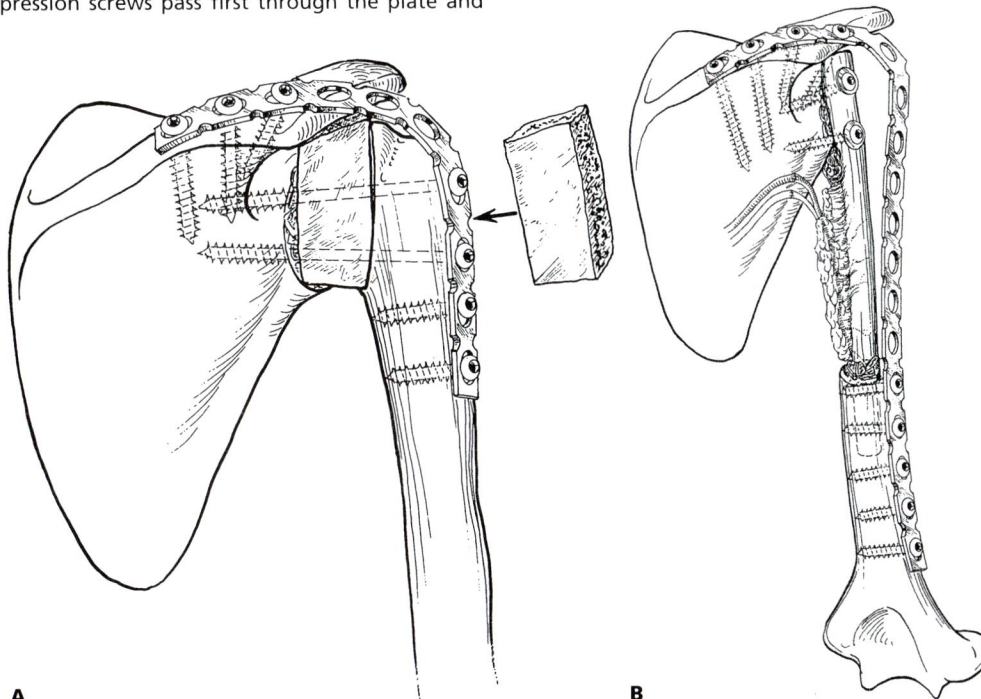

A   B

TECH FIG 3 • **A.** Tricortical bone graft can be placed between the humerus and glenoid when there is proximal humeral deficiency. **B.** Vascularized graft is used for defects greater than 6 cm. (From Iannotti JP, Williams GR, eds. Disorders of the Shoulder: Diagnosis and Management, ed 2. Philadelphia: Lippincott Williams & Wilkins, 2007:689.)

PEARLS AND PITFALLS

Preoperative counseling	▪ The concept of shoulder arthrodesis is difficult for most patients to understand. The most practical way to help them understand is to have them speak with a patient who has undergone the procedure.
Position of fusion	▪ It is important not to place the arm in excessive abduction, because this can lead to increased periscapular pain when the patient rests the arm at the side. ▪ Excessive internal rotation can prevent the patient from reaching his or her mouth or pocket.
Increasing fusion rates	▪ When positioning the arm for arthrodesis, it is important to move the humerus proximal to maximize contact between the undersurface of the acromion and proximal humerus, thereby increasing the surface area available for fusion. ▪ Partially-threaded screws are placed from the plate, through the humerus, and into the glenoid using lag screw technique to increase compression at the glenohumeral joint.
Prominent hardware	▪ The acromion can be notched laterally to decrease any prominence of the hardware in this area. ▪ Even in the presence of extensive deltoid atrophy, the muscle fibers help to protect the hardware, so it is important to reattach the deltoid to the acromion and cover as much of the plate as possible. ▪ If the hardware is removed, the patient should be informed that there is an initial risk of humeral fracture because of the increase in stress on the screw holes.

POSTOPERATIVE CARE

▪ In the operating room, after the procedure, a pillow is placed between the patient's arm and chest, and the arm is then wrapped to the chest with a swathe.

▪ A radiograph is obtained in the recovery room to verify position of the internal fixation.

▪ A thermoplastic orthosis is applied on the day after surgery and adjusted as needed.

▪ Patients usually are discharged from the hospital on the second postoperative day and maintained in the orthosis for 6 weeks.

▪ If, at 6 weeks, there are no radiographic signs of loosening of the hardware, the patient may progress to a sling.

▪ Another radiograph is obtained at 3 months. If there are no signs of loosening, thoracoscapular strengthening and mobilization exercises are initiated.

▪ Glenohumeral arthrodesis places significant stress on the periscapular musculature. The rehabilitation process is slow, and a recovery period of 6 to 12 months should be expected.

OUTCOMES

▪ After successful arthrodesis, the patient usually can reach the mouth, opposite axilla, belt buckle, and side pocket. The patient cannot work or reach overhead, and cannot reach the back pocket or a bra strap, and perineal care often is very difficult using the fused shoulder.

▪ Richards et al.[3] assessed the ability to perform specific activities of daily living in 33 patients following glenohumeral arthrodesis.

▪ Patient satisfaction was highest in those patients undergoing the procedure for a brachial plexus injury, osteoarthritis, and failed total shoulder arthroplasty.

▪ Cofield and Briggs[4] reported their results for glenohumeral fusion with internal fixation in 71 patients. Eighty-two percent of the patients felt that they benefited from the procedure, and 75% were able to perform activities that involved reaching their trunk.

▪ Scalise and Iannotti[5] analyzed the results of arthrodesis in seven patients following failed prosthetic arthroplasty. Five of the seven patients eventually achieved fusion. Four patients required additional bone-grafting procedures in an attempt to achieve union, and two of these patients ultimately had a persistent nonunion despite the additional procedures.

COMPLICATIONS

▪ Nonunion
▪ Prominent hardware
▪ Malposition
▪ Infection
▪ Humeral shaft fracture

REFERENCES

1. Barr J, Freiberg JA, Colonna PC, et al. A survey of end results on stabilization of the paralysed shoulder. Report of the Research Committee of the American Orthopaedic Association. J Bone Joint Surg 1942;24:699–707.
2. Cofield RH, Briggs BT. Glenohumeral arthrodesis. J Bone Joint Surg Am 1979;61A:668–677.
3. Richards RR, Beaton DE, Hudson AR. Shoulder arthrodesis with plate fixation: A functional outcome analysis. J Shoulder Elbow Surg 1993;2:225–239.
4. Rowe CR. Re-evaluation of the position of the arm in arthrodesis of the shoulder in the adult. J Bone Joint Surg Am 1974;56A:913–922.
5. Scalise JJ, Iannotti JP. Glenohumeral arthrodesis after failed prosthetic shoulder arthroplasty. J Bone Joint Surg Am 2008;90A:70–77.

Hemiarthroplasty, Total Shoulder Arthroplasty, and Biologic Glenoid Resurfacing for Glenohumeral Arthritis With an Intact Rotator Cuff

Gerald R. Williams

DEFINITION

■ Glenohumeral arthritis is characterized by loss of articular cartilage and varying degrees of soft tissue contracture, rotator cuff dysfunction, and bone erosion, depending on the underlying arthritic condition.

■ The results of surgical treatment are largely dependent on the integrity of the rotator cuff; therefore, glenohumeral arthritides are often subdivided on this basis.

■ Common arthritic and related conditions that generally involve an intact or reparable rotator cuff include osteoarthritis, posttraumatic arthritis, and avascular necrosis.

■ Although some patients with inflammatory arthritides such as rheumatoid arthritis have intact or reparable rotator cuffs, the rotator cuff is torn or dysfunctional in many patients. When reference is made to patients with inflammatory arthritis in this section, it pertains to the subset of patients in whom the cuff is intact or reparable.

ANATOMY

■ The pertinent surgical anatomy can be divided into bone, ligaments, muscles, and neurovascular structures.

■ Normal osseous relationships include humeral head center, thickness, and radius of curvature, humeral neck–shaft angle, humeral head offset, glenohumeral offset, greater tuberosity-to-acromion distance, greater tuberosity-to-humeral-head distance, glenoid radius of curvature, glenoid size, glenoid version, and glenoid offset (**FIG 1**).[14,22]

■ Humeral head radius and thickness are variable and correlate with patient size. Mean humeral head radius is about 24 mm, with a range of 19 to 28 mm. Mean humeral head thickness is about 19 mm, with a range of 15 to 24 mm.[14,22]

■ The ratio of humeral head thickness to humeral head radius of curvature is remarkably constant at about 0.7 to 0.9, regardless of patient height or humeral shaft size.[14,22]

■ The center of the humeral head does not coincide with the projected center of the humeral shaft. The distance between the center of the humeral head and the central axis of the intramedullary canal is defined as the humeral head offset and is about 7 to 9 mm medial and 2 to 4 mm posterior (**FIG 2**).[2,22]

■ Humeral retroversion averages 20 to 30 degrees, with a wide range of about 20 to 55 degrees.[2,14,22] The vertical distance between the highest point of the humeral articular surface and the highest point of the greater tuberosity (ie, head to greater tuberosity height) is about 8 mm and shows a relatively small range of interspecimen variability.[14]

■ Humeral neck–shaft angle is defined as the angle subtended by the central intramedullary axis of the humeral shaft and the base of the articular segment and shows substantial individual variation. The average neck–shaft angle is 40 to 45 degrees (130–135) degrees, with a range of 30 to 55 (120–145) degrees.[2,14,22]

■ Pertinent musculotendinous anatomy includes the deltoid, pectoralis major, conjoined tendon of the coracobrachialis and short head of the biceps, rotator cuff, and long head of the biceps.

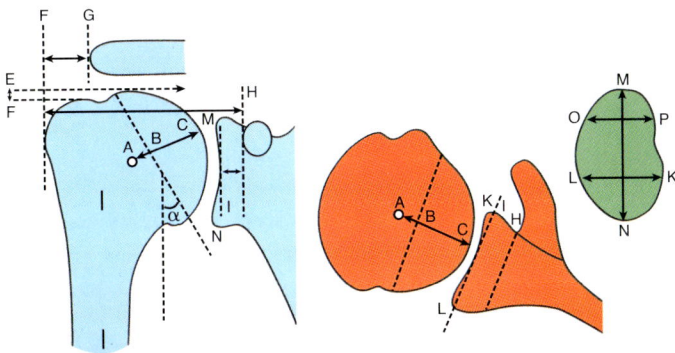

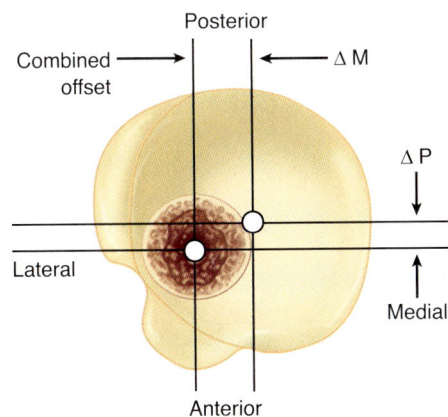

FIG 1 • The normal glenohumeral anatomical relationships. (Adapted from Iannotti JP, Gabriel JP, Schneck SL, et al. The normal glenohumeral relationships: an anatomical study of one hundred and forty shoulders. J Bone Joint Surg Am 1992;74A:491–500.)

FIG 2 • The humeral head center, on average, lies 2 to 4 mm posterior and 7 to 9 mm medial to the projected center of the intramedullary canal. (Adapted from Boileau P, Walch G. The three-dimensional geometry of the proximal humerus: implications for surgical technique and prosthetic design. J Bone Joint Surg Br 1997;79B:857–865.)

- Ligamentous structures that are potentially important in the surgical management of glenohumeral arthritis include the coracoacromial ligament and the glenohumeral capsular ligaments. In many cases of glenohumeral arthritis with an intact cuff, the anterior and inferior capsular ligaments are contracted, resulting in restriction of external rotation and posterior humeral head subluxation.

- Neurovascular structures are abundant and subject to potential injury during shoulder arthroplasty. The axillary artery and all of its branches, especially the anterior humeral circumflex, posterior humeral circumflex, and the subscapular arteries, are particularly vulnerable.

- The entire brachial plexus traverses the anterior aspect of the shoulder and is subject to traction and other injuries. The two most pertinent nerves are the axillary nerve and the musculocutaneous nerve.

- The axillary nerve is a terminal branch of the posterior cord of the brachial plexus and is composed primarily of motor fibers from the fifth and sixth cervical roots. It descends the anterior surface of the subscapularis to the inferior aspect of the joint capsule, where it courses through the quadrilateral space to enter the posterior aspect of the shoulder.

- The musculocutaneous nerve is one of the terminal branches of the lateral cord of the brachial plexus that is anterior and lateral to the axillary nerve. It typically pierces the conjoined tendon of the coracobrachialis and short head of the biceps about 5 cm distal to the tip of the coracoid. However, this course is variable and the entry point into the conjoined tendon can be as proximal as 2 cm.

PATHOGENESIS

- The biologic basis for glenohumeral arthritis is not known. However, the loss of articular cartilage associated with primary osteoarthritis, posttraumatic arthritis, avascular necrosis, and other arthritides is, in some way, the result of imbalance in the normal cycle of cartilage damage and repair.

- In some cases of posttraumatic arthritis, catastrophic cartilage damage associated with single-event or repetitive trauma overwhelms the shoulder's cartilage repair mechanisms and arthritis ensues.

- Primary osteoarthritis may be associated with mechanical factors such as glenoid hypoplasia and increased retroversion. However, in many cases, no cause is evident. The final common pathway involves a release of degradative enzymes such as collagenase, gelatinase, and stromelysin, and a variety of inflammatory mediators, which further damage the cartilage and eventually the underlying bone.

- A detailed discussion of the pathogenesis of avascular necrosis is beyond the scope of this chapter. However, the development of glenohumeral arthritis in this condition is likely the result of advanced cartilage damage following collapse of the humeral head. Involvement of glenoid articular cartilage does not occur until the later stages of the disease, when the irregular humeral head has been articulating with the previously normal glenoid surface.

- Rheumatoid arthritis is characterized by activation of the immune system that leads to an influx of lymphocytes into the joint and synovial tissue, with subsequent release of a variety of cytokines, destructive enzymes, and mediators of inflammation such as interleukins and tumor necrosis factor. This autoimmune response is thought to be important in perpetuating joint destruction.[25]

NATURAL HISTORY

- Glenohumeral arthritis of any type is characterized by progressive stiffness, pain, and loss of function.

- Patients with primary osteoarthritis and many types of posttraumatic arthritis develop progressive loss of external rotation, posterior subluxation, and posterior glenoid bone loss. Large osteophyte formation, especially on the inferior humeral neck, is common. Full-thickness rotator cuff tears are distinctly uncommon and occur in 5% to 10% of patients.

- Rheumatoid arthritis results in progressive regional osteopenia, central glenoid bone erosion, and rotator cuff tears. The prevalence of full-thickness rotator cuff tears in patients with rheumatoid arthritis of the shoulder is 25% to 40%.[27] However, rotator cuff dysfunction and substantial partial tearing are extremely common.

PATIENT HISTORY AND PHYSICAL FINDINGS

- Patients with glenohumeral arthritis will give a history of chronic (years) shoulder pain and restricted motion, often with a recent (months) exacerbation. Posttraumatic arthritis is typically associated with a history of prior injury, such as fracture or dislocation, or surgery.

- Pain is often worse with activity and usually interferes with sleep. Neck pain, distal radiation below the elbow, and numbness and paresthesias in the fingers and hand are uncommon and should suggest other potential causes of shoulder pain, such as cervical stenosis or cervical radiculopathy.

- Bilateral involvement is common in primary osteoarthritis. Contralateral symptoms are often present, but to a lesser extent.

- Physical findings in patients with glenohumeral arthritis and an intact rotator cuff include:
  - Posterior joint line tenderness, especially in osteoarthritis associated with posterior subluxation[20]
  - Generalized atrophy or flattening of the shoulder from long-term lack of function
  - Posterior prominence of the humeral head in cases of posterior subluxation
  - Symmetrical loss of active and passive range of motion (**FIG 3**)
  - Disproportionate loss of external rotation in comparison to other motions, especially in osteoarthritis or after capsulorrhaphy arthropathy[20]
  - Increased pain with passive stretch of the capsule at the end range of motion, especially external rotation
  - Intact neurologic function, except in rare patients with prior neurologic injury from trauma or surgery

IMAGING AND OTHER DIAGNOSTIC STUDIES

- Glenohumeral arthritis is a radiographic diagnosis. Routine radiographs should include anteroposterior (AP) views in internal and external rotation and an axillary view.

- Radiographic findings in primary osteoarthritis include subchondral sclerosis and cyst formation, osteophyte formation, and asymmetrical posterior joint space narrowing (**FIG 4A,B**).[20]

- In cases of posttraumatic arthritis, radiographs may reveal retained hardware.

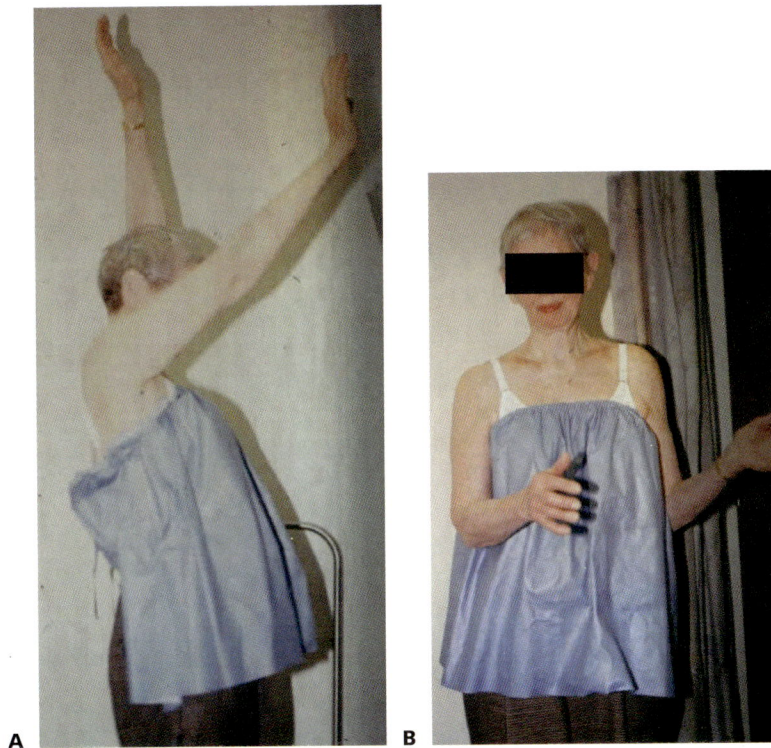

A

B

FIG 3 • The hallmark of glenohumeral osteoarthritis is symmetrical loss of both active and passive range of motion (**A**), especially external rotation (**B**).

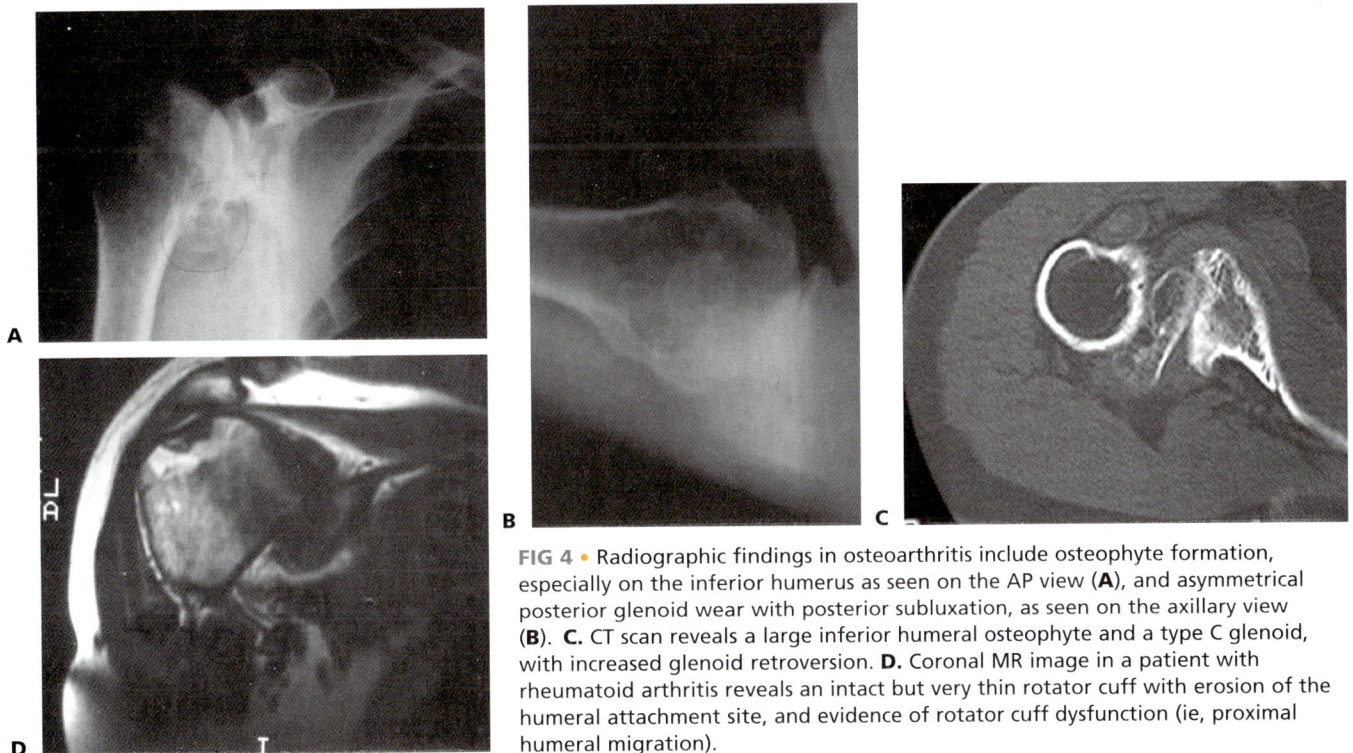

A

B

C

D

FIG 4 • Radiographic findings in osteoarthritis include osteophyte formation, especially on the inferior humerus as seen on the AP view (**A**), and asymmetrical posterior glenoid wear with posterior subluxation, as seen on the axillary view (**B**). **C.** CT scan reveals a large inferior humeral osteophyte and a type C glenoid, with increased glenoid retroversion. **D.** Coronal MR image in a patient with rheumatoid arthritis reveals an intact but very thin rotator cuff with erosion of the humeral attachment site, and evidence of rotator cuff dysfunction (ie, proximal humeral migration).

- Glenoid deformity in osteoarthritis has been classified by Walch[29] according to the presence of posterior subluxation and posterior bone deformity:
  - Type A: centered
  - Type B: posteriorly subluxated (B1) and posteriorly subluxated with posterior erosion (B2)
  - Type C: posteriorly subluxated with increased retroversion (hypoplasia)
- Computed tomographic (CT) scans are helpful in quantifying bone loss in patients with posterior subluxation (**FIG 4C**).
- MRI is useful in patients with rheumatoid arthritis to determine rotator cuff integrity (**FIG 4D**).
- Electromyography may be used in patients suspected of having posttraumatic or postsurgical nerve injuries.
- Medical consultation is warranted in patients with substantial comorbidities.

DIFFERENTIAL DIAGNOSIS

- Frozen shoulder
- Posttraumatic or postsurgical infection
- Cervical stenosis
- Cervical radiculopathy
- Neoplasm

NONOPERATIVE MANAGEMENT

- Avoiding activities that are painful or place an undue strain on the shoulder, such as weight lifting, is important.
- Nonsteroidal anti-inflammatory medications may be helpful in reducing pain and inflammation.
- In patients with rheumatoid arthritis, rheumatologic consultation for maximizing medical treatment is helpful.
- Glucosamine chondroitin and other nutritional supplements may reduce the pain associated with arthritis, despite the relative lack of standardized data.
- Intra-articular corticosteroid injections are almost always helpful, but the relief is often only temporary.
- Hyaluronic acid derivatives are not yet approved by the U.S. Food and Drug Administration for use in the shoulder but may be of benefit in the future.
- Therapeutic exercises should be used judiciously. Stretching to maintain flexibility may be helpful, but vigorous exercises may increase pain.

SURGICAL MANAGEMENT

- Surgical options are considered when pain and dysfunction justify surgical intervention, nonoperative management has failed, medical comorbidities do not preclude surgery, and the patient is willing to accept the risks of surgery and the responsibility of postoperative rehabilitation and activity limitations.
- Nonprosthetic options such as arthroscopic or open débridement are indicated in patients who are too young and active for any type of prosthetic replacement.
- Prosthetic options include hemiarthroplasty, hemiarthroplasty plus biologic resurfacing, and total shoulder replacement.
- Total shoulder replacement with a polyethylene glenoid component provides the most predictable pain relief but has the disadvantage of progressive polyethylene wear and eventual component loosening.[26]
- Hemiarthroplasty can be successful in providing pain relief, especially with minimal glenoid involvement or concentric glenoid wear. However, progressive glenoid erosion is likely and may require revision to total shoulder replacement.
- Hemiarthroplasty with resurfacing of the glenoid with biologic materials such as meniscal allograft, capsular or fascia lata autograft, fascia lata allograft, dermal allograft, Achilles tendon allograft, or xenograft materials has been performed, particularly in patients too young or active for a polyethylene glenoid component.[3,21,30]
- The additional benefit of biologic resurfacing of the glenoid over hemiarthroplasty alone has not been clearly demonstrated, nor has its durability been confirmed.[10]
- Hemiarthroplasty may be accomplished by replacement or resurfacing of the humeral head.
- Replacement of the humeral head is most commonly accomplished with a prosthetic head that is anchored to the shaft with a stem. However, more recently, humeral head replacements have been developed that are fixed to the metaphysis without violation of the diaphyseal canal.
- The relative indications for hemiarthroplasty, hemiarthroplasty with biologic resurfacing, and total shoulder arthroplasty are controversial, vary among surgeons, and must be individualized according to patient age, activity level, and bone deformity, among other factors.
- Similarly, the type of implant can be individualized according to patient factors and surgeon preference.
- Concentricity of the joint, without subluxation, likely improves prosthetic performance in all circumstances. Therefore, fixed subluxation should be corrected when possible. Options include contracture release and correction of bone deformity with some combination of asymmetric reaming, bone grafting, and specialized components.
- General principles that summarize procedural and implant indications in patients with glenohumeral arthritis and an intact or reparable cuff include the following:
  - Total shoulder arthroplasty is preferred with adequate glenoid bone, age greater than 50, and sedentary or moderate activity levels.
  - Hemiarthroplasty is favored in patients with normal or minimally involved glenoids, inadequate glenoid bone, age of 50 or under, and activity levels that include weight lifting or other strenuous activity.
  - Biologic resurfacing of the glenoid may be added to hemiarthroplasty but may also fail in patients who participate in heavy weight lifting or other strenuous activity.
  - When substantial reaming or resurfacing of the glenoid is planned, the procedure is facilitated by removing the humeral head rather than resurfacing it. Currently stemmed implants are most popular, but implants with metaphyseal fixation may be useful in patients with adequate bone quality.
  - Humeral resurfacing is useful when hemiarthroplasty is indicated in the absence of substantial glenoid deformity. Resurfacing preserves humeral bone and obviates the need to address humeral head–humeral canal offset.
  - These principles are merely guidelines and should be individualized.
- The following sections will cover the technical aspects of humeral resurfacing, humeral replacement, humeral replacement combined with biologic glenoid resurfacing with allograft lateral meniscus, and total shoulder arthroplasty. Glenoid bone grafting is beyond the scope of this chapter and will not be covered.

Preoperative Planning

- Preoperative radiographs and CT scans should be reviewed to quantify humeral subluxation (especially posterior in osteoarthritis) and glenoid bone loss. This will identify the need for asymmetric glenoid reaming.
- If the goals of asymmetric reaming are to correct glenoid deformity and to contain all fixation appendages of the glenoid component within the glenoid vault, the extent of reaming should be limited to about 5 mm or 15 degrees. If greater correction is desired, arrangements for glenoid bone grafting should be made.
- Preoperative radiographs should be templated to gain an appreciation of the humeral head size, canal diameter, and neck–shaft angle. In patients with highly varus (115–120 degrees) or valgus (145–150 degrees) neck–shaft angles in whom cementless fixation of a stemmed implant is planned, alterations in the level of the humeral cut or the use of a prosthesis with neck–shaft angle variability will be required.
- MRI scans should be read for substantial rotator cuff abnormalities in rheumatoid patients and others suspected of having rotator cuff tears.
- All other relevant preoperative data should be reviewed, including consultations from medical colleagues. The presence of all surgical implants and instruments should be verified.
- Passive range of motion should be measured intraoperatively, before positioning, to determine the need for contracture release. In particular, the degree of passive external rotation loss may dictate the method of subscapularis reflection and repair.
- Subscapularis shortening is typically not a substantial factor in passive external rotation loss, unless the patient has had a prior subscapularis shortening or tightening procedure (eg, Putti-Platt or Magnuson-Stack) or the contracture is particularly severe (eg, external rotation of −30 degrees or more) and longstanding.
- Methods of managing the subscapularis include intratendinous incision and anatomic repair, lesser tuberosity osteotomy and anatomic repair, lateral tendinous release with medial advancement, and Z-lengthening.
- Recent evidence suggests that lesser tuberosity osteotomy is associated with better subscapularis function than soft tissue reflection and repair.[12,23] However, randomized comparison data are not currently available. In addition, a recent study documents good postoperative subscapularis function with tenotomy and soft tissue repair.[4]
- My current preference for subscapularis management in primary shoulder arthroplasty is lesser tuberosity osteotomy and anatomic repair, with the following exceptions:
  - Rheumatoid arthritis with substantial erosion of the subscapularis attachment site on MRI
  - History of a subscapularis shortening or tightening procedure (eg, Putti-Platt or Magnuson-Stack procedure)
  - Passive external rotation of less than −30 degrees
- If lesser tuberosity osteotomy is not performed, lateral detachment with medial reattachment is most often adequate. Subscapularis Z-lengthening is rarely required.

Positioning

- Shoulder arthroplasty is performed with the patient in the semirecumbent position (**FIG 5A**). The hips should be flexed about 30 degrees to prevent the patient from sliding down the table; the knees should be flexed about 30 degrees to relax tension on the sciatic nerves; the back should be elevated 35 to 40 degrees.
- The entire shoulder should be lateral to the edge of the table to allow adduction and extension of the arm (**FIG 5B**). This is

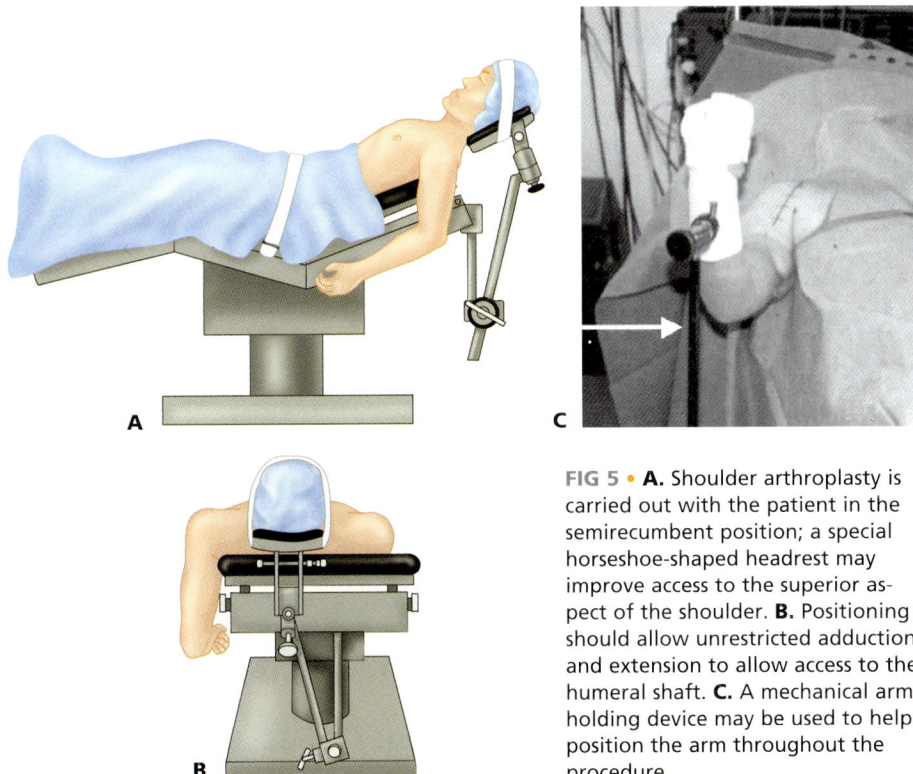

FIG 5 • **A.** Shoulder arthroplasty is carried out with the patient in the semirecumbent position; a special horseshoe-shaped headrest may improve access to the superior aspect of the shoulder. **B.** Positioning should allow unrestricted adduction and extension to allow access to the humeral shaft. **C.** A mechanical arm-holding device may be used to help position the arm throughout the procedure.

required for safe access to the humeral canal and can be accomplished by positioning the patient as far toward the operative side of the table as possible or by using a specialized table with removable cutouts behind the shoulders.

■ A specialized padded, horseshoe-shaped headrest may be helpful in facilitating access to the superior aspect of the shoulder.

■ An adjustable mechanical arm holder (McConnell Orthopedic Mfg. Co., Greenville, TX, or Tenet Medical Engineering, Inc., Calgary, Alberta, CA) is helpful for positioning the arm. Alternatively, a padded Mayo stand can also be used (**FIG 5C**).

Approach

■ The most common approach for shoulder arthroplasty is the deltopectoral approach popularized by Neer.[20] The advantages are preservation of the deltoid origin and insertion, extensibility, and excellent humeral exposure. The need for posterior deltoid retraction, especially in muscular men, can make posterior glenoid exposure difficult and can lead to injury of the cephalic vein, the deltoid itself, or the brachial plexus.

■ The superior or anterosuperior approach was popularized by MacKenzie[19] and involves access to the shoulder by reflecting the anterior deltoid from the acromion. Advantages include excellent anterior and posterior glenoid exposure and a lower incidence of axillary nerve traction injuries than the traditional deltopectoral approach. Disadvantages include nonextensibility, difficult medial and inferior humeral exposure, and potential deltoid dehiscence.

■ Modifications of these exposures include the addition of a clavicular osteotomy and extensive takedown of the deltoid origin to aid in exposure for difficult cases.[13,24]

■ The deltopectoral approach is the most commonly used approach for primary arthroplasty with an intact or reparable cuff and will be used in all subsequent sections of this chapter.

HUMERAL RESURFACING

Superficial Dissection

■ A deltopectoral incision is made from the tip of the coracoid toward the deltoid insertion.

■ The cephalic vein is taken laterally with the deltoid and the pectoralis major is taken medially.

■ The upper 1 cm of the pectoralis major may be released to improve visualization of the inferior aspect of the joint, but this is not always needed.

Deep Dissection

■ The clavipectoral fascia is incised lateral to the conjoined tendon of the short head of the biceps and coracobrachialis and is carried superiorly to the coracoacromial ligament, which does not require excision or release to attain adequate exposure.

■ Digital palpation is used to verify the position of the axillary nerve, which is protected throughout the procedure. The musculocutaneous nerve is usually not easily palpable within the surgical field but can be palpated when its entrance is close to the tip of the coracoid. This should be noted so that excessive retraction of the conjoined tendon can be avoided.

■ With the conjoined tendon retracted medially and the deltoid laterally, the arm is placed in slight external rotation to expose the anterior humeral circumflex artery and veins. These are clamped and coagulated or ligated to avoid inadvertent injury and bleeding during the case.

■ The arm is placed in slight internal rotation and the long head of the biceps is exposed from the superior border of the pectoralis major to the supraglenoid tubercle by incising its investing soft tissue envelope and the rotator interval capsule. The long head of the biceps is tenodesed to the upper border of the pectoralis major using two nonabsorbable sutures and is then released proximal to this tenodesis site and excised from the supraglenoid tubercle.

Lesser Tuberosity Osteotomy

■ A large (2 inch) curved osteotome is used to perform a lesser tuberosity osteotomy (**TECH FIG 1A**). The goal is to obtain a 0.5- to 1-cm-thick, noncomminuted fragment with which to reflect the subscapularis.

■ This is most easily accomplished by placing the blade of the osteotome at the base of the bicipital groove with one hand, palpating the most anterior extent of the tuberosity with the index finger of the other hand, and allowing an assistant to strike the osteotome while the surgeon directs it.

■ Once the osteotomy is completed, a large straight osteotome is placed in the osteotomy and is rotated about its long axis to free the osteotomy fragment from any adjacent soft tissue attachments.

■ A large Cobb elevator is then placed in the osteotomy to lever the fragment anteriorly. This further frees the fragment from the underlying capsule and allows sectioning of the superior glenohumeral ligament attachment.

■ The fragment should now be freely mobile. Three 1-mm nonabsorbable sutures are passed around the lesser tuberosity fragment through the bone–subscapularis tendon junction for traction and later reattachment (**TECH FIG 1B,C**).

■ The arm is externally rotated to expose the most inferior portion of the subscapularis muscle. This may require a right-angle retractor for the pectoralis major. The muscle belly is incised superficially, in line with its fibers, about 1 cm superior to its most inferior border.

■ A blunt elevator is used to dissect the interval between the subscapularis and the underlying capsule. Once this interval is adequately developed, a scalpel is placed between the subscapularis and capsule. With the lesser tuberosity pulled anteriorly, the scalpel is passed laterally so that is exits inferior to the fragment. This is continued from inferior to superior to release the subscapularis and

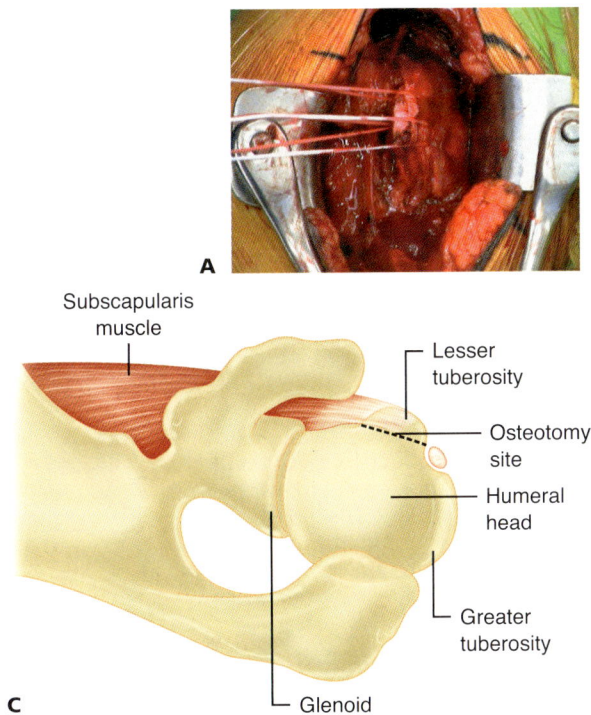

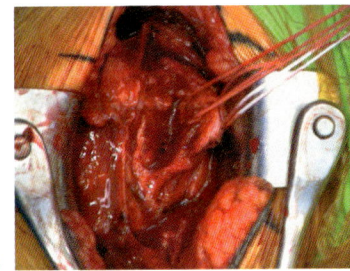

TECH FIG 1 • **A.** A lesser tuberosity osteotomy is performed using a large curved osteotome placed in the base of the bicipital groove and driven medially to produce a lesser tuberosity fragment about 0.5 to 1.0 cm thick. **B,C.** A lesser tuberosity osteotomy has been performed in this right shoulder. **B.** After the fragment has been mobilized from the surrounding soft tissues, three heavy nonabsorbable sutures are placed around the fragment at the bone–tendon junction. **C.** The fragment is then reflected medially and the subscapularis and the accompanying lesser tuberosity are separated from the underlying capsule and retracted medially. (**A**: Adapted from Gerber C, Pennington SD, Yian EH, et al. Lesser tuberosity osteotomy for total shoulder arthroplasty: surgical technique. J Bone Joint Surg Am 2006; 88A[Suppl 1]:170–177.)

lesser tuberosity from the underlying anterior and inferior capsule.

Capsular Release and Osteophyte Excision

- Once released, the subscapularis and attached lesser tuberosity are retracted medially to expose the anterior capsule. A blunt elevator is passed between the remaining inferior 1 cm of subscapularis and the inferior capsule to create a space for a blunt Hohmann retractor. This is used to retract and protect the axillary nerve during inferior capsular release and excision.
- The anterior capsule is released from the anatomic neck of the humerus, starting superiorly and extending inferiorly, well past the 6 o'clock position. This is facilitated by gradually flexing and externally rotating the adducted humerus.
- The humerus is then delivered into the wound with simultaneous adduction, extension, and external rotation (**TECH FIG 2A**). All humeral osteophytes are removed using a combination of rongeurs and osteotomes (**TECH FIG 2B**). This allows identification of the anatomic neck and the peripheral extent of the native articular surface.

Humeral Preparation

- Accurate placement of the central guide pin is the most important portion of the resurfacing procedure. This guide pin fixes the center and inclination of the articular surface in all planes. Once the guide pin is anatomically positioned, the remainder of the procedure is only a matter of choosing the appropriately sized head and placing it at he appropriate depth.

- The pin should penetrate the head at its geometric center and should be advanced slightly through the lateral cortex at an angle that is perpendicular to the plane defined by the periphery of the native articular margin (ie, the anatomic neck).

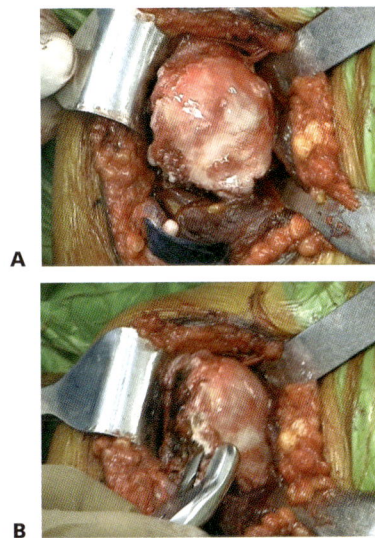

TECH FIG 2 • **A.** The humerus is delivered into the wound with simultaneous adduction, extension, and external rotation in this right shoulder. Retractors include a Brown deltoid retractor superiorly, a large Darrach retractor medially, and a blunt Hohmann retractor anteroinferiorly on the calcar. **B.** All humeral osteophytes are removed at this stage to identify the anatomic neck.

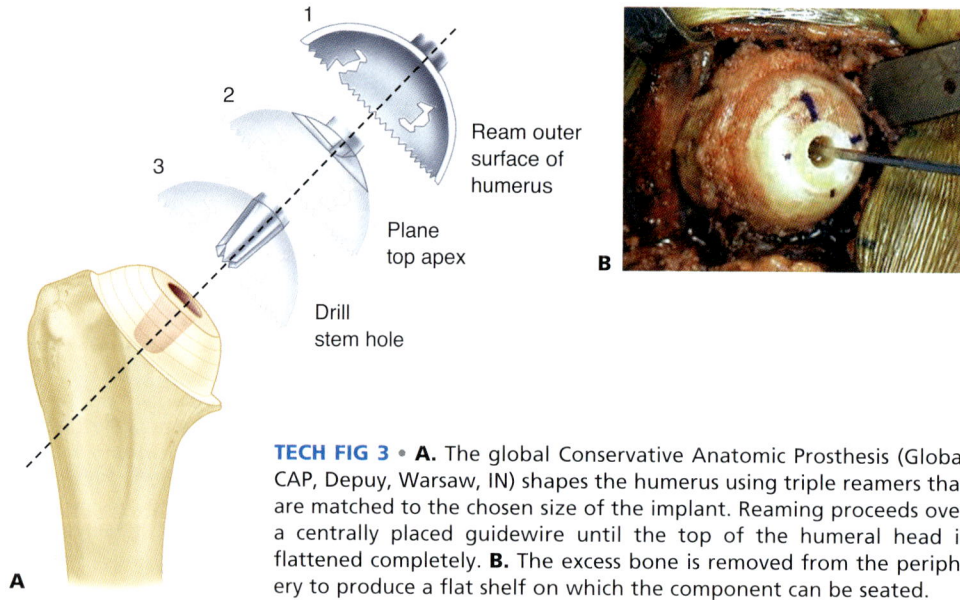

TECH FIG 3 • **A.** The global Conservative Anatomic Prosthesis (Global CAP, Depuy, Warsaw, IN) shapes the humerus using triple reamers that are matched to the chosen size of the implant. Reaming proceeds over a centrally placed guidewire until the top of the humeral head is flattened completely. **B.** The excess bone is removed from the periphery to produce a flat shelf on which the component can be seated.

- In some systems, there are guides that can assist in accurate pin placement. The guides usually are hemispherical and cannulated centrally so that the edge of the guide is positioned parallel to the articular margin in the visual center of the head.
- Once the surgeon is satisfied with pin placement, shaping of the humeral head to fit the deep surface of the resurfacing implant can commence.
- Reamers are selected based on the anticipated size of the prosthetic humeral head, which is, in turn, decided through a combination of preoperative templating and intraoperative measurements.
- Proper selection of humeral head radius and thickness (ie, neck length) is critical and there is a tendency to choose a head that is too large.
- The appropriate reamer is selected and the humerus is reamed until the reamer bottoms out on the humerus (**TECH FIG 3**). There is a tendency to underream. Reaming can continue to within 2 to 3 mm of the rotator cuff reflection superiorly.
- Trial implants are placed over the guide pin onto the reamed humeral surface. Circumferential contact is verified.
- The central punch is placed over the guide pin and driven into the humeral metaphysis to prepare it for the central peg of the prosthetic head.

Glenoid Inspection, Capsular Excision, and Release

- The guide pin is removed and the glenoid is exposed by placing a humeral head retractor within the joint and retracting the humeral head posteriorly. Care should be taken not to damage the reamed surface of the humerus.
- The axillary nerve is protected and the anteroinferior capsule is excised. If the labrum is present, it is left in place. The posterior capsule is released.

- Substantial glenoid reaming should not be required, as these patients are treated with humeral head resection and a stemmed implant in my practice.

Humeral Component Placement and Lesser Tuberosity Repair

- The humerus is redelivered into the wound and the appropriate humeral resurfacing implant is placed and impacted into position (**TECH FIG 4**). Care should be taken to ensure that the implant is completely seated. This requires removal of excess bone from around the periphery of the projected seating point of the implant.
- Two small bone anchors are placed in the humerus medial to the osteotomy but lateral to the humeral prosthetic edge. The sutures on the anchors are passed in a mattress configuration through the subscapularis tendon from deep to superficial at the bone–tendon junction. The sutures are clamped but not tied yet.
- With the humerus reduced and the arm in neutral rotation, the deep limbs of the three sutures previously passed around the lesser tuberosity are passed through the cancellous bone of the osteotomy bed as far laterally

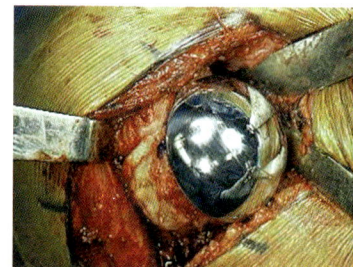

TECH FIG 4 • The final implant is impacted onto the prepared humeral surface and complete seating is verified by visualizing the periphery of the implant sitting flush against the peripheral shelf created on the humerus by the reaming process.

as possible, deep to the bicipital groove and out the lateral cortex of the humerus using a large, cutting free needle. A new needle is used for each pass and the sutures are clamped but not tied.

- The clamps on these three sutures are pulled laterally to hold the lesser tuberosity in a reduced position. The rotator interval is then closed laterally with a 1-mm non-absorbable suture.
- After the rotator interval suture is tied, the three interfragmentary sutures are tied, followed by the sutures from the anchors. This provides a secure lesser tuberosity and subscapularis repair.

- Passive motion achievable without undue tension on the subscapularis repair is noted for guidance of postoperative rehabilitation.

Wound Closure

- A drain is placed deep to the deltoid and is brought out through a separate stab wound, distal to the axillary nerve.
- The wound is closed in layers with interrupted absorbable sutures in the subcutaneous tissues and a running subcuticular monofilament suture.

HEMIARTHROPLASTY

- Hemiarthroplasty with head resection is performed when concentric glenoid reaming is required.
- The techniques of superficial and deep dissection, lesser tuberosity osteotomy, capsular release, and osteophyte excision are the same as described previously.

Humeral Head Resection

- The humeral head is removed with a saw at or near the anatomic neck (**TECH FIG 5A**). This can be accomplished freehand or with intramedullary or extramedullary guides.
- Retroversion of the cut in my practice is prescribed by the plane of the periphery of the native articular surface (ie, native retroversion). A small amount of bone (2 to 3 mm) can be left medial to the supraspinatus insertion (**TECH FIG 5B**).

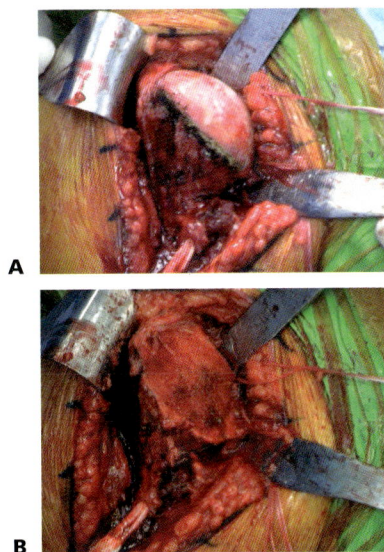

TECH FIG 5 • **A.** After removal of all osteophytes, the location of the anatomic neck is marked with an electrocautery. This can be done freehand or using an external guide. **B.** The humerus is cut in native retroversion, leaving 2 to 3 mm of bone medial to the supraspinatus insertion.

- The neck–shaft angle of the humeral cut is determined by the type of implant used.
- With fixed neck–shaft angle devices, the cut should precisely fit the neck–shaft angle of the selected device.
- With variable neck–shaft angle implants there is more flexibility in osteotomy angle, especially if the variability of the implant neck–shaft angle is infinite within a range.
- Preoperative templating should identify the patient with an extreme varus (less than 125) or valgus (greater than 145 degrees) neck–shaft angle.
- In cases of extreme varus, use of a fixed-angle cementless stem will require a humeral cut that is more valgus than the native neck–shaft angle.
  - The cut exits superiorly 2 to 3 mm medial to the cuff reflection and inferiorly through the native head. This will leave a small portion of the native head in place, even after the inferior osteophyte is removed.
- In cases of extreme valgus, use of a fixed-angle cementless stem will require a humeral cut that is more varus than the native neck–shaft angle.
  - The cut exits inferiorly at the native articular margin and superiorly through the native head. This will leave a small portion of the native head medial to the cuff reflection.
- Alternatively, the cut can be made along the native neck–shaft angle and a variable neck–shaft angle device can be used to fit the native neck–shaft angle.
- The size of the humeral head is estimated by placing trial humeral heads on the cut surface of the osteotomy.

Glenoid Exposure, Capsular Excision, and Surface Preparation

- With the humeral head resected, a Fukuda ring retractor is placed within the joint and the humerus is retracted posteriorly.
- A reverse, double-pronged Bankart retractor is placed on the scapular neck anteriorly, between the anterior capsule and the subscapularis.
- A blunt Hohmann retractor is placed along the anteroinferior portion of the scapular neck to retract and protect the axillary nerve, and the anterior and inferior capsule is excised.

TECHNIQUES

- The posterior capsule is released unless preoperative posterior humeral subluxation of greater than 25% was present, in which case the posterior capsule is preserved.
- The labrum is excised circumferentially to expose the entire periphery of the glenoid. If greater than 25% posterior humeral subluxation was present preoperatively, care is taken to preserve the posterior capsular attachment to the glenoid.
- The glenoid is sized with a sizing disk. The previously estimated humeral head size may give some idea of the glenoid size.
- The center of the glenoid is marked and a centering drill hole for the glenoid reamer is drilled.
- The orientation of this drill hole should be perpendicular to the estimated reamed surface. This can be estimated using preoperative CT measurements of the amount of posterior glenoid bone loss.
- The glenoid is reamed until a concentric surface is obtained.

Humeral Preparation and Component Placement

- The humerus is redelivered into the wound and the humeral canal is reamed with sequentially larger reamers until light purchase is obtained within the intramedullary canal.
- A box osteotome that corresponds to the final reamer size is passed into the humerus to cut the footprint of the humeral implant.
- A broach that corresponds to the size of the box osteotome and final canal reamer is placed to the appropriate depth.
- The system I use allows either a fixed 135-degree neck–shaft angle or an infinitely variable neck–shaft angle within 120 to 150 degrees (Global AP, Depuy, Warsaw, IN).
- Therefore, a collar is screwed into the broach that creates a 135-degree neck–shaft angle. A calcar reamer is placed over the collar and, if the reamer is nearly parallel to the osteotomy surface, it is used to plane the surface to 135 degrees so that an implant with a fixed neck–shaft angle of 135 degrees can be used.
- A trial humeral head is placed over the collar, it is rotated into the offset position that provides the most symmetrical coverage of the humeral metaphysis, and the collar is locked to the broach.
- If the planes of the calcar reamer and the osteotomy surface are not nearly parallel, a variable neck–shaft angle implant will be used. The 135-degree collar is removed and a trial ball taper fitted with a humeral head trial is inserted into the broach. The trial head and ball taper are placed into the position that provides symmetrical coverage of the humeral metaphysis, and the taper is locked to the broach.
- With the trial humeral head locked into position, the remaining humeral osteophytes are removed so that the humeral bone is flush with the humerus around the entire periphery.
- Assuming the humerus has been reduced and adequate soft tissue tension and stability have been verified, the

trial broach is removed and the real implant is assembled with either a fixed 135-degree taper or a variable ball taper in the same position as the trial.
- A nonabsorbable suture is passed around the neck of the prosthesis and the prosthesis is impacted into the humerus with the two ends of the suture protruding anteriorly.
- The humerus is then reduced.

Lesser Tuberosity Repair

- The technique for lesser tuberosity repair is the same as described for humeral resurfacing, except that the suture that was placed around the prosthetic neck before impaction into the humerus takes the place of the suture anchors that were placed in the anterior humerus between the osteotomy bed and the lateral extent of the resurfacing prosthesis (**TECH FIG 6A**).
- Therefore, the osteotomy is stabilized with three suture groups:
    - The three interfragmentary sutures from the lesser tuberosity to the osteotomy bed
    - The rotator interval closure suture at the superior aspect of the osteotomy
    - The suture from the prosthetic through the bone–tendon junction (**TECH FIG 6B**)
- The technique for wound closure is identical to that described for humeral resurfacing.

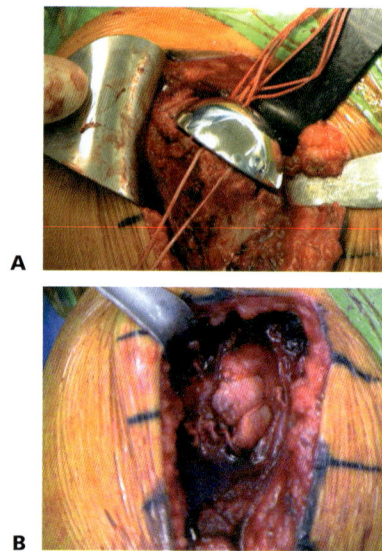

TECH FIG 6 • A. The final implant is seated and any remaining bone prominences are removed. The three interfragmentary sutures around the lesser tuberosity are visible posterior to the prosthesis. The strands from the suture that was placed around the neck of the prosthesis can be seen exiting the space between the prosthetic humeral head and the anterior humeral metaphysis. **B.** The lesser tuberosity has been repaired with a superior side-to-side suture in the lateral rotator interval, the three interfragmentary sutures tied over the bicipital groove, and the medial suture passed from the prosthetic neck through the bone–tendon junction.

HEMIARTHROPLASTY WITH BIOLOGIC RESURFACING (LATERAL MENISCAL ALLOGRAFT)

- All techniques are the same as described earlier for humeral resurfacing and hemiarthroplasty, except that placement of the allograft requires maximum glenoid exposure.
- The allograft can be grossly sized using glenoid sizing disks. It is prepared by suturing the anterior and posterior horns together.
- The glenoid surface should be concentric in order for biologic resurfacing with meniscal allograft to be successful. Therefore, reaming to correct glenoid bone deficiency (eg, posterior wear) should be performed before placing the allograft.
- If the labrum can be preserved, it can be used to anchor the allograft to the glenoid.
- Often, the labrum is absent or too degenerative to dependably hold sutures. Under these circumstances,

absorbable suture anchors are used to attach the allograft around the periphery of the glenoid. Four to six anchoring points should be used, depending on the size of the glenoid (**TECH FIG 7A**).

- The sutures are passed into the periphery of the ring-shaped allograft above the wound at appropriate positions (**TECH FIG 7B**). The allograft is then shuttled down the sutures onto the glenoid surface and the sutures are tied (**TECH FIG 7C**).[30]
- If there is no bleeding bone exposed from reaming, drilling a few holes through the subchondral surface into the glenoid cavity may assist in decompressing the glenoid vault and providing progenitor cells that can assist in healing.

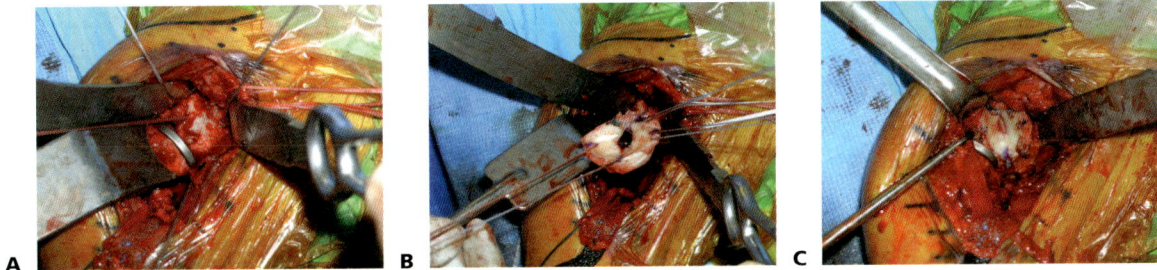

TECH FIG 7 • **A.** The glenoid in this right shoulder is exposed with a Fukuda retractor posteriorly, a large Darrach retractor anteriorly on the neck of the scapula, and a single-prong Bankart retractor posterosuperiorly. Anchors have been placed in the four quadrants of this small glenoid. **B.** The meniscal allograft has been sutured into a ring and sutures from the previously placed anchors are passed through the meniscal allograft above the joint. **C.** The allograft is then transported down the sutures onto the glenoid surface and the sutures are tied. (From Williams G. Hemiarthroplasty and biological resurfacing of the glenoid. In: Zuckerman JD, ed. Advanced Reconstruction: Shoulder. Rosemont, IL: AAOS, 2007:545–556.)

TOTAL SHOULDER ARTHROPLASTY

- All techniques are the same as described earlier for humeral resurfacing and hemiarthroplasty except for placement of the glenoid component.
- Concentric glenoid reaming is an important step in glenoid resurfacing that improves initial seating and stability. This is accomplished by drilling a pilot hole in the center of the glenoid (**TECH FIG 8A**). Special glenoid reamers are used to ream concentrically around the center pilot hole (**TECH FIG 8B**).
- After the surface of the glenoid has been reamed concentrically, the anchoring holes for the glenoid component are created. Both pegged and keeled components are available. The technique described is for an off-axis pegged system (anchor peg glenoid, Depuy, Warsaw, IN).
- The center hole for the larger fluted central peg is drilled, followed by the holes for the three peripheral

pegs (**TECH FIG 8C**). Penetration of any of the peripheral holes is uncommon but should be noted so that a bone plug from the humeral head can be placed before filling the hole with cement.

- A trial glenoid component is placed and complete seating and stability are verified.
- The holes are irrigated and dried.
- Bone cement is placed into the three peripheral holes using a syringe to pressurize the cement column. Any holes that required bone grafting from drill perforation should not receive pressurized cement.
- The glenoid component is impacted into position and can be held with digital pressure until the cement hardens (**TECH FIG 8D**).

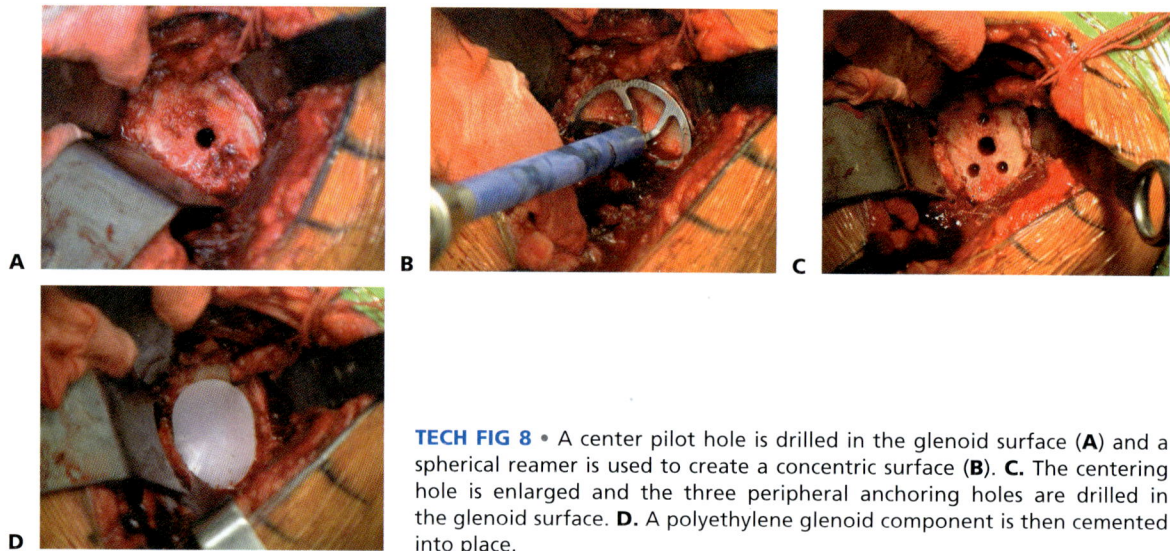

TECH FIG 8 • A center pilot hole is drilled in the glenoid surface (**A**) and a spherical reamer is used to create a concentric surface (**B**). **C.** The centering hole is enlarged and the three peripheral anchoring holes are drilled in the glenoid surface. **D.** A polyethylene glenoid component is then cemented into place.

PEARLS AND PITFALLS

Imaging	▪ Radiographic evaluation must include a quantification of glenoid version, asymmetrical wear, and available bone stock. This requires either a perfect axillary lateral or cross-sectional study, preferably a CT scan.
Patient selection	▪ Glenoid components should be used cautiously if at all in young (ie, under 50) or active patients. The use of biologic resurfacing is controversial and may not offer any advantage over hemiarthroplasty alone.
Patient positioning	▪ Safe access to the humerus during humeral preparation and component placement requires maximum humeral adduction. Therefore, patient positioning must prevent interference from the edge of the operating table.
Glenoid exposure	▪ Adequate glenoid exposure requires accurate humeral resection, humeral osteophyte excision, and adequate capsular excision and releases.
Humeral preparation	▪ Do not over-externally rotate or overream. This may lead to periprosthetic fracture.
Nerve management	▪ Know the position of the axillary nerve and protect it throughout the procedure. Avoid excessive traction on the conjoined tendon, especially if the musculocutaneous nerve is close to the tip of the coracoid. Take the arm out of extreme positions whenever possible.

POSTOPERATIVE CARE

▪ Early rehabilitation (6 weeks)
- ▪ The goals of rehabilitation during the first 6 weeks after surgery are to maximize passive range of motion and to allow healing of the subscapularis or lesser tuberosity.
- ▪ The safe range of glenohumeral motion that prevents excessive tension on the subscapularis is identified intraoperatively.
- ▪ This range of passive motion is performed starting the first postoperative day.
- ▪ In general, uncomplicated shoulder arthroplasty will allow passive elevation to 140 degrees and passive external rotation to 40 degrees. If there is concern for the subscapularis repair, elevation and external rotation can be dropped to 130 and 30 degrees, respectively. If the tissue is poor quality, one may even drop the limits to 90 degrees of elevation and 0 degrees of external rotation.
- ▪ These exercises are performed for 6 weeks postoperatively, in combination with pendulum exercises.
- ▪ The sling may be discontinued at home after the first week or 10 days, when the hand can be used as a helping hand for daily activities.
- ▪ Active elevation above 90 degrees is delayed until 6 weeks postoperatively.

▪ Midterm rehabilitation (6 to 12 weeks)
- ▪ During midterm rehabilitation, active range of motion is encouraged, passive stretching is instituted, and strengthening exercises for the rotator cuff, deltoid, and scapular stabilizers are pursued.
- ▪ Active assisted range of motion within the limits of pain is accomplished with an overhead pulley and 3-foot stick.
- ▪ This is progressed to active range of motion as tolerated.
- ▪ End-range stretching in all planes is begun and progressed.
- ▪ Strengthening exercises with the Theraband commence when active range of motion is maximized.

▪ Late rehabilitation (12 to 24 weeks)
- ▪ Strengthening exercises for the rotator cuff, deltoid, and scapular stabilizers continue throughout the late stage of rehabilitation.
- ▪ Patients will be functional with most daily activities, except at the extremes of motion.
- ▪ Total arm strengthening and gradual return to activities are encouraged.

- Although improvement in function will continue for about 1 year, the vast majority of improvement from formal rehabilitation will be seen in the first 24 weeks (6 months).

OUTCOMES

- Resurfacing
  - Reports of resurfacing arthroplasty are relatively sparse. Most data come out of a single institution.
  - In general, the results parallel the results of hemiarthroplasty. In one series of 103 patients with 5 to 10 years of follow-up, constant scores for patients with osteoarthritis undergoing total shoulder arthroplasty and hemiarthroplasty were 93.7% and 73.5% respectively. Lucency around the humeral component was 30.7%, and 1.9% required revision.[17]
  - In another series of patients with osteoarthritis undergoing resurfacing, hemiarthroplasty was found to be similar to total shoulder replacement.[16]
- Hemiarthroplasty
  - Neer's original article on replacement for osteoarthritis in 1974 included primarily hemiarthroplasties. Over 90% of patients had good or excellent results.[20]
  - The addition of concentric glenoid reaming to encourage the formation of a biologic membrane to resurface the glenoid has been reported by Matsen et al.[8,18] The authors note that similar pain relief and function are possible with this procedure but that patients may take longer than total shoulder replacement patients to reach maximum improvement. In addition, in one of their series, 3 of 37 patients were no better or worse after the surgery.[18]
  - Additional studies have stressed the importance of concentricity of the glenoid in attaining a successful result as well as the relative difficulty in converting a painful hemiarthroplasty to total shoulder replacement.[5]
  - In addition, progressive, painful glenoid erosion can be associated with hemiarthroplasty.
  - Survivorship of hemiarthroplasty in one series decreased substantially with increasing follow-up, with 92%, 83%, and 73% survival at 5, 10, and 15 years, respectively.[26]
- Hemiarthroplasty with biologic resurfacing
  - Although descriptions of this procedure exist before 1993, Burkhead popularized the concept of combining hemiarthroplasty with biologic glenoid resurfacing.[3]
  - A more recent report from Krishnan et al[15] with long-term follow-up revealed only 5 of 39 patients with unsatisfactory results. Moreover, the patient population was relatively young and active.
  - Elhassan et al[10] reported poor results in 13 patients undergoing hemiarthroplasty with biologic glenoid resurfacing. Ten of 13 patients required revision to total shoulder arthroplasty at a mean of 14 months after hemiarthroplasty.
  - Two additional studies,[21,30] one with a minimum 2-year follow-up,[30] confirm good early pain relief and return of function in young active patients undergoing hemiarthroplasty and glenoid resurfacing with lateral meniscal allograft. Both emphasize the importance of articular concentricity and offer data that may be interpreted to question the durability of the allograft.
- Total shoulder arthroplasty
  - Many studies document consistent improvement in pain and function with total shoulder arthroplasty.

- Several studies document better pain relief and, in some cases, better function with total shoulder arthroplasty in comparison to hemiarthroplasty. Survivorship of total shoulder arthroplasty in patients with an intact or reparable cuff is 84% to 88% at 15 years.[9,26]

COMPLICATIONS

- The reported complication rate after shoulder arthroplasty is 12% to 14.7%.[1,6,31] One series reports a decrease in the complication rate with time, which may be explained by glenoid and humeral component loosening in only one shoulder.[6]
- Complications include:
  - Instability
  - Rotator cuff tear
  - Ectopic ossification
  - Glenoid component loosening
  - Intraoperative fracture
  - Nerve injury
  - Infection
  - Humeral component loosening

REFERENCES

1. Bohsali KI, Wirth MA, Rockwood CA Jr. Complications of total shoulder arthroplasty. J Bone Joint Surg Am 2006;88A:2279–2292.
2. Boileau P, Walch G. The three-dimensional geometry of the proximal humerus: implications for surgical technique and prosthetic design. J Bone Joint Surg Br 1997;79:857–865.
3. Burkhead WZ Jr. Hemiarthroplasty with biologic resurfacing of the glenoid for glenohumeral arthritis. J Shoulder Elbow Surg 1993;2:29.
4. Caplan JL, Whitfield B, Neviaser RJ. Subscapularis function after primary tendon to tendon repair in patients after replacement arthroplasty of the shoulder. J Shoulder Elbow Surg 2009;18:193–198.
5. Carroll RM, Izquierdo R, Vazquez M, Blaine TA, et al. Conversion of painful hemiarthroplasty to total shoulder arthroplasty: long-term results. J Shoulder Elbow Surg 2004;13:599–603.
6. Chin PY, Sperling JW, Cofield RH, et al. Complications of total shoulder arthroplasty: are they fewer or different? J Shoulder Elbow Surg 2006;15:19–22.
7. Clavert P, Millett PJ, Warner JJ. Glenoid resurfacing: what are the limits to asymmetric reaming for posterior erosion? J Shoulder Elbow Surg 2007;16:843–848.
8. Clinton J, Franta AK, Lenters TR, et al. Nonprosthetic glenoid arthroplasty with humeral hemiarthroplasty and total shoulder arthroplasty yield similar self-assessed outcomes in the management of comparable patients with glenohumeral arthritis. J Shoulder Elbow Surg 2007;16:534–538.
9. Deshmukh AV, Koris M, Zurakowski D, et al. Total shoulder arthroplasty: long-term survivorship, functional outcome, and quality of life. J Shoulder Elbow Surg 2005;14:471–479.
10. Elhassan B, Ozbaydar M, Diller D, et al. Soft-tissue resurfacing of the glenoid in the treatment of glenohumeral arthritis in active patients less than fifty years old. J Bone Joint Surg Am 2009;91A:419–424.
11. Gerber C, Pennington SD, Yian EH, et al. Lesser tuberosity osteotomy for total shoulder arthroplasty: surgical technique. J Bone Joint Surg Am 2006;88A(Suppl 1 Pt 2):170–177.
12. Gerber C, Yian EH, Pfirrmann CA, et al. Subscapularis muscle function and structure after total shoulder replacement with lesser tuberosity osteotomy and repair. J Bone Joint Surg Am 2005;87A:1739–1745.
13. Gill DR, Cofield RH, Rowland C. The anteromedial approach for shoulder arthroplasty: the importance of the anterior deltoid. J Shoulder Elbow Surg 2004;13:532–537.
14. Iannotti JP, Gabriel JP, Schneck SL, et al. The normal glenohumeral relationships: an anatomical study of one hundred and forty shoulders. J Bone Joint Surg Am 1992;74A:491–500.
15. Krishnan SG, Nowinski RJ, Harrison D, et al. Humeral hemiarthroplasty with biologic resurfacing of the glenoid for glenohumeral arthritis: two to fifteen-year outcomes. J Bone Joint Surg Am 2007;89A:727–734.

16. Levy O, Copeland SA. Cementless surface replacement arthroplasty (Copeland CSRA) for osteoarthritis of the shoulder. J Shoulder Elbow Surg 2004;13:266–271.

17. Levy O, Copeland SA. Cementless surface replacement arthroplasty of the shoulder: 5- to 10-year results with the Copeland mark-2 prosthesis. J Bone Joint Surg Br 2001;83B:213–221.

18. Lynch JR, Franta AK, Montgomery WH Jr, et al. Self-assessed outcome at two to four years after shoulder hemiarthroplasty with concentric glenoid reaming. J Bone Joint Surg Am 2007;89A: 1284–1292.

19. MacKenzie D. The antero-superior exposure for total shoulder replacement. Orthop Traumatol 1993;2:71–77.

20. Neer CS. Replacement arthroplasty for glenohumeral osteoarthritis. J Bone Joint Surg Am 1974;56A:1–13.

21. Nicholson GP, Goldstein JL, Romeo AA, et al. Lateral meniscus allograft biologic glenoid arthroplasty in total shoulder arthroplasty for young shoulders with degenerative joint disease. J Shoulder Elbow Surg 2007;16(5 Suppl):S261–S266.

22. Pearl ML, Volk AG. Coronal plane geometry of the proximal humerus relevant to prosthetic arthroplasty. J Shoulder Elbow Surg 1996;5:320–326.

23. Qureshi S, Hsiao A, Klug RA, et al. Subscapularis function after total shoulder replacement: results with lesser tuberosity osteotomy. J Shoulder Elbow Surg 2008;17:68–72.

24. Redfern TR, Wallace WA, Beddow FH. Clavicular osteotomy in shoulder arthroplasty. Int Orthop 1989;13:61–63.

25. Rodnan G, Schumacher H, Zvaifler N. Rheumatoid arthritis. In Rodnan GP, Schumacher H, Zvaifler N, eds. Primer on the Rheumatic Diseases. Atlanta: Arthritis Foundation, 1983: 38–48.

26. Sperling JW, Cofield RH, Rowland CM. Neer hemiarthroplasty and Neer total shoulder arthroplasty in patients fifty years old or less: long-term results. J Bone Joint Surg Am 1998;80: 464–473.

27. Thomas BJ, Amstutz HC, Cracchiolo A. Shoulder arthroplasty for rheumatoid arthritis. Clin Orthop Relat Res 1991;265: 125–128.

28. Torchia ME, Cofield RH, Settergren CR. Total shoulder arthroplasty with the Neer prosthesis: long-term results. J Shoulder Elbow Surg 1997;6:495–505.

29. Walch G, Badet R, Boulahia A, et al. Morphologic study of the glenoid in primary glenohumeral osteoarthritis. J Arthroplasty 1999;14(6):756–760.

30. Wirth MA. Humeral head arthroplasty and meniscal allograft resurfacing of the glenoid. J Bone Joint Surg Am 2009;91A: 1109–1119.

31. Wirth MA, Rockwood CA Jr. Complications of shoulder arthroplasty. Clin Orthop Relat Res 1994;307:47–69.

Hemiarthroplasty and Total Shoulder Arthroplasty for Glenohumeral Arthritis With an Irreparable Rotator Cuff

Frederick A. Matsen III, Steven B. Lippitt, and Ryan T. Bicknell

DEFINITION

- *Glenohumeral arthritis* is defined as loss of the normal articular cartilage covering of the humeral head and glenoid fossa.
- An irreparable rotator cuff defect is one in which a durable attachment of detached cuff tendons to the tuberosity cannot be re-established.
- The association of glenohumeral arthritis and irreparable rotator cuff defects occurs in several distinct clinical situations, each of which has unique features and specific treatment options.
- The key points in managing these conditions are to define the following:
  - The pathology
  - The deficits in comfort and function experienced by the patient
  - The options for reconstruction
  - The benefits and risks of each of the treatment options

ANATOMY

- The glenohumeral articulation normally is covered with hyaline articular cartilage. The glenoid fossa is a spherical concavity that is deepened because the cartilage is thicker at the periphery and the glenoid rim is surrounded by a fibrocartilaginous labrum. The humeral head is a convexity that fits into this concavity.
- The rotator cuff is a synthesis of the tendons of the subscapularis, supraspinatus, infraspinatus, and teres minor with the subjacent glenohumeral capsule.
- The rotator cuff tendons insert into the humerus just lateral to the articular cartilage and at the base of the tuberosities.
  - The spherical proximal humeral convexity is formed by the smooth blending of the cuff tendons with the tuberosities.
  - The radius of the proximal humeral convexity is the radius of the humeral head plus the thickness of the rotator cuff tendons.
- The coracoacromial arch is a spherical concavity consisting of the undersurface of the acromion and the coracoacromial ligament. The proximal humeral convexity fits into this concavity.
- The glenohumeral joint is normally stabilized by the concavity compression mechanism:
  - The rotator cuff muscles compress the humeral head into the glenoid fossa.
  - The deltoid compresses the proximal humeral convexity into the coracoacromial arch.

PATHOGENESIS

- Loss of glenohumeral articular cartilage can be caused by osteoarthritis, rheumatoid arthritis, neurotrophic arthritis, septic arthritis, traumatic arthritis, avascular necrosis, and iatrogenic arthritis.
- It also can arise from abrasion of the unprotected humeral head on the undersurface of the coracoacromial arch in chronic rotator cuff deficiency, a situation that often is referred to as *rotator cuff tear arthropathy*.
- Defects in the rotator cuff tendons arise when loads are applied to the tendon insertion that are greater than the strength of the tendon attachment to the tuberosity.
  - These defects typically begin at the anterior undersurface of the supraspinatus tendon.
  - Age, systemic disease, corticosteroid injections, and smoking are among the factors that weaken the insertional strength of the rotator cuff tendons, making them more susceptible to tearing and wear.
- When the superior rotator cuff is deficient, the radius of the proximal humeral convexity is decreased by the thickness of the cuff tendon.
- The loss of the spacer effect of the cuff tendon allows the humeral head to translate superiorly under the active pull of the deltoid until the uncovered head contacts the coracoacromial arch.
- The intact coracoacromial arch can provide secondary superior stability to the uncovered humeral head.
  - The upward translation of the humeral head necessary to contact the arch slackens the deltoid, however, reducing its effectiveness in elevation of the arm.
- The coracoacromial arch can be compromised by progressive abrasion with the uncovered humeral head. It also can be compromised by acromioplasty and section of the coracoacromial ligament.
- Compromise of the coracoacromial arch coupled with a substantial rotator cuff defect permits anterosuperior escape of the humeral head on deltoid contraction.
  - This anterosuperior escape eliminates the fulcrum needed for the deltoid to elevate the arm.
- The inability of a functioning deltoid to elevate the arm because of slackening and lack of a fulcrum is known as *pseudoparalysis*.

NATURAL HISTORY

- Rotator cuff deficiency and arthritis can occur individually or together.
  - In most cases of osteoarthritis, the rotator cuff is functionally intact.
  - In most cases of rheumatoid arthritis, the rotator cuff may be thinned but usually is functionally intact.
- In rotator cuff tear arthropathy, the integrity of the cuff, the articular cartilage, and the coracoacromial arch all characteristically degenerate in a progressive manner.

- Some surgeons attempt to improve the comfort and functions of individuals with rotator cuff problems by performing an acromioplasty and coracoacromial ligament section.
  - Unless cuff function is durably restored, this sacrifice of the coracoacromial arch predisposes the shoulder to anterosuperior escape.
- The rotator cuff mechanism can be damaged in the process of humeral head resection during shoulder arthroplasty.
- Individuals who have had a shoulder arthroplasty may tear their rotator cuff in a fall or while lifting.
- When a prosthesis is used to reconstruct a complex proximal humeral fracture, the tuberosities may fail to unite, resulting in the functional equivalent of rotator cuff deficiency.

PATIENT HISTORY AND PHYSICAL FINDINGS

- Rotator cuff tendons fail by some combination of applied load and degeneration ("tear" and "wear").
  - There need be no history of a traumatic episode, especially in older individuals who give a history of progressive loss of comfort, strength, and ability to perform functions of their daily living. These are the persons whose condition may progress to cuff tear arthropathy.
  - By contrast, individuals with acute traumatic rotator cuff tears from the application of substantial load do not typically progress to cuff tear arthropathy.
- In patients with massive atraumatic cuff deficiency, it is important to seek historical evidence of factors that may weaken the cuff, such as systemic disease, cortisone injections, antimetabolic medications, and smoking.
  - Osteoarthritis often presents without a history of injury. Instead, it presents as progressive stiffness, pain, and loss of function.

- Rheumatoid arthritis of the shoulder presents in the context of this systemic condition.
- Important elements of the history are the patient's self-assessment of shoulder comfort and function (such as the simple shoulder test) and an assessment of the patient's goals for treatment.
- The integrity of the principal rotator cuff tendons is determined by the isometric strength of each of the three primary muscles in defined positions.
  - Supraspinatus integrity: weakness (ie, strength grade 3 or less) indicates a full-thickness supraspinatus tear.
  - Infraspinatus integrity: weakness (ie, strength grade 3 or less) indicates a large, full-thickness rotator cuff tear, extending into the infraspinatus.
  - Subscapularis integrity: weakness (ie, strength grade 3 or less) indicates a full-thickness subscapularis tear.
- Defects in the rotator cuff often can be palpated just anterior to the acromion while the shoulder is passively rotated.
- Chronic cuff defects usually are accompanied by atrophy of the muscles attached to the deficient tendons.
- Cuff degeneration often is associated with subacromial crepitus on passive rotation of the humerus beneath the coracoacromial arch.
- Cuff tear arthropathy often is associated with a substantial subacromial effusion.
- Superior instability is demonstrated by having the patient relax the shoulder, hanging it at the side, and then actively contracting the deltoid while the examiner notes superior translation of the humeral head until it contacts the coracoacromial arch (**FIG 1A,B**).
- Anterosuperior escape is the exaggerated form of superior instability that results when the coracoacromial arch is compromised (**FIG 1C,D**).

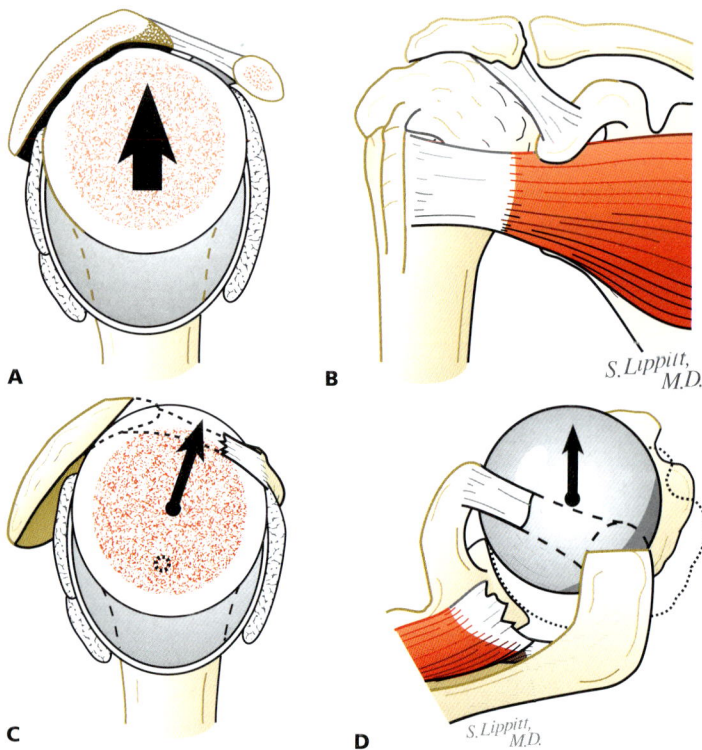

FIG 1 • **A,B.** Characteristic findings of cuff tear arthropathy, including superior displacement of the humeral head, "femoralization" of the proximal humerus, and "acetabularization" of the coracoacromial arch. In such a case, a conventional hemiarthroplasty, possibly using a special cuff tear arthropathy (CTA) head, may be considered. **C,D.** Anterosuperior escape of the humeral head resulting from surgical compromise of the coracoacromial arch. In such a case, a conventional arthroplasty will not provide stability, and a Delta (DePuy, Warsaw, IN) or reverse prosthesis may be considered. (Copyright Steven B. Lippitt, MD.)

IMAGING AND OTHER DIAGNOSTIC STUDIES

- An anteroposterior plain radiograph in the plane of the scapula may reveal:
  - Decreased acromio–humeral distance, signaling the absence of the normally interposed supraspinatus tendon
  - "Femoralization" of the proximal humerus (ie, rounding off of the tuberosities so that the proximal humerus is spherical) as well as other changes in humeral anatomy (**FIG 2A,B**)
  - "Acetabularization" of the acromion-coracoid-glenoid socket (ie, sculpting of a concavity matching the femoralized proximal humerus)
  - The amount of superior and medial erosion of the acromion and upper glenoid
- A true axillary view (**FIG 2C,D**) may reveal:
  - The degree of medial glenoid erosion, ie, the amount of glenoid bone stock available for reconstruction
  - The presence of anterior or posterior glenoid erosion and humeral subluxation, indicating a more complex pattern of instability
- An anteroposterior (AP) view of the proximal humerus with the arm in 30 degrees of external rotation with respect to the x-ray beam may reveal:
  - The approximate size of the humeral medullary cavity that may be used in prosthetic reconstruction
  - Any humeral deformities that may affect prosthetic reconstruction
- We do not routinely use either CT or MRI scans, but they may be useful in clarifying the pathology.
  - CT scans may help with:
    - Defining glenoid bone volume and deformities
    - Defining the glenohumeral relationships
  - MRI scans may help with:
    - Determining the condition of the different rotator cuff tendons
    - Determining the condition of the different rotator cuff muscles
    - The volume and location of fluid in the joint
    - Other pathology, such as tumor or avascular necrosis
- Factors suggesting that the cuff defect is likely to be irreparable include:
  - Insidious, atraumatic onset of cuff deficiency
  - Advanced age of the patient
  - History of repeated corticosteroid injections
  - Systemic illness
  - History of smoking
  - Previous unsuccessful attempts at rotator cuff repair
  - Muscle atrophy
  - Superior displacement or superior instability of the glenohumeral joint
  - Anterosuperior escape
  - Pseudoparalysis

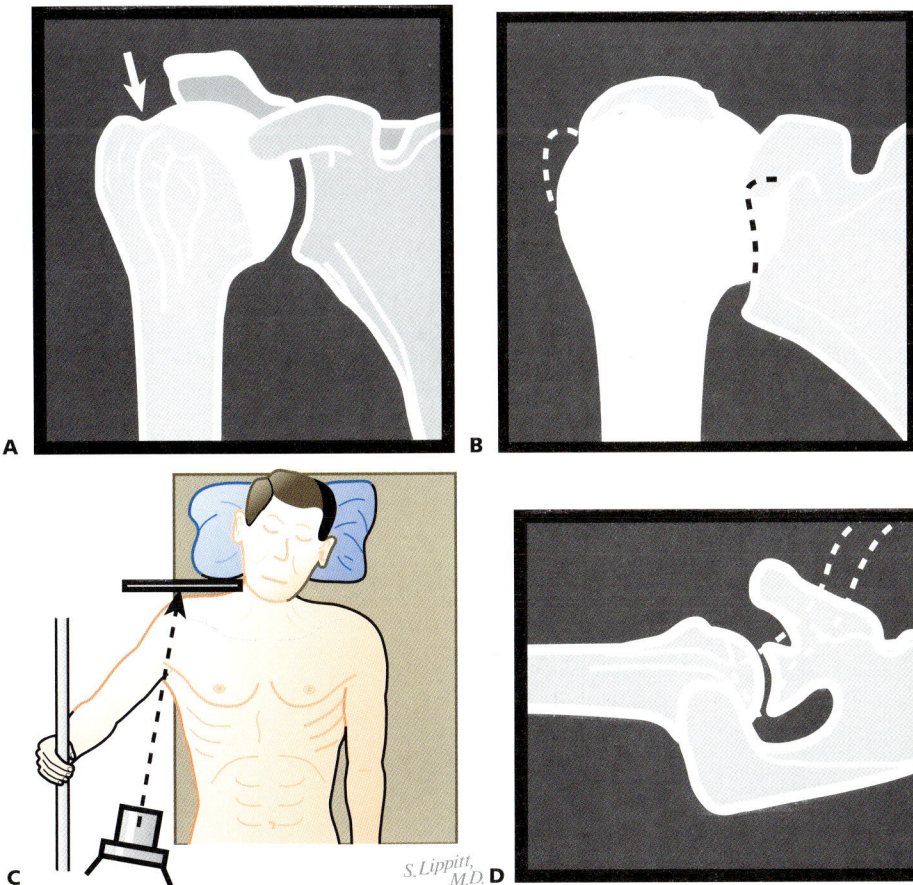

FIG 2 • **A.** Normal glenoid and normal head–glenoid relationship are seen on this AP radiograph in the plane of the scapula. **B.** Superior glenoid erosion and upward displacement of the head are seen on this AP radiograph in the plane of the scapula. This demonstrates "femoralization" of the proximal humerus and "acetabularization" of the coracoacromial arch. **C,D.** A proper axillary view will reveal anterior, posterior, or medial glenoid erosion. (Copyright Steven B. Lippitt, MD.)

DIFFERENTIAL DIAGNOSIS

- Milwaukee shoulder
- Neurotrophic (Charcot) arthropathy
- Septic arthritis
- Nonseptic inflammatory arthropathy

NONOPERATIVE MANAGEMENT

- An acute rotator cuff tear is a matter of relative urgency, but a chronic cuff defect coupled with glenohumeral arthritis provides the opportunity for nonoperative management, including:
    - Range-of-motion exercises in an attempt to resolve the stiffness that may accompany this condition (eg, the four-quadrant stretching program)
    - Gentle progressive strengthening exercises for the deltoid and the rotator cuff musculotendinous units that remain intact (eg, the two-hand progressive supine press)
- Mild nonnarcotic analgesics may be useful in symptom control.
- However, injections of corticosteroids into the shoulder may compromise the integrity of the remaining tendons and increase the risk of infection.

SURGICAL MANAGEMENT

Preoperative Planning

- Consideration of surgical management is based on the type of involvement (Table 1), the patient's overall health and well-being, and the risk–benefit ratio in trying to meet the patient's goals for treatment.
- With each of the procedures, the patient must be well-informed and give informed consent to the risk of infection, neurovascular injury, pain, stiffness, weakness, fracture, instability, loosening of components, anesthetic complications, and the possible need for revision surgery.

Conventional Hemiarthroplasty, Total Shoulder Arthroplasty, and Special Hemiarthroplasty

- Use AP radiograph in the plane of the scapula and axillary view to identify medial, superior, anterior, posterior, or inferior glenoid erosion.
- Use AP humeral radiograph to estimate the size and fit of the humeral component (**FIG 3**).
- Give prophylactic antibiotics.

Delta or Reverse Arthroplasty:

- Use AP radiograph in the plane of the scapula and transparent glenoid template to estimate the most inferior position of the glenoid that will result in the inferior screw being contained in the thick bone of the scapular axillary border.
- Use AP humeral radiograph to estimate the size and fit of the diaphyseal and metaphyseal humeral components.

Positioning

- All procedures can be performed in the beach chair position. This position is comfortable and safe for the patient, and allows good access for the anesthesiologist and the surgeon.
- The patient is positioned and secured with the glenohumeral joint at the edge of the operating table.
- The forequarter is doubly prepped, and the arm is draped so it can be moved freely.

Approach

- Although some surgeons advocate a deltoid-incising lateral approach, we prefer the deltopectoral approach, because it is effective, familiar, versatile, safe, and extensile.
- Each procedure strives to completely preserve and protect the deltoid and the axillary nerve.
- Each procedure includes a complete mobilization of the humeroscapular motion interface with resection of all scar,

Table 1	Types of Arthritis and Irreparable Rotator Cuff Defects and Their Characteristic Features						
Glenohumeral Joint Surface	**Rotator Cuff**	**Register (Glenohumeral Joint Alignment)**	**Active Elevation**	**Coracoacromial Arch**	**Anterior Superior Escape**	**Deltoid**	**Surgical Significance**
Arthritic	Irreparable supraspinatus	Glenohumeral joint aligned	>90 degrees, but weak	Intact	Absent	Intact	Consider conventional hemi- or total shoulder arthroplasty
Arthritic	Irreparable supraspinatus	Superior displacement with acromiohumeral stability	>90 degrees, but weak	Intact	Absent	Intact	Consider conventional or special (eg, CTA) hemi-arthroplasty
Arthritic	Irreparable supraspinatus and infra-spinatus	Superior displacement without acromiohumeral stability	<45 degrees	Compromised	Present	Intact	Consider Delta or reverse arthroplasty
Arthritic	Irreparable supraspinatus and infra-spinatus	Superior displacement without acromiohumeral stability	<45 degrees	Compromised	Present	Severe compromise	No good surgical options
Failed prosthetic	Irreparable supraspinatus and infra-spinatus	Superior displacement without acromiohumeral stability	<45 degrees	Compromised	Present	Intact	Consider Delta or reverse arthroplasty

CTA, cuff tear arthropathy.

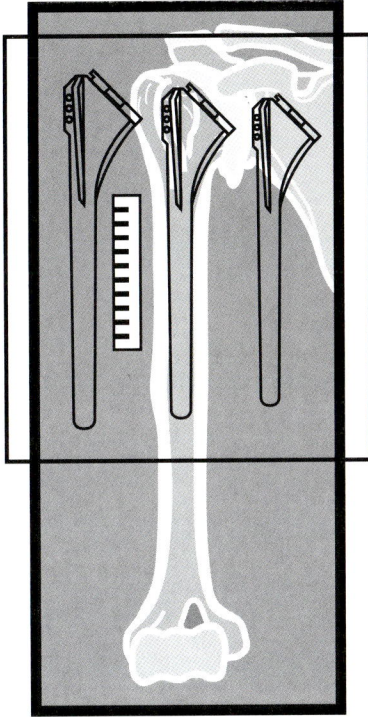

FIG 3 • Templating view of the humerus taken with the arm in 30 degrees of external rotation with respect to the x-ray beam and with a magnification marker. (Copyright Steven B. Lippitt, MD.)

suture, and suture anchors from previous surgical procedures, and hypertrophic bursa.

- This débridement permits complete assessment of the surgical anatomy.
- The integrity of the acromion and coracoacromial ligament is assessed and preserved.
- The subscapularis and subjacent capsule are incised from their attachment to the humerus at the lesser tuberosity.
- A 360-degree subscapularis release is carried out while the axillary nerve is protected.
- One of two types of reconstruction is selected:
  - Anatomic arthroplasty, with one of the following:
    - Hemiarthoplasty using a conventional prosthesis
    - Total glenohumeral arthroplasty
    - Hemiarthroplasty with a special head (eg, Delta CTA [cuff tear arthropathy; DePuy, Inc., Warsaw, IN])
  - Delta or reverse arthroplasty
- At the conclusion of the arthroplasty, the subscapularis is repaired to the bone of the cut humeral surface adjacent to the lesser tuberosity using six sutures of no. 2 nonabsorbable suture passed through drill holes.
- A suction drain is placed just anterior to the subscapularis and led out through a long subcutaneous track to exit the skin of the lateral arm.
- Dry sterile dressings are applied.
- Continuous passive motion is used for 36 hours for all reconstructions except for the Delta or reverse arthroplasty.
- After the Delta arthroplasty, the arm is immobilized for 36 hours.

CONVENTIONAL HEMIARTHROPLASTY, TOTAL SHOULDER ARTHROPLASTY, AND SPECIAL HEMIARTHROPLASTY

Incision and Approach

- Create a deltopectoral incision.
- Lyse adhesions and remove bursa from the humeroscapular motion interface.
- Verify irreparability of the rotator cuff tear and resect useless tendon tissue. If useful cuff elements remain, tag for later reattachment.
- Incise susbscapularis and capsule from insertion to lesser tuberosity, preserving maximal length of tendon.
- Release inferior capsule from humerus.
- Identify axillary nerve.
- Perform a 360-degree subscapularis release.

Humeral Preparation and Implant Sizing

- Insert progressively larger reamers into the canal, stopping at the first endocortical bite (**TECH FIG 1A**).
- Resect the humeral head in 30 degrees of retroversion and 45 degrees with the long axis of the shaft (**TECH FIG 1B**).
- Measure height and diameter of the curvature of the resected head (**TECH FIG 1C**).
- Mince bone of the humeral head to make autogenous graft.
- If the glenoid is rough and eroded medially, but not superiorly, and if the infraspinatus and subscapularis are

intact or robustly reconstructable, and if the patient has soft glenoid bone (as in rheumatoid arthritis), consider inserting a prosthetic glenoid component.

- Using minced autogenous bone from the humeral head, perform impaction autografting of the humeral canal so that the prosthetic stem will achieve a snug press-fit (**TECH FIG 1D**).
- If a partial rotator cuff repair can be carried out, perform that before definitive sizing of component, because repair may diminish the room available for the prosthesis (**TECH FIG 1E**).
- If glenoid arthroplasty has been performed, select the humeral head prosthesis with the appropriate diameter of curvature for the glenoid.
  - If glenoid arthroplasty has not been performed, select the humeral head prosthesis with the diameter equal to that of the resected head.

Component Placement

- With the trial component in position, resect any prominent tuberosity that may abut against the coracoacromial arch on elevation of the arm (**TECH FIG 2A,B**).
- Consider a special humeral head (eg, CTA head) to cover the area of the greater tuberosity (**TECH FIG 2C**).

TECHNIQUES

TECHNIQUES

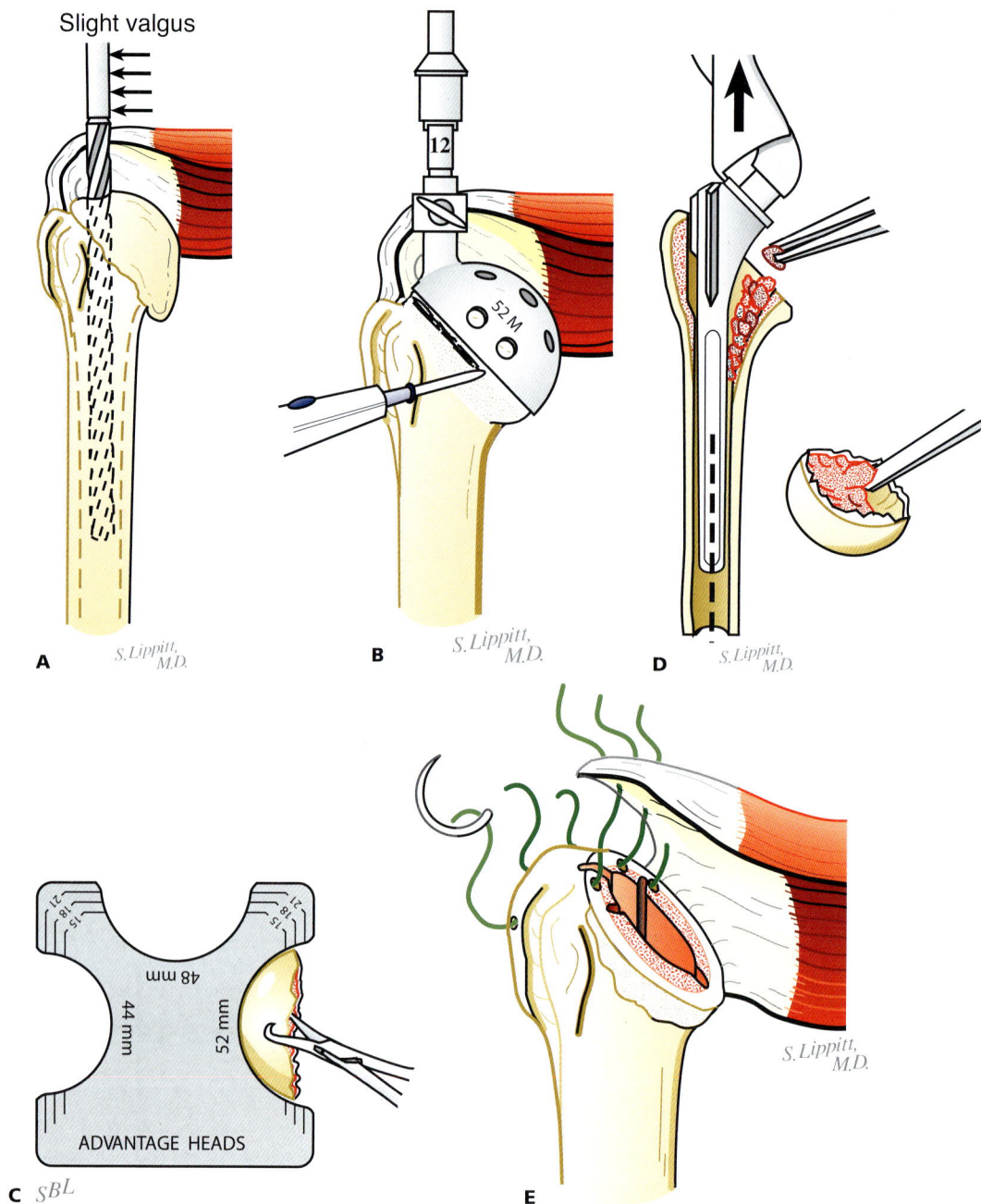

TECH FIG 1 • A. Reaming the humerus until the first endocortical bite is achieved. **B.** Marking the humeral osteotomy at 45 degrees with the reamed axis of the shaft and in 30 degrees of retroversion. Care must be taken to protect the rotator cuff in making the osteotomy. **C.** Measuring the resected head to determine the diameter of curvature and the height. **D.** Impaction grafting of the medullary canal to achieve a secure press-fit without jeopardizing the strength of the diaphyseal cortex. **E.** Partial repair of the rotator cuff to the edge of the resected humerus. (Copyright Steven B. Lippitt, MD.)

- Select the humeral head height that, on trial reduction, allows 40 degrees of external rotation with the subscapularis approximated, 50% posterior translation on the posterior drawer test, and 60 degrees of internal rotation when the arm is abducted to 90 degrees (**TECH FIG 2D–G**).
- Place six no. 2 nonabsorbable sutures in the anterior humeral neck cut for reattachment of the subscapularis (**TECH FIG 2H**).
- Assemble the definitive humeral prosthesis.
- Insert the prosthesis in the impaction-grafted medullary canal.

Final Contouring and Wound Closure

- Ensure smooth passage of the proximal humerus beneath the coracoacromial arch. If abutment occurs, perform smoothing on the humeral side, preserving the integrity of the arch.
- Repair the subscapularis.
- Insert drain.
- Close the deltopectoral interval.
- Perform subcutaneous and skin closure.
- Apply sterile dressings.

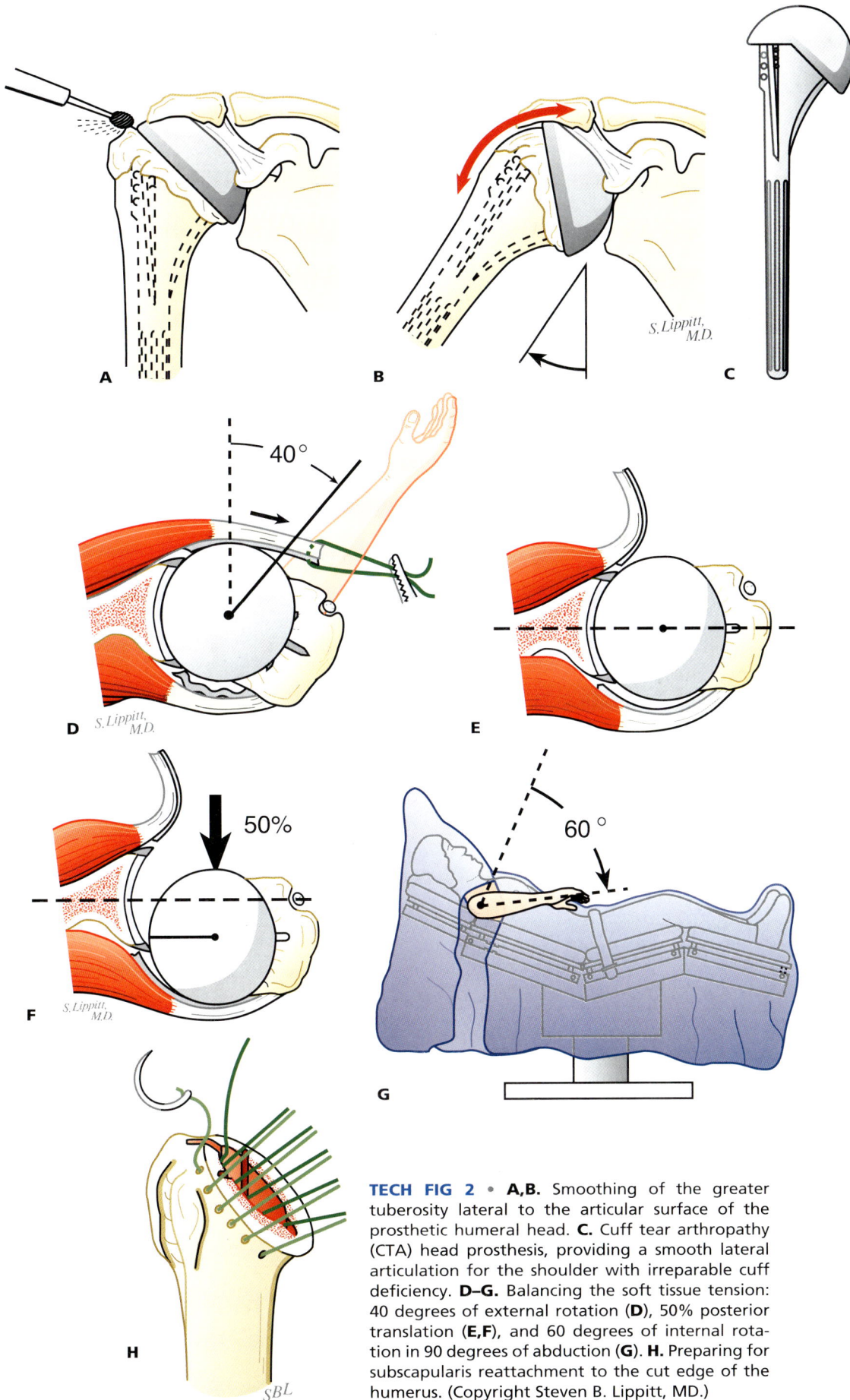

TECH FIG 2 • A,B. Smoothing of the greater tuberosity lateral to the articular surface of the prosthetic humeral head. **C.** Cuff tear arthropathy (CTA) head prosthesis, providing a smooth lateral articulation for the shoulder with irreparable cuff deficiency. **D–G.** Balancing the soft tissue tension: 40 degrees of external rotation (**D**), 50% posterior translation (**E,F**), and 60 degrees of internal rotation in 90 degrees of abduction (**G**). **H.** Preparing for subscapularis reattachment to the cut edge of the humerus. (Copyright Steven B. Lippitt, MD.)

TECHNIQUES

DELTA OR REVERSE ARTHROPLASTY

Incision and Approach

- Make a deltopectoral incision.
- Lyse adhesions and remove bursa from the humeroscapular motion interface, protecting deltoid, acromion, and residual cuff tissue.
- Verify irreparability of the rotator cuff tear and resect useless tendon tissue.
- Tag any potentially reparable elements of the cuff that are identified, for later use.
- Incise the subscapularis and capsule from insertion to lesser tuberosity, preserving maximal length of the tendon.
- Release the inferior capsule from the humerus.
- Identify the axillary nerve.
- Perform a 360-degree subscapularis release.

Humeral Preparation

- Insert humeral resection guide stem into medullary canal (**TECH FIG 3A**).
- Resect humeral head in zero degrees of retroversion (**TECH FIG 3B**).
- When the arm is pulled distally, the plane of the humeral cut should pass just below the inferior glenoid.

Glenoid Preparation

- Dissect the capsule from the anterior glenoid down to and around the inferior pole so that the upper axillary border of the scapula can be palpated and seen, releasing the origin of the long head of the triceps as necessary.
- Check radiographs and exposed glenoid to identify abnormal glenoid anatomy (eg, superior, inferior, anterior, posterior, inferior or medial erosion, as well as defects from previous surgery [such as earlier arthroplasty]).
  - Note the relation of the inferior glenoid lip to the axillary border of the scapula.
- Remove the labrum and cartilage from the glenoid.
- Mark a point 13 mm anterior to the posterior rim of the glenoid and 19 mm superior to the inferior glenoid rim.

- Drill the guidewire into the glenoid at this point (**TECH FIG 4A**).
- Place the metaglene of the Delta prosthesis (**TECH FIG 4B**) over this guidewire, with the peg laterally, to verify the appropriateness of this center point.
  - The inferior aspect of the metaglene should align with a line extended from the axillary border of the scapula.
- When the rim of the metaglene is flush with the extrapolated axillary border, remove the metaglene and drill a central hole with the step drill (**TECH FIG 4C**).
- Ream the glenoid conservatively, removing only enough bone to make the surface relatively flat and making sure the reamer handle remains perpendicular to the face of the glenoid (**TECH FIG 4D**).

Metaglene Placement

- Insert the metaglene peg into the central hole (**TECH FIG 5A**).
- Palpate the anterior and posterior aspects of the axillary border of the scapula and rotate the metaglene so the inferior screw hole is centered over the axillary border.
  - Recall that the inferior locking screw makes a 16-degree angle with the central peg.
  - Using a drill guide, drill a hole for the inferior locking screw, checking frequently to ensure that the drill is in bone by pushing on the drill while it is not rotating.
  - Use a 2-mm drill bit unless the bone is hard (**TECH FIG 5B**).
- At least 36 mm of intraosseous drilling should be achieved.
  - If not, re-examine rotation of the metaglene with respect to the axillary border (**TECH FIG 5C**).

Screw Fixation

- Insert the inferior locking screw (**TECH FIG 6A**).
- Drill and insert the superior locking screw using similar technique (**TECH FIG 6B,C**).

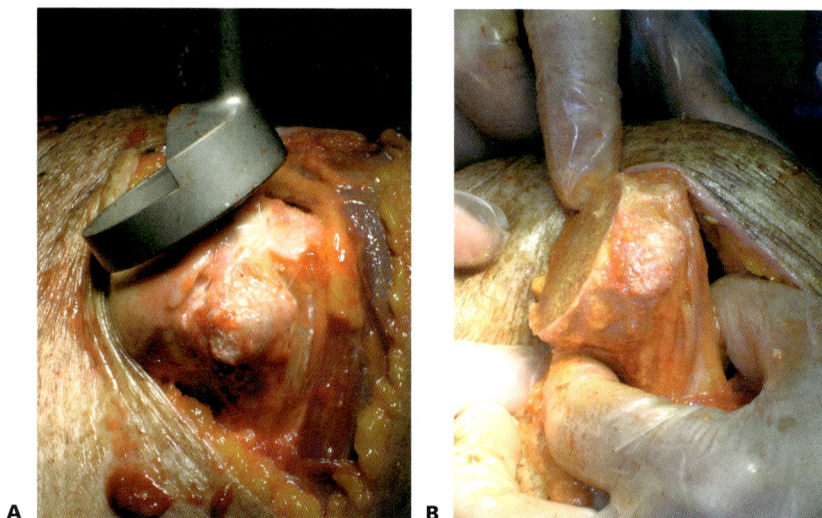

TECH FIG 3 • **A.** Humeral resection guide inserted for cut at 0 degree of retroversion. **B.** Resected humerus after removal of osteophytes. (Copyright Frederick A. Matsen, MD.)

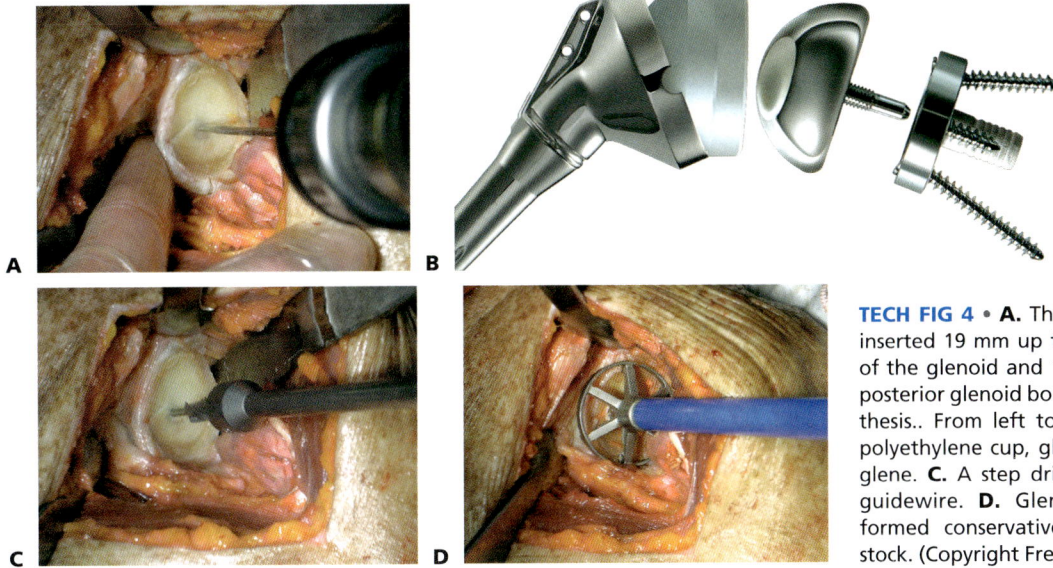

TECH FIG 4 • A. The glenoid guidewire is inserted 19 mm up from the inferior edge of the glenoid and 13 mm anterior to the posterior glenoid border. **B.** The Delta prosthesis.. From left to right: humeral stem, polyethylene cup, glenosphere, and metaglene. **C.** A step drill is inserted over the guidewire. **D.** Glenoid reaming is performed conservatively to preserve bone stock. (Copyright Frederick A. Matsen, MD.)

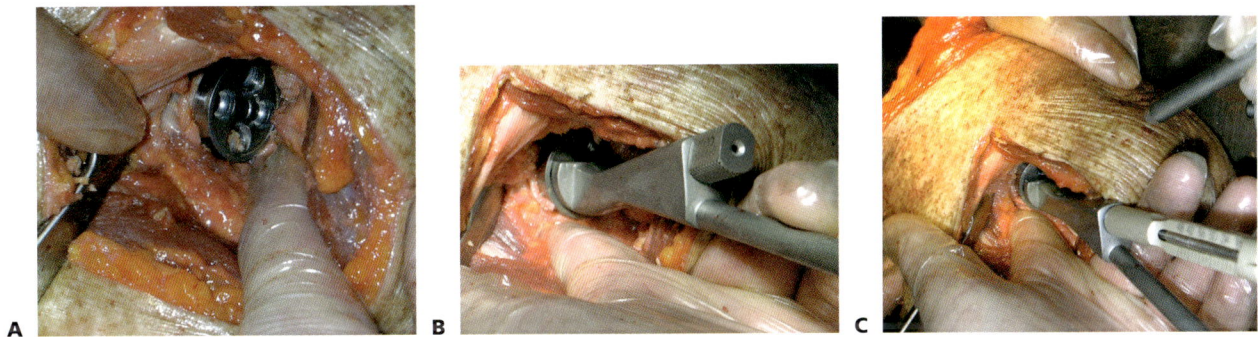

TECH FIG 5 • A. Inserting the metaglene, noting its flush position with the inferior glenoid. **B.** Drill guide aligned with the axillary border of the scapula. **C.** Verifying the intraosseous position of the inferior drill hole by direct palpation. (Copyright Frederick A. Matsen, MD.)

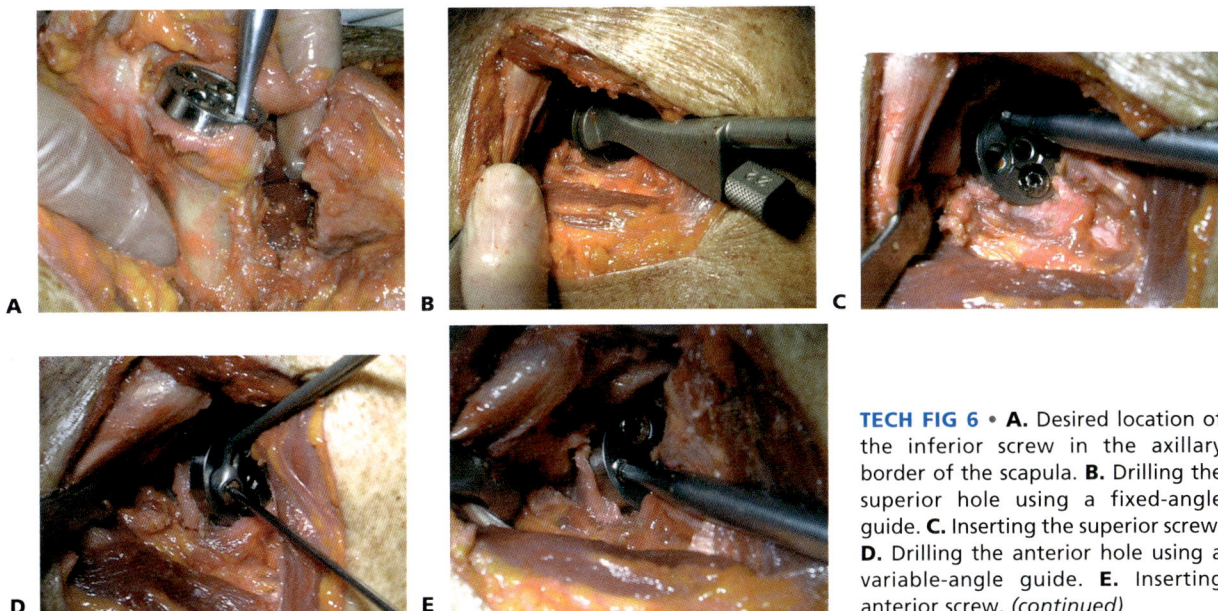

TECH FIG 6 • A. Desired location of the inferior screw in the axillary border of the scapula. **B.** Drilling the superior hole using a fixed-angle guide. **C.** Inserting the superior screw. **D.** Drilling the anterior hole using a variable-angle guide. **E.** Inserting anterior screw. *(continued)*

TECHNIQUES

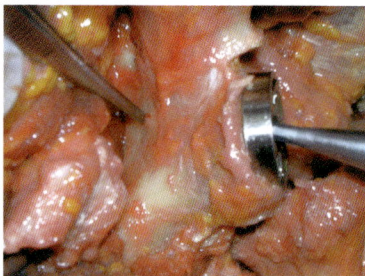

F

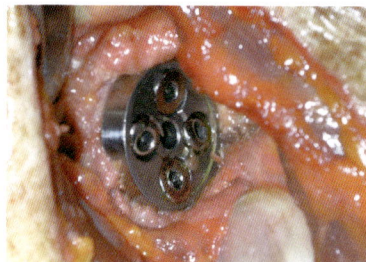

G

TECH FIG 6 • *(continued)* **F.** The desired position of the anterior screw exiting deep in the subscapularis fossa. **G.** Four screws in place in the metaglene. (Copyright Frederick A. Matsen, MD.)

- Drill and insert the anterior nonlocking screw, guiding orientation by palpating the anterior glenoid neck (**TECH FIG 6D–F**).
- Drill and insert the posterior nonlocking screw (**TECH FIG 6G**).
- Once screws have been placed, check the security of metaglene fixation.
- Insert a trial glenosphere onto the metaglene.
- Inspect the inferior aspect of the glenoid, removing any bone that may abut against the humeral polyethylene component.
  - Adequacy of bone resection can be verified by placing a trial polyethylene humeral component over the glenosphere and making sure it can be adducted fully, recalling that the humeral cup makes a 65-degree angle with the humeral shaft.

Humeral Preparation

- Prepare the humeral canal in a manner that preserves bone stock by insertion of progressively larger reamers until cortical contact is just achieved (**TECH FIG 7A,B**).

- Insert a trial stem with a metaphyseal reamer guide in 0 degrees of rotation (**TECH FIG 7C**).
- Ream the metaphysis until bone purchase is achieved (**TECH FIG 7D**).

Trial Placement

- Perform trial reduction of the prepared humerus (without trial components) to see if the reamed metaphysis can be reduced to the glenosphere, indicating that the humeral resection is adequate (**TECH FIG 8A**).
- Assemble and insert the trial humeral component in 0 degrees of retroversion with a 3-mm trial plastic component (**TECH FIG 8B**).
- Reduce the joint (**TECH FIG 8C,D**) and check for:
  - Medial abutment of plastic against the axillary border of the glenoid
  - Stability
  - Range of motion
  - Minimal (<2 mm) distraction on distal traction
- If the joint cannot be reduced, consider lowering the humeral component position by sequentially resecting small amounts of humeral bone.

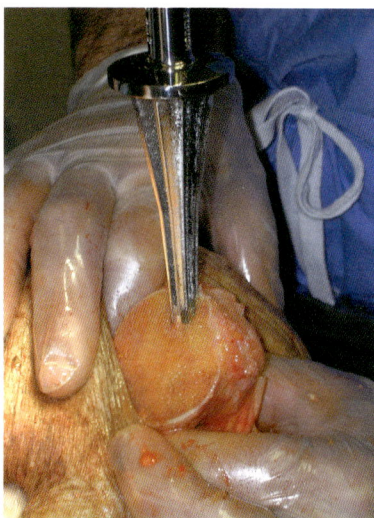

A

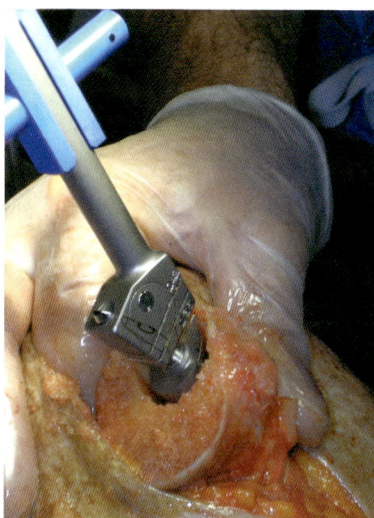

C

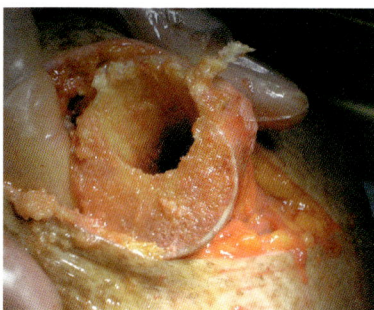

B

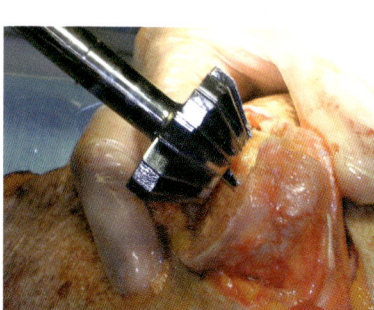

D

TECH FIG 7 • **A.** Medullary reaming of the humerus using a lateral starting point. **B.** Reamed medullary canal of the humerus. **C.** Inserting the metaphyseal reaming guide in 0 degrees of retroversion to the depth appropriate for the 36-mm prosthesis. **D.** Reaming the metaphysis over the metaphyseal reaming guide. (Copyright Frederick A. Matsen, MD.)

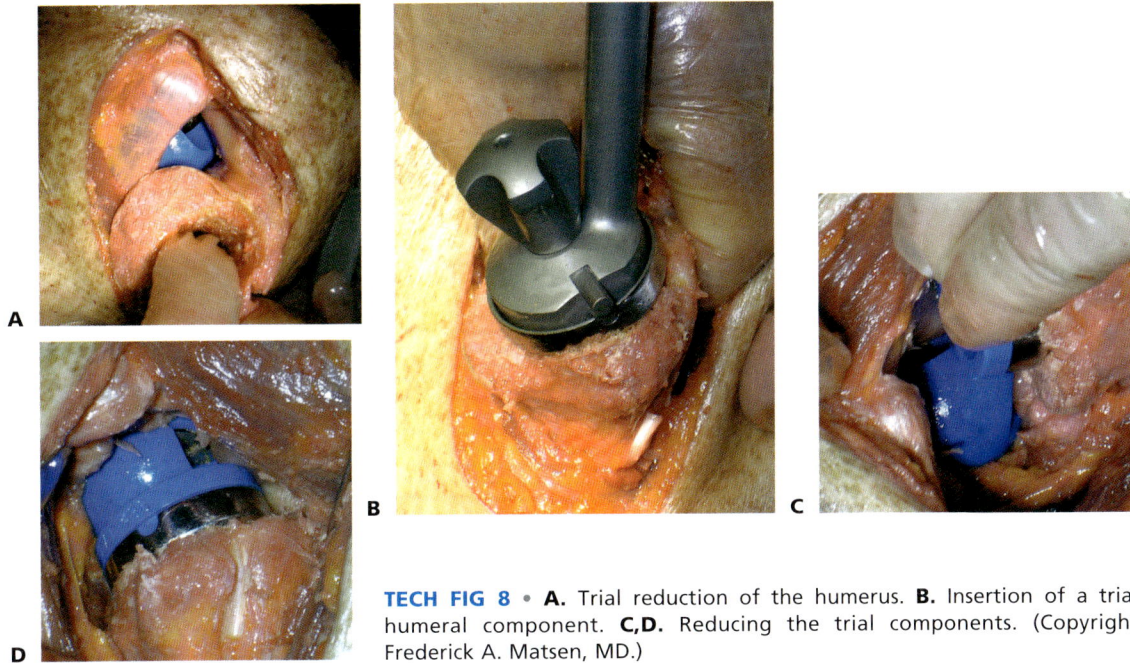

TECH FIG 8 • **A.** Trial reduction of the humerus. **B.** Insertion of a trial humeral component. **C,D.** Reducing the trial components. (Copyright Frederick A. Matsen, MD.)

Final Component Placement

- Insert the glenosphere into the metaglene, making sure it is aligned to avoid cross-threading and making sure it is fully seated.
- Securely assemble the definitive humeral component with a strong crescent wrench.
- Brush and irrigate the humeral medullary canal.
- Insert a cement restrictor 13 cm distal to the lateral aspect of the humeral cut.
- Place six drill holes and no. 2 nonabsorbable sutures in the anterior neck cut for later reattachment of the subscapularis.
- Repair the posterior cuff, if possible.
- Cement the assembled humeral component in 0 degrees of retroversion without a polyethylene insert.
- Trial different heights of polyethylene liners, starting with 3 mm, reducing shoulder to discover the height that

allows for reduction but less than 2 mm of distraction, checking again for abutment of adducted plastic against the lateral glenoid bone inferiorly.
- Insert the definitive polyethylene component, making sure it seats fully.
- Irrigate the wound completely.
- Reduce the joint.

Wound Closure

- Repair the subscapularis to sutures previously placed at the anterior neck cut.
- Place a suction drain.
- Close the deltopectoral interval, close the subcutaneous layer, and close the skin with staples.
- Apply dry sterile dressings and an axillary pad.

PEARLS AND PITFALLS

Glenohumeral arthritis is a chronic condition, so there is no rush to surgical judgment.	• Try gentle range-of-motion and deltoid-strengthening exercises.
Individuals with these conditions often are elderly and frail.	• Perform a thorough preoperative assessment and minimize surgical risk factors before surgery.
In revision surgery, especially revision arthroplasty, be aware of indolent infection, especially with *Staphylococcus epidermidis* and *Propionibacter acnes*.	• Obtain multiple intraoperative cultures for these organisms and hold cultures for 2 weeks.
In "irreparable" cuff tears, the cuff often is partially reparable	• At surgery, seek subscapularis and infraspinatus elements that are reparable.
Tissues are fragile in these patients	• Treat deltoid, acromion, glenoid, and humeral bone gently.
Patients with irreparable cuff tears and arthritis are prone to effusions and postsurgical hematomas	• Drain the surgical site and rehabilitate slowly.

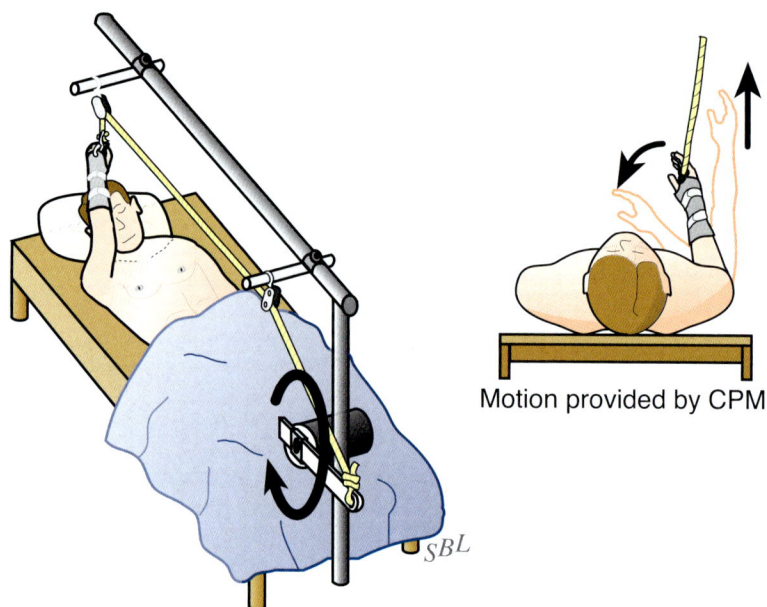

Motion provided by CPM

FIG 4 • Continuous passive motion. (Copyright Steven B. Lippitt, MD.)

POSTOPERATIVE CARE

- Hemiarthroplasty with a conventional prosthesis, total glenohumeral arthroplasty, or hemiarthroplasty with a special head (eg, CTA)
  - Institute a continuous passive motion (**FIG 4**) and early active assisted motion protocol as soon as possible postoperatively (unless major partial cuff repair has been carried out).
  - Elevation of the arm to 140 degrees is achieved before the patient leaves the medical center.
  - For 6 weeks, external rotation is limited to what was easily achievable on the operating table.
  - Gentle progressive strengthening exercises, including the supine press, usually are started at 6 weeks.
- Delta or reverse arthroplasty
  - Institute hand-gripping and active elbow flexion postoperatively.
  - Motion is withheld for 36 hours to minimize the risk of hematoma formation.
  - Gentle activities, such as eating, are started at 36 hours, followed by the slow, progressive addition of other activities, reminding the patient of the need for the shoulder bones and muscles to have time to remodel to their new loading patterns.
  - Avoid lifting anything heavier than 1 pound for 3 months.

OUTCOMES

- The highly variable patient characteristics, shoulder pathology, and surgical techniques make general statements about functional and prosthetic survival difficult.
  - For this reason, a conservative approach to surgery is advised.

COMPLICATIONS

- Systemic perioperative
  - Anesthetic complications
  - Deep venous thrombosis
  - Atelectasis
  - Cardiac events
- Local perioperative
  - Intraoperative fracture of humerus, glenoid, acromion
  - Axillary nerve or plexus injury
  - Deltoid injury
- Postoperative
  - Hematoma
  - Infection
  - Dislocation
  - Failure of tissue repair
  - Fracture of humerus, glenoid, acromion
  - Prosthetic loosening
  - Pain
  - Weakness
  - Failure to regain function

REFERENCES

1. Boileau P, Watkinson D, et al. Neer Award 2005. The Grammont reverse shoulder prosthesis: Results in cuff tear arthritis, fracture sequelae, and revision arthroplasty. J Shoulder Elbow Surg 2006;15: 527–540.
2. Boileau P, Watkinson DJ, et al. Grammont reverse prosthesis: Design, rationale, and biomechanics. J Shoulder Elbow Surg 2005;14 (1 Suppl S):147S–161S.
3. Frankle M, Levy JC, et al. The reverse shoulder prosthesis for glenohumeral arthritis associated with severe rotator cuff deficiency: a minimum two-year follow-up study of sixty patients' surgical technique. J Bone Joint Surg Am 2006;88A(Suppl 1 Pt 2):178–190.
4. Frankle M, Siegal S, et al. The reverse shoulder prosthesis for glenohumeral arthritis associated with severe rotator cuff deficiency: a minimum two-year follow-up study of sixty patients. J Bone Joint Surg Am 2005;87A:1697–1705.
5. Guery J, Favard L, et al. Reverse total shoulder arthroplasty. Survivorship analysis of eighty replacements followed for five to ten years. J Bone Joint Surg Am 2006;88A:1742–1747.
6. Harman M, Frankle M, et al. Initial glenoid component fixation in reverse total shoulder arthroplasty: a biomechanical evaluation. J Shoulder Elbow Surg 2005;14(1 Suppl S):162S–167S.

7. Mahfouz M, Nicholson G, et al. In vivo determination of the dynamics of normal, rotator cuff-deficient, total, and reverse replacement shoulders. J Bone Joint Surg Am 2005;87A(Suppl 2):107–113.

8. Matsen FA III, Lippitt SB. Shoulder Surgery: Principles and Procedures. Philadelphia: WB Saunders, 2003.

9. Neyton L, Walch G, et al. Glenoid corticocancellous bone grafting after glenoid component removal in the treatment of glenoid loosening. J Shoulder Elbow Surg 2006;15:173–179.

10. Nyffeler RW, Werner CM, et al. Biomechanical relevance of glenoid component positioning in the reverse Delta III total shoulder prosthesis. J Shoulder Elbow Surg 2005;14:524–528.

11. Nyffeler RW, Werner CM, et al. Analysis of a retrieved Delta III total shoulder prosthesis. J Bone Joint Surg Br 2004;86B:1187–1191.

12. Rockwood CA, Matsen FA III, Wirth MA, et al, eds. The Shoulder, ed 3. Philadelphia: WB Saunders, 2004.

13. Werner CM, Steinmann PA, et al. Treatment of painful pseudoparesis due to irreparable rotator cuff dysfunction with the Delta III reverse-ball-and-socket total shoulder prosthesis. J Bone Joint Surg Am 2005;87A:1476–1486.

Chapter 27

Pectoralis Major Repair

Matthew D. Pepe, Bradford S. Tucker, and Carl Basamania

DEFINITION

- Pectoralis major ruptures are injuries to the one of the largest and strongest muscles of the shoulder region.
- Injuries can be divided into complete and partial tears.
  - Complete tears typically occur at the tendon-to-bone junction and involve both heads.
  - Partial tears can occur to either the sternocostal or the clavicular head.
  - Both types may also occur at the musculotendinous junction or the muscle itself.

ANATOMY

- The pectoralis major is a broad triangular muscle that originates from the medial clavicle, anterior sternum, costal cartilages to the sixth rib, and external obliques.
- It inserts into the proximal humerus on the lateral edge of the bicipital groove. It has two distinct heads: the smaller clavicular head and the larger sternocostal head.
- The pectoralis major tendon is about 5 cm long. The insertion site has two distinct laminae. The clavicular head is anterior and distal and is about 1 cm long, and the sternocostal head inserts posterior and is 2.5 cm long.[3]
- The sternocostal head spirals 180 degrees on itself, inserting posterior to the clavicular head, creating a rolled inferior surface that is the axillary fold (**FIG 1**).
- The function of the pectoralis major varies depending on the division. Its primary function is to adduct the humerus and its secondary role is to forward flex and internally rotate. The clavicular head primarily forward flexes and horizontally adducts. The sternocostal head internally rotates and adducts.

PATHOGENESIS

- Pectoralis major ruptures typically occur when a powerful eccentric or concentric forward flexion or adduction load to the humerus (such as heavy bench pressing) occurs. The final 30 degrees of humeral extension disproportionally stretches the inferior fibers of the sternocostal head, putting it at a mechanical disadvantage and predisposing it to injury. The inferior fibers fail first, followed by progression toward the clavicular head.
- Ruptures may also occur when a traction injury such as rapid extension, abduction, or external rotation force is applied to the extremity (such as catching oneself during a fall).
- Injuries to the muscle belly can also be caused by a direct blow, which can result in hematoma formation.
- Patients often hear or feel a rip or tear in the shoulder region, feel a burning pain, and occasionally hear a pop.
- Younger patients (under 30 years) tear at the tendon–bone insertion, whereas patients over 30 tend to tear at the musculotendinous junction.
- Swelling and ecchymosis occur from several hours to days after the injury in the lateral chest wall, upper arm, or axilla.
- Medial muscle retraction along with loss of the axillary fold may not be evident for several days until the swelling subsides.
- Anabolic steroids weaken the muscle–tendon unit, making patients more susceptible to tears.[1]

NATURAL HISTORY

- Weakness of the affected shoulder in adduction, forward flexion, and internal rotation can be expected with nonoperative treatment of full-thickness tears of both heads or of partial tears of the sternocostal head.
- Isokinetic strength testing has demonstrated 25% to 50% deficits of strength in adduction and internal rotation in preoperative patients and people treated nonoperatively.[3,4,9]
- Cosmetic deformity occurs secondary to the loss of the tendon in the axillary fold as well as from the medial retraction that occurs during contraction of the muscle.
- Partial tears will elicit a variable degree of weakness and deformity, depending on the amount and location of tendon torn.

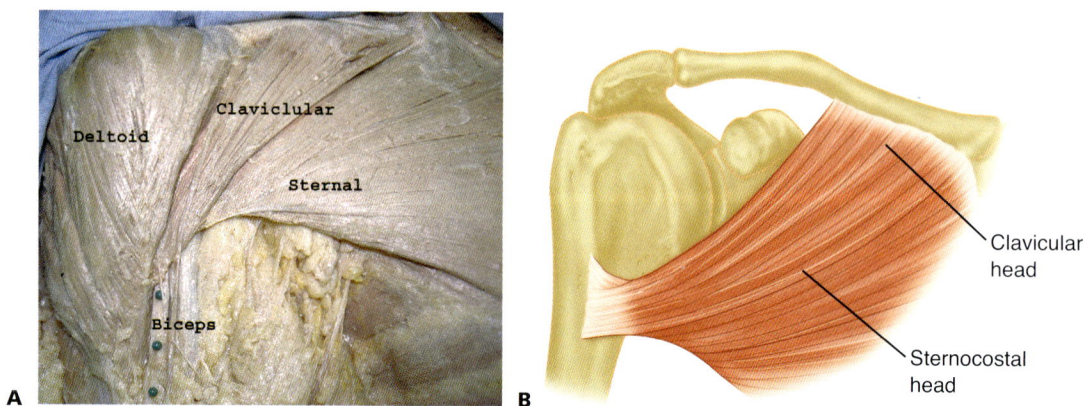

FIG 1 • **A.** Anatomy of the pectoralis major. Two distinct heads are clearly demonstrated. **B.** The clavicular portion of the tendon inserts anterior and distal. The sternocostal lamina inserts posterior and proximal.

■ The initial pain and cramping that occurs during contraction of the pectoralis major usually subsides in 2 to 3 months.
■ Patients treated nonoperatively for full-thickness tears will complain of weakness and fatigue with recreational and occupational activities as well as the cosmetic deformity.

PATIENT HISTORY AND PHYSICAL FINDINGS

■ A previous history of pain is not typical.
■ The patient's occupation and involvement in sports and weight-lifting activities are important in decision making regarding treatment.
■ Physical examination initially will yield painful range of motion of the shoulder and arm. When the swelling subsides, patients typically have full range of motion of the glenohumeral joint.
■ Swelling and ecchymosis are variable depending on the chronicity and the degree of the tear.
■ Isometric or resisted adduction and forward flexion will show the loss of the tendon in the axillary fold and medial retraction of the pectoralis muscle.
■ The examiner should instruct the patient to hold the arm at 90 degrees of abduction, and the anterior head of the deltoid will be accentuated. If the arm is held in forward flexion, the clavicular head will be accentuated (**FIG 2A**).
■ Having patients press their hands together in front of their body for isometric adduction allows inspection of both sides at the same time and simultaneous palpation (**FIG 2B**).
■ Manual strength testing will demonstrate weakness in adduction and forward flexion.

IMAGING AND OTHER DIAGNOSTIC STUDIES

■ A standard shoulder radiographic series is obtained to rule out fractures, avulsions, or signs of instability.

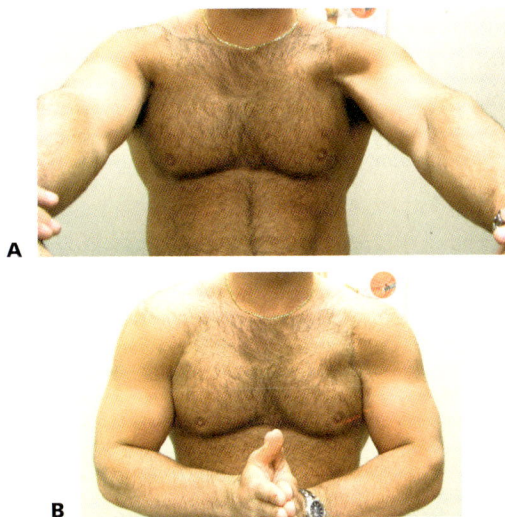

FIG 2 • **A.** Resisted forward flexion demonstrates the intact clavicular head and the defect from the ruptured sternocostal head. The retracted sternocostal head is evident. **B.** Isometric adduction demonstrating the normal contour of the right pectoralis major compared with the medially retracted left sternocostal head.

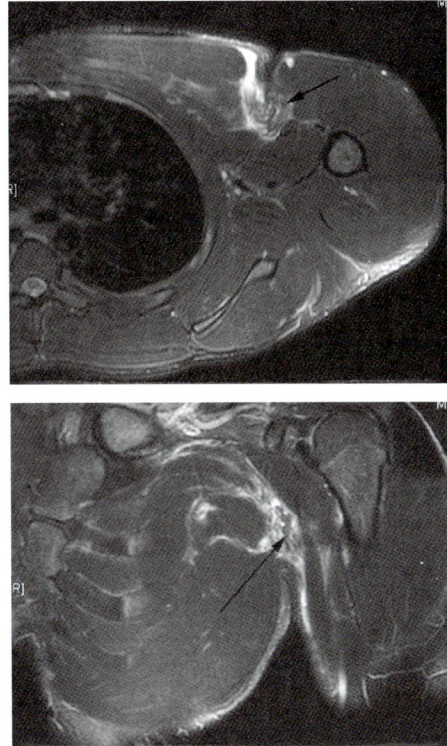

FIG 3 • Axial and coronal T2-weighted MRIs.

■ An MRI of the chest, with attention to the pectoralis major tendon, may be obtained to evaluate the location of the tear or assist in making the diagnosis.[6,11] It has been shown to be beneficial in differentiating musculotendinous junction ruptures from tendinous avulsions and may change the treatment strategy.[11] It is difficult, however, to distinguish between complete and partial ruptures (**FIG 3**).
■ Ultrasound may be used to identify the location and severity of the tear. Results, however, are user-dependent.

DIFFERENTIAL DIAGNOSIS

■ Rotator cuff tears
■ Proximal biceps tear
■ Anterior shoulder instability
■ Deltoid rupture
■ Latissimus dorsi tear
■ Brachial plexus injury

NONOPERATIVE MANAGEMENT

■ Nonoperative treatment is indicated for medial tears, intramuscular tears, or tears at the musculotendinous junction in some people. Also, nonoperative treatment should be considered in low-demand patients with complete or partial distal tendon ruptures.
■ Nonoperative treatment begins with a sling for the first 7 to 10 days. Ice should be applied intermittently for the first 72 hours.
■ Gentle active assisted range of motion is then begun, avoiding aggressive external rotation, abduction, or extension stretching in the initial phases.
■ Strength training is typically initiated at 6 to 8 weeks. Depending on the level of occupational or sporting demands, patients may return between 8 and 12 weeks.

■ Strength deficits of 25% and 50% can be expected with nonoperative treatment.[5]

SURGICAL MANAGEMENT

■ Pectoralis major repair is recommended for all complete distal tears, partial distal tears in high-demand patients, and musculotendinous junction tears in high-demand patients with large defects.

■ A direct tendon-to-bone repair with heavy, nonabsorbable sutures is performed for complete distal tears and sternocostal tears.

■ A side-to-side repair is used for musculotendinous junction tears.

Preoperative Planning

■ A standard examination under anesthesia of the glenohumeral joint is performed to evaluate for instability.

Positioning

■ The patient is placed in the 30-degree modified beach chair position. The shoulder and arm are prepared free. A shoulder positioning device is helpful, but not necessary, to position the arm during surgery (**FIG 4**).

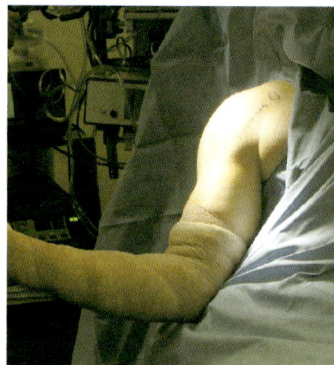

FIG 4 • Operative setup. The patient is placed in the beach chair position with the arm draped free.

Approach

■ An anterior approach to the shoulder and proximal humerus is used—the internervous plane between the axillary nerve of the deltoid and the superior and inferior pectoral nerves of the pectoralis major.

TECHNIQUES

PECTORALIS MAJOR REPAIR USING DRILL HOLES

■ Our preferred technique for direct primary repair of the pectoralis major tendon is to attach the tendon directly to the humeral cortex using drill holes.

■ A limited 4- to 5-cm deltopectoral incision is made (**TECH FIG 1A**). The cephalic vein is identified and retracted laterally with the deltoid.

■ The biceps tendon is identified, gaining access to the insertion of the pectoralis major just lateral to the biceps tendon in the proximal humerus. In cases of musculotendinous junction tears or partial tears, the entire tendon or a portion of it will be intact.

■ Medial dissection is then performed to identify the retracted tendon. The sternocostal and clavicular heads are identified as well as the location of the tendon or musculotendinous junction tear.

■ In cases of complete tears, the tendon is typically retracted medially and folded upon itself, identifiable by palpation.

■ A traction suture is placed in the tendon, and stepwise gentle blunt mobilization of the muscle and tendon is performed.

■ The excursion of the tendon is then tested. Even in cases of chronic tears, the tendon can typically be mobilized to reach the humerus without difficulty.

■ The tendon edge is freshened with a scalpel. A no. 5 braided, nonabsorbable suture is used in a Bunnell or modified Mason-Allen locking stitch in the end of the tendon (**TECH FIG 1B**). Two or three sutures are used, spaced about 1 cm apart, depending on the width of the tendon.

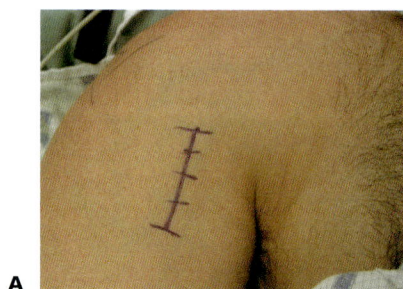

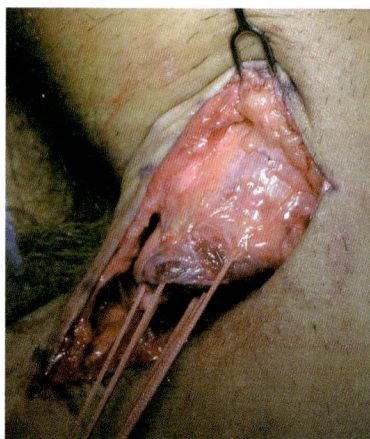

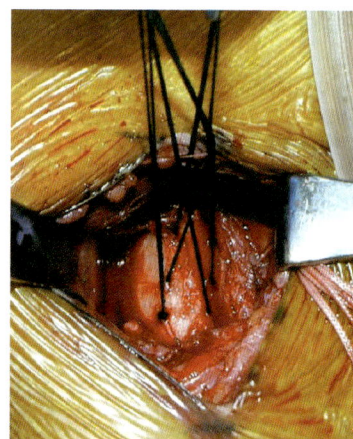

TECH FIG 1 • Drill hole technique. **A.** Limited deltopectoral incision. **B.** Modified Mason-Allen stitch in tendon edge. **C.** Drill hole placement with 2-0 Vicryl sutures placed. (*continued*)

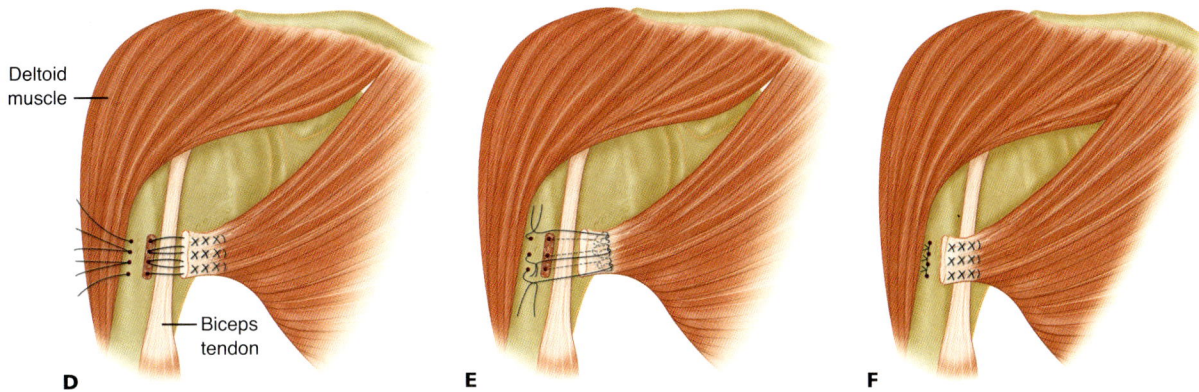

TECH FIG 1 • (*continued*) **D.** Bunnell technique with sutures passed and ready to tie. The central holes are shared by two sutures. **E.** Suture passage when modified Mason-Allen stitch is used. The deep suture is passed through the drill holes. **F.** Bunnell technique after suture tying.

- The insertion site lateral to the biceps tendon is decorticated with a burr.
- A commercially available drill can be used to drill the proximal and distal sets of holes. A bridge of 8 to 10 mm is adequate secondary to the thickness of the humerus.
  - The holes usually need to be overdrilled with a 2-mm drill bit, as the humeral cortex is extremely strong and thick.
- A needle with a matching radius of curvature is then used to pass a 2-0 looped Vicryl passing suture (**TECH FIG 1C**). Each corresponding suture is passed using the 2-0 Vicryl passing suture.

- The central drill holes are shared by the upper and lower respective sutures in a horizontal mattress configuration for the Bunnell technique (**TECH FIG 1D**).
- If a modified Mason-Allen stitch was used, the deep suture is passed through the drill hole and the knot tied on the upper surface of the tendon (**TECH FIG 1E**).
- The sutures are then tied with the arm in adduction and internal rotation to ensure apposition of the tendon to the humerus (**TECH FIG 1F**).
- Alternatively, the drill holes may be made freehand and the sutures passed with either a free needle or a loop of 24-gauge wire.

PECTORALIS MAJOR REPAIR USING SUTURE ANCHORS

- The musculotendinous unit is mobilized in the same way as described for drill hole repair. The humeral cortex is decorticated with a burr.
- Two or three suture anchors are then placed in the humeral insertion, spaced 1 cm apart. The sutures are passed in a Kessler mattress stitch through the distal pectoralis tendon (**TECH FIG 2**).
- One limb is passed in a simple fashion. This is used as the post during tying so the knot slides and apposes the tendon to the humerus without the knot lying in the repair site.
- Metallic anchors loaded with braided, nonabsorbable no. 5 sutures are used, as the humeral cortex in this region may be too thick to accept an absorbable anchor.

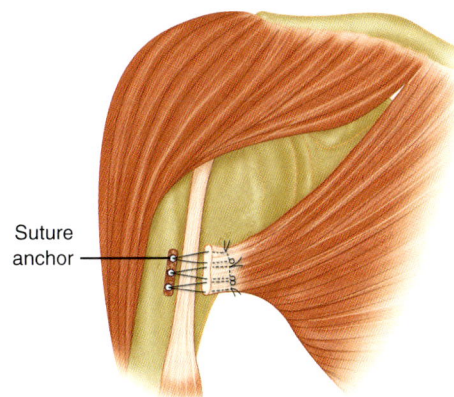

TECH FIG 2 • Suture anchor technique: placement of sutures and passage through the tendon edge.

MUSCULOTENDINOUS JUNCTION REPAIRS

- Multiple figure 8 or modified Kessler sutures of a no. 2 braided, nonabsorbable suture are used on both the superficial and deep layers.
- The quality of the repair depends on the strength and the amount of tendon left on the muscular side.

PEARLS AND PITFALLS

Indications for repair	■ A discussion and risk–benefit analysis is necessary in patients with partial and musculotendinous junction ruptures.
Tendon mobilization	■ Medial dissection is required to free the perimuscular adhesions in chronic ruptures. The neurovascular bundle is rarely at risk.
Suture passing	■ Using a commercially available matched drill and needle facilitates suture passage through the humerus (CurvTek). Because of the thickness of the humerus, overdrilling the holes makes needle passage easier.
Chronic tears	■ Repair of pectoralis major ruptures is feasible up to 5 years after the injury. The outcome of chronic repairs is not as good as that of acute repairs, with residual weakness as the most common complaint.

POSTOPERATIVE CARE

■ The arm is kept in a sling for 6 weeks postoperatively. It is removed from the sling one or two times daily for gentle, progressive passive and active assisted range of motion of the shoulder, elbow, wrist, and hand.

■ The extremes of abduction and external rotation are avoided for the first 6 weeks. At this time, the sling is removed and unrestricted movement is allowed. In addition, strengthening is begun.

■ Return to full activities is generally achieved between 3 and 5 months.

OUTCOMES

■ There are no large prospective or randomized studies in the literature comparing operative and nonoperative treatment. Results are universally good with acute repairs (within 8 weeks).

■ Park and Espiniella[7] in 1970 evaluated 30 patients with pectoralis major ruptures. The results were 90% good to excellent results with operative repair versus 75% with nonoperative treatment.

■ McEntire and colleagues[5] in 1972 compared operative and nonoperative treatment in 11 patients. Again, operative repair had a more favorable outcome at 88% versus 83%, with a higher ratio of excellent to good results.

■ Zenman and coworkers[10] in 1979 reviewed nine athletes with pectoralis major ruptures. Four patients were treated with surgical repair and had excellent results. All five of the patients treated nonoperatively had residual weakness, and two were dissatisfied with their outcome.

■ Kretzler and Richardson[3] in 1989 reported on their results after repair of 16 distal tendon tears. Eighty-one percent regained full motion and strength. Two repairs that occurred 5 years after the injury had persistent weakness.

■ Wolfe and colleagues[9] in 1992 evaluated 14 patients with pectoralis major ruptures, half of whom were treated with operative repair. Cybex strength testing demonstrated normal strength in the repaired patients, with persistent weakness in the unrepaired group.

■ Jones and Matthews[2] in 1988 reviewed the literature and concluded that acute repair within 7 days has 57% excellent and 30% good results. Repair in the setting of a chronic tear yielded 0% excellent and 60% good results. They concluded that although chronic repair is possible even up to 5 years after the injury, the outcome is not as good as an acute repair, with a high likelihood of persistent weakness and cosmetic deformity.

■ Schepsis and colleagues[8] in 2000 found that operatively repaired patients (both acute and chronic) had significantly better outcomes than conservatively treated patients.

■ There are no studies to date documenting rerupture after repair.

COMPLICATIONS

■ Complications are relatively infrequent after pectoralis major repair. One patient experienced loss of abduction.[3] Another patient had ulnar-sided hand paresthesias of unknown etiology that spontaneously resolved.[8]

■ There have been several reports of complications in the elderly after rupture and nonsurgical management. One patient needed a blood transfusion. Two died of sepsis from an infected hematoma. Myositis ossificans developed in one patient 4 months after rupture.

REFERENCES

1. Hunter MB, Shybut GT, Nuber G. The effect of anabolic steroid hormones on the mechanical properties of tendons and ligaments. Trans Orthop Res Soc 1986;11:240.
2. Jones MW, Matthews JP. Rupture of the pectoralis major in weightlifters: a case report and review of the literature. Injury 1988; 19:219.
3. Kretzler HH, Richardson AB. Rupture of the pectoralis major muscle. Am J Sports Med 1989;17:453.
4. Liu J, Wu J, Chang S, Chou Y, et al. Avulsion of the pectoralis major tendon. Am J Sports Med 1992;20:366–368.
5. McEntire JE, Hess WE, Coleman SS. Rupture of the pectoralis major muscle: a report of eleven injuries and review of fifty-six. J Bone Joint Surg Am 1972;54A:1040–1046.
6. Miller MD, Johnson DL, Fu FH, et al. Rupture of the pectoralis major muscle in a collegiate football player: use of magnetic resonance imaging in early diagnosis. Am J Sports Med 1993;21: 475–477.
7. Park JY, Espiniella LJ. Rupture of the pectoralis major muscle: a case report and review of the literature. J Bone Joint Surg Am 1970; 52A:577.
8. Schepsis AA, Grafe MW, Jones HP, et al. Rupture of the pectoralis major muscle: outcome after repair of acute and chronic injuries. Am J Sports Med 2000;28:9–15.
9. Wolfe SW, Wickiewicz TL, Cavanaugh JT. Ruptures of the pectoralis major muscle: an anatomic and clinical analysis. Am J Sports Med 1992;20:587.
10. Zenman SC, Rosenfeld RT, Liscomb PR. Tears of the pectoralis major muscle. Am J Sports Med 1979;7:343.
11. Zvijac JE, Schurhoff MR, Hechtman KS, et al. Pectoralis major tears: correlation of magnetic resonance imaging and treatment strategies. Am J Sports Med 2006;34:289–294.

Jon J. P. Warner and Bassem Elhassan

DEFINITION

- The snapping scapula syndrome first was described by Boinet in 1867.[14]
- It is characterized by painful scapular motion with associated crepitus during scapulothoracic motion, with or without a clear history of injury or trauma.
- It has also been referred to as *scapulothoracic bursitis, retroscapular creaking, superior scapular syndrome*, and *retroscapular pain*.[3,7,11,14]
- The associated audible crepitus, which can be tactile in most instances, has been described by Milch and Burman[11] as a tactile-acoustic phenomenon, possibly generated secondary to an abnormality in the scapulothoracic interval.
- This crepitus is divided into three classes, based on the volume of the sound produced.[10]
  - The first group is considered physiologic, with what is described as a "gentle friction" sound.
  - The second group, which includes most patients with the snapping scapular syndrome, features a louder grating sound.
  - The third group is defined by a loud snapping noise that is considered pathologic in most cases.

ANATOMY

- The scapulothoracic articulation consists of the interface between the anterior aspect of the scapula and the ribs in the posterior aspect of the convex thoracic chest wall (**FIG 1**).
- This articulation is cushioned by several muscles, specifically the subscapularis and the serratus anterior.
- In addition, two major and four minor bursae have been described in the scapulothoracic articulation[6,7,23] (Fig 1).
  - The two major bursae are the infraserratus bursa, located between the serratus anterior muscle and the chest wall, and the supraserratus bursa, located between the serratus anterior and the subscapularis muscles.
  - The four minor bursae are distributed as follows: two at the superomedial angle of the scapula, one at the inferior angle of the scapula, and one at the medial base of spine of the scapula, underlying the trapezius muscle.
- While the major bursae have been found consistently in cadaveric and clinical studies, those of the minor bursae were not.[3,19,20]

PATHOGENESIS

- Incongruence of the scapulothoracic articulation has been postulated to be the main cause of the snapping scapular syndrome, which may or may not be associated with bony anomalies of this region.[13,17]
- Maltracking or dynamic compression of the scapulothoracic articulation has been postulated as a main etiology of this syndrome, because it leads to irritation of the bursa secondary to pathologic contact between the ribs and the superior angle of the scapula.[4,22]
  - This maltracking is considered to be a soft tissue cause of snapping scapula syndrome, which has been reported in cases of subscapularis atrophy secondary to glenohumeral fusion and long thoracic nerve palsy.[11,24]
  - Clinical studies and histologic findings of muscle intrafascicular fibrosis, bursitis, edema, and shoulder girdle muscle atrophy support this hypothesis.[7,17]
- Bony or skeletal causes of snapping scapula syndrome are rare. These include scapular osteochondromas and exostoses (**FIG 2**), anterior angulation of the scapula, scapula fracture, scapular tubercle of Luschka, skeletal abnormalities of the vertebrae (omovertebral bone), and abnormal angulations and tumors of the ribs.[10,11,21]

NATURAL HISTORY

- Patients with snapping scapula syndrome usually complain of pain around the shoulder girdle.
- This pain most often is secondary to bursitis in the scapulothoracic articulation. Constant motion irritates the soft tissues, leading to inflammation and a cycle of chronic bursitis and scarring.

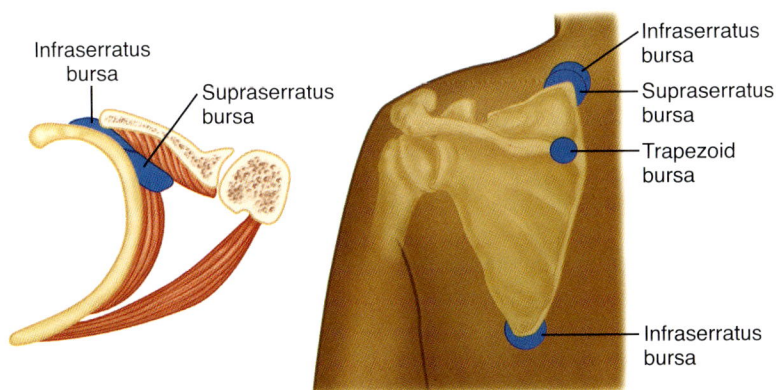

FIG 1 • Four different bursae are shown—two infraserratus, one supraserratus, and one trapezoid bursae.

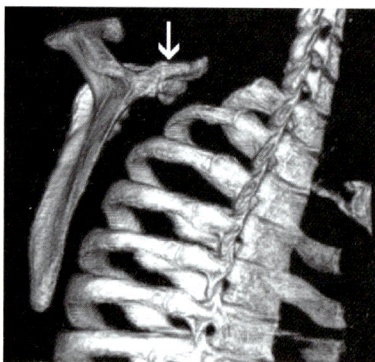

FIG 2 • An osteochondroma (*arrow*) of the superomedial angle of the scapula may, rarely, be the cause of snapping scapula syndrome.

- The chronic inflammation of the bursae will lead to fibrotic, scarred, and tough bursal tissues that can lead to mechanical impingement and pain with motion, resulting in further inflammation.
- Once the patient reaches this level of chronic bursal inflammation, the symptoms rarely subside by themselves without trial of rest and physical therapy.
- In many cases, especially when the cause of snapping is skeletal, surgical intervention becomes essential to manage this problem.

PATIENT HISTORY AND PHYSICAL FINDINGS

- Patients with scapulothoracic bursitis report a history of pain in the shoulder or neck with overhead activities for months or years and often have a history of repetitive overuse in work or recreation or a history of trauma.
- A history of neck injury, shoulder injury or fracture, or previous shoulder surgery should be ruled out.
- Audible or palpable crepitus may accompany the symptoms with scapulothoracic motion; this is another indication for the location of the symptomatic inflamed bursa.
- Some patients report a family history of the disorder and have bilateral symptoms.
- Localized tenderness is an indication for the site of scapulothoracic bursitis.
- Improvement of symptoms by lifting the scapula off the chest wall helps localize the source of pathology to the scapulothoracic articulation.
- Diagnosis is confirmed if significant relief or even elimination of the pain occurs when local anesthetic and corticosteroids are injected in the scapulothoracic bursa under the superomedial border of the scapula.
- The examiner also must assess soft tissue tightness, muscle strength, and flexibility around the involved shoulder.
  - Special attention should be directed to rule out tight trapezius, pectoralis minor, or levator scapula muscles, as well as weakness of any of the scapular muscles, specifically the serratus anterior and the trapezius.
- In patients with winging of the scapula, a careful neuromuscular examination should be performed to differentiate true winging from compensatory pseudo-winging that might originate from a painful scapulothoracic articulation.

IMAGING AND OTHER DIAGNOSTIC STUDIES

- Radiologic studies should include an anterior-posterior (AP) and tangential (Y) views of the shoulder, to identify bony abnormalities in the scapula and ribs (**FIG 3A**).
- A CT scan may be needed for more bony definition. Its role, with or without three-dimensional reconstruction, is still debated,[9,13] but in patients with suspected bony skeletal abnormality, the CT scan might be helpful (**FIG 3B**).
- Fluoroscopy could be used to visualize the snapping during simulated shoulder motion.
- MRI can identify the location and size of the inflamed bursa, but its usefulness is debated. The senior author does not believe that the MRI is necessary and has never ordered it in any of his cases.
- Nerve conduction and electromyography studies are useful if a neurologic injury is suspected as the reason for scapula winging.

DIFFERENTIAL DIAGNOSIS

- Soft tissue lesions, such as atrophied muscle
- Fibrotic muscle
- Anomalous muscle insertion
- Subscapular elastofibroma. This tumor is nonneoplastic and appears to form in response to repetitive injury or microtrauma. Most patients who have this tumor complain of a palpable mass rather than pain.
- Cervical spondylosis and radiculopathy
- Periscapular muscle strain
- Glenohumeral pathology

NONOPERATIVE MANAGEMENT

- The initial management of snapping scapula syndrome, once the diagnosis has been made, is conservative.
- Rest, activity modification, and nonsteroidal anti-inflammatory medications should be started.
- Next, physical therapy should be initiated to restore the normal kinematics of the shoulder and prevent it from sloping.
- Weakness in the serratus anterior, even if subtle, may lead to tilting of the scapula forward, thus increasing the friction and rubbing of the upper medial pole of the scapula on the thoracic ribs. This will cause irritation and inflammation of the scapulothoracic bursae.
- Therapy should emphasize periscapular muscle strengthening, particularly the serratus anterior and subscapulari, which can elevate the scapula off the chest wall when they are hypertrophied.[1,17]
- Taping, a figure-8 harness, scapulothoracic bracing, or postural training can serve to minimize shoulder sloping and thoracic kyphosis.
- Injection of corticosteroid and local anesthetic into the scapulothoracic bursa can be diagnostic and also may be therapeutic and helpful in the rehabilitation program.
- There is no consensus on how long the patient should be kept on trial of physical therapy. The underlying diagnosis is important. In general, a 3- to 6-month trial is a good estimate.
- If the diagnosis is certain, no structural anatomic lesion is present, and the patient has failed 3 to 6 months of appropriate conservative treatment, then surgical options should be considered.
- The threshold to proceed to surgical intervention also should be much lower if the patient has a real structural lesion such as a bony exostosis or an osteochondroma.

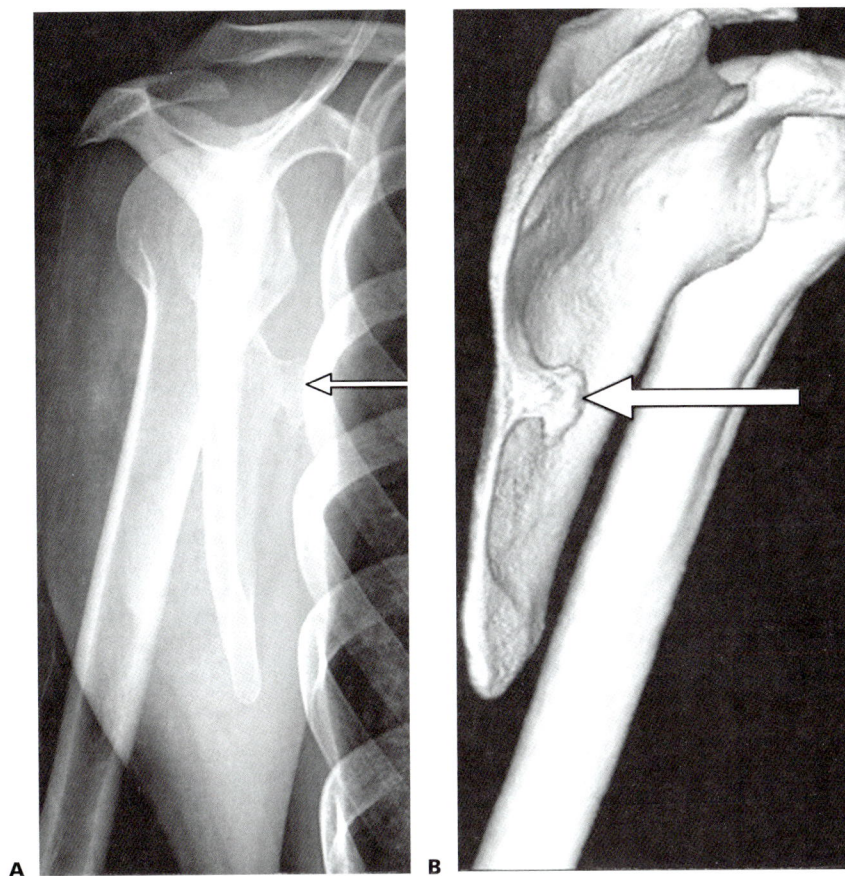

FIG 3 • **A.** A Y-scapular view showing a prominent osteochondroma (*arrow*) of the body of the scapula, causing symptomatic snapping. **B.** A three-dimensional CT scan shows the bony anatomy in more detail. The arrow points to the same osteochondroma.

SURGICAL MANAGEMENT

Preoperative Planning

- All radiographs are reviewed before surgery.
- The decision to operate is made based on relief of pain with anesthetic injection into the scapulothoracic region in patients who failed conservative management, or in patients who have symptomatic snapping scapula syndrome secondary to structural lesion.
- The different surgical approaches, as well as the technique that the surgeon decides to perform, are discussed with the patient before surgery.

Positioning

- The patient is positioned in the prone position for both arthroscopic and open techniques (**FIG 4**).
- The involved arm is placed in internal rotation against the patient's lower back (chicken-wing position). This will cause the scapula to wing out from the thorax and make the superomedial angle more prominent.
- The surgeon stands on the side opposite the scapula to be operated to get the best access to the surgical field.

Approach

- Multiple surgical approaches are available that can decompress the impingement in the superomedial region of the scapula.

- These include open surgical decompression, arthroscopic surgical decompression, or a combination of the two approaches.
- Each of these approaches may include bursectomy alone, bony resection of the superomedial aspect of the scapula alone, or a combination.

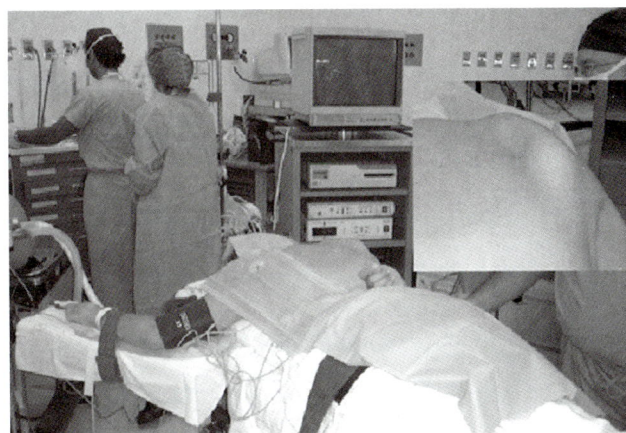

FIG 4 • The operating room setup for arthroscopic scapulothoracic bursectomy. The patient is positioned prone with the hand of the involved shoulder placed behind the back in order to lift the scapula off the chest wall.

OPEN DECOMPRESSION

- A longitudinal incision is made along the medial scapular edge (**TECH FIG 1A**).
- Subcutaneous undermining is performed to expose the superior portion of the scapula, from the level of the scapula spine to the superomedial angle of the scapula.
- Splitting and elevation of the trapezius in line with its fibers is performed at the level of the scapular spine, and

the superomedial edge of the scapula is exposed (**TECH FIG 1B**).

- The levator scapulae and rhomboids are detached from the superior and medial edge of the scapula to expose the upper scapula border (**TECH FIG 1C**).
- Care is taken not to dissect into the rhomboids or fully detach them so as not to injure the dorsal scapular nerve,

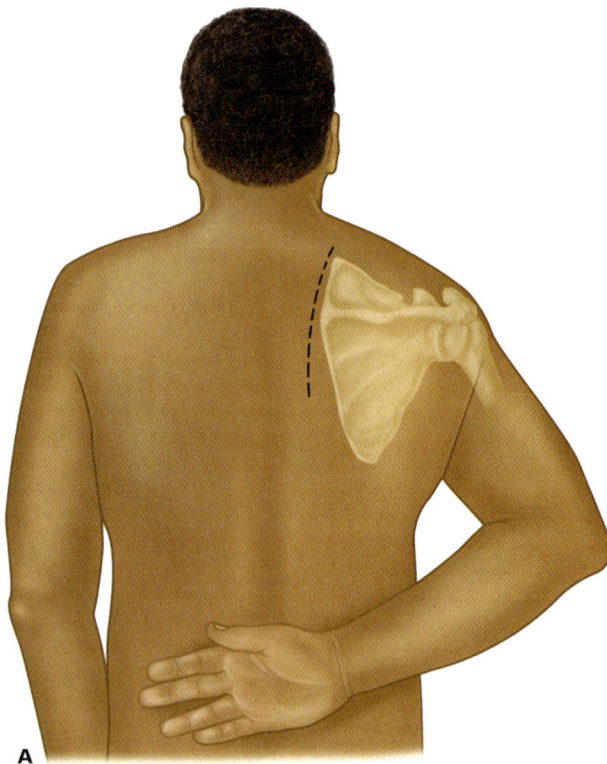

A

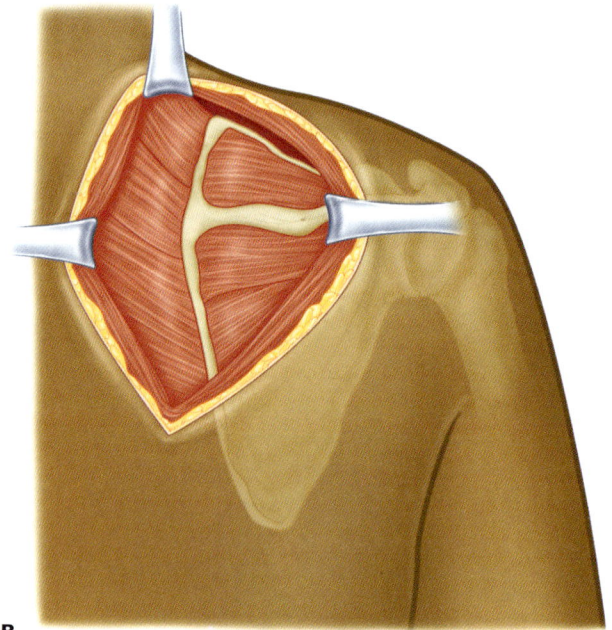

B

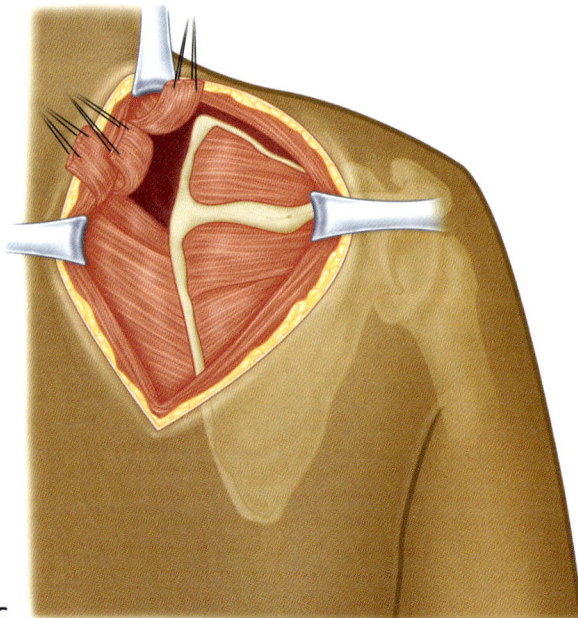

C

TECH FIG 1 • **A.** Patient positioned prone with hand positioned behind back to lift the scapula off the chest wall. The surgical incision is placed over the medial border of the scapula, centered over the level of the scapula spine. **B.** The trapezius is split along its fibers, and the levator scapulae, the rhomboids, and the posterior surface of the scapula are exposed. **C.** The levator scapulae, rhomboid major, and rhomboid minor are detached from their insertion on the scapula and tagged with sutures. *(continued)*

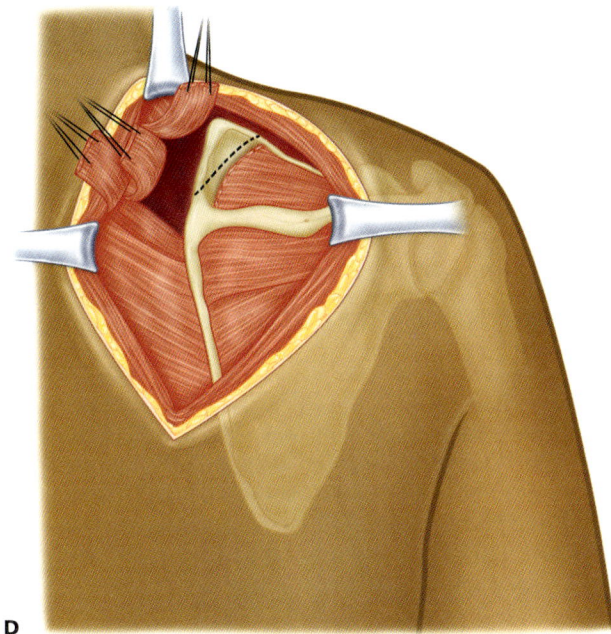

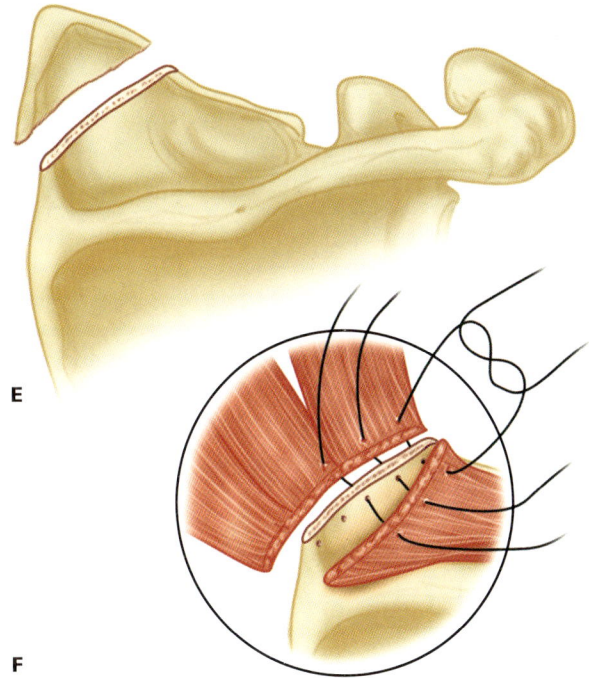

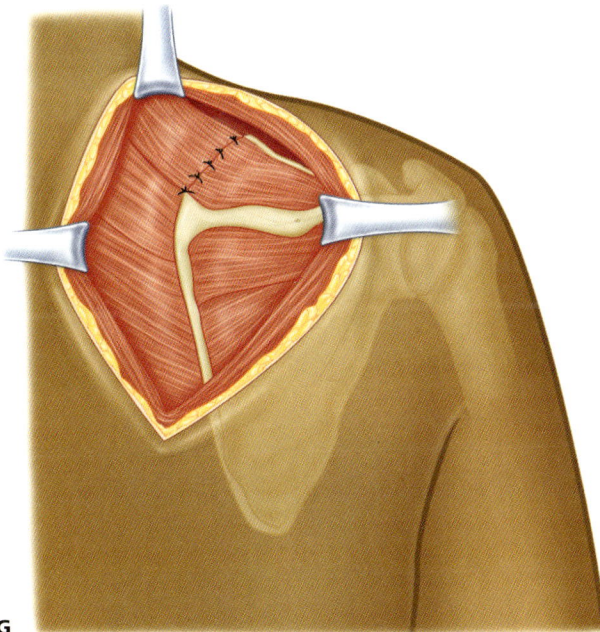

TECH FIG 1 • *(continued)* **D,E.** Resection of the superomedial border of the scapula. **F.** The detached muscles are reattached to the scapula through drill holes. **G.** The final repair of the detached levator scapulae and rhomboids.

which usually is located 2 cm medial to the medial scapular edge.

- The serratus anterior muscle is left intact.
- A retractor is placed underneath the scapula to lift it away from the thoracic ribs.
- The scapulothoracic bursa is identified against the ribs, underneath the serratus anterior muscle.
- A clamp is used to grasp the bursa, and sharp excision of it is performed from superior to inferior.
- Subperiosteal elevation of the muscles around the superomedial border of the scapula, including the supraspinatus, infraspinatus, subscapularis, and serratus

anterior muscles, is performed with the use of electocautery to expose 1 to 2 cm of bone (**TECH FIG 1D**).

- This exposed portion of the superomedial portion of the scapula is resected with use of an oscillating saw (**TECH FIG 1E**).
- Once the bony resection is accomplished, drill holes are placed into the upper-medial border of the scapula in order to reattach the muscles to their anatomic insertion (**TECH FIG 1F**) using a no. 2 nonabsorbable braided suture (**TECH FIG 1G**).
- The skin is closed with absorbable subcuticular suture.

ARTHROSCOPIC BURSECTOMY

- Positioning is the same as in open decompression.
- Placement of the arm in the chicken-wing position results in scapula winging and protraction off the posterior thorax, which facilitates the entry of the arthroscopic instruments in the bursal space.
- Standard arthroscopic portals are used.
- The initial "safe" portal is placed at the level of the scapular spine, 2 cm medial to the scapular edge, to avoid injury to the dorsal scapular nerve and artery (**TECH FIG 2A**).
- The scapulothoracic space is localized with a spinal needle and distended with approximately 30 mL of saline, and the portal is created.
- A blunt obturator is inserted into the scapulothoracic (subserratus) bursa between the posterior thoracic wall and the serratus anterior muscle.
- Care should be taken to avoid overpenetration through the serratus anterior into the subscapular space or through the chest wall.
- A 30-degree arthroscope is inserted into the scapulothoracic space, which was distended with fluid infiltration.
- Use of a fluid pump is optional. Our preference is to use an arthroscopy pump but keep the pressure low, at around 30 mm Hg, to minimize fluid extravasation.
- A spinal needle is used to localize the second portal under direct visualization.

- This portal is inserted, in most instances, in line with and approximately 4 cm distal to the first portal.
- A bipolar radiofrequency device and a motorized shaver are introduced into a 6-mm cannula through the lower portal, and used to resect the bursal tissue. Because the inflamed scapulothoracic bursa is a potential source of bleeding during arthroscopic shaving, the radiofrequency device becomes particularly useful to minimize bleeding in these tissues (**TECH FIG 2B**).
- A methodic approach to resection should be followed, because there are no real landmarks.
- Ablation of tissues should be performed from medial to lateral and then from inferior to superior.
- The surgeon should be ready to switch portals and should have a 70-degree athroscope ready to facilitate visualization. A probe can be used to palpate the scapula and serratus muscle superiorly and the ribs and intercostal muscles inferiorly.
- An additional superior portal may be placed as needed. We prefer not to use this portal, because it may place the accessory spinal nerve, transverse cervical artery, and dorsal scapular neurovascular structures at risk.
- After complete bursectomy is performed, the arthroscopic instruments are withdrawn, and skin closure is performed with absorbable subcuticular sutures.

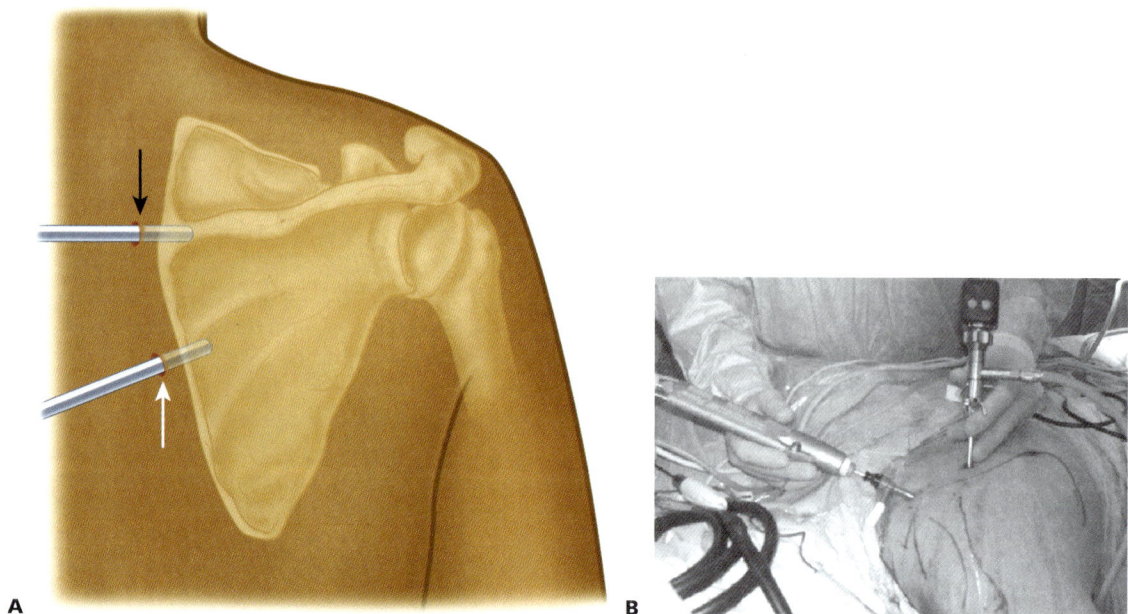

TECH FIG 2 • A. Locations of the arthroscopic portals. A proximal (safe) portal (*black arrow*) is placed 2 cm medial to the spine of the scapula. A distal portal (*white arrow*) is placed in line with and 4 cm distal to the proximal portal. **B.** Sites of portal placement. The shaver and the camera can be placed interchangeably in either portal for viewing and shaving.

ARTHROSCOPIC BURSECTOMY AND PARTIAL SUPEROMEDIAL SCAPULECTOMY

- First, all the steps for arthroscopic bursectomy are followed.
- After the bursa has been completely resected, the superomedial angle of the scapula is localized by palpation through the skin.
- Detachment of the conjoined insertion of the levator scapulae, supraspinatus, and rhomboids is performed with the use of the radiofrequency device.
- A motorized shaver and a burr are used to perform a partial scapulectomy. We do not attempt to repair the periosteal sleeve; it is allowed to heal through scarring.
- The rest of the steps are the same as those for arthroscopic bursectomy.

ARTHROSCOPIC BURSECTOMY AND OPEN PARTIAL SUPEROMEDIAL SCAPULECTOMY

- The decision to perform the superomedial scapular bony resection through a small skin incision rather than through the arthroscope may be made either before surgery or at the time of surgery.
- If full definition of the superomedial border of the scapula becomes difficult because of swelling from the arthroscopic fluid, then bony resection is performed through a small skin incision.
- A 4- to 6-cm incision is performed obliquely over the superomedial border of the scapula (see Tech Fig 1A).
- The trapezius muscle is split, and the levator scapulae and rhomboids are detached from the superomedial angle (see Tech Fig 1B,C).
- The superomedial angle of the scapula is resected. Then the levator scapulae and rhomboids are repaired to the superior scapula through drill holes (see Tech Fig 1D).
- Skin closure is performed with absorbable subcuticular sutures.

PEARLS AND PITFALLS

Indications	▪ Appropriate history, physical examination, and review of radiographs should be done. ▪ Diagnostic injection is very helpful to confirm the diagnosis and predict a good surgical outcome.
Contraindications to arthroscopic decompression	▪ Symptoms that originate from the trapezoid bursa. This bursa is superficial to the scapulothoracic space, and, therefore, removing it will not remove the pathologic tissue.
Positioning	▪ Patient prone, with hand of the affected shoulder behind the back to elevate and protract the scapula. ▪ Surgeon should be standing by the opposite shoulder.
Open decompression	▪ Avoid suprascapular notch during bony resection. ▪ It is essential to reattach the detached muscles to the scapula through bony drill holes.
Arthroscopic decompression	▪ Use a spinal needle for localization of the scapulothoracic space. ▪ Care should be taken to avoid over-penetration through the serratus anterior into the subscapular space or through the chest wall. ▪ Use of a bipolar radiofrequency device is essential to avoid bleeding from the inflamed bursa. ▪ Complete bursectomy should be performed.

POSTOPERATIVE CARE

- After open decompression and a combined arthroscopic and open approach:
  - The patient is kept in a sling, and gentle, passive range of motion is started early after surgery and continued for 4 weeks.
  - After 4 weeks, active range of motion is started.
  - Strengthening is allowed at 8 to 12 weeks.
- After arthroscopic decompression:
  - The patient is kept in a sling and allowed passive and active assisted range-of-motion exercises immediately after surgery.
  - After 4 weeks, isometric exercises are started.
  - Strengthening of the periscapular muscles begins by 8 weeks.

OUTCOMES

- No published reports have compared the outcomes of different surgical techniques of scapulothoracic decompression.

- The outcome of open decompression, as reported in the literature, has been good.[7,12,17,18]
- No large series have been published reporting the outcome of arthroscopic scapulothoracic decompression for symptomatic snapping scapular syndrome.
- Early results from small series of patients who underwent arthroscopic decompression seem promising, with minimal morbidity and early return to work.[2,5,8,15,16]

COMPLICATIONS

- Recurrence of symptoms secondary to incomplete resection
- Pneumothorax
- Iatrogenic injury to the neurovascular structures around the superomedial border of the scapula
- Aggressive bony resection risking injury to the suprascapular nerve through the notch
- Insufficiency of the scapular muscles due to detachment after surgery

REFERENCES

1. Carlson HL, Haig AJ, Stewart DC. Snapping scapula syndrome: three case reports and an analysis of the literature. Arch Phys Med Rehabil 1997;78:506–511.
2. Chan BK, Chakrabarti AJ, Bell SN. An alternative portal for scapulothoracic arthroscopy. J Shoulder Elbow Surg 2002;11:235–240.
3. Ciullo JV, Jones E. Subscapular bursitis: conservative treatment of "snapping scapula" or "wash-board syndrome." Orthop Trans 1992–1993;16:740.
4. Glousman R, Jobe F, Tibone J, et al. Dynamic electomyographic analysis of the throwing shoulder with glenohumeral instability. J Bone Joint Surg Am 1988;70A:220.
5. Harper GD, McIlroy S, Bayley JI. Arthroscopic partial resection of the scapula for snapping scapula: a new technique. J Shoulder Elbow Surg 1999;8:53–58.
6. Kolodychuk LB, Reagan WD. Visualization of the scapulothoracique articulation using an arthroscope: A proposed technique. Orthop Trans 1993–1994;17:1142–1148.
7. Kuhn JE, Plancher KD, Hawkins RJ. Symptomatic scapulothoracique crepitus and bursitis. J Am Acad Orthop Surg 1998;6:267–272.
8. Lehtinen JT, Cassinelli E, Warner JJ. The painful scapulothoracic articulation. Clin Orthop Relat Res 2004;423:99–105.
9. Manske RC, Reiman MP, Stovak ML. Nonoperative and operative management of snapping scapula. Am J Sports Med 2004;32:1554–1565.
10. Milch H. Partial scapulectomy for snapping of the scapula. J Bone Joint Surg Am 1950;32A:561–566.
11. Milch H, Burman MS. Snapping scapula and humerus varus: report of six cases. Arch Surg 1933;26:570–588.
12. Morse BJ, Ebraheim NA, Jackson WT. Partial scapulectomy for snapping scapula syndrome. Orthop Rev Relat Res 1993;22:1141–1144.
13. Mozes G, Bickels J, Ovadia D, et al. The use of three-dimensional computed tomography in evaluating snapping scapula syndrome. Orthopedics 1999;22:1029.
14. Parsons TA. The snapping scapula syndrome and subscapular exostoses. J Bone Joint Surg Br 1973;55B:345–349.
15. Pavlik A, Ang K, Coghlan J, et al. Arthroscopic treatment of painful snapping of the scapula by using a new superior portal. Arthroscopy 2003;19:608–611.
16. Pearse EO, Bruguera J, Massoud S, et al. Arthroscopic management of the painful scapula. Arthroscopy 2006;22:755–761.
17. Percy EL, Birbrager D, Pitt MJ. Scapping scapula: a review of the literature and presentation of 14 patients. Can J Surg 1988;31:248.
18. Richards RR, McKee MD. Treatment of painful scapulothoracic crepitus by resection of the superomedial angle of the scapula: a report of three cases. Clin Orthop Relat Res 1989:247:111–116.
19. Ruland LJ III, Ruland CM, Matthews LS. Scapulothoracic anatomy for the arthroscopist. Arthroscopy 1995;11:52.
20. Sisto DJ, Jobe FW. The operative treatment of scapulothoracic bursitis in professional pitchers. Am J Sports Med 1986;14:192.
21. Strizak AM, Cowen MH. The snapping scapula syndrome: a case report. J Bone Joint Surg Am 1982;64A:941–942.
22. Warner JJ, Micheli LJ, Arslanian LE, et al. Scapulothoracic motion in normal shoulder and shoulders with glenohumeral instability and impingement syndrome. A study using Moire topographic analysis. Clin Orthop Relat Res 1992;(285):191.
23. Williams JJ, Micheli LJ, Arslanian LE, et al. Scapulothoracic motion in normal shoulders with glenohumeral instability and impingement syndrome. A study using Moire topographic analysis. Clin Orthop Relat Res 1992;285:191–198.
24. Wood VE, Verska JM. The snapping scapula in association with the thoracic outlet syndrome. Arch Surg 1989;124:1335–1337.

Eden-Lange Procedure for Trapezius Palsy

Jonathan H. Lee and William N. Levine

DEFINITION

- Trapezius palsy results from a disruption of cranial nerve (CN) XI, also known as the *spinal accessory nerve.*
- Because the trapezius is innervated exclusively by CN XI, any disruption causes trapezius palsy.
- Spinal accessory nerve palsy is a rare but well-described complication of cervical lymph node biopsy.[15,17]
- The trapezius plays an integral part in stabilization of the scapula, and dysfunction leads to painful shoulder disability.
- Nonoperative treatment, including strengthening of the functioning thoracoscapular muscles, does not provide satisfactory clinical results.[2,4]
- Transfer of the levator scapulae, rhomboid major, and rhomboid minor (Eden-Lange procedure, or triple transfer) is an accepted technique for this difficult problem.[16]
- The procedure was first described by Eden[5] in 1924 and then corroborated by Lange[9] in 1951 and Francillon[7] in 1955, all reporting satisfactory short-term results. Further modifications have improved on the initial procedure.[1]
- Lateral transfer of the insertions of the three muscles allows the scapula to be stabilized in a position of abduction and anterior flexion.[15]

ANATOMY

- The trapezius muscle is broad and superficial, taking its origin from the C7–T12 spinous processes and inserting on the acromion, clavicle, and spine of the scapula (**FIG 1A**).
- Its function is to elevate and rotate the scapula; absence of the trapezius leads to lateral winging of the scapula.
- In the posterior cervical triangle, CN XI is located in the subcutaneous tissue; this superficial location renders it susceptible to damage during procedures such as cervical lymph node biopsy.
- Functionally, the trapezius can be divided into three separate parts: upper, middle, and lower.
- The upper portion consists of descending fibers and functions as an aid to suspension of the shoulder girdle, allowing shrugging of the shoulder. The middle portion consists of transverse fibers and contributes to abduction and rotation of the inferior angle of the scapula. The ascending fibers of the lower portion (along with the serratus anterior) anchor the scapula to the chest wall.
- Scapular winging occurs in both spinal accessory and serratus anterior palsy. In serratus palsy, the inferior angle of the scapula is noted to rotate medially (**FIG 1B**), whereas in trapezius palsy, the scapula rotates laterally (**FIG 1C,D**).

PATHOGENESIS

- Paralysis of the trapezius most often results from injury to the spinal accessory nerve during cervical lymph node biopsy.[13]
- Other causes include trauma (including traction injuries) or injuries from other surgical procedures, such as radical neck dissection.[1]

- In one instance, a CN XI palsy was reported to have occurred after a viral infection.[13]
- Idiopathic CN XI paralysis also has been reported.[6]
- Patterson[11] reported trapezius palsy after acromioclavicular and sternoclavicular dissociation.
- Even rarer causes include post-carotid endarterectomy and post-catheterization of the internal jugular vein.[3]
- In most cases, patients report pain and present with visible deformity and dysfunction of the shoulder girdle.

NATURAL HISTORY

- Trapezius palsy most often results from iatrogenic causes, as noted earlier, and, if left untreated, will lead to progressively worsening altered biomechanics and pain of the shoulder girdle.
- Radiating arm pain is thought to be the result of traction on the brachial plexus caused by drooping of the shoulder girdle.[13]

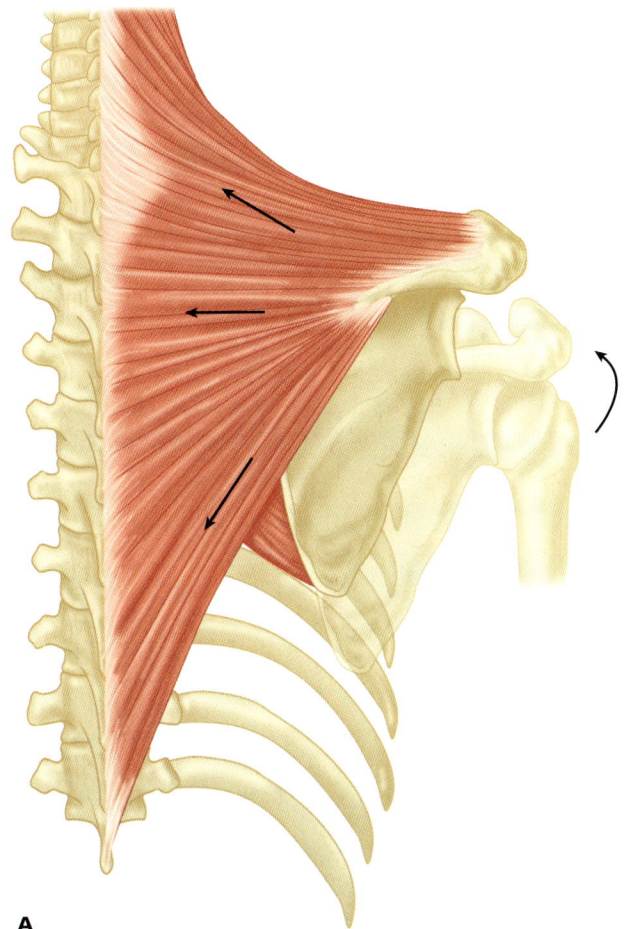

FIG 1 • A. Schematic of the three parts of the normal trapezius muscle: upper, middle, and lower. *(continued)*

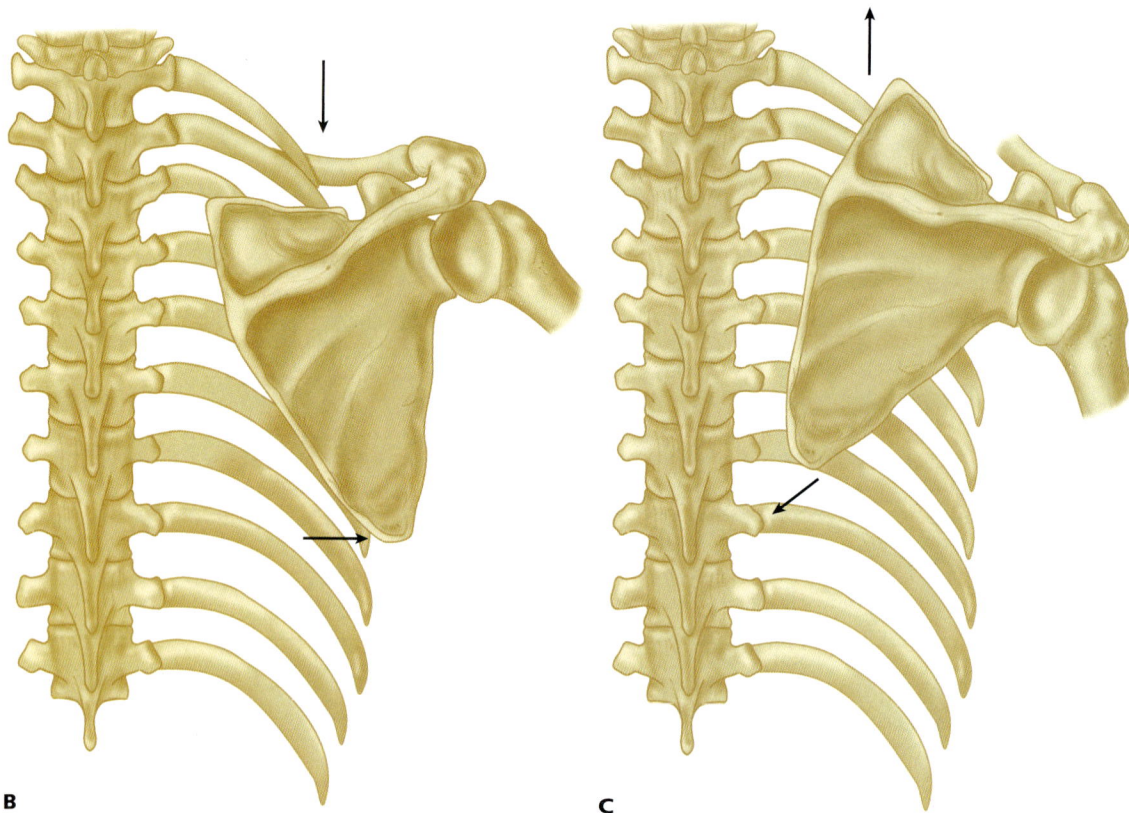

B   C

FIG 1 • *(continued)* **B.** Schematic of trapezius palsy, demonstrating lateral scapular winging and shoulder drooping. **C.** Schematic of serratus anterior palsy, demonstrating medial scapular winging.

■ Although nonoperative management can provide reduction of pain, it does not lead to return of function, and patients treated without surgery usually go on to progressive shoulder dysfunction.

■ Typically, the initial presentation is acute shoulder pain without palsy, with weakness of anterior elevation and abduction appearing after a few days (with slow diminution of pain). Atrophy of the trapezius becomes clinically apparent after a few weeks.[16]

PATIENT HISTORY AND PHYSICAL FINDINGS

■ Altered mechanics of the entire shoulder girdle are possible with trapezius palsy.

■ The classic winging of the scapula seen in CN XI palsy is characterized by downward and lateral translation of the scapula.

■ The patient should be observed from behind so comparison can be made with the contralateral side.

■ Signs unique to CN XI palsy include lateral winging of the scapula (**FIG 2A**), an asymmetric neckline, pain, weakness of shoulder abduction, and forward elevation.[14] Visible atrophy of the trapezius muscle should be noted[16] (**FIG 2B**).

■ Symptoms include weakness made worse by prolonged use of the arm, a feeling of a heavy arm, and a dull pain radiating from the scapula to the forearm (and occasionally with radiation to the hand). The radiation of pain is described as mimicking thoracic outlet syndrome (medial aspect of the upper limb). Pain typically is made worse by abduction of the shoulder as

well as forward elevation.[16] Some patients also reported paresthesias in the distribution of the auricular nerve (posterolateral side of the neck).[16]

■ Patients also often state that the arm feels difficult to control.[13]

■ It should be noted, however, that occasionally patients are pain free and present only with winging and drooping of the scapula.

■ Range of motion is decreased in elevation as well as abduction, and typically is limited to 90 degrees.[13] Teboul et al[16] report average active abduction of 78 degrees (range 30 to 140 degrees), and active forward flexion of 110 degrees (range 50 to 180 degrees). As a result, overhead activities are not possible, nor is shrugging of the shoulder.

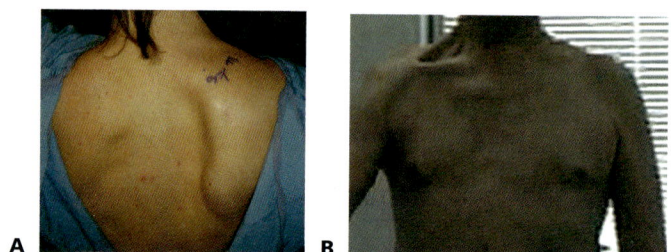

A   B

FIG 2 • **A.** Patient with a trapezius palsy demonstrating characteristic scapular winging. **B.** Anterior sternocleidomastoid muscle wasting due to the spinal accessory nerve palsy.

- External rotation of the shoulder and elbow flexion are not affected by CN XI lesions.[16]
- Reports of stiffness and passive range of motion are somewhat contradictory in the literature. Romero and Gerber[13] state that patients did not always present with a stiff shoulder but passive range of motion typically was decreased. On the other hand, Teboul et al[16] report that patients often presented with stiffness but with no deficit in passive range of motion.
- Often, the diagnosis of CN XI dysfunction is one of exclusion, and it is not until an unsuccessful trial of physical therapy that a patient is referred for an electrodiagnostic study and spinal accessory nerve palsy is confirmed.
- The necessity for electrodiagnostic testing is an issue of debate in the literature. Romero and Gerber[13] state that this testing is not necessary to establish the diagnosis of CN XI palsy, but that it can be a valuable tool if other nerve lesions are suspected. Setter et al[14] advocate electrodiagnostic testing as part of the initial workup.
- Evaluate the scapula for signs of lateral translation by asking patient to perform a wall push-up.
- Spinal accessory nerve (CN XI) palsy also affects the sternocleidomastoid muscle.

IMAGING AND OTHER DIAGNOSTIC STUDIES

- A standard five-view shoulder series (including true AP views of the glenohumeral joint in neutral, external, and internal rotation; as well as a scapular Y and axillary view) is required for every patient, although osseous pathology typically is not associated with CN XI palsy.
- MRI is not necessary, although it could be useful to assess the degree of fatty atrophy of the trapezius muscle as well as to help rule out any associated pathology such as rotator cuff injury.
- Electrodiagnostic testing is recommended in every case, according to Setter et al.[14] Not only will an EMG help confirm the diagnosis of spinal accessory nerve palsy, but it also will serve as confirmation that the muscles to be used in the transfer procedure are functioning normally.

DIFFERENTIAL DIAGNOSIS

- Missed diagnosis of spinal accessory nerve palsy is the rule,[13] most likely owing to the rare nature of the condition.
- Other possible types of shoulder dysfunction that may confuse the issue include serratus palsy and rotator cuff pathology.
- It is crucial to be able to differentiate between spinal accessory nerve (trapezius) palsy and long thoracic nerve (serratus) palsy. In serratus palsy, the inferior angle of the scapula rotates medially, whereas in trapezius palsy, the inferior angle of the scapula rotates laterally.

NONOPERATIVE MANAGEMENT

- Typically, if the injury is not detected within 6 months (after which point nerve repair usually is not recommended), a 12-month trial of nonoperative treatment is recommended.[14]
- Due to possible compensation by the levator scapulae, the impact of injury to the spinal accessory nerve must be determined individually for each patient.[8]
- Maxillofacial surgeons have reported that 30% to 49% of patients do not exhibit any clinical symptoms after radical neck dissection where the spinal accessory nerve is sacrificed.[10]

- If the CN XI palsy is symptomatic, pain sometimes can be relieved after a course of nonoperative treatment, but satisfactory return to function cannot be achieved.
- Strengthening of the remaining scapulothoracic muscles does not compensate for the trapezius deficit, and, in one study, patients who elected nonoperative management could not elevate their arms above the horizontal.[13]
- One study has reported favorable results with nonoperative management in sedentary or elderly persons because discomfort was alleviated.[12]

SURGICAL MANAGEMENT

- If trapezius palsy is detected early, microsurgical repair or reconstruction of the nerve can be considered. Timing of the repair attempt is controversial; some authors believe that repair should only be attempted if diagnosis is confirmed within 6 months of injury,[14] whereas other surgeons advocate repair up to 20 months from the time of the nerve insult.[16]
- In patients with spontaneous spinal accessory palsy for whom conservative treatment has not been helpful, some authors advocate proceeding directly to muscle transfer reconstruction, because nerve procedures have produced poor results.[15]
- Patients who have failed nerve repair attempt or conservative therapy should be considered surgical candidates for the Eden-Lange procedure, the current procedure of choice for stabilization of the scapula after CN XI palsy.
- Timing of the Eden-Lange procedure also is controversial. Typically, however, reconstructive surgery is recommended if more than 12 months has elapsed since the injury.[17]
- The goal of the Eden-Lange procedure is to reconstruct the three parts of the trapezius muscle. Because the rhomboid major and minor and levator scapulae have medial insertions, they are not capable of stabilizing the scapula unless they are transferred laterally.[16]

Preoperative Planning

- It is imperative to have appropriate preoperative discussions with the patient so that he or she understands the procedure, the postoperative rehabilitation program, and the timeframe within which improvement should be expected.

Positioning

- The patient is placed in the lateral decubitus position with thoracic, pubic, and sacral supports.[15,16] The entire upper extremity, including the shoulder girdle, should be draped free (**FIG 3**).

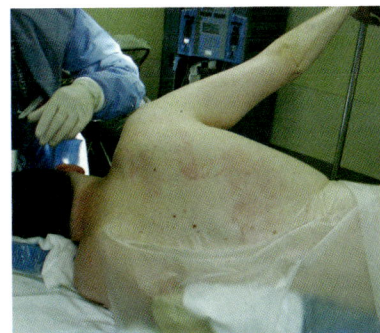

FIG 3 • The patient is placed in the lateral decubitus position with the entire extremity draped free.

EXPOSURE

- Teboul et al[16] describe an incision starting from the spine of the scapula and progressing along its medial angle up to a point 2 cm above the inferior angle of the scapula (**TECH FIG 1A**).
- The trapezius is then divided and retracted, and the three muscles of interest (the levator scapulae, rhomboid major, and rhomboid minor) are identified and dissected and marked with vessel loops (**TECH FIG 1B**).
- The supraspinatus and infraspinatus must be elevated 3 to 5 cm to expose their respective fossae for transfer of the rhomboids[16] (**TECH FIG 1C**).

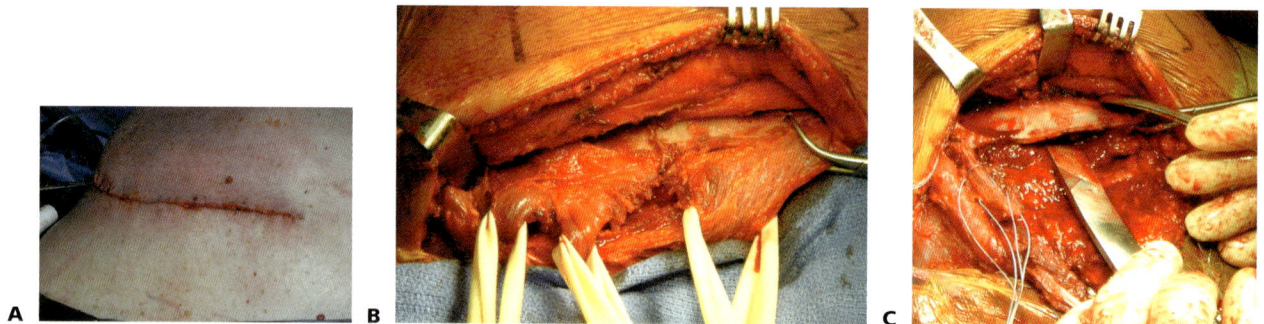

TECH FIG 1 • A. The major incision is made along the medial border of the scapula, extending superiorly to allow exposure to the levator scapula, rhomboid minor, and rhomboid major for their planned transfers. **B.** The levator scapula, rhomboid minor, and rhomboid major are identified and individually released from their scapular attachment sites for lateral transfer. **C.** The supraspinatus and infraspinatus are elevated at least 5 cm medially to allow appropriate exposure of the scapula.

RHOMBOID TRANSFER

- A series of transosseous mattress sutures are placed in anticipation of transferring the rhomboids. At least four mattress sutures are used in the infraspinous fossa (**TECH FIG 2A**) and two in the supraspinous fossa.
- The rhomboids are advanced about 3 cm laterally and attached to the scapula with heavy, nonabsorbable transosseous sutures (**TECH FIG 2B**).

Modification

- Bigliani et al[1] proposed a modification of the procedure in which the rhomboid minor is transferred cephalad to the scapular spine, thereby closing the gap between the rhomboid minor and the levator scapulae (**TECH FIG 3**).
- In this modification, the new position of the rhomboid minor more efficiently substitutes for the middle part of the trapezius.

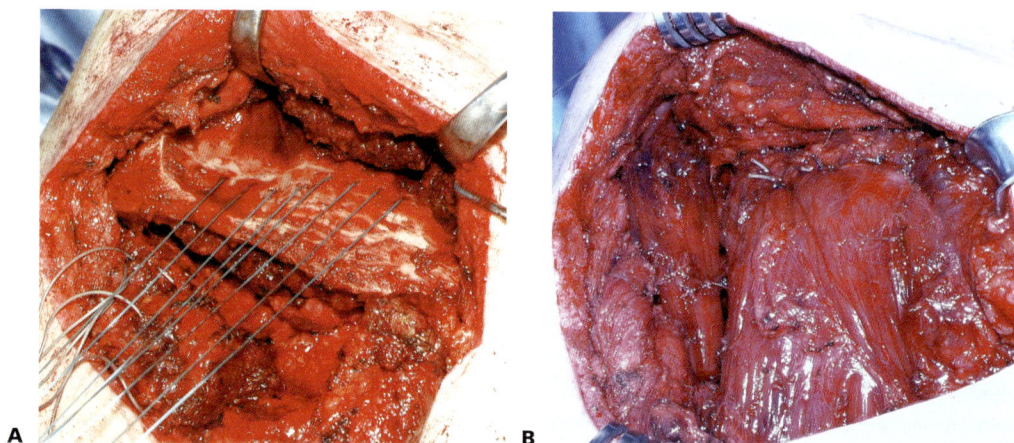

TECH FIG 2 • A. A series of drill holes are made, and transosseous sutures are placed in preparation for securing the transferred muscles. **B.** The rhomboid minor and major are transferred to the supra- and infraspinous fossae, respectively.

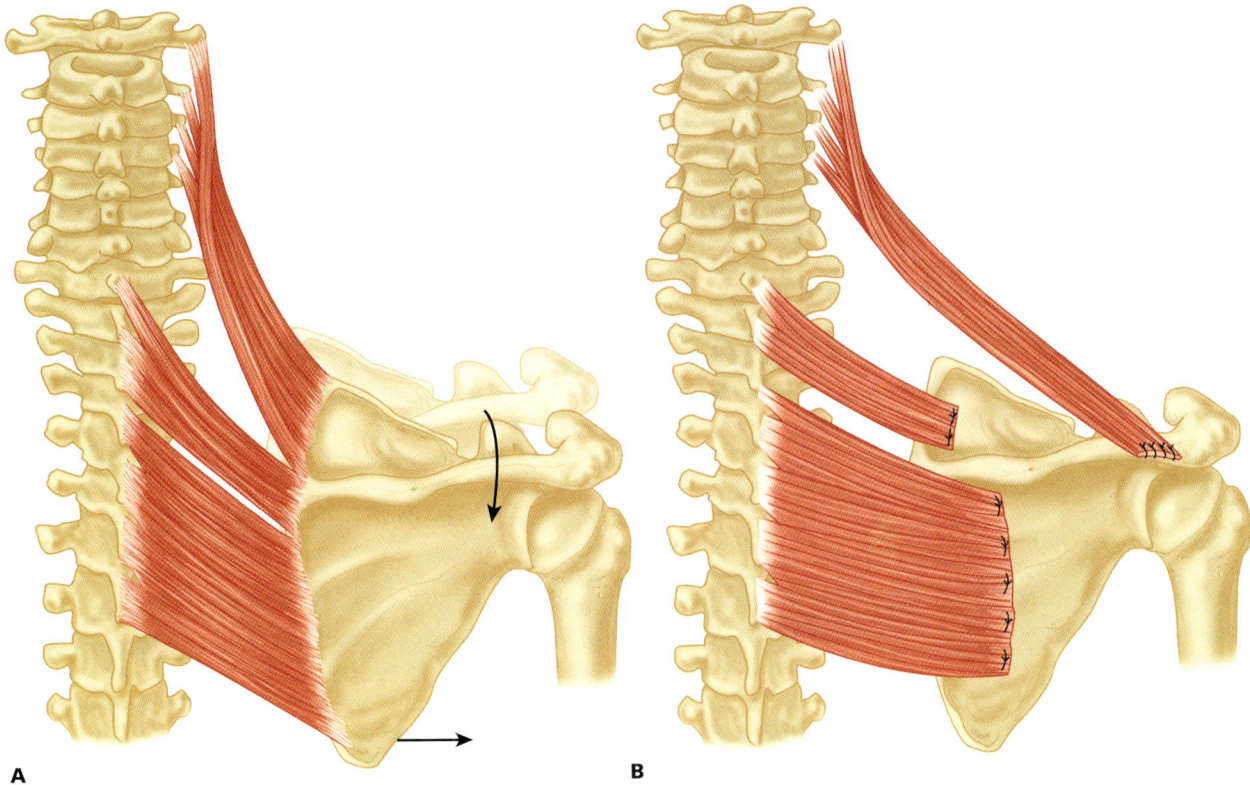

TECH FIG 3 • **A.** Normal position of the levator scapula, rhomboid minor, and rhomboid major on the medial border of the scapula. **B.** Lateral transfer of the levator scapula, rhomboid minor, and rhomboid major. This modification includes transfer of the rhomboid minor to the supraspinatus fossa.

LEVATOR TRANSFER AND WOUND CLOSURE

- A second incision is made about 5 to 7 cm from the posterolateral corner of the acromion for transfer of the levator scapulae (**TECH FIG 4A**).
- Care must be taken to ensure that the levator has been dissected laterally enough to allow tension-free excursion to the scapular spine (**TECH FIG 4B**). The levator is then transferred subcutaneously and affixed with a series of heavy nonabsorbable sutures.
- The infraspinatus muscle is then sutured over the new rhomboid muscle insertions and, finally, the wounds are closed in layers.

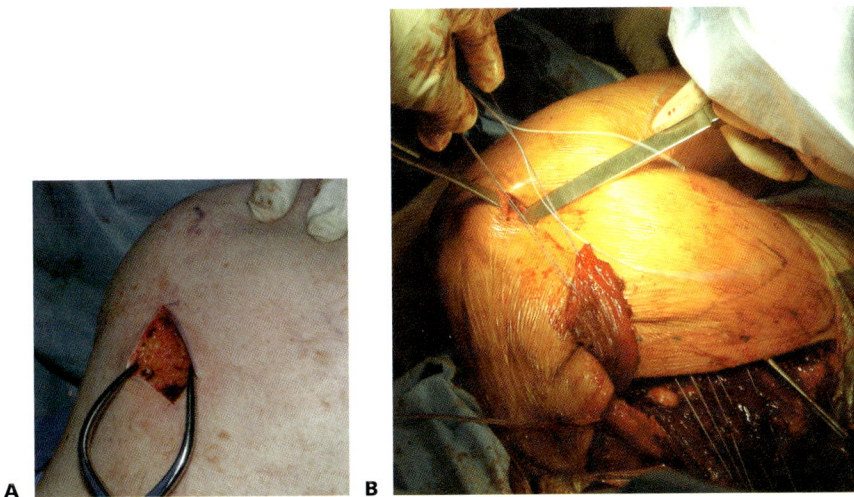

TECH FIG 4 • **A.** The second incision is made 5 to 7 cm medial to the posterolateral corner of the acromion for transfer of the levator scapula muscle. **B.** Excursion of the levator is confirmed before the muscle is subcutaneously tunneled to the planned transfer site.

TECHNIQUES

PEARLS AND PITFALLS

Rhomboid transfer	■ Separate the rhomboid minor from the rhomboid major so they can be transferred separately. ■ The infraspinatus and supraspinatus are elevated from their respective fossae for approximately 5 cm. This modification of the original procedure permits the rhomboid minor to be transferred to a position that better substitutes for the action of the middle trapezius. ■ Care should be taken to prevent injury to the suprascapular nerve, which lies on the deep surface of the supraspinatus muscle.
Levator transfer	■ Dissect the levator scapula far enough laterally to allow tension-free transfer to the scapular spine. ■ Avoid iatrogenic injury to the transverse cervical artery and the dorsal scapular nerve, which run superficial and deep, respectively, to the levator scapulae and then terminate into the deep surface of the rhomboids near their insertion onto the scapula. ■ A tunnel is created through the atrophied trapezius, in line with its upper fibers, for passage of the tagged levator scapulae. ■ The levator should not be transferred too far laterally, because this can cause a web-like deformity in the neck. A good position is 5 to 7 cm from the posterior lateral corner of the acromion.

POSTOPERATIVE CARE

■ Most authors advocate immobilization for 6 weeks postoperatively, followed by initiation of physical therapy (passive and active).[13,14,16]

■ Romero and Gerber[13] prefer an abduction splint, whereas Teboul et al[16] suggest securing the arm to the chest with an elastic bandage.

■ Our routine postoperative protocol is to use a foam wedge or orthosis for the first 4 weeks, keeping the arm in 60 to 70 degrees of abduction. We encourage early passive range of motion above the wedge or orthosis to prevent stiffness (forward elevation to 130 degrees and external rotation to 40 degrees in the first 4 weeks).

■ At 4 weeks, the wedge is discontinued, and gentle strengthening exercises are added. We have designed a progressive strengthening program that uses rubber tubing, free weights, and medicine ball throws to achieve dynamic scapular stability. All of the exercises in the protocol are designed to strengthen the transferred levator scapula and rhomboids.

OUTCOMES

■ The Eden-Lange procedure produces satisfactory results for the difficult problem of trapezius palsy.

■ In a study in which 16 patients were reviewed at a mean follow-up of 32 years, clinical outcomes were noted to be excellent in 9 patients, fair in 2 patients, and poor in 1 patient (as determined by Constant score).[13] Some patients with outcomes that were less than satisfactory also had dorsal scapular and long thoracic lesions.

■ Romero and Gerber[13] describe a radiographic outcomes measure that uses an AP radiograph to measure the angle between a line drawn between the cranial and caudal ends of the glenoid with a vertical axial line. This measurement was compared to the contralateral side, and no statistical differences were found.

■ Another recent study[16] concluded that muscle transfer should be performed only after previous nerve repair surgery had failed or when more than 20 months has elapsed since the injury was incurred. In this series of 7 patients treated with the Eden-Lange procedure (the other 20 patients were treated with nerve surgery), results were excellent in 3 patients, good in 1 patient, and poor in 3 patients. Teboul et al[16] state that two factors are most predictive of a poor result following reconstructive surgery: if the patient is older than 50 years or the lesion is caused by radical neck dissection, penetrating injury, or spontaneous palsy.

COMPLICATIONS

■ Complications associated with the Eden-Lange procedure, in addition to the usual surgical risks, include failed integration of the transferred muscles with resultant continued dysfunction. Such a complication is discussed rarely, and we were only able to find one report of a failure of muscle integration.[16]

■ Patient compliance with strict immobilization for the first 6 weeks after surgery is important to avoid pull-out of the transferred muscles, especially the rhomboids, which, unlike the levator scapulae, are not attached to their new scapular insertion with the tendo-osseous interface intact.

■ Initial complications do not seem to be the problem with the Eden-Lange procedure; rather, the primary complication appears to be later effects of functional outcome falling short of expectations.

■ Iatrogenic dysfunction resulting from no longer having a physiologic levator scapula or rhomboids is not, to our knowledge, discussed in the literature. However, because the origin of these muscles is merely being transposed more laterally, it does not appear that the Eden-Lange procedure creates a new problem while fixing the old one.

■ In cases of failure of the procedure, where pain and dysfunction continue, scapulothoracic arthrodesis can be performed as a salvage procedure.

REFERENCES

1. Bigliani LU, Compito CA, Duralde XA, et al. Transfer of the levator scapulae, rhomboid major, and rhomboid minor for paralysis of the trapezius. J Bone Joint Surg Am 1996;78:1534–1540.
2. Bigliani LU, Perez-Sanz JR, Wolfe IN. Treatment of trapezius paralysis. J Bone Joint Surg Am 1985;67:871–877.
3. Burns S, Herbison GJ. Spinal accessory nerve injury as a complication of internal jugular vein cannulation. Ann Intern Med 1996;125:700.
4. Dunn AW. Trapezius paralysis after minor surgical procedures in the posterior cervical triangle. South Med J 1974;67:312–315.
5. Eden R. Zur behandlung der trapeziuslahmung mittels muselplastik. Deutsche Zeitschr Chir 1924;184:387–397.
6. Eisen A, Bertrand G. Isolated accessory nerve palsy of spontaneous origin. A clinical and electromyographic study. Arch Neurol 1972; 27:496–502.
7. Francillon MR. Zur Behandlung de Accesoriuslahmung. Schweiz Med Wochenschr 1955;33:787–788.

8. Kondo M, Shiro T, Yamada M. Changes of the tilting angle of the scapula following elevation of the arm. In Bateman JE, Walsh RP, eds. Surgery of the Shoulder. Philadelphia: BC Decker, 1984:136–138.

9. Lange M. Die Behandlung der irreparablen Trapeziuslahmung. Langenbecks Arch Klin Chir 1951;270:437–439.

10. Leipzig B, Suen JY, English JL, et al. Functional evaluation of the spinal accessory nerve after neck dissection. Am J Surg 1983;146:526–530.

11. Patterson WR. Inferior dislocation of the distal end of the clavicle: a case report. J Bone Joint Surg Am 1967;49A:1184–1186.

12. Pelissier J, Lopez S, Herisson C, et al. [Shoulder pain and trapezius paralysis: Evaluation of a rehabilitation protocol.] Rev Rhum Mal Osteoartic 1990;57:319–321. In French.

13. Romero J, Gerber C. Levator scapulae and rhomboid transfer for paralysis of trapezius: The Eden-Lange procedure. J Bone Joint Surg Br 2003;85B:1141–1145.

14. Setter KJ, Voloshin I, Bigliani LU. Operative treatment of spinal accessory nerve palsy. Techniques in Shoulder and Elbow Surgery 2004;5:25–36.

15. Teboul F, Bizot P, Kakkar R, et al. Surgical management of trapezius palsy. J Bone Joint Surg Am 2005;87(Suppl 1):285–291.

16. Teboul F, Bizot P, Kakkar R, et al. Surgical management of trapezius palsy. J Bone Joint Surg Am 2004;86A:1884–1890.

17. Wiater JM, Bigliani LU. Spinal accessory nerve injury. Clin Orthop Relat Res 1999;368:5–16.

Chapter 30

Pectoralis Major Transfer for Long Thoracic Nerve Palsy

Raymond A. Klug, Bradford O. Parsons, and Evan L. Flatow

DEFINITION

- Long thoracic nerve palsy leads to classical scapular winging because of weakness of the serratus anterior muscle (**FIG 1**).
  - Other types of winging include trapezius winging and rhomboid winging.
- Lesions of the long thoracic nerve can range from paresis to complete paralysis, leading to varying degrees of shoulder dysfunction.
- The serratus anterior muscle functions to stabilize the scapula against the chest wall, thus providing a fulcrum for the humerus to push against while moving the arm in space.[3,4]
  - Without this fulcrum, shoulder elevation is weakened, which leads to inability to use the arm in forward activities.
  - Forward elevation of the shoulder is most severely affected, followed by shoulder abduction.

ANATOMY

- The serratus anterior is a large broad muscle that covers the lateral aspect of the thorax. It has digitations that take origin from the upper nine ribs, pass deep to the scapula, and insert on the medial aspect of the scapula.[15]
- The muscle has three divisions.[5]
  - The first division consists of one slip and takes origin from the first two ribs. This division runs slightly upward and inserts on the superior angle of the scapula.
  - The second division is made up of three slips from the second, third, and fourth ribs, and inserts on the anterior surface of the medial border of the scapula.
  - The third division, which consists of the inferior five slips from ribs five through nine, inserts on the inferior angle of the scapula. Because this division has the longest course it has the longest lever-arm and the most power for scapular rotation.
- The serratus anterior muscle stabilizes the scapula against the chest wall, creating a fulcrum for the proximal humerus to lever against while moving the arm in space.
  - The serratus anterior protracts and upwardly rotates the glenoid.
  - Its direction of pull brings the inferomedial border of the scapula anteriorly. The inferior border of the scapula is pulled forward with forward elevation of the arm. This causes the glenoid to tip posteriorly and allow full forward elevation without impingement.
  - With weakness of the serratus anterior muscle, the scapula translates superiorly and medially, and the inferior border rotates medially and dorsally (**FIG 2A**).
- The serratus anterior muscle is innervated by the long thoracic nerve, which arises from the ventral rami of cervical roots C5–7.
  - The C5 and C6 roots pass through the scalenus medius muscle and merge before they receive a branch from C7.
  - The nerve enters the axillary sheath at the level of the first rib and travels posteriorly in the axilla.
  - It then passes over a prominence in the second rib and descends along the lateral chest wall, where it enters the serratus anterior fascia and then the muscle itself (**FIG 2C**).[5,15]
- The total length of the nerve is about 24 cm, and there are several possible points of injury.
  - Proximally, as well as distally along the chest wall, the nerve is susceptible to injury because of its superficial location.
  - The nerve is tethered in the axillary sheath, which places it on stretch with forward elevation of the arm.

PATHOGENESIS

Scapular Winging

- Scapular winging may be due to primary, secondary, or voluntary causes.[8]
- Primary scapular winging can be divided into neurologic, bony, and soft tissue types.
  - Neurologic disorders, which are most common, include:
    - Long thoracic nerve palsy (serratus anterior weakness)
    - Spinal accessory nerve palsy (trapezius weakness)
    - Dorsal scapular nerve palsy (rhomboid weakness)
    - Trapezius weakness winging may be distinguished from serratus winging by the position and direction of scapular laxity (see Fig 2A,B).
  - Bony abnormalities include osteochondromas of the scapula or fracture malunion.
  - Soft tissue disorders include:
    - Soft tissue contractures, causing winging
    - Muscular disorders such as fascioscapulohumeral dystrophy

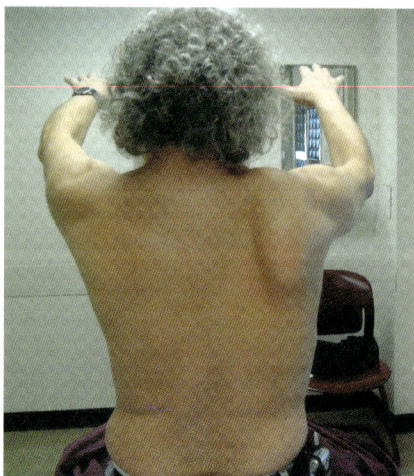

FIG 1 • Clinical photograph of serratus winging.

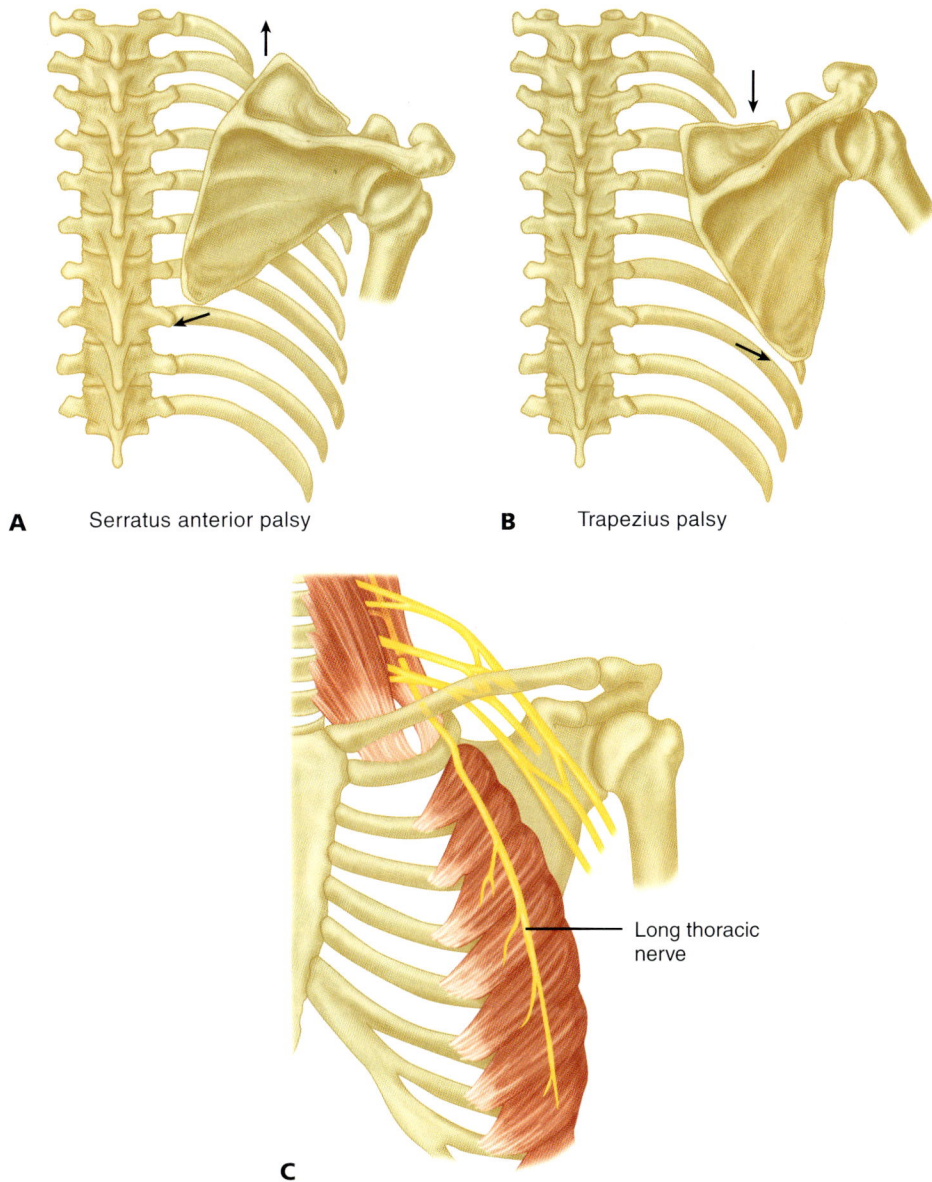

A Serratus anterior palsy

B Trapezius palsy

C

FIG 2 • A,B. Resting position of the scapula with serratus anterior and trapezius palsy. **C.** Superficial location of the long thoracic nerve.

- Congenital absence or traumatic rupture of the parascapular muscles
  - Scapulothoracic bursitis
- Secondary winging may occur following disorders of the glenohumeral joint. The most common causes are multidirectional and posterior instability.
- The sequence of events leading to secondary scapular winging due to primary shoulder pathology is as follows:
  - Primary glenulohumeral or subacromial pathology, *leading to*
  - Limited glenulohumeral motion, *leading to*
  - Increased compensatory scapulothoracic motion, *leading to*
  - Increased demand on periscapular muscles, *leading to*
  - Fatigue of periscapular muscles—serratus, trapezius, and rhomboids—*leading to*
  - Secondary scapular winging

- Voluntary winging may occur in psychiatric patients or for secondary gain.

Long Thoracic Nerve Palsy

- Long thoracic nerve palsy is the most common cause of serratus dysfunction resulting in symptomatic scapular winging, especially in those patients who fail nonoperative management and are being considered for pectoralis tendon transfer.[1]
- Long thoracic nerve palsy has been reported to result from idiopathic, iatrogenic, viral, compressive, or traumatic (blunt or penetrating) causes.[15]
- Most injuries are neurapraxic, due to blunt trauma.
  - Lesions also may occur through entrapment of the fifth or sixth cervical roots at the level of the scalenus medius, during traction over the second rib, or with traction and compression at the inferior angle of the scapula with general anesthesia or prolonged abduction of the arm.

- Iatrogenic injuries may occur during radical mastectomy, first rib resection, or transaxillary sympathectomy, or during surgical positioning.[6]
- Other less common causes include viral illnesses, Parsonage-Turner syndrome, isolated long thoracic neuritis, immunizations, or C7 nerve root lesions.
  - Often, the cause is idiopathic, with a questionable history of trauma or viral illness.

Pathoanatomy

- A mechanical advantage is gained by stabilization of the scapula against the chest wall.
  - With loss of this mechanical advantage, forward elevation against resistance is decreased owing to scapulothoracic motion.
- Additional types of shoulder pathology can result secondary to stabilization of the scapula:
  - Impingement due to relative anterior rotation of the acromion (**FIG 3**)
  - Weakness due to loss of mechanical advantage in forward elevation
  - Adhesive capsulitis from disuse
- With complete paralysis of the serratus anterior, complete forward elevation and abduction greater than 110 degrees are not possible.[3,15]

NATURAL HISTORY

- As mentioned previously, most injuries to the long thoracic nerve are neurapraxic from stretch of the nerve or blunt trauma.
- Most cases resolve spontaneously without operative intervention within 12 months, although maximal recovery may take up to 24 months.[2,7,9]
- The exception to this rule is injury due to nerve laceration from penetrating trauma or iatrogenic injury.

PATIENT HISTORY AND PHYSICAL FINDINGS

- A thorough history (including previous illnesses, procedures and interventions, hand dominance, and activity level) and complete examination of the shoulder and back are essential.

- Treatment often is delayed, and diagnosis may become apparent only after failed treatment for other disorders.
  - Furthermore, patients may develop secondary stiffness from disuse, and this may be the primary complaint.
- Patients often present with vague complaints of shoulder pain or weakness with overhead activities.
  - Because winging may be subtle, the patient must be undressed from the waist up, viewed from the back, and tested with provocative maneuvers such as resisted forward elevation and pushups against a wall.
- Pain may come from several sources, making diagnosis of long thoracic nerve palsy based on pain distribution difficult.
  - Compensatory overuse of the remaining scapulothoracic musculature may cause pain localized posteriorly about the scapula.
  - Patients may present with impingement-type pain with forward elevation.
  - In secondary winging, pain may result from an underlying diagnosis such as glenohumeral instability.
  - With severe pain, long thoracic neuritis or Parsonage-Turner syndrome should be considered.
- Physical examination usually reveals classic winging, with the scapula translated medially and the inferior border rotated toward the midline (see Fig 1).
- Patients may present with varying degrees of weakness of forward elevation of the arm.
  - Resisted testing may accentuate winging, as will having the patient do a pushup against a wall.
  - Weakness of forward elevation may be decreased by manual scapular stabilization against the chest wall by an examiner, the so-called "scapular stabilization test."[13]

IMAGING AND OTHER DIAGNOSTIC STUDIES

- Plain radiographs of the shoulder, cervical spine, and chest should be part of the workup.
  - Although radiographs rarely are diagnostic, bony abnormalities such as osteochondromas, cervical spondylosis, or scoliosis may be evident.
  - CT or MRI scans may be helpful in these situations, but are often not necessary.

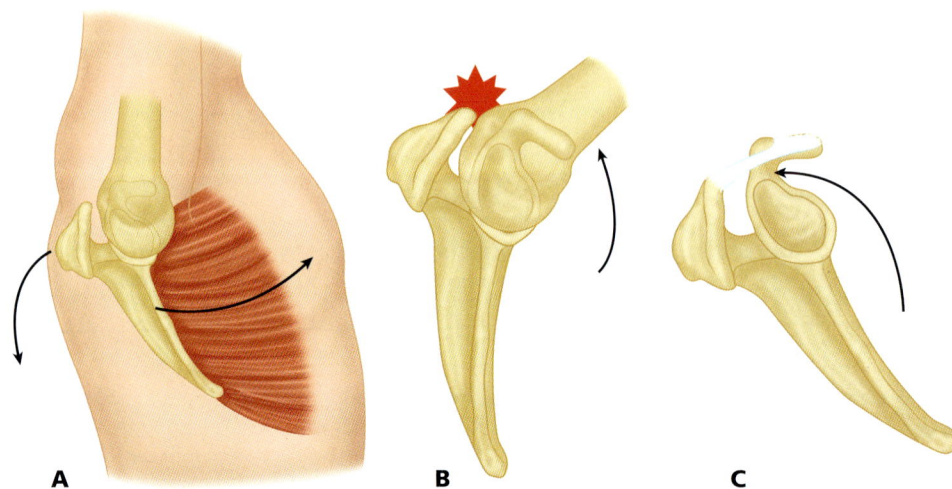

A   **B**   **C**

FIG 3 • Normal and abnormal scapular kinematics and its relationship to subacromial impingement syndrome.

■ Electromyographic and nerve conduction velocity studies are useful in confirming the diagnosis as well as following patients clinically.

■ Additionally, in idiopathic cases or where dystrophy is suspected, these tests may be helpful in ruling out other neuromuscular disorders (such as fascioscapulohumeral dystrophy) that may preclude muscle transfer as an option for scapular stabilization.

■ Serial studies every 3 months are recommended.

■ Studies should include cervical roots, brachial plexus, and the spinal accessory nerve.

DIFFERENTIAL DIAGNOSIS

■ Rotator cuff tear
■ Fracture malunion
■ Glenohumeral instability
■ Impingement
■ Acromioclavicular joint disease
■ Biceps tendinitis
■ Neurologic disorders
■ Suprascapular nerve entrapment
■ Scoliosis
■ Scapular osteochondroma

NONOPERATIVE MANAGEMENT

■ Whether idiopathic, viral, or compressive, almost all cases of serratus winging from long thoracic palsy resolve spontaneously within 1 to 2 years.[2,7,9]

■ Without a clear history of penetrating trauma, all patients initially should be treated conservatively (**FIG 4**).

■ Physical therapy should consist of range-of-motion exercises to avoid secondary glenohumeral stiffness.

■ Braces and orthotics that have been designed to stabilize the scapula to the chest wall may provide symptomatic relief. Their use is controversial, however, and many patients find them cumbersome.

■ Some authors have recommended bracing to decrease continued traction on the nerve.[14]

SURGICAL MANAGEMENT

■ Patients for whom nonoperative treatment has failed and who have persistent symptomatic scapular winging are candidates for surgical stabilization.

■ Patients often are given up to 24 months to recover nerve and muscle function before surgical repair is considered.

■ However, Fery[2] has reported that up to 25% of patients with serratus anterior paralysis may fail nonoperative treatment.

■ Patients who have penetrating trauma or iatrogenic injury, where a long thoracic nerve transection is suspected, may be indicated for acute nerve exploration and repair.

■ Historically, three different procedures have been used to treat patients with symptomatic serratus anterior dysfunction: scapulothoracic fusion, static stabilization procedures, and dynamic muscle transfers.

■ Scapulothoracic fusion is mainly a salvage procedure, sometimes used in patients with previous failures or in patients with dystrophies, such as fascioscapulohumeral dystrophy, where multiple muscles may be affected.

■ Static stabilization uses fascial slings or tethers to help stabilize the scapula.

■ These procedures have fallen out of favor because the slings may gradually stretch out, with subsequent loss of scapular stability.

■ Dynamic muscle transfers, first described by Tubby[12] in 1904, have been found to offer the optimal recovery and result in nearly normal scapulothoracic motion.

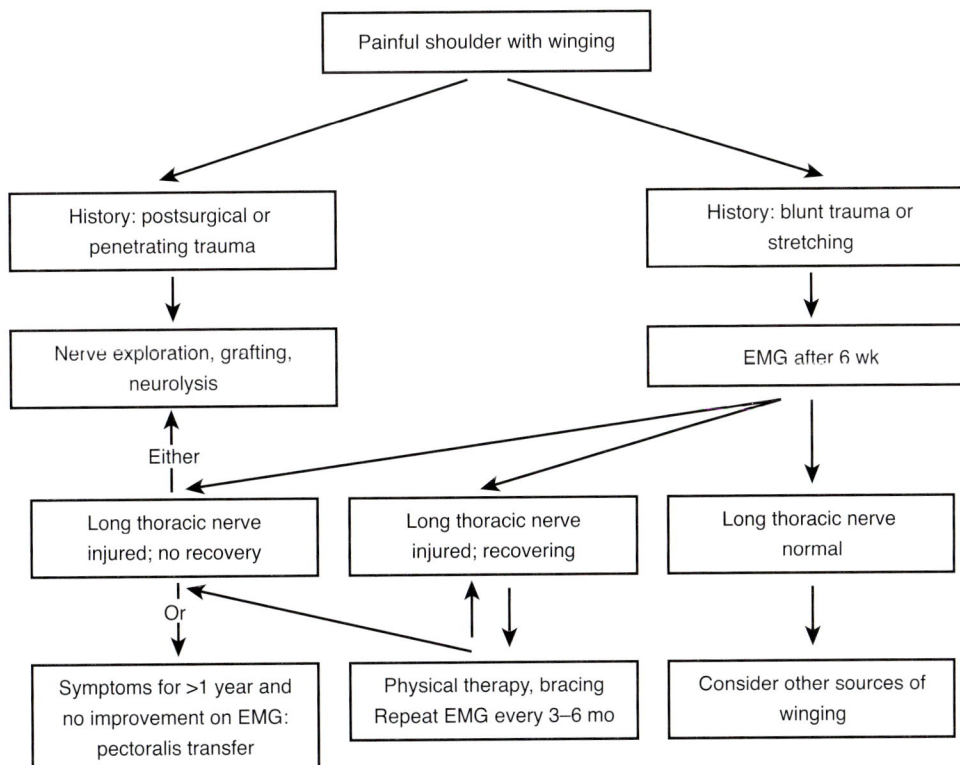

FIG 4 • Algorithm for treatment of serratus palsy. EMG, electromyography. (Adapted from Kuhn JE. The scapulothoracic articulation: anatomy, biomechanics, pathophysiology, and management. In: Iannotti JP, Williams GR Jr., eds. Disorders of the Shoulder: Diagnosis and Management, ed 2. Philadelphia: Lippincott Williams & Wilkins, 2007:1058–1086.)

- Numerous different transfers have been described, but most surgeons currently perform a transfer of the sternal head of the pectoralis major to the inferior angle of the scapula to reconstruct the function of the deficient serratus anterior.
  - The sternal head of the pectoralis is preferred because it has good excursion and similar power to the serratus, and its fiber orientation is similar to that of the serratus.[1,2]

Preoperative Planning

- Preoperative planning should include a discussion with the patient regarding allograft versus autograft augmentation of the pectoralis transfer.
  - Typical options include contralateral fascia lata or semitendinosus autograft, or semitendinosus allograft.
- A tendon stripper is needed for autograft harvest if desired.
- A 5-mm round trip burr or drill bit is needed to fashion a tunnel through the inferior angle of the scapula.
- Heavy nonabsorbable suture (no. 2 or no. 5) is needed to attach the pectoralis transfer and prepare the graft augmentation.

Patient Positioning

- The patient is placed supine in the beach chair position, with care taken to leave access to the midline posteriorly and anteriorly.
  - A pad is placed behind the midline of the thorax to improve posterior exposure.
  - The forequarter is draped free with the entire scapula in the surgical field.
- A pneumatic arm positioner (Spider Limb Positioner, Tenet Medical Engineering, distributed by Smith & Nephew Endoscopy, Andover, MA) is helpful during the procedure to maintain position of the extremity.
- If fascia lata or semitendinosus autograft is to be harvested, the lower extremity must be prepped and draped free as well.

Approach

- The following section describes our preferred technique for transfer of the sternal head of the pectoralis major to the inferior angle of the scapula for serratus anterior dysfunction.

EXPOSURE

- A 10- to 15-cm incision is made in the axillary crease posterior to the lateral border of the scapula (**TECH FIG 1A**).
- The deltopectoral interval is developed, and the cephalic vein is retracted laterally.
- The pectoralis tendon is identified at its humeral insertion.
- The sternal head, which lies deep to the clavicular head, is identified and isolated bluntly (**TECH FIG 1B,C**).
  - Often, abduction and external rotation of the extremity is helpful in exposing the sternal head.

- The sternal head insertion is released sharply from the humerus, taking care not to damage the underlying long head of the biceps tendon or the clavicular head of the pectoralis major (**TECH FIG 1D,E**).
- Traction sutures are placed into the sternal head tendon, and the muscle belly is freed of adhesions medially.

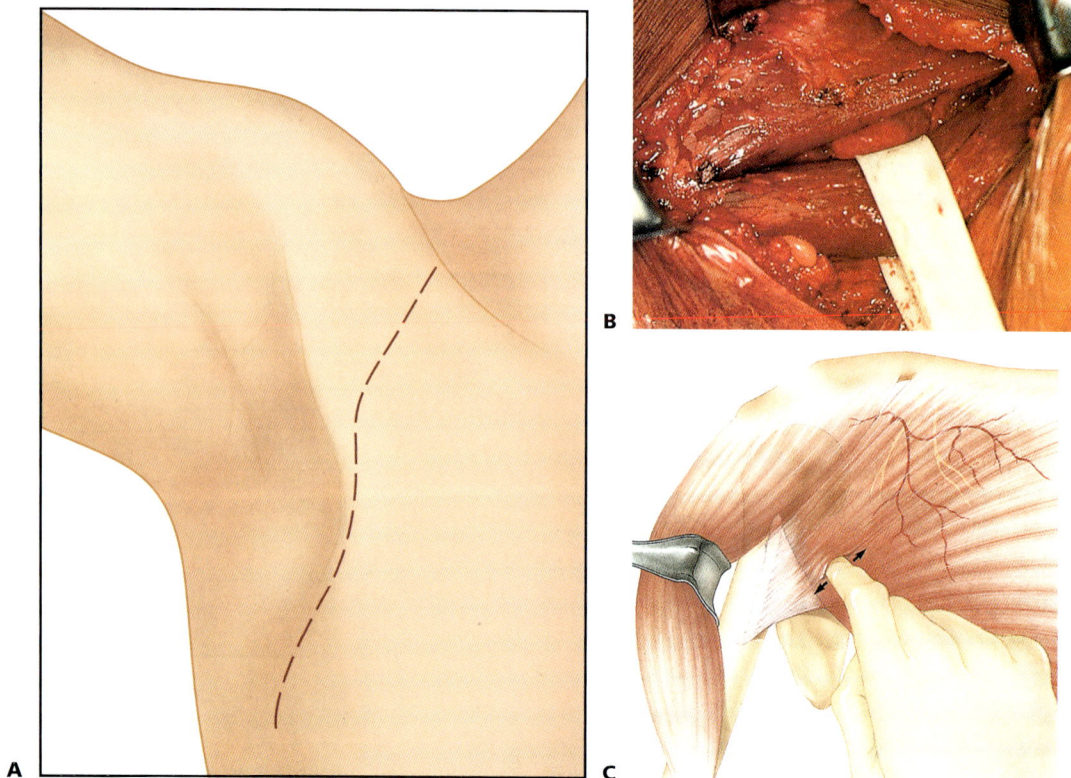

TECH FIG 1 • A. Axillary incision used for pectoralis major transfer. **B,C.** The sternal head, which lies deep to the clavicular head, is identified and isolated bluntly. *(continued)*

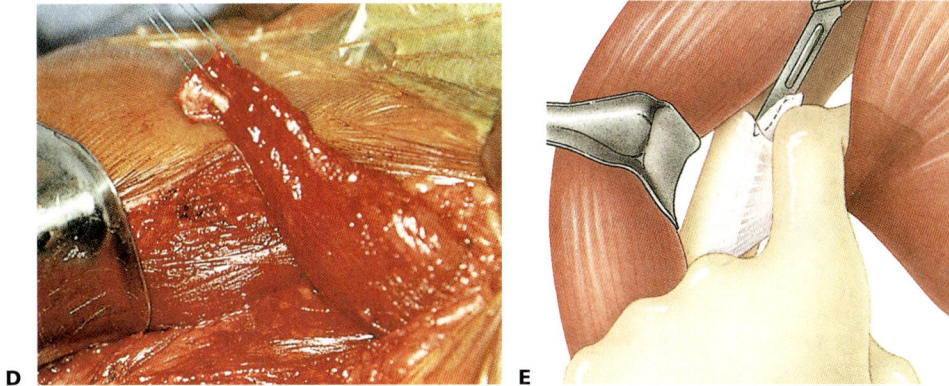

TECH FIG 1 • *(continued)* **D,E.** The sternal head insertion is released sharply from the humerus, taking care not to damage the underlying long head of the biceps tendon or the clavicular head of the pectoralis major. (**B–E:** from Post M. Orthopaedic management of neuromuscular disorders. In: Post M, Flatow EL, Bigliani LU, Pollack RG, eds. The Shoulder: Operative Technique. Philadelphia: Lippincott Williams & Wilkins, 1998:201–234.)

GRAFT HARVESTING

- At this point, attention is turned to the fascia lata harvest, or preparation of the allograft tendon.
  - For fascia lata harvest, two small incisions (2 to 3 cm) are made on the lateral aspect of the thigh, about 20 cm apart.
  - After incision, the fascia lata is exposed and cleaned with an elevator between the two incisions.
  - Once the fascia lata is identified and isolated, a tendon stripper is used to harvest a graft approximately 6 cm × 20 cm.

- The graft is then folded over itself and tubularized using heavy, nonabsorbable suture.
- Once prepared, the graft is woven into the sternal head tendinous origin and secured with heavy, nonabsorbable suture (**TECH FIG 2**).

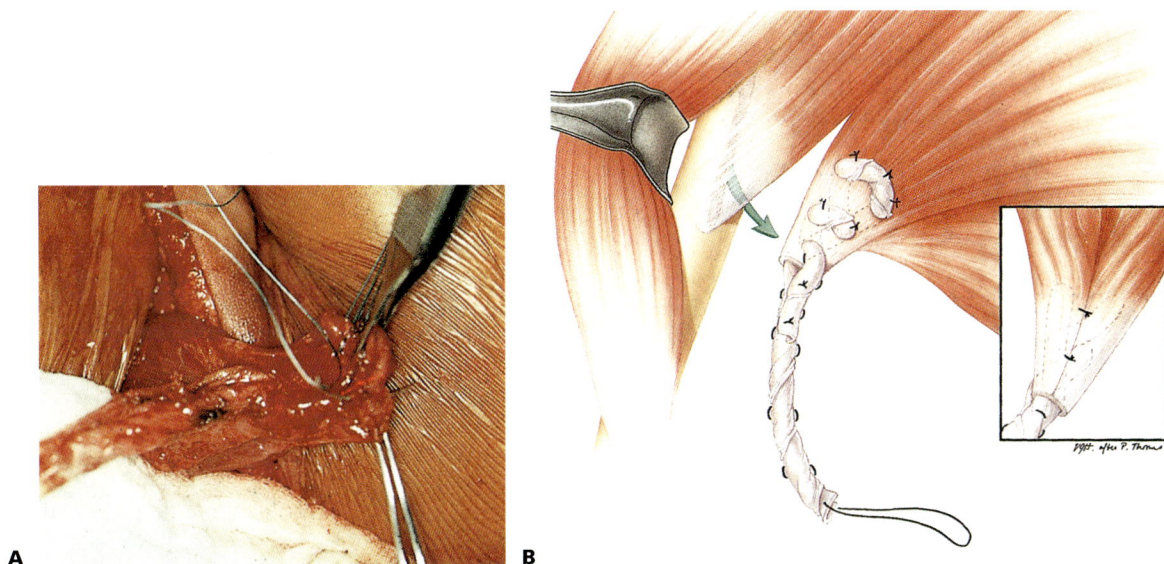

TECH FIG 2 • Once prepared, the graft is woven into the sternal head tendinous origin and secured with heavy, nonabsorbable suture. (From Post M. Orthopaedic management of neuromuscular disorders. In: Post M, Flatow EL, Bigliani LU, et al, eds. The Shoulder: Operative Technique. Philadelphia: Lippincott Williams & Wilkins, 1998:210–234.)

TECHNIQUES

SCAPULAR EXPOSURE, PREPARATION, AND TENDON ATTACHMENT

- After the pectoralis tendon and graft are ready, the scapula is exposed.
- The inferior angle of the scapula is identified and exposed by blunt dissection along the chest wall.
- The latissimus dorsi and teres major tendons are retracted distally, and the lateral neurovascular structures are avoided by staying medial.
- Once the inferior angle of the scapula is identified, it is exposed subperiosteally, and a 6- to 8-mm burr hole is made 2 cm from the lateral and inferior border of the scapula.
- The graft is then passed through the bone hole from anterior to posterior, tensioning the graft while reducing the scapula on the chest wall, so that the native pectoralis tendon is flush with the bone tunnel.
- The graft is then looped through the hole in the inferior scapula and sutured to itself using heavy, nonabsorbable suture (**TECH FIG 3**).
  - It is necessary to ensure that native pectoralis tendon is brought to the scapula, because the tendon graft may stretch over time.

TECH FIG 3 • The graft is looped through the hole in the inferior scapula and sutured to itself using heavy, nonabsorbable suture. (From Post M. Orthopaedic management of neuromuscular disorders. In: Post M, Flatow EL, Bigliani LU, et al, eds. The Shoulder: Operative Technique. Philadelphia: Lippincott Williams & Wilkins, 1998:210–234.)

- The wound is then closed in layers over a drain.
- The extremity is placed in a sling and a scapulothoracic orthosis, which maintains pressure on the scapula against the chest wall.

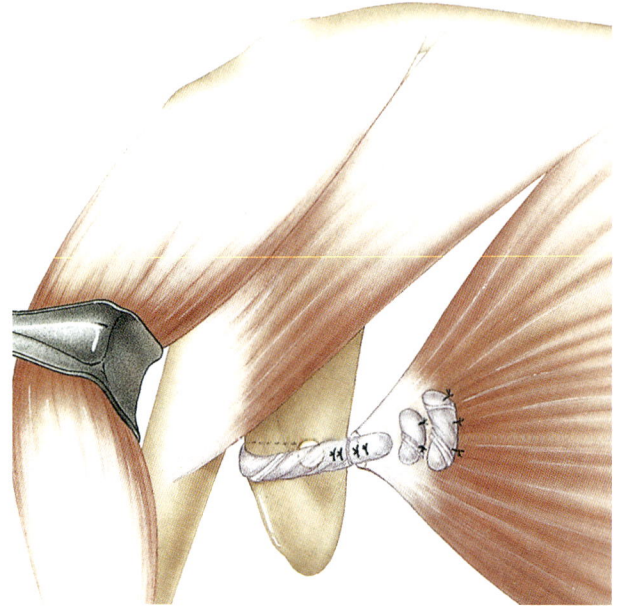

PEARLS AND PITFALLS

- Electromyography is helpful in identifying patients with dystrophy or other palsies, which may preclude the possibility of a sternal head transfer for serratus anterior dysfunction.
- Patients with blunt trauma or idiopathic etiologies initially should be managed nonoperatively, because most will recover serratus anterior function.
- The sternal head lies deep to the clavicular head, and positioning the arm in abduction and external rotation can help identify the insertion of the tendon.
- When approaching the inferior scapula, care is taken to stay medial while retracting the latissimus and teres major distally, because the neurovascular structures are lateral.
- The scapula should be reduced to the chest wall by an assistant before tensioning the pectoralis transfer.
- Avoid scapular fracture by keeping the osseous tunnel a minimum of 1 cm away from the scapular borders.
- The sternal head is lengthened by autograft or allograft, but it is critical to have native, living pectoralis tendon attached directly to the inferior scapula. The auto- or allograft is meant for augmentation.

POSTOPERATIVE CARE

- Patients are kept immobilized in the sling and orthosis for 6 weeks.
- After 6 weeks, range-of-motion exercises are begun, and the brace is discontinued.
- Strengthening exercises are begun as motion returns.
- Patients are restricted from heavy lifting or manual labor for 6 months.

OUTCOMES

- Most series of sternal head transfer for serratus anterior dysfunction and scapular winging report good to excellent results

with improvement in function, relief of pain, and correction of winging.
- Post[11] reported on eight patients treated with sternal head transfer with excellent results.
- Connor et al[1] reported on 11 patients, 10 of whom (91%) had significant improvement in pain and function and relief of winging.
- Warner and Navarro[13] reported that seven of eight patients had excellent results, with the only unsatisfactory outcome following a deep infection.
- Conversely, Noerdlinger et al[10] reported that of 15 patients treated, only 7 (47%) had good to excellent results. They found that those patients who lacked external rotation at follow-up

had poorer results, and that more aggressive therapy regarding rotation may be needed.

COMPLICATIONS

- Seroma and infection[13]
- Neurovascular injury
- Scapular fracture through bone tunnel
- Shoulder stiffness[10]
- Graft loosening and loss of tension[11]

REFERENCES

1. Connor PM, Yamaguchi K, Manifold SG, et al. Split pectoralis major transfer for serratus anterior palsy. Clin Orthop Relat Res 1997; 341:134–142.
2. Fery A. Results of treatment of anterior serratus paralysis. In Post M, Morrey BF, Hawkins R, eds. Surgery of the Shoulder. St. Louis: Mosby-Year Book, 1990:325–329.
3. Gregg JR, Labosky D, Harty M, et al. Serratus anterior paralysis in the young athlete. J Bone Joint Surg Am 1979;61A:825–832.
4. Inman VT, Saunders JB, Abbott LC. Observations on the function of the shoulder joint. J Bone Joint Surg 1944;26:1–30.
5. Jobe CM. Gross anatomy of the shoulder. In Rockwood CA Jr, Matsen FA III, eds. The Shoulder. Philadelphia: WB Saunders, 1998:34–94.
6. Kauppila LI, Vastamaki M. Iatrogenic serratus anterior paralysis. Long-term outcome in 26 patients. Chest 1996;109:31–34.
7. Kuhn JE, Hawkins RJ. Evaluation and treatment of scapular disorders. In Warner JJ, Iannotti JP, Gerber C. Complex and Revision Problems in Shoulder Surgery. Philadelphia: Lippincott-Raven, 1997:357–376.
8. Kuhn JE, Plancher KD, Hawkins RJ. Scapular winging. J Am Acad Orthop Surg 1995;3:319–325.
9. Leffert RD. Neurologic problems. In Rockwood CA Jr, Matsen FA III, eds. The Shoulder. Philadelphia: WB Saunders, 1998:965–988.
10. Noerdlinger MA, Cole BJ, Stewart M, et al. Results of pectoralis major transfer with fascia lata autograft augmentation for scapula winging. J Shoulder Elbow Surg 2002;11:345–350.
11. Post M. Pectoralis major transfer for winging of the scapula. J Shoulder Elbow Surg 1995;4:1–9.
12. Tubby AH. A case illustrating the operative treatment of paralysis of the serratus magnus by muscle grafting. Br Med J 1904;2:1159–1160.
13. Warner JJ, Navarro RA. Serratus anterior dysfunction. Recognition and treatment. Clin Orthop Relat Res 1998;349:139–148.
14. Watson CJ, Schenkman M. Physical therapy management of isolated serratus anterior muscle paralysis. Phys Ther 1995;75:194–202.
15. Wiater JM, Flatow EL. Long thoracic nerve injury. Clin Orthop Relat Res 1999;368:17–27.

Shadley C. Schiffern and Sumant G. Krishnan

DEFINITION

- Refractory disorders of the scapulothoracic articulation have been reported to result in debilitating pain and dysfunction that may require surgical management.
- The most common clinical presentation, scapular winging,[12] was first reported in the published literature in 1723, and several etiologies for scapular winging have been documented since then.
- Soft tissue operations (eg, pectoralis major tendon transfer) have had reported success in stabilizing the dyskinetic scapula in appropriate patients.
- Despite successful clinical outcomes, a population of patients experience recurrent symptomatic scapular winging even after pectoralis major transfer.[6,10,12]
  - Several authors[5,7,10,12] report that arthrodesis is the treatment of choice for these failed muscle transfers. For failed pectoralis transfer or significant (ie, irreducible) fixed winging, scapulothoracic arthrodesis can be a successful salvage operation for these patients.[14]

ANATOMY

- The scapula is positioned over the posterolateral aspect of the rib cage, overlying ribs 1 to 7. It is suspended from the sternum by the clavicle anteriorly and plays an important role in positioning the upper extremity for proper function.
- The lateral scapula includes the glenoid fossa for articulation with the humeral head.
- The scapula provides an attachment for 16 muscles, which help maintain it in functional positions. It articulates on the thoracic cavity, allowing rotation, protraction, and retraction.
- A thin bursal layer separates the scapula from the underlying ribs.

PATHOGENESIS

- Dysfunction of the scapulothoracic articulation has been well documented in the peer-reviewed literature.
- The most common manifestation of scapulothoracic dysfunction is symptomatic scapular winging[7,12] (**FIG 1**).
  - Traumatic injuries to the serratus anterior muscle or the long thoracic nerve have been reported to cause symptomatic winging.[7,8,11,12,19,20]
  - Atraumatic etiologies, such as neuralgic amyotrophy, polio, and the muscular dystrophies, also may produce disabling scapular winging.[1,2,4,5,8,10,15,16]
  - Intolerable winging also has been demonstrated in association with other bony abnormalities (eg, rib or scapular osteochondromas and malunited scapular fractures) or soft tissue lesions (eg, scapular-stabilizing muscle contractures, muscle avulsions, and scapulothoracic bursitis).[3,11,12]
  - Recent authors[18] have reported a significant incidence of scapular winging secondary to glenohumeral joint lesions such as rotator cuff tears and glenohumeral instability (especially posterior and multidirectional instability).

- The scapulothoracic articulation also is a potential source of debilitating pain in the shoulder girdle.
  - Several authors[9,13,17,18] have documented the incidence of painful scapulothoracic crepitus ("snapping scapula" syndrome) and scapulothoracic bursitis.
  - Painful crepitus can be due to interposed muscle, fibrous and granulomatous lesions, or bony incongruity associated with osteochondromata, fractures, scoliosis, or kyphosis.[13]

NATURAL HISTORY

- Most patients who present with symptomatic scapular winging, scapulothoracic pain, or crepitus respond to nonoperative measures.
- A subset of this patient population, however, experiences complex scapulothoracic dysfunction or pain refractory to conservative measures.

PATIENT HISTORY AND PHYSICAL FINDINGS

- Patients presenting with scapulothoracic disorders typically complain of debilitating pain, shoulder dysfunction, or scapulothoracic crepitus.
- Physical findings commonly include scapular winging, crepitus, alterations in normal scapulohumeral rhythm, or neurologic deficits.
- Physical examination should focus on the resting posture of the scapula, as well as its dynamic position.
  - Both scapulae should be observed and palpated while the arms are elevated or while the patient performs a wall push-up. These dynamic tests may make subtle winging more obvious.
  - The pattern of winging distinguishes between serratus anterior dysfunction (long thoracic nerve) or trapezius palsy (spinal accessory nerve).

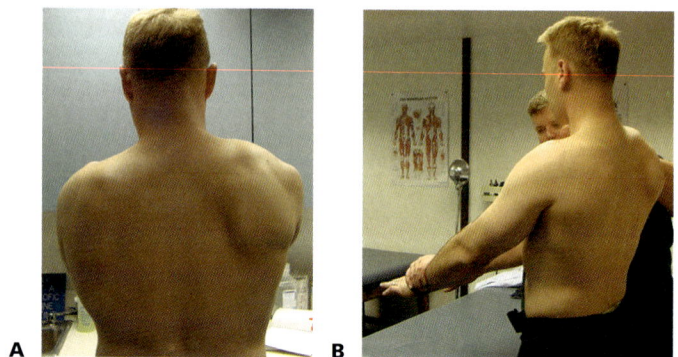

A **B**

FIG 1 • **A.** Moderate dynamic scapular winging demonstrated with slow forward elevation of the arms in the frontal plane. **B.** The same patient demonstrating marked medial winging with the resisted elevation at 30 degrees.

- The more common medial winging is consistent with serratus anterior dysfunction, whereas lateral winging is observed in trapezius palsy.
- Further assessment includes the scapula stabilization test to assess for fixed or correctable winging. This test is crucial in determining fixed versus reducible winging. It demonstrates the amount of discomfort the patient has and indicates the extent to which reduction of the scapula will relieve that discomfort.
- Painful crepitus localized to the scapulothoracic region is verified by diagnostic injection, in which 1% lidocaine is injected beneath the medial border of the scapula into the scapulothoracic bursa. Improvement in pain may be noted in the examination room, further supporting the diagnosis.

IMAGING AND OTHER DIAGNOSTIC STUDIES

- Standard plain radiographs of the shoulder, including anteroposterior views in internal and external rotation, axillary lateral views, and scapula Y views are obtained to evaluate the status of the clavicle, acromioclavicular joint, glenohumeral joint, and bony contour of the scapula.
- CT scans, including axial images and reformatted coronal and sagittal images, provide further detail, and may be required to assess scapula morphology and the presence of exostoses or deformity.
- Electromyography and nerve conduction velocity are important to verify neurologic dysfunction of the long thoracic or spinal accessory nerves.

DIFFERENTIAL DIAGNOSIS

- Long thoracic nerve palsy
- Spinal accessory nerve palsy
- Glenohumeral joint derangement with secondary scapular winging
- Scapulothoracic bursitis
- Snapping scapula
- Scapular exostosis or osteochondroma

NONOPERATIVE MANAGEMENT

- Nonoperative treatment is the cornerstone of management of scapulothoracic dysfunction.
- Therapeutic modalities involve supervised scapular–stabilizer and glenohumeral stretching and strengthening, the judicious use of oral anti-inflammatory medications, and selective cortisone injections.

SURGICAL MANAGEMENT

- Patients who have failed an extensive nonoperative course are candidates for surgical treatment.
- Surgical options for scapulothoracic dysfunction include:
  - Arthroscopic or open decompression and bursectomy or medial border scapulectomy for painful crepitus
  - Split pectoralis major tendon transfer for dynamic winging
  - Scapulothoracic arthrodesis
- Surgical indications for scapulothoracic arthrodesis include the following clinical situations:
  - For patients with disabling pain associated with crepitus, failure of previous resection of the superomedial border of the scapula is an indication for fusion.

- For patients with disabling pain associated with fixed scapular winging or failed pectoralis transfer, indications for fusion include:
  - Significant winging
  - Difficulty in reducing the scapula with the "scapular stabilization test"
  - Significant pain relief (>75%) that substantially improved function during a scapular stabilization test

Preoperative Planning

- Preoperative anesthesia consultation is recommended. We use general anesthesia with a double-lumen endotracheal tube to allow for selective deflation of the ipsilateral lung during wire passage.

Positioning

- Patients are placed in the prone position.
- Care is taken to pad all bony prominences.
- The entire involved arm, scapula, and ipsilateral posterior iliac crest are prepped and draped to the midline of the spine (**FIG 2**).
  - It is essential that the entire arm be prepped and draped in the surgical field to allow for appropriate manipulation of the scapula and accurate placement of the scapula on the rib cage for fusion.

Approach

- A direct approach to the scapulothoracic articulation along the medial border of the scapula is used. This approach allows excellent exposure of the underlying ribs and undersurface of the scapula. The superficial location of the scapula makes this approach relatively straightforward.

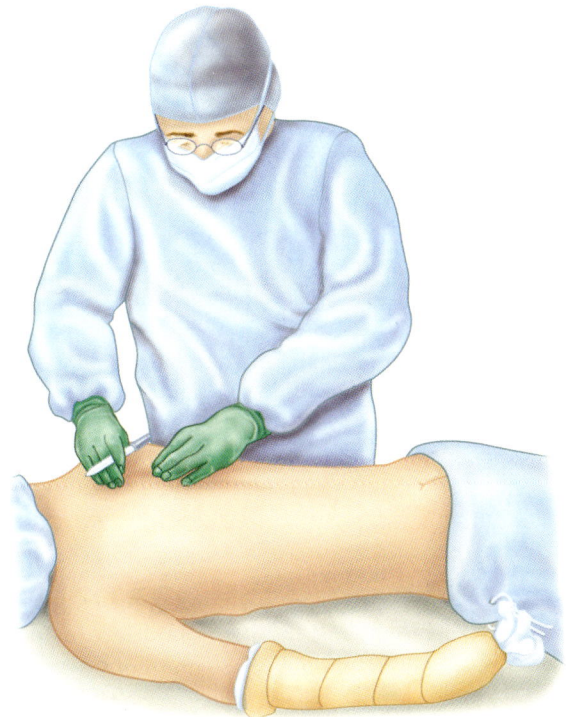

FIG 2 • Patient in the prone position. The surgical preparation must include the entire arm and the back, extending medially past the midline of the spine and inferiorly to include the posterior superior iliac crest.

EXPOSURE

- The incision is placed along the medial border of the scapula from just superior to the scapular spine to the inferior angle.
- The superficial fascia is incised, and the trapezius muscle is identified and retracted medially (**TECH FIG 1A**). The rhomboid muscles are incised off the medial edge of the scapula and are tagged for reattachment before closure (**TECH FIG 1B**).
- With the rhomboid muscles elevated, a rake retractor can be placed on the anterior surface of the medial

scapular border to retract the medial scapula away from the rib cage (**TECH FIG 1C**).
- About one third of the musculature of the serratus anterior and the subscapularis is resected from medial to lateral off the anterior surface of the scapula to allow for a wide fusion surface (**TECH FIG 1D**).
- Care must be taken to avoid resecting the subscapularis beyond the midline of the scapula to prevent denervation.

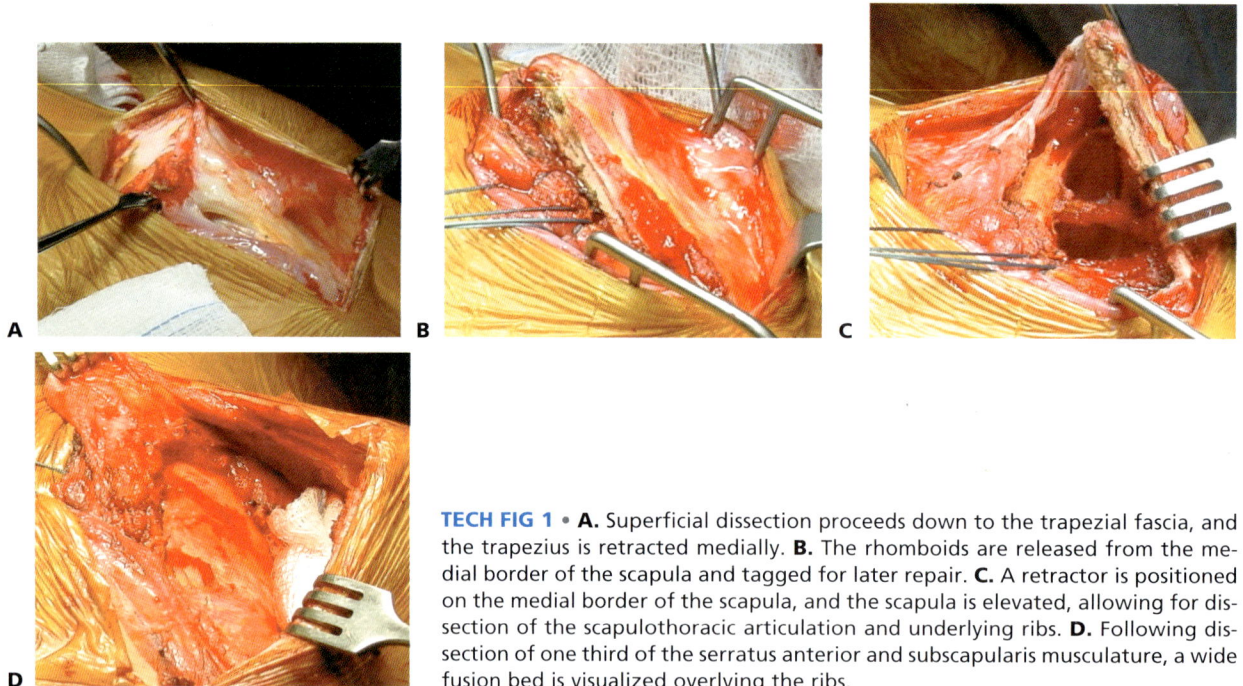

TECH FIG 1 • **A.** Superficial dissection proceeds down to the trapezial fascia, and the trapezius is retracted medially. **B.** The rhomboids are released from the medial border of the scapula and tagged for later repair. **C.** A retractor is positioned on the medial border of the scapula, and the scapula is elevated, allowing for dissection of the scapulothoracic articulation and underlying ribs. **D.** Following dissection of one third of the serratus anterior and subscapularis musculature, a wide fusion bed is visualized overlying the ribs.

BONY PREPARATION

- The anterior surface of the scapula is now roughened slightly with a burr (**TECH FIG 2A**). Care must be taken during this maneuver to avoid thinning the medial border excessively, because that could lead to fracture during hardware fixation.
- Next, the scapula is reduced to the rib cage in approximately 20 to 25 degrees of external rotation from the midline to maximize subsequent shoulder range of motion (most notably elevation and external rotation).
- If patients demonstrated concomitant multidirectional glenohumeral instability with a symptomatic inferior component, the scapula is rotated externally 35 to 40 degrees from the midline to use the inferior glenoid rim to buttress against inferior translation.

- The ribs corresponding to the decorticated anterior surface of the scapula are identified, and the scapula is again retracted to allow for rib preparation.
  - Depending on the size and configuration of the scapula, three or four ribs typically will be used in the fusion (usually the third to sixth ribs).
- The periosteum is incised carefully in a longitudinal direction and stripped off each rib (**TECH FIG 2B,C**).
- The ribs are minimally roughened with a burr down to bleeding bone.
- It is essential to remove all areas of soft tissue between the scapula and rib cage to permit maximum bony contact between the anterior surface of the scapula and the ribs (**TECH FIG 2D**).

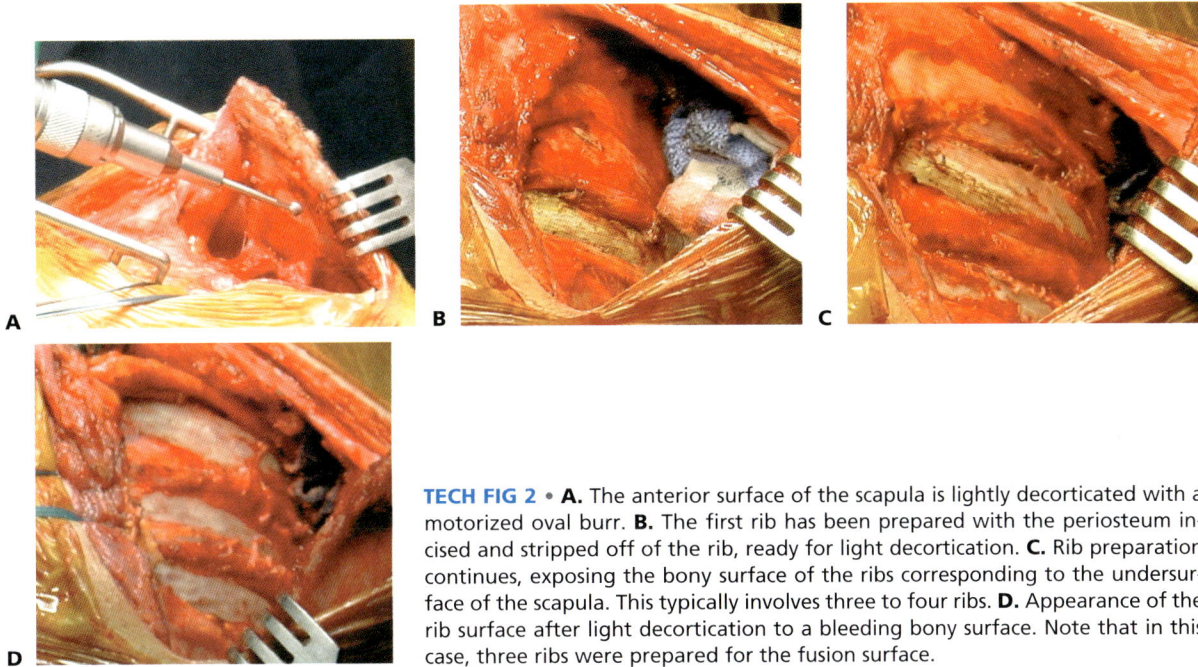

TECH FIG 2 • **A.** The anterior surface of the scapula is lightly decorticated with a motorized oval burr. **B.** The first rib has been prepared with the periosteum incised and stripped off of the rib, ready for light decortication. **C.** Rib preparation continues, exposing the bony surface of the ribs corresponding to the undersurface of the scapula. This typically involves three to four ribs. **D.** Appearance of the rib surface after light decortication to a bleeding bony surface. Note that in this case, three ribs were prepared for the fusion surface.

WIRE PASSAGE AND PLACEMENT OF SEMITUBULAR PLATE

- At this time, the involved lung is deflated before cerclage wires are passed around the ribs, to minimize trauma to the lung fields.
- Using rib and periosteal dissectors, a cerclage wire with a minimum diameter of 1.5 mm is passed carefully around each of the exposed ribs at the level where the medial border of the scapula will be placed on the rib cage (**TECH FIG 3A,B**).

- After passage of the cerclage wires, a one-third semitubular large fragment plate (usually with 5 or 6 holes, depending on the size of the scapula) is lined up on the posterior aspect of the medial border of the scapula (the thickest part of the scapula; **TECH FIG 3C**).
- A 3-mm burr is used to make holes through the scapula corresponding to the holes in the semitubular plate (**TECH FIG 3D**).

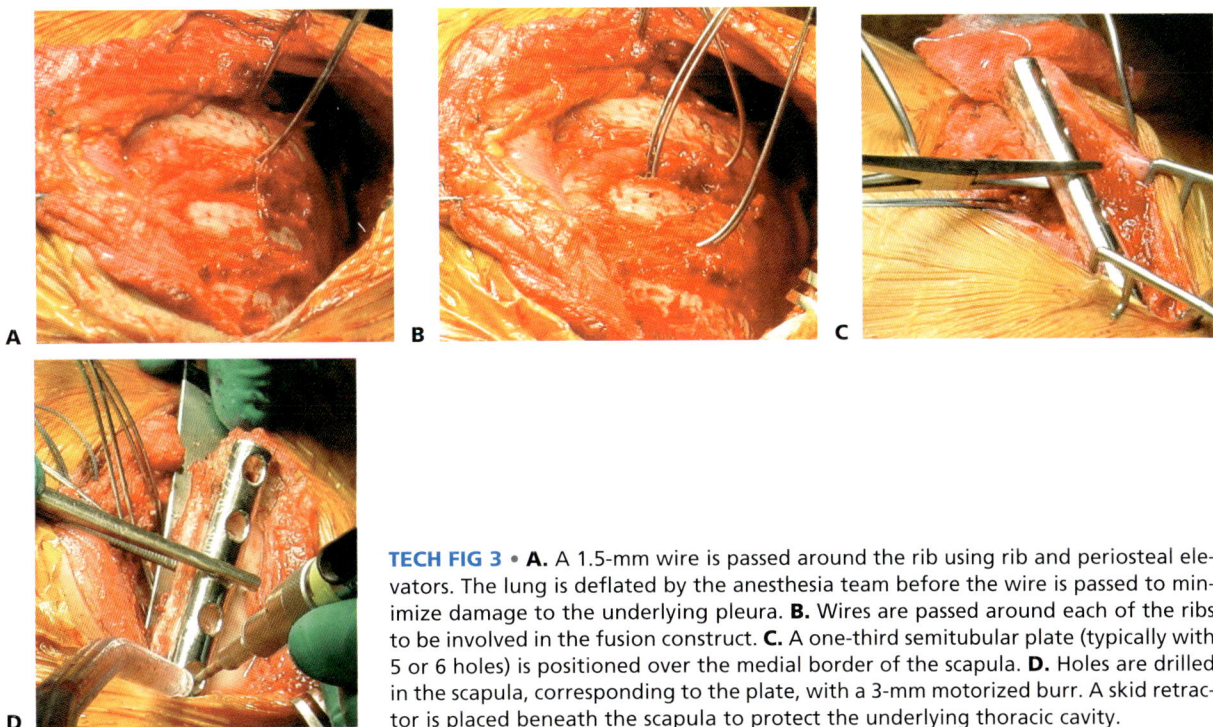

TECH FIG 3 • **A.** A 1.5-mm wire is passed around the rib using rib and periosteal elevators. The lung is deflated by the anesthesia team before the wire is passed to minimize damage to the underlying pleura. **B.** Wires are passed around each of the ribs to be involved in the fusion construct. **C.** A one-third semitubular plate (typically with 5 or 6 holes) is positioned over the medial border of the scapula. **D.** Holes are drilled in the scapula, corresponding to the plate, with a 3-mm motorized burr. A skid retractor is placed beneath the scapula to protect the underlying thoracic cavity.

REDUCTION AND PLATE FIXATION

- Cancellous bone is now harvested from the posterior iliac crest in routine fashion through a separate incision paralleling the path of the cluneal nerves.
  - If more bone graft is desired, either allograft cancellous chips or a synthetic bone graft substitute can be added.
- The wires are now passed through the scapula and semitubular plate (**TECH FIG 4A**), and the bone graft is placed between the scapula and ribs.

- The scapula is reduced to the underlying ribs (**TECH FIG 4B**), and the wires are sequentially tightened with the scapula held in 20 to 25 degrees of external rotation from the midline (**TECH FIG 4C,D**).
  - The semitubular plate allows uniform stress distribution once the wires are tightened (**TECH FIG 4E,F**).
- The wires are cut, and attention is turned to closure of the wound (**TECH FIG 4G**).

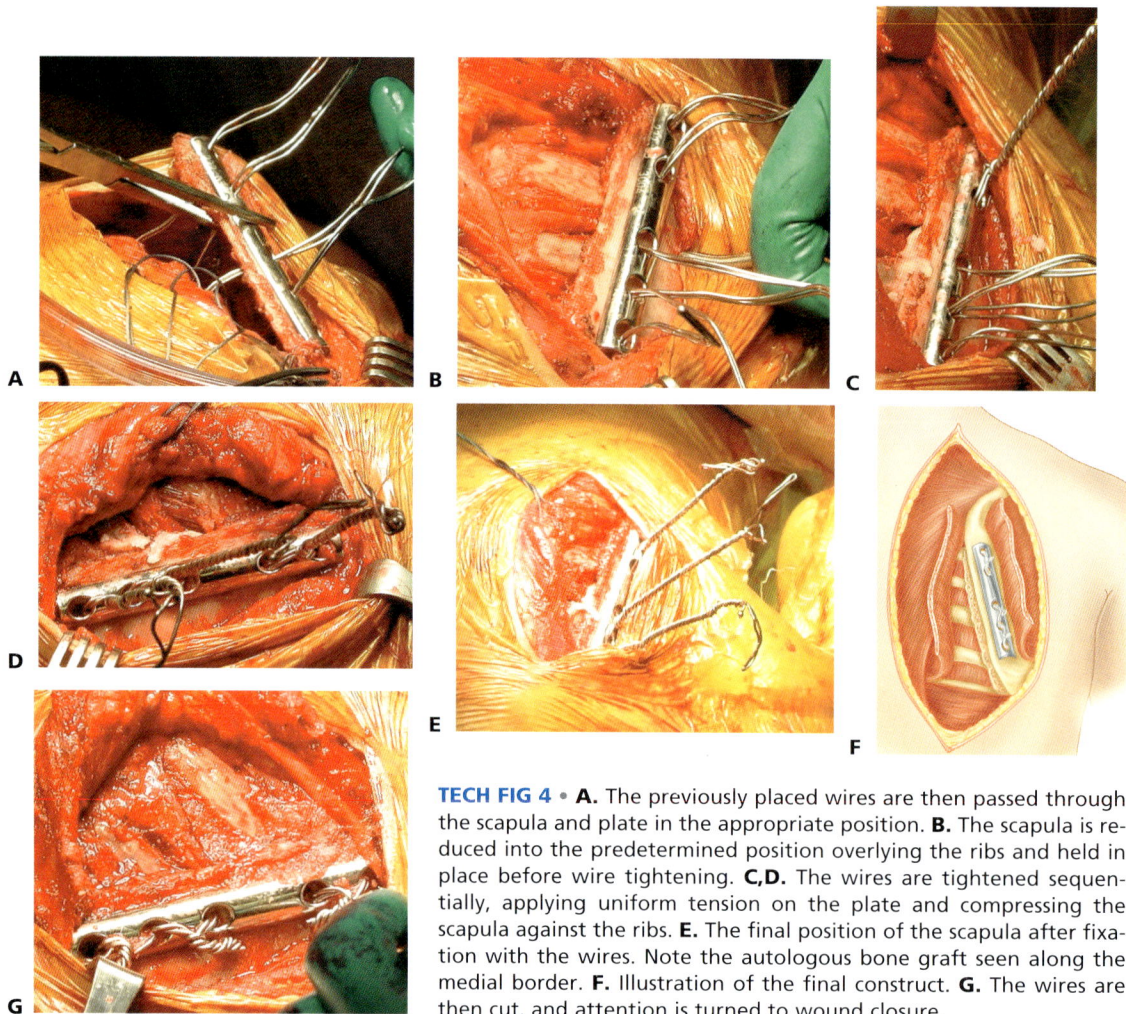

TECH FIG 4 • A. The previously placed wires are then passed through the scapula and plate in the appropriate position. **B.** The scapula is reduced into the predetermined position overlying the ribs and held in place before wire tightening. **C,D.** The wires are tightened sequentially, applying uniform tension on the plate and compressing the scapula against the ribs. **E.** The final position of the scapula after fixation with the wires. Note the autologous bone graft seen along the medial border. **F.** Illustration of the final construct. **G.** The wires are then cut, and attention is turned to wound closure.

TECHNIQUES

WOUND CLOSURE AND CHEST TUBE PLACEMENT

- The lung is reinflated, and irrigation is used to assess for a pneumothorax, which may be present.
- The rhomboids are then reattached to the medial aspect of the scapula (**TECH FIG 5**), and the subcutaneous tissue and skin are closed in the usual fashion.
- A thoracotomy tube is inserted if necessary, both to treat any associated pneumothorax and to drain any reactive pleural effusion that may develop postoperatively.

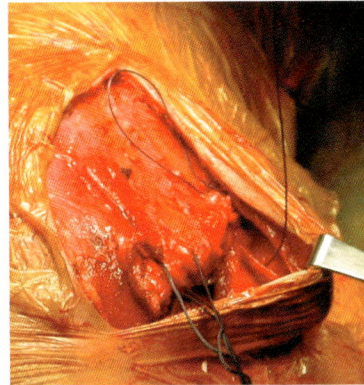

TECH FIG 5 • The rhomboids are repaired securely to the medial border of the scapula. This provides adequate coverage of the hardware.

PEARLS AND PITFALLS

Avoiding pulmonary complications	■ Use double-lumen tube and deflate lung ■ Meticulous subperiosteal passage of rib cerclage wires ■ Thoracotomy tube when necessary
Avoiding hardware complications and nonunion	■ Minimum size for wire is 1.50 mm ■ Use posterior iliac crest autograft ■ Use cancellous autograft ■ Immobilize in "gunslinger" or similar brace
Avoiding neurologic complications	■ Prevention of intercostal neuralgia by minimizing trauma to intercostal nerves is the best method to reduce neurologic complications.
Avoiding wound complications	■ Infection is rare, but surgeons must maintain vigilance.

POSTOPERATIVE CARE

- The patient is placed in a "gunslinger" brace, immobilizing the arm in neutral rotation (**FIG 3**), and a postoperative chest radiograph is obtained to document any hemo- or pneumothorax.
- If a chest tube has been placed, it is removed 1 or 2 days postoperatively, depending on chest tube outputs and pulmonary status.
- Patients are immobilized in the brace for 12 weeks.

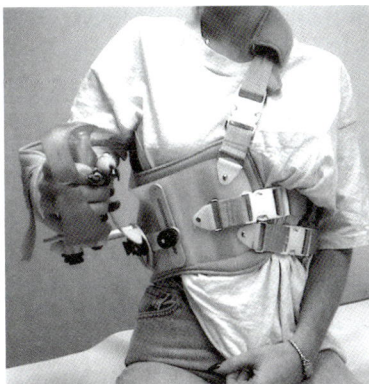

FIG 3 • "Gunslinger" brace with the arm positioned in neutral rotation.

- Rehabilitation is commenced at 12 weeks with a gentle passive range-of-motion program that emphasizes forward elevation and external rotation.
- Three weeks later, the patient is progressed to an active range-of-motion program.
- A strengthening program involving resisted exercises is begun 6 weeks after the gunslinger brace is removed.

OUTCOMES

- Despite the significant complication rate (nearly 50%) that accompanies scapulothoracic arthrodesis, this operation has been documented to provide improvements in both pain and functional disability.
- A high level of patient satisfaction when patients are chosen appropriately and expert surgical technique is used can make this operation rewarding for both patient and surgeon.
- In one series of 23 patients undergoing scapulothoracic fusion, mean ASES scores improved from 35.8 to 40.1. Postoperative pain scores decreased from mean 5.5 to 4.7. Mean patient satisfaction was 9.5 out of 10 for the surgical procedure, and 91% of patients reported that they would undergo the procedure again.[14]

COMPLICATIONS

- Complications are not uncommon with this procedure and have been reported to be as high as 50% in some series.[14]

- The most commonly cited complications associated with this procedure include:
  - Pneumothorax
  - Hemothorax
  - Hardware complications, including wire breakage, nonunion, and pseudoarthrosis
  - Neurologic complications, including intercostal neuralgia
  - Wound complications, including infection or wound dehiscence

REFERENCES

1. Bunch WH, Siegel IM. Scapulothoracic arthrodesis in fascioscapulohumeral muscular dystrophy. J Bone Joint Surg Am 1993;75A:372–376.
2. Connor PM, Yamaguchi K, Manifold SG, et al. Split pectoralis major for serratus anterior palsy. Clin Orthop Relat Res 1997;341:134–142.
3. Cooley LH, Torg JS. "Pseudowinging" of the scapula secondary to subscapular osteochondroma. Clin Orthop Relat Res 1982;162:119–124.
4. Fery A. Results of treatment of anterior serratus paralysis. In: Post M, Morrey BF, Hawkins RJ, eds. Surgery of the Shoulder. Philadelphia: Mosby, 1990:325–329.
5. Foo CL, Swann M. Isolated paralysis of the serratus anterior. A report of 20 cases. J Bone Joint Surg Br 1983;65B:552–556.
6. Freedman L, Munro RR. Abduction of the arm in the scapular plane: scapular and glenohumeral movements. J Bone Joint Surg Am 1966;48A:1503–1510.
7. Gozna ER, Harris WR. Traumatic winging of the scapula. J Bone Joint Surg Am 1979;61A:1230–1233.
8. Gregg JR, LaBosky D, Harty M, et al. Serratus anterior paralysis in the young athlete. J Bone Joint Surg Am 1979;61A:825–832.
9. Harper GD, McIlroy S, Bayley JIL, et al. Arthroscopic partial resection of the scapula for snapping scapula: a new technique. J Shoulder Elbow Surg 1999;8:53–57.
10. Hawkins RJ, Willis RB, Litchfield RB. Scapulothoracic arthrodesis for scapular winging. In Post M, Morrey BF, Hawkins RJ, eds. Surgery of the Shoulder. Philadelphia: Mosby, 1990:340–349.
11. Hays JM, Zehr DJ. Traumatic muscle avulsion causing winging of the scapula. J Bone Joint Surg Am 1981;63A:495–497.
12. Kuhn JE, Plancher KD, Hawkins RJ. Scapular winging. J Am Acad Orthop Surg 1995;3:319–325.
13. Kuhn JE, Plancher KD, Hawkins RJ. Symptomatic scapulothoracic crepitus and bursitis. J Am Acad Orthop Surg 1998;6:267–273.
14. Krishnan SG, Hawkins RJ, Michelotti JD, et al. Scapulothoracic arthrodesis: indications, technique, and results. Clin Orthop Relat Res 2005;435:126–133.
15. Marmor L, Bechtol CO. Paralysis of the serratus anterior due to electric shock relieved by transplantation of the pectoralis major muscle: A case report. J Bone Joint Surg Am 1963;45:156–160.
16. Perlmutter GS, Leffert RD. Results of transfer of the pectoralis major tendon to treat paralysis of the serratus anterior muscle. J Bone Joint Surg Am 1999;81A:377–384.
17. Richards RR, McKee MD. Treatment of painful scapulothoracic crepitus by resection of the superomedial angle of the scapula. Clin Orthop Relat Res 1989;247:111–116.
18. Strizak AM, Cowen MH. The snapping scapula syndrome. J Bone Joint Surg Am 1982;64A:941–942.
19. Warner JJP, Navarro RA. Serratus anterior dysfunction. Clin Orthop Relat Res 1998;349:139–148.
20. Wiater JM, Flatow EL. Long thoracic nerve injury. Clin Orthop Relat Res 1999;368:17–27.

Chapter 32

Suprascapular Nerve Decompression

Andreas H. Gomoll and Anthony A. Romeo

DEFINITION

- Suprascapular nerve (SSN) entrapment is an uncommon cause for shoulder pain and weakness. It was initially described by Koppel and Thompson.[11]
- SSN entrapment typically occurs at the suprascapular or spinoglenoid notch and presents with symptoms ranging from diffuse shoulder pain to weakness and atrophy of the supraspinatus and infraspinatus muscles.

ANATOMY

- The SSN arises from the upper trunk of the brachial plexus, with contributions from C5 and C6 (rarely also C4), and provides branches to the supraspinatus and infraspinatus muscles. It also carries afferent fibers from the glenohumeral joint and rarely also cutaneous fibers from the lateral aspect of the shoulder.
- The nerve traverses two potential compression points, at the suprascapular notch and spinoglenoid notch (**FIG 1**), and is accompanied by the suprascapular artery and vein.
- At the suprascapular notch, the nerve runs in a fibroosseous canal formed by the scapular notch and the transverse scapular ligament. Generally, the nerve runs under the ligament, but it is occasionally accompanied by a branch of the main vessels, which course over the ligament.
- The suprascapular notch is approximately 4.5 cm medial to the posterolateral corner of the acromion and 3 cm medial to the glenoid rim (supraglenoid tubercle). The spinoglenoid notch is approximately 1.8 cm medial to the glenoid rim and 2.5 cm inferomedial to the supraglenoid tubercle.[3]
- Several anatomic studies have described the presence of a spinoglenoid ligament (inferior transverse scapular ligament) at the spinoglenoid notch in 3% to 60% of specimens,[5,6] but its role in nerve entrapment at this level is controversial.

PATHOGENESIS

- The most common site of entrapment is at the suprascapular notch, where it can be compressed by a thickened or ossified transverse scapular ligament.
- The relative confinement of the nerve at the suprascapular notch also places it at risk for injury due to traction, such as seen either in acute trauma or repetitive overhead activities such as volleyball, tennis, or weightlifting.
- Compression from labral ganglions can also occur, typically at the spinoglenoid notch.[1] These cysts can develop as the result of labral tears that allow fluid extravasation but block backflow, similar to a one-way valve.
- More recently, traction injury to the nerve has been described as the result of massive, retracted tears of the posterosuperior cuff.[2]
- Direct or indirect trauma leading to SSN neuropathy has been described as the result of shoulder dislocation, proximal humerus fracture, or scapular fracture.

- Iatrogenic injury to the SSN can occur during distal clavicle resection, positioning during spine surgery, transglenoid drilling for instability repair, shoulder arthrodesis, or the posterior approach to the glenohumeral joint.

NATURAL HISTORY

- The natural history depends on the presence or absence of a space-occupying lesion as the cause of SSN neuropathy.
    - Without compression by a mass, most patients will improve with time and supervised physical therapy.[8]
    - Conversely, the presence of a mass, such as a cyst or ganglion, usually results in failure of conservative management and will require decompressive surgery.
- The natural history of periarticular ganglion cysts in the shoulder is controversial, but they are thought to persist and enlarge with time.[9] In rare instances, spontaneous resolution of ganglion cysts has been documented.

PATIENT HISTORY AND PHYSICAL FINDINGS

- SSN neuropathy secondary to compression at the suprascapular notch typically presents as a dull pain in the posterior

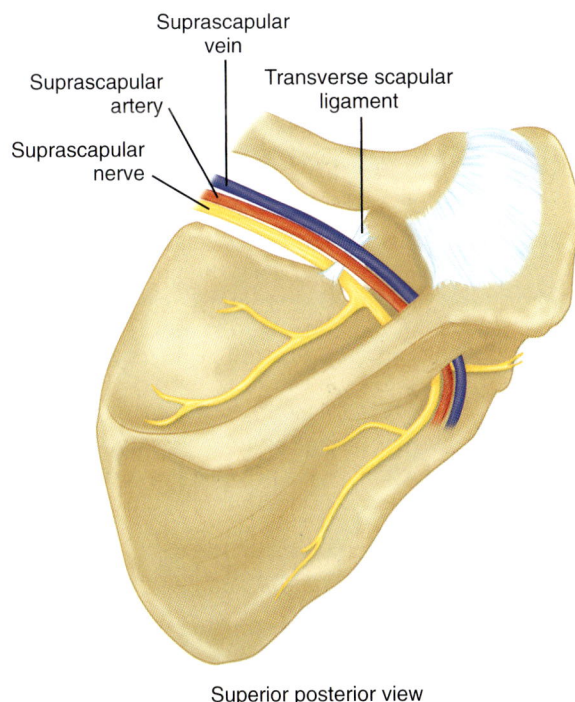

FIG 1 • Anatomy of the suprascapular nerve (SSN). The SSN is accompanied by the suprascapular artery and vein, which course over the transverse scapular ligament (TSL), while the nerve passes underneath. All three then traverse the spinoglenoid notch.

Superior posterior view

Labels: Suprascapular vein; Suprascapular artery; Suprascapular nerve; Transverse scapular ligament

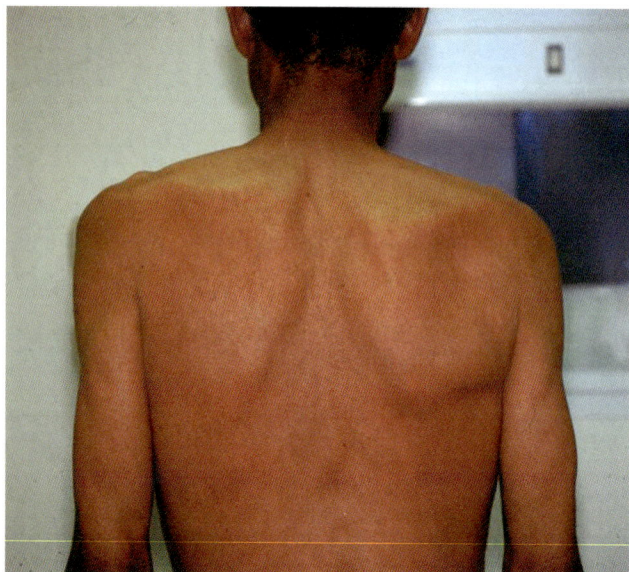

FIG 2 • Posterior photograph of a patient with right infraspinatus muscle wasting secondary to suprascapular nerve entrapment at the spinoglenoid notch.

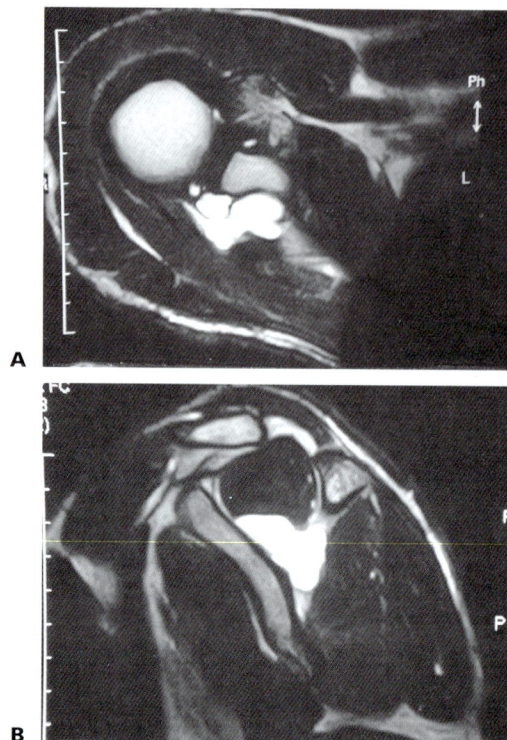

FIG 3 • T2-weighted MR images depicting axial (**A**) and oblique (**B**) sagittal views showing a cyst in the area of the spinoglenoid notch.

and lateral shoulder, but the pain can also be referred to the anterior chest wall, lateral arm, and ipsilateral neck. Compression at the spinoglenoid notch is often comparatively pain-free and presents with isolated infraspinatus atrophy (**FIG 2**).

▪ The patient often provides a history of acute or repetitive trauma to the shoulder, such as a fall on the outstretched hand, or activities such as volleyball, tennis, or weightlifting.

▪ There appears to be an increased incidence of isolated infraspinatus atrophy in asymptomatic volleyball players. This typically responds well to conservative measures.

▪ Depending on the chronicity and degree of compression, varying amounts of weakness in abduction and external rotation can be detected on physical examination.

▪ In longstanding compression, atrophy of the supraspinatus and infraspinatus can be observed.

▪ Atrophy, if present, may assist in differentiating compression at the suprascapular notch from that at the spinoglenoid level, since supraspinatus atrophy occurs only with the former.

▪ Palpation of the spinoglenoid notch and cross-body adduction may reproduce the patient's symptoms.

▪ It is important to exclude other potential sources of pain, such as the cervical spine, acromioclavicular joint, or rotator cuff.

IMAGING AND OTHER DIAGNOSTIC STUDIES

▪ An anesthetic injection into the suprascapular notch can be diagnostic if it results in complete but transient pain relief.

▪ Stryker notch views, or anteroposterior radiographs of the scapula, with a 15- to 30-degrees caudally directed beam, provide visualization of the suprascapular notch. Alternatively, a CT scan can provide good osseous detail in cases of posttraumatic deformity or ossification of the transverse scapular ligament.

▪ MRI can reveal a superior or posterior labral tear and the presence of a ganglion in the area of the suprascapular or

spinoglenoid notch (**FIG 3**). Ganglion cysts present as homogeneous masses with low signal intensity on T1-weighted images and high signal intensity on T2-weighted images.

▪ Electromyography and nerve conduction studies can often provide a conclusive diagnosis by showing denervation potentials, fibrillations, spontaneous activity, and prolonged motor latencies in the supraspinatus or infraspinatus, depending on the level of entrapment.

DIFFERENTIAL DIAGNOSIS

▪ Cervical radiculopathy
▪ Glenohumeral instability
▪ Rotator cuff pathology
▪ Acromioclavicular joint arthrosis

NONOPERATIVE MANAGEMENT

▪ Initial treatment for SSN neuropathy in the absence of a space-occupying lesion is conservative and will lead to near-complete resolution of symptoms in most cases.

▪ Complete resolution of pain and weakness can take more than 1 year.

▪ Supervised physical therapy, followed by a self-directed home exercise program, should consist of range-of-motion exercises, as well as strengthening of the rotator cuff muscles, the deltoid, and the periscapular musculature, including the trapezius, rhomboids, and serratus musculature. Restoring proper scapular function is beneficial in recovery and may prevent recurrence of the injury.

▪ Image-guided cyst aspiration has shown success in about half of patients, with persistence or recurrence in the other half.[9,12]

SURGICAL MANAGEMENT

- Surgical treatment is indicated in patients who have failed to respond to 6 to 12 months of nonoperative measures and continue to have significant pain and dysfunction. SSN neuropathy secondary to a mass is best treated with decompression, and evaluation and potential repair of the glenoid labrum.
- Other sources for shoulder pain and dysfunction should be ruled out if the mass is smaller than 1 cm in diameter or is not directly compressing the neurovascular bundle.

Preoperative Planning

- Oblique sagittal MR imaging allows visualization of the SSN in the supraspinatus fossa, the spinoglenoid notch, and the infraspinatus fossa.
  - If a space-occupying lesion is present, this imaging will assist in preoperative planning by delineating the exact position of the mass and determining whether it is confined to the supraspinatus or the infraspinatus fossa or involves both areas.
- A paralabral ganglion or cyst that is confined to one area, especially when associated with a labral tear or other intra-articular pathology, is often amenable to arthroscopic decompression.
- We have found it useful first to perform a diagnostic shoulder arthroscopy and potential treatment of intra-articular pathology, followed by arthroscopic or open decompression of the SSN.
- Arthroscopic decompression has the potential advantages of treating associated intra-articular lesions, such as labral tears and avoiding the morbidity associated with open procedures.

Positioning

- Either the beach chair or the lateral decubitus position can be used.

OPEN DECOMPRESSION

Approach to the Suprascapular Notch

- Decompression of the suprascapular nerve at the suprascapular notch is best achieved through a trapezius-splitting approach.
  - The anterior approach requires a more complex dissection and therefore carries a higher risk of neurovascular complications. It also offers incomplete visualization of the SSN posterior to the notch and is generally not recommended.
- A saber-type skin incision following the Langer lines is performed over the top of the shoulder. The incision begins posteriorly at the distal third of the scapular spine and extends anteriorly to a point 2 cm medially off the acromioclavicular joint (**TECH FIG 1A**).
- A transverse skin incision parallel to the scapular spine can be chosen instead but produces a less cosmetic scar.
- The trapezius fascia and muscle is divided in line with its fibers for a distance of 5 cm.
- Abduction of the arm decreases tension on the muscle, which if necessary can be elevated off the scapular spine for an extensile exposure.
- The supraspinatus muscle is bluntly dissected off the anterior aspect of the suprascapular fossa and retracted posteriorly to provide access to the suprascapular notch (**TECH FIG 1B**).

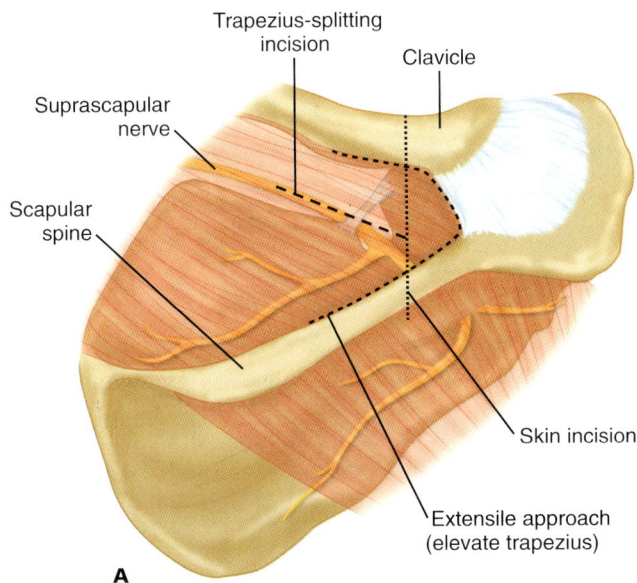

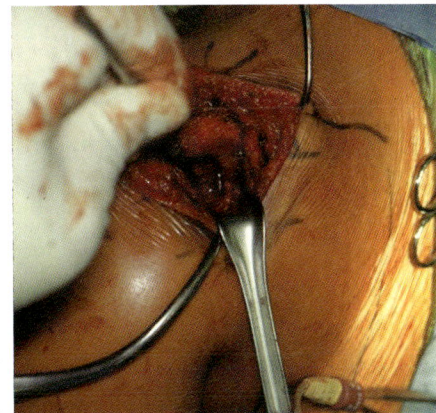

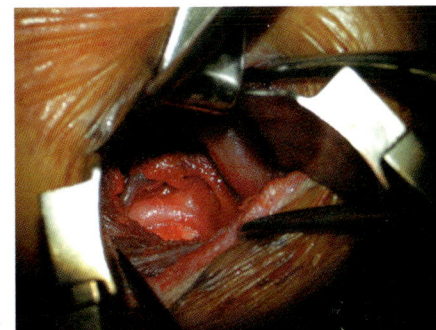

TECH FIG 1 • Schematic and intraoperative photograph demonstrating suprascapular nerve release at the suprascapular notch. **A.** The trapezius muscle is split in line with its fibers. **B.** The supraspinatus muscle is bluntly dissected off the suprascapular fossa and retracted to expose the suprascapular notch. **C.** The transverse scapular ligament has been released.

■ The overlying suprascapular artery and vein are gently retracted to expose the transverse scapular ligament.

■ A small right-angle clamp can be used to bluntly dissect under the ligament and protect the underlying nerve while the ligament is transected with a scalpel.

■ Occasionally the nerve is still tethered after release of the transverse ligament, requiring careful resection of the medial aspect of the suprascapular notch. The resected edge of the bone must be smooth at the completion of the procedure.

■ If the trapezius was detached during the approach, it should be sutured back to the bone of the scapular spine. If the muscle was only split in line with its fibers, it is reapproximated with interrupted, absorbable sutures.

Approach to the Spinoglenoid Notch

■ The posterior approach provides direct visualization of the suprascapular nerve at the spinoglenoid notch.

■ A longitudinal skin incision is centered approximately 4 cm medial to the posterolateral corner of the acromion, approximately 5 cm in length. Following Langer lines provides a cosmetically acceptable scar.

■ The underlying fascia and deltoid muscle is split in line with its fibers beginning at the level of the scapular spine and extending 5 cm distal from the posterior acromion (**TECH FIG 2A**). A stay suture placed at the distalmost extent of the incision protects against propagation of the split, which carries a risk of injury to the axillary nerve.

■ The infraspinatus is identified, dissected off the scapular spine, and retracted inferiorly (**TECH FIG 2B**).

■ Commonly, a small area of vascular fibrous tissue is encountered posterior to the site of the spinoglenoid notch, covering the suprascapular neurovascular structures.

■ If a ganglion is present, the contents of the cyst should be removed along with the wall (**TECH FIG 2C**).

■ A spinoglenoid ligament, if present, should be excised.

■ Decompression is complete when the SSN can be followed along its entire length from the spinoglenoid notch until it arborizes into its infraspinatus branches (**TECH FIG 2D**).

■ The infraspinatus muscle is allowed to return to its anatomic position.

■ The deltoid muscle and fascia is reapproximated with interrupted, absorbable sutures.

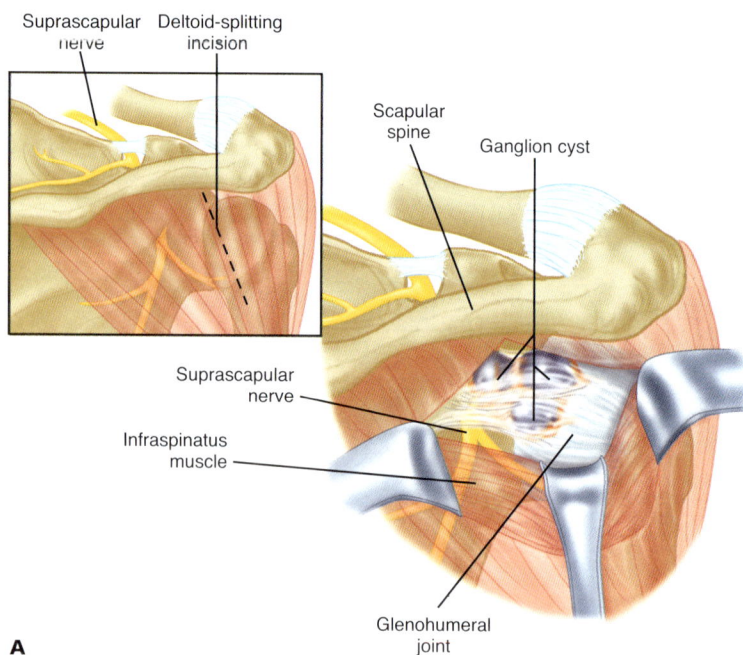

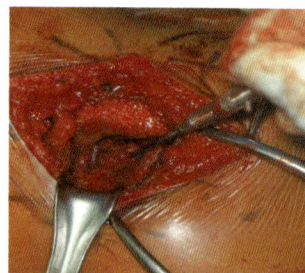

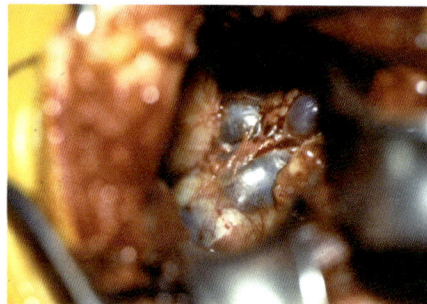

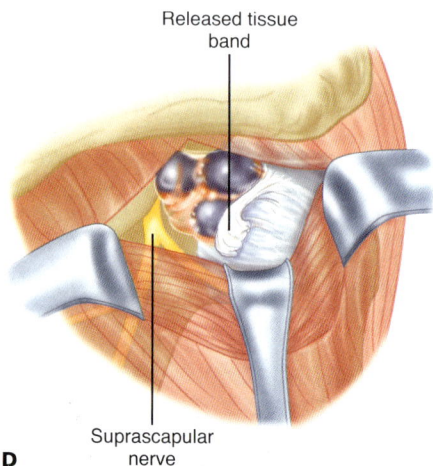

TECH FIG 2 • Schematics and intraoperative photographs showing suprascapular nerve release at the spinoglenoid notch. **A.** The deltoid muscle is split in line with its fibers, beginning about 4 cm medial to the posterolateral corner of the acromion. **B.** The spinoglenoid notch has been exposed. The retractors displace the infraspinatus muscles posteriorly and inferiorly. **C.** A multilobulated ganglion cyst. **D.** The suprascapular nerve is now visible after the soft tissue band has been divided.

ARTHROSCOPIC DECOMPRESSION

Approach to the Suprascapular Notch

- Routine glenohumeral arthroscopy is performed to assess concomitant pathology, especially tears of the superior-posterior labrum.
- The subacromial bursa is resected, extending more medially than what is usual for subacromial decompression.
  - The bursectomy should allow adequate visualization from the acromioclavicular (AC) joint and coracoid anteriorly to the scapular spine posteriorly.
- The coracoid is palpated with a probe or switching stick, which can also be used to bluntly dissect the surrounding soft tissues to expose the coracoclavicular ligaments.
  - Alternatively, the ligaments can be found approximately 15 mm medial to the AC joint and then followed inferiorly to their insertion on the coracoid.
- The conoid ligament attaches to the coracoid just laterally to the suprascapular notch. Fibers of the conoid ligament are in continuity with the transverse scapular ligament.

- The suprascapular notch is typically covered by the supraspinatus muscle and fat, complicating visualization of the neurovascular bundle (**TECH FIG 3A**).
- An accessory portal is created approximately 2 cm medial to the standard Neviaser portal along a line that bisects the angle formed between the clavicle and spine of the scapula. An 18-gauge spinal needle helps with correct positioning of the portal (**TECH FIG 3B**).
- Use of a switching stick or smooth trocar through this accessory portal allows careful, blunt dissection of the fat to expose the suprascapular vessels coursing over the transverse scapular ligament, which presents as glistening white fibers.
- Once adequate visualization has been achieved, the nerve is protected with a probe or small trocar while the overlying ligament is cut with the arthroscopic scissors as far lateral as possible (**TECH FIG 3C–E**).
- The SSN is probed to ensure adequate decompression; any residual compression from the bony structures can be removed with the arthroscopic burr.

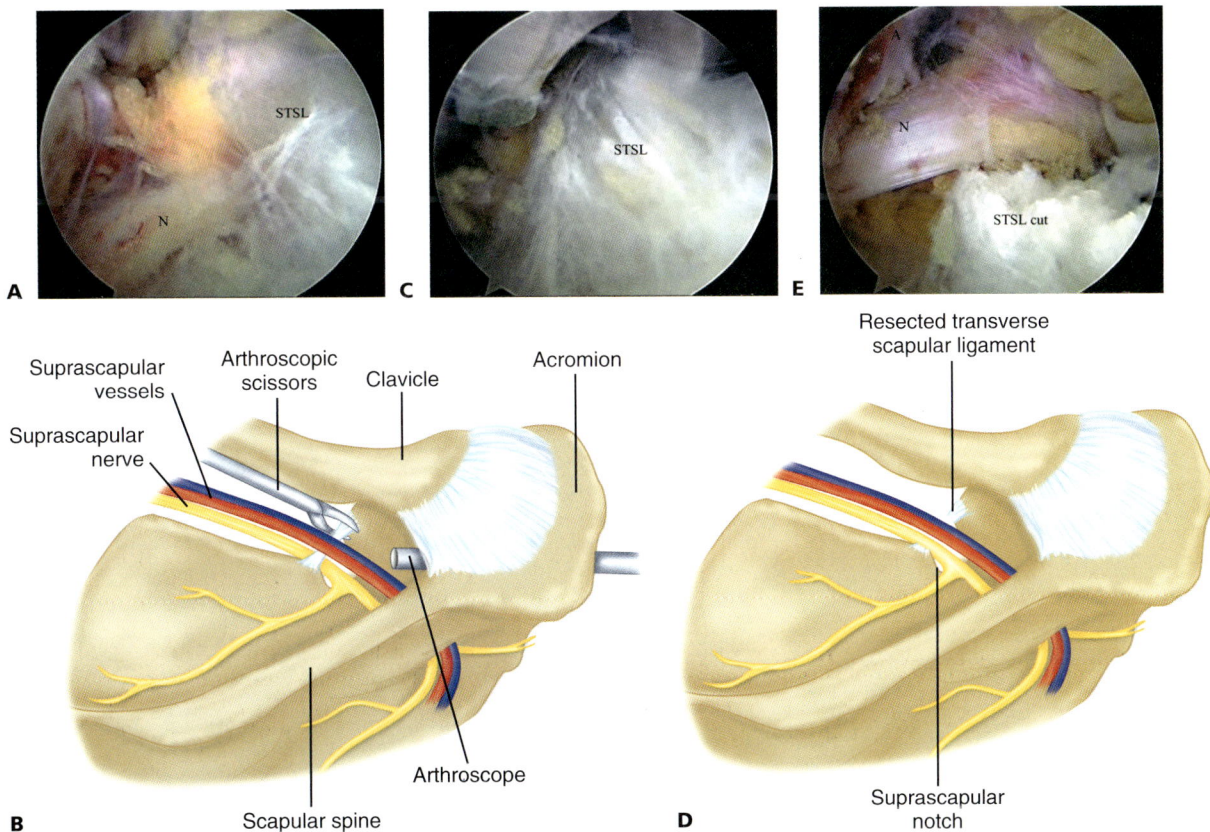

TECH FIG 3 • Schematic and arthroscopic images showing arthroscopic suprascapular nerve release at the suprascapular notch. **A.** After soft tissue removal, the nerve (N) can be visualized underneath the superior transverse scapular ligament (STSL). A blunt trocar is retracting the overlying vessel. **B.** The arthroscope is positioned in the lateral portal and the instruments are introduced through a superior portal, medial to the standard Neviaser portal. **C.** Arthroscopic scissors positioned to cut the STSL. **D,E.** The ligament has been released. *A,* artery. (**A,C,E**: Courtesy of Dr Laurence Higgins.)

Approach to the Spinoglenoid Notch

- Ganglion cysts associated with labral tears are most commonly located at the spinoglenoid notch. They often extend into the infraspinatus fossa.
- With an intact labrum, the joint capsule above the superior-posterior labrum is incised, beginning posterior to the biceps root and extending posteriorly for 2 to 3 cm.
- After incision of the capsule, the fibrous raphe between the supraspinatus and infraspinatus seen lateral to the spinoglenoid notch provides a useful landmark.
- The spinoglenoid notch can be palpated with an arthroscopic instrument, providing a bony landmark that can be correlated with the cyst position as seen on preoperative MR imaging.

- An accessory posterolateral portal is placed after first establishing correct orientation with an 18-gauge spinal needle.
- Similar to open decompression, fibrovascular tissue covers the neurovascular bundle and has to be bluntly dissected with a switching stick or similar tool through the accessory portal before the nerve can be visualized.
- The SSN is positioned medially, in direct contact with the bone of the spinoglenoid notch; the vascular structures are positioned laterally and closer to the glenoid.
- Ganglion cysts are typically located posterior to the nerve and should be removed completely, including the lining.
- After cyst removal, the nerve should be inspected for any additional sites of compression.

POSTOPERATIVE CARE

- The arm is immobilized in a sling for 2 or 3 days for comfort.
- Pendulum exercises commence on postoperative day 1, and active motion is increased as tolerated.

OUTCOMES

- Nonoperative treatment is successful in 80% of patients without space-occupying lesions.[8]
- Open decompression with release of the transverse scapular ligament improved pain and weakness in 73% to 87% of patients.[4,13]

- Reports on the outcomes of arthroscopic decompression are rare, but outcomes seem to approach the success rate of open approaches.

COMPLICATIONS

- Damage to the suprascapular nerve and vessels
- Damage to the spinal accessory nerve if mobilization of the trapezius muscle is carried out far medially
- Incomplete decompression, especially in rare cases of compression at both suprascapular and spinoglenoid notch

PEARLS AND PITFALLS

Arthroscopic decompression	▪ Hemostasis and visualization can be improved by increasing the fluid pressure to 50 mm Hg and using an electrothermal device to cauterize bleeders. ▪ The decompression should be performed before treatment of any concomitant pathology to avoid further complicating this procedure owing to fluid extravasation and swelling. ▪ A 70-degree scope is sometimes helpful to visualize the notch. ▪ Visualization should be performed through the lateral portal, with posterior and accessory medial working portals.

REFERENCES

1. Aiello I, Serra G, Traina GC, et al. Entrapment of the suprascapular nerve at the spinoglenoid notch. Ann Neurol 1982;12:314–316.
2. Albritton MJ, Graham RD, Richards RS II, et al. An anatomic study of the effects on the suprascapular nerve due to retraction of the supraspinatus muscle after a rotator cuff tear. J Shoulder Elbow Surg 2003;12:497–500.
3. Bigliani LU, Dalsey RM, McCann PD, et al. An anatomical study of the suprascapular nerve. Arthroscopy 1990;6:301–305.
4. Callahan JD, Scully TB, Shapiro SA, et al. Suprascapular nerve entrapment: a series of 27 cases. J Neurosurg 1991;74:893–896.
5. Cummins CA, Anderson K, Bowen M, et al. Anatomy and histological characteristics of the spinoglenoid ligament. J Bone Joint Surg Am 1998;80:1622–1625.
6. Demaio M, Drez D Jr, Mullins RC. The inferior transverse scapular ligament as a possible cause of entrapment neuropathy of the nerve to the infraspinatus: a brief note. J Bone Joint Surg Am 1991;73A: 1061–1063.
7. Lafosse L, Tomasi A. Technique for endoscopic release of suprascapular nerve entrapment at the suprascapular notch. Tech Shoulder Elbow 2006;7:1–6.
8. Martin SD, Warren RF, Martin TL, et al. Suprascapular neuropathy: results of non-operative treatment. J Bone Joint Surg Am 1997;79A: 1159–1165.
9. Piatt BE, Hawkins RJ, Fritz RC, et al. Clinical evaluation and treatment of spinoglenoid notch ganglion cysts. J Shoulder Elbow Surg 2002;11:600–604.
10. Romeo AA, Rotenberg DD, Bach BR Jr. Suprascapular neuropathy. J Am Acad Orthop Surg 1999;7:358–367.
11. Thompson W, Kopell H. Peripheral entrapment neuropathies of the upper extremity. N Engl J Med 1959;260:1261–1265.
12. Tirman PF, Feller JF, Janzen DL, et al. Association of glenoid labral cysts with labral tears and glenohumeral instability: radiologic findings and clinical significance. Radiology 1994;190:653–658.
13. Vastamaki M, Goransson H. Suprascapular nerve entrapment. Clin Orthop Relat Res 1993;297:135–143.

Open Reduction and Internal Fixation of Supracondylar and Intercondylar Fractures

Joaquin Sanchez-Sotelo

PATIENT HISTORY AND PHYSICAL FINDINGS

- Distal humerus fractures occur in two age groups:
  - Younger patients who sustain high-energy trauma
  - Older patients with underlying osteopenia
- Comminution is the dominant feature of supracondylar and intercondylar fractures and complicates internal fixation.
- The goals of the initial evaluation are to:
  - Understand the fracture pattern.
  - Determine the existence of previous symptomatic elbow pathology.
  - Determine the extent of associated soft tissue (open fractures).
  - Identify associated musculoskeletal or neurovascular injuries.

IMAGING AND OTHER DIAGNOSTIC STUDIES

- Elbow radiographs in the anteroposterior and lateral planes are the first imaging studies obtained and should be carefully scrutinized to identify the fracture lines and fragments as well as the extent of comminution.
  - A complete understanding of the fracture pattern is difficult to obtain based only on simple radiographs because of the complex geometry of the distal humerus and fragment overlapping (**FIG 1A,B**).
- CT with three-dimensional reconstruction is extremely helpful, especially in the more complex cases. It allows the surgeon to look for specific fractured fragments at the time of fixation, facilitating accurate fracture reduction (**FIG 1C,D**).

- Traction radiographs obtained in the operating room with the patient under anesthesia just before surgery also can be helpful, especially if a CT scan is not available.

SURGICAL MANAGEMENT

- Internal fixation is the treatment of choice for most fractures of the distal humerus.
- Modern fixation techniques seem to benefit from:
  - Fixation strategies designed to improve the mechanical stability of the construct
  - Use of precontoured periarticular plates
  - Use of screws locked to the plates
- Elbow arthroplasty should be considered in elderly patients with previous elbow pathology or in very low, comminuted fractures in patients with osteopenia.
- The goal of the internal fixation technique is to achieve a construct stable enough to allow immediate unprotected motion without fear of redisplacement.[12] This can be attained in most distal humerus fractures—even the most complex—provided the following principles are adhered to (**FIG 2**):
  - Plates used for internal fixation are applied so that fixation in the distal fragments is maximized.
  - Distal screw fixation contributes to stability at the supracondylar level, where true interfragmentary compression is achieved.

Approaches

- Adequate exposure is necessary to achieve satisfactory reduction and fixation.
- Subcutaneous transposition of the ulnar nerve is associated with a decreased incidence of postoperative ulnar neuropathy.

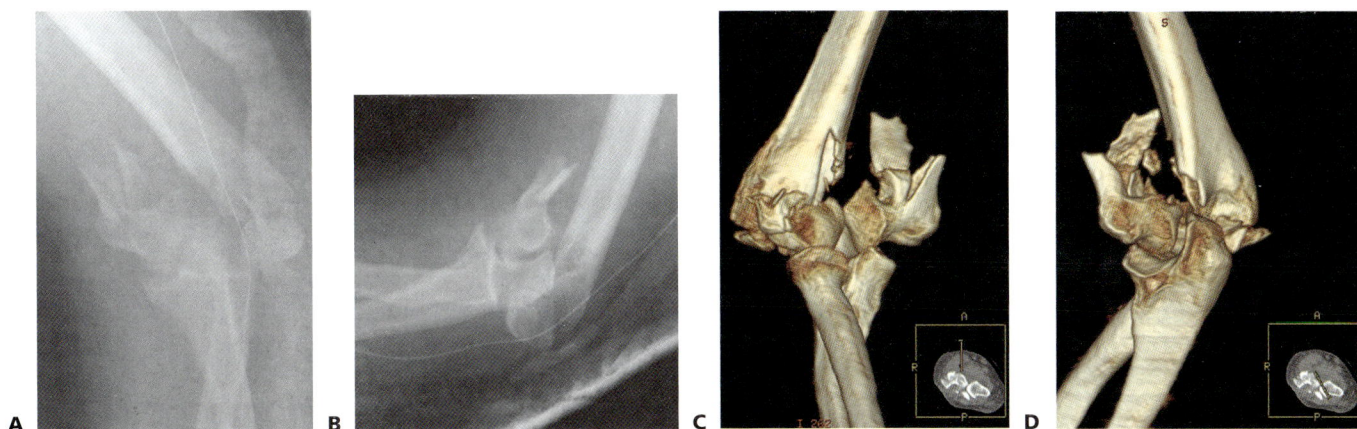

FIG 1 • **A,B.** AP and lateral radiographs showing a comminuted intra-articular supraintercondylar fracture of the distal humerus. The complexity of the fracture is difficult to appreciate fully because of the geometry of the distal humerus, fracture comminution, and fragment overlapping. **C,D.** The use of CT with three-dimensional reconstruction and surface rendering helps understand the fracture configuration and anticipate the surgical findings.

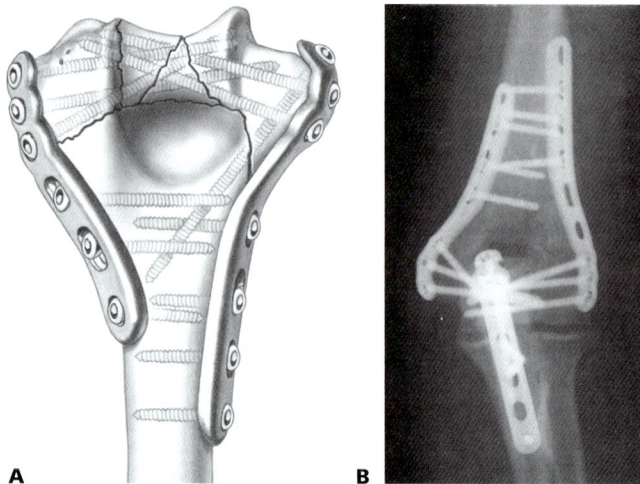

FIG 2 • A. Internal fixation using two parallel medial and lateral plates allows maximal fixation of the plates in the distal fragments and increased stability at the supracondylar level. **B.** This postoperative AP radiograph shows anatomic reduction of a complex distal humerus fracture and stable fixation using the principles and technique described in this chapter. The olecranon osteotomy was fixed with a plate. (**A:** Copyright Mayo.)

- Most fractures require mobilization of the extensor mechanism of the elbow through an olecranon osteotomy, triceps reflection, or triceps split.
- Simple fractures occasionally may be addressed working on both sides of the triceps without mobilization of the extensor mechanism.
- Olecranon osteotomy is the preferred surgical approach for internal fixation for most distal humerus fractures.[11]
  - Advantages
    - Provides excellent exposure
    - Offers the potential of bone-to-bone healing, thereby limiting the risk of triceps dysfunction
  - Disadvantages
    - Complications: nonunion, intra-articular adhesions
    - Hardware removal may be needed.
    - Limits the ability for intraoperative conversion to elbow arthroplasty
    - May devitalize the anconeus muscle
    - The proximal ulna cannot be used as a template to judge reduction and motion.
- Triceps reflection and triceps split[8] allow preservation of the intact ulna.
  - Avoids complications related to olecranon osteotomy
  - Facilitates intraoperative conversion to total elbow arthroplasty
  - Allows use of the proximal ulna as a template for reduction of the distal humerus articular surface
  - Allows assessment of extension deficit after fracture fixation, which is especially useful in fractures requiring metaphyseal shortening
- Bilaterotricipital approach[1]
  - Goals and indications
    - The goal is to provide adequate exposure for fracture fixation without violating the extensor mechanism.
    - This approach is used only for the more simple fracture patterns (eg, extra-articular or simple intra-articular distal humerus fractures [AO/OTA A, C1, C2]) or when elbow arthroplasty is being considered.
  - Advantages
    - This approach avoids complications related to the extensor mechanism.
    - No postoperative protection is needed.
    - Surgical time is decreased.
  - Disadvantage
    - The procedure provides limited exposure of the articular surface.

TECHNIQUES

SURGICAL APPROACH

Olecranon Osteotomy

- Chevron osteotomy provides increased stability (**TECH FIG 1A**).
- The distal apex of the chevron osteotomy is centered with the bare area of the olecranon articular surface.
- The anconeus is divided with electrocautery in line with the lateral limb of the osteotomy.
  - Alternatively, the anconeus may be preserved by dissecting it free on its distal aspect and reflecting it proximally attached to the proximal ulnar fragment.[2]
- Start the osteotomy with a thin oscillating saw.
- Complete the osteotomy with an osteotome.
  - Decreases risk of damage to the articular cartilage on ulna and humerus
  - Creates irregularities at the opposing cut surfaces, which may increase interdigitation
- Mobilize the fragment to facilitate exposure (**TECH FIG 1B**).
- Fixation (**TECH FIG 1C**)

- Some biomechanical studies support the combination of a 7.3-mm cancellous screw and tension band over either a screw alone or K-wires plus tension band; others have found no differences.
- The author's preferred method uses K-wires plus a tension band.
- If screw fixation is planned, drill and tap the ulna before performing the osteotomy.
- Plate fixation is preferred by some.
  - It provides improved fixation, but the risk of wound complications is increased.

Triceps Reflection and Triceps Split

- Bryan-Morrey triceps-sparing approach (**TECH FIG 2**)
  - The triceps is elevated from the medial intermuscular septum.
  - The forearm fascia and periosteum are incised just lateral to the flexor carpi ulnaris.
  - The triceps, forearm fascia, and anconeus are elevated in continuity from medial to lateral.

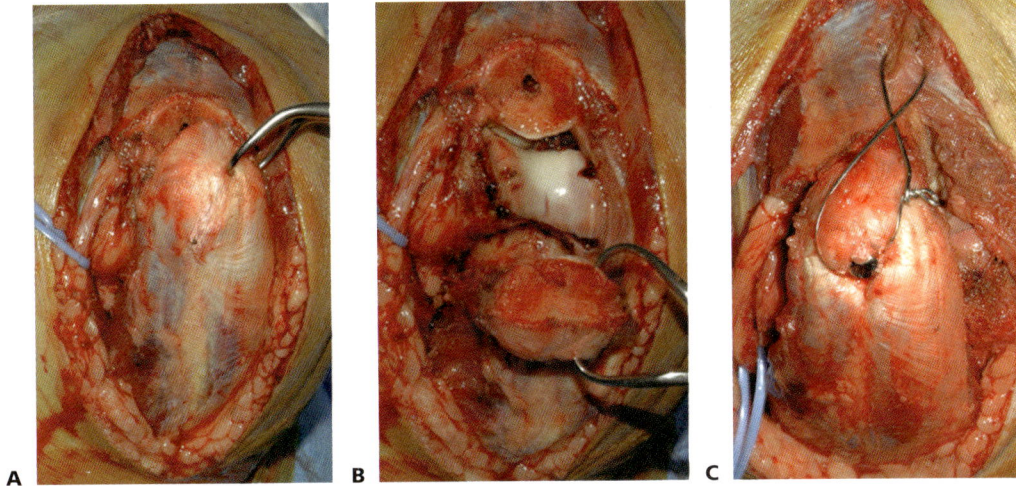

TECH FIG 1 • Olecranon osteotomy provides an excellent exposure for distal humerus fracture fixation. **A.** A chevron osteotomy is initiated with a microsagittal saw and completed with an osteotome. Drilling and tapping before performing the osteotomy facilitates fixation of the osteotomy if screw fixation is selected. **B.** Proximal mobilization of the osteotomized fragment and triceps allows ample exposure of the articular surface and columns. **C.** Fixation may be performed with a cancellous screw and tension band, wires and a tension band, or a plate.

- The anterior bundle of the medial collateral ligament and the lateral ulnar collateral ligament must be preserved to avoid postoperative instability.
- Mayo-modified extensile Köcher approach
  - The triceps is elevated from the lateral intermuscular septum.
  - The triceps and anconeus are elevated in continuity from lateral to medial.

- As noted earlier, the anterior bundle of the medial collateral ligament and the lateral ulnar collateral ligament must be preserved to avoid postoperative instability.

Bilaterotricipital Approach

- The triceps is elevated from the medial and lateral intermuscular septae.
- Lateral dissection can be extended anterior to the anconeus muscle (**TECH FIG 3**).
- Arthrotomy is performed posterior to the medial collateral ligament and lateral collateral ligament complex.

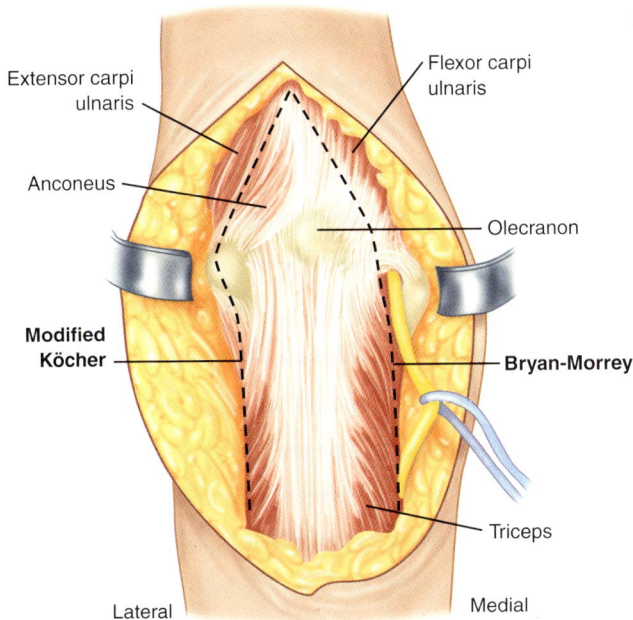

TECH FIG 2 • The extensor mechanism (ie, triceps, anconeus, and forearm fascia) may be elevated off the ulna subperiosteally in continuity from medial to lateral (Bryan-Morrey approach) or from lateral to medial (Mayo-modified extensile Köcher approach).

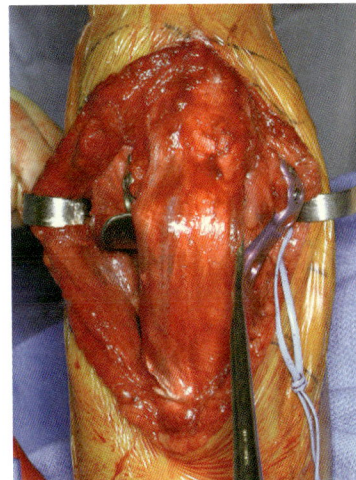

TECH FIG 3 • Fractures with no or limited articular involvement may be fixed working on both sides of the triceps. As shown in this image, the extensor mechanism is left mostly undisturbed.

INTERNAL FIXATION

Technical Objectives

- Screws in the distal fragments (articular segment) should be placed according to the following principles:
  - Every screw should pass through a plate.
  - Each screw should engage a fragment on the opposite side that also is fixed to a plate.
  - As many screws as possible should be placed in the distal fragments.
  - Each screw should be as long as possible.
  - Each screw should engage as many articular fragments as possible.
  - The screws should lock together by interdigitation within the distal segment, thereby rigidly linking the medial and lateral columns together, creating an architectural structure similar to that of an arch or dome.
- Plates are used for fixation.
  - Plates should be applied such that compression is achieved at the supracondylar level for both columns.
  - Plates must be strong enough and stiff enough to resist breaking or bending before union occurs at the supracondylar level.

Provisional Assembly of the Articular Surface and Plate Placement

- Reduce the articular surface fragments anatomically.
  - The proximal ulna and radial head may be used as templates.
- Rotational alignment should be carefully assessed.
- Use smooth K-wires to maintain the reduction provisionally (**TECH FIG 4A**).
  - Two 2.0-mm smooth wires introduced at the medial and lateral epicondyles facilitate provisional placement of the plates and can be replaced by screws later.

- Fine-threaded wires or absorbable pins may be used for definitive fixation of small fracture fragments.
- Medial and lateral plates are placed so that one of the distal holes of each plate slides over the medial and lateral 2.0-mm smooth wires introduced at the medial and lateral epicondyles (**TECH FIG 4B**).
- One cortical screw is loosely introduced into a slotted hole of each plate to hold the plates in place; use of slotted holes for these screws facilitates later adjustments in plate positioning.

Articular and Distal Fixation

- Two or more distal screws are inserted through the plates medially and laterally. As noted, the screws should be as long as possible and engage the opposite column.
  - Before screw application, a large bone clamp is used to compress the articular fracture lines, unless there is comminution of the articular surface.
- The two 2.0-mm smooth pins may be replaced with distal screws without previous drilling, to avoid accidental breakage of the drill when contacting the other screws. Usually, these last screws will interdigitate with the previously applied distal screws, thereby increasing the stability of the construct (**TECH FIG 5**).

Supracondylar Compression and Proximal Plate Fixation

- The proximal screw on one side is backed out, and a large bone clamp is applied distally on that side and proximally on the opposite side to apply maximum compression at the supracondylar level. Compression is maintained by application of one proximal screw in the compression mode (**TECH FIG 6A,B**).
- The same steps are followed on the opposite side.

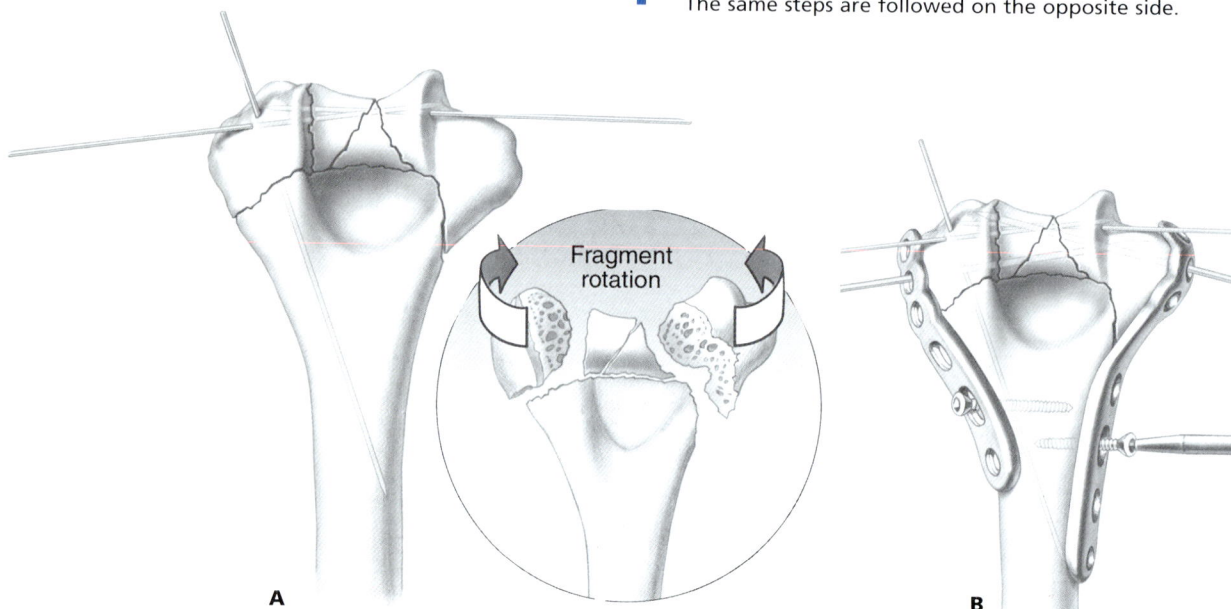

TECH FIG 4 • **A.** Anatomic reduction of the articular surface is maintained provisionally with fine wires placed so that they will not interfere with plate and screw application. **B.** The medial and lateral plates are held in place provisionally with two distal 2.0-mm pins (which later will be replaced by screws) and two proximal screws through an oval hole to allow small adjustments in plate positioning. (Copyright Mayo.)

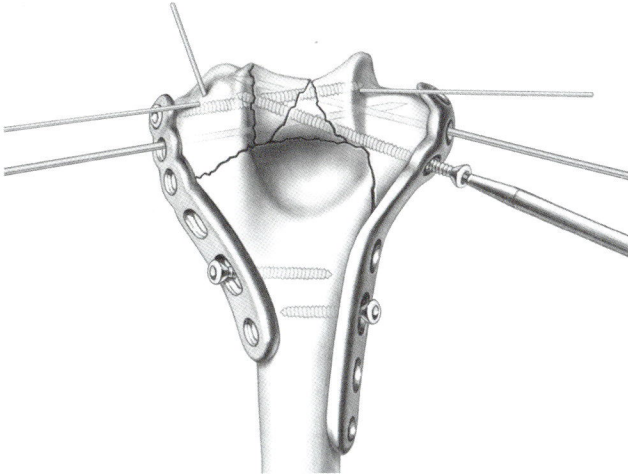

- The remaining diaphyseal screws are then introduced, providing additional compression as they push the undercontoured plates to gain intimate contact with the underlying bone (**TECH FIG 6C,D**).
- Small posterior fragments can be fixed with threaded wires or absorbable pins.
- Provisional wires are removed.
- The elbow is put through range of motion. Motion should be smooth. If extension is limited, the tip of the olecranon may be removed.

TECH FIG 5 • Maximal distal plate anchorage is then achieved by insertion of multiple long screws through the plates and into the distal fragments. Usually the screws from the medial and lateral directions will engage, creating an interlocked structure that increases fracture stability. (Copyright Mayo.)

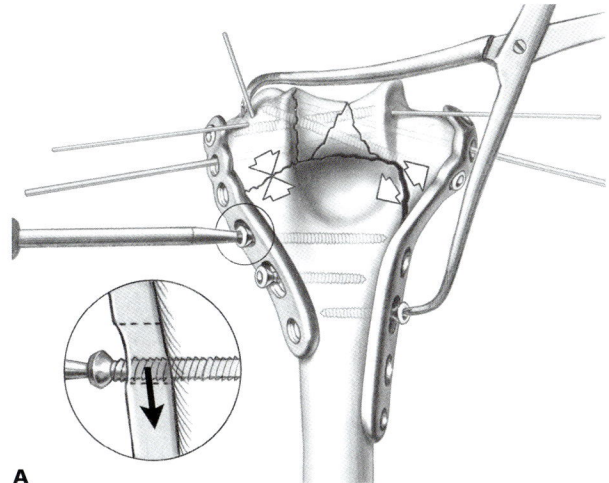

A

TECH FIG 6 • **A,B.** Supracondylar compression is achieved with the use of a large clamp, insertion of screws in the compression mode, and slight undercontouring of the plates. The same technique is applied laterally and medially. **C.** Internal fixation of a complex distal humerus fracture. (**A,B:** Copyright Mayo.)

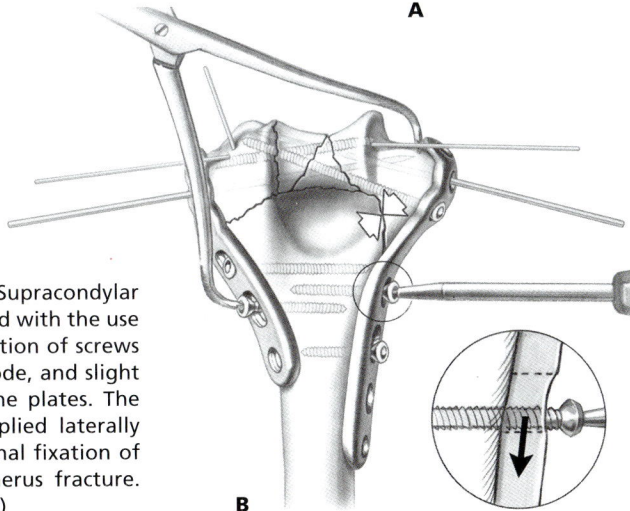

B

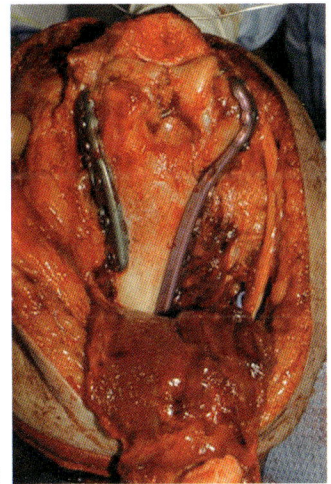

C

SUPRACONDYLAR SHORTENING

- In cases with supracondylar comminution (ie, bone loss), compression at the supracondylar level cannot be achieved unless the humerus is shortened into a nonanatomic reduction that will provide adequate bone contact (**TECH FIG 7A,B**).
  - The humerus may be shortened between a few millimeters and 2 cm with only minor losses in extension strength.[9]
- Bone is trimmed from the diaphysis to ensure adequate bone contact with the distal fragments.

- The distal fragments are translated proximally and anteriorly. Anterior translation is necessary to create room for the radial head and the coronoid in flexion.
- The fracture is fixed in the desired position using the technique described previously.
- A new deep and wide olecranon fossa is created by removing bone from the distal and posterior aspect of the diaphysis (**TECH FIG 7C**). Otherwise, extension will be restricted.

TECHNIQUES

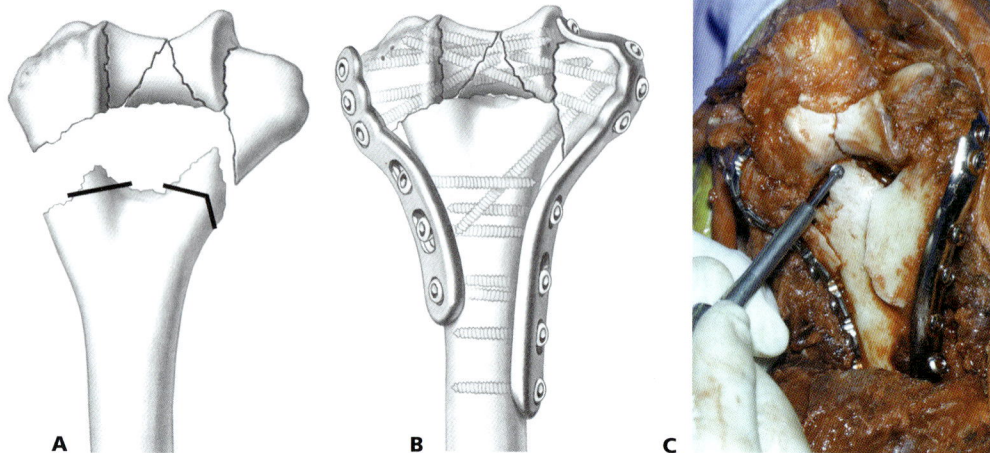

TECH FIG 7 • In cases of severe supracondylar comminution, adequate interfragmentary contact and compression takes priority over anatomic reduction. The humerus may be shortened anywhere from a few millimeters to 2 cm by trimming the bony spikes of the diaphysis (**A**), advancing the distal segment proximally and anteriorly, and fixing it in a nonanatomic fashion (**B**). **C.** The olecranon fossa is recreated in this case by removing bone from the posterior aspect of the diaphysis with a burr. (**A,B:** Copyright Mayo.)

PEARLS AND PITFALLS

Olecranon osteotomy	▪ Position the apex of the osteotomy distally. ▪ Use a thin oscillating saw to minimize bone loss. ▪ If plate fixation is preferred, consider drilling the holes for the plate before beginning the osteotomy. This facilitates plate fixation of the osteotomy at the conclusion of the surgery. ▪ Similarly, if tension band fixation with an intramedullary screw is preferred, predrill the screw hole.
Triceps reflection and triceps split	▪ Subperiosteal detachment of the extensor mechanism is critical to preserve its thickness and facilitate a strong reattachment. ▪ Reproduce anatomic reattachment of the extensor mechanism. ▪ Use heavy nonabsorbable suture (no. 5 Ethibond [Ethicon, Inc., Somerville, NJ] or no. FiberWire [Arthrex, Inc., Naples, FL]) through bone. ▪ Protect extension against resistance for 6 weeks.
Bilaterotricipital approach	▪ Separate the triceps from the underlying medial and lateral joint capsules. ▪ Resect the posterior capsule and fat pad to improve visualization.

POSTOPERATIVE MANAGEMENT

▪ After closure, the elbow is placed in a bulky noncompressive dressing with an anterior plaster splint to maintain the elbow in extension, and the upper extremity is kept elevated.

▪ Motion is initiated according to the extent of soft tissue damage. Motion usually can be initiated on the first or second postoperative day, but it may be necessary to wait for several days in the case of open fractures or severe soft tissue damage.

▪ Most patients benefit from a program of continuous passive motion for the first week or two after fixation; some may benefit from a longer period of passive motion.

▪ When postoperative motion fails to progress as expected, a program of patient-adjusted static flexion and extension splints is implemented.

▪ Treatment with indomethacin or single-dose radiation to the soft tissues shielding the fracture site may be considered for patients with high risk of heterotopic ossification, such as those with associated head or spinal trauma as well as those who require several surgeries in a short period of time.

OUTCOMES

▪ The results of internal fixation for fractures of the distal humerus using modern techniques are summarized in Table 1.

▪ The results of the different studies are difficult to interpret, because the severity of the injuries included cannot be compared, and there may be variations in the accuracy of range-of-motion measurements.

▪ Improvements in fixation techniques have resulted in a decreased rate of hardware failure and nonunion, but range of motion is not reliably restored in every patient.

COMPLICATIONS

▪ Infection

▪ Nonunion

▪ Stiffness, with or without heterotopic ossification

▪ Need for removal of the hardware used for fixation of the olecranon osteotomy

▪ Posttraumatic osteoarthritis or avascular necrosis requiring interposition arthroplasty or elbow replacement

Table 1   Results of Internal Fixation for Distal Humerus Fractures Affecting the Humeral Columns

Study	No.	Mean Age (Range) (y)	Follow-up (mo)	Fracture Type (no.) (AO Classification)	Open	Mean Degrees ROM (range)	Overall results	Complications (no.)	Reoperations (no.)
Jupiter et al[5]	34	57 (17–79)	70 (25–139)	C1 (13) C2 (2) C3 (19)	14 (41%)	76% achieved at least 30–120	79% satisfactory*	Nonunion (2) Refracture (1) Olecranon osteotomy nonunion (2) Class II HO (1) Ulnar neuropathy (4) Median neuropathy (1)	Hardware removal (24) Capsulectomy (3) HO removal (1) Nerve decompression (4)
Henley et al[4]	33	32 (15–61)	18.3	C1 (23) C2 (8) C3 (2)	14 (42%)	Mean extension, 19; mean flexion 126	92% satisfactory* (only 25 patients evaluated)	Hardware failure (5) Infection (2) Olecranon osteotomy nonunion (2) Class II HO (2)	Repeat ORIF (2) TBW removal (6) Olecranon osteotomy repeat ORIF (2)
Sanders et al[14]	17	51 (12–85)	>24	C1 (4) C2 (3) C3 (10)	7 (41%)	108 (55–140)	76% satisfactory*	Delayed union (2) Infection (2) Pulmonary embolism (1) Ulnar neuropathy (1)	Hardware removal (3) Ulnar nerve decompression (1)
McKee et al (closed fractures)[7]	25	47 (19–85)	37 (18–75)	C (25)	None	108 (55–140)	Mean DASH: 20 (0–55)	Ulnar neuritis (3) Transient radial nerve palsy (1) Nonunion (1) Malunion (1)	TBW removal (3) Repeat ORIF (1) Elbow release (2)
McKee et al (open fractures)[6]	26	44 (17–78)	51 (10–141)	C1 (5) C2 (13) C3 (8)	100%	97 (55–140)	Mean DASH 23.7 (0–57.5) 60% satisfactory MEPS	Septic nonunion (1) Delayed union (4) Transient radial nerve palsy (1)	Repeat ORIF (3)
Pajarinen et al[10]	21	44 (16–81)	24 (10–41)	C1 (6) C2 (12) C3 (3)	5 (24%)	107 (98–116)	56% satisfactory OTA	Deep infection (1) Nonunion (2) Traumatic nerve injuries (3) Olecranon osteotomy nonunion (1)	Repeat ORIF (2)
Gofton et al[3]	23	53 (16–80)	45 (14–89)	C1 (3) C2 (11) C3 (9)	7 (30%)	122 (extension loss 19 ±12, flexion 142 ± 6)	Mean DASH: 12 (0–38) Subjective satisfaction: 93% 87% satisfactory MEPS	Deep infection (1) Olecranon osteotomy nonunion (2) Class II HO (3) Avascular necrosis (1) Reflex sympathetic dystrophy (1) Capitellar nonunion (1)	Olecranon osteotomy repeat ORIF (2) Elbow release (3) Capitellar ORIF (1)
Soon et al[15]	15	43 (21–80)	12 (2–27)	B (3) C1 (4) C2 (4) C3 (4)	None	109 (45–145)	86% satisfactory MEPS	Transient ulnar neuritis (2) Hardware failure (3) Nonunion (1)	Total elbow arthroplasty (1) Repeat ORIF (3) Elbow manipulation or release (4)
Sanchez-Sotelo et al[13]	32	58 (16–99)	24 (12–60)	A3 (3) C2 (4) C3 (25)	13 (44%)	Mean extension: 26 (0–55) Mean flexion: 124 (80–150)	83% satisfactory MEPS	Delayed union (1) Ulnar neuropathy (6) Class II HO (5) Infection (1)	Wound débridement or coverage (4) Bone grafting (1) HO removal (4) HO removal and distraction arthroplasty (1) Triceps reconstruction (1)

Class II HO, heterotopic ossification restricting motion; DASH, Disabilities of the Arm, Shoulder and Hand questionnaire; MEPS, Mayo Elbow Performance Score; ORIF, open reduction and internal fixation; OTA, Orthopedic Trauma Association rating; ROM, range of motion; TBW, tension band wiring.
* According to the Jupiter rating system.

REFERENCES

1. Alonso-Llames M. Bilaterotricipital approach to the elbow. Its application in the osteosynthesis of supracondylar fractures of the humerus in children. Acta Orthop Scand 1972;43:479–490.
2. Athwal GS, Rispoli DM, Steinmann SP. The anconeus flap transolecranon approach to the distal humerus. J Orthop Trauma 2006;20:282–285.
3. Gofton WT, Macdermid JC, Patterson SD, et al. Functional outcome of AO type C distal humeral fractures. J Hand Surg Am 2003;28:294–308.
4. Henley MB, Bone LB, Parker B. Operative management of intra-articular fractures of the distal humerus. J Orthop Trauma 1987;1:24–35.
5. Jupiter JB, Neff U, Holzach P, et al. Intercondylar fractures of the humerus. An operative approach. J Bone Joint Surg Am 1985;67:226–239.
6. McKee MD, Kim J, Kebaish K, et al. Functional outcome after open supracondylar fractures of the humerus. The effect of the surgical approach. J Bone Joint Surg Br 2000;82B:646–651.
7. McKee MD, Wilson TL, Winston L, et al. Functional outcome following surgical treatment of intra-articular distal humeral fractures through a posterior approach. J Bone Joint Surg Am 2000;82A:1701–1707.
8. Morrey BF. Anatomy and surgical approaches. In: Morrey BF, ed. Joint Replacement Arthroplasty. Philadelphia: Churchill-Livingstone, 2003:269–285.
9. O'Driscoll SW, Sanchez-Sotelo J, Torchia ME. Management of the smashed distal humerus. Orthop Clin North Am 2002;33:19–33.
10. Pajarinen J, Bjorkenheim JM. Operative treatment of type C intercondylar fractures of the distal humerus: Results after a mean follow-up of 2 years in a series of 18 patients. J Shoulder Elbow Surg 2002;11:48–52.
11. Ring D, Gulotta L, Chin K, et al. Olecranon osteotomy for exposure of fractures and nonunions of the distal humerus. J Orthop Trauma 2004;18:446–449.
12. Sanchez-Sotelo J, Torchia ME, O'Driscoll SW. Principle-based internal fixation of distal humerus fractures. Tech Hand Upper Extremity Surg 2001;5:179–187.
13. Sanchez-Sotelo J, Torchia ME, O'Driscoll SW. Complex distal humeral fractures: internal fixation with a principle-based parallel-plate technique. J Bone Joint Surg Am 2007;89A:961–969.
14. Sanders RA, Raney EM, Pipkin S. Operative treatment of bicondylar intraarticular fractures of the distal humerus. Orthopedics 1992;15:159–163.
15. Soon JL, Chan BK, Low CO. Surgical fixation of intra-articular fractures of the distal humerus in adults. Injury 2004;35:44–54.

Asif M. Ilyas and Jesse B. Jupiter

DEFINITION

- Capitellar fractures are uncommon, accounting for less than 1% of all elbow fractures and 6% of all distal humerus fractures.[3]
- They often are associated with radial head fractures and posterior elbow dislocations.
- A classification system for capitellar fractures has been proposed by Bryan and Morrey[3] and modified by McKee:
  - Type 1: complete fractures of the capitellum[11]
  - Type 2: superficial subchondral fractures of the capitellar articular surface[22]
  - Type 3: comminuted fractures[2]
  - Type 4: coronal shear fractures that include a portion of the trochlea as well as the capitellum as one piece[17] (**FIG 1**)
- Ring and Jupiter[21] have proposed a new classification, expanding on the growing understanding that isolated capitellum fractures are rare and often are involved as part of articular shear fractures of the distal humerus. The classification includes five anatomic components:
  - The capitellum and lateral aspect of the trochlea
  - The lateral epicondyle
  - The posterior aspect of the lateral column
  - The posterior aspect of the trochlea
  - The medial epicondyle

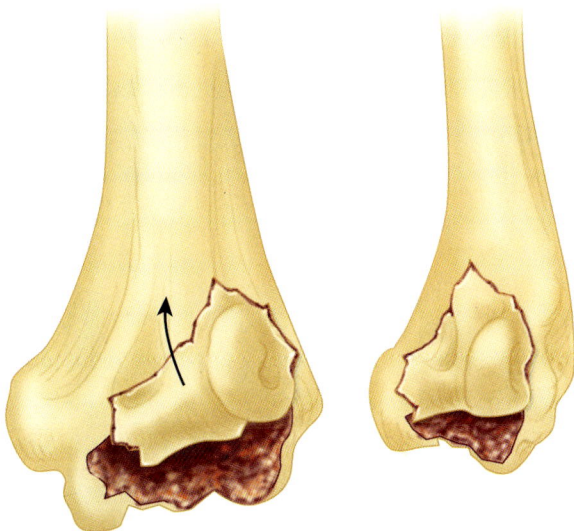

FIG 1 • Type 4 coronal shear fractures of the distal humerus. (Adapted from McKee MD, Jupiter JB, Bosse G, et al. Coronal shear fractures of the distal end of the humerus. J Bone Joint Surg Am 1996;78A:49–54.)

ANATOMY

- The two condyles of the distal humerus diverge from the humeral shaft to form the lateral and medial columns, which support the trochlea between them. The anterior aspect of the lateral column is covered with articular cartilage, forming the capitellum. Distally, these two condyles can be visualized as forming a triangle at the end of the humerus.
- The capitellum is the first epiphyseal center of the elbow to ossify.
- It is covered by articular surface anteriorly but devoid of it posteriorly.
- The capitellum is directed distally and anteriorly at an angle of 30 degrees to the long axis of the humerus.
- The radial head rotates on the anterior surface of the capitellum in elbow flexion and articulates with its inferior surface in elbow extension.
- The lateral collateral ligament inserts next to the lateral margin of the capitellum.
- The blood supply of the capitellum is derived posteriorly. It arises from the lateral arcade, which is the anastomosis of the radial collateral arteries of the profunda brachii and the radial recurrent artery.[23]

PATHOGENESIS

- Capitellar fractures usually result from a fall on an outstretched hand or forearm as the radial head impacts the capitellum on impact.
- Capitellar–trochlear shear fractures involve impaction of the radial head against the lateral column of the distal humerus in a semi-extended position, resulting in a shearing mechanism of the distal humerus.
- Fracture fragments vary in size and displace superiorly and anteriorly into the radial fossa, resulting in impingement with elbow flexion.

NATURAL HISTORY

- Capitellar fractures occur almost exclusively in adults. These fractures do not occur in children, because in that age group the capitellum is largely cartilaginous, and a similar mechanism of injury would instead cause a supracondylar or lateral condyle fracture.
- Capitellar fractures are more common in females, a finding that has been attributed to the higher carrying angle of the elbow.
- Elderly patients of both genders are more susceptible to capitellum and complex capitellar–trochlear shear fractures because of the metabolic susceptibilities of osteoporosis.
- Displaced fractures that go untreated can have a poor outcome owing to progressive loss of motion and posttraumatic arthrosis.

PATIENT HISTORY AND PHYSICAL FINDINGS

- Symptoms of capitellar fractures are similar to those of radial head fractures, including pain and swelling along the lateral elbow and pain with elbow motion.
- Although there may be variable loss of forearm rotation, loss of flexion and extension is common, often accompanied by crepitus and pain.
- The association of concomitant radial head fractures and ligamentous injuries with capitellar fractures is high.[18]
- The shoulder and wrist should be examined for concomitant injury.

IMAGING AND OTHER DIAGNOSTIC STUDIES

- Standard radiography is inadequate for accurate assessment of capitellar fractures.
- Lateral radiographs are best for obtaining an initial evaluation of capitellar fractures.
- Anteroposterior views do not reliably show the fracture, because the outline of the distal humerus is not consistently affected.
- The radial head–capitellum view can help identify fractures of the capitellum. This view is a lateral oblique projection taken with the x-ray beam pointing 45 degrees dorsoventrally, thereby eliminating the ulno- and radiohumeral articulation shadows.[10]
  - A type 1 fracture appears as a semilunar fragment sitting superiorly with its articular surface pointing up and away from the radial head in most cases.
  - Type 2 fractures are more difficult to diagnose, depending on the amount of subchondral bone accompanying the articular fragment. They may appear as a loose body lying in the superior part of the joint.
  - Type 3 fractures display variable amounts of comminution.
  - Coronal shear fractures show a characteristic "double arc" sign on lateral radiographic views (**FIG 2A**).
- CT scans are necessary for delineating the fracture pattern and should be performed in all cases.
  - CT scanning of the elbow should be done at 1- to 2-mm intervals using axial or transverse cuts.
- Three-dimensional (3D) CT reconstructions provide the best detail and ability to appreciate the anatomic orientation of the fracture patterns and should be ordered if 3D imaging is available (**FIG 2B,C**).

DIFFERENTIAL DIAGNOSIS

- Radial head fracture
- Distal humeral lateral condyle fracture
- Elbow dislocation

NONOPERATIVE MANAGEMENT

- Truly nondisplaced and isolated capitellum fractures can be splinted for 3 weeks, followed by protected motion. We do not advocate nonoperative management for any other type of capitellum fracture.
- Closed reduction techniques, which have been described in the literature, should be performed with caution, and only complete anatomic reduction should be accepted.[4,19]
- Capitellar–trochlear shear fractures should not be treated nonoperatively because of their inherent instability and articular incongruity.

SURGICAL MANAGEMENT

- The goal of surgery is anatomic reduction and fixation of the fracture to allow for early motion without mechanical block.
  - Long-term goals are pain-free and maximal motion with minimal stiffness.
- Capitellar fractures are uncommon, and the wide array of treatment options presented in the literature is based on relatively small series.
  - Treatment options include closed reduction,[4,19] open excision,[1,8,16] open reduction and internal fixation (ORIF), and arthroplasty.[5,9]
- With the improvement in techniques for fixation of small fragments and management of articular surfaces, ORIF has become the mainstay of treatment.
  - Advantages of ORIF include restoration of anatomy and stability.
  - Disadvantages include stiffness and failed fixation.
- In elderly patients, we do consider total elbow arthroplasty for complex intra-articular distal humerus fractures.
  - Advantages include early return to function and motion.
  - Disadvantages include functional limitations.

Preoperative Planning

- Before proceeding with surgery, a thorough understanding of the fracture and its orientation should be obtained with the help of a CT scan, and, if possible, 3D reconstructions.

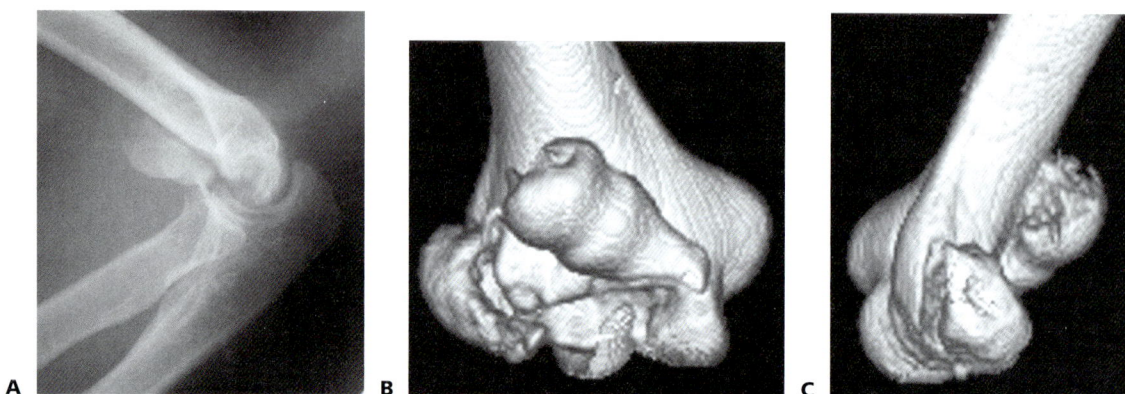

FIG 2 • **A.** Characteristic "double arc" sign on lateral radiographs of coronal shear fractures. **B,C.** 3D CT reconstructions of a coronal shear fracture of the distal humerus.

■ The timing of surgery is important. Fractures preferably should be approached within 2 weeks, before osseous healing sets in, but after swelling has gone down.

■ Ensure that the necessary implants and hardware are available.

■ Reduction and fixation of the fracture will require K-wires, articular or headless screws, and small-fragment AO screws.

■ An image intensifier should be used during surgery to confirm reduction of the fracture and proper positioning of implanted hardware.

Positioning

■ General anesthesia is recommended.

■ The patient usually is positioned supine on the operating table, with a radiolucent hand table.

■ Alternatively, a lateral or prone position can be considered, with the anterior surface of the elbow supported by a padded bolster to use the universal posterior approach.

Approach

■ Either a lateral or posterior midline incision should be used, depending on the nature of the fracture, followed by a lateral approach into the elbow joint.

■ Multiple intervals that can be exploited in the lateral approach to the elbow.

■ We advocate the Köcher approach, which uses the interval between the extensor carpi ulnaris and the anconeus and affords greater protection of the posterior interosseous nerve.

■ To increase exposure, the origin of the extensor carpi ulnaris (ECU), extensor digitorum communis, and extensor carpi radialis longus can be raised off of the lateral epicondyle anterior to its interval with the triceps.

■ In many cases, a capsular violation has occurred. This can be exploited and used as the interval to expose the fracture, thereby avoiding the need to cause an additional soft tissue defect.

CAPITELLAR FRACTURES

Exposure

■ The incision should begin 2 cm proximal to the lateral epicondyle and extend 3 to 4 cm distal toward the radial neck.

■ If no large soft tissue or capsular defect is present, a direct lateral Köcher approach between the anconeus and ECU interval is recommended.

■ The common extensor origin is sharply raised off the lateral epicondyle and reflected anteriorly to expose the lateral elbow joint.

■ Care must be taken to avoid damage to the radial nerve traveling between the brachialis and brachioradialis.

■ Often the lateral ligamentous complex will be avulsed from the distal aspect of the humerus, with or without some aspect of the lateral epicondyle.

■ This ligamentous violation can be exploited to improve exposure by hinging open the joint on the medial collateral ligament with a varus stress.

■ The capitellar fracture usually is displaced proximally and rotated and has no soft tissue attachments.

Reduction and Fixation

■ The fragment is reduced under direct visualization, held with reduction tenaculums, and provisionally fixed with 0.045-inch K-wires from an anterior-to-posterior direction.

■ Internal fixation options include fixation from posterior to anterior with AO cancellous screws or from either direction with headless compression screws.

■ Cancellous screws are best for fracture fragments with a large subchondral component, as in type 1 fracture fragments. However, extending the dissection posteriorly around the lateral column theoretically increases the risk of osteonecrosis (**TECH FIG 1**).

■ Headless compression screws, such as the Herbert screw, are best for fragments with less subchondral

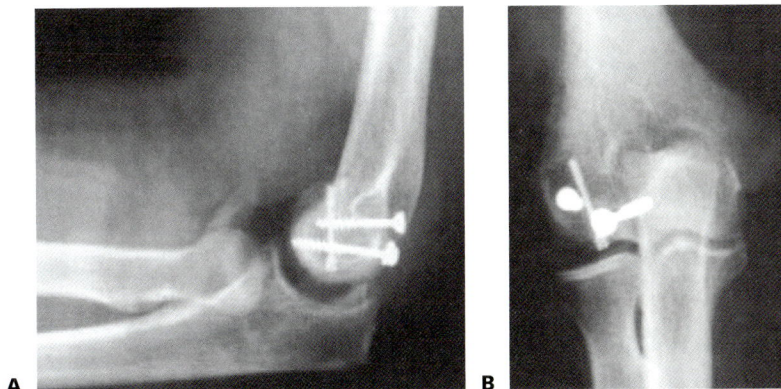

TECH FIG 1 • Fixation of a type 1 capitellum fracture with a headless screw anteriorly and AO screws from posterior to anterior.

TECHNIQUES

bone, such as type 2 and small type 1 fracture fragments. The head of the screw must be buried below the articular surface.

- Excision of fracture fragments is recommended in type 2 fractures with small, thin articular pieces and type 3 comminuted fractures where the fragments are not amenable to internal fixation.

- Fragment reduction and hardware position should be confirmed by image intensifier.

- Unrestricted forearm rotation and elbow flexion–extension without mechanical block or catching should be confirmed intraoperatively.

- If the lateral collateral ligament is found to be avulsed, it should be repaired back to the lateral epicondyle with drill holes and nonabsorbable no. 2 suture or suture anchors.

- The capsule should be closed.

- The retracted extensor origin should be relaxed and closed to the surrounding soft tissue.

CAPITELLAR–TROCHLEAR SHEAR FRACTURES

Exposure

- A posterior midline incision should be made, and full-thickness flaps should be raised medially and laterally off of the extensor mechanism.
  - This incision provides extensile exposure, access to both sides, and ease of osteotomy if necessary (**TECH FIG 2A**).

- Beginning medially, the ulnar nerve should be decompressed in situ behind the medial epicondyle (**TECH FIG 2B**).

- Returning laterally, the interval between the anconeus and the ECU should be developed. In many cases, a capsular violation can be exploited (**TECH FIG 2C**).

- The common extensor origin, including the ECU, extensor digitorum communis, and extensor carpi radialis longus, is then sharply raised off the lateral epicondyle and reflected anteriorly to expose the lateral elbow joint and improve visualization medially.

- Care must be taken to avoid injury to the radial nerve proximally as it travels between the brachialis and brachioradialis, and to the posterior interosseous nerve distally when raising the ECU anteriorly. This may be done by keeping the forearm pronated.

- In many cases, the lateral epicondyle will have avulsed off of the distal humerus, and this traumatic osteotomy can be exploited.
  - Otherwise, a formal lateral epicondyle osteotomy can be performed to enhance visualization while maintaining the integrity of the lateral ligamentous complex.

- Additionally, an olecranon osteotomy may be performed to improve visualization and fixation of fractures extending medially and posteriorly.

- The fracture fragments should now be visualized and accounted for. They are most commonly displaced proximally and internally rotated (**TECH FIG 2D**).

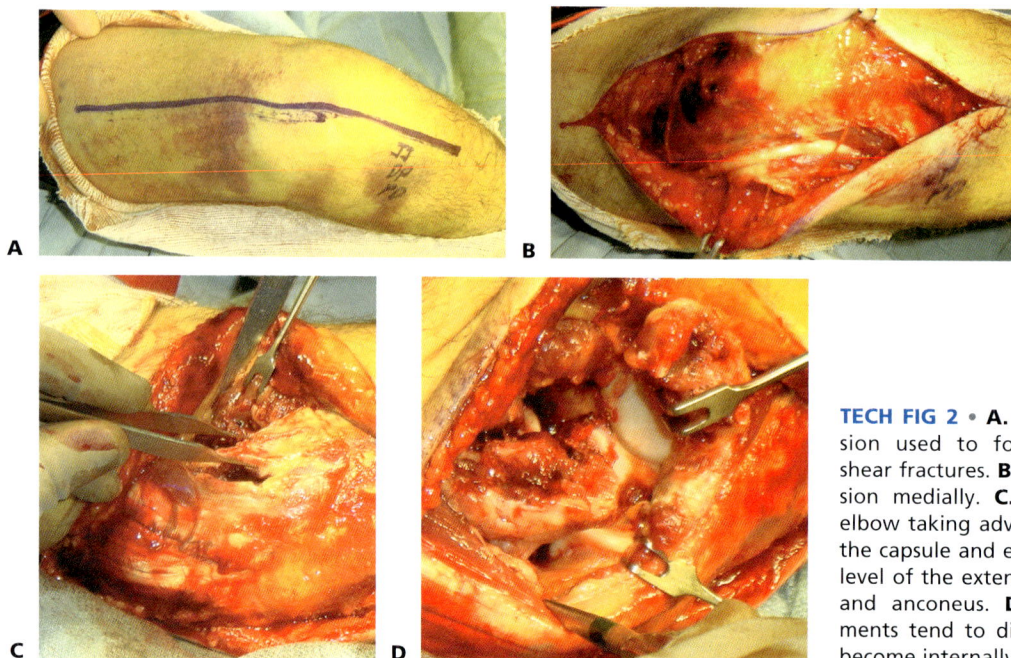

TECH FIG 2 • A. Posterior midline incision used to for capitellar–trochlear shear fractures. **B.** Ulnar nerve compression medially. **C.** Lateral approach to elbow taking advantage of violation of the capsule and extensor muscles at the level of the extensor carpi ulnaris (ECU) and anconeus. **D.** The fracture fragments tend to displace proximally and become internally rotated.

Reduction and Fixation

- The fragment is reduced under direct visualization, held with reduction tenaculums, and provisionally fixed with 0.045-inch K-wires from anterior to posterior (**TECH FIG 3A**).
- Inability to reduce the fracture anatomically may represent fracture impaction, requiring either disimpaction or bone grafting, or both.
- Options for internal fixation include fixation from posterior-to-anterior with AO screws or from either direction with headless compression screws.
- Cancellous screws are best when the fracture fragment has a large subchondral component, but they make it necessary to extend the dissection posteriorly around the lateral column, theoretically increasing the risk of osteonecrosis.

- Headless compression screws, such as the Herbert screw, are best for fragments with less subchondral bone and provide the added benefit that they can be used in either direction, anteriorly or posteriorly. Diligence must be maintained to confirm that the head of the screw is buried below the articular surface when placed anteriorly.
- Fragment reduction and hardware position should be confirmed by image intensifier.
- Unrestricted forearm rotation and elbow flexion–extension without mechanical block or catching should be confirmed intraoperatively.
- The lateral epicondyle, if avulsed or osteotomized, should be repaired with a tension band technique or plate and screws (**TECH FIG 3A,B**).
- The capsule should be closed.
- The interval and released extensor origin should be relaxed and closed to the surrounding soft tissue.

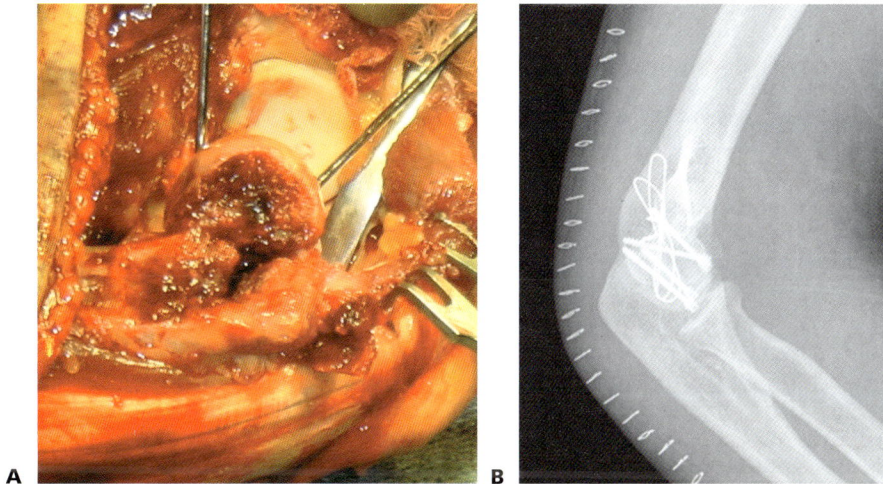

TECH FIG 3 • **A.** The fracture is reduced and pinned with 0.045-inch K-wires. **B.** Postoperative radiographs illustrate repair of the lateral epicondyle and fracture fixation.

PEARLS AND PITFALLS

Diagnosis	▪ Diligence should be paid to identifying concomitant injuries such as dislocations, radial head fractures, and ligamentous instability.
Imaging	▪ Plain radiographs are insufficient, and a CT scan should be performed routinely. ▪ Order 3D reconstructions if possible.
Nonoperative management	▪ Nonoperative management should be chosen cautiously. Anatomic and stable reduction of the fracture is necessary. Otherwise, a painful elbow with restricted motion may result. ▪ We do not recommend nonoperative management of any capitellar–trochlear shear fractures.
Surgical management	▪ A straight posterior skin incision will allow ulnar nerve decompression and fracture fixation. ▪ Lateral epicondyle osteotomy can enhance exposure. ▪ Inability to reduce the fracture anatomically may represent impaction of the lateral column and require disimpaction or bone grafting. ▪ Excision of comminuted fragments that cannot be fixed internally is preferred over nonanatomic reduction and malunion. ▪ Concomitant fractures and ligamentous injuries should be treated simultaneously to optimize outcomes.
Postoperative management	▪ Stable fixation should be sought to allow for early motion. ▪ Heterotopic ossification is common after elbow fractures, and prophylaxis with nonsteroidal anti-inflammatory drugs should be considered.

TECHNIQUES

POSTOPERATIVE CARE

▪ If secure fixation has been obtained, immediate mobilization can be initiated postoperatively.

▪ If fixation is tenuous, splint or cast the elbow for 3 to 4 weeks, followed by active and assisted range-of-motion exercises.

OUTCOMES

▪ Focusing initially on outcomes after ORIF of types 1 and 2 capitellar fractures, multiple small series have shown good results using Herbert screws in an anterior to posterior direction.[6,13,14,20]

▪ More recently, Mahirogullari et al[15] reported on 11 cases of type 1 capitellum fractures treated with Herbert screws, which yielded 8 excellent and 3 good results. They recommended fixation in a posterior-to-anterior direction with at least two Herbert screws.

▪ Reported outcomes on type 4 capitellar–trochlear shear fractures are limited. McKee et al[17] originally described this pattern and reported on 6 cases.

　▪ Each case involved an extended lateral Köcher approach and fixation with Herbert screws from an anterior to posterior direction. Good or excellent results were achieved in all cases, with average elbow motion of 15 to 141 degrees, and forearm rotation of 83 degrees pronation and 84 degrees supination.

▪ Ring and Jupiter examined 21 cases of articular fractures of the distal humerus treated with Herbert screw fixation and found 4 excellent results, 12 good results, and 5 fair results.

　▪ All of the fractures healed and had an average range of motion of 96 degrees. No ulnohumeral instability, arthrosis, or osteonecrosis was reported.

　▪ The authors stressed the importance of proper evaluation of these fractures and awareness that apparent capitellum fractures often are complex articular fractures of the distal humerus.[21]

▪ Dubberley et al[7] further subclassified type 4 fractures in their series of 28 cases. They achieved an average range of motion of flexion–extension of 25 degrees less than the contralateral elbow and 4 degrees of supination–pronation less than the contralateral elbow.

　▪ Two comminuted cases required conversion to a total elbow arthroplasty.

　▪ Varied fixation methods were used, including Herbert screws, cancellous screws, absorbable pins, and supplementation with K-wires.

COMPLICATIONS

▪ The most common complication of capitellar fractures is loss of elbow motion and residual pain. The compromised motion most commonly is manifested in loss of flexion and extension.

▪ Ulnar neuropathy has been noted after ORIF, and some recommend routine ulnar nerve decompression.[21]

▪ Osteonecrosis may occur from the initial fracture displacement or surgical exposure. Blood is supplied to the capitellum from a posterior to anterior direction and may be compromised by surgical dissection.

　▪ In symptomatic cases in which revascularization after fixation has not occurred, delayed excision is indicated.

▪ Malunions may occur when the patient has delayed seeking treatment, when inadequate reduction or loss of closed reduction occurs, or after ORIF. Malunions result in loss of motion and may require excision of the fragment and soft tissue releases.

▪ Nonunions may occur, although this is uncommon. They most likely result secondary to inadequate reduction or lack of revascularization of the fragment.

REFERENCES

1. Alvarez E, Patel M, Nimberg P, et al. Fractures of the capitellum humeri. J Bone Joint Surg Am 1975;57A:1093–1096.
2. Broberg MA, Morrey BF. Results of delayed excision of the radial head after fracture. J Bone Joint Surg Am 1986;68A:669–674.
3. Bryan RS, Morrey BF. Fractures of the distal humerus. In: Morrey BF, ed. The Elbow and Its Disorders. Philadelphia: WB Saunders, 1985:302–399.
4. Christopher F, Bushnell L. Conservative treatment of fractures of the capitellum. J Bone Joint Surg 1935;17:489–492.
5. Cobb TK, Morrey BF. Total elbow arthroplasty as primary treatment for distal humerus fractures in elderly patients. J Bone Joint Surg Am 1997;79A:826–832.
6. Collert S. Surgical management of fracture of the capitulum humeri. Acta Orthop Scand 1977;48:603–606.
7. Dubberley JH, Faber KJ, Macdermid JC, et al. Outcome after open reduction and internal fixation of capitellar and trochlear fractures. J Bone Joint Surg Am 2006;88A:46–54.
8. Fowles JV, Kassab MT. Fracture of the capitulum humeri: treatment by excision. J Bone Joint Surg Am 1975;56A:794–798.
9. Garcia JA, Myulka R, Stanley D. Complex fractures of the distal humerus in the elderly: the role of total elbow replacement as primary treatment. J Bone Joint Surg Br 2002;84B:812–816.
10. Greenspan A, Norman A. The radial head, capitellum view: useful technique in elbow trauma. AJR Am J Roentgenol 1982;138:1186–1188.
11. Hahn NF. Fall von einer besonderes Varietat der Frakturen des Ellenbogens. Z Wund Geburt 1853;6:185.
12. Jupiter JB, Neff U, Ragazzoni P, et al. Unicondylar fractures of the distal humerus: an operative approach. J Orthop Trauma 1988;2:102–109.
13. Lansinger O, Mare K. Fracture of the capitulum humeri. Acta Orthop Scand 1981;52:39–44.
14. Liberman N, Katz T, Howard CV, et al. Fixation of capitellar fractures with Herbert screws. Arch Orthop Trauma Surg 1991;110:155–157.
15. Mahirogullari M, Kiral A, Solakoglu C, et al. Treatment of fractures of the humeral capitellum using Herbert screws. J Hand Surg Eur Vol 2006;31:320–325.
16. Mazel MS. Fracture of the capitellum. J Bone Joint Surg 1935;17:483–488.
17. McKee MD, Jupiter JB, Bosse G, et al. Coronal shear fractures of the distal end of the humerus. J Bone Joint Surg Am 1996;78A:49–54.
18. Milch H. Fractures and fracture-dislocations of the humeral condyles. J Trauma 1964;13:882–886.
19. Ochner RS, Bloom H, Palumbo RC, et al. Closed reduction of coronal fractures of the capitellum. J Trauma 1996;40:199–203.
20. Richards RR, Khoury GW, Burke FD, et al. Internal fixation of capitellar fractures using Herbert screw: a report of four cases. Can J Surg 1987;30:188–191.
21. Ring D, Jupiter JB, Gulotta L. Articular fractures of the distal part of the humerus. J Bone Joint Surg Am 2003;85A:232–238.
22. Steinthal D. Die isolirte Fraktur der eminentia Capetala in Ellengogelenk. Zentralk Chir 1898;15:17.
23. Yamaguchi K, Sweet FA, Bindra R, et al. The extraosseous and intraosseous arterial anatomy of the adult elbow. J Bone Joint Surg Am 1997;79A:1653–1662.

Chapter 35

Open Reduction and Internal Fixation of Radial Head and Neck Fractures

Anshu Singh, George Frederick Hatch III, and John M. Itamura

DEFINITION

- The radial head is distinctive in anatomy and function with unique considerations regarding the diagnostic and treatment options available to the surgeon.
- Radial head and neck fractures are the most common elbow fractures in adults, representing 33% of elbow fractures.
- The original Mason classification was modified by Johnson, then Morrey. Hotchkiss proposed that the classification system be used to provide guidance for treatment. It has poor intraobserver and interobserver reliability (**FIG 1**).[9]
  - Type I fractures are nondisplaced and offer no block to pronation and supination on examination.
  - Type II fractures have displaced marginal segments that block normal forearm rotation. We only include fractures with three or fewer articular fragments, which meet criteria for fractures that can be operatively reduced and fixed with reproducibly good results.
  - Type III fractures are comminuted or impacted articular fractures that are optimally managed with prosthetic replacement.
  - Type IV fractures are associated with elbow instability and should never be resected in the acute setting.

ANATOMY

- The radial head is entirely intra-articular. It has two articulations, one with the humerus, via the radiocapitellar joint, and another with the ulna, via the proximal radioulnar joint (PRUJ).
  - The radiocapitellar joint has a saddle-shaped articulation allowing both flexion and extension as well as rotation.
  - The PRUJ, constrained by the annular ligament, allows rotation of the radial head in the lesser sigmoid notch of the proximal ulna.
    - To avoid creating a mechanical block to pronation and supination, implants must be limited to a 90-degree arc (the "safe zone") outside the PRUJ (**FIG 2**).[4]

- Blood supply to the radial head is tenuous, with a major contribution from a single branch of the radial recurrent artery in the safe zone and minor contributions from both the radial and interosseous recurrent arteries, which penetrate the capsule at its insertion into the neck (**FIG 3**).[13]
- There is considerable variability in the shape of the radial head, from nearly round to elliptical, as well as variability in the offset of the head from the neck.
- The anterior band of the medial collateral ligament (MCL) is the primary stabilizer to valgus stress. The radial head, a secondary stabilizer, maintains up to 30% of valgus resistance in the native elbow. Therefore, in cases where the MCL is ruptured:
  - A radial head that is not reparable should be replaced with a prosthesis and not excised given its biomechanical importance.
  - It may be prudent to protect a repaired radial head from high valgus stress during early range of motion by placing a hinged external fixator.
- The radial head also functions in the transmission of axial load, transmitting 60% of the load from the wrist to the elbow.[10] This is a crucial consideration when the interosseous membrane is disrupted in the Essex-Lopresti lesion.[5] Resection of the radial head in this setting results in devastating longitudinal radioulnar instability, proximal migration of the radius, and possible ulnar-carpal impingement.

PATHOGENESIS

- Radial head fractures result from trauma. A fall on an outstretched hand with the elbow in extension and the forearm in pronation produces an axial or valgus load (or both) driving the radial head into the capitellum, fracturing the relatively osteopenic radial head.
  - Loading at 0 to 35 degrees of extension causes coronoid fractures.
  - Loading at 0 to 80 degrees of extension produces radial head fractures.

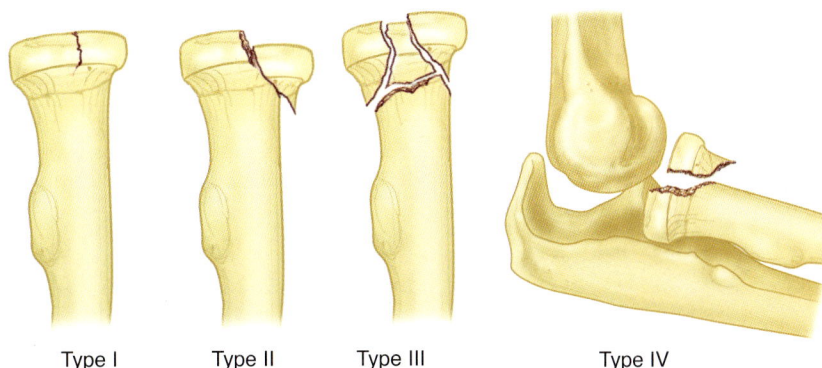

Type I   Type II   Type III   Type IV

FIG 1 • The modified Mason classification for radial head fractures.

Pronation   Neutral   Supination

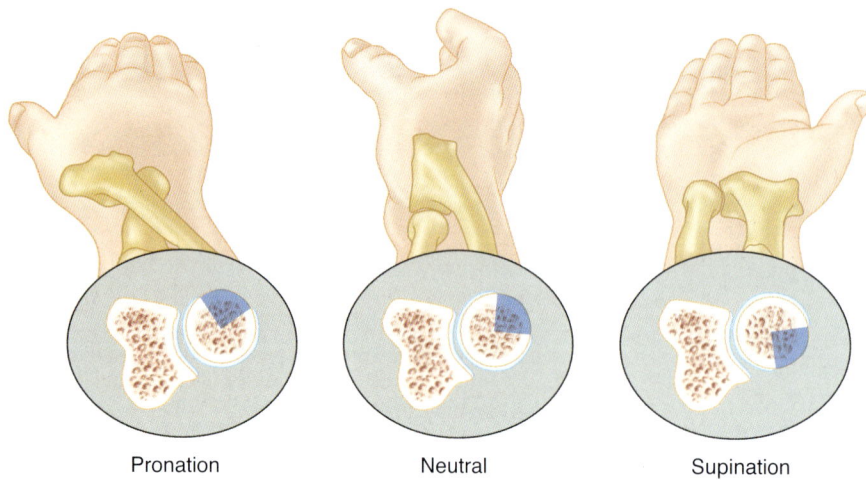

FIG 2 • The "safe zone" is a roughly 90-degree arc of the radial head that does not articulate with the ulna in the proximal radioulnar joint with full supination and pronation. With the wrist in neutral rotation, the safe zone is anterolateral.

■ Associated soft tissue injuries can lead to considerable complications, including pain, arthrosis, stiffness, and disability:
  ■ MCL injury in 50%
  ■ Lateral ligament disruption in about 80%
  ■ Capitellar bone bruises in 90%[8]
  ■ Capitellar cartilage defects in about 50%

■ The axial loading may also rupture the interosseous membrane, causing longitudinal radioulnar instability with dislocation of the distal radioulnar joint (DRUJ) (**FIG 4**).

■ The "terrible triad" injury results from valgus loading of the elbow, disrupting the MCL or lateral ulnar collateral ligament and fracturing the radial head and coronoid process.

NATURAL HISTORY

■ Results are mixed regarding the efficacy of radial head excision for treatment of radial head fracture. Good or fair results may be possible, with a few caveats:

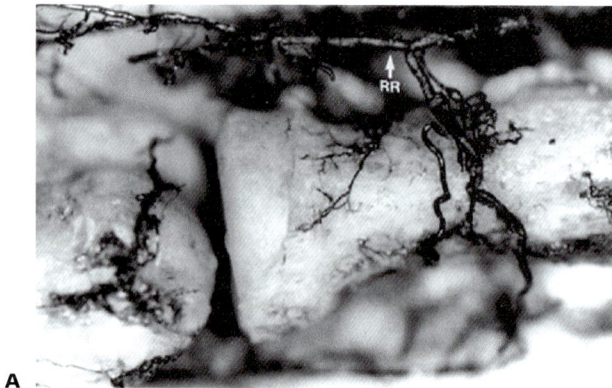

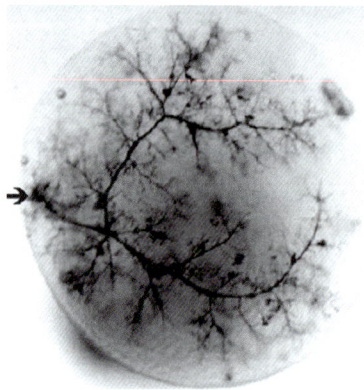

FIG 3 • **A.** The radial recurrent artery, a branch of the radial artery, provides the main blood supply to the radial head. **B.** In most cadaveric specimens, a branch of the radial recurrent penetrates the radial head in the safe zone. (From Yamaguchi K, Sweet FA, Bindra R, et al. The extraosseous and intraosseous arterial anatomy of the adult elbow. J Bone Joint Surg Am 1997;79A:1653–1662.)

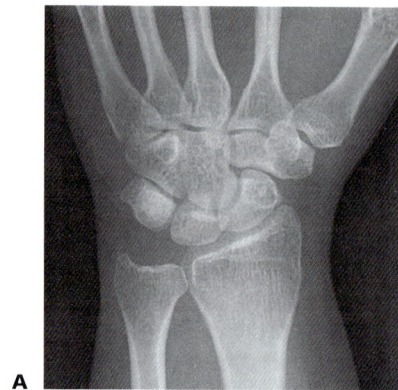

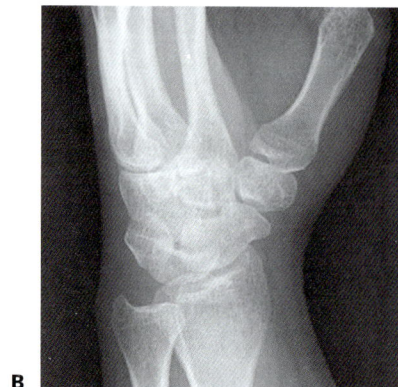

FIG 4 • **A.** AP radiograph of the wrist in cases of longitudinal radioulnar instability (the Essex-Lopresti lesion). Subtle shortening of the radius is demonstrated. **B.** Lateral radiograph of the wrist may show dorsal subluxation of the distal ulna.

- There is a demonstrable increase in ulnar variance at the wrist and increased carrying angle.
- 10% to 20% loss of strength is expected.
- It is contraindicated in the face of associated soft tissue injuries.

■ Radiographic, but usually clinically silent, degenerative changes such as cysts, sclerosis, and osteophytes occur radiographically in about 75% of elbows after radial head excision (**FIG 5**).

■ Results of excision are poor in patients with concomitant MCL, coronoid, or interosseous membrane injury.

- Radial head resection should be reserved for patients with low functional demands or limited life expectancy, and when the surgeon has excluded elbow instability with a fluoroscopic examination.

■ Delayed excision of the radial head after failed nonoperative management may be considered with modest increase in function; it has shown 23% fair or poor results at 15 years of follow-up.[3] Other studies suggest that there is no difference between delayed and primary excision.[6]

■ Although open reduction and fixation of a comminuted fracture can be attempted, a large series by experienced elbow surgeons found that fixation of a radial head with more than three articular fragments is fraught with poor results.[11]

■ Nonanatomic reduction of the shaft or joint may result in limited range of motion due to a cam effect in the PRUJ, but no literature or prospective studies indicate what parameters are "acceptable."

PATIENT HISTORY AND PHYSICAL FINDINGS

■ The history typically involves a fall on an outstretched hand followed by pain and edema over the lateral elbow, accompanied by limited range of motion.

■ The examiner should note the patient's activity level and profession.

■ Physical examination should include neurovascular status and examination of the skin to look for medial ecchymosis, which may suggest injury to the MCL.

- A detailed examination of the elbow must include bony palpation of the medial and lateral epicondyles, olecranon process, DRUJ, and radial head, as well as the squeeze test

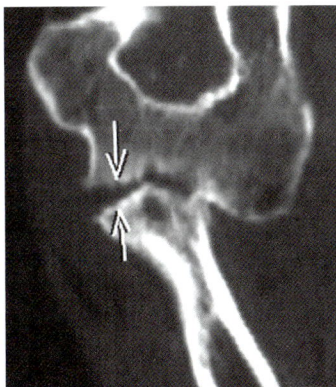

FIG 5 • A CT scan demonstrating symptomatic posttraumatic arthrosis with cyst formation in the ulnohumeral articulation after radial head resection.

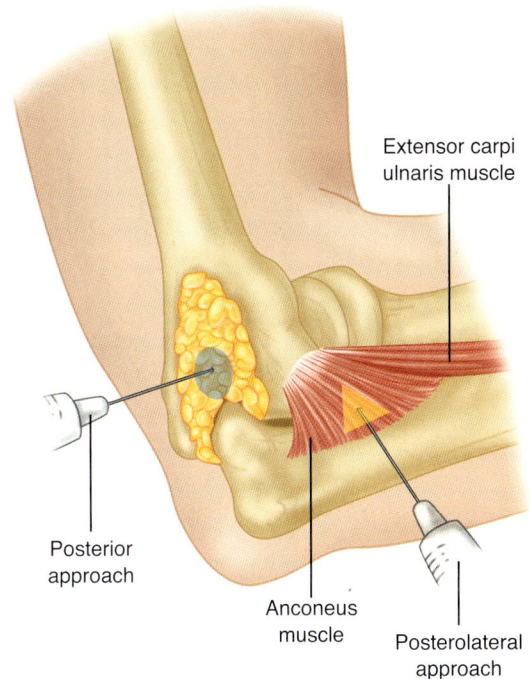

FIG 6 • The elbow joint can be aspirated and injected through the posterior and posterolateral approaches. They are equally effective and should be used based on soft tissue injury.

of the interosseous membrane and DRUJ to screen for potential longitudinal instability.

- Varus and valgus stress testing, with or without fluoroscopy, can indicate injury to the anterior band of the MCL or to the lateral ulnar collateral ligament, respectively.

■ Range-of-motion and stress examinations are vital to proper decision making and may obviate the need for advanced imaging if performed correctly with adequate anesthesia. If omitted, this will lead to undiagnosed associated injuries and may result in flawed decision making.

- In the emergency department or office, adequate anesthesia may be obtained by aspirating hematoma, then injecting the elbow joint with 5 mL of local anesthetic and examining the elbow under fluoroscopy. This may be performed by the traditional lateral injection in the "soft spot" or posteriorly into the olecranon fossa (**FIG 6**).[12]

- If operative intervention is clearly indicated, this examination can be performed under a general anesthetic, provided the surgeon and patient are prepared for a change in operative plan as dictated by the examination.

- Normal values are 0 to 145 degrees of flexion–extension, 85 degrees of supination, and 80 degrees of pronation. The examiner should check for a bony block to motion.

IMAGING AND OTHER DIAGNOSTIC STUDIES

Radiography

■ Anteroposterior (AP), lateral, and oblique views are the standard of care, but they underestimate or overestimate joint impaction and degree of comminution (**FIG 7A,B**).

- A radiocapitellar view with forearm in neutral and at 45 degrees cephalad gives an improved view of the articular surfaces.

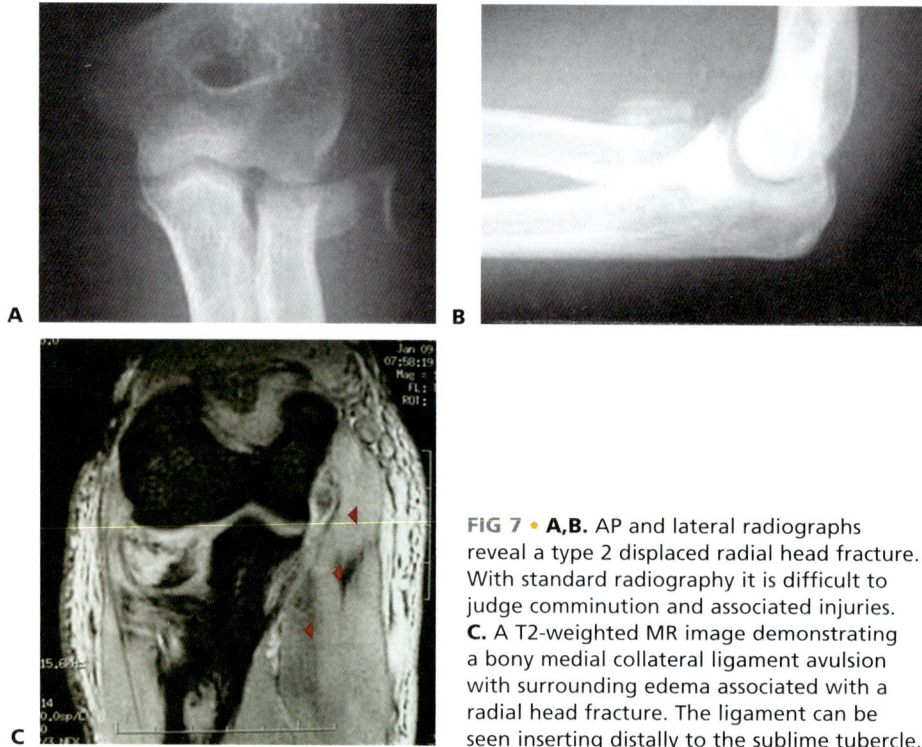

FIG 7 • **A,B.** AP and lateral radiographs reveal a type 2 displaced radial head fracture. With standard radiography it is difficult to judge comminution and associated injuries. **C.** A T2-weighted MR image demonstrating a bony medial collateral ligament avulsion with surrounding edema associated with a radial head fracture. The ligament can be seen inserting distally to the sublime tubercle.

■ If the examination reveals wrist or forearm tenderness, the examiner should have a low threshold for obtaining bilateral wrist posteroanterior (PA) views to rule out an Essex-Lopresti lesion.

Magnetic Resonance Imaging

■ Magnetic resonance imaging (MRI) is a useful adjunct to physical examination for evaluating associated injuries such as collateral ligament tears, chondral defects, and loose bodies,[8] but it is not routinely indicated (**FIG 7C**).

DIFFERENTIAL DIAGNOSIS

■ Simple elbow dislocation
■ Distal humerus fracture
■ Olecranon fracture
■ Septic elbow

NONOPERATIVE MANAGEMENT

■ The standard protocol for treating radial head fractures is shown in FIGURE 8.

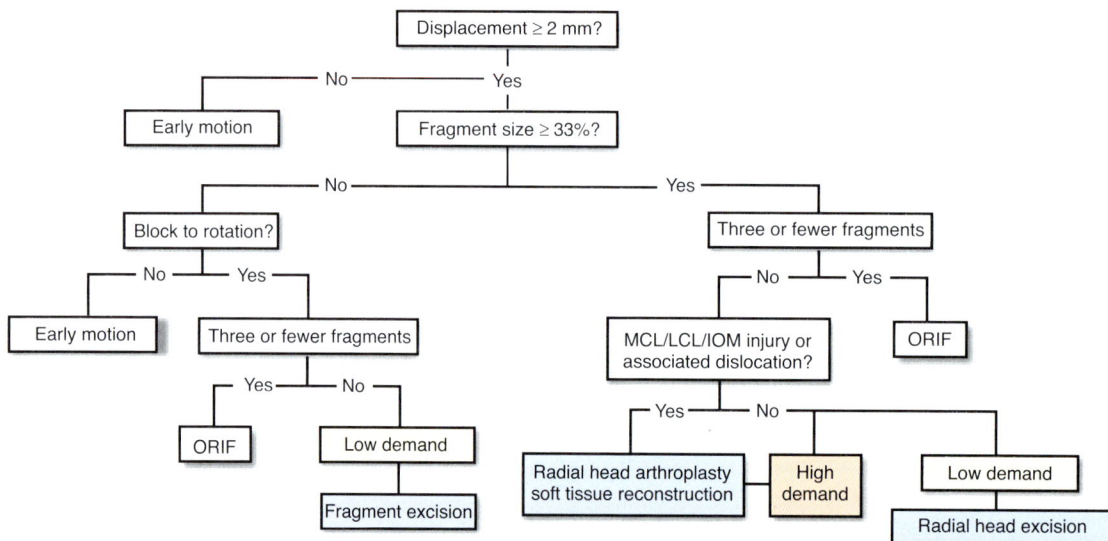

FIG 8 • Treatment algorithm for radial head fractures.

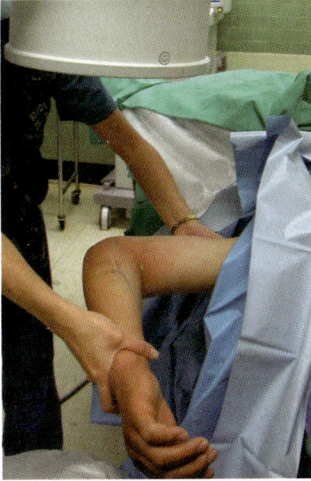

FIG 9 • Intraoperative photograph demonstrating the fluoroscopic examination. This is crucial to proper decision making and may be performed just before operative management.

■ Conservative management, with a week of sling immobilization followed by range of motion once the acute pain resolves, it is the treatment of choice in nondisplaced radial head fractures, where universally good and excellent results have been reported.
■ Nonoperative management is also the treatment of choice in fractures with less than 2 mm of displacement, with minor head involvement, and without bony blockage to range of motion.
   ■ A 7-day period of cast or splint immobilization is followed by aggressive motion after the inflammatory phase.
■ Our current practice for fractures that are more than 2 mm displaced is to determine whether there is a blockage of motion on fluoroscopic examination.
   ■ If there is maintenance of at least 50 degrees of both pronation and supination, we recommend conservative treatment.
   ■ If there is a blockage or instability, excision, fixation, or arthroplasty is recommended based on patient factors and instability.
■ A recent report regarding the long-term results of nonoperative management (similar to that described) of 49 patients with radial head fractures encompassing over 30% of the joint surface and displaced 2 to 5 mm revealed that 81% of patients had no subjective complaints and minimal loss of motion versus the uninjured extremity. Only one patient had daily pain.[1]

SURGICAL MANAGEMENT

Preoperative Planning

■ It is essential to review all radiographs and, most importantly, perform thorough history, physical, and fluoroscopic examinations before making an incision.
   ■ The presence of instability or associated fractures warrants a more extensile approach (**FIG 9**).

Positioning

■ Positioning depends on the planned approach and the surgeon's preference.
   ■ We prefer the patient supine with the affected extremity brought across the chest over a bump to allow access to the posterolateral elbow.
   ■ A tourniquet is placed high on the arm.

Approach

■ Two approaches, the extensile posterior (Boyd) and posterolateral (Köcher), will be presented (**FIG 10**).
■ The extensile posterior (Boyd) approach[2] with an interval between the ulna and anconeus allows for excellent visualization compared to traditional approaches. This versatile approach facilitates ORIF or arthroplasty of the radial head if the fracture proves to be more comminuted than preoperative imaging would predict. It can be easily accessed through a universal extensile incision that allows the surgeon to address ligamentous injuries in addition to the radial head fracture.

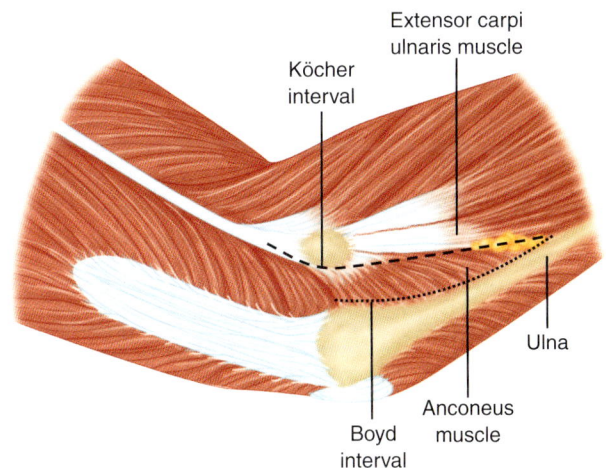

FIG 10 • Surgical intervals for the Boyd approach and the Köcher approach.

BOYD APPROACH

■ An 8-cm straight longitudinal incision is made just lateral to the olecranon (**TECH FIG 1A**).
■ Full-thickness skin flaps are developed bluntly over the fascia.
■ The fascia is longitudinally incised in the interval between the anconeus and ulna (**TECH FIG 1B**).
■ The anconeus is dissected off the ulna, elevating proximal to distal to preserve the distal vascular pedicle. Great care is taken not to violate the joint capsule or

lateral ulnar collateral ligament by using blunt fashion (**TECH FIG 1C**).
■ The lateral ulnar collateral ligament and annular ligament complex are sharply divided and tagged from their insertion on the crista supinatorus of the ulna. The radial head and its articulation with the capitellum are now evident (**TECH FIG 1D**).
■ After repair or replacement, the ligaments are repaired to their insertion with suture anchors.

TECHNIQUES

TECHNIQUES

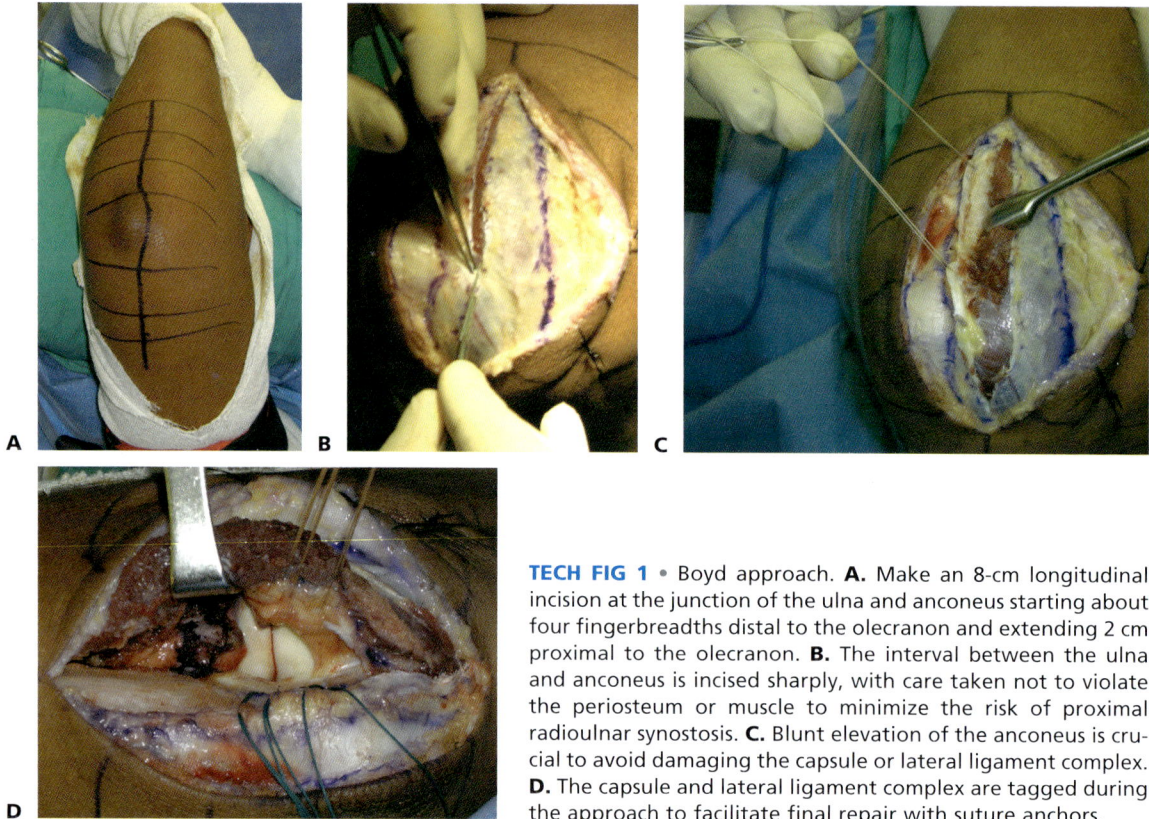

TECH FIG 1 • Boyd approach. **A.** Make an 8-cm longitudinal incision at the junction of the ulna and anconeus starting about four fingerbreadths distal to the olecranon and extending 2 cm proximal to the olecranon. **B.** The interval between the ulna and anconeus is incised sharply, with care taken not to violate the periosteum or muscle to minimize the risk of proximal radioulnar synostosis. **C.** Blunt elevation of the anconeus is crucial to avoid damaging the capsule or lateral ligament complex. **D.** The capsule and lateral ligament complex are tagged during the approach to facilitate final repair with suture anchors.

KÖCHER APPROACH

- The traditional posterolateral (Köcher) approach between the anconeus and extensor carpi ulnaris is cosmetic and spares the lateral ulnar collateral ligament.
  - We recommend not using an Esmarch tourniquet to allow visualization of penetrating veins that help identify the interval.
- A 5-cm oblique incision is made from the posterolateral aspect of the lateral epicondyle obliquely to a point three fingerbreadths below the tip of the olecranon in line with the radial neck (**TECH FIG 2A**).
- The radial head and epicondyle are palpated and the fascia is divided in line with the skin incision.

- The Köcher interval is identified distally by small penetrating veins and bluntly developed, revealing the lateral ligament complex and joint capsule (**TECH FIG 2B**).
- The anconeus is reflected posteriorly and the extensor carpi ulnaris origin anteriorly. The capsule is incised obliquely anterior to the lateral ulnar collateral ligament (**TECH FIG 2C,D**).
- The proximal edge of the annular ligament may also be divided and tagged, with care taken not to proceed distally and damage the posterior interosseous nerve.

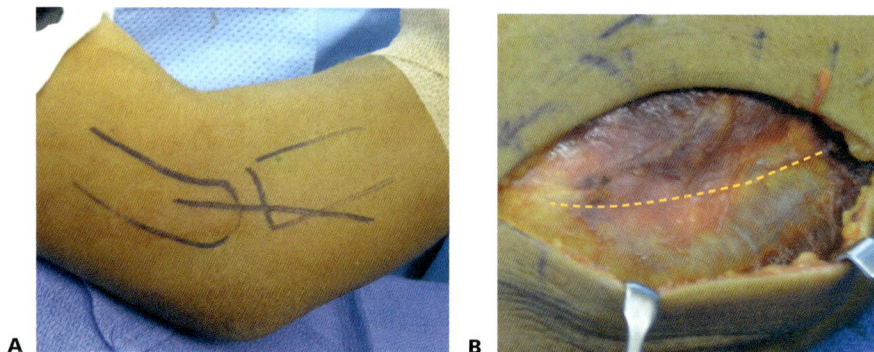

TECH FIG 2 • Köcher approach. **A.** The skin incision proceeds distally from the posterolateral aspect of the lateral epicondyle to the posterior aspect of the proximal radius. **B.** Full-thickness flaps are made and the fascial interval between the extensor carpi ulnaris and anconeus muscles is identified. *(continued)*

TECHNIQUES

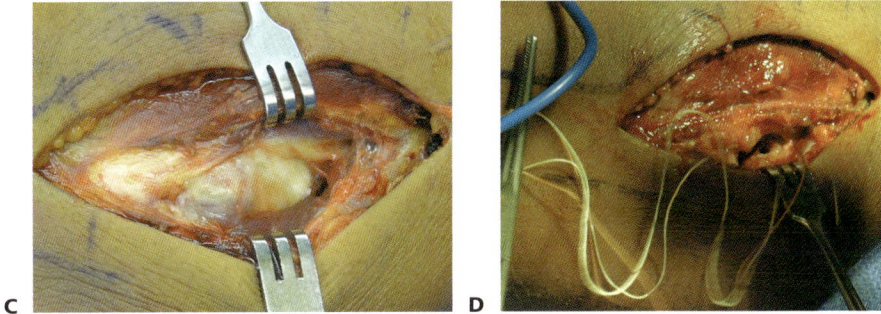

TECH FIG 2 • *(continued)* **C.** With longitudinal incision of the fascia and blunt division of the muscles, the joint capsule is evident. **D.** The capsule is longitudinally incised and the fascia is tagged with figure 8 stitches for later anatomic repair.

FRACTURE INSPECTION AND PREPARATION

- The fracture is now visible (**TECH FIG 3**).
- The wound is irrigated and loose bodies are removed.
- The forearm is rotated to obtain a circumferential view of the fracture and appreciate the safe zone for hardware placement.
- If comminution (more than three pieces) is evident at this step, we elect to replace the radial head.

TECH FIG 3 • Here the fractured radial head fragment has violated the lateral capsule, indicating a high-energy injury. The proximal radius is now exposed for fixation or prosthetic replacement.

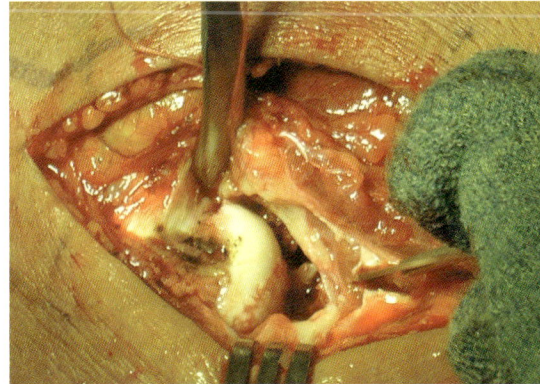

REDUCTION AND PROVISIONAL FIXATION

- Any joint impaction is elevated and the void filed with local cancellous graft from the lateral epicondyle.
- The fragments are reduced provisionally with a tenaculum and held with small Kirschner wires placed out of the zone where definitive fixation is planned.
- It is acceptable to place this temporary fixation in the safe zone (**TECH FIG 4**).

TECH FIG 4 • We prefer to use 0.062-inch Kirschner wires placed outside the zone of planned definitive fixation to provisionally hold the reduction.

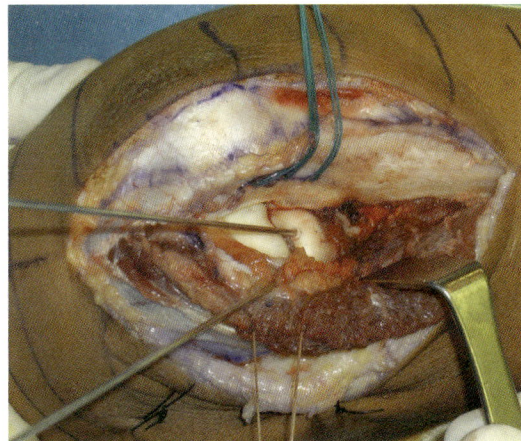

TECHNIQUES

FIXATION

- There are many options for definitive fixation[7]:
  - One or two countersunk 2.0-mm or 2.7-mm AO cortical screws perpendicular to the fracture (**TECH FIG 5A**)
  - Mini-plates (**TECH FIG 5B**)
  - Small headless screws
  - Polyglycolide pins
  - Small threaded wires
- We prefer to use two small parallel screws for isolated head fractures. For fractures with neck extension, we prefer AO 2.0-mm or 2.7-mm mini-plates along the safe zone.

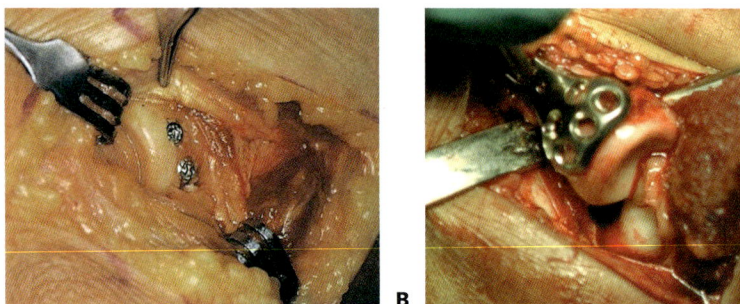

TECH FIG 5 • A. Two screws are placed in the safe zone perpendicular to the fracture. **B.** A plate is placed on a radial neck fracture.

CLOSURE

- Any releases or injury to the annular ligament or lateral ulnar collateral ligament must be repaired anatomically. Drill holes with transosseous sutures are a proven method, but most authors now use suture anchors with reproducible results.
- Skin closure is performed in standard fashion with drains at the surgeon's discretion. Small hemovac drains are routinely pulled on postoperative day 1.

PEARLS AND PITFALLS

Protection of the posterior interosseous nerve	▪ Pronation of the forearm moves the posterior interosseous nerve away from the operative field during posterior approaches. ▪ Dissection should remain subperiosteal.
Comminution	▪ We have a low threshold for excision or arthroplasty in the setting of comminution.
Fluoroscopy	▪ A fluoroscopy unit should be available for examination under anesthesia before sterile preparation.
Hardware	▪ Prosthetic radial head replacement should be discussed with the patient as an option and should be available in the room should the fracture prove to be comminuted. ▪ A hinged external fixator should be available if instability may be an issue.
Examination	▪ A thorough fluoroscopic examination is the most important factor in deciding what treatment is appropriate. To obtain a true lateral we recommend abducting the arm and externally rotating the shoulder while placing the elbow on the image intensifier.

POSTOPERATIVE CARE

- The elbow is immobilized in a splint for 7 to 10 days.
- Active range of motion is allowed as soon as tolerable. Supervised therapy may be considered if the patient is not making adequate progress.
- Associated injuries may call for more protected range of motion.
- Light activities of daily living are allowed at 2 weeks, with increased weight bearing at 6 weeks.

RESULTS

- The results of open reduction and internal fixation depend both on host factors such as the type of fracture, smoking, compliance, demand, as well as surgical and rehabilitation protocols.
  - In uncomplicated fractures, over 90% satisfactory results can be expected.
  - Complications and resultant secondary procedures will be more likely in cases with undiagnosed instability and associated injury.

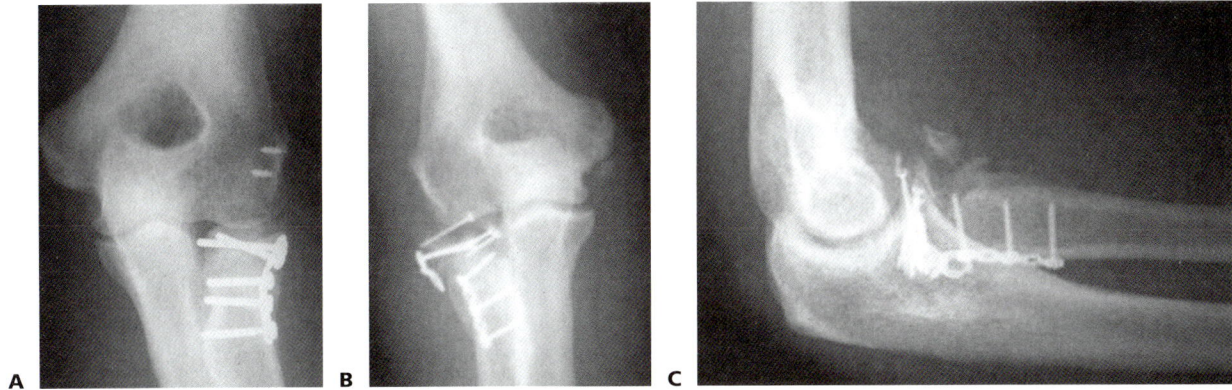

FIG 11 • A. AP radiograph demonstrating a screw penetrating the proximal radioulnar joint. **B,C.** Although these low-profile implants were apparently well placed, this patient went on to develop avascular necrosis with fragmentation of the radial head.

COMPLICATIONS

- Stiffness is the most common complication, with loss of terminal extension, supination, and pronation being most evident.
- Arthritis of the radiocapitellar joint or proximal radioulnar joint
- Heterotopic ossification
- Symptomatic hardware may require secondary removal (**FIG 11A**).
- Infection
- Early and late instability from missed or failed treatment of associated injuries
- The rate of avascular necrosis is about 10%, significantly higher in displaced fractures. This is expected given that the radial recurrent artery inserts in the safe zone where hardware is placed. This is generally clinically silent.
- Loss of reduction
- Nonunion (**FIG 11B,C**)

REFERENCES

1. Akesson T, Herbertsson P, Josefsson PO, et al. Primary nonoperative treatment of moderately displaced two-part fractures of the radial head. J Bone Joint Surg Am 2006;88A:1909–1914.
2. Boyd HB. Surgical exposure of the ulna and proximal third of the radius through one incision. Surg Gynecol Obstet 1940;71:86–88.
3. Broberg MA, Morrey BF. Results of delayed excision of the radial head after fracture. J Bone Joint Surg Am 1986;68A:669–674.
4. Caputo AE, Mazzocca AD, Sontoro VM. The nonarticulating portion of the radial head: Anatomic and clinical correlations for internal fixation. J Hand Surg Am 1998;23A:1082–1090.
5. Essex-Lopresti P. Fractures of the radial head with distal radioulnar dislocation. J Bone Joint Surg Br 1951;33B:244–250.
6. Herbertsson P, Josefsson PO, Hasserius R, et al. Fractures of the radial head and neck treated with radial head excision. J Bone Joint Surg Am 2004;86A:1925–1930.
7. Ikeda M, Sugiyama K, Kang C, et al. Comminuted fractures of the radial head: comparison of resection and internal fixation. J Bone Joint Surg Am 2006;88A:11–23.
8. Itamura J, Roidis N, Vaishnav S, et al. MRI evaluation of comminuted radial head fractures. J Shoulder Elbow Surg 2005; 14:421–424.
9. Morgan SJ, Groshen SL, Itamura JM, et al. Reliability evaluation of classifying radial head fractures by the system of Mason. Bull Hosp Jt Dis 1997;56:95–98.
10. Morrey BF, An KN, Stormont TJ. Force transmission through the radial head. J Bone Joint Surg Am 1988;70A:250–256.
11. Ring D, Quintero J, Jupiter JB. Open reduction and internal fixation of fractures of the radial head. J Bone Joint Surg Am 2002;84A: 1811–1815.
12. Tang CW, Skaggs DL, Kay RM. Elbow aspiration and arthrogram: an alternative method. Am J Orthop 2001;30:256.
13. Yamaguchi K, Sweet FA, Bindra R, et al. The extraosseous and intraosseous arterial anatomy of the adult elbow. J Bone Joint Surg Am 1997;79A:1653–1662.

Yishai Rosenblatt and Graham J. W. King

DEFINITION

- Radial head fractures are the most common fracture of the elbow and usually can be managed either nonoperatively or with open reduction and internal fixation.
- Radial head arthroplasty is indicated for unreconstructable displaced radial head fractures with an associated elbow dislocation or a known or possible disruption of the medial collateral, lateral collateral, or interosseous ligaments.[16]
- Most comminuted radial head fractures have an associated ligament injury, so radial head excision without replacement is uncommonly indicated in the setting of an acute radial head fracture.
- Biomechanical studies have shown that the kinematics and stability of the elbow are altered by radial head excision, even in the setting of intact collateral ligaments,[15] and are improved with a metallic radial head arthroplasty.[19,23]
- Radial head replacement is also indicated to treat posttraumatic conditions such as radial head nonunion and malunion and to manage elbow or forearm instability after radial head excision.

ANATOMY

- The radial head has a circular concave dish that articulates with the spherical capitellum and an articular margin that articulates with the lesser sigmoid notch of the ulna.
- The articular dish has an elliptical shape that varies considerably in size and shape and is variably offset from the axis of the radial neck.
- There is a poor correlation between the size of the radial head and the medullary canal of the radial neck, making a modular implant desirable for an optimal fit.[18]
- Elbow stability is maintained by joint congruity, capsuloligamentous integrity, and an intact balanced musculature.
- The radial head is an important valgus stabilizer of the elbow, particularly in the setting of an incompetent medial collateral ligament, which is the primary stabilizer against valgus force.
- The radial head is also important as an axial stabilizer of the forearm and resists varus and posterolateral rotatory instability by tensioning the lateral collateral ligament.
- The radial head accounts for up to 60% of the load transfer across the elbow.[11]
- The lateral ulnar collateral ligament is an important stabilizer against varus and posterolateral rotational instability of the elbow and should be preserved or repaired after radial head arthroplasty (**FIG 1**).

PATHOGENESIS

- Displaced radial head fractures typically result from a fall on the outstretched arm.
- Axial, valgus, and posterolateral rotational patterns of loading are all thought to be potentially responsible for these fractures.

- Injuries of the medial collateral or lateral collateral ligament or the interosseous ligament are typically associated with comminuted displaced unreconstructable radial head fractures.[6]
- In more severe injuries, dislocations of the elbow and forearm and fractures of the coronoid, olecranon, and capitellum can occur and further impair stability.

NATURAL HISTORY

- Long-term follow-up studies suggest a high incidence of radiographic arthritis with radial head excision, although the incidence of symptomatic arthritis varies widely between series.[4,13,14]
- Biomechanical data have demonstrated an alteration in the kinematics, load transfer, and stability of the elbow after radial head excision[3,15] that may lead to premature cartilage wear of the ulnohumeral joint and secondary pain due to arthritis.
- Metallic radial head replacement in elbows with intact ligaments restores the kinematics and stability similar to that of a native radial head and has been shown to provide good clinical and radiographic outcome in most patients at medium-term follow-up; however, long-term outcome studies are lacking.[3]

PATIENT HISTORY AND PHYSICAL FINDINGS

- The mechanism of injury is typically a fall on the outstretched hand.
- The patient will complain of pain and limitation of elbow or forearm motion.

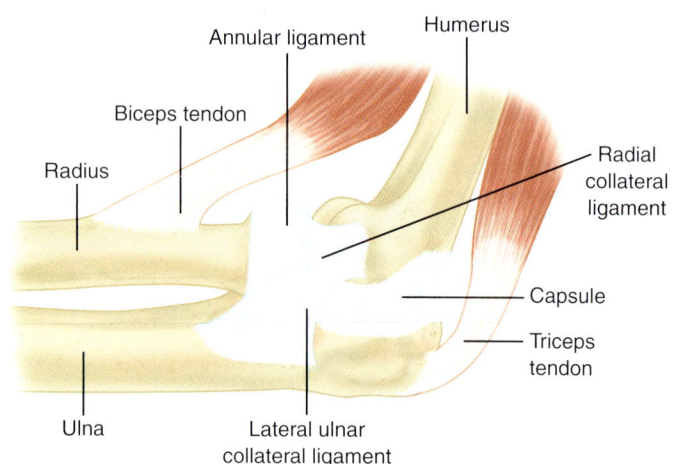

FIG 1 • The ligaments on the lateral aspect of the elbow include the lateral ulnar collateral ligament, the radial collateral ligament, and the annular ligament. The lateral ulnar collateral ligament is an important stabilizer against varus and posterolateral rotational instability of the elbow and should be preserved or repaired after radial head arthroplasty.

- A history of forearm or wrist pain should be sought.
- Inspection may reveal ecchymosis along the forearm or medial aspect of the elbow. Deformity may be evident if there is an associated dislocation.
- Careful palpation of the radial head, the medial and lateral collateral ligaments of the elbow, the interosseous ligament of the forearm, and the distal radioulnar joint should be performed. Local tenderness over one or all of these structures implies a possible derangement of the relevant structure.
- Since associated injuries of the shoulder, forearm, wrist, and hand are common, these areas should be carefully examined.
- Range of motion, including forearm rotation and elbow flexion–extension, should be evaluated. The presence of palpable and auditory crepitus should be noted.
- Loss of terminal elbow flexion and extension is expected as a consequence of a hemarthrosis in acute fractures, while loss of forearm rotation typically is caused by a mechanical impingement.
- A careful neurovascular assessment of all three major nerves that cross the elbow should be performed.
- The examiner should observe for localized or diffuse swelling in the elbow. Effusion represents hemarthrosis due to intra-articular fracture.
- The examiner should compare active and passive range of motion to the uninjured side. Reduced range of motion may be a result of hemarthrosis or mechanical block from a broken fragment. Intra-articular injection of a local anesthetic helps differentiate between reduced range of motion due to a mechanical block versus pain inhibition.
- The examiner should look for varus–valgus instability. Any gapping on the medial or lateral side beneath the examiner's hand is noted. Positive findings suggest mediolateral collateral ligament insufficiency. Typically, this test is positive only when performed under a general anesthetic.
- The lateral pivot shift test is performed. Positive apprehension or a clunk that is seen or felt when the ulna and radius reduce on the humerus suggests posterolateral rotatory instability.

IMAGING AND OTHER DIAGNOSTIC STUDIES

- Anteroposterior (AP), lateral, and oblique elbow radiographs, with the x-ray beam centered on the radiocapitellar joint, usually provide sufficient information for the diagnosis and treatment of radial head fractures.
- Bilateral posteroanterior radiographs of both wrists in neutral rotation should be performed to evaluate ulnar variance in patients with wrist discomfort or a comminuted radial head fracture, since there is a higher incidence of an associated interosseous ligament injury in these patients.[6]
- Computed tomography with sagittal, coronal, and 3D reconstructions may assist with preoperative planning and can help the surgeon predict whether a displaced radial head fracture can be repaired with open reduction and internal fixation or if an arthroplasty will likely be needed.

DIFFERENTIAL DIAGNOSIS

- Acute radial head fractures
- Other fractures or dislocations about the elbow (eg, supracondylar, capitellar, coronoid, osteochondral fractures)
- Radial head nonunion or malunion, posttraumatic arthritis
- Congenital dislocation of the radial head
- Forearm or elbow instability

- Lateral epicondylitis
- Rheumatoid arthritis or osteoarthritis
- Synovitis, inflammatory or infectious
- Tumors

NONOPERATIVE MANAGEMENT

- The indications for surgical management of radial head fractures are not well defined in the literature. Fragment size, number of fracture fragments, degree of displacement, and bone quality influence decision making regarding the optimal management.
- Nondisplaced fractures or small (less than 33% of radial head) minimally displaced fractures (less than 2 mm) can be treated with early motion with an excellent outcome in the majority of patients.
- Associated injuries and a block to motion are also important factors to consider when deciding between nonoperative and surgical management.

SURGICAL MANAGEMENT

- Small displaced fractures that cause painful crepitus or limited motion are managed with fragment excision if they are too small (typically less than 25% of the diameter of the radial head) or osteopenic to be internally fixated.
- Larger displaced fractures are typically managed with ORIF with good outcomes in most patients.
- Radial head fractures that are displaced but too comminuted to be anatomically reduced and stably fixed and that are too large to consider fragment excision (involve more than a quarter to a third of the radial head) should be managed by radial head excision with or without arthroplasty.
- Patients who are known to have, or are likely to have, an associated ligamentous injury of the elbow or forearm should have a radial head arthroplasty because radial head excision is contraindicated (**FIG 2**).
- The decision as to what fracture is reconstructable depends on surgeon factors (eg, experience), patient factors (eg, osteoporosis), and fracture factors (eg, fragment number and size, comminution, associated soft tissue injuries). The final decision is often made only at the time of surgery.
- Other indications for radial head arthroplasty include radial head nonunion or malunion, primary or secondary management of forearm or elbow instability (eg, Essex-Lopresti injury), rheumatoid arthritis or osteoarthritis, and tumors.

Preoperative Planning

- Currently available devices include spacer implants, press-fit and ingrowth stems, and bipolar and ceramic articulations.
- Silicone radial head implants offer little in the way of axial or valgus stability to the elbow and have been complicated by a high incidence of implant wear, fragmentation, and silicone synovitis leading to generalized joint damage. As a result, they have fallen out of favor and have been replaced by metallic implants.
- Most metallic radial head implants that have been developed and used to date employ a monoblock design, making size matching suboptimal and implant insertion often difficult because of the need to subluxate the elbow to allow for insertion of these devices.[10]
- Recently, modular metallic radial head prostheses have become available with separate heads and stems, allowing improved size matching of the native radial head and neck[18] and easier placement in the setting of competent lateral ligaments.[17]

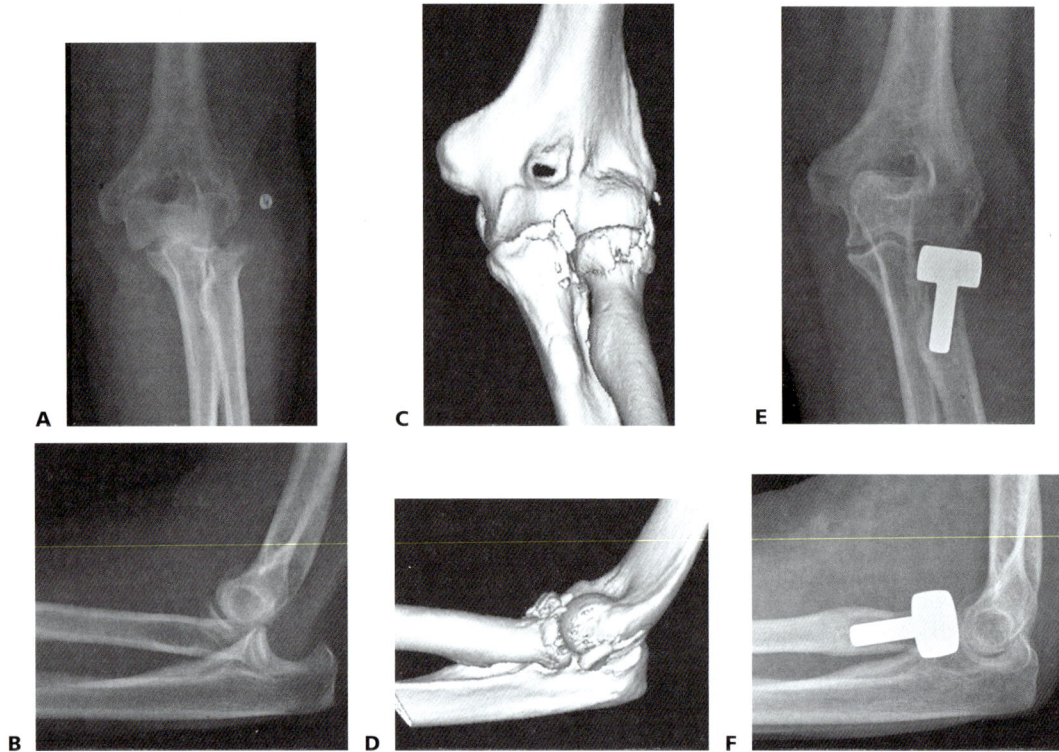

FIG 2 • **A,B.** AP and lateral radiographs of a 54-year-old woman who sustained a posterolateral elbow dislocation associated with a comminuted fracture of the radial head and coronoid—the "terrible triad." **C,D.** Preoperative 3D reconstruction images demonstrating a comminuted radial head fracture with a small undisplaced coronoid fracture. **E,F.** Postoperative radiographs after modular radial head arthroplasty (Evolve, Wright Medical Technology, Arlington, TN) and repair of the lateral collateral ligament. Medial collateral ligament and coronoid repairs were not required since the elbow was sufficiently stable at the end of the procedure. A good functional outcome was achieved at the final follow-up.

■ Precise implant sizing and placement are critical with these devices to ensure correct capitellar tracking and to avoid a cam effect with forearm rotation, which may cause premature capitellar wear due to shearing of the cartilage and stem loosening due to increased loading of the stem–bone interface.

■ Preoperative radiographic templating of the contralateral normal radial head should be employed in the setting of a secondary radial head replacement but is not needed for acute fractures because the excised radial head is available for accurate implant sizing.

Positioning

■ The patient is placed supine on the operating table and a sandbag is placed beneath the ipsilateral scapula to assist in positioning the arm across the chest.

■ Alternatively, the patient can be positioned in a lateral position with the affected arm held over a bolster.[2]

■ Prophylactic intravenous antibiotics are administered.

■ General or regional anesthesia is employed.

■ A sterile tourniquet is applied.

TECHNIQUES

SURGICAL APPROACH

■ A midline posterior elbow incision is made just lateral to the tip of the olecranon (**TECH FIG 1A**).

■ A full-thickness lateral fasciocutaneous flap is elevated on the deep fascia. This extensile incision decreases the risk of cutaneous nerve injury and provides access to the radial head, coronoid, and medial and lateral collateral ligaments for the management of more complex injuries (**TECH FIG 1B**).[8,22]

■ Alternatively, a lateral skin incision centered over the lateral epicondyle and passing obliquely over the radial head can be used (see Tech Fig 1A).

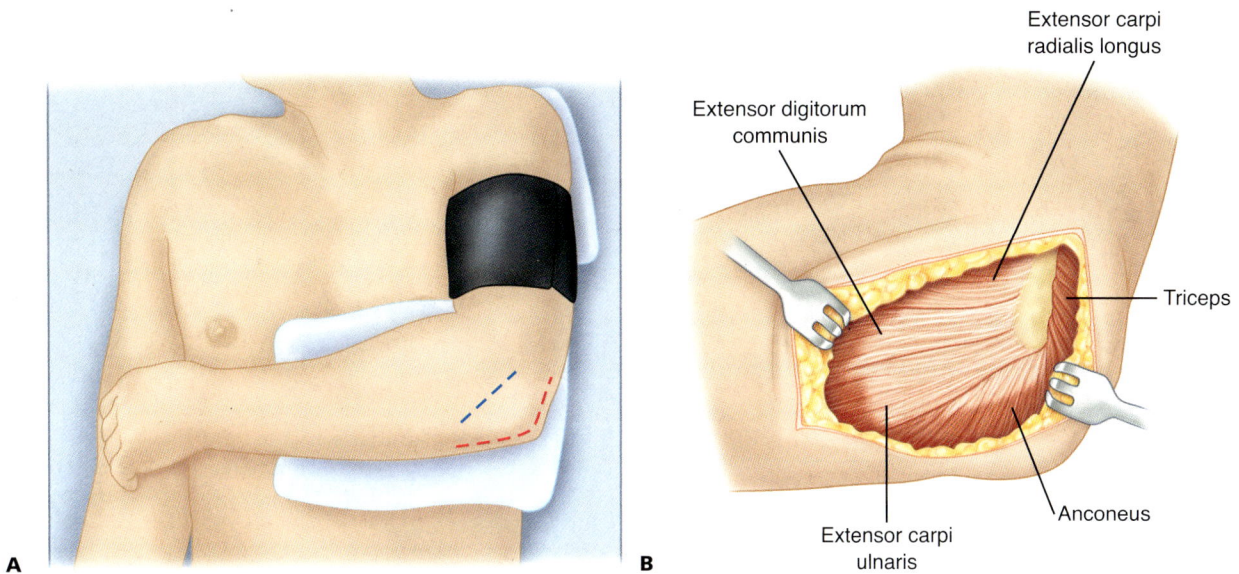

TECH FIG 1 • A. The patient is placed supine on the operating table and a sandbag is placed beneath the ipsilateral scapula to assist in positioning the arm across the chest. The posterior incision is indicated in red. Alternatively, a lateral skin incision centered over the lateral epicondyle and passing obliquely over the radial head can be used (blue). **B.** A midline posterior elbow incision made just lateral to the tip of the olecranon. A full-thickness lateral fasciocutaneous flap is elevated on the deep fascia. This extensile incision allows access to both the lateral and medial aspects of the elbow, in case of more complex injuries, and reduces the incidence of cutaneous nerve injury.

COMMON EXTENSOR SPLIT

- The extensor digitorum communis tendon is identified.
  - The landmarks for this plane are a line joining the lateral epicondyle and the tubercle of Lister.
- The extensor digitorum communis tendon is split longitudinally at the middle aspect of the radial head, and the underlying radial collateral and annular ligaments are incised (**TECH FIG 2A**).
  - Dissection should stay anterior to the lateral ulnar collateral ligament to prevent the development of posterolateral rotatory instability (see Fig 1).
  - The forearm is maintained in pronation to move the posterior interosseous nerve more distal and medial during the surgical approach.[7]
- If further exposure is required:
  - The humeral origin of the radial collateral ligament and the overlying extensor muscles are elevated anteriorly off the lateral epicondyle to improve the exposure if needed (**TECH FIG 2B**).
  - Release of the posterior component of the lateral collateral ligament can be considered, but careful ligament repair is required at the end of the procedure in order to restore the varus and posterolateral rotatory stability of the elbow.[9]

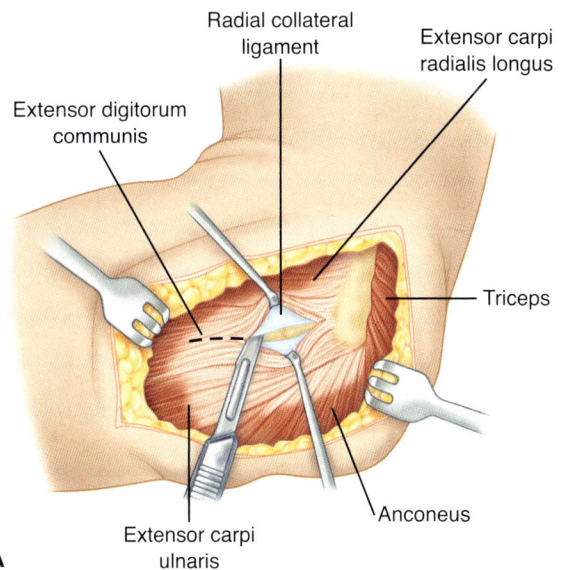

TECH FIG 2 • A. The extensor digitorum communis tendon is split longitudinally at the middle aspect of the radial head and the underlying radial collateral and annular ligaments are incised. The forearm is pronated to protect the posterior interosseous nerve. *(continued)*

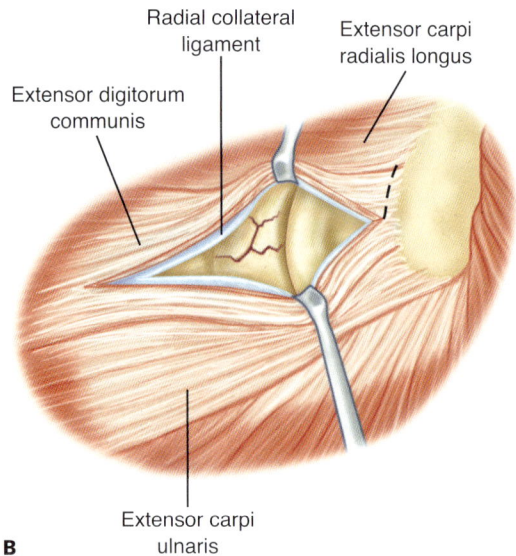

TECH FIG 2 • *(continued)* **B.** The humeral origin of the radial collateral ligament and the overlying extensor muscles are elevated anteriorly off the lateral epicondyle to improve the exposure if needed.

PREPARATION OF THE RADIAL HEAD AND NECK

- All fragments of the radial head are removed, as well as a minimal amount of radial neck at a right angle to the medullary canal, to make a smooth surface for seating of the prosthetic radial head.
  - Complete fragment excision can be confirmed with the use of an image intensifier.
- The capitellum is evaluated for chondral injuries or osteochondral fractures.
- The radial head prosthesis is sized in one of several ways:
  - The resected radial head is reassembled in the provided sizing template to assist in the accurate sizing of the prosthesis (**TECH FIG 3A–C**).
  - The diameter of radial head prosthesis should be based on the size of the articular dish. This is typically 2 mm smaller than the outer diameter of the excised radial head.

- Alternatively, if the radial head has been previously excised, radiographic templating of the contralateral normal radial head may be used to determine the appropriate diameter and height of the radial head implant.
- If the native radial head is in between available implant sizes, the implant diameter or thickness should be downsized.
- The radial neck is delivered laterally using a Hohmann retractor carefully placed around the posterior aspect of the proximal radial neck (**TECH FIG 3D**).
  - An anteriorly based retractor should be avoided because of the risk of injury from pressure on the posterior interosseous nerve.
- The medullary canal of the radial neck is reamed using hand reamers until cortical contact is encountered.
  - A trial stem one size smaller than the rasp is inserted to achieve a nontight press-fit.

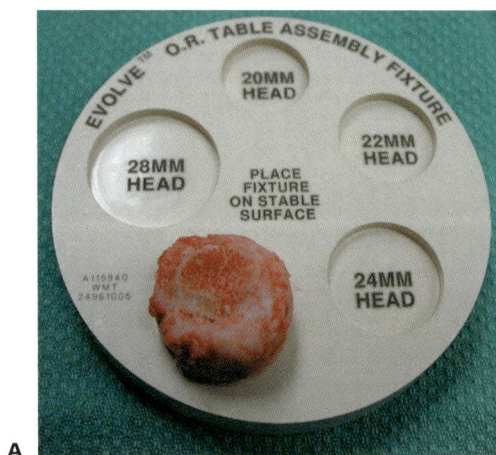

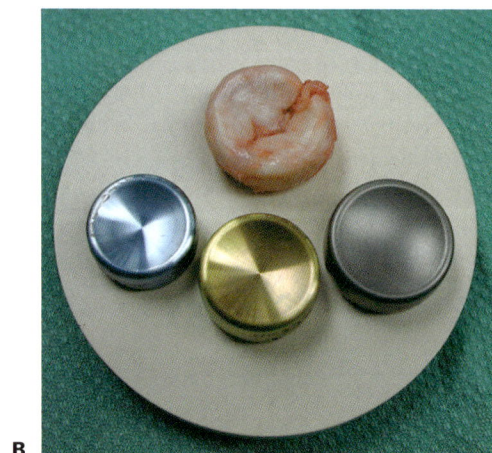

TECH FIG 3 • The resected radial head is reassembled in the provided sizing template (**A**) to assist in the accurate sizing of the prosthesis in terms of diameter (**B**) *(continued)*

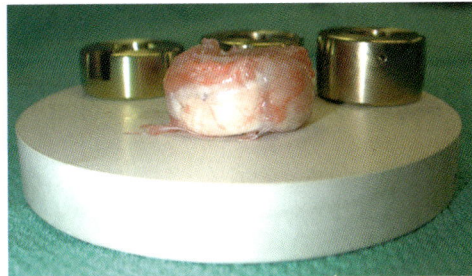

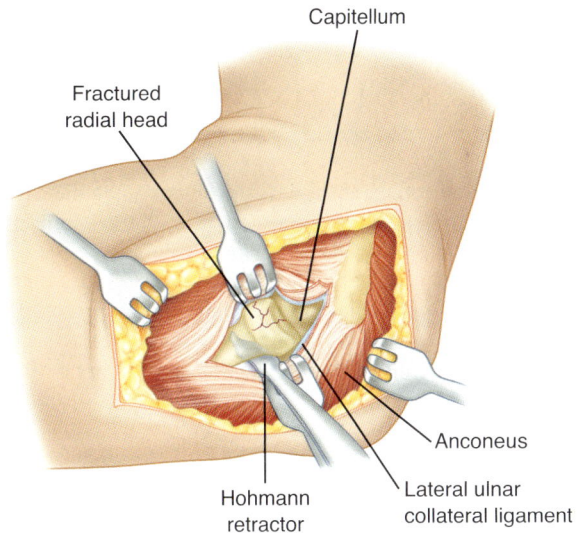

Capitellum

Fractured
radial head

Anconeus

Hohmann
retractor

Lateral ulnar
collateral ligament

C

D

TECH FIG 3 • *(continued)* and height (**C**), and to ensure that all the fragments have been removed from the elbow. **D.** The radial neck is delivered laterally using a Hohmann retractor carefully placed around the posterior aspect of the proximal radial neck. An anteriorly based retractor should be avoided because of the risk of injury to the posterior interosseous nerve.

RADIAL HEAD REPLACEMENT

- A trial head is inserted onto the stem, and the diameter, height, tracking, and congruency of the prosthesis are evaluated both visually and with the aid of an image intensifier.
  - The radial head prosthesis should articulate at the same height as the radial notch of the ulna and about 1 mm distal to the tip of the coronoid (**TECH FIG 4A**).
  - The alignment of the distal radioulnar joint, ulnar variance, as well as the width of the lateral and medial portions of the ulnohumeral joint, are checked and compared to the contralateral wrist and elbow, respectively, under fluoroscopy.
  - Overlengthening the radiocapitellar joint with a radial head implant that is too thick should be avoided

to reduce the risk of cartilage wear on the capitellum from excessive pressure; a nonparallel medial ulnohumeral joint space that is wider laterally is suggestive of overstuffing.
  - Some modular and bipolar implants allow insertion of the stem first, then placement of the head onto the stem with coupling in situ, which significantly reduces the surgical exposure needed (**TECH FIG 4B**).
- If the prosthesis is maltracking on the capitellum with forearm rotation, a smaller stem size should be trialed to ensure that the articulation of the radial head with the capitellum is controlled by the annular ligament and articular congruency and not dictated by the proximal radial shaft.

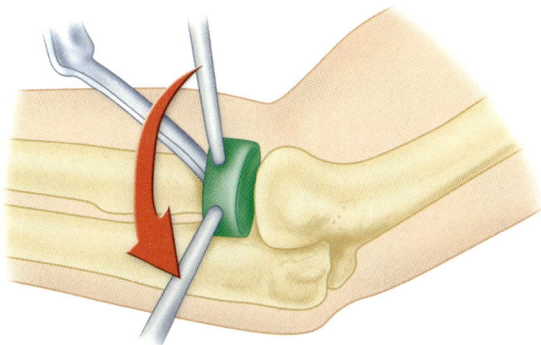

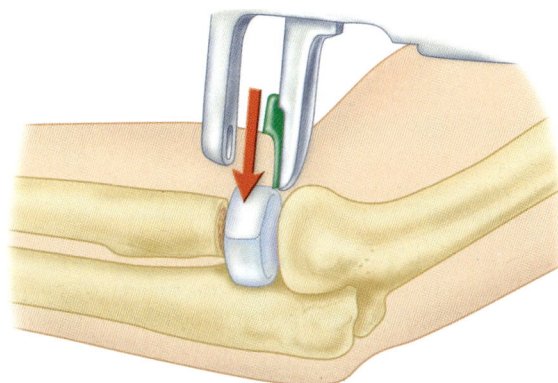

A

B

TECH FIG 4 • **A.** A trial stem is inserted. A trial head is inserted onto the stem and the diameter, height, tracking, and congruency of the prosthesis are evaluated both visually and with the aid of an image intensifier. **B.** Some modular and bipolar implants allow insertion of the stem first, then placement of the head onto the stem with coupling in situ, which significantly reduces the surgical exposure needed.

TECHNIQUES

LATERAL SOFT TISSUE CLOSURE

- After radial head replacement, the lateral collateral ligament and extensor muscle origins are repaired back to the lateral condyle.
- If the posterior half of the lateral collateral ligament is still attached to the lateral epicondyle, then the anterior half of the lateral collateral ligament (the annular ligament and radial collateral ligament) and extensor muscles are repaired to the posterior half using interrupted absorbable sutures (**TECH FIG 5A**).
- If the lateral collateral ligament and extensor origin have been completely detached either by the injury or surgical exposure, they should be securely repaired less equalize to the lateral epicondyle using drill holes through bone and nonabsorbable sutures or suture anchors.

- A single drill hole is placed at the axis of motion (the center of the arc of curvature of the capitellum) and connected to two drill holes placed anterior and posterior to the lateral supracondylar ridge.
- A locking (Krackow) suture technique is employed to gain a secure hold of the lateral collateral ligament and common extensor muscle fascia (**TECH FIG 5B–D**).
- The ligament sutures are pulled into the holes drilled in the distal humerus using suture retrievers and the forearm is pronated, and varus forces are avoided, while tensioning the sutures before tying (**TECH FIG 5E**).
- The knots should be left anterior or posterior to the lateral supracondylar ridge to avoid prominence.

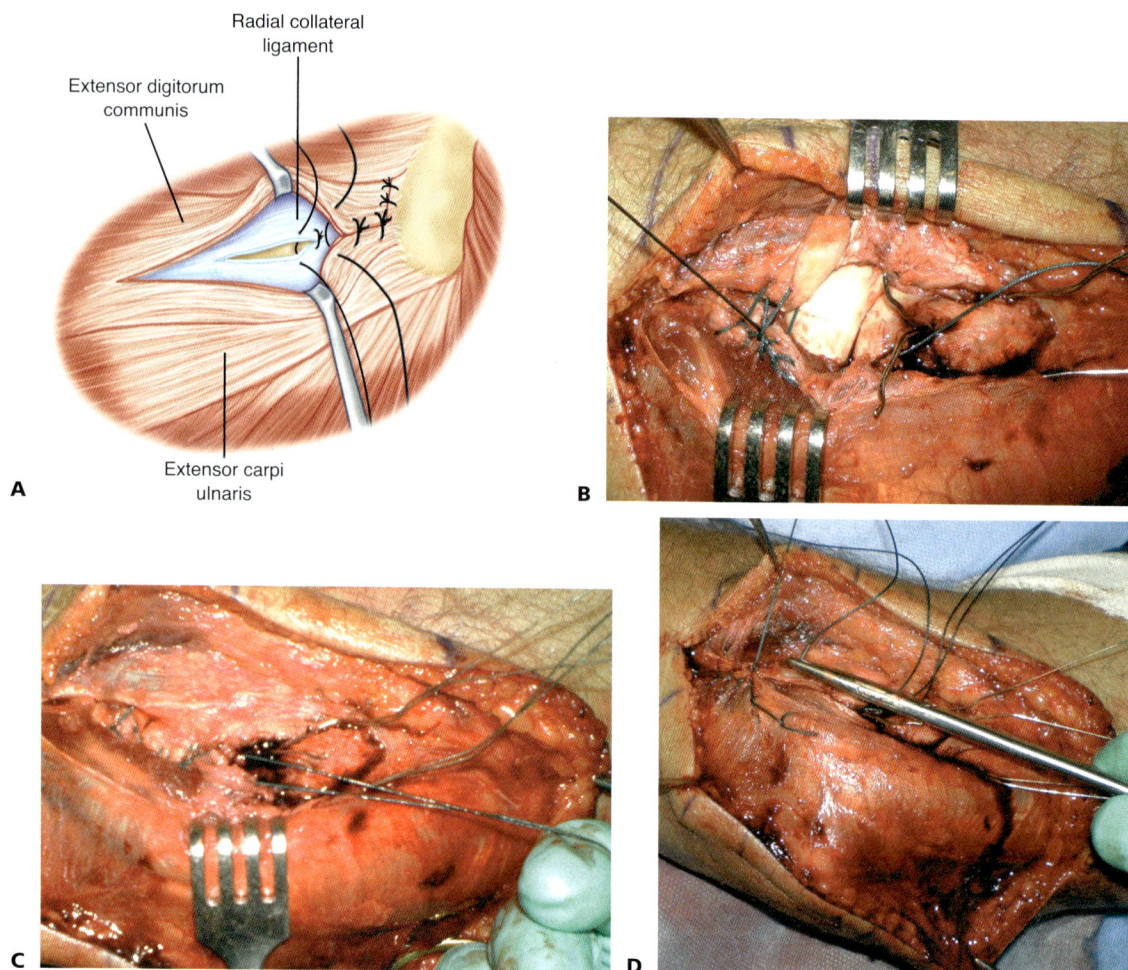

TECH FIG 5 • **A.** If the posterior half of the lateral collateral ligament is still attached to the lateral epicondyle, then the anterior half of it (the annular ligament and radial collateral ligament) and extensor muscles are repaired to the posterior half using interrupted absorbable sutures. *ECU*, extensor carpi ulnaris; *EDC*, extensor digitorum communis. **B–D.** If the lateral collateral ligament and extensor origin have been completely disrupted by the injury or detached by the surgical exposure, they should be securely repaired to the lateral epicondyle. A single drill hole is placed at the center of the arc of curvature of the capitellum and connected to two drill holes placed anterior and posterior to the lateral supracondylar ridge. A locking (Krackow) suture technique is employed to gain a secure hold of the lateral collateral ligament (**B**) as well as of the annular ligament (**C**). **D.** A second stitch is used in a similar manner to repair the common extensor muscle fascia. *(continued)*

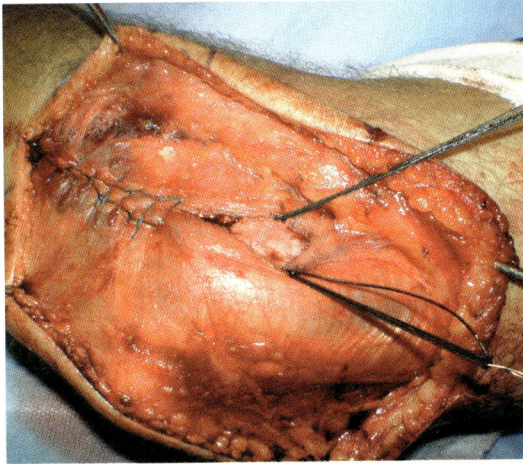

E

TECH FIG 5 • *(continued)* **E.** The sutures are pulled into the holes drilled in the distal humerus using suture retrievers, tensioned while keeping the forearm pronated and while avoiding varus forces, and eventually tied over the lateral supracondylar ridge.

COMPLETION

- After replacement arthroplasty and lateral soft tissue closure, the elbow should be placed through an arc of flexion–extension while carefully evaluating for elbow stability in pronation, neutral, and supination.[2]
- Pronation is generally beneficial if the lateral ligaments are deficient,[9] supination if the medial ligaments are deficient,[1] and neutral position if both sides have been injured.

- In patients who have an associated elbow dislocation, additional repair of the medial collateral ligament and flexor pronator origin should be performed if the elbow subluxates at 40 degrees or more of flexion.
- Tourniquet deflation and hemostasis should be secured before wound closure.

KÖCHER APPROACH

- Alternatively, the radial head may be approached by using the Köcher interval[20] between the extensor carpi ulnaris and anconeus.
- The fascial interval between these muscles is identified by noting the diverging direction of the muscle groups and small vascular perforators that exit at this interval (**TECH FIG 6**).
- Care should be taken to preserve the lateral ulnar collateral ligament, which is vulnerable as the dissection is carried deeper through the capsule.

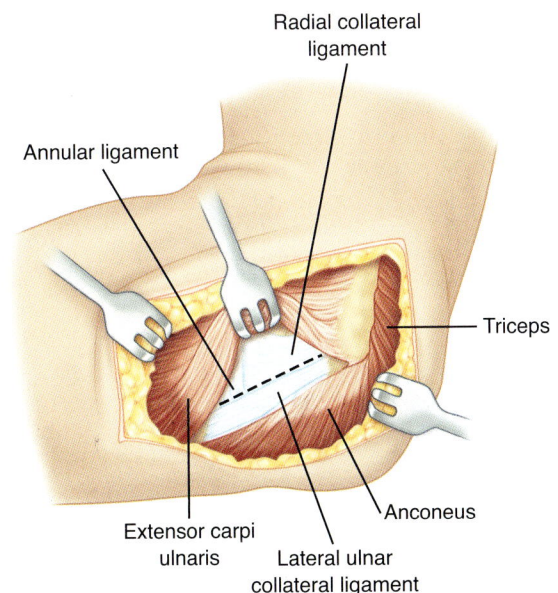

TECH FIG 6 • The extensor carpi ulnaris is elevated anteriorly and an arthrotomy is performed at the midportion of the radial head. Care should be taken to preserve the lateral ulnar collateral ligament, which is vulnerable as the dissection is carried deeper through the capsule.

PEARLS AND PITFALLS

Indications	▪ Displaced unreconstructable fracture of the radial head with known or probable associated medial or lateral collateral or interosseous ligament injury
Pearls	▪ A preoperative radiographic template of the contralateral native radial head should be used in the setting of a secondary radial head replacement.
	▪ Dissection should stay anterior to the lateral ulnar collateral ligament to prevent the development of posterolateral rotatory instability.
	▪ The radial head should be sized based on the diameter of the articular dish and thickness of the excised radial head.
	▪ The radial head implant is typically 2 mm smaller than the outer diameter of the radial head.
	▪ Radial head articular surface height should be at the level of the proximal radioulnar joint.
	▪ If the radial head does not track well on the capitellum, the stem should be downsized.
	▪ If the native radial head is in between implant sizes, the implant should, in general, be downsized.
	▪ Intraoperative fluoroscopy is used to assess the alignment of the radiocapitellar and distal radioulnar joints and to avoid overlengthening of the radius.
Pitfalls	▪ Hohmann retractors should not be used around the anterior aspect of the radial neck and the forearm should be kept pronated to avoid damage to the posterior interosseous nerve.
	▪ The surgeon should avoid overstuffing the thickness or diameter of the radial head because of the risk of capitellar wear and pain. Filling the gap between the capitellum and radial neck is not a useful landmark for prosthesis thickness because lateral soft tissues are often deficient owing to the surgical exposure or initial injury.

POSTOPERATIVE CARE

▪ The elbow with stable ligaments should be splinted using anterior plaster slabs in extension and elevated for 24 to 48 hours to diminish swelling, decrease tension on the posterior wound, and minimize the tendency to develop a flexion contracture.

▪ In the setting of a more tenuous ligamentous repair or the presence of some residual instability at the end of the operative procedure, the elbow should initially be splinted in 60 to 90 degrees of flexion in the optimal position of forearm rotation to maintain stability.

▪ Perioperative antibiotics are continued for 24 hours postoperatively.

▪ Indomethacin 25 mg three times daily for 3 weeks may be considered in patients undergoing radial head arthroplasty to decrease postoperative pain, reduce swelling, and potentially lower the incidence of heterotopic ossification.

▪ Indomethacin should be avoided in elderly patients and those with a history of peptic ulcer disease, asthma, known allergy, or other contraindications to anti-inflammatory medications.

▪ For an isolated radial head replacement treated with a lateral ulnar collateral ligament-sparing approach, active range of motion should be initiated on the day after surgery.

  ▪ A collar and cuff with the elbow maintained at 90 degrees is employed for comfort between exercises.

  ▪ A static progressive extension splint is fabricated for nighttime use for patients without associated ligamentous disruptions and is employed for a period of 12 weeks. The splint is adjusted weekly as extension improves.

  ▪ In patients with associated elbow dislocations or residual instability, extension splinting is not implemented until 6 weeks after surgery.

▪ Patients with associated fractures, dislocations, or ligamentous injuries should commence active flexion and extension motion within a safe arc 1 day postoperatively.

  ▪ Active forearm rotation is performed with the elbow in flexion to minimize stress on the medial or lateral ligamentous injuries or repairs.

  ▪ Extension is performed with the forearm in the appropriate rotational position—that is, pronation if the lateral ligaments are deficient,[9] supination if the medial ligaments are deficient,[1] and neutral position if both sides have been injured.

  ▪ A resting splint with the elbow maintained at 90 degrees and the forearm in the appropriate position of forearm rotation is employed for 3 to 6 weeks.

▪ Passive stretching is not permitted for 6 weeks to reduce the incidence of heterotopic ossification.

▪ Strengthening exercises are initiated once the ligament injuries and any associated fractures have adequately healed, usually at 8 weeks postoperatively.

OUTCOMES

▪ Silicone radial head arthroplasty, while initially successful in many patients,[5,24] has fallen out of favor because of problems with residual instability and arthritis, implant fracture, and silicone synovitis due to particulate debris.[25]

▪ While the short- and medium-term results of metallic radial head implants are encouraging, there is a paucity of literature demonstrating the long-term outcome with respect to loosening, capitellar wear, and arthritis.

▪ Metallic radial head replacement in elbows with intact ligaments restores the kinematics and stability similar to that measured with a native radial head. Moreover, when the fractured radial head occurs in combination with ligamentous and soft tissue disruption, a metallic prosthesis restores elbow stability, with only mild residual deficits in strength and motion.

▪ Moro et al[21] reported the functional outcome of 25 cases managed with a metallic radial head arthroplasty for unreconstructable fractures of the radial head at an average follow-up of 39 months. The results were rated as 17 good or excellent, 5 fair, and 3 poor.

  ▪ The radial head prosthesis restored elbow stability when the fractured radial head occurred in combination with a dislocation of the elbow, rupture of the medial collateral ligament, fracture of the coronoid, or fracture of the proximal ulna.

  ▪ There were mild residual deficits in strength and motion, and no patient required removal of the implant.

- Harrington et al[12] reported their experience with metallic radial head arthroplasty in 20 patients at an average follow-up of 12 years. The results were excellent or good in 16 and fair or poor in 4.
- Improvements in radial head arthroplasty designs, sizing, and implantation techniques may lead to improved outcomes for unreconstructable radial head fractures.

COMPLICATIONS

- Posterior interosseous nerve injury can occur as a consequence of dissection distal to the radial tuberosity and placement of anterior retractors around the distal radial neck.
- Infection
- Loss of motion, mainly terminal extension due to capsular contracture, heterotopic ossification, or retained cartilaginous or osseous fragments
- Prosthetic loosening or polyethylene wear
- Capitellar wear and pain due to implant overstuffing
- Complex regional pain syndrome
- Instability or recurrent dislocations of the elbow due to an inadequate or failed ligament repair
- Osteoarthritis of the capitellum as a consequence of articular cartilage damage from the initial injury, from component insertion, from persistent instability, or due to loading from a radial head implant that is too thick.

REFERENCES

1. Armstrong AD, Dunning CE, Faber KJ, et al. Rehabilitation of the medial collateral ligament-deficient elbow: an in vitro biomechanical study. J Hand Surg Am 2000;25A:1051–1057.
2. Bain GI, Ashwood N, Baird R, et al. Management of Mason type III radial head fractures with a titanium prosthesis, ligament repair, and early mobilization. J Bone Joint Surg Am 2005;87A:136–147.
3. Beingessner DM, Dunning CE, Gordon KD, et al. The effect of radial head excision and arthroplasty on elbow kinematics and stability. J Bone Joint Surg Am 2004;86A:1730–1739.
4. Boulas HJ, Morrey BF. Biomechanical evaluation of the elbow following radial head fracture: comparison of open reduction and internal fixation versus excision, Silastic replacement and non-operative management. Ann Chir Main 1998;17:314–320.
5. Carn RM, Medige J, Curtain D, et al. Silicone rubber replacement of the severely fractured radial head. Clin Orthop Relat Res 1986;209:259–269.
6. Davidson PA, Moseley JB Jr, Tullos HS. Radial head fracture: a potentially complex injury. Clin Orthop Relat Res 1993;297:224–230.
7. Diliberti T, Botte MJ, Abrams RA. Anatomical considerations regarding the posterior interosseous nerve during posterolateral approaches to the proximal part of the radius. J Bone Joint Surg Am 2000;82A:809–813.
8. Dowdy PA, Bain GI, King GJ, et al. The midline posterior elbow incision: an anatomical appraisal. J Bone Joint Surg Br 1995;77B:696–699.
9. Dunning CE, Zarzour ZD, Patterson SD, et al. Muscle forces and pronation stabilize the lateral ligament deficient elbow. Clin Orthop Relat Res 2001;388:118–124.
10. Gupta GG, Lucas G, Hahn DL. Biomechanical and computer analysis of radial head prostheses. J Shoulder Elbow Surg 1997;6:37–48.
11. Halls AA, Travill A. Transmission of pressures across the elbow joint. Anat Rec 1964;150:243–248.
12. Harrington IJ, Sekyi-Otu A, Barrington TW, et al. The functional outcome with metallic radial head implants in the treatment of unstable elbow fractures: a long-term review. J Trauma 2001;50:46–52.
13. Ikeda M, Oka Y. Function after early radial head resection for fracture: a retrospective evaluation of 15 patients followed for 3–18 years. Acta Orthop Scand 2000;71:191–194.
14. Janssen RP, Vetger J. Resection of the radial head after Mason type III fracture of the elbow. J Bone Joint Surg Br 1998;80B:231–233.
15. Jensen SL, Olsen BS, Sojbjerg JO. Elbow joint kinematics after excision of the radial head. J Shoulder Elbow Surg 1999;8:238–241.
16. Johnston GW. A follow-up of one hundred cases of fracture of the head of the radius with a review of the literature. Ulster Med J 1962;31:51–56.
17. King GJ. Management of radial head fractures with implant arthroplasty. J Am Soc Surg Hand 2004;4:11–26.
18. King GJ, Zarzour ZD, Patterson SD, et al. An anthropometric study of the radial head: implications in the design of a prosthesis. J Arthroplasty 2001;16:112–116.
19. King GJ, Zarzour ZD, Rath DA, et al. Metallic radial head arthroplasty improves valgus stability of the elbow. Clin Orthop Relat Res 1999;368:114–125.
20. Köcher T. Textbook of Operative Surgery. London: Adam and Charles Black, 1911.
21. Moro JK, Werier J, MacDermid JC, et al. Arthroplasty with a metal radial head for unreconstructible fractures of the radial head. J Bone Joint Surg Am 2001;83A:1201–1211.
22. Patterson SD, Bain GI, Mehta JA. Surgical approaches to the elbow. Clin Orthop Relat Res 2000;370:19–33.
23. Pomianowski S, Morrey BF, Neale PG, et al. Contribution of monoblock and bipolar radial head prostheses to valgus stability of the elbow. J Bone Joint Surg Am 2001;83A:1829–1834.
24. Swanson AB, Jaeger SH, La Rochelle D. Comminuted fractures of the radial head: the role of silicone-implant replacement arthroplasty. J Bone Joint Surg Am 1981;63A:1039–1049.
25. Vanderwilde RS, Morrey BF, Melberg MW, et al. Inflammatory arthritis after failure of silicone rubber replacement of the radial head. J Bone Joint Surg Br 1994;76B:78–81.

Chapter 37

Open Reduction and Internal Fixation of Olecranon Fractures

David Ring

DEFINITION

- Fracture of the olecranon process is common, usually displaced, and nearly always treated operatively.
- Important injury characteristics include displacement, comminution, and subluxation or dislocation of the elbow, and all are accounted for in the Mayo classification (**FIG 1**).[6]
- Fracture-dislocations of the olecranon can be anterior (trans-olecranon) or posterior (the most proximal type of posterior Monteggia according to Jupiter and colleagues[3]) in direction.[2,3,9,10]
- Open injuries are unusual.

ANATOMY

- The greater sigmoid notch of the ulna is formed by the coronoid and olecranon processes and forms a nearly 180-degree arc capturing the trochlea.
- The region between the coronoid and olecranon articular facets is the nonarticular transverse groove of the olecranon, a common location of fracture and a place where precise articular reduction is not critical.
- The triceps has a broad and thick insertion from just superior to the point of the olecranon and the tip of the olecranon process that can be used to enhance fixation of small, osteoporotic, or fragmented fractures and can be split longitudinally, if needed, when applying a plate.

PATHOGENESIS

- Fractures of the olecranon are most often the result of a direct blow to the point of the elbow, but occasionally they result from indirect forces during a fall on the outstretched hand.

NATURAL HISTORY

- Stable nondisplaced or minimally displaced fractures are uncommon.
- The majority of olecranon fractures are displaced and benefit from operative treatment.
- The occasional untreated displaced simple olecranon fracture demonstrates a slight flexion contracture, some weakness of extension, no arthrosis, and little if any pain.
- In contrast, undertreated or poorly treated fracture-dislocations lead to severe arthrosis with or without instability.
- Even well-treated complex injuries are at risk for stiffness, heterotopic ossification, arthrosis, and occasionally nonunion.

PATIENT HISTORY AND PHYSICAL FINDINGS

- Knowledge of the characteristics of the patient (age, gender, medical health) and the injury (mechanism, energy) will help the surgeon understand the injury and determine optimal treatment.
- First the patient is assessed for life-threatening injuries (ATLS protocol) and any medical problems that may have contributed to the injury.

- A secondary survey is performed to identify any other fractures, ipsilateral arm injuries in particular.
- The skin is carefully inspected for any wounds associated with the fracture.
- The pulses are palpated, capillary refill inspected, and an Allen test performed if necessary.
- Peripheral nerve function is assessed.
- Patients with high-energy injuries, particularly those with ipsilateral wrist or forearm injuries, are at risk for compartment syndrome. If the clinical examination is suggestive or unreliable (owing to problems with mental status), compartment pressure monitoring should be performed.

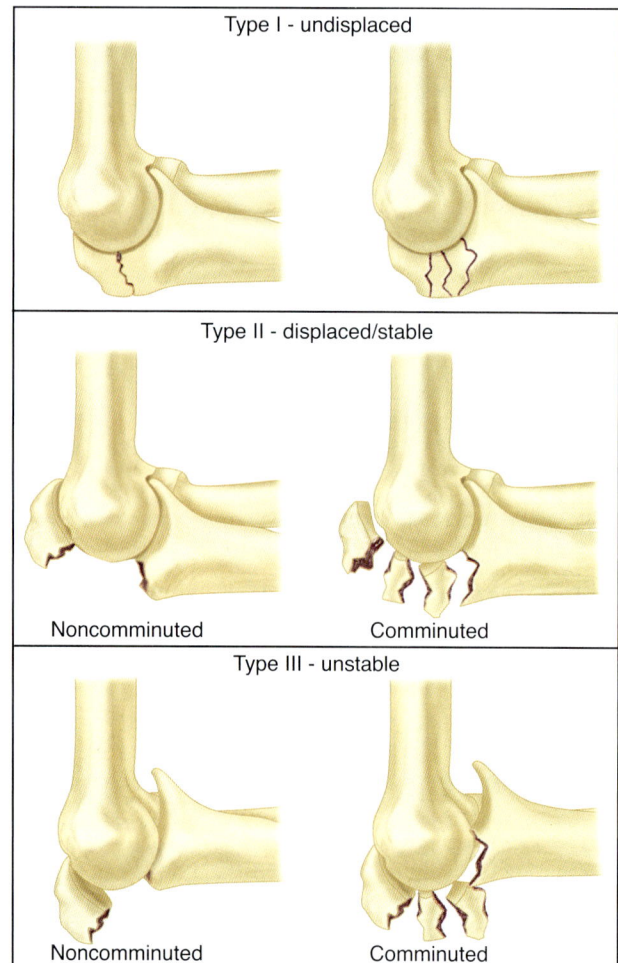

FIG 1 • The Mayo classification of olecranon fractures accounts for the factors that will influence treatment decisions: displacement, comminution, and dislocation or subluxation of the articulations.

IMAGING AND OTHER DIAGNOSTIC STUDIES

- Anteroposterior (AP) and lateral radiographs are used for initial characterization of the injury.
- Radiographs after reduction or splinting, or oblique views can be useful.
- Computed tomography (CT) is useful for characterization of fracture-dislocations. In particular, 3D CT reconstructions can be useful for assessment of the coronoid and radial head.

DIFFERENTIAL DIAGNOSIS

- Elbow dislocation
- Monteggia and Essex-Lopresti fracture-dislocations of the forearm
- Distal humerus fracture

NONOPERATIVE MANAGEMENT

- Nonoperative management is appropriate for the rare fracture of the olecranon that is less than 2 millimeters displaced with the elbow flexed 90 degrees.
- Four weeks of splint immobilization followed by active assisted mobilization of the elbow will usually result in a healed fracture and good elbow function.

SURGICAL MANAGEMENT

- The vast majority of olecranon fractures are displaced and merit operative treatment.

- Transverse, noncomminuted fractures not associated with fracture-dislocation are treated with tension band wiring.[4,8]
- Comminuted fractures and fracture-dislocations are treated with dorsal contoured plate and screw fixation.[1–3]
- The treatment of fracture-dislocations requires attention to the coronoid, radial head, and lateral collateral ligament.[2,9–11]

Preoperative Planning

- The fracture characteristics that determine treatment are defined on radiographs and CT.
- Templating the surgery with tracings of the radiographs is a useful way of running through the surgery in detail before performing it, familiarizing oneself with the anatomy, anticipating problems, and ensuring that all of the implants and equipment that might be necessary are available.

Positioning

- In most patients a lateral decubitus position with the arm over a bolster or support is best.
- Some patients with fracture-dislocations that require both medial and lateral access may be positioned supine with the arm supported on a hand table.
- A sterile pneumatic tourniquet is used.

Approach

- A dorsal longitudinal skin incision is used.

TENSION BAND WIRING

Reduction and Kirschner Wire Fixation

- Blood clot and periosteum are cleared from the fracture site to facilitate reduction.
- Limited periosteal elevation is performed at the fracture site to monitor reduction.
- A large tenaculum clamp is used to secure the fracture in a reduced position (**TECH FIG 1A,B**). A drill hole can be made in the dorsal cortex of the distal fragment to facilitate clamp application.

- Two 1.0-mm smooth Kirschner wires are drilled across the fracture site (**TECH FIG 1C**).
  - If these are drilled obliquely from dorsal proximal to volar distal, they will exit the anterior ulnar cortex distal to the coronoid process, providing an anchoring point of cortical bone to limit the potential for pin migration.
  - In anticipation of later impaction of the proximal ends of the wires, the Kirschner wires should be retracted 5 to 10 mm after drilling through the anterior ulnar cortex.

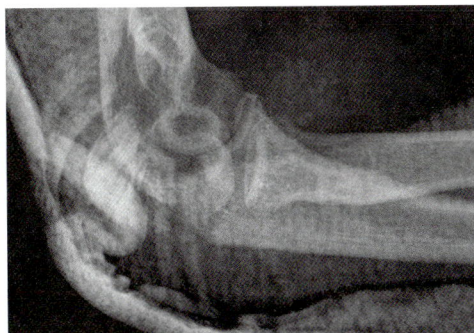

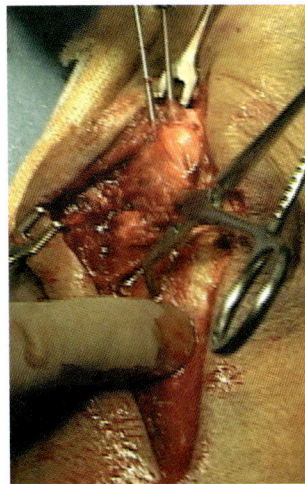

TECH FIG 1 • **A.** A lateral radiograph with the arm in plaster shows a transverse, noncomminuted fracture of the olecranon. **B.** An open reduction is held with a fracture reduction forceps. *(continued)*

TECHNIQUES

TECHNIQUES

C

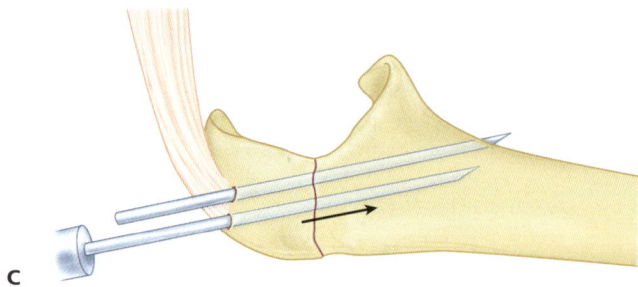

TECH FIG 1 • *(continued)* **C.** Two 1-mm Kirschner wires are drilled obliquely across the fracture site so that they exit the anterior ulnar cortex distal to the coronoid process. (**A,B:** Copyright David Ring, MD.)

Wiring

- The apex of the ulnar diaphysis just distal to the flat portion of the proximal ulna is drilled with a 2.0-mm drill, with or without prior subperiosteal dissection.
  - When two wires are used, a second drill hole is made a centimeter more distal.
- If one wire is used, it should be 18 gauge. My preference is to use two 22-gauge stainless steel wires to limit the size of the knots, which may diminish implant prominence. The wires are passed through the drill holes. A large-bore needle can be used to facilitate passage of the wire through the drill hole (**TECH FIG 2A**).
- The two tension wires are each passed over the dorsal ulna in a figure 8 fashion, then around the Kirschner wires, and underneath the insertion of the triceps tendon using a large-bore needle (**TECH FIG 2B**).

- Each wire is tensioned both medially and laterally by twisting the wire with a needle holder (**TECH FIG 2C,D**).
  - This should be done to take up slack only. These small wires will break if they are firmly tightened, which is not necessary.
  - The tightening should be done in a place that will make the wire knots less prominent.
  - After tightening the knots are trimmed and bent into the soft tissues to either side.
- The Kirschner wires are then bent 180 degrees and trimmed.
- These bent ends are then impacted into the proximal olecranon, beneath the triceps insertion, using an osteotome (**TECH FIG 2E–H**).

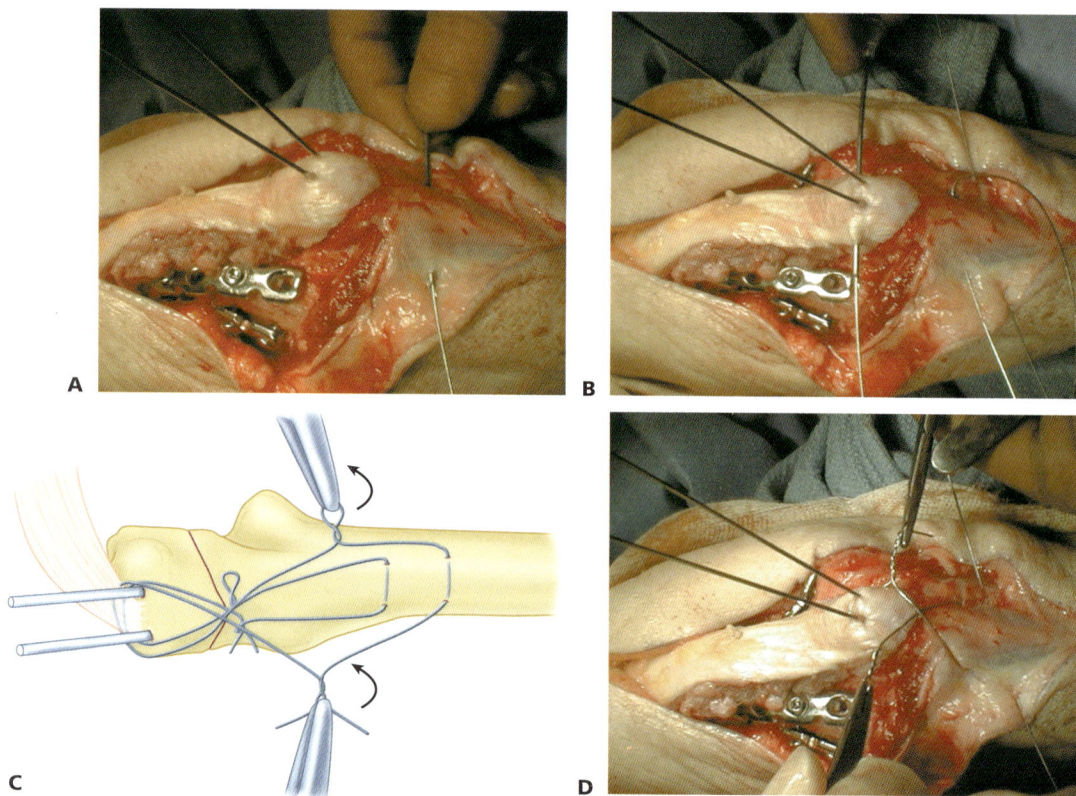

A

B

C

D

TECH FIG 2 • **A.** Two 22-gauge stainless steel tension wires are passed in a figure 8 fashion through drill holes in the ulnar shaft. **B.** They engage the triceps insertion proximally. **C,D.** The wires are tensioned on both sides. These do not need to be tight, but simply snug, with all slack taken up. Attempts to tighten these smaller 22-gauge wires will break them. *(continued)*

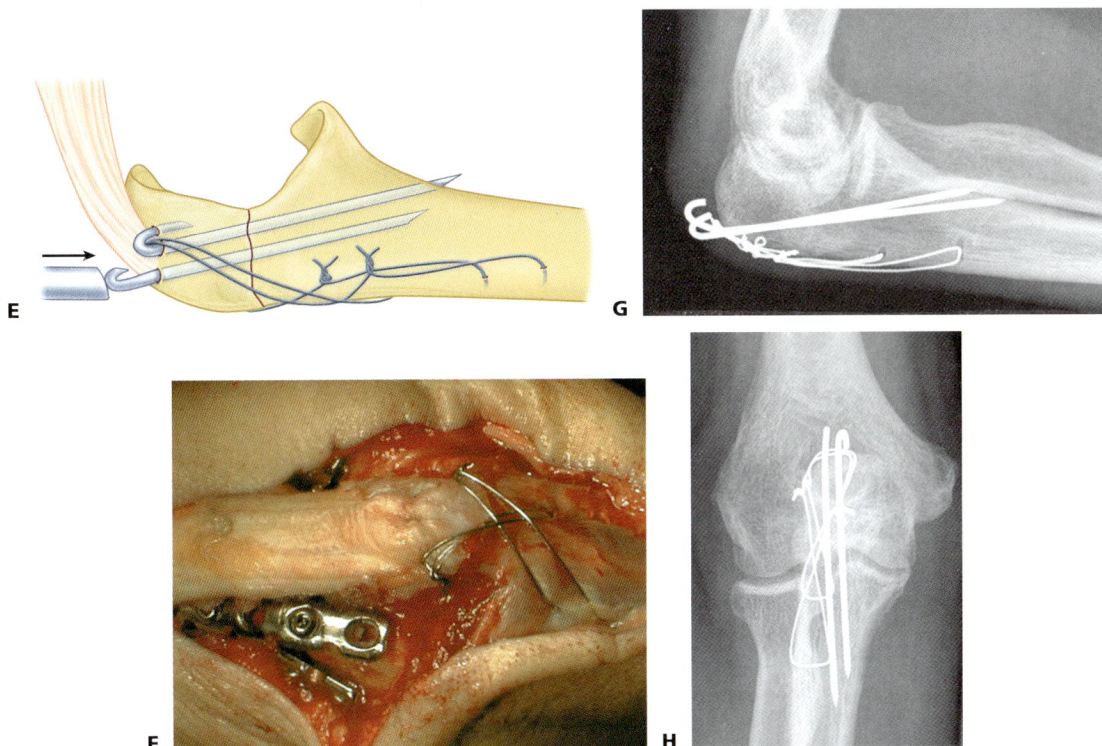

TECH FIG 2 • *(continued)* **E.** The proximal ends of the Kirschner wires are bent 180 degrees and impacted into the olecranon process, beneath the triceps insertion. **F.** The resulting fixation has a relatively low profile and is unlikely to migrate. **G,H.** Even these small wires are strong enough for active exercises to regain elbow motion. (**A,B,D,F–H:** Copyright David Ring, MD.)

PLATE AND SCREW FIXATION OF OLECRANON FRACTURES

- Contour the plate to wrap around the proximal aspect of the olecranon or use a precontoured plate (**TECH FIG 3A–C**).
- A straight plate will have only two or three screws in metaphyseal bone proximal to the fracture.
- Bending the plate around the proximal aspect of the olecranon provides additional screws in the proximal fragment. The most proximal screws can be very long, crossing the fracture line into the distal fragment. In some cases,

these screws can be directed to engage one of the cortices of the distal fragment, such as the anterior ulnar cortex.

- A plate contoured to wrap around the proximal ulna can be placed on top of the triceps insertion. Alternatively, the triceps insertion can be incised longitudinally and partially elevated medially and laterally sufficiently to allow direct plate contact with bone.
- If the proximal (olecranon) fragment is small, fragmented, or osteoporotic, it can be useful to add a figure

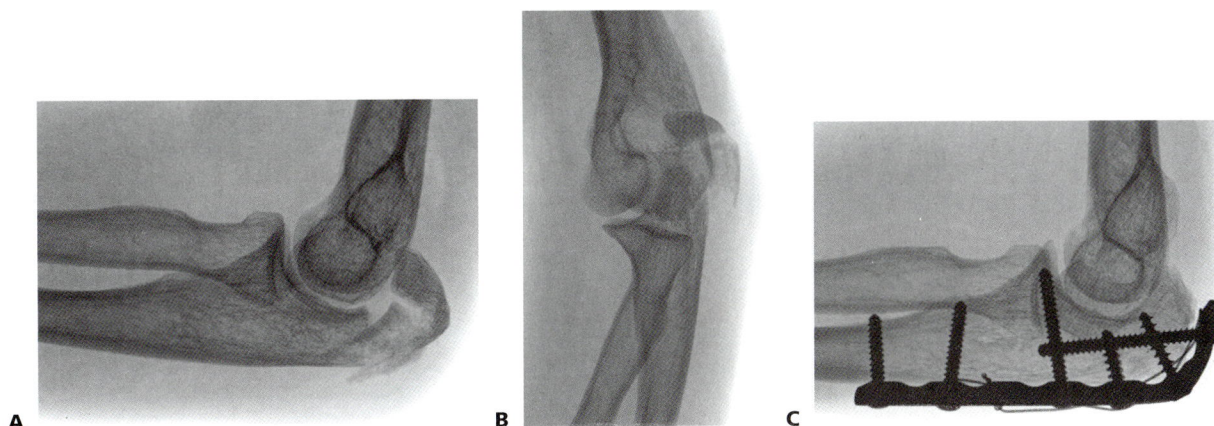

TECH FIG 3 • **A.** A lateral radiograph illustrates a comminuted olecranon fracture with a small proximal olecranon fragment. **B.** An oblique view shows the fragmentation. **C.** A 3.5-mm limited-contact dynamic compression plate and screws contoured to wrap around the dorsal surface of the olecranon is used for fixation. *(continued)*

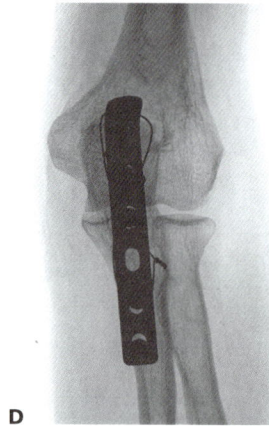

TECHNIQUES

TECH FIG 3 • *(continued)* **D.** A 22-gauge stainless steel wire engages the triceps insertion—this is useful when the olecranon fragment is small, fragmented, or osteopenic. (Copyright David Ring, MD.)

8 tension wire that engages the triceps insertion and passes over the top of the plate and around one of the screws at the metaphyseal level.

- Distally, a dorsal plate will lie directly on the apex of the ulnar diaphysis. The muscle need only be split sufficiently to gain access to this apex—there is no need to elevate the muscle or periosteum off either the medial or lateral flat aspect of the ulna.

- No attempt is made to precisely realign intervening fragmentation—once the relationship of the coronoid and olecranon facets is restored and the overall alignment is restored, the remaining fragments are bridged, leaving their soft tissue attachments intact.
  - Bone grafts are rarely necessary if the soft tissue attachments are preserved.

- If the olecranon fragment is small, osteoporotic, or fragmented, a wire engaging the triceps insertion should be used to reinforce the fixation (**TECH FIG 3D**).
  - The plate and screws will serve to hold the coronoid and olecranon facets in proper alignment and bridge fragmentation, and the wire will help ensure fixation even if screw purchase is lost.

PLATE AND SCREW FIXATION OF FRACTURE-DISLOCATIONS OF THE OLECRANON

Exposure

- In the setting of a fracture-dislocation of the olecranon (**TECH FIG 4A**), fractures of the radial head and coronoid process can be evaluated and often definitively treated through the exposure provided by the fracture of the olecranon process.
  - With little additional dissection, the olecranon fragment can be mobilized proximally as one would do

with an olecranon osteotomy, providing exposure of the coronoid through the ulnohumeral joint.

- If the exposure of the radial head through the posterior injury is inadequate, a separate muscle interval (eg, Köcher or Kaplan intervals) accessed by the elevation of a broad lateral skin flap can be used.

- If the exposure of the coronoid is inadequate through posterior injury and olecranon fracture, a separate medial or lateral exposure can be developed.

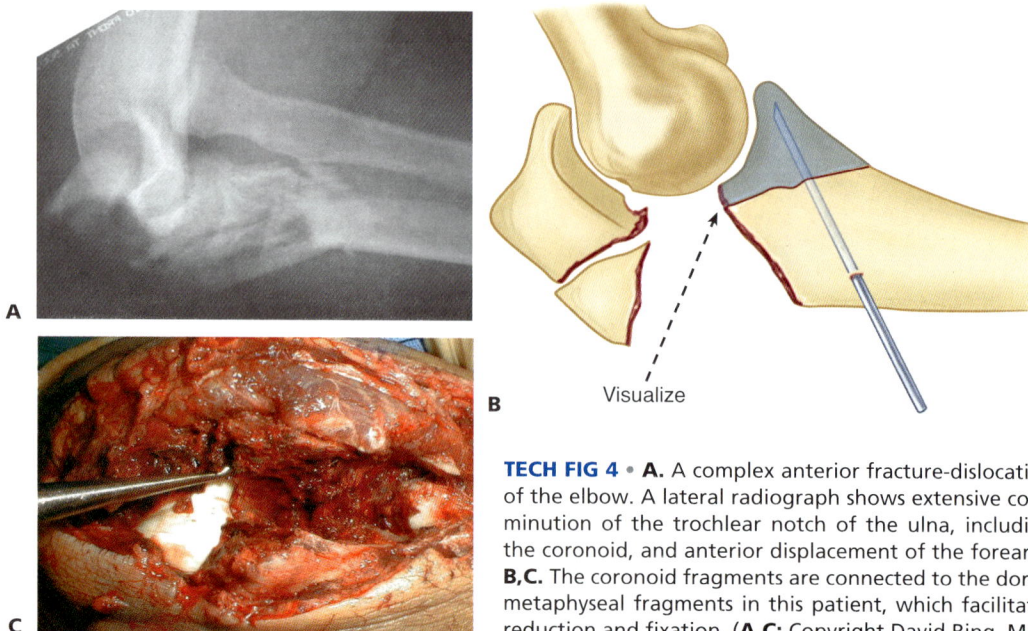

TECH FIG 4 • **A.** A complex anterior fracture-dislocation of the elbow. A lateral radiograph shows extensive comminution of the trochlear notch of the ulna, including the coronoid, and anterior displacement of the forearm. **B,C.** The coronoid fragments are connected to the dorsal metaphyseal fragments in this patient, which facilitates reduction and fixation. (**A,C:** Copyright David Ring, MD.)

- A medial exposure, between the two heads of the flexor carpi ulnaris, or by splitting the flexor-pronator mass more anteriorly, or by elevating the entire flexor–pronator mass from dorsal to volar, may be needed to address a complex fracture of the coronoid, particularly one that involves the anteromedial facet of the coronoid process.
- When the lateral collateral ligament is injured, it is usually avulsed from the lateral epicondyle. This facilitates repair that can be performed using suture anchors or suture placed through drill holes in the bone.
- The fracture of the coronoid can often be reduced directly through the elbow joint using the limited access provided by the olecranon fracture (**TECH FIG 4B,C**).

Fixation

- Provisional fixation can be obtained using Kirschner wires to attach the fragments either to the metaphyseal or diaphyseal fragments of the ulna, or to the trochlea of the distal humerus when there is extensive fragmentation of the proximal ulna.
- An alternative to keep in mind when there is extensive fragmentation of the proximal ulna is the use of a skeletal distractor (a temporary external fixator; **TECH FIG 5A**).
  - External fixation applied between a wire driven through the olecranon fragment and up into the trochlea and a second wire in the distal ulnar diaphysis can often obtain reduction indirectly when distraction is applied between the pins.
  - Definitive fixation can usually be obtained with screws applied under image intensifier guidance.
- The screws are placed through the plate when there is extensive fragmentation of the proximal ulna.
- A second, medial plate may be useful when the coronoid is fragmented.
- If the coronoid fracture is very comminuted and cannot be securely repaired, the ulnohumeral joint should be protected with temporary hinged or static external fixation, or temporary pin fixation of the ulnohumeral joint, depending on the equipment and expertise available.
- A long plate is contoured to wrap around the proximal olecranon (**TECH FIG 5B**).
  - A very long plate should be considered (between 12 and 16 holes), particularly when there is extensive fragmentation or the bone quality is poor.
- When the olecranon is fragmented or osteoporotic, a plate and screws alone may not provide reliable fixation.
  - In this situation, it can be useful to use ancillary tension wire fixation to control the olecranon fragments through the triceps insertion (**TECH FIG 5C**).

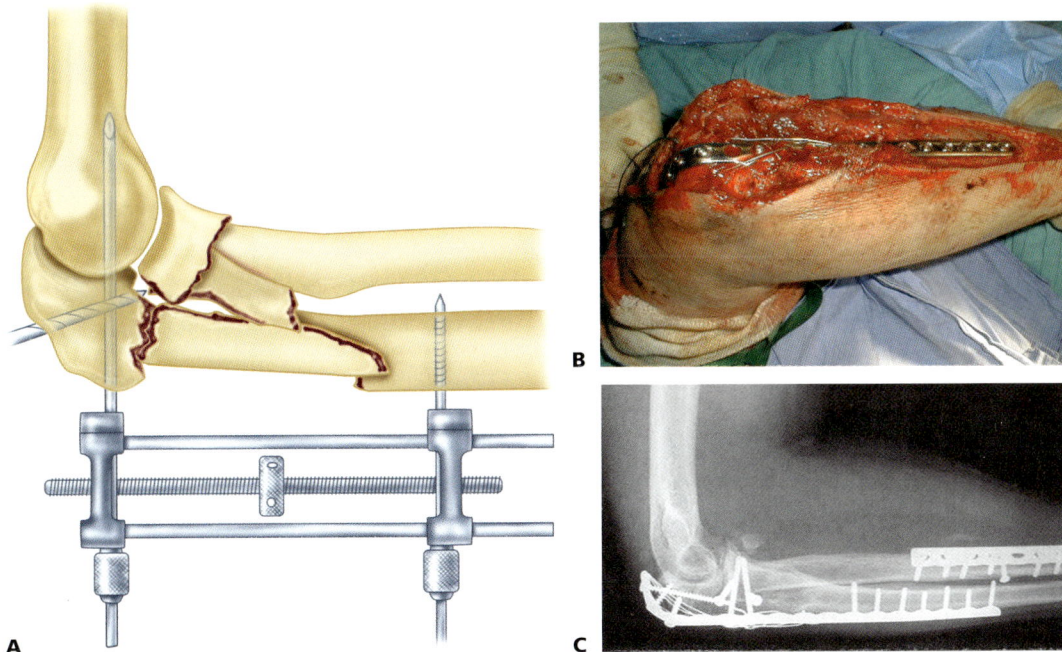

TECH FIG 5 • A. When there is diaphyseal comminution, a temporary external fixator may be useful. **B.** A long, 3.5-mm limited-contact dynamic compression plate is used for fixation. A 22-gauge stainless steel wire is used to enhance fixation of the comminuted olecranon fragments. **C.** The comminution extending into the diaphysis heals with the bridging plate. The trochlear notch is restored with good elbow function. (**B,C:** Copyright David Ring, MD.)

PEARLS AND PITFALLS

Prominence of olecranon hardware	■ The use of two small (22-gauge) wires rather than one large one will results in smaller knots. Care taken to place the Kirschner wires below the triceps insertion and impacting them into bone will limit prominence and the potential for migration.[5,8]
Narrowing of trochlear notch	■ The surgeon should not use a tension wire alone on a comminuted fracture. An intact articular surface to absorb compressive forces with active motion is mandatory for tension band wiring to be effective.
Plate loosening	■ The surgeon should use a dorsal plate contoured to wrap around the olecranon, providing a greater number of screws and screws at different, nearly orthogonal angles. Use of a medial or lateral plate should be avoided.[10,11]
Loss of fixation of the proximal (olecranon) fragment	■ Screw fixation alone should not be trusted if the fragment is small, fragmented, or osteoporotic. A tension wire engaging the triceps insertion should be added.
Failure to recognize a complex injury	■ The surgeon should be vigilant for subluxation or dislocation of the elbow, fracture of the coronoid or radial head, and injury to the lateral collateral ligament. When identified, each injury is treated accordingly. The olecranon and proximal ulna is always secured with a plate and screws.

POSTOPERATIVE CARE

■ When good fixation is obtained (which occurs in most patients), active assisted and gravity-assisted elbow and forearm exercises can be initiated immediately after surgery. A delay of several days for comfort is reasonable.

■ If the lateral collateral ligament was repaired, the patient must be instructed not to abduct the shoulder for the first month.

■ If the fixation is tenuous, it is reasonable to immobilize the arm in a splint for a month or so before beginning exercises.

OUTCOMES

■ Nonunion is nearly unheard of after simple olecranon fractures, and early implant failure is usually due to noncompliance.[6]

■ The appeal of tension band wiring has been limited by prominence of the implants; however, if the techniques described herein are followed, few patients will request a second surgery specifically for implant removal.[8]

■ Macko and Szabo pointed out that it was initial implant prominence and not migration that led to implant-related problems after tension band wiring of olecranon fractures.[5]

■ In any case, a second surgery for implant removal is not unreasonable, and it may not be appropriate to consider this a complication.

■ Some surgeons have considered plate-and-screw fixation of simple, noncomminuted olecranon fractures.[1] However, plates can also cause symptoms, and if only a few screws can be placed in the olecranon fragment, particularly in the setting of fragmentation or osteoporosis, it may be preferable to use the soft tissue attachments to enhance fixation rather than relying on implant–bone purchase alone.

■ Medial and lateral plates have been associated with early failure, malunion, and nonunion in the treatment of complex proximal ulna fractures.[10,11]

■ Dorsal plates perform better, but the elbow is often compromised in the setting of such complex injuries.

COMPLICATIONS

■ Implant loosening
■ Implant breakage
■ Nonunion
■ Malunion
■ Instability
■ Arthrosis

REFERENCES

1. Bailey CS, MacDermid J, Patterson SD, et al. Outcome of plate fixation of olecranon fractures. J Orthop Trauma 2001;15:542–548.
2. Doornberg J, Ring D, Jupiter JB. Effective treatment of fracture-dislocations of the olecranon requires a stable trochlear notch. Clin Orthop Relat Res 2004;429:292–300.
3. Jupiter JB, Leibovic SJ, Ribbans W, et al. The posterior Monteggia lesion. J Orthop Trauma 1991;5:395–402.
4. Karlsson M, Hasserius R, Besjakov J, et al. Comparison of tension-band and figure-of-eight wiring techniques for treatment of olecranon fractures. J Shoulder Elbow Surg 2002;11:377–382.
5. Macko D, Szabo RM. Complications of tension-band wiring of olecranon fractures. J Bone Joint Surg Am 1985;67A:1396–1401.
6. Morrey BF. Current concepts in the treatment of fractures of the radial head, the olecranon, and the coronoid. J Bone Joint Surg Am 1995;77A:316–327.
7. O'Driscoll SW, Jupiter JB, Cohen M, et al. Difficult elbow fractures: pearls and pitfalls. AAOS Instruct Course Lect 2003;52:113–134.
8. Ring D, Gulotta L, Chin K, et al. Olecranon osteotomy for exposure of fractures and nonunions of the distal humerus. J Orthop Trauma 2004;18:446–449.
9. Ring D, Jupiter JB, Sanders RW, et al. Trans-olecranon fracture-dislocation of the elbow. J Orthop Trauma 1997;11:545–550.
10. Ring D, Jupiter JB, Simpson NS. Monteggia fractures in adults. J Bone Joint Surg Am 1998;80A:1733–1744.
11. Ring D, Tavakolian J, Kloen P, et al. Loss of alignment after surgical treatment of posterior Monteggia fractures: salvage with dorsal contoured plating. J Hand Surg Am 2004;29A:694–702.

Chapter 38

Management of Simple Elbow Dislocation

Bradford O. Parsons

DEFINITION

- Simple elbow dislocation is a dislocation of the ulnohumeral joint without concomitant fracture.
- Complex instability denotes the presence of a fracture associated with dislocation.
- The elbow is the second most commonly dislocated large joint (excluding phalanx dislocations and so forth).

PATHOANATOMY

- Elbow stability is conferred by both the osseous anatomy as well as the ligamentous anatomy.
- Primary stabilizers of the ulnohumeral joint include the osseous architecture of the joint, including the coronoid process and greater sigmoid notch of the ulna, and the trochlea of the humerus.
  - The anterior band of the medial collateral ligament (aMCL) and the lateral ulnar collateral ligament (LUCL) are the primary ligamentous stabilizers of the elbow.[9,12]
  - The aMCL originates on the anterior inferior face of the medial epicondyle and inserts on the sublime tubercle of the ulna.
  - The LUCL originates from an isometric point on the lateral supracondylar column and traverses across the inferior aspect of the radial head, inserting on the supinator crest of the ulna.[8]
- Secondary stabilizers include the radial head and dynamic constraints such as the flexor and extensor muscles of the forearm.
  - The anterior joint capsule is also felt to play a role in ulnohumeral stability.
- O'Driscoll[12] has proposed the term "posterolateral rotatory instability" (PLRI) to describe the series of pathologic events that result in ulnohumeral dislocation.
  - PLRI is felt to start with disruption of the LUCL and progresses medially with tearing of the anterior and posterior capsules. This allows the ulna to "perch" on the distal humerus. Further soft tissue or osseous injury results in dislocation[13] (**FIG 1A**).
    - Most traumatic injuries to the LUCL result in avulsion of the ligament from the lateral humerus (**FIG 1B**).
  - As forces continue from lateral to medial across the joint, the anterior and posterior capsular tissues and eventually the MCL may be disrupted.
    - It is possible to dislocate the ulnohumeral joint with disruption of the LUCL and preservation of the aMCL.[12]
- Common fractures that occur with elbow dislocation include radial head or neck and coronoid fractures, although any fracture about the elbow may be observed.
  - Radial head fractures are usually readily apparent on plain radiographs.
  - Coronoid fractures may be subtle, and even a "fleck" of coronoid is often a hallmark of a more significant injury

(eg, "terrible triad" injury), and its importance should not be underestimated.
- Recently, a variant of elbow instability termed postero-*medial* rotatory instability (PMRI) has been described, which is a consequence of LUCL injury and medial coronoid facet fracture. This injury pattern is most commonly observed *without* radial head fracture, making it potentially very subtle on plain radiographs. A computed tomography (CT) scan can delineate this injury in detail and should be obtained if any suspicion exists (**FIG 1C–E**).[2,11]

ETIOLOGY AND CLASSIFICATION

- Most elbow dislocations occur with a fall on an outstretched arm.
- Forces of valgus, extension, supination, and axial load across the joint can result in the ulna rotating away from the humerus, disrupting lateral–anterior soft tissues initially, and dislocating the elbow.
- Simple elbow dislocations are classified by the direction of displacement of the ulna in reference to the humerus, with posterolateral dislocation the most common.
  - Less common variants include anterior, medial, or lateral dislocations.

PATIENT HISTORY AND PHYSICAL FINDINGS

- History is aimed at determining the timeline and mechanism of injury, frequency of dislocations, and previous treatment.
- Unlike the shoulder, recurrent instability of the elbow is rare after an initial simple dislocation that was treated expediently.
  - Recurrent instability is more common in association with fractures (eg, the "terrible triad" injury).
  - Chronic instability, although rare in the United States, does occasionally occur, and management often requires reconstructive surgery or elbow replacement. Closed treatment is rarely successful in these patients.
- Iatrogenic injury of the LUCL (during procedures such as open tennis elbow release or radial head fracture management) is a known cause of recurrent PLRI. However, these patients often complain of subtle lateral elbow pain due to subluxation of the joint with activities, such as rising from a chair, but rarely have recurrent dislocation.
- Examination at the time of injury requires attention to the neurovascular anatomy.
  - Nerve injury can occur after elbow dislocation, and a thorough neurologic examination of the extremity is mandatory before any treatment of the dislocation.
    - Most nerve injuries are neuropraxia that often resolve.
    - The ulnar nerve is most frequently involved, although median or radial nerve injury may also occur.[14]
  - The dislocated elbow has obvious deformity, with the elbow often held in a varus position and the forearm supinated.

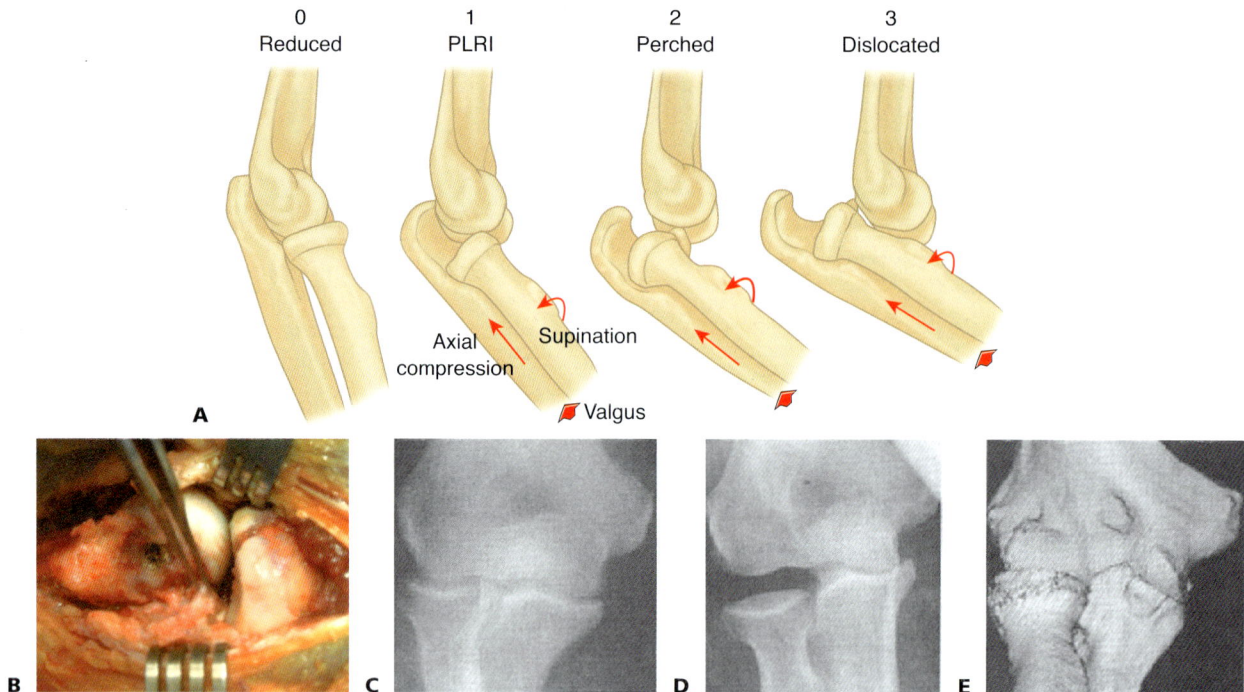

FIG 1 • A. Posterolateral rotatory instability follows a typical progression of disruption, allowing the joint to become perched and then dislocate as soft tissue injury progresses. **B.** Intraoperative photograph demonstrating avulsion of the origin of the lateral ulnar collateral ligament (LUCL) after traumatic dislocation of the elbow. The origin of the LUCL and the extensor muscles are avulsed as one layer, held by the forceps. **C–E.** Posteromedial rotatory instability is a variant of elbow instability in which the elbow dislocates, rupturing the LUCL, and the medial coronoid sustains an impaction fracture **C,D**. In this injury pattern, the radial head remains intact, making appropriate diagnosis of the severity of the injury difficult on standard radiographs. CT scans help better delineate the injury pattern. **E.** Impaction fracture can be seen on the 3D CT reconstruction. (**A:** Adapted from O'Driscoll SW, Morrey BF, Korinek S, et al. Elbow subluxation and dislocation: a spectrum of instability. Clin Orthop Relat Res 1982;280:194. **C–E:** Copyright the Mayo Foundation, Rochester, MN.)

■ After initial reduction, the neurovascular status of the limb is re-evaluated. Loss of neurologic function after closed reduction is rare but can be an indication for surgical exploration to rule out an entrapped nerve.

■ Stability of the joint is assessed based on the amount of extension obtainable and association of pronation or supination with instability (see the treatment algorithm section).

　■ It is helpful to evaluate the stability throughout the elbow range of motion while the patient is still anesthetized, as this may guide treatment (examination under anesthesia).

　■ Stressing of the lateral soft tissues is performed with the lateral pivot-shift maneuver, which can be performed under anesthesia and with fluoroscopic imaging[12] (**FIG 2**).

　　■ This test can be used to assess the degree of posterolateral rotatory instability, and may aid in determining treatment.

■ Medial ecchymosis may be a sign of an aMCL injury, and often is apparent 3 to 5 days after dislocation when the MCL has been injured.

IMAGING AND OTHER DIAGNOSTIC STUDIES

■ Standard orthogonal radiographs of the elbow are obtained before and after reduction to assess for fracture and confirm relocation of the joint.

　■ Congruency of the trochlea–ulna and radial head–capitellum is assessed.

■ Valgus stress views, once the joint is reduced, may help demonstrate an aMCL injury.

　■ With the elbow flexed 30 degrees and the forearm in pronation, a valgus stress is placed under fluoroscopic evaluation to see if the medial ulnohumeral joint opens compared to the resting state.

■ Varus stress views are often not helpful.

■ CT scans with 3D reconstructions are obtained in any situation where a fracture may be suspected, as it is critical to identify PMRI variants or subtle coronoid fractures, which may be an indication for surgical management.

■ Magnetic resonance imaging (MRI) is usually not necessary in the management of simple dislocation, although if questions regarding the integrity of the MCL exist, an MRI can delineate this structure well.

NONOPERATIVE MANAGEMENT

■ Most simple dislocations may be managed nonoperatively with splinting or bracing, guided by the degree of instability determined during the examination under anesthesia after reduction.[12]

■ Once reduced, elbow stability is assessed during flexion–extension in neutral forearm rotation.

　■ If the elbow is stable throughout an arc of motion, it is immobilized in a sling or splint for 3 to 5 days for comfort and then range-of-motion exercises are begun.

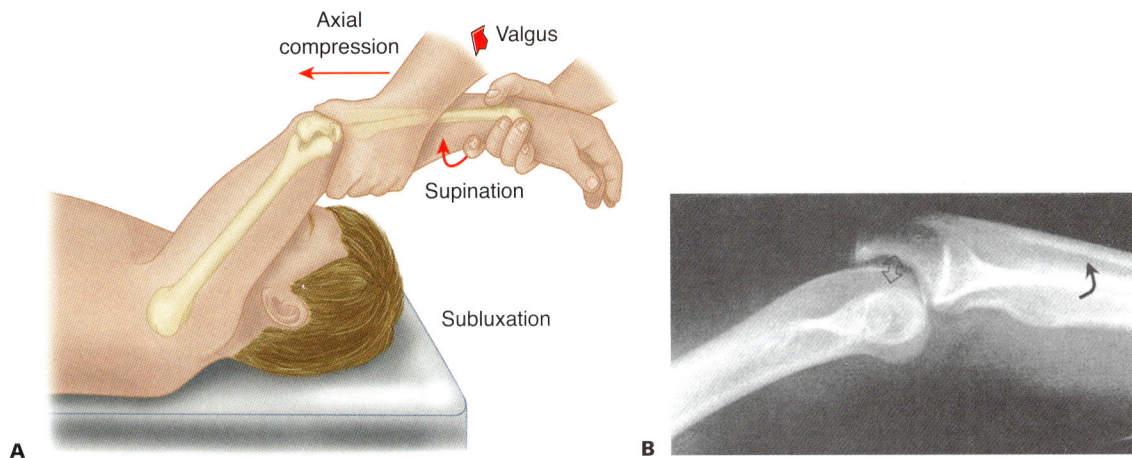

FIG 2 • A. The lateral pivot-shift maneuver is performed with the patient's arm positioned overhead, and a supination–valgus stress is applied. As the elbow is brought into flexion the joint reduces, often with a clunk. **B.** When performed under fluoroscopy, subluxation of the radial head posterior to the capitellum can be observed, consistent with posterolateral rotatory instability. (**B:** From O'Driscoll SW, Bell DF, Morrey BF. Posterolateral rotatory instability of the elbow. J Bone Joint Surg Am 1991;73A:440–446.)

■ If instability is present in less than 30 degrees of flexion, the forearm is pronated and stability is reassessed.
  ■ If pronation confers stability, then a hinged orthosis that maintains forearm pronation is used, after 3 to 5 days of splinting, to allow protected range of motion.
■ Elbows that sublux (confirmed by fluoroscopic imaging) in less than 30 degrees of flexion and pronation of the forearm are managed with a brief period of splinting, followed by a hinged orthosis that controls rotation of the forearm and has an extension block.
■ Elbows that are unstable in more than 30 degrees of flexion and pronation often are managed surgically.
■ Hinged bracing is maintained for 6 weeks, with progressive advancement of extension and rotation, as allowed by stability of the joint.
  ■ Weekly radiographs are needed to ensure maintenance of a congruent joint during the first 4 to 6 weeks.
■ After 6 weeks bracing is discontinued and terminal stretching to regain motion is used if flexion contractures exist.

SURGICAL MANAGEMENT

Indications

■ Surgical management is indicated in elbows that are unstable, even when placed in flexion (more than 30 degrees) and pronation, elbows that recurrently sublux or dislocate during the treatment protocol, or those with associated fractures ("complex" instability).
■ Management of simple dislocation requires repair or reconstruction of those ligamentous injuries resulting in instability. By definition, simple dislocation occurs without fracture.
■ An algorithmic approach to ligament repair is used to stabilize the elbow. The LUCL is felt to be the primary lesion of dislocation, and therefore this ligament is addressed first, followed by assessment of stability.
■ The LUCL usually avulses from its origin during dislocation, and therefore most often can be repaired after acute injury.
  ■ Repair may be performed via bone tunnels in the humerus or with suture anchors, depending on the surgeon's preference.

■ Reconstruction of the LUCL is rarely needed in acute management but is more commonly needed in chronic instability.
  ■ Reconstruction, when necessary, uses autograft (either palmaris or gracilis) or allograft.
■ Often, repair or reconstruction of the LUCL confers stability, even in the face of MCL injury, as the intact radial head is a secondary stabilizer to valgus instability.
■ Persistent instability after LUCL repair is rare and is more commonly observed with fracture-dislocations or chronic instability.
  ■ If persistent instability exists, the MCL is repaired or reconstructed, a hinged external fixator is placed, or both are performed.
■ This section will discuss the surgical technique of LUCL repair and reconstruction.

Preoperative Planning

■ Planning should include the possibility of reconstruction of the LUCL using autograft, which will be harvested at surgery, or by having allograft available.
  ■ If autograft is to be harvested, a tendon stripper is needed.
  ■ For allograft we routinely use semitendinosus tendon.
■ A hinged external fixator should be available in the rare case that the elbow remains unstable after ligamentous repair or reconstruction.
■ 2.0- and 3.2-mm drill bits or burrs are used to make bone tunnels for LUCL repair or reconstruction.
  ■ Alternatively, some surgeons prefer suture anchor repair of ligament avulsions; if desired, these should be available.
■ Fluoroscopy is useful for confirming reduction and is required for placement of a hinged external fixator.
■ A sterile tourniquet is used if exposure of the proximal humerus is necessary for placement of proximal external fixator pins.

Patient Positioning

■ Patients are positioned supine with the arm on a radiolucent hand table.

TECHNIQUES

- A small bump is placed under the scapula to aid in arm positioning.
- The forequarter is draped free to ensure the entire brachium is kept in the surgical field.

- If hamstring autograft is to be used for LUCL, the leg should be draped free and a bump is placed under the hemipelvis to aid in exposure.

LATERAL ULNAR COLLATERAL LIGAMENT REPAIR

Surgical Approach and Arthrotomy

- Tourniquet control is used during this procedure.
- Two different surgical approaches are used to manage elbow instability.
- Often, a posterior midline skin incision can be used to gain access to both the medial and lateral aspects of the joint; therefore, it is a very extensile approach to the elbow.
- Alternatively, a "column" incision, centered over the lateral epicondyle, may be used (**TECH FIG 1A**). If medial-sided exposure is needed, a similar "column" incision may be made over the medial epicondyle to gain access.
- There are benefits to both approaches, and currently no data exist delineating which approach is better.
  - For simple dislocation we routinely use a lateral column approach.
- After skin incision, skin flaps are raised anteroposterior at the level of the deep fascia.
- Often the lateral soft tissues are avulsed off the epicondyle, exposing the joint. Occasionally, however, the extensor origin is intact with an underlying ligament injury.
  - If the extensor muscles are intact, the interval between the extensor carpi ulnaris (ECU) and anconeus (the Köcher approach), which directly overlies the LUCL, is used. This interval is often readily identified by the presence of a "fat stripe" in the deep fascia (**TECH FIG 1B**).
- The elbow joint is then exposed by incising the proximal capsule along the lateral column of the humerus, continuing distally along the radial neck (through the supinator muscle and underling capsule) in line with the ECU–anconeus interval.
  - The posterior interosseous nerve (PIN) is at risk with this exposure, and therefore the forearm is kept in pronation to protect the PIN.

- The radiocapitellar joint and coronoid are inspected to confirm no fractures are present and that no soft tissue is interposed in the joint, preventing reduction.
- Once the joint is clear of debris, the ability to obtain a concentric reduction is confirmed with fluoroscopy.

Ligament Repair

- The origin of the LUCL is identified.
  - Often, the LUCL is avulsed from the isometric point on the lateral capitellum, and the origin can be identified by a "fold" of tissue on the deep surface of the capsule (**TECH FIG 2A**).
- Starting at the origin, a running no. 2 nonabsorbable Krackow locking suture is placed along the anterior and posterior aspect of the ligament. Once placed, the suture–ligament construct is tensioned to confirm the integrity of the insertion onto the ulna.
  - A common mistake is to start the repair at the level of the proximal origin of the superficial tissue, which is not the origin of the LUCL but part of the extensor origin.
- The isometric origin on the humerus is then identified in the center of the capitellum, not the lateral epicondyle (**TECH FIG 2B,C**).
  - Confirmation of the isometric point is made by clamping the limbs of the running suture at the point of isometry and then flexing and extending the elbow to confirm proper placement.
- A 2.0-mm burr is used to make a humeral bone tunnel.
  - It is critical to make the most anterior aspect of the bone tunnel at the isometric point, not the center of the tunnel, as this small translation can result in a lax LUCL repair (**TECH FIG 2D**).
- Two "exit" tunnels (in a Y configuration), one anterior and one posterior to the lateral column, are then made

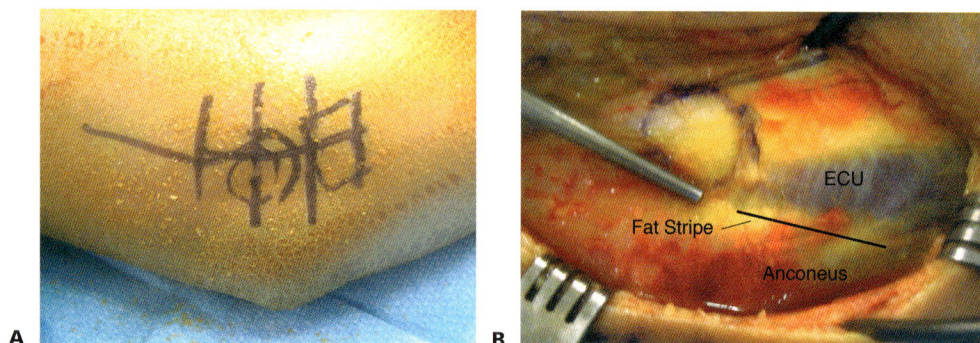

A   B

ECU
Fat Stripe
Anconeus

TECH FIG 1 • **A.** Lateral column skin incision. The lateral incision is centered over the epicondyle and radiocapitellar joint and is often the primary incision, as the lateral ulnar collateral ligament (LUCL) rupture is thought to be the primary injury in simple dislocations. **B.** The deep interval between the extensor carpi ulnaris and anconeus is used to gain exposure to the joint. This is often identified by a "fat stripe" in the fascia. Care should be taken not to violate the LUCL, which traverses in line with this interval deep to the fascia and supinator muscle.

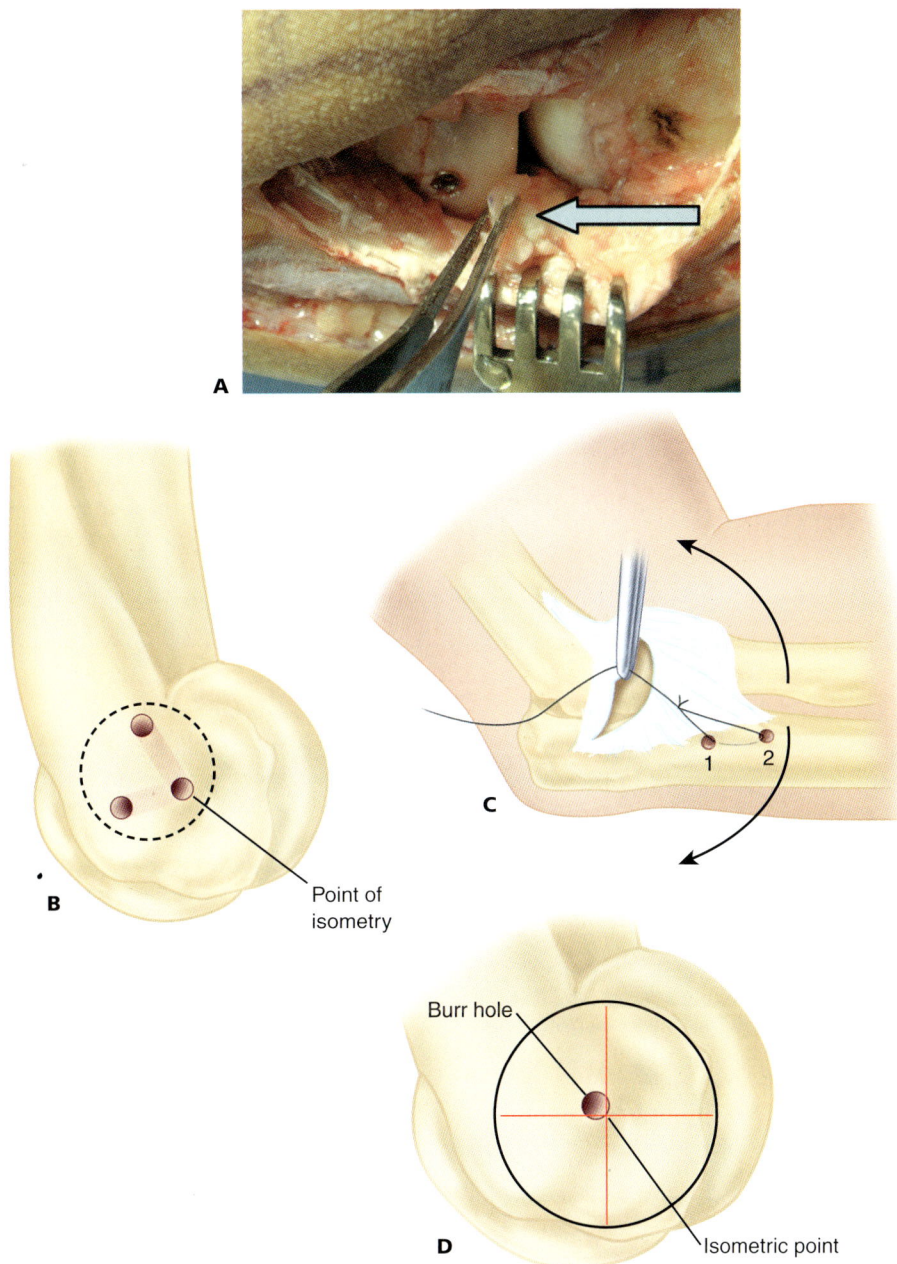

TECH FIG 2 • **A.** The origin of the lateral ulnar collateral ligament (LUCL), which often avulses during elbow dislocation, is identified by a "fold" of tissue on the deep surface of the capsule. The isometric point of the joint is in the center of rotation of the capitellum (**B**), and confirmation is made using the previously placed sutures in the ligament remnant to ensure that an isometric repair will be obtained (**C**). **D.** It is important to make the humeral tunnel so that the most anterior aspect of the tunnel is placed at the isometric point. Exit holes for the humeral tunnel are made anterior and posterior to the lateral supracondylar ridge (**B**).

with a 2.0-mm drill bit or burr, connected to the distal humeral tunnel at the isometric point.

- Once the humeral tunnels are completed, the limbs of the running suture are passed through the humeral tunnels.
- The joint is concentrically reduced with fluoroscopic confirmation and the LUCL repair sutures are then tied with the joint reduced and the elbow in 30 degrees of flexion and neutral rotation.

- The elbow is ranged through an arc of motion to assess stability, with careful attention placed on the radial head's articulation with the capitellum, looking for posterior sag in extension, indicating either a lax LUCL or a nonisometric repair.
- If the elbow is stable through an arc of motion, the extensor origin is repaired with interrupted, heavy (no. 0) nonabsorbable suture and the skin is closed in layers.

TECHNIQUES

LATERAL ULNAR COLLATERAL LIGAMENT RECONSTRUCTION

- Occasionally, the native LUCL is damaged beyond repair (more often with iatrogenic PLRI than with primary instability) or attenuated after recurrent or chronic elbow instability, and reconstruction is necessary.
- Autograft palmaris or gracilis or allograft may be used.
- Autograft and allograft options should be discussed with the patient and decisions made preoperatively. We routinely use semitendinosus allograft unless the patient desires autograft.
- This section will cover the technique of ligament graft reconstruction once tendon graft has been harvested.

Bone Tunnel Preparation

- We use a "docking" technique, similar to those described for MCL reconstruction,[1] for LUCL reconstruction.
- The insertion of the LUCL is at the supinator crest of the ulna, and reconstruction begins with creation of the ulnar tunnels at the supinator crest.
- Reflecting the supinator origin from the ulna posterior to the radial head exposes the supinator crest.
   - The forearm is held in pronation to protect the PIN.
- Once the crest is exposed, the ulnar tunnel is made at the level of the radial head using two 3.4-mm burr holes placed 1 cm apart. Care is taken to connect the holes using small curettes or awls without fracturing the roof of the tunnel (**TECH FIG 3**).
- Once the ulnar tunnel is made, a suture is placed in the tunnel to aid in graft passage and to help identify the isometric point on the humerus, similar to the technique described with ligament repair.
- Once the isometric origin on the humerus is confirmed, humeral bone tunnels are made as mentioned in the LUCL repair section.
   - With LUCL reconstruction the isometric tunnel is deepened to about 1 cm to allow graft docking.
   - Further, the docking tunnel is widened using a 3.4-mm burr to be able to accept both limbs of the graft.
   - It is important to widen the docking hole anterior and proximal to the isometric point, as the most posterior aspect of the tunnel needs to be at the isometric point.

Graft Preparation

- One end of the graft is freshened and tubularized using a no. 2 nonabsorbable suture in a running Krackow fashion.
- The graft is then passed through the ulnar bone tunnels using the passage suture previously placed.
- The limb of the graft with locking suture is then fully docked into the humeral origin, and the joint is reduced.
- The final length of the graft is determined by tensioning the graft and identifying the point at which the free limb of the graft meets the isometric origin. This point is marked on the graft.
   - Care should be taken to ensure appropriate graft tension and length by fully docking the first limb and then marking the free limb at the point of initial contact with the humerus, thereby allowing some overlap of graft limbs in the humeral tunnel but minimizing the likelihood of slack in the final construct.
- The marked graft end is then freshened and tubularized in an identical fashion as the other limb.

Final Reconstruction

- Once the graft is placed and ready for final tensioning and fixation, the capsule and remnant of the LUCL is repaired back to the humerus in an effort to make the ligament reconstruction extra-articular, if possible.
- Each limb of the graft is then placed into the isometric docking tunnel on the humerus with corresponding limbs from each locking suture exiting the proximal humeral tunnels.
   - Both limbs of locking suture from one end of the graft are passed through one proximal tunnel in the humerus, followed by the limbs from the other end of the graft through the second proximal tunnel.
- The joint is then reduced and the graft is finally tensioned to ensure there is no slack and neither graft end has "bottomed out" in the humeral docking tunnel.
- The locking sutures are then tied together over the lateral column of the distal humerus with the joint concentrically reduced in 30 degrees of flexion and neutral rotation.
- The joint is then ranged and stability assessed. If the joint is stable, no further reconstruction is necessary and the extensor muscles are repaired using a nonabsorbable interrupted stitch, followed by skin closure.

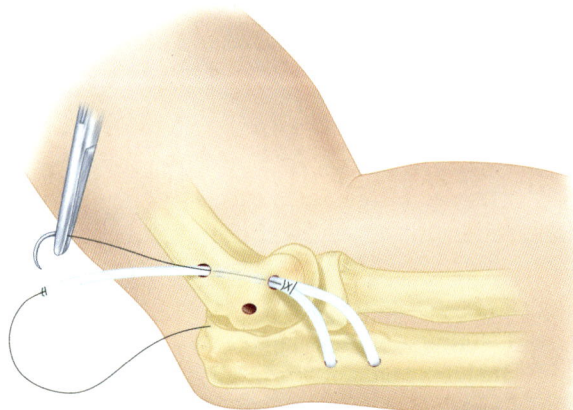

TECH FIG 3 • The insertion of the lateral ulnar collateral ligament is the supinator crest of the ulna. Reconstruction uses an ulnar tunnel in the supinator crest made at the level of the radial head. Holes are made about 1 cm apart and connected to form a tunnel.

HINGED EXTERNAL FIXATION

- A hinged fixator may be necessary in chronic dislocations, some fracture-dislocations, or rarely in patients with persistent instability after LUCL repair or reconstruction for simple dislocation.[4,16]
- Once any soft tissue blocking reduction is removed and a concentric reduction can be obtained, the fixator is placed.
- All hinged elbow fixators are constructed around the axis or rotation of the elbow to allow range of motion to occur while maintaining a concentric reduction.
  - Most implants are built around an axis pin, placed in this center of rotation.
  - The center of rotation is identified as the center of the capitellum on a lateral aspect of the elbow, and on the medial side it is just anteroinferior to the medial epicondyle, in the center of curvature of the trochlea (**TECH FIG 4**).
  - The axis pin is placed through both of these points, parallel to the joint surface, and the position is confirmed by fluoroscopy.

- After placement of the axis pin, the humeral and ulnar pins are placed after confirmation of concentric reduction of the elbow is made.
- Once the external fixator is fully constructed, the elbow is taken through an arc of motion and maintenance of reduction is confirmed.
- Fixators are kept on for 6 to 8 weeks.
- Meticulous pin care is necessary to minimize pin tract infections or loosening.

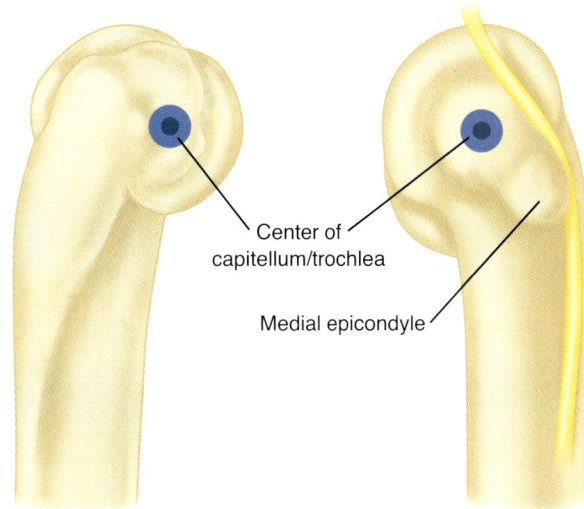

Center of capitellum/trochlea

Medial epicondyle

TECH FIG 4 • The center of rotation of the elbow, along which an axis pin for hinged fixators is placed, is identified by the center of the capitellum and just anteroinferior to the medial epicondyle.

PEARLS AND PITFALLS

- LUCL avulsion is the primary ligamentous injury in most simple dislocations of the elbow.
- If the radial head and coronoid are intact (as is the case in a simple dislocation), the MCL rarely needs to be repaired or reconstructed, as the radial head acts as a secondary stabilizer in the elbow with a repaired lateral ligament complex.
- The LUCL origin can be identified by a capsular fold of tissue. This is the point at which repair sutures should be placed, not at the origin of the more superficial extensor tendons.
- The isometric origin of the LUCL is in the center of the capitellum, as projected onto the lateral column, and repair or reconstruction needs to be brought to this point to have an isometric ligament.
- Bone tunnels in the humerus for repair or reconstruction are made so the anteroinferior aspect of the tunnel is at the isometric origin.
- A hinged external fixator may be necessary in management of elbow dislocation, especially chronic or recurrent situations, and should be available.
- All hinged fixators are constructed around the axis of rotation of the elbow, identified by a line between the isometric point on the lateral capitellum and the center of rotation of the trochlea on the medial aspect of the joint.
- Stiffness is the most common adverse sequela of elbow dislocation, and therefore range of motion should be started as soon as soft tissue and skin healing allows, with care taken to avoid varus or valgus stress.

POSTOPERATIVE CARE

- After operative stabilization without external fixation, the elbow is splinted in flexion for 3 to 5 days to allow wound healing.
- Range-of-motion exercises are then begun in flexion, extension, and rotation, with care taken to avoid varus or valgus stress.
  - A hinged orthosis can be helpful in protecting the ligament repair or reconstruction.
- Active and passive motion is continued for 6 weeks, when strengthening is added.

- Residual contractures, often loss of extension, can be managed with static splinting and terminal stretching.

OUTCOMES

- Most series have reported the results of closed management of simple dislocation.
  - Mehlhoff and colleagues[7] reported the results of 52 simple dislocations managed, with most patients having normal elbows. Length of immobilization, especially greater then 3 weeks, was found to be more likely to result in persistent loss of extension.

■ Similarly, Eygendaal and colleagues[3] reported the long-term results of 50 patients after closed management of simple dislocations. Sixty-two percent of patients described their elbow function as good or excellent, and 24 of 50 (48%) patients had loss of extension of 5 to 10 degrees.

■ Some series have examined the surgical management of PLRI, often as a result of recurrent instability after traumatic dislocation.

■ Nestor and colleagues[10] reported the results of 11 patients with recurrent PLRI managed with either repair or reconstruction of the LUCL. Ten of 11 (91%) remained stable and 7 of 11 (64%) had an excellent result.

■ More recently, Sanchez-Sotelo and colleagues[15] reported the results of 44 patients treated for recurrent PLRI (9 occurred after simple dislocation). Thirty-two (75%) of the patients had an excellent result by Mayo score.

■ Lee and Teo[5] found that in patients with chronic PLRI, reconstruction offered more predictable outcomes over repair.

COMPLICATIONS

■ Stiffness[3,7]
■ Heterotopic ossification[6]
■ Neurovascular injury[14]
■ Recurrent instability[3,7]
■ Compartment syndrome
■ Hematoma or infection

REFERENCES

1. Dodson CC, Thomas A, Dines JS, et al. Medial ulnar collateral ligament reconstruction of the elbow in throwing athletes. Am J Sports Med 2006;34:1926–1932.
2. Doornberg JN, Ring DC. Fracture of the anteromedial facet of the coronoid process. J Bone Joint Surg Am 2006;88A:2216–2224.
3. Eygendaal D, Verdegaal SH, Obermann WR, et al. Posterolateral dislocation of the elbow joint: relationship to medial instability. J Bone Joint Surg Am 2000;82A:555–560.
4. Jupiter JB, Ring D. Treatment of unreduced elbow dislocations with hinged external fixation. J Bone Joint Surg Am 2002;84A:1630–1635.
5. Lee BP, Teo LH. Surgical reconstruction for posterolateral rotatory instability of the elbow. J Shoulder Elbow Surg 2003;12:476–479.
6. Linscheid RL, Wheeler DK. Elbow dislocations. JAMA 1965;194:1171–1176.
7. Mehlhoff TL, Noble PC, Bennett JB, et al. Simple dislocation of the elbow in the adult. Results after closed treatment. J Bone Joint Surg Am 1988;70A:244–249.
8. Morrey BF, An KN. Functional anatomy of the ligaments of the elbow. Clin Orthop Relat Res 1985;201:84–90.
9. Morrey BF, Tanaka S, An KN. Valgus stability of the elbow: a definition of primary and secondary constraints. Clin Orthop Relat Res 1991;265:187–195.
10. Nestor BJ, O'Driscoll SW, Morrey BF. Ligamentous reconstruction for posterolateral rotatory instability of the elbow. J Bone Joint Surg Am 1992;74A:1235–1241.
11. O'Driscoll SW. Acute, recurrent, and chronic elbow instabilities. In: Norris TR, ed. Orthopaedic Knowledge Update: Shoulder and Elbow 2. Rosemont, IL: American Academy of Orthopaedic Surgeons, 2002:313–323.
12. O'Driscoll SW, Bell DF, Morrey BF. Posterolateral rotatory instability of the elbow. J Bone Joint Surg Am 1991;73A:440–446.
13. O'Driscoll SW, Morrey BF, Korinek S, et al. Elbow subluxation and dislocation: a spectrum of instability. Clin Orthop Relat Res 1992;280:186–197.
14. Rana NA, Kenwright J, Taylor RG, et al. Complete lesion of the median nerve associated with dislocation of the elbow joint. Acta Orthop Scand 1974;45:365–369.
15. Sanchez-Sotelo J, Morrey BF, O'Driscoll SW. Ligamentous repair and reconstruction for posterolateral rotatory instability of the elbow. J Bone Joint Surg Br 2005;87B:54–61.
16. Tan V, Daluiski A, Capo J, et al. Hinged elbow external fixators: indications and uses. J Am Acad Orthop Surg 2005;13:503–514.

Open Reduction and Internal Fixation of Fracture-Dislocations of the Elbow With Complex Instability

Jubin B. Payandeh and Michael D. McKee

DEFINITION

- Simple dislocations of the elbow can most often be treated successfully with closed means: reduction and short-term immobilization followed by early motion.
- Fracture-dislocations of the elbow are more troublesome in that they often require operative intervention.
- Fractures associated with elbow dislocations often involve the radial head and coronoid. When both are combined with dislocation, this is termed the "terrible triad."
- The principle of treating fracture-dislocations of the elbow is to provide sufficient stability through reconstruction of bony and ligamentous restraints such that early motion can be instituted without recurrent instability.
- Failure to achieve this will result in either recurrent instability or severe stiffness after prolonged immobilization.

ANATOMY

- Posterolateral dislocations of the elbow are associated with disruption of the medial and lateral collateral ligaments.
- The medial collateral ligament (MCL) is the primary stabilizer to valgus stress (**FIG 1**).
- The lateral collateral ligament (LCL) is the primary stabilizer to posterolateral rotatory instability. Most often the disruption is from the lateral epicondyle, leaving a characteristic bare spot. Less commonly, the ligament may rupture mid-substance.[5] Secondary restraints on the lateral side that may also be disrupted are the common extensor origin and the posterolateral capsule.
- Radial head fractures have been classified by Mason:
  - Type I: small or marginal fracture with minimal displacement
  - Type II: marginal fracture with displacement
  - Type III: comminuted fractures of the head and neck[2]
- Coronoid fractures have been classified by Regan and Morrey[9] (**FIG 2**):
  - Type I: tip fractures (not avulsions)
  - Type II: less than 50% of the coronoid
  - Type III: more than 50% of the coronoid
    - The insertion of the MCL is at the base of the coronoid and it may be involved in type III fractures[1]

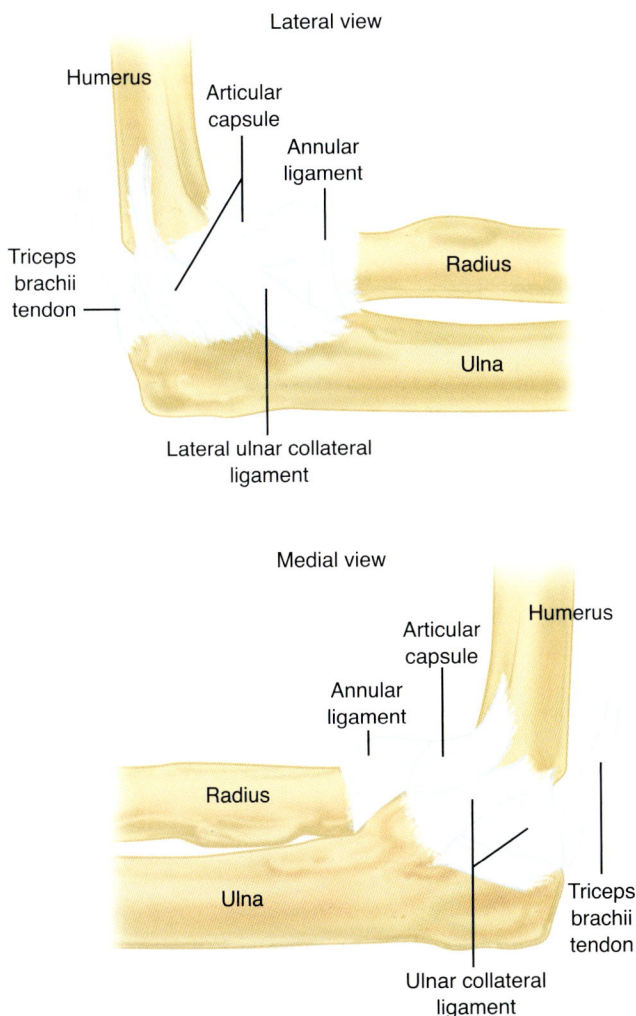

FIG 1 • The medial and collateral ligament complexes of the elbow. Note their points of attachment on the distal humerus and proximal ulna.

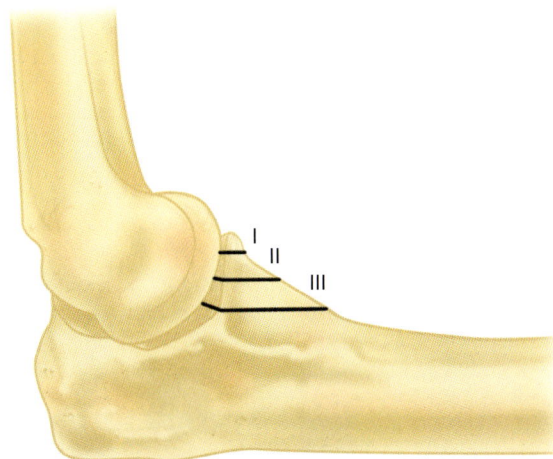

FIG 2 • Lateral view of the elbow depicting the different types of coronoid fractures.

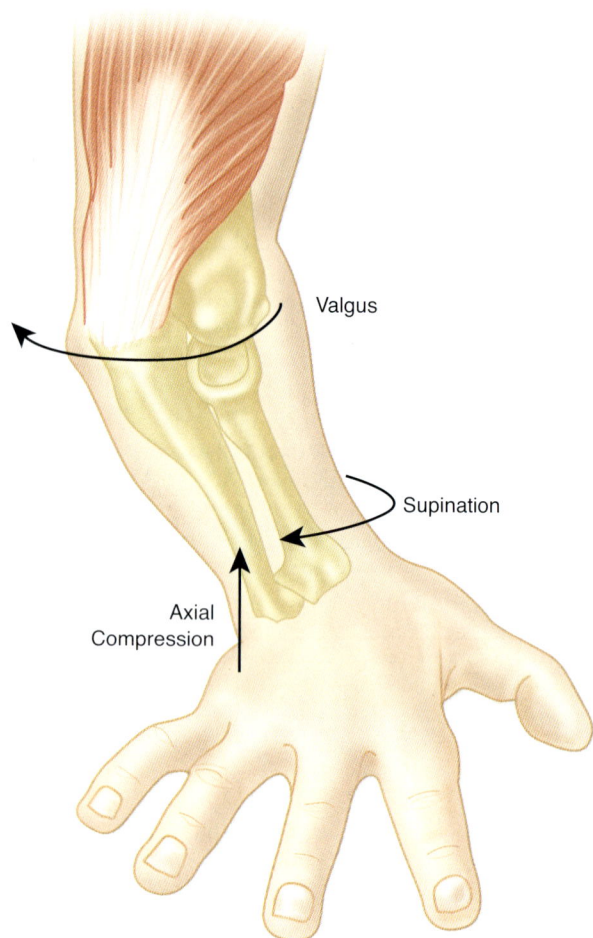

FIG 3 • Typical mechanism of elbow fracture dislocation. Note the forces at play on the elbow.

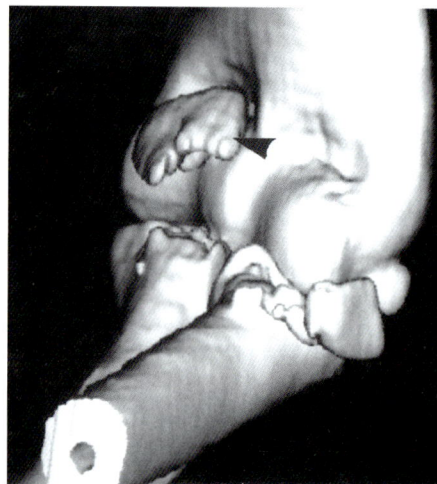

FIG 4 • Three-dimensional CT reconstruction of "terrible triad" injury. The *arrow* represents the large coronoid fragment anterior to the elbow. (From Pugh DMW, Wild LM, Schemitsch EH, et al. Standard surgical protocol to treat elbow dislocations with radial head and coronoid fractures. J Bone Joint Surg Am 2004;86A:1122–1130.)

PATHOGENESIS

- Fracture-dislocations of the elbow occur during falls onto an outstretched hand, falls from a height, motor vehicle accidents, or other high-energy trauma (**FIG 3**).
- Typically there is a hyperextension and valgus stress applied to the pronated arm.

NATURAL HISTORY

- Elbow dislocations with associated coronoid or radial head fractures have a poor natural history. Redislocation or subluxation is likely with closed treatment.
- Treatment of the radial head fracture by excision alone in the context of an elbow dislocation has a high rate of failure due to recurrent instability.
- Problems of recurrent instability, arthrosis, and severe stiffness lead to poor functional results.[10]

PATIENT HISTORY AND PHYSICAL FINDINGS

- Fracture-dislocations of the elbow are acute and traumatic, so the history should be straightforward.
- It is not unusual for these injuries to occur with high-energy trauma, so a diligent search for other musculoskeletal and systemic injuries must accompany evaluation of the elbow. The ipsilateral shoulder and wrist should be evaluated.
- The evaluation and documentation of peripheral nerve and vascular function in the injured extremity is critical.

IMAGING AND OTHER DIAGNOSTIC STUDIES

- High-quality plain radiographs in the anteroposterior (AP) and lateral plane should be obtained before and after closed reduction.
  - Cast material can obscure bony detail after closed reduction.
- If there is any evidence of forearm or wrist pain associated with the elbow injury, these should be imaged as well.
- Computed tomography (CT) scans with reformatted images and 3D reconstructions are helpful in understanding the configuration of bony injuries and are helpful in treatment planning (**FIG 4**).

DIFFERENTIAL DIAGNOSIS

- Radial head or neck fractures without associated dislocation
- Coronoid fracture associated with posteromedial instability. This results from a varus force and is associated with rupture of the LCL. The radial head is not fractured, making diagnosis more difficult.

NONOPERATIVE MANAGEMENT

- Initial treatment involves closed reduction and splinting with radiographs to confirm reduction (**FIG 5**).
- If reduction cannot be maintained because of bone or soft tissue injury, repeated attempts at closed reduction should not be attempted. This is thought to contribute to the formation of heterotopic ossification.
- The ability of nonoperative management to meet treatment goals in these situations is rare and surgery is indicated in almost all cases.

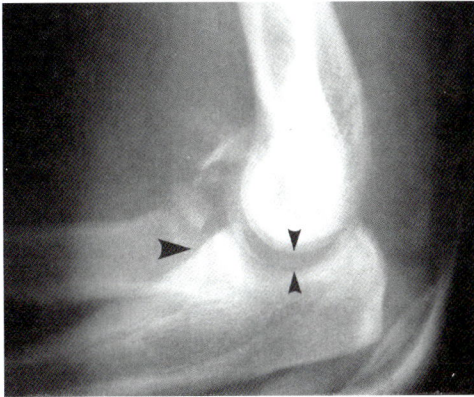

FIG 5 • Radiograph revealing nonconcentric reduction after closed reduction. The *small arrows* highlight the nonconcentric reduction of the ulnohumeral joint. (From Pugh DMW, Wild LM, Schemitsch EH, et al. Standard surgical protocol to treat elbow dislocations with radial head and coronoid fractures. J Bone Joint Surg Am 2004;86A:1122–1130.)

SURGICAL MANAGEMENT

- The goals of surgery are to obtain and maintain a concentric and stable reduction of the ulnohumeral and radiocapitellar joint such that early motion within a flexion–extension arc of 30 to 130 degrees can be initiated. Early motion is key to avoid elbow stiffness and resultant poor function.
- Management of elbow dislocations with associated radial head and coronoid fractures should follow an established protocol (Table 1) that has produced reliable results.[8]
- The radial head is an important secondary stabilizer of the elbow to valgus stress and posterior instability.[7]
    - It is also a longitudinal stabilizer of the forearm to proximal translation.
    - If fractured in this setting, it must be fixed or replaced, as excision leads to recurrent instability and unacceptable results.[10]

Preoperative Planning

- Before surgery, the surgeon must ensure that the proper equipment and implants are available.

Table 1	**Treatment Protocol for Elbow Dislocation With Associated Radial Head and Coronoid Fractures**

Step	Action
1	Fix the coronoid fracture
2	Fix or replace the radial head
3	Repair the lateral collateral ligament
4	Assess elbow stability within 30 to 130 degrees of flexion–extension with the forearm in full pronation
5	If the elbow remains unstable, consider fixing the medial collateral ligament
6	Failing this, apply a hinged external fixator to maintain concentric reduction and allow for early motion

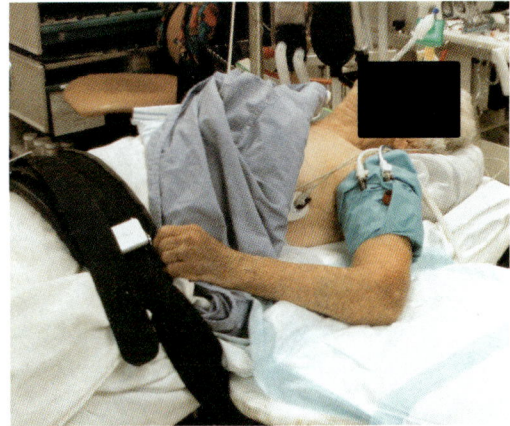

FIG 6 • Patient positioned supine with hand table.

- Coronoid fractures are fixed with small fragment or cannulated screws of appropriate size.
- Radial head and neck fracture fixation is accomplished with small fragment plates and screws.
    - We often use countersunk Herbert screws to fix articular head fragments.
    - A metallic, modular radial head implant system should be available if primary osteosynthesis cannot be achieved.
- An image intensifier is helpful during surgery. Films confirming concentric reduction and the proper positioning of implanted hardware should always be obtained before leaving the operating room.
- In rare instances in which bony and ligamentous repair fails to restore sufficient elbow stability, dynamic hinged external fixation is used.
    - This is a highly specialized technique that may not be appropriate for all surgeons.
    - In that case, static external fixation and patient referral is an appropriate alternative.

Positioning

- Most commonly, the patient is positioned supine on the operating table under general anesthesia.
- The operative limb is supported on a hand table and a tourniquet is applied to the upper arm before preparation and draping (**FIG 6**).
- Alternatively, the lateral decubitus position can be used with the operative limb supported by a padded bolster. This position is used if hinged fixation is deemed likely.

Approach

- The lateral approach is the workhorse for treatment of these injuries where the coronoid, radial head, and LCL can be addressed. A direct lateral incision with the patient supine and the arm on a hand table is used.
- Landmarks and skin incision are shown in FIGURE 7A.
- The surgeon should use the traumatic dissection that occurred at the time of injury to gain exposure of the elbow.
- Typically the LCL has been avulsed from the lateral distal humerus, leaving a bare spot (**FIG 7B**).[8]
- Some cases require a medial approach as well for either medial ligament reconstruction or plating of a coronoid

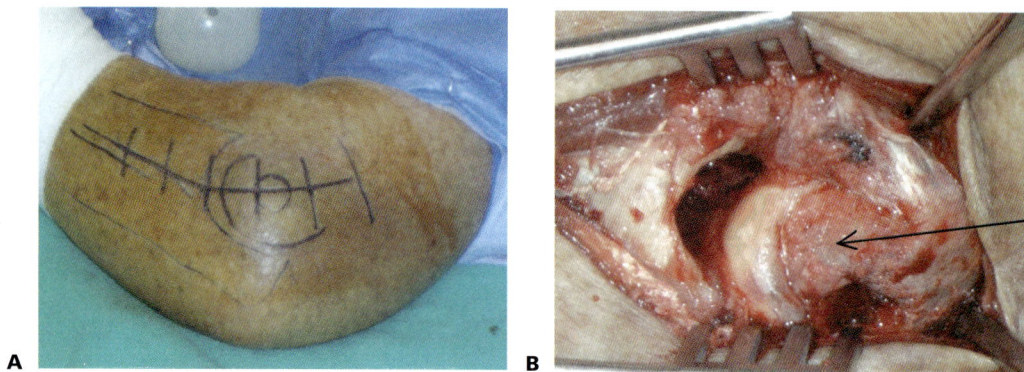

FIG 7 • **A.** Landmarks and skin incision. The underlying bones have been represented and the position of the lateral skin incision is marked with the *hashed line*. **B.** Avulsion of lateral collateral ligament. The *arrow* is pointing to the bare spot on the distal lateral humerus where the lateral collateral ligament complex has been avulsed.

fracture. This can be accomplished through a second medial incision.

- The ulnar nerve is at risk in this approach and should be identified and protected. The common flexor origin is split distal to the medial epicondyle to expose the coronoid medially.

- Alternatively, a posterior skin incision can be used with elevation of full-thickness flaps at the fascial level to approach both laterally and medially.
  - The patient can be placed in the lateral decubitus position or supine with the arm across the chest for this approach.

TECHNIQUES

LATERAL EXPOSURE

- Make an incision along the lateral supracondylar ridge of the humerus curving at the lateral epicondyle toward the radial head and neck.
- At the fascial level, elevate full-thickness flaps and insert a self-retaining retractor (**TECH FIG 1**).
- Split the common extensor origin in line with its fibers.
- Make use of the traumatic dissection that occurred at the time of injury.
  - Most commonly, the LCL will have avulsed from the distal humerus, leaving a bare spot. The common extensor origin is avulsed as well two thirds of the time.[7]
- Reconstruction occurs in an orderly fashion from deep to superficial.
- If the radial head is to be replaced, its excision provides excellent exposure of the coronoid through the lateral approach.
  - If, on the other hand, it is to be fixed, set free fragments aside to allow access to the coronoid.

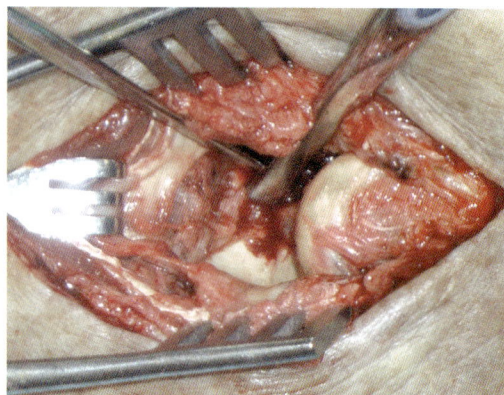

TECH FIG 1 • Lateral approach. In this case, the radial neck was fractured and the head has been removed. An excellent view of the coronoid is achieved. Here a type I coronoid fracture is present.

ORIF OF CORONOID FRACTURE

Type I Coronoid Fractures

- For type I fractures, we recommend fixation with a nonabsorbable (no. 2 braided) suture passed through the anterior elbow capsule just above the bony fragment (**TECH FIG 2**).
- Two parallel drill holes are made from the dorsal surface of the ulna through a separate small incision and directed toward the coronoid tip. These are made with a small drill or Kirschner wire.
- Once the suture is passed through the capsule, its ends are brought out each of the drill holes and tied over the ulna to plicate the anterior elbow capsule.
- The suture ends can be retrieved through the drill holes using an eyeleted Kirschner wire, a Keith needle, or a suture retriever.

TECHNIQUES

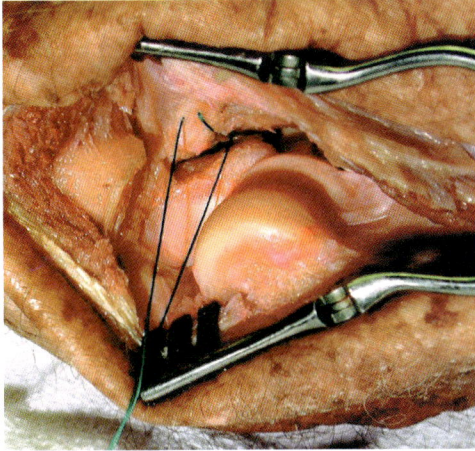

TECH FIG 2 • Suture fixation of a type I coronoid fracture. The suture is passed through the anterior capsule above the coronoid. Its ends will be passed through the proximal ulna and tied over the dorsal surface. This type of fixation is used if the coronoid fragment is too small to accept a screw. (From McKee MD, Pugh DM, Wild LM, et al. Standard surgical protocol to treat elbow dislocation with radial head and coronoid fractures. J Bone Joint Surg Am 2005;87A:22–32.)

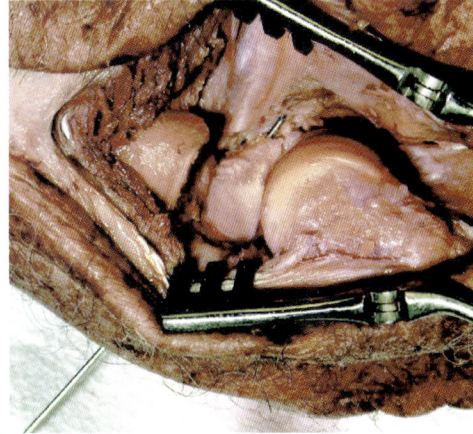

TECH FIG 3 • Coronoid fracture held reduced with Kirschner wire. (From McKee MD, Pugh DM, Wild LM, et al. Standard surgical protocol to treat elbow dislocation with radial head and coronoid fractures. J Bone Joint Surg Am 2005; 87A:22–32.)

Type II and III Coronoid Fractures

- Type II and III coronoid fractures can be fixed with one or two cannulated screws. Regular, partially threaded, cancellous screws can also be used.
- Once the fracture has been débrided such that it can be anatomically reduced, pass a guidewire from the dorsal surface of the proximal ulna such that it exits at the fracture site.
    - Back the guidewire up until it is just buried, and reduce the fracture.
- Hold the fragment reduced with a pointed instrument such as a dental pick and advance the wire across the fracture site into the fragment (**TECH FIG 3**). If there is enough space, insert a second wire across the fracture.

- Once one or two guidewires are in place, they are replaced with appropriate-length screws, cannulated or regular. It is critical to tap the fragment before screw placement to avoid splitting the fragment on screw insertion.
- Coronoid fractures that are comminuted may be difficult to treat. Typically, the largest fragment with articular cartilage is fixed.
- If screw fixation is not possible or access is difficult due to an intact radial head, the coronoid can also be addressed through a medial approach.
    - A medial incision along the supracondylar ridge is used.
    - The ulnar nerve is identified and protected.
    - The common flexor origin is split to gain access to the coronoid on the proximal ulna.
    - From the medial side, a buttress or spring plate can be used to secure a comminuted fracture.

RADIAL HEAD OR NECK FRACTURE

- Radial head fracture is addressed after treatment of the coronoid injury because once the head is fixed or replaced, access to the coronoid from the lateral approach is limited.
- The decision to fix a radial head is largely based on the fracture configuration. If fracture comminution is limited such that the head is in two or three fragments, reduction and fixation is usually possible.
    - Fractures that are comminuted or with articular surface damage require replacement.
- Expose the head and neck as necessary for fracture reduction and fixation by extending the Köcher interval.
- The posterior interosseous nerve is at risk during more distal radial neck exposures. Its distance from the operative site can be maximized by keeping the forearm in full pronation.

ORIF of Radial Head Fractures

- For radial head fragments, reduce and hold the fragment to the intact head with a pointed reduction clamp.
- We secure the fragments with Herbert screws. The fragments can be held temporarily with a 2-mm Kirschner wire and then replaced with a Herbert screw.
    - If the screw is inserted through articular cartilage, its head must be countersunk.
- Radial neck fractures, once reduced, can be held provisionally with a Kirschner wire.
- Definitive fixation is with a small fragment T plate over the "safe zone" (**TECH FIG 4**).
    - Care is taken to not injure the posterior interosseous nerve while exposing the shaft or by trapping it under the plate distally.
- If the radial head cannot be reconstructed, it is replaced.

TECHNIQUES

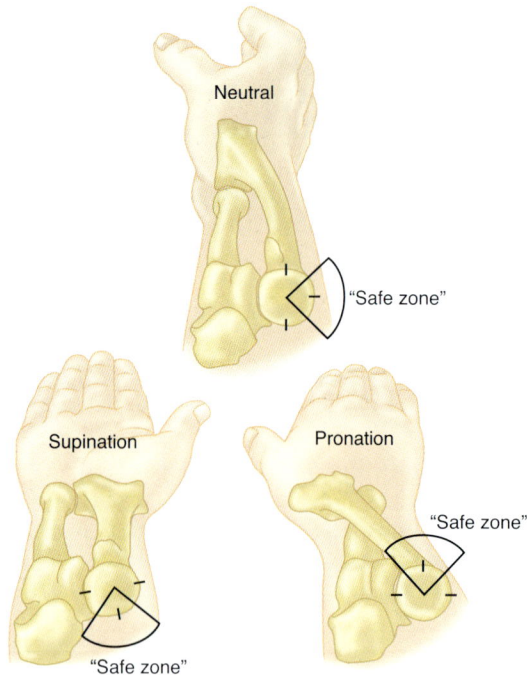

TECH FIG 4 • The "safe zone" for plating radial neck fractures. The 90-degree arc outlined does not articulate with the proximal ulna throughout the full range of forearm rotation. Plating a radial neck fracture in this zone will not interfere with rotation.

Radial Head Replacement

- The replacement used must be metallic as silicone implants are inadequate both biomechanically and biologically.[6]
  - We use a modular implant such that the stem diameter can be varied independent of the head diameter and thickness.

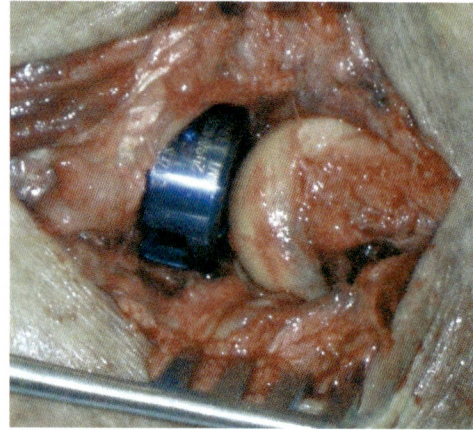

TECH FIG 5 • Radial head implant. An appropriately sized radial head implant has been inserted. It is held reduced with the forearm in full pronation. Note the anatomic alignment with the capitellum.

- If required, cut the proximal radius at the level of the neck with a micro-sagittal saw.
- Ream the canal of the proximal radius to cortical bone with sequentially larger reamers.
- Radial head size can be judged by assembling the fractured fragments that have been removed. In general, downsizing the head slightly is recommended such that the elbow joint is not overstuffed.
- A trial implant should be inserted to test stability and motion. Elbow range of motion, both flexion–extension and forearm rotation, should be checked. View the articulation between the proximal radius and ulna to see if the diameter of the implant seems appropriate.
- Once satisfied with sizing, the definitive implant is inserted (**TECH FIG 5**).

REPAIR OF THE LATERAL COLLATERAL LIGAMENT COMPLEX

- Repair of the LCL complex is critical to re-establish elbow stability (**TECH FIG 6A**).
- It is most often avulsed from the distal humerus. Its anatomic attachment point is slightly posterior to the lateral epicondyle at the center of the arc of the capitellum.

- The LCL is a discrete structure deep to the common extensor origin, which runs from the lateral epicondyle to the supinator crest of the ulna (**TECH FIG 6B**).
- Use a no. 2, braided, nonabsorbable suture for the repair.

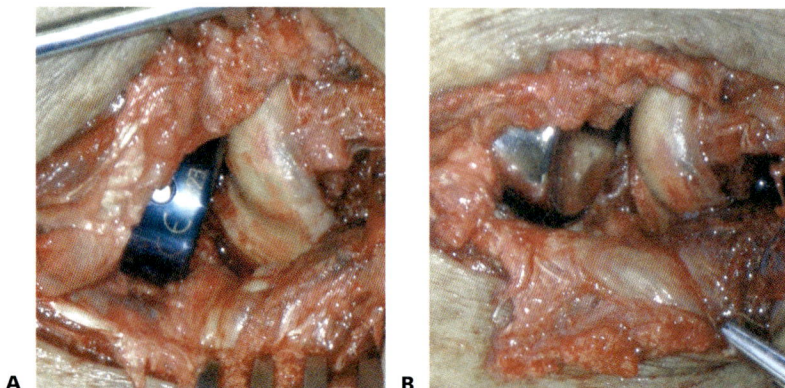

TECH FIG 6 • **A.** Elbow instability associated with deficient lateral collateral ligament. Without repair of the lateral collateral ligament, the radial head subluxes into a posterolateral position with forearm supination. Note that the radial head and capitellum are no longer in normal alignment. **B.** The lateral collateral ligament is held by the forceps. It is a distinct structure easily identified in this acutely injured elbow. (*continued*)

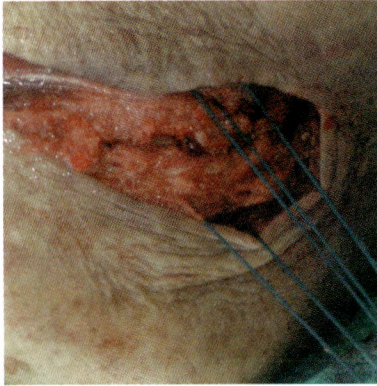

C

TECH FIG 6 • (*continued*) **C.** Sutures passed for lateral collateral ligament repair.

- The ligament can be reattached to the distal humerus through bone tunnels or using suture anchors. We prefer bony tunnels.
- Using a drill, Kirschner wire, or pointed towel clip, make holes in the distal lateral humerus above the epicondyle.
- Pass the suture through the holes and into the lateral ligament such that it will tighten on tying the sutures.
- At least two, preferably three, sutures through bone are required. Pass, cut, and snap all of the sutures (**TECH FIG 6C**).
  - Ensure that the elbow is now held in 90 degrees of flexion and full forearm pronation.
  - Incorporate the more superficial common extensor origin in the repair.
- Tie the sutures once they have all been passed and then close the lateral wound in layers.

PERSISTENT INSTABILITY

- On occasion, repair of the coronoid, radial head, and LCL from the lateral approach is insufficient to restore elbow stability such that early motion may be initiated.
- In these cases, further efforts must be made to obtain such stability.
- Repair of the MCL through a separate medial incision is one option if a lateral approach has been used for coronoid and radial head fracture fixation.
  - Alternatively, a posterior skin incision can be used with full-thickness flaps created to access both sides. Positioning the patient in the lateral decubitus position facilitates this approach.
- A deep approach to the medial aspect of the elbow puts the ulnar nerve at risk, and it must be identified and protected during the procedure.
- Usually the MCL is torn in its mid-substance. Suture repair of this is often unsatisfying. Using a graft to replace the MCL is not recommended in the acute injury setting.
- If elbow stability remains insufficient, applying a hinged fixator is the final option.[3]
  - If the hinge is not available or the surgeon is not familiar with its use, a static fixator can be applied to maintain elbow reduction.

Hinged External Fixation

- Application of the hinged fixator starts with the insertion of a guide pin through the center of elbow rotation.

- Insert the pin from medial to lateral starting at the medial epicondyle through a small incision and protect the ulnar nerve. The pin should be directed through the center of the capitellum.
- After pin insertion, the elbow is held reduced while the frame is assembled around it.
- The hinge slides over the guide pin on either side of the elbow. Three-quarter rings are attached proximal and distal to the elbow.
- Insert two half-pins in the humerus above the elbow through small open incisions over the posterior surface by bluntly spreading the triceps fibers.
- Insert two half-pins in the ulna over its subcutaneous border dorsally.
- Attach the pins to the rings and tighten all parts of the hinged fixator.
- Verify that the elbow remains reduced in the frame through 30 to 130 degrees of motion. The forearm is maintained in pronation to protect the lateral ligament repair.
- Lock the elbow at 90 degrees in the hinge for the initial postoperative course.
- Obtain plain radiographs in the operating room before the conclusion of the procedure.

PEARLS AND PITFALLS

Indications	▪ Elbow dislocations with associated fractures of the coronoid or radial head must be recognized as complex dislocations. They usually require surgical treatment.
Goals of treatment	▪ The goals are to obtain a concentric reduction with sufficient elbow stability such that early range of motion is possible, and to avoid persistent instability, elbow stiffness, and arthritis.
Coronoid fractures	▪ Repair of coronoid fractures is technically demanding but necessary for successful treatment.
Radial head	▪ The surgeon should be prepared to replace the radial head if necessary with a metal, modular prosthesis. ▪ Excision alone is not an option.

Lateral ligaments	■ Repair of the lateral ligaments is important to impart the necessary stability for early motion and to avoid late posterolateral rotatory instability.
Physiotherapy	■ It is important to emphasize to the patient the need to be diligent with rehabilitation and exercises, as this will have a great effect on the end result.

POSTOPERATIVE CARE

■ The injured elbow is placed in a well-padded plaster splint at 90 degrees of flexion and full pronation. The patient is given a sling for comfort.

■ AP and lateral radiographs are obtained in the operating room to ensure congruent reduction and verify hardware placement.

■ The patient typically stays in hospital one night to receive adequate analgesia and prophylactic antibiotics.

■ We do not routinely give prophylaxis for heterotopic ossification unless the patient has a concomitant head injury: in this case, indomethacin 25 mg three times a day is prescribed with a cytoprotective agent for 3 weeks.

■ The patient returns to our clinic at 7 to 10 days postoperatively for staple removal. The splint is typically removed at this point.

■ Range-of-motion exercises are initiated at this time under the supervision of a physiotherapist.

■ Active and active-assisted flexion–extension between 30 and 130 degrees and forearm rotation with the elbow at 90 degrees of flexion is initiated.

■ A lightweight resting splint is made for the injured elbow that is removed for hygiene and physiotherapy.

■ The patient returns at 4, 8, and 12 weeks after surgery for clinical review with plain radiographs. Thereafter the interval of clinic visits is widened, but we follow our patients out to 2 years.

■ At 4 weeks we allow unrestricted range of motion and at 8 weeks unrestricted strengthening.

■ Evidence of fracture union is usually present between 6 and 8 weeks.

■ Progress with range of motion can be slow and frustrating for the patient but does not plateau until 1 year of follow-up.

OUTCOMES

■ Following the protocol outlined for fracture-dislocations of the elbow should yield satisfactory functional results.

■ Pugh et al[8] reported the results of this treatment protocol for 36 elbows at 34 months.

  ■ The flexion–extension arc averaged 112 degrees and rotation 136 degrees.

  ■ Fifteen patients had excellent results, 13 good, 7 fair, and 1 poor by the Mayo Elbow Performance Score.

  ■ Eight patients had a complication requiring reoperation.

COMPLICATIONS

■ The most likely complication after treatment is unacceptable elbow stiffness with a resultant nonfunctional range of motion.

  ■ An acceptable range is 30 to 130 degrees of flexion.

■ At about 1 year after surgery, once motion has plateaued, patients are candidates for release with hardware removal if they are not happy with their range of motion and the flexion–extension arc is less than 100 degrees.

  ■ This is done through the lateral approach with an anterior and posterior capsulectomy plus manipulation under anesthesia.

  ■ A radial head implant in place can be downsized to improve motion, but it should not be simply removed. The lateral ligament complex is preserved.

  ■ In our series, this was necessary in 11% of cases.[8]

■ Synostosis around the elbow is another possible cause of rotational forearm stiffness.

  ■ A resection can be planned to improve motion.

  ■ CT scanning preoperatively helps to define the extent of the lesion. Resection is technically demanding.

■ Superficial and deep wound infection is possible after repair. Immediate and aggressive treatment is recommended with antibiotics initially and irrigation with débridement if rapid improvement is not seen.

■ Persistent instability is rare but may occur despite best efforts at repair.

■ Posttraumatic arthritis may be a long-term problem.

REFERENCES

1. Cage DJ, Abrams RA, Callahan JJ, et al. Soft tissue attachments of the ulnar coronoid process: an anatomic study with radiographic correlation. Clin Orthop Relat Res 1995;320:154–158.
2. Mason ML. Some observations on fractures of the head of the radius with a review of one hundred cases. Br J Surg 1954;42:123–132.
3. McKee MD, Bowden SH, King GJ, et al. Management of recurrent, complex instability of the elbow with a hinged external fixator. J Bone Joint Surg Br 1998;80B:1031–1036.
4. McKee MD, Pugh DM, Wild LM, et al. Standard surgical protocol to treat elbow dislocation with radial head and coronoid fractures. J Bone Joint Surg Am 2005;87A:22–32.
5. McKee MD, Schemitsch EH, Sala MJ, et al. The pathoanatomy of lateral ligamentous disruption in complex elbow instability. J Shoulder Elbow Surg 2003;12:391–396.
6. Moro JK, Werier J, MacDermid JC, et al. Arthroplasty with a metal radial head for unreconstructable fractures of the radial head. J Bone Joint Surg Am 2001;83A:1201–1211.
7. Morrey BF, Tanaka S, An KN. Valgus stability of the elbow: a definition of primary and secondary constraints. Clin Orthop Relat Res 1991;265:187–195.
8. Pugh DMW, Wild LM, Schemitsch EH, et al. Standard surgical protocol to treat elbow dislocations with radial head and coronoid fractures. J Bone Joint Surg Am 2004;86A:1122–1130.
9. Regan W, Morrey B. Fractures of the coronoid process of the ulna. J Bone Joint Surg Am 1989;71:1248–1254.
10. Ring D, Jupiter JB, Zilberfarb J. Posterior dislocation of the elbow with fractures of the radial head and coronoid. J Bone Joint Surg Am 2002;84A:547–551.

Chapter 40

Monteggia Fractures in Adults

Matthew L. Ramsey

DEFINITION

- This injury was initially reported by Giovanni Monteggia in 1814 as a fracture of the ulna associated with an anterior dislocation of the radial head.[6]
- The term "Monteggia lesions" was coined by Bado to describe any fracture of the ulna associated with a dislocation of the radiocapitellar joint.[1]
- The Bado classification of Monteggia lesions,[1] with the Jupiter subclassification of type II fractures,[4] is shown in Table 1.
- Equivalent injuries in adults
  - Variable pathology that is thought to be equivalent to injuries classified by the Bado system
  - Equivalent injuries do not always fall within the traditional definition of a Monteggia fracture in that they do not always have a concomitant radiocapitellar dislocation. Therefore, it can be argued that these injuries are not necessarily equivalent to Monteggia fractures.
  - Type I and II injuries are the only ones that have equivalent injury patterns.

PATHOGENESIS

- The exact mechanism of injury for Monteggia fractures is controversial.
- Proposed mechanisms of injury for type I injuries include the following:
  - Direct blow to the posterior aspect of the elbow
  - Fall on outstretched arm with hyperpronated hand (forearm pronation levers radial head anteriorly)
  - Fall on outstretched arm
  - Violent contraction of biceps pulling radial head anteriorly
- Proposed mechanism for type II injuries: hypothesized to occur when a supination force tensions the ligaments that are stronger than bone
- Proposed mechanism for type III injuries: direct blow to the inside of the elbow with or without rotation

PATIENT HISTORY AND PHYSICAL FINDINGS

- The initial examination should systematically evaluate:
  - Skin integrity
  - Neurovascular status of the extremity
  - Bony injury
- Ulna fracture
  - Injury pattern
    - Noncomminuted
    - Comminution
    - Associated injury to key structural elements of the ulna (coronoid, olecranon)
- Radial head injury
  - Isolated dislocation without fracture
  - Radial head or neck fracture

IMAGING AND OTHER DIAGNOSTIC STUDIES

- Plain radiographs (**FIG 1**): Orthogonal radiographs of the elbow, forearm, and wrist are required.
  - Ulna fracture is easily identified.
  - Radial head fracture or dislocation can be subtle, especially if radial head dislocation reduces.
- Computed tomography (CT) scans can be helpful to determine the extent of the bony injury and the location of fracture fragments. They are particularly helpful in fractures involving the coronoid, olecranon, and radial head.
- 3D CT reconstructions provide information on the spatial relationship of fracture fragments in comminuted fractures.

DIFFERENTIAL DIAGNOSIS

- Isolated ulna fracture
  - Nightstick fracture
  - Olecranon fracture
- Fracture-dislocation of the elbow ("terrible triad" injury)
- Transolecranon fracture-dislocation

NONOPERATIVE MANAGEMENT

- Monteggia fracture-dislocations in the adult population are generally treated surgically.
- Improved fixation methods and surgical technique have remarkably improved the results of surgery, making it a more reliable treatment option.

SURGICAL MANAGEMENT

Preoperative Planning

- The timing of surgery depends on the condition of the soft tissues and the availability of necessary equipment and personnel.
- The surgeon should define all injuries that need to be addressed.
- Equipment requirements:
  - Small fragment plates and screws or anatomic plating system
  - Minifragment system
  - Threaded Kirchner wires
  - Radial head replacement
- Bone graft (allograft or autograft)

Patient Positioning

- Lateral decubitus position with the arm over a padded arm support (**FIG 2**)
- Supine positioning is an alternative approach (although it is not preferred because of difficulty in maintaining the arm across the chest). If this approach is used, a saline bag under the ipsilateral shoulder will help keep the arm across the chest.

Table 1	Bado Classification of Monteggia Lesions, With Jupiter Subclassification of Type II Fractures

Type	Description	Illustration
I	Anterior dislocation of the radial head with fracture of the diaphysis of the ulna with anterior angulation of the ulna fracture (most common type of lesion)	
II	Posterior or posterolateral dislocation of the radial head with fracture of the ulnar diaphysis with posterior angulation of the ulna fracture	
IIA	Fracture at the level of the trochlear notch (ulna fracture involves the distal part of the olecranon and coronoid)	
IIB	Ulna fracture is at the metaphyseal–diaphyseal junction, distal to the coronoid	
IIC	Ulna fracture is diaphyseal	
IID	Comminuted fractures involving more than one region	

Table 1   *(continued)*

Type	Description	Illustration
III	Lateral or anterolateral dislocation of the radial head with fracture of the ulnar metaphysis	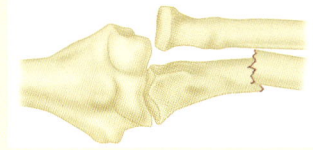
IV	Anterior dislocation of the radial head with a fracture of the proximal third of the radius and ulna at the same level	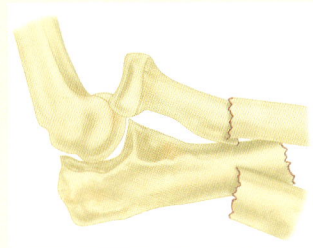

Adapted from Bado J. The Monteggia lesion. Clin Orthop Relat Res 1967;50:717; and Jupiter JB, Leibovic SJ, Ribbans W, et al. The posterior Monteggia lesion. J Orthop Trauma 1991;5:395–402.

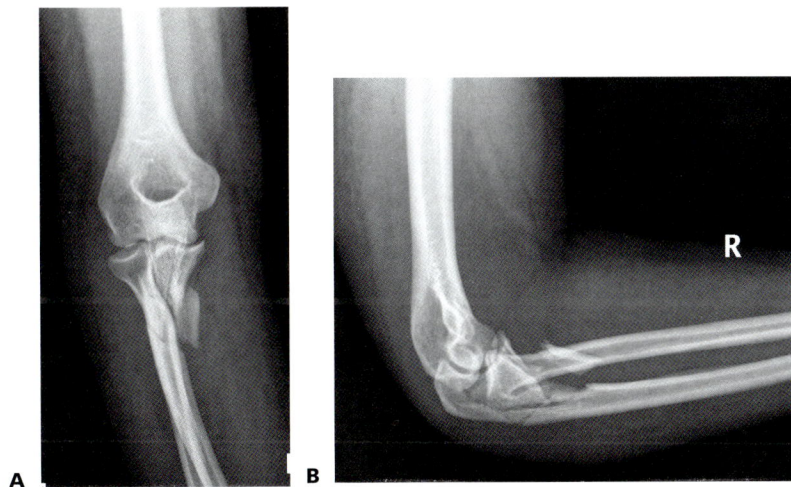

FIG 1 • Plain AP and lateral radiographs typically demonstrate fracture pattern.

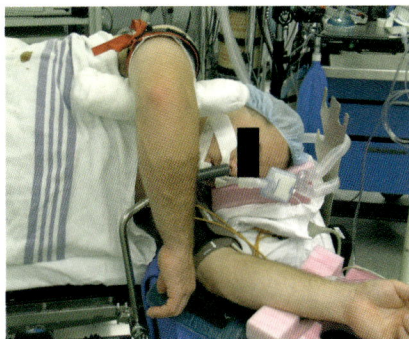

FIG 2 • Lateral decubitus positioning is preferred.

TECHNIQUES

SURGICAL APPROACH

- A midline posterior skin incision is placed lateral to the tip of the olecranon (**TECH FIG 1A**).
- Subcutaneous flaps are elevated on the fascia of the forearm. The medial antebrachial cutaneous nerve does not need to be identified if dissection is performed on the fascia of the flexor–pronator muscles since it is mobilized with the medial skin flap.
- The interval between the flexor carpi ulnaris (FCU) and anconeus is developed along the subcutaneous border of the ulna to expose the fracture site. The amount of

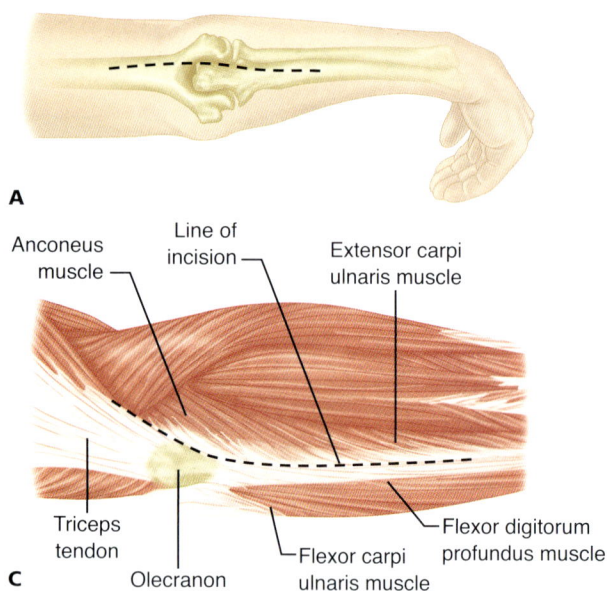

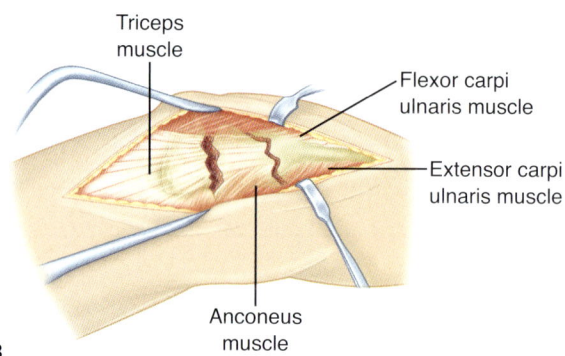

dissection required for exposure is dictated by the fracture pattern and the type of fixation to be used (**TECH FIG 1B**).
- If the radial head needs to be addressed surgically, the anconeus can be mobilized more extensively through a Boyd approach (**TECH FIG 1C**). If the ulna fracture permits, the radial head can be fixed through the fracture bed of the ulna before definitive fixation of the ulna. Once the ulna is fixed, access to the radial head is not possible.

TECH FIG 1 • **A.** Posterior midline incision positioned just off the lateral aspect of the olecranon. **B.** Deep surgical interval uses the internervous plane between the anconeus and flexor carpi ulnaris. **C.** Exposure of the radial head can be accomplished by releasing the anconeus from the humerus and reflecting it proximally to expose the radial head.

RADIAL HEAD MANAGEMENT

- Radial head fractures are typically fixed before the ulna fracture is addressed. If the lesser sigmoid notch of the ulna is involved, determining radial length if radial head replacement is required can be difficult. Therefore, fractures are generally fixed before the ulna while replacement may need to be performed after ulnar fixation is completed in order to establish appropriate radial head sizing.
- Reconstructable fractures of the radial head are fixed (**TECH FIG 2A,B**).
- Unreconstructable fractures of the radial head are replaced (**TECH FIG 2C**).

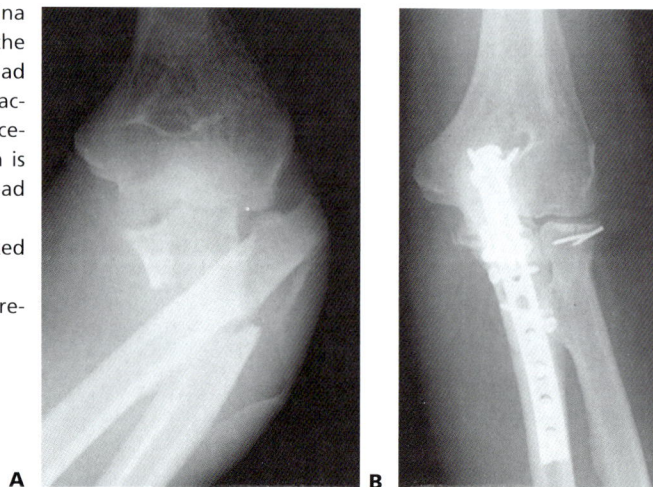

TECH FIG 2 • **A,B.** Preoperative and postoperative radiographs demonstrating open reduction and internal fixation of the radial head component of the Monteggia fracture. (*continued*)

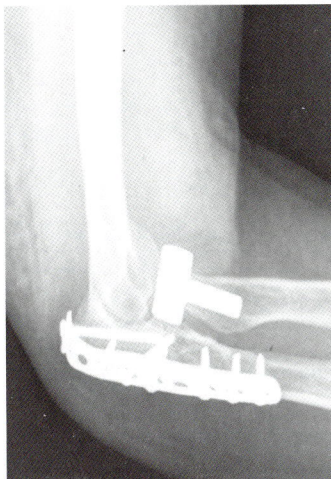

C

TECH FIG 2 • (*continued*) **C.** Postoperative radiograph of a Monteggia fracture in which the radial head fracture needed to be replaced.

ULNA FRACTURE FIXATION

No Articular Involvement of the Ulnohumeral Joint

- Ulna fractures distal to the coronoid can be plated laterally or on the subcutaneous border of the ulna.
- Lateral plate placement is preferred by some to prevent hardware prominence.

Articular Involvement of the Ulnohumeral Joint

- Fractures extending proximal to the coronoid require the plate be placed on the subcutaneous border of the ulna to accommodate the complex geometry of this region.
- In general, the ulna fracture is reconstructed from distal to proximal. Ensure that any associated injury to the coronoid is identified and addressed.
- The fracture is reconstructed by fixing the distal fragments; this may require interfragmentary fixation or subarticular Kirchner wires (**TECH FIG 3A**). As fixation progresses proximally, reconstruction of the coronoid and greater sigmoid notch is performed. Particular attention is directed at anatomic reconstruction of the articular surface.
- Coronoid involvement with a Monteggia fracture-dislocation often extends distally into the volar cortex of the ulna, as opposed to the axial-plane fracture patterns characterized by Regan and Morrey[9] (**TECH FIG 3B**).
- Larger fragments can be definitively fixed with antegrade lag screws from the dorsal aspect of the ulnar or can be provisionally fixed with threaded wires and ultimately definitively fixed once the plate is applied to the dorsal aspect of the ulna.
- Coronoid fracture exposure can typically be obtained through the olecranon fracture. If this does not provide sufficient exposure, the FCU can be elevated from the dorsal aspect of the ulna.
- The final fragment to be fixed is the olecranon fragment. The attached triceps will obscure fracture reduction if reduced before distal reconstruction (**TECH FIG 3C**).

- Definitive fixation is performed with a dorsal plate. The triceps is partially split to allow the proximal aspect of the plate to oppose the olecranon (**TECH FIG 3D**).

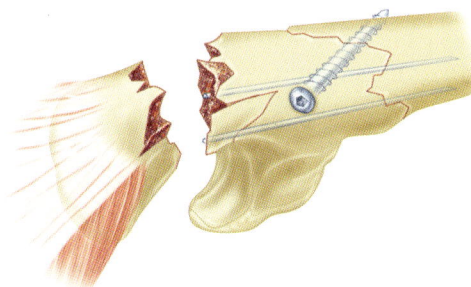

A

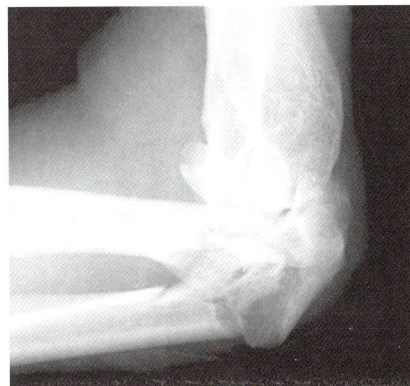

B

TECH FIG 3 • **A.** Monteggia fractures with articular involvement should be fixed distal to proximal. Fixation may require intramedullary Kirschner wires or interfragmentary fixation. **B.** Coronoid fracture often extends into the volar cortex of the ulnar. (*continued*)

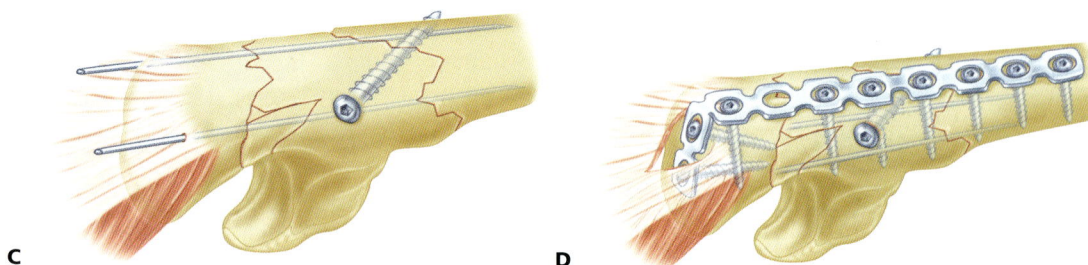

C   **D**

TECH FIG 3 • (*continued*) **C.** The olecranon fragment with attached triceps is reduced and provisionally held with medial and lateral Kirschner wires pending definitive fixation. **D.** Final fixation for most Monteggia fractures is with a rigid plate applied to the dorsal cortex.

WOUND CLOSURE

- The tourniquet is deflated and hemostasis is obtained.
- The fascia between the FCU and anconeus is closed with interrupted absorbable 0 or 1 suture.
- Subcutaneous tissues are closed with 3-0 absorbable suture and skin is closed with staples.
- I prefer to close the wound over a drain placed in the subcutaneous tissues to avoid hematoma.
- A well-padded dressing is applied and an anterior splint is placed with the elbow in full extension.

PEARLS AND PITFALLS

Indications	▪ Monteggia fracture-dislocations in adults require surgical intervention.
Goals of treatment	▪ The first goal is to restore ulnar length and location of the radial head. When the articulation is involved, the goal is to obtain a concentric reduction with sufficient elbow stability that early range of motion is possible. ▪ The second goal is to avoid complications that compromise function.
Ulna fractures	▪ Fractures distal to the coronoid need only to be fixed such that ulnar length is re-established. ▪ When plating these fractures, avoiding malreduction of the ulna is critical to reduction of the radial head. Failure to re-establish ulnar geometry can result in persistent subluxation or dislocation of the radial head (**FIG 3**). ▪ Fractures involving the articulation require stable fixation to re-establish a competent joint.
Radial head	▪ Radial head fractures are fixed or replaced.
Physical therapy	▪ Early range of motion is the goal of treatment but may be delayed if fixation is questionable.

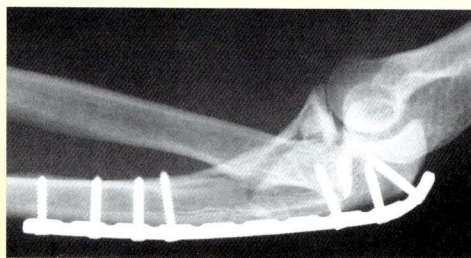

FIG 3 • Malunion of the ulna with resulting apex dorsal angulation results in dislocation of the radial head.

POSTOPERATIVE CARE

- The arm is splinted in full extension to take pressure off the posterior soft tissues.
- If a drain is used, the splint and dressing are removed when the drain output is less than 30 mL in 8 hours. If no drain is used, the dressing is removed on postoperative day 1.
- Active or active-assisted flexion and gravity-assisted extension is begun once the surgical dressings are removed.
- If fixation is tenuous because of poor-quality bone or comminution, mobilization is delayed.

OUTCOMES

- Historically, the results of operative treatment of Monteggia fracture-dislocations have been unpredictable.[3,7,8,11]
- The advent of rigid internal fixation has improved the results of operative treatment.[2,4,7]
- Certain factors have been associated with a poor clinical result[5]:
  - Bado type II injury
  - Jupiter type IIa injury
  - Fracture of the radial head
  - Coronoid fracture
  - Complications requiring further surgery

COMPLICATIONS

- Complications associated with Monteggia fracture-dislocations occur with frequency. A multicenter study evaluating Monteggia fracture-dislocations in adults demonstrated complications in 43% of the patients treated, with an unsatisfactory outcome in 46% of the patients treated.[10]
- Radial nerve palsy
  - Most commonly posterior interosseous nerve
  - Causes of injury include:
    - Compression at the arcade of Frosche
    - Direct trauma
    - Traction with lateral displacement of the radial head
- Most common with type III fractures
  - Complete resolution typically occurs.
- Malunion
  - Most common in type II fractures with volar comminution that is not appreciated or addressed

- If radial head subluxation persists, malunion must be considered.
- Nonunion
  - Causes of nonunion include:
    - Infection
    - Inadequate internal fixation
  - Compression plate fixation required, particularly if fracture is comminuted
  - Semitubular and reconstruction plates are not structurally strong enough.
- Radioulnar synostosis
  - Seen with high-energy injuries with associated comminution
  - Higher incidence if radial head fracture associated with ulna fracture at the same level
  - Boyd approach implicated since the radius and ulna are exposed through the same incision

REFERENCES

1. Bado J. The Monteggia lesion. Clin Orthop Relat Res 1967;50:71.
2. Boyd H, Boals J. The Monteggia lesion: a review of 159 cases. Clin Orthop Relat Res 1969;66:94–100.
3. Bruce H, Harvey JJ, Wilson JJ. Monteggia fractures. J Bone Joint Surg Am 1974;56A:1563–1576.
4. Jupiter JB, Leibovic SJ, Ribbans W, et al. The posterior Monteggia lesion. J Orthop Trauma 1991;5:395–402.
5. Konrad GG, Kundel K, Kreuz PC, et al. Monteggia fractures in adults: long-term results and prognostic factors. J Bone Joint Surg Br 2007;89B:354–360.
6. Monteggia GB. *Instituzioni Chirurgiche*. 2nd ed. Milan: G. Masperp, 1813–1815.
7. Reckling F. Unstable fracture-dislocations of the forearm (Monteggia and Galeazzi lesions). J Bone Joint Surg Am 1982;64A:857–863.
8. Reckling FW, Cordell LD. Unstable fracture-dislocations of the forearm: the Monteggia and Galeazzi lesions. Arch Surg 1968;96:999–1007.
9. Regan W, Morrey B. Fractures of the coronoid process of the ulna. J Bone Joint Surg Am 1989;71A:1348–1354.
10. Reynders P, De Groote W, Rondia J, et al. Monteggia lesions in adults: a multicenter Bota study. Acta Orthop Belg 1996;62(Suppl 1):78–83.
11. Speed J, Boyd H. Treatment of fractures of ulna with dislocation of the head of radius (Monteggia fracture). JAMA 1940;115:1699–1705.

Lateral Collateral Ligament Reconstruction of the Elbow

Jason A. Stein and Anand M. Murthi

DEFINITION

- Lateral collateral ligament (LCL) injuries most often occur after significant elbow trauma, most commonly dislocation.
- Attenuation of the LCL can also occur after multiple surgeries to the lateral side of the elbow and after multiple corticosteroid injections[4] and has recently been reported to occur in patients who have residual cubitus varus after malunion of supracondylar humerus fractures.[7]
- Significant injury to the LCL complex can result in posterolateral rotatory instability (PLRI).

ANATOMY

- The LCL is made up of four major components: the lateral ulnar collateral ligament (LUCL), also called the radial ulnohumeral ligament (RUHL); the radial collateral ligament proper (RCL); the annular ligament; and the accessory collateral ligament (**FIG 1**).
- The ligaments originate from a broad band over the lateral epicondyle, deep to the extensor muscle mass, and separate distally into more discrete structures.
- The RUHL is the most important stabilizer against PLRI, and it attaches distally on the supinator crest of the ulna.[6]
- The RCL is more anterior and primarily resists varus stress.
- The annular ligament sweeps around the radial head and stabilizes the proximal radioulnar joint.
- The capsule acts as a static stabilizer, especially at the anterior portion, while the arm is extended.
- The anconeus and extensor muscle groups act as dynamic stabilizers.

PATHOGENESIS

- Multiple studies have shown that injury to the LCL can lead to PLRI, which is the first stage in elbow instability that can lead to frank elbow dislocation.

- It is controversial whether injury to the RUHL alone can lead to PLRI or whether further injury to the LCL complex is necessary.[5]
- When the forearm is supinated and slightly flexed, a valgus stress with an attenuated LCL causes the ulnohumeral joint to rotate, compresses the radiocapitellar joint, and ultimately causes the radial head to subluxate or dislocate posteriorly.

NATURAL HISTORY

- PLRI is not a new condition, but it has only recently been described and studied.
- The prevalence and natural history of this condition are currently not known.

PATIENT HISTORY AND PHYSICAL FINDINGS

- Patients typically report trauma but may have had recurrent lateral epicondylitis or previous surgery.
- Elderly patients may not have frank dislocation of the elbow, but 75% of patients younger than 20 years report elbow dislocation.[5]
- Patients report mechanical-type symptoms (clicking, popping, and slipping) during elbow supination and extension and rarely report recurrent dislocations.
- Physical examination can be difficult; provocative tests are described below. It is often necessary to conduct these tests with the patient under anesthesia or with the aid of fluoroscopy.
  - Inspection for effusion: With acute injuries, effusion is likely to be present, but in more chronic situations, it may be absent.
  - Range of motion (ROM): Locking of the elbow could represent loose bodies; stiffness may indicate intrinsic capsular contracture.

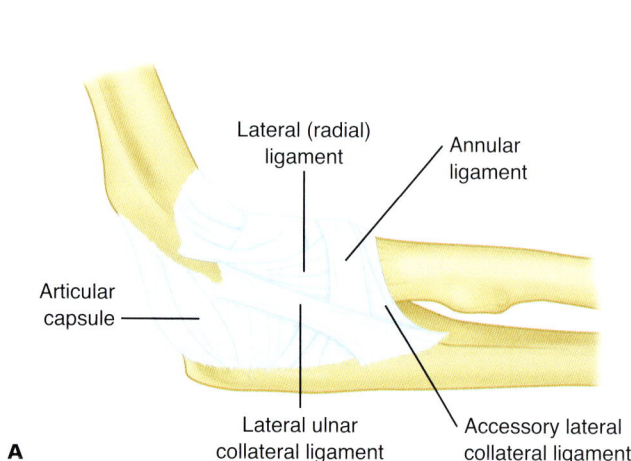

FIG 1 • **A.** The lateral collateral ligament complex is made up of four major components: the lateral ulnar collateral ligament, also called the radial ulnohumeral ligament; the radial collateral ligament proper; the annular ligament; and the accessory collateral ligament. **B.** Osseous anatomy of the lateral collateral ligament insertion.

■ Supine lateral pivot-shift test: When the elbow is slightly flexed, the radial head can be palpated to subluxate or frankly dislocate, and as the elbow flexes past 40 degrees, it relocates, often with a palpable clunk.[6] This test is difficult to perform on an awake patient because often apprehension is felt and the patient does not allow the test to continue.

■ Prone pivot-shift test: Radial head or ulnohumeral subluxation constitutes a positive test, same as the supine lateral pivot-shift test. Examination under anesthesia may be required.

■ Push-up test: Reproduction of the patient's symptoms of apprehension during supination and not pronation constitutes a positive test. Inability to complete the push-up also constitutes a positive test.

■ Chair push-up: Elicited pain constitutes a positive test.

■ Table-top relocation test: Elicited pain or apprehension as the elbow reaches 40 degrees constitutes a positive test.

■ Elbow drawer test: Ulnohumeral subluxation constitutes a positive test.

■ A thorough examination of the elbow should also be completed to rule out other injuries.

■ Valgus instability with the forearm in pronation and 30 degrees of flexion suggests medial collateral ligament (MCL) injury.

■ Lateral epicondylitis or radial tunnel syndrome can present with tenderness over the proximal extensor mass and with resisted extension of the wrist (Thompson test) and long finger.

■ Loose bodies may present with crepitus or locking of the elbow during ROM.

IMAGING AND OTHER DIAGNOSTIC STUDIES

■ Standard anteroposterior (AP) and lateral view radiographs often indicate normal findings but may reveal small lateral epicondyle avulsion fractures and radiocapitellar wear.

■ Stress AP and lateral view radiographs may reveal widening of the ulnohumeral joint and posterior subluxation of the radial head (**FIG 2A**).

■ Magnetic resonance imaging (MRI), especially with intra-articular contrast enhancement, may reveal injuries to the LCL complex. The proximal extensor mass requires attention (**FIG 2B**).

■ Diagnostic arthroscopy of the elbow can be performed, although we do not recommend routine diagnostic arthroscopy for this injury.

■ The drive-through sign occurs when the scope can easily be "driven through" the lateral gutter into the ulnohumeral joint from the posterolateral portal.

■ The pivot-shift test also can be performed during arthroscopy, and the radial head will subluxate posteriorly.

DIFFERENTIAL DIAGNOSIS

■ Lateral epicondylitis
■ Loose bodies
■ Elbow fracture-dislocation
■ MCL injury
■ Radial head dislocation

NONOPERATIVE MANAGEMENT

■ If the injury is diagnosed early, immobilization in a hinged elbow brace in pronation for 4 to 6 weeks may prevent chronic instability.[3]

■ Removable neoprene sleeves may offer support.

■ A trial of elbow extensor strengthening can be performed.

SURGICAL MANAGEMENT

Indications

■ Recurrent symptomatic PLRI despite nonoperative treatment

Preoperative Planning

■ All imaging studies should be reviewed and informed consent obtained.

■ An examination of the elbow should be performed with the patient under anesthesia, especially the pivot-shift test.

■ If there is any doubt regarding the diagnosis, a pivot-shift test should be performed under fluoroscopy.

Positioning

■ The patient is placed supine on the operating room table.

■ The arm can be placed on an arm board or across the patient's chest with a sterile tourniquet applied to the upper arm and the entire arm draped free (**FIG 3**).

■ During the approach, the forearm should be pronated to protect the posterior interosseous nerve.

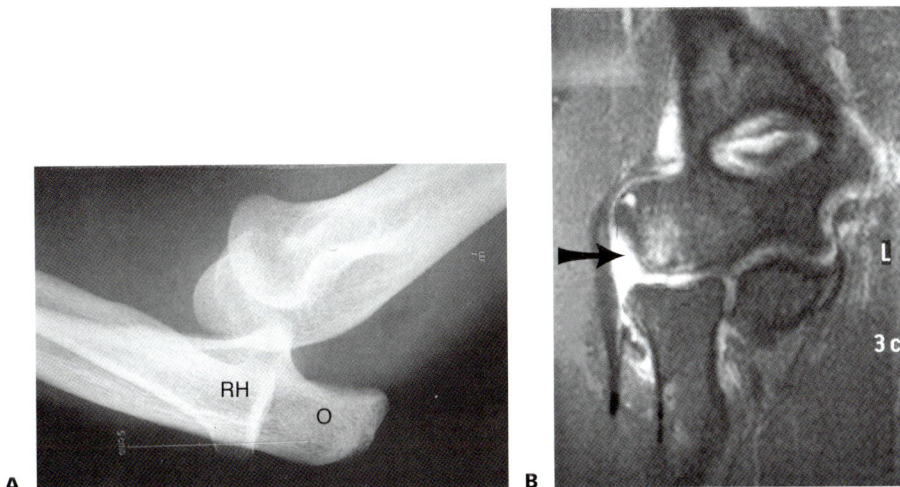

FIG 2 • **A.** Lateral view stress radiograph reveals complete ulnohumeral and radial head (*RH*) rotatory instability. *O*, olecranon. **B.** Coronal oblique view magnetic resonance image of elbow (with contrast enhancement). Lateral collateral ligament disruption can be seen (*arrow*).

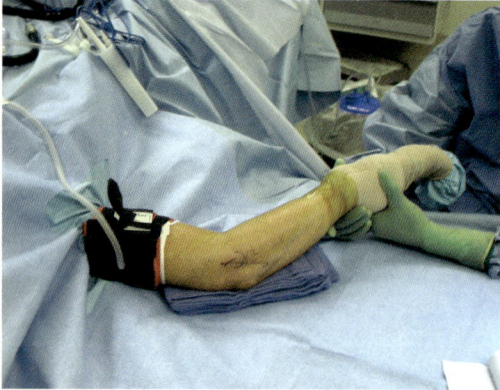

Approach

- The main approach is the Köcher interval between the anconeus and extensor carpi ulnaris muscles.
- This can be accomplished through a lateral skin incision or through a utilitarian posterior incision.
  - A posterior incision should be considered if a medial approach will also be needed to repair concomitant ligamentous or bony injury.

FIG 3 • The patient is placed supine on the operating room table. The arm is placed on an arm board with a sterile tourniquet applied to the upper arm and the entire arm draped free. During the approach, the forearm should be pronated to protect the posterior interosseous nerve.

FIGURE 8 YOKE TECHNIQUE

Surgical Approach

- A 10-cm incision is made over the Köcher interval.
  - The interval between the anconeus and the extensor carpi ulnaris is developed, and the remainder of the LCL complex is identified along with the supinator crest and the lateral epicondyle.
- The lateral epicondyle and 2 cm of the supracondylar ridge are exposed.

Tunnel Placement

- Two drill holes for the graft insertion site are made in the ulna.
  - One is drilled near the tubercle of the supinator crest (palpate in supination and varus stress), the other 1.25 cm proximal to that, near the insertion of the annular ligament (**TECH FIG 1A**).
- A suture is passed through the two holes and tied to itself. The suture is then held up against the lateral epicondyle as the elbow is ranged in flexion and extension to determine its isometric point.

- The isometric ligament insertion occurs at the point where the suture does NOT move.
- The isometric point is usually more anteroinferior than expected (**TECH FIG 1B,C**).
- A Y-shaped tunnel is made with the base exiting at the isometric point.
  - The hole is widened to accept a three-ply graft. (Palmaris longus is usually harvested; if not present, gracilis or allograft is used.) A 16-cm graft is usually sufficient.

Graft Passage and Tensioning and Wound Closure

- The graft is passed through the ulnar tunnel with enough length to just reach the isometric point.
  - The end is then sutured to the long end of the graft (the Yoke stitch).
  - The long end is then passed through the isometric point and exits the superior humeral tunnel (**TECH FIG 2A**).

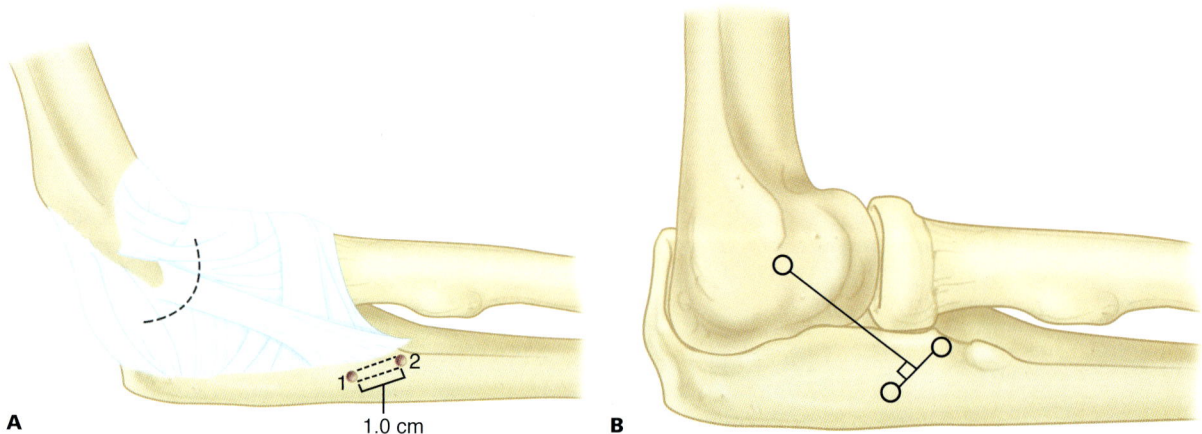

TECH FIG 1 • **A.** Two drill holes for the graft insertion site are made in the ulna. One is drilled near the tubercle of the supinator crest (palpate while varus and supination applied); the other is drilled 1.25 cm proximal, near the insertion of the annular ligament. *1*, proximal hole near insertion of annular ligament; *2*, tubercle of supinator crest. **B.** The ulnar holes should lie perpendicular to the intended direction of the lateral ulnar collateral ligament. *(continued)*

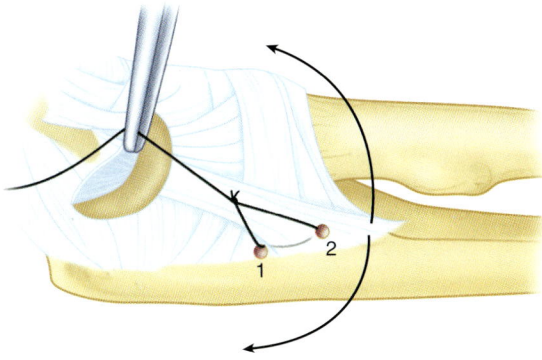

TECH FIG 1 • *(continued)* **C.** A suture is passed through the two holes and tied to itself. The suture is then held up with a hemostat against the lateral epicondyle as the elbow is ranged in flexion and extension to determine its isometric point. No movement occurs if the suture is at the isometric point.

- The long end is wrapped around the supracondylar ridge and passed through the distal tunnel, exiting back through the isometric point and into the ulnar tunnel.
  - The graft is then tensioned in 40 degrees of flexion, full pronation, and axial tension.
  - If the graft is not long enough to reach the ulnar tunnel, it can be sutured back to itself (**TECH FIG 2B**).
- The reconstruction can be reinforced by weaving a no. 2 Fiberwire suture (Arthrex, Inc., Naples, FL) from distal to proximal through the course of the figure 8, thus sewing the graft to itself.
- Plicate the anterior and posterior capsule as needed.
- The extensor origin is repaired to the lateral epicondyle, and the extensor carpi ulnaris fascia is reapproximated to the anconeus muscle with absorbable sutures.

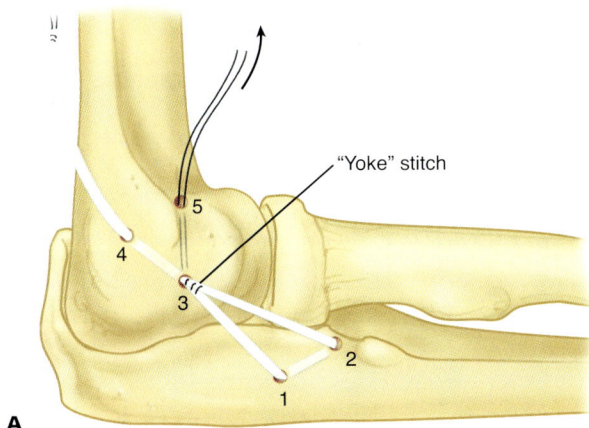

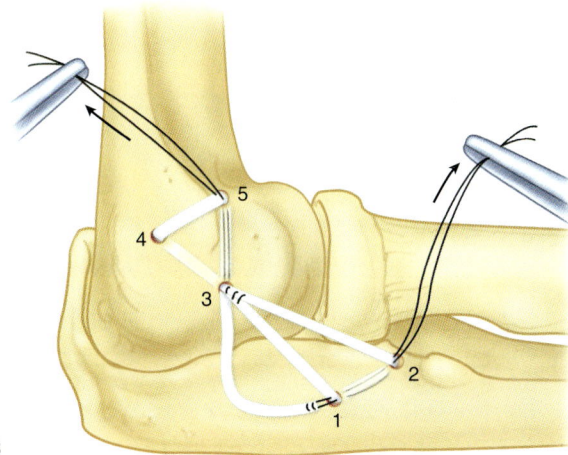

TECH FIG 2 • **A.** A Y-shaped tunnel is made with the base exiting at the isometric point (3). The hole is widened to accept a three-ply graft. The tendon graft is passed through the ulnar tunnel (1→2) with enough length to just reach the isometric point. The end is then sutured to the long end of the graft (the Yoke stitch). The long end is then passed through the isometric point and exits the superior humeral tunnel (3→4). **B.** The long end is then passed through the distal tunnel, exiting back through the isometric point (5→3) and into the ulnar tunnel (3→1→2). The graft is then tensioned in 40 degrees of flexion, full pronation, and axial tension. If the graft is not long enough to reach the ulnar tunnel, it can be sutured back to itself.

SPLIT ANCONEUS FASCIA TRANSFER

- We have developed a reproducible technique for LCL reconstruction that has proved biomechanical strength and reproducibility.
- Advantages include using only local autograft tissue and the minimal creation of bone tunnels.[1,2]

Surgical Approach

- A 6- to 8-cm skin incision is made over the Köcher interval, exposing the underlying Köcher interval between the extensor carpi ulnaris and anconeus (**TECH FIG 3A,B**).

- The interval between the anconeus and extensor carpi ulnaris muscles is developed, taking care to preserve the remainder of the underlying LCL complex.
  - The annular ligament, lateral epicondyle, and 2 cm of supracondylar ridge are isolated (**TECH FIG 3C**).

Graft Preparation

- The anconeus and distal triceps fascia are isolated in continuity. A 1.0-cm-wide by 8.0-cm-long band of fascia is mobilized off the underlying muscle, leaving the ulnar insertion intact (**TECH FIG 4A,B**).

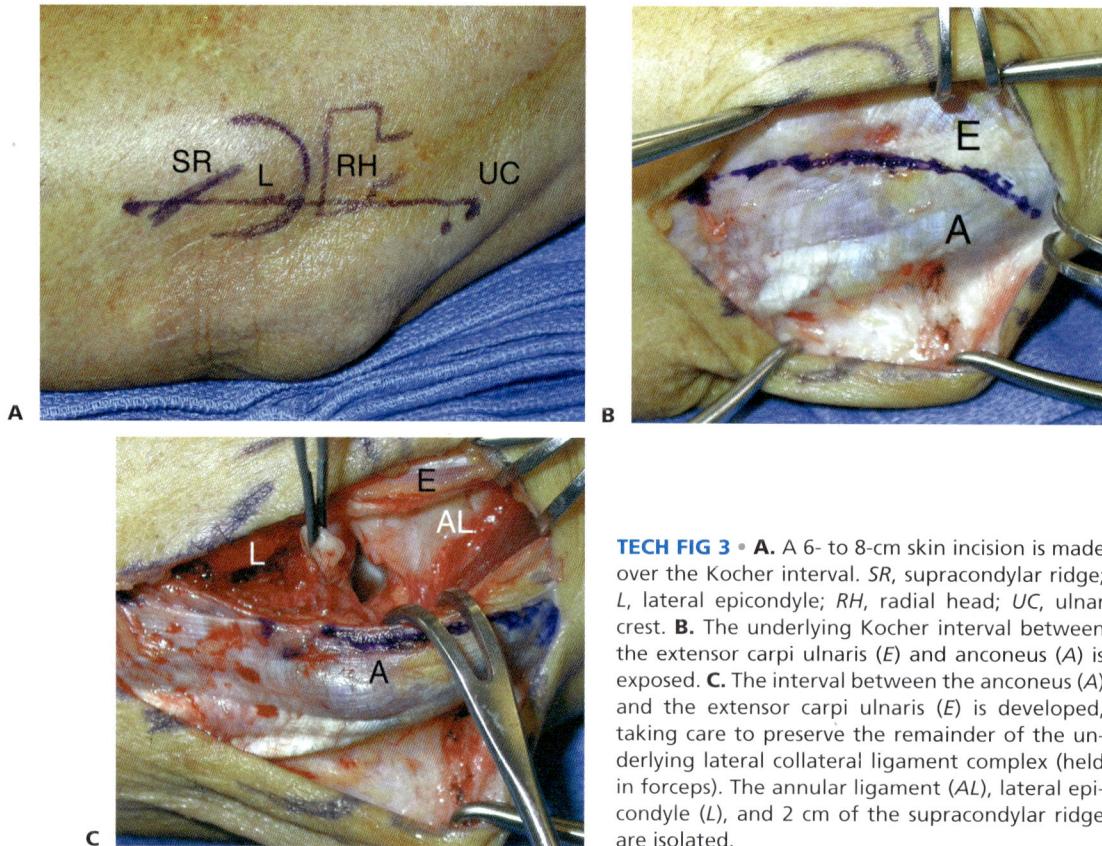

TECH FIG 3 • **A.** A 6- to 8-cm skin incision is made over the Kocher interval. *SR*, supracondylar ridge; *L*, lateral epicondyle; *RH*, radial head; *UC*, ulnar crest. **B.** The underlying Kocher interval between the extensor carpi ulnaris (*E*) and anconeus (*A*) is exposed. **C.** The interval between the anconeus (*A*) and the extensor carpi ulnaris (*E*) is developed, taking care to preserve the remainder of the underlying lateral collateral ligament complex (held in forceps). The annular ligament (*AL*), lateral epicondyle (*L*), and 2 cm of the supracondylar ridge are isolated.

- The band is then divided longitudinally into two bands of equal width (**TECH FIG 4C**).
- The anterior band is passed through an incision just distal to the annular ligament while the posterior band is passed under the anconeus muscle (**TECH FIG 4D**).
- The isometric point of the lateral epicondyle is then located by holding the two bands against the epicondyle while ranging the elbow (**TECH FIG 4E**).
- The final lengths of the fascial bands are estimated by holding the bands along their respective paths. The bands are then trimmed appropriately to prevent them from "bottoming out" prematurely in the humeral docking tunnel.

- Separate Krackow sutures are placed in each band with no. 0 FiberWire suture.

Tunnel Preparation

- A 5-mm round burr is used to create a 1.5-cm-long (depth) docking tunnel into the humerus at the isometric point. A 1-mm side-cutting burr is then used to make anterior and posterior bone bridge holes. The holes are separated by 1.5 cm. Individual suture lassos are placed from proximal to distal into the docking tunnel from the separate humeral tunnels (**TECH FIG 5**).

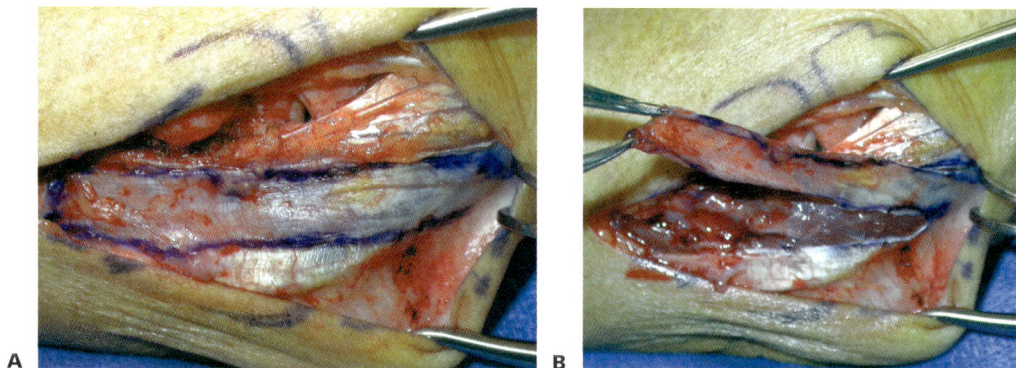

TECH FIG 4 • **A.** The anconeus and distal triceps fascia are isolated in continuity. **B.** A 1.0-cm-wide by 8.0-cm-long band of fascia is mobilized off the underlying muscle, leaving the ulnar insertion. *(continued)*

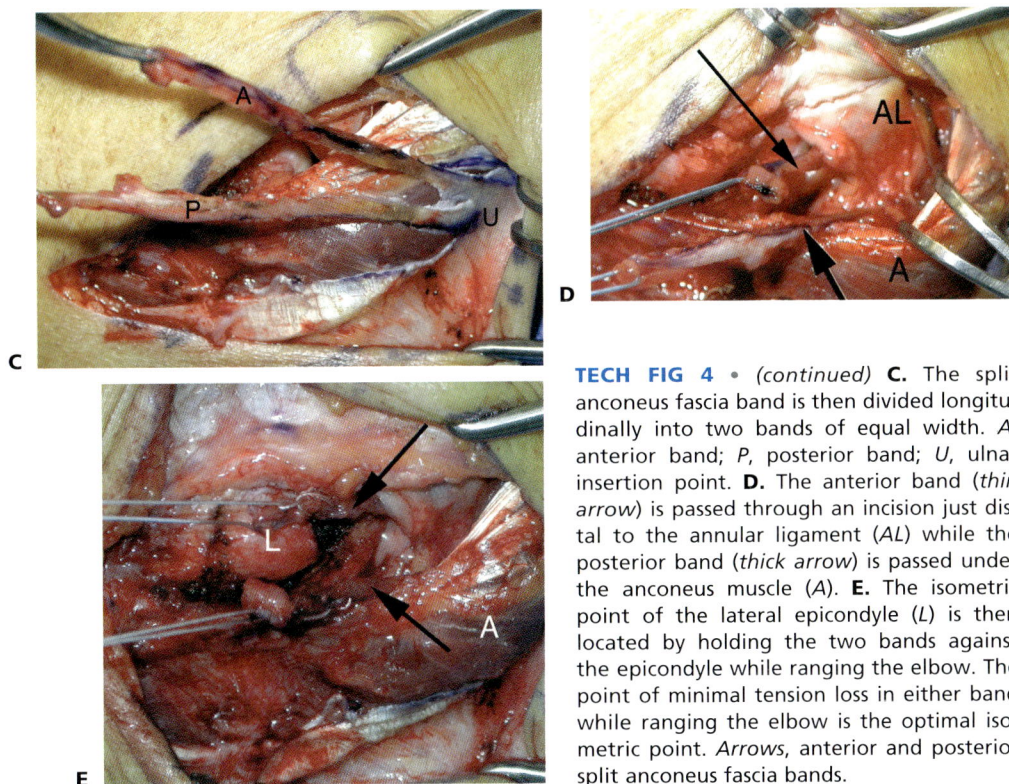

TECH FIG 4 • *(continued)* **C.** The split anconeus fascia band is then divided longitudinally into two bands of equal width. *A,* anterior band; *P,* posterior band; *U,* ulnar insertion point. **D.** The anterior band (*thin arrow*) is passed through an incision just distal to the annular ligament (*AL*) while the posterior band (*thick arrow*) is passed under the anconeus muscle (*A*). **E.** The isometric point of the lateral epicondyle (*L*) is then located by holding the two bands against the epicondyle while ranging the elbow. The point of minimal tension loss in either band while ranging the elbow is the optimal isometric point. *Arrows,* anterior and posterior split anconeus fascia bands.

Graft Passage and Tensioning and Wound Closure

- The anterior band sutures are brought out the anterior humeral exit hole by using suture passers. The posterior band passes superficial to the annular ligament, and its sutures are brought out the posterior humeral exit tunnel.
- The ends of the fascial bands are docked into the humeral tunnel, and the grafts are tensioned with the elbow in 40 degrees of flexion, in full pronation, and with a valgus stress.
- The sutures are then tied over the bony bridge on the supracondylar ridge (**TECH FIG 6A**).
- The extensor origin is then repaired to the lateral epicondyle and the extensor carpi ulnaris fascia is reapproximated to the anconeus muscle with absorbable sutures.
- The skin is closed with a running subcuticular suture (**TECH FIG 6B**).

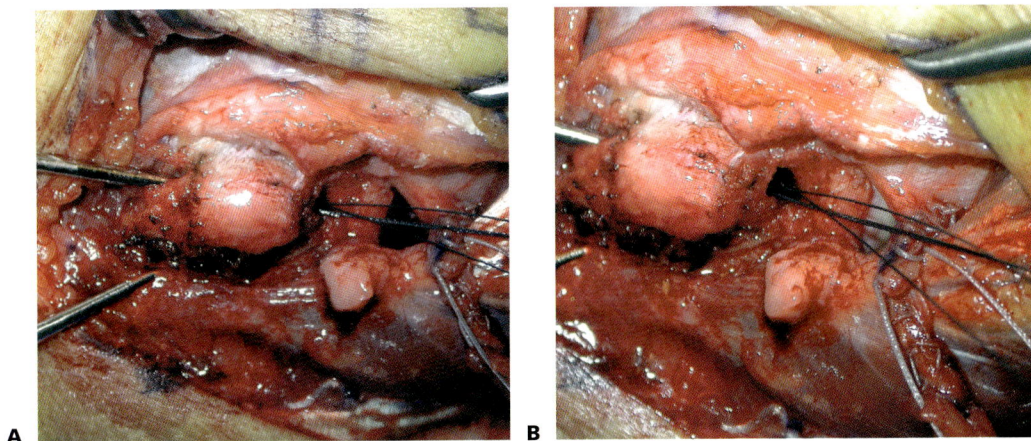

TECH FIG 5 • **A.** Suture lassos passed through exit holes out distal docking tunnel. *SCR,* supracondylar ridge. **B.** Suture lasso wires exiting docking tunnel.

TECHNIQUES

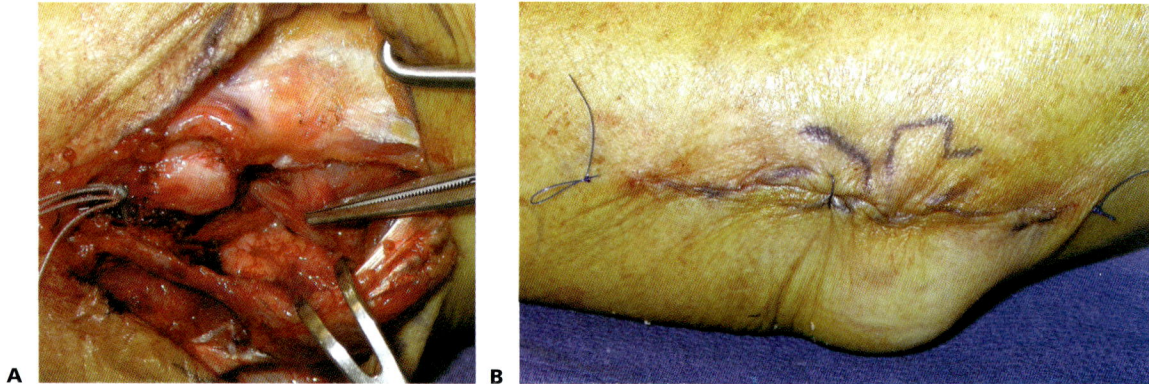

TECH FIG 6 • A. The ends of the fascial bands are docked into the humeral tunnel, and the grafts are tensioned with the elbow in 40 degrees of flexion, full pronation, and valgus stress. Sutures are then tied over the bony bridge on the supracondylar ridge (clamp on posterior band). **B.** The incision is closed with subcuticular suture.

DOCKING TECHNIQUE

- As previously discussed, the Köcher approach is used for the docking technique.
- Preparation of the ulnar drill holes is described in the section on the figure 8 yoke technique elsewhere in this chapter.
- A 5-mm round burr is used to create a 1.5-cm-long (depth) docking tunnel into the humerus at the isometric point. A 1-mm side-cutting burr is then used to make anterior and posterior bone bridge holes. The holes are separated by 1.5 cm. Individual suture lassos are placed from proximal to distal into the docking tunnel from the separate humeral tunnels (see Tech Fig 5).
- After passage of the graft through the ulnar tunnels, the final lengths of the two graft strands are estimated by holding the strands against the docking tunnel with the arm in the "reduced" position of 40 degrees of flexion, full pronation, and axial tension.

- The strands are then trimmed appropriately to prevent the strands from "bottoming out" prematurely in the humeral docking tunnel.
  - Separate Krackow sutures are placed in each graft strand with no. 0 FiberWire suture for 1 cm.
- The anterior graft strand sutures are brought out the anterior humeral exit hole by using suture passers. The posterior graft strand sutures are brought out the posterior humeral exit tunnel.
- The ends of the humeral graft portion are docked into the humeral tunnel, and the grafts are tensioned with the elbow in 40 degrees of flexion, in full pronation, and with a valgus stress.
- The sutures are then tied over the bony bridge on the supracondylar ridge.
- Standard incision closure is performed.

DIRECT REPAIR

- As previously discussed, the Köcher approach is used for direct repair.
- If the LCL complex is intact but avulsed from its ulnar or humeral attachments (or both), it can be directly repaired to its correct anatomic location with suture anchors or bone tunnels.
- A running locked no. 2 FiberWire suture is placed into the detached LCL complex and repaired back to its origin on the lateral epicondyle through the anterior and posterior drill holes (**TECH FIG 7**).
- A careful repair of the extensor origin and the interval between the anconeus and the extensor carpi ulnaris is performed.

TECH FIG 7 • Primary lateral ulnar collateral ligament repair. Running locked suture placed through detached lateral ulnar collateral ligament. A relaxing incision can be made at its attachment to the base of the annular ligament. Repair through drill holes in the lateral epicondyle.

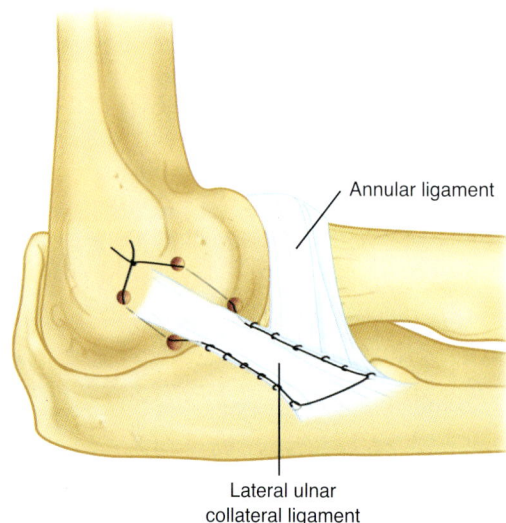

Annular ligament

Lateral ulnar collateral ligament

PEARLS AND PITFALLS

Indications	■ Iatrogenic causes (eg, "tennis elbow" surgery) very common ■ Careful history and physical examination to exclude other pathologic conditions ■ History of numerous lateral elbow corticosteroid injections
Split anconeus fascia technique: exposure	■ Isolate Köcher interval; fatty stripe within interval. ■ Anconeus fibers oblique to extensor carpi ulnaris ■ Identify LCL disruption. ■ Isolate annular ligament; protect posterior interosseous nerve.
Splint anconeus fascia preparation	■ Be careful to harvest long enough fascial band (proximal to humeral bone tunnels). ■ Be careful not to detach from ulnar insertion. ■ Isolate LCL complex isometric point of origin. ■ Harvest fascial band in line with old LUCL.
Figure 8 yoke technique	■ Carefully isolate isometric point on lateral epicondyle, usually more anterior and inferior; err on inferior placement. ■ Make ulnar tunnel perpendicular to direction of LUCL. ■ Chamfer bone tunnels to prevent graft impingement and breakage.
Bone tunnel preparation	■ Maintain sufficient bony bridge between tunnels. ■ Smooth edges to prevent graft irritation.
Arm position for final graft tensioning	■ 40 degrees of elbow flexion ■ Full pronation ■ Axial load, valgus stress

POSTOPERATIVE CARE

■ Stage I (0 to 3 weeks)
  ■ Elbow immobilization in posterior splint or brace at 40 degrees of flexion
  ■ Wrist and hand isometrics as tolerated
  ■ Shoulder active and passive ROM
■ Stage II (3 to 6 weeks)
  ■ Hinged elbow brace or orthoplast splint, with limits set by surgeon
  ■ Begin flexor–pronator isometrics
  ■ Continue with wrist and hand strengthening
  ■ Continue shoulder as above
  ■ Active-assisted ROM: 20 to 120 degrees of flexion; keep forearm pronated at all times
■ Stage III (6 to 12 weeks)
  ■ Discontinue immobilization
  ■ Passive ROM and active-assisted ROM to full motion, including supination
  ■ Begin unrestricted strengthening of flexor–pronators and extensors
■ Stage IV (3 to 6 months)
  ■ Avoid varus stress to elbow and ballistic movement in terminal elbow ranges
  ■ Begin shoulder strengthening with light resistance (emphasis on cuff)
  ■ Start total body conditioning
  ■ Terminal elbow stretching in flexion and extension
  ■ Resistive elbow exercises as tolerated

OUTCOMES

■ Nestor et al[5] have shown successful functional outcomes in patients using the figure 8 reconstruction technique with reproducible results.

■ Our early experience with the split anconeus fascia reconstruction technique has shown excellent results, with no failures to date in 22 patients at an average follow-up of 2 years. All elbows have achieved stability without loss of motion.

COMPLICATIONS

■ Recurrent elbow instability
■ Elbow stiffness
■ Infection
■ Graft harvest site morbidity (if remote autograft is used for reconstruction)
■ Humerus stress fracture through bone tunnels
■ Ulnar stress fracture through bone tunnels
■ Bone bridge compromise

REFERENCES

1. Chebli CA, Murthi AM. Lateral collateral ligament complex: anatomic and biomechanical testing. 73rd Annual Meeting and Scientific Program of the American Academy of Orthopaedic Surgeons, Chicago, March 2006.
2. Chebli CM, Murthi AM. Split anconeus fascia transfer for reconstruction of the elbow lateral collateral ligament complex: anatomic and biomechanical testing. 22nd Open Meeting of the American Shoulder and Elbow Surgeons. Chicago, IL, March 2006.
3. Cohen MS, Hastings H II. Acute elbow dislocation: evaluation and management. J Am Acad Orthop Surg 1998;6:15–23.
4. Kalainov DM, Cohen MS. Posterolateral rotatory instability of the elbow in association with lateral epicondylitis: a report of three cases. J Bone Joint Surg Am 2005;87A:1120–1125.
5. Nestor BJ, O'Driscoll SW, Morrey BF. Ligamentous reconstruction for posterolateral rotatory instability of the elbow. J Bone Joint Surg Am 1992;74A:1235–1241.
6. O'Driscoll SW, Bell DF, Morrey BF. Posterolateral rotatory instability of the elbow. J Bone Joint Surg Am 1991;73A:440–446.
7. O'Driscoll SW, Spinner RJ, McKee MD, et al. Tardy posterolateral rotatory instability of the elbow due to cubitus varus. J Bone Joint Surg Am 2001;83A:1358–1369.

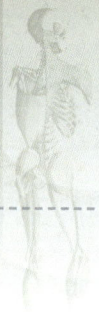

Chapter 42

Ulnohumeral (Outerbridge-Kashiwagi) Arthroplasty

Filippos S. Giannoulis, Alexander H. Payatakes, and Dean G. Sotereanos

DEFINITION

- Primary osteoarthritis of the elbow is a relatively uncommon but limiting disorder that affects mostly middle-aged men who use the upper extremity in a repetitive fashion. Typically, patients are heavy manual workers or athletes. Osteoarthritis affects the elbow less frequently than other major joints.
- Early stages of arthritis of the elbow may be characterized primarily by pain at the extremes of motion, with some loss of terminal extension and flexion. Some patients present with pain carrying an object with the arm in extension. More advanced stages may present with pain and crepitus throughout the range of motion, stiffness, or locking. Rotation of the forearm may be spared, depending on radiohumeral involvement.
- Radiographs show osteophyte formation on the coronoid and olecranon but relatively preserved joint space at the early stages. More advanced stages may be associated with significant joint space narrowing.
- Multiple operative techniques have been described for treatment of primary osteoarthritis of the elbow: débridement arthroplasty, interposition arthroplasty, the Outerbridge-Kashiwagi procedure, arthroscopic débridement, and total elbow replacement.
  - Ulnohumeral (Outerbridge-Kashiwagi) arthroplasty was first described in 1978 and became popular a few years later. It is based on a posterior approach to the elbow, removal of olecranon spur and bony overgrowth of the olecranon fossa, and drilling of a hole in this fossa with a trephine to expose the anterior capsule and excise the coronoid osteophyte.

ANATOMY

- The elbow joint consists of three separate articulations: the ulnohumeral, the radiocapitellar, and the proximal radioulnar joints.
- The elbow has two main functions: position the hand in space and stabilize the upper extremity for motor activities and power.
- The normal range of elbow flexion–extension is 0 to 150 degrees and normal forearm pronation–supination is 80 and 80 degrees.
- A 100-degree flexion–extension arc of motion, from 30 to 130 degrees, is quoted for normal activities of daily living. Functional forearm rotation is quoted as 100 degrees, with 50 degrees pronation and 50 degrees supination.
- The condyles articulate at the elbow joint, as the trochlea medially and the capitellum laterally. The articular surface is angled about 30 degrees anterior to the axis of the humeral shaft and has a slight valgus position, about 6 degrees, compared to the epicondylar axis.

- The coronoid fossa and the olecranon fossa, just proximal to the articular surface, accommodate the coronoid process and olecranon process of the ulna in the extremes of flexion and extension, respectively.
- The olecranon and coronoid process coalesce to form the greater sigmoid notch, the articulating portion of the proximal ulna. It is often not completely covered with articular cartilage centrally.

PATHOGENESIS

- Symptomatic osteoarthritis of the elbow has been found to affect about 2% of the general population and represents only 1% to 2% of all patients diagnosed with degenerative arthritis.
- It has a predilection for males, with a ratio of 4 or 5 to 1. It is most commonly seen in middle-aged and older patients.
- The majority of patients experience symptoms in their dominant extremity.
- The exact etiology of primary degenerative elbow arthritis is still unknown. It is generally attributed to overuse. About 60% of patients report employment or hobbies or sports requiring repetitive use of the limb. The few younger patients who present likely have a predisposing condition such as osteochondritis dissecans.
- There are characteristic pathologic changes that occur within the elbow joint: osteophyte formation on the olecranon, olecranon fossa, coronoid, and coronoid fossa.
  - In early stages the joint space is relatively preserved. The periarticular bone is typically hard.
  - Very often, loose bodies may be present into the joint and cause clicking or locking of the elbow, or both.
  - Capsular contracture and fibrosis of the anterior capsule contribute to loss of extension.

NATURAL HISTORY

- Early stages of primary osteoarthritis of the elbow are characterized by pain at the extremes of motion and some loss of terminal extension and flexion. As the severity of the arthritis progresses, pain, stiffness, and loss of range of motion increase.
- When symptoms do not improve with nonoperative treatment, surgical intervention is indicated.
- Because osteoarthritis is a progressive disease, symptoms and pathologic condition may recur. The most common problem is recurrence of impingement pain and flexion contractures.
- Prognostic factors include the etiology of arthritis, the degree of motion loss, mid-arc versus end-range discomfort, the presence of loose bodies, mechanical symptoms, and the presence or absence of cubital tunnel syndrome.

PATIENT HISTORY AND PHYSICAL FINDINGS

- The typical patient with primary degenerative elbow arthritis is a man older than 45 years of age, exposed to repetitive manual labor, who presents with pain at the end ranges of motion, especially in extension.
- Younger patients also may provide a history of sports such as weightlifting, boxing, and other throwing-intensive activities. Arthritic elbows in athletes frequently will include a spectrum of pathologic changes, such as loose bodies and bone spurs.
- Some patients report a history of chronic use of crutches or wheelchairs.
- The chief complaint is pain, especially terminal extension pain, as a result of mechanical impingement.
  - Patients usually feel pain while carrying objects with the elbow in full extension.
  - The intensity of pain is mild to moderate and only occasionally is described as severe.
  - Pain is not usually noted in the mid-range of motion until later stages of arthritis.
- Loss of motion is the most common presenting symptom.
  - Loss of extension is often partially the result of posterior olecranon and humeral osteophytes or anterior capsule contracture.
  - Loss of flexion is secondary to osteophytes on the coronoid or its fossa and to loose bodies.
  - Supination–pronation is not restricted or is only minimally restricted, owing to limited involvement of the radiohumeral joint.
- Catching or locking may be present with articular incongruity, or when loose bodies are present.
- Crepitus may be present throughout the range of motion.
- Swelling may occur but is not typical.
- Ulnar nerve symptoms may also be present owing to excessive osteophyte formation. They should actively be sought out because they may influence treatment decisions and even direct the surgical approach.
- Physical examination may reveal a positive Tinel sign and a positive elbow flexion test, with decreased sensation and weakness in the ulnar nerve distribution. Cubital tunnel syndrome may be present in up to 20% of patients.

IMAGING AND OTHER DIAGNOSTIC STUDIES

- Anteroposterior (AP), lateral, and oblique radiographs (**FIG 1**) are diagnostic and illustrate characteristic features of the condition.
  - The AP view should be taken with the beam perpendicular to the distal humerus for distal humerus pathology and perpendicular to the radial head for proximal forearm pathology. These views will show ossification and osteophyte formation of the olecranon and coronoid fossa.
  - The lateral view should be taken in 90 degrees of flexion with the forearm in neutral rotation. This view will show an anterior osteophyte on the coronoid fossa and process and a posterior osteophyte on the olecranon fossa and process.
  - The lateral oblique view provides better visualization of the radiocapitellar joint, medial epicondyle, and radioulnar joint.
  - The medial oblique view provides better visualization of the trochlea, olecranon fossa, and coronoid tip.
  - A cubital tunnel view may be useful if there is ulnar nerve symptomatology.
- A lateral tomogram and computed tomography are helpful for preoperative planning to assess the presence and location of loose bodies and subtle osteophyte formation (especially in earlier stages).

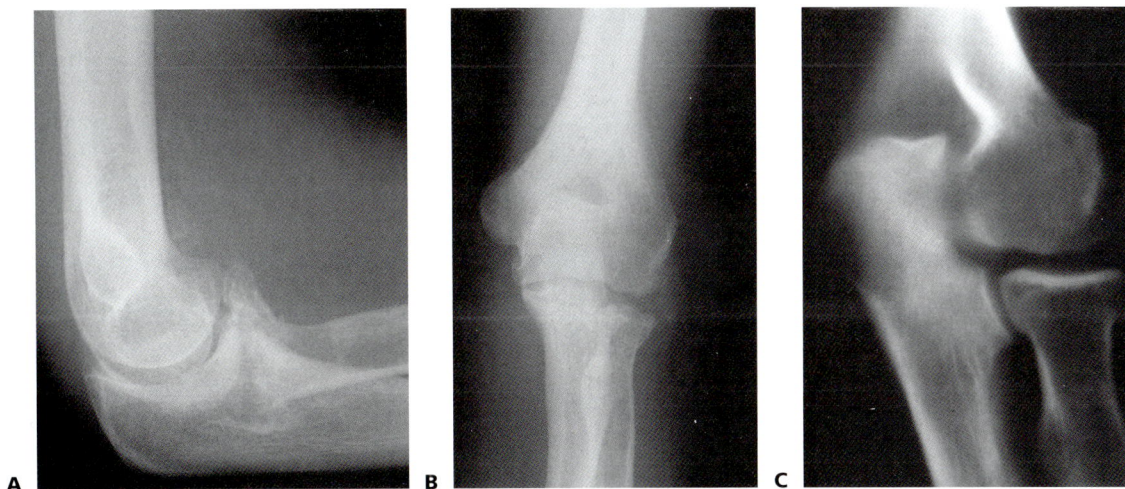

FIG 1 • A. Lateral radiograph of a 50-year-old heavy laborer's elbow. The patient had severe pain at the extremes of motion. The radiograph reveals characteristic osteophytes of the olecranon and of the coronoid process. **B.** AP radiograph of the elbow (same patient). This view shows ossification and osteophytes of the olecranon and coronoid fossa. **C.** Lateral oblique radiograph. This view provides better visualization of the radiocapitellar and radioulnar joint. There is an osteophyte at the tip of the olecranon, which causes pain during full extension.

DIFFERENTIAL DIAGNOSIS

- Posttraumatic arthritis
- Rheumatoid (inflammatory) arthritis

NONOPERATIVE MANAGEMENT

- Nonoperative treatment may be helpful in the early stages.
- Patients should limit activities that require heavy elbow use.
- Physical therapy is used to maintain range of motion and strength. Modalities such as heat and cold may be effective.
- Nonsteroidal anti-inflammatory drugs can decrease pain and are of some value. Intra-articular corticosteroid injections may also improve symptoms, but their benefits are usually temporary.
- Avoidance of pressure on the cubital tunnel and avoidance of prolonged elbow flexion are recommended if ulnar nerve symptoms are present.

SURGICAL MANAGEMENT

- Surgical treatment is indicated when symptoms do not improve with appropriate nonoperative management.
- The procedure is indicated in patients with pain in terminal extension or flexion (or both), radiographic evidence of coronoid or olecranon osteophytes (or both), ulnar neuropathy, and functional limitations due to pain or loss of motion.
- The procedure is contraindicated in patients with pain throughout the entire arc of motion, marked limitation of motion with an arc of less than 40 degrees, or severe involvement of the radiohumeral or proximal radioulnar joints.

Preoperative Planning

- It is very important to carefully review all radiographs (AP, lateral, oblique) before surgery to assess the severity of arthritic changes and evaluate for the presence of loose bodies. A lateral tomogram or CT scan may assist in this evaluation. Care should be taken not to overlook any loose bodies, as these may lead to persistent mechanical symptoms postoperatively.
- Specific attention should be paid to the presence of ulnar nerve pathology. If present, this must be addressed at the time of the procedure.

Positioning

- There are two options for positioning:
  - The patient may be positioned in the lateral decubitus position with the elbow flexed at 90 degrees and resting on an armrest.

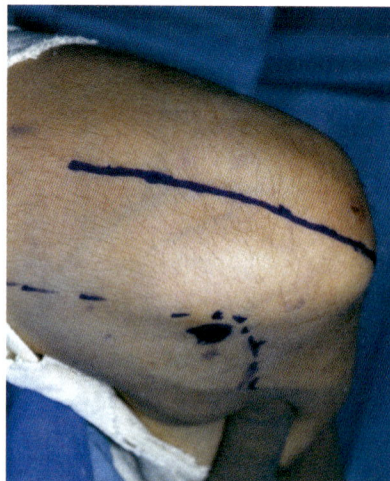

FIG 2 • With the patient in the lateral decubitus position, the elbow is flexed at 90 degrees and is resting on pillows (authors' preferred method). A posterior approach is used via a straight skin incision, which extends distally about 4 cm and proximally 6 to 8 cm from the tip of the olecranon. Note the marked medial epicondyle.

- Alternatively, the patient may be placed supine with a sandbag underneath the scapula. The elbow is flexed at 90 degrees and brought across the chest. The patient is rotated about 35 degrees for better access to the posterior aspect of the affected elbow.

Approach

- A posterior approach is used. The incision is straight, starting 6 to 8 cm proximal to the tip of the olecranon and extending 4 cm distal to the olecranon (**FIG 2**).
- Dissection is carried down to the triceps fascia.
- The triceps tendon can be split or reflected. In the original description, the triceps muscle is split along the midline, exposing the posterior aspect of the elbow to the lateral and medial supracondylar ridges. Alternatively, the medial margin of the triceps tendon may be reflected from the olecranon.
- The decision to reflect or to split the tendon can be determined based on the size of the distal part of the triceps and the need to explore and decompress the ulnar nerve. If the muscle is very bulky, reflection will not provide adequate exposure.

EXPOSURE

- After the skin incision is made, the subcutaneous tissue is reflected from the medial aspect of the triceps.
- The ulnar nerve is identified and decompressed at the cubital tunnel if there is evidence of ulnar nerve pathology.
- The triceps muscle–tendon unit is split longitudinally or reflected.

- The triceps is elevated from the posterior aspect of the distal humerus by blunt dissection using a periosteal elevator.
- A capsulotomy is then performed (**TECH FIG 1**).

TECHNIQUES

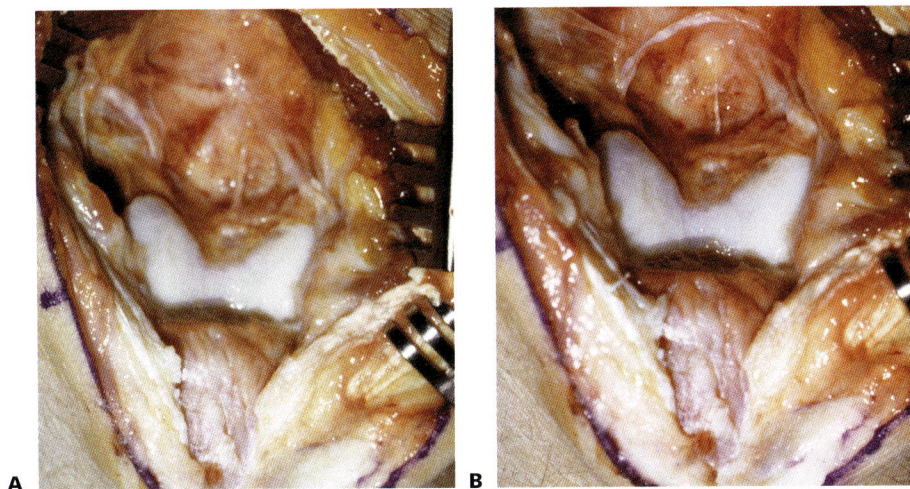

TECH FIG 1 • The triceps muscle has been split to expose the posterior joint. The prominent olecranon osteophyte and the tip of the olecranon process are then removed. The initial cut should be made with an oscillating saw to provide optimal orientation. The osteotomy of the olecranon is completed with an osteotome parallel to each face of the trochlea.

OSTEOPHYTE REMOVAL AND OLECRANON RESECTION

- To minimize impingement in extension, the posterior osteophyte and the tip of the olecranon are removed using an oscillating saw. An osteotome is then used to complete the resection. The orientation of the osteotomy should be parallel to each face of the trochlea.

- A rongeur is used to smooth the edges.
- A hole is drilled in the olecranon fossa to gain access to the anterior elbow compartment and the coronoid process. This requires removal of osteophytes around the olecranon fossa (**TECH FIG 2**).

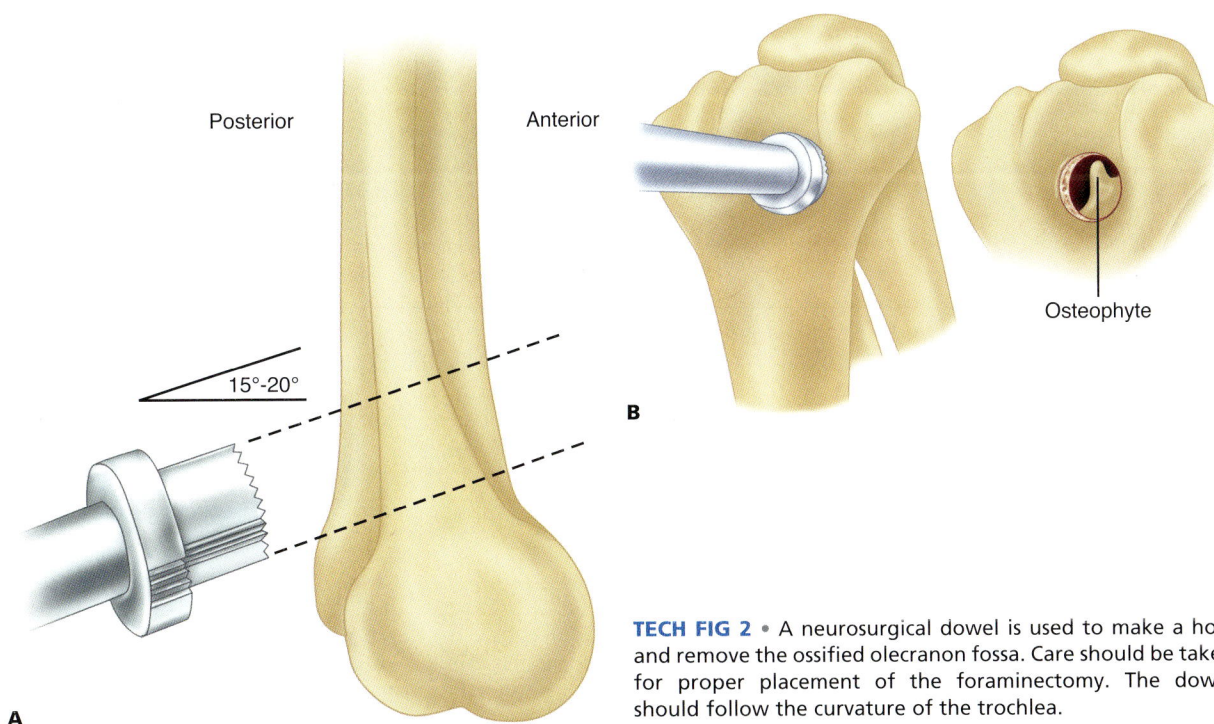

TECH FIG 2 • A neurosurgical dowel is used to make a hole and remove the ossified olecranon fossa. Care should be taken for proper placement of the foraminectomy. The dowel should follow the curvature of the trochlea.

FORAMINECTOMY

- A 1.5-cm neurosurgical dowel is applied to a reaming drill bit, and a drill hole is developed. Proper placement of this foraminectomy is of great importance. The dowel should follow the curvature of the trochlea.

- Once the foraminectomy is complete, a core of bone is removed from the distal humerus. This may include osteophytes from the anterior aspect of the joint (**TECH FIG 3A,B**).

TECHNIQUES

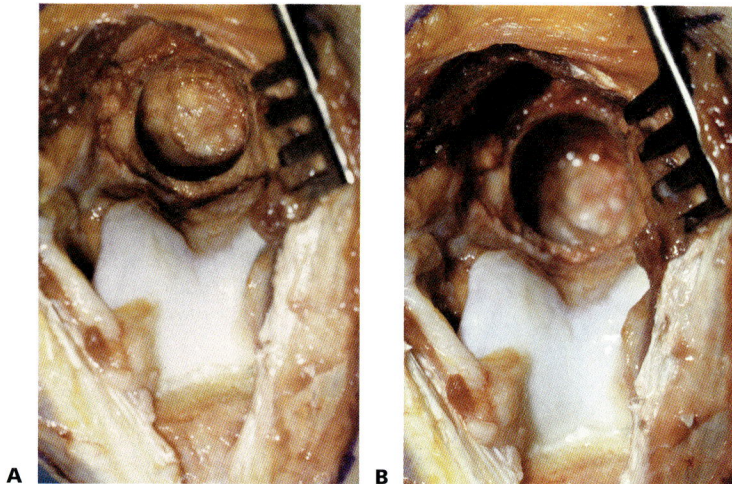

TECH FIG 3 • **A,B.** Once the foraminectomy is completed, the core of bone is removed from the distal humerus. This allows access to the anterior elbow compartment and to the coronoid. At this time, loose bodies of the anterior compartment may be identified and removed. **C.** With maximum elbow flexion, the anterior osteophyte from the coronoid process is removed, using a curved osteotome. **D.** An instrument is then introduced through the foramen and the osteophyte and a portion of the coronoid are removed.

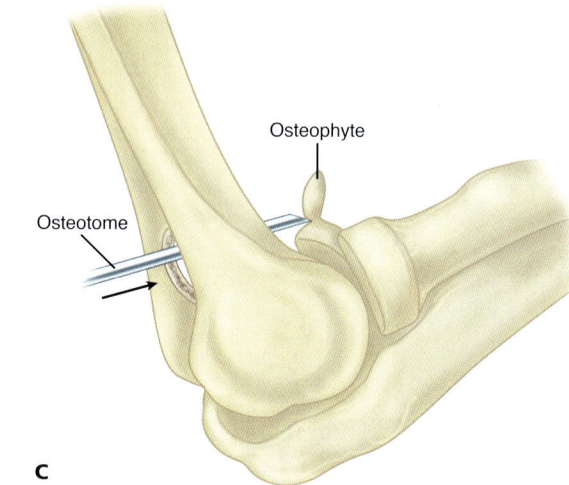

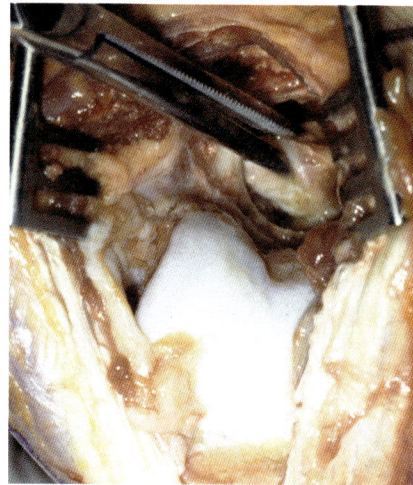

- This hole is used to clean debris and remove loose bodies from the anterior aspect of the elbow (**TECH FIG 3C,D**).
- With maximum elbow flexion, the anterior osteophyte from the coronoid process is removed using a curved osteotome.
- Occasionally it is necessary to strip the anterior capsule from the anterior humerus using a blunt periosteal elevator, to regain better extension.

- Care must be taken to ensure that no osteophytes or loose bodies are overlooked.
- Bone wax is used to cover the margins of the foramen, and Gelfoam is inserted into the defect to fill the dead space.
- The wound is meticulously irrigated and closed in standard fashion.
- The elbow is carefully manipulated to maximize the total arc of motion.

PEARLS AND PITFALLS

Indications	■ Primary osteoarthritis of the elbow presenting with pain at the extremes of motion due to osteophyte formation on the olecranon or coronoid process (or both) and in the olecranon or coronoid fossa (or both)
Contraindications	■ Severe involvement of the radiohumeral joint ■ Pain throughout the entire arc of motion
Assessment	■ Careful selection of patients is important. ■ Appropriate imaging studies should be obtained to identify all loose bodies or osteophytes. A preoperative lateral tomogram may be indicated. ■ The surgeon should always evaluate for coexisting ulnar nerve pathology, which should be addressed during surgery.
Operation	■ Proper placement of foraminectomy ■ Meticulous inspection of posterior and anterior aspects of the joint ■ Removal of all loose bodies and osteophytes

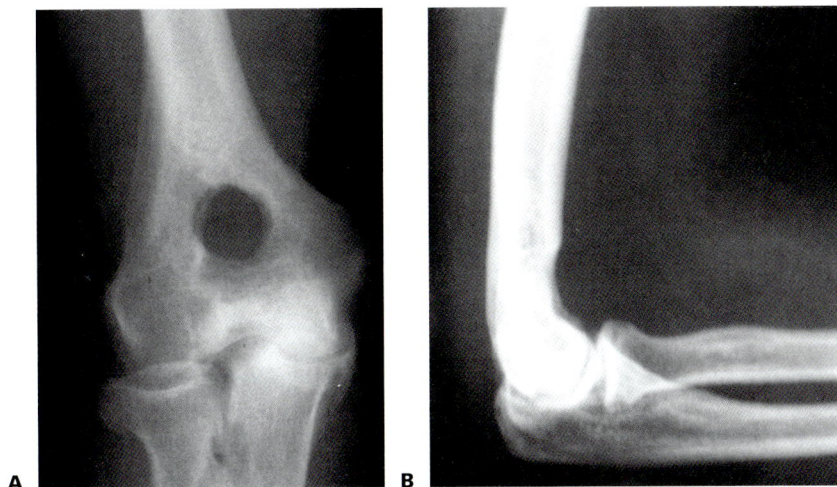

FIG 3 • AP and lateral radiographs after ulnohumeral arthroplasty has been performed. The hole of the foraminectomized distal humerus can be easily seen. There are no osteophytes of the olecranon and coronoid process and the patient has gained a much better arc of motion without pain.

POSTOPERATIVE CARE

■ A splint is applied with the elbow in 15 degrees of extension for 1 week.
■ Active range of motion is allowed 7 to 10 days after surgery.
■ The patient is re-evaluated at 3 weeks, 6 weeks, and 3 months after surgery.
■ Continuous passive motion can be initiated on the day of surgery and is discontinued after 3 weeks.

OUTCOMES

■ A review of the literature shows satisfactory results in over 80% of patients.
■ Satisfactory pain relief is achieved in about 90% of patients.
■ Extension improves by about 10 to 15 degrees and flexion improves by about 10 degrees. Overall improvement in the motion arc is about 20 to 25 degrees (**FIG 3**).
■ There have been no reports of postoperative instability.

COMPLICATIONS

■ The complication rate for this procedure is very low, in contrast to most reconstructive procedures of the elbow.
■ The recurrence rate is less than 10%.
■ Iatrogenic ulnar nerve palsy is unusual, but can occur as a result of overzealous use of retractors intraoperatively.
■ Improper placement of the foraminectomy may result in a column fracture.

REFERENCES

1. Antuna SA, Morrey BF, Adams RA, et al. Ulnohumeral arthroplasty for primary degenerative arthritis of the elbow. J Bone Joint Surg Am 2002;84A:2168–2173.
2. Forster MC, Clark DI, Lunn PG. Elbow osteoarthritis: prognostic indicators in ulnohumeral debridement—the Outerbridge-Kashiwagi procedure. J Shoulder Elbow Surg 2001;10:557–560.
3. Kashiwagi D. Intra-articular changes of the osteoarthritic elbow, especially about the fossa olecrani. J Jpn Orthop Assoc 1978;52:1367–1382.
4. Kashiwagi D. Outerbridge-Kashiwagi arthroplasty for osteoarthritis of the elbow. In Kashiwagi D, ed. Elbow joint. Proceedings of the International Congress, Kobi, Japan. Amsterdam: Elsevier Science Publishers, 1986:177–188.
5. Minami M, Kato S, Kashiwagi D. Outerbridge-Kashiwagi's method for arthroplasty of osteoarthritis of the elbow: 44 elbows followed for 8–16 years. J Orthop Sci 1996;1:11–15.
6. Morrey BF. Primary degenerative arthritis of the elbow: treatment by ulnohumeral arthroplasty. J Bone Joint Surg Br 1992;74B:409–413.
7. Morrey BF. Primary degenerative arthritis of the elbow: ulnohumeral arthroplasty. In: Morrey BF, ed. The Elbow and Its Disorders. Philadelphia: WB Saunders, 2000:799–808.
8. Morrey BF. Ulnohumeral arthroplasty. In: Morrey BF, ed. Master Techniques in Orthopaedic Surgery: The Elbow. New York: Raven Press Ltd, 1994:277–289.
9. O'Driscoll SW. Elbow arthritis: treatment options. J Am Acad Orthop Surg 1993;1:106.
10. Tsuge K, Mizuseki T. Debridement arthroplasty for advanced primary osteoarthritis of the elbow. J Bone Joint Surg Br 1994;76B:641–646.
11. Tsuge K, Murakami T, Yasunaga Y, et al. Arthroplasty of the elbow: twenty years experience of a new approach. J Bone Joint Surg Br 1987;69B:116–120.
12. Vingerhoeds B, Degreef I, De Smet L. Debridement arthroplasty for osteoarthritis of the elbow (Outerbridge-Kashiwagi procedure). Acta Orthop Belg 2004;70:306–310.

Chapter 43

Lateral Columnar Release for Extracapsular Elbow Contracture

Leonid I. Katolik and Mark S. Cohen

DEFINITION

- Extrinsic elbow contracture refers to elbow stiffness secondary to fibrosis, thickening, and, occasionally, ossification of the elbow capsule and periarticular soft tissues.
- In contrast to intrinsic contracture, the articular surface is either uninvolved or minimally involved, without the presence of intra-articular adhesions or articular cartilage destruction.
- While a distinction is made between extrinsic and intrinsic causes of contracture, these entities often overlap.

ANATOMY

- The elbow is a compound uniaxial synovial joint comprising three highly congruous articulations.
- The ulnohumeral joint is a ginglymus, or hinge, joint. The radiocapitellar and proximal radioulnar joints are gliding joints.
- All three articulations exist within a single capsule and are further stabilized by the proximity of the articular surface and capsule to the intracapsular ligaments and overlying extracapsular musculature.

PATHOGENESIS

- The propensity for elbow stiffness after even trivial elbow trauma is well recognized. After even seemingly trivial injuries, the capsule can undergo structural and biochemical alterations leading to thickening, decreased compliance, and loss of motion.
- Causes of extrinsic elbow contracture include capsular contracture, damage to and fibrosis of the flexor–extensor muscular origins, collateral ligament scarring, heterotopic bone, and skin contracture.
- Prolonged immobilization after trauma may be a separate risk factor for the development of stiffness.

NATURAL HISTORY

- Little consensus exists regarding the natural history of capsular contracture. It is felt that appropriate recognition and treatment of acute elbow injuries, avoidance of prolonged immobilization, and early active range of motion may limit the severity of posttraumatic extrinsic contracture.
- Patients typically do not tolerate elbow stiffness well since adjacent joints do not provide adequate compensatory motion.
  - Morrey[10] showed that the performance of most activities of daily living requires a functional arc of motion from 30 to 130 degrees.
  - Vasen and colleagues[11] have demonstrated that volunteers with uninjured elbows may adapt to a functional arc of motion from 70 to 120 degrees to perform 12 tasks of daily living.
  - Patients typically request treatment for elbow contracture when loss of extension approaches 40 degrees and flexion does not exceed 120 degrees.
  - Patients who do not improve with a concerted effort at nonoperative treatment often require surgical release.

- Stiffness of the elbow typically is incited by soft tissue trauma, hemarthrosis, and the patient's response to pain. Elbow trauma may cause tearing and contusion of the periarticular soft tissues. The patient typically holds the injured elbow in a flexed position to reduce pain. A fibrous tissue response then ensues within the hematoma and damaged muscular tissues. This fibrous tissue may ossify. In addition, overly aggressive therapy may further exacerbate these injuries, potentiating the cycle of pain, swelling, and limitation in motion that leads ultimately to frank contracture.
- Collateral ligament injury may contribute to contracture. Primary fibrosis may develop within the collateral ligaments because of the initial injury. Alternatively, secondary fibrosis may result from immobilization and scar formation.
- Significant injury to the anterior joint capsule and the overlying brachialis muscle may also result in capsular hypertrophy and fibrotic reaction contributing to ankylosis. This is particularly common in association with fracture-dislocations of the elbow.

PATIENT HISTORY AND PHYSICAL FINDINGS

- The cause of contracture should generally be easily elucidated from the history. Particular notation should be made of concomitant injuries, including closed head injury or associated burn injury.
- The duration and possible progression of symptoms should be noted.
- The impact of the contracture on the patient's upper extremity function and any limitations in activities of daily living should be noted.
- Any previous treatment for contracture should be elucidated. This should include the appropriateness, duration, and results of prior physical therapy, splinting, intra-articular injections, and surgeries.
- For patients with prior elbow surgery, the presence and type of any residual internal fixation devices should be noted. In addition, attention should be paid to any remote history of elbow infection.
- Physical examination should include a general physical examination as well as a detailed examination of the involved extremity.
  - Attention must be paid to the examination of the skin and soft tissue envelope about the elbow, with notation made of prior incisions, skin grafts, flaps, or areas of wound breakdown.
- Elbow motion should be measured with a goniometer and active and passive motion should be compared.
- Notation should be made whether motion improves with the forearm in full pronation, which may suggest posterolateral rotatory instability. This effectively "spins" the forearm away from the humerus, causing gapping of the ulnohumeral joint and posterior subluxation of the radial head from the

capitellum. While frank dislocation is not possible in the unanesthetized patient, guarding is effectively a positive sign.

■ While rare, symptomatic incompetence of the ulnar collateral ligament may elucidated by examination.

■ Strength of the involved limb should be assessed, as a joint without adequate strength is unlikely to maintain motion after release.

■ Since many posttraumatic and inflammatory contractures about the elbow are associated with ulnar nerve symptoms, a careful neurologic examination should be performed. A positive Tinel test over the cubital tunnel as well as a positive elbow flexion test should increase the suspicion for concomitant ulnar nerve pathology.

IMAGING AND OTHER DIAGNOSTIC STUDIES

■ Anteroposterior (AP) and lateral radiographs are often all that is needed for preoperative planning (**FIG 1**).

■ Cross-sectional imaging with computed tomography is helpful in visualizing the articular surfaces, particularly after fracture.

   ■ We advocate the use of computed tomography for preoperative planning in cases of moderate to severe heterotopic ossification.

■ Extracapsular contracture is typically not painful through the remaining arc of motion and is not painful at rest. If pain is a significant component of the patient's symptoms, serologic workup for infection, including a complete blood count, erythrocyte sedimentation rate, and C-reactive protein, is indicated.

DIFFERENTIAL DIAGNOSIS

■ Conversion disorder
■ Infection
■ Inflammatory arthropathy
■ Intracapsular contracture

NONOPERATIVE MANAGEMENT

■ Alternative measures to improve elbow stiffness include conservative modalities to decrease joint swelling and inflammation and relax or stretch contracted soft tissues. For protracted swelling, edema control sleeves, ice, elevation, active motion (including the forearm, wrist, and hand), and oral agents such as anti-inflammatory medication can be useful.

■ A short-term oral prednisone taper can be very effective in difficult cases. In addition, one can consider an intra-articular cortisone injection to decrease inflammation and joint synovitis.

■ Rarely, when patients exhibit guarding and involuntary co-contraction, biofeedback may be a helpful adjunct.

■ Dynamic splints, which apply a constant tension to the soft tissues, may be helpful.

■ Patient-adjusted static braces appear to be more effective. These braces use the principle of passive progressive stretch, allowing for stress relaxation of the soft tissues. They are applied for much shorter periods of time and are better tolerated by patients.

SURGICAL MANAGEMENT

■ To improve elbow flexion, one must release any soft tissue structures posteriorly that might be tethering the joint. These include the posterior joint capsule and the triceps muscle and tendon, which can become adherent to the humerus.

   ■ Any bony or soft tissue impingement also must be removed anteriorly, including osteophytes off the coronoid process and any bony or soft tissue overgrowth in both the coronoid and radial fossae.

   ■ There must be a concavity above the humeral trochlea to accept both the coronoid centrally and the radial head laterally for full flexion to occur.

■ Similarly, to improve elbow extension, posterior impingement must be removed between the olecranon tip and the olecranon fossa.

   ■ Anteriorly, any tethering soft tissues must be released, namely the anterior joint capsule and any adhesions between the brachialis and the humerus.

Preoperative Planning

■ All radiographic studies should be reviewed.
■ The presence and type of any retained implants is noted.
■ Range-of-motion and pivot-shift testing is performed under anesthesia as well as under live fluoroscopy.

Positioning

■ Patients are positioned supine with the arm on a hand table.
■ The patient's torso is brought to the edge of the operating table to ensure adequate elbow exposure for fluoroscopic imaging.
■ A towel bump may be placed under the medial elbow.

Approach

■ A direct posterior skin incision or a lateral incision is used.
   ■ A direct posterior incision has been criticized for an increased propensity toward postoperative seroma formation.

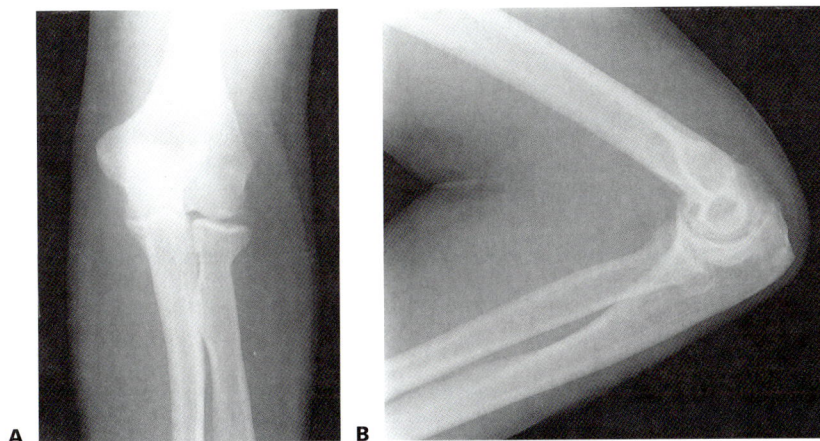

FIG 1 • Routine preoperative AP (**A**) and lateral (**B**) radiographs are obtained in all cases. Contracture may occur after subtle injury. This patient developed stiffness after nonoperative treatment of a nondisplaced radial neck fracture.

TECHNIQUES

■ It has the advantage of being a utilitarian incision that allows access to the medial and lateral sides simultaneously.

■ Advantages to the lateral exposure include its simplicity, less extensor and flexor–pronator disruption, and access to all three joint articulations.

■ The main disadvantage of the lateral exposure is the inability to address the ulnar nerve when indicated.

■ The deep interval for exposure of the anterior capsule lies between the extensor carpi radialis longus (ECRL) proximally and the extensor carpi radialis brevis (ECRB) distally. Posterior access is achieved between the triceps and the humerus.

SURGICAL APPROACH

■ The procedure can be performed under general anesthesia or under regional anesthesia with a long-acting regional block.

■ For the posterior incision, care is taken to avoid placing the line of incision directly over the prominence of the olecranon. Full-thickness fasciocutaneous flaps are elevated laterally to expose the extensor muscle mass.

■ For a lateral incision, an extended Köcher approach is used, beginning along the lateral supracondylar ridge of the humerus and passing distally in the interval between the anconeus and the extensor carpi ulnaris (ECU).

POSTERIOR RELEASE

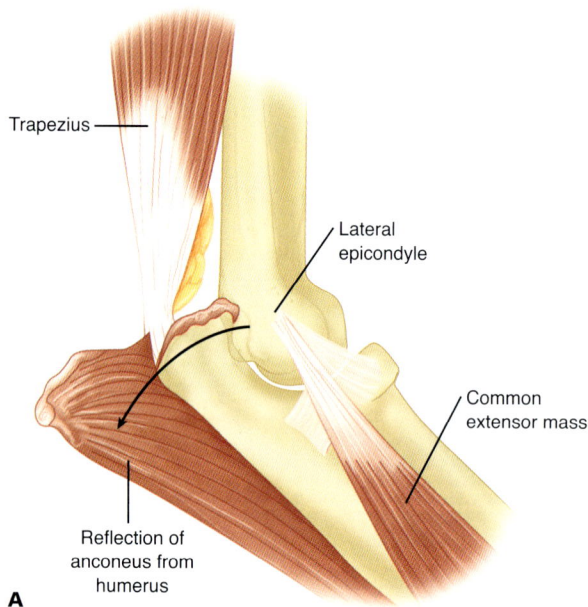

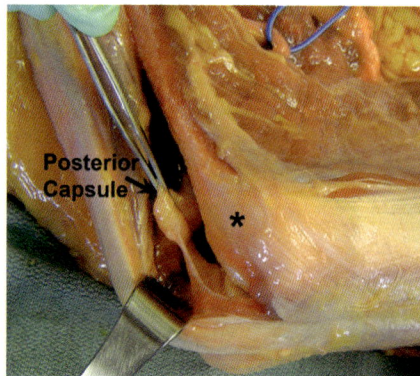

■ The Köcher interval between the anconeus and ECU is developed.

■ The anconeus is reflected posteriorly in continuity with the triceps. This exposes the posterior and posterolateral joint capsule (**TECH FIG 1A,B**).

■ A triceps tenolysis is carried out with an elevator, releasing any adhesions between the muscle and the posterior humerus. The humeroulnar joint is identified posteriorly and the olecranon fossa is cleared of any fibrous tissue or scar that would restrict terminal extension. The tip of the olecranon is removed if there was evidence of overgrowth or impingement (**TECH FIG 1C**).

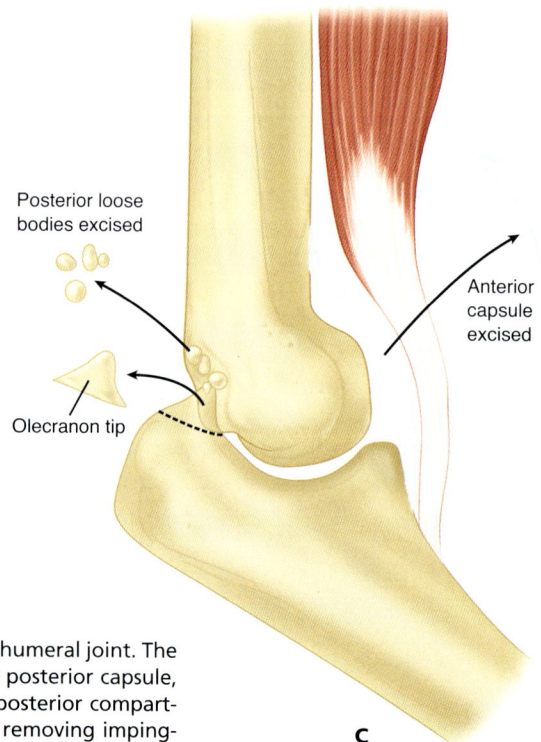

TECH FIG 1 • A,B. Exposure of the lateral and posterior ulnohumeral joint. The anconeus and triceps are reflected posteriorly, exposing the posterior capsule, olecranon tip, and olecranon fossa. **C.** Visualization of the posterior compartment permits débridement of the posterior joint, including removing impinging tissue of osteophytes in the olecranon fossa and the tip of the olecranon.

- The posterior aspect of the radiocapitellar joint is inspected after excision of the elbow capsule just proximal to the conjoined lateral collateral and annular ligament complex through the "soft spot" on the lateral side of the elbow. The proximal edge of this complex lies along the proximal border of the radial head.

ANTERIOR RELEASE

- Once the posterior release is completed, dissection is carried anteriorly. The anterior interval proximally is between the lateral supracondylar column and the brachioradialis and ECRL. Distally the interval is between the ECRL and extensor digitorum communis (EDC) (**TECH FIG 2A**).
- The brachialis is then mobilized off the humerus and anterior capsule with an elevator, releasing any adhesions between the muscle and the anterior humerus (**TECH FIG 2B**).
- The brachioradialis and ECRL released from the lateral supracondylar ridge of the humerus (**TECH FIG 2C**).
- This dissection is continued distally between the ECRL and ECRB, allowing exposure of the anterior capsule with preservation of the lateral collateral ligament and the origins of the ECRB, the EDC and minimi, and the ECU from the lateral epicondyle.

- Dissection is then carried out beneath the elbow capsule between the joint and the brachialis. The capsule is excised as far as the medial side of the joint.
- The radial and coronoid fossae are cleared of fibrous tissue and the tip of the coronoid is removed if overgrowth or impingement was noted in flexion. Loose bodies are removed (**TECH FIG 2D,E**).
- After release of the anterior capsule, gentle extension of the elbow with applied pressure usually brings the joint out to nearly full extension.
- In longstanding cases of contracture, the brachialis muscle can be tight, inhibiting full terminal elbow extension. This myostatic contracture can be stretched for several minutes during the procedure and requires attention at subsequent physiotherapy (**TECH FIG 2F**).

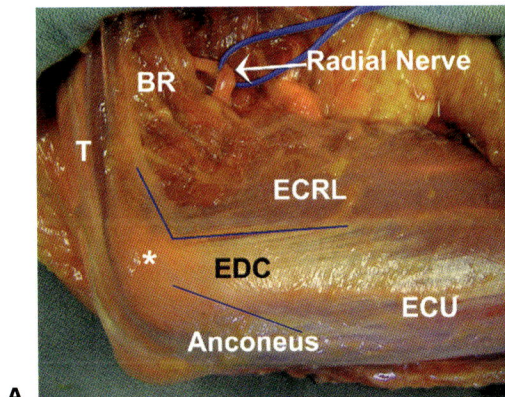

A

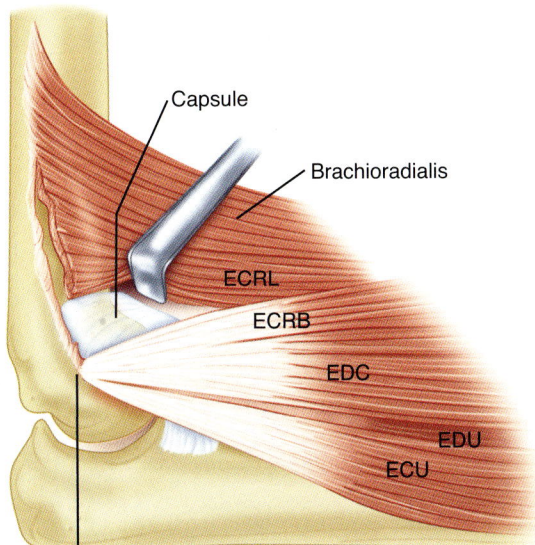

B Lateral epicondyle

TECH FIG 2 • A. The lateral view of a dissected elbow. Blue lines mark the fascial intervals for access to the anterior and posterior aspect of the joint, which leaves the extensor carpi ulnaris (ECU), extensor digitorum communis (EDC), and extensor carpi radialis longus (ECRL) origins intact as well as the underlying lateral collateral ligament complex. The anterior elbow capsule is exposed by releasing the extensor carpi radialis longus from the lateral supracondylar ridge. Distally the exposure continues between the ECRL and ECRB. *T,* triceps; *BR,* brachioradialis. **B,C.** The anterior exposure for release. The anterior capsule is exposed by detaching the humeral origin of the ECRL proximally and the interval between the ECRL and ECRB distally. The brachialis is released from the anterior capsule. The capsule should be visualized all the way over to the medial joint with all muscle reflected anteriorly. *(continued)*

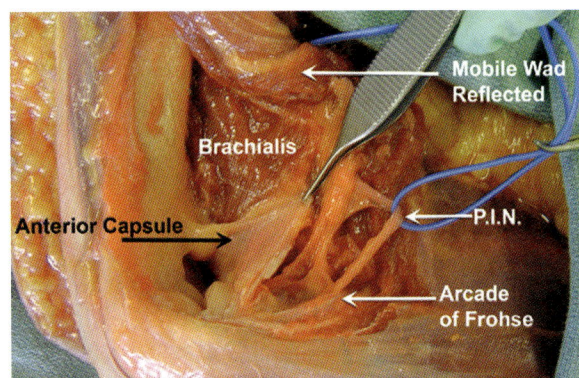

C

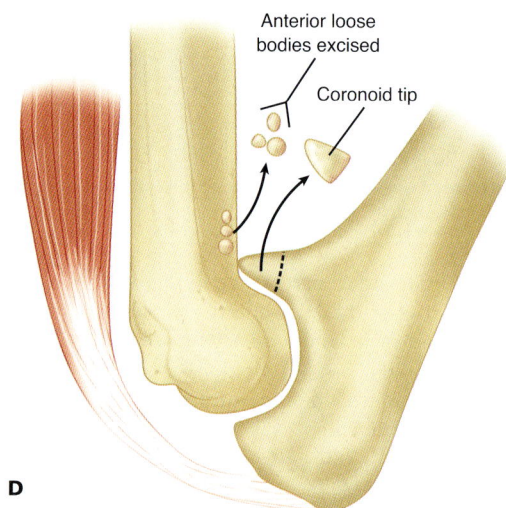

Anterior loose bodies excised

Coronoid tip

D

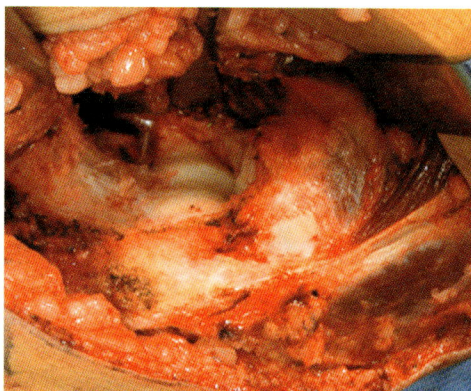

E

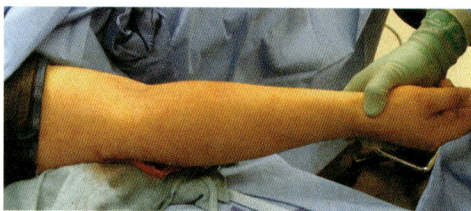

F

TECH FIG 2 • *(continued)* **D,E.** Anterior compartment débridement removes the tip of the coronoid and clears the coronoid and radial fossae. **F.** Intraoperative extension after contracture release.

PEARLS AND PITFALLS

Indications	■ The importance of prolonged postoperative rehabilitation cannot be stressed enough. A program of active and passive range of motion, weighted elbow stretches with wrist weights, formal therapy, and patient-adjusted elbow bracing is common for 3 to 6 months after surgery. ■ Postoperative gains may easily be lost in the patient who is not fully committed to rehabilitation or who does not have access to regular supervised therapy.
Ulnar nerve	■ Patients with preoperative signs and symptoms of ulnar nerve irritability should undergo neurolysis and transposition of the ulnar nerve. Although no strict guidelines exist, patients with preoperative flexion less than 100 degrees generally undergo concurrent ulnar nerve release even in the absence of preoperative symptoms.
Median nerve and brachial artery	■ These structures are generally well protected by the brachialis muscle. Their safety is increased if dissection proceeds in the interval between the elbow capsule and the brachialis.
Radial nerve injury	■ The posterior interosseous nerve may be encountered as extracapsular dissection proceeds distal to the radiocapitellar joint. Care must be taken with more distal dissection, and a firm understanding of neural anatomy is mandatory before attempting capsular release. Except in cases of significant anterolateral heterotopic ossification, we do not routinely dissect and isolate the radial nerve from proximal to distal.
Iatrogenic posterolateral rotatory instability	■ Instability may be induced with overly aggressive dissection about the lateral condyle. Care should be taken to stay anterior to the origin of the extensor carpi radialis brevis.

POSTOPERATIVE CARE

■ Although several rehabilitation programs may be effective, we have found continuous passive motion, begun immediately in the recovery room and used continuously until the following morning, to be helpful in maintaining the motion gained at surgery (**FIG 2A**).

■ Formal therapy is begun on postoperative day 1.

■ The dressing is removed and edema control modalities (eg, an edema sleeve or Ace wrap, ice) are used to limit swelling.

■ Active and gentle passive elbow motion is combined with intermittent continuous passive motion.

■ To help maintain extension, weighted passive stretches using a two-pound wrist weight with the arm extended over a bolster are performed several times daily for 10 to 15 minutes as tolerated.

■ Because the collateral ligaments are not released at surgery, no restrictions are typically placed on therapy.

■ Static progressive elbow bracing is begun early in the postoperative period. The brace is worn for about 30 minutes, two

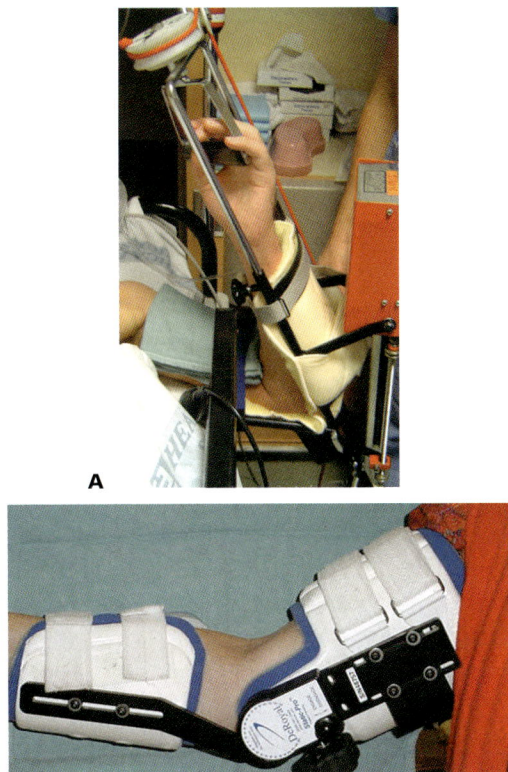

FIG 2 • **A.** Elbow continuous passive motion device. **B.** Patient-adjusted static elbow brace.

or three times a day. Flexion and extension are alternated based on the preoperative deficit and the early progress of the elbow (**FIG 2B**).

- A nonsteroidal anti-inflammatory agent (Indocin) is commonly prescribed as a prophylaxis against heterotopic ossification for several weeks postoperatively. This also helps to limit inflammation of the joint and soft tissues during rehabilitation.
- Patients are typically discharged home on postoperative day 1. Home therapy is performed daily thereafter, including active and passive exercises, continuous passive motion, weighted stretches, and patient-adjusted bracing.
  - Progress should be closely monitored by a therapist who is familiar with the protocol. The physician must also follow these patients closely.
- Although the bulk of ultimate elbow motion is gained during the first 6 to 8 weeks, patients can continue to make gains in terminal flexion and extension for several months postoperatively. This is especially true for elbow flexion.
- Continuous passive motion is typically discontinued at 3 to 4 weeks, but bracing is continued for several months as required. As long as the patient is able to obtain full elbow flexion and extension once per day (eg, in the brace), a favorable prognosis exists with respect to the ultimate outcome if vigilance is maintained.

OUTCOMES

- In appropriate patients, release of the contracted elbow can be a reliable and satisfying procedure with predictable results.
- We reviewed our results for 22 patents treated for posttraumatic elbow stiffness using a soft tissue release of the elbow through a lateral approach. The average length of follow-up was 29 months.
  - Total elbow motion improved in all subjects. Extension increased from an average of 39 ± 10 degrees preoperatively to 8 ± 6 degrees at follow-up. Elbow flexion increased from 113 ± 18 degrees preoperatively to 137 ± 9 degrees at follow-up. Thus, total ulnohumeral joint motion increased an average of 55 degrees (P <0.001).
  - Elbow pain, as determined by visual analogue scales, decreased in all patients. Elbow function, as determined by standardized scales, also significantly improved.
  - Radiographic analysis revealed no patients with regrowth of excised osteophytes or loose bodies at follow-up.

COMPLICATIONS

- Ulnar nerve
  - The most common complication after elbow release surgery involves the ulnar nerve. This may be related in part to improved elbow flexion after surgery, as ulnar nerve tension increases with flexion. This may precipitate symptoms in a nerve that is already subclinically compromised.
  - Patients with preoperative signs and symptoms of ulnar nerve irritability should undergo neurolysis and transposition of the ulnar nerve.
  - Although no strict guidelines exist, patients with preoperative flexion less than 100 degrees generally undergo concurrent ulnar nerve release even in the absence of preoperative symptoms.
- Median nerve and brachial artery
  - Although generally well protected by the brachialis muscle, these structures are at risk with anterior dissection. Their safety is increased if dissection proceeds in the interval between the elbow capsule and the brachialis.
  - In addition, transient median neuritis is known to occur in our practices after release. This is likely due to stretch of the median nerve with extension of the severely contracted elbow.
- Radial nerve injury
  - The posterior interosseous nerve may be encountered as extracapsular dissection proceeds distal to the radiocapitellar joint.
  - Except in cases of significant anterolateral heterotopic ossification, the radial nerve does not typically require identification.
- Persistent stiffness
  - The importance of prolonged postoperative rehabilitation cannot be stressed enough. A program of active and passive range of motion, weighted elbow stretches with wrist weights, formal therapy, and patient-adjusted elbow bracing is common for 3 to 6 months after surgery. All of our patients meet preoperatively both with the therapists at our home institutions as well as with their local therapists.

REFERENCES

1. Cohen MS, Hastings H. Post-traumatic contracture of the elbow: operative release using a lateral collateral sparing approach. J Bone Joint Surg Br 1998;80B:805–812.
2. Cohen MS, Hastings H. Capsular release for contracture of the elbow: operative technique and functional results. Orthop Clin North Am 1999;30:133–139.
3. Cohen MS, Hastings, H. Rotatory instability of the elbow: the anatomy and role of the lateral stabilizers. J Bone Joint Surg Am 1997;79A:225–233.

4. Gates HS, Sullivan FL, Urbaniak JR. Anterior capsulotomy and continuous passive motion in the treatment post-traumatic flexion contracture of the elbow. J Bone Joint Surg Am 1992;74A:1229–1234.

5. Green DP, McCoy H. Turnbuckle orthotic correction of elbow flexion contractures after acute injuries. J Bone Joint Surg Am 1979;61A:1092–1095.

6. Jupiter JB, O'Driscoll SW, Cohen MS. The assessment and management of the stiff elbow. AAOS Instr Course Lect 2003;52:93–112.

7. Kasparyan NG, Hotchkiss RN. Dynamic skeletal fixation in the upper extremity. Hand Clin 1997;13:643–663.

8. Mansat P, Morrey BF. The column procedure: a limited lateral approach for extrinsic contracture of the elbow. J Bone Joint Surg Am 1998;80A:1603–1615.

9. Modabber MR, Jupiter JB. Current concepts review: reconstruction for posttraumatic conditions of the elbow joint. J Bone Joint Surg Am 1995;77A:1431–1446.

10. Morrey BF. Post-traumatic contracture of the elbow: operative treatment, including distraction arthroplasty. J Bone Joint Surg Am 1990;72A:601–618.

11. Vasen AP, Lacey SH, Keith MW, Shaffer JW. Functional range of motion of the elbow. J Hand Surg Am 1995;20(2):288–292.

Extrinsic Contracture Release: Medial Over-the-Top Approach

Pierre Mansat, Aymeric André, and Nicolas Bonnevialle

DEFINITION

- Multiple techniques have been described for the release of elbow contractures. The medial approach has the advantages of direct access to both the anterior and posterior aspects of the ulnohumeral joint, and direct visualization of the ulnar nerve.
- Medial-based releases were initially proposed by Wilner,[24] whose technique involved medial epicondylectomy and wide dissection.
  - Weiss[23] subsequently has described splitting the flexor pronator mass rather than complete release of the flexor pronator mass.
  - Hotchkiss[12] popularized this approach to deal with extrinsic contracture of the elbow and ulnar nerve involvement.
  - Itoh et al[10] and Wada et al[22] underlined the importance of the posterior oblique band of the medial collateral ligament as a critical structure to identify and release if an extension contracture exists.

ANATOMY

- The medial compartment of the elbow includes the medial side of the ulnohumeral joint, the medial collateral ligament, the flexor–pronator mass, the ulnar nerve, and the medial antebrachial cutaneous nerve (**FIG 1A**).
- The medial ulnohumeral joint is composed of the medial column, the medial epicondyle, the medial side of the proximal aspect of the ulna, and the coronoid process.
- The medial collateral ligament consists of three parts: anterior, posterior, and transverse segments (**FIG 1B**).
  - The anterior bundle is the most discrete component, the posterior portion being a thickening of the posterior capsule, and is well defined only in about 90 degrees of flexion.
  - The transverse component appears to contribute little or nothing to elbow stability.
  - The medial collateral ligament originates from a broad anteroinferior surface of the epicondyle but not from the condylar elements of the trochlea just inferior to the axis of rotation.[18] The ulnar nerve rests on the posterior aspect of the medial epicondyle, but it is not intimately related to the fibers of the anterior bundle of the medial collateral ligament itself.
- The flexor–pronator mass includes the pronator teres, the most proximal of the flexor pronator group; the flexor carpi radialis, which originates just inferior to the origin of the pronator teres at the anteroinferior aspect of the medial epicondyle; the palmaris longus muscle, which arises from the medial epicondyle and from the septa it shares with the flexor carpi radialis and flexor carpi ulnaris; the flexor carpi ulnaris, which is the most posterior of the common flexor tendons originating from the medial epicondyle and from the medial border of the coronoid and the proximal medial aspect of the ulna; and the flexor digitorum superficialis, which is the deepest from the common flexor tendon but superficial to the flexor digitorum profundus.

IMAGING AND OTHER DIAGNOSTIC STUDIES

- Diagnosis of the contracture is usually made by identifying a characteristic history and performing a physical examination.
- Joint involvement is confirmed by plain radiographs. The anteroposterior (AP) view gives good visualization of the joint line, but the lateral view demonstrates osteophytes on the coronoid and at the tip of the olecranon, even when the joint space is preserved.
- The details of the extent of the involvement are best observed on computed tomography.
- Transverse imaging by magnetic resonance imaging (MRI) has little utility in our practice.

NONOPERATIVE MANAGEMENT

- Several options have been proposed for the treatment of elbow contracture.
- Nonoperative treatment with mobilization of the elbow through the use of alternating flexion and extension splints[17] or dynamic splints[8] sometimes provides a good result if it is begun soon after the contracture develops.
- Manipulation with the patient under anesthesia has also been recommended, but loss of motion and ulnar nerve injury have been reported.[6]
- Recently, botulinum toxin has been used to release muscle contracture in order to improve elbow rehabilitation.[20]
- Nonoperative treatment usually is successful only for extrinsic stiffness that has been present for 6 months or less, however, and the results are unpredictable. With failure of nonoperative treatment, surgical release may be indicated. Some reports of this being done through an arthroscopic procedure recently appeared. Most surgeons employ an open procedure, and several have been described.

SURGICAL MANAGEMENT

Indications

- Contracture release
- Stiff elbow
- Degenerative arthritis with anterior and posteromedial osteophytes
- Ulnar nerve symptoms

Advantages

- Allows exposure, protection, and transposition of the ulnar nerve
- Preserves the anterior band of the medial collateral ligament
- Affords access to the coronoid with intact radial head

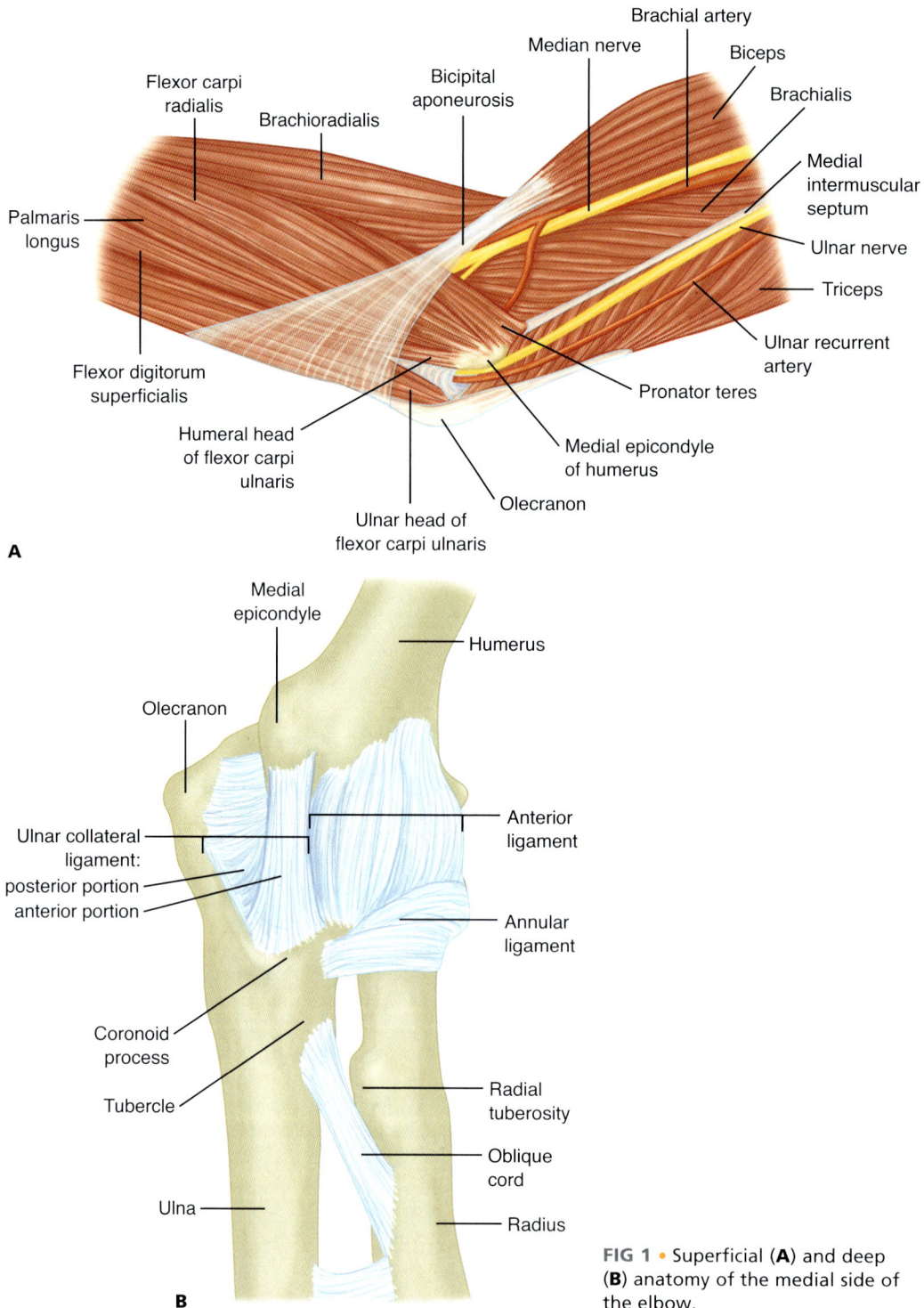

FIG 1 • Superficial (**A**) and deep (**B**) anatomy of the medial side of the elbow.

Disadvantages

- Difficulty in removing heterotopic bone on the lateral side of the joint
- Affords poor access to radial head

Preoperative Planning

- Before surgery, the decision must be made to approach the capsule from the lateral or medial aspect.
  - If the ulnar nerve is to be addressed or there is extensive medial or coronoid arthrosis, the medial approach is of value.

- If the radiohumeral joint is involved or if a simple release is all that is required, the lateral "column" procedure is carried out.

Positioning

- The patient is usually positioned supine, supported by an elbow or a hand table.
- Two folded towels should be placed under the scapula.
- A sterile tourniquet is positioned.

- To expose the posterior joint, the patient's shoulder should have fairly free external rotation; otherwise, the arm should be positioned over the chest.

Approach

- The skin incision may be a posterior skin incision or a midline medial one (**FIG 2**).
- The key to this exposure is identification of the medial supracondylar ridge of the humerus.
- At this level, the surgeon can locate the medial intermuscular septum, the origin of the flexor–pronator muscle mass, and the ulnar nerve.
- This site also serves as the starting point of the anterior and posterior subperiosteal extracapsular dissection of the joint.

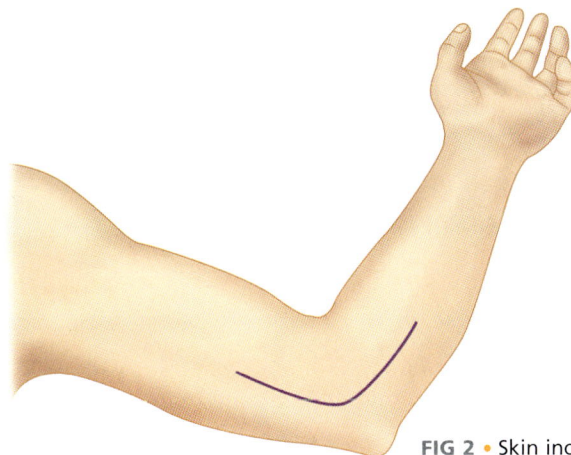

FIG 2 • Skin incision.

EXPOSING THE ULNAR NERVE AND THE MEDIAL FASCIA

- Once the medial intermuscular septum is identified, the medial antebrachial cutaneous nerve is identified, traced distally, and protected.
  - The branching pattern varies, however, so it is occasionally necessary to divide the nerve to gain full exposure and to adequately mobilize the ulnar nerve, especially in revision surgery.
  - If this is necessary, the nerve is divided as proximally as the skin incision will allow, ensuring that the cut end lies in the subcutaneous fat (**TECH FIG 1**).
- If previously anterior transposition was performed, the ulnar nerve should be fully identified and mobilized before proceeding.

- The surgeon must be prepared to extend the previous incision proximally, as necessary.
- In this setting, the nerve is often flattened over the medial flexor–pronator muscle mass, or it can "subluxate" to a posterior position.
- This dissection requires patience and may take considerable time. Dissection of the nerve needs to be carried distally far enough to allow the nerve to sit in the anterior position without being kinked distal to the epicondyle.
- The septum is excised from the insertion on the supracondylar ridge to the proximal extent of the wound, usually about 5 to 8 cm.
  - Many of the veins and perforating arteries at the most distal portion of the septum require cauterization.

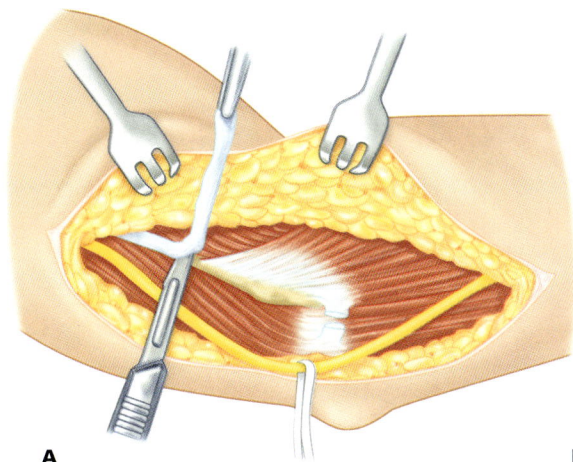

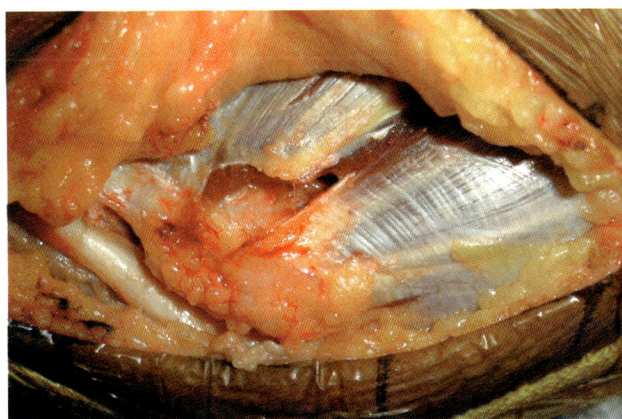

A　　　　　　　　　　　　　　　　　**B**

TECH FIG 1 • Exposure of the ulnar nerve and medial fascia.

EXPOSING THE ANTERIOR CAPSULE FOR EXCISION AND INCISION

- Once the septum has been excised, the flexor–pronator muscle mass should be divided parallel to the fibers, leaving roughly a 1.5-cm span of flexor carpi ulnaris tendon attached to the epicondyle (**TECH FIG 2A,B**).

- The surgeon then returns the supracondylar ridge and begins elevating the anterior muscle with a Cobb elevator.

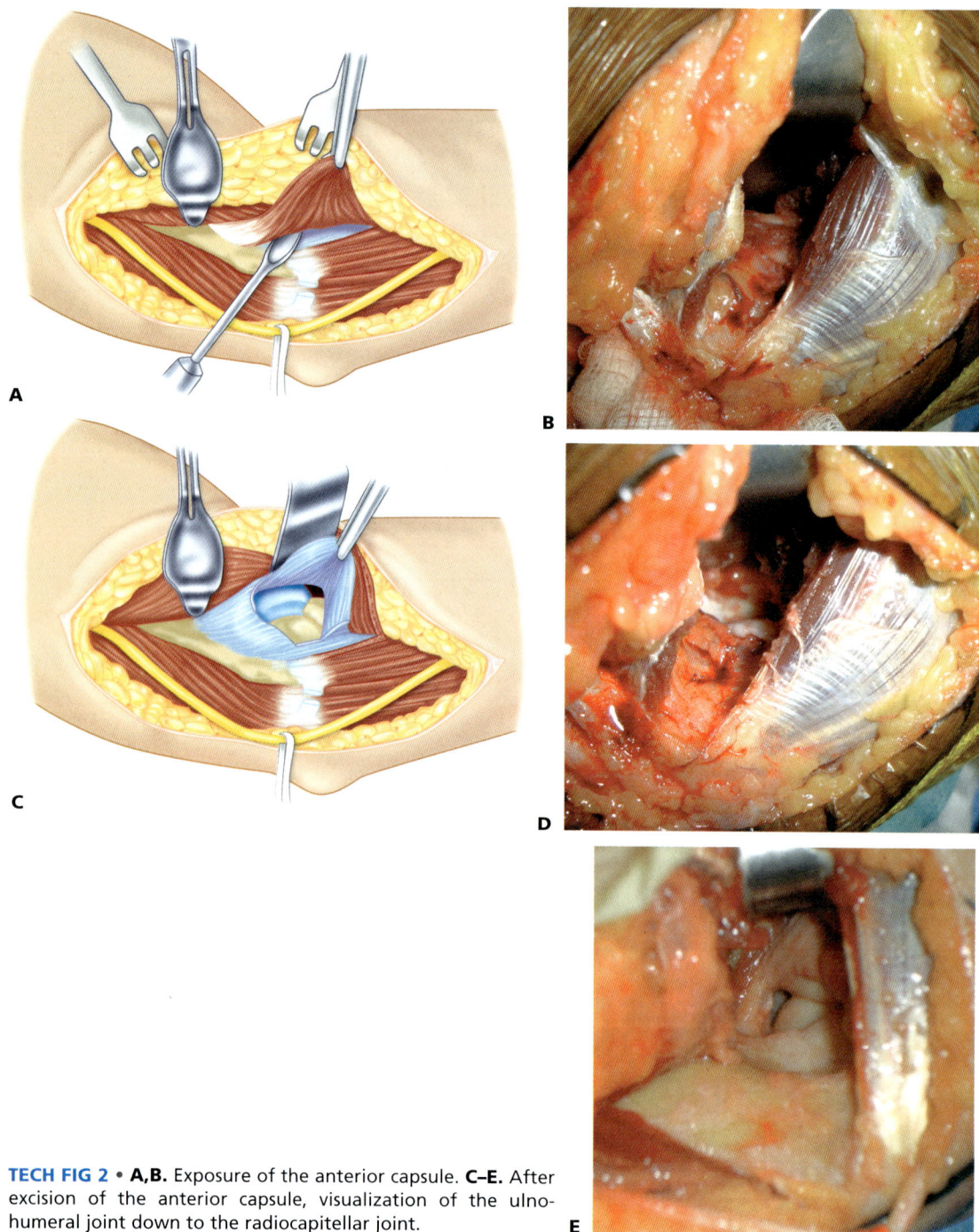

TECH FIG 2 • A,B. Exposure of the anterior capsule. **C–E.** After excision of the anterior capsule, visualization of the ulnohumeral joint down to the radiocapitellar joint.

- Subperiosteally, the anterior structures of the distal humeral region proximal to the capsule are elevated to allow placement of a wide Bennett retractor. As the elevator moves from medial to lateral, the handle of the elevator is lifted carefully, keeping the blade of the elevator along the surface of the bone.
  - When heterotopic ossification along the lateral distal humerus is profuse, the radial nerve is at risk if it is entrapped in the scar on the surface of the bone.
  - A separate approach to the lateral side is sometimes needed.
- The median nerve, brachial vein, and artery are superficial to the brachialis muscle.

- A small cuff of tissue of the flexor–pronator origin can be left on the supracondylar ridge as the muscle is elevated. This facilitates reattachment during closing.
- A proximal, transverse incision in the lacertus fibrosus may also be needed to adequately mobilize this layer of muscle.
- Once the Bennett retractor is in place and the medial portion of the flexor–pronator has been incised, the plane between muscle and capsule should be carefully elevated.
  - As this plane is developed, the brachialis muscle is encountered from the underside. This muscle should be kept anterior and elevated from the capsule and anterior surface of the distal humerus.

TECHNIQUES

- Finding this plane requires careful attention.
- The dissection of the capsule from the brachialis muscle proceeds both laterally and distally.
- At this point, it is helpful to feel for the coronoid process by gently flexing and extending the elbow. The first few times that this approach is used, the coronoid seems quite deep and far distal.
    - A deep, narrow retractor is often helpful to allow the operator to see down to the level of the coronoid.
- The extreme anteromedial corner of the exposure deserves special comment.
    - In a contracture release, the anteromedial portion often requires release.
    - To see this area, a small, narrow retractor can be inserted to retract the medial collateral ligament, pulling it medially and posteriorly.
    - This affords visualization of the medial capsule and protection of the anterior medial collateral ligament.

- The anterior capsule should be excised (**TECH FIG 2C–E**) to the extent that that is practical and safe.
    - When first performing this procedure, it is helpful first to incise the capsule from the medial to the lateral aspect along the anterior surface of the joint.
    - Once this edge of the capsule is incised, it can be lifted and excised as far distally as is safe. From this vantage, and after capsule excision, the radial head and capitellum can be visualized and freed of scar, as needed.
- In cases of primary osteoarthritis of the elbow, removing the large spur from the coronoid is crucial.
    - Using the Cobb elevator, the brachialis muscle can be elevated anteriorly for 2 cm from the coronoid process.
    - With the elevator held in position, protecting the brachialis but anterior to the coronoid, the large osteophyte can be removed with an osteotome.
    - The brachialis insertion is well distal to the tip of the coronoid.

EXPOSING AND EXCISING THE POSTERIOR CAPSULE AND BONE SPURS

- The posterior capsule of the joint is exposed. The supracondylar ridge is again identified (**TECH FIG 3**).
    - Using the Cobb elevator, the triceps is elevated from the posterior distal surface of the humerus.
    - The exposure should extend far enough proximal to permit use of a Bennett retractor.
- The posterior capsule can be separated from the triceps as the elevator sweeps from proximal to distal. The posterior medial joint line should also be identified, as it is often involved by osteophytes or heterotopic bone.

- In contracture release, the posterior capsule and posterior band of the medial collateral ligament should be excised.
- The medial joint line up to the anterior band of the medial collateral ligament should also be exposed and the capsule excised. This area is the floor of the cubital tunnel.
- In contracture release and in primary osteoarthritis, the tip of the olecranon usually must be excised to achieve full extension.
    - The posteromedial joint line is easily visualized, but the posterolateral side must also be carefully palpated to ensure clearance.

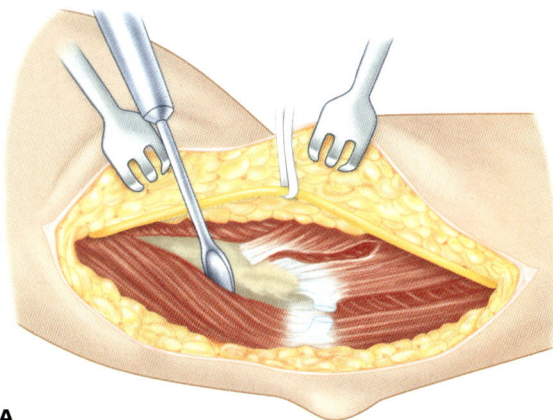

TECH FIG 3 • Exposure of the posterior compartment.

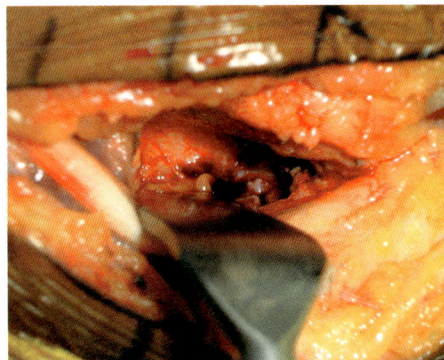

ULNAR NERVE TRANSPOSITION

- After being reattached to the medial supracondylar region, the ulnar nerve should be transposed and secured with a fascial sling to prevent posterior subluxation.
    - The sling can be fashioned by elevating two overlapping rectangular flaps of fascia or by using a medially based flap attached to the underlying subcutaneous tissue.

- Once this maneuver is completed, the nerve must not be compressed or kinked.
- The joint should be flexed and extended to ensure that the nerve is free to move.

TECHNIQUES

CLOSURE

- The flexor–pronator mass should be reattached to the supracondylar ridge with nonabsorbable braided 1-0 or 0 suture.
  - If a large enough cuff of tissue was left on the medial epicondyle, no holes need be drilled in bone.
  - Otherwise, drill holes in the edge of the supracondylar ridge can be made to secure the flexor–pronator mass (**TECH FIG 4**).

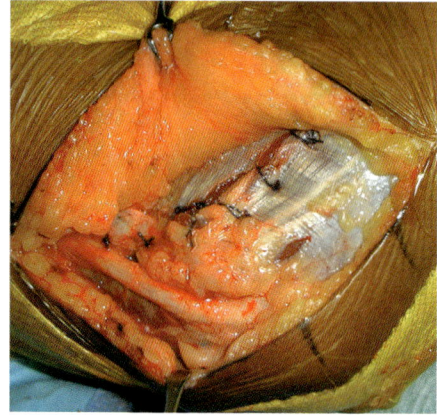

TECH FIG 4 • Closure.

PEARLS AND PITFALLS

Wrong incision	▪ Identification of the medial supracondylar ridge
Injury to the medial antebrachial cutaneous nerve	▪ Identification of the medial antebrachial cutaneous nerve
Injury to the ulnar nerve	▪ Identification, mobilization, and protection of the ulnar nerve
Disinsertion of the flexor–pronator mass from the medial epicondyle	▪ The flexor–pronator muscle mass should be divided parallel to the fibers.
Injury to the anterior vessels and nerves	▪ A Bennett retractor is placed between the anterior muscle and the capsule.
Section of the anterior band of the medial collateral ligament	▪ A small, narrow retractor is inserted to retract the medial collateral ligament, pulling it medially and posteriorly.

POSTOPERATIVE CARE

- If the neurologic examination findings in the recovery room are normal, a brachial plexus block is established and maintained with a continuous pump through a percutaneous catheter.
  - The arm is elevated as much as possible, and mechanical continuous passive motion exercise is begun the day of surgery and adjusted to provide as much motion as pain or the machine itself allows.
  - After 2 days the plexus block is discontinued, and, at day 3, the continuous passive motion machine is stopped.
- Physical therapy is not used, but a detailed program of splint therapy is prescribed.
  - Adjustable splints are prescribed, depending on the motion before and after the procedure. The splints include a hyperextension or a hyperflexion brace, or both.
  - A detailed discussion regarding heat, ice, and anti-inflammatory medication, along with a visual schedule for bracing, is provided.
  - During the first 3 months, the patient sleeps with the splint adjusted to maximize flexion or extension, whichever is more needed; it should not be so uncomfortable as to prevent sleeping for at least 6 hours.
  - Because the principal objective is to gain motion but to avoid pain, swelling, and inflammation, routine use of an anti-inflammatory medication is prescribed.
- Therapy with splints is continued for about 3 months, during which time the patient is seen at 2- to 4-week intervals, if possible.
- After 4 weeks, an arc of about 80 degrees of motion is obtained, and the amount of time that each splint is worn is gradually decreased.
- Splinting at night is continued for as long as 6 months if flexion contracture tends to recur when the splint is not used.
- Patients are advised that it may take a year to realize full correction.

OUTCOMES

- Recent reports on the results of surgical arthrolysis reveal an absolute gain in the flexion–extension arc between 30 and 60 degrees.[1,3–5,7,9–11,14–16,19,21]
  - A functional arc of motion between 30 and 130 degrees is obtained in more than 50% of cases, and some improvement in motion in more than 90% of the cases has been reported in the literature.[1,3–5,7,9–11,14–16,19,21]
  - In Europe, a combined lateral and medial approach has been used for many years, and gains in flexion arc have averaged between 40 and 72 degrees (in about 400 procedures).[1,3,7,14] Some preferred a posterior extensile approach if medial and lateral exposures are anticipated.
  - The importance of sequential release of tissues has been emphasized, based on an experience with 44 of 46 patients

(95%) who were satisfied with such an approach.[13] The preoperative arc improved from 45 to 99 degrees.

■ The authors emphasize the need to release the exostosis and the collateral ligament when contracted, especially noting the need to release the posterior portion of the medial collateral ligament and decompress the ulnar nerve when ulnar nerve symptoms exist preoperatively.[13]

■ Using a medial approach, Wada et al[22] obtained improvement of the mean arc of movement of 64 degrees. A functional arc of flexion–extension (30 to 130 degrees) was obtained in 7 of the 14 elbows. None of the patients developed symptoms related to the ulnar nerve. According to those authors, the medial approach has several advantages over both the anterior and lateral approaches:

■ Pathologic changes in the posterior oblique bundle of the medial collateral ligament can be observed and excised under direct vision.

■ Anterior and posterior exposure is possible through one medial incision, through which a complete soft tissue release and excision of part of the olecranon and coronoid process can be undertaken if necessary. Additional lateral exposure is indicated only if the medial approach has proved to be inadequate.

■ In the medial approach, the ulnar nerve is routinely released and protected under direct vision, which decreases the risk of damage.

COMPLICATIONS

■ A most important emerging consideration of the proper treatment of elbow stiffness is the vulnerability of the ulnar nerve.

■ The most common cause of failure of treatment has been in patients whose preoperative ulnar nerve symptoms were not appreciated or addressed, or patients in whom ulnar nerve symptoms developed postoperatively without adequate treatment. This is attributable to traction neuritis caused by the abrupt increase in elbow flexion or extension during the operation.

■ Even in the absence of preoperative neurologic symptoms, the nerve may be compromised subclinically and become symptomatic as elbow motion increases after surgery. Therefore, all patients who have stiff elbows must be evaluated for the presence or absence of ulnar nerve symptoms.

■ Antuna et al[2] recommended that elbows with preoperative flexion limited to 90 to 100 degrees in which we expect to improve the motion by 30 or 40 degrees must be treated with inspection and often prophylactic decompression or translocation of the nerve, depending on the appearance of the nerve once the surgical procedure is finished.

■ Furthermore, all patients with preoperative ulnar nerve symptoms, even if they are mild, are treated with mobilization of the nerve.

■ These authors stated that manipulation of the elbow in the early postoperative period must be avoided if the nerve has not been decompressed or translocated.

REFERENCES

1. Allieu Y. Raideurs et arthrolyses du coude. Rev Chir Orthop 1989; 75(Suppl I):156–166.
2. Antuna SA, Morrey BF, Adams RA, et al. Ulnohumeral arthroplasty for primary degenerative arthritis of the elbow: long-term outcome and complications. J Bone Joint Surg Am 2002;84A:2168–2173.
3. Chantelot C, Fontaine C, Migaud H, et al. Etude retrospective de 23 arthrolyses du coude pour raideur post-traumatique: facteurs prédictifs du résultat. Rev Chir Orthop 1999;85:823–827.
4. Cikes A, Jolles BM, Farron A. Open elbow arthrolysis for posttraumatic elbow stiffness. J Orthop Trauma 2006;20:405–409.
5. Cohen MS, Hastings H II. Posttraumatic contracture of the elbow: operative release using a lateral collateral ligament sparing approach. J Bone Joint Surg Br 1998;80B:805–812.
6. Duke JB, Tessler RH, Dell PC. Manipulation of the stiff elbow with patient under anesthesia. J Hand Surg Am 1991;16:19–24.
7. Esteve P, Valentin P, Deburge A, et al. Raideurs et ankyloses posttraumatiques du coude. Rev Chir Orthop 1971;57(Suppl I):25–86.
8. Gelinas JJ, Faber KJ, Patterson SD, et al. The effectiveness of turnbuckle splinting for elbow constractures. J Bone Joint Surg Br 2000; 82B:74–78.
9. Husband JB, Hastings H. The lateral approach for operative release of post-traumatic contracture of the elbow. J Bone Joint Surg Am 1990;72A:1353–1358.
10. Itoh Y, Saegusa K, Ishiguro T, et al. Operation for the stiff elbow. Int Orthop 1989;13:263–268.
11. Mansat P, Morrey BF. The "column procedure": a limited surgical approach for the treatment of stiff elbows. J Bone Joint Surg Am 1998;80A:1603–1615.
12. Mansat P, Morrey BF, Hotchkiss RN. Extrinsic contracture: the column procedure, lateral and medial capsular releases. In Morrey BF, ed. The Elbow and Its Disorders, 3rd ed. Philaelphia: WB Saunders, 2000:447–456.
13. Marti RH, Kerkhoffs GM, Maas M, et al. Progressive surgical release of a posttraumatic stiff elbow: technique and outcome after 2–18 years in 46 patients. Acta Orthop Scand 2002;73:144–150.
14. Merle D'Aubigne R, Kerboul M. Les opérations mobilisatrices des raideurs et ankylose du coude. Rev Chir Orthop 1966;52:427–448.
15. Morrey BF. Post-traumatic contracture of the elbow: operative treatment, including distraction arthroplasty. J Bone Joint Surg Am 1990; 72A:601–618.
16. Morrey BF. The posttraumatic stiff elbow. Clin Orthop Relat Res 2005;431:26–35.
17. Morrey BF. The use of splints for the stiff elbows. Perspect Orthop Surg 1990;1:141–144.
18. O'Driscoll SW, Horii E, Morrey BF. Anatomy of the attachment of the medial ulnar collateral ligament. J Hand Surg Am 1992;17:164.
19. Park MJ, Kim HG, Lee JY. Surgical treatment of post-traumatic stiffness of the elbow. J Bone Joint Surg Br 2004;86B:1158–1162.
20. Rosenwasser M. Sequellae of fractures of the elbow. 11th Trauma Course, AIOD, Strasbourg, 2005.
21. Urbaniak JR, Hansen PE, Beissinger SF, et al. Correction of posttraumatic flexion contracture of the elbow by anterior capsulotomy. J Bone Joint Surg Am 1985;67A:1160–1164.
22. Wada T, Ishii S, Usui M, et al. The medial approach for operative release of post-traumatic contracture of the elbow. J Bone Joint Surg Br 2000;82B:68–73.
23. Weiss AP, Sachar K. Soft tissue contractures about the elbow. Hand Clin 1994;10:439–451.
24. Wilner P. Anterior capsulectomy for contractures of the elbow. J Int Coll Surg 1948;11:359–361.

Chapter 45

Total Elbow Arthroplasty for Rheumatoid Arthritis

Bryan J. Loeffler and Patrick M. Connor

DEFINITION

- Rheumatoid arthritis (RA) is a chronic, systemic, inflammatory condition of unknown etiology affecting 1% to 2% of the population.
  - It affects females two to three times as frequently as males, and the incidence increases with age, typically peaking between 35 and 50 years of age.
- Peripheral joints are often affected in a symmetric pattern.
- The elbow is affected in about 20% to 70% of patients with RA, with a wide spectrum of severity.
  - Ninety percent of these patients also have hand and wrist involvement, and 80% also have shoulder involvement.
- Juvenile rheumatoid arthritis (JRA) is diagnosed based on the presence of arthritis, synovitis, or both in at least one joint lasting for more than 6 weeks in an individual less than 16 years old.
- Compared with adult-onset RA, JRA is complicated by severe osseous destruction, deformity, and soft tissue contractures.

PATHOGENESIS

- The cause of RA is unknown.
  - Infectious etiologies have been proposed, but no microorganism has been proven to be causative.
  - Genetic and twin studies have demonstrated that a genetic predisposition clearly exists, and the disease is also associated with autoimmune phenomena.
- In patients with RA, numerous cell types, including B lymphocytes, CD4 T cells, mononuclear phagocytes, neutrophils, fibroblasts, and osteoclasts, have been shown to produce abnormally high levels of various cytokines, chemokines, and other inflammatory mediators.
- The result is inflammatory-mediated proliferation of synovial tissue, leading to soft tissue and finally bony destruction.

NATURAL HISTORY

- Overall, the disease progresses from predominantly soft tissue (synovial) inflammation to articular cartilage damage and ultimately subchondral and periarticular bone destruction.
- Manifestations of RA are initiated by synovitis and synovial hyperplasia resulting in pannus formation. This correlates with a boggy, inflamed elbow that is painful and with limited range of motion.
- Synovial proliferation coupled with joint capsule distention may produce a compressive neuropathy with pain, paresthesias, or weakness in the ulnar or radial nerve distributions, or both.
- Degeneration may progress to ligamentous erosion or disruption, or both. Clinically, the patient experiences progressive instability as ligamentous integrity is compromised.
  - It may affect the annular ligament and produce radial head instability with anterior displacement.

- Eventually the medial and lateral collateral ligament complexes may be disrupted, thus causing further instability.
- Prolonged synovitis leads to erosion of the cartilage followed by subchondral cyst and marginal osteophyte formation; the result is end-stage arthritis.
- End-stage disease is marked by severe damage to subchondral bone and gross joint instability. At this stage, patients typically have a painful, weak, and functionally unstable elbow.

PATIENT HISTORY AND PHYSICAL FINDINGS

- Patients typically describe a history of a swollen, tender, and warm elbow with diminished and painful range of motion.
  - This may be accompanied by a report of progressively declining function, constitutional complaints, and often polyarticular involvement.
- In early stages of the disease, the elbow may appear more boggy, with impressive soft tissue swelling and erythema about the elbow.
- As the disease progresses to later stages, soft tissue swelling may become less prominent, and the elbow becomes more stiff and painful.

Differences in Examination Findings Between Rheumatoid Arthritis and Juvenile Rheumatoid Arthritis

- Elbows affected by JRA obviously occur in younger patients as compared with elbows affected by RA.
- Patients with JRA also have stiffer elbows and therefore typically do not have instability.
- Often JRA patients have more joints affected by the rheumatoid process, but they also demonstrate a greater tolerance for pain.

IMAGING AND OTHER DIAGNOSTIC STUDIES

- Anteroposterior (AP) and lateral radiographs of the elbow are obtained to assess the degree of rheumatoid involvement and for preoperative planning (**FIG 1**). No further studies are typically required.

Classification

- Although several classification systems have been proposed, the most commonly used is the Mayo Radiographic Classification System (Table 1).[6]
  - It allows monitoring of disease progression and often correlates well with clinical examination findings and patients' functional limitations.
  - The grading system is based on bone quality, joint space, and bony architecture and delineates four grades of progression in order of increasing severity.

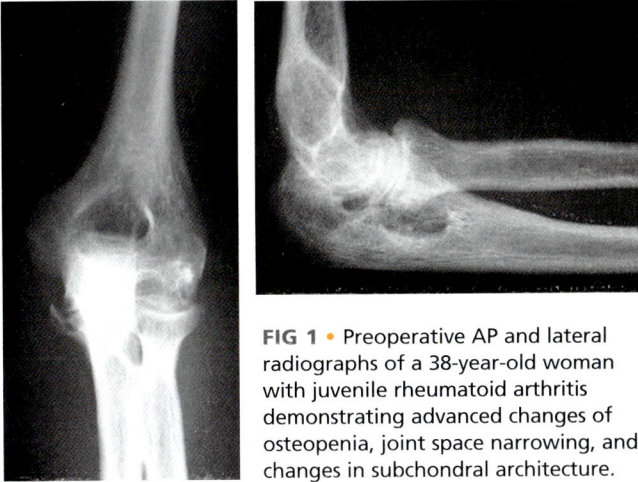

FIG 1 • Preoperative AP and lateral radiographs of a 38-year-old woman with juvenile rheumatoid arthritis demonstrating advanced changes of osteopenia, joint space narrowing, and changes in subchondral architecture.

DIFFERENTIAL DIAGNOSIS

- Calcium pyrophosphate deposition disease
- Osteoarthritis
- Polymyalgia rheumatica
- Psoriatic arthritis
- Systemic lupus erythematosus
- Fibromyalgia

NONOPERATIVE MANAGEMENT

- Optimal care of the patient with RA requires a team-based approach between the orthopaedic surgeon, rheumatologist, and physical therapists to coordinate the full gamut of nonsurgical and surgical treatment options.

Medical Therapy

- The medical management of RA continues to evolve at an impressive rate.
- The mainstays of medical therapy are the classes of drugs known as disease modifying antirheumatic drugs (DMARDs).
  - These include older agents such as gold salts as well as newer agents such as methotrexate, sulfasalazine, anti-tumor necrosis factor (anti-TNF) medications, and other immunomodulators. Such medications may be given alone or as part of combination therapy.
- Other medications prescribed to abate symptoms include nonsteroidal anti-inflammatories (NSAIDs) and steroids.
- Judicious use of intra-articular steroid injections also plays a role in symptom management.
- The importance of early referral to a rheumatologist for medical management cannot be overemphasized. Aggressive management of the synovitis can limit or delay the onset and severity of joint involvement. The most reliable and effective responses to the DMARDs are observed with therapy initiated in the early stages of the disease.

Physical Therapy

- The goal of physical therapy is to encourage range of motion, functional strength, and maintenance of activities of daily living. This is accomplished by activity modification, rest, ice, and gentle exercise.
- The primary objective of nonoperative management of the rheumatoid elbow is to minimize soft tissue swelling and to optimize range of motion, as preoperative range of motion is often predictive of postoperative total arc of motion after arthroscopic synovectomy as well as total elbow arthroplasty.

SURGICAL MANAGEMENT

- Surgical management of the rheumatoid elbow primarily consists of synovectomy and total elbow arthroplasty.

Surgical Management of the Elbow Before Total Elbow Arthroplasty

- For early disease states, excellent clinical results may be achieved with synovectomy performed using open or arthroscopic techniques.
- The goal of synovectomy is to relieve pain and swelling. Although this procedure has not necessarily been shown to alter the natural history of the disease, it reliably produces symptomatic relief for 5 or more years in the majority of cases performed on elbows in the early stages of the disease process.[3]
- The arthroscopic approach is advantageous over the more traditional open approach in that it is less invasive, is associated with less perioperative morbidity, and also allows predictable access to the sacciform recess. When open synovectomy is performed, the radial head must be excised to access and completely débride the diseased synovial tissue that exists in this region.
- Open synovectomy has traditionally been accompanied by radial head excision due to (1) ubiquitous radiocapitellar and proximal radioulnar joint articular destruction and (2) the need to surgically expose the sacciform recess for the requisite complete synovectomy.
  - It has been shown that routine radial head excision may predispose some patients with RA to increasing valgus elbow instability due to the loss of the stabilizing effect of the radial head (particularly if the medial collateral ligament is adversely affected by the rheumatoid process).[7]
  - Now that the entire synovial proliferation around the radial neck can be accessed arthroscopically, a combined arthroscopic radial head excision is performed only in patients with stable elbows and preoperative elbow symptoms with forearm rotation. Otherwise, a complete arthroscopic synovectomy is performed without excising the radial head.
- In addition, the minimally invasive nature of an arthroscopic approach yields the potential advantages of less pain, faster recovery with earlier range of motion, and a lower rate of infection compared with an open procedure.
- An arthroscopic anterior capsular release may be performed at the time of the arthroscopic synovectomy to improve elbow extension. A posterior olecranon-plasty may also be performed to re-establish normal concavity of the olecranon fossa.
- Posteromedial capsule release should be avoided to prevent the risk of iatrogenic ulnar nerve injury. If an elbow requires a release of the posterior capsule to regain elbow flexion (typically those with 100 degrees or less of preoperative flexion), then the surgeon should consider performing an open ulnar nerve decompression and subcutaneous transposition followed by complete posterior capsule release (including the posteromedial band of the medial collateral ligament).

Table 1	Mayo Radiographic Classification System		
Grade	**Radiographic Appearance**	**Description**	**Implications**
I		Synovitis in a normal-appearing joint with mild to moderate osteopenia	Often correlates with impressive soft tissue swelling on clinical examination
II		Loss of joint space, but maintenance of the subchondral architecture	Varying degrees of soft tissue swelling are present
III		Marked by complete loss of joint space	The synovitis has "burned out" and the elbow is typically more stiff
IIIA		Bony architecture is maintained	
IIIB		Associated bone loss	
IV		Severe bony destruction	Patients often have severe pain and functional limitations; functional instability may also be present if the joint's bony architecture is destroyed.
V		Presence of bony ankylosis of the ulnohumeral joint	Most commonly seen with juvenile rheumatoid arthritis

(Adapted from Morrey BF, Adams RA. Semiconstrained arthroplasty for the treatment of rheumatoid arthritis of the elbow. J Bone Joint Surg Am 1992;74A:479–490; and from Connor PM, Morrey BF. Total elbow arthroplasty in patients who have juvenile rheumatoid arthritis. J Bone Joint Surg Am 1998;80A:678–688.)

Total Elbow Arthroplasty

- This procedures is indicated primarily for advanced (grade III or IV) RA of the elbow in patients with significant pain and limitations in activities of daily living.
- Absolute contraindications include active infection, upper extremity paralysis, and a patient's refusal or inability to abide by postoperative activity restrictions.
- Relative contraindications include presence of infection at a remote site and a history of infected elbow or elbow prosthesis.

Preoperative Planning

- AP and lateral radiographs of the elbow are reviewed to assess humeral bow and medullary canal diameter as well as angulation and diameter of the ulnar medullary canal.
  - Preoperative radiographic templates may be helpful to assess preoperative radiographic magnification.
- In particular for JRA patients, the canal width may be very small, and therefore the surgeon must ensure that appropriately sized implants as well as intramedullary guidewires and reamers are available.
- If an ipsilateral total shoulder arthroplasty has been performed or is anticipated, use of a 4-inch humeral implant and a humeral cement restrictor should be considered.
- Preoperative limitations in forearm rotation may be due in part to ipsilateral distal radioulnar joint pathology. Thus, radiographs should also be obtained on the ipsilateral shoulder and wrist.

Implant Selection for Total Elbow Arthroplasty

- Implant options have traditionally been classified as linked (semiconstrained) or unlinked.
  - These terms are being used with decreasing frequency, however, as unlinked implant designs have been developed that have precisely contoured components that create a degree of constraint.
  - Linked, semiconstrained implants have about 7 degrees of varus–valgus "play" and 7 degrees of axial rotation, while unconstrained implants consist of unlinked, resurfacing components.
  - The stability of unconstrained implants depends on soft tissue and ligamentous integrity, while such tissues may be destroyed by the rheumatoid inflammatory process or surgically released with semiconstrained implants without compromising stability.
- Although no prospective comparisons between linked (semiconstrained) and unlinked implants have yet been performed, both appear to have similar survivorship records.
  - The semiconstrained design is preferred because it is equally effective in pain relief and in improving range of motion and function, while preserving stability without an observed increase in aseptic loosening.[5]
  - The Techniques section below focuses on implantation of a linked (semiconstrained) implant.

Sequence and Timing of Total Elbow Arthroplasty in the Patient with Polyarticular Involvement

- Because RA typically affects multiple joint articulations, the timing of elbow arthroplasty should be considered with regard to the need for arthroplasties of other joints.

- In general, the most disabling articulation should be addressed first. In the case of equivocal involvement in the elbow and a lower extremity joint in which arthroplasty is planned, the surgeon must consider the postoperative effects of surgery and plan accordingly.
- If total elbow arthroplasty is performed first, at least 3 to 6 months should pass before lower extremity reconstruction is performed to allow adequate healing in the elbow. If the lower extremity will be addressed first, total elbow arthroplasty should be delayed until assistive ambulatory devices, which may put strain on the elbow, are no longer required.
  - Patients with total elbow arthroplasty should not weight bear with crutches. A walker may be used, provided it does not increase strain on the elbow. This may be achieved by raising the walker's arm rests to an appropriate height such that when the forearms are placed on the arm rests, the elbow may not be extended beyond 90 degrees of flexion.

Assessment of the Cervical Spine

- Because nearly 90% of patients with RA have cervical spine involvement, about 30% of whom have significant subluxation, the cervical spine must be evaluated before any surgery in which intubation is likely.
  - Cervical spine radiographs should be routinely obtained.
  - If patients have neck pain, decreased range of motion, myelopathic symptoms, or radiographic evidence of instability, a magnetic resonance imaging (MRI) study should be ordered with concomitant referral to a spine surgeon to consider addressing the cervical spine pathology before elbow surgery.

Temporary Cessation of Medications Before Total Elbow Arthroplasty

- Tumor necrosis factor (TNF) inhibitors affect the immune system and have been found to increase the risk of developing a prosthetic joint infection.
  - In general, anti-TNF agents are typically stopped for a short period before surgery and for about 2 weeks after surgery to reduce the risk of perioperative morbidity.
- Patients on chronic NSAIDs should stop taking those medications about 2 weeks before surgery to reduce the risk of increased bleeding.
- For patients on chronic steroids, stress-dose steroids may be required perioperatively.
- Communications with the patient's rheumatologist and the anesthesiologist are imperative to coordinate these efforts.

Positioning

- Intravenous antibiotics are administered 30 to 60 minutes before the incision.
- The patient is placed in a supine position on the operating table with a rolled towel under the ipsilateral scapula.
- The entire operative extremity and shoulder girdle is prepared and draped; a sterile tourniquet is placed.
- The arm is exsanguinated and the tourniquet inflated.

Approach

- Although multiple approaches may be used, the Bryan-Morrey approach (triceps–anconeus "slide") is preferred.

INCISION AND EXPOSURE

- A straight incision, measuring about 15 cm, is made centered between the lateral epicondyle and the tip of the olecranon.
- The ulnar nerve is carefully identified and isolated along the medial aspect of the triceps.
- Proximal neurolysis of the nerve is achieved by incising the fascia from the medial head of the triceps to the medial intermuscular septum and then mobilized to beyond its first motor branch distally by splitting the cubital tunnel retinaculum, which includes the band of Osborne (the fascia between the two heads of the flexor carpi ulnaris [FCU]) and the FCU fascia (**TECH FIG 1A,B**).
- The intermuscular septum is excised and a deep pocket of subcutaneous tissue over the flexor pronator group distally and anterior to the triceps proximally is created.
  - The nerve is then anteriorly transposed into this subcutaneous tissue pocket; it must be protected throughout the operation.
- An incision is then made over the medial aspect of the ulna between the anconeus and FCU. The anconeus is subperiosteally elevated off the ulna.
- The medial aspect of the triceps is then retracted along with the fibers of the posterior capsule to tension the Sharpey fibers at their ulnar insertion (**TECH FIG 1C,D**).

- These fibers are then sharply dissected, and the triceps in continuity with the anconeus is reflected from medial to lateral (**TECH FIG 1E**).
- The lateral ulnar collateral ligament complex is released from its humeral attachment, thus allowing the extensor mechanism to be completely reflected to the lateral aspect of the humerus (**TECH FIG 1F**).
- If ulnohumeral ankylosis is present, as is sometimes the case in JRA patients, a saw or osteotome may be necessary to re-establish the joint line and to create the osteotomy at the appropriate center of rotation of the ulnohumeral joint.
- The elbow is then progressively flexed, exposing the medial collateral ligament, which is then released subperiosteally from its humeral attachment (**TECH FIG 1G**).
- The tip of the olecranon is removed with a rongeur or oscillating saw, depending on the quality of the bone, and the humerus is then externally rotated and the elbow fully flexed to adequately expose the articulating surfaces of the humerus, ulna, and radial head.

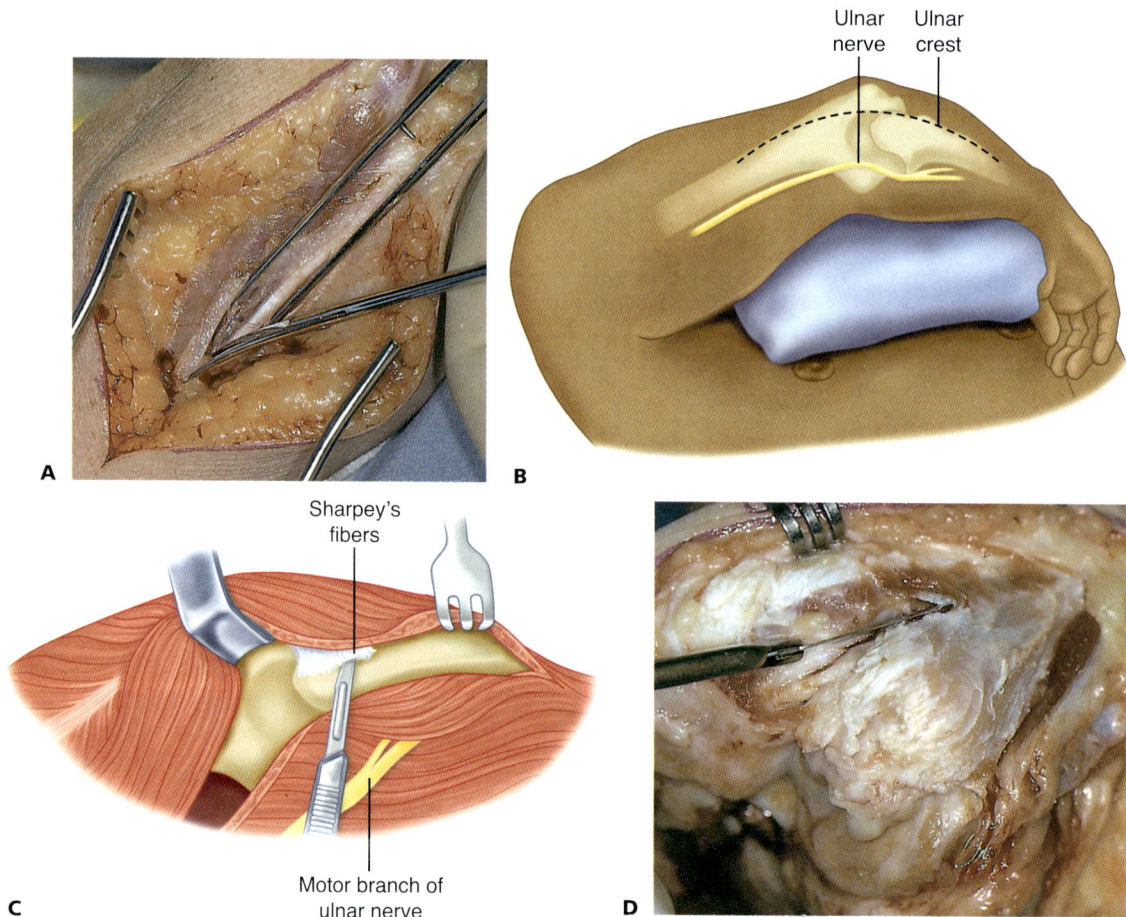

TECH FIG 1 • A,B. The ulnar nerve is identified along the medial border of the triceps, and a vessel loop is placed. **C,D.** Under tension, the medial and ulnar border of the triceps (**C**) and the anconeus (**D**) are incised from their insertions into the olecranon. *(continued)*

TECHNIQUES

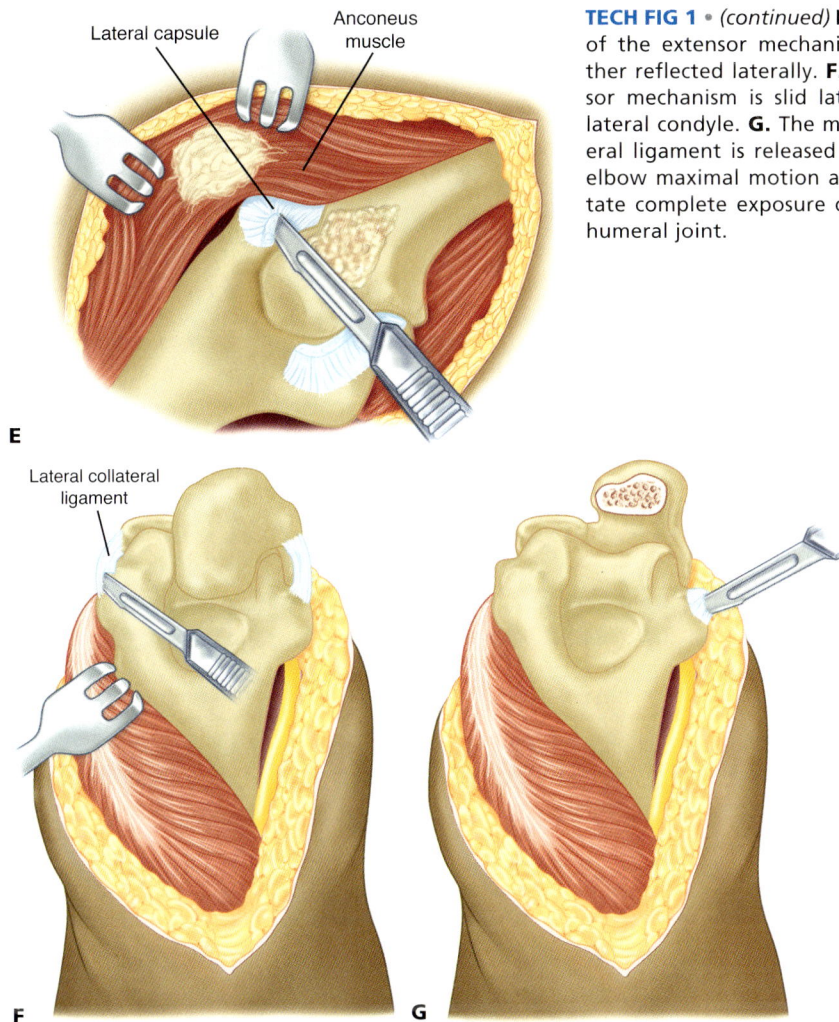

TECH FIG 1 • *(continued)* **E.** The fibers of the extensor mechanism are further reflected laterally. **F.** The extensor mechanism is slid lateral to the lateral condyle. **G.** The medial collateral ligament is released to give the elbow maximal motion and to facilitate complete exposure of the ulnohumeral joint.

Labels in figure: Lateral capsule, Anconeus muscle, Lateral collateral ligament

HUMERAL PREPARATION

- The midportion of the trochlea is then removed, with an oscillating saw if the bone is dense or with a rongeur if the bone is soft, up to the roof of the olecranon fossa.
- The removed bone should be preserved for the anterior, distal humeral bone graft needed later in the procedure (**TECH FIG 2A**).
- The roof of the olecranon is entered with a rongeur or burr, and a small twist reamer is then used to identify the humeral medullary canal (**TECH FIG 2B,C**).
- For patients with severe stiffness, the effect of humeral shortening should be considered.
  - Hughes et al[4] developed a biomechanical model that demonstrated that resecting 1 cm or less of humeral bone has little effect on triceps strength.
    - With the elbow in 30 degrees of flexion, resecting 1 to 2 cm reduced triceps strength by 17% to 40%, while shortening of 3 cm reduced extension strength by 63%.
    - Therefore, the humerus should not be shortened by greater than 2 cm.

- An alignment stem is then placed down the canal. The handle of the alignment stem is then replaced by the humeral cutting jig (**TECH FIG 2D,E**).
- An oscillating saw is used to make oblique cuts along the edges of the jig, with the tip of the saw pointing away from the midline of the humerus to avoid cross-hatching at the junction of the column and the olecranon fossa (**TECH FIG 2F**).
  - Care must be taken as this area may be very thin in patients with RA, and thus susceptible to fracture.
- With the midportion of the trochlea removed, a thin rasp or intramedullary guide is used to again identify the humeral canal.
  - Progressive 6-inch rasps are typically used unless an ipsilateral shoulder arthroplasty has been performed or is planned (**TECH FIG 2G**).
    - In these cases, consider using a 4-inch humeral component.
- The anterior capsule is completely subperiosteally released from the anterior aspect of the humerus to accommodate the flange of the humeral component and to allow unencumbered postoperative elbow extension.

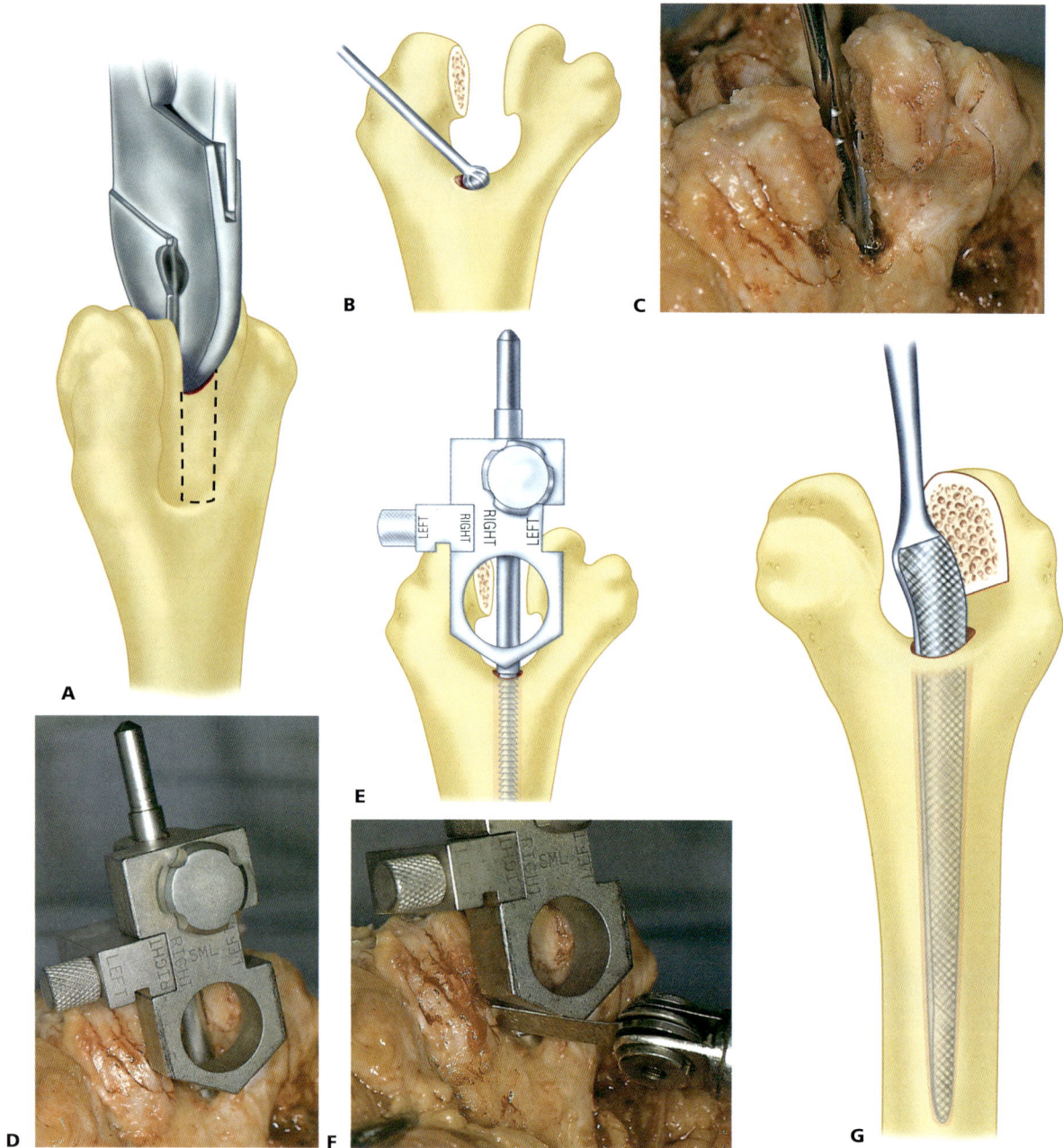

TECH FIG 2 • A. For soft bone, a rongeur is used to remove the midportion of the trochlea. **B.** A burr is used to enter the roof of the olecranon. **C.** Then a twist reamer is used to identify the medullary canal. **D,E.** The humeral cutting jig is aligned as a template for removal of the distal humeral articulation. **F.** An oscillating saw is placed at an oblique angle to the jig to accurately remove the articulating surface of the distal humerus while avoiding cross-hatching of the supracondylar columns. **G.** An appropriately sized rasp is used for the humeral canal.

TECHNIQUES

ULNAR PREPARATION

- It is important to fully expose the greater sigmoid notch.
- A high-speed burr is angled 45 degrees relative to the axis of the ulnar shaft at the junction of the sigmoid fossa and coronoid to identify the ulnar medullary canal (**TECH FIG 3A,B**).
- Again, a twist reamer is used to further identify the canal, and an appropriately sized ulnar rasp is then inserted.
- The ulnar bow should be acknowledged and palpated while inserting the ulnar rasps to avoid ulnar perforation.
  - During advancement of the rasp, it is important to maintain proper rotation of the rasp so that the handle is perpendicular to the flat, dorsal aspect of the proximal ulna (**TECH FIG 3C,D**).
- Alternatively, reaming should be considered if the canal is very small, as may be the case in JRA patients.

- The ulnar canal is thus prepared, and the ulnar component is inserted to the depth such that the center of the ulnar component is midway between the tips of the olecranon and coronoid to reproduce the elbow's axis of rotation (**TECH FIG 3E**).
- A rongeur is then used to remove the tip of the coronoid.
- Because proximal radioulnar arthritis is ubiquitous in patients with RA and JRA, and the Conrad-Morrey total elbow arthroplasty does not require proximal radioulnar and radiocapitellar reconstruction, a radial head excision is performed.
- This may be performed by rotating the forearm and using a rongeur to progressively excise the radial head from an axial orientation, while holding the elbow in full flexion.

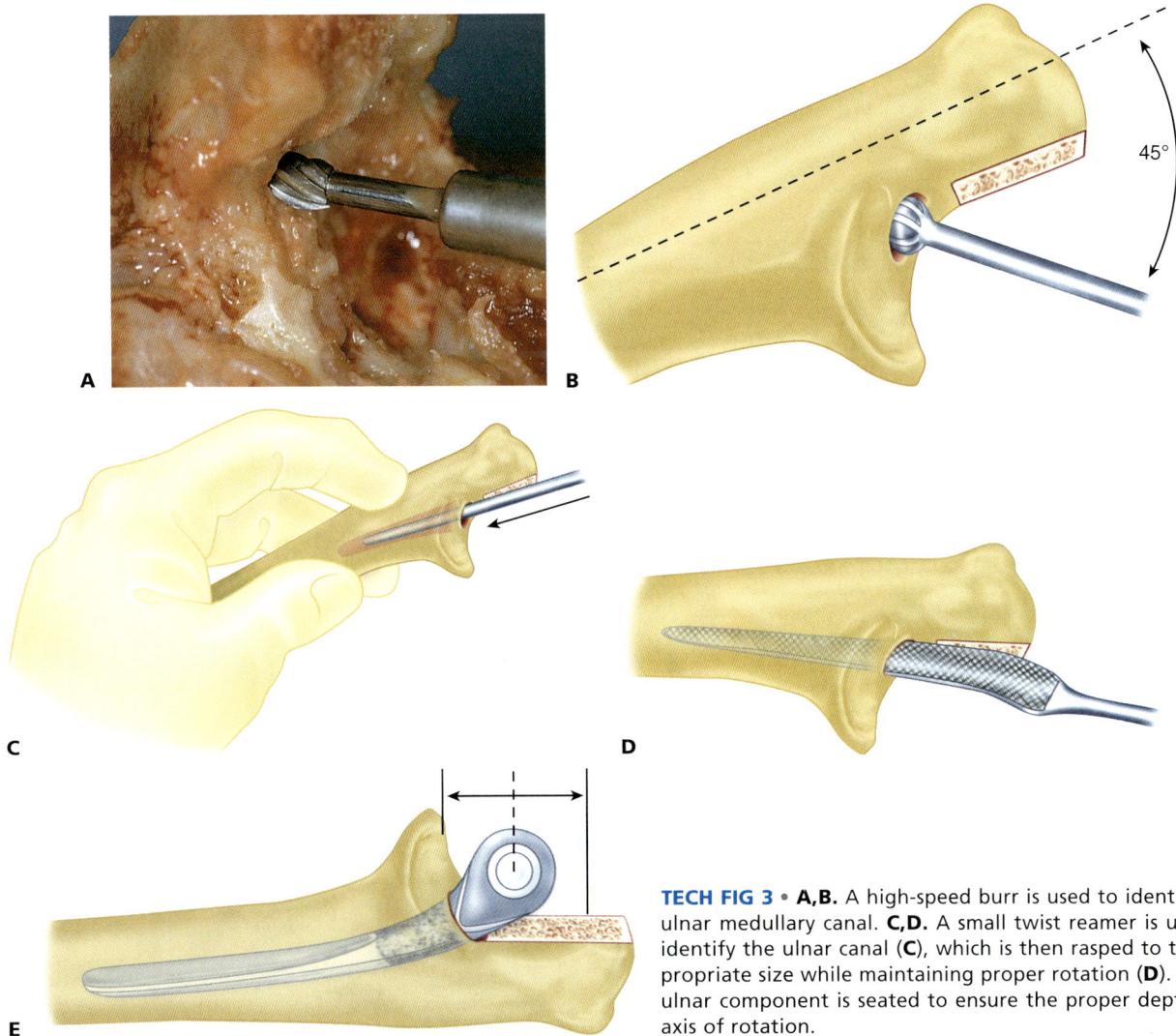

45°

TECH FIG 3 • A,B. A high-speed burr is used to identify the ulnar medullary canal. **C,D.** A small twist reamer is used to identify the ulnar canal (**C**), which is then rasped to the appropriate size while maintaining proper rotation (**D**). **E.** The ulnar component is seated to ensure the proper depth and axis of rotation.

TECHNIQUES

TRIAL REDUCTION

- The humeral component is then inserted and a trial reduction is performed.
- Range of motion is tested and should be full without limitation in the flexion–extension plane.
  - If range of motion is limited owing to inadequate soft tissue release, this should be addressed at this time.
- The components should also be evaluated for bony impingement, which may commonly occur posteriorly (olecranon impingement on the humerus) or anteriorly (coronoid tip on the anterior flange of the humeral component; **TECH FIG 4**).
  - Any impinging bone should be removed with a rongeur.
- After satisfactory trial reduction, the provisional components are removed.

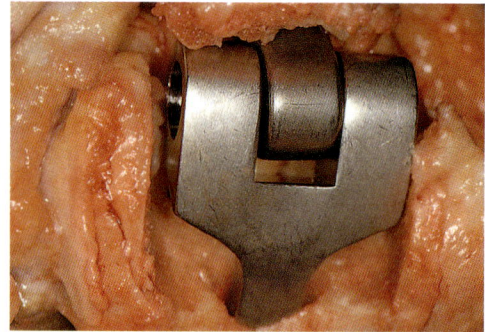

TECH FIG 4 • A trial reduction of the components is performed and range of motion is assessed to evaluate for bony impingement.

CEMENTING

- Both medullary canals are then pulse lavaged and dried.
- Based on the trial components used, the length of the cement applicator is measured to equal that of the humeral component.
  - The tip of the applicator is cut at this level to ensure appropriate depth of the cement down the humeral canal (**TECH FIG 5**).

- It is recommended that cementing of the components be performed simultaneously.
  - Two packs of cement with antibiotics are mixed and injected with a runny consistency.
  - The humeral cement is placed first, followed by the ulnar cement and then the ulnar component.
  - Remove excess cement.

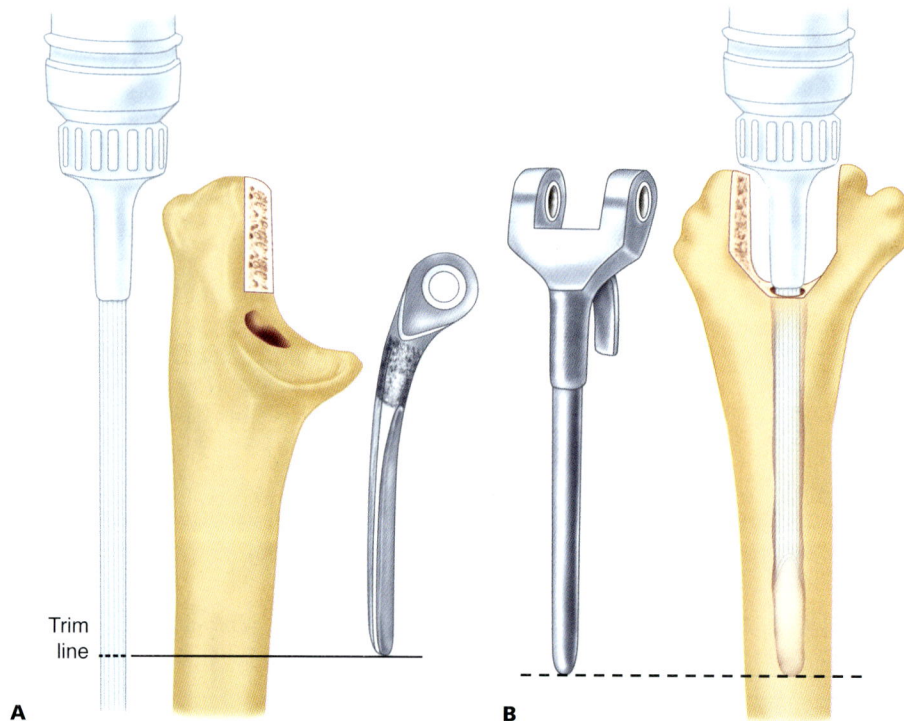

Trim line ----

A   B

TECH FIG 5 • Simultaneous cementing of the humeral and ulnar medullary canals is recommended.

TECHNIQUES

HUMERAL COMPONENT AND BONE GRAFT

- A small (about 2 cm × 2 cm and 2- to 4-mm thick) piece of the removed trochlea is used for the anterior bone graft.
- This bone graft is wedged between the anterior aspect of the humerus and the flange as the humeral component is placed (**TECH FIG 6**).
- This provides the humeral component with rotational stability as well as additional stability in the AP plane.
- Once again, excess cement is removed at this time.

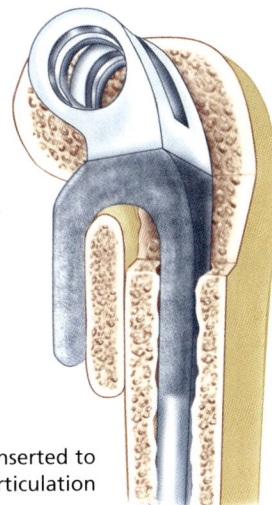

TECH FIG 6 • The humeral component is inserted to the optimal depth that allows proper articulation with the ulnar component.

ASSEMBLY AND IMPACTION

- The components are then linked with the use of two interlocking cross-pins, which are placed from opposite directions (**TECH FIG 7A**).
- If humeral bowing or a small canal exists, a slight bow can be placed in the proximal aspect of the humeral component to ensure proper fit (**TECH FIG 7B,C**).
- After coupling the prosthesis, the components must be seated; the elbow is flexed to 90 degrees and the humeral component is then impacted such that the dis-

tal aspect of the humeral component is roughly at or slightly proximal to the contour of the distal capitellum (**TECH FIG 7D,E**).
- Range of motion is checked and a full arc of motion is confirmed.
- The elbow is taken through several arcs of flexion--extension to "normalize" the rotational version of components to one another.
- Hold the elbow in full extension until the cement cures.

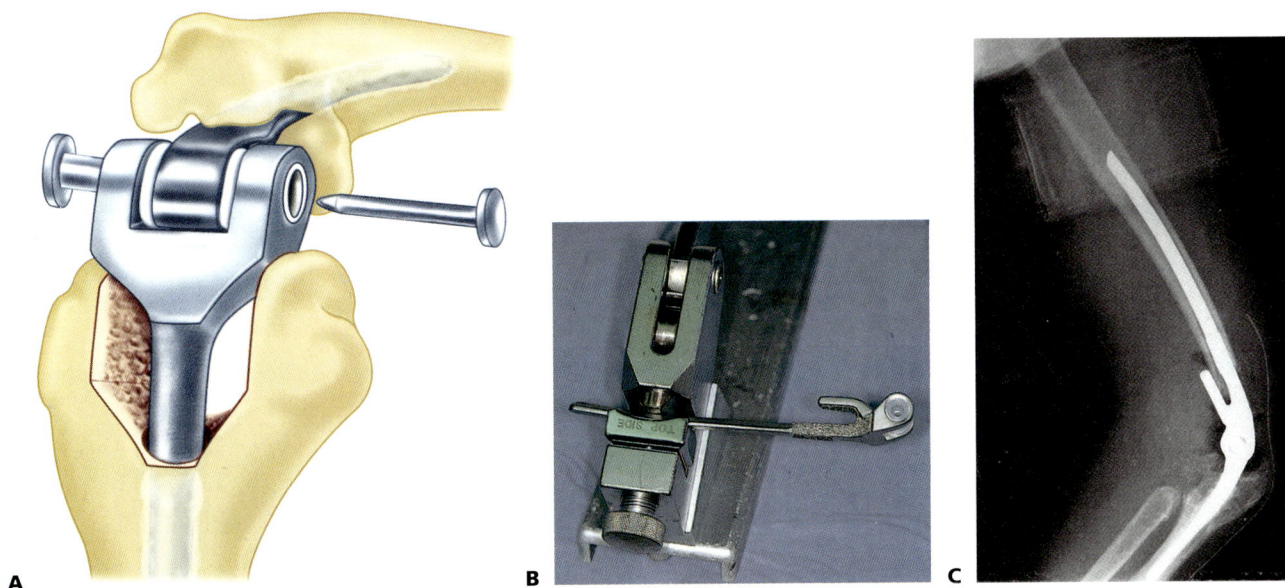

A

B

C

TECH FIG 7 • **A.** The ulnar and humeral components are linked by two interlocking cross-pins, which are placed from opposite sides. **B,C.** A slight bow may be created in the proximal aspect of the humeral component if humeral bowing or a small canal is present. *(continued)*

TECHNIQUES

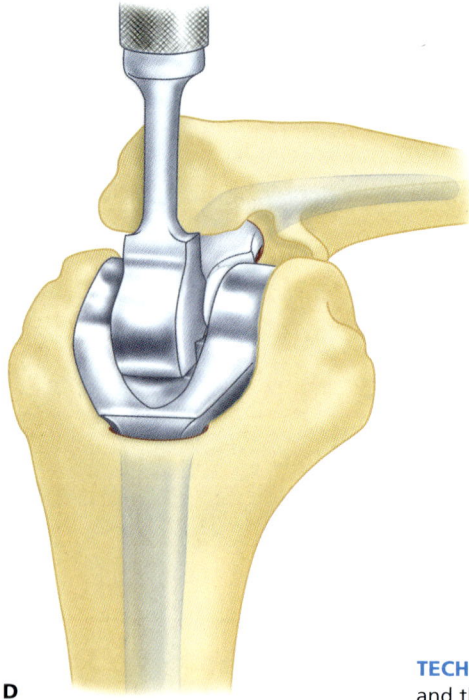

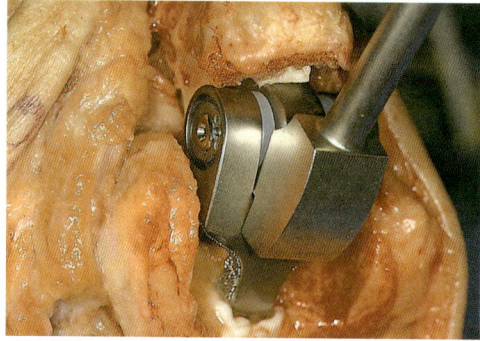

TECH FIG 7 • *(continued)* **D,E.** The elbow is flexed to 90 degrees and the humeral component is then impacted.

TRICEPS REATTACHMENT

- Small cruciate and transverse drill holes are placed through the olecranon at the site of triceps reattachment, and a heavy, nonabsorbable suture is placed on a Keith needle and then brought through the distal medial cruciate drill hole and out the proximal lateral hole (**TECH FIG 8A–C**).
- The elbow is flexed to about 60 degrees and the extensor mechanism is reduced over the tip of the olecranon; consider slightly overreducing the extensor mechanism medially to minimize the potential for postoperative lateral subluxation.
- The suture is woven through the triceps tendon in a locking, crisscross pattern such that the suture emerges at the proximal medial hole (**TECH FIG 8D**).

- The suture is then passed through this hole and out the distal medial hole such that it is located directly across from the initial suture end.
- These suture ends are then passed again through the forearm extensor fascia and tied together.
- Two reinforcing sutures are then passed through the transverse holes and extensor fascia before being tied together.
- Avoid knots directly over the subcutaneous border of the proximal ulna.
- The tourniquet is then deflated and hemostasis is achieved.
- The medial soft tissue extensor mechanism is then reapproximated.

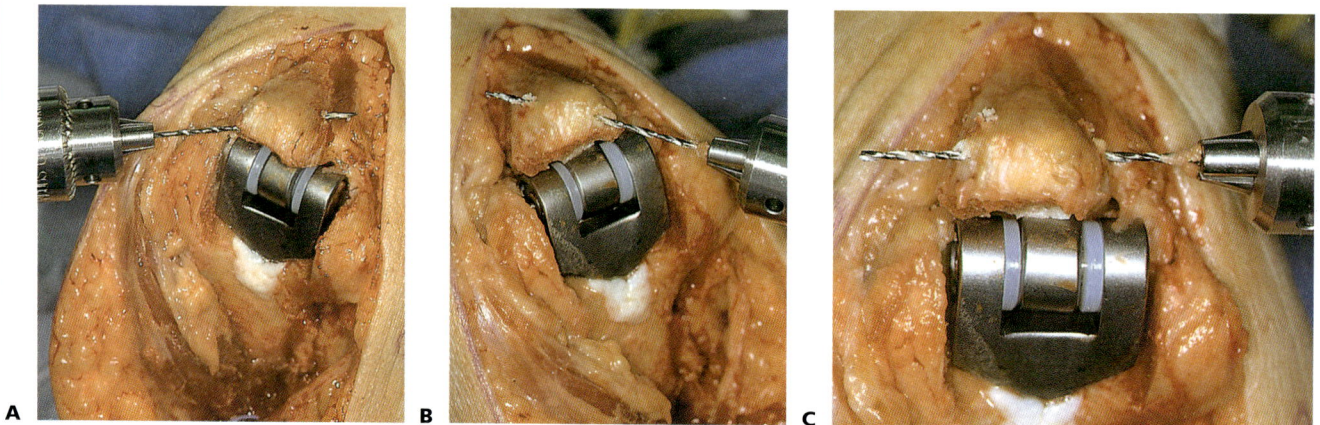

TECH FIG 8 • Cruciate (**A,B**) and transverse (**C**) drill holes are placed in the ulna for triceps reattachment. *(continued)*

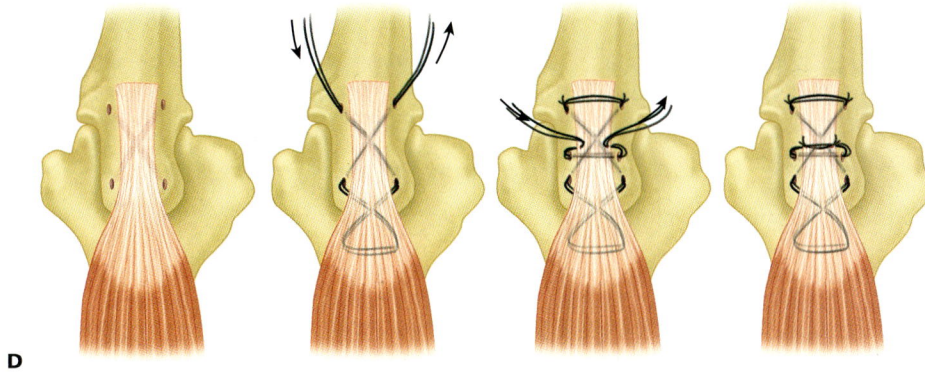

TECH FIG 8 • *(continued)* **D.** Suture is passed through the proximal ulna and then woven through the triceps tendon before being tied together.

ULNAR NERVE TRANSPOSITION AND WOUND CLOSURE

- The protected nerve is in the subcutaneous tissue pocket previously created, and dermal sutures are placed to protect and secure the nerve (**TECH FIG 9**).
- Wounds are closed in layers, and a drain is placed. Staples are used to close the skin.
- A volar splint is placed with the elbow in full extension, making sure to adequately pad the anterior aspect of the splint both proximally and distally to prevent skin breakdown.

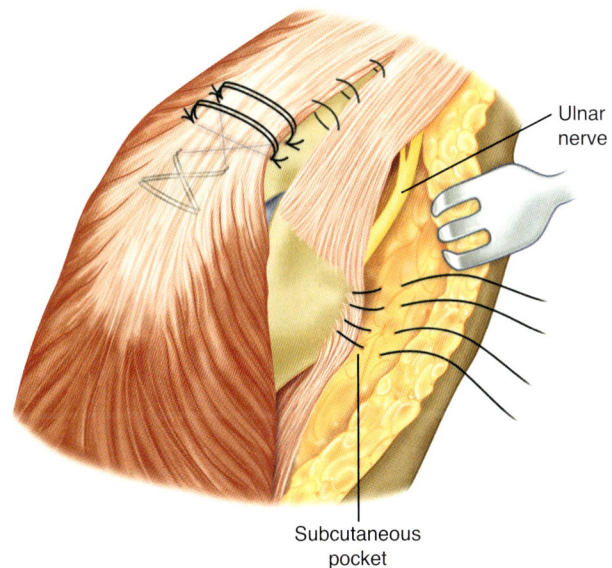

TECH FIG 9 • The ulnar nerve is transposed into the subcutaneous tissue of the medial epicondylar region and secured with sutures in the dermal layer.

PEARLS AND PITFALLS

Approach and exposure	▪ Take your time with the Bryan-Morrey approach; maintaining subperiosteal elevation of the extensor mechanism will make for a better postoperative extensor mechanism repair. ▪ Obtain complete ulnohumeral dissociation before bony preparation. This includes complete releases of the lateral ulnar collateral ligament and medial collateral ligament complexes, and a complete anterior capsule release. ▪ Consider reflection of common flexors or extensors if severe deformities or arthrofibrosis is present.
Humeral preparation	▪ Shorten the humerus by 1 cm or less to augment postoperative range of motion without compromising strength. ▪ Use a burr distally to open up the humeral canal if needed, rather than forcing with rasps.
Radial and ulnar preparation	▪ Excise the radial head and the tip of the coronoid. ▪ Always palpate the ulna and consider the ulnar bow before ulnar preparation to avoid perforation. ▪ Have guidewires and reamers (5.0, 5.5, 6.0, 6.5) available if needed.
Cementing	▪ Review the cement technique and order mentally before proceeding; use cement that does not rapidly set.
Triceps reattachment	▪ Overreduce the triceps–anconeus repair medially.
Postoperative care	▪ Use a postoperative extension splint for 24 to 36 hours. ▪ Make all efforts to reduce postoperative swelling.

POSTOPERATIVE CARE

- Postoperatively, the anteriorly placed splint maintains the elbow in full extension for about 24 to 36 hours.
- The elbow is elevated overnight and on postoperative day 1.
- The drain is removed on postoperative day 1 or when output is less than 30 mL in an 8-hour period.
- After splint removal, open-chain active-assisted range of motion is allowed. A formal physical therapy consultation is not usually required.
- The patient is restricted to no pushing and no overhead activities for 3 months to protect the triceps. In addition, no repetitive lifting of objects heavier than 5 pounds and no lifting greater than 10 pounds in a single event is allowed for life.
- A collar and cuff are provided for comfort.

OUTCOMES

- Successful outcomes for total elbow arthroplasty are judged based on relief of pain and improved range of motion, stability, and function.
  - The Mayo Elbow Performance Score assigns numeric values to each of these categories to produce scores for each of these criteria as well as an overall score.[6] Outcomes are often compared using this system.
- Total elbow arthroplasty for RA
  - In the largest study with the longest follow-up in the literature, Gill and Morrey[2] reported 86% good or excellent results with a 13% reoperation rate on 69 patients with RA treated with a semiconstrained total elbow arthroplasty. Forty-four of these patients were followed for more than 10 years.
  - The prosthetic survival rate was 92.4% at 10 years of follow-up, thus approaching the success of lower extremity arthroplasty.
- Total elbow arthroplasty for JRA
  - Connor and Morrey[1] reported 87% good or excellent results on 19 patients (24 elbows) followed for a mean of 7.4 years.
    - The mean improvement in the Mayo Elbow Performance Score was 59 points, 96% had little or no pain, and there was no evidence of loosening in any prostheses at the latest follow-up.
  - The mean flexion–extension arc of motion improved by only 27 degrees (from 67 to 90 degrees) in this study, but these outcomes were reported before shortening of the humerus for severely contracted elbows was routinely performed.

COMPLICATIONS

- Infection
- Aseptic loosening
- Mechanical failure
  - Short term
  - Long term
- Ulnar nerve injury
- Triceps weakness or avulsion
- Ulnar component fracture
- Ulnar fracture
- Wound healing problems

REFERENCES

1. Connor PM, Morrey BF. Total elbow arthroplasty in patients who have juvenile rheumatoid arthritis. J Bone Joint Surg Am 1998;80A:678–688.
2. Gill DR, Morrey BF. The Coonrad-Morrey total elbow arthroplasty in patients who have rheumatoid arthritis: a ten- to fifteen-year follow-up study. J Bone Joint Surg Am 1998;80A:1327–1335.
3. Horiuchi K, Momohara S, Tomatsu T, et al. Arthroscopic synovectomy of the elbow in rheumatoid arthritis. J Bone Joint Surg Am 2002;84A:342–347.
4. Hughes RE, Schneeberger AG, An KN, et al. Reduction of triceps muscle force after shortening of the distal humerus: a computational model. J Shoulder Elbow Surg 1997;6:444–448.
5. Little CP, Graham AJ, Karatzas G, et al. Outcomes of total elbow arthroplasty for rheumatoid arthritis: comparative study of three implants. J Bone Joint Surg Am 2005;87A:2439–2448.
6. Morrey BF, Adams RA. Semiconstrained arthroplasty for the treatment of rheumatoid arthritis of the elbow. J Bone Joint Surg Am 1992;74A:479–490.
7. Rymaszewski LA, Mackay I, Amis AA, et al. Long-term effects of excision of the radial head in rheumatoid arthritis. J Bone Joint Surg Br 1979;66B:109–113.

Chapter 46

Elbow Replacement for Acute Trauma

Srinath Kamineni

DEFINITION

- Most comminuted elbow fractures have significant associated soft tissue injuries, which are often of equal or greater importance to the bony element.
- The key point in determining how to treat acute elbow fractures is to assume that all fractures will be anatomically reduced and fixed.
- An acute elbow replacement should be considered only if it is felt that open reduction and internal fixation is unlikely to achieve a predictably good functional outcome.
- In the vast majority of cases, elbow replacements for the treatment of acute fractures should be limited to the physiologically elderly patient with low demands and osteoporotic bone stock.

ANATOMY

- The bony anatomy of the elbow consists of the distal humerus, proximal ulna, and proximal radius.
- Important soft tissue stabilizers include the medial and lateral ligamentous complexes and surrounding musculature, especially the brachialis, common flexor and common extensor masses, and triceps.
- The ulnar nerve is tethered to the medial condylar–epicondylar fragment by the cubital tunnel retinaculum distally and the arcade of Struthers proximally.

PATHOGENESIS

- Elbow injuries are often the result of direct impact—for example, a direct blow on the elbow during a fall.
- Knowing the energy of the fracture is important to gauge the likelihood of associated injuries.
- Less energy is required to create a comminuted fracture in elderly and osteoporotic individuals, but muscular injuries of the triceps and brachialis are common, with a subsequent influence on the functional outcome.
- The ulnar nerve displaces with the medial fragment. As a consequence, the nerve may kink, leading to a local nerve injury. Nerve lacerations are an uncommon consequence of comminuted distal humeral fractures.

NATURAL HISTORY

- Most distal humeral fractures are treatable with either open reduction and internal fixation (ORIF) or nonoperative management. The challenging fracture subgroups are those that involve the articular surfaces and are comminuted.
- Many direct and indirect soft tissue complications may ensue, including neurovascular entrapment,[2,6] muscle tears leading to myositis ossificans,[6,11,15] and soft tissue contracture with joint stiffness.
- There is some evidence to suggest that congruently reducing and fixing a comminuted intra-articular distal humeral fracture

does not eliminate the risk of posttraumatic arthritis,[7] although, where possible, ORIF should remain the primary goal.

PATIENT HISTORY AND PHYSICAL FINDINGS

- The physical examination (**FIG 1**) should be performed gently in the presence of fractures, especially when comminution suggests the possibility of neurovascular injury if the examination is too vigorous.
- A complete examination of the elbow should also include evaluation of associated injuries. It should begin away from the elbow, progressing toward it.
- The following associated injuries should be ruled out:
  - Distal radial and scaphoid fractures: Since the most common mechanism of injury is a fall onto an outstretched hand, the energy transfer of the fall begins in the extended wrist, through the distal radius and scaphoid. Direct palpation of the distal radius should be done and anatomic snuffbox tenderness should be elicited. Palpation of the scaphoid tubercle and ulnar and radial deviation of the wrist may also identify a scaphoid injury.
  - Distal radioulnar joint disruption: Ballottement of the ulnar head should be done in the volar and dorsal directions, in pronation and supination. A disrupted joint is often painful with such ballottement, and the ulnar head may be prominent with the forearm in pronation.
  - Fracture extension beyond the elbow: The examiner should palpate the ulna shaft, along its subcutaneous border, from the wrist to the olecranon.
  - Interosseous membrane injury: Palpating the interval between the bones of the forearm is not a sensitive examination but can raise suspicion for an Essex-Lopresti injury,

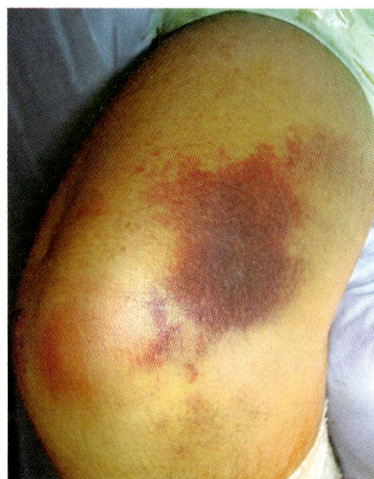

FIG 1 • Typical appearance of an elbow with an underlying fracture with extensive swelling and bruising.

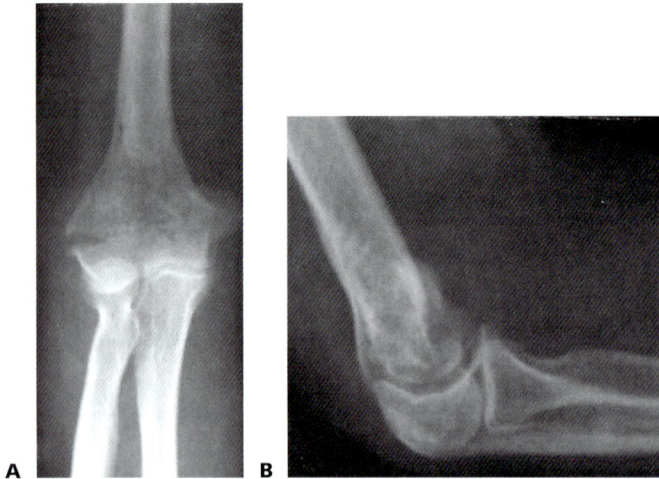

FIG 2 • Standard AP and lateral plain radiographs.

leading to further imaging. If an interosseous membrane disruption is present, this will influence the type of implant used for elbow replacement (one with a radial head replacement), but the pathology is not commonly described.

IMAGING AND DIAGNOSTIC STUDIES

- Plain radiographs, including anteroposterior (AP) and lateral views (**FIG 2**) of the elbow and both wrists, should be obtained. The elbow view may have to be taken in a protective splint or plaster back-slab for patient comfort.
- Elbow radiographs will allow initial assessment of the degree of comminution and may indicate the presence of decreased bone mineral density.
- Bilateral wrist views will indicate the presence of an axial (interosseous membrane) injury if the ulnar head is in positive variance compared to the contralateral uninjured wrist.
- Plain tomograms are of use in improving the understanding of the fracture configuration, but an alternative would be a computed tomography (CT) scan. With the latter the surgeon can view a three-dimensional reconstruction, which is a useful surgical planning tool.
- If there is evidence on physical examination of a neurologic injury, it is prudent to document its extent with a carefully performed neurologic examination.

DIFFERENTIAL DIAGNOSIS

- Nonunion
- Ligamentous disruption
- Fracture-dislocation

NONOPERATIVE MANAGEMENT

- The "bag-of-bones" technique is a nonoperative method of treatment described by Eastwood that encourages the compressive molding of the comminuted distal humeral fracture fragments.
- Subsequent rehabilitation with collar and cuff support achieves substandard but acceptable results only in the elderly and debilitated group of patients who have almost no demand on elbow function.
- This type of treatment does not achieve acceptable results with respect to stability and strength in younger patients.

SURGICAL MANAGEMENT

Open Reduction and Internal Fixation

- ORIF has been widely documented for comminuted fractures of the distal humerus.
- Some reported series demonstrate good results with fixation of such challenging fractures, with better results predominantly in the younger age groups.[12,16] Rarely are good results achieved in the elderly, osteoporotic group.[7]
- Many series report less-than-satisfactory outcomes in the elderly treated by operative fixation.[12]
- A direct comparison of internal fixation to primary total elbow replacement in the elderly osteoporotic group revealed that replacement produced no poor results and no need for revision surgery at 2 years of follow-up. The internal fixation group produced three poor results requiring revision to a total elbow replacement.[4]

Elbow Arthroplasty

- When a distal humerus fracture is not reconstructable, arthroplasty becomes a valid treatment option.
- Elbow replacement following a failed attempt at fixation has proven to have a significantly worse outcome than if the arthroplasty was performed initially.[3]
- There are a number of studies that support the concept of an acute total elbow arthroplasty in select patients with comminuted fractures of the distal humerus.[1,3,9]
- The more traditional form of replacement for the elderly and low-demand population with an unreconstructable distal humerus fracture is the total elbow arthroplasty.
- A more recent innovation has been the replacement of the distal humerus (hemiarthroplasty) to preserve an intact ulna and radial head.[13] This procedure is not FDA approved and so should be considered experimental and not for general consideration, especially since the elbow joint is variable and highly congruent in its topography, which differs from many of the standard implants used for acute fractures.

Indications and Contraindications

- Indications for acute total elbow arthroplasty
  - Comminuted, unreconstructable distal humerus fracture
  - Physiologically elderly patient
  - Low-demand patient
- Indications for acute elbow hemiarthroplasty
  - Unreconstructable distal humeral fracture (C3)
  - Unreconstructable combined fractures of capitellum and trochlea
  - Very low bicondylar T fracture of distal humerus
    - Young patient
    - Active patient
  - Repairable or intact collateral ligaments (may require reconstruction of the medial and lateral supracondylar columns)
  - Repairable or intact radial head
- Absolute contraindications for acute joint replacement
  - Infection (overt)
  - Lack of soft tissue coverage (skin, muscle)
- Relative contraindications for acute joint replacement
  - Infection in distant body part
  - Contaminated wound
  - Neurologic injury involving the elbow flexors

Preoperative Planning

- Standard radiographs should be obtained (AP and lateral).
- If doubt exists regarding the ability to anatomically repair the fracture, then a CT scan should be requested to assess the degree of comminution and the fracture line orientation.
- An assessment of humeral shaft bone loss is important in planning the implant design that might be considered. If the degree of loss is greater than the articular condylar fragments, an implant that has the ability to restore humeral length will be more appropriate. If an unreconstructable fracture of the humeral articular surfaces without humeral shaft bone loss is encountered, an implant with the ability to resurface the articular surfaces as a hemiarthroplasty or a resurfacing ulnotrochlear replacement can be considered, but the former implantation technique should be regarded as an off-label and experimental procedure.
- Humeral shaft length loss of 2 cm can be tolerated and standard implants used.
- Humeral shaft length loss of greater than 2 cm can be restored with implant designs with anterior flanges, especially those with extended flanges that allow restoration of humeral length.
- The surgeon should assess the intramedullary canal dimensions of the humerus and ulna. This will help to plan the requirement of extra-small diameter.
- Neurovascular status of the limb should be fully assessed and documented in the clinical notes.

Patient Positioning

- Two methods of patient positioning can be used, depending on surgeon comfort and the access required:
  - Supine: The arm is draped for maximum maneuverability. During the procedure the arm is supported on a large rolled towel placed on the patient's upper thorax, carefully avoiding the endotracheal tube, stabilized by an assistant. In this position the surgeon stands on the side of the patient's injured limb (**FIG 3A**).
  - Lateral decubitus: The arm is positioned on an arm support, thereby minimizing the need for an assistant, but this set-up is less maneuverable. In this position the surgeon stands on the opposite side of the patient's injured limb (**FIG 3B**).

Surgical Approach

- Two main surgical approaches are useful for acute total elbow arthroplasty:

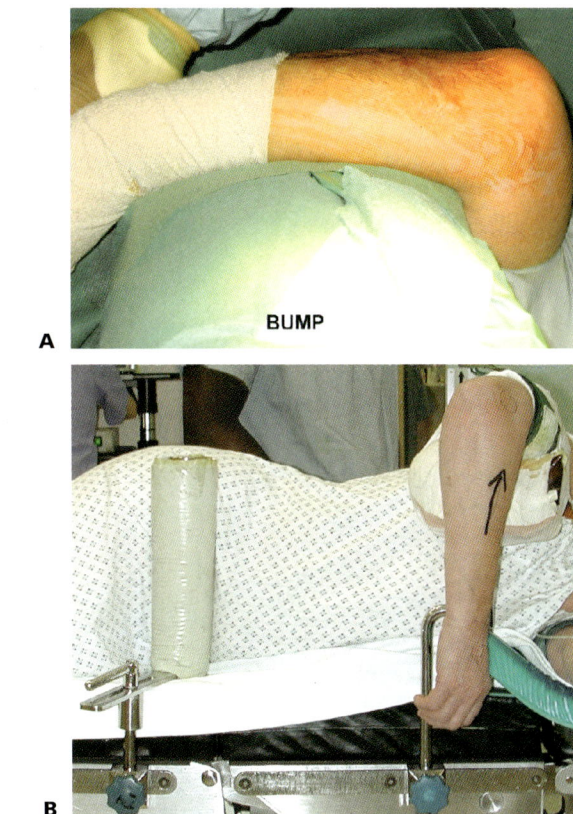

FIG 3 • **A.** Patient positioned in a supine position. The elbow is isolated and placed on a roll of towel placed on the patient's chest, and stabilized by an assistant. The surgeon must take care to avoid the neck and anesthetic equipment. **B.** Patient positioned in a lateral decubitus position with the elbow draped over an arm support.

- Triceps-splitting approach
- Bryan-Morrey approach
- The triceps should be carefully managed in either approach, and it often has a thin tendon, especially in older patients and those with rheumatoid arthritis. The triceps tendon should be dissected from the olecranon with a small curved scalpel blade, maintained perpendicular to the interface between the tendon and bone.

INCISION AND DISSECTION

- Make a midline longitudinal skin incision (**TECH FIG 1A**), with a gentle curve to avoid the olecranon weight-bearing prominence. Extend the incision 5 cm distal to and proximal to the prominence of the olecranon tip.
- Develop the full-thickness medial and lateral skin flaps (**TECH FIG 1B**) and define the medial and lateral borders of the triceps (**TECH FIG 1C,D**).
- At the medial border, define and partially neurolyse the ulnar nerve, and mark and handle it with a tied vessel loop (without an attached hemostat, since its constant weight may cause inadvertent nerve injury) (**TECH FIG 1E**).
- With the nerve visualized and handled to safety, remain in the medial gutter to extend the dissection distally to define the medial fracture fragment. Transect the medial collateral ligament in its entirety, and remove all soft tissue from this bony fragment and remove the latter (**TECH FIG 1F**).

TECHNIQUES

TECHNIQUES

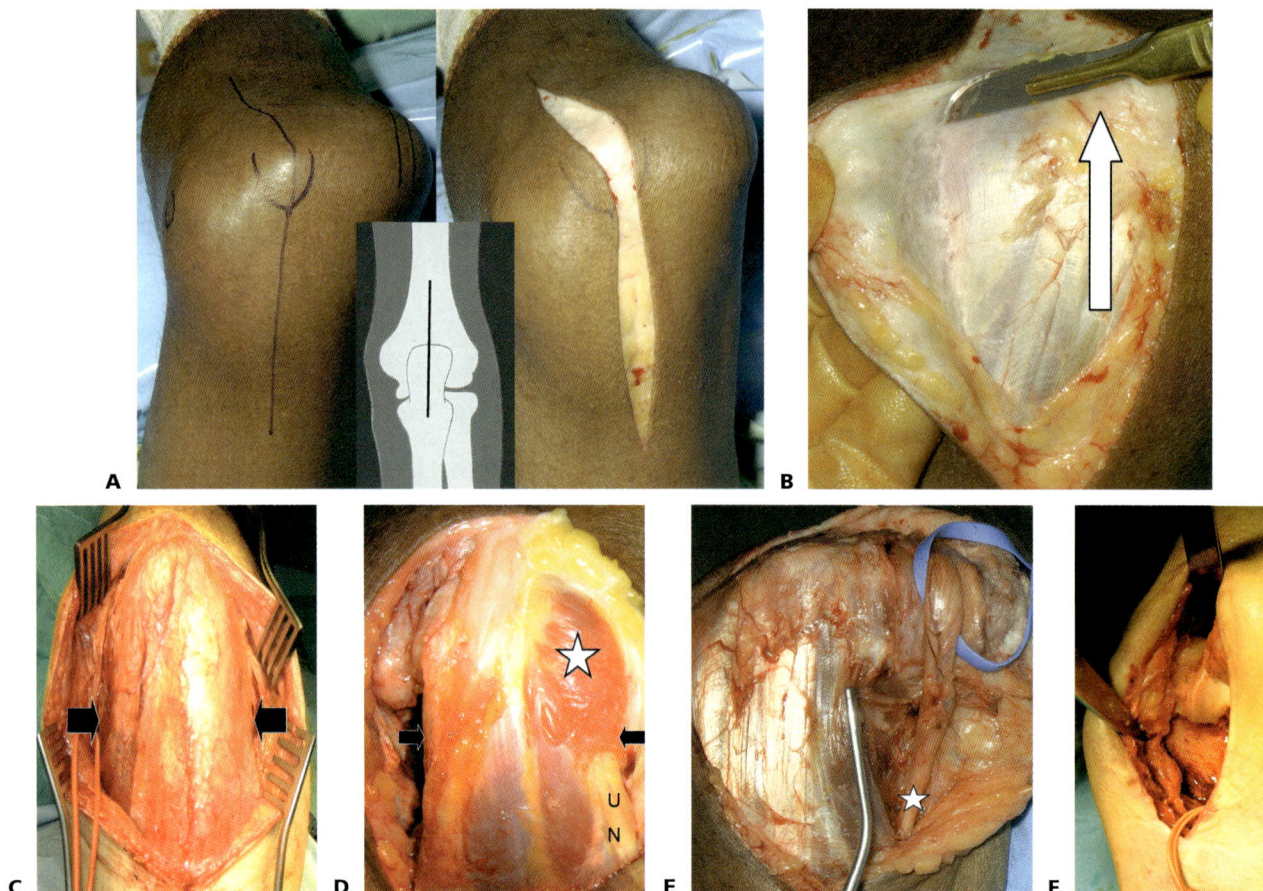

TECH FIG 1 • **A.** Skin incision is posterior longitudinal, with or without a small diversion to avoid the "point" of the olecranon. **B.** Raising the skin should aim to maintain the full thickness of the flaps by using the "flat knife" technique. **C.** The medial and lateral borders of the triceps are defined (*arrows*). **D.** This patient had an anconeus epitrochlearis (*star*) in relation to the ulna nerve (UN). **E.** A vessel loop is used to maneuver the nerve without an attached clip. **F.** The medial fragment of the fracture is removed once all the soft tissues are released from it, and the nerve is gently retracted to ensure tension-free removal.

TRICEPS MANAGEMENT

Triceps Preserving

- With the ulnar nerve gently medially retracted, use a periosteal elevator to define the plane between the triceps and the posterior humerus, from the medial to the lateral border, exiting posterior to the lateral intermuscular septum. Use this elevator to lift the triceps, with blunt dissection, by sliding the shaft of the elevator proximal and distal in the interface (**TECH FIG 2A**).
- Develop the lateral triceps–lateral intermuscular septum margin and resect the lateral fracture fragments, having firstly cleared them of soft tissue attachments (**TECH FIG 2B**).
  - While in the lateral corridor, visualize the radial head and resect sufficient head to prevent abutment on the prosthesis.
- From the lateral margin of the humeral shaft, raise the brachialis from 2 to 3 cm of the anterior surface.

Modified Bryan-Morrey Approach

- Preserving the integrity of the triceps insertion makes component insertion more difficult. An alternative approach for managing the triceps is to reflect it from the tip of the olecranon from medial to lateral, thereby improving exposure (**TECH FIG 3**).
- Define the medial triceps border and dissect the ulna nerve free from its connections, while protecting it in a vessel loop. The nerve is transposed into a subcutaneous pocket.
- The medial triceps is dissected to its ulna attachment. Release the triceps from the medial condylar fragments and transect the medial collateral ligament. Free the medial fragments from soft tissue attachments and remove the medial fragments between the triceps and a gently anteriorly retracted ulnar nerve.

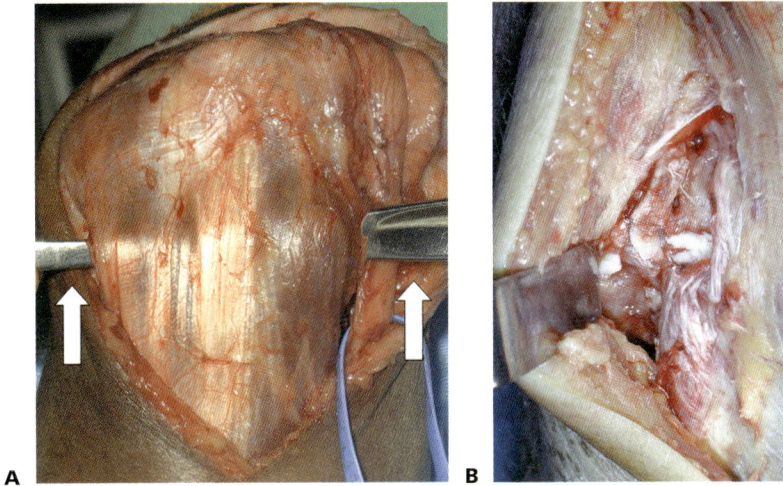

TECH FIG 2 • **A.** A periosteal elevator is introduced between the triceps and the humeral shaft and the two structures are separated by sliding the elevator proximally and then distally to the level of the triceps insertion. **B.** The lateral corridor is defined and lateral fragments are removed.

- Develop the interval between the anconeus and flexor carpi ulnaris along the subcutaneous border of the ulna.
- The triceps tendon is sharply elevated from the olecranon, in continuity with the anconeus, and subluxed laterally. Take care to release the Sharpey fibers adjacent to the bone in order to retain the flap thickness. Further access is

afforded by raising the anconeus from its ulnar attachment while maintaining its attachment distally.

- As the triceps is reflected laterally, the lateral condylar fragments are identified and removed by releasing the lateral collateral ligament and common extensor tendon.

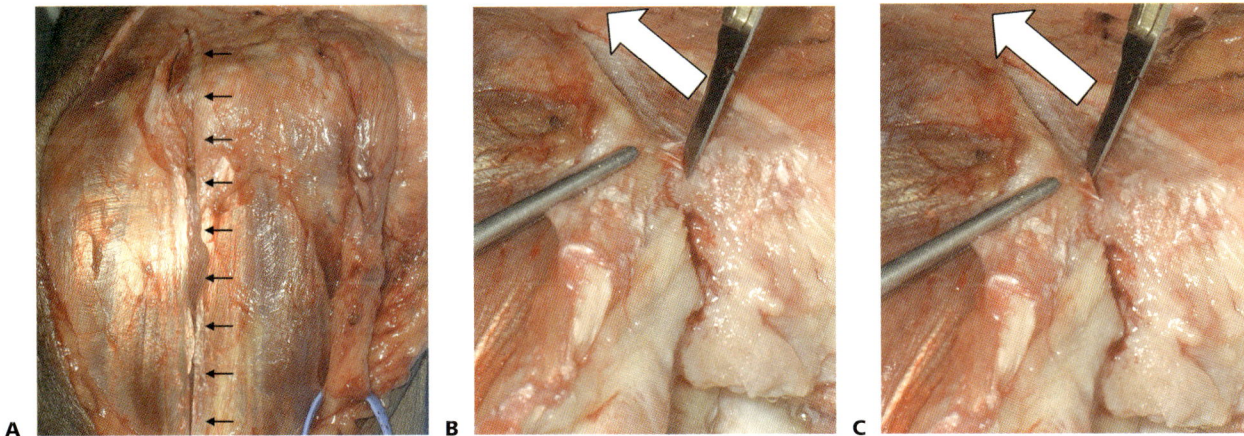

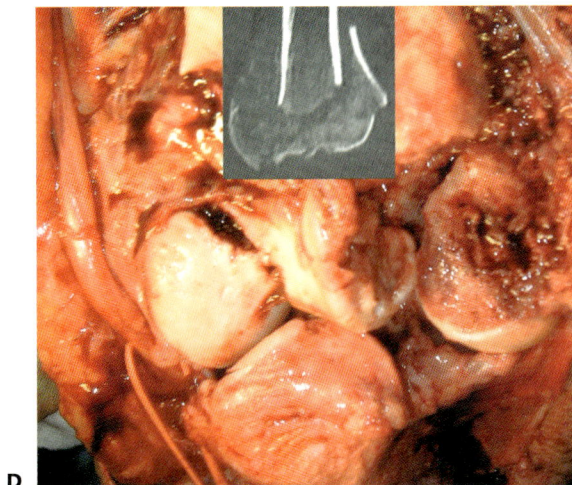

TECH FIG 3 • **A.** The triceps is split through its central tendon, in line with the fibers. The tendinous portion is dissected from the olecranon to gain access to the ulna. **B,C.** To dissect the Sharpey fibers off the ulna, the surgeon uses the scalpel parallel to the ulna surface and maintains the release directly adjacent to the bone. **D.** Comminuted distal humeral fracture in an osteoporotic elderly woman, with CT imaging confirming significant articular comminution. This is the view through the triceps split.

BONE PREPARATION

- Identify the olecranon fossa (if any part of it still exists). This landmark is the seating point for the base of the anterior flange of the Coonrad-Morrey humeral component (**TECH FIG 4A**). If the olecranon fossa is not present owing to a greater degree of comminution, an extended-flange humeral component can be used.
- Release the anterior capsule and any soft tissue from the anterior surface of the distal humerus. This provides a site for the anterior humeral bone graft.
- The posterior flat surface of the humerus is identified since this plane approximates the axis of rotation of the

distal humerus (**TECH FIG 4B**). Humeral canal preparation is completed with the canal broaches provided with the implant system being used.
- The ulnar canal preparation commences with removal of the tip of the olecranon. The intramedullary canal is entered at the base of the coronoid (**TECH FIG 4C,D**).
- The entry point is enlarged up toward the coronoid with a burr to allow easier component insertion without cortical abutment, which leads to malalignment (**TECH FIG 4E**).

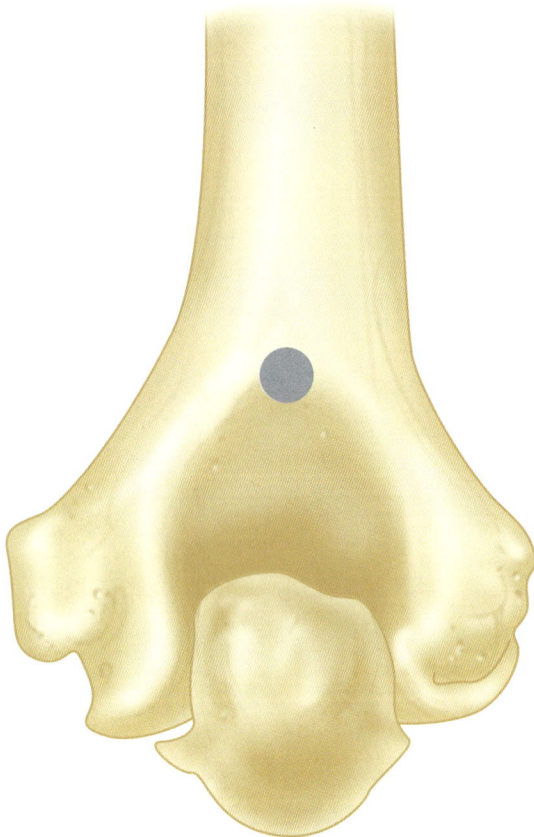

A

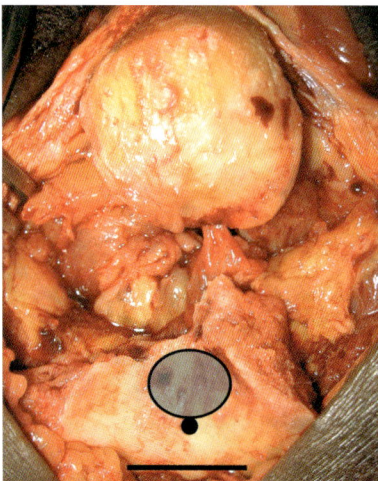

B

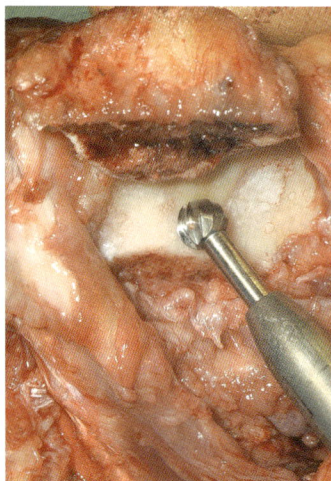

C

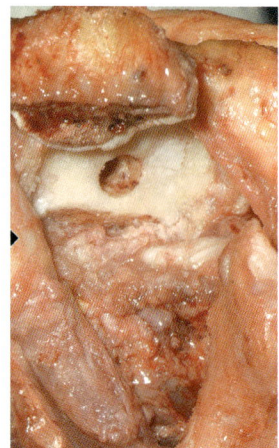

D

TECH FIG 4 • A. The humeral component entry point, the apex of the olecranon fossa, is identified and humeral canal preparation is commenced by opening the canal with a bone nibbler or burr. **B.** The posterior flat surface of the humeral shaft is identified and the component is aligned. **C,D.** Ulnar canal preparation is commenced by opening the canal at the base of the coronoid process with a drill or burr. *(continued)*

E

F

Olecranon   Coronoid

G

H

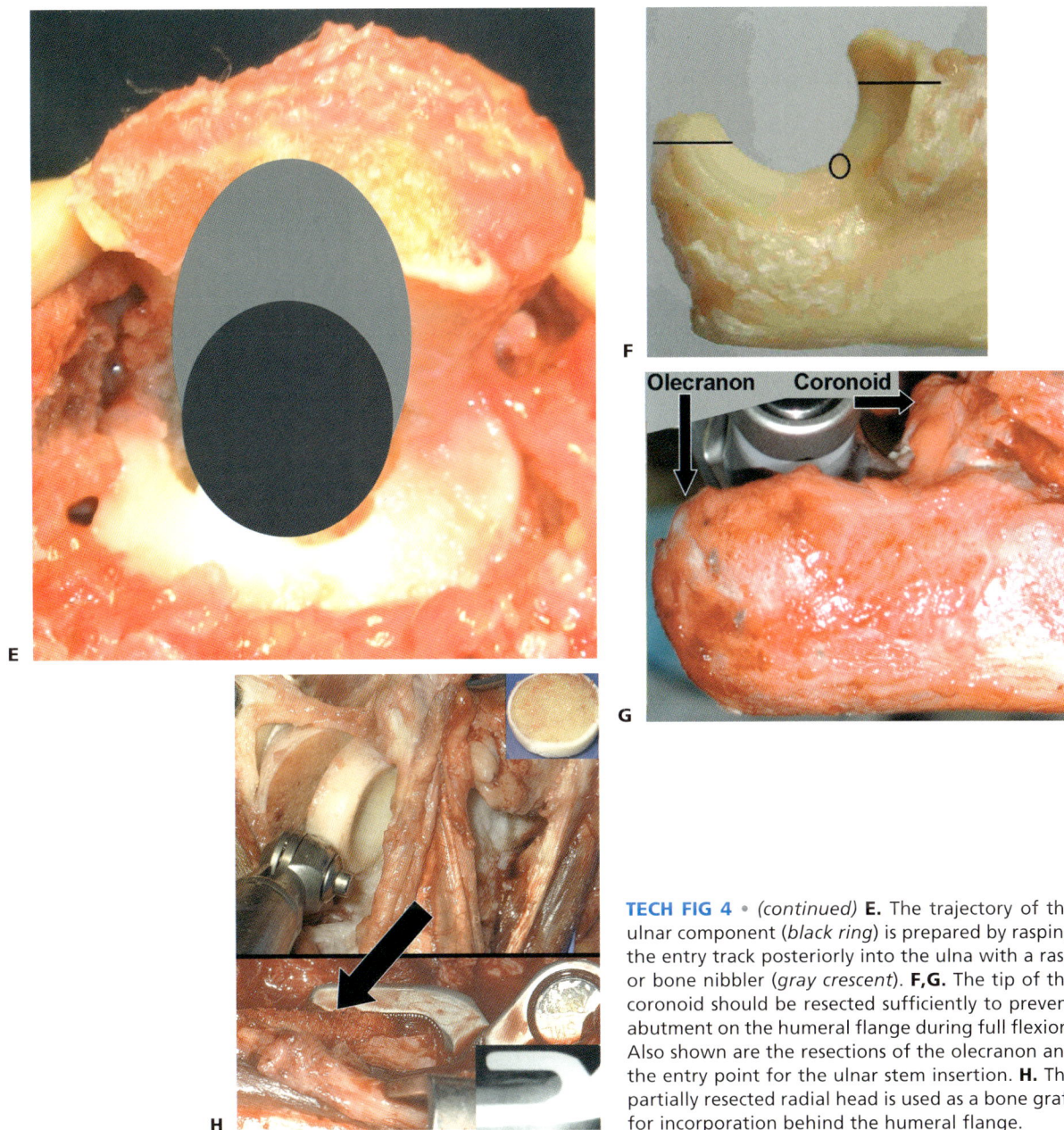

TECH FIG 4 • *(continued)* **E.** The trajectory of the ulnar component (*black ring*) is prepared by rasping the entry track posteriorly into the ulna with a rasp or bone nibbler (*gray crescent*). **F,G.** The tip of the coronoid should be resected sufficiently to prevent abutment on the humeral flange during full flexion. Also shown are the resections of the olecranon and the entry point for the ulnar stem insertion. **H.** The partially resected radial head is used as a bone graft for incorporation behind the humeral flange.

- During intramedullary preparation, the broaches must parallel the subcutaneous border of the ulna. This ensures that the track of insertion of the ulna parallels the intramedullary canal.

- The tip of the coronoid is removed to avoid impingement during terminal flexion (**TECH FIG 4F,G**).
- The radial head does not need to be resected if there is no disease of the proximal radioulnar joint (**TECH FIG 4H**).

IMPLANT INSERTION AND TENSIONING

- With the canal preparation completed (**TECH FIG 5A**), including pulse lavage of the medullary canals and cement restrictor placement, implant insertion can commence (**TECH FIG 5B,C**).
- Humeral insertion
  - When bone loss is at or below the level of the olecranon fossa, standard humeral insertion can occur. If bone loss occurs above the olecranon fossa

(greater than 2 cm), then humeral length must be restored.
- Prepare a wedge-shaped bone "cookie" for placement behind the humeral flange.
- Inject antibiotic cement into the humerus.
- When inserting the humeral component, place the bone graft behind the anterior flange. Because the humeral condyles have been resected, the implant can

TECHNIQUES

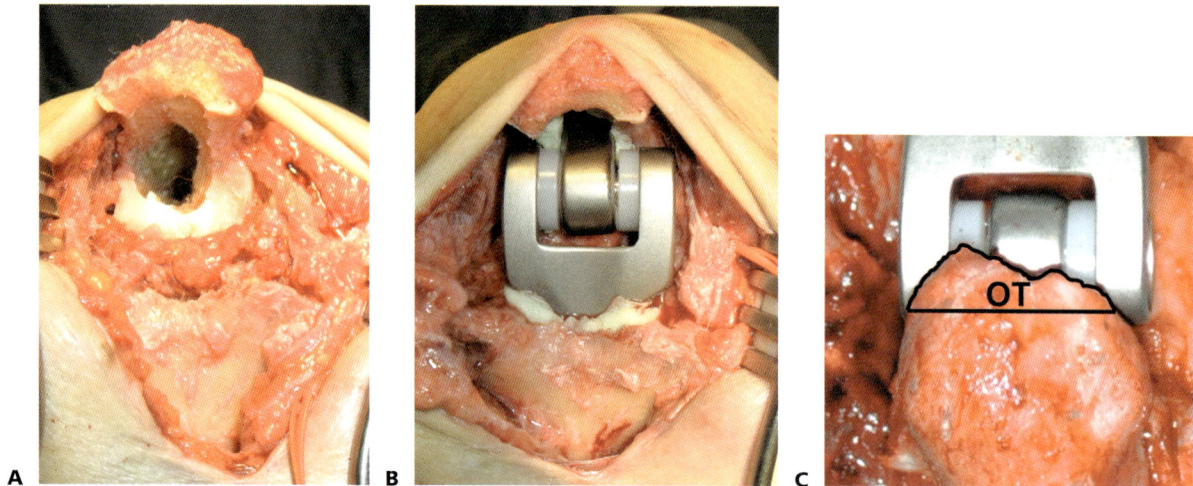

TECH FIG 5 • **A.** The prepared bony surfaces, with the fracture fragments removed, and just before implantation. **B.** The linked Coonrad-Morrey replacement is cemented and linked in situ. **C.** If in terminal extension there is abutment of the tip of the olecranon on the implant, the surgeon resects the olecranon tip (OT) but should not approach the triceps insertion footprint.

- be completely seated and coupled once the cement has hardened.
- Maintain the component orientation relative to the posterior flat surface of the distal humerus.
- Seat the component and flange until the flange is completely engaged with the anterior cortex.

- Ulnar component insertion
  - Inject antibiotic cement into the ulnar canal.
  - The ulnar component is inserted such that the axis of rotation is recreated and the implant is perpendicular to the dorsal flat surface of the olecranon.

TRICEPS REATTACHMENT

- The triceps is reattached using a nonabsorbable suture in a running locking mode (eg, running Krakow stitch) to achieve predictable purchase (TECH FIG 6A,B).
- Avoid capturing large amounts of triceps muscle fibers within the locking loops.
- The triceps tendon should be reattached to the flat of the olecranon process, not to the tip (TECH FIG 6C,D). Pass the sutures through bone tunnels (oblique crossing) that begin on the periphery of the flat reattachment area of the olecranon (TECH FIG 6E).
- Avoid tying the sutures directly over the midline of the proximal ulna, which is a source of painful symptoms and may require knot removal. Place the knot under the anconeus.
- When tensioning the triceps at reattachment, place the elbow at 30 to 45 degrees of flexion while tying the knot.
- Use a separate absorbable suture to "cinch" the triceps footprint onto the reattachment area (TECH FIG 6F).

TECH FIG 6 • **A,B.** A running locking stitch is used to improve triceps purchase when reattaching the muscle to the ulna. **A.** An example of a running locking stitch on either side of the split tendon. **B.** A locking stitch that locks both sides of the split together with one continuous locking suture. It is then reinforced with a reversed across-split locking suture. *(continued)*

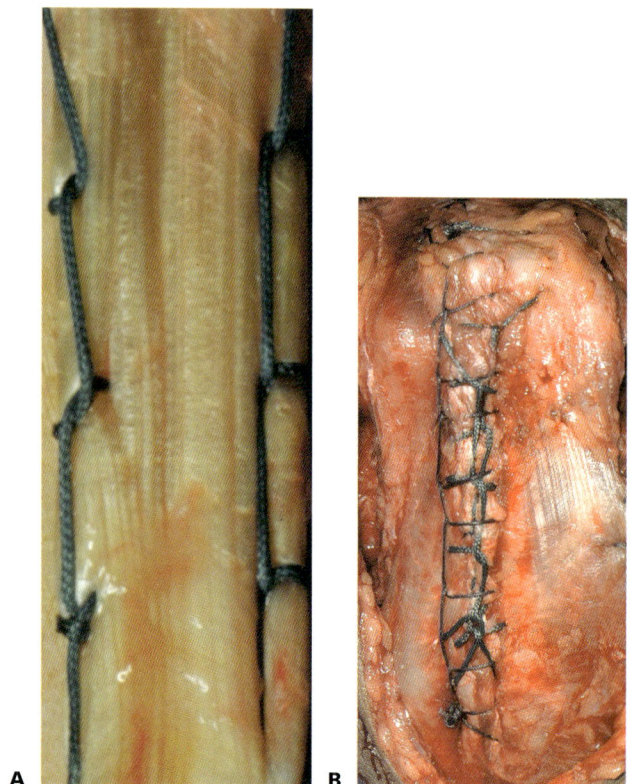

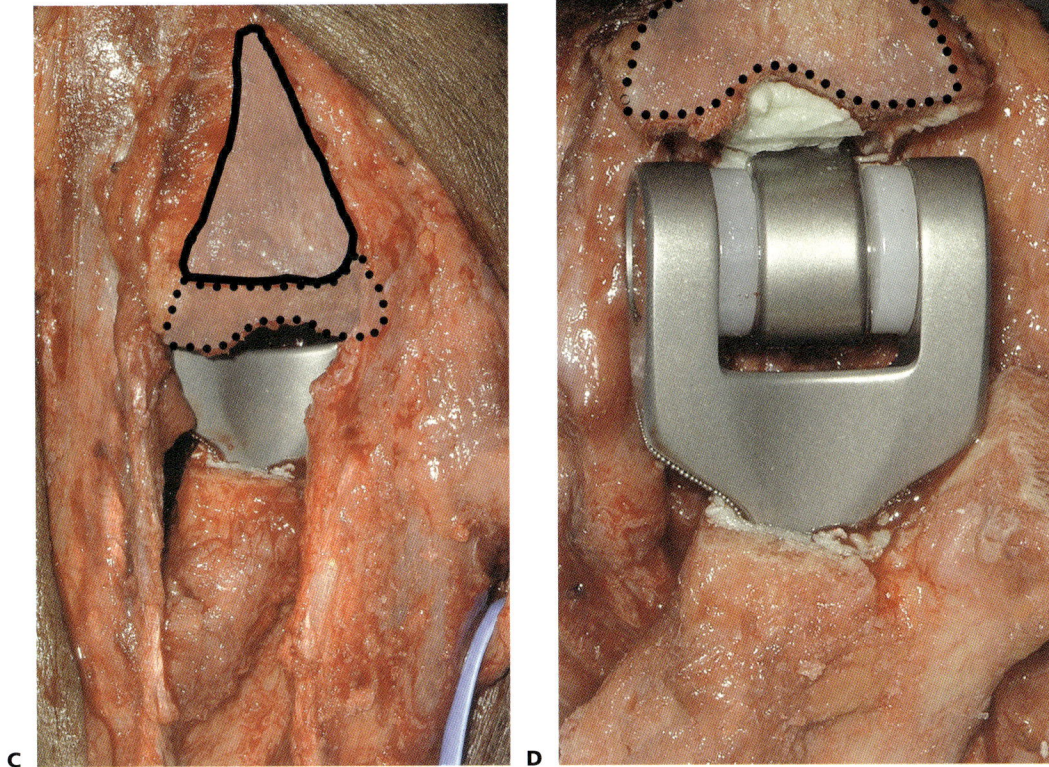

C D

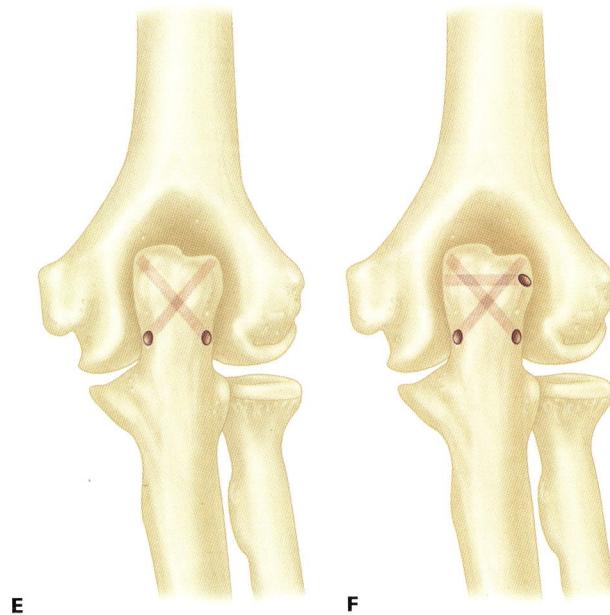

E F

TECH FIG 6 • *(continued)* **C,D.** The triceps footprint to which reattachment should be attempted is predominantly on the flat part of the ulna or olecranon process, and not the tip, which is resected to prevent posterior abutment. **E.** Drill holes (1.5 to 2 mm) are oriented in a crossing fashion to secure the triceps to the footprint area. **F.** A separate "cinch" suture is used to increase the security and the area of contact between the triceps and the ulna, thereby improving healing potential.

WOUND CLOSURE

- The ulnar nerve is transposed into an anterior subcutaneous location.
- Reapproximate the triceps to the flexor and extensor masses with absorbable suture. Do not overtighten this repair, as it will restrict motion.

- The use of a subcutaneous drain is a matter of surgeon preference. However, there is no literature demonstrating the efficacy of a postoperative drain in preventing hematoma.

PEARLS AND PITFALLS

Indications	▪ A complete history and physical examination should be performed, with specific questions about any bone mineral density problems and healing tendency. ▪ Care must be taken to address associated pathology at the elbow, wrist, and shoulder.
Planning	▪ The surgeon should attempt fracture osteosynthesis when physiologically the patient has adequate bone stock and demand on the elbow. ▪ Arthroplasty should be available in the physiologically older and lower-demand patient, with a view to converting the decision to an acute arthroplasty if the osteosynthesis potential is tenuous.
Exposure	▪ Initial definition and protection of the ulnar nerve are important. Careful dissection of the nerve from the cubital tunnel restraints will allow freedom to move the nerve without risking traction injury during the remainder of the procedure. ▪ If the exposure involves removing the triceps from its ulnar attachment (Bryan-Morrey or TRAP approach), the site of Sharpey fiber attachment should be marked and reattached anatomically. ▪ During a tendon-splitting approach, the distal triceps tendon should be split within the structure of the tendon and should not involve the muscular belly.
Inspection	▪ A thorough inspection of the ulna and radial articular surface should be performed to investigate the possibility of a hemiarthroplasty replacement in the appropriately selected younger patient. ▪ The surgeon should observe the state of the ulnar nerve and muscles around the elbow (especially triceps and brachialis); this will help to explain altered nerve function in the former, and weakness and possible myositis ossificans and stiffness in the latter.
Bone preparation	▪ If the humeral columns are intact, then an attempt at preservation should be made, with their extensor and flexor mass attachments, during a total elbow replacement.
Implantation	▪ When planning length and implantation, the surgeon should pay careful attention to the tension and lever arms of the main motor drivers; the brachialis and triceps need some tension to function well, but if over-tensioned the elbow will be stiff and if under-tensioned the elbow will be weak.
Wound closure	▪ Drains should not be used because of the superficial nature of the elbow and the risk of deep infection. However, the surgeon should pay close attention to hemostasis, and for the first 12 hours a moderately tight bandage should be used to avoid hematoma formation. The dressing is reduced the next day.
Rehabilitation	▪ With triceps reattachment, the surgeon should be cautious to avoid overzealous rehabilitation for fear of compromising triceps healing, with subsequent avulsions or extension weakness.

POSTOPERATIVE CARE

▪ A volar plaster or thermoplastic splint is used to maintain the elbow in full extension for the first several days. This avoids tension on the incision and on the triceps reattachment.
▪ The arm is elevated on pillows or with a Bradford sling overnight to prevent edema.
▪ Nonsteroidal anti-inflammatories are avoided because of their detrimental effects on tissue healing (bone to tendon and bone to bone).
▪ On the second day after surgery the dressing is removed and the compliant patient should commence gentle active antigravity flexion, with passive gravity-assisted extension.
▪ Graduated and targeted motion is prescribed, with greater than 90 degrees of elbow flexion attempted after 5 weeks. This allows sufficient time for the triceps to adhere and heal (incompletely) to the ulna. Aggressive flexion too early may result in triceps avulsion or pull-out. Triceps antigravity exercises can commence after 5 weeks.
▪ Always, at each patient interaction, the surgeon should reiterate the restrictions of use with an elbow arthroplasty: limited internal (varus) and external (valgus) rotatory torques, 2-pound repetitive and 10-pound single-event lifting.

COMPLICATIONS

▪ Triceps avulsion
▪ Stiffness
  ▪ Overlengthened implantation
  ▪ Overtensioned triceps reattachment

  ▪ Overzealous closure of triceps to flexor–extensor compartments
  ▪ Inadequate soft tissue release
▪ Impingement
  ▪ Radial head on humeral component (distal yolk)
  ▪ Coronoid on humeral component (anterior yolk)
  ▪ Olecranon process on posterior humerus
▪ Deep venous thrombosis
▪ Infection
▪ Periprosthetic fracture
  ▪ Osteoporotic bone
  ▪ Stem–canal mismatched sizes
  ▪ Stem–canal mismatched curvature
  ▪ Inadequate opening for ulna component at coronoid base
▪ Ulna nerve neuropathy or injury

OUTCOMES

▪ Cobb and Morrey[1] reported 15 excellent and 5 good results, with one patient with inadequate data, in a cohort of patients with acute distal humeral fractures (average age 72 years) at 3.3 years of follow-up.
▪ Ray et al[14] reported 5 excellent and 2 good functional results in a group of patients with an average age of 81 years at 2 to 4 years of follow-up.
▪ Gambirasio et al[5] reported excellent functional results in a cohort of 10 elderly patients with osteoporotic intra-articular fractures.

▪ Frankle et al[4] compared the outcomes of patients over age 65 with comminuted intra-articular distal humeral fractures treated with ORIF versus acute total elbow replacements. The ORIF group had 8 excellent results, 12 good results, 1 fair result, and 3 poor results, with 3 patients requiring conversion to elbow replacement. All 12 acute primary elbow replacements achieved excellent (n = 11) or good (n = 1) results.

▪ Kamineni and Morrey[8] reported an average Mayo Elbow Performance Score (MEPS) of 93/100 in a series of 49 acute distal humeral fractures (average patient age 67 years) at 7 years of follow-up. The average arc of motion was 107 degrees.

▪ Lee et al[10] reported seven acute elbow replacements for distal humeral fractures in patients with an average age of 73 years. The average arc of motion was 89 degrees and the average MEPS was 94/100 at an average follow-up of 25 months.

REFERENCES

1. Cobb TK, Morrey BF. Total elbow arthroplasty as primary treatment for distal humeral fractures in elderly patients. J Bone Joint Surg Am 1997;79A:826–832.
2. Faierman E, Wang J, Jupiter JB. Secondary ulnar nerve palsy in adults after elbow trauma: a report of two cases. J Hand Surg Am 2001;26A:675–678.
3. Frankle MA, Herscovici D Jr, DiPasquale TG, et al. A comparison of open reduction and internal fixation and primary total elbow arthroplasty in the treatment of intraarticular fractures of the distal humerus in women older than 65 years. J Shoulder Elbow Surg 1999;9:455.
4. Frankle MA, Herscovici D Jr, DiPasquale TG, et al. A comparison of open reduction and internal fixation and primary total elbow arthroplasty in the treatment of intraarticular distal humerus fractures in women older than age 65. J Orthop Trauma 2003;17:473–480.
5. Gambirasio R, Riand N, Stern R, Hall JE. Total elbow replacement for complex fractures of the distal humerus: an option for the elderly patient. J Bone Joint Surg Br 2001;83B:974–978.
6. Holmes JC, Skolnick MD, et al. Untreated median-nerve entrapment in bone after fracture of the distal end of the humerus: postmortem findings after forty-seven years. J Bone Joint Surg Am 1979;61A:309–310.
7. Huang TL, Chiu FY, Chuang TY, et al. The results of open reduction and internal fixation in elderly patients with severe fractures of the distal humerus: a critical analysis of the results. J Trauma 2005;58:62–69.
8. Kamineni S, Morrey BF. Distal humeral fractures treated with non-custom total elbow replacement. J Bone Joint Surg Am 2004;86A:940–947.
9. Kamineni S, Morrey BF. Distal humeral fractures treated with non-custom total elbow replacement: surgical technique. J Bone Joint Surg Am 2005;87A:41–50.
10. Lee KT, Lai CH, Singh S. Results of total elbow arthroplasty in the treatment of distal humerus fractures in elderly Asian patients. J Trauma 2006;61:889–892.
11. Mohan K. Myositis ossificans traumatica of the elbow. Int Surg 1972;57:475–478.
12. Pajarinen J, Bjorkenheim JM. Operative treatment of type C intercondylar fractures of the distal humerus: results after a mean follow-up of 2 years in a series of 18 patients. J Shoulder Elbow Surg 2002;11:48–52.
13. Parsons M, O'Brien R, Hughes JS. Elbow hemiarthroplasty for acute and salvage reconstruction of intra-articular distal humerus fractures. Tech Shoulder Elbow Surg 2005;2:87–97.
14. Ray PS, Kakarlapudi K, Rajsekhar C, et al. Total elbow arthroplasty as primary treatment for distal humeral fractures in elderly patients. Injury 2000;31:687–692.
15. Thompson HC 3rd, Garcia A. Myositis ossificans: aftermath of elbow injuries. Clin Orthop Relat Res 1967;50:129–134.
16. Zhao J, Wang X, Zhang Q. Surgical treatment of comminuted intra-articular fractures of the distal humerus with double tension band osteosynthesis. Orthopedics 2000;23:449–452.

Management of Primary Degenerative Arthritis of the Elbow: Linkable Total Elbow Replacement

Bassem Elhassan, Matthew L. Ramsey, and Scott P. Steinmann

DEFINITION

- Primary degenerative arthritis of the elbow is an uncommon problem.[1]
  - It occurs in less than 2% of the population[29] and principally affects the dominant extremity in middle-aged manual laborers.[1,3,17,23,29]
  - The disorder predominates in men and is rarely seen in women, with an incidence of 4 to 5:1.[8]
  - The dominant extremity is involved in 80% to 90% of symptomatic patients. Bilateral involvement of the elbow is noted in 25% to 60% of patients.[6]
  - It has also been reported in people who require continuous use of a wheelchair or crutches, in athletes, and in patients with a history of osteochondritis dissecans of the elbow.[21,25]
- The pattern of pathologic changes in primary degenerative arthritis is different than the age-related changes of the distal humerus and the radiohumeral joint.[6,26]
- The current understanding of the disease process in primary degenerative arthritis has led to treatment algorithms designed to address the pathologic process short of joint replacement.
- The role of total elbow arthroplasty (TEA) for patients with primary degenerative arthritis of the elbow is limited, in large part because of the younger age and increased activity levels of patients with this condition.

PATHOGENESIS

- The exact pathogenesis of primary osteoarthritis of the elbow is still unknown. It is generally believed that overuse plays a key role in the onset of the disease process. However, younger patients with this disease often have predisposing conditions such as osteochondritis dissecans.[11]
- The degenerative changes of the elbow joint are usually more advanced in the radiohumeral joint, where bare bone is often in wide contact, and the capitellum appears to have been shaved obliquely (**FIG 1**).[6]
  - This is due to the high axial, shearing, and rotational stresses at this articulation, which result in marked erosion of the capitellum and hypertrophic callus formation in a skirt-like pattern on the radial neck.[32]
- The ulnohumeral joint is usually less involved in the beginning of the disease process, but involvement becomes more pronounced with more advanced disease.[21]
  - The central aspect of the ulnohumeral joint is characteristically spared. The anterior and posterior involvement of this joint is usually manifested by fibrosis of the anterior capsule in the form of a cord-like band and hypertrophy of the olecranon.
  - Osteophytes are seen over the olecranon, especially medially, the coronoid process, and the coronoid fossa.

- These changes in the radiohumeral and ulnohumeral joints lead to the loss and fragmentation of the cartilaginous joint surfaces with distortion, cyst formation, and bone sclerosis.[2]
  - Kashiwagi[9] noted that the early stage of the disease is characterized by small, round bony protuberances; the early stage progresses into various shapes of osteophytes and bony sclerosis with more advanced cases.
  - Suvarna and Stanley[30] reported on the progressive fibrosis of the local marrow, increased thickness of all the bony components of the olecranon fossa, and increases in anterior and posterior fibrous tissues.

PATIENT HISTORY AND PHYSICAL FINDINGS

- Despite considerable radiographic severity, many patients with osteoarthritis of the elbow report minimal symptoms.[11]
- Trauma rarely underlies the onset of degenerative arthritis. However, trivial injury often brings the problem to the patient's attention.
- Characteristic manifestations of primary degenerative arthritis of the elbow are well described.[22,24] These include:
  - Progressive loss of motion

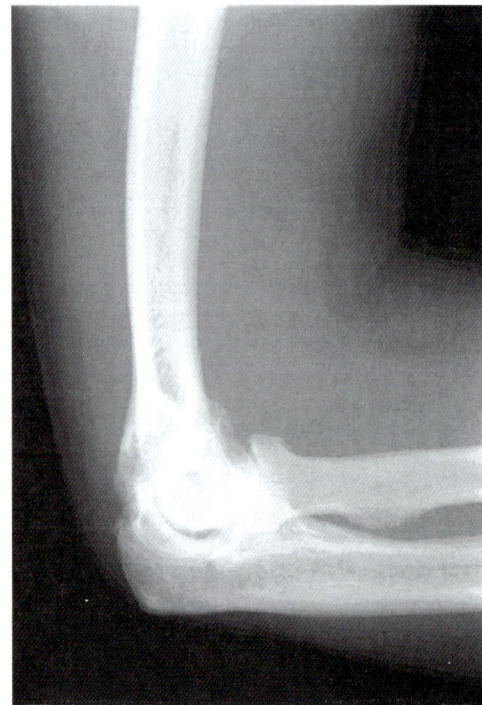

FIG 1 • Lateral view of right elbow, showing advanced osteoarthritis specifically involving the radiocapitellar joint. Notice osteophyte formation anteriorly and posteriorly.

- Mechanical symptoms of locking and catching caused by intra-articular loose bodies (occurs in about 10% of patients)[9]
- Pain at the extremes of motion due to mechanical impingement of osteophytes (pain occurs most frequently at terminal extension, although about 50% of patients also have pain during terminal flexion)
- Pain throughout the arc of motion indicates significant involvement of the ulnohumeral joint; this typically occurs late in the disease process.
- Ulnar neuropathy
  - Medial joint pain in patients with advanced osteoarthritis of the elbow might be the first manifestation of ulnar neuropathy.
  - Up to 20% of patients with primary osteoarthritis of the elbow have some degree of ulnar neuropathy.[1]
  - The proximity of the ulnar nerve to the arthritic posteromedial aspect of the ulnohumeral joint makes it susceptible to impingement.
  - The expansion of the capsule as a result of synovitis and the presence of osteophytes in that area of the joint result in direct compression and ischemia of the ulnar nerve.
  - Acute onset of cubital tunnel syndrome in patients with osteoarthritis of the elbow might be also the first manifestation of a medial elbow ganglion.[10]
- Radiocapitellar symptoms: With more progressive disease, the patients may have pain with forearm rotation and throughout the range of elbow motion. This could lead to disability in this patient population as well in the older laborers who extensively use their upper extremity.[6,16,33]

PHYSICAL FINDINGS

- Physical examination findings depend on the extent of the patient's disease.
- Range of motion
  - The flexion-extension arc will demonstrate loss of extension greater than flexion and will average about 30 to 120 degrees.
    - The midrange of the flexion–extension arc is typically pain-free in the early stages of the disease.
  - A painful midrange of motion and crepitus indicate more extensive involvement of the ulnohumeral joint.
  - The arc of pronation–supination is rarely affected early in the disease process. Involvement of the proximal radioulnar and radiohumeral joint later in the disease process may limit forearm rotation.
- Forced motion at the extremes of flexion and extension will often cause pain, particularly in extension.
- Ulnar nerve symptoms need to be thoroughly evaluated. Symptoms of ulnar neuropathy associated with primary degenerative arthritis of the elbow include:
  - Decreased sensation and weakness
  - Positive Tinel sign at the cubital tunnel
  - Positive elbow hyperflexion test

IMAGING AND OTHER DIAGNOSTIC STUDIES

- Some characteristic radiographic features are seen on the anteroposterior and lateral radiographs of the elbow:
  - Radiocapitellar narrowing (noted in 25% to 50% of patients)
  - Ossification and osteophyte formation in the olecranon fossa in almost all patients with osteoarthritis of the elbow[15,21]
  - Osteophyte formation of the coronoid and olecranon processes
  - Loose bodies and fluffy densities might be observed filling the coronoid and olecranon fossae (**FIG 2A,B**).
  - Radiographs do not allow for accurate visualization of all osteophytes.
- A cubital tunnel view is obtained if there is ulnar nerve irritation to look for impinging osteophytes or loose bodies.[4,6,7]
- Computed tomography (CT) helps in delineating the detailed structural anatomy of the articular surface of the elbow with an accurate determination of the locations of the osteophytes and loose bodies (**FIG 2C**).
  - When contemplating surgical treatment of the osteoarthritic elbow, a CT is quite helpful for determining which osteophytes need to be removed.

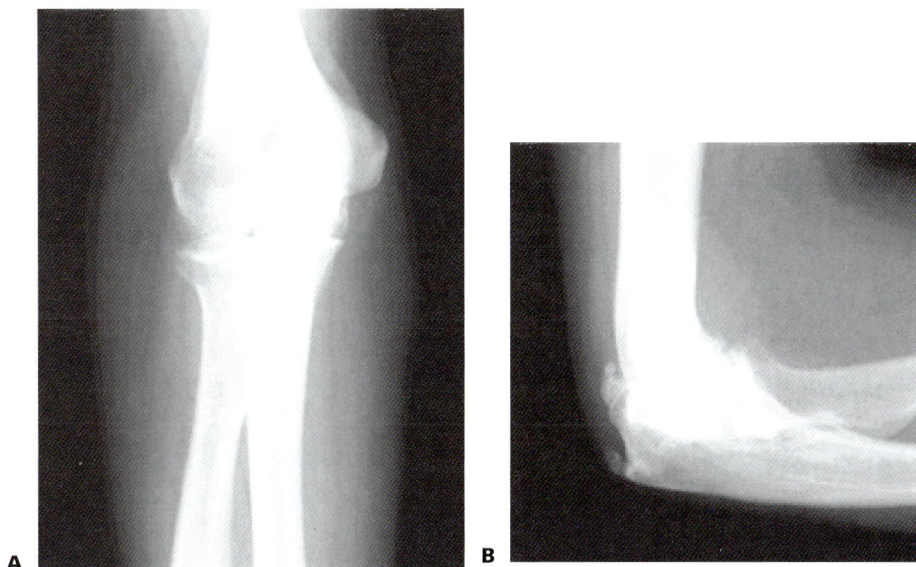

FIG 2 • A,B. Anteroposterior and lateral views of a right osteoarthritic elbow show narrowing of the joint line and subchondral sclerosis, with formation of osteophytes in the coronoid, capitellar, and olecranon fossae. *(continued)*

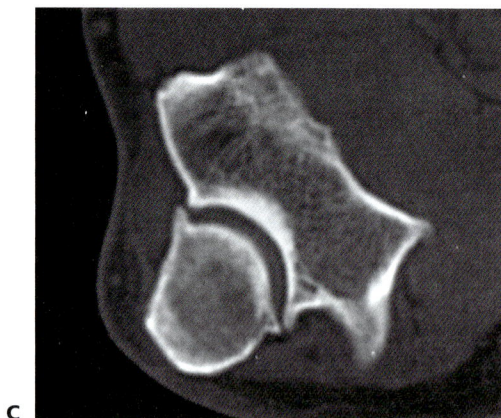

FIG 2 • *(continued)* **C.** Computed tomography of the elbow demonstrating marginal osteophytes on the ulna and olecranon fossa.

- Three-dimensional reconstructions provide additional detail on osteophytic deformity and facilitate preoperative planning of removal.
- MRI does not provide any useful information in primary osteoarthritis of the elbow and is rarely indicated.

NONOPERATIVE MANAGEMENT

- Because of their young age, most patients with primary osteoarthritis of the elbow tend to be active and involved in manual labor, which will place a great demand on any kind of prosthetic replacement.
- Early in the course of the disease, treatment by nonsurgical measures should be followed.[21]
  - This consists of activity modification, physical therapy, anti-inflammatory medications, and possibly steroid injection or visco-supplementation.[13]

SURGICAL MANAGEMENT

Indications

- If nonoperative treatment fails to improve symptoms, surgery may be indicated.
- Several surgical options exist for the management of primary degenerative arthritis of the elbow. Surgery is directed toward addressing the pathology contributing to the predominant complaints of the patient.
- The surgical techniques depend on:
  - Degree of osteophyte formation
  - Degree and direction of motion loss
  - Associated loose bodies
  - Associated ulnar nerve symptoms
  - Degree of ulnohumeral involvement resulting in pain through the midrange of motion

Arthroscopic Débridement

- Arthroscopic management of degenerative arthritis of the elbow is discussed in detail in Chapter SM-22.
- In general, arthroscopic débridement for degenerative arthritis of the elbow can be performed for moderate to severe disease when there are no midrange symptoms, indicating limited involvement of the ulnohumeral joint.
- Advantages of arthroscopy include the ability to visualize the entire joint and limited morbidity from surgery.
  - Savoie et al reported good results with extensive arthroscopic débridement involving capsular release, fenestration of the distal part of the humerus, and removal of osteophytes.[28]

- Disadvantages of arthroscopy include potential neurovascular injury and difficulty assessing the normal anatomic relationships, resulting in inadequate débridement, compared with open débridement and release.
- Contraindications to arthroscopic treatment include altered neurovascular anatomy, limited surgical expertise, and advanced involvement of the ulnohumeral joint.

Open Débridement

- Open débridement can be performed for all patients with primary degenerative arthritis of the elbow.
- Open joint débridement should be considered in patients with advanced disease or when the treating surgeon has limited experience with arthroscopic techniques.
- Options for open débridement of the elbow include:
  - Outerbridge-Kashiwagi arthroplasty (see Chap. SE-42)
  - Lateral column approach for débridement (see Chap. SE-43)
  - Medial over-the-top approach for débridement (see Chap. SE-44)

Total Elbow Arthroplasty

- TEA for the treatment of primary osteoarthritis of the elbow is performed sparingly in carefully selected patients. In general, the patient population with primary degenerative arthritis of the elbow includes relatively young men who are physically active in their occupation and want to remain so. TEA is contraindicated in high-demand patients.
- The indications for TEA for primary degenerative arthritis of the elbow include patients older than 65 years with low physical demands and a painful arc of motion. These patients should have attempted and failed all other appropriate treatment options.

Implant Choices

- Unlinked (resurfacing) and linked (semiconstrained) designs may be appropriate in patients with primary degenerative arthritis of the elbow.
- The current literature supports the use of linked implant designs for primary degenerative arthritis. However, osteoarthritis may be the best indication for the use of an unlinked implant.
- Linked implants
  - Current linked designs with a semiconstrained, loose-hinged articulation allow varying degrees of varus–valgus motion and rotational laxity (**FIG 3A**).
  - Muscle activation about the elbow protects against excessive loading, thereby reducing aseptic loosening.

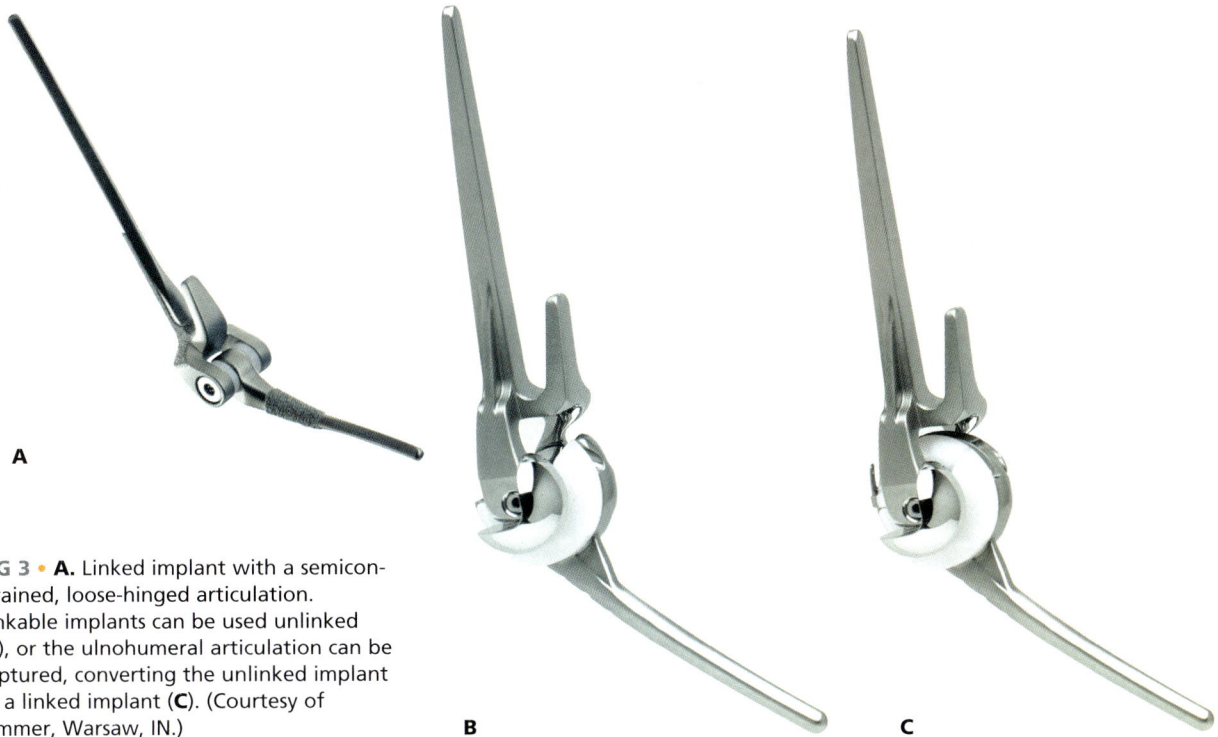

FIG 3 • **A.** Linked implant with a semiconstrained, loose-hinged articulation. Linkable implants can be used unlinked (**B**), or the ulnohumeral articulation can be captured, converting the unlinked implant to a linked implant (**C**). (Courtesy of Zimmer, Warsaw, IN.)

- Unlinked implants
  - Anatomic requirements for the use of unlinked implants include:
    - Competence of the medial and lateral collateral ligaments
    - Minimal deformity of the subchondral architecture
    - Integrity of the medial and lateral supracondylar columns
  - Maintenance of the collateral ligaments and surrounding muscles helps absorb forces across the elbow, thereby reducing stress on the bone–cement interface. This has the theoretical, but unproven, advantage of offloading stresses on the implant.
  - Some authors believe that this potential advantage may allow this implant type to be used in a higher-demand patient population. However, this potential advantage is yet unproven. Therefore, the indications for total elbow replacement are still limited in this patient population to patients willing to adopt low physical demands.
  - The major complication of unlinked implants is instability.
  - If an unlinked implant is considered in this patient population, the ability to convert to a linked replacement (linkable) has obvious advantages.
- Linkable implants
  - These devices permit implantation in an unlinked fashion, taking advantage of the benefits of an unlinked design (**FIG 3B**).
  - The ulnohumeral articulation can be captured, thereby converting the unlinked implant to a linked implant by placing an ulnar cap on the ulnar component (**FIG 3C**). This can be performed at the time of implantation of the unlinked implant if stability cannot be established or at a point distant to the initial implantation if instability becomes an issue.

Patient Positioning

- The patient is positioned supine on the operating room table with a bump under the ipsilateral scapula. The arm is positioned across the chest and supported on a bolster (**FIG 4**).
- A tourniquet is applied to the arm. The use of a sterile tourniquet increases the "zone of sterility" and allows removal for more proximal exposure if needed.

Approach

- The surgical technique for linked arthroplasty is discussed in other chapters. Please refer to these chapters for the specific technical details of implantation of a linked, semiconstrained implant. This chapter will discuss an unlinked total elbow system, which can be converted to a linked implant if required for stability.

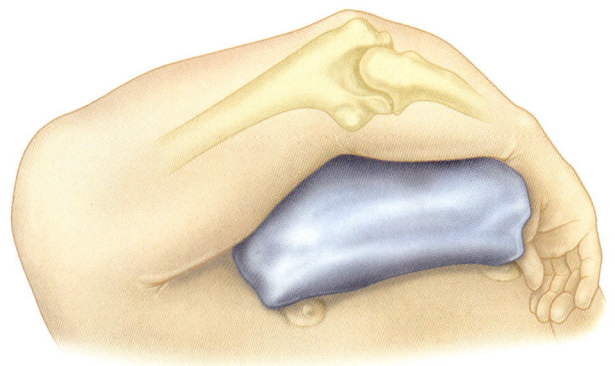

FIG 4 • Patient positioning with the arm across the chest supported on a bolster.

TECHNIQUES

SURGICAL EXPOSURE

- A straight posterior, midline incision placed just off the medial tip of the olecranon is used (**TECH FIG 1**).
- Full-thickness flaps are elevated. The extent of flap elevation is based on how the triceps is to be managed surgically.
- The ulnar nerve is identified, protected with help of a Penrose drain, and transposed anteriorly.

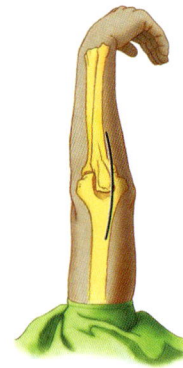

TECH FIG 1 • Straight posterior midline skin incision is placed off the medial aspect of the olecranon. (Courtesy of Tornier, Inc., Edina, MN.)

TRICEPS MANAGEMENT

- Surgical management of the triceps is a matter of surgeon preference. The general methods of triceps management are triceps-sparing, triceps-reflecting, and triceps-splitting approaches.
  - Triceps-sparing approaches leave the triceps attached to the tip of the olecranon. The advantage of this type of approach is that it prevents triceps weakness postoperatively, but it sacrifices surgical exposure.
  - Triceps-reflecting approaches subperiosteally elevate the triceps from its attachment on the ulna; it must be carefully reattached and protected postoperatively. However, surgical exposure is facilitated with these approaches.
  - Triceps-splitting approaches violate the attachment of the triceps to the ulna yet provide the advantages of improved visualization of the joint.
- Triceps-splitting approach
  - A triceps-splitting approach is performed by completing a midline split in the triceps muscle and tendon,

which is carried distally onto the ulna along the subcutaneous border of the ulna between the anconeus and the flexor carpi ulnaris (**TECH FIG 2A**).

- The medial triceps is elevated in continuity with the flexor carpi ulnaris while the lateral triceps is elevated in continuity with the anconeus. Care must be taken when elevating the medial triceps flap. The medial triceps attachment to the triceps is tenuous in comparison to the lateral triceps flap, which is much more robust.
- The medial collateral ligament (anterior bundle) and lateral collateral ligament complex are tagged and released from their humeral attachment (**TECH FIG 2B**).
- The shoulder is externally rotated and the elbow is flexed, allowing the ulna to separate from the humerus (**TECH FIG 2C**).

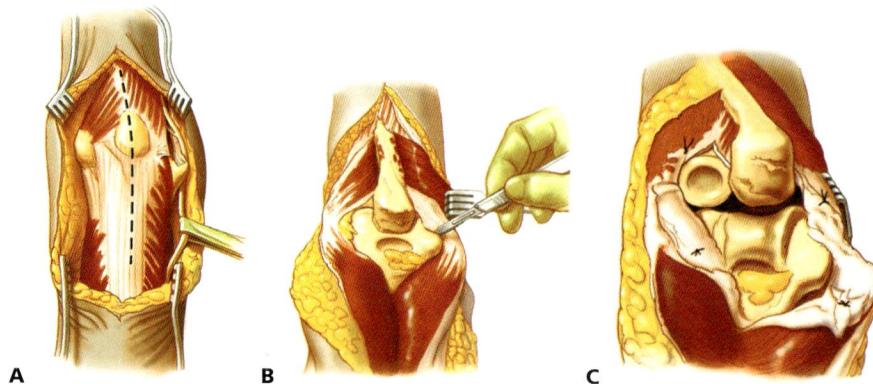

TECH FIG 2 • **A.** Triceps-splitting approach carried from the subcutaneous border of the ulna proximally into the triceps tendon. The medial and lateral triceps are subperiosteally elevated from the olecranon. **B.** The medial and lateral collateral ligaments are released from their humeral attachment and tagged for later repair. **C.** The elbow is dislocated with flexion of the joint, allowing the ulna to separate from the humerus. This separation provides exposure for component insertion. (Courtesy of Tornier, Inc., Edina, MN.)

IMPLANTATION

Humeral Preparation

- Sizing of the implant to the patient's native anatomy is critical. Trial spools should be compared to the distal humerus and the proximal radioulnar joint for appropriate sizing (**TECH FIG 3A,B**). If the native joint size is between spool sizes, the smaller spool is selected.
- The medial and lateral points of the axis of rotation through the distal humerus are determined and an axis pin is placed through these two points, thereby replicating the axis. A drill guide aids in reproducing these points (**TECH FIG 3C**).
- The central portion of the distal humerus articulation is removed, the intramedullary canal is opened, and a rod is placed in the intramedullary canal. The axis pin is replaced to determine the offset of the intramedullary canal relative to the flexion–extension axis (**TECH FIG 3D,E**).
- A distal humeral cutting block is used to precisely prepare the distal humerus relative to the intramedullary canal and the flexion–extension axis (**TECH FIG 3F,G**).
- The humeral canal is sequentially broached to the size selected for the articular spool.

Ulnar Preparation

- Preparation of the ulna is based on the flexion–extension axis of the proximal radius and ulna. The selected size spool is attached to the cutting guide, and the guide is tightened with set screws (**TECH FIG 4A**). Care must be taken to maintain the relationship of the trochlea and capitellar portions of the spool with the native greater sigmoid notch and radial head.

- A bell saw is used to resect a small portion of the articular surface and subchondral bone of the ulna (**TECH FIG 4B**).
- If the radial head is going to be replaced, a sagittal saw is used to resect the radial head through the cutting guide. The canal is broached and a trial radial head component is inserted.
- The ulnar canal is opened and sequentially broached to the same size as the selected humeral component.

Component Placement

- If the replacement is going to be unlinked, a short ulnar component can be used. If the implant is going to be linked, a standard (longer) stem is selected. If a standard ulnar component is going to be used, flexible reamers may be required to prepare the ulna.
- Trial reduction is performed to assess the alignment, stability, and tracking of the components.
- If the components are going to be inserted unlinked, the collateral ligaments are reattached to the anatomic origin through the humeral implant. An accessory box stitch could be placed through the ulna and humeral component to support the collateral ligament repair.
- The canals are lavaged and cement restrictors are placed in the humerus and ulna.
- Antibiotic-impregnated cement is injected into the canals. Methylene blue is added to the cement to facilitate cement removal if required in the future.

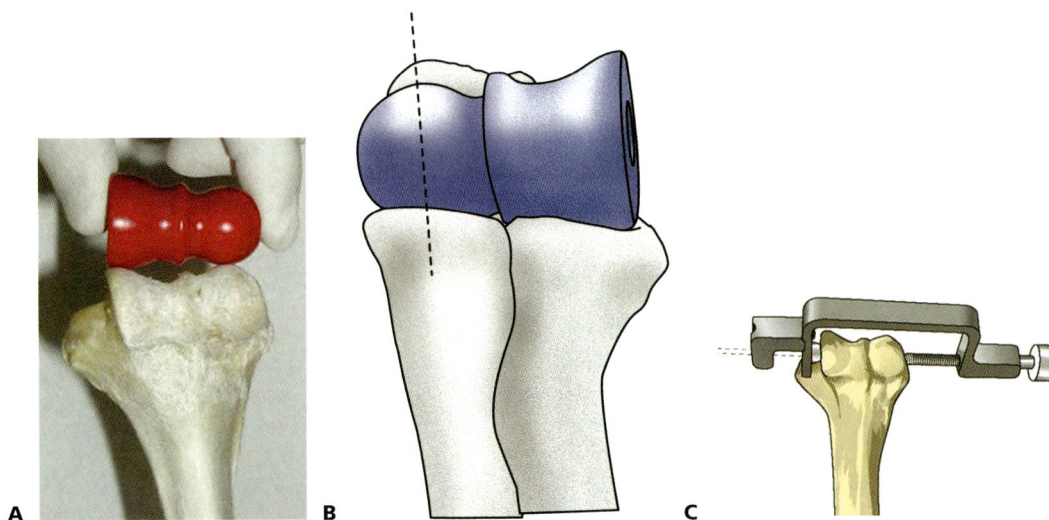

TECH FIG 3 • The anatomic spool is sized against the native distal humerus (**A**) and the proximal radioulnar articulation (**B**). **C.** The native flexion–extension axis is determined. A drill guide assists in accurately establishing the flexion–extension axis. Next, the offset of the distal humeral articulation with respect to the intramedullary canal is determined. *(continued)*

TECHNIQUES

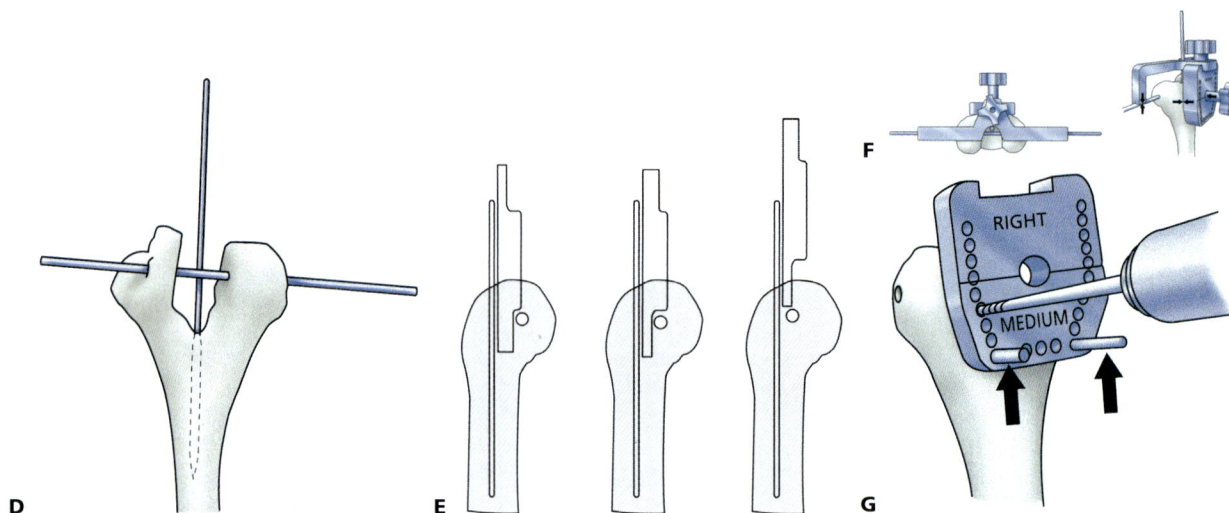

TECH FIG 3 • (continued) **D.** The relationship between the axis of flexion–extension and the intramedullary canal is determined. **E.** Measurement guides are used to determine whether the offset is anterior, posterior, or neutral. **F.** A cutting block is placed relative to the flexion–extension axis. **G.** The cutting block is fixed to the humerus with pins and the guide is removed. Once all of the holes are drilled, the cutting block is removed and the holes are connected with an oscillating saw. (Courtesy of Tornier, Inc., Edina, MN.)

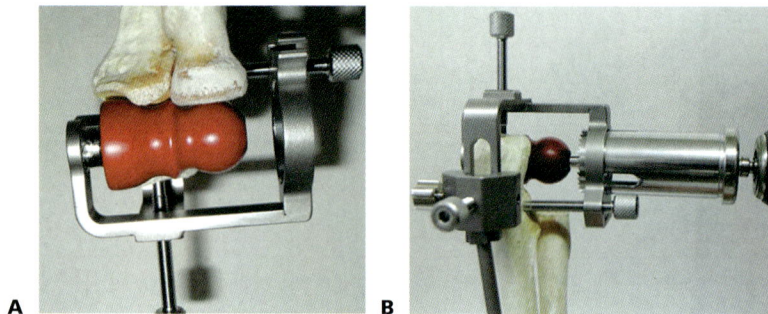

TECH FIG 4 • **A.** The selected anatomic spool is attached to the ulnar cutting jig. The set screws are tightened, taking care to ensure the anatomic spool stays firmly opposed to the native radius and ulna. **B.** With the ulnar cutting guide properly aligned, a bell saw is used to prepare the proximal ulna. The radial head can also be removed using the same cutting jig. (Courtesy of Tornier, Inc., Edina, MN.)

LIGAMENT REPAIR

- A locking stitch is used to repair the collateral ligaments through the cannulated humeral bolt (**TECH FIG 5A**).

- Further support is achieved using a cerclage stitch passed through the humeral bolt and a transverse drill hole in the ulna (**TECH FIG 5B**).

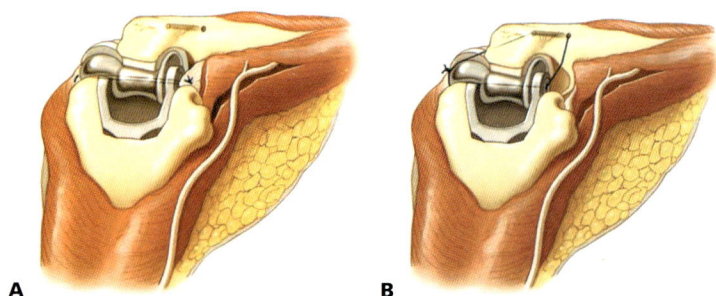

TECH FIG 5 • **A.** The medial and lateral collateral ligaments are reattached to the epicondyles using a locking stitch that is passed through the cannulated humeral screw. **B.** The collateral ligament repair is reinforced with a box stitch passed through the cannulated humeral screw and a transverse hole placed through the proximal ulna. (Courtesy of Tornier, Inc., Edina, MN.)

TECHNIQUES

TRICEPS REPAIR

- Triceps repair is crucial for the stability of unlinked devices.
- The triceps is reattached through two crossing drill holes and one transverse drill hole in the olecranon.
- A grasping suture (Krackow stitch) is used and passed through the crossing drill holes.
- A cerclage stitch is passed through the transverse drill hole around the triceps attachment (**TECH FIG 6**).

TECH FIG 6 • The triceps is repaired to the ulna through drill holes. The split in the triceps and between the anconeus and flexor carpi ulnaris is closed side to side with interrupted or running suture. (Courtesy of Tornier, Inc., Edina, MN.)

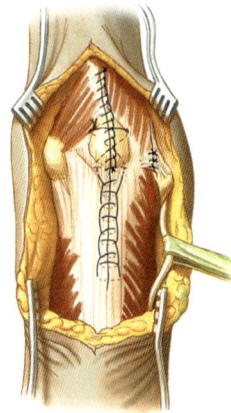

WOUND CLOSURE

- The ulnar nerve is transposed into an anterior subcutaneous pouch.
- The wound is closed over a drain placed in the subcutaneous position.

POSTOPERATIVE CARE

- The arm is placed in a well-padded postoperative dressing and the arm is immobilized in about 90 degrees of flexion for the first several days.
- A resting elbow splint at 90 degrees with the wrist included is fabricated before discharge to protect the soft tissue repair while it heals.

OUTCOMES

- Most studies in the literature reporting on TEA involve large numbers of patients, mostly with rheumatoid arthritis or other inflammatory pathologies but very few patients with primary osteoarthritis.
  - This makes it difficult to make accurate conclusions on the value of this treatment option for this population of patients.[5,14,20,27]
  - There are few studies in the English literature reporting specifically on the outcome and complications of TEA as a treatment option for patients with primary osteoarthritis of the elbow.[4,13]
- Kozak[13] reported on the Mayo clinic experience.
  - Over a 13-year period, only 5 of 493 patients (<1%) who underwent TEA had the procedure performed for primary osteoarthritis of the elbow.
  - A linked Coonrad-Morrey implant (Zimmer, Warsaw, IN) was used in three patients and an unlinked Pritchard elbow resurfacing system (ERS) (DePuy, Warsaw, IN) was used in the other two patients.
    - The average age of the patients was 67 and follow-up ranged from 37 to 121 months.
    - Two minor and four major complications were reported in four elbows, two of which required revision.

  - This rate of complications, according to the authors, is much higher than the rate of complications reported in TEA performed for other reasons in the same institution during the same period of time, including revision TEA, posttraumatic arthritis, nonunion of distal humerus, and rheumatoid arthritis.[12,18,19]
- Espag et al[4] reported on 11 Souter-Strathclyde cemented unlinked primary TEAs in 10 patients with osteoarthritis of the elbow.
  - The diagnosis was primary osteoarthritis of the elbow in nine patients and posttraumatic osteoarthritis in two patients.
  - The average age of the patients was 66 years; mean follow-up was 68 months.
  - Only one patient required revision after 97 months for ulnar component loosening.
  - All patients reported good symptomatic relief of pain and a significant increase in range of motion, and all patients considered the procedure to be successful.
  - The authors compared these results with the result of Souter-Strathclyde TEA used in patients with rheumatoid arthritis.[27,31]
  - The revision rate in their series (9%) performed for ulnar component loosening compares favorably with the revision rate with the rheumatoid patients (5% to 21%), in which the main indications for revision included dislocation, and perioperative fracture.
    - The authors attributed the decrease in the incidence of peri- and postoperative fracture to the good amount of bone stock in patients with primary osteoarthritis of the elbow, which makes the risk of fracture very minimal.
    - As evident from this review, the outcome studies of TEA in patients with primary osteoarthritis of the elbow are very limited. The above-mentioned studies included a

small number of patients, and no final recommendation could be drawn at this time.

■ It is hoped that a greater understanding of elbow anatomy and kinematics will lead to advances in prosthetic design and surgical technique.

  ■ The newer anatomic unlinked implants may improve the outcome of elbow replacement in younger patients.[7]

  ■ More outcome studies are needed on these implants or any other modern implants before openly recommending elbow replacement in younger active patients with primary osteoarthritis of the elbow.

REFERENCES

1. Antuna SA, Morrey BF, Adams RA, et al. Ulnohumeral arthroplasty for primary degenerative arthritis of the elbow: long-term outcome and complications. J Bone Joint Surg Am 2002;84A:2168–2173.
2. Bullough PG. Atlas of Orthopedic Pathology, 2nd ed. New York: Gower Medical Publishing, 1992;10:4–10.
3. Doherty M, Preston B. Primary osteoarthritis of the elbow. Ann Rheum Dis 1989;48:743–747.
4. Espag MP, Black DL, Clark DI, et al. Early results of the Souter-Strathclyde unlinked total elbow arthroplasty in patients with osteoarthritis. J Bone Joint Surg Br 2003;85B:351–353.
5. Ewald FC. Total elbow replacement. Orthop Clin North Am 1975;3:685–696.
6. Goodfellow JW, Bullough PG. The pattern of aging of the articular cartilage of the elbow joint. J Bone Joint Surg Br 1967;49B:175–181.
7. Gramstad GD, King GJ, O'Driscoll SW, et al. Elbow arthroplasty using a convertible implant. Tech Hand Up Extrem Surg 2005;9:153–163.
8. Kahiwagi D. Intra-articular changes of the osteoarthritis of the elbow. Orthop Clin North Am 1995;26:691–706.
9. Kashiwagi D. Osteoarthritis of the elbow joint: intra-articular changes and the special operative procedure, Outbridge-Kashiwagi method (O-K method). In: Kashiwagi D, ed. Elbow Joint. Amsterdam: Elsevier Science Publishers Biomedical Division, 1985:177–188.
10. Kato H, Hirayama T, Minami A, et al. Cubital tunnel syndrome associated with medial elbow ganglia and osteoarthritis of the elbow. J Bone Joint Surg Am 2002;84A:1413–1419.
11. Kellgren JH, Larence JS. Radiological assessment of osteoarthrosis. Ann Rheum Dis 1957;16:494–501.
12. King GJW, Adams RA, Morrey BF. Total elbow arthroplasty: revision with use of a non-custom semiconstrained prosthesis. J Bone Joint Surg Am 1997;79A:394–398.
13. Kozak TK, Adams RA, Morrey BF. Total elbow arthroplasty in primary osteoarthritis of the elbow. J Arthroplasty 1998;13:837–842.
14. Kraay MJ, Figgie MP, Inglis AE, et al. Primary semiconstrained total elbow arthroplasty. J Bone Joint Surg Br 1994;76B:636–640.
15. London JT. Kinematics of the elbow. J Bone Joint Surg Am 1981;63A:529–535.
16. Meachim G. Age changes in articular cartilage. Clin Orthop Relat Res 1969;64:33–44.
17. Mintz G, Fraga A. Severe osteoarthritis of the elbow in foundry workers. Arch Environ Health 1973;27:78–80.
18. Morrey BF, Adams RA, Bryan RS. Total replacement for post-traumatic arthritis of the elbow. J Bone Joint Surg Br 1991;73B:607–612.
19. Morrey BF, Adams RA. Semiconstrained elbow replacement arthroplasty for distal humeral non-union. J Bone Joint Surg Br 1995;77B:67–72.
20. Morrey BF, Bryan RS, Dobyns JH, et al. Total elbow arthroplasty. J Bone Joint Surg Am 1981;81A:80–84.
21. Morrey BF. Primary degenerative arthritis of the elbow. J Bone Joint Surg Br 1992;74B:409–413.
22. O'Driscoll SW. Arthroscopic treatment for osteoarthritis of the elbow. Orthop Clin North Am 1995;26:691–706.
23. O'Driscoll SW. Elbow arthritis: treatment options. J Am Acad Orthop Surg 1993;1:106–116.
24. Ogilvie-Harris DJ, Schemitsch E. Arthroscopy of the elbow for removal of loose bodies. Arthroscopy 1993;9:5–8.
25. Oka Y. Debridement for osteoarthritis of the elbow in athletes. Int Orthop 1999;23:91–94.
26. Ortner DJ. Description and classification of degenerative bone changes in the distal joint surfaces of the humerus. Am J Phys Anthrop 1968;28:139–155.
27. Rozing P. Souter-Strathclyde total elbow arthroplasty. J Bone Joint Surg Br 2000;82B:1129–1134.
28. Savoie FH III, Nunley PD, Field LD. Arthroscopic management of the arthritic elbow: indications, technique, and results. J Shoulder Elbow Surg 1999;8:214–219.
29. Stanley D. Prevalence and etiology of symptomatic elbow osteoarthritis. J Shoulder Elbow Surg 1994;3:386–389.
30. Suvarna SK, Stanley D. The histologic changes of the olecranon fossa membrane in primary osteoarthritis of the elbow. J Shoulder Elbow Surg 2004;13:555–557.
31. Trail IA, Nuttal D, Stanley JK. Survivorship and radiological analysis of the standard Souter-Strathyclyde total elbow arthroplasty. J Bone Joint Surg Br 1999;81B:80–84.
32. Tsuge K, Mizuseki T. Debridement arthroplasty for advanced primary osteoarthritis of the elbow: results of a new technique used for 29 elbows. J Bone Joint Surg Br 1994;76B:641–646.
33. Wadworth TG. Osteoarthritis. In: Wadworth TG, ed. The Elbow. Edinburgh: Churchill Livingstone, 1982:292–293.

Chapter 48

Surgical Management of Traumatic Conditions of the Elbow

Matthew L. Ramsey

DEFINITION AND PATHOGENESIS

■ Posttraumatic conditions of the elbow represent a variety of disorders involving the elbow as a result of previous injury. Included among the posttraumatic conditions are:
  ■ Posttraumatic arthritis
    ■ Primary pathology involves posttraumatic degeneration of the articular surface.
    ■ Secondary pathologies can include contracture, loose bodies, and heterotopic bone.
  ■ Nonunion of the distal humerus
    ■ Total elbow arthroplasty (TEA) is considered when reconstruction of the nonunion is deemed impossible or undesirable.
  ■ Dysfunctional instability of the elbow
    ■ This is a special clinical situation where the fulcrum for stable elbow function is lost. The forearm may be dissociated from the brachium (**FIG 1**).
  ■ Chronic instability (dislocation)
    ■ Chronic ligamentous instability of the elbow can lead to articular degeneration, particularly in the elderly, osteopenic patient.
■ Treatment for posttraumatic conditions is individualized depending on the underlying pathology as well as the functional demands and age of the patient.

PATIENT HISTORY AND PHYSICAL FINDINGS

■ The patient history is directed at gaining information about the initial injury, treatments undertaken, complications of treatment, presenting complaints, and patient expectations.
  ■ Detailed investigation of the patient's symptoms should include questions regarding the degree of pain, presence of instability or stiffness, and mechanical symptoms of catching, or locking.
■ The physical examination of the elbow should follow a systematic approach:
  ■ Inspection of the elbow
    ■ Presence and location of previous skin incisions or persistent wounds
    ■ Alignment of the extremity at rest
    ■ Prominent hardware
  ■ Range of motion (ROM)
    ■ Active ROM is assessed and compared to the opposite side. The degree of motion, smoothness of motion, and feel of the endpoint are established.
    ■ Normal active ROM varies, but it should be symmetrical with the opposite unaffected side. Range of motion should be from near full extension (may have hyperextension) to 130 to 140 degrees of flexion. Normal forearm rotation is an arc of 170 degrees, with slightly more supination than pronation.
    ■ Functional ROM has been defined as a flexion–extension arc from 30 degrees to 130 degrees and a

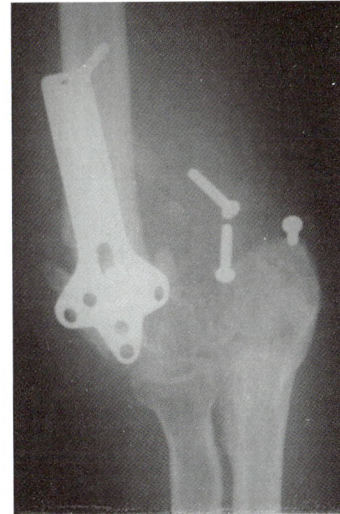

FIG 1 • Radiograph demonstrating dissociation of the forearm from the brachium in a patient with an inadequately treated fracture of the distal humerus with resultant nonunion.

pronation–supination arc from 50 degrees of pronation and 50 degrees of supination.[10]
    ■ Passive range of motion (PROM) is then assessed and compared to the active motion arc.
  ■ Palpation of the elbow should systematically review all of the bony and soft tissue structures of the elbow.
    ■ The ulnar nerve needs to be carefully assessed. If previously surgically manipulated, its location should be identified if possible.
    ■ Motor function of the elbow should be assessed, in particular the flexor (biceps and brachialis) and extensor (triceps) function.

IMAGING AND OTHER DIAGNOSTIC STUDIES

■ Orthogonal radiographic views of the elbow are mandatory (**FIG 2**).
  ■ A good lateral radiograph can typically be obtained.
  ■ A useful anteroposterior (AP) radiograph can be difficult, particularly if the patient has significant flexion contracture. A poor AP radiograph can make assessment of the joint space difficult, typically resulting in overestimating the amount of joint destruction.
■ Oblique radiographs can be helpful in obtaining more detail.
■ CT scans are particularly helpful in assessing the integrity of the bone and establishing whether the joint space is reasonably preserved.
  ■ Three-dimensional reconstructions provide a better understanding of any deformity.
■ Magnetic resonance imaging is rarely needed in the assessment of a posttraumatic joint and is therefore used sparingly.

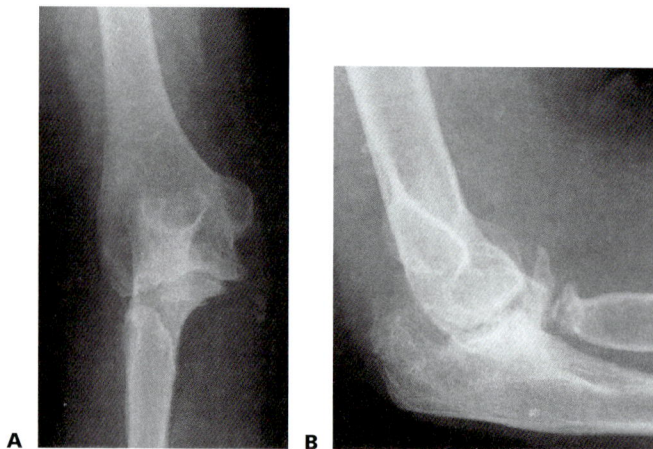

FIG 2 • AP and lateral radiographs of the elbow in a patient with posttraumatic arthritis of the elbow.

DIFFERENTIAL DIAGNOSIS

- Nonunion or malunion of the distal humerus
- Posttraumatic stiffness of the elbow
- Chronic dislocation of the elbow

NONOPERATIVE MANAGEMENT

- The success of nonoperative management depends on specific features of the pathology and the motivation and goals of the patient.
- Activity modification is used to reduce the forces across the elbow.
- Range of motion of the elbow should be maintained. Aggressive efforts to regain lost motion can aggravate the joint.
- External bracing is occasionally used to support an unstable extremity. However, in general, bracing is poorly tolerated and functionally limiting.

SURGICAL MANAGEMENT

- Surgical management of traumatic conditions of the elbow is directed at addressing the underlying cause of disability and should take into consideration the patient's age, physical requirements, and expectations.

Surgical Options

Interposition Arthroplasty[2,7]

- Indications
  - Patients with pain or loss of range of motion who have failed to respond to nonoperative management
  - Posttraumatic arthritis in patients who are either too young for TEA or who are unwilling to accept the functional restrictions with TEA
  - The patients who do best following interposition are those with painful loss of motion when there is no requirement for aggressive, heavy use of the extremity.
- Contraindications
  - Active infection (septic arthritis with persistent infection)
  - Grossly unstable elbow
  - Marked angular deformity
  - Pain without associated functional loss

- Inadequate bone stock
- Patients unable or unwilling to follow postoperative instructions

Total Elbow Replacement[3–5,8,11,14,15]

- Patients with posttraumatic conditions of the elbow tend to be younger than other patients undergoing TEA.
- In this group of patients, TEA should be considered in patients who:
  - Have failed to respond to appropriate nonoperative management
  - Are not appropriate candidates for other surgical options
  - Are willing to adopt a more sedentary lifestyle
  - Have no absolute contraindications to the procedure

Preoperative Planning

Interposition Arthroplasty

- Graft options
  - Achilles tendon allograft has the advantage of no donor site morbidity. It can also be used to reconstruct the collateral ligaments if necessary.
  - Dermis or fascia lata autogenous graft
  - Dermal tissue allograft
- Revision
  - The salvage for a failed interposition arthroplasty is a TEA.[1]
  - Interposition arthroplasty should not be undertaken unless the surgeon is comfortable performing a total elbow replacement in the face of failure.

Total Elbow Replacement

- Implants are described in terms of their physical linkage (linked, unlinked, or linkable) and based on their constraint (constrained, semiconstrained, minimally constrained).
  - Linkage is determined by whether the components are physically linked.
  - Constraint is a more poorly defined quality of the implant. It depends on the geometry of the implant and its interaction with stabilizing soft tissues about the elbow.[6]
- Implant selection in posttraumatic arthritis
  - Linked (semiconstrained) designs: Linked implants have the advantage of being universally applicable to all posttraumatic conditions of the elbow.
  - Unlinked designs: The requirement for the use of unlinked designs in posttraumatic conditions of the elbow is integrity of the collateral ligaments and limited deformity such that normal anatomic relationships can be re-established.
  - Linkable designs: Linkable designs have been developed to take advantage of the features of an unlinked implant while capturing the universal applicability of the linked implants. They can be converted from unlinked to linked either at the time of an initial surgery if stability cannot be conferred or remotely if instability becomes an issue postoperatively.

Positioning

- Interposition arthroplasty
  - Supine with the arm across the chest and a bump under the ipsilateral shoulder
  - Alternatively, the lateral decubitus position with the arm over an arm holder
- Total elbow replacement

■ Patients are placed supine on the operating table with a bump under the ipsilateral shoulder. The arm should be freely mobile through the shoulder to allow manipulation of the joint throughout surgery. The arm can then be placed across the body on a bump or externally rotated through the shoulder and flexed at the elbow (**FIG 3**).

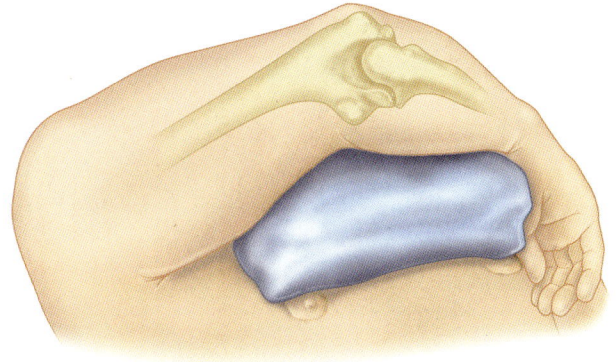

FIG 3 • Patient positioning for total elbow arthroplasty with the arm across the body supported on a bolster.

TECHNIQUES

INTERPOSITION ARTHROPLASTY

■ Posterior skin incision: Develop medial and lateral subcutaneous flaps.
■ Isolate and transpose the ulnar nerve.
■ Perform deep exposure to the elbow through an extensile Köcher approach.[9] The triceps can be partially released from the ulna to allow the triceps–anconeus composite to be mobilized (**TECH FIG 1A**).
■ Mobilize the common extensor group from the anterior capsule and release it proximally with the extensor carpi radialis longus.
■ Isolate the lateral ulnar collateral ligament and release it from its humeral origin (**TECH FIG 1B**). Perform an anterior and posterior capsular release. Supination of the forearm allows the ulna to be rotated away from the humerus. Attempt to leave the medial collateral ligament intact as it will improve postoperative stability.
■ Inspect the cartilage surfaces. If more than 50% of the articular surface is involved, surgery proceeds to interposition.
■ If extensile exposure is required, the extensile Köcher approach can be expanded to a triceps-reflecting anconeus pedicle (TRAP) approach (**TECH FIG 1C,D**).[13]
■ Reshape the distal humerus to conform to the olecranon. Remove the cartilage from the distal humerus and smooth the bone, but avoid aggressive resection of bone (**TECH FIG 1E**).
■ Prepare the interposition tissue. The graft of choice is up to the surgeon, but there is a growing experience with allograft Achilles tendon. In addition to being a robust graft source, it allows for reconstruction of one or both collateral ligaments (**TECH FIG 2A**).
■ Place drill holes across the supracondylar region from anterior to posterior (**TECH FIG 2B**). These drill holes are placed at the medial aspect of the trochlea, above the trochlear sulcus, at the lateral margin of the trochlea, and at the lateral aspect of the capitellum.
■ Drape the interposition tissue over the distal humerus and secure it with sutures placed through the graft from front to back. If there is collateral ligament insufficiency, the tails of the graft (especially when using Achilles tendon) can be fashioned to reconstruct the collateral ligaments (**TECH FIG 2C**).
■ Leave the radial head intact, especially if medial collateral ligament reconstruction is performed, to contribute to the valgus stability of the elbow.
■ Repair the lateral collateral ligament through drill holes at the center of rotation laterally. Do not tie the ligament until the external fixator is securely applied.

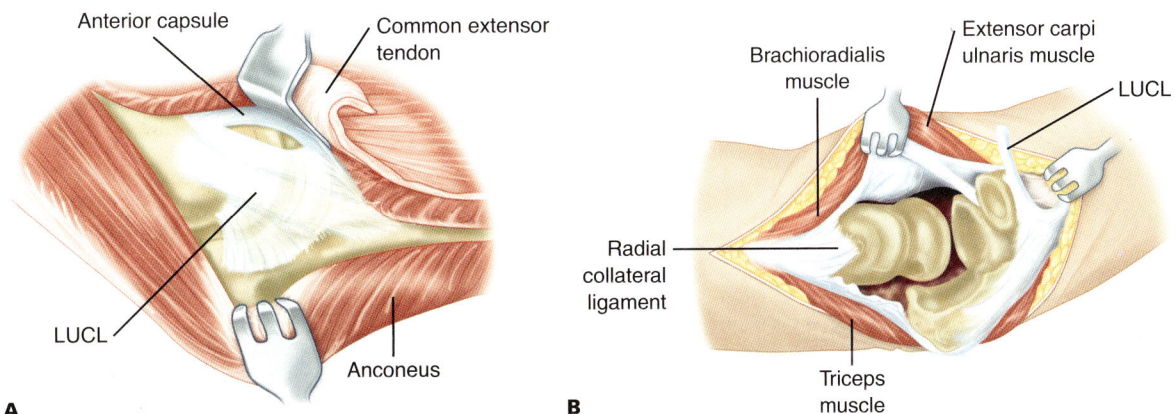

A   **B**

TECH FIG 1 • A. Extensile Köcher approach to the lateral elbow. The anconeus and triceps are elevated off the posterolateral capsule while the common extensor group is elevated off the anterior capsule. Exposure can be extended posteriorly with partial release of the triceps from the lateral aspect of the olecranon. **B.** Deep extensile exposure requires release of the lateral collateral ligament and anterior and posterior capsule. *(continued)*

TECHNIQUES

C

D

E

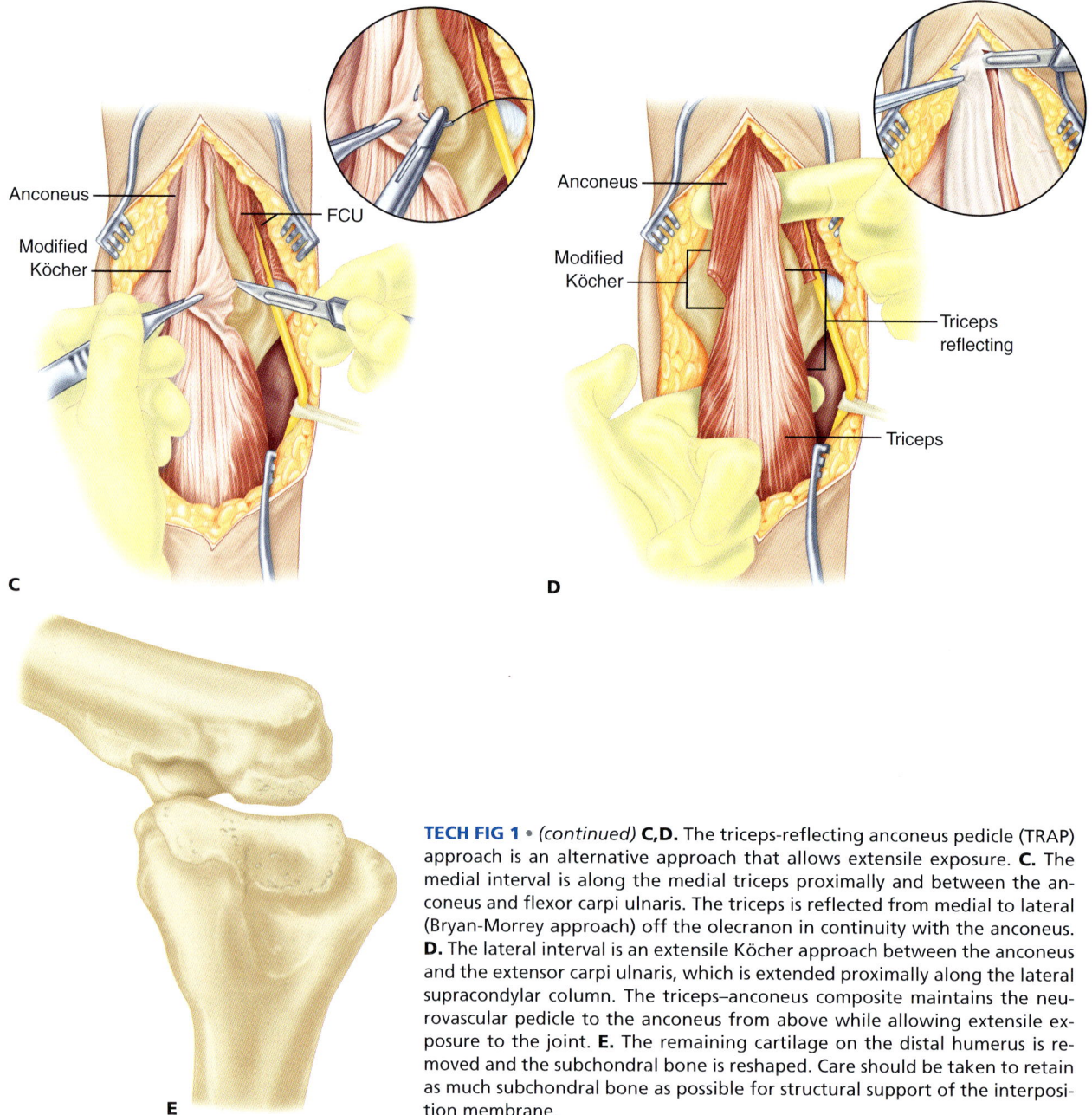

TECH FIG 1 • *(continued)* **C,D.** The triceps-reflecting anconeus pedicle (TRAP) approach is an alternative approach that allows extensile exposure. **C.** The medial interval is along the medial triceps proximally and between the anconeus and flexor carpi ulnaris. The triceps is reflected from medial to lateral (Bryan-Morrey approach) off the olecranon in continuity with the anconeus. **D.** The lateral interval is an extensile Köcher approach between the anconeus and the extensor carpi ulnaris, which is extended proximally along the lateral supracondylar column. The triceps–anconeus composite maintains the neurovascular pedicle to the anconeus from above while allowing extensile exposure to the joint. **E.** The remaining cartilage on the distal humerus is removed and the subchondral bone is reshaped. Care should be taken to retain as much subchondral bone as possible for structural support of the interposition membrane.

Hinged Elbow External Fixator

- Apply a hinged external fixator to protect the interposed graft and to stabilize the joint while soft tissue healing occurs.
- The axis of rotation of the elbow is defined by bony landmarks about the lateral and medial joint (**TECH FIG 3A**).
  - The center of rotation at the lateral elbow is the center point of an arc defined by the articular surface of the capitellum.
  - The center of rotation at the medial elbow is defined by tightly distributed instantaneous centers of rotation approximated by a point at the anterior inferior aspect of the medial epicondyle.
- Establish an axis pin coincident with the lateral and medial centers of rotation. This is the foundation for construction of the fixator.

- The type of fixator used dictates the method of pin insertion relative to the axis pin. Fixator systems that allow the humeral and ulnar pins to be placed independently and than assembled to the axis pin are easiest for the surgeon with limited experience (**TECH FIG 3B**).
- When placing the humeral pin, take care to avoid injury to the neurovascular structures.
  - Pins in the proximal humerus are placed through the anterolateral aspect of the deltoid distal to the axillary nerve.
  - Pins in the midshaft of the humerus are placed in the anterolateral humerus to avoid the radial nerve, which lies posteriorly.
- Ulnar pins are placed along the posterolateral aspect of the ulna.

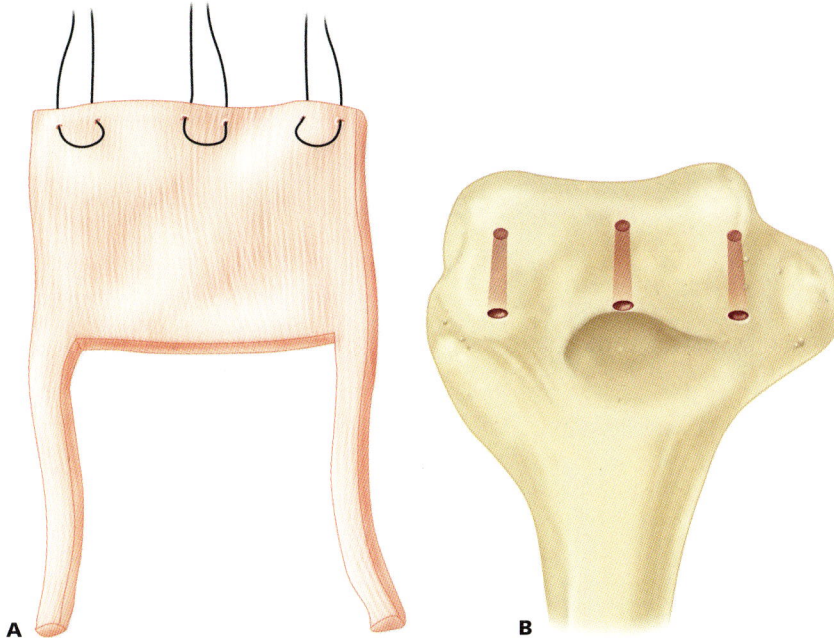

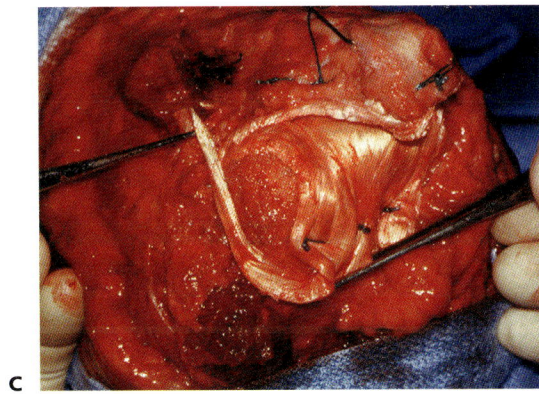

TECH FIG 2 • **A.** The interposition membrane is prepared with mattress sutures placed distally. The Achilles tendon allograft also permits reconstruction of the collateral ligaments if necessary. **B.** Drill holes are placed from posterior to anterior across the supracondylar region to secure the interposition graft. **C.** The interposition membrane is secured to the distal humerus. If necessary, the graft can be fashioned to reconstruct the collateral ligaments. (From Morrey BF, Larson AN. Interposition arthroplasty of the elbow. In: Morrey BF, Sanchez-Sotelo J, eds. *The Elbow and Its Disorders,* 4th ed. Philadelphia: Elsevier; 2009: Figure 69–6.)

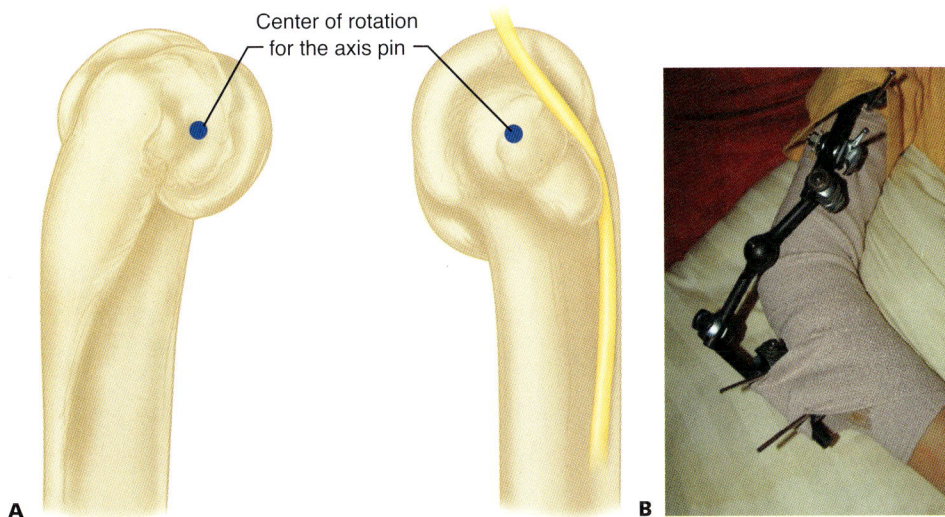

Center of rotation for the axis pin

TECH FIG 3 • **A.** Drawing demonstrating the center of rotation on the lateral and medial side of the elbow. **B.** Photograph demonstrating a hinged external fixator. The humeral and ulnar pins are independently attached to the hinge.

TECHNIQUES

- A bar is fixed to the humeral and another bar is fixed to the ulnar pins.
- The hinge is loosely attached to the humeral and ulnar bars.

- The joint is reduced and ligament reconstruction, if necessary, is completed.
- With the joint reduced, the fixator is tightened. If desired, distraction can be applied.

TOTAL ELBOW REPLACEMENT

Surgical Approach

- A straight posterior skin incision placed off the medial aspect of the olecranon is preferred. Previous incisions may modify the location of the incision. Regardless of the incision used, deep access to the medial and lateral aspect of the joint is essential.
- Identify the ulnar nerve. If not previously handled surgically, the nerve is transposed anteriorly. If the nerve was previously transposed, it only needs to be identified, but not formally dissected unless the position of the nerve places it at risk during surgery.

Triceps Management

- Triceps-reflecting approaches are preferred over triceps-sparing approaches for posttraumatic conditions. Posttraumatic scarring and deformity can make a triceps-sparing approach difficult unless a nonunited distal humeral segment is to be resected.
- A Bryan-Morrey approach is typically performed (**TECH FIG 4A,B**).[9] The medial aspect of the triceps is developed proximally while the interval between the anconeus and flexor carpi ulnaris (FCU) is developed distal to the olecranon. The triceps is reflected from medially to laterally in continuity with the anconeus. Release of the lateral and medial collateral ligaments completes the exposure and allows separation of the ulna from the humerus.

- A modification of the Bryan-Morrey approach involves release of the triceps insertion onto the ulna through an extra-articular osteotomy of the dorsal tip of the ulna (**TECH FIG 4C,D**).[16] The rationale for this modification relates to the recognized complication of triceps insufficiency that occurs with soft tissue release of the triceps. The osteotomy affords several advantages:
  - Bone-to-bone healing of the osteotomy is more reliable than soft tissue healing of the triceps to the ulna.
  - Failure of the osteotomy to heal can be identified radiographically and addressed early.

Deep Dissection

- Release the collateral ligaments and capsule (**TECH FIG 5**). This permits the ulna to be separated from the humerus. If ligamentous integrity is necessary (ie, unlinked arthroplasty) then the lateral ulnar collateral ligament and medial collateral should be tagged with plans at reattachment via bone tunnels in the humerus during closure.
- Release contracted muscles (flexor–pronator and common extensor) to correct deformity, which can result in maltracking of the TEA. Release the scarring about the elbow sufficiently to gain unencumbered access to the humerus and ulna for component implantation.
- The tip of the olecranon can be removed to better visualize the trochlea.

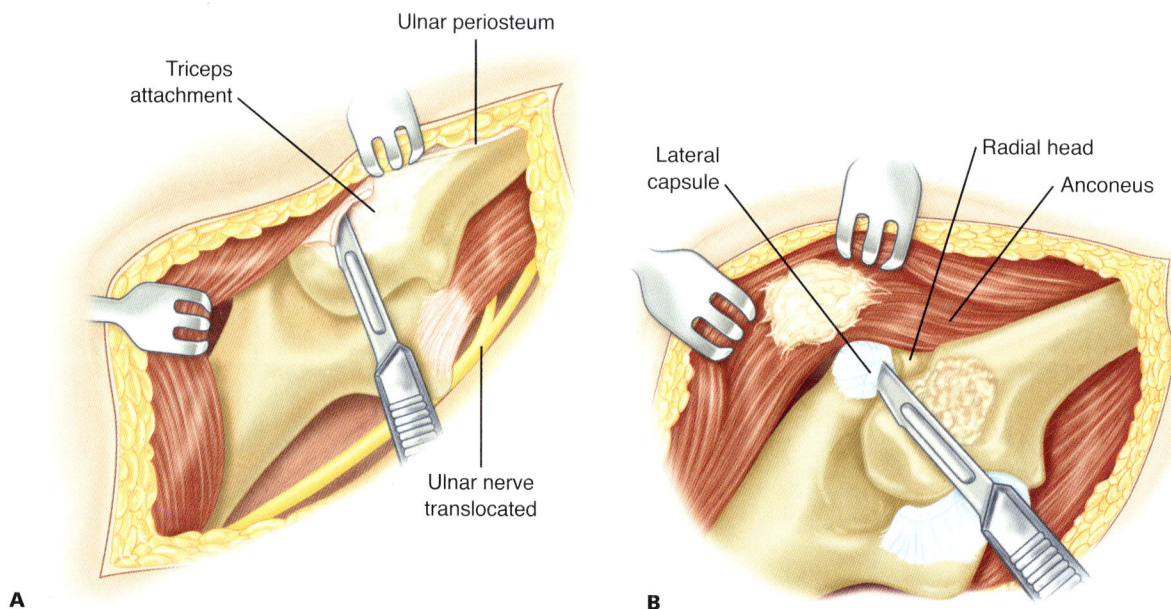

A **B**

TECH FIG 4 • **A,B.** Bryan-Morrey triceps-reflecting approach. **A.** The triceps insertion is released in continuity with the anconeus from medial to lateral. **B.** Further dissection allows the collateral ligaments to be released. *(continued)*

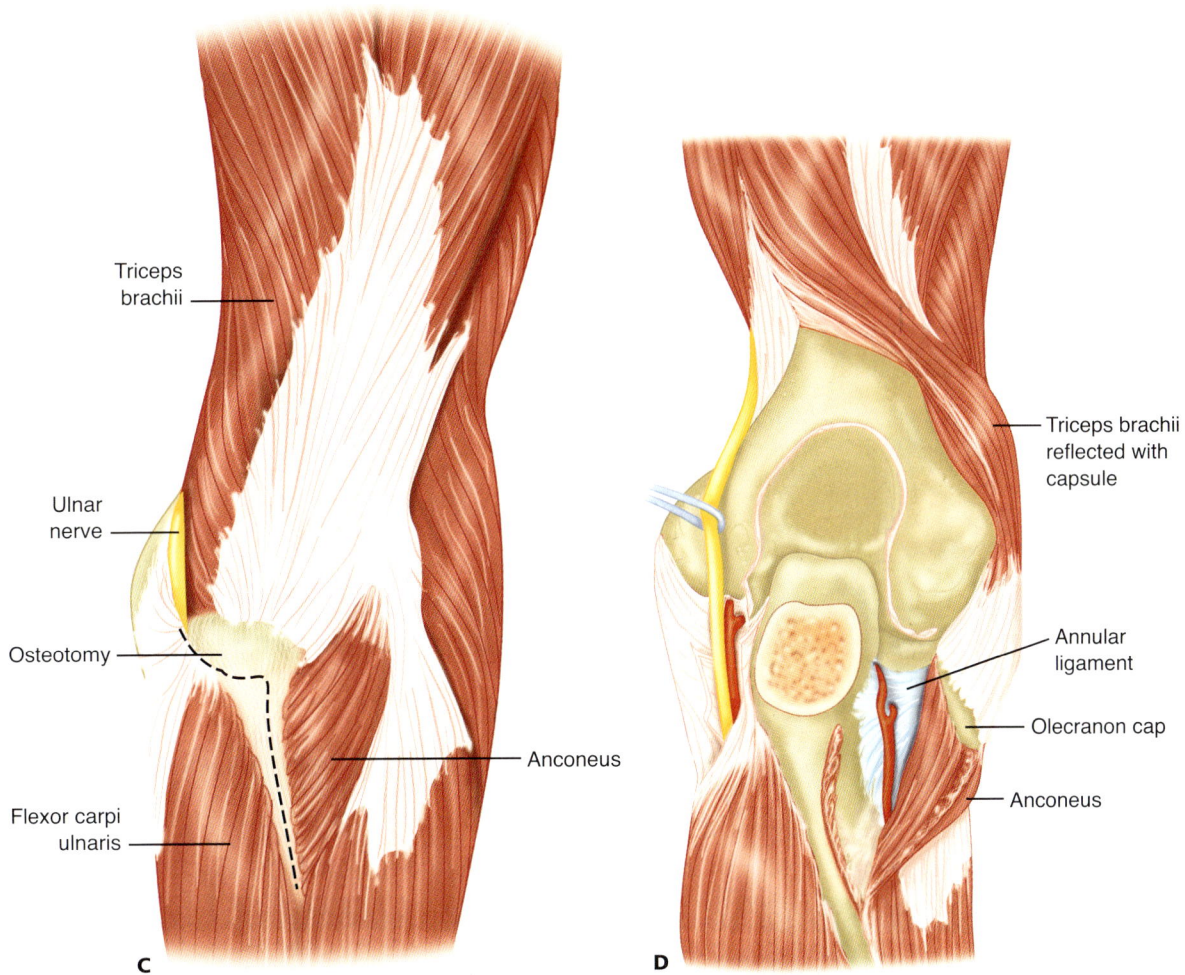

Triceps
brachii

Ulnar
nerve

Osteotomy

Anconeus

Flexor carpi
ulnaris

C

Triceps brachii
reflected with
capsule

Annular
ligament

Olecranon cap

Anconeus

D

TECH FIG 4 • *(continued)* **C,D.** The osteo-anconeus flap approach. The triceps is reflected from medial to lateral in the distal interval between the flexor carpi ulnaris and anconeus.

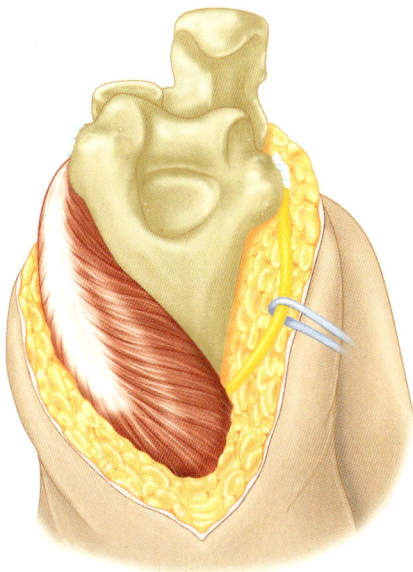

TECH FIG 5 • An extra-articular osteotomy of the tip of the olecranon is performed, leaving the triceps attached to the fragment. The shoulder is externally rotated and the elbow is hyperflexed to allow separation of the ulna from the humerus.

Component Insertion and Completion

- Insertion of total elbow implants is performed in standard fashion and is described in Chapter SE-45.
- After component insertion, the triceps mechanism is repaired through bone tunnels in the ulna. When a sliver of bone is taken with the triceps insertion, transverse tunnels are made. Each limb of nonabsorbable suture is tied over the top of the triceps and bone fragment. An additional cerclage suture is brought through one of the two transverse tunnels and is brought around the tip of the olecranon, incorporating the triceps insertion. This suture counters the pull of the triceps.
- The anconeus is repaired to the flexor carpi ulnaris fascia. Similarly, the medial triceps is repaired to the flexor–pronator group.
- Subcutaneous ulnar nerve transposition is routinely performed.
- A subcutaneous drain is placed and wound closure is performed.

PEARLS AND PITFALLS

Indications	▪ Interposition arthroplasty is considered in patients with a stable elbow and limited, painful ROM. ▪ TEA is considered in carefully selected patients if other nonoperative and operative measures have been exhausted.
Goals of treatment	▪ Regardless of the treatment undertaken, the goal of treatment is a pain-free, functional arc of motion.

Interposition arthroplasty	▪ Predictors of poor outcome:
	  ▪ Painful, mobile elbow
	  ▪ Preoperative instability
	  ▪ Need to reconstruct both the medial and lateral ulnar collateral ligaments at the time of interposition
	▪ Maintain the fixator for at least 4 weeks (preferably 6 weeks).
	▪ Meticulous pin care is required.

TEA	▪ Ulnar nerve transposition in all cases ▪ Triceps-reflecting approach, especially when the joint is very stiff ▪ Release both the medial and lateral collateral ligaments. ▪ Release the flexor–pronator and common extensor, particularly if there is significant preoperative deformity.

POSTOPERATIVE MANAGEMENT

Interposition Arthroplasty

▪ ROM is started as quickly as allowed by the condition of the soft tissues. In general, immediate motion is preferred. However, the prerequisite is a quiet soft tissue envelope. ROM may be assisted with a continuous passive motion machine if desired.

▪ Patients are taught pin care, which is performed daily at home.

▪ Patients are seen at 10 to 14 days postoperatively for staple removal and wound check and every 2 weeks thereafter until pin removal.

▪ The external fixator is left in place for about 4 to 6 weeks and then removed in the operating room with assessment of elbow stability and motion under anesthesia.

  ▪ I prefer to wait 6 weeks to allow collateral ligament healing since instability is the most common complication after fixator removal.

▪ Rehabilitation is continued, focusing on obtaining a functional ROM.

Total Elbow Replacement

▪ The elbow is immobilized in full extension in a well-padded anterior splint.

▪ The arm is elevated on pillows or suspended from an IV pole to reduce swelling.

▪ The splint is removed 24 to 48 hours after surgery.

▪ Gentle active ROM is begun in flexion, pronation, and supination. Active extension is avoided for 6 weeks to protect the triceps repair. However, gravity-assisted extension or passive extension is permitted.

▪ In general, formal physical therapy is rarely required to regain ROM. However, it may be beneficial in patients who struggle to regain their ROM. The general timeline of therapy is:

  ▪ Phase I (0 to 6 weeks): Protect the soft tissue and begin protected active-assistive ROM.

  ▪ Phase II (6 to 12 weeks): Continue to improve ROM. Begin strengthening exercises and encourage functional use of the arm.

  ▪ Phase III (12 to 16 weeks): Return to normal functional activities within the restrictions for TEA.

▪ Postoperative stiffness may be helped with splinting. Static splinting is preferred over dynamic splinting.

▪ Restrictions: Lifetime limitations of the operated extremity include 2- to 5-pound repetitive lifting and 10-lb single-event restriction.

OUTCOMES

Interposition Arthroplasty

▪ The most predictable results for interposition occur in patients presenting with:

  ▪ Stiffness and pain preoperatively

  ▪ Stable elbow

  ▪ One or no ligament reconstruction required at surgery

▪ Poor results are noted when:

  ▪ Pain is the only presenting complaint

  ▪ Elbow is unstable

  ▪ Reconstruction of both the medial and lateral collateral ligaments is needed at the time of interposition

▪ Most studies report a 70% satisfaction rate among patients with respect to pain relief; 80% of patients regain a functional ROM.

▪ Cheng and Morrey[2] found that 67% of patients treated for rheumatoid arthritis had satisfactory relief of pain, and 75% of patients treated for osteoarthritis were satisfied at 5-year follow-up.

Total Elbow Arthroplasty

▪ Patients undergoing TEA for posttraumatic conditions of the elbow tend to be younger and have higher demand.

▪ TEA for posttraumatic conditions of the elbow is associated with improved clinical outcomes.

▪ A higher complication rate is noted for posttraumatic conditions compared to other indications for TEA.

▪ Mechanical complications such as component fracture and increased polyethylene bushing wear are more common.

Causes of increased complications include:

- Multiple previous surgeries
- Deformity of the elbow requiring realignment of the extremity through the implant

COMPLICATIONS

Interposition Arthroplasty

- Complications of interposition arthroplasty include:
  - Instability
  - Infection
  - Ulnar neuropathy
  - Resorptive bone loss
  - Heterotopic bone formation
- Complications related to the external fixator include:
  - Superficial pin tract infections
  - Deep infection (osteomyelitis)
  - Pin breakage
- In the literature, complications have been reported to occur in up to 25% of patients.

Total Elbow Replacement

- TEA for traumatic conditions is associated with a high complication rate. Major complications include:
  - Infection
    - Current reports indicate an infection rate of 2% to 5% for primary TEA.
    - Higher infection rates are noted with posttraumatic arthritis and a history of prior surgery.
  - Loosening
  - Triceps insufficiency (an underrecognized problem)
  - Neurologic injury (incidence of transient ulnar neuropathy as high as 26% and permanent nerve injury up to 10%)
  - Wound complications
    - Associated with prior surgery
    - Manage wound by immobilizing in extension postoperatively; use a subcutaneous drain to avoid hematoma formation. A significant postoperative hematoma should be evacuated.
  - Periprosthetic fracture (can occur intraoperatively or postoperatively; incidence ranges from 1% to 23%)

REFERENCES

1. Blaine TA, Adams R, Morrey BF. Total elbow arthroplasty after interposition arthroplasty for elbow arthritis. J Bone Joint Surg Am 2005;87A:286–292.
2. Cheng SL, Morrey BF. Treatment of the mobile, painful arthritic elbow by distraction interposition arthroplasty. J Bone Joint Surg Am 2000;82A:233–238.
3. Figgie MP, Inglis AE, Mow CS, et al. Salvage of non-union of supracondylar fracture of the humerus by total elbow arthroplasty. J Bone Joint Surg Am 1989;71A:1058–1065.
4. Figgie HE III, Inglis AE, Ranawat CS, et al. Results of total elbow arthroplasty as a salvage procedure for failed elbow reconstructive operations. Clin Orthop Relat Res 1987;219:185–193.
5. Inglis AE, Inglis AE Jr, Figgie MM, et al. Total elbow arthroplasty for flail and unstable elbows. J Shoulder Elbow Surg 1997;6:29–36.
6. Kamineni S, O'Driscoll SW, Urban M, et al. Intrinsic constraint of unlinked total elbow replacements: the ulnotrochlear joint. J Bone Joint Surg Am 2005;87A:2019–2027.
7. Larson AN, Morrey BF. Interposition arthroplasty with an Achilles tendon allograft as a salvage procedure for the elbow. J Bone Joint Surg Am 2008;90A:2714–2723.
8. Moro JK, King GJ. Total elbow arthroplasty in the treatment of posttraumatic conditions of the elbow. Clin Orthop Relat Res 2000;370:102–114.
9. Morrey BF. Surgical exposures of the elbow. In: Morrey BF, Sanchez-Sotelo J, eds. The Elbow and its Disorders, 4th ed. Philadelphia: Saunders Elsevier, 2009:115–142.
10. Morrey BF, Askew LJ, Chao EY. A biomechanical study of normal functional elbow motion. J Bone Joint Surg Am 1981;63A:872–877.
11. Morrey BF, Schneeberger AG. Total elbow arthroplasty for posttraumatic arthrosis. AAOS Instr Course Lect 2009;58:495–504.
12. Nolla J, Ring D, Lozano-Calderon S, et al. Interposition arthroplasty of the elbow with hinged external fixation for post-traumatic arthritis. J Shoulder Elbow Surg 2008;17:459–464.
13. O'Driscoll SW. The triceps-reflecting anconeus pedicle (TRAP) approach for distal humeral fractures and nonunions. Orthop Clin North Am 2000;31:91–101.
14. Ramsey ML, Adams RA, Morrey BF. Instability of the elbow treated with semiconstrained total elbow arthroplasty. J Bone Joint Surg Am 1999;81A:38–47.
15. Schneeberger AG, Adams R, Morrey BF. Semiconstrained total elbow replacement for the treatment of post-traumatic osteoarthrosis. J Bone Joint Surg Am 1997;79A:1211–1222.
16. Wolfe SW, Ranawat CS. The osteo-anconeus flap: an approach for total elbow arthroplasty. J Bone Joint Surg Am 1990;72A:684–688.

Chapter 49

Elbow Arthrodesis

Mark A. Mighell and Thomas J. Kovack

BACKGROUND

- Elbow arthrodesis is a rarely performed orthopaedic procedure.
- It is mainly performed for severe joint destruction due to:
  - Posttraumatic arthrosis
  - Instability
  - Infection
- Historically, it is performed for a tuberculous infection of the elbow.[1]
- Early fusion rates are about 50%.[1]
- With modern techniques, fusion rates approach 50% to 100%.[3,9]
- Arthrodesis of the elbow results in greater functional disability than arthrodesis of the ankle, hip, or knee joints.
- Satisfactory shoulder function is a prerequisite, even though it does not compensate for loss of motion in the elbow.[2]
- Compensatory motion is seen more in the spinal column and wrist.
- A functional hand is also desirable when performing arthrodesis of the elbow.
- No optimal position for arthrodesis exists.
  - The position of fusion is dictated by the needs of the patient.

PATIENT HISTORY AND PHYSICAL FINDINGS

- Skin and soft tissue defects are evaluated.
- The surgeon should evaluate the need for bone graft or soft tissue coverage before arthrodesis.
- If soft tissue coverage is necessary, a plastic surgery consultation is recommended.
- Shoulder, wrist, and spinal column motion is evaluated.
- Neurologic and motor deficits are documented.
- Blood flow to the hand is determined.
- The quality and quantity of bone available for fusion are assessed.

IMAGING AND OTHER DIAGNOSTIC STUDIES

- Standard radiographs of the elbow are obtained.
- Computed tomography (CT) scans of the elbow are obtained for more detailed bony anatomy.
- If infection is suspected:
  - Blood work is obtained for complete blood count, sedimentation rate, and C-reactive protein.
  - The joint is aspirated or an indium scan is performed.

SURGICAL MANAGEMENT

- The elbow is one of the most difficult joints to fuse because of the long lever arm and strong bending forces across the fusion site.
- Arthrodesis should be considered a salvage procedure when no other satisfactory surgical option exists.

Indications

- Septic and tuberculous arthritis
- Sequela of septic arthritis
- Complex war injuries (with large bone and soft tissue defects)
- Young healthy laborers with posttraumatic arthritis who are too young for total elbow arthroplasty
- Posttraumatic arthrosis or severe instability
- Pseudarthrosis
- Severely comminuted intra-articular fractures of the distal humerus with joint destruction
- Chronic osteomyelitis
- Failed elbow arthroplasty
- Failed internal fixation for nonunions

Contraindications

- Massive bone loss preventing successful arthrodesis
- Massive soft tissue loss not amenable to flap reconstruction
- Compromised function of the ipsilateral shoulder, wrist, and spinal column

Preoperative Planning

- The best elbow position is controversial, although the literature suggests between 45 and 110 degrees.
  - Historically, 90 degrees is accepted as the best position.
- Factors for choosing the best position include:
  - Gender
  - Occupation
  - Hand dominance
  - Functional requirements
  - Associated joint involvement
  - Unilateral versus bilateral arthrodesis
  - Patient preference
- One to 3 weeks before surgery, the elbow to be fused is braced or casted in various angles.
  - Generally acceptable angles include:
    - Male: dominant arm at 90 degrees
    - Females seem to prefer lower angles of 40 to 70 degrees.
    - Ninety to 110 degrees is better for personal hygiene.
    - Forty to 70 degrees is better for extrapersonal needs and activities.
    - Bilateral elbow arthrodesis: dominant arm at 110 degrees, nondominant arm at 65 degrees
- Soft tissue coverage is evaluated.
- Flap coverage or skin grafts are performed before arthrodesis.
- If soft tissue coverage is required, the joint is stabilized with an external fixator.
- The surgeon should consider bulk graft with demineralized bone matrix and cancellous allograft or autograft.

- For large bone defects, autograft cancellous bone is preferable.
- Antibiotics are given 30 minutes before the incision.
- General anesthesia is used.
- An axillary or interscalene block can be used.

Special Instruments

- Large fragment locking set (4.5-mm locked narrow plate)
- A 3.5-mm locked plate may be substituted in smaller patients.
- Sterile goniometer
- Plate press

- High-speed burr
- Power drill
- Osteotomes
- Oscillating saw
- Kirschner wire set

Patient Positioning

- A tourniquet is placed as high on the arm as possible. A sterile tourniquet is required to increase the zone of sterility.
- The patient is placed in the lateral decubitus position with the operative arm resting on a padded arm rest.

SURGICAL APPROACH

- Mark existing surgical scars and use prior incisions.
- Use a direct posterior approach for the elbow.
  - An anterior approach may be needed if the tissue is compromised posteriorly.
- If flap coverage is present, a plastic surgeon may be required for exposure.
  - Flaps with vascular pedicles can be located with Doppler.

- Create full-thickness flaps right down to the bone.
  - Split the triceps tendon longitudinally.
  - Carry the triceps split distally in the interval between the flexor carpi ulnaris (FCU) and the anconeus.
- Identify the ulnar nerve and make sure it remains protected.
  - Identify neurovascular structures in known areas before following structures through areas of heavy scar tissue.

ARTHRODESIS

Osteotomy and Fracture Reduction

- Expose the dorsal surface of the distal humerus and proximal ulna.
- Use osteotomes to "fish-scale" the exposed bone.
- Open the medullary canal of the humerus and ulna.
- Perform a step-cut osteotomy of the proximal ulna and distal humerus to increase the surface area for fusion (**TECH FIG 1A**).
- Contour the bone so that it can be reduced at the appropriate angle chosen for arthrodesis.
  - It is often necessary to excise the radial head to allow for adequate reduction of the humerus and ulna.
- Reduce the distal humerus to the proximal ulna.
  - Confirm the fusion angle with a sterile goniometer (**TECH FIG 1B**).
  - Provisionally hold the reduction at the desired angle with 1.6-mm Kirschner wires.

Screw and Plate Fixation

- Drill from distal to proximal for lag screw insertion (**TECH FIG 2A**).
  - Use two or three lag screws whenever possible.

- Apply the 4.5-mm locking plate posteriorly, prebent at the chosen angle of arthrodesis (**TECH FIG 2B**).
  - A long plate should be selected with a minimum of 10 to 14 holes.
  - A plate press is easier to use than bending irons.
- The plate functions as a neutralization device.
  - All compression is achieved with the lag technique employed for screw placement.
- The plate is pulled down to the bone and secured with cortical screws before adding locked screws.
- Use at least one locked screw proximal and distal to the fusion site to increase the torsional strength of the construct (**TECH FIG 2C**).

Completion

- Check the position and fixation of the construct intraoperatively with fluoroscopy.
- The final construct should compress well at the fracture site.
  - The plate should conform securely to the bone at the desired angle of fusion (**TECH FIG 3A**).
- Irrigate and close the wound.
  - Place one or two deep flat drains.
- Final radiographs should be taken intraoperatively (**TECH FIG 3B,C**).

TECHNIQUES

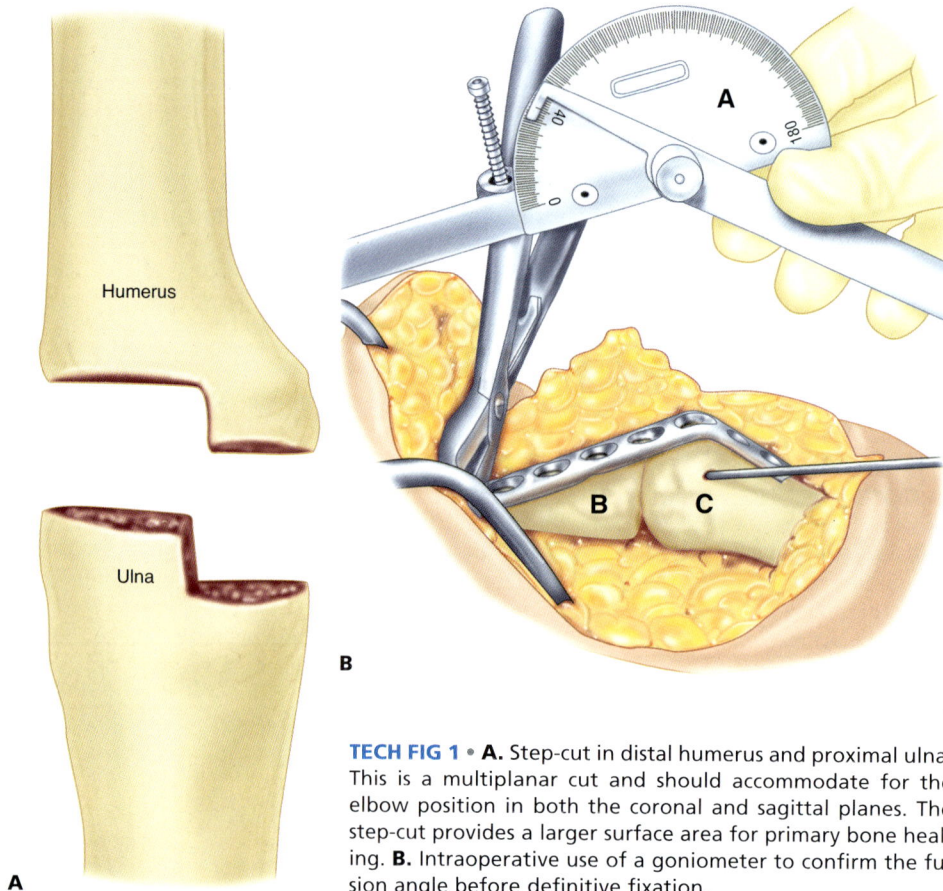

TECH FIG 1 • **A.** Step-cut in distal humerus and proximal ulna. This is a multiplanar cut and should accommodate for the elbow position in both the coronal and sagittal planes. The step-cut provides a larger surface area for primary bone healing. **B.** Intraoperative use of a goniometer to confirm the fusion angle before definitive fixation.

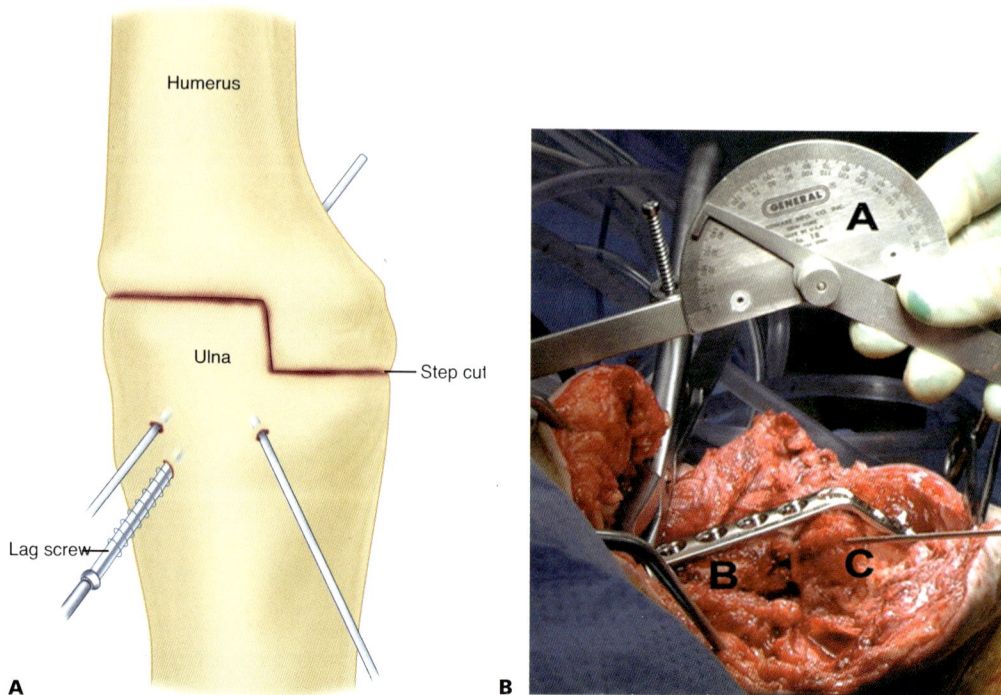

TECH FIG 2 • **A.** Placement of lag screw. Screws are placed from distal to proximal in a crossed configuration. Two or three lag screws are placed before plate application. Provisional fixation is obtained with Kirschner wires and the fusion position is measured with a goniometer. **B.** Plate placement after the fusion angle has been confirmed. *(continued)*

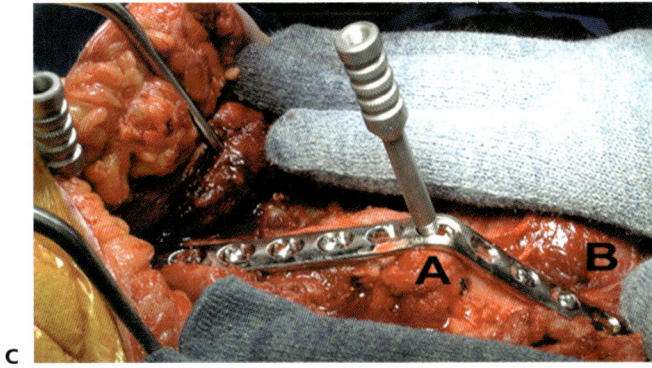

TECH FIG 2 • *(continued)* **C.** A guide for locking the screw through the plate and across the step-cut osteotomy. Compression must be achieved before locking screws are placed. *A,* distal humerus; *B,* proximal ulna.

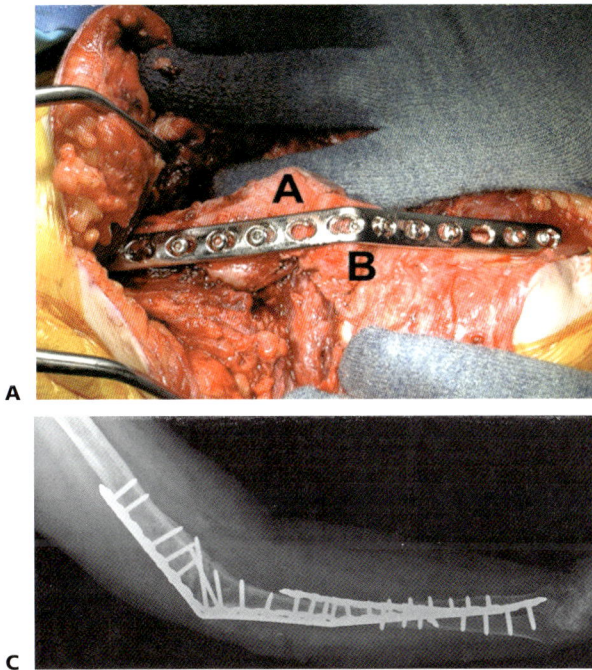

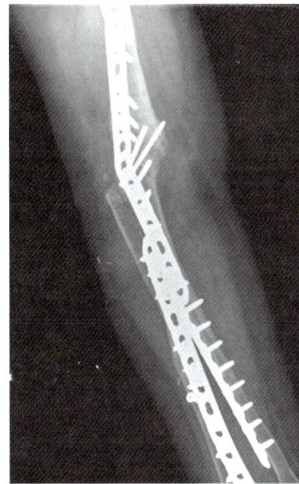

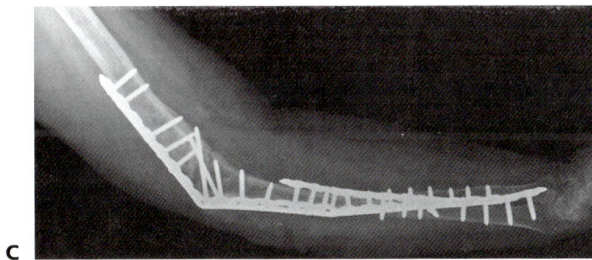

TECH FIG 3 • **A.** Completed elbow arthrodesis using step-cut osteotomy and 3.5-mm locking plate and lag screw technique. *A,* distal humerus; *B,* proximal ulna. **B,C.** AP and lateral postoperative radiographs of left elbow fusion using step-cut osteotomy and locked plating technique.

PEARLS AND PITFALLS

- Step-cut bone to increase the surface area for healing.
- Place lag screws in both vertical and horizontal planes to increase compression.
- Keep dorsal tissue flaps at full thickness, including the periosteum.
- Use lag technique to compress the bone ends.
- Never identify neurovascular structures in areas of extensive surgical scarring. Work from known to unknown surgical fields.
- Open the medullary canal to facilitate blood flow.
- Select a plate of sufficient length to span the fusion site. Longer plates are desirable.
- Never place locking screws before reduction and compression of the bone ends.
- Keep patients in a cast for at least 4 months, until fusion occurs, depending on radiographs.

POSTOPERATIVE CARE

- Drains are removed before hospital discharge.
- Intravenous antibiotics are continued for 48 hours or longer, depending on intraoperative cultures.
- Sutures or staples are removed at 2 weeks.
- The arm is placed in a long-arm cast at the 2-week visit.
- The patient is placed in serial casts for at least 4 months.
- Cast application is continued until there is radiographic evidence of union.

REFERENCES

1. Arafiles RP. A new technique of fusion for tuberculous arthritis of the elbow. J Bone Joint Surg Am 1981;63A:1396–1400.
2. Beckenbaugh RD. Arthrodesis. In: Morrey BF, ed. The Elbow and its Disorders, ed 3. Philadelphia: WB Saunders, 2000:731–737.
3. Bilic R, Kolundzic R, Bicanic G, et al. Elbow arthrodesis after war injuries. Military Med 2005;170:164–166.
4. Irvine GB, Gregg PJ. A method of elbow arthrodesis: brief report. J Bone Joint Surg Br 1989;71B:145–146.
5. McAuliffe JA, Burkhalter WE, Ouellette EA, et al. Compression plate arthrodesis of the elbow. J Bone Joint Surg Br 1992;74B:300–304.
6. Morrey BF, Askew LJ, Chao EY, et al. A biomechanical study of normal functional elbow motion. J Bone Joint Surg Am 1981;63A: 872–877.
7. Nagy SM, Szabo RM, Sharkey NA. Unilateral elbow arthrodesis: the preferred position. J South Orthop Assoc 1999;8:80–85.
8. O'Neill OR, Morrey BG, Tanaka S, et al. Compensatory motion in the upper extremity, after elbow arthrodesis. Clin Orthop Relat Res 1992;281:89–96.
9. Orozco JR. A new technique of elbow arthrodesis. Int Orthop 1996;20:92–93.
10. Presnal BP, Chillaq KJ. Radiohumeral arthrodesis for salvage of failed total elbow arthroplasty. J Arthroplasty 1995;10:699–701.
11. Rashkoff E, Burkhalter WE. Arthrodesis of the salvage elbow. Orthopedics 1986;9:733–738.
12. Tang C, Roidis N, Itamura J, et al. The effect of simulated elbow arthrodesis on the ability to perform activities of daily living. J Hand Surg Am 2001;26A:1146–1150.

Exam Table for Hand, Wrist, and Forearm

Examination	Technique	Illustration	Grading & Significance
Abductor pollicis brevis muscle test	Abduction of thumb against resistance with palpation of thenar muscle		MRC grading. If weak, the surgeon should consider a median nerve lesion.
Advancing Tinel sign	Percussion along course of a nerve in a distal to proximal direction		During percussion, the patient notes a tingling sensation in the sensory distribution of the nerve. Detects regenerating (unmyelinated) axons. Serial progression of a Tinel sign distally is useful to monitor axon progression after nerve repair or injury.
Allen test	The patient is asked to actively open and close the hand to create blanching in the palm. With the hand tightly closed, the examiner occludes the radial and ulnar arteries. The examiner releases one artery and watches for reperfusion and then repeats, releasing the other artery.		Reperfusion should occur within a few seconds. If it does not, then that artery does not provide good flow to the hand. If, for example, the radial artery is dominant (ie, the ulnar artery does not reperfuse the hand), then injury to this vessel during the procedure could lead to ischemia of the hand.
Anatomic snuffbox palpation	The examiner palpates the anatomic snuffbox between the first and third extensor compartment tendons while moving the wrist from radial to ulnar deviation.		Pain at the articular–nonarticular junction of the scaphoid may be the result of periscaphoid synovitis, scaphoid instability, radial styloid arthrosis, or scaphoid fracture or nonunion.
Boyes oblique retinacular ligament tightness test	The examiner passively extends the proximal interphalangeal (PIP) joint and evaluates distal interphalangeal (DIP) motion. Tightness of the oblique retinacular ligaments of Landsmeer is evaluated by assessing the relative degree of resistance to active and passive DIP joint flexion with the PIP joint held in maximum extension by the examiner.		In a positive test, passive extension of the PIP joint will result in extension of the DIP joint. Increased resistance to active and passive DIP joint flexion with the PIP joint held in extension signifies relative tightness of the oblique retinacular ligaments (ORLs) of Landsmeer, signifying a potential subacute or chronic central slip injury. Continued shortening of the ORLs will result in a boutonnière deformity.

(continued)

1

Examination	Technique	Illustration	Grading & Significance
Bunnell intrinsic tightness test	While holding the metacarpophalangeal (MCP) joint in extension, the examiner assesses the degree of resistance to passive PIP joint flexion. The test is repeated with the MCP joint held in flexion.		Intrinsic tightness results in limited passive flexion of the PIP joint when the MCP joint is held extended. Extrinsic tightness results in limited PIP joint passive flexion when the MCP joint is held flexed.
Carpal supination reduction test	The examiner applies dorsally directed pressure to the volar aspect of the supinated ulnar carpus.		The ulnar carpus will be supinated and the distal ulna prominent, signifying an ulnar extrinsic ligament injury. Reduction is noted visually after application of the force.
Carpal tunnel compression test	The examiner applies direct compression to the median nerve at the level of the carpal tunnel for 60 seconds or until symptomatic.		Reproduction of symptoms in the median nerve distribution is consistent with carpal tunnel syndrome.
Carpometacarpal (CMC) distraction test	The examiner distracts the thumb and palpates the CMC joint.		Reproduction of pain confirms the CMC joint as a site of disease or inflammation.
CMC grind test	The examiner axially compresses the thumb and applies flexion, extension, circumduction, and rotation.		Usually crepitus is appreciated starting with stage II disease, but it is more predictable in stage III or IV disease. A positive test is suggestive of degenerative thumb CMC joint disease.
Cross-finger test	The patient is asked to cross the long and index fingers.		The test is positive if the patient cannot cross the fingers. This test demonstrates weakness of dorsal and palmar interossei.
Cubital tunnel Tinel sign	The ulnar nerve is percussed around the elbow.		A positive test results in radiating paresthesias into the ulnar nerve distribution of the hand. This test may not be specific for ulnar nerve pathology.

Examination	Technique	Illustration	Grading & Significance
Distal radioulnar joint (DRUJ) compression test	The examiner compresses the ulnar head against the sigmoid notch while holding the patient's mid-forearm and passively rotating.		Positive or negative. A positive test is exacerbation of pain, which suggests arthritis or instability; dorsal or palmar subluxation may be noted.
DRUJ press test	With both wrists pronated, the patient rises from a chair using the affected hand and wrist or pushes downward on a tabletop.		Increased depression of the ulnar head on the affected side results in a "dimple sign" indicating instability. Pain without increased ulnar head depression may indicate a triangular fibrocartilage complex tear.
DRUJ stability test	With the elbow flexed 90 degrees, the examiner grasps the radius over its distal third with one hand and holds the ulna head between the index finger and thumb with the other hand. The examiner displaces the ulna volarly and dorsally in neutral rotation, full supination, and full pronation. The sides are compared.		Substantially less stability than is noted on the opposite side or pain at extremes of rotation may correlate with symptomatic DRUJ instability related to triangular fibrocartilage complex or ligamentous instability. Palpable crepitus at the DRUJ may be indicative of DRUJ arthrosis. Instability Grading Scale: 0: normal; about 1 cm of motion in neutral, no motion at extremes of rotation I: <0.5 cm of motion at extremes. Firm endpoint. II: >0.5 cm of motion at extremes with soft endpoint but no dislocation III: reduced joint before stress with dislocation of the DRUJ at extremes IV: dislocated joint. "Mushy" feeling with stressing joint.
Extensor carpi ulnaris (ECU) subluxation test	The patient is asked to ulnarly deviate the wrist while actively pronating and supinating. The examiner palpates the ECU tendon at and just proximal to the ulnar groove with the patient's wrist in supination, mild flexion, and ulnar deviation. The sides are compared.		Passively subluxatable versus actively subluxatable. Click versus no click. Pain with subluxation versus no significant pain with subluxation. If the tendon dislocates with passive supination, palmar flexion, and ulnar deviation the ECU is grossly unstable. If the addition of ECU contraction is required for frank dislocation, some inherent stability remains. Pain with subluxation is a critical finding when contemplating surgical treatment.

(continued)

Examination	Technique	Illustration	Grading & Significance
Elbow flexion test	The elbow is fully flexed with the forearm supinated for 60 seconds or until symptoms develop.		The test is positive for cubital tunnel syndrome if the patient's symptoms are reproduced in the ulnar nerve distribution while holding this position.
Elsen test	The patient's injured PIP joint is flexed 90 degrees over the edge of a table. The patient is asked to actively extend the PIP joint against resistance. The examiner palpates for active middle phalanx extension and simultaneous extension rigidity of the DIP joint.		A positive test is consistent with a complete central slip disruption at any time frame. No extension force is felt associated with the middle phalanx but DIP joint rigidity is readily perceived secondary to the effects of the lateral bands. This test will not necessarily detect a partial central slip injury.
Extensor apparatus examination	The examiner observes and palpates the extensor tendon and sagittal bands at MCP and PIP.		The examiner should look for: 1. Tenderness adjacent to MCP 2. Tendon subluxation at MCP 3. Swan-neck deformity Rules out extensor mechanism abnormalities, which may cause overlapping signs or symptoms.
Flexor digitorum profundus (FDP) examination	The patient is asked to flex the DIP with the PIP joint blocked in extension.		FDP function present or absent. Loss of active DIP flexion suggests disruption or loss of FDP function.
Flexor digitorum superficialis (FDS) examination	The patient is asked to flex the finger with the adjacent digits held in extension.		FDS function present or absent. Loss of active PIP flexion suggests disruption or loss of FDS function.

Examination	Technique	Illustration	Grading & Significance
Finger cascade	The examiner observes the position of the fingers with the patient at rest.		Loss of the normal cascade suggests disruption or loss of function of the flexor tendons.
Finkelstein maneuver	With palpation along the first dorsal compartment, the thumb is flexed and the wrist is ulnarly deviated.		Pain indicates DeQuervain tenosynovitis.
Flexor tendon contracture	The wrist and metacarpophalangeal joints are extended, and the examiner assesses extension of the interphalangeal joints.		With flexor tendon contracture there will be limited extension of the interphalangeal joints.
Foveal sign	The examiner palpates the ulnocarpal joint in the interval between the ulnar styloid and the flexor carpi ulnaris tendon.		Pain is indicative of triangular fibrocartilage complex pathology.
Froment sign	The patient is asked to pinch a piece of paper between the index and thumb. Then the examiner attempts to pull the paper out. Both hands are tested simultaneously.		Positive if paper is held only by flexing the thumb interphalangeal joint. This results from recruitment of the flexor pollicis longus and paralysis of the adductor pollicis, usually from an ulnar nerve disorder.

(continued)

Examination	Technique	Illustration	Grading & Significance
Grip strength	The Jamar Dynometer can be used to objectively measure grip strength. The patient's elbow is placed in 90 degrees of flexion and the forearm and wrist in neutral. The recorded value is the average of three maximal attempts with the dynamometer set on the third station.		Findings are compared to the contralateral side. Decreased strength in association with physical findings can be indicative of wrist pathology. The presence of pain in the central aspect of the wrist with attempted grip has been associated with scapholunate ligament disruption. Mean grip strength for males is 103 to 104 for the dominant extremity and 92 to 99 for the non-dominant extremity. Mean grip strength for females is 62 to 63 for the dominant extremity and 53 to 55 for the non-dominant extremity.
Lichtman Midcarpal Shift Test	With the hand pronated and the forearm stabilized, the examiner positions the wrist in 15 degrees ulnar deviation. The examiner grabs the patient's hand and exerts palmar pressure on the distal capitate. The examiner axially loads and ulnarly deviates the wrist. The procedure is repeated for radial deviation.		No characteristic clunk to severe clunk with pain. Midcarpal instability.
Love pin test	The head of a pin or paperclip is gently pressed against the tender area to localize the pain.		Locates a glomus tumor. In subungual tumors, the pin is placed on the nail plate at various locations to find the tumor.
Lunotriquetral (LT) compression test	Compression is applied in the ulnar snuffbox to give a radially directed force across the LT joint.		Pain with this maneuver may indicate pathology at the LT or triquetral hamate joints.
Lumbrical muscle contracture	An intrinsic tightness test is performed with the fingers radially or ulnarly deviated. Alternatively, the test can be performed with the DIP joint flexed as well as the PIP joint.		With lumbrical contracture, there is less passive flexion of the PIP joint with the finger deviated or with the DIP joint flexed in comparison to intrinsic testing. If present, this suggests lumbrical muscle contracture as part of the pathology.

Examination	Technique	Illustration	Grading & Significance
LT ballottement (Reagan) test	The examiner secures the lunate between the thumb and index finger of one hand and the pisotriquetral unit with the other hand. Anterior and posterior stress is applied across the LT joint.		The test is positive if increased antero-posterior laxity and pain are present. Pain and instability are indicative of LT ligament tear or arthrosis.
LT shear (Kleinman) test	The forearm is placed in neutral rotation and the elbow on the examination table. The examiner's contralateral thumb is placed over the dorsum of the lunate. With the lunate supported, the examiner's ipsilateral thumb loads the pisotriquetral joint from the palmar aspect, creating a shear force at the LT joint.		Positive with pain, crepitance, and abnormal mobility of the LT joint
LT Shuck test	The examiner stabilizes the pisotriquetral joint while passively ulnarly and radially deviating the wrist. Findings are compared with the contralateral wrist.		In a positive test the patient experiences a painful click as the lunate and triquetrum slide abnormally. It signifies a LT ligament injury.
Metacarpophalangeal (MCP) and proximal interphalangeal (PIP) joint instability testing	The individual MCP or PIP joints are tested by the examiner grasping the patient's finger and then applying a valgus and then a varus stress with the joint extended and flexed. The resultant motion is compared to the contralateral side. Differences in laxity indicate ligamentous instability.		Grade 1: No difference in joint line opening compared to the contralateral joint Grade 2: Notable opening of the joint line compared to the contralateral joint, but a solid "endpoint" is reached Grade 3: Complete opening of the radial or lateral joint line with valgus or varus stress. No endpoint can be discerned. Attempts at hyperextension of the digit at the PIP of the MCP joints can identify volar plate instability and the propensity of the digit to subluxate or dislocate.
Mill test	With the elbow flexed, the forearm slightly pronated, and the wrist slightly extended, the patient actively supinates against resistance.		Pain either at the epicondyle or radiating distally along the extensor carpi radialis brevis represents a positive test. Increasing strain in an inflamed or degenerative tendon causes pain.
Palpation of LT interval	The LT joint is deeply palpated dorsally and slightly distal to the site of the 4–5 arthroscopy portal.		Point tenderness indicates LT interosseous ligament injury or triangular fibrocartilage complex pathology.

(continued)

Examination	Technique	Illustration	Grading & Significance
Palpation of scapholunate (SL) interval	The SL joint is deeply palpated dorsally and 1.5 cm distal to the tubercle of Lister (slightly distal to the 3–4 arthroscopy portal). Alternatively, the examiner palpates the third metacarpal, moving proximally until a depression is felt. Just proximal to this cavity is the SL joint, which is palpable between the second and fourth dorsal extensor compartments.		Point tenderness may indicate SL interosseous ligament injury, scaphoid injury, ganglion cyst, or Kienbock disease.
Phalen test	The patient's wrist is placed in maximum flexion and the elbow in extension for 60 seconds or until symptomatic.		Reproduction of symptoms in the median nerve distribution indicates carpal tunnel syndrome.
Piano key sign	The radius is stabilized with one hand. The ulna is passively translated dorsally and volarly with the opposite hand. This test is performed in pronation, neutral, and supination, and findings are compared to the opposite side.		A positive result is characterized by painful laxity in the affected wrist compared with the contralateral wrist, suggesting DRUJ synovitis related to instability. "Winging" is associated with loss of structural support at the DRUJ and may indicate a complete peripheral tear of the triangular fibrocartilage complex. Depression and rebounding of the ulnar head is a positive finding.

Examination	Technique	Illustration	Grading & Significance
Pisotriquetral shear test	The examiner's thumb is placed over the pisiform and a circular grinding motion and dorsally directed pressure are applied.		Crepitus and pain over pisotriquetral joint. Pisotriquetral arthritis.
Scaphoid ballottement test	The scaphoid is grasped with one hand and the lunate with the other. The scaphoid is then balloted anteroposteriorly. Anteroposterior translation is compared to the contralateral side.		Pain and increased anteroposterior laxity are highly suggestive of SL instability.
Scaphoid shift test (Watson)	Dorsally directed pressure is exerted on the patient's volar scaphoid tuberosity (distal pole) by the examiner's ipsilateral thumb while the wrist is passively moved from ulnar to radial deviation by the examiner's contralateral hand. The distal pole of the scaphoid is stabilized with the wrist in ulnar deviation, and then the examiner passively radially deviates the wrist. Next the pressure on the distal pole is removed and the examiner feels for relocation of the scaphoid into the scaphoid facet of the distal radius. Findings are compared with the contralateral wrist.		The scaphoid normally flexes as the wrist goes from ulnar to radial deviation. The examiner's thumb prevents scaphoid flexion and in scapholunate dissociation, the proximal scaphoid pole subluxates dorsally out of the scaphoid fossa, causing pain. When the thumb is released from the distal pole of the scaphoid, there may be a palpable or audible clunk, signifying spontaneous reduction of the scaphoid back into the scaphoid fossa. This clunk may be present in 11% of asymptomatic wrists. It is the presence of pain along with the clunk that is diagnostic for scapholunate ligament disruption. If only pain is present and no clunk is felt, a sprain or a partial tear of the scapholunate ligament is likely. This test is not terribly specific and may be positive in patients with hyperlaxity, synovitis, occult ganglia, and radioscaphoid impingement or arthritis.
Supination test (Ouellette)	With the forearm mildly pronated, the examiner uses their contralateral hand to stabilize the distal ulna and their ipsilateral hand to secure the pisotriquetral unit and with that hand exert a supination force on the ulnar carpus along with compression across the ulnocarpal joint. The examiner listens for clicks and clunks.		Pain, instability and the presence of clicks or clunks are compared to the contralateral wrist. Graded from stable to unstable. The examiner should note the presence of clicks and clunks in both wrists. Abnormal supination of carpus in relation to the forearm.
Thompson test	With the elbow extended, the wrist in slight extension, and the digits in a fist, the patient extends the wrist against the examiner.		Pain either at the lateral epicondyle or radiating distally along the extensor carpi radialis brevis is indicative of inflamed or degenerative tendon.

(continued)

Examination	Technique	Illustration	Grading & Significance
Thumb MCP joint collateral ligament stability test	The metacarpal is stabilized between the examiner's thumb and index finger of one hand and the proximal phalanx is stabilized between the examiner's thumb and index finger of the other hand. Radially or ulnarly directed forces are applied with the joint flexed 30 to 35 degrees and with the joint extended. Findings are compared with the uninjured thumb. Use of a digital block is sometimes helpful to obtain an accurate assessment.		Grade 0: No significant instability Grade 1, Mild: <25 degrees of opening Grade 2, Moderate: <30 degrees of difference versus the contralateral thumb Grade 3, Severe: Gross instability, without a solid endpoint in both flexion and extension. Consistent with a complete disruption of the proper and accessory collateral ligaments. Severe collateral ligament injury is uncommon in conjunction with volar plate instability but must be recognized and treated where indicated.
Trigger digit evaluation	A digit is placed along the volar aspect of the thumb or finger, proximal to the MP joint, and the patient is asked to flex and extend the digit.		Reproduction of pain, triggering, or locking of the thumb indicates trigger thumb as a cause.
Ulnocarpal (triangular fibrocartilage complex) compression test	The examiner ulnarly deviates, pronates, and axially loads the wrist. Passive pronation and supination may be added.		A click or snap reproducing pain and symptoms is a positive test and consistent with triangular fibrocartilage complex, LT, and midcarpal pathology. This maneuver will also be painful if ulna impaction syndrome is present.
Volar plate stability	The metacarpal is stabilized between the examiner's thumb and index finger of one hand and the proximal phalanx is stabilized between the examiner's thumb and index finger of other hand. Hyperextension force is applied.		0 = No hyperextension; 1 = Mild, definite endpoint; 2 = moderate, soft endpoint; 3 = severe, gross instability. Volar instability must be recognized and treated appropriately to maximize outcomes.
Wartenberg sign	The patient is asked to extend the fingers.		The sign is considered positive if the small finger assumes an abducted posture with finger extension. This sign is the result of palmar interossei weakness resulting in unopposed ulnar pull of the extensor digiti quinti.

Exam Table for Shoulder and Elbow

Examination	Technique	Illustration	Grading & Significance
Shoulder			
Active forward flexion	Patient attempts to actively bring the arm forward above his or her head.		Normal active flexion is 170–180 degrees. Limited active forward flexion is indicative of possible large rotator cuff tear. Patients with function at or above shoulder level are more likely to have improved active forward flexion postoperatively.
Active external rotation	With arms at the patient's side and the elbows flexed to 90 degrees, the patient is asked to maximally externally rotate the arms.		Less active external rotation on the affected side. Decreased external rotation on affected side indicates partial or complete loss of infraspinatus function due to tear involvement or muscle dysfunction.
Abduction strength testing	The arm is placed in 90 degrees abduction in the scapular plane. The patient is asked to resist downward force.		Tests deltoid muscle strength: full strength, decreased strength, or unable to maintain position against gravity. Weak deltoid suggests less postoperative active range of motion secondary to inadequate strength.
External rotation lag sign	Arm is passively placed in maximal external rotation and then released. Patient is asked to maintain the arm in external rotation.		Inability to maintain maximal external rotation ($\geq$20 degree lag sign) suggests the tear extends well into the infraspinatus.

(continued)

Examination	Technique	Illustration	Grading & Significance
External rotation strength testing	Arm is placed in maximal external rotation and patient is asked to resist internal rotation force.		Full-strength resistance suggests no infraspinatus tear involvement. Weakness suggests progressive infraspinatus involvement or dysfunction.
Lift-off test	Patient places the dorsum of the hand against the lumbar region of the back and attempts to lift the hand from the back and hold it.		Inability to lift the hand from the back is a positive result. Indicates subscapularis muscle weakness or tear.
Belly press test (Napoleon test)	The patient is asked to keep the palm of his or her hand on the abdomen with the wrist extended and the shoulder flexed and in maximal internal rotation while the examiner attempts to forcefully pull the patient's hand off the abdomen.		A positive belly-press test occurs when the patient must flex the wrist and extend the arm to maintain the palm on the abdomen. This indicates subscapularis muscle weakness or tear.
Modified belly press	With palm on abdomen, the patient is asked to bring the elbow forward, in front of the plane of the body.		Inability to perform action demonstrates dysfunctional or torn subscapularis tendon and a higher rate of clinical failure with muscle transfer.
Bear hug test	The hand of the affected side is placed on the opposite shoulder with the fingers extended and the elbow elevated forward. The patient resists as the examiner attempts to lift the hand off the shoulder.		If the examiner can lift the hand off the shoulder, then the patient likely has a partial or complete tear of the upper subscapularis tendon. This is perhaps the most sensitive test for a subscapularis tear.
Wall push-up	The patient is asked to perform a wall push-up by placing the hands at shoulder level on a wall and doing a push-up.		The scapula is carefully evaluated for signs and severity of medial or lateral translation.
Impingement sign	With the patient upright, the examiner fixes the scapula to prevent it from moving and then brings the arm into full forward elevation with some force.		A positive test is pain during this maneuver. Forcing the fully forward elevated arm against the fixed scapula helps to localize the finding to the rotator cuff.

Examination	Technique	Illustration	Grading & Significance
Palm-down abduction test	With the scapula stabilized by the examiner, the arm is internally rotated and then elevated forcibly in the plane of the scapula.		A positive test produces pain with the maneuver. By internally rotating the arm, the supra- and anterior infraspinatus tendons are placed directly under the coracoacromial arch. Elevating the arm in the scapular plane when it is in internal rotation compresses these tendons against the undersurface of the acromion.
Coracoid impingement	The arm is forward flexed to 90 degrees, internally rotated, and adducted.		Reproduction of pain or a painful click indicates a positive test. A positive test is indicative of impingement of the coracoid onto the subscapularis.
Apprehension test	The arm is placed in 90 degrees of abduction. The arm is slowly brought into external rotation and extension.		Apprehension, not simply pain, is required for a positive apprehension test. The apprehension test has a sensitivity of 72% and specificity of 96% for anterior instability. Positive anterior apprehension can be associated with anterior labral injuries. Patient feels a sensation of instability with the arm in the at-risk position. Sensation of pain suggests internal impingement, not instability.
Anterior load and shift test	The patient is positioned supine with the arm in 20 degrees abduction, 20 degrees flexion, and neutral rotation. With axial load to reduce the humeral head, an anterior force is applied to the arm.		0 = no translation; 1+ = to the anterior rim; 2+ = over the rim but spontaneously reduces; 3+ = dislocation of the humeral head that locks over the anterior rim. Indicates anterior instability.
Load and shift test	If the right shoulder is examined, the examiner's left hand grasps the humeral shaft with the fingers anterior and the thumb posterior. The examiner's right hand grasps the forearm and positions the arm in the plane of the scapula in 40 to 60 degrees of abduction and neutral rotation. An axial load is applied to the humerus through the forearm and the examiner's left hand displaces the humeral head anteriorly. The degree of displacement of the humeral head on the glenoid rim is noted.		Grade 0: Little or no movement Grade 1: Shift to edge of glenoid Grade 2: Shift over edge of glenoid but spontaneously reduces Grade 3: Shift over edge of glenoid but does not spontaneously relocate This is difficult to perform in the awake patient in clinic but sensitive when the patient is under anesthesia.
Miniaci bony apprehension test	The arm is placed in approximately 45 degrees of abduction. With external rotation, there is development of apprehension.		Apprehension with lower degrees of abduction indicates a significant and symptomatic bony contribution to the instability.

(continued)

Examination	Technique	Illustration	Grading & Significance
Sulcus sign	An inferior force is applied to the arm at the side.		0 = no translation; 1+ = <1 cm; 2+ = 1–2 cm; 3+ = >3 cm. Indicates an inferior component of instability.
Biceps resistance test (Speed's test)	With the patient's arm at 90 degrees of forward elevation, a downward force is applied to the arm while the patient tries to resist that force.		A positive test is pain along the tendon of the long head of the biceps. Pain during this maneuver indicates involvement of the long head of the biceps tendon.
Speed's test	The arm is abducted to 90 degrees and brought forward 45 degrees while the forearm is supinated and the elbow extended. The patient then resists a downward force.		If the maneuver produces pain or tenderness, the test is positive. A positive test may indicate bicipital pathology, although the test is not specific.
Yergason test	The elbow is flexed to 90 degrees. The patient attempts to supinate the arm from a pronated position while the examiner resists.		The patient will experience pain as the biceps tendon subluxes out of the groove with a positive test. A positive test indicates biceps instability.
Scapula stabilization test	When winging is observed, a hand is placed to stabilize the scapula in a reduced position, and the patient then elevates the arm.		The examiner should assess for fixed scapula winging versus reducible winging as well as improvement in arm elevation and comfort with the scapula reduced. This is crucial in determining fixed versus reducible winging.

Examination	Technique	Illustration	Grading & Significance
Selective injection with local anesthetic and corticosteroid	The involved arm is placed on the back to lift the scapula off the chest wall. The injection is given in the scapulothoracic bursa under the superomedial border of the scapula.	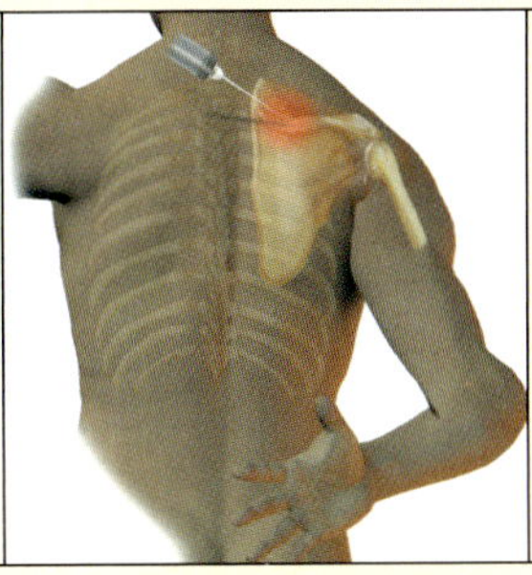	Significant pain relief or elimination of the pain confirms the diagnosis.

Elbow

Examination	Technique	Illustration	Grading & Significance
Range of motion (ROM), elbow	Active and passive ROM (flexion–extension of the elbow, rotation of the forearm) is compared to the uninjured side. Palpable and auditory crepitus should be noted.	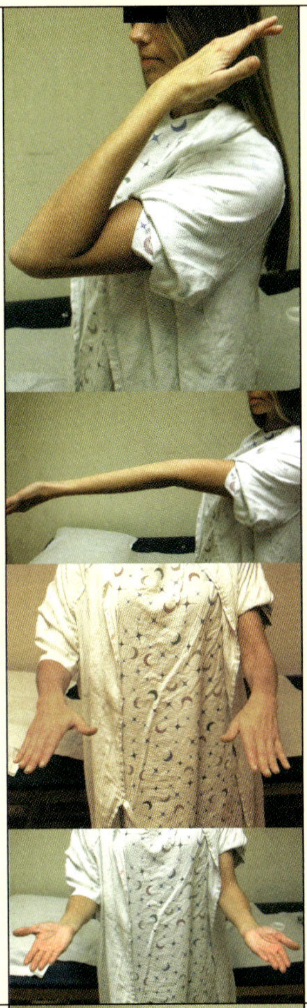	Normal values: 0 to 145 degrees of flexion–extension, 85 degrees of supination, and 80 degrees of pronation. The examiner should check for perching on the lateral view. Locking of the elbow could represent loose bodies. Stiffness may indicate intrinsic capsular contracture.
Effusion	The examiner palpates the anconeus triangle (radial head [RH], lateral epicondyle [L], and olecranon tip [O]) and lateral gutter, noting prominence of lateral epicondyle, gutter effusion, or subcutaneous atrophy from prior corticosteroid injections.	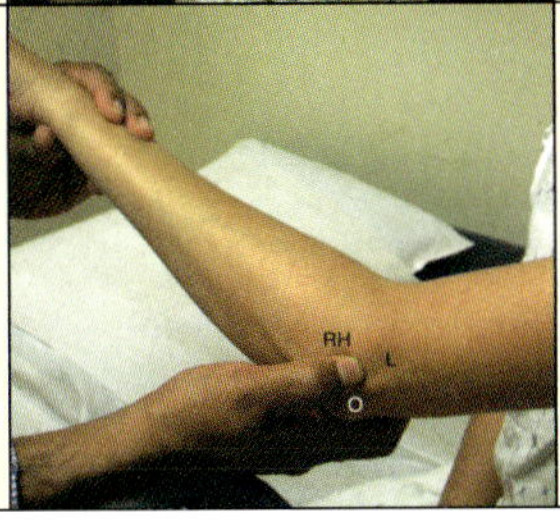	It is difficult to estimate the amount of fluid, but the presence of an effusion should be noted and may represent hemarthrosis due to intra-articular fracture, radiocapitellar wear, or ligamentous disruption. In acute injuries an effusion should be present; in more chronic situations it may be absent.

(continued)

Examination	Technique	Illustration	Grading & Significance
Supine lateral pivot-shift test	Patient is supine, with arm extended overhead and supinated. The examiner stabilizes the humerus with one hand and applies a valgus force with the other as the elbow is taken from extension to flexion.		When the elbow is slightly flexed the radial head can be palpated to subluxate or frankly dislocate; as the elbow flexes past 40 degrees, it will relocate, often with a palpable clunk. This test is difficult to perform on an awake patient; often apprehension will be felt and the patient will not allow the test to continue. Examination under anesthesia may be required.
Prone pivot-shift test	Placing the patient prone with the arm hanging over the table stabilizes the humerus and leaves one of the examiner's hands free to palpate the radial head.		A positive test reveals radial head or ulnohumeral subluxation. Same as pivot-shift test.
Elbow drawer test	With the patient in prone position, the humerus is stabilized with one arm while a distraction force is placed on the forearm to sublux the ulnohumeral joint.		A positive test reveals ulnohumeral subluxation.
Push-off test	From a seated position the patient attempts to push off from the armrests. Pain or apprehension is suggestive of lateral ligamentous insufficiency.		A positive test will reproduce the patient's symptoms of apprehension during supination and not pronation. Inability to complete the push-up is a positive test. A positive test indicates a posterolateral rotatory insufficiency.

Examination	Technique	Illustration	Grading & Significance
Table-top relocation test	The symptomatic hand/arm is placed on the lateral edge of a table. The patient is asked to perform push-up with the elbow pointing laterally. The maneuver is repeated with the examiner's thumb stabilizing the radial head during press-up. The maneuver is once again repeated without the examiner's thumb in place.		A positive test elicits pain or apprehension as the elbow reaches 40 degrees.
Varus stress test	Stabilize the humerus and stress the elbow in supination and slight flexion.		A positive test indicates injury to the anterior band of the medial collateral ligament.
Valgus stress test	The examiner stabilizes the humerus and stresses the lateral ulnar collateral ligament in slight flexion.		A positive test indicates injury to the lateral ulnar collateral ligament.
Medial collateral ligament shear test	Patient places the contralateral arm under the injured elbow and grasps the thumb of the symptomatic extremity. With the elbow maximally flexed the patient applies a valgus load to the elbow as he or she brings it out into extension.		A positive test will localize pain to the medial elbow, suggesting an incompetent ulnar collateral ligament.

(continued)

Examination	Technique	Illustration	Grading & Significance
Squeeze test	Deep palpation of interosseous membrane and distal radioulnar joint		This test screens for potential longitudinal instability.
Tinel's test	Percussion of the ulnar nerve proximal to or across the cubital tunnel		A positive test elicits pain at the site of percussion and paresthesias in an ulnar nerve distribution distally, which indicates ulnar neuropathy at the elbow.
Elbow flexion test	With the patient seated, the elbows are maximally flexed and the wrists held in neutral. Reproduction of paresthesias in an ulnar nerve distribution distally within 1 minute is a positive test.		A positive test indicates ulnar neuropathy at the elbow.

INDEX

Page numbers followed by *f* and *t* indicated figures and tables, respectively.

CCS0610

WS00010224

FOR
REFERENCE ONLY

REMOVED
FROM
STOCK